The American Psychiatric Publishing

Textbook of
CLINICAL PSYCHIATRY

FOURTH EDITION

The American Psychiatric Publishing

Textbook of
CLINICAL PSYCHIATRY

FOURTH EDITION

Edited by

Robert E. Hales, M.D., M.B.A.
Joe P. Tupin Professor and Chair,
Department of Psychiatry and Behavioral Sciences,
University of California, Davis School of Medicine
Medical Director, Sacramento County Mental Health Services,
Sacramento, California

Stuart C. Yudofsky, M.D.
D.C. and Irene Ellwood Professor and Chairman,
Department of Psychiatry and Behavioral Sciences,
Baylor College of Medicine
Chief of Psychiatry Services, The Methodist Hospital,
Houston, Texas

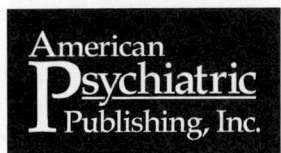

American Psychiatric Publishing, Inc.

Washington, DC
London, England

Diagnostic criteria included in this textbook are reprinted, with permission, from *Diagnostic and Statistical Manual of Mental Disorders*, 4th Edition, Text Revision. Copyright © 2000, American Psychiatric Association.

Typeset in Adobe's Revival, Caecilia, and Formata

Manufactured in the United States of America on acid-free paper
07 06 05 04 03   5 4 3 2 1
Fourth Edition

American Psychiatric Publishing, Inc.
1400 K Street, N.W.
Washington, DC 20005
www.appi.org

Library of Congress Cataloging-in-Publication Data
The American Psychiatric Publishing textbook of clinical psychiatry / edited by Robert
E. Hales, Stuart C. Yudofsky.-- 4th ed.
    p. ; cm
  Rev. ed. of: The American Psychiatric Press textbook of psychiatry / edited by Robert
E. Hales, Stuart C. Yudofsky, John A. Talbott. c1999.
  Includes bibliographical references and index.
  ISBN 1-58562-032-7 (alk. paper)
    1. Psychiatry. I. Title: Textbook of clinical psychiatry. II. Hales, Robert E. III.
Yudofsky, Stuart C. IV. American Psychiatric Press textbook of psychiatry.
  [DNLM: 1. Mental Disorders. 2. Psychiatry. WM 140 A5126 2003]
RC454 .A419 2003
616.89--dc21

                                                                                    2002067896

British Library Cataloguing in Publication Data
A CIP record is available from the British Library.

We dedicate the Fourth Edition of
Textbook of Clinical Psychiatry to

John C. Nemiah, M.D.
Gifted psychoanalyst, dedicated teacher
Brilliant writer, inspired editor
Gracious mentor, consummate role model, and generous friend

Herbert Pardes, M.D.
Tireless, effective worker for all patients who suffer from psychiatric disorders
Visionary leader of psychiatrists and other physicians
Esteemed colleague and devoted friend

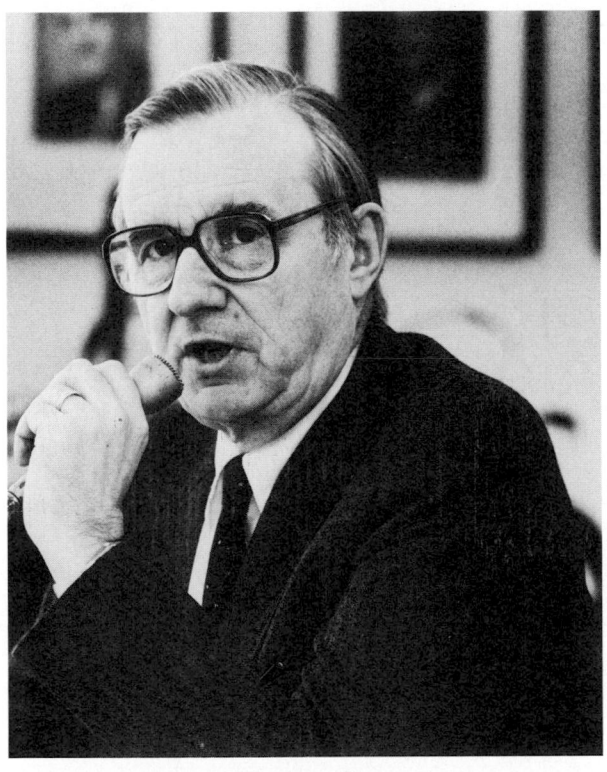

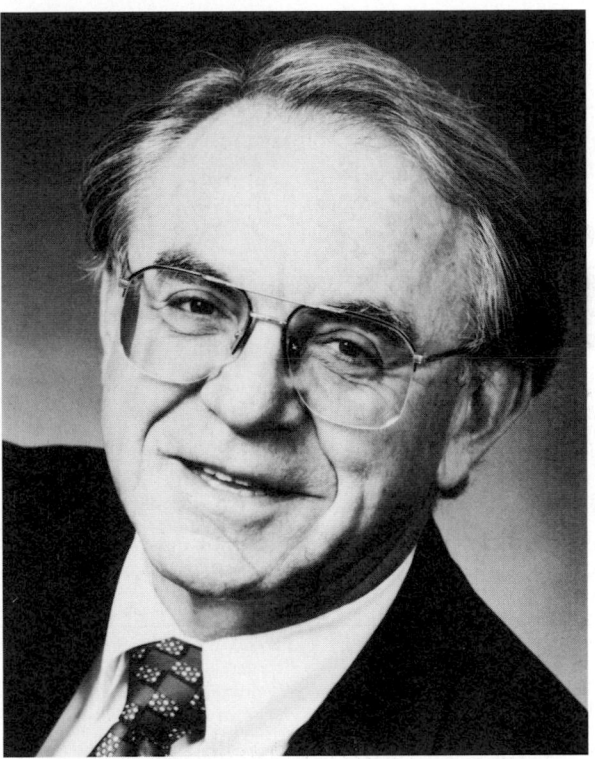

John C. Nemiah, M.D.
Professor of Psychiatry Emeritus,
Harvard Medical School and
Dartmouth Medical School;
Editor Emeritus,
The American Journal of Psychiatry

Herbert Pardes, M.D.
President and Chief Executive Officer,
New York–Presbyterian Healthcare System;
Former Vice President for Health Affairs,
Dean of the Faculty of Medicine, and
Chairman, Department of Psychiatry,
Columbia University College of Physicians and Surgeons

Contents

PART I

Theoretical Foundations and Assessment

PART IV

Special Clinical Topics

Contributors

Nancy C. Andreasen, M.D., Ph.D.
Andrew H. Woods Professor of Psychiatry and Director of the Mental Health Clinical Research Center, Department of Psychiatry, University of Iowa College of Medicine, Iowa City, Iowa

Charles E. Bailey, M.D.
Medical Director, CNS Healthcare, Orlando, Florida

Aaron T. Beck, M.D.
University Professor, Department of Psychiatry, University of Pennsylvania School of Medicine, Philadelphia, Pennsylvania

Judith V. Becker, Ph.D.
Professor of Psychology and Psychiatry, Department of Psychology, University of Arizona College of Medicine, Tucson, Arizona

C. Christian Beels, M.D., M.S.
Faculty, Ackerman Institute for the Family, New York, New York

Edward Bein, Ph.D.
Research Professor, San Francisco State University's Center for Community Research; and Adjunct Faculty Member, Wright Institute, Berkeley, California

Robert I. Berkowitz, M.D.
Associate Professor of Psychiatry, Division of Child and Adolescent Psychiatry, Department of Psychiatry, The University of Pennsylvania School of Medicine, The Children's Hospital of Philadelphia, Philadelphia, Pennsylvania

Donald W. Black, M.D.
Professor of Psychiatry, Department of Psychiatry, University of Iowa College of Medicine, Iowa City, Iowa

Dan G. Blazer, M.D., Ph.D.
J.P. Gibbons Professor of Psychiatry, Duke University School of Medicine, Durham, North Carolina

Howard C. Blue, M.D.
Assistant Clinical Professor of Psychiatry, Department of Psychiatry, Yale University School of Medicine, New Haven, Connecticut

James A. Bourgeois, O.D., M.D.
Associate Professor of Clinical Psychiatry and Behavioral Sciences and Director of the Psychiatry Consultation-Liaison Service, University of California, Davis School of Medicine, Sacramento, California

Michael Brook, B.S.
Postgraduate Researcher, Department of Psychiatry and Behavioral Sciences, University of California, Davis School of Medicine, Sacramento, California

Vivien K. Burt, M.D., Ph.D.
Professor of Psychiatry and Director of the Women's Life Center at the University of California, Los Angeles Neuropsychiatric Institute and Hospital, Los Angeles, California

Stephen F. Butler, Ph.D.
Senior Vice President, Inflexxion, Newton, Massachusetts

T. Carroll-Ghosh, M.D.
Associate Clinical Professor of Psychiatry, University of California, San Francisco School of Medicine, San Francisco; and Medical Director, Behavioral Health, HealthNet Federal Services, San Diego, California

John F. Clarkin, Ph.D.
Professor of Clinical Psychology in Psychiatry, Department of Psychiatry, Weill Medical College of Cornell University, The New York–Presbyterian Hospital—Westchester Division, White Plains, New York

Paul D. Cox, M.D.
Associate Clinical Professor of Psychiatry and Behavioral Sciences, University of California, Davis School of Medicine, Sacramento, California

Stephen J. Cozza, M.D.
Associate Professor of Psychiatry and Vice Chairman of the Department of Psychiatry, F. Edward Hébert School of Medicine, Uniformed Services University of the Health Sciences, Bethesda, Maryland; and Chief, Department of Psychiatry, Walter Reed Army Medical Center, Washington, D.C.

Glen C. Crawford, M.D.

Assistant Professor of Psychiatry, F. Edward Hébert School of Medicine, Uniformed Services University of the Health Sciences; and Staff Child and Adolescent Psychiatrist, Department of Psychiatry, National Naval Medical Center, Bethesda, Maryland

C. Deborah Cross, M.D.

Director, Inpatient Service, Elmhurst Hospital, Queens, New York

Robert Davies, M.D.

Assistant Professor of Psychiatry, University of Colorado School of Medicine, Denver, Colorado

Amelia N. Dubovsky, B.A.

Graduate Student, Premedical Studies, Columbia University, New York, New York

Steven L. Dubovsky, M.D.

Professor of Psychiatry and Medicine and Vice Chair of the Department of Psychiatry, University of Colorado School of Medicine, Denver, Colorado

Mina K. Dulcan, M.D.

Professor of Psychiatry and Pediatrics, Head of the Department of Child and Adolescent Psychiatry, and Margaret C. Osterman Professor of Child Psychiatry, Children's Memorial Hospital; and Professor of Psychiatry and Behavioral Sciences, Northwestern University Medical School, Chicago, Illinois

Allen R. Dyer, M.D., Ph.D.

Professor of Psychiatry and Behavioral Sciences, Department of Psychiatry, East Tennessee State University, Johnson City, Tennessee

Marc D. Feldman, M.D.

Professor, Department of Psychiatry and Behavioral Neurobiology, and Vice Chair of Clinical Services, University of Alabama at Birmingham, Birmingham, Alabama

Eric A. Fertuck, Ph.D.

Fellow of Psychology in Psychiatry, Department of Psychiatry, Weill Medical College of Cornell University, The New York–Presbyterian Hospital—Westchester Division, White Plains, New York

Laurie Fields, Ph.D.

Assistant Clinical Professor of Psychiatry and Behavioral Sciences, University of California, Davis School of Medicine, Sacramento, California

Richard J. Frances, M.D.

Clinical Professor of Psychiatry, New York University School of Medicine, New York, New York; Adjunct Professor of Psychiatry, University of Medicine and Dentistry of New Jersey, Newark, New Jersey; and President and Medical Director, Silver Hill Hospital, New Canaan, Connecticut

John E. Franklin Jr., M.D., M.Sc.

Associate Professor of Psychiatry and Director of Addiction Psychiatry, Northwestern University Medical School, Evanston, Illinois

Glen O. Gabbard, M.D.

Professor and Director, Baylor Psychiatry Clinic, Department of Psychiatry and Behavioral Sciences, Baylor College of Medicine; and Training and Supervising Analyst, Houston-Galveston Psychoanalytic Institute, Houston, Texas

G. Davis Gammon, M.D.

Clinical Assistant Professor, Child Study Center, Yale University School of Medicine, New Haven, Connecticut

Donald C. Goff, M.D.

Associate Professor of Psychiatry, Harvard Medical School; and Director, Schizophrenia Program, Massachusetts General Hospital, Boston, Massachusetts

Carlos A. González, M.D.

Assistant Clinical Professor of Psychiatry, Yale University School of Medicine, New Haven, Connecticut

Ezra E. H. Griffith, M.D.

Professor of Psychiatry and African-American Studies, Yale University School of Medicine, New Haven, Connecticut

John G. Gunderson, M.D.

Professor of Psychiatry, Harvard Medical School, Boston; and Director, Psychosocial Research Program, McLean Hospital, Belmont, Massachusetts

Robert E. Hales, M.D., M.B.A.

Joe P. Tupin Professor and Chair, Department of Psychiatry and Behavioral Sciences, University of California, Davis School of Medicine; and Medical Director, Sacramento County Mental Health Services, Sacramento, California

Katherine A. Halmi, M.D.

Professor of Psychiatry, Weill Medical College of Cornell University, White Plains, New York

Victoria C. Hendrick, M.D.
Assistant Professor of Psychiatry, Director of the Pregnancy and Postpartum Mood Disorders Program, and Assistant Director, Women's Mood Disorders Research Program, University of California, Los Angeles Neuropsychiatric Institute and Hospital, Los Angeles, California

Margaret E. Hertzig, M.D.
Professor of Psychiatry, Payne Whitney Clinic, Department of Psychiatry, Weill Medical College of Cornell University, New York, New York

Donald M. Hilty, M.D.
Associate Professor of Clinical Psychiatry and Behavioral Sciences, University of California, Davis School of Medicine; and Medical Director, Sacramento County Mental Health Treatment Center, Sacramento, California

Beng-Choon Ho, M.R.C.Psych.
Assistant Professor of Psychiatry and Clinical Director of the Mental Health Clinical Research Center, Department of Psychiatry, University of Iowa College of Medicine, Iowa City, Iowa

Eric Hollander, M.D.
Professor of Psychiatry and Director of Clinical Psychopharmacology, Department of Psychiatry, Mount Sinai School of Medicine, New York, New York

Bradley R. Johnson, M.D.
Assistant Professor of Psychiatry, University of Arizona College of Medicine, Tucson; and Chief of Psychiatry, Arizona Community Protection and Treatment Center, Phoenix, Arizona

Steven A. King, M.D., M.S.
Clinical Professor of Psychiatry, New York University School of Medicine; and Co-Director, Pain Center, Hospital for Joint Diseases–Orthopaedic Institute, New York, New York

James A. Knowles, M.D., Ph.D.
Associate Professor of Clinical Psychiatry, Columbia University College of Physicians and Surgeons, Columbia Genome Center, New York State Psychiatric Institute, New York, New York

Steven Koontz, B.S.
Social Worker, Capital District Psychiatric Center, Albany, New York

David J. Kupfer, M.D.
Thomas Detre Professor and Chairman, Department of Psychiatry, University of Pittsburgh School of Medicine, Pittsburgh, Pennsylvania

Martin H. Leamon, M.D.
Assistant Professor of Clinical Psychiatry and Behavioral Sciences, University of California, Davis School of Medicine, Sacramento, California

Hanna Levenson, Ph.D.
Director, Brief Psychotherapy Program, California Pacific Medical Center; and Director, Levenson Institute for Training, San Francisco, California

James L. Levenson, M.D.
Professor of Psychiatry, Medicine, and Surgery, Vice Chair of the Department of Psychiatry, and Chair of the Division of Consultation-Liaison Psychiatry, Medical College of Virginia, Virginia Commonwealth University, Richmond, Virginia

Avram H. Mack, M.D.
Fellow, Columbia University College of Physicians and Surgeons; and Resident Psychiatrist, New York State Psychiatric Institute, New York, New York

José R. Maldonado, M.D.
Assistant Professor and Chief, Medical and Forensic Psychiatry Section, and Director, Medical Psychotherapy Clinic, Department of Psychiatry and Behavioral Sciences, Stanford University School of Medicine; and Medical Director, Consultation/Liaison Service, Stanford University Medical Center, Stanford, California

Lauren B. Marangell, M.D.
Associate Professor of Psychiatry, Director, Mood Disorders Research, and Director, Clinical Psychopharmacology, Department of Psychiatry, Baylor College of Medicine, Houston, Texas

John C. Markowitz, M.D.
Associate Professor of Psychiatry, Weill Medical College of Cornell University, New York–Presbyterian Hospital; Lecturer in Psychiatry, Columbia University College of Physicians and Surgeons; and Research Psychiatrist, New York State Psychiatric Institute, New York, New York

Stephen S. Marmer, M.D., Ph.D.
Assistant Clinical Professor, University of California, Los Angeles Neuropsychiatric Institute, Department of Psychiatry and Biobehavioral Medicine, University of California, Los Angeles; and Senior Faculty, Southern California Psychoanalytic Institute, Los Angeles, California

Merry N. Miller, M.D.
Professor and Chair, Department of Psychiatry and Behavioral Sciences, East Tennessee State University, Johnson City, Tennessee

John M. Morihisa, M.D.
Professor of Psychiatry, Albany Medical College, Capital District Psychiatric Center, Albany, New York

Thomas L. Morrison, Ph.D.
Professor of Psychiatry and Behavioral Sciences, University of California, Davis School of Medicine, Sacramento, California

Jeffrey Newcorn, M.D.
Associate Professor of Psychiatry and Director of the Child Psychiatry Division, Division of Child and Adolescent Psychiatry, Department of Psychiatry, Mount Sinai School of Medicine, New York, New York

Thomas C. Neylan, M.D.
Assistant Professor in Residence, University of California, San Francisco School of Medicine and Veterans' Affairs Medical Center, San Francisco, California

Katharine A. Phillips, M.D.
Associate Professor of Psychiatry, Brown University School of Medicine; and Director, Body Dysmorphic Disorder Program, Butler Hospital, Providence, Rhode Island

Charles W. Popper, M.D.
Clinical Instructor in Psychiatry, Harvard Medical School, Boston; and Associate Child Psychiatrist, McLean Hospital, Belmont, Massachusetts

Michael Precioso, Ph.D.
Assistant Professor of Psychiatry, Albany Medical College, Capital District Psychiatric Center, Albany, New York

Stephen Price, M.D.
Associate Professor of Psychiatry, Albany Medical College, Capital District Psychiatric Center, Albany, New York

Charles F. Reynolds III, M.D.
Professor of Psychiatry and Neurology and Director of the Mental Health Clinical Research Center for Late-Life Mood Disorders, University of Pittsburgh School of Medicine, Pittsburgh, Pennsylvania

Stephen C. Scheiber, M.D.
Adjunct Professor of Psychiatry, Northwestern University Medical School, Chicago, Illinois; Adjunct Professor of Psychiatry, Medical College of Wisconsin, Milwaukee, Wisconsin; and Executive Vice President, American Board of Psychiatry and Neurology, Deerfield, Illinois

Charles L. Scott, M.D.
Assistant Professor of Clinical Psychiatry and Chief of Forensic Psychiatry, Department of Psychiatry and Behavioral Sciences, University of California, Davis School of Medicine, Sacramento, California

Jeffrey S. Seaman, M.S., M.D.
Clinical Assistant Professor in Psychiatry, University of Texas Health Sciences Center at San Antonio; and Director, Consultation-Liaison Service, Department of Psychiatry, Wilford Hall Medical Center, Lackland Air Force Base, San Antonio, Texas

Mark E. Servis, M.D.
Associate Professor of Clinical Psychiatry and Behavioral Sciences and Vice Chair for Education, Department of Psychiatry and Behavioral Sciences, University of California, Davis School of Medicine, Sacramento, California

Theodore Shapiro, M.D.
Professor of Psychiatry and Professor of Psychiatry in Pediatrics, Payne Whitney Clinic, Department of Psychiatry, Weill Medical College of Cornell University, New York, New York

Edward K. Silberman, M.D.
Clinical Professor of Psychiatry and Human Behavior and Director of Residency Education, Department of Psychiatry and Human Behavior, Jefferson Medical College of Thomas Jefferson University Hospital, Philadelphia, Pennsylvania

Jonathan M. Silver, M.D.
Clinical Professor of Psychiatry, New York University School of Medicine; and Assistant Director for Clinical Services and Research, Department of Psychiatry, Lenox Hill Hospital, New York, New York

Daphne Simeon, M.D.
Associate Professor of Psychiatry, Mount Sinai School of Medicine, New York, New York

Robert I. Simon, M.D.
Clinical Professor of Psychiatry and Director of the Program in Psychiatry and Law, Department of Psychiatry, Georgetown University School of Medicine, Washington, D.C.

David Spiegel, M.D.
Willson Professor and Associate Chair of Psychiatry and Behavioral Sciences, Department of Psychiatry and Behavioral Sciences, Stanford University School of Medicine, Stanford, California

James J. Strain, M.D.
Professor of Psychiatry, Mount Sinai School of Medicine/New York University Medical Center Health Service, New York, New York

Kenneth J. Tardiff, M.D., M.P.H.
Professor of Psychiatry and Public Health and Director of the Division of Epidemiology, Department of Psychiatry, Weill Medical College of Cornell University, New York, New York

Michael E. Thase, M.D.
Professor of Psychiatry, University of Pittsburgh School of Medicine, Pittsburgh, Pennsylvania

Robert J. Ursano, M.D.
Professor of Psychiatry and Neuroscience and Chairman of the Department of Psychiatry, F. Edward Hébert School of Medicine, Uniformed Services University of the Health Sciences, Bethesda, Maryland

Bruce S. Victor, M.D.
Associate Clinical Professor of Psychiatry, University of California, San Francisco School of Medicine, San Francisco, California

Sophia Vinogradov, M.D.
Associate Professor of Psychiatry, University of California, San Francisco School of Medicine, San Francisco, California

Scott A. West, M.D.
President and Chief Executive Officer, CNS Healthcare, Orlando, Florida

Jesse H. Wright, M.D., Ph.D.
Professor of Psychiatry and Associate Chairman of the Department of Psychiatry and Behavioral Sciences, University of Louisville School of Medicine, Louisville, Kentucky

Irvin D. Yalom, M.D.
Professor Emeritus of Psychiatry and Behavioral Sciences, Department of Psychiatry and Behavioral Sciences, Stanford University, Stanford, California

Shirley Yen, Ph.D.
Assistant Professor, Department of Psychiatry and Human Behavior, Brown University School of Medicine, Providence, Rhode Island

Stuart C. Yudofsky, M.D.
D.C. and Irene Ellwood Professor and Chairman, Department of Psychiatry and Behavioral Sciences, Baylor College of Medicine; and Chief of Psychiatry Services, The Methodist Hospital, Houston, Texas

Sean H. Yutzy, M.D.
Associate Professor of Psychiatry and Director of Forensic Services, Department of Psychiatry, Washington University School of Medicine, St. Louis, Missouri

Preface

The fourth edition of *The American Psychiatric Publishing Textbook of Clinical Psychiatry* has undergone more comprehensive and significant change than any previous edition. Although it remains a one-volume, clinically oriented textbook of psychiatry that has been crafted for use primarily by advanced psychiatry residents and practicing psychiatrists, it remains a standard educational reference for physicians of other specialties, such as family practice, internal medicine, pediatrics, and neurology. With the burgeoning psychiatric knowledge gained during the 1990s, the size of the *Textbook* grew from 1,344 pages and 38 chapters in 1988 to 1,790 pages and 50 chapters in 1999. We decided that it was time to refocus the *Textbook* back to its original mission: to be the finest one-volume, clinically oriented textbook in the field; hence, the name change of this edition to the *Textbook of Clinical Psychiatry*. Accordingly, we eliminated 10 chapters for the fourth edition, but because of the significant growth in research in psychiatry, the total number of pages was reduced only slightly, to 1,758. At the same time, we added a chapter on interpersonal therapy, because the efficacy of this therapy in treating a number of psychiatric disorders, especially depression, has been established through rigorous research. Chapters are intended to be scholarly and authoritative, while being of practical, clinical utility for treating patients.

We have maintained close contact with many of the professionals who purchased the 1988, 1994, and 1999 editions of the *Textbook* and have benefited from their comments and suggestions.

Work on the fourth edition began in earnest in early 2000. This edition represents the culmination of a nearly 3-year effort to provide the most useful and up-to-date clinical information in the field. Of the original 61 contributors from the first edition, 30 remain. However, 58 new contributors have been added in the 13 years since the first edition was published. For this edition, the total number of contributors is 88. All chapters have been updated to include the latest references and research findings, and selected chapters have been completely rewritten by new authors. An important feature of *The American Psychiatric Publishing Textbook of Clinical Psychiatry* is the combination of senior and junior authors for selected chapters. For instance, Chapter 9, "Schizophrenia and Other Psychotic Disorders," is authored by Nancy Andreasen, M.D., Ph.D., Editor-in-Chief of the *The American Journal of Psychiatry*, and Professor Donald Black, M.D. For this edition Drs. Andreasen and Black added a new co-author, Assistant Professor Beng-Choon Ho, M.R.C.Psych. Similarly, Chapter 11, "Anxiety Disorders," features Professor Eric Hollander, M.D., together with a newly promoted Associate Professor, Daphne Simeon, M.D. We have found that the addition of more junior authors has infused the chapters with new research insights and fresh and expanded perspectives on the subject matter. The senior authors have been able to temper these new ideas with their considerable wisdom and vast research and clinical experience. We believe that these collaborations enrich the appeal of the chapters to readers at all levels of educational and clinical experience. We also believe that these collaborations have enriched the diversity and quality of material presented in the *Textbook*. We express sincere gratitude to our dear colleague and friend—noted author, educator, and psychoanalyst, Glen O. Gabbard, M.D.—for writing such an inspirational and edifying introduction for this edition.

A companion volume for the *Textbook* is being prepared. *Essentials of Clinical Psychiatry*, which includes the 20 most clinically relevant chapters from the *Textbook*, is being designed for third- and fourth-year medical students, junior psychiatry residents, and residents in other specialties, especially neurology, family practice, and internal medicine. This book will be published in 2004.

All chapters were reviewed by a member of our editorial board and by the editors. We are grateful to our long-term collaborator, John A. Talbott, M.D., for serving as Chair of the Editorial Board. John has been a great colleague and friend these past 18 years. The editorial board includes prominent psychiatrists who were actively involved in reviewing chapters within their respective areas of expertise.

In the first two editions, we included two appendixes: the complete diagnostic criteria from the *Diagnostic and Statistical Manual of Mental Disorders* and excerpts from the *American Psychiatric Glossary*. However, as many readers have reported to us, these appendixes added another 125 pages to an already large book, and we wanted to maintain the *Textbook* as a one-volume text. Consequently, readers who purchased the third edition received a CD-ROM instead. Readers who purchase this edition will receive on CD-ROM the Electronic DSM-IV-TR Plus, Version 1.0, which includes the full text of DSM-IV-TR; the APA Practice Guidelines; the complete *American Psychiatric Glossary*, Seventh Edition; the *Principles of Medical Ethics With Annotations Especially Applicable to Psychiatry*, and *Opinions of the Ethics Committee on the Principles of Medical Ethics With Annotations Especially Applicable to Psychiatry*. The advantage of the CD-ROM is that the contents are fully searchable by disorder, code, or phrase and replete with cross-references and hypertext links. The CD-ROM will also give readers the options of reading the text, printing selected material, and adding it to their own databases.

We thank many people for their invaluable assistance with the fourth edition of *The American Psychiatric Publishing Textbook of Clinical Psychiatry*. First, we are grateful to the outstanding authors who produced exceptional chapters and who labored to respond with good humor to our many editorial suggestions and critiques of their chapters. Our distinguished editorial board worked closely with us in designing a clinically focused and scientifically substantiated volume. Herbert Pardes, M.D., provided us with a conceptual framework in organizing and updating the book. He provided us with an overview of where psychiatry was, where it is today, and where it is going. Because of his considerable positive influence on our careers, this edition is dedicated to him and to the equally outstanding John C. Nemiah, M.D., Editor Emeritus of *The American Journal of Psychiatry* and a long-term supporter and friend.

The outstanding staff at APPI has been highly encouraging and effective with all aspects of this project. Ron McMillen, CEO, and Carol Nadelson, M.D., former Editor-in-Chief and CEO, have been perennially insightful and invaluable to the concept, organization, and content of all editions of the *Textbook*. Claire Reinburg, former Editorial Director, assisted us with key structural elements of the book and many related administrative matters, which were continued without interruption by the equally exceptional John McDuffie. Pam Harley, Managing Editor, Books Department, coordinated the entire production process with the Project Editor, Jennifer Wood, who had the daunting challenge of overseeing the line-by-line editing of all the manuscripts. Special thanks go to Anne Barnes, Graphics and Prepress Manager, who designed and coordinated the layout of the book, and to Judy Castagna, Production Manager, for ensuring that the book itself is manufactured at the highest standards of quality. Thanks also go to Kathy Stein, the highly competent Director of Financial and Business Operations, and the always pleasant and helpful Robin Simpson, Acquisitions Coordinator, who aided us with numerous administrative and technical requirements for the publication of this edition. Finally, Bob Pursell, Director of Sales and Marketing, has organized an outstanding program for publicizing our *Textbook* to the field through various promotional efforts.

The organizational headquarters for this edition of *Textbook of Clinical Psychiatry* was located at the University of California, Davis School of Medicine in Sacramento. Tina Coltri-Marshall, Editorial Assistant, handled all the correspondence and the majority of the calls to our authors and editorial board members. Her dedication and commitment to the publication of this edition are greatly appreciated and were invaluable. We simply could not have accomplished a project of this magnitude and complexity without her. Tina is the best!

We would also like to thank our wives, Dianne Hales and Beth Yudofsky, and our four daughters, Julia Hales and Elissa, Lynn, and Emily Yudofsky, for their support and understanding over the past 3 years, especially during evenings and on weekends.

Finally, and of most importance, we acknowledge the many people with psychiatric disorders, their families, and those who have dedicated their lives to caring for them through clinical service, research, and education. These brave and exemplary people have provided us with the inspiration, motivation, and knowledge for the crafting of this textbook.

Robert E. Hales, M.D., M.B.A.
Sacramento, California

Stuart C. Yudofsky, M.D.
Houston, Texas

Introduction

Glen O. Gabbard, M.D.

Now in its fourth edition, *The American Psychiatric Publishing Textbook of Clinical Psychiatry* has become a classic in the field. To the editors' credit, they have continued to define psychiatry broadly. As the selection of chapters and chapter authors reflects, psychiatrists engage in a plethora of diverse activities: prescribing medication; administering electroconvulsive therapy; conducting individual, group, and conjoint therapies; testifying in court; contributing to the understanding of public health issues such as violence and suicide; expanding our knowledge of how culture contributes to psychopathology; and examining the interface of genetics and environment in shaping what makes us human. The biopsychosocial model made famous by Engel (1982) is applicable to all of medicine. However, the model reaches its ultimate fulfillment in contemporary psychiatry. Psychiatrists are also distinct from all other mental health professionals in that their knowledge and training allow them to be the ultimate integrators of the biological and psychosocial perspectives underlying diagnostic understanding and treatment.

I stress that *The American Psychiatric Publishing Textbook of Clinical Psychiatry* continues to cast its net broadly because in our managed care era, the biopsychosocial model is increasingly relegated to political lip service. Psychiatrists are often limited to doing brief medication checks, whereas psychosocial interventions, such as psychotherapy, are provided by nonpsychiatric mental health professionals. This fragmentation of the patient into a mind and a brain, or a psychology and a biology, insidiously undermines the integrative thrust of psychiatry. Reductionism in either a psychological or a biological direction risks an incomplete picture of the patient.

One survey of practitioners suggested that 55% of patients currently receive both medication and psychotherapy (Pincus et al. 1999). In the most recent Practice Research Network survey (American Psychiatric Association Practice Research Network Update 2000), only one-third of psychiatric patients were not receiving some type of psychotherapy. Hence, most psychiatric patients receive both medication and psychotherapy, but the education of psychiatrists in the integration of both modalities is in jeopardy. In her anthropological study of American psychiatry, Luhrmann (2000) noted how the juggernaut of managed care has intensified ideological tension between biomedical and psychosocial psychiatry: "These approaches are presented in different lectures, taught by different teachers, associated with different patients, learned in different settings. The new policies have sharply enhanced that separation and severely truncated the psychotherapeutic side" (p. 247).

Prominent voices in American psychiatry (Detre and McDonald 1997; Lieberman and Rush 1996) proposed new models for the field that explicitly call for dramatic reduction in the provision of psychotherapy by psychiatrists. Under these proposals, psychiatry would be reshaped in a biologically reductionistic direction. Psychotherapy is often regarded as a luxury that is not cost-effective. In fact, the cost is well worth the benefit it provides in many cases because the provision of psychotherapy may save money by reducing other costs, such as hospitalization (Gabbard et al. 1997).

By its inclusiveness, this encyclopedic textbook of psychiatry stresses that a broad knowledge of both psychology and neuroscience is the essence of psychiatric practice and the basis on which treatment decisions are ideally based. Like surgeons, who are trained to know when they should *not* operate, psychiatrists are trained to know when they should *not* prescribe, and their knowledge allows them to think about patients from the dual perspective of both biology and psychology in all clinical encounters (Gabbard and Kay 2001).

Several decades ago, considerable concern was expressed that medication and psychotherapy might be incompatible. Some worried that prescribing psychotropic agents might interfere with the patient's capacity to make use of psychotherapy. Concerns such as these have largely disappeared from the current psychiatric landscape as a result of a common clinical observation that medication often enhances the patient's reflective capacities. Indeed, a growing research literature suggests that for most major psychiatric disorders, a combination of medication and various psychotherapies may produce better results than either modality alone. For patients with bulimia nervosa, those who receive both cognitive-behavioral therapy and an antidepressant experience greater reduction in binge eating and depression symptoms than those who receive either modality alone (Walsh et al. 1997). For persons with schizophrenia, the combination of psychoeducational family therapy and antipsychotic medication produces dramatic improvements in the relapse rate, compared with either treatment alone (Hogarty et al. 1991; Zhang et al. 1994).

Similar advantages of combined treatments have been demonstrated in chronic forms of depression (Keller et al. 2000) and for elderly depressed patients (Reynolds et al. 1999). In the case of major depression, medication appears to provide rapid relief from acute distress, whereas psychotherapeutic interventions may provide broad and enduring change in vocational and social areas.

The advantage of combining treatments is also clear in some anxiety disorders. The combination of cognitive-behavioral therapy and imipramine for the treatment of panic disorders shows clear advantage at long-term follow-up over either treatment alone (Barlow et al. 2000). Combining behavior therapy and imipramine for specific phobia and social phobia results in superior efficacy compared with the results in patients who have received only behavior therapy or imipramine (Mavissakalian 1993).

Not all psychiatric disorders have been subject to rigorous trials involving combined treatment versus single treatments. Moreover, clinical experience suggests that all patients do not require both psychotherapy and pharmacotherapy. However, an overriding concern in psychiatric education is that even when medication alone is the chosen treatment, psychotherapeutic management is essential to ensure compliance with the medication regimen. Whether the treatment is psychotherapy or pharmacotherapy, a solid therapeutic alliance is essential. In a classic study (Krupnick et al. 1996), trained raters scored the therapeutic alliance for depressed patients who were placed in one of four treatments: 16 weeks of cognitive-behavioral therapy, 16 weeks of interpersonal therapy, imipramine plus clinical management, or placebo plus clinical management. The researchers concluded that the therapeutic alliance was just as important for pharmacotherapy as for psychotherapy. In fact, the strength of the therapeutic alliance accounted for more of the variance in treatment outcomes (21%) than the treatment method itself (1%) (Krupnick et al. 1996).

This dichotomization of mind and brain has long been associated with the view in psychiatry that psychotherapy is a treatment for "psychologically based" disorders, whereas medication should be used to treat "brain-based" disorders. This polarized view is increasingly specious as we come to realize that psychotherapy works by its impact on the brain. Kandel (1998, 1999) elaborated on how psychotherapeutic interventions may work at the synaptic and intracellular levels. Psychotherapy can be viewed as one example of how environmental experience alters gene expression (Kandel 1999).

Psychotherapy has an effect on biology, and medication has an effect on psychology. What we know as "mind" can be understood as the activity of the brain (Andreasen 1997). Nevertheless, mental states are not easily reducible to neural states, and the language of psychology and the language of biology involve two different levels of discourse when working with the patient (Edelson 1984; Reiser 1985). The biopsychosocial psychiatrist must be conceptually bilingual to provide comprehensive treatment.

The one-person treatment model demands that the psychiatrist think in terms of both a dysfunctional brain and a psychologically distressed human being. Docherty et al. (1977) termed this dual role *bimodal relatedness*, akin to the physicist who must simultaneously think in terms of particles and waves. In one appointment with the patient, the psychiatrist must be capable of shifting from a more or less objective and observational perspective to an empathic, intersubjective (but no less scientific) approach. Although this balancing act is challenging, it is also the essence of good medical and psychiatric practice and epitomizes Engel's biopsychosocial model. The psychiatrist, like any good physician, treats the whole person.

Many psychiatrists find this integration daunting and prefer to think in reductionistic terms. It is to the benefit of our field that editors Hales and Yudofsky have not succumbed to the siren song of reductionism. In their auspicious choice to be integrative and inclusive, they provide a road map for psychiatry in the twenty-first century that both trainees and experienced clinicians would be well advised to follow.

Glen O. Gabbard, M.D.
Professor and Director,
Baylor Psychiatry Clinic,
Department of Psychiatry and Behavioral Sciences,
Baylor College of Medicine;
Training and Supervising Analyst,
Houston-Galveston Psychoanalytic Institute,
Houston, Texas

References

American Psychiatric Association Practice Research Network Update: Are Psychiatrists Providing Psychotherapy to Their Patients? Washington, DC, American Psychiatric Association Practice Research Network, Spring 2000

Andreasen NC: Linking mind and brain in the study of mental illnesses: a project for a scientific psychopathology. Science 275:1586–1593, 1997

Barlow DH, Gorman JM, Shear MK, et al: Cognitive-behavioral therapy, imipramine, or their combination for panic disorder: a randomized controlled trial. JAMA 283:2529–2536, 2000

Detre T, McDonald MC: Managed care and the future of psychiatry. Arch Gen Psychiatry 54:201–204, 1997

Docherty JP, Marder SR, van Kammen DP, et al: Psychotherapy and pharmacotherapy: conceptual issues. Am J Psychiatry 134:529–533, 1997

Edelson M: Hypothesis and Evidence in Psychoanalysis. Chicago, IL, University of Chicago Press, 1984

Elkin I, Shea MT, Watkins JT, et al: National Institute of Mental Health Treatment of Depression Collaborative Research Program: general effectiveness of treatments. Arch Gen Psychiatry 64:532–539, 1989

Engel GL: Sounding board: the biopsychosocial model and medical education. Who are to be the teachers? N Engl J Med 306:802–805, 1982

Gabbard GO, Kay J: The fate of integrated treatment: whatever happened to the biopsychosocial psychiatrist? Am J Psychiatry 158:1956–1963, 2001

Gabbard GO, Lazar SG, Hornberger J, et al: The economic impact of psychotherapy: a review. Am J Psychiatry 154:147–155, 1997

Hogarty GE, Anderson CM, Reiss DJ, et al: Family psychoeducation, social skills training, and maintenance chemotherapy in the aftercare treatment of schizophrenia, II: two-year effects of a controlled study on relapse and adjustment. Arch Gen Psychiatry 48:340–347, 1991

Kandel ER: A new intellectual framework for psychiatry. Am J Psychiatry 155:457–469, 1998

Kandel ER: Biology and the future of psychoanalysis: a new intellectual framework for psychiatry revisited. Am J Psychiatry 156:505–524, 1999

Keller MG, McCullough JP, Klein DN, et al: A comparison of nefazodone, the cognitive behavioral analysis system of psychotherapy, and their combination for the treatment of chronic depresson. N Engl J Med 342:1462–1470, 2000

Krupnick JL, Sotsky SM, Simmens S, et al: The role of therapeutic alliance in psychotherapy and pharmacotherapy outcome: findings in the National Institute of Mental Health Treatment of Depression Collaborative Research Program. J Consult Clin Psychol 64:532–539, 1996

Lieberman JA, Rush AJ: Redefining the role of psychiatry in medicine. Am J Psychiatry 153:1388–1397, 1996

Luhrmann TM: Of Two Minds: The Growing Disorder in American Psychiatry. New York, Alfred A. Knopf, 2000

Mavissakalian MR: Combined behavior and pharmacological treatment of anxiety disorders, in American Psychiatric Press Review of Psychiatry, Vol 12. Edited by Oldham JM, Riba MB, Tasman A. Washington, DC, American Psychiatric Press, 1993, pp 565–584

Pincus HA, Zarin DA, Tanielian TL, et al: Psychiatric patients and treatments in 1997: findings from the American Psychiatric Association Practice Research Network. Arch Gen Psychiatry 56:441–449, 1999

Reiser MF: Converging sectors of psychoanalysis and neurobiology: mutual challenge and opportunity. J Am Psychoanal Assoc 33:11–34, 1985

Reynolds CF III, Frank E, Perel JM, et al: Nortriptyline and interpersonal psychotherapy as maintenance therapies for recurrent major depression: a randomized controlled trial in patients older than 59 years. JAMA 281:39–45, 1999

Walsh BT, Wilson GT, Loeb KL, et al: Medication and psychotherapy in the treatment of bulimia nervosa. Am J Psychiatry 154:523–531, 1997

Zhang M, Wang M, Li J, et al: Randomized controlled trial of family interventions for 78 first-episode male schizophrenic patients: an 18-month study in Suzhou, Jiangsu. Br J Psychiatry 165(suppl):96–102, 1994

PART

I

Theoretical Foundations and Assessment

CHAPTER 1

Genetics

James A. Knowles, M.D., Ph.D.

The field of psychiatric genetics has made significant advances and is poised for more in the next few years. As described in this chapter, many reports of genetic linkage have now been replicated when examined in independent samples. These include, but are not limited to, linkages on chromosome arms 1q, 5q, 6p, 6q, 8p, 10p, 13q, 15q, and 22q in schizophrenia and chromosome arms 1q, 4p, 10p, 10q, 12q, 13q, 18p, 18q, 21q, and 22q in manic-depressive (bipolar) illness. During the decade preceding these findings, most of the positive results in the field were not replicated in follow-up studies by either the original investigator or other groups. Because replication of a linkage finding is the best proof that it is real, the above findings represent a significant advance in the field and should lead to the identification of DNA sequence variations that increase an individual's risk of developing a psychiatric disorder. It is hoped that identifying the cellular and molecular pathways altered by these DNA sequence variations will facilitate a basic understanding of the pathogenesis of these disorders, enable investigators to conduct studies of the environmental factors that interact with each gene to modify an individual's risk for disease, and allow for rational drug design to develop better pharmaceutical treatments. In the more distant future, gene therapies for some of the disorders may be possible.

Underlying the recent successes in psychiatric genetics are advances in the field of human genetics, such as the cloning by virtue of genomic position of many of the genes for the mendelian disorders; the Human Genome Project, including the sequencing of the human genome;

and the localization of loci for genes for the complex disorders. As of November 2001, there are 13,118 established gene loci (Online Mendelian Inheritance in Man: http://www3.ncbi.nlm.nih.gov/Omim/Stats/mimstats.html), and through the year 2000, 1,112 disease genes have been discovered that cause 1,430 clinical diseases (some genes cause more than one disease) (Peltonen and McKusick 2001).

At present, almost all of the 1,430 clinical genetic diseases in humans are disorders that are transmitted in patterns that can be predicted from knowledge of how genetic information is transmitted to offspring during meiosis (Mendel's laws). The identification of the genes that cause three relatively common diseases—cystic fibrosis (CF, an autosomal recessive disease); neurofibromatosis, type I (NF1, an autosomal dominant disease); and Duchenne muscular dystrophy (DMD, an X-linked disease)—illustrates the power of human genetics to determine the cause of human disease. In each of these mendelian disorders, the techniques of molecular biology were used to 1) determine the chromosomal location of the disease gene, 2) isolate the gene itself, 3) identify the disease-causing mutation, and 4) produce the abnormal protein product of the disease gene in vitro for further study. Unlike the mendelian disorders mentioned above, the psychiatric disorders do not have clear-cut inheritance patterns and are therefore classified as some of the "complex" genetic disorders. In addition, the psychiatric disorders do not have etiological homogeneity, well-defined (or for that matter stable) phenotypes, or reproducibly associated chromosomal rearrangement syn-

This work was supported by grants from the National Institute of Mental Health (RO1-MH60912, RO1-MH50214), National Institute on Drug Abuse (RO1-DA12190, DA12853), National Institute on Aging (RO1-AG15473), and the National Alliance for Research on Schizophrenia and Depression.

dromes, all of which make finding the disease genes considerably more difficult.

Help for this difficulty comes in the form of the Human Genome Project. Started in 1985 with the goal of determining the complete sequence of the human genome by 2005, the project is ahead of schedule, and draft sequences (94%–96%) of the genome were published in 2001 from both public (Lander et al. 2001) and private (Venter et al. 2001) groups. This remarkable achievement has produced a number of insights. Although the final number is not yet known, humans appear to have between 30,000 and 40,000 genes. This number is markedly lower than the 100,000 genes that the genome was thought to contain based on DNA hybridization experiments and is only twice the number in a roundworm or a fruit fly and only six times as many as yeast, a unicellular organism; however, the genes in humans appear to be more complex. Most of the evolutionarily new genes code for neuronal function, tissue-specific developmental regulation, and the immune system. Of the approximately 3 billion base pairs (bp) in the human genome, 1% of the DNA is exons of genes, 24% is introns of genes, and 75% is intergenic. Two random chromosomes differ on average about once in every 1,000 bp, so there are approximately 3 million differences per individual, while most people are 99.999% identical. Most of this genetic variation is in the form of single nucleotide polymorphisms (SNPs), and more than 4 million SNPs are currently available in the public databases (see next paragraph). One last major finding of the draft genome sequence that has direct relevance to psychiatric genetics is that the mutation rate is twice as high in males as in females. It is tempting to speculate that the recently observed increase in the risk of schizophrenia with advancing paternal age (Malaspina et al. 2001) is connected with the higher mutation rate in males.

Other benefits from the Human Genome Project have been the complete DNA sequences of more than 40 bacterial genomes (http://www.ncbi.nlm.nih.gov/COG), yeast, roundworm, and fruit fly. The DNA sequencing of the mouse, rat, and pufferfish genomes are in progress and will provide comparative information that will be necessary to understand the functioning of the human genome. Draft versions of the human genome can be viewed on-line at http://www.ncbi.nlm.nih.gov/cgi-bin/Entrez/map_search or http://genome.ucsc.edu/. Other information about the Human Genome Project can be accessed through the Web page of the National Center for Biotechnology Information at http://www.ncbi.nlm.nih.gov/.

With these resources, the genes responsible for several of the complex disorders have now been isolated or localized. The best success has been in the field of cancer genetics, in which multiple genes for the different forms of cancer have been isolated. For instance, analysis of families with multiple individuals who developed breast cancer revealed that the disorder had a complex mode of inheritance. However, when only those families with a young age at onset were examined, an autosomal dominant mode of inheritance was observed (Newman et al. 1988). This led to the linkage of the breast cancer 1 gene (BRCA1) to chromosome 17 (Hall et al. 1990), the subsequent cloning of the gene (Miki et al. 1994), and the detection of more than 130 disease-causing mutations in the gene (Couch and Weber 1996). Since then, a second breast cancer gene, BRCA2, has been localized to chromosome 13 and cloned (Wooster et al. 1994, 1995). There also have been several large-scale genome-wide scans for linkage to the complex disorders of diabetes (Davies et al. 1994), multiple sclerosis (Ebers et al. 1996; Haines et al. 1996b; Kuokkanen et al. 1996; Sawcer et al. 1996), and asthma (The Collaborative Study on the Genetics of Asthma [CSGA] 1997; Xu et al. 2001). In all of these cases, there is a direct biological test for the presence or absence of the disorder (e.g., pathology, blood glucose). The work in type 2 diabetes mellitus has led to the possible identification of calpain-10 as a disease gene, one of the first for a polygenic form of a disorder, although more work needs to be done to confirm the finding (Horikawa et al. 2000). Genetic linkage studies in psychiatry are expected to be more difficult due to the diagnostic uncertainties of our field. Nonetheless, there is great excitement over the prospects of the next few years.

Psychiatric Genetics: Aims and Methods

At the core of psychiatric genetics has been the investigation of the genetic contribution to psychiatric disorders. These core studies, however, have led researchers into many related areas, such as the search for environmental etiological factors, the refinement of psychiatric nosology, the investigation of normal and abnormal psychological and behavioral traits, and the development of effective methods for the prevention and treatment of psychiatric disorders.

Aims

The goals of genetic investigation in psychiatry are as follows:

1. To establish and specify the genetic component of the etiology of psychiatric syndromes and thus determine a) to what extent a psychiatric disorder is genetically caused, b) the DNA variation that underlies the genetic contribution, c) the biopsychosocial abnormalities associated with the gene or genes involved, and d) the processes by which genetic abnormalities lead to symptoms.

2. To establish and specify the nongenetic component of the etiology of psychiatric syndromes and thus identify environmental factors that, acting independently of or interacting with vulnerable genotypes, produce or increase the likelihood of a disorder.

3. To validate the boundaries of diagnostic entities and subtypes within entities by determining a) the similarities in genetic variations between disorders, or between subtypes of a disorder, to establish groupings of genetically related disorders (e.g., a schizophrenia spectrum) or to split disorders established on clinical phenomenology (e.g., different subtypes of schizoaffective disorder); and b) the characteristics (e.g., severity, subject's age at onset) of a disorder that increase its heritability, thereby helping to identify diagnostic boundaries that more closely correspond to biological boundaries.

4. To specify the genetic contribution to traits and psychological symptoms, independent of their role as components of defined psychiatric syndromes.

5. To develop methods of preventing or treating psychiatric disorders based on knowledge of genetic and environmental factors in their etiology. These methods include genetic counseling, alteration of the necessary/permissive environment for persons at risk, and gene therapy.

Methods

Research methods have evolved for each of the aims of genetic investigation. Over the past two decades, the methodologies have been especially productive in determining to what extent a psychiatric disorder is genetically caused (Table 1–1). New techniques hold the promise of determining the location, nature, and product of the genetic contribution to many disorders. Genetic investigation of a psychiatric disorder attempts to answer a sequence of questions:

- Is the illness familial?
- Is this familiality caused by genetic factors?
- What are the various clinical expressions of the abnormal gene(s)?
- What are the earliest manifestations of this predisposition to illness?
- What environmental variables increase or decrease the chances of predisposed individuals developing the disorder?
- What is the mode of transmission?
- Where is (are) the abnormal gene(s)?
- What is the biological, physiological, and psychological outcome of the genetic abnormality?

Different techniques, each with their own advantages and disadvantages, as described below, are used to attempt to answer these questions.

Is the Illness Familial?—Family Risk Studies and Epidemiological Studies

Family risk studies are designed to determine to what extent an illness runs in families because all genetic illnesses have increased rates of illness among relatives (although not all familial traits are genetic [e.g., language]). Research by the pioneers of psychiatric genetics in the early part of the twentieth century found that rates of schizophrenia and bipolar illness were higher among family members of affected individuals than in the general population. As diagnostic criteria have been developed and validated, such studies have continued, both for the psychoses and for other diagnostic entities (schizophrenia [Kendler et al. 1985], affective disorders [Andreasen et al. 1987], panic disorder [Noyes et al. 1986], simple phobias [Fyer et al. 1990], and anorexia nervosa [Gershon et al. 1984]).

The methodology of conducting such studies has developed to meet higher research standards. In those studies conducted in the early part of the twentieth century, nonrepresentative hospitalized cases were sampled, and the collection of data on family members was indirect. Diagnoses were made on the basis of global clinical impressions by investigators who were not blind to the diagnoses of other family members. The results were then compared with control subjects diagnosed by other investigators.

The current state-of-the-art family risk study does the following:

1. Samples patients (termed *probands* or *index cases*) in a nonbiased way to obtain a sample representative of all patients with the disorder.

2. Either interviews family members directly or obtains detailed descriptions of a family member's illness through records and multiple informants.

3. Arrives at diagnoses while blind to the disease status of the index case.

4. Uses operationalized diagnostic criteria (such as those in DSM-IV-TR; American Psychiatric Association 2000]).

TABLE 1–1. Evidence in support of genetic transmission of various psychiatric disorders

Illness	Genetic transmission supported by			
	Family risk studies	**Twin studies**	**Adoption studies**	**Molecular studies**
Schizophrenia	+	+	+	+
Bipolar disorder	+	+	+	+
Major depression	+	+	(+)	+
Panic disorder and agoraphobia	+	+		+
Generalized anxiety disorder	+	+		
Simple phobia	+	+		
Social phobia	+	+		
Obsessive-compulsive disorder	(+)	+		+
Posttraumatic stress disorder		+		
Anorexia nervosa	+	+		+
Briquet's syndrome/somatization disorder and sociopathy	+	(+)	+	
Alcoholism	+	(+)	+	+
Personality disorders				
Antisocial	+			
Schizotypal	+	+		+
Borderline		+		
Avoidant	+			
Dependent	+			
Alzheimer's disease	+	(+)		+

Note. Evidence discussed, with references, in text. + = most or all findings support genetic transmission; (+) = some findings support genetic transmission, but others do not.

5. Demonstrates reliability in both the information gathering and the diagnostic processes.
6. Compares the data on familial psychopathology, using appropriate statistical analyses, with the rate of psychopathology in the family members of a matched control group investigated simultaneously with the same methodology.

Investigations that use these techniques not only have supported the original studies showing the familial nature of many psychiatric illnesses but also have yielded much more precise estimates of the prevalence of various forms of psychopathology among relatives. From these studies the concepts of a spectrum of illnesses related to schizophrenia, an affective disorder spectrum, and associations between clinically distinct disorders such as anorexia nervosa and affective disorders have emerged.

Calculation of the extent of psychiatric disorders among the relatives of probands begins with the rates as determined through the process of family interviews. Because some family members will not have passed through the age at risk for the disorder, it would be an underestimate of the eventual rate of psychopathology among relatives to assume that these individuals will remain well. Therefore, the data usually are reported in terms of *lifetime morbid risk*, which is an estimate of the eventual rate of illness among relatives, were they to be followed through the age at risk. Various methods are used to calculate lifetime morbid risk, all based on knowledge of the cumulative incidence of cases for a certain disorder through the life span. A simple method, the *Weinberg abridged method*, determines morbid risk by dividing the number of ill relatives by a new denominator (called a *bezugsziffern*). This denominator is determined by counting all relatives, then subtracting out the relatives below the age at risk, and subtracting out one-half of the number of relatives within the age at risk (Gottesman and Shields 1982). A more precise method used in modern studies is that of *survival analysis*, which is used to plot the time of onset of the disorder among relatives and, through this, to estimate the proportion of relatives who eventually will be affected (Kalbfeish and Prentice 1980). If the cumulative incidence of a disorder is not known, as is currently the case, for example, with most personality disorders, lifetime morbid risk calculations cannot legitimately be made.

When the lifetime morbid risks for first-degree relatives of ill and control probands are determined, a *relative risk* for first-degree relatives of ill probands can be calculated. As seen in Table 1–2, which is based on

TABLE 1–2.   Relative risk for psychiatric disorders

Disorder	Relative risk	Reference
Bipolar disorder	24.5	Weissman et al. 1984a
Schizophrenia	18.5	Kendler et al. 1985
Bulimia nervosa	9.6	Kassett et al. 1989
Panic disorder	9.6	Crowe et al. 1983
Alcoholism	7.4	Merikangas 1989
Generalized anxiety disorder	5.6	Noyes et al. 1987
Anorexia nervosa	4.6	Strober et al. 1985
Simple phobia	3.3	Fyer et al. 1990
Social phobia	3.2	Fyer et al. 1993
Somatization disorder	3.1	Cloninger et al. 1986
Major depression	3.0	Weissman et al. 1984a
Agoraphobia	2.8	Crowe et al. 1983

Note.   Other studies may have relative risk ratios that differ considerably from those in these studies, especially if different diagnostic criteria were used. However, the methodological soundness of studies referenced here prompted our selection of them for discussion in the text and in this comparison.

selected methodologically sound studies, this relative risk varies from approximately 3 to 25 for the psychiatric disorders studied, indicating significant familial aggregation for all of them. From these data, it appears that bipolar disorder, schizophrenia, bulimia nervosa, panic disorder, and alcoholism are the most familial.

As noted earlier, however, such rates of illness may be influenced by environmental conditions shared by family members. Thus, the extent to which a disorder is familial cannot be immediately taken as an indication of the extent to which it is genetically determined. Family studies are quite good for ruling out a genetic basis of a disorder but can only provide support, not proof, of the existence of heritable factors. There also may be *assortative mating*, which is the tendency for those with a psychiatric disorder to mate preferentially, usually with those who have similar psychopathology, or in other nonrandom ways, thus increasing the likelihood of the children inheriting a genetic predisposition to the disorder beyond what would be the case were only one parent affected. Unless recognized, this could lead to a familial pattern that overestimates the genetic effect.

Large-scale epidemiological studies, such as the National Institute of Mental Health (NIMH) Epidemiologic Catchment Area (ECA) study (Robins et al. 1984) and the National Comorbidity Survey (NCS; Kessler et al. 1994), can contribute to the value and interpretation of the familial data. With the use of structured interview schedules and standardized diagnostic criteria, estimates of the population prevalence of disorders can be determined and compared with the data obtained from the family studies. Some studies blend the techniques of epidemiology and family risk, studying geographic, ethnic, or cultural isolates (Egeland et al. 1987; Gusella et al. 1983).

In isolated populations, we expect greater genetic homogeneity for the psychiatric disorder present because all or most cases of the disorder may stem from a common progenitor who is the single source of the pathogenic gene(s). In addition, higher environmental homogeneity is likely, and because the variation of a trait explained by genetic factors is the sum of the environmental and genetic factors, decreasing the environmental variance increases the genetic variance. There also may be a higher prevalence of certain disorders in such populations. These elevated rates may be caused by an increased frequency of the abnormal genotype or a higher rate of expression of the gene (i.e., increased penetrance). Isolated kindreds showing a high incidence of the disorder provide the best samples for the segregation and linkage analytic techniques, described later, that can identify and localize a potent genetic contributory factor.

Do Genetic Factors Contribute to the Illness?— Twin and Adoption Studies

After a psychiatric disorder has been found to be familial, twin and adoption studies are used to dissect the relative contributions of genetics and environment to the etiology of the disorder.

Twin studies.   Twin studies examine the concordance, or the coincidence, of a disorder in monozygotic, genetically identical (MZ), and in dizygotic, fraternal (DZ) twins, the latter sharing, on average, one-half of their genes, as do siblings.[1] One strategy involves comparing concordance in MZ pairs and same-sex DZ pairs. If only the rearing environment has predisposed an index case to illness, then the co-twin, whether MZ or DZ, also should be at risk, and the rates for both MZ and DZ twins should be elevated (compared with the population rate) and equal. If, on the other hand, pathogenic genes have predisposed the index twin to illness, then an MZ co-twin would be at a higher risk than would a DZ co-twin. The concordance rate for MZ twins would be higher than that for DZ twins, and the latter should be similar to the concordance rate for siblings.

One assumption of this strategy is that the MZ and DZ twins have the same degree of similarity of the familial environment—in other words, that MZ twins do not share more environmental similarity than do DZ twins in ways that would increase the MZ concordance for psychiatric disorders. It is obvious that in some ways MZ twins are treated more similarly (e.g., being dressed alike). It is also clear that in many families MZ twins receive very similar emotional and attitudinal input from their parents. However, to indicate the complexity of this issue, evidence indicates that the temperamental characteristics of the MZ twins (which may be genetic in origin) generate this similarity in rearing. The available empirical evidence does support the assumption of an equal environment in both female (Kendler et al. 1993d) and male (Xian et al. 2000b) twin pairs.

Because it is difficult to determine the degree to which shared environment could account for the increased MZ concordance rates of twins raised in the same home, studies of twins raised apart in uncorrelated (i.e., randomly assigned) environments would be useful. Ideally, the concordance rates of MZ and DZ pairs raised apart could be compared, but even having only such a sample of MZ twins would allow for comparison of their concordance rates with those of MZ twins raised in the same home. Systematic samples of such twins are difficult to obtain, however, and case reports of concordance are more likely to be noted and published than are those of discordant pairs.

A third way to use the concordance rates for twins to address the question of genetic versus environmental factors is to examine the extent to which MZ twins are discordant for a disorder. Given that MZ twins are genetically identical, any degree of discordance implies that

there are nongenetic etiological factors that can either produce or unmask the disorder. For example, these findings could result from "phenocopies," cases that appear to have the disorder in question but have an environmentally determined, pathogenically distinct illness that mimics the genetically determined disease. Another possibility is that environmental conditions might be necessary to add to or to interact with genetic factors to produce the illness, leading to MZ twins being both predisposed genetically for the disorder but discordant on the basis of having experienced different environments. Huntington's disease has a nearly 100% MZ concordance rate, whereas common psychiatric disorders such as schizophrenia and bipolar disorder have rates that approximate 50% and 65%, respectively.

The twin strategies described produce quantitative data that are tempting to translate into estimates of the extent to which a disorder is genetically caused. The *heritability* of a psychiatric disorder is defined as the portion of a trait's variation in the population that is accounted for by genetic factors. Two types of heritability have been defined: *broad-sense heritability*, the portion accounted for by all genetic influences, and *narrow-sense heritability*, the portion accounted for by additive genetic variance only. Broad-sense heritability is calculated by doubling the difference in rates of concordance observed in the MZ and DZ twin pairs for a disease or trait. For instance, if the concordance rates found in a twin study of schizophrenia were 47.5% and 17.5% for MZ and DZ twin pairs, respectively, then the estimated broad-sense heritability would be 60% [$2 \times (47.5 - 17.5)$]. Broad-sense heritability includes the influence of gene dominance and epistasis (interactions between genes), whereas narrow-sense heritability estimates the amount of genetic influence that is likely to be passed on to offspring.

Questions regarding the interpretation of MZ twin concordance rates may be resolved by another twin strategy, the study of the offspring of discordant MZ twins. If the ill twin has a purely environmentally caused disorder, then the offspring of the well co-twin should not be at elevated risk (unless he or she is exposed to the pathogenic environmental insults that his or her aunt or uncle, but not his or her parent, experienced). On the other hand, if the ill and well twins share a genetic predisposition to the illness, but one had not experienced certain precipitating or contributing environmental insults, then

---

[1]There are two methods of calculating concordance: pairwise and probandwise. In the pair method, every pair is counted only once; in the proband method, pairs are counted twice if each twin was an ill proband sampled for the study independently, and this usually results in somewhat higher concordances. Many geneticists regard the latter method as preferable because the rates can be compared with population rates (Gottesman and Shields 1982). In this chapter, probandwise rates are given unless otherwise noted.

the well co-twin will be a carrier of liability for the illness, and his or her offspring will be at elevated risk. This strategy was pioneered by Fischer (1971) and extended by Gottesman and Bertelsen (1989), who found that the offspring of nonschizophrenic MZ co-twins and the offspring of their ill co-twins had an equal morbid risk for the illness, suggesting that much of the discordance between the twins could be attributed to differential exposure to environmental factors.

Adoption studies. Adoption studies are based on the knowledge that adoption separates the two major influences parents have on their children, namely, genes and rearing. It offers researchers a naturalistic "experiment" that has the potential to answer the questions of whether a disorder is familial because of genetic transmission or the shared environment. Four types of adoption studies have been used:

1. *Adoptee study method:* the study of adopted-away children of a parent with a disorder.
2. *Cross-fostering strategy:* the study of children born of nondisordered parents adopted into a family with a disordered parent.
3. *Adoptee's family method:* the study of the adoptive and the biological relatives of disordered adoptees.
4. *MZ twins reared apart:* the study of MZ twins reared apart, as discussed previously (see "Twin Studies").

Such research is much easier to conceptualize than to execute. State-of-the-art investigations using these strategies must use systematic sampling, adoptee control subjects, careful attention to make diagnoses blind to the diagnosis of the index case, and operationalized diagnostic criteria. Pioneering studies were done by Rosenthal, Kety, Wender, and Schulsinger with later collaboration by Kendler in an investigation of schizophrenia in a Danish sample. Adoption studies have been done for mood disorders, alcoholism, drug abuse, sociopathy, attention-deficit/hyperactivity disorder, and other psychiatric conditions as well as for IQ and personality variables.

Although adoption offers an ideal separation of genetic from environmental influences, this research has methodological pitfalls. Because few children are adopted away immediately after birth, usually some familial environmental influences of undetermined significance exist that are difficult to measure. Also, "environment" does not begin at birth; the uterine environment of an affected mother may be significant in the transmission of the illness, which may be examined by comparing the risk to the children of affected mothers with the risk to the children of affected fathers or, in the adoptee's family method, the risk to paternal half-siblings compared with maternal half-siblings.

Another major difficulty stems from the unusual nature of adoption itself. The types of parents or the circumstances that lead parents to give up their children may alter the representative nature of the sample. Thus, the investigator comparing the adopted-away children of ill parents with the adopted-away children of "normal" control subjects must accept the fact that the control parents might themselves be ill in some way and that the rates of psychiatric illness in both groups of adoptees might be unusually high. Similarly, the investigator studying the biological and adoptive parents of adoptees with disorders cannot legitimately use differences in the rates of illness between these two groups to prove a genetic hypothesis, given that adoptive parents are often psychiatrically screened by adoption agencies. Thus, the biological relatives of the disordered adoptees and the biological relatives of the control adoptees must be compared, again encountering the problem of high rates of psychopathology among the control relatives.

These methodological difficulties, unless they can be overcome by removing ill probands from the control group, tend to lead to a rejection or minimization of the genetic hypothesis (a *type II error*). Thus, it is somewhat surprising that so many adoption studies have yielded results strongly supportive of genetic factors in the etiology of psychiatric disorders but not surprising that the diagnostic evaluations from these studies have been strongly contested because of the high rates of illness diagnosed among the control subjects.

What Are the Various Clinical Expressions of the Abnormal Gene(s)?—Spectrum Studies

In most of the family studies done on the major psychiatric disorders, investigators have found an increase not only in the disorder in question but also in other types of psychopathology. At times, this increase has been in milder or related syndromes of the major disorder, such as dysthymia in the relatives of patients with major depression or unipolar depression in the relatives of patients with bipolar disorder. In other illnesses, more distant syndromes have appeared—an increase in mood disorders in the relatives of patients with eating disorders and in sociopathy in the relatives of patients with somatization disorder.

As evidence has accumulated suggesting that genetic factors account for the increased familial incidence of the major psychiatric disorders, the hypothesis has been put forth that the other syndromes found to be increased among relatives are also the result of this same genetic predisposition. This concept has been expressed as the "spectrum" of disorders related to, for example, schizophrenia or bipolar disorder. As discussed below, the former is said to include schizotypal personality, paranoid personality, schizoaffective disorder (by DSM-III-R [American Psychiatric Association 1987] criteria), and atypical psychosis; the latter, bipolar II disorder, recurrent major depressive disorder, cyclothymia, dysthymia, schizoaffective disorder (Research Diagnostic Criteria [RDC; Spitzer et al. 1978] bipolar type), and possibly others.

The diagnostic trend in American psychiatry, first prominently represented in DSM-III (American Psychiatric Association 1980) and continued in the subsequent editions, has been to narrow the boundaries of Axis I disorders and to develop alternative categories (e.g., atypical psychosis, psychosis not otherwise specified) for less severe or mixed-symptom cases. It was hoped that these restrictions would produce more symptomatically and etiologically homogeneous categories, an especially appropriate development for the study of treatment effects and biological markers, for which a sample of "pure" cases could thus be recruited.

For many types of genetic studies, however, determining who in the family is ill and who is well, for all family members, is often of the utmost importance. Studies attempting to determine the mode of transmission (i.e., segregation analysis) and linkage studies are most obviously affected by misclassification. Because problems are posed by both overinclusion and overexclusion, the issue of which phenotypic syndromes are manifestations of the genotype is essential. In practice, the spectrum of disorders found in the current or prior studies to be increased in the family members of index cases, as compared with similarly diagnosed control families, is often entered into one or more data analyses as alternative manifestations of the genotype. In genetic research studies, then, the spectrum concept is not only developed but also employed.

This use of spectrum findings has problems. Even if the assumption of genetic relatedness between the disorders is correct, some of the individual cases may be genetically connected and some may not. (Consider, for example, the various causes of major depression among relatives of a patient with bipolar disorder.) Also, there may not be a direct genetic link between the disorders, even if there is a familial association. The syndromes in the spectrum may be the result of environmental influences associated with index families (e.g., the effect of early parental depression or suicide on children), or, even if genetically caused, they may be the product of assortative mating. (Consider, for example, the case of sociopathic individuals mating with schizophrenic or depressed patients, leading to increased sociopathy in the offspring.)

The problems of using spectrum diagnoses become even greater when this genetic causation is assumed to apply in a clinical situation. For heterogeneous illnesses, the etiological factors most often at work in index families may not be those represented in the population at large. Thus, whereas a schizophrenic patient's first-degree relative with a schizotypal personality disorder may very likely share the genetic predisposition to schizophrenia, the schizotypal individual without such a family history may be much less likely to have this same genetic makeup. The determination of the extent to which a spectrum illness is associated with the "index" disorder must include identification of that spectrum illness in family studies of other index disorders and in family studies that take the spectrum diagnosis as the index disorder. An example of this process has occurred with schizotypal personality disorder, first described as occurring in the families of schizophrenic patients and thus classified as part of the schizophrenic spectrum. In addition, an equal increase of schizotypal personality disorder in the families of mood disorder patients has been shown (Squires-Wheeler et al. 1989). Family studies of schizotypal disorder itself have shown increased rates of both schizotypal personality disorder and schizophrenia in relatives of schizotypal personality disorder probands (Battaglia et al. 1995).

What Are the Early Manifestations of and Environmental Risk Factors for the Illness?—High-Risk Studies

High-risk research, or the study of children at risk, is a strategy that begins with a factor of known or putative importance for the development of psychopathology and examines, through controlled studies, the influence of that factor on exposed infants or children. Such a design has been used to delineate the effects of maternal alcohol consumption during pregnancy on low birth weight. It also has been used to identify the early development of psychopathology among the offspring of parents with psychiatric disorders. This strategy entails selection of parent probands with an accurately diagnosed disorder, evaluation of psychopathology in the co-parents, and usually a longitudinal evaluation of the children with a battery of psychological and biological measures, as well as a record of environmental conditions during development. These studies can investigate 1) presymptomatic differences between the high-risk group and the control group and whether such abnormalities predict later psychopathology, 2) early manifestations of psychopathology in subjects who later develop the same disorder that their parents experienced, 3) the childhood psychopathological syndromes that may be genetically related to the adult psychiatric disorders of either or both parents, and 4) environmental variables that are associated with the development of illness in the genetically predisposed group.

Investigating presumably predisposed individuals in the well state for hidden psychological or physiological differences that could play a role in their development of the illness (e.g., psychological or physiological differences in the response of sons of alcoholic parents to alcohol) avoids one of the major pitfalls of studies of already ill individuals—namely, that abnormalities found in ill subjects may be sequelae of the illness or of its treatment rather than aspects of an intrinsic vulnerability. Investigations of the first manifestations of an illness (such as attentional deficits in the children of schizophrenic parents) may be helpful in establishing the nature of a genetically determined "core deficit" in evolving illnesses such as schizophrenia. Examining the rates of specific childhood disorders in the at-risk group (e.g., the rates of separation anxiety in the children of parents with panic disorder) can establish links between childhood and adult syndromes in the same way that family and adoption studies can identify a spectrum of adult disorders with a possibly shared genetic causation.

In high-risk studies, the environment can be controlled (Nagler 1985), but it is usually studied by evaluation of the influence of spontaneously occurring environmental events in a genetically predisposed population. These events could be those with a predisposing potential, such as parental loss, or those that might protect a vulnerable individual, such as experiences of competence and success. This application of high-risk studies parallels the study of discordant MZ twins for environmental variables that account for their discordance.

Major problems in the execution and interpretation of high-risk studies include the influence of co-parent psychopathology that may not be randomized because of assortative mating, the large sample of children that must be studied in low-prevalence disorders such as schizophrenia to achieve meaningful statistical results, the difficulty of identifying pathogenic environmental stressors when these are nonspecific and cumulative, and the difficulty of elucidating the influence of any environmental variable when it is not known who among the offspring are truly genetically predisposed. In the future, when DNA variations have been found that are clearly thought to increase the risk of developing a psychiatric disorder, a new generation of high-risk studies will explore the early manifestations of the variation and the influence of environmental factors in the offspring and relatives of probands.

What Is the Mode of Transmission?— Segregation Analysis

When family, twin, and adoption studies show that genetic factors play a role in the pathogenesis of a disorder, then *segregation analysis* can be used to attempt to determine the mode of transmission of these genetic factors. This is done by studying the pattern of inheritance of the disorder in a collection of families and comparing it with known patterns of inheritance. Mutations at any single gene are inherited in a dominant or recessive manner and may be autosomal or sex-linked. If the disorder is transmitted in families in one of these patterns, it is likely due to a single gene.

For example, approximately 50% of the offspring of parents affected with one of the dominant monogenic disorders (Huntington's disease or acute intermittent porphyria) are themselves affected. Affected offspring always have an affected parent (unless the offspring's condition represents a new mutation, which is rare). If a group of families with a particular disorder all have this pattern of transmission, then the disorder is caused by a single dominant gene. For the recessive disorders (e.g., phenylketonuria or cystic fibrosis), each affected individual will have unaffected parents who must nonetheless be carriers, and approximately 25% of the offspring of two carrier parents will be affected. Often, the incidence of consanguineous marriages (inbreeding) is increased in these families. In the sex-linked recessive disorders (e.g., hemophilia), all of the daughters of an affected father are unaffected carriers, and 50% of their sons in turn will be affected. Furthermore, no father-to-son transmission occurs.

Segregation analysis was originally developed as a test for recessive inheritance: segregation ratios in sibships were observed and compared with the 25% affected:75% unaffected ratio predicted by Mendel's first law. Subsequently, this modest approach has been expanded into a sophisticated mathematical analysis. Qualitative notions such as dominant and recessive inheritance have given way to quantitative estimates of gene frequency, gene transmission probability, and genotype penetrance. Moreover, the laws of mendelian inheritance have been replaced by models for single-gene transmission that incorporate intermediate types of gene effect. When these estimates and models are varied, they predict different phenotypic resemblances between different classes of relatives (MZ twins, DZ twins, full sibs, half sibs, and parents and offspring). These predictions are then statistically compared with the observed concordance between relatives, allowing the investigator to determine "best-fit" models. If there is an extremely close fit between the predictions and the observations, then the model's mode of inheritance and quantitative estimates are supported. If even the best-fit model for a certain mode of transmission shows little resemblance to the observed concordances, then it can be ruled out as a possible mode of transmission. However, it is important to note that segregation analysis relies on pooled data from many nuclear families and assumes genetic homogeneity across these families. This assumption is not always warranted (disorders may be phenotypically identical but etiologically distinct) and may lead to spurious results, such as the false rejection of monogenic transmission.

Unfortunately, segregation analyses of common psychiatric disorders do not confirm one of the simple mendelian or sex-linked patterns described above (Matthysse and Kidd 1976). For this reason, the psychiatric disorders belong to the group of "complex" (i.e., nonmendelian) genetic disorders. Other complex genetic disorders are hypertension and diabetes. Complex patterns can arise from multiple genetic phenomena. The first of these is *genetic heterogeneity*. If a disorder can be caused by an abnormal gene at two (or more) genetic loci, and one of these causes the disorder in a recessive pattern and the other in a dominant pattern, then a segregation analysis of all those with the disorder will support neither model. Genetic heterogeneity is suspected because it has been shown in so many other medical disorders for which the genetics have been determined. Complex patterns also may occur because of environmental influences. There may be individuals who have the disorder but do not have any genetic predisposition. These individuals are said to have a *phenocopy* of the genetic form of the disorder. Likewise, individuals who carry the disease gene may not have the disorder because of *reduced penetrance* of the gene. The psychiatric disorders are thought to show many of the above phenomena, complicating segregation analysis. All of the major psychiatric disorders can be mimicked by medical illnesses; thus, other phenocopies, indistinguishable clinically, are suspected.

Another cause of complex inheritance patterns is termed *polygenic* or *multifactorial inheritance*. These cause disease when multiple genes, none of which has a very strong effect itself, interact with one another to cause the disorder (polygenic inheritance) or when multiple genes (some of which might have a major effect) and various environmental factors all contribute (multifactorial inheritance [Kidd 1981]). Because polygenic and multifactorial models have many variables, they produce a wide variety of possible values for familial concordances and thus can often fit quite closely with the observed data. In other words, monogenic disorders can be characterized by specific segregation ratios (i.e., rates of disorder in relatives), whereas polygenic disorders cannot. However, newer methods of segregation analysis that use Monte Carlo Markov Chain methods may provide insights into how many genes contribute to polygenic traits or disease (Daw et al. 1999).

A few predictions that stem from polygenic models differ from those of monogenic models. In polygenic disorders (e.g., cleft lip/palate), relatives of affected probands are at greater risk for being affected with increasing severity of illness in the proband and with greater numbers of other affected relatives. In addition, risk of illness drops off precipitously as one moves from MZ twins to first- and second-degree relatives (Risch 1990), and affected relatives are often found on both maternal and paternal sides (Gottesman and Shields 1982). Also, monogenic disorders tend to have low population prevalences. This suggests that common diseases (i.e., those occurring in more than 1% of the population) are likely to be polygenic, as are many traits that have been genetically studied (e.g., intelligence, height, skin color).

In summary, segregation analysis has shown that most psychiatric disorders do not show a simple monogenic pattern of any variety. This finding leads to increased consideration of (but not proof for) polygenic inheritance and of confounding factors such as heterogeneity, reduced penetrance, and phenocopies. The technique may be of more value if more discrete disorders are discovered or if it is used to study the genetics of specific symptoms or physiological phenomena.

Where Is the Abnormal Gene?—Genetic Linkage Analysis and Association Studies

Two general approaches to discovering genetic factors responsible for the pathogenesis of disease have been used: *genome scans followed by subsequent positional cloning* and *candidate gene association studies*. In the first approach, the broad chromosomal location of an abnormal gene is identified, perhaps containing hundreds of genes, without reference to the abnormal protein for which it codes, by the use of a genome scan and genetic linkage analysis (described in the next paragraph). Additional genetic analysis can then lead to a smaller region and eventually to the DNA variation(s) that underlie the disease. Researchers using the positional cloning approach have elucidated the pathogenesis of hundreds of genes for the mendelian genetic disorders, including cystic fibrosis, NF1, DMD, and the early-onset forms of familial Alzheimer's disease.

Genetic linkage analysis is a technique based on exceptions to Mendel's second law (Cox and Suarez

1985; Suarez and Cox 1985). This empirical observation, also known as the *law of independent assortment*, states that alleles (specific gene configurations) at different genetic loci are inherited independently of one another. This clearly applies to loci lying on different chromosomes. This law also often applies to loci lying on the same chromosome because of the exchange of genetic material between homologous chromosomes that occurs during the meiotic phase of gametogenesis in a process known as *crossing over*. To illustrate this phenomenon (Figure 1–1), consider the possible gametes (i.e., reproductive cells) that may result from the mating of two parents, one of whom is heterozygous at two loci, A and B, on a given paired chromosome (a_1b_1/a_2b_2), and the other who is homozygous at both loci (a_2b_2/a_2b_2). In the absence of crossing over, the gametes that are produced include only a_1b_1 and a_2b_2. If crossing over occurs between loci A and B, two new gametes, known as *recombinants*, are produced by the mother (a_1b_2 and a_2b_1), and alleles at loci A and B may appear to be assorting independently in this family, even though they are on the same chromosome.[2] Consequently, within a given pedigree, the parental gametes (in the example above, a_1b_1 and a_2b_2) will be disproportionately represented if loci A and B are located near each other, and alleles at these loci will appear to violate Mendel's second law. Loci A and B may then be said to be "linked" (Figure 1–1). By extension, if linkage can be established between a hypothetical disease locus and a marker locus with known chromosomal location, then the approximate location of the disease locus can be inferred, and, ultimately, the disease gene can be isolated.

Several approaches are available for determining linkage between disease and marker loci. One approach, known as the *likelihood method* (Morton 1955), may be used to examine the cosegregation of the disease and marker phenotypes within a pedigree; determine the probability (likelihood [L]) of achieving the observed distribution of phenotypes, given estimates for the proportion of recombinant gametes among gametes (i.e., the recombination fraction), θ, ranging from 0.0 to 0.5 (the latter representing no linkage); and calculate the odds ratio (defined as the ratio $L[\theta]\backslash L[\theta=0.5]$)—that is, the relative likelihood of the evidence for linkage versus the evidence for no linkage. By convention, the odds ratio is expressed as its base 10 logarithm (known as the *lod score*) so that linkage data from several families can be

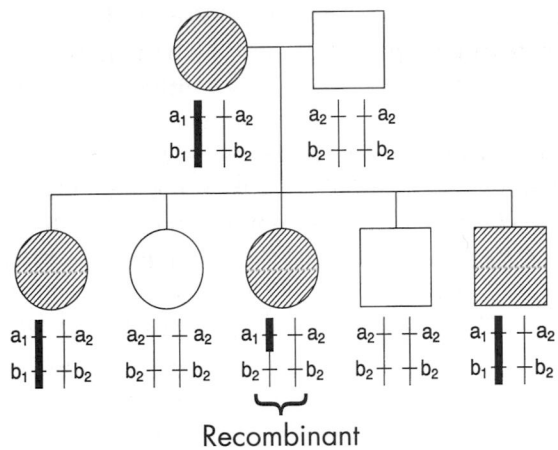

FIGURE 1–1. Genetic linkage and recombination.

Depicted is a hypothetical family (*circles*: females; *squares*: males) transmitting an autosomal dominant disease. The disease locus A (containing either the defective allele a_1 or its normal counterpart a_2) lies close to a marker locus B (containing marker alleles b_1 and b_2). The mother is affected with the disease (*shaded symbol*) and is heterozygous at both the disease and the marker loci. The father is unaffected (*open symbol*) and is homozygous at both loci. Because the disease and marker loci are genetically linked (i.e., they lie near each other), crossing over rarely occurs between them. Most children who inherit the disease allele a_1 also receive the b_1 marker allele from their mother. Occasionally, a recombination event (i.e., "crossing over") occurs in the mother, and she transfers a chromosome bearing the b_2 marker allele along with the disease allele (as occurred in the daughter labeled "recombinant"). The frequency of such recombinants increases as the distance between the disease and marker locus increases.

pooled and their respective contributions added to obtain a combined probability of linkage. For monogenic diseases that have mendelian patterns of inheritance, when the lod score at the best estimate of θ (best being defined as that estimate that yields the highest lod score) is greater than +3, linkage is confirmed; when it is less than –2, linkage is rejected. The lod scores required to confirm or reject linkage for the psychiatric disorders need to be of greater magnitude because of the complex pattern of inheritance. Corrections for the testing of multiple disease models are also required.

If some, but not all, families have linkage to a marker, a statistical test can be performed to determine whether there is evidence for genetic heterogeneity within a disorder. This appears to be the case with Charcot-Marie-Tooth disease (peroneal muscular atrophy). Once linkage

---

[2]However, crossing over rarely occurs between loci lying near one another. The frequency with which recombination results is about proportional to the distance between the affected loci. For example, a recombination frequency of 1% per meiosis corresponds to a functional distance of 1 centimorgan and a physical distance of approximately 1 million DNA base pairs.

is established, knowledge of the genotype can then permit presumptive presymptomatic identification of affected persons in individual pedigrees at risk for the disease, given appropriate information about family members.

Although the likelihood method is a statistically powerful approach for detecting linkage, it relies on several assumptions that may not be warranted. These assumptions include random mating, no association between particular disease and marker alleles within the population, and genetic homogeneity of the illness across pedigrees. Also included is specification of genetic parameters (i.e., mode of inheritance, gene frequencies, and genotype penetrances) for both the disease and the marker loci. To circumvent these problems, several nonparametric methods for finding genetic loci have been developed. In general, these methods trade the need to specify a genetic model for the ability to detect linkage under a known model with the likelihood method. The first of these, the *affected sib-pair method* (Suarez et al. 1978), posits that siblings who are both affected with a genetic disorder should be identical in the region of the genome that causes the disorder. In the other areas of the genome, the siblings should, on average, share one-half of their genetic material. Multiple sib pairs are tested, and the number of pairs who are identical for a given marker provides a statistical measure of support for linkage. This method makes no assumptions about mode of inheritance. By sampling only sib pairs in which both members are clearly affected, it avoids considering either ambiguous cases or well individuals. (For disorders with reduced penetrance, the latter may be genetically vulnerable but are thought to represent instances of recombination.) The sib-pair method, despite its advantages, is also plagued with certain limitations. Although it can use information from sibships, it is forced to disregard other information present in extended pedigrees and does not provide an estimate of genetic distance to the disease. It is also nearly equivalent to a parametric analysis assuming complete penetrance and a recessive mode of inheritance. Although it is most powerful in detecting linkage in rare, recessive disorders, this technique may only be powerful enough to detect linkage in major psychiatric disorders if the illness is linked to a marker locus for most families (Goldin and Gershon 1988).

In the likelihood and affected sib-pair methods, linkage refers to a correlation between two loci, not to their associated alleles within families. *Candidate gene genetic association studies* look for correlations between certain alleles at a locus and the population of individuals with a disease. Although certain allele pairings of linked loci are likely to be disproportionately represented within any given kindred, as recombination occurs, this eventually will result in an even distribution of disease-marker allele combinations within the population at large. When the disease gene and marker loci are relatively far apart, such distribution will occur over the course of a few generations. On the other hand, if marker loci are close to a mutation that has spread through the population, this equilibrium may not have occurred.[3] Thus, an association between a disease and a particular allele within the population (linkage disequilibrium) suggests that the location of the disease gene and the marker locus is within a small genetic region. The advantage of this method over linkage analysis is that it may be sensitive to genes with small phenotypic effects. The drawbacks of this method are that the ability to detect a genetic association declines rapidly as genetic distance increases and that this method, like linkage analysis, is affected by genetic heterogeneity. The choice of the genetic control group is also critical. If those with the illness are from genetic backgrounds that differ from those of the control subjects with whom they are compared, the observed differences in allele frequencies may be due to racial differences rather than to differences in disease status (*population stratification*). Newer statistical approaches have been developed to address this potential artifact.

Historically, various marker loci have been used for genetic linkage mapping. The first markers were blood antigens from both erythrocytes (ABO, Rh, MNS) and leukocytes (human leukocyte antigen [HLA]) that could be measured serologically; serum proteins and isoenzymes that could be measured electrophoretically; and common anomalies such as color blindness. The major shortcomings of these marker loci were their paucity (about 30 known) and their irregular distribution throughout the genome. In the early 1980s, the first markers using DNA polymorphisms, the restriction fragment length polymorphisms (RFLPs), came into use. The RFLP markers detect variations in DNA sequence that cause the presence or absence of sites for enzymes that cut specific sequences of DNA (i.e., restriction endonucleases). Because a restriction endonuclease site is either present or absent in a given chromosome (i.e., there are only two possible alleles), the RFLP markers limit the frequency of heterozygotes to 50%. The varia-

---

[3]It has been estimated that approximately 69 generations, or 2,000 years, are necessary for the frequency of an allele combination to go to half of its equilibrium value for two loci that are separated by 1 centimorgan.

tion in DNA sequence that underlies most RFLPs is an SNP (discussed below).

Driven by the reduced information available from having only two alleles and the cumbersome technique required to generate the RFLP data (i.e., Southern blots), a second generation of polymorphic DNA markers, *microsatellites* or *simple sequence repeats*, were developed and mapped to the various chromosomes. These markers use the naturally occurring variations in the length of dinucleotide (also tri-, tetra-, pentanucleotide) DNA repeat sequences. For example, an individual might have the DNA sequence ...GATT(CA)$_{12}$GCTA... on one of his homologous chromosome pairs and the DNA sequence ...GATT(CA)$_{16}$GCTA... on the other. After these DNA fragments have been selectively amplified 100,000-fold by the polymerase chain reaction (PCR) with radioactive nucleotides, they can be separated by length (32 bp vs. 40 bp) and detected by autoradiography. The inheritance of these fragments can then be followed up in families who have the disease of interest (Figure 1–2). The microsatellite markers have multiple alleles (e.g., [CA]$_{12}$ to [CA]$_{30}$) and therefore ensure that pedigree members are quite likely to be heterozygous for the marker loci. As illustrated in Figure 1–1, individuals who are heterozygous at a marker locus are essential for linkage studies. At the current microsatellite loci, 65%–85% of the individuals will be heterozygous. These markers are also widely and uniformly distributed in the human genome (approximately every 6 kilobases), and genotypes for the pedigree members can be determined in a day or two with the PCR. High-density maps of each chromosome have been made using more than 8,000 of these markers (Broman et al. 1998).

The third generation of polymorphic markers is the SNPs (single nucleotide polymorphisms). In these single base-pair variations, one chromosome might have a "G," whereas another has an "A" embedded in a stretch of identical DNA sequence. As mentioned earlier, SNPs that occur in the cutting sites of restriction endonucleases cause RFLPs. In humans, two unrelated genomes are estimated to differ every 1 in 500 to 1 in 1,000 bp. Given the estimated size of the human genome of 3 billion base pairs, approximately 3 million DNA sequences are nonidentical between two unrelated individuals, and 90% of this variation are SNPs. With the sequencing of the human genome, 4.2 million SNPs are available in the public databases as of May 16, 2002 (http://www.ncbi.nlm.nih.gov/SNP/overview.html). Although the microsatellite markers have more alleles and this provides more information for linkage analyses, the biallelic nature of the SNP markers makes automated computer scoring of alleles much more reliable. The SNP markers are also much more common, so it is possible to overcome the lack of information from any one SNP by doing multiple SNPs in a given gene so that the higher laboratory throughput of SNP genotypes provides more information than the microsatellite markers. In addition, some of the SNPs will be the actual DNA variation that influences phenotypic traits, and this increases the power to detect them. Last, the high density of the SNP markers will enable genomewide association studies in which hundreds of thousands of SNP markers are genotyped in a collection of pedigrees (Risch and Merikangas 1996).

Problems of Diagnosis and Classification in Genetic Investigations

Most genetic studies are greatly impeded by any ambiguity in knowing who has and who does not have the illness being studied. For example, accurate diagnosis of all family members is essential for all forms of segregation analysis and for almost all molecular genetic studies. (Changes in the diagnoses of pedigree members can have profound effects on the evidence for linkage, as described later for studies of bipolar disorder.)

The various versions of research diagnostic criteria developed for psychiatric disorders have not solved the diagnostic problems that exist for genetic investigation. These criteria often exclude ambiguous cases rather than clarify their status. Also, although reliable criteria have been constructed for many psychiatric disorders, validation of the diagnostic categories as specific entities has not been established.

The high prevalence of psychiatric disorders and the existence of many known medical disorders that can produce the major psychiatric syndromes (e.g., the various "symptomatic schizophrenias") are reasons to believe that most psychiatric diagnostic categories are clinical syndromes, identifying patients with a variety of etiological abnormalities. A diagnosis of Huntington's disease or DMD is known to specify a group with a specific etiology and pathogenesis, whereas a diagnosis of schizophrenia or major depressive disorder is not. If the diagnostic entities that psychiatry has established are not etiologically homogeneous, then searching for the modes of transmission or genetic linkages of these disorders may be likened to the genetic study of pneumonia, renal failure, or dropsy. Thus, even the most reliable criteria available for psychiatric disorders, validated to the best of our current ability, may fail to identify certain individuals with the disease

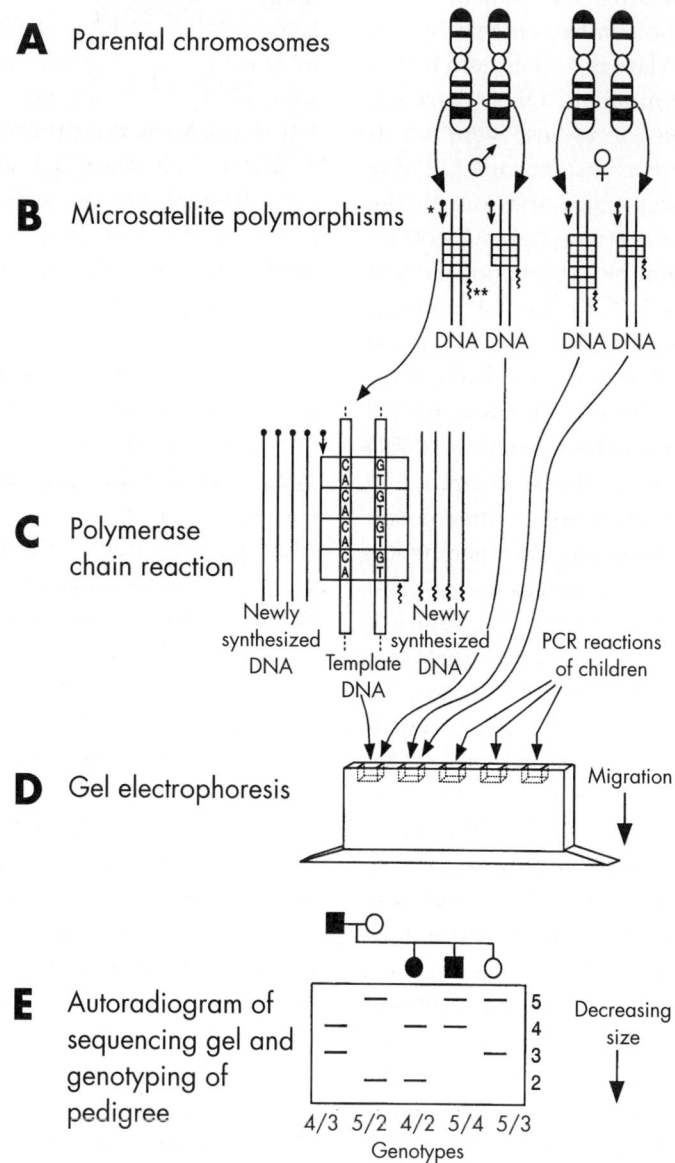

A Parental chromosomes

B Microsatellite polymorphisms

DNA DNA   DNA DNA

C Polymerase chain reaction

Newly synthesized DNA   Template DNA   Newly synthesized DNA   PCR reactions of children

D Gel electrophoresis   Migration

E Autoradiogram of sequencing gel and genotyping of pedigree

5
4
3
2

Decreasing size

4/3 5/2 4/2 5/4 5/3

Genotypes

FIGURE 1–2.   Schematic representation of a microsatellite marker.

Note.   A) Autosomal homologous chromosome pairs from parents in a pedigree to be genotyped. B) The DNA sequence on the long arm of the chromosome is examined in greater detail, revealing the variable repeating DNA sequence termed a *microsatellite marker*. For a dinucleotide repeat, each box represents two nucleotides (e.g., CA). Differing numbers of repeats of this dinucleotide are frequently found in different individuals. The example shows a father with four and three repeats and a mother with five and two repeats. (This is a simplification; most commonly there are 15–20 repeats.) C) Using DNA primers (* and **), one of which is radiolabeled, and a heat-stable DNA polymerase, repetitive cycles of DNA denaturation and replication exponentially amplify (105-fold) the DNA sequence bound by the primers. This process is termed the *polymerase chain reaction* (PCR) and is shown for only one of the two chromosomes of the father. Because the length of the fragment amplified is bounded by the primers, which are attached to nonrepeating sequences outside the microsatellite region, the length of the product of this reaction from each chromosome will be determined by the number of repeats. D) The amplified DNA fragments are separated on the basis of size by gel electrophoresis. E) The presence of the bands is determined by autoradiography. Individuals have two bands that correspond to the lengths of the amplified fragments. Each band is a marker for this region of the long arm of its own chromosome. The inheritance of these fragments can then be followed through all members of a pedigree whose DNA is available for the PCR reaction. Genotypes for each of the members of the hypothetical pedigree are shown under the autoradiogram. If an autosomal dominant disease is depicted by solid symbols, allele 4 would be linked to the disorder in this pedigree. This linkage, if statistically significant, indicates that the microsatellite marker is located close to the disease gene.

(especially those with milder or deviant forms) and also may fail by identifying as affected some individuals with a "similar disease" (if there are multiple diseases that lead to a common clinical picture).

Most psychiatric disorders are probably complex in origin, with multiple interacting genetic and environmental contributors (i.e., polygenetic or multifactorial inheritance). In these cases, for linkage studies to succeed, the diagnostic schema must identify a group in which most patients share some specific abnormal genetic component, and this may not be the case with the current nomenclature. Psychiatric nosology has of course aimed at identifying illnesses with the specificity needed by genetic analysis, and it has explored the validity of various diagnostic systems by using broad versus narrow definitions, exclusion criteria, definitions of "functional impairment" and "secondary cases," and correction factors for diagnostic instability. The relative failure of this attempt may be inevitable for a nosology based on clinical phenomenology, and greater knowledge of the biological pathogenesis of psychiatric disorders may be necessary. To make use of the new advances in genetic methodology, psychiatry may need to discover subtypes of current diagnostic categories that have one or more specific measurable biochemical or physiological traits (e.g., precipitation of panic attacks with lactate infusion, association of schizophrenia with deviant eye tracking) in addition to the symptoms of the illness. This development may be fostered by the emerging advances in neuroradiography, neurophysiology, neurochemistry, and the specification of cognitive deficits.

However, certain aspects of psychiatric disorders will continue to make accurate diagnosis problematic, such as late age at onset, intermittent expression of symptoms, variation in symptoms over time (e.g., major depressive disorder becoming bipolar disorder), and the influence of environmental factors on the emergence (i.e., penetrance) of these disorders or in producing phenocopies. Also, as discussed earlier in the subsection "What Are the Various Clinical Expressions of the Abnormal Gene(s)?—Spectrum Studies," all the major conditions have mild or intermediate forms (e.g., schizotypal personality disorder, schizoaffective disorder), and such cases may at times represent *formes frustes* that are genetically associated with the major disorder. There are benefits to counting these cases as affected in genetic studies, but even more etiological heterogeneity is likely in these milder and intermediate syndromes than in the major ones, and considering such cases as affected can result in misleading results regarding specific genetic determinations (such as mode of transmission or linkage).

Genetics of Psychiatric Disorders

Schizophrenia

Family Studies

Beginning with the pioneering work of Rudin (1916), Kallmann (1946), and others in the Berlin school, the past 80 years have witnessed more than 20 studies examining the risk of schizophrenia in the relatives of more than 5,000 affected individuals. These studies have consistently reported elevated morbid risks for schizophrenia in the first-degree relatives of schizophrenic probands (parents, mean = 5.6%; sibs, 10.1%; children, 12.8%) compared with those in the general population (0.9%), which suggests that schizophrenia is familial (Gottesman and Shields 1982). Later studies that have satisfied modern criteria for the collection of family data have corroborated these earlier findings (Kendler 1986). The relatively lower risk to parents is at odds with mendelian inheritance—all first-degree relatives, sharing 50% of their genes, should show equal risk—but may reflect the reproductive fitness effects.

It would appear that schizophrenia, both broadly and narrowly defined, is familial. Furthermore, schizoaffective disorder (as defined in DSM-III-R), paranoid personality disorder, atypical psychosis, and schizotypal personality disorder also aggregate in the relatives of schizophrenic probands, indicating the possible boundaries of the phenotypic spectrum (Kendler et al. 1985). Additional studies have extended this boundary to other clinical conditions (qualitative phenotypes) and clinical and subclinical signs (quantitative phenotypes). It appears that even bipolar disorder may be elevated in the relatives of schizophrenic probands, at least in some families (Pope and Yurgelun-Todd 1990)—possibly those with schizophrenia "spectrum conditions" (Baron and Gruen 1991)—or if the mood disorder is associated with psychotic symptoms (Decina et al. 1991; Tsuang and Lyons 1989).

Quantitative, clinically apparent phenotypes that are elevated in the relatives of schizophrenic probands include 1) positive symptoms measured by the Thought Disorder Index (Shenton et al. 1989); 2) negative symptoms measured by the Scale for the Assessment of Negative Symptoms (Tsuang et al. 1991); 3) neuropsychological signs such as deficits in abstraction (as measured by the Wisconsin Card Sorting Test) and in short-term verbal memory (Franke et al. 1992; Tsuang et al. 1992); and 4) neurological soft signs (Kinney et al. 1991).

Subclinical phenotypes that are elevated in the relatives of schizophrenic probands include 1) disturbances in thinking, social relatedness, volition, and affective expressivity as measured by a psychometric index derived from the Minnesota Multiphasic Personality Inventory (MMPI) (Moldin et al. 1990a); 2) eye movement dysfunction on smooth pursuit (Clementz et al. 1990; Curtis et al. 2001; Holzman and Levy 1977) and visual fixation tasks (Amador et al. 1995); 3) impairments in suppression of the 50 msec preattentional component (P50) of the auditory evoked potential in a conditioning testing paradigm (Clementz et al. 1998; Waldo et al. 1991); and 4) attentional disturbances as measured by the Continuous Performance Test (CPT) (Keefe et al. 1997), the Forced-Choice Span of Apprehension Task (SPAN), and the Digit Symbol Substitution Test (DSST) (Laurent et al. 2000).

Family studies also have provided clues to the genetic boundaries of other psychotic and related disorders. Thus, both schizophrenia and bipolar disorder may be elevated in the relatives of probands with schizoaffective disorder (Coryell and Zimmerman 1988; Gershon et al. 1988), psychotic affective illness may be elevated in the relatives of patients with schizophreniform disorder (Pulver et al. 1991), and schizophrenia may be elevated in the relatives of patients with schizotypal personality disorder (Battaglia et al. 1995; Lyons et al. 1994). A meta-analysis of the relative risk to first-degree relatives of probands with schizophrenia from three large independent family studies found odds ratios of developing schizophrenia, schizotypal personality disorder, and other nonaffective psychoses of 16, 5, and 4, respectively (Kendler and Gardner 1997).

Family studies may help in elucidating etiologically homogeneous subgroupings in schizophrenia. For example, specific environmental exposures, structural brain abnormalities, and/or age at onset may predict more or less "familial" forms of the disorder: probands who had obstetrical complications may be at lower familial risk than those who did not (Bersani et al. 1995). Similarly, the siblings of the probands with a negative family history have greater ventricular enlargement (Silverman et al. 1998). One exception to this may be males with very early onset, who may be at elevated familial risk (Pulver et al. 1990). Similarly, females with especially early onset (<22 years) may be at elevated familial risk (Sham et al. 1994). Age at onset has not been associated with familial risk of illness in all studies; for example, the epidemiologically based County Roscommon study found no such association (Kendler et al. 1996a). Prognostic features may predict other types of familial risk: for example, probands with good social, occupational, and residential outcome may have elevated family risks for unipolar illness (Kendler and Tsuang 1988).

On the other hand, family studies may help to eliminate nongenetic subgroupings. For example, in one study, paranoid versus nonparanoid subtypes of schizophrenia neither bred true nor could be distinguished by differential rates of schizophrenia or mood disorder in the relatives of probands (Kendler et al. 1988). Likewise, there may be no individual symptoms in probands that result in differential risk for schizophrenia in relatives (Alda et al. 1989; Kendler et al. 1994).

Finally, family studies performed on special populations may shed light on (epigenetic) etiological factors contributing to disease expression. The recent observation of a 4- to 15-fold increase in the morbid risk for schizophrenia among siblings of (British-born) second-generation African Caribbean schizophrenic probands compared with the siblings of their white counterparts (Hutchinson et al. 1996; Sugarman and Craufurd 1994) suggests the interaction of a particularly vulnerable genetic background with risk-conferring environmental factors, in a phenomenon known as *phenotype amplification* (Weiss 1993).

Thus, family studies have done much to define the (clinical and subclinical) schizophrenia spectrum, clarify the nosological status of other psychotic disorders to schizophrenia, and address the issues of etiological heterogeneity and etiology. These studies have confirmed that schizophrenia is familial. It bears emphasizing, however, that even well-designed family studies cannot distinguish between genetic and environmental influences on familial aggregation of a disorder such as schizophrenia. Other strategies, including twin and adoption studies, are needed.

Twin Studies

If genetic factors are important in schizophrenia, we would expect that MZ and DZ co-twins of probands with schizophrenia would differ in their risk for the disorder. In fact, this has been consistently observed since the initial twin studies of Luxenberger conducted almost 60 years ago. Up to 1986, 817 MZ twin pairs and 1,016 same-sex DZ twin pairs were studied, with weighted mean probandwise concordances of 59.2% and 15.2%, respectively, and therefore a broad-sense heritability of 88% (Kendler 1986). Nonetheless, estimates of probandwise concordance have varied, possibly reflecting differences in diagnostic criteria, case sampling, and zygosity assessment across studies (Walker et al. 1991). For example, broader diagnoses and more severe illness in probands—fewer positive symptoms, more negative symptoms, poorer premorbid social competence (Dworkin et al. 1988; Onstad et al. 1991)—both yield higher concordance rates. A more recent meta-analysis of five recent large studies that used explicit operational diagnostic criteria found DSM-III-R schizophrenia concordances of 50% for MZ and 4% for DZ pairs and found the best fit to a model with a narrow-sense heritability of 88% (83% using ICD-10 [World Health Organization 1992] diagnoses) (Cardno and Gottesman 2000).

In addition to establishing the importance of genetic factors, estimates of concordance also may shed light on the boundaries of schizophrenia; by identifying which operational definition of schizophrenia maximizes the difference between MZ and DZ concordance rates, investigators may determine a genetically validated definition of the disorder. In a reanalysis of the Maudsley twin study reported by Gottesman and Shields (1972), the maximum difference in rates occurred when DSM-III schizophrenia, affective disorder with mood-incongruent delusions, atypical psychosis, and schizotypal personality disorder were considered affected (Farmer et al. 1987). However, it is likely that not all of the genetic factors of these disorders are shared because one analysis of the Finnish twin sample that tested a multiple threshold model in which schizophrenia has the highest liability and affective and other psychoses have a lower liability found no support for the model (Cannon et al. 1998).

To summarize, the risk of schizophrenia in MZ co-twins of affected probands is at least three times that in DZ co-twins and some 40–60 times the risk in the general population. Just as noteworthy, however, is that only approximately half of MZ twin pairs are concordant for schizophrenia despite genetic identity. Monochorionic MZ twins are more likely to be concordant than are dichorionic MZ twins, perhaps because the former share not only identical genes but also a similar in utero environment (J.O. Davis et al. 1995). Although many non-schizophrenic MZ co-twins of affected probands show a variety of psychiatric disorders, including "neurotic" and character disorders and "schizoid" conditions, many (up to 43% in one series [Fischer 1971]) appear to have no psychiatric disorder. Moreover, the offspring of non-schizophrenic MZ co-twins may be at as high a risk for schizophrenia as are the offspring of their affected siblings (Fischer 1971; Gottesman and Bertelsen 1989; Kringlen and Cramer 1989), implying that these co-twins carry the schizophrenic genotype despite their "normal" appearance. These findings argue against phenocopies as the sole explanation for MZ twin discordance in schizophrenia. (An additional argument against phenocopies is that discordant and concordant MZ twin pairs do not differ with respect to family risk, nor do they differ in birth order, birth weight, or condition at birth [Onstad et al. 1992].) These findings also suggest a range of phenotypes compatible with the schizophrenic genotype and suggest an additive (or interactive) relation between genes and epigenetic (environmental) factors in the pathogenesis of the disorder.

Discordant MZ twins also provide a clue to timing of these epigenetic factors and their effect on brain development. Differences between discordant MZ twins in dermatoglyphic patterns established in utero have suggested that a second-trimester environmental stressor combines with genetic risk in a "two-hit" model of disease pathogenesis (Bracha et al. 1992; Rosa et al. 2000). Other studies of discordant MZ twin pairs have shown differences in left hemisphere hypodensity on computed tomography (CT) scan (Reveley et al. 1987); smaller anterior pes hippocampi on magnetic resonance imaging (MRI) (Suddath et al. 1990); and diminished activation of the dorsolateral prefrontal cortex while performing the Wisconsin Card Sorting Test, as measured by regional cerebral flood flow (Weinberger et al. 1992), smooth pursuit eye tracking (Litman et al. 1997), and electroencephalogram patterns (Stassen et al. 1999).

Adoption Studies

All four varieties of adoption study have been applied to schizophrenia: adoptee study method, cross-fostering, adoptee's family method, and the study of MZ twins reared apart (see discussion of adoption studies earlier in this chapter). Despite varying methodology, these studies have consistently suggested a role for genetic influences in schizophrenia.

The adoptee study method was initially used by Heston (1966), who found a significantly greater risk for schizophrenia among the offspring of schizophrenic mothers separated at birth than among the adopted-away offspring of control mothers. This finding was replicated in a Danish sample by Rosenthal et al. (1968) in a study that has withstood blind reanalysis with DSM-III criteria and in a Finnish sample by Tienari et al. (2000) in a study that has incorporated modern techniques such as direct, blind interview of adoptees and detailed examination of adoptive families, the latter permitting an analysis of genotype-environmental interactions.

The sole cross-fostering study to date found equivalent rates of severe psychiatric illness among adoptees from biological parents without psychiatric illness, regardless of whether their adoptive parents had schizophrenia: both adoptee groups had rates of illness significantly lower than those in a group of adoptees from biological parents with schizophrenia and related disorders (Wender et al. 1974). In addition to providing evidence for the etiological importance of genetic factors in schizophrenia, this cross-fostering study argues against a causative role for rearing factors associated with parent psychosis, except, perhaps, in the presence of a susceptible genotype.

The adoptee's family method has been used in a series of studies conducted by Kety and colleagues in Denmark. They found that schizophrenia and related disorders were more common in the biological relatives of 34 schizophrenic adoptees (13 of 150 vs. 3 of 156, $P<0.01$), whereas the rates for these disorders did not differentiate the adoptive relatives of either adoptee group, being low in both. The Danish adoption study has withstood reanalysis with DSM-III criteria (Kendler and Gruenberg 1984) and has been replicated with a second cohort of 41 index and control adoptees (Kety 1988). The biological relatives of schizophrenic adoptees have shown higher rates not only of schizophrenia but also of DSM-III diagnosed schizotypal and paranoid personality disorders, again expanding the boundaries of the schizophrenic syndrome (Kendler and Gruenberg 1984). Overall, the biological relatives of schizophrenic adoptees have shown a 10-fold increase in risk for schizophrenia and spectrum disorders over the biological relatives of control subjects (Kety et al. 1994).

Finally, two studies of MZ twins reared apart have shown high pairwise concordance for schizophrenia, providing further evidence for a genetic component in the etiology of this disorder (Gottesman and Shields 1982).

High-Risk Studies

High-risk studies have examined both early characteristics that distinguish the offspring of schizophrenic parents from control subjects and premorbid features that predict which of those offspring will go on to develop schizophrenia. By age 1 year, high-risk infants were more likely than control infants to show "anxious" attachment behavior and sensorimotor deficits. By age 2 years, they were seen to be more passive and less attentive in play. Later, they had less social competence. These findings have been taken as evidence of an inherited neurointegrative defect in schizophrenia (Fish 1977, 1987; Fish et al. 1992; Marcus et al. 1987). Alternatively, the findings might reflect developmental delays caused by obstetrical complications (such as low birth weight), which frequently befall schizophrenic mothers. In fact, psychopathology at age 6 years (especially among males) has been associated with low socioeconomic status, low Apgar score, and neonatal neurological abnormality (McNeil and Kaij 1987).

Older high-risk children have shown defective emotional rapport and disturbed cognition in unblinded clinical interviews (Parnas et al. 1982), diminished attention on measures such as the CPT (Watt et al. 1984) and the digit cancellation task (Mirsky et al. 1995), and greater impairment on the aforementioned psychometric index derived from the MMPI (Moldin et al. 1990b). These abnormalities support the Bleulerian notion of a primary affective, associational, and attentional disturbance in schizophrenia. Moreover, because these abnormalities characterize high-risk individuals who go on to develop either schizophrenia or schizotypal personality disorder, they support the genetic relatedness of these disorders. Because the abnormalities described herein affect only about 10%–25% of high-risk offspring (Watt et al. 1984), they appear to be somewhat removed from a core monogenic defect (if present) in schizophrenia. On the other hand, smooth pursuit eye movement dysfunction has been reported to characterize approximately 50% of the teenaged children of schizophrenic parents and thus may more closely reflect the schizophrenic diathesis (Mather 1985).

Premorbid psychosocial predictors of schizophrenia (vs. schizotypal personality disorder) among adopted-away high-risk children have included communication deviance within the adoptive family (Tienari et al. 1994). Such observations do not clarify, however, whether this intrafamilial deviance is causative of, or reactive to, greater psychopathology among juvenile adoptees destined to develop more severe psychopathology in adulthood. Premorbid physiological predictors of adult schizophrenia among high-risk children have included obstetrical complications; soft neurological signs such as impaired balance, left-right confusion, and motor overflow in childhood; and autonomic hypoarousal in adolescence (Cannon et al. 1990). Moreover, adult correlates of schizophrenia (vs. schizotypal personality disorder) among high-risk offspring have included ventricular enlargement (especially of the third ventricle) on CT scan (Cannon et al. 1994; Dykes et al. 1992; Schulsinger et al. 1984). It is tempting to speculate that these clinical and radiological findings reflect a common perinatal neurological insult that contributes to disease expression. This speculation is supported not only by prospective studies of high-risk individuals but also by retrospective studies of schizophrenic patients (Hultman et al. 1997) and by studies of discordant MZ twins. In these studies, poorer outcome has been associated with the triad of obstetrical complications, neurological dysfunction, and ventricular enlargement (the latter perhaps reflecting primarily enlargement *ex vacuo* of the temporal horn of the lateral ventricle in association with smaller anterior pes hippocampi). Nonetheless, many of these findings await replication and should be viewed with caution.

Mode of Inheritance

Several models for the genetic transmission of schizophrenia have been proposed, including monogenic/single major locus, oligogenic, and polygenic/multifactorial models. For example, Böök (1953) was able to account for observed frequencies of schizophrenia in a geographical isolate in northern Sweden by proposing a dominant gene (with gene frequency of 0.07) with homozygous penetrance of 100% and limited heterozygous penetrance (20%). Similarly, Karlsson (1988) suggested that a dominant gene with reduced penetrance (25%) could account for most cases of schizophrenia in Iceland. The reproductive disadvantage of schizophrenia (Larson and Nyman 1973), however, would seem to select strongly against a dominant gene.

A recessive monogenic model (with reduced penetrance) predicts that the incidence of schizophrenia among the offspring of two schizophrenic parents would be comparable to the probandwise concordance for MZ twins, and, in fact, this is what has been observed (Kringlen 1978). Similarly, a recessive model could allow for the maintenance of the abnormal gene in the population, despite reduced reproductive fitness of those individuals with the illness (Erlenmeyer-Kimling and Paradowski 1966). Normal rates of consanguinity in most families with schizophrenia, however, argue against recessive transmission of the disorder (Rosenthal 1970; but see Chaleby and Tuma 1987 regarding special populations).

Sex-linked models have been proposed by DeLisi and Crow (1989), who suggested that a schizophrenia susceptibility gene might reside on the X chromosome on the basis of sex differences in the clinical presentation of the illness, with a later onset and more benign course in women perhaps attributable to demonstration of random inactivation of X chromosomes carrying mutant alleles. Alternatively, these authors argued X chromosome inheritance on the basis of cytogenetic anomalies (including X chromosome aneuploidies—XXY, XXX—as well as a fragile site at Xq27) associated with schizophrenia-like psychoses. They attributed the observation that schizophrenia appears to be transmitted on the X chromosome in some families, and, given cases of male-to-male transmission, on an autosome in others, to be compatible with a susceptibility gene for the disorder residing in the "pseudoautosomal" region of the sex chromosomes (i.e., a region of sequence homology between X and Y chromosomes wherein recombination may occur during male meiosis [Burgoyne 1982]). "Pseudoautosomal" transmission would predict an increased frequency of same-sex sibling pairs affected with schizophrenia when illness is inherited through the paternal lineage, and, in fact, this

has been observed (Crow et al. 1989).

Monogenic models, however, have difficulty accounting for the sharp drop in risk for schizophrenia as one moves from MZ twins to first- and second-degree relatives. Oligogenic models involving the epistatic interaction of two or three gene loci may better account for these data (Risch 1990). Likewise, monogenic models are hard pressed to account for the observed increased risk of schizophrenia in relatives, given either increased severity in the proband or a greater number of other affected relatives (Gottesman and Shields 1982). These observations, on the other hand, are compatible with a polygenic/multifactorial model. Furthermore, O'Rourke et al. (1982) argued against a single-locus, two-allele model by citing its inability to account for the observed distribution in the rates of schizophrenia among four classes of relatives of schizophrenia probands (parents, siblings, and MZ and DZ co-twins) in 21 studies meeting criteria of adequacy. Finally, several segregation analyses have similarly rejected monogenic models or, at least, have been unable to reject polygenic models (Risch and Baron 1984; Tsuang et al. 1982; Vogler et al. 1990). Finally, multiple genomewide searches for schizophrenia have been performed with linkage analysis, and the presence of a single major gene has not been observed.

These results are compatible, however, with a so-called mixed model involving a major locus in the setting of a multifactorial background (Tsuang et al. 1991). Moreover, they do not preclude the possibility that major loci underlie certain aspects of the schizophrenia phenotype. Thus, admixture analysis, a strategy complementary to segregation analysis that examines the population distribution of a quantitative phenotype for multimodality (each mode presumably reflecting the mean phenotypic consequence of a particular genotype), has provided preliminary evidence for a major gene underlying the aforementioned psychometric index derived from the MMPI (Moldin et al. 1990c) and smooth pursuit eye movement dysfunction (Clementz et al. 1992).

Linkage Analysis

In the past decade, several genetic loci have been implicated in the pathogenesis of schizophrenia. There have been partially replicated findings of loci on chromosome arms 1q, 5q, 6p, 6q, 8p, 10p, 13q, 15q, and 22q (reviewed in Baron 2001). Note that several of these loci overlap with those observed for bipolar disorder (see section "Mood [Affective] Disorders" later in this chapter). In addition, there have been nonreplicated reports of linkage to loci on chromosome arms 3p and 5p. Although none of these regions has yet to yield a gene for schizophrenia, the hopes are high that at least some of the regions contain genes for schizophrenia that will be isolated in the next several years. The replicated findings are discussed in some detail below, followed by a brief mention of the nonreplicated findings. Numerous investigations also have been undertaken of various candidate genes for schizophrenia by linkage, genetic association, and direct DNA sequencing. Some of these studies also are discussed. This area has been recently reviewed (O'Donovan and Owen 1999).

Chromosome arm 1q. There is strong evidence for the presence of at least one and possibly two loci for schizophrenia on 1q. The best evidence for a locus for schizophrenia on 1q (and all other chromosomes) comes from a genome scan of 22 Canadian pedigrees, which produced a lod score of 6.50 with a recessive model and a narrow disease model between markers *D1S1653* and *D1S1679* on 1q21–22 (Brzustowicz et al. 2000). Two other genome scans have reported evidence for a gene in this region (Gurling et al. 2001; Shaw et al. 1998). The expression of one gene in this region, regulator of G-protein signaling 4 (*RGS4*), was significantly decreased in the prefrontal cortex of schizophrenic subjects as compared with control subjects, but no mutations in the coding region were observed (Mirnics et al. 2001). *HKCa3/KCNN3* is another candidate gene that maps to the region (1q21) and codes for a potassium channel. There was an initial report of positive genetic association of this gene to schizophrenia (Dror et al. 1999) that has not been replicated in most subsequent studies. A linkage signal detecting either the same locus or a second locus on 1q has been observed in a sample of 221 families from Finland in the region of markers *D1S2709* and *D1S245* (1q32–41), some 55–75 cM telomeric to the 1q21–22 region with lod scores of 2.3–3.2 (Ekelund et al. 2001). Of interest, *D1S2709* lies within the *DISC1* (disrupted in schizophrenia 1) gene, which is interrupted by a balanced translocation (1;11)(q42;q14.3) that cosegregates with schizophrenia in a large Scottish pedigree that also contains individuals with major and bipolar depression (Millar et al. 2000).

Chromosome arm 5q. Evidence for a locus that contributes vulnerability to schizophrenia in this region was first observed by a German research group during a genome scan for schizophrenia (Schwab et al. 1997). In their initial scan, they observed a lod score of 1.8 for the marker *IL9* on 5q in 14 German families. This was followed up by examining 40 additional families with other markers in the region. Multipoint analyses of the affected sib pairs in the sample gave a lod score peak of 1.8 at

marker *D5S399* (2 cM telomeric to *IL9*), which decreased to 1.3 when 4 families from the original 14 were removed (Schwab et al. 1997). By itself, this result is not suggestive of linkage, but additional support for a gene in the region came from a study of 265 Irish pedigrees by researchers at the Medical College of Virginia (Straub et al. 1997). They obtained a pairwise lod score of 3.04 for marker *D5S393* (same location as *D5S399*), using a recessive genetic model and assuming genetic heterogeneity. This locus (if it is real) appears to be segregating in 10%–25% of the Irish pedigrees. Analysis of the Irish data with multipoint methods gave a score of similar magnitude but moved the most likely location of the gene 12 cM closer to the centromere (Straub et al. 1997). This entire region (5q21–q31) is distinct from the 5q11.2–13.3 linkage that was reported earlier (Sherrington et al. 1988) but was not replicated (Gurling 1992; McGuffin et al. 1990).

Chromosome arm 6p. In the summer of 1994, researchers at Medical College of Virginia informed other groups working on the genetics of schizophrenia that they had positive lod scores on 6p22–24, allowing many groups to publish their findings together in November 1995. The group at Medical College of Virginia found evidence for a locus that contributed to a vulnerability to schizophrenia in 15%–30% of their 265 pedigrees of Irish descent (Straub et al. 1995). They got their highest lod score (3.51) with *D6S296*, which is located telomeric to HLA, with an intermediate definition of affectedness (schizophrenia, poor-outcome schizoaffective disorder, schizotypal personality disorder, and other nonaffective psychotic disorders).

As noted, several other groups reported their findings at the same time. Some of these studies found positive lod scores on 6p, although not with the same markers or phenotypic diagnoses as in the Medical College of Virginia study (Antonarakis et al. 1995; Bailer et al. 2000; Moises et al. 1995a; Schwab et al. 1995a, 2000). Another study found evidence of linkage to the severity of positive symptoms in the same region (Brzustowicz et al. 1997). Two other studies published at the same time did not find evidence of a gene for schizophrenia on 6p (Gurling et al. 1995b; Mowry et al. 1995) nor did two later studies (Garner et al. 1996; Riley et al. 1996). The genetic region that is positive in the original and replication studies spans about 40 cM of 6p that goes as far centromeric as the HLA locus.

In a large collaborative study designed to pool data from 14 research groups (713 pedigrees) with five microsatellite markers from the region, a suggestion of linkage to 6p was observed (Schizophrenia Linkage Collaborative Group for Chromosomes 3, 6, and 8 1996). A lod score of 2.19 was observed in the new sample using MAPMAKER/SIBS (a multipoint sib-pair analysis) and a narrow definition of affectedness (schizophrenia or schizoaffective disorder). When the Medical College of Virginia was added back in, the score increased to 2.68. These scores are not conclusive for linkage to a schizophrenia gene in the region but are suggestive (Lander and Kruglyak 1995). Unfortunately, this large study only tested markers in the region that was positive in the original report (Straub et al. 1995) and hence did not cover the entire region flanking the HLA locus.

Chromosome arm 6q. The first report of possible linkage of schizophrenia to 6q21–22 used two independent samples of 63 and 87 sib pairs and found evidence of linkage to both ($P = 0.00024$ and 0.0004, respectively) with markers *D6S416* and *D6S424*, which are 14 cM apart (Cao et al. 1997). The same group found further support for a locus in this region in another sample (Martinez et al. 1999). In a meta-analysis of 734 informative multiplex pedigrees (824 independent affected sibling pairs from 8 groups) that investigated linkage to 5q, 6q, 10p, and 13q, the locus on 6q was the best supported with a maximum lod score of 3.1 (Levinson et al. 2000).

Chromosome arm 8p. During the course of a genome scan for genetic factors for schizophrenia using 520 markers and 57 pedigrees, researchers at Johns Hopkins University found evidence for loci on chromosomes 3 and 8 (Pulver et al. 1995). Markers *D8S133* and *D8S136* (9 cM apart) gave maximum lod scores of 2.35 with a dominant and 2.20 with a recessive "affected only" analysis model using a narrow diagnostic model (schizophrenia or schizoaffective disorder). Affected sib-pair analysis found four markers in the region that gave P values of <0.001. Analysis of an additional 51 pedigrees continued to support the region (Blouin et al. 1998), and recent subtyping of these families into those with schizophrenia spectrum personality disorders found the strongest genomewide linkage support to the region (Pulver et al. 2000).

These findings have been replicated by other research groups (Kendler et al. 1996b; Kunugi et al. 1996) and in a large collaborative study (see "Chromosome Arm 6p" earlier in this chapter) (Schizophrenia Linkage Collaborative Group for Chromosomes 3, 6, and 8 1996). In the collaborative study, a lod score of 2.22 was obtained in the replication sample using a recessive model and assuming genetic heterogeneity with marker *D8S261*. When the replication sample was combined with the Johns Hopkins University data, the score at this marker

increased to 3.06 under the same analysis model. In both cases, the maximum lod score was obtained when the proportion of families linked to the marker was about 20%. A nonparametric sib-pair analysis gave a peak of 2.73 centered on marker *D8S133* in the combined dataset. The region also has been replicated in a sample of 21 Canadian pedigrees with a lod score of 3.49 (Brzustowicz et al. 1999).

Chromosome arm 10p. In a genome scan of the 43 pedigrees with 50 independent sib pairs collected by the NIMH Genetics Initiative, the best evidence of linkage was observed with markers *D10S1423* (lod score = 3.4) and *D10S582* (lod score = 3.2) on 10p11–15 (Faraone et al. 1998). The existence of a locus in this location is supported by two other groups (Schwab et al. 1998; Straub et al. 1998) and by the meta-analysis described above (Levinson et al. 2000).

Chromosome arm 13q. Positive lod scores have been observed on 13q14.1–q32 in a collection of 13 multiplex families (11 United Kingdom/2 Japanese) in the region of the serotonin type 2A (5-HT$_{2A}$) receptor gene locus (Lin et al. 1995). A lod score of 1.61 was obtained with marker *D13S144* under a dominant genetic model and the assumption of genetic heterogeneity. A multipoint analysis assuming that 40% of the families are linked yielded a maximum lod score of 2.0 near marker *D13S128* (about 30 cM telomeric from *D13S144*). A follow-up by the same group indicated that it is the Caucasian families that are linked to this region (Lin et al. 1997). In a genome scan of 54 pedigrees, the strongest evidence of linkage was observed for markers in 13q42 with a maximum lod score assuming heterogeneity and a dominant model of inheritance of 4.5 (Blouin et al. 1998). A lod score of 4.42 using a recessive model has been observed in 21 Canadian families (Brzustowicz et al. 1999). Positive findings for this region also have been observed for bipolar and panic disorders (see "Mood [Affective] Disorders").

Chromosome arm 15q. Linkage to 15q13–15 has been observed with two different phenotypic models. Strong evidence of linkage (lod score = 5.3) to the P50 auditory sensory gating response was found with an autosomal dominant model to markers on 15q13–14 in nine families (Freedman et al. 1997). Only moderately positive lod scores were observed if schizophrenia, rather than P50 status, was used as the phenotype for the analysis. This region contains the α7-nicotinic cholinergic receptor gene, and further study has found genetic association to the gene in other pedigrees (Freedman et al. 2001). The other positive findings in the region were found in a genome scan of 12 families that had a high density of the periodic catatonic subtype of schizophrenia (Stober et al. 2000). This group found a nonparametric lod score of 3.57 ($P = 0.000026$) to markers in the region, and parametric analysis with a dominant model also was positive.

Chromosome arm 22q. The first region of the genome that was found to contain replicable loci for potential genes for schizophrenia is 22q. Researchers at Johns Hopkins University obtained a lod score of 2.85 in 39 families using a dominant genetic model with marker *IL2RB* (Pulver et al. 1994c). At the same time, a group at the University of Utah had completed a genome scan for schizophrenia with 9 families and obtained a lod score of 2.07 with marker *D22S276* and a recessive genetic model (Coon et al. 1994). An initial attempt to replicate the finding by the Johns Hopkins University and three other groups was unsuccessful (Pulver et al. 1994a).

Since that time, multiple groups have found some evidence for the presence of a locus for schizophrenia in the region (Moises et al. 1995b; Polymeropoulos et al. 1994; Schwab et al. 1995b; Vallada et al. 1995a, 1995b), whereas others have not (Kalsi et al. 1995). In the largest collaborative study, 11 research groups genotyped their samples for marker *D22S278* (296 sib pairs) and found evidence of allele sharing among affected siblings ($P = 0.001 - 0.006$) (Gill et al. 1996).

Other evidence supporting the presence of a gene for schizophrenia on 22q comes from the observation that affected individuals have a high rate of hemizygous microdeletions in the 22q11 region (Karayiorgou et al. 1995). In addition, these microdeletions overlap with the minimal genetic region containing the gene(s) for velocardiofacial syndrome. This is of interest because individuals with velocardiofacial syndrome have an extremely high rate of schizophrenia (Pulver et al. 1994b), and individuals with schizophrenia have a high rate of velocardiofacial syndrome dysmorphic features (Beatty et al. 1996).

Nonreplicated regions reported. Several regions of the genome have been implicated as harboring a gene for schizophrenia in individual studies. Examination of 5p in a collection of 12 families identified one large family, of Puerto Rican descent, that appeared to be linked to 5p14.1–p13.1. A two-point analysis using marker *D5S111* gave a lod score of 3.72 for the family with an autosomal dominant genetic model. A multipoint genetic analysis with other markers in the region raised the score to 4.37. The other pedigrees in the collection did not support linkage to the region (Silverman et al. 1996).

Another linkage approach to the genetic dissection of the psychiatric diseases is to use physiological measures that correlate with the disorder. In eight pedigrees, researchers from Germany found linkage of eye tracking dysfunction to markers on 6p (lod score = 3.51 to *D6S271*) on the centromeric side of the HLA complex (most of the 6p findings described earlier find evidence of linkage telomeric to HLA), assuming autosomal dominant transmission (Arolt et al. 1996). Increasing the number of families to 10 raised the lod score to 3.70 (Arolt et al. 1999). Linkage analysis using various models of schizophrenia gave only moderately positive lod scores to 6p in this pedigree collection (Arolt et al. 1996). If replicated, these studies may represent the future of psychiatric genetics because finding the genes for related phenotypes that are inherited in a mendelian manner should be straightforward.

Genetic Association Studies of Schizophrenia

Many candidate genes have been tested for linkage disequilibrium to schizophrenia in genetic association studies. There are currently more than 100 published association studies. Most of these studies examined candidate genes in the dopaminergic and serotonergic pathways and have not found convincing evidence of an association (O'Donovan and Owen 1999). As an example, one of the most studied loci, the dopamine D_3 receptor, has been observed to be associated with schizophrenia in some studies (Asherson et al. 1996; Crocq et al. 1992; Ebstein et al. 1997a; Kennedy et al. 1995; Mant et al. 1994; Nimgaonkar et al. 1996; Tanaka et al. 1996), whereas no association is seen in others (Chen et al. 1997; Nothen et al. 1993; Rietschel et al. 1996; Sabate et al. 1994; Saha et al. 1994). A meta-analysis of more than 5,000 subjects did find suggestive evidence of a genetic association ($P = 0.0002$) but with a very small odds ratio (1.23) for homozygosity at this locus (Williams et al. 1998). A very similar strength finding has been observed with a thymidine to cytosine SNP at nucleotide 102 in the 5-HT_{2A} receptor gene (Inayama et al. 1996; Williams et al. 1997).

Other Approaches

Several other approaches have been taken to help identify genetic factors for schizophrenia and subsequently elucidate the pathophysiological role of the molecular variations. The patterns of expression of thousands of genes can now be assayed simultaneously with microarray technology. In its simplest form, up to 10,000 complementary DNA (cDNA) clones of various genes are individually spotted onto glass microscope slides, and then this array is incubated with fluorescently labeled RNA from a brain region of interest. The RNA molecules in solution find their cDNA clones in the array, and the amount of hybridization can be determined by laser scanning. When the level of expression of more than 7,000 genes in the prefrontal cortex area 9 was examined in six matched pairs of schizophrenic and control subjects using microarrays, 4.8% of the transcripts were thought to be differentially expressed (half up and half done) (Mirnics et al. 2000). The overall data were analyzed after separating them into 250 groups related to metabolic or functional pathways, enzymes, or brain-specific functions. Most of the groups showed no difference in expression, but the expression of the presynaptic secretory machinery, γ-aminobutyric acid (GABA) and glutamate transmission, energy metabolism, growth factors, and receptor groups was thought to differ. The presynaptic secretory machinery gene group, which also includes molecules related to membrane trafficking, showed the most robust findings, with 18% of these genes having decreased expression at the 99% confidence level in the schizophrenia brains relative to control brains, although different genes were downregulated in each subject (Mirnics et al. 2000). These results suggest that "altered function of proteins controlling the 'mechanics' of synaptic transmission" is central to the pathogenesis of schizophrenia (Mirnics et al. 2000).

Once a putative gene for schizophrenia has been identified, further study is needed to understand how variation in the DNA sequence leads to an increased risk for the disorder. One way is to engineer mice that have a complete absence of the gene (knockout) or with specific variations introduced into the mouse genome (site-directed mutagenesis) and then study the effect of this manipulation on the behavior of the mice. For most of the current neuropsychiatric candidate genes, knockout mice have been created and are currently under active study. Another approach is to study individuals with genotypic variation at a putative disease locus and attempt to correlate with behaviors, traits, or endophenotypes. Genetic association studies of schizophrenia and an SNP that causes an amino acid change at position 158 (valine to methionine) of the catechol-O-methyltransferase (COMT) gene on chromosome 22, and consequently a three- to fourfold difference in the enzymatic activity of the protein, have been equivocal. However, when 175 individuals with schizophrenia, 219 of their unaffected siblings, and 55 control subjects were tested with the Wisconsin Card Sorting Test and the results stratified by COMT genotype (Met/Met, Met/Val, Val/Val), 4% of the variance of the perseverative errors was accounted for, *even in the normal control group* (Egan et al. 2001). Individuals with each genotype were then assayed with functional MRI and a working memory task, and genotype predicted the efficiency of prefrontal processing (Egan et al. 2001). Innovative technologies and approaches like those outlined here are likely needed to unravel the effect of genotype on the phenotype of schizophrenia.

Mood (Affective) Disorders

Since the major mood disorders—bipolar disorder and major depression (also called unipolar depressive disorder)—were derived from the concept of bipolar illness 30 years ago, they have been found to be highly familial in several European and American studies. First-degree relatives of bipolar probands have an elevated morbid risk for both bipolar and major depressive illness, whereas relatives of major depression probands have an elevated risk for major depression but not bipolar disorder (Weissman et al. 1984a). In these studies, there have been inconsistent findings of increased rates of alcoholism and sociopathy among relatives. Schizoaffective disorder, especially schizoaffective disorder with manic symptoms, also has frequently been found to be associated with a high rate of bipolar disorder among relatives.

In addition to finding these high familial rates of mood disorder, some studies have found that the risk for family members and the morbid risk in the population have increased for those born in later versus earlier decades of the twentieth century (Gershon et al. 1987; Klerman et al. 1985). This has been termed an *age-period-cohort effect*, and it has been found to be present in many countries (Weissman et al. 1992). The cause of this ominous trend is undetermined.

The results of a very large NIMH collaborative study (2,226 interviewed relatives) that used the RDC (Spitzer et al. 1978), as reported by Andreasen et al. (1987) for interviewed relatives, are summarized in Table 1–3. These data confirm the above findings. This study also found that schizoaffective probands with depressive features had a somewhat elevated rate (2.5%) of schizophrenia in first-degree relatives and a zero prevalence of bipolar I disorder. These findings were quite different from those for schizoaffective disorder, bipolar type, providing evidence that certain types of schizoaffective disorder may not be related to bipolar disorder. In this study, the authors decided to report rates of illness rather than morbid risk figures because the age and sex distributions across relative groups were similar, and the presence of the age-period-cohort effect could prevent accurate morbid risk calculations.

TABLE 1–3. National Institute of Mental Health Collaborative Study of Affective Disorders: rates of illness in interviewed first-degree relatives

Diagnoses in relatives (%)	Diagnosis of proband					
	Bipolar I	Bipolar II	Unipolar	Schizoaffective–depressive	Schizoaffective–bipolar	Schizophrenia
Bipolar I	3.9	4.2	22.8	0.2	0.5	1.0
Bipolar II	1.1	8.2	26.2	0	0.4	0.4
Unipolar	0.6	2.9	8.4	20.3	0.2	0.3
Schizoaffective—depressed	0	3.7	21.0	0	0	2.5
Schizoaffective—bipolar	3.6	5.8	25.4	0	0.7	0.7

Source. Data from Andreasen et al. 1987.

Many other family studies also have attempted to use variations in the rate of affected relatives to validate subtypes of major depression. This is an effort, in part, to find a phenotype(s) that could be a discrete illness and correspond to mendelian inheritance patterns or show linkage to genetic markers. This search has investigated various definitions of endogenous depression, pharmacological response, severity of illness, suicidality, the presence of psychotic features, rapid cycling, associated illnesses (e.g., alcoholism, anxiety disorder), decreased rapid eye movement (REM) latency, early age at onset, and recurrent episodes. Except for the last three, most of these factors have not been consistently shown to increase familial risk. In two studies, reduced REM latency also was associated with higher familial rates (Giles et al. 1988; Mendlewicz et al. 1989). In addition, early age at onset (before age 20) has been shown, in more than six studies with depressed and/or bipolar probands, to be associated with an increased rate of illness among adult relatives two- to threefold (vs. relatives of other depressed probands). The increase is even greater for early-onset cases among relatives (Kupfer et al. 1989; Rice et al. 1987b; Weissman et al. 1984b). The corresponding increase in a study of prepubertal depression was 14-fold (Weissman et al. 1988). Last, two family studies (Bland et al. 1986; Rice et al. 1987a) reported increased familial risk for probands with recurrent major depressive disorder. Age at onset and recurrence appear to act independently to increase risk. When probands had recurrent disease and an age at onset below the sample median (about 50), their relatives had more than five times higher risk of major depressive disorder than did relatives of later-onset, single-episode probands (Bland et al. 1986).

Similar efforts to distinguish subtypes of major depression, but beginning with the differences in familial background rather than proband characteristics, were made by G. Winokur et al. (1975). In this work, patients with major depression who have a first-degree relative with bipolar disorder are considered bipolar disorder related, whereas others with major depression are divided into *familial pure depressive disorder* (i.e., first-degree relative with affective illness), *depressive spectrum disease* (i.e., first-degree relative with alcoholism or antisocial personality), and *sporadic depressive disease* (i.e., no family history of depression, antisocial personality, or alcoholism). Additional studies that used this typology have found a more favorable short-term (i.e., 6-month) outcome with pure depressive disorder, and those subjects with depressive spectrum disease were found to have less severe depression (but more alcoholism and social maladjustment) on long-term (i.e., 11-year) follow-up.

Twin studies have supported the importance of genetic factors in the transmission of the major mood disorders. Summed data from early twin studies that did not distinguish between bipolar disorder and major depression give a 65% pairwise concordance rate for MZ twin pairs and a 14% rate for DZ pairs (Nurnberger and Gershon 1982). The MZ rate for bipolar disorder is higher than that for major depression, but the study sample sizes are much smaller. One of the studies that found the highest heritability of bipolar disorder observed, using strict criteria, a pairwise concordance rate for MZ pairs of 58% compared with 17% for DZ pairs in a total of 110 pairs (broad-sense heritability of 82%) (Bertelsen et al. 1977). A meta-analysis of five twin studies of major depression, with a starting sample of more than 21,000 individuals, estimated that the additive genetic contribution to developing the disorder was 37%, and the rest of the variance was explained by individual-specific environmental effects, whereas none was attributable to shared familial environmental effects (Sullivan et al. 2000). Two recent twin studies of major depression suggested that the heritability of major depression is higher in females than in males (Bierut et al. 1999; Kendler et al. 2001b), particularly when using a broad disease definition, but this was not observed in the meta-analysis.

The few adoption studies of major mood disorders have produced somewhat conflicting data that are confounded by differences in sampling. The one study of adopted-away offspring found that the children of mothers with bipolar disorder or major depression had a higher rate of major mood disorder than did the adopted-away children of mothers with other psychiatric conditions (Cadoret 1978). Mendlewicz and Rainer (1977) found a significantly increased risk for affective illness in the biological parents of bipolar adoptee probands, compared with their adoptive parents or with the biological parents of control subjects. Wender et al. (1986) studied a group of adoptees with mixed mood disorder diagnoses (bipolar, unipolar, neurotic depression, "affect reaction") and found an increase in suicide and some mood disorders among their biological, but not their adoptive, relatives when each was compared with his or her corresponding control subject. Conversely, von Knorring et al. (1983), in a similar design, found no differences between the biological parent groups and noted an excess of psychiatric illness in the adoptive parents of the index cases, who were primarily adoptees with nonbipolar depression.

Many psychiatric disorders have been associated with bipolar disorder and/or major depression in family and twin studies, so an "affective disorder spectrum" is thought to include dysthymia, cyclothymia, schizoaffective disorder (RDC), alcoholism, and eating disorders. Newer studies convincingly add attention-deficit/hyperactivity disorder, nicotine addiction, and even migraine to this list. In addition, certain personality traits, such as rigidity, appear to be increased among relatives (Maier et al. 1992). However, preferential mating between those persons with mood disorders, plus the frequency of secondary depressions complicating almost all severe illnesses, makes it difficult to determine whether these associations actually reflect joint etiological determinants.

High-risk studies of children of parents with major mood disorders have quite consistently found high rates of social and psychiatric impairment. Controlled studies of specific diagnoses have noted an increased prevalence of major depression, conduct disorder, attention-deficit/hyperactivity disorder, anxiety disorder, substance abuse, and school problems, as well as poorer social functioning, among these children. The age at onset of depression in these high-risk offspring was earlier (mean age = 12–13) than among depressed control subjects whose parents were not depressed (mean age at onset = 16–17).

Research on the mode of transmission of the mood disorders is an area of great current activity and interest. One hypothesis that has been repeatedly tested is that major depression and bipolar disorder are, respectively, mild and severe forms of the same disorder, either by being on the same continuum of liability to illness (polygenic or multifactorial model) or by being phenotypic variants of the same (abnormal) genotype at a single major locus. The prevalence data from family studies usually have been consistent with multiple-threshold polygenic models, but some data sets have been equally consistent with multiple-threshold single major locus models. Pedigree and segregation analysis, which are more powerful techniques, have tended to reject single autosomal locus transmission, but the best fitting genetic model in the largest segregation analysis of bipolar disorder was to a dominant, mendelian major locus (Spence et al. 1995). In contrast, a segregation analysis on the Amish pedigrees could rule out autosomal dominant transmission under some circumstances (Pauls et al. 1995a). Another segregation analysis failed to correspond well to either multifactorial-polygenic or single major locus models, leading the authors to conclude that bipolar disorder, although highly familial, has a "complex" mode of transmission (Rice et al. 1987b). Likewise for major depression, segregation analyses have not resolved the mode of inheritance. Two older studies found evidence of a single major locus effect with nonmendelian transmission probabilities (Price et al. 1987; Rice et al. 1987a), whereas a newer study of early-onset, recurrent depression (before age 25) found evidence for nonmendelian inheritance of a recessive single major locus effect with a narrow diagnosis (recurrent major depressive disorder) and evidence for a mendelian codominant major locus with residual parental and spousal effects with a broader diagnostic definition (Marazita et al. 1997).

The first reported linkage findings in psychiatry used pedigrees collected from the Old Order Amish, a genetically isolated population living in Lancaster County, Pennsylvania, descendant from 30 progenitors who emigrated from Europe in the early eighteenth century. Strong genetic linkage was reported between a locus conferring a strong predisposition to bipolar disorder and two RFLP DNA polymorphisms located on 11p15: the cellular oncogene Ha-*ras*-1 and the insulin locus. The analyses showed lod scores of 3 or more for both of these markers within a wide range of penetrance and allele frequency values, further strengthening the findings (Egeland et al. 1987). Shortly after this study came a report of linkage of bipolar disorder to a region of the X chromosome (Xq28) (Baron et al. 1987), finding close linkage of bipolar disorder to the phenotypic markers color blindness and glucose-6-phosphate dehydrogenase in a series of Sephardic pedigrees from Israel. The maximum cumulative lod scores ranged from 7.52 (assuming homogeneity) to 9.17 (assuming heterogeneity). These findings confirmed some prior studies of bipolar disorder that had suggested linkage with the Xg locus and color blindness. Together, the Egeland and Baron studies indicated two separate genetic forms of the illness (i.e., genetic heterogeneity).

Unfortunately, these promising early findings were reversed or have not been confirmed. A reanalysis of an updated and extended version of the Old Order Amish pedigree showed no evidence for linkage to the same Ha-*ras*-1 and insulin loci on chromosome 11 (Kelsoe et al. 1989). Part of the change in lod score was the result of a key pedigree member who linked two large branches of the pedigree developing bipolar illness. Numerous studies on other pedigrees for chromosome 11 linkage similarly failed to find evidence for linkage, and a second Old Order Amish study concluded that it could exclude the possibility of linkage, at least for genes on 11p (Pauls et al. 1991). Similarly, the existence of the early X-chromosome-linked subtype of bipolar disorder also has not been upheld. One linkage report supported X linkage at Xq27 (Mendlewicz et al. 1987); however, an extension and reevaluation of the Israeli pedigrees with RFLP DNA markers found very little support for linkage to Xq28 and no support for linkage to Xq27 (Baron et al. 1993).

Since that time, multiple genome scans of bipolar disorder have been performed, and there are now multiple regions of interest on different chromosomes. The regions with the best support for containing a disease gene for bipolar disorder are 1q25–32, 4p16, 10p14, 10q25–26, 12q23–24, 13q31–32, 18p11, 18q21–23, 21q22, 22q11–13, and Xq24–28 (reviewed in more detail in Baron 2002). Note that several of these loci overlap with those observed for schizophrenia.

Chromosome Band 1q25–32

A genome scan of 22 pedigrees with a high density of bipolar disorder from the United States with 607 microsatellite markers found a multipoint lod score of 2.67 ($P = 0.00022$) and a single-locus lod score of 2.37 with marker *GATA124F08* with a dominant model (Detera-Wadleigh et al. 1999), which is located close to *D1S245*-one marker linked to the Finnish schizophrenia families (see subsection "Chromosome Arm 1q" earlier in this chapter). This region is somewhat centromeric to the translocation breakpoint (1q42) observed in a Scottish pedigree that is linked to schizophrenia, bipolar disorder, and recurrent major depression with a lod score of 7.1

(Blackwood et al. 2001) but closer to a fragile site on 1q32 that has been observed in bipolar patients (Turecki et al. 1995).

Chromosome Band 4p16

In a study of 12 pedigrees, marker *D4S394* gave a positive lod score (4.1) in one of the families under a dominant model (Blackwood et al. 1996). The score remained positive, under the assumption of genetic heterogeneity, when the other families were added in but did not increase further. Positive lod scores in the region also have been seen in three other studies (Detera-Wadleigh et al. 1999; Ewald et al. 1998b; Polymeropoulos and Schaffer 1996). In addition, when the genome scan data of the Old Order Amish were analyzed to look for genes that are "protective" against the development of bipolar disorder, the best support was for 4p16, with a nonparametric analysis score from 4.05 ($P = 0.00052$) (Ginns et al. 1998).

Chromosome Band 10p14

A genome scan of 97 families from the NIMH Genetics Initiative collection found the best support for a gene near *D10S1423* on 10p14, with a lod score of 2.5 (Foroud et al. 2000). This is the same region of chromosome 10 that has been linked to schizophrenia (see "Chromosome Arm 10p" earlier in the chapter).

Chromosome Band 10q25–26

A study of 75 families (66 from Germany) found the best support for a locus at marker *D10S217* (lod score = 2.86) with a dominant model (Cichon et al. 2001). Support has been observed for the region in a genome scan (Kelsoe et al. 2001).

Chromosome Band 12q23–24

A genome scan of a large pedigree with 120 living members from the relatively genetically homogeneous population of the Saguenay–Lac St. Jean area of Quebec found an nonparametric linkage score of 3.92 using the nonparametric analyses program GENEHUNTER with marker *D12S82* located on 12q (Morissette et al. 1999). A second peak of 2.5 was observed at marker *D12S86*, some 40 million bp telomeric. For this analysis, the large pedigree had to be broken up into smaller units, and other tests showed the possibility of intrafamilial genetic heterogeneity in the large pedigree. A second pedigree from the region with 34 members was mildly supportive of linkage to the region (Morissette et al. 1999). Three additional studies have observed positive linkage to the telomeric region (Dawson et al. 1995b; Detera-Wadleigh et al. 1999; Ewald et al. 1998a). In addition, cosegregation of Darier's disease and bipolar disorder has been observed (Craddock et al. 1994), and the gene for this disorder maps between the two peaks, and has been identified (*ATP2A2*), but mutations in *ATP2A2* have not been observed in individuals with bipolar disorder (Jacobsen et al. 2001).

Chromosome Band 13q31–32

A multipoint lod score of 3.5 ($P = 0.000028$) was observed on chromosome arm 13q (*D13S1252-S1271*) as the best score in a genome scan of 22 pedigrees (see "1q25–32" earlier in this chapter) (Detera-Wadleigh et al. 1999). Lod scores greater than 2 also were observed in a genome scan of 20 pedigrees from the United States with the nearby markers *D13S225* and *D13S796* (Kelsoe et al. 2001). This region is of particular interest because positive findings also have been observed for schizophrenia and panic disorders.

Chromosome Bands 18p11 and 18q21–23

During the course of a genomewide search for loci for bipolar illness, Berrettini et al. (1994a) noticed that markers in the pericentromeric region of chromosome 18 gave positive lod scores in some of their families (although the overall combined lod scores were negative). This occurred with both dominant and recessive genetic models. Analyses with nonparametric methods (affected sib pairs and Affected Pedigree Member) gave positive results and suggested the presence of a locus in the region. Since then, multiple other groups have tested markers on chromosome 18. The data from some of these groups replicate the finding (De Bruyn et al. 1996; Maier et al. 1995; Stine et al. 1995), whereas others have not found evidence for genes on chromosome 18 when they specifically examined the region (Pauls et al. 1995c) or in the course of a genome scan (Blackwood et al. 1996; Ginns et al. 1996). Of note is the work of a group at Johns Hopkins University, who noticed an excess of maternally transmitting families (parent-of-origin effect) in their pedigree series (McMahon et al. 1995). When the group stratified their chromosome 18 linkage results on the basis of the sex of the transmitting parent, they found evidence of linkage to the pericentromeric region in all pedigrees (thus replicating the initial finding) and evidence of a new locus on 18q in the paternal pedigrees (Stine et al. 1995). The pedigrees in the original report were then divided according to the sex of the transmitting parent, and linkage was observed in the paternal but not the maternal pedigree (Gershon et al. 1996). Evi-

dence for yet another locus on chromosome 18, this time much closer to the telomere (18q22–q23), was found in two pedigrees collected from Costa Rica (Freimer et al. 1996) and six pedigrees from Utah (Coon et al. 1996). In the Costa Rican study, seven markers in the 18q22–q23 region gave lod scores greater than 1.0, and a shared DNA marker haplotype was seen in 23 of 26 of the bipolar I individuals in the study. So, at this time, it appears likely that there is at least one, and possibly more, genetic locus for bipolar disorder located on chromosome 18. Close examination of one candidate gene in the pericentromeric region was negative (Ram et al. 1997).

Chromosome Band 21q22

At about the same time as the original chromosome 18 linkage report, researchers at Columbia University reported a lod score of 3.41 for one large family with bipolar disorder using marker *PFKL* on 21q22.3 (Straub et al. 1994). Five of the other 46 families studied gave positive lod scores for markers in the region, but the total lod score summed over all 47 families was negative. Follow-up studies by the same group have continued to support a locus in this region (Liu et al. 2001). In another study, Gurling et al. (1995a) used marker *D21S171* (near *PFKL*) and obtained a maximum lod score of 1.28 (with 35% of the families linked) in a collection of 23 pedigrees under the assumption of genetic heterogeneity. This group also saw moderately positive lod scores to the tyrosine hydroxylase (*TH*) locus on 11p15.5 (Smyth et al. 1996). TH is located near the Ha-*ras*-1 locus implicated in the Amish study, and some (Meloni et al. 1995; Perez de Castro et al. 1995), but not all (Gill et al. 1991; Inayama et al. 1993; Korner et al. 1994; Souery et al. 1996), studies of the locus have found an allelic association to bipolar disorder. When an admixture analysis was performed that assumed that a family was linked to *either TH* or *D21S171* locus, a lod score of 3.58 was obtained (Gurling et al. 1995a). Another group investigated the 21q region with 18 markers in 22 pedigrees and found significant sharing of alleles between affected sib pairs for markers near *PFKL* (Detera-Wadleigh et al. 1996). In addition, the allele sharing was "more impressive" in the maternally transmitting pedigrees (Detera-Wadleigh et al. 1996). However, like all the other positive loci observed in psychiatric genetics, not every study of the region has been positive (Byerley et al. 1995).

Chromosome Band 22q11–13

In the same region where linkage has been observed for schizophrenia, Detera-Wadleigh et al. (1999) found a suggestion of linkage to the region of markers *D22S689* and *D22S685* for bipolar disorder (multipoint lod score = 2.1, $P = 0.00094$). The best lod score (3.84) of a genome scan of 20 pedigrees by Kelsoe et al. (2001) was for the nearby marker *D22S278*. Using an animal model of psychotic mania, methamphetamine treatment of rats, changes in brain expression of thousands of genes were assayed with microarrays. One of the genes, G protein–coupled receptor kinase 3 (*GRK3*), maps to 22q11–13, and tests of the expression of the protein found decreased expression in cell lines from patients that correlated with disease severity (Niculescu et al. 2000).

Chromosome Band Xq24–28

A Finnish research group reported linkage of a large pedigree to markers on Xq24–q27.1 (Pekkarinen et al. 1995). They obtained lod scores between 1.3 and 3.5, depending on the phenotypic and genetic models used. In addition, they found a shared marker haplotype, 20 cM in length, in all members of the pedigree with bipolar or schizoaffective disorder. Lod scores between 1.23 and 1.34 also have been observed on the X chromosome in a large collaborative study of bipolar illness (NIMH Genetics Initiative Bipolar Group 1997).

Genetic Association Studies of Depression

There have been numerous genetic association studies of bipolar disorder and several of major depression. Meta-analyses of some of these are presented here, as the details are available in three recent reviews (Kato 2001; Malhi et al. 2000; Nurnberger and Foroud 2000). Given that selective serotonin reuptake inhibitors specifically inhibit the serotonin transporter (5-HTT), this gene has been studied extensively in mood disorders (eight positive and seven negative reports). Two polymorphisms in the gene have been most frequently investigated: a 44-bp insertion in the promoter of the gene (5-HTTLPR) that affects expression (insertion = long allele, that has increased expression) and a variable number of tandem repeats (VNTR) polymorphism in intron 2. A meta-analysis of 739 control subjects, 392 bipolar disorder patients, and 275 major depression patients for 5-HTTLPR found significant association to the short, less active allele, with odds ratios of about 1.2 in bipolar disorder, major depression, or bipolar disorder plus major depression, but no association was seen with the VNTR (Furlong et al. 1998a). There is also evidence that variation at 5-HTTLPR is predictive of response to selective serotonin reuptake inhibitors (see section "Psychopharmacogenetics" later in this chapter). Meta-analyses of a dinucleotide microsatellite repeat in intron 2 of the *MAOA* gene were marginally significant ($P = 0.02$) for

association to bipolar disorder and suggested an odds ratio of 1.5–2.6 for some alleles at the locus (Furlong et al. 1999a; Preisig et al. 2000). Meta-analyses for variation in the genes encoding tyrosine hydroxylase (*TH*; Furlong et al. 1999b; Turecki et al. 1997), tryptophan hydroxylase (*TPH*; Furlong et al. 1998c), the D$_2$ dopamine receptor (Furlong et al. 1998b), and *COMT* (Biomed European Bipolar Collaborative Group 1997) found no association to bipolar disorder or major depression (*COMT* was bipolar disorder only).

Trinucleotide Expansion and Genetic Anticipation

It also has been suggested that bipolar illness displays the phenomena of *genetic anticipation* (earlier onset or greater severity of illness with each succeeding generation in a pedigree) (McInnis et al. 1993; Petronis and Kennedy 1995). However, it is always difficult to discern between genetic anticipation and an ascertainment bias. In disorders in which the molecular basis of the genetic anticipation is understood (i.e., Huntington's disease, fragile X syndrome, spinal and bulbar muscular atrophy), an expanding trinucleotide repeat sequence is responsible. This has prompted a search for evidence of expanding trinucleotide repeat sequences in bipolar illness (Jain et al. 1996; O'Donovan et al. 1995, 1996; Rubinsztein et al. 1996; Sasaki et al. 1996a; Vincent et al. 1996). Although some of these studies are positive in populations, no study has demonstrated cosegregation of an expanding trinucleotide sequence in a pedigree.

Anxiety Disorders

The NIMH epidemiological study of 1-year prevalence rates found anxiety disorders, at 12.6%, to be the most common category of illness (Regier et al. 1993). Diagnostic terms and concepts in the area of anxiety disorders have changed considerably over the past decade, diminishing the relevance of older studies in this area. However, whenever studied, "anxiety neurosis" was found to be highly familial, with up to two-thirds of families showing cases in first-degree relatives. Studies that used DSM-III-R diagnostic categories have reported increased familial rates for panic disorder and agoraphobia, generalized anxiety disorder, simple and social phobias, and obsessive-compulsive disorder (OCD).

Panic Disorder

Several family studies have found a higher rate of panic disorder in the relatives of probands who have the disorder than in the relatives of control subjects. This has been seen consistently in all studies, many of which are from different countries. The relative risk to first-degree relatives of panic disorder probands ranged between 2.6- and 20-fold (Crowe et al. 1980, 1983; Maier et al. 1993; Mendlewicz et al. 1993; Noyes et al. 1986; Weissman et al. 1993), with a median value of 7.8-fold (Knowles and Weissman 1995). Most of these studies were done on samples ascertained from treatment settings, and so this relative risk may reflect a more severe form of panic disorder. As an example of this type of study, Crowe et al. (1983) found a 17.3% risk for panic disorder in first-degree relatives and an additional risk of 7.4% for "probable panic disorder" (i.e., two or three rather than four criterion symptoms). Control rates were 1.8% and 0.4%, respectively. In a family study of agoraphobia, Noyes et al. (1986) found high risk for panic disorder (definite plus probable) both in the relatives of panic disorder probands (17.3%) and in the relatives of agoraphobic probands (8.3%), compared with 4.2% in the relatives of control subjects. They also found that the risk for agoraphobia was increased among the relatives of agoraphobic probands (11.6%), but not the relatives of panic disorder probands (1.9%), when compared with control subjects (4.2%). All agoraphobic probands and relatives had panic attacks as well. In both of these studies, the risk of panic disorder and/or agoraphobia among female relatives was two to three times higher than that for male relatives. Neither study showed an increased rate of generalized anxiety disorder in the relatives of the index cases. Noyes et al. and Crowe et al. concluded that their findings are consistent with agoraphobia being a more severe variant of panic disorder. However, this is at odds with the observation that agoraphobia is more common than panic disorder in the general population (Kessler et al. 1994; Wittchen et al. 1998)

Individuals with panic disorder are more sensitive to the anxiogenic effects of multiple substances, including cholecystokinin (CCK), lactate, and inhaled carbon dioxide. Family studies of carbon dioxide sensitivity have been performed and have shown a larger increase in anxiety symptoms in the first-degree relatives of panic disorder patients as compared with healthy control subjects (Coryell 1997; Perna et al. 1995; van Beek and Griez 2000). Some evidence indicates that this response is specific to panic disorder and social phobia but not the other anxiety disorders (Caldirola et al. 1997). A segregation analysis suggested that the response to carbon dioxide might be transmitted as a single major locus (Cavallini et al. 1999b).

The possibility of a genetic relation between adult and childhood anxiety disorders has been prompted by the high rates of separation anxiety and school phobia reported by adults with panic disorder. Some available family studies have shown elevated rates of separation anxiety in the children of parents with panic disorder or agoraphobia, but others have concluded that childhood school phobias are related to adult neurotic illness in general rather than specifically to adult agoraphobia. Recently, a systematic, blind, case-control, high-risk study of the children of parents with panic disorder, major depression, both, or neither was published (Biederman et al. 2001). Offspring of the parents with panic disorder were more likely to have separation anxiety disorder, panic disorder, and agoraphobia, regardless of the presence of depression in the parents. Offspring of the parents with major depression were more likely to have social phobia, separation anxiety disorder, major depression, and disruptive behavior disorders, regardless of the presence of panic disorder in the parents. A genetic relation between panic disorder and mood disorders, particularly bipolar disorder, also is likely because the presence of panic disorder in families with bipolar disorder was more tightly linked to chromosome 18 in one study (MacKinnon et al. 1998). Similarly, some evidence suggests that the relatives of panic disorder probands may have a higher rate of alcohol abuse. The studies that have investigated the comorbidity between these disorders have not provided a clear answer to the degree of genetic overlap, and the final determination of this will probably await the cloning of disease genes for each of the disorders.

Several twin studies of panic disorder have been done. The earliest were performed by Torgersen (1983, 1990) and Skre et al. (1993), who found broad-sense heritability estimates between 30% and 62%. The higher estimates of heritability are likely to be overestimates because of the absence of observed DZ pairs concordant for panic disorder in the early studies. Since then, two large twin studies of panic disorder have been performed. The first was a population-based study of 2,163 females (1,033 twin pairs) from the Virginia Twin Registry with a mean age of 30 years (Kendler et al. 1993b). Of the 2,163 twins, 5.8%, 10.9% (166 twin pairs), 4.6%, and 7.6% met lifetime criteria for clinician-narrow, clinician-broad, computer-narrow, and computer-broad diagnoses, respectively. The estimate of narrow-sense heritability was 46%, 32%, 0%, and 37% for the clinician-narrow, clinician-broad, computer-narrow, and computer-broad diagnoses, respectively. This estimate of narrow-sense heritability for panic disorder (30%–40%) is markedly less than that observed for schizophrenia, autism, and major mood disorder (Plomin et al. 1994). A subsequent study indicated that there was little overlap with the genes responsible for generalized anxiety disorder in this population (Kendler et al. 1995). In contrast, in a study of 3,362 male twin pairs from the Vietnam Era Twin Registry, additive genetic factors appear to account for 43.4% of the risk for panic attacks and 37.2% for generalized anxiety disorder of 1 month's duration. The best fitting bivariate model predicted that approximately half of this additive genetic effect was shared in common between panic and generalized anxiety disorder (Scherrer et al. 2000).

Three groups have published genome scans of panic disorder and/or agoraphobia. The group at Columbia University found the strongest support for a recessive locus on 7p15 (lod score = 1.7) in 23 families (Knowles et al. 1998) and a dominant locus on 13q (lod score = 4.2) in 45 families when the affected phenotype for the analysis was either panic disorder, mitral valve prolapse, serious headache, thyroid problems, or kidney or bladder problems (Weissman et al. 2000). The group at Iowa University also found their highest scores on 7p15 (lod score = 2.2–3.0) in 23 families, but this was with a dominant model (Crowe et al. 2001). The Yale University group found a lod score of 2.0 on chromosome 1 using a dominant model of inheritance and 20 families (Gelernter et al. 2001). In this same region, a dominant lod score of 1.1 was observed in the Iowa scan. In addition, the Yale group found a lod score of 2.0 on chromosome arm 11p with a marker in the CCK B receptor (CCKBR) gene (discussed later in this section), but no signal was observed in the other two scans.

A partial genome scan, focusing on regions of the human genome that are homologous to regions of the mouse genome that are thought to contain quantitative trait loci for anxiety phenotypes, found evidence of linkage to 10q (lod score = 2.38) and 12q13 (nonparametric test, $P = 0.006$) in one large pedigree with 99 members (Smoller et al. 2001). Very high lod scores (up to 5.0) have been observed between a large (10–17 Mb), polymorphic duplication of 15q24–26 (DUP25) and a combined phenotype of panic disorder, agoraphobia, social phobia, simple phobia, and joint laxity in a population of Spanish ethnicity (Gratacos et al. 2001). All patients with panic disorder with or without agoraphobia in seven pedigrees and 68 of 70 (97%) panic patients in a second sample had the duplication as compared with 7% of Centre d'Etudes du Polymorphisme Humain (CEPH) control individuals. The duplication probably arises somatically because only about 60% of an individual's cells have it. It is hypothesized that overexpression, because of the presence of the extra copies, of one or more of the 23 genes in the region is responsible for panic disorder.

Multiple candidate genes have been examined and show no association to panic disorder (TH, adrenergic receptors, pro-opiomelanocortin, D_2 dopamine receptor gene [DRD2] and D_4 dopamine receptor gene [DRD4], GABAB1R, serotonin and dopamine transporters) (Crawford et al. 1995; Crowe et al. 1987; Deckert et al. 1997; Hamilton et al. 1999, 2000a; Mutchler et al. 1990; Sand et al. 2000; Schmidt et al. 1993; Wang et al. 1992). However, positive associations have been observed for the adenosine receptor 2A, the monoamine oxidase A (MAOA) gene, and genes in the CCK system. Deckert et al. (1998, 1999) observed positive genetic associations with panic disorder and the adenosine receptor 2A and MAOA genes; however, the latter finding was not replicated in another sample (Hamilton et al. 2000b), but this study may not have had sufficient power. Genetic association of panic disorder and a polymorphism in the promoter of the CCK gene has been observed in one study (Wang et al. 1998) but not in two others (Hamilton et al. 2001; Kennedy et al. 1999). The latter two studies also examined the CCKBR gene, and Kennedy et al. observed an association, in a case-control study, but this was not found in the family-based study by Hamilton et al. Last, genetic association between the human homologue of the Drosophila white gene and panic has been observed (Nakamura et al. 1999), but this locus has not been studied by others.

Obsessive-Compulsive Disorder

The results of family studies of OCD are inconsistent. No increase in strict OCD was found among relatives in studies by Hoover and Insel (1984), McKeon and Murray (1987), and Black et al. (1992). However, each of these studies found high family rates of other psychiatric disorders, described as depressive and neurotic disorders, anxiety disorders, or "a more broadly defined OCD." The one study that showed a significant familial increase in OCD began with child and adolescent probands and reported a 25% incidence among fathers plus 9% among mothers (Lenane et al. 1990). In contrast to the earlier studies, more recent family studies of OCD do suggest a familial component to the disorder (Nestadt et al. 2000b; Nicolini et al. 1993; Pauls et al. 1995b). In the Nicolini et al. and Pauls et al. studies, the relative risk of OCD to relatives of OCD probands was four- to fivefold higher than the risk to relatives of control subjects, and there appeared to be an increased risk to relatives of probands with an early age at onset. These latter findings, when considered with work of Lenane et al., support the hypothesis that early-onset OCD, like early-onset mood disorder, is more highly familial. Substantial comorbidity of Gilles de la Tourette's syndrome is seen with OCD, and family studies suggest a shared genetic diathesis (Barr and Sandor 1998; Leckman and Chittenden 1990).

For OCD, Carey and Gottesman (1981) found significant MZ-DZ differences (87% vs. 47%, respectively, giving a heritability estimate of 80%), which is similar to results found earlier in a Japanese investigation and others. These twin studies of OCD indicate that genetic factors may be involved. One of the environmental factors that might interact with a genetic vulnerability is poststreptococcal autoimmunity (pediatric autoimmune neuropsychiatric disorders associated with streptococcal infections) (Leonard and Swedo 2001). Several segregation analyses of OCD have suggested that a single major locus, possibly dominant, best accounted for the familial aggregation (Cavallini et al. 1999a; Nestadt et al. 2000a; Nicolini et al. 1991).

One genome scan for early-onset OCD has been performed and found a peak 9 cM from the telomere of the short arm of chromosome 9. Investigation of the neuronal and epithelial glutamate transporter *EAAC1* gene in the region was negative (Veenstra-VanderWeele et al. 2001). Candidate gene association studies of OCD and the *DRD2*, *DRD3*, and *DRD4* genes, as well as the *5HT2B* and *5HT2C* genes, have had negative results. Two studies reported positive associations of the long allele of the VNTR polymorphism in 5-HTTLPR (Bengel et al. 1999; McDougle et al. 1998) but not in three others (Billett et al. 1997; Frisch et al. 2000; Kinnear et al. 2000). A genetic association between an allele at the *COMT* gene and males with OCD has been reported (Karayiorgou et al. 1997, 1999). Other groups observed an association between homozygosity (Schindler et al. 2000) or heterozygosity (Niehaus et al. 2001) at the locus or no association in a small sample (Ohara et al. 1998).

Other Anxiety Disorders (Generalized Anxiety Disorder, Phobias, and Posttraumatic Stress Disorder)

Family studies of generalized anxiety disorder, simple phobias, and social phobia, but not posttraumatic stress disorder (PTSD), have found familial aggregation. Noyes et al. (1987) noted that the increased rates of generalized anxiety disorder were specific and that they were not found among the relatives of patients with panic disorder. Fyer et al. (1990) reported a rate of 31% for simple phobia in first-degree relatives compared with 11% in control subjects (relative risk = 3.3). For social phobia, two studies (Fyer et al. 1993; T. Reich et al. 1988) found a threefold increase in this disorder in the relatives of probands, the latter reporting rates of 16% vs. 5% in the control group. When subtypes of social phobia were studied, an

approximately 10-fold increase in the rate of generalized social phobia (and avoidant personality disorder), but not discrete and nongeneralized social phobia, was observed in the first-degree relatives of patients with social phobia of each respective subtype as compared with the relatives of control subjects (Stein et al. 1998a). There is extensive comorbidity of these disorders in probands (Goisman et al. 1995; Goldenberg et al. 1996), but the disorders "breed true" when the families of probands without comorbidity are studied (Fyer et al. 1995). Finally, no increase in PTSD was found in the families of PTSD probands studied (using family history methodology) by Davidson et al. (1989); however, a family history of depression increased the risk to develop PTSD after rape (Davidson et al. 1998).

Hettema et al. (2001) conducted a twin study of generalized anxiety disorder, finding a heritability of about 15%–20% in both males and females, with no evidence of sex-specific genetic factors. Kendler et al. (1992) also found evidence for a significant genetic contribution to agoraphobia, social phobia, and animal phobia in a study of female twins (heritabilities of 30%–40%). The influence of genetic factors increases when the unreliability of a single assessment is accounted for (Kendler et al. 1999). Another study of 1,344 twins from the Missouri Adolescent Twin Study found that social phobia had a heritability of 28%, and these genetic factors overlap completely with those that predispose individuals to major depression (Nelson et al. 2000). In the Virginia Twin Registry sample, such overlap was observed (Kendler et al. 1993a). In males, the heritabilities of all fears were somewhat lower (25%–37%), and there was some evidence for common genetic risk factor(s) for all phobias and other phobia-specific genetic risk factors (Kendler et al. 2001a). In contrast to the family studies, True et al. (1993) reported that genetic factors provided a substantial contribution to all the symptoms of PTSD. Furthermore, one common genetic loading accounts for 15% of the variance to develop PTSD (and 55% and 25% of the variance to develop alcohol and drug dependence, respectively), and PTSD-specific genetic factors account for 20% (total 35%) (Xian et al. 2000a). In addition, evidence indicates that genetic factors may influence one's exposure to trauma (Lyons et al. 1993).

There are few molecular genetic studies of these disorders as yet. The genes encoding the 5-HTT and 5-HT$_{2A}$ receptor have been examined in 17 pedigrees with 122 samples segregating social phobia, and no linkage was observed (Stein et al. 1998b). As mentioned earlier in the "Panic Disorder" subsection, duplication of a portion of chromosome 15 may predispose to social and simple phobia (Gratacos et al. 2001). A study of anxiety disorders in a Japanese sample found no evidence of association to COMT (Ohara et al. 1998). There is one report of genetic association between PTSD and the A1 allele of the *DRD2* gene (Comings et al. 1996), but this has not been replicated in another study (Gelernter et al. 1999b).

Eating Disorders

In 9 of 10 family studies of anorexia nervosa performed between 1983 and 1998, the only cases of anorexia nervosa that were observed were in relatives of anorexia nervosa probands. In the largest family study of the eating disorders, 1,831 relatives of 504 probands (152 pure anorexia nervosa, pure 171 bulimia nervosa, and 181 screened subjects without eating disorders), the relative risk to first-degree relatives of anorexia nervosa and bulimia nervosa probands for developing anorexia nervosa was 11.3 and 12.3, respectively, as compared with the first-degree relatives of the control subjects (Strober et al. 2000). In addition, the relative risk of bulimia nervosa for relatives of anorexia nervosa and bulimia nervosa probands was 4.2 and 4.4, respectively. Taken together, this suggests that the two disorders share a familial (possibly genetic) etiological factor; however, the absence of the observation of cases of combined anorexia nervosa and bulimia nervosa in the families is not consistent with this hypothesis (Strober et al. 2000).

Comorbid major depression and anorexia nervosa has been observed in clinical population studies, and increased rates of major depression have been observed in the first-degree relatives of anorexia nervosa probands (Strober et al. 1990). It is unclear if this comorbidity is due to a common familial factor (Lilenfeld et al. 1998; Wade et al. 2000).

The heritabilities of anorexia nervosa and bulimia nervosa have been reported to range from 0% to 70% and 0% to 83%, respectively (Fairburn et al. 1999). However, recent studies of anorexia nervosa have found heritabilities of 58% for a broad definition of anorexia nervosa in the Virginia Twin Registry (Wade et al. 2000) and 88% when the earlier studies of Holland et al. (1988) were reanalyzed (Bulik et al. 2000). Similar reanalyses of the Virginia and Australian twin data found estimates of heritability of bulimia nervosa of 83% and 59%, respectively, and estimated the shared family environment contribution at 0% (Bulik et al. 2000). A segregation analysis of 141 families with eating disorders found evidence of autosomal dominant transmission if OCD was included along with anorexia nervosa and bulimia nervosa in the analysis (Cavallini et al. 2000).

Investigations have been made of multiple candidate genes for association to the eating disorders. Negative results have been observed for β_3-adrenergic receptor (*ADRB3*); *DRD4*; *DRD3*; leptin (*LEP*); melanocortin MC4 receptor (*MC4R*); pro-opiomelanocortin (*POMC*); *NPYR1*; 5-HT$_{1D\beta}$ (*HTR1B*), 5-HT$_{2C}$ (*HTR2C*), and 5-HT$_7$ (*HTR7*) receptors; and *TPH* (reviewed in Hinney et al. 2000). A positive association of bulimia nervosa to the short allele of a VNTR polymorphism that affects the expression of the serotonin transporter was reported (Di Bella et al. 2000), but this was not observed in two other studies of anorexia nervosa and the gene (Hinney et al. 1997b; Sundaramurthy et al. 2000). Other single studies have found associations between anorexia nervosa and the agouti-related protein gene (Vink et al. 2001), *COMT* (Frisch et al. 2001), the uncoupling protein locus (Campbell et al. 1999), and the estrogen β receptor (Rosenkranz et al. 1998) and therefore need to be examined in other samples. An association between the A allele of the −1438 G/A SNP upstream of the 5-HT$_{2A}$ (*HTR2A*) gene and anorexia nervosa has been observed in four studies (Collier et al. 1997; Enoch et al. 1998; Nacmias et al. 1999; Sorbi et al. 1998), but not in three others (Campbell et al. 1998; Hinney et al. 1997a; Ziegler et al. 1999). A meta-analysis of six of the studies (excluding Hinney et al.) found no evidence of an association (Ziegler et al. 1999), but further studies in family-based samples are warranted.

Drug Dependence

Alcoholism has been shown to be highly familial in many studies, which, as reviewed by Merikangas (1989), show the risk to first-degree relatives to be increased approximately sevenfold. This work has been extended to other drugs of abuse, with most having an eightfold increased risk to first-degree relatives (Merikangas et al. 1998). A similar study of the siblings of the probands in the Collaborative Study on the Genetics of Alcoholism (COGA) found similar results (Bierut et al. 1998). Both studies found evidence of specific transmission of risk for each drug of abuse, in addition to general factors that predispose to all drugs.

Several adoption studies also provide evidence that genetic factors, as well as environmental ones, are involved in the etiology of alcoholism. Goodwin (1979) showed that alcoholism in the biological parents predicted alcoholism in their male offspring, even when the offspring were raised by unrelated adoptive parents. Cadoret et al. (1980) reported similar results. The results for female offspring were less clear. Goodwin (1979) found elevated rates of alcoholism among both the adopted-away daughters of alcoholic persons and the control adoptees, whereas Cadoret et al. (1985) found higher rates in the daughters of the index cases compared with control subjects. Data from a large Swedish sample also support a genetic predisposition to alcoholism in both women and men (Bohman et al. 1981; Cloninger et al. 1981), as well as the possible importance of certain environmental factors (such as lower occupational status of the adoptive father). In the COGA study, the risk of alcoholism in siblings of females with alcoholism was observed to be slightly higher than for siblings of males with alcoholism, suggesting a higher genetic predisposition in the females (T. Reich et al. 1998). In all of these studies, alcoholism in the adoptive environment was not shown to increase the risk for alcoholism among the adoptees. However, another study (Cadoret et al. 1985) found that alcoholism in the adoptive family more broadly defined (to include all adoptive first- and second-degree relatives) increased the rates of alcohol abuse among adoptees. The Swedish study also identified two potential subtypes of alcohol abuse, "milieu-limited" (type 1) and "male-limited" (type 2); type 2 families have a more heritable, severe, earlier-onset form of alcoholism that is associated with criminality (Bohman et al. 1987). However, not all the features of these subtypes have been observed in a subsequent study (Irwin et al. 1990).

Twin studies support the hypothesis that the substance abuse disorders are very heritable and that genetic factors predispose to abuse in general and to specific substances. In one very large twin study of 3,372 male twin pairs from the Vietnam Era Twin Registry, the proportions of the variance to developing drug abuse to marijuana, stimulants, sedatives, heroin, and psychedelics were 33%, 33%, 27%, 54%, and 26%, respectively (Tsuang et al. 1998). For marijuana and stimulants, about one-third of the genetic variance was due to drug-specific factors, whereas for heroin, 70% of the genetic variance was specific to the drug. These results are similar to what has been observed in family studies (see earlier discussion in this section). Alcoholism also has been shown to have a significant genetic diathesis in most twin studies. For instance, in a study of 4,097 twin pairs of both sexes from the Virginia Twin Registry, the estimated proportion of population variation in liability attributed to genetic factors was similar in both women (55%–66%) and men (51%–56%), and there was little evidence of shared familial nongenetic factors (Prescott et al. 1999). In addition, it appeared that genetic factors influencing alcoholism did not completely overlap between the sexes. This is consistent with the animal work in alcoholism (see later discussion in this section). Furthermore, these sex-specific genetic factors appear to overlap with those that

predispose individuals to developing major depression (Prescott et al. 2000). Substantial overlap between the genetic factors for alcoholism and nicotine use (heritability of 50%–70% in many studies) has been observed in three twin studies (Hettema et al. 1999; Swan et al. 1997; True et al. 1999). Last, overlap between the genetic factors for major depression and nicotine use has been observed in females (Kendler et al. 1993c), making it very likely that a set of genes exist that predispose to major depression, nicotine dependence, and alcoholism, and they may act in a sex-specific fashion.

There are multiple molecular studies of the substance abuse disorders, and discussion of all of them is beyond the scope of this chapter. These studies have been reviewed recently (Enoch and Goldman 2001; Vanyukov and Tarter 2000). The only known genes that influence the development of a substance abuse disorder encode alcohol dehydrogenase (*ADH2*), which metabolizes ethanol to acetaldehyde, and aldehyde dehydrogenase (*ALDH2*), which converts acetaldehyde to acetate (Radel and Goldman 2001). Acetaldehyde is toxic, and genetic variations that increase its synthesis or decrease its breakdown cause a reaction of facial flushing, headache, palpitations, hypotension, tachycardia, nausea, and vomiting. Such variants have been observed in the Asian population and appear to be protective against developing alcoholism (Thomasson et al. 1991).

Most of the candidate gene work on substance abuse has been on the genes in the dopamine pathway, given its role in reward behavior and addiction (Koob and Nestler 1997). One early finding was an association of alcoholism (especially with severe medical complications) with an SNP located 13,000 bases downstream of the *DRD2* gene (*Taq* A_1 allele) (Blum et al. 1990). These findings are controversial because most subsequent studies did not find a statistically significant association (Bolos et al. 1990; Chen et al. 1996; C.C. Cook et al. 1996; Edenberg et al. 1998; Gelernter et al. 1991; Heinz et al. 1996; Lu et al. 1996). Two meta-analyses of the data (Gelernter et al. 1993; Uhl et al. 1993) came to very different conclusions (i.e., the *DRD2* locus accounts for one-half of the genetic variance vs. has no effect), because each group excluded a portion of the available data.

The *DRD1*, *DRD3*, *DRD4*, *DRD5*, *DAT1*, and *MAOA* genes have been studied for genetic association, and these largely negative results are reviewed in Vanyukov and Tarter (2000). The µ opiate receptor has been studied in substance abuse and alcoholism with positive results in some (Hoehe et al. 2000; Town et al. 1999), but not all, studies (Bergen et al. 1997; Gelernter et al. 1999a; Sander et al. 1998).

Multiple candidate genes for nicotine use have been

investigated. One population-based genetic association study found that individuals with a least one null allele for cytochrome P450 2A6 (*CYP2A6*), the gene that encodes the enzyme that metabolizes nicotine to nicotine iminium, seemed to significantly reduce the risk of cigarette dependence (Pianezza et al. 1998), although the accuracy of the genotyping has been questioned (Oscarson et al. 1998). Other studies of nicotine use have examined the *TH*, *DAT1*, *DRD4*, *DRD5*, *SLC6A3*, and *CHRNB2* genes, but there are no replicated positive findings from methodologically sound studies.

Genome scans have been performed for alcohol and nicotine dependence. A genome scan of 105 families from the COGA study found evidence for a linkage of chromosomes 1, 2, and 7 (highest lod score = 3.49) and for a protective locus on chromosome 4, which contains the *ADH* gene cluster (T. Reich et al. 1998). More recent analysis suggests that the locus on chromosome 1 predisposes to both alcoholism and major depression (Nurnberger et al. 2001), which is what was predicted by the family and twin study discussed earlier. A second genome scan of 172 sibling pairs from a Southwestern American Indian tribe found evidence for loci on both chromosomes 4 (lod score = 2.9), which contains the *GABAB1* gene, and 11 (lod score = 3.1), which contains the genes for *TH* and *DRD4* (Long et al. 1998). One genome scan has been published for nicotine dependence, and this study of 130 families from New Zealand and an additional 91 families from Virginia found the strongest evidence for linkage on chromosome 2 (lod score = 2.63) (Straub et al. 1999), and weaker signals were detected on chromosomes 4, 10, 16, 17, and 18.

An additional molecular genetic approach that has worked particularly well in understanding the biology of substance abuse is the use of animal models. Berrettini et al. (1994b) were able to map three loci in mice for oral morphine preference by breeding mice from progenitor strains that differed in their morphine preference. The effect of one of these loci, on mouse chromosome 10, could be replicated in another sample, and the linked region contains a good candidate gene, the μ opiate receptor (Alexander et al. 1996). Two sex-specific loci for alcohol preference in mice also have been mapped (Melo et al. 1996). Interestingly, the locus for alcohol preference in female mice demonstrates *genomic imprinting* (is only active when passed from one parental line—in this case from the mother). Neither locus for alcohol preference overlaps with the three loci for morphine preference, suggesting that the genetic basis for different addictive disorders is distinct.

Suicide and Impulsive Behavior

Many family studies have found familial clustering of suicide attempts and completions. This has been observed in studies of completers that used either friends (Shafii et al. 1985), individuals from the community (Brent et al. 1996), or nonsuicidal diagnostically matched control subjects (Tsuang 1983). Although it is difficult to control for the psychiatric comorbidity that also runs in the families of the victims, Brent et al. (1996) found a fourfold increased risk of suicide attempts and completions in the relatives of suicide probands as compared with the relatives of control subjects from the community. In the Amish, 73% of suicides occur in 16% of the pedigrees, even though some of the nonsuicide pedigrees are just as severely affected with bipolar disorder (Egeland and Sussex 1985). This pattern of increased risk to relatives of suicide probands as compared with relatives of control subjects, even beyond the risk conferred by an Axis I disorder, is also seen for relatives of suicide attempters.

Several lines of evidence suggest that a portion of this familial clustering is due to genetic factors. One study of 176 twin pairs found 11% (7 of 62) of MZ and 1% (2 of 114) of DZ twin pairs to be concordant for suicide (Roy et al. 1991). Another study found concordance rates of attempted suicide among co-twins of suicide victims to be 38% (10 of 26) for MZ and 0% (0 of 9) for DZ twin pairs (Roy et al. 1995). The largest twin study of suicide behavior interviewed 2,718 twin pairs and found the best estimate of heritability of reporting any suicidal ideation, persistent thoughts, and suicide plans or attempts to be about 44% and that of reporting serious attempts to be 55% (Statham et al. 1998). Adoption studies of suicide provide additional support for the hypothesis that there are genetic factors (Schulsinger et al. 1979; Wender et al. 1986).

Many studies have suggested that there is a disorder of serotonin metabolism in both the trait of impulsivity and suicidal behavior. With this theoretical basis, an SNP in intron 7 of the gene for TPH, the rate-limiting enzyme in the synthesis of serotonin, was examined for genetic association to a group of violent alcoholic Finnish offenders and arsonists (Nielsen et al. 1994). The frequency of the "U" allele was 0.32 in the 36 individuals who had made a suicide attempt and 0.54 in the 34 who did not ($P = 0.016$), suggesting an association between the "L" allele and a history of attempted suicide. This study also examined the relation between cerebrospinal fluid 5-hydroxyindoleacetic acid concentration and TPH genotype and found a highly significant association ($P = 0.0036$) between the two in impulsive but not nonimpulsive or control subjects (Nielsen et al. 1994). Most, but not all, subsequent studies have found genetic association to the intron 7 SNP, but often to the other allele, suggesting that this SNP is not the disease-predisposing variant but may be in linkage disequilibrium with one. Additional SNPs now have been found in and around the gene, and studies that have genotyped multiple polymorphisms and then formed haplotypes have implicated the 5′ (Turecki et al. 2001) and 3′ (Abbar et al. 2001) regulatory regions of the gene, particularly in those who made violent suicide attempts.

Other genes in the serotonergic system also have been investigated. 5-HTTLPR has been investigated by several groups. No genetic association (Geijer et al. 2000; Russ et al. 2000; Zalsman et al. 2001), association to the "L" allele (Du et al. 1999), and association to the "S" allele all have been observed (Bondy et al. 2000; Courtet et al. 2001). In some of the studies, the results were stronger in patients with violent attempts, suggesting that the potential association might be due to a predisposition to violence rather than suicide. The genes for 5-HT$_{1B}$ and 5-HT$_{2A}$ also have been investigated, but no clear genetic associations to suicide were found.

Perhaps the clearest link between a genetic mutation and a human behavior causing a psychiatric illness comes from the study of Brunner's syndrome in a large Dutch family (Brunner et al. 1993b). This X-linked syndrome is characterized by borderline mental retardation along with aggressive and violent impulsive behavior in affected males. Some of these behaviors include arson, exhibitionism, and attempted rape and suicide. A linkage study of the X chromosome found a lod score of 3.69 at the *MAOA* gene locus, and 24-hour urinalysis of three affected males showed abnormal monoamine metabolism (Brunner et al. 1993b). Subsequent analysis of the *MAOA* gene revealed that affected males in the family have a cytosine to thymidine mutation at position 936, changing a glutamine codon to a termination codon, and cell culture assays showed the lack of *MAOA* enzymatic activity in the affected males (Brunner et al. 1993a). Further proof of the effect of this gene on behavior comes from the finding of aggressive behavior in a transgenic mouse strain in which the *MAOA* gene was deleted (Cases et al. 1995).

Somatoform Disorders and Sociopathy

Hysteria was not accepted as a diagnostic term in DSM-III, but most of the components of the concept were included in the DSM-III-R section on somatoform disorders, which includes somatization, conversion, and somatoform pain disorders as well as hypochondriasis. Histrionic personality disorder, one of the most important "faces" of hysteria, was put into the personality disorders section, where it resides close to antisocial personality disorder but far from those disorders presenting medical symptomatology. Studies of hysteria as well as its component parts have continued, and the accumulated data on the genetic relationships of all these disorders and antisocial personality disorder are considered here.

The DSM-IV-TR criteria for somatization disorder are a shortened and simplified version of the criteria for *Briquet's syndrome*, a term coined by Samuel Guze (1970) and other researchers at Washington University. These investigators attempted to delineate a syndrome of multiple somatic complaints that are without a demonstrable organic basis while avoiding the confusion and pejorative connotations of the term *hysteria*. Most of the studies reviewed here are of Briquet's syndrome rather than of somatization disorder because this latter concept is relatively new. Studies have shown strong overlap of the two concepts but also the possibility of greater severity and/or greater homogeneity for patients meeting the full Briquet's criteria, as indicated by higher rates of familial aggregation. The prevalence of Briquet's syndrome in first-degree female relatives has been found to be 7.7%, compared with 2.5% in control subjects (Cloninger et al. 1986).

The connection between Briquet's syndrome and antisocial personality disorder was first recognized by finding the coincidence of these two disorders in many samples, especially among women. (Histrionic personality disorder has been associated with these two disorders as well.) Family studies have repeatedly shown a link, most consistently by finding Briquet's syndrome among female relatives of probands (male or female) who are sociopaths or criminals, but also by finding elevated rates of sociopathy in the first-degree relatives of Briquet's or somatization subjects (Lilienfeld et al. 1986).

Adoption studies have given support more to genetic than to environmental determinants of the intraindividual and familial associations between these disorders. Some studies that used the adoptee study method showed an increase in somatic symptoms without medical explanation, as well as antisocial symptoms, among female adoptees of biological parents with antisocial personality. The largest study, which used the adoptee's family method, comprising 144 female adoptee "somatizers"(identified by having two or more sick leaves per year), identified two types of the disorder, each having a link to a form of criminality among the subjects' fathers. One type, termed *diversiform somatization*, was linked to a syndrome of alcoholism plus criminal behavior in biological fathers, with the finding of increased alcohol abuse among adoptive fathers as well. The other type, *high-frequency somatizers*, had biological fathers with a recurrent history of arrest for violent crimes but no history of alcoholism and no increase in psychopathology among adoptive fathers (Cloninger et al. 1984).

Older twin studies of hysteria found higher MZ than DZ rates of concordance, but the pairwise MZ rates were low enough (averaging 21%) to question the importance of genetic factors. A newer twin study examined a mixed group of somatoform disorders and found an MZ concordance of 29% and a DZ concordance of 10% for the group of disorders as a whole (Torgersen 1986). In this study, the co-twins had an increased prevalence of generalized anxiety disorder as well, raising the question of a genetic connection between these disorders. Data on criminality or antisocial personality among the twins were not reported.

Multifactorial models of transmission allow for the possibility of linking clinically discrete illnesses on a continuum of shared liability. Such a model was proposed by Cloninger et al. (1975), in which Briquet's syndrome in women, sociopathy in men, and sociopathy in women were considered increasingly severe expressions of the same multifactorial determinants. This model adequately fits the available data on the risks to first-degree relatives of probands with the various disorders.

Most twin and adoption studies of criminality and antisocial personality have focused on the transmission of these conditions per se and their relation with alcohol abuse rather than on their relation with somatization disorder. A genetic component has consistently been supported (Cloninger and Gottesman 1987), as well as environmental factors. The largest of these studies (Bohman et al. 1982) delineated two types of criminality, each showing genetic predisposition without significant overlap. One was associated with alcoholism and more violent, repeated offenses. The other, associated with petty crimes, appeared to be caused by a genetic predisposition independent of alcoholism as well as by environmental factors that differed for the two sexes. The specific nature of gene–environment interaction has been investigated, revealing the importance of exposure to alcoholism, antisocial behavior, and other factors associated with low socioeconomic status for those who are genetically predisposed (Cadoret et al. 1995).

Personality Disorders and Quantitative Behavioral Traits

Many more genetic studies of Axis I disorders than of Axis II disorders have been done, and the two most extensively studied personality disorders, antisocial and schizotypal, have already been reviewed in this chapter.

Because personality can be described by so many attributes, researchers have worked to condense these into a few "dimensions," usually by factor analytic techniques. Those that have emerged as most replicable and most used in genetic studies are extraversion and neuroticism, as originally derived by Eysenck (1981). The dimensions of *harm avoidance* (anxiety proneness vs. risk taking), *reward dependence* (social attachment vs. disgust), and *novelty seeking* (impulsivity vs. slowness to anger), as defined by Cloninger (1986, 1987), plus the additional dimensions of persistence, self-directedness, cooperativeness, and self-transcendence added subsequently (Cloninger et al. 1993), as assessed by the Tridimensional Personality Questionnaire (TPQ), are also widely used. The seven-dimension TPQ data can be associated with the respective DSM-III-R personality disorder diagnoses (Svrakic et al. 1993).

The extensive family, twin, and adoption studies of extraversion and neuroticism give strong evidence for a genetic effect, but the extent of the genetic contribution, measured as heritability estimates, is greater in twin studies (40%–60%) than in family studies, in which values of approximately one-half those in twin studies have been reported. A possible interpretation, as discussed by Plomin et al. (1990), is nonadditive genetic variance, an allelic interaction that makes identical twins quite alike but does not "breed true" for first-degree relatives, because only one of the alleles can be passed on from a parent.

Following the specification of diagnostic criteria for personality disorders in DSM-III and DSM-III-R, a few family studies have now been reported for the disorders. J.H. Reich (1989) found avoidant and dependent personality disorders to be significantly familial, and this held true for the disorders when grouped as Cluster C ("anxious cluster") as well. In a later report, J. Reich (1991) found that the increase in anxious cluster personality diagnoses among relatives also was found for probands with mixed anxiety and depression who did not have personality disorders. Relatives of Cluster B ("flamboyant cluster") personality disorders showed a high level of personality disorder psychopathology but of a diverse nature. Borderline personality disorder also has been found to be modestly familial. We have already discussed the familiality of Cluster A personality disorders in the earlier section on schizophrenia.

At present, there are no positive molecular genetic studies of the personality disorders, but there are now several reports of genes responsible for a portion of the genetic variance of some of the personality dimensions. Increased novelty seeking, one of the dimensions of the TPQ, was associated with the 7 repeat allele in exon 3 of the *DRD4* gene in a study of 124 unrelated Israeli subjects (Ebstein et al. 1996). This has been replicated in a study of 315 individuals (mostly male) from the United States that used data from the Neuroticism, Extroversion, and Openness (NEO) personality inventory to reconstruct the TPQ scale (Benjamin et al. 1996). Variation at the *DRD4* gene was estimated to account for 3%–4% of the variance in the novelty-seeking trait, which is estimated to about 40% genetic (Heath et al. 1994); therefore, about 10% of the genetic variance has been accounted for. Subsequent studies have not, for the most part, replicated these findings (reviewed in Paterson et al. 1999). More recent studies of the *DRD4* gene have found an association to novelty seeking with a polymorphism in the promoter region (–521 C/T) that appears to cause an approximately twofold variation in transcription of the gene in a model system (Okuyama et al. 2000; Ronai et al. 2001), suggesting that variation in other locations of the gene may be important.

Loci for another dimension of the TPQ, harm avoidance, have been uncovered in a genome scan of 758 pairs of siblings in 177 nuclear families of alcoholic persons (Cloninger et al. 1998). A lod score of 3.2 was observed for a locus that accounted for 38% of the total variance to harm avoidance using markers on 8p21–23. Genetic interactions with loci on 21q21–22.1, 11, and 20 also were observed and might account for most of the genetic variance of harm avoidance. This work awaits replication. One locus that was not observed in the genome scan was the gene for the serotonin transporter (*SLC6A4*) on 17q12. An earlier study of 505 individuals had found a genetic association between a polymorphism in the regulatory region of the gene and the neuroticism scale of the NEO personality inventory ($P = 0.002$) and the anxiety scale of Cattell's personality inventory ($P = 0.023$) (Lesch et al. 1996). These results have been replicated in some (Du et al. 2000; Greenberg et al. 2000; Katsuragi et al. 1999; Mazzanti et al. 1998), but not all, subsequent studies (Ebstein et al. 1997b; Gustavsson et al. 1999; Nakamura et al. 1997).

Neuropsychiatric Disorders

The neuropsychiatric disorders—Gilles de la Tourette's syndrome, Huntington's disease, Lesch-Nyhan syndrome, Parkinson's disease—are well covered in the companion *The American Psychiatric Publishing Textbook of Neuropsychiatry and Clinical Neurosciences*, 4th Edition (Yudofsky and Hales 2002). Alzheimer's disease is also well covered there, but because it is one of the "complex" genetic disorders and because there has been success in finding the disease genes for some forms of the disorder, it is discussed here.

Approximately 10% of the population older than 65 years and 45% of those older than 85 years are affected with Alzheimer's disease. Epidemiological studies report an increased prevalence of dementia in the family members of Alzheimer's patients. Family studies are hindered by the late age at onset because individuals can die from other conditions or develop a dementia from a different etiology. Family studies in Alzheimer's disease have been well reviewed by St. George-Hyslop et al. (1989): estimates of the increase in Alzheimer's disease risk to family members vary widely and may be small (10%–14.4% for parents; 3.8%–13.9% for siblings). Life table studies that adjust for deaths not due to Alzheimer's disease find that the risk of Alzheimer's disease may be as high as 50% in family members by age 90 and only 10% in control subjects (Breitner et al. 1986; Mohs et al. 1987). These analyses support the hypothesis that there could be an autosomal gene for Alzheimer's disease with an age-dependent penetrance, which was subsequently borne out. Farrer et al. (1989), however, who also factored in diagnostic uncertainties, found a risk of only 24% to first-degree relatives by age 93 and of 16% to control subjects by age 90. The increased family prevalence of Alzheimer's disease may occur predominantly in an early-onset group (Heston 1981), although it may be that such cases are just more easily ascertained.

Twin studies for Alzheimer's disease have been difficult to perform because the number of twin pairs that survive until the age at onset of the disorder is low. The concordance rates observed in some twin studies are quite similar in MZ and DZ pairs (about 40%) (R.H. Cook et al. 1981; Embry and Bruyland 1985; Jarvik et al. 1980; Nee et al. 1987). A more recent study of veterans found concordance rates of 21% (4 of 19) for MZ and 11% (2 of 19) for DZ twin pairs, suggesting a small genetic component to the disorder (Breitner et al. 1995), but a large study in Norway found a heritability of 60% (Bergem et al. 1997).

The best support for a genetic diathesis on the predisposition to Alzheimer's disease comes from the finding of four genes, all of which affect the production or deposition of amyloid, that cause or influence the development of the disorder. Familial Alzheimer's disease is classified as either early- (mean family age at onset<60 years,<5% of all familial Alzheimer's disease) or late-onset disease. Early-onset familial Alzheimer's disease tends to be transmitted in an autosomal dominant fashion, and three genes that cause this form of the disorder have been found (*APP*, *PS1*, and *PS2*). The occurrence of neuropathological changes indicative of Alzheimer's disease by age 40 in individuals with Down syndrome initially directed the search for an Alzheimer's disease locus to chromosome 21. The gene for amyloid precursor protein (*APP*), which has 19 exons, is located on this chromosome. Parts of exons 16 and 17 of the *APP* gene encode amyloid, a 39–43 amino acid peptide, which is the major constituent of the senile plaques of Alzheimer's disease. Several groups reported evidence for an Alzheimer's disease gene linked to the pericentromeric region of chromosome 21, especially in early-onset families (David et al. 1988; Goate et al. 1989; St. George-Hyslop et al. 1987; Van Broeckhoven et al. 1988). However, linkage was not found in all pedigrees (Pericak-Vance et al. 1988; Roses et al. 1988; Schellenberg et al. 1988). Subsequently, Hardy and colleagues (Goate et al. 1991) identified a mutation in the APP gene that cosegregated with Alzheimer's disease in two unrelated chromosome 21–linked early-onset families. A search of the early-onset familial Alzheimer's disease pedigrees has led to the identification of multiple disease mutations in *APP*. These mutations flank the amyloid peptide coding sequence, suggesting that they cause improper cleavage of *APP*. Two mutations in the amyloid coding sequences cause cerebral hemorrhage either with or without dementia. The *APP* mutations are thought to account for about 5% of early-onset familial Alzheimer's disease (St. George-Hyslop et al. 1990).

Presenilin 1 (*PS1*), located on chromosome 14, was the second gene for early-onset Alzheimer's disease to be found. Schellenberg et al. (1992) initially described linkage to chromosome arm 14q in nine early-onset (mean age at onset < 52 years) pedigrees (maximum lod score = 9.15). This was quickly replicated by others (Mullan et al. 1992; St. George-Hyslop et al. 1992; Van Broeckhoven et al. 1992), and the gene was subsequently cloned (Sherrington et al. 1995). The *PS1* gene is a 467 amino acid protein with 7–10 hydrophobic transmembrane domains. More than 64 different mutations in *PS1* have been observed, and these account for about 75% of early-onset familial Alzheimer's disease. *PS1* is also an essential gene in mice that is required for normal pattern formation via the Notch signaling pathway during early development (Shen et al. 1997; Wong et al. 1997). The presenilin 2 (*PS2*) gene was cloned by homology to *PS1* and mapped to chromosome 1 (Levy-Lahad et al. 1995a), right into a region where a locus for Alzheimer's disease in the Volga Germans had been mapped (Levy-Lahad et al. 1995b). A missense mutation was then observed in the German pedigrees (Levy-Lahad et al. 1995a) and subsequently an Italian pedigree (Rogaev et al. 1995). Both *PS1* and *PS2* are thought to be aspartyl proteases, called γ-secretases, that cleave APP into the 42 amino acid form of the amyloid peptide (Aβ1–42) (Esler and Wolfe 2001). Mutations in either of the presenilin gene products then increase the production of the Alzheimer's disease causing Aβ1–42.

A susceptibility locus for late-onset Alzheimer's disease was localized to 19q13.2 by linkage analysis in a genome scan (Pericak-Vance et al. 1991). This region contained multiple candidate genes, and one of these, the apolipoprotein E (*APOE*) gene, was found to be associated with late-onset Alzheimer's disease. The frequency of the *APOE* ε4 allele was 0.50 in late-onset Alzheimer's disease cases as compared with 0.16 in age-matched control subjects (Saunders et al. 1993). This association has been replicated in more than 100 laboratories (Roses 1996). Although a genetic association is a population correlation, and therefore not proof of causation, several aspects of the *APOE* ε4 allele support the hypothesis that it is the disease susceptibility locus. There is a dose effect of the ε4 alleles, there may be a protective effect of the ε2 allele, the association is seen in multiple ethnic groups, and *APOE* modifies the effect of some of the early-onset Alzheimer's disease genes (Levy-Lahad and Bird 1996). Compared with the common ε3/ε3 genotype, individuals with one ε4 allele are at a 3- to 4-fold increased risk, and individuals with two ε4 alleles are at 7- to 19-fold increased risk. This increased risk appears to act by causing an earlier age at onset of the illness, with each ε4 lowering the age at onset by 7–9 years in late-onset familial Alzheimer's disease (Strittmatter et al. 1993). However, individuals with one ε4 allele have only a 25%–40% chance of developing Alzheimer's disease. Likewise, individuals with no copies of the ε4 allele are still at risk for developing the illness. This lack of sensitivity and specificity limit the use of *APOE* testing as a diagnostic or predictive test, and it is not currently recommended (Jarvik et al. 1995).

An oligogenic segregation analysis has suggested that between four and seven loci contribute to load, with several that may have as large an effect as *APOE* (Warwick et al. 2000). One of these loci may be located on chromosome 12. A genome scan of 16 families with Alzheimer's disease and a follow-up sample of 38 families found evidence of linkage to the short arm of chromosome 12 (lod scores = 2.7–3.5 with various methods) (Pericak-Vance et al. 1997). The possibility of a gene (or possibly two) in this area of the genome is further supported by additional studies by the same group (Scott et al. 1999, 2000) and others (Mayeux et al. 2002; Rogaeva et al. 1998; Wu et al. 1998). There are conflicting data about whether the finding is stronger or weaker in families without an *APOE4* allele. The initial linkage findings led to the investigation of α2-macroglobulin (*A2M*), a ligand for the apolipoprotein E receptor, LRP, as a positional candidate gene. When a 5-bp deletion polymorphism in an intron with no known biological function was investigated in a sample of 109 families, a 3.5-fold increased risk of Alzheimer's disease ($P = 0.001$) was conferred by having the deletion. A test of genetic association also was highly significant ($P = 0.00009$). These findings appeared to be independent of the effect of the *APOE* locus. Attempts to replicate these findings have been equivocal (Dow et al. 1999; Rogaeva et al. 1999; Romas et al. 2000a; Rudrasingham et al. 1999). Less support has been observed for an association with a second polymorphism in the *A2M* gene that causes a change in the coding sequence of the protein.

In addition to a locus on chromosome 12, other studies have suggested the presence of one or two loci on chromosome 10. The first of these loci is located on 10q21, near marker *D10S1225*, and was identified by both a two-stage genome scan of the genome with 429 Alzheimer's disease sib pairs (lod scores = 3.8–4.8) (Myers et al. 2000) and independently using the quantitative trait of plasma Aβ42 in five pedigrees (lod score = 3.93) (Ertekin-Taner et al. 2000). Linkage also has been observed to markers about 30 cM (~30 million bp) away from *D10S1225*, near the gene for the insulin-degrading enzyme, which is involved in the degradation of Aβ peptides (Bertram et al. 2000), but it is unclear if this gene is the same as or different from the one detected with *D10S1225*.

More than 40 different candidate genes have been examined for genetic association to Alzheimer's disease, and these are reviewed in Schellenberg et al. (2000). Most of the genes are candidates based on known interactions in the pathways of amyloid synthesis, processing, or degradation. One of the most frequently studied has been the α$_1$-antichymotrypsin gene because it may be a modifier of the *APOE* locus. There has not been consistent replication (DeKosky et al. 1996; Gilfix and Briones 1997; Haines et al. 1996a; Kowalska et al. 1996; Morgan et al. 1997; Muller et al. 1996; G.M. Murphy Jr. et al. 1996; Nacmias et al. 1996; Talbot et al. 1996) of the initial genetic association (Kamboh et al. 1995). The early-onset disease genes also have been examined in the late-onset form of the disease. For instance, a polymorphism in an intron of the *PS1* gene has been associated with late-onset familial Alzheimer's disease (Wragg et al. 1996). This has been replicated in some (Higuchi et al. 1996; Kehoe et al. 1996) but not all studies (Romas et al. 2000b; Scott et al. 1996).

Psychopharmacogenetics

Psychopharmacogenetics refers to the study of genetic differences in the behavioral response to pharmacological agents. Behavioral differences may result from both phar-macokinetic variability (i.e., genetic differences in the absorption and degradation of drugs) and pharmacodynamic variability (i.e., genetic differences in tissue sensitivity to drugs). It is hoped that these differences can be used to predict the efficacy and possibility of an adverse event of various pharmacological agents.

Most psychopharmacogenetic studies have focused on the antidepressants and neuroleptics. Plasma levels of one of the tricyclics, nortriptyline, appear to be under genetic control: MZ twins have more comparable concentrations than DZ twins following identical oral doses (Alexanderson et al. 1969). Variation in the *CYP2D6* and *CYP2C19* genes alters the metabolism of many tricylic antidepressants (and some selective serotonin reuptake inhibitors), and dose reductions have been suggested for individuals who carry alleles that make them poor metabolizers of these agents (Kirchheiner et al. 2001), and these genotypes can be determined with microarrays (G.M. Murphy et al. 2001). Plasma levels of the monoamine oxidase inhibitor phenelzine also are under genetic control: a polymorphism in the hepatic enzyme *N*-acetyltransferase that is responsible for degradation of the drug has been identified and appears to be inherited in a mendelian fashion. Individuals with the less active isoenzyme ("slow acetylators") appear to be more prone to side effects from phenelzine (Price-Evans et al. 1965) and, in at least one study, have shown greater therapeutic response to moderate doses of the drug. Also, evidence suggests that the tendency to respond to a specific class of antidepressants is familial (Franchini et al. 1998; O'Reilly et al. 1994; Pare et al. 1962). Although this might reflect the aforementioned pharmacokinetic differences in the rates of metabolism of these drugs, it is equally plausible that there are genetically distinct biological types of depression associated with different drug responses. Also, several studies suggest that variation in 5-HTTLPR may predict response to selective serotonin reuptake inhibitors. In the first study, 102 individuals with psychotic depression were treated with fluvoxamine with or without pindolol and also genotyped for the 5-HTTLPR polymorphism. Individuals homozygous for the short form of the polymorphism (s/s) did not respond as quickly or as well as those with genotypes of l/s and l/l if treated with fluvoxamine alone (Smeraldi et al. 1998). All three genotypic groups responded the same in the fluvoxamine plus pindolol treatment group. These findings have been replicated with both fluvoxamine (Zanardi et al. 2001) and paroxetine (Pollock et al. 2000; Zanardi et al. 2000) in patients with nonpsychotic depression. A small study of individuals with bipolar disorder who became manic when treated with selective serotonin reuptake inhibitors also found an association to the short allele of 5-HTTLPR (Mundo et al. 2001). Variation at the *TPH* gene also has been reported to affect the speed of response to fluvoxamine or paroxetine, and again this difference is ameliorated by the addition of pindolol (Serretti et al. 2001a, 2001b).

Studies of neuroleptic response have suggested that among patients with schizophrenia, haloperidol nonresponders (Silverman et al. 1987) or delayed responders (Sautter et al. 1993) are more likely than other schizophrenic patients to have relatives with schizophrenia spectrum disorders. A substantial amount of work has been performed investigating the association of genetic factors with clozapine response and side effects. Ten studies examined the effect of variation in the 5-HT$_{2A}$ (*HTR2A*) gene on clozapine response, and the results were mixed. A meta-analysis of the studies prior to 1999 found a significant association of the *C102* allele to nonresponse to clozapine based on the data from all studies, but this was nonsignificant when the first positive study was removed (Arranz et al. 1998). Meta-analysis of another polymorphism in the gene, His452Tyr, also showed significant association, albeit with a smaller sample. More recent studies continue to support the association of *HTR2A* and clozapine response (Joober et al. 1999; Yu et al. 2001). Studies of other serotonin receptor genes and the *DRD3* and *DRD4* genes have not produced consistently positive associations with response (Pickar and Rubinow 2001). A study of 133 responders and 67 nonresponders to clozapine with 19 polymorphisms in 10 genes found that a combination of 6 polymorphisms in the genes encoding 5-HT$_{2A}$, 5-HT$_{2C}$, 5-HTT, and H2 was successful in predicting response 77% of the time ($P=0.0001$) with a sensitivity of 95% (Arranz et al. 2000). This study will need replication before a panel of polymorphisms can be used clinically. Genetic factors also appear to be important in the likelihood of developing an agranulocytotic reaction to the atypical neuroleptic clozapine. Lieberman et al. (1990) found increased frequencies of the HLA antigens B38, DR4, and DQw3 in Ashkenazi Jews who developed agranulocytosis. Further work has supported the association of HLA-B38 and clozapine-induced agranulocytosis (Meged et al. 1999; Valevski et al. 1998). Last, genetic variations in the *DRD3* and *HTR2C* genes have been associated with akathisia and tardive dyskinesia (Eichhammer et al. 2000; Segman et al. 2000).

Genetic Counseling

With the increasing awareness among patients, families, psychiatrists, and the general public of the genetic aspects of psychiatric illness, interest in genetic counseling has developed. However, the aims of those seeking genetic counseling for psychiatric disorder are manifold, and these, as well as the data and techniques involved, must be understood by physicians before attempting such an endeavor or referring patients for it.

It is often not the patient who seeks genetic counseling; or, if such is the case, it may be at the insistence of others. Family members and prospective spouses frequently ask for genetic information 1) to learn about the risk for themselves or their offspring, 2) to obtain advice on decisions of marriage or pregnancy, 3) to gain an understanding of a devastating illness in a family member, or 4) to reduce their sense of guilt or to ascribe guilt to others. Patients themselves, when they do seek this type of help, usually do so in the context of an ongoing therapeutic relationship. They may be seeking to understand the cause of their illness, to discover the implications it has for their descendants (present and future), or to determine whether it is "curable."

The components, or stages, of counseling as described by Tsuang (1978) are as follows:

- Diagnosis
- Family history
- Estimation of the risk of recurrence
- Evaluation of the aims, intelligence, and emotions of the counselee
- Helping the counselee understand the risk of recurrence in the context of the burden of the disorder
- Formation of a plan of action
- Follow-up

Accurate diagnosis is essential, and careful review of the patient's history as well as diagnostic interviews with relatives may reveal diagnostic issues that have genetic implications (e.g., depressive disorder with early onset, or "symptomatic schizophrenia" from temporal lobe epilepsy).

With the diagnosis established, there are various methods of estimating the risk of recurrence. Risk rates for siblings, offspring, and other classes of relatives, such as those presented in this chapter, are available. These, however, are averages that are known not to apply under certain circumstances. For example, the risk for schizophrenia is increased in families by severity of the proband's illness, the presence of schizophrenic relatives besides the proband, and psychiatric illness in the proband's mate (Gottesman and Shields 1982). More sophisticated analyses can take into account information such as the number of ill relatives, subclinical or "spectrum" illnesses, and the age at risk for onset of illness, but such computerized programs need to assume an underlying mode of transmission. The mode of transmission is not known for most psychiatric disorders, and such assumptions can affect risk estimates greatly (up to 10-fold). Thus, establishing accurate risk estimates in family members for most psychiatric disorders is not currently possible, and counseling must proceed in the face of considerable uncertainty.

Although we lack knowledge of the mode of transmission and the ability to identify family members at risk for the psychiatric disorders, this is not true for all genetic disorders. Before the gene for Huntington's disease was found, this disease was known to have autosomal dominant transmission and to be closely linked to a marker for a DNA polymorphism, *G8* (or *D4S10*). It is illustrative to see how estimation of risk proceeded under these circumstances, which may apply to other late-onset disorders if efforts to establish linkage are successful. Although all individuals could be typed for the *G8* marker, this by itself was not conclusive regarding risk status. It was necessary to know which *G8* allele was linked to the Huntington's disease gene in the patient's parents. This determination was made by knowing the marker and illness status of parents, uncles and aunts, and members of a third generation (e.g., grandmother) who had lived through the age at risk. When this information was not available, it could (at times) be reconstructed from the other family members. Even with full information on the pedigree, knowledge of the presence of the Huntington's gene was not assured because of the possibilities of 1) recombination (crossover) occurring between the marker and the pathological gene and 2) heterogeneity, in which case the marker is not informative regarding the presence of the gene. Thus, even in this disease with full penetrance, known dominant inheritance, and a closely linked marker, complicated calculations had to be done to determine the probability of being an affected individual. Fortunately, a computerized linkage program exists by which accurate assignments can be made, with the caveat that the program assumes no heterogeneity (Ott 1974).

The genetic counselor, especially one who is psychiatrically trained, has an opportunity to provide much important aid beyond estimating the risks of recurrence. This includes evaluating and helping the counselee, especially by reducing the amount of misinformation, confusion, guilt, and fear regarding the illness. The counselor also may be able to offer a plan with the potential for reducing or preventing the transmission of the illness but should recognize that counseling, although often successful in its educational goals, is unlikely to affect reproductive decisions (Kessler 1989). In doing this work, the counselor must combine the skills of geneticist, internist, psychiatrist, psychotherapist, marital counselor, and family therapist. Within psychiatry and in other fields, especially pediatrics, expertise and training programs have developed in this area, and such specialized training is a prerequisite for success in this task.

Toward the Future

The past 5 years have witnessed the discovery of specific gene abnormalities underlying or associated with some neuropsychiatric disorders (such as presenilin and apolipoprotein E4 in Alzheimer's disease), as well as the detection of replicated linkage results in many others. Building on these promising results and on advances in clinical, molecular, and statistical genetics, it is anticipated that the next 5 years will witness the realization of a least some of the goals of psychiatric genetics, including identification of specific susceptibility genes, clarification of the pathophysiological processes whereby these genes lead to symptoms, establishment of epigenetic factors that interact with these genes to produce disease, validation of nosological boundaries that more closely reflect the actions of these genes, and development of effective preventive and therapeutic interventions based on genetic counseling, gene therapy, and modification of permissive or protective environmental influences.

Gene Discovery

Although genetically "simple" mendelian disorders usually are associated with rare, disease-causing mutations in affected individuals, the genetically "complex" disorders, such as those in psychiatry, are likely associated with relatively common genetic variants, which enhance the likelihood of disease in affected individuals either by being more prevalent, by working in concert with common variants at other loci, or both.

The identification of common genetic variants that are neither necessary nor sufficient to produce disease requires different clinical resources than those that have been successfully used in the identification of rare disease mutations. Linkage analyses have to rely on very large samples (approaching several thousand affected subjects and/or affected sibling pairs); perforce this has led to increasing reliance on collaboration among research groups. Large, multisite collaborative studies are ongoing to collect large numbers of pedigrees affected with nearly all the disorders discussed in this chapter. There is recognition that significantly increased efficiency may be achieved by characterizing affected subjects by continuous, rather than categorical, phenotypes (Moldin et al. 1991); by selectively studying affected sibling pairs that are maximally discordant for the phenotype of interest (Risch and Zhang 1995); or by employing linkage disequilibrium strategies in genetically isolated and homogeneous populations (Risch and Merikangas 1996). Although relatively isolated populations, like that of Finland, have been a boon to the identification of genes underlying "simple" disorders (those with allele frequencies as large as 0.005) (Hastbacka et al. 1990), such populations still may have too many founders to assume that all individuals with a given "complex" disorder carry a specific, clonal disease-predisposing allele, a necessary condition for linkage disequilibrium to be detectable (Weiss 1995). It may be necessary to study even more extremely isolated populations, in which the present-day population can be thought of as one very large pedigree. In such a population, disease-predisposing alleles are likely to be clonal, and relatively few genetic and environmental factors may contribute to disease etiology.

Such studies will be facilitated by remarkable advances in molecular genetics and the Human Genome Project. As mentioned in the introduction to this chapter, a draft of the genome sequence has been produced (2001) and has given some insights into the nature of the genome. These insights have implications for the identification of disease-predisposing DNA sequence variations (Collins and McKusick 2001; Peltonen and McKusick 2001). Having a complete list of all the human genes and proteins provides thousands of new drug targets for the psychiatric diseases. One of the largest advances for gene discovery is the availability of multiple polymorphic genetic markers (principally SNPs) in every gene. This will allow genetic investigation of every gene for genetic association to a particular disorder, if necessary. Just as important, it will enable the construction of genomewide linkage disequilibrium maps that will outline the genealogy of chromosomal segments in human subpopulations and enable testing of a smaller number of SNPs to detect disease associations. Once the variation in the DNA sequences has been correlated with the phenotypic variations of psychiatric disorders, personality traits, and drug response, then individualized diagnosis, prevention, and treatment may be possible.

Pathophysiology

Progress in molecular genetics and computational genomics also should help elucidate the complex pathophysiological links between genotype and phenotype. Approaches such as microarrays and highly automated 2-D gel electrophoresis may reveal coordinated changes in expression between several cDNAs or proteins following drug treatment or in the disease state. Once disease-predisposing mutations are found, transgenic animal models not only serve to underscore a causal role for particular gene mutations but also should clarify the neuroanatomical, neurochemical, and neurophysiological concomitants of such mutations. These approaches should become increasingly tenable as we move from the gene mapping to the "complete genomics" era.

Epigenesis

Parallels between neuropsychiatric disorders and other medical conditions suggest potential mechanisms for gene-environment interactions and the methods by which such interactions might be elucidated. For example, schizophrenia bears many similarities to type 1 diabetes mellitus: both disorders are associated with a modest increase in risk to first-degree relatives (λ_s of 15), an intermediate concordance among MZ twins (approximately 50%), and a combined effect of several major susceptibility loci. Perhaps the most important of these loci for type 1 diabetes mellitus is the class II major histocompatibility complex (MHC) locus (Davies et al. 1994), governing, among other things, the host response to viral infection. Not surprisingly, infection by a common agent, *Coxsackievirus*, and molecular mimickry between viral and host antigens, has been implicated in the pathogenesis of type 1 diabetes mellitus (Solimena and De Camilli 1995). Insofar as several studies have suggested a role for both the class II MHC locus (Nimgaonkar et al. 1995) and viral infection (Kaufmann and Ziegler 1987) in schizophrenia, a similar mechanism may be involved (Wright et al. 1995). The availability of suitable cohorts of subjects with schizophrenia, such as those originally identified through the landmark Child Health and Development Study (1959–1966), who have been followed up since early in gestation, and on whom both subject DNA and maternal prenatal serum samples have been obtained, should permit questions of class II MHC variation and specific intrauterine viral exposure to be directly answered.

Nosology

As genetic variations underlying neuropsychiatric disorders are revealed, our notions of the boundaries between these disorders may need to be revised. With only linkage results in hand, we already have indications that disorders such as bipolar disorder and schizophrenia, once thought to be distinct, in fact overlap. Thus, some groups studying bipolar disorder have found linkage in the same region of chromosome 6 implicated in schizophrenia; conversely, other groups studying schizophrenia have found evidence for linkage in the same region of chromosome 18 implicated in bipolar disorder. In addition, as mentioned earlier in this chapter, many of the replicated findings for both disorders identify the same chromosomal regions. Likewise, linkage analyses of panic disorder have found positive lod scores in some of the same chromosomal regions, corroborating path analyses that suggest an overlap between mood and anxiety disorders. The possibility of a continuum between bipolar disorder and schizophrenia has been debated since the time of Kraepelin. Perhaps these disorders do lie on a continuum, or share some, but not all, of a set of epistatic loci. Regardless of how, we can be certain that the lines between diagnostic categories will need to be redrawn as their molecular bases become clear.

Prevention and Treatment

As the molecular mechanisms underlying neuropsychiatric disorders become clearer, points of potential clinical intervention also will become apparent. These may be divided into those involving primary, secondary, and tertiary prevention, referring to interventions that prevent disease, prevent its evolution, or prevent its complications, respectively. Among primary preventive interventions are genetic counseling and gene therapy. Preconceptional decision making will need to change, as genetic counseling takes stock of complex disorders for which risks are relative, susceptibilities are multiple, and outcomes are uncertain. Prospects for gene therapy of disorders that afflict the postmitotic brain, once thought impossible, now appear real. Highly selective, neurotropic, defective viral vectors (e.g., *adenoviruses* and *herpesviruses*) have emerged as likely agents for wild-type gene transfer into the nervous system (Kaplitt and Makimura 1997). The possibility that gene transfer into the central nervous system might be effective has gained support from the observation that certain "stemlike" neural cells retain their pleuripotentiality until late in development (Snyder et al. 1997). Among secondary preventive interventions are targeted environmental manipulations in at-risk subjects, that is, reductions in exposure to relevant epigenetic factors, be they viruses, nutritional deficiencies, or early losses, in individuals with particular genetic susceptibilities. Ironically, in this regard, the very complexities that vex the study of complex disorders bode well for their treatment. Finally, the long delay between in utero exposure and adult onset for many neuropsychiatric disorders provides a large window for tertiary preventive interventions. For example, pharmacological

studies of animal models of schizophrenia, such as those involving perinatal damage to the anterior hippocampus, suggest that early intervention with anticonvulsants may forestall the development of limbic dopaminergic supersensitivity (and presumably "positive" symptoms), whereas epidemiological studies of patients with schizophrenia suggest that early intervention, after the development of "positive" symptoms, with neuroleptic or electroconvulsive therapy may forestall the development of "negative" symptoms.

Progress in human genetics in general, and psychiatric genetics in particular, is occurring at an ever-increasing pace. No doubt, only some of the future developments that we have suggested will be borne out, and other, unimagined developments will occur. We need only consider the disparity between the depiction of the late twentieth century evident in early science fiction films and our current reality to know that prognostication is a clumsy art, at best. Nonetheless, we can be certain that the next few years will be enormously revealing and gratifying for psychiatric genetics.

References

Abbar M, Courtet P, Bellivier F, et al: Suicide attempts and the tryptophan hydroxylase gene. Mol Psychiatry 6:268–273, 2001

Alda M, Dvorakova M, Zvolsky P, et al: Genetic aspects in chronic schizophrenia: morbidity risks and contributory factors. Schizophr Res 2:339–344, 1989

Alexander RC, Heydt D, Ferraro TN, et al: Further evidence for a quantitative trait locus on murine chromosome 10 controlling morphine preference in inbred mice (letter). Psychiat Genet 6:29–31, 1996

Alexanderson B, Price-Evans DA, Sjoqvist F: Steady-state plasma levels of nortriptyline in twins: influence of genetic factors and drug therapy. BMJ 4:764, 1969

Amador XF, Malaspina D, Sackeim HA, et al: Visual fixation and smooth pursuit eye movement abnormalities in patients with schizophrenia and their relatives. J Neuropsychiatry Clin Neurosci 7:197–206, 1995

American Psychiatric Association: Diagnostic and Statistical Manual of Mental Disorders, 3rd Edition. Washington, DC, American Psychiatric Association, 1980

American Psychiatric Association: Diagnostic and Statistical Manual of Mental Disorders, 3rd Edition, Revised. Washington, DC, American Psychiatric Association, 1987

American Psychiatric Association: Diagnostic and Statistical Manual of Mental Disorders, 4th Edition, Text Revision. Washington, DC, American Psychiatric Association, 2000

Andreasen NC, Rice J, Endicott J, et al: Familial rates of affective disorder: a report from the National Institute of Mental Health Collaborative Study. Arch Gen Psychiatry 44:461–469, 1987

Antonarakis SE, Blouin JL, Pulver AE, et al: Schizophrenia susceptibility and chromosome 6p24–22. Nat Genet 11:235–236, 1995

Arolt V, Lencer R, Nolte A, et al: Eye tracking dysfunction is a putative phenotypic susceptibility marker of schizophrenia and maps to a locus on chromosome 6p in families with multiple occurrence of the disease. Am J Med Genet 67:564–579, 1996

Arolt V, Lencer R, Purmann S, et al: Testing for linkage of eye tracking dysfunction and schizophrenia to markers on chromosomes 6, 8, 9, 20, and 22 in families multiply affected with schizophrenia. Am J Med Genet 88:603–606, 1999

Arranz MJ, Munro J, Sham P, et al: Meta-analysis of studies on genetic variation in 5-HT2A receptors and clozapine response. Schizophr Res 32:93–99, 1998

Arranz MJ, Munro J, Birkett J, et al: Pharmacogenetic prediction of clozapine response. Lancet 355:1615–1616, 2000

Asherson P, Mant R, Holmans P, et al: Linkage, association and mutational analysis of the dopamine D3 receptor gene in schizophrenia. Mol Psychiatry 1:125–132, 1996

Bailer U, Leisch F, Meszaros K, et al: Genome scan for susceptibility loci for schizophrenia. Neuropsychobiology 42:175–182, 2000

Baron M: Genetics of schizophrenia and the new millennium: progress and pitfalls. Am J Hum Genet 68:299–312, 2001

Baron M: Manic-depression genes and the new millennium: poised for discovery. Mol Psychiatry 7:342–358, 2002

Baron M, Gruen RS: Schizophrenia and affective disorder: are they genetically linked? Br J Psychiatry 159:267–270, 1991

Baron M, Risch N, Hamburger R, et al: Genetic linkage between X chromosome markers and bipolar affective illness. Nature 326:289–292, 1987

Baron M, Freimer NF, Risch N, et al: Diminished support for linkage between manic depressive illness and X-chromosome markers in three Israeli pedigrees. Nat Genet 3:49–55, 1993

Barr CL, Sandor P: Current status of genetic studies of Gilles de la Tourette syndrome. Can J Psychiatry 43:351–357, 1998

Battaglia M, Bernardeschi L, Franchini L, et al: A family study of schizotypal disorder. Schizophr Bull 21:33–45, 1995

Beatty B, Squires J, Weksberg R, et al: Velocardiofacial syndrome and schizophrenia. Am J Hum Genet Suppl 59:A87, 1996

Bengel D, Greenberg BD, Cora-Locatelli G, et al: Association of the serotonin transporter promoter regulatory region polymorphism and obsessive-compulsive disorder. Mol Psychiatry 4:463–466, 1999

Benjamin J, Li L, Patterson C, et al: Population and familial association between the D4 dopamine receptor gene and measures of novelty seeking. Nat Genet 12:81–84, 1996

Bergem AL, Engedal K, Kringlen E: The role of heredity in late-onset Alzheimer disease and vascular dementia: a twin study. Arch Gen Psychiatry 54:264–270, 1997

Bergen AW, Kokoszka J, Peterson R, et al: Mu opioid receptor gene variants: lack of association with alcohol dependence. Mol Psychiatry 2:490–494, 1997

Berrettini WH, Ferraro TN, Goldin LR, et al: Chromosome 18 DNA markers and manic-depressive illness: evidence for a susceptibility gene. Proc Natl Acad Sci U S A 91:5918–5921, 1994a

Berrettini WH, Ferraro TN, Alexander RC, et al: Quantitative trait loci mapping of three loci controlling morphine preference using inbred mouse strains. Nat Genet 7:54–58, 1994b

Bersani G, Taddei I, Venturi P, et al: Familial occurrence and obstetric complications in siblings discordant for schizophrenia. Minerva Psichiatrica 36:127–132, 1995

Bertelsen A, Harvald B, Hauge M: A Danish twin study of manic-depressive disorders. Br J Psychiatry 130:330–351, 1977

Bertram L, Blacker D, Mullin K, et al: Evidence for genetic linkage of Alzheimer's disease to chromosome 10q. Science 290:2302–2303, 2000

Biederman J, Faraone SV, Hirshfeld-Becker DR, et al: Patterns of psychopathology and dysfunction in high-risk children of parents with panic disorder and major depression. Am J Psychiatry 158:49–57, 2001

Bierut LJ, Dinwiddie SH, Begleiter H, et al: Familial transmission of substance dependence: alcohol, marijuana, cocaine, and habitual smoking: a report from the Collaborative Study on the Genetics of Alcoholism. Arch Gen Psychiatry 55:982–988, 1998

Bierut LJ, Heath AC, Bucholz KK, et al: Major depressive disorder in a community-based twin sample: are there different genetic and environmental contributions for men and women? Arch Gen Psychiatry 56:557–563, 1999

Billett EA, Richter MA, King N, et al: Obsessive compulsive disorder, response to serotonin reuptake inhibitors and the serotonin transporter gene. Mol Psychiatry 2:403–406, 1997

Biomed European Bipolar Collaborative Group: No association between bipolar disorder and alleles at a functional polymorphism in the COMT gene. Br J Psychiatry 170:526–528, 1997

Black DW, Noyes R Jr, Goldstein RB, et al: A family study of obsessive-compulsive disorder. Arch Gen Psychiatry 49:362–368, 1992

Blackwood DH, He L, Morris SW, et al: A locus for bipolar affective disorder on chromosome 4p. Nat Genet 12:427–430, 1996

Blackwood DH, Fordyce A, Walker MT, et al: Schizophrenia and affective disorders: cosegregation with a translocation at chromosome 1q42 that directly disrupts brain-expressed genes: clinical and P300 findings in a family. Am J Hum Genet 69:428–433, 2001

Bland RC, Newman SC, Orn H: Recurrent and nonrecurrent depression: a family study. Arch Gen Psychiatry 43:1085–1089. 1986

Blouin JL, Dombroski BA, Nath SK, et al: Schizophrenia susceptibility loci on chromosomes 13q32 and 8p21. Nat Genet 20:70–73, 1998

Blum K, Noble EP, Sheridan PJ, et al: Allelic association of human dopamine D2 receptor gene in alcoholism. JAMA 263:2055–2060, 1990

Bohman M, Sigvardsson S, Cloninger CR: Maternal inheritance of alcohol abuse: cross-fostering analysis of adopted women. Arch Gen Psychiatry 38:965–969, 1981

Bohman M, Cloninger CR, Sigvardsson S, et al: Predisposition to petty criminality in Swedish adoptees, I: genetic and environmental heterogeneity. Arch Gen Psychiatry 39:1233–1241, 1982

Bohman M, Sigvardsson S, Cloninger R, et al: Alcoholism: lessons from population, family and adoption studies. Alcohol Alcohol Suppl 1:55–60, 1987

Bolos AM, Dean M, Lucas-Derse S, et al: Population and pedigree studies reveal a lack of association between the dopamine D2 receptor gene and alcoholism. JAMA 264:3156–3160, 1990

Bondy B, Erfurth A, de Jonge S, et al: Possible association of the short allele of the serotonin transporter promoter gene polymorphism (5-HTTLPR) with violent suicide. Mol Psychiatry 5:193–195, 2000

Böök JA: A genetic neuropsychiatric investigation of a North Swedish population. Acta Genetica Medica Statistica 4:1–100, 1953

Bracha HS, Torrey EF, Gottesman II, et al: Second-trimester markers of fetal size in schizophrenia: a study of monozygotic twins. Am J Psychiatry 149:1355–1361, 1992

Breitner JCS, Murphey EA, Folstein MF: Familial aggregation of Alzheimer dementia, II: clinical genetic implications of age dependent onset. J Psychiatr Res 20:45–55, 1986

Breitner JCS, Welsh KA, Gau BA, et al: Alzheimer's disease in the National Academy of Sciences—National Research Council Registry of Aging Twin Veterans, III: detection of cases, longitudinal results, and observations on twin concordance. Arch Neurol 52:763–771, 1995

Brent DA, Bridge J, Johnson BA, et al: Suicidal behavior runs in families: a controlled family study of adolescent suicide victims. Arch Gen Psychiatry 53:1145–1152, 1996

Broman KW, Murray JC, Sheffield VC, et al: Comprehensive human genetic maps: individual and sex-specific variation in recombination. Am J Hum Genet 63:861–869, 1998

Brunner HG, Nelen M, Breakefield XO, et al: Abnormal behavior associated with a point mutation in the structural gene for monoamine oxidase A. Science 262:578–580, 1993a

Brunner HG, Nelen MR, van Zandvoort P, et al: X-linked borderline mental retardation with prominent behavioral disturbance: phenotype, genetic localization, and evidence for disturbed monoamine metabolism. Am J Hum Genet 52:1032–1039, 1993b

Brzustowicz LM, Honer WG, Chow EW, et al: Use of a quantitative trait to map a locus associated with severity of positive symptoms in familial schizophrenia to chromosome 6p. Am J Hum Genet 61:1388–1396, 1997

Brzustowicz LM, Honer WG, Chow EW, et al: Linkage of familial schizophrenia to chromosome 13q32. Am J Hum Genet 65:1096–1103, 1999

Brzustowicz LM, Hodgkinson KA, Chow EW, et al: Location of a major susceptibility locus for familial schizophrenia on chromosome 1q21-q22. Science 288:678–682, 2000

Bulik CM, Sullivan PF, Wade TD, et al: Twin studies of eating disorders: a review. Int J Eat Disord 27:1–20, 2000

Burgoyne PS: Genetic homology and crossing-over in the X and Y chromosomes of mammals. Hum Genet 61:85–90, 1982

Byerley W, Holik J, Hoff M, et al: Search for a gene predisposing to manic-depression on chromosome 21. Am J Med Genet 60:231–233, 1995

Cadoret RJ: Evidence for genetic inheritance of primary affective disorder in adoptees. Am J Psychiatry 135:463–466, 1978

Cadoret RJ, Cain CA, Grove WM: Development of alcoholism in adoptees raised apart from alcoholic biologic relatives. Arch Gen Psychiatry 37:561–563, 1980

Cadoret RJ, O'Gorman TW, Troughton E, et al: Alcoholism and antisocial personality: interrelationships, genetic and environmental factors. Arch Gen Psychiatry 42:161–167, 1985

Cadoret RJ, Yates WR, Troughton E, et al: Genetic–environmental interaction in the genesis of aggressivity and conduct disorders. Arch Gen Psychiatry 52:916–924, 1995

Caldirola D, Perna G, Arancio C, et al: The 35% CO_2 challenge test in patients with social phobia. Psychiatry Res 71:41–48, 1997

Campbell DA, Sundaramurthy D, Markham AF, et al: Lack of association between 5-HT2A gene promoter polymorphism and susceptibility to anorexia nervosa (letter). Lancet 351:499, 1998

Campbell DA, Sundaramurthy D, Gordon D, et al: Association between a marker in the UCP-2/UCP-3 gene cluster and genetic susceptibility to anorexia nervosa. Mol Psychiatry 4:68–70, 1999

Cannon TD, Mednick SA, Parnas J: Antecedents of predominantly negative- and predominantly positive-symptom schizophrenia in a high-risk population. Arch Gen Psychiatry 47:622–632, 1990

Cannon TD, Mednick SA, Parnas J, et al: Developmental brain abnormalities in the offspring of schizophrenic mothers, II: structural brain characteristics of schizophrenia and schizotypal personality disorder. Arch Gen Psychiatry 51:955–962, 1994

Cannon TD, Kaprio J, Lonnqvist J, et al: The genetic epidemiology of schizophrenia in a Finnish twin cohort: a population-based modeling study. Arch Gen Psychiatry 55:67–74, 1998

Cao Q, Martinez M, Zhang J, et al: Suggestive evidence for a schizophrenia susceptibility locus on chromosome 6q and a confirmation in an independent series of pedigrees. Genomics 43:1–8, 1997

Cardno AG, Gottesman II: Twin studies of schizophrenia: from bow-and-arrow concordances to Star Wars Mx and functional genomics. Am J Med Genet 97:12–17, 2000

Carey G, Gottesman II: Twin and family studies of anxiety, phobic, and obsessive disorders, in Anxiety: New Research and Changing Concepts. Edited by Klein DF, Rabkin J. New York, Raven, 1981, pp 117–136

Cases O, Seif I, Grimsby J, et al: Aggressive behavior and altered amounts of brain serotonin and norepinephrine in mice lacking MAOA. Science 268:1763–1766, 1995

Cavallini MC, Pasquale L, Bellodi L, et al: Complex segregation analysis for obsessive compulsive disorder and related disorders. Am J Med Genet 88:38–43, 1999a

Cavallini MC, Perna G, Caldirola D, et al: A segregation study of panic disorder in families of panic patients responsive to the 35% CO2 challenge. Biol Psychiatry 46:815–820, 1999b

Cavallini MC, Bertelli S, Chiapparino D, et al: Complex segregation analysis of obsessive-compulsive disorder in 141 families of eating disorder probands, with and without obsessive-compulsive disorder. Am J Med Genet 96:384–391, 2000

Chaleby K, Tuma TA: Cousin marriages and schizophrenia in Saudi Arabia. Br J Psychiatry 150:547–549, 1987

Chen CH, Chien SH, Hwu HG: Lack of association between TaqI A1 allele of dopamine D2 receptor gene and alcohol-use disorders in Atayal natives of Taiwan. Am J Med Genet 67:488–490, 1996

Chen CH, Liu MY, Wei FC, et al: Further evidence of no association between Ser9Gly polymorphism of dopamine D3 receptor gene and schizophrenia. Am J Med Genet 74:40–43, 1997

Cichon S, Schmidt-Wolf G, Schumacher J, et al: A possible susceptibility locus for bipolar affective disorder in chromosomal region 10q25–q26. Mol Psychiatry 6:342–349, 2001

Clementz BA, Sweeney JA, Hirt M, et al: Pursuit gain and saccadic intrusions in first-degree relatives of probands with schizophrenia. J Abnorm Psychol 99:327–335, 1990

Clementz BA, Grove WM, Iacono WG, et al: Smooth-pursuit eye movement dysfunction and liability for schizophrenia: implications for genetic modeling. J Abnorm Psychol 101:117–129, 1992

Clementz BA, Geyer MA, Braff DL: Poor P50 suppression among schizophrenia patients and their first-degree biological relatives. Am J Psychiatry 155:1691–1694, 1998

Cloninger CR: A unified biosocial theory of personality and its role in the development of anxiety states. Psychiatric Developments 4:167–226, 1986

Cloninger CR: A systematic method for clinical description and classification of personality variants: a proposal. Arch Gen Psychiatry 44:573–588, 1987

Cloninger CR, Gottesman II: Genetic and environmental factors in antisocial behavior disorders, in The Causes of Crime: New Biological Approaches. Edited by Mednick SA, Moffitt TE, Stack SA. New York, Cambridge University Press, 1987, pp 92–109

Cloninger CR, Reich T, Guze SB: The multifactorial model of disease transmission, III: familial relationship between sociopathy and hysteria (Briquet's syndrome). Br J Psychiatry 127:23–32, 1975

Cloninger CR, Bohman M, Sigvardsson S: Inheritance of alcohol abuse: cross-fostering analysis of adopted men. Arch Gen Psychiatry 38:861–868, 1981

Cloninger CR, Sigvardsson S, von Knorring A-L, et al: An adoption study of somatoform disorders, II: identification of two discrete somatoform disorders. Arch Gen Psychiatry 41:863–871, 1984

Cloninger CR, Martin RL, Guze SB, et al: A prospective follow-up and family study of somatization in men and women. Am J Psychiatry 143:873–878, 1986

Cloninger CR, Svrakic DM, Przybeck TR: A psychobiological model of temperament and character. Arch Gen Psychiatry 50:975–990, 1993

Cloninger CR, Van Eerdewegh P, Goate A, et al: Anxiety proneness linked to epistatic loci in genome scan of human personality traits. Am J Med Genet 81:313–317, 1998

Collier DA, Arranz MJ, Li T, et al: Association between 5-HT2A gene promoter polymorphism and anorexia nervosa (letter). Lancet 350:412, 1997

Collins FS, McKusick VA: Implications of the Human Genome Project for medical science. JAMA 285:540–544, 2001

Comings DE, Muhleman D, Gysin R: Dopamine D2 receptor (DRD2) gene and susceptibility to posttraumatic stress disorder: a study and replication. Biol Psychiatry 40:368–372, 1996

Cook CC, Palsson G, Turner A, et al: A genetic linkage study of the D2 dopamine receptor locus in heavy drinking and alcoholism. Br J Psychiatry 169:243–248, 1996

Cook RH, Schneck SA, Clark DB: Twins with Alzheimer's disease. Arch Neurol 38:300–301, 1981

Coon H, Jensen S, Holik J, et al: Genomic scan for genes predisposing to schizophrenia. Am J Med Genet 54:59–71, 1994

Coon H, Hoff M, Holik J, et al: Analysis of chromosome 18 DNA markers in multiplex pedigrees with manic depression. Biol Psychiatry 39:689–696, 1996

Coryell W: Hypersensitivity to carbon dioxide as a disease-specific trait marker. Biol Psychiatry 41:259–263, 1997

Coryell W, Zimmerman M: The heritability of schizophrenia and schizoaffective disorder: a family study. Arch Gen Psychiatry 45:323–327, 1988

Couch FJ, Weber BL: Mutations and polymorphisms in the familial early onset breast cancer (BRCA1) gene; Breast Cancer Information Core. Hum Mutat 8:8–18, 1996

Courtet P, Baud P, Abbar M, et al: Association between violent suicidal behavior and the low activity allele of the serotonin transporter gene. Mol Psychiatry 6:338–341, 2001

Cox NJ, Suarez BK: Linkage analysis for psychiatric disorders, II: methodological considerations. Psychiatric Developments 3:369–382, 1985

Craddock N, McGuffin P, Owen M: Darier's disease cosegregating with affective disorder (letter; comment). Br J Psychiatry 165:272, 1994

Crawford F, Hoyne J, Diaz P, et al: Occurrence of the Cys311 DRD2 variant in a pedigree multiply affected with panic disorder. Am J Med Genet 60:332–334, 1995

Crocq M-A, Mant R, Asherson P, et al: Association between schizophrenia and homozygosity at the dopamine D3 receptor gene. J Med Genet 29:858–860, 1992

Crow TJ, DeLisi LE, Johnstone EC: Concordance by sex in sibling pairs with schizophrenia is paternally inherited: evidence for a pseudoautosomal locus. Br J Psychiatry 155:92–97, 1989

Crowe RR, Pauls DL, Slymen DJ, et al: A family study of anxiety neurosis: morbidity risk in families of patients with and without mitral valve prolapse. Arch Gen Psychiatry 37:77–79, 1980

Crowe RR, Noyes R, Pauls DL, et al: A family study of panic disorder. Arch Gen Psychiatry 40:1065–1069, 1983

Crowe RR, Noyes R Jr, Persico AM: Pro-opiomelanocortin (POMC) gene excluded as a cause of panic disorder in a large family. J Affect Disord 12:23–27, 1987

Crowe RR, Goedken R, Samuelson S, et al: Genomewide survey of panic disorder. Am J Med Genet 105:105–109, 2001

Curtis CE, Calkins ME, Grove WM, et al: Saccadic disinhibition in patients with acute and remitted schizophrenia and their first-degree biological relatives. Am J Psychiatry 158:100–106, 2001

David F, Clerget F, Lucote G: Familial Alzheimer's disease (FAD): cosegregation between alleles at the D21S11 DNA marker and the FAD gene in a particular pedigree. J Neurol 235:485–486, 1988

Davidson J, Smith R, Kudler H: Familial psychiatric illness in chronic posttraumatic stress disorder. Compr Psychiatry 30:339–345, 1989

Davidson JR, Tupler LA, Wilson WH, et al: A family study of chronic post-traumatic stress disorder following rape trauma. J Psychiatr Res 32:301–309, 1998

Davies JL, Kawaguchi Y, Bennett ST, et al: A genome-wide search for human type 1 diabetes susceptibility genes. Nature 371:130–136, 1994

Davis JO, Phelps JA, Bracha HS: Prenatal development of monozygotic twins and concordance for schizophrenia. Schizophr Bull 21:357–366, 1995

Daw EW, Heath SC, Wijsman EM: Multipoint oligogenic analysis of age-at-onset data with applications to Alzheimer disease pedigrees. Am J Hum Genet 64:839–851, 1999

Dawson E, Parfitt E, Roberts Q, et al: Linkage studies of bipolar disorder in the region of the Darier's disease gene on chromosome 12q23-24.1. Am J Med Genet 60:94–102, 1995b

De Bruyn A, Souery D, Mendelbaum K, et al: Linkage analysis of families with bipolar illness and chromosome 18 markers. Biol Psychiatry 39:679–688, 1996

Decina P, Mukherjee S, Lucas L, et al: Patterns of illness in parent-child pairs both hospitalized for either schizophrenia or a major mood disorder. Psychiatry Res 39:81–87, 1991

Deckert J, Catalano M, Heils A, et al: Functional promoter polymorphism of the human serotonin transporter: lack of association with panic disorder. Psychiatr Genet 7:45–47, 1997

Deckert J, Nothen MM, Franke P, et al: Systematic mutation screening and association study of the A1 and A2a adenosine receptor genes in panic disorder suggest a contribution of the A2a gene to the development of disease. Mol Psychiatry 3:81–85, 1998

Deckert J, Catalano M, Syagailo YV, et al: Excess of high activity monoamine oxidase A gene promoter alleles in female patients with panic disorder. Hum Mol Genet 8:621–624, 1999

DeKosky ST, Aston CE, Kamboh MI: Polygenic determinants of Alzheimer's disease: modulation of the risk by alpha-1-antichymotrypsin. Ann N Y Acad Sci 802:27–34, 1996

DeLisi LE, Crow TJ: Evidence for a sex chromosome locus for schizophrenia. Schizophr Bull 15:431–440, 1989

Detera-Wadleigh SD, Badner JA, Goldin LR, et al: Affected-sib-pair analyses reveal support of prior evidence for a susceptibility locus for bipolar disorder, on 21q. Am J Hum Genet 58:1279–1285, 1996

Detera-Wadleigh SD, Badner JA, Berrettini WH, et al: A high-density genome scan detects evidence for a bipolar-disorder susceptibility locus on 13q32 and other potential loci on 1q32 and 18p11.2. Proc Natl Acad Sci U S A 96:5604–5609, 1999

Di Bella DD, Catalano M, Cavallini MC, et al: Serotonin transporter linked polymorphic region in anorexia nervosa and bulimia nervosa. Mol Psychiatry 5:233–234, 2000

Dow DJ, Lindsey N, Cairns NJ, et al: Alpha-2 macroglobulin polymorphism and Alzheimer disease risk in the UK. Nat Genet 22:16–17, 1999

Dror V, Shamir E, Ghanshani S, et al: hKCa3/KCNN3 potassium channel gene: association of longer CAG repeats with schizophrenia in Israeli Ashkenazi Jews, expression in human tissues and localization to chromosome 1q21. Mol Psychiatry 4:254–260, 1999

Du L, Faludi G, Palkovits M, et al: Frequency of long allele in serotonin transporter gene is increased in depressed suicide victims. Biol Psychiatry 46:196–201, 1999

Du L, Bakish D, Hrdina PD: Gender differences in association between serotonin transporter gene polymorphism and personality traits. Psychiatr Genet 10:159–164, 2000

Dworkin RH, Lenzenweger MF, Moldin SO, et al: A multidimensional approach to the genetics of schizophrenia. Am J Psychiatry 145:1077–1083, 1988

Dykes KL, Mednick SA, Machon RA, et al: Adult third ventricle width and infant behavioral arousal in groups at high and low risk for schizophrenia. Schizophr Res 7:13–18, 1992

Ebers GC, Kukay K, Bulman DE, et al: A full genome search in multiple sclerosis. Nat Genet 13:472–476, 1996

Ebstein RP, Novick O, Umansky R, et al: Dopamine D4 receptor (D4DR) exon III polymorphism associated with the human personality trait of novelty seeking. Nat Genet 12:78–80, 1996

Ebstein RP, Macciardi F, Heresco-Levi U, et al: Evidence for an association between the dopamine D3 receptor gene DRD3 and schizophrenia. Hum Hered 47:6–16, 1997a

Ebstein RP, Gritsenko I, Nemanov L, et al: No association between the serotonin transporter gene regulatory region polymorphism and the Tridimensional Personality Questionnaire (TPQ) temperament of harm avoidance. Mol Psychiatry 2:224–226, 1997b

Edenberg HJ, Foroud T, Koller DL, et al: A family based analysis of the association of the dopamine D2 receptor (DRD2) with alcoholism. Alcohol Clin Exp Res 22:505–512, 1998

Egan MF, Goldberg TE, Kolachana BS, et al: Effect of COMT Val108/158 Met genotype on frontal lobe function and risk for schizophrenia. Proc Natl Acad Sci U S A 98:6917–6922, 2001

Egeland JA, Sussex JN: Suicide and family loading for affective disorders. JAMA 254:915–918, 1985

Egeland JA, Gerhard DS, Pauls DL, et al: Bipolar affective disorders linked to DNA markers on chromosome 11. Nature 325:783–787, 1987

Eichhammer P, Albus M, Borrmann-Hassenbach M, et al: Association of dopamine D3-receptor gene variants with neuroleptic induced akathisia in schizophrenic patients: a generalization of Steen's study on DRD3 and tardive dyskinesia. Am J Med Genet 96:187–191, 2000

Ekelund J, Hovatta I, Parker A, et al: Chromosome 1 loci in Finnish schizophrenia families. Hum Mol Genet 10:1611–1617, 2001

Embry C, Bruyland S: Presumed Alzheimer's disease beginning at different ages in two twins. J Am Geriatr Soc 33:61–62, 1985

Enoch MA, Goldman D: The genetics of alcoholism and alcohol abuse. Current Psychiatry Reports 3:144–151, 2001

Enoch MA, Kaye WH, Rotondo A, et al: 5-HT2A promoter polymorphism-1438G/A, anorexia nervosa, and obsessive-compulsive disorder. Lancet 351:1785–1786, 1998

Erlenmeyer-Kimling LE, Paradowski W: Selection and schizophrenia. American Naturalist 100:651–665, 1966

Ertekin-Taner N, Graff-Radford N, Younkin LH, et al: Linkage of plasma Abeta42 to a quantitative locus on chromosome 10 in late-onset Alzheimer's disease pedigrees. Science 290:2303–2304, 2000

Esler WP, Wolfe MS: A portrait of Alzheimer secretases—new features and familiar faces. Science 293:1449–1454, 2001

Ewald H, Degn B, Mors O, et al: Significant linkage between bipolar affective disorder and chromosome 12q24. Psychiatr Genet 8:131–140, 1998a

Ewald H, Degn B, Mors O, et al: Support for the possible locus on chromosome 4p16 for bipolar affective disorder. Mol Psychiatry 3:442–448, 1998b

Eysenck HJ: A Model for Personality. New York, Springer, 1981

Fairburn CG, Cowen PJ, Harrison PJ: Twin studies and the etiology of eating disorders. Int J Eat Disord 26:349–358, 1999

Faraone SV, Matise T, Svrakic D, et al: Genome scan of European-American schizophrenia pedigrees: results of the NIMH Genetics Initiative and Millennium Consortium. Am J Med Genet 81:290–295, 1998

Farmer AE, McGuffin P, Gottesman II: Twin concordance for DSM-III schizophrenia: scrutinizing the validity of the definition. Arch Gen Psychiatry 44:634–641, 1987

Farrer LA, O'Sullivan DM, Cupples A, et al: Assessment of genetic risk for Alzheimer's disease among first-degree relatives. Ann Neurol 25:485–493, 1989

Fischer M: Psychoses in the offspring of schizophrenic monozygotic twins and their normal co-twins. Br J Psychiatry 118:43–52, 1971

Fish B: Neurobiologic antecedents of schizophrenia in children: evidence for an inherited, congenital neurointegrative defect. Arch Gen Psychiatry 34:1297–1313, 1977

Fish B: Infant predictors of the longitudinal course of schizophrenic development. Schizophr Bull 13:395–409, 1987

Fish B, Marcus J, Hans SL, et al: Infants at risk for schizophrenia: sequelae of a genetic neurointegrative defect; a review and replication analysis of pandysmaturation in the Jerusalem Infant Development Study. Arch Gen Psychiatry 49:221–235, 1992

Foroud T, Castelluccio PF, Koller DL, et al: Suggestive evidence of a locus on chromosome 10p using the NIMH Genetics Initiative bipolar affective disorder pedigrees. Am J Med Genet 96:18–23, 2000

Franchini L, Serretti A, Gasperini M, et al: Familial concordance of fluvoxamine response as a tool for differentiating mood disorder pedigrees. J Psychiatr Res 32:255–259, 1998

Franke P, Maier W, Hain C, et al: Wisconsin Card Sorting Test: an indicator of vulnerability to schizophrenia? Schizophr Res 6:243–249, 1992

Freedman R, Coon H, Myles-Worsley M, et al: Linkage of a neurophysiological deficit in schizophrenia to a chromosome 15 locus. Proc Natl Acad Sci U S A 94:587–592, 1997

Freedman R, Leonard S, Gault JM, et al: Linkage disequilibrium for schizophrenia at the chromosome 15q13–14 locus of the alpha7-nicotinic acetylcholine receptor subunit gene (CHRNA7). Am J Med Genet 105:20–22, 2001

Freimer NB, Reus VI, Escamilla M, et al: An approach to investigating linkage for bipolar disorder using large Costa Rican pedigrees. Am J Med Genet 67:254–263, 1996

Frisch A, Michaelovsky E, Rockah R, et al: Association between obsessive-compulsive disorder and polymorphisms of genes encoding components of the serotonergic and dopaminergic pathways. Eur Neuropsychopharmacol 10:205–209, 2000

Frisch A, Laufer N, Danziger Y, et al: Association of anorexia nervosa with the high activity allele of the COMT gene: a family based study in Israeli patients. Mol Psychiatry 6:243–245, 2001

Furlong RA, Ho L, Walsh C, et al: Analysis and meta-analysis of two serotonin transporter gene polymorphisms in bipolar and unipolar affective disorders. Am J Med Genet 81:58–63, 1998a

Furlong RA, Coleman TA, Ho L, et al: No association of a functional polymorphism in the dopamine D2 receptor promoter region with bipolar or unipolar affective disorders. Am J Med Genet 81:385–387, 1998b

Furlong RA, Ho L, Rubinsztein JS, et al: No association of the tryptophan hydroxylase gene with bipolar affective disorder, unipolar affective disorder, or suicidal behaviour in major affective disorder. Am J Med Genet 81:245–247, 1998c

Furlong RA, Ho L, Rubinsztein JS, et al: Analysis of the monoamine oxidase A (MAOA) gene in bipolar affective disorder by association studies, meta-analyses, and sequencing of the promoter. Am J Med Genet 88:398–406, 1999a

Furlong RA, Rubinsztein JS, Ho L, et al: Analysis and metaanalysis of two polymorphisms within the tyrosine hydroxylase gene in bipolar and unipolar affective disorders. Am J Med Genet 88:88–94, 1999b

Fyer AJ, Mannuzza S, Gallops MS, et al: Familial transmission of simple phobias and fears: a preliminary report. Arch Gen Psychiatry 47:252–256, 1990

Fyer AJ, Mannuzza S, Chapman TF, et al: A direct interview family study of social phobia. Arch Gen Psychiatry 50:286–293, 1993

Fyer AJ, Mannuzza S, Chapman TF, et al: Specificity in familial aggregation of phobic disorders. Arch Gen Psychiatry 52:564–573, 1995

Garner C, Kelly M, Cardon L, et al: Linkage analyses of schizophrenia to chromosome 6p24-p22: an attempt to replicate. Am J Med Genet 67:595–610, 1996

Geijer T, Frisch A, Persson ML, et al: Search for association between suicide attempt and serotonergic polymorphisms. Psychiatr Genet 10:19–26, 2000

Gelernter J, O'Malley S, Risch N, et al: No association between an allele at the D2 dopamine receptor gene (DRD2) and alcoholism. JAMA 266:1801–1807, 1991

Gelernter J, Goldman D, Risch N: The A1 allele at the D2 dopamine receptor gene and alcoholism: a reappraisal. JAMA 269:1673–1677, 1993

Gelernter J, Kranzler H, Cubells J: Genetics of two mu opioid receptor gene (OPRM1) exon I polymorphisms: population studies, and allele frequencies in alcohol- and drug-dependent subjects. Mol Psychiatry 4:476–483, 1999a

Gelernter J, Southwick S, Goodson S, et al: No association between D2 dopamine receptor (DRD2) "A" system alleles, or DRD2 haplotypes, and posttraumatic stress disorder. Biol Psychiatry 45:620–625, 1999b

Gelernter J, Bonvicini K, Page G, et al: Linkage genome scan for loci predisposing to panic disorder or agoraphobia. Am J Med Genet 105:548–557, 2001

Gershon ES, Schreiber JL, Hamovit JR, et al: Clinical findings in patients with anorexia nervosa and affective illness in their relatives. Am J Psychiatry 141:1419–1422, 1984

Gershon ES, Hamovit JH, Guroff JJ, et al: Birth-cohort changes in manic and depressive disorders in relatives of bipolar and schizoaffective patients. Arch Gen Psychiatry 44:314–319, 1987

Gershon ES, DeLisi LE, Hamovit J, et al: A controlled family study of chronic psychoses: schizophrenia and schizoaffective disorder. Arch Gen Psychiatry 45:328–336, 1988

Gershon ES, Badner JA, Detera-Wadleigh SD, et al: Maternal inheritance and chromosome 18 allele sharing in unilineal bipolar illness pedigrees. Am J Med Genet 67:202–207, 1996

Giles DE, Biggs MM, Rush AJ, et al: Risk factors in families of unipolar depression, I: psychiatric illness and reduced REM latency. J Affect Disord 14:51–59, 1988

Gilfix BM, Briones L: Absence of the A1252G mutation in alpha 1-antichymotrypsin in a North American population suffering from dementia. J Cereb Blood Flow Metab 17:233–235, 1997

Gill M, Castle D, Hunt N, et al: Tyrosine hydroxylase polymorphisms and bipolar affective disorder. J Psychiatr Res 25:179–184, 1991

Gill M, Vallada H, Collier D, et al: A combined analysis of D22S278 marker alleles in affected sib-pairs: support for a susceptibility locus for schizophrenia at chromosome 22q12; Schizophrenia Collaborative Linkage Group (Chromosome 22). Am J Med Genet 67:40–45, 1996

Ginns EI, Ott J, Egeland JA, et al: A genome-wide search for chromosomal loci linked to bipolar affective disorder in the Old Order Amish. Nat Genet 12:431–435, 1996

Ginns EI, St Jean P, Philibert RA, et al: A genome-wide search for chromosomal loci linked to mental health wellness in relatives at high risk for bipolar affective disorder among the Old Order Amish. Proc Natl Acad Sci U S A 95:15531–15536, 1998

Goate AM, Haynes AR, Owen MJ, et al: Predisposing locus for AD on chromosome 21. Lancet 1:352–355, 1989

Goate AM, Chartier-Harlin MC, Mullan M, et al: Segregation of a missense mutation in the amyloid precursor protein gene with familial Alzheimer's disease. Nature 349:704–706, 1991

Goisman RM, Goldenberg I, Vasile RG, et al: Comorbidity of anxiety disorders in a multicenter anxiety study. Compr Psychiatry 36:303–311, 1995

Goldenberg IM, White K, Yonkers K, et al: The infrequency of "pure culture" diagnoses among the anxiety disorders. J Clin Psychiatry 57:528–533, 1996

Goldin LR, Gershon ES: Power of the affected-sib-pair method for heterogeneous disorders. Genet Epidemiol 5:35–42, 1988

Goodwin DW: Alcoholism and heredity: a review and hypothesis. Arch Gen Psychiatry 36:57–61, 1979

Gottesman II, Bertelsen A: Confirming unexpressed genotypes for schizophrenia: risks in the offspring of Fischer's Danish identical and fraternal discordant twins. Arch Gen Psychiatry 46:867–872, 1989

Gottesman II, Shields J: Schizophrenia and Genetics: A Twin Vantage Point. New York, Academic Press, 1972

Gottesman II, Shields J: Schizophrenia: The Epigenetic Puzzle. Cambridge, England, Cambridge University Press, 1982

Gratacos M, Nadal M, Martin-Santos R, et al: A polymorphic genomic duplication on human chromosome 15 is a susceptibility factor for panic and phobic disorders. Cell 106:367–379, 2001

Greenberg BD, Li Q, Lucas FR, et al: Association between the serotonin transporter promoter polymorphism and personality traits in a primarily female population sample. Am J Med Genet 96:202–216, 2000

Gurling HM: New microsatellite polymorphisms fail to confirm chromosome 5 linkage in Icelandic and British schizophrenia families. Paper presented at the American Psychopathological Association Meeting, New York, March 1992

Gurling H, Smyth C, Kalsi G, et al: Linkage findings in bipolar disorder. Nat Genet 10:8–9, 1995a

Gurling H, Kalsi G, Hui-Sui Chen A, et al: Schizophrenia susceptibility and chromosome 6p24-22. Nat Genet 11:234–235, 1995b

Gurling HM, Kalsi G, Brynjolfson J, et al: Genomewide genetic linkage analysis confirms the presence of susceptibility loci for schizophrenia, on chromosomes 1q32.2, 5q33.2, and 8p21-22 and provides support for linkage to schizophrenia, on chromosomes 11q23.3-24 and 20q12.1-11.23. Am J Hum Genet 68:661–673, 2001

Gusella JF, Wexler NS, Conneally PM, et al: A polymorphic DNA marker genetically linked to Huntington's disease. Nature 306:234–238, 1983

Gustavsson JP, Nothen MM, Jonsson EG, et al: No association between serotonin transporter gene polymorphisms and personality traits. Am J Med Genet 88:430–436, 1999

Guze SB: The role of follow-up studies: their contribution to diagnostic classification as applied to hysteria. Seminars in Psychiatry 2:392–402, 1970

Haines JL, Pritchard ML, Saunders AM, et al: No association between alpha 1–antichymotrypsin and familial Alzheimer's disease. Ann N Y Acad Sci 802:35–41, 1996a

Haines JL, Ter-Minassian M, Bazyk A, et al: A complete genomic screen for multiple sclerosis underscores a role for the major histocompatibility complex; The Multiple Sclerosis Genetics Group. Nat Genet 13:469–471, 1996b

Hall JM, Lee MK, Newman B, et al: Linkage of early onset familial breast cancer to chromosome 17q21. Science 250:1684–1689, 1990

Hamilton SP, Heiman GA, Haghighi FG, et al: Lack of genetic linkage or association between a functional serotonin transporter polymorphism and panic disorder. Psychiatr Genet 9:1–6, 1999

Hamilton SP, Haghighi F, Heiman GA, et al: Investigation of dopamine receptor (DRD4) and dopamine transporter (DAT) polymorphisms for genetic linkage or association to panic disorder. Am J Med Genet 96:324–330, 2000a

Hamilton SP, Slager SL, Heiman GA, et al: No genetic linkage or association between a functional promoter polymorphism in the monoamine oxidase-A gene and panic disorder. Mol Psychiatry 5:465–466, 2000b

Hamilton SP, Slager SL, Helleby L, et al: No association or linkage between polymorphisms in the genes encoding cholecystokinin and the cholecystokinin B receptor and panic disorder. Mol Psychiatry 6:59–65, 2001

Hastbacka J, Kaitila I, Sistonen P, et al: Diastrophic dysplasia gene maps to the distal long arm of chromosome 5. Proc Natl Acad Sci U S A 87:8056–8059, 1990

Heath AC, Cloninger CR, Martin NG: Testing a model for the genetic structure of personality: a comparison of the personality systems of Cloninger and Eysenck. J Pers Soc Psychol 66:762–775, 1994

Heinz A, Sander T, Harms H, et al: Lack of allelic association of dopamine D1 and D2 (TaqIA) receptor gene polymorphisms with reduced dopaminergic sensitivity to alcoholism. Alcohol Clin Exp Res 20:1109–1113, 1996

Heston LL: Psychiatric disorders in foster home reared children of schizophrenic mothers. Br J Psychiatry 112:819–825, 1966

Heston LL: Genetic studies of dementia: with emphasis on Parkinson's disease and Alzheimer's neuropathology, in The Epidemiology of Dementia. Edited by Mortimer JA, Schuman LM. New York, Oxford University Press, 1981, pp 101–117

Hettema JM, Corey LA, Kendler KS: A multivariate genetic analysis of the use of tobacco, alcohol, and caffeine in a population based sample of male and female twins. Drug Alcohol Depend 57:69–78, 1999

Hettema JM, Prescott CA, Kendler KS: A population-based twin study of generalized anxiety disorder in men and women. J Nerv Ment Dis 189:413–420, 2001

Higuchi S, Muramatsu T, Matsushita S, et al: Presenilin-1 polymorphism and Alzheimer's disease. Lancet 347:1186, 1996

Hinney A, Ziegler A, Nothen MM, et al: 5-HT2A receptor gene polymorphisms, anorexia nervosa, and obesity. Lancet 350:1324–1325, 1997a

Hinney A, Barth N, Ziegler A, et al: Serotonin transporter gene-linked polymorphic region: allele distributions in relationship to body weight and in anorexia nervosa. Life Sci 61:295–303, 1997b

Hinney A, Remschmidt H, Hebebrand J: Candidate gene polymorphisms in eating disorders. Eur J Pharmacol 410:147–159, 2000

Hoehe MR, Kopke K, Wendel B, et al: Sequence variability and candidate gene analysis in complex disease: association of mu opioid receptor gene variation with substance dependence. Hum Mol Genet 22:2895–2908, 2000

Holland AJ, Sicott N, Treasure J: Anorexia nervosa: evidence for a genetic basis. J Psychosom Res 32:561–571, 1988

Holzman PS, Levy DL: Smooth-pursuit eye movements and functional psychoses: a review. Schizophr Bull 3:15–27, 1977

Hoover CF, Insel TR: Families of origin in obsessive-compulsive disorder. J Nerv Ment Dis 172:207–215, 1984

Horikawa Y, Oda N, Cox NJ, et al: Genetic variation in the gene encoding calpain-10 is associated with type 2 diabetes mellitus. Nat Genet 26:163–175, 2000

Hultman CM, Ohman A, Cnattingius S, et al: Prenatal and neonatal risk factors for schizophrenia. Br J Psychiatry 170:128–133, 1997

Hutchinson G, Takei N, Fahy TA, et al: Morbid risk of schizophrenia in first-degree relatives of white and African-Caribbean patients with psychosis. Br J Psychiatry 169:776–780, 1996

Inayama Y, Yoneda H, Sakai T, et al: Lack of association between bipolar affective disorder and tyrosine hydroxylase DNA marker. Am J Med Genet 48:87–89, 1993

Inayama Y, Yoneda H, Sakai T, et al: Positive association between a DNA sequence variant in the serotonin 2A receptor gene and schizophrenia. Am J Med Genet 67:103–105, 1996

Irwin M, Schuckit M, Smith TL: Clinical importance of age at onset in type 1 and type 2 primary alcoholics. Arch Gen Psychiatry 47:320–324, 1990

Jacobsen NJ, Franks EK, Elvidge G, et al: Exclusion of the Darier's disease gene, ATP2A2, as a common susceptibility gene for bipolar disorder. Mol Psychiatry 6:92–97, 2001

Jain S, Leggo J, Delisi LE, et al: Analysis of thirteen trinucleotide repeat loci as candidate genes for schizophrenia and bipolar affective disorder. Am J Med Genet 67:139–146, 1996

Jarvik GP, Wijsman EM, Kukull WA, et al: Interactions of apolipoprotein E genotype, total cholesterol level, age, and sex in prediction of Alzheimer's disease: a case-control study. Neurology 45:1092–1096, 1995

Jarvik LF, Ruth V, Matsuyama SS: Organic brain syndrome and aging: a six-year follow-up of surviving twins. Arch Gen Psychiatry 37:280–286, 1980

Joober R, Benkelfat C, Brisebois K, et al: T102C polymorphism in the 5HT2A gene and schizophrenia: relation to phenotype and drug response variability. J Psychiatry Neurosci 24:141–146, 1999

Kalbfeish JD, Prentice RL: The Statistical Analysis of Failure Time Data. New York, Wiley, 1980

Kallmann FJ: The genetic theory of schizophrenia. Am J Psychiatry 103:309–322, 1946

Kalsi G, Brynjolfsson J, Butler R, et al: Linkage analysis of chromosome 22q12–13 in a United Kingdom/Icelandic sample of 23 multiplex schizophrenia families. Am J Med Genet 60.298–301, 1995

Kamboh MI, Sanghera DK, Ferrell RE, et al: APOE*4–associated Alzheimer's disease risk is modified by alpha 1–antichymotrypsin polymorphism. Nat Genet 10:486–488, 1995

Kaplitt MG, Makimura H: Defective viral vectors as agents for gene transfer in the nervous system. J Neurosci Methods 1:125–132, 1997

Karayiorgou M, Morris MA, Morrow B, et al: Schizophrenia susceptibility associated with interstitial deletions of chromosome 22q11. Proc Natl Acad Sci U S A 92:7612–7616, 1995

Karayiorgou M, Altemus M, Galke BL, et al: Genotype determining low catechol-O-methyltransferase activity as a risk factor for obsessive-compulsive disorder. Proc Natl Acad Sci U S A 94:4572–4575, 1997

Karayiorgou M, Sobin C, Blundell ML, et al: Family based association studies support a sexually dimorphic effect of COMT and MAOA on genetic susceptibility to obsessive-compulsive disorder. Biol Psychiatry 45:1178–1189, 1999

Karlsson JL: Partially dominant transmission of schizophrenia in Iceland. Br J Psychiatry 152:324–329, 1988

Kassett JA, Gershon ES, Maxwell ME, et al: Psychiatric disorders in the first-degree relatives of probands with bulimia nervosa. Am J Psychiatry 146:1468–1471, 1989

Kato T: Molecular genetics of bipolar disorder. Neurosci Res 40:105–113, 2001

Katsuragi S, Kunugi H, Sano A, et al: Association between serotonin transporter gene polymorphism and anxiety-related traits. Biol Psychiatry 45:368–370, 1999

Kaufmann CA, Ziegler RJ: The viral hypothesis of schizophrenia, in Receptors and Ligands in Psychiatry. Edited by Sen AK, Lee T. Cambridge, England, Cambridge University Press, 1987, pp 187–208

Keefe RSE, Silverman JM, Mohs RC, et al: Eye tracking, attention, and schizotypal symptoms in nonpsychotic relatives of patients with schizophrenia. Arch Gen Psychiatry 54:169–176, 1997

Kehoe P, Williams J, Lovestone S, et al: Presenilin-1 polymorphism and Alzheimer's disease: the UK Alzheimer's Disease Collaborative Group (letter). Lancet 347:1185, 1996

Kelsoe JR, Ginns EI, Egeland JA, et al: Re-evaluation of the linkage relationship between chromosome 11p loci and the gene for bipolar affective disorder in the Old Order Amish. Nature 342:238–243, 1989

Kelsoe JR, Spence MA, Loetscher E, et al: A genome survey indicates a possible susceptibility locus for bipolar disorder on chromosome 22. Proc Natl Acad Sci U S A 98:585–590, 2001

Kendler KS: Genetics of schizophrenia, in American Psychiatric Association Annual Review, Vol 5. Edited by Frances AJ, Hales RE. Washington, DC, American Psychiatric Press, 1986, pp 25–41

Kendler KS, Gardner CO: The risk for psychiatric disorders in relatives of schizophrenic and control probands: a comparison of three independent studies. Psychol Med 27:411–419, 1997

Kendler KS, Gruenberg AM: An independent analysis of the Danish adoption study of schizophrenia, VI: the relationship between psychiatric disorders as defined by DSM-III in the relatives and adoptees. Arch Gen Psychiatry 41:555–564, 1984

Kendler KS, Tsuang MT: Outcome and familial psychopathology in schizophrenia. Arch Gen Psychiatry 45:338–346, 1988

Kendler KS, Gruenberg AM, Tsuang MT: Psychiatric illness in first-degree relatives of schizophrenic and surgical control patients: a family study using DSM-III criteria. Arch Gen Psychiatry 42:770–779, 1985

Kendler KS, Gruenberg AM, Tsuang MT: A family study of the subtypes of schizophrenia. Am J Psychiatry 145:57–62, 1988

Kendler KS, Neale MC, Kessler RC, et al: The genetic epidemiology of phobias in women: the interrelationship of agoraphobia, social phobia, situational phobia, and simple phobia. Arch Gen Psychiatry 49:273–281, 1992

Kendler KS, Neale MC, Kessler RC, et al: Major depression and phobias: the genetic and environmental sources of comorbidity. Psychol Med 23:361–371, 1993a

Kendler KS, Neale MC, Kessler RC, et al: Panic disorder in women: a population-based twin study. Psychol Med 23:397–406, 1993b

Kendler KS, Neale MC, MacLean CJ, et al: Smoking and major depression: a causal analysis. Arch Gen Psychiatry 50:36–43, 1993c

Kendler KS, Neale MC, Kessler RC, et al: A test of the equal-environment assumption in twin studies of psychiatric illness. Behav Genet 23:21–27, 1993d

Kendler KS, Neale MC, Heath AC, et al: A twin-family study of alcoholism in women. Am J Psychiatry 151:707–715, 1994

Kendler KS, Walters EE, Neale MC, et al: The structure of the genetic and environmental risk factors for six major psychiatric disorders in women: phobia, generalized anxiety disorder, panic disorder, bulimia, major depression, and alcoholism. Arch Gen Psychiatry 52:374–383, 1995

Kendler KS, Karkowski-Shuman L, Walsh D: Age at onset in schizophrenia and risk of illness in relatives: results from the Roscommon Family Study. Br J Psychiatry 169:213–218, 1996a

Kendler KS, MacLean CJ, O'Neill FA, et al: Evidence for a schizophrenia vulnerability locus on chromosome 8p in the Irish Study of High-Density Schizophrenia Families. Am J Psychiatry 153:1534–1540, 1996b

Kendler KS, Karkowski LM, Prescott CA: Fears and phobias: reliability and heritability. Psychol Med 29:539–553, 1999

Kendler KS, Myers J, Prescott CA, et al: The genetic epidemiology of irrational fears and phobias in men. Arch Gen Psychiatry 58:257–265, 2001a

Kendler KS, Gardner CO, Neale MC, et al: Genetic risk factors for major depression in men and women: similar or different heritabilities and same or partly distinct genes? Psychol Med 31:605–616, 2001b

Kennedy JL, Billett EA, Macciardi FM, et al: Association study of dopamine D3 receptor gene and schizophrenia. Am J Med Genet 60:558–562, 1995

Kennedy JL, Bradwejn J, Koszycki D, et al: Investigation of cholecystokinin system genes in panic disorder. Mol Psychiatry 4:284–285, 1999

Kessler RC, McGonagle KA, Zhao S, et al: Lifetime and 12-month prevalence of DSM-III-R psychiatric disorders in the United States: results from the National Comorbidity Survey. Arch Gen Psychiatry 51:8–19, 1994

Kessler S: Psychological aspects of genetic counseling, VI: a critical review of the literature dealing with education and reproduction. Am J Med Genet 34:340–353, 1989

Kety SS: Schizophrenic illness in the families of schizophrenic adoptees: findings from the Danish national sample. Schizophr Bull 14:217–222, 1988

Kety SS, Wender PH, Jacobsen B, et al: Mental illness in the biological and adoptive relatives of schizophrenic adoptees: replication of the Copenhagen Study in the rest of Denmark. Arch Gen Psychiatry 51:442–455, 1994

Kidd KK: Genetic models for psychiatric disorders, in Genetic Research Strategies for Psychobiology and Psychiatry. Edited by Gershon ES, Matthysse S, Breakefield XO, et al. Pacific Grove, CA, Boxwood Press, 1981, pp 369–382

Kinnear CJ, Niehaus DJ, Moolman-Smook JC, et al: Obsessive-compulsive disorder and the promoter region polymorphism (5-HTTLPR) in the serotonin transporter gene (SLC6A4): a negative association study in the Afrikaner population. Int J Neuropsychopharmacol 3:327–331, 2000

Kinney DK, Yurgelun-Todd DA, Woods BT: Hard neurologic signs and psychopathology in relatives of schizophrenic patients. Psychiatry Res 39:45–53, 1991

Kirchheiner J, Brosen K, Dahl ML, et al: CYP2D6 and CYP2C19 genotype-based dose recommendations for antidepressants: a first step towards subpopulation-specific dosages. Acta Psychiatr Scand 104:173–192, 2001

Klerman GL, Lavori PW, Rice J, et al: Birth cohort trends in rates of major depressive disorder among relatives of patients with affective disorder. Arch Gen Psychiatry 42:689–693, 1985

Knowles JA, Weissman MM: Panic disorder and agoraphobia, in American Psychiatric Press Review of Psychiatry, Vol 14.

Edited by Oldham JM, Riba MB. Washington, DC, American Psychiatric Press, 1995, pp 383–404

Knowles JA, Fyer AJ, Vieland VJ, et al: Results of a genome-wide genetic screen for panic disorder. Am J Med Genet 81:139–147, 1998

Koob GF, Nestler EJ: The neurobiology of drug addiction. J Neuropsychiatry Clin Neurosci 9:482–497, 1997

Korner J, Rietschel M, Hunt N, et al: Association and haplotype analysis at the tyrosine hydroxylase locus in a combined German-British sample of manic depressive patients and controls. Psychiatr Genet 4:167–175, 1994

Kowalska A, Danker-Hopfe H, Wender M, et al: Association between the PI*M3 allele of alpha 1–antitrypsin and Alzheimer's disease? A preliminary report. Hum Genet 98:744–746, 1996

Kringlen E: Adult offspring of two psychotic parents, with special reference to schizophrenia, in The Nature of Schizophrenia. Edited by Wynne LC, Cromwell RL, Matthysse S. New York, Wiley, 1978, pp 9–24

Kringlen E, Cramer G: Offspring of monozygotic twins discordant for schizophrenia. Arch Gen Psychiatry 46:873–877, 1989

Kunugi H, Curtis D, Vallada HP, et al: A linkage study of schizophrenia with DNA markers from chromosome 8p21–p22 in 25 multiplex families. Schizophr Res 22:61–68, 1996

Kuokkanen S, Sundvall M, Terwilliger JD, et al: A putative vulnerability locus to multiple sclerosis maps to 5p14–p12 in a region syntenic to the murine locus Eae2. Nat Genet 13:477–480, 1996

Kupfer DJ, Frank E, Carpenter LL, et al: Family history in recurrent depression. J Affect Disord 17:113–119, 1989

Lander ES, Kruglyak L: Genetic dissection of complex traits: guidelines for interpreting and reporting linkage results. Nat Genet 11:241–247, 1995

Lander ES, Linton LM, Birren B, et al: Initial sequencing and analysis of the human genome. Nature 409:860–921, 2001

Larson CA, Nyman GE: Differential fertility in schizophrenia. Acta Psychiatr Scand 49:272–280, 1973

Laurent A, Biloa-Tang M, Bougerol T, et al: Executive/attentional performance and measures of schizotypy in patients with schizophrenia and in their nonpsychotic first-degree relatives. Schizophr Res 46:269–283, 2000

Leckman JF, Chittenden EH: Gilles de la Tourette's syndrome and some forms of obsessive-compulsive disorder may share a common genetic diathesis. Encephale 16:321–323, 1990

Lenane MC, Swedo SE, Leonard H, et al: Psychiatric disorders in first degree relatives of children and adolescents with obsessive compulsive disorder. J Am Acad Child Adolesc Psychiatry 29:407–412, 1990

Leonard HL, Swedo SE: Paediatric autoimmune neuropsychiatric disorders associated with streptococcal infection (PANDAS). Int J Neuropsychopharmacol 4:191–198, 2001

Lesch KP, Bengel D, Heils A, et al: Association of anxiety-related traits with a polymorphism in the serotonin transporter gene regulatory region. Science 274:1527–1531, 1996

Levinson DF, Holmans P, Straub RE, et al: Multicenter linkage study of schizophrenia candidate regions on chromosomes 5q, 6q, 10p, and 13q: Schizophrenia Linkage Collaborative Group III. Am J Hum Genet 67:652–663, 2000

Levy-Lahad E, Bird TD: Genetic factors in Alzheimer's disease: a review of recent advances. Ann Neurol 40:829–840, 1996

Levy-Lahad E, Wasco W, Poorkaj P, et al: Candidate gene for the chromosome 1 familial Alzheimer's disease locus. Science 269:973–977, 1995a

Levy-Lahad E, Wijsman EM, Nemens E, et al: A familial Alzheimer's disease locus on chromosome I. Science 269:970–973, 1995b

Lieberman JA, Yunis J, Egea E, et al: HLA-B38, DR4, DQw3 and clozapine-induced agranulocytosis in Jewish patients with schizophrenia. Arch Gen Psychiatry 47:945–948, 1990

Lilenfeld LR, Kaye WH, Greeno CG, et al: A controlled family study of anorexia nervosa and bulimia nervosa: psychiatric disorders in first-degree relatives and effects of proband comorbidity. Arch Gen Psychiatry 55:603–610, 1998

Lilienfeld SO, VanValkenburg C, Larntz K, et al: The relationship of histrionic personality disorder to antisocial personality and somatization disorders. Am J Psychiatry 143:718–722, 1986

Lin MW, Curtis D, Williams N, et al: Suggestive evidence for linkage of schizophrenia to markers on chromosome 13q14.1–q32. Psychiatr Genet 5:117–126, 1995

Lin MW, Sham P, Hwu HG, et al: Suggestive evidence for linkage of schizophrenia to markers on chromosome 13 in Caucasian but not Oriental populations. Hum Genet 99:417–420, 1997

Litman RE, Torrey EF, Hommer DW, et al: A quantitative analysis of smooth pursuit eye tracking in monozygotic twins discordant for schizophrenia. Arch Gen Psychiatry 54:417–426, 1997

Liu J, Juo SH, Terwilliger JD, et al: A follow-up linkage study supports evidence for a bipolar affective disorder locus on chromosome 21q22. Am J Med Genet 105:189–194, 2001

Long JC, Knowler WC, Hanson RL, et al: Evidence for genetic linkage to alcohol dependence on chromosomes 4 and 11 from an autosome-wide scan in an American Indian population. Am J Med Genet 81:216–221, 1998

Lu RB, Ko HC, Chang FM, et al: No association between alcoholism and multiple polymorphisms at the dopamine D2 receptor gene (DRD2) in three distinct Taiwanese populations. Biol Psychiatry 39:419–429, 1996

Lyons MJ, Goldberg J, Eisen SA, et al: Do genes influence exposure to trauma? A twin study of combat. Am J Med Genet 48:22–27, 1993

Lyons MJ, Toomey R, Faraone SV, et al: Comparison of schizo-typal relatives of schizophrenic versus affective probands. Am J Med Genet 54:279–285, 1994

MacKinnon DF, Xu J, McMahon FJ, et al: Bipolar disorder and panic disorder in families: an analysis of chromosome 18 data. Am J Psychiatry 155:829–831, 1998

Maier W, Lichtermann D, Minges J, et al: Personality traits in subjects at risk for unipolar major depression: a family study perspective. J Affect Disord 24:153–163, 1992

Maier W, Lichtermann D, Minges J, et al: A controlled family study in panic disorder. J Psychiatr Res 27(suppl 1):79–87, 1993

Maier W, Hallmayer J, Zill P, et al: Linkage analysis between pericentrometric markers on chromosome 18 and bipolar disorder: a replication test. Psychiatr Res 59:7–15, 1995

Malaspina D, Harlap S, Fennig S, et al: Advancing paternal age and the risk of schizophrenia. Arch Gen Psychiatry 58:361–367, 2001

Malhi GS, Moore J, McGuffin P: The genetics of major depressive disorder. Current Psychiatry Reports 2:165–169, 2000

Mant R, Williams J, Asherson P, et al: Relationship between homozygosity at the dopamine D3 receptor gene and schizophrenia. Am J Med Genet 54:21–26, 1994

Marazita ML, Neiswanger K, Cooper M, et al: Genetic segregation analysis of early onset recurrent unipolar depression. Am J Hum Genet 61:1370–1378, 1997

Marcus J, Hans SL, Nagler S, et al: Review of the NIMH Israeli Kibbutz-City Study and the Jerusalem Infant Development Study. Schizophr Bull 13:425–438, 1987

Martinez M, Goldin LR, Cao Q, et al: Follow-up study on a susceptibility locus for schizophrenia on chromosome 6q. Am J Med Genet 88:337–343, 1999

Mather JA: Eye movements of teenage children of schizophrenics: a possible inherited marker of susceptibility to the disease. J Psychiatr Res 19:523–532, 1985

Matthysse SW, Kidd KK: Estimating the genetic contribution to schizophrenia. Am J Psychiatry 133:185–191, 1976

Mayeux R, Lee JH, Romas SN, et al: Chromosome 12 mapping of late-onset Alzheimer disease among Caribbean Hispanics. Am J Hum Genet 70:237–243, 2002

Mazzanti CM, Lappalainen J, Long JC, et al: Role of the serotonin transporter promoter polymorphism in anxiety related traits. Arch Gen Psychiatry 55:936–940, 1998

McDougle CJ, Epperson CN, Price LH, et al: Evidence for linkage disequilibrium between serotonin transporter protein gene (SLC6A4) and obsessive compulsive disorder. Mol Psychiatry 3:270–273, 1998

McGuffin P, Sargeant M, Hetti G, et al: Exclusion of a schizophrenia susceptibility gene from the chromosome 5q11–q13 region: new data and a reanalysis of previous reports. Am J Hum Genet 47:524–535, 1990

McInnis MG, McMahon FJ, Chase GA, et al: Anticipation in bipolar affective disorder. Am J Hum Genet 53:385–390, 1993

McKeon P, Murray R: Familial aspects of obsessive-compulsive neurosis. Br J Psychiatry 151:528–534, 1987

McMahon FJ, Stine OC, Meyers DA, et al: Patterns of maternal transmission in bipolar affective disorder. Am J Hum Genet 56:1277–1286, 1995

McNeil TF, Kaij L: Swedish high-risk study: sample characteristics at age 6. Schizophr Bull 13:373–381, 1987

Meged S, Stein D, Sitrota P, et al: Human leukocyte antigen typing, response to neuroleptics, and clozapine-induced agranulocytosis in Jewish Israeli schizophrenic patients. Int Clin Psychopharmacol 14:305–312, 1999

Melo JA, Shendure J, Pociask K, et al: Identification of sex-specific quantitative trait loci controlling alcohol preference in C57BL/6 mice. Nat Genet 13:147–153, 1996

Meloni R, Leboyer M, Bellivier F, et al: Association of manic-depressive illness with tyrosine hydroxylase microsatellite marker. Lancet 345:932, 1995

Mendlewicz J, Rainer JD: Adoption study supporting genetic transmission in manic depressive illness. Nature 268:327–329, 1977

Mendlewicz J, Simon P, Sevy S, et al: Polymorphic DNA marker on X chromosome and manic depression. Lancet 1:1230–1232, 1987

Mendlewicz J, Sevy S, deMaertelaer V: REM sleep latency and morbidity risk of affective disorders in depressive illness. Neuropsychobiology 22:14–17, 1989

Mendlewicz J, Papadimitriou G, Wilmotte J: Family study of panic disorder: comparison with generalized anxiety disorder, major depression, and normal subjects. Psychiatr Genet 3:73–78, 1993

Merikangas KR: Genetics of alcoholism: a review of human studies, in Genetics of Neuropsychiatric Diseases. Edited by Wetterberg I. London, England, Macmillan, 1989, pp 269–280

Merikangas KR, Stolar M, Stevens DE, et al: Familial transmission of substance use disorders. Arch Gen Psychiatry 55:973–979, 1998

Miki Y, Swensen J, Shattuck-Eidens D, et al: A strong candidate for the breast and ovarian cancer susceptibility gene BRCA1. Science 266:66–71, 1994

Millar JK, Wilson-Annan JC, Anderson S, et al: Disruption of two novel genes by a translocation co-segregating with schizophrenia. Hum Mol Genet 9:1415–1423, 2000

Mirnics K, Middleton FA, Marquez A, et al: Molecular characterization of schizophrenia viewed by microarray analysis of gene expression in prefrontal cortex. Neuron 28:53–67, 2000

Mirnics K, Middleton FA, Stanwood GD, et al: Disease-specific changes in regulator of G-protein signaling 4 (RGS4) expression in schizophrenia. Mol Psychiatry 6:293–301, 2001

Mirsky AF, Ingraham LJ, Kugelmass S: Neuropsychological assessment of attention and its pathology in the Israeli cohort. Schizophr Bull 21:193–204, 1995

Mohs RC, Breitner JCS, Silverman JM, et al: Alzheimer's disease: morbid risk among first-degree relatives approximates 50% by 90 years of age. Arch Gen Psychiatry 44:405–408, 1987

Moises HW, Yang L, Kristbjarnarson H, et al: An international two-stage genome-wide search for schizophrenia susceptibility genes. Nat Genet 11:321–324, 1995a

Moises HW, Yang L, Li T, et al: Potential linkage disequilibrium between schizophrenia and locus D22S278 on the long arm of chromosome 22. Am J Med Genet 60:465–467, 1995b

Moldin SO, Gottesman II, Erlenmeyer-Kimling L, et al: Psychometric deviance in offspring at risk for schizophrenia, I: initial delineation of a distinct subgroup. Psychiatr Res 32:297–310, 1990a

Moldin SO, Rice JP, Gottesman II, et al: Psychometric deviance in offspring at risk for schizophrenia, II: resolving heterogeneity through admixture analysis. Psychiatr Res 32:311–322, 1990b

Moldin SO, Rice JP, Gottesman II, et al: Transmission of a psychometric indicator for liability to schizophrenia in normal families. Genet Epidemiol 7:163–176, 1990c

Moldin SO, Gottesman II, Rice JP, et al: Replicated psychometric correlates of schizophrenia. Am J Psychiatry 148:762–767, 1991

Morgan K, Morgan L, Carpenter K, et al: Microsatellite polymorphism of the alpha 1-antichymotrypsin gene locus associated with sporadic Alzheimer's disease. Hum Genet 99:27–31, 1997

Morissette J, Villeneuve A, Bordeleau L, et al: Genome-wide search for linkage of bipolar affective disorders in a very large pedigree derived from a homogeneous population in Quebec points to a locus of major effect on chromosome 12q23-q24. Am J Med Genet 88:567–587, 1999

Morton NE: Sequential tests for the detection of linkage. Am J Hum Genet 7:277–318, 1955

Mowry BJ, Nancarrow DJ, Lennon DP, et al: Schizophrenia susceptibility and chromosome 6p24–22. Nat Genet 11:233–234, 1995

Mullan M, Houlden H, Windelspecht M, et al: A locus for familial early onset Alzheimer's disease on the long arm of chromosome 14, proximal to the alpha 1-antichymotrypsin gene. Nat Genet 2:340–342, 1992

Muller U, Bodeker RH, Gerundt I, et al: Lack of association between alpha 1-antichymotrypsin polymorphism, Alzheimer's disease, and allele epsilon 4 of apolipoprotein E. Neurology 47:1575–1577, 1996

Mundo E, Walker M, Cate T, et al: The role of serotonin transporter protein gene in antidepressant-induced mania in bipolar disorder: preliminary findings. Arch Gen Psychiatry 58:539–544, 2001

Murphy GM Jr, Yang L, Yesavage J, et al: Rate of cognitive decline in Alzheimer's disease is not affected by the alpha-1-antichymotrypsin A allele or the CYP2D6 B mutant. Neurosci Lett 217:200–202, 1996

Murphy GM, Pollock BG, Kirshner MA, et al: CYP2D6 genotyping with oligonucleotide microarrays and nortriptyline concentrations in geriatric depression. Neuropsychopharmacology 25:737–743, 2001

Mutchler K, Crowe RR, Noyes R Jr, et al: Exclusion of the tyrosine hydroxylase gene in 14 panic disorder pedigrees. Am J Psychiatry 147:1367–1369, 1990

Myers A, Holmans P, Marshall H, et al: Susceptibility locus for Alzheimer's disease on chromosome 10. Science 290:2304–2305, 2000

Nacmias B, Tedde A, Latorraca S, et al: Apolipoprotein E and alpha 1-antichymotrypsin polymorphism in Alzheimer's disease. Ann Neurol 40:678–680, 1996

Nacmias B, Ricca V, Tedde A, et al: 5-HT2A receptor gene polymorphisms in anorexia nervosa and bulimia nervosa. Neurosci Lett 277:134–136, 1999

Nagler S: Overall design and methodology of the Israeli high-risk study. Schizophr Bull 11:31–37, 1985

Nakamura M, Ueno S, Sano A, et al: Polymorphisms of the human homologue of the Drosophila white gene are associated with mood and panic disorders. Mol Psychiatry 4:155–162, 1999

Nakamura T, Muramatsu T, Ono Y, et al: Serotonin transporter gene regulatory region polymorphism and anxiety-related traits in the Japanese. Am J Med Genet 74:544–545, 1997

Nee LE, Eldridge R, Sunderland T, et al: Dementia of the Alzheimer type: clinical and family study of 22 twin pairs. Neurology 37:359–363, 1987

Nelson EC, Grant JD, Bucholz KK, et al: Social phobia in a population-based female adolescent twin sample: co-morbidity and associated suicide-related symptoms. Psychol Med 30:797–804, 2000

Nestadt G, Lan T, Samuels J, et al: Complex segregation analysis provides compelling evidence for a major gene underlying obsessive-compulsive disorder and for heterogeneity by sex. Am J Hum Genet 67:1611–1616, 2000a

Nestadt G, Samuels J, Riddle M, et al: A family study of obsessive-compulsive disorder. Arch Gen Psychiatry 57:358–363, 2000b

Newman B, Austin MA, Lee M, et al: Inheritance of human breast cancer: evidence for autosomal dominant transmission in high-risk families. Proc Natl Acad Sci U S A 85:3044–3048, 1988

Nicolini H, Hanna G, Baxter L, et al: Segregation analysis of obsessive-compulsive and associated disorders: preliminary results. Ursus Med 1:25–28, 1991

Nicolini H, Weissbecker K, Mejia JM, et al: Family study of obsessive-compulsive disorder in a Mexican population. Arch Med Res 24:193–198, 1993

Niculescu AB III, Segal DS, Kuczenski R, et al: Identifying a series of candidate genes for mania and psychosis: a convergent functional genomics approach. Physiological Genomics 4:83–91, 2000

Niehaus DJ, Kinnear CJ, Corfield VA, et al: Association between a catechol-O-methyltransferase polymorphism and obsessive-compulsive disorder in the Afrikaner population. J Affect Disord 65:61–65, 2001

Nielsen DA, Goldman D, Virkkunen M, et al: Suicidality and 5-hydroxyindoleacetic acid concentration associated with a tryptophan hydroxylase polymorphism. Arch Gen Psychiatry 51:34–38, 1994

Nimgaonkar VL, Rudert WA, Zhang XR, et al: Further evidence for an association between schizophrenia and the HLA DQB1 gene locus. Schizophr Res 18:43–49, 1995

Nimgaonkar VL, Sanders AR, Ganguli R, et al: Association study of schizophrenia and the dopamine D3 receptor gene locus in two independent samples. Am J Med Genet 67:505–514, 1996

NIMH Genetics Initiative Bipolar Group: Genomic survey of bipolar illness in the NIMH Genetics Initiative pedigrees: a preliminary report. Am J Med Genet 74:227–237, 1997

Nothen MM, Cichon S, Propping P, et al: Excess of homozygosity at the dopamine D3 receptor gene in schizophrenia not confirmed. J Med Genet 30:708–709, 1993

Noyes R Jr, Crowe RR, Harris EL, et al: Relationship between panic disorder and agoraphobia: a family study. Arch Gen Psychiatry 43:227–232, 1986

Noyes R Jr, Clarkson C, Crowe RR, et al: A family study of generalized anxiety disorder. Am J Psychiatry 144:1019–1024, 1987

Nurnberger JI Jr, Foroud T: Genetics of bipolar affective disorder. Current Psychiatry Reports 2:147–157, 2000

Nurnberger JI Jr, Gershon ES: Genetics, in Handbook of Affective Disorders. Edited by Paykel ES. New York, Guilford, 1982, pp 126–145

Nurnberger JI Jr, Foroud T, Flury L, et al: Evidence for a locus on chromosome 1 that influences vulnerability to alcoholism and affective disorder. Am J Psychiatry 158:718–724, 2001

O'Donovan MC, Owen MJ: Candidate-gene association studies of schizophrenia. Am J Hum Genet 65:587–592, 1999

O'Donovan MC, Guy C, Craddock N, et al: Expanded CAG repeats in schizophrenia and bipolar disorder. Nat Genet 10:380–381, 1995

O'Donovan MC, Guy C, Craddock N, et al: Confirmation of association between expanded CAG/CTG repeats and both schizophrenia and bipolar disorder. Psychol Med 26:1145–1153, 1996

O'Reilly RL, Bogue L, Singh SM: Pharmacogenetic response to antidepressants in a multicase family with affective disorder. Biol Psychiatry 36:467–471, 1994

O'Rourke DH, Gottesman II, Suarez BK, et al: Refutation of the general single locus model for the etiology of schizophrenia. Am J Hum Genet 34:630–649, 1982

Ohara K, Nagai M, Suzuki Y, et al: No association between anxiety disorders and catechol-O-methyltransferase polymorphism. Psychiatry Res 80:145–148, 1998

Okuyama Y, Ishiguro H, Nankai M, et al: Identification of a polymorphism in the promoter region of DRD4 associated

with the human novelty seeking personality trait. Mol Psychiatry 5:64–69, 2000

Onstad S, Skre I, Torgersen S, et al: Subtypes of schizophrenia—evidence from a twin-family study. Acta Psychiatr Scand 84:203–206, 1991

Onstad S, Skre I, Torgersen S, et al: Birthweight and obstetric complications in schizophrenic twins. Acta Psychiatr Scand 85:70–73, 1992

Oscarson M, Gullsten H, Rautio A, et al: Genotyping of human cytochrome P450 2A6 (CYP2A6), a nicotine C-oxidase. FEBS Lett 438:201–205, 1998

Ott J: Estimation of the recombination fraction in human pedigrees: efficient computation of the likelihood for human linkage. Ann Hum Genet 26:588–597, 1974

Pare CMB, Ress L, Sainsbury MJ: Differentiation of two genetically specific types of depression by the response to antidepressants. Lancet 2:1240–1343, 1962

Parnas J, Schulsinger F, Schulsinger H, et al: Behavioral precursors of schizophrenia spectrum: a prospective study. Arch Gen Psychiatry 39:658–664, 1982

Paterson AD, Sunohara GA, Kennedy JL: Dopamine D4 receptor gene: novelty or nonsense? Neuropsychopharmacology 21:3–16, 1999

Pauls DL, Gerhard DS, Lacy LG, et al: Linkage of bipolar affective disorders to markers on chromosome 11p is excluded in a second lateral extension of Amish pedigree 110. Genomics 11:730–736, 1991

Pauls DL, Bailey JN, Carter AS, et al: Complex segregation analyses of Old Order Amish families ascertained through bipolar I individuals. Am J Med Genet 60:290–297, 1995a

Pauls DL, Alsobrook JP II, Goodman W, et al: A family study of obsessive-compulsive disorder. Am J Psychiatry 152:76–84, 1995b

Pauls DL, Ott J, Paul SM, et al: Linkage analyses of chromosome 18 markers do not identify a major susceptibility locus for bipolar affective disorder in the Old Order Amish. Am J Hum Genet 57:636–643, 1995c

Pekkarinen P, Terwilliger J, Bredbacka P, et al: Evidence of a predisposing locus to bipolar disorder on Xq24–q27.1 in an extended Finnish pedigree. Genome Res 5:105–115, 1995

Peltonen L, McKusick VA: Genomics and medicine: dissecting human disease in the postgenomic era. Science 291:1224–1229, 2001

Perez de Castro I, Santos J, Torres P, et al: A weak association between TH and DRD2 genes and bipolar affective disorder in a Spanish sample. J Med Genet 32:131–134, 1995

Pericak-Vance MA, Yamaoka LH, Haynes CS, et al: Genetic linkage studies in Alzheimer's disease families. Exp Neurol 102:271–279, 1988

Pericak-Vance MA, Bebout JL, Gaskell PC Jr, et al: Linkage studies in familial Alzheimer disease: evidence for chromosome 19 linkage. Am J Hum Genet 48:1034–1050, 1991

Pericak-Vance MA, Bass MP, Yamaoka LH, et al: Complete genomic screen in late-onset familial Alzheimer disease: evidence for a new locus on chromosome 12. JAMA 278:1237–1241, 1997

Perna G, Cocchi S, Bertani A, et al: Sensitivity to 35% CO_2 in healthy first-degree relatives of patients with panic disorder. Am J Psychiatry 152:623–625, 1995

Petronis A, Kennedy JL: Unstable genes—unstable mind. Am J Psychiatry 152:164–172, 1995

Pianezza ML, Sellers EM, Tyndale RF: Nicotine metabolism defect reduces smoking (letter). Nature 393:750, 1998

Pickar D, Rubinow K: Pharmacogenomics of psychiatric disorders. Trends Pharmacol Sci 22:75–83, 2001

Plomin R, DeFries JC, McClearn GE: Behavioral Genetics: A Primer, 2nd Edition. San Francisco, CA, WH Freeman, 1990

Plomin R, Owen MJ, McGuffin P: The genetic basis of complex human behaviors. Science 264:1733–1739, 1994

Pollock BG, Ferrell RE, Mulsant BH, et al: Allelic variation in the serotonin transporter promoter affects onset of paroxetine treatment response in late-life depression. Neuropsychopharmacology 23:587–590, 2000

Polymeropoulos MH, Schaffer AA: Scanning the genome with 1772 microsatellite markers in search of a bipolar disorder susceptibility gene. Mol Psychiatry 1:404–407, 1996

Polymeropoulos MH, Coon H, Byerley W, et al: Search for a schizophrenia susceptibility locus on human chromosome 22. Am J Med Genet 54:93–99, 1994

Pope HG Jr, Yurgelun-Todd D: Schizophrenic individuals with bipolar first-degree relatives: analysis of two pedigrees. J Clin Psychiatry 51:97–101, 1990

Preisig M, Bellivier F, Fenton BT, et al: Association between bipolar disorder and monoamine oxidase A gene polymorphisms: results of a multicenter study. Am J Psychiatry 157:948–955, 2000

Prescott CA, Aggen SH, Kendler KS: Sex differences in the sources of genetic liability to alcohol abuse and dependence in a population-based sample of U.S. twins. Alcohol Clin Exp Res 23:1136–1144, 1999

Prescott CA, Aggen SH, Kendler KS: Sex-specific genetic influences on the comorbidity of alcoholism and major depression in a population-based sample of US twins. Arch Gen Psychiatry 57:803–811, 2000

Price RA, Kidd KK, Weissman MM: Early onset (under age 30 years) and panic disorder as markers for etiologic homogeneity in major depression. Arch Gen Psychiatry 44:434–440, 1987

Price-Evans DA, Davison K, Pratt RTC: The influences of acetylator phenotype on the effects of treating depression with phenelzine. Clin Pharmacol Ther 6:430–433, 1965

Pulver AE, Brown CH, Wolyniec P, et al: Schizophrenia: age at onset, gender and familial risk. Acta Psychiatr Scand 82:344–351, 1990

Pulver AE, Brown CH, Wolyniec P, et al: Psychiatric morbidity in the relatives of patients with DSM-III schizophreniform disorder: comparisons with the relatives of schizophrenic

and bipolar disorder patients. J Psychiatr Res 25:19–29, 1991

Pulver AE, Karayiorgou M, Lasseter VK, et al: Follow-up of a report of a potential linkage for schizophrenia on chromosome 22q12–q13.1: part 2. Am J Med Genet 54:44–50, 1994a

Pulver AE, Nestadt G, Goldberg R, et al: Psychotic illness in patients diagnosed with velo-cardio-facial syndrome and their relatives. J Nerv Ment Dis 182:476–478, 1994b

Pulver AE, Karayiorgou M, Wolyniec PS, et al: Sequential strategy to identify a susceptibility gene for schizophrenia: report of potential linkage on chromosome 22q12–q13.1: part 1. Am J Med Genet 54:36–43, 1994c

Pulver AE, Lasseter VK, Kasch L, et al: Schizophrenia: a genome scan targets chromosomes 3p and 8p as potential sites of susceptibility genes. Am J Med Genet 60:252–260, 1995

Pulver AE, Mulle J, Nestadt G, et al: Genetic heterogeneity in schizophrenia: stratification of genome scan data using cosegregating related phenotypes. Mol Psychiatry 5:650–653, 2000

Radel M, Goldman D: Pharmacogenetics of alcohol response and alcoholism: the interplay of genes and environmental factors in thresholds for alcoholism. Drug Metab Dispos 29:489–494, 2001

Ram A, Guedj F, Cravchik A, et al: No abnormality in the gene for the G protein stimulatory alpha subunit in patients with bipolar disorder. Arch Gen Psychiatry 54:44–48, 1997

Regier DA, Narrow WE, Rae DS, et al: The de facto US mental and addictive disorders service system: Epidemiologic Catchment Area prospective 1-year prevalence rates of disorders and services. Arch Gen Psychiatry 50:85–94, 1993

Reich JH: Familiality of DSM-III dramatic and anxious personality clusters. J Nerv Ment Dis 177:96–100, 1989

Reich J[H]: Using the family history method to distinguish relatives of patients with dependent personality disorder from relatives of controls. Psychiatr Res 39:227–237, 1991

Reich T, Cloninger CR, Van Eerdewegh P, et al: Secular trends in the familial transmission of alcoholism. Alcoholism 12:458–464, 1988

Reich T, Edenberg HJ, Goate A, et al: Genome-wide search for genes affecting the risk for alcohol dependence. Am J Med Genet 81:207–215, 1998

Reveley MA, Reveley AM, Baldy R: Left cerebral hemisphere hypodensity in discordant schizophrenic twins: a controlled study. Arch Gen Psychiatry 44:625–632, 1987

Rice JP, Endicott J, Knesevich MA, et al: The estimation of diagnostic sensitivity using stability data: an application to major depressive disorder. J Psychiatr Res 21:337–345, 1987a

Rice JP, Reich T, Andreasen NC, et al: The familial transmission of bipolar illness. Arch Gen Psychiatry 44:441–447, 1987b

Rietschel M, Nothen MM, Albus M, et al: Dopamine D3 receptor Gly9/Ser9 polymorphism and schizophrenia: no increased frequency of homozygosity in German familial cases. Schizophr Res 20:181–186, 1996

Riley BP, Rajagopalan S, Mogudi-Carter M, et al: No evidence for linkage of chromosome 6p markers to schizophrenia in southern African Bantu-speaking families. Psychiatr Genet 6:41–49, 1996

Risch N: Linkage strategies for genetically complex traits, I: multilocus models. Am J Hum Genet 46:222–228, 1990

Risch N, Baron M: Segregation analysis of schizophrenia and related disorders. Am J Hum Genet 36:1039–1059, 1984

Risch N, Merikangas K: The future of genetic studies of complex human diseases. Science 273:1516–1517, 1996

Risch N, Zhang H: Extreme discordant sib pairs for mapping quantitative trait loci in humans. Science 268:1584–1589, 1995

Robins LN, Helzer JE, Weissman MM, et al: Lifetime prevalence of specific psychiatric disorders in three sites. Arch Gen Psychiatry 41:949–958, 1984

Rogaev EI, Sherrington R, Rogaeva EA, et al: Familial Alzheimer's disease in kindreds with missense mutations in a gene on chromosome 1 related to the Alzheimer's disease type 3 gene. Nature 376:775–778, 1995

Rogaeva E, Premkumar S, Song Y, et al: Evidence for an Alzheimer disease susceptibility locus on chromosome 12 and for further locus heterogeneity [see comments]. JAMA 280:614–618, 1998

Rogaeva EA, Premkumar S, Grubber J, et al: An alpha-2-macroglobulin insertion-deletion polymorphism in Alzheimer disease. Nat Genet 22:19–22, 1999

Romas SN, Mayeux R, Rabinowitz D, et al: The deletion polymorphism and Val1000Ile in alpha-2-macroglobulin and Alzheimer disease in Caribbean Hispanics. Neurosci Lett 279:133–136, 2000a

Romas SN, Mayeux R, Tang MX, et al: No association between a presenilin-1 polymorphism and Alzheimer's disease. Arch Neurol 57:699–702, 2000b

Ronai Z, Barta C, Guttman A, et al: Genotyping the -521C/T functional polymorphism in the promoter region of dopamine D4 receptor (DRD4) gene. Electrophoresis 22:1102–1105, 2001

Rosa A, Fananas L, Bracha HS, et al: Congenital dermatoglyphic malformations and psychosis: a twin study. Am J Psychiatry 157:1511–1513, 2000

Rosenkranz K, Hinney A, Ziegler A, et al: Systematic mutation screening of the estrogen receptor beta gene in probands of different weight extremes: identification of several genetic variants. J Clin Endocrinol Metab 83:4524–4527, 1998

Rosenthal D: Genetic Theory and Abnormal Behavior. New York, McGraw-Hill, 1970

Rosenthal D, Wender PH, Kety SS, et al: Schizophrenics' offspring reared in adoptive homes. J Psychiatr Res 6:377–391, 1968

Roses AD: Apolipoprotein E alleles as risk factors in Alzheimer's disease. Annu Rev Med 47:387–400, 1996

Roses AD, Pericak-Vance MA, Dawson DV, et al: Standard likelihood and sib pair analyses in late onset Alzheimer's disease, in The Molecular Biology of Alzheimer's Disease (Current Communications in Molecular Biology). Edited by Davis P, Finch C. New York, Cold Spring Harbor Laboratory, 1988, pp 180–186

Roy A, Segal NL, Centerwall BS, et al: Suicide in twins. Arch Gen Psychiatry 48:29–32, 1991

Roy A, Segal NL, Sarchiapone M: Attempted suicide among living co-twins of twin suicide victims. Am J Psychiatry 152:1075–1076, 1995

Rubinsztein DC, Leggo J, Crow TJ, et al: Analysis of polyglutamine-coding repeats in the TATA-binding protein in different human populations and in patients with schizophrenia and bipolar affective disorder. Am J Med Genet 67:495–498, 1996

Rudin E: Zur Vererbung und Neuenstehung der Dementia Praecox. Berlin, Germany, Springer-Verlag, 1916

Rudrasingham V, Wavrant-De Vrieze F, Lambert JC, et al: Alpha-2 macroglobulin gene and Alzheimer disease. Nat Genet 22:17–19, 1999

Russ MJ, Lachman HM, Kashdan T, et al: Analysis of catechol-O-methyltransferase and 5-hydroxytryptamine transporter polymorphisms in patients at risk for suicide. Psychiatry Res 93:73–78, 2000

Sabate O, Campion D, d'Amato T, et al: Failure to find evidence for linkage or association between the dopamine D3 receptor gene and schizophrenia. Am J Psychiatry 151:107–111, 1994

Saha N, Tsoi WF, Low PS, et al: Lack of association of the dopamine D3 receptor gene polymorphism (BalI) in Chinese schizophrenic males. Psychiatr Genet 4:201–204, 1994

Sand PG, Godau C, Riederer P, et al: Exonic variants of the GABA(B) receptor gene and panic disorder. Psychiatr Genet 10:191–194, 2000

Sander T, Gscheidel N, Wendel B, et al: Human mu-opioid receptor variation and alcohol dependence. Alcohol Clin Exp Res 22:2108–2110, 1998

Sasaki T, Billett E, Petronis A, et al: Psychosis and genes with trinucleotide repeat polymorphism. Hum Genet 97:244–246, 1996a

Saunders AM, Strittmatter WJ, Schmechel D, et al: Association of apolipoprotein E allele epsilon 4 with late-onset familial and sporadic Alzheimer's disease. Neurology 43:1467–1472, 1993

Sautter F, McDermott B, Garver D: Familial differences between rapid neuroleptic response psychosis and delayed neuroleptic response psychosis. Biol Psychiatry 33:15–21, 1993

Sawcer S, Jones HB, Feakes R, et al: A genome screen in multiple sclerosis reveals susceptibility loci on chromosome 6p21 and 17q22. Nat Genet 13:464–468, 1996

Schellenberg GD, Bird TD, Wijsman EM, et al: Absence of linkage of chromosome 21q21 markers to familial Alzheimer's disease. Science 241:1507–1510, 1988

Schellenberg GD, Bird TD, Wijsman EM, et al: Genetic linkage evidence for a familial Alzheimer's disease locus on chromosome 14. Science 258:668–671, 1992

Schellenberg GD, D'Souza I, Poorkaj P: The genetics of Alzheimer's disease. Current Psychiatry Reports 2:158–164, 2000

Scherrer JF, True WR, Xian H, et al: Evidence for genetic influences common and specific to symptoms of generalized anxiety and panic. J Affect Disord 57:25–35, 2000

Schindler KM, Richter MA, Kennedy JL, et al: Association between homozygosity at the COMT gene locus and obsessive compulsive disorder. Am J Med Genet 96:721–724, 2000

Schizophrenia Linkage Collaborative Group for Chromosomes 3, 6, and 8: Additional support for schizophrenia linkage on chromosomes 6 and 8: a multicenter study. Am J Med Genet 67:580–594, 1996

Schmidt SM, Zoega T, Crowe RR: Excluding linkage between panic disorder and the gamma-aminobutyric acid beta 1 receptor locus in five Icelandic pedigrees. Acta Psychiatr Scand 88:225–228, 1993

Schulsinger F, Kety SS, Rosenthal D, et al: A family study of suicide, in Origin, Prevention and Treatment of Affective Disorders. Edited by Schou M, Stromgren E. New York, Academic Press, 1979, pp 277–287

Schulsinger F, Parnas J, Petersen ET, et al: Cerebral ventricular size in the offspring of schizophrenic mothers: a preliminary study. Arch Gen Psychiatry 41:602–606, 1984

Schwab SG, Albus M, Hallmayer J, et al: Evaluation of a susceptibility gene for schizophrenia on chromosome 6p by multipoint affected sib-pair linkage analysis. Nat Genet 11:325–327, 1995a

Schwab SG, Lerer B, Albus M, et al: Potential linkage for schizophrenia on chromosome 22q12–q13: a replication study. Am J Med Genet 60:436–443, 1995b

Schwab SG, Eckstein GN, Hallmayer J, et al: Evidence suggestive of a locus on chromosome 5q31 contributing to susceptibility for schizophrenia in German and Israeli families by multipoint affected sib-pair linkage analysis. Mol Psychiatry 2:156–160, 1997

Schwab SG, Hallmayer J, Albus M, et al: Further evidence for a susceptibility locus on chromosome 10p14-p11 in 72 families with schizophrenia by nonparametric linkage analysis. Am J Med Genet 81:302–307, 1998

Schwab SG, Hallmayer J, Albus M, et al: A genome-wide autosomal screen for schizophrenia susceptibility loci in 71 families with affected siblings: support for loci on chromosome 10p and 6. Mol Psychiatry 5:638–649, 2000

Scott WK, Roses AD, Haines JL, et al: Presenilin-1 polymorphism and Alzheimer's disease (letter). Lancet 347:1560, 1996

Scott WK, Grubber JM, Abou-Donia SM, et al: Further evidence linking late-onset Alzheimer disease with chromosome 12. JAMA 281:513–514, 1999

Scott WK, Grubber JM, Conneally PM, et al: Fine mapping of the chromosome 12 late-onset Alzheimer disease locus: potential genetic and phenotypic heterogeneity. Am J Hum Genet 66:922–932, 2000

Segman RH, Heresco-Levy U, Finkel B, et al: Association between the serotonin 2C receptor gene and tardive dyskinesia in chronic schizophrenia: additive contribution of 5-HT2Cser and DRD3gly alleles to susceptibility. Psychopharmacology (Berl) 152:408–413, 2000

Serretti A, Zanardi R, Cusin C, et al: Tryptophan hydroxylase gene associated with paroxetine antidepressant activity. Eur Neuropsychopharmacol 11:375–380, 2001a

Serretti A, Zanardi R, Rossini D, et al: Influence of tryptophan hydroxylase and serotonin transporter genes on fluvoxamine antidepressant activity. Mol Psychiatry 6:586–592, 2001b

Shafii M, Carrigan S, Whittinghill JR, et al: Psychological autopsy of completed suicide in children and adolescents. Am J Psychiatry 142:1061–1064, 1985

Sham PC, Jones P, Russell A, et al: Age at onset, sex, and familial psychiatric morbidity in schizophrenia: Camberwell Collaborative Psychosis Study. Br J Psychiatry 165:466–473, 1994

Shaw SH, Kelly M, Smith AB, et al: A genome-wide search for schizophrenia susceptibility genes. Am J Med Genet 81:364–376, 1998

Shen J, Bronson RT, Chen DF, et al: Skeletal and CNS defects in presenilin-1–deficient mice. Cell 89:629–639, 1997

Shenton ME, Solovay MR, Holzman PS, et al: Thought disorder in the relatives of psychotic patients. Arch Gen Psychiatry 46:897–901, 1989

Sherrington R, Brynjolfsson J, Petursson H, et al: Localization of a susceptibility locus for schizophrenia on chromosome 5. Nature 336:164–167, 1988

Sherrington R, Rogaev EI, Liang Y, et al: Cloning of a gene bearing missense mutations in early onset familial Alzheimer's disease. Nature 375:754–760, 1995

Silverman JM, Mohs RC, Davidson M, et al: Familial schizophrenia and treatment response. Am J Psychiatry 144:1271–1276, 1987

Silverman JM, Greenberg DA, Altstiel LD, et al: Evidence of a locus for schizophrenia and related disorders on the short arm of chromosome 5 in a large pedigree. Am J Med Genet 67:162–171, 1996

Silverman JM, Smith CJ, Guo SL, et al: Lateral ventricular enlargement in schizophrenic probands and their siblings with schizophrenia-related disorders. Biol Psychiatry 43:97–106, 1998

Skre I, Torgersen S, Lygren S, et al: A twin study of DSM-III-R anxiety disorders. Acta Psychiatr Scand 88:85–92, 1993

Smeraldi E, Zanardi R, Benedetti F, et al: Polymorphism within the promoter of the serotonin transporter gene and antidepressant efficacy of fluvoxamine. Mol Psychiatry 3:508–511, 1998

Smoller JW, Acierno JS Jr, Rosenbaum JF, et al: Targeted genome screen of panic disorder and anxiety disorder proneness using homology to murine QTL regions. Am J Med Genet 105:195–206, 2001

Smyth C, Kalsi G, Brynjolfsson J, et al: Further tests for linkage of bipolar affective disorder to the tyrosine hydroxylase gene locus on chromosome 11p15 in a new series of multiplex British affective disorder pedigrees. Am J Psychiatry 153:271–274, 1996

Snyder EY, Park KI, Flax JD, et al: Potential of neural "stem-like" cells for gene therapy and repair of the degenerating central nervous system. Adv Neurol 72:121–132, 1997

Solimena M, De Camilli P: Coxsackieviruses and diabetes [published erratum appears in Nat Med 1:272, 1995]. Nat Med 1:25–26, 1995

Sorbi S, Nacmias B, Tedde A, et al: 5-HT2A promoter polymorphism in anorexia nervosa (letter). Lancet 351:1785, 1998

Souery D, Lipp O, Mahieu B, et al: Excess tyrosine hydroxylase restriction fragment length polymorphism homozygosity in unipolar but not bipolar patients: a preliminary report. Biol Psychiatry 40:305–308, 1996

Spence MA, Flodman PL, Sadovnick AD, et al: Bipolar disorder: evidence for a major locus. Am J Med Genet 60:370–376, 1995

Spitzer RL, Endicott J, Robins E: Research Diagnostic Criteria: rationale and reliability. Arch Gen Psychiatry 35:773–782, 1978

Squires-Wheeler E, Skodol AE, Bassett A, et al: DSM-III-R schizotypal personality traits in offspring of schizophrenic disorder, affective disorder, and normal control parents. J Psychiatr Res 23:229–239, 1989

St George-Hyslop PH, Tanzi RE, Polinsky RJ, et al: The genetic defect causing familial Alzheimer's disease maps on chromosome 21. Science 235:885–890, 1987

St George-Hyslop PH, Myers R, Haines JL, et al: Familial Alzheimer's disease: progress and problems. Neurobiol Aging 10:417–425, 1989

St George-Hyslop PH, Haines JL, Farrer LA, et al: Genetic linkage studies suggest that Alzheimer's disease is not a single homogeneous disorder. Nature 347:194–197, 1990

St George-Hyslop P, Haines J, Rogaev E, et al: Genetic evidence for a novel familial Alzheimer's disease locus on chromosome 14. Nat Genet 2:330–334, 1992

Stassen HH, Coppola R, Gottesman II, et al: EEG differences in monozygotic twins discordant and concordant for schizophrenia. Psychophysiology 36:109–117, 1999

Statham DJ, Heath AC, Madden PA, et al: Suicidal behaviour: an epidemiological and genetic study. Psychol Med 28:839–855, 1998

Stein MB, Chartier MJ, Hazen AL, et al: A direct-interview family study of generalized social phobia. Am J Psychiatry 155:90–97, 1998a

Stein MB, Chartier MJ, Kozak MV, et al: Genetic linkage to the serotonin transporter protein and 5HT2A receptor genes excluded in generalized social phobia. Psychiatry Res 81:283–291, 1998b

Stine OC, Xu J, Koskela R, et al: Evidence for linkage of bipolar disorder to chromosome 18 with a parent-of-origin effect. Am J Hum Genet 57:1384–1394, 1995

Stober G, Saar K, Ruschendorf F, et al: Splitting schizophrenia: periodic catatonia-susceptibility locus on chromosome 15q15. Am J Hum Genet 67:1201–1207, 2000

Straub RE, Lehner T, Luo Y, et al: A possible vulnerability locus for bipolar affective disorder on chromosome 21q22.3. Nat Genet 8:291–296, 1994

Straub RE, MacLean CJ, O'Neill FA, et al: A potential vulnerability locus for schizophrenia on chromosome 6p24–22: evidence for genetic heterogeneity. Nat Genet 11:287–293, 1995

Straub RE, MacLean CJ, O'Neill FA, et al: Support for a possible schizophrenia vulnerability locus in region 5q21–31 in Irish families. Mol Psychiatry 2:148–155, 1997

Straub RE, MacLean CJ, Martin RB, et al: A schizophrenia locus may be located in region 10p15-p11. Am J Med Genet 81:296–301, 1998

Straub RE, Sullivan PF, Ma Y, et al: Susceptibility genes for nicotine dependence: a genome scan and followup in an independent sample suggest that regions on chromosomes 2, 4, 10, 16, 17 and 18 merit further study. Mol Psychiatry 4:129–144, 1999

Strittmatter WJ, Saunders AM, Schmechel D, et al: Apolipoprotein E: high-avidity binding to beta-amyloid and increased frequency of type 4 allele in late-onset familial Alzheimer disease. Proc Natl Acad Sci U S A 90:1977–1981, 1993

Strober M, Morell W, Burroughs J, et al: A controlled family study of anorexia nervosa. J Psychiatr Res 19:239–246, 1985

Strober M, Lampert C, Morrell W, et al: A controlled family study of anorexia nervosa: evidence of familial aggregation and lack of shared transmission of affective disorders. Int J Eat Disord 9:239–253, 1990

Strober M, Freeman R, Lampert C, et al: Controlled family study of anorexia nervosa and bulimia nervosa: evidence of shared liability and transmission of partial syndromes. Am J Psychiatry 157:393–401, 2000

Suarez BK, Cox NJ: Linkage analysis for psychiatric disorders, I: basic concepts. Psychiatric Developments 3:219–243, 1985

Suarez BK, Rice J, Reich T: The generalized sib pair IBD distribution: its use in the detection of linkage. Ann Hum Genet 42:87–94, 1978

Suddath RL, Christison GW, Torrey EF, et al: Anatomical abnormalities in the brains of monozygotic twins discordant for schizophrenia. N Engl J Med 322:789–794, 1990

Sugarman PA, Craufurd D: Schizophrenia in the Afro-Caribbean community. Br J Psychiatry 164:474–480, 1994

Sullivan PF, Neale MC, Kendler KS: Genetic epidemiology of major depression: review and meta-analysis. Am J Psychiatry 157:1552–1562, 2000

Sundaramurthy D, Pieri LF, Gape H, et al: Analysis of the serotonin transporter gene linked polymorphism (5-HTTLPR) in anorexia nervosa. Am J Med Genet 96:53–55, 2000

Svrakic DM, Whitehead C, Przybeck TR, et al: Differential diagnosis of personality disorders by the seven-factor model of temperament and character. Arch Gen Psychiatry 50:991–999, 1993

Swan GE, Carmelli D, Cardon LR: Heavy consumption of cigarettes, alcohol and coffee in male twins. J Stud Alcohol 58:182–190, 1997

Talbot C, Houlden H, Craddock N, et al: Polymorphism in AACT gene may lower age of onset of Alzheimer's disease. Neuroreport 7:534–536, 1996

Tanaka T, Igarashi S, Onodera O, et al: Association study between schizophrenia and dopamine D3 receptor gene polymorphism. Am J Med Genet 67:366–368, 1996

The Collaborative Study on the Genetics of Asthma (CSGA): A genome-wide search for asthma susceptibility loci in ethnically diverse populations. Nat Genet 15:389–392, 1997

Thomasson HR, Edenberg HJ, Crabb DW, et al: Alcohol and aldehyde dehydrogenase genotypes and alcoholism in Chinese men. Am J Hum Genet 48:677–681, 1991

Tienari P, Wynne LC, Moring J, et al: The Finnish adoptive family study of schizophrenia: implications for family research. Br J Psychiatry 23(suppl):20–26, 1994

Tienari P, Wynne LC, Moring J, et al: Finnish adoptive family study: sample selection and adoptee DSM-III-R diagnoses. Acta Psychiatr Scand 101:433–443, 2000

Torgersen S: Genetic factors in anxiety disorders. Arch Gen Psychiatry 40:1085–1089, 1983

Torgersen S: Genetics of somatoform disorders. Arch Gen Psychiatry 43:502–505, 1986

Torgersen S: Comorbidity of major depression and anxiety disorders in twin pairs. Am J Psychiatry 147:1199–1202, 1990

Town T, Abdullah L, Crawford F, et al: Association of a functional mu-opioid receptor allele (+118A) with alcohol dependency. Am J Med Genet 88:458–461, 1999

True WR, Rice J, Eisen SA, et al: A twin study of genetic and environmental contributions to liability for posttraumatic stress symptoms. Arch Gen Psychiatry 50:257–264, 1993

True WR, Xian H, Scherrer JF, et al: Common genetic vulnerability for nicotine and alcohol dependence in men. Arch Gen Psychiatry 56:655–661, 1999

Tsuang MT: Genetic counseling for psychiatric patients and their families. Am J Psychiatry 135:1465–1475, 1978

Tsuang MT: Risk of suicide in the relatives of schizophrenics, manics, depressives, and controls. J Clin Psychiatry 44:396–400, 1983

Tsuang MT, Lyons MJ: Drawing the boundary of the schizophrenia spectrum: evidence from a family study, in Schizophrenia: Scientific Progress. Edited by Schultz SC, Tamminga CA. New York, Oxford University Press, 1989, pp 23–27

Tsuang MT, Bucher KD, Fleming JA: Testing the monogenic theory of schizophrenia: an application of segregation analysis to blind family study data. Br J Psychiatry 140:595–599, 1982

Tsuang MT, Gilbertson MW, Faraone SV: Genetic transmission of negative and positive symptoms in the biological relatives of schizophrenics, in Positive vs. Negative Schizophrenia. Edited by Marneros A, Tsuang MT, Andreasen N. New York, Springer-Verlag, 1991, pp 265–291

Tsuang MT, Faraone SV, Kremen W, et al: Familial connections with deficit syndrome. Paper presented at the 145th annual meeting of the American Psychiatric Association, Washington, DC, May 2–7, 1992

Tsuang MT, Lyons MJ, Meyer JM, et al: Co-occurrence of abuse of different drugs in men: the role of drug-specific and shared vulnerabilities. Arch Gen Psychiatry 55:967–972, 1998

Turecki G, De AC, Smith M, et al: Type I bipolar disorder associated with a fragile site on chromosome 1. Am J Med Genet 60:179–182, 1995

Turecki G, Rouleau GA, Mari J, et al: Lack of association between bipolar disorder and tyrosine hydroxylase: a meta-analysis. Am J Med Genet 74:348–352, 1997

Turecki G, Zhu Z, Tzenova J, et al: TPH and suicidal behavior: a study in suicide completers. Mol Psychiatry 6:98–102, 2001

Uhl G, Blum K, Noble E, et al: Substance abuse vulnerability and D2 receptor genes. Trends Neurosci 16:83–88, 1993

Valevski A, Klein T, Gazit E, et al: HLA-B38 and clozapine-induced agranulocytosis in Israeli Jewish schizophrenic patients. Eur J Immunogenet 25:11–13, 1998

Vallada H, Curtis D, Sham PC, et al: Chromosome 22 markers demonstrate transmission disequilibrium with schizophrenia. Psychiatr Genet 5:127–130, 1995a

Vallada HP, Gill M, Sham P, et al: Linkage studies on chromosome 22 in familial schizophrenia. Am J Med Genet 60:139–146, 1995b

van Beek N, Griez E: Reactivity to a 35% CO2 challenge in healthy first-degree relatives of patients with panic disorder. Biol Psychiatry 47:830–835, 2000

Van Broeckhoven C, van Hul W, Backhoven H, et al: The familial Alzheimer gene is located close to the centromere of chromosome 21 (abstract). Am J Hum Genet 43:A205, 1988

Van Broeckhoven C, Backhoven H, Cruts M, et al: Mapping of a gene predisposing to early onset Alzheimer's disease to chromosome 14q24.3. Nat Genet 2:335–339, 1992

Vanyukov MM, Tarter RE: Genetic studies of substance abuse. Drug Alcohol Depend 59:101–123, 2000

Veenstra-VanderWeele J, Kim SJ, Gonen D, et al: Genomic organization of the SLC1A1/EAAC1 gene and mutation screening in early onset obsessive-compulsive disorder. Mol Psychiatry 6:160–167, 2001

Venter JC, Adams MD, Myers EW, et al: The sequence of the human genome. Science 291:1304–1351, 2001

Vincent JB, Klempan T, Parikh SS, et al: Frequency analysis of large CAG/CTG trinucleotide repeats in schizophrenia and bipolar affective disorder. Mol Psychiatry 1:141–148, 1996

Vink T, Hinney A, van Elburg AA, et al: Association between an agouti-related protein gene polymorphism and anorexia nervosa. Mol Psychiatry 6:325–328, 2001

Vogler GP, Gottesman II, McGue MK, et al: Mixed-model segregation analysis of schizophrenia in the Lindelius Swedish pedigrees. Behav Genet 20:461–472, 1990

von Knorring A-L, Cloninger CR, Bohman M, et al: An adoption study of depressive disorders and substance abuse. Arch Gen Psychiatry 40:943–950, 1983

Wade TD, Bulik CM, Neale M, et al: Anorexia nervosa and major depression: shared genetic and environmental risk factors. Am J Psychiatry 157:469–471, 2000

Waldo MC, Carey G, Myles-Worsley M, et al: Codistribution of a sensory gating deficit and schizophrenia in multi-affected families. Psychiatr Res 39:257–268, 1991

Walker E, Downey G, Caspi A: Twin studies of psychopathology: why do the concordance rates vary? Schizophr Res 5:211–221, 1991

Wang Z, Crowe RR, Tanna VL, et al: Alpha 2 adrenergic receptor subtypes in depression: a candidate gene study. J Affect Disord 25:191–196, 1992

Wang Z, Valdes J, Noyes R, et al: Possible association of a cholecystokinin promotor polymorphism (CCK-36CT) with panic disorder. Am J Med Genet 81:228–234, 1998

Warwick DE, Payami H, Nemens EJ, et al: The number of trait loci in late-onset Alzheimer disease. Am J Hum Genet 66:196–204, 2000

Watt NF, Anthony EJ, Wynne LC, et al (eds): Children at Risk for Schizophrenia: A Longitudinal Perspective. Cambridge, England, Cambridge University Press, 1984

Weinberger DR, Berman KF, Suddath R, et al: Evidence of dysfunction of a prefrontal-limbic network in schizophrenia: a magnetic resonance imaging and regional cerebral blood flow study of discordant monozygotic twins. Am J Psychiatry 149:890–897, 1992

Weiss KM: Genetic Variation and Human Disease. Cambridge, England, Cambridge University Press, 1993, pp 229

Weiss KM: Genetic Variation and Human Disease: Principles and Evolutionary Approaches. Cambridge, England, Cambridge University Press, 1995

Weissman MM, Members of the Cross-National Collaborative Group: The changing rate of major depression: cross-national comparisons. JAMA 268:3098–3105, 1992

Weissman MM, Gershon ES, Kidd KK, et al: Psychiatric disorders in the relatives of probands with affective disorders: the Yale University-National Institute of Mental Health Collaborative Study. Arch Gen Psychiatry 41:13–21, 1984a

Weissman MM, Wickramaratne P, Merikangas KR, et al: Onset of major depression in early childhood: increased familial loading and specificity. Arch Gen Psychiatry 41:1136–1143, 1984b

Weissman MM, Warner V, Wickramaratne P, et al: Early onset major depression in parents and their children. J Affect Disord 15:269–277, 1988

Weissman MM, Wickramaratne P, Adams PB, et al: The relationship between panic disorder and major depression: a new family study. Arch Gen Psychiatry 50:767–780, 1993

Weissman MM, Fyer AJ, Haghighi F, et al: A potential panic disorder syndrome: clinical and genetic linkage evidence. Am J Med Genet 96:24–35, 2000

Wender PH, Rosenthal D, Kety SS, et al: Crossfostering: a research strategy for clarifying the role of genetic and experiential factors in the etiology of schizophrenia. Arch Gen Psychiatry 30:121–128, 1974

Wender PH, Kety SS, Rosenthal D, et al: Psychiatric disorders in the biological and adoptive families of adopted individuals with affective disorders. Arch Gen Psychiatry 43:923–929, 1986

Williams J, McGuffin P, Nothen M, et al: Meta-analysis of association between the 5-HT2a receptor T102C polymorphism and schizophrenia (letter). EMASS Collaborative Group. European Multicentre Association Study of Schizophrenia. Lancet 349:1221, 1997

Williams J, Spurlock G, Holmans P, et al: A meta-analysis and transmission disequilibrium study of association between the dopamine D3 receptor gene and schizophrenia. Mol Psychiatry 3:141–149, 1998

Winokur G, Cadoret R, Baker M, et al: Depressive spectrum disease versus pure depressive disease: some further data. Br J Psychiatry 127:75–77, 1975

Wittchen HU, Reed V, Kessler RC: The relationship of agoraphobia and panic in a community sample of adolescents and young adults. Arch Gen Psychiatry 55:1017–1024, 1998

Wong PC, Zheng H, Chen H, et al: Presenilin 1 is required for Notch 1 and Dll1 expression in the paraxial mesoderm. Nature 387:288–292, 1997

Wooster R, Neuhausen SL, Mangion J, et al: Localization of a breast cancer susceptibility gene, BRCA2, to chromosome 13q12–13. Science 265:2088–2090, 1994

Wooster R, Bignell G, Lancaster J, et al: Identification of the breast cancer susceptibility gene BRCA2. Nature 378:789–792, 1995

World Health Organization: The ICD-10 Classification of Mental and Behavioral Disorders. Geneva, Switzerland, World Health Organization, 1992

Wragg M, Hutton M, Talbot C: Genetic association between intronic polymorphism in presenilin-1 gene and late-onset Alzheimer's disease: Alzheimer's Disease Collaborative Group. Lancet 347:509–512, 1996

Wright P, Takei N, Rifkin L, et al: Maternal influenza, obstetric complications, and schizophrenia. Am J Psychiatry 152:1714–1720, 1995

Wu WS, Holmans P, Wavrant-DeVrieze F, et al: Genetic studies on chromosome 12 in late-onset Alzheimer disease [see comments]. JAMA 280:619–622, 1998

Xian H, Chantarujikapong SI, Scherrer JF, et al: Genetic and environmental influences on posttraumatic stress disorder, alcohol and drug dependence in twin pairs. Drug Alcohol Depend 61:95–102, 2000a

Xian H, Scherrer JF, Eisen SA, et al: Self-reported zygosity and the equal-environments assumption for psychiatric disorders in the Vietnam Era Twin Registry. Behav Genet 30:303–310, 2000b

Xu J, Meyers DA, Ober C, et al: Genomewide screen and identification of gene-gene interactions for asthma-susceptibility loci in three U.S. populations: Collaborative Study on the Genetics of Asthma. Am J Hum Genet 68:1437–1446, 2001

Yu YW, Tsai SJ, Yang KH, et al: Evidence for an association between polymorphism in the serotonin-2A receptor variant (102T/C) and increment of N100 amplitude in schizo-phrenics treated with clozapine. Neuropsychobiology 43:79–82, 2001

Yudofsky SC, Hales RE: The American Psychiatric Publishing Textbook of Neuropsychiatry and Clinical Neurosciences, 4th Edition. Washington, DC, American Psychiatric Publishing, 2002

Zalsman G, Frisch A, Bromberg M, et al: Family based association study of serotonin transporter promoter in suicidal adolescents: no association with suicidality but possible role in violence traits. Am J Med Genet 105:239–245, 2001

Zanardi R, Benedetti F, Di Bella D, et al: Efficacy of paroxetine in depression is influenced by a functional polymorphism within the promoter of the serotonin transporter gene. J Clin Psychopharmacol 20:105–107, 2000

Zanardi R, Serretti A, Rossini D, et al: Factors affecting fluvox-amine antidepressant activity: influence of pindolol and 5-HTTLPR in delusional and nondelusional depression. Biol Psychiatry 50:323–330, 2001

Ziegler A, Hebebrand J, Gorg T, et al: Further lack of association between the 5-HT2A gene promoter polymorphism and susceptibility to eating disorders and a meta-analysis pertaining to anorexia nervosa. Mol Psychiatry 4:410–412, 1999

CHAPTER 2

Normal Child and Adolescent Development

Theodore Shapiro, M.D.

Margaret E. Hertzig, M.D.

The current focus in modern psychiatry on descriptive nomenclatures, diagnosis, and treatment does not necessarily include a developmental point of view. On the other hand, there are strong historical and clinical reasons why any student of personality and pathology within a medical framework should be interested in what is known about the normal developmental process—its stages, phases, inhibitions, impediments, and deviances. Moreover, the roots of the inquiry are within medicine and within psychiatry in particular.

Historical Background

As far back as the Enlightenment, psychiatrists such as Pinel recorded longitudinal histories from patients in the French asylums in and about Paris. Pinel's understanding that psychopathology in adulthood may have something to do with life history or past social circumstance is deeply ingrained in the notion of "humane treatment" that followed. He struck the chains of the insane just as the ideas of the Quaker layman William Tuke, about treating patients without physical restraints, took hold in England. In the United States, Adolf Meyer, founder of the concept of psychobiology, emphasized the life event chart as a mainstay of clinical knowledge.

While these trends in general psychiatry held sway, Freud (1905/1953), at the beginning of the twentieth century, elaborated the idea that the first 5 years of life had a determining effect on later psychopathology and development. Whether one reads this as a strict rule of early influence or more loosely as a complementary series

of intrinsic and extrinsic weightings, the view certainly echoed a trend that became a part of the medical mentality, adumbrated by the poet Wordsworth, who wrote "The child is father to the man."

From a more general medical vantage point, because there was so much to be learned about normal developmental processes for well baby care and so many skills to be gained in dealing with children of all ages, a more specialized training seemed to be required. As a result, pediatrics was split off from general medicine. Most pediatricians consider themselves practitioners of developmental medicine. Thus, the notions of developmental medicine and developmental psychiatry are the historical roots from which specific areas of knowledge and skill have grown. Such increased awareness has compelled us to look at normal growth and development as a key component of our work as well as an essential basis for etiological thought.

There are also important historical roots outside of medicine that have determined, in part, how we think about development. The language of developmental psychology derives from Darwin's linking of variation in forms of life to their survival value in evolution. Darwin's formulations then led to Ernst Haeckel's biogenetic law that "ontogeny recapitulates phylogeny." This series of events, barely skimmed here, served to turn biologists and physicians into students of embryology. Indeed, the language of embryology has been adopted in the literature of developmental psychology and medicine. Concepts such as maturation, development, differentiation, pleiomorphism, and organizers all have been borrowed from embryology and have enriched our understanding of how children start to be, beginning with gametization, embryogenesis, and then birth and progressing to later developmental stages that can be observed and staged. In fact, the same terms used in embryology have been adapted for use in psychosocial development.

Developmental Principles

The starting point for our understanding of the general principles of development is the Darwinian notion of small brood in conjunction with prolonged caretaking because of the relative immaturity of those structures that permit independent survival. Freud (1905/1953), working from this viewpoint, was then able to conceive of the neuroses as an accrual of the prolonged dependency and caring necessary for the human infant before independence, and ultimately survival, could be ensured.

The terms *growth*, *maturation*, and *development*, although used imprecisely in common parlance, connote a direction from more global reactiveness to more specified reactiveness and from a less complex organization to a more complex state of organization (Table 2–1). *Growth* usually refers to the simple accretion of tissue (i.e., an increase in size or in the number of cells). Changes in height and weight are examples of growth. *Maturation* is a convenient fiction that has a somewhat teleological implication of a direction toward which the individual is headed in accord with his or her functions, abilities, structures, and competencies. In its most narrow meaning, the term suggests that there is a natural unfolding of genetic potential toward an end that is known as "maturity." This end can come about in average, expectable environments given the premise that the organism has average species-specific biological equipment. The concept does not invoke the variation that may occur in certain special ecologies. *Development*, on the other hand, includes whatever the maturational potential provides plus the variations in social and environmental influence. This concept refers to the changing structure of behavior and thought over time.

Many of the issues of developmental psychology and psychiatry concern the limiting factors that will prevent, alter, or render maturation sequences retarded or deviant. Normative studies suggest a cephalocaudal developmental sequence, with the head end of the organism at the beginning of life presenting as a more highly differentiated functional entity than the tail end. Biological forces such as myelinization of the central long tracts progressing from head to toe help us to understand that regardless of the cultural variation in the early months, most human children begin to walk between the ages of 10 and 18 months (Gesell and Amatruda 1947). This will occur whether the infant is bound to a pallet by its Native American mother or is permitted to kick free in an apartment in New York. Similarly, along with the achievement of that motor landmark, the landmarks of language development occur in a lockstep sequence. However, to add complexity, each line of development may mature independently, such as in a limited cerebral palsy affecting only the small section of the cortex that controls limb motor pathways.

Moreover, no matter what language is spoken by the parent, most 1-year-olds acquire the equivalent designations "Mama," "Dada," and one additional word. By 18 months the 20- to 50-word vocabulary is expressed in single-word utterances (Gesell and Amatruda 1947). By the time the child is 2 years old, he or she usually can string together two- and sometimes three-word utterances with some competence in grammatical formatting. Such vocalizations appear as telegraphic utterances in which the small units of meaning that signify past, plural, etc., known as *grammatical morphemes*, are omitted. The addition of grammatical morphemes occurs next, as toddlers take on the job of making sentences (R. Brown 1973). This maturational sequence does not mean that children do not make errors, but they do seem to be capable of forming the language units appropriately. The errors that are made derive from overgeneralization of grammatical rules and are not random.

From the developmental vantage, these maturational regularities are acted on by social nurturing influences; the achievements are not entirely innate. For example, if a child is tied down or forced to remain recumbent, the maturational event of walking surely will be delayed because of muscular disuse. Nonetheless, walking is a somewhat irrepressible landmark, given biologically normal equipment and the opportunity to exercise. Similarly, although the capacity for language and grammar may be built in, children will not achieve speech and language in the usual manner if they are deaf or if they are not spoken to. Moreover, it is impossible that children growing up in a German-speaking world, for example, will speak Italian or vice versa. Thus, environment has a significant influence on the developmental sequence of *what language* is spoken rather than *that a language is spoken*.

Differentiation and Integration

Maturation within individual systems also requires that we consider another central theme in development, *differentiation*. Just as the blastosphere differentiates into endoderm, ectoderm, and mesoderm, and these further

TABLE 2–1. Developmental principles (examples in each domain)

	Neurological	Biobehavioral	Intrapsychic	Social
Growth	Increasing length of neuronal axon; dendritic proliferation			
Maturation	Myelinization of axons	Palmar to pincer grasp; supine to prone; increasing axial control—sitting to walking	Fantasy level concerns—body themes to resolution of Oedipus complex; fearing loss of mother to fearing loss of love	Move from parent to peers and increasing intimacy
Development	Functional feedback of experience on selective dendritic proliferation	Acquisition of the speech of surround grafted on language universals	Using experience with others as feedback to relations, social referencing	Increasing arena of interactions, including peers
Differentiation	Neuronal specificity by regions; special senses; selective neurotransmitter areas	Pincer grasp; lexical discrimination and specificity	Appreciation of qualities of object that distinguish it from others; social smile to separation anxiety	Specificity of peer preferences; social group formation and selectivity
Integration	Increasing interhemispheric tracts; establishment of cerebral dominance	Grasp what is seen; syntactic organization; word-meaning	Good objects can be bad; affective regulation of impulse	Increasing capacity to adapt from one group to others

mature into more highly differentiated tissues, so, analogously, do psychological and social systems differentiate. The newborn infant's grasp reflex traverses a known series of steps to its final form in the distinctively human pincer grasp. Although the newborn can distinguish between patterned visual stimuli, it is only later that colors, shapes, forms, and faces become meaningfully differentiated as familiar, hostile, friendly, or frightening. In a psychological sense, the general arousal of infants differentiates selectively into responses signifying that the child distinguishes between human and nonhuman, mother and nonmother, friend and foe.

Integration also emerges between and among the varying senses. In the beginning the eye sees what impinges on it; the hand grasps that which is put into it. At 3 or 4 months, if the child sees the hand and the thing to be grasped in the same visual field, he or she will grasp. It is not until some time later that the child reaches for that which he or she sees even if the hand is not in the visual field. The ultimate capacities to, for example, shoot a basket, hit a ball, draw in imitation of nature, and tap out a tune require higher levels of integration between and among the senses and the motor apparatus. At a psychological level, the capacity to put together good and bad experiences with a person and also to change set in relation to varying exposures requires integration. As the infant, showing more differentiated and inte-

grated functioning, moves from the more global apprehension of the world, he or she may also lose some functions that were natively available. There is evidence, for example, that the infant can make distinctions between phonetic forms at 4 months, but he or she loses this ability when such forms become no longer useful in the language that is spoken (Eimas et al. 1971). By 6 months, infants pay special selective attention to phonemes that characterize the speech they hear (Kuhl 1992).

Hierarchic Reorganization and Critical Periods

As each stage unfolds, the question arises as to whether it could unfold without the child having had to pass through the prior stage. *Epigenesis* is the concept of sequential steps influencing subsequent steps. Each stage in that model is highly dependent on resolution of the experiences of the prior stage. The epigenetic vantage point permits, but it does not necessarily include, another model that is known as *hierarchic reorganization*. Heinz Werner (1957) introduced this concept to indicate that development not only can be conceived of as linear, but perhaps also may involve changing structures over time that permit alterations in organization that are not the logical or necessary outcome of prior stages.

Instead, each new integration of biological and neuronal function meshes with psychocognitive capacities that are more than the sum of their parts. Each stage is truly a new structure permitting functions and adaptations that are not easily predicted from their precursors. These reorganizations permit the next level of behavior and competence as the child pulls himself or herself along the chronological ladder. However, there is evidence to suggest both linear and discontinuous progression in the developmental course.

Invoking a hierarchically reorganized sequence permits consideration of a concept known as *critical periods*, which has been stressed by ethologists. Critical periods require that an environmental releaser stimulate the emergence of a developmental capacity that is inborn and ready for use only within a limited time period. If no release occurs, the function is said to *involute*. Such releasers may not adequately describe the way in which human biological development takes place (Schneirla and Rosenblatt 1961). The time lines are not as critically limited as in other mammals, and thus we should be cautious in applying data across species. Reorganization may occur in hierarchic fashion on the basis of independent neural and cognitive lines of maturation rather than by requiring that the organism go through certain specific and critical experiences. Indeed, Schneirla and Rosenblatt (1961) indicated that some species require continuous biological influence to effect social behavior (which is known as *biosocial organization*). Other species obey rules of recency, and earliest experience may not be as prolonged in its influence (which is known as *psychosocial organization*). In one extreme case, a child who had not been spoken to from 18 months to 15 years was taught sufficient language to converse, to make her needs known, and to carry out basic communication (Curtiss 1981). However, in this cruel "experiment," the child had been bound and abused.

The foregoing describes an emergent child. However, recent data support the idea of a *competent* infant (Spelke 1998). This does not mean an infant that is fully functional at birth, but rather one that has many functions in place, even during the first 6 months. The readiness of the preformed structures is then enhanced by experience, and the central nervous system (CNS) dendritic proliferation reinforces the connections that account for later competence. New methods of inquiry have increased our knowledge of the basic substructures that subsume the many functions of the young organism.

Developmental Psychologies

It should be evident by now that there are various approaches to the study of development, each of which is based on different sets of data derived from looking at children using different observational techniques. All developmentalists explore questions of how children move from point A to point B over time. Indeed, what follows will necessarily indicate that the formulations available about developmental stages are all bound by a particular method. The empirical support for each stage is highly dependent on the experimental method used, and therefore there is not one developmental psychology, but rather a number of developmental psychologies, each of which is identified by the unique ideas of a particular investigator or technique of observation.

In terms of the psychiatric outlook, most psychiatrists are well versed in the retrospective reconstructive attitude of the Freudian developmental system. However, early psychoanalysts did not observe children, except as a derivative aspect of the genetic point of view. The *genetic point of view* was Freud's attempt to retrospectively divine the infantile roots of adult behavior and pathology. His assumptions of polymorphously perverse infantile sexuality and the maturational sequences described in libido theory were based on retrospective reconstructions of how men and women seem to organize their fantasy lives. Later psychoanalytic thinkers (e.g., Mahler et al. 1975; Spitz 1965) looked at children directly and created their own developmental systems that elaborated Freud's system.

The behavioral vantage point, which was well outlined in the initial work of Watson (1919) and then B.F. Skinner (1953), is based on learning theory and takes a Lockean philosophical position in which experience is said to be inscribed on a blank slate of mind, thereby transforming it. No competence becomes possible that is not learned. Furthermore, nothing can be learned that is not within the capacity of the species, which in turn determines the limits of responsiveness. The virtue of a learning model for development is that such a model can be empirically apprehended and there is little inferred substructure and very few intervening variables.

Jean Piaget, the most important progenitor of modern cognitive psychology, introduced a complex system during the first half of the twentieth century suggesting that experience alone cannot account for the child's understanding of the world (Piaget and Inhelder 1969). In fact, Piaget set out to determine how intelligent behavior evolves. Calling himself a "genetic epistemologist" concerned only with non–affect-laden behavior, he addressed the issue of how children strategically arrive at right or wrong answers by means of their native capacities and regularized sequence of stages.

The normative developmental theory of Arnold Gesell (Gesell and Amatruda 1947) is more closely related to those of the learning theorists, but within the medical framework. Gesell attempted to unify the biological and neurodevelopmental principles that were available at that time from embryogenesis and the normative sequences of observed behaviors. His work was an important precursor to the concepts of normative stage–phase capacities and behaviors. Gesell's studies inspired others to examine large numbers of children "cross-sectionally" in order to find out what they do at each chronological age. These findings were then used to determine the limits of normal distribution and deviance within the range of the tasks presented. These cross-sectional, normative approaches established the essential empirical basis from which more highly theoretical proposals emerged.

Normative, cross-sectional studies, however, do not tell how one progresses (i.e., the process) throughout the longitudinal cycle from one stage to another. *Longitudinal studies* more easily address such issues. Although longitudinal studies are not generally reported in terms of how child A responds at point X and then at point Y, investigators in such studies do have the potential to do just that: to track developmental facts in individual subjects at varying stages, looking for outcomes from past behaviors and checking on retrospective suggestions.

Human development has always been studied by analogy. Investigators become impatient because of the longevity of humans and look for quicker ways of determining sequencing and invariance. Thus, animal models are employed, and in human development, analogy and homology to ethological studies of nonhuman species are sought. The effects of imprinting, inborn response systems, and species-specific releasers have been well studied in various animals. However, outside the ethological frame, other animal observers (Harlow 1960; Schneirla and Rosenblatt 1961) have questioned ideas such as critical periods and have produced more interesting models that do not depend as heavily on postulates of innateness. Rather, such models suggest that each emergent behavior can be tracked to precursor experiences and that the essence of a developmental analysis involves just such an exploration. However, a number of major human developmental theories, such as that of John Bowlby's (1969, 1973, 1980) attachment model, have grown out of work with nonhuman species.

Thus, to study normal development we have to inquire about developmental paths and investigative biases, models, and tools. In this brief outline of the central developmental positions, our interest is in these issues in the context of the needs of physicians and psychiatrists. In addition, another matter will become apparent. Many mechanisms and processes are postulated as

maturational, but a central concern remains for developmental psychology to determine *what* moves the individual from stage to stage—what pilot guides both biological and social adaptations. Such process variables tend to be less prominent than observed landmarks and behaviors.

The most influential points of view are described in their essentials to introduce the beginning developmentalist to some of the language and theory of each developmental system. We discuss as representative developmental positions the psychoanalytic perspective and the work of Piaget, Gesell, and Bowlby.

Psychoanalytic Developmental Viewpoint

The psychoanalytic view of childhood (Table 2–2) derives from two sources. The first source (i.e., *genetic*) uses retrospective and reconstructive inferences about the patient's past to construct a coherent and plausible sequenced history. The other source (i.e., *developmental*), based on the prospective studies by psychoanalytically oriented observers, attempts to observationally flesh out the models of development derived from the genetic point of view. Thus, we can distinguish initially between genetic and developmental aspects of psychoanalytic theory.

The Freudian Perspective

Freud's initial view of childhood as a period of polymorphously perverse infantile sexuality grew out of his observation that adult disorder reveals certain constant, compelling features. Adult sexuality consists not only of coitus and gametization, but of erotic arousal that depends on stimulation of various bodily zones. Perverse activity and normal foreplay both led to arousal and orgasmic behavior. In Freud's view, neurotic individuals did not dare think about the things that perverse individuals perpetrated. On these grounds, Freud suggested that repression was the prime mechanism that both hid and modified early sexual thoughts from the conscious minds of neurotic individuals. Libido theory was introduced to describe the maturational sequence that children were expected to traverse en route to adulthood. The theory included the active and passive aims of children seen retrospectively in relation to their primary objects, mother and father. These aims became what Erikson (1963) called the enactments and fantasies of the tragedies and comedies that occur around the orifices of the body.

Psychopathology at this early stage of theorizing was viewed by Freud as the result of either a fixation at (i.e., an arrest in the progress of psychosexual maturation) or

TABLE 2–2. Psychoanalytic theories of development

Period	Freud	Erikson	Spitz	Mahler	Stern
Infancy (approximately 0–12 months)	Oral	Trust vs. mistrust	Smiling response (1st organizer, 6 weeks); stranger anxiety (2nd organizer, 7 months)	Normal autism (0–2 months), normal symbiosis (2–6 months), separation-individuation; subphase 1, differentiation (6–10 months)	Sense of an emergent self (throughout life span); sense of a core self (2 months throughout life span); sense of a subjective self (7 months throughout life span)
Toddler (approximately 12–36 months)	Anal	Autonomy vs. shame and doubt	"No" (3rd organizer, 15 months)	Subphase 2, practicing period (10–15 months); subphase 3, rapprochement (16–24 months); subphase 4, consolidation and resolution (24–36 months)	Sense of a verbal self (15 months throughout life span)
Preschool (approximately 3–5 years)	Phallic Oedipal	Initiative vs. guilt Initiative vs. guilt			
School-age (approximately 5–12 years)	Latency	Industry vs. inferiority			
Adolescence (approximately 12 years and up)		Identity vs. role confusion			

a regression to (i.e., a symbolic or functional return to earlier ways of acting or thinking) one or another of these stages. As Erikson (1963), in his recasting of Freud, noted, the body zones and modes of function are analogous to other behaviors in life. For example, ingesting and spitting out as bodily acts were thought to become introjection and projection as mental defenses, and so forth. Although this sequence is looked at by many as the essence of Freudian psychology, it refers only to the content analysis of thought and fantasy and is, as Freud noted, his mythology and less significant to his later, more mature developmental theorizing.

Freud finally took up a strongly developmental position in response to the challenge thrown before him by Otto Rank, who wrote that birth anxiety was at the center of symptom formation. In 1926, Freud developed his last, and most sophisticated, major developmental theory (Freud 1926/1959b). He suggested that anxiety only breaks through to consciousness when successful repression does not take place and that anxiety functions as a signal that a dangerous situation is at hand in response to the emergence of specific thoughts as they threaten to break into consciousness. Freud posited a hierarchy of threats that humans have to evaluate and cope with during early childhood. Helplessness is the first signal of danger. Separation, occurring somewhere between 7 and 24

months, follows, and then castration anxiety (or body integrity anxiety) takes over from the third to the sixth years. Finally, danger of punishment by guilt ensues from an internalized value system embodied in the superego, which is an agency of the tripartite mind of the new structural model. Thus, at each stage of development the danger takes on a different configuration. The progression moves, as Freud (1926/1959b) suggests, from fear of loss of the object to fear of loss of the love of the object, with, in this instance, the mental object being a representation of the mother. This progression from concrete to abstract is also consistent with cognitive models that do not derive from Freud's dynamic formulation.

It should be noted, however, that Freud recognized that the Oedipus complex consists of a recasting of the prior preoedipal determinants and considered it to be a nucleus of conflict around which neurosis forms. Thus, his model was both epigenetic, as Erikson noted, and discontinuous in its invocation of the principle of hierarchic reorganization. The Oedipus complex becomes a watershed of prior developmental lines because its formation takes into consideration the ambivalent love and hate, the active and passive aims, toward parents of a child growing up in a family. Boys in the oedipal phase unconsciously desire their mother's undivided love and attention and wish to dispense with their competitive father. This configuration in normal girls (the Electra complex) involves their wish for undivided love from their father and their disavowal of their mother. These configurations vary greatly, leading to other permutations and combinations that evolve into pathological personality formation.

The Perspective of Ego Psychology

Freud's work was followed by empirical observations by others who moved away from depth psychology toward what was called *ego psychology*. The observational model began to take hold around the work of Rene Spitz and then Margaret Mahler, each of whom was at the center of a larger array of contributors who observed children.

Spitz's genetic field theory.   Rene Spitz's (1965) genetic field theory was derived from direct observation of infants. He invoked the concept of the "organizer" in the development of human behavior, and there are three organizers that have significance for the differentiation process. The concept of an organizer was derived from the embryological model that prescribes a formative fixing element in maturation that interferes with the pluripotentiality of protoplasm. Although this theory has an essentially maturational thrust, there also are important considerations of how the environment interacts with the biological tendencies.

Spitz's first organizer, the *smiling response*, includes a consistent and repeatable social smile in response to a full face or a moving oval with darkened areas representing eyes. The format of the human face entailed here suggests that this is the first "not-me" object to be appreciated by an infant. This maturational landmark links outside experience and autonomous function, supporting the notion of a regularly responsive internalization en route to what psychoanalysts call *object constancy*.

The next organizer, the *stranger response*, occurs at about 7 months. The child now turns away from the stranger with apprehension, terminating what Anna Freud (1965) has called the period of *need satisfying object*. This second organizer marks the attachment to a specific other. Curiously, studies suggest that the fear response is linked to facial expression and that the amygdala is the CNS site of this discrimination (K.M. Thomas et al. 2001).

The third organizer, the *development of the signal for no*, then signifies a fully internalized and individuated human toddler who now can undo with a verbal signal. According to Spitz, the toddler is now an agency and center of will separate from the mother. Indeed, the development of a capacity to negate or undo a prior verbal imposition is used to study executive function.

Mahler's separation-individuation theory.   Spitz's ideas received further observational support in the later work of Margaret Mahler et al. (1975). Mahler's separation-individuation theory continues the process of development into the postuterine period, involving the "hatching" of human consciousness, with the toddler as a separate, discrete autonomous agency. In Mahlerian terms the child moves from an autistic to a symbiotic stage in which he or she is initially enmeshed psychologically with the mother as though he or she were not separate from the mother.

The separation-individuation process includes a number of substages that equip the child with various capacities enabling him or her to develop the ego strengths necessary for adaptation. During the *differentiation* subphase, psychological birth occurs under the rubric of hatching, which is characterized by a permanently alert sensorium in which visual and manual examination of the external world become central. Next emerges the *practicing subphase*, which is characterized by increased curiosity. In Greenacre's (1957) picturesque phrasing, "the love affair with the world" begins. The child now appears as if he or she were omnipotent and as if an internal agency were not dissociated from an external agency. Only with the understanding that the mother is separate, during the next subphase, does the child arrive at what is called *object constancy*. Relative independent action can take place after the child is able to keep a stable mental image of the important caregiver.

Mahler's process of separation-individuation is an attempt to offer a psychoanalytic theory of development that is paralleled by fantasy formation matching the Freudian libido phases. When object constancy ensues at about 25 months to 3 years, the child is on his or her way toward independence, just as the three organizers proposed by Spitz provide the basis for later differentiation in that system.

Anna Freud's multilinear theory.   Anna Freud (1974) described a series of developmental lines that are central to the modern psychoanalytic view. These developmental lines suggest multilinearity in development, as Heinz Werner posited, but also offer an easy clinical frame from which to look at development. Roughly summarized, the child moves 1) from being nursed to rational eating, 2) from wetting and soiling to bowel and bladder control, 3) from egocentricity toward companionship with peers, 4) from play to the capacity to work, 5) from physical to mental pathways of discharge of drives, 6) from animate to inanimate objects, and 7) from irresponsibility to guilt. One can infer from these observations and their variations that a central theme evolves concerning how the child organizes behavior in an affective climate and in relation to others. This has become the observational groundwork of what now is called *object relations theory* in psychoanalysis, in which the object referred to is the child's mental representation of significant adults such as parents.

Other developmental frameworks do not consider these matters at such a molecular level of personal meaning. Cognitive and cross-sectional developmental schemes tend to exclude consideration of affect and conation (motive, will). (Later in this chapter the more recent nonpsychoanalytic theories of affect development are considered.) Within Freudian theory, moral development was viewed as the result of Oedipus complex resolution. However, more recent work (Buchsbaum and Emde 1990) has clearly shown that even 36-month-old children make moral judgments and have various responses to narrative that was designed to stimulate conflict over negative parental injunctions.

Development of Self

In recent years psychoanalytic theory has turned toward self psychology. Daniel Stern (1985) offered developmental empirical data delineating the emergence from a core sense of self to a verbal self within the evolving matrix of mother–infant communication. This model uses the new turn toward ideas such as the co-construction of monologues and the interdependence of emotional and cognitive developmental structures.

Normative Cross-Sectional Development

Cross-sectional developmental observers determine what children can do at varying ages and seek to construct sequential maps consisting of stages. Gesell's (see Gesell and Amatruda 1947) cross-sectional scheme (Table 2–3) is of interest because it was developed within a medical framework. Gesell divided behavior into four sectors: motor, adaptive, language, and personal-social. He tracked these behavioral observations over the long period of infancy and described a normative timetable. The essential question asked is, Does the child at age X achieve behavior in accord with what most children at age X can do? Gesell's organizing principle was neurodevelopmental integrity. He watched the child in the supine and prone positions give way to the sitting position and then to the standing and walking position. Nonetheless, Gesell matched Freud when he stated that the developmental span that lies between birth and 5 years is formative and of major significance for the entire life of the human organism. He also averred strongly that prenatal

fetal development has continuing relevance for the postnatal period and that the behaviors that one sees early can be organized into a developmental quotient for each sector. The developmental quotient (i.e., maturational age divided by chronological age and then multiplied by 100 [$(MA/CA) \times 100$]) gives a rough index of what the child tested can do at each stage. These developmental quotients are only roughly related to later measures of IQ (intelligence quotient), but they are relevant for detecting retardation and also deviance during the first 3 years.

Other cross-sectional schemes of childhood pertain largely to the development of intelligence. At the beginning of the twentieth century, the French sought to determine what sort of schooling children might best accommodate to if they were selected for some vital adaptive functions that could be called intelligence. Binet (1905) invented the IQ measure for that purpose. His test was revised in the United States as the Stanford-Binet Intelligence Test, which has been in continuous use as the IQ standard ever since. It has become, with revisions, a normative outline of what children are, on the average, capable of at each age.

Most studies of development rest on cross-sectional visions similar to the IQ and Gesell's developmental quotient, but the most recent studies of cross-sectional behavior have tried to include a large sector of behaviors other than verbal behavior. Thus, the Wechsler Intelligence Scale for Children (WISC; Wechsler 1949) was designed to include both verbal and performance scales. The most recent revision (WISC-III; Wechsler 1991) provides us with a broader understanding of the child's general adaptiveness that may be subsumed under intelligent behavior. The latest revisions provide updated norms for American youth whose primary language is English. The Wechsler Preschool and Primary Scale of Intelligence (WPPSI; Wechsler 1989) is an adaptation of the WISC for children from 3 to 6 years of age.

Piagetian Cognitive Development

Intelligent behavior received a new definition from the pioneering work of Piaget (1952; Piaget and Inhelder 1969) during the 1920s (Table 2–4). Piaget took a unique stance when he noted that getting the right answer is only one aspect of intelligence. He confessed that the affective component of development was of lesser interest to him; he wished instead to understand *how it is that children come to know what they seem to know*. In other words, what processes do children use to arrive at right or even wrong answers? Piaget found the regularities in sequence that permit abstract intelligent behavior. He sought to make intelligent behavior understandable by

TABLE 2–3. Landmarks of normal behavioral development—the revised Gesell developmental schedules

Age	Motor (gross/fine)	Adaptive	Language	Personal/Social
4 weeks	Tonic neck reflex position; rotates head when prone; makes alternating crawling movements	Responds to sound; follows moving objects to midline	Small throaty noises	Regards face; reduces activity
8 weeks	Symmetric posture seen; head bobbingly erect	Follows moving objects past midline	Vocalizes in response to social stimulation; sustained "cooing"	Follows moving person; smiles responsively
16 weeks	Symmetric posture predominates; holds head balanced; hands engage in midline; rolls to prone	Looks at object in hand	Laughs and squeals; "talks" to people/toys spontaneously	Initiates social smile; smiles and vocalizes at mirror; discriminates strangers (20 weeks)
28 weeks	Sits unsupported with hands up (1 minute); gets to hands and knees	One hand reach and grasp of toy; transfers toy	Vocalizes "m-m-m" when crying; understands name (32 weeks)	Gets feet to mouth; tries to obtain toys out of reach
40 weeks	Sits indefinitely with hands free (36 weeks); pulls to stand (36 weeks); cruises; lets self down; inferior pincer grasp	Matches two objects in midline; uncovers toy (44 weeks)	"Mama" or "Dada" and two "words" with meaning; responds to "no-no"	Initiates "pat-a-cake" and "peek-a-boo"; holds own bottle (36 weeks); helps in dressing; gives toy on request (44 weeks)
52 weeks	Picks up object from floor from standing position; walks several steps; helps turn pages (56 weeks)	Releases toy; imitates scribble; puts round block in formboard spontaneously	Six "words"; uses jargon	Points for wants; hugs doll; offers toy to image in mirror
15 months	Walks alone, seldom falls; walks up stairs, one hand held; creeps down; hurls ball; builds tower of three blocks	Spontaneous scribble; gets toy with stick after demonstration	10–19 words; knows one body part	Feeds self with spoon (spills); says "Thank you"; seeks help; pulls adult's hand to show
18 months	Walks down stairs, one hand held; builds tower of four blocks	Imitates stroke of crayon; places three blocks in formboard after demonstration	20–29 words including names of siblings, friends, relatives; combines two to three words ("daddy go"); asks for more food and drink	Gets spoon to mouth right side up; passes empty dish; echoes two or more last words; imitates mother/father sweeping, hammering, etc.
24 months	Jumps, both feet off floor; kicks large ball on request; builds tower of seven blocks	Imitates vertical stroke; imitates circular scribble; inserts circle, square, triangle in formboard spontaneously	50+ words; uses I and you; three- to four-word sentences; uses plurals	Occasionally indicates toilet needs; calls self me; helps put things away
30 months	Alternates feet going up stairs; rides tricycle using pedals; turns pages singly; builds tower of nine blocks	Names own drawing; imitates horizontal stroke, circle; adapts to rotation of formboard; repeats two digits (1–3 trials)	Eight- to nine-word sentences; carries tune; uses he and she correctly; relates events of 2–3 days ago	Pours from glass to glass; keeps time to music; pulls up pants; puts shoes on; names self in mirror
36 months	Alternates feet going down stairs; throws ball overhand; builds tower of 10 blocks	Copies vertical and horizontal stroke; copies circle; imitates cross, repeats three digits (1–3 trials); imitates bridge	Uses and or but; recites all of a song; knows up and down; follows three commands (three of the following: on, under, in back of, in front of, beside); knows two colors	Fully toilet trained; understands taking turns; plays with other children; washes and dries hands; knows front from back
48 months	Stands on one foot (4–8 seconds); skips on one foot only	Draws person with two parts; adds three parts to incomplete man	Follows four commands	Laces shoes; cooperates with children; goes on errands
60 months	Skips using feet alternately; walks on tiptoe	Adds eight parts to incomplete man; copies square (54 months) and triangle; counts 10 objects pointing; prints first name	Names penny, nickel, dime; describes pictures; asks meanings of words; gives first and last name	Dresses and undresses with little assistance; dresses up in adult clothes; ties a bow

TABLE 2–4. Piagetian stages of cognitive development

I. Sensorimotor intelligence
   A. Reflex looking and grasping (0–1 months)
   B. Primary circular reactions; the acquisition of new schemas centered on the infant's own body (1.0–4.5 months)
   C. Secondary circular reactions; new schema include events of objects in the external environment (4–9 months)
   D. Object permanence (9–12 months)
   E. Tertiary circular reactions; active searching for novel events (12–18 months)
   F. Beginning reasoning; mental trial and error replaces trial and error in action (18 months to 2 years)
II. Representative intelligence and the period of concrete operations
   A. Preoperational representations
      1. Appearance of symbolic function and the beginning of internalized actions (2.0–3.5 years)
      2. Representational organizations based on static configurations or on assimilation to one's own action (4.0–5.5 years)
      3. Meticulated representational regulation (5.5–7.0 or 8.0 years)
   B. Concrete operations
      1. Simple operations—classifications, seriations, term-by-term correspondence (8–10 years)
      2. Whole system—Euclidean coordinates, projective concepts, simultaneity (9–11 years)
III. Representative intelligence and formal operations
   A. Hypothetical deductive logic and combinatorial operations (11–14 years)
   B. Structure of lattice and the group of four transformations: identity, negation, reciprocity, and correlativity (13–14 years)

virtue of emergent cognitive structures.

Piaget proposed that the infant is born with two kinds of reflexes: those that remain fixed through life and those that are plastic in response to experience. The experiential world impinges on the child reflexively, and gradually a mental organization, called a *schema*, develops around repeated interactions. The *process* of development remains the same throughout life, but the *structures* change. The repeated process involves a reexperiencing in *assimilation*, but the assimilative schemas can change as they *accommodate*, leading to *adaptation*. For Piaget, assimilation is the incorporation into existing schemas of a structure of action that the subject judges to be equivalent. Accommodation, in turn, occurs when the schema must change to appreciate new objects and differentiate them from old assimilatory forms. Around this universal complementary functional format, the child then passes

through four stages: sensorimotor, preoperational, concrete operational, and formal operational.

During the *sensorimotor stage*, no behavior and its schema are separated into sensory and motor components. A thing to be acted on is appreciated as the thing acted on. It does not exist as a sensorily discrete entity without action. It is as though the infant were constantly embedded in a trial-and-error world. Werner and Kaplan (1963) describe this as the period of "things of action."

As the infant strips away the motor component, he or she can, between the ages of 18 months and 2 years, maintain a stable mental representation and create a representational world. This inaugurates the *preoperational period*, during which things are worked on in accord with how effective the child is.

The *concrete operational stage*, from 7 to 14 years, introduces a series of functional components suggesting that behavior becomes more rule-governed and that the rules permit decentering. When the child decenters, he or she loses his or her literal egocentricity—that is, he or she can generalize. However, he or she cannot yet generalize from data. Conservation becomes possible, and change in surface appearance does not necessarily signify basic change as in the concepts of volume or weight. Reversal operations may become possible, and trial and error are superseded by mental work employed to solve problems in one's mind, as in equation reversibility.

The later stage, that of *formal operations*, involves reasoning from empirical observations that then can be abstracted as general rules that can be used to dictate future actions. The child is now sufficiently decentered to take on another's vantage point, and reversibility is well established. The rules of logic of language are established. Piaget wrote also about imagination and dreams and about language itself. He looked at these functions as having various logical structures.

The intelligence of the mature human is a far cry from the intelligence described in the sensorimotor period. Most recently, neo-Piagetians have discovered that the stages outlined are not as rigid as stated and that empirical design may render some of the earlier judgments false, but that the regularities of sequence seem valid.

Ethological Development

Bowlby (1969) was the first to build a human developmental psychology based on a melding of psychoanalytic and ethological literature. His exposure to children separated from parents during World War II provided the human impetus for his theoretical work (Bowlby 1952), as did his experiences with adolescents with conduct disorder. Bowlby recognized the nature of human ties as an organizing precursor to later mature development. His work paralleled the work of Spitz (1945) and others, who also studied separation, and extended his own earlier observations of affectively deprived delinquents who suffered early separation. Bowlby noted that there were strong reactive effects consequent to separation from the mother or her surrogate.

Bowlby (1969) reviewed the nature of the maternal tie, establishing what he called a component instinctual response system that bore some similarity to Freud's 1905 theory. The infant is described as having five components that make up attachment behavior. Experiences are integrated to create a unified mental representation. The activated reflexes of *sucking, clinging,* and *following* have representation in other species, but are also present in the human. *Crying* and *smiling* achieve their ends by reciprocal maternal behavior: they bring the mother to the child. Each of these component instincts is considered to be an inborn response activated by an external caregiver (e.g., the mother). The evolutionary basis for this attachment is accounted for in the survival value and the natural selection for these responses.

Borrowing from the work of Harlow, Lorenz, and Tinbergen, among others, Bowlby then suggested that the responses to separation could be systematized. *Protest, despair,* and *grief* were repeatedly observed on separation, and then, if these responses were carried on too long, *denial of need* ensued. These behaviors serve as negative indicators that the normal process of the attached state has been interrupted. This work has been seminal in producing further empirical study of time of attachment, bonding and separation, and strange situation paradigms by which investigators explore attachment (see the "Affective-Interactive Organization" subsection later in this chapter).

These major frames of reference for development have given rise to myriad further work. We only touch on some new and derivative formats to alert the reader who may wish to pursue the topic further.

Longitudinal studies have been with us since the early diarists of language development. However, few of them have made as much impact as has the New York Longitudinal Study. This study group initially followed 133 middle-class children from 85 families, beginning in 1956. The observational data were organized in terms of nine variables: activity level, regularity, approach/withdrawal, adaptability, intensity, threshold, mood, distractibility, and persistence. Although somewhat removed from direct observation, the variables have good interrater reliability and give us a profile of reactivity for an individual child. The important work of relating these "temperamental variables," as they are called, to outcome in the "difficult child syndrome" or in relation to later personality development is ongoing (A. Thomas and Chess 1989). Such work holds promise as a developmental vantage point that should be integrated with later studies of character.

The work on affective development has provided yet another perspective (M. Lewis and Michelson 1983).

As noted earlier, although we have not exhausted the varying developmental vantage points currently used, those discussed provide a framework of empirically based or theoretically sound systems from which we can judge our new observations of developmental process.

We now traverse the developmental span from birth to preadolescence and then consider adolescence separately, in order to provide an overview of physical, neurological, sensorimotor, and cognitive development. Following this, we discuss the development of emotion in an interpersonal context. Finally, we will look at adolescence as a way station between middle childhood and adulthood that offers the integrations necessary for later life. Although we stress the early years, a truly developmental perspective includes the entire life span.

Normal Growth and Development: Birth to Prepuberty

Neurodevelopmental and Cognitive Organization

Biodevelopmental Reorganizations in the First 2 Years of Life

Although the human infant is born with a largely prewired nervous system, with many capacities designed for survival already built into the organism (Stern 1985), recent neuroscientific studies focus on delineating the mechanisms through which the brain changes with experience (Garraghty et al. 1998; Merzenich and Jenkins 1993). The issue of plasticity has been discussed mainly at the synaptic level. Variations in the environment seem to influence the CNS and neuronal networks largely through increases and decreases in the proliferation of synaptic connections and dendritic growth. We are accustomed to the idea that muscles grow stronger and senses are sharpened by use and that they atrophy by disuse. CNS growth during the early years seems to obey similar laws, with appropriate consideration for maturational differentiation and integration of pathways. While these processes are taking place, there also is evidence of discontinuities in neurodevelopment. There is a general proliferation of neural connections through the sixth and seventh year of life, followed by a decline, so that at puberty the network appears less dense (but not, however, as sparse as that found in the human brain at birth) (Huttenlocher 1979).

Neuroimaging methods have provided an altogether different level of analysis of plasticity. Instead of individual synapses, more recent research focuses on the question of how experience influences the set of neural areas active within a task and their time course of activation. Changes on the electroencephalogram (EEG), clinical neurological status, and cognitive levels also can be cited to document periods of radical change. These latter observations have led to formulations on the psychobehavioral level known as *discontinuities in development*, or as *biodevelopmental shifts* by other developmentalists intent on bringing the behavioral level into relation with the substrate (Emde et al. 1976; Shapiro and Perry 1976; Werner 1957). There is a correspondence between certain behavioral events at some stages and other parameters of biological study (Posner and Rothbart 2000).

Neurological organization. The first suggestion of a biodevelopmental shift occurs at the time of the first social organizer, the social smile, described by Spitz as signaling the recognition of an external stimulus of the human face as a releaser. The EEG becomes reorganized at a physiological level. Moreover, the rapid heartbeat of early infancy during disposition of attention gives way to slowing of the heartbeat with attentive staring after 2 months. This biodevelopmental shift thus can be documented at a number of physiological levels as well as at the behavioral level.

Similar concepts have been promulgated regarding the variation in state in early development as measured in sleep–wake cycles and reflected in the organization of REM (rapid eye movement) patterns. The six or seven regularly recurring REM periods during adult sleep only gradually emerge, evolving from early infancy (less than 3 months), when light sleep (Stages 1 and 2) dominates the EEG (Roffwarg et al. 1966). Moreover, sleep EEGs of premature infants show that up to 70% of sleep time is spent in a Stage 1 REM pattern. Sleep spindles appear only at 3–4 months, and by 3 months the infantile form of going to sleep that is characterized by rapid shifts from Stage 1 to Stage 4 recedes. These changes parallel the behavioral characteristics known as *settling*, when 70% of babies become night sleepers, rescinding their former pattern of waking at 3- to 4-hour intervals. By the end of the first year of life, the adult pattern of sleep is established on a physiological level. This event has been matched on an observational level because of the concordance of rapid eye movements with restlessness and other motor and respiratory patterns that are associated with varying stages of sleep.

Motoric behavior. Gesell's observation of the functional significance of attaining upright posture derives from an evolutionary perspective. He emphasized the capacity to turn over, sit upright, and, finally, use bipedal locomotion as developmental markers of maturation. These achievements are signs of the integration of CNS structures. Not only do they subsume the progression from cephalic dominance to the importance of manual dexterity and locomotion in human children, but they also mark the growing capacity of the child to become separate from the caretaking parent on the grounds of motor competence and, later, linguistic abilities, which then provide the bases of psychological independence.

The timetable for the emergence of motor milestones is well established. Behaviorally the infant at birth lies in a "fencer" position (tonic neck reflex) and during alert wakeful times can be stimulated to focus, grasp, and respond reflexively to rooting and sucking, all of which are adaptive for survival. These behaviors later give way to lying in a supine position and beginning to use both hands for grasping and mouthing objects as hand–mouth integrations become possible. The flailing hand sometimes scratches the infant's face as he or she tries to once again find his or her mouth. It almost seems as if there is an early dysmetria until the linkage becomes regular. Only by 10 months does the infant grasp objects in both hands and bring them to the midline. Symmetrical use of limbs and axial support become essential to the child's being able to turn over at 4 months and, ultimately, to achievement of the sitting position at 6 months.

More recently, study of the acquisition of motor skills has moved beyond the descriptive to consideration of the processes by which infants and children learn to control their bodies. Infants are surrounded by multisensory information that fuels the engines of developmental change as they learn to act in both social and physical worlds. During their waking hours, infants are watching, listening, feeling, and generating movements and experiencing the consequences of their activities. Processes of exploration and selection, together with the ability to generate behavior, provide a variety of perceptual-motor experiences resulting both in increasingly controlled action sequences and the establishment of ever more complex integrations between information deriving from all sense systems, including the motor senses (Thelen 1995).

Linguistic behavior. The vocal apparatus is used to produce protolinguistic expressions attracting the environment to the child while the child is incorporating the vocalizations of the surround. Even at this stage, infants seem to be prepared to selectively attend to congruent visual and acoustic signals (MacKain et al. 1983). Infants' babbling begins to take on meaning and significance as it differentiates into the speech of their mothers. Sapir (1921) suggested that in the beginning the child is overheard. Overheard expressive vocalizations in infancy, usually beginning with vowel sounds and gutturals, have been operationally divided into comfort and discomfort series based on the assumption that they have social significance (M.M. Lewis 1936). Infants move from expression to appeal to propositioning.

We now understand that the child is well prepared for phonetic distinctions in that he or she can discriminate phonetic contrasts during the first 4 months (Eimas et al. 1971). This refinement may undergo both specialization and involution as development proceeds so that distinctions that are selectively important in one's language flourish, whereas others disappear (Kuhl 1992). For example, the *r/l* distinction is lost in Japanese, although it is available in infants, and can be retaught only with difficulty to adult native Japanese speakers. The *t/d* distinction is available in infancy but may be lost in some language groups. The outcome of the intrusion of experience on early language and speech competence guarantees that the phonetic shape of words becomes specialized in accord with the community heard by the child. Surprisingly, most languages are made up of only 25–30 discrete phonemes that serve as the building blocks of more complex forms (Shapiro 1979).

Cognitive behavior.   On a cognitive level, infants of ages 3–6 months show evidence of interest in hidden objects that then reappear (Bower et al. 1970). The work of Spelke (1998) insistently reminds us of how the 0- to 6-month-old infant has skills of discrimination and anticipation and knowledge of the world. However, the cognitive substructures that subsume representational reality and thus constancy are still thought to be dependent on the achievement of the passage through the sensorimotor period to the preoperational and early concrete operational stages.

During this first year of development, the child is undergoing major cognitive shifts in his or her capacity to apprehend the external environment in a manner consonant with commonsense cultural reality. As noted, the period from birth to 18 months, from the standpoint of the development of intelligent action, concerns the development of a representational reality that spans the six stages of sensorimotor intelligence, as described by Piaget and discussed later. Although these stages are disputed by some, they do offer a plan of ontogenetic progress that helps heuristically to comprehend the infant's world.

The first and second stages refer to *heterologous and practical groups* in which no behavior pattern relative to vanished objects is observed and each event in time and space does not seem to be connected to its contiguous event. It is as if the experience is fragmented, or cut into frames. As noted, sensory impressions are intimately entwined with motor activity—hence the term *sensorimotor intelligence*. In fact, paradoxically, our adult concept of a distinctive perceptual sensory experience apart from motor activity should be viewed as an achievement of development. We would have to project ourselves into our distant past to realize the intimate entwinement of the two. An adult analogy to the infant's plight might be cited in the opposite sequence. We try to learn a new motor skill by first intellectually trying to grasp it. Only later do we do it as a motor automatism (e.g., our fingers "remember" the tune when we play a piano). Recent work indicates that earliest memories are stored as procedural sequences, only later to be translated into nominal and verbal propositions. The latter changes are related to hippocampal development (Cohen et al. 1985).

The third stage of cognitive development is presumed when the child *extends movements already started*, which indicates that there is some sense of "thing permanence" so that, for example, the child follows the trajectory of the dropped ball to a vanishing point.

The fourth stage is characterized by *reversible operations* of seeking and finding with an active search for the vanished object. However, the child is not yet able to take into account the *sequential displacements* that go on out of sight. Thus, the infant may search as an extension of the motor act already begun.

By the fifth stage, *objective groups* are established and there is some sense of the permanence of the object that is extended into the sixth and final stage, that of *representative groups*. Only then can the child imagine invisible displacements. The "thing" finally exists as a mental property, naively but practically assumed to be in the world. Bishop Berkeley's demand that things exist only as they are perceived bears some resemblance to Piaget's notion of early developmental reality. Things thus become objectified as development proceeds, and during this last stage, from age 16 to 18 months, "things" are freed of their motor components. The child can begin to mentally retrace movements. The possibility of a mental world has become established on purely cognitive grounds.

Although Piaget's scheme does not refer to emotional systems, Heinz Werner, inferring a more holistic view of development, refers to the sensorimotor-affective world of the infant. More recent work on affect and attachment will be addressed in a later section of this chapter. It is sufficient at this juncture, however, to note that the establishment of a representational world has some bearing on other matters of representations that *do* touch emotions. For example, how does the child represent the mother? How does the child keep an image alive as a mental property even in the absence of a stimulus? What are the precursors to fantasying, imagining, and, finally, projecting the future? These features are abstracted in Piaget's model into the minimum set of achievements that are required in the mental schemata that lead to the accession of well-established representations of the external world. The alternation between *assimilating* a new event into a preexisting mental schema and then having that schema *accommodate* as a new structure now ready to receive other experiences is a process that goes on throughout the life span, carrying the child to the *preoperational period* of age 2–7 years.

Toddler and Preschool Years: Language and Cognition

A toddler's life is replete with rapid changes in phenomenal behavior. He or she is animated, lively, striking out for independence, beginning to speak, and certainly comprehending. Representational play begins to appear, as does rapidly advancing hand-eye manipulation. From 3 years of age on, the toddler can begin to copy geometric forms, name them, and progressively begin to represent the human figure. The 3-year-old, full of exuberance, is also a language user. He or she can participate at table and can behave in limited social situations. Attendance at nursery school, with its routinized group demands of sharing and taking turns, becomes possible. Fantasy pretend play emerges in the early socialization process as well.

During the preoperational period, the child is still not able to decenter or imagine the vantage point from different positions in a room. There is no conservation of weight or volume and no cardinality of number or reversibility.

Piaget concentrated on the regularities in sequence of developmental achievement. Moreover, he proposed that children are active in their learning. However, qualitative differences between stages may not be as clear-cut as formerly thought. An uncanny experiment suggests that some abilities are present early but must reemerge later during the age period of 2–6 years with new cognitive underpinnings. If one puts a cube in an infant's mouth and then presents different shaped objects visually, the child focuses on the cube. Other synesthesias have been described as well. Certain children at 3 or 4 years of age can solve some conservation problems, but these problems must be presented in language that is appropriate to the age. This indicates that perhaps some of the failures and difficulties of younger children are due to the kind of language that was used in the initial experiments. Egocentricity, too, in the taking of other vantages may be more confounded by the language of the experimenter than Piaget thought.

In summary, the model proposed by Piaget and associates requires modifications to preserve some of its developmental principles. In addition, Piagetian staging must take into account the role of affects. Only a few aspects of staging that are specifically affected by human affective tone will be discussed in this section.

For example, social referencing (Klinnert et al. 1986) is one area in which an early relationship influences cognitive performance. A young child who is capable of crawling (i.e., age 8 months and older) can recognize a "visual cliff" (i.e., an illusion that there is a drop-off, although a transparent Plexiglas plate covers the drop). The child stops crawling at the cliff margin. However, if the mother is at the other end encouraging him or her, the child will proceed in accord with the afforded confidence (perhaps a sign of Erikson's basic trust). This permission indicates that cognitive perceptual and neurodevelopmental capacity may be qualified on the grounds of early facial recognition of affects and socialization. This hypothesis offers a fascinating possibility for a review of adaptation not only as an achievement of cognitive significance but also as the neural basis of understanding the emotional surround (K.M. Thomas et al. 2001).

As the child moves into the toddler years, much of what takes place in the cognitive sphere well into the beginnings of school rests on the acquisition of language and communicative ability. The emotional and social climate of learning also becomes very important, and we tend to take the neurodevelopmental aspects and cognitive aspects more for granted until the changes that occur at ages 6 and 7 years. Language competence and performance develop at a rapid pace. The 2-year-old rapidly achieves telegraphic speech of two words, which indicates his or her understanding that some words are more important than others when a message is to be conveyed. The child then adds grammatical morphemes (i.e., small endings on words that signify tense, person, etc.) (R. Brown 1973). These rapid shifts occur sequentially, in an orderly manner, in accord with the language that is spoken. By 3 years of age the child is a fairly competent speaker, with a three- to six-word mean length of utterance (MLU)—a circumstance that most competent adult speakers would be pleased to achieve if they were traveling in a foreign country and wished to have reasonable talking grasp of the commonplace aspects of living and expression of needs among that language group.

These linguistic feats have their precursors in the capacity to designate. Werner and Kaplan (1963) described the progression from reaching to grasping to pointing and, finally, to designating verbally by single words. These early words may stand for full sentences. Indeed, it was formerly thought that the first 50-word corpus consisted of only nouns. However, some children have a higher concentration of prepositions and verbs that refer to rather complicated concepts (Nelson 1981). Moreover, what we thought of as concreteness during the 1- to 3-word stage may represent a more canny understanding of the world than our prior understanding would admit. It has been argued by some linguist-developmentalists that one-word utterances are indeed phrases (or at least refer to phrases), although the child has a constraint on his or her capacity to form longer phrases. Certainly there is general agreement that the child may imitate before he or she comprehends, and that production follows. Thus, there is a greater constraint developmentally on expression production than on understanding. A most remarkable finding that undoes some of the mechanical presuppositions about language development concerns the early detection of narrative lines in children's learning, even with children at age 2 or 3 years (Bretherton 1989; Nelson 1986). Events are organized into scripts that aid in mastery at each stage.

The remarkable achievement of deixis suggests a very early capacity to distinguish a "this" from a "that," or "I" from "you" from "me." These distinctions are regularly achieved by age 2 years. Similarly, concreteness begs for explanation. The child of limited vocabulary who designates his or her dog "Rex" may then see a horse or a sheep and call either "Rex." The child is not acting concretely, nor is ignorance a factor. A more parsimonious explanation is that the child has an essential understanding of quadrupedia.

Nonetheless, the child may exhibit concreteness in other ways because of a limited understanding of the nuances of language. This is most apparent in the adult concept of the *joke*. Jokes told by 5- to 10-year-olds tend to be puns or restatements of naughty words and are not very funny to adults. The child practices with the laughter that goes with the presumed joke. He or she also seems to thrive on repetition, but it is certain that the adult sense of the word "joke" is not achieved.

Although the cognitive and neurodevelopmental capacities necessary for independence may be present before 7 years of age, the maturity of the mental apparatus and judgments about the world are not sufficient for the child to take his or her place in the larger social world. We have instituted nursery schools for day care and kindergartens since the late nineteenth century, but these are generally places where socialization occurs and manipulative skills are stressed. Even as such schooling has taken hold, we are forced to recognize variation in temperament as attributes to be considered in the interactive process. Kagan et al. (1989) described quiet, vigilant, and restrained children at 2 years of age as constituting a distinctive group with physiological correlates. The children in this group negotiate the interpersonal world more cautiously and require special attention lest they become overanxious. Although such variation is apparent early in life and may persist, most cultures have decided that formal schooling should take place somewhere between 6 and 7 years. This landmark, among others, marks the seventh year (plus or minus 1 year) (Shapiro and Perry 1976).

The Second Biodevelopmental Shift

Every level of study, from the neurodevelopmental to the cognitive and social, suggests that there is a hierarchic reorganization at age 7 years that would correspond to a second biodevelopmental shift. The brain attains its adult format and reaches the asymptote of its maximum weight at 7 years. Neuronal dendrites are most dense at this age. Moreover, it is after age 7 that children begin to understand that their feelings, intuitions, and thoughts may be of interest to others and, more important, may be thought about by others. Recent work on the relevance of the concept of a theory of mind has been used to record phenomena related to our ability to conceptualize others' mentalizing as different from our own. Children of age 7 have had the experience of viewing the actions of others in terms of separate motivation, and they can infer feelings. They also seem to begin to understand cause-and-effect relationships between objects, events, and situations, and they can begin to understand concepts such as ambivalence. Children at this age begin to show understanding of conservation and reversibility as noted earlier. They can grasp the concept of conservation of weight (despite how much a piece of clay is distorted in shape), of volume (despite container shape), or of number (despite, for example, the length of a line of coins).

Although children ages 7 years and older can do all these things, they may also develop social rigidities. They become rulebound and even moralistic about rules, outreasoning their parents in accord with the rules they have been taught. They chastise parents for smoking or for minor infractions of the law. They make statements such as, "I didn't learn it this way!" Yet, although they expect devotion and rigor from their parents, children this age sometimes break rules too.

Children at this age are exceedingly fickle in friendships, but at the same time demand absolute allegiance. "Best friends" may turn out to be different individuals each day. Children during this period tend to set up clubs with complicated rule structures and debate (what would be the equivalent of Robert's Rules of Order). These clubs may consist of two or at most five individuals, thus making everyone a leader or officer.

Rituals are also rampant despite the achievement of formal cognitive landmarks. In their monumental work *Lore and Language of School Children*, Opie and Opie (1959) indicated how the development of children's games and jump-rope rhymes traversed the English-speaking world by oral transmission. The similarities in games across natural boundaries are remarkable. Latency is a period when games are paramount and when persistence at games and collecting are central concerns; 8- to 12-year-olds collect anything from baseball cards to paper clips, and commercial firms exploit that trait.

We know that in this stage inner life goes on, but it seems to become subsumed under tasks that are of highly practical and personal appeal. The period that Freud called *latency* and that is now more neutrally named *middle childhood* becomes a time of mastering a great number of facts and skills. The period through fourth grade is considered by many educators to be a time of skill development in preparation for the application of reading, arithmetic, and writing to those creative activities that are to ensue. Self-righteousness and preoccupation with being admired and cared for, and acceptance of the ministrations of parents, are the hallmark of this stage in normal environments. On the other hand, persistence of difficulty in going to sleep, righteous indignation, and other irrationally dictated activities may be manifest in the same time period and setting in which these new maturities are developing.

Historically the period from age 7 years on has been recognized as a watershed. The Roman Catholic Church designated 7 years as the age of reason. It is a time when children in modern cultures begin first grade (or "real" school). During the eighteenth and nineteenth centuries this period was a time of apprenticeship away from the home. The language and motor capacities of these youngsters were so cultivated that during the Industrial Revolution heavy work and exploitation also were possible. Children were used for many tasks. Their size (cognitive capacities permitting) prompted their use as chimney sweeps and as laborers in mines, leading to the later development of child labor laws to legislate against the abuse that was permitted by such exploitation.

The beginning signs of puberty and the special socialization that Harry Stack Sullivan (1953, p. 245) called "chumship" (i.e., during the juvenile years between 10 and 14) mark the end of latency. The child then becomes ready to move on to adolescence. The physiological underpinnings of preadolescence and adolescence are marked by growth spurts, body configuration changes, and changes toward sexual readiness for procreation. The physiological and neurological bases are matched also by cognitive changes in the variable attainment of abstract reasoning. Thus, we have ample reason to believe that puberty is a biological event. Socialization changes also during this period. If one looks historically to the period prior to universal public education, many youngsters, barely pubescent, went off to the university or to seek their fortune or the like. For example, Benjamin Franklin at age 12 became an apprentice in a print shop in Philadelphia. Others went west to the Allegheny mountains and later to the Great Plains and the Rockies. The further characteristics of social maturation and development in this period will be dealt with later in the section on adolescence.

Affective-Interactive Organization

The Newborn Infant

The human infant is born into a social world. From the very first moments of life the infant's physical characteristics and behavioral patterns attract the caring attention of the people in its environment. Bowlby (1969), beginning with observations of children separated from their parents during World War II, has expanded our vision of the determinants of attachment between caregiver and child, through observations of humans in part but also of ethological systems across species. Drawing on work with primates, ungulates, and nonmammalian species, Bowlby proposed that attachment originates in inherited species-characteristic behavior called *inborn response systems*. The appeal of the very young—what Darwin (1872) called "babyness"—is universal. The infant's physical appearance—its tininess, largish head with prominent forehead, small face, big eyes, chubby cheeks and small mouth, coupled with its small body, uncoordinated movement patterns, occasional smiles, brightening of the eyes, and vocalizations and cries—stimulates the interest and concern of parents. By clinging, sucking, vocalizing, crying, smiling, and following, the infant brings or keeps the caregiver close. Human babies initially follow with their eyes, cling as part of a grasp reflex, and suck to obtain nutrition needed for survival. The behavioral patterns of the newborn ensure the proximity of the caretaker that is necessary for sheer physical survival. Indeed, it is the survival value of these systems that makes them relevant to the socialization process.

Among these inborn response systems, *affectivity* is essential. For the first 2 months of life, the care of the infant is primarily concerned with the regulation and stabilization of sleep–wake and hunger–satiation cycles. The parents of newborns are focused on the tasks of responding to signals of distress: of feeding, changing, and getting the infant to sleep. Parents accomplish these tasks through behaviors that are social as well as physical; they rock, stroke, talk, and sing to the baby in their efforts to comfort and soothe. These caregiving activities intensify parental attachment.

Recent research contributions have led to major revisions in our understanding of the capacities of the newborn to perceive, assimilate, organize, and respond to social stimuli. Rather than occupying a state of "normal autism," essentially unrelated to others (Mahler et al. 1975) and shielded by a "stimulus barrier" (Freud 1920/ 1959a), it has become increasingly clear that the newborn infant seeks sensory stimulation in periods of quiet alertness. The world of the newborn is not the blooming, buzzing confusion postulated by William James. Between birth and 2 months of age, infants select out the movement and size attributes of visual stimuli. As noted earlier, these very young infants are capable of recognizing similarities and differences not only within sense systems but across sensory modalities as well. By 6 weeks of age babies tend to look more closely at faces that speak, and in experimental situations they focus longer on faces that move in ways consistent with, rather than discrepant from, a simultaneously presented auditory stimulus. Thus, infants appear to have an innate general capacity to take information received in one sensory modality and translate it into another sensory modality, a capacity referred to as *amodal perception* (Stern 1985; Karmiloff-Smith 1995).

Infants can perceive persons as unique forms from the very beginning. Newborns act differently when scanning live faces than when scanning inanimate patterns; they vocalize more and their movement patterns are smoother and more coordinated (Brazelton et al. 1974). Neonates have consistently been shown to be able to discriminate the mother's voice from that of another woman reading the same material (DeCasper and Fifer 1980), and infants as young as 2 days have been found to be able to reliably imitate an adult model who either smiled, frowned, or showed a surprise face (Field et al. 1982). Moreover, by 6 weeks of age infants display evidence of delayed imitation. Infants presented with a person who pulled his tongue in and out repeatedly, pushed out their tongues when viewing the same person, this time with lips closed, after an interval of 24 hours. Such behaviors were not generated in response to new faces seen for the first time (Meltzoff and Moore 1994).

Babies are particularly receptive to the ways in which people interact with them. When babies cry, fret, gaze, or vary their facial expressions, parents and other caregivers characteristically look with widened eyes and raised eyebrows (i.e., "baby faces") and speak in high-pitched voices with exaggerated rhythm (i.e., "baby talk" or "motherese"). It is the rhythmic features of the acoustic signal itself, with its exaggerated prosodic contours, that initially holds the attention of infants (Kaplan et al. 1995). Mothers have little difficulty in deciding whether their babies are content or distressed, and only somewhat more difficulty in attaching specific affective labels to facial expressions (Pannabecker et al. 1980). Izard (1982), in analyzing film records of neonates, has reliably differentiated facial expressions of interest, joy, distress, disgust, surprise, and anger. The behavior repertoire of even the youngest of infants includes an emotional component (i.e., emotional expression).

Emergence of Emotional Experience

Modern theorists of emotional development distinguish between emotional state, emotional expression, and emotional experience. In the structural analysis of emotions proposed by M. Lewis and Michelson (1983), *emotional state* refers to internal changes in somatic and/or physiological activity, and *emotional expression* to observable changes in face, body, voice, and activity level that occur when the CNS is activated by emotionally salient stimuli. *Emotional experience* refers to the consequences of the cognitive appraisal and interpretation of perceived emotional states and expression. Although some investigators have used emotional expression as an indicator of emotional state (Izard 1982), others have pointed out that the two are not necessarily congruent. However, neither state nor observable expression is connected in a one-to-one relationship with emotional experience. Emotional experiences require a sense of self—an "I" to evaluate changes in "me"—as well as the cognitive capacity to perceive, discriminate, recall, associate, and compare. From this perspective, the very young baby's emotional expressions tell us little of his or her emotional experience. Nevertheless, parents and others respond to the infant's emotional expressions as if they were reflections of subjective experience. By interpreting and evaluating emotional expression, the social environment provides the rules by which children come to learn to evaluate and interpret—in other words, to experience—

their own behaviors and states.

Thus, the infant is a social being from the first moments of extrauterine life, with innate capacities that permit him or her to function as an active partner in the social interactions that occur within the context of the regulation of physiological functions. In Stern's (1985) view, an emergent sense of self—in relation to others—is present from birth: "[Infants] never experience a period of total self/other undifferentiation, [and] there is no confusion between self and other in the beginning or at any point during infancy" (p. 10). The affects, perceptions, sensorimotor events, memories, and other cognitions that accompany social interactions become increasingly integrated over time, providing a framework for the further elaboration of both a sense of self and an awareness of and attachment to others.

Even though newborn infants have the capacity to deal with the stimulation afforded by the external world and can become deeply engaged in and related to social stimuli, their tolerance is limited. During the first 2 months of life, the baby is in a state of quiet alertness for only very short periods of time. Gesell and Amatruda (1947) noted that the 4-week-old child sleeps for as many as 20 hours each day. Often it is only in the late afternoon (typically between 4 and 6 o'clock) that there is a more sustained opportunity for social interaction.

By 2 months of age, biobehavioral transformations affecting the nature and quality of social interactions are well underway (Emde et al. 1976; Spitz 1965). Sleep and activity cycles have stabilized, motor patterns are more mature, and altered visual scanning patterns permit new strategies for attachment to the world. Symmetry, complexity, and novelty are becoming salient attributes of visual stimuli. Learning occurs more rapidly and more inclusively. The perceptual preferences for the human face and voice, present at birth, are fully operative. The social smile is well established, vocalizations directed at persons entering the infant's range of vision have begun, and mutual gaze is actively sought.

The period between 2 and 7 months is perhaps the most exclusively social period of life. The baby is described as liking people to pay attention, talk, or sing to him or her. The spontaneous behavior of adults—"baby talk" and "baby faces"—is well matched to the infant's perceptual biases, with the result that the infant can maximally attend to the adult social stimulus. Typically, caregivers repeat their exaggerated facial expressions, gestures, and vocalizations with minor variations, which serve to regulate the infant's level of arousal and excitation within a tolerable range. Infants, too, are able to regulate their level of social engagement, using gaze aversion to cut out stimulation that has risen above an optimal

range, and vocalizations and alterations of facial expression to invite new levels of stimulation when excitation has fallen too low. As a consequence the baby gains experience with both self-regulation and the regulation of the behavior of others.

Infants draw on these daily life experiences to consolidate a sense of a core self as a separate, cohesive, bounded physical unit. For Stern (1985) there is no symbiotic-like phase as Mahler proposed. Between 2 and 6 or 7 months, babies come to recognize their own agency—that is, they are increasingly able to recognize relations between actions and reactions, to engage in voluntary activities, and to anticipate the consequences of such activities, both for themselves and for others. Moreover, the infant has a growing capacity to register motoric and perceptual events, together with their concomitant affects, in memory (Stern 1985).

Emergence of Seventh-Month Wariness (Stranger Anxiety)

The development of a core sense of self is paralleled by an increasing ability to engage in social discriminations. Gesell (Gesell et al. 1974) noted that the 16-week-old baby displays a marked interest in the father and also in young children. Between 4 and 6 months, the baby begins to respond to more than one person at a time and appears to enjoy being handed from one familiar person to another.

At about this time a wariness of strangers first becomes apparent (Schaffer and Emerson 1964). The baby appears cautious and watchful in the presence of strangers. Often wariness is combined with expressions of interest and curiosity. Although facial expressions of fear begin to be noted at 6 months of age (Cicchetti and Sroufe 1978), outright fear in the presence of a stranger is not regularly observed until somewhat later (8–12 months), and even then it is dependent on the situation. Expressions of fear are least likely to occur if the infant is with a parent, if there is a familiarization period, and if the stranger's approach is mediated by a toy or game. Fear is most likely when strangers intrude rapidly and seek to pick up the infant (Bretherton and Ainsworth 1974; Horner 1980; Rheingold and Eckerman 1973).

Historically, expressions of wariness and fear in the presence of strangers have been referred to as "stranger anxiety." This has been designated as the second organizer by Spitz, as noted earlier. The baby is also beginning to be most demanding of attention from a particular person, most often, as Gesell pointed out, "the one who feeds him" (Gesell and Ilg 1949, p. 115), and is more readily comforted by this person when distressed.

Affective Attunement

When infants are between 7 and 9 months of age, Stern (1985) suggested, the sense of self undergoes further reorganization to include a capacity to share certain subjective experiences—in particular, attention, intention, and affective states. Infants of 9 months appear to be capable of joint attention. Not only will they visually follow the direction of the mother's pointing finger beyond her hand to the target, but after their gaze reaches the target they will look back at the mother and appear to use the feedback from her face to confirm that they have arrived at the intended goal. Similarly, babies at this time are increasingly capable of communicating intention and of sharing affective experiences.

Stern (1985) provided rich behavioral descriptions of the process of affective sharing that characterizes attunement. *Attunement* refers to that dimension of the caregiver's behavior that matches not behavior per se, but rather some aspect of the behavior that appears to underscore the baby's feeling state. In attunements, the matching is largely cross-modal—that is, the modality of expression used by the mother to match the infant's behavior is different from that used by the infant. For example, a 9-month-old boy bangs his hand on a soft toy, setting up a steady rhythm and smiling with pleasure and exuberance. Mother falls into his rhythm and says, "Kaaa-bam, kaaa-bam," with the "bam" falling on the stroke and the "kaaa" accompanying the upswing of his arm. These experiences play a role in the infant coming to recognize that internal feeling states are forms of human experience that are shareable with others. The baby's behavior is also beginning to be influenced by the emotional expressions of others—a phenomenon called *social referencing*. As noted above, investigators (Klinnert et al. 1986) have demonstrated that a baby of 8 months of age or older can be induced to cross a visual cliff if his or her mother smiles, but will turn away if she assumes a fearful facial expression. Taken together, Stern's sense of a core self and his sense of intersubjective self correspond to what self psychologists term the *subjective* or *existential self*—the "me" (Harter 1983).

Selective Attachment

By 10 months of age most infants not only exhibit wariness of strangers but also have developed selective attachments to a small number (usually three or four) of specific persons. Children become attached not only to their mothers, but to fathers, siblings, other relatives, baby-sitters, and family friends. However, there is usually a marked hierarchy among these various attachments, with the mother at the top. Once attachment has developed, babies actively seek proximity and contact with the mother, particularly when faced with an unfamiliar or frightening situation. When they are with their mother, they tend to comfortably play and explore the environment, but when mother is out of sight, the infants will very likely follow or protest, either immediately or after a short while. The term *separation anxiety* has been used to describe the distress exhibited by the baby when mother is unavailable. Also, according to Bowlby (1969), the visible distress of separation is a manifestation not only of anxiety but of depression occasioned by the loss of a love object. When this situation is considered in terms of the structural theory of emotions proposed by M. Lewis and Michelson (1983), it is not clear that the baby who exhibits wariness or fear of strangers, or protests the departure of an attachment figure, actually experiences anxiety and/or depression. The 10-month-old baby is just beginning to develop the capacity to engage in the cognitive self-appraisal of his or her emotional states and expressions.

The Strange Situation

Ainsworth et al. (1978) developed a research method for assessing the quality of attachment in 12- to 18-month-old children. The *strange situation procedure* involves a set series of 3-minute separations and reunions with a caregiver and with a stranger in an unfamiliar room. Children who show mild protest following the departure, who seek the mother when she returns, and who are easily placated by her (about two-thirds of a sample of middle-class 1-year-old American children) are considered as the most *securely attached*. Infants who do not protest maternal departure and who do not approach the mother when she returns (about one-quarter of the sample) are characterized as *avoidant*. Children who become markedly upset by departure and who resist the mother's efforts to comfort them when she returns (about a tenth of the sample) are described as *resistant* or *anxiously attached*.

The classification derives from Bowlby's (1969) proposal that the biological "purpose" of attachment is to provide emotional security and social autonomy. He theorized (Bowlby 1973, 1980) that experience with primary caretakers leads to expectations and beliefs ("working models") about the self and relationships with others. However, attachment patterns are not immutable or independent of subsequent experience. The development of measures of the quality of attachment from the preschool period to adulthood (Bar-Haim et al. 2000; Main et al. 1985) make it possible to examine continuities and discontinuities over time. Changes in attachment status occur in one-quarter to one-third of subjects followed from infancy through early adulthood (Hamilton 2000; Waters et al. 2000), suggesting that experiences beyond infancy influence adult security. Adverse life events, including loss of a parent through death or divorce, life-threatening illness of parent or child, parental psychiatric illness, and physical or sexual abuse by a family member, are associated with the persistence of "insecure" attachment as well as with changes from "secure" to "insecure" attachment status.

Babies designated as showing "secure" attachments tend later to exhibit greater social competence and better peer relationships and to experience fewer negative life events (Sroufe and Fleeson 1984). Moreover, a caregiver's own experience and attitude toward attachment are highly predictive of the toddler's attachment status (Fonagy et al. 1991). An "insecure" attachment early in life does not inevitably predict the later emergence of psychopathology. Rather, varying patterns of attachment in infancy are initiating conditions that frame the ways in which relationships develop over time. Thus, early experience does not cause later pathology in a linear way, but it does have significance as a result of the complex, transactional nature of development. Prior history is both past and part of current content, and as such it plays a role in both the selection and interpretation of subsequent experience and in the use of available environmental supports (Sroufe et al. 1999).

The behavior of children in the "strange situation" may also be considered from the perspective of individual differences in temperamental organization (Kagan 1984). Temperament is commonly considered to reflect biologically rooted individual differences in behavioral tendencies that are present early in life and are relatively stable across various situations over the course of time (Bates 1989). Temperamental constructs have been operationalized somewhat differently by different investigators (Buss and Plomin 1984; Rothbart and Goldsmith 1985). In the New York Longitudinal Study, A. Thomas and Chess (Chess and Thomas 1984; A. Thomas and Chess 1977) identified nine categories of temperament that describe how children behave in daily life situations:

1. Activity level
2. Rhythmicity (regularity of biological functions)
3. Approach or withdrawal to new situations
4. Adaptability in new or altered situations
5. Sensory threshold of responsiveness to stimuli
6. Intensity of reaction
7. Quality of mood
8. Distractibility
9. Attention span/persistence

These categories cluster as follows:

1. The *easy child* pattern is characterized by regularity, positive approach responses to new stimuli, high adaptability to change, and expressions of mood that are only mild or moderate in intensity and predominantly positive.
2. The *difficult child* pattern, at the opposite end of the temperamental spectrum, is characterized by irregularity in biological functions, negative withdrawal responses to new situations, nonadaptability or slow adaptability to change, and intense, frequently negative expressions of mood.
3. The *slow-to-warm-up child* is characterized by a combination of negative responses of mild intensity to new situations with slow adaptability after repeated contact. Kagan et al.'s (1989) inhibited child belongs in this group.

Although difficult children composed only 10% of the New York Longitudinal Study sample, 70% of those who were classified as difficult during the first 3 years of life developed clinically evident behavior problems during early and middle childhood (A. Thomas and Chess 1977).

The 1-year-old child's behavior in the strange situation provides a prototype for many of the social developmental changes during the next 2 years. The child's capacity to physically explore the environment, to engage in social interactions, to comfort himself or herself, and to derive comfort from others in the absence of the mother increases dramatically. In Mahler's view (Mahler et al. 1975), these events occur as a consequence of a process of *separation-individuation* during which the mother comes to be perceived as a separate person while the child realizes his or her capabilities as an independent and autonomous entity who can function effectively in the mother's absence.

Separation-Individuation

In the period between approximately 10 and 16 months, the child devotes considerable energy to practicing locomotor skills and exploring the environment. Early in this period, the infant will search for the absent mother or repeat "Mama." Later the child shows a greater tolerance for separation and may seem unconcerned with the mother's whereabouts. Mahler calls this the *practicing subphase* (Mahler et al. 1975). Although having some mental representation of mother that is comforting in her absence, the infant also frequently seeks to reestablish bodily or visual contact with her. This behavior has become known as *refueling*, as it is considered a restorative process that provides the child with sufficient energy to further practice newly found skills and explore the environment.

Between 16 and 24 months, ambivalence is often intense. The child seems to want to be united with but at the same time be separate from the mother. Temper tantrums, whining, sad moods, and intense separation reactions are at their peak. Mahler suggests that during this *rapprochement subphase* the mental image of mother is considered to be insufficiently strong to provide comfort in periods of upset, leading the child to cling to the mother and to displace anger onto another caregiver.

Between 24 and 36 months, *negativism, willfulness,* and *contrariness* give way to a new realization of social demands. Disappointment, frustration, and absence of mother become better tolerated as the child's mental representation of the mother develops more stability. Not only is the mother clearly perceived as a separate person in the outside world, but the internal representations of her "good" and "bad" aspects are more solidly integrated. The availability of a secure and reliable internal representation of mother affords comfort when she is absent and facilitates the child's increasing ability to engage in independent activities and more flexible personal relations.

Between 18 months and 3 years, the development of language contributes to the further organization of the sense of self and the sense of others. Language provides the self and others with a new medium for exchange with which to create shared meanings. With the advent of what Stern (1985) refers to as the "verbal self," children begin to see themselves objectively. By 18 months of age they are able to recognize themselves in mirrors, still pictures, and videotapes (M. Lewis and Brooks-Gunn 1979). By 2 years they begin to use "I" to refer to themselves, and shortly thereafter to call other people "you." Genetic, prenatal-hormonal, pubertal-hormonal, and socialization factors all contribute to the determination of subsequent sexual status and orientation (Money 1987), but for most children, core gender identity becomes psychologically established as well and is manifested in gender role behaviors. Thus, the achievements of locomotion, language, sense of self, and core gender all seem to coordinate a growing child's sense of separateness.

Lewis (M. Lewis and Michelson 1983; M. Lewis et al. 1989) suggested that the emergence of a categorical self and the corresponding ability to categorize others facilitate the acquisition of social knowledge of emotions and the development of the complex emotional experiences that accompany the social emotions of empathy, guilt, embarrassment, and shame. Children as young as 18 months display a beginning understanding of the goals

and intentions of others (Meltzoff 1995), and by 2 years of age, some children are capable of empathic behavior and show some cognitive understanding of the emotions of others (Borke 1971).

Emotions in Toddlers and Middle Childhood

Children can discriminate among pictures depicting different emotions earlier than they can label them, although some 2-year-old children can produce verbal labels for emotional behaviors such as crying and laughter. The recognition and labeling of the basic emotions of joy, sadness, anger, and fear develop earlier than those of emotions such as contempt and shame. By 2 years of age, children can dissimulate emotions and pretend to assume emotional states. Between 2 and 4 years of age, children produce increasingly appropriate facial expressions when provided with a verbal label, and between 3 and 4 years they begin to be able to designate what emotions are appropriate to particular situations (M. Lewis and Michelson 1983). Emotional experiences become increasingly clearly defined through the interaction of children with their social environment.

By 3 years of age, children have developed a well-articulated sense of both the subjective self and the objective self, or, to use the terminology of M. Lewis and Brooks-Gunn (1979), the *existential* self and the *categorical* self. Children at this age have well-established social relations with members of their immediate families and are beginning to expand their social horizons beyond the confines of home. Nevertheless, if a stranger is present or the situation is otherwise stressful, children of 3 years may still become upset at separation from mother. The advent of language facilitates the capacity for symbolic play reflective of daily life experiences, as well as the identification and sharing of affective states. Affective displays come under increasing control. Affects are beginning to be socialized, and the complex experiences of guilt, embarrassment, and shame begin to be elaborated. Children come to know the names of their feelings and when to display what affects and increasingly to experience empathy (Bretherton and Ainsworth 1974).

Between 3 and 5 years of age, the concept of a private self that is not observable by others begins to be elaborated. Expressed emotions, which encompass a full range of affects, fluctuate easily at age 4 but have become more stable by age 5. The ability to use language to distinguish among affects expands, as does the capacity to identify situation-appropriate emotions. Conversational reference to feelings and mental states expands during the preschool period (J.R. Brown et al. 1996). Children begin to elaborate a "theory of mind" as they become increasingly adept at inferring what it is that others know and feel (Baron-Cohen 1989). As the capacity for "mind reading" develops, so does the ability to engage in deception, teasing, and cooperative play with a division of roles and a sharing of goals (Dunn 1996).

Relationship patterns become more complicated, and rivalries, jealousies, secrets, and envy begin to emerge. Fantasies become increasingly complex when compared with earlier scripts and include aggressive and sexual elements as well as concerns about separation and loss of love. Behavioral differentiation of the sexes is minimal when children are observed or tested individually. Sex differences emerge primarily in social situations, and their nature varies with the gender composition of dyads and groups. Tendencies to prefer same-sex playmates can be seen among 3-year-olds, and preferences increase in strength and are maintained at a high level between the ages of 6 and at least 11 (Maccoby 1990).

The period of middle childhood is marked by changes in the ability to regulate and modulate affects. Six-year-olds can be highly emotional, and angry outbursts are frequent. By age 7, children may appear to be moody and sulky and complain that no one likes them and that people are mean and unfair. By age 8, children are described as impatient and demanding, frequently bursting into tears or laughing uproariously. Humor begins to play a role in the modulation of affects. A sense of right and wrong emerges, and children may feel guilty and inwardly unhappy and frankly sad if they have failed to live up to a standard. First-graders have come to appreciate that they cannot change—say, become an animal or a child of the opposite sex—and that the self is continuous from past to future (Guardo and Bohan 1971). As they progress through primary school, children become increasingly capable of emotional deception—that is, the ability to display an emotion different from their underlying feelings (Saarni 1979).

During this period children are also interested in defining their place in the family and in relation to other family members. Children fluctuate between love for family and worries about not belonging. Fantasies of having been adopted and having rich and powerful natural parents are frequent. This is referred to as the *family romance fantasy*. The relationship between siblings is distinctive in its emotional power and intimacy. Studies of siblings throughout childhood and adolescence report a marked range of individual differences between sibling pairs in measures of friendliness, conflict, rivalry, and dominance. Moreover, such dimensions are relatively independent of one another. Maternal behavior (particularly *differences* in the mother's behavior toward her two children), the children's ages, the difference in age

between them, and their temperament all contribute significantly to differences between sibling pairs (Stocker et al. 1989).

Not only do relationships between siblings differ in different families, but the personality characteristics of children growing up in the same family are also often strikingly dissimilar. Plomin and Daniels (1987) have suggested that within-family differences—the nonshared environment—may be more important than between-family differences in their effects on the developing child.

During middle childhood, interests in relationships with peers and teachers expand. Childhood games with rules emerge, as does a capacity for intimacy with a "best friend." However, the two sexes engage in fairly different kinds of activities and games. Boys play in somewhat larger groups, on the average, and their play is rougher and more expansive. Boys more often play in streets and other public places, whereas girls more often congregate in private homes or yards. Girls tend to form close, intimate friendships with one or two other girls, and these friendships are marked by the sharing of confidences. Boys' friendships are more oriented around mutual interests in activities. The breakup of girls' friendships is usually accompanied by more intense emotional reactions than is the case for boys.

Different interactive styles develop in same-sex groups. Boys in their groups are more likely than girls in all-girl groups to interrupt one another, refuse to comply with another child's demand, heckle a speaker, or call another child names. Girls in all-girl groups are more likely than boys to express agreement with what another speaker has just said, pause to give another girl a chance to speak, and acknowledge a point made by another speaker. There is more conflict in boys' groups, and when conflict occurs, girls are more likely to use "conflict-mitigating strategies," whereas boys more often use threats of physical force. Although boys appear to be more concerned with issues of dominance, their confrontational style does not necessarily impede effective group functioning, as evidenced by their ability to cooperate with teammates in sports. Moreover, when interacting among themselves, girls are not unassertive. Rather, while pursuing their own ends, they simultaneously strive to tone down coercion and dominance to bring about agreement and restore or maintain group functioning (Maccoby 1990).

Between 9 and 10 years of age, children still define themselves in terms of concrete objective categories such as address, physical appearance, possessions, and play activities. Self-criticism is prominent, but children are also beginning to be able to accept jokes by others about themselves. The concept of family continues to be important to most children, although they often prefer to be either on their own, with friends, or with other adults who, like the parents, may serve as role models. There are well-developed capacities for empathy, love, compassion, and sharing, as well as outbursts of person-directed anger, self-evaluative depression, and self-centered righteousness. Children increasingly evaluate their own behavior; they may be disgusted or apprehensive about their own actions and guilty and ashamed about past behaviors. New affects around sexual differences begin to emerge. Children begin to experience both excitement and shyness in relation to sexual themes, and shame becomes a prominent guide to action, heralding the onset of puberty and entry into adolescence.

Adolescence

What is Adolescence?

Adolescence has come to represent the developmental bridge between middle childhood or latency and adulthood. It also marks a discontinuity in development based on biological, psychological, and social factors that set this period apart from both childhood and adulthood. Regrettably, in the minds of many, development ends here. However, modern theorists suggest that developmental processes continue throughout the life cycle and that each phase or period may be subjected to a developmental analysis. In that sense this chapter on development is incomplete. Among the developmental stages, adolescence has gathered a questionable, if not bad, reputation, second only to the terror that the "terrible twos" elicit in young parents. Adolescence stands out because of the disruptions in behavior, the moodiness, and the difficulties in living, as well as the conflicts and strife with families that have been considered normative.

These popular opinions are striking in view of the fact that adolescence is relatively new on the developmental scene, partly so because there remains some uncertainty as to how to define adolescence and whether adolescence existed in preindustrial society or exists in non-Western communities (Ariès 1962; Esman 1990; Stone and Church 1957). From a sociological vantage point, the rites of passage that mark the terminus of childhood are well known. They include initiation rights of religion and society in the form of confirmation, bar mitzvah, hunting tasks, scarification, and penile subincision that permit entry into the adult community of men and women in various cultures. These rituals mark entry into adulthood rather than into an intermediate phase. On the other hand, in some communities as distant as pre-Periclean Greece, there was a clear distinction between the young man (i.e., the *ephebus*) and the marriageable nubile girl and those who became fully procreative members of the community. Indeed, sociologists sometimes look at adolescence as consisting of an alienated group of a certain age who are defined by exclusion. Neither children nor adults, they are partially excluded from both of these more dominant communities. More recent work seeks to define adolescence as a distinct subculture with its own lore and rules.

Although some would like to see adolescence as equivalent to puberty (see "Puberty" section below), it would be hard to justify that it simply is puberty. Nonetheless, growing into one's primary and secondary sexual characteristics is one of the essential tasks of adolescence. To this we might add the psychological and social adaptations that are secondary to external as well as bodily biological demands. Thus, our definition of adolescence will have to be tailored to three factors: the biological, the social, and the psychological demands of the period.

Puberty

Biologically, *puberty* refers to attaining the capacity to procreate as a mature member of a species. The appropriate growth and development of the external genitalia and of the ovaries and testes and their products, the ovum and sperm becoming viable and ready for fertilization and the formation of a gamete, are essential for survival. The notion of puberty as a phase in the biological life cycle is more important from a psychosocial vantage point because the external characteristics (i.e., secondary sexual characteristics) of both sexes become prominent social signs. In females puberty occurs 2 years earlier than in males, and the first signs are breast buds, followed by the growth of pubic and axillary hair and the attainment of a feminine body habitus with broadening of the hips (Tanner 1968). In the United States, girls achieve menarche at a mean age of 12.7 years (Zacharias et al. 1970), with 5% beginning at 11–11.5 years, 25% at 12–12.5 years, and 60% by age 13. Nine percent of normal females experience menarche up to 5 years after the beginning of breast development. A height spurt also begins to take place at age 11 that peaks at 12 and then falls off at 14 or 15. Menarche is frequently followed by irregular anovulatory periods for 12–18 months before a more regular menstrual cycle ensues. The task of adapting to the new bodily format soon encroaches on and influences psychological content and becomes an important feature of social adaptation (Tanner 1968).

In boys, the height spurt begins somewhat later, at age 12, peaking at around 14 years, and begins to fall by age 16 or 17. Correspondingly, the penis and the testes are already on their way to achieving adult size and form. The pubic escutcheon and axillary hair likewise begin to be prominent, as does the masculine habitus, and there is deepening of the voice.

In both sexes these primary and secondary sexual changes correspond to activation of hypothalamic functions that in turn stimulate the gonadotropic hormones of the pituitary. These hormones stimulate both estrogen and luteinizing hormone at the periphery as well as testosterone, especially in boys. The changes are thought to be coordinated with maturation of the hypothalamic cells. They become less sensitive to the feedback-dampening effect of circulating sex hormones. In males, nocturnal emissions are observed to occur about a year after the secondary sexual characteristics develop and mark the beginning of the capacity to procreate.

In the CNS, dendritic connections attain their adult levels, dropping back from the high density of proliferation seen at about age 7 (see "The Second Biodevelopmental Shift" subsection earlier in this chapter). Encephalographic changes also occur by age 14 when mature alpha-rhythm patterns become well established.

The regular trend toward earlier puberty, especially in girls, in European and American populations has been attributed to better diet. There is also some suggestion that menarche and physical maturity may have long historical cycles so that the early onset of puberty in our time may be a temporary event. However, the data available do suggest that during the 1880s the average onset of menarche was 15–16 years; by 1925 it was 13–14.

Cognitive Organization in Adolescence

While these bodily changes are taking place, intellectual and cognitive developments keep pace. Piaget (1952) suggested that operational intelligence gained at age 7 is advanced to *abstract* intelligence in adolescence. The adolescent is now ready to mature into formal operations, leaving concrete operations behind. For example, instead of the adolescent girl suggesting to her mother that she ought to be able to wear lipstick because all the other girls do, she could now argue that given her maturity, exemplified by new competence, and her age, she ought to be able to make decisions about lipstick in the same way she is permitted to make other decisions. The march of sophisticated reasoning involving causal and combinatorial thought establishes the abstract attitude.

Achievement of the landmark of abstract intelligence, however, does not occur as uniformly at the age of 14 as previously thought. There are data to suggest that only 10% of 14-year-olds, and 35% of 16- to 17-year-olds, achieve formal operations. Sixty percent of those classified as gifted adolescents attain formal operations. This latter figure is in sharp contrast to the average adult population, in which 25%–33% attain formal operations (Dulit 1972). These developments in both cognitive and biological maturation provide the groundwork and raw material for varied psychosocial problems and have given rise to the many observations that make up the concept of adolescence.

Social Determinants of Adolescence

The features to be discussed are more prominent now than in the early years of our nation. In the West, during the early nineteenth century in the United States, formal education did not continue into the young adult years for many. At the attainment of puberty, which coincided with the capacity to work or to become an independent earner, one could also start a new life. What we now consider the adolescent years coincided with young adulthood, and youths adopted the adventuresome spirit that has been romanticized in the popular history of this region. Moreover, the social significance of adolescence did not take hold until economic gain became attached to long periods of education and continuation of economic dependency.

Indeed, one of the by-products of adolescence is the conflict experienced by biologically mature organisms who are still dependent on family support both socially and psychologically. Such conflict does not seem to abate when education is financed by the state or by socialist governments. Thus, with the attainment of more leisure time, urbanization, and the increased need for a service work force over the need for manual labor, there has been an increasing necessity for specialized education and training. A full-blown "social adolescence" has been developed that implies psychological components as well.

Psychiatrists must attend to these issues not only because they may find themselves treating adolescents but also because adolescent themes and conflicts persist into adulthood. Moreover, as we consider the social determinants of adolescence, we must also keep abreast of changing social patterns that may affect youngsters from ages 12 to 18. For example, what are the effects of a shift away from the nuclear family and a divorce rate that has exceeded 50%?

Directly related to the latter issue is the fact that there are more than 8 million one-parent families in the United States. In addition, divorce rates peak early in the first 2 years of marriage but then again just when families are rearing young teenagers. Other social forces involving the women's movement have changed family patterns, with both parents going out to work and women beginning or finishing their education just as their children can begin to be physically, but not psychologically, able to care for themselves. The latter condition shifts the time allotments of families so that time for intimacy, commiseration, and exchanges of all sorts may be curtailed. There is no doubt that poverty continues to have a major effect as well. Sociopathy, drug use, and legal entanglements associated with psychiatric disorder have much higher representation in the lower-socioeconomic-status classes. During the 1990s, many communities began to embrace the offspring, natural and adopted, of those gay and lesbian couples who choose to raise children. Many communities still do not. The tensions of familial and community aims have their effect on the adolescent in a manner yet to be discovered.

Thus, biological and social factors converge to create adolescence. But how do these factors affect the psychological unfolding of these older children?

Psychology of Adolescence: Normative Studies

Among the earlier psychoanalytic writers, Freud himself described the treatment of a late adolescent, Dora (Freud 1905/1953). It was during treatment with this patient, as Freud later realized, that he developed the concept of *countertransference*. Perhaps it was apt that an adolescent developmental process should have caused the early psychotherapist to have to ask about how his own feelings affected his actions.

Adolescence was largely ignored by analysts until Anna Freud (1946) described a rapid oscillation between excess and asceticism during adolescence. She viewed the rapid swings of behavior and mood as secondary to the surgent effect on behavior of the drives stimulated by sexual maturity and the hormones of puberty. The instability of the newly stressed defenses against impulse was seen as the ego's contribution to the erratic behaviors being manifested.

This view of adolescence as tumult and turmoil colored the vantage point of subsequent investigators. In fact, Erikson's (1959) concept of *adolescent turmoil* and his concomitant notion of *identity diffusion* became the hallmarks of our view of normal adolescence. Although Erikson cautioned that diffusion was a maladaptive, temporary state, he implied that we all traverse the stage more or less. Later developmental normative studies

employing the direct observation of adolescents have shown less turmoil and upheaval than formerly thought. Only now do we generally accept the formulations of Offer and Offer (1975), who showed that, by and large, adolescence is more quiescent than was formerly thought. Because their work is of landmark proportions, we will review it briefly.

Offer and Offer studied two Midwestern middle- and upper-middle-class community high schools. Their findings, although based on only adolescent males, were later extended and verified by others (see Emde 1985; Hauser et al. 1991; Oldham 1978). The young men in Offer and Offer's sample were 14 years old and entering high school in 1962. Those individuals who were within at least one standard deviation from the mean in 9 of 10 scales of personal and social adjustment were the subjects of the study. Sixty-one adolescents were then studied more intensively by a questionnaire technique and were followed well into later life to determine outcome. To convey the advantaged status of the sample, it is worth noting that 74% went to college during the first year after high school graduation. They came largely from intact families, and through the 8 years of study, from 1962 to 1970, there were no serious drug problems or any major delinquent activity, and no one was arrested for political sit-ins. The group showed no visible generational gap or difference in basic values from their parents. (An earlier study of young women at Bennington College in Vermont [Newcomb 1943] under the tutelage of their less-conventional teachers adopted radical political stances; however, 10 years later, having returned to their home communities, these women had reverted to conservative values similar to those of their parents.)

The findings from this study suggest that even after environmental influence from powerful social forces such as an educational milieu, early and long exposure to parental values has significant effects on long-term adaptation. Possibly relating to Offer's finding of stability, these effects on long-term adaptation are added testimony to the heightened impressionability of late teenagers under special cultural conditions that then give way, under the social temptations of middle-class ease, as new family responsibilities supersede more carefree adolescence.

Varieties of Adolescent Psychological Development

The Offers found three developmental routes, which they designated as *continuous growth* (23% of the sample), *surgent growth* (35%), and *tumultuous growth* (21%). The remaining 21% were not easily classified but were closer to the first two categories than the third. In the *continuous growth* group, major separation, death, and severe illness were less frequent. Parents were described as encouraging independence, and the adolescents showed a capacity for what were described as good human relationships. They were able to achieve Eriksonian intimacy and to display shame and guilt and had few problems of major intrapsychic complexity as far as the methods of investigation could provide. The *surgent* group were "late bloomers," as the term implies. They were not as action-oriented as the first group and were given to more frequent depressive and anxious moments. They were often successful but tended to be less introspective and reported more areas of disagreement between parents about child raising. Finally, the *tumultuous* group reported recurrent self-doubt and conflict with their families and came from less stable backgrounds. Academically this group preferred the arts, humanities, and social sciences to professional and business careers.

The results of studies such as the Offers' (Offer 1969; Offer and Offer 1975; Offer and Sabshin 1974) and those by Block and Haan (1971) and Vaillant (1977) tend to negate the notion that turmoil is necessary for adolescent development.

Block (Block and Haan 1971) extended the observations of the Berkeley longitudinal sample and showed a persistence of character style as individuals develop. A Q-sort technique was used as a study measure of repeat reliability. This approach showed repeated differences between men and women in those studies where both sexes were considered. However, certain important cohort effects and temporal cultural demands may have affected the outcomes. (For example, the Bennington study [Newcomb 1943] might be repeated during our current historical period to verify the effect seen in that group.) Block divided the data of the study sample into "changers" and "nonchangers" to refer to correlations across time, below and above the mean. Adolescent changers in their 30s appeared more unsure of themselves, were tenser and more guarded, and felt they were still working on problems. A factor-analytic approach was also used to render additional information. The 84 males and 86 females in the study were divided into five and six types, respectively. Among the males the following groups were isolated:

1. Ego-resilient adolescents
2. Belated adjusters (who seem very similar to Offer's surgent group)
3. Vulnerable overcontrollers
4. Anomic extroverts (who seem to have less inner life and relatively uncertain values)

5. Unsettled undercontrollers (who are given to impulsivity)

The categories represented by these individuals are not meant to refer to pathological entities but rather to styles of adaptation.

Block divided the cohort of females into the following:

1. Female prototypes (obeying stereotyped descriptions of what the authors thought of as feminine in the 1980s)
2. Cognitive types (who tend to be intellectualized in the way in which they negotiate problems)
3. Hyperfeminine repressors (who are close in description to persons with hysterical personality disorders)
4. Dominating narcissists
5. Vulnerable undercontrollers
6. Lonely independents

As students of development, we recognize the culture-bound stereotypes used.

There is some suggestion that identity formation in both boys and girls is the result of more than learning to be like mothers and fathers, and that sex-linked role characteristics result from how parents of one sex act toward the parents of the opposite sex as well. Hauser and his colleagues (1991) at Harvard studied a sample of 133 14-year-olds longitudinally. Almost half the sample had been inpatients in a psychiatric hospital. However, these authors' mode of study did not show crucial differences in the outcome of this largely middle-class group through their teen years. An ego scale was used that describes stages in maturation with designations such as preconformist, conformist, and postconformist. The authors found three paths of progression from the steady conformist group: early, advanced, and dramatic. This central group of progressive development represents the "team players" of adolescence and constitutes one-third of the group. Only six teenagers attained the level designated as a stage of integrity and conscience, the highest level on the scale. Their parental environment was of a model sort, but as a group they did not differ significantly from the steady conformists in the measures taken.

The research of Hauser is based on Eriksonian and ego psychological constructs that have also been incorporated into further work concerning the role of the extended environment on identity formation in adolescence. A recent Dutch survey (Meeus and Dekoviic 1995) explored relational, school, and occupational identity in 12- to 14-year-olds and 21- to 24-year-olds. Relational identity is the earliest to consolidate, and occupational roles follow. As one would expect in these age groups, peer influence is the most significant factor in role definition, with only a minor influence from parents. The identity construct also has been studied in terms of competence in adolescents. Masten et al. (1995) have shown that romantic and job competence become important in the 17- to 23-year-old group in addition to school, social and conduct dimensions in the 8- to 12-year-old groups. Not surprisingly, antisocial behavior interferes with academic and job competence throughout adolescence. The longitudinal Duneden Study in New Zealand (Fergusson and Lynskey 1996) showed that the most resilient 16-year-olds studied had higher IQs, demonstrated lower association with delinquent peers, and were less novelty seeking.

Studies such as those discussed above tend to emphasize the overriding effect of socioeconomic status, family intactness, and presumed genetic endowment as central to adequate adolescent progression.

Developmental Themes of Adolescence

In addition to the data presented, clinical wisdom accumulated over three-quarters of a century suggests that adolescents must negotiate a series of issues before they emerge as adults. These issues can be grouped into eight themes in the developmental process, as shown in Table 2–5.

TABLE 2–5.   Developmental themes of adolescence

Dependence vs. independence
License vs. intellectualized control
Family vs. peer group
Normalization vs. privacy
Idealization vs. devaluation
Identity, role, and character
Sexuality: identity, role, and partner
  Masturbation/mutual pleasure
Reshuffling of defenses (style)

Dependence Versus Independence

The *dependence/independence* interaction refers to the intrapsychic struggle for a sense of emancipation from the nuclear family that permits goals to be formed as a personal claim. This struggle has both biological and social roots and has implications for the capacity for species survival through procreation and the development of intimacy outside of the family. Adolescents feel that they must extricate themselves from the caretaking hold of parents. They see their elders as either exacting gratitude or inducing guilt and shame as internal controls over individual action. On the other hand, these actions may

strike families as egocentric and selfish.

In contrast to nuclear families, children growing up in collectivist societies, where the group rather than the parents is the controlling social force, find it very difficult to move into the larger society where independent individualized action seems to be required (Ainsworth 1962). The notion of an individual achiever and self-starter seems to be related to social values, and these values then become the prominent dynamism in regard to what Blos (1985) called a *second separation-individuation phase*, in which biological, motor, and social equipment are developed to the point that a youth can take his or her place in society and begin to move away from the dependent relationships with parents. This is achieved only with ambivalence and conflict in many families, not only because of the actual social pull toward dependency, but because of the psychological pull that bespeaks the adolescent's wish for continued indulgence and caretaking without contingent sense of obligation. The narcissistic entitlement of some adolescents when frustrated yields rage that is hard to control.

License Versus Intellectualized Control

The conflict between *license* and *intellectualized control* is probably best exemplified by Anna Freud's descriptions during the 1930s of the oscillation in behaviors of adolescents. Adolescence may be a period of experimentation regarding sexuality, drug use, general disobedience, and other opportunities seen as temptations. Newly formed cognitive skills also permit intellectuality to be used as a controlling mechanism both on a defensive basis and as an interpersonal tool to resist indulgence of wishes and to help define one's goals during adolescence. It should be clear that these themes will of necessity overlap as they form an interpenetrating substrate for behavioral motives. Adolescents themselves have become fond of describing each other by employing distinctions that refer to various behavioral outcomes. The *nerd* and the *head* are some of the most commonly employed. The *nerd* is typified as compliant, socially awkward, and overly intellectualized and is oblivious to temptations. In sharp contrast, the *head* is someone who has permitted himself or herself to drink or use drugs in excess or become oblivious to or defiant of external or internal controls supposedly defined for his or her well-being. In each of these extremes the adolescent is at the mercy of strong peer influence. Surveys such as that of Trent et al. (1996) consistently show that external perceptions drive adolescents. However, they are more important for male scholastic and athletic performance, whereas young women maintain a stronger internal model, again reinforcing impressions about the psychological and personality differences between young men and women. Gilligan's (1982) qualitative study of the difference in conscience as seen in boys and girls shows teen girls to be more considerate of context and circumstance and more compassionate than the rule-governed conscience of boys.

Family Versus Peer Group

The third theme, *group formation* in adolescence, is intimately related to the first two themes. Large or small peer group formation brings the adolescent's attempt at removal from family life into sharp focus. Whether this removal is used as a substitution for or regression from family life depends on how the group is used and how the adolescent determines his or her role in that group. During the juvenile period just prior to adolescence, or in early adolescence, Sullivan (1953) described the "chumship" as a time of same-sex social companionship and interest in which sharing and comparing of personal secrets take place. During this initial small-group formation, the adolescent is gradually made aware that companionship, companionableness, and the inner life can somehow now be translated into intimate relations with same-age, same-sex peers for developmental advantage. These small groups of two then gradually develop into larger groups during the early adolescent phase.

Phenomenologically, young women begin to wear the same clothes and share the same style, and young men belong to a team and exhibit the common expressions of individuality in pairs, bringing to light a kind of twinning effect (Burlingham 1945) that then proceeds into larger group formation. The larger groups may be clubs, teams, or social groups that are designed for the adolescent to share athletic or social interests. Such groups are usually self-governed as principles of self-determination and responsibility are learned. The resilient 16-year-olds in the Duneden Study mentioned previously (Fergusson and Lynskey 1996) had all the prosocial traits that would exclude them from excessive novelty seeking and bad peers.

The generation of small groups into dispirited or isolated groups of individuals who seek mutual support as families begin to fail is an expression of both progressive socialization and sometimes antisocial forces. If these new social groups take on an antifamily stance or become indifferent to the values of the community, they may become degenerated groups or gangs. However, each adolescent in the group may then bolster his or her individual pride in the new group identity. New peer leadership is established as well that seems to the adolescent to be more caring and more responsive to his or her needs than parents have been in the past. This radical split occurs most commonly among those adolescents with disrupted families or in lower socioeconomic groups, or when social values have broken down. A recent study of 221 African American adolescents in ninth through twelfth grade showed the important positive effect of peer support when stress was high. Racial identity seemed to be less significant in this study (McCreary et al. 1996). The issue of license for groups or gangs becomes a public concern when illicit drugs, drag racing, public sexual display, or harassment of "grownups" or elderly people are at the forefront. All of these activities bring youngsters together either in a common mockery of the adult community or in upholding the idea that there is adequate mutual support apart from one's family, sometimes mimicking a kind of Robin Hood mentality. The latter may be a distortion or a realistic protest taking the form of, for example, the following statement: "You have exploited us and have been indifferent to our needs for so long, we will now be indifferent to your values and exploit and confront you." The escape from conscience is thus justified. Among girls the adolescent breakaway from the family may center on romantic fantasies that another peer's parent(s) is more ideal than one's own parent(s). This *family romance* fantasy, which seems to be universal among both sexes at ages 6 and 7, is revived in adolescence. It may be expressed more prominently among girls in our culture, taking hold in the special chumship period during which younger adolescent women engage in a twinning reaction with a same-sex peer. Together the young women plan together, discuss crushes, and plot strategies about romantic concerns. The sense of community that is generated sometimes expands into threesomes, foursomes, and small group formation, or is manifested in better-organized group activities such as dancing, gymnastics, or intellectual clubs. In the last quarter of the twentieth century we witnessed a greater tendency of opposite-sex friendships and chumships and earlier incursion on groups by heterosexual pairing than had been seen earlier in that century.

During the 1990s and into the new millennium, we have witnessed the effect of the new technology and the media on adolescents. Chat rooms and films have brought adolescents together in a new way, exploiting their sexual interests and curiosities and gratifying their need for contact and community while ignoring intimacy. New terms such as "hooking up" are designations for casual sexual contact, but the practice is not new. Nonetheless, the adolescent culture is newly abuzz with the search for immediate gratification, with many validations for their actions in film and television. We do not know the long-term effects of such reinforcement on institutions such as marriage and family and on social responsibility. Teen pregnancy is high but still predominates in the lower socioeconomic stratum, calling forth the same predictors of social pathology as in prior generations.

Normalization Versus Privacy

The *normalizing function of adolescent community* must be contrasted with the need for privacy. These two issues are sometimes, but not always, in opposition to each other. The normalizing function addresses issues of what the adolescent can tell a peer, what is private, and what the adolescent must feel is either sacred to the family or sacred to himself or herself. Recent studies of peer acceptance and friendships in 542 ninth graders show that one friend is sufficient to ensure high self-esteem scores (Bishop and Inderbitzen 1995). However, such correlations do not attest to the priority of friendship or of self-esteem in this conjunction. The tempting possibility of sharing a special or "weird" fantasy with somebody involves risk taking for the adolescent and is an essential part of learning where he or she fits into the expanding world. The common language of adolescence (i.e., "sociolects") that becomes segregated from the adult's language (Shapiro 1985) is a startling representation of a search for group cohesion by excluding others. "Trading dozens" among ghetto blacks and "Valley speak," imported from the West Coast, are examples of when adolescents try new forms that segregate themselves from an adult world that has not fully taken them in.

Even as the adolescent clings to groups, he or she also craves privacy. The closed door, secret telephone conversations, chat rooms, instant messages, diaries, and music blasting through earphones are but a few examples of how the adolescent counteracts the urge to tell with the need to hide. Being alone with one's thoughts, the sense of working one's problem through in one's head, writing poetry, and simply indulging one's feelings further exemplify how intellectualized or sentimental and brooding the adolescent may become.

We have ample recent examples from the gay rights movement to suggest that some young men and women understand early—in their eleventh to fifteenth year—that their homosexual impulses are dominant, and yet their ability to "come out" continues to be under social and familial constraints. Some of these children may become even more private for a time; yet others have been able to find peers with whom they can express their interests and share their concerns. It is perhaps more the case than not that, whatever one's sexual preference, adolescence is a time for seeing how others feel about the same ideas or of becoming ashamed with the conviction that one's thoughts are unnatural. Acceptance of a gay or lesbian adolescent by his or her family, although not universal, is becoming more common.

Idealization Versus Devaluation

While attempting to normalize his or her experience, the adolescent often spends a great deal of time in *idealizing and devaluing adults or peers*. Crushes, pinups, and hero worship are the hallmark of the adolescent. Indeed, sometimes one's parent or parents may be temporarily idealized. The usual, expected adolescent sequence involves devaluing one's parents while idealizing a public figure or special teacher. Such idealization and devaluation, however, are fragile and frequently lose their power as rapidly as they are constructed. The slightest hurt or presumed injury is significant. A crush on a teacher or the longing wish to be a superstar quarterback or a prima ballerina may help the young adolescent to take the appropriate steps in the fulfillment of building ego ideals against which his or her own developmental progress may be measured. At the same time, the need to devalue parents permits a psychological means of discounting their authority, separating the adolescent from oedipal longing and also permitting him or her to move away from the family urgings and toward goals nourished and encouraged outside the family. As these processes are taking hold, the adolescent is also beginning to establish his or her own character or identity.

Identity, Role, and Character

Identity, *role*, and *character* have been associated in the developmental literature with the name of Erik Erikson (1963), who contended that "the sense of ego identity... is the accrued confidence that the inner sameness and continuity prepared in the past are matched by the sameness and continuity of one's meaning for others, as evidenced in the tangible promise of a 'career'" (pp. 261–262). The adolescent seeks to establish continuity with the past and to mentally work over the various and sometimes fragmentary idealizations and identifications to ultimately form a coherent unity in character. Thus, identity not only extends backward but is projected forward in the form of establishment of goals, aims, and anticipated career and lifestyle. Sexual identity, sense of self, and role in the community are also part of the concept.

Identity usually is not viewed as being equivalent to character, but, on the other hand, it contains many of the elements that might be addressed under concepts such as character and personality. It is important to note that adolescence is a period involving the rapid establishment of these presumed structures. If a failure occurs, there may be a functional breakdown akin to what Erikson called identity diffusion, a condition that is marked by doubt, confusion, insecurity, and aimlessness. Once these particular structures become more consistently established, the adolescent may then move into the next stage of development to adulthood. Regrettably, concepts such as temperament have not been empirically well linked to later character and personality. Moreover, there is no strong evidence that Axis II personality disorder diagnoses are easily made in adolescence because of the rapid changes occurring.

Sexuality: Identity, Role, and Partner

Sexuality may be seen as a substructure of identity, but it is important during the adolescent period not only in terms of role establishment but in terms of matching one's core sexual identity with sexual role and sexual object choice. Blos (1985) posited, on clinical grounds, that the early phases of sexual functioning are characterized by a recrudescence of masturbation, especially in males. In fact, masturbation becomes a frequently used channel for discharging tension as a generalized activity to relieve anxiety. It is only as the teenager moves into the second part of adolescence (ages 15–20) that this overuse of masturbation as a discharge channel gives way to more differentiated sexual activity guided by fantasies about others with a clearer determination of mental partners in pleasure. Whether this object is heterosexual or homosexual, the maturational thrust is in the direction of permitting one's sexuality to be expressed as a bid for an affiliation that ultimately will bind affection and bodily pleasure.

One of the important aspects of masturbatory activity in adolescence concerns the idiosyncratic establishment of the masturbation fantasy created to satisfy many features of past problems and current understanding. In short, the adolescent can in fantasy be active and passive, sadistic and compliant, tender and vigorous, male and female. In fact, he or she can be an observer or exhibitor as well. The imagery of the masturbation fantasy may make up a core personality feature, because the personal organization of the fantasy points to the central conflicts of that person's life. This view has been expressed specifically by Laufer (1976) in the notion of a *central masturbation fantasy.*

As adolescents move into the world and attempt to express their sexuality, they seek a person who more or less matches their mental object. Adolescents then attempt to work out the varying aspects of what is arousing and what creates a human interaction and brings the elements of satisfaction and security together. Sexual experimentation may take place. According to large epidemiologically based questionnaire studies, there may be an initial temporary homosexuality expressed transiently that then gives way to heterosexuality. Following this, a relative fixity of pattern of sexual choices is established. Adolescence is a time of dating, going together, and experimentation with others. Even if sexual intercourse or its arousing foreplay is not accomplished, it is on the mind of the adolescent. If there is sexual enactment during the periods of turmoil and rebellion, developmental conflicts concerning dependence and independence, license and intellectualization, and removal from family groups in favor of the sexual alliance are the themes of the enactment. For example, cohabitation in spite of family or religious restriction may be simultaneously a sexual act, a rebellion against authority, and a need for community. Choosing someone who is the opposite of one's mother or father in appearance or removed from one's ethnic group may be an example of reaction formation in the face of threatened oedipal impulses. On the other hand, choices too close to home may have the same meaning of oedipal patterning and dependency. It is of maximum importance to understand that sexuality, like any other of the areas discussed, can be used in the service of either expression of wish or defense during the formative adolescent years. The biological underpinnings of sexual orientation are now being carefully studied, but which specific genes and hormones are significant is as yet uncertain.

As children move into adolescence, the patterns they developed in their childhood same-sex groups are carried over into cross-sex encounters. People of both sexes are faced with a relatively unfamiliar situation to which they must adapt. Young men, accustomed to counterdominance and competitive reactions to their own power assertions, may find themselves relating to women who agree with them and otherwise offer enabling responses. Young women, in interactions with men, are less likely to receive the reciprocal agreement and opportunities to talk that they have learned to expect from other women. Whereas the behavior of men in mixed-sex and same-sex groups tends to be similar, women's behavior in mixed groups is more complex. Some women become more like men as tradition would describe them—raising their voices, interrupting, and otherwise becoming more assertive than they would be when interacting with women only. Others appear to act as they do in same-sex groups, sometimes in exaggerated form, and may end up speaking less and smiling more than they would in a women's group.

Although patterns of mutual influence can become more symmetrical in intimate male–female dyads, the distinctive styles of the two sexes still persist (Maccoby 1990). On balance, the interactive styles of girls and women appear to put them at a disadvantage in cross-sex encounters, a factor of increasing importance as more and more women enter the workplace in traditionally male occupations. Moreover, the centrality of interdependence and caring relationships in the lives of girls and women tends to be viewed pejoratively by those persons, including many women themselves, who stress the importance of self-actualization through competitive success (Gilligan 1982).

Two recent surveys (De Gaston et al. 1996; Harvey and Spigner 1995) are relevant to our understanding: Among 1,800 junior high school students, females remain less likely than males to have had "sex" and show a greater commitment to abstinence and believe that early contact is more detrimental to future goal attainment. Moreover, a survey of 1,026 high school students suggests that sexually active males were also more likely to use alcohol and have higher levels of stress, were less likely to use seat belts, and were more likely to engage in fist fights and to worry about AIDS. Those girls who had engaged in sex also used alcohol and cigarettes and had higher levels of stress.

Reshuffling of Defenses (Style)

In the beginning of adolescence there is a tendency to project outward and to make adaptations that are alloplastic (i.e., externalized). The world, not the adolescent's inner wishes or aims, becomes the reason why the adolescent acts the way he or she does. Blame is placed outside of the individual; responsibility for actions are seen as exterior to the self. This tendency toward denial and projection has led some investigators to suggest that the adolescent acts in a way that may be dystonic to consensual reality. In other adolescents identifications take hold early in a firmer way, and reaction formations and repression begin to help the individual to cut loose from earlier oedipal ties. We begin to see in adolescents a clear establishment of defensive operations in line with productive work and adaptation using their idealized images as guides to planning future aims.

Style of functioning again may be related to temperament and how various traits help or hinder the adolescent's adaptive stance as he or she plans for the future. Thus, the characterizations of adolescence as a developmental step and a developmental epoch seem to be in line with the sum of developmental tasks that must be accomplished. Erikson wrote that adolescence is a time of life when work and sexuality must be linked and pregenital arousal and procreative aims converge. Others have described how reconciliations of the period concern not only the past and the future but also the issues that are involved in identity formation and goal setting.

Erikson's contribution to our understanding that adolescence is not the end of the developmental line has been echoed by others as well (see, e.g., Vaillant 1977), producing more extensive visions of what development looks like *in later life*. These issues, which do not fall within the scope of this chapter, are discussed elsewhere. Although this chapter ends with adolescence, developmental psychology is a state of mind of the observer—a point of view. Developmental analysis can be carried out to discover the stage-specific aspects of each age and how the individual acts and experiences throughout the life cycle.

Summary

There are strong historical and clinical reasons to recommend psychiatric interest in the process of normal development. General principles of development derive from the Darwinian proposal that small broods require prolonged caretaking. Growth, maturation, and development are the cornerstones of the process resulting in mature adaptive functioning and adult organization. The course of development is characterized by differentiation and by integrations among neurological, psychological, and social systems. Each new integration and hierarchic reorganization yields a new structure that offers new functions and adaptations. Development proceeds continuously, as well as discontinuously, as evidenced by biodevelopmental shifts. Rather than a single developmental psychology, the delineation of developmental process is method-bound. Psychoanalytic, Piagetian, Gesellian, and Bowlbyan stances are exemplars of representative positions. Any psychiatric problem can be approached from a developmental standpoint weighing risk and protective factors, as well as from a sequenced analysis of the evolution of disorder.

The psychoanalytic view of childhood initially derived from retrospective and reconstructive inferences. Freud suggested that repression was the prime mechanism that both hid and modified the postulated polymorphously perverse infantile sexual thoughts from the conscious minds of neurotic individuals. Freud introduced libido theory to describe the maturational mental sequence that children traversed. He also posited a hierarchy of danger signals that children have to evaluate and cope with: helplessness during the first months of life; separation between 7 and 12 months; castration or body integrity anxiety from ages 3 to 6 years; and, finally, danger of punishment by guilt ensued from an internalized value system (i.e., the superego). As development proceeds, the danger assumes a different configuration, progressing from *fear of loss of the object* to *fear of loss of the love of the object*. For Freud, the Oedipus complex represents a watershed of prior developmental lines and a focal configuration for conflict.

Later psychoanalysts directly observed children. Spitz postulated three organizers and their functions in the development of human behavior: 1) the smiling response linking external and internal events; 2) the stranger response marking attachment to a specific other; and 3) the development of the signal "No" reflecting a fully internalized and individualized human toddler who has become an agency of will separate from the mother. The separation-individuation process includes a number of substages that culminate in attachment and object constancy leading to independent action. Anna Freud posited developmental lines that describe how a child organizes behavior in an affective climate in relation to others.

Contributions from nonpsychoanalytic developmentalists include the following:

1. Gesell, in his normative developmental theory, attempted to unify principles derived from embryogenesis and normative sequences of observed behaviors. Four areas of behavior—motor, adaptive, language, and personal-social—were tracked during infancy and childhood, and a normative timetable was described that established an empirical basis for theory construction.
2. Piaget approached development from the perspective of understanding how it is that children come to know what they seem to know. He described the sensorimotor, preoperational, concrete operational, and formal operational stages through which the infant and child pass on the road to abstract intelligent behavior.
3. Bowlby constructed a human developmental psychology by melding psychoanalytic and ethological concepts, directing attention to both the biological and the social components of attachment, which have been expanded by a network of experimental paradigms.

These considerations provide a framework for the examination of the physical, neurological, sensorimotor, cognitive, and affective development from birth to preadolescence. Adolescence is considered a way station to the further integrations necessary to adult life introduced by the Industrial Revolution.

The human infant is born with a largely prewired nervous system, and many capacities designed for survival are already built into the organism—hence the designation *the competent infant*. Motor functions develop in a cephalocaudal direction. Reflexive behaviors gradually become reorganized so that by 10 months the infant grasps objects in both hands and brings them to the midline. Symmetrical use of limbs and axial support are essential precursors for the achievement of turning over at 4 months, sitting at 6 months, and standing and walking by the end of the first year of life. Motor and cognitive behaviors as well depend on maturation and feedback to the CNS. Although prewiring is the basis of some achievements, dendritic proliferation and pruning are also necessary, and these are dependent on experience.

During the first year of life the child undergoes major cognitive shifts in his or her capacity to apprehend the external environment on the way to the achievement of object permanence. The vocal apparatus is used to produce protolinguistic expressions attracting the environment to the child. Infants selectively attend to congruent visual and acoustic signals. By the end of the first year of life the child can use several single words communicatively. Language competence and performance develop at a rapid pace. The 2-year-old rapidly moves from telegraphic speech of two-word phrases to the achievement of a three- to six-word mean length of utterance by 3 years of age.

Throughout the toddler and preschool years the child changes in behavior. A 3-year-old is a language user and can behave appropriately in limited social situations, attend nursery school, cooperate with routines and demands for sharing and taking turns, and participate in fantasy pretend play.

The human infant is born into a social world with capacities to perceive, assimilate, organize, and respond to social stimuli—capacities that permit him or her to function as an active partner in the social interaction. During the first year, caregivers regulate infants' level of arousal and excitation by varying facial expression, gestures, and vocalization. Infants regulate their level of social engagement through gaze aversion, vocalization, and facial expression. They gain experience with both self and other regulation and come to recognize their own agency.

By 7 months, wariness of strangers is apparent (so-called stranger anxiety). Between 7 and 9 months of age, joint attention emerges, as well as attunement and social referencing. By 10 months of age, selective attachments to specific individuals have developed. The strange situation procedure has been used to assess the quality of attachment in 12- to 20-month-old children. Approximately two-thirds of children are securely attached, as evidenced by their seeking proximity with mother and using her as a source of comfort after separation. These children tend to exhibit greater social competence and better peer relationships during nursery school.

Between 10 and 16 months of age, the child devotes considerable energy and skill to locomotor activity and exploration. Infants will search for the absent mother or call for her (i.e., *refueling* in Mahlerian terms). Between 16 and 24 months, ambivalence is often intense. Later, as the child's mental representation of mother becomes more stable, separation is more easily tolerated. The availability of a secure and reliable internal representation of mother facilitates the child's increasing ability to engage in independent activities.

Data deriving from studies of neurodevelopmental cognitive and social organization suggest that there is a discontinuity at 7 years that corresponds to a second biodevelopmental shift. Neuronal dendrites are most dense at age 7. It is after age 7 that children begin to understand that their feelings, intuitions, and thoughts may be of interest to others. Children of this age begin to infer feelings and to understand cause-and-effect relationships between objects, events, and situations, and concepts such as ambivalence. Children of 7 years and older are initially rule-bound and even moralistic. Friendship patterns are frequently reorganized. The period of middle childhood is a time of skill development in preparation for application to the more creative aspects of learning in the future. Adolescence has come to represent the developmental bridge between middle childhood and adulthood. Biological, psychological, and social factors set it apart. Puberty refers to achievement of capacity to procreate as a mature member of a species. The external characteristics—secondary sexual characteristics—of both sexes become prominent social signs. Simultaneously, intellectual and cognitive capacities expand, too. Adolescents become capable of formal operations and the achievement of abstract intelligence.

Early psychoanalytically informed studies marked adolescence as a period of turmoil. Later developmental normative studies based on the direct observation of adolescents have identified developmental paths that are less dramatic. Nevertheless, adolescents must negotiate a series of issues before they can emerge as adults. The following themes characterize the developmental process during adolescence: dependence versus independence; license versus intellectualized control; family versus peer group; normalization versus privacy; idealization versus devaluation; the achievement of identity, role, and char-acter; sexuality; and the reshuffling of defenses (style). New technological advances in computers and the media provide a challenge for the next generation. Development does not stop with the attainment of adult status. Developmental analysis can be carried out at any age to discover the stage-specific aspects of each period and to define how the individual acts and experiences throughout the life cycle.

References

Ainsworth MDS: The effects of maternal deprivation: a review of findings and controversy in the context of research strategy, in Deprivation of Maternal Care: A Reassessment of Its Effects. Public Health Papers No 14. Geneva, World Health Organization, 1962

Ainsworth MDS, Blehar MD, Waters E, et al: Patterns of Attachment: A Psychological Study of the Strange Situation. Hillsdale, NJ, Lawrence Erlbaum, 1978

Ariès P: Centuries of Childhood: A Social History of Family Life. Translated by Baldick R. New York, Alfred A Knopf, 1962

Bar-Haim Y, Sutton DB, Fox NA, et al: Stability and change of attachment at 14, 24, and 58 months of age: behavior, representation, and life events. J Child Psychol Psychiatry 41:381–388, 2000

Baron-Cohen S: The autistic child's theory of mind: a case of specific developmental delay. J Child Psychol Psychiatry 30:285–298, 1989

Bates JE: Concepts and measures of temperament, in Temperament in Childhood. Edited by Kohnstamm GA, Bates JE, Rothbart MK. New York, Wiley, 1989

Binet A: New methods for the diagnosis of the intellectual level of the subnormals. L'Annee Psychologique 12:191–244, 1905

Bishop JA, Inderbitzen HM: Peer acceptance and friendship: an investigation of their relation to self-esteem. Journal of Early Adolescence 15:476–489, 1995

Block J, Haan N: Lives Through Time. Berkeley, CA, Bancroft Books, 1971

Blos P: Son and Father: Before and Beyond the Oedipus Complex. New York, Free Press, 1985

Borke H: Interpersonal perception of young children: egocentrism or empathy. Developmental Psychology 5:263–269, 1971

Bower T, Broghton J, Moore M: Infant responses to approaching objects. Percept Psychophys 9:193–196, 1970

Bowlby J: Maternal Care and Mental Health. Geneva, Switzerland, World Health Organization, 1952

Bowlby J: Attachment and Loss, Vol 1: Attachment. New York, Basic Books, 1969

Bowlby J: Attachment and Loss, Vol 2: Separation: Anxiety and Anger. New York, Basic Books, 1973

Bowlby J: Attachment and Loss, Vol 3: Loss: Sadness and Depression. New York, Basic Books, 1980

Brazelton TB, Koslowski B, Main N: The origins of reciprocity: the early mother-infant interaction, in The Effect of the Infant on Its Caregiver. Edited by Lewis M, Rosenblum L. New York, Wiley, 1974, pp 49–76

Bretherton I: Pretense: the form and function of make-believe play. Developmental Review 9:383–401, 1989

Bretherton I, Ainsworth MDS: Responses of one-year-olds to a stranger in a strange situation, in The Origins of Fear. Edited by Lewis M, Rosenblum LA. New York, Wiley, 1974, pp 131–164

Brown JR, Donelan-McCall N, Dunn J: Why talk about mental states? The significance of children's conversations, with friends, siblings and mothers. Child Dev 67:836–849, 1996

Brown R: A First Language: The Early Stages. Cambridge, MA, Harvard University Press, 1973

Buchsbaum HK, Emde RN: Play narrations in thirty-six month old children: early moral development and family relationships. Psychoanal Study Child 40:129–155, 1990

Burlingham DT: The fantasy of having a twin. Psychoanal Study Child 1:205–210, 1945

Buss AH, Plomin R: Temperament: Early Developing Personality Traits. Hillsdale, NJ, Lawrence Erlbaum, 1984

Chess S, Thomas A: Origins and Evolution of Behavior Disorders From Infancy to Early Adult Life. New York, Brunner/Mazel, 1984

Cicchetti D, Sroufe LA: An organizational view of affect: illustration from the study of Down's syndrome infants, in The Development of Affect. Edited by Lewis M, Rosenblum LA. New York, Plenum, 1978, pp 309–335

Cohen NJ, Eichenbaum H, Deacedo BS, et al: Different memory systems underlying acquisition of procedural and declarative knowledge. Ann N Y Acad Sci 444:54–71, 1985

Curtiss S: Dissociations between language and cognition: cases and implications. J Autism Dev Disord 11:15–30, 1981

Darwin C: The Expression of the Emotions in Man and Animals. London, England, J Murray, 1872

DeCasper A, Fifer W: Of human bonding: newborns prefer their mothers' voices. Science 208:1174–1176, 1980

De Gaston JF, Week S, Jensen L: Understanding gender differences in adolescent sexuality. Adolescence 31:217–231, 1996

Dulit E: Adolescent thinking à la Piaget: the formal stage. Journal of Youth and Adolescence 4:281–301, 1972

Dunn J: The Emanuel Miller Memorial Lecture 1995: Children's relationships: bridging the divide between cognitive and social development. J Child Psychol Psychiatry 37:507–518, 1996

Eimas PD, Squeland ER, Josczyk P, et al: Speech perception in infants. Science 171:303–306, 1971

Emde RN: From adolescence to midlife: remodeling the structure of adult development. J Am Psychoanal Assoc 33(suppl):59–112, 1985

Emde RN, Gaensbauer T, Harmon R: Emotional Expression in Infancy: A Bio-Behavioral Study. New York, International Universities Press, 1976

Erikson E: Growth and Crises of the Healthy Personality. New York, International Universities Press, 1959

Erikson E: Childhood and Society, 2nd Edition, Revised and Expanded. New York, WW Norton, 1963

Esman A: Adolescence and Culture. New York, Columbia University Press, 1990

Fergusson DM, Lynskey MT: Adolescent resiliency to family adversity. J Child Psychol Psychiatry 37:281–292, 1996

Field M, Woodson R, Greenberg R, et al: Discrimination and imitation of facial expressions by neonates. Science 218:179–181, 1982

Fonagy P, Steele H, Steele M: Maternal representations of attachment during pregnancy predict the organization of infant–mother attachment at one year of age. Child Dev 62:891–905, 1991

Freud A: The Ego and the Mechanisms of Defense. New York, International Universities Press, 1946

Freud A: The Assessment of Normality in Childhood. New York, International Universities Press, 1965

Freud A: A psychoanalytic view of developmental psychopathology. Journal of the Philadelphia Association for Psychoanalysis 1:7–17, 1974

Freud S: Three essays on the theory of sexuality (1905), in The Standard Edition of the Complete Psychological Works of Sigmund Freud, Vol 7. Translated and edited by Strachey J. London, England, Hogarth Press, 1953, pp 123–245

Freud S: Beyond the pleasure principle (1920), in The Standard Edition of the Complete Psychological Works of Sigmund Freud, Vol 18. Translated and edited by Strachey J. London, England, Hogarth Press, 1959a, pp 1–64

Freud S: Inhibitions, symptoms and anxiety (1926), in The Standard Edition of the Complete Psychological Works of Sigmund Freud, Vol 20. Translated and edited by Strachey J. London, England, Hogarth Press, 1959b, pp 75–175

Garraghty PE, Churchill JD, Banks MK: Adult neural plasticity: similarities between two paradigms. Current Directions in Psychological Science 7:87–91, 1998

Gesell AL, Amatruda CS: Developmental diagnosis, in Normal and Abnormal Child Development: Clinical Methods and Psychiatric Applications, 2nd Edition. New York, Hoeber, 1947, pp 3–14

Gesell AL, Ilg FL: Child Development: An Introduction to the Study of Human Growth. New York, Harper & Row, 1949

Gesell AL, Ilg FL, Ames LB: The Infant and Child in the Culture of Today: the Guidance of Development in Home and Nursery School. New York, Harper & Row, 1974

Gilligan C: In a Different Voice: Psychological Theory and Women's Development. Cambridge, MA, Harvard University Press, 1982

Greenacre P: The childhood of the artist. Psychoanal Study Child 12:57–58, 1957

Guardo CJ, Bohan JB: Development of a sense of self-identity in children. Child Dev 42:1909–1921, 1971

Hamilton CE: Continuity and discontinuity of attachment from infancy through adolescence. Child Dev 71:690–694, 2000

Harlow HF: Primary affectional patterns in primates. Am J Orthopsychiatry 30:676–684, 1960

Harter S: Developmental perspectives on the self-system, in Handbook of Child Psychology, Vol 4: Socialization, Personality, and Social Development. Edited by Hetherington EM. New York, Wiley, 1983, pp 275–385

Harvey SM, Spigner C: Factors associated with sexual behavior among adolescents: a multivariate analysis. Adolescence 30:253–264, 1995

Hauser ST, Powers S, Noam GG: Adolescents and Their Families. New York, Free Press, 1991

Horner TM: Two methods of studying stranger reactivity in infancy: a review. J Child Psychol Psychiatry 21:203–219, 1980

Huttenlocher PR: Synaptic density in human frontal cortex: developmental changes and effects of aging. Brain Res 163:195–205, 1979

Izard CE: Measuring Emotions in Infants and Children. Cambridge, England, Cambridge University Press, 1982

Kagan J: The Nature of the Child. New York, Basic Books, 1984

Kagan J, Reznick JS, Gibbons J: Inhibited and uninhibited types of children. Child Dev 60:838–845, 1989

Kaplan PS, Goldstein MH, Huckeby ER, et al: Habituation, sensitization, and infants' responses to Motherese speech. Dev Psychobiol 28:45–57, 1995

Karmiloff-Smith A: Annotation: the extraordinary cognitive journey from foetus through infancy. J Child Psychol Psychiatry 36:1293–1313, 1995

Klinnert MD, Emde RN, Butterfield P, et al: Social referencing: the infant's use of emotional signals from a friendly adult with mother present. Developmental Psychology 22:427–432, 1986

Kuhl P: Linguistic experience alters phonetic perception in infants by six months. Science 255:606–608, 1992

Laufer M: The central masturbation fantasy, the final sexual organization, and adolescence. Psychoanal Study Child 31:297–316, 1976

Lewis M, Brooks-Gunn J: Social Cognition and the Acquisition of Self. New York, Plenum, 1979

Lewis M, Michelson L: Children's Emotions and Moods: Developmental Theory and Measurement. New York, Plenum, 1983

Lewis M, Sullivan MW, Stanger C, et al: Self development and self consciousness emotions. Child Dev 60:146–156, 1989

Lewis MM: Infant Speech. New York, Harcourt Brace, 1936

Maccoby EE: Gender and relationships: a developmental account. Am Psychol 45:513–520, 1990

MacKain K, Studdert-Kennedy M, Spieker S, et al: Infant intermodal speech perception is a left-hemisphere function. Science 219:1347–1349, 1983

Mahler MS, Pine F, Bergman A: The Psychological Birth of the Human Infant: Symbiosis and Individuation. New York, Basic Books, 1975

Main M, Kaplan N, Cassidy J: Security in infancy, childhood and adulthood: a move to the level of representation. Monogr Soc Res Child Dev 50 (1–2, Ser No 209 [Growing Points of Attachment Theory and Research; Bretherton I, Waters E, eds.):66–106, 1985

Masten AS, Coatsworth JD, Neemann J, et al: The structure and coherence of competence from childhood through adolescence. Child Dev 66:1635–1659, 1995

McCreary ML, Slavin LA, Berry EJ: Predicting problem behavior and self-esteem among African American adolescents. Journal of Adolescent Research 11:216–234, 1996

Meeus W, Dekoviic M: Identity development, parental and peer support in adolescence: results of a national Dutch survey. Adolescence 30:931–944, 1995

Meltzoff AN: Understanding the intentions of others: re-enactment of intended acts by 18-month-old children. Developmental Psychology 31:838–850, 1995

Meltzoff AN, Moore MK: Imitation, memory and the representation of persons. Infant Behavior and Development 17:83–99, 1994

Merzenich MM, Jenkins MM: Cortical representations of learned behaviors, in Memory Concepts. Edited by Anderson P, Hvalby O, Paulsen O, et al. Amsterdam, The Netherlands, Elsevier, 1993, pp 437–451

Money J: Sin, sickness, or status? Homosexual gender identity and psychoneuroendocrinology. Am Psychol 42:384–399, 1987

Nelson K: Individual differences in language development. Developmental Psychology 17:170–187, 1981

Nelson K: Event Knowledge: Structure and Function in Development. Hillsdale, NJ, Lawrence Erlbaum, 1986

Newcomb TM: Personality and Social Change. New York, Dryden Press, 1943

Offer B, Offer JB: From Teenage to Young Manhood: A Psychological Study. New York, Basic Books, 1975

Offer D: The Psychological World of the Teenager: A Study of Normal Adolescent Boys. New York, Basic Books, 1969

Offer D, Sabshin M: Normality: Theoretical and Clinical Concepts of Mental Health, Revised Edition. New York, Basic Books, 1974

Oldham DG: Adolescent turmoil: a myth revisited, in Adolescent Psychiatry: Developmental and Clinical Studies, Vol 6. Edited by Feinstein SC, Giovacchini PL. Chicago, IL, University of Chicago Press, 1978, pp 267–279

Opie I, Opie P: The Lore and Language of School Children. London, England, Oxford University Press, 1959

Pannabecker BJ, Emde RN, Johnson W, et al: Maternal perceptions of infant emotions from birth to 18 months: a preliminary report. Paper presented at the International Conference of Infant Studies, New Haven, CT, April 1980

Piaget J: The Origins of Intelligence in Children. Translated by Cook M. New York, International Universities Press, 1952

Piaget J, Inhelder B: The Psychology of the Child. New York, Basic Books, 1969

Plomin R, Daniels D: Why are children in the same family so different from one another? Behav Brain Sci 10:1–16, 1987

Posner MI, Rothbart MK: Developing mechanisms of self-regulation. Dev Psychopathol 12:427–441, 2000

Rheingold HL, Eckerman CO: Fear of the stranger: a critical examination, in Advances in Child Development and Behavior, Vol 8. Edited by Reese HW. New York, Academic, 1973, pp 186–223

Roffwarg H, Muzio J, Dement W: Ontogenetic development of the human sleep-dream cycle. Science 152:604–619, 1966

Rothbart MK, Goldsmith HH: Three approaches to the study of infant temperament. Developmental Review 5:237–260, 1985

Saarni C: Children's understanding of display rules for expressive behavior. Dev Psychol 15:424–429, 1979

Sapir E: Language: An Introduction to the Study of Speech. New York, Harcourt, Brace & World, 1921

Schaffer HR, Emerson PE: The development of social attachments in infancy. Monogr Soc Res Child Dev 29(Ser No 94), 1964

Schneirla TC, Rosenblatt JS: Behavioral organization and genesis of the social bond in insects and mammals. Am J Orthopsychiatry 31:223–253, 1961

Shapiro T: Clinical Psycholinguistics. New York, Plenum, 1979

Shapiro T: Adolescent language: a diagnostic clue to and group identity values and treatment, in Adolescent Psychiatry. Edited by Sugar M. Chicago, IL, University of Chicago Press, 1985, pp 297–311

Shapiro T, Perry R: Latency revisited: the age 7 plus or minus 1. Psychoanal Study Child 31:79–105, 1976

Skinner BF: Science and Human Behavior. New York, Macmillan, 1953

Spelke ES: Nativism, empiricism and the origins of knowledge. Infant Behavior and Development 21:181–200, 1998

Spitz RA: Hospitalism: an inquiry into the genesis of psychiatric conditions in early childhood. Psychoanal Study Child 1:53–74, 1945

Spitz RA: The First Year of Life: A Psychoanalytic Study of Normal and Deviant Development of Object Relations. New York, International Universities Press, 1965

Sroufe LA, Fleeson J: Attachment and the construction of relationships, in Relationships and Development. Edited by Hartup W, Rubin Z. New York, Cambridge University Press, 1984, pp 51–71

Sroufe LA, Carlson EA, Levy AK, et al: Implications of attachment theory for developmental psychopathology. Dev Psychopathol 11:1–13, 1999

Stern DN: The Interpersonal World of the Infant: A View From Psychoanalysis and Developmental Psychology. New York, Basic Books, 1985

Stocker C, Dunn J, Plomin R: Sibling relationships: links with child temperament, maternal behavior, and family structure. Child Dev 60:715–727, 1989

Stone L, Church J: Adolescence as a cultural phenomenon, in Childhood and Adolescence. New York, Random House, 1957, pp 438–443

Sullivan HS: Interpersonal Theory of Psychiatry. Edited by Perry HS, Gawel ML. New York, WW Norton, 1953

Tanner JM: Growth of bone, muscle and fat during childhood and adolescence, in Growth and Development of Mammals. Edited by Lodge ME. London, England, Butterworths, 1968

Thelen E: Motor development: a new synthesis. Am Psychol 50:79–95, 1995

Thomas A, Chess S: Temperament and Development. New York, Brunner/Mazel, 1977

Thomas A, Chess S: Temperament and personality, in Treatment in Childhood. Edited by Kohnstamm GA, Bates JE, Rothbart MK. New York, Wiley, 1989, pp 249–262

Thomas KM, Drevets WC, Whalen PJ, et al: Amygdala response to facial expressions in children and adults. Biol Psychiatry 49:309–316, 2001

Trent L, Cooney G, Russell G, et al: Significant others' contribution to early adolescents' perceptions of their competence. British Journal of Educational Psychology 66:95–107, 1996

Vaillant GE: Adaptation to Life. Boston, MA, Little, Brown, 1977

Waters E, Merrick S, Treboux D, et al: Attachment security in infancy and early adulthood: a twenty-year longitudinal study. Child Dev 71:684–689, 2000

Watson J: Psychology From the Standpoint of a Behaviorist. Philadelphia, PA, JB Lippincott, 1919

Wechsler D: Wechsler Intelligence Scale for Children. New York, The Psychological Corporation, 1949

Wechsler D: Wechsler Preschool and Primary Scale of Intelligence Manual. New York, Harcourt Brace Jovanovich, 1989

Wechsler D: Wechsler Intelligence Scale for Children, III. New York, Harcourt Brace Jovanovich, 1991

Werner H: Comparative Psychology of Mental Development. New York, International Universities Press, 1957

Werner H, Kaplan B: Symbol Formation. New York, Wiley, 1963

Zacharias L, Wurtman RJ, Shatzoff M: Sexual maturation in contemporary American girls. Am J Obstet Gynecol 108:833–846, 1970

Glossary

Accommodation   A functional aspect of Piaget's model of cognitive development. Accommodation occurs when existing schemas (mental organization) differentiate into new structures ready for new psychic elements.

Assimilation   A functional aspect of Piaget's model of cognitive development that refers to the incorporation of a sensorimotor schema that is repeated with new experiences judged to be equivalent into existing mental organizations.

Adolescence   The developmental period between middle childhood (i.e., latency) and adulthood, characterized by puberty and psychological and social discontinuities in development.

Biosocial organization   Social behavior determined by biological determinants, such as pheromones emanating from a queen ant or bee. The biological agent is active throughout life.

Core self   The self as a cohesive, bounded, psychophysical unit, a dawning sense of which begins to emerge by 2 months of age and becomes consolidated by 30 months (see Stern 1985).

Critical period   Time frame during which an environmental releaser stimulates the emergence of a developmental capacity that is inborn. If no release occurs, that function is said to *involute*. Concept derives from ethological study of nonmammalian species. Among mammals, however, time lines are not as critically limited; therefore, caution must be exercised in applying data across species.

Development   The changing structure of behavior and thought over time. Development includes whatever is provided by maturational potential plus variations in social and environmental influences.

Differentiation   The move from more global reactions to increasingly individuated processes within systems that occurs in the course of maturation and development.

Ego psychology   A psychoanalytic model and movement that superceded depth Id psychology in the late 30s and has persisted. It is to be distinguished from self psychology, intersubjectivity, and object relations theory. Anna Freud may be said to have begun the idea with *The Ego and the Mechanisms of Defense* (A. Freud 1946), and Hartmann, Kris, and Lowenstein were major exponents of the model in the 1950s and 1960s. Its focus is on the ego as an organizing mediator between drive and reality.

Epigenesis   A description of how early sequential steps influence subsequent steps in development. In this linear model of development, each stage is dependent on the resolution of the experiences of the prior stage.

Gender identity   An individual's belief and self-awareness of being male or female. Gender identity is generally established by age 3 years and is usually determined by the sex in which an individual is reared independent of biological factors.

Growth   Biologically, simple accretion of tissue or increase in size or in the number of cells. Change over time in height and weight is an example of growth. Metaphorically, used for describing development.

Hierarchic reorganization   Changes in organization that are not the logical or necessary outcome of prior stages. In this nonlinear model of development, each new integration of biological and neuronal function meshes with psychocognitive capacities so that the result is more than the sum of the parts. Each new stage is a new structure that permits qualitatively different functions and adaptations (see Werner 1957).

Integration   The increasing complexity of relations between and among the senses and the motor apparatus that occurs in the course of maturation and development. Can be applied to psychological functions as well.

Latency   In psychoanalytic theory, the period between the resolution of the Oedipus complex and the onset of puberty during which the drives are relatively quiescent. More neutrally described as middle childhood, this is a period of skill and social development and increasing ability to regulate and modulate affects.

Lines of development   Anna Freud's proposal that in the course of development the child moves 1) from being nursed to rational eating; 2) from incontinence to bowel and bladder control; 3) from egocentricity toward companionship with peers; 4) from play to a capacity for work; 5) from physical to mental pathways of discharge of drives; 6) from animate to inanimate objects; and 7) from irresponsibility to guilt. Symptoms are viewed as regressions or arrests in these lines.

Maturation   The natural unfolding of genetic potential toward an end characterized by full functioning.

Object constancy   The capacity of the developing child (2–3 years) to maintain a stable mental image of the important caregiver in his or her absence.

Organizer   A behavior identified by Spitz as being analogous to an embryonic organizer in general biology. These behaviors are the smiling response (2 months), the stranger response (7 months), and the signal for "No" (around 2 years).

Practicing Subphase of Mahler's theory of the process of separation-individuation (10–16 months) during which the child "practices" newly found locomotor and psychological skills and actively explores his or her environment with exuberance.

Psychosocial organization Social behavior is primarily determined by early experience and its organizational effect in memory rather than by ongoing biological processes.

Puberty Attainment of the capacity to procreate as a mature member of a species (see Tanner 1968).

Rapprochement Subphase of Mahler's theory of the process of separation-individuation (16–24 months) during which temper tantrums, whining behavior, moodiness, and intense separation reactions are at their peak.

Separation-individuation Mahler's descriptive theory of the process by which the baby becomes a separate, discrete, and autonomous toddler.

Social referencing The ability of the baby, established during the final quarter of the first year of life, to respond behaviorally to the emotional expressions of others. Crawling babies can be induced to cross a "visual cliff" (i.e., an illusion that there is a drop-off, although a transparent Plexiglas plate covers the drop) if their mother smiles in encouragement and will turn away if the mother assumes a fearful facial expression. Eye gaze for permission is a later behavioral organizer.

Sensorimotor The first stage of Piaget's model of cognitive development, in which the ability to maintain a stable mental representation and to create a representative world matures. During this stage, sensory and motor behaviors are fused.

Appendix

Major Names in Developmental Psychiatry

Ainsworth, Mary   Canadian-educated American psychologist, collaborator and student of John Bowlby, who developed the strange situation procedure, a laboratory method for assessing the quality of attachment in 12- to 18-month-old children, and fostered further empirical study of attachment research paradigms.

Bowlby, John   British psychiatrist and psychoanalyst, known as the "father of attachment," who was the first to build a human developmental psychology that melded the psychoanalytic and ethological literature. Bowlby recognized the nature of human ties as an organizing precursor to later mature development. His work stimulated further empirical study of attachment, bonding, and separation.

Erikson, Erik Homburger   German-born American psychoanalyst who proposed that personality development takes place through a series of crises that must be overcome and internalized by the individual as he or she passes through eight stages of development from infancy to old age. Additional interests included social psychology and the interactions of psychology with history, politics, and culture. Erikson is best known for his work on identity in adolescents.

Freud, Anna   Psychoanalyst of children, daughter of Sigmund. She introduced play therapy, ego defenses, and developmental lines as significant ideas in child development.

Freud, Sigmund   Viennese founder of psychoanalysis, a treatment and theoretic system that has influenced a century of thought. Freud introduced the idea of polymorphous perverse infantile sexuality and created interest in childhood experience as the basis for adult neurosis.

Gesell, Arnold   American psychologist and pediatrician whose pioneering studies of normal physical and mental development resulted in the establishment of a schedule describing the motor, adaptive, language, and personal/social achievements of infants and young children from birth through 5 years of age. Gesell's normative schedule has been adapted as the Denver Developmental Screen, which is widely used by pediatricians.

Mahler, Margaret   Originally a Hungarian pediatrician, she became an American psychoanalyst and was responsible for the introduction of separation-individuation theory, which was based on direct observation of children in a systematic manner.

Main, Mary   Berkeley University of California Professor of Psychology who introduced the Adult Attachment Interview, an instrument that uses narrative analysis based on Gricean constructs to determine an adult's attachment status.

Piaget, Jean   Swiss psychologist who was one of the first to make a systematic study of the acquisition of understanding in children. Piaget described four stages of development: sensorimotor stage, preoperational stage, concrete operational stage, and formal operational stage. Self-designated as a "genetic epistemologist," he fathered development of cognitive psychology known as the Geneva School.

Skinner, Burrhus Frederic   American psychologist whose work profoundly influenced psychology during the second half of the twentieth century. Skinner's principles of operant conditioning provide the basis for much of modern-day behavior therapy.

Spitz, Rene   A European psychoanalyst who spent most of his professional life in the United States, Spitz studied infants in institutions and mother–infant interaction empirically. He was responsible for the term *anaclitic depression* and the earliest theories of infant ego development. Spitz spent his last years at the University of Colorado, where he influenced Robert Emde.

Stern, Daniel   American psychoanalyst and developmental investigator of mother–infant interaction using microanalytic observational techniques. Stern introduced the terms *motherhood constellation* and *attunement* and has had a significant impact on late-twentieth-century infant research and theory.

Watson, John Broadus   American psychologist whose work in the early years of the twentieth century earned him the title "Founder of Behaviorism." Watson defined psychology as the "science of behavior" and sought to develop a behavioral theory of emotions. His studies of "Little Albert" demonstrated the artificial conditioning of emotional responses in children.

CHAPTER 3

Theories of the Mind and Psychopathology

Stephen S. Marmer, M.D., Ph.D.

In this new era of scientific psychiatry, do we really need a theory of the mind? Is it not a hope that our field will soon have facts that will settle the claims of competing theories and resolve whether the concept of mind as apart from brain has a meaningful place in psychiatry? Impressed as we are by the advances in biological psychiatry and neuroscience, is the psychological mind still even a viable concept? As posed by Goodman (1997) in a thoughtful article,

> Psychiatry occupies a uniquely integrative position among the scientific disciplines. It addresses both physical and mental aspects of human functioning, and uses both of the separate sets of methods that characterize each realm....More than any other discipline, psychiatry has the potential to be an integrative science that weaves together in one fabric various broad perspectives on the human being: biological, behavioral, psychodynamic, interpersonal, and social.... Psychiatry's comprehensiveness, however, bears the seeds of its crisis. Psychiatry as a unitary structure rests on the relationship between physical and mental, a fundamental duality that defines a schism within psychiatry between its physically oriented components (the biological and behavioral) and its mentally oriented components (the psychodynamic, interpersonal, and social). This schism threatens the integrity of psychiatry as a science. (pp. 357–358) (See also Ghaemi and Oepen 1994; Maunder 1995.)

It is not the purpose of this chapter to resolve the mind–body dilemma. However, in devoting a chapter to theories of the mind, this textbook affirms that the mind has an important place in modern psychiatry.

Competing theories are not new in science in general or in psychiatry in particular. Historians and philosophers of science such as Popper (1959, 1962), Kuhn (1970),

and Fleck (1979) have written eloquently on the role of theory in all science. For them, the course of science is necessarily marked by communities of thinkers who invent hermeneutically useful theories or paradigms that reflect underlying world views. These paradigms determine ways to think about the topic in question.

Theories are not limited to subjects such as psychiatry. Fleck points out that theories colored the perception of what we might otherwise think of as the hard science of bacteriology. For its ability to organize an approach to a field, theory is indispensable. In our era, theories are regarded as useful if they are confirmed by data, if they aid in our understanding of the subject being studied, or if they stimulate helpful questions, experiments, or observations. In this sense, theories are neither true nor false; instead, they are more or less useful in interpreting available data or in leading to new information.

In this chapter, I address psychological or mental theory. Current thinking in the biology of the mind or in the genetics of psychopathology is discussed elsewhere in this textbook (see Knowles, Chapter 1). Since the last edition of this textbook, no new theories have risen to the top of our thinking.

To put these theories into perspective, one can turn to the dawn of modern psychiatry, nearly 200 years ago. At the beginning of the nineteenth century, psychiatric patients were just beginning to be considered legitimate "objects" of study. Personality was still viewed under one theory or another as an immutable matter of innate biology. Severe psychopathology was still treated mainly by sequestering patients, and milder psychopathology was still generally regarded as either moral weakness or malingering. Severe psychopathology was the focus of psychiatry, exemplified best by the work of Emil Kraepelin, who classified major mental disorders. Milder psychopathological states generally came to the attention not of psychiatrists but of general physicians and neurologists. This makes understandable the historical irony that the most influential theory of personality was created not by a psychiatrist but by a neurologist: Sigmund Freud.

The theories under discussion represent the ways ingenious investigators made sense out of human behavior. These theories emphasize various data, assume different notions of what constitutes proof or verification, reckon development of the personality according to different factors and timetables, place greater or lesser emphasis on either the biological sphere or the experiential sphere, offer different ideas about the mutability of personality and psychopathology, and therefore lead to different schools of treatment. A theory of the mind and its psychopathology in fact has several components, including concepts of development and of normality, ideas of how the mind works and even of what constitutes the mind, and determinations of treatment technique.

Theories of mind and psychopathology also position themselves variously along certain continua. For example, how much is psychopathology the result of deficiencies, or the absence of ingredients necessary for emotional health, and how much the result of conflict, whether between persons or within the individual? How much is psychopathology the result of actual historical events and how much the result of fantasy? How much influence shall be placed on constitutional factors, on the maturational stage of development, on ordinary learned experience, or on extraordinary traumatic events? How much is out of our awareness, and how much is within the realm of cognition? Answers to these questions lead in turn to treatment choices and further questions: How much does treatment rely on interpretation, and how much on education, exhortation, or a nonspecific healing presence? How much is treatment dependent on the transference and how much on the real relationship?

In a brief chapter such as this, each point of view is presented in an oversimplified, sometimes schematic manner that will not do justice to every subtlety. However, there may be some merit in surveying the entire forest. Although some theories are more ambitious than others, none can yet lay claim to explaining everything. Every generation accumulates experiences with patients that were not adequately addressed by the prior generation's theories. These various theories are best appreciated when the reader makes an effort to see the world through the eyes and theories of each theorist, on the assumption that no great thinker is either wholly right or wholly wrong.

This chapter traces the development of the major modern theories of the mind, starting with the mainstream of psychoanalysis, from Freud through those who questioned, revised, or modified his theories but stayed within the tradition of psychoanalysis.

Next the chapter turns to theories that offer notions of mental structure with a parallel psychodynamic tradition of their own, including the modern rediscovery of trauma.

The chapter closes with a look at some behavioral and cognitive theories that overlap with but in many ways are different from the psychodynamic perspective.

Psychoanalytic Tradition

Freud's Theories

So powerful is the influence of the theories of Sigmund Freud that it is nearly impossible to think about personality or about psychotherapy absent of Freudian considerations. Even the proponents of most alternative theories accept parts of the Freudian legacy that were hotly contested a century ago.

It is more proper to regard Freud as having offered a series of complementary theories, for although he revised his work often during his lifetime and corrected certain emphases, he never fully withdrew earlier versions of his work.

Prepsychoanalytic Theories

Many biographers have commented on the relevance of Freud's work in physiology and neurology to his psychoanalytic theorizing (Ellenberger 1970; Greenberg and Mitchell 1983; Grunbaum 1984; Jones 1953, 1955, 1957; Laplanche and Pontalis 1973; Ricoeur 1970; Wollheim 1971). Although Freud's teachers focused on physiology and not on personality, their metaphors became Freud's organizing principles for his studies of the mind. Strong influences were Helmholz, from whom Freud learned to pattern psychological theories after physical ones, and who focused particularly on matters of the distribution of energy; Brucke, who also emphasized the concept of conservation of energy; Meynert, who bridged Freud's interests in neuroanatomy and its behavioral consequences; and Charcot, whose work in hysteria opened for Freud the path that would eventually lead to psychoanalysis. Freud also borrowed heavily from the great neurologist Hughlings Jackson.

From Helmholz, Brucke, and Meynert, Freud evolved his emphasis on discharge of drives, his principle of constancy, his notion of the theory of repression, and the concept of psychic energy, all anchored in the images of electrical and hydraulic science prevalent in that era. From Charcot, he gained an interest in hysteria and hypnosis. From Jackson, he gleaned an approach to the relation between mental structure and function.

Charcot legitimized for Freud the study of patients with hysteria. Older theories held that such patients were either malingering or had a "wandering uterus." Charcot rejected these theories in favor of an emphasis on the link between symptoms and traumatic events. He noted that hysterical symptoms followed popular rather than anatomically correct malfunction of sensation or movement. For example, a patient might develop numbness of the hand in the popular understanding of glove anesthesia rather than the anatomically correct distribution of the median and ulnar nerves. This meant that symbolic factors were very important in hysteria. Furthermore, Charcot established the role that hypnosis played in the treatment of hysteria. For him, hysteria was caused by trauma in susceptible individuals, yet because ideas rather than neuroanatomy determined the nature of the hysterical patient's symptoms, the condition also was receptive to influence by treatment in the realm of ideas. Words, concepts, and symbols, which entered into the formation of symptoms, therefore, could be curative.

The work of the great neurologist Hughlings Jackson constitutes a neglected inspiration for Freud's work in three critical areas. This can be seen in Freud's prepsychoanalytic monograph "On Aphasia" (S. Freud 1891/1953). From Jackson's thoughts on dynamic associationism grew the concept of psychoanalytic free association. From the maintenance of early memories in the brain grew the concept of regression. And from Jackson's evolutionary theories of brain development came Freud's own theory of psychological stages of development.

This protopsychoanalytic phase culminated with two major works. The first was *Studies on Hysteria* (1893–1895), which was coauthored with Josef Breuer (Breuer and Freud 1893–1895/1955). The second was *Project for a Scientific Psychology* (begun and largely left unfinished in 1895 but not published until 1950; S. Freud 1950/1966). It was Freud's ambitious attempt to link experience, behavior, memory, and motivation into a single neurophysiological system. Unfortunately, even the biology of our age is inadequate to explain such matters comprehensively,[1] and Freud had to abandon his quest.

Freud's theory of hysteria at that time implied a the-

ory of the mind. At first, Freud thought that hysteria was caused by actual events, generally traumatic, the memories of which do not fade away in the usual fashion. After a traumatic event, painful memory is repressed. However, because of a memory's powerful emotional charge, hysterical phenomena are the direct result of reproductions or enactments of the traumatic event. "Hysterics," Freud noted, "suffer mainly from reminiscences" (Breuer and Freud 1893–1895/1955, p. 71). Breuer and Freud used hypnosis to help their patients rid themselves of pathological memories. They did so through a process called *abreaction*, the vivid reliving of the memories and emotions of a past, previously repressed event.

The results of abreaction, however, forced Freud to expand his theory. First, cure rarely came from a single abreaction of a single memory. Every symptom had a multiplicity of "overdetermined" causes. This concept, which is explained more fully later in this chapter (see section "Overdetermination"), means that most symptomatology stems from many layered causes rather than a single simple direct one. Second, Freud was an indifferent hypnotist, and some patients (Elisabeth von R. chief among them) found that talking freely was more effective. Some patients developed powerful emotional attachments to their doctors, which would eventually lead Freud to elaborate his theory of *transference*. Finally, Freud developed the theory that actual traumatic events, generally seductions, were not at the root of hysteria, although he never totally abandoned this view as a possibility in selected cases. This turned Freud from an exploration of actual traumatic experience toward an exploration of the world of inner fantasy. (For a vigorous dissenting minority view, see Masson 1984.) These latter two revisions, transference and fantasy, heralded central aspects of what was to become *psychoanalysis*.

Early theory of defense.   In his early theories, Freud made three important breakthroughs. First, Freud moved away from Charcot's trauma theory to one emphasizing fantasy. Second, Freud revised his thinking on the relation between memory and symptoms. Charcot had emphasized that trauma itself caused hysteria in susceptible individuals. In *The Neuro-Psychoses of Defence*, S. Freud (1894/1962) stated that it was not the trauma itself but rather the defense against the recollection of the memory of the trauma and its affects that caused neurotic symptoms. Predisposition or susceptibility was

---

[1]For example, Panksepp (1998) stated, "Although I have tried to clarify the neural foundations of affective experience in mammals, the actual manifestations of the neural circuits within living brains are so complex that many centuries of work will be needed to reveal how emotional systems really operate" (p. 319).

deemphasized. What was defended against was the linkage of the memory and the affect.

Third, Freud expanded the range of conditions that his method could study. For Charcot, the field was limited to hysteria. Freud added obsessional neurosis to that list and soon expanded it to include phobia as well. He was then prepared to make certain distinctions between these conditions. Freud theorized that in hysteria disturbing emotions or affects underwent a process he called *conversion* to a motor or sensory symptom. These symptoms were chosen symbolically so that the person could remove unpleasant or traumatic ideas from consciousness. In hysteria, the body did the talking and feeling so that the individual could forget. *Obsessional neurotic* persons used different defenses to solve the same problem of ridding their minds of unpleasant emotions or memories. Obsessional neurotic patients could not "convert" to body symptoms. Instead, in those patients, both the affect and the memory data remained in consciousness. To rid themselves of their disturbing effect, they became separated from each other: the idea was rendered empty of affect, and the affect was displaced onto a different, "false" idea that became the clinical obsessional symptom. Freud moved from a simple trauma theory to a theory of defense that applied not just to hysteria but also to a wide variety of symptomatic situations. Moving from a directly causal trauma theory to one that used the concept of defense enriched Freud's notion of mental life as the arena in which psychopathology takes place (see also S. Freud 1896/1962).

Topographical Model

From his prepsychoanalytic era, Freud recognized that the bulk of psychic life lies outside of consciousness. It was his major contribution to psychiatric thinking to elaborate and illuminate unconscious mental life. Freud himself regarded this contribution as one of the two hypotheses fundamental to his psychoanalytic theory. The second, related hypothesis was that of *psychic determinism*, which held that all mental events were causally linked to others in an associative network. Both hypotheses trace their origins back to the *Project* and to the work on aphasia, which stressed associative links and considered the spatial topography of the brain. Freud's work with dreams bolstered and modified his topographic model. These were presented in a systematic way in the famous Chapter VII of *The Interpretation of Dreams* (S. Freud 1900/1953).

The *topographical model* introduces the three "areas" of the mind: conscious, preconscious, and unconscious (Table 3–1). The conscious mind was already conceptualized within existing psychiatric and neurological theories. The enduring significance of the topographical model was to define unconscious mental processes as the field of psychoanalytic investigation and treatment. Freud's first concept of unconscious processes has been called the *descriptive unconscious*. By this, Freud was referring to the fact that mental life could not be limited to conscious or cognitive processes alone. The fact that comatose patients could report registering events that took place while they had been unconscious was enough to suggest that mental life continued even during periods when consciousness was interrupted. Similar proofs included the phenomena of posthypnotic suggestion, the very act of dreaming, and patients with dual or multiple personality. The preconscious, which contained mental content that was not at that moment conscious, would be grouped with the unconscious, from this descriptive point of view. The concept of the *descriptive unconscious*, which filled in the gaps in mental life and accounted for well-observed phenomena such as sleep or coma, predates Freud and aroused relatively little controversy.

Elaborating on these concepts, Freud asserted that forces are at work that keep mental processes and mental content unconscious or that work to push the content of the unconscious into consciousness (S. Freud 1915b/ 1957, 1915c/1957). These forces constitute the *dynamic unconscious*. It is not merely that there is a neutral continuity of mental life at all times. Rather, the placement of mental content in consciousness or in the unconscious is a matter of the relative strength of powerful forces. Evidence of the power of these forces could be taken from examples of what S. Freud (1901/1960) called the "psychopathology of everyday life" in his work of the same name. Examples would be a slip of the tongue that betrays one's true feelings in a setting in which polite dissembling would be in order or a behavior that reveals deeper disavowed feelings, such as a bridegroom stopping at a green light on the way to his wedding. In the clinical setting, Freud contended, resistance to remembering is evidence that forces are at work to keep mental content out of the patient's awareness. Yet the memories, ideas, and affects that are repressed exert their effect through symptoms that symbolically express what was to remain unconscious. The relation of conscious, preconscious, and unconscious to each other is set forth in Table 3–1.

Here a number of questions arise. Does the barrier between consciousness and the dynamic unconscious lie in the unconscious or within consciousness? What is the content of the unconscious? Does energy flow toward keeping things unconscious, or does it flow in the direction of pushing toward emergence in consciousness? Herein lie some issues for psychoanalytic theory that

TABLE 3–1. The topographical model

	Operating system	Motivation principle	Descriptive position	Dynamic position	"System" position
Conscious	Secondary process	Reality principle	Within awareness	Not repressed; easily accessible	Word oriented; denotative; linear; time bound; declarative
Preconscious	Secondary process	Reality principle	Outside of awareness	Not repressed; can have relatively easy access when attention is focused	Word oriented; denotative; linear; time bound; can be poetic
Unconscious	Primary process	Pleasure principle	Outside of awareness	Repressed; difficult access; available in dreams and symptoms	Image oriented; connotative; nonlinear; not time bound; symbolic

caused Freud to expand and eventually revise his topographical model.

Freud was not completely consistent in his use of terms. At times, it seems as though he asserted that only ideas, in the form of stored memory, exist in the unconscious but are robbed of their energy by having been repressed. At other times, Freud asserted that drives, wishes, and affects exist in the unconscious, with powerful energy that must be met by equally powerful repressive energy to keep them unconscious. At times, it is only that which had once been conscious and was later repressed that fills the unconscious. At other times, Freud argued that most of mental content starts in the unconscious, with only a small portion emerging in consciousness. How Freud's later theory of drives and his eventual development of the structural model solve some of these questions is seen in a subsequent subsection of this chapter (see "The Structural Model").

Perhaps even more important than the dynamic unconscious is the theory of the *system unconscious*. The system unconscious, which Freud abbreviated as the system UCs, works by a different internal logic than does the conscious mind. In this theory, consciousness, or more properly the system conscious (system Cs), is linked to sensation and perception, as well as to speech and the association with words. The apparatus of perception records events, which are then stored as representations, or mnemonic images. The storage system arranges these images in a chronological sequence and also into an associative system that connects related subjects. This unconscious storage system records *thing-presentations* that are related to, but are not exactly the same as, memory traces but that may be linked to other thing-presentations according to the various affects and attributes that the thing-presentation possesses. In addition to mne-

monic images, mental representations of the drives, or instincts, may be stored. Associative links are made by means of a logic system specific to the system UCs, called *primary process.*

Primary process. Primary process is the set of rules that govern the workings of the system UCs. Primary process is motivated by what S. Freud (1915c/1957) first called the *unpleasure principle* and later renamed the *pleasure principle*. In the pleasure principle, unpleasure is avoided at all times, and drives seek to be discharged (i.e., satisfied or relieved). Thus, under the pleasure principle, the motivation of the system UCs is to fulfill wishes and to discharge instinctual drives. Attachment to a particular mental content moves freely from one association to another, in what is called a *mobile cathexis*, a terribly awkward neologism describing the concept of investment or binding of psychic energy. In primary process, time flows equally in both directions, permitting the blending of past, present, and future; an idea and its opposite may coexist, and mental contents are condensed and displaced freely.

Condensation is the representation of multiple ideas, memories, and affects in a single symbol. *Displacement* is the operation of taking attributes, affects, or aspects of one thing and attaching them to another. *Symbolization* is often listed as a third attribute of primary process. Because the system UCs operates on the basis of thing-presentations, symbols rather than words constitute its language.

Secondary process. The so-called system preconscious (or system PCs) and the system conscious (Cs) work by the rules of *secondary process*. The basic motivating force in secondary process is the *reality principle*, according to which gratification is delayed for other purposes. This delay of gratification required by the reality principle is made possible by, and in turn makes possible, delays in discharge of drives. Thus, psychic energy is more highly bound and less mobile. A consequence of this is that attention moves more slowly from one thing to another in the associative path of secondary process. What has come to be known as *Aristotelian logic* is followed: time moves in forward linear direction, contradictions may not exist simultaneously, and thinking is more concerned with the content and logic of ideas than with their emotional intensity. The vocabulary of the system PCs and the system Cs consists of both thing-presentations and *word-presentations*. Freud felt that an indispensable ingredient of consciousness was this linkage between the imagistic, visual thinking of thing-presentations and the linguistic, auditory thinking of word-presentations. This notion underlies the emphasis on psychoanalysis as a "talking cure" and on the power of verbal associations and verbal interpretations. It is precisely because thing-presentations, governed by the primary process in the system UCs, can be translated into verbal word-presentations, governed by secondary process in the system Cs, that conscious verbal influences can gradually assert transforming control over the unconscious part of mental life.

The topographical model does not imply an anatomical correlation in the brain, although Freud always left that possibility open. It would be misleading, for example, to equate hemispheric specialization (i.e., right brain and left brain) with primary and secondary process, but it reminds us of the kind of metaphors Freud was using. One metaphor often used has to do with *topographical regression*. Because of their unique structure in which perception is stored in what Freud called *mnemic images*, dreams reveal how topographical regression returns us to the imagistic unconscious mentation that resembles the original perception. Dreams give us special access to unconscious memories and feelings. This, in turn, leads us to a further consideration of dreams and dreaming.

Dreams and dreaming. Dreams have always had a special place in the development of psychoanalytic theory, and Freud said that whenever he began to doubt the direction of his work, he would return to the bedrock of dream theory for renewed certainty. He called dreams "the Royal Road to the Unconscious." Through the analysis and self-analysis of dreams, Freud discovered the main points of his theory.

Dreams, according to Freud (S. Freud 1900/1953, 1917[1915]/1957), were the outstanding example of unconscious mental activity. Dreamers reported what Freud called the *manifest dream:* the conscious rendition of what the dreamer had experienced during the act of dreaming. But even manifest dreams revealed imagistic content, with improbable actions, and frequent blending of past and present. Freud theorized that every dream contains several elements: *day residue*, which consists of the memories of events of the preceding day that retain unconscious emotional charge, and *nocturnal stimuli*, which may be noises within the area where the dreamer is sleeping or may be enteroceptive awareness of bodily states (e.g., a full bladder). These relatively conscious elements are blended with *unconscious wishes* and the childhood memories associated with such wishes. Together, these constitute the *latent dream*.

In the process of sorting through the day residue and the nocturnal stimuli, the associative files to repressed unconscious childhood (or *infantile*) wishes are stimulated. With the ability of the system UCs to make rapid associative links via the mobile cathexis of primary process, elements from different periods can easily be mixed. Because the dreamer is asleep, motoric discharge for these infantile drives and wishes is blocked; topographical regression occurs, producing a dream experienced as a visual hallucination. The mere fact of exposure to these otherwise repressed wishes ordinarily would create anxiety, and in so doing might awaken the dreamer. The system UCs disguises the dream by using its intrinsic abilities of condensation and displacement, together with the symbolization inherent in dream images. The disguised dream affords the dreamer maximum expression of forbidden infantile wishes with minimum discovery. In this respect, dreams work the same way as Freud understood neurotic symptoms to work. They are both *compromise formations*, which simultaneously express and disguise, reveal and conceal, the underlying unconscious mental content, with its memories, associations, and drives.

The process of turning the latent dream into the manifest dream is called *dream work*. To the initial actions of condensation, displacement, and symbol formation is added the transformation of the dream after the dreamer awakens. This smoothing out of the logical contradictions in the dream to make it conform more to the rules of secondary process and conscious narration is called *secondary elaboration* or *secondary revision*.

Dream interpretation. The psychoanalytic approach to understanding a dream involves reversing the disguises of this dream work. Under the assumption of psychic determinism, every part of the dream comes into being for a reason related to the latent content of the dream and the dream censorship. Through the process of free association, the dreamer inexorably will be led back across the associative network to the original repressed memories and drives that stimulated the dream in the first place.

The reliance on free association to understand dreams places emphasis on the individual's personal use of symbols. Although dreamers from a common culture or era have similarities that would lead them to use common symbols, Freud emphasized that it was the individual's own personal free associations, not a standardized "dream dictionary," that would lead to the latent dream meaning.

Overdetermination. The emphasis on the overdetermined nature of the mind constitutes one of the most important differences between psychoanalysis and other popular theories of psychology. Psychoanalytic theory holds that no single explanation can account for what is seen in human behavior. Matters such as the stage of development, the symbolic meaning, the alignment of sibling order, and parental unconscious issues all go into determining whether a particular event will turn out the way it did. Kaufmann (1980) gives a particularly apt example when analyzing why an accident takes place:

> Why did it happen? The road was icy at that point. And the driver of the small car was in a great hurry because he was late for a crucial appointment, because the person who had promised to pick him up had not come. And his reflexes were slower than usual because he had had hardly any sleep that night because his mother had died the day before. And just before the accident his attention was distracted for one crucial second by a very pretty girl on the side of the road who reminded him of a girl he had once known. Yet he might have regained control of his car if only a truck had not come toward him just as he skidded into the left lane. The truck driver might have managed not to hit him, but.... If we add that the truck driver had just gone through a red light and was, moreover, going much faster than the legal speed limit, [one] might discount as irrelevant everything said before the three dots and be quite content to explain the accident simply in terms of the truck driver's two violations. *He* caused the accident. But that does not rule out the possibility that the other driver had a strong death wish because his mother had died, or that he punished himself for looking at an attractive girl the way he did so soon after his mothers death, or that the person who had let him down was partly to blame. (pp. 279–280)

The overlapping of multiple causes, combining conscious and unconscious factors, mixing internal and external actions and motivations, is one of the hallmarks of the psychoanalytic view of the mind, originally forced on the theory by the failure of recovery of simple single memories to cure patients.

Instinctual Drives

Earlier in his work, Freud explained the cause of psychopathology in terms of his theory of trauma, particularly sexual trauma. When that theory was no longer tenable, Freud continued to preserve the central role of sexuality in the genesis of neurosis. He was able to reason that his patients had not universally been traumatized, but rather they universally had sexual fantasies. This conclusion Freud deduced from his patients' dreams and associations and most importantly from the transference.

Transference, which is described more fully later in this chapter (see subsection "Transference"), is the phenomenon whereby feelings and relationships from the past bend our perceptions and reactions in the present. For Freud, it was the capacity of individuals under the influence of transference to recreate their fantasies within the treatment situation that made him downplay actual trauma and emphasize fantasy in his theory of neurosis.

Some confusion has arisen over the terms *instinct* and *drive*. Outside of psychoanalysis, the term *instinct* designates hereditary "prewiring" found in essentially the same form in all members of a given species. Such "wiring" is highly specific and related to innate recognition patterns and trigger mechanisms. *Drive* indicates a general innate need that can induce a variety of pathways for satiation from several objects of satisfaction. The tendency to fly south for the winter would be an instinct, and hunger would be a drive in this usage. Freud himself preserved this distinction in the original German (see S. Freud 1915a/1957), but his translators elected to render *Trieb* as "instinct" rather than "drive," thus causing the aforementioned confusion. Many modern authors attempt to get around this by using the term *instinctual drives*.

Instinctual drives are the form that physiological forces take in mental life. When the organism is stimulated, instinctual drives must be discharged. Instinctual drives of all types become mentally significant as psychic energy. This energy has an innate tendency toward discharge but may become attached (or *cathected*) to various mental representations on its way to achieving ultimate discharge; or it may become bound or redirected.

Every instinctual drive has a pressure (or quantitative strength), a source, an object, and an aim. Because it was the maldischarge of sexual instinct that presented itself clinically in his earliest patients, Freud turned his attention to those instinctual drives first. Noting the frequency of childhood sexual fantasies, Freud postulated that sexuality begins not at puberty, as the then-prevailing view had it, but in childhood. For the adult, the source of sexual energy was excitation of the genital area, the aim was genital orgasm, and the object was a person who possessed the complementary genitals of the opposite sex. Matters were not so simple with childhood sexuality.

Sexuality can be broken down into component instincts (S. Freud 1905/1953) (Table 3–2). The first would be sucking. The pleasure that the infant gets from sucking is considered by Freud to be sexual in nature. The source is the sucking reflex, and the aim is to suck. The object is at first the infant himself or herself, and the sucking is thus termed *autoerotic*. Soon the infant distinguishes the differences between sucking at the breast and autoerotic sucking. This is the phase of *orality*. In this phase, the erotogenic zone is the mouth, and the aim is not only to nurse at the breast but also to do all the things that a mouth is capable of doing, such as taking in, savoring, swallowing, digesting, and (later) biting, spitting, and remaining closed. As the child matures, the principal erotogenic zone moves to *anal* and *urethral* areas. Once again, what starts as direct pleasure in the sensation of urination and defecation generalizes to pleasure in what those zones can do, including things such as retaining, controlling, making orderly, expelling, and withholding. Sexuality next organizes in the *phallic stage*. This will be dealt with more fully in the "Theories of Development" subsection later in this chapter. Finally, childhood sexuality is bound during *latency*, when its energy is stripped for the next half-dozen or so years of its intense pleasurable affect and displaced onto other activities. This displacement makes it possible for the child during latency to become absorbed with the cognitive tasks of school. Sexuality again reappears in its direct form in the true *genital phase*, which begins with puberty and goes on to adulthood.

Freud justified expanding his notion of sexuality beyond that of adult heterosexual intercourse for several reasons. There was the evidence of his early patients and their fantasies of childhood sexual experiences and yearnings. There also was evidence from cases of child analysis such as "Little Hans" (S. Freud 1909a/1955), whose overt interest in sexual matters and whose childhood sexual ideas seemed to confirm Freud's own views (see also S. Freud 1907/1959, 1908/1959). The transference, in which things that were not explicitly sexual in themselves took on intense sexual charge, also provided further evidence. Still further justification for Freud's expanded notion of sexuality could be found in the perversions, in which Freud asserted that the component instincts were displayed in variations of aim and object. In the perversions, oral and anal sexual component instincts and the variability of object choices could be seen clearly in the practices associated with adult perversions. Finally, Freud noted the component instincts in normal foreplay: *oral sexuality*, such as visual stimulation and kissing; *anal sexuality*, such as mastery, control, and domination and the switching back and forth between activity and passivity; and *phallic sexuality*, with its focus on the penis itself, concomitant with exhibitionistic activity and an emphasis on exaggerated masculine and feminine roles. These component instincts seen in foreplay lead to and heighten genital sexuality if the participants are normally sexually healthy.

TABLE 3–2. Psychosexual stages of development

Phase	Subphase	Aggressive component	Object relations	Adult manifestation
Oral	Receptive	To consume	Autoerotic, with little awareness of mother as separate person	Trust, curiosity, greed, insatiability. Good is seen as reposing outside self
	Aggressive	To devour entirely	Breast and mother experienced as hostile when infant is hungry	Envy—the resentment of another who has something good
Anal	Expulsive	To project and to eliminate or be rid of	Others seen as objects to contain what is bad in us	Bad seen as inside
	Retentive	To control and hoard	Others seen as objects to control or be controlled by	Mastery, control, punctuality, parsimony, perfectionism, orderliness, shame, diminished emotionality
Phallic		Exhibitionism, to be admired	Others seen as competitors or as audience to be won over	Grandiosity, teasing, fame seeking, competitive, achievement oriented

In expanding the concept of sexuality, Freud did not "make everything sexual." He was very explicit about the fact that his was not a theory of pansexuality. There was always an alternative category of instincts. In the earlier stages of Freud's work, the opposing categories of instincts were sexuality, also called *libido*, and life-preservation, also called *ego instincts*. At birth, these two are joined in the *anaclitic* relationship between infant and mother. That is, the sexual pleasure in sucking is joined with the survival instinct in sucking. Freud hypothesized that, at first, the infant cannot distinguish between autoerotic sucking, the hallucination of the breast, and the real experience of sucking at the breast. As the infant makes this distinction, the survival ego instinct and the pleasurable libidinal activity of the sexual instinct undergo a disjunction, which, in turn, makes possible the beginnings of object relations (discussed later in this chapter).

Death instinct.   The subject of the *death instinct* has been difficult and controversial for the psychoanalytic tradition. Summaries of psychoanalysis (e.g., Brenner 1955; Fenichel 1945) generally give this concept a brief, dry dismissal. Because it was important to S. Freud (1920/1955), we attempt briefly to see why he was drawn to proposing it and what he meant by it.

Freud acknowledged the hypothetical nature of his theory of instinctual drives: "The theory of the instincts is so to say our mythology.…In our work we cannot for a moment disregard them, yet we are never sure that we are seeing them clearly" (S. Freud 1933[1932]/1964, p. 95). But the view that instinctual life consisted of libido in opposition to ego instincts was not satisfactory. It did not adequately explain phenomena such as sadism, masochism (S. Freud 1924a/1961), or negative therapeutic reaction (i.e., when the patient gets worse the closer the treatment gets to the heart of the patient's issues). Nor could such a view explain the extremes of melancholia, excessively aggressive behavior in patients, or the symptoms of traumatic neurosis.

To further understand the dilemma Freud faced, we should review his reliance on the pleasure principle as demonstrated in his theory of dreams. Recall that dreams were regarded by Freud as the disguised fulfillment of an infantile wish. According to the pleasure principle, unacceptable anxiety-producing wishes emerge from the unconscious during sleep and are transformed by the mechanism of dream work into a manifest dream that allows the dreamer to continue to sleep by taking anxiety below the threshold of awakening. The purpose of the dream is to bring pleasure through maximum tolerable expression of a wish. If dreams were under the influence of the pleasure principle alone, how then could we explain the persistent existence of painful traumatic dreams repeated over and over again? We cannot unless we go "beyond the pleasure principle" (S. Freud 1920/ 1955) to another principle. In this second principle—the *nirvana principle*—the individual uses drive discharge to reestablish quiescence and erects barriers to stimuli to restore and maintain an undisturbed state. The pleasure principle explains the rules governing the operation of libido, and the nirvana principle explains and underlies the operation of the death instinct.

The new instinctual drive was unfortunately named the *death instinct*, but it actually consisted of three elements:

1. Aggression and the tendency to create destruction and disorder
2. The compulsion to repeat, which went beyond the notion of attempting mastery or restitution, but in which patterns and memories were repeated even without constructive purpose
3. The establishment of stimulus barriers to achieve a state of quiescence

All three elements were seen to arise independent of the pleasure principle, but "luckily," as S. Freud (1933[1932]/1964) noted, "the aggressive instincts are never alone but always alloyed with the erotic ones" (p. 111).

The death instinct, then, is a broad concept that Freud used to explain the clinical phenomena of ambivalence, aggression, sadism, masochism, and severe melancholia. The death instinct is governed by the nirvana principle, which establishes stimulus barriers to create a state of quiescence. In the ultimate state of quiescence, of course, the individual would no longer be alive; hence, Freud's ill chosen term, *death instinct*.

The role of instinct theory.   Instinctual drives have had diminished importance within the psychoanalytic tradition, especially since the 1950s. The ego instincts have resurfaced in some respects in the theories of ego psychologists and in Kohut's work on self psychology. Followers of those schools have tended to place the acquisition and maintenance of a coherent self in a position of primacy relative to the sexual or libidinal instinctual drives.

The notion of death instincts as a regulator of stimulus barriers of isolation and quiescence according to the nirvana principle has not been taken up as a major point by any of Freud's followers. Most of them have also thought that the genesis of aggression did not require the existence of an independent instinctual drive. Some theorists view aggression as the natural forcefulness of any drive, and others view aggression as a secondary reaction to frustration. The death instinct expressed in terms of innate aggression has been most fully elaborated by Melanie Klein and her followers, who elevated it to a position of equality, or perhaps even primacy, and made it a centerpost of their theory.

The theory of instinctual drives led Freud back to the defenses, which had been known prior to 1900 but which were rediscovered as Freud studied the vicissitudes of instinctual drives (S. Freud 1915a/1957). His study of instinctual drives also led to further investigation of the topics of narcissism and object relations.

Narcissism and Object Relations

The subjects of narcissism and object relations emerged naturally from Freud's instinct theory. Freud had indicated that every instinctual drive has a source, an aim, and an object. The object of an instinct is that through which the instinct is able to achieve its aim. It seems that Freud is implying that objects serve the purpose of providing satisfactory ways of achieving satisfaction for instinctual drives. Clearly the pleasure-seeking aspects predominate. However, as soon as we begin to look carefully at what is involved in satisfaction of instincts, the situation becomes more complicated because our way of relating to objects, although initially instinctually driven, soon becomes separated from the initial instinctual need. For example, consider the fact that at the beginning the infant has a pleasure-seeking drive for oral sexual satisfaction by sucking at the breast and a survival need to suckle at the breast. His or her way of relating to the breast is through the modality of swallowing or incorporation. Although things start this way, it soon becomes clear that the mode of oral incorporation is our way of relating to objects in the external world.

Instincts start out in their component forms. Sexuality, for example, is expressed orally, tactilely, and visually and is only later consolidated into a multifaceted whole. By the same token, the objects of these component instincts also start out as *part objects*. In other words, mother, a whole object, is broken down by the infant into face, arms, breast, and so forth. These, in turn, are broken down further into good face, when mother is smiling, and bad face, when mother is scowling. Development progresses as drives become progressively more consolidated and objects also become progressively more whole. The biologically driven instinctual needs merge during the phase called *genital organization*. One of the most important signs of emerging maturity in childhood is the transformation of relationships with part objects (e.g., breast, face) into relationships with complex whole objects (mother as total person) who can be understood and experienced to have both good and bad qualities.

Modern theories date these tasks earlier in development than did Freud, who conceived of component instincts as consolidating and of part objects as yielding to whole objects during the oedipal period. Most theorists now see these trends beginning by the second or third year of life, with some investigators arguing that the process starts within the first year.

The notion of object relations tends to emphasize the interplay or interrelationship between the subject and the object. On the one hand, objects are entirely fungible. One is as good as another as long as it can fulfill an instinctual aim. Presumably for a newborn, any nipple would be equally as good and any bottle or any formula equally as good. On the other hand, during the course of development, the modes of relating to objects and our specific history with them leave a trail in our identity that is not at all fungible but highly particular. Freud, on the one hand, thought that objects were the easiest part of a drive complex to vary, and yet, on the other hand, he indicated that we never actually find objects but that we indeed only refind them. This is certainly true when we observe the ways that marital choices rework the object relations (part and whole) that we have with the internalized images of our parents, which affect our own identity and our ability to love others.

It is to be emphasized that the interest in object relations does not imply that everything is contained in the real relationship. The psychoanalytic tradition demands that object relations be thought of in terms of internal fantasy life as well as the real relationship. This is a point of distinction between psychoanalytic and interpersonal schools.

In object relations, the infant starts in a state of autoerotism, with all libido attached to the self and an obliviousness to external objects. As the ego develops, there is a stage of primary narcissism in which the individual is concerned with and in love with himself or herself. From this stage, the child moves to a state of object relatedness that starts out as anaclitic or need related but in the course of frustration of these needs returns for defensive purposes to a focus on the self, called *secondary narcissism*. In secondary narcissism, the individual makes object choices of persons like himself or herself. These later object choices are narcissistic object choices in that we are drawn to people who are like the way we would want to be or who in some respect help define who we are. It is for this reason that in "Mourning and Melancholia," Freud (1917[1915]/1957) pointed out that when we lose a connection to a person in whom we had strong emotional investment, especially if that connection was ambivalent and our relationship narcissistic, "the shadow of the object falls upon the ego" (p. 249). We are then ever after influenced by our lost narcissistically held object.

Primary narcissism (S. Freud 1914a/1957) is a state in which the infant takes himself or herself and his or her perceptions as a love object. This stage precedes the full acknowledgment of the external world as having a reality of its own beyond the infant. If development proceeds optimally, the child will become less self-absorbed and less omnipotent and will develop the capacity to love others for themselves. The child also will retain some reserve of primary narcissism to fuel self-confidence and self-esteem. In unfavorable development, which can come from neglect, conflict, or trauma, the child's ties to others will be narcissistic. In lieu of legitimate self-esteem, the child will develop narcissistic ties to others based on their ability to do things for the child or to maintain his or her self-esteem. Such a child grows into an adult who relies on others to define his or her self-image, indeed his or her very being.

Anxiety

As Freud originally conceived it, anxiety resulted from an accumulation of sexual tension or dammed-up libido. Freud then believed that neurosis originated in the holding back from libido. Observing that neurosis was accompanied by anxiety, he drew the conclusion that anxiety was transformed libido. And frequently when Freud found in his clinical experience that his patients had a more normal sexual life, indeed many of their symptoms did in fact disappear. Later in his thinking, Freud began to consider some of the differences between realistic anxiety and neurotic anxiety, anxiety as an affect, anxiety as a physiological reaction, and anxiety as connected with fear and fright. Anxiety can be bodily movements, an awareness of unpleasure, and an autonomic reaction.

In "Inhibitions, Symptoms and Anxiety," S. Freud (1926/1959) concluded that psychological anxiety was in fact a signal phenomenon and that neurotic anxiety starts as the remembrance of realistic anxiety. A real danger is one that threatens a person with an external reality. A neurotic danger is one that threatens him or her from a fantasy or from an instinctual internal demand. If an individual feels overwhelmed, he or she is placed in a traumatic situation. Also, if the person feels overwhelmed by an object on whom he or she depends for instinctual satisfaction or for survival, he or she is in a traumatic situation. Each stage of life has age-appropriate determinants

of anxiety, beginning with the fear of birth and moving through the fear of separation from the mother and the fear of castration. The fear of the superego is experienced initially as fear of its anger or punishment, and then as fear of its loss of love, and ultimately as fear of death. Generally speaking, when faced with a realistic anxiety, we fight or we flee. Faced with an internal neurotic anxiety, we generally act against the internal source; thus, we displace the anxiety by doing something with the drive to make it no longer dangerous to us.

Various forms of neurotic anxiety express themselves as phase-appropriate or age-appropriate prototypes, but earlier ones continue to underlie later ones, and later fears can revive earlier ones. This accounts for great complexity in our neurotic lives and is in turn accounted for by the fact that time flows in both directions in primary process. Indeed, anxiety produces repression and other defenses rather than repression producing anxiety. The various transference neuroses can be understood in terms of the type of neurotic anxiety from which they emerged. Freud, for instance, suggested that there was a connection between hysteria and the fear of loss of love, between phobia and the fear of castration, and between obsessional neurosis and the superego. Tracing the course of anxiety then became no less important than tracing the nature of the instinctual drives themselves. The shift of interest from the drive itself to the way in which the anxiety about the drive is handled laid the groundwork for the next main change in Freud's work, the structural model.

The Structural Model

In the structural model, Freud proposed the division of the mind into id, ego, and superego. Why was it necessary to introduce this new theory? There had always been some sort of ego in prior theories, but its attributes and definition were different in various eras. The ego was a synonym for the mental self, the agency that exerted control over drives and defenses, including the ego-produced dream censorship and dream work. The ego was the organ of perception and the organizer of the filing system of mnemonic images and memories, and, as we have seen, the ego was involved in primary and secondary narcissism. In addition, the ego was the source of the ego instincts of self-preservation.

In the earliest days of psychoanalytic theory, the ego had at its command the ability to engage in a variety of defenses, but in the middle stages of his theorizing, Freud principally emphasized repression. In fleshing out his idea of repression, Freud saw that energy was needed to press against unconscious ideas in their striving to reach consciousness. Freud sometimes called this process *anticathexis* or *countercathexis*. To be most effective, this countercathexis had to operate out of awareness. But if it too was unconscious, what was doing the repressing? The question of the locus of the operation of repression, the awareness of the multiple forms of defense, early notions of the ego ideal and of identification, and the fact that psychopathology depended at least as much on management of instinctual drives as on the drives themselves all converged to bring about a major rethinking of the operations of the mind. Structural theory is an attempt to find a better explanation for the various operations of the mind.

It should once again be emphasized that Freud never abandoned the topographical model. The structural and topographical points of view are neither incompatible nor exactly complementary. They are two different approaches to understanding the mechanisms of mental functioning.

What is the sense in which there could be mental structures? Freud certainly did not postulate that ego, id, and superego were physical or corporeal, having any particular locus. A good example of a noncorporeal structure from ordinary life would be the "free press." In the United States, there is a tradition of free expression and also specific provisions of the Bill of Rights that uphold a free press. The concept of a free press, however, goes beyond the physical structures of newspaper plants and radio and television studios and goes beyond the words of the Constitution physically preserved in historical archives. Other countries may have the same hardware, and some even have the same words in their constitutions, but they do not have a "free" press. This noncorporeal structure is a combination of long-standing precedent, patterns of behavior, procedural mechanisms, symbolic meaning, and the interweaving of all of these into the definition of who we are as a country.

In like manner, the ego is heir to history—within a culture, within a specific family, and within an individual—which builds up over years. It is protected by defense mechanisms analogous to the procedural mechanisms of a country, which are institutionalized and become more than the materialist or corporeal reality on which they rest. The ego is no more a collection of neurons than the free press is a collection of newspaper, ink, and metal; nor is the ego any more located in a specific area of the brain than could we identify the free press as existing in certain cities located on certain streets. Both are anchored in a corporeal, material reality, but both are noncorporeal structures or institutions.

According to the structural theory, the organism starts out as a poorly organized collection of drives. These drives are initially intensely physiologically driven. During this phase, the need to survive and the path to pleasure lean on each other. According to the original version of the structural theory, the ego does not exist at this phase, but the potential for the ego to exist begins immediately with perception. In fact, the ego owes its origin to and starts out from its activity of perception. In the course of perceiving, the ego discerns differences between internal and external; differences between pleasurable and unpleasurable; and differences between those perceptions that can be changed by body movement, those that can be made to disappear solely through mental acts, and those that the organism cannot influence. Thus, the ego starts out as a function of the body that defines the mental image of the body, which is what Freud meant by saying that first and foremost the ego is a bodily ego.

One way the ego learns the difference between internal and external is through the sense of touch. This unique sensory modality is the earliest one in which the ego is simultaneously the organ that does the touching and the organ that is aware that it is being touched. Touching one's own skin thus becomes the beginning of learning who one is and what one's boundaries are. The distinction between the hallucinated dream or wish for the breast and the actual breast constitutes another way of distinguishing between internal and external, between real and hallucinated. The feeling of satiation that comes from the hallucinated breast does not last, in contrast to the feeling of satiation that comes from the real breast. Dreamed or wished mental content comes and goes for internal reasons. The mother and other objects in the world come and go of their own external volition. Thus, the ego, in the course of its formation, begins to establish the *reality principle*. Rooted in perception, the ego is also anchored in reality, whereas the id, rooted in drives, is anchored in the pleasure principle.

The goal and mission of the id is to provide maximum pleasure through maximum fulfillment of the instinctual drives. The goal of the ego is to attain clarity of perception, accuracy of interpretation of the perceptions, and the greatest possible consonance with reality. Early on, the id learns, so to speak, that the hallucinations, dreams, and wishes of the pleasure principle are not ultimately as satisfying as the accuracy of the perceptions of the reality principle. The id forms an alliance with the ego, subordinating itself and its energy to the ego in return for the ego's help in focusing the organism's behaviors around the reality principle for maximum satisfaction of instinctual drives. Thus, during this period of cooperation, the ego gains enormous strength from the id.

The reality principle requires binding of cathexis,

which is another way of saying that drive discharge must be postponed, deferred, or redirected in order to meet the constraints of reality. The pleasure principle works on the basis of primary process, with mobile cathexis and rapid movement from one strategy to another so as to get immediate gratification. Thus, although the ego and the id start out as allies, they frequently find themselves working at cross purposes, with the impatient id wanting immediate results and the cautionary ego insisting on delay. The ego's "weapon" against the id could be the refusal to cooperate for the purpose of achieving the id's goals. To do so, however, would defeat the ego's goals as well. After all, the reality principle is also a more sophisticated and comprehensive version of the pleasure principle. The ego too wishes gratification. Through its capacity to understand time and to delay discharge, the ego understands that the shortest path is not always the most efficient one. The ego then inflicts anxiety on the id, creating pain (Freud preferred the term *unpleasure*) for the id. The avoidance of such unpleasure is a paramount consideration for the id. One can say, in somewhat anthropomorphic terms, that the id starts out wanting fulfillment; finds an ally in the ego, which has access to valuable perceptions; and engages in cooperation with the perceptual ego to accomplish its ends. However, the id, having soon enough given more power to the ego than it originally anticipated, now finds itself the recipient of unpleasure from its ally.

In the course of its evolution, the ego deals with an environment that more than any other single thing consists of the actions of the parents. The ego needs the parents and their cooperation and alliance every bit as much as the id needed the ego's perceptual cooperation. Thus, the successful pursuit of its mission to maximize pleasure according to the constraints of the reality principle requires that the ego understand and ultimately mold itself to the actions of the parents. In doing so, the ego becomes like the parents through identification. It needs the parents, but the parents, being separate individuals, are not always available. The ego takes the parents in and then has permanent mental representations of these important figures on which it can rely in their absence.

The expectations of the parents for the organism and the ego's knowledge of what it needs to do to get the maximum cooperation from the parents form the basis of the *ego ideal*. The realistic awareness of those things that bring the ego unpleasure and diminish the cooperation between the ego and the parents becomes the basis of the *superego*.

The superego is initially an auditory superego, coming from the auditory perception of the word "no." The ego finds itself in relation to the ego ideal and superego in very much the position in which the id found itself in relation to the ego earlier. The superego and ego ideal enforce a reality principle of an advanced form, a kind of moral reality principle rather than a purely perceptual reality principle, on the ego. In similar fashion, the ego offers some of its energy to the superego for maximum clarity of moral reality. The superego in turn uses its capacity to inflict anxiety to keep the ego in line. Thus, we have a finely tuned network: the ego relates to an id driven by the pleasure principle, to a superego driven by identifications (e.g., mother, father), and to reality.

The superego starts out as harsh because the cognitive ability of the young child to understand the subtleties of the reason for prohibitions is absent. For example, the early, or "archaic," superego is extremely harsh because the small infant about to stick his or her finger into an electrical outlet is greeted with a loud "No!" from the parent, who might in addition slap the child's hand. The superego then is blunt, direct, harsh, and unequivocal. The archaic superego is incapable of a calm lecture on the dangers of electricity, but over the course of time, a more mature superego might indeed function like that. It is postulated that in the resolution of the oedipal phase, the ego ideal and the harsh archaic superego blend to form a more mature superego, containing both punitive and loving elements, guiding the individual both for what not to do to avoid unpleasure and for what to do to gain maximum pleasure and self-regard.

The strength and harshness of the superego do not rest on the actual harshness or gentleness of the parents during the oedipal period. Rather, the superego is an amalgam of real parental prohibitions, real parental approval, the ability of the child to overcome splitting defenses (see section "Splitting" later in this chapter), the nature and power of the child's drives and fantasies, and the style with which the child metabolizes those fantasies.

The foregoing account is highly simplified and somewhat anthropomorphic. It also conveys the impression that the ego, the superego, and the id become distinctly different from one another. This is extremely far from what S. Freud (1926/1959) had in mind, as is evident in the following passage from "Inhibitions, Symptoms and Anxiety":

> [Some misunderstanding] is due to our having taken abstractions too rigidly and attended exclusively now to the one side and now to the other of what is in fact a complicated state of affairs. We were justified, I think, in dividing the ego from the id.... *On the other hand the ego is identical with the id, and is merely a specially differentiated part of it* ....if a real split has occurred between the two, the weakness of the ego becomes apparent. But if the ego remains bound up with the id and indistinguishable from it, then it displays its

strength. The same is true of the relation between the ego and the super-ego. In many situations the two are merged; and as a rule we can only distinguish one from the other when there is a tension or conflict between them. In repression the decisive fact is that the ego is an organization and the id is not. *The ego is, indeed, the organized portion of the id.* We should be quite wrong if we pictured the ego and the id as two opposing camps. (p. 97; emphasis added)

Freud was struggling to show that although there were in some respects no differences at all between ego and id, and that indeed they were parts of each other, a key difference had to do with the ways in which they were organized. The ego is the organized aspect of the id. The superego is a further organized aspect of the ego and thus the id too. At times, it appears as though the ego is stronger than the id, in that it can cause repression and can inflict anxiety. Yet the ego is also powerless over the id. They react against each other and yet they are the same as each other, one being organized more along the lines of secondary process and the reality principle and the other being organized more along the lines of primary process and the pleasure principle (Figure 3–1).

It is also important to remember that from the point of view of the descriptive unconscious, most of the functions of ego, superego, and id are unconscious. Occasionally, bits of the id emerge in consciousness and a bit more of the ego and the superego is also accessible to consciousness. From the point of view of the dynamic unconscious, ego, id, and superego also are largely unconscious. Their forces interact with one another out of ordinary awareness, although occasionally transparent dreams or the product of years of analysis results in some of that interaction reaching consciousness.

The concepts of the topographical model can be applied to the structural model. The ego operates mostly by secondary process (which is in the system Cs), even though most of the ego is out of daily awareness (which puts it in the descriptive preconscious). The id operates mostly by primary process (found in the system UCs) and is also unconscious from the descriptive point of view. The superego operates by both primary and secondary process. Figure 3–1 is an attempt to depict these relationships graphically.

Under the influence of the structural theory, the attention of psychoanalysis moved away from instinctual drives to the workings of each individual ego as it dealt with drives and anxiety to achieve maximum adaptation.

Mechanisms of Defense

It is a psychoanalytic cliché that the ego serves three harsh masters: the id, the superego, and reality. It is also

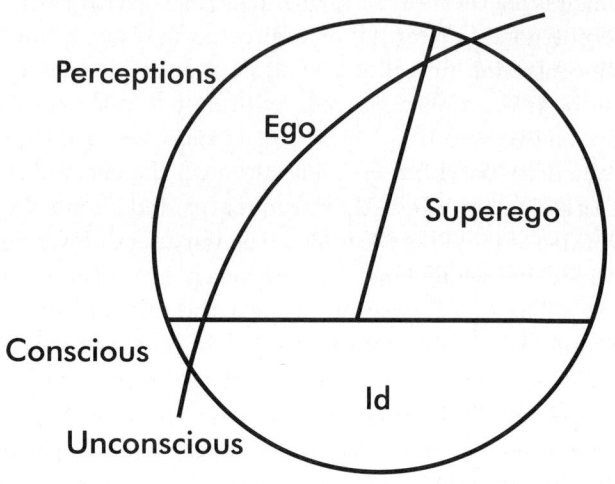

FIGURE 3–1. The structural model.

The barriers between the three "structures" are semipermeable. Most of the id is unconscious, more of the superego is available to consciousness, and still more of the ego is conscious. However, for all three the bulk of activity goes on without consciousness. Because the ego has direct access to perception, it develops reality testing. However, it must serve "three harsh masters": the superego, the id, and reality.

emphasized that the ego is the executive of the organism in charge of the task of balancing the competitive needs of all of the other systems. In so doing, the ego acts as an organ of perception and of cognition, and as a regulator of internal mental life, all in the service of achieving the maximum amount of gratification consistent with its role as executor of the id. The ego itself grows largely as a result of layers of identifications and internal mental representations of the important figures to whom it has been exposed, particularly the parents and other members of the immediate family, who over the course of time and healthy development become *depersonified,* transforming their role from that of organized memory files of the original person to aspects of the ego itself.

To function smoothly, the ego has to have a set of automatic operations with which to deal with the competing memories, perceptions, external realistic needs, drives, and anxieties that it faces. These automatic operations by which the ego balances its competing interests are known as *defense mechanisms.*

In psychoanalytic theory, some confusion has arisen as to the differences among defense mechanisms, defenses, defensive operations, and defensive behaviors. Some authors have long lists, whereas others have short lists; some lists are simpler and more streamlined, whereas others are more highly elaborated and complex. For instance, the primary process rules of condensation, displacement, and symbolization could be viewed as defense mechanisms or alternatively as operations that permit defense mechanisms to function. The important concept to remember is that each defense mechanism uses capacities of the mind to alter mental content.

How many defense mechanisms are there? Some have contended that there is only one defense mechanism, namely repression, and that all other mechanisms are means by which repression is carried out. Authors add or subtract defenses according to the slant of their particular theoretical point of view.

Sigmund Freud listed nine defense mechanisms, and Anna Freud (1936/1946) slightly modified the list, adding a tenth, "which pertains rather to the study of the normal than to that of neurosis: sublimation, or displacement of instinctual aims. So far as we know at present the ego has these ten different methods at its disposal in its conflicts with instinctual representatives and affects" (p. 47).

Bibring et al. (1961) generated a "glossary of defenses" that contained 24 basic mechanisms and 15 more complex ones. Vaillant (1977) discussed pathological defense mechanisms and adaptive coping mechanisms, expanding the list manyfold.

However we organize the list, it is important to remember that defenses not only ward off unacceptable mental content but also are themselves mental content with accompanying fantasies (Schafer 1968; Wallerstein 1983). Defenses also yield pleasure by allowing a degree of discharge while simultaneously warding off the drive through negation or fantasy. We must analyze in detail the fantasy contained within any particular defense, remembering as well that there can be defenses not only against unwelcome mental contents but also against other defenses (Waelder 1936). Thus, defenses exist in hierarchical layers.

Anna Freud attempted to correlate stages of psychic development with the coming into existence of different defenses but did not entirely succeed in her classification. Masterson and Rinsley, Kernberg, and others have attempted to continue this work. This approach is particularly important when each kind of psychopathology has its characteristic specific clusters of defenses. For example, in hysteria, repression and conversion are prominent defenses. In obsessive-compulsive disorder, isolation, reaction formation, regression, and undoing are the primary mechanisms. In paranoia and psychosis, introjection and projection are the primary mechanisms of defense. If one can know the diagnosis, one can infer the defense mechanisms most likely to be encountered in the treatment. Conversely, if one observes certain defensive operations in action, one can infer the diagnosis. One also can predict the form in which the transference will unfold by knowing the principal defense mechanisms used by a particular patient.

The classical defense mechanisms as enumerated by Anna Freud are briefly discussed in the following subsections (Table 3–3).

Repression. Repression is the defense that keeps from consciousness unwanted affects, memories, or drives. Repression requires permanent energy against the emergence of unwelcome mental content into awareness. The countercathexis takes place on an unconscious basis. The equilibrium between the pressure of the repression to reach consciousness and the countercathexis to keep it unconscious is a fluid one, and the countercathexis of the ego is always in danger of being diminished, such as occurs in sleep and which permits dreams to become part of mental content. When something is successfully repressed, it is barred from access to consciousness, but it is also no longer amenable to further modification by the ego and can take on a life of its own in the form of a symptom complex or a portion of character structure.

Regression. When the defense of regression is used, we return to an earlier level of maturational functioning. We see mild regression in medically ill patients and in college students when they return home on vacations. An example that Sigmund Freud gave was that of a patient who transformed his phallic-level rivalry with his father into the fantasy of being orally devoured by a father figure in the children's story "The Gingerbread Man." In this case, the patient regressed to an earlier level of development and an earlier conceptualization of his interactions with the significant objects in his life in an effort to return to a state that was associated with less anxiety but in fact expressed his anxiety over his relationship in a more primitive way.

Isolation. Isolation separates affect from memory. This defense mechanism is frequently used by obsessional persons and, in its more common form, consists of both ideational content and affect having access to consciousness, but not at the same time. What is blocked is the link between ideational content and affect. In its extreme forms, patients who use isolation may be unable to feel too much emotion of any kind. Thoughts or affects are treated as though they were untouchable and therefore require distance. An example is a patient talking about a painful event with a bland emotional expression.

Reaction formation. In reaction formation, another defense mechanism frequently found in obsessional persons, affects are transformed into their opposites, and ambivalence is resolved in the opposite manner from which it arises. For example, "I don't love this; I hate it," or, "I am not interested in gratifying a dangerous wish; I

TABLE 3–3. Classical defenses

Repression	Keeping unwanted affects, memories, and drives from consciousness, allowing them to remain in our behavior outside of awareness. Mechanism by which we "forget" unpleasant information or feelings.
Regression	Returning to an earlier level of maturational functioning.
Isolation	Separating link between affect and memory. Often used by obsessive-compulsive patients.
Reaction formation	Transforming affects into their opposites (e.g., "I don't love this; I hate it"). Often used by obsessive-compulsive patients.
Undoing	Attempting to nullify or atone for forbidden fantasy, affect, or memory. Used by obsessive-compulsive patients.
Projection	Sending an unacceptable thought or feeling away and attributing it to an external source (e.g., "I don't hate him; he hates me"). Often used by paranoid patients. *Projective identification* is a more primitive version in which identity is ascribed to another, generally in a relationship in which the other accepts the projection.
Identification	Taking attributes of important others into our own selves. This can either be part of normal growth or be pathological, depending on maturational level. *Introjection* is the style of identification that takes in another person's identity as a foreign body. *Incorporation* is more advanced, taking on another's characteristics. *Identification* is most advanced; we become like others by acquiring their attributes, which we can then modify.
Turning against	Taking an impulse intended to be expressed toward someone else and directing it against oneself (e.g., biting your tongue by "accident" when you feel like saying something hostile toward another person).
Reversal	Taking an impulse and reversing its polarity (e.g., changing sadistic feelings into masochistic ones or transforming the active role into the passive role).
Denial	Invalidating an unpleasant or unwanted piece of information and living life as though it did not exist. Seen in many patients with addictions who do not acknowledge the consequences of their behavior. Differs from repression in that there is slight consciousness, but a piece of reality is being denied, not just mental content.
Splitting	Keeping "good objects," pleasurable affects, and good memories apart from "bad objects," unpleasurable affects, and bad memories. Early in life, this defense keeps infants from having good experiences drowned out by bad ones. Later, it prevents people from experiencing others as multifaceted, complex whole objects possessing both good and bad characteristics. Often seen in borderline personality disorder patients.
Sublimation	Turning our drives, affects, and memories into healthy and creative outcomes.

am interested in seeing to it that the fulfillment of these dangerous wishes never comes to pass." A historical example of reaction formation in action would be that of the nineteenth-century British statesman who, in reaction to his own lust, spent frequent evenings in the red-light district of London importuning prostitutes to give up their wayward lives. This outward set of behaviors permitted him to be in the company of prostitutes while denying forbidden desires by transforming them into what would look like their opposite.

Undoing. In undoing, a behavior is engaged in or a series of fantasies are indulged in that atone for a forbidden fantasy, affect, or memory (S. Freud 1909b/1955). A clinical example of undoing would be engaging in hand-washing rituals to atone for fantasies of soiling. The way in which undoing might enter character structure as a permanent defense is illustrated by the clinical vignette of a hyperconscientious physician who double- and triple-checked every detail of his patients' care with

a devotion that made family life incompatible with professional life. During the course of analysis, it was discovered that this physician was spending a lifetime undoing the consequences of childhood murderous fantasies against his younger sibling during his mother's pregnancy. These fantasies had to be atoned for when the sibling was born with a severe birth defect. In this example, the defense became part of the character structure and had both an adaptive and a pathological meaning.

Projection. Projection is a complex defense mechanism that can operate at a more primitive or a more advanced level. Projection involves the fantasy of spitting, throwing, or in some other way hurling from ourselves some unacceptable mental content. The schematic prototype would be "I don't hate him; he hates me," an example in which the affect is disowned and, through displacement, projected onto someone else (S. Freud 1911/1958, 1921/1955, 1922/1955). This defense mechanism is prevalent in paranoia. The advantage for the person who is using projection is that he or she rids himself or herself of unwelcome thoughts and affects; the disadvantage, however, is that the projecting person then lives in a merciless world in which others harbor the unacceptable affects and fantasies that he or she wishes to disown. These individuals become purified of their bad fantasies, but then it appears that everyone else has those same bad intentions toward them. Once the affect is projected, one's ability to modify the content of the projection is severely diminished.

Projective identification. Projective identification is another form of projection, thought to be more primitive by Melanie Klein and her followers who elaborated it. It can best be understood by means of an example. A husband is plagued by feelings of incompetence. When he comes home, he scans the house for any sign that it is his wife and not himself who has the identity of the incompetent one. He attacks her on flimsy pretext to attain the position of the self-righteously competent spouse stuck with an incompetent wife. He has projected an entire piece of his identity onto her. When projective identification occurs in an intimate or empathic relationship, the recipient of the projection feels altered by it. In this example, the wife may not only feel attacked but also actually take on the identity of incompetence projected onto her. When projective identification occurs in a treatment setting, the close and careful analysis of it within the transference and the study of the countertransference reactions evoked in the analyst form a significant portion of Kleinian theory and technique (Klein et al. 1973; Segal 1973).

Introjection and identification. A great deal of confusion arises here because identification is both a defense and a normal mechanism of growth. Important objects are taken in to avoid the pain of losing or being separated from them. When the identification is primitive, it is called *introjection*, more closely resembling unconscious imitation. When a child develops a low frustration tolerance and becomes irritable as a result of an angry parent's interactions, the child is "swallowing whole" this image of the angry parent and growing into it himself or herself. When the characteristics of a parent become the child's own in a way that allows the child to modify them as he or she matures, this is *identification*. Incorporation entails partial blending of the external object and the self. Identification implies eventual depersonification in which the traits of the individual no longer remain bound to specific memories but are acquired as genuine traits of one's own. Thus, identification can be more or less healthy, more or less a part of normal growth and development, or more or less pathological, depending on its type.

Turning against the self. As originally elaborated in the vicissitudes of the instincts, any drive can be directed toward its object or turned back against the self or both at once. This is the basis of secondary narcissism and explains how sadism and masochism can be two sides of the same coin. Turning against the self is illustrated in the following clinical vignette:

> A 5-year-old boy was bragging to his uncle about how superior his father was to his uncle. When the father showed disapproval, the boy became quiet. A few moments later, the boy, who was ordinarily quite well coordinated, tripped and hurt his head against the side of a table. Analysis of the event revealed that the boy's rivalry with his father had undergone a reaction formation and a projection as follows: "I'm not better than my father. My father is better than you. And it is not I who have a rivalry with my father; it is my uncle who has a rivalry with my father." When both of these mechanisms were not successful in binding the child's unacceptable thoughts because of the father's disapproval, the young boy turned his competitive aggression against himself and tripped.

This vignette also illustrates that defense mechanisms rarely appear in pure form and usually appear in clusters.

Reversal. The difficult-to-understand defense of reversal is the process by which the aim of an instinct is transformed into its opposite, as in activity changing to passivity or passivity changing into activity. It is part of the elaboration of how sadism and masochism can alternate with each other. It is a defense very closely related to turning against the self.

Denial. Denial is the invalidation of an unpleasant or unwanted piece of information and involves living one's life as though it did not exist. It is a more severe form of defense related to repression. It denies access to consciousness but is more thoroughgoing and costly in that a piece of reality has to be not only ignored as in repression but also actually invalidated. Thus, reality testing is diminished. Milder forms of denial may exist in transient ways, such as when one continues to refer to a recently deceased member of the family in the present tense. A patient who built a decorative fountain requiring strenuous work the weekend after he was told that he had advanced coronary artery disease would be engaging in a stronger form of denial. Frequently, denial is easiest to spot in its more nearly conscious forms, as in the case of the alcoholic person who denies the existence of the illness because he never drinks before 5:00 P.M. The persis-

talk because of embarrassment, fear of retribution, or some other fantasy and then would not disclose that that was the reason. Now resistance is less a noun and more a gerund. Resistance means that the patient is in the act of resisting (Schafer 1973). What is he or she resisting? The patient is resisting the ongoing nature of the analytic process of unfolding of the transference, free communication of mental content, and free flow of affect. Or he or she is trying to transform the relationship into something other than analysis by turning it into a friendship, into advice giving, or into problem solving.

Interpretation.   Interpretation is the articulation on the part of the analyst, and eventually on the part of the patient, of the connections and meaning of what is going on during the process of analysis. Interpretations are strongest and most comprehensive when, as in the example given earlier, they link the historical past to the current life situation and to phenomena within the analysis such as the transference.

To the extent that a treatment relies on the interpretation of transference and resistance, it comes closer to psychoanalysis. To the extent that it relies more on explanation, on theory, on construction of the historical past in lieu of the unfolding of the transference, on formulas for decoding rather than living through defense mechanisms, it moves into the realm of psychoanalytic psychotherapy or psychodynamic psychotherapy. To the extent that it focuses more on confrontation, on specific problem solving, or on teaching of techniques, it becomes more cognitive or behavior therapy. To the extent that the patient comes to treatment for direct solutions to problems, it most closely resembles counseling.

Followers of Freud

There is by no means unanimity among current psychoanalysts. Intramural dispute has taken place among a profusion of schools of thought. While correcting and revising the work of Freud and adding new perspectives of their own, many theorists have stayed within the psychoanalytic tradition, viewing themselves as resting on the foundation of Freud's work and having the same ambitious goals to understand the entire structure of a person's mind. I therefore regard them as falling broadly within the psychoanalytic tradition (Table 3–5).

We now turn to four areas of psychoanalytic theory left largely unfinished by Freud: *object relations and the self, development, character structure,* and the *rediscovery of trauma.* I blend the historical approach with a survey of the modern state of affairs in each of these four main areas.

Object Relations and the Self

Sigmund Freud had included a theory of object relations in his classical theory. Instincts had a source, an aim, and an object. The oedipal period depended on the actual relationship with the parents, and in "Mourning and Melancholia," Freud (1917[1915]/1957), attempting to distinguish between the depression of normal mourning and the pathological depression of melancholia, talked about the influence of object relations. The word *object*, of course, is in contrast to the word *subject*. Critics of psychoanalysis who point to use of the term *object relations* and contend that therefore psychoanalysis is not concerned with human beings simply misunderstand the usage of this term.

In "Mourning and Melancholia," Freud said that ordinarily when a significant object is lost to us, we enter a period of mourning, but that if the object relation was more of a narcissistic object choice than a true object relation, and if it was filled with intense ambivalence, then "the shadow of the object falls upon the ego." In other words, through identification we take in qualities of the object that then influence our ego state. To put it yet another way, the infant starts in an autoerotic state and moves through the anaclitic relationship to a state of object relation. The baby loves the mother. To the extent that the mother is excessively disappointing or to the extent that the baby is incapable of mastering its ambivalence, the baby will retreat into a state of secondary narcissism. In that case, its relationship with the mother confuses self and object. The mother is recognized only to the extent to which she fulfills the needs of the baby. Thus, a narcissistic object choice develops, in which others are not viewed in their own right but rather in terms of the extent to which they fulfill our needs. Thus, when they are lost, we have to incorporate them into ourselves in order not to feel that we are lost. Then the negative half of the ambivalence that we felt toward the object we now direct toward the self, hence melancholia.

Notwithstanding his acknowledgment of the importance of object relations, Freud primarily developed the instinctual drive portion of his theory, and he never completed the elaboration of his object relational theory—a task that was left to his successors (Greenberg and Mitchell 1983; Sutherland 1980).

Klein.   Melanie Klein (see Klein et al. 1973) paid substantial attention to the process of pathological identification and to the fate of the incorporated object. In the strictest sense, she was not an object relations theorist in that she still believed that the primary motive for human behavior was drive discharge. She placed her emphasis on

TABLE 3–5. Followers of Freud who remained within the psychoanalytic tradition

Klein	Emphasis on aggression as a primary drive. Splitting and projective identification seen as most important defenses. Developmental stages known as "paranoid position" and "depressive position" are compressed into first 6 months of life. Technique focuses on patient's projective identification toward the therapist. Countertransference reactions are presumed to be elicited by the patient's projections.
Fairbairn	First true object relations theorist. Postulated that primary drive is to seek connections with objects. Holds that the ego is present from birth in a pristine state. This pristine ego then fragments into a "libidinal ego," associated with excitement and an "antilibidinal ego" associated with negativity toward the self.
Winnicott	Held that one cannot think of a baby psychologically in the absence of a mother. In development, the child does not need perfection, merely "good enough" to align with the infant's needs. We use "transitional objects," or experiences and things that are neither self nor other, to help us define our place in the world. For a child, one such object might be a blanket; for adults, they might be music, religion, or creativity. If all goes well, we develop the "capacity to be alone," that is, the secure sense of self that permits us to be content in ourselves while also relating to others in a way that does not blur our identity. If not, we develop a "false self" to meet our parents' pathology, thus obscuring our "true self." Technique relies on creating a "holding environment" in which the true self can emerge safely.
Kohut	Founder of "self psychology." Development seen not as psychosexual but as the growth of a cohesive and stable sense of self. This is nurtured by "mirroring," a process by which the child builds worth and self-esteem as reflected in the eyes of his or her parents. "Selfobjects" are the mental constructions by which we define ourselves in terms of how we are perceived by others. Technique relies on mirroring and affective attunement, the process by which the therapist shows empathic connection with the patient's emotional state. Kohut rejected interpretations based on theoretical constructs and insisted on "experience-near" interpretations related to the immediate feelings experienced in the session. His theory of transference holds that patients do not distort per se, but rather are reacting to subtle interactions initiated by the therapist. His theory has further evolved into the school of "intersubjectivity." This holds that the patient and therapist jointly create a field in which the patient's transference meets the therapist's countertransference. It is in navigating this field that growth is supposed to take place.
Kernberg	Blends object relations perspective with more classical structural theory. There is an emphasis on the ways affect, self-representation, and object relations interact as a triad. Classifies character pathology according to hierarchies of defense (see Table 3–4). Elaborated the concept of borderline personality organization. Technique emphasizes earlier interpretation of aggression and negative transference.

the discharge of the aggressive drives and seemed to give them primacy over the libidinal drives, but, in any event, drives constituted the motivation for the individual. Klein was less concerned with the source and the aim and more concerned with the object of the drives. Noting the child's tendency to split experience into good and bad, Klein postulated that the child first has relations with part objects and that only later in development does the child have relations with whole objects. Her theory said that this tendency to engage in projective identification, to get rid of our unwelcome impulses and our unwelcome incorporation of part objects, causes our internal mental life to be populated by monstrous, distorted, and incomplete versions of objects. Thus, the more pathological splitting there was, the more split we would be in our internal mental life and the more vulnerable to ongoing distortion.

Fairbairn. W. R. D. Fairbairn was the first true object-relations theorist insofar as he postulated that the primary drive was object seeking (Fairbairn 1972). Whereas Freud thought that the drive was primary and the objects were interchangeable, Fairbairn thought that the objects were primary and the drives were interchangeable. If, for Freud, anyone could satisfy the baby's hunger, for Fairbairn, we were given hunger so that we could have a reason to make a human bond. For Fairbairn, the ego is present at birth. Because it is immature and it cannot tolerate the intensity of stimuli, this pristine ego is then rendered asunder, splitting into a libidinal ego (which has an association with the exciting object) and an antilibidinal ego (which has an association with a rejecting object). The course of maturity, then, is to undo the split and reintegrate into a more robust central ego.

Winnicott. D. W. Winnicott did not offer a full theory, but he is grouped with the object-relations theorists because of many important contributions. Winnicott pointed out that it is neither conceptually nor clinically proper to conceive of a baby without the mother as well. This viewpoint restored an interpersonal balance to psychoanalysis. A "good-enough" mother (Winnicott 1965) will respond to the baby's communications, meeting his or her needs within an optimal zone of frustration and gratification. Imposing her own needs, a pathological mother will force the baby to create a "false self" to protect its "true self." On the other hand, a mother who accepts increasing autonomy in gradual stages permits the child to have his or her own agenda while remaining dependent on her. Under such circumstances, the child can be himself or herself in the presence of a mother who can be herself while they are still together. Winnicott called this "the capacity to be alone" in the presence of someone else.

Winnicott (1953) also postulated an intermediate stage of separation-individuation during which the infant relates to "transitional objects" that are neither self nor other but form an intermediate zone. This intermediate zone initially may take the form of a blanket or a toy but remains with us throughout life as a phenomenon to help us deal with our aloneness and separation in the universe. Thus, in mature adult life, music, scientific creativity, and religion constitute transitional phenomena or transitional experiences that are neither self nor object but act as a link between the two (see Winnicott 1966).

Kohut.   Although he would not have grouped himself in the object-relations school, Heinz Kohut also placed emphasis on the relationship between self and object. Kohut (1971) postulated two lines of development, one involving the libido and conflict and the other involving the development of the self. Kohut stated that two kinds of transferences that are found in patients with narcissi are keys to the understanding of stages of development through which individuals pass on their way to developing a cohesive self. The development of a cohesive self requires optimal empathy that consists of mirroring and idealization. *Mirroring* is the experience wherein children define themselves by observing themselves in the gleam in their mother's eye. Kohut believed that the development of a cohesive self is more important than the vicissitudes of instincts. *Self psychology*, the school of thought that grew out of Kohut's theories, holds that the cohesive self can manage its drives.

Kohut's sensitivity to absences of phase-appropriate mirroring and idealization led him to emphasize deficiencies of emotional nutrients over conflicts as a cause of pathology. The narcissistic dilemma comes from object relations that were arrested in a phase during which others are seen in terms of how they help to define us. Kohut (1977) characterized this phase with the term *selfobjects*.

Kohut also stressed the paramount need for psychoanalysis to operate on the basis of empathy. Interpretations based on instinctual drives or ego structures are *experience-distant* and therefore not as useful as ones based on awareness of subjective feelings, especially of

vulnerability, that are *experience-near*. Transference was not seen as a phenomenon whereby the patient distorts reality but rather the way the patient experiences (perhaps with exaggerated intensity, but not without basis) the interaction between doctor and patient.

Kohut's earlier contributions described transferences that recapitulated deficient aspects of the child's development. With the introduction of selfobjects, a new school within psychoanalysis began. At first, Kohut tried to bridge earlier theories of libido with his newer theory of the self by postulating two separate tracks for development. As time went on, this dual-track theory was dropped, and the theory of the self took over.

As a theory, self psychology emphasized the absence of crucial "emotional vitamins" as the main pathogenic feature of childhood. On the assumption that "a well-regulated self can manage its drives," repair of an incoherent self was seen as the task of psychotherapy. Interpretation of childhood manifestations in adult action came to be seen as less important than empathic understanding of the transference-expressed needs of the patient at that moment. Affective attunement between patient and therapist superseded interpretations that looked for historical causes, and deficiency superseded conflict.

In an earlier era, psychoanalysis might not have been able to live harmoniously with self psychology. Just as Fairbairn had turned psychoanalytic theory upside down when he made libido a derivative of object seeking, self psychology had the same effect when it made conflict and drives secondary to deficiency and the formation of a coherent self. However, by the 1970s, psychoanalysis had become a broader tradition and could embrace both object relations and self psychology.

As self psychology has matured, new emphasis has been focused on the intersubjective nature of psychotherapy (Kohut 1984; Stolorow and Brandschaft 1987; Stolorow and Lachmann 1980). This new focus has influenced technique. Therapists influenced by self psychology are more likely to take personal responsibility for their patient's negative affects in the transference and are more likely to address the patient's experience of hurt than the patient's active role in his or her life frustrations (Fine and Fine 1990). In an illustrative clinical vignette, a female patient was engaged to a man toward whom she felt extremely ambivalent. He reminded her of her father, with whom there was much conflict. The death of her mother when the patient was quite young had made intimacy and commitment extremely difficult and frightening even though it was desperately sought. One day she returned in tears from a weekend with her fiancé: they had broken up after days of fighting, initiated largely by her. When the therapist interpreted her ambivalence, her conflicts over closeness, and her provocations that precipitated this breakup, the patient interrupted to say, "Everything you say may be true, but you could at least start by telling me you were sorry for the grief I'm suffering."

A theorist of self psychology might point to this vignette as an example of a patient's need for empathy to correct a childhood deficiency left by the death of her mother. A Kleinian might choose to emphasize the patient's hostility in provoking an argument with her fiancé or her wish to distance the fiancé to save both parties from the destruction inherent in intimacy. A more "classical" therapist might explore the patient's ambivalent relationship with her father and its influence on the relationship with the fiancé. These differences in emphasis and sequence have stimulated vigorous discussion among different subschools within the psychoanalytic tradition.

In another important distinction, a Kleinian would see aggression as a principal organizing force in character and psychopathology and would view aggressive drives as innate. Kohut and the self psychologists see aggression as the result of frustration and interpret the frustration rather than the aggression itself. This brings us to Kernberg, who sees affect and aggression as central to psychodynamics.

Kernberg.   One of Otto Kernberg's (1976) contributions to object-relations theory was to emphasize that affect, self-representation, and an object representation always appear together. One cannot analyze any one without knowing about the others.

The infant is born unable to distinguish between internal and external and is only able to distinguish between pleasurable and unpleasurable experience. This is the logical consequence of the fact that the infant spends most of the day sleeping and the majority of sleep dreaming. Therefore, at first the child has difficulty distinguishing between realistic experiences and dreamed or hallucinated experiences. However, the infant can distinguish between experiences that feel good and experiences that feel bad. This is the origin of what I term *passive splitting*, so called because it occurs as a result of the maturational phase of the infant rather than an affirmative mental effort. One of the positive consequences of passive splitting is that there is an opportunity for good images to be accumulated. For an infant, bad experiences feel more powerful than good experiences, and therefore passive splitting helps to preserve the integrity of good experiences. Eventually, as the infant begins to distinguish between inner and outer, he or she develops active splitting, based on the fear that if the good and the bad were to get too close together, the bad would indeed

destroy the good. Finally, the infant, growing into a child, begins to be aware of whole objects, to distinguish between internal and external (due to the ascendancy of the reality principle), and to fuse good and bad. This fusion into a whole self and a whole object coincides with the maturation of the superego and the fusion of the old, archaic superego and the ego ideal. Tremendous energy is liberated as a result of this fusion because the energy necessary to keep splits apart can now be used for other purposes.

It is at this point coinciding with the end of rapprochement and beginning with the object-constancy phase, and also coinciding with the oedipal phase of classical theory, that the individual moves from the splitting hierarchy of defenses to the repression hierarchy of defenses. Kernberg's theory is further elaborated on later in the section on character pathology.

Theories of Development

It is known that the child grows both physically and cognitively in phases after birth until he or she reaches adulthood. Developmental theories assume that psychological growth also proceeds in phases, and the emotional capability of the child and his or her capacity for dealing with mental content, even the definition of what constitutes mental content, change according to the maturational stage. Developmental arrests, fixation points, and points of regression have an effect on the development of the particular psychological system at greatest risk at any given age. The correlation of psychopathology in adults with the developmental stage of presumed trauma during childhood was an important extension of the concept that childhood events influence adult states.

A variety of developmental systems have been proposed by persons within the psychoanalytic tradition (Figure 3–2). Some of these systems have been full-fledged theories, and others have been simply limited observations or partial theories about substages of development. I introduce the main theories of development in this subsection and then discuss their application to adult psychopathology in the subsection ""Psychopathology and Character States" later in this chapter.

The classical theory of Freud and Abraham.   The classical theory initiated by Sigmund Freud (1905/1953, 1925/1961) and elaborated by Karl Abraham (1968) has already been alluded to and is presented here briefly. At birth, the infant is in a state of autoerotism. The development of the libido at this point is such that the infant is attached only to itself, for a psychological sense of self per se does not yet exist. The ego instinct for survival and

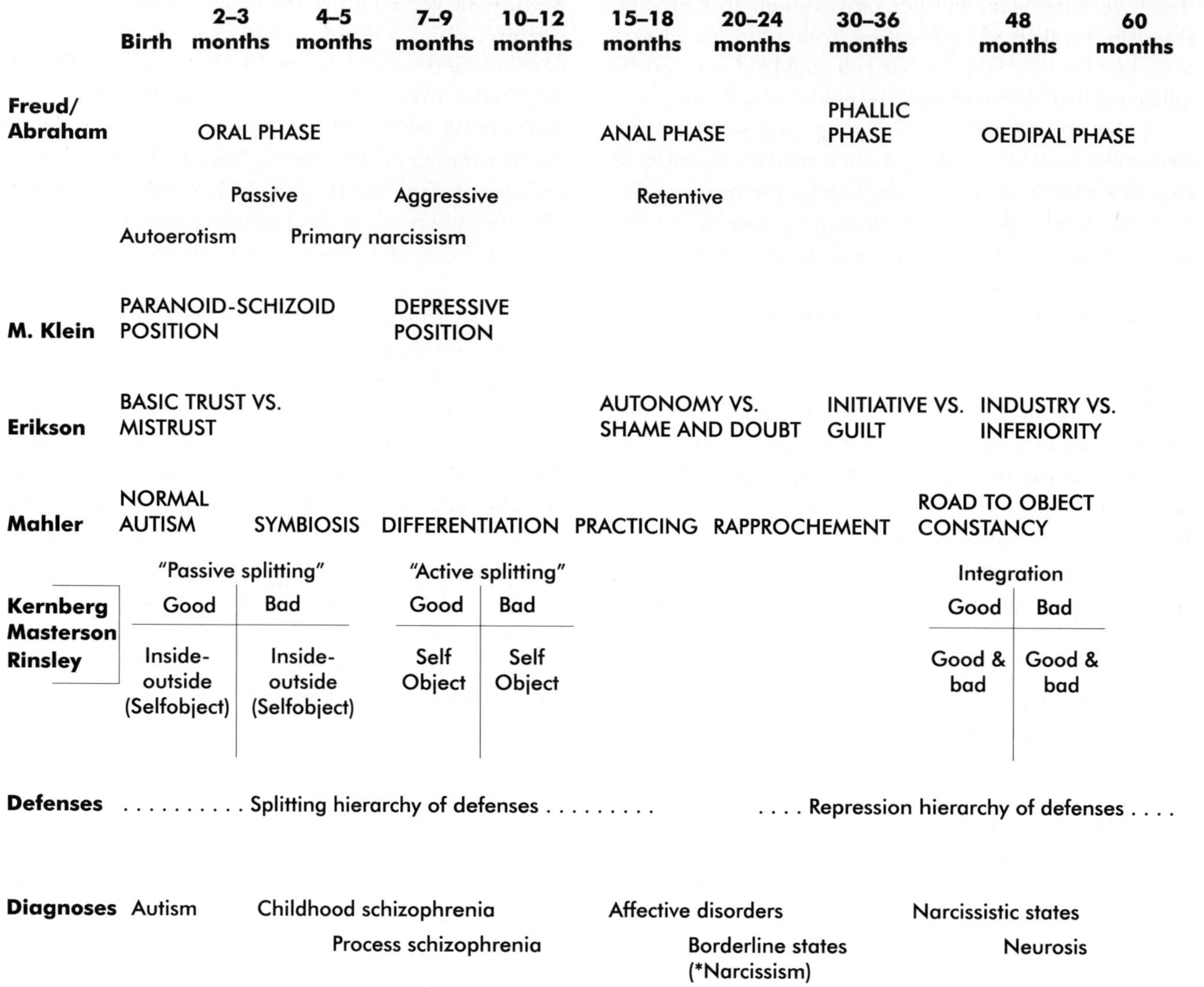

	Birth	2–3 months	4–5 months	7–9 months	10–12 months	15–18 months	20–24 months	30–36 months	48 months	60 months
Freud/ Abraham		ORAL PHASE				ANAL PHASE		PHALLIC PHASE	OEDIPAL PHASE	
			Passive	Aggressive		Retentive				
	Autoerotism		Primary narcissism							
M. Klein	PARANOID-SCHIZOID POSITION			DEPRESSIVE POSITION						
Erikson	BASIC TRUST VS. MISTRUST					AUTONOMY VS. SHAME AND DOUBT		INITIATIVE VS. GUILT	INDUSTRY VS. INFERIORITY	
Mahler	NORMAL AUTISM		SYMBIOSIS	DIFFERENTIATION		PRACTICING	RAPPROCHEMENT		ROAD TO OBJECT CONSTANCY	

Kernberg / Masterson / Rinsley

"Passive splitting"		"Active splitting"		Integration	
Good	Bad	Good	Bad	Good	Bad
Inside-outside (Selfobject)	Inside-outside (Selfobject)	Self Object	Self Object	Good & bad	Good & bad

Defenses . . . . Splitting hierarchy of defenses . . . . Repression hierarchy of defenses . . . .

Diagnoses

Autism	Childhood schizophrenia		Affective disorders		Narcissistic states
		Process schizophrenia		Borderline states (*Narcissism)	Neurosis

FIGURE 3–2.   Theories of development.

This figure is an approximate display of each listed author's developmental scheme for comparison with other authors' schemes. The phases shown do not have exact correlation with age (i.e., this figure is not to be read in columns). The phases overlap, and neighboring phases may coexist. The theories of each author are not presented as exact equivalents of the similar-age stages of other authors. The diagnoses listed at the bottom are those that some developmental theorists believe match essential developmental fixations and arrests with future child and adult psychopathology.

the libidinal instinct for pleasure are intertwined, and the child starts with an anaclitic relationship with the mother. In other words, libido leans on survival. Gradually, through the experience of frustration as well as the emergence of the ego and the beginnings of the reality principle associated with the maturation of perception, the child begins to recognize that a distinction exists between internal and external, and a rudimentary form of object relations emerges.

The child's first main modality for relating is oral, meaning literally the mouth, lips, and tongue importantly involved in nursing. But orality also includes taking in of perceptions and "swallowing" the world of sensory perceptions. If there is excessive frustration, the child will retreat from early object-relatedness and establish a state of secondary narcissism. If frustration is moderate and optimal, the child will begin to recognize bit by bit that the objects of the world are not under his or her full control, nor is he or she under their full control. As the organism matures, libidinal interest leaves the initial oral phase and enters an aggressive oral phase in which swallowing and taking in are replaced by biting and spitting. The child learns to say no, and this signals a crucial step in the differentiation of the child from others and the growing establishment of a sense of self (see Spitz 1965).

The libido then moves to the anal phase in which questions of control over bodily contents and the nature of bodily contents are paramount. These issues are both literal in terms of weaning and toilet training and metaphorical in terms of the functions that an anus is supposed to fulfill—namely, control of time, delay of discharge, containment, making sure that everything is in its proper place, yielding to authority, and making judgments about whether one's internal contents are good or bad. Difficulties in this area will result in fixation at the anal phase and yield an anal character type, with overemphasis on parsimony, orderliness, and obstinacy. Disorders characterized by obsessive-compulsive behaviors are thought to result from fixations at the anal phase.

The third phase of development is the phallic phase, expressed by interest in the penis itself, which, according to the classical theory, results in exhibitionism for boys and a feeling of envy and inferiority for girls. Most modern theorists working within the psychoanalytic tradition have importantly modified this aspect of the classical theory.

Exhibitionism and its grandiosity lead to a heightened rivalry with the same-sex parent and usher in the oedipal phase. This oedipal period shows its earliest beginnings in 3- to 4-year-olds and culminates in 5- to 6-year-olds.

The oedipal phase was seen as preeminent in neurosis because it is 1) the culmination of childhood libidinal development, 2) a multiperson interaction on which future social relatedness is based, and 3) the hypothesized period of solidification for the superego—the time when gender identity is fixed and sexual object choice is decided. Moving from a two-person to a three-person world was momentous because it prepared the child to relinquish the fantasy of centrality in the universe. Conventions of society, values of culture, the ability to share, and the roots of sublimation all converge at this time. Oedipal issues were believed to be universal and would eventually emerge in every psychoanalysis. Neurosis was believed to be crystallized at this time. A latency period follows, interrupted by puberty and followed by adolescence.

Klein and Fairbairn. Melanie Klein did not have a full-fledged theory of development; however, she took issue with the classical theory on some important points. Klein believed that the critical issue at birth was not autoerotism but what she originally called the paranoid position and what she later, under the influence of Fairbairn, renamed the *paranoid-schizoid position*. By that, Klein meant that from birth the infant relies heavily on mechanisms of introjection, projective identification, and splitting and sees the world in terms of what she called *part objects*. Aggression is preeminent and uncontrollable and cannot be neutralized. If successful, the child then moves to the depressive position by age 6 months when

the realization occurs that objects are not entirely split but that they are indeed whole and when the realization of the imperfection of the world and of the power of aggression takes hold. Thus, the ego and superego are present, for Klein, at an extremely early age, as are precursors of the oedipal period. No stages of development are postulated beyond the depressive position of 6 months.

Fairbairn (1972) believed that the ego is present from birth and that the child is object seeking, not pleasure seeking. According to Fairbairn, a child is born with a pristine ego, but because of conflict, the child is forced to split off the unacceptable object relations and ego states. Thus, an "id" is created as a result of splitting the pristine ego and repressing the libidinal ego and its associated exciting objects. A "superego" is created by splitting off the antilibidinal ego and its associated rejecting objects. To the extent that these splits are deep and profound, the remaining central ego is impoverished and depleted with little in the way of mature object relations. The task of treatment and of maturity becomes restoring as much as possible to the central ego and reducing the libidinal ego and its exciting objects and the antilibidinal ego and its rejecting objects.

Bowlby. John Bowlby is a British psychoanalyst whose interest in early development was heightened by his duties dealing with displaced children during World War II. Drawing on his knowledge and interest in ethology, Bowlby, agreeing with Fairbairn that the child at birth was object seeking, asserted that there was a primary independent bonding drive that was not anaclitic, leaning on physiological survival, but autonomous and independent and had phases of its own. Bowlby (1958) offered five responses that make up attachment behavior: sucking, clinging, following, crying, and smiling, which are behavior patterns specific to humans. Working quasi-independently but synergistically, each one has a specific trajectory and reaches its height during different months of the first 3 years of life. The components of attachment behavior influence the development of the cognitive sphere as well as the formation of character structure.

In Bowlby's theory, parent–child relationships are central, and object relations have as much importance as instinctual drives.

Balint and Guntrip. Michael Balint (1968) described a stage of development in his more severely disturbed patients in which they developed a *basic fault*. Balint adopted this term to indicate that some form of integration was missing in much the way an earthquake fault line would indicate the lack of integration of tectonic plates.

The problem was one of integration, of something missing, rather than drives that were frustrated in their inability to find expression. Balint thought that this basic fault was caused by a failure of fit between the response of the mother and the needs of the child. Those persons who have this basic fault will slip into one of two types of object relations: *ocnophilia*, in which the relationships with others are filled with great intensity and deep dependence, or *philobatism*, in which objects are avoided and the inner world is intensely clung to. These two developmental alternatives then characterize the organizing principles for the reaction to the inadequate mother–child relationship.

Harry Guntrip (1974), the main disciple of Fairbairn, expanded the notion of philobatism in terms of his theory of schizoid phenomena. He also saw development as progressing according to degree and type of dependency rather than drive discharge.

Erikson. Another ambitious theory of development was offered by Erik Erikson (1963). He postulated eight phases of development, spanning the entire life and serving as nodal points for adaptation to the age-appropriate requirements of any phase of development. He modified the concept of libidinal distribution by the concept of zones and modes. *Zone* refers to the organ system or cluster of physical and conceptual skills that the person has to deal with in that particular phase of development. *Mode* refers to the manner in which the developmental task is undertaken. For example, applying Erikson's notion of zones and modes to Freud and Abraham's oral phase, one might say that the zone is the mouth and perhaps also the nerve endings of the perceptual system. The mode is that of taking in, of swallowing, and of digesting, spitting, or vomiting. When the oral mode is emphasized, we have issues of dependency and of neediness, hunger, and starvation that might operate quite independent of the oral zone.

Instead of using bodily zones to serve as signposts for his theory, Erikson chose the developmental task that exists at any particular age. *Basic trust versus mistrust* is the stage of acquisition of sense that the universe is reliable and that our most important object relations are consistent and available. *Autonomy versus shame and doubt* addresses how much control of our body and our thinking we can attain and how much we will be a disappointment to those around us and to ourselves. The phase of *initiative versus guilt* coincides with the issues of the oedipal phase for Freud and Abraham. During the stage of *industry versus inferiority*, the child deals with latency and school. During puberty and adolescence is the phase of *identity versus role confusion*, our opportunity to clarify

issues of personal identity and own our own internal representations. This is sometimes referred to as *depersonification*. Psychopathology around areas of identity confusion appears at this time. The young adulthood phase of *intimacy versus isolation* opens the task of rediscovering attachment and mature bonding. In midadulthood, the issue is *generativity versus stagnation*, and in maturity the questions concern *ego integrity versus despair*.

Another point that Erikson made is the interactive nature between the child and the parent. Ordinarily it is assumed that it is the parent who raises the child, but Erikson emphasized that the relationship goes in two directions:

> Babies control and bring up their families as much as they are controlled by them; in fact, we may say that the family brings up the baby by being brought up by him. Whatever reaction patterns are given biologically and whatever schedule is predetermined developmentally must be considered to be a series of *potentialities for changing patterns of mutual regulation.* (Erikson 1963, p. 69)

Erikson's phases of development were regarded as very important when initially promulgated but have not been given much attention by mainstream psychoanalysis in recent years.

Mahler. Probably the most influential and important developmental theory since Freud and Abraham's is that proposed by Margaret Mahler (see Mahler et al. 1975). For Mahler, the issue was not the progress of libidinal development but rather phases of separation and individuation. The key question of development was, "To what extent does the infant, who is originally born without identity, acquire a sense of separate identity?" Mahler's early work with severely disturbed children led her to investigate this area. Her theory has become the modern classic theory of psychoanalysis, accepted in its essential form by most psychoanalysts, although current investigators are beginning to question certain aspects of it (see Siegel 1999; Stern 1985).

Normal autism. During the period from birth to 2 months, sleeplike states of the newborn and very young infant far outweigh states of arousal and are reminiscent of the primal states that prevailed during intrauterine life.

Symbiosis. The enhanced awakening and the increased perceptual experience of the infant permit a gradual distinction between what is inside and what is outside, and what is pleasurable and what is unpleasurable. Mahler believed that the mechanism of splitting arises in its first form during this phase. The essential feature of this phase is an omnipotent fusion with the representation of the mother and a delusion of a common boundary between two physically separate individuals. The symbiotic phase reaches its peak at about age 4–5 months, when it starts to decline as the beginnings of differentiation emerge.

Differentiation.   Differentiation coincides with a more permanently alert sensorium, as the infant awakens from his or her postnatal state and becomes more aware of the world. Mahler called this the *hatching process*. The infant's attention during the first few months had been primarily inward; now it becomes more outward. At this phase, transitional objects become important. At about 7–8 months, the infant is beginning to move away from the mother but can do so only for brief periods and then has to check back with the mother visually or tactilely. At about 8 months, the infant becomes acutely aware of the difference between familiar people like mother and those who are not familiar. This is called the *stranger reaction* or, in more severe cases, *stranger anxiety*. Its proper timing indicates progress of the differentiation phase.

Practicing.   Practicing occurs from about 10 months to 16–18 months. As Mahler et al. (1975, p. 71) said, "During these precious six to eight months...the world is the junior toddler's oyster.... Narcissism is at its peak! The child's first upright independent steps mark the onset of the practicing period par excellence with substantial widening of his world and of reality testing." The enormous expansion of the child's ability to be autonomous during this phase creates a state of imperviousness to disappointment that makes the child appear to be in love with the world.

Rapprochement.   The child's ability to walk and to move away from the mother, together with the beginning of representational cognition (which is the precursor of speech), makes the child a much more separate and autonomous person. By 18 months, the infant has matured to a sufficient degree to recognize in a new way his or her helplessness and dependency. During the practicing phase, the child had been preoccupied with all of the new skills he or she was acquiring that permitted greater separation. Now there is a change in emotional life, with greater susceptibility to frustration, greater fears of object loss, and more awareness of separation and consequently greater anxiety. Mahler believed that the child alternates between periods of great need for closeness and periods of need for distance. During this subphase, the child will need to be refueled by intimate bodily contact and also by language and other kinds of communication. He or she will shadow the mother and will dart away and then come back and dart away again.

Here the mother's attitude is extremely important, as well as that of the father, whose role expands considerably during this phase. The mother who rejects the child for having become more independent will make that child feel that further autonomy is dangerous. The child must not regard the mother as an extension of himself or herself, and the mother must not regard the child as an extension of herself. In this phase, Mahler believed that a structuralization of the ego occurs and a coherent self is established. If mother and child have a fluent moving back and forth within an optimal range of closeness and distance, the child will gradually learn that it is safe and rewarding to move toward greater autonomy and that he or she can do so without fear of losing the relationship with the mother and father. Disturbances in this phase leave the child confused about autonomy; lacking a solid, cohesive self; and preoccupied with the dangers of separation—all of which might result in a clinging, dependent pattern or in a pattern of defiant, defensive disengagement.

Object constancy.   Mahler called the next subphase the consolidation of individuality and the beginnings of emotional object constancy. This stage begins at 24–30 months and lasts in a major way for 2–3 more years and in a subtler way for the rest of one's life. In this subphase, the child takes the progressive steps toward object integration, affective stability, and a synthesis between the previously separated good and bad experiences.

Masterson (1981) and Rinsley (1980) have been important contributors in working out the correlation between Mahler's phases of separation-individuation and adult psychopathology.

Infant observation.   Psychoanalytic theories of development come from two sources: reconstructions based on inferences made through interpretation of the transference in the psychoanalytic setting and direct naturalistic and experimental observations of infants by a host of researchers. Compelling work has emerged in this latter area and has been integrated by Daniel Stern (1985). He challenged some of Mahler's conceptions about symbiosis and autism, holding that even at birth the child is aware of surroundings and intensely interested in them. Stern postulated four senses of self that emerge during the first 12–18 months of life:

1. A sense of an emergent self in the period from birth to about 2 months

2. A sense of a core self that arises from about 2–3 months to 7–9 months

3. A sense of a subjective self from about 9–15 months, with intersubjective relatedness

4. A sense of a verbal self from about 15–18 months, with emphasis on verbal relatedness

Stern believed that there must be a greater correlation between the data of child observation and those of psychoanalysis.

Psychopathology and Character States

The weakest part of psychoanalytic theory is that of psychopathology. Psychoanalysts have generally striven to understand the entire workings of the mind. Symptoms are regarded as signs of malfunction of internal mental processes rather than as diagnostic entities themselves. Psychoanalysis attempts to understand and unravel the mysteries of the entire personality, not just seek symptomatic relief of the state for which the patient originally presented. Furthermore, the symptom may in itself be a defense against more severe underlying difficulties. Hence, a phenomenological approach has never played the important role for psychoanalysis that it has for psychiatry in general. Nevertheless, certain pathological states have been discussed at length and constitute clinical elaborations rather than a theory of psychopathology itself.

When Freud began treating patients, most of whom presented with hysteria (S. Freud 1905[1901]/1953), he found that the repression of unacceptable mental content was the central feature causing the symptoms. He postulated that the symptom was like a dream in that it was a compromise formation that allowed partial expression of a repressed idea or affect. The obvious therapeutic course, therefore, was to make the unconscious conscious. This Freud could do relatively quickly, and in the early days of psychoanalysis, treatment was very brief, perhaps sometimes only a few weeks in length. Over time, it became increasingly clear that symptoms could not be separated from character structure. The shift from analyzing id content to analyzing ego mechanisms solidified this change of emphasis from symptom neurosis to character.

Abraham (1968) attempted to organize character according to the presumed stage of development that was malformed. Wilhelm Reich (1972) tended to classify character according to the predominant form that the neurosis took. Thus, for Reich there were phallic characters, passive characters, dependent characters, obsessional characters, hysterical characters, and so on. The goal, according to Reich, was to strive for a genital character. Reich's extremely important contribution to psychoanalysis was to emphasize the way in which character structure reveals itself directly and indirectly in the transference, which helped to shift psychoanalytic technique away from interpreting mental *content* in favor of interpreting mental *process*. The style with which the patient defends against mental content becomes equally important and in some cases more important than the content that is being defended against.

Anna Freud (1936/1946) attempted to link stages of development, clusters of defenses, and character types. Workers in the psychoanalytic tradition have isolated particular clusters of patients who were of interest to them and elaborated their character structure. For example, Balint and Guntrip were interested in patients with severe psychopathology and invented categories to describe them. Soon inconsistencies were found within seemingly similar psychopathology groups.

Hysterical neurosis was presumed to be based on repression of unwelcome sexual content. Obsessional neurosis was presumed to involve fixation at the anal phase and the development of symptoms that sought to get rid of unwelcome aggression and anal erotism. But individuals seeking treatment who come with apparently similar symptom pictures respond vastly differently to analysis. In the 1950s, patients who received diagnoses of hysteria were found to fall into at least two clusters, one of which had a more infantile or oral version and the other of which had the more classical oedipal disturbance. Similar confusion arose with patients who had an unusual degree of narcissism. Sigmund Freud (1924[1923]/1961, 1924b/1961) had originally equated this condition with psychosis, indicating that the transference neuroses could be treated with analysis but that the narcissistic neuroses were refractory to analysis because of an intractable inability to move from narcissistic object-choice to true object relations, a move that is a necessary precursor for development of the transference neurosis. However, some investigators began to have success with such patients, whereas others noted that narcissistic features emerged in treatment of the patients who did not originally present with them. The same thing happened with severely regressed patients. In the 1950s and 1960s, some psychoanalytic investigators believed that certain patients with psychotic symptoms were treatable with psychoanalysis; others believed that similar patients could be treated with modified psychoanalysis; still others maintained that such severe psychopathology was beyond the ken of psychoanalytic treatment. Clearly, there was some confusion in the psychoanalytic nomenclature to account for this disparity of findings.

The clarification of the borderline and narcissistic

states, primarily by Kernberg and Kohut in the 1960s and 1970s, has been extremely helpful in reducing this confusion, although another decade or two may have to pass for accumulation of data not adequately explained by these theories. Nevertheless, it is one of Kernberg's greatest contributions to have rethought the question of character pathology and to have offered his scheme of hierarchies of character states.

Classification of character states. To understand an individual patient, one has to conduct a careful review of systems based on the patient's functional capacities and style of mental action. Within each of these categories, one can make judgments about diagnosis and presumed underlying dynamics. One must understand six main areas to classify properly a patient's character pathology (summarized in Table 3–6, as derived from Kernberg's [1976] work). As a commentary on this organization, Table 3–7 provides a "psychoanalytic review of systems" in the form of questions to be raised in evaluating a patient's character structure and psychopathology.

Diagnoses. Having done a review of systems, one will reduce the likelihood of mistakenly being drawn astray by overreliance on the presenting symptoms. There is a spectrum of character pathology, from the individual who is primarily psychotic through persons with low, medium, and high levels of character structure, up through persons in the normal range. Those persons with borderline and narcissistic disorders, those who have an infantile personality, those with multiple sexual perversions without stable object relations or ongoing partners, hypomanic persons, schizoid persons, those persons with a paranoid personality, some persons who abuse substances, and those persons who are antisocial, chaotic, and impulse-ridden all fall into the category of low character function and severe character pathology. Passive-aggressive persons, sadomasochistic persons, some of the better-functioning infantile and hysteroid-type persons, many persons with narcissistic personalities, some persons with borderline disorders, some persons with some of the more stable sexual deviations with relatively stable object relations, some cyclothymic persons, and some persons who abuse substances, particularly those who abuse substances that are not illegal such as food and alcohol, all fall into the category of medium character function. The higher level of character function includes the persons with hysterical characters, obsessive-compulsive persons, depressive-masochistic persons, and the assortment of neurotic persons whose complaints are lack of sufficient creativity, difficulties in achieving intimacy, and inability to sustain creativity.

Borderline and narcissistic states. Although there is general agreement that the borderline and narcissistic states are related to each other, investigators in the field have considerable differences of opinion with regard to the details of these two states. Kohut wrote almost as if to imply that in his conceptualization nearly all of these patients have narcissistic disorders, and the tiny few who are so badly damaged that they cannot be treated with psychoanalysis are consigned to the borderline category. Kernberg seemed to conceptualize these persons primarily as having the mechanisms of borderline personality organization and suggested that perhaps some of the most well-functioning group who have the lowest levels of aggression resemble those patients whom Kohut referred to as narcissistic. Masterson and Rinsley believed that there are many more borderline patients than there are narcissistic ones. Rinsley believed that the fixation point for narcissism is late in the rapprochement phase (18–30 months) because these are patients who generally have a higher level of function and more signs of maturity. Masterson believed that the predominance of grandiosity in these patients indicates that they are fixated in the practicing phase (10–15 months), as though stuck in the grandiose time warp characteristic of that phase.

The significance of one's point of view is that it will influence the sequence in which interpretations are given. For instance, Masterson advocated confrontation for borderline patients and interpretation for narcissistic patients because the borderline patients lack a sense of identity and therefore will coalesce around the clarifying aspect of a confrontation, whereas the narcissistic patients will disintegrate if their fragile hold on well-being is punctured. Finally, the DSM system, starting with DSM-III (American Psychiatric Association 1980), which introduced the diagnosis of borderline personality disorder, merged the more descriptive approach of Gunderson (1984; Gunderson and Kolb 1976; Gunderson et al. 1975) with the more psychodynamic approach of Kernberg (1975) (Marmer and Fink 1994).

Two clinical illustrations. The following clinical vignettes illustrate the usefulness of Kernberg's review of systems approach for character pathology:

David was an extremely disturbed 23-year-old man when he first came into treatment. He appeared disheveled, his clothes did not match, and he had recently been fired from a menial job because he was unable to follow simple instructions. He had taken 5 years to barely graduate from the university with the lowest possible grade point average. At school, he had spent most of his time cloistered in his room, even urinating in empty soda bottles that he would empty at

TABLE 3–6. A classification of character states

Category	Psychotic organization	Low level of organization	Medium level of organization	Higher level of organization	Healthy organization
Instinctual development		Preponderance of pathological condensation of genital and pregenital strivings, with excess primitive aggression	Pregenital, especially oral; regression and fixation points predominate	Genital primacy attained	
Ego and its defenses	Lack of good, consistent reality testing	Splitting and related defenses (e.g., primitive dissociation, denial, idealization, devaluation, omnipotence, projective identification) Excessive splitting impairs ego's synthetic function; Direct expression of instincts is linked with defenses; Self not cohesive or integrated; mix of grandiose and contemptible and shameful	Uses repression-type defenses, but reverts to splitting-type defenses under stress; Reaction formations coexist with partial expression of rejected impulses; Inconsistent self	Repression and related defenses (e.g., intellectualization, rationalization, undoing, projection); Inhibitions and reactive traits predominate; Constricted ego	Considerable conflict-free energy; Sublimation
Superego		Archaic unintegrated superego precursors	Lack of integration; sadistic, with overidealization in ego ideal	Integrated, although severe, harsh, and perfectionistic	Less severe superego, more realistic ego ideal, integration between them
Internalized object relations	Difficulty distinguishing between self and object; Fusion, symbiosis, or autistic thinking	Part objects predominate, object constancy not fully established; inability to love an object who frustrates; self not stable; good and bad self-images not integrated; identity diffusion; inner world inhabited by caricatures of good and bad aspects of important objects	Stable self and object world, but with severe conflictual relationships; may fragment under severe stress	Stable self, stable representational world; whole objects predominate	Mostly whole objects and a consistent, cohesive self
Affect		Impaired capacity for guilt or mourning; basis for self-evaluation constantly fluctuating between harsh criticism and overidealized aspirations of grandiose notions	Severe mood swings (according to relationship with superego and ego ideal)	Can experience guilt and mourning; wider range of affects; Sexual and aggressive drives partially inhibited	Wide range of possible affects; Excellent anxiety tolerance and frustration threshold

TABLE 3–6. A classification of character states *(continued)*

Category	Psychotic organization	Low level of organization	Medium level of organization	Higher level of organization	Healthy organization
		Impulsive; contradictory repetitive behaviors seen	"Structured impulsivity"	Can have fairly deep and stable object relations, with genuine concern; considerable empathy; better anxiety tolerance	Good empathic powers; able to love and to mourn
		Sadistic, polymorphously perverse infantile drives	Modest empathy; slight anxiety tolerance		
		Little empathy; little conflict-free energy; very poor tolerance of affects, especially anxiety			
Interpersonal		Relationships tend to be need-gratifying or threatening; chronic work failure and creative failure; not nurturing to others when under stress	Lasting, although turbulent relationships, sometimes promising intimacy that cannot be sustained	Moderate impairment of social adaptation; problems may appear only in closest relationships (e.g., spouse, children)	
Diagnostic groups		Infantile personality	Passive-aggressive, sado-masochistic	Hysterical characters, obsessive-compulsive, depressive-masochistic persons	
		Many of the narcissistic disorders	Better-functioning infantile and hysteroid types		
		Most borderline patients	Many narcissistic, some borderline persons		
		Antisocial, as-if, chaotic, impulse-ridden, inadequate, and self-mutilating	Persons with stable sexual deviations with relatively stable object relations		
		Persons with multiple sexual perversions, especially those without stable object relations or ongoing partners	Cyclothymic persons		
		Paranoid personalities, hypomanic, schizoid	Some persons who abuse substances (especially food and alcohol)		
		Some persons who abuse substances (including gambling, eating, alcohol, and drugs)			

TABLE 3–7. A psychoanalytic review of systems

Instinctual development

Where are the instinctual drives?

Is there a predominance of early oral or anal fixation?

Is the patient's experience oralized or analized?

Is there an enormity of aggression?

Is there a lack of fusion of aggression and libido, or has a degree of fusion of instincts been achieved?

Has the person made it to a primarily genital level?

To what extent has the individual attained primacy of secondary process?

Is the person capable of a bound cathexis, or is all psychic energy subject to mobile cathexis and the need for instantaneous discharge?

Has the capacity to delay been achieved?

Ego and defenses

Does the individual primarily use splitting and the related defenses of projective identification, primitive dissociation, denial, idealization, devaluation, and omnipotence?

Does excessive splitting impair the ego's synthetic function?

Do the defenses primarily express and only incidentally conceal the underlying drives? Or, does the individual use repression-type defenses, reverting to the splitting when only under stress? Or, does the person use primarily the repression defenses such as intellectualization, rationalization, undoing, projection, and reaction formation with primarily inhibitions and a constricted ego?

How much conflict-free energy is there?

To what extent is there a cohesive self?

How much does the individual vacillate between grandiose states and contemptible, shameful states?

Superego

Does the individual primarily have the features of an archaic, unintegrated superego precursor with extremely harsh prohibitions and an excessively lofty and grandiose ego ideal?

Is there a more integrated, still sadistic superego that is moderately harsh and an overidealized ego ideal but not one that is too grandiose? Or, is there an integrated although harsh and perfectionistic superego? (In healthier states, the superego is less severe and more realistic, and there is considerable integration between the superego and the ego ideal. The person can feel praise for himself or herself as well as punishment.)

Object relations

Does the individual have difficulty distinguishing between inside and outside, between self and object?

In the clinical setting or in the pathological situation of the symptoms, does one see fusion, symbiosis, or autistic defenses?

Do part objects predominate without object constancy being fully established?

Is there an inability to love an object who frustrates?

Is the self stable or not?

Do good and bad images become integrated?

How diffuse is identity?

To what extent is the inner world inhabited by caricatures or aspects of important objects rather than whole objects? (If there is primarily a whole object world and a consistent, cohesive self, then object relations have advanced to a more mature degree.)

Affects

Is there a wide range of affective expression or a very narrow one?

Is the individual impulsive?

Are contradictory repetitive behaviors seen?

Is the individual sadistic?

Does the affect fluctuate between overly harsh criticism and overly idealized grandiosity?

Is there cyclothymia?

Does the individual have empathy?

Can the individual experience guilt and mourning?

Can the individual have deep, stable object relations with genuine concern?

How much tolerance is there for anxiety, or to what extent must anxiety be instantaneously discharged?

Interpersonal relationships

Is there an attainment of social adaptation?

Are there lasting relationships, or do the relationships promise intimacy but cannot be sustained?

Is the individual nurturing to others when under stress? Or do relationships constantly alternate between need gratification and threatening rejection?

2:00 A.M. when he was confident no one would see him. He had a delusional numerology system for the date of his birth and fantasies that the clouds were giving him messages. He was in an extremely anxious state and appeared defiant and hostile when he first came to see me. Based on his symptoms, one might have wondered if he were either schizophrenic or severely borderline. However, a more careful evaluation found that he had a much wider range of affect, that he had a profound consistent relationship with mythical parents (humanistic authors whose works he had read and cherished throughout a very disturbed high school and college period), and that he had had several lifelong friends who had remained friendly with him through the course of his illness. In the sessions, he showed a warm, gentle sense of humor. All of these factors coexisted with the extremely severe psychopathology with which he presented. Consequently, I made the diagnosis of a medium level of character pathology and felt safe in initiating a psychoanalytic treatment.

In contrast, Peter was a successful musician and composer. He had had several hit songs and had written scores for television. His presenting symptom was panic attacks that began when his parents were given lifetime career achievement awards in a related profession. His own self-diagnosis was that of a severe anxiety reaction centered around oedipal issues. However, very early in the transference, the predominance of severe splitting and projective identification and idealization was manifest. Both in the transference and in Peter's marriage, part objects predominated. Good and bad images of himself were not integrated, and his mood fluctuated in a cyclothymic manner according to whether he was in alignment with his grandiose ego ideal or his extremely harsh, punitive superego. Although he had occasional use of repression hierarchy defenses (such as intellectualization, reaction formation, and undoing), splitting predominated. He had an outwardly stable marriage, but his lack of ability to delay and the excess of primitive aggression were revealed both in the compulsive nature of his sexual behavior and in his inability to tolerate any frustration. Therefore, it was not surprising when in the second year of psychoanalytic psychotherapy a transference psychosis emerged with a full-fledged delusion regarding my influence over his mind and body, and in the office Peter experienced hallucinations of me in the appearance of the devil.

This latter case example illustrates the converse of David's case: a patient whose underlying character structure was much more pathological than the apparent level of adaptation indicated by his initial presenting symptoms. These two cases also illustrate the kinds of patients that are addressed within the psychoanalytic tradition and the extent to which underlying character pathology is more important than phenomenological diagnosis.

Rediscovery of Trauma

The most exciting development for theory of the mind and psychopathology in the 1980s and 1990s was the rediscovery of the role trauma plays in shaping personality and creating symptoms. In some ways, this represented a throwback to the nineteenth century and the days of Charcot and Janet. Many authors (Davis 1990; Edelson 1990; Ellenberger 1970; Erdleyi 1990) have commented on the central role of trauma in the theories of the nineteenth century. The French, most especially Charcot and Janet, observed that acute and chronic trauma was responsible for a wide variety of psychopathology. This observation was the linchpin for Charcot's theory of hysteria and for Janet's notion of the role of dissociation in his theory of the mind. Even Briquet (1859, noted in Loewenstein 1990), whose name is not generally associated with psychodynamic thinking, noted that a substantial number of his patients with somatiza-tion disorder had histories of childhood physical and sexual abuse.

Certain characteristics of the 1980s seem to be responsible for this rediscovery. The posttraumatic stress disorders in the veterans of the war in Vietnam had a dramatic effect on American psychiatrists. The capacity of real trauma to have prolonged influence on symptoms and a debilitating effect on personality and adaptation forced us to rethink our assumptions about the relation between trauma and the ability to function. Long-lasting dissociation and physiological instability in these patients could not be ascribed simply to preexisting conditions or to fantasy.

The recognition of the widespread prevalence of child abuse forced psychiatrists to review all of their former assumptions (Kluft 1990; McDougall 1982; Miller 1984, 1990). From the perspective of physical findings, pediatrics had become aware in the 1970s of the "battered child." In the 1980s, the awareness of the psychiatric findings exploded into public consciousness. Incest was found to be much more frequent than had been believed, and the results of childhood sexual and physical abuse were found to be longer lasting and more profound than previously thought. Several celebrated cases (e.g., the case of Sybil [Schreiber 1973]) became widely known, and interest as well as the index of suspicion grew accordingly.

Terrorism and mind-controlling individuals and cults also drew the attention of psychiatrists worldwide. Whether the survivors of hijacking, hostage taking, kidnapping, or escape from religious or political cults, patients emerging from traumatic scenarios represented certain characteristic findings that challenged the field of psychiatry.

Both acute trauma (Herman 1992; Krystal 1988; Terr 1990; van der Kolk 1987) and chronic trauma (Fish-Murray et al. 1987; Goodwin 1985; Herman 1992; Horowitz 1991; Kluft 1985; Krystal 1988; Niedlerland 1974; Putnam 1985, 1989, 1990; Shengold 1989; Spiegel 1990a, 1990b; Wilbur 1985) can cause psychopathology, and both can warp the formation of personality. Acute trauma is more likely to be limited to the traditional symptoms of posttraumatic stress disorder: flashbacks, numbing, and hypervigilance. Chronic trauma leads to an increase in dissociative defenses that place the memory of the full effect of the trauma at a distance. Somatization may be one result, with physical symptoms expressing the psychic pain of the trauma, as in the phenomenon known as *alexithymia*. The alexithymic person is unable to feel affect as emotions and instead feels it in the form of body sensations (Krystal 1988; Taylor 1987). Memory problems ranging from reduced concentration to amnesia can be another response.

Repetition of the trauma in the form of seeking relationships that replicate abuse patterns constitutes an all too common pattern. For example, one patient who had been sexually abused by both mother and father married an alcoholic man who beat her when he was intoxicated. After her divorce, the patient became intimate with another psychiatric patient whom she had met during a hospitalization. He doused her with lighter fluid and threatened to ignite her when she tried to leave. Later, she married another man who did not abuse her but who did molest the child they had together. Not until she was able to face the full effect of her own childhood was she successful in stopping this ongoing repetition.

Perhaps the most important finding in the rediscovery of trauma was the awareness of the profound effect and widespread nature of the defense of dissociation (see also Chapter 15 of this textbook by Maldonado and Spiegel). Dissociative responses can range from feelings of partial unreality in the form of depersonalization and derealization to profound identity disturbances such as dissociative identity disorder (formerly called multiple personality disorder) (Davis 1990; Edelson 1990; Erdleyi 1990; Kihlstrom and Hoyt 1990; Marmer 1980; Marmer and Fink 1991; Putnam 1985; Spiegel 1990a, 1990b; West 1967; Wilbur 1985). Although at times it appears that Sigmund Freud (1920/1955) thought of dissociation as a basic defense unto itself, we now usually think of dissociation as a defense mechanism combining denial, repression, and isolation to detach the person from unbearable awareness—both ideational and emotional—of trauma and of the person's reaction to it. The effects of growing up in a dissociated state are severe and profound and can interfere with all aspects of cognitive and psychological development. Any part of the experience may be dissociated, or dissociation itself can become an organizing principle. In the latter case, thoughts, affects, body feelings, perceptions, memory, or concentration can be disconnected, singly or in combination. How the individual develops will depend on which combinations of the dissociative process predominate.

The thread that all these responses have in common is the organization of the mind that keeps the traumatic memory and its emotion out of awareness. All people develop the structure of their mind under the influence of nature, nurture, and fate (Masterson 1981; Winnicott 1988). Likewise, all people develop their personalities and their psychopathology in response to conflict, deficiency, and trauma. Traditional psychoanalytic theory emphasizes the concept of conflict, with different mental forces battling against each other and fantasy struggling with reality. Self psychology emphasizes deficiency, not-

ing the effects on the formation of a coherent self when an insufficient supply of empathy is available during childhood. To these viewpoints is now being added an awareness of real trauma and the mind's reaction to it to form symptoms of somatization, alexithymia, flashbacks, numbing, hypervigilance, depersonalization, amnesia, dissociation, and repetition of trauma.

The pendulum of theory has a way of swinging too far in one direction, then too far in the other. Charcot and Janet focused on the innate vulnerability of some persons to real trauma. Freud called our attention to the complex way our fantasies can alter our perceptions and shape our personalities. Kohut and his followers made the question of lack of empathy their theory's fulcrum. Now a new wave of theorists in the tradition of Janet are again reminding us of the pivotal role of trauma. The student of psychiatric theory must remember that conflict and fantasy, deficiency and empathy, and trauma and dissociation are all present in everyone. The art is to see the correct proportion in each person.

The issue of repressed memory.   The renewed interest in trauma has brought about an increase in the reports of traumatic events. Some authors have wondered whether reports of previously repressed memories of trauma and abuse are iatrogenically engendered. For example, Loftus and Ketcham (1994) argued that false memories can be implanted in normal college students, who later recall these memories as if they had happened. They asserted that if false memories can be implanted, then patients' reports of childhood abuse that had previously been repressed might well be false also. This would occur in cases of excessive therapeutic zeal on the part of a therapist committed to the theory of trauma. On the other hand, Williams (1995) and her colleagues reported that repression of documented childhood abuse occurs approximately one-third of the time. She studied cases of childhood abuse seen in hospital emergency departments. Nineteen years later, the victims were interviewed. A third of them had nearly continuous memory of their abuse, a third had intermittently repressed the memories, and a third had no memory at all. At present, our theories of memory have not reconciled the Loftus and the Williams positions (but see Freyd 1996), nor has a complete theory of memory been integrated into our theories of the mind. Freud started out viewing repressed memories as causative for symptoms. Later, he believed that defenses against memories caused symptoms. Still later, he believed that many memories were actually fantasies and that conflicts over fantasies and wishes or drives were the cause of psychopathology. Simple theories that ignore the layered overdetermination of both trauma and fantasy risk missing the richness of each particular patient's presentation. Until we have a more complete theory of memory, the clinician is urged to avoid suggestive techniques when taking a trauma history but also to be open to trauma's real role in psychopathology.

Theories of Dynamic Psychiatry

In the following section, I discuss theorists of dynamic psychiatry whose interest included the total personality and character structure and the interplay of conscious and unconscious forces but who either left the psychoanalytic tradition or were never part of it (Table 3–8). The reader should be aware that the focus has been limited to a few representatives of each group. Many other important figures have not been mentioned. Within the psychoanalytic tradition, these figures include Alexander, Arlow, Bion, Brenner, Federn, Ferenczi, Hartmann, Kris, Loewenstein, Rapaport, Searles, Schafer, Spence, and Spitz. Kohut's and Melanie Klein's complex views have been highly condensed. In the psychodynamic tradition, the work of Allport, Bateson, Beck, Berne, Biswanger, Boss, Frankl, Fromm, Fromm-Reichman, Goldstein, Jackson, Jaspers, George Klein, Klerman, Lewin, Maslow, Masserman, Meyer, Murray, Perls, Rodgers, and others has been omitted.

Jung

Carl Jung was one of the most prolific writers in dynamic psychiatry, with his collected works in the English edition nearly as extensive as those of Freud. Jung is perhaps the only theorist in this group to have a large international following that still refers to its school of thought by a term using his name. Jungians have had only an indirect influence on psychoanalysis, on general psychiatry, and on psychology but have had a large influence in academic settings where psychoanalysis and depth psychology are taken seriously, as well as a substantial influence on psychotherapy in general and their own movement in particular.

Jung originally was a member of Sigmund Freud's circle and was designated by Freud to be his successor as the leader of international psychoanalysis. However, several years after their collaboration began, the two drifted apart permanently and irrevocably. Jung had had a wide background in philosophy, religion, and anthropology, as well as considerable psychiatric experience working with psychotic patients before and after his contact with Freud. The first significant difference between Freud (1925[1924]/1959) and Jung (1961) came on the ques-

tion of libido and psychic energy. Freud had contended that libido was sexual, whereas Jung considered the libido to be the unitary force of psychic energy, not explicitly sexual, nor even limited to being sensual, but something closer to the *elan vital* of Henri Bergson. Both Freud and Jung believed in some kind of principle of constancy, which for Jung took the form of the principles of equivalence and entropy, indicating that psychic energy seeks an equilibrium and that if it is increased in one area, it is depleted in another.

Freud and Jung also disagreed about the nature of the unconscious. For Freud, the content of the unconscious was the product of the individual's personal history. Although the unconscious contained innate drives, its specific content consisted of the introjects, identifications, fantasies, memories, affects, and associations accumulated over a life span. For Jung (1966b), the unconscious mind consisted of a collective unconscious, which was the storehouse of latent memories of our cultural past, our racial memory, the entire history of Homo sapiens, and even prehuman memory. It was shared by all human beings as the psychic residue of evolution. Although Jung did not say that specific racial memories were inherited, the potential to revive them by means of symbols was always present. In contrast to Freud, Jung conceptualized the personal unconscious as constituting only a small portion of the total unconscious. In Jung's view, the ego was similar to the conscious mind.

The structure of the unconscious consisted of component archetypes. Jung (1964) conceptualized them as innate ideas (or preformatting) that ready us for real experiences. For instance, there is an innate idea of the mother that readies us for our real-life experience with our mother. There are innate ideas of father, of hero, of leader, and so forth. These archetypes originate in the mind as a permanent deposit accreted over the generations as the categories into which human symbolic thought is preordained to be experienced. Archetypes are also semiautonomous dynamic systems that can act with partial independence.

Five archetypes stand out and define personality organization (Table 3–9). The *persona* is the outward mask by which the person balances the demands of society with other internal needs. An individual may have both a public and a private persona. *Anima* and *animus* are the feminine and masculine prototypes within each of us. On this issue, Jung agreed with Freud about the innate bisexuality of humans but elaborated it differently. Our understanding of men and women is the effect of the anima or animus in each of us that corresponds to the opposite sex. The *shadow* is the representation of animal instincts that human beings have as their legacy of evolution from

TABLE 3–8. Major dynamic theorists who left the psychoanalytic tradition

	Theoretical contribution	Technique
Jung	Collective unconscious is the theory that we have a common species-wide set of ideas, symbols, and images shared by all. Archetypes are the permanent and innate structures in the collective unconscious that are the categories into which all human symbolic thought is preordained to be experienced. Complexes are clusters of archetypes and defenses.	Jungian technique emphasizes the decoding of archetypical elements in dreams. His technique includes more therapist self-disclosure than does psychoanalysis. The mystical, spiritual, symbolic, and cultural are embraced more than in any other school.
Adler	Aggression and inferiority are key elements in development. All children are said to feel inferior in the presence of adults, setting them on a lifetime quest for mastery over this basic early feeling of inferiority. The balance between their personal striving and getting along with others in a social context is known as *style of life*. Birth order is particularly significant in psychopathology and development.	Less emphasis on the unconscious; more emphasis on encouragement and instruction from the therapist to help the patients balance their style of life.
Rank	The "trauma of birth" is the prototype of all subsequent traumas and for all anxieties about separation. To become separate and to individuate, one must assert his or her will, but doing so creates guilt for what one might have done to others. In addition, individuation reactivates the primal separation anxiety associated with the birth trauma. Finding individuation and will without engendering excessive guilt or separation anxiety is the central dilemma of development and psychopathology.	Shorter, time-limited treatment is emphasized. The content of the sessions is more reality focused and less concerned with unconscious fantasy life.
Horney	Psychopathology is thought to originate in distorted parent–child relationships that are inappropriately repeated throughout life. Three main neurotic strategies are pathological ways of moving toward, away from, or against others. Aggression is held not to be innate but rather a self-protective response to threat or frustration. In the psychology of women, the concept of "penis envy" is rejected.	Flexibility of technique is encouraged. Therapeutic alliance is stressed equally with the transference. Nonspecific factors such as the consistency and reliability of the therapist are thought to be on the same level of importance as interpretations.
Sullivan	Founder of the "interpersonal school" of psychotherapy. The personality in isolation is considered a mere hypothetical concept. All real people live in an interpersonal world. Anxiety arises out of threats to interpersonal security. This creates internal sense of good and bad self. Makes the main human motivation the achievement of a sense of security. Foreshadowing Erikson, Sullivan holds that development takes place throughout the life cycle, from infancy through adulthood.	Flexible technique. Little emphasis on deeper unconscious fantasy. More emphasis on how we feel in the presence of and in relation to others.

lower animals. The shadow concept gives us passion, vitality, and zest as well as our concept of evil, devil, or enemy. The *self* holds everything together and attempts to produce unity, equilibrium, and stability by balancing various archetypes and complexes.

The mind has four functions or operations: thinking, feeling, sensing, and intuiting (Table 3–10). These functions may be directed primarily to the inner world of subjective reality (i.e., introversion) or to the external world of objective reality (i.e., extroversion). *Thinking* is verbal and ideational and consists of logic and reasoning. *Feeling* permits pleasure and pain, anger and joy, and love and loss. It is also the faculty with which we make judgments about good and bad. Through *sensation* we acquire facts. *Intuition* is perception by means of unconscious processes, involving the essence of reality that lies beyond thoughts, perceptions, and feelings. In each individual, these four component functions may be ranked in order of superiority to inferiority according to the strength with which they are developed. Defense mechanisms are limited to repression and sublimation, which leads to the next concept.

TABLE 3–9. Jung's major archetypes

Persona	The face the individual presents to the world. A person may have one persona for the general public and another for intimates.
Anima and Animus	The feminine and masculine aspects of an individual. Both are present in everyone but in varying proportion and balance.
Shadow	The darker animal aspects of the individual. Shadow is responsible both for passion and for evil.
Self	The executive function that holds identity together and attempts to keep other forces in a balanced equilibrium.

TABLE 3–10. Jung's four mental functions

Thinking	Logical reasoning expressed verbally.
Feeling	Affects such as pain, pleasure, love, hate, loss. Also includes the faculty of judgment of good and bad.
Sensation	Our sensory mental apparatus by which we gain information about the world.
Intuition	The process of deriving connections through unconscious mental function.

Note. According to Jung, the balance among these four mental functions is critical in character formation.

Each faculty within the individual and each aspect are either in unity or in opposition, or each acts in compensation for weaknesses in another realm. Thus, the purpose of treatment is to restore balance and promote unity by understanding the component parts. In treatment, therefore, the focus is on understanding the various symbols, all of which are presumed to be present but out of balance in pathology.

In contrast to Freud's psychic determinism is Jung's own view of why events occur. *Causality* explains a present event in terms of the past, and *teleology* explains the present in terms of future potential. Synchronicity is a higher order of causation on the edge between the psychical and the physical worlds and thus blends science with mysticism.

The theory of archetypes and the collective unconscious contrasts with psychoanalytic theories in the interpretation of dreams. In keeping with the ontogenetic point of view emphasizing personal history, Freud held that the dream is the unique idiosyncratic product of the dreamer and reflects an amalgam of current life situations, recent events, and infantile wishes from important periods of childhood. From the phylogenetic perspective,

Jung contended that the dream reveals imbalances in the unity of the self and is understood by identifying the archetypal meaning of the symbols in question.

Critics point to the mystical and stereotyping aspects of Jung's theories and to some of his controversial statements and actions (see Carotenuto 1982; Jung 1934/1966a). Adherents to Jung's theory see it as a comprehensive attempt to understand the individual's use of the universal characteristics of human beings. This theory also has been responsible for technical innovations and modifications practiced within Jungian therapy.

Adler

Alfred Adler was another early member of Freud's circle who also differed with him on the subject of instinctual drives (S. Freud 1925[1924]/1959). He emphasized the importance of aggression and recognition, presaging some of Kohut's work on the self. Adler (1956) concluded that aggression was an innate drive; one not used for the purpose of destruction, but rather with the emphasis on seeking power and recognition. Adler came to this position based on his studies of inferiority, which started out as a narrow concept of organ inferiority and was broadened to include the inevitable feeling of inferiority that every child has when faced with adults who have dominance or adults on whom the children depend. This situation stimulates a perpetual desire to overcome the feelings of inferiority and dependency.

Adler also emphasized that aggression and inferiority were not solely an intrapsychic issue. He believed that every human is born into a family and that every child has a relationship with a mother; therefore, no human development could occur outside of a social context. Thus, for Adler, side by side with the striving for superiority and the innate assertiveness of aggression was also an innate drive for social cooperation and what he called social interest, which balances the personal and selfish interests.

Adler coined the term *style of life*, by which he meant pathways that each individual uses to balance social interest and personal striving. Style of life then is determined partly by the particular inferiorities that a child faced historically as well as the creative self, which also is an innate principle of human life helping the person transcend his or her physical and environmental beginnings.

Adler was particularly interested in the effects of birth order on personality and believed that the oldest, the middle, and the youngest children in a family were likely to be distinctive and predictable. Oldest children are given enormous attention and are suddenly dethroned when the second child is born. Second children are constantly striving to surpass older siblings. Youngest children tend to be spoiled. He also believed that earliest memories were capsulized versions of one's basic orientation in life.

In technique, Adler differed considerably from therapists in the psychoanalytic tradition. For Adler, the goal of treatment was the remaking of the patient's lifestyle, particularly balancing the sense of inferiority, the need to compensate for it, and the social feeling of cooperation. Great emphasis was placed on the therapeutic alliance, which in many respects was regarded as the most important aspect of the treatment. The therapist and the patient together then learned about the patient's history, mostly through reconstruction rather than through the transference. Adler relied a great deal on encouragement and on the nonspecific effects of the therapeutic alliance to reeducate the patient in a proper therapeutic environment, one in which he or she would feel totally accepted and that was thought would lead to a healthier style of life. Such a setting required an optimistic attitude, a belief in the possibility of change, encouragement to be responsible for one's actions, and a high degree of empathy and rapport between therapist and patient.

Rank

Otto Rank was yet another early follower of Freud who stayed within the psychoanalytic tradition for many years but eventually broke with Freud (Ferenczi and Rank 1956). Rank (1973) supplanted the centrality of the Oedipus complex in the formation of neurosis with the centrality of the birth trauma, which in his theory was the basic and original anxiety through which all subsequent anxieties were interpreted. Freud did not deny that there was birth anxiety, but he did not make it central to his theory. For Rank, the trauma of birth then became the paradigm for all separations, and separation anxiety became heir to primal birth anxiety. Infantile sexuality was subordinated to the birth trauma as well. Masochism was seen as the transmuting of the pain of birth into pleasure, and sadism was seen as the expression of anger and retribution by one who has been traumatized by expulsion from the womb.

Individuation became a central principle for Rank. The individual has to define himself or herself and does so by saying no and asserting his or her will. However, the assertion of will results in guilt over the harm done to the person who formerly met the individual's dependency needs. Also, having remembered the trauma of birth, the individual has the fear that he or she will be expelled from the family if his or her individuality is too assertively revealed.

Development proceeds through three stages of individuation. During the first stage, the individual follows biological needs and the values of parents and society. In the second phase, there is a conflict of wills, and the individual seeks to construct his or her own standards. The third stage heralds an autonomous ego capable of creativity.

Rank believed that treatment could proceed more quickly than in traditional psychoanalysis, and in his treatment he emphasized the therapeutic relationship, especially the emotional dynamics revealed within the therapy and the development of new forms of behavior in the therapeutic setting. Rank also emphasized the value of setting time limits for treatment. Treatment goals are to help the patient overcome the birth trauma and all subsequent separations and be able to assert will without fear or guilt. It is recognized that every separation creates great anxiety and that acquisitions of autonomy create the fear of separation. Therefore, the therapist must accept negative reactions from the patient and gently encourage the acquisition of autonomy.

Because of the emphasis on the assertion of will in expressing autonomy, Rank believed that reality had to be introduced relatively early in treatment, and his theory emphasized realistic reexamination of the true life situation—past, present, and future. He also stressed realistic limitations on what the therapeutic situation could provide. Thus, the therapist and the patient learn through practice that it is safe to assert one's will and to be autonomous.

Rank's views addressed legitimate unsolved problems that the psychoanalytic tradition eventually addressed. The importance of separation and individuation and of separation anxiety was acknowledged by Mahler's theories. The role of the therapeutic alliance has been well documented by Greenson (1967) and others. The value of setting limitations for therapy is sometimes accepted in psychoanalytic psychotherapy but not in psychoanalysis (but see also S. Freud 1937/1964). Rank's work is an often unacknowledged source of relevant ideas for psychotherapy.

Horney

Karen Horney was trained in orthodox psychoanalysis and was a teacher at the traditional New York Psychoanalytic Institute. However, she broke with orthodox psychoanalysis, partly for reasons of organization and internal politics but largely for philosophical differences that she had with some of Freud's theories. In particular, she believed that classical psychoanalysis was too mechanistic, too biologically based, and insufficiently humanistic.

Horney (1937, 1950) also had specific differences with Freud regarding the psychology of women. She believed that the concept of penis envy, with its view that the psychology of women depended on their feelings of genital inferiority and jealousy of men, was ill-founded. Horney instead contended that feminine psychology overemphasized the love relationship and that it was not based on anatomy. She also believed that aggression was not innate but was a self-protective mechanism that was stimulated by threats to one's security and added to by experiences of frustration.

Although she left the psychoanalytic tradition and modified psychoanalytic technique, Horney focused on unconscious forces and on the way in which unconscious factors create character structure. According to Horney (1950), neurosis originates in distorted parent–child relationships that are subsequently self-perpetuated throughout life. Neuroses are characterized by the repeated reaction in new situations to the same distortions or reactions that emanated from the original parent–child relationship. These neurotic strategies may involve pathological ways of moving toward people, of moving away from people, and of moving against people. Horney herself presented 10 neurotic needs that were manifestations of these three main ways of living. These were neurotic needs for 1) affection and approval, 2) a partner who will take over one's life, 3) restriction of one's own life, 4) power, 5) exploitation, 6) prestige, 7) admiration, 8) achievement, 9) self-sufficiency, and 10) perfection and unassailability. Three major character defenses act to reduce anxiety and resolve these neurotic needs: self-effacement, expansiveness, and resignation.

Horney's technique of treatment used modified psychoanalysis and psychoanalytic psychotherapy. She encouraged the patient to choose the couch or the face-to-face arrangement and analyzed the choice. Sessions could occur once a week or every day. Free association was important but not central. Transference was still appreciated but stood on equal footing with the therapeutic alliance. Countertransference was regarded as an especially important clue and not simply a sign of an unanalyzed portion of the therapist's personality. Nonspecific factors in the therapeutic alliance, such as the analyst's mere presence, consistency, optimism, acceptance, lack of judgment, and sticking to the task, became therapeutic agents.

Horney's work brought psychoanalytic principles into psychotherapy settings and anticipated some of the modern work on narcissism, narcissistic defenses, and the transference/countertransference valences evoked when working with such defenses.

Sullivan

Harry Stack Sullivan is an important figure, in part because he was the first altogether homegrown major theorist to start an American school of psychodynamic psychotherapy. For him, personality was a hypothetical construct; what was real and actual were relationships. Everything therefore had to be interpreted through the lens of interpersonal relationships (Sullivan 1953). For Sullivan, anxiety is a product of interpersonal threats to security, and repeated interpersonal experiences between child and parent result in the formation of a good "me self" and a bad "me self."

Personifications, the internal representations of the self or other, include affects and grow out of need-satisfying relationships and anxiety in the pursuit of need-satisfying relationships.

In Sullivan's (1953) view, the mind worked on the basis of three different cognitive processes. The earliest was called the *protaxic process*, which was that of raw perception. The *parataxic process* was the next to evolve, and it followed *post hoc ergo propter hoc* logic (i.e., things following each other in time are assumed to be causally related). This was the root of animistic superstitious thinking. The third form, *syntaxic thinking*, consensually validated reality with a symbolic content following something similar to the verbal logic of Freud's secondary process.

Motivations result from tension that arises both out of physiological need and out of anxiety related to maintenance of security. This sense of security was an important feature of Sullivan's work.

Sullivan had his own theory of development. During *infancy*, there is a period of apathy and detachment as well as connection. Good and bad personifications arise, the self-representation is formed, and thinking moves from a protaxic to a parataxic level. In the second phase, called *childhood*, language develops, playmates join parents as important interpersonal figures, gender takes shape, and the inner world is one of dramatizations and preoccupations, which are rehearsals for adulthood. The third phase, the *juvenile stage*, coincides with grammar school and is the period in which the child learns to expand the interpersonal world to group reactions and an orientation to living in society. The fourth phase is *preadolescence*. This very important phase introduces the special same-sex peer or "chum" form of interpersonal relating that becomes the first genuine human relationship not governed by excessive dependency. The fifth phase is that of *early adolescence*, in which heterosexuality and interpersonal gender questions are worked out. The sixth area of development is *late adolescence*, during which time adult responsibility is introduced. Finally, the organism emerges into *adulthood* and continues the cycle by reworking these themes in new interpersonal situations.

Sullivan's emphasis on interpersonal factors balanced the primary intrapsychic focus of Freud by underscoring that an infant cannot exist conceptually or in reality in the absence of the mother. One might say that Winnicott took some of the best points of Sullivan and elaborated them within the psychoanalytic tradition. On the other hand, the interpersonal focus may be criticized for neglecting the depth of fantasy that can take place on an intrapsychic level. Nevertheless, some followers of Sullivan, such as Searles, have become part of the psychoanalytic tradition.

Behavioral and Cognitive Theories[2]

The next set of theories, those involving behavioral and cognitive principles, have evolved out of an entirely different tradition and are based on different notions of how the mind works and even what constitutes the mind. The learning theory that underlies these points of view arises from the laboratory setting of experimental psychology, generating applications for the clinical situation. This approach is in contrast to those of psychoanalysis and dynamic psychiatry, both of which arose in the treatment setting and rely on that same setting for confirmation. Although some philosophers of science (e.g., Grunbaum 1984) take psychoanalysis seriously enough to challenge it to seek independent settings for confirmation of its theories, learning theory has always based its idea of the mind on observation of performance and behavior.

Learning is itself an inference based on the observation of changes in the behavior of an organism. Learning may be inferred from permanent or quasi-permanent changes in behavior that occur under specific circumstances. An organism is influenced by the effect of its behaviors, and its responses reflect that learning. If the organism repeats a certain behavior to attain a particular state, or if the organism stops that behavior to avoid a particular state, then learning may be said to have taken place. This is known within learning theory as *Thorndike's law of effect*.

States associated with behaviors can become reinforcers. A *positive reinforcer* is the occurrence of an event that increases the probability that the antecedent behavior will be repeated. A *negative reinforcer* is the occurrence of an event that decreases the probability that the antecedent behavior will be repeated. *Punishment* is a special type of negative reinforcement that is intended to stop a specific behavior. Those behaviors that need periodic positive reinforcement to be maintained may slowly disappear by means of the phenomenon of *extinction* if the positive reinforcer is removed (see Skinner 1938, 1953). Extinction essentially means that most conditioned responses will eventually fade away if they are not periodically reinforced.

Although some theorists believe that *classical conditioning* is a special case of *operant conditioning*, these two forms are traditionally regarded as separate. In classical conditioning, a stimulus not intrinsically or ordinarily associated with a response may be used to induce that response. The organism "learns" to take the once-neutral stimulus and respond according to the conditioning. Pavlov's famous experiment illustrates this type of conditioning. A dog will salivate when presented with food because of an *unconditioned* physiological reflex response. If a bell, which has no intrinsic power to induce salivation, is rung before the food is presented, the dog will "learn" to salivate when it hears the bell.

Operant conditioning (or instrumental conditioning) occurs as the organism learns that behaviors are associated with positive or negative events. Behaviors in operant conditioning are initiated by the organism, and associated events are less directly linked to immediate physiological reflexes than in classical conditioning.

Behaviors may be "shaped" by introducing reinforcers for successive approximations of the desired behavior. Behaviors may be initiated by the presence of other incompatible states. For example, because anxiety and relaxation cannot occur simultaneously, behavior therapists link relaxation with stimuli that formerly produced anxiety. This method of reciprocal inhibition is used to desensitize phobic patients or persons with posttraumatic states. Behaviors also may be linked in complex chains by adding steps that the organism must perform to reach desired reinforcers. A clinical example might be the treatment of a person afraid of tall buildings. Under a psychoanalytic theory, the symbolic meaning of fear of heights might be explored; it might mean fear of success,

---

[2]The behavioral and cognitive therapists are being reviewed as a group, with some of the important figures being examined but a considerable amount of detail being omitted, including the subtler differences among learning theorists such as Pavlov, Hull, Mowrer, and Tolman, as well as the clinical innovations and contributions of Bandura, Dollard and Miller, and Wolpe, to name but a few.

fear of besting one's father, or some such thing. In a behavioral view of the mind, the underlying symbolic reasons are either thought not to exist or are not relevant to the treatment plan. In systematic desensitization, the patient might first be taught how to relax and then to apply relaxation techniques to pictures of tall buildings. When this is mastered, he or she might be brought to the site of such a building to practice his or her relaxation. Then he or she might go to the second floor and do his or her relaxation exercises. Gradually, he or she might make it up to the highest balcony.

When responding to stimuli during conditioning, the organism is capable of responding to other stimuli that resemble the original one. Stimulus generalization would explain how the dog that responded to a bell might respond similarly to a gong or a chime. Stimulus generalization also may be seen as the explanation learning theory gives to the psychoanalytic phenomenon of the transference. The transference would be an example of stimulus generalization gone amok, with an ordinarily innocuous stimulus from the analyst being erroneously generalized to a traumatic stimulus from the parent during childhood. The response then is the one that was originally "learned" in childhood and then inappropriately enacted in the present situation. For example, under psychoanalytic theory, a patient's overreaction to a doctor's 2-minute lateness might be a transferential re-creation of panic at the chronic lateness of his or her mother during critical phases in childhood. Under learning theory, the same reaction might be seen as a case of stimuli from one circumstance (mother late during childhood) erroneously generalized to another circumstance (doctor 2 minutes late for appointment). From the perspective of learning theory, much psychopathology may be understood as based on errors in *stimulus discrimination* and *stimulus generalization*.

Drives are seen as propelling the organism to reduce its need by finding appropriate responses to stimuli. *Habits* are complex clusters of stimuli and responses. In behavior therapy, psychopathology is seen as persistent habits of learned unadaptive behavior acquired in anxiety-generating situations (Wolpe 1958). The need to respond to the anxiety and to avoid its negative effect maintains psychopathological behaviors.

Thus far, stimuli and responses, and behaviors and reinforcers, have been presented by a theory in which they are linked by contiguity or association. What an organism reacts to is association, not causality. Some learning theorists (e.g., Tolman, Bandura 1974, Dollard and Miller) believe that learning is more than reaction to association by contiguity. They believe that organisms form *cognitive maps* of their environmental situations

through internal representations in the form of thoughts, signs, and symbols. Others (e.g., Skinner and Wolpe) feel that thoughts, perceptions, and even imagination are no different from the musculoskeletal responses and obey the same laws of stimulus, response, reinforcement, and conditioning.

For the first group, learning theory represents another level on which to explain the mind, much as physics may explain chemistry or chemistry may explain biology. For the second group, the psychoanalytic and dynamic theories of this chapter represent unacceptable *mentalism*, or the inference about the existence of the mind in the absence of hard data. Members of the first group assume that there is a mind that organizes learned data. Members of the second group hold that it is not necessary to infer anything beyond complex chains of stimulus and response.

Behavioral and cognitive theorists focus their therapeutic strategies on the pathological behaviors themselves and use a variety of techniques to help the patient unlearn maladaptive behaviors and to inhibit unwanted states such as anxiety. They introduce new learning through techniques such as shaping and modeling, creating—through careful application of positive reinforcement, negative reinforcement, and extinction—new chains of habit and adaptive behavior.

Conclusion

In this chapter, I reviewed theories of the mind and psychopathology from the major psychotherapeutic schools. For most of these perspectives, Freud and psychoanalysis constitute a kind of "basic science" from which the schools make their modifications and their "applied science." Even when large differences exist in theory and practice, most psychotherapeutic schools grew out of or in reaction to that psychoanalytic beginning.

The behavioral and cognitive theories offer one pole that conceptualizes the mind as consisting of large chains of learned responses and another pole that looks for internal cognitive maps. This latter pole is closer to psychoanalysis. It may even be possible to translate the data of the psychoanalytic and psychodynamic schools into learning theory language.

A large group of creative thinkers who were never a part of the psychoanalytic tradition, or else who left it, constitute a psychodynamic tradition of their own. These theories, which range from the more modest to the more ambitious, constitute the major theoretical foundation of eclectic psychotherapy.

The psychoanalytic tradition, although heavily

indebted to Freud, is far from static. Major shifts have taken place over the decades, with emphasis on ego psychology, object relations, development, and the self. Reading about these theories can provide a theoretical basis for understanding patients. Studying these theories can provide a lifetime of deepening understanding of the mechanism of psychotherapy and the workings of the mind in normality and psychopathology.

References

Abraham K: Selected Papers on Psychoanalysis. Translated by Bryan D, Strachey A. New York, Basic Books, 1968

Adler A: The Individual Psychology of Alfred Adler: A Systematic Presentation in Selections From His Writings. Edited by Ansbacher HL, Ansbacher RR. New York, Basic Books, 1956

American Psychiatric Association: Diagnostic and Statistical Manual of Mental Disorders, 3rd Edition. Washington, DC, American Psychiatric Association Press, 1980

Balint M: The Basic Fault. London, England, Tavistock, 1968

Bandura A: Behavior theory and the models of man. Am Psychol 29:859–869, 1974

Bibring GL, Dwyer TF, Huntington DS, et al: A study of the psychological processes in pregnancy and of the earliest mother-child relationship. Psychoanal Study Child 16:9–72, 1961

Bowlby J: The nature of the child's tie to his mother. Int J Psychoanal 39:350–373, 1958

Brenner C: An Elementary Textbook of Psychoanalysis. New York, International Universities Press, 1955

Breuer J, Freud S: Studies on hysteria (1893–1895), in Standard Edition of the Complete Psychological Works of Sigmund Freud, Vol 2. Translated and edited by Strachey J. London, England, Hogarth, 1955, pp 1–319

Briquet P: Traite de l'Hysterie. Paris, France, J Bailliere, 1859

Carotenuto A: A Secret Symmetry. New York, Pantheon, 1982

Davis PJ: Repression and the inaccessibility of emotional memories, in Repression and Dissociation: Implications for Personality Theory, Psychopathology, and Health. Edited by Singer JL. Chicago, IL, University of Chicago Press, 1990, pp 387–403

Edelson M: Defense in psychoanalytic theory: computation or fantasy? in Repression and Dissociation: Implications for Personality Theory, Psychopathology, and Health. Edited by Singer JL. Chicago, IL, University of Chicago Press, 1990, pp 33–60

Ellenberger H: The Discovery of the Unconscious: The History and Evolution of Dynamic Psychiatry. New York, Basic Books, 1970

Erdleyi MH: Repression, reconstruction, and defense: history and integration of the psychoanalytic and experimental frameworks, in Repression and Dissociation: Implications for Personality Theory, Psychopathology, and Health. Edited by Singer JL. Chicago, IL, University of Chicago Press, 1990, pp 1–31

Erikson E: Childhood and Society, 2nd Edition, Revised and Enlarged. New York, WW Norton, 1963

Fairbairn WRD: Psychoanalytic Studies of the Personality. London, England, Routledge and Kegan Paul, 1972

Fenichel O: The Psychoanlaytic Theory of Neurosis. New York, WW Norton, 1945

Ferenczi S, Rank O: The Development of Psycho-Analysis. New York, Dover, 1956

Fine S, Fine E: Four psychoanalytic perspectives: a study of differences in interpretive interventions. J Am Psychoanal Assoc 38:1017–1048, 1990

Fish-Murray CC, Koby EV, van der Kolk BA: Evolving ideas: the effect of abuse on children's thought, in Psychological Trauma. Edited by van der Kolk BA. Washington, DC, American Psychiatric Press, 1987, pp 89–110

Fleck L: Genesis and Development of a Scientific Fact. Chicago, IL, University of Chicago Press, 1979

Freud A: The Ego and the Mechanisms of Defence (1936). Translated by Baines C. New York, International Universities Press, 1946

Freud S: On Aphasia (1891). Translated by Stengel E. New York, International Universities Press, 1953

Freud S: The neuro-psychoses of defence (1894), in Standard Edition of the Complete Psychological Works of Sigmund Freud, Vol 3. Translated and edited by Strachey J. London, England, Hogarth, 1962, pp 41–68

Freud S: Further remarks on the neuro-psychoses of defence (1896), in Standard Edition of the Complete Psychological Works of Sigmund Freud, Vol 3. Translated and edited by Strachey J. London, England, Hogarth, 1962, pp 157–185

Freud S: The interpretation of dreams (1900), in Standard Edition of the Complete Psychological Works of Sigmund Freud, Vol 4. Translated and edited by Strachey J. London, England, Hogarth, 1953

Freud S: The psychopathology of everyday life (1901), in Standard Edition of the Complete Psychological Works of Sigmund Freud, Vol 6. Translated and edited by Strachey J. London, England, Hogarth, 1960

Freud S: Fragment of an analysis of a case of hysteria (1905[1901]), in Standard Edition of the Complete Psychological Works of Sigmund Freud, Vol 7. Translated and edited by Strachey J. London, England, Hogarth, 1953, pp 1–122

Freud S: Three essays on the theory of sexuality, I: the sexual aberrations (1905), in Standard Edition of the Complete Psychological Works of Sigmund Freud, Vol 7. Translated and edited by Strachey J. London, England, Hogarth, 1953, pp 135–172

Freud S: The sexual enlightenment of children (1907), in Standard Edition of the Complete Psychological Works of Sigmund Freud, Vol 9. Translated and edited by Strachey J. London, England, Hogarth, 1959, pp 129–139

Freud S: On the sexual theories of children (1908), in Standard Edition of the Complete Psychological Works of Sigmund Freud, Vol 9. Translated and edited by Strachey J. London, England, Hogarth, 1959, pp 5–226

Freud S: Analysis of a phobia in a five-year-old boy (1909a), in Standard Edition of the Complete Psychological Works of Sigmund Freud, Vol 10. Translated and edited by Strachey J. London, England, Hogarth, 1955, pp 1–149

Freud S: Notes upon a case of obsessional neurosis (1909b), in Standard Edition of the Complete Psychological Works of Sigmund Freud, Vol 10. Translated and edited by Strachey J. London, England, Hogarth, 1955, pp 151–318

Freud S: Psycho-analytic notes on an autobiographical account of a case of paranoia (dementia paranoides) (1911), in Standard Edition of the Complete Psychological Works of Sigmund Freud, Vol 12. Translated and edited by Strachey J. London, England, Hogarth, 1958, pp 1–82

Freud S: Recommendations to physicians practising psycho-analysis (1912), in Standard Edition of the Complete Psychological Works of Sigmund Freud, Vol 12. Translated and edited by Strachey J. London, England, Hogarth, 1958, pp 109–120

Freud S: On beginning the treatment (further recommendations on the technique of psycho-analysis I) (1913), in Standard Edition of the Complete Psychological Works of Sigmund Freud, Vol 12. Translated and edited by Strachey J. London, England, Hogarth, 1958, pp 121–144

Freud S: On narcissism: an introduction (1914a), in Standard Edition of the Complete Psychological Works of Sigmund Freud, Vol 14. Translated and edited by Strachey J. London, England, Hogarth, 1957, pp 67–102

Freud S: Remembering, repeating and working-through (further recommendations on the technique of psycho-analysis II) (1914b), in Standard Edition of the Complete Psychological Works of Sigmund Freud, Vol 12. Translated and edited by Strachey J. London, England, Hogarth, 1958, pp 145–156

Freud S: Instincts and their vicissitudes (1915a), in Standard Edition of the Complete Psychological Works of Sigmund Freud, Vol 14. Translated and edited by Strachey J. London, England, Hogarth, 1957, pp 109–140

Freud S: Repression (1915b), in Standard Edition of the Complete Psychological Works of Sigmund Freud, Vol 14. Translated and edited by Strachey J. London, England, Hogarth, 1957, pp 141–158

Freud S: The unconscious (1915c), in Standard Edition of the Complete Psychological Works of Sigmund Freud, Vol 14. Translated and edited by Strachey J. London, England, Hogarth, 1957, pp 159–215

Freud S: Mourning and melancholia (1917[1915]), in Standard Edition of the Complete Psychological Works of Sigmund Freud, Vol 14. Translated and edited by Strachey J. London, England, Hogarth, 1957, pp 237–260

Freud S: Beyond the pleasure principle (1920), in Standard Edition of the Complete Psychological Works of Sigmund Freud, Vol 18. Translated and edited by Strachey J. London, England, Hogarth, 1955, pp 1–64

Freud S: Group psychology and the analysis of the ego (1921), in Standard Edition of the Complete Psychological Works of Sigmund Freud, Vol 18. Translated and edited by Strachey J. London, England, Hogarth, 1955, pp 65–143

Freud S: Some neurotic mechanisms in jealousy, paranoia and homosexuality (1922), in Standard Edition of the Complete Psychological Works of Sigmund Freud, Vol 18. Translated and edited by Strachey J. London, England, Hogarth, 1955, pp 221–232

Freud S: Neurosis and psychosis (1924[1923]), in Standard Edition of the Complete Psychological Works of Sigmund Freud, Vol 19. Translated and edited by Strachey J. London, England, Hogarth, 1961, pp 147–153

Freud S: The economic problem of masochism (1924a), in Standard Edition of the Complete Psychological Works of Sigmund Freud, Vol 19. Translated and edited by Strachey J. London, England, Hogarth, 1961, pp 155–170

Freud S: The loss of reality in neurosis and psychosis (1924b), in Standard Edition of the Complete Psychological Works of Sigmund Freud, Vol 19. Translated and edited by Strachey J. London, England, Hogarth, 1961, pp 181–187

Freud S: Some psychical consequences of the anatomical distinction between the sexes (1925), in Standard Edition of the Complete Psychological Works of Sigmund Freud, Vol 19. Translated and edited by Strachey J. London, England, Hogarth, 1961, pp 241–258

Freud S: An autobiographical study (1925[1924]), in Standard Edition of the Complete Psychological Works of Sigmund Freud, Vol 20. Translated and edited by Strachey J. London, England, Hogarth, 1959, pp 1–74

Freud S: Inhibitions, symptoms and anxiety (1926), in Standard Edition of the Complete Psychological Works of Sigmund Freud, Vol 20. Translated and edited by Strachey J. London, England, Hogarth, 1959, pp 75–175

Freud S: New introductory lectures on psycho-analysis (1933[1932]) (Lectures XXIX–XXXV), in Standard Edition of the Complete Psychological Works of Sigmund Freud, Vol 22. Translated and edited by Strachey J. London, England, Hogarth, 1964, pp 1–182

Freud S: Analysis terminable and interminable (1937), in Standard Edition of the Complete Psychological Works of Sigmund Freud, Vol 23. Translated and edited by Strachey J. London, England, Hogarth, 1964, pp 209–253

Freud S: An outline of psycho-analysis (1940a[1938]), in Standard Edition of the Complete Psychological Works of Sigmund Freud, Vol 23. Translated and edited by Strachey J. London, England, Hogarth, 1964, pp 139–207

Freud S: Splitting of the ego in the process of defence (1940b[1938]), in Standard Edition of the Complete Psychological Works of Sigmund Freud, Vol 23. Translated and edited by Strachey J. London, England, Hogarth, 1964, pp 271–278

Freud S: Project for a scientific psychology (1950[1895]), in Standard Edition of the Complete Psychological Works of Sigmund Freud, Vol 1. Translated and edited by Strachey J. London, England, Hogarth, 1966, pp 281–397

Freyd JJ: Betrayal Trauma: The Logic of Forgetting Childhood Abuse. Cambridge, MA, Harvard University Press, 1996

Ghaemi SN, Oepen G: Mind-brain theories in psychiatry. Integrative Psychiatry 10:52–57, 1994

Gill MM: The analysis of the transference. J Am Psychoanal Assoc 27(suppl):263–288, 1979

Goodman A: Organic unity theory: an integrative mind-body theory for psychiatry. Theoretical Medicine 18:357–378, 1997

Goodwin J: Post-traumatic symptoms in incest victims, in Post-traumatic Stress Disorder in Children. Edited by Eth S, Pynoos RS. Washington, DC, American Psychiatric Press, 1985, pp 155–168

Greenberg JR, Mitchell SA: Object Relations in Psychoanalytic Theory. Cambridge, MA, Harvard University Press, 1983

Greenson RR: The Technique and Practice of Psychoanalysis, Vol 1. New York, International Universities Press, 1967

Grunbaum A: The Foundations of Psychoanalysis. Berkeley, CA, University of California Press, 1984

Gunderson JG: Borderline Personality Disorder. Washington, DC, American Psychiatric Press, 1984

Gunderson JG, Kolb J: Discriminating features of borderline patients. Am J Psychiatry 135:792–796, 1976

Gunderson JG, Carpenter WT, Strauss JS: Borderline and schizophrenic patients: a comparative study. Am J Psychiatry 132:1257–1264, 1975

Guntrip H: Personality Structure and Human Interaction. New York, International Universities Press, 1974

Herman JL: Trauma and Recovery. New York, Basic Books, 1992

Horney K: The Neurotic Personality of Our Time. New York, WW Norton, 1937

Horney K: Neurosis and Human Growth: The Struggle Toward Self-Realization. New York, WW Norton, 1950

Horowitz MJ (ed): Person Schemas and Maladaptive Interpersonal Patterns. Chicago, IL, University of Chicago Press, 1991

Jones E: The Life and Work of Sigmund Freud, Vol 1. New York, Basic Books, 1953

Jones E: The Life and Work of Sigmund Freud, Vol 2. New York, Basic Books, 1955

Jones E: The Life and Work of Sigmund Freud, Vol 3. New York, Basic Books, 1957

Jung CG: Memories, Dreams, Reflections. New York, Vintage, 1961

Jung CG: Man and His Symbols. New York, Dell, 1964

Jung CG: Zur gegenwartigen Lage der Psychotherapie (1934), qtd in Selesnick S: Psychoanalytic Pioneers. Edited by Alexander F, Eisenstein S, Grotjahn M. New York, Basic Books, 1966a, pp 63–77

Jung CG: Two Essays on Analytical Psychology. Princeton, NJ, Princeton University Press, 1966b

Kaufmann W: Discovering The Mind, Vol 3. New York, McGraw-Hill, 1980, pp 279–280

Kernberg O: Borderline Conditions and Pathological Narcissism. New York, Jason Aronson, 1975

Kernberg O: Object-Relations Theory and Clinical Psychoanalysis. New York, Jason Aronson, 1976

Kihlstrom JF, Hoyt IP: Repression, dissociation and hypnosis, in Repression and Dissociation: Implications for Personality Theory, Psychopathology, and Health. Edited by Singer JL. Chicago, IL, University of Chicago Press, 1990, pp 181–208

Klein M, Heimann P, Isaacs S, et al: Developments in Psycho-Analysis. London, England, Hogarth/Institute of Psycho-Analysis, 1973

Kluft RP (ed): Childhood Antecedents of Multiple Personality. Washington, DC, American Psychiatric Press, 1985

Kluft RP: Introduction, in Incest-Related Syndromes of Adult Psychopathology. Edited by Kluft RP. Washington, DC, American Psychiatric Press, 1990, pp 1–10

Kohut H: The Analysis of the Self: A Systematic Approach to the Psychoanalytic Treatment of Narcissistic Personality Disorders. New York, International Universities Press, 1971

Kohut H: The Restoration of the Self. New York, International Universities Press, 1977

Kohut H: How Does Analysis Cure? Chicago, IL, University of Chicago Press, 1984

Krystal H: Integration and Self-Healing: Affect, Trauma, Alexithymia. Hillsdale, NJ, Analytic Press, 1988

Kuhn TS: The Structure of Scientific Revolutions, 2nd Edition. Chicago, IL, University of Chicago Press, 1970

Laplanche J, Pontalis J-B: The Language of Psycho-Analysis. Translated by Nicholson-Smith D. New York, WW Norton, 1973

Loewenstein RJ: Somatoform disorders in victims of incest and child abuse, in Incest-Related Syndromes of Adult Psychopathology. Edited by Kluft RP. Washington, DC, American Psychiatric Press, 1990, pp 75–107

Loftus E, Ketcham K: The Myth of Repressed Memory: False Memories and Allegations of Sexual Abuse. New York, St Martins Press, 1994

Mahler MS, Pine F, Bergman A: The Psychological Birth of the Human Infant: Symbiosis and Individuation. New York, Basic Books, 1975

Marmer SS: Psychoanalysis of multiple personality. Int J Psychoanal 61:439–459, 1980

Marmer SS: Multiple personality disorder: a psychoanalytic perspective. Psychiatr Clin North Am 14:677–693, 1991

Marmer SS, Fink D: Rethinking the comparison of borderline personality disorder and multiple personality disorder. Psychiatr Clin North Am 17:743–771, 1994

Maunder R: Implications of mind-body theory for integration in psychiatry. Psychiatry 58:85–97, 1995

Masson J: The Assault on the Truth. New York, Farrar, Straus, & Giroux, 1984

Masterson JF: The Narcissistic and Borderline Disorders: An Integrated and Developmental Approach. New York, Brunner/Mazel, 1981

McDougall J: Theaters of the Mind: Illusion and Truth on the Psychoanalytic Stage. New York, Brunner/Mazel, 1982

Miller A: Thou Shalt Not Be Aware: Society's Betrayal of the Child. Translated by Hannum H, Hannum H. New York, Meridian, 1984

Miller A: For Your Own Good: Hidden Cruelty in Child-Rearing and the Roots of Violence. Translated by Hannum H, Hannum H. New York, Noonday Press, 1990

Niedlerland WG: The Schreber Case: Psychoanalytic Profile of a Paranoid Personality. New York, Quadrangle/New York Times Book Co, 1974

Panksepp J: Affective Neuroscience. New York, Oxford University Press, 1998

Popper KR: The Logic of Scientific Discovery. New York, Science Editions, 1959

Popper KR: Conjectures and Refutations: The Growth of Scientific Knowledge. New York, Basic Books, 1962

Putnam FW Jr: Dissociation as a response to extreme trauma, in Childhood Antecedents of Multiple Personality. Edited by Kluft RP. Washington, DC, American Psychiatric Press, 1985, pp 65–97

Putnam FW Jr: Diagnosis and Treatment of Multiple Personality Disorder. New York, Guilford, 1989

Putnam FW Jr: Disturbances of "self" in victims of childhood sexual abuse, in Incest-Related Syndromes of Adult Psychopathology. Edited by Kluft RP. Washington, DC, American Psychiatric Press, 1990, pp 113–131

Rank O: The Trauma of Birth. New York, Harper & Row, 1973

Reich W: Character Analysis, 3rd Edition. New York, Farrar, Straus & Giroux, 1972

Ricoeur P: Freud and Philosophy. New Haven, CT, Yale University Press, 1970

Rinsley DB: Treatment of the Severely Disturbed Adolescent. New York, Jason Aronson, 1980

Schafer R: The mechanisms of defence. Int J Psychoanal 49:49–62, 1968

Schafer R: The idea of resistance. Int J Psychoanal 54:259–285, 1973

Schreiber FR: Sybil. Chicago, IL, Henry Regnery, 1973

Segal H: Introduction to the Work of Melanie Klein. London, England, Hogarth/Institute of Psycho-Analysis, 1973

Shengold L: Soul Murder: The Effects of Childhood Abuse and Deprivation. New York, Fawcett Columbine, 1989

Siegel DJ: The Developing Mind: Toward a Neurobiology of Interpersonal Experience. New York, Guilford, 1999

Skinner BF: The Behavior of Organisms. New York, Appleton-Century-Crofts, 1938

Skinner BF: Science and Human Behavior. New York, Macmillan, 1953

Spiegel D: Hypnosis, dissociation, and trauma: hidden and overt observers, in Repression and Dissociation: Implications for Personality Theory, Psychopathology, and Health. Edited by Singer JL. Chicago, IL, University of Chicago Press, 1990a, pp 121–142

Spiegel D: Trauma, dissociation, and hypnosis, in Incest-Related Syndromes of Adult Psychopathology. Edited by Kluft RP. Washington, DC, American Psychiatric Press, 1990b, pp 247–261

Spitz RA: The First Year of Life: A Psychoanalytic Study of Normal and Deviant Development of Object Relations. New York, International Universities Press, 1965

Stern D: The Interpersonal World of the Infant. New York, Basic Books, 1985

Stolorow R, Brandschaft B: Developmental failure and psychic conflict. Psychoanalytic Psychology 4:241–253, 1987

Stolorow R, Lachmann R: The Psychoanalysis of Developmental Arrests. New York, International Universities Press, 1980

Sullivan HS: The Interpersonal Theory of Psychiatry. Edited by Perry HS, Gawel ML. New York, WW Norton, 1953

Sutherland JD: The British object relations theorists: Balint, Winnicott, Fairbairn, Guntrip. J Am Psychoanal Assoc 28:829–860, 1980

Taylor GJ: Psychosomatic Medicine and Contemporary Psychoanalysis. Madison, WI, International Universities Press, 1987

Terr L: Too Scared to Cry: Psychic Trauma in Childhood. New York, Harper & Row, 1990

Vaillant GE: Adaptation to Life. Boston, MA, Little, Brown, 1977

van der Kolk BA: The psychological consequences of overwhelming life experiences, in Psychological Trauma. Edited by van der Kolk BA. Washington, DC, American Psychiatric Press, 1987, pp 1–30

Waelder R: The principle of multiple function: observations on over-determination. Psychoanal Q 5:45–62, 1936

Wallerstein R: Defense, defense mechanisms, and the structure of the mind. J Am Psychoanal Assoc 31(suppl):201–225, 1983

West LJ: Dissociative reaction, in Comprehensive Textbook of Psychiatry. Edited by Freedman AM, Kaplan HI. Baltimore, MD, Williams & Wilkins, 1967, pp 885–899

Wilbur CB: The effect of child abuse on the psyche, in Childhood Antecedents of Multiple Personality. Edited by Kluft RP. Washington, DC, American Psychiatric Press, 1985, pp 21–35

Williams LM: Recovered Memories of Abuse in Women with Documented Child Sexual Victimization Histories. J Trauma Stress 8:649–673, 1995

Winnicott DW: Transitional objects and transitional phenomena. Int J Psychoanal 34:89–97, 1953

Winnicott DW: The Maturational Processes and the Facilitating Environment. London, England, Hogarth/Institute of Psycho-Analysis, 1965

Winnicott DW: The location of cultural experience. Int J Psychoanal 48:368–372, 1966

Winnicott DW: Human Nature. New York, Schocken Books, 1988

Wollheim R: Sigmund Freud. New York, Viking, 1971

Wolpe J: Psychotherapy by Reciprocal Inhibition. Palo Alto, CA, Stanford University Press, 1958

Suggested Readings

Dollard J, Miller NE: Personality and Psychotherapy. New York, McGraw-Hill, 1950 [*Presents learning theory in a way that can be integrated with a psychodynamic approach.*]

Freud S: Analysis of a phobia in a five-year-old boy (1909a), in Standard Edition of the Complete Psychological Works of Sigmund Freud, Vol 10. Translated and edited by Strachey J. London, England, Hogarth, 1955, pp 1–149

Freud S: Notes upon a case of obsessional neurosis (1909b), in Standard Edition of the Complete Psychological Works of Sigmund Freud, Vol 10. Translated and edited by Strachey J. London, England, Hogarth, 1955, pp 151–318

Freud S: The ego and the id (1923), in Standard Edition of the Complete Psychological Works of Sigmund Freud, Vol 19. Translated and edited by Strachey J. London, England, Hogarth, 1961, pp 1–66 [*Demonstrates the applicability of learning theory to psychotherapy.*]

Freud S: Inhibitions, symptoms and anxiety (1926), in Standard Edition of the Complete Psychological Works of Sigmund Freud, Vol 20. Translated and edited by Strachey J. London, England, Hogarth, 1959, pp 75–175 [*These four papers by Freud demonstrate the breadth of his work. "Analysis of a Phobia in a Five-Year-Old Boy" (known as "Little Hans") and "Notes Upon a Case of Obessional Neurosis" (known as "The Rat Man") show Freud's clinical acumen.*

In The Ego and the Id, Freud clearly explains the structural model. Inhibitions, Symptoms and Anxiety, one of Freud's most important and interesting papers, exposes his thinking process at work.]

Greenberg JR, Mitchell SA: Object Relations in Psychoanalytic Theory. Cambridge, MA, Harvard University Press, 1983 [*Presents the evolution of this line in psychoanalysis.*]

Greenson RR: The Technique and Practice of Psychoanalysis, Vol 1. New York, International Universities Press, 1967 [*A readable introduction to technique.*]

Herman J: Trauma and Recovery. New York, Basic Books, 1992 [*Despite its rather forceful rhetorical tone, the book offers an excellent presentation of the rediscovery of trauma in psychopathology.*]

Jung CG: Man and His Symbols. New York, Dell, 1964 [*Presents the Jungian viewpoint well.*]

Kernberg O: Object-Relations Theory and Clinical Psychoanalysis. New York, Jason Aronson, 1976 [*Dense and difficult reading but presents the modern integration of drives, object relations, development, and psychopathology with great depth in all its complexity.*]

Kohut H: The Restoration of the Self. New York, International Universities Press, 1977 [*This important volume launched self psychology as a separate school within psychoanalysis.*]

Mahler MS, Pine F, Bergman A: The Psychological Birth of the Human Infant: Symbiosis and Individuation. New York, Basic Books, 1975 [*This work presents the modern view of development.*]

Malcolm J: Psychoanalysis, the Impossible Profession. New York, Alfred A Knopf, 1981 [*An outstanding exposition of the discovery of transference, and of the tension between more and less abstinent therapeutic technique.*]

Strachey J: The nature of the therapeutic action of psychoanalysis (1934). Int J Psychoanal 50:275–292, 1969 [*Discussion of how analysis works.*]

Sullivan HS: The Interpersonal Theory of Psychiatry. Edited by Perry HS, Gawel ML. New York, WW Norton, 1953 [*Sets forth the psychodynamic interpersonal view.*]

Glossary

Anal phase   The second phase in Freud's theory of psychosexual development in which toilet training typically occurs. In this phase, the psychological issues are control and mastery.

Anima and Animus   Jung's terms for the feminine and masculine principles found in all people.

Archetype   Jung's concept of built-in mental structures that govern the categories by which our minds work.

Collective unconscious   Jung's concept of a common database and mental structure shared by the entire species or by members of the same race.

Conscious   That part of the mind that is always within our awareness.

Countertransference   Narrowly, this refers to the reaction of the therapist to the patient's transference. More broadly, it refers to the unresolved problems in the personality of the therapist that get in the way of therapy. For the Kleinian school and some others, countertransference is the emotion evoked in the therapist by the patient's projections.

Defense mechanisms   Characteristic techniques and fantasies used by a person to avoid unwelcome or anxiety-provoking mental content.

Depressive position   A Kleinian concept referring to the awareness that one's projections may have damaged a valued object.

Ego   In Freud's structural model, the collection of functions that exerts executive control of the person, balancing his or her desires, conscience, and awareness of reality. Sometimes Freud used this term in this narrower sense; other times he used it as a synonym for "self."

Id   In the structural theory, the largely unconscious part of the mind that contains our urges, drives, and desires.

Instinctual drives   The biological and psychological wants, desires, and aims of our unconscious mind. Freud first divided the drives into the sexual and the self-preservative. Later, he regarded sexuality (or libido) and aggression (the death instinct) as the basic drives.

Narcissism   In normal development, everyone goes through a phase of primary narcissism. As we develop and encounter disappointment, narcissism (known as secondary narcissism) becomes the defense by which we protect our fragile self-esteem. Narcissism entails a brittle, grandiose overvaluation of ourselves.

Object   Not to be confused with things inanimate. *Object* refers to the other people whom an individual subject relates to.

Object relations   The way other real people leave permanent impressions on us. *Object relations* describes our ability to see others as whole or as split into parts.

Oedipal phase   In psychoanalytic theory, the phase in which the child recognizes that mother and father have a relationship with each other independent of the child. To give up the yearning for an exclusive relationship with the mother, boys will identify with father and later in life seek a woman like their mother. The oedipal phase for girls is not as clear but is thought to involve a cementing of the identification with the mother.

Oral phase   The first psychosexual phase of Freud's theory. In the oral phase, the child is oriented around the mouth and everything it can do. Metaphorically, this includes taking in, savoring, swallowing, digesting, regurgitating, spitting, and biting.

Overdetermination   The psychoanalytic concept holding that there are multiple real and fantasy causes for each mental event. In therapeutic technique, the concept of overdetermination cautions us not to make simplistic, reductionistic, or one-dimensional interpretations.

Paranoid-schizoid position   Part of the developmental theory of Klein in which there is the heavy use of splitting, projective identification, and disconnection from the object.

Persona   Jung's term for the outward face we show the world.

Phallic phase   The third phase of Freud's theory of psychosexual development, in which preoccupation with the body, especially the genitals, occurs. It is a phase of competition and exhibitionism as well as insecurity over body image.

Pleasure principle   The motivating process of the "system unconscious." This principle is said to govern the id. It seeks immediate gratification of its desires, regardless of the long-term consequences.

Practicing phase   Mahler's phase in which the child is gaining the ability to walk and the beginnings of speech. During this phase, the child has a "love affair" with the world. It coincides with the months before and after the first birthday.

Preconscious   In the topographical model, this refers to mental content that is not conscious at this particular moment but that could very easily be brought to consciousness by a shift in attention.

Primary process   This is the operating system of the "system unconscious." It is mostly imagistic, connotative, and free flowing. In primary process, time moves in both directions, and logical contradictions can coexist.

Rapprochement Mahler's phase of development that follows the practicing phase. It coincides approximately with the period of 18–36 months. The child moves back and forth between increasing independence and a return to the parent for nurturing and security. The manner in which the parents let this process flow is thought to have a significant effect on development of borderline and narcissistic states.

Reality principle The motivating force of the "system conscious" and the ego. The reality principle takes into account the immediate and long-term consequences of gratifying desire. It is therefore a more sophisticated version of the pleasure principle. Thanks to the reality principle, delayed gratification is possible.

Secondary process This is the operating system of the "system conscious," or conscious mind. Information is understood mostly in verbal form, according to denotation. Time flows in only one direction, and Aristotlean logic is observed.

Self This refers to the individual. For Kohut, the term had the additional significance of referring to the cohesive sense of being that regulates the entire person. For Jung, the term referred to the part of the personality that balances the contradictory archetypes within us.

Shadow Jung's term for the animal side of the person, including both passion and evil.

Structural model Freud's division of the mind into ego, superego, and id.

Superego In the structural model, this refers to the conscience. The archaic superego only punishes. The mature superego both punishes and praises.

Therapeutic alliance Term for the cooperative relationship between the patient and the therapist. The patient agrees to show up regularly and on time and to speak with honesty and without censorship. The therapist agrees to listen with empathy and understanding and to use his knowledge and skill for the exclusive benefit of the patient. Transference and countertransference reactions arise in the course of dynamic therapies. At such times, the strength of the therapeutic alliance can help the therapist and patient alike endure the storms and use them for therapeutic purpose.

Topographic model Freud's theory in which the mind is divided into conscious, preconscious, and unconscious parts. The unconscious is understood in three ways: as a descriptive state, a dynamic state, and an operating system. The operating system is known as primary process.

Transference The experience in a current relationship of affects, fantasies, and anxieties that trace back to an earlier relationship. Transference is ubiquitous but occurs in particularly strong form in dynamic psychotherapy, especially psychoanalysis. The transference is the reliving of a relationship configuration from the past, reexperienced with the therapist.

Unconscious That part of the mind that is out of our current awareness. Descriptively, anything we are not thinking of is unconscious. Dynamically, the unconscious refers to our deep drives and desires. As an operating system, the "system unconscious" is based on the pleasure principle and works on the logic of primary process.

CHAPTER 4

The Psychiatric Interview, Psychiatric History, and Mental Status Examination

Stephen C. Scheiber, M.D.

The medical care health delivery system is changing in a revolutionary fashion. Rapid advances are being made in the understanding of the etiologies of mental disorders. The diagnosis of psychiatric disorders has been undergoing dramatic changes as a reflection of a better understanding of these disorders. Patient education has led to a better-informed public, allowing patients to make treatment choices. Pharmacological advances have resulted in a greater number of options in the treatment of psychiatric disorders. The pharmacology industry has initiated two new strategies: 1) advertising its products directly to "consumers" and 2) enhancing the presence of drug detail salesmen in psychiatric residency training programs and with treating physicians to promote their products. This direct advertising to the public has led to patients' asking for particular products, whether appropriate or not for their specific conditions.

Time allotted for diagnostic evaluations and for psychiatric treatments has been shortened. This has led to the temptation to highlight symptom formation at the expense of understanding patients and their total functioning. Multiple diagnoses with simultaneous treatment for each of the diagnoses—as if they are equally important—has been replacing prioritizing diagnoses and treating a primary disorder. With all these changes, the psychiatric interview remains the essential vehicle for the assessment of the psychiatric patient. The psychiatrist is the medical specialist in psychiatric diagnosis, psychiatric treatment, and understanding interpersonal relationships. The patient reveals what is troubling him or her in the context of a confidential doctor–patient relationship.

The psychiatrist listens and responds, attempting to obtain as clear an understanding as possible of the patient's problems in the context of the patient's culture and environment. The psychiatrist encourages a free-flowing exchange with the patient and then, at the conclusion of the interview, arrives at a diagnostic formulation of the patient's problems. The more accurate the diagnostic assessment, the more appropriate the treatment planning (Halleck 1991).

The *psychiatric history* includes information about the patient as a person, the chief complaint, the present illness, premorbid adjustment, pertinent past history, history of medical illnesses, family history of psychiatric and medical disorders, and a developmental history of the patient. The psychiatrist obtains as much history as needed to arrive at a differential diagnosis. With subsequent interviews, the psychiatrist refines his or her working diagnosis and examines the influences of biological, psychological, cultural, familial, and social factors on the patient's life. During the course of a psychiatric history, the psychiatrist evaluates the patient's perceptions of himself or herself and his or her experiences, the patient's perspectives on his or her problems, the goals of treatment, and the desired treatment relationship.

The *mental status examination* is a cross-sectional summary of the patient's behavior, sensorium, and cognitive functioning. Information pertaining to the mental status of the patient is obtained informally during a psychiatric interview as well as through formal testing. Informal information is based on the psychiatrist's observations of the patient and his or her listening to what the patient says. Categories of such information include appearance and behavior, motor activity, eye contact, mode of relating, mood, affect, quality and quantity of speech, thought content, thought processes, and use of vocabulary.

Formal testing considers orientation, attention and concentration, recent and remote memory, fund of information, vocabulary, abilities to abstract, judgment and insight, and perception and coordination. The need for and specificity of formal testing are based on information and clues derived from the psychiatric interview (Othmer and Othmer 1994).

The Psychiatric Interview

Psychiatric Diagnosis

The single most important method of arriving at an understanding of the patient who exhibits the signs and symptoms of a psychiatric disorder is by the psychiatric interview. Although having many features in common with a medical interview, the psychiatric interview has significant elaborations and departures from the medical interview. In addition to the descriptive features of psychiatric diagnoses, which are detailed in DSM-IV-TR (American Psychiatric Association 2000), the psychiatric interview serves as an entrée into a multidimensional understanding of the patient as a person. The psychiatric interview focuses on multiple areas (Table 4–1).

TABLE 4–1. Areas of focus in the psychiatric interview

1. Patient's psychological makeup
2. How the patient relates to his or her environment
3. Significant social, religious, and cultural influences on the patient's life
4. Conscious and unconscious motivations for the patient's behavior
5. Patient's ego strengths and weaknesses
6. Coping strategies used by the patient
7. Defense mechanisms that are predominant and under what conditions
8. Available support systems and networks for the patient
9. Patient's points of vulnerability
10. Patient's aptitude and achievement

The psychiatric interview is a creative act and is a study of movement and change (Fenichel 1984; Hartmann 1964; Havens 1984; Shea 1998). Common features of both the psychiatric interview and the medical interview include identifying data regarding the patient, the chief complaint, the history of the present illness, sig-

nificant past history, social history, and family history.

Distinctive features of the psychiatric interview include examining feelings about significant events in the individual's life, identifying significant persons and their relationship to the patient in the course of his or her life, and identifying and tracing the major influences on the biological, social, and psychological development of the individual. The interviewer gathers cross-sectional data related to the signs and symptoms of primary psychiatric disorders, such as anxiety disorders, mood disorders, schizophrenic disorders, substance-related disorders and cognitive disorders—that is, those categorized under Axis I of the five axes of DSM-IV-TR. The interviewer simultaneously looks for lifetime patterns of the individual's adaptation and relation to the environment in the form of character traits and, at times, character disorders that are described formally under Axis II of DSM-IV-TR.

In the course of a thorough medical/psychiatric examination, the clinician elicits historical information, including genetic and family predispositions that may influence the type of problems the patient presents, and completes a physical examination with appropriate laboratory, imaging, and electrophysiological examinations to ascertain the patient's medical problems, listed under Axis III of DSM-IV-TR. This part of the examination aids the psychiatrist in assessing the influence of medical disorders on behavior, mood, and cognition. Axes IV and V are used to supplement the psychiatric diagnoses; they estimate, respectively, the severity of psychosocial stressors and the highest level of adaptive functions currently and in the past year. These axes have potential value in planning treatment and assessing the prognosis of the patient's condition.

The psychiatrist in the course of the interview assesses whether the patient exhibits psychotic thinking and/or behavior and whether the patient is harboring suicidal or homicidal thoughts or plans. Safety issues are always foremost in the psychiatrist's evaluation of patients. The patient's capacity to control impulses is also assessed. If in the course of an interview it is determined by the psychiatrist that a patient may be a danger to himself or herself or to others by virtue of a major mental disorder, the psychiatrist is obligated to consider psychiatric hospitalization to protect the patient and/or society. Some states mandate that a psychiatrist notify potential victims of threatened harm revealed during the course of an interview (Halleck 1991).

The psychiatric interview—in addition to eliciting information for the analysis of cross-sectional data to arrive at a formal diagnosis and to obtain information regarding the past growth and development of the individual—is also a potentially healing event in which a patient, a suffering individual with psychiatric signs and symptoms, gains relief from his or her symptoms by revealing himself or herself in the context of a trusting, nonjudgmental relationship with his or her psychiatrist. A variety of mechanisms may be used, including support, insight, and self-disclosure. Key elements in promoting therapeutic aspects of an interview are an openness to sharing information and the ability to listen empathetically within the context of a confidential doctor–patient relationship (Bird 1973; Shea 1998).

During the course of a diagnostic interview, the psychiatrist assesses which of several modalities of therapy could benefit the patient. This assessment is then periodically reviewed and updated. The psychiatrist brings to the interview an in-depth knowledge of normal and abnormal behavior and has a command of psychodynamic principles, using them as a theoretical framework to understand the complexities of the patient's unique personality patterns, major psychological conflicts, use of defense mechanisms, biological assets and deficits, and modes of adapting. The psychiatrist assesses the influences of genetic factors and organic processes on the patient's behavior, thinking, and feeling states. Psychopathology is evaluated as a product of the patient's entire being in the context of biological, social, economic, and cultural, as well as emotional, influences.

Psychiatric interviewing is an art that is learned over time, with practice under the tutelage of supervisors skilled and experienced in teaching the psychiatric interview. A careful, methodical review of interviewing style, technique, and process by a mentor or a peer augments the psychiatric resident/interviewer's learning. Audiovisual aids may also be used to facilitate the process of learning interviewing skills. In addition, educational guidelines, outlines, or manuals of principles and techniques help the resident. Among the topics discussed in training are general considerations about the interview, the physician/patient relationship, and specific interviewing techniques, all discussed below.

General Considerations

Initiation

The initial contact for psychiatric appointments is usually by telephone. Those receiving such calls must be attuned to recognizing psychiatric emergencies and be sensitive to issues of patient confidentiality. As much pertinent information as possible is obtained during the call. This includes the reason for the call, the location of the patient, how the caller can be reached by the psychiatrist, and the urgency of the problem. When the recipient of the call assesses that a psychiatric emergency exists, the call should be transferred immediately to the psychiatrist, if he or she is available. If the psychiatrist is not available, the patient should be referred to an emergency psychiatric facility and the emergency department notified of the patient referral, with as much background information as was gleaned from the caller.

Most calls are not emergencies. The psychiatrist, when returning a call, requires sufficient time to assess several critical subjects (Table 4–2).

TABLE 4–2. Critical subjects to assess when returning patient phone calls

1. What are the circumstances that led to the patient's calling?
2. What are the presenting complaints?
3. Who referred the patient?
4. Is (or was) the patient in treatment with another psychiatrist?
5. What does the patient hope to gain by seeing a psychiatrist?
6. Does the identified problem require the expertise of a psychiatrist?
7. Does the caller need to be referred elsewhere?

The psychiatrist elicits enough information to determine whether the patient is in need of an immediate assessment and examination for a psychiatric hospitalization. If the psychiatrist judges that the patient may need hospitalization, the psychiatrist tells the patient to go to the emergency department. The psychiatrist then either goes to the emergency department or arranges for someone at the emergency department to evaluate (not admit) the caller (Morrison 1993).

If the patient is referred by his or her physician, the psychiatrist inquires about any current medical problems and about medications that the patient is taking. The psychiatrist requests permission to speak to the patient's physician to discuss reasons for the referral and to ascertain whether the physician is requesting consultation so as to better deal with a particular psychiatric problem (e.g., adjustment of dosage of antidepressant medication, compliance problems, level of depression of the patient) or whether the physician is requesting a thorough psychiatric evaluation and ultimate treatment by the psychiatrist.

Coordinating care with a referring physician is important, particularly when there are overlapping medical/psychiatric problems and when medications are prescribed. This coordination is critical in working with primary care physicians. When the patient is referred for a single visit or a limited number of visits, psychiatrists must determine whether it is reasonable to respond to the requests of the referring physician within the time limits that have been predetermined, often by third-party payers. Complicated problems typically require extended evaluations. Many medications will alter the mental status of the patient (e.g., antianxiety agents, antihypertensive agents, anticholinergic drugs). Psychotropic medications can influence medical conditions (e.g., lithium and renal disease). The primary care physician is an excellent source of objective information about the patient. The psychiatrist should welcome as much data as the primary physician can offer regarding the patient's history and mental status. The psychiatrist assures the primary care physician that the patient will be referred back to the physician on conclusion of the evaluation. If the patient agrees to psychiatric treatment, the primary care physician is informed. On conclusion of the evaluation, the psychiatrist sends the referring physician a summary of his or her clinical findings, conclusions, and recommendations.

In initial contacts with a patient, the psychiatrist should ascertain whether the patient's presenting problems are appropriate for the psychiatrist's field of expertise. A patient may call inquiring whether the psychiatrist uses a specific therapeutic method to treat a specific complaint, such as nicotine patches for smoking addictions, hypnosis for memory lapses, or health food store natural herbs or vitamins as substitutes for prescribed medications for depression. If the patient requests a particular treatment and the psychiatrist does not have experience with or believe in the efficacy of that treatment, he or she offers to refer the patient to a colleague with specific expertise. Consumer-minded patients may request an interview with several psychiatrists to assess which one they believe will be most helpful to them.

Initial telephone contacts set the stage for subsequent psychiatric interviews. The psychiatrist exhibits the capacity to be an expert listener who will work to understand the patient and his or her problem. Rapport with a patient begins with the initial contact. In addition to listening to the patient's problems, the psychiatrist advises the patient about what to expect when coming for an evaluation. The patient is told the minimum amount of time that the psychiatrist expects will be needed to do a complete assessment, how much time will be allowed per visit, over what period of time the assessment will be conducted, what the hourly cost will be, the charge for missed appointments, and whether the psychiatrist anticipates being available to treat the patient when the assessment is completed. The psychiatrist inquires about when the patient would be available to come for an evaluation and sets up a time that is mutually agreeable (Table 4–3).

TABLE 4–3. Initial steps of the psychiatric interview

Background information
Reason for call
Location of patient
How caller can be reached
Presenting complaints
Referral source's name and telephone number
Treatment history
Concurrent medical conditions
What patient hopes to gain
Determination of urgency
Primary physician's name and phone number
Expectations
Time for assessment
Cost of evaluation
Purpose of assessment
Psychiatrist's availability for treatment

Requests for appointments with a psychiatrist can also be initiated by third parties, who can include relatives, treating physicians, judges, lawyers, staff of employee health services or student health services, staff of disability evaluation organizations, military superiors, and others. In every instance, it is essential for the psychiatrist to learn what the patient has been told about requests for a psychiatric consultation or evaluation and to find out what the patient expects from seeing a psychiatrist. The purpose of the examination should be explicit. If the purpose is to advise an employer about the patient's psychiatric fitness to continue employment, the psychiatrist advises the employer to inform the patient that this is the purpose and to make sure the patient knows that the psychiatrist's conclusions will be shared with the employer.

If a relative is calling, it is important not only to ascertain what the patient knows of the call but to find out the reasons why the patient is not calling directly. The psychiatrist does everything possible to dissuade a family member from using deception in getting the patient to agree to an appointment. An example of deception would be a parent advising a youngster that he is going for a doctor's appointment to have a thorough examination without mentioning that it is a psychiatric examination (Leventhal and Crofts 1997) or a grown child bringing an elderly parent to a psychiatrist after telling the parent that she is going to have her back pain checked out by a doctor.

Third-party callers should also be advised of what information they can expect following a psychiatric examination. In most instances, no information will be shared without the patient's consent. In the case of a minor, the information may be shared with the parent. If the purpose of an examination is to collect information as an expert witness in a court of law, the patient is advised at the onset of the interview that everything he or she says may be used as part of the psychiatrist's expert testimony in court. In this instance, the usual doctor–patient confidentiality is not in force.

Time

The amount of time set aside for an initial psychiatric outpatient evaluation varies, ranging from 45 minutes for some evaluations to 90 minutes for others. If the evaluation is conducted at the bedside on a medical service, the length of the interview is often shorter because of the patient's medical condition, and more frequent, brief visits may be necessary. In emergency department settings, the evaluation may be prolonged, particularly if hospitalization is in question and supporting data are needed from resources not immediately available, such as from relatives and treating physicians who have to be reached by telephone. If a patient is exhibiting psychotic behaviors during an outpatient appointment, the interview may be abbreviated if, in the judgment of the psychiatrist, prolonging the interview will aggravate the patient's condition. When possible, the psychiatrist should have some flexibility in his or her schedule at the time of an initial interview. In most instances, evaluations for treatment require scheduling additional meetings beyond the initial hour.

Among the psychiatrist's first observations of the patient will be the patient's handling of time. A patient who arrives an hour early for an appointment is usually very anxious. Those arriving very late are often conflicted about coming. Psychiatrists can learn much about patients' handling of time by exploring with patients the reasons for their tardiness. For the patient who is very late, it is important for the psychiatrist not only to explore reasons for tardiness but also to discourage the patient from introducing emotionally charged issues at or near the conclusion of an initial visit, unless the psychiatrist is prepared to stay with the patient beyond the scheduled hour.

Psychiatrists need to be aware and conscious of their own handling of time as well. The psychiatrist, if he or she anticipates being late, should contact the patient, and, as a minimum, the patient should be informed of when he or she may expect the psychiatrist to arrive. If not able to contact the patient beforehand, the psychiatrist after arriving should acknowledge the tardiness and apologize for the delay. Such courtesies are appropriate for nonpsychiatrist physicians as well. Repeated violations of appointment hours by psychiatrists suggest an unresolved problem for them in the doctor–patient relationship and one that they need to explore and correct.

Setting

The most important space consideration for a psychiatric interview is establishing privacy so that the interview proceeds in a setting where confidentiality can be ensured. In academic settings, where audiovisual equipment and one-way viewing mirrors are used for teaching, the patient is owed an explanation by the resident about the purposes for which recording devices are being used. The patient has the right of refusal regarding the use of such devices. Most patients attending a clinic in a teaching institution expect that part of going to such an institution for help will involve using them as teaching aids for residents. The resident's dealing directly and honestly with a patient's questions and concerns is essential and also will enhance the doctor–patient relationship. The resident learns the importance of being sensitive to the patient's reactions to the use of such equipment. For instance, adolescent patients may be reluctant to discuss negative feelings toward their parents or other authority figures in the face of a camera or recording device until they are ensured that such data will not be shared with the parents.

The psychiatrist does everything possible to put the patient at ease during the interview. The setting should be one that promotes comfort for both patient and psychiatrist. The height of chairs should be approximately equal in size so that neither party is looking down on the other. There should be no barriers between the patient and doctor such as a desk, and there should be sufficient light to maximize the psychiatrist's visual observation without glaring light that would disturb the patient. Background sounds should be minimized. Noisy distractions such as bubbling fish tanks, which psychiatrists may like for aesthetic reasons, should not mar the quiet of an interview room, as it may interfere with the patient's concentration.

Special populations and settings require variations from an office setting with comfortable chairs. Hospital bedside consultations are difficult to conduct while ensuring privacy. The psychiatrist should check with the nursing staff to see whether the patient's medical condition will permit his or her being moved to a quiet room to avoid multiple interruptions at the bedside by hospital personnel, visitors, shared bedside telephones, and roommates in semiprivate rooms and ward settings.

For young children, a playroom setup, with toys that children can express themselves with, is preferable for diagnostic interviewing. Much formal training, skill, and experience are needed to appropriately evaluate a child in a playroom setting (Greenspan and Greenspan 1991; Kestenbaum 1997; Robson 1986; Rutter et al. 1988).

In hospital emergency department settings, a quiet room should be available with a mattress and no removable (and potentially dangerous) objects. Such a room will prove to be the safest setting in which to interview a psychotic patient who has exhibited out-of-control behaviors. In addition to privacy and comfort, safety is an important consideration. With a potentially agitated paranoid patient, it is important for the psychiatrist to have unimpeded access to an exit door.

Note Taking

The purpose of taking written notes during a psychiatric interview is so that the psychiatrist has accurate information for preparing the report of the interview. Newly trained psychiatrists, when interviewing, tend to take extensive notes, because they are lacking in knowledge and experience about what is relevant and what is not. For the newly trained psychiatrist who often uses audiovisual aids such as audio- or videotape recorders for supervisory review, these same devices can be used for reviewing databases and can substitute for note taking. Any recording devices need to be in clear view of the patient, and an explanation is to be given to the patient about its use. The patient should be assured that the tapes will be erased after they are reviewed.

The greatest limitation in excessive note taking is that it can inhibit the free flow of exchange between patient and doctor. If the interviewer is preoccupied with note taking, he or she will miss important nonverbal messages and will not pursue important leads in the interview. The psychiatrist might not observe, for example, the patient's tears when the patient is discussing the loss of an important object in his or her life. The interviewer would then miss the opportunity to reflect, "You seem sad when talking about your sister." Another problem with extensive note taking is the failure to notice important aspects of the mental status examination, such as appearance and behavior. The psychiatrist may not notice the patient's becoming fidgety in his chair, tapping his right index fingers on his knees, and exhibiting a malar flush when describing the first date with his girlfriend at age 16 years (Edelson 1980).

If a patient requests that the psychiatrist not take notes, this request should be respected. Patients may react to the relative absence of note taking as well. They may comment, "How can you remember everything I have to say?" Such patients are concerned about whether the psychiatrist values them as individuals and cares about what they are saying. The psychiatrist then reflects these concerns, for example, by commenting, "You wonder whether I value what you are saying."

Notes help psychiatrists remember information accurately. The psychiatrist should record his or her notes, observations, and conclusions as soon after the interview as possible. Prompt recording of data and information while still fresh in the psychiatrist's mind maximizes the accuracy of the information and minimizes distortions and gaps in the database that will result when the psychiatrist delays his or her recording. The psychiatrist should set aside time at the conclusion of the interview to accomplish this task. For the experienced psychiatrist, 5–10 minutes at the conclusion of a 45- to 50-minute interview usually suffices. The newly trained psychiatrist will require additional time.

The notes that are incorporated in the patient's record are necessarily more comprehensive following initial interviews than subsequent ones, because all the data constitute new information. With subsequent interviews, only new, pertinent information needs to be recorded. Psychiatrists need to be particularly sensitive to what information is incorporated into a general hospital chart that is available to multiple caretakers and to third-party reviewers. Only essential information for the overall care of the patient should be included in a general medical chart.

Interruptions

The time set aside and agreed upon for a patient interview is viewed as sacred and protected time for the patient. Calculated measures are taken to discourage interruptions. If the door to the interview room is in an area where others may knock, a sign should be hung on the door with an instruction such as "Do not disturb" or "Interview in progress" or "In session." If someone does knock and the psychiatrist chooses to respond, he or she should go to the door and open it only wide enough for the other party to hear. The psychiatrist positions himself or herself to protect the patient from being seen. The interaction with the person knocking should be as brief as possible.

Incoming telephone calls are screened by a secretary and the callers informed that the psychiatrist is with a patient. Sessions are interrupted only for emergencies. If the psychiatrist must leave, the patient should be informed of when the psychiatrist anticipates returning, if the absence is expected to be brief. Otherwise, the psychiatrist advises the patient when to return. If, at the beginning of an interview, the psychiatrist anticipates that an urgent call may be received during the hour, he or she informs the patient at the beginning of the interview that an interruption may occur and that the psychiatrist will ask the patient to leave during the telephone call. Most patients understand interruptions for emergencies and appreciate feeling that if they were in an emergency situation, the psychiatrist would respond immediately (Bernstein and Bernstein 1980).

Relatives or Friends Accompanying the Patient

When relatives arrive with the patient, the psychiatrist always interviews the patient first and tells relatives that he or she may want to talk with them later. (An exception would be a couple coming for couple evaluation and possible couple therapy.) In the course of the patient's interviews, the psychiatrist can indicate his or her desire to speak with the relatives and can explore the patient's feelings about the psychiatrist's doing so. The patient must grant permission before relatives are interviewed. If the patient refuses, the psychiatrist must respect the patient's wishes. By doing so, the psychiatrist demonstrates that the most valued part of his or her relationship with the patient is confidentiality. Patients must also grant permission before the psychiatrist discusses their case with any other party.

An exception to this rule occurs when the psychiatrist judges the patient to be in imminent danger of hurting himself or herself or others and when the patient refuses voluntary hospitalization. In such an instance, the patient must be told why the psychiatrist is obliged to talk to a third party without the patient's permission.

If the psychiatrist wants to meet with the patient's relatives, he or she must advise the patient whether the meeting will take place with or without the patient present. If in doubt, the psychiatrist chooses to have the patient present. This signals to the patient that the psychiatrist does not want to jeopardize the doctor–patient relationship. This relationship is more important than obtaining additional information that relatives may not want to reveal in the patient's presence. Another advantage of having the patient present is that the psychiatrist can observe the interactions of the patient with the relative(s). The patient's presence also discourages a relative from trying to reveal any information that he or she would prefer that the patient not know and thus avoids the situation in which the relative wants the psychiatrist to keep secrets from the patient. It is possible to enhance the accuracy of diagnoses by a best-estimate procedure. This involves diagnosis made by one clinician on the basis of diagnostic information from a direct interview conducted by another clinician, plus information from medical records and reports from family members. Such an approach may be especially applicable for enhancing the diagnosis of antisocial personality disorder and of alcoholism (Kosten and Rounsaville 1992).

If the psychiatrist chooses to see relatives without the patient present, the ground rule needs to be established with relatives that the psychiatrist is not at liberty to share, without the patient's permission, any information obtained from the patient in confidence but is at liberty to share with the patient any information that relatives reveal. This principle extends beyond the initial visit to subsequent telephone calls that relatives may initiate. If relatives call after an initial visit, it is best for the psychiatrist to inquire first whether the patient has given permission for relatives to call. If not, the psychiatrist suggests that the patient's permission be granted before proceeding. At the beginning of the next contact with the patient, the psychiatrist informs him or her that relatives called.

Sequence

The psychiatrist's first impressions of the patient begin with the initial telephone contact. The formal assessment of the patient begins with the psychiatrist's initial observations of the patient. The psychiatrist observes the patient's appearance and behavior in the waiting area, who is with the patient, how the patient responds when the psychiatrist greets him or her by name, and how the patient responds to a handshake. It is preferable with adult patients to refer to them by their last names during the initial encounter, and then, when they are in the interview room, to inquire what the patient's preference is regarding first- or last-name usage. Referring to geriatric patients by first names without the patients' permission is particularly demeaning and infantilizing.

The psychiatrist then walks with the patient to the interview room and indicates interest in the patient by being friendly but does not make any clinical inquiries or comments until the interviewing room door is closed. The psychiatrist indicates which seat he or she will sit in while offering the patient a choice if there is more than one seat available.

At the beginning of the interview, the psychiatrist encourages the patient to speak as spontaneously and openly as possible about the reasons for his or her coming at this time. The psychiatrist can facilitate this process by briefly summarizing what he or she has learned about the patient and the patient's problems and then saying that he or she would like to hear in the patient's own words what is troubling the patient. An opening inquiry such as "Tell me what brings you here today" encourages the patient to express what currently is troubling him or her.

The psychiatrist establishes a primary posture of listening, allowing the patient to tell his or her story with minimal interruptions or direction. In the early part of the interview, if the patient stops talking, the psychiatrist encourages him or her to continue, using comments such as "Tell me more about [a particular incident]." If the patient describes a significant event in his or her life and expresses no emotion, the psychiatrist inquires, "How do you feel about this?" If the patient describes a disturbing event and starts clenching his or her fists and exhibiting flushing, the psychiatrist inquires about the patient's feelings at the moment. If the patient denies any feelings, the psychiatrist advises him or her that most people would react to similar circumstances with anger. Thus, in the initial part of the interview, the psychiatrist establishes that he or she is interested in not only the chronology of events that led to the patient's coming but also the feelings that accompany such events and encourages the patient's expression of these feelings. At times, when the expression of feelings is too overwhelming for the patient, the psychiatrist must not push the patient beyond his or her tolerance for expressing them. If the patient has had one or more psychiatric hospitalizations, the psychiatrist should learn details about each hospitalization and most particularly the events leading up to the initial hospitalization. It is also key to inquire what was most helpful during a patient's hospitalization as well as what follow-up care was most beneficial.

Throughout the interview the psychiatrist tries to learn how the patient experiences life events and to understand the patient's perceptions of how such events evolve. Once the psychiatrist has a grasp of the essentials of the present illness and accompanying feelings, he or she then shifts the focus to other subjects.

In the middle portion of the interview, the psychiatrist tries to learn about the patient as a person. There are numerous areas of the patient's life to explore: significant relationships, multigenerational family history, current living situation, occupation, avocations, education, value systems, religious and cultural background, military history, social history, medical history, developmental history, sexual history, and legal history, to name a few. The breadth of material requires several interview sessions for the psychiatrist to gather the pertinent data.

The patient will frequently be asked to describe a typical day in his or her life. The psychiatrist tries to establish the patient's highest level of functioning and assesses when current symptoms began to interfere with the patient's functioning. The decision regarding the order in which the psychiatrist inquires about these data is a matter of clinical judgment. The patient usually signifies his or her comfort with particular subjects by raising them in the interview, and the psychiatrist then follows up with questions to get more in-depth information.

As a rule, the psychiatrist moves from areas assumed to be of positive value to those of neutral interest and, finally, to those that the psychiatrist anticipates will be more emotionally charged for the patient. For example, in interviewing an adolescent, the psychiatrist may begin with inquiries regarding activities that the patient enjoys by asking, "What do you do for fun?" The psychiatrist may choose to begin his or her inquiries about school with "Tell me about your favorite subject in school." Inquiries about relationships may be made by starting with a request such as "Tell me about your best friend." The psychiatrist then may proceed to inquiries about family members by saying, "Tell me about your family."

Throughout these initial inquiries, the psychiatrist is ascertaining the patient's strengths and weaknesses and is monitoring the responses to ascertain potential areas of conflict for the patient. The psychiatrist's follow-up inquiries will be guided by the responses to the initial questions. Inquiry may then be made about specific relationships, for example, "How do you get along with your mother? your father? your brother? your sister?" With the latter, the psychiatrist is advised to ask for names and to refer to the siblings in subsequent inquiries by name.

Again, the psychiatrist is guided by the patient's responses in terms of inquiring about areas in which the patient may be reluctant to respond. When inquiring about the sexual history of a boy or man, the psychiatrist begins with, "Do you have a girlfriend?" If yes, the psychiatrist follows with "Tell me about her" and can then inquire about the nature of the relationship. The psychiatrist follows up by asking about specific areas of sexual conduct. Beginning with questions regarding kissing and then petting and then sexual intercourse, the psychiatrist then asks about the patient's feelings in regard to various sexual activities, inquiring about both heterosexual and homosexual interests and relationships. Histories of sexual abuse should be elicited (Morrison 1993). Inquires should also be made about sexually transmitted diseases such as AIDS.

In the concluding portion of the interview, the psychiatrist notes for the patient the remaining time left. The patient is asked whether there are any important areas that he or she has not talked about. The psychiatrist asks whether the patient has any questions, then answers each of the patient's questions. If the psychiatrist has insufficient information to answer a question, he or she tells the patient just that.

At this time the psychiatrist shares with the patient his or her clinical impressions in words that the patient understands, avoiding psychiatric jargon. The psychiatrist then presents a treatment plan to the patient. It is important to ascertain the patient's fiscal status as well as to determine the third-party insurance that will cover the patient's care. It may be that, under the limitations of a managed-care situation, the psychiatrist will have to advise the patient that the tried and true treatment modalities may not be available to him or her because of the limitations of his or her reimbursement system. Psychiatrists have the ethical responsibility to try to assist patients to receive optimal care. On the other hand, patients must decide within the limitations of their fiscal abilities what is feasible for themselves and their families.

If records and information are available from other sources, the psychiatrist requests written permission to obtain medical records from hospitals or other physicians. If the psychiatrist wants to contact others by telephone, he or she obtains permission from the patient before doing so. If the patient is receiving medical care from other physicians, the psychiatrist obtains consent to contact them. If the patient is reluctant to grant permission, the psychiatrist explains his or her reasons for wanting to initiate these contacts. For example, the psychiatrist may want to prescribe medications but, before doing so, wants to be sure that there are no medical contraindications. If the patient was referred by another physician, it is important for the psychiatrist to call the referring physician. The patient may want the psychiatrist to advise him or her about what information the psychiatrist will share with the referring physician. Most patients understand the importance of their care being coordinated by the two physicians when assured that information that is best kept in confidence will not be shared.

For example, a 58-year-old depressed male patient with hypertension and cardiac arrhythmia reveals that he had homosexual relations when he was a teenager. The psychiatrist advises the patient that she would like to prescribe antidepressant medications but, before doing so, wants to confer with the patient's primary physician about the type of cardiac arrhythmia he has had and the current treatment of his cardiovascular problems. The psychiatrist wants to ascertain which antidepressants may be contraindicated because of the patient's cardiac problems, wants to avoid any adverse drug reactions, and wants to choose the most appropriate medication given the patient's combined medical/psychiatric problems. At the same time, the psychiatrist assures the patient that his past sexual life will not be revealed to the primary care physician.

It is important to solicit patients' reactions to as well as agreement with a given treatment plan. Patients are entitled to know the various treatments available for their disorder. The psychiatrist shares with the patient

his or her specific recommendations for treatment and responds to the patient's questions about why the psychiatrist believes these suggestions are best for the patient. If the patient wants an alternative plan, it is best for the psychiatrist to postpone implementation of specific treatment until there is mutual agreement. There is a better likelihood for patient compliance when the patient understands a treatment plan and agrees to it (Table 4–4) (Garrett 1942; Gill et al. 1954; Group for the Advancement of Psychiatry 1961; Leon 1982; Nurcombe and Fitzhenry-Coor 1982; Rutter and Cox 1981; Strupp and Binder 1984; Sullivan 1954; Whitehorn 1944).

TABLE 4–4. Phases of the psychiatric interview

Initial
Chief complaint
Present illness
Feelings about significant events
Middle
Patient as a person
Multigenerational family history
Current living situation
Occupation
Avocations
Education
Value systems
Religions and cultural background
Military history
Social history
Medical history
Developmental history
Sexual history
Typical day
Strengths and weaknesses
Concluding
Time remaining
Important areas not covered
Patient's questions
Sharing clinical impressions
Permission to obtain records
Permission to speak with others
Treatment plan and patient's reaction

The Physician–Patient Relationship

Transference

Transference is a process whereby the patient unconsciously projects his or her emotions, thoughts, and wishes related to significant persons in his or her past onto people in his or her current life and, in the context of the psychiatrist–patient relationship, onto the psychiatrist. The patient is reacting to the psychiatrist as if the psychiatrist were part of the patient's past. Whereas the reaction patterns may have been appropriate in an earlier situation, they are inappropriate when applied to figures in the present, including the psychiatrist. This theoretical construct is borrowed from the psychoanalytic literature.

For example, a 24-year-old male patient notices the long braided hair and blue eyes of the psychiatrist. He starts making several demands of the psychiatrist using a whining voice, without being consciously aware that he is doing so. Such demanding behavior replicates how he behaved in the presence of a significant aunt in his youth with similar physical features, with whom he had a highly dependent relationship and in whose presence he had exhibited similar whining voice intonations.

It is important for the psychiatrist to recognize these patterns and to treat them as distortions, not to respond in kind. An ultimate understanding of such unconscious behaviors is one of the goals of insight-oriented psychotherapy. In the early training of a psychiatrist, the psychiatric supervisor devotes considerable time to the resident's understanding of the process of transference so that the resident will not treat these reaction patterns as personal assaults.

Countertransference

Countertransference is a process whereby the psychiatrist unconsciously projects emotions, thoughts, and wishes from his or her past onto the patient's personality or onto the material that the patient is presenting, thus expressing unresolved conflicts and/or gratifying the psychiatrist's own personal needs. These reactions are inappropriate in the doctor–patient relationship. In this instance, the patient assumes the role of an important person from the psychiatrist's earlier life. This construct is also gleaned from the psychoanalytic literature. In such instances, the psychiatrist mistakenly attributes to the patient feelings and thoughts that are based on the psychiatrist's own life experiences, which can interfere with his or her understanding of the patient.

For example, a male psychiatrist responds inappropriately to an internist's consultation request on a 76-year-old, dying, hospitalized female patient. The psychiatrist has been making twice-daily hour-long bedside visits followed by frequent calls to the patient's internist. The psychiatrist questions the internist's medical care of the patient and recommends antianxiety agents to treat the patient's presumed anxiety. As a child, the psychiatrist had experienced strong attachment to his grandmother, who had died in his childhood home. He unconsciously retained guilt feelings for not doing something to prevent

her death. The psychiatrist's handling of the consultation is in essence an attempt to cope with his own anxieties and guilt about his grandmother's death without consciously realizing that he is doing this or being cognizant of the inappropriateness of his behavior.

The psychiatrist in this case would benefit from consultation with a colleague, who could help clarify the psychiatrist's reaction patterns and guide him toward more appropriate professional behavior.

One of the values of personal psychoanalysis for psychiatrists is to enhance their awareness of their unconsciously motivated behaviors so that they can better use their countertransference reactions to understand their patients. In their training, residents will be helped by a supervisor to examine their countertransference reactions so that these reactions will not interfere with patients' treatment but will aid the residents in understanding their patients.

Therapeutic Alliance

The therapeutic alliance, a third theoretical construct from the psychoanalytic literature, is a process whereby the patient's mature, rational observing ego is used in combination with the psychiatrist's analytic abilities to advance the psychiatrist's understanding of the patient. The basis for such an alliance is the trusting relationship established in early life between the child and the mother, as well as other significant trusting relationships from the patient's past. The psychiatrist encourages the development of this alliance, and both persons must invest in cultivating the alliance so that the patient can benefit. The psychiatrist enhances this alliance by his or her professional conduct and attitudes of caring, concern, and respect.

Psychiatrists accept and respect patients' value systems and their integrity as persons. Without a therapeutic alliance, patients cannot reveal their innermost thoughts and feelings. It is unethical for psychiatrists to exploit patients sexually or to exploit them for personal financial gain by inquiring about investment opportunities from patients knowledgeable about such matters. These are violations of the doctor–patient relationship. Psychiatrists must never victimize patients by exploiting their roles as physician-healers (American Psychiatric Association 2001).

Resistance

Resistance is a theoretical construct that reflects any attitudes or behaviors that run counter to the therapeutic objectives of the treatment. Understanding resistance is critical to the conduct of dynamic psychotherapy. Freud described several types of resistance, including conscious resistance, ego resistance, id resistance, and superego resistance (Table 4–5).

TABLE 4–5. Types of resistance

1. Conscious ego
2. Ego
3. Id
4. Superego

Conscious resistance by patients occurs for a variety of reasons, such as lack of trust of psychiatrists, shame on the part of patients in revealing certain events and aspects of themselves or feelings that they are experiencing, and fear of displeasing or risking rejection by psychiatrists. One form of conscious resistance by patients is silence. The psychiatrist must acknowledge the difficulties the patient is experiencing and encourage the patient to verbalize material that is difficult to express. This should be done in a tactful, sensitive manner.

There are three forms of *ego resistance*: repression resistance, transference resistance and secondary-gain resistance. One form is *repression resistance*, whereby, for mostly unconscious reasons, the same forces that led to the patient's symptoms keep him or her from developing an awareness of the underlying conflicts. A second type of ego resistance, *transference resistance*, can take many forms. Such resistance may occur when the patient projects undesirable feelings onto the psychiatrist and ascribes these feelings to the psychiatrist. This, in turn, can lead to the patient's attacking the psychiatrist, and a negative transference can result. It is critical that the psychiatrist understand the underpinnings of such a transaction and, rather than retaliate, treat the patient's expressions as a resistance. A third type of ego resistance is *secondary-gain resistance*. A patient's symptoms will elicit nurturing responses from significant figures and will gratify his or her dependency needs. Manifestations of this phenomenon are commonly observed on inpatient services. For example, a patient who has been hospitalized 7 days for a cerebral hemorrhage secondary to a cerebral aneurysm shows gradual improvement in healing and has decreased complaints of headaches for 6 days. However, he resumes his complaints to the nurse in the 24 hours before his proposed discharge from the hospital. In addition to gratifying dependency needs, symptoms also serve as attention-seeking devices. Patients unconsciously resist giving up their symptoms. Such resistance must be understood by the patients' caregivers.

Id resistance occurs in psychoanalytic practice when a patient repeatedly brings up the same material in the face of repeated interpretations of the behavior.

Superego resistance occurs most frequently with obsessional, depressed patients who, by virtue of their guilt feelings and self-defeating behaviors, exhibit a need for punishment. Thus, patients continue to exhibit symptoms that serve as punishment, and they are resistant to relinquishing them (Luborsky 1984).

Resistance takes many forms. These include patients' censoring of what they are thinking, intellectualization, generalization, preoccupation with one phase of life, concentration on trivial details while avoiding important topics, affective displays, frequent requests to change appointment times, using minor physical symptoms as an excuse to avoid sessions, arriving late or forgetting appointments, forgetting to pay bills, competitive behaviors with the psychiatrist, seductive behaviors, asking for favors, and acting out (MacKinnon and Michels 1971).

Confidentiality

Psychiatrists are bound by medical ethical principles to not divulge any information revealed to them unless they have patients' consent. They must protect patients and assume responsibility for seeing that no harm will come to patients by virtue of the patients' revealing information about themselves. If patients refuse to give permission to psychiatrists to reveal information, whether it be to a referring physician or for filling out an insurance form, psychiatrists must respect the patients' wishes.

For example, a 32-year-old female patient with borderline personality disorder is referred to a psychiatrist by her internist for evaluation of depressive symptoms. The psychiatrist learns that the patient episodically abuses diazepam, prescribed by her internist, along with alcohol when she is feeling upset. The psychiatrist's assessment is that the combination of these two chemical depressants is contributing to her depressive symptoms. The psychiatrist requests permission to share this assessment with the referring internist, but the patient refuses. The psychiatrist abides by the patient's wishes while advising the patient that this combination is likely to be responsible for contributing to her depressive symptoms. He also suggests that the patient reconsider the refusal to let him share his findings with her internist.

In hospital or clinic settings, the patient is told about the types of information that will be recorded and who may have access to the information. When psychiatrists record information in the general hospital record, they record only data pertinent to the overall care of the patient, such as medications prescribed, and minimize recording personal information that has no relevance to the general medical care of the patient. In general hospital settings, it is preferable to have separate psychiatric records that can be housed and locked in an area separate from the general hospital records, to which only trained psychiatric personnel will have access.

Only when patients are in danger of hurting themselves or others by virtue of their mental illness is the psychiatrist obliged to reveal such information in order to institute involuntary hospitalization.

When third-party carriers are seeking psychiatric information, psychiatrists review with patients the information that has been prepared for the carrier and obtain patients' permission to submit reports.

Interview Technique

Facilitative Messages

The most important component in the psychiatrist–patient relationship is the interest psychiatrists show in their patients. The most important element in the psychiatric interview of patients is for psychiatrists to allow patients to tell their stories in an uninterrupted fashion. Psychiatrists assume an attentive listening posture; they do not ask excessive questions that would interrupt the flow of the interview. Throughout the interview, patients will experience resistance to revealing themselves that is based on the realities of the interview situation as well as on transference issues.

Newly trained psychiatrists often mistakenly believe that sitting in an unresponsive, silent posture emulates a psychoanalyst's approach to a patient and that this is the optimal way to interview a psychiatric patient. On the contrary, residents need to learn a repertoire of interviewing techniques that will facilitate communication as much as possible (Table 4–6). Some of these techniques are described here.

Open-ended questions. An open-ended question reflects a topic that the psychiatrist is interested in exploring but leaves it to the patient to choose the areas he or she believes are relevant and important to share.

Examples of open-ended questions by the psychiatrist are as follows:

> Psychiatrist: Can you tell me about your depression?
> Patient: I've been having crying spells.
> Psychiatrist: Can you describe them?
> Patient: They come on during certain times of the month.
> Psychiatrist: Can you say more about them?
> Patient: They've been troubling me since I was a teenager.
> Psychiatrist: They seem to have been bothering you for a long time; tell me more.

TABLE 4–6. Facilitative messages

Type	Example
Open-ended questions	"Tell me about…"
Reflections	"You're anxious about succeeding."
Facilitation	"Uh-huh."
Positive reinforcement	"Good. That helps me understand you."
Silence	Long pause allowing patient to take distance from verbal material.
Interpretation	"When you can't perform the way you think you should, you try to do something to please."
Checklist questions	"When you feel nervous, do you develop sweaty palms? heart palpitations? rapid breathing? butterflies in your stomach?"
"I want" messages	"We should explore other topics besides your depression. Tell me about your family."
Transitions	"Now that you've told me about your job, tell me what a typical day is like."
Self-disclosure	"When I've been in similar situations, I've felt terrified."

The psychiatrist attempts to get the patient to relate in his or her own words, as much as possible, the most significant aspects of his or her depression. The psychiatrist may return later in the interview to fill in specific details if the patient fails to do so spontaneously. In the example above, the psychiatrist would want to know more about the patient's symptoms, the times of the month that the symptoms appear, and what precipitated their onset when the patient was a teenager, among other issues.

Reflections. The psychiatrist often wants to draw patients' attention to the affective concomitants of their verbal productions. One way of doing this is by rephrasing what the patient has stated and stressing the feelings that accompany a reported event. By restating the patient's verbalizations, the psychiatrist provides the patient with an opportunity to correct any misconceptions that the psychiatrist may have about the patient's condition. This technique is referred to as *reflections*. Examples of reflective responses are as follows:

> Patient: I've been concerned about my job. I used to be able to keep up with my fellow workers. But in the last 3 months they seem to be handling the adjustments to the new computer and I have been unable to do so.
> Psychiatrist: You're concerned about keeping up with new demands and about retaining your job.

Patient: That's right. You know that at 58 you can't concentrate on those new manuals the way the younger people can, and I've been experiencing butterflies in my stomach and sweaty palms these last 3 months.

Psychiatrist: You've been anxious since these changes occurred at work?

Patient: You better believe it! I have not been myself. I've had heart palpitations, shakiness all over my body, and occasionally I've been stuttering.

Psychiatrist: So you'd like help in dealing with your anxieties?

Patient: I sure would.

By reflecting the patient's recent life events and by drawing attention to the principal affective component, in this case anxiety, the psychiatrist demonstrates his or her capacity to understand what the patient has been experiencing and is able to help the patient define the areas they will work on together in treatment.

Facilitation. The psychiatrist uses body language and minimal verbal cues to encourage and reinforce the patient's continuing along a particular line of thought with minimal interruptions in the patient's flow of verbalizations. Examples of these cues include attributes that are frequently ascribed to psychiatrists, such as the nodding of their heads or comments such as "Uh-huh." Other examples of facilitations include raising of eyebrows, cocking of head, leaning toward patients, and verbalizations from the psychiatrist such as "I see," "Go on," "What else?" "Anything more?" and "Proceed." Facilitations indicate to the patient that the psychiatrist is interested in the particular train of thought and that he or she is attentive to what the patient is saying. Excessive reliance on a single facilitation will, however, approach the parody of a psychiatrist and become counterproductive.

Positive reinforcement. The subjects that the psychiatrist explores with the patient are frequently ones that the patient is unaccustomed to talking about and finds difficult to explain. When the patient has struggled with a particular topic and is then able to communicate clearly, the psychiatrist signals his or her approval by using positive reinforcement. An example of such reinforcement would be the following:

Psychiatrist: How do you feel when you can't have an erection?

Patient (blushes): You know—it just doesn't get hard.

Psychiatrist: Do you experience anything else?

Patient (long pause): How do I feel?

Psychiatrist: Yes.

Patient: Oh! I get terribly frustrated and then I get angry.

Psychiatrist: Good. Those are the kinds of feelings I was asking about. That helps a lot for me to better understand what you experience.

In this manner, the psychiatrist encourages the patient to describe sensitive topics and feelings without demeaning the patient for his or her initial response of embarrassment. Positive reinforcement will then encourage the patient to verbalize other emotional states as he or she, along with the psychiatrist, explores other areas of his or her life.

Silence. The judicious use of silence when interviewing a patient is an important component of the psychiatrist's repertoire of interviewing techniques. Silences allow patients to create some distance from what they have been saying and can help them put their thoughts in order or enable them to understand better the psychological meaning and context of what has happened in the interview.

Newly trained psychiatrists are frequently anxious when interviewing patients. One way they deal with their own anxiety is to try to fill any voids in the flow of conversation by asking questions or making comments before patients have had time to digest and process what has been said and to determine what they think or feel. In this situation, patients are denied an opportunity to reflect and to gain an understanding of what they have experienced.

In a similar fashion, patients often try to please the psychiatrist by continuously verbalizing, in the belief that the psychiatrist wants to have them speak continuously. It is often necessary for the psychiatrist to educate patients that silences are desirable. The psychiatrist must also keep in mind that silences can be a form of resistance, and, in such instances, he or she needs to encourage patients to proceed by responding to those silences with "Tell me what you are thinking."

Interpretation. The psychiatrist works with patients to try to help them understand their motivations and the meanings of their thoughts, feelings, and actions. The psychiatrist examines repeated patterns of behaviors and draws inferences regarding these patterns. Such inferences are called *interpretations*. Several interpretation techniques may be used to help patients. The psychiatrist may lead the patient in the direction of self-interpretation by taking certain pieces of data that the patient assumes are unrelated and helping him or her identify certain patterns. The patient can then piece together these seemingly unrelated events and feelings and draw inferences. In another way of interpreting, the psychiatrist both presents the patterns of behavior and draws the inferences for the patient as a tentative hypothesis, which the patient can then either accept or reject. The following are examples of interpretations:

Patient: Based on what I've been telling you, it seems that every time I face new situations, I develop symptoms that reflect my anxieties.
Psychiatrist: Yes, that's what I've observed.

Psychiatrist: You've just shared with me how upset you are when you can't please your mother. What do you make of that?
Patient: Yeah, every time I try to do something to please someone I want to get strokes from and they don't respond the way I want them to, I get frustrated and angry.

Psychiatrist: It appears that when you can't get your own way with women, you resort to seductive behaviors and then you engage in activities that you later regret. How do you see these patterns?
Patient (long pause): I've never realized that before, but it sure seems to fit.

Interpretations allow patients to advance their understanding of their own behaviors and, by helping them to be more conscious of their patterns of behavior, give them the opportunity to choose to behave or react differently when similar events occur in the future. Newly trained psychiatrists, in their anxiousness to please patients and show they understand them, will often overinterpret patients' behavior and reassure them inappropriately and unnecessarily. The timing and appropriate use of interpretation are best learned under supervision.

Checklist questions. The psychiatrist spells out a list of potential responses for a patient when the patient is unable to describe or quantify to the degree of specificity that the psychiatrist believes is important to know in particular situations, as in the following examples:

Patient: This makes me feel dizzy.
Psychiatrist: Can you tell me what you experience? [open-ended]
Patient: You know—I don't like the dizzy sensation.
Psychiatrist: Do you feel light-headed, or do you experience your head spinning, or do you feel that the room is spinning?
Patient: It's more light-headed—like I'm going to faint.

Patient: I get this pain in my stomach.
Psychiatrist: What seems to bring it on? [open-ended]
Patient: It just seems to come any time.
Psychiatrist: Do you experience pain when you have an empty stomach, or is it after meals, or when you feel anxious?

Patient (pause): It seems to be when I'm experiencing tension.

The psychiatrist uses a checklist of questions when open-ended questions do not yield the necessary information and when more specific information than what has been obtained with the open-ended questions is needed. The checklist format is often helpful for elucidating medical problems.

"I want" messages. When the psychiatrist senses that an interview has failed to progress because of the patient's need to focus on a single theme, the psychiatrist asserts that they need to move on to other areas of inquiry. The psychiatrist is firm with the patient that sufficient information has been obtained about the single theme and that he or she understands the patient's concerns and feelings about that particular topic.

Patient (for the fourth time): These voices—do you know what they're doing to me?
Psychiatrist: Yes, I understand how terrifying they are to you, but we must move on to talk about other areas now, and we can return at another time to discuss the voices. How would that be for you?

By asserting his need to move on, the psychiatrist avoids building up his own resentments and averts acting on his own frustrations with the patient.

Transitions. Once sufficient information regarding a particular part of a patient's history is obtained, the psychiatrist then signals to the patient his or her satisfaction with the understanding of that portion of the interview and invites the patient to move on to another area. This technique is referred to as *transitions*, an example of which is as follows:

Psychiatrist: I understand what it is that brings you here. Now, I'd like for you to tell me something about yourself.

Once the psychiatrist believes he knows about the patient as a person, the next transition would be

Psychiatrist: I have a sense of what you're like as a person; tell me how you get along with people.

This could then lead to the next transition:

Psychiatrist: Now that you've told me about your friendships, please tell me about your family.

These transitions allow the psychiatrist to guide the patient from one significant topic to another while signaling to the patient the areas that are important for the psychiatrist to learn about. Once the patient has given clues that he or she is prepared to talk about a particular area, the choice of ordering of topics is best dictated by the patient. The psychiatrist, by keeping attuned to the patient's readiness to discuss a topic, will orchestrate a smooth transition from one topic to another.

Self-disclosure.   The psychiatrist, at times, will judge that it is in the patient's best interest for the psychiatrist to disclose certain thoughts, feelings, or actions about himself or herself. This self-disclosure may be in response to the patient's questions, or it may occur when the psychiatrist believes that sharing his or her own experiences will benefit the patient.

> Patient: I am uncertain about whether a counselor or a psychiatrist is best suited for treating my problems. What kind of training did you have?
> Psychiatrist: I am a graduate of Northwestern Medical School, where I also completed 4 years of residency training, and I'm certified by the American Board of Psychiatry and Neurology.

or

> Psychiatrist: I've experienced similar problems in dealing with what my doctor should reveal to my health insurance carrier about my history. This is how I handled the situation....

Requests on the part of patients for the psychiatrist to reveal himself or herself are best treated in the context of understanding the individual patient. In the first example, the patient may have been exhibiting a resistance to treatment, in which case the psychiatrist's response would have been very different. If judging the patient's question in that way, the psychiatrist would have responded, "You're wondering whether I'm able to help you with your problems." Such resistance will often be presented by the patient in the form of questions such as "How old are you?" Residents need to understand that the patient's meta-message is "Are you experienced enough to treat me?" Residents need to learn to reflect the patient's underlying concerns back to the patient; in the case above, a resident's self-disclosure that he is 28 years old is not going to be helpful and will be counterproductive.

Obstructive Messages

Obstructive messages tend to interfere with the uninterrupted flow of the patient's verbalizations and stand in the way of the establishment of a trusting relationship between psychiatrist and patient (Table 4–7). These communications are interview techniques that should be avoided. Some were learned in medical school, and psychiatric residents need to be coached in how to avoid using them.

TABLE 4–7.   Obstructive messages

Type	Example
Excessive direct questions	Psychiatrist: What's making you sad? Patient: I've lost a girlfriend. Psychiatrist: Do you cry a lot? Patient: Probably not. Psychiatrist: Did you grieve inadequately? Patient: I'm not sure.
Run-on questioning	Psychiatrist: Is there a family history of mental illness such as anxiety disorders, depressive disorders, major psychotic disorders, dementia, drug or alcohol problems, suicide, and/or personality disorders? Patient: Yes.
Preemptive topic shifts	Patient: I feel suicidal. Psychiatrist: Are you feeling despondent? Patient: I'm terribly depressed. Psychiatrist: Are you having trouble with your marriage? Patient: I can't say.
Premature advice	Patient: I have an upset stomach. Psychiatrist: You may want to try antacids and warm milk at bedtime and six meals a day.
False reassurance	Psychiatrist: You need not worry about your phantom pains—lots of persons with amputations experience the same problem.
Doing without explanation	Psychiatrist: I know what your problem is. You're suffering anxiety from too much stress. Cut back your hours of study. Take these pills three times a day. Start eating three meals a day.
Put-down questions	Psychiatrist: How can you continue to complain about your academic inadequacies when you have all A's and just made Phi Beta Kappa?
"You are bad" statements	Psychiatrist: You keep crying when you mention your mother—hysterics are known to do that.
Trapping patients with their own words	Psychiatrist: You just said you were pleased with your progress; now you're complaining that you're still depressed.
Nonverbal messages of resentment	Psychiatrist turns away from patient, shuffles papers on desk, and closes eyes when patient repeats same verbalization.

Excessive direct questions.   Excessive direct questions represent the antithesis of open-ended questions. They occur when the psychiatrist directs the patient to a single response. This technique does not allow the patient to choose those areas that are of greatest concern to him or her. An example of an excessive number of direct questions is as follows:

> Psychiatrist: Are you a sad person?
> Patient: I think so.
> Psychiatrist: Have you been sad since you were a little boy?
> Patient: Perhaps.
> Psychiatrist: Do you lose your appetite when you're sad?
> Patient: Yes.
> Psychiatrist: How much weight do you lose?
> Patient: Around five pounds.
> Psychiatrist: Does being thin make you sad?

The excessive use of direct questions lends itself to the patient's answering only what is on the psychiatrist's list of questions. It presupposes that the psychiatrist alone knows the issues, priorities, and relevant information. The patient thus becomes a passive recipient of the psychiatrist's inquiries and fails to become an equal partner with the psychiatrist.

Run-on questioning.   Rather than giving the patient a chance to respond to a single question, the psychiatrist asks several questions at one time. The patient may not know which question to answer or attempt to condense all the questions into one and respond with a yes or no response. For example:

> Psychiatrist: Now that we have discussed your depression, have you ever felt the opposite of depressed—where you had racing thoughts, where others have trouble keeping up with your thinking? Have you had spending sprees where you run up huge bills on a credit card? Have you had feelings of euphoria, where you feel happier than everyone around you? Have you gone 36 or more waking hours without requiring sleep?
> Patient: No.

The psychiatrist is lumping together for the patient a series of hypomanic signs and symptoms without giving the patient an opportunity to respond to each one. Such run-on questions suggest that there is no interest in the answers to each of the questions being posed.

Preemptive topic shifts.   Rather than responding to the patient's cues about meaningful events, the psychiatrist moves from one topic to another, seemingly insensitive to what is important to the patient, as in the following example:

> Patient (tremulously): I'm feeling very shaky inside.
> Psychiatrist: Tell me how you get along with your mother.
> Patient: I've been having troubles trusting her lately.
> Psychiatrist: And your father?
> Patient: I don't see that much of him.

Rather than focusing on the patient's shaky feelings and exploring this area in depth, the psychiatrist shifts to other areas that he or she wants to cover and fails to investigate issues that are of immediate concern to the patient. The patient is left feeling that the psychiatrist is unconcerned about the patient's troubles. Preemptive topic shifts may be a conscious or unconscious defense by the psychiatrist when he or she is threatened or unhappy with the topic.

Premature advice.   The psychiatrist may assert his or her authority by telling the patient what to do without sufficient information and without engaging the patient in seeking solutions to his or her own problems. The following exchange demonstrates premature advice:

> Patient: I've been having trouble getting to sleep.
> Psychiatrist: You ought to try running 2 miles each evening and drink a warm glass of milk before retiring, and then read a book that doesn't excite you when you go to bed.

Rather than pursuing what may be the etiology of the patient's complaint and getting details of what may be going on in the patient's life, the psychiatrist advances a series of solutions that may be totally inappropriate for the patient. Such premature advice leads the patient to react with resentment and hinders his or her relationship with the psychiatrist (Balint 1972).

False reassurance.   When the psychiatrist tells the patient that something will or will not occur, and either he or she has insufficient information to draw that conclusion or the clinical situation suggests that just the opposite may happen, the psychiatrist is giving the patient false reassurance. Examples of such an obstructive message are as follows:

> Patient: I've been having trouble with my memory.
> Psychiatrist: That occasionally happens with someone your age, and I know it will improve.

> Patient: I've been hospitalized four times in the last 2 years for my schizophrenia. Will it ever go away?
> Psychiatrist: Lots of people get over their schizophrenia, and you need not worry.

In the first instance, the psychiatrist has no basis for knowing that the patient's memories will improve, but tells the patient something that the psychiatrist thinks the patient would want to hear in order to feel better. In the second example, the psychiatrist is advising the patient of something the patient knows is unlikely to happen, and the admonishment not to worry accentuates rather than alleviates the patient's concerns. Such responses serve to undermine the patient's trust in the psychiatrist.

Doing without explanations. When psychiatrists do something to or for patients without reviewing their rationale and without getting the patients' consent, they falsely assume that patients accept their authority without question and are passive recipients of their ministrations. An example of doing without explanations is as follows:

> Patient: So you believe my problem is depression.
> Psychiatrist: Yes, and I'm writing you a prescription for some pills that you should take twice daily for a week and then increase to three a day for the second week. I will have my secretary set you up for a follow-up appointment in 2 weeks. Call me if you have any problems.

The psychiatrist in this example assumes that the patient implicitly trusts the psychiatrist's clinical judgment about diagnosis and about the precise treatment that will aid the patient without any questioning of authority. Other than in life-threatening emergency situations, psychiatrists as physicians are obligated to describe what they plan to do for or to patients and not only to obtain consent in advance but to elicit patients' cooperation as well.

Put-down questions. Although the psychiatrist may pose a question, the underlying message is one of criticism, derision, or annoyance with the patient. Examples of put-down questions include the following:

> Patient (appears disheveled): I can't seem to find work.
> Psychiatrist: How can you expect any employer to hire you when you're dressed that way?

> Patient: I forgot to take my pills.
> Psychiatrist: Don't you ever want to get better?

In the first example, the psychiatrist is expressing his own displeasure with the patient's dress. Although there is no justification for ever attacking a person's appearance, couching disapproval in the form of a question is an indirect way for the psychiatrist to express his own feelings. In the second example, the psychiatrist misuses the questioning mode as a way of dealing with his frustration at the patient's noncompliance with treatment. By virtue of patients' showing up for their appointments, psychiatrists should assume patients want to get better.

"You are bad" statements. In another form of derision of a patient, the psychiatrist, falsely believing that he or she is making an interpretation, makes a statement critical of the patient:

> Patient: You don't seem to know what's wrong with me.
> Psychiatrist: You keep trying to put the burden of your problem on me; you're a passive-dependent personality, and that's how you deal with all your relationships.

The psychiatrist, in this case, uses a diagnostic term to label the patient, which in turn signifies to the patient that being passive-dependent is bad. The psychiatrist places the patient in a defensive posture while falsely believing that he or she is interpreting the patient's behavior. The psychiatrist in this example is also encouraging the patient to play "word games," which often leads to adversarial jousting.

Trapping patients with their own words. The psychiatrist may focus on contradictions in the patient's verbalizations to the point of trapping the patient. An example would be a patient who protests that he is very fond of a teacher whom he describes as not treating him fairly in the classroom. The psychiatrist then traps him in the following manner:

> Psychiatrist: And how do you feel about this teacher who treated you unfairly?
> Patient: I am furious with him.
> Psychiatrist: Now you're contradicting yourself. Before you said how fond you were of him, and now you claim you're furious.
> Patient: You're wrong—I never said that.

At this point, the flow of the interview stops. The patient gets angry and upset that the psychiatrist has trapped him in a contradiction. The patient was initially denying his angry feelings. Confronting the patient with a contradiction in his verbalizations is counterproductive.

Nonverbal messages of resentment. A psychiatrist may be annoyed at or disapprove of a patient's behaviors. Rather than dealing directly with the patient, he or she uses body language to signal disapproval. For example, a patient walks into the psychiatrist's office and ignores "No Smoking" signs. The patient lights up a cigarette. Instead of confronting the patient's behavior, the psychiatrist begins coughing frequently and frowning at the patient. The patient picks up from these nonverbal cues that the psychiatrist is signaling disapproval. The patient believes that the psychiatrist disapproves of her as a patient. Because of the psychiatrist's behavior, the patient experiences diminished self-esteem and feels demeaned (Platt and McMath 1979; Strayhorn 1977).

Specific Interviewing Situations

Psychiatrists learn to adapt their interviewing methods and styles on the basis of multiple variables that any individual patient presents, including particular psychiatric problems.

Interviewing the Delusional Patient

A delusion is a fixed, false belief that the patient holds to even though it has no basis in reality. There are several types of delusions: delusions of persecution, delusions of grandiosity, erotomania, delusions of jealousy, delusions of reference, and somatic delusions. The psychiatrist inquires whether the patient has ever acted on a delusional belief or has plans to do so.

The psychiatrist's examination of the patient's delusional beliefs will yield significant information regarding the patient's underlying psychodynamic conflicts. The psychiatrist can also observe how the patient defends against painful realities in his or her life and uses his or her delusional system as a form of protection. The psychiatrist looks for the precipitating stresses in the patient's life that led to the formation of these delusions.

The delusional patient is most often brought to treatment by third parties against his or her will. It is important for the psychiatrist to empathically acknowledge the patient's wishes not to be a patient, but also to point out how the psychiatrist may be helpful to the patient and to encourage the patient to communicate with him or her.

The most common error for the newly trained psychiatrist is to try to convince the patient with delusions that his or her false beliefs make no logical sense. Such an approach is counterproductive. Instead, the psychiatrist takes a neutral stance with the patient and neither agrees with a delusional belief nor openly challenges its verity. Only at such a point that the patient expresses doubt about a delusion should the psychiatrist support this doubt. Patients usually do not consider their delusions to be a clinical problem. It is preferable for the psychiatrist to focus on other signs and symptoms for which the patient may want help.

Very often, as the patient's overall clinical condition improves, he or she stops talking about his or her delusional beliefs. It is not necessary for the psychiatrist to raise questions about the delusions, even though he or she may be curious about how steadfast the patient is in retaining the delusions.

Interviewing the Depressed and Potentially Suicidal Patient

Depression, one of the most common problems that psychiatrists evaluate and treat in their practice, can be either a primary psychiatric disorder or secondary to medical disorders or other psychiatric disorders. It is frequently part of a dual diagnosis. For every depressed patient, it is imperative that psychiatrists explore the risk of suicide.

The assessment of depression begins with the patient's appearance and behavior. The psychiatrist observes the patient's general demeanor and posture. The patient walks slowly, holding his or her head down, and lacks spontaneity. Some patients present with an anxious or an agitated depression, with the wringing of hands and pacing. Others exhibit a retarded depression, with a paucity of spontaneous movements. The pace of the interview itself is usually slow, with the patient responding to questions with long pauses and short answers. Very often there is a blunted range of facial expressions, and, at other times, the patient may cry or fight back tears. Not all patients will verbalize feeling depressed. They will often give clues through their verbalizations that indicate a sense of giving up and of not wanting to go on. A depressed patient's thinking and verbalizations are also slowed. Voice intonation patterns are often monotonal. Thinking often reveals excessive guilt, feelings of loss of self-esteem and self-confidence, and a general lack of interest in activities that the patient had previously participated in. These patients exhibit low energy, and their social contacts are diminished as well.

Because the patient often has a number of physical manifestations that are part of the depression, the psychiatrist explores problems with sleep, appetite, bowel habits, sexual functioning, and pain syndromes, among others. The psychiatrist explores the nature of these disturbances and how they have interfered with the patient's functioning. The patient is helped to understand that these physical changes are part of the depression. Because the patient often does not associate the physical complaints with depression, this new knowledge can be a relief.

In exploring the origins of a depression, the psychiatrist looks for significant losses and separations in the patient's life. Death or separation from a loved one often leads to depression. The onset of the syndrome of depression is often delayed following a significant loss. The psychiatrist should also explore anniversary phenomena—depression that occurs on the anniversary of a significant loss.

The psychiatrist takes an active role when interviewing the depressed patient. The patient is encouraged to verbalize what he or she is experiencing. The psychiatrist empathizes with the patient's pain and mental anguish. Prolonged silences on the part of the psychiatrist are rarely helpful with these patients and should be discouraged.

The newly trained psychiatrist is often reluctant to inquire about suicide with a depressed patient, fearing that he or she may be planting an idea that the patient may not have had or fearing that the patient will take offense. Psychiatrists' inquiries about suicide are, on the contrary, a relief to patients. It is essential that the psychiatrist find out what kinds of thoughts the patient has had regarding suicide and whether the patient has ever acted on these thoughts, what plans he or she currently has, and what has kept him or her from acting on these plans.

The subject of suicide is introduced with such questions as "Have things ever gotten so bad that you've had thoughts of ending your life?" If the patient answers in the affirmative, the psychiatrist follows with "Tell me about them." In inquiring about past suicidal behavior, the psychiatrist asks, "Have you ever done anything to hurt yourself?" Again, the psychiatrist pursues details. If all the responses are about the past, the psychiatrist inquires about the present with "Have you had any thoughts of ending your life lately?" The interest here is not only in thoughts or actions but also in the patient's ability to control these impulses. To assess this, the psychiatrist inquires, "What is it that has kept you from carrying out your plans?"

By pursuing the topic of suicide, the psychiatrist arrives at a clinical judgment about the imminent danger of suicide in the patient's life. He or she also learns about what suicide means to an individual patient.

Interviewing the Psychosomatic Patient

Patients with psychosomatic illnesses are usually referred by their primary care physician and rarely seek psychiatric consultation on their own. Their greatest fear is that psychiatric consultation is being sought because they are "crazy" or because the primary physician does not believe that they have a legitimate reason for their complaints.

Psychosomatic patients may interpret psychiatric consultation as a signal that their primary physician has given up on them. It is important for the psychiatrist to discuss with the referring physician what the patient has been told about the consultation and to ascertain what clinical questions the referring physician wants the psychiatrist to address in the consultation. Before seeing the patient, the psychiatrist reviews the patient's medical history, including medications and medical procedures and the results of any tests given.

After introducing and identifying himself or herself as a psychiatrist, the consultant psychiatrist reviews with the patient the complaints that led to the patient's seeking care. The psychiatrist then explores with the patient his or her understanding of the reasons for the primary physician's wanting a psychiatric consultation. The psychiatrist establishes his or her interest in the patient's physical complaints as well as any emotional concomitants and also follows up with the patient in clarifying any misunderstandings about the psychiatrist's role as a consultant.

While reviewing the patient's medical history with the patient, the psychiatrist looks for clues to any psychological stresses that may be accompanying the patient's physical symptoms. The psychiatrist checks for autonomic signs of distress during the interview and inquires about the patient's feelings at these points. As the interview progresses, the psychiatrist reviews the specific circumstances that were occurring in the patient's life when he or she first became symptomatic, any significant antecedent events, and the range of feelings that the patient experienced with the onset of the illness.

The psychiatrist inquires about how the patient's symptoms may be interfering with the patient's level of functioning and looks for both the primary and the secondary gains of the symptoms. The psychiatrist explores what the patient feels is wrong with himself or herself, what he or she fears will happen as a result of the illness, and in what ways the symptoms will interfere with the patient's future life.

Because the patient's presenting complaints are physical, the psychiatrist establishes that he or she is interested in these complaints and that in no way is his or her intention to minimize the significance of the complaints. The psychiatrist acknowledges that subjective complaints are real and that his or her inquiries about emotional concomitants are necessary to gain a better understanding of the patient.

The psychiatrist leaves time at the end of the psychiatric consultation visit to answer specific questions that the patient may have or to clarify any misunderstandings. The psychiatrist also summarizes his or her findings and shares any specific recommendations, including return visits to further explore areas not covered in the initial visit. Usually several visits are needed before patients are ready to accept the importance of the impact of emotional reactions on their physical complaints.

Interviewing the Elderly Patient

Elderly patients often need special attention during a psychiatric interview. Psychiatrists usually need to slow the pace of the interview and may need several short interviews instead of one prolonged interview. They need to pay special attention to any physical limitations, whether sensory, motor, coordination, extrapyramidal, or other. For example, hearing-impaired individuals might need to be seated closer to the psychiatrist. The psychiatrist must speak in clear, loud tones for a hearing-impaired elderly patient to be able to understand him or her. Visual impairments such as cataracts and macular degeneration may lead to elderly patients' not being able to clearly see those interviewing them. Unlike younger patients, with whom an initial handshake may and should be the only physical contact, elderly patients may need to have psychiatrists assist with the patients' safely walking in and out of the room, and a gentle pat on the shoulder or a grasping of elderly patients' hands as a signal of reassurance is often indicated.

The physical status of elderly patients needs special attention so that those with cardiac or respiratory limitations are not overly stressed in an individual interview session. The psychiatrist needs to review medications prescribed and those taken over the counter so that he or she is especially attuned to any drug interactions and aware of the influences of these medications on the elderly patient's mental status and behavior.

Interviewing the Violent Patient

Patients exhibiting violent behavior are most frequently seen in a hospital emergency department setting. The police often bring violent patients to the hospital. One of the first judgments that a psychiatrist must make is the safety of removing physical restraints from patients. Before the police remove handcuffs, the psychiatrist makes contact with the patient to assess his or her reality testing and ability to verbalize. If the patient is judged to be unable to communicate verbally or to be out of touch with reality, the psychiatrist, before proceeding with the interview, requests that the patient be placed in a quiet room where he or she may be restrained. Restraints can be physical or chemical. The psychiatrist first talks with a patient who can communicate verbally about whether to remove restraints. If the patient exhibits any hostile or belligerent behavior when the restraints are being removed, the psychiatrist requests that the restraints remain in place until the patient is calmer. The interview is often conducted with a security officer present, as the officer's uniform is often a deterrent to patients' acting out their impulses. The psychiatrist emphasizes to the patient that the restraints are needed both for the patient's safety and for the safety of persons in the immediate area.

The psychiatrist never confronts or challenges a violent patient. The psychiatrist lets the patient know when the psychiatrist is frightened by the patient's behavior, and he or she seeks assistance in placing a potentially violent patient in a safe setting. On inpatient units, a seclusion room is used as a temporary placement for violent patients until their behavior is judged not to be dangerous to themselves or others.

The key factor in the approach to violent patients is safety. The psychiatrist works with available staff to maintain the safety of the patient, the staff, and other patients. At no time should the psychiatrist resort to individual heroics in trying to subdue a violent patient. Each hospital is advised to have an emergency plan of action for the management of violent patients, with nursing personnel trained to respond to help control violent patients' behavior. This plan should be rehearsed at staff meetings from month to month, because personnel may change or may forget procedures (Slaby et al. 1981).

Interviewing Relatives

The importance of obtaining consent from the patient before interviewing relatives was addressed earlier in this chapter. Interviewing relatives can serve several useful functions. The relatives' observations of the patient's presenting problems, their impressions of his or her current living situation, their understanding of the family, their knowledge of the patient's past history, and their recital of developmental milestones can aid in the diagnosis and add to the psychiatrist's understanding of the patient. Relatives can also serve as valuable allies in the treatment process. They can learn to recognize early signs of decompensation and to seek help to prevent further decompensation. They can participate in treatment and aid with compliance, such as with medications, and they can work with the patient and psychiatrist in noting significant changes in the patient's condition. Such changes can include the onset of manic symptoms, suicidal thoughts or behaviors, and psychotic behaviors. The psychiatrist can assess whether couples or family therapy may benefit the patient. The more serious the psychiatric condition, the more likely that the patient will benefit from a relative's participation in assessment and/or treatment. The relative's participation is contingent on the knowledge and agreement that the psychiatrist cannot, without obtaining consent, divulge to a relative any material that the patient presented in confidence to the psychiatrist. On the other hand, the psychiatrist can share any material with the patient that a relative presents. It is of vital importance to consider involving family members and other significant persons in the treatment of most (although not all) patients.

Past History

The previous section on interviewing emphasized the importance of the psychiatrist's pursuing a patient's history according to the leads that the patient presents. However, when recording the material, a specific format is used. This section provides an outline of such a format for the patient's record.

Identification of the Patient

The psychiatrist begins with a brief report of who the patient is, including the following:

- Full name
- Age
- Race
- National/ethnic origin
- Religious affiliation
- Marital status and number of children
- Current employment (past employment, if the patient is unemployed)
- Living situation
- Total number of hospitalizations (and in each case the name of the hospital), including nonpsychiatric hospitalizations
- Total number of hospitalizations for the presenting problem (if the patient has been hospitalized)
- Names and phone numbers of the patient's primary physicians
- Name and phone number of the nearest living relative

Circumstances of Referral

The psychiatrist describes how the patient came to see him or her, who referred the patient, and how the patient was transported. If a patient is referred by a professional, the name and phone number of the referring agent are recorded. If a third party brought the patient, the psychiatrist notes the third party's name and relationship to the patient. The psychiatrist records his or her judgment of the reliability of the third-party informant.

Chief Complaint

The psychiatrist records verbatim the patient's reasons for seeking help at the time of the initial interview. If the patient is too disturbed to verbalize his or her reasons for being seen, a statement from a third party is recorded and the informant is identified. The chief complaint is not always evident in the first interview, particularly in patients with long, complex histories.

History of Present Illness

The psychiatrist records the chronology of events from the onset of symptoms up to the present. With patients who can give a coherent account of their problems, the psychiatrist inquires when the symptoms began. The patient's highest level of functioning is established, and a description is made of how the patient's problems are interfering with his or her optimal functioning. The psychiatrist examines the patient's functioning in the biological, psychological, and social spheres. The psychiatrist documents all the relevant symptoms with which the patient presents. For psychotic patients, psychiatrists need to structure the interview in a way that will obtain the necessary data and to record the data in an organized fashion.

The psychiatrist also notes the precipitating stressors at the time the patient became symptomatic. For psychosomatic patients, a "parallel history" is a useful technique and is considered when patients are unable to make connections between emotional factors and physical complaints. The psychiatrist draws inferences about the influence of emotional factors on the physical symptoms but does not confront the patient with these inferences. Only when the patient gives clues that he or she is ready to look at the influence of emotional factors does the psychiatrist encourage the patient in this direction.

The psychiatrist also assesses the secondary gains of the patient's symptoms but, again, does not confront the patient with his or her findings.

Psychiatric History

The psychiatrist inquires about the first time the patient was aware of any psychiatric problems. The psychiatrist asks whether any help was sought at that time, and, if help was sought, he or she notes the following:

- Who saw the patient and for how long
- The nature of the treatment

- Medications, if any, that were prescribed
- Modality that was helpful (i.e., individual therapy, group therapy, psychopharmacological interventions)
- Length of treatment
- Reason for discontinuing treatment

Significant events such as hospitalizations, as well as information on where they took place, which treatment modalities were used in these settings, and the length of stay and outcomes should also be noted. Contact with previous treating psychiatrists is most helpful in assisting with understanding past evaluations and treatments.

Alcohol and Drug History

The psychiatrist obtains a history from the patient on the consumption of alcohol and drugs. Inquiries are made about the precise amounts that are consumed and the method of administration, whether it be oral (alcohol), by sniffing (cocaine), or by injections (heroin). The frequency of use is noted. The social setting in which the substances are used is recorded. The psychiatrist learns about the patient's reasons for using drugs—that is, for recreational purposes, to treat or mask one's symptoms (e.g., hallucinations or depression), to succumb to peer pressure, or as part of an addiction pattern. Tolerance for drugs such as sedatives or narcotics is ascertained. The psychiatrist asks whether the patient has ever considered drug taking or alcohol consumption a problem. If so, the psychiatrist learns whether the patient has 1) overdosed on drugs, 2) lost consciousness in the past, and 3) ever suffered from withdrawal effects from drugs. Medical, orthopedic, and surgical complications (including head trauma) as a result of drug consumption are recorded. Any previous efforts toward withdrawal from addicting substances are noted, including problems such as delirium tremens with alcohol withdrawal. The psychiatrist also notes whether the patient has been in psychiatric treatment or has been treated in separate chemical dependency programs, including self-help groups.

The effects of alcohol consumption and drug taking on the patient's life are also evaluated. These effects include the patient's ability to maintain employment, his or her ability to maintain social relationships, and whether the patient has had any trouble with the law, such as charges of driving while intoxicated.

The effectiveness of previous therapeutic interventions is assessed. The consideration of dual diagnoses with other DSM-IV-TR Axis I diagnoses is reviewed, along with Axis II considerations.

Collateral histories are often vital, because drug- and alcohol-consuming populations are notorious for histori-

cal distortions, particularly about the amounts consumed.

Family History

The psychiatrist reviews and records a family tree and lists names and ages of living relatives and names, ages, and time of death of deceased relatives. Any emotional problems as well as organic diseases in family members are indicated (Table 4–8).

TABLE 4–8. Pertinent family psychiatric history

Who had sought psychiatric help and their diagnosis, if known
Psychiatric hospitalizations, if any
What treatment modalities were administered
The names of specific drugs taken, if known
The outcome of treatment
Suicidal behaviors or death by suicide

Family histories are particularly useful in families who seem to have a genetic vulnerability for psychiatric or organic diseases, including schizophrenia, major affective disorders, Huntington's chorea, and epilepsy.

The family history also describes who the significant relatives in the patient's life have been, what they were like as persons, how the patient related to them, and what roles they played in the patient's upbringing, as well as a description of current significant relationships. When obtaining information about the family from relatives, the psychiatrist notes the sources and reliability of each of the historians. The psychiatrist is also interested in assessing who the supportive figures currently are in the patient's life.

Personal History

The psychiatrist obtains information on the patient's personal history in order to help determine a psychodynamic formulation of the patient's problems. The psychiatrist seeks to understand the critical past events that have led the patient to be the way he or she is today as a person. The clues regarding relevant areas to explore are gleaned from the patient's presentations of the present illness.

A patient's history is never complete. The organization of the data follows a chronology of life events.

Prenatal Period

The psychiatrist records information on the patient from conception to birth. The principal family members are described, and the environment and the household before the patient was born are noted. Significant data include whether a pregnancy was "planned," whether the baby was "wanted," what the toxicological and nutritional status of the mother was during pregnancy, whether the mother had any medical problems such as infections or obstetrical complications, and what type of prenatal care she received. Particular prenatal wishes are noted, such as whether the parents wanted a boy or a girl, what the parental expectations were for the child when he or she was growing up (e.g., to be an astronaut), whether the child was replacing one lost through a miscarriage or childhood death, and any other special characteristics that were expected of the child. Learning how names were selected and whom the child was named after (if anyone) can give important clues as to parental expectations. The recording of the father's role during the pregnancy and delivery can also yield helpful information. Data about any problems with the delivery, such as a cesarean section and the reasons for it, and any defects at birth are also important to record. Drugs taken by the mother, whether prescribed, over the counter, or illicit, are important to know.

Infancy and Early Childhood Development

The psychiatrist describes the early infant–mother relationship, noting any problems in feeding and sleep patterns, as well as development milestones such as smiling, sitting, standing, and walking. Infantile illnesses or illnesses of the infant's caregivers are noted, as well as how such illnesses may have affected the development of the baby. The psychiatrist also ascertains who the significant people were in the caregiving of the baby and what particular influences each individual had on the child's development.

Symptoms of unusual rocking behaviors, head banging, screaming, thumb sucking, temper tantrums, bed wetting, and nail biting are explored and recorded in detail. Delays of motor activities, speech development, and socialization are noted.

A description is given of each of the siblings at home and of how the early sibling relationships developed. The psychiatrist looks for the caregiving roles of siblings as well as roles in which rivalries, if any, developed.

To assess social development, the psychiatrist examines the child's play activities. Independent behaviors and the capacity to concentrate and to look for social interactions are assessed. The patient's earliest memories and the events and feelings associated are important to record. The psychiatrist also explores favorite childhood stories and the patient's associations with them, as well as favorite activities and favorite people.

Middle Childhood (Ages 3–11)

The psychiatrist, who is interested in the intellectual development of the child, inquires about nursery school experiences and how the child adapted to social situations. The child's reactions to first going off to school and leaving home are noted. The psychiatrist inquires about important figures in the patient's life: schoolteachers, ministers, camp counselors, and childhood friends. The child's recreational, athletic, and cultural activities are explored, as well as how the child would spend a typical day. Explorations regarding academic development include the child's favorite subjects, subjects that he or she excelled in, and those that he or she found difficult. If the child repeated any grades, the reasons for having done so are noted.

The psychiatrist also records any prolonged illnesses, surgeries, and accidents with injuries and the influence of these medical/surgical events on the patient's life. In children who were "accident prone" or had multiple soft-tissue injuries and multiple fractures, the psychiatrist is alerted to the possibility of child abuse. Patterns of neglect are also explored.

Areas that relate to discipline and the types of punishment that were used are also explored. The psychiatrist learns who the figures were who meted out punishment and assesses the effects that these behaviors had on the child's development. The psychiatrist also explores any significant personal losses or separations during this period, such as the death of significant figures and whether there were any parental separations or divorces and remarriages. The emotional impact of these events is also recorded.

Symptoms reflecting emotional distress are noted. These would include enuresis, nail biting, night terrors, and excessive masturbation.

Late Childhood and Adolescence

The teenage years are important transitional years in the development of the individual from a dependent child to an independent adult. The psychiatrist traces biological development in terms of major body changes and their influence on the individual, as well as the child's psychological development and social development. The psychiatrist inquires about the child's interests and activities, participation in organized sports, hobbies, church activities, introduction to civic responsibilities, work history (often beginning with baby-sitting and newspaper delivery routes), social network, and the influence of religious instruction and the commonalities and differences of the child's belief systems with those of his or her family. In addition to noting the grades and achievements in academic work, the psychiatrist further studies the child's academic potential and his or her areas of special interest and the child's relationship with his or her peer group and with people whom the child likes and wants to emulate, such as teachers, coaches, or public figures.

The psychiatrist examines areas that have led to psychological stress, such as problems in relationships with authority figures, with peers, and with siblings. The psychiatrist also inquires about eating disorders, sleep disturbances, periods of depression, self-mutilation, suicidal ideation, alcohol and drug intake, and problems that relate to the personal identity of the teenager.

Adulthood

The psychiatrist explores the patient's capacities for intimacy, development of friendships, social networks, adult educational history, employment record, intellectual pursuits, recreational activities, and avocational interests. The patient's military history, civic responsibilities, religious affiliations, value systems, political involvements, fiscal security, vacation habits, and relationship with his or her family are also reviewed. The psychiatrist documents what the patient's plans are for the future, whether such plans are achievable, and how the patient intends to implement them. The psychiatrist then records the impact of illnesses, both the patient's own and those affecting close relationships and affecting the patient's life.

Sexual History

The psychiatrist inquires about the patient's early life experiences related to sexual development. The patient's childhood sexual playing experiences, such as playing "doctor" and "nurse," observing the genitalia of other children, and fantasies about sexuality as a child, are explored. The psychiatrist notes not only the child's reactions to these fantasies and play activities but also how family members reacted when the child revealed them or was found engaged in them.

The psychiatrist inquires about what and how the patient learned about sexual activities, conception, and pregnancy and who was responsible for the learning. The reactions of the patient's parents to the patient's inquiries about how babies are born are elicited. The psychiatrist also inquires about a history of sexual abuse.

The psychiatrist asks both male and female patients about their experiences in puberty. With female patients, the inquiries begin with menarche. The female patient is asked about who prepared her for menses, what she was told about what to expect, what the meaning of menses

was to the patient, and what the parents' reactions to the menarche were. For both male and female patients, a masturbatory history is obtained with explorations about fantasies that accompanied masturbation. Descriptions of sexual experiences, both heterosexual and homosexual, are elicited, including activities such as kissing, necking, petting, and sexual intercourse.

Attitudes of the patient toward heterosexual and homosexual fantasies and experiences are noted. The psychiatrist also records parental and sibling responses to the adolescent's activities.

The psychiatrist then explores adulthood attitudes and behaviors: the patient's choice of partner, how the couple met, their courting history, their engagement history, premarital sexual activities, their marriage, and (with traditional marriages) their honeymoon. Also recorded are the couple's expectations regarding children, as well as the couple's reactions to childbearing and child rearing and to different stages of development of their children. Marital crises and threats, or actual separations and/or divorces, are also subjects of inquiry. Similar inquiries are made for patients with nontraditional relationships.

Areas of sexual conflict or sexual dysfunctions are examined, such as loss of sexual desire, inability to perform, difficulties with erections and ejaculations, and problems of pain with intercourse or failure to achieve orgasm. The biological, psychological, and social factors influencing these dysfunctions are sought.

Patients will often be reluctant to discuss some, if not all, of these topics regarding sexuality because of accompanying shame, embarrassment, or discomfort. Psychiatrists learn to be nonjudgmental and supportive in exploring the sexual history of their patients.

Medical History

The psychiatrist reviews the patient's medical history, including common as well as chronic childhood illnesses, conditions leading to frequent medical consultation and treatment, and those requiring emergency department visits as well as those leading to hospitalizations. The psychiatrist also reviews the patient's surgical experiences, noting those requiring the administration of anesthesia. The history of accidents and orthopedic interventions is recorded. In addition to the nature and course of each illness, the psychiatrist reviews the impact of these illnesses on the child's growth and development. Inquiries are made about the patient's attitudes toward the professionals who cared for him or her as a child as well as family attitudes toward his or her medical problems.

The psychological meaning of illnesses and interventions is explored in terms of the patient's feelings about injury to body parts, effects on body image, and fears and concerns about invalidism and death. The psychiatrist reviews adult-onset illnesses, medical interventions, and surgical and obstetrical events. The effects of these on the patient's functioning at work and at play, on the families, and on interpersonal relationships are noted. The psychiatrist also assesses the patient's motivations for and capacities to assist in recovery, his or her levels of denial of the effect of serious illnesses on functioning and longevity, and the coping mechanisms that the patient employs. Inquiries are made about support systems that the patient has used to aid in the recovery from past illnesses, including the availability of these systems and the willingness of the patient to use them to help with the current situation (Table 4–9).

Problems With Psychiatric History Taking

One of the most difficult challenges for the newly trained psychiatrist is learning how to conduct a smoothly flowing interview that allows patients to unfold their stories in such a fashion that they feel they are understood. Simultaneously, the psychiatrist is examining for patterns of behaviors so that he or she can construct a multidimensional formulation of the patient's problems while accumulating the necessary facts and chronology of events to arrive at a cross-sectional diagnosis. In addition to a formal diagnosis, the psychiatrist attempts to obtain a keen understanding of what renders the patient unique and individual in terms of personality patterns and how the patient relates to his or her social setting and environment. Therefore, it is essential for psychiatrists not only to learn pertinent facts in patients' histories but also to learn about patterns of behavior.

The art of psychiatric interviewing develops with practice and supervision by skilled mentors. Psychiatric supervisors are well advised not only to listen to residents' verbal reports of their clinical findings but to experience firsthand how residents conduct themselves in interviews with patients. The supervisors may do this by sitting in the room with residents and patients, or they may elect to observe behind a one-way viewing mirror or review video- or audiotapes of an interview. Telemedicine should add another dimension to this type of learning in the future. The supervisors not only coach the residents about transference and countertransference issues but critique the residents' interviewing style and methods and share with residents their observations of the residents' interviewing strengths and areas that need

improvement. It is also important for supervisors to review the recording of observations and to critique the residents' record-keeping abilities (MacKinnon and Yudofsky 1986).

Mental Status Examination

The mental status examination is a description of all the areas of mental functioning of the patient. It serves the same function for psychiatrists as the physical examination does for the primary care physician. Psychiatrists follow a structured format in recording their findings. These descriptive data are then used to support the psychiatrists' diagnostic conclusions. An outline of the component parts of the mental status examination follows (Carlat 1999; Engel 1979; Keller and Manschreck 1981; Lewis 1943; Masserman and Schwab 1974; Menninger 1952; Reiser and Schroder 1980; Small 1981; Sommers-Flanagan and Sommers-Flanagan 1999; Stevenson 1969; Tilley and Hoffman 1981; Trzepacz and Baker 1993; Weitzel et al. 1973).

General Description

Appearance

The psychiatrist records in detail the prominent physical features of an individual such that a portrait of the person could be painted that highlights his or her unique aspects. Included are facial features; hair color, texture, styling, and grooming; height; weight; body shape; cleanliness; neatness; posture; bearing; clothing; jewelry; skin texture, scar formation, and tattoos; level of eye contact; eye movements; facial expressions and mobility; tearfulness; degrees of friendliness; and an estimate of how old the patient looks compared with chronological age. In the report of these findings, poetic license can be used in painting a picture of the person.

Motor Behavior

The psychiatrist describes the patient's gait and freedom of movement, noting the firmness and strength of handshake. The psychiatrist observes any involuntary or abnormal movements such as tremors, tics, mannerisms, lip smacking, akathisias, or repeated stereotyped movements. The pace of movements, whether accelerated or retarded, is also noted. The psychiatrist comments on the purposefulness of movements and takes note of degrees of agitation of the patient as reflected in pacing and hand wringing.

TABLE 4–9. Order of recording psychiatric history

1. Patient identification
   a. Age
   b. Race/ethnicity
   c. Marital status
   d. Gender
   e. Occupation
2. Circumstances of referral
   a. Self
   b. Primary care physician
   c. Family members
   d. Legal authorities
3. Chief complaint (in patient's own words, what problems led to seeing a psychiatrist)
4. History of present illness
   a. When symptoms first began
   b. Setting in which the symptoms occurred
   c. What aggravates the symptoms
   d. What relieves the symptoms
   e. Severity of symptoms
   f. Life events occurring at the time of symptoms
5. Past psychiatric history
   a. First time that the symptoms occurred
   b. Previous hospitalizations
   c. Nature and extent of previous evaluations and results
   d. Types of treatments
   e. Response to treatment
   f. Highest level of functioning since the initial episode

6. Alcohol and drug history
   a. Estimates of quantity of alcohol and mind-altering drugs, including prescription medications
   b. Effects of alcohol and drugs on behavior
   c. History of withdrawal
   d. Loss of consciousness
   e. History of treatments
   f. Prevention measures
7. Family history
   a. Diagnosis and treatment of psychiatric disorders, including substance abuse, in blood relatives
   b. History of suicide in the family
8. Past personal history
   a. Prenatal history
   b. Infancy and early childhood development
   c. Middle childhood
   d. Late childhood and adolescence
   e. Adult history
9. Sexual history
   a. Developmental milestones: menarche, puberty, menopause
   b. Sexual abuse history
   c. Significant relationships: heterosexual and homosexual
   d. Sexual activity, including masturbation, kissing, petting, fondling, and intercourse
   e. History of sexually transmitted diseases and their treatment
10. Medical history
    a. Allergies
    b. History of medical and surgical hospitalizations
    c. Medical conditions diagnosed and treated
    d. Current medications
    e. Names of primary care doctors and specialists

Speech

The psychiatrist listens for the patient's rate of speech, the spontaneity of verbalizations, the range of voice intonation patterns, the volume in terms of loudness, defects with verbalizations such as stammering or stuttering, and any aphasias.

Attitudes

The psychiatrist routinely summarizes how the patient related to him or her in the course of the interview. The psychiatrist not only notes general impressions such as "friendly and cooperative" but focuses on any shifts or changes in attitude during particular points in the interview. An example would be the psychiatrist's noting that when inquiring about a patient's relations with authority figures, the patient related in a "belligerent, hostile, and threatening manner."

It is also helpful for the psychiatrist to keep track of his or her own attitudes toward the patient, whether they be "warm, caring, concerned, and empathic" or "frustrated and angry." Such a summary of the psychiatrist's attitudes can often help in diagnostic formulations as well as in planning treatment strategies.

Emotions

Mood

Mood is the sustained feeling tone that prevails over time for a patient. At times the patient will verbalize this mood. At other times, the psychiatrist will have to inquire about it and even infer the patient's mood from observations of the patient's nonverbal body language. When describing a mood, the psychiatrist records how deeply it is felt, the length of time that it prevails, and how much it fluctuates. Anxious, panicky, terrified, sad, depressed, angry, enraged, euphoric, and guilty are moods frequently described.

Affective Expression

The psychiatrist records his or her observations regarding the range of expression of feeling tones. The predominant expression is described. This may include flat affect, in which there is virtually no visible expression of feelings during the relating of emotionally charged material. This mode of expression has been classically associated with schizophrenia. The incongruity of the expressions with the verbalizations is most striking in schizophrenia and other psychotic disorders. Constricted affects are often seen with depression, lability of mood may be associated with cognitive disorders, and blunting of affect is often seen with dementia. The psychiatrist observes and records the patient's nonverbal behaviors, such as facial mobility, voice intonation patterns, and body movements, to assess affective expression.

Appropriateness

The psychiatrist judges whether the affective tone and expression are appropriate to the subject matter being discussed in the context of the patient's thinking. Disharmonies between affective expression and thought content are worthy of exploration with the patient.

Perceptual Disturbances

Hallucinations and Illusions

A *hallucination* is a perceptual distortion that a patient experiences for which there is no external stimulus. These hallucinations may be auditory (hearing noises or voices that nobody else hears), visual (seeing objects that are not present), tactile (feeling sensations when there is no stimulus for them), gustatory (tasting sensations when there is no stimulus for them), or olfactory (smelling odors that are not present). Hallucinations during the hypnagogic state (the drowsy state preceding sleep) and the hypnopompic state (the semiconscious state preceding awakening) are experiences associated with normal sleep and with narcolepsy.

An *illusion* is a false impression that results from a real stimulus. An example of an illusion is driving down a dry road and observing "water patches" several hundred feet ahead of you, then driving closer and having them disappear.

Depersonalization and Derealization

Depersonalization describes patients' feelings that they are not themselves, that they are strange, or that there is

something different about themselves that they cannot account for. The symptom is associated with a variety of psychiatric disorders.

Derealization expresses patients' feelings that the environment is somehow different or strange but they cannot account for these changes. This perceptual distortion is frequently seen in schizophrenic patients.

Thought Process

The psychiatrist assesses how well a patient formulates, organizes, and expresses his thoughts. Coherent thought is clear, easy to follow, and logical. A formal thought disorder includes all disorders of thinking that affect language, communication of thought, or thought content. Such disorder is often ascribed to the disordered thinking of schizophrenic patients.

Stream of Thought

The psychiatrist records the quantity and rate of the patient's thoughts. The psychiatrist looks for the two extremes, whether a paucity or a flooding of thoughts. He or she also notes whether there is retardation or slowing or whether there is acceleration or racing. When thoughts are so sped up that the psychiatrist has difficulty keeping up with the patient, it is termed a *flight of ideas*.

The psychiatrist also examines the patient for the goal directedness and continuity of the patient's thoughts. Disturbances include circumstantiality, tangential thinking, blocking, loose associations, and perseveration. *Circumstantiality* is a disorder of associations in which the patient exhibits lack of goal directedness, incorporates tedious and unnecessary details, and has difficulty in arriving at an end point. *Tangentiality* describes a thought process in which the patient digresses from the subject under discussion and introduces thoughts that seem unrelated, oblique, and irrelevant. An example of *blocking* is a sudden cessation in the middle of a sentence, at which point a patient cannot recover what he or she has said or complete his or her thoughts. *Loose associations* refers to a jumping from one topic to another with no apparent connection between the topics. *Perseveration* refers to the patient's repeating the same response to a variety of questions and topics, with an inability to change his or her responses or to change the topic.

Marked abnormalities of thought processes include neologisms, word salad, clang associations, and echolalia. A *neologism* is a word that a patient makes up—often a condensation of several words that is unintelligible to another person. *Word salad* is an incomprehensible mixing of meaningless words and phrases. In *clang associations*, the connections between thoughts may be tenuous, and the patient uses rhyming and punning. *Echolalia* describes a patient's irrelevant parroting of what another person has said.

Thought Content (Delusions, Obsessions, Compulsions, Preoccupations, Phobias)

Thought content refers to what the patient talks about. There are specific areas that the psychiatrist inquires about if they are not brought up by the patient. One important area is whether the patient has suicidal thoughts. This is particularly important in patients who signal feelings of helplessness, hopelessness, worthlessness, or giving up.

Delusions are false fixed beliefs that have no rational basis in reality and are deemed unacceptable by the patient's culture. Delusions that cannot be understood by other psychological processes are referred to as *primary delusions*. Examples include thought insertion, thought broadcasting, and beliefs about world destruction. *Secondary delusions* are based on other psychological experiences. These include delusions derived from hallucinations, other delusions, and morbid affective states.

Types of delusions include those of persecution, of jealousy, of guilt, of love, of poverty, and of nihilism.

In addition to the description of delusions, the psychiatrist assesses the degrees of organization of the delusion. The psychiatrist notes ideas of reference and ideas of influence.

The psychiatrist notes any *obsessions* the patient may have. These are marked by repetitive, unwelcome, irrational thoughts that impose themselves on the patient's consciousness and over which he or she has no apparent control. These thoughts are accompanied by feelings of anxious dread and are ego-alien, unacceptable, and undesirable. They are strongly resisted by the patient.

Compulsions, a closely parallel phenomenon, are repetitive, stereotyped behaviors that the patient feels impelled to perform ritualistically, even though he or she recognizes the irrationality and absurdity of the behaviors. Although no pleasure is derived from performing such an act, there is a temporary sense of relief of tension when it is completed.

In addition to describing obsessions and compulsions, the psychiatrist discusses the degree of interference with the patient's functioning. *Preoccupations* are also noted. These reflect the patient's absorption with his or her own thoughts to such a degree that the patient loses contact with external reality. The degree of preoccupation is also observed. Mild forms are reflected in absentmindedness; severe forms can involve suicidal or homicidal ideation

and the autistic thinking of the schizophrenic patient.

Phobias are morbid fears that are reflected by morbid anxiety. They are often not spontaneously conveyed in the interview, and the psychiatrist should make specific inquiries about their presence (Campbell 1981; Stone 1988; Thompson 1979).

Abstract Thinking

Abstract, or categorical, thinking is formed late in the development of thought and reflects the capacity to formulate concepts and to generalize. Several methods are used to test this capacity. These include testing similarities, differences, and the meaning of proverbs. The inability to abstract is referred to as concreteness, which in turn reflects an earlier childhood development of thought. Concreteness of responses on formal testing reflects intellectual impoverishment, cultural deprivation, and cognitive disorders such as dementia. Bizarre and inappropriate responses to proverbs reflect schizophrenic thinking.

An example of testing for similarities is the psychiatrist's asking a patient how a peach and a plum are alike. The patient who responds "They are both fruit" reflects a good ability to abstract. The patient who responds "You bite into each of them" exhibits a form of concreteness. A bizarre response would be "Juice, plum, like peach, you know."

In testing with proverbs, psychiatrists begin with "Do you know what proverbs are? They are sayings that have different meanings for different people. I will tell you a proverb and ask what it means to you. For instance, 'A bird in the hand is worth two in the bush.' What does that mean to you?" A patient's explanation, "It's preferable to gamble on something small that you know you can win than to take the chance of losing it all by going for a long shot" is an example of a good abstract response. A response such as "Having one bird in your hand—you know—is better than having two birds in a bush" is an example of a concrete response. An inappropriate response would be "Birds fly—one bird flies, two birds fly—fly away birdy—chirp, chirp."

Education and Intelligence

Intelligence is best measured in the clinical interview by the patient's use of vocabulary. The expectations of levels of intelligence are influenced by the level of education of the patient. If the patient had dropped out of grade school and exhibits an advanced vocabulary, the psychiatrist concludes that the patient's intelligence exceeds his or her scholastic achievement. Specific testing for intelligence is used only when deficits are anticipated on the basis of the interview.

Concentration

Concentration reflects the patient's ability to focus and to maintain his or her attention on a task. In the interview, troubles with concentration are reflected in the patient's inability to pay attention to the questions that he or she is being asked. He or she may be distracted by external or internal stimuli. When the patient's concentration is impaired, the psychiatrist often has to repeat the questions.

Formal testing for concentration includes serial 7s, in which the patient is asked to subtract 7 from 100 and keep subtracting 7 from each answer. Serial 3s or counting backward from 20 can be substituted if the patient has cognitive difficulties performing serial 7s. If the patient has been asked to do serial 7s repeatedly, he or she should start subtracting from 101 rather than 100 to avoid giving learned responses.

Immediate recall and concentration abilities often overlap. One way to test for immediate recall is to ask the patient to repeat digits forward and backward. The patient is instructed that the psychiatrist is going to recite numbers and then ask the patient to repeat them. The psychiatrist tells the patient, "I am going to recite the numbers 3, 8, 7, and I want you to repeat 3, 8, 7." The psychiatrist recites the numbers 1 second apart and then asks the patient to repeat them. Once the patient understands the instruction, the psychiatrist recites three other numbers, increasing by 1 the number he or she recites until the patient fails to repeat them accurately. If the patient fails to repeat six numbers forward, the psychiatrist then gives a different series of six numbers. If again the patient fails to repeat them, the psychiatrist stops the exercise and records that the patient was able to repeat five digits forward.

The psychiatrist then conducts an exercise with repeating digits backward. The patient is instructed that when the psychiatrist says, "4, 9, 2," he or she wants the patient to respond, "2, 9, 4." Again, the difficulty is increased by adding one digit at a time until the patient fails to repeat the numbers backward on two trials. The psychiatrist then records how many numbers the patient can correctly recite backward.

Orientation (Time, Place, Person, Situation)

Orientation reflects patients' capacities to know who they are, where they are, what date and time it is, and what their present circumstances are. Patients who have deficits in three spheres are commonly suffering from cognitive disorders. Testing for time includes asking the patient the month, the day of the month, the year, the day of the week, and the time of day and the season of the year. Orientation to place includes the patient's knowing the name of the place where he or she is currently located and the name of the city and state. Orientation to person includes the patient's knowing his or her own name and the names and roles of persons in his or her immediate surroundings. Orientation to situation indicates the patient's present circumstances and why he or she finds himself or herself in such circumstances. This is often an important clue toward the competency of individuals to give informed consent. In reversible cognitive disorders such as delirium, the reorientation to person precedes that of place, and the last function recovered is time.

Psychiatrists introduce orientation testing with a question such as "Do you have any difficulties keeping track of time?—For instance, do you know what today's date is? the month? the year? What day of the week is this? Do you know the name of this place? What is your full name? Do you know my name?"

Memory

Remote Memory

Remote memory is the recollection of events from earlier in life. The psychiatrist tests for this function by asking where the patient grew up, where he or she went to school, and what his or her first job was and inquires about significant people from the past (e.g., naming of presidents) and also significant events (e.g., World War II, the Korean War, the Vietnam War).

Recent Past Memory

Recent past memory refers to recalling verifiable events from the past few days. To test for this, the psychiatrist inquires about what the patient ate for breakfast or what he or she read in the newspaper or asks for details about what the patient watched on television the night before.

Recent Memory

Recent or short-term memory is gauged by the patient's capacity to recount what he or she was told 5 minutes after hearing it and being coached to remember it. The psychiatrist tests this capacity by asking the patient to repeat the names of three unrelated objects, then informing him or her that they will go on to discuss other subjects and that in 5 minutes the patient will be asked to name the three objects (Albert 1984; Folstein et al. 1975; Gurland et al. 1976; Taylor et al. 1980; Yudofsky and Hales 1997).

Impulse Control

Impulse control is "the ability to control the expression of aggressive, hostile, fearful, guilty, affectionate, or sexual impulses in situations where their expression should be maladaptive" (MacKinnon and Yudofsky 1986, p. 74). Manifestations of this phenomenon are verbal and/or behavioral. A loss of control can reflect a low frustration tolerance (MacKinnon and Yudofsky 1986; Yudofsky et al. 1986).

Judgment

Judgment refers to the patient's capacity to make appropriate decisions and appropriately act on them in social situations. An assessment of this function is best made in the course of obtaining the patient's history. There is no necessary correlation between intelligence and judgment. Formal testing is rarely helpful. An example of testing would be to ask the patient, "What would you do if you saw a train approaching a broken track?"

Insight

The capacity of the patient to be aware and to understand that he or she has a problem or illness and to be able to review its probable causes and arrive at tenable solutions is referred to as insight. Emotional insight refers to the patient's awareness of his or her motivations, and, in turn, his or her feelings, so that the patient can change long-standing, ingrained patterns of behavior. Self-observation alone is insufficient for insight. Emotional insight must be applied for change to occur (Donnelly et al. 1970; Ross and Leichner 1984).

Reliability

On completion of an interview, the psychiatrist assesses the reliability of the information that has been obtained. Factors affecting reliability include the patient's intellectual endowment, his or her honesty and motivations, the presence of psychosis or organic defects, and the patient's tendency to magnify or understate his or her problems (Table 4–10).

Psychodynamic Formulation

At the conclusion of the interview, history taking, and mental status examination, the psychiatrist documents a psychodynamic formulation of the patient. The psychiatrist describes the key elements of the patient's personal-

TABLE 4–10. The mental status examination

1. General description
   a. Appearance
   b. Motor behavior
   c. Speech
   d. Attitudes
2. Emotions
   a. Mood
   b. Affective expression
   c. Appropriateness
3. Perceptual disturbances
   a. Hallucinations
   b. Illusions
   c. Depersonalization
   d. Derealization
4. Thought process
   a. Stream of thought
   b. Thought content
   c. Abstract thinking
   d. Education and intelligence
   e. Concentration
5. Orientation
6. Memory
   a. Remote memory
   b. Recent past memory
   c. Recent memory
7. Impulse control
8. Judgment
9. Insight

ity structures, principal psychological conflicts, and healthier, adaptive abilities.

The psychiatrist assesses the ego functions of the patient, including defense mechanisms used, regulation and control of drives, relationships to others, self-representation, stimulus regulation, adaptive relaxation, reality testing, and synthetic integration. By reviewing the patient's developmental history, the psychiatrist assesses the patient's typical drives, impulses, wishes, and anxieties at each stage of development. The psychiatrist can then establish the origins of each of the patient's conflicts and how they carry over to successive periods of development. The psychiatrist focuses on the major adaptive problems of the patient and on how earlier developmental deficits help explain the patient's current difficulties (Freud 1936/1946; Pruyser 1979; Wallerstein 1983; Yudofsky et al. 1986).

Psychiatrists thus trace from early development to the present patients' major conflicts, evolving symptoms, character traits, and defenses. They then organize these data in a psychodynamic formulation (MacKinnon and Yudofsky 1986).

Conclusions

The psychiatric interview is unique among medical interviews in its potential to go beyond mere formulation of symptoms and assignment of a diagnosis. When properly conducted, the interview allows for a thorough understanding of a patient and of how presenting problems relate to this particular individual. The interview represents an opportunity to gain an understanding of the patient in multiple dimensions—psychological, social, and biological. The psychiatric interview allows the psychiatrist to understand the patient and his or her illness.

References

Albert M: Assessment of cognitive function in the elderly. Psychosomatics 25:310–313, 316–317, 1984

American Psychiatric Association: Diagnostic and Statistical Manual of Mental Disorders, 4th Edition, Text Revision. Washington, DC, American Psychiatric Association, 2000

American Psychiatric Association: The Principles of Medical Ethics With Annotations Especially Applicable to Psychiatry, 2001 Edition. Washington, DC, American Psychiatric Association, 2001

Balint M: The Doctor, His Patient and the Illness, 2nd Edition. New York, International Universities Press, 1972

Bernstein L, Bernstein RS: Interviewing: A Guide for Health Professionals. New York, Appleton-Century-Crofts, 1980

Bird B: Talking With Patients. Philadelphia, PA, JB Lippincott, 1973

Campbell RJ: Psychiatric Dictionary, 5th Edition. New York, Oxford University Press, 1981

Carlat, DJ: The Psychiatric Interview: A Practical Guide, Philadelphia, PA, Lippincott, Williams & Wilkins, 1999

Donnelly J, Rosenberg M, Fleeson WP: The evolution of the mental status—past and future. Am J Psychiatry 126:997–1002, 1970

Edelson M: Language and medicine, in Applied Psycholinguistics and Mental Health. Edited by Rieber RW. New York, Plenum, 1980, pp 177–204

Engel IM: The mental status examination in psychiatry: origin, use and content. Journal of Psychiatric Education 3:99–108, 1979

Fenichel O: Ego strength and ego weakness, in Collected Papers (Series 2). New York, WW Norton, 1984

Folstein MF, Folstein SW, McHugh PR: "Mini-Mental State": a practical method of grading the cognitive state of patients for the clinician. J Psychiatr Res 12:189–198, 1975

Freud A: The Ego and the Mechanisms of Defense (1936). New York, International Universities Press, 1946

Garrett A: Interviewing: Its Principles and Methods. New York, Family Service Association of America, 1942

Gill M, Newman R, Redich FC: The Initial Interview in Psychiatric Practice. New York, International Universities Press, 1954

Greenspan SI, Greenspan NT: The Clinical Interview of the Child, 2nd Edition. Washington, DC, American Psychiatric Press, 1991

Group for the Advancement of Psychiatry: Initial Interviews. New York, Group for the Advancement of Psychiatry, 1961

Gurland BJ, Copeland L, Sharpe J, et al: The Geriatric Mental Status Interview (GMS). Int J Aging Hum Dev 7:303–311, 1976

Halleck SL: Evaluation of the Psychiatric Patient: A Primer. New York, Plenum, 1991

Hartmann H: Essays on Ego Psychology: Selected Problems in Psychoanalytic Theory. New York, International Universities Press, 1964

Havens LL: The need for tests of normal functioning in the psychiatric interview. Am J Psychiatry 141:1208–1211, 1984

Keller MB, Manschreck TC: The bedside mental status examination—reliability and validity. Compr Psychiatry 22:500–511, 1981

Kestenbaum CJ: The clinical interview of the child, in Textbook of Child and Adolescent Psychiatry, 2nd Edition. Edited by Wiener JM. Washington, DC, American Psychiatric Press, 1997, pp 79–88

Kosten TA, Rounsaville BJ: Sensitivity of psychiatric diagnosis based on the best estimate procedure. Am J Psychiatry 149:1225–1227, 1992

Leon RL: Psychiatric Interviewing: A Primer. New York, Elsevier/North Holland, 1982

Leventhal BL, Crofts ME: The parent interview, in Textbook of Child and Adolescent Psychiatry, 2nd Edition. Edited by Wiener JM. Washington, DC, American Psychiatric Press, 1997, pp 95–102

Lewis NDC: Outlines for Psychiatric Examinations, 3rd Edition. Albany, NY, New York State Department of Mental Hygiene, 1943

Luborsky L: Principles of Psychoanalytic Psychotherapy: A Manual for Supportive-Expressive Treatment. New York, Basic Books, 1984

MacKinnon RA, Michels R: The Psychiatric Interview in Clinical Practice. Philadelphia, PA, WB Saunders, 1971

MacKinnon RA, Yudofsky SC: The Psychiatric Evaluation in Clinical Practice. Philadelphia, PA, JB Lippincott, 1986

Masserman JH, Schwab JJ: The Psychiatric Examination. New York, Intercontinental Medical Books, 1974

Menninger KA: A Manual for Psychiatric Case Study. New York, Grune & Stratton, 1952

Morrison J: The First Interview: A Guide for Clinicians. New York, Guilford, 1993

Nurcombe B, Fitzhenry-Coor I: How do psychiatrists think? Clinical reasoning in the psychiatric interview: a research and education project. Aust N Z J Psychiatry 16:13–24, 1982

Othmer E, Othmer SC: The Clinical Interview Using DSM-IV, Vol 1: Fundamentals. Washington, DC, American Psychiatric Press, 1994

Platt FW, McMath JC: Clinical hypocompetence: the interview. Ann Intern Med 91:898–902, 1979

Pruyser PW: The Psychological Examination: A Guide for Clinicians. New York, International Universities Press, 1979

Reiser DE, Schroder AK: Patient Interviewing: The Human Dimension. Baltimore, MD, Williams & Wilkins, 1980

Robson KS (ed): Manual of Clinical Child Psychiatry. Washington, DC, American Psychiatric Press, 1986

Ross CA, Leichner P: Residents training in the mental status examination. Can J Psychiatry 29:315–318, 1984

Rutter M, Cox A: Psychiatric interviewing techniques, I: methods and measures. Br J Psychiatry 138:273–282, 1981

Rutter M, Tuma AH, Lann IS: Assessment and Diagnosis in Child Psychopathology. New York, Guilford, 1988

Shea SC: Psychiatric Interviewing: The Art of Understanding, 2nd Edition. Philadelphia, PA, WB Saunders, 1998

Slaby AE, Lieb J, Tancredi LR: Handbook of Psychiatric Emergencies: A Guide for Emergencies in Psychiatry, 2nd Edition. Garden City, NY, Medical Examination Publishing, 1981

Small SM: Outline for Psychiatric Examination. East Hanover, NJ, Sandoz Pharmaceuticals, 1981

Sommers-Flanagan R, Sommers-Flanagan J: Clinical Interviewing, 2nd Edition. New York, Wiley, 1999

Stevenson I: The Psychiatric Examination. Boston, MA, Little, Brown, 1969

Stone EM: American Psychiatric Glossary, 6th Edition. Washington, DC, American Psychiatric Press, 1988

Strayhorn JM Jr: Talking It Out: A Guide to Effective Communication and Problem Solving. Champaign, IL, Illinois Research Press, 1977

Strupp HH, Binder JL: Psychotherapy in a New Key: A Guide to Time-Limited Dynamic Psychotherapy. New York, Basic Books, 1984

Sullivan HS: The Psychiatric Interview. Edited by Perry HS, Gawel ML. New York, WW Norton, 1954

Taylor MA, Abrams R, Faber R, et al: Cognitive tasks in the mental status examination. J Nerv Ment Dis 168:167–170, 1980

Thompson MGG (ed): A Resident's Guide to Psychiatric Education. New York, Plenum, 1979

Tilley DH, Hoffman JA: Mental status examination: myth or method? Compr Psychiatry 22:562–564, 1981

Trzepacz PT, Baker RW: The Psychiatric Mental Status Examination. New York, Oxford University Press, 1993

Wallerstein RS: Defenses, defense mechanisms, and the structure of the mind. J Am Psychoanal Assoc 31(suppl):207–225, 1983

Weitzel WD, Morgan DW, Guyden TE, et al: Toward a more efficient mental status examination. Arch Gen Psychiatry 28:215–218, 1973

Whitehorn JC: Guide to interviewing and clinical personality study. Archives of Neurology and Psychiatry 52:197–216, 1944

Yudofsky SC, Hales RE (eds): American Psychiatric Press Textbook of Neuropsychiatry, 3rd Edition. Washington, DC, American Psychiatric Press, 1997

Yudofsky SC, Silver JM, Jackson W, et al: The Overt Aggression Scale for the objective rating of verbal and physical aggression. Am J Psychiatry 143:35–39, 1986

Suggested Readings

Cameron N: Personality Development and Psychopathology: A Dynamic Approach. Boston, MA, Houghton-Mifflin, 1963

Endicott J, Spitzer RL: A diagnostic interview: the Schedule for Affective Disorders and Schizophrenia. Arch Gen Psychiatry 35:837–844, 1978

Enelow AJ, Swisher SN: Interviewing and Patient Care, 2nd Edition. New York, Oxford University Press, 1979

First MB, Spitzer RL, Gibbon M, et al: Structured Clinical Interview for DSM-IV–Clinical Version (SCID-CV). Washington, DC, American Psychiatric Press, 1997

Glossary

Abstract thinking The capacity to formulate concepts and to generalize.

Affect Range of expression of feelings.

Categorical thinking *See* Abstract thinking.

Compulsions Repetitive stereotyped behaviors that patients feel they must perform in a ritualistic fashion even though they are consciously aware of the irrationality and absurdity of the behaviors.

Concentration Ability to focus and maintain attention on a task.

Concrete thought Inability to abstract.

Countertransference A process whereby psychiatrists unconsciously project their emotions, thoughts, and wishes from their past life onto patients' personalities or onto other material that patients are presenting, thus expressing unresolved conflicts and gratifying their own personal needs.

Delusions Fixed false beliefs that patients hold to even though the beliefs have no basis in reality.

Depersonalization Patients' feelings that they are not themselves, that they are strange, or that there is something different about themselves for which they cannot account.

Derealization Patients' feelings that the environment is somehow different or strange in a way for which they cannot account.

Echolalia Irrelevant parroting of another person's words.

Hallucinations A perceptual distortion for which there is no external stimulus.

Illusion False impression resulting from real stimuli.

Impulse control Ability to keep in check the expressions of aggressive, hostile, fearful, guilty, affectionate, or sexual impulses in situations when their expression would be maladaptive.

Insight Capacity to be aware of and understand a problem or illness and be able to review probable causes and arrive at tenable solutions.

Interpretations Inferences that psychiatrists draw from examination of repeated patterns of behavior.

Judgment Capacity to make appropriate decisions and act upon them appropriately in social situations.

Mood Sustained feeling tone that prevails over time for patients.

Neologism Words made up or a condensation of several words that is unintelligible.

Phobia Marked fear reflected by intense anxiety.

Preoccupations Absorption with one's own thoughts to the extent of losing contact with external reality.

Resistance A reflection of any attitudes or behaviors that run counter to the therapeutic objective of treatment.

Therapeutic alliance A process whereby a patient's mature rational observing ego is used in combination with the psychiatrist's analytic abilities to advance the latter's understanding of the patient.

Word salad Incomprehensible mixing of meaningless words and phrases.

CHAPTER 5

Psychological and Neuropsychological Assessment

John F. Clarkin, Ph.D.

Eric A. Fertuck, Ph.D.

The current methodology and content of psychiatric diagnosis, the level of sophistication of treatment planning in regard to both medication and psychosocial interventions, and the nature of the health care delivery system all influence the context that determines the use of psychological tests and rating scales to inform treatment planning. Two major forces have influenced treatment planning in the recent past: 1) the use of a diagnostic system, since 1980, which has been strong on reliability and relatively uneven and weak on validity, and 2) the impact of changes in the priorities and structure of the health care delivery system with its emphasis on cost saving and delivery of services deemed "medically necessary." Psychological assessment has evolved under these influences, resulting in a diversification of this unique form of assessment. What is relatively new at this point in time are 1) the use of instruments to provide data on patients in a managed care system and 2) the assessment of systems of care as a whole.

In this chapter we discuss the objectives, forms, and utility of psychological assessment and provide an outline for considering the main areas of assessment. We review the most valid and established tests within this structure and present a clinical decision tree that relates both to the referral of patients for testing and to the selection of appropriate tests. Also, we review recent developments in the use of psychological testing in managed care and "evidence-based" mental health treatment.

Definition and Development of Psychological Assessment Instruments

Three types of instruments are currently used in the assessment of patient functioning: psychological tests, rating scales, and semistructured interviews (Table 5–1). Psychological tests are standardized methods of sampling behaviors in a reliable and valid way. The test stimuli, the method of presenting these stimuli, and the method of scoring the responses are carefully standardized to ensure reliability. The actual test stimuli can be constructed in numerous ways. For example, test items on the Wechsler Adult Intelligence Scale–Third Edition (WAIS-III; Wechsler 1997), a widely used intelligence test, include factual questions (e.g., "What does ponder mean?"), and each answer is scored 2 (i.e., to contemplate), 1 (i.e., to wonder), or 0 (i.e., to fret). The restandardized Minnesota Multiphasic Personality Inventory–2 (MMPI-2; Butcher et al. 1989), a highly developed and widely used symptom and personality test, consists of questions about presence or absence of specific feelings, thoughts, and experiences (e.g., "I usually feel that life is worthwhile," an item on Scale 2) in a true/false format. Test stimuli on the Rorschach (Rorschach 1949), a widely used projective test of personality styles and characteristics, are amorphous inkblots (Figure 5–1). The patient is asked to tell the examiner what it looks like or what it reminds the patient of. The response is recorded verbatim and scored with a standardized system.

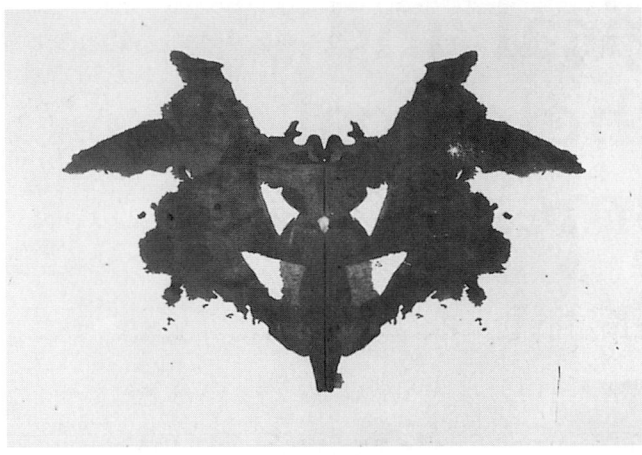

FIGURE 5–1. Rorschach, Card I.

Source.   Reprinted with permission from Rorschach H: *Rorschach Test.* Copyright Verlag Hans Huber AG, Bern, Switzerland, 1921, 1948, 1994.

TABLE 5–1. Three types of psychological assessment instruments

Type	Example
Psychological tests	Wechsler Adult Intelligence Scale–Third Edition (WAIS-III)
	Minnesota Multiphasic Personality Inventory–2 (MMPI-2)
Rating scales	Brief Psychiatric Rating Scale (BPRS)
Semistructured interviews	Structured Clinical Interview for DSM-IV Axis I Disorders (SCID)
	International Personality Disorder Examination (IPDE)

Behavior rating scales are standardized devices that allow various informants or observers (e.g., therapist, nurse on a clinical inpatient unit, relatives, trained observers) to rate the behavior of the patient in specified areas. To aid the observer in a reliable rating of the behavior, anchor points are provided in one of several ways. For example, on the Brief Psychiatric Rating Scale (BPRS; Overall and Gorham 1962), somatic concern, defined as the "degree of concern over present bodily health," is rated by the interviewer on a 7-point scale from "not present" to "extremely severe." Commonly used rating scales, to be discussed later in this chapter, include the BPRS, the Hamilton Rating Scale for Depression

(HRSD; Hamilton 1960, 1967), and the Katz Adjustment Scales (KAS; Katz and Lyerly 1963).

Semistructured interviews are standardized by controlling the questions, including specifying what kind of probes can be used, and standardizing the scoring of the patient's response, often by using rating scales as described above. Although developed for research, these interviews have clinical usefulness in the reliable assessment of diagnostic criteria. As an example of a semistructured interview item, the following is a question from the Structured Clinical Interview for DSM-IV Axis I Disorders (SCID; First et al. 1995): "In the last month, has there been a period of time when you were feeling depressed or down most of the day nearly every day?" The subject's response is rated on a scale from 1 (absent or false), to 2 (subthreshold) to 3 (threshold or true). Useful semistructured interviews include the Schedule for Affective Disorders and Schizophrenia (SADS; Endicott and Spitzer 1979), the SCID, and the International Personality Disorder Examination (IPDE; Loranger 1999).

The science of assessment depends on the development of instruments that meet certain standards. Chief among these standards are those for reliability and various types of validity. Standardization of administration and scoring to minimize the influence of factors unrelated to the area of assessment is essential for establishing reliability. The degree to which a test meets acceptable standards for reliability is evaluated by readministering the test at later times to determine if individual scores remain stable; developing alternative forms of the test that, when compared, provide roughly equivalent scores for an individual; and demonstrating that any subgroup of items from the test yields a score comparable to an equivalent number of items in any other subgroup of items. These procedures for establishing reliability are generally referred to as test–retest reliability, alternate form reliability, and split-half reliability, respectively (Table 5–2).

Demonstration of adequate test reliability is only the first step in test development. It establishes that the test items are sufficiently closely related to one another to provide relatively stable measurements. However, a test's reliability does not guarantee its validity. Establishing a test's validity requires a demonstration that the test measures what it is intended to measure. Three major types of validity can be assessed: content validity, criterion-related validity, and construct validity. *Content validity* can be achieved only if the content of the test can be said to adequately sample the area of interest. For example, an intelligence test must contain items that tap several areas of intellectual functioning, such as knowledge of words, arithmetic ability, abstracting ability,

TABLE 5–2. Types of reliability and validity

Type	Description
	Reliability
Test–retest	Test yields comparable scores at two proximate points in time
Alternate form	Two forms of the same test yield comparable scores
Split-half	Subgroups of items yield comparable score to other subgroups of items
	Validity
Content	Items adequately sample the content area
Criterion related	Test score correlates with other measurements of the same area of activity
Construct	Test measures a theoretical construct and is unrelated to similar but different constructs

knowledge of social conventions, and so forth, in order to meet acceptable standards for content validity. *Criterion-related validity* refers to the test's relationship to independent criteria of an individual's ability in a particular area (i.e., concurrent validity) or to the ability of the test to make predictions about future behavior (i.e., predictive validity). For example, a test of the severity of depressive symptoms would achieve concurrent validity if scores on the test were closely related to a trained observer's rating of the severity of the depression, and would achieve predictive validity if scores on the test were found to be related to the likelihood that a given individual would respond to a specific treatment for reducing depressive symptoms. *Construct validity* can be achieved only by demonstrating that the test specifically measures a theoretical construct of interest and that scores on the test are unrelated to similar areas.

If a clinician needs to determine whether a test will be valid with a patient from another culture, there are specific psychometric procedures the instrument should have undergone. These include translation of the test from English to the patient's native language, subsequent norming and validation of the translated test, and demonstration of the new test's relevance to the target cultural group (Geisinger 1994).

Despite the importance of cultural factors in the assessment process, few tests have been adequately developed to address the test biases that could influence important clinical decisions such as diagnosis, severity of psychopathology, and intelligence/achievement levels. However, the MMPI-2 is an instrument that has been restandardized and normed on adolescents, ethnic minority groups, non-English cultures, and the elderly (Butcher 1998). It is recommended in personality assess-

ment in diverse cultures. Also, intelligence can be assessed in a culturally and linguistically fair manner by using nonverbal tests of intelligence or by utilizing an interpreter during the testing process.

For further information on the general principles of assessment, tests, and test construction, one can consult Anastasi (1982) and Cronbach and Meehl (1955). Also, the Mental Measurements Yearbooks, edited by Buros (1971, 1978), provide excellent reviews of existing instruments. One can also consult Newman and Ciarlo (1994) for criteria that can be used to select instruments for various tasks.

Goals of Assessment

The role of assessment has always been closely linked to the need to conceptualize and implement successful intervention strategies for the remediation of psychological disorders. As a consequence, the goals of assessment should constantly be revised as new treatment methods are developed. Common assessment goals are listed in Table 5–3.

TABLE 5–3. Specific objectives of assessment

1. Clarification of diagnostic uncertainty following clinical interview
2. Specification of the severity of symptoms and other difficulties
3. Assessment of patient strengths (e.g., intelligence, personality traits)
4. Informing differential treatment assignment
5. Role-inducing the patient into a therapeutic stance
6. Monitoring the impact of treatment over time
7. Assessment of barriers to learning for educational planning
8. Assessment of the quality and cost-effectiveness of systems of care
9. Screening for psychiatric disturbance

Diagnostic assessment remains the primary reason for clinical psychiatric referral. DSM-IV (American Psychiatric Association 1994) provides a focus for diagnostic issues and simultaneously capitalizes on and fuels a growing interest in the issues of accurate diagnosis. Much of the research stimulated by the development and implementation of DSM-III (American Psychiatric Association 1980) and its successors focused on the sensitivity and specificity of the diagnostic criteria with the aim of identifying groups of symptoms that are optimally responsive to the growing armamentarium of psychiatric and psychological interventions. This kind of research represented a shift from the idiographic approach, typical of earlier psychiatric research, to a more nomothetic approach. Under the latter approach, the goals of assessment are to relate the individual features of test performance to patterns of performance typical of certain diagnostic groups rather than to highlight the unique aspects of any one individual's performance (Hurt et al. 1991).

For the clinical psychologist, this shift in emphasis suggests that assessment is much more likely to be tailored to specific aspects of the referral and to the salient dimensions of information that constitute the differential. For example, depressed mood is featured as a criterion for a number of DSM-IV disorders, including major depression, atypical depression, bipolar disorder, dysthymia, adjustment disorder with depressed mood, schizoaffective disorder, and borderline personality disorder. Because these different disorders are optimally responsive to different treatments, or because attempts to ameliorate the depressed mood itself may require different intervention strategies for some of these disorders, the goal of differential diagnosis takes on added value. The clinical psychologist, therefore, must carefully choose the instruments for the assessment in light of the need for distinguishing among these disorders.

Differential treatment planning, then, is at the heart of the assessment process and provides the rationale for the diagnostic effort. In the absence of treatment specificity, there is little justification for an intensive focus on diagnosis. Although the science of differential therapeutics is in its infancy, the proliferation of medication and treatment approaches and modalities has spawned a growing literature on the assessment of various characteristics and dimensions that are thought to be essential to the understanding of and rational treatment planning for the various disorders. Often, there is a close relationship between Axis I diagnosis and medication treatment targets (e.g., major depression). The relationship between diagnosis and psychotherapy is likewise closely related with certain Axis I disorders such as anxiety and depression. However, there are many nondiagnostic patient issues that affect the psychotherapeutic selection and process. A recent extensive review of this area suggested that there are six major patient variables that are central to psychotherapy treatment planning: functional impairment, subjective distress, social support, problem complexity and chronicity, reactance, and coping styles (Beutler et al. 2000).

A ready example of this kind of development can be found in the literature on depression. Drawing on the infrahuman learning literature, Beck and Young (1985) have argued that cognitions such as hopelessness, helplessness, and worthlessness are essential for understanding depression. This cognitive theory of depression has been sufficiently well elaborated to lead to the development of rating scales that are sensitive to these cognitions, and to the design of an appropriate treatment approach.

Clinical Decision Tree

With medical care costs soaring in part as a result of indiscriminate use of laboratory tests, a psychiatrist should be clear about the precise areas for assessment before referring a patient for testing. Likewise, clinical psychologists should pursue testing with efficiency and should use instruments that will answer the referral questions with precision, reliability, and validity. Both psychiatrists and psychologists should make use of a clinical decision tree that informs their differential therapeutic procedures.

At the present state of knowledge, we suggest that before referring a patient for assessment, the psychiatrist should complete a semistructured interview (or methodical clinical interview) that elicits information about which DSM-IV criteria (on both Axis I and Axis II) the patient meets. Armed with this diagnostic information, the clinical psychologist can pursue questions about the patient along any one or mix of the axes that we describe in this chapter—symptoms, personality traits, cognitive functioning, psychodynamics, and environment and social adjustment—by selecting and administering tests, interviews, and rating scales with the overall goal of informed differential therapeutics. Which of the five axes the psychologist pursues will depend on which DSM-IV criteria the patient meets and the nature of the pathology that requires further explication.

Psychological assessment currently takes many forms. Depending on the objective of the assessment, the clinician can decide on the types of tests, the number of tests, and the level of expertise required to complete the assessment. By level of expertise, we mean whether the assessment can be conducted by a nonpsychologist clinician or requires the training and expertise of a psychologist. The most common forms of assessment include screening, diagnostic/treatment planning assessment, and neurocognitive/neuropsychological assessment.

Psychological screening is typically done with self-report instruments during the initial evaluation and periodically during and after the treatment process to assess the severity, complexity, and type of distress in a quick, cost-effective manner. The scoring and interpretation of these instruments is straightforward and can be done with reliability and validity by most clinicians. The Symptom Checklist–90—Revised (SCL-90-R; Derogatis 1977, 1983), discussed later in this chapter, is commonly used and recommended for initial and periodic screening in psychiatric settings. If a screening and standard psychiatric interview does not adequately clarify the referral question, referral to a psychologist for more elaborate assessment may be recommended.

The indications for assessment vary with the setting in which the assessment is conducted and the typical patient encountered in that setting. In clinical psychiatric settings, assessment is most often requested to aid in reducing uncertainty regarding diagnosis and in evaluating the severity of specific symptoms or symptom complexes (e.g., depression, suicide intent, thought disorder). Such an assessment plays an important role in providing information on patients that can be usefully generalized by facilitating comparisons between patients or by tracking the severity of symptoms under the impact of treatment. This assessment may form the basis for recommended treatments, help in establishing goals for the general treatment plan, or assist in determining treatment progress and the need for further intervention.

Historically, inpatient settings have focused on the question of differential diagnosis. In day hospital settings, referrals often emphasize the need for assessment of specific cognitive, vocational, and social assets that can be adaptively employed in helping the patient return to full participation in community life.

In general outpatient settings, psychological assessment can uniquely address a variety of clinical issues. Common referral questions include the following:

- *"Does this patient exhibit a thought disorder indicative of a diagnosis of psychosis?"* The answer to this question will clarify whether and what type of medication may be required and the form of psychosocial intervention that is optimal (e.g., an exploratory or supportive psychotherapy).
- *"What is the cognitive ability (e.g., intelligence) of this patient?"* This common referral question will inform clinicians as to whether the patient may require special education and/or whether the patient has the intellectual capacity to benefit from psychosocial interventions, which usually require at least average intelligence.
- *"What type of personality characteristics does this patient have, and how might these affect the patient's ability to utilize treatment—in particular, psychotherapy?"* Factors such as the presence of a personality disorder, a treatment-resistant personality profile, a tendency toward deception, and level of psychological sophistication all can predict treatment dropout, adherence, and success rates. Behavior therapists working in a phobia clinic may be particularly inter-

ested in the interaction between fear and situation so as to successfully plan a program of desensitization. A psychoanalyst may refer a patient for psychological assessment early in treatment to determine the patient's capacity for long-term, psychodynamic psychotherapy and to assess the status of various transference paradigms that would help him or her to tailor the patient's treatment.

Neurocognitive and neuropsychological assessments are increasingly valuable forms of assessment that measure impairments in how patients process information and examine how these impairments might be affected by brain–behavior relationships. In neurology clinics, referral for assessment is frequently made to more specifically identify the nature, degree, and localization of impairment, particularly in children and in elderly persons. Because the symptoms overlap, a common question for referral is, "Is this geriatric patient suffering from dementia or depression?" Different answers to this question will lead to quite different treatment approaches. Another common referral question is, "Is this patient's cognitive profile indicative of possible brain damage such as from a stroke?" Finally, neuropsychological assessment can be used to answer the question, "Does this patient have a learning disability that affects his or her ability to perform academically?" Because of the training in administration, scoring, and interpretation required with neuropsychological batteries, this type of assessment demands the expertise of a clinical psychologist or clinical neuropsychologist and the administration of several tests (a battery) in a reliable and standardized manner. Furthermore, the scoring, interpretation, and synthesis of the information require supervised training. Therefore, these assessments require the expertise of a clinical psychologist, unlike screening assessments.

Cultural Factors in Psychological Assessment

The results from the psychological tests described previously must be carefully considered in the context of the patient's culture, subculture, gender, age, and linguistic competence. The Multicultural Assessment Procedure (MAP; Ridley et al. 1998) is a flexible and pragmatic clinical procedure that allows clinicians to meaningfully incorporate cultural data into the assessment process. The principles of the procedure can be applied to all clinical data, whether from a standard interview or from psychological testing. The four phases of MAP are reviewed in the following paragraphs.

1. *Identify cultural data during the initial interview.* Cultural variables include level of acculturation, economic issues, history of oppression, language, experience of racism and prejudice, sociopolitical issues (e.g., citizenship status, level of political activity), methods of child rearing, religious and spiritual practices, family composition, and cultural values (e.g., attitudes toward time, property, family, work, gender, sexuality, leisure).

2. *Interpret the cultural data.* This phase requires that the clinician arrive at a working hypothesis regarding the impact of cultural variables on the patient's clinical presentation. For example, the suspicion of white culture exhibited by many African American patients can be an adaptive and healthy response to racism in the culture. However, how extreme does such a patient's suspicion need to be before one can diagnose psychopathology? The working hypothesis requires careful consideration of the relative contributions of the patient's current stressors, clinical presentation, experience with racism, psychiatric history, and reality testing.

3. *Incorporate the cultural data.* In this third phase, the working hypothesis is measured against additional data and criteria. This process can include medical evaluation, psychological tests, and DSM-IV diagnostic criteria. For example, does the previously mentioned African American individual meet DSM-IV criteria for schizophrenia, paranoid type, and is his or her MMPI profile consistent with that diagnosis? A yes to both questions would lead the clinician to seriously question the adaptiveness of the suspicious ideation.

4. *Arrive at a sound assessment decision.* Once the working hypothesis has been tested with additional data, the clinician can devise an assessment and treatment plan that meaningfully and fairly incorporates the cultural data. In this manner, the clinician has guarded against cultural bias continuously during the assessment process.

Major Areas of Assessment

To further the overall goal of clinical assessment (i.e., differential treatment planning), one must consider the most important content areas of assessment. The assessment procedures chosen should depend on the nature of the patient's difficulties revealed or suspected during routine psychiatric examination. They should be carried out in the context of the major dimensions of human functioning relevant to diagnosis and treatment planning.

The areas or dimensions of human functioning that seem most central for diagnosis and treatment planning include 1) symptoms and related Axis I disorders, 2) cognitive functioning, 3) personality traits and disorders, 4) psychodynamics, and 5) environmental demands and social adjustment. In the subsections that follow we review the best available instruments in each of these five areas.

Assessment of Axis I Constellations and Related Symptoms

As psychiatric nomenclature has undergone revision, assessment tools have been developed that rely on interviews and self-reports (Table 5–4), providing data that are immediately relevant to diagnosis.

The SADS represents this tradition. Developed in the 1970s at the New York State Psychiatric Institute, the SADS was designed as a semistructured interview instrument to gather information pertinent to the classification of psychiatric disorders. Its primary purpose was to provide information that was sufficient to classify patients into relatively homogeneous subgroups for the purposes of research (Endicott and Spitzer 1979). These classifications were explicated through use of the Research Diagnostic Criteria (RDC; Feighner et al. 1972), which specified explicit symptomatic criteria for 23 psychiatric disorders. These criteria served as the forerunner to DSM-III and have, in the main, been incorporated into that version of psychiatric nomenclature. Using the same semistructured interview format and item rating procedures, Spitzer et al. (1992) developed the Structured Clinical Interview for DSM-IV Axis I Disorders (SCID-I; First et al. 1995), which directly orients the diagnostic process to the Axis I and Axis II categories of the DSM system.

With their explicit focus on psychiatric classification, the SADS and the SCID have acquired all of the problems inherent in adopting the present psychiatric nomenclature as the reference point for assessment. Chief among these problems is the insufficient validation of the diagnostic categories themselves. However, as tools for investigating the range, severity, frequency, and duration of symptomatic disturbance and for training in the formal interview assessment of psychopathology, these instruments are an important part of the assessment armamentarium.

Omnibus Measures of Symptoms

There are a number of instruments that have been developed for the assessment of a wide variety of symptoms (Table 5–5). These measures depend on either self-report or interview methods for data collection.

TABLE 5–4.   Assessment of DSM-IV Axis I disorders

Instrument	General classification	Description	Scoring features
Structured Clinical Interview for DSM-IV Axis I Disorders (SCID-I)	Semistructured interview	3-point rating scales of symptoms	Oriented to diagnosis using DSM-IV

TABLE 5–5.   Instruments for the assessment of symptom patterns

Instrument	General classification	Description	Scoring features
Minnesota Multiphasic Personality Inventory–2 (MMPI-2)	Self-report	566-item checklist, true/false format	T scores for 13 criterion scales
Symptom Checklist–90—Revised (SCL-90-R)	Self-report	90-item checklist, 5-point intensity scales	T scores for 9 symptom clusters
Brief Psychiatric Rating Scale (BPRS)	Clinical interview	16 items, 7-point severity scales	5 factor scores and total scores
Personality Assessment Inventory (PAI)	Self-report	344 items, true/false format	4 validity scales, 10 clinical scales covering symptoms and severe personality disorders
Millon Clinical Multiaxial Inventory–III (MCMI-III)	Self-report	175 items, true/false format	3 validity scales, 22 clinical scales covering Axis I and II areas

Minnesota Multiphasic Personality Inventory.   The MMPI (Hathaway and McKinley 1967) and its successor, the MMPI-2 (Hathaway and McKinley 1989), are probably the most widely used assessment instruments in existence. There are several reasons for the MMPI's extensive use, including its efficiency (the patient spends 1–2 hours taking the test, which can then be computer scored), the extensive data accumulated with the test, its normative base, the use of validity scales that indicate the patient's test-taking attitude, and its impressive cross-cultural validation. Although labeled as a personality test, the MMPI was constructed to assess what are now categorized as Axis I conditions and, to a lesser extent, a few dimensions of personality that are not represented on Axis II.

The MMPI was developed in the 1940s by J. Charnley McKinley, a psychiatrist, and Starke R. Hathaway, a psychologist. Items were generated from lists of psychiatric symptoms and complaints found in the current textbooks of psychiatry and previously constructed personality inventories. Beginning with a large pool of such items, McKinley and Hathaway used the method of contrasting criterion groups to construct several psychopathological scales. For example, a hypochondriasis scale measuring the degree of concern with bodily health was developed on the basis of items frequently endorsed by patients with hypochondriasis uncomplicated by psychosis or other psychiatric disorders. The patients' responses to the MMPI items were contrasted to those of friends or relatives who visited the University Hospitals in Minneapolis. Using this method of criterion-keyed scoring, McKinley and Hathaway constructed nine clinical scales: hypochondriasis (Hs, or Scale 1), depression (D, or Scale 2), hysteria (Hy, or Scale 3), psychopathic deviance (Pd, or Scale 4), masculinity–femininity (Mf, or Scale 5), paranoia (Pa, or Scale 6), psychasthenia (Pt, or Scale 7), schizophrenia (Sc, or Scale 8), and mania (Ma, or Scale 9) (Table 5–6). Items were worded so that persons with an elementary school education could take the test, and norms were established for determining the degree of disturbance typical of psychopathological groups. For example, an item on Scale 2 (i.e., depression) reads as follows: I find it hard to keep my mind on a task or job (True).

In addition to the clinical scales, validity scales were developed to assess the test-taking attitudes of the patient. McKinley et al. (1948) focused on the assessment of defensiveness or of minimizing symptoms and problems (faking good) and maximizing or exaggerating problems (faking bad). Validity scales were constructed to evaluate these dimensions, which are helpful in interpreting the severity of symptomatic complaints on the clinical scales.

The MMPI has been revised and restandardized as the MMPI-2. Revisions include the deletion of objectionable items and the rewording of other items to reflect more modern language usage, as well as the addition of several new items focusing on suicide, drug and alcohol abuse,

TABLE 5–6. Scales of the Minnesota Multiphasic Personality Inventory–2 (MMPI-2)

Scale	Characteristics of high scorers
Validity scales	
Lie	Dishonest, deceptive, and/or defended
Infrequency	Exhibit randomness of responses or psychotic psychopathology
Correction/defensiveness	Defensive through presenting themselves as healthier than they are
Clinical scales	
1. Hypochondriasis	Somatizers, possible medical problems
2. Depression	Dysphoric, possibly suicidal
3. Hysteria	Highly reactive to stress, anxious, and sad at times
4. Psychopathic deviate	Antisocial, dishonest, possible drug abusers
5. Masculinity–femininity	Exhibit lack of stereotypical masculine interests, aesthetic and artistic
6. Paranoia	Exhibit disturbed thinking, ideas of persecution, possibly psychotic
7. Psychasthenia	Exhibit psychological turmoil and discomfort, extreme anxiety
8. Schizophrenia	Confused, disorganized, possible hallucinations
9. Hypomania	Manic, emotionally labile, unrealistic self-appraisal
10. Social introversion	Very insecure and uncomfortable in social situations, timid

Type A behavior, interpersonal relations, and treatment compliance. Restandardization of the norms was based on a randomly solicited national sample of 1,138 males and 1,462 females.

Clinical interpretation of the MMPI-2 is not, however, simply a matter of noting a scale that is high relative to these norms and assigning that diagnosis to the patient (e.g., a patient with a high Sc, or Scale 8, score would not necessarily receive a schizophrenia diagnosis). Instead, relying on an extensive clinical database, typical symptomatic and personality dysfunctions are described on the basis of 2- and 3-point codes (Dahlstrom et al. 1972; Greene 1991; Marks et al. 1974). For example, individuals with a 2–4–8 three-point code (scores above 70 on Scales 2, 4, and 8) are described as typically distrustful of people, keeping others at a distance, afraid of emotional involvement, using projection and rationalization as defenses, argumentative and sensitive to anything that can be construed as a demand, and unpredictable and changeable in behavior and attitudes (Marks and Seeman 1963). Research has indicated that many patients with this code exhibit symptoms that fulfill criteria for borderline personality disorder (Hurt et al. 1985).

Personality Assessment Inventory. The Personality Assessment Inventory (PAI; Morey 1991), focuses on clinical syndromes that have been staples of psychopathological nosology and have retained their importance in contemporary diagnostic practice. Items were written with careful attention to their content validity, which was designed to reflect the phenomenology of the clinical construct across a broad range of severity. An initial pool of 2,200 items was generated from the research literature, classic texts, the DSM, and other diagnostic manuals and from the clinical experience of practitioners who participated in the project. This pool of items was finally reduced to 344 items covering 4 validity scales, 11 clinical syndromes, 5 treatment planning areas, and the 2 major dimensions of the interpersonal complex. All items are rated with a 4-point Likert-type response format. For example, on the borderline scale is the following item: "I'm too impulsive for my own good." Final clinical validation was carried out on the data from 235 subjects from 10 clinical sites and 2 community and 2 college-student samples.

Symptom Checklist–90—Revised. The SCL-90-R (Derogatis 1994) is a relatively recent revision of a much-used self-report instrument designed to provide information about a broad range of complaints typical of individuals with psychological symptomatic distress. Briefer than the MMPI-2 and the PAI, the SCL-90-R contains only 90 items and can be administered in 30 minutes and scored by computer. These items are combined into nine symptom scales: 1) somatization, 2) obsessive-compulsive behavior, 3) interpersonal sensitivity, 4) depression, 5) anxiety, 6) hostility, 7) phobic anxiety, 8) paranoid ideation, and 9) psychoticism. In addition, three global indices are compiled: 1) general severity, 2) positive symptom distress index, and 3) total positive symptoms. The criterion group method was not used in the development of this test. Rather, the content validity and internal consistency of the items guided the construction of the scales.

A companion instrument, the Hopkins Psychiatric Rating Scale (HPRS; Derogatis et al. 1974), can be used to rate material obtained through direct interview of the patient on each of the nine symptom dimensions of the SCL-90-R. No structured interview procedure is associated with the HPRS, so formal training in the interview assessment of psychopathology is essential to the accuracy of the assessment. Eight additional dimensions are covered in the interview.

Brief Psychiatric Rating Scale. Another widely used rating scale for a range of psychiatric symptoms is the Brief Psychiatric Rating Scale (BPRS; Overall and Gorham 1962), which was developed mainly for the assessment of symptoms with an inpatient population. Areas rated include somatic concern, anxiety, emotional withdrawal, conceptual disorganization, guilt, tension, mannerisms and posturing, grandiosity, depressive mood, hostility, suspiciousness, hallucinatory behavior, motor retardation, uncooperativeness, unusual thought content, blunted affect, excitement, and disorientation.

The MMPI-2, PAI, SCL-90-R, HPRS, and BPRS represent efforts to develop procedures for the general assessment of psychopathology that meet standards of test construction. These procedures provide coverage of symptomatically distressing areas that are independent of psychiatric classifications. However, through the extensive use of these procedures in psychiatric settings, a large body of literature has developed that relates the findings of these tests to diagnostic categories favored in such settings.

Specific Areas of Symptomatology

In addition to the omnibus measures of symptomatology, there are a number of instruments that assess one area of symptomatology in depth (Table 5–7). The major constellations of symptoms that may require assessment are 1) substance abuse, including abuse of food, alcohol, and drugs; 2) affects such as anxiety, elation, and depression; 3) thought disorder; and 4) suicidal intentions and behaviors.

Substance abuse. Psychological distress and dysfunction arising from the abuse of a wide variety of substances is perhaps the chief reason for seeking psychological or psychiatric treatment. The treatment of alcoholism, drug abuse, and eating disorders, combined with the income lost, probably consumes more health dollars than does any other group of disorders. Thus, the identification of these disorders deserves careful attention. The threat to the validity of self-report screening instruments to detect substance abuse is such that these instruments should be buttressed by urine screens and interview (Greene and Banken 1995). However, it is helpful to review the instruments that have been used for this purpose. The

prominent instruments in this area are the MacAndrew Alcoholism Scale (MacAndrew 1965), the Addiction Potential Scale from the MMPI-2 (Weed et al. 1992), and Scales B and T from the Millon Clinical Multiaxial Inventory—III (MCMI-III; Millon et al. 1997).

The assessment of substance abuse potential is reflected in omnibus symptom rating scales such as the MMPI-2, which contains an item key, the MacAndrew Alcoholism Scale, for identifying patients who have histories of alcohol abuse or who have the potential to develop problems with alcohol (Hoffmann et al. 1974). A more thorough instrument, the Alcohol Use Inventory (AUI; Horn et al. 1986), is a self-administered test standardized on over 1,200 admissions to an alcoholism treatment program. It contains 24 scales that measure alcohol-related problems and considers the subjects' responses in four separate domains: benefits from drinking, style of drinking, consequences of drinking, and concerns associated with drinking.

Garner has developed an inventory to assess attitudes and behaviors associated with anorexia nervosa. This inventory, the Eating Disorders Inventory–2 (EDI-2; Garner 1992), consists of 91 items rated on 6-point frequency scales. The items were chosen to reflect important clinical aspects of anorexia and were retained if they successfully discriminated between anorexic, normal-weight, and obese males and females. Internal reliability, construct validity, and treatment response data have been reported, and the EDI-2 can be a useful screening instrument for identifying inpatients with potentially serious eating disorders.

Affects. The content, range, and management of emotional expression constitute a symptomatic area of focus for the evaluation of psychopathology and are important in the differential diagnosis of a wide variety of psychiatric disorders. The main affects of interest are anxiety, depression, aggression, and elation.

As one factor in the larger context of the total personality, anxiety can be assessed with the 16–Personality Factor Inventory (16-PF; Cattell et al. 1970), the Eysenck Personality Inventory (EPI; Eysenck and Eysenck 1969), and the Taylor Manifest Anxiety Scale (TMAS; Taylor-Spence and Spence 1966), a scale derived from the MMPI.

Other instruments assess only anxiety or other forms of fearfulness and thus may be more clinically useful as dimensional measures of the severity of anxiety or in the identification of specific situational anxiety that will become the focus of intervention. The Anxiety Status Inventory (ASI) is a rating scale for anxiety developed for clinical use adhering to an interview guide, and the Self-

TABLE 5–7. Instruments for the assessment of specific symptom areas

Instrument	General classification	Description	Scoring features
Substance abuse			
Alcohol Use Inventory	Self-report	228 items rated on 2–6 point scales	17 primary scales in four areas and 7 second-order factor scales
Eating Disorders Inventory–2	Self-report	91 forced-choice items rated on a 6-point frequency scale	8 subscales and 3 provisional scales for issues and features pertinent to eating disorders
Affects			
State–Trait Anxiety Inventory	Self-report	Two 20-item scales, 4-point frequency ratings	Total scores for state and trait anxiety
S-R Inventory of Anxiousness	Self-report	14-item responses on 5-point severity scales to 11 situations	Focus on intensity and quality of situations arousing anxiety
Fear Questionnaire	Self-report	17 items reflecting specific phobias rated on 9-point avoidance scales	Total scores for agoraphobia, social phobia, and blood and injury phobias
Beck Depression Inventory	Self-report	20 items, 4-point intensity scales	Total score
Hamilton Rating Scale for Depression	Clinical interview	17–24 items, 3- to 5-point severity scales	Total score
Manic-State Rating Scale	Observer rating	26 items, each scored for frequency and intensity	Total score
State-Trait Anger Inventory	Self-report		Total scores for state and trait anger
Suicidal behavior			
Suicide Intent Scale	Self-report	15 items, 3-point categorical scales	Total score
Index of Potential Suicide	Self-report or semistructured interview	50 items, 5-point severity scales	Total score and 6 subscores
Reasons for Living Inventory	Self-report	6 factors	Total score
Thought disorder			
Thought Disorder Index	Content rating	22 categories at 4 levels of severity	Total score

Rating Anxiety Scale (SRAS) is a companion self-report instrument, both developed by Zung (1971). Both scales assess a wide range of anxiety-related behaviors: fear, panic, physical symptoms of fear, nightmares, and cognitive effects. These scales are recommended for the serial measurement of the effects of therapy on anxiety states. Hamilton (1959) devised an anxiety rating scale parallel to the HRSD but less frequently used.

The State-Trait Anxiety Inventory (STAI; Spielberger et al. 1976) is a self-report instrument in which patients are asked to report on anxiety in general (i.e., trait) and at particular points in time (i.e., state). The Endler S-R Inventory of Anxiousness (Endler et al. 1962) is a self-report measure of the interaction between the patient's anxiety and environmental situations such as interpersonal, physically dangerous, and ambiguous situations. This instrument has been widely used as a therapy outcome measure and is recommended as an instrument that

may be helpful in tailoring treatment to the specific circumstances of the patient's anxiety.

The Liebowitz Social Anxiety Scale (LSAS; Liebowitz 1987) is a clinician-administered semistructured interview that assesses social phobias. The instrument covers a wide range of fears and avoidance across social and performance situations. The LSAS has potential clinical usefulness in the development of a fear hierarchy and the assessment of treatment progress for patients with social phobias. A similar instrument is the Brief Social Phobia Scale (BSPS; Davidson et al. 1991), an 11-item semistructured interview constructed to assess severity and treatment response of social phobias.

The measurement of the severity of obsessive-compulsive symptoms is often accomplished with the widely used Yale-Brown Obsessive Compulsive Scale (Y-BOCS; Goodman et al. 1989). There are two subscales in this clinician-administered semistructured interview, an obsessions subscale and a compulsions subscale. The instrument has been demonstrated to reliably discriminate between subjects with and without obsessive-compulsive disorder and to be sensitive to change.

A useful self-report instrument for quantifying the presence and severity of posttraumatic stress disorder symptoms is the Posttraumatic Stress Diagnostic Scale (PDS) devised by Foa (1995). This instrument can be used for screening and can be supplemented with an associated clinician-administered structured interview, the Clinician-Administered PTSD Scale (CAPS; Blake et al. 1990), when the accuracy of patient self-report data are in doubt.

The Beck Depression Inventory (BDI; Beck et al. 1988) is probably the most widely used self-report inventory of depression. The original scale was administered in an interviewer-assisted manner, but a later version is completely self-administered. The 21 items of the inventory were selected to represent symptoms commonly associated with a depressive disorder. The rating of each item relies on the endorsement of one or more of four statements listed in order of symptom severity. Item categories include mood, pessimism, crying spells, guilt, self-hate and accusations, irritability, social withdrawal, work inhibition, sleep and appetite disturbance, and loss of libido. The content of the BDI emphasizes pessimism, a sense of failure, and self-punitive wishes. This emphasis is consistent with Beck's cognitive view of depression and its causes. This self-report instrument is frequently used in conjunction with the HRSD, which allows a clinician to rate the severity of depressive symptoms during an interview with the patient. In contrast to the BDI, the HRSD is more systematic in assessing neurovegetative signs. Although only rough interview guidelines for using the HRSD are available, interrater reliability is generally good.

The Manic-State Rating Scale (MSRS; Beigel et al. 1971) is a 26-item observer-rated scale that is useful with patients with bipolar depression. Eleven items reflecting elation–grandiosity and paranoid–destructive features of manic patients have produced the most consistent results and have been applied successfully in the prediction of inpatient lengths of stay (Young et al. 1978). The scale has demonstrated adequate reliability and concurrent validity, and it can detect clinical change (Janowsky et al. 1978). Secunda et al. (1985) have used similar items from several instruments employed in the National Institute of Mental Health Clinical Research Branch Collaborative Program on the psychobiology of depression to develop indices for responsiveness to lithium treatment in manic patients. A newer rating scale, the Internal State Scale (ISS; Bauer et al. 1991), is a self-report instrument that allows individuals to rate the present state of 17 items reflecting bipolar symptomatology.

Aggressive behavior, including aggressive imagery and hostile affect, is an important area in treatment planning both for the individual patient and for the general concepts that the inventory assesses. The Buss–Durkee Hostility Inventory (Buss and Durkee 1957) is a 75-item self-report questionnaire that measures different aspects of hostility and aggression. There are eight subscales: assault, indirect hostility, irritability, negativism, resentment, suspicion, verbal hostility, and guilt. Some norms exist for clinical populations. Megargee et al. (1967) developed an overcontrolled hostility scale using MMPI items. A review of studies involving this scale (Greene 1991) suggests that it can be used to screen for patients who display excessive control of their hostile impulses and are socially alienated. Spielberger has developed a State–Trait Anger Expression Inventory (STAEI; Spielberger 1991; Spielberger et al. 1976) that takes about 15 minutes to complete. This 44-item scale divides behavior into state anger (i.e., current feelings) and trait anger (i.e., disposition toward angry reactions), and the latter area has subscales for angry temperament and angry reaction (sample items: "How I feel right now: I feel irritated"; "How I generally feel: I fly off the handle").

The Overt Aggression Scale–Modified (OAS-M; Coccaro et al. 1991) is a semistructured clinician interview that assesses aggression, irritability, and suicidality in the past week. The OAS-M is intended for outpatients, and it is adapted from the original OAS, which was developed for inpatients (Yudofsky et al. 1986). Given its focus on actual behaviors and the time span of the previous week, the instrument would be most useful in assessing patient change in these areas.

Thought disorder. One approach to the reliable assessment of cognition is the use of semistructured interviews such as the SADS and the SCID. The presence or absence of disorders of thinking such as thought derailment or frank hallucinations or delusions is determined during the course of an extensive interview. There are obvious problems with this approach. Many individuals may not wish to reveal frank delusional experiences, or they may be unaware of the presence of more subtle varieties of disordered thinking. To avoid these pitfalls, an alternative approach is to obtain a sample of the thought process. The test most widely used in examinations for thought disorders has been the Rorschach inkblot test, which was developed by the Swiss psychiatrist Hermann Rorschach. In this test, a relatively ambiguous stimulus (a colored or achromatic "inkblot") is used, and, without additional instruction, individuals are asked to state what the blot looks like to them. Responses are scored for location (i.e., the area of the card that elicits a response), determinants (i.e., form, movement, color, and shading), form quality (i.e., the degree to which percepts are congruent with the area chosen), and content (e.g., human, animal, object). Exner (1974, 1978) has developed a scoring system that attempts to integrate the best aspects of prior systems.

Holzman and his colleagues have published extensively on the relationship of various forms of thought disorder and its severity to psychiatric diagnosis and treatment (Hurt et al. 1983; Johnston and Holzman 1979; Solovay et al. 1986). Although the scoring scheme can be applied to any record of verbal production, its most frequent application has been in the context of verbal records from the administration of such tests as the WAIS-III and the Rorschach. In its present version, the Thought Disorder Index (Solovay et al. 1986) considers 22 forms of thought disturbance ranging across four levels of severity as the basis for a total score. The total score has been found to distinguish psychotic from nonpsychotic patients, and more severe forms of thought disorder have been most frequently associated with schizophrenic disorders. A recent report indicates a strong relationship between the degree of hypertrophy of the left posterior superior temporal gyrus, noticeable with magnetic resonance imaging, and the severity of thought disorder in schizophrenia patients (Shenton et al. 1992).

In addition to the work of Holzman and his colleagues, Harrow and associates have developed another battery, consisting of three tests, to quantify thought disorder. This work has considered patients with clinical diagnoses of schizophrenia, affective disorder, and schizoaffective disorder. In a series of studies, these investigators addressed the persistence of thought disorders in treated groups who had been followed for a period of 2–4 years (Harrow and Quinlan 1985; Marengo and Harrow 1985).

Suicidal behavior. The suicide potential of patients has obvious treatment and management implications for the clinician. Suicidal threats, suicidal planning and/or preparation, suicidal ideation, and recent parasuicidal behavior are all direct indicators of current risk and should be assessed thoroughly and specifically in the clinical interview. In addition, self-report instruments that focus specific and detailed attention on known predictors of suicidal behavior are sometimes clinically useful. Thus, it is recommended that the assessment of suicidal behavior be embedded in an assessment package that involves interview and use of instruments (Bongar 1991).

With that caveat in mind, suicidal assessment instruments that are frequently used include the Beck Hopelessness Scale and the Beck Suicide Intent Scale. In addition, it should be noted that the Koss–Butcher critical item set revised on the MMPI is a list of 22 items that are related specifically to the depressed, suicidal ideation. These critical items should not be seen as scales, but rather as markers of particular item content that might be significant in assessing the individual patient (Butcher 1989).

The Suicide Intent Scale (SIS; Beck et al. 1974), the Index of Potential Suicide (Zung 1974), and the Suicide Probability Scale (SPS; Cull and Gill 1986) are three widely used instruments. A complementary approach has been taken, culminating in the development of the Reasons for Living Inventory (RFL; Linehan et al. 1983). Of practical interest is that the fear-of-suicide subscale in the RFL differentiates between those who have only considered suicide and those who have made previous suicide attempts. Individuals scoring high on reasons for living and on subscales measuring survival and coping skills, responsibility to family, and child-related concerns were less likely to attempt suicide.

Assessment of Cognitive Functioning

The development of clinical assessment procedures for the investigation of brain–behavior relationships has been an active area of psychological investigation. Because impairment to different areas of the brain results in disorders in higher cortical functions in humans, clinical neuropsychology has been able to develop assessment procedures that consider both the localization and the degree of functional impairment as the focus for test development. Present-day neuropsychological assessment procedures in the United States can be traced to the pioneering work begun in the 1930s by such investigators as Ward Halstead and Joseph Wepman at the University of Chicago. These early investigators were concerned with the localization and degree of functional impairment in neurologically impaired populations. In recent years, the extension of these procedures to the assessment of less clearly anatomically based functional disorders characteristic of clinical psychiatric populations has occurred (Clarkin and Mattis 1991).

Application of these procedures beyond the arena in which they were first developed has introduced difficulties in the interpretation of the results of such procedures. These procedures are sensitive to abnormalities of brain function due to the direct alteration of brain tissue. For example, among chronically schizophrenic patients, the degree of neuropsychological dysfunction has been found to be correlated with structural abnormalities on computed tomography scan (Seidman 1983). In other psychiatric groups in which the evidence for structural abnormalities is less clear, the degree to which these disorders interfere with performance on these tests by mechanisms other than structural abnormalities of brain tissue is as yet unclear. There is increasing evidence that some schizophrenic and affective disorders that were traditionally considered functional psychoses may result from as yet poorly understood abnormalities of brain biochemistry (Barchas et al. 1977), and modern imaging techniques such as positron emission tomography and magnetic resonance imaging have begun to produce evidence of alterations in brain functioning that may be relatively specific to traditional functional psychiatric diagnoses. The relationships between these biochemical and neurophysiological findings and the quality and severity of functional impairment identified through neuropsychological assessments remain to be clarified.

In general, one assesses specific cognitive abilities in psychiatric patients for two reasons: 1) to document disorders in cognitive skills referable to primary or concomitant neurogenic disorder (e.g., discriminating between a thought disorder and a language disorder or the mnemonic deficits of a depression versus a dementia), or 2) to document a specific disorder in cognition referable to a specific class of psychiatric disorders (e.g., intrusion into thought of task-irrelevant items in patients complaining of delusional or obsessive ideation, or disturbances in recall in patients with major affective disorders).

Common clinical questions in a psychiatric setting with a neuropsychological focus include 1) differentiation of early dementia versus mild delirium versus depression, 2) toxicity in substance-abusing individuals, 3) cognitive and affective status of an individual post–head injury, and 3) specific learning disabilities in children and adolescents. In clinical psychiatric populations, the possibly confounding influences of behavioral impairment because of the nature and severity of the emotional disturbance and the impact of concurrent pharmacological treatments must be carefully assessed in order to reduce the rate of false-positive diagnoses of organic mental disorder. These factors should be carefully weighed in the context of determining the timing of the assessment and in interpreting the results.

Although the fields of cognitive and experimental psychology may offer an almost limitless number of different cognitive functions capable of being defined and measured in the adult, only a finite number appear, at present, to be clinically useful. In one form or another, most neuropsychological assessments of cognitive pro-

cesses evaluate the presence of disorders in the following abilities: general intelligence, attention and concentration, memory and learning, perception, language, conceptualization, constructional skills, executive motor processes, and affect.

In many clinical settings, the areas of higher cortical functions of interest are assessed by a formal battery of tests. Two such standardized batteries are the Halstead-Reitan (Boll 1981) and the Luria-Nebraska (Golden et al. 1978) neuropsychological batteries (Table 5–8).

The Halstead-Reitan is a composite battery of tests originally developed by Ward Halstead and his former student, Ralph Reitan. In its present form, the Halstead-Reitan Neuropsychological Test Battery consists of five tests that yield seven summary scores and a total impairment index. The five tests are a category test, a tactile perception test, a speech sounds perception test, the Seashore rhythm test, and a finger oscillation test. A group of tests referred to as the allied procedures are frequently included as a part of the total examination. The entire examination typically takes from 4 to 6 hours, depending on the number of ancillary procedures (i.e., intelligence and academic performance) included. The reliability and validity of the tests are well established, and normative data for most comparisons of interest in clinical psychiatric populations are available.

A second widely used battery of procedures has been developed from the work of Luria (1966, 1973). Christensen (1975) was instrumental in bringing Luria's stimuli and procedures to the attention of neuropsychologists outside the former Soviet Union. Golden et al. (1978) have been the primary proponents and developers of a standardized neuropsychological instrument using Christensen's published material. In its present form, the Luria-Nebraska covers the areas of motor function; rhythm (and pitch) skills; tactile and visual functions; receptive and expressive speech; writing, reading, and arithmetic skills; memory; and intelligence. The complete examination consists of 269 items that yield raw scores in each area. Three additional scores for right- and left-hemisphere impairment and a pathognomonic score are also computed. These 14 raw scores are plotted as T scores for the purposes of interscale and interindividual comparison. The current literature on the Luria-Nebraska includes studies in brain-damaged, chronic schizophrenia, and medical control subjects. The results of these studies have established the preliminary validity of the battery; no reliability data have been published.

Both the Halstead-Reitan and the Luria-Nebraska batteries are oriented toward an extensive evaluation of neuropsychological functioning, and in clinical practice they are typically supplemented with instruments that

With increasing use of computer-assisted examinations, a popular continuous performance test developed by Rosvold can be employed (Mirsky and Kornetsky 1964; Rosvold et al. 1956). In this task, the patient is presented with a randomly selected letter in midscreen at fixed intervals and directed to push a button (or press the space bar) when a given letter is presented. The number of hits (i.e., correct responses), misses, false alarms (i.e., the number of times the bar is pressed in response to a nontarget item), and correct rejections is then noted. The advantage to this computer-assisted approach to the measure of attention lies in its flexibility and the accuracy with which responses can be recorded and stimuli presented. The reaction time of each response can be measured and fluctuations in reaction time noted over the duration of the task. Stimulus characteristics such as stimulus duration, speed of presentation, or even size of target and duration of task can be systematically altered. A good deal of clinical research has been conducted using such a procedure to explore the attentional characteristics of children with attention-deficit/hyperactivity disorder.

Research in attentional processes has demonstrated the efficacy of a procedure called "dichotic stimulation" (Kimura 1967), which presents dissimilar auditory stimuli simultaneously to each ear and requires the patient to report both stimuli. Thus the patient might simultaneously hear the number "1" in the right ear and "4" in the left ear. Strings of three such pairs might be presented to the adult patient and he or she asked to report all six digits. The competing stimuli can be matched for such stimulus characteristics as time of onset, offset, peak amplitude, and so forth, making it a very difficult speech sound discrimination task as well as an attentional measure.

Memory Disorders

The memory disorder of particular interest to the clinician is the one that affects "recent" memory and that is generally referable to impairment of limbic system functioning. Operationally, one presents the patient with a specific set of information or events and then diverts his or her attention so that the set cannot be rehearsed; the patient is subsequently required to demonstrate that the target information has been encoded and stored by either reproducing the material or recognizing it among distractor items. Thus, recall of brief paragraphs or reproduction of geometric designs from memory is often used to assess mnemonic processes. Among the most commonly used standard tests of memory are the Wechsler Memory Scale—III (Wechsler 1997), which presents both verbal and nonverbal material as the items to be remembered, and the Benton Test of Visual Retention (Benton 1955), which presents only geometric designs.

Free recall of recent events has been found to be among the most sensitive functions of the memory process. Unfortunately, in many instances free recall has been found to be quite fragile and vulnerable to disruption because of affective arousal, depression, and motivational factors, and therefore may present many "false positives" when being used to discriminate between neurogenic and psychogenic diagnostic considerations. It has been suggested that mechanisms other than free recall might be employed to assess the integrity of encoding and storage processes. Recognition memory techniques, in which the patient is asked to detect a recently presented word or design from among distractor items, have been successfully used to discriminate patients with major affective disorders from those with organic amnesias such as progressive dementia. For example, free recall in patients presenting with a major depression might be quite consonant with recall in patients with Alzheimer's disease, but recognition memory in patients with major depression remains relatively intact.

The well-designed instruments assessing both recall and recognition memory generally present the patient with a list-learning task requiring free recall and, subsequent to that, a recognition memory probe in which the patient must detect the target from among distractor items. Most of the instruments introduce either an interpolated list or a significant time delay before presentation of the final recall and recognition trials. Among the most widely used instruments are the Rey Auditory Verbal Learning Test (Geffen et al. 1990; Rey 1964) and the California Verbal Learning Test (Delis et al. 1987). Several instruments have multiple forms that are useful in the serial examination of patients, for example, the Hopkins Verbal Learning Test (Brandt 1991) and the Mattis–Kovner Verbal Learning Test (Mattis et al. 1978).

It should be noted that neurology patients with focal lesions might present only a verbal or nonverbal recent memory defect, depending on the locus of the lesion. It is therefore only in patients with bilateral or diffuse neurogenic impairment that one finds amnesic disorders in both realms. Thus, both verbal and nonverbal memory must be assessed independently, with the finding of asymmetric dysfunction strongly suggestive of focal neurological impairment.

Perceptual Disorders

Very little evidence exists for a significant prevalence of perceptual deficits in a psychiatric population when care is taken to exclude significant problem-solving components from the task and the presence of concurrent toxic metabolic disorders in the patients. Nonetheless, it is probably a good idea to rule out the presence of perceptual deficits. Visual–perceptual processes can be assessed with tasks such as the Benton Line Orientation Test (Benton et al. 1975), which requires the patient to match a target line at a given orientation to true vertical with alternative lines presented at various orientations. Another such test is the Benton Face Recognition Test (Benton and Van Allen 1968), in which a photograph of a face is presented as the target and the patient is requested to detect this face from among alternatives. In this task the correct face is presented as an identical photograph as well as photographs of the same individual in various profiles. Both of these tests have good validation as measures of the integrity of posterior cerebral, primarily nondominant hemisphere, functioning.

Auditory perception tends to be difficult to assess without hardware. However, at present the fidelity available in small, portable, "Walkman"-type tape players with earphones affords the clinician a wide range of excellent auditory stimuli. Tests such as the Goldman-Fristoe Test of Speech Sound Discrimination (Goldman et al. 1976) allow for the assessment of the efficiency of speech sound detection with and without background noise. The use of dichotic stimulation tests as measures of speech sound discrimination has already been mentioned in the discussion of attentional disorders. Subtests of the Seashore battery of tests of musical abilities (Seashore et al. 1960), especially the timbre discrimination and tonal memory subtests, have been used as measures of auditory perception of nonverbal material.

The study of disorders of somatosensory perception has a long history in the field of psychophysics, and the techniques evolved from this early literature constitute a large part of the standard neurological examination for peripheral and central nervous system (CNS) disorder. Measures of pressure threshold (Von Frey hairs and Semmes-Ghent-Weinstein pressure esthesiometer), two-point discrimination, joint position sense, finger agnosia, finger order and differentiation, graphesthesia, and stereognosis are common assessment procedures for the presence of disorders of parietal lobe functioning.

Language Disorders

Perhaps the most specific index of neurogenic impairment is the presence of a language disorder. For almost all right-handed individuals and half of left-handed individuals, focal or diffuse impairment of the left hemisphere is likely to result in an aphasia (i.e., a disorder of language comprehension and/or usage). The relationship between the nature of the aphasia (e.g., fluent vs. nonfluent) and the locus of cerebral impairment is among the most well documented of brain–behavior relations (Mesulam 1985). Thus, the examination for the aphasias can provide the "hardest" evidence in the mental status exam of the presence and locus of brain impairment. There are, needless to say, many well-constructed tests for aphasia. In general, the aphasia examination consists of specific measures of disorders of linguistic processes well correlated with focal brain lesion. Most such batteries will contain measures of verbal labeling or word-finding skills, language comprehension, imitative speech, and motor–expressive speech. Many such tests also include specific measures of reading and writing. Among the most commonly used multifactorial instruments are the Multilingual Aphasia Examination (Benton and Hamsher 1976), the Neurosensory Center Comprehensive Examination for Aphasia (Spreen and Benton 1977), and the Boston Diagnostic Aphasia Examination (Goodglass and Kaplan 1972). Among the most widely used screening instruments for the assessment of aphasia is the Halstead-Wepman Aphasia Screening Test (Halstead and Wepman 1959).

Conceptualization Disorders

The question of whether or not the patient can assume an abstract attitude is often critical to the diagnosis and the treatment planning. The question arises most often when the differential diagnostic considerations include diffuse brain damage and, to some degree, schizophrenia. Perhaps the most direct measure of the concept of abstract or categorical thinking is the similarities subtest of the WAIS-III, which presents the patient with perceptually dissimilar items and asks him or her to determine the category to which they both belong (e.g., "How are north and west alike?"). Proverb explanation has a long history in the psychiatric mental status examination as a task designed to measure abstract reasoning and is included among the items of the comprehension subtest of the WAIS-III (e.g., "Shallow brooks are noisy"). However, some consider explanation of proverbs too dependent on general intellectual abilities and sociocultural factors to be a specific measure of concretization of thought. Analogical reasoning can also be gauged by using such tasks as the Conceptual Level Analogies Test (Willner 1971) for verbal reasoning and the Raven Progressive Matrices Test (Raven 1960) for nonverbal or spatial analogical reasoning.

Two measures of concept formation arising from the neuropsychological literature have recently been applied to psychiatric patients. The data thus far indicate that schizophrenic patients, like patients with frontal lobe lesions, have particular difficulty with the booklet form of the Category Test (DeFillipis et al. 1979) and the Wisconsin Card Sorting Test (Berg 1948; Heaton and Crowley 1981). Both tests require the patient to induce a concept or rule of organization from patterned visual stimuli. In the Wisconsin Card Sorting Test, which has received the most recent programmatic research attention, the patient is shown a pack of cards depicting colored geometric figures. The patient is required to match the top card with one of four cards that vary as to color, number, or form. As the patient matches his or her card to one of the alternatives, the examiner informs him or her as to the "correctness" of the sort, and the patient then attempts to match the next card correctly. The "rule" of sorting that the examiner reinforces in color, form, or number is changed after the patient correctly sorts 10 cards in a row (indicating that he or she has grasped the rule). The examiner notes the number of concepts correctly induced and the number of perseverative errors in matching.

Constructional Disorders

Perhaps the quickest estimate of the integrity of the CNS can be obtained by asking the patient to draw a complex figure. Posterior sensory, central spatial, and anterior planning, monitoring, and simple motor skills must all be intact, integrated, and appropriately sequenced for this task to be successfully completed. One can alter the degree to which psychological and dynamic factors, and initiative or executive planning, play a role by modulating both task structure and design complexity. For example, asking the patient to draw a person in his or her family requires a maximum level of planning, initiative, and decision making; does not put any limit on the degree of complexity of the figures; and involves a subject matter fraught with complex feelings and attitudes. Patients without structural impairment but with conflictual feelings about family or disordered thinking that affects planning and execution will have difficulty on such tasks. However, asking a patient to draw a clock, setting the hands to a specific time (e.g., 10 minutes to 11:00), also requires complex planning and initiative but without the conflictual overlay. Similarly, asking the patient to copy a complex design (e.g., the Rey-Osterreith figure [Rey 1941]) minimizes initiative and limits (but does not eliminate) planning, but maintains assessment of high levels of spatial constructional skills. Contrasting the patient's figure drawing with his or her clock and copy of geometric figures often allows valid inferences as to presence and locus of CNS impairment and the degree to which affective and psychiatric factors impair otherwise intact cog-

nitive skills. Quite often, construction tasks other than drawing, such as the block design and object assembly subtests of the WAIS-III, are used for the same assessment goals.

Disorders of Executive Motor Skills

In general, in assessing disorders in executive skills, one is alert to the presence of perseveration in motor activity, thought, and affect. Perseveration of motor activity is often elicited by starting the patient on a simple repeated task and then altering one of the motor components. Thus, having the patient perform a simple diadochokinetic task such as alternating palm up/palm down and then presenting as the next task palm up/palm down/fist, may result in repeated performance of only two components of the task. Similarly, asking the patient to write, in script, alternating m's and n's will also elicit simple motor perseveration. Perseveration of thought or set is often quickly elicited by shifting task instruction. For example, in a task developed by Luria (1966) for the assessment of frontal lobe dysfunction, the examiner tells the patient, "When I raise one finger, then you raise one finger, and when I raise two fingers, you raise two fingers." After a number of successful completions, the patient is told, "Now when I raise one finger, you raise two fingers, and when I raise two fingers, you raise one." Patients with dorsolateral frontal lobe lesions have a great deal of trouble with such tasks. The Trail Making Test (Lezak 1969) is a "connect the dots" type of task in which the patient must first connect the dots in ascending numerical order (Trails A), and then connect the dots in an alternating sequence of numbers and letters (e.g., 1 to A to 2 to B to 3 to C, etc.; Trails B). Note is made of both the time to completion and the number of errors.

Disorders in evolving or shifting more complex ideas can also be measured quite accurately. Concept formation tasks such as the booklet form of the Category Test and the Wisconsin Card Sorting Test differ in specific directions and stimuli but present a series of specific examples of a class of events and require the patient to induce the concept or rule of which they are an exemplar. The rule changes over time. Thus, one might observe the patient's failure to induce the first concept or his or her perseveration in the same rule well past its utility. The number of perseveration errors is among the scores obtained on both tests.

Disorders in Motor Skills

Disorders in simple motor skills are among the common concomitants of most toxic–metabolic disorders and of structural lesions of both the extrapyramidal and pyramidal systems. Examination is usually exceptionally brief, and the results are quite reproducible and valid. One can measure line quality parameters of copied geometric drawings (Mattis et al. 1975). One can, in addition, present simple fine motor coordination tasks such as the Purdue Pegboard (Costa et al. 1963) or the Grooved Pegboard. The Purdue Pegboard measures the number of slim cylinders (i.e., pegs) one can insert in a row of holes in 30 seconds. One notes the number of 1) pegs placed with the right hand alone, 2) pegs placed with left hand alone, and 3) pairs of pegs placed with both hands simultaneously. The number of pegs placed simultaneously has proven to be a sensitive measure of frontal dysfunction. The Grooved Pegboard has pegs that contain a flange on one side so that the pegs fit into a keyhole-shaped opening. The keyholes are placed in differing orientations on the board. One notes the total time needed to place all the pegs with each hand alone. Given the greater fine motor component of the grooved pegs, the Grooved Pegboard tends to be a more sensitive measure of tremor than is the Purdue.

Assessment of Personality Traits and Disorders

In developing a treatment plan for a specific patient, the psychiatrist must assess personality traits for various reasons: personality traits or disorders may 1) be the focus of intervention, 2) exacerbate or be related to the incidence of certain symptoms (e.g., depression), or 3) either help or hinder the development of a therapeutic relationship with the patient.

Dimensional Assessment of Personality

The dimensional assessment of personality using psychological tests has been characterized by a nomothetic approach in which specific personality dimensions (e.g., introversion) are assessed. The dimensions chosen for assessment are typically derived from a personality theory, and individuals are expected to show quantitative differences on these various dimensions. The number of items relevant to a particular dimension that are endorsed is thought to reflect important aspects of that individual's personality style. Within the field of personality measurement, much attention has been paid to the generalizability of such measures. Efforts to investigate the relationship between self-report measures of interpersonal behavior and actual behavior in interpersonal situations continue to contribute to the refinement of this important area of psychological assessment. Just as the levels of distress and of awareness of specific problems

are insufficient for determining the capacity to profit from any specific treatment, so, too, is general knowledge about the reported style of interpersonal behavior insufficient for determining the reaction to various interpersonal situations or the ability to modify the style under certain circumstances.

Several widely used and psychometrically sound instruments are available for the assessment of personality (Table 5–9). Such tests include the 16-PF, the EPI, and the California Personality Inventory (CPI; Gough 1956). These instruments were designed for the validation of personality constructs rather than for the assessment of psychopathology, although they have been employed in clinical settings with limited success. These instruments and their designers, however, have not been oriented toward psychopathology, and there is no explicit theory of personality disorder that underlies the interpretation of results from these tests.

The Neuroticism, Extroversion, and Openness Personality Inventory (NEO-PI), a carefully constructed instrument measuring five central facets of personality, has gained in recognition (Wiggins and Pincus 1992), and its clinical use will probably increase. The revised version, the NEO-PI-R (Costa and McCrae 1992), provides a measure of five facets of personality: neuroticism, extraversion, openness, agreeableness, and conscientiousness. Each of the facets also includes six subscales. For example, the six facets of neuroticism include anxiety, anger/hostility, depression, self-consciousness, impulsiveness, and vulnerability. The revised version completes the earlier instrument by providing facet scales for agreeableness and conscientiousness.

In this era of searching for efficient care, some consideration should be given to the use of screening instruments that can be administered rapidly to assess for the potential for personality disorders, disorders that retard and complicate the treatment of Axis I disorders. Four screening instruments deserve consideration: the International Personality Disorder Examination Screen (IPDE-S; Lenzenweger et al. 1997), the Iowa Personality Disorder Screen (Pfohl and Langbehn 1994), the self-directedness subscale from the Temperament and Character Inventory (Cloninger et al. 1993; Svrakic et al. 1993), and a screen for personality disorders developed from the Inventory of Interpersonal Problems (IIP; Pilkonis et al. 1996).

Interpersonal Aspects of Personality

One particular school of personality research that has concerned itself with pathological expressions of personality factors has focused explicitly on interpersonal

TABLE 5–9. Instruments for the assessment of personality traits and disorders

Instrument	General classification	Description	Scoring features
Neuroticism, Extroversion, and Openness (NEO) Personality Inventory—Revised	Self-report	240 items, 5-point scale	Five domain scales and 30 facet scales
16–Personality Factor Inventory	Self-report	3 equivalent forms of 106–187 items each	Scaled scores for 16 personality traits
Eysenck Personality Inventory	Self-report	57 yes/no items, parallel forms	Scores on extraversion and neuroticism
Schedule for Nonadaptive and Adaptive Personality	Self-report	12 primary traits and 3 temperament dimensions	
Dimensional Assessment of Personality Pathology–Basic Questionnaire	Self-report	18 scales	Scores on 18 scales
California Personality Inventory	Self-report	468 items	Scores on 18 scales and 4 special scales
Millon Clinical Multiaxial Inventory—III	Self-report	175 items, true/false format	Base rate scores on 22 clinical scales
Structural Interview for the DSM-IV Personality Disorders	Semistructured interview	3-point rating scales	Yields DSM-IV Axis II diagnoses
International Personality Disorders Examination	Semistructured interview	Semistructured interview for patient and self-report by family member on the patient	Dimensional and categorical scales on DSM-IV Axis II personality disorders
Structural Analyses of Social Behavior	Self-report	36–72 statements of interpersonal behavior rated true/false	Internalized attitudes regarding self and significant others

behavior. Adherents of this view of psychopathology emphasize the centrality of the problems that people experience with others, for it is in this area that all symptoms are activated, reinforced, and (for some persons) caused. The assessment of interpersonal behavior can be central to understanding the patient's social world with its pleasures and disappointments, as well as barriers to success in love and work, and can be used as a forecast of the kind of relationship the patient will form with the clinician.

This interpersonal tradition dates back to psychologist Timothy Leary's circumplex model (Leary 1957). Underlying the expression of all interpersonal styles are the two major orthogonal axes of power and affiliation. Each interpersonal style is seen as involving varying degrees of the expression of power and affiliation leading to 16 modes of interaction. These 16 modes are organized along the circumference of a circle defining eight broad categories that are used in interpersonal diagnosis: ambitious–dominant, gregarious–extroverted, warm–agreeable, unassuming–ingenuous, lazy–submissive, aloof–introverted, cold–quarrelsome, and arrogant–calculating. This system is more than merely descriptive. Theoretically, one is able to predict not only the kind of

interpersonal style that the patient expresses but also the kind of behavior that this style tends to elicit from others. Behavior on one side of the circle tends to elicit from others behaviors on the opposite side of the circle. For example, a patient who is ambitious–dominant tends to elicit lazy–submissive behavior from others. In terms of differential therapeutic treatment planning, this model suggests not only that the patient will behave in a certain fashion but also that this behavior will elicit therapist behavior found on the opposite side of the circle. It has been suggested that interpersonal diagnosis can thus highlight transference and possible countertransference reactions in therapies that are interpersonal in orientation. Furthermore, the theory indicates what kinds of counterbehavior the therapist should engage in to dislodge the patient from his or her predominant mode of interaction.

There are several instruments that have been developed from this basic interpersonal theory. In a series of investigations, Lorr and McNair (1965) generated the most recent version of the Interpersonal Behavior Inventory (IBI). The IBI has been judged to be psychometrically sound and a useful clinical device for the assessment of patient characteristics and therapy outcome (Wiggins

1982). The instrument is a clinical rating by professionals but in principle could be employed in a self-report format. The Interpersonal Style Inventory (ISI; Lorr and Youniss 1973) is a self-report instrument for persons ages 14 years and older. A large number (300) of true/false statements are employed to assess interpersonal involvement, socialization, self-control, stability, and autonomy. Techniques of rational scale construction, including validity factor analyses, were employed. Norms were established based on 1,500 college and high school students.

Also in the same tradition, Benjamin (1974, 1988) developed an instrument for the assessment of interpersonal behavior, the Structural Analysis of Social Behavior (SASB), and a computer-based scoring system marketed under the trade name INTREX, which is self-administered. The SASB can also be used by clinicians to record their impressions about the patient. A related coding scheme has been developed for use by trained observers to record the patient's actual interactions with others, such as family members, during the course of treatment.

Assessment of Personality Disorders

A relatively new approach to the assessment of personality disorders is to construct instruments, either self-report or semistructured interviews, that evaluate the presence or absence of specific personality traits described in Axis II of DSM-IV. DSM-IV neither defines nor develops from any particular theory of personality. Instead, it identifies clusters (in most cases, those with little empirical validation) of personality traits that are considered sufficiently maladaptive to warrant the personality disorder designation. Personality traits are described as enduring patterns of perceiving, relating to, and thinking about the environment and oneself that are exhibited or manifested in a wide range of important social and interpersonal contexts. When these traits are inflexible and maladaptive and cause either significant impairment in social or occupational functioning or subjective distress, they are defined as a personality disorder in DSM-IV. The most promising instruments of this type include the Personality Diagnostic Questionnaire–4 (PDQ-4; Hyler 1994; Hyler et al. 1988), the MCMI-III, the SCID, the Personality Disorder Examination (PDE; Loranger 1988), and the Structural Interview for the DSM-IV Personality Disorders (SIDP-IV; Pfohl et al. 1997).

The PDQ is a self-report inventory of Axis II traits, and the test yields scores on each of the 13 personality disorder categories of DSM-III. Preliminary investigation of the instrument suggests that patients typically report a number of traits and will often meet criteria for several

diagnostic categories; the PDQ may, however, be useful for screening (Hurt et al. 1984).

The MCMI-III is a 175-item true/false self-report instrument that yields scores on 11 personality disorder dimensions closely related to the personality disorder diagnoses of DSM-III Axis II, and 9 clinical syndromes. Probably the major difficulty with this instrument is psychometric in nature, as there is much item overlap in the scales (Wiggins 1982). In the Millon Clinical Multiaxial Inventory—II (MCMI-II; Millon 1987), a revision of the original scale, two new personality disorder scales were introduced and two of the original personality scales were modified. An item-weighting system has been introduced into the MCMI-II to reflect item differences related to the strength of each item's supporting validation data.

There are several new self-report questionnaires that assess personality and personality pathology that have been carefully constructed with attention to psychometric properties. These include the Schedule for Nonadaptive and Adaptive Personality (SNAP; Clark 1993) and the Dimensional Assessment of Personality Pathology–Basic Questionnaire (DAPP-BQ; Schroeder et al. 1994).

There are three semistructured interviews that have been designed to assess, via the patient's report and the clinical judgment of the interviewer, the presence of Axis II disorders: the IPDE, the SIDP-IV, and the Structured Clinical Interview for DSM-IV Axis II Personality Disorders (SCID-II; First et al. 1997).

The IPDE is a semistructured interview that yields both dimensional and categorical scores for DSM-IV Axis II criteria. An important feature of this semistructured interview, which takes approximately 1–2 hours to administer, is that the criteria are assessed in related clusters such as self-concept, affect expression, reality testing, impulse control, interpersonal relations, and work. The interview goes beyond a simple listing of the criteria and in many cases provides multiple questions designed to help the interviewer gain a broad appreciation of the criterion under assessment. A parallel version of the interview has been constructed for use with informants, in recognition of the fact that information from patients themselves, especially around personality issues, may be distorted. Initial reliability data are impressive and validity studies are under way. The instrument is likely to be widely used. In fact, it has been translated into several languages and was used in an international study approved by the World Health Organization and the former Alcohol, Drug Abuse, and Mental Health Administration (Loranger et al. 1991).

The SIDP-IV consists of a semistructured interview form that provides 160 questions pertinent to the diagnostic criteria of Axis II of DSM-III. The questions are organized into 16 assessment areas, such as low self-esteem/dependency, egocentricity, ideas of reference and magical thinking, and hostility/anger. The questions are keyed to the DSM-III criteria for Axis II disorders. A rating form provides a 3-point rating scale for each criterion. Ratings are based on the clinical assessment of the interview data. The authors of the interview recommend that it be used in conjunction with a general psychiatric interview in which major (i.e., Axis I) psychiatric disorders have been diagnosed so that lifelong personality traits can be distinguished from episodic psychiatric disorders. The authors also recommend gathering information from an informant who knows the patient well.

The SCID-II is concerned with the assessment of Axis II personality disorders. The interview format is determined by the DSM-IV disorders and provides no guide for elaborating the assessment of the criteria.

There are several problems with this relatively new approach of assessing personality disorders guided solely by DSM-IV. First, Axis II is neither an empirically nor a theoretically derived compilation of personality traits that lead to, cause, or constitute psychopathology. Rather, it is a somewhat arbitrary collection of traits that are thought to be important markers of pathology. Thus, any instrument guided solely by DSM-IV will leave serious questions of internal consistency, content validity, and construct validity largely unanswered. Most probably, attempts to assess these important test characteristics within the context of DSM-IV are likely to be carried out with these instruments.

Assessment of Psychodynamics

The assessment of factors relevant to psychodynamic and psychoanalytic theory and treatment approaches has a long history in the clinical psychological literature. The development of the "standard battery," including the WAIS-III, the Rorschach, and the Thematic Apperception Test (Table 5–10), has its origins in the efforts of clinical psychologists to provide an assessment of such psychodynamic factors as drives, unconscious wishes, conflicts, and defenses. For those clinicians committed to the psychodynamic model, assessments that focus exclusively on overt behaviors will be less than totally satisfactory.

The importance of providing information about personality dynamics and structure that are outside the conscious awareness of the examinee has been the single most important rationale for the continued use of projective tests. In part, therefore, the value of such assessments varies directly with the degree to which maladaptive and symptomatic behaviors are presumed to be beyond the conscious control of the examinee. A second rationale for the continued use of these tests is that the unstructured nature of the tests provides a singular opportunity to assess the degree to which organization of behavior is dependent on a high degree of structure in the examination procedure itself. The assessment of both of these factors is of clear relevance to a treatment method that attempts to explore and alter unconscious determinants of behavior and that depends for its success on introducing as little structure into the treatment as is realistically possible.

The most widely used assessment procedure for the examination of patients over a range of ego functions and dynamic factors is the Rorschach inkblot test, described earlier. Scoring systems have been developed by many authors, and Exner (1974, 1978) created a scoring system that attempts to integrate the best aspects of earlier systems. From these scores, inferences are drawn concerning the patient's self-image, identity, defensive structure, reality testing, affective control, amount and degree of fantasy life, degree of thought organization, and potential for impulsive acting out.

The Thematic Apperception Test (TAT) is another widely used projective process for assessing the patient's self-concept in relation to others. Originally developed by Murray (1943), the test consists of a set of 30 pictures depicting one or more individuals (Figure 5–2). The patient is asked to make up a story based on each picture. The stories generated are then scored for the individual's needs as reflected in the feelings and impulses attributed to the major character in each story and the interactions with the environment leading to a resolution. As currently used, the stories are most often examined for the patient's self–other concepts as revealed in the interaction and outcome of the story line.

Assessment of Environmental Demands and Social Adjustment

The interaction between the patient and the pressures of the environment is now acknowledged in the standard diagnostic system (DSM-IV; American Psychiatric Association 1994) by a rating on Axis IV. Probably the most substantiated area with empirical data indicating the impact of the patient–environment interaction is the investigation of expressed emotion and its influence on the course of schizophrenia. This work suggests that certain elements in the home environment of a schizophrenic patient can adversely affect the course of the illness. Expressed emotion can be assessed by the Camberwell Family Interview (Brown and Rutter 1966), a 1-hour semistructured interview of a relative of the patient. The

TABLE 5–10. Instruments for the assessment of psychodynamics and patient enabling factors

Instrument	General classification	Description	Scoring features
Rorschach	Unstructured or projective test	10 ambiguous inkblots, responses scored on multiple criteria	Accuracy of form, location, use of color, shading, etc., provide summary scores
Thematic Apperception Test	Unstructured or projective test	30 ambiguous scenes	Affects, outcomes, and other qualities
Minnesota Multiphasic Personality Inventory–2	Self-report	566 item checklist, true/false format	T scores for 13 criterion scales
Symptom Checklist–90—Revised	Self-report	90-item checklist, 5-point intensity scales	T scores for 9 symptom clusters
Millon Clinical Multiaxial Inventory—III	Self-report	175 items, true/false format	Base rate scores for 22 clinical scales

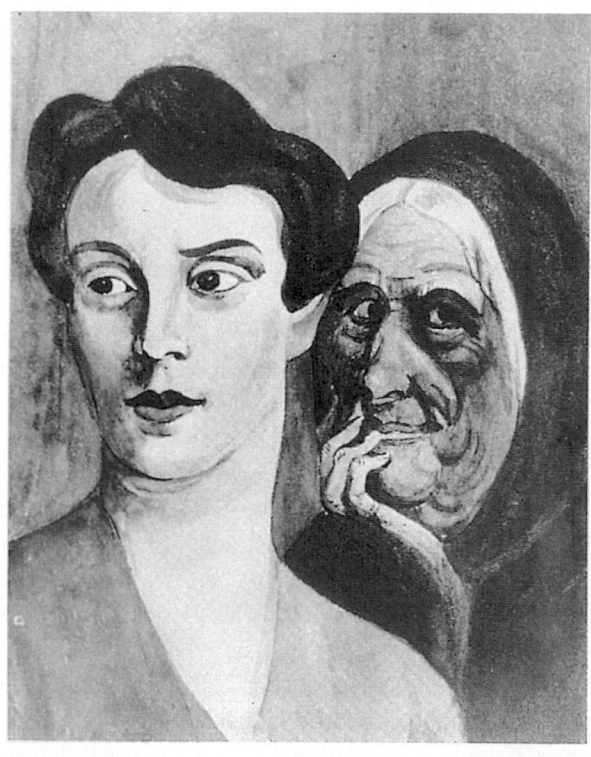

FIGURE 5–2. Thematic Apperception Test, Card 12F.
Source. Reprinted by permission of the publishers from Murray HA: *Thematic Apperception Test.* Cambridge, MA, Harvard University Press, 1943. Copyright 1943 by the President and Fellows of Harvard College; copyright 1971 by Henry A. Murray.

scoring scheme for this instrument is not readily accessible and is therefore not usable in standard clinical situations.

In measuring both stress and the patient's ability to cope with stress, one can assess the stimuli, the individual's response to the stimuli, or the interaction of the person with stressful stimuli (Table 5–11). The Jenkins Activity Survey (JAS; Jenkins et al. 1967) is the proto-

type of an interaction-based measure of stress, focusing on the cognitive and perceptual characteristics of the individual that mediate responses to stress. This instrument has been shown to have predictive validity in studies of reaction to coronary heart disease. The Derogatis Stress Profile (DSP; Derogatis 1982) is helpful in evaluating stimuli from work and home and can be used to assess health, as well as characteristic attitudes and coping mechanisms.

We use the term *social adjustment* to indicate the skill of the individual in handling interpersonal situations, whether at home, in school, or in the work setting. The term social adjustment has been used more narrowly to indicate the community and social adjustment of diagnosed psychiatric patients, who often have severe illnesses such as schizophrenia and major affective disorder (Weissman and Sholomskas 1982). Notable assessment instruments in this area include the Katz Adjustment Scale–Relative's Form (KAS-R; Katz and Lyerly 1963), the Social Adjustment Scale–Self-Report (SAS-SR; Weissman and Bothwell 1976), and the Dyadic Adjustment Scale (DAS; Spanier 1976).

The KAS-R is a relative's self-report inventory of the patient's symptomatic behavior and social adjustment in the community. The scale has sections on symptoms and social behavior, performance of socially expected tasks, relative's expectation for the performance of these tasks, the patient's leisure-time activities, and the relative's satisfaction with the performance of these free-time activities.

The SAS-SR contains 42 questions covering instrumental and affective qualities in role performance, social and leisure activities, relationships with extended family, marital role, parental role, family unit, and economic independence. Norms are available for nonpatient community samples, acutely ill and recovered depressed out-

TABLE 5–11. Instruments for the assessment of environmental stressors

Instrument	General classification	Description	Scoring features
Social Adjustment Scale–Self Report	Self-report	42 questions, rated on 5-point scale of severity	Mean score for 7 areas and an overall score
Dyadic Adjustment Scale	Self-report	31 items, 4 dimensions	Total score
Marital Satisfaction Inventory	Self-report	280 items	T scores on 11 scales

patients, schizophrenic patients, and drug-addicted patients. The Social Support Questionnaire (SSQ; Sarason et al. 1983) is an efficient method for assessing social satisfaction. This instrument provides information about available resources of support and the patient's level of satisfaction with this support system.

The whole area of the quality of marital adjustment is relevant to treatment planning for married individuals with psychiatric disorders such as phobias and mood disorders (Clarkin et al. 1992), as well as those couples who present with marital difficulties. Two useful self-report instruments in this area are the DAS and the Marital Satisfaction Inventory (Snyder et al. 1981).

Assessment of Therapeutic Enabling Factors

Accurate diagnosis is not sufficient for determining optimal specific treatments. Although the patient's diagnosis helps to narrow the focus, optimal treatment planning depends on nondiagnostic factors such as characteristics of the patient that will affect the acceptance, use, and absorption of the treatment that is recommended. Psychological tests can be useful in assessing these dimensions. From a review of the comparative psychotherapy outcome research data (Beutler 1983; Beutler and Clarkin 1990; Gaw and Beutler 1995) one can isolate five areas of assessment: 1) problem severity, 2) motivational distress, 3) problem complexity, 4) resistance potential or reactance level, and 5) coping style.

Problem severity is defined as a continuum of functioning ranging from little impairment to incapacitation. Instruments reviewed in this chapter assessing symptoms and general functioning are appropriate tools for measuring problem severity. Motivational distress is the degree of subjective disturbance experienced by the patient in reference to his or her problems. Motivational distress is important because it motivates help-seeking activity such as psychotherapy in order to reduce discomfort. The Brief Symptom Inventory (BSI; Derogatis 1992) is an efficient method of assessing aspects of patient self-

defined problem severity. The global severity index from the BSI can be used as an estimate of subjective or motivational distress. It is suggested that when the global severity index value exceeds a T score of 63, a treatment that is designed to reduce subjective distress is indicated (Derogatis 1992). If distress levels are low, the clinician must consider whether to confront the patient with the contradiction of low distress in the face of impairment. The MMPI-2 can also be used to assess motivational distress. For example, Scale 7 (psychasthenia [Pt]) is an index of psychological turmoil and discomfort (Graham 1990). Scores above 70 on the F scale may suggest good motivation for treatment. Those whose high scores on the F scale are matched with elevations on the L and K scales tend to resist and react to authority and, inferentially, to therapists.

Problem complexity relates to the pervasiveness and the endurance of the problem. A complex problem is pervasive and enduring; that is, it is chronic and transsituational rather than situation specific. The BSI offers information on the degree to which the problem spreads across symptom domains, as this is one aspect of complexity. The MMPI-2 two-point code types (Graham 1990) and the Axis II indicators from the MCMI-II may also shed light on the spread and chronicity of problems.

Reactance is a construct that comes from social psychology which indicates the degree to which an individual is resistant or oppositional to interpersonal demands such as the recommendations or advice of a mental health professional. One of the most promising instruments for assessing reactance is the Therapeutic Reactance Scale (TRS; Dowd et al. 1991). This is a 28-item self-report instrument for which there have been two normative studies.

Coping style refers to the manner in which an individual manages or deals with anxiety that arises from interpersonal or intrapersonal conflict. The MMPI-2 is useful in defining the patient's coping styles along an internalizing–externalizing dimension. Externalizing patterns are indicated by the Hy, Pd, Pa, and Ma scales. Internalizing coping styles are indicated by the Hs, depression (D), Pt, and social introversion (Si) scales.

Psychological Assessment in the Contemporary Health Care Climate

There is the potential for psychological assessment to become integral to the mental health care system because of its methodological rigor and psychometric sophistication. Rapidly escalating health care costs have forced businesses, legislators, and consumers to identify cost containment as a top priority (Fonagy 1999; Moreland et al. 1994). For better or worse, third-party payers are demanding that services become time-limited, problem-focused, and "medically necessary." Traditional psychological assessment, by these standards, has been seen as a superfluous and unnecessary cost and has therefore been forced to significantly change its focus.

Psychological assessment has survived in this era and will continue to do so insofar as it contributes to cost-containment mechanisms, quality improvement, and consumer satisfaction in health care settings (Moreland et al. 1994). Consequently, certain areas of priority have begun to be addressed in systematic and rigorous ways, the hallmark of sound psychological assessment: 1) treatment planning, 2) ongoing assessment of the impact of treatment and assessment of outcome, 3) quality assurance within and across institutions, and 4) screening for psychiatric disturbance (Ben-Porath 1997; Berman and Hurt 1999; Fonagy 1999).

In the arena of *treatment planning*, psychological assessment can systematically inform clinicians and reviewers about the most cost-effective treatment. Such assessment involves questions such as "What level of care is most appropriate for this patient at this time—inpatient, partial hospital, intensive outpatient, or outpatient?"

Once treatment has begun, routine, standardized psychological assessment can *track the progress and impact of treatment* among individuals and groups. Many efficient, easy to administer omnibus measures have been developed that can quickly (via computerized databases) assess changes in patients' symptoms, behaviors, quality of life, and functional levels during the treatment process. With these data, informed decisions can be made about whether the current treatment is effective or whether another treatment should be considered. Consider, for example, a depressed patient with a BDI score of 24 and few Reasons for Living at the outset of treatment. If these measures were readministered by the clinician at monthly intervals, that clinician would obtain reliable and valid indicators of the impact of treatment.

Possession of such indicators would enable the clinician to communicate convincingly with reviewers about the current treatment's effectiveness and the continued need for treatment.

In regard to the ongoing impact of treatment, outcome assessment addresses the immediate and long-term stability of improvements in patients and groups. At the end of treatment and after, psychological assessment can be utilized to address questions such as "How permanent are the patient's improvements in symptoms of depression?" and "With improvements in mood, has the patient's ability to work and have relationships improved (functional level)?" Insofar as recidivism, relapse, and short-term treatment effects constitute a major financial drain, any health care system serious about containing costs must grapple with long-term outcomes in terms of patients' functional levels after treatment has ended, even if the treatments appear to adequately improve symptoms and behavior in the short term.

At present, *quality assurance* appears to be primarily defined by the satisfaction of the health care consumer; however, it can be argued that this aspect is not, by itself, an adequate measure of quality. Notwithstanding, psychological assessment has the ability to systematically track patient satisfaction for accrediting agencies that require such information (e.g., the Joint Committee on Health Care Accreditation). Ideally, these data can be observed in concert with other outcome data, such as symptoms, behaviors, and quality of life.

Within the past several years, mental health tracking systems have been developed to collect data that is useful for clinicians (treatment planning), administrators (efficiency of clinicians in delivering care), and third-party payers, employers, and accrediting agencies (patient satisfaction and outcome assessment). By gathering systematic and sequential data, these systems provide information for utilization review regarding the need for additional treatment. Such data can also be used to assess clinicians' performance in relation to cost and to identify clinicians who are effective or ineffective in conducting interventions with different types of individuals. Mental health tracking systems focus on patient processes and outcomes of interest to employers as well. These include alleviation of symptom distress, reduction of health care expenses, and reduction of absenteeism.

In summary, the role of the psychological assessment system in determining the cost-effectiveness of treatments for mental and physical health will likely become more prominent in the new century's health care as the demand for rigorous and systematic documentation of treatment effects remains a priority. Given this scenario, one can predict that psychological assessment will continue to evolve to address individual, group, and institutional variables; will become more rapid and focused; will rely heavily on computerized administration, scoring, and database management; and will address not just symptoms and behavior in the short term, but also functional level and quality of life in the long term. In addition, psychological and biological assessments will continue to become more integrated (e.g., neuropsychological assessment). Finally, considering these trends, psychiatrists will need to become better educated and trained regarding the principles and uses of rigorous, empirically sound psychological assessment.

References

American Psychiatric Association: Diagnostic and Statistical Manual of Mental Disorders, 3rd Edition. Washington, DC, American Psychiatric Association, 1980

American Psychiatric Association: Diagnostic and Statistical Manual of Mental Disorders, 4th Edition. Washington, DC, American Psychiatric Association, 1994

Ammons RB, Ammons CH: The Quick Test (QT): provisional manual. Psychol Rep 11:111–161, 1962

Anastasi A: Psychological Testing, 5th Edition. New York, Macmillan, 1982

Barchas JD, Berger PA, Ciaranello RD, et al: Psychopharmacology: From Theory to Practice. New York, Oxford University Press, 1977

Bauer MS, Crits-Christoph P, Ball WA, et al: Independent assessment of manic and depressive symptoms by self-rating: scale characteristics and implications for the study of mania. Arch Gen Psychiatry 48:807–812, 1991

Beck AT, Young JE: Depression, in Clinical Handbook of Psychological Disorders. Edited by Barlow DH. New York, Guilford, 1985, pp 202–244

Beck AT, Schuyler D, Herman I: Development of suicidal intent scales, in The Prediction of Suicide. Edited by Beck AT, Resnick HLP, Lettieri DJ. Bowie, MD, Charles Press, 1974, pp 2045–2056

Beck AT, Steer RA, Brown GK: Beck Depression Inventory Manual, 2nd Edition. San Antonio, TX, Psychological Corporation, 1996

Beigel A, Murphy DL, Bunney WE Jr: The Manic-State Rating Scale: scale construction, reliability, and validity. Arch Gen Psychiatry 25:256–262, 1971

Benjamin LS: Structural analysis of social behavior. Psychol Rev 81:392–425, 1974

Benjamin LS: SASB Short Form User's Manual. Salt Lake City, UT, University of Utah, 1988

Ben-Porath YS: Use of personality assessment instruments in empirically guided treatment planning. Psychol Assess 4:361–367, 1997

Benton AL: Visual Retention Test. New York, Psychological Corporation, 1955

Benton AL, Hamsher K: Multilingual Aphasia Examination. Iowa City, IA, University of Iowa, 1976

Benton AL, Van Allen MW: Impairment in facial recognition in patients with cerebral disease. Cortex 4:344–358, 1968

Benton AL, Hannay HJ, Varney NR: Visual perception of line direction in patients with unilateral brain disease. Neurology 25:907–910, 1975

Berg EA: A simple objective test for measuring flexibility in thinking. J Gen Psychol 39:15–32, 1948

Berman WH, Hurt SW: The implementation of clinical outcomes systems: conceptual and practical issues, in Outcomes in Behavioral Health, Child Health and Social Service Settings. Edited by Mullen E. Washington, DC, National Association of Social Workers Press, 1999

Beutler LE: Eclectic Psychotherapy: A Systematic Approach. New York, Pergamon, 1983

Beutler LE, Clarkin JF: Systematic Treatment Selection: Toward Targeted Therapeutic Interventions. New York, Brunner/Mazel, 1990

Beutler LE, Clarkin JF, Bongar B: Guidelines for the Systematic Treatment of the Depressed Patient. New York, Oxford University Press, 2000

Blake DD, Weathers FW, Nagy LN, et al: A clinician ratings scale for assessing current and lifetime PTSD: the CAPS-1. Behavior Therapist 18:187–188, 1990

Boll TJ: The Halstead-Reitan Neuropsychology Battery, in Handbook of Clinical Neuropsychology. Edited by Filskov SB, Boll TJ. New York, Wiley, 1981, pp 577–607

Bongar B: The Suicidal Patient: Clinical and Legal Standards of Care. Washington, DC, American Psychological Association, 1991

Brandt J: The Hopkins Verbal Learning Test: development of a new memory test with six equivalent forms. The Clinical Neuropsychologist 5:125–142, 1991

Brown GW, Rutter M: The measurement of family activities and relationships: a methodological study. Human Relations 19:241–263, 1966

Buros OK (ed): The Seventh Mental Measurements Yearbook. Highland Park, NJ, Gryphon Press, 1971

Buros OK (ed): The Eighth Mental Measurements Yearbook. Highland Park, NJ, Gryphon Press, 1978

Buss AH, Durkee A: An inventory for assessing different kinds of hostility. J Consult Psychol 21:343–349, 1957

Butcher JN: The Minnesota Report: Adult Clinical System MMPI-2. Minneapolis, MN, University of Minnesota Press, 1989

Butcher JN: Objective study of abnormal personality in cross-cultural settings: the Minnesota Multiphasic Personality Inventory (MMPI-2). J Cross-Cultural Psychol 29:189–211, 1998

Butcher JN, Dahlstrom WG, Graham JR, et al: Manual for the Restandardized Minnesota Multiphasic Personality Inventory (MMPI-2): An Administrative and Interpretive Guide. Minneapolis, MN, University of Minnesota Press, 1989

Cattell RB, Eber HW, Tatsuoka MM: Handbook for the Sixteen Personality Factor Inventory. Champaign, IL, Institute for Personality and Ability Testing, 1970

Christensen AL: Luria's Neuropsychological Investigation: Manual. New York, Spectrum, 1975

Clark LA: Manual for the Schedule for Nonadaptive and Adaptive Personality (SNAP). Minneapolis, MN, University of Minnesota Press, 1993

Clarkin JF, Mattis S: Psychological assessment, in Inpatient Psychiatry: Diagnosis and Treatment, 3rd Edition. Edited by Sederer LI. Baltimore, MD, Williams & Wilkins, 1991, pp 360–378

Clarkin JF, Haas GL, Glick ID: Family and marital therapy, in Handbook of Affective Disorders, 2nd Edition. Edited by Paykel ES. London, England, Churchill Livingstone, 1992, pp 487–500

Cloninger CR, Svrakic DM, Przybeck TR: A psychobiological model of temperament and character. Arch Gen Psychiatry 50:975–990, 1993

Coccaro EF, Harvey PD, Kupsaw-Lawrence E, et al: Development of neuropharmacologically based behavioral assessments of impulsive aggressive behavior. J Neuropsychiatry Clin Neurosci 3:S44–S51, 1991

Costa LD, McCrae RR: NEO PI-R: Professional Manual. Odessa, FL, Psychological Assessment Resources, 1992

Costa LD, Vaughan HG, Levita E, et al: Perdue Pegboard as a predictor of the presence and laterality of cerebral lesions. Journal of Consulting Psychology 27:133–137, 1963

Cronbach L, Meehl P: Construct validity in psychological tests. Psychol Bull 42:281–301, 1955

Cull JG, Gill WS: Suicide Probability Scale (SPS) Manual. Los Angeles, CA, Western Psychological Services, 1986

Dahlstrom WG, Welsh GS, Dahlstrom LE: An MMPI Handbook, Revised Edition, Vols 1 and 2. Minneapolis, MN, University of Minnesota Press, 1972

Davidson JRT, Potts NLS, Richichi EA, et al: The Brief Social Phobia Scale. J Clin Psychiatry 52:48–51, 1991

DeFillipis NA, McCambell E, Rogers P: Development of a booklet form of the Category Test: normative and validity data. J Clin Neuropsychol 1:339–342, 1979

Delis DC, Kramer J, Kaplan E, et al: California Verbal Learning Test (CVLT), Research Edition Manual. New York, Psychological Corporation, 1987

Derogatis LR: The SCL-90R. Baltimore, MD, Clinical Psychometric Research, 1977

Derogatis LR: Self-report measures of stress, in Handbook of Stress. Edited by Goldberger L, Breznitz S. New York, Free Press, 1982, pp 270–294

Derogatis LR: SCL-90-R: Administration, Scoring, and Procedures Manual II. Baltimore, MD, Clinical Psychometric Research, 1983

Derogatis LR: The Brief Symptom Inventory (BSI): Administration, Scoring and Procedures Manual, 2nd Edition. Baltimore, MD, Clinical Psychometric Research, 1992

Derogatis LR: SCL-90-R, Brief Symptom Inventory, and matching clinical rating scales, in Psychological Testing, Treatment Planning, and Outcome Assessment. Edited by Maruish M. New York, Lawrence Erlbaum, 1994

Derogatis LR, Lipman RS, Rickels K, et al: The Hopkins Symptom Checklist (HSCL): a measure of primary symptom dimensions, in Psychological Measurements in Psychopharmacology, Vol 7: Modern Problems of Pharmacopsychiatry. Edited by Pichot P. Basel, Switzerland, S Karger, 1974, pp 79–110

Dowd ET, Milne CR, Wise SL: The Therapeutic Reactance Scale: a measure of psychological reactance. J Consult Clin Psychol 69:541–545, 1991

Endicott J, Spitzer RL: Use of the Research Diagnostic Criteria and the Schedule for Affective Disorders and Schizophrenia to study affective disorders. Am J Psychiatry 136:52–56, 1979

Endler NS, Hunt J McV, Rosenstein AJ: An S-R inventory of anxiousness. Psychol Monogr: Gen Applied 76 (monogr no 536, issue no 17):1–31, 1962

Exner JE Jr: The Rorschach: A Comprehensive System, Vol 1. New York, Wiley, 1974

Exner JE Jr: The Rorschach: A Comprehensive System, Vol 2. New York, Wiley, 1978

Eysenck HJ, Eysenck SB: The Structure and Measurement of Personality. San Diego, CA, RR Knapp, 1969

Feighner JP, Robins E, Guze SB, et al: Diagnostic criteria for use in psychiatric research. Arch Gen Psychiatry 26:57–63, 1972

First MB, Spitzer RL, Gibbon M, et al: Structured Clinical Interview for DSM-IV Axis I Disorders–Patient Edition (SCID-I/P). New York, Biometrics Research Department, New York State Psychiatric Institute, 1995

First MB, Gibbon M, Spitzer RL, et al: User's Guide for the Structured Clinical Interview for DSM-IV Axis II Personality Disorders (SCID-II). Washington, DC, American Psychiatric Press, 1997

Foa EB: Posttraumatic Stress Diagnostic Scale: Manual. Minneapolis, MN, National Computer Systems, 1995

Folstein MF, Folstein SE, McHugh PR: Mini-mental state: a practical method for grading the cognitive state of patients for the clinician. J Psychiatr Res 11:189–198, 1975

Fonagy P: Process and outcome in mental health care delivery: a model approach to treatment evaluation. Bull Menninger Clin 63:288–304, 1999

Garner DM: Eating Disorder Inventory 2: Professional Manual. Odessa, FL, Psychological Assessment Resources, 1992

Gaw KF, Beutler LE: Integrating treatment recommendations, in Integrative Assessment of Adult Personality. Edited by Beutler LE, Berren MR. New York, Guilford, 1995, pp 280–319

Geffen G, Moar KJ, O'Hanlon AP, et al: Performance measures of 16- to 86-year-old males and females on the Auditory Verbal Learning Test. The Clinical Neuropsychologist 4:45–63, 1990

Geisinger KF: Cross-cultural normative assessment: translation adaptation issues influencing the normative interpretation of assessment instruments. Psychol Assess 6:312–314, 1994

Golden CJ, Hammeke TA, Purisch AD: Diagnostic validity of a standardized neuropsychological battery derived from Luria's neuropsychological tests. J Consult Clin Psychol 46:1258–1265, 1978

Goldman R, Fristoe M, Woodcock RW: Auditory Skills Test Battery. Circle Pines, MN, American Guidance Service, 1976

Goodglass H, Kaplan E: Assessment of Aphasia and Related Disorders. Philadelphia, PA, Lea & Febiger, 1972

Goodman WK, Price LH, Rasmussen SA, et al: The Yale-Brown Obsessive Compulsive Scale, I: development, use, and reliability. Arch Gen Psychiatry 46:1006–1011, 1989

Gough HG: California Psychological Inventory. Palo Alto, CA, Consulting Psychologists Press, 1956

Graham JR: MMPI-2: Assessing Personality and Psychopathology. New York, Oxford University Press, 1990

Greene RL: The MMPI-2/MMPI: An Interpretive Manual. Needham Heights, MA, Allyn & Bacon, 1991

Greene RL, Banken JA: Assessing alcohol/drug abuse problems, in Clinical Personality Assessment: Practical Approaches. Edited by Butcher JN. New York, Oxford University Press, 1995, pp 460–474

Halstead WC, Wepman JM: The Halstead-Wepman Aphasia Screening Test. J Speech Hear Disord 14:9–15, 1959

Hamilton M: The assessment of anxiety states by rating. Br J Med Psychol 32:50–55, 1959

Hamilton M: A rating scale for depression. J Neurol Neurosurg Psychiatry 23:51–56, 1960

Hamilton M: Development of a rating scale for primary depressive illness. Br J Soc Clin Psychol 6:278–296, 1967

Harrow M, Quinlan D (eds): Disordered Thinking and Schizophrenic Psychopathology. New York, Gardner, 1985

Hathaway SR, McKinley JC: Minnesota Multiphasic Personality Inventory Manual, Revised Edition. New York, Psychological Corporation, 1967

Hathaway SR, McKinley JC: Minnesota Multiphasic Personality Inventory–2. Minneapolis MN: University of Minnesota Press, 1989

Haxby JV, Raffaele K, Gillete J, et al: Individual trajectories of cognitive decline in patients with dementia of the Alzheimer type. J Clin Exp Neuropsychol 14:575–592, 1992

Heaton RK, Crowley TJ: Effects of psychiatric disorders and their somatic treatments on neuropsychological test results, in Handbook of Clinical Neuropsychology. Edited by Filskov SB, Boll TJ. New York, Wiley, 1981, pp 481–525

Hoffmann H, Loper RG, Kammeier ML: Identifying future alcoholics with MMPI alcoholism scales. Q J Stud Alcohol 35(pt A):490–498, 1974

Horn JL, Wanberg KW, Foster FM: Alcohol Use Inventory. Minneapolis, MN, National Computer Systems, 1986

Hurt SW, Holzman PS, Davis JM: Thought disorder: the measurement of its changes. Arch Gen Psychiatry 40:1281–1285, 1983

Hurt SW, Hyler SE, Frances A, et al: Assessing borderline personality disorder with self-report, clinical interview, or semistructured interview. Am J Psychiatry 141:1228–1231, 1984

Hurt SW, Clarkin JF, Frances A, et al: Discriminate validity of the MMPI for borderline personality disorder. J Pers Assess 49:56–61, 1985

Hurt SW, Reznikoff M, Clarkin JF: Psychological Assessment, Psychiatric Diagnosis, and Treatment Planning. New York, Brunner/Mazel, 1991

Hyler SE: Personality Diagnostic Questionnaire–4. New York, New York State Psychiatric Institute, 1994

Hyler SE, Rieder RO, Williams JBW, et al: The Personality Diagnostic Questionnaire: development and preliminary results. J Personal Disorders 2:229–237, 1988

Janowsky D, Judd L, Huey L, et al: Naloxone effects on manic symptoms and growth-hormone levels (letter). Lancet 2:320, 1978

Jastak S, Wilkinson GS: The Wide Range Achievement Test—Revised. Wilmington, DE, Jastak Associates, 1981

Jenkins CD, Rosenman RH, Friedman J: Development of an objective psychological test for the determination of the coronary-prone behavior pattern in employed men. J Chronic Dis 20:371–379, 1967

Johnston MH, Holzman PS: Assessing Schizophrenic Thinking. San Francisco, CA, Jossey-Bass, 1979

Karzmark P, Heaton RK, Grant I, et al: Use of demographic variables to predict full scale IQ: a replication and extension. J Clin Exp Neuropsychol 7:412–420, 1985

Katz MM, Lyerly SB: Methods for measuring adjustment and social behavior in the community, I: rationale, description, discriminative validity and scale development. Psychological Reports Monograph 13:503–535, 1963

Kimura D: Functional asymmetry of the brain in dichotic listening. Cortex 3:163–178, 1967

Leary T: Interpersonal Diagnosis of Personality. New York, Ronald Press, 1957

Lenzenweger MF, Loranger AW, Korfine L, et al: Detecting personality disorders in a nonclinical population: application of a two-stage procedure for case detection. Arch Gen Psychiatry 54:345–351, 1997

Lezak M: Neuropsychological Assessment. New York, Oxford University Press, 1969

Liebowitz MR: Social phobia. Mod Probl Pharmacopsychiatry 22:141–173, 1987

Linehan MM, Goodstein JL, Nielson SL, et al: Reasons for staying alive when you are thinking of killing yourself: the Reasons for Living Inventory. J Consult Clin Psychol 51:276–286, 1983

Loranger AW: Personality Disorder Examination (PDE) Manual. Yonkers, NY, DV Communications, 1988

Loranger AW: International Personality Disorder Examination (IPDE) Manual. Odessa, FL, Psychological Assessment Resources, 1999

Loranger AW, Hirschfeld RMA, Sartorius N, et al: The WHO/ADAMHA international pilot study of personality disorders: background and purpose. Journal of Personality Disorders 5:296–306, 1991

Lorr M, McNair DM: Expansion of the interpersonal behavior circle. J Pers Soc Psychol 2:823–830, 1965

Lorr M, Youniss RP: An inventory of interpersonal style. J Pers Assess 37:165–173, 1973

Luria AR: Higher Cortical Functions in Man. New York, Basic Books, 1966

Luria AR: The Working Brain: An Introduction to Neuropsychology. Translated by Haigh B. New York, Basic Books, 1973

MacAndrew C: The differentiation of male alcohol outpatients from nonalcoholic psychiatric patients by means of the MMPI. Q J Stud Alcohol 26:238–246, 1965

Marengo J, Harrow M: Thought disorder: a function of schizophrenia, mania, or psychosis? J Nerv Ment Dis 173:35–41, 1985

Marks IM, Seeman W: The Actuarial Description of Abnormal Personality. Baltimore, MD, Williams & Wilkins, 1963

Marks IM, Seeman W, Haller DL: The Actuarial Use of the MMPI With Adolescents and Adults. Baltimore, MD, Williams & Wilkins, 1974

Mattis S: Dementia Rating Scale: Professional Manual. Odessa, FL, Psychological Assessment Resources, 1988

Mattis S, French JH, Rapin I: Dyslexia in children and young adults: three independent neuropsychological syndromes. Dev Med Child Neurol 17:150–163, 1975

Mattis S, Kovner R, Goldmeier E: Different patterns of mnemonic deficits in two organic amnestic syndromes. Brain Lang 6:179–191, 1978

McKinley JC, Hathaway SR, Meehl PE: The MMPI, VI: K scale. Journal of Consulting Psychology 12:20–31, 1948

Megargee EI, Cook PE, Mendelsohn GA: Development and validation of an MMPI scale of assaultiveness in overcontrolled individuals. J Abnorm Psychol 72:519–528, 1967

Mesulam M-M: Principles of Behavioral Neurology. Philadelphia, PA, FA Davis, 1985

Millon T: Millon Clinical Multiaxial Inventory—II: Manual for the MCMI-II. Minneapolis, MN, National Computer Systems, 1987

Millon T, Davis R, Millon C: MCMI-III Manual, 2nd Edition. Minneapolis, MN, National Computer Systems, 1997

Mirsky AF, Kornetsky C: On the dissimilar effects of drugs on the Digit Symbol Substitution and Continuous Performance Tests: a review and preliminary integration of behavioral and physiological evidence. Psychopharmacologia 5:161–177, 1964

Morey LC: Personality Assessment Inventory. Odessa, FL, Psychological Assessment Resources, 1991

Moreland KL, Fowler RD, Honaker LM: Future directions in the use of psychological assessment for treatment planning and outcome assessment: predictions and recommendations, in The Use of Psychological Testing for Treatment Planning and Outcome Assessment. Edited by Maruish ME. Hillsdale, NJ, Lawrence Erlbaum, 1994, pp 581–602

Murray HA: Thematic Apperception Test Manual. Cambridge, MA, Harvard University Press, 1943

Nelson HE: National Adult Reading Test (NART) Test Manual. Berkshire, MA, NFER-Nelson, 1982

Newman FL, Ciarlo JA: Criteria for selecting psychological tests/instruments, in Use of Psychological Testing for Treatment Planning and Outcome Assessment. Edited by Maruish M. Malvern, PA, LEA Publishers, 1994, pp 98–110

Overall JE, Gorham DR: The Brief Psychiatric Rating Scale. Psychol Rep 10:799–812, 1962

Pfohl B, Langbehn D: Iowa Personality Disorder Screen (Version 1.2). Iowa City, IA, University of Iowa, Department of Psychiatry, 1994

Pfohl B, Blum N, Zimmerman M: Structured Interview for DSM-IV Personality (SIDP-IV). Washington, DC, American Psychiatric Press, 1997

Pilkonis PA, Kim Y, Proitetti JM, et al: A screen scale for personality disorders developed from the Inventory of Interpersonal Problems. J Pers Disorders 10:355–369, 1996

Raven JC: Guide to the Standard Progressive Matrices. London, England, HK Lewis, 1960

Rey A: L'examen psychologique dans les cas d'encephalopathie traumatique. Archives de Psychologie 28:286–340, 1941

Rey A: L'Examen Clinique en Psychologique. Paris, France, Presses Universitaires de France, 1964

Ridley CR, Li LC, Hill CL: Multicultural assessment: re-examination, reconceptualization and practical application. Counseling Psychologist 26:827–910, 1998

Rorschach H: Psychodiagnostics. New York, Grune & Stratton, 1949

Rosvold HE, Mirsky AF, Sarason I, et al: A continuous performance test of brain damage. J Consult Clin Psychol 20:343–350, 1956

Sarason IG, Levine HM, Basham RB, et al: Assessing social support: the Social Support Questionnaire. J Pers Soc Psychol 44:127–139, 1983

Schroeder ML, Wormworth JA, Livesley WJ: Dimensions of personality disorder and the five-factor model of personality, in Personality Disorders and the Five-Factor Model of Personality. Edited by Costa PT, Widiger TA. Washington,

DC, American Psychological Association, 1994, pp 117–127

Seashore CE, Lewis D, Saetveit DL: Seashore Measures of Musical Talents, Revised Edition. New York, Psychological Corporation, 1960

Secunda S, Katz M, Swann A, et al: Mania: diagnosis, state measurement, and prediction of treatment response. J Affect Disord 8:113–121, 1985

Seidman IJ: Schizophrenia and brain dysfunction: an integration of recent neurodiagnostic findings. Psychol Bull 94:195–238, 1983

Shenton ME, Kikinis R, Frenc AJ, et al: Abnormalities of the left temporal lobe and thought disorder in schizophrenia: a quantitative magnetic resonance imaging study. N Engl J Med 327:604–612, 1992

Shipley WC: The Institute of Living Scale. Los Angeles, CA, Western Psychological Services, 1946

Snyder DK, Wills RM, Keiser TW: Empirical validation of the Marital Satisfaction Inventory: an actuarial approach. J Consult Clin Psychol 49:262–268, 1981

Solovay MR, Shenton ME, Gasperetti C, et al: Scoring manual for the Thought Disorder Index. Schizophr Bull 12:483–496, 1986

Spanier GB: Measuring dyadic adjustment: new scales for assessing the quality of marriage and similar dyads. Journal of Marriage and the Family 38:15–28, 1976

Spielberger CD: State-Trait Anger Expression Inventory, Revised Research Edition. Odessa, FL, Psychological Assessment Resources, 1991

Spielberger CD, Gorsuch RL, Luchene RE: Manual for the State-Trait Anxiety Inventory. Palo Alto, CA, Consulting Psychologists Press, 1976

Spitzer RL, Williams J, Gibbon M, et al: Structured Clinical Interview for DSM-III-R (SCID): User's Guide. Washington, DC, American Psychiatric Press, 1992

Spreen O, Benton AL: Neurosensory Center Comprehensive Examination for Aphasia. Victoria, BC, University of Victoria, 1977

Svrakic DM, Whitehead C, Przybeck TR, et al: Differential diagnosis of personality disorders by the seven-factor model of temperament and character. Arch Gen Psychiatry 50:991–999, 1993

Taylor-Spence JA, Spence KW: The motivational components of manifest anxiety: drive and drive stimuli, in Anxiety and Behavior. Edited by Spielberger CD. New York, Academic Press, 1966, pp 291–326

Vitaliano PP, Breen AR, Russo J, et al: The clinical utility of the Dementia Rating Scale for assessing Alzheimer patients. J Chronic Dis 37:743–753, 1984

Wechsler D: Wechsler Adult Intelligence Scale—III Administrative and Scoring Manual. San Antonio, TX, Psychological Corporation, 1997

Weed NC, Butcher JN, McKenna T, et al: New measures for assessing alcohol and drug abuse with the MMPI-2: the APS and AAS. J Pers Assess 58:389–404, 1992

Weissman MM, Bothwell S: Assessment of social adjustment by patient self-report. Arch Gen Psychiatry 33:1111–1115, 1976

Weissman MM, Sholomskas D: The assessment of social adjustment by the clinician, the patient, and the family, in The Behavior of Psychiatric Patients: Quantitative Techniques for Evaluation. Edited by Burdock EI, Sudilovsky A, Gershon S. New York, Marcel Dekker, 1982, pp 177–209

Wiggins JS: Circumplex models of interpersonal behavior in clinical psychology, in Handbook of Research Methods in Clinical Psychology. Edited by Kendall PC, Butcher JN. New York, Wiley, 1982, pp 183–221

Wiggins JS, Pincus AL: Personality: structure and assessment. Annu Rev Psychol 43:473–504, 1992

Willner AE: Towards development of more sensitive clinical tests of abstraction: the analogy test. Proceedings of the 78th Annual Convention of the American Psychological Association 5:553–554, 1971

Young RC, Biggs JT, Ziegler VE, et al: A rating scale for mania: reliability, validity and sensitivity. Br J Psychiatry 133:429–435, 1978

Yudofsky SC, Silver JM, Jackson W, et al: The Overt Aggression Scale for the objective rating of verbal and physical aggression. Am J Psychiatry 143:35–39, 1986

Zung WWK: A rating instrument for anxiety disorders. Psychosomatics 12:371–379, 1971

Zung WWK: Index of Potential Suicide (IPS): a rating scale for suicide prevention, in The Prediction of Suicide. Edited by Beck AT, Resnick HLP, Lettieri DJ. Bowie, MD, Charles Press, 1974, pp 221–249

CHAPTER 6

Laboratory and Other Diagnostic Tests in Psychiatry

John M. Morihisa, M.D.

C. Deborah Cross, M.D.

Stephen Price, M.D.

Michael Precioso, Ph.D.

Steven Koontz, B.S.

As we begin a new century of searching for meaning in the complex mechanisms of the human brain, we find ourselves at the crossroads of converging technologies in molecular genetics, brain imaging, and computerized data analysis that will synergistically propel us to the long-sought elucidation of the disease processes that constitute psychiatric illness. In this century, we will build neural-network models of the myriad ways in which the brain malfunctions in each psychiatric disorder, and with these models, we will elaborate enhanced diagnostic and therapeutic tools in our work to alleviate the suffering and devastation of mental illness (Morihisa 2001).

The increased use of biological therapies in psychiatry has resulted in a parallel, enhanced interest in the application of laboratory and diagnostic test evaluations for psychiatric patients. The reasons for this growing interest include an expanding awareness of physical conditions that can produce psychiatric symptoms and the need to use the laboratory to monitor certain psychopharmacological interventions. Additionally, psychiatrists have been accumulating evidence of subtle neurophysiological dysfunction in many psychiatric disorders, and an effort is being made to try to characterize some of these abnormalities. Such research findings have significantly expanded the scope of thinking concerning many disease processes and have raised the hope that if these pathophysiological abnormalities can be clearly elucidated, new and more useful laboratory tests for psychiatry might be developed.

The laboratory and diagnostic test procedures used by psychiatrists today range from those commonly used by physicians (e.g., complete blood count [CBC], chemistry panels, electrocardiography) to those used mainly in psychiatric research (e.g., positron emission tomography [PET]). However, the reader should be aware that the field of laboratory and diagnostic testing in psychiatry will not only be determined by research findings in clinical psychiatry and the neurosciences but also probably be influenced by changing economic realities and by quality assurance and liability issues. Furthermore, medical science is constantly evolving, and no consensus has been achieved concerning many diagnostic approaches. The clinician must ultimately use good clinical judgment in determining an appropriate, comprehensive evaluation for each patient. No chapter or table can provide complete or exhaustive protocols for every patient; rather, this information is meant to be a starting point from which the reader can begin the complicated, complex, and demanding task of customizing the appropriate evaluation for each patient.

The use of laboratory and other diagnostic tests in the evaluation and treatment of psychiatric patients must ultimately be determined by each physician, who can consider the entire unique constellation of clinical elements that characterizes each individual patient. No text or protocol can replace the clinical judgment required of each physician in determining the appropriate selection and interpretation of such tests in the development of an effective diagnostic and therapeutic strategy.

Use of Diagnostic Tests in Detecting Physical Illness in Psychiatric Patients

DSM-IV-TR (American Psychiatric Association 2000) has for many psychiatric diagnoses a common criterion: the necessary exclusion of any underlying physical condition that might account for the patient's symptomatology. Indeed, several studies have found that physical illnesses are quite common among psychiatric patients. In addition, many of these physical disorders have been thought to be causative or exacerbating factors in patients' psychiatric presentation (Hoffman and Koran 1984). Furthermore, it has been suggested that many psychiatric patients with concomitant medical disorders are particularly vulnerable to excessive morbidity because of their medical conditions (Dvoredsky and Cooley 1986).

Initial suspicion of a possible organic component in a patient's psychiatric presentation can come from clues provided by a careful history taking and physical examination. Although there is no complete consensus about which signs and symptoms are most suggestive of organic conditions, several investigators have proposed criteria that they believe might implicate an organic mental disorder. For example, Hoffman and Koran (1984) outlined a table of clues "suggestive" of organic mental disorders (Table 6–1). In addition, Hall et al. (1978) reported that when a review-of-symptoms checklist was used in psychiatric outpatients, patients with four or more positive responses on the checklist had a much higher incidence of abnormal laboratory results than did those who were symptom negative. Many of these abnormal laboratory results were thought to reflect physical conditions that influenced the patients' psychiatric presentation.

For patients known to have (or who are suspected of having) a medical illness, one orders the laboratory tests necessary to work up or follow up the physical condi-

TABLE 6–1. Some clues suggestive of organic mental disorders

1. Psychiatric symptoms after age 40
2. Psychiatric symptoms
   a. During a major medical illness
   b. While taking drugs that can cause mental symptoms
3. History of
   a. Alcohol or drug abuse
   b. Physical illness impairing organ function (neurological, endocrine, renal, hepatic, cardiac, pulmonary)
   c. Taking multiple prescribed or over-the-counter drugs
4. Family history of
   a. Degenerative or inheritable brain disease
   b. Inherited metabolic disease (e.g., diabetes, pernicious anemia, porphyria)
5. Mental signs including
   a. Altered level of consciousness
   b. Fluctuating mental status
   c. Cognitive impairment
   d. Episodic, recurrent, or cyclic course
   e. Visual, tactile, or olfactory hallucinations
6. Physical signs including
   a. Signs of organ malfunction that can affect the brain
   b. Focal neurological deficits
   c. Diffuse subcortical dysfunction, such as slowed speech/mentation/movement, ataxia, incoordination, tremor, chorea, asterixis, dysarthria
   d. Cortical dysfunction (e.g., dysphasia, apraxias, agnosias, visuospatial deficits, or defective cortical sensation)

Source. Reprinted with permission from Hoffman RS, Koran RM: "Detecting Physical Illness in Patients With Mental Disorders." *Psychosomatics* 25:654–660, 1984. Copyright 1984 American Psychiatric Press, Inc.

tion (Hales 1986). Physical conditions not thought to be contributing to the psychiatric presentation also need to be appropriately evaluated because psychiatric patients with concomitant medical problems have been reported to have increased mortality secondary to their medical conditions (Dvoredsky and Cooley 1986; Karasu et al. 1980; Koranyi 1979). In addition, some of the physical conditions initially considered only coincidental to the psychiatric illness might later prove to be etiological or to exacerbate the psychiatric condition. Consultation from other medical specialists might be necessary, but the consultants' impressions and recommendations all require careful scrutiny by the attending psychiatrist, who holds the ultimate responsibility for fitting together the pattern of specialized opinions. Decisions to continue or extend laboratory evaluation are often complex and generally include some type of risk-benefit analysis, as well as consideration of prevailing economic and liability issues. This is not to suggest that a laboratory test that a physician believes might be useful should or should not be used because of primarily economic or legal considerations. Good clinical judgment needs to be the final arbiter for all clinical decisions regarding choice of laboratory and diagnostic testing. Test risks that should be considered (and weighed against the potential benefits of obtaining the test) include possible physical complications, pain, or discomfort (e.g., from repeated venipuncture).

Most clinicians must limit studies according to some assessment of their likely utility in each individual case. Some studies of the use of rather extensive laboratory testing strategies in psychiatric patients have reported that such approaches yield a relatively small amount of useful new information for the clinician (see, e.g., Dolan and Mushlin 1985). However, it can be argued that subclinical physical disorders can cause or possibly exacerbate psychiatric symptoms. Cognitive or behavioral symptoms usually do not signal a specific type of underlying organic problem, but rather suggest an often extensive differential diagnosis.

Studies of medically ill patients and anecdotal reports in the literature have described a wide range of different psychiatric symptoms or syndromes caused by different neuromedical conditions (e.g., Giannini et al. 1978). Additionally, psychiatric symptoms alone usually are inadequate for differentiating the type of underlying medical problem present. For instance, Asaad and Shapiro (1986) outlined organic conditions that can be associated with hallucinations. These organic conditions can include substance abuse disorders, medication psychotoxicity (e.g., secondary to such agents as propranolol and atropine), neurological disorders (e.g., complex partial seizures, central nervous system [CNS] infections), and endocrine and metabolic abnormalities, as well as hallucinations associated with eye and ear diseases (e.g., bilateral hearing loss). Furthermore, many specific organic factors can cause myriad different psychiatric symptom pictures in different patients.

Specific laboratory protocols for some common psychiatric complaints, such as schizophrenia, bipolar disorder, depression, and anxiety, have been proposed (e.g., Expert Consensus Panel for Bipolar Disorder 1996; Expert Consensus Panel for Schizophrenia 1996). The protocols would provide the psychiatric clinician with thorough laboratory and diagnostic tests based on the possible differential diagnosis for the patient's psychiatric complaints. Note that the patients generally would not have any obvious physical signs or symptoms of the possible organic disorder to be evaluated in the laboratory screen. Many of the diagnostic tests ordered would be part of a search for various areas of possible organic dys-

function. The use of these laboratory screening test protocols would require the clinician to become familiar with the often complex organic differential diagnoses for various psychiatric symptoms so that he or she could more meaningfully interpret any discovered laboratory test abnormalities and proceed appropriately. A possible general algorithm for laboratory and diagnostic testing in psychiatric patients is outlined in Figure 6–1.

Screening Tests in Psychiatry

There is incomplete agreement as to what should constitute a "routine" screening laboratory and diagnostic test battery (see Tables 6–2 and 6–3). Some investigators recommend a very brief and selective laboratory and diagnostic test evaluation in patients with no obvious signs or symptoms of physical disease; the choice of tests in this situation is generally based on clinical relevance to the patient's particular condition. Hoffman and Koran (1984) proposed a somewhat more extensive screening battery based on a selection of the available studies of physical disorders in psychiatric patients (see, e.g., Hall et al. 1980). The recommendations include a CBC; automated chemistry panels (including electrolytes, glucose, renal and hepatic functions, and calcium and phosphate levels); thyroid function tests; a screening test for syphilis and for vitamin B_{12} and folate levels; and a urinalysis. Specific thyroid function tests that have been recommended in the past include triiodothyronine (T_3) resin uptake (T_3RU), thyroxine (T_4), and thyroid-stimulating hormone (TSH); however, other thyroid function tests are also available (e.g., T_3 radioimmunoassay [RIA]). Hoffman and Koran (1984) further recommended an electrocardiogram (ECG) and chest X ray as part of the workup because possible cardiopulmonary dysfunction detected by these screening tests could be particularly relevant to an evaluation of a possible organic mental disorder. Additional suggestions for tests to be included in routine screens are a slide test of stool for occult blood, tuberculin skin tests, and an electroencephalogram (EEG) (Hoffman and Koran 1984). Other tests sometimes added to this routine laboratory workup include an erythrocyte sedimentation rate, serum proteins, serum protein electrophoresis, and tests for lupus erythematosus (LE) cells or antinuclear antibodies, as well as urine examinations for substances of abuse, porphyrins, and heavy metals (see Table 6–3). Finally, periodic Papanicolaou tests and mammography for women in appropriate age groups represent important screening procedures for all physicians to remember.

As alluded to earlier in this chapter, some investigators have argued for less extensive, more selective routine

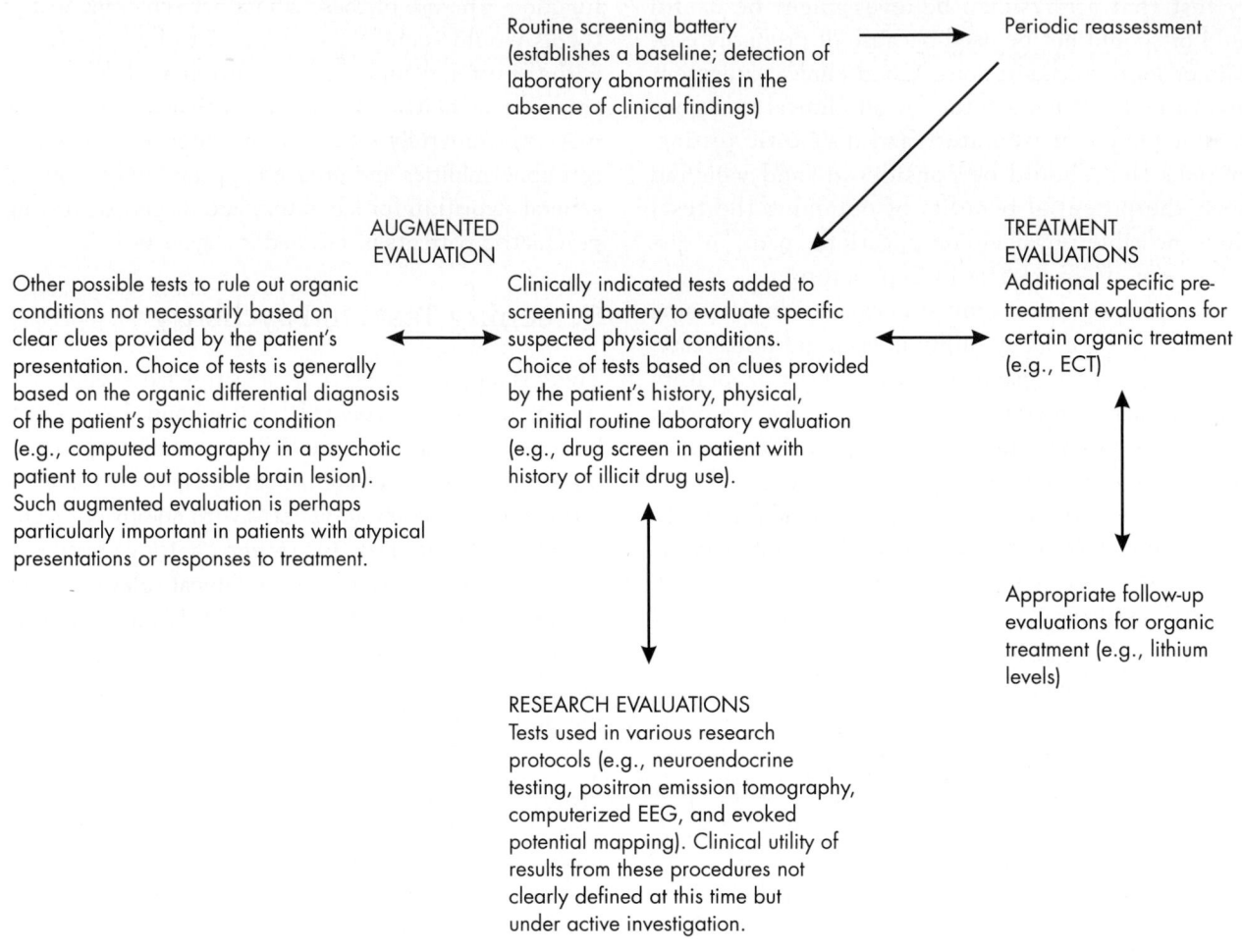

FIGURE 6–1. General guidelines for the use of diagnostic testing in psychiatry.

ECT = electroconvulsive therapy; EEG = electroencephalography.

screening batteries for psychiatric patients who have no signs or symptoms of physical illness. These investigators probably would recommend that many of these previously described laboratory and diagnostic tests be ordered only if indicated by the history, clinical evaluation, or initial laboratory evaluation. For instance, Dolan and Mushlin (1985) studied 250 psychiatric inpatients who had a mean number of routine admission laboratory tests of close to 30. They found that the mean percentage of true positive results from all the laboratory tests performed was only 1.8% and that for only 11 patients (4%) were important medical problems discovered through the routine laboratory testing described by the investigators. Dolan and Mushlin reported that a routine battery—consisting of only a CBC (hemoglobin, hematocrit, white blood cell [WBC] count, and mean cell volume); serum levels of thyroxine, calcium, aspartate aminotransferase (AST), alkaline phosphatase, and syphilis serology; and a urinalysis—would have identified all 11 psychiatric patients whose diagnoses had been made on the basis of

the screening laboratory examination and who required further evaluation.

Note, however, that Dolan and Mushlin addressed only some of the clinical laboratory and diagnostic testing procedures that we have described so far. For instance, their study did not address the value of routine screening with tests such as sedimentation rate, vitamin B_{12} and folate levels, stool tests for occult blood, ECG, EEG, skin testing (e.g., purified protein derivative), and chest X ray. It is hoped that future epidemiological research on large numbers of psychiatric patients will help settle the debate about a selective versus a nonselective screening battery, which should help clinicians better decide which tests would be most appropriate in a "routine" screen for psychiatric patients.

Economic factors and cost–benefit analyses for populations of patients are often taken into consideration in this debate (especially with the increasing emphasis on cost containment in health care). Until some consensus is reached, the psychiatrist must use his or her judgment in

TABLE 6–2. Laboratory and diagnostic tests useful for detecting physical disease in psychiatric patients

Complete blood count[a]

Chemistry panel, including serum electrolytes,[a] glucose,[a] albumin, total protein, blood urea nitrogen,[a] creatinine,[a] calcium, phosphate, aspartate aminotransferase,[a] alanine aminotransferase,[a] alkaline phosphatase,[a] γ-glutamyltransferase,[a] bilirubin,[a] iron, magnesium, serum cholesterol, and triglycerides

Thyroid function tests[a]

Screening test for syphilis (VDRL or rapid plasma reagin)[a]

HIV serology in potentially high-risk patients

Serum vitamin B_{12} and folate levels[a]

Urinalysis (with dipstick for protein and glucose)[a]

Urine toxicology (e.g., for substances of abuse, heavy metals, anabolic steroids)

Urine for uroporphyrins and porphobilinogen

Erythrocyte uroporphyrinogen-1-synthetase

Serum ceruloplasmin

Chest X ray

Electrocardiography

Electroencephalography[a]

Computed tomography or magnetic resonance imaging[a]

Note. The important principles of informed consent should always be applied. Tables 6–2 and 6–3 are not meant to be mutually exclusive. VDRL = Venereal Disease Research Laboratory.

[a]These tests are included in the recommended screening battery for patients with new onset of dementia. Tests considered "supplemental" to the core battery are computed tomography, magnetic resonance imaging, electroencephalography, and lumbar puncture studies. National Institutes of Health Consensus Development Panel: "Differential Diagnosis of Dementing Disease." National Institutes of Health Consensus Development Conference Statement 6:1–9, 1987.

Source. Data from Rosse et al. 1989; Koran et al. 1989; and Sox et al. 1989.

TABLE 6–3. Supplemental laboratory and diagnostic tests for evaluating physical conditions in psychiatric patients

Computed tomography scan

Magnetic resonance imaging scan

Skull films

Electroencephalography

Blood or breath alcohol level

Drug screen (e.g., thin-layer chromatography) and possible confirmatory test(s) for positive results (e.g., chromatography–mass spectroscopy)

Heavy-metal screen

Blood levels of medications

Sedimentation rate

Antinuclear antibodies

Lumbar puncture with cerebrospinal fluid studies

Serum and urine copper levels

Serum ceruloplasmin

HIV testing

Monospot test

Blood cultures

Skin test for tuberculosis or brucellosis

Pregnancy tests

Urine for uroporphyrins

Urine and serum osmolality

Polysomnography

Nocturnal penile tumescence

Evoked potentials

Stool tests for occult blood

Arterial blood gases

Note. The important principles of informed consent should always be applied. Tables 6–2 and 6–3 are not meant to be mutually exclusive.

selecting screening protocols for patients who present without symptoms that mandate a specific laboratory strategy.

Diagnostic Screening Batteries for Geriatric Psychiatric Patients

Regarding the most useful diagnostic test screening battery for geriatric patients, no complete consensus yet seems to exist. For instance, Kolman (1985) reported on a study that attempted to determine whether the number of routine laboratory tests ordered for a geriatric patient population could be decreased without compromising quality of care. The admitting psychiatrist's judgment in deciding which laboratory and diagnostic tests should be performed for a particular patient was evaluated. In this study, Kolman found that the admitting phy-

sicians tended to underestimate the number of tests that would yield an abnormal result.

For a geriatric population, Kolman suggested the use of a fairly extensive routine admission screening protocol: serum hemoglobin; a WBC count; sedimentation rate; serum vitamin B_{12} and folate levels; a biochemical profile, including serum sodium, potassium, bicarbonate, blood urea nitrogen (BUN), calcium, phosphate, alkaline phosphatase, bilirubin, thyroxine, and glucose; a urinalysis (with bacteriological culture, if appropriate); a chest X ray; a skull X ray; and an ECG.

The National Institute on Aging Task Force (1980) recommended a similar test battery for the evaluation of dementia. Their recommendation included a CBC, erythrocyte sedimentation rate, serum electrolytes (sodium, potassium, bicarbonate, chloride, calcium, phosphorus), BUN and glucose, serum bilirubin, serum vitamin B_{12} and folate, thyroid screen, serological test for syphilis, urinalysis (including albumin, glucose, and ketone levels and microscopic examination), stool exam-is suspected that they recently ingested alcohol). Different types of breath alcohol instruments exist (e.g., chemical reagent tube tests, tests using an electrochemical cell that generates a voltage in response to alcohol vapor, and tests that use infrared detectors). Finally, it is often helpful to consult with staff from the laboratory used by the physician about which drug screening and follow-up confirmation tests might be ordered and which specimens should be sent in a specific clinical situation.

Laboratory Evaluation for Environmental Toxins

Exposure to several different environmental toxins has been associated with various behavioral abnormalities. Possible environmental toxins with behavioral consequences include the heavy metals, such as mercury, lead, manganese, thallium, and arsenic. In the case of suspected heavy-metal exposure (e.g., through industrial or toxic waste contamination), a determination of blood or urinary concentrations of these metals might be helpful (DeLisi 1984). The clinician should remain alert to the possibility of poisoning by these metals as well as other environmental toxins (e.g., organophosphate insecticides) associated with behavioral aberrations. The appropriate laboratory tests should be ordered when the possibility of such environmental toxin exposure is high. Care must be taken to avoid possible artifactual contamination of the sample. For instance, if capillary blood is drawn from the fingertips of small children in the evaluation of possible lead poisoning, the risk of contamination from the skin is reduced if proper washing procedures are used.

Computed Tomography and Magnetic Resonance Imaging in Clinical Psychiatry

Computed tomographic scanning of the head offers the clinician cross-sectional X-ray images of the brain from multiple brain levels (both cortical and subcortical). The procedure has been available for general clinical use by psychiatrists since the mid-1970s and is most often used in the evaluation of patients with suspected structural brain abnormalities (e.g., tumor, subdural hematoma, stroke, abscess). An example of a single cross-sectional CT scan image is presented in Figure 6–2. Guidelines to help clinicians in deciding when to order structural brain-imaging studies such as a CT scan for psychiatric patients have ranged from very specific, limited indications to a broad spectrum of symptoms and presentations (see Table 6–6). Larson et al. (1986) recommended ordering a CT scan in psychiatric patients with focal neurological

findings, whereas others have indicated that the presence of an abnormal EEG result in psychiatric patients also would be a good indication for ordering a CT scan. Weinberger (1984) expanded on these two possible indications and recommended obtaining a CT scan in psychiatric patients whose clinical presentation includes any of the following: confusion, dementia of unknown cause, first episode of a psychosis of unknown etiology, movement disorder of unknown etiology, diagnosis of anorexia nervosa, prolonged catatonia, or first episode of major affective disorder or personality change after age 50. Emsley et al. (1986) extended these recommendations to include ordering CT scans for any patient with a history of alcohol abuse, craniocerebral trauma, or seizures.

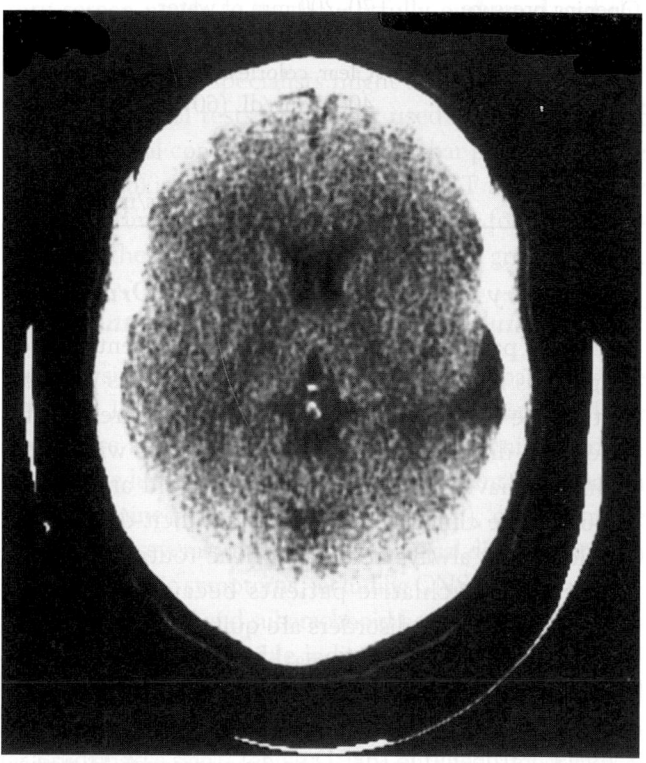

FIGURE 6–2. Computed tomographic scan of the head without contrast material.

Image for a single brain level shown. Note hypodense area in the left temporal region adjacent to the skull. Intravenous injection of a standard roentgenographic contrast medium may be used to enhance a computed tomographic study for improved visualization of certain brain lesions (e.g., recent stroke, tumors, infections, abscesses).

MRI of the brain (Figure 6–3) can usefully supplement or replace CT in certain clinical situations because some lesions are better appreciated on MRI than on CT scan (Table 6–7). The MRI usually is superior to CT scan when lesions are suspected in the posterior fossa, brain stem, or temporal and apical areas of the brain because

TABLE 6–6. Possible indications for structural brain-imaging procedure (computed tomography or magnetic resonance imaging) in psychiatric practice

Focal neurological findings
Abnormal electroencephalogram findings
Unknown etiology in cases of
   Confusion
   First episode of psychosis
   Movement disorder
   Anorexia nervosa
   Prolonged catatonia
   First affective episode after age 50
Personality change after age 50
Alcohol dependence
History of head trauma
History of seizures
Impaired cognition on mental status examination

Source. Data from Rosse et al. 1989.

the surrounding bone can distort the CT image (Jaskiw et al. 1987) or obstruct visualization (Figure 6–4). Indeed, the CT scan, with its excellent visualization of bone and calcifications, has an important utility in the evaluation of trauma and pathological processes involving calcification. The ability to differentiate between gray and white matter, as well as CSF, gives MRI a distinct advantage over CT. Furthermore, MRI provides superior delineation of the pathology of and changes associated with demyelinating disease and is, as well, of special value in the investigation of pathology in the cervical spinal cord and the cervicomedullary junction (Jacobson 1988). MRI has an advantage for patients who require multiple scans over time because there is no ionizing radiation and there are no known adverse effects of MRI studies at present. However, MRI is contraindicated in patients with ferromagnetic structures or devices that may be adversely affected by powerful magnetic fields, such as aneurysm clips (Morihisa 1991). In addition, because of the length of time needed to complete the scan and the confining nature of the machine, some patients may be psychologically or medically unable to tolerate the procedure. Finally, the utility of nonspecific CT and MRI findings can sometimes be enhanced through the strategic use of specific neuropsychological tests to further characterize and localize pathological findings.

Electroencephalogram

The EEG measures brain electrical activity from electrodes placed on the scalp in standardized positions (usually conforming to the International 10–20 system of scalp electrode placement). The electrical activity that can be detected by the EEG scalp electrodes is presumed to originate primarily in neurons in the uppermost cortical cell layers. The amplitude and frequency of the electrical activity are graphically recorded on paper by ink markers for multiple areas of the brain surface as oscillating lines with different peaks and troughs, giving rise to the EEG tracing. The EEG frequencies have been divided into the following bands: beta activity ($\geq$13 Hz), alpha rhythm (between 8 and 13 Hz), theta activity (between 4 and 8 Hz), and delta activity (<4 Hz) (see Figure 6–5). The EEG is used primarily in the evaluation of epilepsy and other neurological disorders (e.g., neoplasm, trauma, stroke, metabolic or degenerative disease). The clinical reading of the EEG involves the visual inspection of, usually, large amounts of EEG tracings for certain EEG abnormalities, which can be divided as follows (Figure 6–5):

1. Dysrhythmias, such as isolated bursts of slow activity or spikes, as can be seen in the epilepsies
2. Asymmetries of the EEG recording from comparable parts of the head
3. Suppression of EEG amplitude (as in subdural hematoma or brain death)
4. EEG slowing (e.g., delta activity in an awake tracing, as can be seen in delirium; see Nunez 1981)

Most important, it should be noted that the effective use of an EEG recording depends on the skill and training of the electroencephalographer who reads and interprets the EEG data.

Some investigators have recommended that the EEG be a part of the routine screening battery for psychiatric patients (e.g., Hoffman and Koran 1984), especially patients with suspected organic mental disorder. In cases in which the patients have episodic behavioral disturbances that are possibly epileptic in nature, Goodin and Aminoff (1984) noted that a normal initial EEG alone cannot be used to completely exclude a diagnosis of epilepsy. Repeat EEGs or 24-hour ambulatory recordings can be obtained. Hall et al. (1980) suggested the utility of the sleep-deprived EEG, which they believe is more sensitive than a routine EEG. The role of augmenting the EEG with nasopharyngeal (NP) leads is unclear. Some researchers and clinicians, such as Sternberg (1986), suggested that NP leads can increase the diagnostic yield of the EEG, but a study by Ramani et al. (1985) called into question the value of the EEG supplemented with NP leads in psychiatric patients. In patients with a possible diagnosis of schizophrenia, a protocol described by Grebb et al. (1986) suggests obtaining a sleep-deprived EEG, preferably with NP leads, especially if it is the

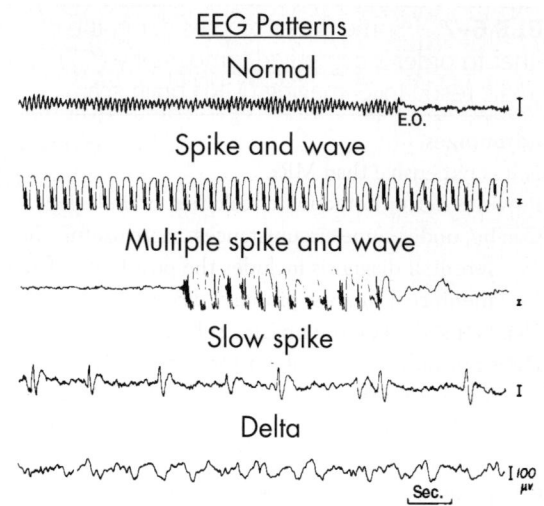

FIGURE 6–5. Some examples of electroencephalogram (EEG) abnormalities.

Top tracing demonstrates alpha rhythm, which attenuates with eye opening (E.O.) and is then replaced by lower amplitude beta rhythm. *Source.* Reprinted with permission from Nunez PL: *Electric Fields of the Brain.* New York, Oxford University Press, 1981, p. 234. Copyright 1981 Oxford University Press.

ciated with normal penile rigidity. Computerized tumescence monitoring devices are available that quantitate both penile base and tip expansion as well as rigidity (Bradley et al. 1985). NPT studies can be a part of a polysomnographic evaluation. The absence of adequate erectile function during nocturnal sleep lends some diagnostic support to an organic etiology of a patient's impotence. However, abnormal NPT studies suggestive of an organic etiology have been reported in association with major depression (Thase et al. 1987).

Evoked potentials. Evoked potential (EP) testing involves the measurement of specific brain electrical responses to discrete sensory stimuli. The evoking stimulus can be visual (VEP), auditory (AEP), or somatosensory (SEP). In the process of EP testing, the subject is repeatedly exposed to certain stimuli (e.g., flashing lights), and the evoked brain electrical responses are added together and averaged by a computer to remove background, non-stimulus-related activity. The result is a characteristic waveform (the EP), which generally consists of negative and positive peaks spread along a time axis, measured in milliseconds (msec). The "early" peaks (or components) are often defined as peaks occurring within the first 50 msec poststimulus. Middle peaks occur 50–250 msec poststimulus, and late peaks encompass those occurring after 250 msec. At this time, EP

testing can theoretically help the psychiatrist in differentiating between some organic and functional complaints (e.g., in the evaluation of hysterical blindness using VEP). A brain-stem AEP might be ordered in cases of suspected psychogenic deafness or used in the evaluation of an unresponsive, mute, catatonic patient. Such a study would assess the integrity of the brain-stem structures involved in the processing of auditory stimuli. Demyelinating conditions such as multiple sclerosis also can be usefully evaluated with certain EP testing procedures.

Various abnormalities of different EPs in certain psychiatric disorders have been described, including abnormalities of the early, middle, and late EP components (Shagass 1977; Buchsbaum 1977; Roth 1977, respectively). However, none of these findings have been clearly demonstrated to be characteristic of any specific psychiatric disorders, and their diagnostic potential is the subject of investigation. Ford et al. (2001) used event-related potentials to investigate the hypothesis that auditory hallucination in patients with schizophrenia is misidentified inner speech and reported abnormal auditory cortical responsiveness that might provide support for this model. EP studies are unique in their ability to provide information on certain aspects of cortical processing that occur on the order of milliseconds.

Laboratory Evaluation of Some Psychiatric Organic Therapies

As Hall and Beresford (1984) pointed out, one of the goals of the initial laboratory workup is to help provide useful baseline information for the patient who is likely to receive psychotropic medications. Many of the organic treatments are associated with adverse reactions that might be detected by changes in certain laboratory or other diagnostic test values (e.g., increasing liver function test values suggesting hepatotoxicity from a medication, or electrocardiographic changes reflecting potential cardiac toxicity from a psychotropic agent). It is therefore important to have baseline test values on a patient who is about to be exposed to an organic therapy so that future changes from these baseline values, possibly reflecting drug toxicity, can be properly assessed.

When a specific psychotropic agent is being used, more information about potentially useful laboratory tests, drug–drug interactions, and possible side effects and contraindications should be reviewed in other more comprehensive publications, such as the *Physicians' Desk Reference* and textbooks of psychopharmacology.

Tricyclic Antidepressants, Antipsychotics, and Benzodiazepines

In general, there is no absolute consensus concerning standardized protocols for the pretreatment evaluation of most biological treatments in psychiatry. However, some important examples are presented. For instance, because of the risk of agranulocytosis with clozapine, the U.S. Food and Drug Administration (FDA) standards for patients taking this medication include a baseline and then weekly WBC counts for the first 6 months of continuous treatment with clozapine. Thereafter, the FDA standard indicates biweekly WBC counts for those patients who continue to have acceptable WBC levels. Another example would be that for patients about to start taking tricyclic antidepressants (TCAs), antipsychotics, or benzodiazepine medications. Gelenberg (1983) recommended laboratory tests only as clinically indicated, based on consideration of each patient's medical history, physical examination, history of adverse drug reactions, and knowledge of the potential adverse effects from the biological therapy to be used. For example, an ECG should be ordered in a patient with a significant history of cardiac pathology who is about to begin taking an antidepressant or some of the antipsychotics because some of these medications have been associated with potentially significant ECG abnormalities (especially the TCAs and the antipsychotic thioridazine). Generally, in the case of certain drugs that have been associated with ECG abnormalities (e.g., QTc prolongation by drugs such as mesoridazine, droperidol, pimozide, thioridazine, and ziprasidone) or in situations in which drug-drug interactions can affect plasma levels, prudent monitoring for ECG changes can justify costs by enhancing patient safety. In the absence of a history of cardiac pathology, one might consider obtaining an ECG in a man older than 30 or a woman older than 40 who has not had one in the past year and is about to start taking a psychotropic medication that has been associated with potential cardiotoxicity (Gelenberg 1983). In addition, it seems advisable to order liver function tests in patients with a history of liver disease who are about to start taking certain psychotropics metabolized by the liver. The clinician might need to have a lower threshold for ordering diagnostic tests in patients belonging to populations at greater risk for adverse reactions from some of the organic therapies (e.g., pediatric, geriatric, or chronically ill patients). Likewise, the follow-up laboratory evaluation for some of these organic therapies also might need to be more extensive in such vulnerable patient populations. Again, the clinician needs to be aware of the major potential adverse reactions of the organic therapies he or she uses and

should use this knowledge to help guide the pretreatment and follow-up laboratory test evaluations. For instance, because of the risk of seizure for patients taking clozapine, some clinicians obtain EEGs in these patients before treatment. Furthermore, an EEG study might be of particular value during the course of treatment if high dosages of clozapine are contemplated.

In the following subsections, we present more specific guidelines for the pretreatment and follow-up evaluations of the patient about to begin treatment with lithium carbonate, an anticonvulsant, or electroconvulsive therapy (ECT). Of course, many of the broad principles previously described for choosing appropriate diagnostic tests for a particular patient also apply to the patient about to begin each of these treatments.

Tricyclic Antidepressant Blood Levels

There seems to be incomplete agreement regarding the usefulness of plasma TCA levels (Kocsis et al. 1986; Simpson et al. 1983). The American Psychiatric Association (APA) Task Force on the Use of Laboratory Tests in Psychiatry (1985) concluded that plasma-level measurements of imipramine, desmethylimipramine (desipramine), and nortriptyline are unequivocally useful in certain situations. Situations in which a TCA blood level might be ordered include those involving 1) patients with questionable compliance, 2) patients with a poor response to a "typical" antidepressant dose, 3) patients who experience side effects at a very low dose, 4) patients who are potentially very sensitive to side effects (e.g., medically ill or geriatric patients), and 5) patients for whom treatment is urgent and who require potentially therapeutic blood levels in as short a time possible (e.g., the severely suicidal patient).

Note that TCA blood levels are generally obtained about 9–12 hours after the last dose (usually in the morning after a nighttime dose). In addition, steady-state blood levels of the TCA are reportedly not achieved until about 5 days after either initiating the medication or changing the medication dose. The utility of plasma-level determinations for antidepressants other than those just outlined remains under investigation.

Pretreatment Lithium Evaluation

Lithium can have several potentially significant adverse affects, including those on the thyroid gland, kidney, heart, and developing fetus, as well as a usually benign elevation of the WBC count. Recommended pretreatment diagnostic evaluations often include a CBC with differential, serum electrolytes, BUN, serum creatinine, signs or symptoms of bone marrow suppression are present (e.g., petechiae, pallor, undue weakness, fever, infection). If hematological abnormalities appear on the laboratory examination, the hematological studies should be repeated more often until the results approach baseline. Of course, appropriate decisions must always be made concerning the need to discontinue the medication depending on the clinical significance of such abnormalities.

Minor decreases in the WBC count often occur in patients taking carbamazepine. Post (1984) suggested guidelines for carbamazepine discontinuation that include a WBC count of less than 3,000, erythrocyte count of less than $4.0 \times 10_6$ mm$_3$, hemoglobin less than 11 mg/dL, platelets less than 100,000, reticulocyte count of less than 0.3%, and serum iron greater than 150 mg/dL. It should be noted that the hematological thresholds for drug discontinuation outlined in the *Physicians' Desk Reference* are more conservative. Hyponatremia has been associated with carbamazepine therapy, so the clinician should order periodic serum electrolytes or when the clinical situation so warrants. Furthermore, periodic monitoring of hepatic function might be required, especially in patients with known hepatic dysfunction. Finally, carbamazepine blood levels should be carefully monitored because this drug can increase its metabolism through induction of liver enzymes (Schatzberg et al. 1997, p. 210).

Patients taking valproate need evaluation of their hepatic function (e.g., liver function tests) before initiating treatment and frequently thereafter, particularly in the first 6 months of therapy (*Physicians' Desk Reference* 1998, p. 425). During treatment with valproate, a CBC with differential and platelet count should be periodically completed as well as annual cardiac risk profiles (including high-density lipoprotein). Increases in ammonia levels can reflect hepatotoxicity and require careful monitoring of any changes in mental status (e.g., evidence of encephalopathy). Decreases in serum fibrinogen and albumen also can reflect hepatotoxic processes associated with valproic acid.

Antipsychotic Blood Levels

Methodologies for the laboratory measurement of blood antipsychotic levels include gas-liquid chromatography (GLC), HPLC, GC-MS, fluorimetry, RIA, and radioreceptor assay (Creese and Synder 1977). Therapeutic levels and ranges for some of the antipsychotics have been reported (P.J. Perry 2000; P.J. Perry and Miller 1993; Van Putten et al. 1992) and implemented, but universally accepted standardized protocols concerning the use of therapeutic levels or ranges for all the neuroleptics

have not yet been firmly established. Interesting findings relevant to the clinical use of antipsychotic blood levels include the reports of low correlations between prescribed neuroleptic dose and subsequent serum neuroleptic levels (highlighting individual variation) and reports that low neuroleptic levels for any given neuroleptic often help identify those patients who are most likely to relapse. However, it also has been reported that patients with persistent psychotic symptoms generally have neuroleptic levels indistinguishable from those of patients who are in remission (Brown and Laughren 1983). Furthermore, it has been argued that a significant and consistent correlation between plasma levels and therapeutic response is a requirement for the monitoring of plasma concentrations of a particular drug to have clinical utility (P.J. Perry 2000).

Although consensus guidelines for the use of antipsychotic blood levels have not been comprehensively established, examples of possible current uses of this laboratory test might include the assessment of patient compliance or the evaluation of patients taking medication but possibly achieving only low serum levels or, conversely, toxically high levels. There may be some other specific situations in which antipsychotic blood levels might be of some value, such as the assessment of certain drug interactions. An example of this was described by Arana et al. (1985), who noted a decrease in plasma haloperidol levels in patients taking both haloperidol and carbamazepine. These authors therefore suggested that blood haloperidol level monitoring might be useful for patients taking both haloperidol and carbamazepine, especially in the context of clinical deterioration after the initiation of carbamazepine.

This is an area of active research because the determination of accurate therapeutic ranges of antipsychotic drugs holds the potential to enhance response rates and decrease the time needed to achieve clinical response.

Electrocardiographic Monitoring of Patients Taking Psychotropics

Psychotropic medications, including the TCAs, antipsychotics, and carbamazepine, have been associated with various electrocardiographic changes. The most frequently alluded to changes are those representing a slowing of atrioventricular conduction in the heart—for example, as reflected by a widening of the QT or QRS interval on the ECG. Significantly, malignant arrhythmias have been reported in some patients taking TCAs and thioridazine. Indeed, torsade de pointes and sudden death have reportedly been caused by pimozide, sertindole, droperidol, and haloperidol according to a comprehensive review article by Glassman and Bigger (2001); these authors also suggested that the greatest risk for torsade de pointes and sudden death is with thioridazine and that widespread experience with ziprasidone will empirically clarify the safety of this medication. Prolongation of the QT interval corrected for rate (QTc) has been reported with a significant number of nonpsychiatric medications as well as with psychiatric drugs, and drug–drug interactions always should be considered. It has been suggested that a lengthening of the QT interval may prolong the period of cardiac vulnerability to potentially life-threatening arrhythmias. Patients who seem at particularly high risk for developing these potentially lethal arrhythmias are those with preexisting "excessively" prolonged QT intervals or those who develop "excessive" QT prolongation during drug treatment (Flugelman et al. 1985), as well as patients with already compromised cardiac function. Perhaps in these cases ECGs obtained both before and during administration of certain psychotropic drugs associated with electrocardiographic changes would be most crucial, but in general, the prudent use of monitoring ECG changes in patients taking medications that can adversely affect the cardiac system would enhance patient safety, particularly in medications with more limited experience such as ziprasidone. Schwartz and Wolf (1978) reported that when the QTc exceeds 0.440 seconds, the risk of sudden cardiac death is increased because of ventricular tachycardia or ventricular fibrillation. Beresford et al. (1986) argued that it is difficult to predict which psychiatric patients taking psychotropic medications will develop widened QT intervals. They suggest that the clinician must evaluate each patient case by case and maintain a low threshold for seeking cardiology consultation.

Some other applications of the ECG for psychiatric patients are worth mentioning. In the situation of TCA overdose, it has been reported that a widened QRS interval (e.g., > 0.10 seconds) is more reliable for determining the degree for potential TCA-induced cardiac morbidity and toxicity than is an antidepressant blood level (Boehnert and Lovejoy 1985). Additionally, with the increasing use of β-blockers for certain psychiatric conditions, the clinician should realize that β-blockers are contraindicated in patients with sinus bradycardia or evidence of certain cardiac conduction abnormalities.

Laboratory Evaluation Prior to Electroconvulsive Therapy

Certain laboratory and diagnostic tests are commonly completed before a patient begins ECT. The pretreatment workup often includes a CBC, blood chemistries (e.g., chem-20 profile), a urinalysis, a chest X ray, spinal X rays, and an ECG (Sakauye 1986). In addition, a CT scan and an EEG might be ordered if indicated by medical history or by the physical, neurological, or mental status examination. Spinal X rays are currently ordered less often than in the past because of the reportedly lower incidence of orthopedic complications associated with the contemporary administration of ECT (e.g., with the routine use of succinylcholine as part of the ECT procedure). Routine pre-ECT screening for abnormal pseudocholinesterase activity is probably not mandatory because inherited or acquired deficiency of pseudocholinesterase is reportedly quite rare. Indications for possibly obtaining measures of plasma pseudocholinesterase activity include a history of prolonged succinylcholine-induced apnea in the patient or in a blood relative (Nelson and Burritt 1986). A possible pre-ECT laboratory evaluation is outlined in Table 6–10. In patients with significant medical histories or medical conditions that might cause complications during ECT, a medical consultation would be prudent.

TABLE 6–10. Suggested laboratory evaluation before administering electroconvulsive therapy

Complete blood count
Blood chemistries (chem-20 profile)
Chest X ray
Spinal X ray
Urinalysis
Electrocardiogram

Biological Marker Research

Neuroscience investigators continue to search for meaningful laboratory and diagnostic tests for *functional* psychiatric disorders. These functional, or idiopathic, disorders are psychiatric conditions for which a clear causative or contributing neuropathophysiological lesion has yet to be identified. The proposed tests are also referred to as "biological markers," and these markers might have some potential future uses to psychiatrists and neuroscientists, including assistance in improving our understanding of the underlying neurobiology of functional disorders, in making an accurate psychiatric diagnosis, in arriving at the most appropriate treatment plan, in assessing prognosis, and in identifying patients who are at potential risk for developing a psychiatric disorder who might benefit from preventive measures. These biological marker tests have been receiving increasing attention in the psychiatric literature. The tests encompass a wide range of procedures, including neuroendocrine challenge tests, brain-imaging techniques, and the quantitative and qualitative laboratory evaluation of CNS active substances or other relevant samplings obtained from the urine, blood, CSF, and peripheral tissues. Some difficulties associated with the markers studied to date have been problems with sensitivity, specificity, reliability, and possible contamination from artifactual influences (e.g., concurrent illnesses, medication effects, and normal individual variation among patients). Currently, because of these and other problems, none of the markers yet seem to have the sensitivity and specificity that would make them clearly useful in routine clinical practice.

Neuroendocrine Testing

Neuroendocrine testing research in psychiatry currently includes measurements of basal hormone levels as well as neuroendocrine challenge tests. Basal endocrine evaluation includes blood measurements of certain hormone levels (e.g., thyroid function testing or serum cortisol levels) or measurement of certain hormone metabolites in the urine (e.g., urine ketosteroid measurements). Although frank endocrine dysfunction (as manifested by blood hormonal levels outside norms accepted by most endocrinologists) is known to be associated with various organic mental disorders, demonstration of a clear relation between subtle differences in basal measurements (still within established normal ranges) in psychiatric patients remains an elusive goal of ongoing research. Of course, thorough endocrine laboratory testing should be performed if the clinician suspects underlying endocrine disease. A possible example of the utility of basal hormonal measurements to the psychiatric clinician is the patient with a rapid-cycling bipolar disorder. Both clinical and subclinical hypothyroidism (e.g., as manifested by an elevated serum TSH level) have been reported to be associated with a significant proportion of these patients (Cho et al. 1979; Cowdry et al. 1983). In addition, severe depression has been associated with a hypersecretion of cortisol (i.e., hypercortisolism) as well as a possible loss of the normal diurnal variation of cortisol secretion (Allen et al. 1987). A lower prevalence of hypercortisolism has been reported in patients with schizophrenia (Roy et al. 1986).

Dexamethasone Suppression Test

The dexamethasone suppression test (DST) has been one of the most actively investigated of the neuroendocrine challenge tests used in psychiatric research. In fact, this test enjoyed a brief period during which it was used by some psychiatrists in their routine clinical practice, outside an established research setting. This was the result of the considerable excitement surrounding the possibility that the DST might be a useful marker for endogenous melancholic depression (Carroll 1984). Some investigators proposed that the DST could detect some of the subtle abnormalities of the hypothalamic-pituitary-adrenal axis that had been hypothesized to be present in patients with depression.

In a commonly described version of the DST (Allen et al. 1987; Carroll 1984), the patient received 1 mg of dexamethasone orally at 11:00 P.M. Blood was drawn over the next 24 hours, generally at 8:00 A.M., 4:00 P.M., and 11:00 P.M. The test result was considered abnormal, or positive, if the postdexamethasone serum cortisol level equaled or exceeded approximately 5 mg/dL, although this cutoff point varied somewhat among different laboratories and investigators. In addition, different laboratories used different cortisol measurement methodologies with different accuracies and reliability for measuring serum cortisol.

Although extensive research has been devoted to the evaluation of the clinical application of this test, its role in clinical psychiatry is unclear. When it has been used to try to assist in the diagnostic assessment of melancholic depression, major limitations in the use of the DST have included problems with test sensitivity (reflecting accurate identification of those with depression) and specificity (reflecting correct identification of those who do not have major depression). Significant limitations in specificity have been noted when the DST is used in patients with other psychiatric disorders. Moreover, artifactual contamination has been reported from variables such as weight loss, certain medical illnesses (e.g., uncontrolled diabetes mellitus), acute psychiatric hospitalization, certain medications (e.g., steroids, estrogens, phenytoin, carbamazepine, indomethacin, barbiturates), and individual differences in the metabolism of dexamethasone (Allen et al. 1987; Arana et al. 1985; Carroll 1986). Such confounding variables will greatly limit any potential clinical application that might be delineated for this test. The DST does not appear to be appropriate for routine screening of psychiatric patients (Carroll 1986). Indeed, it remains to be determined whether this test can increase incrementally the ability to diagnose or treat depression. Moreover, a normal DST result is probably without specific clinical utility.

In conclusion, the DST remains a research tool, and attempts to delineate a specific clinical application will require further investigation. One possible use of the DST may lie in its potential for providing biological subtypes and prognostically meaningful subgroups. For example, preliminary evidence has suggested that the DST may prove useful in predicting relapse in some patients treated for depression (Nemeroff and Evans 1984).

Thyrotropin-Releasing Hormone Stimulation Test

The thyrotropin-releasing hormone stimulation test (TRHST) has been proposed as a potential biological marker of mood disorders (Loosen and Prange 1982). In a commonly described version of this test, an endocrine challenge of 500 μg of TRH was administered intravenously to a patient. Serum values of TSH were obtained just prior to the TRH administration, as well as 15, 30, 60, and 90 minutes after the TRH was given. (TRH normally stimulates the pituitary to release TSH.) A change in the TSH serum value from before TRH administration (i.e., baseline TSH) to after TRH administration was determined (called TSH). A "blunted" response was regarded as a change in TSH values (or ΔTSH)/5–7 μIU/mL.

In major depression, a blunted TSH response to TRH has been reported to occur about 25% of the time (Loosen and Prange 1982). Similar responses also have been noted in patients with alcoholism, bulimia, borderline personality, and panic disorder, all of which are illnesses that have been hypothesized as possibly being related to mood disorders (Roy-Byrne et al. 1986). The reader should note that hyperthyroidism is also associated with a blunted TSH response to TRH, although there are generally also abnormalities of some of the baseline thyroid function tests (e.g., TSH, T_4, T_3RU). In another possible use of the TRHST, Targum et al. (1984) suggested that treatment-resistant depressed patients with an "augmented" TSH response (e.g., > 30 μIU/mL) might benefit from thyroid hormone medication added to their antidepressant regimen. Targum et al. (1992) also reported variability of responses to the TRH test in depressed and nondepressed elderly subjects.

In addition, it has been suggested that the TRHST combined with the DST might identify more patients with mood disorder than would either test used alone (Extein at al. 1981). More research will be required to clarify whether this is so. Like the DST, the TRHST is a useful research approach, but its clinical utility requires further investigative clarification.

Other Neuroendocrine Challenge Tests

Other neuroendocrine research diagnostic tests include serum growth hormone responses to pharmacological challenges such as dopamine, apomorphine, dextroamphetamine, clonidine, and insulin-induced hypoglycemia, as well as serum prolactin changes secondary to challenges by substances such as apomorphine, TRH, and methadone. A sample of findings in this area includes the reports of blunted growth hormone responses to insulin-induced hypoglycemia in patients with major depression and reports that apomorphine-induced prolactin suppression is greater in depressed patients than in patients with schizophrenia or in psychiatrically normal control subjects (Allen et al. 1987; Meltzer et al. 1984). Another neuroendocrine challenge test perhaps related to the DST is the corticotropin-releasing hormone (CRH) stimulation test. CRH is normally released by the hypothalamus and acts on the pituitary to cause a release of corticotropin. P.W. Gold et al. (1986) reported that depressed patients had basal hypercortisolism that was associated with a decreased responsiveness of corticotropin to an intravenous challenge with CRH. Roy et al. (1986) reported that patients with schizophrenia generally had basal cortisol blood levels as well as corticotropin responses to CRH challenge that were similar to those of psychiatrically normal control subjects.

All of these tests remain research tools at this time. Their most significant potential contribution to our understanding of psychiatric disorders may lie in their possible utility in the development of biologically based diagnostic and prognostic subtyping strategies.

Brain Imaging

Whereas the proposed neuroendocrine tests largely provide an indirect measure of brain activity (e.g., through central effects on endocrine function), brain-imaging techniques have the potential for providing a more direct window on the functioning of the living human brain. Functional brain-imaging techniques include computerized electroencephalography and EP mapping, PET, single photon emission computed tomography (SPECT), and regional cerebral blood flow (rCBF). MRI and CT are structural brain-imaging techniques that can provide an anatomical view of the living human brain. Over the past decade, software and technical advances in MRI have allowed this technique to "evolve" into new functional brain-imaging approaches: magnetic resonance spectroscopy (MRS), blood-oxygenation-level-dependent functional MRI (BOLD fMRI), and dynamic fMRI. Technical advances have made the coregistration of functional and structural brain images commonly available in research settings, allowing the proliferation of the combined use of complementary (Morihisa and McAnulty 1985) brain-imaging techniques.

Positron Emission Tomography

Whereas computerized EEG mapping provides information about brain electrical activity presumably arising from only the uppermost cortical cell layers, PET allows for the direct visualization of both cortical and subcortical (e.g., limbic system) brain functioning. Different aspects of brain functioning can be evaluated, including CBF, brain oxygen use, and certain aspects of brain glucose metabolism, as well as some specific CNS neurotransmitter system functions.

In preparation for a PET scan, a positron-emitting element (e.g., fluorine-18 [^{18}F], carbon-14 [^{14}C], carbon-11 [^{11}C]) is incorporated into a biologically significant compound, which is introduced into the body (usually intravenously). The compound used determines which brain function will be visualized. For example, when ^{18}F-labeled deoxy-D-glucose is used, it allows for the visualization of certain aspects of brain glucose metabolism. Other examples of radionuclides used include etorphine or carfentanil citrate labeled with ^{11}C, which allows for the visualization of brain opiate receptor activity, as well as ^{18}F-labeled N-methylspiroperidol, ^{11}C-labeled ^{3}N-methylspiperone, and ^{11}C-labeled raclopride, which permit the visualization of dopamine receptor function. The evaluation of the utility and accuracy of using different radiopharmaceuticals to assess certain neurotransmitter system functions is an area of very active investigation and some controversy. In addition, inhalation of the radionuclide oxygen-15 (^{15}O) allows for the direct visualization of oxygen use in the brain.

The distribution of these compounds after they enter the brain is determined by an array of detectors that surround the head. The detectors are sensitive to gamma rays that are formed after the positrons emitted by the radionuclides collide with electrons in the brain, resulting in the generation of coincident gamma rays in opposite (180°) directions. Data collected by the detectors are relayed to a computer, which uses the detection of these two coincident gamma rays to calculate the amount of radionuclide at different locations in the brain and produce the PET brain image.

Some PET findings in patients with schizophrenia and bipolar disorder have included reports of abnormalities of the anteroposterior gradient of glucose use (Buchsbaum 1986; Buchsbaum et al. 1984), as well as decreased absolute glucose use in the frontal lobes in schizophrenia (Wolkin et al. 1985). R.E. Gur et al. (1987) did not find "hypofrontality" in the schizophrenic patients studied but reported higher subcortical/cortical glucose metabolism ratios for patients with schizophrenia as compared with psychiatrically normal control subjects. Another study used radioisotopes capable of binding to brain dopamine D_2 receptors; D_2 receptors in the caudate nucleus were elevated in patients with schizophrenia compared with psychiatrically normal control subjects (Wong et al. 1986), although there is a lack of consensus in the literature concerning this finding. In another PET study, Tamminga et al. (1992) reported abnormalities of the limbic system, particularly the hippocampus, in schizophrenia. R.E. Gur et al. (1995) found that left midtemporal metabolism was relatively higher in schizophrenic patients and that this finding varied with clinical subtypes. These PET findings in schizophrenia are generally consistent with a theory of dysfunction of neural networks involving temporal limbic structures and associated prefrontal cortex. However, attempts to correlate metabolic findings with clinical variables have thus far failed to achieve any consensus. The disparity in research design and focus has contributed to the difficulty in comparing and integrating the wide spectrum of findings. The multiplicity of findings in brain-imaging research in schizophrenia also may reflect the heterogeneity of this disorder. Furthermore, in mood disorders, there have been functional imaging reports of abnormalities of temporal lobes and in particular the prefrontal cortex (Ketter et al. 1994).

More recently, a series of exciting PET studies have exploited cognitive neuroscience strategies to investigate schizophrenia. Holcomb et al. (2000) used ^{15}O PET and a tone recognition task and found evidence that patients with schizophrenia cannot optimally use frontocingulate systems during a demanding task. Ragland et al. (2001) used PET CBF and reported abnormalities of left frontotemporal activation during word encoding and retrieval in patients with schizophrenia. Finally, Meyer-Lindenberg et al. (2001) used PET and an innovative functional neuroimaging analytic method that can characterize cortical functional connectivity and found a pattern of abnormal frontotemporal interactions in schizophrenia, which may become the basis for a trait marker (see Figure 6–6).

In an elegant application of the PET radioligands [^{11}C]raclopride to assess striatal D_2 receptor occupancy and [^{11}C]FLB 457 to assess extrastriatal D_2 receptor occupancy, Talvik et al. (2001) found no support for regional selectivity as a proposed mechanism of action for clozapine. Meyer et al. (2001) used the PET radioligand [^{11}C]DASB to ascertain serotonin receptor occupancy during treatment with paroxetine and citalopram and reported 80% occupancy, which might have significance for therapeutic efficacy.

Drevets et al. (1999) conducted a PET study that used the highly selective serotonin type 1A (5-HT$_{1A}$)

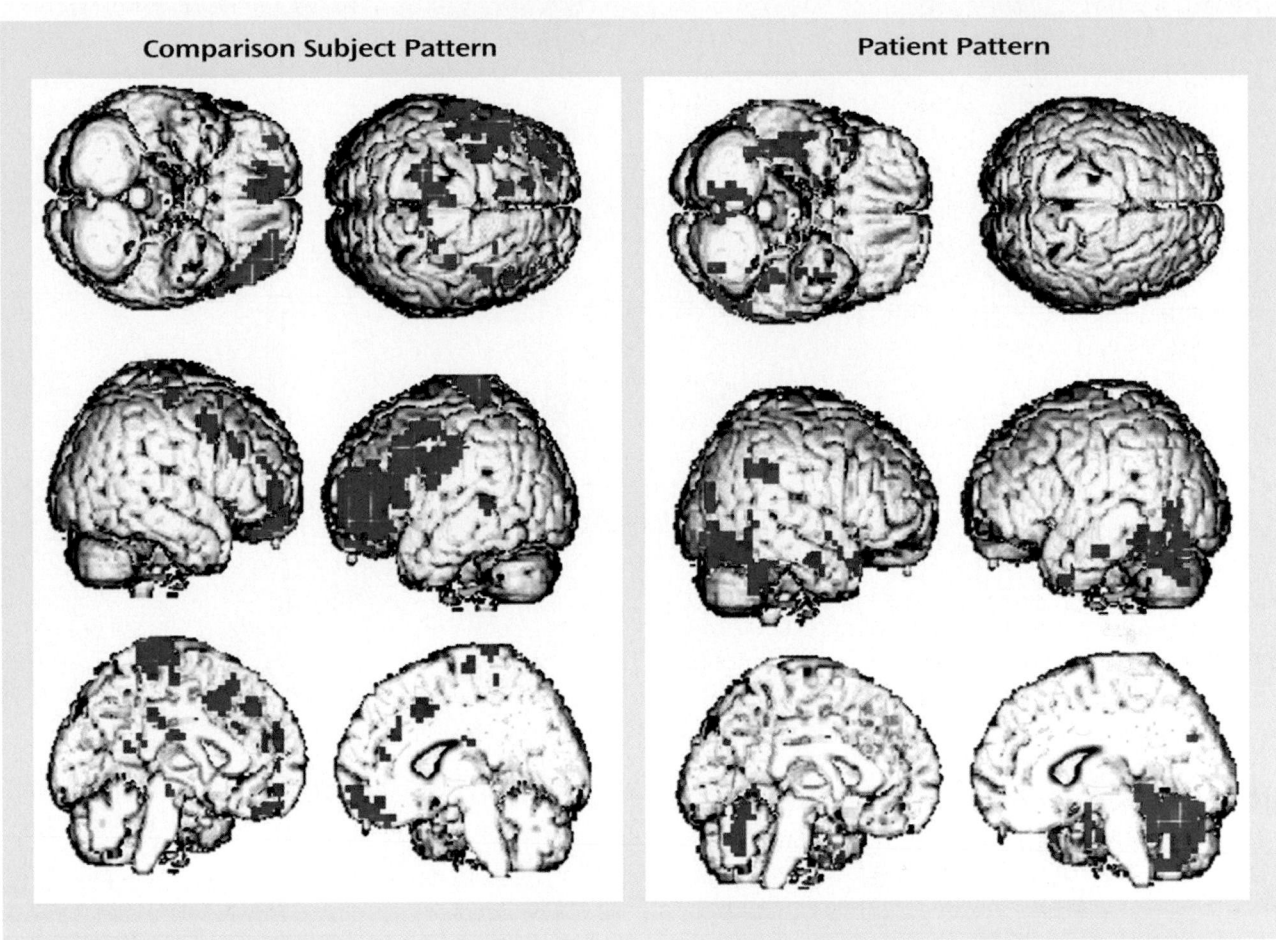

FIGURE 6–6. Map of the eigenimage ("functional connectivity") pattern that best differentiated patients from control subjects.

This image shows that brains of control subjects exhibit a pattern of regional coactivation particularly involving lateral frontal cortex and cingulate cortex, whereas the patients' pattern most characteristically involves the cerebellum and temporal cortex, particularly the hippocampal/parahippocampal region.

receptor radioligand [carbonyl-^{11}C]WAY-100635 to study depression (Drevets 2001) and found that 5-HT$_{1A}$ receptor binding was decreased. Kennedy et al. (2001) used [^{18}F]fluorodeoxyglucose PET to investigate depression and reported further evidence for a dysfunction in corticolimbic circuitry. Saxena et al. (2001) used [^{18}F]fluorodeoxyglucose PET to compare cerebral metabolic patterns of major depressive disorder and obsessive-compulsive disorder. Finally, Nobler et al. (2001) used PET to assess regional brain metabolism after ECT and found evidence of decreased neuronal activity in some cortical regions, which may provide clues to ECT's antidepressant effect.

PET studies have not yet shown sufficient sensitivity or specificity to elaborate a definitive role in psychiatric practice. As is the case for most brain-imaging applications, PET is most accurately considered a research tool in the investigation of classical psychiatric disorders.

Single Photon Emission Computed Tomography

SPECT can generate cross-sectional images from multiple levels of the brain and can therefore visualize the CNS in three dimensions (as can PET). SPECT uses radionuclides that emit gamma radiation (i.e., photons). These photons are measured by gamma detectors containing sodium iodide scintillation crystals. Information may then be calculated about the location in the brain and the relative amount of radionuclide at that locus. Different radiopharmaceuticals can be used to investigate different parameters of brain function. For example, qualitative measures of rCBF have been obtained with iodine-123 (^{123}I)-labeled iodoamphetamine, and quantitative measures of rCBF have been obtained with xenon-133. Technetium (Tc) 99m hexamethylpropyleneamine oxime (HMPAO) has been used in SPECT rCBF studies as well. One radiopharmaceutical currently being evalu-

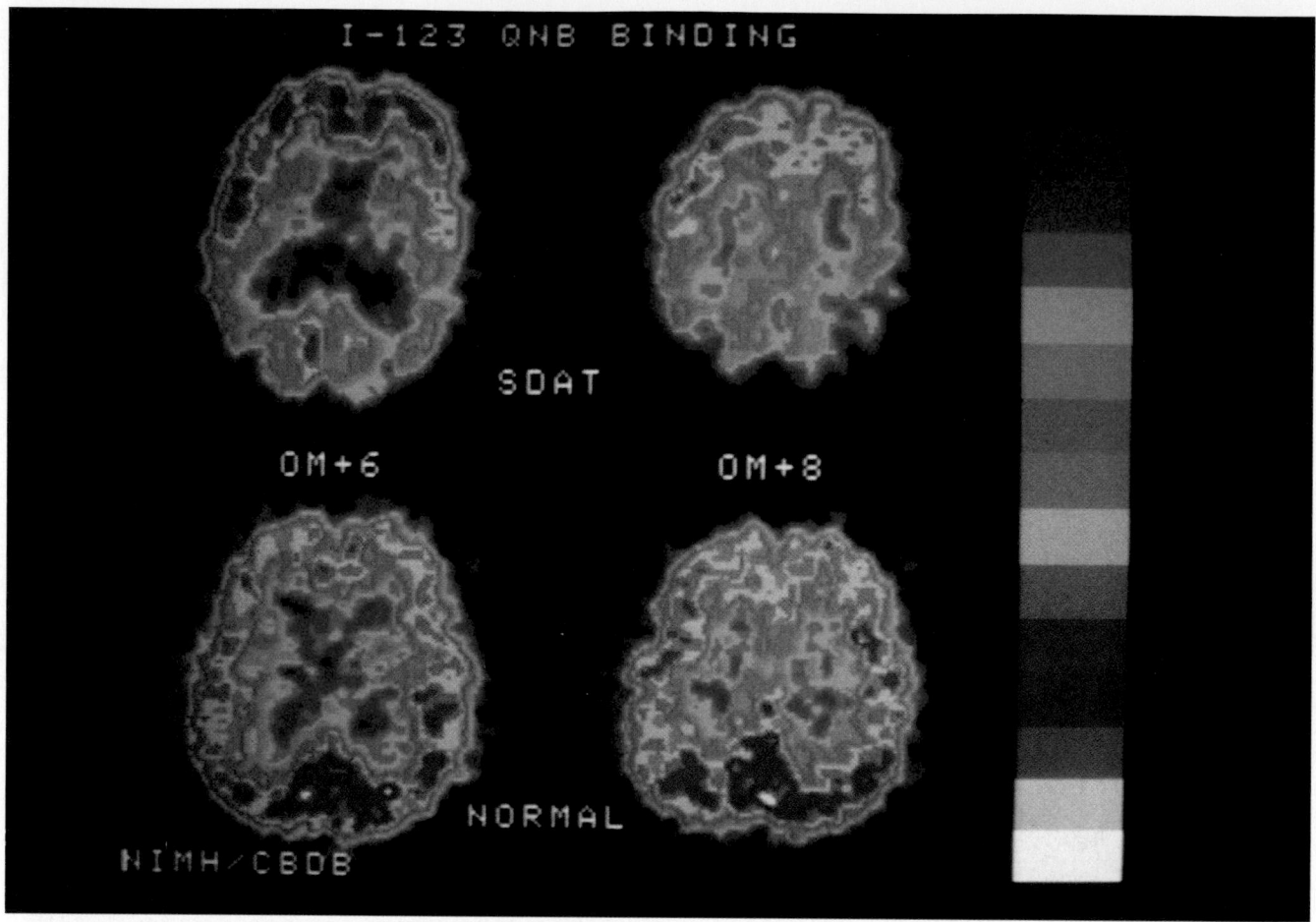

FIGURE 6–7. A single photon emission computed tomography (SPECT) image of two subjects using the radiopharmaceutical iodine-123 [^{123}I]-labeled 3-quinuclidinyl-4-iodobenzilate (QNB).

The *bottom two* images represent a normal control subject, and the *top two* images represent a subject with primary degenerative dementia of the Alzheimer type.

Source. Courtesy of Daniel R. Weinberger, M.D., Clinical Brain Disorders Branch, National Institute of Mental Health, Bethesda, MD.

ated as a putative window on muscarinic receptor activity is ^{123}I-labeled 3-quinuclidinyl-4-iodobenzilate (QNB). Weinberger et al. (1992a) studied patients with Alzheimer's disease (AD) with both [^{123}I]-QNB SPECT, a measure of muscarinic receptor availability (Figure 6–7), and [^{18}F]-2-fluoro-2-deoxyglucose PET to investigate the potential utility of using both types of functional brain-imaging approaches in the study of this disorder (Figure 6–8).

For classic psychiatric disorders, there is insufficient evidence that SPECT can yet provide the sensitivity or specificity required for the development of new diagnostic or prognostic approaches (Morihisa 1991). One of the confounding variables in any attempt to consolidate SPECT findings into clinically meaningful protocols is that a significant discrepancy exists between the investigational capabilities of many SPECT systems currently in use. Nevertheless, recently developed research-grade SPECT systems feature improved resolution that can

rival that of PET scans, and some investigations have suggested that this modality may provide valuable research information in some disease entities.

Regional Cerebral Blood Flow

In rCBF, blood flow to various regions of the brain is evaluated. To accomplish this, a metabolically inert radioactive substance (usually xenon-133) is introduced into the body (usually through inhalation). The radioactive substance is carried by the blood to various parts of the brain, and radiation emanating from the brain is picked up by detectors surrounding the skull. This method of investigation of brain function depends on the close linkage between CBF and cerebral metabolism (i.e., increased activity of a certain part of the brain is normally associated with an increase in blood flow to the area). The procedure can be performed with the subject at rest or engaging in mental activity (Figure 6–9). Unfortunately,

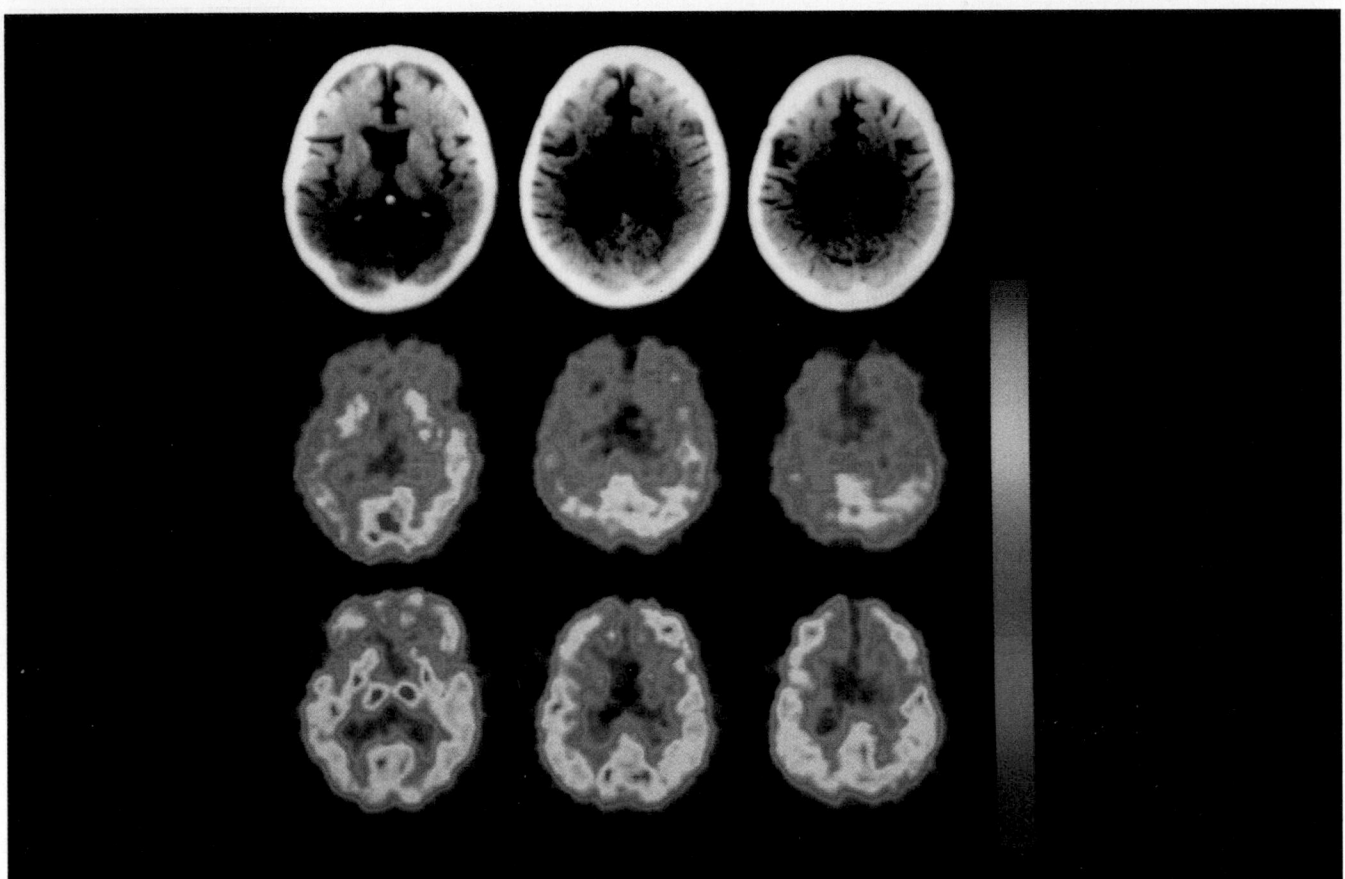

FIGURE 6–8. Magnetic resonance imaging, iodine-123 [^{123}I]-labeled 3-quinuclidinyl-4-iodobenzilate (QNB) single photon emission computed tomography (SPECT), and fluorine-18 [^{18}F]-labeled fluorodeoxyglucose positron emission tomography (PET) are demonstrated for a subject with a clinical diagnosis of Pick's disease–type dementia.
Note the relative hypoactivity of the prefrontal and temporal regions.
Source. Courtesy of Daniel R. Weinberger, M.D., Clinical Brain Disorders Branch, National Institute of Mental Health, Bethesda, MD.

unlike PET or SPECT, rCBF using the xenon-133 inhalation technique cannot delineate blood flow in subcortical structures.

Ingvar and Franzen (1974) reported on rCBF studies in patients with schizophrenia. They found decreased blood flow in frontal brain regions in these patients, which they did not find in their alcoholic control subjects. More recently, Weinberger et al. (1986) reported that schizophrenic subjects failed to show increased blood flow to the dorsolateral prefrontal cortex during challenge by the Wisconsin Card Sorting Test, a task that is thought to require the functional integrity of the dorsolateral prefrontal cortex and has been shown to be associated with increased blood flow to the dorsolateral prefrontal cortex in nonschizophrenic subjects (see Figure 6–9). This work provided the basis for a neurodevelopmental theory for the pathogenesis of schizophrenia (Weinberger 1987) and focused investigational interest on the dorsolateral prefrontal cortex (Morihisa and Weinberger 1986). Furthermore, work by Weinberger et al. (1992b) has extended this theory to implicate dysfunction of a prefrontal-limbic neural network in schizophrenia.

Computed Tomography

In CT, multiple X rays are taken through the CNS that provide the basis for the elaboration of cross-sectional images of the brain. Possible indications for the use of CT in the organic workup of psychiatric patients have already been described in this chapter. Again, when CT is used in this manner, it is generally in an effort to rule out neurological lesions, such as CNS neoplasms, that might be causing or contributing to the psychiatric symptomatology. Indeed, it would appear that it is in the evaluation of classic neurological disease processes that structural imaging techniques such as CT and MRI have their most significant utility in clinical psychiatry (Morihisa 1991).

Scientific investigators have used CT to identify several subtle structural abnormalities in the CNS of

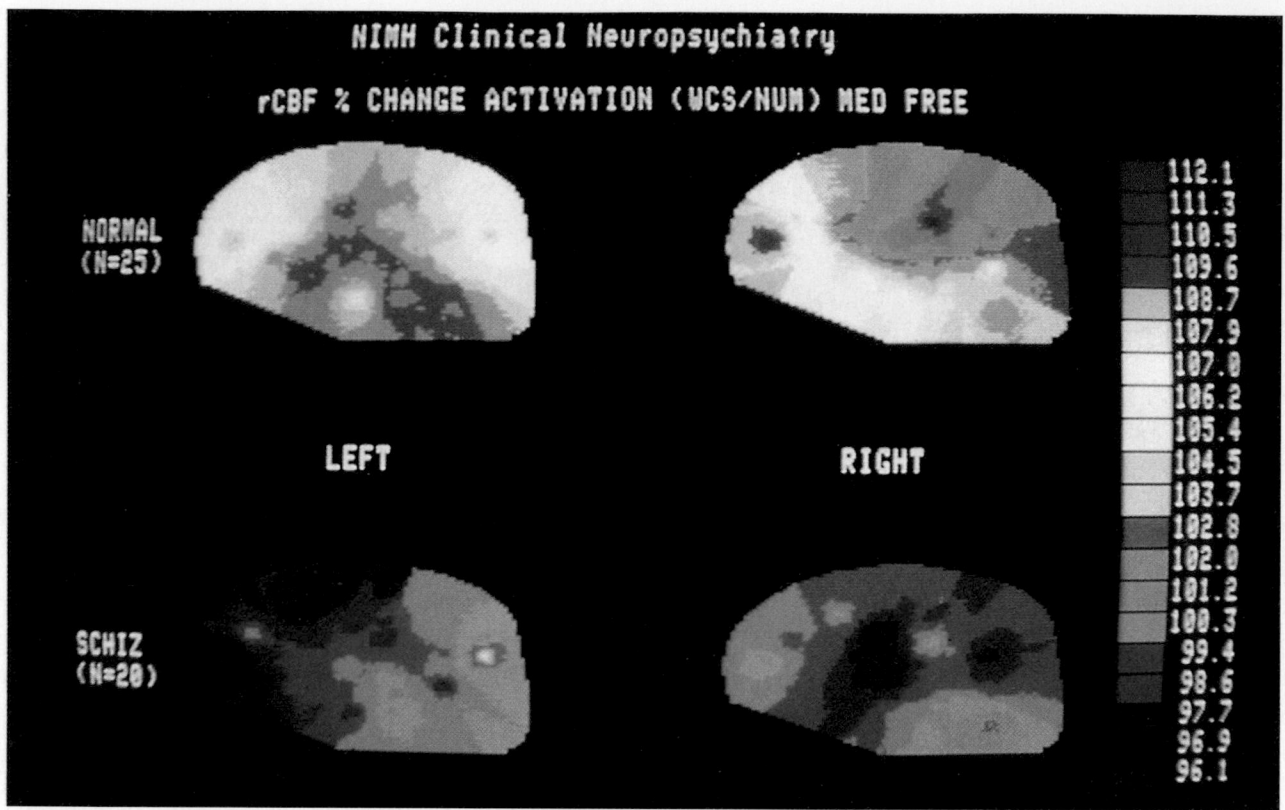

FIGURE 6–9. Topographic map of the regional distribution of cerebral blood flow (CBF) percent change in a group of patients with schizophrenia (*bottom*) versus control subjects (*top*), comparing two cognitive challenge tasks: a number-matching task and the Wisconsin Card Sorting (WCS) Test.

Note that in the control group, blood flow to the frontal cortex is increased during the WCS Test, whereas in the schizophrenic patients, it is not.
Red denotes the greatest amounts of CBF change from the baseline number task that controls for CBF during a cognitive activation task.
Source. Courtesy of Daniel R. Weinberger, M.D., Clinical Brain Disorders Branch, National Institute of Mental Health, Bethesda, MD.

patients with primary psychiatric disorders. Findings have included increased ventricular-to-brain (VBR) ratios in patients with schizophrenia (Weinberger et al. 1979), cortical atrophy, and third ventricle enlargement in schizophrenia (Nasrallah et al. 1985). A growing body of research suggests that the structural findings in schizophrenia are the result of abnormal neurodevelopment (Weinberger 1987, 1995).

An extensive scientific effort has been under way to attempt to correlate these structural findings with clinically relevant variables, but it has thus far failed to delineate clearly any parameters that can significantly enhance our current diagnostic or treatment approach to classic psychiatric disorders. There may be an association between enlarged ventricles in schizophrenia and several variables, including medication response, negative symptoms (Pearlson et al. 1984), and cognitive impairment (Johnston et al. 1976). The attempt to elaborate the clinical meaning of these findings is further confounded by the fact that enlarged ventricles have been reported in other psychiatric illnesses, including eating disorders,

alcoholism, bipolar disorder, dementia (Coffman 1989; Fogel and Faust 1987), and depression (Nasrallah et al. 1989). Thus, it is clear that this finding is neither pathognomonic nor even characteristic of a single psychiatric disorder (Morihisa 1991). Further research will be required to move us from our present stage of reporting statistically significant findings, based on intergroup comparisons, to the next stage of clearly established clinical correlates before we can achieve a consensus concerning the use of these data in the clinical practice of psychiatry.

Magnetic Resonance Imaging

The technique of MRI provides three-dimensional visualization of the brain's structure in axial, sagittal, and coronal planes by measuring the differential distribution of hydrogen nuclei, mainly in the water and fat of the brain. In the MRI technique, a magnetic field (usually 0.5–1.5 tesla in strength) is applied to the brain, and the spinning nuclei of hydrogen become aligned in accordance with this field. These nuclei are then exposed to brief pulses of a second field created by a radio frequency coil that causes nuclei to precess as well as spin. These pulses must "broadcast" on the characteristic resonant frequency (Larmor frequency) of hydrogen. Following the pulse, the nuclei return to their previously aligned positions and in doing so emit a characteristic electromagnetic pattern. MRI detects this characteristic signal with a radio frequency receiver. The imposition of a magnetic gradient allows spatial information to be acquired. The return over time of these hydrogen nuclei to their previously aligned positions is termed relaxation. T1 and T2 (relaxation times) are measures of the rate of this return of nuclei to their original state. Adjustments in transmission parameters can emphasize (i.e., weight) certain informational characteristics in the image. For example, a T1-weighted scan generally provides the best gray/white matter differentiation and anatomical delineation, whereas a T2-weighted scan generally provides superior discrimination of brain tissue abnormalities (Morihisa 1991).

MRI studies of schizophrenia have successfully replicated the work of previous CT investigations, extending findings of frontal lobe abnormalities (Andreasen et al. 1994) and significantly highlighting a compelling focus on regional abnormalities of the temporal lobes (Suddath et al. 1989).

It has been thought that only a subpopulation of all patients with schizophrenia have significantly enlarged ventricles compared with a psychiatrically normal control population. However, MRI research on monozygotic twins discordant for schizophrenia (Suddath et al. 1990) has raised the possibility that enlarged ventricular size may be found to be more pervasive than originally thought. In this research, the twin with schizophrenia usually had ventricular enlargement when compared with his or her unaffected twin, a uniquely powerful control who shares the same genome (Weinberger 1995; Figure 6–10). Thus, it is possible that with appropriate controls or sufficiently elegant research paradigms, ventricular enlargement may be found to be present in a greater percentage of patients with schizophrenia than previously reported. A related finding in monozygotic twins discordant for schizophrenia was identified by using $H_2{}^{15}O$ PET rCBF, in which the twin with schizophrenia had decreased metabolic activity in the dorsolateral prefrontal cortex compared with the unaffected twin (Figure 6–11) (D.R. Weinberger, personal communication, July 1997).

In patients with mood disorders, there have been structural research reports of increased ventricular size and reductions in the temporal lobe and the prefrontal region (Ketter et al. 1994). In addition, there have been reports of subcortical leukoencephalopathy or periventricular hyperintensities seen in some patients with mood disorder. The significance of these findings has yet to be elucidated (Nasrallah et al. 1989). Nevertheless, exciting efforts are being made (Steffen and Krishnan 1998) to delineate the potentially meaningful clinical correlates of MRI findings in mood disorders with intention of further expanding the frontiers of psychiatric classification by proposing new biologically based diagnostic subtypes. For example, citing a growing body of evidence, including findings of MRI hyperintensities, Sackeim (2001) argued that the evolving consensus is that there is a vascular basis for at least a subgroup of patients with late-life depression. Finally, Taylor et al. (2001) used MRI diffusion tensor imaging and reported evidence that MRI hyperintensities are associated with damage to brain tissue structure.

Employing advances in technology, researchers use MRS to image brain function, as reflected by differences in brain chemistry, for compounds that contain phosphorus-31, carbon-13, sodium-23, fluoride-19, and hydrogen, as well as the element lithium-7. In this manner, in vivo investigations of certain neurotransmitters, lipid metabolism, electrolyte balance, amino acid metabolism, high-energy phosphate metabolism, and carbohydrate metabolism may be pursued (Keshavan et al. 1991). In addition, drug studies of compounds incorporating carbon-13, lithium-7, or fluoride-19 may be possible (Guze 1991). An MRS study using phosphorus-31 (Pettegrew et al. 1991) investigated CNS membrane phospholipid metabolism as well as high-energy phosphate metabolism in the dorsal prefrontal cortex in schizophrenia. The authors interpreted their results as suggestive of hypoactivity in this region and also speculated that abnormalities of cell membranes may play a role in the pathogenesis of schizophrenia (Pettegrew et al. 1991). In 1996, a multi-slice proton MRS imaging (H-MRSI) study (Bertolino et al. 1996) investigated the regional neurochemical concentrations of N-acetyl aspartate (NAA), choline-containing compounds (CHO), and creatinine/phosphocreatinine in schizophrenia. These investigators (Bertolino et al. 1996, 1998) reported reductions of relative signal intensities of NAA in the dorsolateral prefrontal cortex and hippocampal regions and interpreted (Bertolino et al. 1996) these findings as suggestive of neuronal pathology, consistent with a neurodevelopmental theory of dysfunction in temporal limbic and associated prefrontal cortical neural networks in schizophrenia. Figure 6–12 shows MRS data of a psychiatrically normal control subject with the associated MRI structural image. More recently, Callicott et al. (2000b) reported that in schizophrenia, decreased NAA, which indicates decreased neuronal integrity, in the dorsal prefrontal cortex is predic-

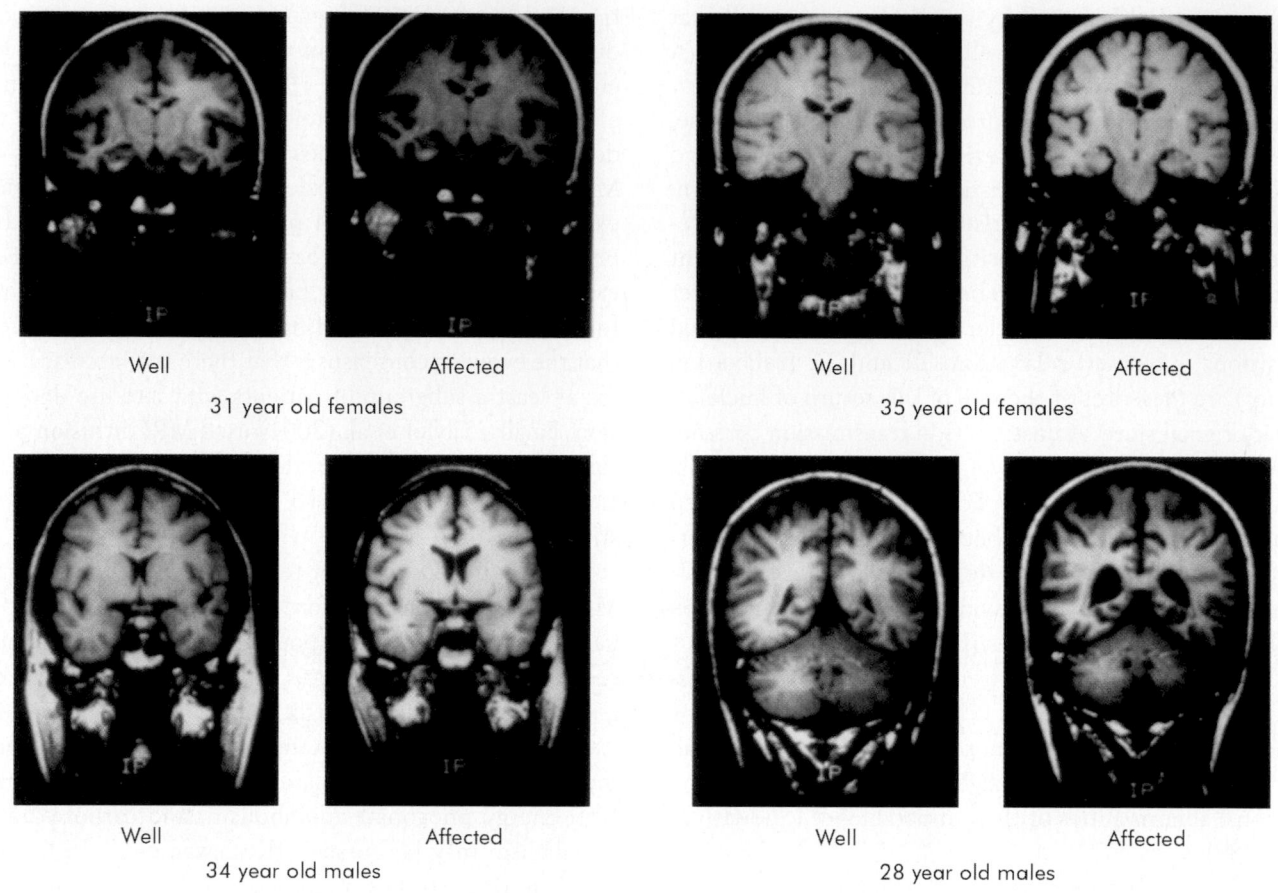

FIGURE 6–10. Paired magnetic resonance imaging (MRI) scans from four sets of monozygotic twins discordant for schizophrenia.

Note that in each case the affected twin has greater ventricular size than does the well twin.

Source. Reprinted with permission from Weinberger DR: "From Neuropathology to Neurodevelopment." *Lancet* 346:552–557, 1995.

tive of negative symptoms. The use of MRS-NAA measures as a putative measure of neuronal pathology in concert with functional imaging modalities has been proposed to enhance our confidence that abnormal brain imaging findings do indeed correlate with brain pathology (Callicott 2001).

Functional Magnetic Resonance Imaging

fMRI is an increasingly available technique that is minimally invasive and offers superior spatial/temporal resolution compared with SPECT and PET (Table 6–11). Moreover, fMRI avoids exposure to ionizing radiation and thereby raises the possibility of multiple functional studies. One such fMRI approach, BOLD fMRI, exploits the paramagnetic properties of deoxygenated hemoglobin (David et al. 1994). Another approach, dynamic MRI, employs signal enhancement by use of contrast materials such as gadopentetate dimeglumine.

Because of the low signal-to-noise ratio of most fMRI studies, undetected or uncorrected movement artifact can easily invalidate findings and represents a significant limitation in the application of fMRI in psychiatric research.

In 1996, Ramsey et al. compared a PET technique ($H_2{}^{15}O$ PET rCBF) with a three-dimensional BOLD fMRI technique to investigate the potential utility of fMRI. Also, Breiter et al. (1996) used fMRI and reported an increase in limbic system activation elicited by subject-specific stimuli in patients with obsessive-compulsive disorder. By 1999, Callicott et al. was using fMRI to investigate prefrontal cortex activation in healthy subjects over a dynamic range of working memory, thereby expanding our knowledge base concerning the full spectrum of normal brain function, as did Erin Hazlett et al. (2001) in an fMRI study of healthy subjects with an auditory cognitive task (see Figure 6–13).

Carter et al. (2001) used an event-related fMRI technique to study anterior cingulate cortex activity and found evidence consistent with changes in the internal monitoring of performance, an element of executive function, in patients with schizophrenia. In a preliminary

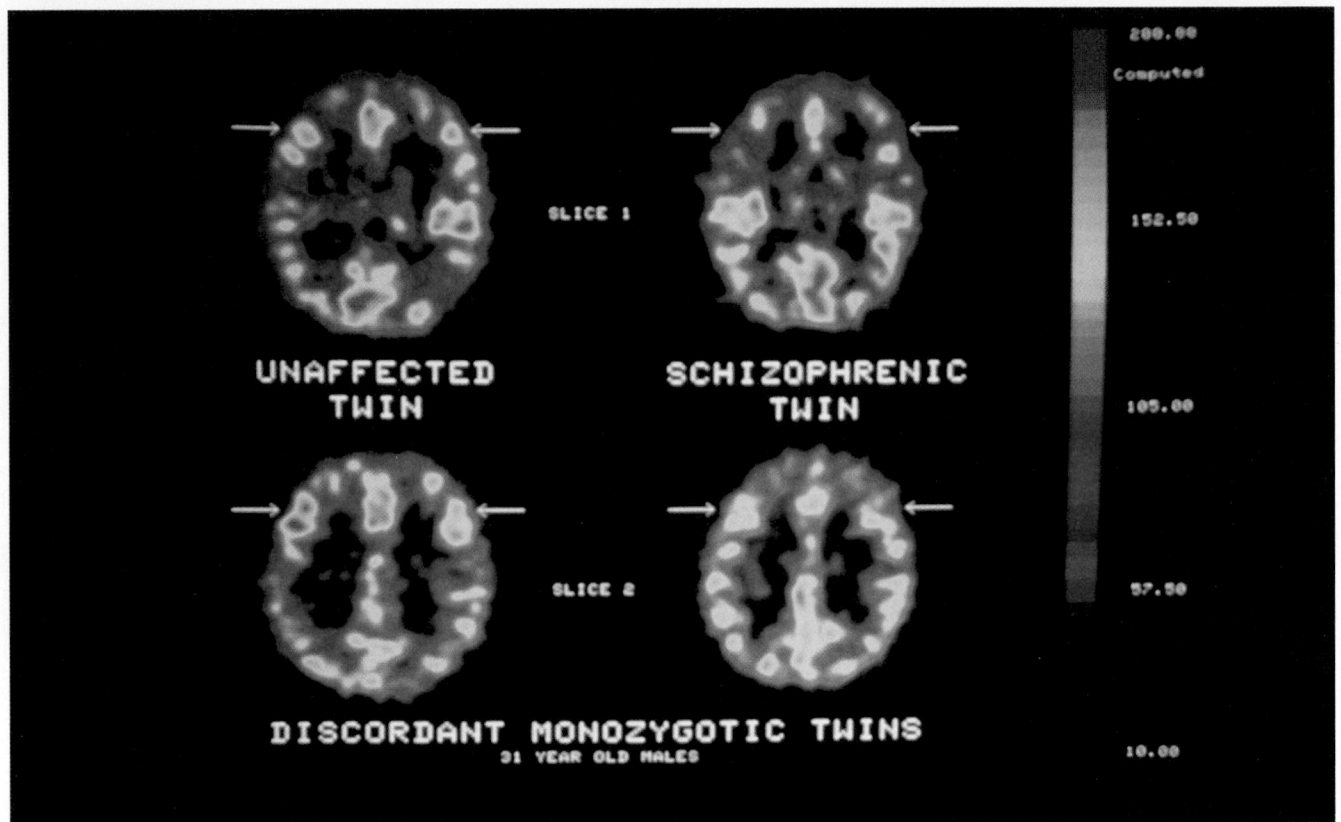

FIGURE 6–11. $H_2{}^{15}O$ positron-emission tomography (PET) regional cerebral blood flow (rCBF) scan of a pair of twins discordant for schizophrenia.

Note that the area of the dorsolateral prefrontal cortex (see *arrows*) is relatively decreased in the twin with schizophrenia compared with the unaffected twin.

Source. Courtesy of Daniel R. Weinberger, M.D., Clinical Disorders Branch, National Institute of Mental Health, Bethesda, MD.

TABLE 6–11. Research advantages of fMRI imaging over SPECT, PET, and rCBF

fMRI avoids exposure to ionizing radiation.

fMRI is increasingly available and does not need a source of radiopharmaceuticals as do SPECT, PET, and rCBF.

fMRI offers superior spatial/temporal resolution than SPECT, PET, and rCBF.

fMRI does not have the same degree of limitations on multiple studies that SPECT, PET, and rCBF have.

Note. fMRI = functional magnetic resonance imaging; PET = positron emission tomography; rCBF = regional cerebral blood flow; SPECT = single photon emission computed tomography.

study, Kircher et al. (2001) used fMRI to investigate a correlation between neural activity in Wernicke's area and the severity of formal thought disorder in patients with schizophrenia. Wible et al. (2001) used fMRI and reported data that suggested an abnormality of early auditory processing in schizophrenia. Menon et al. (2001) used fMRI and reported findings that suggested basal ganglia dysfunction in schizophrenia.

As has been the case in PET investigations, fMRI studies have used a wide variety of cognitive tasks and have, in addition, examined several motor tasks. These studies have reported a multitude of abnormalities of activation in schizophrenia, which have contributed further evidence for neurocircuitry dysfunction involving several anatomical structures, including the prefrontal cortex (Callicott et al. 2000a; Volz et al. 1999; Yurgelun-Todd et al. 1996), limbic system (Phillips et al. 1999), and temporal cortex (Woodruff et al. 1997).

Although many early fMRI studies focused on schizophrenia, other clinical entities have been investigated. For example, Rubia et al. (1999) used fMRI to investigate attention-deficit/hyperactivity disorder and found evidence of abnormal activation of prefrontal systems during a higher-order motor control task.

Indeed, some researchers (Pine 2001) believe that fMRI may be uniquely powerful in the delineation of the underlying pathophysiology of psychiatric disorders, particularly in a pediatric context, with its avoidance of ionizing radiation and limited known risks. For example, a

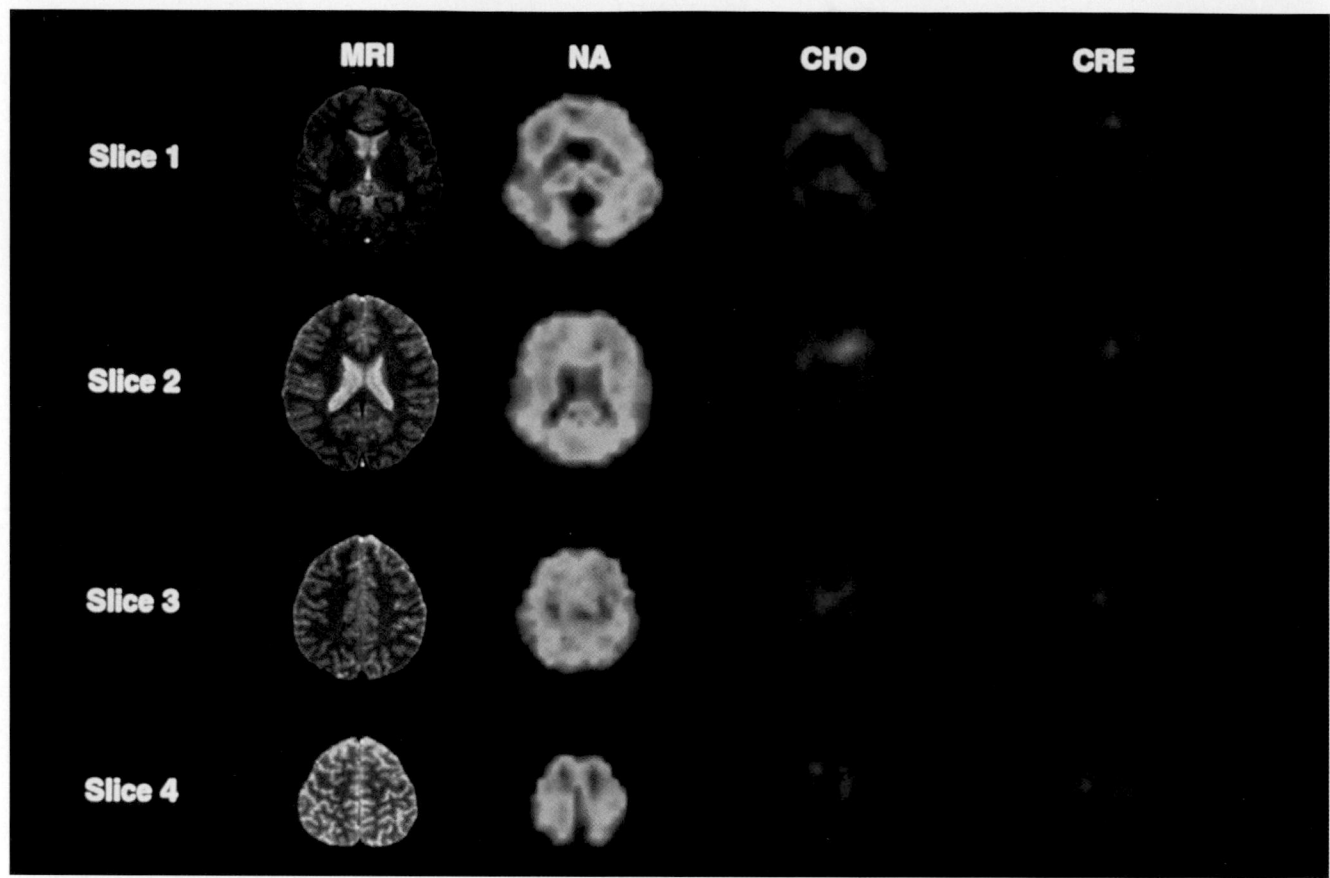

FIGURE 6–12.   Magnetic resonance spectroscopy data of a psychiatrically normal control subject at four slice levels with the associated magnetic resonance imaging (MRI) structural image.

Signal intensities for *N*-acetyl aspartate (NA), choline-containing compounds (CHO), and creatinine/phosphocreatinine (CRE) are shown.
Source.   Courtesy of Daniel R. Weinberger, M.D., Clinical Brain Disorders Branch, National Institute of Mental Health, Bethesda, MD.

recent study (Thomas et al. 2001) that used fMRI reported that children with depression and children with anxiety disorders manifested abnormalities of amygdala function, further adding to the growing body of neuroscience findings concerning the amygdala's role in assigning emotional significance to sensory stimuli.

fMRI has opened a new era of functional brain-imaging investigations in psychiatry (Morihisa 2001) and promises exciting and clinically important synergies with cognitive neuroscience and molecular genetic research.

Genetic Markers

One of the most promising areas of research in the medical sciences is the hunt for the genetic basis of disease. The concept of disease-related alleles that are specific gene variants (Barondes 1999) as an important part of the origins of disease processes has sharply focused the attention of medical scientists and captured the imagination of the general public. Furthermore, it is anticipated that from an understanding of the molecular and biochemical

ramifications of these genetic variations, a host of new engineered drug therapies, diagnostic tests, and more efficacious preventive strategies will evolve.

However, to anticipate the likely timeline for development of such new diagnostic tests, it is important to understand some problematic differences between causative gene variants that are sufficient to cause diseases such as Huntington's disease, which have mendelian dominant patterns of inheritance, and susceptibility gene variants that confer only enhanced vulnerability for complex diseases such as diabetes, schizophrenia, and bipolar disorder (Barondes 1999).

The expression of complex diseases, such as schizophrenia, depends on the contribution of multiple (polygenic) susceptibility genes combined with the necessary environmental factors. Simply put, a complex interplay between nature and nurture (Rutter and Plomin 1997) is necessary for most major psychiatric illnesses, such as schizophrenia and bipolar disorder, to occur in any individual. However, to date in psychiatry, there have been a good number of reports of linkage but very limited repli-

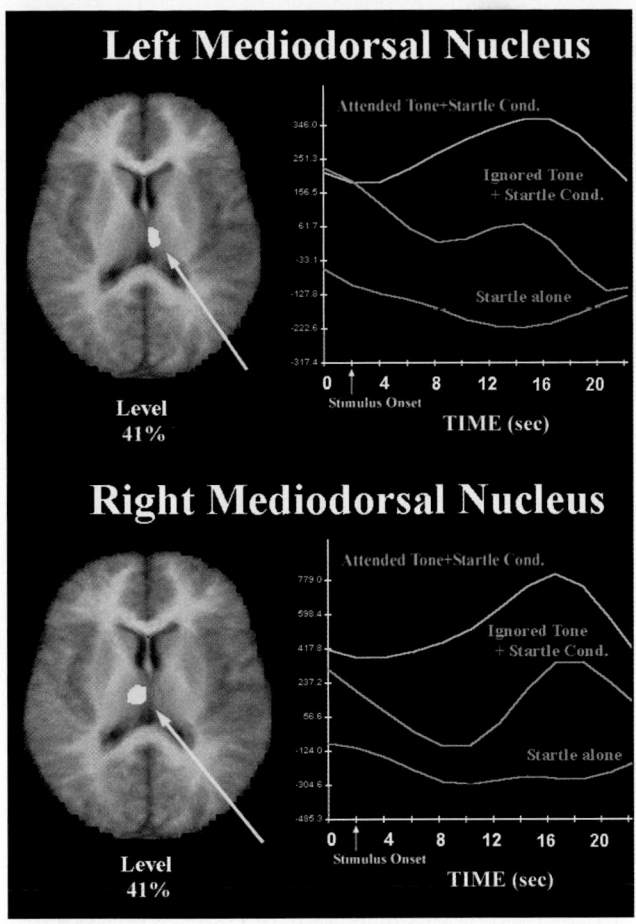

FIGURE 6–13. Statistical fMRI maps comparing cognitive activation during an attention task in the left (*top image*) and right (*bottom image*) mediodorsal nucleus.

In the figure, greater activation was observed in the mediodorsal nucleus during an attended prepulse inhibition condition than during an ignored or baseline condition. This figure demonstrates coregistration of functional MRI (fMRI) images and structural MRI scans and extends our knowledge of the mediodorsal nucleus, which is an important association nucleus of the thalamus and has reciprocal connections to the prefrontal cortex.

cation across studies (DeLisi and Crow 1999). Indeed, it is likely that larger samples, using allele sharing linkage techniques and studies of allelic association (Farmer et al. 2000; Owen and Craddock 1996) in concert with advances in statistical methodology and computing power, will be required to elucidate all the susceptibility genes of the major psychiatric disorders. Furthermore, not only must all susceptibility genes and their complex interactions be elucidated, but the relevant environmental risk factors also must be identified and their interplay with genetic-based vulnerabilities clearly understood before complex disease processes may be predicted with certainty (Farmer et al. 2000; Owen and McGuffin 1997). Thus, the anticipated diagnostic predictive value of many susceptibility gene tests (e.g., the apolipoprotein

E [APOE] test for AD) for complex diseases such as schizophrenia is currently thought to be low (Farmer et al. 2000). Indeed, the Nuffield Council on Bioethics (1998) recommended that genetic testing for susceptibility genes that offer low predictive or diagnostic certainty should be discouraged unless there are clear medical benefits (Farmer et al. 2000). This recommendation addresses only one of a number of challenging ethical, economic, medical, and research questions that have been raised by the prospect of eventually elucidating the genetic information that underlies disease processes. These concerns include issues of confidentiality for individuals as well as their relatives; informed consent, including a true understanding of the usually limited benefits to an individual and the potentially significant psychological risks; and the usually rare possibility of precise diagnostic prediction for participants. In addition, the commercialization of genetic research raises several problematic issues, including whether patients should share in potentially large profits from research based on their genetic information (Farmer et al. 2000).

The search for the genetic basis of AD is instructive as to the challenges and complexity as well as some of the current limitations of genetic marker research. AD is both a complex and a heterogeneous (i.e., different combinations of multiple susceptibility genes can contribute to the manifestation of this illness in different groups of people) disorder. Current research suggests that only about half of the cases of the approximately 5% of AD that are early onset are caused by autosomal dominant mutations in the β-amyloid protein precursor (APP) of chromosome 21, the presenilin-1 gene on chromosome 14, and the presenilin-2 gene on chromosome 1, whereas for the remaining 95% of cases that are late-onset AD, several polymorphisms such as the *APOE* gene on chromosome 19 and α_2-macroglobulin have been reported that confer increased vulnerability for AD (Blacker and Tanzi 1998; Tanzi 2000). However, neither *APOE* nor α_2-macroglobulin is necessary or sufficient for the development of AD and therefore is thought to have limited value as a predictive test for AD and cannot be used in place of an appropriate neurological diagnostic evaluation (Blacker and Tanzi 1998). Indeed, both the American College of Medical Genetics/American Society of Human Genetics Working Group on ApoE and Alzheimer's Disease (in 1995) and the National Institute on Aging/Alzheimer's Association Working Group (in 1996) recommended that *APOE4* (the 4 allele of the *APOE* gene confers enhanced AD vulnerability) not be used as a predictive test for AD (Blacker and Tanzi 1998).

Thus, most genetic tests for diseases of particular

interest to psychiatry remain primarily powerful research tools that will help to lay the groundwork for the future advances in our understanding of the pathogenesis of these disorders. In a timely review article by Liddell et al. (2001), current information is given about the complex challenges of advising relatives of the genetic risk of AD. For the relatively few families with autosomal dominant AD, the authors report that a DNA diagnosis can be obtained in about 70% of the cases, but for the vast majority of patients, an accurate risk prediction cannot be obtained (Liddell et al. 2001). Indeed, these authors argue that *APOE* genotyping is not an appropriate predictive test and provides minimal diagnostic information. Perhaps most important, Liddell et al. (2001) emphasized the importance of referring cases of familial AD to a regional center for medical genetics.

Nevertheless, recent reports of genetic findings in psychiatric illness are both compelling and tantalizing in their potential implications for the future direction of psychiatry. For example, in a review of the molecular genetics of bipolar disorder, Craddock and Jones (2001) reported that the great majority of research investigations indicate that polygenic interactions with environmental factors account for most cases of bipolar disorder and that although specific genes have not been conclusively identified, regions of interest on some chromosomes are areas of active investigation. For example, McMahon et al. (2001) reported findings that further support a genetic linkage between chromosome arm 18q and bipolar disorder and provide "preliminary support for bipolar II disorder as a genetically valid subtype."

In an excellent discussion of genes, environment, and schizophrenia, Tsuang et al. (2001) stated that research from family and twin and adoption studies provides compelling evidence of the importance of genetic factors in schizophrenia, and advances in scientific methodology have focused attention on regions of interest on several chromosomes. Kendler (2001), in an overview of twin studies of psychiatric illnesses, raised compelling issues concerning gene–environment interactions and discussed the mechanism of an external pathway of gene action in which genes influence an individual's social environment (e.g., degree of social support and level of risk of stressful events in life).

Some examples of recent genetic research include a report on the molecular epidemiology of alcohol dependence that discussed the interactions between genetic and environmental risk factors (Heath et al. 2001), evidence for a loci (gene or genes) on chromosome 1 that may be associated with alcoholism or depression (Nurnberger et al. 2001), a meta-analysis supporting a small but real association between attention-deficit/hyperactivity disorder and the 7-repeat allele of the dopamine D_4 receptor gene (Fara-

one et al. 2001), an investigation suggesting that variations in the *DRD2* gene may affect neuroleptic response (Schafer et al. 2001), a recent study at the messenger RNA (mRNA) level (Dracheva et al. 2001) reporting abnormal expression of the N-methyl-D-aspartate (NMDA) receptor subunits in elderly patients with schizophrenia, and a brief report suggesting an association between the *Taq*IA *DRD2* polymorphism and a predisposition to neuroleptic malignant syndrome (Suzuki et al. 2001).

One of the most intriguing genetic marker strategies for investigating this complex phenomenon has proposed that brain imaging may be able to identify biological phenotypes that might provide the basis for alternative classification systems for genetic linkage and association studies that could facilitate the characterization of genetic susceptibility to mental illnesses (Callicott 2001) and lead to more efficacious treatment strategies and preventive measures, as well as a deeper understanding of the underlying pathophysiology of these devastating illnesses.

Biochemical Markers

The laboratory has been increasingly used by physicians from all specialties to help detect, confirm, or rule out diagnoses of various physical conditions. There has also been the hope that the quantitative laboratory could similarly be used by psychiatrists and neuroscientists to help in the evaluation of patients with functional disorders. Research scientists have used various strategies in their search for quantitative laboratory applications to psychiatry, including the examination of various potentially relevant compounds found in the blood, urine, and spinal fluid, as well as the examination of CNS enzyme and receptor systems also found in tissues outside the brain (e.g., blood platelets, lymphocytes, skin fibroblasts). An example of a potential spinal fluid marker for dementia of the Alzheimer's type (DAT) is the CSF test for neural thread protein. The test measures an approximately 20-kD protein, which is reported to be increased in DAT compared with control subjects without DAT (de la Monte et al. 1992). Other potential CSF tests for DAT include measurement of tau protein (e.g., Burger nee Buch et al. 1999; Jensen et al. 1995) and amyloid β-protein (Pirttila et al. 1994).

Body fluid markers include molecular compounds found in the plasma, serum, urine, and CSF that are of particular interest to psychiatrists. Some of the biochemical markers that have been studied include neurotransmitter substances thought to be relevant to the pathogenesis of some psychiatric disorders (e.g., dopamine, serotonin, and norepinephrine), their metabolites (e.g., homovanillic acid, 5-hydroxyindoleacetic acid, and 3-methoxy-4-

hydroxyphenylglycol), various neuropeptides (e.g., endorphins, enkephalins), and biological compounds such as immunoglobulins (e.g., IgM) and plasma melatonin. Overall, most of the studies have yielded mixed results. Furthermore, advances in the fields of molecular genetics, cognitive neuroscience, and brain imaging have made possible the elaboration of putative endophenotypes, which have opened up compelling new pathways of investigation. Kendler (2001) skillfully explained the concept and power of endophenotypes by explaining that if one assumes an "etiologic cascade from DNA to clinical phenotype," then an endophenotype would reflect "processes in that cascade more proximal to gene expression than the clinical phenotype itself" (p. 1012).

Additional Research Diagnostic Studies in Psychiatry

Polysomnography

Polysomnography, besides having demonstrated utility in the evaluation of sleep disorders (e.g., narcolepsy, sleep apneas), also has been used in the search for potential biological markers of psychiatric disorder. An interesting example of a research finding in this area includes the report by Kupfer et al. (1978) of an increase in the overall amount of rapid eye movement and a shortened rapid eye movement latency period in patients with major depression. Polysomnographic findings in schizophrenia include reports of decreased amounts of Stages II, III, and IV sleep (Grebb et al. 1986).

Neuro-Ophthalmological Markers

The study of unusual eye movement patterns found more commonly among psychiatric patients than among psychiatrically normal control subjects also has been an area of research for potential biological markers. One measure of an abnormal voluntary eye movement has been the evaluation of smooth pursuit eye movement (SPEM). The SPEM abnormality consists of a larger number of jerky eye movements (saccades) during the tracking of a smoothly moving object. Various eye-tracking tasks and recording techniques have been used. SPEM dysfunction has been reported in up to 85% of schizophrenic patients, 40% of bipolar patients, and about 8% of the psychiatrically normal population (Holzman 1985; Holzman et al. 1984).

Computerized Electroencephalography and Evoked Potential

In computerized EEG and EP mapping, computers are used to amass and process large quantities of electrophys-

iological data. The computers analyze the data in various ways and graphically present the data in two-dimensional, color-coded maps of brain electrical activity. The brain electrical activity is measured in a manner similar to that used in the conventional EEG, although extra scalp electrode positions might be used to augment the conventional International 10–20 system of electrode placement depending on the type of computerized topographic system used. Computerized topographic systems can generally display data within a graphic outline of the head as if viewed from above or in profile. (Separate maps for the left and right hemispheres are produced.) Computerized EEG and EP have yet to show clear clinical utility in the diagnosis of classical psychiatric illnesses such as schizophrenia and major depression, and they are most appropriately considered research tools at this time. Research investigations that used computerized EEG and EP approaches have added to the body of evidence suggesting brain abnormalities in schizophrenia (Morihisa 1990).

Although this brain-imaging technique has high chronological resolution (a window measured in milliseconds for EPs) and is relatively economical, it is limited by a relatively poor spatial resolution for data collected from electrodes placed on the scalp and by vulnerability to a variety of artifacts (e.g., medication, muscle, and eye movement artifacts). However, ongoing advances in computer applications and the use of specialized test paradigms may enhance the utility of this research approach (Boutros et al. 2001; Hughes and John 1999).

Magnetoencephalography

Magnetoencephalography (MEG) is a technique for measuring brain electrical activity (Lopes da Silva and Van Rotterdam 1982). MEG exploits the fact that the electrical activity of the neurons of the brain generates very weak magnetic fields. When a very sensitive instrument is used to measure these generated magnetic fields, the magnetic energy is converted back into an electrical signal. The detection of these very weak fields currently requires the use of a super quantum interference device (SQUID) that must be super cooled.

The MEG can measure electrical activity in all areas of the brain (e.g., both cortical and subcortical brain tissues), in contrast to the conventional EEG and computerized EEG and EP, which are thought to reflect largely cortical surface electrical activity. The MEG is totally noninvasive, and the patient is exposed to no gamma or X radiation. Despite innovative investigations, major advances in the widespread application of this approach in psychiatric research may need to await significant refinements in MEG technology.

Conclusion

The use of laboratory and diagnostic tests in psychiatry is a rapidly evolving area. This process is most clear in the evaluation of possible organic disorders of the CNS in psychiatric patients as well as in patients who are beginning or continuing treatment with a psychotropic medication. However, controversies exist concerning the extent to which screening batteries should be used in psychiatric patients who do not have signs or symptoms of an organic condition, as well as the exact clinical utility of some psychotropic drug levels. Nevertheless, regardless of the type or number of tests used, the clinician should be sensitive to the fact that many of these tests are associated with varying degrees of discomfort, expense, and risk of adverse effects. In addition, abnormal laboratory results can at times lead to other procedures that might be associated with unnecessary danger and expense. Good clinical judgment needs to be the final arbiter when choosing any laboratory or other diagnostic tests for a particular patient.

No biological markers for any classic psychiatric disorders (such as major depression, schizophrenia, or bipolar disorder) have yet been confirmed as having a clearly defined utility in routine clinical practice. Nevertheless, psychiatrists and clinical neuroscientists continue their search for biological markers that will be useful to clinicians in making diagnostic, treatment, and prognostic determinations for psychiatric patients. The promise of research involving potential biological markers is that they may help elucidate the underlying pathophysiology of psychiatric illness, suggest useful new diagnostic approaches and subtyping strategies, and lead to more efficacious treatment approaches. However, although rapidly evolving technical advances have provided a wealth of new data, many new challenges in the areas of managing and interpreting this information have been created. Innovative software developments (e.g., Andreasen et al. 1992) and image analysis methods (Drevets 2000) have extended the utility of many of these techniques. However, major advances in new technologies, such as MRS and fMRI, represent the leading edge in the normal maturational process of applying brain imaging techniques to psychiatry (Morihisa 2001). Furthermore, a uniquely exciting convergence of synergies is evolving between molecular biology, genetic research, brain imaging, and new statistical methodologies that will welcome in a new era of knowledge about healthy brain function, the mechanisms of disease, unimagined innovations in therapeutic intervention, and exceptionally efficacious strategies for prevention.

Caveats

When assessing research reports in brain imaging and laboratory testing, it is useful to view the findings as only statistically significant. Often these abnormalities are subtle and can only be appreciated when a group of patients are compared with a group of matched control subjects. The findings should therefore be seen primarily as possible evidence that the measured phenomenon is relevant to the specific disease process. These exciting investigational achievements through laboratory and brain-imaging research, however, have not as yet been able to provide an innovative new basis for the comprehensive diagnostic categorization of classic psychiatric disorders such as schizophrenia and unipolar depression. Indeed, we have not yet even achieved incremental validity. In other words, there is as yet no definitive evidence that any psychiatric laboratory test or brain-imaging measure can provide a comprehensive and clearly incremental improvement to the existent approach to the clinical diagnosis of classic psychiatric illnesses (Morihisa 1991). (This caveat, of course, excludes the important use of these tests to rule out or identify organic processes such as are associated with classic neurological disorders—e.g., dementia, CNS neoplasms, and demyelinating disorders—endocrine disorders, or general medical disorders, as well as the workup and monitoring of biological therapies.) However, Callicott (2001) sagely pointed out that the most rewarding application of brain-imaging techniques may be in the identification of specific neuropathology and dysfunctional neurocircuitry rather than in the attempt to elaborate pathognomonic findings. This concept may apply to varying degrees to much of biological research in psychiatry.

Furthermore, one of the most significant obstacles in psychiatric research in this area is our inadequate investigation and understanding of the range of normal brain function. For example, the finding in normal adults of sex differences in resting regional cerebral glucose metabolism (R.C. Gur et al. 1995) has significant ramifications for the interpretation of functional studies of psychiatric disorders.

Moreover, as we explore new avenues of investigation and identify putative endotypes, we will likely find that issues of diagnosis, treatment, and prevention become more complex and filled with ethical and philosophical challenges. Indeed, a final caveat would be that we must be careful that our advances in biotechnology are paralleled by equally efficacious advances in medical ethics and medical economics. For example, the recent developmental evolution of the field of immunology may provide an instructive warning against any expectation of quick, clear, and concise clinical applications. The explosion of research investigations in the immunological sciences has led to a rapidly expanding knowledge base concerning disease processes, which has made the clinical practice of medicine far more complex and demanding rather than providing simplification or rapid definitive therapeutic interventions (Morihisa 1991). In a similar fashion, we should expect that findings in the clinical neurosciences will raise far more questions in the short run than they will provide immediate, clear resolution of vexing diagnostic and therapeutic challenges.

Nevertheless, the evolving alliance between brain imaging, molecular genetics, and the cognitive (Carter 2001) and basic neurosciences raises the possibility of identifying dysfunctional neural networks in psychiatric illnesses that may eventually provide the basis for enhanced diagnostic, prognostic, and treatment approaches in diseases such as schizophrenia and depression (Morihisa 2001).

References

Allen CB, Davis BM, Davis KL: Psychoendocrinology in clinical psychiatry, in American Psychiatric Association Annual Review, Vol 6. Edited by Hales RE, Frances AJ. Washington, DC, American Psychiatric Press, 1987, pp 188–209

Amdisen A: Monitoring lithium dose levels: clinical aspects of serum lithium estimation, in Handbook of Lithium Therapy. Edited by Johnson FN. Lancaster, England, MTP Press, 1980, p 179

American College of Medical Genetics/American Society of Human Genetics Working Group on ApoE and Alzheimer's Disease: Statement on use of apolipoprotein E testing for Alzheimer's disease. JAMA 274:1627–1629, 1995

American Psychiatric Association: Diagnostic and Statistical Manual of Mental Disorders, 4th Edition, Text Revision. Washington, DC, American Psychiatric Association, 2000

American Psychiatric Association Task Force on the Use of Laboratory Tests in Psychiatry: Tricyclic antidepressants—blood level measurements and clinical outcome: an APA Task Force report. Am J Psychiatry 142:155–162, 1985

Andreasen NC, Cohen G, Harris G, et al: Image processing for the study of brain structure and function: problems and programs. J Neuropsychiatry Clin Neurosci 4:125–133, 1992

Andreasen NC, Flashman L, Flaum M: Regional brain abnormalities in schizophrenia measured with magnetic resonance imaging. JAMA 272:1768–1769, 1994

Arana GW, Baldessarini RJ, Ornsteen M: The dexamethasone suppression test for diagnosis and prognosis in psychiatry:

commentary and review. Arch Gen Psychiatry 42:1193–1204, 1985

Asaad G, Shapiro B: Hallucinations: theoretical and clinical overview. Am J Psychiatry 143:1088–1097, 1986

Barondes SH: An agenda for psychiatric genetics. Arch Gen Psychiatry 56:549–552, 1999

Beresford TP, Wilson F, Hall RCW, et al: Q-T prolongation in psychiatric outpatients. Psychosomatics 27:497–500, 1986

Bertolino A, Nawroz S, Mattay V, et al: Regionally specific pattern of neurochemical pathology in schizophrenia as assessed by multislice proton magnetic resonance spectroscopic imaging. Am J Psychiatry 153:1554–1563, 1996

Bertolino A, Callicott JH, Elman I, et al: Regionally specific neuronal pathology in untreated patients with schizophrenia: a proton magnetic resonance spectroscopic imaging study. Biol Psychiatry 43:641–648, 1998

Bezchlibnyk-Butler KZ, Jeffries JJ (eds): Clinical Handbook of Psychotropic Drugs. Seattle, WA, Hogrefe & Huber, 2001

Blacker D, Tanzi RE: The genetics of Alzheimer disease; current status and future prospects. Arch Neurol 55:294–296, 1998

Boehnert MT, Lovejoy FH: Value of the QRS duration versus the serum drug level in predicting seizures and ventricular arrhythmias after an acute overdose of tricyclic antidepressants. N Engl J Med 313:474–479, 1985

Boutros NN, Miano AP, Hoffman RE, et al: EEG monitoring in depressed patients undergoing repetitive transcranial magnetic stimulation. J Neuropsychiatry Clin Neurosci 13:197–205, 2001

Bradley WE, Timm GW, Gallagher JM, et al: New method for continuous measurement of nocturnal penile tumescence and rigidity. Urology 26:4–9, 1985

Breiter HC, Rauch SL, Kwong KK, et al: Functional magnetic resonance imaging of symptom provocation in obsessive-compulsive disorder. Arch Gen Psychiatry 53:595–606, 1996

Brown WA, Laughren T: Serum neuroleptic levels in the maintenance treatment of schizophrenia. Psychopharmacol Bull 19:76–78, 1983

Buchsbaum MS: The middle evoked response components and schizophrenia. Schizophr Bull 3:93–104, 1977

Buchsbaum MS: Brain imaging in the search for biological markers in affective disorder. J Clin Psychiatry 47(suppl):7–10, 1986

Buchsbaum MS, DeLisi LE, Holcomb HH, et al: Anteroposterior gradients in cerebral glucose use in schizophrenia and affective disorders. Arch Gen Psychiatry 41:1159–1166, 1984

Burger nee Buch K, Padberg F, Nolde T, et al: Cerebrospinal fluid tau protein shows a better discrimination in young old (<70 years) than in old old patients with Alzheimer's disease compared with controls. Neurosci Lett 277:21–24, 1999

Callicott JH: Functional brain imaging in psychiatry: the next wave, in Advances in Brain Imaging. Edited by Morihisa JM. (Review of Psychiatry Series, Vol 20, No 4; Oldham JM and Riba MB, series eds). Washington, DC, American Psychiatric Publishing, 2001, pp 1–24

Callicott JH, Mattay VS, Bertolino A, et al: Physiological characteristics of capacity constraints in working memory as revealed by functional MRI. Cereb Cortex 9:20–26, 1999

Callicott JH, Bertolino A, Mattay VS, et al: Physiological dysfunction of the dorsolateral prefrontal cortex in schizophrenia revisited. Cereb Cortex 10:1078–1092, 2000a

Callicott JH, Bertolino A, Egan MF, et al: A selective relationship between prefrontal N-acetylaspartate measures and negative symptoms in schizophrenia. Am J Psychiatry 157:1646–1651, 2000b

Carroll BJ: Dexamethasone suppression test, in Handbook of Psychiatric Diagnostic Procedures, Vol 1. Edited by Hall RCW, Beresford TP. New York, SP Medical & Scientific Books, 1984, pp 3–28

Carroll BJ: Informed use of the dexamethasone suppression test. J Clin Psychiatry 47(suppl):10–12, 1986

Carter CS: Cognitive neuroscience: the new neuroscience of the mind and its implications for psychiatry, in Advances in Brain Imaging. Edited by Morihisa JM. (Review of Psychiatry Series, Vol 20, No 4; Oldham JM and Riba MB, series eds). Washington, DC, American Psychiatric Publishing, 2001, pp 25–52

Carter CS, Macdonal AW, Ross LL, et al: Anterior cingulate cortex activity and impaired self-monitoring of performance in patients with schizophrenia: an event-related fMRI study. Am J Psychiatry 158:1423–1428, 2001

Cho JT, Bone S, Dunner DL, et al: The effect of lithium treatment on thyroid function in patients with primary affective disorder. Am J Psychiatry 136:115–116, 1979

Coffman JA: Computed tomography in psychiatry, in Brain Imaging: Applications in Psychiatry. Edited by Andreasen NC. Washington, DC, American Psychiatric Press, 1989, pp 1–65

Cowdry RW, Wehr TA, Zis AP, et al: Thyroid abnormalities associated with rapid-cycling bipolar illness. Arch Gen Psychiatry 40:414–420, 1983

Craddock N, Jones I: Molecular genetics of bipolar disorder. Br J Psychiatry 178:S128–S133, 2001

Creese I, Synder SH: A simple and sensitive radioreceptor assay for antischizophrenic drugs in blood. Nature 270:180–182, 1977

David A, Blamire A, Breiter H: Functional magnetic resonance imaging (editorial). Br J Psychiatry 164:2–7, 1994

de la Monte SM, Volcier L, Hauser SL, et al: Increased levels of neuronal thread protein in cerebrospinal fluid of patients with Alzheimer's disease. Ann Neurol 32:733–742, 1992

DeLisi LE: Use of the clinical laboratory, in Biomedical Psychiatric Therapeutics. Edited by Sullivan JL, Sullivan PD. Boston, MA, Butterworth Publishers, 1984, pp 89–119

DeLisi L, Crow T: Chromosome Workshops 1998: current state of psychiatric linkage. Am J Med Genet 88:215–219, 1999

Dolan JG, Mushlin AI: Routine laboratory testing for medical disorders in psychiatric inpatients. Arch Intern Med 145:2085–2088, 1985

Dracheva S, Marras SAE, Elhakem SL, et al: N-Methyl-D-aspartic acid receptor expression in the dorsolateral prefrontal cortex of elderly patients with schizophrenia. Am J Psychiatry 158:1400–1410, 2001

Drevets WC: Neuroimaging studies of mood disorders. Biol Psychiatry 48:813–829, 2000

Drevets WC: Neuroimaging studies of major depression, in Advances in Brain Imaging. Edited by Morihisa JM. (Review of Psychiatry Series, Vol 20, No 4; Oldham JM and Riba MB, series eds). Washington, DC, American Psychiatric Publishing, 2001, pp 123–170

Drevets WC, Frank E, Price JC, et al: PET imaging of serotonin 1A receptor binding in depression. Biol Psychiatry 46:1375–1387, 1999

Dvoredsky AE, Cooley HW: Comparative severity of illness in patients with combined medical and psychiatric diagnoses. Psychosomatics 27:625–630, 1986

Emsley RA, Gledhill RF, Bell PSH, et al: Indications for CAT scans of psychiatric patients (letter). Am J Psychiatry 143:1199, 1986

Expert Consensus Panel for Bipolar Disorder: Treatment of bipolar disorder. J Clin Psychiatry 57(suppl 12A), 1996

Expert Consensus Panel for Schizophrenia: Treatment of schizophrenia. J Clin Psychiatry 57(suppl 12B), 1996

Extein I, Pottash ALC, Gold MS: Thyrotropin-releasing hormone test in the diagnosis of unipolar depressives. Psychiatry Res 5:311–316, 1981

Faraone SV, Doyle AE, Mick E, et al: Meta-analysis of the association between the 7-repeat allele of the dopamine D4 receptor gene and attention deficit hyperactivity disorder. Am J Psychiatry 158:1052–1057, 2001

Farmer AE, Owen JM, McGuffin P: Bioethics and genetic research in psychiatry. Br J Psychiatry 176:105–108, 2000

Feinsilver DL: Psychiatric diagnostic procedures in the emergency department, in Handbook of Psychiatric Diagnostic Procedures, Vol 1. Edited by Hall RCW, Beresford TP. New York, SP Medical & Scientific Books, 1984, pp 315–330

Flugelman MY, Tal A, Pollack S, et al: Psychotropic drugs and long QT syndromes: case reports. J Clin Psychiatry 46:290–291, 1985

Fogel BS, Faust D: Neurologic assessment, neurodiagnostic tests, and neuropsychiatry in medical psychiatry, in Principles of Medical Psychiatry. Edited by Stoudemire A, Fogel BS. Orlando, FL, Grune & Stratton, 1987, pp 37–77

Ford JM, Mathalon DH, Kalba S, et al: Cortical responsiveness during inner speech in schizophrenia: an event-related potential study. Am J Psychiatry 158:1914–1916, 2001

Gabel RH, Barnard N, Norko M, et al: AIDS presenting as mania. Compr Psychiatry 27:251–254, 1986

Garber HJ, Weinberg JB, Buonammo FS, et al: Use of magnetic resonance imaging in psychiatry. Am J Psychiatry 145:154–171, 1988

Gelenberg AJ: Laboratory tests for patients taking psychotropic drugs. Massachusetts General Hospital Newsletter 6:5–7, 1983

Gelenberg AJ: Carbamazepine (Tegretol) for manic depressive illness: an update. Massachusetts General Hospital Newsletter 8:21–24, 1985

Giannini AJ, Black HR, Goettsche RL: Psychiatric Psychogenic and Somatopsychotic Disorders Handbook. Garden City, NY, Medical Examination Publishing, 1978

Glassman AH, Bigger JT: Antipsychotic drugs: prolonged QTc interval, torsade de pointes, and sudden death. Am J Psychiatry 158:1774–1782, 2001

Gold MS, Dackis CA: Role of the laboratory in the evaluation of suspected drug abuse. J Clin Psychiatry 47(suppl):17–23, 1986

Gold PW, Loriaux DL, Roy A, et al: Response to corticotropin-releasing hormone in the hypercortisolism of depression and Cushing's disease: physiologic and diagnostic implications. N Engl J Med 314:1329–1335, 1986

Goodin DS, Aminoff MJ: Does the interictal EEG have a role in the diagnosis of epilepsy? Lancet 1:837–839, 1984

Grebb JA, Weinberger DR, Morihisa JM: Electroencephalogram and evoked potential studies of schizophrenia, in Handbook of Schizophrenia, Vol 1: The Neurology of Schizophrenia. Edited by Nasrallah HA, Weinberger DR. Amsterdam, The Netherlands, Elsevier, 1986, pp 121–140

Gur RC, Mozley LH, Mozley PD, et al: Sex differences in regional cerebral glucose metabolism during a resting state. Science 267:528–531, 1995

Gur RE, Resnick JM, Alavi A, et al: Regional brain function in schizophrenia, I: a positron emission tomography study. Arch Gen Psychiatry 44:119–125, 1987

Gur RE, Mozley PD, Resnick SM, et al: Resting cerebral glucose metabolism in first-episode and previously treated patients with schizophrenia relates to clinical features. Arch Gen Psychiatry 52:657–667, 1995

Guze BH: Magnetic resonance spectroscopy: a technique for functional brain imaging. Arch Gen Psychiatry 48:572–574, 1991

Hales RE: The diagnosis and treatment of psychiatric disorders in medically ill patients. Mil Med 151:587–595, 1986

Hall RCW, Beresford TP: Laboratory evaluation of newly admitted psychiatric patients, in Handbook of Psychiatry Diagnostic Procedures, Vol 1. Edited by Hall RCW, Beresford TP. New York, SP Medical & Scientific Books, 1984, pp 255–314

Hall RCW, Popkin MK, Devaul RA, et al: Physical illness presenting as psychiatric disease. Arch Gen Psychiatry 35:1315–1320, 1978

Hall RCW, Gardner ER, Stickney SK, et al: Physical illness manifesting as psychiatric disease, II: analysis of a state hospital inpatient population. Arch Gen Psychiatry 37:989–995, 1980

Hart RG, Easton JD: Carbamazepine and hematological monitoring. Ann Neurol 11:309–312, 1982

Hazlett EA, Buchsbaum MS, Tang CY, et al: Thalamic activation during an attention-to-prepulse startle modification paradigm: a functional MRI study. Biol Psychiatry 50:281–291, 2001

Heath AC, Madden PAF, Bucholz KK, et al: Towards a molecular epidemiology of alcohol dependence: analyzing the interplay of genetic and environmental risk factors. Br J Psychiatry 178:S33–S40, 2001

Hoffman RS, Koran LM: Detecting physical illness in patients with mental disorders. Psychosomatics 25:654–660, 1984

Holcomb HH, Lahti AC, Medoff DR, et al: Brain activation patterns in schizophrenic and comparison volunteers during a matched-performance auditory recognition task. Am J Psychiatry 157:1634–1645, 2000

Holzman PS: Eye movement dysfunctions and psychosis. Int Rev Neurobiol 27:179–205, 1985

Holzman PS, Solomon CM, Levin S, et al: Pursuit eye movement dysfunctions in schizophrenia: family evidence for specificity. Arch Gen Psychiatry 41:136–139, 1984

Hughes JR, John ER: Conventional and quantitative electroencephalography in psychiatry. J Neuropsychiatry Clin Neurosci 11:190–208, 1999

Ingvar DH, Franzen G: Abnormalities of cerebral blood flow distribution in patients with chronic schizophrenia. Acta Psychiatr Scand 50:425–462, 1974

Jacobson HG: Magnetic resonance imaging of the central nervous system: Council on Scientific Affairs Report of the Panel on Magnetic Resonance Imaging. JAMA 259:1211–1222, 1988

Jaskiw GE, Andreasen NC, Weinberger DR: X-ray computed tomography and magnetic resonance imaging in psychiatry, in American Psychiatric Association Annual Review, Vol 6. Edited by Hales RE, Frances AJ. Washington, DC, American Psychiatric Press, 1987, pp 260–299

Jefferson JW, Greist JH, Ackerman DC: Lithium Encyclopedia for Clinical Practice, 2nd Edition. Washington, DC, American Psychiatric Press, 1987

Jenike MA: Should lumbar puncture be part of the workup for dementia? Massachusetts General Hospital Newsletter: Topics in Geriatrics 4:21–23, 1985

Jensen M, Basun H, Lannfelt L: Increased cerebrospinal fluid tau in patients with Alzheimer's disease. Neurosci Lett 186:189–191, 1995

Johnston EC, Crow TJ, Frith CD, et al: Cerebral ventricular size and cognitive impairment in schizophrenia. Lancet 2:924–926, 1976

Karasu TB, Waltzman SA, Lindenmayer J-P, et al: The medical care of patients with psychiatric illness. Hosp Community Psychiatry 31:463–472, 1980

Kendler KS: Twin studies of psychiatric illness; an update. Arch Gen Psychiatry 58:1005–1014, 2001

Kennedy SH, Evans KR, Kruger S, et al: Changes in regional brain glucose metabolism measured with positron emission tomography after paroxetine treatment of major depression. Am J Psychiatry 158:899–905, 2001

Keshavan MS, Kapur S, Pettegrew JW: Magnetic resonance spectroscopy in psychiatry: potential, pitfalls, and promise. Am J Psychiatry 148:976–985, 1991

Ketter TA, George MS, Ring AA: Primary mood disorders: structural and resting functional studies. Psychiatr Ann 24:637–642, 1994

Kircher TT, Liddle PF, Brammer MJ, et al: Neural correlates of formal thought disorder in schizophrenia. Arch Gen Psychiatry 58:769–774, 2001

Kocsis JH, Hanin I, Bowden C, et al: Imipramine and amitriptyline plasma concentrations and clinical response in major depression. Br J Psychiatry 148:52–57, 1986

Kolman PBR: Predicting the results of routine laboratory tests in elderly psychiatric patients admitted to hospital. J Clin Psychiatry 46:532–534, 1985

Koran LM, Sox HC Jr, Marton KI, et al: Medical evaluation of psychiatric patients, 1: results in a state mental health system. Arch Gen Psychiatry 46:733–740, 1989

Koranyi EK: Morbidity and rate of undiagnosed physical illnesses in a psychiatric clinic population. Arch Gen Psychiatry 36:414–419, 1979

Kupfer DJ, Foster FG, Coble P, et al: The application of EEG sleep for the differential diagnosis of affective disorders. Am J Psychiatry 135:69–74, 1978

Larson EB, Reifler BV, Sumi SM, et al: Diagnostic tests in the evaluation of dementia: a prospective study of 200 elderly outpatients. Arch Intern Med 146:1917–1922, 1986

Liddell MB, Lovestone S, Owen MJ: Genetic risk of Alzheimer's disease: advising relatives (review article). Br J Psychiatry 178:7–11, 2001

Loosen PT, Prange AJ Jr: Serum thyrotropin response to thyrotropin-releasing hormone in psychotic patients: a review. Am J Psychiatry 139:405–416, 1982

Lopes da Silva F, Van Rotterdam A: Biophysical aspects of EEG and MEG generation, in Electroencephalography: Basic Principles: Clinical Applications and Related Fields. Edited by Niedermeyer E, Lopes da Silva F. Baltimore, MD, Urban & Schwarzenberg, 1982, pp 15–26

McMahon FJ, Simpson SG, McInnis MG, et al: Linkage of bipolar disorder to chromosome 18q and the validity of bipolar II disorder. Arch Gen Psychiatry 58:1025–1031, 2001

Meltzer HY, Kolakowska T, Fang VS, et al: Growth hormone and prolactin response to apomorphine in schizophrenia and the major affective disorders: relation to duration of illness and depressive symptoms. Arch Gen Psychiatry 41:512–519, 1984

Menon V, Anagnoson RT, Glover GH, et al: Functional magnetic resonance imaging evidence for disrupted basal ganglia function in schizophrenia. Am J Psychiatry 158:646–649, 2001

Meyer JH, Wilson AA, Ginovart N, et al: Occupancy of serotonin transporters by paroxetine and citalopram during treatment of depression: a [11C] DASB PET imaging study. Am J Psychiatry 158:1843–1849, 2001

Meyer-Lindenberg AM, Poline JB, Kohn PD, et al: Evidence for abnormal cortical functional connectivity during working memory in schizophrenia. Am J Psychiatry 158:1809–1817, 2001

Morihisa JM: Brain-imaging approaches in psychiatry: early developmental considerations. J Clin Psychiatry 51(suppl):44–46, 1990

Morihisa JM: Advances in neuroimaging technologies, in Medical Psychiatric Practice. Edited by Stoudemire A, Fogel BS. Washington, DC, American Psychiatric Press, 1991, pp 3–28

Morihisa JM (ed): Advances in Brain Imaging (Review of Psychiatry Series, Vol 20, No 4; Oldham JM and Riba MB, series eds). Washington, DC, American Psychiatric Publishing, 2001

Morihisa JM, McAnulty GB: Structure and function: brain electrical activity mapping and computed tomography in schizophrenia. Biol Psychiatry 20:3–19, 1985

Morihisa JM, Weinberger DR: Is schizophrenia a frontal lobe disease? An organizing theory of relevant anatomy and physiology, in Can Schizophrenia Be Localized in the Brain? Edited by Andreasen NC. Washington, DC, American Psychiatric Press, 1986, pp 17–36

Nasrallah HA, Jacoby CG, Chapman S, et al: Third ventricular enlargement on CT scans in schizophrenia: association with cerebellar atrophy. Biol Psychiatry 20:443–450, 1985

Nasrallah HA, Coffman JA, Olson SC: Structural brain imaging findings in affective disorders: an overview. J Neuropsychiatry Clin Neurosci 1:21–26, 1989

National Institute on Aging/Alzheimer's Association Working Group: Apolipoprotein E genotyping in Alzheimer's disease. Lancet 347:1091–1095, 1996

National Institute on Aging Task Force: Senility reconsidered: treatment possibilities for mental impairment in the elderly. JAMA 244:259–263, 1980

Nelson TC, Burritt MF: Pesticide poisoning, succinylcholine-induced apnea, and pseudocholinesterase. Mayo Clin Proc 61:750–755, 1986

Nemeroff CB, Evans DL: Correlation between the dexamethasone suppression test in depressed patients and clinical response. Am J Psychiatry 141:247–249, 1984

Nobler MS, Oquendo MA, Kegeles LS, et al: Decreased regional brain metabolism after ECT. Am J Psychiatry 158:305–308, 2001

Nuffield Council on Bioethics: Mental Disorder and Genetics: The Ethical Context. London, England, Nuffield Council on Bioethics, 1998

Nunez PL: Electric Fields of the Brain: The Neuroleptics of EEG. New York, Oxford University Press, 1981

Nurnberger JI, Foroud T, Flury L, et al: Evidence for a locus on chromosome 1 that influences vulnerability to alcoholism and affective disorder. Am J Psychiatry 158:718–724, 2001

Owen MJ, Craddock N: Modern molecular genetic approaches to complex traits: implications for psychiatric disease. Mol Psychiatry 1:21–26, 1996

Owen MJ, McGuffin P: Genetics and psychiatry. Br J Psychiatry 171:201–202, 1997

Pearlson GD, Garbacz DJ, Breakey WR, et al: Lateral ventricular enlargement associated with persistent unemployment and negative symptoms in both schizophrenia and bipolar disorder. Psychiatry Res 12:1–9, 1984

Perry PJ: Therapeutic drug monitoring of atypical antipsychotics: is it of potential clinical value? CNS Drugs 13:167–171, 2000

Perry PJ, Miller DD: Clinical use of clozapine plasma concentrations, in Clinical Use of Neuroleptic Plasma Levels. Edited by Marder SR, Davis JM, Janicak PG. Washington, DC, American Psychiatric Press, 1993, pp 85–100

Perry S, Jacobsen P: Neuropsychiatric manifestations of AIDS-spectrum disorders. Hosp Community Psychiatry 37:135–142, 1986

Pettegrew JW, Keshavan MS, Panchalingam K, et al: Alterations in brain high-energy phosphate and membrane phospholipid metabolism in first-episode, drug-naive schizophrenics: a pilot study of the dorsal prefrontal cortex by in vivo phosphorus 31 nuclear magnetic resonance spectroscopy. Arch Gen Psychiatry 48:563–568, 1991

Phillips ML, Williams L, Senior C, et al: A differential neural response to threatening and non-threatening negative facial expressions in paranoid and non-paranoid schizophrenics. Psychiatric Research: Neuroimaging 92:11–31, 1999

Physicians' Desk Reference, 52nd Edition. Montvale, NJ, Medical Economics Company, 1998

Pine DS: Functional magnetic resonance imaging in children and adolescents: implications for research on emotion, in Advances in Brain Imaging. Edited by Morihisa JM. (Review of Psychiatry Series, Vol 20, No 4; Oldham JM and Riba MB, series eds). Washington, DC, American Psychiatric Publishing, 2001, pp 53–82

Pirttila T, Kim KS, Mehta PD, et al: Soluble amyloid beta-protein in the cerebrospinal fluid from patients with Alzheimer's disease, vascular dementia and controls. J Neurol Sci 127:90–95, 1994

Post RM: Clinical approaches to the treatment resistant manic and depressive patient, in Psychopharmacology in Practice: Clinical and Research Update 1984. Bethesda, MD, Foundation for Advanced Education in the Sciences, 1984, pp 23–54

Pryse-Phillips W, Murray TJ: Essential Neurology, 3rd Edition. New York, Medical Examination Publishing Company, 1986

Ragland JD, Gur RC, Raz J, et al: Effect of schizophrenia on frontotemporal activity during word encoding and recognition: a PET cerebral blood flow study. Am J Psychiatry 158:1114–1125, 2001

Ramani V, Loewenson RB, Torres F: The limited usefulness of nasopharyngeal EEG recording in psychiatric patients. Am J Psychiatry 142:1099–1100, 1985

Ramsey NF, Kirby BS, Gelderen PV, et al: Functional mapping of human sensorimotor cortex with 3D BOLD fMRI correlates highly with H_2 ^{15}O PET and CBF. J Cereb Blood Flow Metab 16:755–764, 1996

Rosse RB, Giese AA, Deutsch SI, et al: Concise Guide to Laboratory and Diagnostic Testing in Psychiatry. Washington, DC, American Psychiatric Press, 1989

Roth WT: Late event-related potentials and psychopathology. Schizophr Bull 3:105–120, 1977

Roy A, Pickar D, Doran A, et al: The corticotropin-releasing hormone stimulation test in chronic schizophrenia. Am J Psychiatry 143:1393–1397, 1986

Roy-Byrne PP, Uhde TW, Rubinow DR, et al: Reduced TSH and prolactin response to TRH in patients with panic disorder. Am J Psychiatry 143:503–507, 1986

Rubia K, Overmeyer S, Taylor E, et al: Hypofrontality in attention deficit hyperactivity disorder during higher-order motor control: a study with functional MRI. Am J Psychiatry 156:891–896, 1999

Rutter M, Plomin R: Opportunities for psychiatry from genetic findings. Br J Psychiatry 171:209–219, 1997

Sackeim HA: Brain structure and function in late-life depression, in Advances in Brain Imaging. Edited by Morihisa JM. (Review of Psychiatry Series, Vol 20, No 4; Oldham JM and Riba MB, series eds). Washington, DC, American Psychiatric Publishing, 2001, pp 83–121

Sakauye KM: A model for administration of electroconvulsive therapy. Hosp Community Psychiatry 37:785–788, 1986

Saxena S, Brody AL, Ho ML, et al: Cerebral metabolism in major depression and obsessive-compulsive disorder occurring separately and concurrently. Biol Psychiatry 50:159–170, 2001

Schafer M, Rujescu D, Giegling I, et al: Association of short-term response to haloperidol treatment with a polymorphism in the dopamine D2 receptor gene. Am J Psychiatry 158:802–804, 2001

Schatzberg AF, Cole JO, DeBattista C: Manual of Clinical Psychopharmacology, 3rd Edition. Washington, DC, American Psychiatric Press, 1997

Schwartz P, Wolf S: QT interval prolongation as prediction of sudden death in patients with myocardial infarction. Circulation 57:1074–1077, 1978

Shagass C: Early evoked potentials. Schizophr Bull 3:80–92, 1977

Simpson GM, Pi EH, White K: Plasma drug levels and clinical response to antidepressants. J Clin Psychiatry 44:27–34, 1983

Sox HC Jr, Koran LM, Sox CH, et al: A medical algorithm for detecting physical disease in psychiatric patients. Hosp Community Psychiatry 40:1270–1276, 1989

Sramek JJ, Baumgartner WA, Tallos JA, et al: Hair analysis for detection of phencyclidine in newly admitted psychiatric patients. Am J Psychiatry 142:950–953, 1985

Steffens DC, Krishnan KRR: Structural neuroimaging and mood disorders: recent findings, implications for classification, and future directions. Biol Psychiatry 43:705–712, 1998

Sternberg DE: Testing for physical illness in psychiatric patients. J Clin Psychiatry 47(suppl):3–9, 1986

Suddath RL, Casanova MF, Goldberg TE, et al: Temporal lobe pathology in schizophrenia: a quantitative magnetic resonance imaging study. Am J Psychiatry 46:464–472, 1989

Suddath RL, Christison GW, Torrey EF: Cerebral anatomical abnormalities in monozygotic twins discordant for schizophrenia. N Engl J Med 322:789–794, 1990

Suzuki A, Kondo T, Otani K, et al: Association of the Taq 1 A polymorphism of the dopamine D2 receptor gene with predisposition to neuroleptic malignant syndrome. Am J Psychiatry 158:1714–1716, 2001

Talvik M, Nordstom AL, Nyberg S, et al: No support for regional selectivity in clozapine-treated patients: a PET study with [C11] raclopride and [C11] FLB 457. Am J Psychiatry 158:926–930, 2001

Tamminga CA, Thaker GK, Buchanan R, et al: Limbic system abnormalities identified in schizophrenia using positron emission tomography with fluorodeoxyglucose and neocortical alterations with deficit syndrome. Arch Gen Psychiatry 49:522–530, 1992

Tanzi RE: Unraveling the genetics of Alzheimer disease. American Society for Experimental Neurotherapeutics Abstracts. Arch Neurol 57, 2000

Targum SD, Greenberg RD, Harmon RL, et al: Thyroid hormone and the TRH stimulation test in refractory depression. J Clin Psychiatry 45:345–346, 1984

Targum SD, Marshall LE, Fischman P: Variability of TRH test responses in depressed and normal elderly subjects. Biol Psychiatry 31:787–793, 1992

Taylor WD, Payne ME, Ranga Rama Krishnan K, et al: Evidence of white matter tract disruption in MRI hyperintensities. Biol Psychiatry 50:179–183, 2001

Thase ME, Reynolds CF, Glanz LM, et al: Nocturnal penile tumescence in depressed men. Am J Psychiatry 144:89–92, 1987

Thomas KM, Drevets WC, Dahl RE, et al: Amygdala response to fearful faces in anxious and depressed children. Arch Gen Psychiatry 58:1057–1063, 2001

Tsuang MT, Stone WS, Faraone SV: Genes, environment and schizophrenia. Br J Psychiatry 178:S18–S24, 2001

Van Putten T, Marder SR, Mintz J, et al: Haloperidol plasma levels and clinical response: a therapeutic window relationship. Am J Psychiatry 149:500–505, 1992

Volz H, Gaser C, Hager F, et al: Decreased frontal activation in schizophrenics during stimulation with the Continuous Performance Test: a functional magnetic resonance imaging study. Eur Psychiatry 14:17–24, 1999

Weinberger DR: Brain disease and psychiatric illness: when should a psychiatrist order a CAT scan? Am J Psychiatry 141:1521–1527, 1984

Weinberger DR: Implications of normal brain development for the pathogenesis of schizophrenia. Arch Gen Psychiatry 44:660–669, 1987

Weinberger DR: From neuropathology to neurodevelopment. Lancet 346:552–557, 1995

Weinberger DR, Torrey EF, Neophytides AN, et al: Lateral cerebral ventricular enlargement in chronic schizophrenia. Arch Gen Psychiatry 36:735–739, 1979

Weinberger DR, Berman KF, Zec RF: Physiologic dysfunction of dorsolateral prefrontal cortex in schizophrenia, I: regional cerebral blood flow evidence. Arch Gen Psychiatry 43:114–124, 1986

Weinberger DR, Jones D, Reba RC, et al: A comparison of FDG PET and IQNB SPECT in normal subjects and in patients with dementia. J Neuropsychiatry Clin Neurosci 4:239–248, 1992a

Weinberger DR, Berman KF, Suddath R, et al: Evidence of dysfunction of a prefrontal-limbic network in schizophrenia: a magnetic resonance imaging and regional cerebral blood flow study of discordant monozygotic twins. Am J Psychiatry 149:890–897, 1992b

Wible CG, Kubicki M, Yoo SW, et al: A functional magnetic resonance imaging study of auditory mismatch in schizophrenia. Am J Psychiatry 158:938–943, 2001

Williams W: Psychogenic erectile impotence a useful or a misleading concept? Aust N Z J Psychiatry 19:77–82, 1985

Wolkin A, Jaeger J, Brodie JD, et al: Persistence of cerebral metabolic abnormalities in chronic schizophrenia as determined by positron emission tomography. Am J Psychiatry 142:564–571, 1985

Wong DF, Wagner HN, Tune LE, et al: Positron emission tomography reveals elevated D2 dopamine receptors in drug-naive schizophrenics. Science 234:1558–1563, 1986

Woodruff PWR, Wright IC, Bullmore ET, et al: Auditory hallucinations and the temporal cortical response to speech in schizophrenia: a functional magnetic resonance imaging study. Am J Psychiatry 154:1676–1682, 1997

Yurgelun-Todd DA, Waternaux CM, Cohen BM, et al: Functional magnetic resonance imaging of schizophrenic patients and comparison subjects during word production. Am J Psychiatry 153:200–205, 1996

P A R T

II

Psychiatric Disorders

Delirium, Dementia, and Amnestic Disorders

James A. Bourgeois, O.D., M.D.

Jeffrey S. Seaman, M.S., M.D.

Mark E. Servis, M.D.

Delirium, dementia, and amnestic disorders are classified with other disorders of memory and other cognitive functions in DSM-IV-TR (American Psychiatric Association 2000). As a group, they represent psychiatric disturbances formerly described as exclusively due to "organic" as opposed to "functional" etiological factors. As research into the etiology and treatment of other psychiatric disorders has progressed, the artificial distinction between *organic* (an anachronistic term in current clinical practice) and *functional* psychiatric illness has blurred substantially. Nonetheless, these cognitive disorders generally have clear structural and functional disturbances in brain function as their primary causes. In addition, however, psychological factors may be of great importance in the patient's experience of symptoms and his or her behavioral and emotional response to illness. Delirium, dementia, and the amnestic disorders make clear the need for psychiatric evaluation based on the biopsychosocial model of psychiatric illness.

In the management of cognitive disorders, there is a high likelihood of psychiatrist involvement with other specialty physicians in the often-complex medical and surgical presentations of these patients. Thorough evaluation of psychiatric, neurological, general medical/surgical, and psychosocial variables is essential to render appropriate care. One cognitive disorder may predispose a patient to other cognitive disorders. For example, it is common to discover that a patient with delirium also has a preexisting dementia. Although delirium, dementia, and amnestic disorders are discussed in this chapter as separate pathological entities, the alert physician must be mindful of the possible comorbidity of more than one cognitive disorder in a given patient.

Recent research and clinical developments have enabled advances in pathophysiology, prevention efforts, and treatments for delirium, dementia, and amnestic disorders. Interventions are now available to significantly reduce the suffering caused by and at times improve the clinical outcomes of these disorders. Skill in management of these disorders is expected of all psychiatrists and is the sine qua non of those practicing consultation-liaison psychiatry.

Delirium

Two millennia ago, physicians understood delirium. They knew it occurred in hypo- and hyperactive forms (*lethargus* and *phrenitis*), attributed both forms to brain disease, and recommended both physiological and psychological treatments (Lipowski 1991). In modern times, varying terms have been used for delirium, such as *acute confu-*

The author of the "Delirium" and "Dementia" portions of this chapter (J.A.B.) is grateful to Michael G. Wise, M.D., for his thoughtful review and editorial suggestions.

sional disorder, *metabolic encephalopathy*, and *intensive care unit (ICU) psychosis*. The term chosen was often more dependent on the specialty of the physician than it was on the clinical picture itself. In psychiatry, Lipowski (1983) led the effort to remedy this by reintroducing the term *delirium* in DSM-III (American Psychiatric Association 1980), departing from the more inclusive term *organic mental disorder* used in DSM-II (American Psychiatric Association 1968). The use of explicit diagnostic criteria in both DSM-III and DSM-IV (American Psychiatric Association 1994) also helped to provide standards for researchers and clinicians alike. Additionally, the American Psychiatric Association's (APA's) scientifically grounded "Practice Guideline for the Treatment of Patients With Delirium" (American Psychiatric Association 1999) further enhanced consensus. Even more recently, the reemergence of delirium as a "distinct pathophysiological and clinical entity" (Brown 2000) has enabled exciting new opportunities for both research and clinical management.

Definition

Delirium is an acute, potentially reversible brain dysfunction manifested by a syndromal array of neuropsychiatric symptoms. Engel and Romano (1959) called delirium a "syndrome of cerebral insufficiency," analogous to cardiac or renal insufficiency. They were the first to assert that delirium not only complicated the treatment of concurrent systemic illnesses but also carried a real risk of irreversible brain damage in its own right. In other words, Engel and Romano essentially proposed that delirium is both a disease and a syndrome—a "new" conceptualization fundamental to a full understanding of delirium.

Clinical Features

Delirium is not always a "fortunate complication" of being hospitalized and seriously ill. For those who retain some awareness of their delirious episode, the experience can be a very unpleasant event. Certainly, the disturbing symptomatology can wreak havoc on the emotions and duties of the families and staff caring for the patient.

DSM-IV-TR Diagnosis of Delirium

The DSM-IV-TR diagnostic criteria for delirium require a disturbance in *consciousness/attention* and a change in *cognition* that develop *acutely* and tend to *fluctuate* (Table 7–1). Lipowski (1983, 1987) characterized delirium as a disorder of attention, wakefulness, cognition, and motor behavior. The disruption of attention is often

considered the core symptom. Patients struggle to sustain attentional focus, are easily distracted, and often vary in their level of alertness. Sleep and wake cycles are disrupted as well, with patients often having grossly fragmented sleep and loss of normal circadian rhythm. The impairment in cognition can be across a wide spectrum—from subtle to overt and from focal to global. Deficits can occur in perception, memory, language, processing speed, and executive functioning. The reported frequencies of these clinical features are shown in Table 7–2.

TABLE 7–1. DSM-IV-TR diagnostic criteria for delirium due to…*[indicate the general medical condition]*

A. Disturbance of consciousness (i.e., reduced clarity of awareness of the environment) with reduced ability to focus, sustain, or shift attention.

B. A change in cognition (such as memory deficit, disorientation, language disturbance) or the development of a perceptual disturbance that is not better accounted for by a preexisting, established, or evolving dementia.

C. The disturbance develops over a short period of time (usually hours to days) and tends to fluctuate during the course of the day.

D. There is evidence from the history, physical examination, or laboratory findings that the disturbance is caused by the direct physiological consequences of a general medical condition.

Coding note: If delirium is superimposed on a preexisting vascular dementia, indicate the delirium by coding 290.41 vascular dementia, with delirium.

Coding note: Include the name of the general medical condition on Axis I, e.g., 293.0 delirium due to hepatic encephalopathy; also code the general medical condition on Axis III.

Delirium Subtypes

Delirium subtypes have been described. One subtype may be a subsyndromal variant (Levkoff et al. 1992; Lowy et al. 1973; Meagher and Trzepacz 1998). Little is known about this subtype, although it may be a prodromal or residual condition. Consistent with the ancient descriptions of phrenitis and lethargis, hyperactive and hypoactive subtypes have been reported. Liptzin and Levkoff (1992) characterized delirious patients with restlessness, hypervigilance, rapid speech, irritability, and combativeness as *hyperactive*, whereas those showing slowed speech and kinetics, apathy, and reduced alertness were designated *hypoactive*. Hypoactive patients tend to have more severe cognitive disturbances (Koponen et al. 1989c) and a poorer prognosis (Liptzin and Levkoff 1992; Reyes et al. 1981; Weddington 1982). The reported occurrence of the hyperactive subtype has

TABLE 7–2. Range of reported frequencies of clinical features of delirium

Clinical features	Range (%)
Poor attention/vigilance	100
Clouding of consciousness	100
Disorientation	43–100
Disorganized thinking/thought disorder	95
Diffuse cognitive impairment	77
Poor memory	64–90
Language disorder	41–93
Sleep disturbance	25–96
Delusions	18–68
Mood lability	43–63
Psychomotor changes	38–55
Perceptual changes/hallucinations	17–55

Source. Adapted with permission from Meagher DJ, Trzepacz PT: "Delirium Phenomenology Illuminates Pathophysiology, Management, and Course." *Journal of Geriatric Psychiatry and Neurology* 11:150–156, 1998.

ranged from 9% to 31%, the hypoactive type from 19% to 72%, and a mixed type from 33% to 54% (Breitbart et al. 1997; Francis et al. 1990; Liptzin and Levkoff 1992; Meagher et al. 1998).

Meagher and Trzepacz (1998) further hypothesized that specific delirium subtypes portend different precipitants and causes. Two examples are the hypoactive presentation in hepatic encephalopathy and the hyperactive or mixed forms in alcohol and sedative withdrawal. To examine this hypothesis, Meagher et al. (1998) subdivided patients into three precipitant categories—1) low perfusion, 2) drug related, and 3) infectious or metabolic—and then followed these patients during hospitalization. The patients with drug-related delirium were the youngest and had the highest total Delirium Rating Scale (DRS; Trzepacz et al. 1988b) scores, those with the low-perfusion form were more likely to be hypoactive, and distinguishable "DRS patterns" emerged among the three groups. This study confirmed that unique symptom patterns define the various subtypes, which in turn could reflect slightly different pathophysiological processes.

Etiopathogenesis

One key to sustained progress in understanding delirium is a refutation of the misleading model wherein delirium is believed to be caused by the comorbid systemic disease. Delirium is itself a disease. Comorbid systemic diseases may precipitate delirium, but they do not cause it. A campfire analogy may help to clarify this proposed model. The flammability of the wood is the baseline vulnerability, the matches are the precipitants, the fire is the etiopathogenic engine, and finally, the light and heat are the cognitive and behavioral manifestations of delirium. In this section, the "fire," or "core," of the disease will be explored.

Neuronal Integrity

Engel and Romano (1959) initiated the search to understand the basis of delirium. In their view, the functional integrity of the neuron was paramount; they even hypothesized that disturbances in oxygen and glutamate metabolism could be key. More recently, two clinician-scientists, Trzepacz (1994) and Brown (2000), have led the effort to extend Engel and Romano's work (American Psychiatric Association 1999).

The cornerstone of the Brown (2000) theory is the notion that it is the relationship between the limited energy reserves of the neuron and the varying resilience of different neuronal populations that underlies the behavioral and cognitive changes seen in delirium. In other words, Brown hypothesized, the development of delirium is initiated and then sustained through the selective and progressive dysfunction of specific neurotransmitters and neural circuits. Fundamentally, Brown (2000) noted that cerebral insufficiency is intimately linked to relative deficits in oxygen (O_2) and energy metabolism.

Role of Oxygen

The clinical importance of oxygen in the pathogenesis of delirium was demonstrated in several studies. Aakerlund and Rosenberg (1994) reported that postthoracotomy patients who developed delirium had lower postoperative O_2 saturations compared with patients who did not develop delirium, and supplemental O_2 successfully treated these cases. Another study (Rosenberg and Kehlet 1993) found a strong correlation between mental function on postoperative days 3 and 7 and the O_2 saturations on the second postoperative night. The importance of oxidative metabolism is also evident in patients with delirium associated with sepsis. These patients have lower hemoglobin, lower cerebral blood flow (CBF), lower metabolic rate for O_2, and lower cerebral O_2 delivery compared with control subjects (Maekawa et al. 1991). Even among healthy young adults, concentration and short-term learning is degraded when the partial pressure of oxygen (PaO_2) drops to 45–60 mm Hg, and frank delirium reliably occurs at a PaO_2 of 35–45 mm Hg (Gibson et al. 1981). Delirium would likely have developed at a higher PaO_2 had this study been in a less robust population such as the elderly, who have less compensatory reserves.

Cardiovascular and Respiratory Reserves

A broad decline in cardiovascular and respiratory reserves occurs with age. By age 85, vital capacity is reduced by 30%–40% and the arterial–alveolar gradient widens; by age 90, basal PaO_2 drops to 70 mm Hg, the ventilatory response to acute hypoxia is blunted, and maximum heart rate and cardiac output are decreased (Pack and Millman 1988). Oxygen delivery to the brain in times of increased metabolic stress can also be limited by the reduced capacity for compensatory changes in carotid and vertebral vessel dynamics due to vasculopathy. In part for these reasons, the frail elderly patient can be viewed as being exquisitely vulnerable to sliding into "brain insufficiency" (Tune 1991)—much like patients with "brittle" congestive heart failure.

Oxygen Demand and Anemia

Brown (2000) noted that the hospitalized patient's homeostasis is additionally threatened by the increased O_2 demand from acute illness and fever (Fink 1997; Weissman et al. 1984). Anemia, which further limits O_2 delivery to the brain, is also commonly encountered among hospitalized surgery patients and the chronically ill. Often, the clinical threshold to transfuse is based on providing a baseline minimum for the brain and kidneys. Although the "baseline minimum" hematocrit may be enough to keep the brain alive and to avoid watershed strokes, critically, it may not be enough to support normal function, particularly for the delirious patient with limited cerebral reserve. As will be shown, keeping the brain alive but not at an adequate functional level can have dire consequences.

Anoxia

In further exploring the role of oxidative metabolism in the development of delirium, Brown (2000) referred to research on anoxic encephalopathy. According to studies in this area, inadequate aerobic metabolism results in an inability to maintain ionic gradients (Somjen and Aitken 1984), leading to abnormal neurotransmitter synthesis, release, and metabolism (Gibson et al. 1981); anoxic depolarization and "spreading depression" of neuronal function (Balestrino et al. 1989); and increased production and decreased disposal of neurotoxins (D.W. Choi et al. 1989; Globus et al. 1988a; Kirsch et al. 1989). Brown (2000) hypothesized that delirium might share these events, and thus, addressing these consequences of inadequate aerobic metabolism could provide more precise targets for physiological interventions.

Although a complete understanding of anoxic encephalopathy is not yet available, numerous details are known. When oxygen delivery to brain tissue falls, sodium and calcium flood into the cells, and potassium flows out secondary to failure of ATPase pumps (Siesjo 1984). The calcium influx accelerates the activity of tyrosine hydroxylase (Carmen and Wyatt 1977), which converts tyrosine to 3,4-dihydroxyphenylalanine (DOPA), thus enabling more dopamine production, and uncouples oxidative phosphorylation in brain mitochondria (Kirsch et al. 1989), thus disabling adenosine triphosphate (ATP) production. Importantly, the calcium influx also stimulates neurotransmitter release and thus anoxic depolarization (Balestrino et al. 1986) and activates intraneuronal catabolic enzymes (D.W. Choi et al. 1989). The sodium influx is believed to contribute to anoxic depolarization via cell swelling (Balestrino 1995). The duration of anoxic depolarization has been linked to the reversibility of brain damage from cerebral ischemia (Balestrino and Somjen 1986). Anoxic depolarization could be an underlying mechanism for some of the chronic morbidity and functional decline seen in delirium survivors. One study demonstrated that a traditional delirium treatment (dopamine antagonist) effectively protected brain tissue in a hypoxic encephalopathy model by delaying the anoxic depolarization (Balestrino and Somjen 1986).

Additionally, research has demonstrated the selective vulnerability (Somjen et al. 1990) concept, which Brown (2000) suggested was applicable to delirium as well. Small interneurons with minimal energy requirements (e.g., γ-aminobutyric acid [GABA] neurons) are more resilient to relative anoxia than are larger neurons with long axons to support (e.g., dopamine neurons). The hippocampus is known to be very sensitive to cerebral ischemia (Benveniste et al. 1984). On the basis of the data from spreading depolarization in hypoxia, Brown (2000) hypothesized that a similar pattern of regional brain insufficiency could occur in delirium. He posited that the hippocampus fails first, followed by the neocortex, the subcortical nuclei, the brain stem, the cortical gray matter, and finally the cerebellum.

Additional Selective Mechanisms

Further support for the role of selective vulnerability in delirium comes from animal models. In one hypoxic encephalopathy model, dopamine release was shown to increase 500-fold, whereas GABA release was increased only fivefold (Globus et al. 1988a). This massive increase in dopamine results from a breakdown in ATP-dependent transporters (decreased reuptake) during anoxic depolarization (Pulsinelli and Duffy 1983) as well as decreases in metabolism through the reduced activity of the O_2-dependent catechol-O-methyltransferase (Gibson et al. 1981). Another potential mechanism underlying the increase in dopamine is reduced activity of dopamine-β-hydroxylase. This enzyme is also O_2 dependent; thus, in hypoxic conditions, less dopamine is converted to norepinephrine (Gibson et al. 1981). Another animal model of encephalopathy (sepsis) also demonstrated these higher dopamine levels, particularly in the striatum, hippocampus, mesencephalon, and pons-medulla (Freund et al. 1986).

A decreased redox (nicotinamide adenine dinucleotide, NAD [oxidized form]:NADH [reduced form]) state rather than ATP depletion itself may link the failure in energy metabolism to neurotransmitter abnormalities (Gibson et al. 1981). Supportive of this notion, the decrease in acetylcholine (ACh) during hypoxia has been shown to be proportional to the decline in the NAD:NADH ratio (Gibson and Blass 1976). Additional work to clarify the roles of these two mechanisms in delirium is needed.

In hypoxic conditions, the metabolism of dopamine, but not of other catecholamines, shifts to more toxic oxidative pathways, generating cytotoxic quinones (Graham 1978). Interestingly, preexisting lesions of the substantia nigra have been found to protect projection areas during hypoxia (Globus et al. 1986). For these toxic agents to injure neurons, they first must overwhelm the cell's protective mechanisms—for example, superoxide dismutase, catalase, glutathione peroxidase, and reduced glutathione (Graham 1984). It would be of clinical interest to examine whether these protective systems are reduced in patients at high risk for delirium and, as Brown (2000) posited, whether these toxic metabolites are related to the permanent cognitive sequelae of delirium.

Research in hepatic encephalopathy may also offer insight into the etiopathogenesis of delirium. Specifically, ATP and phosphocreatine depletion occur in this disease (Bluml et al. 1998; Kosenko et al. 1994; Schenker et al. 1967). In addition, astrocytes have been demonstrated to have decreased oxygen consumption in response to increased levels of ammonia (Albrecht et al. 1987), perhaps indicating a progressive effect of ammonia or glutamate toxicity on astrocyte activity. As with hypoxic encephalopathy, ATP depletion does not by itself appear to fully explain neuronal dysfunction in hepatic encephalopathy. The neurotoxicity of ammonia is also mediated by N-methyl-D-aspartate (NMDA) receptor activation (Felipo et al. 1998), which in turn further increases ATP consumption. Nonetheless, NMDA inhibitors exist that can prevent glutamate-induced neuronal death without affecting ATP levels (Marcaida et al. 1995). Additionally,

dopamine excess may be necessary for glutamate to exert its toxic effect (Globus et al. 1988b). Brown (2000) hypothesized that this massive dopamine excess may play a central facilitating role in activating the high-threshold NMDA receptors. Interestingly enough, glutamate excess is also seen in hypoxia (Benveniste et al. 1984; Globus et al. 1988a).

Finally, a global shift of CBF and cerebral metabolic rate from cortical to subcortical areas (Lockwood et al. 1991) occurs in hepatic encephalopathy patients. Within the cortex, regional differences in CBF in subclinical hepatic encephalopathy patients have also been reported (Trzepacz 1994). The largest reduction in CBF was identified in the right dorsolateral prefrontal cortex. These shifts may be linked to alterations in levels of tryptophan (Rodriguez et al. 1987)—the precursor to the cerebral vasoconstrictor serotonin (5-hydroxytryptamine [5-HT]). Indeed, the metabolites of 5-HT and of dopamine (homovanillic acid) were found to be elevated in the cerebrospinal fluid (CSF) of patients with hepatic encephalopathy (Knell et al. 1974).

Neurotransmitter Roles

Regarding specific changes in neurotransmitters in delirium, the two most accepted are a reduction in ACh activity and an excess of dopamine activity (Trzepacz 2000). ACh has long been known to be decreased in delirium (Itil and Fink 1966) as well as in hypoxia (Gibson and Blass 1976). Attention, cognitive functioning, and memory are heavily dependent on ACh (Trzepacz 2000). Both human (Itil and Fink 1966) and animal (Trzepacz et al. 1992) models of delirium have utilized anticholinergic medications to induce delirium with the resultant hyperactivity, psychosis (humans), cognitive impairment, and electroencephalogram (EEG) slowing.

Dopamine is considered to have important roles in attention, mood, motor activity, perception (Trzepacz 2000), and executive functioning. Excess dopamine agonism can lead to delirium, as seen with drugs such as L-dopa or cocaine. Agonists of dopamine have also been shown to cause EEG slowing despite motoric hyperactivity (Ongini et al. 1985). Moreover, interplay between dopamine and ACh exists, as evidenced experimentally by the finding that D_2 antagonists enhance ACh release (Ikarashi et al. 1997) and clinically by the utility of antipsychotics in reversing anticholinergic-precipitated delirium (Itil and Fink 1966).

Among other neurotransmitters, serotonin levels may have an inverse relationship with hypoactive or hyperactive delirium subtypes (Brown 2000). Serotonin receptor subtypes have differential effects in either stimulating or inhibiting ACh release via the median raphe–basal forebrain tract (summarized in Trzepacz 2000). Levels and circadian rhythms of somatostatin, β-endorphin, and cortisol (Koponen and Riekkinen 1990; Koponen et al. 1989a; McIntosh et al. 1985) have also been suggested to be disrupted in delirium.

Neuroanatomic Loci

Although there is no single neuroanatomic locus for delirium, studies and case reports consistently identify prefrontal and right-sided brain dysfunction (Doyle and Warden 1996; Koponen et al. 1989b; Trzepacz 2000). Trzepacz (2000) suggested that further evidence for right-sided brain dysfunction comes from cognitive testing (visuospatial attention and visual memory) implicating the right side of the brain as well as the higher prevalence of delirium in bipolar disorder patients (also believed to lateralize to the right). Nonetheless, in a recent prospective study comparing stroke patients who became delirious with those who did not, there were no differences found between lesion location and delirium rates (Henon et al. 1999). Overall, although delirium is associated with specific brain regions (i.e., bifrontal and right prefrontal cortex, right anterior thalamus, right posterior parietal cortex, basal ganglia, and lingual gyrus), lesions anywhere can precipitate delirium (Trzepacz 2000).

Epidemiology

Inpatient Studies

Delirium is epidemic among hospitalized patients, especially in the elderly. Inouye (1998) estimated that delirium annually complicated the hospitalizations of 2.3 million elderly Americans, was present for about 17 million inpatient days, and cost Medicare alone 4 billion dollars, excluding the substantial postdischarge morbidity costs. Inpatient studies have reported a delirium prevalence of 12%–40% among geriatric patients (Francis and Kapoor 1992; Hodkinson 1973; Inouye and Charpentier 1996; Inouye et al. 1993, 1998; Johnson et al. 1990; O'Keeffe and Lavan 1997; Rockwood 1989; Schor et al. 1992; Thomas et al. 1988), 10%–15% across patients of all ages (Cameron et al. 1987; Erkinjuntii et al. 1986), 13% among patients on a geriatric psychiatric ward (Koponen et al. 1989c), and 37% among postoperative patients (Dyer et al. 1995). Delirium has been found to be even more common in elderly patients with hip fractures (41%, Marcantonio et al. 2000; 61%, Gustafson et al. 1988), hospitalized AIDS patients (57%, Fernandez et al. 1989), terminally ill cancer patients (46%, Gagnon et al.

2000; 85%, Massie et al. 1983), and patients undergoing stem-cell transplantation (73%, Fann et al. 2000). Besides the 38% of geriatric inpatients reported as having delirium in one study (Levkoff et al. 1992), an additional 33% were recognized to have a "subsyndromal delirium." Thus, a total of 71% had some or all of the features of delirium during hospitalization.

Diagnostic and Liaison Challenges

As consultation psychiatrists can attest, most delirium cases either are never diagnosed (Cameron et al. 1987; Elie et al. 2000; Francis et al. 1988, 1990; Levin 1951; Rockwood et al. 1994; Thomas et al. 1988) or are misdiagnosed (Armstrong et al. 1997; Golinger et al. 1987; Nicholas and Lindsey 1995). Inouye (1994) suggested that delirium is so common in the ICUs that some providers have accepted it as an inevitable and even a natural event in hospitalized elderly patients. Diagnosis can also be difficult because some delirious patients remain "fluent" despite marked cognitive impairment (C.A. Ross et al. 1991). Delirium, of course, can also fluctuate. A patient may be in a "lucid interval" for the physician's visit and yet be frankly delirious at other times. Furthermore, because delirium still is often viewed as a syndrome caused by the patient's systemic illness(es), nonpsychiatric physicians may feel reluctant to consult a psychiatrist for help. Hence, it often seems that only the troublesome behavioral cases generate consultation requests or receive delirium-specific treatment (Engel and Romano 1959; Meagher et al. 1996). Opportunities clearly exist, then, for consultation-liaison psychiatrists to actively educate their physician colleagues and assist in the management of delirium.

Clinical Evaluation

History

The diagnosis of delirium is relatively straightforward for the trained clinician (Table 7–3). A thorough history is fundamental and provides the majority of the diagnostic information. In addition, a meticulous approach with good "situational awareness" is required of the diagnostician, because several potential factors can obscure the clinical picture. For one, the referral problem may be characterized as psychosis, depression, noncompliance, or unruly behavior. The perspective of the consultation psychiatrist may facilitate clarification of the clinical question. Furthermore, the consultant may be called later in the course of a delirium and thus must retrospectively search for history and hospital course data.

Central to the history gathering is establishing what the

TABLE 7–3. Evaluation of delirium

Standard
Complete history
Medication review
Neurological examination
Vital signs
Bedside testing: Mini-Mental State Examination, Trails B,
  Clock drawing, a test for vigilance, days of the week backward
As clinically warranted
Laboratory work: Complete blood count, electrolytes, blood
  urea nitrogen, creatinine, glucose, calcium, pulse oximetry or
  arterial blood gas, urinalysis, drug screens, liver function tests
  with serum albumin, cultures, cerebrospinal fluid examina-
  tion
Tests: Chest X ray, electrocardiogram, brain imaging, electro-
  encephalogram

patient's premorbid baseline is, whether a recent change occurred, and when. Not only is this information key in distinguishing delirium from dementia, it may also identify precipitants. Prime sources of information are those who have known the patient for some time, such as family members and outpatient physicians, as well as the nurses and technicians of the inpatient treatment team. Review of the patient's current medical or surgical illness is also essential. Assessment of the treatment environment with a focus on variables that could affect sensory deprivation or disorientation is helpful as well (Francis and Kapoor 1990). These variables may include visual or hearing aids; light, dark, and noise cycles; communication efforts and assistive devices; familiar versus unfamiliar caretakers, objects, and routines; and depersonalization factors.

Medication Review

Every delirium evaluation warrants a medication review that includes current and recently discontinued drugs, whether prescription, over-the-counter, herbal, or illicit. Medications with anticholinergic properties should be discontinued or substituted as possible. The potential for drug–drug interactions should be reviewed on an individual basis. Such adverse interactions include both pharmacodynamic (e.g., toxic synergies such as meperidine with a monoamine oxidase inhibitor [MAOI], agonist–antagonist combinations such as L-dopa and an antipsychotic) and pharmacokinetic effects (e.g., cytochrome P450 system inductions or "bottlenecks," competition for serum protein binding, renal function). Similarly, consideration of the unique metabolism or medication sensitivity in special populations—such as the young, the old, and the malnourished (Dickson 1991), as well as those with HIV or with renal or liver compromise—is a necessity.

Interview and Observation

The interview itself should focus on establishing a global image of the patient's cognitive functioning. It is helpful to observe for decreased attention capacity, psychosis, short-term memory deficits, disorientation, executive dysfunction (problems with disinhibition, perseveration, sequencing, planning, organizing, response inhibition), and changes in mood or kinetics. Bedside exams (e.g., the A test for vigilance) and tests sensitive for frontal lobe dysfunction (e.g., Trails B, clock drawing) are quick and easy to administer. In regard to Folstein et al.'s (1975) Mini-Mental State Examination (MMSE; Figure 7–1), one study (C.A. Ross et al. 1991) reported the mean MMSE score to be 14.3 for delirious patients, versus 29.6 for control subjects. The most sensitive items were the serial 7s, orientation, and recall memory. Another study found the MMSE to correlate with EEG findings in delirious patients (Koponen et al. 1989c). Unfortunately, the MMSE is not particularly sensitive (33%) in identifying delirium (Trzepacz et al. 1986). Tests such as the MMSE are valuable, however, for following the course of a delirium. Indeed, Tune and Folstein (1986) reported serial improvement in MMSE scores with delirium resolution. Another potential benefit of these bedside tests is that they provide objective demonstration of cognitive dysfunction for colleagues who may not have initially appreciated the covert deficits.

Rating Scales

The use of diagnostic and rating tools may also be warranted. These tools are invaluable for research and are useful for psychiatrists (Zou et al. 1998), other physicians, and "physician extenders" (e.g., physician's assistants, nurse practitioners) as well. Several of the commonly used and validated instruments are the DRS and the Delirium Rating Scale—Revised–98 (DRS-R-98; Trzepacz et al. 1988b, 2001), the Confusion Assessment Method (CAM; Inouye et al. 1990), the Memorial Delirium Assessment Scale (Breitbart et al. 1997), and the Delirium Symptom Interview (Albert et al. 1992).

Neurological Examination

Unexplained or new focal neurological signs beyond cognitive disturbances are atypical in delirium and warrant discussion with a neurologist. Neuroimaging should be considered for patients with head injuries, focal findings, cancer, stroke risk, AIDS, and atypical presentations (e.g., young, healthy, lack of identifiable precipitants). Abnormalities on neuroimaging—such as periventricular

MINI-MENTAL STATE EXAMINATION AND INSTRUCTIONS

Patient _____
Examiner _____
Date _____

Maximum score	Score	Orientation
5	( )	What is the (year) (season) (date) (day) (month)?
5	( )	Where are we: (state) (county) (town) (hospital) (floor)?

Registration

3	( )	Name 3 objects: 1 second to say each. Then ask the patient all 3 after you have said them. Give 1 point for each correct answer. Then say them until he/she learns all 3. Count trials and record. Trials _____

Attention and Calculation

5	( )	Serial 7s. 1 point for each correct. Stop after 5 answers. Alternatively spell "world" backwards.

Recall

3	( )	Ask for the 3 objects repeated above. Give 1 point for each correct.

Language

9	( )	Name a pencil, and watch (2 points) Repeat the following "No ifs, ands, or buts." (1 point) Follow a 3-stage command: "Take a paper in your right hand, fold it in half, and put it on the floor." (3 points)

Read and obey the following:

Close your eyes (1 point)
Write a sentence (1 point)
Copy design (1 point)

Total score

Assess level of consciousness along a continuum

Alert   Drowsy   Stupor   Coma

(continued)

FIGURE 7–1. Mini-Mental State Examination.

Source. Reprinted with permission from Folstein MF, Folstein SE, McHugh PR: "Mini-Mental State": A Practical Method for Grading the Cognitive State of Patients for the Clinician. *Journal of Psychiatric Research* 12:189–198, 1975. The copyright in the Mini Mental State Examination is wholly owned by the MiniMental LLC, a Massachusetts limited liability company. For information about how to obtain permission to use or reproduce the Mini Mental State Examination, please contact John Gonsalves Jr., Administrator of the MiniMental LLC, at 31 St. James Avenue, Suite 1, Boston, MA 02116; (617) 587-4215.

MINI-MENTAL STATE EXAMINATION AND INSTRUCTIONS

Orientation

1. Ask for the date. Then ask specifically for parts omitted, e.g., "Can you also tell me what season it is?" One point for each correct.
2. Ask in turn "Can you tell me the name of this hospital?" (town, county, etc.). One point for each correct.

Registration

Ask the patient if you may test his memory. Then say the names of 3 unrelated objects, clearly and slowly, about one second for each. After you have said all 3, ask him to repeat them. This first repetition determines his score (0–3) but keep saying them until he can repeat all 3, up to 6 trials. If he does not eventually learn all 3, recall cannot be meaningfully tested.

Attention and Calculation

Ask the patient to begin with 100 and count backwards by 7. Stop after 5 subtractions (93, 86, 79, 72, 65). Score the total number of correct answers.

If the patient cannot or will not perform this task, ask him to spell the word "world" backwards. The score is the number of letters in correct order, e.g., dlrow = 5, dlorw = 3.

Recall

Ask the patient if he can recall the 3 words you previously asked him to remember. Score 0–3.

Language

Naming: Show the patient a wrist watch and ask him what it is. Repeat for pencil. Score 0–2.

Repetition: Ask the patient to repeat the sentence after you. Allow only one trial. Score 0 or 1.

3-Stage command: Give the patient a piece of plain blank paper and repeat the command. Score 1 point for each part correctly executed.

Reading: On a blank piece of paper print the sentence "Close your eyes," in letters large enough for the patient to see clearly. Ask him to read it and do what it says. Score 1 point only if he actually closes his eyes.

Writing: Give the patient a blank piece of paper and ask him to write a sentence for you. Do not dictate a sentence; it is to be written spontaneously. It must contain a subject and verb and be sensible. Correct grammar and punctuation are not necessary.

Coding: On a clean piece of paper, draw intersecting pentagons, each side about 1 in., and ask him to copy it exactly as it is. All 10 angles must be present and 2 must intersect to score 1 point. Tremor and rotation are ignored.

Estimate the patient's level of sensorium along a continuum, from alert on the left to coma on the right.

FIGURE 7–1. Mini-Mental State Examination. *(continued)*

Source. Reprinted with permission from Folstein MF, Folstein SE, McHugh PR: "Mini-Mental State": A Practical Method for Grading the Cognitive State of Patients for the Clinician. *Journal of Psychiatric Research* 12:189–198, 1975. The copyright in the Mini Mental State Examination is wholly owned by the MiniMental LLC, a Massachusetts limited liability company. For information about how to obtain permission to use or reproduce the Mini Mental State Examination, please contact John Gonsalves Jr., Administrator of the MiniMental LLC, at 31 St. James Avenue, Suite 1, Boston, MA 02116; (617) 587-4215.

---

white matter disease, varying degrees of cortical atrophy, and ventricular enlargement—are common among the delirious elderly (Koponen et al. 1987, 1989b), although they are often described as "chronic, age-related changes." The cortical atrophy could in turn be considered a marker of reduced cerebral reserve. Indeed, the degree of generalized cortical atrophy has been more closely linked to delirium risk than focal cortical lesions alone (Tsai and Tsuang 1979).

Laboratory Tests

Laboratory tests are important but are not the foundation of a delirium evaluation. Tests are thus warranted on an individually tailored basis (Inouye 1998). Not only is such a practice fiscally responsible, it also avoids the error of pursuing clinically irrelevant and/or false-positive test abnormalities. Evaluations may include a complete blood count, electrolytes, blood urea nitrogen, creatinine, glucose, calcium, pulse oximetry or arterial blood gas, and urinalysis. Other tests commonly obtained are urine drug screens, liver function tests with serum albumin, cultures, chest X ray, and electrocardiogram (ECG). CSF examination should also be considered for cases in which meningitis or encephalitis is suspected as well as for atypical cases of delirium.

Electroencephalogram

Utilizing the EEG, Romano and Engel (1944) first demonstrated delirious patients had progressive disorganization of rhythms and generalized slowing (Figure 7–2). Specifically, delirious patients have slowing of the peak and average frequencies, in addition to increased theta and delta but decreased alpha rhythms (Koponen et al. 1989d). This same pattern of EEG slowing has been elicited in an animal model of delirium (Trzepacz et al. 1992) by decreasing ACh or increasing dopamine activity

(Keane and Neal 1981). The pattern is also seen in humans with hypoxic encephalopathy (Bauer 1982). Interestingly, the EEG changes correlate with cognitive dysfunction and memory and attention deficits, but not with psychomotor subtype (Koponen et al. 1989d; Trzepacz 1994). It is also important to realize that there are instances when the EEG may be read as "normal" in delirium, but is actually *abnormal* for the individual patient when compared with previous EEG—particularly for those patients whose baseline EEGs reside in the fast range (Pro and Wells 1977; Trzepacz and Wise 1997).

In contrast to the EEG changes observed in delirium, patients with sedative-withdrawal delirium are known to have a pattern characterized by low-voltage fast activity (Kennard et al. 1945). Other than in connection with drug intoxication or drug-withdrawal delirium, however, there are only very rare reports of low-voltage fast activity in hyperactive delirium (Pro and Wells 1977).

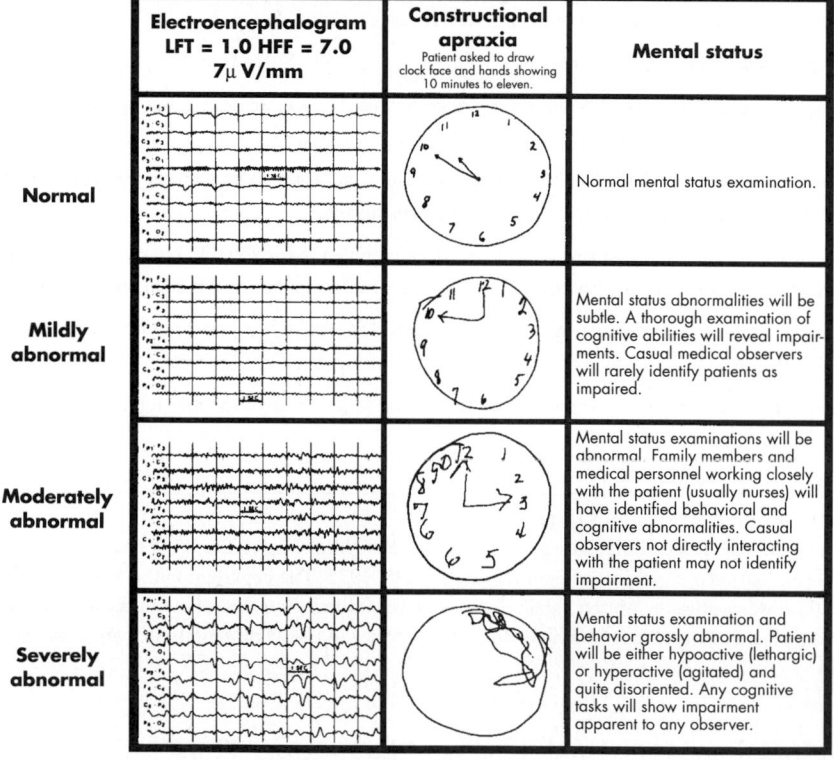

FIGURE 7–2. Comparison of electroencephalogram, constructional apraxia, and mental status in delirium.

In clinical practice, the EEG is only rarely used, as it is not necessary for the diagnosis of delirium and has limited specificity. EEG changes normalize before cognitive dysfunction clears (Trzepacz et al. 1992), whereas cognitive testing remains sensitive throughout the course of the delirium (Trzepacz et al. 1988a). Additionally, nondelirious elderly patients can exhibit EEG slowing, particularly if they have dementia (Obrist 1979). On the other hand, improved differentiation between dementia and delirium can be achieved with quantitative EEG (Jacobson et al. 1993a, 1993b).

Differential Diagnosis

Frequently, delirium needs to distinguished from dementia. Dementia has an insidious rather than an acute onset, features chronic memory and executive disturbances, and—unless it is Lewy body dementia or there is a superimposed delirium—tends not to fluctuate. A nondelirious dementia patient typically has intact attention and alertness; in addition, dementia is characterized by impoverished speech and thinking, as opposed to the confused or disorganized pattern seen in delirium. "Beclouded dementia" describes delirium that develops in a patient who already has dementia. Beclouded dementia should be approached like any other case of delirium (Trzepacz et al. 1998), albeit with the understanding that such patients are highly sensitive to precipitants and medications, in part because of a diminished cerebral reserve.

Other possibilities to consider in the differential diagnosis include drug intoxication, schizophrenia, and Bell's mania. A thorough history, physical examination, and toxicology screen should identify most intoxication cases. Stimulants, hallucinogens, and dissociative drugs are commonly abused agents capable of mimicking delirium. It is worth noting that agents such as mescaline and lysergic acid diethylamide (LSD) do not cause diffuse slowing like that seen in delirium (Engel and Romano 1959). The first episode of a psychotic disorder can also be difficult to differentiate from delirium, particularly if the mental status change developed acutely without a prolonged prodrome. Attentional difficulties, disorganization, and diffuse cognitive dysfunction can occur in both illnesses. If no localizing neurological abnormalities are present in an otherwise healthy young person, and no identifiable deliriogenic precipitants are found, a trial of antipsychotics and observation may suffice. If the cause was delirium, it typically clears rapidly in this population. On the other hand, if the negative signs of schizophrenia persist with residual delusions or hallucinations but attention and cognitive function improve, the illness is likely to be the first episode of a primary psychotic disorder. Another rare possibility to consider is brief psychotic disorder, a poorly understood condition that can be associated with various stressors (e.g., sleep deprivation). Finally, Bell's mania is a syndrome presenting as an extreme manic episode that also has the cognitive and attentional disturbances of delirium. History gathering is essential in diagnosing this illness, which is best treated with both antipsychotics and mood-stabilizing agents or electroconvulsive therapy (ECT) (Fink 1999).

Risk Factors: Precipitants and Baseline Vulnerability

A measure of confusion exists in the literature regarding what constitutes a cause versus a risk factor of delirium. For example, the terms *cause*, *risk factor*, *associated conditions*, and *underlying etiology* were used interchangeably in the APA practice guideline (American Psychiatric Association 1999). It is recommended that *cause* be reserved for the underlying cerebral etiopathology of the disease of delirium, even though that etiopathology has not yet been fully elucidated. *Precipitant* should be used to subsume risk factors that are generally transient or acute (e.g., a medication effect, a urinary tract infection). Finally, *baseline vulnerability* is best suited to describe risk factors that by definition are more chronic and innate to the patient (e.g., age, vision impairment, dementia). Thus, it is proposed that numerous and widely varying precipitants can activate the disease of delirium in susceptible (high baseline vulnerability) patients (O'Keeffe 1999).

One of the most common precipitants of delirium is medication. Indeed, numerous medications across many classes have been noted to precipitate delirium (Brown and Stoudemire 1998). The anticholinergic activity of a medication has been shown to correlate with its propensity to cause delirium (Beresin 1988; Blazer et al. 1983; Golinger et al. 1987). A 1992 study (Tune et al.) in fact, found that 14 of the 25 drugs most commonly prescribed for elderly patients (furosemide, digoxin, Dyazide, Lanoxin, dipyridamole, theophylline, warfarin, prednisone, nifedipine, isosorbide dinitrate, codeine, cimetidine, captropril, and ranitidine) had detectable anticholinergic effects. Moreover, 10 of those drugs result in anticholinergic levels sufficient to create memory and attentional deficits in healthy elderly subjects (Miller et al. 1988). A recent report noted that a serum level of anticholinergic activity (SAA) above 20 pmol/mL atropine equivalents confers a risk for delirium (Mussi et al. 1999). Therefore, although a single medication may have a low SAA, the combined effect of several such medications (Tune et al.

1992) may precipitate delirium in a susceptible individual.

Prospective studies have identified many other precipitants and baseline risks for delirium (Table 7–4). Two of the most frequently reported are pre-existing cognitive decline and advanced age. Inouye and Charpentier (1996) separated out baseline risks present at admission (e.g., poor vision, preexisting cognitive impairment) from precipitants affecting patients after admission (e.g., new medications, new-onset respiratory insufficiency). They found that robust patients with less baseline vulnerability ("more cerebral reserve") were more resilient to new precipitants following admission (Figure 7–3). The reverse was true as well: the more baseline vulnerability a patient had, the higher the likelihood that he or she would develop delirium if the fragile homeostasis ("less cerebral reserve") was stressed with additional precipitants.

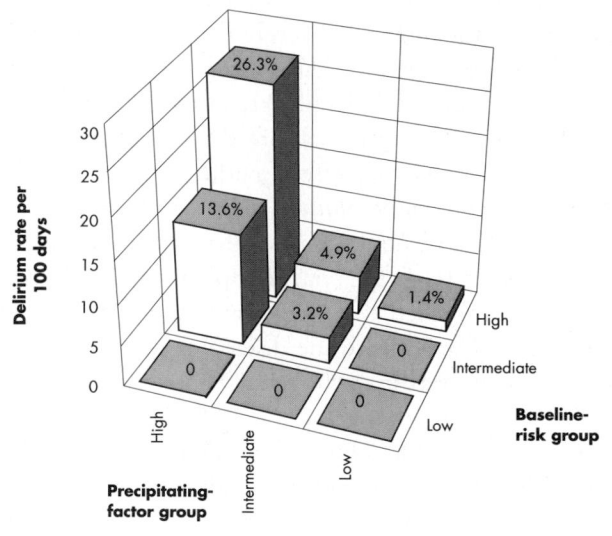

FIGURE 7–3. Interrelationship of baseline and precipitating factors.

Source. Adapted with permission from Inouye SK, Charpentier PA: "Precipitating Factors for Delirium in Hospitalized Elderly Persons: Predictive Model and Interrelationship With Baseline Vulnerability." *JAMA* 275:852–857, 1996. Copyright 1996 American Medical Association.

Prognosis

Mortality

Lipowski (1983) described delirium as a "grave prognostic sign," and a wealth of published data support this view. Essentially, delirium independently predicts substantial morbidity and helps to identify patients with higher mortality risks. Published studies have reported a wide range (5.6%–65%) of death rates for delirious inpatients (Bleasdale and Singleton 1997; Cameron et al.

TABLE 7–4. Prospectively identified risk factors for delirium

Risk factor	Study*
Dementia/preexisting cognitive impairment	(3), (4), (5), (6), (7), (8), (10), (12)
Elderly age	(1), (3), (5), (6), (9), (10), (12)
Alcohol/sedative withdrawal	(7), (6), (9)
Illness severity	(4), (8)
Blood urea nitrogen/creatinine > 18	(8), (4)
Abnormal sodium, potassium, or blood glucose levels	(4), (6)
Anticholinergics	(11)
Vision or hearing impairment	(8)
Hypoxia	(1)
Windowless intensive care unit	(2)
Use of a bladder catheter	(13)
More than 3 new medications begun	(13)
Malnutrition	(13)
Psychoactive medications used	(4)
Thoracic or aortic aneurysm surgery	(6)
Preexisting cerebral atrophy	(3)
Fever	(4)
Fracture or infection	(5)

Note. *1 = Foy et al. 1995; 2 = L.M. Wilson 1972; 3 = Henon et al. 1999; 4 = Francis et al. 1990; 5 = Schor et al. 1992; 6 = Marcantonio et al. 1994; 7 = Pompei et al. 1994; 8 = Inouye et al. 1993; 9 = Williams-Russo et al. 1992; 10 = Rockwood 1989; 11 = M.P. Rogers et al. 1989; 12 = Gustafson et al. 1988; 13 = Inouye and Charpentier 1996.

1987; Francis and Kapoor 1992; Francis et al. 1990; Gustafson et al. 1988; Guze and Daengsurisri 1967; Henon et al. 1999; Inouye et al. 1998; Kelly et al. 2001; Koponen et al. 1989c; Levkoff et al. 1992; Liptzin and Levkoff 1992; Marcantonio et al. 1994; O'Keeffe and Lavan 1997; Rabins and Folstein 1982; Rockwood 1993; Thomas et al. 1988; Trzepacz et al. 1985; van Hemert et al. 1994; Varsamis et al. 1972; Weddington 1982). When the most robust studies were combined in a meta-analysis (Cole and Primeau 1993), patients with delirium were reported to have an average 1-month mortality of 14.2% (vs. 4.8% in control subjects) and a 6-month mortality of 22.2% (vs. 10.6% in control subjects). One study found the mortality risk to be higher, even after multivariate analysis, for patients whose delirium failed to improve and/or was rated as severe (Kelly et al. 2001). Delirium also independently predicted a shorter survival time in cancer patients receiving palliative care (Caraceni et al. 2000). In contrast, several other studies have not found delirium to independently affect mortality (Dolan et al. 2000; Francis and Kapoor 1992; Levkoff et al. 1992;

O'Keeffe and Lavan 1997). In regard to delirium subtypes, patients with the hyperactive subtype had better prognoses than those with the hypoactive subtype (Liptzin and Levkoff 1992; Reyes et al. 1981). This difference could be due to variability in age, illness severity, or mobility between the subtypes. Another possible explanation relates to the increased medical and nursing attention that hyperactive patients tend to generate (Liptzin and Levkoff 1992; Meagher et al. 1996).

Morbidity

Delirium independently leads to poor clinical outcomes. The length of hospital stay (LOS) was found to be longer (Francis et al. 1990; Levkoff et al. 1992), and the loss of independent living more common (Francis and Kapoor 1992; Marcantonio et al. 2000; O'Keeffe and Lavan 1997), among patients who had been delirious. These differences persist even after control for variables such as illness severity, preexisting chronic cognitive impairment, and activities of daily living (ADL) status. In contrast, one study (Inouye et al. 1998) found that delirium independently predicted increased nursing home placements and decreased ability to perform ADL (as also noted by O'Keeffe and Lavan 1997; Marcantonio et al. 2000) but not increased LOS alone. Overall, a meta-analysis (Cole and Primeau 1993) found that patients with delirium had a mean LOS of 20.7 days (vs. 8.9 days for control subjects) and a rate of independent living 6 months after admission of 56.8% (vs. 91.7% in control subjects). The higher LOS has in turn been shown to increase health care costs for delirious patients (Franco et al. 2001).

Patients who experience delirium during hospitalization have less functional improvement 2 years after orthopedic surgery, experience a higher rate of major postoperative and hospital-acquired complications, and do less well in rehabilitation compared with patients without delirium (Dolan et al. 2000; Gustafson et al. 1988; Marcantonio et al. 1994, 2000; O'Keeffe and Lavan 1997; M.P. Rogers et al. 1989). Complications such as falls, incontinence, pulled intravenous lines, and uncooperativeness have been shown to be the proximate causes of increased LOS and placement problems (Saravay et al. 2000). Thus, delirium is not just a marker of poor prognosis but is actually a vital determinant of hospital outcomes (Inouye et al. 1998).

Duration

Average delirium episodes of 3–13 days have been reported, although 20 days was the mean in a sample of patients with "beclouded" dementia (Koponen et al. 1989c). Persistence beyond 7 (40%, Gustafson et al.

1988), 14 (20%, O'Keeffe and Lavan 1997), 20 (25%, Manos and Wu 1997), or 30 days (13%, Siroi 1988; 31%, Marcantonio et al. 2000) is not uncommon. Additionally, patients with hypoactive delirium have been shown to have longer episodes than those with the mixed or hyperactive subtypes (Kelly et al. 2001). Studies have also noted that some delirium symptoms persist at time of discharge in as many as 60%–96% of elderly patients who experienced delirium during their stay (Levkoff et al. 1992; Kelly et al. 2001; Rockwood 1993). Furthermore, in a recent study, stem cell transplant patients who had previously been delirious were later found to have more residual or new cognitive impairment well after the delirium had resolved (Fann et al. 2001). These findings suggest that delirium can resolve completely, resolve gradually, or transition to a more permanent cognitive disorder.

Persistent Cerebral Damage

Some investigators have suggested that the long-term morbidity and incomplete symptom resolution could be due to cerebral damage from the disease of delirium (Engel and Romano 1959; O'Keeffe 1999; O'Keeffe and Lavan 1997). Others have speculated that delirium may unmask a subtle, previously unidentified dementia that would account for most of the functional and progressive decline (Francis and Kapoor 1992; Koponen et al. 1989c). To examine this question, a recent prospective study followed elderly patients without preexisting diagnoses of dementia for 2 years after their initial episode of delirium (Rahkonen et al. 2000). Dementia was newly diagnosed in 27% after the resolution of their delirium, and by the 2-year point, a total of 57% of the patients had been diagnosed with dementia. Alternatively, Inouye et al. (1998) argued that the residual symptoms of delirium might themselves contribute to the observed morbidity (institutionalization, functional decline). All of these theories are potentially valid, and they may well function together to explain delirium's permanent sequelae.

Treatment and Prevention

Ideally, therapies can be matched more precisely to the neuropathology once the basis of delirium is better understood. Although new approaches can be proposed, traditional treatments remain the mainstay in the management of delirium.

Nonpharmacological Interventions

Among traditional treatments, nonpharmacological techniques clearly have a role in the management of delirium. Interventions have included reorientation, maintenance of circadian cycles, enhancement of communication, minimization of sensory deprivation and depersonalization, and reinforcement of cognitive functioning (American Psychiatric Association 1999; Inouye 1998; McCartney and Boland 1993). A recent effort, "The Elder Life Program," used nonpharmacological interventions targeted specifically toward delirium precipitants (Table 7–5; Inouye et al. 1999). In this preventive model, delirium developed in 9.9% of the treatment group versus 15% of the usual-care control group. The cost of the program was $327 per patient; it saved an average of $6,341 for each patient who did not develop delirium.

Pharmacotherapy

Although environmental manipulations and supportive care are important, medications offer further advantages. First, interventions directed at delirium precipitants should be instituted (e.g., antibiotics for urinary tract infection). Unless the delirium clears very rapidly or is mild, the concurrent use of delirium-specific treatments is also recommended. Antipsychotic medications are not just for behavioral management, as some have suggested, but rather are disease-specific treatments for delirium. Elevated dopamine levels are known to occur in delirium; thus, the use of dopamine-receptor antagonists is logical. Although further study is needed, patients with the nonagitated, hypoactive subtype of delirium may be among the most important to treat with delirium-specific medication (Platt et al. 1994), considering their poor prognosis (Liptzin and Levkoff 1992; Reyes et al. 1981).

Haloperidol is the most studied and most widely accepted treatment for delirium. The APA practice guideline (American Psychiatric Association 1999) supports haloperidol as a first-line agent for delirium because of its minimal anticholinergic effects, minimal sedation or orthostasis, low likelihood of extrapyramidal side effects (EPS) with intravenous use, and flexibility in dosing and administration with oral, intramuscular, and intravenous routes. Both oral and intravenous forms have been used for more than 40 years and have an extensive track record of safety and efficacy in even the most ill medical and surgical patients (Ayd 1978; Cassem and Sos 1978; Fernandez et al. 1989; Massie et al. 1983; Stiefel and Holland 1991). Haloperidol has also been proven clearly superior to benzodiazepines alone in delirium (Breitbart et al. 1996).

Oral haloperidol peaks in 4–6 hours, whereas intravenous doses offer onset of action within 5–20 minutes (Settle and Ayd 1983). The recommended dose (American Psychiatric Association 1999) is 1–2 mg every 2–4 hours as needed, with further titration until desired

effects are seen. Once stabilized, patients are often transitioned to a twice-daily or a daily bedtime oral dose, which is then continued or slowly tapered until the delirium has resolved. AIDS patients are sensitive to developing EPS (Breitbart et al. 1988; Swenson et al. 1989); thus, low doses of haloperidol or atypical antipsychotics with lower EPS risk are recommended. Doses of 0.25–1 mg twice a day are recommended when haloperidol or risperidone are used in the elderly (Zayas and Grossberg 1998).

In severe delirium refractory to boluses, continuous haloperidol infusions of 3–25 mg/hour have been used safely (Fernandez et al. 1988; Riker et al. 1994), although the APA practice guideline suggested a ceiling of 5–10 mg/hour. ECG monitoring is recommended with continuous infusion because of concerns about torsades des pointes, although no specific dose threshold has been designated (American Psychiatric Association 1999; Hunt and Stern 1995; Sharma et al. 1998; Zee-Cheng et al. 1985). Awareness and management of risk factors for QTc (hypokalemia, hypomagnesemia, bradycardia, congenital long-QT syndrome, preexisting cardiac disease, and drug–drug interactions) is advised (Gury et al. 2000). Therefore, even though the association between haloperidol use and torsades des pointes is unclear (Trzepacz and Wise 1997), QTc intervals beyond 450 msec or 25% over baseline should prompt a cardiology consultation, a dosage reduction, or discontinuation of the antipsychotic agent (American Psychiatric Association 1999). Another agent that has been used for intractable hyperactive delirium is propofol. It decreases CBF and is associated with hypotension; its use requires intubation and artificial ventilation (Mirenda and Broyles 1995).

Of the atypical antipsychotics, risperidone (Sipahimalani and Masand 1997), quetiapine (Torres et al. 2001), and olanzapine (Passik and Cooper 1999; Sipahimalani and Masand 1998) have been reported to treat delirium successfully and safely in small case series. Parenteral olanzapine (B. Jones et al. 2001; Wright et al. 2001), when available, may provide further benefits in the treatment of delirium, such as fast onset, reduced EPS, and minimal concerns about QTc interval changes.

Among other potential medications, droperidol has also been used for delirium (Frye et al. 1995). This faster-acting butyrophenone is more sedating, more hypotensive, and has more effect on QTc lengthening than does haloperidol (Gury et al. 2000). Most other antipsychotics (e.g., chlorpromazine, thioridazine) can be used to treat delirium, but, in general, they are not the best choices because of their associated anticholinergic, hypotensive, and excess sedation effects in addition to

TABLE 7–5. Risk factors for delirium and intervention protocols

Targeted risk factor and eligible patients	Standardized intervention protocols
Cognitive impairment[a] All patients, protocol once daily; patients with baseline MMSE score of <20 and orientation score of <8, protocol three times daily	Orientation protocol: board with names of care-team members and day's schedule; communication to reorient to surroundings Therapeutic activities protocol: cognitively stimulating activities three times daily (e.g., discussion of current events, structured reminiscence, word games)
Sleep deprivation All patients; need for protocol assessed once daily	Nonpharmacological sleep protocol: at bedtime, warm drink (milk or herbal tea), relaxation tapes or music, and back massage Sleep-enhancement protocol: unitwide noise-reduction strategies (e.g., silent pill crushers, vibrating beepers, and quiet hallways) and schedule adjustments to allow sleep (e.g., rescheduling of medications and procedures)
Immobility All patients; ambulation whenever possible, and range-of-motion exercises when patient is chronically nonambulatory, bed- or wheelchair-bound, or immobilized (e.g., because of an extremity fracture or deep venous thrombosis) or has been prescribed bed rest	Early mobilization protocol: ambulation or active range-of-motion exercises three times daily; minimal use of immobilizing equipment (e.g., bladder catheters, physical restraints)
Visual impairment Patients with <20/70 visual acuity on binocular near-vision testing	Vision protocol: visual aids (e.g., glasses or magnifying lenses) and adaptive equipment (e.g., large illuminated telephone keypads, large-print books, fluorescent tape on call bell), with daily reinforcement of their use
Hearing impairment Patients with <7 of 12 whispers on Whisper Test	Hearing protocol: portable amplifying devices, earwax disempaction, and special communication techniques, with daily reinforcement of these adaptations
Dehydration Patients with ratio of blood urea nitrogen to creatinine of >17, screened for protocol by geriatric nurse–specialist	Dehydration protocol: early recognition of dehydration and volume repletion (i.e., encouragement of oral intake fluids)

Note. [a]Orientation score consists of first 10 items on the Mini-Mental State Examination (MMSE).
Source. Adapted with permission from Inouye SK, Bogardus ST Jr, Charpentier PA, et al.: "A Multicomponent Intervention to Prevent Delirium in Hospitalized Older Patients." *New England Journal of Medicine* 340:669–676, 1999. Copyright 1999, Massachusetts Medical Society. All rights reserved.

concerns about EPS and QTc lengthening. Pimozide, an antipsychotic with calcium-blocking properties (thus potentially cardiotoxic), may be worth further study. Because calcium plays a crucial role in anoxic depolarization, agents with dopamine and calcium-channel blockade could potentially have a unique therapeutic niche in delirium (Mark et al. 1993). In a recent study, intravenous administration of ondansetron, a 5-HT$_3$ antagonist, produced a dramatic and safe reversal of agitation within 10 minutes in delirious patients (Bayindir et al. 2000). Replication of this new finding in a double-blind, placebo-controlled format with use of a delirium-specific rating scale is warranted.

Cholinergic agents would seem to be a logical treatment option as well, although little research has been done with them. Physostigmine has been successfully used to treat anticholinergic toxicity, including the associated delirium, although its side effects preclude routine use (American Psychiatric Association 1999). Among newer agents, rivastigmine was described as reversing a nonanticholinergic delirium in a single case report (Fischer 2001). On the other hand, tacrine toxicity was reported to precipitate delirium in a patient with Alzheimer's disease (AD; Trzepacz et al. 1996). Hence, further study is needed to explore the potential role of acetylcholinesterase (AChE) inhibitors in the treatment of delirium.

Prevention

An attractive intervention in the management of delirium is prevention (Inouye 1998; Lipowski 1983). Several studies have identified and tracked risk factors with which to develop predictive instruments, also called risk-stratification models (Eden et al. 1998; Francis et al. 1990; Inouye and Charpentier 1996; Inouye et al. 1993; Marcantonio et al. 1994). Four risk factors—vision impairment, severe illness, preexisting cognitive impairment, and dehydration—were used in one predictive model (Inouye et al. 1993). Nine percent of the low-risk patients (i.e., those with none of the four factors) later developed delirium, compared with 23% of those with one or two factors and 83% of those with three or four factors.

Ideally, patients could be quickly screened for delirium in the emergency department (Monette et al. 2001) and also scored with a predictive model. Patients would be eligible for prophylactic interventions if judged to be at high risk for developing delirium. Such screening practices would be much like what is currently done to reduce the risks of other illnesses (e.g., subcutaneous heparin for pulmonary-embolus prophylaxis, benzodiazepines for alcohol-withdrawal prophylaxis). Candidates for preventive interventions would include low-dose antipsychotics, targeted protocols such as those employed in the Elder Life Program (Inouye et al. 1999), supplemental oxygen (Aakerlund and Rosenberg 1994), or close monitoring for and correction of hypoxemia, hypotension, electrolyte imbalance, and anemia (Marcantonio et al. 1994). Such preventive efforts could lessen the substantial morbidity and mortality associated with delirium and reduce associated costs as well.

Finally, as interventions for cerebral ischemia advance, it would seem reasonable to explore their use in delirium as well. Agents such as carnitine can reduce glutamate-induced neuronal death by increasing the affinity of glutamate for metabotropic mGluR5 receptors (Felipo et al. 1998), thus interfering with the neurotoxic effect of NMDA receptor activation. Exogenous phosphocreatine delays ATP depletion during hypoxia and doubles the latency of anoxic depolarization, which is intimately linked to brain damage in hypoxia. Protection against neuronal swelling may improve resilience to hypoxia (Balestrino 1995). Efforts to decrease brain metabolic requirements, as well as levels of glutamate inhibitors, NMDA receptor antagonists, calcium antagonists, and free-radical scavengers, have also been suggested (Kirsch et al. 1989; Kornhuber and Weller 1997).

Summary

Delirium is both a neuropsychiatric syndrome and a disease. Many different precipitants can trigger delirium in susceptible populations. New hypotheses suggest that specific, recurring pathological changes in neuronal metabolism occur in delirium. Clarifying the etiopathogenesis of delirium and then directly applying this knowledge with targeted interventions and preventive strategies are the next steps in improving the care of delirious patients.

Dementia

The dementias are a heterogeneous group of psychiatric disorders characterized by loss of previous levels of cognitive, executive, and memory (anterograde and/or retrograde) function in a state of full alertness. The loss of socioeconomic productivity and burdens to family caregivers are profound. Dementia is most common in the elderly; with the increasing age of the population, the prevalence of dementia is expected to double by 2030 (Doraiswamy et al. 1998).

Dementia directly increases health care expenditures and complicates the management of comorbid medical conditions (Weiner et al. 1998). Patients with dementia have increased rates of institutionalization and mortality (Baldereschi et al. 1999). The average duration from diagnosis to death is 3–10 years (Doraiswamy et al. 1998).

The biopsychosocial management of dementia is an integral part of primary care, neurology, and psychiatry practice. Dementia uniquely challenges the psychiatrist's diagnostic, psychopharmacological, and psychotherapeutic skills. Because of the progressive nature of most dementias, the likelihood of physician involvement in medicolegal matters such as institutionalization and determination of decreased cognitive capacity for decision making is high. Although the typical course of most dementias is progressive cognitive and functional decline until death, physicians are now urged to view the dementias as treatable illnesses. Contemporary advances in psychopharmacology equip the physician with a greater range of medications to maximize function, delay disease progression, and minimize disruption to patients and caregivers. Early identification of cases is now imperative, given that prompt evaluation and diagnosis facilitates early use of cognition-enhancing and neuroprotective therapies and supportive care to the patient and family (Doraiswamy et al. 1998; Haley 1997). Thorough evaluation and management of comorbid systemic and neuropsychiatric illness is essential to foster the best clinical outcomes.

Clinical Features of the Dementias

DSM-IV-TR Classification of Dementias

According to DSM-IV-TR, core features of the dementias include multiple cognitive deficits (anterograde and/or retrograde memory impairment and aphasia, apraxia, agnosia, or disturbance in executive functioning) that cause impairment in role functioning and represent a significant decline (American Psychiatric Association 2000). Dementia subtypes specified in DSM-IV-TR are shown in Table 7–6. Although the dementias share core features, specific dementia syndromes differ in terms of the sequence of presentation of these and additional associated clinical features.

TABLE 7–6. Diagnostic features of the dementias

Features common to all dementias:
Multiple cognitive deficits that do not occur exclusively during the course of delirium, including memory impairment and aphasia, apraxia, agnosia, or disturbed executive functioning that represent a decline from previous level of functioning and impair role functioning

Dementia of the Alzheimer's type, additional features:
Gradual onset and continuing cognitive decline, deficits are not due to other central nervous system, systemic, or substance-induced conditions and not better attributed to another Axis I disorder

Vascular dementia, additional features:
Focal neurological signs and symptoms or laboratory/radiological evidence indicative of cerebrovascular disease etiologically related to deficits

Dementia due to other general medical conditions, additional features:
Clinical evidence that cognitive disturbance is direct physiological consequence of one of the following: HIV, head trauma, Parkinson's disease, Huntington's disease, Pick's disease, Creutzfeldt-Jakob disease, or another general medical condition (includes Lewy body dementia)

Substance-induced persisting dementia, additional features:
Deficits persist beyond usual duration of substance intoxication or withdrawal with clinical evidence that deficits are etiologically related to the persisting effects of substance use

Dementia due to multiple etiologies, additional feature:
Clinical evidence that the disturbance has more than one etiology

Dementia not otherwise specified, additional feature:
Dementia that does not meet criteria for one of the specified types above

Source. Adapted with permission from American Psychiatric Association: *Diagnostic and Statistical Manual of Mental Disorders,* 4th Edition, Text Revision. Washington, DC, American Psychiatric Association, 2000. Copyright 2000 American Psychiatric Association.

Cortical and Subcortical Dementias

A distinction is made between dementias with primarily cortical and those with primarily subcortical pathology (Table 7–7). Whereas all dementias exhibit the same core clinical features, cortical and subcortical dementias often differ in their specific clinical presentation. Cortical dementia is characterized by prominent memory impairment (recall and recognition), language deficits, apraxia, agnosia, and visuospatial deficits (Doody et al. 1998; Meyer et al. 1995; Paulsen et al. 1995b). Subcortical dementia features greater impairment in recall memory, decreased verbal fluency without anomia, bradyphrenia (slowed thinking), depressed mood, affective lability, apathy, and decreased attention/concentration (Doody et al. 1998; Paulsen et al. 1995a, 1995b). Cortical dementias generally lack prominent motor signs, while subcortical dementias typically feature such signs (Geldmacher and Whitehouse 1997). The cortical–subcortical dichotomy is not absolute, however, because aphasia, apraxia, and agnosia (in isolation) have a low sensitivity in distinguishing cortical from subcortical dementia, and several dementia types may express both cortical and subcortical features at some point in the course of illness (Kramer and Duffy 1996). In addition, neuropsychological assessment may more readily identify dementia than discriminate between cortical and subcortical types (Paulsen et al. 1995a).

TABLE 7–7. Cortical and subcortical dementia types

Cortical dementias
    Dementia of the Alzheimer's type
    Frontotemporal dementia, including dementia due to Pick's disease
    Dementia due to Creutzfeldt–Jakob disease
Subcortical dementias
    Dementia due to HIV
    Dementia due to Parkinson's disease
    Dementia due to Huntington's disease
    Dementia due to multiple sclerosis
Dementias with cortical and subcortical features
    Vascular dementia (formerly multi-infarct dementia)[a]
    Vascular dementia (poststroke dementia)[a]
    Lewy body variant of Alzheimer's disease[a]
    Lewy body dementia[a]

Note. [a]Relative amount of cortical and subcortical features is dependent on location of neuropathology.

Cortical Dementias

Dementia of the Alzheimer's type (DAT), the most common dementia, is estimated to affect nearly 2 million white Americans (Hy and Keller 2000). There is an important conceptual and semantic distinction between the DSM-IV-TR diagnoses of DAT and AD (Rabins et al. 1997). DAT is a clinical diagnosis, based on the findings of insidious onset and gradual, steady progression of cognitive deficits. Because symptoms and signs consistent with DAT may be present with *other* types of neuropathology, a clinical diagnosis of AD should only be made after medical evaluation fails to reveal other causes for the dementia symptoms (Rabins et al. 1997). Even so, the clinical diagnosis of AD can only be *definitively* validated by microscopic examination of neural tissue, typically at autopsy, for characteristic AD neuropathology (Rabins et al. 1997). A *clinical* diagnosis of AD (after ruling out other dementia causes) is pathologically validated in 70%–90% of cases (Rabins et al. 1997). These distinctions should be kept in mind by the reader, because many literature references use the terms *Alzheimer's disease* or *Alzheimer's dementia* interchangeably and somewhat presumptively to describe cases that have not yet gone to autopsy. For simplicity, in this chapter the abbreviation DAT is used to refer to the clinical illness that is not yet validated by autopsy, and AD is used for literature addressing neuropathologically validated Alzheimer's disease. Established and proposed risk factors for DAT are shown in Table 7–8 (Evans et al. 2000; Guo et al. 2000; Hall et al. 2000; Helmer et al. 1999; Merchant et al. 1999; Moceri et al. 2000; Ott et al. 1999; Plassman et al. 2000; Whalley et al. 2000; Zubenko et al. 1996, 1999).

TABLE 7–8. Established and proposed risk factors for dementia of the Alzheimer's type

Increased age
Female gender
Head trauma
Small head size
Family history
Low childhood intelligence
Limited education
Childhood rural residence
Large sibships
Smoking
Never having married
Depression
Diabetes mellitus
Increased total cholesterol
Increased platelet membrane fluidity
Apolipoprotein E (APOE) ε4 allele on chromosome 19
Abnormalities on chromosomes 1, 6, 12, 14, and 21
Trisomy 21

Amnesia and other cognitive symptoms may be present early in the disease, although poor insight regarding memory loss is common. Decreased sense of smell with a lack of awareness of the deficit may predict the onset of DAT (Devanand et al. 2000). Decreased visual attention may be a key factor in cognitive impairment (Rizzo et al. 2000). The patient may become spatially disoriented and wander aimlessly. Apraxias for self-care behaviors may be evident. Deficits in memory, concentration, attention, and executive functions eventually render the patient unable to maintain employment or safely operate a motor vehicle.

Mood symptoms that occur before cognitive deficits may represent a prodromal state (Berger et al. 1999). Depressive disorders have been reported in up to 86% of patients with DAT, with a median estimate of 19% (Katz 1998). Depression is more common in mild DAT, whereas psychosis is more common in moderate to severe DAT (Mega et al. 1996; Rabins et al. 1997; Rao and Lyketsos 1998). Apathy is frequently a symptom; apathy, agitation, dysphoria, and aberrant motor behavior all increase with illness progression and increasing cognitive impairment (Kuzis et al. 1999; Mega et al. 1996). Disinhibited social and sexual behavior, assaultiveness, and inappropriate laughter or tearfulness are common. Evening agitation ("sundowning") may be a notably disruptive symptom. Other motor symptoms include motor slowing, EPS, gait disturbances, dysarthria, myoclonus, and seizures (Goldman et al. 1999; Rabins et al. 1997). Parkinsonian symptoms are associated with a more rapid progression of the disease (R.S. Wilson et al. 2000).

Psychosis is present in up to 40% of patients with DAT (Mega et al. 1996; Paulsen et al. 2000). The early appearance of psychosis or EPS correlates with more rapid cognitive decline (Levy et al. 1996; Paulsen et al. 2000). Visual hallucinations are the most common perceptual disturbance (Class et al. 1997). Physical aggression often accompanies hallucinations, while verbal aggression is associated with delusions (Aarsland et al. 1996). The prevalence of delusions in DAT is high as 73%; delusions of persecution, theft, reference, and jealousy are common (Rao and Lyketsos 1998). Depression, behavioral disturbances, and psychosis are often recurrent (Levy et al. 1996).

The neuropathology of AD includes β-amyloid deposits, neuritic plaques, and neurofibrillary tangles (NFTs) (Figure 7–4) (Felician and Sandson 1999; Jellinger 1996). Amyloid precursor protein (APP, coded on chromosome 21) is cleaved by proteases (β and γ secretases), producing insoluble β-amyloid (Felician and Sandson 1999; Haass and De Strooper 1999; Jellinger 1996). APP processing may be partially controlled by cholinergic mechanisms (Small 1998b). Inhibition of β and γ secretases and presenilin proteins 1 and 2 (proteins coded for on chromosomes 1 and 14, respectively, which appear to modulate secretase activity) may decrease cleavage of APP, thereby decreasing production of insoluble β-amyloid (Haass and De Strooper 1999).

β-Amyloid activates macrophages and microglia, producing inflammation that accelerates neuronal damage, although β-amyloid has itself been reported to be toxic to cultured neurons (Breitner 1996; Smits et al. 2000). Oxidative stress appears to increase the rate of neuronal death; this process may be blocked by vitamin E (Felician and Sandson 1999). Increased CSF prostaglandin E2 (PGE2) has been found in AD, supporting the possibility that prostaglandin production may play a significant role in the pathogenesis of AD; this process might be blocked by the use of nonstero idal anti-inflammatory drugs (NSAIDs) (Montine et al. 1999). Amyloid deposition in cerebral vessels is also seen (Cummings et al. 1998a).

Diffuse plaques are β-amyloid depositions without surrounding neuronal degeneration (Felician and Sandson 1999). Neuritic plaques (a core of β-amyloid surrounded by dystrophic neurites) are surrounded by immune-activated microglia and reactive astrocytes (Felician and Sandson 1999; Smits et al. 2000). Neuritic plaque density is increased in several regions of the cortex, hippocampus, entorhinal cortex, amygdala, and cerebral vessels in AD and continues to increase with disease progression (Felician and Sandson 1999; Haroutunian et al. 1998).

NFTs, intraneuronal bundles of phosphorylated tau proteins, are an early pathological change in the hippocampus, amygdala, and entorhinal cortex (Felician and Sandson 1999). Dementia severity is proportional to the density of NFTs (Felician and Sandson 1999; Jellinger 1996). With accumulated neuron damage, presynaptic terminal density is decreased (Cummings et al. 1998a). The pathophysiological events in AD are represented schematically in Figure 7–5 (Felician and Sandson 1999).

CSF markers for AD include decreased β-amyloid and increased tau protein, AD7c–neuronal thread protein, the light subunit of the neurofilament protein (NFL) and nerve growth factor; increased CSF tau may discriminate between AD and depression (Hock et al. 2000; Hulstaert et al. 1999; Kahle et al. 2000; Rosengren et al. 1999). Increased NFL levels have also been reported in frontotemporal dementia and vascular dementia (Rosengren et al. 1999).

The apolipoprotein E (APOE) ε4 allele on chromosome 19 affects the rate of β-amyloid production and the clinical manifestations of AD in a dose-dependent fashion; homozygotes have a higher risk and faster rate of decline than heterozygotes and noncarriers (Caselli et al. 1999; Craft et al. 1998; Felician and Sandson 1999). Adults without dementia who carried the APOE ε4 allele were found to exhibit decreased verbal memory performance and minor hippocampal damage (Bottino and Almeida 1997; Small et al. 1999). Nondemented carriers of the APOE ε4 allele show greater (presumably compensatory) brain activation during memory-activation tasks on functional magnetic resonance imaging (fMRI); these subjects had a subsequent decline in memory 2 years later (Bookheimer et al. 2000). The effect of the APOE ε4 allele on the risk and course of dementia has been found to be absent in patients over age 85 years (Juva et al. 2000). The APOE ε2 allele may confer protection against AD, whereas the APOE ε3 allele appears to not affect AD risk (Rebeck and Hyman 1999).

The hippocampus is an early locus of pathology in AD. There is a correlation between hippocampal neuron and volume loss and an increase in hippocampal NFTs (Bobinski et al. 1996). This suggests that hippocampal atrophy in AD is due to primary neurofibrillary pathology, as hippocampal volume decreases were not correlated with an increased density of amyloid plaques. Volumetric measurements of the hippocampus on magnetic resonance imaging (MRI) predict memory loss in both normal aging and AD (Jack et al. 2000; Petersen et al. 2000). The hippocampus also features granulovacuolar degeneration in AD (Cummings et al. 1998a).

Central cholinergic hypofunction follows neuronal loss in the nucleus basalis of Meynert, medial septum, and diagonal band of Broca (collectively part of the cholinergic basal forebrain), clinically correlating with decreased attention and memory (Felician and Sandson 1999; Small 1998b; Whitehouse 1998). Decreased central AChE activity has been found on positron emission tomography (PET) scanning in AD (Kuhl et al. 1999). With progression of AD, a deficiency in central cholinergic function leads to a relative hyperdopaminergic condition correlating with the emergence of psychotic symptoms (Rao and Lyketsos 1998). The connections between the hippocampus and adjacent temporal lobe structures and those between the basal forebrain and the rest of the cortex suffer disproportionate degeneration in AD (Geula 1998). Reciprocal connections between the hippocampus and entorhinal cortex are notably disrupted by a high concentration of NFTs in AD (Geula 1998).

Other neurotransmitter systems affected in AD include serotonin (neuronal loss and NFTs in the dorsal raphe and central septal nucleus) and norepinephrine (similar changes in the locus coeruleus) (Felician and Sandson 1999). In one study, acute depletion of tryptophan led to an abrupt further decrease in cognitive

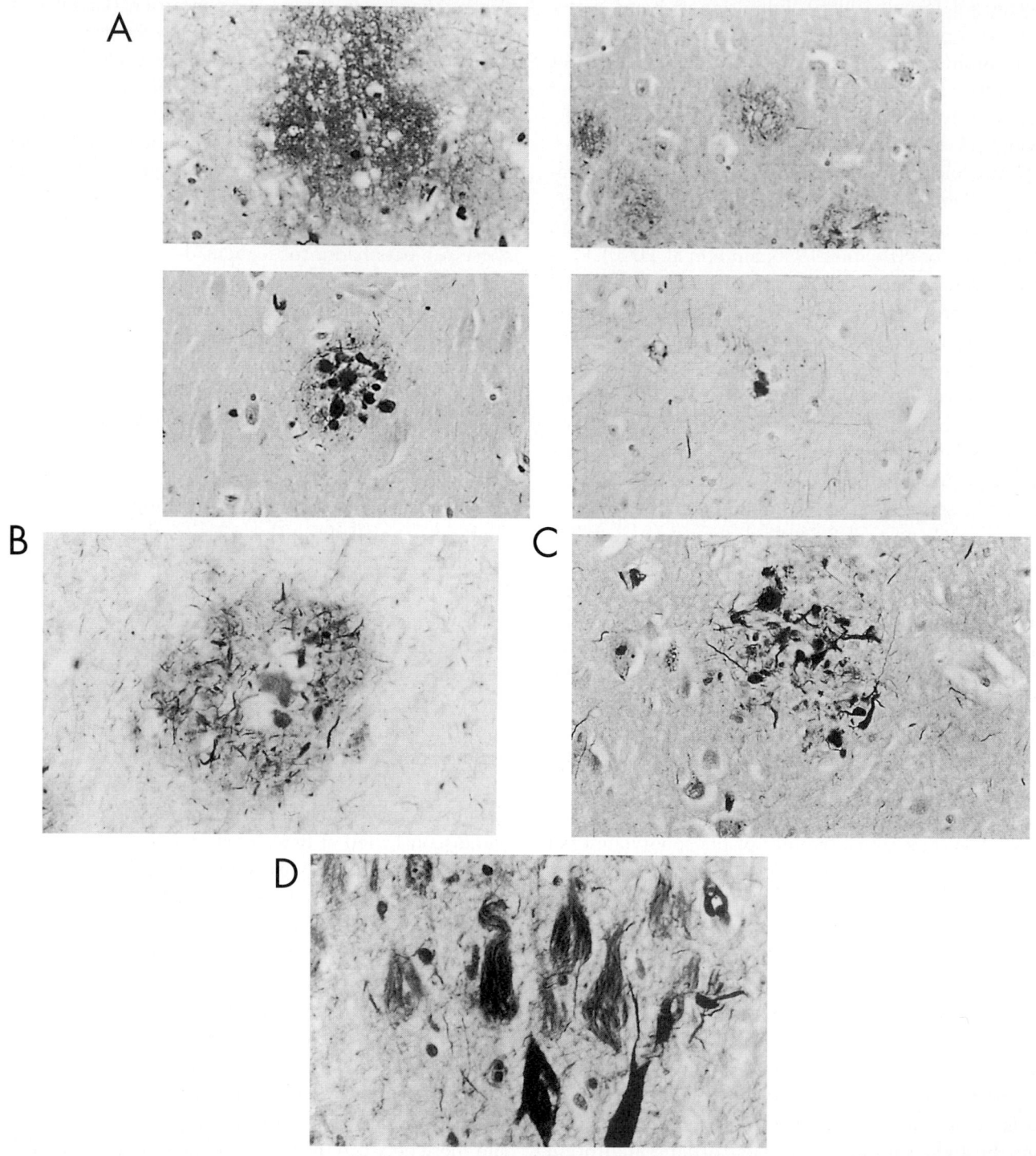

FIGURE 7–4. Alzheimer's disease. Histopathology figures of β-amyloid plaques, neuritic plaques, and neurofibrillary tangles.

A, Four recognized stages of neuritic plaque development revealed by the Bielschowsky silver technique. *Top left:* Diffuse plaque composed mostly of beta-amyloid (Aβ) peptide without increased density of neurites. *Top right:* Primitive plaque consisting of Aβ peptide accumulation and increased numbers of nonenlarged neurites. *Bottom left:* Mature plaque with a densely stained central Aβ amyloid core surrounded by greatly enlarged, dystrophic neurites. *Bottom right:* Burned-out (end-stage) plaque consisting of an isolated mass of Aβ amyloid. **B,** The classic, mature neuritic plaque, about 100 μm in diameter, containing a pale staining amyloid core at its center that is surrounded by a halo of dystrophic (enlarged) neurites. Bielschowsky silver technique. **C,** A mature neuritic plaque with enlarged, dystrophic neurites but no amyloid core. **D,** High magnification view of neurofibrillary tangles, which appear coarse and stain darkly by the Bielschowsky silver technique.

Source. Reprinted with permission from Davis RL, Robertson DM (eds): *Textbook of Neuropathology,* 3rd Edition, Baltimore, MD, Williams & Wilkins, 1997. Copyright 1997 Williams & Wilkins.

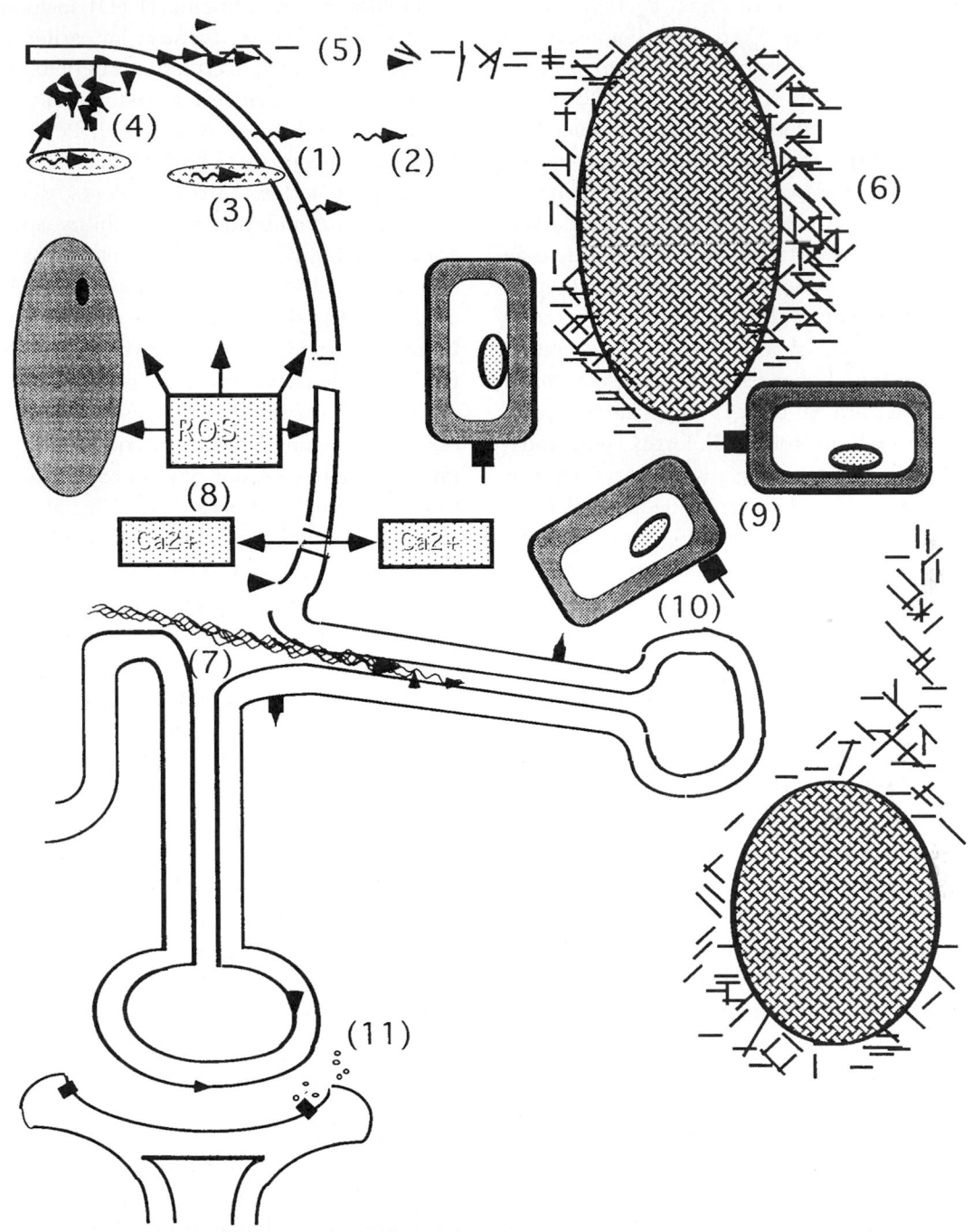

FIGURE 7–5. Schematic view of the main pathologic events in Alzheimer's disease.

Amyloid precursor protein or APP (1) is released into the media after cleavage by α-secretase to form the soluble α APP (2). Conversely, APP may be internalized (3) and cleaved by β- and γ-secretases to form β-amyloid (AB) fragments (4). The protein AB aggregates (5) in fibrillar nonsoluble material to compose the core of the neuritic plaque (6). Neurofibrillary tangles form (7). The neurotoxicity of tau and amyloid results in oxidative stress, with increased intracellular reactive oxygen species (ROS), and disruption of structures involved in ion homeostasis such as ion-motive adenosine triphosphatases (8). Inflammatory responses with reactive glial cells (9) lead to production of cytokines and complement. Possibly playing key roles are membrane receptors such as class A scavenger receptor or receptor for advanced glycation end products (10). Global decrease occurs in neurotransmitters, including acetylcholine (11). *Potential pharmacological targets:* β-amyloid protein metabolism (1–5) and aggregation (6); tau protein metabolism (7); oxidative stress, acting via calcium channels (8); inflammatory response (9, 10); neurotransmitter modulation (11); and neuroprotection.

Source. Reprinted with permission from Felician O, Sandson TA: "The Neurobiology and Pharmacotherapy of Alzheimer's Disease." *Journal of Neuropsychiatry and Clinical Neuroscience* 11:19–31, 1999. Copyright 1999 American Psychiatric Press, Inc.

function in AD, suggesting that cognitive deficits follow decreased cholinergic and serotonergic function (Porter et al. 2000). In another study, AD patients demonstrated lower 5-HT$_{2A}$ receptor binding in the anterior cingulate, prefrontal cortex, and sensorimotor cortex on PET scanning, consistent with serotonergic neuronal degeneration (Meltzer et al. 1999). Depressed AD patients have a more dramatic loss of norepinephrine (Small 1998b).

Later stages of AD affect various areas of the cortex, forming the anatomic substrates for clinical deficits in construction, language, and problem solving (Paulsen et al. 1995b). Delacourte et al. (1999) demonstrated a temporal and spatial sequence of neurofibrillary degeneration in AD as follows: initial changes in the transentorhinal cortex; then the entorhinal cortex, hippocampus, anterior inferior and medium temporal cortex, polymodal association areas, unimodal areas, and primary motor or sensory areas; and, finally, all remaining neocortical areas. Volumes of the hippocampus, parahippocampal gyrus, fusiform gyrus, medial inferior and superior temporal gyrus, and cortex have been shown to be smaller in patients with AD than in control subjects (Bottino and Almeida 1997).

Reduced activation of the bilateral midinferotemporal and posterior inferotemporal regions on fMRI has been reported in normal subjects at high genetic risk for AD (Smith et al. 1999). In the parietal cortex, patients with AD were found to have decreased glucose metabolism both at rest and following stimulation, whereas the relatively more preserved areas of the visual and auditory cortex showed decreased glucose metabolism only under stimulation (Pietrini et al. 1999). Reduced temporoparietal cortex blood volume has also been reported (Harris et al. 1996). Functional impairment of the parietal-occipital cortex has been demonstrated in a study examining visuospatial perception in AD (Tetewsky and Duffy 1999). Abnormal occipital cortex function has been reported in AD on the basis of reduced regional cortical blood flow observed during PET scanning (Mentis et al. 1996).

Higher educational attainment may lead to cognitive reserve that operates to forestall the clinical onset of memory decline in incipient AD (Stern et al. 1999). This was demonstrated by Mori et al. (1997), who showed that greater brain volume and higher intellectual function serve as a "reserve" against dementia, a finding supported in a subsequent study (Coffey et al. 1999). The "cognitive reserve" concept was also supported in a study using PET scanning (Alexander et al. 1997). For equal levels of dementia severity, patients with higher levels of premorbid intellectual function showed greater decreases in cerebral metabolism in the prefrontal, premotor, and left superior parietal association areas.

Frontotemporal dementia (FTD), including dementia due to Pick's disease, features an earlier age at onset, executive dysfunction, attentional deficits, and personality changes with relatively spared memory and visuospatial functions (Duara et al. 1999; Perry and Hodges 2000). Patients may exhibit "childlike" exuberance, "catastrophic" reactions to trivial events, decreased social awareness, disinhibition, distractibility, aphasia, perseveration, carbohydrate cravings, and frontal lobe release signs and may have a poorer response to cholinesterase inhibitors than do patients with AD (Duara et al. 1999; Neary et al. 1998). Consensus criteria for the diagnosis of FTD have been developed that include the following core diagnostic features: insidious onset and gradual progression, early decline in social interpersonal conduct, early impairment in regulation of personal conduct, early emotional blunting, and early loss of insight (Neary et al. 1998). Neuropathological findings in FTD are restricted to the frontal and anterior temporal lobes and include characteristic Pick inclusion bodies, NFTs, and ballooned cells, all containing tau protein (Jellinger 1996; H.R. Morris et al. 1999).

Dementia due to Creutzfeldt–Jakob disease (CJD), also called "spongiform encephalopathy," is a prion-mediated infection. It manifests as a rapidly progressive cortical dementia accompanied by myoclonus and may first appear with psychosis (Dunn et al. 1999; Zerr et al. 2000). In patients with CJD, the EEG shows a characteristic pattern of repetitive sharp waves or slow spikes followed by synchronous triphasic sharp waves (Dunn et al. 1999; Zerr et al. 2000). In classic CJD, the cortex is diffusely affected, with a general loss of cortical substance and a spongy, atrophic appearance (Dunn et al. 1999).

Subcortical Dementias

Dementia due to HIV initially manifests as decreased psychomotor and information-processing speed, verbal memory, learning efficiency, and fine motor function with later cortical symptoms of decreased executive function, aphasia, apraxia, and agnosia (Maldonado et al. 2000). In advanced stages, ataxia, spasticity, increased muscle tone, and incontinence may develop (Maldonado et al. 2000). Dementia has been reported in up to 30% of HIV-positive patients, may present early in the course of illness, increases suicide risk, and may compromise compliance with antiviral regimens (Cohen and Jacobson 2000; Maldonado et al. 2000). Recent estimates of the incidence of dementia due to HIV are somewhat lower, possibly due to the neuroprotective effects of early, aggressive antiviral treatment (d'Arminio Monforte et al.

2000; Goodkin et al. 2001). Dementia due to HIV results from neurotoxicity mediated by HIV-infected macrophages (which serve as the site for viral replication) (McDaniel et al. 2000; Smits et al. 2000). Intravenous drug abuse and prominent psychomotor slowing are associated with greater macrophage activation and rapid decline (Bouwman et al. 1998).

Dementia due to Parkinson's disease (PD) is seen in as many as 60% of patients with PD and features brady-phrenia, apathy, poor retrieval memory, decreased verbal fluency, and attention deficits (Levy and Cummings 2000; Marsh 2000). Although dementia due to PD is classified as a primarily subcortical dementia, cortical symptoms of executive dysfunction, visuospatial impairment, agnosia, anomia, aphasia, and apraxia may be seen in patients with PD dementia who develop cortical Lewy bodies (Hurtig et al. 2000; Levy and Cummings 2000; Marsh 2000). Increased age, greater severity of neurological symptoms, and the APOE ε2 allele have been associated with an increased risk of dementia in patients with PD (Harhangi et al. 2000; Hughes et al. 2000). Cognition may improve with treatment for the common comorbid mood disorders (Levy and Cummings 2000). Psychosis can be induced by antiparkisonian treatment of the motor symptoms of PD (Rabins et al. 1997). In one study, the siblings of PD patients with dementia were shown to have a dramatically elevated risk of AD, suggesting a genetic aggregation of the two conditions (Marder et al. 1999). Dementia due to PD features deposition of α-synuclein or tau protein in the substantia nigra and commonly involves Lewy bodies in the substantia nigra, cortex, and subcortex, with resulting deficits in dopaminergic, noradrenergic, cholinergic, and serotonergic neurotransmission (Levy and Cummings 2000; Marsh 2000; H.R. Morris et al. 1999).

Dementia due to Huntington's disease (HD) features impairments in retrieval memory, cognitive speed, concentration, verbal learning, and cognitive flexibility (Ranen 2000). With progression, more global impairment in memory, visuospatial function, and executive function may follow (Ranen 2000). These patients have a high risk for personality change, irritability, aggressive behavior, and suicide (Ranen 2000; Rosenblatt and Leroi 2000). Dementia due to HD carries a high risk for comorbid depression and adverse anticholinergic side effects of tricyclic antidepressants (TCAs) (Rosenblatt and Leroi 2000). HD dementia results from cell loss in primary sensory and association areas, entorhinal cortex, caudate nucleus, and putamen (Jellinger 1996; Ranen 2000).

Dementia due to multiple sclerosis is seen in as many as 65% of multiple sclerosis patients (Schwid et al. 2000). Clinical features include deficits in memory,

attention, information-processing speed, learning, and executive functions; language and verbal intelligence are relatively spared (Schwid et al. 2000). Cognitive impairment may present early in the course of multiple sclerosis, and progression is roughly proportional to the number of central nervous system (CNS) demyelinating lesions (Schwid et al. 2000).

Dementias with Cortical and Subcortical Features

Vascular dementia (VaD) broadly includes dementias resulting from vascular pathology that have as a final common pathway the loss of functional cortex. Because VaD exists on a continuum extending from the essentially subcortical pathology formerly described as "multi-infarct dementia" to the primarily cortical pathology in "poststroke dementia" (i.e., dementia following a single stroke), it is problematic to attempt to fit all vascular dementias (thus inclusively defined) into the "cortical versus subcortical" dichotomy. This already problematic distinction between multi- and single-infarct dementias is further obscured by the inclusion of dementia following a single stroke within the classification of VaD in much clinical literature (Kaye 1998). In other literature, the term *vascular dementia* generally refers to dementia following multiple infarcts. Even DSM-IV is somewhat equivocal on this issue; the heading of "Vascular Dementia (Formerly Multi-Infarct Dementia)" would implicitly exclude dementia following a single stroke, yet the detailed diagnostic criteria for VaD in DSM-IV would include it (American Psychiatric Association 1994). A reasonable (albeit cumbersome) solution would be for clinicians to describe all dementias due to vascular pathology as "vascular dementia," with further specification as "multi-infarct" or "poststroke" as appropriate to the clinical situation, remaining mindful of the semantic imprecision in the clinical literature.

Additionally, the boundary between AD and the broad category of VaD is itself quite permeable. Cerebral infarcts in established AD are associated with greater overall severity of dementia and poorer neuropsychological testing performance (Heyman et al. 1998). The distinction between AD and VaD is further complicated by the findings of Zhu et al. (2000) that mild dementia and cognitive impairment are themselves associated with an increased risk of stroke in subjects over age 75 years.

Multi-infarct VaD is characterized by abrupt onset, decreased executive functioning, gait disturbance, affective lability, and parkinsonian symptoms (S.H. Choi et al. 2000; Patterson et al. 1999). Risk factors include increased age, hypertension, diabetes mellitus, atherosclerotic heart disease, hypertriglyceridemia, and hyperlipidemia (Curb et al. 1999; G.W. Ross et al. 1999). Because the cognitive deficits follow a series of discrete lesions, progression is "stepwise" with relative stability of cognitive status between vascular insults, as opposed to the gradual progression of deficits seen in AD. The progression of multi-infarct VaD may be affected by risk factor modification and antiplatelet therapy (Rabins et al. 1997). Lesions are generally located in the subcortical nuclei, frontal lobe white matter, thalamus, and internal capsule and are associated with a characteristic appearance on MRI of periventricular hyperintensities on the T2 images (Figure 7–6) (S.H. Choi et al. 2000; Doody et al. 1998). However, periventricular hyperintensities are also seen in normal aging and in other types of dementia and thus, in isolation, represent a nonspecific finding (Smith et al. 2000). Diffusion-weighted MRI has been shown to be a more sensitive method of evaluating small-vessel ischemic disease in VaD (S.H. Choi et al. 2000).

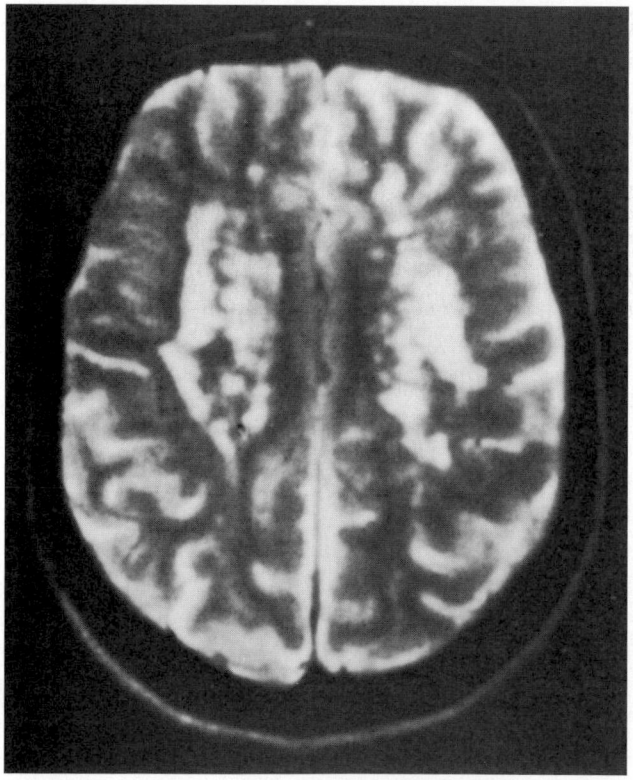

FIGURE 7–6. T2 magnetic resonance image (MRI) of vascular dementia, multi-infarct type in a patient with diabetes mellitus and hypertension.

The bilateral, symmetrical pattern of white matter lesions is characteristic of small vessel arterial disease. Enlarged sulci are consistent with associated perenchymal loss.

Source. Reprinted with permission from Yock DH: *Imaging of CNS Disease: A CT and MRI Teaching File.* St. Louis, MO, Mosby–Year Book, Inc., 1991.

Poststroke VaD—dementia occurring as the acute or subacute consequence of a single stroke—may be difficult to clearly distinguish from multi-infarct VaD that follows a series of vascular events. Poststroke dementia is associated with apraxia, neglect, hemianopsia, facial paralysis, and extremity weakness (de Koning et al. 1998). Poststroke VaD was found to independently increase the risk of stroke recurrence (Moroney et al. 1997). Poststroke dementia was found in 24% of a series of 300 stroke patients (de Koning et al. 1998). Left-hemisphere lesions were associated with a decreased incidence of poststroke dementia, whereas hemorrhagic stroke carried an increased risk of subsequent dementia. Of the dementias seen in this study, 25% were AD plus VaD (inclusively defined) and the remaining 75% were probable VaD. Another study found poststroke dementia in 26% of a series of 453 patients (Desmond et al. 2000). Of these poststroke dementias, 57% were VaD (broadly defined) and 38% were AD. Major dominant-hemisphere stroke, left-hemisphere location, internal carotid artery distribution, diabetes mellitus, prior cerebrovascular accident (CVA), older age, less education, and nonwhite race were found to be risk factors for poststroke dementia (Desmond et al. 2000). Major depression is common with poststroke dementia, with anterior left-hemisphere stroke posing the highest risk (Robinson 1998). The risk for poststroke dementia associated with major depression is highest in the first year (Robinson 1998). Deficits in orientation, language, visuoconstruction, and executive functions are common but may improve with treatment of the poststroke depression (Robinson 1998).

Lewy body variant (LBV) of AD and Lewy body dementia (LBD) have a significant degree of overlap and may be difficult to differentiate clinically (Hansen et al. 1990). The more general term *dementia with Lewy bodies* is often used to denote the continuum of LBV, LBD, and dementia due to PD (Gomez-Isla et al. 1999; Jellinger 1996). The heterogeneity of symptoms and classification has made diagnostic specificity problematic (Lopez et al. 1999).

Clinically, LBV and LBD share the common features of fluctuation of mental status, visual hallucinations, delusions, depression, and EPS (Hansen et al. 1990; Heyman et al. 1999; Lopez et al. 2000a; Weiner et al. 1996). Visual hallucinations occur even with mild levels of cognitive impairment (Ballard et al. 2001). In comparison with AD, LBV exhibits greater deficits in attention, verbal fluency, and visuospatial functioning and increased parkinsonian symptoms (Hansen et al. 1990; Heyman et al. 1999; Lopez et al. 2000a; McKeith et al. 2000; Weiner et al. 1996). LBV has also been associated with more rapid cognitive decline, earlier institutionalization, and shorter survival time (Lopez et al. 2000a; Olichney et al. 1998). The clinical distinction between LBV and AD may be more apparent in the moderate/severe stages of dementia (Lopez et al. 2000b). LBD also features impaired executive functioning, disinhibited social behavior, syncope, and increased sensitivity to antipsychotic agents (manifested by drowsiness, further cognitive decline, and neuroleptic malignant syndrome) (Litvan and McKee 1999; McKeith et al. 2000). Progression is usually more rapid in LBD than in AD, although psychotic symptoms in LBV and LBD may be improved by treatment with cholinesterase inhibitors (Ballard et al. 2001; Levy and Cummings 2000).

A similar degree of overlap is seen in the neuropathology of LBV and LBD. Pathologically, LBV is characterized by the presence of Lewy bodies (intraneuronal eosinophilic inclusion bodies) in subcortical and cortical structures in addition to AD neuropathology (Figure 7–7) (Gomez-Isla et al. 1999; Hansen et al. 1990; Rabins et al. 1997). LBV has a lower density of NFTs in the neocortex than does AD (Heyman et al. 1999). LBV exhibits pallor of the substantia nigra; greater neuronal cell loss in the locus coeruleus, substantia nigra, and substantia innominata; and medial temporal lobe spongiform vacuolization (Hansen et al. 1990). LBD also features subcortical and cortical Lewy bodies, with a relative absence of NFTs and other AD neuropathology (Gomez-Tortosa et al. 1999; Litvan and McKee 1999). Relatively less atrophy of temporal lobe structures is seen in LBD than in AD or VaD (Barber et al. 2000; McKeith et al. 2000). Occipital lobe metabolic rates in LBD have been found to be lower than those in AD, a finding that correlates with the prominence of visual hallucinations in LBD (Ishii et al. 1998). That CSF tau protein levels are normal in LBD further distinguishes it from AD (Kanemaru et al. 2000). Both LBV and LBD are characterized by a marked loss of choline acetyltransferase (ChAT) activity, independent of AD pathology, and show more ChAT activity loss than does pure AD (Tiraboschi et al. 2000).

Epidemiology

Dementia Types

The risk of dementia increases exponentially with age, from 1% under age 65 years to 25%–50% over age 85 (Rabins et al. 1997; Jorm and Jolley 1998). The annual risk of dementia is 0.5% between ages 60 and 69 years, 1% between 70 and 74 years, 2% between 75 and 79 years, 3% between 80 and 84 years, and 8% thereafter (Rabins et al. 1997). The prevalence of dementia was found to be 3.9% for patients over the age of 60 in a general hospital population (Lyketsos et al. 2000a). The risk for patients between ages 60 and 64 years was 2.6%; this risk increased to 8.9% for those over 85 years. Dementia was associated with a 40% increase in inpatient LOS. Dementia was found in 68% of African American nursing home residents (Class et al. 1996). The subtypes seen were DAT (48%), VaD (9%), substance-induced dementia (3%), PD (1%), and other types (7%). Reported estimates of the relative frequency of the different dementia types in study populations of dementia patients include 50%–90% DAT, 8%–20% VaD, and 7%–26% LBD, with other subtypes less common (Lyketsos et al. 2000b; Parnetti 2000; Small 1998a). There is an estimated overlap of 20% between DAT and VaD, referred to as mixed dementia (Small 1998a). Reversible dementias are estimated to account for 1%–10% of dementias; examples of potentially reversible dementias are shown in Table 7–9 (Gliatto and Caroff 2001; Rabins et al. 1997; Small 1998a; Tager and Fallon 2001).

Comorbidity and Differential Diagnosis

The patient with cognitive impairment may have psychiatric illnesses other than or in addition to dementia. Clinical history and examination need to be focused to consider these other diagnostic possibilities. The psychiatric differential diagnosis of dementia is shown in Table 7–10.

Delirium

Dementia increases the risk for delirium from numerous systemic conditions (e.g., urinary tract infections, pneumonia, dermatological infections, dehydration, constipation), both after surgery and as a side effect of medications, particularly anticholinergic medication (Rabins et al. 1997). Delirium in the elderly patient with dementia may present with decreased psychomotor activity (Daniel 2000). Episodes of delirium may be more prolonged in dementia. Given that aberrant motor behaviors, such as repetitive pacing, are uncommon in early dementia, their presence in a patient with mild dementia is suggestive of a superimposed delirium (Mega et al. 1996). Digit span and memory registration, although preserved until late in the course of dementia, may be initially impaired in delirium (Small 1998a). Hallucinations are more common in delirium than in dementia. EEG may be helpful in differentiating delirium from dementia, because an abnormal EEG is more suggestive of delirium. Onset of symptoms following a medical illness, a recent change in medication, or some other perturbation is strongly suggestive of delirium.

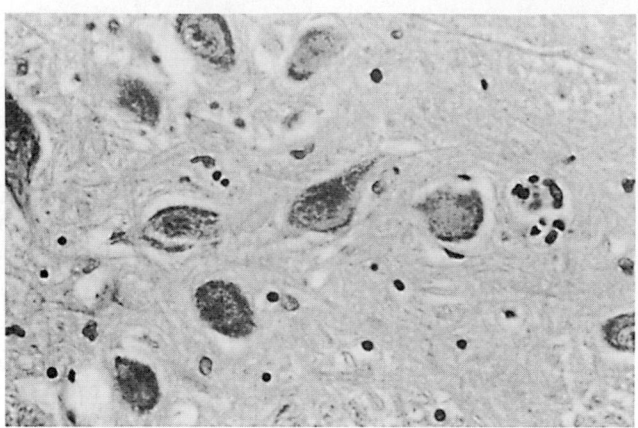 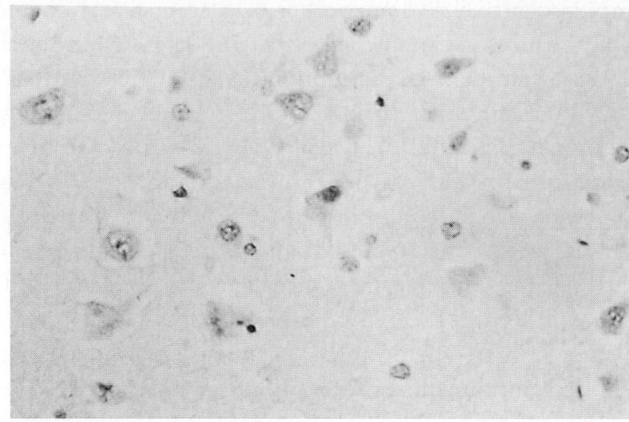

FIGURE 7–7. Histopathology figures, Lewy body variant of Alzheimer's disease.

In this demented patient, the number of plaques and tangles in the neocortex were borderline for the diagnosis of Alzheimer's disease. *Left*, The substantia nigra showed a moderate degree of nerve cell loss and small numbers of Lewy bodies. *Right*, Ubiquitin immunohistochemistry revealed multiple Lewy bodies in nerve cells of the cingulate gyrus.

Source. Reprinted with permission from Davis RL, Robertson DM (eds): *Textbook of Neuropathology*, 3rd Edition. Baltimore, MD, Williams & Wilkins, 1997. Copyright 1997 Williams & Wilkins.

TABLE 7–9. Potentially reversible etiologies of dementia

Structural central nervous system factors
   Vascular dementia
   Head trauma
   Subdural hematoma
   Normal-pressure hydrocephalus
   Multiple sclerosis
Psychiatric illness
   Major depression
   Substance dependence
Systemic/metabolic factors
   Hypothyroidism
   Hypercalcemia
   Hypoglycemia
   Thiamine, niacin, B_{12} deficiency
   Renal failure
   Hepatic failure
   Medications
Infectious diseases
   HIV
   Central nervous system infection

TABLE 7–10. Psychiatric differential diagnosis of dementia

Delirium
Mood disorders
Amnestic disorders
Substance use disorders
Psychotic disorders
Mental retardation

Mood Disorders

Depressed patients may appear to have cognitive impairment, a phenomenon described as "pseudodementia." Such patients will often have a history of mood disorders (Raskind 1998). Although pharmacological treatment of the mood disorder can improve cognitive function, the improvement may be incomplete and/or temporary (Butters et al. 2000; Raskind 1998). Depressed dementia patients may communicate their mood state indirectly, with agitation and insomnia, rather than through specific mood complaints (Small 1998a). Depressed dementia patients may underreport the severity of their depressive symptoms relative to the observations of caregivers. Depressive disorders coexisting with dementia can increase the use of inpatient psychiatric inpatient resources beyond that for either condition alone (Kales et al. 1999). Patients with depression plus dementia have a high rate of depression in first-degree relatives, independent of any family risk for dementia (Strauss and Ogrocki 1996).

Amnestic Disorders

Amnestic disorders can be profoundly impairing, but the diagnosis of dementia requires impairment in other spheres of mental activity beyond loss of memory function. Conditions characterized by "pure" amnesia (e.g., carbon monoxide poisoning, Wernicke's encephalopathy, transient global amnesia) should be considered.

Substance Abuse/Dependence

Substance use disorders can lead to dementia, especially following a long history of alcohol dependence. Active management of substance abuse and dependence should be accomplished in the context of other psychiatric interventions for substance-dependent dementia patients.

Psychotic Disorders and Mental Retardation

Schizophrenia will very rarely be first diagnosed in an elderly patient and will feature prominent psychotic symptoms at the onset of illness, not after several years of cognitive losses. Mental retardation, while increasing the risk for dementia (e.g., trisomy 21), represents a stable state of decreased cognitive function.

Clinical Evaluation

History

A clinical history should first be obtained from the patient directly, initially without the presence of other family members (Doraiswamy et al. 1998). History taking should address recent cognitive function; examples include function at work, at home, while driving, and while performing other high-risk activities (Patterson et al. 1999). A complaint of memory loss may be predictive of a later diagnosis of DAT, even without demonstrable memory deficits on initial clinical examination (Geerlings et al. 1999). A personal and family history of psychiatric illness should be obtained, specifically to include dementia and neurological illness with high risk for dementia. Because the patient is most reliable in the early stages of illness, the physician should then separately interview family members and synthesize the separate histories obtained to derive the most balanced view of the patient's functioning (Cummings and Masterman 1998).

The medical history should address all chronic illnesses, with particular attention to systemic conditions that increase risk for DAT, VaD, and other dementia types. Specific examples of such chronic illnesses include hypertension, diabetes mellitus, hyperlipidemia, PD, multiple sclerosis, and prior CVA (Geldmacher and Whitehouse 1997). Recent illnesses that may put the patient at risk for delirium also need to be explored. The medication history should address both psychotropic and nonpsychotropic medications taken before the onset of the cognitive and behavioral symptoms (Doraiswamy et al. 1998). The use of nonprescription medications (especially antihistamines and sedatives) and herbal preparations also needs to be explored.

The social history should address the patient's living circumstances, presence of supportive family members and/or of other significant persons living nearby, financial and insurance resources, participation in social activities, and personal relationships. Collateral history obtained from family members should focus on concerns about the patient's cognitive function and overt behavior. Problematic symptoms such as paranoia, agitation, physical violence, and inattentive and dangerous operation of dangerous machinery need to be addressed, as well as access to weapons and any threats made to self or others. Any complaint of neglect or abuse, or any physical examination findings suggestive of inappropriate care, should be reported promptly to the agency responsible for performing onsite evaluation of neglect or abuse of adults. Aggressive and/or delusional patients may be at greatest risk of such maltreatment (Cummings and Masterman 1999). Dementia patients are also at increased risk for syncope and loss of consciousness, which can result in head trauma, hip fracture, or other injuries. Any report of falls in dementia patients requires a full evaluation for injuries.

Mental Status Examination

Formal assessment of cognitive function must be added to routine evaluation of mood and affect, level of consciousness, psychomotor activity, speech production, thought content, and thought processes. It is recommended that the clinician use a cognitive assessment instrument such as the MMSE (see Figure 7–1). A score of 24 or less on the MMSE, when correlated with clinical findings, is highly suggestive of dementia, but education and other patient-specific variables must be taken into close account (Patterson et al. 1999). A cutoff score of 22 is advised in the elderly nursing home population; the MMSE may overestimate dementia in patients with less education, age older than 85, or a history of depression (Dufouil et al. 2000; Grigoletto et al. 1999; Nadler et al. 1995). Conversely, patients with high levels of education and other evidence of premorbid high intellectual function may score in the "unimpaired" range on the MMSE despite decreased functional status (Doraiswamy et al. 1998; Small 1998a). Serial administrations of the MMSE can quantify the progress or stability of dementia; a typical decline in MMSE scores in DAT is 2–4 points per year (Folstein et al. 1975; Rabins et al. 1997). An alternative dementia rating scale is the Alzheimer's Disease Assessment Scale (ADAS; Mohs and Cohen 1988; Rosen et al. 1984), a 21-item scale that scores both cognitive and noncognitive items to derive the degree of impairment. Depression rating scales (e.g., the Hamilton Rating Scale for Depression [Hamilton 1960], the Geriatric Depression Scale [Yesavage et al. 1983]) are recommended to assist in distinguishing dementia from depression and in monitoring response to antidepressants (Katz

1998). Suicide risk increases in the elderly population, and clinical assessment of other suicide risk factors (e.g., substance abuse, isolation, past suicidal behavior, access to weapons) needs to be integrated into the physician's clinical examination.

Physical Examination

Assessment of vision and hearing should not be overlooked (Doraiswamy et al. 1998). Relative sensory deprivation due to uncorrected vision and/or hearing deficits can cause spuriously poor performance on formal cognitive testing. Loss of visual acuity and severe cognitive impairment in patients with DAT can increase visual hallucinations (Chapman et al. 1999). Neurological examination should include assessment of gait, frontal lobe release signs, movement disorders, sensory function, and focal neurological deficits (Doraiswamy et al. 1998; Grossberg and Lake 1998). Physical examination should address signs of metabolic illnesses, marginal hygiene, poor nutritional status, weight loss, and dehydration.

Laboratory Tests

Laboratory tests may be modified on a case-by-case basis. Tests to consider are shown in Table 7–11 (Doraiswamy et al. 1998; Grossberg and Lake 1998; Patterson et al. 1999; Rabins et al. 1997). Serum drug levels of medications associated with altered mental status (e.g., TCAs, anticonvulsants, digitalis, antiarrhythmics) should be obtained if clinically indicated. A 12-lead ECG should be considered, especially if there is a history of cardiac and/ or vascular disease.

TABLE 7–11. Laboratory tests for dementia workup

Electrolytes, blood urea nitrogen, creatinine, calcium
Liver-associated enzymes
Glucose
Complete blood count
Thyroid profile with thyroid-stimulating hormone assay
Erythrocyte sedimentation rate, antinuclear antibody panel
Prothrombin time/partial thromboblastin time
B_{12} and folate
Syphilis serology
Urinalysis and urine toxicology
Pulse oximetry
Medication levels (e.g., tricyclic antidepressants, anticonvulsants, digitalis, antiarrhythmics)

When CJD is suspected, CSF samples should be obtained for testing for the neuronal proteins 14-3-3 and γ-enolase (Dunn et al. 1999; Zerr et al. 2000). CJD is characterized by a classic EEG appearance of repetitive sharp waves or slow spikes followed by synchronous triphasic sharp waves, although the six different phenotypes of this illness may present with different combinations of EEG findings (Dunn et al. 1999; Zerr et al. 2000). Lumbar puncture should also be considered if there is a clinical suspicion of normal-pressure hydrocephalus, metastatic carcinoma, or unusually early onset and/or rapid progression of deficits (Small 1998a). Other laboratory tests to consider in specific cases include serum ammonia, heavy metals, and cortisol; carotid Doppler studies; chest X ray; and mammography (Patterson et al. 1999; Rabins et al. 1997).

Neuroimaging

Although there may be a relatively low yield, it is recommended that computed tomography (CT) or MRI be considered to evaluate dementia (Doraiswamy et al. 1998; Small and Leiter 1998). One consensus panel recommends CT in the presence of age younger than 60 years, rapid cognitive decline, less than a 2-year duration of illness, head trauma and associated neurological symptoms, history of cancer, history of bleeding disorder and/ or anticoagulant therapy, incontinence, gait disturbance, atypical cognitive symptoms, or localizing neurological signs (Patterson et al. 1999). The American College of Radiology recommends MRI more highly than CT in cases of suspected dementia (American College of Radiology 1996). Contrast-enhanced CT and gadolinium-enhanced MRI are recommended less highly. In cases of suspected DAT, hippocampal atrophy may serve as a sensitive early marker for cognitive decline (Figure 7–8) (Bottino and Almeida 1997; Jack et al. 2000; Petersen et al. 2000; Scheltens 1999). When more quantitative techniques for assessing hippocampal size and appearance become more widely available, they are likely to increase specificity (Small 1998a).

Cortical atrophy and ventriculomegaly do not by themselves confirm dementia and, in isolation, are not specific findings (Doraiswamy et al. 1998; Small 1998a). Progressive cerebral atrophy and ventriculomegaly are more likely in DAT than in VaD and have been reported to correlate with declines in performance on the MMSE (Fox et al. 1999; Meyer et al. 1995; Patterson et al. 1999). If initial neuroimaging reveals hippocampal and/ or cortical atrophy that correlates with the clinical presentation and gradual course of DAT, then serial neuroimaging to follow progress is not routinely necessary. Periventricular hyperintensities on MRI may be seen in DAT as well as in VaD; their significance in DAT is unclear, as they may not correlate independently with

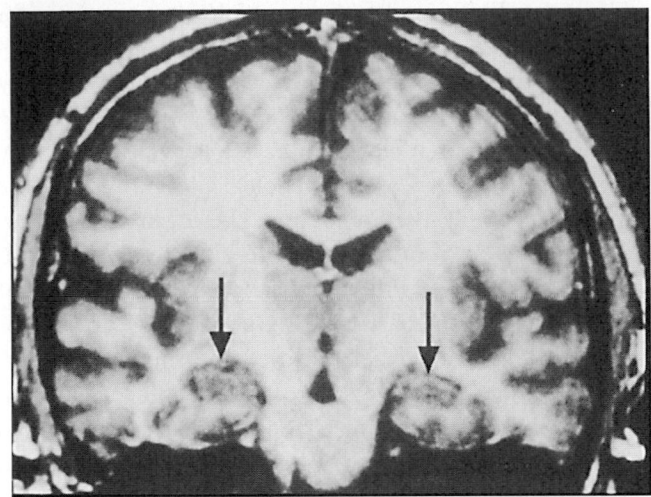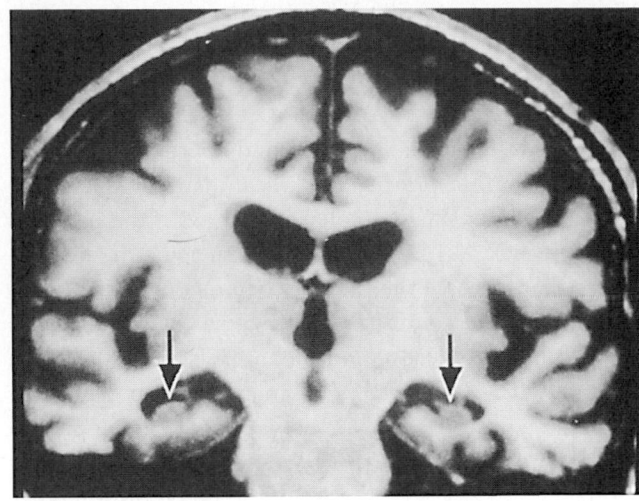

FIGURE 7–8. Magnetic resonance image (MRI) of hippocampal volume (*arrows*) in a normal subject (*left*) and a patient with Alzheimer's disease and hippocampal atrophy (*right*).

Source. Reprinted with permission from Foster NL, Minoshima S, Kuhl DE: "Brain Imaging in Alzheimer Disease," in *Alzheimer Disease*, 2nd Edition. Edited by Terry RD, Katzman R, Bick KL, et al. Philadelphia, PA, Lippincott Williams & Wilkins, 1999, p. 69, Figures 2A & 2B. Copyright 1999, Lippincott Williams & Wilkins.

cognitive changes (Doody et al. 1998; Smith et al. 2000). Overreliance on MRI findings may lead to an overdiagnosis of VaD and a relative underdiagnosis of DAT (Rabins 1998). Decreased white matter volume has been associated with DAT (Smith et al. 2000). If initial imaging shows white matter lesions typical of VaD that correlate with clinical findings, a follow-up CT or MRI could be considered if the patient later presents with an abrupt decrease in mental status suggestive of delirium and/or a new CVA. Diffusion-weighted MRI, which has been shown to be more sensitive than CT in imaging the ischemic small-vessel disease in VaD, may be used to monitor progression of these patients (S.H. Choi et al. 2000). Functional neuroimaging (e.g., single photon emission computed tomography [SPECT], PET scanning), although not currently widely available, holds promise in the evaluation of the cortical pathology of dementia, particularly when combined with genetic assessment of patients at risk for clinical dementia (Small 1998a). Functional neuroimaging techniques may reveal a specific pattern of parietal and temporal deficits in DAT that could lead the physician to consider earlier treatment with antidementia pharmacotherapy (Small and Leiter 1998).

Multidisciplinary Referrals

Neuropsychological consultation may be helpful in early dementia cases when cognitive deficits are subtle on clinical examination (Tschanz et al. 2000). Recall, delayed recall, verbal fluency, and visuomotor ability deficits are predictive of dementia (Bottino and Almeida 1997). Neuropsychological assessment may be especially useful in patients in whom the capacity for autonomy (e.g., driving, medical informed consent) appears equivocal on interview alone. Executive dysfunction (especially when confirmed by neuropsychological assessment) may correlate significantly with loss of capacity for decision making (Marson et al. 1999).

Social work intervention may be of substantial benefit. Family therapy can assist the patient and family to adjust to the reduced social expectations and impairments of the patient. Social workers may facilitate patient and family access to supportive social services to assist the patient in staying with his or her family, to secure institutional placement, and to explore funding sources for institutional care.

Psychiatric nurses may be invaluable in the area of home visitation and outreach. A system of care in which the psychiatric nurse calls on the patient at home may be established for patients with dementia. The psychiatric nurse assesses mental status, helps with the management of psychotropic medications, and evaluates the residence for safe living circumstances, which may help to avoid unneeded hospitalization and to forestall nursing home placement.

Occupational, recreational, and physical therapy may be very helpful with in vivo assessment of the patient's ability to function safely and independently in various physical and social environments, as part of a comprehensive patient safety evaluation (Grossberg and Lake 1998). Occupational therapists may assist in assessment of the patient's ability to drive safely.

Management

Clinical Management

Attention to comorbid systemic and neuropsychiatric illnesses is the first priority in clinical management of the dementia patient. Close collaboration with the patient's other physician(s) is essential for managing medical illnesses that increase the risk for cognitive deficits. Examples include the neurologist in the case of a patient with PD or multiple sclerosis and the internist in the case of a patient with VaD or HIV. Management of pain may decrease agitated behavior in patients with dementia (Geda and Rummans 1999). Psychopharmacological approaches to anxiety, psychotic, and mood disorders are discussed in detail below (see "Pharmacotherapy" later in this section). Substance abuse interventions consisting of medical detoxification, participation in Alcoholics Anonymous or other 12-Step recovery programs, judicious use of agonist therapies, and close attention to comorbid substance-induced mood and anxiety disorders is necessary in the dementia patient with comorbid substance abuse or dependence.

Early, frank discussion of diagnosis, prognosis, and management, with clinical follow-ups scheduled at least every 3 months, are advised. Every visit should include an evaluation of whether the patient can still safely live at home. More-frequent visits should be scheduled to monitor response and side effects when psychotropic medications are prescribed. Supportive psychotherapy may assist the patient in dealing with grief and loss. Admission to a psychiatry inpatient unit skilled in dealing with dementia patients may be needed for severely regressed, suicidal, violent, or psychotic patients, especially if complex psychopharmacological regimens and/or ECT are considered (Rabins et al. 1997).

Psychoeducation can be very valuable, especially for family caregivers (Grossberg and Lake 1998). *The 36-Hour Day: A Family Guide to Caring for Persons with Alzheimer's Disease, Related Dementing Illnesses, and Memory Loss in Later Life* (Mace and Rabins 1981) is often helpful to both patients and families. Support and advocacy groups are available through the Alzheimer's Association (1-800-621-0379; www.alz.org) (Rabins et al. 1997). The Alzheimer's Association can facilitate patient enrollment in the Safe Return Program, a nationwide program that assists in the identification and return of dementia patients who wander. The patient should always carry and/or wear identification (e.g., a Medic-Alert bracelet) and can be registered with the local police department. Physicians should inform caregivers of the increased risk of depression in primary caregivers of dementia patients and facilitate respite opportunities for caregivers (Grossberg and Lake 1998; Haley 1997).

Environmental and behavioral management may include provision of adequate lighting, music, access to pets, and appropriate levels of psychological stimulation. Because of the decreased psychological flexibility of the dementia patient, the home should be organized to allow for simplicity of routines, with prominent display of calendars, schedules, and the photographs and names of people close to the patient. Events that trigger problematic behaviors should be identified and minimized (Parnetti 2000). For safety, childproofing devices may be considered. Vehicle keys, power tools, and sharp household objects should be secured. Weapons should be removed from the home or at least be secured in a locked cabinet. Bright-light therapy may improve the sleep patterns of agitated elderly dementia patients with sleep–wake cycle disturbances (Lyketsos et al. 1999).

Institutional placement is often a painful decision for the family, patient, and physician. To many patients, the loss of the home environment, even when clearly necessary to preserve safety, is a devastating experience that usually leads to further confusion, behavioral regression, and increased risk of depression. The lack of or loss of a primary caregiver may predict earlier institutionalization (Patterson et al. 1999). The physician should make every reasonable effort to maintain the patient in his or her home environment. An important intervention is respite care for caregivers. Various respite models to consider include in-home caregivers (e.g., the visiting nurse model) and adult day care centers/senior centers (in which the patient attends a supervised therapeutic environment for the business day and returns home at night).

However, the patient may ultimately regress to a point at which life without 24-hour supervision is not safe. Specific examples of behaviors that cannot safely be managed at home include assaultive or threatening behavior, leaving dangerous appliances on inappropriately, continuing to drive despite prohibitions, and an inability to maintain feeding, drinking, dressing, and toileting functions. When placement is necessary, an institution that specializes in the care of dementia patients is advised. A secured unit may be required to prevent wandering. Treatment models emphasizing behavioral modification can decrease agitated behavior and minimize the need for pharmacological therapy and physical restraint (Teri et al. 2000). Physicians and family members should clarify with nursing home facilities what degree of medical morbidity can be managed in these institutions, as medical illnesses may lead to more frequent changes in care setting, promoting further behavioral regression with each change of venue.

Legal issues should be addressed early in the course of the illness, while the patient can still direct his or her wishes. These matters include the completion of medicolegal documents such as living wills, durable powers of attorney, and advance directives (Grossberg and Lake 1998). The physician may be asked to comment on the patient's capacity to make legally binding decisions. Neuropsychological testing may be of help. The capacity for medical decision making needs to be considered as well. The physician is advised to thoroughly evaluate the patient's clinical status at the time a medical decision is needed to ensure that the patient understands the implications of his or her medical choices. A retrospective study on dementia patients followed in clinical research protocols found that it was very useful to complete durable powers of attorney in the mild-to-moderate stage of DAT (Dukoff and Sunderland 1997).

Driving and the operation of other dangerous machinery is often a point of great contention. Many patients will maintain the motor skills for driving despite showing substantial cognitive deficits on the clinical interview and on formal mental status testing (Rabins 1998). Even in mild dementia, the statistical risk of motor vehicle accidents is increased (Dubinsky et al. 2000). Physicians are advised to acquaint themselves with the disclosure laws regarding notification of dementia diagnoses to state motor vehicle departments (Rabins 1998). A road competency test may be advisable (Grossberg and Lake 1998). A useful clinical guideline to consider is that driving is not advised whenever a dementia diagnosis leads the clinician to institute pharmacotherapy for dementia and/or when the MMSE score is less than 24. Other contraindications could be the presence of paranoia, agitation, or assaultive behavior.

Pharmacotherapy

Anticholinesterase agents act through inhibition of AChE, increasing the net amount of synaptic ACh available for neurotransmission (Table 7–12) (Taylor 1998). Anticholinesterase agents are advised early in the course of DAT and may reduce the rate of cognitive decline (Farlow 2000). Although their effects may be relatively modest, more often involving a slowing of decline than a reversal of cognitive losses, they represent a major breakthrough in psychopharmacology.

Anticholinesterase agents should also be considered (along with antipsychotics) in managing dementia-related psychotic symptoms (Rao and Lyketsos 1998). These agents can also be safely combined with antidepressants, thus leading to greater symptomatic improvement, given that catecholamine abnormalities may be related to some of the symptoms of dementia (Tune and Sunderland 1998). Cholinergic side effects seen with anticholinesterase agents include nausea, abdominal discomfort, vomiting, loose stools, muscle cramps, muscle weakness, increased sweating, and bradycardia (Ringman and Cummings 1999). AChE inhibitors should be discontinued before surgery in which succinylcholine may be used, because of the risk of prolonged paralysis (Ringman and Cummings 1999).

Anticholinesterase agents may also be used for other dementing illnesses (e.g., dementia due to PD, LBV, LBD, and CJD; mixed VaD and DAT); they may be particularly helpful with the psychotic symptoms of LBV and LBD (Cummings and Masterman 1998). Combination regimens consisting of an anticholinesterase agent and other agents more directly protective against neuronal degeneration (e.g., antioxidants, anti-inflammatory agents, hormones) with psychotropic medications (to address specific neuropsychiatric symptoms) are emerging as treatment for DAT (Cummings et al. 1998a; Farlow and Evans 1998). Tacrine, donepezil, rivastigmine, and galantamine are U.S. Food and Drug Administration (FDA)–approved for DAT, and metrifonate, eptastigmine, and controlled-release physostigmine are under investigation. Although tacrine has been associated with hepatotoxicity, the other agents have not.

Tacrine is taken four times daily, from an initial dose of 10 mg four times a day with dose increases every 6 weeks to a maximum of 160 mg/day (Felician and Sandson 1999). Dosages greater than 80 mg/day may delay nursing home placement (Knopman et al. 1996). About 50% of patients taking tacrine develop increases in liver-associated enzymes, usually within 12 weeks after starting treatment; 25% of patients have increases above three times the upper limit of the reference range (Soares and Gershon 1995). Weekly monitoring of liver-associated enzymes for the first 18 weeks of therapy and every 3 months thereafter is recommended (Class et al. 1997; Soares and Gershon 1995). Because of concerns about increased liver-associated enzymes, tacrine is now used infrequently.

Donepezil is started at 5 mg/day, which may be increased to 10 mg/day in 1–6 weeks. It has been shown to slow the rate of decline of or to improve cognitive performance in mild to moderate DAT (S.L. Rogers et al. 1998). Donepezil has been found to maintain improvements in cognition when continued for up to 98 weeks (S.L. Rogers and Friedhoff 1998). In addition, emotional and behavioral symptoms of dementia may improve (Weiner et al. 2000). Donepezil may help to delay higher-cost interventions associated with disease progression (Neumann et al. 1999).

TABLE 7–12. Dementia pharmacotherapy

Medication class	Target symptom(s)	Starting dose	Maximum dose
Cholinesterase inhibitors	Decreased cognition, delusions, hallucinations		
Tacrine		10 mg four times a day	40 mg four times a day
Donepezil		5 mg/day	10 mg/day
Rivastigmine		1.5 mg twice a day	6 mg twice a day
Galantamine		4 mg twice a day	12 mg twice a day
Antioxidants	Decreased cognition		
Alpha-tocopherol		1,000 IU twice a day	
Selegiline		5 mg/day	10 mg/day
Antidepressants	Depression, irritability, anxiety		
Fluoxetine		10 mg/day	40 mg/day
Paroxetine		10 mg/day	40 mg/day
Sertraline		25 mg/day	200 mg/day
Citalopram		10 mg/day	40 mg/day
Venlafaxine (extended release)		37.5 mg/day	350 mg/day
Nefazadone		50 mg/day	300 mg twice a day
Trazodone		25 mg/day at bedtime	400 mg/day at bedtime
Bupropion		37.5 mg twice a day	200 mg twice a day
Anxiolytic	Anxiety, irritability		
Buspirone		5 mg three times a day	20 mg three times a day
Anticonvulsants	Irritability, agitation		
Carbamazepine		100 mg/day	[a]
Valproate		125 mg/day	[b]
Antipsychotics	Delusions, hallucinations, disorganized thoughts, agitation		
Risperidone		0.25 mg/day at bedtime	3 mg/day at bedtime
Olanzapine		2.5 mg/day at bedtime	10 mg/day at bedtime
Quetiapine		25 mg/day at bedtime	100 mg twice a day
Additional medications (consider as adjunctive therapy on case-by-case basis)			
Psychostimulants			
Nonsteroidal anti-inflammatory drugs			
Antiplatelet agents			
Hormones			
Highly active antiretroviral therapy (HAART)			

Note. [a]Upper limit of dose to give serum drug level of 8–12 ng/mL; [b]Upper limit of dose to give serum drug level of 50–60 ng/mL.

Rivastigmine is a cholinesterase inhibitor with effects on both AChE and butyrylcholinesterase (BuChE) (Spencer and Noble 1998; Stahl 2000). Because of its effects on BuChE, it is theoretically of additional benefit in advanced DAT, when glial proliferation leads to greater CNS concentrations of BuChE (Stahl 2000). Rivastigmine is highly selective for the hippocampus and cortex (Spencer and Noble 1998). Because it is not metabolized through the hepatic cytochrome P450 isoenzyme system, it has little likelihood of problematic drug–drug interac-

tions (Spencer and Noble 1998). Rivastigmine is started at 1.5 mg twice daily for 2 weeks; the dosage may be gradually raised every 2 weeks to a maximum recommended dose of 6 mg twice daily. Doses from 3 to 6 mg twice a day have a beneficial effect on cognitive and functional status (Spencer and Noble 1998).

Galantamine is a cholinesterase inhibitor that also allosterically modulates nicotine cholinergic receptors, theoretically further enhancing ACh release (Raskind et al. 2000; Stahl 2000). This agent may enhance the release of other CNS neurotransmitters important in dementia (Stahl 2000), thereby leading to further improvements in emotional and behavioral symptoms. Galantamine is initially started at 4 mg twice a day, with dosage increases to 8 mg twice daily and 12 mg twice daily after 4-week intervals. A 6-month study of galantamine showed that a 24-mg daily dose was associated with improved cognitive and global function (Raskind et al. 2000). Another trial of galantamine for DAT found doses of 16 or 24 mg/day to be associated with benefits in cognitive, behavioral, and functional status (Tariot et al. 2000).

Metrifonate, a prodrug, is converted to the active anticholinesterase metabolite 2,2,-dimethyl dichlorovinylphosphate (DDVP). Metrifonate is reported to be selective for the G1 monomer of AChE, which is relatively spared in DAT (Ringman and Cummings 1999). It is not metabolized by the hepatic cytochrome P450 enzyme system, has few drug–drug interactions, and is minimally protein bound (J.C. Morris et al. 1998; Raskind et al. 1999). Metrifonate dosages of 30–60 mg/day were associated with improved cognitive, behavioral, and global clinical function in mild to moderate DAT (Farlow et al. 1999; J.C. Morris et al. 1998). A 26-week study of metrifonate at 50 mg/day showed beneficial effects on cognition, ADL, psychiatric and behavioral disturbances, and global level of function (Raskind et al. 1999). Another study compared maintenance doses of 0.2 mg/kg/day (10–20 mg/day), 0.3 mg/kg/day (15–25 mg/day), and 0.65 mg/kg/day (30–60 mg/day) for 10 weeks and found dose-related improvements in cognitive and global function (Cummings et al. 1998b).

Eptastigmine is a cholinesterase inhibitor with a lower risk of peripheral cholinesterase inhibition in comparison with donepezil and metrifonate (Imbimbo et al. 1999). A trial of eptastigmine for DAT showed significant improvement in cognitive, functional, and clinical status, with a dose of 20 mg three times daily superior to 15 mg thrice daily (Imbimbo et al. 1999). A dose-dependent neutropenic effect was noted, however, which may limit this agent's clinical utility.

Physostigmine is a centrally active cholinesterase inhibitor (Thal et al. 1999). A 24-week trial of physostigmine (controlled-release preparation) 30 or 36 mg day for DAT revealed enhanced cognitive and global levels of function in the treated groups (Thal et al. 1999).

The antioxidants selegiline and α-tocopherol (vitamin E) are used for their neuroprotective effects. Selegiline (a selective monoamine oxidase B [MAO-B] inhibitor) 5–10 mg/day is used in mild to moderate DAT for its antioxidant properties and its effect of increasing CNS catecholamine levels (Sano et al. 1997; Tolbert and Fuller 1996).

Selegiline may have a positive effect on both cognition and behavior (Lawlor et al. 1997; Tolbert and Fuller 1996). A minimum of 12 weeks is needed for an adequate trial (Tolbert and Fuller 1996). A tyramine-restricted diet is not required at doses up to 10 mg/day. Selegiline must be used cautiously because of its risk of drug–drug interactions and orthostatic hypotension (Sano et al. 1997). Its use is contraindicated with selective serotonin reuptake inhibitors (SSRIs), TCAs, and meperidine (Rabins et al. 1997).

α-Tocopherol 1,000 IU twice daily may slow the progression of moderate DAT, as its antioxidant properties may protect against neuronal damage caused by amyloid deposition (Felician and Sandson 1999). α-Tocopherol has been reported to protect against the development of VaD as well (G.W. Ross et al. 1999). In addition, it has been associated with decreased coagulation function in patients with vitamin K deficiency (Rabins et al. 1997). Either selegiline or α-tocopherol may delay a poor outcome in dementia (e.g., death, institutionalization, inability to perform ADL), although no current evidence demonstrates benefits from combining them (Sano et al. 1997).

Antipsychotics are indicated for paranoid thinking, hallucinations, delirium, and agitation (Alexopoulos et al. 1998; Lanctot et al. 1998; Rabins 1998). Initial doses in elderly patients with dementia should be less than those used in younger patients because of the risks of sedation and further cognitive decline. Although conventional antipsychotic agents are often used as first-line treatment for agitation, they are associated with frequent adverse side effects in patients with dementia (Alexopoulos et al. 1998; Daniel 2000).

The atypical antipsychotic agents risperidone, olanzapine, and quetiapine are recommended in dementia with agitation and psychosis because of their greater tolerability and lower risk of EPS and neuroleptic malignant syndrome (Daniel 2000; De Deyn et al. 1999). Reduced starting and maximum dosages (e.g., risperidone dosage range of 0.25–3 mg/day at bedtime) are recommended to minimize side effects (Class et al. 1997; Daniel 2000). Nighttime dosing is preferred, as sleep is facilitated and the risk of daytime sedation is minimized. Risperidone dosages ranging from 0.75 to 1.75 mg/day were associated with only a 2.6% risk of tardive dyskinesia at 1-year follow-up (Jeste et al. 2000). In patients with feeding tubes or other limitations affecting their use of solid medications, risperidone elixir can be considered. Suggested dosages for olanzapine are 2.5–10.0 mg/day at bedtime; quetiapine dosages can range from 25 mg/day at bedtime to 100 mg twice daily (Daniel 2000). Olanzapine has been shown to attenuate the emergence of psychosis in DAT (Clark et al. 2001).

Follow-up monitoring should include examination for medication-induced movement disorders with the Assessment of Involuntary Movements Scale. If problems with compliance lead the physician to consider depot antipsychotics, reduced doses (e.g., fluphenazine decanoate 1.25–3.75 mg im monthly) can be considered (Rabins et al. 1997). In the United States, the use of antipsychotic medication in nursing home patients with dementia is regulated by the Omnibus Budget Reconciliation Act of 1987, which requires clear documentation of clinical indications and consideration of alternative interventions (Rabins et al. 1997). Dosage decreases or trial discontinuations of antipsychotics should be considered as the illness progresses. Atypical antipsychotics may still be indicated even in severe dementia; in one study, risperidone 1 mg/day led to improvement in objective behavioral measures (particularly decreased aggression) without further decrements in cognitive function or self-care (Katz et al. 1999).

Antidepressants should be used for comorbid depressive disorders, depressive and anxiety symptoms that do not qualify for a full depressive or anxiety disorder diagnosis, sleep disturbances, and agitation (Borson and Raskind 1997; Raskind 1998). Because of their generally benign side-effect profile and their effectiveness, SSRIs are the preferred class of antidepressants in dementia patients and should be started at lower doses than in healthy adults (Alexopoulos et al. 1998; Katz 1998). Initial doses can be doubled after 2–4 weeks if necessary, and a trial should continue for at least 12 weeks once the usual adult dose has been reached (Class et al. 1997). Paroxetine has more clinically significant anticholinergic activity than the other SSRIs and should be used with caution. SSRIs may also have utility in managing sexual disinhibition in dementia (Stewart and Shin 1997).

Other antidepressants to consider include bupropion, trazodone, and venlafaxine extended release (Alexopoulos et al. 1998; Class et al. 1997). Blood pressure must be monitored in patients using venlafaxine because of the risk of hypertension. TCAs should be used with caution in dementia because of the cognitive toxicity that may result from anticholinergic side effects (Katz 1998; Petracca et al. 1996). "Pseudodementia" due to depression should be managed with antidepressants and follow-up cognitive assessment.

Psychostimulants as adjunctive therapy with antidepressants may be considered for refractory mood symptoms and/or apathy; methylphenidate 2.5–5 mg/day is a recommended starting dose (Rabins et al. 1997). ECT should be considered for cases of treatment-refractory depression; however, because of the risk for post-ECT delirium and amnesia, ECT treatments should be given no more frequently than twice per week with unilateral electrode placement (Rabins et al. 1997).

Anxiolytics may be used for anxiety or agitation. Because of the high risk of further memory impairment, sedation, and falls, physicians should avoid the use of benzodiazepines in dementia patients (Rabins et al. 1997). The clinician might consider buspirone 5 mg thrice daily and increase doses gradually to an upper limit of 20 mg three times a day (Alexopoulos et al. 1998; Class et al. 1997).

Anticonvulsants may be indicated for agitated and aggressive behavior or for emotional lability (Class et al. 1997). A recommended starting dose of carbamazepine for the elderly patient with dementia is 100 mg/day, which can be titrated to achieve a serum drug level of 8–12 ng/mL (Rabins et al. 1997). Carbamazepine has been shown to help control agitation and aggression in dementia (Tariot et al. 1998). Side effects include ataxia, sedation, confusion, and (rarely) bone marrow suppression (Rabins et al. 1997).

Divalproex sodium can be started at 125 mg/day and titrated upward to yield a serum drug level of 50–60 ng/mL (Rabins et al. 1997). Divalproex sodium is associated with gastrointestinal distress, ataxia, and (rarely) hepatotoxicity or bone marrow suppression (Rabins et al. 1997). Monitoring of complete blood count and of liver-associated enzymes is recommended with the use of carbamazepine and valproate (Rabins et al. 1997). Trials of antipsychotics, antidepressants, anxiolytics, or anticonvulsants for agitated behavior should be continued for a minimum of 1 month in mildly agitated patients and up to 9 months for severely agitated dementia patients (Alexopoulos et al. 1998).

NSAIDs (e.g., indomethacin 100–150 mg/day) may delay disease progression in dementia, based on the lower risk for DAT in patients with rheumatoid arthritis and/or chronic NSAID use (Anthony et al. 2000; Breitner 1996). There is some evidence that NSAIDs may decrease the role of inflammation in the production of neuritic plaques and NFTs by suppressing microglial activation (Felician and Sandson 1999; Mackenzie 2000).

Antiplatelet therapy and/or ergot mesylates (e.g., hydergine 3 mg/day initially to a maximum of 9 mg/day) may be considered for cases of VaD and may stabilize or improve cognitive function (Meyer et al. 1995). Hydergine may be associated with nausea and other gastrointestinal symptoms; its use is contraindicated in patients with psychotic symptoms (Rabins et al. 1997).

Hormones may have an adjunctive role in dementia. Estrogen may improve blood flow in cerebral vessels and may also have more direct neuroprotective effects (Birge

1997). Female patients with DAT have been shown to have lower levels of endogenous estrogen (Manly et al. 2000). A large meta-analysis of the effects of postmenopausal hormone replacement on cognition concluded that hormone replacement therapy produced improvement in verbal memory, vigilance, reasoning, and motor speed in women with menopausal symptoms (LeBlanc et al. 2001). Estrogen replacement has been associated with decreased dementia risk but has not been shown to be beneficial in short-term use in DAT (Henderson et al. 2000; LeBlanc et al. 2001; Schneider et al. 1996; Wang et al. 2000; Waring et al. 1999). Medroxyprogesterone may be used to manage disinhibited sexual acting-out behavior in male patients with AD (Rabins et al. 1997).

Future exploration in pharmacotherapy will likely target DAT but would be expected to have applicability to other dementia types as well. Areas of active interest include neurotrophic factors (e.g., nerve growth factor), modification of amyloid metabolism (likely targeting the activities of APP), and reduction of oxidative stress and inflammation (Aisen and Davis 1997).

Highly active antiretroviral therapy (HAART) for the underlying HIV infection is an essential part of the management of HIV dementia and can reverse cognitive losses (Cohen and Jacobson 2000; Maldonado et al. 2000; McDaniel et al. 2000). The cognitive effects of HAART may be further enhanced in combination with ibuprofen (Gendelman et al. 1998). Psychostimulants may be helpful in HIV-associated fatigue and decreased concentration and memory (Maldonado et al. 2000; McDaniel et al. 2000). Addition of the antioxidant OPC-14117 or the platelet-activating-factor antagonist lexipafant to an antiretroviral regimen may improve cognitive function in HIV patients with cognitive impairment (Schifitto et al. 1999; The Dana Consortium on the Therapy of HIV Dementia and Related Cognitive Disorders 1997).

Summary

The dementias are a heterogeneous group of clinical syndromes, unified by their common findings of deterioration in cognitive and executive functions. Physicians need to be alert to the need for a thorough history, targeted evaluation, and psychopharmacological and psychosocial management in patients with these clinical syndromes. Modern clinical interventions, including anticholinesterase agents in concert with other psychopharmacological agents, should be aggressively used early in the disease process to maintain the patient's cognitive functional status. Advances in basic science research point to possible new directions in the pathophysiology and psychopharmacological management of this major public health problem.

Amnestic Disorders

Amnestic disorders are characterized by a loss of memory due to the direct physiological effects of a general medical condition or due to the persisting effects of a substance. The amnestic disorders share a common symptom presentation of memory impairment but are differentiated by etiology. Amnestic disorders are secondary syndromes caused by systemic medical illness, primary cerebral disease or trauma, substance use disorders, or adverse medication effects. The impairment must be sufficient to compromise social and occupational functioning, and it should represent a significant decline from the previous level of functioning.

Epidemiology

Few data are available on the prevalence and incidence of amnestic disorders (Harper et al. 1995). Memory impairment due to head trauma is probably the most common etiology, with more than 500,000 patients hospitalized annually in the United States for head injury. Alcohol abuse and associated thiamine deficiency is a historically common etiology, but recent studies suggest that the incidence of alcohol-induced amnestic disorders is decreasing, whereas that of amnestic disorders due to head trauma is increasing (Kopelman 1995).

Etiology

The DSM-IV-TR diagnostic classification for amnestic disorders is based on etiology. Amnestic disorders can be diagnosed as resulting from a general medical condition (Table 7–13), as due to the effects of a substance (Table 7–14), or as "not otherwise specified." The most common etiologies are listed in Table 7–15 and usually involve bilateral damage to areas of the brain involved in memory. These areas include the dorsomedial and midline thalamic nuclei, the hippocampus, the amygdala, the fornix, and the mammillary bodies. Unilateral damage may sometimes be sufficient to produce memory impairment, particularly in the case of left-sided temporal lobe and thalamic structures (Benson 1978). Several iatrogenic causes, such as medication effects, ECT, and the ICU setting, lack clearly identified neuroanatomic damage (C. Jones et al. 2000).

TABLE 7–13. DSM-IV-TR diagnostic criteria for amnestic disorder due to...*[indicate the general medical condition]*

A. The development of memory impairment as manifested by impairment in the ability to learn new information or the inability to recall previously learned information.
B. The memory disturbance causes significant impairment in social or occupational functioning and represents a significant decline from a previous level of functioning.
C. The memory disturbance does not occur exclusively during the course of a delirium or a dementia.
D. There is evidence from the history, physical examination, or laboratory findings that the disturbance is the direct physiological consequence of a general medical condition (including physical trauma).

    Specify if:
        Transient: if memory impairment lasts for 1 month or less
        Chronic: if memory impairment lasts for more than 1 month

Coding note: Include the name of the general medical condition on Axis I, e.g., amnestic disorder due to head trauma; also code the general medical condition on Axis III.

TABLE 7–14. DSM-IV-TR diagnostic criteria for substance-induced persisting amnestic disorder

A. The development of memory impairment as manifested by impairment in the ability to learn new information or the inability to recall previously learned information.
B. The memory disturbance causes significant impairment in social or occupational functioning and represents a significant decline from a previous level of functioning.
C. The memory disturbance does not occur exclusively during the course of a delirium or a dementia and persists beyond the usual duration of substance intoxication or withdrawal.
D. There is evidence from the history, physical examination, or laboratory findings that the memory disturbance is etiologically related to the persisting effects of substance use (e.g., a drug of abuse, a medication).

Code [Specific substance]–induced persisting amnestic disorder:
    (291.1 alcohol; 292.83 sedative, hypnotic, or anxiolytic; 292.83 other [or unknown] substance)

Clinical Features

Patients with amnestic disorders either are impaired in their ability to learn and recall new information (anterograde amnesia) or are unable to recall previously learned material (retrograde amnesia). The deficits in short-term or recent memory seen in anterograde amnesia can be assessed by asking the patient to recall three objects after a 5-minute distraction. Whereas anterograde amnesia is

TABLE 7–15. Causes of amnestic disorders

Head trauma
Wernicke-Korsakoff syndrome
Alcohol-induced blackouts
Benzodiazepines
Barbiturates
Intrathecal methotrexate
Methylenedioxymethamphetamine (MDMA; "Ecstasy")
Seizures
Herpes simplex encephalopathy
Kluver-Bucy syndrome
Electroconvulsive therapy
Carbon monoxide poisoning
Heavy metal poisoning
Hypoxia
Hypoglycemia
Cerebrovascular disorders
Cerebral neoplasms

nearly always present, retrograde amnesia is more variable and depends on the location and severity of brain damage. Both immediate recall (as tested by digit span) and remote memory for distant past events are usually preserved. Memory for the physical traumatic event that caused the deficit is often lost. Orientation may be impaired, because it is dependent on the ability to store information regarding time, date, location, and circumstance. The patient may therefore present as confused and disoriented, but without the fluctuation in level of consciousness associated with delirium. Orientation to self is nearly always preserved in amnestic disorders.

Most patients with amnestic disorders lack insight into their deficits and may vehemently deny the presence of memory impairment despite clear evidence to the contrary. This lack of insight may lead to anger, accusations, and occasionally agitation. More commonly, patients present with apathy, lack of initiative, and diminished affective expression suggestive of altered personality function.

Confabulation is often associated with amnestic disorders. Confabulation is characterized by responses to questions that not only are inaccurate but also are often so bizarre and unrealistic as to appear psychotic. Historically, confabulation was considered to represent an attempt by these patients to "cover up" their deficits in memory, but this explanation is probably overly simplistic. The presence and degree of confabulation are usually correlated not with the severity of memory deficits but rather with the loss of self-corrective and monitoring functions, as seen in bifrontal lobe disease (Benson 1978; Mercer et al. 1977; Stuss et al. 1978). Confabulation in amnestic disorders is usually seen during the early stages of the illness and tends to disappear over time.

The onset of amnesia may be sudden or gradual, depending on etiology. Head trauma, vascular events, and specific neurotoxic exposures such as carbon monoxide poisoning are associated with acute mental status changes. Prolonged substance use, sustained nutritional deficiency, and chronic neurotoxic exposures may produce a more gradual and sustained decline in memory function, eventually leading to a clinically diagnosable impairment.

Selected Amnestic Disorders

Head Injury

Severe neurological and psychiatric symptoms can result from head injury, even in the absence of radiological evidence of structural damage. Amnesia following head injury typically includes both anterograde (or ongoing) amnesia and retrograde amnesia for a period ranging from a few minutes to several years before the injury. As anterograde amnesia fades and the patient regains the ability to learn and recall new information, retrograde amnesia "shrinks," usually remaining only for the very short period (seconds to minutes) before the injury. A prolonged retrograde amnesia is an indication of ongoing anterograde amnesia, whereas a short period of retrograde amnesia is associated with recovery (Benson and McDaniel 1991). Severe injuries may result in permanent deficits, although some recovery of memory function can be seen up to 24 months after head trauma.

Korsakoff's Syndrome

Korsakoff's syndrome is an amnestic disorder caused by thiamine deficiency, usually associated with excessive, prolonged ingestion of alcohol. It can occur in other malnourished conditions, such as marasmus, gastric carcinoma, and HIV (Kopelman 1995). Korsakoff's syndrome is associated with an acute phase of illness—known as Wernicke's encephalopathy—that presents with ophthalmoplegia, peripheral neuropathy, ataxia, nystagmus, and delirium. Although these acute neurological symptoms respond to aggressive thiamine repletion, a residual, persistent amnestic syndrome usually remains. The associated neuroanatomic abnormalities in Korsakoff's syndrome include bilateral sclerosis of the mammillary bodies (Benson 1978) and punctate lesions of the gray nuclei in the periventricular regions of the third and fourth ventricles and the sylvian aqueduct (Victor et al. 1989). Some investigators have questioned whether there are distinctive pathophysiological differences between Wernicke–Korsakoff syndrome and the cognitive impairment and dementia due to chronic alcohol neurotoxicity (Blansjaar and van Dijk 1992; Bowden 1990; Jernigan et al. 1991). Given the high prevalence of missed diagnoses of Wernicke–Korsakoff syndrome and the insidious, progressive course of the illness, in which each episode gives rise to cumulative damage, all alcohol-dependent patients should be treated with thiamine (Blansjaar and van Dijk 1992).

Transient Global Amnesia

Transient global amnesia is a form of amnestic disorder characterized by an abrupt episode of profound anterograde amnesia and a variable inability to recall events that occur during the episode. These episodes typically last for only a few minutes or hours, ending with a rapid, spontaneous restoration of intact cognitive function. Mean duration of the amnestic period is 4.2 hours; periods greater than 12 hours are exceptional. The patient's level of consciousness and orientation to self are unaffected during the episode (Fisher and Adams 1958; Shuping et al. 1980). Patients are often bewildered and confused during the episodes and may ask repeated questions about their circumstances. No data are available to suggest that transient global amnesia is associated with focal neurological features or with any comorbid psychiatric illness. Transient global amnesia is more common in men and usually occurs after age 50. The etiology is unclear, but most experts believe that it is associated with cerebrovascular disease and episodic vascular insufficiency of the mesial temporal lobe. Other etiologies of transient global amnesia, including brain tumors, cardiac arrhythmias, migraine, thyroid disorders, polycythemia vera, epilepsy, and myxomatous mitral valvular disease, have also been reported (Hodges and Warlow 1990a; Pai and Yang 1999). The most common angiographic findings are in the vertebrobasilar system, specifically occlusion or stenosis of the posterior cerebral artery (Mathew and Meyer 1974). Transient global amnesia generally has a good prognosis, with only 8% of patients experiencing a second episode (Hodges and Warlow 1990b).

Benzodiazepine Persisting Amnestic Disorder

Several medications have been associated with amnestic syndromes, with benzodiazepines receiving the most attention. Benzodiazepines can cause anterograde amnesia and may interfere with memory consolidation and retrieval. Risk factors include high dose, intravenous administration, and use of high-potency, short-half-life agents such as triazolam (Scharf et al. 1987). These effects may be enhanced by the concurrent use of alcohol

(Linnoila 1990; Roth et al. 1984). The resulting memory impairment is not associated with the degree of sedation or psychomotor impairment (Roache and Griffiths 1985).

Differential Diagnosis

Memory deficits seen in amnestic syndromes are frequently a feature of delirium and dementia. In delirium, the memory disturbance is accompanied by a disturbed level of consciousness and usually fluctuates with time. More pervasive signs of cerebral dysfunction, such as difficulty focusing or sustaining attention, are present. In dementia, memory impairment is accompanied by additional cognitive impairments such as aphasia, apraxia, agnosia, and disturbances in executive functioning.

In dissociative or psychogenic forms of amnesia, the memory loss usually does not involve deficits in learning and recalling new information. Patients typically present with a circumscribed inability to recall previously learned and personal information, often regarding the patient's own identity or a traumatic or stressful event. These deficits persist even as the patient continues to function normally in the present. Interestingly, changes in limbic function are observed on PET in patients with psychogenic amnesia (Yasuno et al. 2000). Patients with malingering or factitious disorders can present with amnestic symptoms that also fit the profile for dissociative amnesia. Systematic memory testing of these patients will often yield inconsistent results.

Treatment

As in delirium and dementia, the primary goal of treatment in amnestic disorders is to identify and treat the underlying cause or pathological process. There are no definitively effective treatments for amnestic disorder that are specifically aimed at reversing apparent memory deficits. Fortunately, these deficits are often temporary—as in transient amnestic syndromes—or are partially or completely reversible—as in head trauma, thiamine deficiency, or anoxia. Acute management should include continuous reorientation of the patient by means of verbal redirection, clocks, calendars, and familiar stimuli. Individual supportive psychotherapy for the patient, and family counseling to assist and educate caregivers, is also helpful. Chronic reversible amnestic syndromes may be managed with cognitive rehabilitation and therapeutic milieus intended to promote recovery from brain injury (Kashima et al. 1999). More severe and permanent deficits may require supervised living environments to ensure appropriate care.

Conclusions

The cognitive disorders represent a heterogeneous group of clinical syndromes with the common denominator of disturbances in memory and other cognitive functions. Psychiatrists need to be mindful of the broad differential diagnosis of patients presenting with cognitive impairment. Thorough history taking; directed mental status testing; use of laboratory tests, EEG, and neuroimaging; and a willingness to creatively employ psychopharmacological and behavioral interventions based on an application of the biopsychosocial model are advised for the care of these patients. It is likely that future neuroscientific, pharmacological, and neuroimaging research will yield further options for diagnosis, treatment, and prevention of cognitive impairment.

References

Aakerlund LP, Rosenberg J: Postoperative delirium: treatment with supplemental oxygen. Br J Anaesth 72:286–290, 1994

Aarsland D, Cummings JL, Yenner G, et al: Relationship of aggressive behavior to other neuropsychiatric symptoms in patients with Alzheimer's disease. Am J Psychiatry 153:243–247, 1996

Aisen PS, Davis KL: The search for disease-modifying treatment for Alzheimer's disease. Neurology 48(suppl 6):S35–S41, 1997

Albert MS, Levkoff SE, Reilly C, et al: The delirium symptom interview: an interview for the detection of delirium symptoms in hospitalized patients. J Geriatr Psychiatry Neurol 5:14–21, 1992

Albrecht J, Wysmyk-Cybula U, Rafalowska U: Cerebral oxygen consumption in experimental hepatic encephalopathy: different responses in astrocytes, neurons, and synaptosomes. Exp Neurol 97:418–422, 1987

Alexander GE, Furey ML, Grady CL, et al: Association of premorbid intellectual function with cerebral metabolism in Alzheimer's disease: implications for the cognitive reserve hypothesis. Am J Psychiatry 154:165–172, 1997

Alexopoulos GS, Silver JM, Kahn DA, et al: Treatment of agitation in older patients with dementia. A Postgraduate Medicine Special Report. Minneapolis, MN, McGraw-Hill, 1998, pp 1–88

American College of Radiology Appropriateness Criteria for Imaging and Treatment Decisions Pocket Guide, Vols 1 and 2. Reston, VA, American College of Radiology, 1996

American Psychiatric Association: Diagnostic and Statistical Manual of Mental Disorders, 2nd Edition. Washington, DC, American Psychiatric Association, 1968

American Psychiatric Association: Diagnostic and Statistical Manual of Mental Disorders, 3rd Edition. Washington, DC, American Psychiatric Association, 1980

American Psychiatric Association: Diagnostic and Statistical Manual of Mental Disorders, 4th Edition. Washington, DC, American Psychiatric Association, 1994

American Psychiatric Association: Practice guideline for the treatment of patients with delirium. Am J Psychiatry 156(suppl):1–20, 1999

American Psychiatric Association: Diagnostic and Statistical Manual of Mental Disorders, 4th Edition, Text Revision. Washington, DC, American Psychiatric Association, 2000

Anthony JC, Breitner JCS, Zandi PP, et al: Reduced prevalence of AD in users of NSAIDs and H2 receptor antagonists. Neurology 54:2066–2071, 2000

Armstrong SC, Cozza KL, Watanabe KS: The misdiagnosis of delirium. Psychosomatics 38:433–439, 1997

Ayd FJ: Intravenous haloperidol therapy. International Drug Therapy Newsletter 13:20–23, 1978

Baldereschi M, Di Carlo A, Maggi S, et al: Dementia is a major predictor of death among the Italian elderly. Neurology 52:709–713, 1999

Balestrino M: Pathophysiology of anoxic depolarization: new findings and a working hypothesis. J Neurosci Methods 59:99–103, 1995

Balestrino M, Somjen GG: Chlorpromazine protects brain tissue in hypoxia by delaying spreading depression-mediated calcium influx. Brain Res 385:219–226, 1986

Balestrino M, Aitken PG, Somjen CG: The effects of moderate changes of extracellular K+ and Ca2+ on synaptic and neural function in the CA1 region of the hippocampal slice. Brain Res 377:229–239, 1986

Balestrino M, Aitken PG, Somjen CG: Spreading depression-like hypoxic depolarization in CA1 and fascia dentata of hippocampal slices: relationship to selective vulnerability. Brain Res 497:102–107, 1989

Ballard CG, O'Brien JT, Swann AG, et al: The natural history of psychosis and depression in dementia with Lewy bodies and Alzheimer's disease: persistence and new cases over 1 year of follow-up. J Clin Psychiatry 62:46–49, 2001

Barber R, Ballard C, McKeith IG, et al: MRI volumetric study of dementia with Lewy bodies: a comparison with AD and vascular dementia. Neurology 54:1304–1309, 2000

Bauer G: Cerebral anoxia, in Electroencephalography: Basic Principles, Clinical Applications and Related Fields. Edited by Niedermayer E, Lopes da Silva F. Baltimore, MD, Urban & Schwarzenberg, 1982, pp 319–324

Bayindir O, Akpinar B, Can E, et al: The use of the 5-HT3-receptor antagonist ondansetron for the treatment of post-cardiotomy delirium. J Cardiothorac Vasc Anesth 14:288–292, 2000

Benson DF: Amnesia. South Med J 71:1221–1228, 1978

Benson DF, McDaniel KD: Memory disorders, in Neurology in Clinical Practice, Vol 2. Edited by Bradley WG, Daroff RB, Fenichel GM, et al. Boston, MA, Butterworth-Heinemann, 1991, pp 1389–1406

Benveniste H, Drejer J, Schousboe A, et al: Elevation of the extracellular concentrations of glutamate and aspartate in rat hippocampus during transient cerebral ischemia monitored by intracerebral microdialysis. J Neurochem 43:1369–1374, 1984

Beresin E: Delirium in the elderly. J Geriatr Psychiatry Neurol 1:127–143, 1988

Berger A-K, Fratiglioni L, Frosell Y, et al: The occurrence of depressive symptoms in the preclinical phase of AD: a population-based study. Neurology 53:1998–2002, 1999

Birge SJ: The role of estrogen in the treatment of Alzheimer's disease. Neurology 48(suppl 7):S36–S41, 1997

Blansjaar BA, Van Dijk JG: Korsakoff minus Wernicke syndrome. Alcohol Alcohol 27:435–437, 1992

Blazer DG, Federspiel CF, Ray WA, et al: The risk of anticholinergic toxicity in the elderly: a study of prescribing practices in two populations. J Gerontol 38:31–35, 1983

Bleasdale GJ, Singleton SJ: Causes and prognosis of delirium in elderly patients admitted to a district general hospital. Age Ageing 26:423–427, 1997

Bluml S, Zuckerman E, Tan J, et al: Proton-decoupled 31P magnetic resonance spectroscopy reveals osmotic and metabolic disturbances in human hepatic encephalopathy. J Neurochem 71:1564–1576, 1998

Bobinski M, Wegel J, Wisniewski HM, et al: Neurofibrillary pathology-correlation with hippocampal formation atrophy in Alzheimer disease. Neurobiology of Aging 17:909–919, 1996

Bookheimer SY, Strojwas MH, Cohen MS, et al: Patterns of brain activation in people at risk for Alzheimer's disease. N Engl J Med 343:450–456, 2000

Borson S, Raskind MA: Clinical features and pharmacologic treatment of behavioral symptoms of Alzheimer's disease. Neurology 48(suppl 6):S17–S24, 1997

Bottino CM, Almeida OP: Can neuroimaging techniques identify individuals at risk of developing Alzheimer's disease? Int Psychogeriatr 9:389–403, 1997

Bouwman FH, Skolasky RL, Hes D, et al: Variable progression of HIV-associated dementia. Neurology 50:1814–1820, 1998

Bowden SC: Separating cognitive impairment in neurologically asymptomatic alcoholism from Wernicke-Korsakoff syndrome: is the neuropsychological distinction justified? Psychol Bull 107:355–366, 1990

Breitbart W, Marotta R, Call P: AIDS and neuroleptic malignant syndrome. Lancet 2:1488–1489, 1988

Breitbart W, Marotta R, Platt MM, et al: A double-blind trial of haloperidol, chlorpromazine, and lorazepam in the treatment of delirium in hospitalized AIDS patients. Am J Psychiatry 153:231–237, 1996

Breitbart W, Rosenfeld B, Roth A, et al: The memorial delirium assessment scale. J Pain Symptom Manage 13:128–137, 1997

Breitner JCS: The role of anti-inflammatory drugs in the prevention and treatment of Alzheimer's disease. Ann Rev Med 47:401–411, 1996

Brown TM: Basic mechanisms in the pathogenesis of delirium, in The Psychiatric Care of the Medical Patient, 2nd Edition. Edited by Stoudemire A, Fogel BS, Greenberg DB. New York, Oxford University Press, 2000, pp 571–580

Brown TM, Stoudemire A: Psychiatric Side Effects of Prescription and Over-the-Counter Medications. Washington, DC, American Psychiatric Press, 1998

Butters MA, Becker JT, Nebes RD, et al: Changes in cognitive functioning following treatment of late-life depression. Am J Psychiatry 157:1949–1954, 2000

Cameron DJ, Thomas RI, Mulvihill M, et al: Delirium: a test of the Diagnostic and Statistical Manual III criteria on medical inpatients. J Am Geriatr Soc 35:1007–1010, 1987

Caraceni A, Nanni O, Maltoni M, et al: Impact of delirium on the short term prognosis of advanced cancer patients. Italian Multicenter Study Group on Palliative Care. Cancer 89:1145–1149, 2000

Carmen JS, Wyatt RJ: Calcium and malignant catatonia. Lancet 2:1124–1125, 1977

Caselli RJ, Graff-Radford NR, Reiman EM, et al: Preclinical memory decline in cognitively normal apolipoprotein E epsilon-4 homozygotes. Neurology 53:201–207, 1999

Cassem NH, Sos J: Intravenous use of haloperidol for acute delirium in intensive care settings. Paper presented at 131st Annual Meeting of the American Psychiatric Association, Washington, DC, May 1978

Chapman FM, Dickinson J, McKeith I, et al: Association among visual hallucinations, visual acuity, and specific eye pathologies in Alzheimer's disease: treatment implications. Am J Psychiatry 156:1983–1985, 1999

Choi DW, Weiss JH, Koh JY, et al: Glutamate neurotoxicity, calcium, and zinc. Ann N Y Acad Sci 568:219–224, 1989

Choi SH, Na DL, Chung CS, et al: Diffusion-weighted MRI in vascular dementia. Neurology 54:83–89, 2000

Clark WS, Street JS, Feldman PD, et al: The effects of olanzapine in reducing the emergence of psychosis among nursing home residents with Alzheimer's disease. J Clin Psychiatry 62:34–40, 2001

Class CA, Unverzagt FW, Gao S, et al: Psychiatric disorders in African American nursing home residents. Am J Psychiatry 153:677–681, 1996

Class CA, Schneider L, Farlow MR: Optimal management of behavioural disorders associated with dementia. Drugs Aging 10:95–106, 1997

Coffey CE, Saxton JA, Ratcliff G, et al: Relation of education to brain size in normal aging: implications for the reserve hypothesis. Neurology 53:189–196, 1999

Cohen MAA, Jacobson JM: Maximizing life's potential in AIDS: a psychopharmacologic update. Gen Hosp Psychiatry 22:375–388, 2000

Cole MG, Primeau FJ: Prognosis of delirium in elderly hospital patients. Can Med Assoc J 149:41–46, 1993

Craft S, Teri L, Edland SD, et al: Accelerated decline in apolipoprotein E-epsilon 4 homozygotes with Alzheimer's disease. Neurology 51:149–153, 1998

Cummings JL, Masterman DL: Assessment of treatment-associated changes in behavior and cholinergic therapy of neuropsychiatric symptoms in Alzheimer's disease. J Clin Psychiatry 59(suppl 13):23–30, 1998

Cummings JL, Vinters HV, Cole GM, et al: Alzheimer's disease: etiologies, pathophysiology, cognitive reserve, and treatment opportunities. Neurology 51(suppl 1):S2–S17, 1998a

Cummings JL, Cyrus PA, Bieber F, et al: Metrifonate treatment of the cognitive deficits of Alzheimer's disease. Neurology 50:1214–1221, 1998b

Curb JD, Rodriguez BL, Abbott RD, et al: Longitudinal association of vascular and Alzheimer's dementia, diabetes, and glucose tolerance. Neurology 52:971–975, 1999

Daniel DG: Antipsychotic treatment of psychosis and agitation in the elderly. J Clin Psychiatry 61(suppl 14):49–52, 2000

d'Arminio Monteforte A, Duca PG, Vago L, et al: Decreasing incidence of CNS AIDS-defining events associated with antiretroviral therapy. Neurology 54:1856–1859, 2000

De Deyn PP, Rabheru K, Rasmussen A, et al: A randomized trial of risperidone, placebo, and haloperidol for behavioral symptoms of dementia. Neurology 53:946–955, 1999

de Koning I, van Kooten F, Dippel DWJ, et al: The CAMCOG: a useful screening instrument for dementia in stroke patients. Stroke 29:2080–2086, 1998

Delacourte A, David JP, Sergeant N, et al: The biochemical pathway of neurofibrillary degeneration in aging and Alzheimer's disease. Neurology 52:1158–1165, 1999

Desmond DW, Moroney JT, Paik MC, et al: Frequency and clinical determinants of dementia after ischemic stroke. Neurology 54:1124–1131, 2000

Devanand DP, Michaels-Marston KS, Liu X, et al: Olfactory deficit in patients with mild cognitive impairment predict Alzheimer's disease at follow-up. Am J Psychiatry 157:1399–1405, 2000

Dickson LR: Hypoalbuminemia in delirium. Psychosomatics 32:317–323, 1991

Dolan MM, Hawkes WG, Zimmerman SI, et al: Delirium on hospital admission in aged hip fracture patients: prediction of mortality and 2-year functional outcomes. J Gerontol 55:M527–M534, 2000

Doody RS, Massman PJ, Mawad M, et al: Cognitive consequences of subcortical magnetic resonance imaging changes in Alzheimer's disease: comparison to small vessel ischemic vascular dementia. Neuropsychiatry Neuropsychol Behav Neurol 11:191–199, 1998

Doraiswamy PM, Steffens DC, Pitchumoni S, et al: Early recognition of Alzheimer's disease: What is consensual? What is controversial? What is practical? J Clin Psychiatry 59(suppl 13):6–18, 1998

Doyle M, Warden D: Use of SPECT to evaluate postcardiotomy delirium (letter). Am J Psychiatry 153:838–839, 1996

Duara R, Barker W, Luis CA: Frontotemporal dementia and Alzheimer's disease: differential diagnosis. Dement Geriatr Cogn Disord 10(suppl 1):37–42, 1999

Dubinsky RM, Stein AC, Lyons K: Practice parameter: risk of driving and Alzheimer's disease (an evidence-based review). Neurology 54:2205–2211, 2000

Dufouil C, Clayton D, Brayne C, et al: Population norms for the MMSE in the very old: estimates based on longitudinal data. Mini-Mental State Examination. Neurology 55:1609–1613, 2000

Dukoff R, Sunderland T: Durable power of attorney and informed consent with Alzheimer's disease patients: a clinical study. Am J Psychiatry 154:1070–1075, 1997

Dunn NR, Alfonso CA, Young RA, et al: Creutzfeldt-Jakob disease appearing as paranoid psychosis. Am J Psychiatry 156:2016–2017, 1999

Dyer CB, Ashton CM, Teasdale TA: Postoperative delirium: a review of 80 primary data-collection studies. Arch Intern Med 155:461–465, 1995

Eden BM, Foreman MD, Sisk R: Delirium: comparison of four predictive models in hospitalized critically ill elderly patients. Applied Nursing Research 11:27–35, 1998

Elie M, Rousseau F, Cole M, et al: Prevalence and detection of delirium in elderly emergency room department patients. Can Med Assoc J 163:977–981, 2000

Engel GL, Romano J: Delirium: a syndrome of cerebral insufficiency. J Chronic Dis 9:260–277, 1959

Erkinjuntii T, Wikstrom J, Palo J, et al: Dementia among medical inpatients: evaluation of 2000 consecutive admissions. Arch Intern Med 146:1923–1926, 1986

Evans RM, Emsley CL, Gao S, et al: Serum cholesterol, APOE genotype, and the risk of Alzheimer's disease: a population-based study of African Americans. Neurology 54:240–242, 2000

Fann JR, Roth-Roemer S, Burington B, et al: Delirium in patients undergoing hematopoietic stem cell transplantation: epidemiology, risk factors, and outcomes. Symposium presented at the annual meeting of the Academy of Psychosomatic Medicine, Palm Springs, CA, November 2000

Fann JR, Burington B, Roth-Roemer S, et al: Delirium and affective and cognitive outcomes in patients undergoing stem cell transplantation. Ann Behav Med 23(suppl):S064, 2001

Farlow M: New approaches in assessing delay of progression of Alzheimer's disease (pp 795–798), in Geula C, Farlow M, chairs: Alzheimer's disease: translating neurochemical insights into clinical benefits (Academic Highlights). J Clin Psychiatry 61:791–802, 2000

Farlow MR, Evans RM: Pharmacologic treatment of cognition in Alzheimer's dementia. Neurology 51(suppl 1):S36–S44, 1998

Farlow MR, Cyrus PA, Nadel A, et al: Metrifonate treatment of AD: influence of APOE genotype. Neurology 53:2010–2016, 1999

Felician O, Sandson TA: The neurobiology and pharmacotherapy of Alzheimer's disease. J Neuropsychiatry Clin Neurosci 11:19–31, 1999

Felipo V, Hermenegildo C, Montoliu, et al: Neurotoxicity of ammonia and glutamate: molecular mechanisms and prevention. Neurotoxicology 19:675–682, 1998

Fernandez F, Holmes VF, Adams F, et al: Treatment of severe, refractory agitation with a haloperidol drip. J Clin Psychiatry 49:239–241, 1988

Fernandez F, Levy JK, Mansell PW: Management of delirium in terminally ill AIDS patients. Int J Psychiatry Med 19:165–172, 1989

Fink M: Cytopathic hypoxia in sepsis. Acta Anaesthesiol Scand 110(suppl):87–95, 1997

Fink M: Delirious mania. Bipolar Disord 1:54–60, 1999

Fischer P: Successful treatment of nonanticholinergic delirium with a cholinesterase inhibitor (letter). J Clin Psychopharmacol 21:118, 2001

Fisher CM, Adams RD: Transient global amnesia. Trans Am Neurol Assoc 83:143–146, 1958

Folstein MF, Folstein SE, McHugh PR: "Mini-Mental State": a practical method for grading the cognitive state of patients for the clinician. J Psychiatr Res 12:189–198, 1975

Fox NC, Scahill RI, Crum WR, et al: Correlations between rates of brain atrophy and cognitive decline in AD. Neurology 52:1687–1689, 1999

Foy A, O'Connell D, Henry D, et al: Benzodiazepine use as a cause of cognitive impairment in elderly hospital inpatients. J Gerontol 50A:M99–M106, 1995

Francis J, Kapoor WN: Delirium in hospitalized elderly. J Gen Intern Med 5:65–79, 1990

Francis J, Kapoor WN: Prognosis after hospital discharge of older medical patients with delirium. J Am Geriatr Soc 40:601–606, 1992

Francis J, Strong S, Martin D, et al: Delirium in elderly general medical patients: common but often unrecognized. Clin Res 36:711A, 1988

Francis J, Martin D, Kapoor WN: A prospective study of delirium in hospitalized elderly. JAMA 263:1097–1101, 1990

Franco K, Litaker D, Locala J, et al: The cost of delirium in the surgical patient. Psychosomatics 42:68–73, 2001

Freund HR, Muggia-Sullam M, LaFrance R, et al: Regional brain amino-acid and neurotransmitter derangements during abdominal sepsis and septic encephalopathy in the rat. Arch Surg 121:209–216, 1986

Frye MA, Coudreaut MF, Hakeman SM, et al: Continuous droperidol infusion for management of agitated delirium in an intensive care unit. Psychosomatics 36:301–305, 1995

Kales HC, Blow FC, Copeland LA, et al: Health care utilization by older patients with coexistent dementia and depression. Am J Psychiatry 156:550–556, 1999

Kanemaru K, Kameda N, Yamanouchi H: Decreased CSF amyloid beta 42 and normal tau levels in dementia with Lewy bodies. Neurology 54:1875–1876, 2000

Kashima H, Kato M, Yoshimasu H, et al: Current trends in cognitive rehabilitation for memory disorders. Keio J Med 48:79–86, 1999

Katz IR: Diagnosis and treatment of depression in patients with Alzheimer's disease and other dementias. J Clin Psychiatry 59(suppl 9):38–44, 1998

Katz IR, Jeste DV, Mintzer JE, et al: Comparison of risperidone and placebo for psychosis and behavioral disturbances associated with dementia: a randomized, double-blind trial. J Clin Psychiatry 60:107–115, 1999

Kaye JA: Diagnostic challenges in dementia. Neurology 51(suppl 1):S45–S52, 1998

Keane PE, Neal H: The effect of injections of dopaminergic agonists into the caudate nucleus on the electrocortigram of the rat. J Neurosci Res 6:237–241, 1981

Kelly KG, Zisselman M, Cutillo-Schmitter T, et al: Severity and course of delirium in medically hospitalized nursing facility residents. Am J Geriatr Psychiatry 9:72–77, 2001

Kenard MA, Bueding E, Wortis WB: Some biochemical and electroencephalographic changes in delirium tremens. Q J Stud Alcohol 6:4–14, 1945

Kirsch J, Diringer M, Borel C, et al: Brain resuscitation: medical management and innovations. Crit Care Nurs Clin North Am 1:143–154, 1989

Knell AJ, Davidson AR, Williams R, et al: Dopamine and serotonin metabolites in hepatic encephalopathy. BMJ 1:549–551, 1974

Knopman D, Schneider L, Davis K, et al: Long-term tacrine (Cognex) treatment: effects on nursing home placement and mortality. Neurology 47:166–177, 1996

Kopelman MD: The Korsakoff syndrome. Br J Psychiatry 166:154–173, 1995

Koponen H, Riekkinen PJ: A longitudinal study of beta-endorphin-like immunoreactivity in delirium, II: changes at the acute stage and at one-year follow-up. Acta Psychiatr Scand 20:501–505, 1990

Koponen H, Hurri L, Stenback U, et al: Acute confusional states in the elderly: a radiological evaluation. Acta Psychiatr Scand 76:726–731, 1987

Koponen H, Stenback U, Mattila E, et al: Cerebrospinal fluid somatostatin in delirium. Psychol Med 19:605–609, 1989a

Koponen H, Hurri L, Stenback U, et al: Computed tomography findings in delirium. J Nerv Ment Dis 177:226–231, 1989b

Koponen H, Stenback U, Mattila E, et al: Delirium among elderly persons admitted to a psychiatric hospital: clinical course during the acute stage and one-year follow-up. Acta Psychiatr Scand 79:579–585, 1989c

Koponen H, Partanen J, Paakkonen A, et al: EEG spectral analysis in delirium. J Neurol Neurosurg Psychiatry 52:980–985, 1989d

Kornhuber J, Weller M: Psychogenicity and N-methyl-D-aspartate receptor antagonism: implications for neuroprotective pharmacology. Biol Psychiatry 41:135–144, 1997

Kosenko E, Kaminsky Y, Grau E, et al: Brain ATP depletion induced by acute ammonia intoxication in rats is mediated by activation of NMDA receptor and Na+, K+ ATPase. J Neurochem 63:2172–2178, 1994

Kramer JH, Duffy JM: Aphasia, apraxia, and agnosia in the diagnosis of dementia. Dementia 7:23–26, 1996

Kuhl DE, Koeppe RA, Minoshima S, et al: In vivo mapping of cerebral acetylcholinesterase activity in aging and Alzheimer's disease. Neurology 52:691–699, 1999

Kuzis G, Sabe L, Tiberti C, et al: Neuropsychological correlates of apathy and depression in patients with dementia. Neurology 52:1403–1407, 1999

Lanctot KL, Best TS, Mittman N, et al: Efficacy and safety of neuroleptics in behavioral disorders associated with dementia. J Clin Psychiatry 59:550–561, 1998

Lawlor BA, Aisen PS, Green C, et al: Selegiline in the treatment of behavioural disturbance in Alzheimer's disease. Int J Geriatr Psychiatry 12:319–322, 1997

LeBlanc ES, Janowsky J, Chan BKS, et al: Hormone replacement therapy and cognition: systematic review and meta-analysis. JAMA 285:1489–1499, 2001

Levin M: Delirium: a gap in psychiatric teaching. Am J Psychiatry 107:689–694, 1951

Levkoff SE, Evans DA, Liptzin B, et al: Delirium: the occurrence of and persistence of symptoms among elderly hospitalized patients. Arch Intern Med 152:334–340, 1992

Levy ML, Cummings JL: Parkinson's disease, in Psychiatric Management in Neurological Disease. Edited by Lauterbach EC. Washington, DC, American Psychiatric Press, 2000, pp 41–70

Levy ML, Cummings JL, Fairbanks LA, et al: Longitudinal assessment of symptoms of depression, agitation, and psychosis in 181 patients with Alzheimer's disease. Am J Psychiatry 153:1438–1443, 1996

Linnoila MI: Benzodiazepines and alcohol. J Psychiatr Res 24(suppl 2):121–127, 1990

Lipowski ZJ: Transient cognitive disorders (delirium, acute confusional states) in the elderly. Am J Psychiatry 140:1426–1436, 1983

Lipowski ZJ: Delirium (acute confusional states). JAMA 258:1789–1792, 1987

Lipowski ZJ: Delirium: how its concept has developed. Int Psychogeriatr 3:115–120, 1991

Liptzin B, Levkoff SE: An empirical study of delirium subtypes. Br J Psychiatry 161:843–845, 1992

Litvan I, McKee A: Clinicopathologic case conference. J Neuropsychiatry Clin Neurosci 11:107–112, 1999

Lockwood AH, Yap EW, Rhoades HM, et al: Altered cerebral blood flow and glucose metabolism in patients with liver disease and minimal encephalopathy. J Cereb Blood Flow Metab 11:331–336, 1991

Lopez OL, Litvan I, Catt KE, et al: Accuracy of four clinical diagnostic criteria for the diagnosis of neurodegenerative dementias. Neurology 53:1292–1299, 1999

Lopez OL, Wisniewski S, Hamilton RL, et al: Predictors of progression in patients with AD and Lewy bodies. Neurology 54:1774–1779, 2000a

Lopez OL, Hamilton RL, Becker JT, et al: Severity of cognitive impairment and the clinical diagnosis of AD with Lewy bodies. Neurology 54:1780–1787, 2000b

Lowy FH, Engelsmann F, Lipowski ZJ: Study of cognitive functioning in a medical population. Compr Psychiatry 14:331–338, 1973

Lyketsos CG, Veiel LL, Baker A, et al: A randomized, controlled trial of bright light therapy for agitated behaviors in dementia patients residing in long-term care. Int J Geriatr Psychiatry 14:520–525, 1999

Lyketsos CG, Shepard J-M, Rabins PV: Dementia in elderly persons in a general hospital. Am J Psychiatry 157:704–707, 2000a

Lyketsos CG, Steinberg M, Schantz JT, et al: Mental and behavioral disturbances in dementia: findings from the Cache County Study on Memory in Aging. Am J Psychiatry 157:708–714, 2000b

Mace NL, Rabins PV: The 36-Hour Day: A Family Guide to Caring for Persons with Alzheimer's Disease, Related Dementing Illnesses, and Memory Loss in Later Life. Baltimore, MD, The Johns Hopkins University Press, 1981

Mackenzie IRA: Anti-inflammatory drugs and Alzheimer-type pathology in aging. Neurology 54:732–734, 2000

Maekawa T, Fujii Y, Sadamitsu D, et al: Cerebral circulation and metabolism in patients with septic encephalopathy. Am J Emerg Med 9:139–143, 1991

Maldonado JL, Fernandez F, Levy JK: Acquired immunodeficiency syndrome, in Psychiatric Management in Neurological Disease. Edited by Lauterbach EC. Washington, DC, American Psychiatric Press, 2000, pp 271–295

Manly JJ, Merchant CA, Jacobs DM, et al: Endogenous estrogen levels and Alzheimer's disease among postmenopausal women. Neurology 54:833–837, 2000

Manos PJ, Wu R: The duration of delirium in medical and postoperative patients referred for psychiatric consultation. Ann Clin Psychiatry 9:219–226, 1997

Marcaida G, Minana MD, Grisolia S, et al: Lack of correlation between glutamate-induced depletion of ATP and neuronal death in primary cultures of cerebellum. Brain Res 695:146–150, 1995

Marcantonio ER, Goldman L, Mangione CM, et al: A clinical predictive rule for delirium after elective noncardiac surgery. JAMA 271:134–139, 1994

Marcantonio ER, Flacker JM, Michaels M, et al: Delirium is independently associated with poor functional recovery after hip fracture. J Am Geriatr Soc 48:618–624, 2000

Marder K, Tang M-X, Alfaro B, et al: Risk of Alzheimer's disease in relatives of Parkinson's disease patients with and without dementia. Neurology 52:719–724, 1999

Mark BZ, Krunkel EJ, Fabi MB, et al: Pimozide is effective in delirium secondary to hypercalcemia when other neuroleptics fail. Psychosomatics 34:446–450, 1993

Marsh L: Neuropsychiatric aspects of Parkinson's disease. Psychosomatics 41:15–23, 2000

Marson DC, Annis SM, McInturff B, et al: Error behaviors associated with loss of competency in Alzheimer's disease. Neurology 53:1983–1992, 1999

Massie MJ, Holland J, Glass E: Delirium in terminally ill cancer patients. Am J Psychiatry 140:1048–1050, 1983

Matthew RJ, Meyer JS: Pathogenesis and natural history of transient global amnesia. Stroke 5:303–311, 1974

McCartney JR, Boland R: Understanding and managing behavioral disturbances in the ICU. J Crit Illn 8:87–97, 1993

McDaniel JS, Chung JY, Brown L, et al: Practice guideline for the treatment of patients with HIV/AIDS. Work Group on HIV/AIDS. American Psychiatric Association. Am J Psychiatry 157(11 suppl):1–62, 2000

McIntosh TK, Bush HL, Yeston NS, et al: Beta-endorphin, cortisol, and postoperative delirium: a preliminary report. Psychoneuroendocrinology 10:303–313, 1985

McKeith IG, Ballard CG, Perry RH, et al: Prospective validation on consensus criteria for the diagnosis of dementia with Lewy bodies. Neurology 54:1050–1058, 2000

Meagher DJ, Trzepacz PT: Delirium phenomenology illuminates pathophysiology, management, and course. J Geriatr Psychiatry Neurol 11:150–156, 1998

Meagher DJ, O'Hanlon D, O'Mahony E, et al: A study of environmental strategies in the study of delirium. Br J Psychiatry 168:512–515, 1996

Meagher DJ, O'Hanlon D, O'Mahony E, et al: Relationship between etiology and phenomenologic profile in delirium. J Geriatr Psychiatry Neurol 11:146–149, 1998

Mega M, Cummings JL, Fiorello T, et al: The spectrum of behavioral changes in Alzheimer's disease. Neurology 46:130–135, 1996

Meltzer CC, Price JC, Mathis CA, et al: PET imaging of serotonin type 2A receptors in late-life neuropsychiatric disorders. Am J Psychiatry 156:1871–1878, 1999

Mentis MJ, Horwitz B, Grady CL, et al: Visual cortical dysfunction in Alzheimer's disease evaluated with a temporally graded "stress test" during PET. Am J Psychiatry 153:32–40, 1996

Mercer B, Wepner W, Gardner H, et al: A study of confabulation. Arch Neurol 34:429–433, 1977

Merchant C, Tang M-X, Albert S, et al: The influence of smoking on the risk of Alzheimer's disease. Neurology 52:1408–1412, 1999

Meyer JS, Muramatsu K, Mortel KF, et al: Prospective CT confirms differences between vascular and Alzheimer's dementia. Stroke 26:735–742, 1995

Miller PS, Richardson JS, Jyu CA, et al: Association of low serum anticholinergic levels and cognitive impairment in elderly presurgical patients. Am J Psychiatry 145:342–345, 1988

Mirenda J, Broyles G: Propofol as used for sedation in the ICU. Chest 108:539–548, 1995

Moceri VM, Kukull WA, Emanuel I, et al: Early life risk factors and the development of Alzheimer's disease. Neurology 54:415–420, 2000

Mohs RC, Cohen L: Alzheimer's Disease Assessment Scale (ADAS). Psychopharmacol Bull 24:627–628, 1988

Monette J, Galbaud du Fort G, Fung SH, et al: Evaluation of the Confusion Assessment Method (CAM) as a screening tool for delirium in the emergency room. Gen Hosp Psychiatry 23:20–25, 2001

Montine TJ, Sidell KR, Crews BC, et al: Elevated CSF prostaglandin E2 levels in patients with probable AD. Neurology 53:1495–1498, 1999

Mori E, Hirono N, Yamashita H, et al: Premorbid brain size as a determinant of reserve capacity against intellectual decline in Alzheimer's disease. Am J Psychiatry 154:18–24, 1997

Moroney JT, Bagiella E, Tatemichi TK, et al: Dementia after stroke increases the risk of long term stroke recurrence. Neurology 48:1317–1325, 1997

Morris HR, Lees A, Wood NW: Neurofibrillary tangle parkinsonian disorders—tau pathology and tau genetics. Mov Disord 14:731–736, 1999

Morris JC, Cyrus PA, Orazem J, et al: Metrifonate benefits cognitive, behavioral, and global function in patients with Alzheimer's disease. Neurology 50:1222–1230, 1998

Mussi C, Ferrari R, Ascari S, et al: Importance of serum anticholinergic activity in the assessment of elderly patients with delirium. J Geriatr Psychiatry Neurol 12:82–86, 1999

Nadler JD, Relkin NR, Cohen MS, et al: Mental status testing in the elderly nursing home population. J Geriatr Psychiatry Neurol 8:177–183, 1995

Neary D, Snowden JS, Gustafson L, et al: Frontotemporal lobar degeneration: a consensus on clinical diagnostic criteria. Neurology 51:1546–1554, 1998

Neumann PJ, Hermann RC, Kuntz KM, et al: Cost-effectiveness of donepezil in the treatment of mild or moderate Alzheimer's disease. Neurology 52:1138–1145, 1999

Nicholas LM, Lindsey BA: Delirium presenting with symptoms of depression. Psychosomatics 36:471–479, 1995

Obrist WD: Electroencephalographic changes in normal aging and dementia, in Brain Function in Old Age. Edited by Hoffmeister F, Mhuller C. New York, Springer-Verlag, 1979, pp 102–111

O'Keeffe ST: Delirium in the elderly. Age Ageing 28:5–8, 1999

O'Keeffe ST, Lavan J: The prognostic significance of delirium in older hospital patients. J Am Geriatr Soc 45:174–178, 1997

Olichney JM, Galasko D, Salmon DO, et al: Cognitive decline is faster in Lewy body variant than in Alzheimer's disease. Neurology 51:351–357, 1998

Ongini E, Caporali MG, Massotti M: Stimulation of dopamine D1 receptors by SKF 38393 induces EEG desynchronization and behavioral arousal. Life Sci 37:2327–2333, 1985

Ott A, Stolk RP, van Harskamp F, et al: Diabetes mellitus and the risk of dementia: the Rotterdam Study. Neurology 53:1937–1942, 1999

Pack AI, Millman RP: The lungs in later life, in Pulmonary Diseases and Disorders, 2nd Edition. Edited by Fishman AP. New York, McGraw-Hill, 1988, pp 80–90

Pai M, Yang S: Transient global amnesia: a retrospective study of 25 patients. Chinese Med Journal 62:140–144, 1999

Parnetti L: Therapeutic options in dementia. J Neurol 247:163–168, 2000

Passik SD, Cooper M: Complicated delirium in a cancer patient successfully treated with olanzapine. J Pain Symptom Manage 17:219–223, 1999

Patterson CJS, Gauthier S, Bergman H, et al: The recognition, assessment, and management of dementing disorders: conclusions form the Canadian Consensus Conference on Dementia. Can Med Assoc J 160(suppl):S1–S14, 1999

Paulsen JS, Salmon DP, Monsch AU, et al: Discrimination of cortical from subcortical dementias on the basis of memory and problem-solving tests. J Clin Psychol 51:48–58, 1995a

Paulsen JS, Butters N, Sadek JR, et al: Distinct cognitive profiles of cortical and subcortical dementia in advanced illness. Neurology 45:951–956, 1995b

Paulsen JS, Salmon DP, Thal LJ, et al: Incidence of and risk factors for hallucinations and delusions in patients with probable AD. Neurology 54:1965–1971, 2000

Perry RJ, Hodges JR: Differentiating frontal and temporal variant frontotemporal dementia from Alzheimer's disease. Neurology 54:2277–2284, 2000

Peskind ER: Pharmacologic approaches to cognitive deficits in Alzheimer's disease. J Clin Psychiatry 59(suppl 9):22–27, 1998

Petersen RC, Jack CR, Xu Y-C, et al: Memory and MRI-based hippocampal volumes in aging and AD. Neurology 54:581–587, 2000

Petracca G, Teson A, Chemerinski E, et al: A double-blind placebo-controlled study of clomipramine in depressed patients with Alzheimer's disease. J Neuropsychiatry Clin Neurosci 8:270–275, 1996

Pietrini P, Furey ML, Alexander GE, et al: Association between brain functional failure and dementia severity in Alzheimer's disease: resting versus stimulation PET study. Am J Psychiatry 156:470–473, 1999

Plassman BL, Havlik RJ, Stefens DC, et al: Documented head injury in early adulthood and risk of Alzheimer's disease and other dementias. Neurology 55:1158–1166, 2000

Platt MM, Breitbart W, Smith M, et al: Efficacy of neuroleptics for hypoactive delirium. J Neuropsychiatry 6:66, 1994

Pompei P, Foreman M, Rudberg MA, et al: Delirium in hospitalized older persons: outcomes and predictors. J Am Geriatr Soc 42:809–815, 1994

Porter RJ, Lunn BS, Walker LLM, et al: Cognitive deficit induced by acute tryptophan depletion in patients with Alzheimer's disease. Am J Psychiatry 157:638–640, 2000

Pro JD, Wells CE: The use of the electroencephalogram in the diagnosis of delirium. Diseases of the Nervous System 38:804–808, 1977

Pulsinelli WA, Duffy TE: Regional energy balance in rat brain after transient forebrain ischemia. J Neurochem 40:1500–1503, 1983

Rabins PV: Alzheimer's disease management. J Clin Psychiatry 59(suppl 13):36–38, 1998

Rabins PV, Folstein MF: Delirium and dementia: diagnostic criteria and fatality rates. Br J Psychiatry 140:149–153, 1982

Rabins PV, Blacker D, Bland A, et al: Practice guideline for the treatment of patients with Alzheimer's disease and other dementias of late life. American Psychiatric Association. Am J Psychiatry 154(suppl):1–39, 1997

Rahkonen T, Luukkainen-Markkula R, Paanila S, et al: Delirium episode as a sign of undetected dementia among community dwelling elderly subjects: a 2 year follow up study. J Neurol Neurosurg Psychiatry 69:519–521, 2000

Ranen NG: Huntington's disease, in Psychiatric Management in Neurological Disease. Edited by Lauterbach EC. Washington, DC, American Psychiatric Press, 2000, pp 71–92

Rao V, Lyketsos CG: Delusions in Alzheimer's disease: a review. J Neuropsychiatry Clin Neurosci 10:373–382, 1998

Raskind MA: The clinical interface of depression and dementia. J Clin Psychiatry 59(suppl 10):9–12, 1998

Raskind MA, Cyrus PA, Ruzicka BB, et al: The effects of metrifonate on the cognitive, behavioral, and functional performance of Alzheimer's disease patients. J Clin Psychiatry 60:318–325, 1999

Raskind MA, Peskind ER, Wessel T, et al: Galantamine in AD: a 6-month randomized, placebo controlled trial with a 6-month extension. The Galantamine USA-1 Study Group. Neurology 54:2261–2268, 2000

Rebeck GW, Hyman BT: Apolipoprotein E and Alzheimer disease, in Alzheimer Disease, 2nd Edition. Edited by Terry RD, Katzman R, Bick KL, et al. Philadelphia, PA, Lippincott Williams & Wilkins, 1999, pp 339–346

Reyes RL, Bhattacharyya AK, Heller D: Traumatic head injury: restlessness and agitation as prognosticators of physical and psychological improvement in patients. Arch Phys Med Rehabil 62:20–23, 1981

Riker RR, Fraser GL, Cox PM: Continuous infusion of haloperidol controls agitation in critically ill patients. Crit Care Med 22:433–440, 1994

Ringman JM, Cummings JL: Metrifonate: update on a new antidementia agent. J Clin Psychiatry 60:776–782, 1999

Rizzo M, Anderson SW, Dawson J, et al: Visual attention impairments in Alzheimer's disease. Neurology 54:1954–1959, 2000

Roache JD, Griffiths RR: Comparison of triazolam and pentobarbital: performance impairment, subjective effects, and abuse liability. J Pharmacol Exp Ther 234:120–133, 1985

Robinson RG: The Clinical Neuropsychiatry of Stroke: Cognitive, Behavioral, and Emotional Disorders Following Vascular Brain Injury. New York, Cambridge University Press, 1998

Rockwood K: Acute confusion in elderly medical patients. J Am Geriatr Soc 37:150–154, 1989

Rockwood K: The occurrence and duration of symptoms in elderly patients with delirium. J Gerontol 48:M162–M166, 1993

Rockwood K, Cosway S, Stolee P, et al: Increasing the recognition of delirium in elderly patients. J Am Geriatr Soc 42:252–256, 1994

Rodriguez G, Testa R, Celle G, et al: Reduction in cerebral blood flow in subclinical hepatic encephalopathy and its correlation with plasma-free tryptophan. J Cereb Blood Flow Metab 7:768–772, 1987

Rogers MP, Liang MH, Daltroy LH, et al: Delirium after elective orthopedic surgery: risk factors and natural history. Int J Psychiatry Med 19:109–121, 1989

Rogers SL, Friedhoff LT: Long-term efficacy and safety of donepezil in the treatment of Alzheimer's disease: an interim analysis of the results of a US multicentre open label extension study. Eur Neuropsychopharmacol 8:67–75, 1998

Rogers SL, Farlow MR, Doody RS, et al: A 24-week, double-blind, placebo-controlled trial of donepezil in patients with Alzheimer's disease. Neurology 50:136–145, 1998

Romano J, Engel GL: Delirium, part 1: electroencephalographic data. Archives of Neurology and Psychiatry 51:356–377, 1944

Rosen WG, Mohs RC, Davis KL: A new rating scale for Alzheimer's disease. Am J Psychiatry 141:1356–1364, 1984

Rosenberg J, Kehlet H: Postoperative mental confusion-association with postoperative hypoxemia. Surgery 114:76–81, 1993

Rosenblatt A, Leroi I: Neuropsychiatry of Huntington's disease and other basal ganglia disorders. Psychosomatics 41:24–30, 2000

Rosengren LE, Karlsson J-E, Sogren M, et al: Neurofilament protein levels in CSF are increased in dementia. Neurology 52:1090–1093, 1999

Ross CA, Peyser CE, Shapiro I, et al: Delirium: phenomenologic and etiologic subtypes. Int Psychogeriatr 3:135–147, 1991

Ross GW, Petrovich H, White LR, et al: Characterization of risk factors for vascular dementia: the Honolulu-Asia Aging Study. Neurology 53:337–343, 1999

Roth T, Roehrs R, Wittig R, et al: Benzodiazepines and memory. Br J Clin Pharmacol 18:45–49, 1984

Sano M, Ernesto C, Thomas RG, et al: A controlled trial of selegiline, alpha-tocopherol, or both as treatment for Alzheimer's disease. The Alzheimer's Disease Cooperative Study. N Engl J Med 336:1216–1222, 1997

Saravay SM, Kaplowitz M, Zeman D, et al: The chronology of the mental versus the behavioral and procedural manifestations of delirium and dementia and their impact on length of stay. Presented at the annual meeting of the Academy of Psychosomatic Medicine, Palm Springs, CA, November 2000

Scharf MB, Saskin P, Fletcher K: Benzodiazepine-induced amnesia: clinical laboratory findings. J Clin Psychiatry Monogr 5:14–17, 1987

Scheltens P: Early diagnosis of dementia: neuroimaging. J Neurol 246:16–20, 1999

Schenker S, McCandless DW, Brophy E, et al: Studies on intracerebral toxicity of ammonia. J Clin Invest 46:838–848, 1967

Schifitto G, Sacktor N, Marder K, et al: Randomized trial of the platelet-activating factor antagonist lexiphant in HIV-associated cognitive impairment. Neurology 53:391–396, 1999

Schneider LS, Farlow MR, Henderson VW, et al: Effects of estrogen replacement therapy on response to tacrine in patients with Alzheimer's disease. Neurology 46:1580–1584, 1996

Schor JD, Levkoff SE, Lipsitz LA, et al: Risk factors for delirium in hospitalized elderly. JAMA 267:827–831, 1992

Schwid SR, Weinstein A, Wishart HA, et al: Multiple sclerosis, in Psychiatric Management in Neurological Disease. Edited by Lauterbach EC. Washington, DC, American Psychiatric Press, 2000, pp 249–270

Settle EC, Ayd FJ: Haloperidol: a quarter century of experience. J Clin Psychiatry 44:440–448, 1983

Sharma ND, Rosman HS, Padhi D, et al: Torsades de pointes associated with intravenous haloperidol in critically ill patients. Am J Cardiol 81:238–240, 1998

Shuping JR, Rollinson RD, Toole JF: Transient global amnesia. Ann Neurol 7:281–285, 1980

Siesjo BK: Cerebral circulation and metabolism. J Neurosurg 60:883–908, 1984

Sipahimalani A, Masand PS: Use of risperidone in delirium: case reports. Ann Clin Psychiatry 9:105–107, 1997

Sipahimalani A, Masand PS: Olanzapine in the treatment of delirium. Psychosomatics 39:422–430, 1998

Siroi F: Delirium: 100 cases. Can J Psychiatry 33:375–378, 1988

Small GW: Differential diagnosis and early detection of dementia. Am J Geriatr Psychiatry 6:S26–S33, 1998a

Small GW: The pathogenesis of Alzheimer's disease. J Clin Psychiatry 95(suppl 9):7–14, 1998b

Small GW, Leiter F: Neuroimaging for diagnosis of dementia. J Clin Psychiatry 59(suppl 11):4–7, 1998

Small GW, Chen ST, Komo S, et al: Memory self-appraisal in middle-aged and older adults with the apolipoprotein E-4 allele. Am J Psychiatry 156:1035–1038, 1999

Smith CD, Andersen AH, Kryscio RJ, et al: Altered brain activation in cognitively intact individuals at high risk for Alzheimer's disease. Neurology 53:1391–1396, 1999

Smith CD, Snowdon DA, Wang H, et al: White matter volumes and periventricular white matter hyperintensities in aging and dementia. Neurology 54:838–842, 2000

Smits HA, Boven LA, Pereira CF, et al: Role of macrophage activation in the pathogenesis of Alzheimer's disease and human immunodeficiency virus type I–associated dementia. Eur J Clin Invest 30:526–535, 2000

Soares JC, Gershon S: THA: historical aspects, review of pharmacological properties and therapeutic effects. Dementia 6:225–234, 1995

Somjen GG, Aitken PG: The ionic and metabolic responses associated with neuronal depression of Leao's type in cerebral cortex and hippocampal formation. An Acad Bras Cienc 56:495–504, 1984

Somjen GG, Aitken PG, Balestrino M, et al: Spreading depression-like depolarization and selective vulnerability of neurons. Stroke 21(suppl):III179–III183, 1990

Spencer CM, Noble S: Rivastigmine: a review of its use in Alzheimer's disease. Drugs Aging 13:391–411, 1998

Stahl SM: The new cholinesterase inhibitors for Alzheimer's disease, part I: their similarities are different. J Clin Psychiatry 61:710–711, 2000

Stiefel F, Holland J: Delirium in cancer patients. Int Psychogeriatr 3:333–336, 1991

Stern Y, Albert S, Tang M-X, Tsai W-Y: Rate of memory decline in AD is related to education and occupation: cognitive reserve? Neurology 53:1942–1947, 1999

Stewart JT, Shin KJ: Paroxetine treatment of sexual disinhibition in dementia. Am J Psychiatry 154:1474, 1997

Strauss ME, Ogrocki PK: Confirmation of an association between family history of affective disorder and the depressive syndrome in Alzheimer's disease. Am J Psychiatry 153:1340–1342, 1996

Stuss DT, Alexander MP, Lieberman A, et al: An extraordinary form of confabulation. Neurology 28:1166–1172, 1978

Swenson JR, Erman M, Labell J, et al: Extrapyramidal reactions: neuropsychiatric mimics in patients with AIDS. Gen Hosp Psychiatry 11:248–253, 1989

Tager FA, Fallon BA: Psychiatric and cognitive features of Lyme disease. Psychiatr Ann 31:173–181, 2001

Tariot PN, Erb R, Podgorski CA, et al: Efficacy and tolerability of carbamazepine for agitation and aggression in dementia. Am J Psychiatry 155:54–61, 1998

Tariot PN, Solomon PR, Morris JC, et al: A 5-month, randomized, placebo-controlled trial of galantamine in AD. Neurology 54:2269–2276, 2000

Taylor P: Development of acetylcholinesterase inhibitors in the therapy of Alzheimer's disease. Neurology 51(suppl 1):S30–S35, 1998

Teri L, Logsdon RG, Peskind E, et al: Treatment of agitation in AD: a randomized, placebo controlled clinical trial. Neurology 55:1271–1278, 2000

Tetewsky SJ, Duffy CJ: Visual loss and getting lost in Alzheimer's disease. Neurology 52:958–965, 1999

Thal LJ, Ferguson LM, Mintzer J, et al: A 24-week randomized trial of controlled-release physostigmine in patients with Alzheimer's disease. Neurology 52:1146–1152, 1999

The Dana Consortium on the Therapy of HIV Dementia and Related Cognitive Disorders: Safety and tolerability of the antioxidant OPC-14117 in HIV-associated cognitive impairment. Neurology 49:142–146, 1997

Thomas RI, Cameron DJ, Fahs MC: A prospective study of delirium and prolonged hospital stay. Arch Gen Psychiatry 45:937–940, 1988

Tiraboschi P, Hansen LA, Alford M, et al: Cholinergic dysfunction in diseases with Lewy bodies. Neurology 54:407–411, 2000

Tolbert SR, Fuller MA: Selegiline in treatment of behavioral and cognitive symptoms of Alzheimer disease. Ann Pharmacother 30:1122–1129, 1996

Torres R, Mittal D, Kennedy R: Use of quetiapine in delirium: case reports. Psychosomatics 42:347–349, 2001

Trzepacz PT: The neuropathogenesis of delirium: a need to focus our research. Psychosomatics 35:374–391, 1994

Trzepacz PT: Is there a final common neural pathway in delirium? Focus on acetylcholine and dopamine. Seminars in Clinical Neuropsychiatry 5:132–148, 2000

Trzepacz PT, Wise MG: Neuropsychiatric aspects of delirium, in The American Psychiatric Press Textbook of Neuropsychiatry, 3rd Edition. Edited by Yudofsky SC, Hales RE. Washington, DC, American Psychiatric Press, 1997, pp 447–470

Trzepacz PT, Teague GB, Lipowski ZJ: Delirium and other mental disorders in a general hospital. Gen Hosp Psychiatry 7:101–106, 1985

Trzepacz PT, Maue FR, Coffman G, et al: Neuropsychiatric assessment of liver transplantation candidates: delirium and other psychiatric disorders. Int J Psychiatry Med 7:101–111, 1986

Trzepacz PT, Brenner RP, Coffman G, et al: Delirium in liver transplantation candidates: discriminant analysis of multiple test variables. Biol Psychiatry 24:3–14, 1988a

Trzepacz PT, Baker RW, Greenhouse J: A symptom rating scale for delirium. Psychiatry Res 23:89–97, 1988b

Trzepacz PT, Leavitt M, Congioli K: An animal model for delirium. Psychosomatics 33:404–414, 1992

Trzepacz PT, Ho V, Mallavarapu H: Cholinergic delirium and neurotoxicity associated with tacrine for Alzheimer's dementia. Psychosomatics 37:299–301, 1996

Trzepacz PT, Mulsant BH, Amanda Dew M, et al: Is delirium different when it occurs in dementia? A study using the delirium rating scale. J Neuropsychiatry Clin Neurosci 10:199–204, 1998

Trzepacz PT, Mittal D, Torres R, et al: Validation of the Delirium Rating Scale—Revised—98: comparison with the delirium rating scale and cognitive test for delirium. J Neuropsychiatry Clin Neurosci 13:229–242, 2001

Tsai L, Tsuang MT: The Mini-Mental State Test and computerized tomography. Am J Psychiatry 136:436–439, 1979

Tschanz JT, Welsh-Bohmer KA, Skoog I, et al: Dementia diagnosis from clinical and neuropsychological data compared: the Cache County study. Neurology 54:1290–1296, 2000

Tune LE: Postoperative delirium. Int Psychogeriatr 3:325–332, 1991

Tune LE, Folstein MF: Post-operative delirium. Adv Psychosom Med 15:51–68, 1986

Tune LE, Sunderland T: New cholinergic therapies: treatment tools for the psychiatrist. J Clin Psychiatry 59(suppl 13):31–35, 1998

Tune LE, Carr S, Hoag E, et al: Anticholinergic effects of drugs commonly prescribed for the elderly: potential means for assessing risk of delirium. Am J Psychiatry 149:1393–1394, 1992

van Hemert AM, Vandermast RC, Hengeveld MW, et al: Excess mortality in general hospital patients with delirium: a 5-year follow-up of 519 patients seen in psychiatric consultation. J Psychosom Res 38:339–346, 1994

Varsamis J, Zuchowski T, Maini KK: Survival rates and causes of death in geriatric psychiatric patients. Can Psychiatr Assoc J 17:17–22, 1972

Victor M, Adams RD, Collins GH: The Wernicke-Korsakoff Syndrome and Related Neurologic Disorders Due to Alcoholism and Malnutrition, 2nd Edition. Philadelphia, PA, FA Davis, 1989

Wang PN, Liao SQ, Liu RS, et al: Effects of estrogen on cognition, mood, and cerebral blood flow in AD: a controlled study. Neurology 54:2061–2066, 2000

Waring SC, Rocca WA, Petersen RC, et al: Postmenopausal estrogen replacement therapy and risk of AD: a population-based study. Neurology 52:965–970, 1999

Weddington WW: The mortality of delirium: an underappreciated problem? Psychosomatics 23:1232–1235, 1982

Weiner MF, Risser RC, Cullum M, et al: Alzheimer's disease and its Lewy body variant: a clinical analysis of postmortem verified cases. Am J Psychiatry 153:1269–1273, 1996

Weiner M, Powe NR, Weller WE, et al: Alzheimer's disease under managed care: implications from Medicare utilization and expenditure patterns. J Am Geriatr Soc 46:762–770, 1998

Weiner MF, Martin-Cook K, Foster BM, et al: Effects of donepezil on emotional/behavioral symptoms in Alzheimer's disease patients. J Clin Psychiatry 61:487–492, 2000

Weissman C, Kemper M, Damask M, et al: Effect of routine intensive care interactions on metabolic rate. Chest 86:815–818, 1984

Whalley LJ, Starr JM, Athawes R, et al: Childhood mental ability and dementia. Neurology 55:1455–1459, 2000

Whitehouse PJ: The cholinergic deficit in Alzheimer's disease. J Clin Psychiatry 59(suppl 13):19–22, 1998

Williams-Russo P, Urquhart BL, Sharrock NE, et al: Post-operative delirium: predictors and prognosis in elderly orthopedic patients. J Am Geriatr Soc 40:759–767, 1992

Wilson LM: Intensive care delirium: the effect of outside deprivation in a windowless unit. Arch Intern Med 130:225–226, 1972

Wilson RS, Bennett DA, Gilley DW, et al: Progression of parkinsonian signs in Alzheimer's disease. Neurology 54:1284–1289, 2000

Wise MG, Gray KF, Seltzer B: Delirium, dementia and amnestic disorders, in The American Psychiatric Press Textbook of Neuropsychiatry, 3rd Edition. Edited by Yudofsky SC, Hales RE. Washington, DC, American Psychiatric Press, 1999, pp 317–362

Wright P, Birkett M, David SR, et al: Double-blind, placebo-controlled comparison of intramuscular olanzapine and intramuscular haloperidol in the treatment of acute agitation in schizophrenia. Am J Psychiatry 158:1149–1151, 2001

Yasuno F, Nishikawa T, Nakagawa Y, et al: Functional anatomical study of psychogenic amnesia. Psychiatry Res 99:43–57, 2000

Yesavage JA, Brink TL, Rose TL, et al: Development and validation of a geriatric depression screening scale: a preliminary report. J Psychiatr Res 17:37–49, 1983

Zayas EM, Grossberg GT: The treatment of psychosis in late life. J Clin Psychiatry 59(suppl):5–10, 1998

Zee-Cheng CS, Mueller CE, Siefert CF, et al: Haloperidol and torsades de pointes (letter). Ann Intern Med 102:418, 1985

Zerr I, Schultz-Schaeffer WJ, Giese A, et al: Current clinical diagnosis in Creutzfeldt-Jakob disease: identification of uncommon variants. Ann Neurol 48:323–329, 2000

Zhu L, Fratiglioni L, Guo Z, et al: Incidence of stroke in relation to cognitive function and dementia in the Kungsholmen Project. Neurology 54:2103–2107, 2000

Zou Y, Cole MG, Primeau FJ, et al: Detection and diagnosis of delirium in the elderly: psychiatric diagnosis, confusion assessment method, or consensus diagnosis? Int Psychogeriatr 10:303–308, 1998

Zubenko GS, Hughes HB, Stiffler JS: Neurobiological correlates of a putative risk allele for Alzheimer's disease on chromosome 12q. Neurology 52:725–732, 1999

Zubenko GS, Tepley I, Winwood E, et al: Prospective study of increased platelet membrane fluidity as a risk factor for Alzheimer's disease: results at 5 years. Am J Psychiatry 153:420–423, 1996

Substance Use Disorders

Avram H. Mack, M.D.

John E. Franklin Jr., M.D., M.Sc.

Richard J. Frances, M.D.

Accounts of use and abuse of substances, including alcohol, coca leaves, opium, and cannabis, are as old as civilization. Physicians, philosophers, theologians, poets, and politicians have long debated the merits and harmful effects of such substances. In the United States, substance use disorders constitute a tremendous medical and social challenge: 13.8% of all Americans will have an alcohol-related substance use disorder in their lifetimes, an estimated 14.8 million Americans were current users of illicit drugs in 1999, and the monetary cost to the nation, including the related aspects of crime, absenteeism, and treatment, is estimated to be greater than $275 billion annually. Those in every category of health care—physicians, nurses, psychologists, social workers, alcohol and drug counselors, and rehabilitation therapists—and students in all of these areas are constantly faced with treatment choices and options that are critical to the care of patients with substance use disorders. In recent decades, advances in communication, technology, and medicine have led to production of new drugs, wider distribution and marketing of drugs produced in many parts of the world, and new routes of administration of drugs that have long been available. Fueled by widespread demand in the United States, there has been increased cocaine production in and distribution from Latin America. Thus, substance use disorders are significant conditions that can be understood via the biopsychosocial model.

The Disease Model of Addiction

Models for the definition of a disease or a disorder abound in medicine; they may focus on the lack of homeostasis, discomfort, difference from the norm, discernible biological components, response to biological treatment, or lack of perfect health; definitions can be narrow or broad, culturally defined or not, relatively stable or changing over time. In this context, more than in any other area of medicine, the validity of substance use disorders has been challenged. Some critics have reductionistically asserted that substance abuse is simply a moral problem in which the choice to abuse a substance deserves shame and punishment more than empathy and treatment. Others assume that addiction is simply excessive or compulsive use of one or another substance. In current models, three (probably intertwined) aspects of the addictions are seen as central to their understanding as diseases: 1) addiction is the compulsion to use the substance, 2) addiction is a "brain disease," and 3) addiction is a chronic medical disorder.

That addiction is a "compulsion" means that the individual uses the substance at all costs, even in the face of severe negative consequences. The evidence that there is a biological component to addiction is growing. There is a basis for a genetic vulnerability to abuse of particular substances; there are biological markers in such vulnerable persons. Furthermore, research is focusing on the long-term changes in synaptic architecture and alterations in neurotransmitter physiology that may form the basis of the position that the brain of the addicted patient is different as a result of his or her excessive use—a difference that creates and maintains the compulsion to use (Leshner 1997). By no means should this perspective diminish the social, environmental, or personal aspects of addiction. Biological aspects are important at least in that they lend support to the disease model of addiction.

Another development is the conceptualization of addiction as a chronic medical disease. Addictions have chronic courses characterized by multiple relapses from abstinence to use. The individual abuser suffers from complications of use and also from social and economic problems as a result of abuse. More and more those involved in the treatment of the addictions have compared substance use disorders with other chronic medical disorders such as diabetes mellitus, arthritis, and asthma—diseases that we can treat but perhaps never entirely cure, and in which relapses are to be expected, especially as they relate to choices patients make. In this view, the former cocaine abuser who relapses after entering the environment in which he previously used the drug is analogous to the child with asthma who walks into a smoky room and develops an attack (O'Brien and McLellan 1996).

If one accepts this view, a logical conclusion might be that society ought to stop the moralizing about substance abuse that has impeded the recognition of, research of, and care for these disorders for generations. It is hoped that society will rid itself of the view that dependence and abuse are the "fault" of the individual and will instead emphasize personal responsibility in seeking and accepting treatment. After all, in our legal system individuals are for the most part held accountable for acts committed during intoxication. The "compulsion" position could lead to a greater emphasis on treatment rather than punishment, a reduction in overly harsh sentencing such as that mandated by the Rockefeller Laws in New York State, and use of drug courts and sentencing alternatives that emphasize treatment for nonviolent drug crimes. On the other hand, these concepts might be misconstrued as implying that abuse, dependence, or even relapse are acceptable and that abstinence is irrelevant, which could lead to legalization of drug use. Most addiction and legal experts are against legalization because it would result in increased drug availability, increased drug use, and increased prevalence and complications of addictions.

Neurobiology of the Addictions: Clinical Implications of Research Findings

Advances in cellular and molecular biology have been staggering over the past decade, and this is no less the case in psychiatry and the addictions. There is increasing evidence that craving and addiction to virtually all substances of abuse are related to the dopaminergic systems in the brain—especially the mesolimbic reward system and the areas to which it projects: the limbic system and the orbitofrontal cortex (Leshner and Koob 1999). This even has been seen in the case of cannabinoids (Diana et al. 1998), and it may be the result not simply of homeostatic adaptations of neurons but even of neural plasticity and synaptic rearrangement that follow from activation of particular signal transduction pathways between stimulus and gene expression. Thus addiction is not only a degenerative disease or a lesion but also a learned process in which long-term memory occurs (inappropriately) at the molecular level. Such a view diminishes the personal role in relapse (O'Brien and McLellan 1996), an assessment with which many clinicians and self-help groups will adamantly disagree. A full discussion of the burgeoning science of addiction is beyond the scope of this clinically oriented chapter; the reader is referred to more extensive manuscripts on this topic (Kreek 2000; Volkow and Fowler 2000; Volkow et al. 2001).

General Epidemiology of Substance Use Disorders

Substance use disorders are likely the most prevalent of all types of medical and mental disorders, and they cost society greatly. There are a number of studies from which we have gathered most of our data on substance use disorders: the Drug Abuse Warning Network (DAWN; Office of Applied Studies 2000a), which provides ongoing surveillance data; the Monitoring the Future study, an ongoing study of substance abuse among American high school and college students and young adults (Johnston et al. 2001); the National Household Survey (NHS; Office of Applied Studies 2000b); the Epidemiologic Catchment Area study (ECA; Regier et al. 1990); and the National Comorbidity Survey (NCS; Kessler et al. 1997). Despite massive efforts in interdiction, prevention, and treatment, substance abuse is not waning in the United States; complications of abuse make it a problem of great magnitude. There are a number of factors that hinder efforts to reduce use.

Medical and psychiatric problems associated with substance use disorders produce morbidity and mortality that hamper efforts to treat these disorders. Such problems include the effects of intoxication, overdose, and withdrawal and the consequences of chronic use: malnutrition, poor self-care, injection of unknown substances, cognitive disorder, endocarditis, and HIV among intravenous drug users. Fortunately, the newest antiretroviral medications have effected a decline in the prevalence and incidence of HIV contracted by intravenous drug use (Des Jarlais et al. 2000), but in general the medical, psychiatric, and dental complications of substance abuse pose a serious challenge both for those attempting to become sober and for their caretakers.

Systems of care can impede proper treatment. Many psychiatric halfway houses will not accept alcoholics, and halfway houses for substance abusers will often not accept patients on medications. Confrontational methods useful in therapeutic communities and self-help groups may be detrimental to those with more severe psychiatric illness. The full-service facilities with psychiatric treatment and rehabilitation are expensive; however, they represent a healthy integration of treatment approaches. Managed care has driven a number of clinical changes, including the forging of health care systems that attempt to save money by coordinating care and reducing unnecessary spending or interventions. The emphasis is on outpatient care, including outpatient detoxification. In recent years, managed care has reduced the amount spent on addiction treatment by 75%, and many of the cuts have been detrimental to good care.

Finally, despite efforts at interdiction, the Internet has become an important tool with which those who abuse drugs can obtain information about drugs of abuse: how to get them, how to hide them, how to grow plants, who to buy from and who not to buy from, and where the interdiction agencies are concentrating their energies and attention (Halpern and Pope 2001).

In 1999, 14.8 million Americans were current users of illicit drugs, an increase from 13.6 million in 1998 (Office of Applied Studies 2000b). An estimated 3.6 million Americans met diagnostic criteria for dependence on illicit drugs in 1999, and 1.1 million of these were ages 12–17 years (Office of Applied Studies 2000b). Between 1997 and 1998, drug abuse deaths reported to DAWN increased from 9,565 to 10,091 (Office of Applied Studies 2000a). Use varies by age to a great degree, and the rates of use are changing.

The most recent data show that, in general, use by adolescents ages 12–17 years is declining: 11.4% in 1997, 9.9% in 1998, and 9.0% in 1999. The rate was highest (16.3%) in 1979, declined to 5.3% in 1992, and has fluctuated since. Unfortunately, at the same time, use by young adults (ages 18–25 years) has increased, from 14.7% in 1997 to 18.8% in 1999 (Office of Applied Studies 2000b). Between 1997 and 1998, there was no change in the proportion of youth ages 12–17 years who reported that using cigarettes, marijuana, cocaine, or alcohol was risky, nor were there changes in this population's perceptions regarding ease of obtaining marijuana (56%) or heroin (21%) (Office of Applied Studies 2000b).

Measures of the monetary cost of the addictions include per capita consumption, lifetime and point prevalence, morbidity and mortality, fetal effects of drugs, health care costs, and total cost of lost work time. The actual monetary cost to the nation is estimated to be greater than $275 billion annually, which includes the related aspects of crime, absenteeism, and treatment. Also, 30%–55% of the mentally ill have a substance use disorder, a circumstance that greatly multiplies the cost of treating primary mental illness.

Alcohol

At least 9 million Americans are alcohol dependent, and another 6 million abuse alcohol. The ECA study concluded that 13.8% of Americans will have an alcohol-related substance use disorder at some time in their lives. The current annual costs attributed to alcohol abuse are $166.5 billion, almost double the annual cost of the late 1980s (Harwood et al. 1998). The rate of frequent drinking among pregnant women, even when controlled for social characteristics, was approximately 4 times higher in 1995 than in 1991 (3.5% in 1995 and 0.8% in 1991) (Centers for Disease Control and Prevention 1997a).

Although consumption of alcoholic beverages is illegal for those under 21 years of age, 10.4 million current drinkers were ages 12–20 years in 1999. Of this group, 6.8 million engaged in binge drinking, including 2.1 million who would also be classified as heavy drinkers. No statistically significant changes in the rates of underage drinking have occurred since 1994.

Morbidity and mortality secondary to alcohol depend on the culture and nationality of the user. In America, the average person over age 14 years consumes 2.77 gallons of absolute alcohol annually, an amount less than in Russia, France, Scandinavia, and Ireland but more than in Islamic and Mediterranean cultures or in China. In the United States, approximately 10% of persons who drink consume half of all the alcohol sold. With suicide ranking as the eighth leading cause of death in 1998 and liver disease the tenth (Murphy 2000), the estimate that 100,000 deaths per year are alcohol related is of importance. Alcoholism is the leading risk factor for cirrhosis even though less than 10% of alcoholic persons develop the disease. About 25% of general hospital admissions involve problems related to chronic alcohol use (e.g., cirrhosis, cardiomyopathy) or withdrawal (e.g., seizures, pneumonia, liver failure, subdural hematomas).

There is a high association between alcohol and violence. The suicide rate in persons with alcoholism is about 5%–6%, which is much higher than in the general population. Alcohol is a risk factor for violence. Nearly

50% of violent deaths in the United States are linked with alcohol (Institute of Medicine 1999), and in Eastern European nations alcohol is involved in 33% of all deaths in the 15- to 29-year age group (World Health Organization 2001). In the United States the proportion of traffic fatalities that were alcohol related was 38.5% in 1997 (Centers for Disease Control and Prevention 1999a).

Sedatives, Hypnotics, and Anxiolytics

Since 1976 there has been a decline in the abuse of benzodiazepines and sedative–hypnotics. Abuse of these agents is related to the high prevalence of anxiety disorders. Barbiturate overdoses, once frequently the cause of emergency room visits, have decreased with the declining popularity of barbiturate prescription. Barbiturates have been replaced by benzodiazepines, which are relatively safer. Abuse of the substances in this category is often iatrogenically induced.

Opioids

An estimated 149,000 persons used heroin for the first time in 1999. Between 1994 and 1999, the rate of initiation for youths was at its highest level since the early 1970s (Office of Applied Studies 2000b). The estimated number of current heroin users was 68,000 in 1993, 117,000 in 1994, 196,000 in 1995, 216,000 in 1996, 325,000 in 1997, 130,000 in 1998, and 200,000 in 1999 (Office of Applied Studies 2000b). Lifetime heroin prevalence estimates have ranged from 2.3 million in 1979 to 1.7 million in 1992, 2 million in 1997, and 2.4 million in 1998 (Office of Applied Studies 2000b). The ECA study showed that opioid use was greater in males, with a male:female ratio of between 3:1 and 4:1. Heroin abuse is usually a problem in urban males and in the 18- to 25-year-old group. A higher incidence of nonmedical use of opioids other than heroin (e.g., "painkillers") is found among whites (12% versus 7% for minorities). The rate of heroin abuse among minorities is twice as high as that in the general population—a figure that may be skewed because whites account for fewer admissions to public facilities and because there may be many white middle-class addicts who do not respond to surveys. Greater psychopathology is found in cultural groups in which heroin is less endemic. Among lifetime heroin users, the proportion who had ever smoked, sniffed, or snorted heroin increased from 55% in 1994 to 75% in 1998, yet during the same period, the proportion who had ever injected heroin remained relatively unchanged (49% in 1994; 54% in 1998) (Office of Applied Studies 2000b).

Cocaine

Cocaine use reached a peak of 5.7 million persons (3.0% of the population) in 1985. In 1999 an estimated 1.5 million (0.7%) Americans ages 12 and older were current users of cocaine (Office of Applied Studies 2000b). The highest current cocaine use in 1998 was for those ages 18–25 years. The estimated number of current crack cocaine users was 413,000 in 1999 (Office of Applied Studies 2000b). In 1998 current cocaine use rates were 1.3% for blacks, 1.3% for Hispanics, and 0.7% for whites. Use increased significantly among Hispanics between 1997 and 1998, from 0.8% to 1.3% (Office of Applied Studies 2000b). Cocaine use is inversely related to education. Cocaine use is highest among the unemployed; in 1998 3.4% of unemployed adults (ages 18 and older) were current cocaine users. More men than women use cocaine.

Amphetamines

The estimated number of persons who have tried methamphetamine is 4.7 million (Office of Applied Studies 2000b). The diversion and abuse of amphetamines, which are often prescribed in the treatment of narcolepsy, weight disorders, attention-deficit/hyperactivity disorder (ADHD), and depressive disorders, peaked in the 1960s. With better control, rates of legal use, diversion, and illegal use declined. Yet a substantial increase in use occurred in the 1990s, especially in California. Amphetamine-related admissions to publicly funded treatment programs increased from 14,000 in 1992 to 53,000 in 1997 (Office of Applied Studies 2000b). Methamphetamine-related emergency department episodes more than tripled, from 4,900 in 1991 to 17,400 in 1994 (Centers for Disease Control and Prevention 1995). From 1991 to 1994, the number of methamphetamine-related deaths nearly tripled, from 151 to 433, and most were in persons who were 26–44 years old (66%), male (80%), and white (80%). Nearly all deaths involved at least one other drug, most often alcohol (30%), heroin (23%), or cocaine (21%) (Office of Applied Studies 2000a).

Phencyclidine and Ketamine

PCP abuse is epidemic in certain areas of the United States and is often associated with violent and bizarre behavior. It reached a nadir in the 1980s but has become more popular again.

Ketamine has quickly become a major substance of abuse, especially among youth and young adults. It was first added to the Monitoring the Future survey in 2000, when the prevalence of ketamine abuse was 1.6%, 2.1%, and 2.5% in grades 8, 10, and 12, respectively (Johnston et al. 2001).

Hallucinogens

In 1999 there were an estimated 1.2 million new hallucinogen users, and the rate of current use was 0.4% (Office of Applied Studies 2000b). To date there exist 12 natural hallucinogens and more than 100 synthetic hallucinogens. Lysergic acid diethylamide (LSD) is thought to have achieved its greatest popularity in the 1960s and 1970s; however, it is once again becoming popular in some high school communities. Some students have discovered that LSD is not easily detectable in urine samples. Although few new drugs of the indolealkylamine derivatives (of which LSD is one) have been synthesized, a steady flow of new ("designer") phenylalkylamine derivatives has appeared, including the ring-substituted amphetamines such as MDA, MDMA (old and new "Ecstasy"), and MDEA.

MDMA first appeared at "raves" around 1995. It has grown in popularity and is increasingly implicated in deaths. Its use and perceived availability have moved from cities in the Northeast to all areas of the United States. MDMA is mainly used among youth and young adult groups. Between 1999 and 2000, the prevalence of MDMA use increased by 3.1%, 5.4%, and 8.2% among students in grades 8, 10, and 12, respectively. The perceived availability of MDMA has risen dramatically, whereas the perception of risk or disapproval has changed little in recent years (Johnston et al. 2001). Compared with other drugs, MDMA is strongly and significantly associated with high-risk sexual behaviors among gay males in dance clubs in New York City (Klitzman et al. 2000).

Cannabis

Worldwide, cannabis may be the most widely abused illicit substance of all; in the United States it accounts for 75% of all illicit drug use. Marijuana use peaked among adolescents in the 1970s, but it continues to be a gateway drug for other substances of abuse. The number of individuals using marijuana for the first time in the United States was estimated at 2.3 million in 1999. Frequent users were estimated to number 6.8 million in 1998, significantly more than in 1995 (5.3 million) (Office of Applied Studies 2000b). Among females, the age at first use is declining even as the prevalence of secondary problems is rising (Greenfield and O'Leary 1999). The prevalence of current marijuana use among adolescents more than doubled between 1992 and 1995, from 3.4% to 8.2%. About 1 in 12 adolescents ages 12–17 years (8.3%) were current marijuana users in 1998 (Office of Applied Studies 2000b). The prevalence of marijuana use in youth peaked in 1979 at 14.2%, declined to 3.4% in 1992, then climbed to 8.2% in 1995 and has fluctuated near that point since then (7.1 in 1996, 9.4% in 1997, and 8.3% in 1998) (Office of Applied Studies 2000b).

Nicotine

Tobacco is the leading cause of preventable morbidity and mortality in the United States. Approximately 430,000 deaths annually (Centers for Disease Control and Prevention 1999b) are attributable to tobacco use. The prevalence of use is increasing: in 1999 an estimated 30.2% of Americans (66.8 million) used cigarettes, an increase from the number in 1998 (27.7%, 60 million).

Tobacco use is tied to race and ethnicity: prevalence of use in 1999 was significantly higher among American Indians/Alaska Natives (43.1%) than among most other groups, including non-Hispanic blacks (26.6%), non-Hispanic whites (31.9%), Hispanics (24.4%), and Asians/Pacific Islanders (18.6%). Use is higher among persons living below the poverty level (33.3%) than among those at or above that level (24.6%). Although cigarette use is decreasing in men, it has increased in women.

It is alarming that of the 2.1 million Americans who began smoking cigarettes in 1997, more than 50% were younger than age 18 years (Office of Applied Studies 2000b). Among adults ages 18–25 years, the rate rose from 34.6% in 1994 to 41.6% in 1998 and fell to 39.7% in 1999 (Office of Applied Studies 2000b). In a 1999 Centers for Disease Control and Prevention survey, 70.4% of all students reported having smoked at least once in their life (Centers for Disease Control and Prevention 2000). In 1999 youths ages 12–17 who currently smoked cigarettes were 7.3 times more likely to use illicit drugs and 16 times more likely to drink heavily than were their nonsmoking peers.

Inhalants

Inhalant use stabilized in 1996 after increasing for 4 years, according to the National High School Senior and Young Adult Survey (Johnston et al. 1997). Fortunately, annual prevalence has declined in grades 8 through 12 as the view that these agents are dangerous has increased. Inhalants tend to be used by socioeconomically deprived males 13–15 years old and in certain subcultures (e.g., American and Mexican Indians). Inhalant intoxication has been linked with aggressive, disruptive, antisocial behavior as well as with poor performance in school, increased family disruption, and abuse of other drugs.

Polysubstance Problems

Polysubstance abuse—with combined use of alcohol, heroin, cocaine, methadone, and/or tobacco—is on the rise. In the ECA study, 30% of alcoholic individuals also met criteria for another substance use disorder. The ECA study found that the most common comorbid psychiatric condition was another substance use disorder: nicotine dependence.

Use of combinations of substances has been especially noted in young and female patients. Teenagers tend to progress from alcohol and tobacco use to marijuana use and use of barbiturates, codeine, or other opioids before abusing heroin. Deaths related to overdose are more commonly associated with combinations of alcohol, depressants, and heroin than with cocaine, which has recently received greater public attention. Of note, treatment for one substance usually has the effect of lowering the use of others (e.g., a methadone maintenance program reduces comorbid cocaine abuse).

Substance-Related Disorders: DSM-IV-TR Definitions and Diagnostic Categories

In DSM-IV (American Psychiatric Association 1994) and DSM-IV-TR (American Psychiatric Association 2000), disorders related to substances are divided into two groups. The first, *substance use disorders*, contains substance dependence and substance abuse. The second group, *substance-induced disorders*, encompasses substance intoxication and substance withdrawal as well as other cognitive or psychiatric symptoms that are judged to be a direct physiological consequence of a substance.

DSM-IV-TR provides generic definitions of *dependence*, *abuse*, *intoxication*, and *withdrawal*, as well as various specific definitions for substance-induced syndromes. The reader is referred to DSM-IV-TR for full and detailed definitions of each diagnostic category. This section discusses particular issues in the definition of the more complex conditions.

The following general points are important when considering a DSM-IV-TR substance-related disorder diagnosis:

1. In DSM-IV-TR, the term *substance* can refer to a drug of abuse, a medication, or a toxin, and it need not be limited to those that are "psychoactive."

2. "Organic" is a term absent from DSM-IV-TR. The conditions previously designated "substance-induced organic mental disorders" are now classified in the substance use disorders section. DSM-IV-TR does distinguish substance-induced *mental* disorders from substance-induced disorders that are due to a general medical condition and those that have no known etiology.

3. DSM-IV-TR diagnoses require the presence of "clinically significant distress and impairment in social, occupational, or other important areas of functioning."

4. DSM-IV-TR diagnoses require that the symptoms not be due to a general medical condition and not be better accounted for by another mental disorder.

Substance Use Disorders

Substance Dependence

Dependence is a state of cognitive, behavioral, and physiological features that, together, signify continued use despite significant substance-related problems. It is a pattern of repeated self-administration that can result in tolerance, withdrawal, and compulsive drug-taking behavior. In DSM-IV-TR a patient must exhibit at least 3 behaviors from a 7-item, polythetic criteria set over a 12-month period (Table 8–1). Although neither tolerance nor withdrawal is necessary or sufficient for a diagnosis of substance dependence, a past history of tolerance or withdrawal is usually associated with a more severe clinical course. *Tolerance*—the need for greatly increased amounts of a substance to produce a desired effect or a greatly diminished effect with constant use of the same amount of the substance—may be difficult to discern by history when the substance used is of unknown purity. In such situations, quantitative laboratory tests may help. *Withdrawal* occurs when blood or tissue concentrations of a substance decline in an individual who had maintained prolonged heavy use of the substance. In this state, the person will likely take the substance to relieve or to avoid unpleasant withdrawal symptoms.

According to DSM-IV-TR, dependence can be further specified as mild, moderate, or severe, and remission may be noted to be early partial, early full, sustained full, or sustained partial. The presence or absence of tolerance or withdrawal, other signs of "physiological dependence," current use of agonist therapy, and placement in a controlled environment may also be specified.

Substance Abuse

In DSM-IV-TR, substance *abuse* includes continued use despite significant problems caused by the use in those who do not meet criteria for substance dependence.

TABLE 8–1. DSM-IV-TR criteria for substance dependence

A maladaptive pattern of substance use, leading to clinically significant impairment or distress, as manifested by three (or more) of the following, occurring at any time in the same 12-month period:

(1) tolerance, as defined by either of the following:
   (a) a need for markedly increased amounts of the substance to achieve intoxication or desired effect
   (b) markedly diminished effect with continued use of the same amount of the substance
(2) withdrawal, as manifested by either of the following:
   (a) the characteristic withdrawal syndrome for the substance (refer to Criteria A and B of the criteria sets for withdrawal from the specific substances)
   (b) the same (or a closely related) substance is taken to relieve or avoid withdrawal symptoms
(3) the substance is often taken in larger amounts or over a longer period than was intended
(4) there is a persistent desire or unsuccessful efforts to cut down or control substance use
(5) a great deal of time is spent in activities necessary to obtain the substance (e.g., visiting multiple doctors or driving long distances), use the substance (e.g., chain-smoking), or recover from its effects
(6) important social, occupational, or recreational activities are given up or reduced because of substance use
(7) the substance use is continued despite knowledge of having a persistent or recurrent physical or psychological problem that is likely to have been caused or exacerbated by the substance (e.g., current cocaine use despite recognition of cocaine-induced depression, or continued drinking despite recognition that an ulcer was made worse by alcohol consumption)

Specify if:
With Physiological Dependence: evidence of tolerance or withdrawal
   (i.e., either Item 1 or 2 is present)
Without Physiological Dependence: no evidence of tolerance or withdrawal (i.e., neither Item 1 nor 2 is present)
Course specifiers:
Early Full Remission
Early Partial Remission
Sustained Full Remission
Sustained Partial Remission
On Agonist Therapy
In a Controlled Environment

"Failure to fulfill major role obligations" is a criterion. To fulfill an abuse criterion, the substance-related problem must have occurred repeatedly or persistently during the same 12 months. The criteria for abuse do not include tolerance, withdrawal, or compulsive use (Table 8–2).

TABLE 8–2. DSM-IV-TR criteria for substance abuse

A. A maladaptive pattern of substance use leading to clinically significant impairment or distress, as manifested by one (or more) of the following, occurring within a 12-month period:
   (1) recurrent substance use resulting in a failure to fulfill major role obligations at work, school, or home (e.g., repeated absences or poor work performance related to substance use; substance-related absences, suspensions, or expulsions from school; neglect of children or household)
   (2) recurrent substance use in situations in which it is physically hazardous (e.g., driving an automobile or operating a machine when impaired by substance use)
   (3) recurrent substance-related legal problems (e.g., arrests for substance-related disorderly conduct)
   (4) continued substance use despite having persistent or recurrent social or interpersonal problems caused or exacerbated by the effects of the substance (e.g., arguments with spouse about consequences of intoxication, physical fights)
B. The symptoms have never met the criteria for substance dependence for this class of substance.

Substance abuse cannot be applied to caffeine and nicotine. The term *abuse* should not be used as a blanket term for "use," "misuse," or "hazardous use."

Substance-Induced Disorders

Substance Intoxication

Substance *intoxication* (Table 8–3) is a reversible syndrome caused by recent exposure to a substance. It is often associated, and may be concurrently diagnosed, with substance abuse or dependence. The category does not apply to nicotine. Different substances (sometimes even different substance classes) may produce identical symptoms during intoxication. DSM-IV-TR allows specification of the presence of "perceptual disturbances" in intoxication by some substances.

Substance Withdrawal

Substance *withdrawal* (Table 8–4) is a behavioral, physiological, and cognitive state caused by cessation of, or reduction in, heavy and prolonged substance use. Perhaps all withdrawing individuals crave the substance to reduce withdrawal symptoms. Signs and symptoms vary according to the substance used; most symptoms are the opposite of those observed in intoxication by the same substance. Withdrawal is usually associated with substance

TABLE 8–3. DSM-IV-TR criteria for substance intoxication

A. The development of a reversible substance-specific syndrome due to recent ingestion of (or exposure to) a substance. **Note:** Different substances may produce similar or identical syndromes.
B. Clinically significant maladaptive behavioral or psychological changes that are due to the effect of the substance on the central nervous system (e.g., belligerence, mood lability, cognitive impairment, impaired judgment, impaired social or occupational functioning) and develop during or shortly after use of the substance.
C. The symptoms are not due to a general medical condition and are not better accounted for by another mental disorder.

TABLE 8–4. DSM-IV-TR criteria for substance withdrawal

A. The development of a substance-specific syndrome due to the cessation of (or reduction in) substance use that has been heavy and prolonged.
B. The substance-specific syndrome causes clinically significant distress or impairment in social, occupational, or other important areas of functioning.
C. The symptoms are not due to a general medical condition and are not better accounted for by another mental disorder.

dependence. DSM-IV-TR allows for specification of "perceptual disturbances" in withdrawal from some substances.

Substance-Induced Mental Disorders

Diagnosis of a substance-induced mental disorder requires evidence of intoxication or withdrawal. Some disorders can persist after the substance has been eliminated from the body, but symptoms lasting more than 4 weeks after acute intoxication or withdrawal are considered manifestations either of a primary mental disorder or of a substance-induced persisting disorder. The differential diagnosis is complicated: withdrawal from some substances (e.g., sedatives) may partially mimic intoxication with others (e.g., amphetamines). That a syndrome (e.g., depression with suicidal ideation) is caused by a substance (e.g., cocaine) in no way diminishes its clinical import. In most cases, intoxication and withdrawal are distinguished from substance-induced disorders of the same class because symptoms in the latter disorders are in excess of those usually associated with intoxication or withdrawal from the substance and are severe enough to warrant independent clinical attention.

Alcohol

Alcohol Use Disorders

Although some groups have referred to alcohol dependence as "alcoholism," the term has no operational definition. It is important to distinguish alcohol abuse from dependence because the prognostic consequences of the two are different: whereas the alcohol-abusing person has some chance of drinking in a controlled manner, the alcohol-dependent person *must* become abstinent. Of course, it is difficult to predict which abusers will go on to dependence. Abstinence is the safest course and prevents progression to dependence in those likely to do so.

Alcohol Dependence

The DSM-IV-TR diagnostic criteria for alcohol dependence follow those for other substance disorders as delineated in Table 8–1. Specifying the presence of physiological dependence has prognostic value because it indicates a more severe clinical course (Schuckit et al. 1998), especially when withdrawal rather than tolerance is the basis on which physiological dependence is diagnosed.

Alcohol Abuse

Alcohol abuse requires fewer symptoms than does dependence and is diagnosed only if dependence has been ruled out. A person's drinking when driving and a physician's drinking before seeing patients are two examples of alcohol abuse (i.e., substance use that jeopardizes a person's ability to fulfill major role obligations). The development of medical and psychiatric complications related to alcohol use also helps in making the diagnosis.

Alcohol-Induced Disorders

Alcohol Intoxication

Alcohol intoxication is time-limited and reversible, with onset depending on tolerance, amount ingested, and amount absorbed. It is affected by interactions with other substances, by medical status, and by individual variation. Table 8–5 lists blood alcohol levels and corresponding clinical features of a nonhabituated patient. For a habituated patient, chronic alcoholic presentation can vary greatly. Intoxication stages range from mild inebriation to anesthesia, coma, respiratory depression, and death. Relative to degree of tolerance, increasing blood alcohol levels can lead to euphoria, mild coordination problems, ataxia, confusion, and decreased consciousness, and then, with blood alcohol levels greater than 0.4

TABLE 8–5. Blood alcohol level (BAL) and typical clinical presentation in the nontolerant, alcohol-intoxicated patient

BAL (mg/dL)	Clinical presentation
30	Attention difficulties (mild), euphoria
50	Coordination problems, driving is legally impaired
100	Ataxia, drunk driving
200	Confusion, decreased consciousness
>400	Anesthesia, ?coma, ?death

mg% (milligrams per 100 mL of blood), to anesthesia, coma, and death. Yet chronic heavy drinkers maintain high blood alcohol levels with fewer effects. Alcohol intoxication may affect heart rate and electroencephalogram (EEG) readings and may cause nystagmus; slowed reaction times; and behavioral changes such as mood lability, impaired judgment, impaired social or occupational functioning, cognitive problems, and disinhibition of sexual or aggressive impulses. Alcohol intoxication closely resembles sedative, hypnotic, or anxiolytic intoxication. Individual and cultural variations of tolerance may influence symptom presentation. Other neurological conditions, such as cerebellar ataxia from multiple sclerosis, may mimic some of the physiological signs and symptoms of alcohol intoxication. "Alcohol idiosyncratic intoxication" is not present in DSM-IV-TR but could be diagnosed as alcohol use disorder not otherwise specified (NOS). It should be noted that the odor of alcohol should not discount the possibility that more than one substance has been used.

Alcohol Withdrawal

Any relative drop in an individual's blood alcohol level can precipitate withdrawal, even during continued alcohol consumption. Features of withdrawal include coarse tremor of hands, tongue, or eyelids; nausea or vomiting; malaise or weakness, autonomic hyperactivity; orthostatic hypotension; anxiety, depressed mood, or irritability; transient hallucinations (generally poorly formed) or illusions; headache; and insomnia. The generalized tremor, which is coarse and of intermediate frequency (5–7 Hz), can worsen with motor activity or emotional stress; it is most likely to be observed on extension of the hands or tongue. Often patients complain only of feeling shaky inside. Careful attention should be paid to vital signs in a suspected alcoholic individual. Symptoms peak 24–48 hours after the last drink and subside in 5–7 days even without treatment. Insomnia and irritability may last 10 days or longer. The withdrawal symptoms may precipitate a relapse. Major motor seizures ("rum fits") occur and are more likely to develop in those with a history of epilepsy and those with other medical illnesses, malnutrition, fatigue, and depression.

Alcohol Intoxication Delirium or Withdrawal Delirium

Delirium tremens (DTs) can result from alcohol withdrawal or intoxication. It is a condition that differs from uncomplicated withdrawal in that it is a delirium that may include abnormal perceptions, agitation, terror, insomnia, mild fever, or autonomic instability. A wide variation of presentations can occur, from quiet confusion, agitation, and peculiar behavior lasting several weeks to marked abnormal behavior, vivid terrifying delusions, and other disorders of perception. Hallucinations may be auditory and of a persecutory nature, or they may be kinesthetic, such as tactile sensations of crawling insects. DTs can appear suddenly, but it usually occurs gradually 2–3 days after cessation of drinking, with peak intensity on day 4 or 5. It is usually benign and short-lived: the majority of cases subside after 3 days; subacute symptoms may last 4–5 weeks. Although early reports stated that up to 20% of cases may end fatally, later reports have found that the fatality rate may be less than 1%. DTs is associated with infections, subdural hematomas, trauma, liver disease, and metabolic disorders, and if death occurs amid DTs, the cause is usually infectious fat emboli or cardiac arrhythmias (usually associated with hyperkalemia, hyperpyrexia, and poor hydration). DTs generally occurs in withdrawing alcoholics with 5–15 years of heavy drinking.

Alcohol Withdrawal Seizures

Alcohol lowers the seizure threshold. Alcohol withdrawal seizures that are not a part of DTs generally occur between 7 and 38 hours after the last alcohol use in chronic drinkers; the average is about 24 hours after the last drink. Half of these seizures occur in bursts of two to six grand mal seizures. A total of 10% of all chronic drinkers endure a grand mal seizure; of these, one-third go on to DTs and 2% go on to status epilepticus. Focal seizures suggest a focal lesion, which may indicate trauma or epilepsy. Hypomagnesemia, respiratory alkalosis, hypoglycemia, and increased intracellular sodium have been associated with these seizures. Serum magnesium should be tested in alcoholic patients who develop seizures. These seizures have important prognostic value in predicting a complicated withdrawal period.

Alcohol-Induced Persisting Dementia

Prolonged and heavy use of alcohol may be followed by dementia. Diagnosis is confirmed by its presence at least 3 weeks after ending alcohol intake. In this condition, unlike alcohol-induced persisting amnestic disorder, cognitive impairment affects more than memory function and no cause other than alcohol is found.

Alcohol-Induced Persisting Amnestic Disorder (Korsakoff's Syndrome)

Thiamine (vitamin B_1) deficiency associated with prolonged heavy use of alcohol produces alcohol-induced persisting amnestic disorder (i.e., Korsakoff's syndrome) with its associated neurological deficits (peripheral neuropathy, cerebellar ataxia, and myopathy). Korsakoff's syndrome often follows acute Wernicke's encephalopathy (confusion, ataxia, nystagmus, ophthalmoplegia, and other neurological signs). As Wernicke's subsides, severe impairment of anterograde and retrograde memory remains; confabulation is common. Early treatment of Wernicke's encephalopathy with large doses of thiamine may prevent Korsakoff's syndrome. Unlike the case with other dementias, intellectual function is preserved in alcohol-induced persisting amnestic disorder.

Alcohol-Induced Psychotic Disorder With Delusions or Hallucinations

The hallucinatory form of alcohol-induced psychotic disorder is far more common than the delusional form. Hallucinosis presents with vivid and persistent hallucinations usually within 48 hours after reduction of alcohol in dependent patients. Auditory or visual hallucinations can occur. The disorder may last several weeks or months. Hallucinations may range from sounds (e.g., clicks, roaring, humming, ringing bells, chanting) to threatening or derogatory voices. One derogatory remark may proceed to relentlessly persistent auditory accusations and commands by several voices. Patients usually respond with fear, anxiety, and agitation. Diagnosis is usually made on the basis of a history of heavy alcohol use, absence of formal thought disorder, and lack of psychosis in the personal or family history. In the majority of cases, the symptoms recede in a few hours to days, the patients fully realizing that the perceptions were imaginary. Rarely, patients develop a quiet, chronic, paranoid delusional state indistinguishable from frank schizophrenia, from which remission would not be expected after 6 months. Overall, differential diagnosis includes DTs, withdrawal syndrome, paranoid psychosis, and borderline transient psychotic episodes. In contrast to DTs, these hallucinations usually occur in a clear consciousness. Lack of autonomic symptoms differentiates the syndrome from withdrawal.

Alcohol-Induced Sexual Dysfunction

Alcohol broadly affects reproductive function, generally in proportion to the magnitude of use. Contrary to myth, both men and women have decreased sexual function when alcohol dependent.

Blackouts

Blackouts are periods of amnesia during periods of intoxication (with most central nervous system [CNS] depressants) despite a state of consciousness that seems normal. They may occur in nonalcoholic persons during heavy drinking or at any time during alcohol dependence. Severity and duration of use correlate with blackout occurrence.

Sedatives, Hypnotics, and Anxiolytics

The sedative, hypnotic, and anxiolytic substances include the benzodiazepines, the carbamates (e.g., glutethimide, meprobamate), the barbiturates (e.g., secobarbital), and the barbiturate-like hypnotics (e.g., methaqualone). This class includes all prescription sleeping medications (e.g., chloral hydrate and paraldehyde) and almost all prescription anxiolytics. The nonbenzodiazepine anxiolytics (e.g., buspirone, gepirone) are not included. Polysubstance abusers frequently self-medicate with sedatives to treat undesirable effects of cocaine or amphetamine. Definitions for this class of drugs follow the generic DSM-IV-TR definitions of abuse and dependence presented in Tables 8–1 through 8–3. This class of substances produces secondary clinical syndromes that generally parallel those secondary to alcohol, but their pharmacokinetics differ from alcohol in important ways. It is important to distinguish legitimate use of these medications from adaptation and maladaptive habituation and from illegal use.

Sedative, Hypnotic, or Anxiolytic Use Disorders

Sedative, Hypnotic, or Anxiolytic Dependence

A diagnosis of dependence should be considered only when, in addition to having physiological dependence, the individual using the substance shows evidence of a range of problems (e.g., an individual who has developed drug-seeking behavior to the extent that important activities are given up or reduced to obtain the substance). In this substance class, degree of physical dependence is closely related to dosage and length of use. An individual who has abruptly discontinues benzodiazepines that were taken for long periods of time at prescribed and therapeutic doses may have evidence of tolerance and withdrawal in the absence of a diagnosis of substance dependence.

Sedative-, Hypnotic-, or Anxiolytic-Induced Disorders

Sedative, Hypnotic, or Anxiolytic Intoxication

Memory impairment is a prominent feature of sedative, hypnotic, or anxiolytic intoxication and is most often characterized by an anterograde amnesia that resembles "alcoholic blackouts," which can be quite disturbing to the individual. As with other CNS depressants, one (or more) of the following signs develop during, or shortly after, sedative, hypnotic, or anxiolytic use: slurred speech, incoordination, unsteady gait, nystagmus, impairment in attention or memory, or stupor or coma.

Sedative, Hypnotic, or Anxiolytic Withdrawal

This characteristic syndrome develops in response to a decrease in intake after regular use. Even low-dose diazepam (5–10 mg) over time can result in significant withdrawal upon abrupt cessation. Benzodiazepine abuse can reach several hundred milligrams of diazepam or its equivalent. Individuals who tolerate these dosages are dependent and require active substance abuse treatment with medications. As with alcohol, withdrawal here includes two or more symptoms such as autonomic hyperactivity, tremor, insomnia, anxiety, nausea, vomiting, and psychomotor agitation. Relief on administration of any sedative–hypnotic agent supports a diagnosis of withdrawal. Grand mal seizures occur in 20%–30% of untreated individuals. The withdrawal syndrome produced by substances in this class may present as a life-threatening delirium. In severe withdrawal, perceptual disturbances can occur (if the person's reality testing is intact and his or her sensorium clear, the specifier "with perceptual disturbances" should be noted). The timing and severity of the syndrome depends on the substance and its pharmacokinetics and pharmacodynamics. Symptoms may develop more slowly for drugs with longer half-lives than for those with shorter half-lives. There may be additional longer-term symptoms at a much lower level of intensity that persist for several months. As with alco-

hol, lingering withdrawal symptoms (e.g., anxiety, moodiness, trouble sleeping) can be mistaken for non–substance-induced anxiety or depressive disorders (e.g., generalized anxiety disorder).

Sedative, Hypnotic, or Anxiolytic Withdrawal Delirium

Sedative, hypnotic, or anxiolytic withdrawal delirium is characterized by disturbances in consciousness and cognition, with visual, tactile, or auditory hallucinations. When delirium is present, withdrawal delirium should be diagnosed instead of withdrawal.

Opioids

Opioid Use Disorders

Opioid Dependence

Most individuals with opioid dependence have significant tolerance and experience withdrawal on abrupt discontinuation. The diagnosis requires the presence of features that reflect either compulsive use without legitimate medical purpose or use of doses that are greatly in excess of those needed for pain relief.

Opioid Abuse

Dependence, rather than abuse, should be considered when problems related to opioid use are accompanied by evidence of tolerance, withdrawal, or compulsive behavior related to the use of opioids.

Opioid-Induced Disorders

Opioids are less likely than most other drugs of abuse to produce psychiatric symptoms and in fact may reduce such symptoms. Opioid intoxication and opioid withdrawal are distinguished from the other opioid-induced disorders because the symptoms in the other disorders are in excess of those usually associated with intoxication or withdrawal and are severe enough to warrant independent clinical attention.

Opioid Intoxication

The magnitude of the behavioral and physiological changes that result from opioid use depends on the dose of the drug as well as the characteristics of the user. Symptoms of intoxication usually last as long as the half-life of the drug. Intoxication is marked by miosis or, if severe, by mydriasis (due to anoxia). Drowsiness, slurred speech, and impairment in attention and memory are other signs. Aggression and violence are rarely seen. When hallucinations occur in the absence of intact reality testing, a diagnosis of opioid-induced psychotic disorder, with hallucinations, should be considered. Intoxication by alcohol, sedatives, hypnotics, or anxiolytics resembles opioid intoxication but does not produce miosis or a response to a naloxone challenge.

Opioid overdose is an emergent situation that can be quickly diagnosed: It presents as coma, shock, and pinpoint pupils (dilation in severe cases) and depressed respiration that may lead to death. It rapidly responds to naloxone (Narcan), an opioid receptor antagonist; thus, a lack of response to naloxone undermines a presumed diagnosis of opioid overdose. However, if other classes of drugs are responsible for the altered mental state, naloxone will produce only partial improvement. Opioid intoxication is best distinguished from alcohol and sedative intoxication by the presence of pupillary constriction and laboratory studies.

Opioid Withdrawal

Opioid withdrawal is a syndrome that follows a relative reduction in heavy and prolonged use. The syndrome begins within 6–8 hours after the last dose and peaks at 48–72 hours; symptoms disappear in 7–10 days. It includes signs and symptoms that are opposite the acute agonist effects: lacrimation, rhinorrhea, pupillary dilation, piloerection, diaphoresis, diarrhea, yawning, mild hypertension, tachycardia, fever, and insomnia. A flulike syndrome subsequently develops, with complaints, demands, and drug seeking. Although intense, uncomplicated withdrawal is usually not life-threatening unless a severe underlying disorder, such as cardiac disease, is present. The anxiety and restlessness associated with opioid withdrawal resemble symptoms seen in sedative, hypnotic, or anxiolytic withdrawal. However, opioid withdrawal is also accompanied by rhinorrhea, lacrimation, and mydriasis, which are not seen in sedative-type withdrawal (see Table 8–6 for the DSM-IV-TR criteria set).

Neonatal Opioid Withdrawal

Withdrawal occurs in 60%–94% of neonates of opioid-addicted mothers. The baby may appear normal at birth, but signs may appear 12–24 hours later and may persist for months. The syndrome can include hyperactivity, tremors, seizures, hyperactive reflexes, gastrointestinal dysfunction, respiratory dysfunction, and autonomic signs (yawning, sneezing, sweating, nasal congestion, increased lacrimation, and fever). Over months, infants may appear anxious, hard to please, hyperactive, and emotionally labile.

TABLE 8–6. DSM-IV-TR diagnostic criteria for opioid withdrawal

A. Either of the following:
  (1) cessation of (or reduction in) opioid use that has been heavy and prolonged (several weeks or longer)
  (2) administration of an opioid antagonist after a period of opioid use
B. Three (or more) of the following, developing within minutes to several days after Criterion A:
  (1) dysphoric mood
  (2) nausea or vomiting
  (3) muscle aches
  (4) lacrimation or rhinorrhea
  (5) pupillary dilation, piloerection, or sweating
  (6) diarrhea
  (7) yawning
  (8) fever
  (9) insomnia
C. The symptoms in Criterion B cause clinically significant distress or impairment in social, occupational, or other important areas of functioning.
D. The symptoms are not due to a general medical condition and are not better accounted for by another mental disorder.

Cocaine

Cocaine can be administered in the form of coca leaves (chewed); coca paste (smoked); cocaine hydrochloride powder (inhaled or injected); and cocaine alkaloid, "freebase," or "crack" (smoked). "Speedballing"—mixing cocaine and heroin—is particularly dangerous due to potentiation of respiratory depressant effects. Cocaine-induced states should be distinguished from the symptoms of schizophrenia (paranoid type), bipolar and other mood disorders, generalized anxiety disorder, and panic disorder.

Cocaine Use Disorders

Cocaine Dependence

Exposure to cocaine can quickly produce dependence. An early sign is a growing difficulty resisting the drug. With cocaine's short half-life, frequent use is needed to keep "high." Complications of chronic use are common and include paranoia, aggression, anxiety, depression, and weight loss. Tolerance occurs with repeated use (by any route of administration). Withdrawal symptoms, particularly dysphoria, can be seen but are usually transitory and associated with high-dose use.

Cocaine Abuse

The intensity and frequency of cocaine use are less in abuse than in dependence. Episodes of clinically significant use often occur around paydays or special occasions, leading to a pattern of brief periods (hours to days) of heavy use and longer periods (weeks to months) of nonsignificant use or abstinence. Dependence, rather than abuse, should be considered when use is accompanied by tolerance, withdrawal, or compulsive behavior related to obtaining and using the drug.

Cocaine-Induced Disorders

Cocaine Intoxication

Cocaine intoxication is a state that develops during, or shortly after, cocaine use. After an initial "high," intoxication produces one or more of the following behavioral or psychological changes: euphoria with enhanced vigor, gregariousness, hyperactivity, restlessness, hypervigilance, interpersonal sensitivity, talkativeness, anxiety, tension, alertness, grandiosity, stereotyped or repetitive behavior, anger, and impaired judgment, and, in the case of chronic intoxication, affective blunting with fatigue or sadness and social withdrawal. These features occur with two or more of the following signs and symptoms: tachycardia or bradycardia; pupillary dilation; elevated or lowered blood pressure; perspiration or chills; nausea or vomiting; evidence of weight loss; psychomotor agitation or retardation; muscular weakness, respiratory depression, chest pain, or cardiac arrhythmias; and confusion, seizures, dyskinesias, dystonias, or coma. Cocaine's stimulant effects (e.g., euphoria, tachycardia, hypertension, psychomotor activity) are seen more commonly than its depressant effects (e.g., sadness, bradycardia, hypotension, psychomotor retardation), which emerge only with chronic high-dose use. In humans, binges are highly reinforcing and may lead to psychosis or death. Cocaine's effects on the noradrenergic system are significant and in the overdose setting are associated with muscular twitching, rhabdomyolysis, seizures, cerebrovascular accidents, myocardial infarctions, arrhythmias, and respiratory failure.

Intravenous or freebase use greatly intensifies cocaine's rush. Used intravenously, cocaine's half-life is less than 90 minutes, with euphoric effects lasting 15–20 minutes. Most cocaine is hydrolyzed to benzoylecgonine, which may be detected in the urine for up to 36 hours. Metabolism is slowed when cocaine is combined with alcohol, in which case there is a 18- to 25-fold greater chance of death than for cocaine alone. Smoked freebase has an onset of intense euphoria within seconds because it passes directly from the lungs to the systemic circulation. Euphoric effects depend on concentration and on the slope of the peak concentration (Karan et al. 1998).

Tolerance to cocaine's euphoric effects develops during a binge; however, there is less tolerance for adverse experiences such as increasing anxiety, panic, or frank delirium. With prolonged cocaine administration, a transient delusional psychosis simulating paranoid schizophrenia can be seen. Usually the symptoms remit, although heavy, prolonged use or predisposing psychopathology may lead to persisting psychosis. In general, higher dosages differentiate overdose from intoxication. Often, amphetamine or phencyclidine intoxication can be distinguished from cocaine intoxication only through toxicological studies.

Cocaine Withdrawal

Cocaine withdrawal is accompanied by dysphoric mood, irritability, anxiety, fatigue, insomnia or hyposomnia, vivid and unpleasant dreams, and psychomotor agitation. Anhedonia and drug craving may be present. Withdrawal occurs more than 24 hours after cessation of use and generally peaks in 2–4 days (although irritability and depression may continue for months). Acute withdrawal symptoms are often seen after periods of repetitive high-dose use. These periods are characterized by intense and unpleasant feelings of lassitude and depression, perhaps with suicidal ideation, and generally require days of rest and recuperation. EEG abnormalities may be present.

Cocaine Intoxication Delirium

Cocaine intoxication delirium may occur within 24 hours of use. It may produce tactile and/or olfactory hallucinations; violent or aggressive behavior is more frequent. It is self-limited and usually resolves after 6 hours.

Cocaine-Induced Psychotic Disorder, With Delusions

Cocaine-induced psychotic disorder with delusions is characterized by rapidly developing persecutory delusions that may be accompanied by body-image distortion, misperception of people's faces, formication, and aggression or violence.

Amphetamines

This drug class includes substances with a substituted-phenylethylamine structure (e.g., amphetamine, dextroamphetamine, methamphetamine ["speed"]) and those that have amphetamine-like action but are structurally different (e.g., methylphenidate and most agents used as appetite suppressants).

Amphetamine Use Disorders

Signs and symptoms of amphetamine use parallel those of cocaine, although effects may last longer than in cocaine. Patterns of use involve oral administration (predominantly in pill form) and resemble those for cocaine, with binge episodes alternating with "crash" symptoms. Peripheral sympathomimetic effects may be quite potent.

Amphetamine-Induced Disorders

Amphetamine Intoxication

Amphetamine intoxication follows use of amphetamine or a related substance. Behavioral and psychological changes are accompanied by at least two of the following: tachycardia or bradycardia, mydriasis, hyper- or hypotension, perspiration or chills, nausea or vomiting, weight loss, psychomotor agitation or retardation, muscular weakness, respiratory depression, and chest pain. Confusion, arrhythmias, seizures, dyskinesias, dystonias, or coma may follow. The state begins no more than 1 hour after use, depending on the drug and method of delivery. "Perceptual disturbances" should be specified when hallucinations or illusions occur without delirium and with intact reality testing. If hallucinations or illusions are accompanied by impaired reality testing, the diagnosis "amphetamine-induced psychotic disorder, with hallucinations" should be considered. Amphetamine psychosis can resemble acute paranoid schizophrenia, frequently with visual hallucinations.

Differential Diagnosis of Amphetamine-Induced Disorders

Amphetamine-induced disorders may resemble primary mental disorders. A very difficult differential diagnosis is that between amphetamine-induced psychosis and schizophrenia (Flaum and Shultz 1996). Intoxication with cocaine, hallucinogens, or phencyclidine may cause a similar picture and sometimes can only be distinguished from amphetamine intoxication by urine or serum toxicology, although mydriasis, history of recent drug use, and speed of onset are giveaways. Amphetamine dependence or abuse should be distinguished from dependence or abuse involving cocaine, phencyclidine, or hallucinogens.

Phencyclidine and Variants

Originally an anesthetic, phencyclidine (PCP; "angel dust," the "PeaCe" pill) has become a street drug with epidemic use in some urban areas. Variations include ketamine (Ketalar) and the thiophene analogue of PCP (TCP). These substances can be used orally or intravenously and can be smoked and inhaled. PCP is often mixed with other substances such as amphetamines, cannabis, cocaine, or hallucinogens.

Phencyclidine Use Disorders

Phencyclidine Dependence

PCP dependence may have a rapid onset, and its effects are generally unpredictable. Although the DSM-IV-TR diagnostic criteria for PCP dependence include the first 7 items of the generic definition of substance dependence, criteria 2a and 2b may not apply, given that a clear-cut withdrawal pattern is difficult to establish. As with hallucinogens, adverse reactions to PCP may be more common among individuals with preexisting mental disorders.

Phencyclidine Abuse

PCP abusers may fail to fulfill important role obligations because of intoxication. They may use the drug in situations where its use is physically hazardous. There may be recurrent social or interpersonal problems (due to intoxicated behavior or due to a chaotic lifestyle), legal problems, or arguments with significant others.

Phencyclidine-Induced Disorders

Phencyclidine Intoxication

Intoxication begins by 5 minutes and peaks within 30 minutes. It produces affective instability, stereotypies, bizarre aggression, altered perception, disorganization, and confusion. Signs include hypertension, numbness, muscular rigidity, ataxia, and, at high dosages, hyperthermia and involuntary movements, followed by amnesia and coma, analgesia, seizures, and respiratory depression at the highest doses (i.e., >20 mg). Milder intoxication usually resolves after 8–20 hours; however, because of PCP's fat solubility, this state may persist for many days. Mydriasis and nystagmus (vertical more than horizontal) are characteristic of PCP use and help confirm the diagnosis. Perceptual disturbances should be specified if present.

Phencyclidine-Induced Psychotic Disorder

Psychosis, the most common PCP-induced disorder, may occur in predisposed individuals. It may be indistinguishable from a psychotic episode. Chronic psychosis may occur, along with long-term neuropsychological deficits.

Differential Diagnosis of Phencyclidine-Induced Disorders

PCP-induced disorders may resemble primary mental disorders. Recurring episodes of psychotic or mood symptoms due to PCP may mimic schizophrenia or mood disorders. The fact of PCP use establishes a role for the substance in producing the mentally disordered state but does not rule out the co-occurrence of other primary mental disorders. Also, although a rapid onset of symptoms also suggests PCP intoxication rather than a mental disorder, it may be that PCP use uncovers psychiatric syndromes in individuals with preexisting disease. Course and the absence of a history of the disorder may aid in this differentiation. Drug-related violence or impaired judgment may co-occur with, or may mimic aspects of, conduct disorder or antisocial personality disorder. Again, a history of conduct disorder may help to clarify this differentiation. PCP users often use other drugs; thus, comorbid abuse or dependence on other substances must be considered.

Hallucinogens

This diverse group of substances includes indoleamine derivatives (LSD, morning glory seeds); phenylalkylamine derivatives (mescaline, "STP" [2,5-dimethoxy-4-methylamphetamine], and ring-substituted amphetamines—MDA [methylenedioxyamphetamine; old "ecstasy"], MDMA [methylenedioxymethamphetamine; new "Ecstasy"], MDEA [methylenedioxyethamphetamine]); indole alkaloids (psilocybin, DMT [dimethyltryptamine]); and miscellaneous other compounds. Excluded from this group are PCP and cannabis/delta-9-tetrahydrocannabinol (THC). Hallucinogens are usually taken orally, although dimethyltryptamine is smoked, and use by injection does occur.

Hallucinogen Use Disorders

Hallucinogen Dependence

No specific criteria exist for hallucinogen dependence; in addition, some of the generic DSM-IV-TR substance dependence criteria do not apply, and others require qualification. Hallucinogen use is often limited to only a few times a week, even among individuals who meet the full criteria for hallucinogen dependence. Although tolerance to the euphoric and psychedelic effects of hallucinogens develops rapidly, tolerance to the autonomic effects (mydriasis, hyperreflexia, hypertension, increased body temperature, piloerection, and tachycardia) does not. Cross-tolerance exists between LSD and other hallucinogens (e.g., psilocybin, mescaline). Withdrawal has not been demonstrated, but clear reports of "craving" after stopping hallucinogens are known. Some MDMA users describe a "hangover" the day after use that includes insomnia, fatigue, drowsiness, sore jaw muscles from teeth clenching, loss of balance, and headaches. Some of the reported adverse effects may be due to adulterant or substitute substances such as strychnine, PCP, or amphetamine.

Hallucinogen-Induced Disorders

Hallucinogen Intoxication

In hallucinogen intoxication, perceptual changes occur alongside full alertness during or shortly after hallucinogen use. Changes include subjective intensification of perceptions, depersonalization, derealization, illusions, hallucinations, and synesthesias. DSM-IV-TR criteria require the presence of at least two of the seven listed physiological signs. At low doses, the perceptual changes often do not include hallucinations. Synesthesias (a blending of senses) may result in sounds being "seen." Hallucinations are usually visual, often involving geometric forms, but sometimes involving persons and objects. Auditory or tactile hallucinations are rare. Reality testing is usually preserved. Hallucinogen intoxication should be differentiated from amphetamine or PCP intoxication. Toxicological tests are helpful in making this differential. Intoxication with anticholinergics (e.g., trihexyphenidyl) can produce hallucinations, but such states are often associated with fever, dry mouth and skin, flushed face, and visual disturbances.

Hallucinogen-Induced Psychotic Disorder

Hallucinogen-induced psychotic disorder may be brief or may lead into a long-lasting psychotic episode that is difficult to distinguish from schizophreniform disorder.

Hallucinogen Persisting Perception Disorder

Hallucinogen persisting perception disorder ("flashbacks") following cessation of hallucinogen use involves the reexperiencing of one or more of the same perceptual symptoms experienced while originally intoxicated. The disorder is usually fleeting, but in rare cases it may be more lasting and persistent. It may involve noticing "visual" trails, intensified flashes of colors, auditory or visual hallucinations, and false perceptions of movement. Symptoms may be triggered by stress, drug use (including that of other drugs such as cannabis), emergence into a dark environment, or even by intention. If the person's interpretation of the etiology of the state is delusional, the diagnosis is psychotic disorder NOS. Hallucinogen intoxication is distinguished from flashbacks by temporal relation to use. Also, in hallucinogen persisting perception disorder, the individual does not believe that the perception represents external reality, whereas a person with a psychotic disorder often believes that the perception is real. Hallucinogen persisting perception disorder may be distinguished from migraine, epilepsy, or a neurological condition through a neuro-ophthalmological history, physical examination, and appropriate laboratory evaluation.

Cannabis

The most commonly used substances in this class are marijuana, hashish, and purified THC. Although usually smoked, these substances may also be mixed with food and eaten.

Cannabis Use Disorders

Cannabis Dependence

Dependence is marked by daily, or almost daily, compulsive cannabis use. Tolerance to most of the effects of cannabis has been reported in chronic users, but these patients do not generally develop physiological dependence, and this is not a criterion for diagnosis in DSM-IV-TR. Withdrawal after heavy use is not clinically significant.

Cannabis Abuse

Abuse is characterized by episodic cannabis use with maladaptive behavior. When significant levels of tolerance are present or when psychological or physical problems are associated with cannabis in the context of compulsive use, dependence should be considered rather than abuse.

Cannabis-Induced Disorders

Cannabis Intoxication

Cannabis intoxication includes effects of the drug, which primarily depend on the interaction of drug, person, and setting (route of administration, pharmacodynamics, and pharmacokinetics). Intoxication peaks 10–30 minutes after smoking cannabis and lasts about 3 hours; metabolites may have a half-life of approximately 50 hours. Because most cannabinoids are fat soluble, their effects may occasionally persist or recur for 12–24 hours due to a slow release from fatty tissue or to enterohepatic circulation. Intoxication includes euphoria, anxiety, suspiciousness or paranoid ideation, sensation of slowed time, impaired judgment, and social withdrawal. Inappropriate laughter, panic attacks, and dysphoric affect may occur. Adverse reactions may be more common in those with psychiatric disorders or those frightened about the drug-taking situation. At least two of the following signs develop within 2 hours of use: 1) conjunctival infection, 2) increased appetite, 3) dry mouth, and 4) tachycardia. For differentiation, note that intoxication with alcohol or with a sedative, hypnotic, or anxiolytic substance usually decreases appetite, increases aggressive behavior, and produces nystagmus or ataxia. At low doses, hallucinogen intoxication may resemble cannabis intoxication. PCP intoxication is much more likely to cause ataxia and aggressive behavior. DSM-IV-TR provides a specifier for intoxication "with perceptual disturbances," although if hallucinations occur without intact reality testing, "substance-induced psychotic disorder, with hallucinations" should be diagnosed.

Cannabis-Induced Delusional Disorder

Cannabis-induced delusional disorder is a syndrome (usually with persecutory delusions) that develops shortly after cannabis use. It may be associated with marked anxiety, depersonalization, and emotional lability and may be misdiagnosed as schizophrenia. Subsequent amnesia for the episode can occur.

Cannabis-Induced Mental Disorders

Cannabis-induced mental disorders are diverse. Chronic cannabis use can cause a syndrome resembling dysthymic disorder. Acute adverse reactions to cannabis should be differentiated from panic, major depressive disorder, delusional disorder, bipolar disorder, or paranoid schizophrenia.

Nicotine

Nicotine has euphoric effects and reinforcement properties similar to those of cocaine and opioids. Its effects can follow use of all forms of tobacco, including prescription medications (nicotine gum and patch).

Nicotine Use Disorder

Nicotine Dependence

For nicotine, some of the generic DSM-IV-TR substance dependence criteria do not appear to apply, and others need qualification. *Tolerance* can refer either to the absence of nausea, dizziness, and other characteristic symptoms despite the use of substantial amounts or to a diminished effect observed with continued use of the same amount of the substance. In assessing a patient for nicotine dependence, it should be recalled that spending a great deal of time attempting to procure nicotine is generally rare. An example of giving up important social, occupational, or recreational activities is the avoidance of an activity because it occurs in a smoking-restricted area.

Nicotine-Induced Disorders

Nicotine Withdrawal

Nicotine withdrawal develops after abrupt cessation of, or reduction in, nicotine use following a prolonged period (at least several weeks) of daily use. The withdrawal syndrome includes four or more of the following: dysphoric or depressed mood; insomnia; irritability, frustration, or anger; anxiety; difficulty concentrating; restlessness or impatience; decreased heart rate; and increased appetite or weight gain. Heart rate decreases by 5–12 beats per minute in the first few days after cessation, and weight increases an average of 2–3 kg in the year after cessation. Mild withdrawal may occur after switching to low-tar/low-nicotine cigarettes or after discontinuing the use of chewing tobacco, nicotine gum, or patches.

Differential Diagnosis of Nicotine-Induced Mental Disorders

The symptoms of nicotine withdrawal overlap with those of other withdrawal syndromes; caffeine intoxication; anxiety, mood, and sleep disorders; and medication-induced akathisia. Symptom reduction in response to replacement of nicotine confirms the diagnosis.

Inhalants

This class of inhaled substances includes the aliphatic and aromatic hydrocarbons found in substances such as gasoline, glue, paint thinners, and spray paints. Less commonly used are the halogenated hydrocarbons (in cleaners, correction fluid, spray-can propellants) and other volatile compounds containing esters, ketones, and glycols.

Inhalant Use Disorders

It is usually difficult to determine the exact substance responsible for an inhalant use disorder. Diagnosis is always confirmed by toxicology. Although there may be subtle differences in the effects of the compounds, not enough is known about their effects to distinguish among them. Indeed, these drugs may be used interchangeably, and use may depend on availability and experience. Nonetheless, all of the substances in this class are capable of producing dependence, abuse, and intoxication. There are no specific criteria sets for dependence or abuse of inhalants, in part because of uncertainty in regard to the existence of tolerance or withdrawal syndromes. A possible withdrawal syndrome beginning 24–48 hours after cessation of use and lasting from 2 to 5 days has been described, with symptoms including sleep disturbances, tremor, irritability, diaphoresis, nausea, and fleeting illusions.

Inhalant-Induced Disorders

Inhalant Intoxication

Inhalant intoxication involves clinically significant maladaptive behavioral or psychological changes (e.g., belligerence, assaultiveness, apathy, impaired judgment, impaired social or occupational functioning) that develop during or shortly after exposure. The maladaptive changes are accompanied by signs that include dizziness or visual disturbances (blurred vision or diplopia), nystagmus, incoordination, slurred speech, unsteady gait, tremor, and euphoria. Higher doses of inhalants may lead to the development of lethargy and psychomotor retardation, generalized muscle weakness, depressed reflexes, stupor, or coma.

Differential Diagnosis of Inhalant-Induced Disorders

Inhalant-induced disorders may be characterized by symptoms that resemble primary mental disorders. Mild to moderate intoxication from inhalants can be similar to intoxication caused by alcohol, sedatives, hypnotics, or anxiolytics. Chronic users are likely to use other substances frequently and heavily, further complicating the diagnosis. History of the drug used and characteristic findings (including odor of solvent or paint residue) may help differentiate inhalant intoxication from other substance intoxications. Rapid onset and resolution may also differentiate inhalant intoxication from other mental disorders and neurological conditions. Industrial workers may occasionally be accidentally exposed to volatile chemicals and suffer physiological intoxication. The category "Other Substance-Related Disorders" should be used for such toxin exposures.

Caffeine

Caffeine is widely used in the form of coffee, tea, cola, chocolate, and cocoa and also through use of over-the-counter analgesics, cold preparations, and stimulants.

Caffeine Use Disorders

There is no DSM-IV-TR diagnosis for caffeine dependence or abuse. Although withdrawal headaches may occur, they are usually not severe enough to require treatment.

Caffeine-Induced Disorders

Caffeine Intoxication

Caffeine intoxication can lead to restlessness, nervousness, excitement, insomnia, flushing, diuresis, and gastrointestinal complaints. Doses leading to intoxication can vary. At high doses, there can be psychosis, arrhythmias, and psychomotor agitation. Mild sensory disturbances can occur at higher doses; at massive doses, grand mal seizures and respiratory failure can result. In persons who have developed tolerance, intoxication may not occur despite high caffeine intake.

DSM-IV-TR recognizes other caffeine-induced disorders such as anxiety disorder and sleep disorder, and there is a category for caffeine-related disorder NOS.

Differential Diagnosis of Caffeine-Induced Disorders

Caffeine-induced mental disorders must be differentiated from medical conditions that mimic intoxication. The temporal relationship of the symptoms to increased caffeine use or to abstinence from caffeine helps to establish the diagnosis. Manic episodes; panic disorder or generalized anxiety disorder; amphetamine intoxication; sedative, hypnotic, or anxiolytic withdrawal or nicotine withdrawal; sleep disorders; and medication-induced side effects (e.g., akathisia) can cause a clinical picture similar to that of caffeine intoxication.

Other (or Unknown) Substance-Related Disorders

The DSM-IV-TR category of other (or unknown) substance-related disorders encompasses symptoms of dependence, abuse, intoxication, withdrawal, delirium, psychosis with delusions, psychosis with hallucinations, persisting dementia or amnesia, mood disturbance, anxiety, sexual dysfunction, or disordered sleep that result either from use of a substance whose identity is unknown at the time of the patient's presentation or from use of a substance belonging to a group not large enough to warrant its own category. Examples of the latter include amyl nitrate, anticholinergics, γ-hydroxybutyrate (GHB), corticosteroids, anabolic steroids, antihistamines, antiparkinsonian agents, and others.

GHB, a schedule I substance, is a CNS depressant that is used in some countries (but not the United States) as an anesthetic. It is structurally related to γ-aminobutyric acid (GABA). It is increasingly used worldwide as a recreational drug by party and nightclub attendees and bodybuilders, and it may also be used as a "date rape" drug. It has been marketed to bodybuilders as a growth-hormone releaser. Known as "liquid Ecstasy," GHB increases CNS dopamine levels and has effects in the endogenous opioid system. GHB toxicity includes coma, seizures, respiratory depression, vomiting, anesthesia, and amnesia (Centers for Disease Control and Prevention 1997b). The drug is missed by routine diagnostic urine screens. Although full recovery usually occurs, the toxic state is life-threatening and may be complicated by severe muscular pathology leading to rhabdomyolysis and myoglobinuria (Graeme 2000). An increasing number of reports have described clinically significant states of withdrawal from GHB (Craig et al. 2000).

Polysubstance Dependence

The DSM-IV-TR category of polysubstance dependence is used when, within the past year, the individual has repeatedly used at least three classes of substances (excepting nicotine and caffeine) without one predominating. Dependence is global and not for any one drug. Patients often downplay their use of these secondary drugs and a thorough substance use history is always essential to ensure attention to all substances the patient is using, not simply the one he or she identifies as "the problem."

Often one drug is used to counterbalance the side effects or to potentiate the effects of another drug. "Speedballing"—ingestion of the intravenous combination of heroin and cocaine—is lethal but is known to mitigate cocaine dysphoria. Glutethimide (Doriden) and cocaine are often combined, potentiating respiratory depression. Pentazocine (Talwin) and diphenhydramine (Benadryl)—the "T's and Blues"—are prescription medications that produce intoxication when combined. Virtually any combination of alcohol and other drugs is seen. Use of marijuana is often so pervasive in this population that it is not perceived as a drug of abuse.

Clinical Diagnosis of Substance Use Disorder

Substance-abusing patients present with medical, neurological, and psychiatric disturbances that require careful, systematic assessment. The extreme complexity of differential diagnosis in this population should instill some degree of humility and conservatism. Cautious management with a careful review of the medical, psychiatric, and substance abuse histories; physical and mental status examinations; laboratory tests; and third-party information can clarify the diagnoses. In some cases, however, etiology can be elucidated only with time and observation.

Signs and Symptoms

Diagnosing and caring for substance-abusing patients requires attention to physical signs and symptoms. At the outset it should be noted that when attempting to differentiate among overdose, withdrawal, chronic brain disease, and psychiatric diagnoses, one should rule out or treat life-threatening conditions first. For example, tachycardia and fever may indicate infection, withdrawal, or drug toxicity. An abnormal pulse may indicate intoxication with sympathomimetic drugs, withdrawal from CNS depressants, or arrhythmia from overdose. Bradycardia could indicate opioid intoxication, severe head trauma, or cardiac conduction delays. Abnormal pupil size or occulogyric movements can help clarify various drug overdose situations. Pinpoint pupils in a comatose patient may signal opioid overdose. Mydriasis is associated with sympathomimetic intoxication. Gaze palsies, confusion, and ataxia could be due to thiamine deficiency leading to Wernicke's encephalopathy. Nystagmus occurs in PCP intoxication. Physical examination can detect fresh needle marks, recent alcohol intake, or nasal irritation from cocaine or inhalant abuse. Of course, drug-abusing patients frequently have comorbid medical and neurological conditions that affect mental and physical status, such as AIDS dementia, seizures, head trauma, and infections, and these should be considered.

Markedly altered mental status, evidence of recent substance intake, and reliable corroborating history can aid in distinguishing between withdrawal, chronic brain disease, and functional diagnoses. Diagnosis may be delayed or provisional in patients with a known chronic substance abuse history, an unreliable recent history, or a history of major psychiatric symptoms. Long-standing brain disease can confound diagnosis. Alcohol-induced dementia and postconcussive head syndromes can sensitize the brain to react to minor substance abuse with dramatic and unpredictable results. In such patients, many things are happening at once. It is important to provide a safe environment; to protect the patient and others from harm; and to ensure basic airway, respiratory, and cardiac support until a basic diagnostic workup can be completed.

Countertransference and Diagnosis

Substance-abusing patients with histrionic, paranoid, borderline, or antisocial features may present with an exacerbation of primitive defenses (e.g., projection, projective identification, and splitting during intoxication). These patients may be belligerent, distrustful, unappreciative, uncooperative, or violent, making management and history taking difficult. Because of the strong countertransference reactions such patients evoke, inappropriate diagnostic and treatment decisions may ensue. Before making an unusual treatment decision or participating in uncharacteristic behavior with a patient, consultation with another expert may be useful, and sometimes a team approach is especially helpful. Countertransference feelings should not be ignored but rather should be used to help clarify diagnosis. Frequently, obnoxious, uncooperative, or destructive behavior or apparent personality problems are time limited and related to the substance-induced state. They may reflect the patient's fear and low self-esteem or may quickly resolve on detoxification.

Psychiatric Comorbidity

Dual-diagnosis patients have a substance abuse disorder and another major psychiatric diagnosis. The connections between the two may be manifold (Vaillant 1993). Major psychiatric disorders may precede the development of substance abuse, develop concurrently with substance abuse, or manifest secondarily to substance abuse. Psychiatric disorders may precipitate the onset or modify the course of a substance use disorder. Psychiatric disorders and substance abuse may present as independent conditions. Thus, it is difficult at any one time to differentiate symptoms of withdrawal, intoxication, and secondary cognitive, affective, perceptual, or personality changes from underlying psychiatric disorders. Among the major psychopathologies, the reported odds ratios for comorbid substance use were 2 for major depressive disorder, 3 for panic disorder, 5 for schizophrenia, and 7 for bipolar illness (Regier et al. 1990). Important tools in differential diagnosis include careful history taking, particularly in terms of the course or sequence of symptoms, and laboratory studies. Information obtained from third parties is critical as well.

Affective Disorders

Regardless of the patient's expectation or experiences of euphoria during chronic use, chronic major depression occurs late in the course of addiction. This may be the result of altered neurochemistry, hormonal or metabolic changes, chronic demoralization, or grief from personal losses, or it may result from the stresses of the addictive lifestyle. Chronic heroin use often leads to lethargy and social withdrawal. Sustained alcohol use generally produces depression and anxiety, although brief periods of euphoria may still occur.

It is vitally important to differentiate alcohol-induced depressive disorder from primary depressive disorder. According to a study conducted in a large population of alcoholic patients, primary major depressive episodes were more likely to occur in patients who were female, white, and married; who had had experience with fewer drugs and less treatment for alcoholism; who had attempted suicide, and who had a close relative with a major mood disorder (Schuckit et al. 1997). Although most individuals with alcoholism will not have an independent diagnosis of major depressive disorder, other less severe depressive disorders may persist in a large proportion of alcoholic persons after cessation of drinking. Drinking may be more of a problem during a hypomanic or manic phase of a bipolar disorder than during a depressed phase. In most cases, depressive symptomatology subsides after 3–4 weeks of abstinence and usually needs no pharmacological intervention. Use of antidepressants is indicated after a drug-free period, and abstinence is required for these agents' efficacy. The presence of untreated major depression in a patient with primary alcoholism or of secondary alcoholism in a patient with primary depressive disorder worsens prognosis.

There is considerable evidence that depression is higher in active opioid users than in the population and may subside with abstinence. The prevalence of major depression ranges from 17% to 30% in heroin-addicted persons and is considerably higher among methadone clients. Affective disorders have ranged as high as 60% among opioid abusers. Depressive episodes often are mild, may be related to treatment seeking, and frequently are stress related. In one study, depression was found to be a poor prognostic sign at 2.5-year follow-up in opioid-addicted patients, except in those with coexistent antisocial personality, in whom depression improved prognosis (Brooner et al. 1997).

Affective disorders have been concurrently diagnosed in 30% of cocaine addicts, with a significant proportion of these patients having bipolar or cyclothymic disorder. Bipolar manic patients may use cocaine to heighten feelings of grandiosity. The profound dysphoric mood related to cocaine binges will resolve in the majority of cocaine addicts. A minority of patients may have underlying unipolar or bipolar disorder, which needs to be treated separately. This abstinence dysphoria may be secondary to depletion of brain catecholamines (e.g., dopamine) or to alteration in neural receptors, with resultant postsynaptic supersensitivity. Some authors suggest that comorbid cocaine abuse constitutes a robust predictor of poor outcome among depressed alcoholic persons.

Psychosis

Psychotic symptomatology can result from the use of a wide range of psychoactive substances: alcohol, cocaine, PCP, hallucinogens, stimulants, and inhalants. As noted previously, all of these substances can cause "organic" syndromes that mimic various functional psychiatric syndromes. Opioids, however, have shown some antipsychotic properties.

The relationship between schizophrenia and substance abuse is complex. Various studies have shown that 50%–60% of schizophrenia patients and 60%–80% of bipolar patients abuse substances (Schneier and Siris 1987). The role of substance abuse in precipitating or altering the course of an underlying schizophrenic disorder is unclear. Substance abuse may trigger the reappearance of symptoms that were previously well controlled by medication. Alcohol, marijuana, hallucinogen, or cocaine abuse may produce psychotic symptoms that persist only in vulnerable individuals. It may be that schizophrenia patients seek out certain types of drugs for self-medication and for self-treatment of medication side effects. Persons with schizophrenia also use tobacco and caffeine more often than do control populations. Tobacco use has been associated with lowering of blood levels of neuroleptics and leads to a need for higher-than-average doses of neuroleptics for symptom control. Schizophrenia patients may seek out drugs that increase their chances of experiencing psychotic episodes to feel a sense of mastery or to experience merging. They may be attempting to counteract dysphoria or the negative symptoms of their disease and may use stimulants to allow themselves to feel more intensely. They may be treating the extrapyramidal or sedative side effects of neuroleptic medications. Schizophrenic patients who abuse stimulant drugs may also be treating an independent underlying affective disorder. Substance abuse may provide these patients with an experience of control over unpredictable states of consciousness or may offer such patients an alternative identity—that of substance abuser—that may be more palatable and be perceived as carrying less stigma than that of schizophrenia.

Anxiety Disorders

Generalized anxiety disorder, posttraumatic stress disorder, panic disorder, and phobic disorder are overrepresented in substance abuse patients, especially abusers of CNS depressants. One study of alcoholic patients reported general anxiety disorder in 9% and phobias in 3%, prevalences significantly higher than those in the general population (Ross et al. 1988). Posttraumatic stress disorder has been related to the high rates of alcoholism in Vietnam veterans who saw active duty. Panic disorder has been found in 5% of alcoholic inpatients (Kushner et al. 1990). Use of high doses of benzodiazepines (up to 1,000 or 1,500 mg diazepam equivalent) has been reported in patients with underlying anxiety disorders and very high tolerance to benzodiazepines. These patients are often very difficult to treat because of the complex interaction between the anxiety and the substance abuse disorder. In the treatment of substance-addicted patients with anxiety disorders, benzodiazepines should be avoided if possible. Specific treatment of underlying anxiety disorders may include typical and low-dose atypical antipsychotics, antidepressants, monoamine oxidase inhibitors (MAOIs), buspirone, gabapentin, or propranolol (see "Treatment of Substance Use Disorders").

Neuropsychiatric Impairment

Chronic abuse of alcohol, sedatives, or inhalants has been well correlated with chronic brain damage and neuropsychological impairment. These impairments may be obvious (as in alcohol dementia or Korsakoff's syndrome) or relatively mild and detectable only by neuropsychological testing. Cognitive impairment may be short lived and recede after 3–4 weeks of abstinence, may improve gradually over several months or years of abstinence, or be permanent. Damage to brain tissue due to alcohol has been shown by abnormal computed tomography (CT) scan findings (cortical atrophy—which may reverse as well; see "Laboratory Tests and Diagnostic Instruments"), altered EEG (decreased alpha activity), and altered evoked potentials (decreased P3 component). In the case of benzodiazepines, however, the cognitive impairment may be reversible (Salzman et al. 1992).

Natural Histories of Substance Abuse

Alcohol

The signs and symptoms of alcoholism can be strikingly consistent among individuals in the late stages of the disease. Nonetheless, bearing in mind the concept of "case heterogeneity," there appear to be subtypes of alcoholics that may present with different ages at onset, underlying etiologies, degrees of hereditary influence, social and cultural backgrounds, and natural outcomes. Thus, it is important to understand alcoholism as a disease that assumes many different patterns and is characterized by relapses. Vaillant's (1996) longitudinal studies of alcoholic patients found that some drink until death, others stop drinking, and still others display a pattern of long abstinence followed by relapses. Large-scale outcome studies suggest that approximately 30% of alcoholic persons will at some point in the course of their illness achieve stable abstinence without any form of treatment (Armor et al. 1978). This percentage improves in some studies to approximately 70% with some form of treatment.

Types of Alcoholism

Jellinek (1960) was the first to describe subgroups of alcoholics. More recently, Cloninger et al. (1988) described two subtypes of alcoholism. In persons with type I alcoholism, heavy drinking generally starts after age 25 years and is reinforced by external circumstances. These individuals have greater ability to abstain for long periods of time and frequently feel loss of control, guilt, and fear about their alcohol dependency. In contrast, persons with type II alcoholism generally have an early onset—before age 25 years—and show spontaneous alcohol-seeking behavior regardless of external circumstances. Fights and arrests are common with these individuals, and they rarely experience feelings of loss of control, guilt, or fear about their alcohol dependency. These two groups may differ in terms of response to antirelapse medication and in amounts of platelet monoamine oxidase B (MAO-B).

Medical Complications

Gastrointestinal effects. Alcohol use can promote hepatic pathology. Fatty liver deposits occur in anyone with sufficient alcohol intake. Alcoholic hepatitis has a 5-year mortality rate of 50%. Cirrhosis occurs in only 10% of alcoholic persons, yet 11,000 die from liver disease annually. Of patients with chronic pancreatitis, 75% have an alcohol use disorder. Alcohol dissolves mucus and irritates the gastric lining, which contributes to bleeding. Every alcoholism patient should have a stool guaiac as part of a complete physical examination (Lieber 1995). In the acute, subacute, and chronic stages of alcohol use, hepatic dysregulation is present, albeit in differing patterns: in the acute (intoxicated) stage, there is inhibition of the metabolism of other molecules, such as medications (including substances of overdose); in the subacute phase, there is induction of liver cytochrome P450 (CYP) enzymes, increasing the metabolism of other molecules; and finally, in the cirrhotic state with portacaval shunting, there is again reduced metabolism of other systemic molecules (Weller and Preskorn 1984).

Hematological effects. Alcoholism is part of the differential diagnosis for anemia, especially megaloblastic anemia. Alcohol impairs immune function and promotes oropharyngeal, esophageal, gastric, hepatic, and pancreatic cancer. Patients with oral cancer tend to delay seeking treatment longer than most other cancer patients. Early detection is particularly crucial in these diseases.

Endocrinological effects. Sexual function is affected indirectly through alcohol's impact on the limbic system and the hypothalamic-pituitary-adrenal axis. Alcohol affects male sexual function and fertility both directly via effects on testosterone levels and indirectly through testicular atrophy. Relatively increased levels of estrogen lead to gynecomastia and body-hair loss in men. In women there may also be severe gonadal failure, affecting secondary sexual characteristics, reducing menstruation, and producing infertility.

Neurological effects. Alcoholism increases blood pressure and is associated with increased risk of cerebrovascular accidents. Alcoholic cerebellar degeneration is a slowly evolving condition encountered in patients with a long-standing history of excessive use. Alcoholic peripheral neuropathy is characterized by a stocking-and-glove paresthesia with decreased reflexes and autonomic nerve dysfunction. Other long-term neurological effects of alcoholism include central pontine myelinolysis, Marchiafava-Bignami disease, and muscular pathology. CT studies have shown that brain changes resulting from alcohol use may be reversible in as little as 3 weeks' time (Trabert et al. 1995).

Cardiovascular effects. The relationship between alcohol and cardiovascular health and disease is complex and is the focus of much study. Alcoholic cardiomyopathy can develop after 10 or more years of drinking. Absti-

nence contributes to recovery in those cases in which the damage is not too extensive. For heavy drinkers, alcohol increases the risk of cardiomyopathy, heart failure, and poor postmyocardial infarction survival. Moderate (defined as 1–20 ounces per month) use of alcohol, on the other hand, may have beneficial effects on both the risk of heart failure in the elderly (Abramson et al. 2001) and postinfarction survival in the general population (Mukamal et al. 2001). However, these effects may be brittle (moderate, beneficial use might quickly become pathologic), and no consensus recommendation yet exists for moderate use of alcohol.

Genetics: Familial Studies and High-Risk Populations

That alcoholism occurs in families was established by Jellinek and Jolliffee and confirmed by twin, adoption, and split-sibling studies. Yet neither the mode of transmission nor the genotype or phenotype transmitted is known. Some studies have suggested that tolerance to alcohol is the transmitted trait. Others have proposed that what is transmitted is a vulnerability to a particular substance, such that the affected proband might become addicted after only one exposure (Schuckit et al. 1998). Further lines of research in the genetics of the addictions will address variability among patients in terms of vulnerability and course.

Biological Markers

Biological markers are physiological findings associated with alcoholism that may help us to identify high-risk individuals before the onset of abuse, recognize dependence when it exists, and follow the course of the disease. Several promising markers have been found (Table 8–8). Identifying children at high risk for alcoholism or substance abuse has been a major research thrust. One group's findings have included evidence of decreased subjective feelings of intoxication and less impairment of motor performance with alcohol ingestion in not-yet-alcoholic children of alcoholic parents. This group also reported less body sway or static ataxia with alcohol challenge and less change in cortisol and prolactin levels in comparison with control subjects (Schuckit 1987).

A finding among abstinent alcoholics and sons of alcoholics is an alteration of normal auditory brain-stem potentials. The p300 event-related potential (ERP)—the voltage of the third positive EEG wave in response to this stimulus—is of low amplitude in alcoholic persons and abstinent young sons of alcoholic men. Increased alpha-wave activity with alcohol exposure in alcoholic versus control subjects has also been reported (Table 8–7).

TABLE 8–7. Possible markers of alcoholism in biological sons of alcoholics

Decreased subjective feelings of intoxication
Less impairment of motor performance
Less body sway
Less static ataxia
Less change in cortisol and prolactin findings
Low P3 amplitude (electroencephalogram)
Increased alpha wave activity

These findings might be more valid for visual than for auditory stimuli (Polich and Bloom 1999). Controversy exists regarding whether alcoholic individuals have low platelet MAO-B activity (which may be even more apparent in type II alcoholism than in type I).

Finally, prospective longitudinal studies of sons of alcoholics have reported some evidence of poor neuropsychological performance in areas such as categorizing, organization, planning, abstracting, and problem-solving ability. Tarter and Edwards (1988) suggested that ADHD or conduct disorder may predispose toward alcoholism and may be an expression of an underlying inherited temperament. Risk taking, sensation-seeking individuals are thought to be at particularly high risk for alcoholism.

Sedatives, Hypnotics, and Anxiolytics

The course of CNS depressant abuse/dependence varies from long prodromal periods of use with benzodiazepines or hypnotics to more rapid onset of addiction with barbiturates to episodic abuse with other CNS depressants such as methaqualone (Quaalude) or ethchlorvynol (Placidyl). Combinations of CNS depressants with alcohol or opioids can potentiate the level of intoxication, leading to respiratory depression and mortality. Chronic sedative abuse can produce "blackouts" and neuropsychological damage similar to that experienced by alcoholic patients (Tonne et al. 1995). In patients originally using sedatives for anxiety, there will be an initial anxiety rebound on discontinuation that typically is similar to sedative withdrawal in terms of course and symptomatology.

Opioids

Psychosocial Features

Opioid abuse is often endemic to economically disadvantaged communities with high unemployment, low family stability, and increased tolerance of criminality. These social stressors may result in hopelessness, low self-esteem, poor self-concept, and identification with drug-involved role models. There exists a clear association between heroin use and crime. Where poverty and high unemployment are prevalent, individuals may perceive little risk from drug experimentation, and conventional scare tactics are ineffective. Alienation from social institutions such as school, increased social deviancy, and impulsivity are high-risk characteristics. The overwhelming majority of inner-city community members, however, are not opioid users.

Adverse Physical Effects

Impurities and contaminated needles may lead to endocarditis, septicemia, pulmonary emboli, pulmonary hypertension, skin infections, hepatitis B, and HIV. Death rates in young addicts are increased 20-fold by infection, homicide, suicide, overdose, and AIDS. Opioid overdose should be suspected in any undiagnosed coma patient.

Progression

The course of heroin addiction generally involves a 2- to 6-year interval between regular use of heroin and seeking of treatment. Early experimentation with opioids may not lead to addiction, but once addiction develops, a lifelong pattern of use and relapse frequently ensues. A preexisting personality disorder may be a factor in drug use progression. The need to secure the drug predisposes the addict to participate in crime.

The Self-Medication Hypothesis

The self-medication hypothesis suggests that the individual self-selects drugs on the basis of preexisting personality and ego impairments. Khantzian (1997) found a strong interaction between dominant dysphoric feelings and drug preference, and he emphasized an "antirage property to opioids" that provides a pharmacological solution or defense against overwhelming anger resulting from either deficient ego defenses or low frustration tolerance.

Cocaine

Natural Course

The time from first intranasal use to cocaine addiction is about 4 years in adults, but it may be only 1.5 years in adolescents. Both groups may progress faster with more potent cocaine derivatives (e.g., "crack"). Most addicts describe initial use as fun. At some point in the experience, however, it becomes joyless and compulsive. Because of the high cost of cocaine, financial and legal problems may be the first indication of trouble before other signs of dependence develop. The activating properties of the drug become more prominent as the euphoria wanes. Consumption of cocaine, initially consumed in public places such as bars and at parties, may become an isolated, alienating experience, associated with considerable paranoia. Most casual cocaine users do not become dependent.

Cocaine is associated with violence. In 20% of suicides in New York City in the 1990s, it had been used immediately prior to death (Marzuk et al. 1992), and other studies have found cocaine in the urine of homicide victims, in those arrested for murder, and in overdose deaths. In cocaine-induced fatalities, the average blood concentration is 6.2 mg/L (Spiehler and Reed 1985).

Adverse Medical Effects

Chronic cocaine use depletes all neurotransmitters and leads to increased receptor sensitivity to dopamine and norepinephrine, which is associated with depression, fatigue, poor attention to self-care, poor self-esteem, poor libido, and mild parkinsonism. Tolerance to cocaine occurs. Psychosis, an attention-deficit syndrome, and/or stereotypies may result from continued use. There is evidence of cerebrovascular disease secondary to chronic use (Bartzokis et al. 1999).

Death may occur even in recreational, low-dose users. Other acute complications include agitation, diaphoresis, tachycardia, subarachnoid hemorrhage, metabolic and respiratory acidosis, arrhythmias, grand mal seizures, and respiratory arrest. Myocardial infarction is produced by coronary vasoconstriction with tachycardia. Malnutrition, severe weight loss, and dehydration often result from cocaine binges. Chronic complications of intranasal abuse include nasoseptal defects due to vasoconstriction, nasal stuffiness or "the runs" due to vasodilation, and dental neglect due to cocaine's anesthetic properties. Intravenous use may produce endocarditis, septicemia, HIV spread, local vasculitis, hepatitis B, emphysema, pulmonary emboli, and granulomas. Cocaine injection sites are characterized by prominent ecchymoses; opioid users more frequently show needle marks. Freebase cocaine has been associated with decreased pulmonary exchange and with persisting pulmonary dysfunction.

Pregnant women who use cocaine may have increased risks for abruptio placenta and neonatal tachycardia (Volpe 1992), and babies of cocaine-using mothers have been shown to have decreased interactive behavior on Brazelton scales. Further research is being conducted to study the teratogenicity of cocaine in infants. Fortunately, there have been few long-term developmental effects ascribed to cocaine itself (Frank et al. 2001).

Amphetamines

Amphetamine abuse may start as attempts at weight loss or energy enhancement. Amphetamine abuse by intravenous administration can present with the same medical complications seen with other drugs. Amphetamines are similar to cocaine in regard to signs, symptoms, and long-term sequelae.

Phencyclidine and Ketamine

Chronic psychotic episodes are reported following use of PCP. Use of PCP may lead to chronic neuropsychological deficits. PCP use may occur in conjunction with other substances, and its abuse may be associated with similar risk factors. Cases of "pure" PCP abuse have been reported in individuals with significant psychopathology; however, it is difficult to distinguish drug effects from premorbid personality. PCP intoxication produces specific autonomic sequelae that are both sympathomimetic and cholinergic, as well as poor function of the cerebellar system, including horizontal nystagmus, ataxia, and dizziness.

Ketamine, originally used as an anesthetic, and its active metabolite norketamine act at many CNS receptor sites, including the NMDA receptor. The drug is taken intranasally or orally and has a fast effect to get to "K land," as its dissociative effects are called. With the drug's elimination half-life of 2 hours, its effects last approximately 30 minutes. Ketamine has been known to produce psychosis in normal individuals (Krystal et al. 1994). The acute effects can be serious. Neurological toxicity includes nystagmus, mydriasis, agitation, delirium, hypertonus, rigidity, hallucinations, and seizures. Movement disturbances are common and include dystonia, ataxia, and bizarre posturing of limbs and facial expression. Rhabdomyolysis can ensue. Cardiovascular toxicity is consistent with sympathetic stimulation and includes tachycardia, palpitations, and hypertension. Respiratory arrest or apnea can occur, and there is a risk of aspiration. In cases of death from overdose, pulmonary edema has been noted.

Although long-term sequelae have not been well studied, flashbacks and cognitive disorder are known to occur in ketamine abuse (Jansen 1993).

Hallucinogens

Most hallucinogens can produce acute adverse effects. The "bad trip" is a syndrome of anxiety, panic, dysphoria, and paranoia that occurs during the period of intoxication. Because the syndrome can lead to suicide ideation and attempts, its recognition is important. There is no recognized withdrawal syndrome from this class of medications. Hallucinogen use can also lead to chronic effects, including prolonged psychotic states that resemble psychosis or mania. However, syndromes that last longer than 4–6 weeks are generally thought to represent underlying primary psychiatric disease rather than conditions secondary to these substances. Flashbacks are another potential chronic sequelae of hallucinogens.

Hallucinogens have been noted to produce flashback experiences in 15%–30% of chronic users. Prevalence of flashbacks increases with the number of times the individual seeks medical attention except during acute intoxication or disturbing flashbacks that may be precipitated by other substances such as marijuana. Most strikingly, some of the drugs in this class have produced permanent parkinsonism in users by selective destruction of the substantia nigra.

MDMA ("Ecstasy")

MDMA, a serotonin releaser and uptake inhibitor, is metabolized by CYP 2D6. Its long-term depletion of serotonin seen in animals may lead to downregulation of serotonin receptors and an overall reduction in serotonin neurons in humans. Indeed, in humans using MDMA, reduced serotonin transporter binding has been demonstrated. MDMA can produce a state that resembles cocaine toxicity: fulminant hepatotoxicity, disseminated intravascular coagulation, cardiotoxicity, hyperthermia, rhabdomyolysis, and acute respiratory distress syndrome (Jonas and Graeme-Cook 2001). Over the long term, cognitive deficits do occur, especially in terms of memory (McCann et al. 1999).

Cannabis

Marijuana abuse tends to begin in adolescence. The use of alcohol, nicotine, or cocaine may be associated with marijuana abuse. Marijuana is described as a stepping stone to other illegal drugs. Although many people experiment with marijuana, actual abuse patterns tend to be associated with introduction to youth drug subcultures, low parental monitoring, parental substance abuse, and abuse of drugs by peers.

Chronic Psychological Effects

Generally, the adverse effects of marijuana are not treated in the medical setting. Mild anxiety, depression, and paranoia are frequent occurrences. Several neuropsychological changes and deficits have been identified with marijuana intoxication. Decreases in complex reaction-time tasks, digit-code memory tasks, fine-motor function, time estimation, the ability to track information over time, tactual form discrimination, and concept formation have been found. Undesirable physical effects include conjunctivitis, dry mouth, and lightheadedness. Emotional symptoms of anxiety, confusion, fear, and increased dependency can progress to panic or frank paranoid pathology. Marijuana can also exacerbate depression.

Chronic Physical Effects

There is increasing evidence that marijuana abuse creates at least some long-term adverse physical effects. For example, several biochemical findings have been reported. Marijuana has been studied in relationship to human male and female fertility, cell metabolism and protein synthesis, normal cell division, and spermatogenesis. Cannabis smoke contains carcinogens similar to those in tobacco smoke, and chronic marijuana abuse may predispose the user to chronic obstructive lung disease and pulmonary neoplasm. Cannabis also increases heart rate and blood pressure, an effect that may be critical in patients with cardiovascular disease. Chronic marijuana abuse may lead to gynecomastia in men. There is some evidence of a marijuana withdrawal syndrome; however, this requires further investigation.

Nicotine

Course

Nicotine addiction frequently presents as a relapsing condition. Experimentation usually begins in adolescence. Environmental influences are important; peer tobacco use, parental tobacco use, and use of other substances are contributing factors. Relapse may be evident during periods of high stress, anxiety or maladjustment, poor social support, or low confidence. There is a strong association between alcohol and smoking. Often, alcoholic individuals can stop drinking but cannot stop smoking at the same time. Many substance treatment programs essentially ignore tobacco; however, it is a major health risk and should be addressed at some point. Factors associated with poor long-term outcomes include poor overall adjustment, low social support, environmental stress, exposure to people who continue to smoke, ignorance of the dangers of cigarette smoking, and higher use or tolerance.

Adverse Medical Sequelae

At this time, the associations between tobacco use and coronary vascular disease, chronic obstructive lung disease, lung cancer, oral cancers, and hypertension are well known. There is growing evidence of nicotine's dose-dependent link to cataracts in men. Nicotine tends to increase liver drug metabolism and thus may lower the levels of medications metabolized by the liver. Psychotropic medications, including neuroleptics and antidepressants, may have lower blood levels in smokers, in some cases resulting from nicotine's induction of CYP enzymes.

Inhalants

Course

Inhalant users are predominantly socioeconomically deprived young males ages 13–15 years. American and Mexican Indians and teenagers in the Southwest have been found to have a high prevalence. Amyl nitrite was popular in the 1970s in the homosexual population. Nitrous oxide may be prevalent among certain health personnel, especially dentists. Most users tend to cease their use after a relatively short period of time and may go on to abuse other psychoactive substances. There is a fairly strong association between aggressive, disruptive, and antisocial behavior and inhalant intoxication.

Adverse Medical Effects

Deaths have been reported from CNS respiratory depression, cardiac arrhythmia, and accidents. Long-term damage to bone marrow, kidneys, liver, neuromuscular tissue, and the brain have been reported. Evidence from CNS single photo emission computed tomography (SPECT) studies show the presence of abnormal perfusion in the brains of former users (Kucuk et al. 2000).

Laboratory Tests and Diagnostic Instruments

Laboratory Testing

There are many reasons to use laboratory studies in the treatment of substance use disorders. These include the need to supplement an incomplete or missing drug history, to correlate clinical state with drug levels, to make a differential diagnosis, as part of follow-up or assessment, for forensic purposes, in athletic competition, to ensure public safety, for detection of relapse, and the fact that drug use declines when serious testing is in place. The importance of urine and blood level screening cannot be overstressed as a means to provide collateral evidence of substance abuse problems. The sensitivity and accuracy of blood and urine screening has improved with the addition of gas chromatography to more routine screening techniques. A general toxicology screen includes a blood alcohol level.

Selection of Toxicological Tests and Pharmacokinetics

The choice of test requires consideration of what to sample, the half-life of the suspected substance, the significance of biotransformation of the suspected substance, and the test's sensitivity, specificity, and cost. Knowledge of the half-life of various drugs is helpful in interpreting results. For example, the half-life of 4 oz of orally administered ethyl alcohol will be 1–2 hours. A blood alcohol level of 200 mg/dL would indicate recent heavy intake and most likely current intoxication. A negative paper chromatography screen for cocaine in a man admitted for a 2-day history of paranoid, delusional behavior will not rule out abuse, because cocaine has a relatively short half-life (it clears in 24–36 hours) and because paper chromatography has a low sensitivity (Gold and Dackis 1986). On the other hand, marijuana, which is highly fat soluble, has a relatively long half-life and can be detected in the urine in heavy users up to 3 weeks after last use.

Urine Drug Screens

Urine drug screen results usually are reported as either positive or negative for any particular drug. Most routine urine screens cover the major drugs of abuse. Specificity and sensitivity are lower with thin-layer chromatography and immunoassay techniques. More sophisticated and sensitive quantitative testing with gas chromatography/mass spectrometry (GC/MS) can be done with certain drugs (e.g., marijuana) if urine from the original sample is positive. Urine drug screens generally are not useful in court because they do not answer the question of degree of intoxication. For general hospital purposes, urine drug screens are imperative in certain situations. Urine drug screening should be routine in cases of coma of unknown cause, in atypical psychiatric presentations, with agitated and confused patients, in persons with known drug histories, or in those with physical evidence of substance abuse. In high-risk populations or in areas where drugs may be epidemic (e.g., certain inner-city general hospitals), urine drug screening should be routinely done for psychiatric admission. To ensure the validity and reliability of urine screen results, direct observation of voiding may be indicated. Finally, it should be noted that morning urine samples are often contaminated and should be avoided if possible.

Blood Screening Tests

Suspicion of alcoholism or substance abuse may be heightened with corroborating laboratory evidence from blood studies (Table 8–8), which are often useful in forensic cases. Elevated mean corpuscular volume (MCV) and elevated liver function tests such as serum glutamic-oxaloacetic transaminase (SGOT), serum glutamic-pyruvic transaminase (SGPT), and lactate dehydrogenase (LDH) may signal alcohol abuse. Elevated serum gamma-glutamyl transpeptidase (SGGT) is a particularly sensitive indicator of alcoholic liver disease; it is a sensitive measure of liver enzyme induction. More than 70% of heavy drinkers have an elevated SGGT (>40 units per liter). Alcoholic patients have a 4 to 10 times higher rate of abnormal SGGT when they are actively drinking than when they are abstinent. As an indicator of heavy alcohol consumption, SGGT has a sensitivity of 70% and a specificity of 90%. SGOT is elevated (>45 units/mL) in 30%–60% of alcoholic persons, with a sensitivity of 80%. Irwin et al. (1988) reported preliminary evidence that increases over baseline abstinence of 20% for SGGT and of 50% for SGOT may reflect heavy drinking even if the increased values fall within the normal range; thus, such increases may be an indicator of relapse.

Increased MCV, a measure of red blood cell size (>95 μ in males, 100 μ in females), is found with certain nutritional deficiencies (e.g., folate or B_{12}) or can be associated with alcohol's direct effect on bone marrow cell production. Increased MCV is found in 45%–90% of alcoholics, whereas only 1%–5% of nonalcoholics demonstrate elevated MCVs (Holt et al. 1981) (and should be differentiated from B_{12} or folate deficiencies).

Attempts are being made to develop laboratory profiles that will serve as better markers for early detection of alcohol problems. For example, the combination of abnormal SGGT and MCV identifies 90% of alcoholics in the general medical population, compared with 70%–80% when MCV or SGGT is used alone (Lumeng 1986). Unfortunately, these panels' high rates of false-negative and false-positive results render them unacceptable for clinical use other than screening at this time. Finally, decreased serum albumin, B_{12}, or folic acid may be evidence of prolonged malnutrition secondary to alcohol or substance abuse. Positive hepatitis B and HIV testing and bacteremia may indicate past or present intravenous use. Laboratory findings consistent with pancreatitis, hepatitis, bone marrow suppression, or certain types of infection may be clues to underlying alcoholism.

The detection of carbohydrate-deficient transferrin (CDT) will be increasingly important in detecting relapse as well as heavy alcohol use. Although this test (usually the percentage CDT TIA) is available in many research laboratories in the United States, it has not achieved widespread clinical use to date. This is lamentable, because the test is superior to SGGT in detecting relapse or recent heavy use (Schmidt et al. 1997). Since their pathogeneses differ, concurrent abnormal CDT and SGGT results are powerful indicators of alcohol abuse or dependence. Nonetheless, even that combination may be less sensitive than the CAGE alone when applied in the emergency department (Reynaud et al. 2001).

Other Studies

Although experience is accumulating with the use of sweat, hair, and saliva as laboratory specimens, their clinical reliability remains unknown. Breathalyzer tests are simple, do not require an invasive procedure, provide immediate results, and are widely used. Imaging studies of the liver, spleen, and brain and an EEG may be useful in the diagnosis of substance abuse as well.

Meaning of Test Results

Qualitative presence of drugs indicates prior exposure but not necessarily current intoxication or impairment. Reaching the truth involves asking questions like the following:

- What test method was used?
- Did the assay analyze for the drug, its metabolite, or both?
- What is the cutoff threshold? (The laboratory should be called if this is unclear.)
- Was the time of sample collection close to the time of exposure?

False positives. In some cases false positives are quite possible. A false positive is almost impossible when using

---

TABLE 8–8. Laboratory findings associated with alcohol abuse

Blood alcohol level
Positive breathalyzer
Elevated mean corpuscular volume
Elevated SGOT, SGPT, LDH
Elevated SGGT (particularly sensitive)
Elevated carbohydrate-deficient transferrin
Decreased albumin, B_{12}, folic acid (due to malnutrition)
Increased uric acid, elevated amylase, and evidence of bone marrow suppression

Note. LDH = lactate dehydrogenase; SGGT = serum gamma-glutamyl transpeptidase; SGOT = serum glutamic-oxaloacetic transaminase; SGPT = serum glutamic-pyruvic transaminase.

thin-layer chromatography (TLC), because this technique has high specificity (although poor sensitivity) for both drugs and their metabolites, and because color dyes increase specificity. In radioimmunoassay (RIA) or enzyme multiplied immunoassay technique (EMIT), two sensitive tests, chemically similar compounds may cross-react, producing false positives. And, as each antibody has a particular affinity, the specificity of each test should be evaluated. Immunoassays can be confirmed by chromatography, and vice versa. False-positive results for cocaine can be produced by fluconazole and local anesthetics, for opioids by chlorpromazine, poppy seeds, dextromorphan, ofloxacin, and rifampin, for cannabis by dronabinol and naproxen, and for benzodiazepines by oxaprozin have been reported (Ellenhorn 1997; Shearer et al. 1998).

False negatives. False negatives occur more easily than do false positives, perhaps because once a specimen tests negative, it is not tested further. Negative TLC results are not conclusive, however. Cutoffs may be too high for RIA or enzyme immunoassay (EIA). When the suspicion for substance use is strong, the clinician should repeat the test and should consult the laboratory regarding whether more sensitive drug-screening procedures, such as GC/MS, are available.

Diagnostic Instruments

Attempts to construct a psychological profile of the substance abuser have generally failed. Early psychodynamic theorists described addictive behavior as related to oral regressive defense mechanisms. More recently, theorists have postulated ego disturbances, difficulty with affect regulation, and defective self-care mechanisms. Pathological dependency, feelings of inadequacy, and counterdependency feelings of bravado have all been described in substance-abusing patients. Cognitive theorists have hypothesized that tension and stress reduction, positive expectancy of mood elevation, and increased perception of self-adequacy all play a role in psychoactive substance abuse. No one personality causes any substance use disorder; thus, other screening instruments are of high importance.

Diagnostic Research Instruments

The need for better standardized diagnostic research instruments in psychiatry has produced structured interviews that have been helpful in identifying alcoholism in large epidemiological studies. These instruments are also used to identify other psychiatric disorders. The Schedule for Affective Disorders and Schizophrenia (SADS; Endicott and Spitzer 1978), which is based on the Research Diagnostic Criteria (RDC; Feighner et al. 1972), is a forerunner to the Diagnostic Interview Schedule (DIS; Regier et al. 1988). The DIS is based on DSM-IV criteria and is designed to be administered by trained lay interviewers. The Structured Clinical Interview for DSM-IV Axis II Personality Disorders (SCID-II; First et al. 1997) is a more recent structured interview based on DSM-IV criteria that can also be used in making DSM-IV personality disorder diagnoses. These instruments have proven to be fairly reliable in establishing DSM-IV and RDC psychoactive substance abuse diagnoses. However, the anxiety, antisocial, and depression sections of these diagnostic instruments may be less useful in the psychoactive substance–using population.

Several instruments designed for research purposes are available that sensitively measure attributes of alcohol abuse. The Alcohol Use Inventory (AUI; Horn et al. 1986) is a 17-item, self-administered questionnaire that assesses 1) perceived benefits of alcohol, 2) problems concomitant to alcohol use, 3) disruptive consequences of drinking, and 4) the patient's concern about his or her use of alcohol and the extent to which the patient acknowledges having a drinking problem (Warburg and Horn 1985). The Alcohol Dependence Scale (ADS; Skinner and Horn 1984) is a brief 10-question instrument assessing physical dependence.

Dimensional Scales

Dimensional personality profile scales such as the Minnesota Multiphasic Personality Inventory (MMPI; Hathaway and McKinley 1967) and the Symptom Checklist–90 (SCL-90; Derogatis et al. 1973) have been useful in substance abuse populations. In the hands of a skilled interpreter, common findings of elevated scores on the hysteria, paranoia, antisocial, and depression subscales can augment initial clinical impressions. A markedly elevated schizophrenia scale score or evidence of male or female identity confusion may occasionally be expected. Valid profiles may indicate that the patient is dissimulating. Although its usefulness is limited to augmentation of a good clinical diagnostic interview, the MMPI may be helpful in charting improvement over time. Because of the time-limited systemic effects of alcohol, patients' symptoms frequently begin to clear after 3 or 4 weeks of abstinence, and this is reflected in the test. Personality subscales may improve as the acquired substance abuse–related personality attributes abate. Conversely, serious psychiatric problems may also be unmasked following drug removal. Frequently, damage to personality structure improves, but recovery may not be total. The MacAndrew Alcoholism Scale (MacAndrew

1965) is a subset scale of the MMPI that has been widely used in identifying alcoholism. The MacAndrew scale is a 48-question true/false scale that can correctly identify 82% of alcoholics. Although this scale has shown promise, recent studies have highlighted some of its limitations in the general medical population.

Diagnostic Screening Devices

Several instruments are available that are designed to measure various aspects of alcohol and other substance abuse. The majority of these instruments are not based on research criteria but have been found to be clinically useful in identifying psychoactive substance abuse. Two widely used alcoholism screening tests are the Michigan Alcoholism Screening Test (MAST) (Table 8–9) and the CAGE questionnaire (Table 8–10). These tests have the advantage of being self-administered, brief screens that can point the way for further study. The MAST is a 25-question form. The short MAST (SMAST) is a 13-item scale that correlates .90 with the MAST. The MAST has a test–retest reliability in excess of .85. The sensitivities of the MAST and the SMAST are approximately .90 and .70, respectively. The proportion of nonalcoholics correctly identified as such averages .74 for the MAST. These tests screen for the major psychological, social, and physiological effects of alcoholism. One new screening instrument for alcoholism, the TWEAK, has been found to be particularly helpful in screening female drinkers (Russel et al. 1991).

Addiction Severity Index

The Addiction Severity Index (ASI) developed by McLellan et al. (1981) has proven to be a useful instrument in the substance abuse population, particularly in treatment outcome research. The ASI establishes a scale and scoring system for the severity of need for treatment in seven major areas: 1) medical status, 2) employment–support status, 3) drug use, 4) alcohol use, 5) legal status, 6) family social relationships, and 7) psychiatric status. This dimensional approach is most helpful for identification of treatment needs in the process of attempting to match patients with specific treatments. Administration can be done by any trained person and will take approximately 50–60 minutes. An ASI geared for teenagers is now available as well (Kaminer et al. 1991).

Treatment of Substance Use Disorders

The treatment of the various substance use disorders spans many different clinical situations created by different substances. Nonetheless, except for some overdose, intoxication, and withdrawal states that require very specific pharmacological and supportive measures, there is much overlap among the treatments for substance use disorders. With naltrexone as an early example, many investigators have begun to apply modalities established for one substance to the treatment of use disorders of other substances (e.g., disulfiram for cocaine; Petrakis et al. 2000). Notwithstanding the standards contained in the American Psychiatric Association's "Practice Guideline for the Treatment of Patients With Substance Use Disorders" (American Psychiatric Association 1995), the American Society of Addiction Medicine's *Patient Placement Criteria for the Treatment of Substance-Related Disorders* (American Society of Addiction Medicine 1996), and the National Institute on Drug Abuse's "Principles of Drug Addiction Treatment" (National Institute on Drug Abuse 1999), facts about optimal treatment combinations await valid and well-constructed outcome research, and clinicians often must use various modalities simultaneously in order to tailor care to an individual patient.

As in any part of the practice of medicine, the clinician's choices of treatment are enhanced by a careful history, by mental status and physical examinations, by diagnostic formulation, and by confirmatory evidence from laboratory tests and third-party sources.

Treatment of substance use disorders can be extremely difficult. Helping the patient to acknowledge that he or she has a problem and to accept help are the two most important steps in treatment, as recognized both by self-help groups and by research in motivational interviewing and stages of awareness (Prochaska et al. 1992). These steps are frequently difficult to take because of the nature of addictive disorders, which leads to denial, lying, and neuropathology. Both patient and therapist may struggle with the stigma of substance disorders and with accepting that the patient has an illness. Most patients will wish to achieve controlled use and will have difficulty accepting the therapist's standard of abstinence as the goal for treatment. Patients frequently feel hopeless about ever achieving sustained abstinence and need to be encouraged that the goal is attainable. Seeing others who are recovering and accumulating personal experience of increasing periods of abstinence can bring renewed hope. Harm-avoidance approaches such as needle exchange, relapse prevention, and continuance of pharmacological and psychotherapeutic modalities for patients with comorbidity can be combined with a long-range goal of abstinence.

TABLE 8–9. The Michigan Alcoholism Screening Test (MAST)

Points	Question	Yes	No
(0)	0. Do you enjoy a drink now and then?	___	___
(2)	1. Do you feel you are a normal drinker? (By normal we mean you drink less than or as much as most other people.) [Negative response is alcoholic response]	___	___
(2)	2. Have you ever awakened the morning after some drinking the night before and found that you could not remember a part of the evening?	___	___
(1)	3. Does your wife, husband, parent, or other near relative ever worry or complain about your drinking?	___	___
(2)	4. Can you stop drinking without a struggle after one or two drinks? [Negative response is alcoholic response]	___	___
(1)	5. Do you ever feel guilty about your drinking?	___	___
(2)	6. Do friends or relatives think you are a normal drinker? [Negative response is alcoholic response]	___	___
(0)	7. Do you ever try to limit your drinking to certain times of the day or to certain places?	___	___
(2)	8. Are you always able to stop drinking when you want to? [Negative response is alcoholic response]	___	___
(2)	9. Have you ever attended a meeting of Alcoholics Anonymous?	___	___
(1)	10. Have you gotten into physical fights when drinking?	___	___
(2)	11. Has your drinking ever created problems between you and your wife, husband, a parent, or other relative?	___	___
(2)	12. Has your wife or husband (or other family members) ever gone to anyone for help about your drinking?	___	___
(2)	13. Have you ever lost friends because of your drinking?	___	___
(2)	14. Have you ever gotten into trouble at work or school because of drinking?	___	___
(2)	15. Have you ever lost a job because of drinking?	___	___
(2)	16. Have you ever neglected your obligations, your family, or your work for 2 or more days in a row because you were drinking?	___	___
(1)	17. Do you drink before noon fairly often?	___	___
(2)	18. Have you ever been told you have liver trouble? Cirrhosis?	___	___
(2)	*19. After heavy drinking, have you ever had delirium tremens (DTs), severe shaking, or heard voices or seen things that really were not there?	___	___
(5)	20. Have you ever gone to anyone for help about your drinking?	___	___
(5)	21. Have you ever been in a hospital because of drinking?	___	___
(2)	22. Have you ever been a patient in a psychiatric hospital or on a psychiatric ward of a general hospital where drinking was part of the problem that resulted in hospitalization?	___	___
(2)	23. Have you ever been seen at a psychiatric or mental health clinic or gone to any doctor, social worker, or clergyman for help with any emotional problem where drinking was part of the problem?	___	___
(2)	**24. Have you ever been arrested for drunk driving, driving while intoxicated, or driving under the influence of alcoholic beverages? (If YES, How many times?___)	___	___
(2)	**25. Have you ever been arrested or taken into custody—even for a few hours—because of other drunk behavior? (If YES, How many times? ___)	___	___

Note. *Five points for DTs; **two points for each arrest.

Scoring system: In general, 5 points or more would place the subject in an "alcoholic" category. 4 points would suggest alcoholism, 3 points or less would indicate the subject is not alcoholic.

The MAST scoring system is very sensitive at the 5-point level and it tends to find more people alcoholics than anticipated. However, it is a screening test and should be sensitive at its lower levels.

Source. Reprinted with permission from Selzer ML: "The Michigan Alcoholism Screening Test: The Quest for a New Diagnostic Instrument." *American Journal of Psychiatry* 127:1653–1658, 1971. Copyright 1971 American Psychiatric Association.

General Principles

The following points are general principles to provide the basis for treatment of substance use disorders:

- *Case heterogeneity:* Patients are individuals and vary in terms of substance(s) used, pattern of use, clinical severity, functional impairment, secondary medical conditions, psychiatric comorbidity, strengths, vulner-

TABLE 8–10. CAGE screen for diagnosis of alcoholism

"Have you ever…"
C thought you should CUT back on your drinking?
A felt ANNOYED by people criticizing your drinking?
G felt GUILTY or bad about your drinking?
E had a morning EYE OPENER to relieve hangover or nerves?
Score total positive responses:
2–3: High index of suspicion
4: Pathognomonic

Source. Reproduced with permission from Ewing JA: "Detecting Alcoholism: The CAGE Questionnaire." *JAMA* 252:1905–1907, 1984. Copyright 1984 American Medical Association.

abilities, and social and environmental context. Thus, no one treatment works for all individuals.

- *Phases of treatment:* Active treatment progresses; it does not all happen at once. Begin with comprehensive assessment and move to treatment of intoxication or withdrawal, development of treatment plan, and enactment of plan. The amount of time in treatment is a critical prognostic factor.

- *Comprehensive treatment:* Assessment and treatment must both take into account all aspects of the individual's life and illness. Collateral sources of information are extremely important in assessment. Coexisting psychiatric and medical conditions should be treated concurrently in an integrated manner. Treatment programs should assess for HIV, hepatitis, tuberculosis, and other infectious diseases and should provide education to help patients to reduce their risk of contracting communicable diseases.

- *Treatment plans:* Goals should include the reduction of use, the achievement of abstinence, the reduction of relapse, and rehabilitation and recovery. Treatment status must be continually reviewed, reassessed, and updated.

- *Viewing relapse:* Relapses occur, and all treatment plans must assess for them. They do not always imply a treatment failure. Treatment must continue, but it must address the need for increased surveillance. Abstinence may sometimes seem an impossible goal (e.g., in the elderly), but reductions in morbidity and mortality follow any reduction in substance use, making the effort worthwhile (Marlatt and Gordon 1985).

Maintaining the Therapeutic Alliance

The therapeutic alliance may be one of the clinician's most important tools. Given that patients with substance problems often grew up in families with substance disorders, their propensity to have typical transference resis-

tances to treatment and to evoke countertransference reactions in the therapist is not surprising. These countertransference reactions can either facilitate or negate treatment, depending on how they are handled (Group for the Advancement of Psychiatry 1998). Therapists who are well informed and well trained and who understand and are in touch with their own feelings are more helpful to patients and less likely to experience "burnout" (Frances and Alexopoulos 1982b). We can think of 10 attributes and attitudes that are helpful in maintaining the therapeutic alliance with substance disorder patients (Table 8–11). (For further reading, see Frances et al. 2001.)

TABLE 8–11. Attributes and attitudes helpful in working with patients with substance disorders

1. Respect for the provision of a caring and compassionate relationship
2. Informed optimism
3. The capacity to tolerate one's own anxiety, pain, frustration, and depression
4. Flexibility and open-mindedness
5. Good knowledge of general psychiatry; resourcefulness and creativity
6. Intellectual curiosity
7. Wisdom
8. Persistence and patience
9. The capacity to listen, to hear both what is and what is not said, and to act accordingly
10. Honesty ands integrity (in the therapist and in the treatment team)

1. The most crucial nonspecific variable is an attitude of respect for the provision of a caring and compassionate relationship. Often underestimated, a concern for patients and a willingness to form an active therapeutic alliance (with some degree of therapeutic zeal but without overidentification) are crucial to working with patients who have substance disorders. An empathic capacity to feel the patient's experience and yet maintain objectivity is crucial. Following a tradition in psychotherapy (which goes back to Ferenczi and Alexander) of taking an active role and of creating an environment in which a patient can achieve comfort and growth is desirable. This includes an ability to confront with concern as well as to provide emotional support appropriately. It does not mean playing a real sexual or parental role or taking on a contrived position that is not genuinely felt by the therapist. It is important that the

ness training are also valuable. The following are two important approaches to relapse prevention:

- *Reduction of guilt and shame:* The clinician expects the patient to see relapse neither as an "all-or-none" act nor as an unforeseeable or unavoidable event. Relapse—defined as a change in one's resolution to change—is a fairly common experience that we all have at times. Relapse, then, is a fact of everyday life. Understanding this may prevent the patient's feeling that he or she has totally failed and that all is lost if a return to use occurs. Marlatt and Gordon (1985) coined the term *abstinence-violation effect* to describe the view that once use occurs, it must inevitably lead to pretreatment levels of use. Guilt, shame, a sense of lack of control, feelings of being trapped, and the absence of a contingency plan to minimize damage may escalate a return to drug use. The immediate benefits of drug use may overshadow the realization of the negative long-term consequences.
- *Practicing of social skills:* Identifying personal strengths, past coping behaviors, and environmental supports is important. Examples of coping mechanisms when faced with temptation or drug use include calling a friend or sponsor, leaving the setting, and refusing the next drink. Relapse prevention may require complete avoidance of high-risk situations and cues, especially in the early stages of recovery. Later on in the process, some avoidable high-risk situations can be mastered with alternative coping skills. Social skills training has also been used in prevention. In some situations, however, it may be advisable to avoid cues at all cost (e.g., having a "crack" addict not return to a setting where cocaine is being used).

Predictors of Successful Treatment Outcome

Treatment outcome is better in those with high socioeconomic stability, antisocial personality, a lack of psychiatric and medical problems, and a negative family history for alcoholism. A history of Alcoholics Anonymous (AA) participation, a stable work and marriage history, and a lack of legal history are correlated with better outcome. Most studies of treatment settings have not differentiated outcome by treatment setting.

Differential Therapeutics

Despite developments in treatment outcome research, choice of the most appropriate treatments for addicted patients is still largely based on the conventional wisdom of clinical considerations. In choosing treatment combinations, clinicians need to take into account that many patients have an additional psychiatric illness, that multiple addiction is frequent, and that selection should fit the unique needs of the patient (Perry et al. 1984). Other factors to be considered include medical and psychiatric illness, illness severity, individual patient characteristics, culture, availability of treatment resources, and awareness of the differential therapeutics of concomitant psychiatric disorders. Recent advances in biobehavioral approaches to psychiatric disorders (i.e., cognitive-behavioral and psychodynamic individual approaches; group and family treatment) need to be considered as well. Integration of 12-Step approaches such as Alcoholics Anonymous (AA) and Narcotics Anonymous (NA) is also widely recommended.

Matching Treatments to Patients

In the past it was easy to apply the finding that longer inpatient stays are more likely to lead to full or partial abstinence of alcohol follow-up and reduced relapse rates. But today there are more treatment options and more pressure for efficiency. This is especially important for patients with substance use disorders and psychiatric disorders. In a series of classic studies, McLellan et al. (1997) found that matching problems to treatment services improved treatment effectiveness and led to good overall effectiveness for alcohol treatment. Patients with severe psychiatric problems did poorly regardless of modality or treatment setting. Patients with legal problems did poorly in inpatient programs. Patients with the least severe psychiatric problems did well in both inpatient and outpatient settings. Those patients with psychiatric problems in the middle range of severity usually also had employment or family problems, needed inpatient care, and improved when psychiatric services were also provided.

Because all patients are individuals with specific, unique problems, the field continues its attempts to create a differential therapeutics. However, it is often difficult to demonstrate differential treatment outcomes with different approaches.

To expand the number of people treated for addictions, a number of studies have explored provision of opioid replacement treatment in noninstitutional settings, especially in terms of buprenorphine and methadone. It is important to increase the number of treatment sites, because the organized, approved programs in central locations reach only 14% of patients with opioid dependence. Dual-diagnosis patients deserve comprehensive, integrated treatment. Outpatient care for such patients must include aggressive outreach, case management, and a longitudinal, stagewise, motivational approach to substance abuse treatment.

Treatment Settings

Inpatient Treatment

Inpatient treatment is indicated in the presence of major medical and psychiatric problems and their complications; severe withdrawal symptoms such as DTs or seizures; failure to benefit from trials of outpatient treatment; inability of family, friends, or AA members to provide an adequate social support network for abstinence; or polysubstance addiction requiring medical management. For most other patients, a trial of outpatient treatment is indicated before hospitalization unless complications are present. Most patients prefer outpatient treatment because it is less disruptive and more cost-effective than inpatient treatment. Inpatient detoxification is followed by outpatient treatment or by inpatient rehabilitation.

The choice of inpatient rehabilitation in a freestanding substance recovery program, a freestanding inpatient psychiatric hospital, or a general hospital psychiatric unit depends on the severity of additional psychiatric and medical problems. Patients with the most severe psychiatric illness may need to be treated on a locked general hospital inpatient psychiatric unit before transfer to a MICA (mental illness, chemical abuse) treatment unit.

Treatment outcome is related to length of treatment in that patients who complete day hospital substance abuse rehabilitation and then go on to participate in self-help groups are likely to have lower rates of alcohol and cocaine use during follow-up. Furthermore, the beneficial effect of self-help-group participation does not appear to be strictly the result of motivation or some other patient characteristic.

Outpatient Treatment

Outpatient treatment delivery ranges from the individual substance abuse therapist to a day or evening addiction treatment program to the primary care provider; all may utilize techniques employed in inpatient treatment programs. Indications for outpatient alcohol detoxification include high motivation and good social support, no previous history of DTs or seizures, brief or nonsevere recent binges, no severe medical or psychiatric problems or polyaddiction, and previous successful outpatient detoxifications.

Treatment of Clinical Situations

Overdose

Overdose is properly treated in the emergency department by a medical team. Table 8–13 outlines the major medical complications and treatment approaches to various drug overdoses (The Medical Letter 1996). Because several drugs are slowly absorbed, the minimal time for observation of a suspected drug overdose should be 4 hours. Exact time of ingestion is often difficult to ascertain reliably. If there is good evidence that a specific drug was ingested, a call to the poison control center is suggested, and transfer to an emergency department is the next step. The first clinical task is to ensure the adequacy of the airway, breathing, and circulation (i.e., the ABCs), which includes assessment of airway patency, respiratory rate, blood pressure, and pulse. Outside of the hospital, cardiopulmonary resuscitation (CPR) may be lifesaving. In the medical setting, almost every overdose with loss of consciousness or any case of coma with unknown etiology should receive 50 mg of dextrose 5% in water (D5W) and 0.4 mg of naloxone, which may need to be repeated. Prompt response provides evidence for hypoglycemia, opioid overdose, or alcohol overdose. D5W should not be given first in Wernicke's encephalopathy because glucose can further suppress thiamine stores. Other basic measures include diazepam treatment for status epilepticus and treatment of metabolic acidosis.

Elimination Methods

Our emphasis here is on general parameters (Table 8–14); the reader is referred elsewhere for technical information on elimination (Goldberg et al. 1986). Gastric emptying is appropriate only for orally ingested drugs. One absolute contraindication to gastric emptying is in cases of caustic ingestion. Ipecac syrup induces vomiting in approximately 30 minutes; to reduce the risk of aspiration, it should be given only to patients who are awake and alert. Ipecac should be administered even after spontaneous emesis, because full gastric emptying may not have been accomplished. Gastric lavage entails flushing the upper gastrointestinal tract with water. This technique is attempted only on a patient whose airway is secured by intubation. Placed in the stomach, activated charcoal serves as an absorbent to remove toxic substances, and it may reduce reabsorption of substances from the duodenum. When ingested substances are weak acids or bases, forced diuresis can be attempted in patients with functioning kidneys. Dialysis is generally a heroic measure to save a life. It is more

TABLE 8–13. Management of overdose

Drug	Major complications[a]	Antidote or specific treatment	Potential lethal dose
Acetaminophen	Hepatotoxicity peaks at 72–96 hours. Complete recovery generally in 4 days, but injury worse for alcoholic patients. Mortality: 1%–2%	Acetylcysteine	140 mg/kg
Alcohol	Respiratory depression	None	350–700 mg (serum)
Amphetamines	Seizures	None; avoid neuroleptics	20–25 mg/kg
Short-acting barbiturates	Respiratory depression	None	>3 g
Long-acting barbiturates	Respiratory depression	None	>6 g
Benzodiazepine	Sedation, respiratory depression, hypotension, coma	Flumazenil reverses effects (but it may induce withdrawal in the dependent)	—
Carbon monoxide	Headaches, dizziness, weakness, nausea, vomiting, diminished visual acuity, tachycardia, tachypnea, ataxia, and seizures are all possible. Other manifestations include hemorrhages (cherry red spots on the skin), metabolic acidosis, coma, and death.	Hyperbaric oxygen	—
Cocaine	Peak toxicity 60–90 minutes after use leads to systemic sympathomimesis and seizures, acidosis. Followed by cardiopulmonary depression, perhaps pulmonary edema. Treatment of acidosis, seizures, and hypertension is imperative.	Naloxone (empirically)	—
Nonbenzodiazepine hypnotics	Delirium, extrapyramidal side effects	None	Varies with tolerance
Hydrocarbons	Gastrointestinal, respiratory, and central nervous system compromise	None	—
Opioids	Miosis, respiratory depression, obtundation, pulmonary edema, delirium, death	Naloxone Nalmefene helpful	Varies with tolerance
Phencyclidine/ketamine	Hypertension, nystagmus, rhabdomyolysis	None; forced diuresis should not be attempted in cases of phencyclidine overdose with suspected rhabdomyolysis.	
Phenothiazines	Anticholinergic effects, extrapyramidal side effects, cardiac effects	Phenothiazine overdose should be monitored for 48 hours for cardiac arrhythmia. Lidocaine may be necessary for treatment of cardiac arrhythmia, norepinephrine for hypotension, sodium bicarbonate for metabolic acidosis, and phenytoin for seizures.	150 mg/kg
Salicylates	Central nervous system, acidosis	None	500 mg/kg
Tricyclic antidepressants	Cardiac effects, hypotension, anticholinergism	None	35 mg/kg
Hallucinogens	Ring-substituted amphetamines, even lysergic acid diethylamide/mescaline, may lead to rhabdomyolysis, hyperthermia, hyponatremia	Temperature reduction, dantrolene	
Inhalants	Cardiotoxicity—arrhythmias	Cardiac monitoring	

Note. ªSee "Overdose" for descriptions of overdose states.

likely to be successful if the ingested drug is one that is in the plasma, minimally bound to tissue, or cleared poorly through the kidney. Dialysis has been especially valuable with alcohol, amphetamine, and aspirin overdose. Hypoperfusion is an extracorporeal blood-filtering technique similar to dialysis that uses a different type of membrane filtration. This technique has been especially useful in barbiturate overdose; it may, however, lead to thrombocytopenia.

Intoxication

Most simple intoxication does not come to medical attention. Those cases that do present to the emergency department should be screened carefully for medical problems such as subdural hematoma, meningitis, HIV, or endocarditis with embolization. Support measures include interrupting substance absorption, providing a safe environment, decreasing sensory stimulation, and allowing the safe passage of time. A calm, nonthreatening manner should be employed, with clear communication and reality orientation. Attempts to reason with most intoxicated patients will not be fruitful; in cases of hallucinogen abuse, however, individuals can frequently be "talked down" from pathological intoxication.

Alcohol

There is no proven amethystic (i.e., anti-drunkenness) agent that can hasten the cessation of alcohol intoxication (not even strong black coffee or cold showers). There has been no shortage of experimental approaches to delaying absorption or decreasing metabolism and elimination, and both opioid antagonists (including naloxone) and CNS stimulants have also been studied as means of protecting against dangerous effects of intoxication. The safe passage of time is currently the only effective measure to reverse acute intoxication.

Opioids

No specific measures are generally needed to treat opioid intoxication. If a life-threatening overdose is suspected, prompt treatment with naloxone is necessary (see previous "Overdose" section and Table 8–13).

Cocaine and Amphetamines

Cocaine abusers often self-medicate with CNS depressants to antagonize the dysphoric stimulant properties of the drug. For severe agitation, benzodiazepines such as diazepam or lorazepam may be helpful. If frank psychosis persists, low-dose haloperidol (2–5 mg) may be helpful, and the dose should be adjusted as necessary to control symptoms; however, haloperidol will also decrease the seizure threshold and should be used with caution. MAOIs should be avoided, as they inhibit the degradation of cocaine and can produce a hypertensive crisis.

Phencyclidine

The fundamental goal in treating the violence associated with PCP intoxication is to ensure the safety of all parties. When a patient becomes threatening, strong physical presence of at least five people is needed for physical containment. Benzodiazepines (e.g., diazepam) are superior to neuroleptics in the treatment of agitation, but neuroleptics such as haloperidol are better for PCP toxic psychosis. Enhancement of excretion is helpful with gastric lavage if the drug was taken orally, or by acidification of the urine if systemically administered. For lasting problems, ECT may be indicated.

Ketamine

As previously discussed, ketamine intoxication is a serious state and can include psychosis; delirium; dissociation; neuromuscular, peripheral, and CNS manifestations; respiratory dysfunction; cardiotoxicity; and movement abnormalities. In severe cases, intensive and supportive care is needed. For milder cases, monitoring for and treatment of rhabdomyolysis is necessary, and sedation with a short-acting benzodiazepine is helpful (Graeme 2000)

Cannabis

Cannabis intoxication generally needs no formal treatment. The occasional severe anxiety attacks or acute paranoid episodes can be handled with reality orientation. In rare cases, severe anxiety may warrant treatment with a benzodiazepine, and low-dose haloperidol or olanzapine may be helpful for cannabis-induced psychosis.

Hallucinogens

For most hallucinogens, patients can be "talked down" with reality orientation and reassurance. Benzodiazepines may help to provide sedation. This approach is adequate for mild cases of intoxication with MDMA; however, overdose, especially with MDMA, can lead to hyperpyrexia, dehydration, tachycardia, and even neuroleptic malignant syndrome, arrhythmias, seizures, cerebrovascular accidents, coma, disseminated intravascular coagulation, or death and should be treated in a medical setting.

TABLE 8–14. Overdose-elimination methods

Drug	Ipecac syrup	Forced diuresis	Gastric lavage	Activated charcoal	Hemodialysis	Hemoperfusion
Acetaminophen	Yes	Yes (alkaline)	Yes	No	No	No
Alcohol	No	No	Yes	Yes	Yes	No
Amphetamines	Yes	Yes (acid)	Yes	Yes	Yes	NA
Barbiturates	NA	Only for long-acting	NA	Yes	NA	Yes
Benzodiazepines	Yes	No	Yes	Repeated	NA	NA
Carbon monoxide	No	No	No	No	No	No
Cocaine	No	No	No	No	No	No
Nonbenzodiazepine hypnotics	Yes	No	Yes	Yes	NA	NA
Hydrocarbons	Yes	NA	Yes	NA	NA	NA
Opioids	NA	NA	Yes if orally ingested	NA	NA	NA
Phencyclidine/ ketamine	Only severe	Not in rhabdomyolysis (avoid in renal failure)	Only severe	Yes	NA	NA
Phenothiazines	Yes	NA	Yes	Yes	NA	NA
Salicylates	Yes	Yes (alkaline)	Yes	Yes	Yes	NA
Tricyclic antidepressants	NA	NA	NA	Repeated	No	No

Note. NA = not applicable.

Inhalants

Inhalant intoxication can vary in its presentation and need for active treatment. The main principle is protection of the individual from harm and from harming others; symptoms are usually time limited.

Gamma-Hydroxybutyrate

GHB may be the cause of many unidentified emergency cases in which the presentation may include CNS depression, aggressive behavior, seizures, myoclonus, nystagmus, tunnel vision, incontinence, bradycardia followed by tachycardia, respiratory depression, apnea, nausea or vomiting, hypothermia, flushing, or diaphoresis. In most cases, all signs resolve in 2–7 hours and improve with supportive care (Graeme 2000).

Withdrawal

Alcohol Withdrawal/Detoxification

Setting: inpatient versus outpatient. For treatment of alcohol use disorders, patients with delirium, low IQ, Wernicke's encephalopathy, trauma history, neurological symptoms, medical complications, psychopathology requiring medication, DTs, or alcoholic seizures or hallucinosis are probably best evaluated and treated in an inpatient setting. Polysubstance abuse, poor compliance, poor family support, inability to get from home to place of treatment, a chaotic or unstable home situation, and an environment in which the patient is continually exposed to others who abuse substances all predict a poor outcome for outpatient detoxification. Yet outpatient detoxification can be appropriate: approximately 95% of patients have only mild-to-moderate withdrawal symptoms. Supportive care without pharmacological intervention is adequate for a significant number of these patients, and even when medication is needed, it can be given in an outpatient setting. Outpatient care reduces costs, allows the patient to continue to function in his or her environment, and provides time for the therapist to evaluate the patient's motivation for treatment.

Treatment: pharmacological versus nonpharmacological. Most withdrawing alcohol users do not have major medical problems, but the best approach is conservative psychopharmacological management. Use of medication for the prevention of DTs or seizures is a top priority, to avoid not only discomfort or death but also the acceleration of cognitive decline secondary to repeated uncontrolled withdrawal. Thus, pharmacological detoxification is warranted for those with significant signs of withdrawal, a clear history of severe daily dependence or

high tolerance, codependence on other CNS depressants, or a past history of DTs or seizures. Medical complications (e.g., infections, trauma, metabolic or hepatic disorders) indicate pharmacological treatment. Physical and subjective discomfort should be minimized. Pharmacological care enhances compliance and provides an alcohol-free interval that may help the patient commit to treatment. Negative countertransference of staff members can result in withholding of appropriate medication. There should be little to no concern that this treatment will make the alcoholic a benzodiazepine abuser. Nonpharmacological detoxification is for patients with mild symptoms or a withdrawal history and mild-to-moderate dependence. Patients are housed for 3–4 days in a supportive, safe environment with rest and nutrition and are detoxified without medication. This environment helps patients to regulate and structure their lives again. Close monitoring of patients for complications and adequate medical backup are needed for detoxification.

Pharmacological Withdrawal

For all patients withdrawing from alcohol, careful monitoring of vital signs, physical signs, and subjective symptoms must be done at least every 4 hours while the patient is awake (Table 8–15). Several objective rating scales and some subjective scales (e.g., Clinical Institute Withdrawal Assessment [CIWA; Sullivan et al. 1989] for those without general medical complications) are used to monitor the withdrawal state. Pharmacological detoxification essentially involves substituting a drug that is cross-tolerant with alcohol and slowly withdrawing it from the body. For withdrawing patients with mental status alterations due to conditions other than alcohol (e.g., other substances, general medical or surgical conditions), detoxification remains a priority. Indeed, for those withdrawing from both opioids and alcohol, benzodiazepines might be given in preference to methadone in order to substitute for the alcohol while avoiding excessive sedation.

Benzodiazepine treatment. Many agents somewhat benefit the withdrawal state, but the benzodiazepines, with their agonist effect at the GABA receptor, are currently the best medications for alcohol detoxification. With adequate benzodiazepine coverage, complications of alcohol withdrawal are extremely rare. At usual doses, benzodiazepines produce little respiratory depression and a have good margin of safety between effective dose and overdose. Chlordiazepoxide (Librium) and diazepam (Valium), the most commonly used benzodiazepines, are long acting. Once a sufficient dose has been given, these drugs can be expected to "self-taper" without the need

TABLE 8–15. Medical workup for alcohol withdrawal

Routine lab tests	Complete blood count with differential, serum electrolytes, liver function tests including bilirubin, blood urea nitrogen, creatinine, fasting blood sugar, prothrombin time, cholesterol, triglycerides, calcium, magnesium, albumin, total protein, hepatitis B surface antigen, B_{12}, folate, stool guaiac, urinalysis, serum and urine toxic screens, chest X ray, electrocardiogram
Ancillary tests	Computed tomography, electroencephalogram, gastrointestinal series, HIV test, Venereal Disease Research Laboratory test

TABLE 8–16. Benzodiazepine treatment for alcohol withdrawal

Outpatient	Chlordiazepoxide 25–50 mg po qid on first day, 20% decrease over 5 days, daily visits
Inpatient	1. Choose agent: diazepam or chlordiazepoxide—Give initial loading dose then monitor objectively every 2–4 hours using vital signs or Clinical Institute Withdrawal Assessment (CIWA) scale or both
	2. Give additional dose every 2–4 hours as needed: chlordiazepoxide 25–50 mg (maximum 400 mg/24 hours), diazepam 5–10 mg (maximum 100 mg/24 hours), oxazepam 15–30 mg, or lorazepam 1 mg
	3. Count total dose needed for stabilization of signs
	4. Total divided by 4 is amount to give four times a day
	5. Taper daily total about 25% over 3 days—continue no more than 10 days
	6. Use adjunctive treatments
	7. And: thiamine 100 mg 4 times a day, folate 1 mg 4 times a day, multivitamin each day, $MgSO_4$ 1 g IM every 6 hours for 2 days if seizures occur (or carbamazepine or valproate).

for further dosing. The intermediate-half-life benzodiazepines (e.g., lorazepam [Ativan], oxazepam [Serax]), which have a lesser risk of accumulation and overdose, are useful in patients with hepatic disease, delirium, dementia, or pulmonary disease or those who are older. Lorazepam also has the advantages of primarily renal clearance and reliable intramuscular absorption. Table 8–17 shows treatment protocols for benzodiazepine treatment of alcohol withdrawal. In all cases, thiamine 100 mg orally or intramuscularly, folic acid 1–3 mg, and multivitamins should also be added. When indicated, naltrexone or disulfiram (Antabuse) can be added after physical examination, electrocardiogram, and blood work are completed, in the absence of contraindications such as arrhythmias, heart disease, severe hepatic disease, esophageal varices, pregnancy, or epilepsy (discussed later) and after at least 72 hours since last ingestion of alcohol.

Suppression of withdrawal symptoms is not a substitute for systematic detoxification. A conservative 5- to 7-day regimen (Table 8–16) promotes comfort, reduces complications, provides structure, and helps most patients cope cognitively and emotionally with the initial treatment. Uncomplicated detoxification treatment of this length rarely occurs on an inpatient unit because of cost pressures, and inpatient alcohol detoxification is often condensed to 3 days. Outpatient detoxification for uncomplicated alcohol dependence can be accomplished with chlordiazepoxide 25 mg administered four times a day decreasing to zero within 4–5 days. Inpatient withdrawal from alcohol is accomplished with chlordiazepoxide (Librium) orally 25–100 mg four times daily, with 25–50 mg every 2 hours as needed for positive withdrawal signs. Doses can be held if the patient appears intoxicated. Both regimens should include thiamine 50–100 mg orally or intramuscularly, multivitamins, and

folate 1–3 mg/day. Naltrexone is usually added 5 days after detoxification.

Adjuncts to benzodiazepines. The direct GABA agonism of benzodiazepines may be insufficient in the treatment of three important potential features of alcohol withdrawal:

- *Protection from seizures:* Consideration of patients at imminent risk of withdrawal seizures or DTs should be a part of all detoxification strategies. We do not regularly provide patients with prophylactic doses of antiepileptics unless they have a history of a seizure disorder. Even those who have previously had seizures during withdrawal do not routinely receive preventive anticonvulsants. Gabapentin, which is renally excreted and which lacks significant drug–drug interactions, cognitive effects, and abuse potential, is an ideal medication for this indication. Phenytoin was previously used for this purpose, and valproate may be used as well. Magnesium sulfate (1 g four times a day for 2 days) is also useful.
- *Alleviation of autonomic nervous system (ANS) signs:* Both β-blockers (e.g., propranolol) and α-blockers (e.g., clonidine) may alleviate ANS signs and symp-

toms that occur during withdrawal. The usual dose of propranolol is 10 mg every 6 hours as needed; that for clonidine is 0.5 mg two to three times a day as needed.

- *Treatment of psychotic features:* Neuroleptics are helpful for delirium, delusions, and hallucinations. Haloperidol 0.5–2.0 mg can be administered intramuscularly every 2 hours.

Withdrawal From Other CNS Depressants

Withdrawal from benzodiazepines, barbiturates, and other depressants often requires pharmacological detoxification. This is true for benzodiazepines used at high doses for short periods and for benzodiazepines used at low-to-medium doses for long periods (i.e., months, years). Conservative treatment requires slow withdrawal over many days or weeks. The effects of benzodiazepine withdrawal generally can be covered with chlordiazepoxide or diazepam (long half-life). A standard benzodiazepine detoxification regimen is outlined in Table 8–17. If the abuse history is unreliable or difficult to ascertain, a pentobarbital tolerance test can be used to find a starting dose (Table 8–18). For most patients with benzodiazepine addictions, detoxification is best done on an inpatient unit. However, for those who have used low doses of benzodiazepines for long periods, detoxification can be accomplished on an outpatient basis with 6–12 weeks of gradual reduction, during which time added support and education are helpful. Offering the option of an as-needed dose to avoid feeling trapped is fine. The worst symptoms occur at the lowest doses and during the first week without any medication. All parties should be prepared: the stress of that week may last a year. One study demonstrated a beneficial effect of imipramine that is begun prior to withdrawal from long-term benzodiazepine use (Rickels et al. 2000).

TABLE 8–17. Benzodiazepine detoxification

1. Establish usual maintenance dose from history or via pentobarbital tolerance test (Table 8–18).
2. Divide maintenance dose into equivalent as-needed doses of diazepam and administer first 2 days.
3. Decrease diazepam dose 10% each day thereafter.
4. Administer diazepam 5 mg every 6 hours as needed for signs of increased withdrawal.
5. When diazepam dose approaches 10% of original dose, reduce dose slowly over 3–4 days, then discontinue.

After detoxification, referral should be made to AA/NA and Al-Anon. For those who originally presented with anxiety, rebound can be expected. Nonbenzodiazepine alternatives for anxiety might include CBT, exercise, relaxation, or psychotherapy. One in eight patients detoxifying from CNS depressants will develop severe anxiety that requires treatment with medications and/or CBT.

Many CNS depressants (e.g., glutethimide [Doriden]) are abused episodically and do not require formal detoxification. For barbiturate or methaqualone abuse, detoxification is necessary. Barbiturates can be detoxified with either a long-acting benzodiazepine or a long-acting barbiturate, such as phenobarbital.

In some cases there is a need to substitute one CNS depressant for another. Most such "cross-tapers" occur over 3 weeks and use clonazepam. In week 1, use clonazepam 0.5 mg at bedtime and the previously used drug on an as-needed basis. In week 2, discontinue the previously used drug. In week 3, reduce the clonazepam to zero. This regimen requires inpatient admission in the case of barbiturate use, polysubstance abusers, or outpatient failures. The pentobarbital tolerance test (see Table 8–19) should be used to set the initial dose when dosage of use is unknown.

Alprazolam (Xanax) is uniquely less amenable to drug substitution; breakthrough seizures have been reported despite adequate coverage with chlordiazepoxide. Alprazolam detoxification should include an estimation of daily use and a slow withdrawal over a several-week period. Clonazepam has also been successfully used in alprazolam detoxification.

Opioid Withdrawal/Detoxification

Opioid detoxification may be needed to interrupt an opioid use disorder. Patients with these disorders rarely bring themselves to treatment; rather, their presentation for treatment may coincide with interrupted supply, overdose, or attempted self-detoxification. Methadone detoxification can be difficult due to its long half-life and chronic place in patients' lives.

The detoxification approach most commonly used for opioids involves the substitution and tapering of a long-acting opioid. An equivalent dose of methadone is substituted for the drug. For most heroin addicts, 20 mg of methadone is adequate, and the patient should be reevaluated every 2–4 hours for additional dosage. Once a stable dose is achieved, methadone should be decreased over 4–14 days, usually by 5 mg/day. As an aid in determining the initial dose, ratios of pure drug to methadone are as follows: heroin:methadone, 2:1; morphine sulfate:methadone, 4:1; oxycodone:methadone, 12:1; meperidine:methadone, 20:1; and codeine:methadone, 50:1.

TABLE 8–18. Pentobarbital tolerance test

Patient condition after test dose	Degree of tolerance	Estimated 24-hour pentobarbital requirement (mg)
Asleep but arousable	None or minimal	None
Drowsy; slurred speech; ataxia; marked intoxication	Definite but mild	400–600
Comfortable; fine lateral nystagmus only	Marked	600–1,000
No signs of effect; abstinence signs persist	Extreme	1,000–1,200 or more: In this case, give 100 mg every 2 hours until mild intoxication is produced (to a maximum of 500 mg). Multiply the amount that produced mild intoxication by 4 to obtain the estimated 24-hour dose of pentobarbital, and convert this amount to phenobarbital equivalents (100 mg of pentobarbital is equivalent to 30 mg phenobarbital). Give that phenobarbital dose for 2 days, then taper by 30 mg per day or 10% per day, whichever is less.

Note. For benzodiazepine discontinuation: see clinical response 1 hour after 200-mg test dose of pentobarbital.

Another approach is to slowly taper the abused drug over time. Although such a method is clearly untenable for illicit drugs, detoxification from a prescription medication such as codeine could be accomplished in this way. A drug dose consisting of an estimation of the daily use is mixed with 30 mg cherry syrup and given every day over 7–10 days, with the amount of added drug decreased daily. A low dose (25–50 mg) of thioridazine (Mellaril) concentrate can be added to reduce subjective discomfort.

Opioid detoxification can be accomplished with clonidine as the sole agent. Clonidine is an α_2-adrenergic agonist (see "Psychopharmacological Modalities") that has been shown effectively to suppress signs and symptoms of autonomic sympathetic activation during withdrawal (it has been less successful in decreasing the subjective discomfort of withdrawal). The chances of successful clonidine detoxification increase with mild dependence, higher motivation, and inpatient treatment. It is given orally on the first day at a dosage range of 0.1–0.3 mg three times a day (maximum 1.2 mg) and increased on the third day to 0.4–0.7 mg three times a day for a total detoxification period of 10–14 days. In appropriate patients, naltrexone can be started during the clonidine detoxification, as described in Table 8–19 (O'Connor et al. 1995). Clonidine's major side effects are hypotension and sedation; vital signs should be monitored carefully for patients receiving this agent. Outpatient detoxification with clonidine may be performed with highly motivated patients (O'Connor et al. 1997). Lofexidine, a centrally acting α_2-adrenergic agonist, may be comparable to clonidine but is not yet U.S. Food and Drug Administration (FDA)–approved for this purpose.

Rapid and ultrarapid detoxification. Rapid and ultrarapid detoxification methods employ opioid antagonists as well as adjuncts such as clonidine, sedation, and even general anesthesia. Offered at few institutions, these approaches are used for patients in transition to antagonist therapy. Unfortunately, ultrarapid detoxification involves the increased risks of anesthesia, is performed without rehabilitation, and is expensive.

Opioid detoxification adjuncts. Detoxification using clonidine as an adjunct should take 5–6 days; it is unlikely to help beyond 14 days. Clonidine can be administered transdermally via a patch. Use of clonidine at night should be avoided. Benzodiazepines are helpful for insomnia. At low doses (2–4 mg/day), buprenorphine is useful as a partial agonist because it blocks withdrawal, but at larger doses it decreases respiratory drive. Other drugs helpful during withdrawal include dicyclomine (Bentyl) for gastrointestinal pain, nonsteroidal anti-inflammatory drugs for myalgias, and antiemetics.

Cocaine, Cannabis, Hallucinogen, and Inhalant Detoxification

There are no specific pharmacological detoxifications for these substances. General support measures are usually adequate. Benzodiazepines may help the cocaine-withdrawing patient but have the potential for abuse. Other medications that may help alleviate the symptoms of cocaine abstinence include desipramine, which is superior to lithium, carbamazepine, and other antidepressants; and perhaps buprenorphine, when opioids are part of the problem. Suicide precautions should be taken for patients who are depressed or psychotic.

TABLE 8–19. Ambulatory opioid detoxification medication protocols

9-Day protocol	\multicolumn{4}{l}{9-Day clonidine detoxification ending with induction of naltrexone 50 mg/day}
	Day 1	Days 2, 3, and 4	Days 5, 6, and 7	Days 8 and 9
Clonidine	0.1–0.2 mg Maximum dose: 1 mg	0.1–0.2 mg po four times a day as needed Maximum dose: 1.4 mg	Taper to zero	Zero
Naltrexone				Day 8: 25 mg Day 9: 50 mg

5-Day protocol	\multicolumn{2}{l}{5-Day clonidine detoxification ending with induction of naltrexone 50 mg/day}
	Days 1 and 2	Days 3, 4, and 5
Clonidine	Preload: 0.2–0.4 mg three times a day Maximum dose: 1.2 mg	Taper to zero
Oxazepam	Preload: 30–60 mg	Zero
Naltrexone	Day 1: 12.5 mg Day 2: 25 mg	50 mg po each day

For inhalant-induced psychosis, carbamazepine has efficacy comparable to that of haloperidol but lacks haloperidol's risk of extrapyramidal side effects or lowering of seizure threshold (Hernandez-Avila et al. 1998).

The dangerous amphetamine-like state caused by ring-substituted amphetamine hallucinogens (MDMA, MDA) should be closely monitored Supportive treatment should include hydration and monitoring for hyperpyrexia, and perhaps administration of dantrolene. The sympathomimetic state produced by LSD and mescaline calls for similar monitoring and support. Anxiety in patients experiencing these states requires reassurance and reorientation. Usually restraint can be avoided. To treat the psychological sequelae of hallucinogens, benzodiazepines are superior to typical neuroleptics.

Nicotine Withdrawal

A number of guidelines for smoking cessation have been produced (American Psychiatric Association 1996). Relapse, unfortunately, is the rule within 3 months. The primary care provider's assistance is essential. Compliance with the nicotine patch is greater than for nicotine chewing gum. Bupropion SR (Zyban) is helpful. Scheduled dosing may be better than as-needed dosing. A nasal spray is also available but is not first line. Neither fluoxetine nor clonidine is helpful.

Opioid Maintenance Treatment

Opioid agonist substitution is the key to maintenance treatment. Methadone is the standard, but new agents such as buprenorphine and levo-alpha acetyl methadol (LAAM) are effective in this attempt to interrupt the addict's lifestyle, promote stability and employment, reduce intravenous drug use and its risk of hepatitis B or HIV, and reduce criminal activity. Methadone is a long-acting (half-life = 24–36 hours), cross-tolerant opioid that curbs extreme fluctuation in serum opioid levels and blunts the euphoric response to illicit heroin. Given once daily, methadone provides a structure for rehabilitation. Starting doses are usually 20–40 mg, depending on the degree of dependence, and may require an increase to 120 mg/day. Maintenance at doses of 70 mg and above leads to fewer relapses. NA-oriented rehabilitation approaches or therapeutic communities may exclude patients on methadone. Debate surrounds the substitution model, but the positive effects of methadone are vital to a subset of patients.

A large number of patients have successfully interrupted a drug lifestyle through methadone maintenance. Unfortunately, only 20%–25% of addicted persons receive this treatment. It is primarily indicated for "hardcore addicts" and for patients who are HIV-positive, pregnant, or have a history of legal problems. Methadone maintenance is contraindicated for persons less than age 16 years, those scheduled to be jailed within 30–45 days, and those with a history of abusing the medicine. Many opioid-addicted persons have compromised liver function caused by alcohol abuse or hepatitis, and methadone may be contraindicated with severe liver damage. Many individuals have been on methadone for several years. When withdrawal is indicated, it should be done slowly to minimize discomfort; this is often a protracted affair. Generally, the medication should not be decreased more than 10% per week. Below 10–20 mg of methadone, subjective symptoms of withdrawal may intensify and may necessitate a further decrease in the rate of withdrawal to 3% per week.

LAAM and buprenorphine are two agents that are used like methadone but that may be superior because they require less frequent dosing. One large study found that methadone, LAAM, and buprenorphine produced similar results in terms of both opioid and cocaine relapse prevention and patient ratings of severity of opioid craving, and also relapse on cocaine (R.E. Johnson et al. 2000). LAAM, a methadone derivative, is another long-acting μ agonist, and its use in maintenance is similar to that of methadone; however, LAAM and its metabolites have a longer half-life and need less-frequent dosing. LAAM 60–100 mg three times weekly is equivalent to methadone 50–100 mg daily. LAAM may become rarely used in the coming years due to its adverse cardiovascular effects. Buprenorphine is a mixed agonist–antagonist that has lower addictive properties, fewer withdrawal symptoms, and lower overdose risk (because of its antagonist properties) relative to methadone. Its efficacy in reducing illicit drug use has been documented (Ling et al. 1998).

Iatrogenic withdrawal from opioid agonist treatment often leads to relapse. A repetitive cycle of frequent detoxifications of methadone with subsequent relapses can be avoided by maintaining methadone. It is useful to remember the half-lives of the opioids: morphine sulfate, 2–3 hours; methadone, 15–25 hours; and LAAM, 55 hours. LAAM need be given only 3 times per week, and on cessation there should be no withdrawal for 72–96 hours.

Antagonist Maintenance

Naltrexone is an opioid antagonist (see "Psychopharmacological Modalities") that, when used regularly, can lead to gradual extinction of drug-seeking behavior. For opioid relapse prevention, naltrexone is usually given as a 25- to 50-mg/day dose over the initial 5–10 days, then gradually increased to 50–100 mg daily or thrice weekly. High rates of treatment refusal and treatment dropout limit its use to highly motivated individuals with a good prognosis who are likely to do well in a variety of treatment options and with whom there is a good treatment alliance. Naltrexone can be used in the outpatient setting over the long term. It is valuable in abstinence-oriented treatment. If administered to a person who has used opioids in the past 7 days, naltrexone may induce withdrawal; the clinician should determine the risk of this situation.

Polysubstance Abuse

Detoxification. Polysubstance abuse makes detoxification more difficult, because the presence of multiple substances greatly confuses the clinical picture. In the case of concurrent withdrawal from CNS depressants and opioids, detoxification of the former is the priority because of the life-threatening nature of CNS-depressant withdrawal and the long duration of opioid detoxification. Also, combining benzodiazepines and methadone creates a risk for overdose and requires close patient monitoring and dose adjustments as needed. Simultaneous detoxification from different substance classes can greatly increase physical or psychological discomfort and lead to higher rates of elopement or relapse.

Integrating treatment approaches. Polysubstance abuse has been inadequately addressed in the treatment system. Drug and alcohol programs are often separately funded. Alcohol counselors may lack the training or interest to treat polysubstance use. Until recently, AA groups had difficulty integrating younger polysubstance abusers into their membership. Unfortunately, a "my addiction is better than your addiction" attitude can develop. In clinical settings, such attitudes must be confronted with education and greater tolerance of social differences among patients. Exclusively alcoholic middle-aged white males, once common in treatment facilities, are today outnumbered by a younger, polyaddicted, and more heterogeneous population with additional psychiatric problems.

Treatment Modalities

The finding in other areas of psychiatry that combination psychotherapy and pharmacotherapy is more effective long term than either modality alone has been replicated in the field of substance abuse treatment, specifically with regard to the positive effects of naltrexone in the treatment of alcoholism (S.S. O'Malley et al. 1996) and the negative effects of discontinuing methadone maintenance in opioid addiction (Sees et al. 2000). Cognitive-behavioral therapy (CBT) is an effective treatment for depression in alcoholism (R.A. Brown et al. 1997).

Psychosocial Treatments

Addiction treatment is not simply "counseling." CBT, interpersonal therapy (IPT), dialectical behavior therapy (DBT), motivational interviewing, and psychodynamically oriented psychotherapy are important treatment modalities, although their effects often require time. There are data that show that psychotherapy combined with certain psychopharmacological treatments is more efficacious than either alone (Anton et al. 1999). Notwithstanding, there are some cases in which medication is essential.

Individual Therapy

Individual therapy can be conducted alone or with other modalities such as pharmacotherapy, 12-Step programs, and family and group treatments. Abstinence is an important measure of efficacy and should be considered a goal and a means to treatment success. Treatments range from psychodynamically-informed supportive and expressive treatment to cognitive-behavioral treatment. Individual treatments are especially indicated when patients face bereavement, loss, or social disruption and have targeted problems (e.g., anxiety disorders, panic disorders). Brief interventions are sometimes effective and are worth a try, especially in primary care settings; however, many patients require long-term care and follow-up.

Initiating Individual Treatment: The Therapeutic Contract

At the outset, the therapist should concentrate on helping the patient accept that he or she has a problem and that treatment is needed to achieve and maintain sobriety. A contract with the patient should specify a clear goal of abstinence; specify treatment frequency and modality, including psychopharmacological treatment if indicated; set limits regarding the continuation of treatment despite continued substance use; and specify the participation of significant others in the patient's social network and arrangements regarding fees and time.

The Individual Psychotherapies

Psychodynamically-oriented therapy. Psychodynamically-oriented individual treatment is for patients with problems relating to identity, separation and individuation, affect regulation, self-governance, and self-care. For those with addictive disorders and other neurotic problems, psychodynamically oriented therapy requires psychological mindedness; a capacity for honesty, intimacy, and identification with the therapist; average to superior intelligence; economic stability; high motivation; and a willingness to discuss conflict. In such patients, expressive psychotherapy may lead to deepening of the capacity to tolerate depression and anxiety without substance use. When patients are not abstinent, however, exploratory treatment may do more harm than good, with reactivation of painful conflicts leading to further drinking and regression (Frances et al. 2001). Formal psychoanalysis is contraindicated in early phases of addictive treatment, especially in those who are actively drinking. With abstinence, however, some patients respond well to insight-oriented psychotherapy.

Cognitive-behavioral therapy. CBT has been modified for treatment of substance use disorders (Wright et al. 1993). The assumption is that abuse and dependence on substances is a learned behavior and can be changed. It is a treatment in which the patient works to identify and modify maladaptive thought patterns resulting in feelings that lead to use. CBT is very helpful for relapse prevention, as well as for patients who are substance dependent or sociopathic or who suffer from primary psychiatric symptoms. It has been helpful for prevention of relapse to cocaine.

Dialectical behavior therapy. DBT is a comprehensive, behaviorally oriented treatment designed for highly dysfunctional patients who meet the criteria for borderline personality disorder. Many of these criteria are characteristic of drug abusers and of some of the problems encountered in the treatment of drug abusers, especially when various treatments are combined. The basic challenge of the DBT therapist is in balancing validation and acceptance treatment strategies with problem-solving procedures, including contingency management, exposure-based techniques, cognitive modification, and skills training. DBT has been shown to be more effective than treatment-as-usual in treating drug abuse in women with borderline personality disorder (Linehan et al. 1999).

Motivational enhancement therapy. Motivational enhancement therapy is a directive, empathic, patient-centered counseling approach that addresses the patient's ambivalence and denial. Ideally, it will help motivate the patient and will make brief interventions more effective by taking the patient through stages of denial and cooperation. Implemented at the right stage, motivational interventions by primary care physicians can substantially contribute to recovery (Prochaska et al. 1992; Samet et al. 1996).

Group Therapy

Group therapy is frequently the principal treatment modality used for addictive disorders. Groups offer opportunities for resocialization, practicing of social skills and object relatedness, and impulse control; they foster an identity as a recovering person and facilitate acceptance of abstinence. They support self-esteem and reality testing. Groups for addicted patients have the advantage of providing a homogeneous issue—dealing with addictions—that can be used as a jumping-off point for discussing other problems that members may share.

Various group formats have been found useful in treatment of substance use disorders, including assertiveness training groups; couples groups; and groups for self-control, for ego strength, for self-concept, and for mood problems (e.g., anxiety, depression). Groups may be used to assist in problem solving, to focus on specific behavioral problems, and to help patients see that others have similar issues. They may be psychodynamically oriented, problem solving, or confrontational; they may offer couples therapy or occupational counseling. Treatment programs frequently employ didactic groups, which may aid in retention of patients in treatment, promote cohesiveness, and foster acceptance of longer-term rehabilitation. Although group modalities have primarily been used for alcohol problems, they may be especially effective for relapse prevention in cocaine dependence.

Network Therapy

Network therapy involves creation of a support group—consisting of family and friends who are not themselves addicted—that is tailored to the patient's needs. It uses a CBT approach regarding environmental triggers, makes use of community reinforcement, and emphasizes the support of the patient's social network as essential to recovery (Galanter et al. 1993). Network therapy can be a useful adjunct to individual therapy or AA.

Family Evaluation and Therapy

A family evaluation is warranted for all substance use disorder patients; information and aid from the family is crucial for both diagnosis and treatment. Often it is family members who have been most affected by a patient's problems. The family system is usually made to accommodate the patient's drinking and may to some degree reinforce it. In many cases, it is confrontation by family members that provides the initial stimulus for the patient to seek treatment, and family confrontation may be important in helping the patient to remain in treatment.

Family treatment is frequently indicated in substance abuse treatment, especially for families in which considerable support is available to the patient. Children of alcoholic parents may benefit from family evaluation and treatment. Family treatments based on the concept of "the alcoholic system" focus on the correction of dysfunctional patterns of interactional behavior within the family and measure success not only by the achievement of abstinence but also by improvement in the family's level of functioning. Techniques used by family therapists include conjoint family therapy, marital therapy groups, and conjoint hospitalization for married couples. The efficacy of these techniques has been documented (Edwards and Steinglass 1995).

Self-Help

Every clinician needs to be thoroughly familiar with the work of the 12-Step self-help programs: AA, Al-Anon, NA, Cocaine Anonymous, Gamblers Anonymous, and Overeaters Anonymous (this includes having personally attended meetings of both AA and Al-Anon so as to be in touch with their patients' experiences). There is a small but growing body of evidence documenting the efficacy of AA. Self-help may also be very important for cocaine abuse and dependence. Peer-led groups have been helpful as well (Galanter 2000).

AA was established in 1935 by Bill Wilson and Dr. Robert Smith in Akron, Ohio, in part in response to the lack of available medical treatment for alcoholism. It had its roots in the Oxford movement (later the moral rearmament movement) and a Jungian emphasis on spirituality. AA has grown into an international network that includes more than 2 million members in the United States and 185,000 groups worldwide. The major message of the organization is that people with alcohol problems can help one another achieve sobriety through a spiritual program that includes recognition of alcoholism as an illness, acceptance of one's powerlessness over alcohol, and dependence on some source of change beyond the self. AA is a voluntary, self-supporting fellowship that avoids any self-serving political or economic activity. Al-Anon is a program parallel to AA that includes self-help for the family. Other family-oriented programs include Alateen, for teenage users and teenage children of alcoholics, and groups for adult children of alcoholics.

How It Works

A 12-Step program involves a series of steps and traditions that rely heavily on self-honesty, sobriety, group process, humility, provision of successful role models, self-care, and the destigmatizing of alcoholism as an illness. Although a 12-Step program is frequently recommended in conjunction with a variety of other treatment approaches, for many patients the program may suffice as the sole treatment for a substance use disorder. On average, members attend approximately 4 meetings per week, although in the early stages many attend daily meetings for 3 months. Patients with multiple addictions may attend several different 12-Step programs or groups. The various types of meetings include open ones that the interested public may attend, closed meetings, beginners' meetings, discussion groups, and homogeneous groups. Although groups vary in style, most generally have a warm, family feel and a sense of acceptance, mutual help, and understanding. The assumption is that alcoholics intuitively understand and can identify with universal problems faced by other alcoholics and can share feelings in a group. An emphasis on mutual help through assisting others with the same problem has contributed widely to the success of this group, and a large part of the spirituality of the program is embedded in its members' generosity of time and energy. A system of sponsorship of new members by veteran AA attendees and the creation of a support network of exchanged telephone numbers are important aspects of AA membership. AA provides an opportunity for people to experience relatedness, gain structure, test values, exercise judgment, practice honesty, find acceptance, and regain hope.

New Developments in 12-Step Programs

Although AA began solely for patients with alcoholism and originally consisted mainly of white, middle-class men, recent years have seen many people seeking help earlier in their illness, and many more members are women. An expansion into a younger population, with more dual addictions and with additional psychiatric problems, has led to a greater attention to groups and their specific needs. Subgroups have developed for alcoholic persons who are gay or lesbian, physicians, adult children of alcoholics, atheists or agnostics, HIV-positive, or dually diagnosed. Meetings can be found in most major cities throughout the world and are essential for alcoholics who travel.

Referrals to 12-Step Programs

The therapist may take an active role in referring patients to 12-Step programs as well as in monitoring and interpreting resistances to regular attendance. The physician can have the patient call AA directly from his or her office or may make the call for the patient in order to select a meeting. Information about AA is easily obtainable from the Online Intergroup of Alcoholics Anonymous (OIAA; see http://www.aa-intergroup.org/). Clinicians should address concerns or negative responses experienced by patients in their first AA meetings. Initially patients may be socially avoidant or may have difficulty understanding AA. Patients who react negatively to the spirituality elements of AA or who feel criticized or unaccepted in AA because of their use of psychiatric medications or their polysubstance abuse will need support. Patients should be encouraged to obtain an AA sponsor.

Counseling

Certified alcohol and drug addiction counselors have increasingly played prominent roles in substance treatment programs. They are involved in every phase of treatment, including evaluation, psychoeducation, individual and group counseling, and aftercare. For relapse prevention, counselors frequently provide support, advice, and valuable information regarding treatment and 12-Step programs.

Education

Most programs include education about the effects of alcohol and drugs on the abusing person and on the family, treatment alternatives, and relapse prevention. Education reduces fear, guilt, and shame; supports the medical model; and provides hope. Lectures, discussion groups, films, books, and homework assignments are an important part of the work of treatment and help keep patients productively engaged during treatment.

Psychopharmacological Modalities

In the treatment of substance use disorders, medications may be prescribed for detoxification, for treatment of comorbid psychiatric disorders or of complicating neuropsychological and medical disorders, for aversive treatment (e.g., disulfiram in alcoholic patients), for attenuation of craving or euphoria (e.g., naltrexone), or for psychological ego support. Generally, these medications are used as adjuncts to psychosocial treatment and education. Physicians should have a clear understanding of the differential diagnosis and natural history of substance abuse disorder and of the limitations of medication, as well as knowledge of drug–drug interactions and medication side effects.

Naltrexone

The superior efficacy of naltrexone (ReVia) for alcohol relapse prevention is well documented (Volpicelli et al. 1992). When administered at 50 mg/day for 3 months, this agent usually prevents relapse. Opioid-receptor functioning is thought to be related to the etiology of alcohol dependence. Opioid μ-receptor antagonists reduce alcohol use overall, likely by blocking release of dopamine in the nucleus accumbens.

Naltrexone's original indication was in the prevention of opioid relapse. As an opioid-receptor antagonist, it causes withdrawal symptoms in persons with opioid intoxication. Because of these effects, many opioid detoxification protocols employ slow induction of naltrexone in conjunction with outpatient clonidine treatment (summarized in Table 8–19). Naltrexone's primary indication is daily relapse prevention, for which the usual dose is 50 mg/day.

Methadone and Levo-Alpha Acetyl Methadol (LAAM)

Methadone has a dose-dependent effect on concurrent use of opioids and cocaine. High doses (65 mg/day) may be the most effective. A stable dose need not be altered except in the case of changes in pharmacokinetics due to emesis; use of phenytoin, rifampin, barbiturates, carbamazepine, or tricyclic antidepressants; heavy labor; or alcohol intoxication. LAAM is a long-acting opioid agonist with used, like methadone, for maintenance. It has a longer half-life than methadone and thus may have the advantage of needing to be taken only 3 times a week.

Buprenorphine

Buprenorphine (Buprenex/Subutex) is a mixed opioid μ agonist–antagonist that has been demonstrated to be more effective than placebo in the treatment of opioid dependence (R.E. Johnson et al. 1995). Buprenorphine shows promise for both opioid detoxification and opioid maintenance. Suboxone, a buprenorphine–naloxone 4:1 combination sublingual tablet, is nearing FDA approval for use in opioid detoxification and maintenance. The naloxone in Suboxone discourages illegal injection street use because it precipitates withdrawal. It is hoped that regulatory approval of buprenorphine will make detoxification treatment more accessible than is now the case with methadone detoxification, because that individual physicians will be able to prescribe buprenorphine. Buprenorphine's long duration of action means that it can be given three times a week instead of daily. A number of strategies for detoxification from buprenorphine have been established (Bickel et al. 1997).

Disulfiram

Disulfiram (Antabuse) is a medication adjunct in the treatment of recovering alcoholics. It is an aversive treatment that enhances motivation for continued abstinence by making the "high" unavailable, thus discouraging impulsive alcohol use. Disulfiram is a potent reversible inhibitor of aldehyde dehydrogenase. Aldehyde dehydrogenase is an enzyme that metabolizes acetaldehyde, the first metabolite of alcohol. Inhibition of this step produces a buildup of acetaldehyde, resulting in toxicity, which consists of nausea, vomiting, cramps, flushing, and vasomotor collapse. Disulfiram has relatively mild side effects, including sedation, halitosis, skin rash, and temporary impotence. More-serious side effects—such as peripheral neuropathy, seizures, optic neuritis, and psychosis—occur only rarely. Disulfiram appears to have a catecholamine effect, which may contribute to the alcohol reaction and make its use contraindicated with MAOI

use. It also may inhibit the metabolism of other medications, including anticoagulants, phenytoin, and isoniazid, leading to higher-than-expected serum levels of these medications. In addition, disulfiram has adverse interactions with cough syrups. Its use should be avoided in patients with hepatic disease, peripheral neuropathy, renal failure, and cardiac disease, as well as in pregnancy. Other contraindications include medical conditions that would be greatly exacerbated by a disulfiram–alcohol reaction, such as liver disease, esophageal varices, heart disease, heart failure, emphysema, and peptic ulcer disease. Disulfiram should be avoided in anyone likely to become pregnant. Psychiatric contraindications include psychosis and severe depression. Disulfiram can exacerbate psychosis; depressed suicidal patients may deliberately precipitate a disulfiram reaction.

Initial doses of disulfiram are 250–500 mg/day. It can be administered in an oral suspension. Subcutaneous implantation is not clinically available. Doses can be adjusted downward to 125 mg if sedation or other side effects are excessive or in those with relative contraindications. Patients should be informed about the rationale of disulfiram use, the disulfiram–alcohol reaction, and common side effects.

Treatment facilities vary in their use of and attitudes toward disulfiram. Some AA-oriented programs may discourage the use of any medication and may see disulfiram as an unnecessary psychopharmacological crutch. Many programs use disulfiram as an adjunctive tool in promoting abstinence. Although there has not been convincing evidence that disulfiram use affects long-term outcomes globally, disulfiram has been shown to be useful in certain subtypes of alcoholism, often when it can be administered by a patient's significant other. Socially stable adult alcoholics and affluent, married, less-sociopathic patients with compulsive tendencies have the best results with disulfiram.

Lithium

Lithium is an integral component in the treatment of substance use disorders in the presence of an underlying primary bipolar or cyclothymic disorder. Its use may dampen or abort extreme mood swings or indirectly affect substance intake. Manic or hypomanic episodes have been linked with increased alcohol or cocaine use. Patients with lithium-responsive depression have a propensity to abuse alcohol or cocaine. Lithium has also been associated with decreased subjective experience of intoxication, exacerbation of deficits in cognitive and motor function during intoxication, and reduced alcohol consumption. Caution should be exercised when prescribing lithium to those who are actively abusing substances or who demonstrate poor compliance with treatment. Such patients need to be hospitalized to ensure abstinence and to manage titration of proper doses. Lithium has no documented usefulness in uncomplicated alcohol abuse or dependence. For adolescents with bipolar disorder and secondary substance dependence, lithium is efficacious for both disorders (Geller et al. 1998).

Antidepressants

Antidepressants do not directly alter substance use disorders but are important adjuncts in the treatment of patients with primary mood disorders. Determination of which antidepressant to use follows consideration of the type of depression present and the side-effect profile of the medications, as well as recognition that judgment, impulse control, and cognition may be impaired in alcoholic patients in early recovery. Extreme caution should be used when prescribing MAOIs for depression in alcoholic patients, especially in view of the fact that wine contains tyramine. Also, intoxication may further impair judgment and increase the risk of using tyramine-containing products. There is evidence that fluoxetine is not helpful for primary cocaine dependence. Venlafaxine, a broad-spectrum antidepressant, may be a safe, well-tolerated, rapidly acting, and effective treatment for patients with a dual diagnosis of depression and cocaine dependence. However, venlafaxine's potential to cause diastolic hypertension at higher doses mandates monitoring of blood pressure.

Dopamimetics

Although few data support their effectiveness, dopamimetic agents are commonly used to treat cocaine dependence and withdrawal. It had previously been hypothesized that because cocaine's effects are dopamine-related, and because dopamine depletion is associated with cocaine craving, a dopamimetic substance such as bromocriptine might have some value during the acute onset of abstinence (first 3–4 days) by diminishing cocaine craving. However, studies have failed to justify this application of bromocriptine, and we do not recommend its use in cocaine substance-related disorders. Amantadine has likewise not been found to affect cocaine dependence, and trials of pergolide (a mixed D_1–D_2 agonist) failed to detect differences from placebo in terms of reducing cravings in cocaine-dependent patients (Malcolm et al. 2000).

Clonidine

Clonidine's use in opioid detoxification was discussed earlier (see "Opioid Withdrawal/Detoxification" subsection earlier in this chapter). Clonidine has also been reported to be helpful in alcohol withdrawal. There have been case reports of the successful use of clonidine for patients with hallucinogen persisting perception disorder (Lerner et al. 1998).

Valproate

Valproate is used in the treatment of bipolar disorder. Moderate doses of valproate (producing an average blood level of approximately 70 mg/L) in alcoholic patients without significant hepatic disease do not cause significant adverse effects on white blood cell count, platelet count, or liver transaminase level (Sonne and Brady 1999). Liver function should be established prior to onset of therapy with this medicine.

Carbamazepine

Although previously felt to be helpful for symptoms of cocaine withdrawal, recent studies have failed to find carbamazepine to be effective for this indication (Cornish et al. 1995).

Gabapentin

Gabapentin had been heralded as a major advance in alcohol relapse prevention, but this promise has not been realized in studies. As a mood stabilizer or an anticonvulsant, it is efficacious and is useful in alcoholism because it is not hepatically metabolized, does not bind to plasma proteins, does not induce liver enzymes, and is renally eliminated without any metabolism.

Adrenergic Blockers

Using propranolol, a β-blocker, to reduce β-adrenergic signs in alcohol withdrawal is controversial and not routinely advocated. β-Blockers are contraindicated in cocaine intoxication and withdrawal.

Neuroleptics

Neuroleptics have no place in the treatment of primary alcoholism. They lower the seizure threshold and carry the long-term risk of tardive dyskinesia. However, they can be very helpful in managing psychosis across a wide spectrum of toxic drug reactions. Neuroleptics can be used adjunctively with benzodiazepines in the treatment of delirium, including DTs. They are the primary treatment of choice in alcohol hallucinosis. Among the newer neuroleptics, olanzapine appears to be as effective as haloperidol in the treatment of cannabis-induced psychotic disorder and is associated with a lower rate of extrapyramidal side effects (Berk et al. 1999).

Benzodiazepines

Benzodiazepines are the treatment of choice for alcohol or benzodiazepine detoxification. They work through the GABA receptor and are very effective in suppressing anxiety symptoms. They also produce tolerance with psychological and physical dependence. Benzodiazepines are generally contraindicated in any substance use disorder except when used for detoxification, for manic patients acutely, or very selectively in compliant abstinent patients with anxiety disorders in whom other treatments have failed.

A common clinical dilemma involves the substance use disorder patient who has an underlying anxiety disorder, often in conjunction with high-dose benzodiazepine abuse. These patients may experience a relapse of their anxiety disorder symptoms following detoxification from CNS depressants. Such an anxiety disorder is often difficult to distinguish from other underlying disorders, anxiety symptoms associated with chronic subacute withdrawal, reactive fear, and anxiety about withdrawal. After detoxification, these patients may be extremely anxious and dysphoric. The impulse to relieve this suffering may lead clinicians to reinstate addictive substances, which can lead to a poor outcome. Effective use of other, perhaps more specific, treatment modalities, including selective serotonin reuptake inhibitors (SSRIs), desipramine, or MAOIs for panic and a neuroleptic for psychotic disorders or SSRIs, buspirone, gabapentin, or adrenergic blockers for generalized anxiety may be helpful. Setting firm limits on the use of psychoactive substances is necessary. Nonetheless, benzodiazepines can occasionally be used as an intervention of last resort in treatment-compliant anxious patients who maintain sobriety.

Buspirone

Buspirone (BuSpar) is an anxiolytic with no CNS depressant activity. Clinical studies to date have demonstrated little abuse potential or withdrawal syndrome for this agent. It apparently does not potentiate the effects of alcohol. Buspirone is a useful adjunct in the treatment of generalized anxiety or transient anxiety in some substance abusers. However, it has the disadvantage of slow onset of efficacy (up to 3 weeks) and is thus of little use in transient anxiety disorders.

Acamprosate

This new medication has great promise in alcohol relapse prevention (Sass et al. 1996). It crosses the blood–brain barrier, is chemically similar to amino-acid neurotransmitters, and acts at the NMDA receptor to reduce withdrawal's glutamatergic hyperactivity. It is dose dependent and has no abuse potential. Giving acamprosate to those dependent on alcohol will not lead to an acute withdrawal syndrome. Acamprosate is not metabolized but rather is renally excreted and should be given with caution to those with renal disease. A starting dose is 2–3 g/day in divided doses, and common side effects include diarrhea and headache.

Ondansetron

Ondansetron, a selective 5-HT$_3$ receptor antagonist, has shown promise in reducing overall alcohol intake, specifically among those with type I alcoholism (see Cloninger et al. 1988), and in diminishing the subjective positive effects of alcohol (B.A. Johnson et al. 2000). Its widespread use awaits further study.

Special Issues in Treatment

Patients With Mental Illness and Substance Abuse

Most psychiatric patients have more than one psychiatric diagnosis, and the most frequent comorbid diagnosis is a substance use disorder. Every patient with a substance use disorder needs a careful psychiatric assessment and treatment plan. Conversely, a thorough substance use history is an essential part of all psychiatric interviews. Interactions between substance use disorders and other psychiatric diagnoses must be integrated into treatment planning. Substance use disorders may be comorbid with disorders of mood, anxiety, personality, sexual orientation, "organic" disorders, schizophrenia, and anorexia nervosa. Substance use disorders can mask, mimic, or result from a wide variety of psychiatric and medical disorders. The psychiatrist provides an understanding of substance use disorders in relation to other psychiatric illness and determines the course of action at the most appropriate level, be it psychosocial or medical.

Longitudinal, adoption, epidemiological, and family studies have not definitively settled the old questions about the causes and effects of and the relationships between psychopathology and addictive behavior. Most studies support the idea that the inherited predisposition to addiction is independent of other psychiatric disorders. The trait of addiction may be primary to psychiatric illness, may develop as a way of coping with other problems, or may coexist with other psychiatric disorders. Treatment planning for mentally ill patients with addictions depends on flexibility and a broad understanding both of psychiatry and of substance abuse.

Patients With Dual Diagnosis

Complex interactions between psychopathology and addictions are difficult to separate clinically because of overlapping signs and symptoms resulting from intoxication, withdrawal, mixed drug reactions, adverse drug responses, medical conditions, and the organic and psychosocial effects of substance use on affective state, anxiety, or personality. The addition of other Axis I, II, and III disorders to a substance use disorder greatly complicates diagnosis and makes treatment more difficult. Treatment of addictions in patients with psychiatric illness is further complicated by a risk of violence toward self or others (associated with anxiety); by irritation, anger, impulsivity, and poor reality testing (in intoxication or withdrawal states); and by aggressivity (with use of cocaine, hallucinogens, PCP, or alcohol).

Personnel in fields of mental health and substance abuse treatment should have the rudimentary knowledge to screen patients properly and to develop a treatment plan that adequately addresses patients' needs. Model programs have been developed around the country to integrate psychiatric and substance abuse treatment. However, the dual-diagnosis patient often falls through the cracks of the treatment system. Severe psychiatric disorders often preclude full treatment in substance abuse clinics or self-help groups. Confrontational techniques and self-exposure, used in some substance abuse programs, may exacerbate psychiatric symptoms. Special AA and NA groups are being formed for dual-diagnosis or "double trouble" patients. Patients with severe psychiatric disorders receive substantial benefit from additional professional psychiatric therapy. Some patients, especially those with frank psychosis or suicidal ideation, require primary psychiatric settings (e.g., day hospital or inpatient setting). However, use of such settings should not preclude addressing substance abuse issues. Attendance at AA or NA meetings should be arranged if possible. An addiction psychiatrist should be available—preferably as part of a multidisciplinary team approach—in psychiatric facilities with a high number of dual-diagnosis patients.

A discussion of the treatment of dual-diagnosis patients would not be complete without a review of some of the pressing social needs of these patients. Often, dual-diagnosis patients have alienated family, friends, and treatment personnel. The need for adequate housing, health care, and follow-up is imperative. Residential facilities are needed to ease the transition of these patients into society. Coordination of the various agencies is required. Talbott (1981) discussed the case management approach extensively. There is evidence that "wrap-around," or integrated, care is helpful (Ries and Comtois 1997). Substance abuse facilities refuse admission to psychiatric patients, and psychiatric facilities reject patients with a history of substance abuse.

Psychiatric patients who abuse drugs present a interesting dilemma when it comes to choosing psychopharmacological treatment with other abusable medications. For example, patients with ADHD who abuse cocaine are at high risk for treatment failure or dropout. Notwithstanding the understandable controversy regarding the use of stimulants in substance abusers, sustained-release methylphenidate (Ritalin) may be helpful in this population.

Rehabilitation

The rehabilitation model, pioneered in substance abuse treatment, has become an important organizing paradigm for a variety of categories of psychiatric illness. It combines self-help, counseling, education, relapse prevention, group treatment, a warm and supportive environment, and emphasis on a medical model geared toward reducing stigma and blame. Most treatment units are highly structured, insist on an abstinence goal, and offer lectures, films, and discussion groups as part of a complete cognitive and educational program. Patients frequently become active 12-Step members and are encouraged to continue in aftercare.

A highly skilled professional team with available consultation is needed to integrate counseling; cognitive-behavioral treatment; relapse prevention strategies; interpersonal, family, and group therapy; applied or brief psychodynamically oriented psychotherapy; social network approaches; education; and occupational and recreational therapy. Inpatient programs previously allotted 5–7 days for detoxification and 3–6 weeks for rehabilitation; now, however, portions of these treatment components are often done in halfway houses in outpatient settings, and hospital stays of 3–12 days are more common. Longer stays are indicated for adolescents and for patients with greater severity of illness, dual diagnoses, or severe medical problems.

The rehabilitation model emphasizes the provision of opportunities for patients to practice social skills and gain control over impulses, using the highly structured program as an auxiliary superego. Self-honesty and expression of feelings are encouraged. The program promotes the use of higher-level defenses (e.g., intellectualization) and actively confronts more primitive defenses (e.g., denial, splitting, projection), especially when these defenses are used in relation to the issue of abstinence (Frances and Alexopoulos 1982a).

Rehabilitation treatment can take place in freestanding rehabilitation facilities, MICA units, general hospitals, inpatient programs, organized outpatient day and evening hospitals, therapeutic communities, and halfway houses. Addiction day treatment programs utilize many of the same techniques employed in inpatient treatment programs. They are staffed by interdisciplinary teams who develop individualized treatment plans. Organized outpatient alcohol programs may provide a range of treatment modalities of varying intensities. These programs are less restrictive than hospitalization and may be useful as part of an aftercare plan.

Aftercare

On discharge from an inpatient or an organized outpatient program, aftercare must be part of the follow-up plan. Referral to a 12-Step program often complements other treatment, although self-help groups may suffice for some faithfully attending individuals. We recommend at least 2 years of follow-up care after the start of abstinence.

Treatment and Consultation in the Medical Setting

It has been estimated that 25%–50% of general hospital admissions are related to complications of substance use (Moore et al. 1989). A high index of suspicion may assist the health care provider in detecting hidden substance use disorders. There may be further advantages in confronting the addictive process during a medical crisis, when denial may be lessened or can be easily counteracted by irrefutable medical evidence. Alcoholism may be diagnosed on the basis of its associated medical problems, which include liver disease, pancreatitis, anemia, certain types of pneumonia, delirium, dementia, gastric ulcers, esophageal varices, tuberculosis, or symptoms mimicking psychiatric syndromes.

Admission Workup

Detailed alcohol and substance histories should be taken on admission from every patient in the general hospital setting. Information should be gathered in a straightforward manner in concert with the rest of the medical history. When substance use problems do exist, answers may be vague, evasive, or aggressively defensive. In early

abuse, some patients may be surprised by the connection between their substance use and their current medical problems. Health professionals should be knowledgeable regarding the components of a basic alcohol and substance history (Table 8–20). In the presence of denial, resistance, organicity, and psychiatric symptoms, a consultation with an addiction specialist may be helpful in making a diagnosis. Third-party sources such as family or friends may be necessary to obtain crucial information. For example, additional corroboration would be needed in the assessment of prior alcohol abuse in a man who, on admission 2 days earlier for routine surgery, denied any alcohol abuse but now appears to be in early DTs. The psychoactive substance abuse history should involve a systematic review of all the major drug classes. Often, patients will not consider a particular substance a "drug." For example, when asked "Do you abuse drugs?," a 30-year-old woman who had been smoking marijuana every day since college took offense. The question seemed to her a pejorative one; she did not perceive marijuana as a drug. Because of her lack of knowledge and particular view of the stigma of drug abuse, she did not provide the desired information.

TABLE 8–20. Components of a basic alcohol and substance use history

Chief complaint
Current medical signs and symptoms
Substance abuse review of systems for all substances of abuse
Dates of first use, regular use, longest period of sobriety and overall life condition during sobriety, pattern, amount, frequency, time of last use, route of administration, circumstances of use, reactions to use
Medical history, medications, HIV and tuberculosis status
History of past substance abuse treatment, response to treatment, history of complications secondary to substances
Psychiatric history
Family history of psychiatric disease and substance use
Legal history
Object relations history
Personal and social history
Review of collected data (chart, family, primary care physician)

Specific Substance History Taking

The patient's experience with drug classes such as alcohol, opioids, cocaine and other stimulants, tranquilizers, hallucinogens, marijuana, inhalants, and over-the-counter medication should be systematically ascertained. Use and possible abuse of prescription medications should be covered. The history should include the type of liquor or the specific drug, the amount, the pattern or frequency

Substance **Sub**

TABLE 8-2 | trib
nou:
Earlier onset | Mar
More severe | susp
Less consiste | pati
Poor academ | und
More antisoc | ety,
Poorer progn | mar

of use, and time of last use; such historical information may be very important in distinguishing various organic mental states. The route of administration (oral, intravenous, or via pulmonary inhalation) may have important health consequences. For example, HIV screening should be conducted for the vast majority of intravenous drug users presenting for admission in the general hospital setting. If alcohol abuse is suspected, symptoms of physical dependence must be actively pursued. Missing such information can be life-threatening.

A history of early-morning tremors or shakes, a subjective need for a drink to calm the nerves, elevated pulse and blood pressure, or a known past history of alcohol-related seizures or DTs should signal the need for pharmacological detoxification. Polysubstance abuse may mask underlying physical dependence on one prominent psychoactive substance (e.g., opioids in "speedballing" or "hits," alcohol dependence secondary to cocaine addiction). Past history of hospitalization for motor vehicle accidents, accidental injuries, or substance-related violence should be sought in addition to any history of treatment for alcohol or other substance abuse problems.

Psychiatric Consultation in the General Hospital

Consultation requests from general hospital departments may involve straightforward requests for substance abuse evaluation or more cryptic requests for evaluation of brain pathology, mood disorders, or acting-out behavior. Requests may consist of solicitations for help in treating overdose or withdrawal, making an initial diagnosis, engaging patients in the therapeutic process, evaluating pain medications, assessing a patient for organ transplant, or managing special patients (e.g., trauma and burn patients, pregnant substance abusers). Often the patients who are being evaluated are perceived as being manipulative, demanding, and unappreciative. In reality, they can indeed present as such. It is important not to disavow the staff's real feelings but rather to provide a framework for an understanding of the addictive process that can make those feelings meaningful and tolerable. The clinician's self-awareness of feelings evoked by patients not only is diagnostic at times but also may relieve the guilt of retaliatory fantasies. Few people enter the medical profession to dislike their patients. Having such feelings surface within themselves may be intolerable to some house staff. In affective illnesses, the presence of overwhelming affects may focus attention away from a concomitant addictive process. In cases of organicity, important historical information may simply be forgotten. Table 8–21 offers general guidelines for approaching this patient

TABLE 8-21. General considerations in approach to consultation

Have a high suspicion for drug abuse and obtain collected data

Obtain serum and urine toxicology screens as soon as possible to admission

Know general principles of detoxification and its differential therapeutics

Realize that detoxification often needs to be tailored to individual medical patients

Recall that when treating polysubstance dependence, sedative withdrawal occurs first

Use challenge tests or estimate conservatively when considering initial detoxification dose

Recognize drug–drug interactions and effects of medications on mental status examination

Always differentiate psychopathology, substance-induced disorders, and medical disorders

Each consultation request should be reviewed to clearly ascertain what is being requested. Frequently, such review requires a call to the referring physician. Questions of confidentiality may arise with patients in regard to their substance abuse. Generally, confidentiality issues must be discussed and handled appropriately. Because honesty is one of the core treatment tools for an addictive disease process, conspiracies or secrets regarding substance abuse are not advisable.

Assessing the Chart

For the consultant, reviewing the medical chart in detail is essential, not only to elicit important information about admitting signs and symptoms, third-party statements, and mental status, but also to piece together divergent clues of substance abuse in a fresh manner. Pertinent laboratory work, X rays, EEG, CT scans, and the like should be reviewed. Suggestions for additional laboratory work (e.g., magnesium levels in a patient with a history of DTs) should be made.

The Interview

If the consultation request is for assessment of a substance abuse problem, that purpose should be clearly stated to the patient early in the interview. The referring physician can be asked to join the interview if that seems appropriate. In writing up findings, it is best that the consulting clinician provide a short summary containing his or her impressions of the reason for the consultation, the patient's identifying information, a brief history of the present illness, past history, medical complications, medications currently and pre-

tects caregivers and patients alike (Perlman et al. 1995). The need for continued patient education and treatment and for a heightened awareness of risks associated with these diseases is great.

Treatment Approaches to Specific Populations

Women

There are unfortunate differences between sexes in the epidemiology, course, treatment, and stigma of substance use disorders. In the United States, the ratio of alcoholism in males compared with females is 3:1 (the contribution of culture is illustrated by the fact that in Korea the ratio is 1:28). This ratio is equal to that for most other substances, with the exception of prescription drugs, which women disproportionately abuse (Warner et al. 1995). Women are underrepresented in substance abuse treatment, where their special needs are often not addressed. Women suffer greater secondary medical morbidity from substance abuse than do men (Ashley et al. 1977). The dangers of fetal alcohol syndrome and HIV transmission add to the clinical significance of substance use disorders in women.

Women's abuse is mostly discovered in nonviolent situations, such as through their EAPs, in family interventions, or in medical evaluations. Women more frequently present with coexisting panic, anxiety, mood, and eating disorders than do men. Female alcohol abusers also have a later onset of abuse, have a more rapid progression of abuse, abuse less total alcohol, and have higher rates of comorbid psychopathology; furthermore, in comparison with male alcohol abusers, they are more likely to have a "significant other" who is also a substance abuser. They also tend to have a history of sexual or physical abuse and to date the onset of their substance use disorder to a stressful event.

In particular, women with alcohol use disorders are more likely to attempt and less likely to complete suicide than are men with these disorders. Among these women there is a higher mortality rate by all causes. For cocaine use disorders, the disease progresses more rapidly in women than in men, women's use is less than that of males, women more often have a spouse who is also an abuser, and there is a greater likelihood of a suicide attempt.

Biological Effects

Compared with men, women have a higher blood alcohol level per pound of body weight per alcoholic drink; in addition, blood alcohol level effects in women fluctuate over the course of the menstrual cycle (the perimenstrual time is often marked by heavier consumption). In addition to having a lower tolerance for alcohol, women tend to have a more "telescoped" course of the chronic effects of excessive drinking, including cirrhosis of the liver, compared with men. These differences may be partially explained by the fact that men have greater amounts of alcohol dehydrogenase in the gastric mucosa. Thus, alcohol's neurotoxic effects may be greater in women than in men (Hommer et al. 2001).

Psychiatric Comorbidity

Whereas psychiatric comorbidity in substance-abusing men most often involves ADHD and antisocial personality disorder, comorbid psychopathology in women with substance use disorders more often involves anxiety (particularly posttraumatic stress disorder), mood, and eating disorders (Kessler et al. 1995). Alcohol abuse as self-medication for anxiety or depression is much more frequent in women than in men and it may replace self-medication with benzodiazepines.

Treatment Issues

In general, although alcoholism and drug abuse treatment for women is similar in many ways to that for men, treatment for women must be tailored to address pathophysiological differences and to provide a perception of safety. Women's groups and special programs and residences for women in rehabilitation programs are beneficial because women in traditional treatment programs may feel intimidated and outnumbered by men and often experience discomfort when talking about sexual abuse and sexual issues in mixed groups. Special treatment considerations include watching especially closely for sedative–hypnotic dependence, anxiety disorders and depression, and hypersensitivity to stigma; helping women deal with abusive spouses; and instilling an awareness of fetal alcohol and drug effects. Having contact with recovered alcoholic women role models and working with female professionals may also facilitate improved self-esteem.

The care of women with substance use disorders who are of childbearing age requires particular attention. Careful use of medication in women of this group includes awareness of important risks and benefits. Inpatient treatment poses special problems for young mothers, and few programs exist in which women can have their children with them during hospitalization. There are also increased fears of loss of custody in alcoholic women and increased needs for child care services. Women frequently have economic problems that can make it more difficult for them to obtain good treatment, and women with alcoholism are often married to addicted men, who may not facilitate—or who may actively hinder—their achievement of recovery. A woman may need to separate from an addicted, abusing spouse to get well, and may depend on sober women friends and positive female role models for help in remaining abstinent. General guidelines for the care of addicted women are presented in Table 8–24 (Blume 1998).

TABLE 8–24. Special considerations in women's substance use treatment

---

Psychiatric assessment for comorbid disorders; date of onset for each (primary/secondary)

Attention to past history and present risk of physical and sexual assault

Assessment of prescription drug abuse/dependence

Comprehensive physical examination for physical complications and comorbid disorders

Need for access to health care (including obstetric care)

Psychoeducation to include information on substance use in pregnancy

Child-care services for women in treatment

Parenting education and assistance.

Evaluation and treatment of significant others and children

Positive female role models (among treatment staff; friends, self-help)

Attention to guilt, shame, and self-esteem issues

Assessment and treatment of sexual dysfunction

Attention to the effects of sexism in the previous experience of the patient (e.g., underemployment, lack of opportunity, rigid sex roles)

Avoidance of iatrogenic drug dependence

Special attention to the needs of minority women, lesbian women, and those in the criminal justice system

---

Problems Secondary to Addiction in Women

General medical conditions. Women who abuse substances are at risk of developing a number of specific general medical conditions, and, compared with men, when they develop such secondary conditions (e.g., alcoholic cardiomyopathy, cirrhosis) (Urbano-Marquez et al. 1995), the conditions progress more quickly and have higher morbidity, a phenomenon known as "telescoping." Women alcohol abusers are at greater risk than nonabusers of developing breast cancer (Longnecker et al. 1988). Thus, female substance use disorder patients need comprehensive primary care assessment (Table 8–24).

AIDS. HIV has produced a growing pandemic whose effects are seen every day among women with substance use disorders. A special concern of women is the possibility of contracting AIDS through intercourse with HIV-positive men who are intravenous drug users or bisexual. Compared with non–substance-using women, women who use substances may take more risks, may have poorer self-care, may be more at risk of being forced into exposure to HIV, and may less frequently insist on safe sex. Women of childbearing age who are intravenous drug users are at very high risk and need careful counseling.

Sexual and reproductive function. Sexual function is affected by almost all drugs of abuse. Despite its reputation, alcohol is not an aphrodisiac; sexual function improves with sobriety (Gavaler et al. 1995). Heroin disrupts ovulation. The treatment of neonates for methadone withdrawal is a common procedure; thus, methadone use is not an absolute contraindication to pregnancy (H.L. Brown et al. 1998).

Fetal alcohol syndrome. The incidence of fetal alcohol syndrome is approximately 1–3 in 1,000 live births in the United States overall and as high as 1 in 100 births in some Eskimo villages (Institute of Medicine 1995). Typical signs of fetal alcohol syndrome include low birthweight, growth deficiency with delayed motor development, mental retardation and learning problems, and other, less severe fetal alcohol behavioral effects. No safe alcohol level during pregnancy has been established, and dangers are dose dependent.

Children and Adolescents

The use, abuse, treatment, and prevention of substance use disorders in children and adolescents are of grave concern; not the least because the prevalence of substance disorders is rising, the age at first use is dropping, and the morbidity and mortality of youth with substance use disorders is increasing. Substance abuse can interfere with natural growth and normal interaction and development, including relationships with peers, performance in school, and attitudes toward law and authority, and can have both acute and chronic systemic effects.

It is difficult to diagnose substance dependence in adolescents because of the reduced likelihood of observing signs and symptoms of withdrawal, which typically occur later in addiction. Compared with adult substance abusers, adolescents are less likely to report withdrawal symptoms, have shorter periods of addiction, and may recover more rapidly from withdrawal. Specific practice parameters have been developed for the treatment of substance use disorders in children and adolescents (Bukstein 1997).

Epidemiology

According to the latest figures from the Substance Abuse and Mental Health Services Administration (SAMHSA) National Household Survey, there was a slight decrease in drug abuse by adolescents (12–17 years old) during 1997, 1998, and 1999, from 11.4% to 9.9% to 9.0%, respectively. However, this reduction follows a stark increase in abuse that began in 1992, when the rate of past-month usage among youth ages 12–17 years reached a low of 5.3% (from a high of 16.3% in 1979). Since 1995, when the rate climbed to 10.9%, the past-month usage rate has fluctuated from 9% to 11% (see www.samhsa.gov/OAS/NHSDA/98Summ). Furthermore, the age at which drugs or alcohol is first used has dropped, such that as of 1994, more than 50% of students in grade 6 reported having tried alcohol or other illicit substances (P.M. O'Malley et al. 1995). Racial and ethnic differences are apparent among child and adolescent substance abusers: in one report, African American students had the lowest rates of illicit substance use in general, Hispanic students had the highest usage rates at grade 8, and white students had the highest at grade 12. However, Hispanic adolescents were found to use more cocaine, heroin, and steroids at grade 12 compared with the other groups (Bachman et al. 1991). Thus, the problem is wide, growing, and complex.

Early Detection in Adolescents

Signs of adolescent drug use include a drop in school performance, irritability, apathy, mood change (including depression), poor self-care, weight loss, oversensitivity to questions about drinking or drugs, and sudden changes in friends. Substance use screening in adolescents should include routine medical examinations before camp or in school. The use of urinalysis may help confirm a diagnosis whenever there is reason to raise the question. These efforts are vital, because it is increasingly recognized that a younger age at onset of addiction is associated with a poorer outcome, including alcohol-related harm (physical damage, illness, or violence), and a greater potential for clinically significant use (DeWit et al. 2000).

Contributing Factors

Peer group, school environment, age, geography, race, values, family attitudes toward substance abuse, risk-seeking temperament, and biological predisposition are all contributing factors to adolescent substance abuse. Nonusing adolescents are more likely to describe close relationships with their parents than are users. They are more likely to be comfortably dependent on their parents and are closer to their families than are users, who report themselves as independent and distant. Users more frequently indicate that they do not want to be like their parents and do not feel they need their parents' approval; they may disavow a desire for affection from their parents. Frequently, adolescents with substance abuse problems have a positive family history for chemical dependence. Genetic studies indicate a strong hereditary predisposition to alcoholism. However, if offspring of alcoholic parents do not abuse substances by age 21, they are unlikely to do so after that point.

Families

Families play a more important role for adolescents than for adult substance abusers and are an important part of treatment. Parents and family members of adolescent abusers may be less resistant to being involved in treatment because the adolescent usually resides with them and the parents may feel responsible for their child's behavior. When parents themselves are actively addicted, the challenges of treatment are greater. Compared with adults, adolescents are less likely to enter treatment to avoid incarceration; rather, they are usually pushed into treatment by their families, by schools, and by pediatricians and family physicians. Children of divorced parents have a particularly high risk for substance abuse.

Mentally Ill Adolescents With Substance Abuse Disorders

To some extent, all childhood psychiatric disorders are associated with substance use disorders. Likewise, most adolescents in substance treatment programs have mental health problems, which can include conduct disorder, affective disorder, ADHD, anxiety disorders, eating disorders, and other Axis I conditions as well as frequent Axis II diagnoses of passive-aggressive personality or borderline or narcissistic personality disorder. Of note, methylphenidate treatment of ADHD in adolescents significantly reduces the risk of developing substance abuse in later life (Biederman et al. 1997).

The risk of morbidity and mortality by various avenues must be assessed in this population. Careful history taking in regard to thoughts of and attempts at suicide as well as impulsive, thrill-seeking, or risk-taking behavior is crucial. In the presence of a family history of suicide or depression, psychosis, isolation from family and friends, previous suicide attempts, clear-cut plans of suicide, or a violent means of carrying out the plan, the risk of suicide is increased. Substance use disorders are major risk factors for suicide among adolescents. Substance abuse in adolescents is frequently associated with risk-taking behavior linked to the spread of HIV infection. Substance use in adolescents may also directly and indirectly affect the immune system. Sexual abuse of children and adolescents is not uncommon in families with substance use disorders and may also increase the risk of HIV infection in families where an HIV-positive substance user is present. The severe medical consequences of MDMA abuse by adolescents have become increasingly apparent (Jonas and Graeme-Cook 2001).

Clinical Settings

Assessment. Assessment of the adolescent must be comprehensive. It requires a careful history of both patient and family, including where and when drugs are used, under what circumstances, dosages used, and what drug effects and reactions have occurred. Parents should be asked about the adolescent's behavior, including personality changes, school performance and absenteeism, change in peers, presence of rebelliousness, and the number of occasions they thought their adolescent was intoxicated. Parents' reactions to the adolescent's drug use, whether confrontation has been tried, and the adolescent's responses to confrontation are important. Parental and sibling use history is also important. Gathering histories from schools, pediatricians, clergy, and probation officers can be helpful as well. The clinician should be aware of the possibility of denial by the adolescent or family.

Clinical management issues. The treatment of adolescents requires both structure and flexibility. Awareness of the possibility of contraband stashes and the necessity for intermittent urine screening are important in inpatient treatment programs to monitor compliance. Most programs place great emphasis on a therapeutic milieu with individualized treatment planning. A warm, supportive environment with an organized structure increases motivation and maximizes positive interactions with the peer group. Adolescent programs rely heavily on peer-support groups, family therapy, organized education, education on drug abuse, 12-Step programs such as AA and Alateen, vocational programs, patient–staff meetings, and activity therapy. Programs that do best with adolescents encourage openness and spontaneous expression of feelings, allow patients to engage in independent decision making, have counselors help patients solve their real problems, use cognitive and behavioral approaches and relaxation techniques, have experienced counselors and staff, and frequently employ the support of volunteers. Cognitive-behavioral approaches have been modified for adolescents, and treatment manuals are available for guidance in the use of this efficacious modality (Kaminer 1994).

Substance intoxication or substance-induced psychosis. Intoxication with drugs or alcohol in adolescents may lead to disinhibition, violence, and medical complications. Strategies to manage these crises include a quiet, supportive environment, which can lessen the chance of the child or adolescent acting out in a violent manner, and sometimes addition of benzodiazepines or atypical antipsychotics. However, one should generally avoid the use of sedatives in adolescents, because benzodiazepines lead to greater disinhibition and increase the possibility of violent acting out. Clinical support staff may be needed to approach potentially violent adolescents and to have an additional quieting effect. Emergency-room checks for weapons are very important with adolescents, and police should be involved if the adolescent is carrying a weapon.

Treatment settings. Inpatient or residential treatment is indicated for adolescents who have a drug problem that has interfered with their ability to function in school, work, and home environments and who have been unable to maintain abstinence through outpatient treatment. Low motivation for change, a disruptive home life, frequent acting out, involvement with the juvenile justice system, and additional psychiatric or medical problems all may be reasons for inpatient treatment. Depression, suicidality, hyperactivity, chemical dependence, and overdoses of drugs are additional indications. Adolescents frequently require longer hospital stays than adults because of greater problems with creating dispositions, more resistance to treatment, greater difficulty of controlling acting out in outpatient therapy, and greater severity of family problems.

Treatment outcome for adolescents is worse than for adults. Predictors of treatment completion include greater severity of alcohol abuse; worse abuse of drugs other than alcohol, nicotine, or cannabis; a higher degree of internalizing problems; and lower self-esteem (Blood and Cornwall 1994).

Psychopharmacology

When considering pharmacological interventions in this population, great care and attention are essential. Disulfiram is seldom used in adolescents. Although withdrawal from alcohol is rarely clinically significant in this population, it should be monitored and treated as in adults. Methadone is generally avoided in adolescents (Hopfer et al. 2001).

Relapses

Relapse prevention with adolescents is often more difficult than with adults, and total abstinence is difficult to achieve. Tough rules regarding relapse are less likely to be effective in adolescent treatment services, where adolescents may be looking for a means of escaping treatment. With adolescents, a slip needs to be understood as a symptom of the problem; the patient should not be rejected because of a relapse. Relapses may lead to adjustment of treatment plans and may require rehospitalization.

To prevent relapses, discharge planning must include outpatient treatment for drug abuse and frequent attendance at self-help support groups. Family or group treatments may be added to individual treatment, depending on need. Urine screens for drugs and alcohol are often part of a comprehensive outpatient plan. Adolescents may also need halfway houses, residential treatment centers, and, in some instances, long-term inpatient psychiatric care.

The Elderly

Substance abuse in the elderly may be the continuation of a lifelong pattern or a reaction to losses of ego or bodily integrity. The scope of substance use disorders in this population is poorly studied, and cultural factors likely create differences among groups. The incidence of alcoholism is lower (perhaps because persons with chronic alcoholism die prematurely), but the abuse of prescription drugs is common. Finally, age-related changes in the pharmacokinetics of prescribed medications compound the severe consequences of substance abuse in the elderly.

Special Problems in Detection

Diagnosis is difficult in the elderly for many reasons. Denial is common, and impairments in social and occupational functioning (including legal problems) may be hard to discern in retirees. It may be difficult to distinguish the consequences of substance use, such as cognitive impairments, from aging or from neurodegenerative disease. The adverse effects of heavy alcohol use on sleep, sexual functioning, and cognitive ability augment the changes that usually occur with aging or with the use of multiple medications. It is essential to keep in mind at all times that elderly alcoholics (especially males) are at a very high risk of suicide. Regular screening for alcohol-related disorders should be instituted. The MAST is a valid measure among elderly outpatients (Hirata et al. 2001).

Complications

The usual pharmacokinetic changes that accompany aging include a relatively increased volume of distribution, greater CNS sensitivity to toxic substances, alterations in protein binding, and changes in hepatic and renal metabolism and excretion (Salzman 1998). Alcohol complicates these problems. Its hepatic effects may lead to either higher or lower bioavailability of medications. Alcohol's depressant effects may further contribute to major depression and cognitive impairment. For some elderly drinkers, there is a loss of tolerance, which leads to greater effects with smaller doses. Alcohol-induced persisting dementia is not reversible but does not progress further on cessation of drinking (Saunders et al. 1991). Thiamine deficiency is a common etiology of dementia in elderly alcoholic persons, and thiamine repletion should be instituted promptly to prevent Wernicke's encephalopathy.

Treatment Issues

Substance abuse treatment for the elderly requires greater creativity, flexibility, and sensitivity to the needs of this population. Geriatric patients may need to be protected from threatening and acting-out behaviors of younger patients. Older patients also require somewhat less confrontation and a higher degree of support, and more attention should be given to work with family members. The consequences of divorce are likely to also be greater in this group, and spouses are less likely to do well if left because of a drinking problem rather than for some other reason. Table 8–25 offers general guidelines for treatment of alcoholism in elderly persons.

TABLE 8–25. Guidelines for care of the elderly substance abuser

Avoid disulfiram

Use short-acting benzodiazepines

Remember that elderly patients are less likely to achieve full abstinence

Consider the patient's life experiences

Institute thiamine repletion

Prescription Drug Abuse

Abuse of prescription drugs is common in the elderly (Abrams and Alexopoulos 1988). Abuse of benzodiazepines and other hypnotics is common among women. Cognitive decline may lead to unintentional misuse. Nursing home patients are sometimes overmedicated to reduce disruptiveness. Abusers of prescription medications may require hospitalization to discontinue use.

Chronically Ill, Disabled, and Homeless Patients

Patients with chronic substance dependence are a group with a wide range of substances of use, demographic characteristics, comorbid medical and psychiatric conditions, and exposure to treatment. Historically, chronic patients have been severely stigmatized, which has led to prejudice with regard to allocation of resources and handling of benefits and disability. This population may need a wide range of services and links with other programs in the community. Programs need to be culturally relevant and to meet local realities of communities. The cognitive impairment associated with chronic substance use is likely to affect the ability of patients to handle cognitive treatment programs. This population is the one most often in need of long-term institutional treatment.

Chronic Psychiatric Comorbidity With Substance Abuse

Chronic mental illness frequently contributes to the chronicity and severity of substance abuse problems. Facilities that combine psychiatric treatment with substance abuse rehabilitation techniques are often unavailable to these patients. Severely disturbed abusers may be shunned by drug rehabilitation units. Confrontational methods and overemphasis on abstinence, which may lead to underuse of appropriate psychotropic medication, can be detrimental to mentally ill substance abusers.

Chronic Substance Abuse in the Multidisabled and Physically Handicapped

Physically disabled individuals may have relatively easier access to prescription drugs, and physicians may too readily prescribe medications to alleviate their own feelings of guilt or futility. Alternatively, patients with multiple disabilities are more likely to suffer from pain, and this can lead to iatrogenic addiction. Disabled individuals who feel frustrated and angry at being dependent, isolated, and discriminated against by society may be more prone to depression, anxiety, low motivation, and low self-esteem—and consequent self-medication.

Blind and visually impaired patients may have problems coping with their impairments, and this may contribute to substance abuse. There may be greater denial of the existence of substance abuse problems within the deaf community because deaf individuals with substance use problems may fear stigmatization from having an additional problem. Adequate sign language terms to symbolize drunkenness or sobriety may be lacking. Innovative treatment programs have been developed that use simultaneous translators in groups to mainstream deaf patients through alcohol rehabilitation programs.

The problems of substance abuse in patients with spinal cord injuries are significant. The spinal cord problems may have been caused by substance abuse in the first place; physical problems such as decubitus ulcers are caused by immobility and poor nutrition, which may be worsened by substance abuse. Treatment programs tailored to alcoholic patients with spinal cord injuries are needed that provide physical rehabilitation, group psychotherapy, and 12-Step recovery groups.

The Mentally Retarded Substance Abuser

Mildly retarded (IQ 60–85) patients are concrete in their thinking, easily manipulated, and may have problems learning from experience. Most of these patients live in the community and may attempt to socialize in neighborhood bars, which are viewed as warm and nonjudgmental. There may be a wish to feel accepted as part of a group. Alcohol and substance abuse are seen as a means of improving socialization. Treatment and prevention efforts need to take into account the special needs of this population. Poor verbal skills may make it more difficult for mentally retarded substance abusers to benefit from AA and NA meetings and from group programs that involve cognitive approaches and education about drug abuse. An emphasis on providing acceptance, warmth, and emotional support is especially important in working with this population. If these patients are able to learn that they cannot drink safely and if simple messages of not drinking are reinforced, they may do very well in treatment.

Homeless Patients With Addictions

The homeless population is no longer principally composed of "skid row" alcoholics or single, older, chronically alcoholic men (Koegel and Burnam 1988). The population is now younger and includes an increasing number of women; in addition, as many as 90% have a primary psychiatric diagnosis. In several different urban samples in the United States, 20%–60% of homeless patients reported alcohol dependence (Koegel and Burnam 1988). Social isolation, legal problems, and stigma all serve as barriers to obtaining care. Clinics that work with homeless substance abusers struggle with trying to get basic social support services for their clients, with adequate provision for meals and a place to live.

Minorities

Substance abuse is a critical problem in subsets of minority populations (Franklin 1998). Substance use disorders have a major impact on overall life expectancies in blacks, Hispanics, and Native Americans. Black teenagers report less alcohol abuse than do their white peers; in their 20s and 30s, however, their rates of abuse are comparable to those of whites and they suffer a disproportionate amount of medical (cirrhosis, esophageal cancer, and AIDS), psychological, and social sequelae. Excessive alcohol consumption is reported among rural and urban Native Americans.

Targeting Treatment

Programs designed for middle-class white Americans may not be equally applicable to minorities. Treatment programs in minority communities should be sensitive to culture as well as the disabling social problems in many of these communities that likely contribute to the high rates of substance use disorders. Although the biopsychosocial approach is equally valid in minority populations, social factors such as poor education, unemployment, low job skills, racism, and substance-abusing peer role models are additional important etiological factors that must be addressed in any culturally sensitive program. Recognition of and cooperation with indigenous cultural institutions such as churches is necessary. Historically, blacks have had less access to treatment, and cutbacks in funding of social agencies may create further barriers to care. Family treatment approaches are especially valuable in the Hispanic community, and respect for cultural diversity is essential in drug treatment programs. Treatment in minority communities generally must focus more on the extended family. Treatment programs and AA meetings must be flexible and responsive to cultural norms.

Cultural Patterns

Some Native Americans have in their culture the tradition of the "drinking party," in which alcohol is consumed to excess and disinhibited behavior is sanctioned. Hispanics have the notion of machismo, wherein manhood is equated with the ability to hold one's liquor. If a man is able to provide for his family, alcoholism may be well tolerated. In many cultures, alcohol consumption is seen as a celebration of life and is an integral part of holidays and festivals. However, problems resulting from alcohol are shameful.

We must also recognize the heterogeneity within minority communities. For example, African Americans in the rural South may have different cultural norms compared with blacks of West Indian descent. In addition, minority women may have particular roles and treatment issues that are not prevalent among women in the majority population. In family therapy with Hispanic groups (e.g., families), attention to issues related to respect and machismo leads to good results. When unmet needs are identified in specific minority groups—for example, substance abuse problems in Native Americans—we must discover the causes and attempt to address them (Novins et al. 2000).

References

Abrams RC, Alexopoulos GS: Substance abuse in the elderly: over-the-counter and illegal drugs. Hosp Community Psychiatry 39:822–823, 1988

Abramson JL, Williams SA, Krumholz HM, et al: Moderate alcohol consumption and risk of heart failure among older persons. JAMA 285:1971–1977, 2001

American Psychiatric Association: Diagnostic and Statistical Manual of Mental Disorders, 4th Edition. Washington, DC, American Psychiatric Association, 1994

American Psychiatric Association: Practice guideline for the treatment of patients with substance use disorders: alcohol, cocaine, opioids. Am J Psychiatry 152(suppl):1–59, 1995

American Psychiatric Association: Practice guideline for the treatment of patients with nicotine dependence. Am J Psychiatry 153(suppl):1–31, 1996

American Psychiatric Association: Diagnostic and Statistical Manual of Mental Disorders, 4th Edition, Text Revision. Washington, DC, American Psychiatric Association, 2000

American Society of Addiction Medicine: Patient Placement Criteria for the Treatment of Substance-Related Disorders, 2nd Edition. Chevy Chase, MD, American Society of Addiction Medicine, 1996

Anton RF, Moak DH, Waid LR, et al: Naltrexone and cognitive behavioral therapy for the treatment of outpatient alcoholics: results of a placebo-controlled trial. Am J Psychiatry 156:1758–1764, 1999

Armor DJ, Polish SM, Stambul HB: Alcoholics and Treatment. New York, Wiley, 1978

Ashley MJ, Olin JS, LeRiche WH, et al: Morbidity in alcoholics: evidence for accelerated development of physical disease in women. Arch Intern Med 137:883–887, 1977

Bachman JG, Wallace JM Jr, O'Malley PM: Racial/ethnic differences in smoking, drinking, and illicit drug use among American high school seniors, 1976–89. Am J Public Health 81:372–377, 1991

Bartzokis G, Beckson M, Hance DB, et al: Magnetic resonance imaging evidence of "silent" cerebrovascular toxicity in cocaine dependence. Biol Psychiatry 45:1203–1211, 1999

Berk M, Brook S, Trandafir AI: A comparison of olanzapine with haloperidol in cannabis-induced psychotic disorder: a double-blind randomized controlled trial. Int Clin Psychopharmacol 14:177–180, 1999

Berlakovich GA, Steininger R, Herbst F, et al: Efficacy of liver transplantation for alcoholic cirrhosis with respect to recidivism and compliance. Transplantation 58:560–565, 1994

Bickel WK, Amass L, Higgins ST, et al: Effects of adding behavioral treatment to opioid detoxification with buprenorphine. J Consult Clin Psychol 65:803–810, 1997

Biederman J, Wilens T, Mick E, et al: Is ADHD a risk factor for psychoactive substance use disorders? Findings from a four-year prospective follow-up study. J Am Acad Child Adolesc Psychiatry 36:21–29, 1997

Blood L, Cornwall A: Pretreatment variables that predict completion of an adolescent substance abuse treatment program. J Nerv Ment Dis 182:14–19, 1994

Blume S: Addictive disorders in women, in Clinical Textbook of Addictive Disorders, 2nd Edition. Edited by Frances RJ, Miller SI. New York, Guilford, 1998

Botvin GJ, Baker E, Dusenbury L, et al: Long-term follow-up results of a randomized drug abuse prevention trial in a white middle-class population. JAMA 273:1106–1112, 1995

Bouckoms A, Hackett TP: Pain patients, in MGH Handbook of General Hospital Psychiatry, 4th Edition. Edited by Cassem NH. St Louis, MO, Mosby-Year Book, 1997, pp 367–415

Brooner RK, King VL, Kidorf M, et al: Psychiatric and substance use comorbidity among treatment seeking opioid abusers. Arch Gen Psychiatry 54:71–80, 1997

Brown HL, Britton KA, Mahaffey D, et al: Methadone maintenance in pregnancy: a reappraisal. Am J Obstet Gynecol 179:459–463, 1998

Brown RA, Evans DM, Miller IW, et al: CBT for depression in alcoholism. J Consult Clin Psychol 65:715–726, 1997

Bukstein O: Practice parameters for the assessment and treatment of children and adolescents with substance use disorders. J Am Acad Child Adolesc Psychiatry 36:140S–156S, 1997

Centers for Disease Control and Prevention: Increasing morbidity and mortality associated with abuse of methamphetamine: United States, 1991–1994. MMWR Morb Mortal Wkly Rep 44:882–886, 1995

Centers for Disease Control and Prevention: Alcohol consumption among pregnant and childbearing-aged women: United States, 1991 and 1995. MMWR Morb Mortal Wkly Rep 46:346–350, 1997a

Centers for Disease Control and Prevention: Gamma hydroxybutyrate use: New York and Texas, 1995–1996. JAMA 277:1511, 1997b

Centers for Disease Control and Prevention: Alcohol involvement in fatal motor-vehicle crashes—United States, 1997–1998. MMWR Morb Mortal Wkly Rep 48:1086–1087, 1999a

Centers for Disease Control and Prevention: Cigarette smoking among adults—United States, 1997. MMWR Morb Mortal Wkly Rep 48:993–996, 1999b

Centers for Disease Control and Prevention: Trends in cigarette smoking among high school students, United States, 1991–1999. MMWR Morb Mortal Wkly Rep 49:755–758, 2000

Cloninger CR, Sigvardsson S, Bohman M: Childhood personality predicts alcohol abuse in young adults. Alcoholism: Clinical and Experimental Research 12:494–505, 1988

Cornish JW, Maany I, Fudala PJ, et al: Carbamazepine treatment for cocaine dependence. Drug Alcohol Depend 38:221–227, 1995

Craig K, Gomez HF, McManus JL, et al: Severe gamma-hydroxybutyrate withdrawal: a case report and literature review. J Emerg Med 18:65–70, 2000

Derogatis LR, Lipman RS, Covi L: The SCL-90: an outpatient psychiatric rating scale. Psychopharmacol Bull 9:13–28, 1973

Des Jarlais DC, Marmor M, Friedman P, et al: HIV incidence among injection drug users in New York City, 1992–1997: evidence for a declining epidemic. Am J Public Health 90:352–359, 2000

DeWit DJ, Adlaf EM, Offord DR, et al: Age at first alcohol use: a risk factor for the development of alcohol disorders. Am J Psychiatry 157:745–750, 2000

Diana M, Melis M, Muntoni AL, et al: Meso-limbic dopaminergic decline after cannabinoid withdrawal. Proc Natl Acad Sci U S A 95:10269–10273, 1998

Edwards ME, Steinglass P: Family therapy treatment outcomes for alcoholism. J Marital Fam Ther 21:475–509, 1995

Ellenhorn MJ: Ellenhorn's Medical Toxicology, Diagnosis, and Treatment of Human Poisoning, 2nd Edition. Baltimore, MD, Williams & Wilkins, 1997

Endicott J, Spitzer RL: A diagnostic interview: the Schedule for Affective Disorders and Schizophrenia. Arch Gen Psychiatry 35:837–844, 1978

Feighner JP, Robins E, Guze SB, et al: Diagnostic criteria for use in psychiatric research. Arch Gen Psychiatry 26:57–63, 1972

First MB, Gibbon M, Spitzer RL, et al: User's Guide for the Structured Clinical Interview for DSM-IV Axis II Personality Disorders (SCID-II). Washington, DC, American Psychiatric Press, 1997

Flaum M, Schultz SK: When does amphetamine-induced psychosis become schizophrenia? Am J Psychiatry 153:812–815, 1996

Frances RJ, Alexopoulos GS: The inpatient treatment of the alcoholic patient. Psychiatr Ann 12:386–391, 1982a

Frances RJ, Alexopoulos GS: Patient management and education; getting the alcoholic into treatment. Physician and Patient 1:9–14, 1982b

Frances R, Borg L, Mack A, et al: Individual treatment: psychodynamics and the treatment of substance-related disorders, in Treatments of Psychiatric Disorders, 3rd Edition. Edited by Gabbard GO. Washington, DC, American Psychiatric Press, 2001, pp 827–838

Frank DA, Augustyn M, Knight WG, et al: Growth, development, and behavior in early childhood following prenatal cocaine exposure: a systematic review. JAMA 285:1613–1625, 2001

Franklin J: Minority populations, in Clinical Textbook of Addictive Disorders, 2nd Edition. Edited by Frances RJ, Miller SI. New York, Guilford, 1998

Galanter M: Self help treatment for combined addiction and mental illness. Hosp Community Psychiatry 51:877–879, 2000

Galanter M, Keller D, Dermatis H: Network therapy for addiction: assessment of the clinical outcome of training. Am J Psychiatry 150:28–36, 1993

Gavaler JS, Rizzo A, Rossaro L, et al: Sexuality of alcoholic women with menstrual cycle function: effects of duration of alcohol abstinence. Alcohol Clin Exp Res 17:778–781, 1995

Geller B, Cooper TB, Sun K, et al: Double-blind and placebo-controlled study of lithium for adolescent bipolar disorders with secondary substance dependency. J Am Acad Child Adolesc Psychiatry 37:171–178, 1998

Gold MS, Dackis CA: Role of the laboratory in the evaluation of suspected drug abuse. J Clin Psychiatry 47:17–23, 1986

Goldberg MJ, Spector R, Park GD, et al: An approach to the management of the poisoned patient. Arch Intern Med 146:1381–1385, 1986

Graeme KA: New drugs of abuse. Emerg Med Clin North Am 18:625–636, 2000

Greenfield SF, O'Leary G: Sex differences in marijuana use in the United States. Harv Rev Psychiatry 6:297–303, 1999

Group for the Advancement of Psychiatry: Addiction treatment; avoiding pitfalls: a case approach. GAP Report 142. Washington, DC, American Psychiatric Press, 1998

Halpern J, Pope HG: Hallucinogens on the Internet: a vast new source of underground drug information. Am J Psychiatry 158:481–483, 2001

Harwood H, Fountain D, Livermore G, et al: The Economic Costs of Alcohol and Drug Abuse in the United States, 1992. Washington, DC, National Institute on Drug Abuse and National Institute on Alcohol Abuse and Alcoholism, 1998

Hathaway SR, McKinley JC: Minnesota Multiphasic Personality Inventory Manual, Revised Edition. New York, Psychological Corporation, 1967

Hernandez-Avila CA, Ortega-Soto HA, Jasso A, et al: Treatment of inhalant-induced psychotic disorder with carbamazepine versus haloperidol. Psychiatr Serv 49:812–815, 1998

Hirata ES, Almeida OP, Funari RR, et al: Validity of the Michigan Alcoholism Screening Test (MAST) for the detection of alcohol-related problems among male geriatric outpatients. Am J Geriatr Psychiatry 9:30–34, 2001

Holt S, Skinner M, Israel Y: Early identification of alcohol abuse, II: clinical and laboratory indicators. Can Med Assoc J 124:1279–1294, 1981

Hommer DW, Momenan R, Kaiser E, et al: Evidence for a gender-related effect of alcoholism on brain volumes. Am J Psychiatry 158:198–204, 2001

Hopfer CJ, Mikulich SK, Crowley TJ: Heroin use among adolescents in treatment for substance use disorders. J Am Acad Child Adolesc Psychiatry 39:1316–1323, 2001

Horn JL, Warburg KW, Foster FM: Alcohol Use Inventory. Minneapolis, MN, National Computer Systems, 1986

Institute of Medicine: Fetal alcohol syndrome: research base for diagnostic criteria, epidemiology, prevention, and treatment. Washington, DC, National Academy Press, 1995

Institute of Medicine: Workshop Summary. The Role of Co-Occurring Substance Abuse and Mental Illness in Violence: Division of Neuroscience and Behavioral Health, Institute of Medicine. Washington, DC, National Academy Press, 1999

Irwin M, Baird S, Smith TL, et al: Use of laboratory tests to monitor heavy drinking by alcoholic men discharged from a treatment program. Am J Psychiatry 145:595–599, 1988

Jansen KLR: Nonmedical use of ketamine. BMJ 306:601–602, 1993

Jellinek EM: The Disease Concept of Alcoholism. New Haven, CT, Hillhouse Press, 1960

Johnson BA, Roache JD, Javors MA, et al: Ondansetron for reduction of drinking among biologically predisposed alcoholic patients: a randomized controlled trial. JAMA 284:963–971, 2000

Johnson RE, Eissenberg T, Stitzer ML, et al: A placebo controlled clinical trial of buprenorphine as a treatment for opioid dependence. Drug Alcohol Depend 40:17–25, 1995

Johnson RE, Chutuape MA, Strain E, et al: A comparison of levomethadyl acetate, buprenorphine, and methadone for opioid dependence. N Engl J Med 343:1290–1297, 2000

Johnston LD, O'Malley PM, Bachman JG: National Annual High School Senior and Young Adult Survey. Washington, DC, U.S. Government Printing Office, 1997

Johnston LD, O'Malley PM, Bachman JG: Monitoring the Future National Survey Results on Adolescent Drug Use: Overview of Key Findings, 2000 (NIH Publ No 01-4923). Bethesda, MD, National Institute on Drug Abuse, 2001

Jonas MM, Graeme-Cook FM: A 17-year-old girl with marked jaundice and weight loss. N Engl J Med 344:591–599, 2001

Kaminer Y: Adolescent Substance Abuse: A Comprehensive Guide to Theory and Practice. New York, Plenum, 1994

Kaminer Y, Bukstein O, Tarter RE: The Teen-Addiction Severity Index: rationale and reliability. Int J Addict 26:219–226, 1991

Kandel D, Faust R: Sequence and stages in patterns of adolescent drug use. Arch Gen Psychiatry 32:923–932, 1975

Karan LD, Haller DH, Schnoll SH: Cocaine and stimulants, in Clinical Textbook of Addictive Disorders, 2nd Edition. Edited by Frances RJ, Miller SI. New York, Guilford, 1998

Kessler RC, Sonnega A, Bromet E, et al: Posttraumatic stress disorder in the National Comorbidity Survey. Arch Gen Psychiatry 52:1048–1060, 1995

Kessler RC, Crum RM, Warner LA, et al: Lifetime co-occurrence of DSM-III-R alcohol abuse and dependence with other psychiatric disorders in the National Comorbidity Survey. Arch Gen Psychiatry 54:313–321, 1997

Khantzian EJ: The self-medication hypothesis of substance use disorders: a reconsideration and recent applications. Harv Rev Psychiatry 4:231–244, 1997

Klitzman RL, Pope HG, Hudson JI: MDMA ("ecstasy") abuse and high risk sexual behaviors among 169 gay and bisexual men. Am J Psychiatry 157:1162–1164, 2000

Koch M, Banys P: Liver transplantation and opioid dependence. JAMA 285:1056–1058, 2001

Koegel P, Burnam A: Alcoholism among homeless adults in the inner city of Los Angeles. Arch Gen Psychiatry 45:1011–1018, 1988

Kreek MJ: Methadone-related opioid agonist pharmacotherapy for heroin addiction. History, recent molecular and neurochemical research and future in mainstream medicine. Ann N Y Acad Sci 909:186–216; 2000

Krystal JH, Karper LP, Seibyl JP, et al: Subanesthetic effects of the noncompetitive NMDA antagonist, ketamine, in humans: psychotomimetic, perceptual, cognitive, and neuroendocrine responses. Arch Gen Psychiatry 51:199–214, 1994

Kucuk NO, Kilic EO, Ibis E, et al: Brain SPECT findings in long term inhalant abuse. Nucl Med Commun 21:769–773, 2000

Kushner MG, Sher KJ, Beitman BD: The relation between alcohol problems and the anxiety disorders. Am J Psychiatry 147:685–695, 1990

Lerner AG, Finkel B, Oyfee I, et al: Clonidine treatment for hallucinogen persisting perception disorder. Am J Psychiatry 155:1460, 1998

Leshner AI: Addiction is a brain disease and it matters. Science 278:45–47, 1997

Leshner AI, Koob GF: Drugs of abuse and the brain. Proc Assoc Am Physicians 111:99–108, 1999

Lieber CS: Medical disorders of alcoholism. N Engl J Med 333:1058–1065, 1995

Linehan MM, Schmidt H 3rd, Dimeff LA, et al: Dialectical behavior therapy for patients with borderline personality disorder and drug-dependence. Am J Addict 8:279–292, 1999

Ling W, Charuvastra C, Collins JF, et al: Buprenorphine maintenance treatment of opiate dependence: a multicenter, randomized clinical trial. Addiction 93:475–486, 1998

Longnecker MP, Berlin JA, Orza MJ, et al: A meta-analysis of alcohol consumption in relation to breast cancer. JAMA 260:652–656, 1988

Lumeng L: New diagnostic markers of alcohol abuse. Hepatology 6:742–745, 1986

MacAndrew C: The differentiation of male alcohol outpatients from nonalcoholic psychiatric patients by means of the MMPI. Q J Stud Alcohol 26:238–246, 1965

Malcolm R, Kajdasz DK, Herron J, et al: A double-blind, placebo-controlled outpatient trial of pergolide for cocaine dependence. Drug Alcohol Depend 60:161–168, 2000

Marlatt GA, Gordon JR: Relapse Prevention: Maintenance Strategies in the Treatment of Addictive Behaviors. New York, Guilford, 1985

Marlatt GA, Baer JS, Kivlahan DR, et al: Screening and brief intervention for high-risk college student drinkers: results from a 2-year follow-up assessment. J Consult Clin Psychol 66:604–615, 1998

Marzuk PM, Tardiff KL, Leon AC, et al: Prevalence of cocaine use among residents of New York City who committed suicide during a one-year period. Am J Psychiatry 149:371–375, 1992

McCann UD, Mertl M, Eligulashvili V, et al: Cognitive performance in (+/–) 3,4-methylenedioxymethamphetamine (MDMA, "ecstasy") users: a controlled study. Psychopharmacology (Berl) 143:417–425, 1999

McGill V, Kowal-Vern A, Fisher SG: The impact of substance use on mortality and morbidity from thermal injury. J Trauma 38:931–934, 1995

McLellan AT, Luborsky L, Woody GE, et al: Are the "addiction-related" problems of substance abusers really related? J Nerv Ment Dis 169:232–239, 1981

McLellan AT, Grissom GR, Zanis D, et al: Problem-service matching in addiction treatment: a prospective study in 4 programs. Arch Gen Psychiatry 54:730–735, 1997

Moore RD, Bone LR, Geller G, et al: Prevalence, detection, and treatment of alcoholism in hospitalized patients. JAMA 261:403–407, 1989

Mukamal KJ, Maclure M, Muller JE, et al: Prior alcohol consumption and mortality following acute myocardial infarction. JAMA 285:1965–1970, 2001

Murphy SL: Deaths: Final Data for 1998: National Vital Statistics Reports, 48(11). Hyattsville, MD, National Center for Vital Statistics, 2000

National Institute on Drug Abuse: Principles of Drug Addiction Treatment: A Research-Based Guide (NIH Publication 00-4180). Rockville, MD, National Institute on Drug Abuse, 1999

Novins DK, Beals J, Sack WH, et al: Unmet needs for substance abuse and mental health services among northern plains American Indian Adolescents. Psychiatr Serv 51:1045–1047, 2000

O'Brien CP, McLellan AT: Myths about the treatment of addiction. Lancet 347:237–240, 1996

O'Connor PG, Waugh ME, Carrol KM, et al: Primary care-based ambulatory opioid detoxification: the results of a clinical trial. J Gen Intern Med 10:255–260, 1995

O'Connor PG, Carroll KM, Shi JM, et al: Three methods of opioid detoxification in a primary care setting. A randomized trial. Ann Intern Med 127:526–530, 1997

Office of Applied Studies: Drug Abuse Warning Network, Annual Medical Examiner Data, 1998. Rockville, MD, Substance Abuse and Mental Health Services Administration, 2000a

Office of Applied Studies: National Household Survey on Drug Abuse. Rockville, MD, Substance Abuse and Mental Health Services Administration, 2000b

O'Malley PM, Johnston LD, Bachman JG: Adolescent substance use. Epidemiology and implications for public policy. Pediatr Clin North Am 42:241–260, 1995

O'Malley SS, Jaffe AJ, Chang G, et al: Six-month follow-up of naltrexone and psychotherapy for alcohol dependence. Arch Gen Psychiatry 53:217–224, 1996

Perlman DC, Saloman N, Perkins MP, et al: Tuberculosis in drug users. Clin Infect Dis 21:1263–1264, 1995

Schizophrenia and Other Psychotic Disorders

Beng-Choon Ho, M.R.C.Psych.

Donald W. Black, M.D.

Nancy C. Andreasen, M.D., Ph.D.

Schizophrenia is perhaps the most enigmatic and tragic disease that psychiatrists treat, and perhaps also the most devastating. It is one of the leading causes of disability among young adults (Table 9–1). Schizophrenia strikes at a young age so that, unlike patients with cancer or heart disease, patients with schizophrenia usually live many years after onset of the disease and continue to suffer its effects, which prevent them from leading fully normal lives—attending school, working, having a close network of friends, marrying, or having children. In a study commissioned by the World Health Organization and the World Bank, schizophrenia ranked as the ninth leading cause of disability in people ages 15–44 years worldwide, and fourth in developed countries (Murray and Lopez 1996).

Apart from its effect on individuals and families, schizophrenia creates a huge economic burden for society. A study at the National Institute of Mental Health calculated the total cost of schizophrenia in 1991 at $65 billion (Wyatt et al. 1995). Nearly two-thirds was attributed to the indirect cost of family caregiving, lost wages, and losses due to early death from suicide, and the remainder went for treatment, public assistance, and other direct costs. Not taken into account is the enormous social and psychological anguish schizophrenia causes to patients and their families. Despite its emotional and economic costs, schizophrenia has yet to receive sufficient recognition as a major health concern or the necessary research support to investigate its causes, treatments, and prevention. Large private foundations (e.g., the Dana Foundation, the National Association for Research in Schizo-

phrenia and Affective Disorder [NARSAD]) have been working to meet these needs, however, indicating a groundswell of public awareness of the importance of schizophrenia that parallels that surrounding Alzheimer's disease a decade earlier.

The decade of the 1980s was a period of reassessment. Earlier optimism about the treatment of schizophrenia had been prompted by the introduction of neuroleptics and the community mental health movement. Deinstitutionalization took hold, and large numbers of people with schizophrenia were released from hospitals. Optimism gradually led to pessimism as it became clear that neuroleptics had a limited ability to control the symptoms of schizophrenia and also exposed patients to health risks with long-term exposure to the drugs. Moreover, many discharged patients could not function in the community and had to be returned to state hospitals or residential care facilities. Others became homeless or were trapped by the "revolving door" of frequent, brief hospitalizations.

Having perhaps promised too much, during the 1990s clinicians and researchers interested in schizophrenia initially found themselves embattled. This resulted in a period of regrouping and reassessment that has led to a more realistic, integrated, and multifaceted approach to understanding this complex disorder. In these early years of the twenty-first century, a new era of guarded optimism has emerged. Clinicians have agreed that the best treatment approaches combine medication with various forms of psychosocial care, and researchers have pioneered methods to integrate genetics, neurochemistry,

TABLE 9–1. Ten leading causes of disability at ages 15–44 years, 1990

Rank	Disease or injury	Disease burden[a]
World		
1	Unipolar major depression	10.25
2	Tuberculosis	4.69
3	Road traffic accidents	4.68
4	Alcohol use	3.54
5	Self-inflicted injuries	3.49
6	Bipolar disorder	3.15
7	War	3.13
8	Violence	3.09
9	Schizophrenia	2.99
10	Iron-deficiency anemia	2.98
Developed regions		
1	Unipolar major depression	12.27
2	Alcohol use	8.88
3	Road traffic accidents	8.60
4	Schizophrenia	4.91
5	Self-inflicted injuries	4.28
6	Bipolar disorder	3.63
7	Drug use	2.96
8	Obsessive-compulsive disorders	2.68
9	Osteoarthritis	2.65
10	Violence	2.44

Note. [a]% total disability-adjusted life year.

Source. Adapted from Murray CJL, Lopez AD: *The Global Burden of Disease: A Comprehensive Assessment of Mortality and Disability From Diseases, Injuries, and Risk Factors in 1990 and Projected to 2020.* Cambridge, MA, Harvard University Press, 1996 (Table 5.4).

and neuropathology. Rapidly evolving techniques in brain imaging and histopathology have provided a major boost to work in schizophrenia, assisted by concomitant advances in descriptive phenomenology, methods of classification, and epidemiology. The neuroscience community has joined together to identify the neural mechanisms of this important disease, promising that it may ultimately be understood at the systems, cellular, and molecular levels. Finally, after many years of "me too" antipsychotics with similar pharmacological profiles, "atypical" medications have been introduced that are more effective for some patients and better tolerated.

Historical Overview

Schizophrenia and related disorders have been recognized in almost all cultures and described throughout much of recorded time. "Mania" or "phrensy" were generic terms that referred to a broad range of psychotic illnesses beginning in classical times. Literary portrayals, such as the madness of Orestes in the *Oresteia* of Aeschylus or the mumblings of Poor Tom in *King Lear*,

make it clear that serious psychoses have been recognized even by lay people for many years. More technical descriptions appear in books such as Reginald Scot's *Discoveries of Witchcraft* in the sixteenth century or the classic psychiatric writings of Pinel in the eighteenth century (Andreasen 1984).

Although others before him, such as Kahlbaum, had circled around the topic of distinct subtypes of psychosis, Emil Kraepelin (1856–1926) is usually credited with delineating schizophrenia, principally on the basis of course and outcome. He observed that among the seriously mentally ill whom he treated in Dorpat and later in Heidelberg and Munich, some began to have symptoms such as delusions and emotional withdrawal at a relatively early age and that these patients were likely to have a chronic and deteriorating course. Kraepelin worked closely with his colleague Alzheimer, who also studied patients with serious cognitive impairment and deterioration beginning at a later age; this condition is now referred to as Alzheimer's disease. The patients whom Kraepelin (1919) studied, in contrast, developed their "dementia" at an early age, and Kraepelin therefore chose to distinguish these patients from the late-onset dementias by referring to them as having *dementia praecox*. Kraepelin was also instrumental in separating dementia praecox not only from Alzheimer's disease but also from a third group of illnesses, which he referred to as "manic-depressive illness." Manic-depressive illness differed from dementia praecox in that it had an age at onset distributed throughout life and a more episodic and less deteriorating course and outcome.

The importance of distinguishing between dementia praecox and manic-depressive illness quickly gained wide acceptance because of its prognostic utility and remains one of the most important distinctions in modern psychiatry. At the urging of Eugen Bleuler (1857–1939), dementia praecox was eventually renamed *schizophrenia*. Bleuler, who also honed his clinical and diagnostic skills through the close observation of large numbers of patients over long periods of time, was convinced that cross-sectional symptoms were more important defining features of schizophrenia than were course and outcome. He stressed that the fundamental and unifying abnormality in schizophrenia was cognitive impairment, which he conceptualized as a "splitting" or "loosening" in the "fabric of thought." He believed that "thought disorder" was the essential and pathognomonic symptom of schizophrenia and named the illness after this symptom: *schizophrenia*, or the fragmenting of mental capacities. He also believed that affective blunting, peculiar and distorted thinking (autism), avolition, impaired attention, and conceptual indecisiveness (ambivalence) were nearly equally important. Bleuler referred to this group of symptoms as "fundamental," whereas other symptoms such as delusions and hallucinations were regarded as "accessory," since they could occur in other disorders such as manic-depressive illness. Further, he pointed out that some patients with schizophrenia improve substantially although without a full recovery (or *restitutio ad integrum*), whereas others have a relatively chronic course. Finally, he noted that some patients begin to experience symptoms of schizophrenia as late as their 30s and 40s. For all these reasons, the term schizophrenia seems preferable to dementia praecox.

After the publication of his classic textbook *Dementia Praecox, or the Group of Schizophrenias* in 1911, Bleuler's ideas enjoyed increasing acceptance and became an influential description of schizophrenia in most of Europe, England, and the United States for decades. Several generations of psychiatrists were taught to recite the Bleulerian "Four A's" (occasionally expanded to five or six in order to reflect more accurately what Bleuler actually said): associations, affect, autism, and ambivalence. Thought disorder, or associative loosening, was considered to be the most important among these. Unlike delu-

sions and hallucinations, Bleulerian fundamental symptoms are on a continuum with normality and can be present in relatively mild forms; some, such as ambivalence, are common in healthy persons. Consequently, the influence of Bleuler led to an increasingly broad definition and conceptualization of schizophrenia as psychiatry gathered strength and momentum during the postwar years and through the 1950s and 1960s. This phenomenon was particularly apparent in the United States, where concepts such as "latent schizophrenia" and "pseudoneurotic schizophrenia" became popular (Black and Bofelli 1989). These concepts were reflected in the initial editions of the *Diagnostic and Statistical Manual of Mental Disorders*, published by the American Psychiatric Association. The first edition (American Psychiatric Association 1952) emphasized intrapsychic mechanisms rather than classes of disease, whereas the second edition (American Psychiatric Association 1968) shifted the emphasis to classification, but without listing specific criteria.

By the late 1960s, a number of factors intervened to introduce a climate of change. Studies of comparative diagnostic practices in the United States, England, and other nations alerted American psychiatrists to the fact that their diagnostic habits were out of step. For example, the United States/United Kingdom diagnostic project (Cooper et al. 1972) set out to determine why the prevalence of schizophrenia was greater in New York than London, while the reverse was true for manic-depressive illness. The investigators discovered that the same patients received different diagnoses in different countries due to conceptual and theoretical differences between their respective diagnostic systems. At about the same time, findings were reported from the International Pilot Study of Schizophrenia (World Health Organization 1975), in which schizophrenia was studied in nine countries. The major finding to emerge was that similar criteria were used in seven of the nine countries, but broader criteria were used in the United States and the Soviet Union.

In the context of these studies, an interest in reliable diagnosis emerged, leading to the development of structured interviews such as the Present State Examination (Wing et al. 1967) and operational diagnostic criteria such as the St. Louis Criteria (Feighner et al. 1972) developed at Washington University. Structured interviews required the definition of a symptom in a way that would ensure close agreement among clinicians and were accompanied by the development of operational diagnostic criteria in which definitions were spelled out in a clear and objective way. Bleulerian symptoms, with their breadth and imprecision, did not lend themselves well to such techniques. On the other hand, the use of delusions and hallucinations as defining features emphasized phenomena that are clearly abnormal and relatively easy to identify. The Present State Examination helped to introduce the concepts of the German psychiatrist Kurt Schneider (1887–1967) and his emphasis on "first-rank symptoms" to the English-speaking world. These forces helped reshape the concept of schizophrenia into one of a relatively severe psychotic disorder, bringing it closer to the original ideas of Kraepelin, but lacking Kraepelin's emphasis on a longitudinal definition that used course and outcome as a diagnostic guide.

Finally, and perhaps more importantly, the development of effective treatments such as neuroleptics, antidepressants, and, eventually, lithium carbonate made diagnosis an important clinical issue. If a patient with bipolar disorder or major depression were misdiagnosed with schizophrenia because of an excessively broad diagnostic concept, that patient might be deprived of the most appropriate treatment available, potentially condemned to an unnecessarily chronic course of illness, and perhaps condemned to needlessly suffer permanent and irreversible medication side effects.

As this brief historical overview indicates, the concept of schizophrenia has varied enormously over time and space. Kraepelin's definition was concise and narrow. For him, dementia praecox was an illness with a characteristic age at onset in the teens or early 20s that had a relatively poor outcome and led much of the time to relatively severe cognitive and emotional impairment. Kraepelin believed that the disorder would eventually be understood in terms of neuropathological mechanisms in the brain because of this clinical course. Although he emphasized the importance of cognitive impairment (i.e., "dementia"), he did not choose any single symptom as characteristic or pathognomonic; rather, his description of the clinical phenomenology stresses a mixture of delusions, hallucinations, motor signs and symptoms, emotional blunting, avolition, and social isolation. The introduction of Bleulerian ideas simultaneously broadened the concept and stressed the importance of symptoms that affected cognition, emotion, and volition. The emphasis on Schneiderian symptoms in the 1970s reintroduced yet another set of cross-sectional symptoms, specific delusions and hallucinations, which were quite different from the Bleulerian symptoms.

All of these developments led to a reassessment of how schizophrenia and other mental disorders were diagnosed, culminating in the third edition of the *Diagnostic and Statistical Manual of Mental Disorders* (DSM-III; American Psychiatric Association 1980), which enumerated specific criteria for all recognized psychiatric disorders. DSM-III and its revision (DSM-III-R; American Psychiatric Association 1987) represented a convergence of these various points of view. The criteria included the Kraepelinian emphasis on course through the requirement that the illness be present for at least 6 months, the emphasis on specific delusions and hallucinations thought important by Schneider, and the emphasis on the importance of fundamental Bleulerian symptoms (thought disorder in the form of associative loosening or incoherence and affective blunting).

The DSM-III and DSM-III-R compromise stirred debate among investigators interested in understanding the pathophysiology and etiology of schizophrenia. New technologies, such as molecular genetics or brain imaging, reemphasized the importance of careful and precise definition of the disease, as had occurred with the introduction of neuroleptics. Geneticists interested in familial patterns of transmission wondered whether the DSM-III and DSM-III-R definitions, with their requirement of florid psychotic symptoms, were too narrow to pick up subclinical cases in family pedigrees. They considered whether the concept of schizophrenia should be expanded to include nonpsychotic forms (e.g., simple and latent schizophrenia, and "schizotaxia"), much as Bleuler originally suggested (Tsuang et al. 2000). Studies of the neurobiology of schizophrenia, made possible by brain imaging and postmortem-brain banks, blurred the distinction between schizophrenia and "organic" disorders. Nearly four decades of psychopharmacological treatment of schizophrenia demonstrated that florid psychotic symptoms are probably not the core defining features after all, since crippling negative or deficit symptoms persist and seem fundamental, much as Bleuler observed. These observations have now been given more weight in DSM-IV (American Psychiatric Association 1994) and DSM-IV-TR (American Psychiatric Association 2000). Research conducted in the 1980s, as well as field trials conducted specifically for the Task Force on DSM-IV, showed that deficit symptoms can be reliably defined and should be considered as core features of the disorder.

Diagnosis

Several sets of operational criteria were developed in the United States during the 1970s to increase the reliability of diagnosis. The St. Louis Criteria developed in 1972 include both longitudinal and cross-sectional criteria designed to identify schizophrenic patients with poor prognosis. The criteria require the exclusion of affective illness, drug abuse, or alcoholism and exclusion of cases of less than 6 months' duration. The Research Diagnostic Criteria (RDC; Spitzer et al. 1978) were introduced later and differ from the St. Louis criteria mainly in emphasis on course of illness. The St. Louis criteria require 6 months of continuous illness, whereas the RDC require only a 2-week history. These two sets of criteria were instrumental in the development of DSM-III in 1980 and DSM-III-R in 1987 and include definitions of schizophrenia requiring both longitudinal and cross-sectional features.

The concept of including both cross-sectional and longitudinal features remains in DSM-IV-TR, but more prominence is given to Bleulerian fundamental symptoms, reconceptualized as disorganized or negative symptoms. According to DSM-IV-TR, schizophrenia consists of the presence of characteristic positive or negative symptoms of at least 1 month in duration (unless successfully treated); deterioration in work, interpersonal relations, or self-care; continuous signs of the disturbance for at least 6 months; the ruling out of schizoaffective disorder and mood disorder with psychotic features; the determination that the disturbance is not due to a general medical condition or the direct physiological effects of a substance; and, finally, if autistic disorder or another pervasive developmental disorder is present, prominent hallucinations or delusions have also been present for at least 1 month. Schizophrenia is further classified according to course of illness as shown in Table 9–2.

If an illness otherwise meets the criteria but has a duration of at least 1 month but less than 6 months, it is termed a *schizophreniform disorder*. If it has lasted less than 4 weeks, it may be classified as either a brief psychotic disorder or a psychotic disorder not otherwise specified, which is a residual category for psychotic disturbances that cannot be better classified.

Changes made in the diagnostic criteria of schizophrenia from DSM-III to DSM-IV are shown in Table 9–3. The major changes involve the description of and time requirement for active-phase symptoms, the introduction of the concept of negative symptoms, the deletion of the age at onset criterion, various exclusions, and the expansion of choices for classification of course.

Differential Diagnosis

Schizophrenia remains a clinical diagnosis that rests on historical information and a careful mental status examination, and there are no predictable laboratory abnormalities that are diagnostic of the disorder. The first step in diagnosis is to take a careful history and perform a physical examination to exclude psychoses with known medical causes. Psychotic symptoms have been found to result from substance abuse (e.g., hallucinogens, phencyclidine, amphetamines, cocaine, alcohol); intoxication due to commonly prescribed medications (e.g., corticosteroids, anticholinergics, levodopa); infectious, metabolic, and endocrine disorders; tumors and mass lesions; and temporal lobe epilepsy. Atypical presentations such as a relatively acute onset, clouding of the sensorium, or onset occurring after age 30 years demand careful investigation.

Routine laboratory tests may be helpful in ruling out potential medical causes. Common screening tests include a complete blood count (CBC), urinalysis, liver enzymes, serum creatinine, blood urea nitrogen (BUN), thyroid function tests, and serological tests for evidence of an infection with syphilis or HIV. Other tests will be indicated in selected patients, such as a serum ceruloplasmin to rule out Wilson's disease. Electroencephalography (EEG), computed tomography (CT), or magnetic resonance imaging (MRI) may be useful in selected cases to rule out alternate diagnoses, such as a tumor or mass lesion or epilepsy.

The major task in differential diagnosis involves separating schizophrenia from schizoaffective disorder, mood disorder with psychotic features, delusional disorder, or a personality disorder. To rule out schizoaffective disorder and psychotic mood disorders, major depressive or manic episodes should have been absent during the active phase, or the mood episode should have been brief relative to the total duration of the psychotic episode. Unlike delusional disorder, schizophrenia is characterized by bizarre delusions, and hallucinations are common. Patients with personality disorders, particularly those in the "eccentric" cluster (e.g., schizoid, schizotypal, and paranoid personality), may be indifferent to social relationships and display restricted affect, may have bizarre ideation and odd speech, or may be suspicious and hypervigilant, but they do not have delusions, hallucinations, or grossly disorganized behavior. Furthermore, patients with schizophrenia may develop other symptoms, such as a profound thought disorder, behavioral disturbances, and enduring personality deterioration. These symptoms are uncharacteristic of the mood disorders, delusional disorder, or the personality disorders.

Depersonalization disorder and sometimes panic disorder are accompanied by feelings of unreality, such as that one's mind and body are separate; however, insight is generally well preserved, and hallucinations and delusions are absent. The rituals occurring in a patient with obsessive-compulsive disorder may result in bizarre behavior, but they are performed to relieve anxiety, and not in response to delusional beliefs.

TABLE 9–2. DSM-IV-TR diagnostic criteria for schizophrenia

A. *Characteristic symptoms:* Two (or more) of the following, each present for a significant portion of time during a 1-month period (or less if successfully treated):
  (1) delusions
  (2) hallucinations
  (3) disorganized speech (e.g., frequent derailment or incoherence)
  (4) grossly disorganized or catatonic behavior
  (5) negative symptoms, i.e., affective flattening, alogia, or avolition
  Note: Only one Criterion A symptom is required if delusions are bizarre or hallucinations consist of a voice keeping up a running commentary on the person's behavior or thoughts, or two or more voices conversing with each other.

B. *Social/occupational dysfunction:* For a significant portion of the time since the onset of the disturbance, one or more major areas of functioning such as work, interpersonal relations, or self-care are markedly below the level achieved prior to the onset (or when the onset is in childhood or adolescence, failure to achieve expected level of interpersonal, academic, or occupational achievement).

C. *Duration:* Continuous signs of the disturbance persist for at least 6 months. This 6-month period must include at least 1 month of symptoms (or less if successfully treated) that meet Criterion A (i.e., active-phase symptoms) and may include periods of prodromal or residual symptoms. During these prodromal or residual periods, the signs of the disturbance may be manifested by only negative symptoms or two or more symptoms listed in Criterion A present in an attenuated form (e.g., odd beliefs, unusual perceptual experiences).

D. *Schizoaffective and Mood Disorder exclusion:* Schizoaffective disorder and mood disorder with psychotic features have been ruled out because either (1) no major depressive, manic, or mixed episodes have occurred concurrently with the active-phase symptoms; or (2) if mood episodes have occurred during active-phase symptoms, their total duration has been brief relative to the duration of the active and residual periods.

E. *Substance/general medical condition exclusion:* The disturbance is not due to the direct physiological effects of a substance (e.g., a drug of abuse, a medication) or a general medical condition.

F. *Relationship to a Pervasive Developmental Disorder:* If there is a history of autistic disorder or another pervasive developmental disorder, the additional diagnosis of schizophrenia is made only if prominent delusions or hallucinations are also present for at least a month (or less if successfully treated).

Classification of longitudinal course (can be applied only after at least 1 year has elapsed since the initial onset of active-phase symptoms):
  Episodic With Interepisode Residual Symptoms (episodes are defined by the reemergence of prominent psychotic symptoms);
    also specify if: **With Prominent Negative Symptoms**
  Episodic With No Interepisode Residual Symptoms
  Continuous (prominent psychotic symptoms are present throughout the period of observation); *also specify if:*
    With Prominent Negative Symptoms
  Single Episode In Partial Remission; *also specify if:*
    With Prominent Negative Symptoms
  Single Episode In Full Remission
  Other or Unspecified Pattern

Other psychiatric disorders also must be ruled out, including schizophreniform disorder, brief psychotic disorder, factitious disorder with psychological symptoms, and malingering. If symptoms persist for more than 6 months, schizophreniform disorder can be ruled out. The history of how the illness presents will help to rule out brief psychotic disorder, since schizophrenia generally has an insidious onset and there are usually no precipitating stressors. Factitious disorder may be difficult to delineate from schizophrenia, especially when the patient is knowledgeable about mental illness or is medically trained, but careful observation should enable the clinician to make the distinction between real or feigned psychosis. Likewise, a malingerer could attempt to simulate schizophrenia, but careful observation will help to distinguish the disorders. With the malingerer, there will be evidence of obvious secondary gain, such as avoiding incarceration, and the history may suggest antisocial personality disorder. The differential diagnosis for schizophrenia is summarized in Table 9–4.

Clinical Findings

Clinical manifestations of schizophrenia and schizophreniform disorders are diverse and can change over

TABLE 9–3. Differences among DSM-III, DSM-III-R, and DSM-IV/DSM-IV-TR criteria for schizophrenia

DSM-III	DSM-III-R	DSM-IV/DSM-IV-TR
Characteristic active-phase symptoms	Characteristic active-phase symptoms for 1 week or more	Characteristic active-phase symptoms 1 month or more (less if treated)
Deterioration in functioning	Impairment in functioning	Social/occupational dysfunction
Duration at least 6 months or more (including active phase)	Duration at least 6 months or more (including active phase)	Duration at least 6 months or more (including active phase)
Depression and mania ruled out	Schizoaffective disorder and psychotic mood disorder ruled out	Schizoaffective disorder and psychotic mood disorder ruled out
Organic mental disorder and mental retardation ruled out	Organic mental disorder ruled out	Effects of substance or general medical condition ruled out
Onset before age 45	Autistic disorder ruled out	If there is a history of pervasive developmental disorder, prominent delusions, hallucinations must also be present for at least 1 month (or less if successfully treated)
Classification of course	Classification of course	Classification of course
Subchronic (>6 months but <2 years)	Subchronic (>6 months but <2 years)	Episodic with interepisode residual symptoms
Chronic (>2 years)	Chronic (>2 years)	Episodic with no interepisode residual symptoms
Subchronic with acute exacerbation	Subchronic with acute exacerbation	Continuous
Chronic with acute exacerbation	Chronic with acute exacerbation	Single episode in partial remission
In remission	In remission	Single episode in full remission
	Unspecified	Other or unspecified pattern

TABLE 9–4. Differential diagnosis of schizophrenia

Psychiatric illness	General medical illness	Drugs of abuse
Psychotic mood disorders	Temporal lobe epilepsy	Stimulants (e.g., amphetamine, cocaine)
Schizoaffective disorder	Tumor, stroke, brain trauma	Hallucinogens (e.g., phencyclidine)
Brief reactive psychosis	Endocrine/metabolic disorders (e.g., porphyria)	Anticholinergics (e.g., belladonna alkaloids)
Schizophreniform disorder	Vitamin deficiency (e.g., B$_{12}$)	Alcohol withdrawal delirium
Delusional disorder	Infectious (e.g., neurosyphilis)	Barbiturate withdrawal delirium
Induced psychotic disorder	Autoimmune (e.g., systemic lupus erythematosus)	
Panic disorder	Toxic (e.g., heavy metal poisoning)	
Depersonalization disorder		
Obsessive-compulsive disorder		
Personality disorders (e.g., "eccentric" cluster)		
Factitious disorder with psychological symptoms		
Malingering		

time. Because of their variety, it has been said that to know schizophrenia is to know psychiatry. Whereas many symptoms are obvious, such as hallucinations, others such as affective blunting or incongruity are relatively subtle and can be easily missed by a casual observer.

Various methods have been developed to describe and classify the multiplicity of symptoms in schizophre-

nia. Traditionally, schizophrenia is considered to be a type of "psychosis," yet the definition of psychosis has been elusive. Older definitions stressed the subjective and internal psychological experience and defined psychosis as an "impairment in reality testing." More recently, psychosis has been defined objectively and operationally as the occurrence of hallucinations and delusions. Because schizophrenia is characterized by so many different types of symptoms, clinicians and scientists have tried to simplify the description of the clinical presentation by dividing the symptoms into subgroups. The most widely used subdivision classifies the symptoms as positive and negative.

Positive and Negative Symptoms

The concept of positive and negative symptoms was originally formulated by the British neurologist John Hughlings Jackson (1931). Jackson believed that positive symptoms reflected release phenomena occurring in more phylogenetically advanced brain regions, due to injury to the brain at a more primitive level. Negative symptoms, on the other hand, simply represented a "dissolution," or a loss of brain function. Current definitions of positive and negative symptoms are an amplification of these earlier ideas.

Positive symptoms, including hallucinations, delusions, marked positive formal thought disorder (manifested by marked incoherence, derailment, tangentiality, or illogicality), and bizarre or disorganized behavior reflect a distortion or exaggeration of functions that are normally present. For example, hallucinations are a distortion or exaggeration of the function of the perceptual systems of the brain: the person experiences a perception in the absence of an external stimulus.

Negative symptoms reflect a deficiency of a mental function that is normally present. For example, some patients display *alogia* (i.e., marked poverty of speech, or poverty of content of speech). Others show *affective flattening, anhedonia/asociality* (i.e., inability to experience pleasure, few social contacts), *avolition/apathy* (i.e., anergia, impersistence at work or school), and *attentional impairment*. These negative or deficit symptoms not only are difficult to treat and respond less well to neuroleptics than positive symptoms, but they are also the most destructive because they render the patient inert and unmotivated. The schizophrenic patient with prominent negative symptoms may be able to raise his or her performance under supervision but cannot maintain it when supervision is withdrawn.

Recent research suggests that these symptoms reflect dimensions rather than discrete categories of psychopathology and that there are probably three dimensions rather than two (Andreasen et al. 1995; Arndt et al. 1995; Bilder et al. 1985; Liddle et al. 1989). Positive symptoms can be further divided into dimensions of psychoticism (i.e., delusions and hallucinations) and disorganization (i.e., disorganized speech and behavior and inappropriate affect). Negative (or deficit) symptoms

represent a third dimension. The relationship between these three dimensions and their underlying pathophysiology continues to be studied and discussed (Andreasen et al. 1995).

Crow (1980) proposed a method for classifying schizophrenic patients on the basis of the presence of positive or negative symptoms. He has designated schizophrenic patients with mostly positive symptoms as Type I and those with mostly negative symptoms as Type II. However, in practice patients generally display a mixture of both positive and negative symptoms (Andreasen et al. 1990b).

The frequency of these and other common symptoms reported in 111 schizophrenic patients is presented in Table 9–5.

The Psychotic Dimension

This symptom dimension refers to two classic "psychotic" symptoms that reflect a patient's confusion about the loss of boundaries between himself or herself and the external world: hallucinations and delusions. Both symptoms reflect a "loss of ego boundaries": the patient is unable to distinguish between his or her own thoughts and perceptions and those that he or she obtains by observing the external world.

Hallucinations have sometimes been considered the hallmark of schizophrenia. Although hallucinations may occur in a variety of other disorders, including mood and organic disorders, they remain important symptoms of schizophrenia and schizophreniform disorders. *Hallucinations* are perceptions experienced without an external stimulus to the sense organs that have qualities similar to a true perception (e.g., intensity, location). They are usually experienced as originating in the outside world, or within one's own body, but not within the mind as through imagination. Hallucinations vary in complexity and in sensory modality. Schizophrenic patients commonly have auditory, visual, tactile, gustatory, or olfactory hallucinations, or a combination of several types. Auditory hallucinations are the most frequent type observed in schizophrenia and may be experienced as noises, music, or more typically "voices." Voices may be mumbled or may sound clear and distinct, and words, phrases, or sentences may be heard. Hallucinations may be inferred when the patient appears to be talking in response to the voices and may whisper, mutter incomprehensibly, talk normally, or shout out loud. Visual hallucinations may be simple or complex and include flashes of light or the image of persons, animals, or objects; they may be smaller or larger than a true perception. They may be experienced as being located outside the field of vision such as being behind the head and are usually

TABLE 9–5. Frequency of symptoms in 111 patients with schizophrenia

Symptom	%	Symptom	%
Negative symptoms		**Positive symptoms**	
Affective flattening		**Hallucinations**	
Unchanging facial expression	96	Auditory	75
Decreased spontaneous movements	66	Voices commenting	58
Paucity of expressive gestures	81	Voices conversing	57
Poor eye contact	71	Somatic-tactile	20
Affective nonresponsivity	64	Olfactory	6
Inappropriate affect	63	Visual	49
Lack of vocal inflections	73	**Delusions**	
Alogia		Persecutory	81
Poverty of speech	53	Jealous	4
Poverty of content of speech	51	Guilt, sin	26
Blocking	23	Grandiose	39
Increased response latency	31	Religious	31
Avolition–apathy		Somatic	28
Impaired grooming and hygiene	87	Delusions of reference	49
Lack of persistence at work or school	95	Delusions of being controlled	46
Physical anergia	82	Delusions of mind reading	48
Anhedonia–asociality		Thought broadcasting	23
Few recreational interests/activities	95	Thought insertion	31
Little sexual interest/activity	69	Thought withdrawal	27
Impaired intimacy/closeness	84	**Bizarre behavior**	
Few relationships with friends/peers	96	Clothing, appearance	20
Attention		Social, sexual behavior	33
Social inattentiveness	78	Aggressive-agitated	27
Inattentiveness during testing	64	Repetitive-stereotyped	28
		Positive formal thought disorder	
		Derailment	45
		Tangentiality	50
		Incoherence	23
		Illogicality	23
		Circumstantiality	35
		Pressure of speech	24
		Distractible speech	23
		Clanging	3

Source. Adapted from Andreasen 1987.

reported in normal color. Olfactory and gustatory hallucinations are often experienced together, leading to unpleasant tastes and odors. Tactile hallucinations (or *haptic* hallucinations) may be experienced as sensations of being touched or pricked, electrical sensations, or even a sensation of insects crawling under the skin, which is called *formication*. Tactile hallucinations may occur as feelings of body organs being pulled upon and distended, and sexual stimulation may be experienced. Schizophrenic patients in all cultures experience hallucinations, although they may differ in frequency and type, depending on the patient's experience and background (Ndetei and Vadher 1984).

Delusions involve a disturbance in inferential thinking rather than perception. Delusions are firmly held beliefs that are untrue; the judgment of "untrueness" must always be made within the context of the person's educational and cultural background. Delusions occurring in patients with schizophrenia may have somatic, grandiose, religious, nihilistic, or persecutory themes (Table 9–6). None is specific to schizophrenia, and like hallucinations, delusions tend to be culturally based. For example, a patient in the United States may worry about persecution by the Central Intelligence Agency or Federal Bureau of Investigation; a Bantu or Zulu might worry about persecution by spirits or demons.

TABLE 9–6. Varied content in delusions

Delusions	Foci of preoccupation
Grandiose	Possessing wealth or great beauty or having a special ability (e.g., extrasensory perception); having influential friends; being an important figure (e.g., Napoleon, Hitler)
Nihilistic	Belief that one is dead or dying; belief that one does not exist or that the world does not exist
Persecutory	Being persecuted by friends, neighbors, or spouses; being followed, monitored, or spied on by the government (e.g., the FBI, the CIA) or other important organizations (e.g., the Catholic Church)
Somatic	Belief that one's organs have stopped functioning (e.g., that the heart is no longer beating) or are rotting away; belief that the nose or other body part is terribly misshapen or disfigured
Sexual	Belief that one's sexual behavior is commonly known; that one is a prostitute, a pedophile, or a rapist; that masturbation has led to illness or insanity
Religious	Belief that one has sinned against God; that one has a special relationship to God or some other deity; that one has a special religious mission; that one is the Devil or is condemned to burn in Hell

Certain types of auditory hallucinations and delusions were considered symptoms of the first rank by Schneider. These symptoms share the common feature that all represent an intrusion of "personal space" by some outside influence: an extreme example of the loss of personal boundaries and the difficulty in distinguishing between internal experiences and the external world.

First-rank hallucinations were described by Schneider (1959) as prolonged, clearly audible voices, often commenting upon a person's actions or arguing with each other about the patient or repeating aloud the patient's thoughts (Mellor 1970). First-rank delusions were those of thought broadcasting, thought withdrawal, thought insertion, or delusions of passivity (i.e., being controlled as if a puppet). More recent work suggests that only approximately 20% of schizophrenia patients experience first-rank symptoms. Furthermore, first-rank symptoms are not specific to schizophrenia, but are also present in many patients with psychotic mood disorders (Andreasen and Akiskal 1983). These symptoms have not proven useful in predicting treatment response or outcome in schizophrenia (Table 9–7 provides a list of common first-rank symptoms).

Several unusual delusions have been described that are often part of a schizophrenic illness. In the *Capgras syndrome*, a patient believes that a person closely related to him or her has been replaced by a double. (This belief was the theme of the 1950s "B" horror movie *Invasion of the Body Snatchers*.) In the *Fregoli syndrome*, a patient identifies a familiar person in various other people he or she encounters. The patient may maintain that although there is no physical resemblance between the familiar person and others, they are nonetheless psychologically identical. *Cotard's syndrome* is characterized by the belief that one of the patient's bodily organs (e.g., brain, bowel) has changed in some impossible way, has stopped functioning, or has even disappeared.

The Disorganization Dimension

The disorganization dimension includes disorganized speech, disorganized or bizarre behavior, and incongruous affect.

Disorganized speech, or *thought disorder*, was regarded as the most important symptom of schizophrenia by Bleuler. Historically, types of thought disorder have included associative loosening, illogical thinking, overinclusive thinking, and loss of ability to engage in abstract thinking. A standard set of definitions for various types of thought disorder has been developed (Andreasen 1979) that stresses objective aspects of language and communication (which are empirical indicators of "thought"), such as derailment, poverty of speech, poverty of content of speech, or tangential replies. All have been found to occur frequently in both schizophrenia and mood disorders. Manic patients often have a thought disorder characterized by tangentiality, derailment (loose associations), and illogicality. Depressed patients manifest thought disorder less frequently than manic patients, but often display a poverty of speech, tangentiality, or circumstantiality. Other types of formal thought disorder include perseveration, distractibility, clanging, neologisms, echolalia, and blocking; with the possible exception of clanging in mania, none appears to be disorder specific. An example of speech from a patient with a prominent thought disorder (particularly derailment) follows:

Let's see, there was one I would have liked if it wasn't for the instructor, well I go along with him, he was always wanting me to do the worse in class, it seemed like, and I'd always get bad, the grade, in my grading, and he tried to make other people like they were good enough to be in Hollywood or something, you know I'd be the last one down the ladder. That, that's the way they wanted the grading to be in the first place accord-

TABLE 9–7. Schneider's first-rank symptoms

First-rank symptoms	Comments
Delusions	
1. Delusional percept	A concept delineated by Jaspers in which a normal perception takes on delusional meaning and has immense personal significance to the patient.
2. Thought withdrawal	Delusions of control, including delusions of thoughts being withdrawn, inserted or broadcast to others; delusions of being influenced to do things or want things the patient does not wish to do and does not want, delusions of being made to feel emotions or sensations (often sexual) that are not the patient's own.
3. Thought insertion	
4. Thought broadcast	
5. "Made" volitional acts	
6. "Made" impulses	
7. Made" affect	
8. Outside influences playing on body	
Auditory hallucinations	
9. *Gedankenlautwerden*	Audible thoughts or thought echo.
10. Voices conversing with each other	Patient may be referred to in the third person.
11. Voices giving running commentary	

ing to whose, theirs, they, they have all different reasons that I, I, I think that they use that they want one, won't come out. (Andreasen 1984, p. 61)

Because these various forms of thought disorder are inferred from listening to patients speak, the concept of disorganized speech has evolved and appears as such in the diagnostic criteria.

Disorganized or *catatonic motor behavior* is another aspect of this dimension. Many patients with schizophrenia display various motor disturbances and changes in social behavior. Abnormal motor behaviors range from catatonic stupor to excitement. In a catatonic stupor, the patient may be immobile, mute, and unresponsive, and yet remain fully conscious. A patient may exhibit uncontrolled and aimless motor activity while in a state of catatonic excitement. Some patients manifest *waxy flexibility* (flexibilitas cerea), in which they allow themselves to be placed in uncomfortable positions, which are maintained without apparent distress. Schizophrenic patients sometimes assume bizarre or awkward postures and maintain them for long periods, such as squatting for hours, which would cause obvious discomfort to most people.

Several disorders of movement that occur in schizophrenia need to be distinguished from drug-induced extrapyramidal side effects of antipsychotics and tardive dyskinesia (Manschreck et al. 1982). These include *stereotypies*, which are repeated movements that are not goal directed such as rocking; *mannerisms*, which are normal goal-directed activities that appear to have social significance but are either odd in appearance or out of context, such as grimacing or repeatedly running a hand through one's hair. *Mitgehen* is seen when the slightest

pressure causes the patient's limbs to move in the direction of the push, despite being told to resist the pressure. Less common symptoms are *echopraxia*, which is imitating the movements and gestures of another person; *automatic obedience*, which is carrying out simple commands in a robotlike fashion; and *negativism*, which is refusing to cooperate with simple requests for no apparent reason. Many schizophrenic patients display ritualistic behaviors resembling those seen in obsessive-compulsive disorder, such as repetitive hand washing, checking, arranging, or counting (Fenton and McGlashan 1986). Some schizophrenic patients develop compulsive water drinking, which can lead to water intoxication necessitating careful attention to fluid and electrolyte balance (deLeon et al. 1994).

Antipsychotic medications are often associated with various extrapyramidal side effects (EPS) as well as tardive dyskinesia, all of which are discussed in Chapter 24. Many schizophrenic patients were reported to display EPS or spontaneous involuntary movements before antipsychotics became available (Chatterjee et al. 1995). The presence of spontaneous EPS has been linked to poorer treatment response and negative symptoms. When tardive dyskinesia is present, schizophrenic patients are often unaware of their involuntary movements. Even when the abnormal movements are pointed out, the patient may remain unconcerned (Caracci et al. 1990).

Deterioration of social behavior often develops along with social withdrawal. Patients may neglect themselves and become messy or unkempt; wear dirty, unmended, or inappropriate clothing; and ignore or neglect their cluttered, untidy surroundings. Patients may develop other odd behaviors, breaking social conventions by exhibiting crude table manners, foraging through garbage bins, or shouting obscenities. It has been estimated that between one-third and one-half of today's "homeless" persons have schizophrenia (Susser et al. 1989).

Incongruity of affect is the third component of the disorganization dimension. Patients may smile inappropriately when speaking of neutral or sad topics, or giggle for no apparent reason. This symptom should not be confused with the nervous smiling or giggling that sometimes occurs in anxious patients. Affective incongruity should only be considered a symptom of schizophrenia when it occurs in the context of other characteristic symptoms.

The Negative Dimension

DSM-IV-TR lists three negative symptoms as characteristic of schizophrenia: alogia, affective blunting, and avolition. Other negative symptoms that are common in schizophrenia include anhedonia and attentional impairment (Andreasen 1982; Andreasen and Olson 1982).

Alogia is characterized by a diminution in the amount of spontaneous speech, a tendency to produce speech that is empty or impoverished in content when the amount is adequate. It is the external expression in language of the impoverishment of thought that occurs in many patients with schizophrenia. Patients may have great difficulty in producing fluent responses to questions. Instead, they tend to say little or reply concretely. For example, if asked, "What brought you to the hospital?" the patient may reply, "A car."

Affective flattening or blunting is a reduced intensity of emotional expression and response. It is manifested by unchanging facial expression, decreased spontaneous movements, poverty of expressive gestures, poor eye contact, lack of vocal inflections, and slowed speech.

Anhedonia, or the inability to experience pleasure, is also very common. Many patients describe themselves as feeling emotionally empty. They are no longer able to enjoy activities that previously gave them pleasure, such as playing sports or seeing family or friends. Their awareness that they have lost the capacity to enjoy themselves may be a source of great psychological pain.

Avolition is a loss of the ability to initiate goal-directed behavior and carry it through to completion. Patients seem to have lost their will or drive. They may initiate a project and then abandon it for no apparent reason. They may take a job, go to work for a few days or weeks, and then fail to appear or wander aimlessly away while at work. This symptom is sometimes interpreted as laziness, but in fact it represents the loss or diminution of basic drives and the capacity to formulate and pursue long-range plans.

Attentional impairment is reflected in the inability to concentrate or focus on a task or a question. Patients may complain of feeling bombarded by stimuli that they cannot process or filter; this in turn causes them to feel confused or to experience fragmented thoughts.

The negative symptoms of schizophrenia and the symptoms of depression are somewhat similar, making differential diagnosis of depression and schizophrenia difficult in some patients. Significant depressive symptoms occur in up to 60% of patients with schizophrenia (Guze et al. 1983), leading to substantial distress, prompting suicidal behavior in some patients, and compromising what little energy and motivation the patient has. Antipsychotic medication itself may induce what appears to be depression but is actually a drug-induced akinesia. This "depression" may go away when the dosage of antipsychotic is reduced or an anticholinergic medication is added (King et al. 1995). The International Classification of Diseases, Tenth Revision (ICD-10; World Health Organization 1992), recognizes a category called "postpsychotic depression," a full-blown depression occurring after the acute phase symptoms have fully resolved. In DSM-IV-TR, a postpsychotic depression, or a major depression occurring in a patient with well-established schizophrenia, is diagnosed as a depressive disorder not otherwise specified.

The following case example (adapted from Andreasen 1984, pp. 57–58) illustrates many of the symptoms found in schizophrenia and shows the profound impact of negative symptoms.

Case Example 1

Ronald, a 42-year-old unmarried man, had lived in a state hospital more or less continuously since the death of his last surviving parent 5 years earlier. As a youngster, his family noted that he was extremely shy and withdrawn. Although clearly attached to them, he did not enjoy hugging, kissing, or other expressions of affection. In school, he tended to be solitary, and although he functioned at an average level, his parents considered him bright and creative because he read a great deal, had a large vocabulary, and enjoyed various intellectual games. He was also preoccupied with inventing things. In high school, he invented a new alphabet that was supposed to be more phonetically functional than the one currently in use. Although he tried to explain its basic principles, no one seemed to understand it. Sometimes his parents were unable to determine whether he was difficult to understand because he was so much smarter than they or whether his thinking was simply disorganized.

During high school Ronald did not participate in any activities, had no friends, and never dated. He entered college, but dropped out with failing grades at the end of his first semester. He returned home to live with his parents, but despite repeated efforts to get him out of the house and into various types of jobs, he was never able to persist and perform any task dependably. He became increasingly absorbed in a fantasy world and spent much of his time involved in "intergalactic communication." He claimed to receive messages from an unknown galaxy in a special language that only he was able to understand. These messages, which he heard as if they were voices talking to him inside his head, would describe events in the distant galaxy of Atan. As he grew older, he seemed to lose interest in discussing this inner world and his inner voices with anyone. Never interested in appearance, he became disheveled. He had to be encouraged by his parents to wear clean clothing, to bathe, and to shave. He tended to select rather bizarre attire and hairstyles and preferred to wear long underwear, overalls, and a baseball cap placed backwards.

Ronald was briefly hospitalized after he returned home from college and placed on antipsychotic medication, which helped minimally. He was unable to follow through on tasks, developed extreme social withdrawal, and became fully preoccupied with his fantasy world. After the death of his mother when he was 32, he again required hospitalization. High doses of antipsychotic medication appeared to help temporarily, but had no lasting benefit. He was 36 when his father died. He lived at home alone for the next year, but was eventually rehospitalized after complaints from neighbors brought him to the attention of community agencies. He had been living in the house for the past year without ever having done laundry, taken out the garbage, or washed the dishes. The house gradually had filled with rotting food, debris, and old newspapers. He was placed in a chronic care facility because he was unable to function independently.

Cognitive Impairment as the Fundamental Deficit

Many thinkers, beginning with both Kraepelin and Bleuler, have considered schizophrenia to be a neurocognitive disorder, with the various signs and symptoms reflecting the downstream effects of a fundamental cognitive deficit. This fundamental cognitive deficit was highlighted in the original name *dementia praecox* and the later name *schizophrenia* ("fragmented mind"). Schizophrenia poses special challenges to the development of cognitive models because of its breadth and diversity of symptoms. The symptoms include nearly all cognitive domains: perception (hallucinations), inferential thinking (delusions), fluency of thought and speech (alogia), clarity and organization of thought and speech ("formal thought disorder"), motor activity (catatonia), emotional expression (affective blunting), ability to initiate and complete goal-directed behavior (avolition), and ability to seek out and experience emotional gratifi-

cation (anhedonia). Not all these symptoms are present in any given patient, however, and none is pathognomonic of the illness. An initial survey of the diversity of symptoms might suggest that multiple brain regions are involved, in a spotty pattern much as once occurred in neurosyphilis. In the absence of visible lesions and known pathogens, however, investigators have turned to the exploration of models that could explain the diversity of symptoms by a single cognitive mechanism. Several leading cognitive neuroscientists and psychiatrists have developed models that can explain the symptoms based on a fundamental cognitive deficit. The convergent conclusions of these different models are striking.

Approaching schizophrenia from the background of cognitive psychology, Frith (1992) divided the symptoms of schizophrenia into three broad groups or dimensions: 1) disorders of willed action (which lead to symptoms such as alogia and avolition), 2) disorders of self-monitoring (which lead to symptoms such as auditory hallucinations and delusions of alien control), and 3) disorders in monitoring the intentions of others ("mentalizing") (which lead to symptoms such as "formal thought disorder" and delusions of persecution). Frith believes that all these are special cases of a more general underlying mechanism: a disorder of consciousness or self-awareness that impairs the ability to think with "meta-representations" (higher order abstract concepts that are representations of mental states) (Frith 1992). Frith and colleagues are currently testing this conceptual framework using positron emission tomography (PET) (see "Functional Circuitry and Functional Neuroimaging").

Approaching schizophrenia from a background that blends lesion studies and single-cell recordings in nonhuman primates to study cognition, Goldman-Rakic (1994) has proposed a model suggesting that the fundamental impairment in schizophrenia is an inability to guide behavior by representations, often referred to as a defect in working memory. *Working memory*, or the ability to hold a representation "online" and perform cognitive operations using it, permits individuals to respond in a flexible manner, to formulate and modify plans, and to base behavior on internally held ideas and thoughts rather than being driven by external stimuli (Goldman-Rakic 1987). A defect in this ability can explain a variety of symptoms of schizophrenia. For example, the inability to hold a discourse plan in mind and monitor speech output leads to disorganized speech and thought disorder; the inability to maintain a plan for behavioral activities could lead to negative symptoms such as avolition or alogia; the inability to reference a specific external or internal experience against associative memories (mediated by cortical and subcortical circuitry involving frontal/parietal/temporal regions and the thalamus) could lead to an altered consciousness of sensory experience that would be expressed as delusions or hallucinations. The model also explains the perseverative behavior observed in studies using the Wisconsin Card Sorting Test and is consistent with the compromised blood flow to the prefrontal cortex in these patients (Weinberger 1987). Overall, Goldman-Rakic's work supports a model that suggests a major role for prefrontal regions and their multiple distributed cortical, thalamic, and striatal connections in a fundamental cognitive function, representationally guided behavior, that permits organisms to adapt flexibly to a changing environment and to achieve temporal and spatial continuity between past experiences and present and future actions.

Using techniques originally derived from neurophysiology, Braff and colleagues have developed another complementary model. This model begins from the perspective of techniques used to measure brain electrical activity, particularly various types of evoked potentials, and hypothesizes that the core underlying deficit in schizophrenia involves information processing and attention (Braff 1993). This model derives from the empirical clinical observation that patients with schizophrenia frequently complain that they are bombarded with more stimuli than they can interpret (McGhie and Chapman 1961). Consequently, they misinterpret (i.e., have delusions), confuse internal with external stimuli (hallucinations), or retreat to safety (negative symptoms such as alogia, anhedonia, or avolition). Early interpretations of this observation drew on the Broadbent filter theory and postulated that patients had problems with early stages in serial order processing that led to downstream effects such as psychotic or negative symptoms (Broadbent 1958). As serial models have been supplanted by distributed models, the deficit may be better conceptualized in terms of resource allocation: Patients cannot mobilize attentional resources and allocate them to relevant tasks.

Andreasen and colleagues have used the clinical presentation of schizophrenia as a point of departure, postulating that the symptoms arise from "cognitive dysmetria." This refers to impaired connectivity between frontal, cerebellar, and thalamic regions as a consequence of a neurodevelopmental defect or perhaps a series of them (Andreasen et al. 1994a, 1994b; Crespo-Facorro et al. 1999b; Nopoulos et al. 1997; Swayze et al. 1990; Wiser et al. 1998). Motor dysmetria has been observed in schizophrenia since its original description by Kraepelin, and "soft signs" of poor coordination are reported in more contemporary studies (Gupta et al. 1995a; Kraepelin 1919). More injurious, however, is the related "cognitive dysmetria," which produces "poor coordination" of

mental activities (Andreasen et al. 1996). The word *metron* literally means "measure": a person with schizophrenia has a fundamental deficit in taking measure of time and space and in making inferences about interrelationships between himself or herself and others, or between past, present, and future. He or she cannot accurately time input and output and therefore cannot coordinate the perception, prioritization, retrieval, and expression of experiences and ideas. This model has received extensive support from work with MRI and PET (see "Neuroanatomy and Structural Neuroimaging" and "Functional Circuitry and Functional Neuromaging").

The common thread in these observations, gleaned from very different starting points, is that schizophrenia reflects a disruption in a fundamental cognitive process that affects a specific circuitry in the brain. Various research teams may use different terminology and somewhat different concepts—meta-representations, representationally guided behavior, information processing/attention, cognitive dysmetria—but they convey a common theme. The cognitive dysfunction in schizophrenia is an inefficient temporal and spatial referencing of information and experience as the person attempts to determine boundaries between self and not-self and to formulate effective decisions or plans that will guide him or her through the small-scale (speaking a sentence) or large-scale (finding a job) maneuvers of daily living. This capacity is sometimes referred to as *consciousness*.

Using diverse technologies and techniques—PET scanning, animal models, lesion methods, single-cell recordings, evoked potentials—the investigators also converge on similar conclusions about the neuroanatomic substrates of the cognitive dysfunction. All agree that it must involve distributed circuits rather that a single specific "localization," and all suggest a key role for interrelationships among prefrontal cortex, other interconnected cortical regions, and subcortical regions, particularly the thalamus and striatum. Animal models are being developed based on knowledge of this circuitry and the fundamental cognitive process, which can be applied to understanding the mechanism of drug actions and to the development of new medications.

Clinical Validity of Cognitive Models

The clinical validity of these cognitive models of schizophrenia is supported by a variety of studies using neuropsychological testing. One crucial question addressed by these studies is whether patients with schizophrenia experience cognitive deterioration over time, as occurs in Alzheimer's disease, or whether the cognitive impairment is stable. The bulk of the evidence supports the latter.

Premorbidly, patients with schizophrenia have subtle deficits in information processing tasks or on neuropsychological tests and have a slightly lower IQ than their siblings and peers (Aylward et al. 1984; Hyde et al. 1994). Following the onset of clinical disorder, mild deterioration occurs in cognitive functioning and neuropsychological test results (Hoff et al. 1991). There is little additional deterioration beyond that resulting from the normal aging process, even for patients who have been ill for more than 50 years. In a study of 74 schizophrenic patients in five age cohorts (i.e., 18–29, 30–39, 40–49, 50–59, 60–69 years), results from a battery of neuropsychological tests were abnormal across all age cohorts (Hyde et al. 1994). Research has also shown that both young and old schizophrenic patients exhibit a similar pattern of deficits (Bilder et al. 1991). This body of work suggests that there is little evidence of a progressive decline in cognitive function during the course of schizophrenia.

Neuropsychological impairment is not restricted to a small subset of patients; measurable impairment is present in 40%–60% of schizophrenic patients (Goldberg et al. 1988). Cognitive impairment tends to be generalized but is most pronounced for cognitive tasks involving attention, memory, and executive functions (Mohamed et al. 1999). Braff et al. (1991) found in a sample of 40 schizophrenic patients selective deficits in tests of complex reasoning, psychomotor speed, new learning, incidental memory, and both motor and sensory–perceptual abilities. Neuropsychological impairment has been linked with enlarged cerebral ventricles (Keilp et al. 1988), negative or deficit forms of schizophrenia (Buchanan et al. 1994), and the presence of neurological soft signs (Flashman et al. 1996).

Other Symptoms

Lack of Insight

Lack of insight is common in schizophrenia. Patients often deny they are ill or abnormal, and insist their hallucinations and delusions are real. Poor insight is one of the most difficult symptoms to treat and often persists even when other symptoms (e.g., hallucinations) respond to medication. Orientation and memory are generally preserved, unless impaired by the patient's psychotic symptoms, inattention, or distractibility.

Soft Signs

Nonlocalizing *soft signs* occur in a substantial proportion of patients with schizophrenia and include abnormalities in stereognosis, graphesthesia, balance, and proprioception (Gupta et al. 1995a). Although their clinical significance is unclear, their presence may reflect dysfunction in areas of motor coordination, integrative sensory function, and ordering complex motor tasks. In one study (Krakowski et al. 1989), violent schizophrenic patients were more likely to exhibit neurological soft signs than were nonviolent patients.

Vegetative Functions

Some patients display disturbances of sleep, sexual interest, or other bodily functions. Various disrupted sleep measures have been reported in schizophrenia, but decreased delta sleep with diminished stage 4 is the most consistent finding (Neylan et al. 1992). Schizophrenic patients often have little interest in sexual activity and may derive little or no pleasure from sexual experiences (Lyketsos et al. 1983).

Immune System Function

Disturbed immune functioning has been reported in schizophrenia and includes abnormalities of circulating lymphocytes, peripheral and/or cerebrospinal fluid immunoglobulin and interferon levels, and the production of antibrain antibodies. In one study (McAllister et al. 1989), patients with schizophrenia were more likely than control subjects to show an increase in the subpopulation of CD5+ β-lymphocytes, cells that have been demonstrated to be increased in patients with certain autoimmune disorders such as rheumatoid arthritis. In another study (Ganguli et al. 1995), patients with schizophrenia had decreased interleukin-2 production, which is also characteristic of autoimmune disease.

Premorbid Personality

Several early writers including Kraepelin and Bleuler observed that patients with schizophrenia often had abnormal premorbid personalities. In a review of early studies of personality and schizophrenia, Cutting (1985) reported that premorbid schizoid traits were present in one-fourth of schizophrenic patients, but one-sixth had a range of other personality disturbances. Consistent with this review, a study of 52 chronic schizophrenic patients from the Iowa 500 sample (Pfohl and Winokur 1983) found 35% to meet criteria for a DSM-III personality disorder premorbidly; 44% of these personality disorders were schizoid, and the rest were a mixture of avoidant, paranoid, histrionic, compulsive, and other personality disorders. Poor premorbid adjustment has been shown to correlate with early disease onset, poor overall prognosis, negative symptoms, cognitive deficits, and poor social functioning (Gupta et al. 1995b).

Substance Abuse and Smoking

Comorbid alcohol and drug abuse is common in patients with schizophrenia and occurs at rates exceeding that found in the community (Dixon et al. 1991). Drug-taking schizophrenic patients tend to be younger and are more likely to be male than non–drug-taking schizophrenic patients. They also have poorer medication compliance, higher rates of rehospitalization, and poorer adjustment and treatment response than patients without such abuse or dependence (Drake et al. 1989). Some researchers believe that schizophrenic patients abuse drugs in an attempt to self-medicate, to treat their medication side effects (i.e., drug-induced akinesia), or to lessen their amotivation and avolition. Cigarette smoking is also very common, and in one study nearly three out of four schizophrenic patients smoke (Goff et al. 1992). Smoking increases neuroleptic metabolism and consequently may be associated with the need for higher neuroleptic dosages.

Subtypes of Schizophrenia

DSM-IV-TR recognizes five classic subtypes of schizophrenia: 1) paranoid, 2) disorganized, 3) catatonic, 4) undifferentiated, and 5) residual (Table 9–8). The main purposes of subtyping are to improve predictive validity, to help the clinician select treatments and predict outcome, and to help the researcher delineate homogeneous subtypes. However, these goals remain largely unfulfilled. The reliability and validity of the classic subtypes are poor. Data from the International Pilot Study of Schizophrenia also failed to substantiate their usefulness (Strauss and Carpenter 1981). Furthermore, many patients seem to fit several of these subtypes during the course of their illness.

Hence, other subtyping strategies have been investigated, including paranoid versus nonparanoid forms, deficit versus nondeficit, Kraepelinian versus non-Kraepelinian, and early versus late onset. In validating the paranoid/nonparanoid subtypes, Kendler et al. (1984) found that across all four diagnostic systems (i.e., DSM-III, RDC, ICD-9, and the Tsuang–Winokur criteria [Tsuang and Winokur 1974]), patients with the paranoid subtype had better short- and long-term outcomes than nonparanoid patients (hebephrenic or undifferentiated subtypes). There was also moderate stability and reliability of subtype diagnosis at follow-up, with the paranoid subtype being the most stable and reliable (Kendler et al. 1985b). However, these subtypes did not appear to "breed true" within families (Kendler et al. 1988). Carpenter et al.

(1988) proposed dividing schizophrenia into deficit and nondeficit forms based on the presence or absence of "primary enduring negative symptoms." A body of literature has accumulated in support of the reliability and validity of this construct (M.A. Roy et al. 2001). The deficit syndrome represents a promising strategy for reducing the heterogeneity of schizophrenia, identifying more-homogeneous subgroup(s), and enhancing the power of research design at each level of inquiry (Carpenter et al. 1999a).

Paranoid Schizophrenia

Kraepelin was the first to identify a paranoid subtype of schizophrenia, in which patients had bizarre and fragmented delusions and, ultimately, personality deterioration. The concept of a paranoid subtype was included in the first edition of DSM (American Psychiatric Association 1952) and has continued to the present. The paranoid subtype is characterized by a preoccupation with one or more delusions and/or frequent auditory hallucinations; disorganized speech/behavior, catatonic behavior, and flat or inappropriate affect are not prominent.

In contrast to other subtypes, patients with paranoid schizophrenia have an older age at onset, better premorbid functioning, and a better outcome. They are more likely to marry and have better occupational functioning than patients with other subtypes (Fenton and McGlashan 1991; Winokur et al. 1974).

Disorganized Schizophrenia

Disorganized schizophrenia was first described in 1871 by Ewald Hecker, who used the term *hebephrenia*. This subtype is characterized by disorganized speech and behavior and flat or inappropriate affect; it does not meet criteria for catatonic schizophrenia. Generally, delusions and hallucinations, if present, are fragmentary, unlike the well-systematized delusions of the paranoid schizophrenic. Hebephrenia typically has an early onset that begins with the insidious development of avolition, affective flattening, deterioration of habits, and cognitive impairment, as well as delusions and hallucinations (Winokur et al. 1974). Hebephrenic patients are also reported to have a greater family history of psychopathology, poorer premorbid functioning, and poorer long-term prognosis with continuous illness than patients with paranoid schizophrenia (Fenton and McGlashan 1991). Clinically, hebephrenic patients often seem silly and childlike. They sometimes grimace or giggle inappropriately or appear self-absorbed (Figure 9–1). Mirror gazing is commonly described in these patients.

TABLE 9–8. DSM-IV-TR subtypes of schizophrenia

Subtype	Criteria	Associated features
Paranoid	Preoccupation with one or more delusions or frequent auditory hallucinations. Relative preservation of cognitive functioning and affect. None of the following is prominent: disorganized speech, disorganized or catatonic behavior, flat or inappropriate affect.	Often associated with unfocused anger, anxiety, argumentativeness, or violence. Stilted, formal quality or extreme intensity of interpersonal interactions may be seen.
Disorganized	All of the following are prominent: disorganized speech; disorganized behavior; flat or inappropriate affect. The criteria are not met for catatonic type.	Silly and childlike behavior is common; associated with extreme social impairment, poor premorbid functioning, and poor long-term functioning.
Catatonic	The clinical picture is dominated by at least two of the following: Motoric immobility as evidenced by catalepsy (including waxy flexibility) or stupor Excessive motor activity (that is apparently purposeless and not influenced by extreme stimuli) Extreme negativism (an apparently motiveless resistance to all instructions or maintenance of a rigid posture against attempts to be moved) or mutism Peculiarities of voluntary movement as evidenced by posturing (voluntary assumption of inappropriate or bizarre postures), stereotyped movements, prominent mannerisms, or prominent grimacing Echolalia or echopraxia	Marked psychomotor disturbance present (stupor or agitation), and unusual motor disturbances may be present. May need medical supervision due to malnutrition, exhaustion, hyperpyrexia, or self-injury. Sodium amobarbital interview may be helpful diagnostically.
Undifferentiated	Symptoms meeting criterion A are present, but criteria are not met for paranoid, disorganized, or catatonic types.	Probably the most common presentation in clinical practice.
Residual	Absence of prominent delusions, hallucinations, disorganized speech, and grossly disorganized or catatonic behavior Continuing evidence of the disturbance, as indicated by the presence of negative symptoms or two or more symptoms listed in criterion A for schizophrenia, present in an attenuated form (e.g., odd beliefs, unusual perceptual experiences)	Active-phase symptoms (i.e., psychotic symptoms) are not present, but patient still exhibits emotional blunting, eccentric behavior, illogical thinking, and mild loosening of associations.

Catatonic Schizophrenia

In 1874 Karl Kahlbaum used the term *catatonia* to describe a disorder with abnormal motor, sensory, and verbal symptoms including verbigeration, mutism, negativism, stereotyped movements, waxy flexibility, and decreased sensitivity to pain (Magrinat et al. 1983). Kraepelin, and later Bleuler, considered catatonia a subtype of schizophrenia. This tradition was continued to the present, and in DSM-IV-TR catatonic schizophrenia is defined as a type of schizophrenia dominated by at least two of the following: motoric immobility as evidenced by catalepsy or stupor, extreme agitation, extreme negativism or mutism, peculiarities of voluntary movement (e.g., stereotypies, mannerisms, grimacing), and echolalia or echopraxia (Figure 9–2). Compared with other subtypes, patients with catatonic schizophrenia tend to have the earliest age at onset, the most chronic course, and the poorest social and occupational functioning (Kendler et al. 1994b). This subtype of schizophrenia is reportedly less common than in the past, at least in developed countries (Sartorius et al. 1986).

Isolated catatonic symptoms are often found in other subtypes of schizophrenia, in other psychotic disorders,

1998; Rabinowitz et al. 2000) all indicate that patients with schizophrenia have deficits across a range of developmental domains, including delays in motor and speech development, and a preference for solitary play. School-teachers were able to distinguish "preschizophrenic" children (i.e., those who would later develop schizophrenia) as having greater social maladjustment; social withdrawal, aggression, and anxiety were most frequently observed (Done et al. 1994 ; Olin et al. 1995). Poor school performance has also been well documented in these children—repeating a grade, requiring special assistance, participating and attaining less in extracurricular activities, and having lower IQ and educational scores (Bearden et al. 2000; M. Cannon et al. 1999; T.D. Cannon et al. 2000; David et al. 1997; Davidson et al. 1999; Done et al. 1994; Isohanni et al. 1998; Jones et al. 1994; Offord 1974; Rabinowitz et al. 2000).

It has been estimated that these childhood behavioral and neuromotor antecedents are present in approximately one-third of schizophrenia patients. Onset of the schizophrenia syndrome itself may be insidious or abrupt, although schizophrenia generally begins with a *prodromal phase* characterized by social withdrawal and other subtle changes in behavior and emotional responsiveness. A patient may be seen as remote, aloof, emotionally detached, or even odd or eccentric. The onset of subtle thought disturbances and impaired attention may also occur at this stage. The prodrome varies in length, but typically lasts from months to years (Carpenter and Buchanan 1994).

The prodrome is followed by an *active phase* in which psychotic symptoms predominate. At this point, clinical disorder becomes evident, and a diagnosis of schizophrenia can usually be made. This phase is characterized by florid hallucinations and delusions, which alarm friends and family members and often lead to medical intervention. A *residual phase* follows the resolution of the active phase and is similar to the prodrome. Psychotic symptoms may persist during this phase, but at a lower level of intensity, and they may not be as troublesome to the patient. Active-phase symptoms may occur episodically ("acute exacerbations"), with variable levels of remission seen between episodes. The frequency and timing of these episodes is unpredictable, although stressful situations may precede these relapses, or in some instances, drug abuse (Linszen et al. 1994). Relapses are often preceded by changes in thought, feeling, or behavior noticed by the patient and family members. Symptoms preceding relapse include dysphoria, seclusiveness, sleep disturbance, anxiety, and ideas of reference (Herz 1985). Through this process patients accrue increased levels of morbidity in the form of residual or persistent symptoms

and decrements in function from their premorbid status. Relatively severe psychosis is continuous and unrelenting in some patients. The course of schizophrenia is shown in Figure 9–3.

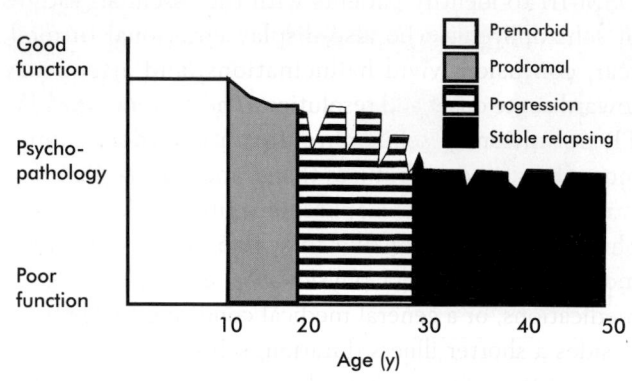

FIGURE 9–3. The natural history of schizophrenia is portrayed.
Source. Reprinted with permission from Lieberman JA: "Atypical Antipsychotic Drugs as a First-Line Treatment of Schizophrenia: A Rationale and Hypothesis." *Journal of Clinical Psychiatry* 57(Suppl 11):68–71, 1996. Copyright 1996 Physicians Postgraduate Press.

There is a tendency for the symptoms of schizophrenia to evolve. Patients may show a preponderance of positive symptoms early in their illness but gradually develop more negative or deficit symptoms. In a longitudinal study of 52 patients with schizophrenia (Pfohl and Winokur 1983), 85% were reported to have persecutory delusions of some type at index hospitalization, but after 10 years of illness only 50% had such delusions; after 20 years of illness, only 40% had persecutory delusions. This trend was true for hallucinations and motor symptoms as well. On the other hand, these investigators found that negative symptoms such as avolition, asociality, and affective flattening increased in frequency during the same period of time. There is some evidence that schizophrenia may plateau at about 5 years without further deterioration (Carpenter and Strauss 1991).

Outcome

The clinical course and outcome in schizophrenia has been studied and debated since Kraepelin first described dementia praecox as chronic and progressive, leading inevitably to severe impairment. Hegarty et al. (1994) summarized the outcome of 51,800 schizophrenic patients from 320 studies reported in the psychiatric literature between 1895 and 1992. Followed an average of nearly 6 years, 40% of patients were considered improved. Improvement was essentially defined as recovery, remission, or being well with minimal symptoms. They reported that outcome was much better when patients were diagnosed according to diagnostic symptoms with broad criteria (47% improved), rather than narrow criteria (27% improved). Further, the proportion of patients who improved was greater after the midcentury mark than before (49% versus 35%), perhaps reflecting a broadened concept of schizophrenia as well as improved treatment. Since 1975 the rate of favorable improvement has fallen to 36%, perhaps reflecting the impact of the reemergence of narrowed diagnostic criteria.

Several long-term follow-up studies have been published using contemporary American definitions of schizophrenia. The two best known are the Iowa 500, which used the St. Louis criteria, and the Chestnut Lodge study, which used the DSM-III criteria. The findings of these studies are remarkably similar (McGlashan 1984; Tsuang et al. 1979). In the Iowa 500 study, 186 schizophrenic patients admitted to the University of Iowa Psychiatric Hospital between 1934 and 1944 were followed up in the early 1970s. Twenty percent of patients with schizophrenia were reported to be psychiatrically well at follow-up, but 54% had incapacitating psychiatric symptoms; 21% were married or widowed, but 67% had never married; 34% lived in their own home or with a relative, but 18% were in mental institutions; 35% were economically productive, but 58% had never worked. The group experienced excess mortality from both natural and unnatural causes, and more than 10% committed suicide. In a recent reanalysis of this seminal study, Winokur and Tsuang (1996) report that only two of the schizophrenic patients followed up were completely free of symptoms (i.e., had "zero symptoms"). They conclude that whereas a patient may be considered improved and is able to work and to live independently, he or she is unlikely to be free of all symptoms.

In the Chestnut Lodge study, 163 schizophrenic patients discharged from the private hospital between 1950 and 1975 were followed up in the early 1980s. Whereas 37% were living in a hospital or sheltered environment, only 28% were living independently; 26% had been employed 50% of the follow-up period or better; 41% were considered continuously incapacitated, and only 6% had recovered. McGlashan (1984) noted that roughly two-thirds of the schizophrenic patients were functioning marginally or worse at follow-up and that 7% had killed themselves during the interim.

However, Riecher-Rossler and Rossler (1998) contend that many of these outcome studies have major methodological problems, particularly with regard to sample selection biases that lead to underrepresentation of patients with both the best and the worst outcomes. Therefore, findings from such studies may not generalize to the real world. In their literature review, which focused on five prospective studies that used representative catchment-area-based first-admitted or first-contact samples, Riecher-Rossler and Rossler concluded that whereas the course of schizophrenia is far from uniform, many patients with schizophrenia have a relatively good outcome and will avoid progressive deterioration. Significant improvement is possible, albeit years or decades after the first manifestations of psychosis. The illness process begins with nonspecific signs that occur long before first hospitalization and before the first occurrence of psychotic symptomatology.

Predicting Outcome

Although a variety of prognostic factors have been reported (Jonsson and Nyman 1984; McCabe et al. 1972; McGlashan 1986; Vaillant 1964), prediction of outcome remains a difficult task. Research has shown that definitions of schizophrenia that exclude patients with mood symptoms or those having a duration of illness under 6 months generally predict a poor prognosis. This is because these relatively restrictive definitions exclude patients with mood disorder, schizophreniform disorder, or schizoaffective disorders, who tend to have better outcomes. Perhaps the best study of outcome prediction was the International Pilot Study of Schizophrenia (World Health Organization 1975), in which psychiatrists in nine different countries participated. Regression analysis showed the five most powerful predictors of poor outcome to be social isolation, long duration of episode, history of past psychiatric treatment, being unmarried, and having a history of behavioral problems in childhood such as truancy and tantrums. The investigators also found that all 47 potential predictors accounted for only 38% of the variance. A summary of commonly reported prognostic factors is shown in Table 9–10.

Other Factors That Affect Outcome

Cultural Factors

Cross-cultural studies have shown that schizophrenic patients living in less developed countries tend to have better outcomes than those in more developed countries. This unexpected finding was reported in the International Pilot Study of Schizophrenia (World Health Organization 1975), which demonstrated that the average outcome was considerably better in the developing countries (Colombia, India, and Nigeria) than in the industri-

TABLE 9–10. Features associated with good and poor outcome in schizophrenia

Feature	Good outcome	Poor outcome
Age	Older	Younger
Gender	Female	Male
Social class	High	Low
Marital history	Married	Never married
Family history of schizophrenia	Negative	Positive
Perinatal complications	Absent	Present
Transcultural factors	Developing nations	Industrialized nations
Premorbid functioning	Good	Poor
Onset	Acute	Insidious
Duration	Short	Chronic
Sensorium	Clouded	Clear
Symptoms/subtypes	Paranoid subtype	Deficit syndrome
Affective symptoms	Present	Absent
Neurological functioning	Normal	Soft signs present
Neurocognition	Normal	Abnormal
Structural brain abnormalities	None	Present

alized countries (Czechoslovakia, Denmark, United Kingdom, United States, and the former Soviet Union). Despite extensive follow-up treatment available in industrialized countries, a high proportion of their patients had additional psychotic episodes not seen in the patients in developing countries. Although there were no important differences in the initial symptoms and other characteristics of the patients at the nine study sites, the possibility cannot be dismissed that these differences in outcome were due to unrecognized differences in the types of patients seeking treatment. One explanation is that the schizophrenic patient is better accepted in less developed countries, has fewer external demands, and is more likely to be taken care of by interested family members. The same finding emerged from a comparison of outcomes of schizophrenia in London and Mauritius (Murphy and Raman 1971).

Gender

Women with schizophrenia appear to have a more favorable outcome than men in treatment response, social functioning, and overall prognosis. A study of 121 schizophrenic patients in England (D.C. Watt et al. 1983) found that at a 5-year follow-up, 62% of women had a good outcome as compared with 35% of men. Women also had better housing, probably due to the fact that they were less likely than men to live alone or to be institutionalized. A similar study of 278 schizophrenic patients in Germany (Angermeyer et al. 1989) found women to have fewer rehospitalizations and shorter lengths of stay.

Epidemiology

Schizophrenia presents a challenge to the epidemiologist, due to disagreements about the definition of its core features and the breadth of its spectrum. The development of operational criteria, such as those in DSM-IV-TR, has provided greater specificity for the diagnosis of schizophrenia and has resulted in a more cautious use of the concept. This has led to a reassessment of earlier epidemiological studies that generated rates based on older conceptualizations of schizophrenia. Despite these advances, case identification remains an ongoing problem among epidemiologists. Efforts to standardize the diagnosis have met with some success, such as with the Present State Examination used in the International Pilot Study of Schizophrenia and the Composite Interview Diagnostic Instrument used in the National Comorbidity Study (Kessler et al. 1994).

Prevalence and Incidence

In a comprehensive review, Eaton et al. (1988) reported that the median point prevalence of schizophrenia was 3.2 per 1,000 (range 0.6–8.3). The median lifetime prevalence rate was 4.4 per 1,000 (range 1.7–7.0). *Point prevalence* includes all identified cases at a given point in time. *Lifetime prevalence*, or "disease expectancy," includes the proportion of persons studied who have ever experienced the disorder up to the time of assessment. The type of prevalence measure reported (i.e., point, lifetime) appears not to strongly influence the rate, presumably due to the chronic nature and low incidence of schizophrenia (Eaton 1985). In the National Comorbidity Study, in which lay-interviewed patients evidencing symptoms of psychosis were reinterviewed by a psychiatrist, the lifetime rate for schizophrenia was 0.14% (Bromet et al. 1995). This rate is much lower than that reported in the Epidemiologic Catchment Area study (1.3% lifetime; Robins et al. 1984). That finding was based on results of the lay-administered Diagnostic Interview Schedule, an instrument with relatively poor reliability for the diagnosis of schizophrenia (Anthony et al. 1985).

A review of annual incidence rates of schizophrenia (Eaton et al. 1988) show a median rate of 0.20 per 1,000 (range 0.11–0.70). *Incidence* is the number of new cases that arise in a given time per unit of population. (A simple formula, prevalence = incidence × duration, shows the relationship between these two parameters.) Because incidence does not confound the rate of occurrence with duration, many investigators find it a more useful measure for etiological studies, although both measures are helpful for planning health services. A World Health Organization study (Jablensky et al. 1992) involving 10 research sites showed that incidence rates were remarkably similar across the various sites. A reported decline in the incidence rate of schizophrenia has been debated, as some researchers believe that new cases are less frequent than many decades ago (Eaton 1991). It is likely that any apparent rate decline is tied to changing diagnostic practices that favor more restrictive definitions such as that in DSM-IV-TR.

Age at Onset and Sex Ratio

Schizophrenia typically begins in early adulthood, but can develop at any age including early childhood (Beitchman 1985). Both Bleuler and Kraepelin reported an earlier onset for men than women, a finding confirmed by subsequent research. In one study (Loranger 1984), mean age at onset was 21.4 years for men and 26.8 years for women. Mean age at first treatment occurred 5 and 7 years later, respectively. A total of 9 of 10 males, but only 2 of 3 females, had developed schizophrenia by age 30. Onset after age 35 occurred in 17% of women, but in only 2% of men. The reason women develop schizophrenia later than men remains a mystery, but it is apparently not an artifact resulting from women having a more sheltered existence that conceals their illness. Kendler et al. (1996) concluded that environmental or developmental factors probably account for the variation seen in the age at onset in schizophrenia.

Early epidemiological studies showed approximately equal rates of schizophrenia for men and women, but the broad concept of schizophrenia used in the past may have led to the inclusion of a disproportionate number of women with mood disorders. Lewine et al. (1984) analyzed the effect of using six different diagnostic systems on the male-to-female ratio of schizophrenia among 387 inpatients. Diagnostic criteria that present a broad concept of schizophrenia, such as the New Haven schizophrenia index, yielded equal rates of schizophrenia among men and women. Diagnostic systems with more stringent criteria, such as the Research Diagnostic Criteria, yielded a greater male-to-female ratio.

Marital Status and Reproduction

Patients with schizophrenia are more likely to remain single than are patients in other diagnostic groups. This is particularly true in male patients (Eaton 1985), which can probably be explained by the fact that women tend to be younger than men when first married and are less likely to have experienced an initial psychotic episode. From a cultural perspective, women have traditionally been less active in initiating relationships, which may account for some of the difference.

Early researchers tended to find low rates of fertility and reproduction among patients with schizophrenia (Kallman 1938). This finding can probably be explained by several factors including lack of interest in social relations, general apathy, low sex drive, and lack of opportunity for a sexual relationship due to hospitalization or institutionalization. Rates of reproduction in patients with schizophrenia have probably increased since deinstitutionalization, although they likely remain lower than those found in the general population (Erlenmeyer-Kimling 1978). The lower rates of fertility and fecundity are more pronounced among males (Nimgaonkar 1998; Nimgaonkar et al. 1997). The persistence of the disease in spite of low fertility rates is an intriguing fact that may suggest a contribution from environmental factors and/or a particular type of genetic transmission (e.g., recessive, low penetrance).

Socioeconomic Status

Patients with schizophrenia generally have low social status. Eaton (1985) reviewed 17 studies of incidence of treated schizophrenia that included indicators of social class. The highest rate of schizophrenia was found in the lowest social class in 15 of the studies. Earlier studies suggested that lower social class status seen in schizophrenic patients probably results from the "downward drift" in socioeconomic status they experience due to the debilitating effects of their symptoms, which impair social and occupational functioning.

Ethnicity and Race

Jablensky and Sartorius (1975) concluded from a literature review that except for a high rate found by Böök in
north Sweden (10.8 per 1,000) and a low rate reported
by Eaton and Weil for the Hutterite sect in the United
States (1.1 per 1,000), prevalence rates for schizophrenia
are relatively similar worldwide. Pockets of high prevalence have been reported in areas of the Istrian peninsula
in Croatia, on the western coast of Ireland, among Canadian Catholics, and among the Tamils of southern India.
Low prevalence has been reported among American Old
Order Amish, in the aboriginal tribes of Taiwan, and in
the native population in Ghana. Although early studies in
the United States suggested a higher rate of schizophrenia in African Americans than in whites, this finding was
probably due to a systematic bias to overdiagnose schizophrenia in blacks (Mukherjee et al. 1983).

Mortality and Morbidity

Research has long shown increased mortality in patients
with schizophrenia (Simpson and Tsuang 1996). In the
past, high death rates were attributed to both natural and
unnatural causes. Before modern medical and psychiatric
treatments were available, many patients suffered the ill
effects of prolonged psychiatric symptoms leading to malnutrition or dehydration or were exposed to tuberculosis
and other infectious diseases in large institutions. Because
general medical and psychiatric care has improved, high
death rates in patients with schizophrenia are now due
primarily to suicide and accidents. In one study (Black
and Fisher 1992), schizophrenic patients showed a near
threefold increase over expected mortality. Those at risk
for premature death were patients younger than 40 years
and who were in their first few years of follow-up.

Based on early epidemiological studies, patients with
schizophrenia were once thought to have some immunity
from cancer. Recent research shows that although cancer
death rates in general are not different than expected,
there is evidence of lower risk for lung cancer despite
high rates of smoking in those patients (Black and
Winokur 1986; Gulbinat et al. 1992). There is evidence,
too, that rheumatoid arthritis is less common in patients
with schizophrenia (Eaton et al. 1992) than among persons in the general population, although the reason for
this association is unknown.

Suicide and Suicidal Behavior

Patients with schizophrenia are at high risk for suicidal
behavior. Nearly one-third will attempt suicide (Allebeck

et al. 1987), and about 1 in 10 will complete suicide
(Tsuang 1978). Between 2% and 3% of suicide completers have schizophrenia (Barraclough et al. 1974). Risk
factors for suicide include male gender, age less than 30
years, living alone, unemployment, chronic relapsing
course, prior depression, past treatment for depression,
depression during the last episode of illness, history of
substance abuse, and recent hospital discharge (Allebeck
et al. 1987; A. Roy 1982). Schizophrenic patients with
the paranoid subtype and those with a high level of education appear to be at greater risk for suicide (Fenton and
McGlashan 1991), perhaps due to the patients' feelings
of inadequacy and hopelessness, fear of disintegration,
and a realization that desired expectations will never be
met. Unlike other psychiatric patients who commit suicide, patients with schizophrenia may fail to communicate their suicidal intentions and may act impulsively,
complicating any effort at intervention (Breier and Astrachan 1984).

Violence and Criminality

Until quite recently it was thought that mentally ill persons were not predisposed to violent behavior (Teplin
1985). In the Epidemiologic Catchment Area study
(Swanson et al. 1990), however, patients with schizophrenia had rates of violent behavior five times higher
than persons without mental illness, although the rate
was about one-half that seen in persons with alcohol
abuse or dependence. Schizophrenic patients with coexisting alcoholism are even more likely to commit violent
acts, including homicide, than patients not abusing substances (Modestin and Ammann 1996). The severely
mentally ill have high rates of conviction for criminal
offenses and incarceration, although many of the offenses
have been called "survival crimes," such as shoplifting
and petty thievery thought due to homelessness or deinstitutionalization (Csillag 1993). To some extent violent
behavior may be a function of the stage of a schizophrenic
patient's illness (e.g., in response to persecutory delusions) and remains one of the primary reasons for hospitalization.

Treatment Delays and
Utilization of Health Services

Studies of first-episode psychosis from around the world
have consistently shown that there is a time lag averaging
1–2 years between the onset of psychotic symptoms and
initiation of treatment (McGlashan 1999). Although the
reasons for the treatment delay remain unclear (Ho and
Andreasen 2001), its implications for service delivery

and outcome are increasingly being recognized (Lieberman and Fenton 2000). Based on the pioneering work of Falloon (1992) and McGorry et al. (1996), programs dedicated to detecting patients at the prodrome stage of the disorder and reducing treatment delays have shown much promise. However, currently available methods of screening for schizophrenia still have moderately high false-positive rates. Furthermore, whether earlier treatment leads to better outcome has yet to be established (Ho and Andreasen 2001). More research is still needed before the potential of secondary prevention can be realized.

Although many patients with schizophrenia delay seeking treatment, they consume a disproportionate share of general medical and psychiatric services after entry into the health care system. According to information from the Monroe County Psychiatric Case Register, schizophrenia accounted for 16.4% of the treatment population in 1975, but 47.6% of psychiatric inpatient days and 36.9% of new state hospital inpatient admissions (Babigian 1984). Schizophrenic patients 65 years and older utilized a disproportionate share of hospitalization days, especially at state facilities, whereas those aged 25–44 years had the highest rate of acute hospitalization episodes.

National Institute of Mental Health data show schizophrenia to be the first or second most frequent diagnosis for admissions to various types of psychiatric inpatient services, ranging from 21% for private hospitals to 38% for state and county hospitals, with a length of stay averaging 18–42 days, respectively. There were over 1.6 million admissions of schizophrenic patients to inpatient facilities in 1980 (Taube and Barrett 1985). Results from the Epidemiologic Catchment Area study (Shapiro et al. 1984) showed that nearly 78% of schizophrenic patients surveyed had health care visits during the previous 6 months; 45% of visits were for mental health care. Patients with schizophrenia tended to obtain mental health care from specialists rather than from general medical providers, which indicates the severity of the illness, since the opposite was true for most nonpsychotic disorders.

Pathophysiology and Etiology

The development of multiple competing theories about the cause of schizophrenia parallels its history. Early theories were shaped by limited knowledge about the nature of mental illness and inadequate research methods. There is still disagreement about the relative contribution of genetic and nongenetic factors to the development of schizophrenia, despite advances in psychiatric nosology, epidemiology, and genetics. Recent work, however, has emphasized the importance of the interaction of both genetic and nongenetic factors in disease expression.

Consensus now exists among many investigators that schizophrenia is best conceptualized as a "multiple-hit" illness similar to cancer. Individuals may carry a genetic predisposition, but this vulnerabilty is not "released" unless other factors also intervene. Although most of these factors are considered environmental, in the sense that they are not encoded in DNA and could potentially produce mutations or influence gene expression, most are also biological rather than psychological and include factors such as birth injuries or nutrition. Current studies of the neurobiology of schizophrenia examine a multiplicity of factors, including genetics, anatomy (primarily through structural neuroimaging), functional circuitry (through functional neuroimaging), neuropathology, electrophysiology, neurochemistry and neuropharmacology, and neurodevelopment.

Genetics

Evidence for a hereditary contribution to schizophrenia is based on family studies, twin studies, and studies of adoptees. As early as 1916, Rudin reported an increased prevalence of dementia praecox among the siblings of affected probands. Subsequent family studies have confirmed an increased prevalence of schizophrenia and related disorders in family members, with risk related to the number of shared genes of family members with the schizophrenic proband. Summaries of individual family studies have shown siblings of schizophrenic patients to have a near 10% lifetime risk of developing schizophrenia, while children who have one parent with schizophrenia have a 5%–6% lifetime risk (Gottesman and Shields 1982). The risk of a family member developing schizophrenia markedly increases when two or more family members have the illness, with a lifetime expectancy of schizophrenia of 17% for those with one sibling and one parent with schizophrenia and up to 46% in children of two parents with schizophrenia. These findings strongly support the familial nature of schizophrenia, but do not confirm a genetic over a familial environmental cause.

Twin studies and adoption studies allow a natural experimental paradigm to separate the genetic and environmental effects of familial associations. Despite varying methods, twin studies have been remarkably consistent in demonstrating high concordance rates for monozygotic twins (Farmer et al. 1987; Gottesman and Shields 1982). Rates have averaged 46% as compared with 14% in dizygotic twins across multiple studies, with only one negative twin study (Tienari 1963). However, the failure of monozygotic twins to be 100% concordant suggests that a hereditary component may be necessary but is insufficient to cause schizophrenia and that environmental factors are also important.

Adoption studies present another paradigm for evaluating genetic influences in familial illness. Heston (1966) examined grown children of mothers with schizophrenia who had been adopted and compared them with control adoptees whose mothers had no psychiatric disorder. He found a nearly 17% age-corrected morbidity risk of schizophrenia in the adoptees of schizophrenic mothers, a figure similar to those reported family studies of children of mothers with schizophrenia not given up for adoption; no control adoptees had schizophrenia. The best-known adoption study was conducted in Denmark using a national psychiatric case register and a register of adoptions. Kety et al. (1975) reported that schizophrenia and *schizophrenia spectrum disorders* were more common in the biological relatives of index adoptees who had schizophrenia than in the biological relatives of mentally healthy control adoptees. Schizophrenia spectrum disorders include personality disorders that share certain characteristics with schizophrenia, such as paranoid ideas or eccentric behavior, without meeting full syndromal criteria. A blind reanalysis of the data (Kendler and Gruenberg 1984) using DSM-III criteria essentially replicated the original results. An adoption study in Finland (Tienari 2000) has shown similar results. Thus, adoption studies have demonstrated that having a schizophrenic parent increases the risk in offspring not only for schizophrenia, but also for spectrum disorders such as schizotypal personality.

Mode of inheritance of schizophrenia has also been studied, mainly by using mathematical modeling of pedigrees and twin and adoption study data. Proposed modes of inheritance include a single-gene model and a polygenic model. A simple Mendelian model of transmission involving a single dominant or recessive gene is not clearly present in the pedigrees of most probands who suffer from schizophrenia, although a single gene is possible if one assumes incomplete penetrance and dominant transmission (Slater 1958), or if eye-tracking dysfunction (i.e., abnormal smooth-pursuit eye movement) is considered an expression of schizophrenia (Holzman et al. 1988). However, polygenic models of inheritance are consistent with published family and twin data (Gottesman and Shields 1982); they are also consistent with genetic studies finding increased risk in families with more than one schizophrenic member and increased risk in first-degree relatives of more severely ill probands

compared to less severely ill probands (Rice and McGuffin 1985). Polygenic models may provide a better explanation of the persistence of schizophrenia in light of the reduced fertility characteristic of the disorder. Sufficient data do not presently exist to definitively support or reject either single gene or polygenetic models.

The molecular genetic techniques described in Chapter 1 are now being used in attempts to pin down mode of inheritance and to locate a "schizophrenia gene" (or genes). The task is complicated by the lack of biological traits or vulnerability markers specific to schizophrenia, as well as clinical heterogeneity. Research has implicated segments on several chromosomes (e.g., chromosomes 6, 8, 11, 13, and 22) as regions where "schizophrenia genes" are likely to be located (Moldin and Gottesman 1997; Pulver 2000). The short arm of chromosome 6 is one of the most consistently replicated regions (Crowe et al. 1991; Schizophrenia Collaborative Linkage Group 1996; Schwab et al. 1995; Wang et al. 1995). The nonreplications do not rule out involvement of a particular gene region in some families and may indicate only that schizophrenia is genetically heterogeneous. Efforts to link schizophrenia to particular gene regions will undoubtedly continue at a rapid pace (Bassett 1998).

Some evidence also suggests that schizophrenia may show the phenomenon of *anticipation:* increasingly severe onset at earlier ages within multigeneration affected families (Gorwood et al. 1996). Anticipation has been observed in other neuropsychiatric disorders, including Huntington's disease, fragile X syndrome, and myotonic dystrophy. In these disorders, increasing proliferation of trinucleotide repeats at the disease locus in successive generations correlated with anticipation. Although there is no evidence of large trinucleotide repeats in schizophrenia (Petronis et al. 1996), the occurrence of anticipation in schizophrenia may provide some clues as to its specific genetic loci and mechanisms (Petronis and Kennedy 1995).

Neuroanatomy and Structural Neuroimaging

Since the early work of Kraepelin, Alzheimer, and Nissl in the late nineteenth and early twentieth centuries, many psychiatrists have been convinced that patients with schizophrenia have some type of structural brain abnormality (Kraepelin 1919). Early pneumoencephalographic and neuropathological studies provided partial support for this hypothesis (Storey 1966), but in recent years new technology has been able to support it more fully. When Johnstone et al. (1976) first described the use of the technique to study brain abnormalities in chronic schizophrenia, their report elicited considerable controversy, but the finding of ventricular enlargement in schizophrenia has now been confirmed by numerous CT studies and is perhaps the best-replicated finding in psychiatry (Andreasen et al. 1982, 1990c; Weinberger et al. 1979, 1980). This early work with CT, conducted during the 1980s, firmly established that schizophrenia is a brain disorder with a measurable structural component that can be observed at the gross anatomic level when groups of patients are pooled together, averaged, and compared with healthy volunteer control subjects.

Cerebral ventricular enlargement is the most consistently replicated finding, but sulcal enlargement or abnormalities in cortical or subcortical subregions are also reported. Although these findings cannot be explained on the basis of such factors as treatment with medications, they may be explained in part by gender, because it may be predominantly a male effect (Flaum et al. 1990). Examination of ventricular size in patients with schizophrenia and healthy subjects over a broad age range suggest that enlargement does not progress over time at a greater rate in schizophrenic patients than normally and that structural brain abnormalities are present from the outset (Andreasen et al. 1990a; Nopoulos et al. 1995a). Although not all studies show exactly the same correlates, there is substantial evidence to suggest that ventricular enlargement is associated with poor premorbid functioning, negative symptoms, poor response to treatment, and cognitive impairment. CT scan abnormalities may have some clinical significance, but they are not diagnostically specific; similar abnormalities are seen in other disorders such as Alzheimer's disease or alcoholism.

MRI has now largely supplanted CT as a clinical and research tool. Its particular advantage lies in its ability to distinguish gray and white matter, allowing the size of particular brain regions and structures to be measured. MRI has permitted investigators to move from asking, "Is there a grossly measurable brain abnormality in schizophrenia?" to asking, "Is a specific region or group of regions affected?" Many candidate regions have been explored, but none has been conclusively confirmed. The conflicting reports appear to largely reflect the growing maturity of this method of study. Early reports used relatively primitive techniques such as area measurements on single slices and manual tracing. More recent studies apply automated volumetric measures that have greater power and sophistication.

The earliest MRI study reported a selective decrease in the frontal cortex, in addition to smaller cerebral and intracranial size, and it suggested that this combination of findings was consistent with a neurodevelopmental process in which the brain failed to grow normally, rather than with a neurodegenerative process (Andreasen et al. 1986). Many subsequent studies examined the issue of brain size; a recent meta-analysis examining all available studies of intracranial size ($N = 18$) and brain volume ($N = 27$) has confirmed a small but highly statistically significant difference between patients and control subjects in both brain and intracranial volume (Ward et al. 1996).

A decrease in frontal lobe size has been less consistently replicated, although hypotheses about a dysfunction of the frontal cortex continue to be widely discussed, particularly in functional imaging studies (see "Functional Circuitry and Functional Neuroimaging"). The prefrontal cortex performs a large array of higher cortical functions that are disrupted in schizophrenia (e.g., "executive functions," abstract thinking, working memory), making it an attractive candidate for study. Yet it is also a large and functionally diverse brain region that was difficult to measure accurately prior to the recent development of three-dimensional acquisition procedures with MRI and volume-rendering techniques that permit visualization of cortical surface anatomy (Figure 9–4) and parcellation of the frontal lobe into functionally distinct areas (Figure 9–5; Crespo-Facorro et al. 1999a). Studies that used relatively sophisticated measurement techniques have shown decreased frontal size in both chronic and first episode patients (Andreasen et al. 1994a; Breier et al. 1992; Nopoulos et al. 1995a). If all studies are pooled, however, negative studies are as frequent as positive ones (for a review, see Shenton et al. 1997). More recent studies have examined specific subregions within the frontal cortex, and both volumetric and morphological differences between schizophrenia patients and healthy control subjects have been reported (Crespo-Facorro et al. 2000; Szeszko et al. 1999).

MRI has also been used to explore possible abnormalities in other specific brain subregions, such as the thalamus, amygdala/hippocampus, temporal lobes, or basal ganglia. Several studies have indicated that the size of temporal regions is decreased in schizophrenia and that there may even be a relatively specific abnormality in the superior temporal gyrus or planum temporale that is correlated with the presence of hallucinations or formal thought disorder (Barta et al. 1990; Shenton et al. 1992).

The thalamus is relatively difficult to measure reliably using MRI because it is composed of multiple nuclei, is a mixture of gray and white matter, and has relatively fuzzy borders as visualized on nearly all types of MRI sequences. Nonetheless, it has been noted to have a decreased size in several studies, and a novel application of image averaging and subtraction methods has indicated that this structure shows the greatest effect size difference when patients are compared to control subjects

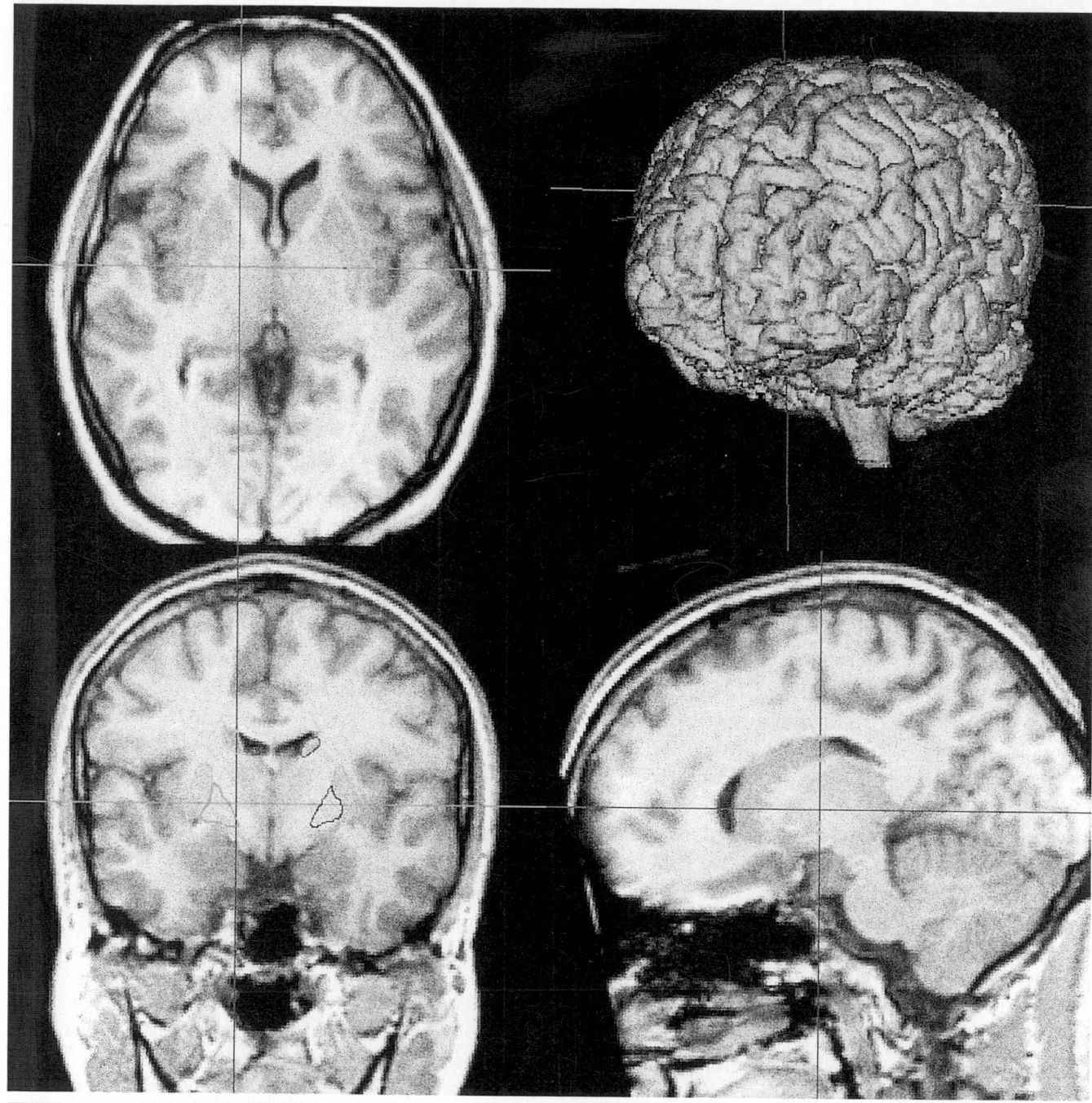

FIGURE 9–4. Magnetic resonance image (MRI) scan showing how three-dimensional acquisition procedures and volume-rendering techniques permit visualization of cortical surface anatomy.

Source. Photo courtesy of N.C. Andreasen, M.D., Ph.D.

(Andreasen et al. 1994b). Like the prefrontal cortex, the thalamus is also an interesting candidate region for schizophrenia; although the precise functions of the various thalamic nuclei are still being mapped, it is clearly a major relay station that could serve functions such as gating or filtering or even generating input and output, because it receives afferent input and sends efferent output from and to widely distributed cortical and primary sensory and motor regions.

Sophisticated image analysis techniques have been developed to measure the total volume of gray matter, white matter, and cerebrospinal fluid (CSF), and these have also been applied to the study of schizophrenia (Cohen et al. 1992; Gur and Pearlson 1993; Harris et al. 1999; Lim et al. 1996). Figure 9–6 shows an image in which the MRI data have been reclassified in these three tissue types to permit quantitative measurement. Most studies consistently show a decrease in total brain tissue

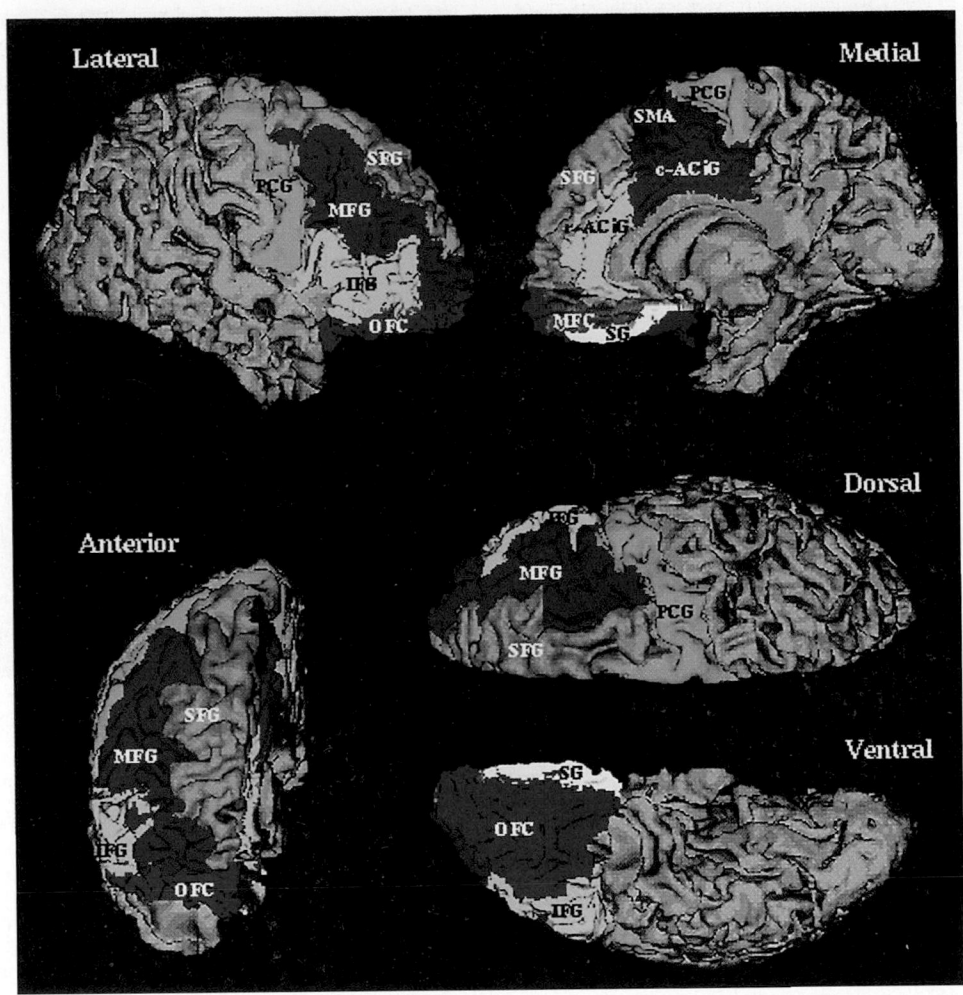

FIGURE 9–5.   Five views of the three-dimensional-rendered brain on which the different frontal subregions have been displayed in distinctive colors.

Note.   c-ACiG = caudal anterior cingulate gyrus; r-ACiG = rostral anterior cingulate gyrus; IFG = inferior frontal gyrus; MFC = medial frontal cortex; MFG = middle frontal gyrus; OFC = orbitofrontal cortex; PCG = precentral gyrus; SFG = superior frontal gyrus; SG = straight gyrus; SMA = supplementary motor area.

volume in schizophrenia as well as an increase in CSF in the ventricles and on the brain surface. Most studies that have evaluated the relative changes in gray and white matter have found a selective decrease in cortical gray matter, although some have also found white matter decreases as well (Breier et al. 1992; Schlaepfer et al. 1994; Zipursky et al. 1994).

MRI studies have also provided some confirmation for neurodevelopmental theories of schizophrenia apart from the observation of decreased intracranical volume and decreased tissue discussed above. Various developmental anomalies are seen by MRI in some patients suffering from schizophrenia. The most consistently reported is an increased frequency of large cavum septi pellucidi, a midline anomaly reflecting a fusion failure of the septal leaflets (S.W. Lewis and Mezey 1985; Nopou-

los et al. 1996, 1997) In addition, partial callosal agenesis (a severe midline anomaly) appears to be modestly increased in schizophrenia (Swayze et al. 1990). Finally, findings that reflect abnormalities in neuronal migration (e.g., gray matter heterotopias) are also seen with increased incidence, although only in a small number of patients (Nopoulos et al. 1995b).

Finally, longitudinal MRI assessments of brain morphology in first-episode schizophrenia patients have revealed that structural abnormalities are present by the time that patients present for treatment. In general, there is little evidence for subsequent progressive neurodegeneration, although a subset of poor-outcome patients may show worsening ventricular enlargement over time (K.L. Davis et al. 1998; Lieberman et al. 2001).

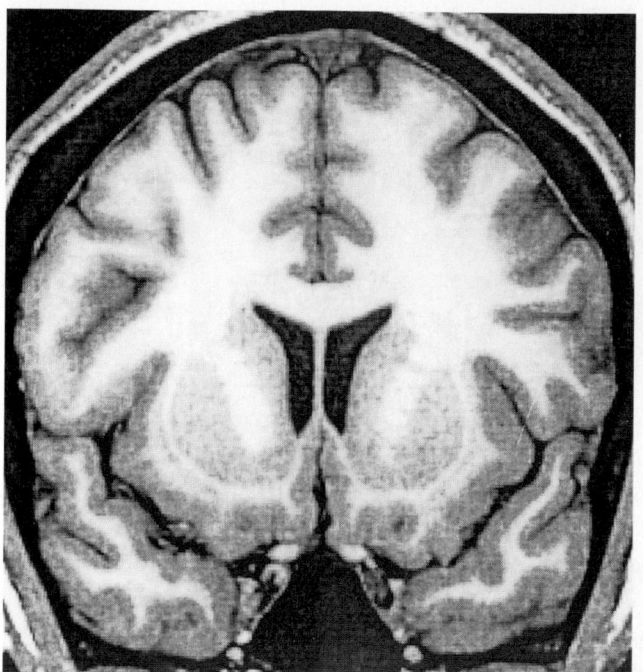 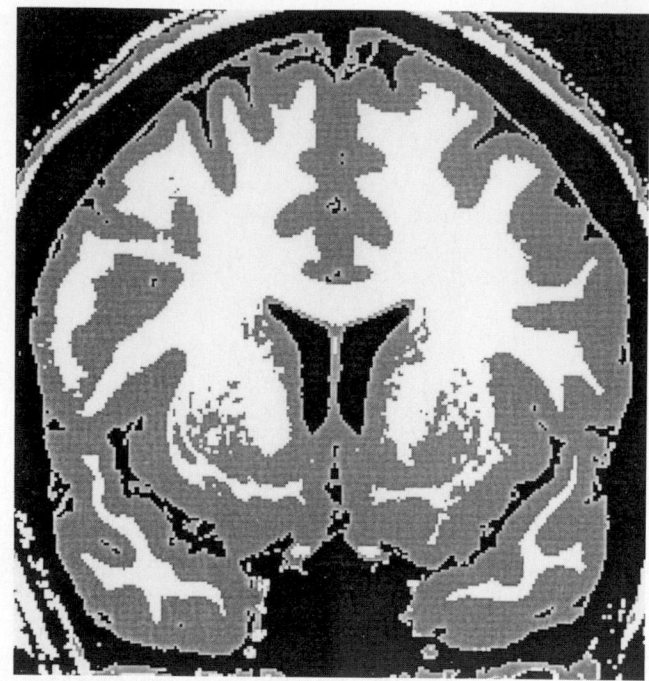

FIGURE 9–6. Magnetic resonance imaging scan showing how magnetic resonance data can be reclassified to permit quantitative measurement of gray matter, white matter, and cerebrospinal fluid.

A, A conventional magnetic resonance scan. B, Tissue composition of the brain after it has been classified as gray matter, white matter, and cerebrospinal fluid.

Source. Photo courtesy of N.C. Andreasen, M.D., Ph.D.

Functional Circuitry and Functional Neuroimaging

Beginning with the work of Ingvar and Franzen (1974), studies of regional cerebral blood flow (rCBF) have been used to explore the possibility of functional or metabolic abnormalities in schizophrenia (Andreasen et al. 1992). Data from these studies suggested that patients with schizophrenia had a relative "hypofrontality," which was associated with prominent negative symptoms. Since that early work, functional imaging studies have become more sophisticated, and it is now clear that PET can be used to explore the functional circuitry used by healthy individuals while they perform a variety of mental tasks and to identify circuits that are dysfunctional in schizophrenia. Much of this work has been facilitated by the maturation of the $^{15}O\ H_2O$ technique with PET. $^{15}O\ H_2O$ is a tracer with a very short half-life (around 2 minutes), which permits investigators to do multiple repeated scans (usually 6–12) with differing cognitive tasks during a short time period (around 2 hours). This permits the dissection of the components of cognitive activities (e.g., memory encoding versus retrieval) and visualization of their associated circuitry.

Current thinking about the mechanisms of schizophrenia, based on functional imaging, postulates a disrup-

tion in distributed functional circuits rather than a single abnormality in a single brain region such as the prefrontal cortex or one of its specific subregions such as the dorsolateral prefrontal cortex. Although no single group of regions has definitely emerged as the "schizophrenia circuit," a consensus is developing concerning some of the nodes that may be involved. They include various subregions within the frontal cortex (orbital, dorsolateral, medial), the anterior cingulate gyrus, the thalamus, several temporal lobe subregions, and the cerebellum.

For example, Frith et al. (1991) began their earliest work by studying *willed action* (their first symptom dimension and analogous to negative symptoms). They tested the neural substrates of willed action by giving subjects tasks for which the correct response is not evident from context, such as verbal fluency or choosing a finger movement. Healthy control subjects activate a frontal circuit during such tasks, whereas patients with schizophrenia show relative decreases in frontal regions and decreases in temporal regions in comparison with normal subjects (Liddle et al. 1992). If the pace of the verbal fluency task is slowed, however, frontal function is similar to normal subjects and only the temporal abnormality remains (Frith 1995). Examination of the correlations between flow in these regions suggests that the normal relationship between them has broken down and that there is abnormal functional connectivity (McGuire and Frith 1996).

More recently this research group completed a systematic study of hallucinations, their second dimension of psychopathology. They assumed that hallucinations are caused by an erroneous attribution of the person's own inner speech to another person, reflecting a defect in self-monitoring. Starting first with healthy subjects, they developed a task that could potentially mimic this mechanism of hallucinations; subjects were asked to perform a sentence completion task and imagine that the response was spoken in another person's voice. They found that this task led to activation of speech production and perception regions, such as Broca's area, the supplementary motor area, and the left superior and middle temporal regions (McGuire et al. 1996a). Applying the same task to people with schizophrenia and comparing hallucinators with nonhallucinators, they found the hallucinators to have decreased flow in the areas used to monitor speech, such as the left middle temporal gyrus and supplementary motor area (McGuire et al. 1996b). They have also examined flow in patients while they were experiencing auditory hallucinations and found activations primarily in subcortical regions (thalamus, striatum), limbic and paralimbic regions (anterior cingulate, parahippocampal gyrus), and cerebellum; they speculate that activity in subcortical regions may generate or moderate hallucinations, whereas the content (e.g., auditory, tactile) may be determined by the specific neocortical regions that are engaged (Silbersweig et al. 1995).

Other research groups have also used functional imaging to explore functional circuitry. Buchsbaum, who conducted the earliest PET studies suggesting hypofrontality (Buchsbaum et al. 1982), more recently measured glucose metabolism in a sample of 20 never-medicated schizophrenic patients and also observed thalamic abnormalities using fluorodeoxyglucose (Buchsbaum et al. 1996). Interestingly, Buchsbaum and colleagues also reported a diminished metabolic rate in the cerebellum in this study.

Andreasen and colleagues have also provided support for abnormalities in multiple frontal subregions, the thalamus, and the cerebellum. In studies comparing first-episode neuroleptic-naïve schizophrenic patients and chronic schizophrenic patients with healthy volunteers during random-episodic silent thought (REST), these investigators observed blood flow abnormalities in medial, orbital, and dorsolateral frontal regions, as well as temporal, cingulate, thalamic, and cerebellar areas (Andreasen et al. 1997; Kim et al. 2000). In another study of practiced and novel recall of complex narrative material, they

observed abnormalities in multiple brain regions, including frontal, thalamic, and cerebellar sites (Andreasen et al. 1996). Andreasen and colleagues have also observed similar abnormalities in schizophrenic patients during episodic memory and semantic/working memory tasks (Crespo-Facorro et al. 1999b; Wiser et al. 1998).

These findings are consistent with the theory that schizophrenia is a disease of multiple distributed circuits in the brain. The disease is characterized by a cognitive dysmetria caused by a disruption in pontine-cerebellar-thalamic-frontal feedback loops (Andreasen 1999; Andreasen et al. 1996, 1998, 1999). The thalamus is a crucial waystation in the brain that has complex interconnections to many other regions. Various parts of the prefrontal cortex (i.e., dorsolateral, orbital, and medial) are connected to it, as are other regions such as the basal ganglia and anterior cingulate. Further, various thalamic nuclei have relay connections to virtually all other parts of the cerebral cortex, including sensory, motor, and association regions. Finally, the cerebellum also projects to multiple cortical regions via thalamic relay nuclei.

The concept of cognitive dysmetria postulates three key nodes in a feedback loop that involves frontal regions, the cerebellum, and the thalamus. Each of these nodes is assumed to have a particular function. The prefrontal node serves the classic "executive function": prioritizing data, placing it within a broad context using information gleaned from other intercommunicating cortical regions, formulating decisions or responses, and initiating their action. The thalamus serves as the filter, receiving sensory information from multiple sources, simplifying it by excluding redundant or extraneous stimuli, and forwarding on the important or relevant information. The cerebellum, which contains half the neurons in the human brain and is composed of cells designed to handle massive amounts of information, may serve as the "metron." That is, it coordinates the information forwarded back to it from cortical regions and sent to it through subcortical and brain stem regions. As a metron, its primary role is to match data within the context of time and space in order to make sure that the correct pieces of information are connected and coordinated with one another.

For example, a person carrying on a conversation must hear and "understand" the words of the other speaker, formulating an interpretation of the speaker's implicit and explicit meaning in order to generate an appropriate reply. In this simple model, the prefrontal cortex does most of the interpretation, whereas the thalamus permits the brain to focus on the conversation itself rather than on the multiple other people that may be nearby or ambient background noise in the room. The thalamus may damp down visual stimulation in order to focus on the auditory stimulation. The cerebellum, acting as the metron or coordinating organ, would be the site where information from the frontal executive and other sensory regions converges and would serve the responsibility of doing extremely rapid online processing, for which it appears to be well designed anatomically. A patient suffering from schizophrenia manifests impaired verbal and social responses in such situations because of a dysfunction in the circuitry that permits prioritizing information, excluding extraneous information, and performing these functions in a rapid, efficient, and well-coordinated manner.

Neuropathology

Schizophrenia, once called the "graveyard of neuropathologists," continues to vex researchers in their efforts to establish its characteristic pathological changes. Although many of the neuropathological findings in schizophrenia remain controversial, histological abnormalities with the strongest evidence include smaller cortical and hippocampal neurons, fewer neurons in the dorsal thalamus, reduced synaptic and dendritic markers in the hippocampus, and absence of gliosis (Harrison 1999).

A better understanding of neurodevelopment has helped shape contemporary postmortem studies (Arnold 1999). During the second trimester neurons in the fetal brain must migrate to the appropriate layers of the cortex, then connect with other groups of neurons to form functional networks. Other developmental processes include excessive proliferation of cells and dendrites, which are subsequently followed by pruning and programmed cell death (apoptosis) of subplate neurons; surviving cells remain as interstitial neurons (or interneurons) of the white matter. The resulting network of neurons and cytoplasmic processes is called the *neuropil*. Several neuropathological studies have supported the idea that schizophrenia could be related to disturbances in any of these phases of brain maturation, ranging from migration to apoptosis. Failure of the cells to migrate to their proper position may show up as ectopic gray matter (Nopoulos et al. 1995b) or neuronal disarray in specific regions of the hippocampus (Conrad et al. 1991; Kovelman and Scheibel 1984). Arnold et al. (1991) reported displacement of neurons and a paucity of neurons in the superficial layers in the rostral and intermediate portions of the entorhinal cortex of the parahippocampal gyrus, which they attributed to faulty neuronal migration. Benes et al. (1991) reported a decreased density of interneurons in the prefrontal, anterior cingulate, and primary motor cortex of the brains of schizophrenic patients, findings that could indicate an accelerated process of neuronal cell death. Akbarian et al. (1996) found selective displacement of interneurons in the frontal lobe cortex, including decreased cell density in the superficial white matter and increased cell density in the deeper white matter, findings also thought consistent with an alteration in the migration of subplate neurons or in the pattern of programmed cell death.

Neuropathology has also been used to explore whether abnormalities can be found in key candidate regions such as the thalamus, prefrontal cortex, and temporal lobe. Pakkenberg (1990) noted decreased cell density in the medial dorsal nucleus of the thalamus, a crucial nucleus that projects to the prefrontal cortex. Thalamic abnormalities have also been noted in other neuropathological studies (Bogerts 1993). Selemon et al. (1995) also demonstrated increased cell packing density in the prefrontal cortex in schizophrenic patients, consistent with a loss of the surrounding neuropil and consequent shrinkage of the interneuronal space. Benes et al. (1998) found decreased number and density of interneurons in a select region of the hippocampal formation.

Thus, a convergence of findings is beginning to emerge from the variable perspectives of structural and functional neuroimaging and neuropathology. These perspectives are all consistent with neurodevelopmental mechanisms and with abnormalities in frontal, temporal, and thalamic regions.

Neurophysiology

Braff (1993) developed a cognitive model of schizophrenia by using neurophysiological paradigms to examine sensory gating. Prepulse inhibition is a technique that measures gating of the startle response that can be triggered by a bright light or loud auditory stimulus; in healthy subjects the startle response can be diminished (inhibited) if a weak prepulse stimulus is delivered in the same modality. Patients with schizophrenia have impaired prepulse inhibition, which occurs across a broad range of stimulus intensities (Grillon et al. 1992). A related paradigm, gating of the P50 evoked potential by a prepulse stimulus, has also been shown to be impaired in schizophrenic patients (e.g., Judd et al. 1992). Waldo et al. (1994) have also shown impairment in P50 gating in unaffected family members of patients with schizophrenia, raising the possibility that this could be used as a trait or vulnerability measure. P50 suppression in healthy individuals is disrupted by amphetamine, an indirect dopamine agonist (Light et al. 1999). Schizophrenia patients receiving atypical neuroleptics show P50 suppression in the normal range, whereas those receiving typical neuroleptics have impaired suppression (Light et al. 2000).

Schizophrenia patients frequently display abnormal smooth-pursuit eye movements (SPEM). This is a disorder of the visual tracking of smoothly moving targets and has been consistently observed in schizophrenic patients for nearly 90 years. Some experts believe that abnormal SPEM may represent a biological marker for schizophrenia, because it has been observed in patients with remitted schizophrenia and schizotypal personality disorder and is more frequently found in relatives of schizophrenic patients than in the general population (Holzman et al. 1984; Thacker et al. 1996). Abnormal SPEM is more common in schizophrenic patients with predominantly negative or deficit symptoms (Ross et al. 1996). A similar abnormality in visual fixation that may have greater familial specificity than SPEM has also been reported (Amador et al. 1991). When administered to healthy individuals, ketamine, an *N*-methyl-D-aspartate (NMDA) antagonist, not only induces schizophrenia-like perceptual and cognitive aberrations but also reproduces some of the SPEM abnormalities characteristic of schizophrenia (Radant et al. 1998; Weiler et al. 2000).

Classical eyeblink conditioning involves the paired presentation of a neutral conditioned stimulus (CS), usually an audio tone, followed by an unconditioned stimulus (US), usually an air puff across the eye. The US evokes an unconditioned response (UR), which is the eyeblink. When the paired CS and US are repeatedly presented, the subject "learns" to blink prior to the US. Abnormalities in classical eyeblink conditioning have been reported in patients with schizophrenia (Sears et al. 2000). The neural circuitry underlying classical eyeblink conditioning depends crucially on the cerebellum, which is increasingly recognized to be important in cognition (Leiner et al. 1986). Disruption in the cortico-cerebellar-thalamic-cortical circuit may produce "cognitive dysmetria" that underlies the syndrome of schizophrenia.

These four neurophysiological measures are candidate phenotypic markers of schizophrenia, and their use in genetic studies and for the early identification of schizophrenia are being investigated. Prepulse inhibition, which can be readily modeled in animals, has also been used to study the effects of medications. It has demonstrated that the cortical-striatal-pallidal-thalamic circuitry plays a key role in modulating startle response in rats. Dopamine agonists such as apomorphine can also lead to loss of sensory gating. Both typical and atypical antipsychotic medications restore prepulse inhibition in apomorphine-treated rats in a profile that correlates with their clinical efficacy. Therefore, prepulse inhibitor may serve as a screen for neuroleptic medications (Swerdlow and Geyer 1993).

Neurodevelopment

Several lines of evidence support the thesis that schizophrenia is a neurodevelopmental disorder resulting from neuronal injury occurring early in life that interferes with normal brain maturation (Andreasen et al. 1986; Feinberg 1982; Weinberger 1987). As described earlier, MRI studies have shown an increased rate of neurodevelopmental brain anomalies in this illness. The observation that perinatal complications often precede the development of severe neurological and psychological disorders, such as cerebral palsy and mental retardation, have led investigators to explore the role of perinatal and obstetrical complications in the etiology of schizophrenia. Schizophrenic patients are more likely to have a history of obstetrical complications than are other psychiatric patients or healthy control subjects (Geddes and Lawrie 1995). Prematurity, oxygen deprivation, and long labor are especially common complications. McNeil and Kaij (1978) observed that among monozygotic twins discordant for schizophrenia, the co-twin with schizophrenia is more likely to have suffered an obstetrical complication. Schizophrenic patients with a history of obstetrical complications are also more likely to exhibit minor physical anomalies (O'Callaghan et al. 1991). Minor physical anomalies (slight anatomic defects of the head, hands, feet, and face) are relatively common in schizophrenia patients and are themselves believed to reflect abnormal neurodevelopment (Green et al. 1994).

Several groups of investigators have looked at the relationship between obstetrical complications and cerebral ventricular size. Turner et al. (1986) reported that ventricular size was positively correlated with obstetrical complications in a small sample of first-episode schizophrenic patients. Pearlson et al. (1985) similarly found that perinatal complications were associated with larger ventricles and earlier age at onset. DeLisi et al. (1986) noted that patients with schizophrenia had larger ventricles than their well siblings and that seven of eight schizophrenic patients with ventricles more than one standard deviation larger than the control mean had a history of obstetrical complications or head injury. These studies suggest that obstetrical complications may contribute to neuronal injury and perhaps predispose to the development of schizophrenia in genetically vulnerable persons.

Throughout the temperate northern latitudes, the birth dates of patients with schizophrenia tend to cluster in the winter months (Hare et al. 1973; Mortensen et al. 1999). This finding suggests that a seasonally varying influence (a viral infection, for example) is acting in utero or in early life to cause neurological injury. Thus, children born during the winter months would be more vulnerable to brain injury due to the increased frequency of viral infections. This was the case in the study by Mednick et al. (1988), who reported that individuals who were in their second trimester of fetal development during a 1957 A2 influenza epidemic in Finland were at a higher risk of hospitalization for schizophrenia than those born in the same months over the previous 6 years. The finding was replicated using data from influenza cases reported to the Ministry of Health in Denmark (Barr et al. 1990). In utero exposure to other infectious agents, including to rubella during the first trimester (Brown et al. 2000b) and to maternal respiratory infections in the second trimester (Brown et al. 2000a), has also been associated with increased risk for schizophrenia.

Rh incompatibility, a form of obstetrical complication, could also be a risk factor for schizophrenia. Hollister et al. (1996) reported that the rate of schizophrenia was much higher in Rh-incompatible men than in Rh-compatible men. The authors suggest that hemolytic disease in the newborn resulting from Rh incompatibility may lead to fetal hypoxia, adversely affecting neurodevelopment. Tying maternal influenza, obstetrical complications, and schizophrenia together, Wright et al. (1995) reported that mothers of schizophrenic patients were more likely than control subjects to report both second-trimester influenza and at least one obstetrical complication.

Another interesting lead into the etiology of schizophrenia concerns nutritional factors during gestation. Susser et al. (1996) looked at the development of schizophrenia after prenatal exposure to the Dutch hunger winter of 1944–1945, when the Nazis imposed a complete food blockade against the populous northeastern section of the Netherlands. The average amount of food eaten was less than 1,000 Kcals per day. The incidence of schizophrenia was increased twofold, suggesting the possibility that malnutrition has a detrimental effect on fetal neurodevelopment. A preliminary study examining the brain morphology of schizophrenia subjects with prenatal exposure to the Dutch hunger winter indicated reductions in intracranial volume, although famine alone was associated with increased white matter hyperintensities regardless of subsequent psychiatric illness (Hulshoff Pol et al. 2000).

Neurochemistry and Neuropharmacology

For many years, the most widely accepted explanation for the biochemical pathophysiology of schizophrenia was the *dopamine hypothesis*, which suggests that the disorder is primarily caused by a functional hyperactivity in the dopamine system (Carlsson 1988; K.L. Davis et al. 1991). Much of the support for the dopamine hypothesis arose from the observation that the efficacy of many of the neuroleptic drugs used to treat schizophrenia was highly correlated with their ability to block dopamine D_2 receptors (Creese et al. 1976; Seeman et al. 1976). Conversely, drugs that enhance dopamine transmission, such as the amphetamines, tend to worsen the symptoms of schizophrenia (Snyder 1972). Therefore, the dopamine hypothesis also suggested that the abnormality in this illness might specifically lie in the D_2 receptors. For many years, the "ideal drug" was thought to be a highly specific D_2 blocker.

Recent work in neuropharmacology and chemical anatomy has demonstrated that there are five types of dopamine receptors, which differ in their cerebral distribution. The D_1 receptor is linked to adenylate cyclase and is located in the cortex and basal ganglia. The D_2 receptor is not linked to adenylate cyclase and is prominent in the striatum. The D_3 and D_4 receptors have a higher distribution in limbic regions. This distribution raises questions about the classic dopamine hypothesis, because limbic regions (or, alternately, frontal or temporal regions) have been the presumed target for neuroleptic drug action, yet D_2 receptors are not densely concentrated in these target regions.

Postmortem brain research has documented an increase in D_2 receptors in the caudate and nucleus accumbens in postmortem brains (Clardy et al. 1993). Other postmortem studies have documented increased dopamine or homovanillic acid in these regions as well as the left amygdala in schizophrenic patients (K.L. Davis et al. 1991). There is a concern, however, that these findings may be an artifact of treatment with antipsychotics. Animal work has shown that antipsychotics produce receptor supersensitivity in response to receptor blockade by increasing the number of D_2 receptors available. Consequently, an increase in D_2 receptors in postmortem brains could be a direct consequence of neuroleptic treatment itself.

Recently, PET has provided another way to assess neurochemical transmission in schizophrenia. This work has involved the use of labeled ligands known to bind to D_2 receptors. Two such ligands—^{3}H-labeled spiperone and ^{11}C-labeled raclopride—are currently used. Spiperone binds to both D_1 and D_2 receptors as well as serotonin sites, but raclopride is highly specific for D_2 receptors. Farde et al. (1985) used this technique to demonstrate D_2 receptor blockade in human beings in vivo, using both healthy control subjects and patients with schizophrenia. Early work (Wong et al. 1986) appeared to confirm the presence of increased D_2 receptors in schizophrenia, but the finding was not verified by subsequent research (Farde et al. 1990). These results have also lessened confidence that D_2 receptors alone could explain the symptoms of schizophrenia.

PET has also been used to measure receptor occupancy, providing an in vivo method for directly observing the mechanisms of pharmacological action. This work, taken together with the development of the highly effective atypical antipsychotics, has shed further doubt on a simple D_2 theory of schizophrenia. As described later in the section on treatment, the new atypicals have a very broad pharmacological profile, blocking 5-HT_2, D_1, and some subtypes of adrenergic receptors as well. One study showed that conventional antipsychotics have prominent D_2 occupancy (78%) and no obvious D_1 occupancy, whereas the atypical antipsychotics showed a 48% occupancy of D_2 receptors and a 38%–52% occupancy of D_1 receptors (Farde et al. 1992). This may help to explain why atypical antipsychotics are much less likely to induce extrapyramidal side effects, because patients with these effects have a higher D_2 receptor occupancy than do those without (Farde et al. 1992).

Alternative biochemical hypotheses have been advanced, in part because of the difficulty in confirming the dopamine hypothesis and in the realization that anti-dopaminergic agents are not always effective. More recent hypotheses also include the role of other neurotransmitter systems (e.g., norepinephrine, serotonin, glutamate, γ-aminobutyric acid [GABA]), neuropeptides, and neuromodulatory substances in the pathophysiology of schizophrenia (Meltzer 1987; VanKammen et al. 1990). The development of the new atypical neuroleptics, which have potent effects on serotonin, provides partial confirmation for the importance of additional neurotransmitter systems in schizophrenia, because they not only cause fewer extrapyramidal side effects than conventional antipsychotics but are more effective as well. The observation that phencyclidine intoxication leads to schizophrenia-like manifestations has also stimulated interest in the NMDA receptor complex and the possible role of glutamate in the pathophysiology of schizophrenia (Javitt and Zukin 1991; Olney and Farber 1995).

Social and Family Factors

Theories about the role of society, urbanization, and stress on the development of mental illness, including schizophrenia, were popular during the 1930s and 1940s. In an early study, Faris and Durham (1939) found higher rates for mental hospital admissions, including admissions for schizophrenia, in central slums than in the suburbs. This finding was replicated in other cities in both the United States and Europe. The conclusion was drawn that schizophrenia was caused by the ill effects of a slum environment, where people were faced with enormous stress from social disorganization, poverty, and the general adversity imposed by poor living conditions. These conditions were believed to produce or "breed" schizophrenia (Hare 1956).

Another explanation soon developed to explain the finding of geographic isolation of the severely mentally ill. The drift hypothesis stated that living in poor areas *resulted from* schizophrenia and was not causal (Wender et al. 1973). Rather, because schizophrenia leads to amotivation, cognitive impairment, poor hygiene, and other symptoms that make it impossible for the person with schizophrenia to maintain employment and survive in middle and upper class structures, persons with schizophrenia drift down in social class as their illness progresses. Subsequent research has supported this view. Silverton and Mednick (1984) found, for example, that patients with schizophrenia have lower social status on average than their parents.

The social isolation frequently experienced by schizophrenic patients has also been suggested as a cause of schizophrenia. However, social isolation typically occurs before illness onset. For reasons of economics and personal choice, persons with schizophrenia tend to live alone, often segregated in certain areas. On the other hand, schizophrenic patients who live with their relatives are more evenly distributed among residential areas (Gerard and Houston 1953) and are less likely to experience downward drift in social class.

Studies of mental illness in immigrants have found a high rate of psychotic disorders (Malzberg 1964), including schizophrenia. Although it was originally believed that the stress of migration caused or contributed to the onset of mental illness, later studies showed that immigrants were more likely to come from low social classes and that immigrant populations were overrepresented with severe mental illness including schizophrenia (Murphy 1977).

Clinical Management

Antipsychotic Medication

Antipsychotic medication has been the mainstay of treatment for schizophrenia since chlorpromazine was introduced in 1952. In fact, these agents are probably responsible in large measure for the deinstitutionalization that occurred in the 1950s and 1960s. Because these medications were so effective, large numbers of patients were able to leave psychiatric hospitals. In 1955, for instance, over one-half million hospital beds were filled by the chronic mentally ill, mainly schizophrenic patients; by the early 1990s the number of beds had been reduced to 103,000 (Lamb 1993).

All antipsychotics are superior to placebo in the treatment of schizophrenia. Controlled studies have not supported use of a specific agent for a specific subtype of schizophrenia, nor is there any benefit from prescribing more than a single antipsychotic at a time. Although these drugs are effective in controlling acute psychosis and provide long-term relapse prevention, they are not curative. The putative mechanism of action of antipsychotic drugs is their ability to block postsynaptic dopamine D_2 receptors in the limbic forebrain. This blockade is thought to initiate a series of events responsible for both acute and chronic therapeutic actions. Whereas these drugs block dopamine D_2 receptors almost immediately, onset of antipsychotic action takes weeks to develop. Recent research findings suggest that clinical response corresponds with the degree of D_2 receptor occupancy (Farde et al. 1992), with increased likelihood of symptomatic improvement when D_2 occupancy exceeds 65% (Kapur et al. 2000). Besides being dopamine-receptor antagonists, these drugs also block noradrenergic, cholinergic, histaminic, and serotonergic receptors to differing degrees, accounting for the unique side-effect profile of each agent.

During the 1990s, several second-generation or "atypical" antipsychotics have been introduced that represent the most important advance in the treatment of schizophrenia since the introduction of chlorpromazine. Clozapine, risperidone, olanzapine, quetiapine, and ziprasidone are now available for clinical use in the United States, and some (except clozapine) have become first-line therapy for schizophrenia. Not only do these second-generation antipsychotics appear to be more effective than first-generation antipsychotics in reducing positive and negative symptoms, but they may also be superior in improving depression (Tollefson et al. 1998) and decreasing cognitive dysfunction in schizophrenia (Keefe et al. 1999). However, two recent meta-analyses have raised questions about the superior efficacy of these newer antipsychotics. Although Leucht et al. (1999) found that olanzapine- and risperidone-treated patients showed greater overall improvement than patients who received conventional antipsychotics, the authors questioned the clinical relevance of the improvement because the effect sizes were modest. Geddes et al. (2000) reported that the advantage for atypical antipsychotics

was observed only when the doses of comparative conventional antipsychotics (haloperidol or chlorpromazine) were relatively high. When the authors analyzed studies in which the mean doses of haloperidol were less than 12 mg/day, the efficacy and dropout rates of the newer atypical antipsychotics were no better than those of lower doses of haloperidol.

Nevertheless, these second-generation antipsychotics still represent a major advance in the treatment of schizophrenia. They are clearly more tolerable than conventional antipsychotics, especially because of their lower propensity to induce extrapyramidal side effects and possibly tardive dyskinesia. Extrapyramidal side effects result from blockade of the nigrostriatal D_2 receptors, and the likelihood of extrapyramidal side effects increases when receptor occupancy exceeds 78% (Kapur et al. 2000). The atypical antipsychotics also block serotonin 5-HT$_{2A}$ receptors in the frontal cortex and striatal system, which may help protect against the development of extrapyramidal side effects as well (Meltzer et al. 1989). However, more recent data from neuroimaging and animal studies suggest that the lower propensity to cause extrapyramidal side effects in this group of antipsychotics may be related to their fast dissociation from D_2 receptors (Kapur and Seeman 2001). Although the atypical antipsychotics are associated with fewer extrapyramidal side effects, other side effects, including weight gain (Allison et al. 1999), impaired glucose tolerance, and dyslipidemia (Goldstein et al. 1999; Henderson et al. 2000), have come to attention. This information poses new challenges for the pharmacotherapy of schizophrenia. The type and severity of these side effects vary among the various second-generation medications.

Another challenge in the treatment of schizophrenia is that approximately 10%–20% of patients respond poorly to antipsychotic drugs, with the quality of response varying from patient to patient (Carpenter and Buchanan 1994). Clozapine remains the "gold standard" in treatment-refractory patients (Chakos et al. 2001). Clozapine was first used in the mid-1970s, but early reports of agranulocytosis in 1%–2% of patients delayed its introduction in the United States. A multicenter clinical trial (Kane et al. 1988) found that about 30% of inpatients with schizophrenia who had failed to respond to traditional antipsychotics responded to clozapine within 4–6 weeks; up to 60% may respond within 4–6 months (Schooler et al. 1995). There is preliminary evidence to suggest that risperidone and olanzapine may also be more effective than conventional antipsychotics in treatment-refractory patients (Conley et al. 1998; Wirshing et al. 1999).

Treatment of Acute Psychosis

Most acutely psychotic schizophrenic patients will respond to a daily dose between 10 and 15 mg of haloperidol (or its equivalent) within several days or weeks (Kane and Marder 1993). Higher dosages of conventional antipsychotics may be needed in some patients, but controlled studies have not shown an advantage to either rapid loading or sustained high dosages. Furthermore, higher dosages will increase the likelihood of adverse side effects. For example, in one study (McEvoy et al. 1991), acutely psychotic schizophrenic patients were given relatively low doses (generally from 2 to 6 mg) of haloperidol for 2 weeks, then randomly assigned to a dosage 2–10 times higher or to the same dosage for another 2 weeks. Higher dosages caused significantly more extrapyramidal side effects, but not greater improvement in measures of psychosis. In another study, Rifkin et al. (1991) found no difference in the response of newly admitted schizophrenic patients given 10 mg, 30 mg, or 80 mg of oral haloperidol for 6 weeks. High dosages of atypical antipsychotics also appear unnecessary. In a fixed-dose trial of risperidone (Marder and Meibach 1994), doses of 2 mg, 6 mg, 10 mg, and 16 mg were compared with doses of 20 mg of haloperidol and placebo. All doses of risperidone were effective in relieving the symptoms of schizophrenia, but the 6-mg dose was the most effective and also proved superior to haloperidol.

Measuring plasma levels of antipsychotic drugs can be helpful in selected cases, but there is little to be gained from routine monitoring. Plasma levels are most useful 1) in patients who have failed to respond to conventional doses, 2) when antipsychotic medications are combined with other drugs that can affect their pharmacokinetics (e.g., carbamazepine), and 3) to assess compliance. The very young, the elderly, or the medically compromised patient with schizophrenia may also benefit from plasma level monitoring. Because of the difficulties involved in correlating plasma levels and response, research results are not entirely consistent. Nonetheless, levels of haloperidol between 5 and 18 ng/mL (P.J. Perry and Smith 1993), levels of fluphenazine between 0.6 and 1.5 ng/mL (Levinson et al. 1995), and levels of clozapine approaching 350 ng/mL (VanderZwaag et al. 1996) appear effective for most patients. Plasma levels of many other antipsychotic drugs can be reliably measured, but attempts to correlate responses with levels have not been successful.

A high-potency conventional antipsychotic (e.g., haloperidol), risperidone (i.e., 4–6 mg daily), or olanzapine (10–20 mg daily) has been recommended as the initial choice for treatment of acute psychosis (American Psychiatric Association 1997). Recent controlled trials have indicated that lower doses of risperidone (2–4 mg daily) are efficacious and are associated with reduced rates of extrapyramidal side effects. The initial starting dose for ziprasidone is 20 mg twice daily with adjustment up to 80–160 mg daily, depending on individual clinical status. The dose–efficacy relationship for quetiapine has been less clear, although 400–600 mg daily is recommended as the therapeutic dose for most patients. If no response is observed after 3–8 weeks, one of the other drugs should be tried. If a patient shows a partial response to the initial antipsychotic at 3 weeks, the trial should be extended another 2–9 weeks (Expert Consensus Guideline Series Steering Committee 1996). In this algorithm, clozapine is a second-line choice because of its expense and propensity to cause agranulocytosis.

Highly agitated patients require rapid control of their symptoms and should be given frequent, equally spaced doses of an antipsychotic drug. High-potency antipsychotic medications (e.g., haloperidol) may be given every 30–120 minutes orally or intramuscularly until the agitation is under control (Dubin et al. 1985). Rarely is more than 20–30 mg of haloperidol required in a 24-hour period, and lower doses are optimal. It is likely that haloperidol's effectiveness in subduing patients results from sedation rather than from any specific antipsychotic effect. Because sedation is desired, a combination of antipsychotic medication and a benzodiazepine may work even better for the rapid control of agitated psychotic patients. In one study (Garza-Trevino et al. 1989), doses of haloperidol (5 mg) and lorazepam (4 mg) were administered and repeated every 30 minutes. Most patients achieved tranquilization after the initial dose. The average time required to achieve a satisfactory response was 60 minutes. Once the patient has calmed down, the benzodiazepine can be gradually withdrawn. Although rapid sedation may also be achieved with administration of droperidol (5–10 mg im) (Slaby and Moreines 1990), the potential side effects of severe hypotension and QT prolongation necessitate caution when using this agent.

Maintenance Therapy

Patients benefiting from short-term treatment with antipsychotic medications are candidates for long-term prophylactic treatment, which has as its goal the sustained control of psychotic symptoms. To minimize the risk of side effects, particularly tardive dyskinesia, an often irreversible movement disorder, the lowest effective antipsychotic dose should be used. In a review of 35 well-designed studies of relapse rates, J.M. Davis et al. (1993)

provided in a day hospital program or contact with a visiting home nurse. Some patients may be self-sufficient and employed, whereas others may require around-the-clock care for extended periods in the hospital. Furthermore, patients may require one type of intervention early in the course of illness and different interventions in later stages, when clinical symptoms have changed. Clinicians must work actively to ensure that patients with schizophrenia receive adequate mental health care and community benefits and are encouraged to develop a close working relationship with their local social service agencies. Although optimal care necessitates the availability of a range of services to fit the needs of the patient, including social, vocational, and housing needs, these services are inadequate in many communities (Lamb 1986). A recent study indicates that the provision of psychosocial treatments for patients with schizophrenia is generally less optimal than provision of pharmacological treatments (Lehman et al. 1998a).

During the past 20 years, significant changes have occurred in the way that treatment of schizophrenia is conceptualized. In the 1960s and 1970s, much emphasis was given to repeated hospital stays for the pharmacological treatment of psychotic episodes. As hospitalizations became briefer and more restricted, the locus of treatment shifted to outpatient settings and the community. At the same time, it became clear that insight-oriented psychotherapy not only was ineffective in treating schizophrenia but also had the potential to worsen its symptoms (Mueser and Berenbaum 1990). Newer psychosocial treatment models have been developed that emphasize the practical resolution of common social and psychological difficulties seen in schizophrenic patients. Meanwhile, older models involving family therapy have received greater prominence. Family interventions are especially important because they have a direct impact on relapse rates. It is now clear that combining pharmacological treatment with psychosocial interventions offers advantages beyond the power of any single approach. Most clinicians understand the importance of integrated treatment approaches. For example, common sense tells us that although medication will not teach patients social skills, or to budget and shop for themselves, it may facilitate learning by diminishing psychotic symptoms.

Locus of Care

Patients with schizophrenia are rarely placed in long-term custodial institutions today, because the locus of care has shifted to outpatient clinics and the community. Patients, their families, and society at large have benefited from this shift, as greater emphasis has been placed on outpatient management and brief hospital stays. Patients are able to achieve greater degrees of independence and have more opportunities to participate in community life. But many communities have been unable to provide the kind of integrated and coordinated system of care that patients need to reduce risk of relapse and enhance functioning.

Hospitalization

Hospitalization is reserved for patients with schizophrenia who pose a danger to themselves or others; patients who refuse to properly care for themselves (e.g., refuse food or fluids); and patients requiring special medical observation, tests, or treatments (Table 9–11). When a patient is a danger to himself or others and refuses to enter the hospital, it is usually necessary to obtain a court order for hospitalization. When hospitalized, schizophrenic patients stay briefly in special psychiatric hospitals or in psychiatric units found in general hospitals. Stays are short (e.g., days to weeks), and the patient is generally returned to the community.

TABLE 9–11. Reasons to hospitalize patients with schizophrenia

When the illness is new, to rule out alternative diagnoses and to stabilize the dose of antipsychotic medication

For special medical procedures such as electroconvulsive therapy

When aggressive or assaultive behavior presents a danger to the patient or others

When the patient becomes suicidal

When the patient is unable to properly care for himself or herself (e.g., refuses to eat or take fluids)

When medication side effects become disabling or potentially life threatening (e.g., severe pseudoparkinsonism, severe tardive dyskinesia, neuroleptic malignant syndrome)

An active ward milieu is superior to a custodial one in the hospital, especially if well structured and not overly stimulating (Maxmen 1984). The following characteristics have been found optimal: small units, short stays, high staff-to-patient ratio, low staff turnover, low percentage of psychotic patients, broad delegation of responsibility with clear lines of authority, low perceived levels of anger and aggression, high levels of support, and a practical problem-solving approach (Ellsworth 1983). Token economies in which patients are provided a high degree of ward structure and are rewarded for desired behaviors seem to be effective in controlling behavior in the hospital, but this improvement often does not generalize to situations outside the hospital.

Partial Hospitalization/Day Treatment

Partial hospitalization programs may provide an alternative to inpatient treatment for acutely psychotic patients or allow for further stabilization following inpatient care. Day treatment programs, on the other hand, provide more continuous structure and support for the more severely impaired patients and assist such patients in maintaining stability within the community and in relapse prevention. Both types of programs generally operate on weekdays, with patients returning home on evenings and weekends. Psychopharmacological management is provided along with psychosocial rehabilitation. With most programs, the services provided and frequency of attendance will be individualized to fit the needs of the patient (Gudeman et al. 1983).

Outpatient Care

The outpatient clinic will be the locus of treatment for most schizophrenic patients and is the most appropriate setting in which to coordinate care. A well-equipped clinic should be able to provide close monitoring of patients for relapse detection and prevention through careful medication management, to provide both individual or group counseling and psychoeducation, to arrange family interventions, and to arrange special programmatic interventions such as social skills training or cognitive rehabilitation. Case managers should be available to help coordinate the patients' care and to help them access governmental programs to which they may be entitled.

Assertive Community Treatment

A treatment modality available in some areas is assertive community treatment (ACT; Stein 1993), which consists of careful monitoring of patients, the availability of mobile mental health teams, and aggressive programming individually tailored to each patient. ACT programs operate 24 hours a day and have been shown to reduce hospital admission rates and to improve quality of life for many schizophrenic patients (i.e., patients report greater satisfaction and are more likely to be employed and living independently). ACT involves teaching patients basic living skills, helping patients work with community agencies, and assisting patients in developing a social support network. Voluntary job placement and supported work settings (i.e., sheltered workshops) are an important part of the program.

Supportive Housing

Appropriate and affordable housing is a major concern for many patients, and depending on the community, options may range from supervised shelters and group homes ("halfway houses") to boarding homes to supervised apartment living. Group homes provide peer support and companionship, along with on-site staff supervision. Supervised apartments offer greater independence with the availability and support of trained staff. Clearly, not all patients with schizophrenia will be able to take advantage of sheltered care residences. Persons with greater levels of impairment may need round-the-clock supervision in a nursing home (Lamberti and Tariot 1995).

Self-Help Organizations

In addition to more formal family interventions, self-help organizations for family members can be enormously beneficial. They provide a forum for family members to obtain information about schizophrenia, to gain encouragement from others, and to learn how to cope with its manifestations. The best-known group in the United States is the Alliance for the Mentally Ill (AMI), and local chapters can be found in many communities. Many other countries have similar national organizations (e.g., the Schizophrenia Fellowship of Canada or Great Britain) that emphasize education, advocacy, mutual support, and self-help.

Specific Psychosocial Interventions

Individual Psychotherapy

The treatment most commonly received by patients with schizophrenia may be the combination of antipsychotic medication with some form of "individual psychotherapy" (Dixon et al. 1999; Fenton 2000). Although intensive psychodynamic- and insight-oriented psychotherapy is generally not recommended, the form of individual psychotherapy that psychiatrists employ when providing pharmacological treatment typically involves a synthesis of various psychotherapeutic strategies and interventions. These include problem solving, reality testing, psychoeducation, and supportive and cognitive-behavioral techniques anchored on an empathetic therapeutic alliance with the patient. The specific approach or combination of approaches used often depends on the patient's clinical condition. The goals of such individual psychotherapy are to improve medication compliance, enhance social and occupational functioning, and prevent relapse. Although combining some form of individual psychotherapy with pharmacological management may seem clinically prudent, there is little to no evidential basis regarding its efficacy.

In contrast, there is a growing body of evidence of the efficacy of cognitive-behavioral therapy (CBT) in schizophrenia, particularly for ameliorating residual psychotic symptoms (Sensky et al. 2000; Tarrier et al. 1993). Initial CBT studies focused on changing the schizophrenic patient's abnormal thoughts (e.g., delusions) or his or her responses to them. Through structured and systematic reality testing, CBT allows patients to collaboratively test alternative explanations to their delusional beliefs and to work toward belief modification. Patients also learn various behavioral coping strategies, such as listening to music to mask auditory hallucinations. Recent randomized controlled trials have extended to testing other CBT techniques, including the use of paced activity scheduling and diary recording of mastery and pleasure to target negative symptoms.

Family Interventions

When combined with antipsychotic medication, family therapy has been demonstrated to reduce relapse rates in schizophrenia. Carpenter (1996) reviewed 14 controlled trials and reported that relapse rates ranged from 40% to 53% in the control condition, compared with 6%–23% in the experimental condition (i.e., family therapy). Although family therapy may gain some of its impact through enhanced medication compliance, it may also help to protect the schizophrenic patient from the demands of the "real world" by providing improved social support, structure, and guidance.

Although the exact mechanism of improvement in family therapy is unknown, and no specific approach is better than another (Penn and Mueser 1996), several recommendations can be made. First, families can benefit from education about schizophrenia itself. This should include information about the chronic nature of the disorder and the need for long-term care based on realistic expectations. Education will improve cooperation and compliance of both patient and family. However, education needs to be combined with other family interventions aimed at improving communication and learning to minimize criticism and emotional overinvolvement—interventions that will help to decrease the schizophrenic patient's level of stress. Gaining a more realistic appraisal of the patient's illness and future expectations will reduce expressed emotion, which, as discussed earlier in the chapter, has been shown to lead to schizophrenic relapse. Family therapy also benefits family members and can help to reduce their feelings of anger, frustration, and helplessness. In addition to education and family support, the Schizophrenia Patient Outcomes Research Team further recommends that family psychosocial interventions provide crisis intervention and training in problem-solving skills (Lehman et al. 1998b). Research shows that multiple-family groups may work even better than single-family interventions (McFarlane et al. 1995).

Group Therapy

Group therapy is frequently used with schizophrenic patients to provide emotional support in a setting where a patient can learn social skills and develop friendships. Groups that are most successful are highly structured and set limited goals (Yalom 1983). Traditional group-therapy approaches that encourage self-exploration and the seeking of insight are generally countertherapeutic (Kanas 1985). This is particularly true with psychotic or highly paranoid individuals, who might misinterpret situations that arise in group therapy.

Psychosocial Rehabilitation

Psychosocial rehabilitation is a term used to describe services that aim to restore the patient's ability to function in the community. It may include the medical and psychosocial treatments described above, but it may also involve ways to foster social interaction, to promote independent living, and to encourage vocational performance (Cook et al. 1996). Patients are encouraged to become involved in developing and implementing their rehabilitation plan, which has as its focus enhancing the patient's talents and skills. The goal of psychosocial rehabilitation is to integrate patients back into the community rather than segregating them in separate facilities, as has occurred in the past. In many locations, patient clubhouses are available to promote psychosocial rehabilitation, such as Fountain House, a program in New York City that patients help to run. The organization serves various functions, including providing job training, social and leisure-time activities, residential assistance, and skills training (Beard et al. 1982).

Social Skills Training

Because social and interpersonal skills are generally deficient in patients with schizophrenia, social skills training aims to help the patient develop more appropriate behaviors. This is accomplished by using modeling and social reinforcement and by providing opportunities, both individual and group, to practice the new behaviors. This could be as simple as helping the patient learn to maintain eye contact or as complicated as helping him learn conversational skills. Research has shown that social skills training can significantly enhance social functioning, but probably has little effect on risk of relapse (Marder et al. 1996). The best results appear to occur in patients with early-onset schizophrenia whose social development would have been disrupted by the emergence of illness and in persons who persist in a training program for more than 1 year (Penn and Mueser 1996). However, the generalizability of social skills training remains uncertain, because there has been limited evidence that patients are able to apply their acquired social skills in real-life situations (Heinssen et al. 2000).

Vocational Rehabilitation

Vocational training and support can also be of enormous benefit to patients with schizophrenia in helping to "mainstream" them back into the community. Research shows that vocational interventions can be effective in helping patients find and maintain paid jobs (Lehman 1995). Vocational rehabilitation may involve supported employment, competitive work in integrated settings, and more formal job training programs. The best initial setting may be a simple, repetitive job environment offering both interpersonal distance and on-site supervision, such as that found in a "sheltered workshop." Although some patients will not be employable in any setting because of apathy, amotivation, or chronic psychosis, employment should be encouraged in able patients. A job will serve to improve self-esteem, bring in additional income, and provide a social outlet for the patient (Mackota and Lamb 1989). Gradually, a patient may move toward a more demanding work setting, although the clinician should help the patient develop appropriate goals. Failure will only diminish a patient's already shaky self-esteem and reinforce the "sick" role. Assessment by a vocational guidance counselor will be helpful in matching patients with appropriate jobs by gaining a better understanding of the patient's abilities, aptitudes, and interests.

Cognitive Rehabilitation

Cognitive rehabilitation has as its goal the remediation of abnormal thought processes known to occur in schizophrenia (Penn and Mueser 1996) and uses techniques pioneered in the treatment of brain-injured persons. Work with schizophrenic patients is focused on improving information-processing skills such as attention, memory, vigilance, and conceptual abilities. Early studies have yielded mixed results but suggest that performance on specific tasks (e.g., Wisconsin Card Sorting Test) can be improved. Whether improvement on specific tasks can generalize to other situations and which cognitive deficits are most appropriate targets for rehabilitation still need further study (Bellack et al. 1999).

Alcohol/Drug Abuse Treatment

Alcohol and other drug abuse is a significant problem for many schizophrenic patients and needs to be a focus of concern. Substance abuse or dependence aggravates the symptoms of schizophrenia, leads to medication noncompliance, and undermines other treatment interventions. Abstinence should be encouraged in all patients, and some will need referral for drug detoxification and rehabilitation (Ziedonis and Fisher 1994). Although these services may not be helpful in acutely psychotic or agitated patients, they may be enormously beneficial once the patient has improved and the schizophrenic illness has stabilized. Disulfiram should be used with caution because it inhibits dopamine-β-hydroxylase, increasing the dopamine available to the central nervous system, and may exacerbate psychotic symptoms (Kingsbury and Salzman 1990).

Schizoaffective Disorder

Conceptual Issues

The concept of schizoaffective disorder attempts to define patients who have features of both schizophrenia and affective disorders. Kasanin (1933) coined the term *acute schizoaffective psychosis* to describe patients with acute onset of "emotional turmoil" and distorted perceptions, usually precipitated by a "difficult environmental situation." Although Kasanin believed schizoaffective psychosis to be a subtype of dementia praecox, these patients were different in that they were well adjusted premorbidly, recovered following weeks or months of psychosis, and were able to attain good social and occupational functioning subsequently.

Schizoaffective disorder is an inherently difficult construct because it is an intermediate category that straddles the boundaries of schizophrenia and mood disorder. Confusion surrounding the term has persisted despite operationalized diagnostic criteria. In fact, profound shifts in its definition over the years (i.e., from the Research Diagnostic Criteria [Spitzer et al. 1978] to DSM-III [American Psychiatric Association 1980], DSM-III-R [American Psychiatric Association 1987], DSM-IV [American Psychiatric Association 1994], and ICD-10 [World Health Organization 1992]) may have added to the confusion. Within the current nomenclature, ICD-10 conceptualizes schizoaffective disorder as *episodic*, whereas DSM-IV describes an *uninterrupted* illness in which the characteristic symptoms of schizophrenia are present concurrently with a depressive syndrome, a manic syndrome, or a mixed episode (Table 9–12). During the illness, more than 2 weeks of delusions or hallucinations in the absence of prominent affective symptoms are required, helping to set schizoaffective disorder apart from psychotic depression or mania. In addition, affective symptoms need to be present for a substantial portion of the total duration of the illness so as to differentiate it from schizophrenia, in which mood symptoms are generally present for brief periods. Investigators have found the interrater reliability of the DSM-IV schizoaffective disorder diagnostic category to be low (Maj et al. 2000). The validity of the schizoaffective disorder construct, as well as its division into depressive and bipolar subtypes, has also been questioned (Kendler et al. 1995; Maj et al. 2000).

TABLE 9–12. DSM-IV-TR diagnostic criteria for schizoaffective disorder

A. An uninterrupted period of illness during which, at some time, there is either a major depressive episode, a manic episode, or a mixed episode concurrent with symptoms that meet Criterion A for schizophrenia.
   Note: The major depressive episode must include Criterion A1: depressed mood.
B. During the same period of illness, there have been delusions or hallucinations for at least 2 weeks in the absence of prominent mood symptoms.
C. Symptoms that meet criteria for a mood episode are present for a substantial portion of the total duration of the active and residual periods of the illness.
D. The disturbance is not due to the direct physiological effects of a substance (e.g., a drug of abuse, a medication) or a general medical condition.
Specify type:
   Bipolar Type: if the disturbance includes a manic or a mixed episode (or a manic or a mixed episode and major depressive episodes)
   Depressive Type: if the disturbance only includes major depressive episodes

---

At least five conceptual models have been proposed to explain the coexistence of schizophrenic and affective symptoms in the same person: 1) all schizoaffective patients have "true" schizophrenia with incidental affective symptoms; 2) all schizoaffective patients have "true" affective disorder with incidental schizophrenia symptoms; 3) schizoaffective disorder patients are a heterogeneous group consisting of "true" schizophrenia and "true" mood disorder patients; 4) all schizoaffective patients have both schizophrenia and affective disorder; and 5) schizoaffective disorder represents a distinct third psychotic illness (Brockington and Meltzer 1983). In all likelihood, schizoaffective disorder probably constitutes a heterogeneous group within which some patients have schizophrenia and others have mood disorders.

Epidemiology

Relatively little is known about the incidence, prevalence, demographic factors, or risk factors associated with schizoaffective disorder. This is in part related to differing definitions of schizoaffective disorder used in various studies. The prevalence of schizoaffective disorder has been estimated to be less than 1% in the general population, but the prevalence in patient populations is often much higher. It appears to occur more often in women than in men. Family studies have shown an increased risk for both schizophrenia and mood disorders among the relatives of schizoaffective patients.

Course and Prognosis

The course of schizaffective disorder is variable, with recovery rates ranging widely (between 29% and 83%). Approximately 20%–30% of patients show a deteriorating course with persistent psychotic symptoms, whereas in another 10% of patients the relative prominence of affective and schizophrenic symptoms may shift over time. Psychotic and affective symptoms can be present concurrently or in an alternating fashion. Psychosis can be either mood congruent or mood incongruent. In general, the prognosis of patients with schizoaffective disorder is intermediate between that of schizophrenia and that of affective disorder patients. Some studies have indicated that outcomes in patients with the bipolar subtype of schizoaffective disorder may be more similar to outcomes in those with bipolar affective disorder, whereas outcomes in the depressive subtype are more akin to those in schizophrenia. Predictors of poor outcome in schizoaffective disorder include poor premorbid functioning, insidious onset, absence of a precipitating factor, predominance of psychotic symptoms, early age at onset, poor interepisode recovery, and a family history of schizophrenia.

Pharmacological Management

Systematic pharmacological treatment studies of schizoaffective disorder represent a relatively neglected area of research. Patients with schizoaffective disorder often end up with complex pharmacological regimens as clinicians attempt to target both psychotic and affective symptoms. There is no clear evidence that any one pharmacological strategy is superior to the others, whether during acute or maintenance treatment: antipsychotic monotherapy, mood-stabilizer monotherapy (lithium, carbamazepine, sodium valproate), antidepressant monotherapy, or combinations (antipsychotic with a mood stabilizer, antipsychotic with an antidepressant). Acute treatment usually requires antipsychotics, because most acutely ill patients have prominent psychotic symptoms. With little evidence from controlled studies, the choice of maintenance strategy is often guided by the subtype of schizoaffective disorder; for example, mood stabilizers may be used in patients with the bipolar subtype, antidepressants in those with the depressive subtype, and antipsychotics in patients with persistent psychosis. There is preliminary evidence that atypical antipsychotics may have mood-stabilizing properties, which suggests that this class may provide the ideal monotherapy for patients with schizoaffective disorder (Keck et al. 1999). In patients with treatment-refractory illness, a trial of clozapine should be considered.

Delusional Disorder

Delusional disorder is characterized by the presence of systematized, nonbizarre delusions accompanied by affect appropriate to the delusion. Personality is generally spared, but the delusion may preoccupy and dominate the patient's life.

Historical Overview

The term *paranoia* was used by the Greeks nearly 2,000 years ago to describe insanity or "craziness" and can be literally translated as "a mind beside itself." The term was revived in the early nineteenth century by German psychiatrists who were interested in disorders characterized by delusions of persecution and grandeur (A. Lewis 1970; Tanna 1974). Karl Kahlbaum (1828–1899) first applied the term to a chronic delusional disorder. Kraepelin, like Kahlbaum, was concerned with longitudinal course and gradually altered his formulation of paranoia. By the eighth revision of his *Lehrbuch der Psychiatrie*, he had restricted the term to describe persons with systematized delusions, an absence of hallucinations, and a prolonged course without recovery but not leading to mental deterioration (Kendler 1988). Kraepelin also identified paraphrenia as an intermediate group of paranoid disorders between dementia praecox and paranoia characterized by unremitting systematized delusions and hallucinations without progression to dementia. The latter term is still used in Britain. Both Kraepelin and Bleuler believed that paranoia was a condition distinct from dementia praecox, although unlike Kraepelin, Bleuler maintained that hallucinations occurred in some patients.

Ernst Kretschmer (1888–1964) regarded paranoia as a psychogenic reaction occurring in people with sensitive personalities rather than as an organic illness.

Delusional disorder, as represented in DSM-IV-TR, resembles the definition put forth by Kraepelin in 1912 for paranoia. The original term for this condition, *paranoid disorder*, which was used in DSM-III, has been abandoned because the word *paranoid* is usually construed to mean "persecutory." Because the delusions found in patients with delusional disorders are not restricted to persecutory themes, the former term was no longer believed appropriate. Kendler (1980) has further proposed that in the absence of hallucinations the term *simple delusional disorder* be used, and that when hallucinations are present the term *hallucinatory delusional disorder* be used.

TABLE 9–13. DSM-IV-TR diagnostic criteria for delusional disorder

A. Nonbizarre delusions (i.e., involving situations that occur in real life, such as being followed, poisoned, infected, loved at a distance, or deceived by spouse or lover, or having a disease) of at least 1 month's duration.

B. Criterion A for schizophrenia has never been met. **Note:** Tactile and olfactory hallucinations may be present in delusional disorder if they are related to the delusional theme.

C. Apart from the impact of the delusion(s) or its ramifications, functioning is not markedly impaired and behavior is not obviously odd or bizarre.

D. If mood episodes have occurred concurrently with delusions, their total duration has been brief relative to the duration of the delusional periods.

E. The disturbance is not due to the direct physiological effects of a substance (e.g., a drug of abuse, a medication) or a general medical condition.

Specify type (the following types are assigned based on the predominant delusional theme):

Erotomanic Type: delusions that another person, usually of higher status, is in love with the individual

Grandiose Type: delusions of inflated worth, power, knowledge, identity, or special relationship to a deity or famous person

Jealous Type: delusions that the individual's sexual partner is unfaithful

Persecutory Type: delusions that the person (or someone to whom the person is close) is being malevolently treated in some way

Somatic Type: delusions that the person has some physical defect or general medical condition

Mixed Type: delusions characteristic of more than one of the above types but no one theme predominates

Unspecified Type

Diagnosis

According to DSM-IV (Table 9–13), delusional disorders are characterized by nonbizarre delusions lasting at least 1 month, behavior that is not obviously odd or bizarre apart from the delusion or its ramifications, absence of active phase symptoms that may occur in schizophrenia (e.g., hallucinations, disorganized speech, negative symptoms), and the determination that the disorder is not due to a mood disorder with psychotic features, is not substance induced, and is not due to a medical condition. The core feature, however, is the presence of a well-systematized, often logical, nonbizarre delusion. The term *systematized* indicates that the delusion and its ramifications fit into an all-encompassing, complex scheme that makes sense to the patient. The term *nonbizarre* implies that the delusion involves situations that can occur in real life, such as being followed, and not implausible or impossible situations, such as having all of one's internal organs replaced by those of bug-eyed Martians. Auditory or visual hallucinations, if present, are not prominent. However, olfactory or tactile hallucinations may be present and prominent.

The diagnostic validity of delusional disorder still remains uncertain (Kendler 1980). It may not be a distinct disease entity that is separate from paranoid schizophrenia or from affective disorders. The symptoms of delusional disorder appear to separate into four independent factors: delusions, hallucinations, depressive symptoms, and irritability (Serretti et al. 1999). Although generally less impaired than patients with schizophrenia, patients with delusional disorder did not differ significantly in terms of clinical, demographic, or neuropsychological measures (Evans et al. 1996). Another study found that the diagnosis of delusional disorder was temporally consistent in only about 50% of the patients (Fennig et al. 1996). This suggests that an initial diagnosis of delusional disorder should be considered as provisional, and that patients need to be reassessed longitudinally.

Differential Diagnosis

A careful assessment is necessary in order to rule out other functional or medical causes for the delusions. This workup should include a physical examination to rule out alcohol-, amphetamine-, cocaine-, and other drug-induced conditions; dementia; and infectious, metabolic, and endocrine disorders (Manschreck 1996). Routine lab tests may be indicated depending on the results of the history and physical examination. CT or MRI may be helpful in selected cases, especially when mass lesions are suspected. Symptom onset, course, and associated features are also relevant. Abrupt changes in mood, mental state, or personality strongly suggest a medical origin. Disturbed consciousness, perceptual disturbances, or physical signs (e.g., fever) may point to specific causes. Isolated paranoid symptoms are often an early sign of medical illness and are especially common among elderly inpatients.

The major diagnostic task remains in separating delusional disorder from mood disorders, schizophrenia, and paranoid personality. The chief distinction is that in delusional disorder a full depressive or manic syndrome is absent, developed after the psychotic symptoms, or was brief in duration relative to the duration of the psychotic symptoms. Unlike schizophrenia, delusional disorder is characterized by nonbizarre delusions and generally either no hallucinations or hallucinations that are not prominent. Furthermore, patients with delusional disorder do not typically develop other schizophrenic symptoms such as incoherence or grossly disorganized behavior, and personality is generally preserved. Persons with paranoid personality are suspicious and hypervigilant, but are not delusional.

Associated features of delusional disorder include anger, social isolation and seclusiveness, eccentric behavior, suspiciousness, hostility, and sometimes violence prompted by the delusion (Kennedy et al. 1992). Winokur (1977) reported that patients with delusional disorders frequently develop sexual problems and depression, and described many as overtalkative and circumstantial. Clinical wisdom suggests that many patients become litigious and end up as lawyers' clients rather than as psychiatrists' patients.

Delusional disorder includes the following DSM-IV-TR subtypes:

1. *Erotomanic type* (de Clerambault's syndrome), in which there is a belief that a person, usually of higher status, is in love with the patient
2. *Grandiose type*, in which there is a belief that one is of inflated worth, power, knowledge, or identity or has a special relation to a deity or famous person
3. *Jealous type*, in which the delusion is that one's sexual partner is unfaithful
4. *Persecutory type*, in which there is a belief that one is being malevolently treated in some way
5. *Somatic type*, in which the delusion is that a person has some physical defect, disorder, or disease, such as AIDS
6. *Mixed type*, in which there is more than one characteristic theme and no one theme predominates
7. *Unspecified type*, in which the patient does not fit any of the previous categories or the dominant delusional belief cannot be clearly determined

The DSM-IV-TR diagnosis of shared psychotic disorder is made when two or more persons share a delusion (*folie à deux*).

The following case example illustrates the jealous subtype of delusional disorder:

Case Example 2

Harvey, a 64-year-old electrician, lived with his wife of 43 years. He voluntarily presented for hospital admission, reporting that he was tired of his wife calling him "crazy." His wife reported that Harvey was chronically jealous, and she was unable to reassure him that she was faithful.

Harvey's family of origin was poor, and his father was alcoholic. Nonetheless, he had achieved good grades in school and participated in sport activities, even though he was considered aloof and distant by his peers. After graduating from high school, he married and joined the Army, serving honorably in World War II. He later worked as an electrician, eventually starting his own business. Although hardworking and honest, he had few friends and was viewed as excessively rigid and humorless by his family. Harvey and his wife had three children, all of whom were healthy and emotionally stable.

Several years after returning from the war, Harvey began to suspect his wife of infidelity. Over the following decades he continued to be convinced that his wife was involved with other men. Although he had never seen her with another man, he was convinced of her infidelity by trivial evidence such as frequently washed bed linen, spots on his wife's undergarments, or unfamiliar tire tracks in the driveway. He once accused his wife of placing sleeping pills in his coffee at night so that after he had fallen asleep she could leave the house for a sexual liaison with a lover. Incredibly, he maintained that several times his wife actually had sexual intercourse with another man in the same bed where he lay sleeping. One particular time, he reported awakening to find the bed sheets in disarray and his shorts pulled down to his knees in what he believed was his wife's lover's attempt to harass him. He also claimed that neighbors had commented to him about the large number of men who visited his wife when he was away on business.

His wife became aware of Harvey's suspiciousness and jealousy early in their marriage, and when confronted by him, she steadfastly maintained that there was no basis for the accusations. No amount of reassurance could alter her husband's convictions. She reported that her husband's jealous beliefs would wax and wane, alternating with periods of relative normalcy. While she continued to love and care for her husband, Harvey's wife admitted that the delusional beliefs had strained the marriage and had led to several trial separations.

In the hospital, Harvey was observed to be friendly with his peers and appropriate with the medical staff. He persisted with the belief that his wife had been unfaithful to him. There was no evidence of hallucinations. A trial of antipsychotic medication did not alter his delusion.

Epidemiology

Delusional disorder constitutes from 1% to 4% of psychiatric admissions and from 2% to 7% of admissions for functional psychosis (Kendler 1982). The incidence of first admissions for paranoia was estimated to fall between 1 and 3 per 100,000 per year and the prevalence to fall between 24 and 30 per 100,000 population. Delusional disorder occurs mainly in middle to late adult life, with a peak frequency of first admissions between 35 and 55 years of age. More women than men develop the disorder, and while 60%–75% of patients are married, up to one-third are widowed, divorced, or separated. Persons with delusional disorder are economically and educationally disadvantaged, and immigrants seem especially prone to develop the disorder. They are also more extroverted, dominant, and hypersensitive premorbidly than are schizophrenic patients, who, as discussed earlier in the chapter, are likely to be introverted and schizoid premorbidly. Once established, delusional disorder is generally chronic and lifelong. However, it appears to have a better long-term prognosis than schizophrenia (Opjordsmoen 1989; Winokur 1977). Remission is reported in one-third to one-half of cases (Jorgensen 1994).

Etiology

The cause of delusional disorder is unknown, although it is unlikely that delusional disorders are related to schizophrenia or the mood disorders. The relatives of probands with delusional disorder show increased rates of jealously, suspiciousness, paranoid personality, and delusional disorder over control relatives, but the families have no increase in schizophrenia or mood disorders (Kendler et al. 1982, 1985a; J.A.G. Watt 1985; Winokur 1985).

Other potentially relevant risk factors for delusional disorder include social isolation and immigration. *Prison psychosis* has been described in which persons placed in solitary confinement have developed a paranoid psychosis. *Migration psychoses*, which are often persecutory, have been described in persons migrating from one country to another (although it is reasonable to assume that persons in whom paranoia is prone to develop may be more likely to emigrate than others). *Querulent paranoia*, a special form of paranoia characterized by litigiousness, is believed by Scandinavian investigators to be a psychogenic disorder in which unlucky personal experiences precipitate paranoia in persons with deviant personalities (Astrup 1984).

Clinical Management

Clinical management of the patient with delusional disorder involves establishing the diagnosis, instituting appropriate interventions, and providing follow-up care. Because there are no systematic data comparing treatments in delusional disorder (Munro and Mok 1995), recommendations are based on clinical observation, not empirical evidence. Treatment will most often include both psychotherapy and medication.

Most patients have little insight about their illness and refuse to acknowledge a problem, so an initial obstacle is getting the patient to the physician. This fact might account for the low percentage of cases reported by physicians. Most patients can be treated as outpatients, but hospitalization is necessary if threats of self-harm or harm to others are present. Suicide is uncommon but may occur when the patient becomes depressed and despondent. The potential for violence may exist because some patients will act on their delusions, particularly jealous or erotomanic men. In these cases the target is not random, but specific to the delusional concern. Thus, a clinician caring for a patient with delusional disorder must carefully assess potential for harm to self or others.

Tact and skill are necessary to help persuade a delusional disorder patient to accept treatment. It may help to first convince the patient to receive treatment for depressive or anxiety symptoms and not the delusions. Once a therapeutic relationship is established, a clinician can begin to gently challenge the delusional beliefs by showing how they interfere with the patient's life, but must neither condemn nor collude in the beliefs. The patient should be assured of privacy, and the physician should take care not to discuss confidential matters with the patient's family without the patient's consent. Group therapy is usually not recommended; the patient's chronic suspiciousness and hypersensitivity may lead him or her to misinterpret situations that may arise in the context of group therapy.

Because delusional disorder is relatively uncommon, its treatment with antipsychotic medication has never been properly evaluated; anecdotal evidence suggests that response is poor (Winokur 1977). Antipsychotics may reduce the agitation, apprehension, and anxiety that accompany delusions, but leave the core delusion untouched. Any of the standard antipsychotics can be used, although there is some suggestion that pimozide may produce better results (Munro and Mok 1995). The selection of medication and dosage will depend on the patient's age and the drug's potential side effects. If the patient is helped by the antipsychotic, depot forms of several are available to ensure compliance (e.g., haloperidol decanoate, fluphenazine decanoate). Neuroleptics have been reported to specifically reduce the intensity of the delusions in erotomania and the associated ideas of reference (Segal 1989).

Monohypochondriacal paranoia (i.e., delusional disorder, somatic type) has been reported to respond to the antipsychotic pimozide at doses of 4–8 mg per day (Munro 1992). Selective serotonin reuptake inhibitors have also been reported helpful in reducing the delusional beliefs, as have the atypical antipsychotics clozapine and risperidone.

Antidepressants and anxiolytics may be indicated for accompanying depressive or anxiety syndromes, but have not been systematically evaluated in patients with delusional disorder. ECT has no role in the treatment of delusional disorder, unless it is used to treat a superimposed major depression.

Conclusions

Tremendous progress has been made during the past two decades to better our understanding of schizophrenia, schizophreniform disorder, and delusional disorder. While the introduction of DSM-III criteria in 1980 narrowed the definition for schizophrenia and created a more homogeneous group of subjects for research, some experts believed the narrowing went too far. A reemphasis on negative symptoms of schizophrenia (Bleuler's "fundamental" symptoms) in DSM-IV-TR has added balance to the perhaps too-rigid emphasis on Schneiderian symptoms in the 1970s. Advances in classification and epidemiology have allowed us to reevaluate the distribution of schizophrenia and its risk factors.

The development of brain-imaging techniques such as CT, MRI, SPECT, and PET have enhanced our understanding of schizophrenia. This technology is allowing us to explore the nature and pattern of brain deficits and examine the possibility of symptom localization in schizophrenia. The development of "brain banks" as well as new techniques in histopathology have given renewed emphasis to postmortem research, permitting a more detailed investigation of abnormalities in neurotransmitter systems and in the neuropathology of schizophrenia. While the nosologists and neuroscientists have been clarifying the classification and pathological mechanisms of schizophrenia, geneticists have been amassing large family data sets and applying new methods such as gene mapping that promise to enrich the study of genetic factors in schizophrenia.

Whereas technological advances are helping us to explore the etiology of schizophrenia, knowledge about course and outcome has been enhanced through long-term studies. We have learned that the best treatment approach to schizophrenia combines pharmacological and psychosocial measures. The pharmacological treatment of schizophrenia has been hampered by undue reliance on the well-worn dopamine theory, and investigators are now looking at other neurotransmitter systems that may yield a more complex interactive model of neurotransmission abnormalities that will result in new pharmacological approaches. Meanwhile, newer atypical antipsychotics have become available, helping many patients formerly thought to be treatment refractory to achieve better functioning in the community. New research has highlighted the importance of family interaction models in schizophrenia, leading to more specific psychosocial interventions in the treatment of this disorder.

During the 1990s, the "Decade of the Brain," the drive in psychiatry was to develop a comprehensive understanding of brain function at levels that range from mind to molecule and to determine how aberrations in these normal functions lead to the development of symptoms of mental illness. Progress in the coming decade will be to build on the foundation of current research and enhance our understanding of the pathophysiology and etiology of schizophrenia. Our ultimate goal is to give physicians more powerful tools to treat those who suffer from schizophrenia and, if possible, prevent its development.

References

Akbarian S, Kim JJ, Potkin SG, et al: Maldistribution of interstitial neurons in prefrontal white matter of the brains of schizophrenic patients. Arch Gen Psychiatry 53:428–436, 1996

Allebeck P, Varla A, Kristjansson E, et al: Risk factors for suicide among patients with schizophrenia. Acta Psychiatr Scand 76:414–419, 1987

Allison DB, Mentore JL, Heo M, et al: Antipsychotic-induced weight gain: a comprehensive research synthesis. Am J Psychiatry 156:1686–1696, 1999

Amador XF, Sackheim HA, Mukherjee S, et al: Specificity of smooth pursuit eye movement and visual fixation abnormalities in schizophrenia: comparison to mania and normal controls. Schizophr Res 5:135–144, 1991

American Psychiatric Association: Diagnostic and Statistical Manual of Mental Disorders. Washington, DC, American Psychiatric Press, 1952

American Psychiatric Association: Diagnostic and Statistical Manual of Mental Disorders, 2nd Edition. Washington, DC, American Psychiatric Press, 1968

American Psychiatric Association: Diagnostic and Statistical Manual of Mental Disorders, 3rd Edition. Washington, DC, American Psychiatric Press, 1980

American Psychiatric Association: Diagnostic and Statistical Manual of Mental Disorders, 3rd Edition, Revised. Washington, DC, American Psychiatric Press, 1987

American Psychiatric Association: Diagnostic and Statistical Manual of Mental Disorders, 4th Edition. Washington, DC, American Psychiatric Press, 1994

American Psychiatric Association: Practice guideline for the treatment of patients with schizophrenia. Am J Psychiatry 154(suppl):1–63, 1997

American Psychiatric Association: Diagnostic and Statistical Manual of Mental Disorders, 4th Edition, Text Revision. Washington, DC, American Psychiatric Press, 2000

Andreasen NC: Thought, language, and communication disorders, I: clinical assessment, definition of terms, and evaluation of their reliability. Arch Gen Psychiatry 36:1315–1321, 1979

Andreasen NC: Negative symptoms in schizophrenia: definition and reliability. Arch Gen Psychiatry 39:784–788, 1982

Andreasen NC: The Broken Brain: The Biologic Revolution in Psychiatry. New York, Harper & Row, 1984

Andreasen NC: The diagnosis of schizophrenia. Schizophr Bull 13:9–22, 1987

Andreasen NC: A unitary model of schizophrenia: Bleuler's "fragmented phrene" as schizencephaly. Arch Gen Psychiatry 56:781–787, 1999

Andreasen NC, Akiskal HS: The specificity of Bleulerian and Schneiderian symptoms: a critical reevaluation. Psychiatr Clin North Am 6:41–54, 1983

Andreasen NC, Olson S: Negative versus positive schizophrenia: definition and validation. Arch Gen Psychiatry 39:789–794, 1982

Andreasen NC, Smith MR, Jacoby CG, et al: Ventricular enlargement in schizophrenia: definition and prevalence. Am J Psychiatry 139:292–296, 1982

Andreasen NC, Nasrallah HA, Dunn V, et al: Structural abnormalities in the frontal system in schizophrenia: a magnetic resonance imaging study. Arch Gen Psychiatry 43:136–144, 1986

Andreasen NC, Ehrhardt JC, Swayze VW, et al: Magnetic resonance imaging of the brain in schizophrenia: the pathophysiologic significance of structural abnormalities. Arch Gen Psychiatry 47:35–44, 1990a

Andreasen NC, Flaum M, Swayze VW, et al: Positive and negative symptoms in schizophrenia: a critical reappraisal. Arch Gen Psychiatry 47:615–621, 1990b

Andreasen NC, Swayze VW, Flaum M, et al: Ventricular enlargement in schizophrenia: evaluation with computed tomographic scanning. Arch Gen Psychiatry 47:1008–1015, 1990c

Andreasen NC, Rezai K, Alliger R, et al: Hypofrontality in neuroleptic-naive patients and in patients with chronic schizophrenia: assessment with xenon 133 single-photon emission computed tomography and the Tower of London. Arch Gen Psychiatry 49:943–958, 1992

Andreasen NC, Flashman L, Flaum M, et al: Regional brain abnormalities in schizophrenia measured with magnetic resonance imaging. JAMA 272:1763–1769, 1994a

Andreasen NC, Arndt S, Swayze V, et al: Thalamic abnormalities in schizophrenia visualized through magnetic resonance image averaging. Science 266:294–298, 1994b

Andreasen NC, Arndt S, Alliger R, et al: Symptoms of schizophrenia: methods, meanings, and mechanisms. Arch Gen Psychiatry 52:341–351, 1995

Andreasen NC, O'Leary DS, Cizadlo T, et al: Schizophrenia and cognitive dysmetria: a positron-emission tomography study of dysfunctional prefrontal-thalamic-cerebellar circuitry. Proc Natl Acad Sci U S A 93:9985–9990, 1996

Andreasen NC, O'Leary DS, Flaum M, et al: Hypofrontality in schizophrenia: distributed dysfunctional circuits in neuroleptic-naive patients. Lancet 349:1730–1734, 1997

Andreasen NC, Paradiso S, O'Leary DS: "Cognitive dysmetria" as an integrative theory of schizophrenia: a dysfunction in cortical-subcortical-cerebellar circuitry? Schizophr Bull 24:203–218, 1998

Andreasen NC, Nopoulos P, O'Leary DS, et al: Defining the phenotype of schizophrenia: cognitive dysmetria and its neural mechanisms. Biol Psychiatry 46:908–920, 1999

Angermeyer ML, Goldstein JM, Kuehn L: Gender differences in schizophrenia: rehospitalization and community survival. Psychol Med 19:365–382, 1989

Anthony JC, Folstein M, Romanoski AJ, et al: Comparison of the lay Diagnostic Interview Schedule and a standardized psychiatric diagnosis. Arch Gen Psychiatry 42:667–675, 1985

Arndt S, Andreasen NC, Flaum M, et al: A longitudinal study of symptom dimensions in schizophrenia: prediction and patterns of change. Arch Gen Psychiatry 52:352–360, 1995

Arnold SE: Neurodevelopmental abnormalities in schizophrenia: Insights from neuropathology. Dev Psychopathol 11:439–456, 1999

Arnold SE, Hyman BT, VanHoesen GW, et al: Some cytoarchitectural abnormalities of the entorhinal cortex in schizophrenia. Arch Gen Psychiatry 48:625–632, 1991

Astrup C: Querulent paranoia: a follow-up. Neuropsychobiology 11:149–154, 1984

Aylward E, Walker E, Bettes B: Intelligence in schizophrenia: meta-analysis of the research. Schizophr Bull 10:430–459, 1984

Babigian HM: Schizophrenia: Epidemiology in Comprehensive Textbook of Psychiatry, 4th Edition, Vol 1. Edited by Kaplan HI, Sadock BJ. Baltimore, MD, Williams & Wilkins, 1984, pp 643–650

Baldessarini RJ, Cohen BM, Teicher MH: Significance of neuroleptic dose and plasma level in the pharmacologic treatment of psychosis. Arch Gen Psychiatry 45:79–91, 1988

Barr CE, Mednick SA, Munk-Jorgensen P: Exposure to influenza epidemics during gestation and adult schizophrenia: a 40-year study. Arch Gen Psychiatry 47:869–874, 1990

Barraclough B, Bunch J, Nelson B, et al: A hundred cases of suicide: clinical aspects. Br J Psychiatry 125:355–373, 1974

Barta PE, Pearlson GD, Powers RE, et al: Auditory hallucinations and smaller superior temporal gyral volume in schizophrenia. Am J Psychiatry 147:1457–1462, 1990

Bassett AS: Progress on the genetics of schizophrenia. J Psychiatry Neurosci 23:270–273, 1998

Beard JH, Propst RN, Malamud TJ: The Fountain House model of psychiatric rehabilitation. Psychosocial Rehabilitation Journal 5:47–54, 1982

Bearden CE, Rosso IM, Hollister JM, et al: A prospective cohort study of childhood behavioral deviance and language abnormalities as predictors of adult schizophrenia. Schizophr Bull 26:395–410, 2000

Beitchman JH: Childhood schizophrenia: a review and comparison with adult onset schizophrenia. Pediatr Clin North Am 8:793–814, 1985

Bellack AS, Gold JM, Buchanan RW: Cognitive rehabilitation for schizophrenia: problems, prospects, and strategies. Schizophr Bull 25:257–274, 1999

Benes FM, McSparren J, Bird ED, et al: Deficits in small interneurons in prefrontal and cingulate cortices of schizophrenic and schizoaffective patients. Arch Gen Psychiatry 48:996–1001, 1991

Benes FM, Kwok EW, Vincent SL, et al: A reduction of nonpyramidal cells in sector CA2 of schizophrenics and manic depressives. Biol Psychiatry 44:88–97, 1998

Bilder RM, Mukherjee S, Rieder RO, et al: Symptomatic and neuropsychological components of defect states. Schizophr Bull 11:409–419, 1985

Bilder RM, Lipschutz-Broch L, Reiter G, et al: Neuropsychological deficits in the early course of first-episode schizophrenia. Schizophr Res 5:198–199, 1991

Black DW, Boffeli TJ: Simple schizophrenia: past, present, and future. Am J Psychiatry 146:1267–1273, 1989

Black DW, Fisher R: Mortality in DSM-III-R schizophrenia. Schizophr Res 7:109–116, 1992

Black DW, Winokur G: Cancer mortality in psychiatric patients: the Iowa Record-Linkage Study. Int J Psychiatry Med 16:189–198, 1986

Bleuler E: Dementia Praecox, or the Group of Schizophrenias (1911). Translated by Zinken J. New York, International Universities Press, 1950

Bogerts B: Recent advances in the neuropathology of schizophrenia. Schizophr Bull 19:431–445, 1993

Braff DL: Information processing and attention dysfunctions in schizophrenia. Schizophr Bull 19:233–259, 1993

Braff DL, Heaton R, Kuck J, et al: The generalized pattern of neuropsychological deficits in outpatients with chronic schizophrenia with heterogeneous Wisconsin Card Sorting Test results. Arch Gen Psychiatry 48:891–898, 1991

Breier A, Astrachan BM: Characterization of schizophrenic patients who commit suicide. Am J Psychiatry 141:206–209, 1984

Breier A, Buchanan RW, Elkashef A, et al: Brain morphology and schizophrenia: a magnetic resonance imaging study of limbic, prefrontal cortex, and caudate structures. Arch Gen Psychiatry 49:921–926, 1992

Broadbent DE: Perception and Communication. London, England, Pergamon, 1958

Brockington IF, Meltzer HY: The nosology of schizoaffective psychosis. Psychiatr Dev 1:317–338, 1983

Bromet EJ, Dew MA, Eaton W: Epidemiology of psychosis with special reference to schizophrenia, in Textbook of Psychiatric Epidemiology. Edited by Tsuang MT, Tohen M, Zahner GEP. New York, Wiley-Liss, 1995, pp 283–300

Brown AS, Schaefer CA, Wyatt RJ, et al: Maternal exposure to respiratory infections and adult schizophrenia spectrum disorders: a prospective birth cohort study. Schizophr Bull 26:287–295, 2000a

Brown AS, Cohen P, Greenwald S, et al: Nonaffective psychosis after prenatal exposure to rubella. Am J Psychiatry 157:438–443, 2000b

Buchanan RW, Strauss ME, Kirkpatrick B, et al: Neuropsychological impairments in deficit versus non-deficit forms of schizophrenia. Arch Gen Psychiatry 51:804–811, 1994

Buchsbaum MS, Ingvar DH, Kessler R, et al: Cerebral glucography with positron tomography. Arch Gen Psychiatry 39:251–259, 1982

Buchsbaum MS, Someya T, Teng CY, et al: PET and MRI of the thalamus in never-medicated patients with schizophrenia. Am J Psychiatry 153:191–199, 1996

Cannon M, Jones P, Huttunen MO, et al: School performance in Finnish children and later development of schizophrenia: a population-based longitudinal study. Arch Gen Psychiatry 56:457–463, 1999

Cannon TD, Bearden CE, Hollister JM, et al: Childhood cognitive functioning in schizophrenia patients and their unaffected siblings: a prospective cohort study. Schizophr Bull 26:379–393, 2000

Caracci G, Mukherjee S, Roth SD, et al: Subjective awareness of abnormal involuntary movements in chronic schizophrenic patients. Am J Psychiatry 147:295–298, 1990

Carlsson A: The current status of the dopamine hypothesis of schizophrenia. Neuropsychopharmacology 1:179–186, 1988

Carpenter WT Jr: Maintenance therapy of persons with schizophrenia. J Clin Psychiatry 57(suppl 19):10–18, 1996

Carpenter WT Jr, Buchanan RW: Schizophrenia. N Engl J Med 330:681–690, 1994

Carpenter WT Jr, Strauss JS: The prediction of outcome in schizophrenia, IV: eleven year follow-up of the Washington IPSS Cohort. J Nerv Ment Dis 179:517–525, 1991

Carpenter WT Jr, Heinrichs DW, Wagman AMI: Deficit and nondeficit forms of schizophrenia: The concept. Am J Psychiatry 145:578–583, 1988

Carpenter WT Jr, Hanlon TL, Heinrichs DW, et al: Continuous versus targeted medication in schizophrenic outpatients: outcome results. Am J Psychiatry 147:1138–1148, 1990

Carpenter WT Jr, Arango C, Buchanan RW, et al: Deficit psychopathology and a paradigm shift in schizophrenia research. Biol Psychiatry 46:352–360, 1999a

Carpenter WT Jr, Buchanan RW, Kirkpatrick B, et al: Diazepam treatment of early signs of exacerbation in schizophrenia. Am J Psychiatry 156:299–303, 1999b

Chakos M, Lieberman J, Hoffman E, et al: Effectiveness of second-generation antipsychotics in patients with treatment-resistant schizophrenia: a review and meta-analysis of randomized trials. Am J Psychiatry 158:518–526, 2001

Chatterjee A, Chako SM, Koreen A, et al: Prevalence and clinical correlates of extrapyramidal signs and spontaneous dyskinesia in never-medication schizophrenic patients. Am J Psychiatry 152:1724–1729, 1995

Christison GW, Kirch DG, Wyatt RJ: When symptoms persist: choosing among alternative somatic treatments for schizophrenia. Schizophr Bull 17:217–245, 1991

Clardy JA, Hyde TM, Kleinman JE: Postmortem neurochemical and neuropathological studies in schizophrenia, in Schizophrenia: From Mind to Molecule. Edited by Andreasen NC. Washington, DC, American Psychiatric Press, 1993, pp 123–146

Cohen G, Andreasen NC, Alliger R, et al: Segmentation techniques for the classification of brain tissue using magnetic resonance imaging. Psychiatry Res 45:33–51, 1992

Conley RR, Tamminga CA, Bartko JJ, et al: Olanzapine compared with chlorpromazine in treatment-resistant schizophrenia. Am J Psychiatry 155:914–920, 1998

Conrad AJ, Abebe T, Austin R, et al: Hippocampal pyramidal cell disarray in schizophrenia as a bilateral phenomenon. Arch Gen Psychiatry 48:413–417, 1991

Cook JA, Pickett SA, Razzano L, et al: Rehabilitation services for persons with schizophrenia. Psychiatr Ann 26:97–104, 1996

Cooper JE, Kendall RE, Gurland BJ, et al: Psychiatric Diagnosis in New York and London: A Comparative Study of Mental Hospital Admissions. Institute of Psychiatry, Maudsley Monographs, No 20. London, England, Oxford University Press, 1972

Coryell W, Tsuang MT: Outcome after 40 years in DSM-III schizophreniform disorder. Arch Gen Psychiatry 43:324–328, 1986

Creese R, Burt BR, Snyder SH: Dopamine receptor binding predicts clinical and pharmacologic potencies of antipsychotic drugs. Science 192:81–84, 1976

Crespo-Facorro B, Kim JJ, Andreasen NC, et al: Human frontal cortex: an MRI-based parcellation method. Neuroimage 10:500–519, 1999a

Crespo-Facorro B, Paradiso S, Andreasen NC, et al: Recalling word lists reveals "cognitive dysmetria" in schizophrenia: a positron emission tomography study. Am J Psychiatry 156:386–392, 1999b

Crespo-Facorro B, Kim J, Andreasen NC, et al: Regional frontal abnormalities in schizophrenia: a quantitative gray matter volume and cortical surface size study. Biol Psychiatry 48:110–119, 2000

Crow TJ: Positive and negative schizophrenic symptoms and the role of dopamine. Br J Psychiatry 137:383–386, 1980

Crowe RR, Black DW, Wesner R, et al: Lack of linkage to chromosome 5q11–q13 markers in six schizophrenia pedigrees. Arch Gen Psychiatry 48:357–361, 1991

Csillag C: Denmark: psychiatric offenders. Lancet 341:683–684, 1993

Cutting J: The Psychology of Schizophrenia. London, England, Churchill Livingstone, 1985

David AS, Malmberg A, Brandt L, et al: IQ and risk for schizophrenia: a population-based cohort study. Psychol Med 27:1311–1323, 1997

Davidson M, Reichenberg A, Rabinowitz J, et al: Behavioral and intellectual markers for schizophrenia in apparently healthy male adolescents. Am J Psychiatry 156:1328–1335, 1999

Davis JM, Kane JM, Marder SR, et al: Dose response of prophylactic antipsychotics. J Clin Psychiatry 54(suppl 3):24–30, 1993

Davis KL, Kahn RS, Ko G, et al: Dopamine in schizophrenia: a review and reconceptualization. Am J Psychiatry 148:1474–1486, 1991

Davis KL, Buchsbaum MS, Shihabuddin L, et al: Ventricular enlargement in poor-outcome schizophrenia. Biol Psychiatry 43:783–793, 1998

deLeon J, Verghese C, Tracy JI, et al: Polydipsia and water intoxication in psychiatric patients: a review of the epidemiologic literature. Biol Psychiatry 35:519–530, 1994

DeLisi LE, Goldin LR, Hamovit VR, et al: A family study of the association of increased ventricular size with schizophrenia. Arch Gen Psychiatry 43:48–53, 1986

DeLisi LE, Hoff Al, Kushner M, et al: Left ventricular enlargement associated with diagnostic outcome of schizophreniform disorder. Biol Psychiatry 32:199–201, 1992

Delva NJ, Letemendia FJJ: Lithium treatment in schizophrenia and schizoaffective disorders. Br J Psychiatry 141:387–400, 1982

Dixon L, Haas G, Weiden PJ, et al: Drug abuse in schizophrenic patients: clinical correlates and reasons for use. Am J Psychiatry 148:224–230, 1991

Dixon L, Lyles A, Scott J, et al: Services to families of adults with schizophrenia: from treatment recommendations to dissemination. Psychiatr Serv 50:233–238, 1999

Done DJ, Crow TJ, Johnstone EC, et al: Childhood antecedents of schizophrenia and affective illness: social adjustment at ages 7 and 11. BMJ 309:699–703, 1994

Drake RE, Osher FC, Wallach MA: Alcohol use and abuse in schizophrenia: a prospective community study. J Nerv Ment Dis 177:408–414, 1989

Dubin WR, Waxman HM, Weiss KJ, et al: Rapid tranquilization: the efficacy of oral concentrate. J Clin Psychiatry 46:475–478, 1985

Eaton WW: Epidemiology of schizophrenia. Epidemiol Rev 7:105–126, 1985

Eaton WW: Update on epidemiology of schizophrenia. Epidemiol Rev 13:320–328, 1991

Eaton WW, Day R, Kramer M: The use of epidemiology for risk factor research in schizophrenia: an overview and methodologic critique, in Handbook of Schizophrenia, Vol 3: Nosology, Epidemiology, and Genetics. Edited by Tsuang MT, Simpson JC. Amsterdam, Elsevier Science, 1988, pp 169–204

Eaton WW, Hayward C, Ram R: Schizophrenia and rheumatoid arthritis: a review. Schizophr Res 6:181–192, 1992

Ellsworth RB: Characteristics of effective treatment milieu, in Principles and Practice of Milieu Therapy. Edited by Gunderson JG, Will OA, Mosher LF. New York, Jason Aronson, 1983, pp 87–123

Erlenmeyer-Kimling L: Fertility in psychotics, in Annual Review of the Schizophrenic Syndrome, Vol 5. Edited by Cancro R. New York, Brunner/Mazel, 1978, pp 298–325

Evans JD, Paulsen JS, Harris MJ, et al: A clinical and neuropsychological comparison of delusional disorder and schizophrenia. J Neuropsychiatry Clin Neurosci 8:281–286, 1996

Expert Consensus Guideline Series Steering Committee: Treatment of schizophrenia. J Clin Psychiatry 57(suppl 12B):1–58, 1996

Falloon IR: Early intervention for first episodes of schizophrenia: a preliminary exploration. Psychiatry 55:4–15, 1992

Farde L, Ehrin E, Eriksson E, et al: Substituted benzamides as ligands for visualization of dopamine receptor binding in the human brain by positron emission tomography. Proc Natl Acad Sci U S A 81:3863–3867, 1985

Farde L, Wiesel FA, Stone-Elander S, et al: D2 dopamine receptors in neuroleptic-naive schizophrenic patients: positron emission tomography study with [11C]raclopride. Arch Gen Psychiatry 47:213–219, 1990

Farde L, Nordstrom AL, Wiesel FA, et al: Positron emission tomographic analysis of central D1 and D2 dopamine receptor occupancy in patients treated with classical neuroleptics and clozapine: relation to extrapyramidal side effects. Arch Gen Psychiatry 49:538–544, 1992

Faris REL, Durham HL: Mental Disorder in Urban Areas. Chicago, IL, University of Chicago Press, 1939

Farmer AE, McGuffin P, Gottesman II: Twin concordance for DSM-III schizophrenia: scrutinizing the validity of the definition. Arch Gen Psychiatry 44:634–641, 1987

Feighner JP, Robins F, Guze SB, et al: Diagnostic criteria for use in psychiatric research. Arch Gen Psychiatry 26:57–63, 1972

Feinberg I: Schizophrenia and late maturational brain changes in man. Psychopharmacol Bull 18:29–31, 1982

Fennig S, Craig TJ, Bromet EJ: The consistency of DSM-III-R delusional disorder in a first-admission sample. Psychopathology 29:315–324, 1996

Fenton WS: Evolving perspectives on individual psychotherapy for schizophrenia. Schizophr Bull 26:47–72, 2000

Fenton WS, McGlashan TH: The prognostic significance of obsessive-compulsive symptoms in schizophrenia. Am J Psychiatry 143:437–441, 1986

Fenton WS, McGlashan TH: Natural history of schizophrenia subtypes, I: longitudinal study of paranoid, hebephrenic, and undifferentiated schizophrenia. Arch Gen Psychiatry 48:969–977, 1991

Flashman LA, Flaum M, Gupta S, et al: Soft signs and neuropsychological performance in schizophrenia. Am J Psychiatry 153:526–532, 1996

Flaum M, Arndt S, Andreasen NC: The role of gender in studies of ventrical enlargement in schizophrenia: a predominantly male effect. Am J Psychiatry 147:1327–1332, 1990

Frith CD: The Cognitive Neuropsychology of Schizophrenia. East Sussex, NJ, Lawrence Erlbaum, 1992

Frith C: Functional imaging and cognitive abnormalities. Lancet 346:615–620, 1995

Frith CD, Friston K, Liddle PF, et al: Willed action and the prefrontal cortex in man: a study with PET. Proc R Soc Lond B Biol Sci 244:241–246, 1991

Ganguli R, Brar JS, Chengappa KNR: Mitogen-stimulated interleukin-2 production in never-medicated, first-episode schizophrenic patients. Arch Gen Psychiatry 52:668–672, 1995

Garza-Trevino ES, Hollister LE, Overall JE, et al: Efficacy of combinations of intramuscular antipsychotics and sedative-hypnotics for control of psychotic agitation. Am J Psychiatry 146:1598–1601, 1989

Geddes JR, Lawrie SM: Obstetrical complications and schizophrenia: a meta-analysis. Br J Psychiatry 167:786–793, 1995

Geddes J, Freemantle N, Harrison P, et al: Atypical antipsychotics in the treatment of schizophrenia: systematic overview and meta-regression analysis. BMJ 321:1371–1376, 2000

Gerard DL, Houston LG: Family setting and social etiology of schizophrenia. Psychiatr Q 27:90–101, 1953

Goff DC, Henderson DC, Amico E: Cigarette smoking and schizophrenia: relationship to psychopathology and medication side effects. Am J Psychiatry 149:1189–1194, 1992

Goldberg TE, Kelsoe JR, Weinberger DR, et al: Performance of schizophrenic patients on putative neuropsychological tests of frontal lobe function. Int J Neurosci 42:51–58, 1988

Goldman-Rakic PS: Circuitry of primate prefrontal cortex and regulation of behavior by representational memory, in Handbook of Physiology. Edited by Plum F, Mountcastle V. Bethesda, MD, American Physiological Society, 1987, pp 373–417

Goldman-Rakic PS: Working memory dysfunction in schizophrenia. J Neuropsychiatry Clin Neurosci 64:348–357, 1994

Goldstein LE, Sporn J, Brown S, et al: New-onset diabetes mellitus and diabetic ketoacidosis associated with olanzapine treatment. Psychosomatics 40:438–443, 1999

Gorwood P, Leboyer M, Falissard B, et al: Anticipation in schizophrenia: new light on a controversial problem. Am J Psychiatry 153:1173–1177, 1996

Gottesman II, Shields J: Schizophrenia: The Epigenetic Puzzle. Cambridge, England, Cambridge University Press, 1982

Green MF, Satz P, Christensen C: Minor physical remedies in schizophrenia patients, bipolar patients, and their siblings. Schizophr Bull 20:433–440, 1994

Grillon C, Ameli R, Charney DS, et al: Startle gating deficits occur across prepulse intensities in schizophrenic patients. Biol Psychiatry 32:939–943, 1992

Gudeman JE, Shore MF, Dickey B: Day hospitalization and an inn instead of inpatient care for psychiatric patients. N Engl J Med 308:749–753, 1983

Gulbinat W, Dupont A, Jablensky A, et al: Cancer incidence in schizophrenic patients: results of record linkage studies in three countries. Br J Psychiatry Suppl 18:75–83, 1992

Gupta S, Andreasen NC, Arndt S, et al: Neurological soft signs in neuroleptic-naïve and neuroleptic treated schizophrenic patients and in normal comparison subjects. Am J Psychiatry 152:191–196, 1995a

Gupta S, Rajaprabhakaran R, Arndt S, et al: Premorbid adjustment as a predictor of phenomenological and neurobiological indices of schizophrenia. Schizophr Res 16:189–197, 1995b

Gur RE, Pearlson GD: Neuroimaging in schizophrenia research. Schizophr Bull 19:332–353, 1993

Guze SB, Cloninger CR, Martin RL, et al: A follow-up and family study of schizophrenia. Arch Gen Psychiatry 40:1273–1276, 1983

Hare EH: Mental illness and social conditions in Bristol. J Ment Sci 102:349–357, 1956

Hare EH, Price JS, Slater E: Mental disorder and season of birth. Nature 241:480, 1973

Harris G, Andreasen NC, Cizadlo T, et al: Improving tissue segmentation in MRI: a three-dimensional multispectral discriminant analysis method with automated training class selection. J Comput Assist Tomogr 23:144–154, 1999

Harrison PJ: The neuropathology of schizophrenia. A critical review of the data and their interpretation. Brain 122:593–624, 1999

Hegarty JD, Baldessarini RJ, Tohen M, et al: One hundred years of schizophrenia: a meta-analysis of the outcome literature. Am J Psychiatry 151:1409–1415, 1994

Heinssen RK, Liberman RP, Kopelowicz A: Psychosocial skills training for schizophrenia: Lessons from the laboratory. Schizophr Bull 26:21–46, 2000

Henderson DC, Cagliero E, Gray C, et al: Clozapine, diabetes mellitus, weight gain, and lipid abnormalities: a five-year naturalistic study. Am J Psychiatry 157:975–981, 2000

Herz M: Prodromal symptoms and prevention of relapse in schizophrenia. J Clin Psychiatry 46:22–25, 1985

Heston LL: Psychiatric disorders in foster home reared children of schizophrenic mothers. Br J Psychiatry 112:819–825, 1966

Ho BC, Andreasen NC: Long delays in seeking treatment for schizophrenia. Lancet 357:898–900, 2001

Hoff AL, Riordan H, O'Donnell DW, et al: Cross-sectional and longitudinal neuropsychological test findings in first-episode schizophrenic patients. Schizophr Res 5:197–198, 1991

Hoffman RE, Boutros NN, Hu S, et al: Transcranial magnetic stimulation and auditory hallucinations in schizophrenia. Lancet 355:1073–1075, 2000

Hogarty GE: Depot neuroleptics: the relevance of psychosocial factors—a United States perspective. J Clin Psychiatry 45:36–42, 1984

Hollister JM, Laing P, Mednick SA: Rhesus incompatibility as a risk factor for schizophrenia in male adults. Arch Gen Psychiatry 53:19–24, 1996

Holzman PS, Soloman CM, Levin S, et al: Pursuit eye movement dysfunctions in schizophrenia: family evidence for specificity. Arch Gen Psychiatry 41:136–139, 1984

Holzman PS, Kringlen E, Matthysse S, et al: A single dominant gene can account for eye tracking dysfunction and schizophrenia in offspring of discordant twins. Arch Gen Psychiatry 45:641–647, 1988

Hughlings-Jackson J: Selected Writings. London, England, Hodder & Stoughton, 1931

Hulshoff Pol HE, Hoek HW, Susser E, et al: Prenatal exposure to famine and brain morphology in schizophrenia. Am J Psychiatry 157:1170–1172, 2000

Hyde TM, Nawroz S, Goldberg TE, et al: Is there a cognitive decline in schizophrenia? A cross-sectional study. Br J Psychiatry 164:494–500, 1994

Ingvar DH, Franzen G: Abnormalities of cerebral blood flow distribution in patients with chronic schizophrenia. Acta Psychiatr Scand 50:425–462, 1974

Isohanni I, Jarvelin MR, Nieminen P, et al: School performance as a predictor of psychiatric hospitalization in adult life: a 28-year follow-up in the Northern Finland 1966 Birth Cohort. Psychol Med 28:967–974, 1998

Jablensky A, Sartorius N: Culture and schizophrenia. Psychol Med 5:113–124, 1975

Jablensky A, Sartorius N, Ernberg G, et al: Schizophrenia: manifestation, incidence, and course, in Different Cultures: A World Health Organization Ten-Country Study—Psychological Medicine Monograph Supplement 20. Cambridge, England, Cambridge University Press, 1992

Javitt DC, Zukin SR: Recent advances in the phencyclidine model of schizophrenia. Am J Psychiatry 148:1301–1308, 1991

Johns CA, Thompson JW: Adjunctive treatments in schizophrenia: pharmacotherapies and electroconvulsive therapy. Schizophr Bull 21:607–619, 1995

Johnstone EC, Crow TJ, Frith CD, et al: Cerebral ventricular size and cognitive impairment in chronic schizophrenia. Lancet 2:924–926, 1976

Jones P, Rodgers B, Murray R, et al: Child development risk factors for adult schizophrenia in the British 1946 birth cohort. Lancet 344:1398–1402, 1994

Jonsson H, Nyman AK: Prediction of outcome in schizophrenia. Acta Psychiatr Scand 69:274–291, 1984

Jorgensen P: Course and outcome in dimensional disorders. Psychopathology 27:79–88, 1994

Judd LL, McAdams LA, Budnick B, et al: Sensory gating deficits in schizophrenia: new results. Am J Psychiatry 149:448–493, 1992

Kallman FJ: The Genetics of Schizophrenia. New York, Augustin, 1938

Kanas N: Inpatient and outpatient group therapy for schizophrenic patients. Am J Psychother 39:431–439, 1985

Kane JM: Antipsychotic drug side effects: their relationship to dose. J Clin Psychiatry 46:16–21, 1985

Kane JM, Marder SR: Psychopharmacologic treatment of schizophrenia. Schizophr Bull 19:287–302, 1993

Kane JM, Rifkin A, Woerner M, et al: Low-dose neuroleptic treatment of outpatient schizophrenics, I: preliminary results for relapse rates. Arch Gen Psychiatry 40:893–896, 1983

Kane JM, Honigfeld G, Singer J, et al: Clozapine for the treatment-resistant schizophrenic: a double-blind comparison with chlorpromazine. Arch Gen Psychiatry 45:789–796, 1988

Kapur S, Seeman P: Does fast dissociation from the dopamine D2 receptor explain the action of atypical antipsychotics? A new hypothesis. Am J Psychiatry 158:360–369, 2001

Kapur S, Zipursky R, Jones C, et al: Relationship between dopamine D2 occupancy, clinical response, and side effects: a double-blind PET study of first-episode schizophrenia. Am J Psychiatry 157:514–520, 2000

Kasanin J: The acute schizoaffective psychoses. Am J Psychiatry 13:97–126, 1933

Keck PE, McElroy SL, Strakowski SM: Schizoaffective disorder: role of atypical antipsychotics. Schizophr Res 35:S5–S12, 1999

Keefe RSE, Silva SG, Perkins DO, et al: The effects of atypical antipsychotic drugs on neurocognitive impairment in schizophrenia: a review and meta-analysis. Schizophr Bull 25:201–222, 1999

Keilp TG, Sweeney JA, Jacobsen P, et al: Cognitive impairment in schizophrenia: specific relations to ventricular size and negative symptomatology. Biol Psychiatry 24:47–55, 1988

Kendler KS: The nosological validity of paranoia (simple delusional disorder): a review. Arch Gen Psychiatry 37:699–706, 1980

Kendler KS: Demography of paranoid psychosis (delusional disorder): a review and comparison with schizophrenia and affective illness. Arch Gen Psychiatry 39:890–902, 1982

Kendler KS: Kraepelin and the diagnostic concept of paranoia. Compr Psychiatry 29:4–11, 1988

Kendler KS, Gruenberg AM: An independent analysis of the Danish Adoption Study of Schizophrenia, VI: the relationship between psychiatric disorders as defined by DSM-III in the relatives and adoptees. Arch Gen Psychiatry 41:555–564, 1984

Kendler KS, Gruenberg AM, Strauss JS: An independent analysis of the Copenhagen sample of the Danish Adoption Study of Schizophrenia, III: the relationship between paranoid psychosis (delusional disorder) and the schizophrenia spectrum disorders. Arch Gen Psychiatry 38:985–987, 1982

Kendler KS, Gruenberg AM, Tsuang MT: Outcome of schizophrenic subtypes defined by four diagnostic systems. Arch Gen Psychiatry 41:149–154, 1984

Kendler KS, Masterson CC, Davis KL: Psychiatric illness in first-degree relatives of patients with paranoid psychosis, schizophrenia, and medical illness. Br J Psychiatry 147:524–531, 1985a

Kendler KS, Gruenberg AM, Tsuang MT: Subtype stability in schizophrenia. Am J Psychiatry 142:827–832, 1985b

Kendler KS, Gruenberg AM, Tsuang MT: A family study of the subtypes of schizophrenia. Am J Psychiatry 145:57–62, 1988

Kendler KS, McGuire M, Gruenberg AM, et al: An epidemiologic, clinical, and family study of simple schizophrenia in County Roscommon, Ireland. Am J Psychiatry 151:27–34, 1994a

Kendler KS, McGuire M, Gruenberg AM, et al: Outcome and family study of the subtypes of schizophrenia in the west of Ireland. Am J Psychiatry 151:849–856, 1994b

Kendler KS, McGuire M, Gruenberg AM, et al: Examining the validity of DSM-III-R schizoaffective disorder and its putative subtypes in the Roscommon Family Study. Am J Psychiatry 152:755–764, 1995

Kendler KS, Karkowski-Shuman L, Walsh D: Age at onset in schizophrenia and risk of illness in relatives: results from the Roscommon Family Study. Br J Psychiatry 169:213–218, 1996

Kennedy HG, Kemp LI, Dyer DE: Fear and anger in delusional (paranoid) disorder: the association with violence. Br J Psychiatry 160:488–492, 1992

Kessler R, McGonagle K, Zhao S, et al: Lifetime and 12-month prevalence of DSM-III-R psychiatric disorders in the United States: results from the National Comorbidity Study. Arch Gen Psychiatry 51:8–19, 1994

Kety SS, Rosenthal D, Wender PH, et al: Mental illness in the biologic and adoptive families of adopted individuals who have become schizophrenic: a preliminary report based on psychiatric interviews, in Genetic Research in Psychiatry. Edited by Fieve R, Rosenthal D, Brill H. Baltimore, MD, Johns Hopkins University Press, 1975, pp 147–165

Kim JJ, Mohamed S, Andreasen NC, et al: Regional neural dysfunctions in chronic schizophrenia studied with positron emission tomography. Am J Psychiatry 157:542–548, 2000

King DJ, Burke M, Lucas RA: Antipsychotic drug-induced dysphoria. Br J Psychiatry 167:480–482, 1995

Kingsbury SJ, Salzman C: Disulfiram in the treatment of alcoholic patients with schizophrenia. Hosp Community Psychiatry 41:133–134, 1990

Kissling W (ed): Guidelines for Neuroleptic Relapse Prevention in Schizophrenia. Berlin, Germany, Springer-Verlag, 1991

Kovelman JA, Scheibel AB: A neurohistological correlate of schizophrenia. Biol Psychiatry 19:1601–1621, 1984

Kraepelin E: Dementia Praecox and Paraphrenia. Translated by Barkley RM. Edinburgh, Scotland, E & S Livingstone, 1919

Krakowski MI, Convit A, Jaeger J, et al: Neurologic impairment in violent schizophrenic inpatients. Am J Psychiatry 146:849–853, 1989

Lamb HR: Some reflections on treating schizophrenics. Arch Gen Psychiatry 43:1007–1011, 1986

Lamb HR: Lessons learned from deinstitutionalization in the United States. Br J Psychiatry 162:587–592, 1993

Lamberti JS, Tariot PN: Schizophrenia in nursing home patients. Psychiatr Ann 25:441–448, 1995

Langfeldt G: Schizophreniform States. Copenhagen, Denmark, E Munksguard, 1939

Lehman AF: Vocational rehabilitation in schizophrenia. Schizophr Bull 21:645–656, 1995

Lehman AF, Steinwachs DM, and PORT coinvestigators: Patterns of usual care for schizophrenia: initial results from the Schizophrenia Patient Outcomes Research Team (PORT) Client Survey. Schizophr Bull 24:11–20, 1998a

Lehman AF, Steinwachs DM, and PORT coinvestigators: Translating research into practice: the Schizophrenia Patient Outcomes Research Team (PORT) treatment recommendations. Schizophr Bull 24:1–10, 1998b

Lehmann HE, Wilson H, Deutsch M: Minimal maintenance medication: effect of three dose schedules on relapse rates and symptoms in chronic schizophrenic outpatients. Compr Psychiatry 24:293–303, 1983

Leiner HC, Leiner AL, Dow RS: Does the cerebellum contribute to mental skills? Behav Neurosci 100:443–453, 1986

Leucht S, Pitschel-Walz G, Abraham D, et al: Efficacy and extrapyramidal side-effects of the new antipsychotics olanzapine, quetiapine, risperidone and sertindole compared to conventional antipsychotics and placebo: a meta-analysis of randomized controlled trials. Schizophr Bull 35:51–68, 1999

Levinson DF, Simpson GM, Lo ES, et al: Fluphenazine plasma levels, dosage, efficacy, and side effects. Am J Psychiatry 152:765–771, 1995

Levinson DF, Umapathy C, Musthaq M: Treatment of schizoaffective disorder and schizophrenia with mood symptoms. Am J Psychiatry 156:1138–1148, 1999

Lewine R, Burbach D, Melzer HY: Effect of diagnostic criteria on the ratio of male to female schizophrenic patients. Am J Psychiatry 141:84–87, 1984

Lewis A: Paranoia and paranoid: a historical perspective. Psychol Med 1:2–12, 1970

Lewis SW, Mezey GC: Clinical correlates of septum pellucidum cavities: an unusual association with psychosis. Psychol Med 15:43–54, 1985

Liddle PF, Barnes TRE, Morris D, et al: Three syndromes in chronic schizophrenia. Br J Psychiatry Suppl Nov:119–122, 1989

Liddle PF, Friston KJ, Frith CD, et al: Patterns of cerebral blood flow in schizophrenia. Br J Psychiatry 160:179–186, 1992

Lieberman JA, Fenton WS: Delayed detection of psychosis: causes, consequences, and effect on public health. Am J Psychiatry 157:1727–1730, 2000

Lieberman JA, Kane JM, Sarantakos S, et al: Prediction of relapse in schizophrenia. Arch Gen Psychiatry 44:592–603, 1987

Lieberman JA, Chakos M, Wu H, et al: Longitudinal study of brain morphology in first episode schizophrenia. Biol Psychiatry 49:487–499, 2001

Light GA, Malaspina DM, Geyer MA, et al: Amphetamine disrupts P50 suppression in normal subjects. Biol Psychiatry 46:990–996, 1999

Light GA, Geyer MA, Clementz BA, et al: Normal P50 suppression in schizophrenia patients treated with atypical antipsychotic medications. Am J Psychiatry 157:767–771, 2000

Lim KO, Tew W, Kushner M, et al: Cortical gray matter volume deficit in patients with first-episode schizophrenia. Am J Psychiatry 153:1548–1553, 1996

Linszen DH, Dingemans PM, Lenior ME: Cannabis abuse and the course of recent-onset schizophrenic disorders. Arch Gen Psychiatry 51:273–279, 1994

Lipinsky JF, Zubenko G, Cohen BM, et al: Propranolol in the treatment of neuroleptic-induced akathisia. Am J Psychiatry 141:412–415, 1984

Loranger AW: Sex difference in age at onset of schizophrenia. Arch Gen Psychiatry 41:157–161, 1984

Lyketsos GC, Sakka P, Mailis A: The sexual adjustment of chronic schizophrenics: a preliminary study. Br J Psychiatry 143:376–382, 1983

Mackota G, Lamb HR: Vocational rehabilitation. Psychiatr Ann 19:548–552, 1989

Magrinat G, Danziger JA, Lorenzo IC, et al: A reassessment of catatonia. Compr Psychiatry 24:218–228, 1983

Maj M, Pirozzi R, Formicola AM, et al: Reliability and validity of the DSM-IV diagnostic category of schizoaffective disorder: preliminary data. J Affect Disord 57:95–98, 2000

Malmberg A, Lewis G, David A, et al: Premorbid adjustment and personality in people with schizophrenia. Br J Psychiatry 172:308–313, 1998

Malzberg B: Mental disease among foreign-born in Canada, 1950–1952, in relation to period of immigration. Am J Psychiatry 120:971–973, 1964

Manschreck TC: Delusional disorder: the recognition and management of paranoia. J Clin Psychiatry 57(suppl 3):32–38, 1996

Manschreck TC, Maher BA, Rucklos ME, et al: Disturbed voluntary motor activity in schizophrenic disorder. Psychol Med 12:73–84, 1982

Marder SR, Meibach RC: Risperidone in the treatment of schizophrenia. Am J Psychiatry 151:825–835, 1994

Marder SR, Wirshing WC, Mintz J, et al: Two-year outcome of social skills training and group psychotherapy for outpatients with schizophrenia. Am J Psychiatry 153:1585–1592, 1996

Maxmen JS: Delivery of after care services, in Management of Chronic Schizophrenia. Edited by Caton CLM. New York, Oxford University Press, 1984

McAllister CG, Rapaport MH, Pickar D, et al: Increased number of CD5+ B lymphocytes in schizophrenic patients. Arch Gen Psychiatry 46:890–894, 1989

McCabe MS, Fowler RC, Cadoret RJ, et al: Symptom differences in schizophrenics with good and poor prognosis. Am J Psychiatry 128:1239–1243, 1972

McEvoy JP, Hogarty GE, Steingard S: Optimal dose of neuroleptic in acute schizophrenia. Arch Gen Psychiatry 48:734–745, 1991

McFarlane WR, Lukens E, Link B, et al: Multiple family groups and psychoeducation in the treatment of schizophrenia. Arch Gen Psychiatry 52:679–687, 1995

McGhie A, Chapman J: Disorders of attention and perception in early schizophrenia. Br J Med Psychol 34:103–116, 1961

McGlashan TH: The Chestnut Lodge Follow-Up Study, II: long-term outcome of schizophrenia and the affective disorders. Arch Gen Psychiatry 41:586–601, 1984

McGlashan TH: The prediction of outcome in chronic schizophrenia, IV: the Chestnut Lodge Follow-Up Study. Arch Gen Psychiatry 43:167–176, 1986

McGlashan TH: Duration of untreated psychosis in first-episode schizophrenia: marker or determinant of course? Biol Psychiatry 46:899–907, 1999

McGorry PD, Edwards J, Mihalopoulos C, et al: EPPIC: an evolving system of early detection and optimal management. Schizophr Bull 22:305–326, 1996

McGuire PK, Frith CD: Disordered functional connectivity in schizophrenia. Psychol Med 26:663–667, 1996

McGuire PK, Silbersweig DA, Murray RM, et al: Functional anatomy of inner speech and auditory verbal imagery. Psychol Med 26:29–38, 1996a

McGuire PK, Silbersweig DA, Wright I, et al: The neural correlates of inner speech and auditory verbal imagery in schizophrenia: relationship to auditory verbal hallucinations. Br J Psychiatry 169:148–159, 1996b

McNeil T, Kaij L: Obstetric factors in the development of schizophrenia: complications in the births of three schizophrenics and in reproduction by schizophrenic patients, in The Nature of Schizophrenia: New Approaches to Research and Treatment. Edited by Wynn LC, Cromwell RL, Matthysse S. New York, Wiley, 1978, pp 401–429

Meares A: The diagnosis of prepsychotic schizophrenia. Lancet 1:55–58, 1959

Mednick SA, Machon RA, Hultunen MO, et al: Adult schizophrenia following prenatal exposure to an influenza epidemic. Arch Gen Psychiatry 45:189–192, 1988

Mellor CS: First rank symptoms of schizophrenia. Br J Psychiatry 117:15–23, 1970

Meltzer HY: Biological studies in schizophrenia. Schizophr Bull 13:77–100, 1987

Meltzer HY, Matsubara S, Lee JC: Classification of typical and atypical antipsychotic drugs on the basis of dopamine D1, D2 and serontonin2 pKi values. J Pharmacol Exp Ther 251:238–246, 1989

Modestin T, Ammann R: Mental disorders and criminality: male schizophrenia. Schizophr Bull 22:69–82, 1996

Mohamed S, Paulsen JS, O'Leary D, et al: Generalized cognitive deficits in schizophrenia. Arch Gen Psychiatry 56:749–754, 1999

Moldin SO, Gottesman II: Genes, experience, and chance in schizophrenia: positioning for the 21st century. Schizophr Bull 23:547–561, 1997

Mortensen PB, Pedersen CB, Westergaard T, et al: Effects of family history and place and season of birth on the risk of schizophrenia. N Engl J Med 340:603–608, 1999

Mueser KT, Berenbaum H: Psychodynamic treatment of schizophrenia: is there a future? Psychol Med 20:253–262, 1990

Mukherjee S, Shukla S, Woodle J, et al: Misdiagnosis of schizophrenia in bipolar patients: a multiethnic comparison. Am J Psychiatry 140:1571–1574, 1983

Munro A: Psychiatric disorders characterized by delusions: treatment in relation to specific types. Psychiatr Ann 22:232–240, 1992

Munro A, Mok H: An overview of treatment in paranoia/delusional disorder. Can J Psychiatry 40:616–622, 1995

Murphy HBM: Migration, culture and mental health. Psychol Med 7:677–684, 1977

Murphy HBM, Raman AC: The chronicity of schizophrenia in indigenous tropical people: results of a twelve-year follow-up survey in Mauritius. Br J Psychiatry 118:489–497, 1971

Murray CJL, Lopez AD: The Global Burden of Disease: A Comprehensive Assessment of Mortality and Disability From Diseases, Injuries, and Risk Factors in 1990 and Projected to 2020. Cambridge, MA, Harvard University Press, 1996

Ndetei DM, Vadher A: A comparative cross-cultural study of the frequencies of hallucinations in schizophrenia. Acta Psychiatr Scand 70:545–549, 1984

Neylan TC, van Kammen DP, Kelley ME, et al: Sleep in schizophrenic patients on and off haloperidol therapy: clinically stable versus relapsed patients. Arch Gen Psychiatry 49:643–649, 1992

Nimgaonkar VL: Reduced fertility in schizophrenia: here to stay? Acta Psychiatr Scand 98:348–353, 1998

Nimgaonkar VL, Ward SE, Agarde H, et al: Fertility in schizophrenia: results from a contemporary US cohort. Acta Psychiatr Scand 95:364–369 1997

Nopoulos P, Torres I, Flaum M, et al: Brain morphology in first-episode schizophrenia. Am J Psychiatry 152:1721–1723, 1995a

Nopoulos PC, Flaum M, Andreasen NC, et al: Gray matter heterotopias in schizophrenia. Psychiatry Res 61:11–14, 1995b

Nopoulos P, Swayze V, Andreasen NC: Pattern of brain morphology in patients with schizophrenia and large cavum septi pellucidi. J Neuropsychiatry Clin Neurosci 8:147–152, 1996

Nopoulos P, Swayze V, Flaum M: Cavum septi pellucidi in normals and patients with schizophrenia as detected by MRI. Biol Psychiatry 41:1102–1108, 1997

O'Callaghan E, Larkin C, Kinsella A, et al: Familial, obstetric, and other clinical correlates of minor physical anomalies in schizophrenia. Am J Psychiatry 148:479–483, 1991

Offord DR: School performance of adult schizophrenics, their siblings and age mates. Br J Psychiatry 125:12–19, 1974

Olin SS, John RS, Mednick SA: Assessing the predictive value of teacher reports in a high risk sample for schizophrenia: a ROC analysis. Schizophr Res 16:53–66, 1995

Olney JW, Farber NB: Glutamate receptor dysfunction and schizophrenia. Arch Gen Psychiatry 52:998–1007, 1995

Opjordsmoen S: Delusional disorders, I: comparative long-term outcome. Acta Psychiatr Scand 80:603–612, 1989

Pakkenberg B: Pronounced reduction of total neuron number in mediodorsal thalamic nucleus and nucleus accumbens in schizophrenics. Arch Gen Psychiatry 47:1023–1028, 1990

Pearlson GD, Garbacz DJ, Moberg PJ, et al: Symptomatic, familial, perinatal, and social correlates of computerized axial tomography (CAT) changes in schizophrenics and bipolars. J Nerv Ment Dis 173:42–50, 1985

Peet M, Middlemiss DN, Yates RA: Propranolol in schizophrenia, II: clinical and biochemical aspects of combining propranolol with chlorpromazine. Br J Psychiatry 139:112–117, 1981

Penn DL, Mueser KT: Research update on the psychosocial treatment of schizophrenia. Am J Psychiatry 153:607–617, 1996

Perry JC, Jacobs D: Overview: clinical applications of the Amytal interview in psychiatric emergency settings. Am J Psychiatry 139:552–559, 1982

Perry PJ, Smith DA: Neuroleptic plasma concentrations: an estimate of their sensitivity and specificity as predictors of response, in Clinical Use of Neuroleptic Plasma Levels. Edited by Marder SR, Davis JM, Janicak PG. Washington, DC, American Psychiatric Press, 1993, pp 113–135

Petronis A, Kennedy JL: Unstable genes—unstable mind? Am J Psychiatry 152:164–172, 1995

Petronis A, Bassett AS, Honer WG, et al: Search for unstable DNA in schizophrenia families with evidence for genetic anticipation. Am J Hum Genet 59:905–911, 1996

Pfohl B, Winokur G: The micropsychopathology of hebephrenic/catatonic schizophrenia. J Nerv Ment Dis 171:296–300, 1983

Pollack M, Woerner MG, Goodman W, et al: Childhood development patterns of hospitalized adult schizophrenic and nonschizophrenic patients and their siblings. Am J Orthopsychiatry 36:510–517, 1966

Pulver AE: Search for schizophrenia susceptibility genes. Biol Psychiatry 47:221–230, 2000

Rabinowitz J, Reichenberg A, Weiser M, et al: Cognitive and behavioural functioning in men with schizophrenia both before and shortly after first admission to hospital. Cross-sectional analysis. Br J Psychiatry 177:26–32, 2000

Radant AD, Bowdle TA, Cowley DS, et al: Does ketamine-mediated N-methyl-D-aspartate receptor antagonism cause schizophrenia-like oculomotor abnormalities? Neuropsychopharmacology 19:434–444, 1998

Rice JP, McGuffin P: Genetic Etiology of Schizophrenia and Affective Disorders in Psychiatry, Vol 1. Edited by Michels R, Cavenar JO. Philadelphia, PA, JB Lippincott, 1985

Riecher-Rossler A, Rossler W: The course of schizophrenic psychoses: what do we really know? A selective review from an epidemiological perspective. Eur Arch Psychiatry Clin Neurosci 248:189–202, 1998

Rifkin A, Doddi S, Karajgi B, et al: Dosage of haloperidol for schizophrenia. Arch Gen Psychiatry 48:166–170, 1991

Robins LN, Helzer JE, Weissman MM, et al: Lifetime prevalence of specific psychiatric disorders in three sites. Arch Gen Psychiatry 41:949–958, 1984

Ross DE, Thaker GK, Buchanan RW, et al: Association of abnormal smooth-pursuit eye movements with the deficit syndrome in schizophrenic patients. Am J Psychiatry 153:1158–1165, 1996

Roy A: Suicide in chronic schizophrenia. Br J Psychiatry 141:171–177, 1982

Roy MA, Merette C, Maziade M: Subtyping schizophrenia according to outcome or severity: a search for homogeneous subgroups. Schizophr Bull 27:115–138, 2001

Rudin E: Studien uber Vererbung and Entstehung geistiger storungen I: Zur vererbung and Neuenstehung der Dementia Praecox. Berlin, Germany, Springer-Verlag, 1916

Sartorius N, Jablensky A, Korten A: Early manifestations and first contact incidence of schizophrenia in different cultures: a preliminary report on the evaluation of the WHO Collaborative Study in Determinants of Outcome of Severe Mental Disorders. Psychol Med 16:909–928, 1986

Schizophrenia Collaborative Linkage Group for Chromosomes 3, 6, and 8: Additional support for schizophrenia linkage on chromosomes 6 and 8: a multi-center study. Am J Med Genet 67:580–594, 1996

Schlaepfer TE, Harris GJ, Tien AY, et al: Diseased regional cortical gray matter volume in schizophrenia. Am J Psychiatry 151:842–848, 1994

Schneider K: Clinical Psychopathology. New York, Grune & Stratton, 1959

Schooler NR, Kane JM, Marder SR, et al: Efficacy of clozapine vs. haloperidol in a long-term clinical trial: preliminary findings (abstract). Schizophr Bull 15:165, 1995

Schwab SG, Albus M, Hallmayer J, et al: Evaluation of a susceptibility gene for schizophrenia on chromosome 6p by multipoint affected sib-pair linkage analysis. Nat Genet 11:325–327, 1995

Sears LL, Andreasen NC, O'Leary DS: Cerebellar functional abnormalities in schizophrenia are suggested by classical eyeblink conditioning. Biol Psychiatry 48:204–209, 2000

Seeman P, Lee T, Chau-Wong M, et al: Antipsychotic drug doses and neuroleptic-dopamine receptors. Nature 261:717–719, 1976

Segal JH: Erotomania revisited: from Kraepelin to DSM-III-R. Am J Psychiatry 146:1261–1266, 1989

Selemon LD, Rajkowska G, Goldman-Rakic S: Abnormally high neuronal density in the schizophrenic cortex. Arch Gen Psychiatry 52:805–818, 1995

Sensky T, Turkington D, Kingdon D, et al: A randomized controlled trial of cognitive-behavioral therapy for persistent symptoms in schizophrenia resistant to medication. Arch Gen Psychiatry 57:165–172, 2000

Serretti A, Lattuada E, Cusin C, et al: Factor analysis of delusional disorder symptomatology. Compr Psychiatry 40:143–147, 1999

Shapiro S, Skinner EA, Kessler LG, et al: Utilization of health and mental health services: three Epidemiologic Catchment Area sites. Arch Gen Psychiatry 41:971–978, 1984

Shenton ME, Kikinis R, Jolesz FA, et al: Abnormalities of the left temporal lobe and thought disorder in schizophrenia: a quantitative magnetic resonance imaging study. N Engl J Med 327:604–612, 1992

Shenton ME, Wible CG, McCarley RW: A review of magnetic resonance imaging studies of brain anomalies in schizophrenia, in Brain Imaging in Clinical Psychiatry. Edited by Krishnan KRR, Doraiswamy PM. New York, Marcel Dekker, 1997, pp 297–380

Silbersweig DA, Stern E, Frith C, et al: A functional neuroanatomy of hallucinations in schizophrenia. Nature 378:176–179, 1995

Silverton L, Mednick S: Class drift and schizophrenia. Acta Psychiatr Scand 70:304–309, 1984

Simpson JC, Tsuang MT: Mortality among patients with schizophrenia. Schizophr Bull 22:485–499, 1996

Siris SG, Morgan V, Fagerstrom R, et al: Adjunctive imipramine in the treatment of postpsychotic depression: a controlled trial. Arch Gen Psychiatry 44:533–539, 1987

Siris SG, Bermanzohn PC, Mason SE, et al: Maintenance imipramine therapy for secondary depression in schizophrenia: a controlled trial. Arch Gen Psychiatry 51:109–115, 1994

Slaby AE, Moreines R: Emergency room evaluation and management of schizophrenia, in Handbook of Schizophrenia, Vol 4: Psychosocial Treatment of Schizophrenia. Edited by Herz MI, Keith SJ, Docherty JP. New York, Elsevier, 1990, pp 247–268

Slater E: The monogenetic theory of schizophrenia. Acta Genet Med Gemellol (Roma) 8:50–56, 1958

Snyder SH: Catecholamines in the brain as mediators of amphetamine psychosis. Arch Gen Psychiatry 27:169–179, 1972

Spitzer RL, Endicott J, Robins E: Research diagnostic criteria: rationale and reliability. Arch Gen Psychiatry 35:773–782, 1978

Stein L: A system approach to reducing relapse in schizophrenia. J Clin Psychiatry 54(suppl 3):7–12, 1993

Storey PB: Lumbar air encephalography in chronic schizophrenia: a controlled experiment. Br J Psychiatry 112:135–144, 1966

Stoudemire A: A differential diagnosis of catatonic states. Psychosomatics 23:245–251, 1982

Strakowski SM: Diagnostic validity of schizophreniform disorder. Am J Psychiatry 151:815–824, 1994

Strauss JS, Carpenter WJ: Schizophrenia. New York, Plenum, 1981

Susser E, Struening EL, Conover S: Psychiatric problems in homeless men: lifetime psychosis, substance use, and current disorders in new arrivals at New York City shelters. Arch Gen Psychiatry 46:845–850, 1989

Susser E, Neugebauer R, Hoek H, et al: Schizophrenia after premorbid famine: further evidence. Arch Gen Psychiatry 53:25–31, 1996

Swanson JW, Holtzer CE, Ganju VK, et al: Violence and psychiatric disorder in the community: evidence from the Epidemiology Catchment Area Surveys. Hosp Community Psychiatry 41:761–770, 1990

Swayze VW, Andreasen NC, Ehrhardt JC, et al: Developmental abnormalities of the corpus callosum in schizophrenia. Arch Neurol 47:805–808, 1990

Swerdlow NR, Geyer MA: Clozapine and haloperidol in an animal model of sensorimotor gating deficits in schizophrenia. Pharmacol Biochem Behav 44:741–744, 1993

Szeszko PR, Bilder RM, Lencz T, et al: Investigation of frontal lobe subregions in first-episode schizophrenia. Psychiatry Res 90:1–15, 1999

Tanna VL: Paranoid states: a selected review. Compr Psychiatry 15:453–470, 1974

Targum SD: Neuroendocrine dysfunction in schizophreniform disorder: correlation with 6-month clinical outcome. Am J Psychiatry 140:309–313, 1983

Tarrier N, Beckett R, Harwood S, et al: A trial of two cognitive-behavioral methods of treating drug-resistant residual psychotic symptoms in schizophrenic patients, I: outcome. Br J Psychiatry 162:524–532, 1993

Taube CA, Barrett SA (eds): Mental Health United States 1985 (DHHS Publ No ADM 85–1378). Rockville, MD, National Institute of Mental Health, 1985

Teplin LA: The criminality of the mentally ill: a dangerous misconception. Am J Psychiatry 142:593–599, 1985

Thacker GK, Cassady S, Adami H, et al: Eye movements in spectrum personality disorders: comparison of community subjects and relatives of schizophrenic patients. Am J Psychiatry 153:362–368, 1996

Tienari P: Psychiatric illness in identical twins. Acta Psychiatr Scand Suppl, No 171, 1963

Tienari P, Wynne LC, Moring J, et al: Finnish adoptive family study: sample selection and adoptee DSM-III-R diagnoses. Acta Psychiatr Scand 101:433–443, 2000

Tollefson GD, Sanger TM, Lu Y, et al: Depressive signs and symptoms in schizophrenia: a prospective blinded trial of olanzapine and haloperidol. Arch Gen Psychiatry 55:250–258, 1998

Tsuang MT: Suicide in schizophrenics, manics, depressives, and surgical controls: a comparison with general population suicide mortality. Arch Gen Psychiatry 35:153–155, 1978

Tsuang MT, Winokur G: Criteria for subtyping schizophrenia: clinical differentiation of hebephrenic and paranoid schizophrenia. Arch Gen Psychiatry 31:43–47, 1974

Tsuang MT, Woolson RF, Fleming JA: Long-term outcome of major psychoses, I: schizophrenia and affective disorders compared with psychiatrically symptom-free surgical conditions. Arch Gen Psychiatry 36:1295–1304, 1979

Tsuang MT, Stone WS, Faraone SV: Toward reformulating the diagnosis of schizophrenia. Am J Psychiatry 157:1041–1050, 2000

Turner SW, Toone BK, Brett-Jones JR: Computerized tomographic scan change in early schizophrenia. Psychol Med 16:209–225, 1986

Vaillant GE: Prospective prediction of schizophrenic remission. Arch Gen Psychiatry 11:509–518, 1964

VanderZwaag C, McGee M, McEvoy JP, et al: Response of patients with treatment-refractory schizophrenia to clozapine with three serum level ranges. Am J Psychiatry 153:1579–1584, 1996

VanKammen DP, Peters J, Yao J, et al: Norepinephrine in acute exacerbations of chronic schizophrenia: negative symptoms revisited. Arch Gen Psychiatry 47:161–168, 1990

Wahlbeck K, Cheine MV, Gilbody S, et al: Efficacy of beta-blocker supplementation for schizophrenia: a systematic review of randomized trials. Schizophr Res 41:341–347, 2000

Waldo M, Cawthra E, Adler L, et al: Auditory sensory gating, hippocampal volume, and catecholamine metabolism in schizophrenics and their siblings. Schizophr Res 12:93–106, 1994

Walker E, Lewine RJ: Prediction of adult-onset schizophrenia from childhood home movies of the patients. Am J Psychiatry 147:1052–1056, 1990

Wang S, Sun CE, Walczak CA, et al: Evidence for a susceptibility locus for schizophrenia on chromosome 6pter–p22. Nat Genet 10:41–46, 1995

Ward KE, Friedman L, Wise A, et al: Meta-analysis of brain and cranial size in schizophrenia. Schizophr Res 22:197–123, 1996

Watt DC, Katz K, Shepard M: The natural history of schizophrenia: a five-year prospective follow-up of a representative sample of schizophrenics by means of a standardized clinical and social assessment. Psychol Med 13:663–670, 1983

Watt JAG: The relationship of paranoid states to schizophrenia. Am J Psychiatry 142:1456–1458, 1985

Watt NF: Patterns of childhood social development in adult schizophrenics. Arch Gen Psychiatry 35:160–165, 1978

Watt NF, Stolorow RD, Lubensky AW, et al: School adjustment and behavior of children hospitalized for schizophrenia as adults. Am J Orthopsychiatry 40:637–657, 1970

Watt NF, Anthony EJ, Wynne LC, et al: Children At Risk for Schizophrenia: A Longitudinal Perspective. Cambridge, England, Cambridge University Press, 1984

Weiden PJ, Dixon L, Frances A, et al: Neuroleptic noncompliance in schizophrenia, in Advances in Neuropsychiatry and Psychopharmacology, Vol 1: Schizophrenia Research. Edited by Tamminga CA, Schulz SC. New York, Raven, 1991, pp 285–296

Weiler MA, Thaker GK, Lahti AC, et al: Ketamine effects on eye movements. Neuropsychopharmacology 23:645–653, 2000

Weinberger DR: Implications of normal brain development for the pathogenesis of schizophrenia. Arch Gen Psychiatry 44:660–669, 1987

Weinberger DR, Torrey EF, Neophytides AN, et al: Lateral cerebral ventricle enlargement in chronic schizophrenia. Arch Gen Psychiatry 36:735–755, 1979

Weinberger DR, Bigelow LB, Kleinman JE, et al: Cerebral ventricular enlargement in chronic schizophrenia: an association with poor response to treatment. Arch Gen Psychiatry 37:11–13, 1980

Wender PH, Rosenthal D, Kety SS, et al: Social class and psychopathology in adoptees: a natural experimental method for separating the roles of genetic and experimental factors. Arch Gen Psychiatry 28:318–325, 1973

depends on how it is defined; broader definitions produce significantly higher rates (Akiskal 1995b; Angst 1995). Most prevalence studies require the presence of mania for a bipolar diagnosis to be recorded, but the bipolar II variant, which is characterized by episodes of hypomania but not mania, is more common than the bipolar I variant (Cassano et al. 1989; Simpson et al. 1993). If bipolar spectrum disorders, or subsyndromal and complex forms of bipolar disorder (see "Masked and Subsyndromal Bipolar Disorder"), are also considered (Akiskal 1995b), the incidence of bipolar mood disorder is substantially higher. About 10%–15% of the patients with a diagnosis of unipolar depression will eventually receive a revised diagnosis of bipolar disorder (Olie et al. 1992).

When conservative criteria are used, between 5% and 15% of cases of adult depression are found to be bipolar (Bebbington 1995; Geller et al. 1996). However, Akiskal's group (Cassano et al. 1989) found that one-third of the patients with primary depression met their criteria for bipolar spectrum disorders. The risk of bipolarity is higher in juvenile major depression—at least 20% in depressed adolescents and 32% in depressed children younger than 11 years (Geller et al. 1996). The lifetime rate of classically defined bipolar disorder is relatively consistent across cultures, ranging from 0.3 per 100 in Taiwan to 1.5 per 100 in New Zealand (Weissman et al. 1996).

In all industrialized countries in the world, the incidence of depression, mania, suicide, and psychotic mood disorders has been increasing with every generation born after 1910 (Cross-National Collaborative Group 1992; Klerman 1988; Klerman et al. 1985). The risk of severe and moderate depression increased 10-fold from 1947–1957 to 1957–1972 (Khodorov et al. 1999). For unknown reasons, there was an abrupt jump in the rate of increase for people born after 1940—a true increase in the incidence of mood disorders in subsequent generations (cohort effect) and not a function of better recognition or more help-seeking (Cross-National Collaborative Group 1992; Doris et al. 1999; Klerman 1988; Klerman et al. 1985). Mood disorders not only are becoming more common but also are appearing at an earlier age (especially bipolar mood disorders) (Lasch and Weissman 1990).

In worldwide surveys, depression is the fourth most important cause of disability (Figiel et al. 1998) and the fourth most costly medical illness (Carney and Jackson 1998). Depressed patients spend more time in bed than do patients with diabetes, hypertension, arthritis, or chronic lung disease (Martin et al. 1992) and have as much functional disability as do patients with heart disease (Martin et al. 1992). Primary care physicians spend more time treating depression than hypertension, arteriosclerotic heart disease, and diabetes mellitus.

Suicide is an obvious public health problem that complicates mood disorders more frequently than other conditions. The lifetime risk of suicide in mood disorders is 10%–15% (Barklage 1991; Guze and Robbins 1970; Mueller and Leon 1996), and the risk of attempted suicide was increased 41-fold in depressed patients compared with those with other diagnoses in the Epidemiologic Catchment Area (ECA) survey (Petronis et al. 1990). It is well known that women attempt suicide more frequently than men do, but men are more likely to succeed. In one study, the excess risk of completed suicide in men was entirely accounted for by a higher prevalence of substance abuse in men and a greater likelihood that women have primary responsibility for children younger than 18 (Young et al. 1994). The risk of suicide is high in mania as well as in depression. Patients with mixed bipolar states characterized by a combination of depression, rage, and grandiosity may be more likely to involve others in a suicide attempt—for example, through gunfights with the police. As many as 4% of the people who commit suicide murder someone else first. High levels of distress and hopelessness increase the risk of suicide attempts in adolescents (Fritsch et al. 2000). Neuropsychological deficits are more common in depressed patients who have made high-lethality suicide attempts than in those who have made low-lethality attempts and nonpatients, suggesting that impaired executive function may exist in people at risk for severe suicide attempts (Keilp et al. 2001).

Although many clinicians agree on factors that increase the risk for suicide, formal attempts to predict suicide have been disappointing (Oxley and Van Meter 1996). This is not surprising; suicide is such a rare event (about 11/100,000 in the United States) that a prohibitively large number of patients would have to be followed up prospectively to show that a constellation of features predicted an increased risk. In addition, no consensus exists about how long to follow a depressed patient before a conclusion can be made that suicide will not occur. There may be a statistically significant association between suicide and traditional risk factors such as older age, recent loss, male sex, bipolar depression, psychosis, comorbid substance abuse, history of a suicide attempt (especially if it was dangerous), and family history of suicide, but this association is not necessarily helpful in predicting suicide in an individual patient.

Despite the demonstrated inability of mental health professionals to predict (or prevent) suicide in any systematic manner (H. L. Miller et al. 1984), patients, families, and courts expect them to be able to do so. In an evaluation of immediate suicide risk, factors summarized in Table 10–1 can be considered (Oxley and Van Meter 1996; Pokorny 1993; Young et al. 1994). However, these factors at best suggest increased immediate risk. In addition, the short-term risk tends to fluctuate, and it is not known whether one risk factor is more important than another or how risk factors may interact with one another (Oxley and Van Meter 1996). Given the current state of knowledge, it is probably impossible for anyone to predict with any accuracy the long-term risk of completed suicide.

TABLE 10–1. Factors suggesting an increased risk of suicide

Demographic factors
  Male sex
  Recent loss
  Never married
  Older age
Symptoms
  Severe depression
  Anxiety
  Hopelessness
  Psychosis, especially with command hallucinations
History
  History of suicide attempts, especially if multiple or
    severe attempts
  Family history of suicide
  Active substance abuse
Suicidal thinking
  Presence of a specific plan
  Means available to carry out the plan
  Absence of factors that would keep the patient from
    completing the plan
  Rehearsal of the plan

Mood Disorders in Special Populations

Postpartum depression occurs in about 10% of mothers; risk factors include a history of a mood disorder, unwanted pregnancy, unemployment of the mother, lack of breast-feeding, and the mother as head of the household (J. Hopkins et al. 1984; Warner et al. 1996). Postpartum depression increases the chance of alcohol and illicit drug use in teenaged mothers (Barnet et al. 1995). Some evidence indicates that depression in a mother adversely affects temperament (C. T. Beck 1996) and cognitive development (Hay and Kumar 1995) in the infant. Depressed mothers of preschoolers have more negative perceptions of and interactions with their children (Lang et al. 1996). Depression that begins for the first time in the postpartum period is more likely to have

a bipolar outcome; postpartum psychosis very frequently is a manifestation of bipolar disorder.

Estimates of the prevalence of major depression in elderly people range from 2%–4% in community samples to 12% of medically hospitalized patients to 16% of geriatric patients in long-term care (Blazer and Koenig 1996). Late-onset depression is associated with an increased likelihood of cerebrovascular disease and enlarged ventricles and may be more likely than depression in younger patients to be accompanied by prominent cognitive complaints (Soares and Mann 1997).

Major depressive disorder (MDD) is said to occur in as many as 18% of preadolescents, with no gender differences (Kashani and Nair 1995). However, mood disorders are often underdiagnosed in this population because many clinicians still do not believe that depression occurs in children and because depression may be more difficult to recognize in children than in older patients. Among adolescents, the prevalence of MDD has been reported to be 4.7% in 14- to 16-year-olds (Kashani and Nair 1995). By this age, depression is more common in girls than in boys (Kashani and Nair 1995). In nonclinical samples, up to one-third of the adolescents reported some depressive symptoms (Kashani and Nair 1995). Major depression in adolescents is associated with substance abuse and antisocial behavior, both of which sometimes obscure the affective diagnosis (Kashani and Nair 1995). The lifetime prevalence of bipolar disorder was 0.6% in 150 adolescents who were not psychiatrically referred (Kashani and Nair 1995). As discussed later in this chapter (see "Mood Disorders in Children and Adolescents"), many cases of bipolar disorder in younger patients may be overlooked because mania has not yet appeared or because, when it is present, it is manifested by anxiety, irritability, and attentional and behavioral syndromes that mask the mood disorder.

Economics of Mood Disorders

Depression produces more impairment of physical functioning, role functioning, social functioning, and perceived current health; is associated with more bodily pain; and causes patients to spend more days in bed because of poor health than do hypertension, diabetes, arthritis, and chronic pulmonary disease (Wells et al. 1989). In a study of general medical patients in a health maintenance organization, patients with depressed mood or anhedonia of 2 weeks' duration but with an insufficient number of additional symptoms to meet full criteria for MDD still had 7.7 times as much impairment of social, family, and work functioning as did patients without any depressive symptoms (Olfson

1996). The total cost of depressive disorders in the United States is generally estimated at $44 billion (Hall and Wise 1995). This is equivalent to the total cost of coronary heart disease, a condition that is no more prevalent and less readily treatable than depression. The direct costs of treating depression are about $12 billion, only $890 million of which is accounted for by the price of antidepressants (Hall and Wise 1995). Yet, tremendous effort is being expended by third-party reviewers to get physicians to prescribe less expensive antidepressants. The morbidity cost of depressive disorders in the United States is around $24 billion, and the mortality costs are $8 billion; these costs can be attributed in part to increased accident rates, substance abuse, development of somatic illness such as coronary heart disease, and increased use of medical hospitalization and outpatient treatment (Denollet et al. 2000; Hall and Wise 1995).

Diagnosis

Attempts to classify depression date back to at least the fourth century B.C., when Hippocrates coined the terms *melancholia* (black bile) and *mania* (to be mad). The independent descriptions in 1854 by two French physicians, Falret and Baillarger, of *folie circulaire* and *la folie à double forme* were the first formal diagnoses of alternating episodes of mania and depression as a single disorder (Sedler 1983). At the beginning of the twentieth century, Emil Kraepelin differentiated schizophrenia (dementia praecox) from "manic-depressive insanity" (now called bipolar disorder) on the basis of a deteriorating course of the former and an episodic course of the latter (Akiskal 1996). Kraepelin (1921) believed that manic-depressive insanity was a single illness that included "periodic and circular insanity," mania, and melancholia, although he also acknowledged that in many cases it was difficult to tell the difference between dementia praecox and manic-depressive insanity. Although many of Kraepelin's observations of the symptoms and course of bipolar mood disorder remain accurate, this condition is now known to be complex groups of disorders that share features such as a high rate of recurrence, a greater risk of psychosis, and alternations of mood states but differ in other important respects.

In the United States, DSM-I (American Psychiatric Association 1952) reflected the influence of Adolph Meyer. Meyer believed that psychiatric disorders were reactions to conflict or stress that were more specific to the individual than to the illness. Psychotic mood disorders (e.g., psychotic depressive reaction) were diagnosed on the basis not of hallucinations and delusions but of severity and lack of a precipitant (American Psychiatric Association 1952). In DSM-II (American Psychiatric Association 1968), *involutional melancholia* and *manic-depressive psychosis* were added. The concept of a depressive reaction was maintained as *depressive neurosis*, which was considered a neurotic reaction to an internal conflict or external event. In the absence of a precipitant, a diagnosis of psychotic depressive reaction was made for a single episode and manic-depressive psychosis for recurrent depressive episodes, regardless of whether the patient met traditional criteria for psychosis in use by most clinicians. Alternating depression and elation was called *cyclothymia*, which was classified with the personality disorders on the grounds that it was chronic and was not caused by a specific circumstance. In subsequent editions of DSM (see "Diagnosis and DSM-IV-TR"), mood disorder diagnoses are based on symptom clusters rather than the presence or absence of an identifiable precipitant, because the presence of a precipitant does not demonstrably affect the course or treatment response of mood disorders.

Endogenous and Reactive Depression

The differentiation of depression according to whether a psychosocial precipitant is present is derived from an early distinction between endogenous (vital or melancholic) and reactive depression. In its original use by German descriptive psychiatrists, the term *reactive* referred to a depressed patient's ability to react positively to interactions and events and thus implied the presence of milder symptomatology. As the term was translated into English, however, it came to mean depression that developed in reaction to some external stress, thus implying an association between mild depression and depression in response to stress. In DSM-II, this concept was conserved as *neurotic depressive reaction*. In later informal diagnostic schemes, milder forms of depression in which mood is more responsive to the environment evolved into the concept of *hysteroid dysphoria*, which is a type of depression with atypical symptoms that occurs in a patient with interpersonal sensitivity and a characterological tendency to dramatize (Shea and Hirschfeld 1996). In DSM-III-R (American Psychiatric Association 1987) and DSM-IV (American Psychiatric Association 1994a), the term *atypical depression* (a modifier of a major depressive episode) is more or less equivalent to hysteroid dysphoria and the modern derivative of neurotic depression.

Atypical depression is distinguished by mood reactivity (i.e., the capacity to be cheered up temporarily by positive interactions or events) as well as by severe anergia (leaden paralysis), sensitivity to rejection, self-pity, a reverse diurnal mood swing (depression is worse later in the day), and reverse vegetative symptoms (e.g., increased instead of decreased appetite and sleep) (M.T. Tsuang and Faraone 1996). About 15% of depressive episodes have atypical features. Atypical symptoms are more common in bipolar depression. As is discussed later in this chapter (see section "Antidepressant Medications"), atypical depression appears to respond better to monoamine oxidase inhibitor (MAOI) and selective serotonin reuptake inhibitor (SSRI) antidepressants than to tricyclic antidepressants (TCAs).

In contrast to reactive depression, the term *endogenous depression* referred in the German literature to depression that was unresponsive to the environment and in the American literature to depression with greater severity, more guilt and loss of interest, and typical vegetative symptoms such as decreased appetite and sleep, difficulty concentrating, early-morning awakening, and a diurnal mood swing (depression is worse in the morning) (M.T. Tsuang and Faraone 1996). In DSM-IV, the *melancholic features* specifier retains most of the features of endogenous depression; recent research suggests that "lack of reactivity" and "distinct quality of depressed mood" predict the full syndrome most consistently (K.S. Kendler 1997). However, melancholic depression can appear in response to an obvious precipitant. Endogenous depression has a better response to TCAs than does reactive depression and has a lower rate of response to psychotherapy and placebo (M.T. Tsuang and Faraone 1996).

Recent work has confirmed that the melancholic subtype of major depression is a more severe form of major depression that is associated with more depressive episodes, more symptoms, more impairment, more help-seeking, and more comorbidity with anxiety disorders and nicotine dependence but that is not qualitatively different from nonmelancholic major depression (K.S. Kendler 1997). In twins, the presence of MDD with melancholic features in one twin increased the risk of major depression but not necessarily melancholia in the other twin (K.S. Kendler 1997). Twin studies do not suggest an environmental influence on liability to melancholia in depressed patients (K.S. Kendler 1997). It is also now appreciated that melancholic and atypical depression are not necessarily mutually exclusive.

Diagnosis and DSM-IV-TR

The term *affect* usually refers to the outward and changeable manifestation of a person's emotional tone, whereas *mood* is a more enduring emotional orientation that colors the person's psychology (American Psychiatric Association 1984). However, the change from *affective disorders* in DSM-III to *mood disorders* in DSM-IV does not imply a reconceptualization of what these disorders primarily involve (i.e., dysregulation of mood or dysregulation of affect); the two terms are used interchangeably in DSM-IV.

DSM-IV (and its recent update DSM-IV-TR [American Psychiatric Association 2000]) distinguishes between mood episodes and mood disorders (Fava and Davidson 1996; First et al. 1996). An episode is a period lasting at least 2 weeks during which there are enough symptoms for full criteria to be met for the disorder. The criteria for a major depressive episode are summarized in Table 10–2. Patients with or without a history of mania may have a major depressive episode if they fulfill these criteria, but MDD refers to one or more episodes of major depression in the absence of mania or hypomania (i.e., unipolar depression). A major depressive episode may be modified by additional specifiers for psychotic, melancholic (Table 10–3), and atypical features (Table 10–4).

The interpretation of studies of mood disorders is facilitated by familiarity with several common terms (Fava and Davidson 1996; First et al. 1996). In most treatment studies, *response* is defined as at least 50% improvement, whereas *partial response* is 25%–50% improvement, and *nonresponse* is less than 25% improvement. According to this terminology, patients who are still half as symptomatic as at the beginning of treatment will be considered responders at the end of a treatment study. This is not a trivial point, given that most studies consider improvement rather than remission as the end point. *Remission* is defined as the state of having few or no symptoms of a mood disorder for at least 8 weeks. *Recovery*, the period after remission, is present if no symptoms have been present for more than 8 weeks, and the term implies that the disorder is quiescent. A *relapse* is a return of symptoms during the period of remission, implying continuation of the original episode, whereas *recurrence* is a later return of symptoms (during recovery), suggesting that a new episode has developed. These distinctions can be difficult to make in clinical practice. For example, mild residual symptoms of an initial episode or persistent psychosocial dysfunction may be overlooked or may be attributed to character pathology after improvement of the more dramatic manifestations of an episode, leading to the mistaken conclusion that a return of more severe symptoms represents a new episode rather than an exacerbation of the original episode.

TABLE 10–2. DSM-IV-TR criteria for major depressive episode

A. Five (or more) of the following symptoms have been present during the same 2-week period and represent a change from previous functioning; at least one of the symptoms is either (1) depressed mood or (2) loss of interest or pleasure.

 Note: Do not include symptoms that are clearly due to a general medical condition, or mood-incongruent delusions or hallucinations.

 (1) depressed mood most of the day, nearly every day, as indicated by either subjective report (e.g., feels sad or empty) or observation made by others (e.g., appears tearful). Note: In children and adolescents, can be irritable mood.

 (2) markedly diminished interest or pleasure in all, or almost all, activities most of the day, nearly every day (as indicated by either subjective account or observation made by others)

 (3) significant weight loss when not dieting or weight gain (e.g., a change of more than 5% of body weight in a month), or decrease or increase in appetite nearly every day. Note: In children, consider failure to make expected weight gains.

 (4) insomnia or hypersomnia nearly every day

 (5) psychomotor agitation or retardation nearly every day (observable by others, not merely subjective feelings of restlessness or being slowed down)

 (6) fatigue or loss of energy nearly every day

 (7) feelings of worthlessness or excessive or inappropriate guilt (which may be delusional) nearly every day (not merely self-reproach or guilt about being sick)

 (8) diminished ability to think or concentrate, or indecisiveness, nearly every day (either by subjective account or as observed by others)

 (9) recurrent thoughts of death (not just fear of dying), recurrent suicidal ideation without a specific plan, or a suicide attempt or a specific plan for committing suicide

B. The symptoms do not meet criteria for a mixed episode.

C. The symptoms cause clinically significant distress or impairment in social, occupational, or other important areas of functioning.

D. The symptoms are not due to the direct physiological effects of a substance (e.g., a drug of abuse, a medication) or a general medical condition (e.g., hypothyroidism).

E. The symptoms are not better accounted for by bereavement, i.e., after the loss of a loved one, the symptoms persist for longer than 2 months or are characterized by marked functional impairment, morbid preoccupation with worthlessness, suicidal ideation, psychotic symptoms, or psychomotor retardation.

TABLE 10–3. DSM-IV-TR criteria for melancholic features specifier

Specify if:

With Melancholic Features (can be applied to the current or most recent major depressive episode in major depressive disorder and to a major depressive episode in bipolar I or bipolar II disorder only if it is the most recent type of mood episode)

A. Either of the following, occurring during the most severe period of the current episode:

 (1) loss of pleasure in all, or almost all, activities

 (2) lack of reactivity to usually pleasurable stimuli (does not feel much better, even temporarily, when something good happens)

B. Three (or more) of the following:

 (1) distinct quality of depressed mood (i.e., the depressed mood is experienced as distinctly different from the kind of feeling experienced after the death of a loved one)

 (2) depression regularly worse in the morning

 (3) early morning awakening (at least 2 hours before usual time of awakening)

 (4) marked psychomotor retardation or agitation

 (5) significant anorexia or weight loss

 (6) excessive or inappropriate guilt

TABLE 10–4. DSM-IV-TR criteria for atypical features specifier

Specify if:

With Atypical Features (can be applied when these features predominate during the most recent 2 weeks of a current major depressive episode in major depressive disorder or in bipolar I or bipolar II disorder when a current major depressive episode is the most recent type of mood episode, or when these features predominate during the most recent 2 years of dysthymic disorder; if the major depressive episode is not current, it applies if the feature predominates during any 2-week period)

A. Mood reactivity (i.e., mood brightens in response to actual or potential positive events)

B. Two (or more) of the following features:

 (1) significant weight gain or increase in appetite

 (2) hypersomnia

 (3) leaden paralysis (i.e., heavy, leaden feelings in arms or legs)

 (4) long-standing pattern of interpersonal rejection sensitivity (not limited to episodes of mood disturbance) that results in significant social or occupational impairment

C. Criteria are not met for with melancholic features or with catatonic features during the same episode.

Unipolar and Bipolar Mood Disorders

One of the most important distinctions between mood disorders is the distinction between unipolar and bipolar categories (Leonhard 1987a, 1987b). Unipolar mood disorders are characterized by depressive symptoms in the absence of a history of pathologically elevated mood. In bipolar mood disorders, depression alternates or is mixed with mania or hypomania. Patients who have only had recurrent mania ("unipolar mania") are given the diagnosis of bipolar mood disorder on the assumption that they will eventually develop an episode of depression (M.T. Tsuang and Faraone 1996). DSM-IV-TR criteria for a manic episode are summarized in Table 10–5. Hypomania, a milder form of pathologically elevated mood that can be present for a shorter period before it is diagnosed, is described in Table 10–6. Although most people think of *elation* as a defining characteristic of mania and hypomania, many patients experience only irritability, anxiety, or a dysphoric sense of increased energy, as if they were "crawling out of their skins." This kind of presentation may occur most frequently in women and younger patients with bipolar disorder and in antidepressant-induced hypomania. In DSM-IV-TR, it is noted that mania is a state of increased goal-directed behavior that is pleasurable and has obvious potential for harm; however, behavior in mania is often excessive, disorganized, and dysphoric but not clearly harmful or dangerous (American Psychiatric Association 2000). The physical hyperactivity of chronic hypomania may be characterized primarily by random increases in activity that shifts its focus from moment to moment, and some patients experience more mental than physical overstimulation.

Most authorities agree that the bipolar–unipolar distinction is dichotomous: a patient either is or is not manic. In addition, the course of bipolar disorders differs from that of unipolar disorders (Dubovsky et al. 1989, 1991a; Faedda et al. 1995; Leibenluft et al. 1995; M.T. Tsuang and Faraone 1996; Weissman et al. 1996; Winokur 1995); the differences are summarized in Table 10–7. On closer scrutiny, these distinctions may not be as obvious as they might seem at first. For example, unipolar depression can be psychotic with severe depressive symptoms, and depressive episodes may be highly recurrent without ever being associated with mania. Lithium can increase the effectiveness of antidepressants in unipolar depression, and electroconvulsive therapy (ECT) is effective in treating both mania and depression (Dubovsky and Buzan 1997). Patients with unipolar depression may have symptoms generally associated with bipolar disorder such as agitation, racing thoughts, and overspending. Unipolar and bipolar disorders can aggre-

TABLE 10–5. DSM-IV-TR criteria for manic episode

A. A distinct period of abnormally and persistently elevated, expansive, or irritable mood, lasting at least 1 week (or any duration if hospitalization is necessary).

B. During the period of mood disturbance, three (or more) of the following symptoms have persisted (four if the mood is only irritable) and have been present to a significant degree:
   (1) inflated self esteem or grandiosity
   (2) decreased need for sleep (e.g., feels rested after only 3 hours of sleep)
   (3) more talkative than usual or pressure to keep talking
   (4) flight of ideas or subjective experience that thoughts are racing
   (5) distractibility (i.e., attention too easily drawn to unimportant or irrelevant external stimuli)
   (6) increase in goal-directed activity (either socially, at work or school, or sexually) or psychomotor agitation
   (7) excessive involvement in pleasurable activities that have a high potential for painful consequences (e.g., engaging in unrestrained buying sprees, sexual indiscretions, or foolish business investments)

C. The symptoms do not meet criteria for a mixed episode.

D. The mood disturbance is sufficiently severe to cause marked impairment in occupational functioning or in usual social activities or relationships with others, or to necessitate hospitalization to prevent harm to self or others, or there are psychotic features.

E. The symptoms are not due to the direct physiological effects of a substance (e.g., a drug of abuse, a medication, or other treatment) or a general medical condition (e.g., hyperthyroidism).

   Note: Manic-like episodes that are clearly caused by somatic antidepressant treatment (e.g., medication, electroconvulsive therapy, light therapy) should not count toward a diagnosis of bipolar I disorder.

gate in the same families, and some studies suggest that there are no significant differences between unipolar and bipolar disorder with regard to familial rates of bipolar illness (E.S. Gershon et al. 1982; Weissman et al. 1984; Winokur 1995). Unipolar and bipolar disorders may not be totally distinct because they coaggregate in families. Some of the overlapping features of bipolar and unipolar mood disorders are illustrated in Figure 10–1.

Given that mania and depression are opposites of each other, one would think that only one of the two disorders could be present at a time. However, between 30% and 50% of manic episodes are accompanied by depressive symptoms (Bowden et al. 1995; McElroy et al. 1992). According to DSM-IV-TR, a mixed episode (dysphoric mania) should be diagnosed if the full criteria (except duration) are met for both mania and major

TABLE 10–6. DSM-IV-TR criteria for hypomanic episode

A. A distinct period of persistently elevated, expansive, or irritable mood, lasting throughout at least 4 days, that is clearly different from the usual nondepressed mood.

B. During the period of mood disturbance, three (or more) of the following symptoms have persisted (four if the mood is only irritable) and have been present to a significant degree:
   (1) inflated self-esteem or grandiosity
   (2) decreased need for sleep (e.g., feels rested after only 3 hours of sleep)
   (3) more talkative than usual or pressure to keep talking
   (4) flight of ideas or subjective experience that thoughts are racing
   (5) distractibility (i.e., attention too easily drawn to unimportant or irrelevant external stimuli)
   (6) increase in goal-directed activity (either socially, at work or school, or sexually) or psychomotor agitation
   (7) excessive involvement in pleasurable activities that have a high potential for painful consequences (e.g., the person engages in unrestrained buying sprees, sexual indiscretions, or foolish business investments)

C. The episode is associated with an unequivocal change in functioning that is uncharacteristic of the person when not symptomatic.

D. The disturbance in mood and the change in functioning are observable by others.

E. The episode is not severe enough to cause marked impairment in social or occupational functioning, or to necessitate hospitalization, and there are no psychotic features.

F. The symptoms are not due to the direct physiological effects of a substance (e.g., a drug of abuse, a medication, or other treatment) or a general medical condition (e.g., hyperthyroidism).

   Note: Hypomanic-like episodes that are clearly caused by somatic antidepressant treatment (e.g., medication, electroconvulsive therapy, light therapy) should not count toward a diagnosis of bipolar II disorder.

TABLE 10–7. Differences between unipolar and bipolar depression

Unipolar	Bipolar
Later onset	Earlier onset
Fewer episodes	More episodes
More gradual onset	Acute onset
Female > male	Female = male
More psychomotor agitation	More psychomotor retardation and lethargy
Typical symptoms	Atypical symptoms
Insomnia	Hypersomnia
Lower risk of suicide	Greater risk of suicide
Less frequently accompanied by psychotic symptoms in younger patients	Greater likelihood of psychotic symptoms in younger patients
Antidepressants more effective	Antidepressants less effective
Lithium less effective	Lithium more effective
Family history of depression	Family history of mania and depression
Normal $[Ca^{2+}]_i$	Increased $[Ca^{2+}]_i$

Note. $[Ca^{2+}]_i$ = free intracellular concentration of calcium ions.

The next steps are to decide which modifiers in addition to melancholia and atypical features apply to the episode and then to consider specific subtypes of mood disorders. Some of these subtypes meet criteria for DSM-IV-TR mood disorders with or without symptomatic or course specifiers, and some are commonly recognized syndromes that may not meet formal diagnostic criteria but are nonetheless clinically important.

Major Depressive Disorder

MDD is characterized by one or more major depressive episodes in the absence of mania or hypomania. Depressive syndromes caused by medical illnesses (mood disorder due to a general medical condition) and by medications or psychoactive substances (substance-induced mood disorder) are not considered to be primary mood disorders and do not qualify for a diagnosis of MDD. In DSM-IV-TR, several course specifiers can be applied to the current or most recent depressive episode. These course specifiers (severity, psychosis, degree of remission, chronicity, catatonic features, melancholic features, atypical features, and postpartum onset) are discussed throughout this chapter. DSM-IV-TR provides two additional descriptors for patients with recurrent depressive episodes: with (or without) interepisode recovery and with seasonal pattern.

Although MDD can consist of a single episode, recurrence is the rule rather than the exception. After a single

depression. However, many more patients with one pole of the disorder have some symptoms of the other, as exemplified by exhibitionistic depression with outbursts of rage and decreased need for sleep or by hypomania with suicide attempts and fatigue (McElroy et al. 1992). Dysphoric mania is more common in females and is associated with a greater risk of suicide and a poorer response to lithium (McElroy et al. 1992). There also may be an association between mixed states and very rapid mood swings (ultradian cycling).

Specific Mood Disorders

The identification of an episode of mania and/or depression is the first step in making a comprehensive diagnosis.

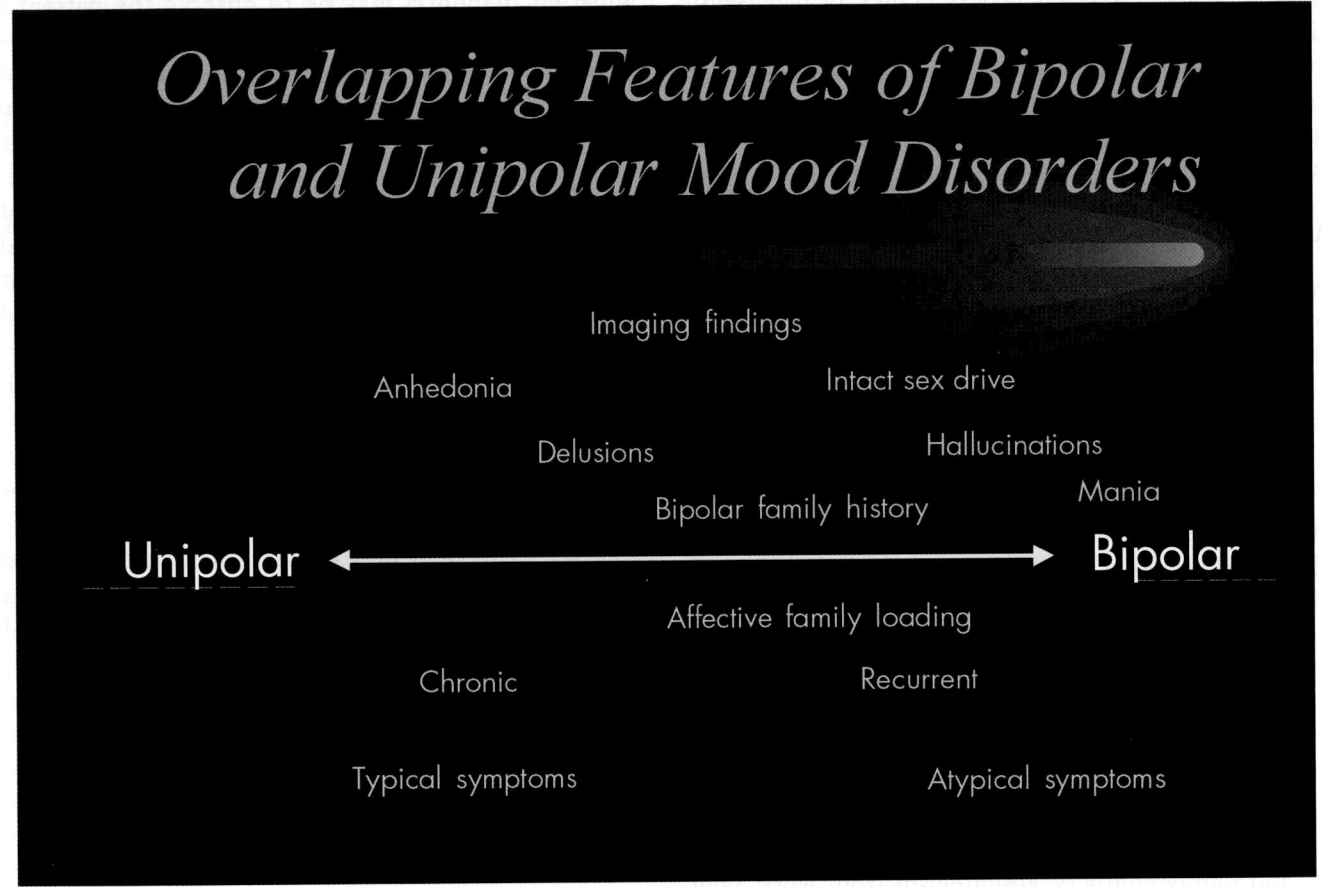

FIGURE 10–1. Overlap of unipolar and bipolar mood disorders.

major depressive episode, the risk of a second episode is about 50%; after a third episode, the risk of a fourth is about 90% (Thase 1990). Each new episode tends to occur sooner and more abruptly, and new episodes often include the same symptoms that previous episodes included, along with new and more severe symptoms. The importance of this tendency of major depression to accelerate over time is discussed later in this chapter (see "Course of Mood Disorders").

DSM-IV-TR specifiers are used to indicate whether a major depressive episode has remitted fully (i.e., no symptoms for at least 2 months), partially (i.e., not enough ongoing depressive symptoms to qualify for a diagnosis of a major depressive episode or no symptoms for less than 2 months), or not at all (i.e., a chronic major depressive episode). Longitudinal course specifiers for MDD indicate whether recurrent major depressive episodes remit completely or partially in between episodes and whether major depressive episodes are superimposed on dysthymia. If one counts only the defining symptoms listed in Table 10–2, these kinds of distinctions may seem relatively uncomplicated. However, recall of depressive symptoms may be greater when a patient feels more

depressed than when depression is less severe (i.e., recall is state dependent). Because the severity of depression tends to fluctuate in all but the most profoundly depressed patients, a history obtained when a patient feels worse may suggest a more chronic illness than may a history obtained when the same patient feels better. One way to clarify whether the first instance represents retrospective amplification of past symptoms in the light of current mood or more accurate recall is to gather additional data from family members and others who have known the patient over time.

Another difficult judgment to make in assessing remission of a major depressive episode is whether the psychology of depression represents residual depression. For example, depression is associated with globally negative thinking such that negative events are attributed to inadequacies in the self and are seen as having pervasive and irreversible consequences (A.T. Beck et al. 1979; Thase 1996). Depressive thinking is derived from rigid, all-or-nothing assumptions such as "If everyone doesn't accept me all the time, no one cares about me at all" or "If I make a mistake, I'm totally incompetent" (Thase 1996). Patients who maintain these attitudes, such as

TABLE 10–8. DSM-IV-TR diagnostic criteria for dysthymic disorder

A. Depressed mood for most of the day, for more days than not, as indicated either by subjective account or observation by others, for at least 2 years. **Note:** In children and adolescents, mood can be irritable and duration must be at least 1 year.

B. Presence, while depressed, of two (or more) of the following:
  (1) poor appetite or overeating
  (2) insomnia or hypersomnia
  (3) low energy or fatigue
  (4) low self-esteem
  (5) poor concentration or difficulty making decisions
  (6) feelings of hopelessness

C. During the 2-year period (1 year for children or adolescents) of the disturbance, the person has never been without the symptoms in Criteria A and B for more than 2 months at a time.

D. No major depressive episode has been present during the first 2 years of the disturbance (1 year for children and adolescents); i.e., the disturbance is not better accounted for by chronic major depressive disorder, or major depressive disorder, in partial remission.
  Note: There may have been a previous major depressive episode provided there was a full remission (no significant signs or symptoms for 2 months) before development of the dysthymic disorder. In addition, after the initial 2 years (1 year in children or adolescents) of dysthymic disorder, there may be superimposed episodes of major depressive disorder, in which case both diagnoses may be given when the criteria are met for a major depressive episode.

E. There has never been a manic episode, a mixed episode, or a hypomanic episode, and criteria have never been met for cyclothymic disorder.

F. The disturbance does not occur exclusively during the course of a chronic psychotic disorder, such as schizophrenia or delusional disorder.

G. The symptoms are not due to the direct physiological effects of a substance (e.g., a drug of abuse, a medication) or a general medical condition (e.g., hypothyroidism).

H. The symptoms cause clinically significant distress or impairment in social, occupational, or other important areas of functioning.

Specify if:
  Early Onset: if onset is before age 21 years
  Late Onset: if onset is age 21 years or older
Specify (for most recent 2 years of dysthymic disorder):
  With Atypical Features

TABLE 10–9. Dysthymic disorder versus major depressive disorder

Dysthymic disorder	Major depressive disorder
2 years' duration	2 weeks' duration
Depressed mood plus two additional symptoms	Depressed mood plus four additional symptoms
More cognitive symptoms	More vegetative symptoms
Mild onset may be followed after 2 years by major depression	Onset may begin with more severe symptoms

MDD) is associated with almost as much impairment as are dysthymic disorder and MDD (Broadhead et al. 1990). Comorbidity with other Axis I disorders and with personality disorders is about equally frequent in the two conditions (Howland 1993; Kocsis 1993; J.C. Perry 1985). Despite dysthymic disorder's being defined as a less severe condition, the prognosis of dysthymic disorder is not substantially different from that of MDD (Wells et al. 1992). Both disorders respond to the same antidepressant and psychotherapeutic regimens (Frances 1993; Kocsis et al. 1989; J. Scott 1992; Stewart et al. 1993).

Chronic MDD and dysthymic disorder may be related to each other in a number of ways. One possibility is that they are separate disorders with overlapping symptoms and with a high rate of comorbidity with each other, with several other conditions (such as anxiety, substance-related, eating, somatoform, and personality disorders), and with chronic medical illnesses (Conte and Karasu 1992; Howland 1993; Marin et al. 1993; J.C. Perry 1985). Another possibility is that dysthymic disorder is an early phase of MDD (Frances 1993), a theory that is suggested by the observation that childhood-onset dysthymic disorder does not persist into adulthood in its original form but is replaced by recurrent MDD and bipolar disorder (Kovacs et al. 1994). Or both disorders may be different presentations over time of the same disturbance of mood, personality traits, and psychosocial functioning, combining chronic low-grade or residual depression with intermittent recurrence of more severe depression.

In the DSM-IV field trials, patients who met criteria for dysthymia on average also reported two-thirds of the symptoms listed in Table 10–10 (Keller et al. 1996). Some of these symptoms are attenuated versions of typical depressive symptoms, whereas others describe global ways of thinking about oneself that overlap with personality traits. A modified version of this symptom list (Table 10–11) was placed in the Appendix to DSM-IV,

to perform social roles (Frances 1993). Even minor depression (a Research Diagnostic Criteria [RDC] condition in which the number of depressive symptoms is insufficient to meet criteria for dysthymic disorder or

TABLE 10–10. Symptoms endorsed by patients meeting DSM-IV-TR criteria for dysthymic disorder

Low self-esteem, feelings of inadequacy
Pessimism, despair, or hopelessness
Social withdrawal
Chronic fatigue or tiredness
Guilt, brooding about the past
Irritability, excessive anger
Decreased activity, effectiveness, or productivity
Difficulty thinking: poor concentration, poor memory, indecisiveness
Generalized loss of interest or pleasure (hypohedonia)

the implication being that these symptoms might end up differentiating dysthymic disorder from MDD (Klein et al. 1996; Shea and Hirschfeld 1996). A recent consensus panel that considered this and five other proposed sets of research criteria for dysthymic disorder supported the presence of dysphoria or gloominess for at least 2 years in adults and 1 year in children, along with at least three of the six symptoms listed in Table 10–11 (Gwirtsman et al. 1997) (as opposed to two of four symptoms in DSM-IV-TR). However, more study is necessary to clarify the value of alternative research criteria for dysthymic disorder (Keller et al. 1996). The overlap between chronic depressive symptoms and personality traits is discussed later in the chapter (see "Subsyndromal Depression").

TABLE 10–11. DSM-IV-TR alternative research criterion B for dysthymic disorder

B. Presence, while depressed, of three (or more) of the following:
  (1) low self-esteem or self-confidence, or feelings of inadequacy
  (2) feelings of pessimism, despair, or hopelessness
  (3) generalized loss of interest or pleasure
  (4) social withdrawal
  (5) chronic fatigue or tiredness
  (6) feelings of guilt, brooding about the past
  (7) subjective feelings of irritability or excessive anger
  (8) decreased activity, effectiveness, or productivity
  (9) difficulty in thinking, reflected by poor concentration, poor memory, or indecisiveness

Minor Depression

Minor depressive disorder is an RDC diagnosis in which the most prominent disturbance is a sustained depressed mood without the full depressive syndrome (Keller et al. 1996). The RDC for minor depression include feeling depressed or down in the dumps for 1 week (probable) or 2 weeks (definite) (Keller et al. 1996). At least two symptoms from a larger symptom list than the list of DSM-IV-TR criteria for MDD and that includes pessimistic attitude and self-pity are required for the diagnosis; impairment or seeking treatment is not required (M.T. Tsuang and Faraone 1996). Minor depression may be chronic, and, like dysthymic disorder, it may be complicated by superimposed major depressive episodes (Keller et al. 1996). In the DSM-IV mood disorders field trial, 3 of 524 subjects met criteria for a lifetime history of minor depression (Keller et al. 1996).

Double Depression

Although it is not a separate DSM-IV-TR diagnosis, double depression, or dysthymic disorder with a superimposed major depressive episode, has been extensively discussed in the literature, and clinicians use the term frequently. The major depressive episode must appear 2 years or more (1 year in children and adolescents) after the onset of dysthymia for double depression to be diagnosed (First et al. 1996). Double depression is far from uncommon in dysthymic patients. Between 68% and 90% of dysthymic patients experience at least one major depressive episode (Thase 1992), and 25%–50% of the patients with MDD have coexisting dysthymic disorder (Hirschfeld 1994; Levitt et al. 1991). It has been estimated that 22%–66% of all patients with unipolar depression have experienced a combination of dysthymia and major depression (Hirschfeld 1994; Keller 1994). A 9-year prospective study found dysthymic disorder with superimposed MDD or recurrent brief depression in 3% of the general population (Hirschfeld 1994).

Compared with major depressive episodes alternating with euthymia (episodic MDD), MDD superimposed on dysthymia has an earlier onset of major depression (Levitt et al. 1991), more severe depressive symptoms (Belsher and Costello 1988; Wells et al. 1992), more psychosocial impairment (Belsher and Costello 1988; Conte and Karasu 1992; Kovacs et al. 1994), a greater risk of suicide (Angst and Wicki 1991), more treatment resistance (Barrett 1984), and more comorbidity (Klein et al. 1988), especially with avoidant and dependent personality disorders (Sanderson et al. 1992). The major depressive episode in double depression is less likely to remit (I.W. Miller et al. 1986; Wells et al. 1992) than that in episodic MDD (i.e., recurrent major depression not superimposed on dysthymia) and is more likely to recur (Levitt et al. 1991). In one report (Belsher and Costello 1988), the relapse rate of major depression after 8 weeks of recovery was 30% for double depression and 4% for episodic MDD. In this study, major depression recurred in 50% of the patients with double depression and 35% of the patients with episodic MDD after 1 year and in 65% and 37%, respectively, after 2 years. The risk of a bipolar outcome also appears greater in double depression: 29% of the patients with double depression in the National Institute of Mental Health Collaborative Study of the Psychobiology of Depression (NIMH-CS) developed hypomania, compared with 9% of the patients with episodic MDD (Keller 1994).

Subsyndromal Depression

Subsyndromal disorders are conditions that partially meet diagnostic criteria for a particular disorder (Jamison 1996). Some subsyndromal forms of unipolar depression such as RDC minor depressive disorder have formal diagnostic criteria, and even though impairment or seeking treatment is not required for the diagnosis, they are associated with clinically important functional impairment (Keller et al. 1996; M.T. Tsuang and Faraone 1996). In the ECA study, one-third of the people using mental health services had subsyndromal mood disorders (Gwirtsman et al. 1997). There is less certainty about the degree to which some constellations of personality traits also may represent subsyndromal forms of chronic depression.

The concept of a depressive temperament or personality representing either a subsyndromal form of depression expressed through the personality, an inherited temperamental disposition, or a "fundamental state" from which more severe depressive episodes emerge later in life was proposed early in this century by Emil Kraepelin and again in the middle of the century by Kurt Schneider (Shea and Hirshfeld 1996). These and other investigators noted that depression is predictably associated with personality traits such as persistent gloominess or despondency (Keller et al. 1996), seriousness (Shea and Hirshfeld 1996), guilt (Keller et al. 1996; Shea and Hirshfeld 1996), lack of self-confidence (Keller et al. 1996; Shea and Hirshfeld 1996), self-denial (Shea and Hirshfeld 1996), conscientiousness (Shea and Hirshfeld 1996), introversion, and neuroticism (Thase 1996). The question that remains to be formally answered is whether such traits are partial expressions of a depressive disorder, manifestations of mildly pathological personality traits mobilized in response to an underlying mood disorder that is less obvious than the overlying personality traits, or markers of a propensity to develop full syndromal mood disorders later in life.

Akiskal (1991, 1994) divided syndromes marked by depressive traits into *subaffective dysthymia*, in which depressive personality traits are caused by chronic sub-

clinical depression, and *character spectrum disorder*, which he considered to be a type of personality disorder in which depressed mood is just one feature of a chronically unhappy and unfulfilled orientation of the personality. As a result of deliberations by the DSM-IV Personality Disorders Work Group, a version of character spectrum disorder is included in the Appendix to DSM-IV as *depressive personality disorder* (Keller et al. 1996). The DSM-IV field trials suggested that this condition "requiring further research" (Table 10–12) was associated with a passive, unassertive style, in the absence of current diagnosable dysthymia, in almost 50% of cases (Keller et al. 1996). Patients thought to have depressive personality disorder were noted to have a tendency to develop dysthymic disorder or MDD after the diagnosis of depressive personality disorder was made, which suggests that the apparent personality disorder might be an early-onset traitlike variant of other depressive disorders. This hypothesis is supported by the existence of a familial association between depressive personality disorder and other depressive disorders (American Psychiatric Association 1994a) and by earlier onset and more depressive episodes in patients with MDD and a premorbid depressive personality than in patients with major depression but without this premorbid temperament (Cassano et al. 1992).

TABLE 10–12. DSM-IV-TR research criteria for depressive personality disorder

A. A pervasive pattern of depressive cognitions and behaviors beginning by early adulthood and present in a variety of contexts, as indicated by five (or more) of the following:
  (1) usual mood is dominated by dejection, gloominess, cheerlessness, joylessness, unhappiness
  (2) self-concept centers around beliefs of inadequacy, worthlessness, and low self-esteem
  (3) is critical, blaming, and derogatory toward self
  (4) is brooding and given to worry
  (5) is negativistic, critical, and judgmental toward others
  (6) is pessimistic
  (7) is prone to feeling guilty or remorseful
B. Does not occur exclusively during major depressive episodes and is not better accounted for by dysthymic disorder.

From a clinical standpoint, defining a personality disorder that overlaps with but is distinct from primary mood disorders has the theoretical benefit of identifying a group of patients who would be expected to have a poor response to typical treatments for depression and a better response to specialized psychotherapeutic approaches.

However, the overlap between abnormal mood and stable personality traits is often so extensive that the two can be indistinguishable (Shea and Hirschfeld 1996). Obviously, many people with diagnoses of MDD and dysthymia meet DSM-IV-TR symptomatic criteria for depressive personality disorder. In one study, 41% of the patients with a major depressive episode were found to meet all criteria for depressive personality disorder, including persistence of symptoms when the full mood disorder was not present (Shea and Hirschfeld 1996).

The effect of an abnormal mood on thinking and behavior is so profound that it can distort most assessments of personality, making it impossible to determine the degree to which a personality disorder is present when a primary mood disorder and a personality disorder appear to coexist. Chronically unstable or depressed mood can intensify pathological defenses and can skew the ways in which a person experiences the self and others (Deitz 1995). On personality inventories, depressed people resemble one another more than they resemble themselves when they are not depressed (Hirschfeld et al. 1989; Loranger et al. 1991). In several studies, more than 50% of the patients (or their relatives) with a diagnosis of borderline personality disorder were found to develop major depression, mania, or hypomania or commit suicide (Akiskal 1984, 1991). This finding could indicate a high rate of comorbidity or an aggravation of pathological personality traits by subclinical mood disorders that are not obvious until they eventually become severe enough to be recognized. Because mild depressive symptoms as well as social impairment can persist after remission of a full depressive syndrome, persistent passivity, negative thinking, low self-esteem, cynicism, and related traits in the absence of a diagnosable mood disorder could represent residual symptoms of a previous episode or prodromal symptoms of another episode rather than a true personality disorder. In the absence of any validated method of distinguishing the two, the most prudent approach for the clinician is to treat depression as vigorously as possible before diagnosing a personality disorder. However, even though features such as negative therapeutic reactions, attachment to a negative view of the self and others, self-destructive motivations, and treatment nonadherence are not necessarily diagnostic of a personality disorder, such tendencies must be addressed because they may interfere with a positive response to even the most straightforward antidepressant regimen.

Psychotic Depression

The term *psychotic depression* (or *delusional depression*) refers to a major depressive episode accompanied by psychotic features (i.e., delusions and/or hallucinations). Some clinicians believe that psychotic depression is relatively uncommon. However, most studies continue to report that 16%–54% of depressed patients have psychotic symptoms (Dubovsky and Thomas 1992). Delusions occur without hallucinations in one-half to two-thirds of the adults with psychotic depression, whereas hallucinations are unaccompanied by delusions in 3%–25% of patients (Dubovsky and Thomas 1992). Half of all psychotically depressed patients experience more than one kind of delusion (Dubovsky and Thomas 1992). Hallucinations occur more frequently than delusions in younger depressed patients and in patients with bipolar psychotic depression (Chambers et al. 1982; Goodwin and Jamison 1991). The common belief that visual and olfactory hallucinations are signs of neurological disease that do not occur commonly in mood disorders has been contradicted by clinical experience with psychotic depression, which shows that auditory and visual hallucinations are equally frequent in psychotic depression and that olfactory and haptic hallucinations may occur in the absence of central nervous system disease (Dubovsky and Thomas 1992).

The classification of psychotic symptoms as mood congruent (i.e., consistent with a depressed or an elated mood) or mood incongruent is complex. Prominent mood-incongruent psychotic symptoms in depressed patients such as delusions of control, along with poor adolescent adjustment, may be associated with a somewhat worse prognosis of psychotic depression (K.S. Kendler 1991; D. Tsuang and Coryell 1993). The RDC, which were used in many earlier studies of psychotic depression, specify a diagnosis of schizoaffective disorder for depressed patients with concurrent mood-incongruent psychotic features. However, bipolar psychotic depression is frequently associated with mood-incongruent psychotic symptoms, some of which may be bizarre and easily mistaken for typical "schizophrenic" symptoms (Akiskal et al. 1983, 1985; McGlashan 1988); a formal thought disorder occurs in at least 20% of psychotically depressed patients (Goodwin and Jamison 1991). Because bipolar illness is overrepresented in psychotic depression (Coryell 1996; Weissman et al. 1988a), it may be bipolar illness and not mood incongruence that contributes to a poorer treatment response in mood-incongruent psychotic depression. In recognition of the uncertain contribution of mood incongruence to the prognosis, DSM-IV-TR requires the existence of psychotic symptoms for 2 or more weeks in the absence of prominent mood symptoms for a diagnosis of schizoaffective disorder, a specifier that seems more consistently associated with a somewhat poorer prognosis of mixed affective and psychotic syndromes than the RDC (Coryell 1996).

Recognizing psychotic symptoms in depressed patients is not always straightforward. If the patient does not seem severely depressed (this can occur in patients with bipolar psychotic depression who have a mixed element of elevated mood and energy that makes them appear less depressed than they feel), the clinician might not inquire about psychotic symptoms in the first place. Some patients do not consider hearing voices, seeing things, paranoia, or ideas of reference to be abnormal and do not report such symptoms. Other patients conceal psychotic symptoms because they do not want to be considered "crazy." To be certain that psychotic symptoms are not present, it may be necessary to ask repeatedly about them, beginning with nonspecific questions such as "Does your mind ever play tricks on you?" and progressing gradually to more specific questions such as "Do you ever hear your name called when there's no one there?" and then "Do you ever hear a voice saying more than your name?"

Psychotic features tend to develop after several episodes of nonpsychotic depression. Once psychotic symptoms occur, they reappear with each subsequent episode, even if depression in later episodes is not as severe. With each recurrence, psychotic symptoms take the same form that they did in previous episodes (e.g., patients with hallucinations have them in the same modality and with the same content from episode to episode) (Dubovsky and Thomas 1992). Relatives of psychotically depressed patients have an increased risk for psychotic depression themselves; and when psychotic depression is present, the content of the psychosis tends to be similar to that of the proband. The families of psychotically depressed patients also have an elevated risk of schizophrenia.

Whereas treatment with both an antipsychotic drug and an antidepressant is usually necessary for a remission of psychotic depression, *antipsychotic* drugs may improve the *depression* and the *antidepressant* may improve *psychosis* (Dubovsky and Thomas 1992). Furthermore, coaggregation of severe mood disorders and schizophrenia exists in families of patients with psychotic depression. These two observations suggest that psychotic depression is not a simple combination of psychosis and depression but rather a complex interaction between the capacity to become psychotic and the capacity to become severely depressed (Dubovsky and Thomas 1992). Depression may have to reach a certain level of severity for psychosis to be expressed; but once psychosis develops, a unique disorder has evolved. Some features in addition to the unique treatment response that distinguish psychotic from nonpsychotic depression include a greater rate of recurrence; a higher suicide risk; more nonsuppression on the dexamethasone suppression test (DST), with higher postdexamethasone cortisol levels; more prominent sleep abnormalities; a level of neuropsychological impairment similar to schizophrenia, and higher ventricular-to-brain ratios (Albus et al. 1996; Coryell 1996; Dubovsky and Thomas 1992). The extent to which the symptoms, course, and treatment response of psychotic depression are a function of psychosis itself or the overrepresentation of bipolar disorder in psychotically depressed patients (Weissman et al. 1988a) has not been studied.

Involutional Depression

As was mentioned earlier in this chapter (see section "Mood Disorders in Special Populations"), first onset of unipolar depression in elderly patients is often associated with cerebrovascular disease, especially on the left side of the brain (whereas late-onset mania is often associated with right-sided disease). Contrary to popular wisdom, depression in women does not begin at the time of menopause, although depression tends to recur over the years with each reproductive event (e.g., menarche, childbirth, menopause) (Dell and Stewart 2000). Because of the likelihood of associated neurological impairment, depression that appears for the first time in the geriatric patient is more difficult to treat than depression that begins earlier in life.

Recurrent Brief Depression

Both RDC (M.T. Tsuang and Faraone 1996) and DSM-IV-TR criteria (First et al. 1996; M.T. Tsuang and Faraone 1996) require 2 weeks of continuous symptoms for a diagnosis of a major depressive episode to be made. Researcher Jules Angst and his colleagues described a depressive disorder called *recurrent brief depression*, in which depressive episodes meet DSM-IV-TR symptomatic but not duration criteria for major depression. Depressive episodes in recurrent brief depression have the same number and severity of symptoms as DSM-IV-TR major depressive episodes but last 1 day to 1 week (Keller et al. 1996). Depressive episodes must recur at least once per month over at least 12 months (not in association with the menstrual cycle) for recurrent brief depression to be diagnosed (Angst and Hochstrasser 1994). Although each acute depressive episode is short-lived, recurrent brief depression carries a high risk of suicide (Lepine et al. 1995), perhaps because of the inevitable return of depression and the repeated drastic contrast between the depressed and well states.

The appendix to DSM-IV listed recurrent brief depressive disorder defined by Angst's criteria as a condition requiring further study because it was thought that not enough data had accumulated to warrant its inclusion as an established diagnosis (American Psychiatric Association 1994a). In the DSM-IV mood disorders field trial, 1.5% of 524 subjects had a lifetime history of recurrent brief depression (Keller et al. 1996), and the 1-year prevalence of recurrent brief depressive disorder was 7% (American Psychiatric Association 1994a). Recurrent brief depression has been found to have rates of comorbidity with panic disorder, generalized anxiety disorder, and substance use disorders that are similar to comorbidity rates with MDD (Keller et al. 1996; Lepine et al. 1995). Recurrent brief depression also has been found often to have a seasonal pattern, with more recurrences in the winter (American Psychiatric Association 1994a; Keller et al. 1996).

One might assume that such a highly recurrent mood disorder likely would eventually have a bipolar outcome (Cassano et al. 1992), and in fact, prophylaxis of brief depressive recurrences is more successful with lithium than with antidepressants (Angst et al. 1990). However, extended follow-up of patients with this condition found that they never developed mania or hypomania (Angst and Hochstrasser 1994; Angst et al. 1990). This important observation suggests that recurrence may be a feature of mood disorders that is more common in, but not restricted to, bipolar subtypes and that lithium may be an antirecurrence as much as an antimanic treatment. The latter point is supported by the capacity of lithium to prevent recurrences of other cyclical and recurrent disorders such as cluster headaches.

Bipolar Subtypes

Bipolar disorder is a mood disorder that is accompanied by episodes of mania and/or hypomania (DSM-IV-TR criteria for manic, hypomanic, and mixed episodes are summarized in Tables 10–5 and 10–6). DSM-IV-TR includes two primary subtypes of bipolar disorder. Bipolar I disorder is characterized by manic episodes with or without episodes of hypomania. In bipolar II disorder, one or more hypomanic episodes occur, but the patient never experiences mania; hypomanic episodes may be milder than depressive episodes (Akiskal 1995b). Evidence that bipolar II disorder is distinct from bipolar I disorder comes from several sources (Akiskal 1996; Bowden 1993; Bowden et al. 1995; Leibenluft 1996; Solomon et al. 1995). Patients with bipolar II disorder never become manic, despite multiple hypomanic episodes. In addition, the bipolar II diagnosis seems to "breed true" in that

patients with this diagnosis have close relatives with hypomania but not mania, whereas patients with bipolar I disorder have some relatives who have had mania and some who have had only hypomania. Rapid cycling, which is described later in this chapter (see subsection "Rapid Cycling"), seems to be more common in bipolar II disorder.

Although bipolar III disorder is not a DSM-IV-TR diagnosis, the term has been used to describe patients with a history of depression who have at least one blood relative with a history of mania (M.T. Tsuang and Faraone 1996), on the grounds that such patients may have a bipolar diathesis that has not yet been expressed. In some circles, *bipolar III* refers to patients with antidepressant-induced mania, and *bipolar IV* is used to describe depressed patients with a family history of mania. In DSM-IV-TR, mania or hypomania that appears in response to treatment with an antidepressant is not counted toward a diagnosis of a bipolar mood disorder, but many clinicians consider antidepressant-induced mania to be an indication of the capacity to develop mania or hypomania spontaneously and therefore a sign of a type of bipolar mood disorder (this seems most likely to be true of children and adolescents [Akiskal 1995a; Strober and Carlson 1982]).

Brief hypomania.   Angst (1995) defined a subtype of hypomania called *brief hypomania*. Brief hypomania consists of the same symptoms as hypomania, but the duration of symptoms is 1–3 days rather than the 4 days or more required by DSM-IV-TR for a diagnosis of hypomania. Angst found that despite the short duration of any episode, brief hypomania has a very high rate of recurrence and produces marked impairment. The prevalence of brief hypomania was 2.28% among patients with bipolar mood disorders in one study (Angst 1995), but further data are needed before diagnostic precision can be achieved for brief manic or hypomanic symptoms. Ultrarapid cycling, which is discussed in the "Ultradian Cycling" subsection later in this chapter, probably would qualify as a condition associated with manic or hypomanic symptoms lasting only a short time but recurring very frequently. Presumably, the difference between ultradian cycling and brief hypomania is that the latter is characterized by euthymia between hypomanic episodes.

Bipolar depression.   Depression in patients with bipolar mood disorders may alternate or be mixed with mania. Classical bipolar depression is characterized by "atypical" symptoms such as hypersomnia, anergia, carbohydrate craving, and psychomotor slowing (Goodwin and Jamison 1991). However, in contrast to atypical unipolar depression, mood in bipolar depression that is not mixed with hypomania usually is not reactive (Mitchell et al. 2001). Especially in younger patients, bipolar depression is more frequently associated with psychotic symptoms (Mitchell et al. 2001). Much of the time, depression and mania are not neatly differentiated states, depressive symptoms being mixed with dysphoric hypomanic symptoms such as anxiety, racing thoughts, insomnia, and exquisite interpersonal sensitivity. By the same token, depressive symptoms are frequently present in mania.

Cyclothymic Disorder

Cyclothymic disorder (cyclothymia) was originally classified as a personality disorder with mood swings that were not clearly manic or depressed. Although most investigators now consider cyclothymic disorder to be a mood disorder, it is still called *cyclothymic personality* in the RDC (M.T. Tsuang and Faraone 1996). As Table 10–13 indicates, DSM-IV-TR cyclothymia can be diagnosed in patients with recurrent hypomanic and depressive symptoms that may not permit a diagnosis of major depression or hypomania. In the RDC, cyclothymia is characterized by recurrent depressed mood lasting several days, alternating with elevated mood with at least two hypomanic symptoms. In both schemes, the patient rarely experiences a normal mood (M.T. Tsuang and Faraone 1996).

Patients with cyclothymia typically experience mood states that alternate between depression, irritability, cheerfulness, and relative normality that last days, weeks, or months (Jamison 1993, 1996). Many complain of unpredictable changes in energy, vague physical symptoms, and a seasonal pattern of mood swings (e.g., depression in the winter) (Jamison 1996). In some studies, 44% of the cyclothymic patients developed hypomania while taking antidepressants, and about one-third developed full-blown hypomanic, manic, or depressive episodes during drug-free follow-up (Akiskal et al. 1977; Jamison 1996). In addition, at least one-third of the time the onset of clear bipolar I or bipolar II mood disorder is preceded by cyclothymia, which usually begins in adolescence or early adulthood (Jamison 1996).

Rapid Cycling

In DSM-IV-TR, *rapid cycling* is a specifier that refers to a bipolar I or bipolar II mood disorder in which four or more episodes of depression and/or mania or hypomania occur per year, with either 2 weeks of normal mood between episodes or a shift directly from one pole to the other (e.g., from mania to depression) with no intervening period of normal mood (American Psychiatric Association 2000). Rapid-cycling bipolar disorder is probably

TABLE 10–13. DSM-IV-TR diagnostic criteria for cyclothymic disorder

A. For at least 2 years, the presence of numerous periods with hypomanic symptoms and numerous periods with depressive symptoms that do not meet criteria for a major depressive episode. **Note:** In children and adolescents, the duration must be at least 1 year.

B. During the above 2-year period (1 year in children and adolescents), the person has not been without the symptoms in Criterion A for more than 2 months at a time.

C. No major depressive episode, manic episode, or mixed episode has been present during the first 2 years of the disturbance.
   Note: After the initial 2 years (1 year in children and adolescents) of cyclothymic disorder, there may be superimposed manic or mixed episodes (in which case both bipolar I disorder and cyclothymic disorder may be diagnosed) or major depressive episodes (in which case both bipolar II disorder and cyclothymic disorder may be diagnosed).

D. The symptoms in Criterion A are not better accounted for by schizoaffective disorder and are not superimposed on schizophrenia, schizophreniform disorder, delusional disorder, or psychotic disorder not otherwise specified.

E. The symptoms are not due to the direct physiological effects of a substance (e.g., a drug of abuse, a medication) or a general medical condition (e.g., hyperthyroidism).

F. The symptoms cause clinically significant distress or impairment in social, occupational, or other important areas of functioning.

not a separate illness but a phase in the evolution of bipolar disorder that may last years but may not be permanent (Kilzieh and Akiskal 2000; Tomitaka and Sakamoto 1994). Rapid cycling may have a lower response to lithium (Kilzieh and Akiskal 2000; Roy-Byrne et al. 1984). Rapid cycling is more common in women and in patients with bipolar II disorder (Leibenluft 1996; Lish et al. 1993) and is more likely to occur after an episode of mania or hypomania than after depression (Altschuler et al. 1995; Post 1988). Additional risk factors for the development of rapid cycling include hypothyroidism, right cerebral hemisphere disease, mental retardation, and use of alcohol and stimulants (Ananth et al. 1993; Leibenluft 1996; Sachs 1996). As many as 60%–90% of patients with rapid cycling have been found to have hypothyroidism, which often is too mild to produce medical morbidity even though it can contribute to mood instability (Bauer et al. 1990; Cowdry et al. 1983). Lithium itself may cause rapid cycling by inducing hypothyroidism (Terao 1993). Correcting subclinical forms of hypothyroidism therefore is an important intervention in rapid cycling (Extein et al. 1985).

A causal role of antidepressants in mania and rapid cycling has been widely debated. A review of records of 535 patients admitted to a general psychiatric inpatient service found that 8.1% required hospitalization because of psychosis or mania that occurred within 16 weeks of starting an antidepressant and remitted rapidly with antidepressant withdrawal (Preda et al. 2001). Antidepressants may contribute to rapid cycling by inducing mania or by speeding up the inherent cyclicity of bipolar mood disorders (Altschuler et al. 1995; Goodwin et al. 1982; Kilzieh and Akiskal 2000; Post 1994; Sachs 1996; Wehr 1993). Although most patients with rapid-cycling bipolar disorder are taking antidepressants, it is difficult to prove that antidepressants are the cause of rapid cycling (Altschuler et al. 1995). Alternative explanations would be that antidepressants are administered more frequently to patients with rapid-cycling and other forms of deteriorating bipolar disorder because depression is prominent or because nothing else is helping or that rapid cycling would have developed with or without an antidepressant. The only way to prove a causal relation would be to follow prospectively matched patients with bipolar mood disorder who were randomly assigned to take antidepressants or placebos, an experiment that is too difficult technically and ethically to be performed. If assessment of the association between starting antidepressants and developing rapid cycling is retrospective, the results are subject to being skewed by state-dependent recall and difficulty remembering the exact onset of complex mood swings. Even in a prospective study, it is difficult to be certain whether rapid cycling that develops after prolonged treatment with an antidepressant was caused by the medication or simply reflected the natural history of the condition.

These issues were addressed to some extent by Altschuler et al. (1995), who defined antidepressant-induced mania and rapid cycling as a change in order of episodes or a first episode of severe mania or cycling appearing within 8 weeks of starting antidepressants. In a literature review, Altschuler et al. (1995) identified 158 patients with bipolar depression in 15 placebo-controlled antidepressant trials in patients with mostly unipolar depression. Within this subgroup, 35% had likely antidepressant-induced mania by the stringent criteria used, the risk being more than 2.5 times as great (72% vs. 28%) for patients who were not also taking lithium. Among the limitations of the literature review were the relatively small number of patients with bipolar mood disorders in each study reviewed, the lack of reliable data from trials of other antidepressants, and the lack of inclusion of hypomania as an antidepressant-induced event. In addition, patients in these studies were not identified as hav-

ing bipolar mood disorders in the first place and might have had a different response to antidepressants than patients with more obvious bipolar disorder.

Altschuler and her colleagues (1995) then used a life-chart method to characterize affective episodes carefully in 51 patients with lithium-refractory bipolar mood disorders, 55% of whom had rapid cycling. Although 82% of the sample developed mania while taking an antidepressant, the investigators concluded that only one-third met their criteria for definite antidepressant-induced mania. One reason for this low rate may have been that their patients had such a high rate of spontaneous affective episodes and so many had taken antidepressants at some point, that it was not possible to detect increases attributable to an antidepressant. The authors found that antidepressant-induced mania increased the risk of rapid cycling by 4.6-fold; 50% of the increase was directly attributable to the use of antidepressants and 50% was assumed to reflect the natural history of bipolar disorder. On the basis of their study and literature review, the authors suggested that continuing antidepressants aggravated rapid cycling, but withdrawing the antidepressant did not necessarily stop cycling. Most ominously, antimanic drugs did not predictably prevent or treat rapid cycling. In a review of patients with refractory bipolar disorder that used a similar methodology, mania was thought to be attributable to antidepressant therapy in 35% of the patients and rapid cycling in 26% (Roy-Byrne et al. 1985).

These results must be considered conservative for several reasons. First, hypomania and more subtle forms of pathologically elevated mood were not considered. Second, only classically defined rapid cycling was considered; other forms of mood cycling (described in the next subsection) may be even more common. Because there is no reason to think that antidepressants must take 8 weeks or less to induce hypomania or mood swings, use of this arbitrary cutoff value may result in overlooking many patients for whom months or even years of antidepressant therapy may be necessary to destabilize mood but who would not develop rapid cycling without antidepressants.

Ultradian Cycling

In a malignant form of rapid cycling called *ultradian cycling* (or *ultrarapid cycling*) (Pazzaglia et al. 1993; Roy-Byrne et al. 1984), patients appear chronically depressed. On close inspection, however, they experience multiple recurrences of mania and depression over the course of hours to days. For example, a patient may wake up feeling emotionally paralyzed and unable to get out of bed. A few hours later, the patient feels so energized that it is impossible to sit still and to refrain from acting impulsively; shortly thereafter, the patient sinks abruptly into suicidal despair. The patient briefly feels relatively well but then flies into a rage when criticized and has command hallucinations. Racing thoughts keep the patient from falling asleep, but once the patient does fall asleep, sleep lasts 14 hours, and the patient is exhausted the next day. Rather than having nonspecific "mood swings," the patient is experiencing distinct but very brief recurrences of bipolar depression, dysphoric hypomania, a mixture of depressive and hypomanic symptoms, and a psychotic energized state, with fleeting euthymia between episodes or an abrupt switch from one pole to the other. Akiskal (1991) called this a "protracted pseudo unipolar mixed state" (p. 161) that fluctuates considerably in intensity and with regard to the kinds of symptoms that predominate. The labile moods and behavior of the patient with ultradian cycling are often mistaken for evidence of borderline personality disorder (Akiskal 1996). Mood swings in such states seem random and disorganized but may be described by a chaos theory model (Kilzieh and Akiskal 2000).

It is not clear whether ultradian cycling is a deteriorated form of rapid cycling or a different condition. However, no evidence indicates that ultradian cycling is a separate bipolar subtype (Kilzieh and Akiskal 2000). The research that has been performed with patients with ultradian cycling suggests that it is even more refractory to treatment than traditionally diagnosed rapid cycling (Pazzaglia et al. 1993; Post 1988). No prospective studies support the assertion that precipitating mania with antidepressants could be followed by ultradian cycling, but ultradian cycling, like rapid cycling, may be preceded by one or more hypomanic episodes (Post 1988, 1990b, 1994). Experience does suggest that the depression of ultradian cycling is aggravated rather than ameliorated by antidepressants (Akiskal 1991; J. Scott 1988).

Mixed Bipolar States

Almost half of bipolar patients experience depressive and manic symptoms at the same time (Freeman and McElroy 1999). Manic symptoms in mixed states usually are dysphoric, with irritability, anxiety, or unpleasant activation rather than elation. Such states can be difficult to distinguish from ultradian cycling, in which moods change so rapidly that they seem to blend into each other, and mixed states and ultrarapid cycling often accompany each other. Both conditions probably represent deterioration of a more organized mood disorder associated at least in some cases with chronic use of antidepressants, and both have similar treatments.

Masked and Subsyndromal Bipolar Disorder

When the features listed in Tables 10–5 and 10–6 are obvious and sustained, the diagnosis of a bipolar mood disorder is straightforward. However, brief mood swings with mixed symptoms that wax and wane rather than clearly remit and recur can be more difficult to identify; as a result, more than one-third of the patients with bipolar disorder were thought to have unipolar depression in one study, even though they had experienced a first episode of mania or hypomania (Ghaemi et al. 2000). Hypomania presenting not as elation but as anxiety attacks, insomnia, difficulty concentrating, irritability, dysphoria, agitation, impulsivity, or hypersexuality can easily be mistaken for an anxiety disorder or a personality disorder. Bipolar depression with mixed dysphoric hypomanic symptoms such as anxiety, restlessness, and agitation may be confused with agitated unipolar depression (Akiskal 1996). Because mania is often associated with a formal thought disorder and with bizarre hallucinations (Goodwin and Jamison 1991), some bipolar psychoses can be confused with excited schizophreniform psychoses.

Subclinical and masked forms of bipolar disorder range from agitated psychoses to temperamental dysregulation of mood (Akiskal 1995b). As is true of subsyndromal depression, subtle forms of bipolar disorders appear characterological. Hyperthymia, which was originally described by J. Delay in 1946, is a chronic pattern of elevated mood that is less obvious than hypomania. Hyperthymic individuals are expansive, dynamic, joyful, and optimistic and have a robust sense of well-being, a decreased need for sleep, decreased appetite, increased energy, increased creativity, and a family history of bipolar disorder (Cassano et al. 1992; Hellekson 1989). Although their social and occupational functioning are not necessarily impaired, hyperthymic people are prone to more blatant episodes of hypomania and depression, and their underlying emotional pressure may alienate others (Hellekson 1989). Some investigators consider hyperthymia to be the premorbid personality style of bipolar disorder (Feline 1993).

Subaffective hypomania may present with personality traits such as arrogance, pushiness, irritability, insensitivity, talkativeness, emotional intensity, interpersonal hypersensitivity, temper tantrums, promiscuity, restlessness, and unpredictability. Never at a loss for a cutting repartee or an excuse, the person may be at the forefront of new movements and groups, only to lose interest after getting everyone else involved. Mixtures of subsyndromal mania and depression are frequently present, as exemplified by wild jokes with a dark or cynical edge, self-destructive thrill seeking, or suicidal humor (McElroy et al. 1992). Bipolar individuals who are chronically high-strung, moody, exhibitionistic, grandiose, hypersensitive, overreactive, and unstable often are thought to have dramatizing personality disorders such as borderline or narcissistic personality disorder. If they seek excitement through stealing or are habitually aggressive, they may appear to have an antisocial personality disorder. Indeed, some diagnostic criteria for borderline personality disorder—unstable, intense relationships; affective instability; inappropriate, intense anger; impulsivity; and recurrent suicidal behavior, for example—also are typical of bipolar mood disorders. In one report, hysteria or sociopathy had previously been diagnosed in two-thirds of the patients with cyclothymia (Akiskal et al. 1977). In another report, 22% of 23 patients with bipolar mood disorders met criteria for a personality disorder (Carpenter et al. 1995). High rates of narcissistic pathology have been noted in people with bipolar mood disorders (Grubb 1997), possibly reflecting subsyndromal grandiosity as well as a chronic attempt to bolster self-esteem that is undermined by feelings of helplessness to control an unpredictable mood. Patients also may attempt to achieve a sense of control over unstable mood and impulsivity by becoming purposefully self-destructive, impulsive, or thrill seeking, as if they wanted to behave in this manner and were not at the mercy of their mood swings. The same motivation can lead to use of substances such as cocaine that further destabilize their moods. Making the distinction between borderline and narcissistic personality disorders and chronic bipolar disorders therefore can be challenging.

Cycloid Psychoses

The cycloid psychoses are a group of disorders that may represent an interaction between the bipolar dimensions of frequent recurrence with interepisode recovery and strong affective coloring with a propensity for psychosis. It is not yet clear whether these disorders are atypical bipolar subtypes or whether they should be classified with brief psychotic disorder, schizoaffective disorder, or schizophreniform disorder or other acute primary psychoses (Pfuhlmann 1998). However, differences have emerged between cycloid psychoses and other psychotic illnesses. For example, patients with cycloid psychosis have more visual hallucinations and "delusional mood" and have a better outcome than do patients with schizoaffective disorder (Maj 1988). Even after years of recurrent illness, patients with cycloid psychosis do not have the same ventricular enlargement seen in imaging studies of patients with schizophrenia (Hoffler et al. 1997). Cycloid psychoses have been associated with different pat-

terns of the P300 auditory evoked potential than either schizophrenia or bipolar disorder (Strik et al. 1997, 1998). Individuals with cycloid psychosis consistently showed normal P300 topographies and latencies but significantly higher amplitudes than did control subjects, a finding not seen in any other psychiatric condition (Strik et al. 1997). An appreciation of cycloid psychoses therefore may eventually expand understanding of the border between psychotic bipolar disorder and other conditions.

The concept of cycloid psychosis dates back at least a century in the European literature. In 1893, Magnan described a recurrent condition characterized by the sudden onset of fluctuating psychotic symptomatology, which he called *bouffées dèlirantes*. In 1928, Kleist coined the term *zykloide Psychosen* and went on to delineate three distinct subtypes. During the 1950s, Leonhard (1957) further differentiated these subtypes as "anxiety-happiness psychosis," "confusion psychosis," and "motility psychosis" (Ban 1990). Features of these subtypes often accompany one another as opposed to appearing in pure form (Perris 1990).

The hallmark of cycloid psychosis is the sudden onset of rapidly changing and polymorphic psychotic and affective symptoms. A degree of confusion is typically present, as well as overwhelming anxiety, mood lability, and mood-incongruent delusions and/or hallucinations. Mood is disorganized, fearful, ecstatic, or transcendent, with ideas of great insight or of having a special mission. Patients may have catatonia-like symptoms, such as extreme excitement or stupor with preserved or even intensified awareness. Cycloid psychoses typically have a rapid onset, with equally abrupt and full resolution of symptoms after variable periods of time.

Epidemiological studies in Sweden have estimated the 1-year incidence for first psychiatric admission for cycloid psychosis to be 5 per 100,000 for women and 3.5 per 100,000 for men, with the lifetime prevalence being less than 1% (approximately half of that for schizophrenia) (Lindvall et al. 1990, 1993). A significant number of cases of postpartum psychoses meet criteria for cycloid psychosis (Pfuhlmann et al. 1998), and a history of cycloid psychosis increases the risk for postpartum psychosis, which is most frequently a bipolar variant (McNeil 1986).

Neuroleptics alone or in combination with lithium have been reported to be effective acutely for single episodes of cycloid psychosis (Perris 1988). In several studies (Maj 1984; Perris 1978; Perris and Smigan 1984), lithium and carbamazepine (Ban 1990) have been reported to reduce recurrences, although it is not clear whether mood stabilizers are effective acutely. ECT has been reported to produce rapid improvement in patients with cycloid psychosis refractory to medications (J.D. Little et al. 2000; Perris 1988).

Seasonal Affective Disorder

Many people living in climates in which there are marked seasonal differences in the length of the day have seasonal changes in mood, sleep, and energy (Hellekson 1989; Kasper et al. 1989). Also, seasonal variations occur in most mood disorders. For example, unipolar depression is more likely to recur in the spring, whereas bipolar depression is more likely to recur in the fall, and mania is more likely to recur during the summer (Barbini et al. 1995). Contrary to popular wisdom, the time of greatest risk of suicide is not during the Christmas holidays but during the months of May and June (Hellekson 1989). The time of the seasonal peak in the incidence of suicide is independent of latitude, but the amplitude of the peak is greatest where the seasonal variation in light is the greatest (Hellekson 1989). Hospital admissions for unipolar depression peak in the spring, whereas admissions for mania peak in the summer (Hellekson 1989). The observations that seasonal variations in mood disorders in the Southern Hemisphere are the reverse of those in the Northern Hemisphere (e.g., more admissions for mania during the winter) and that the pattern of seasonal affective disorder (SAD) is the reverse in the Northern and Southern Hemispheres support the hypothesis that these changes are dependent on variations in available daylight (Hellekson 1989).

SAD was defined by Norman Rosenthal and associates (Hellekson 1989) as a condition that meets criteria for an RDC major affective disorder in which major depression occurs during the fall or winter for at least 2 consecutive years, with remission in the spring or summer. In SAD, depressive episodes cannot be associated with seasonal stressors, and no other Axis I diagnoses can be present. DSM-IV-TR criteria (Table 10–14), which are derived from the criteria of Rosenthal et al. (Hellekson 1989), include additional provisos that hypomania as well as remission of depression may occur during the summer and that seasonal depressive episodes should substantially outnumber nonseasonal episodes (American Psychiatric Association 2000). In DSM-IV-TR, a seasonal pattern is considered to be not a separate diagnosis but an additional specifier of MDD with recurrent depression, bipolar I disorder, or bipolar II disorder. As we noted in the previous paragraph, the well-described pattern of winter depression and summer euthymia or hypomania is reversed in the Southern Hemisphere (Hellekson 1989). In the Northern Hemisphere, reverse SAD, in which patients become depressed in the summer, seems related

TABLE 10–14. DSM-IV-TR criteria for seasonal pattern specifier

Specify if:

With Seasonal Pattern (can be applied to the pattern of major depressive episodes in bipolar I disorder, bipolar II disorder, or major depressive disorder, recurrent)

A. There has been a regular temporal relationship between the onset of major depressive episodes in bipolar I or bipolar II disorder or major depressive disorder, recurrent, and a particular time of the year (e.g., regular appearance of the major depressive episode in the fall or winter).
 Note: Do not include cases in which there is an obvious effect of seasonal-related psychosocial stressors (e.g., regularly being unemployed every winter).

B. Full remissions (or a change from depression to mania or hypomania) also occur at a characteristic time of the year (e.g., depression disappears in the spring).

C. In the last 2 years, two major depressive episodes have occurred that demonstrate the temporal seasonal relationships defined in Criteria A and B, and no nonseasonal major depressive episodes have occurred during that same period.

D. Seasonal major depressive episodes (as described above) substantially outnumber the nonseasonal major depressive episodes that may have occurred over the individual's lifetime.

to seasonal changes in temperature and humidity rather than changes in light (Hellekson 1989).

SAD occurs more frequently in women than in men, with a greater female-to-male ratio than in nonseasonal MDD (Hellekson 1989). SAD occurs in children as well as adults (Hellekson 1989). In a survey of centers specializing in the treatment of SAD (Hellekson 1989), the most common symptoms reported during depressive episodes were sadness, irritability, anxiety, decreased activity, increased appetite with carbohydrate craving, increased weight, increased sleep, daytime drowsiness, work and interpersonal problems, and menstrual difficulties. Symptoms began in November in Washington, D.C., and in late August in Alaska, supporting the role of shortening of the day as the precipitant of winter depression. The mean duration of depressive symptoms across centers was about 5–6 months. More than half the patients had a family history of mood disorder, and many had a family history of SAD.

In some samples, most patients with SAD have summer hypomania and therefore meet criteria for a diagnosis of bipolar II disorder; in other samples, the incidence of hypomania is low (Hellekson 1989). Some of the discrepancy may be a function of the frequency with which increased energy, decreased sleep, and related experiences during the summer are viewed as hypomania or simply relief of depression. More data are needed to determine how frequently SAD is bipolar and how frequently it is unipolar. There is greater agreement about the presence of atypical depressive symptoms in the winter depressions of SAD (Hellekson 1989), features that occur more frequently in bipolar depression.

Secondary Mood Disorders

In some circles, the term *secondary mood disorder* is used to indicate a mood disorder having another cause—for example, a medical illness or substance. To other experts, a secondary mood disorder is a mood disorder that occurs in the context of another disorder, such as schizophrenia or an anxiety disorder, with etiology not necessarily being implied (Knesper 1995; M.T. Tsuang and Faraone 1996). DSM-IV-TR implies causality of secondary mood disorders with the phrases *mood disorder due to a general medical disorder* (mood disorder caused by a medical or surgical illness; see Table 10–15) and *substance-induced mood disorder* (mood disorder caused by a medication or a psychoactive substance; see Table 10–16) ("Drugs That Cause Psychiatric Symptoms" 1993; Long and Kathol 1993). Adrenal steroids in particular frequently induce affective syndromes, with mania developing approximately twice as frequently as depression (Wada et al. 2000).

TABLE 10–15. Some medical conditions that can cause manic or depressive syndromes

Neurological disease	Parkinson's disease, Huntington's disease, traumatic brain injury, stroke, dementias, multiple sclerosis
Metabolic disease	Electrolyte disturbances, renal failure, vitamin deficiencies or excess, acute intermittent porphyria, Wilson's disease, environmental toxins, heavy metals
Gastrointestinal disease	Irritable bowel syndrome, chronic pancreatitis, Crohn's disease, cirrhosis, hepatic encephalopathy
Endocrine disorders	Hypo- and hyperthyroidism, Cushing's disease, Addison's disease, diabetes mellitus, parathyroid dysfunction
Cardiovascular disease	Myocardial infarction, angina, coronary artery bypass surgery, cardiomyopathies
Pulmonary disease	Chronic obstructive pulmonary disease, sleep apnea, reactive airway disease
Malignancies and hematological disease	Pancreatic carcinoma, brain tumors, paraneoplastic effects of lung cancers, anemias
Autoimmune disease	Systemic lupus erythematosus, fibromyalgia, rheumatoid arthritis

The other meaning of secondary mood disorder has been addressed in two ways in DSM-IV-TR. Although it is permissible to make a diagnosis of a mood disorder in a patient with another Axis I disorder such as schizophrenia, chronic affective symptoms that occur exclusively during the course of a psychotic disorder such as schizophrenia and do not meet criteria for an independent mood disorder are not given a separate diagnosis of a depressive disorder (First et al. 1996). The purpose of this approach is to avoid implying meaningless comorbidity. It is also important to distinguish between symptoms that are a component of another disorder and mood disorders that are truly secondary to another condition, which have a poorer treatment response than primary mood disorders (Knesper 1995). On the other hand, a potential problem that can occur if affective symptoms are considered secondary to the psychotic (or other) Axis I illness is that treatment may be directed only toward the "primary" disorder, with insufficient attention to a coexisting mood disorder that might respond to additional specific treatment. Differentiating between comorbidity of a mood disorder with another Axis I condition and affective symptoms that are manifestations of another disorder therefore has important clinical implications.

Mood Disorders in Children and Adolescents

When it was thought that the child's superego was too immature to experience depression or mania (which was considered a defense against depression), childhood depression was thought to be very rare. As a result, DSM-I did not include psychiatric disorders of children, and DSM-II included only behavioral disorders of children. However, it is now known that depression can be diagnosed in children as young as 3 years old. Consequently, DSM-III and DSM-III-R criteria for juvenile mood disorders were similar to those for adult mood disorders except that irritability could substitute for depressed mood, failure to maintain expected weight gain could substitute for weight loss, decreased school performance could substitute for decreased occupational function, and loss of interest in friends and play could substitute for loss of interest or pleasure. Symptom duration for a diagnosis of dysthymia in children and adolescents was established as 1 year as opposed to the required duration of 2 years in adults (Kashani and Nair 1995). These criteria have not been changed substantially in DSM-IV-TR.

Because of continued disagreement about the nature of juvenile mood disorders, estimates of prevalence and

TABLE 10–16. Some substances that can cause mania or depression

Drug	Reaction	Comments
Acyclovir	Psychosis, depression	At high doses
Alcohol	Depression, withdrawal, mania	
Amantadine	Psychosis, mania	More frequent in elderly
Amphetamine-like drugs	Psychosis, mania, anxiety, withdrawal, depression	
Anabolic steroids	Mania, depression, psychosis	
Anticonvulsants	Depression, mania	Usually with high doses or blood levels
Antidepressants	Mania, anxiety; abulia with SSRIs	Mania to hypomania in 0.5%–10% of patients
Asparaginase	Depression, paranoia	May occur frequently
Baclofen	Psychosis, mania, depression	Sometimes with treatment and high doses, but usually with sudden withdrawal
Barbiturates	Depression, excitement	Especially in children and elderly
Benzodiazepines	Depression, psychosis, mania	During treatment and withdrawal
β-Adrenergic blockers	Depression, confusion, mania	With usual doses, including ophthalmological use
Bromocriptine	Mania, psychosis, depression	Not dose related; may persist for weeks after drug is stopped
Bupropion	Mania, psychosis, agitation	Can aggravate schizophrenia
Buspirone	Mania, panic attack	In a few patients
Captopril	Mania, anxiety, psychosis	Especially in depressed patients
Carbamazepine	See "Anticonvulsants"	
Chloroquine	Psychosis, mania	Several reports
Clonidine	Depression	May resolve with continued use
Contraceptives, oral	Depression	In 15% in one study
Corticosteroids	Mania, depression, psychosis	Especially with high doses or withdrawal
Cyclobenzaprine	Mania, psychosis	Several reports
Cycloserine	Anxiety, depression, psychosis	Common
Cyclosporine	Psychosis, mania	Each in one patient
Dapsone	Psychosis, mania, depression	Several reports, even with low doses
Diethyltoluamide	Mania, psychosis	With excessive or prolonged use
Digitalis glycosides	Psychosis, depression	Especially with high doses or blood levels
Diltiazem	Depression, suicidal thoughts	Reported in eight patients
Disopyramide	Psychosis, depression	Within 24–48 hours of starting
Disulfiram	Depression, psychosis	Not related to alcohol reactions
Enalapril	Depression, psychosis	Two reports
Ethionamide	Depression, psychosis	Multiple reports
Etretinate	Severe depression	
Fenfluramine	See "Amphetamine-like drugs"	
Histamine H_2-receptor antagonists	Psychosis, depression, mania	Usually with high doses, more often in elderly, and with renal dysfunction
HMG-CoA reductase inhibitors	Depression	In several patients; may be rare
Interferon-α	Delirium, psychosis, depression, suicidal thoughts, mania	Common adverse effects; depression may be treated with SSRIs
Isocarboxazid	See "Monoamine oxidase inhibitors"	Mania and psychosis in two patients during withdrawal
Isoniazid	Depression, psychosis	Several reports
Isosorbide	Psychosis, depression	In one elderly woman on two occasions
Isotretinoin	Depression	Several reports
Levodopa	Depression, hypomania, psychosis	More common in elderly or with prolonged use
L-Glutamine	Grandiosity, hyperactivity	In two men
Loxapine	Mania	In one man
Mefloquine	Psychosis, depression	Several reports

TABLE 10–16. Some substances that can cause mania or depression *(continued)*

Drug	Reaction	Comments
Methyldopa	Depression, psychosis	Several reports
Metoclopramide	Mania, severe depression, crying	Several reports
Metrizamide	Psychosis, depression	May be prolonged
Metronidazole	Depression, crying, psychosis	Two cases with oral use
Monoamine oxidase inhibitors	Mania, psychosis	
Nalidixic acid	Depression	Rare
Narcotics	Euphoria, dysphoria, depression, psychosis	Usually with high doses
Nifedipine	Irritability, depression	Several reports
Nonsteroidal anti-inflammatory drugs	Psychosis, depression	Not reported with all drugs in this class
Norfloxacin	Depression	
Ofloxacin	Depression, mania	Single reports of each
Penicillin G procaine	See "Procaine derivatives"	
Pergolide	Psychosis, depression	On withdrawal
Phenelzine	See "Monoamine oxidase inhibitors"	
Phentermine	See "Amphetamine-like drugs"	
Phenylephrine	Depression, psychosis	Overuse of nasal spray; single report with oral use
Phenylpropanolamine	See "Amphetamine-like drugs"	
Phenytoin	See "Anticonvulsants"	
Prazosin	Psychosis, depression	In four patients, two had renal failure
Procaine derivatives	Psychosis, depression, anxiety	Many reports, especially with penicillin G procaine
Procarbazine	Mania	In two children
Propafenone	Psychosis, mania	Several reports
Pseudoephedrine	Psychosis, mania	Reported with usual doses in children and with overuse in one adult
Quinacrine	Mania, psychosis	More common with high doses
Reserpine	Depression	Common with >0.5 mg/day
Selegiline	See "Monoamine oxidase inhibitors"	
Sulfonamides	Depression, euphoria	Several reports
Theophylline	Mania, depression	Usually with high serum concentrations
Thiazides	Depression, suicidal ideation	In several patients after weeks to months of use
Thyroid hormones	Mania, depression, psychosis	Initial doses in susceptible patients
Tranylcypromine	See "Monoamine oxidase inhibitors"	Hypomania or mania in up to 10% of depressed patients
Trimethoprim-sulfamethoxazole	Psychosis, depression	Several reports
Valproate	See "Anticonvulsants"	
Vinblastine	Depression	
Vincristine	Depression	
Zidovudine	Mania, psychosis	Reported in two patients

Note. HMG-CoA = hepatic hydroxymethylglutaryl-coenzyme A; SSRI = selective serotonin reuptake inhibitor.

incidence vary. When the Schedule for Affective Disorders and Schizophrenia for School-Aged Children (K-SADS) was administered to 1,710 adolescents age 14–18 years, almost 30% had at least one current depressive symptom, the most common symptoms being depressed mood, disturbed sleep, problems thinking, and anhedonia (Roberts et al. 1995). However, only 2.6% of the sample met full criteria for a current diagnosis of a mood disorder. In contrast to adults in other studies, adolescents in this study who had experienced two episodes of major depression had different symptoms during each episode. Other reports suggested that childhood mood disorders have more familial loading than adult mood disorders and that when children from depressed families become depressed, the depression occurs earlier than does depression in children of families that are not depressed (ages 12–13 years vs. 16–17 years) (Geller et al. 1996). These kinds of findings suggest that inherited factors may be more important in juvenile mood disorders. Mood disorders in younger patients, as in adults, present a definite risk of suicide, as does substance use (Marttunen et al. 1995; Shaffer et al. 1996). The cumulative prevalence of suicide attempts in adolescents is as high as 3% (Shaffer et al. 1996). However, early intervention in childhood and adolescent mood disorders may improve long-term outcome (Duffy 2000).

One area of ongoing investigation is the presentation of bipolar disorder in children and adolescents. Compared with adult bipolar disorder, juvenile bipolar disorder is characterized by more irritability, dysphoria, psychosis, schizophreniform symptoms, hyperactivity, mixed mania, rapid cycling, chronicity, and familial loading (Ballenger et al. 1982; Faedda et al. 1995; Geller et al. 1995). An important question is whether a first episode of major depression in a younger patient is more likely than a first episode in an adult to be the initial presentation of a bipolar mood disorder (i.e., to be followed by the later development of mania or hypomania) (Akiskal 1995a; Kashani and Nair 1995). When conservative criteria are used, between 5% and 15% of the cases of major depression in adults are bipolar (Bebbington 1995; Geller et al. 1996), compared with at least 20% of the cases among adolescents and 32% of the cases among children younger than 11 years (Geller et al. 1996). Features that juvenile major depressive episodes share with bipolar disorder include an early age at onset, equal numbers of males and females affected, mood lability, a high rate of recurrence, prominent irritability and explosive anger suggestive of mixed bipolar episodes, and a relatively poor response to antidepressants (Akiskal 1995a). In addition, juvenile major depressive episodes are often associated with cyclothymic or hyperthymic temperaments (Akiskal 1995a).

The diagnostic challenge implied by these kinds of observations is to identify those juvenile patients with major depressive episodes who are at greater risk for a bipolar outcome and who might have a better ultimate response to mood-stabilizing treatments than to antidepressants. Features of major depressive episodes in younger patients listed in Table 10–17 have been found to increase the likelihood of the eventual occurrence of mania (Akiskal 1995a, 1995b; Strober and Carlson 1982). Although no predictive studies exist regarding the prognostic validity of these features, their regular occurrence in younger patients with bipolar disorder is reason for caution in treating juvenile major depression. One of these factors in particular warrants additional discussion. As we noted earlier, hypomania that occurs only when

TABLE 10–17. Features associated with a bipolar outcome in juvenile major depression

Early onset
Acute onset
Psychotic symptoms, especially hallucinations
Significant psychomotor slowing
Family history of bipolar disorder
Any mood disorder in three consecutive generations
Antidepressant-induced hypomania

antidepressants are being taken is excluded in DSM-IV-TR as a diagnostic criterion for bipolar disorder in adults because not all patients with this experience will become manic spontaneously. However, several small studies of depressed adolescents and children indicate a very high rate of spontaneous mania or hypomania following antidepressant-induced hypomania (Akiskal 1995a, 1995b, 1996).

Difficulty recognizing juvenile bipolar disorder accounts for the recent finding that half of the children who fulfilled diagnostic criteria for mania had received a different diagnosis (Kashani and Nair 1995). A controversial area of diagnostic confusion concerns attention-deficit/hyperactivity disorder (ADHD). Some reports suggest a familial link between juvenile bipolar disorder and ADHD, and these conditions are frequently diagnosed together (Biederman 1995). For example, in a study in which 28% of 270 psychiatric inpatients age 5–18 years who were given the K-SADS met criteria for ADHD, 36% of the patients with ADHD met criteria for nonpsychotic depression, 8% met criteria for an affective psychosis, and 22% met criteria for bipolar disorder (Butler et al. 1995); there was no follow-up to determine how many of the depressed patients developed mania.

Clinical experience also suggests that ADHD and bipolar disorder are often diagnosed in the same patient, but it is not clear whether this means that the two disorders are frequently comorbid or that the symptoms of the two disorders overlap, so that patients who meet criteria for one condition will regularly also meet criteria for the other (Butler et al. 1995). The latter point is illustrated in Table 10–18 (American Psychiatric Association 1994a; Kashani and Nair 1995).

Most patients with bipolar disorder meet virtually all criteria for ADHD, but patients with ADHD do not meet most criteria for bipolar disorder (Geller et al. 1998). For example, elation, depression, decreased need for sleep, hypersomnia, grandiosity, psychosis, and rapid, pressured speech are not characteristic of ADHD (Biederman 1995; Kashani and Nair 1995) except as manifestations of stimulant toxicity. Racing and tangential thinking may be difficult to differentiate from the kind of talkativeness that is encountered in patients with ADHD, but an increased content of thought, especially with multiple coexisting complex ideas and plans, is more suggestive of bipolar disorder than ADHD. Irritability, fighting, and thrill seeking can be encountered in both disorders, but attacks of rage that provoke prolonged organized attacks on others in response to threats to self-esteem and attempts to control the patient are more common in bipolar disorder, as is the kind of grandiosity that leads to fighting multiple opponents, fearlessness in the face of overwhelming odds, and jumping from extreme heights with the belief that one cannot be hurt and a response of hilarity to being injured. Historical elements listed in Table 10–17 are more common in bipolar disorder, although, as we noted earlier, bipolar disorder and ADHD may aggregate in the same families. Finally, bipolar disorder may be more common in tertiary care centers, given that uncomplicated ADHD is usually treated successfully in the offices of pediatricians, family physicians, and psychiatrists who consult to schools.

A study of 140 boys age 6–17 years with diagnoses of ADHD attempted to address the question of symptomatic overlap by rediagnosing patients after specific symptoms of ADHD listed in Table 10–18 had been subtracted (Milberger et al. 1995). Seventy-nine percent of

the patients still met criteria for MDD, 56% met criteria for bipolar disorder, and 75% met criteria for generalized anxiety disorder. One interpretation of these findings is that other disorders may have a sufficient number of characteristics similar to those of ADHD (and each other) to result in diagnostic confusion between these conditions. A positive response to stimulants is often interpreted as evidence in favor of a diagnosis of ADHD, but the effect of stimulants in enhancing attention is not specific to ADHD. In addition, depressed patients with slowed thinking may show improvement of attention with stimulants, and some manic patients have been noted to experience calming and behavioral slowing in response to stimulants (Max et al. 1995). Although no controlled studies have addressed this issue, adolescent and young adult patients are encountered in practice who were apparently treated successfully with stimulants or antidepressants for ADHD, only to develop dysphoric manic symptoms such as increasing irritability, anxiety, impulsivity, thrill seeking, grandiose defiance, mood swings, and psychosis with continued treatment. It is impossible to know whether long-term treatment with stimulants eventually destabilized mood in patients with bipolar disorders misdiagnosed as ADHD or whether the adverse outcome represented the natural progression of bipolar disorder.

TABLE 10–18.   Common features of juvenile bipolar disorder and attention-deficit/hyperactivity disorder

Attention-deficit/hyperactivity disorder	Bipolar disorder[a]
Mood lability, temper outbursts	Mood lability, temper outbursts
Fails to give close attention to detail	(Racing thoughts, impulsivity)
Difficulty sustaining attention	Racing thoughts
Does not listen when spoken to directly	Self-involvement
Does not follow through	(Impulsivity, distractibility, tangential thinking, changeable direction of effort driven by mood swings)
Difficulty organizing tasks and activities	(Disorganization, changeable focus of attention, impulsivity)
Loses things necessary for tasks	(Distractibility, impulsivity)
Easily distracted	Distractibility
Forgetful in daily activities	(Fluctuating interest and motivation)
Fidgets or squirms	(Increased levels of activity)
Leaves seat when remaining seated is expected	Increased energy
Runs about or climbs excessively	Increased activity
Difficulty playing quietly	Increased energy and activity
Often on the go or as if driven by a motor	Increased energy and activity
Talks excessively	Pressure of speech
Blurts out answers before questions have been completed	Racing thoughts
Difficulty awaiting turn	(Impulsivity, increased energy)
Interrupts or intrudes on others	(Impulsivity, grandiose self-centeredness)

Note.   [a]DSM-IV-TR symptoms of bipolar disorder; features of bipolar disorder not formally listed as diagnostic criteria for bipolar disorder are noted in parentheses.

1995). Major depression occurs at increased rates in patients with myocardial infarction, ventricular arrhythmias, and congestive heart failure (Franco-Bronson 1996). Major depression has been found to increase the risk of developing coronary heart disease and to increase mortality after myocardial infarction (Barefoot and Schroll 1996). Hypothyroidism is very common in patients with depression, especially among those with treatment-refractory mood disorders and rapid-cycling bipolar disorder (Franco-Bronson 1996). Much of the hypothyroidism that occurs in depressed patients is caused by thyroiditis, which suggests a link between susceptibility loci for major depression and thyroiditis. There appears to be a similar link between migraine headaches and MDD. In a subgroup analysis of the Baltimore ECA study, the lifetime risk of self-reported migraine headaches was elevated 3.14 times in current major depression (Swartz et al. 2000). Additional medical conditions frequently associated with depression include irritable bowel syndrome, fibromyalgia, chronic fatigue syndrome, acquired immunodeficiency syndrome, renal failure, and autoimmune disease (Franco-Bronson 1996; Gruber et al. 1996).

Several neurological illnesses are also associated with an increased risk of mood disorders (Fann and Tucker 1995). Between 8% and 75% of patients with cerebrovascular accidents develop major depression; in one study, depressed stroke patients had an eightfold risk of mortality compared with matched nondepressed stroke patients (P.L.P. Morris et al. 1993). Anatomical location of the stroke appears to have a marked effect on the prevalence of associated depression: left prefrontal and basal ganglia strokes more frequently result in depressive disorders than do right hemisphere lesions (P.L.P. Morris et al. 1993). Conversely, right hemisphere lesions are often associated with development of secondary mania (Berthier et al. 1996). Cerebrovascular and degenerative disease on the left side of the brain is a common cause of late-onset depression, and disease on the right side of the brain is often associated with late-onset mania (Shulman and Hermann 1999; Simpson et al. 1999). Depression is the most frequent psychiatric complication of Parkinson's disease, possibly because of the participation of the basal ganglia in mood regulation (Klassen et al. 1995).

About 50% of patients with Alzheimer's disease meet criteria for major depression or dysthymia (Petracca et al. 1996). Approximately 2%–3.8% of Alzheimer's disease patients develop mania (Fann and Tucker 1995). Despite the fact that the pattern of dementia is cortical in Alzheimer's disease and subcortical in the dementia syndrome of depression, it can be impossible to distinguish one from the other clinically, and depression can aggravate the dementia of Alzheimer's disease. The interaction of depression and dementia was discussed earlier in this chapter. The incidence of depression is also increased in temporal lobe epilepsy, AIDS, Huntington's disease, traumatic brain injury, spinal cord injury, and multiple sclerosis, and AIDS and traumatic brain injury also can present as mania (Blumer et al. 1995; Fann and Tucker 1995; Kishi and Robinson 1996; T.F. Scott et al. 1996).

Anxiety Disorders

Anxiety is a prominent symptom in as many as 70% of depressed outpatients (Rosenbaum et al. 1995). In addition, comorbidity of specific mood and anxiety disorders has been found consistently in large studies (Weissman et al. 1996). The NIMH-CS, a community survey, found that 32% of the depressed patients had phobias, 31% had panic attacks, and 11% had obsessions or compulsions (Glass et al. 1989). Conversely, major depressive episodes have been reported in 8%–39% of the patients with generalized anxiety disorder, 50%–90% of the patients with panic disorder, 35%–70% of the patients with social phobia, and 33% of the patients with obsessive-compulsive disorder (OCD) (Brawman-Mintzer and Lydiard 1996; Gorman and Coplan 1996). Social phobia has been reported in more than 40% of the patients with MDD (Bruder et al. 1997). Bipolar illness is also more common in patients with panic disorder and OCD (Strakowski et al. 1994).

There are a number of possible associations between mood and anxiety disorders. Many kinds of distress in depressed patients can be referred to as *anxiety* (Bruder et al. 1997), and patients may describe arousal and dysphoria as anxiety at one point and depression at another. Some patients cannot tell the difference between anxiety and depression, and some of the items on mood rating scales such as the HRSD are symptoms of anxiety. Some of the time, anxiety may reflect a separate disorder that occurs at a higher-than-expected rate in depressed patients; this rate may be higher because one disorder lowers the threshold for the expression of the other or because susceptibility to one disorder is linked to susceptibility to the other. Manic overstimulation may be expressed as panic attacks, which can be distinguished from panic disorder by the presence of racing thoughts and a sense of having too much energy. Anxiety in patients with bipolar mood disorders is often an indication of mixed (dysphoric) states.

Alternating emphasis on particular symptoms probably accounts for the observation that a group of patients with depressive disorders followed up prospectively are rediagnosed with anxiety disorders, whereas patients with initial diagnoses of anxiety disorders may receive a later diagnosis of a mood disorder (Kovacs et al. 1989). In some instances, the predominance of one or the other symptom may represent a prodromal phase of a mood disorder in which both anxiety and depression are important symptoms. The extent to which one disorder is emphasized over the other (e.g., depression with secondary anxiety or anxiety with secondary depression) may be more a matter of features that strike the examiner or the patient at a particular moment than of the nature of the illness.

In addition to their comorbidity, depression, mania, and anxiety as dimensions of affective experience have complex overlap and interactions with one another. Anxiety in depressed patients increases severity, chronicity, and impairment associated with depression and makes depression more refractory to treatment; anxiety also increases the risk of suicide in depressed patients, perhaps because it is a marker of higher levels of arousal (Keck et al. 1994; Rudd et al. 1993). Depressed people who are anxious have more anxious people in their families, and they also have more familial loading for depression (Breier et al. 1985; Clayton et al. 1991). In these families, anxiety may be a marker of a risk factor for more severe, treatment-resistant, and/or familial form of depression (K.K. Kendler et al. 1987).

Substance Use Disorders

Major mood disorders have high rates of comorbidity with use of many substances, especially alcohol (Maier et al. 1995b; Weissman et al. 1996). Alcohol abuse or dependence occurs in 50% of unipolar depression patients, 60% of bipolar I disorder patients, and 50% of bipolar II disorder patients (Feinman and Dunner 1996). The ECA study reported that about one-third of the individuals with mood disorders had a comorbid substance use disorder (McDowell and Clodfelter 2001). Comorbid alcoholism worsens the course of both unipolar depression (Hasin et al. 1996) and bipolar disorder (Feinman and Dunner 1996). Conversely, abstinence improves the response of the mood disorder to treatment (Hasin et al. 1996).

The prevalence of depression in individuals with substance dependence is higher in active drinkers, consistent with findings discussed earlier that certain substances can induce depression. In one study (K.M. Davidson 1995), prevalence rates for depression in alcohol-dependent patients decreased from 67% when they were actively drinking to 13% after detoxification. Such findings, as well as studies showing reduced response rates to antidepressants during active alcohol use, have led to the clini-

cal practice of deferring treatment for depression until substance use has been curtailed. However, recent work with substance-dependent adolescents suggested that the presence of depression interferes with the patients' ability to engage in treatment for the substance use disorder (Rao et al. 2000; Riggs et al. 1997) and that antidepressant therapy improves depressive symptoms and may even reduce alcohol consumption in nonabstinent depressed alcoholic patients (McGrath et al. 1996). These observations may support an approach to some patients in which depression and substance use are treated concurrently or depression is treated before patients become fully abstinent.

Use of sedatives by manic patients to tone down dysphoric overstimulation is readily understandable. The reason some patients with bipolar mood disorders use stimulants to induce mania would be obvious if the mania were pleasurable, but substance-induced mania is frequently unpleasant. By purposely making themselves manic, some of these patients may be attempting to achieve a sense of mastery over fluctuations in mood that otherwise feel completely unpredictable and uncontrollable. Patients with mood disorders that are treated acutely with neuroleptics may note blunting of the rewarding properties of cocaine, but chronic neuroleptic therapy, which is common in patients who have been hospitalized for bipolar mood disorders (Sernyak and Woods 1993), may enhance the euphoric effects of cocaine.

Schizophrenia

Major depressive episodes occur in 25%–50% of cases of schizophrenia (American Psychiatric Association 1993). The traditional belief that most of these episodes are "postpsychotic" and involve reactions to awareness of having a severe illness is contradicted by the finding that half of the depressive episodes occurring during the course of schizophrenia develop in the midst of an acute psychotic episode, and the affective component may become apparent only after the psychosis resolves (Dubovsky and Thomas 1992). Fears that administration of antidepressants may aggravate schizophrenia have been contradicted by observations that in all but the most acute psychotic exacerbations, treatment of depression improves the prognosis of comorbid schizophrenia (Dubovsky and Thomas 1992).

Personality Disorders

Between 30% and 70% of depressed patients receive a concurrent diagnosis of a personality disorder (Thase 1996), usually in Cluster B (i.e., borderline, histrionic, and antisocial personality disorder) (Corruble et al. 1996). Similar diagnoses, along with narcissistic personality disorder, are often made in patients with bipolar mood disorders. At the same time, 95% of the personality disorder patients who commit suicide have a comorbid Axis I diagnosis, usually depression (Isometsa et al. 1996). As we noted earlier in this chapter (see "Subsyndromal Depression"), personality disorders may be diagnosed frequently in association with mood disorders because pathological defenses mobilized to deal with abnormal mood mimic character pathology. In support of this possibility, Thase's group (Thase 1996) found that when they reinterviewed depressed patients after successful treatment, the rate of personality disorder was half the rate before treatment.

There are several additional possible explanations for the association between mood and personality disorders (Riso et al. 1996; Thase 1996). One possibility is that certain personality traits or disorders may predispose to mood disorders. For example, an overly dependent patient might be more vulnerable to depression in response to loss of an important source of support. Or chronic mood disorders may skew experience in ways that lead to the development of personality disorders, such as when grandiosity, impulsivity, and expansiveness associated with a bipolar mood disorder become integrated into a patient's habitual behavioral repertoire, leading to histrionic or narcissistic personality traits. Vulnerability to depression and to personality disorders may be inherited or acquired together, or common etiological factors may lead to both mood and personality disorders.

Patients with mood disorders who have comorbid personality disorders have more overall symptomatology and experience worse social adjustment than do mood disorder patients without personality disorders (Carpenter et al. 1995). Depressed patients with personality disorders are less responsive to antidepressants and ECT (Black et al. 1988; Thase 1996). The presence of a comorbid personality disorder also has been found to impair response to interpersonal therapy (IPT) (Thase 1996). However, cognitive-behavioral therapy (CBT) has been reported to be equally effective in depressed patients with and without personality disorders (Shea et al. 1990; Stuart et al. 1992; Thase 1996).

In clinical practice, apparent comorbid personality disorders that actually reflect exaggeration of pathological character traits often are no longer as problematic when the mood disorder responds to treatment. On the other hand, issues related to truly comorbid personality disorders such as self-destructive motivations, negative therapeutic reactions, and attachment to an identity as a depressed person can lead to noncompliance, turning of treatments against the clinician, and other behaviors that interfere with a positive response to treatment. The role of personality disorders is further complicated by a tendency of clinicians to attribute to a personality disorder the failure of depressed patients to respond as expected (Thase 1996). This kind of assessment may be premature if there is not a careful longitudinal assessment including an evaluation of the doctor–patient relationship.

Studies of Inherited Factors

Despite the progress made in DSM-IV and the RDC toward defining homogeneous subtypes of mood disorders, there is enough remaining diversity of phenomenology and comorbidity to complicate studies of etiology. Research investigating causes of mood disorders is often contradictory and incomplete because all relevant features of the disorder are not included in each study.

When interpreting studies of etiological factors in mood disorders, it is important to be aware that it is not likely that there is a single cause of even the most rigidly defined mood disorder. There is no reason to think that any inborn factor causes mood disorders; such factors interact with experiential and other environmental influences to lead to illness. Etiologies considered in a single dimension are no less complex. One abnormal gene may produce an abnormal protein that contributes to a positive symptom, whereas another gene may fail to make a protein that regulates the emergence of the same symptom. A neurotransmitter may set in motion a chain of events that overlaps a second cascade initiated by another neurotransmitter, so that dysfunction of either transmitter can have the same end result. In the same manner, any one of a number of symptoms may be a cue for the entire symptom complex that is clinically called an *affective syndrome*. Bearing these limitations in mind, we consider several areas of research and then attempt to integrate the current state of knowledge about the causes of mood disorders.

Family Studies

Family studies have repeatedly shown that mood disorders are familial (M.T. Tsuang and Faraone 1996). Relatives of people with mood disorders are consistently two to three times as likely to have mood disorders as are relatives of control subjects (E.S. Gershon 1990). If one parent has a bipolar mood disorder, the risk that a child will have a unipolar or bipolar mood disorder is around 28%; if both parents have mood disorders, the risk is two to three times as great (Jamison 1996). Patients with mood disorders also have an elevated familial incidence of substance abuse (Geller et al. 1996), and patients who are depressed and anxious have more relatives who are depressed, anxious, or both (Breier et al. 1985; Gorman and Coplan 1996; K.K. Kendler et al. 1987).

Wealth and political affiliation also run in families, but they are not genetic. One way to begin to determine a genetic contribution is to compare the concordance of mood disorders in first- and second-degree relatives of probands with mood disorders. Because first-degree relatives (parents, children, and siblings) share 50% of their genomes, whereas only 25% of the genes are identical in second-degree relatives (grandparents, uncles, aunts, nephews, and nieces), a greater rate of a mood disorder in first-degree relatives of individuals with the same disorder than in second-degree relatives of these individuals suggests a genetic influence (M.T. Tsuang and Faraone 1996). The expectation of a greater likelihood of mood disorders in first-degree relatives of patients with mood disorders than in second-degree relatives or control populations usually has been confirmed (M.T. Tsuang and Faraone 1996).

Most studies suggest a more prominent familial transmission of bipolar than of unipolar mood disorders, often with affected relatives in consecutive generations. In addition, the age at symptom onset is earlier in bipolar individuals with strongly positive family histories (Johnson et al. 2000). Family members of patients with bipolar disorder are more likely to have bipolar as well as unipolar mood disorders themselves than are family members of patients with unipolar disorder (Jamison 1996). However, the rate of bipolar disorder in the families of the patients with unipolar depression is as much as three to four times the rate in control subjects (E.S. Gershon et al. 1982; Weissman et al. 1984). According to published family studies (E.S. Gershon et al. 1982; M.T. Tsuang and Faraone 1996; Weissman et al. 1984), first-degree relatives of patients with unipolar depression have a risk of unipolar depression of 5.5%–28.4% and a risk of bipolar disorder of 0.7%–8.1%; and first-degree relatives of probands with bipolar disorder have a 4.1%–14.6% likelihood of having a bipolar disorder themselves and a 5.4%–14% likelihood of having unipolar depression. Familial overlap also has been found between schizophrenia and mood disorders (Lyons et al. 2000). As we noted earlier in this chapter (see "Bipolar Subtypes"), bipolar II disorder "breeds true"; that is, bipolar II disorder patients have relatives who are hypomanic but not manic, whereas patients with bipolar I disorder have some relatives who are manic and some who are hypomanic (Jamison 1996).

Twin Studies

Another approach to investigating genetic contributions to mood disorders is to study differences in concordance between monozygotic (identical) and dizygotic (fraternal) twins. Monozygotic twins come from the same egg and have the same genes, whereas dizygotic twins come from different eggs and share 50% of their genes, like any other siblings. A greater concordance rate for a disorder in monozygotic twins than in dizygotic twins suggests a genetic influence because the role of intrauterine and postnatal environments is presumably similar for both kinds of twins (M.T. Tsuang and Faraone 1996). Concordance studies (Jamison 1996; M.T. Tsuang and Faraone 1996) reliably confirmed that the overall risk of mood disorders is three times as great in monozygotic as in dizygotic twins of probands with mood disorders. For bipolar disorder, concordance rates average 0.67–1.00 for monozygotic and 0.20 for dizygotic twins. Concordance rates for unipolar depression are generally 0.50 in monozygotic twins and 0.20 in dizygotic twins. The greater difference in concordance rates between monozygotic and dizygotic twins in bipolar disorder may reflect a greater genetic influence in bipolar disorder.

The assumption that identical twins grow up in identical environments may not be entirely accurate. The phase of division of the egg at which two embryos begin to emerge differs in different monozygotic twin pairs, and this has potential implications for later development of the nervous system. Parents can usually tell monozygotic twins apart, and not all sets of monozygotic twins are exposed to the same interpersonal fields as they grow up. Concordance rates for mood disorders in monozygotic twins reared apart from infancy can help to differentiate genetic influences from potential differences in the postnatal environment. In one study, 8 of 12 monozygotic twins of bipolar mood disorder probands raised apart from their twins had bipolar mood disorders themselves, a rate similar to the concordance rate of monozygotic twins of bipolar mood disorder patients reared with their ill twins (Jamison 1996).

Because concordance rates for mood disorders in twin studies are less than 100%, any genetic factors that are present must interact with environmental influences to create the risk for development of the actual disorder (M.T. Tsuang and Faraone 1996). Reviews of twin studies suggest that 21%–45% of the variance in the risk of depressive disorders can be attributed to genetic factors, and 55%–75% of the variance can be attributed to environmental factors (K.K. Kendler et al. 1992b). A substantial amount (60%) of the effect of genetic factors appears to be direct, but 40% seems to reflect genetic factors that increase the likelihood that people will put themselves in situations that lead to depression (e.g., becoming romantically involved with someone who is likely to leave) (K.K. Kendler et al. 1993). Of stressful life events, losses seem to be most influential (K.K. Kendler et al. 1993).

It was mentioned earlier that patients with major depression and comorbid anxiety have both anxiety and depression in their families. In support of this observation, K.K. Kendler et al. (1992a) reported that 1,033 pairs of female twins had increased concordance for both major depression and generalized anxiety disorder, agoraphobia, and social phobia. K.K. Kendler et al. (1987, 1992a, 1993) hypothesized that some common trait predisposing to anxiety and depression may be inherited and that which one predominates depends on experience.

Adoption Studies

The influence of the environment on the development of mood disorders also can be assessed by examining rates of mood disorders in adoptive and biological families of the people who were adopted in infancy. Most of these studies report that adoptees with mood disorders are more likely to have biological than adoptive relatives with mood disorders (M.T. Tsuang and Faraone 1996). Because rates of bipolar disorder in adoptive families of probands with bipolar disorder are no greater than in the general population, whereas rates of bipolar disorder in the biological families of these adoptees are the same as those in bipolar individuals raised with bipolar family members, adoptive factors have little or no role in bipolar mood disorders (M.T. Tsuang and Faraone 1996). Adoptive studies suggest that genetic factors are also important in determining transmission of unipolar depression, but adoptive (i.e., environmental) mechanisms play an important role; similar findings have emerged for transmission of suicide risk (M.T. Tsuang and Faraone 1996).

Linkage Studies

Less inferential studies of genetic factors examine linkage between biological phenotypes or genetic markers with mood disorders. Presumably, a gene or genes influencing development of the mood disorder would be close to the gene for the phenotype or the genetic marker that aggregates with the mood disorder. Linkage studies are most reliable for disorders that have a single dominant gene mode of transmission with complete penetrance, such as Huntington's disease. Unfortunately, the mode of transmission of most mood disorders is oligogenic, and incom-

plete penetrance and variable expressivity are likely to be the rule (M.T. Tsuang and Faraone 1996). Because the familial pattern of some bipolar mood disorders seems more consistent with a dominant mode of transmission, linkage studies of bipolar families have been most promising.

Red-green color blindness, a recessive X-linked trait, has been repeatedly linked to bipolar mood disorders in about one-third of the cases studied (M.T. Tsuang and Faraone 1996). An X-linked factor near the gene for color blindness would be expected to show mother-to-son transmission, which is observed in some bipolar families. Of three linkage studies involving glucose-6-phosphate dehydrogenase (G6PD) deficiency, the gene for which is thought to be close to the gene for color blindness, findings of one supported and findings of another were highly suggestive of linkage of G6PD deficiency to bipolar disorder (M.T. Tsuang and Faraone 1996). A study of the F9 DNA marker on the X chromosome suggested linkage to bipolar disorder, but studies of other DNA markers from the same region did not indicate such linkage (M.T. Tsuang and Faraone 1996). Results of studies of linkage of bipolar mood disorder to different traits thought to be carried on the X chromosome may not have been more consistent because some bipolar subtypes in some families have X-linkage, whereas others do not. Additional reasons for apparently contradictory findings in linkage studies are discussed later in this section.

Attempts to link human leukocyte antigen (HLA) phenotypes to bipolar mood disorders generally have been unsuccessful (M.T. Tsuang and Faraone 1996). The fact that bipolar disorder and thalassemia minor cosegregated in a family seemed to suggest linkage to a gene on the short arm of chromosome 11 close to the H-ras-1 locus because thalassemia minor is caused by a mutation at that locus (Joffe et al. 1986). This possibility was interesting because H-ras may be involved in the translation of experience into changes in neuronal functioning (Post 1992b). However, these results have not been replicated. An association between bipolar mood disorder and blood type O, the gene for which is on chromosome 9, was found in one report (Lavori et al. 1984). This finding also was of theoretical interest because the ABO blood type gene is close to the gene for dopamine β-hydroxylase; however, additional studies have rejected the concept of linkage of bipolar disorder to ABO markers (M.T. Tsuang and Faraone 1996).

A more specific type of linkage analysis involves restriction fragment length polymorphisms (RFLPs), which are DNA fragments prepared by digestion of chromosomes with restriction endonucleases that break DNA at known nucleotide sequences. Each RFLP contains more than one gene. In a widely publicized RFLP study of bipolar disorder in a large pedigree of Old-Order Amish (Egeland et al. 1987), linkage was found to an RFLP on the short arm of chromosome 11 (11p15), another finding of theoretical interest because this locus is close to the gene for tyrosine hydroxylase, the rate-limiting step in the synthesis of norepinephrine. The model derived from this study suggested a penetrance of about 60%; that is, about 60% of the subjects with a specific allele of the marker had a diagnosis of bipolar disorder. Unfortunately, additional data from patients who did not have the 11p15 marker but developed bipolar disorder appeared to refute the original findings and actually exclude linkage to chromosome 11p15 (Kelsoe et al. 1989), whereas European studies of different pedigrees never showed linkage to 11p15 in the first place (Berrettini et al. 1997).

Studies of other loci have had equally confusing results. An investigation of one family suggested linkage of bipolar disorder to the long arm of chromosome 11, but other work rejected this hypothesis (M.T. Tsuang and Faraone 1996). Suggestions of linkage of bipolar disorder to markers on 21q22.3 in a few families were refuted in later research (Vallada et al. 1996). A study of 310 DNA markers covering about 50% of the genome excluded linkage of bipolar I disorder; bipolar II disorder; schizoaffective disorder, bipolar type; and recurrent unipolar depression to all markers except a marker on the centromeric region of chromosome 18 (Berrettini et al. 1997). However, linkage to chromosome 18 was not confirmed in another study of five families (Maier et al. 1995a).

Genetic markers for bipolar disorder are reported in one study and refuted in another for various reasons (Berrettini et al. 1997; M.T. Tsuang and Faraone 1996). Methodologies used differ substantially, as do diagnostic instruments. Even though bipolar and unipolar mood disorders can run in the same families, they probably have different patterns of familial aggregation, and bipolar II disorder has a different familial pattern than does bipolar I disorder. Yet linkage studies do not distinguish between bipolar I disorder and bipolar II disorder, and many studies group subjects with schizoaffective disorder and even recurrent unipolar depression with patients with bipolar disorder so that there will be enough patients to achieve statistically significant findings. If attempts are made to distinguish between unipolar disorder and bipolar disorder in a linkage study, patients with bipolar disorder who have not yet had a manic episode may be counted as unipolar disorder patients, as apparently happened in the Amish study (Egeland et al. 1987). If patients with subsyndromal bipolar mood dis-

orders are counted as unipolar disorder patients, evidence of an association between a particular marker and bipolar disorder will be diluted. Given the oligogenic nature of most mood disorders, it seems likely that positive associations that are found reflect some dimension of the mood disorder such as recurrence, severity, thought disorder, psychosis, or a comorbid condition such as anxiety, substance use, or ADHD that is subject to genetic influences. Additional methodological issues include possible genetic differences between ethnic groups that are lumped together in genetic studies and flaws in statistical assumptions on which measures of significance are based.

Even if financial and technical barriers to large multicenter studies of homogeneous populations of patients with narrowly defined bipolar or unipolar mood disorders could be overcome and more discrete genetic markers could be used, there are several reasons contradictory findings are likely to continue to emerge from linkage studies. First, there is no reason to believe that only one inherited factor predisposes to a given mood disorder, no matter how much patients with the disorder resemble one another clinically. Any one of a number of genes could produce abnormal proteins that alter a cascade of physiological events at different points to produce the same end result. Another gene might fail to produce a protein with sufficient activity to keep the abnormal cascade from having an effect. The same phenotype therefore could be associated with any one of a number of genotypes. In addition, because people with mood disorders tend to marry each other at a greater-than-random rate (assortative mating), members of the same family are likely to have genetically different mood disorders. Conversely, variable expressivity and penetrance can result in patients with the same gene having phenotypically distinct disorders. Finally, some cases of a mood disorder in a given family may clinically resemble a genetic form of the disorder without there being any genetic contribution at all (phenocopies), whereas spontaneous mutations can result in new cases of a genetic form of mood disorder in the absence of a prominent family history of the disorder.

The implication of these complexities is not that linkage and other genetic studies of mood disorders are invalid but that the genetic component of mood disorders is probably underestimated by the current methodology. Subsequent findings in the Amish study do not mean that there is no linkage between bipolar disorder and 11p15; rather, some cases of bipolar disorder in this population probably do have a genetic contribution at this locus, whereas others do not. Some bipolar disorders probably are X-linked, some are sporadic, and some may have no genetic influence. The degree to which a pathogenic gene is expressed as a mood disorder probably depends on interactions of the gene with experience and with other genes. The earlier the onset of the mood disorder, the less adverse experience is associated with its development; and the greater the incidence of similar mood disorders in consecutive generations in the family, the more important the genetic influence is likely to be.

Imaging Findings

A variety of findings have emerged from structural and brain imaging studies of depressed patients. One of the most consistent generalized brain abnormalities in structural imaging studies of unipolar depression has been enlarged lateral ventricles, which are reported most frequently in late-onset MDD (Soares and Mann 1997). Subcortical white matter and periventricular hyperintensities have been found on magnetic resonance imaging (MRI) in older but not younger unipolar depressed patients. Regional abnormalities most consistently reported in unipolar depression have included decreased size of the caudate, putamen, and possibly the cerebellum. The basal ganglia receive input from medial temporal structures that regulate emotion, such as the amygdala and hippocampus, but there has not been any reliable evidence of abnormalities in the amygdala and hippocampus in mood disorders (Soares and Mann 1997). Reduced frontal lobe volume has been variably reported (Soares and Mann 1997).

Imaging studies in patients with bipolar mood disorders (Geller et al. 1996; Soares and Mann 1997; Woods et al. 1995) have noted enlarged third ventricles at all ages in adults (and in a small sample of children), as well as the same kinds of subcortical white matter and periventricular hyperintensities that are seen in older patients with unipolar depression. White matter hyperintensities on MRI increase with age in patients with bipolar mood disorders but not in control subjects, suggesting an interaction between age and diagnosis (Woods et al. 1995). Bipolar disorder is associated with more subcortical hyperintensities on MRI than is unipolar depression or no mood disorder (Dupont et al. 1995). Because the presence of psychotic symptoms may be correlated with enlarged lateral ventricles in depressed patients and because psychotic features are more frequent in bipolar depression than in unipolar depression, ventricular enlargement in bipolar patients at any age may be linked more closely to psychosis than to bipolarity. However, although enlarged lateral ventricles are

more common in major depression with psychotic features, white matter hyperintensities are not (Soares and Mann 1997). In contrast to unipolar depression, no consistent MRI changes in the frontal lobes have been reported in bipolar mood disorders (Soares and Mann 1997).

Subcortical white matter hyperintensities found in older patients with unipolar depression and patients with bipolar disorder at any age may be better markers of cerebrovascular disease than of the mood disorder (Soares and Mann 1997). This could explain why a greater volume of abnormal white matter in bipolar mood disorder patients is correlated with more cognitive impairment (Dupont et al. 1995). A substrate of neurological dysfunction associated with white matter hyperintensities also could account for an increased risk of delirium with ECT, extrapyramidal side effects with neuroleptic medications, chronicity, and overall poor treatment response in patients with this MRI finding (Dupont et al. 1995; Soares and Mann 1997).

Cerebral Blood Flow Findings

Functional brain imaging with positron emission tomography (PET) and single photon emission computed tomography (SPECT) measures regional cerebral blood flow, which is closely related to regional brain metabolism (Bonne et al. 1996; Gyulai et al. 1997). PET has shown reduced metabolic activity in the frontal lobes (i.e., hypofrontality) in unipolar (Buchsbaum et al. 1997) and bipolar (Gyulai et al. 1997) depression. Antidepressants were found to normalize frontal metabolic activity (Buchsbaum et al. 1997). Asymmetries in cerebral blood flow also have been found in depression, but such findings have been variable (Bonne et al. 1996).

Most, but not all, SPECT studies that used technetium 99m hexamethylpropyleneamine oxime (Tc-99m HM-PAO) have found reduced global cerebral blood flow in depressed patients compared with control subjects, with localized perfusion deficits in frontal, prefrontal, cingulate, temporal, and sometimes parietal and subcortical regions (Bonne et al. 1996). Iodine-123 (^{123}I)-labeled iodoamphetamine-SPECT in 12 rapid-cycling bipolar patients in manic, depressed, and euthymic states showed greater uptake in the right than in the left anterior temporal lobe in both the depressed and the manic phase but not during euthymia, which suggests state-dependent metabolic asymmetry in both poles of abnormal mood (Gyulai et al. 1997). Some functional imaging studies have found hyperactivity of the amygdala, hippocampus, and some temporal structures (Doris et al. 1999).

Electroencephalographic Findings

The same direction of cerebral asymmetry has been found in electroencephalographic studies of major depression, with less left frontal activation and greater right frontal activation (as measured by alpha suppression) in major depression (R.J. Davidson 1992). R.J. Davidson (1992) suggested that reduced left frontal activation is associated with a deficit in approach-related behaviors and that right frontal activation is associated with an increase in withdrawal-related behaviors. The interpretation of electroencephalographic findings is complicated by the fact that depression and anxiety may have additive effects on anterior activation and contradictory effects on parietotemporal electroencephalographic activity (Bruder et al. 1997). Bruder et al. (1997) found less left than right anterior cortical activation in depressed patients with comorbid anxiety disorders but not in depressed patients without anxiety disorders. In contrast, nonanxious depressed patients had less activation at right posterior sites than at left posterior sites. These patterns could reflect differences in mobilization of the stress response in anxious arousal compared with that in depression without anxiety. As is true of genetic studies, such findings illustrate the possibility that abnormalities are linked to specific dimensions of the mood disorder rather than to global diagnosis.

Biological Markers

Clear associations have been established between mood disorders and alterations in biological functioning measurable in the laboratory. Most biological markers are reported more frequently in severe, psychotic, and bipolar mood disorders and in inpatients, who are of course more severely ill. However, few markers have consistently distinguished between bipolar and unipolar mood disorders. Although there has been extensive theorizing on the issue, it is not certain whether well-replicated biological markers reflect a process that is the cause or a result of mood disorders.

Dexamethasone Suppression Test

The DST was initially used to study adrenocortical activity in mood disorders because hypercortisolemia has repeatedly been observed in depressed patients (S.-L. Brown et al. 1994). In the DST, 1 mg of dexamethasone (a synthetic adrenal steroid) is given in the afternoon to provide feedback inhibition of cortisol production by the adrenal cortex, and serum cortisol levels are measured one or more times the following day. Because the assay for cortisol does not read dexamethasone, the level of cortisol the day after dexamethasone administration is a measure of how readily the pituitary-adrenal-cortical axis can be suppressed. Normally, cortisol levels decrease to 5 µg/dL or less with dexamethasone suppression. Hyperactivity at any point between the hypothalamus and the adrenal cortex can be associated with failure of dexamethasone suppression, indicated by higher postdexamethasone cortisol levels (i.e., nonsuppression).

Melancholic major depression is associated with a 40%–50% rate of dexamethasone nonsuppression (S.-L. Brown et al. 1994). The frequency of nonsuppression is higher (80%–90%) in severe and psychotic unipolar depression, in major depression associated with more severe suicide attempts, in inpatients, and in those with a family history of affective disorder (Rush et al. 1997). Bipolar depression and mania have the same frequency of dexamethasone nonsuppression as melancholic unipolar depression (Rush et al. 1997). The DST has been found to be a state variable; DST results convert to normal 1–3 weeks before clinical remission and revert to nonsuppression within 1–3 weeks of clinical relapse (S.-L. Brown et al. 1994; Rao et al. 1997; Rush et al. 1997).

The proximate cause of dexamethasone nonsuppression associated with mood disorders may be hypersecretion of corticotropin-releasing factor (CRF) (S.-L. Brown et al. 1994; Gold et al. 1995), the hypothalamic hormone that stimulates the pituitary to release corticotropin, which in turn stimulates the adrenal cortex to release cortisol. Serotonergic input stimulates secretion of both CRF and corticotropin and participates in inhibition by corticosteroids of CRF and corticotropin (S.-L. Brown et al. 1994). Noradrenergic influences inhibit CRF production but can stimulate release of corticotropin (S.-L. Brown et al. 1994). A functional deficiency of norepinephrine activity and/or an excess of serotonin (5-HT) transmission could contribute to dexamethasone nonsuppression (S.-L. Brown et al. 1994; Rush et al. 1997), the former possibility being supported by a significant correlation between postdexamethasone plasma cortisol and cerebrospinal fluid (CSF) levels of the norepinephrine metabolite 3-methoxy-4-hydroxyphenylglycol (MHPG) in depressed patients in many but not all studies (S.-L. Brown et al. 1994). An entirely different mechanism is suggested by findings of considerable variability in dexamethasone serum levels between patients taking the same dose of the steroid (Devanand et al. 1991b). This observation raises the possibility that in some patients, apparent dexamethasone nonsuppression may actually reflect faster metabolism of dexamethasone, with insufficient levels to provide feedback inhibition of CRF and cortisol production.

Although it may create a window into the physiology of arousal in mood disorders, the DST has not proved useful as a diagnostic tool (Carroll 1986; Pitts 1984). Dexamethasone nonsuppression can be a response to hospitalization, acute illness, dementia, and recent weight loss. Smoking, alcohol use, and medications that accelerate dexamethasone metabolism can make it more difficult to achieve levels of dexamethasone necessary to suppress cortisol and can therefore increase the number of false-positive results in actual clinical practice. Because the 50%–60% of endogenously depressed patients with normal DST results still have a depressive illness, without a clinical evaluation it is not possible to differentiate true-positive from false-positive results. On the other hand, persistent dexamethasone nonsuppression in a patient with remitted major depression may be a marker of increased risk of relapse if treatment is stopped, and very high postdexamethasone cortisol levels (>10 μg/dL) may be a marker of psychosis in depressed patients (Dubovsky and Thomas 1992). The DST has a specificity of 87% and a sensitivity of 48% for distinguishing between melancholic and nonmelancholic depression (Rush et al. 1997), but this is not of great practical importance, given that a positive DST result does not inform treatment of depression.

Thyrotropin-Releasing Hormone Stimulation Test

There are important reasons for interest in thyroid function in mood disorders. As we mentioned earlier, thyroiditis is more common in patients with mood disorders, and hypothyroidism occurs with increased frequency in rapid-cycling bipolar disorder. Thyroid hormones play an important role in the regulation of biological cycles (Cowdry et al. 1983) as well as neurotransmitter (Cowdry et al. 1983; Extein et al. 1982) and receptor function (Bernstein 1992; Cowdry et al. 1983; Stancer and Persad 1982). Thyroid dysfunction can induce abnormal fluctuations of monoaminergic systems involved in mood regulation (Cowdry et al. 1983; Extein et al. 1982), which may occur at normal circulating thyroid hormone levels if central nervous system delivery or processing of thyroid hormones is reduced, levels of thyrotropin or thyrotropin-releasing hormone (TRH) are altered (Bauer and Whybrow 1990), or cycling of the thyroid axis is disrupted (Bauer and Whybrow 1986). TRH (protirelin), the hypothalamic hormone that stimulates release of thyrotropin by the pituitary gland, has direct effects on the central nervous system, including modulation of the actions of serotonin and dopamine, independent of stimulation of the thyroid or pituitary gland (Marangell et al. 1997).

The TRH stimulation test, an assay of the activity of the hypothalamic-pituitary-thyroid axis, involves measuring the increase in thyrotropin several times after the intravenous infusion of a standard dose (usually 500 IU) of protirelin. A TRH-induced increase in thyrotropin greater than around 30 IU/mL is considered hyperactive, indicating reduced feedback inhibition of the pituitary by thyroid hormone, which often indicates hypothyroidism or primary hyperactivity at the level of the pituitary. If thyrotropin increases by less than 5 IU/mL after TRH infusion, the TRH stimulation test result is said to be blunted, in which case feedback inhibition of the pituitary by a hyperactive thyroid gland is excessive or primary pituitary failure has occurred.

About one-third of otherwise euthyroid melancholic depressed patients have been found to have a blunted TRH stimulation test result (Rush et al. 1997). In some studies, this finding has been a state variable, reverting to normal with remission of depression (Rush et al. 1997), whereas in other studies, it has been a trait variable, remaining abnormal after mood normalizes (S.-L. Brown et al. 1994). In most studies, there is at most a modest likelihood that depressed patients with a nonsuppressed DST result will also have a blunted TRH stimulation test result (S.-L. Brown et al. 1994; Rush et al. 1997). Conversely, in one study, 74% of the patients with melancholic major depression or bipolar depression who had a blunted TRH stimulation test result also had nonsuppressed dexamethasone in the DST (Rush et al. 1997).

A blunted TRH stimulation test in melancholic depression is not associated with changes in circulating levels of thyroid hormones, and therefore it is unlikely that the test is a marker of true hyperthyroidism. However, delivery of thyroid hormone to feedback systems in the pituitary and hypothalamus may be excessive. It is also possible that TRH receptors in the pituitary are hypoactive. Chronic overstimulation of these receptors by endogenous TRH might lead to their downregulation but also would result in elevated thyroid hormone levels, so a primary defect in cellular signaling seems more likely. The input of serotonergic and noradrenergic tracts to the pituitary could permit a functional deficiency of norepinephrine activity, or an excess of serotonin transmission could contribute to a blunted TRH stimulation test result (Rush et al. 1997).

Abnormal Sleep

Abnormal sleep is one of the most common symptoms of depression, and the most frequent cause of sleep disorders in patients evaluated at sleep centers is depression (Buysse et al. 1994). Well-replicated changes in sleep architecture in MDD include decreased sleep continuity, more awakenings, decreased rapid eye movement (REM) latency (i.e., decreased length of time between the onset of sleep to the first REM cycle), increased REM density (increased number of REMs per unit of time during REM sleep), increased length of time in REM sleep, and difficulty entering and remaining in slow-wave sleep (McDermott et al. 1997; Rush et al. 1997). Some of the decreased REM latency observed in melancholic depression is primary, and some is secondary to reduced slow-wave sleep, which allows REM sleep to shift to the earlier part of the night (Kupfer 1995). Deficiencies in sleep efficiency and slow-wave sleep may explain why depressed patients sometimes feel tired even if they appear to sleep excessively.

Abnormalities of sleep architecture have been most notable in melancholic depression (Thase et al. 1997a) and in bipolar and psychotic depression, the latter being accompanied by sleep-onset REMs or a REM latency of less than 20 minutes (Dubovsky and Thomas 1992). However, reduced REM latency has not been found in SAD (Hellekson 1989). Polysomnographic sleep measures initially were thought to be trait variables but more recently have been found to persist after clinical remission (Rao et al. 1997; Rush et al. 1997). Results may be contradictory because some findings—such as decreased slow-wave sleep—are trait variables, whereas others—such as decreased sleep continuity, decreased REM latency, and increased phasic REM activity—are state variables (Buysse et al. 1997).

Any single abnormality of sleep architecture is not strongly associated with major depression (Rush et al. 1997; Thase et al. 1997a). For example, reduced REM latency has a false-positive rate of 20%–40% or more (Thase et al. 1997a). However, the triad of reduced REM latency, increased REM density, and decreased sleep efficiency reliably discriminated between patients with MDD and control subjects in a carefully controlled study (Thase et al. 1997a). Even in this study, however, 55% of the depressed outpatients had no abnormalities on any of the three measures, which makes the sleep electroencephalogram a poor diagnostic test (Thase et al. 1997a).

Attempts have been made to correlate polysomnographic findings with treatment outcome in MDD. Treatment with antidepressants delays REM onset, decreases total REM sleep, and shifts slow-wave sleep to earlier in the night (Buysse et al. 1997). When slow-wave sleep occupies a more normal position earlier in the night, patients feel more rested, whereas a shift of REM sleep to the latter part of the night and closer to the time of

awakening can cause patients to remember more of their dreams. When suppression of REM sleep by antidepressants leads to REM rebound, however, dreams may become disturbingly vivid.

As presumed markers of a "biological" influence, sleep findings such as decreased REM latency have been said to predict a poorer response to psychotherapy, although this impression was not confirmed in controlled studies (Thase et al. 1997a). On the other hand, Thase et al. (1997b) found that the triad mentioned earlier of reduced REM latency, increased REM density, and decreased sleep efficiency, but not any single measure, predicted a poorer response to IPT and CBT for major depression. It also has been reported that failure of slow-wave sleep to increase or at least shift to earlier in the night in response to any kind of treatment predicts a higher risk of relapse or recurrence (Buysse et al. 1997).

Hypotheses about mechanisms of the complex changes in sleep architecture in major depression are incomplete. In cases of early-morning awakening and decreased REM latency, there appears to be a phase advance of the sleep–wake cycle, which is driven by the "weak oscillator" that also drives activity–rest cycles, and of the REM sleep cycle, which is dependent on the "strong oscillator" that also controls body temperature. Because muscarinic cholinergic systems increase REM sleep (Poland et al. 1997), cholinergic excess could be one cause of increased REM density and increased time in REM sleep (Rush et al. 1997). However, decreased REM latency also could be a function of noradrenergic deficiency (Poland et al. 1997). Changes in REM sleep may be secondary to a disturbance of non-REM sleep, which is regulated by corticothalamic circuits (Buysse et al. 1997).

Clinical Uses of Biological Tests

Laboratory tests are useful for examining the pathophysiology of mood disorders, but the large numbers of false-positive and false-negative results make them relatively ineffective for diagnosing mood disorders. In addition, no laboratory test can outperform the gold-standard clinical interview to which it is referenced (Somoza and Mossman 1990), and no studies exist in which diagnosis was prospectively predicted by laboratory test alone. A single laboratory test such as the DST can occasionally be used to predict the risk of a relapse if an antidepressant is withdrawn or to increase the index of suspicion of psychosis in refractory depression. However, studies of correlations between multiple tests may create a better window into the complex phenomenology of mood disorders.

The DST, the TRH stimulation test, and sleep electroencephalography can distinguish between melancholic and nonmelancholic major depression but not between bipolar and unipolar depression (Rush et al. 1997). For identifying melancholic depression, a blunted TRH stimulation test result has the greatest specificity and the least sensitivity, whereas shortened REM latency has the greatest sensitivity and the least specificity (Rush et al. 1997). The sensitivity and specificity of any of these tests can be adjusted by altering the cutoff point for a positive test result. For example, using a postdexamethasone cortisol level of 10 μg/dL as a positive result will increase the number of true-positive results as well as the number of false-negative results. However, at least one-fourth of the patients with endogenous major depression show no abnormality on any of the three tests (Rush et al. 1997).

Ultimately, biological tests may prove most useful in identifying specific dimensions of mood disorders that may indicate specific treatments or combinations of them. For example, inhibitors of the hypothalamic-pituitary-adrenal axis might be useful for patients with refractory depression and excessive release of CRF, whereas manipulations of the sleep–wake cycle might be effective for patients with prominent disruptions of the relation between slow-wave and REM sleep. If depressed patients with anxiety were found to have a different pattern of arousal than nonanxious depressed patients, then treatments aimed at arousal mechanisms might be specifically helpful.

Etiology: Biological Factors and Theories

Theories linking disordered physiology to disordered mood go back to at least the fourth century B.C., when Hippocrates hypothesized that mood depends on a balance among the four bodily humors—blood, phlegm, yellow bile, and black bile, found in the heart, brain, liver, and spleen, respectively (Whybrow et al. 1984). Hippocrates proposed that depression was caused by an excess of black bile in the spleen (Leonard 1994). Because the spleen occupied a position in the body analogous to the position of Saturn in the heavens, it was believed that those born under the sign of Saturn were prone to depression. These ideas are the basis of references to an attitude of depressive hostility as *spleen* and to morose people as *saturnine*.

The conviction that there must be some inherent biodynamic alteration in mood disorders has continued to be held over the years (Whybrow et al. 1984). Herman

Boerhaave, a prominent Leiden physician of the eighteenth century, argued that depression was caused by "nervous and melancholy juice." Psychologist William James argued that changes in mood must be accompanied by some form of "chemical action." In his "Project for a Scientific Psychology," Sigmund Freud (1950[1895]/1966) proposed a complex pathophysiological theory based on a hydraulic model of neuronal functioning, which he later abandoned. Modern technology has made it possible to study the "humors" and "melancholy juices" of the twentieth century—biological rhythms, neuroanatomy, neurotransmitters, receptors, and intracellular messengers. However, we will see that, as van Praag (1990) pointed out, "though a lot of biology has been uncovered in mental disorders, most of it seems to be devoid of nosological specificity" (p. 2).

Biological Rhythms

Depressed mood often has a diurnal variation, and episodes may follow a monthly or seasonal pattern of recurrence (S.-L. Brown et al. 1994). Some mood disorders, such as SAD and rapid-cycling bipolar disorder, are defined by their periodicity. Phase advances (i.e., peaking earlier in the day) have been noted in sleep onset, REM sleep, temperature, and hormonal and neurotransmitter rhythms, including those of concentrations of cortisol, serotonin, dopamine, and norepinephrine (S.-L. Brown et al. 1994).

This kind of cyclicity has led to hypotheses of chronobiological causes of mood disorders (S.-L. Brown et al. 1994; Goodwin et al. 1982; Teicher et al. 1997). One such hypothesis is that abnormalities of mood in MDD are related to a phase advance or at least desynchronization of the strong oscillator (which controls rhythms of body temperature, REM sleep, plasma cortisol, and melatonin) with respect to the weak oscillator (which controls the sleep–wake and activity–rest cycles). Loss of predictability of circadian rhythms—with reduced amplitude of rhythms of body temperature, norepinephrine, cortisol, and melatonin—could suggest impaired entrainment of these rhythms. Antidepressants restore normal organization of circadian rhythms and resynchronize the two oscillators, but it is not clear whether this is a therapeutic mechanism or one of a number of markers of overall improvement of psychobiology.

Neuroanatomical Factors

Injury to left frontal anterior cortical or subcortical areas causes secondary depression (Bonne et al. 1996; Soares and Mann 1997), whereas right-sided lesions in the limbic system, temporobasal areas, basal ganglia, and thalamus induce secondary mania (Robinson et al. 1988; Soares and Mann 1997). It is possible that subtle alterations in the structure or function of brain areas that participate in mood regulation could contribute to primary mood disorders. Relevant areas of the brain for this kind of formulation include the prefrontal cortex; subcortical structures such as the basal ganglia, thalamus, and hypothalamus; the brain stem; and white matter pathways connecting these structures to one another and the cerebral cortex (e.g., the limbic-thalamic-cortical circuit and the limbic-striatal-pallidal-thalamic-cortical circuit), and possibly the cerebellum (Soares and Mann 1997). Abnormalities in these areas that could contribute to affective symptoms might be caused by abnormal brain development, vascular injury, aging, or degenerative disease (Soares and Mann 1997).

One finding that suggests a degenerative process in some of these areas is the global brain atrophy that occurs in older patients with unipolar depression and patients with bipolar disorder at all ages. Although some argue that enlarged ventricles and sulci are found more frequently (Elkis et al. 1995) and that the severity of structural brain changes is greater (Soares and Mann 1997) in mood disorders than in schizophrenia, others point out that such findings are found in many different psychiatric and medical illnesses, especially mood disorders, schizophrenia, and Alzheimer's disease (Soares and Mann 1997). The most cogent explanation for apparent structural abnormalities in primary mood disorders is that they identify neuroanatomical substrates that can cause secondary mood disorders in older patients and that contribute to dementia syndromes in interaction with a primary mood disorder. In primary mood disorders, neurological factors may lead to treatment resistance and greater cognitive impairment, but no evidence shows that they are etiological in most cases.

Biogenic Amines

Biologically active (biogenic) amines such as norepinephrine, serotonin, dopamine, and acetylcholine (ACh) are neurotransmitters in brain systems that originate in the brain stem. These systems modulate background activity of multiple neuronal circuits, and abnormal function of biogenic amines has been proposed in mood disorders (Salomon et al. 1997). The monoamine hypothesis, which was first proposed in 1965, holds that monoamines such as norepinephrine and serotonin are deficient in depression and that the therapeutic action of antidepressants depends on increasing synaptic availability of these monoamines (Schildkraut 1965). The monoamine

hypothesis was based on observations that antidepressants block reuptake inhibition of norepinephrine, serotonin, and/or dopamine. However, inferring neurotransmitter pathophysiology from an observed action of a class of medications on neurotransmitter availability is similar to concluding that because aspirin causes gastrointestinal bleeding, headaches are caused by too much blood and the therapeutic action of aspirin in headaches is to cause blood loss.

Additional experience has not confirmed the monoamine depletion hypothesis (S.-L. Brown et al. 1994; Salomon et al. 1997). Monoamine precursors such as tyrosine or tryptophan by themselves do not improve mood. Depletion of serotonin can aggravate depression that has been in remission, but it does not predictably cause depression, and when it does cause depression, the depression is not sustained. Some substances that are monoamine reuptake inhibitors, such as amphetamines and cocaine, do not have reliable antidepressant properties, and antidepressant medications exist (e.g., iprindole, mianserin, mirtazapine, ketanserin) that have no effect on monoamine reuptake. In the case of monoamine reuptake inhibitors that are antidepressants, reuptake inhibition is immediate, whereas the onset of antidepressant effect is delayed a month or more.

Neurotransmitter reuptake inhibition may not predict antidepressants' therapeutic effects, but it does predict side effects (S.-L. Brown et al. 1990, 1994). Norepinephrine is a neurotransmitter in arousal centers such as the locus coeruleus and in the sympathetic nervous system. Medications that increase noradrenergic activity can produce anxiety, tremor, tachycardia, diaphoresis, insomnia, and related symptoms of arousal. Because serotonin influences gastrointestinal motility, cerebral vasomotor tone, appetitive functions, and arousal, serotonin reuptake inhibitors can produce nausea, diarrhea, headaches, appetite loss, sexual dysfunction, sedation, and jitteriness. Dopamine is a neurotransmitter of activation, movement, reward, and blood vessel tone, and dopamine reuptake inhibitors tend to be activating and may elevate blood pressure.

Norepinephrine

Both relative deficiencies and excesses of central noradrenergic activity have been postulated to exist in depression (S.-L. Brown et al. 1994). An early hypothesis was that decreased activity and motivation in depression was related to reduced noradrenergic tone and that hyperactivity in mania was related to noradrenergic excess (Schildkraut 1965). However, reports of increased norepinephrine activity in depression have been more frequent than reports of reduced activity (S.-L. Brown et al. 1994). This is consistent with evidence of high levels of arousal such as the nonsuppressed DST or phase advance of circadian rhythms, which are present even in behaviorally slowed depressed patients.

Unmedicated depressed patients do not show consistent changes in α_1-adrenergic receptor numbers (S.-L. Brown et al. 1994). However, downregulation and hyposensitivity of β and possibly α_2-adrenergic receptors have been reported (S.-L. Brown et al. 1994). In animal studies, chronic antidepressant treatment decreases the number of α_2- and β-adrenergic receptors and increases the density of α_1-adrenergic receptors (S.-L. Brown et al. 1994; Leonard 1994). The first change would increase norepinephrine release, whereas the second would be expected to reduce adrenergic transmission through postsynaptic receptors. However, although some antidepressants downregulate β-adrenergic receptors, ECT upregulates these receptors, and mianserin, an antidepressant in use in Europe, does not affect β-adrenergic receptor density at all (Leonard 1994). Reported actions on other adrenergic receptor subtypes may not be relevant to the therapeutic effect of antidepressants (S.-L. Brown et al. 1994).

Drawing on studies of responsiveness of noradrenergic measures such as plasma MHPG, a norepinephrine metabolite, to mild stresses, Siever and Davis (1985) suggested that depression is associated not with consistently elevated or reduced norepinephrine activity but with uneven responsiveness to stresses that activate noradrenergic stress response systems. Like the heat produced by a furnace that is controlled by a poorly regulated thermostat, baseline noradrenergic activity is excessive, but acute stresses that call for mobilization of the stress response result in inadequate mobilization of additional noradrenergic transmission. The behavioral and affective correlates of this situation would be high levels of baseline anxiety with a sense of "spinning one's wheels" with inability to mount an organized response to important challenges.

Serotonin

Neurons using serotonin, which is phylogenetically the oldest neurotransmitter, originate in raphe (midline) nuclei in the brain stem and project throughout the brain. These connections and interactions make it possible for serotonin to interact with other biogenic amines and to contribute to the regulation of many core psychobiological functions that are disrupted in mood disorders, including mood, anxiety, arousal, vigilance, irritability, thinking, cognition, appetites, aggression, circadian and seasonal rhythms, nociception, and neuroendocrine functions (Coccaro 1989; Grahame-Smith 1992; Leonard 1992; Montgomery and Fineberg 1989; Murphy et al. 1989). Serotonin may serve as a "neurochemical brake" on certain innate behaviors that are normally suppressed, such as aggression, including aggression turned against the self (Benkelfat 1993). Therefore, it is not surprising that serotonergic dysfunction has been implicated in mood disorders and that medications that act on serotonin are useful in the treatment of mood disorders.

Serotonin mediates its diverse actions through multiple receptors with different second messenger signaling mechanisms. At least 15 distinct serotonin receptor subtypes have been identified, many with further functional subtypes (e.g., 5-HT$_{1A}$, 5-HT$_{1D}$) (Dubovsky and Thomas 1995; Kroeze and Roth 1998). More is known about some of these receptors than others (Charney et al. 1990; Dubovsky 1994a; Dubovsky and Thomas 1995). For example, 5-HT$_1$ receptors use cyclic adenosine monophosphate (cAMP) and mediate functions such as body temperature, anxiety, and nociception. Subtypes of the 5-HT$_2$ receptor, which signal via the phosphatidylinositol system (described in the "Second Messengers" subsection later in this chapter), mediate psychosis, mood, sleep, vasomotor tone, and platelet aggregation; 5-HT$_2$ heteroreceptors on postsynaptic dopamine D$_2$ receptors influence activity of postsynaptic D$_2$ receptors. The 5-HT$_3$ receptor is linked directly to an ion channel and influences anxiety, psychosis, and nausea; a 5-HT$_3$ heteroreceptor on limbic dopaminergic neurons helps to mediate substance reward. Because the functions of most other receptors, as well as the action of medications on these receptors, have not been well studied in psychiatry, not all of the roles they play in mood disorders are known.

Several studies have found lower concentrations of 5-hydroxyindoleacetic acid (5-HIAA, the major serotonin metabolite) in the CSF of depressed patients than in the CSF of control subjects (S.-L. Brown et al. 1994). The finding of reduced platelet serotonin uptake in unmedicated major depression (S.-L. Brown et al. 1994; Leonard 1994) could represent hypofunction of a cellular serotonin transporter. If a similar malfunction existed in the brain, it could result in reduced serotonin stores, or reduction of serotonin uptake could be a means of compensating for increased serotonin availability. Decreased binding of [3H]-imipramine, a marker of the serotonin uptake site, has been inconsistently found in platelets of unmedicated depressed patients (S.-L. Brown et al. 1994). Additionally, no change in platelet binding of [3H]-paroxetine, which may be a better marker of the serotonin uptake site, has been found in major depression

(S.-L. Brown et al. 1994). Many platelet serotonin findings may be confounded by seasonal and circadian variations in platelet serotonin uptake (S.-L. Brown et al. 1994). Reduced [^{3}H]-imipramine binding has been found in the brains of depressed patients who died of suicide and of natural causes, but this finding has been inconsistent (S.-L. Brown et al. 1994). A more reliable finding has been increased numbers of platelet 5-HT$_2$ receptor sites, consistent with a reduction in systemic serotonergic activity (McBride et al. 1994). Conversely, with the polymerase chain reaction technique, no association was found between polymorphisms of the 5-HT$_{1A}$ and 5-HT$_{2C}$ receptor genes and depression, mania, delusions, or disorganization in patients with unipolar and bipolar mood disorders (Serretti et al. 2000).

Reduction of central serotonin and its metabolites may not be a marker of depression so much as features that commonly accompany depression. Of seven studies, five reported modestly reduced brain-stem serotonin and 5-HIAA in persons who committed suicide, regardless of diagnosis (Mann et al. 1989). In 10 of 15 studies of CSF 5-HIAA, levels were lower in depressed patients who made a suicide attempt than in those who did not attempt suicide (Mann et al. 1989). Increased binding of labeled markers to 5-HT$_2$ and 5-HT$_{1A}$ receptors in the frontal cortex of individuals who committed suicide suggests that these receptors were upregulated to compensate for decreased synaptic availability of serotonin in suicide (Buchsbaum et al. 1997). A study of 22 drug-free depressed inpatients with a history of a suicide attempt found that current depressive episodes in patients whose past attempts caused more medical damage and were better planned were associated with lower CSF 5-HIAA (but no changes in other neurotransmitter metabolites) than were depressive episodes in patients who had made less lethal and less well planned suicide attempts, which suggests that reduced 5-HIAA may be a marker of seriousness of suicidal ideation (Mann and Malone 1997). In a study of 237 patients with mood disorders and 187 control subjects, a variant of the serotonin transporter gene was associated with violent but not other kinds of suicide attempts (Bellivier et al. 2000).

Reduced central serotonin activity was originally thought to be specific for depression (Meltzer and Lowry 1987) and then for suicidal depression, but this finding appears to be correlated with violent and/or impulsive unpremeditated suicidal behavior, whether the descriptive diagnosis is depression, schizophrenia, behavior disorder, or personality disorder (Lopez-Ibor 1988; Mann et al. 1989; McBride et al. 1994; van Praag et al. 1987). Reduced serotonergic tone is not even restricted to suicidality per se but is also associated with loss of control over many forms of impulsivity and/or aggression, regardless of whether they are directed inward or outward (Coccaro 1989; Linnoila and Virkkunen 1992; Mann et al. 1989; Siever and Trestman 1993).

One strategy to assess serotonergic function indirectly in mood disorders involves depletion of tryptophan, the amino acid precursor of serotonin. Some studies have shown that tryptophan-depleting diets produce acute but brief relapses of depression in patients with remitted depression but no effect in healthy subjects (Salomon et al. 1997). Another indirect approach uses neuroendocrine probes of the serotonin system. For example, the serotonin precursors L-tryptophan and 5-hydroxytryptophan and the serotonin releaser and reuptake inhibitor fenfluramine release hormones under serotonergic control such as cortisol, growth hormone, and prolactin (S.-L. Brown et al. 1994). Findings of blunted release of prolactin in response to tryptophan and fenfluramine in some patients with major depression have been interpreted as indicating primary subsensitivity of postsynaptic serotonin receptors located on prolactin-releasing cells (S.-L. Brown et al. 1994). However, these kinds of neuroendocrine challenges are not selective for serotonergic systems, and variations in methodology limit generalizability of the findings. Studies of prolactin response to serotonergic provocation suggest postsynaptic serotonin receptor subsensitivity in major depression, but cortisol release studies suggest the opposite (S.-L. Brown et al. 1994).

Considered together, studies of serotonin in major depression suggest both hypofunction and hyperfunction (S.-L. Brown et al. 1994; Leonard 1994). Findings such as decreased serotonin and 5-HIAA levels in postmortem brain and CSF studies, brief relapse of depression with diets that deplete serotonin precursors, decreased postsynaptic serotonin receptor sensitivity in depression, and the existence of antidepressant properties of some medications that enhance serotonergic transmission suggest underactivity of serotonin systems. Conversely, decreased platelet serotonin uptake in depression, increased 5-HT$_2$ receptor binding in the frontal cortex of individuals who committed suicide, and reduction of postsynaptic 5-HT$_2$ binding and CSF 5-HIAA by chronic antidepressant treatment suggest increased serotonergic transmission in major depression.

One reason for this uncertainty is that neurobiological and pharmacological studies generally emphasize isolated aspects of serotonin function, although in the intact organism, the activity of this neurotransmitter cannot be separated from the action of other transmitters. For example, serotonin is a cotransmitter with γ-aminobutyric acid (GABA) (Kahn et al. 1990) and norepinephrine

(Jaim-Etcheverry and Zieher 1982). Serotonergic and noradrenergic neurons can take up each other's transmitter, altering the functioning of the parent neuron (Jaim-Etcheverry and Zieher 1982). Serotonergic raphe neurons inhibit noradrenergic neurons in the locus coeruleus (Kahn et al. 1990) and regulate β-adrenergic receptor number and function (Charney et al. 1990). Conversely, agonists of α- and β-adrenergic receptors and GABA$_B$ receptors alter the function of several serotonin receptors (Grahame-Smith 1992).

Many other serotonin interactions have been identified. Raphe serotonergic neurons synapse with nigrostriatal and mesolimbic dopaminergic neurons (Bleich et al. 1990), and dopaminergic neurons have serotonin receptors that permit tonic control of dopamine release in the midbrain, striatum, and nucleus accumbens (Meltzer 1992). Depending on the circumstances, serotonin may facilitate dopamine release in the nucleus accumbens and inhibit dopaminergic activity in the striatum (Meltzer 1992). Serotonergic neurons have glucocorticoid receptors that alter gene transcription, perhaps providing a feedback loop between the stress response and resetting of serotonin function (Leonard 1994).

In evaluating the effect of new serotonergic medications, it is important to bear in mind that there is usually no information about the functional subtypes of the disorders in which they are studied. For example, the SSRIs are not so much specific treatments for MDD as they are for any syndrome of depressed mood, self-destructive behavior, circadian rhythm disturbance, or appetitive dysfunction. Similarly, drugs that antagonize the 5-HT$_2$ receptor, such as clozapine, may have applications in a variety of disorders characterized by dysregulated thought and mood. Until validated rating scales for serotonergic functions are used along with measurements of categorical diagnosis in treatment outcome studies, the precise spectrum of action of serotonergic medications will not be fully explored.

Dopamine

Some investigations have found that CSF concentrations of the dopamine metabolite homovanillic acid (HVA) are lower in patients with major depression than in control subjects and that lower CSF HVA levels are found in more severely depressed patients, but results have not been consistent (S.-L. Brown et al. 1994). The dopamine reuptake inhibitors nomifensine (no longer available), amineptine (available in Europe), and bupropion are antidepressants. Dopaminergic agonists such as bromocriptine and piribedil and the dopamine-releasing stimulants methylphenidate and dextroamphetamine have antide-

pressant properties that make them useful adjuncts in the treatment of depression (S.-L. Brown et al. 1994).

As is true of serotonin, any apparent dopaminergic hypofunction may have a greater effect on dimensions of mood disorders than on specific diagnoses. Because mobilization of goal-directed behavior is mediated by dopamine, underactivity of dopaminergic systems may be related to decreased drive and motivation in depression (S.-L. Brown et al. 1994). Unresponsive dopaminergic systems could be one reason that experience is unrewarding to depressed patients. Hyperactivity of dopaminergic motivational and action systems could be related to manic or psychotic symptoms in mood disorders.

GABA

GABA is the major inhibitory neurotransmitter in the central nervous system. Inadequate GABAergic input to noradrenergic arousal systems could lead to the kind of unrestrained arousal that characterizes mood disorders. Decreased CSF GABA levels have been reported in major depression (Leonard 1994), and some antidepressants increase the number of GABA$_B$ receptor sites in rat brain (Leonard 1994). Benzodiazepines, which increase the affinity of GABA$_B$ receptors for endogenous GABA, usually are thought to aggravate depression, but this class of medications can reduce depressive symptoms in patients who are anxious and depressed. Gabapentin, an anticonvulsant with unclear GABAergic actions, has both anxiolytic and antidepressant actions. Reduction of depression could be secondary to decreased anxiety in these situations. Because GABA$_B$ receptors may act as heteroreceptors on serotonergic terminals in limbic regions (Leonard 1994), in addition to moderating noradrenergic output, any pathophysiological contribution of GABA and any therapeutic effect of GABAergic medications in mood disorders may ultimately be mediated by other neurotransmitter systems.

Acetylcholine

It has been hypothesized that cholinergic transmission, relative to noradrenergic transmission, is excessive in depression and inadequate in mania. Because ACh is a neurotransmitter in structures that mediate withdrawal and punishment such as the periventricular system, cholinergic hyperactivity could increase withdrawal behavior and contribute to depression (Poland et al. 1997). In support of this hypothesis are the findings that cholinergic input reduces REM latency (decreased REM latency is seen in depression); some antidepressants have anticholinergic properties; lecithin, an ACh precursor, and cholinesterase inhibitors such as physostigmine and done-pezil, reduce mania in some patients and sometimes replace mania with depression; and cholinergic rebound following abrupt withdrawal of anticholinergic medications can cause a relapse of depression (Dilsaver and Coffman 1989; Janowsky and Risch 1984; Keshavan 1985). Lithium was thought to induce upregulation of cholinergic receptors, but this finding has been contested (Lerer and Stanley 1985). In contrast to earlier suggestions of the existence of muscarinic receptor supersensitivity in depression, no change in muscarinic receptor number was found in the brains of persons who committed suicide (Kaufmann 1984). Additional objections raised against the cholinergic hypothesis include observations that not all anticholinergic medications are antidepressants; that none of the newer antidepressants is anticholinergic; and that muscarinic receptors were initially considered in testing the hypothesis, although most agents used to test the hypothesis act on nicotinic receptors (Dilsaver and Coffman 1989).

Substance P

Speculations have arisen that substance P could mediate the psychological pain of depression as well as physical pain. Some trials of antagonists of substance P receptors have suggested an antidepressant action, but this finding has not been confirmed, and additional studies are now under way.

Interactions of Neurotransmitter Systems

Early attempts to understand the role of neurotransmitters and their receptors involved the hypothesis that some depressions were characterized by functional norepinephrine deficiency, whereas others were associated with serotonin hypofunction. According to this hypothesis, low norepinephrine depression would respond preferentially to noradrenergic antidepressants, and low serotonin depressions would respond better to treatments that enhance serotonin availability. This prediction was never confirmed, and no evidence of differing "serotonergic" and "noradrenergic" depressive subtypes has emerged (S.-L. Brown et al. 1994). The hypothesis was then revised (termed the *permissive amine hypothesis*) to include the concept that serotonergic deficiency contributed to most cases of depression, some of which had additional noradrenergic dysfunction and others of which did not. This hypothesis would predict that treatments that enhance serotonergic transmission are antidepressants. However, tianeptine—an effective TCA available

in France—enhances serotonin reuptake, reducing available synaptic serotonin (Wilde and Benfield 1995).

These kinds of observations underscore the overlap of dimensional features of depression driven by dysfunction of one or more serotonin systems in interaction with other neurotransmitter systems (S.-L. Brown et al. 1990, 1994; Lopez-Ibor 1988; O'Keane et al. 1992). When arousal associated with noradrenergic excess is sufficient to overwhelm regulation of aggression and impulsivity that has been impaired by suboptimally active serotonin systems, suicide, various forms of outwardly directed aggression, or generalized impulsivity may be the predominant problem, whether the primary diagnosis is a mood disorder, an anxiety disorder, schizophrenia, or a personality disorder. Inadequate function of serotonergic systems that regulate intrusive thought may interact with disturbances of mood to produce ruminative depressive states or racing thoughts that remain stuck on a particular idea. If the interaction is with the consequences of traumatic experiences, the intrusive recall of posttraumatic stress disorder may develop if serotonergic systems that regulate recurrent thoughts and arousal do not function normally. Dysregulation of thought processes is a feature of schizophrenia, and when this interacts with the psychobiology of mood, the same malfunction may figure in psychotic depression, bipolar illness, and schizoaffective disorder.

Traditional single neurotransmitter hypotheses ignore evidence of dysfunction of other neurotransmitters in mood disorders. In addition, none of these hypotheses is readily applicable to bipolar mood disorders. If mania is associated primarily with neurotransmitter changes (e.g., increased norepinephrine and dopaminergic activity) that are the opposites of changes in depression, for example, why are almost 50% of manic patients depressed at the same time they are manic (i.e., mixed mania)? And how could the direction of neurotransmitter activity change so abruptly and rapidly if such activity were driving ultradian cycling?

It is impossible to understand reported neurotransmitter changes in mood disorders without appreciating that all neurotransmitters and receptors that have been studied interact with and influence one another (S.-L. Brown et al. 1994; Leonard 1994). Cotransmission using more than one neurotransmitter in the same neuron is the rule (Jaim-Etcheverry and Zieher 1982; McCormick and Williamson 1989). Most cerebral functions are the result of the converging action of many different neurotransmitters. For example, excitability in the human cortex is regulated by ACh, GABA, norepinephrine, histamine, and purines, in addition to serotonin (McCormick and Williamson 1989). Each of these transmitters may produce more than one postsynaptic signal in the same neuron by activating interacting receptors, and more than one transmitter may induce the same change in postsynaptic neurons. This kind of overlap provides a mechanism for fine-tuning of complex adaptations to multiple kinds of input (McCormick and Williamson 1989).

Such interactions make it unlikely that the pathophysiology of mood disorders can be linked to any single neurotransmitter (S.-L. Brown et al. 1994). Instead, different aspects of the psychobiological malfunctions in mood disorders may be related to different kinds of neurotransmitter dysfunctions (S.-L. Brown et al. 1994; Leonard 1994). For example, disordered noradrenergic function may be related to anhedonia, anxiety, and excessive arousal, whereas loss of dopaminergic function could lead to deficits in mobilizing goal-directed behaviors and emotional incentives. Loss of serotonergic regulation of aggression would be best correlated with violent, dangerous, and/or impulsive suicidal behavior; anxiety; rumination; and appetitive dysfunction, and excessive cholinergic tone could lead to withdrawal and an experience of events as punitive. It is likely that other neurotransmitters and neuromodulators such as neuropeptides and prostaglandins are also dysregulated, contributing to increased intensity of dysphoric affect (S.-L. Brown et al. 1994; Leonard 1994).

Rather than being related to any particular neurotransmitter disturbance, mood disorders may be disorders of the overall cohesiveness of multiple transmitter systems involved in responding to danger. Antidepressant therapies do not affect one of these systems but produce adaptational changes in multiple neurotransmitter systems (Leonard 1994). Greater coordination between affective, cognitive, and behavioral systems associated with these transmitters may be associated with normalization of mental state (S.-L. Brown et al. 1994).

Second Messengers

Simultaneous loss of regulation of multiple neurotransmitter systems, or multiple downstream effects of loss of regulation of a single neurotransmitter system, do not on the surface explain the complex pathophysiology of mood disorders, especially if one must postulate opposing neurotransmitter changes at the same time in patients with mixed bipolar syndromes. Given that there are many neurotransmitters and neuromodulators and many more receptors, an alternative hypothesis is that one or more of the few second messengers that mediate diverse neurotransmitter and receptor actions are poorly regulated. The bidirectional actions of second messengers allow unitary changes in second messenger function to produce diverse changes in transmitter synthesis and

release and in receptor activity, leading to complex neurotransmitter and receptor effects.

Three primary second messenger families (Dubovsky et al. 1992b) have been well studied. cAMP acts as an intracellular messenger by activating protein kinase A, which phosphorylates proteins. The phosphatidylinositol system is a self-recycling cascade of membrane phospholipids in which phosphatidylinositol 4,5-bisphosphate is hydrolyzed to inositol 1,4,5-trisphosphate (IP_3) and diacylglycerol (DG) by phospholipase C (PLC). IP_3 releases calcium ions (Ca^{2+}) from intracellular stores and contributes to the influx of Ca^{2+} from the extracellular space, whereas DG activates a ubiquitous intracellular enzyme called protein kinase C (PKC). In the presence of Ca^{2+}, PKC phosphorylates many enzymes involved in processes implicated in mood disorders. In addition, entry of positively charged calcium ions produces the plateau phase of the action potential. Different receptors may use different second messengers. For example, the α_1-adrenergic receptor primarily uses cAMP signaling, and the dopamine D_2 receptor and 5-HT_2 receptor increase phosphatidylinositol turnover, resulting in an increase in free intracellular Ca^{2+} concentration ($[Ca^{2+}]_i$). The 5-HT_3 and $GABA_A$ receptors are linked directly to ion channels that alter neuronal excitability.

Many second messenger effector systems are linked to their receptors through a guanyl-nucleotide-binding protein (G protein). Receptor occupation leads to hydrolysis of the G protein, which produces the sequence of events that mobilizes second messengers. A single receptor may be associated with more than one G protein, permitting a neurotransmitter to activate more than one second messenger. The same G protein may be associated with more than one receptor, enabling the G protein to integrate signals from different transmitters.

The phosphatidylinositol/Ca^{2+} second messenger system has been of interest to investigators of bipolar mood disorders because of the biphasic action of the intracellular calcium ion (Dubovsky et al. 1992b). $[Ca^{2+}]_i$ is normally regulated very tightly at around 100 nM, or 1/10,000th the Ca^{2+} concentration, in the extracellular fluid. Modest elevations of $[Ca^{2+}]_i$ accelerate many intracellular actions, whereas greater elevations can inhibit the same actions. In addition, the same $[Ca^{2+}]_i$ elevation can inhibit a function in one system and activate another function in some other location. Excessive signaling by this messenger, inhibiting some neuronal processes and activating others at the same time, could explain two aspects of bipolar mood disorders that have been difficult to understand—namely, mixtures of manic and depressive symptoms in the same patient and rapid alternations between mania and depression in rapid-cycling bipolar disorder.

In several studies, $[Ca^{2+}]_i$ was elevated in blood platelets (Dubovsky et al. 1989, 1991a, 1991b, 1992a; Tan et al. 1990) and lymphocytes (Dubovsky et al. 1992a) of affectively ill manic and bipolar depressed patients but not in platelets of unipolar depressed patients, control subjects, or bipolar patients who were euthymic after treatment with various medications or ECT. Serotonin-induced Ca^{2+} mobilization in platelets also was increased in mania (Okamoto et al. 1995). In vitro incubation with lithium (Dubovsky et al. 1991b; Tan et al. 1990) and carbamazepine (Dubovsky et al. 1994; Walden et al. 1992) lowers platelet $[Ca^{2+}]_i$ markedly in ill bipolar patients but not in control subjects or euthymic bipolar patients. Carbamazepine, lithium, and lamotrigine have calcium antagonist properties (Dubovsky 1995a; Walden et al. 1992), and lithium reduces hyperactive phosphatidylinositol turnover, in part by inhibiting a key but not rate-limiting enzyme called *inositol 1-monophosphatase* (E. Friedman et al. 1993; Jope and Williams 1994). Calcium channel blockers such as verapamil and nimodipine have antimanic properties (Dubovsky 1995a).

Excessive intracellular calcium signaling could be caused by increased mobilization of stored intracellular Ca^{2+} (which could result from increased IP_3 production) and/or by increased influx of calcium. Any of these processes could be caused by increased G protein activity. Hyperactivity of G proteins and of G protein–linked PLC has been found in mononuclear leukocytes and platelets of patients with bipolar disorder and in postmortem brain samples of bipolar patients who had died from various causes (Avissar and Schreiber 1992b; E. Friedman et al. 1993; Jope and Williams 1994; Mathews et al. 1997). The additional observations that β, muscarinic, and dopaminergic receptor-coupled G protein activity is reversibly increased in mania (Schreiber and Avissar 2000) and that lithium blunts the G protein response to stimulation in animal studies (Avissar and Schreiber 1992a) suggest that increased Ca^{2+} signaling may be the effector arm of a cascade of intracellular events that begins with G protein hyperactivity and that is corrected with antimanic drugs. Antidepressants may have actions on G proteins and other aspects of the second messenger cascade (Avissar and Schreiber 1992b; Leonard 1994), and ECT was found to normalize reduced stimulatory and inhibitory G protein activity in mononuclear leukocytes of patients with unipolar depression (Avissar et al. 1998).

Other Changes in Intracellular Functioning

A growing understanding of the importance of intracellular mechanisms is stimulating research into additional basic actions of the neuron. One finding is that antidepressants in various classes upregulate expression of messenger RNA of the neuroprotective enzyme superoxide dismutase, indicating that these medications can regulate genetic expression (Li et al. 2000). Studies in animals and in human neuronal tissue suggest that antimanic drugs with structures as diverse as valproate and lithium inhibit PKC in addition to altering genetic expression (Manji et al. 1999). The latter actions include increasing activity of the AP-1 family of transcription factors and of a reporter gene driven by an AP-1 promotor, resulting in increases in expression of proteins regulated by these genes. Additional genes that may be abnormally expressed in mood disorders include the c-*fos* tumor promotor gene and genes for nerve growth factor 1A, glucocorticoid receptors, brain-derived neurotrophic factor, preproenkephalin, and *N*-methyl-D-aspartate receptor subunits (Post 1992b; Shelton 2000).

Etiology: Psychological Factors and Theories

Mood disorders are psychological as well as physiological conditions. As with biological data, there is less disagreement about whether specific psychological dimensions of mood disorders exist than about whether they are etiological. And as is true of biological factors, proving that a particular psychological factor is causal would require prospectively following up people at risk for depression to determine whether those with the factor are more likely to develop a mood disorder. A finding that patients who already have had an affective episode and who have the factor in question are more likely to have a recurrence could simply imply that the factor is a residual symptom of the index episode and not an independent risk factor. Even if expensive and difficult prospective studies of psychological risk factors were conducted, a positive finding would not guarantee that any factors identified were not markers of an underlying biological factor.

Because none of the psychological theories of mania (e.g., that it is a defense against depression) has ever been tested empirically, we focus on psychological hypotheses of depression.

Abnormal Reactions to Loss

Loss is the life event that has been most reliably linked to depression. Sigmund Freud (1917[1915]/1957) pointed out that both grief and depression are reactions to loss, but depressive symptoms include guilt and low self-esteem. On the basis of psychoanalytic experience with depressed patients, Freud believed that grieving turned into depression when the bereaved felt ambivalent about the lost object (i.e., person) and could not tolerate the negative side of the ambivalence. An unconscious attack against an internalized image of the lost object that undermines self-esteem that depends in part on identification with the lost person is manifested as depression. Freud thought that early, unresolved losses made the patient more likely to have difficulty dealing with losses as an adult (Whybrow et al. 1984). Later theorists pointed out that loss of anything that represents a person and that is overvalued or ambivalently viewed—a group, a profession, a cherished belief, or an ideal, for example—can result in depression.

In most studies comparing depressed patients with nondepressed control subjects, childhood loss—especially loss of a parent—has had a positive association with adult depression, which has been temporally associated with a recent loss, separation, or disappointment (Bemporad 1988; Paykel 1982). In primate studies, separation from a mother or from a peer in animals raised with peers reliably results in behavioral depression and in the physiology of human depression; separation depression can be prevented or reversed by use of antidepressants (Kaufman and Rosenblum 1967; Suomi et al. 1978). Separation during infancy from the mother or, in the case of animals raised with peers, from the peer group also notably increases the risk of adult separation depression (Kaufman and Rosenblum 1967; McKinney 1988). Similarly, experience with human infants has shown that early separation can produce a depressive syndrome that predisposes to later depression (Bowlby 1980). Taken together, these kinds of findings suggest a role for loss in the etiology of depression, but the role may involve the physiology as much as the psychology of loss. In particular, disruption of an attachment bond in any primate leads first to distress, which, from an evolutionary standpoint, helps to attract back a parent from whom an infant has been separated. If reunion does not occur promptly, separation distress is replaced by withdrawal, which conserves energy and reduces the chance of attack by a predator (Dubovsky 1997). Early separations may sensitize arousal and withdrawal systems to react excessively to subsequent losses, whether real or symbolic.

Although the association between depression and loss seems reliable, it is not as strong as was originally thought. Not only does loss account for only a relatively small portion of the variance in the risk of depression (Paykel 1982), but losses of one kind or another precede many other medical and psychiatric illnesses (MagPhil and Thomas 1981). Loss, an event that is stressful in itself and that removes an important external source of regulation of disrupted psychology and physiology, may be a more severe instance of a range of stresses that predispose to mood disorders.

Other Psychodynamic Theories

Psychoanalyst Karl Abraham postulated that depression is a manifestation of aggression turned against the self in a patient who is unable to express anger against loved ones (Whybrow et al. 1984). Attacks on the introjected other, who psychologically has become a part of the self, undermine adaptive capacities and produce negative affect. In support of this hypothesis is the fact that many depressed patients have difficulty expressing anger openly, either because they lack self-confidence or because they are afraid of being abandoned by a loved one on whom they are excessively dependent. However, it seems unlikely that anger is converted directly into depression in such individuals because many depressed patients are openly irritable. A more likely explanation is that dependency, sensitivity to loss, and lack of assertiveness lead depressed people to conceal anger, or even differences of opinion with others, until it becomes overwhelming, at which point it intrudes into everyday interactions. This problem may be compounded by intensification of all emotional experience in depression.

A hypothesis first clearly articulated by Edward Bibring is that the central psychological fault in depression is loss of self-esteem (Whybrow et al. 1984). According to this hypothesis, the depression-prone person is an overambitious, conventional individual with unrealistically high ego ideals. Depression represents deflation of self-confidence and vitality within the self that results from failing to live up to internalized standards that are essential to the patient's self-concept. This concept was expanded in self-theory (Kohut 1971), which emphasizes the central role of the self as an organizer and driving force of all mental functions. Without coherence, mental activities are fragmented and ineffective. Without a sense of vitality, there is inadequate psychic fuel for optimism and useful engagement with challenges and stress.

It is traditionally held that the premorbid personality of the depressed patient is perfectionistic, involving high expectations of the self and others. However, this opinion is based primarily on retrospective recall by patients, which is likely to be influenced by patients' current states. Low self-esteem is a symptom of depression, but it has not yet been shown to be a cause. On the other hand, unrealistic expectations and perceptions of the self and others are also invoked in cognitive theories of depression, which use more objective measures and more formal studies of this variable.

Interpersonal Theory

Interpersonal theory emphasizes four basic interpersonal issues: unresolved grief, disputes between partners and family members about roles and responsibilities in the relationship, transitions to new roles such as parent and retired person, and deficits in the social skills that are necessary to sustain a relationship (Klerman et al. 1984). As in other psychodynamic theories, depressed mood and altered biology are hypothesized to be responses to loss or the threat of loss. A psychotherapy derived from interpersonal theory (i.e., IPT), which is described later in this chapter (see subsection "Interpersonal Therapy"), has been found to be effective as a primary treatment for depression and an adjunct in the treatment of bipolar disorder, although this does not prove that the etiological concept behind the psychotherapy is accurate.

Cognitive Theory

Cognitive theory, which is related to hypotheses derived from an earlier construct called *rational emotive therapy*, holds that negative thinking is a cause rather than a result of depression (A.T. Beck et al. 1979, 1985; Thase 1996; Whybrow et al. 1984). According to the cognitive model, early experience leads to the development of global negative assumptions called *schemata*. Depressive schemata involve all-or-nothing assumptions such as

- If I'm not completely happy, I'll be totally miserable.
- If something isn't done exactly right, it's worthless.
- If I'm not perfect, I'm a failure.
- If everyone doesn't love me unconditionally, then no one loves me at all.
- If I'm not in complete control, I'm helpless.
- If I depend on anyone for anything, I'm totally needy.

As long as experience seems to support a schema—for example, if everything a person does seems to work out or if a person never leans on anyone else—mood remains unambivalently positive. However, if something happens to contradict an all-or-nothing assumption, the negative side of the patient's thinking predominates. Failure in one endeavor makes the patient feel like a complete failure, or becoming ill or otherwise requiring assistance results in the patient's thinking, "I'm totally needy" or "I can't do anything for myself." These negative beliefs, or negative cognitions, are supported by self-fulfilling prophecies that reinforce negative thinking. For instance, the patient who feels helpless as a result of not having been able to influence the outcome of a complex and difficult situation stops trying to do anything to deal with later, simpler stresses. When this lack of effort results in subsequent failures, the patient's belief that nothing can be done to influence the environment seems to have been proven. Systematic errors in thinking lead to catastrophic thinking and generalization of single negative events to global negative expectations of the self, the environment, and the future (the "cognitive triad").

Much of the evidence in favor of the cognitive theory of depression comes from demonstrations that psychotherapy based on the theory (i.e., cognitive therapy, discussed in the "Cognitive Therapy" section later in this chapter) is an effective treatment for major depression. However, cognitive therapy is effective even when patients do not express negative cognitions, and any psychotherapy or antidepressant can reverse depression whether or not negative thinking is formally addressed. In addition, all-or-nothing thinking is characteristic of several conditions (e.g., personality disorders) in addition to depression.

Learned Helplessness

A concept related to cognitive theory is *learned helplessness*, which was first clearly shown experimentally by psychologist Martin Seligman (Abramson et al. 1978; Seligman 1975). The classic learned helplessness paradigm involves exposing an animal to an inescapable noxious but harmless stimulus such as a mild electrical shock. At first, the animal attempts to flee from the shock, but when escape proves impossible, it lies down and accepts the shock passively. If the situation is changed so that the animal can escape the stimulus (e.g., if the investigator removes a barrier that was preventing the animal from leaving the portion of the cage where the shock is applied), the animal continues to act as though it cannot get away. The animal cannot be coaxed away from the shock; only forcibly dragging the animal to safety reverses the learned helpless behavior. A second instance of learned helplessness develops more readily than a first episode. Learned helplessness that develops in one situation may generalize to other situations.

Learned helplessness resembles the passive, withdrawn behavior of depression, and resistance to reversing a negative experience is reminiscent of the self-fulfilling negative expectations of depression. Learned helplessness can be demonstrated in humans—for example, by exposing normal subjects to an inescapable noxious sound—and subjects who score higher on depression rating scales develop learned helplessness more readily than do those without depressive symptoms (Abramson et al. 1978). In animals, pretreatment with an antidepressant prevents learned helplessness. Considering all these data,

Tricyclic and tetracyclic antidepressants (Table 10–19) have a three- or four-carbon ring structure (Bech 1993; Kasper et al. 1992; Osser 1993). All of these medications have similar properties. In most cases, either the parent drugs (e.g., desipramine) or their metabolites (e.g., desmethylclomipramine) block norepinephrine reuptake, and some parent drugs (e.g., chlorimipramine, imipramine) block serotonin reuptake. As was mentioned earlier, neurotransmitter reuptake inhibition mainly predicts adverse effects. For example, noradrenergic antidepressants are more likely to cause arousal, diaphoresis, tremor, and insomnia, and serotonergic antidepressants are more likely to produce headaches, gastrointestinal side effects, and sexual dysfunction (Leonard 1994). However, potent serotonin reuptake inhibition of clomipramine (chlorimipramine) makes it the only TCA that is effective in the treatment of OCD.

All TCAs have similar side effect profiles (Glassman and Proud'homme 1993; Preskhorn 1991). A quinidine-like effect makes the TCAs as effective as the type IA antiarrhythmics in the treatment of ventricular tachyarrhythmias; however, these medications can aggravate heart block and have a negative inotropic effect. Tertiary amine TCAs such as imipramine and amitriptyline have more anticholinergic and sedative side effects. The tertiary amines also produce more α_1-adrenergic blockade, resulting in postural hypotension, and more histamine H_1 antagonism, which contributes to sedation and weight gain. These kinds of adverse effects, along with the potential negative effect on memory of anticholinergic side effects, make the tertiary amine TCAs poor choices for older patients and patients with dementia. Nortriptyline and desipramine are better tolerated by older

patients. Nortriptyline definitely has a therapeutic window, and desipramine probably has a therapeutic window (Preskhorn 1991). Aside from a sinusoidal correlation between serum level and clinical response for imipramine and possibly amitriptyline, no other correlations between antidepressant serum level and clinical response have been demonstrated (P.J. Perry et al. 1994). Measuring antidepressant levels (i.e., therapeutic drug monitoring) may be useful in determining whether nonresponse to a high antidepressant dose or adverse effects with a low dose may be due to unexpectedly low or high serum levels (Preskhorn 1991).

Second-generation antidepressants (Table 10–20) are heterogeneous with respect to their structures and actions (Bech 1993; Danish University Antidepressant Group 1986, 1990; Kasper et al. 1992; Lader 1988; Montgomery 1995). Trazodone is primarily a 5-HT$_2$ receptor antagonist with prominent sedative properties. It is frequently used as a hypnotic because its short elimination half-life results in less daytime impairment than that caused by some traditional hypnotics. The same feature means that multiple doses of trazodone are necessary to achieve steady-state concentrations. However, daytime sedation may limit this schedule. In 1 in 6,000 patients taking trazodone, α_1-adrenergic blockade causes priapism. Bupropion is not sedating and does not have anticholinergic or cardiotoxic effects. Unlike the serotonin reuptake inhibitors, bupropion does not have sexual side effects. However, divided doses are necessary, even with the sustained-release form, and doses greater than 450 mg/day are associated with a 5% incidence of seizures, which is a greater problem in bulimic patients.

TABLE 10–19. Tricyclic and tetracyclic antidepressants

Generic name	Trade name	Usual daily dose (mg)	Comments
Amitriptyline	Elavil	150–300	Sedating, anticholinergic; metabolized to nortriptyline
Nortriptyline	Pamelor, Aventyl	75–150	Therapeutic window 50–150 ng/mL
Protriptyline	Vivactil	15–60	Used for sleep apnea
Trimipramine	Surmontil	150–300	As potent as cimetidine as histamine H_2 antagonist
Imipramine	Tofranil	150–300	Reference antidepressant; metabolized to desipramine
Desipramine	Norpramin, Pertofrane	150–300	Therapeutic window in some studies 125–200 ng/mL
Doxepin	Sinequan, Triadapin	100–300	Like trimipramine; useful for treating allergies, esophagitis, peptic ulcer
Amoxapine	Asendin	150–600	A metabolite of loxapine, a neuroleptic; 7-OH metabolite of amoxapine has neuroleptic properties
Maprotiline	Ludiomil	150–225	A tetracyclic antidepressant between imipramine and desipramine in side-effect profile; doses above 225 mg/day associated with increased risk of seizures
Clomipramine	Anafranil	150–250	Only tricyclic effective for obsessive-compulsive disorder; doses above 250 mg/day can cause seizures

TABLE 10–20. Second- and third-generation antidepressants

Generic name	Trade name	Usual daily dose (mg)	Comments
Trazodone	Desyrel	200–600	Divided dose necessary for antidepressant effect
Bupropion	Wellbutrin	200–450	Sustained-release preparation still requires twice-daily dosing; drug can be used to treat SSRI-induced sexual dysfunction
Fluoxetine	Prozac	10–60	Therapeutic window may develop over time, requiring reduction in dose; parent drug has half-life of 3 days; biologically active metabolite has half-life of 6–9 days; drug can be more activating than other SSRIs
Sertraline	Zoloft	50–200	One metabolite with minimal activity
Paroxetine	Paxil	10–40	Anticholinergic properties equivalent to those of nortriptyline
Fluvoxamine	Luvox	100–300	Shorter half-life may necessitate twice-daily dosing for some patients
Citalopram	Celexa	10–40	Fewer pharmacokinetic interactions but similar side effects compared with other SSRIs
Venlafaxine	Effexor	75–375	Effective for refractory depression
Nefazodone	Serzone	200–600	Useful for sleep disorders
Mirtazapine	Remeron	15–45	Could have antiemetic properties; oversedation and weight gain are common

Note. SSRI = selective serotonin reuptake inhibitor.

Five serotonin reuptake inhibitors (see Table 10–20) are available in the United States. Although these medications are called SSRIs, none is truly selective clinically or pharmacologically (Benkelfat 1993; Dubovsky 1994a; Grahame-Smith 1992; Jaim-Etcheverry and Zieher 1982; Lopez-Ibor 1988; McCormick and Williamson 1989; Meltzer 1989, 1992; van Praag et al. 1987; Wilde and Benfield 1995). In addition to being equally effective treatments for major depression, the SSRIs have applications in anxiety disorders, OCD, posttraumatic stress disorder, eating disorders, and any condition associated with dysregulation of functions that are moderated by serotonergic systems, such as unpredictable, unprovoked aggression; recurrent, intrusive thinking; and excessive sexual or appetitive behavior. Although SSRIs are more effective at blocking in vitro reuptake of serotonin than are other neurotransmitters, effectiveness at serotonin reuptake inhibition does not parallel antidepressant potency, and tianeptine, a TCA discussed earlier (see subsection "Interactions of Neurotransmitter Systems"), enhances serotonin reuptake (Wilde and Benfield 1995). Interactions of serotonin with other neurotransmitters make an isolated action on serotonin in the intact nervous system impossible. SSRIs all have similar side effects, including nausea, diarrhea, headache, activation, sedation, and sexual dysfunction. An action on 5-HT$_2$ heteroreceptors located on dopaminergic neurons in the basal ganglia can result in reduced dopaminergic transmission, which is sometimes manifested as emotional blunting and extrapyramidal side effects (Dubovsky and Thomas 1996). Fluoxetine and paroxetine inhibit the cytochrome P450 2D6 isoenzyme, whereas fluvoxamine inhibits the

3A4 isoenzyme. Some interactions that result are elevations of serum levels and elimination half-lives of TCAs, phenothiazines, warfarin, and many other medications by fluoxetine and paroxetine and of triazolobenzodiazepines, haloperidol, and astemizole by fluvoxamine. Additional P450 enzyme inhibitions occur with many of the SSRIs. Citalopram does not have significant effects on the cytochrome P450 system, and the effect of sertraline on this system usually is not clinically important.

Several third-generation antidepressants act on various neurotransmitters and receptors, with or without serotonin reuptake inhibition (Dubovsky 1994a; Montgomery and Fineberg 1989; G. Parker and Blennerhassett 1998; Poirier and Boyer 1999). Treatment with venlafaxine—which inhibits reuptake of serotonin, norepinephrine, and, to a lesser extent, dopamine—has been found to be efficacious in refractory depression. Norepinephrine reuptake inhibition is apparent only at higher doses (i.e., > 150 mg) of this medication. The immediate-release form of venlafaxine requires divided dosing, which is also necessary with higher doses of the sustained-release (XR) form. Venlafaxine can have adverse effects related to all three neurotransmitters affected (e.g., headaches, jitteriness, activation). Mild elevation of diastolic blood pressure can occur; more severe hypertension develops rarely. Rapid discontinuation of venlafaxine has been associated with withdrawal symptoms, including headache, nausea, fatigue, dizziness, dysphoria, rebound depression, and occasionally hallucinations. Nefazodone has serotonin reuptake inhibition and 5-HT$_2$ antagonist properties. Unlike most antidepressants, nefazodone does not suppress REM sleep, and therefore the drug is associated with a lower incidence of disturbing dreams caused by REM rebound. The sedative properties of nefazodone and possibly its effect on slow-wave sleep make nefazodone a useful drug for treating patients with insomnia, but because of its short half-life, divided dosing is required, which can be difficult when patients experience daytime sedation or dizziness. Severe hepatotoxicity has been reported in 18 patients. Mirtazapine, which is related to the antidepressant mianserin, is an antagonist of 5-HT$_2$ and 5-HT$_3$ receptors and norepinephrine presynaptic α_2-adrenergic receptors. Antagonism of 5-HT$_2$ receptors could prove useful for treating psychotic depression (as could also be true of nefazodone), whereas 5-HT$_3$ receptor blockade could have an antiemetic effect. Sedation and weight gain are common adverse effects of mirtazapine.

The MAOIs (Priest et al. 1995; Quitkin et al. 1991; Stewart et al. 1993) may be more frequently effective than TCAs for major depression with atypical features (SSRIs also appear to be more effective than the TCAs for atypical depression, although possibly less effective than the MAOIs). Four MAOIs are currently available in the United States. Phenelzine has more sedative and anticholinergic properties than do the other MAOIs but has probably been most widely used. Reports of the use of tranylcypromine, a more activating MAOI, in bipolar depression have been more consistently positive than those of the use of other antidepressants. L-Deprenyl (selegiline), which is used to treat Parkinson's disease in doses of 10 mg/day and may inhibit the progression of neurological damage as a result of an antioxidant effect, has antidepressant properties at doses of 30–50 mg/day. Isocarboxazid, which was recently rereleased, is less activating than other MAOIs.

The most important limitations to the use of MAOIs have been hypertensive reactions when foods high in content of the pressor monoamine tyramine or sympathomimetic medications are ingested and serotonin syndrome when serotonergic substances such as SSRIs or dextromethorphan are used concurrently. These problems arise because inhibition of the A form of monoamine oxidase (MAO-A) in the small intestine as well as the brain leads to absorption of excessive amounts of tyramine, a pressor amine found in many foods. Systemic inhibition of MAO leads to accumulation of toxic levels of serotonin, another monoamine, when MAOIs are combined with serotonergic substances. Two approaches to minimizing this problem have emerged. The first involves developing medications that are selective for the B form of monoamine oxidase (MAO-B), which is present in high concentrations in the brain but not the gastrointestinal tract. Selegiline is an example of a selective MAOI, but at antidepressant doses, it loses its selectivity, and dietary restrictions must be followed. Moclobemide is a reversible inhibitor of MAO-A that is displaced from the enzyme by tyramine, allowing the tyramine to be metabolized normally. Moclobemide is available in several countries but not in the United States because the manufacturer determined that the patent would expire before the cost of gaining Food and Drug Administration approval could be recovered.

Antipsychotic Medications

As we noted earlier, the response rate of psychotic depression to a combination of an antipsychotic drug and an antidepressant is significantly greater than the response to either one alone. Although most research into the use of antipsychotic medications in psychotic depression has involved the neuroleptics, especially perphenazine, the atypical antipsychotics are often medications of first choice because they are better tolerated and because they have antidepressant as well as antipsychotic properties.

Some patients with severe nonpsychotic depression respond to antidepressants as poorly as do patients with psychotic depression. In an 8-week double-blind, random-assignment trial in 28 patients with recurrent, nonbipolar, nonpsychotic depression that had been resistant to antidepressants, olanzapine or fluoxetine alone produced significantly less improvement than the combination of the two medications (Shelton et al. 2001b). Insufficient data about individual patients were reported to determine whether the results support the hypothesis discussed earlier that dimensions of depression such as severity, cognitive dysfunction, or recurrence may influence response to different treatment combinations.

Novel Medications

Based on the importance of the membrane inositol phosphate system in intracellular signaling involving G proteins and calcium ions, observations that lithium reduces inositol biphosphate turnover by inhibiting inositol-1-phosphatase, and reports of reduced CSF inositol levels in depression (Levine et al. 1995), several small trials of inositol in mood disorders have been conducted. In a 4-week study of 28 patients randomly assigned to 12 g/day of inositol or placebo, improvement in HRSD scores was significantly greater in the inositol group (Levine et al. 1995). In contrast, in another trial involving 22 patients with bipolar depression, the likelihood of a 50% reduction in HRSD scores was greater in patients treated with high doses of inositol than in those given placebo, but the differences were not statistically significant (Chengappa et al. 2000). Double-blind addition of inositol to SSRIs in patients who did not respond to the antidepressants alone did not improve depression (Nemets et al. 1999).

In eight randomized controlled trials, St. John's wort (*Hypericum*) was more effective than placebo but less effective than TCAs in treating major depression of mild to moderate severity (Gaster and Holroyd 2000). A 6-week British study published after these studies randomly assigned 324 outpatients with mild major depression to 150 mg/day of imipramine or 500 mg/day of a standardized preparation of *Hypericum* extract (Remotiv/Imipramine Study Group 2000). Mean HRSD scores decreased by about 50% in both groups, but St. John's wort was better tolerated and more effective in reducing anxiety. The absence of a placebo group, the lack of a complete response in either group, and the relatively mild nature of the depression limited the interpretation of the data. One of these deficiencies was corrected in a more recent 8-week American multicenter study in outpatients with major depression and slightly higher baseline severity of depression who were randomly assigned to placebo or 1,200 mg/day of standardized *Hypericum* extract (Shelton et al. 2001a). Reductions in rating scale scores for depression and anxiety did not differ between the groups. Although St. John's wort usually is well tolerated, it may interact with highly serotonergic antidepressants and MAOIs, and occasional cases of apparent serotonin syndrome have been reported (V. Parker et al. 2001).

Observations of elevated activity of the hypothalamic-pituitary-adrenal axis in major depression noted earlier suggest that medications that inhibit cortisol production or action may be useful. In 28 reports of antiglucocorticoid treatment of Cushing's syndrome, depression improved in as many as 70% of the patients (Wolkowitz and Reus 1999). A few small open trials of CRF inhibitors in refractory depression at least support the possibility that such approaches may reduce some depressive symptoms (Wolkowitz and Reus 1999), although this kind of treatment obviously is not without substantial risks. A report of open clinical experience suggested that mifepristone (RU-486) produced rapid relief of psychotic depression in four of five patients (Clawson 2000). This substance, which was recently released in the United States as an emergency contraceptive and abortifacient, produces its gynecological effect by blocking progesterone receptors, but it also antagonizes cortisol receptors.

S-adenosylmethionine is a product of methionine metabolism that participates in transmethylation, transulfuration, and transaminopropylation. Reports of reduced CSF levels of *S*-adenosylmethionine in depressed patients (Bottiglieri et al. 1990) led to a series of clinical trials of supplemental *S*-adenosylmethionine for depression. Double-blind comparisons of parenteral *S*-adenosylmethionine with placebo and several TCAs suggested efficacy in major depression (Janicak et al. 1988a). Comparisons of high doses of oral *S*-adenosylmethionine with imipramine (De Vanna and Rigamonti 1992) and desipramine (Bell et al. 1994) in depressed inpatients found similar degrees of improvement in all groups, but in the absence of a placebo group, it is difficult to know whether this might have occurred with any substance. Observations of mania induced by *S*-adenosylmethionine (De Vanna and Rigamonti 1992), however, support a possible antidepressant action of this substance. Although data are insufficient to support the use of *S*-adenosylmethionine as a first-line treatment for depression, it may be worth considering for patients who do not do well with standard antidepressants.

Recent studies (Adams et al. 1996; Edwards et al. 1998; Maes et al. 1996; Peet et al. 1998) have suggested decreased concentrations of omega-3 fatty acids and decreased ratios of omega-3 to omega-6 fatty acids in the plasma and erythrocytes of patients with major depression. In some of these studies, severity of depression has been negatively correlated with both red blood cell membrane levels and dietary intake of n-3 polyunsaturated fatty acids (Edwards et al. 1998; Maes et al. 1996). One hypothesis is that alterations of unsaturated fatty acids in depression are related to a nonspecific inflammatory response (Freeman 2000) that has been associated with decreased availability of serum tryptophan (Song et al. 1998). Although alterations of membrane fatty acids could alter membrane fluidity and therefore intracellular signaling, adequate treatment of depression does not seem to alter fatty acid composition (Maes et al. 1999). No placebo-controlled studies have yet shown that treatment with omega-3 fatty acids improves depression.

Electroconvulsive Therapy

Unipolar Depression

ECT is the oldest and most reliable of the modern somatic therapies for mood disorders (Abrams 1988; Dubovsky 1995b). In ECT, a bidirectional square wave lasting about 2 msec is applied through right (nondominant) unilateral or bilateral electrodes to produce a generalized electrical seizure in the brain lasting 20–150 seconds. Although it was initially introduced as a treatment for schizophrenia, ECT is now known to benefit only about 15% of patients with this diagnosis—generally those with an acute illness of relatively brief duration accompanied by affective symptoms, perplexity, catatonia, and a good premorbid adjustment. ECT is most clearly useful in the case of acute major depressive episodes, especially when they are characterized by rapid onset, brief duration, severity, psychosis, motor retardation, catatonia, severe pseudodementia, lack of insight, and inability to tolerate antidepressants (Dubovsky 1995b). ECT is also highly effective in mania and catatonia (Small et al. 1988, 1996). At one time, it was thought that ECT would be inappropriate in the presence of delirium because ECT induces an acute confusional state, but more recent experience indicates that ECT can produce rapid improvement in delirium; motor symptoms of Parkinson's disease also improve with ECT, independent of ECT's effect on depressed mood (American Psychiatric Association 1990; Dubovsky 1986, 1995b; Folkerts 1995). ECT has been found to be safe and effective in children as well as adults (Willoughby et al. 1997).

Evidence has emerged of a relation between the dose of the electrical stimulus and response to ECT; stimulus intensities one to three times the seizure threshold appear to be more reliably effective in major depression (Devanand et al. 1991a; Dubovsky 1995b; Lamy et al. 1994). In routine use, right (nondominant) unilateral ECT usually is used first in the treatment of a major depressive episode because it is associated with a lower risk of cognitive impairment. Bilateral ECT is used in cases of nonresponse to unilateral ECT and as an initial approach in severe depression, psychotic depression, catatonic stupor, Parkinson's disease, and depression in which a smaller number of ECT treatments is desirable (e.g., in cases of high anesthetic risk). Although 6–12 ECT treatments usually are sufficient for major depression, standard practice is to continue treatment until the patient responds; further treatment after this point is unnecessary and may produce intolerable cognitive impairment (Dubovsky 1995b). An early practice of estimating the "dose" in ECT by the number of seizure seconds was not supported by later research (Dubovsky 1995b).

ECT usually is recommended for depressed patients who are refractory to antidepressants because the expectation is that it will be effective when medications were not. Comparisons of patients who received adequate doses of antidepressants (or antidepressant-neuroleptic combinations for psychotic depression) with those who received inadequate medication doses found that about 90% of the latter responded to ECT, whereas the response rate was only about 50% for patients who received adequate antidepressant doses (Devanand et al. 1991a; Piper 1993; Sackeim 1994). The assumption that patients who were unresponsive to a particular antidepressant before ECT respond to that medication after ECT also was contradicted by the same research, which showed that antidepressants are no more effective after ECT than they were before it. However, a patient's ability to tolerate an antidepressant may be enhanced by ECT. Some form of maintenance therapy involving either adequate doses of antidepressants that have not been ineffective previously or continued periodic ECT treatments is necessary to prevent relapse and recurrence of depression (Sackeim 1994; Schwarz et al. 1995). Maintenance ECT is safe and effective in preventing relapse and recurrence and is especially useful in the elderly, who tolerate maintenance pharmacotherapy poorly (Rabheru and Persad 1998).

The most common side effects of ECT are confusion and memory loss, and these effects are more pronounced after bilateral ECT (Aperia 1985; Calev et al. 1989, 1995; Krueger et al. 1992; Pettinati and Rosenberg 1984). Anterograde amnesia is most obvious within 45 minutes of a treatment, but loss of memory of events occurring from a few days to as long as 2 years before ECT (i.e., retrograde amnesia) also occurs. In some cases, personally significant memories from the recent or distant past (i.e., autobiographical memory) may be lost permanently. Most of the time, however, cognitive functioning after recovery from the acute effects of ECT is better than it was before the treatment, probably because of recovery from the cognitive impairment of depression (Calev et al. 1995; Krueger et al. 1992; Prudic et al. 2000; Sackeim et al. 1992). A small group of patients complain of severe cognitive disruption that cannot be demonstrated on objective testing (Prudic et al. 2000). Because these patients also have not had remission of depression, cognitive symptoms may represent residual depressive symptoms or perhaps awareness of subtle deficits that nondepressed individuals would ignore. No evidence from studies of cerebral structure or function shows that ECT as it is currently administered causes brain damage (Coffey et al. 1991; Dubovsky 1995b; Weiner 1984).

Bipolar Disorder

Mania is the third most common indication for ECT (Small et al. 1988), which appears to be the most rapidly effective treatment for mania (H.S. Hopkins and Gelenberg 1994; Small et al. 1996) and the most effective treatment for bipolar depression (Bergsholm et al. 1992; H.S. Hopkins and Gelenberg 1994; Zornberg and Rose 1993). In a review of the published literature on the efficacy of ECT for acute mania, Mukherjee et al. (1994)

found that the overall rate of "remission or marked clinical improvement" was 80% (470 of 589 patients). Interpretation of these composite figures is limited by differences in methodology and outcome measures in the studies reviewed and by the secondhand assessment of data with a nonstandard method. Although some studies found that unilateral ECT was as effective as bilateral ECT (Black et al. 1987), others found bilateral ECT to be more frequently and more rapidly effective (Milstein et al. 1987; Small et al. 1985, 1996), possibly because of shunting of current through the scalp with the Lancaster right (nondominant) unilateral electrode placement, which was used in one study showing superiority of bilateral ECT (Mukherjee et al. 1994). In a prospective study (Schnur et al. 1992), five of eight manic patients had a complete remission with the d'Elia right (nondominant) unilateral electrode placement, which has a greater interelectrode distance, but the number of patients was too small for definitive conclusions to be drawn. Maintenance ECT was as effective as lithium in preventing manic relapse and recurrence in a prospective study and some case series (Avissar and Schreiber 1992b; Bigelow et al. 1981; Jaffe et al. 1991; Sachs 1989).

Repetitive Transcranial Magnetic Stimulation

Unipolar Depression

The hypothesis that the pathophysiology of depression involves in part hypoactivity of the left prefrontal cortex (Triggs et al. 1999) led to the application of a potent local magnetic field over the left prefrontal cortex (George et al. 1997; Mosimann et al. 2000), which induces a localized electrical current perpendicular to the magnetic field. Preliminary studies of motor evoked potential threshold suggested that changes in brain activity may occur at sites remote from the stimulus without a generalized electrical seizure in the brain (Triggs et al. 1999). High-frequency (10–20 Hz) repetitive transcranial magnetic stimulation (rTMS), which increases brain glucose metabolism and regional blood flow, has been found to be more effective in the treatment of major depression than low-frequency (1 Hz) rTMS (Post et al. 1999).

Open studies have found that rTMS produces significant improvement in depressive symptoms in patients with refractory depression (Triggs et al. 1999) but has no effect on mood in nondepressed subjects (Mosimann et al. 2000). A random-assignment crossover comparison of active and sham high-frequency rTMS found that the active treatment reduced HRSD scores by 5 points, whereas HRSD scores increased by 3 points during sham

treatment (George et al. 1997). On the other hand, a 2-week double-blind comparison of "real" and sham rTMS followed by 4 weeks of real rTMS failed to find a difference between the groups because of a high rate of spontaneous improvement in all subjects (C. Loo et al. 1999). Although rTMS is theoretically appealing because it does not have cognitive side effects (Kirkcaldie et al. 1997; J.T. Little et al. 2000), the only important adverse effects being headache and rare seizures, most studies are of very short duration and involve small numbers of subjects, limiting interpretation of the data. However, one study noted persistence of improvement 6 months after rTMS with maintenance antidepressant treatment.

Mechanisms of action of rTMS are unclear. Animal studies reported upregulation of β-adrenergic receptors in the frontal cortex and downregulation of the same receptors in the striatum; rTMS downregulated 5-HT_2 receptors in the frontal cortex (Ben-Shachar et al. 1999). The fact that these receptor effects differ from those of other antidepressant treatments may indicate that rTMS has a different mechanism of action or that receptor actions are not the primary mediators of antidepressant action.

Bipolar Disorder

Data on the potential efficacy of rTMS in bipolar disorder are very sparse, although it shows some promise (Post 1999; Post et al. 1998). A comparison of fast left and right prefrontal rTMS in 16 manic patients found significantly more improvement with right than with left placement, which is the opposite of what has been found in unipolar depression (Grisaru et al. 1998).

Antimanic Drug Therapy

Medications that are used to treat mania (i.e., antimanic drugs) also are used to prevent or reduce the frequency of affective recurrences in bipolar disorder, in which case they are called *mood stabilizers*. Although reliable data from well-designed randomized clinical trials are not available for mood-stabilizing actions of antimanic drugs other than lithium, a consensus panel involving 58 national experts produced strong agreement that antimanic drugs should be used in all phases of the treatment of bipolar disorder, including depression (Sachs et al. 2000).

Lithium, the best studied of the antimanic drugs, has established efficacy as an antimanic and is prophylactic against recurrences of mania and depression in bipolar disorder (Schou 1997). Lithium may reduce depressive recurrences in highly recurrent unipolar depression

(Schou 1995, 1997), and it reduces the risk of suicide in patients with mood disorders (Zarate et al. 1995a). Lithium appears to be most effective in patients with pure (i.e., not mixed) mania, complete remissions between episodes, the absence of rapid cycling, and no requirement for neuroleptics (Bowden 1995; Gelenberg and Hopkins 1993; H.S. Hopkins and Gelenberg 1994; Schou 1997; Zarate et al. 1995a). However, more than 50% of the lithium-treated patients have another affective episode within 2 years (Goldberg et al. 1995), and the prophylactic effect of the drug is attenuated over time in 20%–40% of patients (Goldberg et al. 1995, 1996; Harrow et al. 1990; Post 1990b). Discontinuation of lithium (and probably other mood stabilizers), especially if it is rapid, can result in rebound (i.e., worsening) of the mood disorder as well as refractoriness to the therapeutic effect of the medication in some (H.S. Hopkins and Gelenberg 1994; Post 1990a, 1990b) but not all (Berghofer and Miller-Oerlinghausen 2000) patients.

Lithium doses are adjusted by serum level. Although some studies suggest that trough levels greater than 0.8 mEq/L (0.8 mM) are associated with greater efficacy if more side effects (Gelenberg et al. 1989), other research suggests that levels greater than 0.8 mM may not be more effective than levels of 0.5–0.8 mM, possibly because of greater dropout rates at the higher level (Vestergaard et al. 1998). Common adverse effects of lithium at therapeutic levels include polydipsia, polyuria, hypothyroidism, hyperparathyroidism, tremor, impaired cognitive function, nausea, and weight gain. The last-named side effect, along with interference with signaling of insulin receptors, makes lithium therapy problematic for diabetic patients. Lithium toxicity, which becomes more likely as serum levels exceed 1.5 mM, causes a coarse tremor, ataxia, vertigo, dysarthria, vomiting, delirium, muscle fasciculations, cardiotoxicity, and death. Debate continues about whether chronic lithium therapy causes nephrotoxicity (Schou 1997), but permanent neurotoxicity after lithium intoxication has been reported (Saxena and Maltikarjuna 1988). The 24-hour elimination half-life of chronically administered lithium permits once-daily dosing, which may reduce the frequency of adverse effects.

The anticonvulsants carbamazepine and valproate (divalproex) also have been widely studied as antimanic drugs and mood stabilizers (Bowden 1995; Bowden et al. 1994; Chou 1991; Keck et al. 1992, 1993; McElroy et al. 1996b; Okuma et al. 1990; Post 1988; Post et al. 1993, 1998; Simhandl et al. 1993). Alone or in combination with each other or with lithium, the anticonvulsants may be more frequently effective than lithium in mixed mania, rapid-cycling bipolar disorder, and refractory

bipolar disorder. More-rapid dosage escalation may be possible with valproate than with lithium and carbamazepine, an effect that could result in faster achievement of therapeutic levels and possibly earlier discharge of hospitalized manic patients. However, studies with findings supporting briefer hospitalizations of patients treated primarily with valproate versus those treated with lithium have not been controlled for the fact that valproate became a common treatment for mania at the same time that inpatient length of stay began to decline substantially as a result of managed care, new therapeutic philosophies, and other changes in hospital treatment of mania. Controlled trials support the antimanic action of valproate in mixed states more than that of carbamazepine, and the prophylactic effect of carbamazepine more than valproate (Licht 1998).

One study suggested that the therapeutic level of valproate in the treatment of acute mania may be around 100 μg/mL, which is achieved with daily doses of 750–5,000 mg (Bowden et al. 1994). Therapeutic levels can be achieved quickly through rapid oral loading (Keck et al. 1993). The dosage of carbamazepine (usually 400–1,200 mg/day) is frequently adjusted on the basis of serum level, but no scientific evidence indicates a specific therapeutic level for carbamazepine in epilepsy, let alone mood disorders (Chen 1931; Froscher 1992; Schoenenberger et al. 1995). On the other hand, higher serum levels are associated with more psychomotor impairment from the anticonvulsant (Thompson and Trimble 1983). Valproate often can be administered in one bedtime dose, which facilitates sleep, whereas carbamazepine usually is administered in a divided dose. The practice of obtaining periodic complete blood counts and of withdrawing carbamazepine if the white blood cell count drops below 3,000 will not prevent agranulocytosis because this extremely rare (2 cases in 525,000 patients) event occurs abruptly and is not correlated with the benign gradual decrease in white blood cell count that takes place during the first few months of carbamazepine treatment and then remits in one-third of patients. Routine liver function tests with anticonvulsants are not cost-effective because hepatotoxicity is rarely caused by these drugs and when it is, it can be better identified by clinical observation than by laboratory testing (Hoshino et al. 1995; Verma and Haidukewych 1993). Use of valproate and carbamazepine during pregnancy may be associated with fetal neural tube defects and cognitive deficits (Lindhout and Omtzigt 1992).

Two newer anticonvulsants, lamotrigine and gabapentin, which have been approved in the United States as adjuncts in the treatment of refractory epilepsy (Mattson 1995; M.J. McLean 1995; Messenheimer 1995), have been used recently in clinical settings to treat bipolar illness (Calabrese et al. 1996a; Walden and Hesslinger 1995). Positive effects of lamotrigine and gabapentin on mood were suggested by reports that patients in continuation studies elected more often to continue taking these medications than would be expected on the basis of improved seizure control alone, apparently because of an improved sense of well-being (Messenheimer 1995; Smith et al. 1993). A few case reports and open series have been published in which gabapentin was associated with improvement of mood in bipolar disorder (Cabras et al. 1999; Letterman and Markowitz 1999). However, controlled studies have not confirmed this impression (Ghaemi and Gaughan 2000).

Potential mechanisms of a positive effect of lamotrigine in bipolar disorder include inhibition of glutamate release and calcium channel blockade (Berk 1999; Xie and Hagan 1998). Lamotrigine was found in controlled trials to be useful in bipolar depression (Ghaemi and Gaughan 2000), and a small controlled study suggested efficacy in mania (Berk 1999). In a 48-week open trial of lamotrigine as adjunctive treatment ($n = 60$) or monotherapy ($n = 15$) in patients with bipolar I and bipolar II disorder (Calabrese et al. 1999b), depressed patients had a mean reduction in depression scores of 42%, and patients with hypomania, mania, or a mixed state had on average a 74% reduction in mania rating scores. A group treated with a comparison medication and a placebo group would be necessary to be confident of the long-term efficacy of lamotrigine. In an open study of lamotrigine as an adjunctive (in 60 patients) or primary (in 15 patients) medication, patients with rapid cycling entering the study while depressed had a better response than did patients with predominantly manic symptoms (Bowden et al. 1999). A double-blind study by the same group found that 200 mg/day of lamotrigine monotherapy had a significant antidepressant effect in patients with bipolar depression compared with placebo (Calabrese et al. 1999a). However the efficacy of this medication as a mood stabilizer over extended periods remains to be confirmed, and different conclusions were drawn from a limited patient population.

The novel anticonvulsant zonisamide was thought to have antimanic properties in an open trial (Kanba et al. 1994). Topiramate, another new anticonvulsant, has been used clinically as a mood stabilizer. The only data in favor of this application come from a few case reports and case series (McElroy et al. 2000; Post et al. 1998), and no controlled evidence indicates that it is effective for this indication. Topiramate can be useful as an appetite suppressant for some patients who gain weight on, but otherwise tolerate, other medications. However, it may contribute to mood destabilization in some patients, and cognitive impairment can be a limiting side effect. Oxcarbazepine, an analogue of carbamazepine that appears to have fewer adverse effects and interactions but is as effective as an anticonvulsant (Grant and Faulds 1992), has been used as a mood stabilizer, but no controlled studies of this application have been conducted yet. Two brief studies found equivalence to lithium and haloperidol in the treatment of mania.

The most frequent adverse effects of lamotrigine and gabapentin have been dizziness, headache, diplopia, ataxia, nausea, amblyopia, somnolence, fatigue, ataxia, rash, weight gain, and vomiting (Beydoun et al. 1995; Matsuo et al. 1996; M.J. McLean 1995; Messenheimer 1995; G.L. Morris 1995). The manufacturer raised concerns about dangerous allergic rashes with use of lamotrigine, but the precise risk is not clear. Gabapentin has been reported to induce mania (Hauck and Bhaumik 1995; Lweeke et al. 1999) and was associated with aggressive behavior, hyperactivity, and tantrums in some children, most of whom had ADHD (Lee et al. 1996; Tallian et al. 1996).

Calcium Channel Blockers

Increasing experience with refractory bipolar syndromes has created pressure for the development of alternative treatments for patients who do not tolerate or respond to lithium and the anticonvulsants. Of the various innovative therapies that have been proposed, the best studied are the calcium channel blockers. Double-blind trials of verapamil in manic or hypomanic individuals (Dose et al. 1986; Dubovsky et al. 1986; Garza-Trevino et al. 1992; Giannini et al. 1984, 1985, 1987; Hoschl and Kozemy 1989; Pazzaglia et al. 1993) and a blinded trial of nimodipine in 11 rapidly cycling patients (Pazzaglia et al. 1993; Post et al. 1993) have been reported. In two 4- to 5-week double-blind trials (Garza-Trevino et al. 1992; Hoschl and Kozemy 1989), equivalent antimanic efficacy of verapamil and lithium was found. Verapamil and nimodipine have been noted to have mood-stabilizing properties in some manic and rapidly cycling patients (Barton and Gitlin 1987; Giannini et al. 1987; Goodnick 1995; Manna 1991; Pazzaglia et al. 1993; Wehr et al. 1988). One trial has been reported in which verapamil appeared to be less effective than lithium in the treatment of acute mania (Walton et al. 1996), but the results were limited by small absolute numerical differences between groups in rating scale scores, P values that usually would not be considered significant with the statistical measures used in the study, and the absence of any differences between mania rating scale scores in the lithium and verapamil groups.

open method in most patients, a single-blind discontinuation protocol in only 4 patients, a diverse group of patients likely to have had highly variable courses, and different lengths of thyroxine trials in different patients. To the extent that these high doses of thyroxine did in fact enhance the therapeutic effect of the thymoleptics, it is not clear whether this involved a primary action of the hormone or correction of central hypothyroidism in patients with poor delivery of thyroid hormone to the brain. There is no reason to think that thyroxine by itself has antimanic or mood-stabilizing properties in euthyroid patients. Risks of excessive thyroid replacement include anxiety, atrial fibrillation, and osteoporosis in menopausal women.

Tamoxifen

Tamoxifen, an estrogen receptor antagonist used to prevent breast cancer recurrence, is also an inhibitor of PKC (Manji et al. 1999). In a small, open study, tamoxifen appeared to have antimanic properties (Manji et al. 1999). If a mood-stabilizing action of tamoxifen were reported in larger controlled trials, it could be a useful adjunct in the treatment of refractory bipolar disorder. However, adverse effects of this medication, including precipitating menopause and increasing the risk of uterine cancer, would make it appropriate only for life-threatening refractory illness. Mixed estrogen agonist/antagonist medications such as roloxifene have not been investigated as potential mood-stabilizing agents.

Psychosurgery

Stereotactic subcaudate tractotomy (SST), which involves precise localization of a lesion beneath the caudate nucleus, has been found on unstructured follow-up to benefit 50%–60% of the small number of patients with refractory bipolar disorder who have undergone this procedure (Bridges et al. 1994). In two cohorts of 9 patients each—all patients with continuous cycling refractory to all treatments—who were followed up carefully for 2–13 years after SST, 3 patients were essentially well and required no further treatment, 1 patient had mild residual symptoms, 11 patients continued to have affective episodes but they were less severe, 2 patients committed suicide, and 1 patient's condition was unchanged (Lovett and Shaw 1987; Poynton et al. 1988). Like mood-stabilizing medications, SST was more effective in ameliorating hypomania than depression. Complications of surgery included cognitive deficits in a few patients, schizophreniform symptoms in 1 patient, and partial escape from the beneficial effects of surgery over time in several patients.

Psychotherapy for Mood Disorders

Antidepressants have become the predominant form of treatment for unipolar depression. One report (Roose and Stern 1995) stated that even 29% of 56 patients in psychoanalysis with analytic candidates were taking antidepressants. However, certain psychotherapies have been found to be as effective as antidepressants (Antonuccio et al. 1995), especially in less severe cases of unipolar depression (Sotsky et al. 1991). Two psychotherapies designed specifically for major depression—cognitive therapy (and a variant, CBT) and IPT—have been subjected to controlled research and have been compared with reference antidepressants. However, these studies have several features that complicate interpretation of the results. For example, most studies have involved mildly to moderately depressed nonpsychotic, nonbipolar patients. In addition, comparisons of psychotherapy with medication use imipramine, the standard reference antidepressant, in a fixed-dose protocol. The dropout rate in such protocols is undoubtedly greater than it is for patients taking antidepressants in clinical practice because newer, better-tolerated antidepressants are used and because a component of pharmacotherapy includes increasing the dose in the case of nonresponse, treating side effects, and encouraging compliance. In addition, antidepressant medications and psychotherapies may not be directly comparable because they act on different symptoms, psychotherapy working faster to improve social function and suicidal thinking and medications resulting in a faster onset of improvement of disturbed mood, sleep, and appetite.

In the NIMH Collaborative Research Program (Elkin et al. 1989), unipolar, nonpsychotically depressed patients received a 16-week course of placebo plus "clinical management" (i.e., nonspecific supportive psychotherapy), imipramine plus clinical management, IPT, or CBT. For mildly depressed patients, no active treatment was any more effective than placebo plus clinical management, probably reflecting a high rate of spontaneous improvement or at least fluctuation of symptoms in this population. As depression became more severe, imipramine plus clinical management was found to be consistently superior on the broadest range of outcome measures. IPT was better than a placebo but not as effective as imipramine. CBT was only slightly less effective than IPT, but it was not significantly better than a placebo (Hollon and Fawcett 1995; Hollon et al. 1992). The results suggested that support and no medication might be effective for mild acute depression, whereas more severely depressed patients appear to require antidepressants.

This conclusion is not as straightforward as it might seem. The method of analysis involving the last observation carried forward may have underestimated the efficacy of both psychotherapies, and other research suggests that cognitive-behavioral psychotherapy and IPT are effective for severe depression (Antonuccio et al. 1995; Jarrett 1997; P. McLean and Taylor 1992). However, IPT and behavior therapy may be less effective in melancholic than in nonmelancholic depression (Frank et al. 1992; P. McLean and Taylor 1992). Relapse of depression does not occur as rapidly after discontinuation of psychotherapy as it does after withdrawal of antidepressants, and continuation of psychotherapy after recovery reduces the relapse rate (Evans et al. 1992; Kupfer et al. 1992; Thase and Kupfer 1996; Weissman 1994), as is true of antidepressants. This issue is discussed in more detail in the following sections.

Cognitive Therapy

Cognitive therapy is based on the premise that the negative emotions of depression are reactions to negative thinking derived from dysfunctional global negative attitudes. Patient and therapist work together to identify automatic negative thoughts, correct the pervasive beliefs that generate these thoughts, and develop more realistic basic assumptions (A.T. Beck et al. 1979, 1985). Treatment involves systematically monitoring negative cognitions whenever the patient feels depressed; recognizing the association between cognition, affect, and behavior; generating data that support or refute the negative cognition; generating alternative hypotheses to explain the event that precipitated the negative cognition; and identifying the negative schemata predisposing to the emergence of global negative thinking when one side of an all-or-nothing assumption is disappointed. In the course of examining dysfunctional attitudes, the patient learns to label and counteract information-processing errors such as overgeneralization, excessive personalization, all-or-nothing thinking, and generalizing from single negative events.

For example, after keeping track of what he was thinking at the moment he began to feel depressed, a man might realize that the feeling started after he began thinking "nobody loves me" when his wife did not greet him enthusiastically. This thought might be seen to follow logically from the assumption "If she isn't always happy to see me, she doesn't love me." Two kinds of alternative hypotheses could be generated in considering this cognition. First, the patient's wife may have been preoccupied with something else or may have been happy to see him but did not show it in exactly the way he expected. Second, lack of enthusiasm at one particular moment is not necessarily a sign of generalized disinterest. Eventually, the patient learns to correct the underlying all-or-nothing belief "People either are completely devoted to me or they don't care at all."

The best studied of the psychotherapies for major depression (Thase 1995), cognitive therapy has been compared with nonpharmacological-control conditions for the acute-phase treatment of depression in at least 21 randomized controlled clinical trials (Shea et al. 1988; Thase 1995). In a meta-analysis of 12 suitable studies, cognitive therapy had an overall efficacy rate of 46.6% and was 30.1% more effective than no therapy in waiting-list control subjects (two studies) but was only 9.4% more effective than placebo plus clinical management in the collaborative study mentioned earlier (Elkin et al. 1989). Although early studies reported superiority of cognitive therapy over pharmacotherapy provided by a primary care physician, comparisons with more rigorous pharmacological treatment provided by psychiatrists suggest equivalence of the two treatments for depression of moderate severity (Elkin et al. 1989; Hollon et al. 1992). As we noted earlier, pharmacotherapy was more effective than cognitive therapy in more severely depressed patients in the NIMH Collaborative Study (Elkin et al. 1989). The onset of action of antidepressants has been found to be faster than the onset of action of cognitive therapy (Watkins et al. 1993).

Although some studies suggest that starting treatment with an antidepressant and then adding cognitive therapy (sequential combined therapy) may improve efficacy more than adding antidepressants to cognitive therapy (Bowers 1990; Hollon et al. 1992; Thase 1995), in clinical practice, patients with a poor response to cognitive therapy (or any psychotherapy) alone often respond to addition of antidepressants. Response rates to individual cognitive therapy exceed those to group cognitive therapy (50.1% vs. 39.2%). Modified cognitive therapy has been shown to be effective for hospitalized depressed patients (Stuart and Thase 1994). Depressed patients with personality disorders may be more likely to drop out of cognitive therapy (Persons et al. 1996), but those who remain in treatment can improve as much as patients without Axis II disorders (Stuart et al. 1992).

Monthly cognitive therapy achieved the same level of prophylaxis as continuation pharmacotherapy in one study (Blackburn et al. 1986). In a naturalistic follow-up study of cognitive therapy responders compared with antidepressant responders who had been withdrawn from medication and antidepressant responders treated with continuation pharmacotherapy, cognitive therapy–treated patients relapsed significantly less often than did patients treated initially with antidepressants who were withdrawn from antidepressant monotherapy (21% vs. 50% at 2 years) and at a rate comparable to that for antidepressant-treated patients who continued to take medication (15%) (Evans et al. 1992).

Following successful antidepressant therapy, CBT was shown to reduce the risk of relapse of unipolar depression, at least in the relatively near term, after withdrawal of antidepressants (Akiyoshi et al. 1996). After recovering from at least a third episode of major depression with TCAs or SSRIs administered according to a standardized protocol similar to that in the Frank et al. (1990) study discussed in the next section, 40 patients continued for 3–5 months with full doses of antidepressants, after which they were randomly assigned to pharmacotherapy plus CBT or pharmacotherapy plus "clinical management." Antidepressants were then withdrawn from both groups at a rate of 25 mg of amitriptyline equivalent every other week. All patients were medication free during the last two CBT sessions. CBT included treatment of residual negative cognitions, exposure to reduce anxiety, lifestyle modification, and well-being therapy (a two- to three-session approach to changing attitudes that interfere with positive self-regard, relationships with others, environmental mastery, and personal growth). Patients were followed up for 2 years after CBT was completed.

In this study, CBT but not clinical management resulted in significant improvement of residual symptoms. Over the 2 years of treatment-free follow-up, relapse rates were 25% in the CBT group and 80% in the clinical management group ($P<0.001$). After another 4 years (total follow-up = 6 years after completion of CBT), 50% of the CBT patients and 73% of the clinical management patients had at least one relapse, a nonsignificant difference; however, CBT patients had significantly fewer total episodes (i.e., fewer multiple recurrences) than the clinical management group (mean 0.8 ± 0.95 episodes in CBT vs. 1.7 " 1.3 for clinical management) (Beauchamp et al. 1993). Of course, the question of whether simply continuing the antidepressant would have had a similar prophylactic effect was not addressed. The authors speculated that the short course of CBT (10 vs. the usual 16–20 sessions) was effective because CBT was added after medications had established a remission, at which point CBT was only needed for residual symptoms that might otherwise progress to relapse (Akiyoshi et al. 1996).

Interpersonal Therapy

IPT is designed to improve depression by enhancing the quality of the patient's interpersonal world (Klerman et al. 1984). The treatment begins with an explanation of the diagnosis and treatment options, legitimizing depression as a medical illness. The acute course of treatment is conducted according to a manualized protocol over 12–16 weeks. A protocol for maintenance IPT also has been developed. Through structured assignments, IPT helps the patient to work toward explicit goals related to whichever of the four basic interpersonal problems (unresolved grief, role disputes, transitions to new roles, and social skills deficits) is believed to be important. Role-playing is used to help the patient acquire new interpersonal skills, and structured conjoint meetings are used to help partners to clarify their expectations of each other.

It is frequently claimed that IPT is no more than a specialized form of expressive (psychodynamic) psychotherapy, but there are important differences between the two treatments. Unlike expressive psychotherapy, IPT follows a structured approach outlined in a manual and uses explicit homework assignments. Its focus is exclusively on the present; no systematic attempt is made to explore conflicts related to early experience, to address transference, or to change underlying character structure. IPT may be a more acceptable treatment than medication or cognitive or behavior therapies, at least to younger patients (Banken and Wilson 1992).

In initial randomized clinical trials involving outpatients with nonpsychotic major depression, IPT was superior to amitriptyline in producing improvement in mood, suicidal ideation, and interest, whereas the antidepressant was more effective for appetite and sleep disturbances (DiMascio et al. 1979; Elkin et al. 1989; Schneider et al. 1986; Thase 1995; Weissman et al. 1979). In a comparison with nortriptyline in older patients, IPT was found to be as effective in reducing depressive symptoms, and more IPT-treated patients than nortriptyline-treated patients remained in the study (Schneider et al. 1986). In the collaborative study mentioned earlier comparing IPT, cognitive therapy, imipramine plus clinical management, and placebo plus clinical management, IPT was found to be equivalent to imipramine and cognitive therapy by the end of 16 weeks, but imipramine was more rapidly effective (Elkin et al. 1989; Watkins et al. 1993).

Efficacy as a maintenance treatment as well as acute therapy has been shown for IPT. In a prospective study of 128 patients, each of whom had had at least two previous episodes of recurrent unipolar depression, patients were randomized after remission with treatment with imipramine to one of five treatment conditions: 1) continued monthly IPT with imipramine, 2) monthly IPT with placebo, 3) monthly IPT without medication, 4) imipramine with supportive management, and 5) placebo with supportive management (Frank et al. 1990). Both active-medication conditions were associated with about 80% relapse-free rates at 3-year follow-up. In addition, IPT with or without a placebo more than doubled relapse-free survival rates compared with placebo and supportive management at 3 years (30%–40% vs. 10%). Blind independent ratings of the quality of IPT indicated that patients treated with higher-quality IPT had 2-year relapse-free survival rates comparable with rates among patients treated with imipramine, and 3-year survival rates for patients in the former group were about 40%. Patients receiving IPT of below-average quality had survival rates that were no better than rates for patients receiving a placebo (Frank et al. 1991).

In a subsequent study, 20 patients who had taken imipramine and had remained in remission for the first 3 years of the first study (Frank et al. 1990) were randomized to an additional 2 years of treatment with placebo or continuation of the antidepressant (Kupfer et al. 1992). Of those treated with medication, 82% survived the next 2 years without a depressive recurrence, compared with 33% of those randomized to placebo. Of the latter group, only 11% of those receiving placebo alone survived, whereas 78% of those continuing with monthly IPT and placebo survived. The possibility was not investigated that a "dose" of maintenance IPT that is greater than the monthly sessions used in these studies would have produced even better results. IPT was an effective adjunct to maintenance antidepressants in elderly patients (Reynolds et al. 1995).

Another study involved 180 geriatric patients with recurrent unipolar nonpsychotic depression who were experiencing at least their second lifetime episode of unipolar depression after having been well for 3 years or less (Malawska et al. 1999). Patients were treated openly with weekly IPT and nortriptyline (serum level = 0–120 ng/mL) with or without lithium or perphenazine augmentation until depression remitted (HRSD score = 10 or less). Remitted depression was treated for 16 weeks to ensure stability of remission, after which patients (107 of the 180 who were originally enrolled) whose remissions remained stable were randomly assigned to medication clinic with nortriptyline, medication clinic with placebo, monthly IPT plus nortriptyline, or monthly IPT and placebo. Patients remained in maintenance treatment for 3 years or until recurrence of major depression. All active treatments were significantly better than placebo in pre-venting recurrence. Combined IPT and nortriptyline was superior to IPT and placebo (recurrence rate over 3 years = 20% vs. 64%). The combination of IPT and the antidepressant was most effective in preventing recurrences during the first year of maintenance because this was when most recurrences took place, especially in patients older than 70.

A form of IPT called interpersonal and social rhythm therapy (IPSRT) is under study as an adjunct to thymoleptic medication therapy in the maintenance treatment of bipolar mood disorders (Frank et al. 1994). In addition to interpersonal techniques such as encouraging the expression of grief for the loss of the person the patient was before the illness began and resolving interpersonal conflicts, IPSRT includes a structured approach to normalizing circadian rhythms. The patient first keeps a log that records the timing of 17 zeitgebers (e.g., getting out of bed, eating meals, first interaction with another person, exercising, going to bed). Average times for each of these cues to circadian rhythms are computed, and the patient is helped to keep a regular schedule for each of them.

After 1 year of prospective comparison of IPSRT with supportive psychotherapy, using an education and medication compliance module (each psychotherapy added to standard pharmacotherapy protocols), in patients who had achieved a remission of mania or bipolar depression for at least 4 months, patients treated with IPSRT were significantly more likely to have normalized their schedules of the 17 circadian cues (i.e., their schedules were identical to those of control populations studied with the same instrument) (Frank et al. 1997). No significant clinical differences were found between the IPSRT and the supportive psychotherapy groups after half of this planned 2-year study of a relatively small population had been completed. However, the benefit of adding IPSRT as an adjunctive maintenance treatment probably will require large samples to control for variance in illness and treatment.

Family Therapy

Involvement of the family is a defining characteristic of IPT. Family-focused treatment is a manualized psychoeducational treatment for bipolar disorder, the goal of which is to alter family interactions that interfere with medication adherence and promote affective recurrences. Patients and their relatives are exposed to a series of modules that focus on education about bipolar illness in general and their own symptoms in particular, developing a relapse prevention plan, enhancing communication between patients and their relatives, and solving family problems (Craighead and Miklowitz 2000). A recent study of this adjunctive treatment showed that it was associated with fewer relapses and longer delays before relapses when added to open treatment with mood-stabilizing medications (Miklowitz et al. 2000).

Behavior Therapy

Therapies for depression derived from principles of classic and operant conditioning, social learning theory, and learned helplessness include social learning approaches (Lewinsohn et al. 1984; P.D. McLean 1982), self-control therapy (Rehm 1977), social skills training (Hersen et al. 1984), and structured problem-solving therapy (Nezu 1986). Behavior therapies use education, guided practice, homework assignments, and social reinforcement of successive approximations in a time-limited format, typically over 8–16 weeks. Depressive behaviors such as self-blame, passivity, and negativism are ignored, whereas behaviors that are inconsistent with depression, such as activity, experiencing pleasure, and solving problems, are rewarded. Rewards can include anything that the patient seems to seek out—from attention, to praise, to being permitted to withdraw or complain, to money. Learned helplessness is combated by the therapist's giving patients small, discrete tasks that very gradually become more demanding. For example, the person who feels hopeless about ever finding a job is first given the task of getting a newspaper. The next task is merely to look at the want ads, and only later is a list of possible jobs drawn up and one letter of application written. Each positive experience reinforces a feeling of accomplishment that makes the next task easier. Social skills training teaches self-reinforcement, assertive behavior, and the use of social reinforcers such as eye contact and compliments (Thase 1995).

In a meta-analysis of 10 suitable studies by the Agency for Health Care Policy and Services Research (1993), behavior therapy had an overall intention-to-treat efficacy rate of 55.3% and appeared to have a small advantage in relation to comparison psychotherapies in six studies and to pharmacotherapy in two studies. However, the adequacy of the treatments to which behavior therapy was compared has been questioned (Crits-Christoph 1992; Meterissian and Bradwejn 1989). Behavior therapy has appeared to be as effective in depression (R.A. Brown and Lewinsohn 1984) as it is in other psychiatric disorders (Budman et al. 1988). Group and individual behavior therapies appear to have similar efficacy rates.

Support for the efficacy of maintenance behavior therapy in preventing depressive recurrence is not as well developed as is support for its efficacy as an acute treat-ment (Thase 1995). Some studies comparing behavior therapy with no psychotherapy suggested that the benefits of behavior therapy persist after treatment is discontinued (P.D. McLean and Hakstian 1990; Nezu 1986), whereas other studies did not support this hypothesis (R.A. Brown and Lewinsohn 1984; Gallagher-Thompson et al. 1990). Adding antidepressants to behavior therapy did not enhance the outcome in three randomized outpatient trials of the combination (Hersen et al. 1984; Roth et al. 1982; Wilson 1982), but improvement was more rapid in two of the trials (Roth et al. 1982; Wilson 1982). Antidepressants also may have helped a greater number of more severely depressed patients to remain in trials of behavior therapy (Last et al. 1985; Thase 1995).

Psychodynamic Psychotherapy

At one time, extended and often unstructured psychodynamic psychotherapy was the standard psychotherapy for depression, and some case reports seemed to support its efficacy (Arieti and MacKenzie 1988; Gabbard 1995). With more experience, the utility of nondirective "traditional" psychodynamic approaches as treatments for depression (as opposed to character pathology) was increasingly questioned (Thase 1995). No controlled studies of prolonged psychodynamic psychotherapy or psychoanalysis in mood disorders have been done (Gabbard 1995). Brief dynamic psychotherapies have been applied to depressive disorders (Davenloo 1982; Luborsky 1984; Mann 1973; Strupp and Binder 1984), but they have not been studied as rigorously as have cognitive therapy and IPT (American Psychiatric Association 1993; Gabbard 1995). In eight randomized controlled trials, the utility of brief dynamic therapy has been studied, but methodological considerations limit the conclusions that can be drawn (Gabbard 1995). For example, low response rates (~35%) both to psychotherapy and to treatment with antidepressants raise questions about the adequacy of either treatment and the nature of the samples. In addition, five of the six studies examined the treatments in a group format even though individual therapy is more widely practiced, and the therapy usually was performed by nonprofessional therapists who were not formally trained in brief dynamic therapy (Gabbard 1995).

Motivational Enhancement and Relapse Prevention

Motivational enhancement, a manualized therapy developed for the treatment of substance dependence, has been modified to serve as an adjunctive approach designed to enhance compliance with antidepressant therapy. This is a particularly important problem in primary care practice, in which few depressed patients continue antidepressants for the minimum recommended 6–9 months and even fewer receive maintenance treatment despite the high rate of relapse and recurrence (Lin et al. 1998; G. Simon et al. 1995). A relapse prevention program developed for primary care practices uses motivational enhancement with development of an individualized treatment plan that reviews potential advantages and disadvantages of continuing antidepressants, regular support, and outreach to patients with evidence of symptom return and their primary physicians (Katon et al. 2001). An efficacy study found that primary care patients randomly assigned to a relapse prevention program had greater medication adherence and fewer depressive symptoms but not a reduction in rates of relapse or recurrence over 1 year of follow-up (Katon et al. 2001).

Characteristics of an Effective Psychotherapy for Depression

Even though data from controlled studies of psychotherapy for depression are limited, the characteristics listed in Table 10–21 have repeatedly emerged as distinguishing effective treatments, regardless of the technical details of the therapy (Keller et al. 1996; Thase 1996). Extended, unstructured psychotherapies may be useful for treating associated problems such as personality disorders, but given the lack of data supporting the use of these therapies as primary treatments for depression, more focused, time-limited therapies seem appropriate, at least as initial approaches.

Combining Medications and Psychotherapy

A recent review of two studies of psychodynamic therapy, three trials of behavior therapy, and nine studies of cognitive therapy, all of which added antidepressants during the acute phase of treatment, found only a trend favoring an advantage for combined treatment, mainly because the studies reviewed had insufficient statistical power (Hollon and Fawcett 1995; Kazdin and Bass 1989). Until more informative data become available about mild to moderate unipolar nonpsychotic depression, the recommendation that such depressive episodes be treated initially either with antidepressants or with one of the focused psychotherapies for depression (Klerman et al. 1974) seems reasonable. Some experts suggest that more severe major depressive episodes be treated first with antidepressants alone, so that time is not lost and the expense of psychotherapy is avoided for those

TABLE 10–21. Characteristics of an effective psychotherapy for depression

Time limited
Explicit rationale for treatment shared by patient and therapist
Active and directive therapist
Focus on current problems
Emphasis on changing current behavior
Self-monitoring of progress
Involvement of significant others
Expression of cautious optimism
Problems divided into manageable units with short-term goals
Homework assignments

patients who respond to a single treatment. These experts recommend combining medication and psychotherapy for patients with an inadequate response to either modality, with multiple symptom clusters that might respond differentially to psychotherapy and medication, or with a previously chronic course. More severe cases of depression may be more likely to have a better response to combined pharmacotherapy and psychotherapy than either treatment alone (Doris et al. 1999).

Because addition of IPT to antidepressants reduced the attrition rate from 21% to 8% in the continuation therapy study of patients with recurrent unipolar depression (Frank et al. 1990), psychotherapy should be included in the maintenance treatment of recurrent unipolar depression, even if the index episode was not severe. However, as mentioned earlier, adding psychotherapy to antidepressants may be more efficient than starting both treatments at the same time unless barriers to compliance with medications are identified at the start of treatment or the mood disorder is more severe or complex. Combining thymoleptic (mood-stabilizing) medications with IPSRT and behavioral techniques that reduce expressed emotion in the family shows promise of improving both medication compliance (Cochran 1984) and overall treatment response in bipolar mood disorders (Goodwin and Jamison 1991; Miklowitz 1992; Miklowitz and Goldstein 1990; Miklowitz et al. 1988).

Integrated Treatment of Mood Disorders

Although psychotherapy and antidepressants are equally effective for mild depression (Martin et al. 1992), controlled outpatient studies of nonbipolar depression showed that combined pharmacotherapy and psychotherapy was significantly more effective than psychotherapy alone for severe depression (Martin et al. 1992). A "mega-analysis" involved a meta-analysis of original data of 595 patients with nonbipolar, nonpsychotic MDD enrolled in six standardized treatment protocols in which they received treatment for 16 weeks with either CBT or IPT alone ($n = 243$) or IPT plus an antidepressant ($n = 352$) (Thase et al. 1997b). In mild depression, combined therapy was not significantly more effective than psychotherapy alone. However, in more severe recurrent major depression, combined treatment was significantly more effective. In a comparison of monotherapy with nefazodone, a form of CBT alone, or the combination of the two, the combination was statistically and clinically significantly superior to either treatment alone in producing initial improvement and preventing relapse in patients with chronic depression (Keller et al. 2000).

The American Psychiatric Association (1993) "Practice Guideline for Major Depressive Disorder in Adults" states that successful treatment of mood disorders begins with a careful diagnostic, psychosocial, and medical evaluation and consideration of the patient's treatment preferences. The initial assessment of the patient with a mood disorder (and all subsequent treatment) occurs in the context of a relationship between doctor and patient. This interaction is crucial to the development of a therapeutic alliance (Sexton et al. 1996) in which the patient is engaged in a collaborative enterprise (A.T. Beck et al. 1979). In the NIMH Collaborative Study, the therapeutic alliance significantly affected outcomes of IPT, CBT, active pharmacotherapy, and placebo (Blatt et al. 1996; Krupnick et al. 1996). Treatment dropout rates are less than 10% when a collaborative alliance has been fostered (Frank et al. 1995). Informed consent is an essential component of a therapeutic alliance. Insofar as no treatment is clearly established as superior to other reasonable therapies for most mood disorders, the process of obtaining consent should involve a discussion of alternative therapies, the evidence in favor of and against the treatment course that is being recommended, and the likely outcome of no treatment. Like most aspects of the treatment of mood disorders, informed consent is a dynamic process that should periodically be reevaluated.

Evaluation of risk factors for suicide is essential in all patients with mood disorders (Buzan and Weissberg 1992). Because suicidal patients, especially those with psychotic mood disorders, bipolar illness, or both, may kill someone else before they kill themselves (Dubovsky and Thomas 1992), homicide risk also should be evaluated. Dangerousness is not a static issue but one that evolves with the mood disorder. It is therefore necessary to reevaluate dangerousness to self and others repeatedly throughout the treatment of a mood disorder. It is also important to inquire about nonsuicidal forms of self-destructive behavior, which are particularly common in patients with comorbid mood and personality disorders and in some patients with bipolar mood disorders.

Review of the patient's use of substances that can cause or aggravate depression and mania is another essential component of the evaluation of the patient with a mood disorder. Ongoing debate about the possibility of starting an antidepressant before abstinence has been achieved notwithstanding, it is much more difficult to treat a mood disorder in a patient who is actively using alcohol or illicit drugs. Because the presence of comorbid disorders in addition to substance-related disorders, such as medical illness, panic disorder, eating disorders, OCD, generalized anxiety, social phobia, posttraumatic stress disorder, and personality disorders, can alter prognosis and call for a modification of the treatment, it is also important to diagnose these conditions in patients with mood disorders.

The next important step is to decide whether the mood disorder is unipolar or bipolar. Such a distinction is crucial given the different treatment approaches to the two disorders. When a patient has a clear-cut history of mania, the diagnosis is straightforward; bipolar disorder may be more difficult to identify when a patient has had one or a few depressive episodes without obvious manic or hypomanic symptoms. Clues to bipolarity in a depressed patient are summarized in Table 10–22, although like all other aspects of mood disorders, the bipolar-unipolar distinction is one that may be clarified only with continued observation.

TABLE 10–22. Clues to bipolarity in depressed patients

Highly recurrent depression
Intense anger
Racing thoughts
Mood-incongruent psychotic symptoms
Hallucinations
Thrill seeking
Increased libido with severe depression
Family history of bipolar disorder
Three consecutive generations with mood disorders

Unipolar Major Depressive Disorder

A mildly to moderately severe single major depressive episode without psychotic features can be treated with antidepressants or psychotherapy. However, the longer the duration of the episode or the greater its severity, the more likely an antidepressant is to be needed. Even if formal psychotherapy is not provided, antidepressant prescriptions should at least be accompanied by informed psychological management (Merriam and Karasu 1996). Because the presence of a comorbid personality disorder or perfectionism predicts a poorer response to antidepressants (Blatt 1995; Shea et al. 1990), as well as to briefer psychotherapies (Shea and Hirschfeld 1996; Thase 1996), more intensive forms of psychodynamic psychotherapy may be appropriately added to antidepressants when these factors are present (Conte et al. 1986; Gabbard 1995; I.W. Miller and Keitner 1996), although empirical support for this approach has not yet emerged. Conjoint therapy should be considered for patients with more complicated disorders because interpersonal issues are often important to address and because depressed patients often have depressed people in their families. Treatment of depression in a primary care setting is much less likely to include psychotherapy in any form than is treatment by mental health professionals, which produces better results (Meredith 1996; Schulberg 1996).

As was mentioned earlier, all of the currently available antidepressants are equally effective (Bech 1993; Hollon and Fawcett 1995; Kasper et al. 1992). This is not to say that all antidepressants are equally effective for all patients; many patients who do not respond to one agent will respond to another (Rush and Kupfer 1995). The initial choice of an antidepressant generally depends on history and current symptoms. For example, patients who have had a good response to a particular antidepressant may respond to the same medication again, although an antidepressant that was effective at one point may not be as effective on a second trial. Insomnia associated with depression often improves with remission of depression, but more sedating antidepressants such as doxepin, imipramine, trazodone, mirtazapine, and nefazodone can produce more rapid relief of insomnia, whereas more activating antidepressants such as fluoxetine, bupropion, and tranylcypromine can aggravate insomnia (Neylan 1995). Because of their marked antihistaminic properties, trimipramine and doxepin can be useful for treating allergies and peptic ulcer disease, and nefazodone may be useful for treating fibromyalgia. Newer antidepressants are safer than TCAs in patients with heart block and probably in patients with recent myocardial infarctions (Glassman and Proud'homme 1993). Patients with atypical depression appear to respond most frequently to MAOIs and least frequently to TCAs (which are still more effective than placebos); SSRIs are intermediate in efficacy (Quitkin et al. 1990, 1991; Rabkin et al. 1995).

Once recovery with antidepressant therapy begins, its time course is the same as spontaneous remission, suggesting that antidepressants may speed recovery but not change its natural course (Weiss et al. 1993). One implication of this finding is that antidepressants should be continued acutely at least for at least as long as the depressive episode would be expected to last if it had remained untreated. It may take longer than anticipated in the acute treatment of major depression to produce a complete remission. For example, in a Dutch cohort of 56 patients with MDD treated with pharmacotherapy and psychotherapy (Van Londen et al. 1998), 49% of the patients had a full remission and 45% had a partial remission after 9 months. Over the next 3–5 years, 82% had full remission; 16% of the patients required 2 years to reach a full remission. Over the same period, 41% of the sample had recurrences.

Another investigation randomized patients with chronic major or double depression who were partial responders after 3 months of treatment with either imipramine or sertraline to continuation treatment with the same antidepressant (Carney and Jackson 1998). During the next 4 months, 50% of the sample had remissions, 30% remained partial responders, and 20% underwent a change from partial to no response. This result suggests that partial responders to treatment of chronic depression may respond to an additional 4 months of treatment (Carney and Jackson 1998). After satisfactory responses for 7 months, the responders were randomized to maintenance with sertraline or placebo. Sertraline was clinically and statistically superior to placebo in preventing relapse (Carney and Jackson 1998).

Antidepressant overdose is the most common method of suicide in the United States (Buzan and Weissberg 1992). A large body of clinical experience contradicts a report of a small number of cases in which suicidal ideation was thought to be increased by SSRIs (Teicher et al. 1993) and indicates that the risk of suicide is reduced by all antidepressants, especially SSRIs, which decrease inwardly as well as outwardly directed impulsive aggression (Isacsson et al. 1996; Letizia et al. 1996; Warshaw and Keller 1996). Because the newer antidepressants are safer in overdose than TCAs (Glassman and Proud'homme 1993), SSRIs, venlafaxine, mirtazapine, and nefazodone may be the best initial choices for suicidal patients (Montgomery 1995). Prescribing small quantities of antidepressants to a suicidal patient in an attempt to prevent the patient from taking a lethal overdose causes the patient to make frequent trips to the pharmacy, which may encourage noncompliance and indirectly increase the risk of suicide because depression is undertreated. If the risk of suicide is so great that the physician cannot trust the patient with an antidepressant, the patient should be hospitalized.

Debate continues about the best antidepressant for severe depression. Well-publicized controlled studies found clomipramine to be superior to the SSRIs citalopram and paroxetine in severely depressed inpatients (Danish University Antidepressant Group 1986, 1990). However, not all controlled studies support the hypothesis that TCAs are more effective than SSRIs in more severe forms of unipolar depression (Nierenberg 1994). This issue remains unresolved because detecting a statistically significant difference in the efficacy of two active antidepressants requires more than 350 patients in each treatment group and is otherwise methodologically difficult (Lader 1988). ECT is a particularly appropriate option for patients who are too severely depressed or suicidal to wait for an antidepressant to take effect, patients who cannot tolerate an antidepressant, and patients with associated illnesses that might benefit from ECT, such as delirium or Parkinson's disease (Devanand et al. 1991a; Dubovsky 1995b).

A substantial amount of information has accumulated about the treatment of major depression with psychotic features. Psychotic depression has a very low rate of spontaneous recovery (Kettering et al. 1987) and virtually no response to placebo (Spiker and Kupfer 1988) or psychotherapy alone (Dubovsky and Thomas 1992). Only 0%–46% (average, about 25%–35%) of patients with psychotic depression respond to TCAs (Avery and Lubano 1979; W.H. Nelson et al. 1984), even in high doses (Avery and Lubano 1979; W.H. Nelson et al. 1984; Spiker et al. 1986b); MAOIs do not produce better results (Janicak et al. 1988b). Whereas 19%–48% of psychotically depressed patients recover with antipsychotic medications alone (Spiker et al. 1986a, 1986b), the combination of a neuroleptic and an antidepressant leads to improvement in an average of 70%–80% of patients (Anton and Burch 1986; Aronson et al. 1988; Spiker et al. 1986b). "Combination therapy" involves more than differential treatment of psychosis by the antipsychotic drug and depression by the antidepressant because neuroleptic therapy alone ameliorates depression in some patients, and antidepressants alone ameliorate psychosis in others (Dubovsky and Thomas 1992). Higher neuroleptic doses than those used for schizophrenia may be needed for psychotic depression (Aronson et al. 1987; J.C. Nelson et al. 1986; Spiker et al. 1985, 1986b). Amoxapine, an antidepressant that is a metabolite of the neuroleptic loxatine and has neuroleptic properties of its own, is almost as effective as traditional neuroleptic-antidepressant combinations in psychotic depression (Anton and Burch 1986). Preliminary experience suggests that atypical antipsychotic drugs also may be effective as monotherapy (McElroy et al. 1991). The response rate of psychotic depression is greatest with ECT (Solan et al. 1988).

The antidepressant properties of atypical antipsychotic agents, and their lower risk of neurological side effects, make these medications appealing choices for treating psychotic depression. A review of records of 15 hospitalized patients with discharge diagnoses of unipolar or bipolar depression with psychotic features who were given olanzapine compared with matched patients who took neuroleptics (most in each group also taking antidepressants) found a higher rate of improvement in the patients who received olanzapine (Rothschild et al. 1999). Obviously, controlled prospective trials would be necessary to determine whether atypical antipsychotic drugs may be effective alone or in combination with antidepressants.

Following initial improvement, response to an antidepressant sometimes fades. A review of published double-blind, placebo-controlled trials with at least 20 patients reporting loss of antidepressant efficacy during maintenance treatment found this problem to be reported in 9%–33% of patients (van Luijtelaar et al. 1995). Relapse during the first 12 weeks was thought to reflect loss of an initial placebo response, especially when features of a placebo response such as abrupt, fluctuating improvement were present initially. The authors found 75 reported cases that were thought to reflect tolerance to antidepressants following full remission rather than loss of a placebo effect. Tolerance to antidepressants has been reported with serotonin reuptake inhibitors, heterocyclic antidepressants, and MAOIs.

Several possible mechanisms of tolerance to antidepressants exist (van Luijtelaar et al. 1995). A common problem with antidepressants that induce their own metabolism or are taken along with other medications that induce metabolizing enzymes such as carbamazepine is pharmacokinetic tolerance, or a decline in serum levels below the therapeutic range. This problem is usually corrected with one or more increases in dose until levels remain constant. Pharmacodynamic tolerance is probably caused by intracellular mechanisms that attempt to restore the premorbid state by overriding the response of receptors or other targets to the medication. In this situation, raising the dose of an antidepressant may produce a brief return of therapeutic benefit, but this wears off rapidly and a change in medication or a medication combination is likely to be necessary. Treatment with fluoxetine is sometimes associated with the late development of a therapeutic window, possibly because of accumulation of a long-acting metabolite such as norfluoxetine, levels of which may be negatively correlated with antidepressant efficacy of the parent drug. This problem requires a reduction rather than an increase in dose of the antidepressant.

Certain varieties of treatment-emergent loss of antidepressant benefit require a more global reconsideration of the pharmacological strategy (van Luijtelaar et al. 1995). The most important of these is bipolar depression masquerading as recurrent or fluctuating unipolar depression. The antidepressant is effective initially, but as it accelerates the tendency of bipolar depression to recur as well as its tendency to remit, another episode appears that is mistaken for loss of antidepressant efficacy. A change in the antidepressant produces another remission, but this is inevitably followed by another recurrence, often mixed with dysphoric hypomanic symptoms such as anxiety, intense irritability, racing thoughts, inability to shut one's mind off and get to sleep, overstimulation, or subtle psychotic symptoms. Whereas continuing to change the dose or preparation of the antidepressant produces more recurrences and sometimes more persistent depression, adding a mood-stabilizing medication and gradually withdrawing the antidepressant often eliminates depressive recurrences.

Dysthymic Disorder and Chronic Major Depression

Placebo-controlled trials show that dysthymia responds as well as major depression does to TCAs, SSRIs, MAOIs, and atypical antidepressants such as tianeptine, although rates of noncompliance related to demoralization and intolerance of adverse effects are high (Conte and Karasu 1992; Harrison and Stewart 1993; Keller et al. 1996; Kocsis et al. 1988, 1989). In a comparison of the effect of ECT in 25 patients with double depression and 75 patients with MDD only, Prudic et al. (1993) found that both groups had the same level of improvement in depression rating scale scores. However, patients with double depression had more residual symptoms and were more likely to relapse in the year following ECT, which suggests that the underlying dysthymia had been incompletely treated.

Psychotherapies that have been found useful for treating chronic depressive disorders, albeit creating a less robust response than in acute depression (Keller et al. 1996; Thase et al. 1994), include cognitive therapy, IPT, behavior therapy, CBT, supportive therapy, psychoeducation, and family and marital therapy (Akiskal 1994; Conte and Karasu 1992; Frances 1993; Keitner and Miller 1990). Combining specific psychotherapies with antidepressants produces better results than medication therapy alone in dysthymic patients (Conte and Karasu 1992; Frances 1993; J. Scott 1988). Maintenance pharmacotherapy and psychotherapy are particularly important in reducing the risk of recurrence of dysthymia, as well as that of chronic major depression and double depression.

Recurrent Brief Depression

Only a few studies of the treatment of recurrent brief depression have been done. The data that have emerged suggest that antidepressants are not particularly effective in preventing acute depressive recurrences (Angst et al. 1990). Lithium may reduce recurrences, even though no evidence has emerged of a bipolar outcome in recurrent brief depression (Angst and Hochstrasser 1994). It is not known whether other mood-stabilizing medications might reduce the rate of recurrence of this form of depression, but insofar as all of these medications have antirecurrence as well as antimanic properties, it seems reasonable to consider using them. If recurrent brief depression is considered a mood disorder in which a bipolar trait (i.e., a high rate of recurrence) is combined with a type of depression that is unipolar in its form, the possibility must be considered that chronic use of antidepressants could have the potential to speed up the rate of recurrence of acute depressive episodes. This hypothesis awaits formal testing.

Seasonal Affective Disorder

Artificial bright light is an effective treatment for SAD (Rosenthal et al. 1989) in which rates of remission in published studies range from 36% to 75% (Rosenthal and Oren 1995; Tam et al. 1995). The minimal intensity of light that appears necessary for an antidepressant effect is 2,500 lux (1 lux = 10 foot candles) placed about 1 m from the patient (Rosenthal et al. 1989). At greater intensities of light, a shorter duration of exposure to the light appears necessary. For example, remission rates with a 10,000-lux light unit for 30 minutes are similar to those with 2,500 lux for 2 hours (Tam et al. 1995). To be effective, light must enter the patient's eyes (Rosenthal et al. 1989). The assumption that light acts through retinohypothalamic pathways to normalize a phase delay in melatonin secretion has been questioned (Thalen et al. 1995), although compensatory phase advancing the sleep–wake cycle with morning bright light probably is a mechanism of action in some cases (Rosenthal et al. 1989). A light visor is available that has a lower intensity of light but is closer to the eyes than the standard light box, but the 35%–40% response rate to light-visor treatment is no better than to a placebo (Teicher et al. 1995). Use of an "artificial dawn," in which light of gradually increasing intensity is turned on before the patient wakes up, may be useful but is not as effective as standard light therapy (Tam et al. 1995).

Although some patients respond exclusively to morning light and some respond equally well to light adminis-

1997) and for more subtle mixed states, but divalproex in particular is often not very effective as a primary antidepressant for patients without mixed hypomanic symptoms. Lamotrigine has more obvious antidepressant properties (Sachs et al. 2000); however, because its capacity to stabilize mood at the same time remains to be clearly established, it is probably safer to combine it with a well-established antimanic drug.

When bipolar depression does not remit with treatment with an antimanic drug, the clinician must decide whether to add a second antimanic drug or an antidepressant. Antimanic drugs are not as effective as antidepressants for treating depression and have more adverse effects, but all antidepressants carry the risk of inducing mania and rapid cycling (Akiskal 1994; Peet and Peters 1995; Srisurapanont et al. 1995). In the absence of controlled data, only clinical experience and expert opinion are available to guide the choice between these two courses. Our experience has been that antidepressants do not produce a predictably positive response in bipolar depression with prominent mixed hypomanic symptoms such as profound irritability, decreased sleep without feeling tired during the day, racing thoughts, extreme interpersonal sensitivity, hallucinations, or increased libido. Instead, the antidepressant either provokes more dysphoric hypomania or produces initial improvement followed by more recurrences of mixed bipolar depression. Treatment with a combination of antimanic drugs may produce a remission, or it may at least convert a refractory mixed state to a more uncomplicated bipolar depression with hypersomnia, lethargy, slowed thinking, and lack of interpersonal sensitivity that may respond more predictably to addition of an antidepressant.

The combination of lithium and carbamazepine has been found to have antidepressant properties in some reported cases (Ketter et al. 1995; Post 1988). Verapamil has been used to treat bipolar depression in a few cases (Deicken 1990), but nimodipine may be a more effective treatment for bipolar depression as well as brief recurrent depression (Pazzaglia et al. 1993). Initial experience suggested that lamotrigine and gabapentin may have antidepressant as well as antimanic properties that could prove useful for treating mixed bipolar depression (Calabrese et al. 1996a), but no studies of this indication exist. If psychotic symptoms are present, it may be necessary to add neuroleptic therapy, but continuation of neuroleptic therapy may contribute to depressive recurrences in some cases (Dubovsky and Buzan 1997; Hendrick et al. 1994). As we pointed out earlier, clozapine appears to have distinct mood-stabilizing properties that can be useful in complex ultradian cycling and mixed states (Zarate et al. 1995a, 1996).

It seems clear that antidepressants normally should not be administered to patients with bipolar depression unless an antimanic drug is coadministered (Nolen and Bloenkolk 2000; Sachs et al. 2000). However, the choice of a specific antidepressant in treating bipolar depression is limited by lack of replicated data. The TCAs seem more likely to induce mania and rapid cycling than bupropion, the MAOIs, and the SSRIs (Akiskal 1994; Rosenbaum et al. 1995; Sachs et al. 1994a; Stoll et al. 1994). Stimulants generally are not used as primary antidepressants in unipolar depression because tolerance to their antidepressant action develops, but the rapid onset and short duration of antidepressant effect of stimulants can be useful for treating bipolar depression. Artificial bright light can be a rapidly effective and safe antidepressant for bipolar depression with a seasonal component or with lethargy and oversleeping (Papatheodorou and Kutcher 1995); as is true of stimulants, the short duration of action may make adverse effects on mood wear off more rapidly. The atypical antipsychotic drugs other than clozapine can be useful antidepressants, as can lamotrigine and gabapentin. The most reliable class of antidepressant medication for bipolar depression is probably the MAOIs, particularly tranylcypromine (Ketter et al. 1995; Nolen and Bloenkolk 2000). ECT is the most effective treatment for bipolar depression (Dubovsky 1995b), which is unlike other antidepressant therapies in that it rarely induces mania, and when it does, further ECT usually normalizes mood.

In contrast to unipolar depression, no evidence indicates that continuation of antidepressants after remission of bipolar depression prevents further depressive recurrences (H. Loo and Brochier 1995). In view of the risks of long-term antidepressant therapy, it seems prudent to attempt to withdraw the antidepressant once mood normalizes, while continuing the mood-stabilizing regimen (Sharma et al. 1997). Gradual discontinuation of antidepressants may reduce the risk of rebound of depression. If it becomes necessary to continue treatment with the antidepressant, lower doses may be less likely to destabilize mood. As described later in this chapter (see section "Bipolar Disorder: Maintenance Treatment"), maintenance ECT can prevent recurrences of bipolar depression as well as mania. One model of treatment of bipolar depression is illustrated in Figure 10–3.

Mixed and Rapid-Cycling Bipolar Disorder

Although the response rate of uncomplicated mania to lithium in three recent trials ranged from 59% to 91%, response rates in patients with mixed states were only

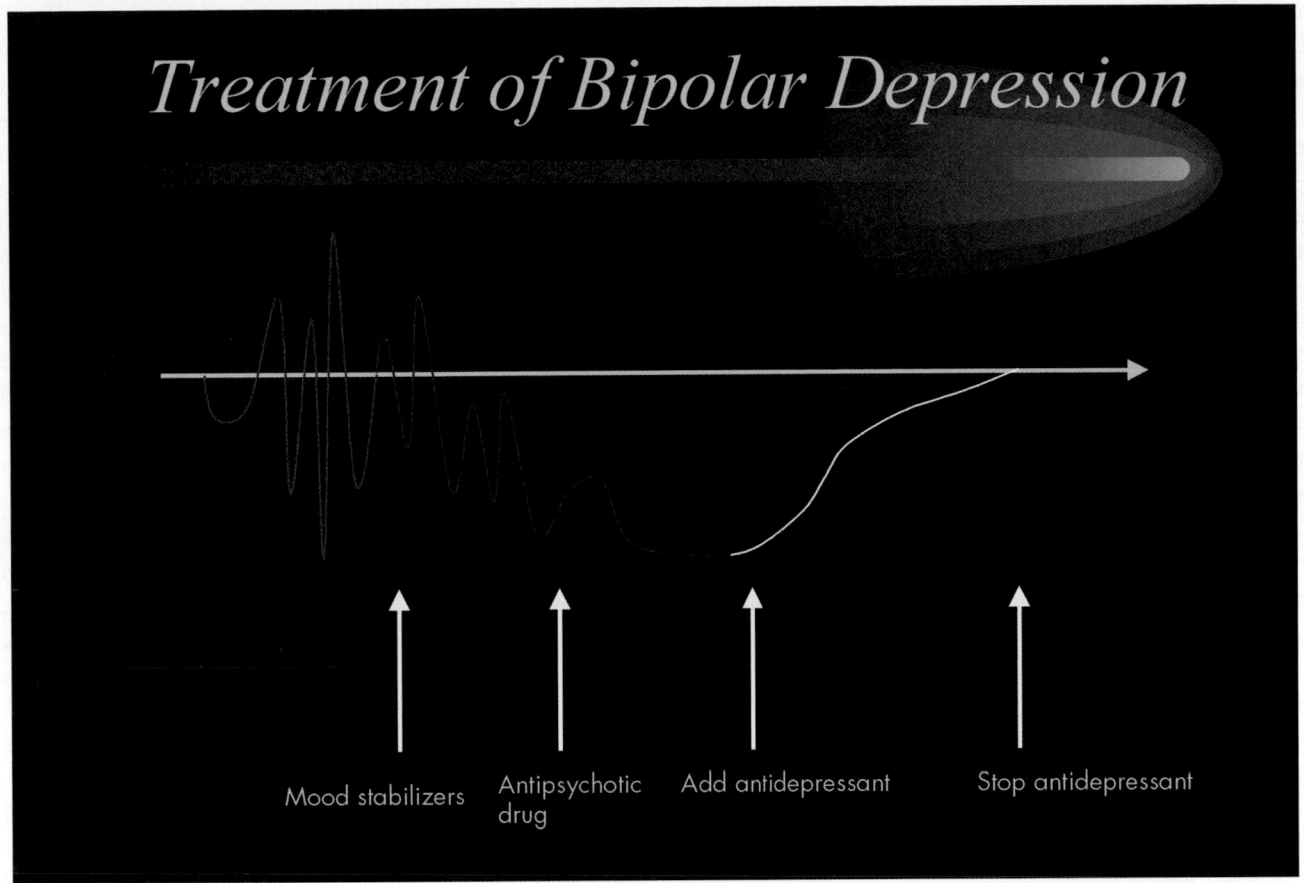

FIGURE 10–3. Treatment of bipolar depression.

29%–43% (S. Gershon and Soares 1997); similar results have been obtained in patients with rapid cycling. Patients with either form of complex mood disorder may have a better response to valproate or carbamazepine (Freeman et al. 1992; Post 1992a; Swann et al. 1997). Valproate appears to be equally effective in rapid- and nonrapid-cycling bipolar disorder (Bowden et al. 1994). A consensus panel recommended valproate as the first choice for treating rapid cycling, followed by carbamazepine and then lithium (Expert Consensus Panel 1996). Additional treatments that have been reported to be useful for some patients with rapid-cycling bipolar disorder include ECT, antimanic combinations, nimodipine, clozapine, and supplementation with suprametabolic doses of thyroxine (Bauer and Whybrow 1990; Baumgartner et al. 1994; Calabrese et al. 1991, 1996b; Expert Consensus Panel 1996; Frye et al. 1996; Goodnick 1995; Pazzaglia et al. 1993; Stancer and Persad 1982; Suppes et al. 1994; Swann 1995; Terao 1993; Wehr et al. 1988). As we mentioned in the previous section, it may be necessary first to use a combination of mood-stabilizing medications, possibly with supplementation with an antipsychotic medication (clozapine can be useful in refractory cases) to

eliminate cycling and mixed hypomanic symptoms, even if this produces stable bipolar depression without any mixed symptoms of activation. The next phase of treatment would involve introduction of an antidepressant, with an attempt to very slowly withdraw the antidepressant when the depression remits and an effort to slowly withdraw the antipsychotic medication, continuing the combination of mood-stabilizing medications.

Bipolar Disorder: Maintenance Treatment

The high rates of affective recurrence and the increasing severity and complexity and more rapid onset of each recurrence (Keller et al. 1993) are reasons to continue a mood-stabilizing regimen after remission of any acute episode of mania or bipolar depression. Treatment response can be assessed over time with the help of a structured mood chart. Post (1992a; Post et al. 1988) and others (Altschuler et al. 1995; Pazzaglia et al. 1993; Roy-Byrne et al. 1984) developed a "life-charting" method that quantifies symptoms and important life events. However, life charting is time-consuming and relies on observations by nursing staff. In everyday outpatient practice, it may be equally helpful to construct with the patient a graph on which specific symptoms are rated one or more times per day on whatever scale makes the most sense (e.g., mood can be rated from −5 for very depressed to +5 for manic, with 0 signifying euthymia). Different symptoms can be indicated by different line colors or styles, and changes in treatment and important events can be noted on the same graph. However it is accomplished, some form of prospective mood charting can be essential in tracking mixtures of depressive, hypomanic, and psychotic symptoms to determine whether to add more mood-stabilizing medications, an antipsychotic drug, or an antidepressant or whether a particular treatment should be withdrawn.

At least 10 double-blind, placebo-controlled studies containing more than 200 patients each reported that lithium substantially reduces the number of manic and depressive recurrences (0%–44% of patients taking lithium had recurrences, compared with 38%–93% of the patients taking placebo) (Goodwin and Jamison 1991; Solomon and Bauer 1993). Serum lithium levels greater than 0.8 mM are sometimes associated with half the recurrence rate of levels less than 0.6 mM, although adverse effects are more common at higher levels (American Psychiatric Association 1994b; Gelenberg et al. 1989). More than 50% of patients experience an affective episode within 6 months of discontinuing lithium therapy, but the risk of recurrence is almost five times as great (median time in remission = 4 months) in patients who discontinue lithium therapy rapidly than in those who taper the drug over several months (median time in remission = 20 months) (Baldessarini et al. 1996). There is no reason to expect different results with discontinuation of other thymoleptics. The prophylactic effect of lithium results in a substantial decrease in suicide rates, which adds 7 years to life expectancy (National Institute of Mental Health 1995). In a study of 405 patients with bipolar mood disorders and 92 with unipolar depression treated in a lithium clinic, the suicide rate increased by 80% if patients left the clinic and discontinued lithium and by 45% if patients left the clinic but continued to take lithium (Kallner et al. 2000).

Carbamazepine was effective as a maintenance treatment in bipolar illness in four published trials; however, lack of a placebo control in three of these trials and only a trend toward superiority of carbamazepine in the only placebo-controlled trial limit the strength of this conclusion (Solomon et al. 1995). Retrospective studies suggest that valproate prevents affective recurrences in bipolar disorder, but only one prospective placebo-controlled study of maintenance with valproate—in which patients were randomized to lithium monotherapy, divalproex monotherapy, or placebo—has been conducted (Solomon et al. 1995). Verapamil and nimodipine have had mood-stabilizing effects in small numbers of cases of bipolar mood disorder with varying degrees of placebo control (Dubovsky 1995a; Dubovsky and Buzan 1997). We reviewed earlier data indicating that mood-stabilizing properties of lamotrigine and the atypical antipsychotic medications have not yet been confirmed.

Case series suggest that combinations of two or three mood stabilizers may provide better affective prophylaxis than can be achieved with monotherapy (Bowden 1996; Expert Consensus Panel 1996). ECT is a highly effective maintenance therapy (Karliner and Wehrheim 1965; Vanelle et al. 1994). Neuroleptics may be necessary adjuncts in the maintenance therapy of psychotic bipolar disorder, although as noted earlier, these medications are thought to increase depressive recurrences in some cases. Clozapine seems more consistently effective as a mood stabilizer (Calabrese et al. 1991; Puri et al. 1995; Zarate et al. 1995b, 1996).

The efficacy of antimanic drugs in preventing recurrences (i.e., as mood stabilizers) has been noted to decline significantly from the first year to the fifth year of treatment (Peselow et al. 1994). Although the evolving physiology of bipolar disorder is probably one important factor in the increasing rate of recurrence with time, the fact that only one-third of outpatients are estimated to remain compliant is at least as important an issue (S. Gershon and Soares 1997). Noncompliance with mood stabilizers occurred in 64% of the patients in the month preceding hospitalization for acute mania in one study (Keck et al. 1996). On follow-up of 140 patients recently hospitalized for bipolar disorder, 51% were partially or totally noncompliant with medications (Keck et al. 1997). Nonadherence, the most common cause of which is denial of illness and the need for treatment, is more common in patients with comorbid substance use disorders (Keck et al. 1996). From a pharmacological standpoint, however, withdrawal of an effective mood stabilizer may result in refractoriness to that medication when it is reintroduced (Post et al. 1991).

Obviously, one important goal of any form of maintenance psychotherapy is to improve medication compliance (Frank et al. 1995; Miklowitz 1992; Miklowitz et al. 2000). IPSRT has been shown to stabilize circadian rhythms, and preliminary evidence suggests that it can enhance the action of mood-stabilizing medications (Frank et al. 1997; Miklowitz and Goldstein 1990). Even if formal IPT and logs of circadian cues are not used, helping the patient to keep regular hours, especially of going to sleep and waking up, and resolving interpersonal and family distress, including unrealistic expectations and high levels of expressed emotion, have an additive effect with mood-stabilizing medications (Frank et al. 1997; Miklowitz and Goldstein 1990; Miklowitz et al. 1988).

Use of Antimanic Drugs in Children and Adolescents

Lithium has not consistently been found to be effective in mania or bipolar depression in younger patients (Geller et al. 1996; Kafantaris 1995). As is true of unipolar depression, higher rates of spontaneous improvement and a high placebo response rate may contribute to the apparent reduced rate of responsiveness to lithium in juvenile bipolar mood disorder. It is also possible that this population requires more frequent dosing or higher serum levels than are required for a thymoleptic response in adults. Anticonvulsants have been the subject of open trials in childhood and adolescent bipolar disorder but not of placebo-controlled studies (Kafantaris 1995; Papatheodorou et al. 1995; Porter 1987). The results of these trials show that valproate and carbamazepine are well tolerated and possibly effective. Verapamil, which is used to treat childhood and adolescent cardiovascular disease, has been used successfully in a few cases of adolescent mania (Kastner and Friedman 1992). Case series and clinical experience indicate that ECT is as effective for treating mania in juvenile patients as it is in adults (Bertagnolli and Borchardt 1990; Carr et al. 1983; Kutcher and Robertson 1995). The course of juvenile bipolar disorder is more chronic than is that of adult bipolar disorder (Lewinsohn et al. 1995), but until empirical data are accumulated, decisions about the balance between potential positive and negative effects of maintenance medications on affective recurrence and intellectual and personality development are matters of opinion and personal experience.

Conclusion

Mood disorders are not unitary illnesses but complex syndromes with distinct etiologies, courses, and treatment responses that ultimately may be better understood through the addition of a more thorough dimensional analysis (e.g., early vs. late onset, comorbidity, disordered thinking, degree of intrusion into the personality) to existing categorical diagnoses and the DSM multiaxial approach. Even the most complete description of an affective episode at one point in time does not fully capture the picture of a mood disorder as it evolves over time. Mood disorders are not static but are dynamic conditions in which each new episode is a function of previous episodes with an evolving course and treatment response (Post 1992b).

As illustrated in Figure 10–4, the evolving course of mood disorders is the result of an incompletely understood interaction of genetics, personality traits, environmental factors, cell biology, and, at times, medication and substance use (Consensus Development Panel 1985; Dubovsky 1997; Post 1990a, 1992b, 1994; Post et al. 1986, 1992, 1996; Thase 1990; Thase and Kupfer 1996). In many cases, initial episodes appear in response to an external stress, usually a loss or separation, or an event that evokes strong arousal or helplessness. The degree to which such events provoke an affective episode depends on their intrinsic severity and on predisposing and protective factors within the individual who experiences them. Mood in early episodes is often more reactive to the environment. Symptoms are less complex, and psychosocial disruption is less complete. The neurobiology of an initial affective episode may be less complex because a single treatment is often effective, and the physiology and the psychology of abnormal mood remits completely with treatment in the absence of substantial genetic loading or overwhelming early adverse experience. If they are not too severe, early depressive episodes respond equally well to environmental manipulation, psychotherapy, or medications. Early uncomplicated hypomanic episodes may respond fully to a single antimanic drug, and it is possible that normalization of circadian rhythms, IPSRT, reduction of expressed emotion in the family, and other psychosocial interventions could be equally effective.

With succeeding affective episodes, the psychobiology of mania and depression becomes more deeply ingrained by processes such as sensitization and kindling, resetting of synaptic connections, and changes in gene expression induced by neurotransmitter, receptor, and second messenger responses to abnormal moods. At this stage, dysregulated affect becomes part of the baseline repertoire of the synapse. At the same time, negative thinking, intrusiveness, arrogance, withdrawal, social ineptitude, irritability, and other manic or depressive behaviors elicit negative input from others, which reinforces feelings of helplessness and solidifies the patient's identity as someone who is unfulfilled, overwhelmed, unpredictable, impulsive, incompetent, or unreliable. As more time is spent in the neurobiology and the psychology of abnormal mood, remissions are less complete and new recurrences develop with less provocation. These episodes are more likely to cause losses than to be caused by them.

Later affective recurrences are more abrupt, more severe, and more complex, as additional systems are recruited into an abnormal state. Additional pressure on

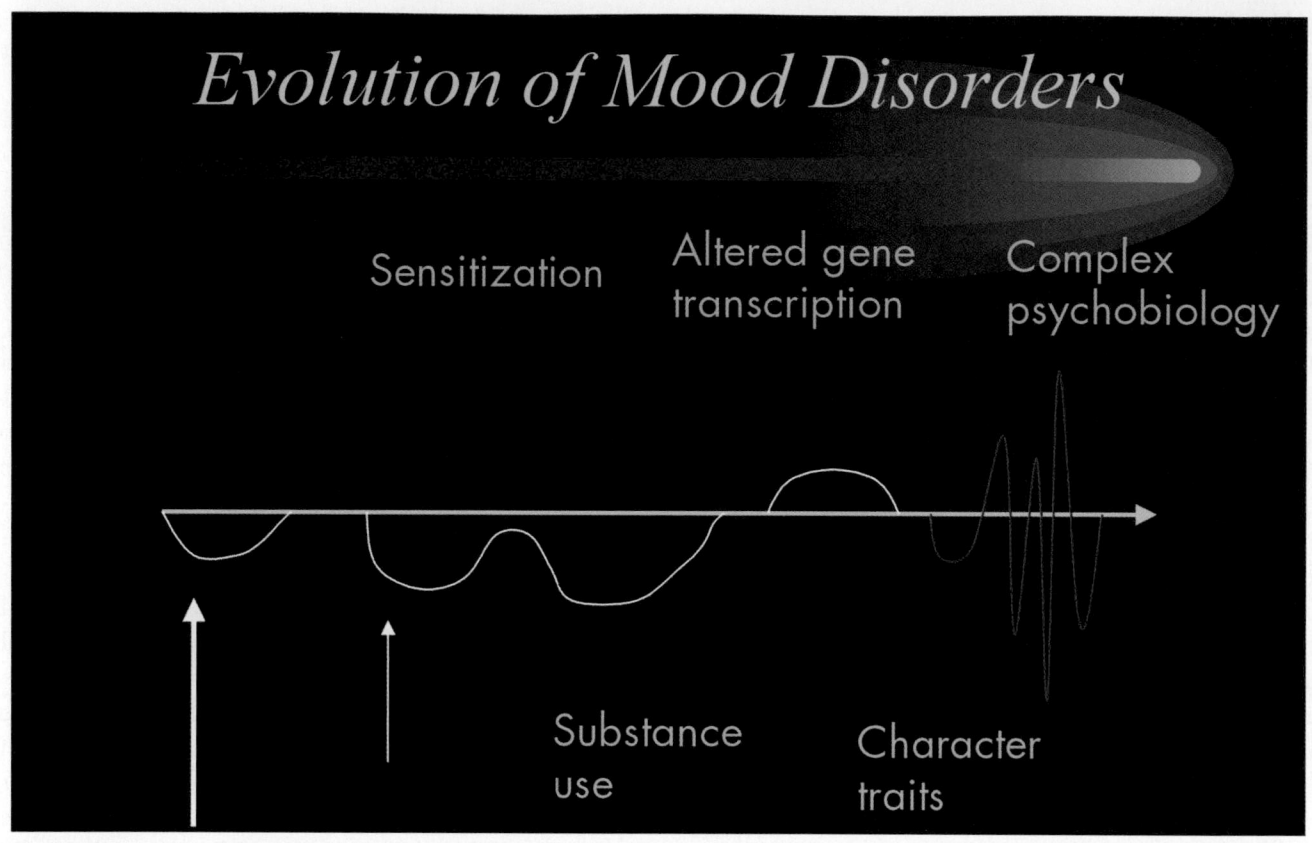

FIGURE 10–4. Evolution of mood disorders.

abnormal systems comes from medications and substances that can elicit affective dysregulation, especially those with stimulating, antidepressant, and pro-psychotic effects such as cocaine, amphetamines, and, in some cases, antidepressants taken for prolonged periods. Environmental manipulations are not as successful at this point because the mood disorder is less responsive to external events. Psychological constellations are less amenable to structured psychotherapies and require more vigorous efforts to become reorganized. In cases in which single medications initially were effective, more complex interventions are necessary to address multiple interacting elements of abnormal cellular function. New medications aimed at second messengers or gene expression may prove useful for treating later-stage mood disorders involving multiple transmitter and receptor systems, and more aggressive and extended forms of psychotherapy may be necessary for mood disorders that have become integrated into the personality.

Similar processes have been well described in other medical disorders. For example, early, small, well-differentiated cancers can be treated with a simple regimen of chemotherapy or radiation. Larger and metastasized cancers are much more complex, with increased expression of genes and proteins that are not normally expressed. Anticancer drugs become less effective as intracellular extrusion mechanisms for these medications are induced, and combinations of treatments acting on different aspects of pathophysiology usually are necessary. Oncologists realize that early, aggressive treatment aimed at a cure can prevent later evolution of an illness, of which the goal of treatment after one or more relapses becomes to control rather than to cure the disease process.

One important implication of the accumulating data about the course of mood disorders is that it is easier to treat early than later episodes of any mood disorder. Complete treatment of early episodes and continuation of effective therapy reduce the risk of later, more refractory episodes. Unfortunately, denial, reluctance to acknowledge needing help because being helped feels like a sign of weakness, pressure from family members who themselves may have mood disorders, and acceptance of a good but incomplete remission make it difficult for people in the early stages of a mood disorder to recognize the seriousness of the illness, let alone treat it. Public education has reduced the stigma of seeking treatment for depression to some extent, but efforts to educate primary care physicians, who are more likely than mental health professionals to encounter patients with mood disorders for the first time, have not been successful in increasing rates of effective recognition, treatment, and, when necessary, referral of these patients for specialty care. Research into strategies for approaching mood disorders in primary care practice is therefore as important as research into new treatment technologies.

References

Abernathy DR, Schwartz JB: Calcium-antagonist drugs. N Engl J Med 341:1447–1457, 2000

Abrams RC: Electroconvulsive Therapy. New York, Oxford University Press, 1988

Abramson LY, Seligman MEP, Teasdale JD: Learned helplessness in humans: critique and reformulation. J Abnorm Psychol 87:49–74, 1978

Adams PB, Lawson S, Sanigorski A, et al: Arachadonic acid to eicosapentaenoic acid ration in blood correlates positively with clinical symptoms of depression. Lipids 31(suppl):S157–S161, 1996

Agency for Health Care Policy and Services Research: Clinical Practice Guideline: Depression in Primary Care, Vol 2: Treatment of Major Depression. Rockville, MD, U.S. Department of Health and Human Services, 1993

Ahlfors UG, Baastrup PC, Dencker SJ: Flupenthixol decanoate in recurrent manic-depressive illness: a comparison with lithium. Acta Psychiatr Scand 64:226–237, 1981

Akiskal HS: The interface of chronic depression with personality and anxiety disorders. Psychopharmacol Bull 20:393–398, 1984

Akiskal HS: Chronic depression. Bull Menninger Clin 240:349–354, 1991

Akiskal HS: Dysthymic and cyclothymic depressions: therapeutic considerations. Compr Psychiatry 55(suppl 4):46–52, 1994

Akiskal HS: Developmental pathways to bipolarity: are juvenile-onset depressions pre-bipolar? J Am Acad Child Adolesc Psychiatry 34:754–763, 1995a

Akiskal HS: Le spectre bipolaire: acquisitions et perspectives cliniques. Encephale 21(Spec No 6):3–11, 1995b

Akiskal HS: The prevalent clinical spectrum of bipolar disorders: beyond DSM-IV. J Clin Psychopharmacol 16(suppl 1):4S–14S, 1996

Akiskal HS, Djenderedjian AM, Rosenthal RH, et al: Cyclothymic disorder: validating criteria for inclusion in the bipolar affective group. Am J Psychiatry 134:1227–1233, 1977

Akiskal HS, Walker P, Puzantian VR, et al: Bipolar outcome in the course of depressive illness. J Affect Disord 5:115–128, 1983

Akiskal HS, Downs J, Jordan P, et al: Affective disorders in referred children and younger siblings of manic-depressives. Arch Gen Psychiatry 42:996–1003, 1985

Akiyoshi J, Isogawa K, Yamada K, et al: Effects of antidepressants on intracellular Ca2+ mobilization in CHO cells transfected with the human 5-HT2C receptors. Biol Psychiatry 39:1000–1008, 1996

Albus M, Hubmann W, Wahlheim C, et al: Contrasts in neuropsychological test profile between patients with first-episode schizophrenia and first-episode affective disorders. Acta Psychiatr Scand 94:87–93, 1996

Altschuler LL, Post RM, Leverich GS: Antidepressant-induced mania and cycle acceleration: a controversy revisited. Am J Psychiatry 152:1130–1138, 1995

Ambrosini PJ, Bianchi MD, Rabinovich H, et al: Antidepressant treatments in children and adolescents, I: affective disorders. J Am Acad Child Adolesc Psychiatry 32:1–5, 1993

American Psychiatric Association: Diagnostic and Statistical Manual: Mental Disorders. Washington, DC, American Psychiatric Association, 1952

American Psychiatric Association: Diagnostic and Statistical Manual of Mental Disorders, 2nd Edition. Washington, DC, American Psychiatric Association, 1968

American Psychiatric Association: Diagnostic and Statistical Manual of Mental Disorders, 3rd Edition. Washington, DC, American Psychiatric Association, 1980

American Psychiatric Association: American Psychiatric Glossary. Washington, DC, American Psychiatric Press, 1984

American Psychiatric Association: Diagnostic and Statistical Manual of Mental Disorders, 3rd Edition, Revised. Washington, DC, American Psychiatric Association, 1987

American Psychiatric Association: The Practice of Electroconvulsive Therapy: Recommendations for Treatment, Training and Privileging. Washington, DC, American Psychiatric Association, 1990

American Psychiatric Association: Practice guideline for major depressive disorder in adults. Am J Psychiatry 150(suppl 4):1–26, 1993

American Psychiatric Association: Diagnostic and Statistical Manual of Mental Disorders, 4th Edition. Washington, DC, American Psychiatric Association, 1994a

American Psychiatric Association: Practice guideline for the treatment of patients with bipolar disorder. Am J Psychiatry 151(suppl 12):1–36, 1994b

American Psychiatric Association: Diagnostic and Statistical Manual of Mental Disorders, 4th Edition, Text Revision. Washington, DC, American Psychiatric Association, 2000

Ananth J, Wohl M, Ranganath V: Rapid cycling patients: conceptual and etiological factors. Neuropsychobiology 27:193–198, 1993

Andreasen NC: Creativity and mental illness: prevalence rates in writers and their first-degree relatives. Am J Psychiatry 144:1288–1292, 1987

Angst J: Clinical course of affective disorders, in Depressive Illness: Prediction of Course and Outcome. Edited by Hedgson T, Daly RJ. Berlin, Germany, Springer, 1988, pp 205–250

Angst J: Epidémiologie du spectre bipolaire. Encephale 21(Spec No 6):37–42, 1995

Angst J, Hochstrasser B: Recurrent brief depression: the Zurich Study. Compr Psychiatry 55(suppl 4):3–9, 1994

Angst J, Wicki W: The Zurich Study, XI: is dysthymia a separate form of depression? Results of the Zurich Cohort Study. Eur Arch Psychiatry Clin Neurosci 240:349–354, 1991

Angst J, Merikangas K, Scheidegger P, et al: Recurrent brief depression: a new subtype of affective disorder. J Affect Disord 19:87–98, 1990

Anonymous: Atypical antipsychotics for treatment of depression in schizophrenia and affective disorders. Collaborative Working Group on Clinical Trial Evaluations. J Clin Psychiatry 59(suppl 12):41–45, 1998

Anton RF, Burch EA: Amoxapine versus amitriptyline combined with perphenazine in the treatment of psychotic depression. Am J Psychiatry 147:1203–1208, 1986

Antonuccio DO, Danton WG, DeNelsky GY: Psychotherapy versus medication for depression: challenging the conventional wisdom with data. Professional Psychology: Research and Practice 26:574–585, 1995

Aperia B: Effects of electroconvulsive therapy on neuropsychological function and circulating levels of ACTH, cortisol, prolactin, and TSH in patients with major depressive illness. Acta Psychiatr Scand 72:536–541, 1985

Arieti S, MacKenzie KR: Psychotherapy of severe depression: recent developments in brief psychotherapy. Am J Psychiatry 39:852–864, 1988

Aronson TA, Shukla S, Hoff A: Continuation therapy after ECT for delusional depression: a naturalistic study of prophylactic treatments and relapse. Convuls Ther 3:251–259, 1987

Aronson TA, Shukla S, Hoff A, et al: Proposed delusional depression subtypes: preliminary evidence from a retrospective study of phenomenology and treatment course. J Affect Disord 14:69–74, 1988

Aronson TA, Shukla S, Hirschowitz J: Clonazepam treatment of five lithium-refractory patients with bipolar disorder. Am J Psychiatry 146:77–80, 1989

Association for Convulsive Therapy: Ambulatory electroconvulsive therapy: report of a task force of the Association for Convulsive Therapy. Convuls Ther 12:42–55, 1996

Avery D, Lubano A: Depression treated with imipramine and ECT: the DeCarolis study reconsidered. Am J Psychiatry 136:559–562, 1979

Avissar S, Schreiber G: Interaction of antibipolar and antidepressant treatments with receptor-coupled G proteins. Pharmacopsychiatry 25:44–50, 1992a

Avissar S, Schreiber G: The involvement of guanine nucleotide binding proteins in the pathogenesis and treatment of affective disorders. Biol Psychiatry 31:435–459, 1992b

Avissar S, Nechamkin Y, Roitman G, et al: Dynamics of ECT normalization of low G protein function and immunoreactivity in mononuclear leukocytes of patients with major depression. Am J Psychiatry 155:666–671, 1998

Baldessarini RJ, Tondo L, Faedda GL, et al: Effects of the rate of discontinuing lithium maintenance treatment in bipolar disorders. Compr Psychiatry 57:441–448, 1996

Ballenger JC, Reus VI, Post RM: The "atypical" clinical picture of adolescent mania. Am J Psychiatry 139:602–606, 1982

Ban TA: Clinical pharmacology and Leonhard's classification of endogenous psychoses. Psychopathology 23:331–338, 1990

Banken DM, Wilson GL: Treatment acceptability of alternative therapies for depression: a comparative analysis. Psychotherapy: Research, Theory, and Practice 29:610–619, 1992

Banov MD, Zarate CA, Tohen M, et al: Clozapine therapy in refractory affective disorders: polarity predicts response in long-term follow-up. Compr Psychiatry 55:295–300, 1994

Barbini B, Di Molfetta D, Gasperini M, et al: Seasonal concordance of recurrence in mood disorder patients. European Psychiatry 10:171–174, 1995

Barefoot JC, Schroll M: Symptoms of depression, acute myocardial infarction, and total mortality in a community sample. Circulation 93:1976–1980, 1996

Barklage NE: Evaluation and management of the suicidal patient. Emergency Care Quarterly 7:9–17, 1991

Barnet B, Duggan AK, Wilson MD, et al: Association between postpartum substance use and depressive symptoms, stress, and social support in adolescent mothers. Pediatrics 96:659–666, 1995

Barrett JE: Naturalistic change after 2 years in neurotic depressive disorders (RDC categories). Compr Psychiatry 25:404–418, 1984

Barton BM, Gitlin MJ: Verapamil in treatment-resistant mania: an open trial. J Clin Psychopharmacol 7:101–103, 1987

Basco MR, Rush AJ: Compliance with pharmacotherapy in mood disorders. Psychiatr Ann 25:269–279, 1995

Bauer MS, Whybrow PC: The effect of changing thyroid function on cyclic affective illness in a human subject. Am J Psychiatry 143:633–636, 1986

Bauer MS, Whybrow PC: Rapid cycling bipolar affective disorder. Arch Gen Psychiatry 47:435–440, 1990

Bauer MS, Whybrow PC, Winokur A: Rapid cycling bipolar affective disorder, I: association with grade I hypothyroidism. Arch Gen Psychiatry 47:427–432, 1990

Baumgartner A, Bauer M, Hellweg R: Treatment of intractable non-rapid cycling bipolar affective disorder with high-dose thyroxine: an open clinical trial. Neuropsychopharmacology 10:183–189, 1994

Beauchamp G, Lavoie P, Elie R: Effect of some stereoisomeric tricyclic antidepressants on 45Ca uptake in synaptosomes from rat hippocampus. Psychopharmacology 110:133–139, 1993

Bebbington R: The epidemiology of bipolar affective disorder. Soc Psychiatry Psychiatr Epidemiol 30:279–292, 1995

Bech P: Acute therapy of depression. Compr Psychiatry 54(suppl 8):18–27, 1993

Beck AT, Rush AJ, Shaw BF: Cognitive Therapy of Depression. New York, Guilford, 1979

Beck AT, Jallon SD, Young JE: Treatment of depression with cognitive therapy and amitriptyline. Arch Gen Psychiatry 42:142–148, 1985

Beck CT: A meta-analysis of the relationship between postpartum depression and infant temperament. Nurs Res 45:225–230, 1996

Bell KM, Potkin SG, Carreon D, et al: S-adenosylmethionine blood levels in major depression: changes with drug treatment. Acta Neurol Scand Suppl 154:15–18, 1994

Bellivier F, Szoke A, Henry C, et al: Possible association between serotonin transporter gene polymorphism and violent suicidal behavior in mood disorders. Biol Psychiatry 48:319–322, 2000

Belsher G, Costello CG: Relapse after recovery from unipolar depression: a critical review. Psychol Bull 104:84–96, 1988

Bemporad JR: Psychodynamic models of depression and mania, in Depression and Mania. Edited by Georgotas A, Cancro R. New York, Elsevier, 1988, pp 167–180

Benazzi F: Olanzapine-induced psychotic mania in bipolar schizo-affective disorder (letter). European Psychiatry 14:410–411, 1999a

Benazzi F: Olanzapine-induced psychotic mania in bipolar schizo-affective disorder. Can J Psychiatry 44:667–668, 1999b

Benkelfat C: Serotonergic mechanisms in psychiatric disorder: new research tools, new ideas. Int Clin Psychopharmacol 8(suppl 2):53–56, 1993

Ben-Shachar D, Gazawi H, Riboyad-Levin J, et al: Chronic repetitive transcranial magnetic stimulation alters beta-adrenergic and 5-HT2 receptor characteristics in rat brain. Brain Res 816:78–83, 1999

Berghofer A, Miller-Oerlinghausen B: Is there a loss of efficacy of lithium in patients treated for over 20 years? Neuropsychobiology 42(suppl 1):46–49, 2000

Bergsholm P, Martinsen EW, Svoen N, et al: Affective disorders: drug treatment and electroconvulsive therapy. Tidsskr Nor Laegeforen 112:2651–2656, 1992

Berk M: Lamotrigine and the treatment of mania in bipolar disorder. Eur Neuropsychopharmacol 9:119–123, 1999

Berk M, Ichim L, Brook L: Olanzapine compared to lithium in mania: a double-blind randomized controlled trial. Int Clin Psychopharmacol 14:339–342, 1999

Bernstein L: Abrupt cessation of rapid-cycling bipolar disorder with the addition of low-dose L-tetraiodothyronine to lithium. J Clin Psychopharmacol 12:443–444, 1992

Berrettini WH, Ferraro TN, Goldin LR, et al: A linkage study of bipolar illness. Arch Gen Psychiatry 54:27–35, 1997

Bertagnolli MW, Borchardt CM: A review of ECT for children and adolescents. J Am Acad Child Adolesc Psychiatry 29:302–307, 1990

Berthier ML, Kulisevsky J, Gironell A: Poststroke bipolar affective disorder: clinical subtypes, concurrent movement disorders, and anatomical correlates. J Neuropsychiatry Clin Neurosci 8:160–167, 1996

Beydoun A, Uthman BM, Sackellares JC: Gabapentin: pharmacokinetics, efficacy, and safety. Clin Neuropharmacol 18:469–481, 1995

Biederman J: Developmental subtypes of juvenile bipolar disorder. Sexual and Marital Therapy 3:227–230, 1995

Bigelow LB, Weinberger DR, Wyatt RJ: Synergism of combined lithium-neuroleptic therapy: a double-blind, placebo-controlled case study. Am J Psychiatry 138:81–83, 1981

Bigger JT, Hoffman BF: Antiarrhythmic drugs, in Goodman and Gilman's The Pharmacological Basis of Therapeutics, 8th Edition. Edited by Gilman AG, Rall TW, Nies AS, et al. New York, Pergamon, 1991, pp 840–873

Black DW, Winokur G, Nasrallah A: Treatment of mania: a naturalistic study of electroconvulsive therapy versus lithium in 438 patients. Compr Psychiatry 48:132–139, 1987

Black DW, Bell S, Hulbert J: The importance of Axis II in patients with major depression. J Affect Disord 14:114–122, 1988

Blackburn I-M: Psychology and psychotherapy of depression. Current Opinion in Psychiatry 7:30–33, 1994

Blackburn I-M, Eunson KM, Bishop S: A two-year naturalistic follow-up of depressed patients treated with cognitive therapy, pharmacotherapy, and a combination of both. J Affect Disord 10:67–75, 1986

Blatt SJ: The destructiveness of perfectionism: implications for the treatment of depression. Am Psychol 50:1003–1020, 1995

Blatt SJ, Sanislow CA, Zuroff DC, et al: Characteristics of effective therapists: further analyses of data from the National Institute of Mental Health Treatment of Depression Collaborative Research Program. J Consult Clin Psychol 64:1276–1284, 1996

Blazer DG, Koenig HG: Mood disorders, in Textbook of Geriatric Psychiatry. Edited by Busse EW, Blazer DG. Washington, DC, American Psychiatric Press, 1996, pp 235–264

Bleich A, Brown S-L, van Praag HM: A serotonergic theory of schizophrenia, in The Role of Serotonin in Psychiatric Disorders. Edited by Brown S-L, van Praag HM. New York, Brunner/Mazel, 1990, pp 183–214

Blumer D, Montouris G, Hermann B: Psychiatric morbidity in seizure patients on a neurodiagnostic monitoring unit. J Neuropsychiatry Clin Neurosci 7:445–456, 1995

Bonne O, Krausz Y, Gorfine M, et al: Cerebral hypoperfusion in medication resistant, depressed patients assessed by Tc99m HMPAO SPECT. J Affect Disord 41:163–171, 1996

Borysewicz K, Borysewicz W: A case of mania following olanzapine administration. Psychiatr Pol 34:299–306, 2000

Bottiglieri T, Godfrey P, Flynn T, et al: Cerebrospinal fluid S-adenosylmethionine in depression and dementia: effects of treatment with parenteral and oral S-adenosylmethionine. J Neurol Neurosurg Psychiatry 53:1096–1098, 1990

Bowden CL: The clinical approach to the differential diagnosis of bipolar disorder. Psychiatr Ann 23:57–63, 1993

Bowden CL: Predictors of response to divalproex and lithium (review). Compr Psychiatry 56(suppl 3):25–30, 1995

Bowden CL: Dosing strategies and time course of response to antimanic agents. Compr Psychiatry 57(suppl 13):4–9, 1996

Bowden CL, Brugger AM, Swann AC: Efficacy of divalproex vs lithium in the treatment of mania. JAMA 271:918–924, 1994

Bowden CL, Calabrese JR, Wallin BA, et al: Illness characteristics of patients in clinical drug studies of mania. Psychopharmacol Bull 31:103–109, 1995

Bowden CL, Calabrese JR, McElroy SL, et al: The efficacy of lamotrigine in rapid cycling and non-rapid cycling patients with bipolar disorder. Biol Psychiatry 45:953–958, 1999

Dell DL, Stewart DE: Menopause and mood: is depression linked with hormone changes? Postgrad Med 108:39–43, 2000

Deltito JA, Moline M, Pollak C, et al: Effects of phototherapy on non-seasonal unipolar and bipolar depressive spectrum disorders. J Affect Disord 23:231–237, 1991

Denollet J, Vaes J, Brutsaert DL: Inadequate response to treatment in coronary heart disease: adverse effects of type D personality and younger age on 5-year prognosis and quality of life. Circulation 102:630–635, 2000

Devanand DP, Sackeim HA, Prudic J: Electroconvulsive therapy in the treatment-resistant patient. Psychiatr Clin North Am 14:905–923, 1991a

Devanand DP, Sackeim HA, Lo E-S, et al: Serial dexamethasone suppression tests and plasma dexamethasone levels. Arch Gen Psychiatry 48:525–533, 1991b

De Vanna M, Rigamonti R: Oral S-adenosyl-L-methionine in depression. Curr Ther Res 52:478–485, 1992

Dilsaver SC, Coffman JA: Cholinergic hypothesis of depression: a reappraisal. J Clin Psychopharmacol 9:173–179, 1989

DiMascio A, Weissman MM, Prusoff BA: Differential symptom reduction by drugs and psychotherapy in acute depression. Arch Gen Psychiatry 36:1450–1456, 1979

Doris A, Ebmeier KP, Shajahan P: Depressive illness. Lancet 354:1369–1375, 1999

Dose M, Emrich HM, Cording-Tommel C: Use of calcium antagonists in mania. Psychoneuroendocrinology 11:241–243, 1986

Drugs that cause psychiatric symptoms. Medical Letter 35:65–70, 1993

Dubovsky SL: Using electroconvulsive therapy for patients with neurological disease. Hosp Community Psychiatry 37:819–825, 1986

Dubovsky SL: Beyond the serotonin reuptake inhibitors: rationales for the development of new serotonergic agents. Compr Psychiatry 55(suppl 2):34–44, 1994a

Dubovsky SL: Why don't we hear more about the calcium antagonists? An industry-academia interaction. Biol Psychiatry 35:149–150, 1994b

Dubovsky SL: Calcium channel antagonists as novel agents for manic-depressive disorder, in The American Psychiatric Press Textbook of Psychopharmacology. Edited by Schatzberg AF, Nemeroff CB. Washington, DC, American Psychiatric Press, 1995a, pp 377–388

Dubovsky SL: Electroconvulsive therapy, in Comprehensive Textbook of Psychiatry/VI, 6th Edition, Vol 2. Edited by Kaplan HI, Sadock BJ. Baltimore, MD, Williams & Wilkins, 1995b, pp 2129–2140

Dubovsky SL: Mind-Body Deceptions. New York, WW Norton, 1997

Dubovsky SL, Buzan RD: Novel alternatives and supplements to lithium and anticonvulsants for bipolar affective disorder. J Clin Psychiatry 58:224–242, 1997

Dubovsky SL, Thomas M: Psychotic depression: advances in conceptualization and treatment. Hosp Community Psychiatry 43:1189–1198, 1992

Dubovsky SL, Thomas M: Beyond specificity: effects of serotonin and serotonergic treatments on psychobiological dysfunction. J Psychosom Res 39:429–444, 1995

Dubovsky SL, Thomas M: Tardive dyskinesia associated with fluoxetine. Psychiatr Serv 47:991–993, 1996

Dubovsky SL, Franks RD, Allen S, et al: Calcium antagonists in mania: a double-blind study of verapamil. Psychiatry Res 18:309–320, 1986

Dubovsky SL, Christiano J, Daniell LC: Increased platelet intracellular calcium concentration in patients with bipolar affective disorders. Arch Gen Psychiatry 46:632–638, 1989

Dubovsky SL, Lee C, Christiano J: Elevated intracellular calcium ion concentration in bipolar depression. Biol Psychiatry 29:441–450, 1991a

Dubovsky SL, Lee C, Christiano J: Lithium decreases platelet intracellular calcium ion concentrations in bipolar patients. Lithium 2:167–174, 1991b

Dubovsky SL, Murphy J, Thomas M, et al: Abnormal intracellular calcium ion concentration in platelets and lymphocytes of bipolar patients. Am J Psychiatry 149:118–120, 1992a

Dubovsky SL, Murphy J, Christiano J, et al: The calcium second messenger system in bipolar disorders: data supporting new research directions. J Neuropsychiatry Clin Neurosci 4:3–14, 1992b

Dubovsky SL, Thomas M, Hijazi A, et al: Intracellular calcium signaling in peripheral cells of patients with bipolar affective disorder. Eur Arch Psychiatry Clin Neurosci 243:229–234, 1994

Duffy A: Toward effective early intervention and prevention strategies for major affective disorders: a review of antecedents and risk factors. Can J Psychiatry 45:338–339, 2000

Dupont RM, Jernigan TL, Heindel W, et al: Magnetic resonance imaging and mood disorders: localization of white matter and other subcortical abnormalities. Arch Gen Psychiatry 52:747–755, 1995

Dwight MM, Keck PE, Stanton SP, et al: Antidepressant activity and mania associated with risperidone treatment of schizoaffective disorder. Lancet 344:554–555, 1994

Edwards R, Peet M, Shay J, et al: Omega-3 polyunsaturated fatty acid levels in the diet and in red blood cell membranes of depressed patients. J Affect Disord 48:149–155, 1998

Egeland JA, Gerhard DS, Pauls D, et al: Bipolar affective disorders linked to DNA markers on chromosome 11. Nature 325:783–787, 1987

Elkin I, Shea MT, Watkins JT, et al: National Institute of Mental Health Treatment of Depression Collaborative Research Program: general effectiveness of treatments. Arch Gen Psychiatry 46:971–982, 1989

Elkis H, Friedman L, Wise A, et al: Meta-analysis of studies of ventricular enlargement and cortical sulcal prominence in mood disorders: comparisons with controls or patients with schizophrenia. Arch Gen Psychiatry 52:735–746, 1995

Emslie GJ, Kennard BD, Kowatch RA: Affective disorders in children: diagnosis and management. J Child Neurol 10(suppl 1):S42–S49, 1995

Esparon J, Kolloori J, Naylor GJ: Comparison of the prophylactic action of flupenthixol with placebo in lithium treated manic-depressive patients. Br J Psychiatry 148:723–725, 1986

Evans MD, Hollon SD, DeRubeis RJ, et al: Differential relapse following cognitive therapy and pharmacotherapy for depression. Arch Gen Psychiatry 49:802–808, 1992

Expert Consensus Panel: Treatment of bipolar disorder. Compr Psychiatry 57(suppl 12A):1–88, 1996

Extein I, Pottash ALC, Gold MS: Does subclinical hypothyroidism predispose to tricyclic-induced rapid mood cycles? Compr Psychiatry 43:290–291, 1982

Extein I, Pottash ALC, Gold MS: Thyroid tests as predictors of treatment response and prognosis in psychiatry. Psychiatric Hospital 16:127–130, 1985

Faedda GL, Baldessarini RJ, Suppes T, et al: Pediatric-onset bipolar disorder: a neglected clinical and public health problem. Sexual and Marital Therapy 3:171–195, 1995

Fann JR, Tucker GJ: Mood disorders with general medical condition. Current Opinion in Psychiatry 8:13–18, 1995

Fava M, Davidson KG: Definition and epidemiology of treatment-resistant depression. Psychiatr Clin North Am 19:179–195, 1996

Fava M, Kaji J: Continuation and maintenance treatments of major depressive disorders. Psychiatr Ann 24:281–290, 1994

Feinman JA, Dunner DL: The effect of alcohol and substance abuse on the course of bipolar affective disorder. J Affect Disord 37:43–49, 1996

Feline A: Les hyperthymies. Encephale 19:103–107, 1993

Fennig S, Craig TJ, Tanenberg-Karant M, et al: Medication treatment in first-admission patients with psychotic affective disorders: preliminary findings on research-facility diagnostic agreement and rehospitalization. Ann Clin Psychiatry 7:87–90, 1995

Figiel GS, Krishnan KRR, Doraiswamy PM: Subcortical structural changes in ECT-induced delirium. J Geriatr Psychiatry Neurol 3:172–176, 1990

Figiel GS, Hassen MA, Zorumski CF, et al: ECT-induced delirium in depressed patients with Parkinson's disease. J Neuropsychiatry Clin Neurosci 3:405–411, 1991

Figiel GS, Epstein C, McDonald WM, et al: The use of rapid-rate transcranial magnetic stimulation (rTMS) in refractory depressed patients. J Neuropsychiatry Clin Neurosci 10:20–25, 1998

Fink M: Electroconvulsive therapy in children and adolescents. Convuls Ther 9:155–157, 1993

First MB, Donovan S, Frances A: Nosology of chronic mood disorders. Psychiatr Clin North Am 19:29–39, 1996

Fitz-Gerald MJ, Pinkofsky HB, Brannon G, et al: Olanzapine-induced mania (letter). Am J Psychiatry 156:1114, 1999

Fochtmann LJ: Animal studies of electroconvulsive therapy: foundations for future research. Psychopharmacol Bull 30:321–344, 1994

Folkerts H: Electroconvulsive therapy in neurologic diseases. Nervenarzt 66:241–251, 1995

Frances AJ: An introduction to dysthymia. Psychiatr Ann 23:607–608, 1993

Franchini J, Zanardi R, Smeraldi E, et al: Early onset of lithium prophylaxis as a predictor of good long-term outcome. Eur Arch Psychiatry Clin Neurosci 249:227–230, 1999

Franco-Bronson K: The management of treatment-resistant depression in the medically ill. Psychiatr Clin North Am 19:329–350, 1996

Frank E, Kupfer DJ, Perel JM, et al: Three-year outcomes for maintenance therapies in recurrent depression. Arch Gen Psychiatry 47:1093–1099, 1990

Frank E, Kupfer DJ, Wagner EF, et al: Efficacy of interpersonal psychotherapy as a maintenance treatment of recurrent depression: contributing factors. Arch Gen Psychiatry 48:1053–1059, 1991

Frank E, Kupfer DJ, Hamer T, et al: Maintenance treatment and psychobiologic correlates of endogenous subtypes. J Affect Disord 25:181–189, 1992

Frank E, Kupfer DJ, Perel JM, et al: Comparison of full-dose versus half-dose pharmacotherapy in the maintenance treatment of recurrent depression. J Affect Disord 27:139–145, 1993

Frank E, Kupfer DJ, Ehlers CL, et al: Interpersonal and social rhythm therapy for bipolar disorder: integrating interpersonal and behavioral approaches. Behav Ther 17:143–149, 1994

Frank E, Kupfer DJ, Siegel LR: Alliance not compliance: a philosophy of outpatient care. Compr Psychiatry 56(suppl 1):11–17, 1995

Frank E, Hlastala S, Ritenour A, et al: Inducing lifestyle regularity in recovering bipolar disorder patients: results from the maintenance therapies in bipolar disorder protocol. Biol Psychiatry 41:1165–1173, 1997

Freeman MP: Omega-3 fatty acids in psychiatry: a review. Ann Clin Psychiatry 12:159–165, 2000

Freeman MP, McElroy SL: Clinical picture and etiologic models of mixed states. Psychiatr Clin North Am 22:535–546, 1999

Freeman TW, Clothier JL, Pazzaglia P, et al: A double-blind comparison of valproate and lithium in the treatment of acute mania. Am J Psychiatry 149:108–111, 1992

Freinhar JP, Alvarez WH: Use of clonazepam in two cases of acute mania. Compr Psychiatry 46:29–30, 1985

Freud S: Mourning and melancholia (1917[1915]), in Standard Edition of the Complete Psychological Works of Sigmund Freud, Vol 14. Translated and edited by Strachey J. London, England, Hogarth, 1957, pp 237–260

Freud S: Project for a scientific psychology (1950[1895]), in Standard Edition of the Complete Psychological Works of Sigmund Freud, Vol 1. Translated and edited by Strachey J. London, England, Hogarth, 1966, pp 281–397

Friedman E, Wang HY, Levinson D, et al: Altered platelet protein kinase C activity in bipolar affective disorder, manic episode. Biol Psychiatry 33:520–525, 1993

Friedman RA: Social impairment in dysthymia. Psychiatr Ann 23:632–637, 1993

Fritsch S, Donaldson D, Spirito A, et al: Personality characteristics of adolescent suicide attempters. Child Psychiatry Hum Dev 30:219–235, 2000

Froscher W: Clinical relevance of the determination of antiepileptic drugs in serum. Wien Klin Wochenschr Suppl 191:15–18, 1992

Frye M, Altschuler LL, Bitran JE: Clozapine in rapid cycling bipolar disorder (letter). J Clin Psychopharmacol 16:87–90, 1996

Gabbard GO: Psychodynamic psychotherapies, in Treatment of Psychiatric Disorders. Edited by Gabbard GO. Washington, DC, American Psychiatric Press, 1995, pp 1205–1220

Gallagher-Thompson D, Hanley-Peterson P, Thompson LW: Maintenance of gains versus relapse following brief psychotherapy for depression. J Consult Clin Psychol 58:371–374, 1990

Garza-Trevino ES, Hollister LE, Overall JE, et al: Efficacy of combinations of intramuscular antipsychotics and sedative-hypnotics for control of psychotic agitation. Am J Psychiatry 146:1598–1601, 1989

Garza-Trevino ES, Overall JE, Hollister LE: Verapamil versus lithium in acute mania. Am J Psychiatry 149:121–122, 1992

Gaster B, Holroyd J: St John's wort for depression: a systematic review. Arch Intern Med 24:152–156, 2000

Gelenberg AJ, Hopkins HS: Report on efficacy of treatments for bipolar disorder. Psychopharmacol Bull 29:447–456, 1993

Gelenberg AJ, Kane JM, Keller MB, et al: Comparison of standard and low serum levels of lithium for maintenance treatment of bipolar disorder. N Engl J Med 321:1489–1493, 1989

Geller B, Sun K, Zimerman B, et al: Complex and rapid-cycling in bipolar children and adolescents: a preliminary study. J Affect Disord 34:259–268, 1995

Geller B, Todd RD, Luby J, et al: Treatment-resistant depression in children and adolescents. Psychiatr Clin North Am 19:253–265, 1996

Geller B, Williams M, Zimerman B, et al: Prepubertal and early adolescent bipolarity differentiate from ADHD by manic symptoms, grandiose delusions, ultra-rapid or ultradian cycling. J Affect Disord 51:81–91, 1998

George MS, Wassermann EM, Kimbrell TA, et al: Mood improvement following daily left prefrontal repetitive transcranial magnetic stimulation in patients with depression: a placebo-controlled crossover trial. Am J Psychiatry 154:1752–1756, 1997

Gerber JS, Nies AS: Antihypertensive agents and the drug therapy of hypertension, in Goodman and Gilman's The Pharmacological Basis of Therapeutics, 8th Edition. Edited by Gilman AG, Rall TW, Nies AS, et al. New York, Pergamon, 1991, pp 784–813

Gershon ES: Genetics, in Manic-Depressive Illness. Edited by Goodwin FK, Jamison KR. New York, Oxford University Press, 1990, pp 373–401

Gershon ES, Hamovit J, Guroff I, et al: A family study of schizoaffective, bipolar I, bipolar II, unipolar and normal control probands. Arch Gen Psychiatry 39:1157–1167, 1982

Gershon S, Soares JC: Current therapeutic profile of lithium. Arch Gen Psychiatry 54:16–18, 1997

Ghaemi SN, Gaughan S: Novel anticonvulsants: a new generation of mood stabilizers? Harv Rev Psychiatry 8:1–7, 2000

Ghaemi SN, Boiman EE, Goodwin FK: Diagnosing bipolar disorder and the effect of antidepressants: a naturalistic study. J Clin Psychiatry 61:804–808, 2000

Giannini AJ, Houser WL, Loiselle RH: Antimanic effects of verapamil. Am J Psychiatry 141:1602–1603, 1984

Giannini AJ, Loiselle RH, Price WA: Comparison of antimanic efficacy of clonidine and verapamil. J Clin Pharmacol 25:307–308, 1985

Giannini AJ, Taraszewski R, Loiselle RH: Verapamil and lithium as maintenance therapy of manic patients. J Clin Pharmacol 27:980–982, 1987

Glass DR, Pilkonis PA, Leber WR, et al: National Institute of Mental Health Treatment of Depression Collaborative Research Program. Arch Gen Psychiatry 46:971–982, 1989

Glassman A, Proud'homme X: Review of the cardiovascular effects of heterocyclic antidepressants. Compr Psychiatry 54(suppl 2):16–22, 1993

Gold PW, Licinio J, Wong ML, et al: Corticotropin releasing hormone in the pathophysiology of melancholic and atypical depression and the mechanisms of action of antidepressant drugs. Ann N Y Acad Sci 77:716–729, 1995

Goldberg JF, Harrow M, Grossman LS: Course and outcome in bipolar affective disorder: a longitudinal follow-up study. Am J Psychiatry 152:379–384, 1995

Goldberg JF, Harrow M, Leon AC: Lithium treatment of bipolar affective disorders under naturalistic followup conditions. Psychopharmacol Bull 32:47–54, 1996

Goodnick PJ: Verapamil prophylaxis in pregnant women with bipolar disorder (letter). Am J Psychiatry 150:1560, 1993

Goodnick PJ: Nimodipine treatment of rapid cycling bipolar disorder. J Clin Psychiatry 56:330, 1995

Goodwin FK, Jamison KR: Manic Depressive Illness. New York, Oxford University Press, 1991

Goodwin FK, Wirz-Justice A, Wehr TA: Evidence that the pathophysiology of depression and the mechanism of antidepressant drugs both involve alterations in circadian rhythms. Adv Biochem Psychopharmacol 32:1–11, 1982

Gorman JM, Coplan JD: Comorbidity of depression and panic disorder. Compr Psychiatry 57(suppl 10):34–41, 1996

Grahame-Smith DG: Serotonin in affective disorders. Int Clin Psychopharmacol 6(suppl 4):5–13, 1992

Grant SM, Faulds D: Oxcarbazepine: a review of its pharmacology and therapeutic potential in epilepsy, trigeminal neuralgia and affective disorders. Drugs 43:873–888, 1992

Green AI, Tohen M, Patel JK, et al: Clozapine in the treatment of refractory psychotic mania. Am J Psychiatry 157:982–986, 2000

Grisaru N, Chudakov B, Yaroslavosky Y, et al: Transcranial magnetic stimulation in mania: a controlled study. Am J Psychiatry 155:1608–1610, 1998

Grubb D: Three Bipolar Women: The Boundary Between Bipolar Disorders and Disorders of the Self. New York, Brunner/Mazel, 1997

Gruber AJ, Hudson JI, Pope HG: The management of treatment-resistant depression in disorders on the interface of psychiatry and medicine. Psychiatr Clin North Am 19:351–369, 1996

Guze SB, Robbins E: Suicide and primary affective disorders. Br J Psychiatry 117:437–438, 1970

Gwirtsman HE, Blehar MC, McCullough JP, et al: Standardized assessment of dysthymia: report of a National Institute of Mental Health conference. Psychopharmacol Bull 33:3–11, 1997

Gyulai L, Alavi A, Broich K, et al: I-123 iofetamine single-photon computed emission tomography in rapid cycling bipolar disorder: a clinical study. Biol Psychiatry 41:152–161, 1997

Hall RC, Wise MG: The clinical and financial burden of mood disorders: cost and outcome. Psychosomatics 36:S11–S18, 1995

Harrison WM, Stewart JW: Pharmacotherapy of dysthymia. Psychiatr Ann 23:638–648, 1993

Harrow M, Goldberg JF, Grossman LS, et al: Outcome in manic disorders: a naturalistic follow-up study. Arch Gen Psychiatry 47:665–671, 1990

Hasin DS, Tsai W-Y, Endicott J, et al: Five-year course of major depression: effects of comorbid alcoholism: the effect of alcohol and substance abuse on the course of bipolar affective disorder. J Affect Disord 37:43–49, 1996

Hauck A, Bhaumik S: Hypomania induced by gabapentin (letter). Br J Psychiatry 167:549, 1995

Hay DF, Kumar R: Interpreting the effects of mothers' postnatal depression on children's intelligence: a critique and re-analysis. Child Psychiatry Hum Dev 25:165–181, 1995

Hellekson C: Phenomenology of seasonal affective disorder: an Alaskan perspective, in Seasonal Affect Disorders and Phototherapy. Edited by Rosenthal NE, Blehar MC. New York, Guilford, 1989, pp 33–43

Hellerstein DJ, Yanowitch P, Rosenthal J, et al: Long-term treatment of double depression: a preliminary study with serotonergic antidepressants. Prog Neuropsychopharmacol Biol Psychiatry 18:139–147, 1994

Hendrick V, Altschuler LL, Szuba MP: Is there a role for neuroleptics in bipolar depression? Compr Psychiatry 55:533–535, 1994

Hersen M, Bellack AS, Himmelhoch JM, et al: Effects of social skills training, amitriptyline, and psychotherapy in unipolar depressed women. Behav Ther 15:21–40, 1984

Hirschfeld RMA: Guidelines for the long-term treatment of depression. Compr Psychiatry 55(suppl 12):61–69, 1994

Hirschfeld RMA, Klerman GL, Lavori P: Premorbid personality assessments of first onset of major depression. Arch Gen Psychiatry 46:345–350, 1989

Hoffler J, Braunig P, Kruger S, et al: Morphology according to cranial computed tomography of first-episode cycloid psychosis and its long-term-course: differences compared to schizophrenia. Acta Psychiatr Scand 96:184–187, 1997

Hollon SD, Fawcett J: Combined medication and psychotherapy, in Treatment of Psychiatric Disorders. Edited by Gabbard GO. Washington, DC, American Psychiatric Press, 1995, pp 1221–1236

Hollon SD, DeRubeis RJ, Evans MD, et al: Cognitive therapy and pharmacotherapy for depression: singly and in combination. Arch Gen Psychiatry 49:774–781, 1992

Hopkins HS, Gelenberg AJ: Treatment of bipolar disorder: how far have we come? Psychopharmacol Bull 30:27–38, 1994

Hopkins J, Marcus M, Campbell SB: Postpartum depression: a critical review. Psychol Bull 95:498–515, 1984

Hoschl C, Kozemy J: Verapamil in affective disorders: a controlled, double-blind study. Biol Psychiatry 25:128–140, 1989

Hoshino M, Heise CO, Puglia P, et al: Hepatic enzymes' level during chronic use of anticonvulsant drugs. Arq Neuropsiquiatr 53:719–723, 1995

Howland RH: General health, health care utilization, and medical comorbidity in dysthymia. Int J Psychiatry Med 23:211–238, 1993

Isacsson G, Bergman U, Rich CL: Epidemiological data suggest antidepressants reduce suicide risk among depressives. J Affect Disord 41:1–8, 1996

Isometsa ET, Henriksson MM, Heikkinen ME: Suicide among subjects with personality disorders. Am J Psychiatry 153:667–673, 1996

Jacob M, Turner L, Kupfer DJ, et al: Attrition in maintenance therapy for recurrent depression. J Affect Disord 6:181–189, 1984

Jaffe RL, Rives W, Dubin WR, et al: Problems in maintenance ECT in bipolar disorder: replacement by lithium. Convuls Ther 7:288–294, 1991

Jaim-Etcheverry G, Zieher LM: Coexistence of monoamines in peripheral adrenergic neurones, in Co-Transmission. Edited by Cuello AC. London, England, Macmillan, 1982, pp 189–207

Jamison KR: Touched With Fire: Manic-Depressive Illness and the Artistic Temperament. New York, Free Press, 1993

Jamison KR: An Unquiet Mind. New York, Knopf, 1995

Jamison KR: Manic-depressive illness, genes, and creativity, in Genetics and Mental Illness: Evolving Issues for Research and Society. Edited by Hall LL. New York, Plenum, 1996, pp 111–132

Janicak PG, Lipinski JF, Davis JM, et al: S-Adenosylmethionine in depression: a literature review and preliminary report. Alabama Journal of Medical Science 25:306–313, 1988a

Janicak PG, Pandey GN, Davis JM, et al: Response of psychotic and nonpsychotic depression to phenelzine. Am J Psychiatry 145:93–95, 1988b

Janowsky DS, Risch SC: Adrenergic-cholinergic balance and affective disorders: a review of clinical evidence and therapeutic implications. Psychiatric Hospital 15:163–171, 1984

Jarrett RB: Comparing and Combining Short-Term Psychotherapy and Pharmacotherapy for Depression. New York, Guilford, 1997

Jarrett RB, Kraft D, Doyle J, et al: Preventing recurrent depression using cognitive therapy with and without a continuation phase: a randomized clinical trial. Arch Gen Psychiatry 58:381–388, 2001

Joffe RT, Horvath Z, Tarvydas I: Bipolar affective disorder and thalassemia minor (letter). Am J Psychiatry 143:933, 1986

John V, Rapp M, Pies R: Aggression, agitation, and mania with olanzapine (letter). Can J Psychiatry 43:1054, 1998

Johnson L, Andersson-Lundman G, Aberg-Wistedt A, et al: Age of onset in affective disorder: its correlation with hereditary and psychosocial factors. J Affect Disord 59:139–148, 2000

Jope RS, Williams MB: Lithium and brain signal transduction systems. Biochem Pharmacol 47:429–441, 1994

Kafantaris V: Treatment of bipolar disorder in children and adolescents. J Am Acad Child Adolesc Psychiatry 34:732–741, 1995

Kahn RS, Kalus O, Wetzler S, et al: The role of serotonin in the regulation of anxiety, in The Role of Serotonin in Psychiatric Disorders. Edited by Brown S-L, van Praag HM. New York, Brunner/Mazel, 1990, pp 129–160

Kallner G, Lindelius R, Petterson U, et al: Mortality in 487 patients with affective disorders attending a lithium clinic or having left it. Pharmacopsychiatry 33:8–13, 2000

Kanba S, Yagi G, Kamijima K, et al: The first open study of zonisamide, a novel anticonvulsant, shows efficacy in mania. Prog Neuropsychopharmacol Biol Psychiatry 18:707–715, 1994

Kaneko S, Takahashi H, Satoh M: The use of Xenopus oocytes to evaluate drugs affecting brain Ca2+ channels: effects of bifemelane and several nootopic agents. Eur J Pharmacol 189:51–58, 1990

Karliner W, Wehrheim HK: Maintenance convulsive treatments. Am J Psychiatry 121:1113–1115, 1965

Kashani JH, Nair J: Affective/mood disorders, in Diagnosis and Psychopharmacology of Childhood and Adolescent Disorders, 2nd Edition. Edited by Weiner JM. New York, Wiley, 1995, pp 229–263

Kasper S, Wehr TA, Bartko JJ, et al: Epidemiological findings of seasonal changes in mood and behavior. Arch Gen Psychiatry 46:823–833, 1989

Kasper S, Fuger J, Moller H-J: Comparative efficacy of antidepressants. Drugs 43(suppl 2):11–23, 1992

Kastner T, Friedman DL: Verapamil and valproic acid treatment of prolonged mania. J Am Acad Child Adolesc Psychiatry 31:271–275, 1992

Katon W, Rutter C, Ludman EF, et al: A randomized trial of relapse prevention of depression in primary care. Arch Gen Psychiatry 58:241–247, 2001

Kaufman IC, Rosenblum LA: The reaction to separation in infant monkeys: anaclitic depression and conservation-withdrawal. Psychosom Med 29:648–675, 1967

Kaufmann CA: Muscarinic binding in suicides. Psychiatry Res 12:47–55, 1984

Kazdin A, Bass D: Power to detect differences between alternative treatments in comparative psychotherapy outcome research. J Consult Clin Psychol 57:138–147, 1989

Keck PE, McElroy SL, Vuckovic A, et al: Combined valproate and carbamazepine treatment of bipolar disorder. J Neuropsychiatry Clin Neurosci 4:319–322, 1992

Keck PE, McElroy SL, Tugrul KC, et al: Valproate oral loading in the treatment of acute mania. J Clin Psychiatry 54:305–308, 1993

Keck PE, Merikangas KR, McElroy SL, et al: Diagnostic and treatment implications of psychiatric comorbidity with migraine. Ann Clin Psychiatry 6:165–171, 1994

Keck PE, McElroy SL, Strakowski SM: Factors associated with pharmacologic noncompliance in patients with mania. J Clin Psychiatry 57:292–297, 1996

Keck PE, McElroy SL, Strakowski SM, et al: Compliance with maintenance treatment in bipolar disorder. Psychopharmacol Bull 33:87–91, 1997

Keilp JG, Sackeim HA, Brodsky BS, et al: Neuropsychological dysfunction in depressed suicide attempters. Am J Psychiatry 158:735–741, 2001

Keitner GI, Miller IW: Family functioning and major depression: an overview. Am J Psychiatry 147:1128–1137, 1990

Keitner GI, Ryan CE, Miller IW, et al: 12-Month outcome of patients with major depression and comorbid psychiatric or medical illness (compound depression). Am J Psychiatry 148:345–350, 1991

Keller MB: Dysthymia in clinical practice: course, outcome and impact on the community. Acta Psychiatr Scand 383(suppl):24–34, 1994

Keller MB, Klerman G, Lavori PW: Long-term outcome of episodes of major depression. JAMA 252:788–792, 1984

Keller MB, Lavori PW, Coryell W, et al: Bipolar I: a five-year prospective follow-up. J Nerv Ment Dis 181:238–245, 1993

Keller MB, Hanks DL, Klein DN: Summary of the DSM-IV mood disorders field trial and issue overview. Psychiatr Clin North Am 19:1–27, 1996

Keller MB, McCullough JP, Klein DN, et al: A comparison of nefazodone, the cognitive behavioral-analysis system of psychotherapy, and their combination for the treatment of chronic depression. N Engl J Med 342:1462–1470, 2000

Kelsoe JR, Ginns EI, Egeland JA, et al: Re-evaluation of the linkage relationship between chromosome 11p loci and the gene for bipolar affective disorder in the old order Amish. Nature 342:238–243, 1989

Kendler KK, Heath AC, Martin NG, et al: Symptoms of anxiety and symptoms of depression: same genes, different environments? Arch Gen Psychiatry 44:451–457, 1987

Kendler KK, Neale MC, Kessler RC, et al: Major depression and generalized anxiety disorder: same genes, (partly) different environments? Arch Gen Psychiatry 49:716–722, 1992a

Kendler KK, Neale MC, Kessler CC, et al: A population-based twin study of major depression in women: the impact of varying definitions of illness. Arch Gen Psychiatry 49:257–266, 1992b

Kendler KK, Kessler CC, Neale MC, et al: The prediction of major depression in women: toward an integrated etiologic model. Am J Psychiatry 150:1139–1148, 1993

Kendler KS: Mood-incongruent psychotic affective illness. Arch Gen Psychiatry 48:362–369, 1991

Kendler KS: The diagnostic validity of melancholic major depression in a population-based sample of female twins. Arch Gen Psychiatry 54:299–304, 1997

Keshavan MS: Benzhexol withdrawal and cholinergic mechanisms in depression. Br J Psychiatry 147:560–564, 1985

Ketter TA, Post RM, Parekh PI, et al: Addition of monoamine oxidase inhibitors to carbamazepine: preliminary evidence of safety and antidepressant efficacy in treatment-resistant depression. Compr Psychiatry 56:471–475, 1995

Kettering RL, Harrow M, Grossman L, et al: The prognostic relevance of delusions in depression: a follow-up study. Am J Psychiatry 144:1154–1160, 1987

Khodorov B, Pinelis V, Vinskaya N, et al: Li+ protects nerve cells against destabilization of Ca2+ homeostasis and delayed death caused by removal of external Na+. FEBS Lett 448:173–176, 1999

Kilzieh N, Akiskal HS: Rapid-cycling bipolar disorder: an overview of research and clinical experience. Psychiatr Clin North Am 22:585–607, 2000

Kinsella JE: Lipids, membrane receptors, and enzymes: effects of dietary fatty acids. JPEN J Parenter Enteral Nutr 14:200S–217S, 1990

Kirkcaldie M, Pridmore S, Reid P: Bridging the skull: electroconvulsive therapy (ECT) and repetitive transcranial magnetic stimulation (rTMS) in psychiatry. Convuls Ther 13:83–91, 1997

Kirkpatrick B, Alphs L, Buchanan RW: The concept of supersensitivity psychosis. J Nerv Ment Dis 180:265–270, 1992

Kishi Y, Robinson RG: Suicidal plans following spinal cord injury: a six-month study. J Neuropsychiatry Clin Neurosci 8:442–445, 1996

Klapheke MM: Clozapine, ECT, and schizoaffective disorder, bipolar type. Convuls Ther 7:36–39, 1991

Klassen T, Verhey FRJ, Rozendaal N: Treatment of depression in Parkinson's disease: a meta-analysis. J Neuropsychiatry Clin Neurosci 7:281–286, 1995

Klein DN, Taylor EB, Harding K, et al: Double depression and episodic major depression: demographic, clinical, family, personality, and socioenvironmental characteristics and short-term outcome. Am J Psychiatry 145:1225–1231, 1988

Klein DN, Kocsis JH, McCullough JP, et al: Symptomatology in dysthymic and major depressive disorder. Psychiatr Clin North Am 19:41–53, 1996

Klein DN, Schwartz JE, Rose S, et al: Five-year course and outcome of dysthymic disorder: a prospective, naturalistic follow-up study. Am J Psychiatry 157:931–939, 2000

Kleist K: Ueber zykloide, paranoide und epileptoide Psychosen und uber die Frage der Degenerationspsychosen. Schweiz Arch Neurol Psychiatr 23:3–37, 1928

Klerman GL: The current age of youthful melancholia: evidence for increase in depression among adolescents and young adults. Br J Psychiatry 152:4–14, 1988

Klerman GL, DiMascio A, Weissman MM, et al: Treatment of depression by drugs and psychotherapy. Am J Psychiatry 131:186–191, 1974

Klerman GL, Weissman MM, Rounsaville BJ, et al: Interpersonal Psychotherapy of Depression. New York, Basic Books, 1984

Klerman GL, Lavori PW, Rice J, et al: Birth-cohort trends in rates of major depressive disorder among relatives of patients with affective disorder. Arch Gen Psychiatry 42:689–693, 1985

Knesper DJ: The depressions of Alzheimer's disease: sorting, pharmacotherapy, and clinical advice. J Geriatr Psychiatry Neurol 8(suppl 1):S40–S51, 1995

Kocsis JH: DSM-IV "major depression": are more stringent criteria needed? Depression 1:24–28, 1993

Kocsis JH, Frances AJ: A critical discussion of DSM-III dysthymic disorder. Am J Psychiatry 144:1534–1542, 1987

Kocsis JH, Frances AJ, Voss C, et al: Imipramine treatment for chronic depression. Arch Gen Psychiatry 45:253–257, 1988

Kocsis JH, Mason BJ, Frances AJ, et al: Prediction of response of chronic depression to imipramine. J Affect Disord 17:255–260, 1989

Koek RJ, Kessler CC: Possible induction of mania by risperidone (letter). Compr Psychiatry 57:174, 1996

Kohut H: The Analysis of the Self. New York, International Universities Press, 1971

Kovacs M, Gatsonis C, Paulauskas SL, et al: Depressive disorders in childhood, IV: a longitudinal study of comorbidity with and risk for anxiety disorders. Arch Gen Psychiatry 46:776–782, 1989

Kovacs M, Akiskal HS, Gatsonis C, et al: Childhood-onset dysthymic disorder: clinical features and prospective naturalistic outcome. Arch Gen Psychiatry 51:365–374, 1994

Kraepelin E: Manic-Depressive Insanity and Paranoia. Translated by Barclay RM. Edinburgh, Scotland, Livingstone, 1921

Kroeze WK, Roth BI: The molecular biology of serotonin receptors: therapeutic implications for the interface of mood and psychosis. Biol Psychiatry 44:1128–1142, 1998

Krueger RB, Sackeim HA, Gamzu ER: Pharmacological treatment of the cognitive side effects of ECT: a review. Psychopharmacol Bull 28:409–424, 1992

Krupnick JL, Sotsky SM, Simmens S, et al: The role of the therapeutic alliance in psychotherapy and pharmacotherapy outcome: findings in the National Institute of Mental Health Treatment of Depression Collaborative Research Program. J Consult Clin Psychol 64:532–539, 1996

Kukopulos A, Reginaldi D, Laddomada P: Course of the manic-depressive cycle and changes caused by treatment. Pharmakopsychiatry Neuropsychopharmakoly 13:156–167, 1980

Kupfer DJ: Sleep research in depressive illness: clinical implications—a tasting menu. Biol Psychiatry 36:391–403, 1995

Kupfer DJ, Frank E, Perel JM: Five-year outcome for maintenance therapies in recurrent depression. Arch Gen Psychiatry 49:769–773, 1992

Kutcher S, Robertson HA: Electroconvulsive therapy in treatment-resistant bipolar youth. J Child Adolesc Psychopharmacol 5:167–175, 1995

Labbate LA, Lafer B, Thibault A, et al: Influence of phototherapy treatment duration for seasonal affective disorder: outcome at one vs. two weeks. Biol Psychiatry 38:747–750, 1995

Lader M: Fluoxetine efficacy vs. comparative drugs: an overview. Br J Psychiatry 153(suppl 3):51–58, 1988

Lamy S, Bergsholm P, d'Elia G: The antidepressant efficacy of high-dose nondominant long-distance parietotemporal and bitemporal electroconvulsive therapy. Convuls Ther 10:43–52, 1994

Lang C, Field T, Pickens J, et al: Preschoolers of dysphoric mothers. J Child Psychol Psychiatry 37:221–224, 1996

Lasch K, Weissman MM: Birth cohort changes in the rate of mania. Psychiatry Res 33:31–37, 1990

Last CG, Thase ME, Hersen M, et al: Patterns of attrition for psychosocial and pharmacologic treatments of depression. Compr Psychiatry 46:361–366, 1985

Lavori P, Keller MB, Roth SL: Affective disorders and ABO blood groups: new data and a reanalysis of the literature using the logistic transformation of proportions. J Psychiatr Res 18:119–129, 1984

Lee DO, Steingard RJ, Cesena M, et al: Behavioral side effects of gabapentin in children. Epilepsia 37:87–90, 1996

Lehtinen V, Joukamaa M: Epidemiology of depression: prevalence, risk factors and treatment situation. Acta Psychiatr Scand 89(suppl):7–10, 1994

Leibenluft E: Women with bipolar illness: clinical and research issues. Am J Psychiatry 153:163–173, 1996

Leibenluft E, Clark CH, Myers FS: The reproducibility of depressive and hypomanic symptoms across repeated episodes in patients with rapid-cycling bipolar disorder. J Affect Disord 33:83–88, 1995

Lenox RH, Modell JG, Weiner S: Acute treatment of manic agitation with lorazepam. Psychosomatics 27(suppl):28–31, 1986

Leonard BE: Sub-types of serotonin receptors: biochemical changes and pharmacological consequences. Int Clin Psychopharmacol 7:13–21, 1992

Leonard BE: Effect of antidepressants on specific neurotransmitters: are such effects relevant to the therapeutic action?, in Handbook of Depression and Anxiety. Edited by den Boer JA, Sitsen JMA. New York, Marcel Dekker, 1994, pp 379–404

Leonhard K: Aufteilung der Endogenen Psychosen. Berlin, Germany, Akademie-Verlag, 1957

Leonhard K: Differential diagnosis and different aetiology of monopolar and bipolar depressions. Psicopatologia 7:277–285, 1987a

Leonhard K: Differential diagnosis and different etiology of monopolar and bipolar phasic psychoses [in German]. Psychiatrie, Neurologie und Medizinische Psychologie 39:524–533, 1987b

Lepine J, Pelissolo A, Weiller E, et al: Recurrent brief depression: clinical and epidemiological issues. Psychopathology 28(suppl 1):86–94, 1995

Lerer B, Stanley M: Does lithium stabilize muscarinic receptors? Biol Psychiatry 20:1247–1248, 1985

Letizia C, Kapik B, Flanders WD: Suicidal risk during controlled clinical investigations of fluvoxamine. Compr Psychiatry 57:415–421, 1996

Letterman L, Markowitz JS: Gabapentin: a review of published experience in the treatment of bipolar disorder and other psychiatric conditions. Pharmacotherapy 19:565–572, 1999

Levine J, Barak Y, Gonzalves M, et al: Double-blind, controlled trial of inositol treatment of depression. Am J Psychiatry 152:792–794, 1995

Levitt AJ, Joffe RT, MacDonald C: Life course of depressive illness and characteristics of current episode in patients with double depression. J Nerv Ment Dis 179:678–682, 1991

Lewinsohn PM, Antonuccio DA, Steinmetz J, et al: The Coping With Depression Course: A Psychoeducational Intervention for Unipolar Depression. Eugene, OR, Castalia Press, 1984

Lewinsohn PM, Klein DN, Seeley JR: Bipolar disorders in a community sample of older adolescents: prevalence, phenomenology, comorbidity, and course. J Am Acad Child Adolesc Psychiatry 34:454–463, 1995

Li XM, Chlan-Fourney J, Juorio AV, et al: Antidepressants up-regulate messenger RNA levels of the neuroprotective enzyme superoxide-dismutase (SOD1). J Psychiatry Neurosci 25:43–47, 2000

Licht RW: Drug treatment of mania: a critical review. Acta Psychiatr Scand 97:387–397, 1998

Lin EH, Katon WJ, Von Korff M, et al: Relapse of depression in primary care: rate and clinical predictors. Arch Fam Med 7:443–449, 1998

Lindenmayer JP, Klebanov R: Olanzapine-induced manic-like syndrome (letter). J Clin Psychiatry 59:318–319, 1998

Lindhout D, Omtzigt JG: Pregnancy and the risk of teratogenicity. Epilepsia 33(suppl 4):S41–S48, 1992

Lindvall M, Hagnell O, Ohman R: Epidemiology of cycloid psychosis. Psychopathology 23:228–232, 1990

Lindvall M, Axelsson R, Ohman R: Incidence of cycloid psychosis: a clinical study of first-admission psychotic patients. Eur Arch Psychiatry Clin Neurosci 242:197–202, 1993

Linnoila M, Virkkunen M: Biologic correlates of suicidal risk and aggressive behavioral traits. J Clin Psychopharmacol 12:19S–20S, 1992

Lish JD, Gyulai L, Resnick SM, et al: A family history study of rapid-cycling bipolar disorder. Psychiatry Res 48:37–46, 1993

Little JD, Ungvari GS, McFarlane J: Successful ECT in a case of Leonhard's cycloid psychosis. J ECT 16:62–67, 2000

Little JT, Kimbrell TA, Wassermann EM, et al: Cognitive effects of 1- and 20-hertz repetitive transcranial magnetic stimulation in depression: preliminary report. Neuropsychiatry Neuropsychol Behav Neurol 13:119–124, 2000

Littlejohn R, Leslie F, Cookson J: Depot antipsychotics in the prophylaxis of bipolar affective disorder. Br J Psychiatry 165:827–829, 1994

London JA: Mania associated with olanzapine (letter). J Am Acad Child Adolesc Psychiatry 37:135–136, 1998

Long TD, Kathol RG: Critical review of data supporting affective disorder caused by nonpsychotropic medication. Ann Clin Psychiatry 5:259–270, 1993

Loo C, Mitchell P, Sachdev P, et al: Double-blind controlled investigation of transcranial magnetic stimulation for the treatment of resistant major depression. Am J Psychiatry 156:946–948, 1999

Loo H, Brochier T: Long-term treatment with antidepressive drugs [in French]. Ann Med Psychol (Paris) 153:190–196, 1995

Lopez-Ibor JL: The involvement of serotonin in psychiatric disorders and behaviour. Br J Psychiatry 153(suppl 3):26–39, 1988

Loranger AW, Lenzenweger MF, Gartner AF, et al: Trait-state artifacts and the diagnosis of personality disorders. Arch Gen Psychiatry 48:720–728, 1991

Lovett LM, Shaw DM: Outcome in bipolar affective disorder after stereotactic tractotomy. Br J Psychiatry 151:113–116, 1987

Lowe MR: Treatment of rapid cycling affective illness (letter). Br J Psychiatry 146:558, 1985

Luborsky L: Principles of Psychoanalytic Psychotherapy: A Manual for Supportive-Expressive Treatment. New York, Basic Books, 1984

Lweeke FM, Bauer J, Elger CE: Manic episode due to gabapentin treatment (letter). Br J Psychiatry 175:291, 1999

Lyons MJ, Huppert J, Toomey R, et al: Lifetime prevalence of mood and anxiety disorders in twin pairs discordant for schizophrenia. Twin Res 3:28–32, 2000

Madhusoodanan S, Brenner R, Araujo L, et al: Efficacy of risperidone treatment for psychoses associated with schizophrenia, schizoaffective disorder, bipolar disorder, or senile dementia in 11 geriatric patients: a case series. Compr Psychiatry 56:514–518, 1995

Maes M, Smith R, Christophe A, et al: Fatty acid composition in major depression: decreased omega-3 fractions in cholesteryl esters and increased C20: 4 omega 6/C20:5 omega 3 ratio in cholesteryl esters and phospholipids. J Affect Disord 38:35–46, 1996

Maes M, Christophe A, Delanghe J, et al: Lowered omega3 polyunsaturated fatty acids in serum phospholipids and cholesteryl esters of depressed patients. Psychiatry Res 85:275–291, 1999

Magnan V: Lecons Cliniques, 2nd Edition. Paris, France, Bataille, 1893

MagPhil PLG, Thomas CB: Themes of interaction in medical students' Rorschach responses as predictors of midlife health or disease. Psychosom Med 43:215–225, 1981

Maier W, Hallmayer J, Zill P, et al: Linkage analysis between pericentrometric markers on chromosome 18 and bipolar disorder: a replication test. Psychiatry Res 59:7–15, 1995a

Maier W, Lichtermann D, Minges J, et al: The relationship between bipolar disorder and alcoholism: a controlled family study. Psychol Med 25:787–796, 1995b

Maj M: Effectiveness of lithium prophylaxis in schizoaffective psychoses: application of a polydiagnostic approach. Acta Psychiatr Scand 70:228–234, 1984

Maj M: Clinical course and outcome of cycloid psychotic disorder: a three-year prospective study. Acta Psychiatr Scand 78:182–187, 1988

Maj M, Veltro F, Pirozzi R, et al: Pattern of recurrence of illness after recovery from an episode of major depression: a prospective study. Am J Psychiatry 149:795–800, 1992

Malawska B, Kulig K, Antkiewicz-Michaluk L, et al: Synthesis, physicochemical properties, anticonvulsant activities, and GABA-ergic and voltage-sensitive calcium channel receptor affinities of alpha-substituted N-benzylamides of gamma-hydroxybutyric acid, part 4: search for new anticonvulsant compounds. Arch Pharm (Weinheim) 332:167–174, 1999

Mandoki MW, Tapia MR, Tapia MA, et al: Venlafaxine in the treatment of children and adolescents with major depression. Psychopharmacol Bull 33:149–154, 1997

Manji HK, Bebchuk JM, Moore GJ, et al: Modulation of CNS signal transduction pathways and gene expression by mood-stabilizing agents: therapeutic implications. J Clin Psychiatry 60(suppl 2):27–39, 1999

Mann J: Time-Limited Psychotherapy. Cambridge, MA, Harvard University Press, 1973

Mann JJ, Malone KM: Cerebrospinal fluid amines and higher-lethality suicide attempts in depressed inpatients. Biol Psychiatry 41:162–171, 1997

Mann JJ, Arango V, Marzuk PM: Evidence for the 5-HT hypothesis of suicide: a review of post-mortem studies. Br J Psychiatry 155(suppl 8):7–14, 1989

Manna V: Disturbi affectivi bipolari e ruolo del calcio intraneuronale: effetti terapeutici del trattamento con cali di litio e/o calcio antagonista in pazienti con rapida inversione di polarita. Minerva Med 82:757–763, 1991

Marangell LB, George MS, Callahan AM, et al: Effects of intrathecal thyrotropin-releasing hormone (protirelin) in refractory depressed patients. Arch Gen Psychiatry 54:214–222, 1997

Marin DB, Kocsis JH, Frances AJ, et al: Personality disorders in dysthymia. J Personal Disord 7:223–231, 1993

Martin M, Figiel GS, Mattingly G, et al: ECT-induced interictal delirium in patients with a history of a CVA. J Geriatr Psychiatry Neurol 5:149–155, 1992

Marttunen MJ, Henriksson MM, Aro HM, et al: Suicide among female adolescents: characteristics and comparison with males in the age group 13 to 22 years. J Am Acad Child Adolesc Psychiatry 34:1297–1307, 1995

Mathews R, Li PP, Young T, et al: Increased $G\alpha_{q/11}$ immunoreactivity in postmortem occipital cortex from patients with bipolar affective disorder. Biol Psychiatry 41:649–656, 1997

Matsuo F, Madsen J, Tolman KG, et al: Lamotrigine high-dose tolerability and safety in patients with epilepsy: a double-blind, placebo-controlled, eleven-week study. Epilepsia 37:857–862, 1996

Mattson RH: Efficacy and adverse effects of established and new antiepileptic drugs. Epilepsia 36(suppl 2):S13–S26, 1995

Max JE, Richards L, Hamdan-Allen G: Case study: antimanic effectiveness of dextroamphetamine in a brain-injured adolescent. J Am Acad Child Adolesc Psychiatry 34:472–476, 1995

McBride PA, Brown RP, DeMeo M: The relationship of platelet 5-HT2 receptor indices to major depressive disorder, personality traits, and suicidal behavior. Biol Psychiatry 35:295–308, 1994

McCabe MS, Norris B: ECT versus chlorpromazine in mania. Biol Psychiatry 12:245–254, 1977

McCormick DA, Williamson A: Convergence and divergence of neurotransmitter action in human cerebral cortex. Proc Natl Acad Sci U S A 86:8098–8102, 1989

McDaniel JS, Musselman DL, Proter MR: Depression in patients with cancer. Arch Gen Psychiatry 52:89–99, 1995

McDermott OD, Prigerson HG, Reynolds CF III, et al: Sleep in the wake of complicated grief symptoms: an exploratory study. Biol Psychiatry 41:710–716, 1997

McDowell DM, Clodfelter RC: Depression and substance abuse: considerations of etiology, comorbidity, evaluation, and treatment. Psychiatr Ann 31:244–251, 2001

McElroy SL, Dessain EC, Pope HG, et al: Clozapine in the treatment of psychotic mood disorders, schizoaffective disorder, and schizophrenia. Compr Psychiatry 52:411–414, 1991

McElroy SL, Keck PE, Pope HG, et al: Clinical and research implications of the diagnosis of dysphoric or mixed mania or hypomania. Am J Psychiatry 149:1633–1644, 1992

McElroy SL, Keck PE, Strakowski SM: Mania, psychosis, and antipsychotics. Compr Psychiatry 57(suppl 3):14–26, 1996a

McElroy SL, Keck PE, Stanton SP, et al: A randomized comparison of divalproex oral loading versus haloperidol in the initial treatment of acute psychotic mania. Compr Psychiatry 57:142–146, 1996b

McElroy SL, Suppes T, Keck PE, et al: Open-label adjunctive topiramate in the treatment of bipolar disorders. Biol Psychiatry 47:1025–1033, 2000

McGlashan TH: Adolescent versus adult onset of mania. Am J Psychiatry 145:221–223, 1988

McGrath PJ, Nunes EV, Stewart JW, et al: Imipramine treatment of alcoholics with primary depression: a placebo controlled clinical trial. Arch Gen Psychiatry 53:232–240, 1996

McKinney WT: Animal models for depression and mania, in Depression and Mania. Edited by Georgotas A, Cancro R. New York, Elsevier, 1988, pp 181–196

McLean MJ: Gabapentin. Epilepsia 36(suppl 2):S73–S86, 1995

McLean PD: Behavior therapy: theory and research, in Short-Term Psychotherapies for Depression. Edited by Rush AJ. New York, Guilford, 1982, pp 19–49

McLean PD, Hakstian AR: Relative endurance of unipolar depression treatment effects: a longitudinal follow-up. J Consult Clin Psychol 58:482–488, 1990

McLean P[D], Taylor S: Severity of unipolar depression and choice of treatment. Behav Res Ther 30:443–451, 1992

McNeil TF: A prospective study of postpartum psychoses in a high-risk group, 1: clinical characteristics of the current postpartum episodes. Acta Psychiatr Scand 74:205–216, 1986

Meltzer HY: Serotonergic dysfunction in depression. Br J Psychiatry 155(suppl 8):25–31, 1989

Meltzer HY: The importance of serotonin-dopamine interactions in the action of clozapine. Br J Psychiatry 160(suppl 17):22–29, 1992

Meltzer HY, Lowry MT: The serotonin hypothesis of depression, in Psychopharmacology: The Third Generation of Progress. Edited by Meltzer HY. New York, Raven, 1987, pp 513–526

Meredith LS: Counseling typically provided for depression: role of clinician specialty and payment system. Arch Gen Psychiatry 53:905–912, 1996

Merriam AE, Karasu TB: The role of psychotherapy in the treatment of depression. Arch Gen Psychiatry 53:301–302, 1996

Messenheimer JA: Lamotrigine. Epilepsia 36(suppl 2):S87–S94, 1995

Meterissian GB, Bradwejn J: Comparative studies on the efficacy of psychotherapy, pharmacotherapy, and their combination in depression: was adequate pharmacotherapy provided? J Clin Psychopharmacol 9:334–339, 1989

Miklowitz DJ: Longitudinal outcome and medication noncompliance among manic patients with and without mood-incongruent psychotic features. J Nerv Ment Dis 180:703–711, 1992

Miklowitz DJ, Goldstein MJ: Behavioral family treatment for patients with bipolar affective disorder. Behav Modif 14:457–489, 1990

Miklowitz DJ, Goldstein MJ, Nuechterlein KH, et al: Family factors and the course of bipolar disorder. Arch Gen Psychiatry 45:225–231, 1988

Miklowitz DJ, Simoneau TL, George EL, et al: Family focused treatment of bipolar disorder: 1-year effects of a psycho-educational program in conjunction with pharmacotherapy. Biol Psychiatry 8:582–592, 2000

Milberger S, Biederman J, Faraone SV, et al: Attention deficit hyperactivity disorder and comorbid disorder: issues of overlapping symptoms. Am J Psychiatry 152:1793–1799, 1995

Miller HL, Coombs DW, Leeper JD, et al: An analysis of the effect of suicide prevention facilities on suicide rates in the United States. Am J Public Health 74:340–343, 1984

Miller IW, Keitner GI: Combined medication and psychotherapy in the treatment of chronic mood disorders. Psychiatr Clin North Am 19:151–171, 1996

Miller IW, Norman WH, Dow MG: Psychosocial characteristics of "double depression." Am J Psychiatry 153:1042–1044, 1986

Miller RJ, Chouinard G: Loss of striatal cholinergic neurons as a basis for tardive and L-dopa-induced dyskinesias, neuroleptic-induced supersensitivity psychosis and refractory schizophrenia. Biol Psychiatry 34:713–738, 1993

Milstein V, Small JG, Klapper MH: Uni- versus bilateral ECT in the treatment of mania. Convuls Ther 3:1–9, 1987

Mitchell PB, Wilhelm K, Parker G, et al: The clinical features of bipolar depression: a comparison with matched major depressive disorder patients. J Clin Psychiatry 62:212–216, 2001

Modell JG, Lenox RH, Weiner S: Inpatient clinical trial of lorazepam for the management of manic agitation. J Clin Psychopharmacol 5:109–113, 1985

Montgomery SA: Selective serotonin reuptake inhibitors in the acute treatment of depression, in Psychopharmacology, The Fourth Generation of Progress. Edited by Bloom FE, Kupfer DJ. New York, Raven, 1995, pp 1043–1051

Montgomery SA, Fineberg N: Is there a relationship between serotonin receptor subtypes and selectivity of response in specific psychiatric illnesses? Br J Psychiatry 155(suppl 8):63–70, 1989

Moos RH, Mertens JR: Patterns of diagnoses, comorbidities, and treatment in late-middle-aged and older affective disorder patients: comparison of mental health and medical sectors. J Am Geriatr Soc 44:682–688, 1996

Morris GL: Efficacy and tolerability of gabapentin in clinical practice. Clin Ther 17:891–900, 1995

Morris PLP, Robinson RG, Samuels J: Depression, introversion and mortality following stroke. Aust N Z J Psychiatry 27:443–449, 1993

Mosimann UP, Rihs TA, Engeler J, et al: Mood effects of repetitive transcranial magnetic stimulation of left prefrontal cortex in healthy volunteers. Psychiatry Res 94:252–256, 2000

Mueller TI, Leon AC: Recovery, chronicity, and levels of psychopathology in major depression. Psychiatr Clin North Am 19:85–102, 1996

Mukherjee S, Rosen AM, Caracci G, et al: Persistent tardive dyskinesia in bipolar patients. Arch Gen Psychiatry 43:342–346, 1986

Mukherjee S, Sackeim HA, Schnur DB: Electroconvulsive therapy of acute manic episodes: a review of 50 years' experience. Am J Psychiatry 151:169–176, 1994

Murad F: Drugs used for the treatment of angina: organic nitrates, calcium-channel blockers, and β-adrenergic agents, in Goodman and Gilman's The Pharmacological Basis of Therapeutics, 8th Edition. Edited by Gilman AG, Rall TW, Nies AS, et al. New York, Pergamon, 1991, pp 764–783

Murphy DL, Zohar J, Benkelfat C: Obsessive-compulsive disorder as a 5-HT subsystem-related behavioural disorder. Br J Psychiatry 155(suppl 8):15–24, 1989

National Institute of Mental Health: Affective Disorders (Mood Disorders): Budget Estimate. Bethesda, MD, National Institute of Mental Health, 1995

Nease DE, Volk RJ, Cass AR: Investigation of a severity-based classification of mood and anxiety symptoms in primary care patients. J Am Board Fam Pract 12:21–31, 1999

Nelson JC, Price LH, Jatlow PI: Neuroleptic dose and desipramine concentrations during combined treatment of unipolar delusional depression. Am J Psychiatry 143:1151–1154, 1986

Nelson WH, Khan A, Orr WW: Delusional depression: phenomenology, neuroendocrine function and tricyclic antidepressant response. J Affect Disord 6:297–306, 1984

Nemets B, Mishory A, Levine J, et al: Inositol addition does not improve depression in SSRI treatment failures. J Neural Transm 106:795–798, 1999

Neylan TC: Treatment of sleep disturbances in depressed patients. Compr Psychiatry 56(suppl 2):56–61, 1995

Nezu AM: Efficacy of a social problem-solving therapy for unipolar depression. J Consult Clin Psychol 54:196–202, 1986

Nierenberg AA: The treatment of severe depression: is there an efficacy gap between SSRI and TCA antidepressant generations? Compr Psychiatry 55(suppl A):55–59, 1994

Nolen WA, Bloenkolk D: Treatment of bipolar depression: a review of the literature and a suggestion for an algorithm. Neuropsychobiology 42(suppl 1):11–17, 2000

Okamoto Y, Kagaya A, Shinno H, et al: Serotonin-induced platelet calcium mobilization is enhanced in mania. Life Sci 56:327–332, 1995

O'Keane V, Maloney E, O'Neill H, et al: Blunted prolactin responses to d-fenfluramine in sociotopathy: evidence for subsensitivity of central serotonergic function. Br J Psychiatry 160:643–646, 1992

Okuma T, Yamashita I, Takahashi R, et al: Comparison of the antimanic efficacy of carbamazepine and lithium carbonate by double-blind controlled study. Pharmacopsychiatry 23:143–150, 1990

Olfson M: Subthreshold psychiatric symptoms in a primary care group practice. Arch Gen Psychiatry 53:880–886, 1996

Olie JP, Brochier T, Bouvet O, et al: La conception actuelle des troubles de l'humeur: incidence sur la prise en charge thérapeutique. Encephale 18(Spec No 1):55–63, 1992

Osser DN: A systematic approach to the classification and pharmacotherapy of nonpsychotic major depression and dysthymia. J Clin Psychopharmacol 13:133–144, 1993

Overall JE, Donachie ND, Faillace LA: Implications of restrictive diagnosis for compliance to antidepressant drug therapy: alprazolam versus imipramine. Compr Psychiatry 48:51–54, 1987

Oxley SL, Van Meter S: The assessment and management of the suicidal patient. Journal of Practical Psychiatry and Behavioral Health 6:327–335, 1996

Papatheodorou G, Kutcher S: The effect of adjunctive light therapy on ameliorating breakthrough depressive symptoms in adolescent-onset bipolar disorder. J Psychiatry Neurosci 20:226–232, 1995

Papatheodorou G, Kutcher SP, Katic M, et al: The efficacy and safety of divalproex sodium in the treatment of acute mania in adolescents and young adults: an open clinical trial. J Clin Psychopharmacol 15:110–116, 1995

Parker G, Blennerhassert J: Withdrawal reactions associated with venlafaxine. Aust N Z J Psychiatry 32:291–294, 1998

Parker V, Wong AH, Boon HS, et al: Adverse reactions to St. John's wort. Can J Psychiatry 46:77–79, 2001

Partonen T, Sihvo S, Lonnqvist JK: Patients excluded from an antidepressant efficacy trial. Compr Psychiatry 57:572–575, 1996

Paykel ES: Handbook of Affective Disorders. New York, Guilford, 1982, pp xii, 699

Pazzaglia PJ, Post RM, Ketter TA, et al: Preliminary controlled trial of nimodipine in ultra-rapid cycling affective dysregulation. Psychiatry Res 49:257–272, 1993

Peet M, Peters S: Drug-induced mania. Drug Saf 12:146–153, 1995

Peet M, Murphy B, Shay J, et al: Depletion of omega-3 fatty acid levels in red blood cell membranes of depressive patients. Biol Psychiatry 43:315–319, 1998

Perris C: Morbidity suppressive effect of lithium carbonate in cycloid psychosis. Arch Gen Psychiatry 35:328–331, 1978

Perris C: The concept of cycloid psychotic disorder. Psychiatric Developments 1:37–56, 1988

Perris C: The importance of Karl Leonhard's classification of endogenous psychoses. Psychopathology 23:282–290, 1990

Perris C, Smigan L: The use of lithium in the long-term morbidity suppressive treatment of cycloid and schizoaffective psychoses, in Psychiatry: The State of the Art, Vol 3: Pharmacopsychiatry. Edited by Pichot P. New York, Plenum, 1984 pp 55–72

Perry JC: Depression in borderline personality disorder: lifetime prevalence at interview and longitudinal course of symptoms. Am J Psychiatry 142:15–21, 1985

Perry PJ, Zeilmann C, Arndt S: Tricyclic antidepressant concentrations in plasma: an estimate of their sensitivity and specificity as a predictor of response. J Clin Psychopharmacol 14:230–235, 1994

Persons JB, Thase ME, Crits-Christoph P: The role of psychotherapy in the treatment of depression. Arch Gen Psychiatry 53:283–290, 1996

Perugi G, Micheli C, Akiskal HS, et al: Polarity of the first episode, clinical characteristics, and course of manic depressive illness: a systematic retrospective investigation of 320 bipolar I patients. J Clin Psychiatry 41:13–18, 2000

Peselow ED, Fieve RR, Difiglia C, et al: Lithium prophylaxis of bipolar illness. Br J Psychiatry 164:208–214, 1994

Petracca G, Teson A, Chemerinski E: A double-blind placebo-controlled study of clomipramine in depressed patients with Alzheimer's disease. J Neuropsychiatry Clin Neurosci 8:270–275, 1996

Petrides G, Dhossche D, Fink M, et al: Continuation ECT: relapse prevention in affective disorders. Convuls Ther 10:189–194, 1994

Petronis KR, Samuels JF, Moscicki EK, et al: An epidemiologic investigation of potential risk factors for suicide attempts. Soc Psychiatry Psychiatr Epidemiol 25:193–199, 1990

Pettinati HM, Rosenberg J: Memory self-ratings before and after electroconvulsive therapy: depression versus ECT induced. Biol Psychiatry 19:539–548, 1984

Pfuhlmann B: Das Konzept der zykloiden Psychosen. Fortschr Neurol Psychiatr 66:1–9, 1998

Pfuhlmann B, Stober G, Franzek E, et al: Cycloid psychoses predominate in severe postpartum psychiatric disorders. J Affect Disord 50:125–134, 1998

Piccinelli M, Wilkinson G: Outcome of depression in psychiatric settings. Br J Psychiatry 164:297–304, 1994

Piper AJ: Tricyclic antidepressants versus electroconvulsive therapy: a review of the evidence for efficacy in depression. Ann Clin Psychiatry 5:13–23, 1993

Pitts FN: Recent research on the DST. Compr Psychiatry 45:380–381, 1984

Poirier MF, Boyer P: Venlafaxine and paroxetine in treatment-resistant depression: double-blind, randomised comparison. Br J Psychiatry 175:12–16, 1999

Pokorny AD: Suicide prevention revisited. Suicide Life Threat Behav 23:1–10, 1993

Poland RE, McCracken JT, Lutchmansingh P, et al: Differential response of rapid eye movement sleep to cholinergic blockade by scopolamine in currently depressed, remitted, and normal control subjects. Biol Psychiatry 41:929–938, 1997

Porter RJ: How to initiate and maintain carbamazepine therapy in children and adults. Epilepsia 28(suppl 3):S59–S63, 1987

Post RM: Approaches to treatment-resistant bipolar affectively ill patients. Clin Neuropharmacol 11:93–104, 1988

Post RM: Non-lithium treatment for bipolar disorder. Compr Psychiatry 51(suppl 8):9–16, 1990a

Post RM: Prophylaxis of bipolar affective disorders. International Review of Psychiatry 2:277–320, 1990b

Post RM: Anticonvulsants and novel drugs, in Handbook of Affective Disorders. Edited by Paykel ES. Edinburgh, Scotland, Churchill Livingstone, 1992a, pp 387–417

Post RM: Transduction of psychosocial stress into the neurobiology of recurrent affective disorder. Am J Psychiatry 149:999–1010, 1992b

Post RM: Mechanisms underlying the evolution of affective disorders: implications for long-term treatment. Washington, DC, American Psychiatric Press, 1994, pp 23–65

Post RM: Comparative pharmacology of bipolar disorder and schizophrenia. Schizophr Res 39:153–158, 1999

Post RM, Rubinow DR, Ballenger JC: Conditioning and sensitisation in the longitudinal course of affective illness. Br J Psychiatry 149:191–201, 1986

Post RM, Roy-Byrne PP, Uhde TW: Graphic representation of the life course of illness in patients with affective disorder. Am J Psychiatry 145:844–848, 1988

Post RM, Leverich G, Altschuler LL, et al: Lithium discontinuation-induced refractoriness: preliminary observations. Am J Psychiatry 149:1727–1729, 1991

Post RM, Weiss SR, Chuang DM: Mechanisms of action of anticonvulsants in affective disorders: comparisons with lithium. J Clin Psychopharmacol 12(suppl 1):23S–35S, 1992

Post RM, Ketter TA, Pazzaglia PJ, et al: New developments in the use of anticonvulsants as mood stabilizers. Neuropsychobiology 27:132–137, 1993

Post RM, Ketter TA, Pazzaglia PJ, et al: Rational polypharmacy in the bipolar affective disorders. Epilepsy Res Suppl 11:153–180, 1996

Post RM, Leverich GS, Denicoff KD, et al: Alternative approaches to refractory depression in bipolar illness. Depress Anxiety 5:175–189, 1997

Post RM, Frye MA, Denicoff KD, et al: Beyond lithium in the treatment of bipolar illness. Neuropsychopharmacology 3:206–219, 1998

Post RM, Kimbrell TA, McCann UD, et al: Repetitive transcranial magnetic stimulation as a neuropsychiatric tool: present status and future potential. J ECT 15:39–59, 1999

Poynton A, Bridges PK, Bartlett JR, et al: Resistant bipolar affective disorder treated by stereotactic subcaudate tractotomy. Br J Psychiatry 152:354–358, 1988

Pozo P, Aleantara AG: Mania-like syndrome in a patient with chronic schizophrenia during olanzapine treatment (letter). J Psychiatry Neurosci 23:309–310, 1998

Preda A, MacLean RW, Mazure CM, et al: Antidepressant-associated mania and psychosis resulting in psychiatric admissions. Compr Psychiatry 62:30–33, 2001

Preskhorn SH: Pharmacokinetics of antidepressants: why and how they are relevant to treatment. Compr Psychiatry 52:4–8, 1991

Prien RF, Caffey EM, Klett CJ: Comparison of lithium carbonate and chlorpromazine in the treatment of mania. Arch Gen Psychiatry 26:146–153, 1972

Priest RG, Gimbrett R, Roberts M, et al: Reversible and selective inhibitors of monoamine oxidase A in mental and other disorders. Acta Psychiatr Scand Suppl 386:40–43, 1995

Privitera MR, Lamberti JS, Maharaj K: Clozapine in a bipolar depressed patient (letter). Am J Psychiatry 150:986, 1993

Prudic J, Sackeim HA, Devanand DP, et al: The efficacy of ECT in double depression. Depression 1:38–44, 1993

Prudic J, Peyser S, Sackeim HA: Subjective memory complaints: a review of patient self-assessment of memory after electroconvulsive therapy. J ECT 16:121–132, 2000

Puri BK, Taylor DG, Alcock ME: Low-dose maintenance clozapine treatment in the prophylaxis of bipolar affective disorder. Br J Clin Pract 49:333–334, 1995

Quitkin FM, McGrath PJ, Stewart JW, et al: Atypical depression, panic attacks, and response to imipramine and phenelzine: a replication. Arch Gen Psychiatry 47:935–941, 1990

Quitkin FM, Harrison W, Stewart JW, et al: Response to phenelzine and imipramine in placebo nonresponders with atypical depression: a new application of the crossover design. Arch Gen Psychiatry 48:319–323, 1991

Rabheru K, Persad E: A review of continuation and maintenance electroconvulsive therapy. Can J Psychiatry 42:476–484, 1998

Rabkin JG, Stewart JW, Quitkin F, et al: Should atypical depression be included as a separate entity in DSM-IV? A review of the research evidence, in DSM-IV Sourcebook. Edited by Widiger TA, Frances AJ, Pincus HA, et al. Washington, DC, American Psychiatric Press, 1995, pp 140–154

Ramasubbu R, Kennedy SH: Factors complicating the diagnosis of depression in cerebrovascular disease, II: neurological deficits and various assessment methods. Can J Psychiatry 39:601–607, 1994

Rao U, McCracken JT, Lutchmansingh P, et al: Electroencephalographic sleep and urinary free cortisol in adolescent depression: a preliminary report of changes from episode to recovery. Biol Psychiatry 41:369–373, 1997

Rao U, Daley SE, Hammen C: Relationship between depression and substance use disorders in adolescent women during the transition to adulthood. J Am Acad Child Adolesc Psychiatry 39:315–322, 2000

Reeves RR, McBride WA, Brannon GE: Olanzapine-induced mania (letter). J Am Osteopath Assoc 98:550, 1998

Rehm LP: A self-control model of depression. Behav Ther 8:787–804, 1977

Reiger DA, Boyd JH, Burke JD: One-month prevalence of mental disorders in the United States. Arch Gen Psychiatry 45:977–986, 1988

Remotiv/Imipramine Study Group: Comparison of St John's wort and imipramine for treating depression: randomised controlled trial. BMJ 321:536–539, 2000

Reynolds CF III, Hoch CC: Differential diagnosis of depressive pseudodementia and primary degenerative dementia. Psychiatr Ann 17:743–748, 1987

Reynolds CF III, Kupfer DJ, Thase ME, et al: Sleep, gender and depression: an analysis of gender effects on the electroencephalographic sleep of 302 depressed outpatients. Biol Psychiatry 28:673–684, 1990

Reynolds CF III, Frank E, Perel JM, et al: Maintenance therapies for late-life recurrent major depression: research and review circa 1995. Int Psychogeriatr 7(suppl):27–39, 1995

Rifkin A, Doddi S, Karajgi B, et al: Dosage of haloperidol for mania. Br J Psychiatry 165:113–116, 1994

Riggs PD, Mikulich S, Coffman L, et al: Fluoxetine in drug-dependent delinquents with major depression: an open trial. J Child Adolesc Psychopharmacol 7:87–95, 1997

Riso LP, Klein DN, Ferro T: Understanding the comorbidity between early onset dysthymia and Cluster B personality disorders: a family study. Am J Psychiatry 153:900–906, 1996

Roberts RE, Lewinsohn PM, Seeley JR: Symptoms of DSM-III-R major depression in adolescence: evidence from an epidemiological survey. J Am Acad Child Adolesc Psychiatry 34:1608–1617, 1995

Robinson RG, Bostan JD, Sarkstein SE, et al: Comparison of mania and depression after brain injury. Am J Psychiatry 145:172–175, 1988

Roose SP, Stern RH: Medication use in training cases: a survey. J Am Psychoanal Assoc 43:163–170, 1995

Rosenbaum JF, Fava M, Nierenberg AA, et al: Treatment-resistant mood disorders, in Treatment of Psychiatric Disorders. Edited by Gabbard GO. Washington, DC, American Psychiatric Press, 1995, pp 1275–1328

Rosenthal NE, Oren DA: Light therapy, in Treatment of Psychiatric Disorders. Edited by Gabbard GO. Washington, DC, American Psychiatric Press, 1995, pp 1263–1273

Rosenthal N, Sack DA, Skwerer RG, et al: Phototherapy for seasonal affective disorder, in Seasonal Affective Disorders and Phototherapy. Edited by Rosenthal NE, Blehar MC. New York, Guilford, 1989, pp 273–294

Ross ED: The aprosodias: functional anatomic organization of the affective components of language in the right hemisphere. Arch Neurol 38:561–569, 1981

Roth D, Bielsky R, Jones M, et al: A comparison of self-control therapy and combined self-control therapy and antidepressant medication in the treatment of depression. Behav Ther 13:133–144, 1982

Rothschild AJ, Bates KS, Boehringer KL, et al: Olanzapine response in psychotic depression. J Clin Psychiatry 60:116–118, 1999

Roy-Byrne PP, Joffe RT, Uhde TW, et al: Approaches to the evaluation and treatment of rapid-cycling affective illness. Br J Psychiatry 145:543–550, 1984

Roy-Byrne PP, Post RM, Uhde TW, et al: The longitudinal course of recurrent affective illness: life chart data from research patients at the NIMH. Acta Psychiatr Scand Suppl 317:1–34, 1985

Rudd MD, Dahm PF, Rajab MH: Diagnostic comorbidity in persons with suicidal ideation and behavior. Am J Psychiatry 150:928–934, 1993

Rush AJ, Kupfer DJ: Strategies and tactics in the treatment of depression, in Treatment of Psychiatric Disorders. Edited by Gabbard GO. Washington, DC, American Psychiatric Press, 1995, pp 1349–1368

Rush AJ, Giles DE, Schlesser MA, et al: Dexamethasone response, thyrotropin-releasing hormone stimulation, rapid eye movement latency, and subtypes of depression. Biol Psychiatry 41:915–928, 1997

Sachs GS: Adjuncts and alternatives to lithium therapy for bipolar affective disorder. Compr Psychiatry 50(suppl 12):31–39, 1989

Sachs GS: Use of clonazepam for bipolar disorder. Compr Psychiatry 51(suppl 5):31–34, 1990

Sachs GS: Treatment-resistant bipolar depression. Psychiatr Clin North Am 19:215–235, 1996

Sachs GS, Lafer B, Stoll AL, et al: A double-blind trial of bupropion versus desipramine for bipolar depression. Compr Psychiatry 55:391–393, 1994a

Sachs GS, Lafer B, Truman CJ, et al: Lithium monotherapy: miracle, myth and misunderstanding. Psychiatr Ann 24:299–306, 1994b

Sachs G, Printz DJ, Kahn DA, et al: The Expert Consensus Guideline Series: Medication Treatment of Bipolar Disorder 2000. Postgrad Med 108(Spec No):1–104, 2000

Sackeim HA: Continuation therapy following ECT: directions for future research. Psychopharmacol Bull 30:501–521, 1994

Sackeim HA, Freeman J, McElhiney M, et al: Effects of major depression on estimates of intelligence. J Clin Exp Neuropsychol 14:268–288, 1992

Sajatovic M: A pilot study evaluating the efficacy of risperidone in treatment-refractory, acute bipolar, and schizoaffective mania (abstract). Psychopharmacol Bull 31:613, 1996

Sajatovic M, DiGiovanni SK, Bastani B, et al: Risperidone therapy in treatment refractory acute bipolar and schizoaffective mania. Psychopharmacol Bull 32:55–61, 1996

Salomon RM, Miller HL, Krystal JH, et al: Lack of behavioral effects of monoamine depletion in healthy subjects. Biol Psychiatry 41:58–64, 1997

Salzman C, Green AI, Rodriguez-Villa F, et al: Benzodiazepines combined with neuroleptics for management of severe disruptive behavior. Psychosomatics 27(suppl):17–21, 1986

Sanderson WC, Wetzler S, Beck AT, et al: Prevalence of personality disorders in patients with major depression and dysthymia. Psychiatry Res 42:93–99, 1992

Santos AB, Morton WA: More on clonazepam in manic agitation. J Clin Psychopharmacol 7:439–440, 1987

Saxena S, Maltikarjuna P: Severe memory impairment with acute overdose lithium toxicity. Br J Psychiatry 152:853–854, 1988

Schaffer CB, Schaffer LC: The use of risperidone in the treatment of bipolar disorder (letter). Compr Psychiatry 57:136, 1996

Schatzberg AF, Nemeroff CB (eds): The American Psychiatric Press Textbook of Psychopharmacology. Washington, DC, American Psychiatric Press, 1998

Schildkraut JJ: The catecholamine hypothesis of affective disorders: a review of supporting evidence. Am J Psychiatry 122:509–514, 1965

Schneekloth TB, Rummans TA, Logan KM: Electroconvulsive therapy in adolescents. Convuls Ther 9:158–166, 1993

Schneider LS, Sloane RB, Staples FR, et al: Pretreatment orthostatic hypotension as a predictor of response to nortriptyline in geriatric depression. J Clin Psychopharmacol 6:172–176, 1986

Schnur DB, Mukherjee S, Sackeim HA, et al: Symptomatic predictors of ECT response in medication-nonresponsive bipolar illness. Compr Psychiatry 53:63–66, 1992

Schoenenberger RA, Tanasijevic MJ, Jha A, et al: Appropriateness of antiepileptic drug level monitoring. JAMA 274:1622–1626, 1995

Schou M: Prophylactic lithium treatment of unipolar and bipolar manic-depressive illness. Psychopathology 28(suppl 1):81–85, 1995

Schou M: Forty years of lithium treatment. Arch Gen Psychiatry 54:9–13, 1997

Schreiber G, Avissar S: G proteins as a biochemical tool for diagnosis and monitoring treatments of mental disorders. Isr Med Assoc J 2(suppl):86–91, 2000

Schulberg HC: Treating major depression in primary care practice: eight-month clinical outcomes. Arch Gen Psychiatry 53:913–919, 1996

Schwarz T, Loewenstein J, Isenberg KE: Maintenance ECT: indications and outcome. Convuls Ther 11:14–23, 1995

Scott J: Chronic depression. Br J Psychiatry 153:287–297, 1988

Scott J: Chronic depression: can cognitive therapy succeed when other treatments fail? Behavioral Psychotherapy 20:25–36, 1992

Scott TF, Allen D, Price TRP: Characterization of major depression symptoms in multiple sclerosis patients. J Neuropsychiatry Clin Neurosci 8:318–323, 1996

Sedler MJ: Falret's discovery: the origin of the concept of bipolar affective illness. Am J Psychiatry 140:1127–1133, 1983

Seligman MEP: Helplessness: On Depression, Development and Death. San Francisco, CA, WH Freeman, 1975

Sernyak MJ, Woods SW: Chronic neuroleptic use in manic-depressive illness. Psychopharmacol Bull 29:375–381, 1993

Serretti A, Lilli R, Lorenzi C, et al: Serotonin-2C and serotonin-1A receptor genes are not associated with psychotic symptomatology of mood disorders. Am J Med Genet 96:161–166, 2000

Severus WE, Ahrens B. Omega-3 fatty acids in psychiatry. Nervenarzt 71:58–62, 2000

Sexton HC, Hembre K, Kvarme G: The interaction of the alliance and therapy microprocess: a sequential analysis. J Consult Clin Psychol 64:471–480, 1996

Shaffer D, Gould MS, Fisher P, et al: Psychiatric diagnosis in child and adolescent suicide. Arch Gen Psychiatry 53:339–348, 1996

Sharma V, Yatham LN, Haslam DR, et al: Continuation and prophylactic treatment of bipolar disorder. Can J Psychiatry 42(suppl 2):92S–100S, 1997

Shea MT, Hirschfeld RM: A chronic mood disorder and depressive personality. Psychiatr Clin North Am 19:103–120, 1996

Shea MT, Elkin I, Hirschfeld RMA, et al: Psychotherapeutic treatment of depression, in American Psychiatric Press Review of Psychiatry. Edited by Frances AJ, Hales RE. Washington, DC, American Psychiatric Press, 1988, pp 235–255

Shea MT, Pilkonis PA, Beckman E, et al: Personality disorders and treatment outcome in the NIMH Treatment of Depression Collaborative Research Program. Am J Psychiatry 147:711–718, 1990

Shelton RC: Intracellular mechanisms of antidepressant drug action. Harv Rev Psychiatry 8:161–174, 2000

Shelton RC, Keller MB, Gelenberg AJ, et al: Effectiveness of St. John's wort in major depression: a randomized controlled trial. JAMA 285:1978–1986, 2001a

Shelton RC, Tollefson GD, Tohen M, et al: A novel augmentation strategy for treating resistant major depression. Am J Psychiatry 158:131–134, 2001b

Shulman KI, Hermann N: Bipolar disorder in old age. Can Fam Physician 45:1229–1237, 1999

Siever LJ, Davis KL: Overview: toward a dysregulation hypothesis of depression. Am J Psychiatry 142:1017–1025, 1985

Siever L, Trestman RL: The serotonin system and aggressive personality disorder. Int Clin Psychopharmacol 8(suppl 2):33–39, 1993

Simhandl CA, Denk E, Thau K: The comparative efficacy of carbamazepine low and high serum level and lithium carbonate in the prophylaxis of affective disorders. J Affect Disord 28:221–231, 1993

Simon AE, Aubry JM, Malky L, et al: Hypomania-like syndrome induced by olanzapine. Int Clin Psychopharmacol 14:377–378, 1999

Simon G, Von Korff M, Wagner E, et al: Patterns of antidepressant use in community practice. Gen Hosp Psychiatry 15:399–408, 1995

Simpson SG, Folstein SE, Meyers DA, et al: Bipolar II: the most common bipolar phenotype? Am J Psychiatry 150:901–903, 1993

Simpson S, Baldwin RC, Jackson A, et al: The differentiation of DSM-III-R psychotic depression in later life from nonpsychotic depression: comparisons of brain changes measured by multispectral analysis of magnetic resonance brain images, neuropsychological findings, and clinical features. Biol Psychiatry 45:193–204, 1999

Singh AN, Catalan J: Risperidone in HIV-related manic psychosis. Lancet 344:1029–1030, 1994

Small JG, Small IF, Milstein V: Manic symptoms: an indication for bilateral ECT. Biol Psychiatry 20:125–134, 1985

Small JG, Klapper MH, Kellams JJ: Electroconvulsive treatment compared with lithium in the management of manic states. Arch Gen Psychiatry 45:727–732, 1988

Small JG, Klapper MH, Milstein V, et al: Comparison of therapeutic modalities for mania. Psychopharmacol Bull 32:623–627, 1996

Smith D, Baker G, Davies G, et al: Outcomes of add-on treatment with lamotrigine in partial epilepsy. Epilepsia 34:312–322, 1993

Soares JC, Mann JJ: The anatomy of mood disorders—review of structural neuroimaging studies. Biol Psychiatry 41:86–106, 1997

Solan WJ, Khan A, Avery DH, et al: Psychotic and nonpsychotic depression: comparison of response to ECT. Compr Psychiatry 49:97–99, 1988

Solhkhah R, Finkel J, Hird S: Possible risperidone-induced visual hallucinations (letter). J Am Acad Child Adolesc Psychiatry 39:1074–1075, 2000

Solomon DA, Bauer MS: Continuation and maintenance pharmacotherapy for unipolar and bipolar mood disorders. Psychiatr Clin North Am 16:515–540, 1993

Solomon DA, Keitner GI, Miller IW, et al: Course of illness and maintenance treatments for patients with bipolar disorder. Compr Psychiatry 56:5–13, 1995

Somoza E, Mossman D: Optimizing REM latency as a diagnostic test for depression using receiver operating characteristic analysis and information theory. Biol Psychiatry 27:990–1006, 1990

Song C, Lin A, Bonaccorso S, et al: The inflammatory response system and the availability of plasma tryptophan in patients with primary sleep disorders and major depression. J Affect Disord 49:211–219, 1998

Sotsky SM, Glass DR, Shea MT, et al: Patient predictors of response to psychotherapy and pharmacotherapy: findings in the NIMH Treatment of Depression Collaborative Research Program. Am J Psychiatry 148:997–1008, 1991

Spiker DG, Kupfer DJ: Placebo response rates in psychotic and nonpsychotic depression. J Affect Disord 14:21–23, 1988

Spiker DG, Weiss JC, Dealy RS, et al: The pharmacological treatment of delusional depression. Am J Psychiatry 142:430–436, 1985

Spiker DG, Perel JM, Hanin I, et al: The pharmacological treatment of delusional depression: part II. J Clin Psychopharmacol 6:339–342, 1986a

Spiker DG, Dealy RS, Hanin I, et al: Treating delusional depressives with amitriptyline. Compr Psychiatry 47:243–246, 1986b

Srisurapanont M, Yatham LN, Zis AP: Treatment of acute bipolar depression: a review of the literature. Can J Psychiatry 40:533–544, 1995

Stancer HC, Persad E: Treatment of intractable rapid-cycling manic-depressive disorder with levothyroxine: clinical observations. Arch Gen Psychiatry 39:311–312, 1982

Stewart JW, McGrath PJ, Quitkin FM: Chronic depression: response to placebo, imipramine, and phenelzine. J Clin Psychopharmacol 13:391–396, 1993

Stoll AL, Mayer PV, Kolbrener M, et al: Antidepressant-associated mania: a controlled comparison with spontaneous mania. Am J Psychiatry 151:1642–1645, 1994

Stoll AL, Severus WE, Freeman MP, et al: Omega3 fatty acids in bipolar disorder: a preliminary double-blind, placebo-controlled trial. Arch Gen Psychiatry 56:407–412, 1999

Strakowski S, McElroy SL, Keck PW Jr: The co-occurrence of mania with medical and other psychiatric disorders. Int J Psychiatry Med 24:305–328, 1994

Strik WK, Fallgatter AJ, Stoeber G, et al: Specific P300 features in patients with cycloid psychosis. Acta Psychiatr Scand 95:67–72, 1997

Strik WK, Ruchsow M, Abele S, et al: Distinct neurophysiological mechanisms for manic and cycloid psychoses: evidence from a P300 study on manic patients. Acta Psychiatr Scand 98:459–466, 1998

Strober M, Carlson G: Bipolar illness in adolescents with major depression. Arch Gen Psychiatry 39:549–555, 1982

Strupp HH, Binder JL: Psychotherapy in a New Key: A Guide to Time-Limited Dynamic Psychotherapy. New York, Basic Books, 1984

Stuart S, Thase ME: Inpatient application of cognitive behavior therapy: a review of recent developments. J Psychother Pract Res 3:284–299, 1994

Stuart S, Simons AD, Thase ME, et al: Are personality assessments valid in acute major depression? J Affect Disord 24:281–290, 1992

Suomi SJ, Seaman SF, Lewis JK: Effects of imipramine treatment of separation-induced social disorders in rhesus monkeys. Arch Gen Psychiatry 35:321–325, 1978

Suppes T, McElroy SL, Gilbert J, et al: Clozapine in the treatment of dysphoric mania. Biol Psychiatry 32:270–280, 1992

Suppes T, Phillips KA, Judd CR: Clozapine treatment of nonpsychotic rapid cycling bipolar disorder: a report of three cases. Biol Psychiatry 36:338–340, 1994

Swann AC: Mixed or dysphoric manic states: psychopathology and treatment. Compr Psychiatry 56(suppl 3):6–10, 1995

Swann AC, Bowden CL, Morris D: Depression during mania. Arch Gen Psychiatry 54:37–42, 1997

Swartz KL, Pratt LA, Armenian HK, et al: Mental disorders and the incidence of migraine headaches in a community sample: results from the Baltimore Epidemiologic Catchment Area Follow-up Study. Arch Gen Psychiatry 57:945–950, 2000

Tallian KB, Nahata MC, Lo W, et al: Gabapentin associated with aggressive behavior in pediatric patients with seizures. Epilepsia 37:501–502, 1996

Tam EM, Lam RWA, Levitt AJ: Treatment of seasonal affective disorder: a review. Can J Psychiatry 40:457–466, 1995

Tan CH, Javors MA, Seleshi E: Effects of lithium on platelet ionic intracellular calcium concentration in patients with bipolar (manic-depressive) disorder and healthy controls. Life Sci 46:1175–1180, 1990

Teicher MH, Glod CA, Cole JO: Antidepressant drugs and the emergence of suicidal tendencies. Drug Saf 8:186–212, 1993

Teicher MH, Glod CA, Oren DA, et al: The phototherapy light visor: more to it than meets the eye. Am J Psychiatry 152:1197–2002, 1995

Teicher MH, Glod CA, Magnus E, et al: Circadian rest-activity disturbances in seasonal affective disorder. Arch Gen Psychiatry 54:124–130, 1997

Terao T: Subclinical hypothyroidism in recurrent mania. Biol Psychiatry 33:853–854, 1993

Thalen BE, Kjellman BF, Morkrid L, et al: Melatonin in light treatment of patients with seasonal and nonseasonal depression. Acta Psychiatr Scand 92:274–284, 1995

Thase ME: Relapse and recurrence in unipolar major depression: short-term and long-term approaches. Compr Psychiatry 51(suppl 26):51–57, 1990

Thase ME: Long-term treatments of recurrent depressive disorders. Compr Psychiatry 53(suppl 9):32–44, 1992

Thase ME: Reeducative psychotherapies, in Treatment of Psychiatric Disorders. Edited by Gabbard GO. Washington, DC, American Psychiatric Press, 1995, pp 1169–1204

Thase ME: The role of Axis II comorbidity in the management of patients with treatment-resistant depression. Psychiatr Clin North Am 19:287–309, 1996

Thase ME, Kupfer DJ: Recent developments in the pharmacotherapy of mood disorders. J Consult Clin Psychol 64:646–659, 1996

Thase ME, Simons AD, McGeary J, et al: Relapse after cognitive behavior therapy of depression: potential implications for longer courses of treatment. Am J Psychiatry 149:1046–1052, 1992

Thase ME, Reynolds CF, Frank E, et al: Response to cognitive-behavioral therapy in chronic depression. J Psychother Pract Res 3:204–214, 1994

Thase ME, Kupfer DJ, Fasiczka AJ, et al: Identifying an abnormal electroencephalographic sleep profile to characterize major depressive disorder. Biol Psychiatry 41:964–973, 1997a

Thase ME, Greenhouse JB, Frank E, et al: Treatment of major depression with psychotherapy or psychotherapy-pharmacotherapy combinations [see comments]. Arch Gen Psychiatry 54:1009–1015, 1997b

Thompson PJ, Trimble MR: Anticonvulsant serum levels: relationship to impairments of cognitive functioning. J Neurol Neurosurg Psychiatry 46:227–233, 1983

Tohen M, Zarate CA, Centorrino F, et al: Risperidone in the treatment of mania. Compr Psychiatry 57:249–253, 1996a

Tohen M, Zarate CA, Centorrino F, et al: Risperidone in the treatment of mania (abstract). Psychopharmacol Bull 31:626, 1996b

Tohen M, Sanger TM, McElroy SL, et al: Olanzapine versus placebo in the treatment of acute mania. Am J Psychiatry 156:702–709, 1999

Tohen M, Jacobs TG, Grundy SL, et al: Efficacy of olanzapine in acute bipolar mania: a double-blind, placebo-controlled study. The Olanzapine HGGW Study Group. Arch Gen Psychiatry 57:841–849, 2000

Tomitaka S, Sakamoto K: Definition and prognosis of rapid cycling affective disorder (letter). Am J Psychiatry 151:1524, 1994

Triggs WJ, McCoy KJ, Greer R, et al: Effects of left frontal transcranial magnetic stimulation on depressed mood, cognition, and corticomotor threshold. Biol Psychiatry 48:1440–1446, 1999

Tsuang D, Coryell W: An 8-year follow-up of patients with DSM-III-R psychotic depression, schizoaffective disorder and schizophrenia. Am J Psychiatry 150:1182–1188, 1993

Tsuang MT, Faraone SV: The inheritance of mood disorders, in Genetics and Mental Illness: Evolving Issues for Research and Society. Edited by Hall LL. New York, Plenum, 1996, pp 79–109

Ulmsten U, Anderson KE, Wingerup I: Treatment of premature labor with the calcium antagonist nifedipine. Arch Gynecol 229:1–5, 1980

Vallada H, Craddock N, Vasquez L, et al: Linkage studies in bipolar affective disorder with markers on chromosome 21. J Affect Disord 41:217–221, 1996

Vanelle J-M, Loo H, Galinowski MD, et al: Maintenance ECT in intractable manic-depressive disorders. Convuls Ther 10:195–205, 1994

Van Londen L, Molenaar RPG, Goerkoop JG, et al: Three- to 5-year prospective follow-up of outcome in major depression. Psychol Med 28:731–735, 1998

van Luijtelaar EL, Ates N, Coenen AM: Role of L-type calcium channel modulation in nonconvulsive epilepsy in rats. Epilepsia 36:86–92, 1995

van Praag HM: Two-tier diagnosing in psychiatry. Psychiatry Res 34:341–351, 1990

van Praag HM, Kahn RS, Asnis GM: Denosologization of biological psychiatry or the specificity of 5-HT disturbances in psychiatric disorders. J Affect Disord 13:1–8, 1987

Verma NP, Haidukewych D: Differential but infrequent alterations of hepatic enzyme levels and thyroid hormone levels by anticonvulsant drugs. Arch Neurol 2:319–323, 1993

Vestergaard P, Licht RW, Brodersen A, et al: Outcome of lithium prophylaxis: a prospective follow-up of affective disorder patients assigned to high and low serum lithium levels. Acta Psychiatr Scand 98:310–315, 1998

Wada K, Yamada N, Suzuki H, et al: Recurrent cases of corticosteroid-induced mood disorder: clinical characteristics and treatment. J Clin Psychiatry 61:261–267, 2000

Walden J, Hesslinger B: Value of old and new anticonvulsants in treatment of psychiatric diseases. Fortschr Neurol Psychiatr 63:320–335, 1995

Walden J, Grunze H, Bungmann D, et al: Calcium antagonistic effects of carbamazepine as a mechanism of action in neuropsychiatric disorders: studies in calcium dependent model epilepsies. Eur Neuropsychopharmacol 2:455–462, 1992

Walter G, Rey J: An epidemiological study of the use of ECT in adolescents. J Am Acad Child Adolesc Psychiatry 36:809–815, 1997

Walton SA, Berk M, Brook S: Superiority of lithium over verapamil in mania: a randomized, controlled, single-blind trial. Compr Psychiatry 57:543–546, 1996

Warner R, Appleby L, Whitton A, et al: Demographic and obstetric risk factors for postnatal psychiatric morbidity. Br J Psychiatry 168:607–611, 1996

Warshaw MG, Keller MB: The relationship between fluoxetine use and suicidal behavior in 654 subjects with anxiety disorders. Compr Psychiatry 57:158–166, 1996

Watkins JT, Leber WR, Imber SD, et al: Temporal course of change of depression. J Consult Clin Psychol 61:858–864, 1993

Wehr TA: Can antidepressants induce rapid cycling? Arch Gen Psychiatry 50:495–496, 1993

Wehr TA, Sack DA, Rosenthal NE, et al: Rapid cycling affective disorder: contributing factors and treatment responses in 51 patients. Am J Psychiatry 145:179–184, 1988

Weiner RD: Does electroconvulsive therapy cause brain damage? Behav Brain Sci 7:1–13, 1984

Weiner RD: Electroconvulsive therapy, in Treatment of Psychiatric Disorders. Edited by Gabbard GO. Washington, DC, American Psychiatric Press, 1995, pp 1237–1273

Weiss SR, Post RM, Anthony P, et al: Contingent tolerance to carbamazepine is not affected by calcium-channel or NMDA receptor blockers. Pharmacol Biochem Behav 45:439–443, 1993

Weissman MM: Psychotherapy in the maintenance treatment of depression. Br J Psychiatry 165(suppl 26):42–50, 1994

Weissman MM, Prusoff BA, DiMascio A, et al: The efficacy of drugs and psychotherapy in the treatment of acute depressive episodes. Am J Psychiatry 136:555–558, 1979

Weissman MM, Prusoff BA, Gammon GD, et al: Psychopathology in the children (ages 6–18) of depressed and normal parents. J Am Acad Child Adolesc Psychiatry 23:78–84, 1984

Weissman MM, Warner V, John K, et al: Delusional depression and bipolar spectrum: evidence for a possible association from a family study of children. Neuropsychopharmacology 1:257–264, 1988a

Weissman MM, Leaf PJ, Bruce ML: The epidemiology of dysthymia in five communities: rates, risks, comorbidity, and treatment. Am J Psychiatry 145:815–819, 1988b

Weissman MM, Bland RC, Canino GJ, et al: Cross-national epidemiology of major depression and bipolar disorder. JAMA 276:293–299, 1996

Wells KB, Stewart A, Hays RD: The functioning and well-being of depressed patients. JAMA 262:914–919, 1989

Wells KB, Burnnam A, Rogers WH, et al: The course of depression in adult outpatients: results from the medical outcomes study. Arch Gen Psychiatry 49:788–794, 1992

Whybrow PC, Akiskal HS, McKinney WT: Mood Disorders: Toward a New Psychobiology. New York, Plenum, 1984, pp 21–42

Wide-Swensson DG, Ingemarsson I, Lunell N, et al: Calcium channel blockade (isradipine) in treatment of hypertension in pregnancy: a randomized placebo-controlled study. Am J Obstet Gynecol 173:872–878, 1996

Wilde MI, Benfield P: Tianeptine: a review of its pharmacodynamic and pharmacokinetic properties, and therapeutic efficacy in depression and coexisting anxiety and depression. Drugs 49:411–439, 1995

Willoughby CL, Hradek EA, Richards NR: Use of electroconvulsive therapy with children: an overview and case report. Journal of Child and Adolescent Psychiatric Nursing 10:11–17, 1997

Wilson PH: Combined pharmacological and behavioral treatment of depression. Behav Res Ther 20:173–184, 1982

Winokur G: Manic-depressive disease (bipolar): is it autonomous? Psychopathology 28(suppl 1):51–58, 1995

Winokur G, Morrison J: The Iowa 500: follow-up of 225 depressives. Br J Psychiatry 123:543–548, 1973

Wolkowitz OD, Reus VI: Treatment of depression with antiglucocorticoid drugs. Psychosom Med 61:698–711, 1999

Woods BT, Yurgelun-Todd D, Mikulis D, et al: Age-related MRI abnormalities in bipolar illness: a clinical study. Biol Psychiatry 38:846–847, 1995

Xie X, Hagan RM: Cellular and molecular actions of lamotrigine: possible mechanisms of efficacy in bipolar disorder. Neuropsychobiology 38:119–130, 1998

Young MA, Fogg LF, Schefner WA, et al: Interaction of risk factors in predicting suicide. Am J Psychiatry 151:434–435, 1994

Zarate CA Jr, Tohen M, Baldessarini RJ: Clozapine in severe mood disorders. Compr Psychiatry 56:411–417, 1995a

Zarate CA Jr, Tohen M, Banov MD, et al: Is clozapine a mood stabilizer? Compr Psychiatry 56:108–112, 1995b

Zarate CA, Tohen M, Baldessarini RJ: Clozapine in severe mood disorders (abstract). Psychopharmacol Bull 31:636, 1996

Zornberg GL, Rose HG: Treatment of depression in bipolar disorder: new directions for research. J Clin Psychopharmacol 13:397–408, 1993

CHAPTER 11

Anxiety Disorders

Eric Hollander, M.D.

Daphne Simeon, M.D.

Anxiety disorders are the most common of all psychiatric illnesses and result in considerable functional impairment and distress. Recent research developments have had a broad impact on our understanding of the underlying mechanisms of illness and treatment response. Working with patients who have an anxiety disorder can be highly gratifying for the informed psychiatrist, because these patients, who are in considerable distress, often respond to proper treatment and return to a high level of functioning. The major anxiety disorders presented in this chapter are panic disorder, generalized anxiety disorder (GAD), social phobia, specific phobias, obsessive-compulsive disorder (OCD), and posttraumatic stress disorder (PTSD). A diagnostic decision tree of the anxiety disorders is presented in Figure 11–1.

If pathological anxiety is induced either by psychoactive substance use or by an Axis III physical illness, it is classified in DSM-IV (American Psychiatric Association 1994) under the anxiety disorders (substance-induced anxiety disorder or anxiety disorder due to a general medical condition, respectively). DSM-III-R (American Psychiatric Association 1987) had lumped any psychopathology associated with medical causes or substance abuse, regardless of its form, under "organic mental disorders." It was hoped that the new DSM-IV format would encourage greater specificity in the differential diagnosis of organic conditions. For what was formerly called *organic anxiety* (i.e., anxiety judged to be due to the direct physiological effects of a general medical condition or a psychoactive substance), DSM-IV allowed specification of the subtype as generalized anxiety, panic attacks, or obsessive-compulsive symptoms.

Panic Disorder

DSM-II (American Psychiatric Association 1968) described an ill-defined condition of *anxiety neurosis*, a term first coined by Freud in 1895 (Breuer and Freud 1893–1895/1955), which included any patient suffering from chronic tension, excessive worry, frequent headaches, or recurrent anxiety attacks. However, subsequent findings suggested that discrete spontaneous panic attacks may be qualitatively dissimilar to other chronic anxiety states. For example, patients with panic attacks were found to be unique in their panic-induction responsiveness to sodium lactate infusion, familial aggregation, development of agoraphobia, and treatment response to tricyclic antidepressants (TCAs). Thus, DSM-III (American Psychiatric Association 1980) and the subsequent DSM-III-R divided the category of anxiety neurosis into panic disorder and GAD.

The DSM-IV-TR (American Psychiatric Association 2000) definition of a panic attack is presented in Table 11–1. Panic disorder is subdivided into panic disorder with and panic disorder without agoraphobia, as in DSM-III-R, depending on whether any secondary phobic avoidance is present (Tables 11–2 and 11–3).

DSM-IV clarified several issues regarding the diagnosis and differential diagnosis of panic disorder that remained obscured in DSM-III-R. Panic attacks are well known to occur not only in panic disorder but also in other anxiety disorders (e.g., specific phobia, social phobia, PTSD). In these other disorders, panic attacks are situationally bound or cued—that is, they occur exclusively within the context of the feared situation. DSM-IV clarified this confusion by explicitly presenting the definition of panic attacks inde-

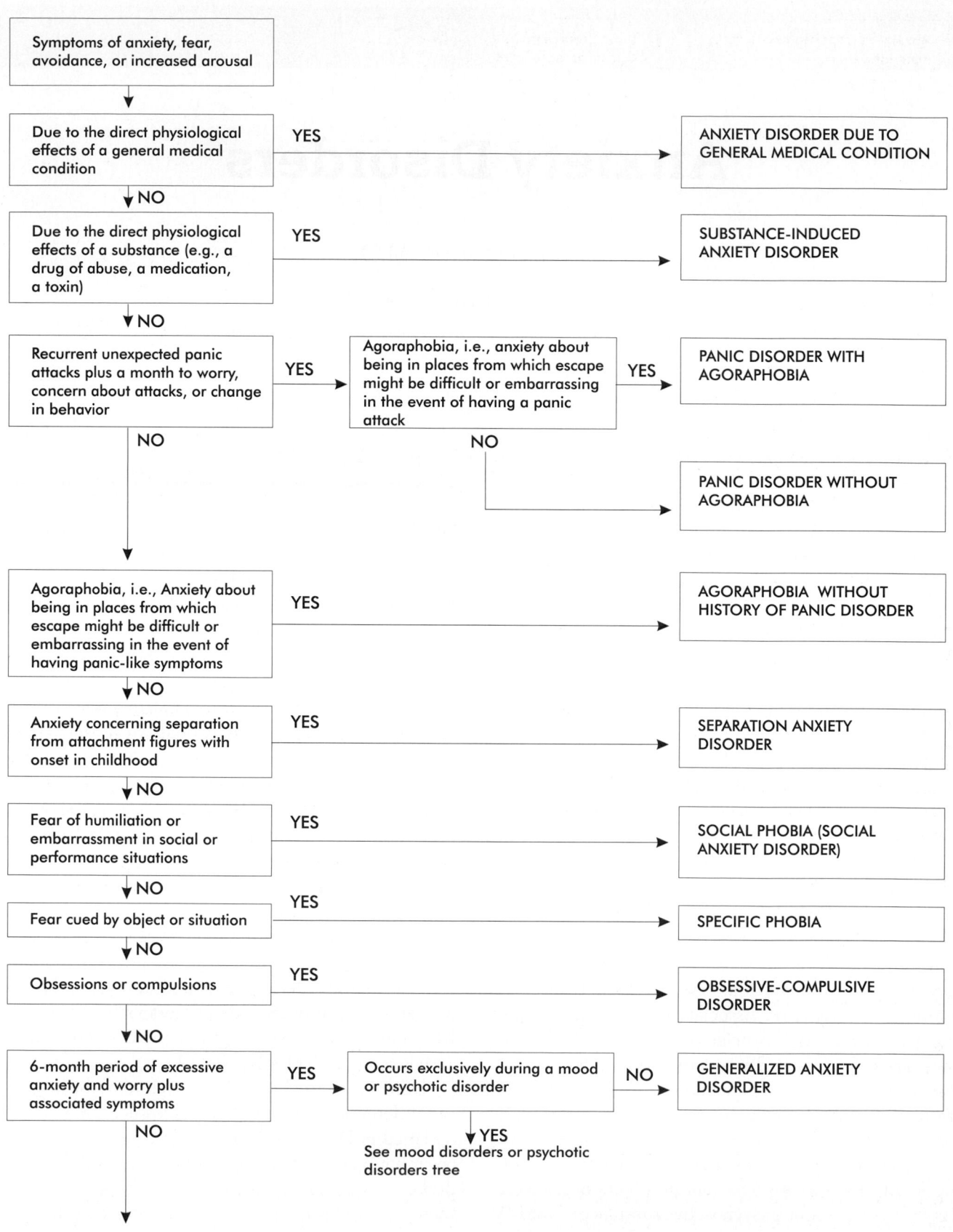

FIGURE 11–1. Diagnostic decision tree for anxiety disorders.

Patients may have more than one disorder and thus must be evaluated for each disorder.

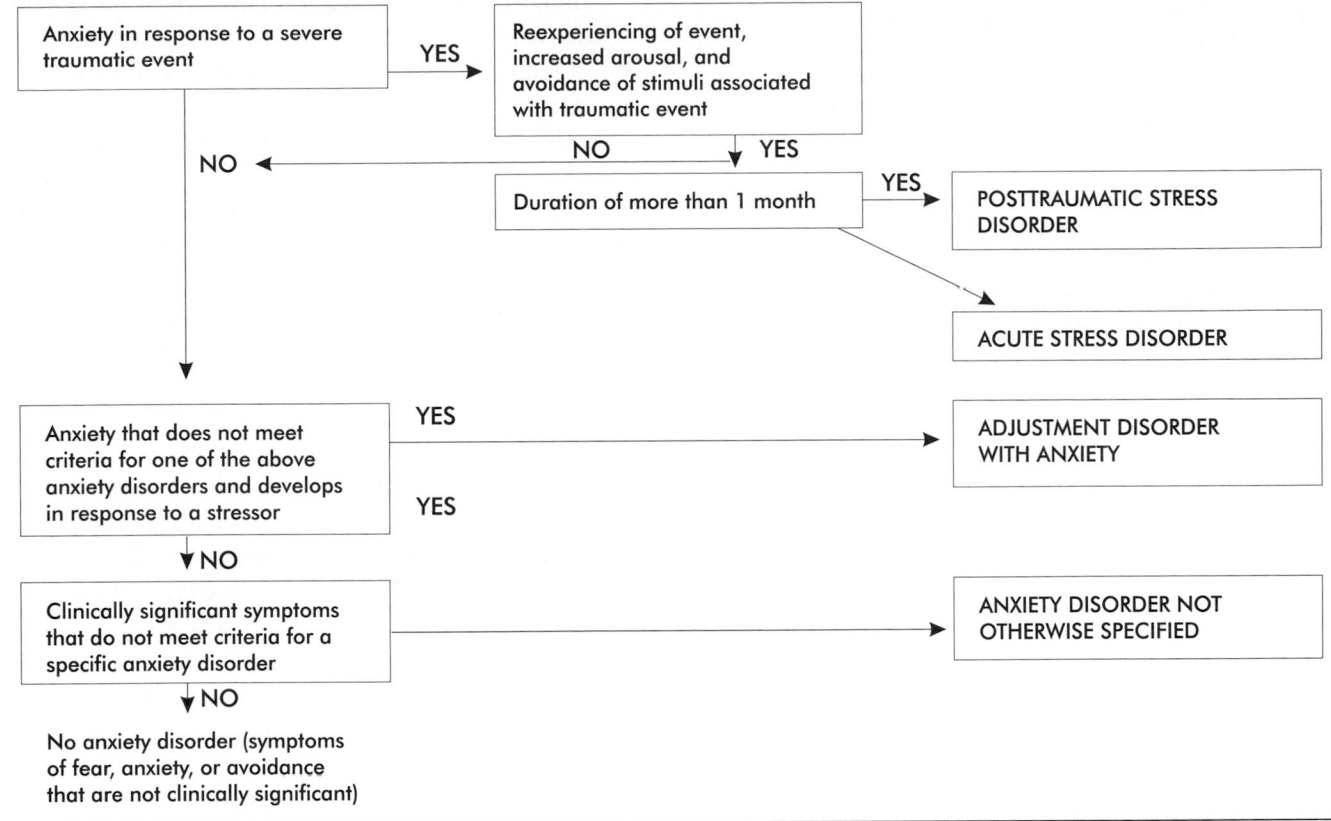

FIGURE 11–1. Diagnostic decision tree for anxiety disorders *(continued)*.
Patients may have more than one disorder and thus must be evaluated for each disorder.

TABLE 11–1. DSM-IV-TR definition of panic attack

A discrete period of intense fear or discomfort in which four (or more) of the following symptoms developed abruptly and reached a peak within 10 minutes:
Palpitations, pounding heart, or accelerated heart rate
Sweating
Trembling or shaking
Sensations of shortness of breath or smothering
Feeling of choking
Chest pain or discomfort
Nausea or abdominal distress
Feeling dizzy, unsteady, lightheaded, or faint
Derealization (feelings of unreality) or depersonalization (being detached from oneself)
Fear of losing control or "going crazy"
Fear of dying
Paresthesias (numbness or tingling sensation)
Chills or hot flushes

pendently of panic disorder (Table 11–1) and specifying that a panic attack can be "unexpected (uncued)," "situationally bound (cued)," or "situationally predisposed."

The differential diagnosis can sometimes become complicated—for example, when, historically, one or several unexpected panic attacks initially occurred in a specific situation, consistent with a diagnosis of panic disorder, but later evolved into a chronic condition in which the attacks were cued exclusively by that situation, or else avoidance of that situation developed because of fear of another attack. Is the diagnosis in such a case panic disorder with agoraphobia or social/specific phobia? DSM-IV retains the distinct diagnoses of panic disorder with agoraphobia, social phobia, and specific phobia and specifies that panic attacks can occur as a feature of all three of these disorders. Therefore, clinical judgment regarding the preponderant clinical pattern is called for in making the differential diagnosis in such cases.

Clinical Description

Onset

In the typical onset of a case of panic disorder, a person is engaged in some ordinary aspect of life when suddenly his heart begins to pound and he cannot catch his breath. The person feels dizzy, light-headed, and faint and is convinced he is about to die. Patients with panic disorder are usually young adults, most likely in the third decade; however, onset may be as late as the sixth decade.

TABLE 11–2. DSM-IV-TR diagnostic criteria for panic disorder with agoraphobia

A. Both (1) and (2):
  (1) recurrent unexpected panic attacks
  (2) at least one of the attacks has been followed by 1 month (or more) of one (or more) of the following:
    (a) persistent concern about having additional attacks
    (b) worry about the implications of the attack or its consequences (e.g., losing control, having a heart attack, "going crazy")
    (c) a significant change in behavior related to the attacks
B. The presence of agoraphobia.
C. The panic attacks are not due to the direct physiological effects of a substance (e.g., a drug of abuse, a medication) or a general medical condition (e.g., hyperthyroidism).
D. The panic attacks are not better accounted for by another mental disorder, such as social phobia (e.g., occurring on exposure to feared social situations), specific phobia (e.g., on exposure to a specific phobic situation), obsessive-compulsive disorder (e.g., on exposure to dirt in someone with an obsession about contamination), posttraumatic stress disorder (e.g., in response to stimuli associated with a severe stressor), or separation anxiety disorder (e.g., in response to being away from home or close relatives).

TABLE 11–3. DSM-IV-TR diagnostic criteria for panic disorder without agoraphobia

A. Both (1) and (2):
  (1) recurrent unexpected panic attacks
  (2) at least one of the attacks has been followed by 1 month (or more) of one (or more) of the following:
    (a) persistent concern about having additional attacks
    (b) worry about the implications of the attack or its consequences (e.g., losing control, having a heart attack, "going crazy")
    (c) a significant change in behavior related to the attacks
B. Absence of agoraphobia.
C. The panic attacks are not due to the direct physiological effects of a substance (e.g., a drug of abuse, a medication) or a general medical condition (e.g., hyperthyroidism).
D. The panic attacks are not better accounted for by another mental disorder, such as social phobia (e.g., occurring on exposure to feared social situations), specific phobia (e.g., on exposure to a specific phobic situation), obsessive-compulsive disorder (e.g., on exposure to dirt in someone with an obsession about contamination), posttraumatic stress disorder (e.g., in response to stimuli associated with a severe stressor), or separation anxiety disorder (e.g., in response to being away from home or close relatives).

Although the first attack generally strikes during some routine activity, several events are often associated with the early presentation of panic disorder. It is not uncommon for the initial panic attack to occur in the context of a life-threatening illness or accident, the loss of a close interpersonal relationship, or a separation from family (e.g., after starting college or accepting a job out of town). Patients developing either hypothyroidism or hyperthyroidism may experience the first flurry of attacks at this time. Attacks also begin in the immediate postpartum period. Finally, many patients have reported experiencing their first attacks while taking drugs of abuse, especially marijuana, lysergic acid diethylamide (LSD), sedatives, cocaine, and amphetamines. However, even when these concomitant conditions are resolved, the attacks often continue unabated. This situation gives the impression that some stressors may act as triggers to provoke the beginning of panic attacks in patients who are already predisposed.

Patients experiencing their first panic attack generally fear that they are having a heart attack or losing their mind. Such patients often rush to the nearest emergency department, where routine laboratory tests, electrocardiography, and physical examination are performed. All that is found is an occasional case of sinus tachycardia, and the patients are reassured and sent home. These patients may indeed feel reassured, and at this point the diagnosis of panic disorder would be premature. However, perhaps a few days or even weeks later they will again have the sudden onset of severe anxiety with all of the associated physical symptoms. Again, they seek emergency medical treatment. At this point, they may be told the problem is psychological, be given a prescription for a benzodiazepine tranquilizer, or be referred for extensive medical workup.

Symptoms

Typically, during a panic attack, a patient will be engaged in a routine activity—perhaps reading a book, eating in a restaurant, driving a car, or attending a concert—when he or she will experience the sudden onset of overwhelming fear, terror, apprehension, and a sense of impending doom. Several of a group of associated symptoms, mostly physical, are also experienced: dyspnea, palpitations, chest pain or discomfort, choking or smothering sensations, dizziness or unsteadiness, feelings of unreality (derealization and/or depersonalization), paresthesias, hot and cold flashes, sweating, faintness, trembling and shaking, and a fear of dying, going crazy, or losing control of oneself. It is clear that most of the physical sensations of a panic attack represent massive overstimulation of the autonomic nervous system.

Attacks usually last from 5 to 20 minutes and rarely as long as an hour. Patients who claim they have attacks that last a whole day may fall into one of four categories. 1) Some patients continue to feel agitated and fatigued for several hours after the main portion of the attack has subsided. 2) At times, attacks occur, subside, and occur again in a wavelike manner. 3) Alternatively, the patient with so-called long panic attacks often has some other form of pathological anxiety, such as severe generalized anxiety, agitated depression, or obsessional tension states. 4) Finally, in some cases, such severe anticipatory anxiety may develop with time in expectation of future panic attacks so that the two may blend together in the patient's description and be difficult to distinguish.

Although many people experience an occasional unexpected attack of panic, the diagnosis of panic disorder is only made when the attacks occur with some regularity and frequency. However, patients with occasional unexpected panic attacks may be genetically similar to patients with panic disorder. A twin study found the best results for genetic linkage when patients with regular panic attacks were included together with patients who had only occasional attacks (Torgersen 1983).

Some patients do not progress in their illness beyond the point of continuing to have unexpected panic attacks. Most patients develop some degree of anticipatory anxiety consequent to the experience of repetitive panic attacks. The patient comes to dread experiencing an attack and starts worrying about doing so in the intervals between attacks. This can progress until the level of fearfulness and autonomic hyperactivity in the interval between panic attacks almost approximates the level during the actual attack itself. Such patients may be mistaken for GAD patients.

It is warranted to draw some further attention to what appears to be the cardinal symptom of panic. Several lines of research evidence indicate that hyperventilation may be the central feature in the pathophysiology of panic attacks and panic disorder. Patients with panic disorder have been shown to be chronic hyperventilators who also acutely hyperventilate during spontaneous and induced panic (the possible etiologies of this symptom are discussed later in this section). This hyperventilation then induces hypocapnia and alkalosis, leading to decreased cerebral blood flow and to the dizziness, confusion, and derealization characteristic of panic attacks. Indeed, signs and symptoms of hyperventilation seem to disappear once a patient with panic disorder has been successfully treated with antipanic medication. Also, behavioral breathing retraining treatments aimed at teaching the patient not to hyperventilate are successful in decreasing the frequency of panic attacks (Clark et al.

1985; Lum 1981), presumably by dampening the ventilatory overreaction that may constitute the hallmark of panic.

Agoraphobia

Agoraphobia frequently develops in response to panic attacks, leading to the DSM-IV diagnosis of panic disorder with agoraphobia. The clinical picture in agoraphobia consists of multiple and varied fears and avoidance behaviors that center around three main themes: 1) fear of leaving home, 2) fear of being alone, and 3) fear of being away from home in situations in which one can feel trapped, embarrassed, or helpless. According to DSM-IV, the fear is one of developing distressing symptoms in situations in which escape is difficult or help is unavailable. Typical agoraphobic fears are of using public transportation (buses, trains, subways, planes); being in crowds, theaters, elevators, restaurants, supermarkets, or department stores; waiting in line; and of traveling a distance from home. In severe cases, patients may be completely housebound, fearful of leaving home without a companion or even of staying home alone.

Most cases of agoraphobia begin with a series of spontaneous panic attacks. If the attacks continue, the patient usually develops a constant anticipatory anxiety characterized by continued apprehension about the possible occasion and consequences of the next attack. Agoraphobic symptoms represent a tertiary phase in the illness. Many patients will causally relate their panic attacks to the particular situation in which the attacks have occurred. They then avoid these situations in an attempt to prevent further panic attacks (Figure 11–2). For example, a man who has had several attacks while taking the train to work may attribute the attacks to the train and, to avoid the train, start driving to work. If he still experiences panic attacks in the morning while driving to work rather than while on the train, he interprets this as a sign that the attacks have spread to driving situations rather than as an indication that they were not caused by the train in the first place. Agoraphobic persons often fear situations that they believe they cannot leave abruptly if an attack occurs, such as crowded rooms, front-row seats, tunnels, bridges, and airplanes. Some individuals continue to have spontaneous panic attacks throughout the course of the illness. In other cases, after the initial phase of the illness, attacks may occur rarely or may occur exclusively when the patient ventures into the feared situation.

One interesting aspect of agoraphobia is the effect of a trusted companion on phobic behavior. Many patients who are unable to leave the house alone can travel long

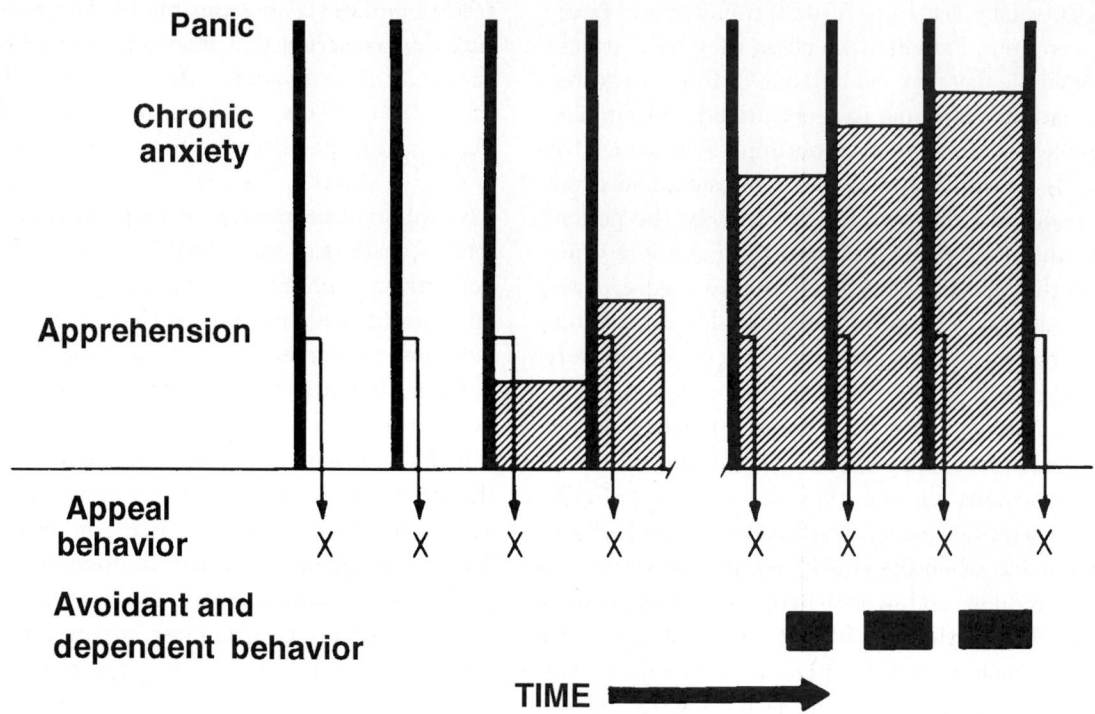

FIGURE 11–2. Development of agoraphobia.

After onset of unexpected panic attacks *(solid bars)*, patient develops acute help-seeking behavior *(X)*, then apprehension culminating in chronic anxiety *(shaded areas)*, and finally agoraphobic behavior *(black blocks)*.

distances and partake in most activities if accompanied by a spouse, family member, or close friend. It is unclear whether vulnerability to panic attacks is actually decreased in this situation or whether the patient feels less helpless and isolated. In addition to panic attacks and chronic anxiety, agoraphobic patients frequently exhibit symptoms of demoralization or secondary depression, multiple somatic complaints, and alcohol or sedative drug abuse.

Character Traits

It has not been clearly established whether particular character types are correlated with panic disorder, and studies are further confounded because the presence of panic disorder may have secondary effects on personality. Noyes et al. (1991) conducted personality follow-up of patients with panic disorder who were treated for panic over 3 years and found that the initial avoidant and dependent traits were to a large extent state related, waning with the treatment of panic. On the other hand, experience leads many clinicians to feel that patients with agoraphobia and panic are more likely to have histories of dependent character traits that predate the onset of panic.

Epidemiology

The National Institute of Mental Health (NIMH) Epidemiologic Catchment Area (ECA) study examined the population prevalence of DSM-III–diagnosed panic disorder using the Diagnostic Interview Schedule (DIS; Regier et al. 1988). The 1-month, 6-month, and lifetime prevalence rates for panic disorder at all five study sites combined were 0.5%, 0.8%, and 1.6%, respectively. Women had a 1-month prevalence rate of 0.7%, which was significantly higher than the 0.3% rate found among men; women also tended to have a greater rise in panic disorder in the age range of 25–44 years, and their attacks tended to continue longer into older age (Regier et al. 1988). The epidemiology of panic disorder appears to be similar in whites and blacks (Horwath et al. 1993).

The relationship between panic disorder and major depression has been questioned in numerous studies because it is well known that the two commonly co-occur. A recent family study found that panic disorder and major depression are clearly distinct disorders, despite their substantial co-occurrence, and panic comorbid with major depression does not segregate in families as a distinct disorder (Weissman et al. 1993).

Etiology

Biological Theories

Several biological theories of panic disorder are prominent in the psychiatric literature. We summarize the evidence for or against some of the most promising of these. Certain agents have a powerful and specific capacity to induce panic, in contrast with other agents that produce prominent physiological changes but fail to induce panic. These findings argue strongly against the notion that panic is a reaction to nonspecific distressing stimuli and suggest more specific biological bases, even if these involve multiple neurochemicals and circuits. The various theories discussed in this subsection need not be viewed as mutually exclusive, but rather as potentially interlocking pieces of a larger puzzle. Neurochemical, imaging, and genetic findings are described as well.

The sympathetic system. Some investigators have found anxiety reactions associated with increases in levels of urinary catecholamines, especially epinephrine. Studies of healthy subjects exposed to novel stress also demonstrate elevations in plasma catecholamine levels (Dimsdale and Moss 1980). Elevated plasma levels of epinephrine are not, however, a regular accompaniment of panic attacks induced in the laboratory (Liebowitz et al. 1985a). It is not clear whether administration of catecholamines can actually provoke anxiety reactions and, if so, whether the reaction is specific to patients with anxiety disorder. Researchers in the 1930s and 1940s did show that epinephrine infusion caused the physical, but not necessarily the emotional, symptoms of anxiety in human subjects, and for many years the possibility that panic attacks are manifestations of massive discharge from the β-adrenergic nervous system had been considered. Frohlich et al. (1969) administered intravenous isoproterenol infusions to patients with a hyperdynamic β-adrenergic circulatory state and produced "hysterical outbursts" that sound similar to panic attacks. In comparison with healthy control subjects, patients with spontaneous anxiety may be more sensitive to the effects of isoproterenol (Rainey et al. 1984).

Gorman et al. (1989b) suggested that the putative panicogenic effect of isoproterenol may be indirect, because isoproterenol does not cross the blood–brain barrier. A peripheral mismatch between induced metabolic demands and actual physiological state may occur and be conveyed to the brain stem, eliciting a panic reaction. The β-adrenergic hypothesis received further support from studies claiming that β-adrenergic–blocking drugs, such as propranolol, have an ameliorative effect on panic attacks and anxiety. When properly designed and con-

trolled studies of β-adrenergic blockers used in specific, well-diagnosed anxiety disorders are reviewed, however, only modest antianxiety effects can actually be demonstrated. No study has ever shown that β-adrenergic blockers are specifically effective in blocking spontaneous panic attacks. For example, intravenously administrated propranolol, in doses sufficient to achieve full peripheral β-adrenergic blockade, is not able to block a sodium lactate–induced panic attack in patients with panic disorder (Gorman et al. 1983). Examination of various autonomic parameters seems to dispel the notion of simple autonomic dysregulation in panic (M.B. Stein and Asmundson 1994). Indeed, global sympathetic activation is not observed in panic disorder patients at rest, nor even during panic attacks in some patients (Wilkinson et al. 1998).

The locus coeruleus has also been implicated in the pathogenesis of panic attacks. This nucleus is located in the pons and contains more than 50% of all noradrenergic neurons in the entire central nervous system. It sends afferent projections to a wide area of the brain, including the hippocampus, amygdala, limbic lobe, and cerebral cortex. Electrical stimulation of the animal locus coeruleus produces a marked fear and anxiety response, whereas ablation of the animal locus coeruleus renders an animal less susceptible to fear response in the face of threatening stimuli (Redmond 1979). In humans, drugs known to be capable of increasing locus coeruleus discharge in animals are anxiogenic, whereas many drugs that curtail locus coeruleus firing and decrease central noradrenergic turnover are antianxiety agents.

Yohimbine challenge was reported to induce greater anxiety and a greater increase in plasma 3-methoxy-4-hydroxyphenylglycol (MHPG), a major noradrenergic metabolite, in patients with frequent panic attacks, compared with patients who have panic attacks less frequently or with healthy control subjects. Such a finding is suggestive of heightened central noradrenergic activity in panic (Charney and Heninger 1984). The results from challenge tests with the α_2-adrenergic agonist clonidine, although difficult to interpret, have suggested noradrenergic dysregulation in panic, with hypersensitivity of some and subsensitivity of other brain α_2-adrenoreceptors. Compared with control subjects, panic disorder patients had heightened cardiovascular responses (Charney et al. 1986; Nutt 1989) but blunted growth hormone (GH) responses (Nutt 1989; Tancer et al. 1993) to clonidine. Dysregulated noradrenergic function, in the form of markedly elevated MHPG volatility in response to clonidine challenge, has been described in patients with panic disorder; it normalizes after treatment with selective serotonin reuptake inhibitors (SSRIs) (Coplan et al. 1997).

However, buspirone, which is also reported to increase locus coeruleus firing, is an anxiolytic medication and has not been reported to induce panic. Examples of medications that curtail locus coeruleus firing include clonidine, propranolol, benzodiazepines, morphine, endorphin, and TCAs. These drugs range from those clearly effective in blocking human panic attacks (e.g., TCAs) to those of more dubious efficacy (e.g., clonidine, propranolol, standard benzodiazepines). Also, controversy exists about the relevance of these animal models. Redmond (1979) and colleagues found abundant evidence that situations that provoke fear and anxiety in laboratory animals are associated with increases both in locus coeruleus discharge and in central noradrenergic turnover. This finding would, of course, support the idea that the locus coeruleus is a kind of generator for anxiety attacks. However, no consistent pattern of increased locus coeruleus discharge is associated with anxiety in animals (S.T. Mason and Fibiger 1979). The locus coeruleus may be involved in arousal and response to novel stimuli rather than in anxiety (Aston-Jones et al. 1984).

The panicogen sodium lactate. Although not without some controversy, sodium lactate provocation of panic attacks has captured much attention as an experimental model for understanding the pathogenesis of spontaneous panic attacks. Lactate-provoked panic is specific to patients with prior spontaneous attacks, closely resembles such attacks, and can be blocked by the same drugs that block natural attacks (Liebowitz et al. 1984a). Cohen and White (1950) first noted that patients with neurocirculatory asthenia, a condition closely related to anxiety disorder, developed higher levels of blood lactate while exercising than did healthy control subjects. This finding stimulated Pitts and McClure (1967) to administer intravenous infusions of sodium lactate to patients with "anxiety" disorder; they found that most of the patients experienced an anxiety attack during the infusion. The subjects all believed that these attacks were quite typical of their naturally occurring attacks. Healthy control subjects did not experience panic attacks during the infusion.

Having been replicated on numerous occasions under proper experimental conditions, the finding that 10 mL/kg of 0.5 molar sodium lactate infused over 20 minutes will provoke a panic attack in most patients with panic disorder but not in healthy control subjects is now a well-accepted fact. The mechanism, however, that may account for the observed biochemical and physiological changes (Liebowitz et al. 1985a) has been the focus of much uncertainty and controversy. Theories have included nonspecific arousal that cognitively triggers

panic; induction of metabolic alkalosis; hypocalcemia; alteration of the NAD:NADH ratio; and transient intracerebral hypercapnia. Of these, transient intracerebral hypercapnia has received considerable interest and validation in recent studies and is discussed later (see "Carbon dioxide hypersensitivity theory" subsection).

GABA–benzodiazepine system. Another area of inquiry that may relate to the biology of panic is the γ-aminobutyric acid (GABA)–benzodiazepine receptor complex; the benzodiazepine receptor is linked to a receptor for the inhibitory neurotransmitter GABA. Binding of a benzodiazepine to the benzodiazepine receptor facilitates the action of GABA, effectively slowing neural transmission. One series of compounds, the β-carbolines, which are inverse agonists of this receptor complex, produce an acute anxiety syndrome when administered to laboratory animals or to healthy human volunteers (Dorow et al. 1983; Skolnick and Paul 1982). On the other hand, benzodiazepines have long been known to be a highly efficacious treatment for panic. The possibility is then raised that either aberrant production of an endogenous ligand or altered receptor sensitivity may occur in patients with panic, interfering with proper benzodiazepine receptor function and causing their symptoms.

There is support for such a theory, although findings in the literature to date have been somewhat contradictory. One study found that patients with panic disorder, compared with healthy control subjects, demonstrated less reduced saccadic eye movement velocity in response to diazepam, suggesting hyposensitivity of the benzodiazepine receptor in panic (Roy-Byrne et al. 1990). The benzodiazepine antagonist flumazenil was found to be panicogenic in panic patients but not in normal control subjects, suggesting a deficiency in an endogenous anxiolytic ligand or altered benzodiazepine receptor sensitivity in panic (Nutt et al. 1990). However, results from another study of flumazenil responses in panic were negative (Strohle et al. 1999).

More recently, imaging studies have consistently revealed alterations in the GABA–benzodiazepine system. Decreased benzodiazepine receptor binding observed on single photon emission computed tomography (SPECT) scanning was found in the hippocampus of patients with panic disorder, and prefrontal cortex binding was also decreased in those subjects who experienced an attack during the scanning (Bremner et al. 2000). These findings could tie in neatly with the current "neurocircuitry of fear" model of panic (described later), in which the amygdala, hippocampus, and prefrontal cortex play a central role in modulating conditioned fear responses. Similarly, a global decrease in benzodiazepine receptor binding, most prominently in the prefrontal cortex and the insula (Malizia et al. 1998), has been observed on positron emission tomography (PET) scans. Finally, a 22% reduction in total occipital GABA levels was recently found in subjects with panic compared with control subjects (Goddard et al. 2001).

The serotonergic system. Although the serotonergic system has not been as extensively investigated in panic in comparison with other neurochemical systems, it is generally thought to be one of the systems that at least indirectly modulate dysregulated responses in panic disorder. Indirect evidence for this is provided by the high efficacy of serotonin reuptake inhibitors in treating panic. It has recently been proposed that serotonergic medications may act by desensitizing the brain's fear network via projections from the raphe nuclei to the locus coeruleus, inhibiting noradrenergic activation; to the periaqueductal gray region, inhibiting freeze/flight responses; to the hypothalamus, inhibiting corticotropin-releasing factor (CRF) release; and possibly directly at the level of the amygdala, inhibiting excitatory pathways from the cortex and the thalamus (Gorman et al. 2000). A recent study of tryptophan, a serotonin (5-hydroxytryptamine [5-HT]) precursor, found that its depletion resulted in increased anxiety and carbon dioxide (CO_2)–induced panic attacks in panic patients but not in comparison subjects (Miller et al. 2000).

Hypothalamic-pituitary-adrenal axis. The hypothalamic-pituitary-adrenal (HPA) system, which is central to an organism's response to stress, would clearly be of interest in panic disorder, in which increased early-life stressful events such as separations, losses, and abuse have been described (Horesh et al. 1997; M.B. Stein et al. 1996; Tweed et al. 1989). However, HPA findings have been inconsistent. Cortisol responses in lactate-induced panic have suggested HPA axis involvement in anticipatory anxiety, as is known to occur in other anxiety and stress states, but not in the actual panic attacks (Hollander et al. 1989). There is some evidence for uncoupling of noradrenergic and HPA axis activity in patients with panic disorder (Coplan et al. 1995). In a recent study, adrenocorticotropic hormone (ACTH) and cortisol responses to CRF challenge were not clearly altered in panic disorder patients compared with healthy subjects (Curtis et al. 1997).

Carbon dioxide hypersensitivity theory. Controlled hyperventilation and respiratory alkalosis do not routinely provoke panic attacks in most patients with panic disorder. Surprisingly, however, giving these patients a mixture of 5% CO_2 in room air to breathe causes panic almost as often as does a sodium lactate infusion (Gorman et al. 1984). This finding has been rather consistently replicated. Similarly, sodium bicarbonate infusion provokes panic attacks in patients with panic disorder at a rate comparable to that induced by CO_2 inhalation (Gorman et al. 1989a).

By what mechanism, then, does 5% CO_2 induce panic? Such a phenomenon may be partially explained by the findings of Svensson and colleagues, who showed that CO_2, when added to inspired air, causes a reliable dose-dependent increase in rat locus coeruleus firing (Elam et al. 1981). Alternatively, patients with panic disorder may have hypersensitive brain-stem CO_2 chemoreceptors in the medulla. Indeed, during the CO_2 induction procedure, patients with panic disorder who experience panic attacks while breathing 5% CO_2 demonstrate a much faster increase in inspiratory drive than do patients without panic disorder or healthy control subjects; inspiratory drive is thought to reflect most directly the brain-stem component of respiratory regulation (Gorman et al. 1988).

Such a model is of interest because it could account for the generally well-established finding that hyperventilation does not cause panic, whereas CO_2, lactate, and bicarbonate do. Infused lactate is metabolized to bicarbonate, which is then converted in the periphery to CO_2. In other words, CO_2 constitutes the common metabolic product of both lactate and bicarbonate. This CO_2 selectively crosses the blood–brain barrier and produces transient cerebral hypercapnia. The hypercapnia then sets off the brain-stem CO_2 chemoreceptors, leading to hyperventilation and panic. Thus, a "false suffocation alarm" theory of panic has been formulated (D.F. Klein 1993) that proposes that patients with panic are hypersensitive to CO_2 because they have an overly sensitive brain-stem suffocation alarm system. In a sense, this condition constitutes the opposite of the hyposensitive suffocation alarm seen in Ondine's curse, a rare illness in which those affected are at risk for suffocating in their sleep. D.F. Klein (1993) proposed that such a theory of panic could explain, for example, the tendency of panic attacks to occur during high-CO_2 states such as deep non–rapid eye movement sleep, premenstrually, and sometimes with relaxation, but not during childbirth, an event otherwise characterized by extreme hyperventilation and potentially catastrophic cognitions.

This theory may be supported by the variety of subtle respiratory dysfunctions that appear to be associated with panic, such as preexisting pulmonary disease, panic disorder patients' chronic tendency to hyperventilate, their increased variance in tidal volume during steady-state respiration, and their greater irregularities in nocturnal breathing (Papp et al. 1993; M.B. Stein et al. 1995a). There is some evidence that irregular breathing patterns are intrinsic to panic patients and are not influenced by induced hyperventilation or cognitive manipulation, suggesting a brain-stem rather than a higher-brain-level dysregulation (Abelson et al. 2001). On the other hand, Gorman et al. (2000) argued, based on several lines of evidence, that brain-stem respiratory centers constitute a secondary mechanism by which panic attack symptoms relating to respiration become manifest, as one of several pathways that are activated by central excitation of the amygdala.

Neurocircuitry of fear. The most recently proposed model of panic attempts to integrate neurochemical, imaging, and treatment findings in the disorder, coupled with mostly preclinical work in the neurobiology of conditioned fear responses (Coplan and Lydiard 1998; Gorman et al. 2000). The model postulates that panic attacks are to a degree analogous to animal fear and avoidance responses and may be manifestations of dysregulation in the brain circuits underlying conditioned fear responses. Panic is speculated to originate in an abnormally sensitive fear network, centered in the amygdala. Input to the amygdala is modulated by both thalamic input and prefrontal cortical projections, and amygdalar projections extend to several areas involved in various aspects of the fear response, such as the locus coeruleus (involved in arousal), the brain stem (respiratory activation), the hypothalamus (activation of the HPA stress axis), and the cortex (cognitive interpretations). This model is thought to explain why a variety of biologically diverse agents have panicogenic properties (by acting at different pathways or neurochemical systems of this network); it is proposed that the respiratory brain-stem nucleus could not be directly triggered by such a variety of agents (Gorman et al. 2000). Thus, dysregulated "cross-talk" between the various neurotransmitter systems previously described, such as serotonergic, noradrenergic, GABA-ergic, CRF, and others, may underlie the pathogenesis of panic (Coplan and Lydiard 1998). This is a very comprehensive and theoretically exciting biological model of panic—which, however, is still in great need of empirical validation.

Genetics. Several family and twin studies of panic disorder have consistently supported the presence of a moderate genetic influence in the expression of panic disorder. Crowe et al. (1983) found a morbidity risk for panic disorder of 24.7% among relatives of patients with panic disorder, compared with a risk of only 2.3% among healthy control subjects. In a study of 32 monozygotic and 53 dizygotic twins, Torgersen (1983) found panic attacks to be five times more frequent in the former than in the latter group. However, the absolute concordance rate in monozygotic twins was 31%, which suggests that nongenetic factors play an important role in the development of the illness. Moderate heritability was also found in a female twin study (Kendler et al. 1993). Individuals with an early onset of the disorder appear to have a much higher familial aggregation of the disorder, possibly suggesting a stronger genetic component in a familial subtype of the disorder, which might better lend itself to molecular genetic studies (Goldstein et al. 1997).

Molecular genetic research on panic disorder has been quite active in recent years and holds promise for the future. However, a whole-genome scan in 23 panic pedigrees did not yield any evidence of linkage (Knowles et al. 1998). Also, there have been several negative studies of putative genetic markers and candidate genes for panic in the last decade, such as a linkage study of eight $GABA_A$ receptor genes (Crowe et al. 1997) and two studies of the serotonin transporter gene (Deckert et al. 1997; Ishiguro et al. 1997). Some studies have yielded positive results for a variety of candidate genes, including the X-linked monoamine oxidase A gene in females (Deckert et al. 1999), the cholecystokinin gene (Wang et al. 1998), the cholecystokinin receptor gene (Kennedy et al. 1999), and the adenosine A2a receptor gene (Deckert et al. 1998). These isolated genetic polymorphisms are best viewed as individual risk factors that possibly increase susceptibility to the disorder but that are not, in and of themselves, necessary or sufficient for phenotypic expression.

Psychodynamic Theories

In this subsection we present the major landmarks in the evolution of psychodynamic theories of anxiety and panic and their relationship to recent biological advances. More lengthy expositions and critiques of the psychoanalytic theories can be referred to by interested readers (Cooper 1985; Michels et al. 1985; Nemiah 1988).

Freud's first theory of anxiety neurosis (id or impulse anxiety). In his earliest concept of anxiety formation, Freud (1895[1894]/1962b) postulated that anxiety stems from the direct physiological transformation of libidinal energy into the somatic symptoms of anxiety, without the mediation of psychic mechanisms. He found evidence for this process in the sexual practices and experiences of patients with anxiety, which were characterized by disturbed sexual arousal and continence and coitus interruptus. He termed such anxiety an "actual neurosis" as opposed to a psychoneurosis, because of the postulated absence of psychic processes. Such anxiety, originating from overwhelming instinctual urges, would today be referred to as id or impulse anxiety.

Over the next several years, Freud started to modify his theory. Although the basic tenet that anxiety stemmed from undischarged sexual energy remained the same, this was no longer posited to be due to external constraints such as sexual dysfunctions. In accordance with Freud's developing topographic theory of the mind, anxiety resulted from forbidden sexual drives in the unconscious being repressed by the preconscious.

Structural theory and intrapsychic conflict. By 1926, with the advent of the structural theory of the mind, Freud's theory of anxiety had undergone a major transformation (Freud 1926/1959). According to Freud, anxiety is an affect belonging to the ego and acts as a signal alerting the ego to internal danger. The danger stems from intrapsychic conflict between instinctual drives from the id, superego prohibitions, and external reality demands. Anxiety acts as a signal to the ego for the mobilization of repression and other defenses to counteract the threat to intrapsychic equilibrium. Inhibitions and neurotic symptoms develop as measures designed to avoid the dangerous situation and to allow only partial gratification of instinctual wishes, thus warding off signal anxiety. In the revised theory then, anxiety leads to repression, instead of the reverse.

Early on, Freud (1895[1894]/1962a) also observed that in the analysis of phobias, nothing is ever found except the emotional state of anxiety. In the case of agoraphobia, we often find the recollection of an anxiety attack; what the patient actually fears is the occurrence of such an attack under the special conditions in which he believes he cannot escape it. This is a succinct description, from more than a century ago, of the development of anticipatory anxiety and agoraphobia after a panic attack. At that time, Freud did not consider phobias to be psychologically mediated. Rather, he understood them, like anxiety neurosis, to be manifestations of a physiologically induced tension state. Undischarged libidinal energy was physiologically transformed into anxiety, which became attached to and partly discharged through objects that were, by their nature or in the patient's prior experience, dangerous.

The intrapsychic conflict model of anxiety continues to constitute a major tenet of contemporary psychoanalytic theory. Psychoanalytic theorists after Freud, such as Melanie Klein (1948) and Joachim Flescher (1955), also made significant contributions to the understanding of the psychodynamic origins of anxiety. Whereas Freud concentrated on the role of sexual impulses and the oedipal conflict in the genesis of anxiety, these theorists drew attention to the role that aggressive impulses and pre-oedipal dynamics can also play in generating anxiety. Since Freud, the psychodynamic literature has to a degree shifted away from formulations that primarily emphasize libidinal wishes and castration fears in understanding phobias such as agoraphobia (Michels et al. 1985). For example, the significance of a trustworthy and safe companion in individuals with agoraphobia could be understood as a simultaneous expression of aggressive impulses toward the companion and a magical wish to protect the companion from such impulses by always being together. Alternatively, excessive fear of object loss and its concomitant separation anxiety could explain both the fear of being away from home alone and the alleviation of this fear when a companion is present.

Although psychoanalytic theories are not universally accepted by psychiatrists today, they remain an invaluable tool in the understanding and treatment of at least some patients. Also, it should be pointed out that Freud's theory of anxiety formation is not incompatible with biological theories of anxiety. Although Freud's first model of anxiety was later overshadowed by the conflictual model, modern biological theories of panic are in many ways more reminiscent of his original physiological formulation. Furthermore, Freud maintained on numerous occasions that biological predispositions to psychiatric symptoms are undoubtedly operant in most conditions and that constitutional factors could play a role in the particular form that neurotic symptoms take in different patients.

Indeed, what psychoanalytic theory does not help us with is a better understanding of the determinants of the various specific forms in which anxiety symptoms manifest themselves. Some patients have anxiety attacks, others have more chronic forms of anxiety, and still others have phobias, obsessions, or compulsions. Freud himself attempted to address this problem of choice of neurosis and partly explained it on the basis of constitutional factors—a concept essentially similar to modern biological notions. In an attempt to reconcile this unpredictability with classical psychodynamic theory, it has been postulated that patients with unconscious conflict and a neural predisposition to panic may manifest their anxiety in the form of panic attacks, whereas individuals without this neural predisposition may manifest milder forms of signal anxiety (Nemiah 1981). Along these more contemporary lines of thinking, a recent psychodynamic study of patients with panic disorder proposed that in patients who are neurophysiologically predisposed to early fearfulness, exposure to parental behaviors that augment this fearfulness may result in disturbances of object relations and persistence of conflicts surrounding dependence and catastrophic fears of helplessness that can be addressed in psychodynamic treatment (Shear et al. 1993).

With the broadening of psychodynamic theory over the decades, different forms of anxiety have been elaborated, such as annihilation anxiety, separation anxiety, anxiety over loss of another's love, castration anxiety, superego anxiety, and id anxiety. In particular, greater emphasis on preoedipal dynamics and research in infant and child development has brought to the forefront attachment theories and the importance of attachment disturbances in the genesis of psychopathology. In the early 1960s, D.F. Klein advanced an etiological theory that agoraphobia with panic attacks may represent an aberrant function of the biological substrate that underlies normal human attachment and threats to it (i.e., separation anxiety). Based on Bowlby's (1973) work on attachment and separation, D.F. Klein (1981) advanced the notion that the attachment of an infant animal or human to its mother is not simply a learned response but rather is genetically programmed and biologically determined. Indeed, 20%–50% of adults with panic disorder and agoraphobia recall manifesting symptoms of pathological separation anxiety, often taking the form of school phobia, when they were children. Furthermore, the initial panic attack in the history of a patient who goes on to develop panic disorder is sometimes preceded by the real or threatened loss of a significant relationship. One systematic study showed the number and severity of recent life events—especially events related to loss—were greater in patients with new-onset panic than in control subjects (Faravelli and Pallanti 1989). A blinded psychodynamic study showed separation anxiety to be a significantly more prevalent theme in the dreams and screen memories of patients with panic disorder than in those of healthy control subjects.

Infant animals demonstrate their anxiety when separated from the mother by a series of high-pitched cries, called distress vocalizations. Imipramine has been found to be effective in blocking distress vocalizations in dogs by Scott (1975) and in monkeys by Suomi et al. (1978). As discussed later, imipramine is a highly effective antipanic drug in adult humans. Hypothesizing a link between adult panic attacks and childhood separation anxiety, Gittelman-Klein and Klein (1971) conducted a study of imipramine treatment for children with school phobia. In these children, fear of separation from their mothers was usually the basis behind refusing to go to school. The drug proved successful in getting the children to return to school. In a related finding, Weissman et al. (1984) found a threefold increase in risk for separation anxiety in children of parents with panic disorder.

Thus, evidence suggests that the same drug that diminishes protest anxiety in higher mammals also reduces separation anxiety in children and blocks panic attacks in adults. This is further confirmation of the link between separation anxiety and panic attacks. Is early separation anxiety linked to agoraphobia or also to panic attacks per se? If imipramine affects panic attacks, and separation anxiety is linked to agoraphobia, then why is imipramine effective in the treatment of school phobia? On the other hand, children with school phobia do not have spontaneous panic attacks, but this could be related to their young age. Perhaps both panic disorder and panic disorder with agoraphobia are linked to a biologically disordered separation mechanism that is responsive to imipramine. This may occur if the retrospective histories of a lesser degree of separation anxiety in patients with panic attacks alone are misremembered.

Contemporary psychoanalysts, in response, have claimed that this neurophysiological and ethological model of a disrupted separation mechanism and panic may be unnecessarily reductionistic (Michels et al. 1985). They point out an inconsistency between the conceptualization of panic attacks as spontaneous and the frequently reported histories of childhood separation anxiety in patients with panic attacks and state that psychological difficulties with separation can also play a role in subsequent vulnerability to panic. On the other hand, contemporary psychoanalysts have also given more credence to the role of biological substrates in the genesis of anxiety symptoms in at least some patients who have developed their anxious personality structure secondary to a largely contentless biological dysregulation, so that although psychological triggers for anxiety may still be found, the anxiety threshold is so low in these patients that it is no longer useful to view the psychological event as etiologically significant (Cooper 1985).

Learning Theories

Behavior or learning theorists hold that anxiety is conditioned by the fear of certain environmental stimuli. If every time a laboratory animal presses a bar it receives a noxious electric shock, the pressing of the lever becomes a conditioned stimulus that precedes the unconditioned stimulus (i.e., the shock). The conditioned stimulus releases a conditioned response in the animal, anxiety, which leads the animal to avoid contact with the lever, thereby avoiding the shock. Successful avoidance of the unconditioned stimulus, the shock, reinforces the avoidant behavior. This leads to a decrease in anxiety level.

By analogy with this animal model, we might say that anxiety attacks are conditioned responses to fearful situations. For example, an infant learns that if his mother is not present (i.e., the conditioned stimulus), he will suffer hunger (i.e., the unconditioned stimulus); thus, he learns to become anxious automatically whenever the mother is absent (i.e., the conditioned response). The anxiety may persist even after the child is old enough to feed himself. Or, to provide another example, a life-threatening situation in someone's life (e.g., skidding in a car during a snowstorm) is paired with the experience of rapid heartbeat (i.e., the conditioned stimulus) and tremendous anxiety. Long after the accident, rapid heartbeat alone, whether during vigorous exercise or minor emotional upset, becomes capable by itself of provoking the conditioned response of an anxiety attack.

Several problems are posed by such a theory. First, although some traumatic situations—for example, thyroid disease, cocaine intoxication, or a life-threatening event such as a suffocation incident—do seem to be paired with the onset of panic disorder, for many patients no such traumatic event can be located. It is noteworthy, however, that a history of traumatic suffocation incidents is found in about 20% of patients with panic disorder, significantly more than in psychiatric comparison subjects (Bouwer and Stein 1997). Given that clinical experience does not support the notion that anxiety disorder patients undergo repeated traumatic events, these patients should be able to extinguish their anxiety. Thus, despite their powerful basis in experimental animal research, learning theories do not seem to explain adequately, in and of themselves, the pathogenesis of human anxiety disorders. However, coupled with a dysregulated biological mechanism or vulnerability that may be linked to the process of fear conditioning in panic, such as altered functioning of the amygdala and related fear circuits (see "Biological Theories" earlier in this chapter), heightened anxiety responses could conceivably persist over time.

It also appears that particular types of information-processing biases contribute to the maintenance of panic, if not its genesis. Compared with control subjects, patients with panic disorder demonstrate an attentional bias toward threatening (versus positive) words (McNally et al. 1997). In addition, a bias in explicit but not implicit memory processes for words denoting physical threat has been demonstrated in patients with panic disorder relative to healthy comparison subjects (Lundh et al. 1997).

Course and Prognosis

The course of illness without treatment is highly variable. At present, there is no reliable way to know which patients will develop, for example, agoraphobia. The illness seems to have a waxing and waning course in which spontaneous recovery occurs, only to be followed months to years later by a new outburst. At the extreme, some patients become completely housebound for decades. Treatment aimed at blocking the occurrence of the attacks, described in detail later in this chapter, is appropriate at any point in the course of the illness when such attacks are occurring. Results are often dramatic. Pharmacological blockade of panic attacks early in the illness, before phobic avoidance has become an ingrained way of life, often leads to complete remission. Even years into the illness, effective disruption of the attacks with medication can lead to resolution of anticipatory anxiety and phobias without other treatment.

However, a substantial number of patients with significant phobic avoidance remain anxious and frightened of confronting feared situations even after the attacks have been blocked. Such patients require other forms of intervention, described elsewhere in this chapter. A 7-year follow-up study examined prognostic factors in naturalistically treated patients with panic disorder. Although patients had generally good outcomes, there were several predictors of poorer outcome, including greater severity of panic attacks and agoraphobia, longer duration of illness, comorbid major depression, separation from a parent by death or divorce, high interpersonal sensitivity, low social class, and single marital status (Noyes et al. 1993). Another long-term outcome study, conducted over a 5-year period, had fairly optimistic findings: at follow-up, 34% of patients were recovered, 46% were minimally impaired, and only 20% remained moderately to severely impaired. The most significant predictor of poor outcome was an anxious–fearful personality type, followed by poor response to initial treatment (O'Rourke et al. 1996). Finally, another large outcome study showed that fewer than 20% of panic disorder patients remained seriously agoraphobic or disabled. Panic attack frequency at baseline, initial medication used, and continuous use of medication (versus intermittent use) were not related to outcome, whereas longer duration of illness and more severe initial avoidance were unfavorable predictors (Katschnig et al. 1995).

An earlier study showed a higher incidence of premature death due to cardiovascular illness and suicide among patients with panic disorder compared with control subjects (Coryell et al. 1982). However, the group of patients studied had all been hospitalized at one point, raising a question as to whether they constituted a more severely ill group of patients than is generally encountered in clinical practice. The increased death rate from cardiovascular illness described in this clinical study was partly supported in an epidemiological investigation by Weissman et al. (1990). In this study, patients with panic disorder had a significantly higher risk for strokes than did patients with other psychiatric disorders, although several methodological limitations were identified. Of note, such medical risks are not routinely evident to clinicians in the usual status of patients undergoing treatment for panic disorder. Most such patients have normal medical workups. The one cardiovascular abnormality that has been found to occur at a higher rate in patients with panic disorder is mitral valve prolapse. This association could conceivably explain a higher incidence of cardiovascular-related death in patients with panic disorder; however, mitral valve prolapse itself is rarely a cause of premature death or major morbidity. One other possible explanation for increased cardiovascular/cerebrovascular risk in patients with panic disorder may be related to aspects of their lifestyle. Such patients tend to live relatively sedentary lives, and some report that vigorous physical exercise precipitates their panic attacks, leading them to avoid exertion of any kind. Heavy cigarette smoking, alcoholism, and poor diets could also contribute to an increased risk in panic patients. Alternatively, left ventricular enlargement and increased risk of thromboembolic events have also been contemplated as possibly accounting for the association (Weissman et al. 1990).

The putative association between panic disorder and increased suicide risk has received much attention in the past decade. Initially it was thought that the association may have been due to the fact that, relative to the general population, patients with panic disorder are more prone to major depressive disorder and to alcoholism at some point in their lives, and in part that theory probably remains valid. However, Allgulander and Lavori (1991) conducted a large retrospective survey in Sweden and found an increased suicide risk in panic disorder in the absence of comorbid diagnoses. Epidemiological data further support this finding. In the ECA study, the lifetime rate of suicide attempts in persons with uncomplicated panic disorder was 7%, about the same as the 7.9% rate for uncomplicated major depression (J. Johnson et al. 1990). However, in a reanalysis of the ECA data that controlled for all comorbidity rather than one disorder at a time, an association between panic and suicide attempts could no longer be shown (Hornig and McNally 1995). In a clinical sample of patients with panic disorder, a 17% incidence of suicide attempts was found for those without comorbid major depression or substance abuse, but these patients did have other comorbidity with some depressive symptoms and/or personality disorder (Lepine et al. 1993). The most recent investigation to examine this issue, a 5-year prospective study, again concluded that panic disorder had no association with suicide in the absence of other risk factors (Warshaw et al. 2000). The ECA study also documented that, apart from suicide risk, there exist a variety of other frequently neglected morbidities associated with panic (Markowitz et al. 1989).

Diagnosis

Physical Signs and Behavior

The diagnosis of panic disorder is made when a patient experiences recurrent panic attacks that are discrete and unexpected and are followed by a month of persistent anticipatory anxiety or behavioral change. These panic attacks are characterized by a sudden crescendo of anxiety and fearfulness, in addition to the presence of at least four physical symptoms. Finally, the attacks cannot be secondary to a known organic factor or due to another mental disorder. However, these diagnoses are not always obvious, and a number of other psychiatric and medical disorders may mimic these conditions (Table 11–4).

Differential Diagnosis

Other psychiatric illnesses. Although the medical conditions that mimic anxiety disorder are usually easily ruled out, psychiatric conditions that involve pathological anxiety can make the differential diagnosis of panic disorder difficult. By far the most problematic is the differentiation of primary anxiety disorder from depression.

TABLE 11–4. Psychiatric and medical differential diagnosis of panic disorders

Psychiatric	
Generalized anxiety disorder	Depersonalization disorder
Depressive disorders	Somatoform disorders
Schizophrenia	Character disorders
Medical	
Hyperthyroidism	Pheochromocytoma
Hypothyroidism	Hypoglycemia
Hyperparathyroidism	True vertigo
Mitral valve prolapse	Drug withdrawal
Cardiac arrhythmias	Alcohol withdrawal
Coronary insufficiency	

Patients with depression often manifest signs of anxiety and may even have frank panic attacks. On the other hand, patients with panic disorder, if untreated for significant amounts of time, routinely become demoralized as the effects of the illness progressively restrict their ability to enjoy a normal life. Further complicating the picture is the fact that some, but not all, studies have shown that patients with anxiety disorder have increased family history of affective disorder.

Although the differentiation of anxiety from depression can at times strain even the most experienced clinician, several points are helpful. Patients with panic disorder generally do not demonstrate the full range of vegetative symptoms seen in depression. Thus, anxious patients usually have trouble falling asleep rather than experiencing early-morning awakening, and they do not lose their appetite. Diurnal mood fluctuation is uncommon in anxiety disorder. Perhaps of greatest importance is the fact that most anxious patients do not lose the capacity to enjoy things or to be cheered up as endogenously depressed patients do.

The distinction between atypical depression and anxiety disorders is even more difficult because of the lack of typical endogenous features in the former. However, although patients with atypical depression can also be cheered up, they tend to slump faster than patients with anxiety disorder. Panic attacks and atypical depression frequently coexist, and coexisting panic attacks may increase the monoamine oxidase inhibitor (MAOI) responsivity of patients with atypical depression (Liebowitz et al. 1984b).

The order of developing symptoms also differentiates depression from anxiety. In cases of panic disorder, anxiety symptoms usually precede any seriously altered mood. Patients can generally recall having anxiety attacks first, then becoming gradually more disgusted with life, and then feeling depressed. In depression, patients usually experience dysphoria first, with anxiety symptoms coming later. However, panic disorder can be complicated by secondary major depression and vice versa.

A few other psychiatric conditions often need to be differentiated from panic disorder. Patients with somatization disorder complain of various physical ailments and discomforts, none of which are substantiated by physical or laboratory findings. Unlike panic disorder patients, somatizing patients present with physical problems that do not usually occur in episodic attacks but are virtually constant.

Patients with depersonalization disorder have episodes of derealization/depersonalization without the other symptoms of a panic attack. However, panic attacks not infrequently involve depersonalization and derealization as prominent symptoms.

Although patients with panic disorder often fear they will lose their minds or go crazy, psychotic illness is not an outcome of anxiety disorder. Reassuring the patient on this point is often the first step in a successful treatment.

Undoubtedly some patients with anxiety disorders abuse alcohol and drugs such as sedatives in attempts at self-medication (Quitkin and Babkin 1982). In one study, after successful detoxification, a group of alcoholic patients with a history of panic disorder were treated with medication to block spontaneous panic attacks (Quitkin and Babkin 1982). These patients did not resume alcohol consumption once their panic attacks were eliminated.

With regard to the agoraphobic component of the disorder, widespread fears and avoidance of being alone or of leaving home can also be seen in paranoid and psychotic states, PTSD, and major depressive disorders. Psychotic states can be differentiated from agoraphobia by the presence of delusions, hallucinations, and thought disorder. Although agoraphobic patients frequently fear that they are going crazy, they do not exhibit psychotic symptoms. Patients with PTSD have a typical history of trauma leading to fear of being alone or of traveling alone following an assault.

Distinguishing between depressive disorders and agoraphobia is more difficult. Patients with depressive disorders and patients with agoraphobia both commonly experience spontaneous panic attacks. Patients with agoraphobia are frequently demoralized and will state that they feel depressed. Close questioning, however, usually does not reveal further vegetative symptoms or a loss of pleasure or interest in activities. Early morning awakening and pervasive anhedonia, which are common symptoms in endogenous depression, are rare in agoraphobia. Agoraphobic individuals will usually say they would love to leave home and engage in a variety of activities if only they could be sure of not panicking. In contrast, depressed individuals usually see no point in going out, because nothing gives them any pleasure and they feel that people will be better off without them.

Patients with atypical depression (i.e., depression characterized by hypersomnia, hyperphagia, extreme low energy, and depressed but reactive mood) frequently have panic attacks but rarely have agoraphobia as part of their life history or current symptoms. Patients with atypical depression and a history of panic attacks may respond preferentially to MAOIs (Liebowitz et al. 1985b).

Hyperthyroidism and hypothyroidism. Both hyperthyroidism and hypothyroidism can present with anxiety unaccompanied by other signs or symptoms. For this reason, it is imperative that all patients complaining of anxiety undergo routine thyroid function tests, including the evaluation of the level of thyroid-stimulating hormone. It should be remembered, however, that thyroid disease can act as one of the predisposing triggers to panic disorder, so that even when the apparently primary thyroid disease is corrected, panic attacks may continue until specifically treated.

Cardiac disease. The relationship of mitral valve prolapse to panic disorder has attracted a great deal of attention over the years. This usually benign condition has been shown by several investigators to occur more frequently in patients with panic disorder than in healthy control subjects. However, screening of patients known to have mitral valve prolapse reveals no greater frequency of panic disorder than is found in the overall population.

Although patients with mitral valve prolapse occasionally complain of palpitations, chest pain, lightheadedness, and fatigue, symptoms of a full-blown panic attack are rare. A comparison of symptoms in mitral valve prolapse and panic disorder is provided in Table 11–5. Panic patients with and without mitral valve prolapse are similar in several important ways. Treatment for panic attacks works regardless of the presence of the prolapsed valve, and patients with both mitral valve prolapse and panic disorder are just as sensitive to sodium lactate as are those with panic disorder alone. Some researchers have speculated that mitral valve prolapse and panic disorder may represent manifestations of the same underlying disorder of autonomic nervous system function (Gorman et al. 1981). Others have suggested that panic disorder, by creating intermittent states of high circulating catecholamine levels and tachycardia, actually causes mitral valve prolapse (Mattes 1981). There are reports that mitral valve prolapse might go away if the panic disorder is maintained under control (Gorman et al. 1981). In a recent meta-analytic study of 21 studies, it was found that there does appear to be a significant association between panic disorder and mitral valve prolapse, although the possibility of publication bias toward favorite positive reports cannot be ruled out (Katerndahl 1993).

In any event, it is clear that the presence of mitral valve prolapse in patients with panic disorder has little clinical or prognostic importance in the management of spontaneous panic attacks. What it may tell us about the underlying etiology of panic disorder is a question currently under vigorous investigation.

Other medical illnesses. Hyperparathyroidism occasionally presents as anxiety symptoms, warranting a

TABLE 11–5. Comparison of symptoms of mitral valve prolapse and panic disorder

Symptoms	Mitral valve prolapse	Panic disorder
Fatigue	+	–
Dyspnea	+	+ +
Palpitations	+ +	+ +
Chest pain	+ +	+
Syncope	+	–
Choking	–	+ +
Dizziness	–	+ +
Derealization	–	+ +
Hot/cold flashes	–	+ +
Sweating	–	+ +
Fainting	–	+ +
Trembling	–	+ +
Fear of dying, going crazy, losing control	–	+ +

Note. + = occasionally; + + = often present; – = rarely present.

serum calcium level determination before definitive diagnosis is made.

Various cardiac conditions can initially present as anxiety symptoms, although, in most cases, the patient's prominent complaints are of chest pain, skipped beats, or palpitations. Ischemic heart disease and arrhythmias, especially paroxysmal atrial tachycardia, should be ruled out by electrocardiography.

Pheochromocytoma is a rare, usually benign tumor of the adrenal medulla that secretes catecholamines in episodic bursts. During an active phase, the patient characteristically experiences flushing, tremulousness, and anxiety. Blood pressure is usually elevated during the active phase of catecholamine secretion but not at other times. Therefore, merely finding a normal blood pressure does not rule out a pheochromocytoma. If this condition is suspected, urine is collected for 24 hours so that a diagnosis can be attempted through determination of catecholamine metabolite concentration. In a study of patients with confirmed pheochromocytoma, about half met criteria for the physical symptoms of panic attacks, but none had panic disorder, because they did not experience terror during the attacks and did not develop anticipatory anxiety or agoraphobia (Starkman et al. 1990).

Disease of the vestibular nerve can cause episodic bouts of vertigo, lightheadedness, nausea, and anxiety that mimic panic attacks. Rather than merely feeling dizzy, patients with disease of the vestibular nerve often experience true vertigo in which the room seems to spin in one direction during each attack. Otolaryngology consultation is warranted when this condition is suspected. Some panic patients complain primarily of dizziness or unsteadiness. Whether these patients are a distinct subgroup with definite neurotological abnormalities is currently under study.

Although many patients believe that their anxiety disorder is caused by reactive hypoglycemia, there is no scientific proof at present that this condition is ever a cause of any psychiatric disturbance. Glucose tolerance tests are not helpful in establishing hypoglycemia as the cause of anxiety, because up to 40% of the normal population will have a random low blood-sugar level during a routine glucose tolerance test. The only convincing way to establish hypoglycemia as a cause of symptoms is to document a low blood-sugar level at the same time the patient is symptomatic. Studies with insulin tolerance tests in panic disorder have yielded negative results.

Treatment

Pharmacotherapy

Antidepressants. When initiating a drug regimen for a patient with panic disorder, it is crucial that the patient understand that the drug will block the panic attacks but may not necessarily decrease the amount of intervening anticipatory anxiety and avoidance, at least initially. For patients with severe anxiety, it can be helpful to initially prescribe a concomitant benzodiazepine, which can be gradually tapered and discontinued after several weeks of antidepressant treatment. It is also important to be aware that some patients with panic disorder display an initial hypersensitivity to antidepressants, whether TCAs or serotonin reuptake inhibitors, during which they complain of jitteriness, agitation, a "speedy" feeling, and insomnia. Although this effect is usually transient, it is unfortunately one of the main reasons that patients opt to discontinue medication early on. Therefore, it is strongly recommended that patients with panic disorder be started on lower doses of antidepressants than would be given to depressed patients.

The central feature in the treatment of panic disorder is the pharmacological blockade of the spontaneous panic attacks. Several classes of medication have been shown to be effective in accomplishing this goal; a summary of the pharmacological treatment of panic disorder is presented in Table 11–6.

The first medications to be widely studied in the treatment of panic disorder were the TCAs, especially imipramine (D.F. Klein 1964; Mavissakalian and Michelson 1986a, 1986b; McNair and Kahn 1981; Sheehan et al. 1980; Zitrin et al. 1980, 1983). Other TCAs, such as

TABLE 11–6. Pharmacological treatment of panic disorder

Selective serotonin reuptake inhibitors (SSRIs)

General indications: first-line, alone or in combination with benzodiazepines if needed; also first choice with comorbid obsessive-compulsive disorder, generalized anxiety disorder, depression, and social phobia

Start at very low doses and increase; response seen with low to moderate doses

Sertraline, paroxetine: U.S. Food and Drug Administration–approved

Fluvoxamine, fluoxetine, citalopram: appear similarly efficacious

Tricyclic antidepressants

General indication: established efficacy, second line if SSRIs fail or are not tolerated

Imipramine: well studied

Clomipramine: high efficacy but not easily tolerated

Desipramine: if patient has low tolerance to anticholinergic side effects

Nortriptyline: if patient is elderly or prone to orthostatic hypotension

Monoamine oxidase inhibitors

General indications: poor response or tolerance of other antidepressants; comorbid atypical depression or social phobia without good SSRI response

Phenelzine: most studied

Tranylcypromine: less sedation

High-potency benzodiazepines

General indications: poor response or tolerance of antidepressants; prominent anticipatory anxiety or phobic avoidance; initial treatment phase until antidepressant begins to work

Clonazepam: longer-acting, less frequent dosing, less withdrawal, first choice

Alprazolam: well studied

Other medications

Other antidepressants: venlafaxine and nefazodone are less studied but seem efficacious

Other options: particularly as augmentation in patients who are refractory or intolerant of all above medications, not well tested to date:

Pindolol: effective augmentation in one controlled trial

Valproate: studied in open trials only

Inositol: studied in open trials only

Clonidine: in open trials, initial response later tended to fade

desipramine, have also been found to be effective, although they have not been studied as extensively as imipramine. Nortriptyline has not been systematically studied, but clinical experience indicates that it is also efficacious and is often better tolerated than other TCAs. The presence of depressed mood is not a predictor or requirement for these drugs to be effective in blocking panic attacks. In recent years, the SSRIs have been shown to be efficacious in treating panic, and because of their several advantages over TCAs, they have become the first-line treatment for panic. TCAs are now reserved, for the most part, for treatment of patients who do not have a good response to, or who do not tolerate, serotonin reuptake inhibitors and related medications.

A standard TCA regimen consists of starting the patient on imipramine, 10 mg/day at bedtime, and increasing the dose by 10 mg every other night until 50 mg is reached. The dosage can be given all at once. Because 50 mg is usually inadequate for full panic blockade, the dosage can then be raised by 25-mg increments every 3 days or by 50-mg increments weekly to as high as 300 mg. Most patients need at least 150 mg daily of a TCA, and, unfortunately, underdosage commonly occurs. In some cases, an imipramine dose over 300 mg is necessary. On "high" imipramine dosing of around 200 mg/day, more than 80% of patients show a marked response in panic attacks (Mavissakalian and Perel 1989). Panic patients not responding to high doses of imipramine should have blood TCA levels measured. Often, blood levels will be disproportionately low for the dose, suggesting rapid metabolism or excretion, malabsorption, or noncompliance. It appears that patients do not show further antipanic responses at combined plasma levels of more than 140 ng/mL (Mavissakalian and Perel 1995). Patients who experience excessive anticholinergic side effects to imipramine can be given desipramine instead. Nortriptyline therapy can be tried in elderly patients or patients who are otherwise very sensitive to orthostatic hypotension.

Results of a number of open and controlled treatment trials have now shown that the potent serotonin reuptake inhibitors are highly effective in the treatment of panic. Given their greater safety and ease of administration in comparison with TCAs, they have become the first-line treatment in panic disorder, either alone or in combination with a benzodiazepine when needed. As a first-line treatment, they also offer the advantage of being effective for several of the common comorbid disorders, such as depression, social phobia, GAD, and OCD.

Although only paroxetine and sertraline are approved by the U.S. Food and Drug Administration (FDA) for this indication, there is no particular reason to think that SSRIs do not all have comparable efficacy in panic. Several controlled trials have documented the efficacy of fluvoxamine at doses up to 150 mg/day (Den Boer 1988; Hoehn-Saric et al. 1993a). Paroxetine has also been demonstrated to be effective in controlled trials, at doses of 20–60 mg daily according to one study (Oehrberg et al. 1995). In another study, however, only the 40-mg daily

dose reached statistically significant superiority over placebo during a 10-week period, whereas the 10-mg and 20-mg doses did not, a finding that highlights the importance of trying higher doses if response to lower doses is inadequate (Ballenger et al. 2000). Not surprisingly, another paroxetine study documented that it was as efficacious as clomipramine in treating panic disorder but better tolerated (Lecrubier et al. 1997). Both medications retained their efficacy during a blinded maintenance period of 9 months, leading to further improvement and highlighting the importance of longer-term treatment (Lecrubier and Judge 1997).

The SSRI sertraline has also been found to be efficacious in treating panic disorder in large controlled trials (Londborg et al. 1998; Pohl et al. 1998). Not only did sertraline markedly decrease the number of panic attacks, it also led to significant improvement in life quality and had a low dropout rate (Pohl et al. 1998). In contrast to the paroxetine study, there was no difference among the three sertraline doses (50, 100, or 200 mg/day) in reducing panic attacks (Londborg et al. 1998). Interestingly, a history of benzodiazepine use does not affect the tolerability of or response to sertraline treatment, regardless of whether the response to the benzodiazepine had been good or bad (Rapaport et al. 2001).

Another SSRI, citalopram, has been shown to be efficacious in treating panic disorder. In an acute 8-week controlled trial, the middle dose of 20–30 mg/day conferred the most advantageous risk–benefit ratio compared with the higher and lower doses used (Wade et al. 1997). In a 1-year controlled maintenance extension of that study, the lowest dose of 10–15 mg/day was not superior to placebo, whereas the middle dose of 20–30 mg/day again showed the best response (Lepola et al. 1998).

Fluoxetine is similarly efficacious in treating panic. Fluoxetine, especially at a daily dose of 20 mg rather than 10 mg, was shown to be superior to placebo in the acute treatment of panic disorder (D. Michelson et al. 1998). Interestingly, this study used a wide range of measures and demonstrated that global improvement was related more to phobia, anxiety, depression, and impairment than to panic attacks per se, again highlighting the importance of looking at the larger picture when assessing change. Over a 6-month maintenance-treatment period, the initial responders to acute fluoxetine treatment demonstrated significant further improvement if randomized to fluoxetine and significant worsening if randomized to placebo (D. Michelson et al. 1999).

Clomipramine, used at doses of 25–200 mg/day titrated to patients' individual responses, appears at least as efficacious—and better tolerated at lower versus higher doses—in treating panic attacks and, to a lesser degree, avoidance (Caillard et al. 1999). Clomipramine is generally less well tolerated than the SSRIs (Lecrubier et al. 1997) and therefore is not routinely used as a first-line treatment in panic.

In one meta-analytic study, serotonin reuptake inhibitors emerged as superior to imipramine and alprazolam in treating panic; however, lower doses of the latter two medications may have partly accounted for this difference (Boyer 1995). Like the TCAs, SSRIs can cause uncomfortable overstimulation in patients with panic disorder if started at the usual doses. It is therefore suggested that treatment be started very cautiously, at 5–10 mg/day for fluoxetine, paroxetine, and citalopram and at 25 mg/day for sertraline and fluvoxamine. The dosage can then be gradually increased to an average dose by weekly adjustments. A moderate or lower daily dose is usually adequate for most patients, as described in the trials above, and high doses are generally not needed and are less well tolerated.

MAOIs are as effective as the TCAs and the SSRIs in treating panic. Both phenelzine and tranylcypromine successfully treat panic, although phenelzine has been studied more extensively. Phenelzine can be started at 15 mg daily in the morning. The dose is then increased by 15 mg every 4–7 days as tolerated, up to a maximum of 60–90 mg daily. If sedation or weight gain is of concern, tranylcypromine may be tried, starting at 10 mg in the morning and increasing by 10 mg every 4 days to a maximum of 80 mg daily. TCAs and serotonin reuptake inhibitors are typically preferred over MAOIs because they are better tolerated and they obviate the need for dietary restrictions and the risk of hypertensive crises. Furthermore, patients who do not respond to monotherapy with a TCA or a serotonin reuptake inhibitor may respond to a combination of the two (Tiffon et al. 1994). However, MAOIs are an option to consider for patients who fail to tolerate or to respond well to other antidepressants. In patients with concomitant atypical depression or social phobia, MAOIs may be an appropriate earlier choice for treatment if SSRIs do not confer adequate results.

Full remission of panic attacks with antidepressants usually requires 4–12 weeks of treatment. Subsequently, the duration of required treatment to prevent relapse is a function of the natural course of panic disorder. The disorder can probably best be characterized as chronic, with an exacerbating and remitting course. Therefore, complete agreement has not been reached regarding the recommended course of treatment. In a naturalistic follow-up study, Noyes et al. (1989) found that most patients with panic disorder initially treated with TCAs had a relatively good prognosis when followed over a few years,

whether they had continued (60% of the sample) or stopped (40% of the sample) taking medication. In a controlled and prospective study with somewhat less optimistic results, a very high relapse rate for panic was found when imipramine therapy was discontinued after 6 months of acute treatment. However, half-dose imipramine at around 80 mg/day was successful in preventing relapse during 1 year of maintenance treatment (Mavissakalian and Perel 1992). Thus, a reasonable recommendation for treating panic patients is to keep them on full-dose medication for at least 6 months to prevent early relapse. Afterward, doses can be tapered to the half-dose level and patients can be followed to ensure that clinical improvement is maintained. Subsequently, the clinician may attempt gradual dosage decreases every few months, as long as the improvement is maintained, to reach a minimal dose at which the patient is relatively symptom free. Some patients may eventually be able to discontinue drug therapy. Other patients may require more chronic maintenance treatment, especially in light of the morbidity and mortality risk that may be associated with the disorder.

Benzodiazepines. Although clinicians prefer to use antidepressants for the first-line treatment of panic, high-potency benzodiazepines are also highly effective in treating the condition. In a large, multicenter treatment study, 82% of patients treated acutely with alprazolam showed at least moderate improvement in panic, compared with 43% of patients taking placebo (Pecknold et al. 1988). Onset of response was rapid, in that significant improvement occurred in the first couple weeks of treatment, and the mean final dosage was 5.7 mg/day (Ballenger et al. 1988). After 8 weeks of acute treatment, medication therapy was gradually discontinued over 4 weeks; 27% of patients experienced rebound panic attacks, and 35% had withdrawal symptoms. After discontinuation, panic outcome for the alprazolam-treated group was not significantly different from that for the placebo group (Pecknold et al. 1988). Clonazepam appears equally promising in the acute treatment of panic according to a large multicenter trial (Rosenbaum et al. 1997). In the acute treatment of panic attacks, the lowest dose of 0.5 mg/day was least efficacious, but doses of 1.0 mg/day or higher (2, 3, and 4 mg/day) were equally efficacious and the lower doses of 1–2 mg/day were better tolerated. Long-term efficacy, possible tolerance and dependency, and difficulties in discontinuing the medication are the main areas of concern in the selection of benzodiazepine treatment. Results of naturalistic follow-up studies of long-term benzodiazepine treatment appear generally optimistic, in that most patients maintain their therapeutic gains without requiring an increase in benzodiazepine dose over time (Nagy et al. 1989; Schweizer et al. 1993).

Benzodiazepines have fewer initial side effects than TCAs and serotonin reuptake inhibitors. However, the general treatment principle is that anxiolytics should be reserved until the different classes of antidepressants have failed, because anxiolytics do pose some risk for tolerance, dependence, and withdrawal. For patients with severe acute distress and disability who may require immediate relief, it may be indicated to start with a benzodiazepine and then replace it with an antidepressant. There is also some evidence that benzodiazepines may be more effective, at least initially, in ameliorating the associated anticipatory anxiety and phobic avoidance, and this may be another indication for their initial use in panic disorder. Systematic comparisons of antidepressants and benzodiazepines in the acute and maintenance treatment of panic disorder have shown that patients treated with alprazolam are significantly more likely to stay in treatment and to experience relief from panic attacks than are patients taking imipramine; the latter drug is associated with worse patient compliance (Schweizer et al. 1993).

Clonazepam should generally be the first choice, because it is longer acting and thus has the advantage of less-frequent twice-daily or even once-daily dosing and less risk of withdrawal symptoms compared with alprazolam. Clonazepam should generally be started at 0.5 mg twice daily and is increased only if needed, usually to a maximum dose of 4 mg/day. Alprazolam is usually started at 0.5 mg four times daily and is gradually increased to an average dose of 4 mg/day, with a range of 2–10 mg/day according to the individual patient. A treatment duration of at least 6 months is recommended, as with the antidepressants. A patient's moods must be followed, because alprazolam may occasionally cause mania and clonazepam can cause depression. Discontinuation must be gradual to prevent withdrawal: 15% of the total dose weekly is generally a safe regimen, but an even slower rate may be required to prevent the recurrence of panic. In a controlled study, one-third of patients were unable to tolerate a gradual discontinuation of alprazolam over 4 weeks after 8 months of maintenance treatment; the strongest predictor of taper failure was initial severity of panic attacks, rather than alprazolam dose (Rickels et al. 1993b). The distinction between actual withdrawal and a simple recrudescence of the original anxiety symptom when the benzodiazepine is stopped remains controversial and can be difficult to make clinically. It has been convincingly shown that the introduction of cognitive-behavioral therapy (CBT) greatly increases the likelihood that patients with panic disorder will be able to successfully reduce and eventually discontinue benzodiazepine dosages (Otto et al. 1993; Spiegel et al. 1994).

Although benzodiazepines are generally safe, with side effects limited mainly to sedation, there is a concern that some patients may develop tolerance or even become addicted to these medications. However, available data indicate that most patients are able to stop taking them without serious sequelae and that the problem of tolerance and dependence is overestimated and probably limited to populations with histories of alcohol or drug addiction or to patients with panic disorder who often increase benzodiazepine usage in unsuccessful attempts at self-medication.

Other medications.   Venlafaxine, found to be efficacious in one controlled study (Pollack et al. 1996), definitely merits further study and consideration when SSRIs do not work well. Nefazodone, a serotonin reuptake inhibitor and serotonin type 2 (5-HT$_2$) antagonist, appears promising in the treatment of panic. Ten of 14 patients (70%) treated openly for 8 weeks with doses of 200–600 mg/day significantly improved (DeMartinis et al. 1996). Nefazodone was again shown to have some efficacy in treating panic disorder in another small open trial (Papp et al. 2000). If these findings are replicated in a larger, controlled study, this medication may hold some benefits in terms of initial anxiogenic response and long-term sexual side effects compared with SSRIs. Panic attacks also receded in four patients treated openly with the combined serotonin and norepinephrine reuptake inhibitor (SNRI) venlafaxine at low doses of 50–75 mg/day (Geracioti 1995).

Buspirone, a 5-HT$_{1A}$ agonist nonbenzodiazepine antianxiety agent, has not been found to be effective in treating panic. Similarly, there is no evidence that β-adrenergic–blocking drugs, such as propranolol, are effective in blocking spontaneous panic attacks. However, if panic attacks occur in a specific social context, such as public speaking, a trial of a β-blocker would be indicated.

Clonidine, which inhibits locus coeruleus discharge, would seem for theoretical reasons to be a good antipanic drug. Although two-thirds of patients in a small series responded initially, the therapeutic effect tends to be lost in a matter of weeks, despite continuation of dose (Liebowitz et al. 1981). A later study confirmed a similar pattern of loss of response during a 10-week trial (Uhde et al. 1989). This loss of response, plus a number of bothersome side effects, makes clonidine a poor initial choice for treatment of panic disorder. However, one controlled study found clonidine to be efficacious for both panic disorder and GAD (Hoehn-Saric et al. 1981).

When response to SSRIs and other antidepressants is inadequate, one augmentation strategy, shown to be effective in a small, blinded trial, may be to add pindolol at 2.5 mg three times a day (Hirschmann et al. 2000).

Valproate may also have some beneficial effects in the treatment of panic attacks (Keck et al. 1993). In one open trial, all of 12 patients were moderately to markedly improved after 6 weeks of treatment, and 11 continued the medication and maintained their gains after 6 months (Woodman and Noyes 1994). Controlled trials however have not been reported. A fairly large controlled trial of another mood stabilizer, gabapentin, at flexible doses of 600–3,600 mg/day showed it to be no better than placebo in treating panic disorder (Pande et al. 2000), although a post hoc analysis revealed some efficacy for gabapentin in the more severely symptomatic patients, suggesting that an augmentation study in refractory panic might be worthwhile.

In a placebo-controlled 4-week trial, inositol, an intracellular second-messenger precursor, was found to be effective in treating panic disorder at a dosage of 12 g/day (Benjamin et al. 1995). This finding has not yet been replicated.

Psychotherapy

Psychodynamic psychotherapy. Even after medication has blocked the actual panic attacks, a subgroup of panic disorder patients remain wary of independence and assertiveness. In addition to supportive and behavioral treatment, traditional psychodynamic psychotherapy might be helpful for some of these patients. Significant unconscious conflict over separations during childhood sometimes appears to operate in patients with panic disorder, leading to a reemergence of anxiety symptoms in adult life each time a new separation is imagined or threatened. Furthermore, it has been found that comorbid personality disorder is the major predictor of continued social maladjustment in patients otherwise treated for panic disorder (Noyes et al. 1990), which suggests that psychodynamic therapy may be an important additional treatment for at least some patients with panic disorder.

Unfortunately, few systematic studies document the efficacy of psychodynamic psychotherapy in panic disorder. Psychodynamically oriented clinicians tend to agree that psychological factors do not appear to be significant in a proportion of patients with panic disorder, and they emphasize the importance of conducting a psychodynamic assessment to determine whether a particular patient may benefit from a psychodynamic treatment component (Gabbard 1990). Moreover, Cooper (1985)

emphasized that in those patients with a predominant biological component to their illness, insistence on dynamic understanding and on responsibility for one's symptoms may be, in the long run, not only useless but potentially harmful, in that it may lead to further damage in self-esteem and strengthened masochistic defenses. However, it is also clear that there are case reports of patients who were successfully treated for panic with psychodynamic therapy or psychoanalysis. A recent controlled study showed that a 15-session course of brief dynamic psychotherapy combined with initial clomipramine treatment led to much lower relapse rates up to 9 months after the medication had been gradually discontinued (Wiborg and Dahl 1996). More recently, an open trial of psychodynamic monotherapy in panic disorder documented clear efficacy for this modality, at least in the selected sample, a finding that emphasizes the need for further controlled studies (Milrod et al. 2000). In the study, 14 patients with panic disorder who were treated for 12 weeks with twice-a-week psychodynamic psychotherapy alone showed significant improvement in panic, anxiety, depression, and overall impairment at the end of the 12 weeks as well as at 6-month follow-up.

Pharmacotherapy is in no way incompatible with behavioral or psychodynamic treatment for patients with panic disorder. The notion that reducing the symptoms of anxiety disorder with medication will disturb a successful psychotherapy has never been convincingly shown and is largely dogmatic. Indeed, successful psychotherapy often cannot take place until the more debilitating aspects of these syndromes have been eliminated pharmacologically.

Supportive psychotherapy. Despite adequate treatment of panic attacks with medication, phobic avoidance may remain. Supportive psychotherapy and education about the illness are necessary in order for the patient to confront the phobic situation. Patients who fail to respond may then need additional psychotherapy, dynamic or behavioral. Encouragement from other patients with similar conditions is often quite helpful.

Cognitive-behavioral therapy. Treatments involving cognitive and behavioral approaches have long focused on phobic avoidance, but more recently, techniques have been developed and shown to be effective for panic attacks per se. In the past few years, interest in cognitive and behavioral therapy for panic has surged, and these approaches have become firmly established in the treatment of this disorder.

The major behavioral techniques for the treatment of panic attacks are breathing retraining, to control both acute and chronic hyperventilation; exposure to somatic cues, usually involving a hierarchy of exposure to feared sensations through imaginal and behavioral exercises; and relaxation training. Cognitive treatment of panic involves cognitive restructuring designed to provide a more benign interpretation for the uncomfortable affects and physical sensations associated with panic. These cognitive-behavioral techniques can be administered in various combinations. The extreme cognitive view is that panic attacks consist of normal physical sensations (e.g., palpitations, slight dizziness) to which patients with panic disorder grossly overreact with catastrophic cognitions. A more moderate view is that although panic patients do have extreme physical sensations such as bursts of tachycardia, they can still help themselves to a significant degree by changing their interpretation of these events from "I am going to die of a heart attack" to "There go my heart symptoms again." Such a theory has received experimental validation: Sanderson et al. (1989) provoked panic attacks in patients with panic disorder via CO_2 inhalation; it was found that when patients had an illusion of control over the inhaled mixture, they experienced significantly fewer and less severe attacks and had less catastrophic cognitions.

Several studies have shown that these various cognitive-behavioral techniques are undoubtedly quite successful in the treatment of panic disorder (Barlow et al. 1989; Beck et al. 1992; L. Michelson et al. 1990; Salkovskis et al. 1986). Group-format cognitive-behavioral treatment for panic has also been shown to be highly successful (Telch et al. 1993). Less is known about the relative or combined efficacy of medications versus that of CBT in the treatment of panic attacks without agoraphobia. In one controlled study, fluvoxamine was significantly beneficial in the acute treatment of panic, whereas cognitive therapy did not surpass placebo in efficacy (D.W. Black et al. 1993). In contrast, another controlled study found cognitive therapy, relaxation, and imipramine to be similarly effective, although cognitive therapy had more lasting effects at 9-month follow-up after treatment was discontinued (Clark et al. 1994). After the initiation of medication treatment for initial symptom control, the introduction of CBT seems greatly to increase the likelihood that a patient will be successful in gradually reducing and eventually discontinuing medication (Otto et al. 1993). Preliminary findings on long-term outcome of panic treated with cognitive-behavioral techniques appear to be favorable, especially in the case of combined cognitive restructuring and exposure, whereas relaxation alone or added to restructuring and exposure does not appear to be helpful and may even be detrimental (Craske et al. 1991). Findings are inconsistent with

regard to whether applied relaxation is equally efficacious or inferior to CBT for controlling panic attacks (Arntz and van den Hout 1996; Ost and Westling 1995).

A recently published multisite controlled study—the largest of its kind conducted to date—compared medication, CBT, and the combination, both acutely and longer term (Barlow et al. 2000), in 312 patients with panic disorder. Subjects were randomly assigned to five different treatment conditions: imipramine alone, CBT alone, combined treatment of imipramine and CBT, placebo medication, and CBT plus placebo. In the initial 3-month acute treatment phase, medication alone and CBT alone had similar efficacy, with limited advantage to combined treatment. For responders treated in the 6-month maintenance phase, imipramine alone produced a higher quality of response in comparison with CBT alone, and more substantial advantage was found than earlier with combined treatment. Finally, at follow-up 6 months after termination of treatment, the results of CBT were found to be the most durable. These results, from this most comprehensive study to date, clearly suggest that both psychotherapy and medication treatment must be seriously considered in treating a patient with panic, each having its advantages and disadvantages.

Treatment of the agoraphobic component of panic disorder. As mentioned previously, there continues to be disagreement in the literature regarding the best treatment method for agoraphobia with panic attacks. Antipanic medication is given to block the occurrence of panic attacks, and its efficacy in this regard is well documented. However, medication alone is often not adequate in patients with significant agoraphobic avoidance. It is generally accepted that some form of treatment involving exposure of agoraphobic patients to the feared situations is necessary for overall improvement. Such exposure may be achieved by various nonspecific methods, such as psychoeducation, reassurance, and supportive therapy (D.F. Klein et al. 1983). However, focused CBT is, on the whole, more successful than nonspecific techniques in reducing agoraphobic avoidance. Consequently, the relative and combined efficacy of medications and CBT for panic with agoraphobia has been the focus of several investigations.

Some studies have not found imipramine to have a significant effect on agoraphobia when given alone or with antiexposure instructions (Marks et al. 1983; Telch et al. 1985), whereas others have shown imipramine alone to decrease phobic avoidance at combined plasma levels of 110–140 ng/mL (Mavissakalian and Perel 1995). Most studies concur that the combination of medication and behavioral treatment (exposure) is superior to either modality alone for treating phobic avoidance (de Beurs et al. 1995; Mavissakalian and Michelson 1986a; Telch et al. 1985; Zitrin et al. 1980).

In summary, antidepressants in combination with cognitive-behavioral treatment should generally be instituted. Combination therapy appears to be superior to either treatment alone. In a large controlled study of alprazolam plus exposure in patients with panic and agoraphobia, the improvement in attacks, anxiety, and avoidance were found to be largely independent of each other, and only early improvement in avoidance predicted global improvement after treatment (Basoglu et al. 1994). Cognitive therapy has been shown to decrease panic attacks but not agoraphobia, whereas exposure reduces agoraphobia but not panic attacks (van der Hout et al. 1994).

Generalized Anxiety Disorder

DSM-IV sharpened the distinction of GAD from "normal" anxiety by specifying that in GAD the worry must be clearly excessive, pervasive, difficult to control, and associated with marked distress or impairment. DSM-IV also clarified that the diagnosis of GAD is excluded when the anxiety or worry occurs exclusively in relation to other major Axis I disorders, and the cumbersome somatic symptom list from DSM-III-R was simplified (Table 11–7).

GAD is the main diagnostic category for prominent and chronic anxiety in the absence of panic disorder. The essential feature of this syndrome, according to DSM-IV, is persistent anxiety lasting at least 6 months. The symptoms of this type of anxiety fall within two broad categories: 1) apprehensive expectation and worry and 2) physical symptoms. Patients with GAD are constantly worried over trivial matters, fearful, and anticipating the worst. Muscle tension, restlessness or a "keyed up" feeling, difficulty concentrating, insomnia, irritability, and fatigue are typical signs of generalized anxiety that also—as a result of a number of studies that attempted to single out the physical symptoms that are the most distinctive and characteristic of GAD—constitute the DSM-IV symptom criteria for GAD. Motor tension and hypervigilance better differentiate GAD from other anxiety states than does autonomic hyperactivity (Marten et al. 1993; Starcevic et al. 1994).

The diagnosis of GAD is made when a patient experiences at least 6 months of chronic anxiety and excessive worry. At least three of six physical symptoms must also be present. Finally, this chronic anxiety must not be sec-

TABLE 11–7. DSM-IV-TR diagnostic criteria for generalized anxiety disorder

A. Excessive anxiety and worry (apprehensive expectation), occurring more days than not for at least 6 months, about a number of events or activities (such as work or school performance).
B. The person finds it difficult to control the worry.
C. The anxiety and worry are associated with three (or more) of the following six symptoms (with at least some symptoms present for more days than not for the past 6 months).   **Note:** Only one item is required in children.
   (1) restlessness or feeling keyed up or on edge
   (2) being easily fatigued
   (3) difficulty concentrating or mind going blank
   (4) irritability
   (5) muscle tension
   (6) sleep disturbance (difficulty falling or staying asleep, or restless unsatisfying sleep)
D. The focus of the anxiety and worry is not confined to features of an Axis I disorder, e.g., the anxiety or worry is not about having a panic attack (as in panic disorder), being embarrassed in public (as in social phobia), being contaminated (as in obsessive-compulsive disorder), being away from home or close relatives (as in separation anxiety disorder), gaining weight (as in anorexia nervosa), having multiple physical complaints (as in somatization disorder), or having a serious illness (as in hypochondriasis), and the anxiety and worry do not occur exclusively during posttraumatic stress disorder.
E. The anxiety, worry, or physical symptoms cause clinically significant distress or impairment in social, occupational, or other important areas of functioning.
F. The disturbance is not due to the direct physiological effects of a substance (e.g., a drug of abuse, a medication) or a general medical condition (e.g., hyperthyroidism) and does not occur exclusively during a mood disorder, a psychotic disorder, or a pervasive developmental disorder.

ondary to another Axis I disorder or a specific organic factor such as medical illness or substance use.

Epidemiology and Comorbidity

Findings on GAD from the ECA study must be interpreted cautiously, because they were assessed only in the second wave of the study and only at three of the five sites. Also, the DIS criteria, in accordance with DSM-III, required only a total of three somatic symptoms and only a 1-month duration of illness and therefore could overestimate the prevalence of GAD relative to current criteria. One-year prevalence rates for the three sites combined were 3.8% without any exclusions, 2.7% when concurrent panic or major depression was excluded, and 1.7%

when any other DSM-III diagnoses were excluded. Lifetime prevalence when panic and major depression were excluded ranged from 4.1% to 6.6%, according to the site. Rates were higher overall in women (Blazer et al. 1991). Another large epidemiological study, the National Comorbidity Survey, assessed DSM-III-R–diagnosed GAD and found it to have a current (past-year) prevalence of 3.1% and a lifetime prevalence of 5.1% in the 15- to 45-year age group, to be twice as common in women as in men, and to have a very high lifetime comorbidity (90%) with a wide spectrum of other psychiatric disorders. Even so, the prevalence and comorbidity patterns of current GAD supported its conceptualization as a distinct disorder. More-recent studies using DSM-IV criteria (Carter et al. 2001) have confirmed a similar epidemiology for GAD, with a 1-year prevalence of 1.5% for threshold GAD and of 3.6% for subthreshold GAD. Higher rates of the disorder were found in women (2.7%) and in the elderly (2.2%). A high degree of comorbidity was again confirmed: 59% for major depression and 56% for other anxiety disorders.

Despite GAD's significant comorbidity with other anxiety and with mood disorders, it has become increasingly evident in recent years that GAD stands as a disorder with its own distinct onset, course, impairment, and prognosis. Epidemiological data have revealed that GAD and depression each show their own statistically significant and independent associations with impairment, of roughly equal magnitude, which cannot be accounted for by comorbidity or sociodemographic variables (Kessler et al. 1999). On certain quality-of-life indexes, individuals with "pure" GAD actually fare worse than those with "pure" major depression (Wittchen et al. 2000).

With regard to Axis II comorbidity, the personality types of patients with GAD have not been well characterized. One study reported that approximately one-third of patients with GAD also suffered from a DSM-III–diagnosed personality disorder, and the most common disorder was dependent personality disorder (Noyes et al. 1987). Avoidant personality disorder also appears to be common in GAD (Mavissakalian et al. 1993). It is not clear, however, whether such personality disorders are primary or consequent to the GAD itself. With regard to personality traits, high levels of mistrust and anger have also been reported in GAD (Mavissakalian et al. 1993).

Biological Theories

Although the neurobiology of generalized anxiety is among the least investigated in the anxiety disorders, advances are now being made. Recent work has focused on brain circuits underlying the neurobiology of fear in animal models and in humans, and on how inherited and acquired vulnerabilities in these circuits might underlie a variety of anxiety disorders. It is speculated that alterations in the structure and function of the amygdala, which are central to fear-related behaviors, may be associated with generalized anxiety. This was supported in a magnetic resonance imaging (MRI) volumetric study comparing children and adolescents with GAD with healthy comparison subjects matched for other general characteristics. GAD children had larger right and total amygdalar volumes, whereas other brain regions were comparable in size between the two groups (DeBellis et al. 2000). The frontal cortex and medial temporal lobe are involved in controlling fear and anxiety, and there is evidence for heightened cortical activity and decreased basal ganglia activity in GAD, possibly accounting for the observed arousal and hypervigilance (Buchsbaum et al. 1987; Wu et al. 1991).

Abnormalities of the GABA–benzodiazepine receptor complex have been implicated in GAD. The benzodiazepine receptor is linked to a receptor for the inhibitory neurotransmitter GABA. Binding of a benzodiazepine to the benzodiazepine receptor facilitates the action of GABA, effectively slowing neural transmission. One series of compounds, the β-carbolines, which are inverse agonists of this receptor complex, produce an acute anxiety syndrome when administered to laboratory animals or to healthy human volunteers (Dorow et al. 1983; Skolnick and Paul 1982). On the other hand, benzodiazepines are well established as an efficacious treatment for GAD. Subjects with GAD have been found to have decreased benzodiazepine receptor density in peripheral blood cells as well as decreased transcriptional mRNA encoding for the receptor, both of which return to normal values with treatment and reduction in anxiety levels (Ferrarese et al. 1990; Rocca et al. 1998). Similarly, benzodiazepine receptor binding has been found to be significantly decreased in the left temporal pole of patients with GAD compared with healthy control subjects (Tiihonen et al. 1997a).

Objective sleep disturbances have been observed using polysomnography and electroencephalogram (EEG) mapping in subjects with GAD, again concordant with CNS hypervigilance and hyperarousal (Saletu et al. 1997). Studies seeking evidence for noradrenergic dysregulation have yielded mixed results. Abelson et al. (1991) reported a blunted GH response to clonidine in patients with GAD compared with healthy control subjects. Plasma norepinephrine and its metabolite were found to be elevated, and α_2-adrenoreceptors decreased, in GAD compared with control subjects (Sevy et al. 1989). Other studies of the noradrenergic system have been negative (Mathew et al. 1981). There is also some evidence of serotonergic dysregulation in GAD, such as heightened anxiety responses to the partial serotonin agonist meta-chlorophenylpiperazine (m-CPP) in patients with GAD compared with control subjects (Germine et al. 1992). Indirect support for serotonergic dysregulation is also derived from the efficacy of buspirone, a 5-HT$_1$ agonist, and nefazodone, a 5-HT$_2$ antagonist, in treating GAD. People with GAD do not show heightened sensitivity to 35% CO_2 inhalation or lactate infusion, as do people with panic, supporting the conceptualization of GAD and panic disorder as two discrete conditions (Cowley et al. 1988; Perna et al. 1999).

There appears to be a genetic component to GAD, albeit a relatively modest one. A 19.5% morbidity risk for GAD was found among relatives of patients with GAD, compared with a 3.5% risk in relatives of healthy control subjects; this may have been somewhat of an overestimate, because the GAD in the relatives was less chronic, less severe, or less likely to receive treatment than that in the probands (Noyes et al. 1987). Torgersen (1983) completed a study of 32 monozygotic and 53 dizygotic twins, and found no monozygotic–dizygotic concordance-rate difference for GAD. However, Kendler et al. (1992a), studying GAD in female twins, determined that the familial component of the disorder was almost entirely genetic, with a modest heritability of about 30%. There have been minimal molecular genetic studies of GAD to date, which require replication, and which have suggested associations to polymorphisms of the dopamine D$_2$ receptor gene (Peroutka et al. 1998), the serotonin transporter gene (Ohara et al. 1999) and dopamine transporter gene (Rowe et al. 1998).

Cognitive Theories

Cognitive hypotheses regarding both the origins and the maintenance of GAD have been thoroughly summarized in recent work (Aikins and Craske 2001). With regard to the origins of generalized anxiety, it has been proposed that insecure attachment relationships, ambivalence toward caregivers, and parental overprotection and lack of emotional warmth may all contribute to later development of anxiety. Regarding mechanisms that may perpetuate GAD, three are summarized. First, worry is used as a strategy for avoiding intense negative affects. Second, worry about unlikely and future threat removes the need to deal with more proximal and realistic threats and limits the capacity to find solutions to more immediate conflicts. Finally, individuals with GAD engage in a certain degree of magical thinking and believe that their worry helps to prevent feared outcomes, thus leading to a neg-

ative reinforcement of the process of worrying. In terms of the etiology of GAD, cognitive theory speculates a relationship either to early cognitive schemas—derived from negative experiences—of the world as a dangerous place (Barlow 1988) or to insecure, anxious early attachments to important caregivers (Cassidy 1995).

There is some evidence that cognitive content in the various anxiety disorders differs in specific ways. Patients with GAD demonstrate more cognitions in the categories of interpersonal confrontation, competence, acceptance, concern about others, and worry over minor matters, whereas patients with panic disorder have more cognitions related to physical catastrophes (Breitholtz et al. 1999). There is also evidence that the process of meta-worry (i.e., worrying about the worrying itself) contributes to the high degree of pathological worry in GAD (Wells and Carter 1999).

In addition, certain information-processing biases may characterize GAD and permit the perpetuation of worry as the central cognitive strategy (Aikins and Craske 2001). These include a bias for threat-related information in implicit memory processes (MacLeod and McLaughlin 1995), selective attentional biases for threatening information (Mogg et al. 1989, 2000), and difficulty in decision making when faced with ambiguity (MacLeod and Cohen 1993).

Course and Prognosis

In contrast with panic disorder, no single, overwhelming event prompts the patient with GAD to seek help. Such patients seem only over time to develop the recognition that their experience of chronic tension, hyperactivity, worry, and anxiety is excessive. Often they will state that there has never been a time in their lives, as long as they can remember, that they were not anxious. GAD appears to be a more chronic condition than panic disorder with fewer periods of spontaneous remission (Raskin et al. 1982; Woodman et al. 1999). Of subjects with GAD followed over a 5-year period, only 18%–35% were found to be in full remission (Woodman et al. 1999; Yonkers et al. 1996). The symptoms of patients with GAD substantially interfere with their lives; these patients have a high degree of professional help seeking and a high use of medications (Wittchen et al. 1994). GAD patients with an earlier onset of anxiety symptoms in the first two decades of life appear to be more impaired overall, to have more severe anxiety that may not be precipitated by specific stressful events, and to have histories of more childhood fears, disturbed family environments, and greater social maladjustment (Hoehn-Saric et al. 1993b). In clinical samples, GAD is frequently comorbid with major depression and other anxiety disorders but still emerges as a clearly distinct entity (Brawman et al. 1993; Wittchen et al. 2000). Abuse of alcohol, barbiturates, and antianxiety medications is also common. Breslau and Davis (1985) showed that if GAD persists for 6 months, as required under the DSM-III-R definition and in the DSM-IV criteria, the comorbidity of depressive disorder will be very high, and the probability of remission over time is lower with comorbid depression (Yonkers et al. 1996). Contrary to panic disorder, which declines with old age, GAD appears to account for many of the anxiety states that arise in late life, often comorbidly with medical illnesses (Flint 1994). In anxious elderly patients, it is particularly important to differentiate generalized anxiety from other anxiety states that could be related to delirium, dementia, psychosis, or depression or that could be manifestations of underlying medical illnesses.

Treatment

Pharmacotherapy

The pharmacological treatment of GAD is summarized in Table 11–8. Although the major changes in diagnostic criteria in consecutive editions of the DSM, the presence of frequent comorbidity, and a tendency to view GAD as a secondary or minor condition hampered past treatment research, pharmacotherapy options have expanded in recent years and will probably continue to do so in the near future. In past years, benzodiazepines have been the first-line treatment of GAD, and they continue to be a first-line option today, despite certain concerns over their chronic use and new medication choices such as buspirone, SSRIs, and SNRIs. Several controlled studies clearly show that chronically anxious patients respond well to benzodiazepines, and all benzodiazepines are probably similarly efficacious in treating GAD (Rickels et al. 1983; Ruiz 1983). There is some evidence that benzodiazepines may be more effective in treating the physical symptoms of anxiety, whereas antidepressants, whether TCAs or SSRIs, may be more effective in treating the psychic symptoms (Hoehn-Saric et al. 1988; Rocca et al. 1997). It has also been suggested that benzodiazepines such as chlordiazepoxide may peak in effectiveness after 4 weeks of treatment, whereas TCAs such as imipramine may be more effective for patients with anxiety over the longer term (Kahn et al. 1986). Although benzodiazepines are generally safe, with side effects limited mainly to sedation and slowed mentation, there is concern that some patients may become tolerant or even addicted to these medications. However, available data indicate that the concern over benzodiazepine abuse in chronically

TABLE 11–8. Pharmacological treatment of generalized anxiety disorder

Venlafaxine extended release

General indications: first-line treatment; U.S. Food and Drug Administration–approved, proven efficacy in large controlled trials; generally well tolerated; once-daily dosing; recommended starting dose is 75 mg/day, which may be adequate for a number of patients

Selective serotonin reuptake inhibitors (SSRIs)

General indications: first-line treatment; proven efficacy for paroxetine in large controlled trials; generally well tolerated; once-daily dosing; recommended starting dose is 20 mg/day, which may be adequate for many patients; SSRIs other than paroxetine have not been extensively tested but are probably efficacious

Benzodiazepines

General indications: well-known efficacy and widely used; all appear similarly efficacious; issues with dependence and withdrawal in certain patients; may be more effective for physical rather than cognitive symptoms of generalized anxiety disorder

Buspirone

General indications: proven efficacy; well tolerated; a trial is generally indicated in all patients; compared with benzodiazepines, requires longer to take effect and is not associated with a "high"; may have less efficacy and be associated with less compliance in the presence of very recent benzodiazepine use

Tricyclic antidepressants

General indications: shown efficacy in few trials; more side effects than benzodiazepines, buspirone, and newer antidepressants; delayed action in comparison with benzodiazepines; may be more effective for cognitive rather than physical symptoms of anxiety

Imipramine: shown efficacy

Trazodone: shown efficacy

Other medications

Nefazodone: one open trial

Mirtazapine: one open trial with comorbid major depression

Clonidine: tends to lose initial response

Propranolol: may be a useful adjuvant in patients with pronounced palpitations and tremor

anxious populations is overestimated, and in reality most patients continue to derive clinical benefits without developing abuse or dependence (Romach et al. 1995). Concerns over addiction are probably justified, for the most part, in individuals with histories of addiction-proneness.

Buspirone, a 5-HT$_{1A}$ agonist nonbenzodiazepine antianxiety agent, may have similar efficacy to the benzodiazepines in treating GAD. Its advantages are a different side effect profile without sedation and the absence of tolerance and withdrawal. Its disadvantage is a slower rate of onset (Rickels et al. 1988), which can lead to early patient noncompliance. Rickels et al. (1988) compared the efficacy of the benzodiazepine clorazepate with that of the nonbenzodiazepine buspirone in the acute, maintenance, and discontinuation treatment of patients with GAD. The two medications had similar efficacy by the fourth week of treatment, and benefits were maintained over a 6-month period, with an approximately 60% reduction of anxiety scores. There was no evidence of tolerance to either medication over the 6-month period. In the first 2 weeks of medication discontinuation, patients who had been on clorazepate had a transient increase of anxiety consistent with withdrawal, whereas buspirone patients did not. Treatment with buspirone is usually started at 5 mg three times a day, and the dose can be increased until a maximum dose of 60 mg/day is reached. A twice-daily regimen is probably as efficacious as a three-times-a-day regimen and easier to comply with.

It has been suggested in the literature that patients previously treated with benzodiazepines may not respond successfully to buspirone (Schweizer et al. 1986). However, a later controlled study refuted this, finding that patients who gradually discontinued lorazepam and were then treated with buspirone in a double-blind fashion did not exhibit benzodiazepine withdrawal or rebound anxiety and did as well with buspirone as they had done with lorazepam (Delle Chiaie et al. 1995). On the other hand, DeMartinis et al. (2000) retrospectively analyzed a large dataset with respect to history of benzodiazepine use prior to a controlled clinical trial. They found that clinical response to buspirone was similar to benzodiazepine response in patients who had never used or remotely used benzodiazepines, but patients who had used benzodiazepines within 1 month of starting the trial had a higher attrition rate and less clinical improvement if randomized to buspirone rather than to benzodiazepine. There is recent evidence, from a controlled trial (Rickels et al. 2000b), that in long-term benzodiazepine users, a successful strategy may be to initiate treatment with buspirone or an antidepressant 1 month before undertaking a gradual 4- to 6-week taper of the benzodiazepine. Other independent predictors of successful benzodiazepine taper were lower initial doses and less severe and chronic anxiety symptoms.

Over the past few years, newer antidepressants have become established as first-line treatments for GAD, as there are now controlled trials documenting their efficacy, and in addition they tend to be well tolerated, require only once-daily dosing, and do not risk abuse and dependence. Three large controlled trials to date have established the efficacy of extended-release venlafaxine, an SNRI, in treating GAD (Davidson et al. 1999; Gelenberg et al. 2000; Rickels et al. 2000a). Venlafaxine at doses of 75, 150, and 225 mg/day was found to be effective in treating GAD in two large, placebo-controlled trials, one trial over an 8-week period (Rickels et al. 2000a) and the other over a 6-month period (Gelenberg et al. 2000). The latter showed an approximately 70% response rate, with benefits appearing as early as the first 2 weeks of treatment. Venlafaxine was generally well tolerated, with nausea, somnolence, and dry mouth being the most common side effects. Neither trial showed differences between the doses of venlafaxine, suggesting it can be started at 75 mg/day for GAD and subsequently increased if clinical improvement is not adequate and side effects permit. In another trial comparing venlafaxine 75–150 mg, buspirone 30 mg, and placebo in nondepressed patients with GAD over an 8-week period, both medications were superior to placebo, and there was weak evidence for possible superiority of venlafaxine over buspirone according to some, but not all, measures (Davidson et al. 1999).

In addition to venlafaxine, the SSRI paroxetine has recently been found to be efficacious in treating GAD in several controlled studies. The first trial (Rocca et al. 1997) found paroxetine 20 mg daily to have similar efficacy to imipramine and benzodiazepine in treating GAD. A large recent trial showed paroxetine at fixed doses of both 20 mg and 40 mg daily to be superior to placebo over an 8-week treatment period, with approximately two-thirds of patients considered responders (Bellew et al. 2000). Additionally, a recent, large, flexible-dosing trial showed that paroxetine in doses ranging from 20 mg to 50 mg daily was superior to placebo in treating GAD over an 8-week period (Pollack et al. 2001). It also showed that about two-thirds of patients who did not respond to the initial 20-mg dose responded to higher doses of 30 mg, 40 mg, or 50 mg daily (McCafferty et al. 2001). Although SSRIs other than paroxetine have not been tested in GAD to date, it is quite possible that they would be efficacious and trials may be under way. Finally, nefazodone was successful in treating GAD in one open trial (Hedges et al. 1996) and mirtazapine was successful in treating GAD in an open trial with comorbid major depression (Goodnick et al. 1999).

Several older studies have shown TCAs to be effective in treating chronically anxious patients independent of the presence of depressive symptoms, although TCA use has largely fallen out of favor recently in light of the newer, better-tolerated antidepressants. In one controlled study comparing imipramine and alprazolam in treating GAD, similar efficacy was found for the two medications, with imipramine acting more on negative affects and cognitions and alprazolam acting more on somatic symptoms (Hoehn-Saric et al. 1988). In another study, imipramine up to 143 mg/day, trazodone up to 255 mg/day, and diazepam up to 26 mg/day were found comparable after 8 weeks of treatment, with about two-thirds of GAD patients experiencing moderate to marked improvement in anxiety. Not surprisingly, during the first 2 weeks of treatment somatic symptoms responded faster to diazepam (Rickels et al. 1993a).

β-Adrenergic–blocking drugs such as propranolol may only be rarely indicated as an adjuvant in patients who experience significant palpitations or tremor. Clonidine, which inhibits locus coeruleus discharge, would seem for theoretical reasons to be a good antianxiety drug. A tendency to lose clinical response, plus a number of bothersome side effects, make clonidine a poor initial choice for treatment. However, one controlled study found clonidine to be efficacious for both panic disorder and GAD (Hoehn-Saric et al. 1981).

Psychotherapy

Research into the psychotherapy of GAD has not been as extensive as for other anxiety disorders. Still, a number of studies exist that clearly show various psychotherapies to be helpful in treating GAD. Given the previously described cognitive profile of GAD, several aspects of the disorder can serve as the foci of psychotherapeutic interventions. These include the heightened tendency to perceive threat, the expectation of low-likelihood catastrophic outcomes, poor problem solving especially in the face of ambivalence or ambiguity, the central feature of worry, and the physical symptoms of anxiety. A variety of treatments have been developed for GAD, including cognitive restructuring, behavioral anxiety management such as relaxation and rebreathing techniques, exposure therapy with or without a cognitive component, and psychodynamic treatment.

CBT is superior to general nondirective or supportive therapy in treating GAD (Chambless and Gillis 1993) and possibly superior to behavior therapy alone (Borkovec and Costello 1993). Cognitive therapy alone may have an edge over behavioral therapy alone according to some studies (Butler et al. 1991), but not others (Ost and Breitholtz 2000). In a study that compared four conditions, behavioral therapy alone, cognitive therapy alone, CBT, and a waiting list control group, all three active treatments were similarly efficacious and superior to the control condition during a follow-up period that lasted up to 2 years. However, the combined CBT group had a much lower dropout rate than the other groups (Barlow

et al. 1992). Another randomized study compared cognitive, analytic, and behavioral management in treating subjects with GAD (Durham et al. 1994). Cognitive therapy emerged as superior, with some edge over behavioral management alone, and significantly better than analytic treatment. Biofeedback is an additional treatment that may have some efficacy in treating GAD (Rice et al. 1993).

Finally, there are minimal data on the use of combined psychotherapy and medication in the treatment of GAD. In one study comparing CBT and benzodiazepine alone, and combined, with placebo (Power et al. 1990), CBT alone or with medication tended to emerge as superior. It appears however that the CBT component of the study was more intensive than the medication treatment, and further studies are clearly needed in this area.

Phobic Disorders: Social Phobia and Specific Phobias

A *phobia* is defined as a persistent and irrational fear of a specific object, activity, or situation that results in a compelling desire to avoid the dreaded object, activity, or situation (i.e., phobic stimulus). The fear is recognized by the individual as excessive or unreasonable in proportion to the actual dangerousness of the object, activity, or situation. Irrational fears and avoidance behavior are seen in a number of psychiatric disorders. However, in DSM-IV the diagnosis of phobic disorder is made only when single or multiple phobias are the predominant aspect of the clinical picture and a source of significant distress to the individual and are not the result of another mental disorder.

Phobias were classified in the first edition of DSM under the rubric "phobic reaction" and in DSM-II as "phobic neurosis." No subtypes were listed in either edition, reflecting the assumption of a qualitative unity implicit in the psychoanalytic model of phobias. DSM-III markedly differed from the previous editions in classifying distinct subtypes of phobias, suggesting a qualitative distinction between these subtypes. This distinction between agoraphobia, social phobia, and miscellaneous specific phobias stemmed from empirical findings, including those of behavioral treatment studies by Marks (1969) and pharmacological treatment studies by D.F. Klein (1964). These three major categories of phobias were maintained in DSM-III-R and subsequently in DSM-IV. In DSM-III-R, agoraphobia was subdivided into panic disorder with agoraphobia and agoraphobia without panic disorder, which emphasizes the primacy of panic when the two conditions coexist. This classification is maintained in DSM-IV.

The major changes in the phobic disorders instituted in DSM-IV, in relation to DSM-III-R, were as follows. In agoraphobia without panic disorder, it is specified that the condition centers on the fear of developing incapacitating symptoms typically in characteristic situational clusters. It is also specified that agoraphobia related to embarrassment over a medical illness is a diagnosis that can be made subject to clinical judgment. The two major changes in social phobia and in specific phobia in DSM-IV are similar for the two disorders. First, it is made explicit that panic attacks can occur as a feature of these phobias, and therefore clinical judgment is required to make the differential diagnosis between panic disorder with agoraphobia and social or specific phobia. Second, specific phobia is now divided into types, because new evidence has accumulated that phenomenology, natural history, and treatment response may differ according to type. The generalized type of social phobia was retained as in DSM-III-R. The DSM-IV-TR diagnostic criteria for agoraphobia without history of panic disorder, social phobia, and specific phobia are presented in Tables 11–9, 11–10, and 11–11, respectively.

In the ECA study, in which trained lay interviewers used the DIS to investigate the prevalence of psychiatric disorders (according to DSM-III criteria) in five cities in the United States, phobias as a group were found to be the most common current psychiatric disorder: 1-month and 6-month prevalence rates were about 6% and 8%, respectively, and lifetime rates averaged 12.5% (Regier et al. 1988). Specific phobias were the most common (11.3% lifetime prevalence), followed by agoraphobia (5.6%) and social phobia (2.7%). Specific phobias were more common in women than in men (14.5 vs. 7.8). Agoraphobia was also more common in women (7.9 vs. 3.2). The prevalence of social phobia was similar in the two genders (2.9 in women vs. 2.5 in men) (Eaton et al. 1991).

TABLE 11–9. DSM-IV-TR diagnostic criteria for agoraphobia without history of panic disorder

A. The presence of agoraphobia related to fear of developing panic-like symptoms (e.g., dizziness or diarrhea).
B. Criteria have never been met for panic disorder
C. The disturbance is not due to the direct physiological effects of a substance (e.g., a drug of abuse, a medication) or a general medical condition.
D. If an associated general medical condition is present, the fear described in Criterion A is clearly in excess of that usually associated with the condition.

TABLE 11–10. DSM-IV-TR diagnostic criteria for social phobia

A. A marked and persistent fear of one or more social or performance situations in which the person is exposed to unfamiliar people or to possible scrutiny by others. The individual fears that he or she will act in a way (or show anxiety symptoms) that will be humiliating or embarrassing. **Note:** In children, there must be evidence of the capacity for age-appropriate social relationships with familiar people and the anxiety must occur in peer settings, not just in interactions with adults.
B. Exposure to the feared social situation almost invariably provokes anxiety, which may take the form of a situationally bound or situationally predisposed panic attack. **Note:** In children, the anxiety may be expressed by crying, tantrums, freezing, or shrinking from social situations with unfamiliar people.
C. The person recognizes that the fear is excessive or unreasonable. **Note:** In children, this feature may be absent.
D. The feared social or performance situations are avoided or else are endured with intense anxiety or distress.
E. The avoidance, anxious anticipation, or distress in the feared social or performance situation(s) interferes significantly with the person's normal routine, occupational (academic) functioning, or social activities or relationships, or there is marked distress about having the phobia.
F. In individuals under age 18 years, the duration is at least 6 months.
G. The fear or avoidance is not due to the direct physiological effects of a substance (e.g., a drug of abuse, a medication) or a general medical condition and is not better accounted for by another mental disorder (e.g., panic disorder with or without agoraphobia, separation anxiety disorder, body dysmorphic disorder, a pervasive developmental disorder, or schizoid personality disorder).
H. If a general medical condition or another mental disorder is present, the fear in Criterion A is unrelated to it, e.g., the fear is not of Stuttering, trembling in Parkinson's disease, or exhibiting abnormal eating behavior in anorexia nervosa or bulimia nervosa.
Specify if:
   Generalized: if the fears include most social situations (also consider the additional diagnosis of avoidant personality disorder)

In the more recent National Comorbidity Survey (Kessler et al. 1994; Magee et al. 1996), which employed DSM-III-R criteria, specific phobias had the same lifetime prevalence (11.3%) as in the ECA study. However, social phobia appeared markedly more prevalent than in the ECA study, with a lifetime occurrence of 13.3%, a 1-year incidence of 7.9%, and a 1-month incidence of 4.5%, and was somewhat more common in women than

TABLE 11–11. DSM-IV-TR diagnostic criteria for specific phobia

A. Marked and persistent fear that is excessive or unreasonable, cued by the presence or anticipation of a specific object or situation (e.g., flying, heights, animals, receiving an injection, seeing blood).

B. Exposure to the phobic stimulus almost invariably provokes an immediate anxiety response, which may take the form of a situationally bound or situationally predisposed panic attack.   **Note:** In children, the anxiety may be expressed by crying, tantrums, freezing, or clinging.

C. The person recognizes that the fear is excessive or unreasonable.   **Note:** In children, this feature may be absent.

D. The phobic situation(s) is avoided or else is endured with intense anxiety or distress.

E. The avoidance, anxious anticipation, or distress in the feared situation(s) interferes significantly with the person's normal routine, occupational (or academic) functioning, or social activities or relationships, or there is marked distress about having the phobia.

F. In individuals under age 18 years, the duration is at least 6 months.

G. The anxiety, panic attacks, or phobic avoidance associated with the specific object or situation are not better accounted for by another mental disorder, such as obsessive-compulsive disorder (e.g., fear of dirt in someone with an obsession about contamination), posttraumatic stress disorder (e.g., avoidance of stimuli associated with a severe stressor), separation anxiety disorder (e.g., avoidance of school), social phobia (e.g., avoidance of social situations because of fear of embarrassment), panic disorder with agoraphobia, or agoraphobia without history of panic disorder.

Specify type:
   Animal Type
   Natural Environment Type (e.g., heights, storms, water)
   Blood-Injection-Injury Type
   Situational Type (e.g., airplanes, elevators, enclosed places)
   Other Type (e.g., fear of choking, vomiting, or contracting an illness; in children, fear of loud sounds or costumed characters)

in men (lifetime 15.5% in women vs. 11.1% in men). Agoraphobia's prevalence was similar to that in the ECA study (lifetime 6.7%, 1-month 2.3%). Median ages at illness onset were 15 years for specific phobias, 16 years for social phobia, and 29 years for agoraphobia. The phobias were highly comorbid with each other, and despite significant functional impairment, only a minority of the individuals interviewed had sought professional help.

Agoraphobia in the absence of panic disorder was traditionally thought to be rare, and thus, for the purposes

of this chapter, agoraphobia is discussed under panic disorder. Agoraphobia without a history of panic attacks is only infrequently encountered in clinical settings, a finding endorsed by most clinical studies and clinicians. Indeed, some investigators believe that an initial panic attack, even if remote or forgotten, is a necessary prerequisite for the development of agoraphobia, according to the model presented in Figure 11–2. However, this conclusion is controversial. For example, in one clinical series of panic disorder with agoraphobia, 23% of patients reported that agoraphobia preceded their initial panic attack (Lelliott et al. 1989), although retrospective biases may cast some doubt on such a finding. Most striking is the high prevalence of agoraphobia without panic reported in epidemiological samples. Based on the ECA study, most new-onset cases of agoraphobia (about two-thirds) occurred without a history of panic attacks (Eaton and Keyl 1990). Such a discrepant finding may, at least in part, be accounted for by an excessively low severity threshold and weaknesses in differential diagnosis in epidemiological assessments.

In this section we discuss two major phobic disorders, social phobia and specific phobias.

Social Phobia

Clinical Description

In social phobia, the individuals' central fear is that they will act in such a way that they will humiliate or embarrass themselves in front of others. Socially phobic individuals fear and/or avoid a variety of situations in which they would be required to interact with others or to perform a task in front of other people. Typical social phobias relate to speaking, eating, or writing in public; using public lavatories; and attending parties or interviews. In addition, a common fear of socially phobic individuals is that other people will detect and ridicule their anxiety in social situations. An individual may have one social fear, a limited number of fears, or numerous social fears. Social phobia is described as generalized if the social fear encompasses most social situations as opposed to being present in circumscribed ones. Generalized social phobia is overall a more serious and impairing condition. Generalized social phobia can be reliably diagnosed as a subtype; afflicted patients have an earlier age at onset, are more often single, and have more interactional fears and greater comorbidity with atypical depression and alcoholism (Mannuzza et al. 1995).

As in specific phobias, the anxiety in social phobia is stimulus-bound. When forced or surprised into the phobic situation, the individual experiences profound anxiety accompanied by various somatic symptoms. Interestingly, different anxiety disorders tend to be characterized by their own constellation of most prominent somatic symptoms. For example, palpitations and chest pain or pressure are more common in panic attacks, whereas sweating, blushing, and dry mouth are more common in social anxiety (Amies et al. 1983; Reich et al. 1988). Actual panic attacks may also occur in individuals with social phobia in response to feared social situations. Blushing is the cardinal physical symptom in social phobia, whereas commonly encountered cognitive constellations include tendencies for self-focused attention, negative self-evaluation regarding social performance, difficulty gauging nonverbal aspects of one's behavior, discounting of social competence in positive interactions, and a positive bias toward appraising others' social performance (Alden and Wallace 1995).

Individuals who have only limited social fears may be functioning well overall and may be relatively asymptomatic unless confronted with the necessity of entering their phobic situation. When faced with this necessity, they are often subject to intense anticipatory anxiety. Multiple social fears, on the other hand, can lead to chronic demoralization, social isolation, and disabling vocational and interpersonal impairment. Alcohol and sedative drugs are often used to alleviate at least the anticipatory component of this anxiety disorder, possibly leading to abuse. In a study that systematically compared individuals with public-speaking phobia and individuals with generalized social phobia, the latter were found to be younger, less educated, and less often employed and to have greater anxiety, depression, and fears of negative social evaluation (Heimberg et al. 1990b).

Epidemiology and Comorbidity

The earliest epidemiological study, the ECA study, first found rather low prevalence for social phobia, 2.8% lifetime (Schneier et al. 1992). However, the assessment of social phobia was incomplete and this number turned out to be an underestimate. Subsequently, the National Comorbidity Survey identified a 13.3% lifetime and 7.9% 1-year prevalence (Magee et al. 1996). Of those, about one-third reported exclusively public-speaking fears, whereas the rest were characterized by at least one other social fear. About one-third had multiple fears qualifying for the generalized type of social phobia, which was found to be more persistent, impairing, and comorbid than the specific public speaking type. However, the two types did not differ in age of onset, family history, and certain sociodemographic variables (Kessler et al. 1998). In a large epidemiological survey of social phobia,

Schneier et al. (1992) found that 70% of those afflicted were women. Mean age at onset was 15, and there was substantial associated morbidity, including greater financial dependency and increased suicidal ideation. Similarly, in a population-based adolescent female twin sample, the lifetime prevalence of social phobia was found to be 16% (Nelson et al. 2000), already carrying at that age a threefold risk for comorbid major depression and a twofold risk for alcohol dependence. Social phobia with comorbid depression was associated with an elevated risk of alcohol problems and suicidality. Epidemiological studies have consistently found significant comorbidity between lifetime social phobia and various mood disorders, with an approximately three- to sixfold higher risk for dysthymia, depression, and bipolar disorder (Kessler et al. 1999b). Social phobia almost always predates the mood disorder, and is a predictor not only of higher likelihood of future mood disorder, but also of more severity and chronicity.

Social phobia can be associated with a variety of personality disorders, in particular avoidant personality disorder (Dyck et al. 2001). In epidemiologically identified probands with social phobia alone, avoidant personality disorder alone, or both, a similarly elevated familial risk of social phobia has been found, suggesting that the Axis I and II disorders may represent dimensions of social anxiety rather than discrete conditions (Tillfors et al. 2001). Indeed, a recent review of the literature comparing generalized social phobia, avoidant personality disorder, and shyness concluded that all three may exist on a continuum (Rettew 2000).

Social phobia, in and of itself, is a highly disabling disorder whose effect on functioning and quality of life has probably been greatly underestimated and hidden in past years. Recent studies (M.B. Stein and Kean 2000) show that persons with social phobia are impaired on a broad spectrum of measures, ranging from dropping out of school to significant disability in whatever their main activity is. They describe dissatisfaction for many aspects of their lives and the quality of their lives is rated as quite low. Importantly, comorbid depression seems to contribute only modestly to these outcomes. Even in preadolescent children, pervasive and serious functional impairment can already be found (Beidel et al. 1999).

Etiology

Psychosocial theories. A number of mechanisms are proposed by learning theories as contributors to the pathogenesis of social phobia (Ost 1987; Stemberger et al. 1995). These include direct exposure to socially related traumatic events, vicarious learning through observing others engaged in such traumatic situations, and information transfer, things that one hears in various contexts regarding social interactions. There is a significant familial component to social phobia, part of which is thought to be heritable (see "Genetics" under "Biological Theories" subsection below) and part acquired. Parents, whether socially anxious themselves or not, might rear socially anxious children through various mechanisms such as lack of adequate exposure to social situations and development of social skills, overprotectiveness, controlling and critical behavior, modeling of socially anxious behaviors, and fearful information conveyed about social situations (Hudson and Rapee 2000). For example, in an experimental paradigm it has been shown that socially ambiguous situations are interpreted favorably by children without socially phobic parents but avoidantly when family input is negative (Dadds et al. 1996).

Parental social phobia is a strong risk factor for social phobia among adolescent offspring, as is parental depression, any other anxiety disorder, any alcohol use disorder, and parental overprotection or rejection; overall family functioning was not predictive (Lieb et al. 2000). Other potential risk factors for social phobia identified in a large epidemiological sample include lack of a close relationship with an adult, not being firstborn for males, parental marital conflict, general parental psychiatric history, moving several times as a child, childhood abuse, running away from home, and doing poorly in school (Chartier et al. 2001). These variables remained largely significant when controlling for comorbidity.

A number of cognitive distortions can be identified in individuals with established social phobia, all centering around various manifestations of a core negative representation of one's social self. There is evidence that individuals with social phobia do not habituate to negative social information as easily as nonanxious control subjects (Amir et al. 2001), have an implicit memory bias for socially threatening information (Amir et al. 2000), show more flexibility in interpreting anxiety symptoms exhibited by others but are more judgmental of their own (Amir et al. 1998b; Roth et al. 2001), produce negative interpretations of ambiguous social events and catastrophic interpretations of mildly negative social events (Stopa and Clark 2000), and have a negative expectation that social success will result in greater future social demands (Wallace and Alden 1997). Children with social phobia, compared with their nonanxious peers, have been found to have social skills deficits, more negative self-talk, less competent social performance with peers, and fewer positive outcomes from peers (Spence et al. 1999). In an information processing paradigm, individuals with social phobia have been found to exhibit higher vigilance and avoidance of threatening information than control subjects (Amir et al. 1998a).

Biological theories. *Genetics.* A strong familial risk for social phobia has been identified, which is believed to be partly heritable and partly environmental. First-degree relatives of probands with generalized social phobia have an approximately 10-fold higher risk for generalized social phobia or avoidant personality disorder (M.B. Stein et al. 1998a). One twin study has not supported a genetic component to social and specific phobia, in contrast to panic disorder, GAD, and PTSD, suggesting environmental causation (Skre et al. 1993). However, in another study of phobias in twins, Kendler et al. (1992b) determined that the familial aggregation of phobias was mostly accounted for by genetic factors, with a modest heritability of 30%–40% depending on the particular phobia. Environmental factors also played a significant role in the development of phobic disorders. An adolescent female twin study estimated the heritability of social phobia to be 28%, with strong evidence for shared genetic vulnerability between social phobia and major depression (Nelson et al. 2000).

The personality trait of behavioral inhibition, which is believed to be largely heritable and becomes manifest and fixed in early childhood (Kagan et al. 1987), is thought to comprise one of the substrates onto which social phobia might develop, also it is neither necessary nor sufficient for the development of the disorder. Behavioral inhibition assessed in toddlerhood has been found, prospectively, to be a strong predictor of social anxiety in adolescence (C. Schwartz et al. 1999). Similarly, behavioral inhibition, in the form of both social avoidance and fearfulness in early high school, prospectively predicted the onset of social phobia 4 years later in adolescence (Hayward et al. 1998). Cross-sectionally, a specific association has been found between childhood shyness and maternal social phobia as opposed to other anxiety disorders (Cooper and Eke 1999).

There are essentially no genetic molecular studies in social phobia. One report found no linkage to the serotonin transporter or 5-HT_{2A} receptor gene in generalized social phobia (M.B. Stein et al. 1998b).

Neurochemistry. Neurochemical studies of social phobia have not been as systematic or as consistently replicated as those in panic disorder, but to date they have implicated a number of neurotransmitter systems, including noradrenergic, GABAergic, dopaminergic, and serotonergic. In one study, patients with social phobia exhibited a blunted GH response to clonidine challenge, suggesting an underlying noradrenergic dysfunction similar to that in patients with panic disorder (Tancer et al. 1993); however, this finding was not replicated in a subsequent study (Tancer et al. 1994). Patients with social phobia also show evidence of altered autonomic responsivity, such as an exaggerated response to the Valsalva maneuver, in comparison with healthy control subjects (M.B. Stein et al. 1994). GABA–benzodiazepine receptor involvement in social phobia is unclear. One study found that the benzodiazepine antagonist flumazenil did not induce a greater surge in anxiety in social phobia patients compared with control subjects (Coupland et al. 2000). However, another study showed significantly decreased peripheral benzodiazepine receptor density in patients with generalized social phobia compared with a healthy control group (M.R. Johnson et al. 1998).

Despite the now-documented efficacy of serotonin reuptake inhibitors in treating social phobia, little is directly known about serotonergic involvement in the disorder. Subjects in one study demonstrated increased cortisol response to fenfluramine suggestive of altered serotonergic sensitivity (Tancer et al. 1994). However, social phobia patients in other studies showed no signs of altered serotonin reuptake sites in platelets (M.B. Stein et al. 1995b) and no abnormalities in the prolactin response to m-CPP (Hollander et al. 1998). Although two studies found normal basal functioning of the HPA axis in patients with social phobia, as measured by basal cortisol levels and the dexamethasone suppression test (Uhde et al. 1994), HPA studies of these patients under conditions of social stress might be more telling. Evidence that social phobia may be associated with decreased central dopaminergic tone includes a report of social phobia triggered by dopamine-blocking agents (Mikkelsen et al. 1981) and successful treatment of social anxiety with the dopamine agonist pergolide (Villareal et al. 2000). Individuals with comorbid panic and social phobia have been found to have decreased levels of the dopamine metabolite homovanillic acid (HVA) in the cerebrospinal fluid (CSF) (M.R. Johnson et al. 1994). Finally, in more definitive recent studies, social phobia was associated with a significant 20% decrease in dopamine transporter site density in the striatum by SPECT (Tiihonen et al. 1997b) and, similarly, with lowered dopamine D_2 receptor binding potential (Schneier et al. 2000).

Neuroimaging. The neuroimaging of social phobia is still in its infancy. One structural imaging study found no volumetric differences in patients with social phobia compared with a healthy control group (Potts et al. 1994), and another found no differences in regional blood flow on SPECT imaging with subjects in a basal resting state (M.B. Stein and Leslie 1996). However, provocation paradigms that evoke social anxiety symptoms during imaging might be expected to have a higher yield in revealing dysfunctional brain circuits in social phobia, and some interesting preliminary findings have been reported in the very few studies of this sort to date. In one small study with a comparison group of healthy control subjects, individuals with social phobia demonstrated a selective higher activation in the amygdala, a center for the emotional processing of fearfulness, in response to emotionally neutral faces presented during functional MRI (Birbaumer et al. 1998). In a PET study using social anxiety–provoking scripts, individuals with social phobia evidenced greater blood flow in the anterior cingulate, the dorsolateral prefrontal cortex, the orbitofrontal cortex, and the insula, areas involved in emotional processing; however, the amygdala was relatively deactivated (Bell et al. 1999). A SPECT study of patients with social phobia imaged before and after treatment with an SSRI showed higher baseline activity in the left temporal cortex and left midfrontal regions in nonresponders compared with responders (Van der Linden et al. 2000). A model similar to that described in panic disorder, involving faulty conditioned fear responses, has also been implicated in other anxiety disorders, each to its specific triggers, including social phobia. Along these lines, a recent study found signal decreases in the amygdala and hippocampus in healthy control subjects presented with the conditioned stimulus of a neutral face associated with an unconditioned stimulus, whereas subjects with social phobia exhibited opposite increased activations in both regions (Schneider et al. 1999).

Course and Prognosis

Social phobia has its onset mainly in adolescence and early adulthood, earlier than agoraphobia, and the course of illness is very chronic. Mean age at onset in two clinical series was 19 years (Amies et al. 1983; Marks and Gelder 1966). Onset of symptoms is sometimes acute (e.g., following a humiliating social experience) but is usually insidious over months or years and without a clear-cut precipitant. Interestingly, in clinical studies, men are equally or even more often affected then women, in contrast to the case in other anxiety disorders. This finding may reflect who is more likely to seek treatment under societal role demands, however, rather than prevalence rates in the population at large.

Social phobia is clearly a chronic and potentially highly impairing condition. It has been found that more than half of patients report significant impairment in some area(s) of their lives, independent of the degree of social support (Schneier et al. 1994; M.B. Stein and Kean 2000). Predictors of good outcome in social phobia are onset after age 11 years, absence of psychiatric comorbidity, and higher educational status (Davidson et al. 1993a). In a recent very large retrospective survey of individuals ages 15–64 years with lifetime social phobia, approximately half of the sample had recovered from their illness at the time of the survey, with a median illness duration of 25 years. Significant predictors of recovery were childhood social context (e.g., no siblings and small-town rearing), onset after age 7 years, fewer symptoms, and either absence of comorbid health problems or depression or occurrence of these conditions before the onset of social phobia (DeWit et al. 1999).

Diagnosis and Differential Diagnosis

Before the diagnosis of phobic disorder can be made, the presence of other disorders that may cause irrational fears and avoidance behaviors must be ruled out. For a complete decision tree of the differential diagnosis of the anxiety disorders, see Figure 11–1.

Avoidance of social situations is seen as part of avoidant, schizoid, and paranoid personality disorders, agoraphobia, OCD, depressive disorders, schizophrenia, and paranoid disorders.

Persons with paranoid disorders fear that something unpleasant will be done to them by others. In contrast, individuals with social phobia fear that they themselves will act inappropriately and cause their own embarrassment or humiliation.

In avoidant personality disorder, the central fear is also of rejection, ridicule, or humiliation by others. The distinction between this entity and generalized social phobia may be conceptual and semantic, and its validity is a subject of dispute. Automatically labeling such patients as having avoidant personalities may lead practitioners away from potentially useful pharmacotherapy and behavioral treatment efforts.

Some agoraphobic patients say that they are afraid they will embarrass themselves by losing control if they panic while in a social situation. These patients are distinguished from patients with social phobia by the presence of panic attacks that also occur in situations not involving scrutiny or evaluation by others.

Interpersonal anxiety or fears of humiliation leading to social avoidance are not diagnosed as social phobia when they occur in the context of schizophrenia, schizo-phreniform or brief reactive psychoses, or major depressive disorder. Patients with psychotic vulnerabilities and massive social isolation or poor interpersonal skills may occasionally be mistaken as having social phobia if seen when they are in nonpsychotic or prepsychotic phases of illness.

Social withdrawal seen in depressive disorders is usually associated with a lack of interest or pleasure in the company of others rather than a fear of scrutiny. In contrast, individuals with social phobia generally express the wish to be able to interact appropriately with others and anticipate pleasure in this eventuality.

Treatment

Pharmacotherapy

The pharmacological treatment of social phobia is summarized in Table 11–12. Several medication options are clearly helpful in social phobia. In performance-type social phobia, several analog (i.e., involving nonclinical samples with performance or social anxiety) studies have shown β-blocker efficacy, particularly when these agents are used acutely before a performance (Brantigan et al. 1982; Hartley et al. 1983; I.M. James et al. 1977, 1983; Liden and Gottfries 1974; Neftel et al. 1982). Many performing artists or public speakers find that β-blockers, taken orally a few hours before stage time, reduce palpitations, tremor, and the "butterfly feeling." Although a variety of β-blockers have been used in studies and are probably efficacious for performance anxiety, the most common ones used are propranolol 20 mg or atenolol 50 mg, taken about 45 minutes before a performance. It also seems that β-blockers are more effective in controlling stage fright, with minimal or no side effects, than are benzodiazepines, which may decrease subjective anxiety but not optimize performance and may have an adverse effect on "sharpness."

Until recently, the MAOIs were the most proven effective medications in treating generalized social phobia. Older studies had shown these drugs to be effective in mixed agoraphobia/social phobia samples (Mountjoy et al. 1977; C. Solyom et al. 1981; L. Solyom et al. 1973; Tyrer et al. 1973). More recently, Liebowitz et al. (1992) conducted a controlled study comparing phenelzine, atenolol, and placebo in the treatment of patients with DSM-III–diagnosed social phobia. About two-thirds of the patients had a marked response to phenelzine at dosages of 45–90 mg/day, whereas atenolol was not superior to placebo. Tranylcypromine in dosages of 40–60 mg/day was also associated with significant improvement in

TABLE 11–12. Pharmacological treatment of social phobia

Selective serotonin reuptake inhibitors (SSRIs)

General indications: first-line treatment; shown efficacy; well tolerated; once-daily dosing; effective for comorbid depression, panic, generalized anxiety disorder, or obsessive-compulsive disorder

Paroxetine: best studied in large controlled trials; U.S. Food and Drug Administration–approved; average dosage 40 mg/day

Fluvoxamine: smaller controlled trials, average dosage 200 mg/day

Sertraline: one controlled trial, 50–200 mg/day

Fluoxetine: open trials

Citalopram: open trials

Monoamine oxidase inhibitors

General indications: demonstrated high effectiveness; may be difficult to tolerate and require dietary restrictions; effective for several comorbid conditions including atypical depression, social phobia, and panic; well worth trying in otherwise refractory patients

Phenelzine: most studied

Tranylcypromine: also effective

Benzodiazepines

General indications: clinically widely used and reportedly efficacious in open trials; generally well tolerated; concerns about dependence and withdrawal in certain patients

Clonazepam: long-acting; efficacy demonstrated in controlled trial

Gabapentin

General indication: found effective in controlled trial, mean dose 2,900 mg/day, consider as augmentation or second-line treatment if inadequate response to or intolerance of SSRIs

Beta-blockers

General indications: highly effective for performance anxiety, taken on an as-needed basis about 1 hour before event; for the most part, not helpful in patients with generalized social phobia

Propranolol, atenolol

Other medications

Buspirone: well tolerated, effective in open but not in controlled trial

Nefazodone: effective in open trial

Venlafaxine: effective in open trial

Bupropion: effective in open trial

Reversible monoamine oxidase inhibitors: moclobemide modestly effective to ineffective, not marketed in U.S.

about 80% of patients with DSM-III–diagnosed social phobia treated openly for 1 year (Versiani et al. 1988). Another study (Gelernter et al. 1991) compared cognitive-behavioral group treatment with phenelzine, alprazolam, and placebo. Although all groups improved significantly with treatment, phenelzine tended to be superior

in regard to absolute clinical response and decreased impairment. Despite their proven efficacy in social phobia, MAOIs are no longer a first-line treatment given their dietary and medication restrictions, potential for hypertensive crises, and frequently poorly tolerated side effects. More recently, there was excitement about the possibility that reversible inhibitors of monoamine oxidase, not yet marketed in the United States, might replace MAOIs in the treatment of social phobia, as they are better tolerated and do not require dietary restrictions. However, findings have been disappointing, and several studies have now shown that moclobemide is at best only very modestly effective, or even ineffective, in social phobia ("The International Multicenter Clinical Trial Group on Moclobemide in Social Phobia," 1997; Noyes et al. 1997; Schneier et al. 1998).

Traditionally, benzodiazepines have held promise and have been used to treat generalized social phobia, despite the usual concerns about their use. Several open trials reported positive results, and in one controlled study, clonazepam at doses of 0.5–3.0 mg/day (mean dosage, 2.4 mg/day) was found to be superior to placebo, with a response rate of 78% and improvement in social anxiety, avoidance, performance, and negative self-evaluation (Davidson et al. 1993b). Alprazolam was also found to be superior to placebo and to have results comparable with those of phenelzine and CBT. However, the alprazolam group had the highest relapse rate 2 months after treatment discontinuation (Gelernter et al. 1991). Given its longer half-life, clonazepam is a better choice than alprazolam. Both medications have the advantages of relatively rapid onset of action and good tolerability. Disadvantages include the potential for abuse, withdrawal, and relapse and a lack of efficacy for comorbid depression. The benzodiazepines would not be considered a first-line treatment for social phobia.

In recent years, newer antidepressants have been tested and have shown efficacy in treating social phobia; as a result, the SSRIs have become the first-line treatment for the disorder. Although investigated to varying degrees, there is no reason to believe that the medications of this class differ in their efficacy for social phobia; all SSRIs are generally well tolerated, are easy to dispense and monitor, and are used in standard doses comparable with those used in depression. Paroxetine is now FDA approved for treating social phobia, its efficacy having been demonstrated in two controlled trials (Baldwin et al. 1999; M.B. Stein et al. 1998c). About one-half to two-thirds of patients with social phobia responded to acute treatment with paroxetine, at average doses of about 40 mg/day. In one controlled trial, fluvoxamine at 150 mg/day for 12 weeks resulted in substantial improvement in

46% of patients, compared with 7% improvement in the placebo group (van Vliet et al. 1994), and this success was subsequently replicated in a larger study with a comparable mean dose of 200 mg/day and a response rate of 43% (M.B. Stein et al. 1999). Of 20 patients treated openly with sertraline for at least 8 weeks, 80% showed some improvement of their social phobia (Van Ameringen et al. 1994), and the efficacy of sertraline was duplicated in a placebo-controlled study at dosages of 50–200 mg/day (Katzelnick et al. 1995). A very recent large 20-week trial of sertraline versus placebo confirmed its efficacy, with flexible dosing up to 200 mg/day and a 53% response rate (Van Ameringen et al. 2001). Similar response rates were found in an open trial of fluoxetine (Van Ameringen et al. 1993) and an open trial of citalopram (Bouwer and Stein 1998).

In addition, other medications seem to hold some promise in treating social phobia. Buspirone, a 5-HT$_{1A}$ agonist, initially appeared promising in an open trial (Schneier et al. 1993), but findings from a subsequent controlled trial were negative (van Vliet et al. 1997). It is conceivable that doses higher than the 30 mg/day employed in the controlled trial may have been more beneficial. An open trial of nefazodone was positive (Van Ameringen et al. 1999), and nefazodone may be a good option in patients who cannot tolerate SSRIs. Similarly, a small open trial of venlafaxine—interestingly, in patients who had not responded to SSRIs—reported positive results (Altamura et al. 1999). Bupropion is the least-studied antidepressant to date, but even it may have some efficacy in social phobia (Emmanuel et al. 1991). Finally, the anticonvulsant gabapentin represents another medication class that has been studied in a controlled setting and therefore merits serious consideration as a second-line agent for patients in whom SSRIs are ineffective or not tolerated. Although gabapentin has not been directly compared with SSRIs, alone or as augmentation, to date, a placebo-controlled trial in patients with social phobia found gabapentin to be superior to placebo at a mean dose of about 2,900 mg/day, with a response rate approaching 40% (Pande et al. 1999).

Cognitive and Behavioral Therapies

Three major cognitive-behavioral techniques are used in the treatment of social phobia: exposure, cognitive restructuring, and social skills training. Exposure treatment involves imaginal or in vivo exposure to specific feared performance and social situations. Although patients with very high levels of social anxiety may need to start out with imaginal exposure until a certain degree of habituation is attained, therapeutic results are not gained until in vivo exposure to the real-life feared situations is done. Social skills training employs modeling, rehearsal, role-playing, and assigned practice to help individuals learn appropriate behaviors and decrease anxiety in social situations, with an expectation that this will lead to more positive responses from others. This type of training is not necessary for all individuals with social phobia and is more applicable to those who have actual deficits in social interacting above and beyond their anxiety or avoidance of social situations. Cognitive restructuring focuses on poor self-concepts, the fear of negative evaluation by others, and the attribution of positive outcomes to chance or circumstance and negative outcomes to one's own shortcomings. It consists of a variety of homework exercises focused on identifying negative thoughts, evaluating their accuracy, and reframing them in a more realistic way.

Results of older studies of behavioral treatments for social phobia were difficult to evaluate because of heterogeneous phobic patient samples, lack of operational definitions of disorder and improvement ratings, and the presentation of outcome data in terms of mean change scores rather than level of achieved functioning. However, in the past decade or so the cognitive-behavioral treatment of social phobia has multiplied and attracted great attention, detailed treatment strategies and approaches have been delineated, and more thorough systematic studies in well-defined clinical populations have emerged.

Recent studies show that exposure, cognitive restructuring, and social skills training may all be of significant benefit in patients with social phobia. In addition, these techniques appear superior to nonspecific supportive therapy, as shown in a randomized controlled study comparing supportive therapy with initial individual cognitive therapy followed by group social skills training (Cottraux et al. 2000). The success of CBT appears to be mediated, at least in part, by a decrease in self-focused attention (Woody et al. 1997). Attempts to correlate patient type (social skills deficits vs. phobic anxiety/avoidance) with preferred treatment modality (social skills training vs. exposure) have not always been fruitful (Wlazlo et al. 1990). Heimberg et al. (1990a) compared cognitive-behavioral group treatment with a credible psychoeducational-supportive control intervention in patients with DSM-III–diagnosed social phobia; both groups got better, but the cognitive-behavioral group showed more improvement, especially in patients' self-appraisal. Finally, it has been suggested that cognitive aspects may be of greater importance in social phobia than in other anxiety or phobic conditions, and therefore cognitive restructuring may be a necessary component to maximize treatment gains. Mattick et al. (1989) reported that combination treatment was superior to either exposure or cognitive restructuring alone in social phobia; cognitive restructuring alone was inferior to exposure alone in decreasing avoidant behavior, but exposure alone did not change self-perception and attitude.

Although long-term outcome is more difficult to assess, studies suggest that CBT leads to long-lasting gains (Turner et al. 1995) and therefore may be of particular significance in this disorder, which tends to have a chronic, often lifetime, course. At this point, it appears that in vivo exposure is a critical component of the treatment, and that the introduction of cognitive restructuring at some point in the treatment contributes to further gains and to their long-term maintenance. Social phobia is a disorder that often starts in the early years, and it is encouraging to know that in prepubertal children, both behavioral therapy consisting of social skills training and anxiety reduction techniques (Beidel et al. 2000) and CBT alone or with the parents (Spence et al. 2000) have been found to be highly effective in controlled trials.

Combination treatment with CBT and medication has also received some attention. It appears that medication alone and CBT alone can have comparable results in the acute treatment of social phobia (Gelernter et al. 1991; Heimberg et al. 1998; Otto et al. 2000). In a rigorous comparison with the medication "gold standard" phenelzine, cognitive-behavioral group therapy was found to have essentially similar efficacy over 12 weeks, although with a longer time to reach response and some inferiority in some of the final measures (Heimberg et al. 1998). Furthermore, the question of the longer-term impact of the two forms of therapy is particularly relevant. In a continuation of the previously described study (Heimberg et al. 1998), responders continued treatment with phenelzine or CBT for a 6-month maintenance phase, and were then followed for an additional 6-month treatment-free phase (Liebowitz et al. 1999). Both treatments maintained their effectiveness for the first 6 months, with phenelzine preserving its slight superiority over CBT. However, after treatment ended, CBT was associated with a greater likelihood of maintaining a good response. Therefore, in a newly presenting patient with social phobia who is reluctant to try medication, it is a very reasonable course of treatment to commence with a CBT trial, while introducing the possibility of later medication treatment.

Other Psychotherapies

In recent years, the successful use of medication and/or behavioral treatments has resulted in psychodynamic therapy for phobias falling out of favor to some degree (Gabbard 1990). However, in those patients in whom underlying conflicts associated with phobic anxiety and avoidance can be identified by the clinician and lend themselves to insightful exploration, psychodynamic therapy may be of benefit. Furthermore, a psychodynamic approach may be valuable in elucidating and resolving the secondary interpersonal ramifications that phobic patients and their partners often become caught up in and that could serve as resistances to the successful implementation of medication or behavioral treatments (Gabbard 1990). In a recent trial of interpersonal psychotherapy adapted for treatment of social phobia, seven of nine patients treated openly for 14 weeks showed significant improvement (Lipsitz et al. 1999a), suggesting that this modality also merits further study.

Specific Phobias

Specific phobias are circumscribed fears of specific objects, situations, or activities. The syndrome has three components: an anticipatory anxiety brought on by the possibility of confrontation with the phobic stimulus, the central fear itself, and the avoidance behavior by which the individual minimizes anxiety. In specific phobia, the fear is usually not of the object itself but of some dire outcome that the individuals believe may result from contact with that object. For example, persons with driving phobia are afraid of accidents; those with snake phobia, that they will be bitten; and those who are claustrophobic, that they will suffocate or be trapped in an enclosed space. These fears are excessive, unreasonable, and enduring, so that although most individuals with specific phobias will readily acknowledge that they know there is really nothing to be afraid of, reassuring them of this does not diminish their fear.

In DSM-IV, for the first time, types of specific phobias were adopted: natural environment (e.g., storms); animal (e.g., insects); blood-injury-injection; situational (e.g., cars, elevators, bridges); and other (e.g., choking, vomiting). The validity of such distinctions is supported by data showing that these types tend to differ with respect to age at onset, mode of onset, familial aggregation, and physiological responses to the phobic stimulus (Curtis and Thyer 1983; Fyer et al. 1990; Himle et al. 1991; Ost 1987). A comparable structure has been found in child and adolescent specific phobia, clustering into three subtypes (Muris et al. 1999).

The general population prevalence of specific phobias is around 10%, and women are affected more than twice as often as men (Magee et al. 1996). In a community study of adolescents, the prevalence of specific phobias was found to be 3.5%, higher in girls than boys, and with significant comorbidity with depressive and somatoform disorders in about one-third of the sample (Essau et al. 2000). Most commonly, individuals never seek treatment for this disorder.

Etiology

Psychodynamic Theory

With the 1909 publication of the case of Little Hans, Freud started to develop a psychological theory of phobic symptom formation (Freud 1909/1955). Little Hans was a 5-year-old boy who developed a phobia of horses. Through an analysis of the boy's conversations with his parents over a period of months, Freud hypothesized that Little Hans's unconscious and forbidden sexual feelings for his mother and aggressive, rivalrous feelings for his father, blocked from discharge because of repression, became physiologically transformed into anxiety, which was then displaced onto a symbolic object, in this case horses, the avoidance of which partly relieved Little Hans's anxiety.

Freud later reconceptualized the case of Little Hans in the context of his evolving structural theory. Freud postulated that phobic symptoms occur as part of the resolution of intrapsychic conflict between instinctual impulses, superego prohibitions, and external reality constraints. Signal anxiety is experienced by the ego when such unconscious impulses threaten to break through. Such anxiety serves to mobilize not only further repression but, in the case of phobia formation, projection and displacement of the conflict onto a symbolic object, which can then be avoided as a neurotic solution to the original conflict.

In the case of Little Hans, sexual feelings for his mother, aggressive feelings toward his father, and the guilty fear of retribution and castration by his father generated anxiety as a signal of oedipal conflict. The conflict became displaced and projected onto an avoidable object, horses, which Little Hans consequently feared would bite him. According to Freud, such a phobic symptom had two advantages. It avoided the ambivalence inherent in Little Hans's original conflict, as he not only hated but also loved his father. It also allowed his ego to cease generating anxiety as long as he could avoid the sight of horses. The cost of this compromise was that Little Hans had become housebound. Psychodynamic work with phobias, then, focuses on the symbolic meanings that the phobic object carries for any individual and the conflicts which is serves to avoid.

Behavioral Theories

In learning theory, phobic anxiety is thought to be a conditioned response acquired through association of the phobic object (i.e., the conditioned stimulus) with a noxious experience (i.e., the unconditioned stimulus). Initially, the noxious experience (e.g., an electric shock) produces an unconditioned response of pain, discomfort, and fear. If the individual frequently receives an electric shock when in contact with the phobic object, then by contiguous conditioning the appearance of the phobic object alone may come to elicit an anxiety response (i.e., conditioned response). Avoidance of the phobic object prevents or reduces this conditioned anxiety and is therefore perpetuated through drive reduction. This classical learning theory model of phobias has received much reinforcement from the relative success of behavioral (i.e., deconditioning) techniques in the treatment of many patients with specific phobias. However, it has also been criticized on the grounds that it is not consistent with a number of empirically observed aspects of phobic behavior in humans.

Models regarding the etiology of specific phobias have been elaborated and critiqued by Fyer (1998). She described that, in order to satisfactorily explain specific phobia, a modified conditioning model would be needed, on four counts. First, many phobic patients do not recall an initial aversive event, suggesting that if such an event had occurred it must be encoded by amygdala-based emotional memory but not by hippocampus-based episodic memory, either because it occurred before age 3 or was encoded under highly stressful conditions. Second, it turns out that a very small number of objects account for most human phobias, suggesting that there may be an evolutionarily wired biological preparedness toward specific stimuli which would be easily conditioned but difficult to extinguish. Third, only a minority of individuals exposed to a certain stimulus develop a phobic reaction, suggesting that additional factors such as genetic vulnerabilities or previous experiences play a role. Fourth, most phobias are resistant to extinction in the absence of specific interventions, despite belief and evidence that there is nothing to fear.

Another model of specific phobias is the nonassociative learning model (Fyer 1998), which is in a sense the converse of the conditioned model above. It proposes that each species has certain innate fears that are part of normal development and that essentially what goes wrong in specific phobia is a failure to habituate over time to these intrinsic developmental fears. This could be due to various processes such as stressful life events, constitutional vulnerabilities or unsafe environments.

Biological Theories

Some interesting recent hypotheses about the origin of phobias have resulted from integration of ethological, biological, and learning theory approaches. Fyer et al. (1990) found high familial transmission for specific phobias, with a roughly threefold risk for first-degree relatives of affected subjects; there was no increased risk for other comorbid phobic or anxiety disorders. However, one twin study did not support a genetic component to specific phobias, suggesting environmental causation (Skre et al. 1993). In a large study of phobias in twins, Kendler et al. (1992b) determined that the familial aggregation of phobias was mostly accounted for by genetic factors, with a modest heritability of 30% to 40% depending on the particular phobia. Environmental factors also played a significant role in the development of phobic disorders.

The neurobiology of specific phobias has barely been studied. Two studies examining response to CO_2 inhalation in subjects with specific phobia have found no differences from healthy subjects and no hypersensitivity as is found in panic disorder (Anthony et al. 1997; Verburg et al. 1994). Brain-imaging studies in specific phobia have been few and inconclusive. One showed no findings during exposure to the phobic stimulus (Mountz et al. 1989), whereas two other studies showed activation of the visual associative cortex (Fredrikson et al. 1993) and the somatosensory cortex (Rauch et al. 1995) suggesting that visual and tactile imagery is one component of the phobic response; findings regarding limbic activation appear equivocal.

The brain circuits mediating conditioned fear have recently been proposed as central to the pathogenesis of a number of anxiety disorders, including specific phobia, although data are extremely limited for this disorder. Such a model is attractive in that it may account for the occurrence of such a highly fearful response to the conditioned phobic stimulus, mediated by the amygdala, without hippocampal or cortically based knowledge or memory of why there is such fear. Studies exposing subjects with specific phobias to masked stimuli (i.e., very brief stimuli that can only be perceived implicitly) have lent partial support to the notion that phobic stimuli, even when not consciously registered, can elicit a subjective or objectively measured fearful response (Ohman and Soares 1994; van den Hout et al. 1997).

Course and Prognosis

Animal phobias usually begin in childhood, whereas situational phobias tend to start later in life. Marks (1969) found the mean age at onset for animal phobias to be 4.4 years, whereas patients with situational phobias had a mean age at onset of 22.7 years. Although systematic prospective studies are limited, it appears that specific phobias follow a chronic course unless treated. A recent study followed up specific phobia 10–16 years after an initial treatment, and found that even among responders with complete initial recovery, about half were clinically symptomatic at follow-up, and none of the patients who had not improved with the initial treatment were any better at follow-up; the study suggests that specific phobias may be resistant to treatment or often do not receive treatment (Lipsitz et al. 1999b).

Treatment

Exposure

The treatment of choice for specific phobias is exposure. The challenge lies in persuading the patient that exposure is worth trying and will be beneficial. Exposure treatments may be divided into two groups, depending on whether exposure to the phobic object is "in vivo" or "imaginal." In vivo exposure involves the patient in real-life contact with the phobic stimulus. Imaginal techniques confront the phobic stimulus through the therapist's descriptions and the patient's imagination.

In both the in vivo and the imaginal techniques, the method of exposure can be graded or ungraded. Graded exposure uses a hierarchy of anxiety-provoking events, varying from least to most stressful. The patient begins at the least-stressful level and gradually progresses up the hierarchy. Ungraded exposure begins with the patients confronting the most stressful items in the hierarchy.

Most exposure techniques have been used in both individual and group settings. In a group setting, both the example and the encouragement of other members are often particularly helpful in persuading the patient to reenter the phobic situation. Techniques may include systematic desensitization, imaginal flooding, prolonged in vivo exposure, and participant modeling and reinforced practice.

Studies thus far have not conclusively shown any one exposure technique to be superior to other techniques or to be specifically indicated for particular phobic subtypes. In those patients whose phobic symptoms include panic attacks, antipanic medication may also be indicated.

Pharmacotherapy

Medications have not been shown to be effective in treating specific phobias. TCAs, benzodiazepines, and β-blockers generally do not appear useful for specific phobias, at least on the basis of the limited number of studies conducted to date. A report of positive results for paroxetine was recently published, however. In this very small controlled trial, 11 patients were randomized to receive either placebo or paroxetine dosages up to 20 mg/day for 4 weeks (Benjamin et al. 2000). The authors reported that 1 of 6 patients responded to placebo and 3 of 5 to paroxetine. Further trials of serotonergic agents may be warranted.

Obsessive-Compulsive Disorder

The essential features of OCD are obsessions or compulsions. The DSM-IV-TR definition and criteria for OCD are presented in Table 11–13.

The terms *obsession* and *compulsion* are sometimes used more broadly to characterize conditions that are not true OCD. Although some activities, such as eating, sexual behavior, gambling, or drinking, when engaged in excessively, may be referred to as "compulsive," these activities are distinguished from true compulsions in that they are experienced as pleasurable and ego-syntonic, although their consequences may become increasingly unpleasant and ego-dystonic over time. Obsessive brooding, ruminations, or preoccupations, typically characteristic of depression, may be unpleasant but are distinguished from true obsessions because they are not as senseless or intrusive and the individual regards them as meaningful although possibly excessive and painful.

The various presentations of OCD are based on symptom clusters. One group includes patients with obsessions about dirt and contamination, patients whose rituals center on compulsive washing and avoidance of contaminated objects. A second group includes patients who engage in pathological counting and compulsive checking. A third group includes purely obsessional patients with no compulsions. Primary obsessional slowness is evident in another group of patients in whom slowness is the predominant symptom; patients may spend many hours every day getting washed, dressed, and eating breakfast, and life goes on at an extremely slow speed. Some patients with OCD, called hoarders, are unable to throw anything out for fear they might someday need something they discarded.

TABLE 11–13. DSM-IV-TR diagnostic criteria for obsessive-compulsive disorder

A. Either obsessions or compulsions:

Obsessions as defined by (1), (2), (3), and (4):

(1) recurrent and persistent thoughts, impulses, or images that are experienced, at some time during the disturbance, as intrusive and inappropriate and that cause marked anxiety or distress

(2) the thoughts, impulses, or images are not simply excessive worries about real-life problems

(3) the person attempts to ignore or suppress such thoughts, impulses, or images, or to neutralize them with some other thought or action

(4) the person recognizes that the obsessional thoughts, impulses, or images are a product of his or her own mind (not imposed from without as in thought insertion)

Compulsions as defined by (1) and (2):

(1) repetitive behaviors (e.g., hand washing, ordering, checking) or mental acts (e.g., praying, counting, repeating words silently) that the person feels driven to perform in response to an obsession, or according to rules that must be applied rigidly

(2) the behaviors or mental acts are aimed at preventing or reducing distress or preventing some dreaded event or situation; however, these behaviors or mental acts either are not connected in a realistic way with what they are designed to neutralize or prevent or are clearly excessive

B. At some point during the course of the disorder, the person has recognized that the obsessions or compulsions are excessive or unreasonable. **Note:** This does not apply to children.

C. The obsessions or compulsions cause marked distress, are time consuming (take more than 1 hour a day), or significantly interfere with the person's normal routine, occupational (or academic) functioning, or usual social activities or relationships.

D. If another Axis I disorder is present, the content of the obsessions or compulsions is not restricted to it (e.g., preoccupation with food in the presence of an eating disorder; hair pulling in the presence of trichotillomania; concern with appearance in the presence of body dysmorphic disorder; preoccupation with drugs in the presence of a substance use disorder; preoccupation with having a serious illness in the presence of hypochondriasis; preoccupation with sexual urges or fantasies in the presence of a paraphilia; or guilty ruminations in the presence of major depressive disorder).

E. The disturbance is not due to the direct physiological effects of a substance (e.g., a drug of abuse, a medication) or a general medical condition.

Specify if:

With Poor Insight: if, for most of the time during the current episode, the person does not recognize that the obsessions and compulsions are excessive or unreasonable

In DSM-IV, OCD is classified among the anxiety disorders because 1) anxiety is often associated with obsessions and resistance to compulsions, 2) anxiety or tension is often immediately relieved by yielding to compulsions, and 3) OCD often occurs in association with other anxiety disorders. However, compulsions decrease anxiety only transiently, and the fears in OCD are distinct in nature from those in other anxiety disorders.

Investigation in the DSM-IV field trial of certain diagnostic disputes regarding OCD led to some changes in criteria and clarifications in DSM-IV. Even though obsessions are typically experienced as ego-dystonic, patients with OCD have a wide range of insight. Although most patients have some degree of insight, about 5% are convinced that their obsessions and compulsions are reasonable (Foa et al. 1995). On the basis on this finding, DSM-IV specified a poor-insight type, which describes a patient who, for most of the time during the current episode, does not recognize that the obsessions and compulsions are excessive or unreasonable. DSM-IV has also made explicit that compulsions can be either behavioral or mental. Mental rituals are encountered in the great majority of patients with OCD and, like behavioral compulsions, are intended to reduce anxiety or prevent harm. Although more than 90% of patients have features of both obsessions and compulsions, 28% are bothered mainly by obsessions, 20% by compulsions, and 50% by both (Foa et al. 1995).

Clinical Description

Onset

OCD usually begins in adolescence or early adulthood but can begin before that time; 31% of first episodes occur between ages 10 and 15 years and 75% develop by age 30 years (A. Black 1974). In most cases, no particular stress or event precipitates the onset of OCD symptoms, and after an insidious onset there is a chronic and often progressive course. However, some patients describe a sudden onset of symptoms. This is particularly true of patients with a neurological basis for their illness. There is evidence of OCD onset associated with the 1920s encephalitis epidemic, abnormal birth events (Capstick and Seldrup 1977), head injury (McKeon et al. 1984), and seizures (Kehl and Marks 1986). Of interest are more recent reports of new onset of OCD during pregnancy (Neziroglu et al. 1992).

Symptoms

Obsessions. Obsessive and compulsive symptoms have been recognized for centuries and were first described in the psychiatric literature by Esquirol in 1838 (Rachman and Hodgson 1980). Obsessional thoughts were defined by Karl Westphal in 1878 as "ideas that in an otherwise intact intelligence, and without being caused by an emotional or affect-like state, against the will of the person… come into the foreground of the consciousness" (Westphal 1878, p. 735).

An obsession is an intrusive, unwanted mental event usually evoking anxiety or discomfort. Obsessions may be thoughts, ideas, images, ruminations, convictions, fears, or impulses and often involve content of an aggressive, sexual, religious, disgusting, or nonsensical nature. Obsessional ideas are repetitive thoughts that interrupt the normal train of thinking, whereas obsessional images are often vivid visual experiences. Much obsessive thinking involves horrific ideas. The person may think of doing the worst possible thing (e.g., blasphemy, rape, murder, child molestation). Obsessional convictions are often characterized by an element of magical thinking, such as "step on the crack, break your mother's back." Obsessional ruminations may involve prolonged, excessive, and inconclusive thinking about metaphysical questions. Obsessional fears often involve dirt or contamination and differ from phobias in that they are present in the absence of the phobic stimulus. Other common obsessional fears have to do with harm coming to oneself or to others as a consequence of one's misdoings, such as one's home catching on fire because the stove was not checked or running over a pedestrian because of careless driving. Obsessional impulses may be aggressive or sexual, such as intrusive impulses of stabbing one's spouse or raping one's child.

Attributing these obsessions to an internal source, the patient resists or controls them to a variable degree, and significant impairment in functioning can result. Resistance is the struggle against an impulse or intrusive thought, and control is the patient's actual success in diverting his or her thinking. Obsessions are usually accompanied by compulsions but may also occur as the main or only symptom. Approximately 10%–25% of patients with OCD are purely obsessional or suffer predominantly from obsessions (Akhtar et al. 1975; Rachman and Hodgson 1980; Welner et al. 1976).

Another hallmark of obsessive thinking involves lack of certainty or persistent doubting. In contrast to manic or psychotic patients, who manifest premature certainty, OCD patients are unable to achieve a sense of certainty between incoming sensory information and internal beliefs. They ask themselves such questions as "Are my hands clean?" "Is the door locked?" "Is the fertilizer poisoning the water supply?" Compulsive rituals such as excessive washing or checking appear to arise from this lack of certainty and constitute misguided attempts to increase certainty.

Compulsions. A compulsive ritual is a behavior that usually reduces discomfort but is carried out in a pressured or rigid fashion. Such behavior may include rituals involving washing, checking, repeating, avoiding, striving for completeness, and being meticulous. Washers represent about 25%–50% of most OCD samples (Akhtar et al. 1975; Rachman and Hodgson 1980; Rasmussen and Tsuang 1986). These individuals are concerned with dirt, contaminants, or germs and may spend many hours a day washing their hands or showering. They may also attempt to avoid contaminating themselves with feces, urine, or vaginal secretions.

Checkers have pathological doubt and thus compulsively check to see whether they have, for example, run over someone with their car or left the door unlocked. Checking often fails to resolve the doubt and in some cases may actually exacerbate it. In the DSM-IV field trial, washing and checking were the two most common groups of compulsions.

Although slowness results from most rituals, it is the major feature of the rare and disabling syndrome of primary obsessional slowness. It may take several hours for the obsessionally slow individual to get dressed or get out of the house. This slowness may be a response to a lack of certainty as well. These patients may have little anxiety despite their obsessions and rituals.

Mental compulsions are also quite common and should be inquired about directly, because they could go undetected if the clinician asks only about behavioral rituals. Such patients, for example, may replay over and over in their minds past conversations with others to make sure they did not somehow incriminate themselves. In the DSM-IV OCD field trials, 80% of patients had both behavioral and mental compulsions, and mental compulsions were the third most common type after checking and washing.

Although distinct symptom clusters exist (washers, checkers, hoarders, those who are purely obsessional, and those with primary slowness), these symptoms may overlap or develop sequentially. One study examined the distribution and grouping of obsessive-compulsive symptoms in about 300 patients with OCD and found that a total of four symptom dimensions accounted for more than 60% of variance: obsessions and checking, symmetry and ordering, cleanliness and washing, and hoarding (Leckman et al. 1997). Such subtypes may prove useful in the future when examining possible genetic, neurobiological or treatment-response heterogeneity in OCD.

Character Traits

Psychoanalytic theorists have suggested that a continuum exists between compulsive personality and OCD. Janet (1908) stated that all obsessional patients have a premorbid personality causally related to the disorder. Freud (1913/1958) noted an association between obsessional neurosis (i.e., OCD) symptoms and personality traits such as obstinacy, parsimony, punctuality, and orderliness.

However, phenomenological and epidemiological evidence suggests that OCD is frequently distinct from obsessive-compulsive personality disorder (OCPD). OCD symptoms are ego-dystonic, whereas obsessive-compulsive personality traits are ego-syntonic and do not involve a sense of compulsion that must be resisted. Epidemiological studies show that obsessive-compulsive character pathology is neither necessary nor sufficient for the development of OCD symptoms. When patients with obsessional traits decompensate, they often develop depression, paranoia, or somatization rather than OCD. Although the older literature suggested the presence of definite obsessional traits in as many as two-thirds of patients with OCD, structured personality assessments were not used. In more recent, standardized evaluations, only a minority of patients with OCD had DSM-III-R–diagnosed OCPD, whereas other personality disorders, such as avoidant or dependent personality disorder, were more common (Thomsen and Mikkelsen 1993). In addition, personality disorders may be more common in the presence of OCD of a longer duration, which suggests that they could be secondary to the Axis I disorder, and criteria for personality disorders may no longer be met after successful treatment of the OCD (Baer and Jenike 1992; Baer et al. 1990). A recent study suggested that a familial spectrum of OCD and OCPD may exist (Samuels et al. 2000).

Epidemiology

OCD was previously considered one of the rarest mental disorders. Early studies suggested a maximum incidence of 5 in 10,000 persons (Woodruff and Pitts 1964). This finding was probably due to clinicians' relative unfamiliarity with the disorder until the past decade, OCD patients' secretiveness about their symptoms, and the fact that the average wait before seeking psychiatric help was 7.5 years (Rasmussen and Tsuang 1986). Current data from the ECA study (described earlier in this chapter) suggest that OCD is quite common, with a 1-month prevalence of 1.3%, a 6-month prevalence of 1.5%, and a lifetime rate of 2.5% (Regier et al. 1988).

In clinical samples of adult OCD, there is a roughly equal ratio of men to women (A. Black 1974). In the ECA epidemiological sample, a slightly higher 1-month prevalence was found for women (1.5%) compared with men (1.1%), which was accounted for in the age range of 25–64 years, but this difference was not significant (Karno et al. 1988; Regier et al. 1988). However, in childhood-onset OCD, about 70% of patients are male (Hollingsworth et al. 1980; Swedo et al. 1989c). This difference seems to be accounted for by the earlier age at onset in males, and it may also suggest partly differing etiologies or vulnerabilities in the two sexes.

Twin and family studies have found a greater degree of concordance for OCD (defined broadly to include obsessional features) among monozygotic twins than among dizygotic twins (Carey and Gottesman 1981), which suggests that some predisposition to obsessional behavior is inherited. There have been no studies of OCD in adopted children or monozygotic twins raised apart. Studies of first-degree relatives of patients with OCD show a higher-than-expected incidence of various psychiatric symptoms and disorders, including obsessive-compulsive symptoms, anxiety disorders, and depression (D.W. Black et al. 1992; Carey and Gottesman 1981; Rapoport et al. 1981). Findings from family studies suggest a genetic link between OCD and Tourette's disorder (Nee et al. 1982). A recent large family study reported that OCD was about fourfold more common in relatives of OCD probands than in control relatives, and this finding was more robust for obsessions. Interestingly, age at onset of OCD in probands was very strongly related to familiality; no OCD was detected in relatives of probands with onset after age 18 years (Nestadt et al. 2000b). This study suggests, as does a similar one of panic disorder, that there may exist a more strongly familial subtype of OCD with an earlier onset. Family studies have also shown that OCD spectrum disorders, such as body dysmorphic disorder, hypochondriasis, eating disorder, and grooming conditions, occur at a higher-than-expected frequency in the relatives of subjects with OCD (Bienvenu et al. 2000).

There are reports demonstrating comorbidity of OCD with schizophrenia, depression, other anxiety disorders such as panic disorder and simple and social phobia, eating disorders, autism, and Tourette's disorder. Epidemiologically, the OCD comorbidity risk for other major psychiatric disorders was found to be fairly high but nondistinctive (Karno et al. 1988). In a clinical sample of schizophrenic and schizoaffective patients, about 8% met criteria for OCD, a finding that highlights the importance of screening for obsessive-compulsive symptoms in such populations, in which detection may be more difficult (Eisen et al. 1997).

Etiology

Psychodynamic Theory

Psychodynamic theory views OCD as residing on a continuum with obsessive-compulsive character pathology and suggests that OCD develops when defense mechanisms fail to contain the obsessional character's anxiety. In this model, obsessive-compulsive pathology involves fixation and subsequent regression from the oedipal to the earlier anal developmental phase. The fixation is presumably due to excessive investment in anal eroticism, resulting from excessive frustrations or gratifications in the anal phase.

Obsessive-compulsive patients are thought to use the defense mechanisms of isolation, undoing, reaction formation, and displacement to control unacceptable sexual and aggressive impulses. The defense mechanisms are unconscious and thus not readily apparent to the patient.

Isolation. Isolation is an attempt to separate the feelings or affects from the thoughts, fantasies, or impulses that are associated with them. An example of isolation is seen in the patient who describes a particularly gruesome thought or fantasy but denies any feelings of anxiety or disgust associated with it.

Undoing. Undoing is an attempt to magically reverse a psychological event, such as a word, thought, or gesture. A real or imagined act can be undone by performing or evoking its opposite (e.g., turning on and then turning off a light switch). For example, a patient who feels he has spent too much money on an item for his own pleasure may attempt to undo this by returning the object or by punishing himself through some other deprivation.

Reaction formation. The defense of reaction formation substitutes an unacceptable unconscious impulse with its opposite. Thus, at moments of heightened anger, a patient who has sadistic impulses to hurt people might behave in a passive or masochistic manner or excessively pronounce his love.

Regression. In OCD, regression is theorized to take place from the genital oedipal phase to the earlier pregenital anal-sadistic phase, which has not been fully relinquished. This regression helps the patient avoid genital conflicts and the anxiety associated with them. Themes characteristic of the anal phase typically reflect conflicts surrounding ambivalence, control, dirt, order, and parsimony.

Ambivalence. In normal development, aggressive impulses are neutralized and loving feelings predominate toward significant objects. In OCD, strong aggressive impulses are thought to reemerge toward love objects, resulting in displaced ambivalence and paralyzing doubts. In addition, the characteristic thought omnipotence results in magical ideation and lack of certainty, such that thoughts of harming someone become confused with action and may lead to a sense of uncertainty regarding whether one has actually harmed someone.

Cognitive and Behavioral Theories

A prominent behavioral model of the acquisition and maintenance of obsessive-compulsive symptoms derives from the two-stage learning theory of Mowrer (1939). In stage 1, anxiety is classically conditioned to a specific environmental event (i.e., classical conditioning). The person then engages in compulsive rituals (escape/avoidance responses) to decrease anxiety. If the individual is successful in reducing anxiety, the compulsive behavior is more likely to occur in the future (stage 2: operant conditioning). Higher-order conditioning occurs when other neutral stimuli such as words, images, or thoughts are associated with the initial stimulus and the associated anxiety is diffused. Ritualized behavior preserves the fear response, because the person avoids the eliciting stimulus and thus avoids extinction. Likewise, anxiety reduction following the ritual preserves the compulsive behavior.

Certain types of cognitions and cognitive processes are highly characteristic of OCD and presumably contribute, if not to the genesis, to the maintenance of the disorder. In particular, negative beliefs about responsibility, especially responsibility surrounding intrusive cognitions, may be a key factor influencing obsessive behavior (Salkovskis et al. 2000). Subjects with OCD also appear to have memory biases toward disturbing themes—for example, better memory for contaminated objects in comparison with control subjects with comparable memory (Radomsky and Rachman 1999). Individuals with OCD who check have been found to have not memory impairments—which presumably could account for the increased checking—but rather decreased confidence in their memory (MacDonald et al. 1997). Deficits in selective attention have been reported in people with OCD, and it has been proposed that such deficits may relate to their diminished ability to selectively ignore intrusive cognitive stimuli (Clayton et al. 1999). Deficits in spatial working memory, spatial recognition, and motor initiation and execution have also been found in OCD (Purcell et al. 1998). In contrast to findings in adults, neuropsychological deficits have not been found in children with OCD, suggesting that OCD symptoms may not interfere with cognition earlier in the illness (Beers et al. 1999).

Biological Theories

Although OCD used to be viewed as having a psychological etiology, a wealth of biological findings that have emerged since the 1980s have rendered OCD one of the most elegantly elaborated psychiatric disorders from a biological standpoint. The association of OCD with a variety of neurological conditions or more subtle neurological findings has been known for some time. Such findings include the onset of OCD following head trauma (McKeon et al. 1984) or von Economo's disease (Schilder 1938); a high incidence of neurological premorbid illnesses in OCD (Grimshaw 1964); an association of OCD with birth trauma (Capstick and Seldrup 1977); abnormalities on EEG (Pacella et al. 1944), auditory evoked potentials (Ciesielski et al. 1981; Towey et al. 1990), and ventricular–brain ratio (VBR) on computed tomography scan (Behar et al. 1984); an association with diabetes insipidus (Barton 1965); and the presence of significantly more neurological soft signs in patients with OCD compared with healthy control subjects (Hollander et al. 1990). Basal ganglia abnormalities were particularly suspected in the pathogenesis of OCD, given that OCD is closely associated with Tourette's disorder (Nee et al. 1982; Pauls et al. 1986), in which basal ganglia dysfunction results in abnormal involuntary movements, as well as with Sydenham's chorea, another disorder of the basal ganglia (Barton 1965; Swedo et al. 1989b). Neuropsychological findings in OCD are also of some interest, although not always consistent; they have suggested abnormalities in memory, memory confidence, trial-and-error learning, and processing speed (Christensen et al. 1992; Galderisi et al. 1996; McNally and Kohlbeck 1993; Otto 1992; Rubenstein et al. 1993).

Advances in neuroimaging techniques have permitted a more sophisticated and elaborate elucidation of the functional anatomy underpinning OCD. In particular, orbitofrontal–limbic–basal ganglia circuits have been implicated in numerous studies. Baxter et al. (1987), in a PET study comparing OCD patients with healthy control subjects, found higher metabolic rates in the orbitofrontal gyri and caudate nuclei in the OCD subjects. Similarly, Swedo et al. (1989a) demonstrated higher metabolic activity in the orbitofrontal and cingulate regions in OCD. Flor-Henry (1983) hypothesized that "the fundamental symptomatology of obsessions is due to a defect in neural inhibition of dominant frontal systems, leading to the inability to inhibit unwanted verbal-ideational mental representations and their corresponding motor sequences" (p. 309). It has been suggested that the severity of obsessive urges correlates with orbitofrontal and basal ganglia activity, whereas the accompanying anxiety is reflected by activity in the hippocampus and cingulate cortex (McGuire et al. 1994). With functional MRI, it has been possible to demonstrate that during the behavioral provocation of symptoms in patients with OCD, significant increases in relative blood flow occur in "real time" in the caudate, cingulate cortex, and orbitofrontal cortex relative to the resting state (Adler et al. 2000; Breiter et al. 1996; Rauch et al. 1994). In addition, higher-resolution MRI techniques have revealed volume abnormalities in a variety of brain regions in OCD subjects, including reduced orbitofrontal and amygdalar volumes (Szeszko et al. 1999), smaller basal ganglia (Rosenberg et al. 1997), and enlarged thalamus (Gilbert et al. 2000).

A certain form of OCD with childhood onset is believed to be related to an autoimmune process secondary to streptococcal infection. In children with this form, enlarged basal ganglia consistent with an autoimmune hypothesis have been found on MRI (Giedd et al. 2000). A particular B lymphocyte antigen, which can be identified by the monoclonal antibody D8/17, is expressed in nearly all patients with rheumatic fever and is thought to be a trait marker for susceptibility to group A streptococcal infection complications. Children with OCD and without a history of rheumatic fever or Sydenham's chorea have now been found to have significantly greater B cell D8/17 expression than control children, which suggests that D8/17 may serve as a marker for susceptibility to childhood-onset OCD (Murphy et al. 1997).

Of great interest are an increasing number of studies that demonstrate not only functional but also structural brain changes after various treatments for OCD. After treatment of OCD with serotonin reuptake inhibitors or with behavior therapy, hyperactivity decreases in the caudate, in the orbitofrontal lobes, and in the cingulate cortex in those patients who have good treatment responses (Baxter et al. 1992; Benkelfat et al. 1990; Perani et al. 1995; Swedo et al. 1992a). Also after successful behavioral treatment, the correlations in brain activity between the orbital gyri and the caudate nucleus decrease significantly, suggesting a decoupling of malfunctioning brain circuits (J.M. Schwartz et al. 1996). In children with OCD, MRI scanning revealed a decrease in initially abnormally large thalamic volumes with successful response to paroxetine treatment (Gilbert et al. 2000). This finding was not replicated in children who responded to CBT (Rosenberg et al. 2000). Magnetic resonance spectroscopy has also revealed a decrease in initially elevated caudate glutamate concentration in children with OCD after successful paroxetine treatment (Rosenberg et al. 2000a).

A neuroethological model of OCD was proposed by Rapoport, Swedo, and their group (Swedo 1989; Wise and Rapoport 1989), based on the hypothesized orbitofrontal–limbic–basal ganglia dysfunction. The basal ganglia act as a gating station that filters input from the orbitofrontal and the cingulate cortex and mediates the execution of motor patterns. Obsessions and compulsions are conceptualized as species-specific fixed action patterns that normally are adaptive but in OCD become inappropriately released, repetitive, and excessive. This could be due to a heightened internal drive state or an increased responsivity to external releasers. For example, OCD behaviors such as excessive washing or saving may be dysregulated manifestations of normal grooming or hoarding behaviors. Studies documenting significant volumetric abnormalities in treatment-naïve children with OCD suggest that a developmentally mediated dysplasia of the ventral prefrontal–striatal circuitry may underlie OCD (Rosenberg and Keshavan 1998).

In parallel with the elucidation of OCD's functional neuroanatomy, the neurochemistry of OCD has received extensive elaboration. Serotonin has been implicated in the mediation of impulsivity, suicidality, aggression, anxiety, social dominance, and learning. Dysregulation of this behaviorally inhibitory neurotransmitter possibly contributes to the repetitive obsessions and ritualistic behaviors seen in OCD patients. Despite some conflicting and nonreplicated data, extensive research has now clearly implicated the serotonergic system in the pathogenesis of OCD. Considerable indirect evidence supporting the role of serotonin in OCD stems from the well-documented antiobsessional effects of potent serotonin reuptake inhibitors such as clomipramine and the SSRIs, in contrast to the ineffectiveness of noradrenergic antidepressants such as desipramine. Furthermore, reduction of OCD symptoms during clomipramine treatment was shown to correlate with a decrease in platelet serotonin level (Flament et al. 1987) and in CSF 5-hydroxyindoleacetic acid (5-HIAA) (Altemus et al. 1992; Swedo et al. 1992b; Thoren et al. 1980b). Although one study reported higher CSF 5-HIAA in patients with untreated OCD compared with healthy control subjects (Insel et al. 1985), this finding has not been replicated (Thoren et al. 1980b).

The use of pharmacological challenge agents to stimulate or block serotonin receptors has also proved fruitful in elucidating the neurochemistry of OCD. Oral m-CPP, a partial serotonin agonist, has been found to transiently exacerbate obsessive-compulsive symptoms in a subgroup of patients with OCD (Hollander et al. 1992; Zohar et al. 1987). Results of studies involving intravenous m-CPP have been mixed (Charney et al. 1988; Pigott et al. 1993). After treatment of the OCD with serotonin reuptake inhibitors such as clomipramine or fluoxetine, m-CPP challenge no longer induced symptom exacerbation (Hollander et al. 1991a; Zohar et al. 1988). A blunted prolactin response to m-CPP challenge has also been found in OCD patients by some investigators (Charney et al. 1988; Hollander et al. 1992) but not others (Zohar et al. 1987). Similarly blunted prolactin responses in OCD have been induced with the serotonin agonist MK-212 (Bastani et al. 1990). Other serotonin agonists, such as tryptophan, fenfluramine, and ipsapirone, or antagonists such as metergoline, have not been shown to induce consistent behavioral or neuroendocrine response abnormalities in patients with OCD (Benkelfat et al. 1989; Charney et al. 1988; Hewlett et al. 1992b; Hollander et al. 1992; Lesch et al. 1991; McBride et al. 1992; Zohar et al. 1987).

In summary, all studies taken together suggest that serotonergic dysregulation in OCD is complex and probably involves variations in receptor function according to brain region and receptor subtypes. Thus, global hyperactivity or hypoactivity of the serotonergic system in OCD is a simplistic formulation. The m-CPP findings may suggest not only hypersensitivity of the serotonin receptors mediating obsessive-compulsive behaviors but also hyporesponsivity of the hypothalamic serotonin receptors mediating prolactin secretion (Hollander et al. 1992).

It also does not appear that serotonergic dysregulation alone can fully explain the neurochemistry of OCD. It is possible that the serotonergic system may, in part, be modulating or compensating for other dysfunctional neurotransmitter systems or neuromodulators. Various neuropeptide abnormalities have begun to be elucidated. Abnormalities in CSF vasopressin (Altemus et al. 1992; Swedo et al. 1992b), CSF somatostatin (Altemus et al. 1993), and CSF oxytocin (Leckman et al. 1994) have been implicated in OCD. With clomipramine treatment, CSF levels of vasopressin and somatostatin tend to decrease whereas oxytocin levels increase (Altemus et al. 1994). All these neuropeptides may be implicated in arousal, memory, and the acquisition and maintenance of conditioned perseverative behaviors. The noradrenergic α_2 agonist clonidine has been reported to induce a transient improvement in OCD symptoms when administered to patients intravenously (Hollander et al. 1991b) or orally (Knesevich 1982), although other noradrenergic challenge findings have been negative (Lucey et al. 1992). Dopaminergic dysregulation has been variously implicated in OCD (Goodman et al. 1990a) through the association between OCD and Tourette's disorder; reports of exacerbation of obsessive-compulsive symptoms with chronic stimulant use; an association between higher pretreatment CSF HVA and good treatment outcome (Swedo et al. 1992b); blunted GH response to the dopamine agonist apomorphine (Brambilla et al. 1997);

and use of dopamine blockers to augment partial treatment response with serotonin reuptake inhibitors (McDougle et al. 1990).

In the past few years, the molecular genetics of OCD, still at its infancy, has been the subject of investigation. Segregation analyses have provided strong support for involvement of a single major gene in OCD (Alsobrook et al. 1999; Nestadt et al. 2000), but even should this be so, the major gene has not been identified to date. A functional polymorphism of the catechol-O-methyltransferase (COMT) gene with low enzymatic activity was initially implicated in a recessive manner in OCD (Karayiorgou et al. 1997, 1999), but the finding has not been consistently replicated (Schindler et al. 2000). Polymorphisms in genes related to serotonin and dopamine transmission, such as the tryptophan hydroxylase gene, the $5-HT_{2A}$ receptor gene, the $5-HT_{2C}$ receptor gene, the serotonin transporter gene, the dopamine receptor D_4 gene, and the dopamine transporter gene, were not shown to be associated with OCD in one study (Frisch et al. 2000). Similarly, no association was found for mutations of the $5-HT_{2B}$ receptor gene (Kim et al. 2000), the tryptophan hydroxylase gene (Han et al. 1999), and the $5-HT_{2C}$ receptor gene (Cavallini et al. 1998). Findings regarding the serotonin transporter gene have been both positive (Bengel et al. 1999) and negative (Billet et al. 1997). The $5-HT_{1D}$ receptor gene has also been implicated in OCD (Mundo et al. 2000a). In summary, then, most molecular research conducted to date has focused on serotonin-related genes and has not yielded clear and replicable findings.

Course and Prognosis

Studies of the natural course of the illness suggest that 24%–33% of patients have a fluctuating course, 11%–14% have a phasic course with periods of complete remission, and 54%–61% have a constant or progressive course (A. Black 1974). Although prognosis of OCD has traditionally been considered to be poor, new developments in behavioral and pharmacological treatments have considerably improved this prognosis. The disorder usually has a major impact on daily functioning, with some patients spending many waking hours consumed with their obsessions and rituals. Patients are often socially isolated, marry at an older age, and have high celibacy rates (this is particularly true of male patients) and low fertility rates. Depression and anxiety are common complications of OCD.

Recently, a major follow-up study reported on the course of OCD in patients followed over a 40-year period in Sweden, from approximately the 1950s to the 1990s (Skoog and Skoog 1999). Findings were more optimistic than one might have expected, with improvement noted in 83% of individuals. Of those, about half were fully or almost fully recovered. Importantly, predictors of worse outcome were earlier age at onset, a more chronic course at baseline, poorer social functioning at baseline, having both obsessions and compulsions, and magical symptoms.

In terms of acute treatment, the presence of hoarding obsessions and compulsions is associated with poorer response to medication treatment (Mataix-Cols et al. 1999).

Diagnosis

Although a variety of biological and neuropsychiatric markers have been associated with OCD, the diagnosis rests solely on the psychiatric examination and history. DSM-IV defines OCD as the presence of either obsessions or compulsions that cause marked distress, are time consuming, or interfere with social or occupational functioning. Although all other Axis I disorders are allowed to be comorbidly present, the OCD symptoms must not be merely secondary to another disorder (e.g., thoughts about food in the presence of an eating disorder, guilty thoughts in the presence of major depression). The diagnosis is usually clear-cut, but occasionally it can be more difficult to distinguish OCD from depression, psychosis, phobias, or severe OCPD.

Differential Diagnosis

Schizophrenia

In some cases the course of OCD may more closely resemble that of schizophrenia, with chronic debilitation, decline, and profound impairment in social and occupational functioning. Sometimes it is difficult to distinguish between an obsession (i.e., contamination) and a delusion (i.e., being poisoned). An obsession is typically ego-dystonic, resisted, and recognized as having an internal origin. A delusion is not resisted and is believed to be external. However, OCD patients may lack insight, and in 12% of cases obsessions may become delusions (Gittleson 1966). Yet longitudinal studies show that OCD patients are not at increased risk of developing schizophrenia (A. Black 1974). Both disorders may exist independently, and DSM-IV allows the diagnosis of both disorders. Thus, the presence of significant obsessive-compulsive symptoms in a patient with schizophrenia warrants separate treatment.

Depression

Patients with OCD frequently have complicating depressions, and these patients may be difficult to distinguish from depressed patients who have complicating obsessive symptoms. Patients with psychotic depression, agitated depression, or premorbid obsessional features that occur before development of depression are particularly likely to develop obsessions (Gittleson 1966). These "secondary" obsessions often involve aggressive themes, but the distinction between primary and secondary obsessions rests on the order of occurrence. In addition, depressive ruminations, in contrast to pure obsessions, are often focused on a past incident rather than a current or future event and are rarely resisted.

Phobic Disorders

A close connection exists between OCD and phobic and anxiety disorders. Patients with OCD who are compulsive cleaners appear very similar to phobic individuals and are often mislabeled "germ phobics." Both have avoidant behavior, both show intense subjective and autonomic responses to focal stimuli, and both are said to respond to similar behavioral interventions (Rachman and Hodgson 1980). Both have excessive fear, although disgust is prominent in OCD patients and not in phobic patients. Also, patients with OCD can never entirely avoid the obsession, whereas phobic patients have more focal, external stimuli that they can successfully avoid.

Patients with OCD who experience high levels of anxiety may describe panic-like episodes, but these are secondary to obsessions and do not arise spontaneously. Unlike panic disorder patients, in OCD patients there is no precipitation of anxiety attack with lactate infusions (Gorman et al. 1985). OCD does, however, appear to have increased comorbidity with simple and social phobia and panic disorder (Rasmussen and Tsuang 1986).

Treatment

Pharmacotherapy

Advances in the pharmacotherapy of OCD have been quite dramatic and have generated a great deal of excitement and optimism for successful treatment of this disorder. What was previously thought to be a rare, psychodynamically laden, and difficult-to-treat illness now appears to have a strong biological component and to respond well to potent serotonin reuptake inhibitors. The pharmacological treatment approach to OCD is summarized in Table 11–14.

Serotonin reuptake inhibitors. The most extensively studied medication for the treatment of OCD is clomipramine, a potent serotonin reuptake inhibitor with weak norepinephrine reuptake blockade. A series of well-

TABLE 11–14. Pharmacological treatment of obsessive-compulsive disorder (OCD)

Serotonin reuptake inhibitors

General indications: first-line treatments; moderate to high doses

Fluoxetine, fluvoxamine, sertraline: efficacy shown in large controlled trials

Paroxetine, citalopram: less studied, similar efficacy

Clomipramine: efficacy shown in multiple controlled trials; may have small superiority over SSRIs; however, typically not used until at least two SSRIs have failed secondary to side effect profile; can be used in low doses in combination with SSRIs in more refractory patients—clomipramine + desmethylclomipramine levels must be closely followed for toxicity

Augmentation strategies

General indications: partial response to SSRIs; presence of other target symptoms

Pimozide: comorbid tic disorders or schizotypal personality

Haloperidol: comorbid tic disorders or schizotypal personality

Risperidone: effective augmentation in controlled trial, regardless of tics or schizotypy

Olanzapine: effective in open trials

Pindolol: effective in controlled trial

Clonazepam: effective in controlled trial; comorbid very high anxiety

Buspirone: one positive trial, three negative

Lithium: ineffective in controlled trial

Trazodone: ineffective in controlled trial

Monoamine oxidase inhibitors: hardly any evidence; ? phenelzine in symmetry obsessions

Other medications

Intravenous clomipramine: efficacy in controlled trial of oral clomipramine–refractory patients

Plasma exchange and intravenous immunoglobulin: effective in children with streptococcus-related OCD

---

controlled double-blind studies have undisputedly documented the efficacy of clomipramine in reducing OCD symptoms (Ananth et al. 1981; Asberg et al. 1982; Flament et al. 1985; Insel et al. 1983; Thoren et al. 1980a). The largest of these was a multicenter trial in which clomipramine was compared with placebo in more than 500 patients with OCD. At an average dose of 200–250 mg/day of clomipramine, the average reduction in OCD symptoms was about 40%, and about 60% of all patients were clinically much or very much improved (Clomipramine Collaborative Study Group 1991). The very low placebo response rate of 2% documents that OCD is a chronic disorder with infrequent spontaneous remissions. Patients should typically be started on 25 mg of clomipramine taken at bedtime, and the dose should then be gradually increased by 25 mg every 4 days or by

50 mg every week, until a maximum dose of 250 mg is reached. Some patients are unable to tolerate the highest dose and may be stabilized on 150 or 200 mg. Improvement with clomipramine is relatively slow, with maximal response occurring after 5–12 weeks of treatment. Some of the more common side effects reported by patients are dry mouth, tremor, sedation, nausea, and ejaculatory failure (in men). The seizure risk is comparable to that of other TCAs and is acceptable in the absence of a neurological history for dosages up to 250 mg/day. Clomipramine is equally effective for OCD patients with pure obsessions and those with rituals, in contrast to behavioral treatments, which are less useful for patients suffering predominantly from obsessions. Although one study found a greater effect of clomipramine compared with placebo only in the most depressed subgroup (Marks et al. 1980), most studies have found strong specific antiobsessional effects irrespective of depressive symptoms (Ananth et al. 1981; Clomipramine Collaborative Study Group 1991; Flament et al. 1985; Insel et al. 1983; Thoren et al. 1980a). Controlled studies have also demonstrated that clomipramine is effective in treating OCD when other antidepressants, such as amitriptyline, nortriptyline, desipramine, and the MAOI clorgyline have no therapeutic effect (Ananth et al. 1981; Insel et al. 1983; Leonard et al. 1989; Thoren et al. 1980a; Zohar and Insel 1987). This finding strongly suggests that improvement in OCD symptoms is mediated through the blockade of serotonin reuptake.

Studies with the SSRIs have further supported this hypothesis in that these agents have turned out to be essentially as efficacious as clomipramine. A controlled study comparing clomipramine and fluoxetine in the treatment of OCD did not find a significant difference in efficacy between the two drugs (Pigott et al. 1990), although the response with fluoxetine appeared somewhat less robust than the response with clomipramine. Similarly, fluvoxamine and clomipramine have been found to have similar efficacy in treating OCD (Mundo et al. 2000b). Numerous large, controlled trials emerged in the 1990s that definitively documented the efficacy of all SSRIs for this disorder. Fluoxetine at dosages of 20–60 mg/day was shown to be superior to placebo in treating OCD, with greater efficacy at higher doses (Montgomery et al. 1993; Tollefson et al. 1994). Similarly, fluoxetine has been shown to be safe and efficacious in treating OCD in children (Riddle et al. 1992).

Fluvoxamine was also found to have a significant antiobsessional effect in several controlled studies (Goodman et al. 1989, 1990b; Jenike et al. 1990a; Perse et al. 1987), with efficacy comparable to that of clomipramine (Freeman et al. 1994; Koran et al. 1996). Goodman and his group (1990b) showed that fluvoxamine is superior to desipramine in treating OCD. In their study, 52% of patients demonstrated marked clinical improvement independent of initial depression. The required daily dose is titrated up to a maximum of 300 mg. The efficacy of fluvoxamine for OCD has also been demonstrated in adolescent patients, at dosages of 100–300 mg/day (Apter et al. 1994). The efficacy of fluvoxamine in the treatment of pediatric OCD (ages 8–17 years) was further confirmed in a multicenter trial that used doses of 50–200 mg/day. Forty-two percent of the subjects were responders (defined as a 25% symptomatic improvement), and the medication was well tolerated; asthenia and insomnia were the most common side effects (Riddle et al. 2001).

Sertraline is another serotonin reuptake inhibitor whose efficacy in OCD has been established. Although an initial placebo-controlled study revealed no beneficial effect (Jenike et al. 1990b), subsequent studies have shown sertraline to be superior to placebo at daily doses ranging from 50 to 200 mg (Chouinard 1992; Greist et al. 1995a; Kronig et al. 1999). In one study, response began to appear as early as the third week of treatment and was firmly apparent by the eighth week (Kronig et al. 1999). Similarly, sertraline has been found to be effective in treating childhood OCD (ages 6–17 years) in a large multicenter trial that used doses up to 200 mg/day. Again, improvement started to appear around the third week, and 42% of children were significantly improved after 12 weeks. The medication was well tolerated overall, the most common side effects being agitation, insomnia, nausea, and tremor (March et al. 1998b).

Although paroxetine and citalopram have not been as extensively studied as other SSRIs in the treatment of adult OCD (Koponen et al. 1997; Montgomery et al. 2001; Mundo et al. 1997; D.J. Stein et al. 2001; Zohar and Judge 1996), they appear to be as efficacious and are widely used at dosages of 20–60 mg/day. There is also limited evidence that citalopram may be helpful in refractory OCD (Bejerot and Bodlund 1998; Marazziti et al. 2001; Pallanti et al. 1999). In open trials of pediatric subjects with OCD, both paroxetine (Rosenberg et al. 1999) and citalopram (Thomsen 1997) have been found to be effective and safe.

Although clomipramine appears to have an edge in documented efficacy for treating OCD, satisfactory systematic comparisons of the various serotonin reuptake inhibitors, balancing benefits and side effects, have not been conducted. Given the similar efficacy of these medications in OCD, an extremely large prospective study would have to be undertaken to demonstrate small but significant differences between the various medications.

Three meta-analytic studies addressed these questions by retrospectively analyzing treatment data from previous trials; results supported a small but significant superiority for clomipramine over the SSRIs (Greist et al. 1995b; Piccinelli et al. 1995; D.J. Stein et al. 1995). However, the clinical applicability of this finding may be limited, because in clinical practice, actual or expected tolerability of different medications often takes precedence over small differences in efficacy. For most patients, the SSRIs are better tolerated than clomipramine (because of clomipramine's strong anticholinergic side effects) and have therefore become the well-established first line of treatment for OCD. If patients do not have a good response to an adequate trial of at least two SSRIs, clomipramine augmentation or monotherapy should be undertaken; the reverse is also true.

Augmentation strategies. It is important to keep in mind that the medication response in OCD is not as dramatic as that in, for example, major depression: a considerable number of patients show a negligible or partial response to the first-line medications described in this section. As a helpful rule of thumb, it is useful to remember that approximately 40%–60% of patients with OCD improve by about 30%–60% with a first-line drug. Thus, various combination and augmentation strategies are often needed to attain a satisfactory response. The most commonly used augmenting agents, unfortunately not always with strong scientific findings supporting their effectiveness, are buspirone, lithium, tryptophan, trazodone, clonazepam, risperidone, olanzapine, pindolol, desipramine, inositol, and the MAOIs. With more rigorous testing in recent years, many of these augmentation strategies no longer look as promising as was initially thought. Still, given the relatively limited treatment options, these strategies are well worth undertaking sequentially, beginning with the most compelling ones. In the following paragraphs we summarize the findings in favor of or against the various augmenting agents for OCD.

Although a small study initially reported similar efficacy for clomipramine alone versus buspirone alone in treating OCD (Pato et al. 1991), three other studies failed to show a significant benefit for buspirone augmentation in clomipramine-treated (Pigott et al. 1992b), fluoxetine-treated (Grady et al. 1993), or fluvoxamine-treated (McDougle et al. 1993b) patients, whereas one study described clinical improvement in 10 of 20 OCD patients who underwent buspirone augmentation of fluoxetine treatment (Jenike et al. 1991a). If buspirone is tried, higher doses of 30–60 mg/day should be aimed for. A controlled study of lithium augmentation of clomipramine did not detect any benefit (Pigott et al. 1991). A controlled study of trazodone monotherapy in OCD likewise found no benefit in comparison with placebo (Pigott et al. 1992a). A controlled crossover study showed clonazepam to be effective in 40% of subjects with OCD who had failed to respond to clomipramine trials (Hewlett et al. 1992a), and clonazepam may also be helpful with the very high anxiety levels frequently associated with OCD (Hewlett et al. 1990). Evidence in support of MAOIs is very weak despite a positive report (Vallejo et al. 1992), possibly with the exception of some benefit for symmetry obsessions from phenelzine (Jenike et al. 1997). A controlled trial of lithium augmentation was negative (McDougle et al. 1991a), as were controlled trials of trazodone monotherapy (Pigott et al. 1992a) and desipramine augmentation of SSRI treatment (Barr et al. 1997). In a small open trial, 10 patients with OCD who had not responded to serotonin reuptake inhibitor trials were treated with inositol augmentation, at 18 mg/day, for 6 weeks; only 3 patients reported clinically significant improvement, leaving inositol also as an option of unclear efficacy (Seedat and Stein 1999).

Antipsychotics are a major medication class that can be successfully used to augment partial response to serotonin reuptake inhibitors in OCD. McDougle et al. (1990) first reported that about 50% of patients with OCD improved noticeably when pimozide was added to fluvoxamine therapy; comorbid tic disorders or schizotypal personality predicted a good response, a finding that supports the hypothesis that the dopaminergic system may be dysregulated in at least a subgroup of patients with OCD (Goodman et al. 1990a). OCD patients with comorbid tic disorders may actually be less responsive to SSRI monotherapy (McDougle et al. 1993a), and they appear to respond well to haloperidol augmentation (McDougle et al. 1994).

In more recent years, atypical antipsychotics have received increasing attention as a major augmentation strategy for OCD, regardless of comorbid tics or schizotypy, and such a strategy is now supported by controlled trials. Risperidone has been used successfully for augmentation in open trials, with good results for horrific mental imagery (Saxena et al. 1996). In another open 8-week trial in which risperidone 3 mg/day was added to an SSRI in 20 patients with refractory OCD, all were described as showing some improvement (Pfanner et al. 2000). More compellingly, a controlled 6-week trial of risperidone in patients refractory to a serotonin reuptake inhibitor found significant improvement in half of the patients (McDougle et al. 2000); this response was not associated with whether tics or schizotypy were present. Four pediatric patients with refractory OCD were also described as responsive to risperidone augmentation

(Fitzgerald et al. 1999). Olanzapine appears to be as promising as risperidone. In a 3-month open augmentation trial with olanzapine in OCD patients unresponsive to fluvoxamine, almost half showed notable improvement (Bogetto et al. 2000). Similarly, benefits were noted in the majority of subjects who had partially responded to an SSRI and were augmented openly with olanzapine for 8 weeks (Weiss et al. 1999). In a probably more refractory sample of nine OCD patients who had failed to respond in more than three serotonin reuptake inhibitor trials, three showed at least a 30% improvement with 8-week open olanzapine augmentation at doses of 2.5–10.0 mg/day (Koran et al. 2000). When considering antipsychotic use, it should be borne in mind that the atypical antipsychotic clozapine has been reported to worsen OCD, possibly because of its particular serotonergic properties, although reports are contradictory (R.W. Baker et al. 1992; Ghaemi et al. 1995). Regardless, clozapine does not appear to be beneficial, at least as monotherapy (McDougle et al. 1995).

Other than antipsychotics, pindolol is the only additional medication proven to be a useful augmentation agent in a controlled study (Dannon et al. 2000). Fourteen patients with treatment-refractory OCD who had not responded to three SSRI trials received paroxetine augmentation with pindolol or placebo for 6 weeks. In comparison with placebo, pindolol at 2.5 mg three times daily was significantly superior in reducing OCD symptoms.

The combination of clomipramine with an SSRI is another strategy commonly used in treating refractory patients. Although clomipramine is generally well tolerated, lower doses of clomipramine should be used and blood levels monitored to avoid toxicity (because clomipramine levels can become markedly elevated) (Szegedi et al. 1996). In one small randomized trial in patients with refractory OCD, citalopram combined with clomipramine led to significantly greater improvement than did citalopram alone (Pallanti et al. 1999).

When oral medications fail to be successful enough in highly refractory patients, other options can be considered, including cognitive-behavioral techniques (which are described later on) and several other biological interventions. Electroconvulsive therapy may also be considered in highly refractory cases, although its efficacy is debatable (Maletzky et al. 1994). Intravenous clomipramine has been successful in some patients who are unresponsive to oral clomipramine (Fallon et al. 1992; Warneke 1985). In a more recent controlled study, intravenously administered clomipramine proved more effective than intravenous placebo in a trial with 54 patients with OCD refractory to oral clomipramine; 58% of patients were responders, and the treatment was safely tolerated (Fallon et al. 1998). Plasma exchange and intravenous immunoglobulin have been found to be effective in lessening symptom severity in children with streptococcal infection–triggered OCD (Perlmutter et al. 1999), but plasma-exchange treatment was found not to help children whose OCD did not have streptococcus-related exacerbations (Nicolson et al. 2000). In extreme cases of refractory, severely impaired OCD patients, neurosurgery can be considered. Jenike et al. (1991b), in a thorough retrospective analysis, estimated that cingulotomy resulted in notable improvement in at least 25%–30% of patients. This response rate was confirmed in a 2-year prospective cingulotomy study (Baer et al. 1995). A comparable response rate of 38% was reported in another study at follow-up 10 years after the sterotactic surgery (Hay et al. 1993). Guidelines for the use of neurosurgical techniques in the treatment of severe, refractory OCD—including selection, documented failed treatments, indications, contraindications, benefits, risks, and workup—have been thoroughly reviewed elsewhere (Mindus and Jenike 1992). A recent review of 29 patients who underwent capsulotomy between 1976 and 1989 at the Karolinska Hospital in Stockholm, Sweden, found localized successful lesioning to the middle of the anterior limb of the internal capsule (Lippitz et al. 1999). Most recently, transcranial magnetic stimulation has been used in OCD and appears to have some promise; however, this technique requires much further study (Greenberg et al. 1997).

Although there are no definitive predictors of medication treatment response, several factors appear to be predictive of a poorer prognosis, including earlier age at onset, longer duration of illness, higher frequency of compulsions, presence of washing rituals, a chronic course, prior hospitalizations, and comorbid avoidant, borderline, and schizotypal as well as multiple personality disorders (Ackerman et al. 1994; Baer and Jenike 1992; Baer et al. 1992; Ravizza et al. 1995). A recent review of 274 patients with OCD found no differences between responsive and nonresponsive subjects in age, gender, age at onset, duration of illness, or symptom subtypes. Responders had a higher incidence of family history of tics, sudden onset of OCD, and an episodic course of illness. Nonresponders had more severe symptoms, poorer insight into their OCD, and comorbid eating disorder (Hollander et al. 2001).

OCD tends to be a chronic illness, and many patients may require ongoing drug treatment to stay well. Long-term continuation of medication treatment generally maintains a good treatment response; this strategy is widely supported in clinical treatment and was validated by a 1-year double-blind maintenance study that used sertraline dosages of 50–200 mg/day (Greist et al. 1995c). In a subsequent study, patients who maintained their response in the latter study were given a second year of open maintenance treatment with sertraline at the same doses, during which they maintained or even slightly improved their gains (Rasmussen et al. 1997). Conversely, in a double-blind discontinuation study of OCD patients who had done well on clomipramine for about 1 year, 90% experienced substantial worsening within 7 weeks (Pato et al. 1988). The same relapse rate of 90% was found in an adolescent OCD group when chronic clomipramine was blindly substituted with 8 weeks of desipramine (Leonard et al. 1991). Again at 1-year follow-up, patients who were randomly assigned to continue fluoxetine rather than be switched to placebo had much lower rates of relapse (Romano et al. 2001). At follow-up several years later, most patients remained symptomatic and required continued pharmacotherapy, with a substantial minority of 20% remaining refractory to multiple treatment regimens (Leonard et al. 1993).

Behavioral Therapy

Behavioral treatments of OCD involve two separate components: 1) exposure procedures that aim to decrease the anxiety associated with obsessions and 2) response prevention techniques that aim to decrease the frequency of rituals or obsessive thoughts. Exposure techniques include systematic desensitization with brief imaginal exposure and flooding (in which prolonged exposure to the real-life ritual-evoking stimuli causes profound discomfort). The ultimate goal of exposure techniques is to decrease the discomfort associated with the eliciting stimuli through habituation. In exposure therapy, the patient is assigned homework exercises, performance of which may require assistance either from the therapist (via home visits) or from family members. Response prevention requires patients to face feared stimuli (e.g., dirt, chemicals) without resorting to excessive hand washing or to tolerate doubt (e.g., "Is the door really locked?") without succumbing to excessive checking. Initial work may involve delaying performance of the ritual, but ultimately the patient works to fully resist the compulsions. The psychoeducation and support of family members can be pivotal to the success of the behavioral therapy, because family dysfunction is prevalent and the majority of parents or spouses accommodate to or are involved in the patients' rituals, possibly as a way to reduce the anxiety or anger that patients may direct at their family members (Calvocoressi et al. 1995; Shafran et al. 1996).

It is generally agreed that combined behavioral techniques (e.g., exposure with response prevention) yield the greatest improvement. It is also generally reported that patients who primarily suffer from obsessions and have few rituals are the least responsive to behavioral treatment, although new behavioral techniques for obsessions may be more promising (Salkovskis and Westbrook 1989). When the combined techniques of in vivo exposure and response prevention were used, up to 75% of ritualizing patients willing and able to undergo the arduous treatment were reported to show significant improvement (Marks et al. 1975). Marks et al. (1988) reported that self-exposure was the most powerful treatment component; however, clomipramine doses in this study were rather low (i.e., 125–150 mg), and therapist-aided exposure was instituted late in the treatment and only briefly. The addition of imaginal exposure to in vivo exposure/response prevention is reported to help maintain treatment gains, perhaps by moderating obsessive fears of future catastrophes (Steketee et al. 1982). Foa et al. (1984) systematically compared in vivo exposure, response prevention, and the two treatments combined. All groups improved, but the combined treatment was superior in decreasing anxiety, rituals, and overall impairment. The proportion of clinical responders, defined as those patients who showed at least 30% improvement with treatment, was 33% for response prevention, 55% for exposure, and 90% for combination treatment. Of interest, this study found that most OCD patients successfully treated with behavior therapy had relapsed at follow-up, which suggests that, just as with medication, long-term behavioral maintenance treatment may be necessary. Predictors of poorer outcome for behavioral treatment of OCD include initial depression, initial OCD severity, longer duration, and lower motivation for treatment (Keijsers et al. 1994). Exposure and response prevention has also been used successfully to treat children and adolescents with OCD, with at least 50% improvement in the vast majority of subjects (Franklin et al. 1998). A maintenance program can be highly effective in helping patients retain the benefits of CBT over several years of follow-up (Marks 1997; McKay 1997).

It is not yet well understood how behavioral techniques compare with medications in treatment of OCD. Also of interest is the question of the degree to which the results of controlled behavioral trials, in which highly selected individuals meeting stringent inclusion criteria are enrolled, generalize to broader community samples. A recent study investigated this important question and found comparable success for exposure and prevention therapy conducted in an outpatient fee-for-service setting (Franklin et al. 2000). In a study comparing behavioral treatment and clomipramine pharmacotherapy in children with OCD, both were similarly helpful, suggesting that nonpharmacological options might be good first-line options in the younger population in an initial attempt to avoid medication (de Haan et al. 1998).

Cognitive Therapy

Another modality that has more recently been advocated in the treatment of OCD is cognitive therapy, which centers on cognitive reformulation of themes related to the perception of danger, estimation of catastrophe, expectations about anxiety and its consequences, excessive responsibility, thought–action fusion, and illogical inferences (Freeston et al. 1996; O'Connor and Robillard 1996; Rachman et al. 1995; vanOppen and Arntz 1994). A review of 15 open and controlled cognitive trials in patients with OCD showed little evidence of improvement overall when cognitive therapy was added to the existing pharmacological and behavioral techniques (I.A. James and Blackburn 1995). However, one controlled study found cognitive therapy's effectiveness to be similar to that of exposure and response prevention in treating OCD (vanOppen et al. 1995).

Combination Therapy

Combination therapy is commonly used and recommended in the treatment of OCD. Unless symptoms are mild or subjects highly motivated to begin with CBT techniques, a common approach used in clinical practice is to start out with medication, attain a degree of improvement that will allow better utilization of CBT, and then possibly attempt some degree of medication taper once CBT has been mastered and observed to be effective. In a recent study testing this commonly used paradigm, it appeared quite effective (Simpson et al. 1999). Patients who remained symptomatic with a 12-week course of an SSRI received a course of exposure and ritual prevention and demonstrated a 50% decrease in their OCD symptoms (Simpson et al. 1999). Another study that compared behavioral or cognitive monotherapy with initial SSRI treatment subsequently complemented with such therapies showed no differences among the treatments. These findings were interpreted as suggesting that psychotherapy alone may be sufficient, at least in this group of subjects (van Balkom et al. 1998). Finally, a meta-analytic comparison study of OCD treatments, after controlling for a number of confounding variables, found that clomipramine, SSRIs, and exposure with response prevention all had comparable results (Kobak et al. 1998).

Other Psychotherapies

Patients with OCD frequently present with symptoms that appear laden with unconscious symbolism and dynamic meaning. However, OCD has generally proven refractory to psychoanalytically oriented, as well as to loosely structured, nondirective exploratory psychotherapies. In contrast to its lack of efficacy in treating chronic OCD, dynamic psychotherapy may be helpful for patients with acute and limited symptoms who are otherwise psychologically minded and motivated to explore their conflicts, as well as in dealing with obsessive character traits of perfectionism, doubting, procrastination, and indecisiveness (Salzman 1985). However, controlled clinical data are not available to support these clinical impressions.

Patients with OCD need supportive treatment even while pharmacotherapy or behavior therapy is being applied. Because of their tendency toward excessive doubt, these patients may require a great deal of reassurance during the early phase of treatment. More active supportive therapy that encourages risk taking helps patients with OCD live with their anxiety, and a focus on the present has been reported to be helpful (Salzman 1985). In addition, psychoeducational support groups for patients and their families have been described as being highly successful in helping treat these patients (D.W. Black and Blum 1992; Tynes et al. 1992).

Posttraumatic Stress Disorder

PTSD was first introduced in DSM-III, its inclusion being spurred in part by the increasing recognition of posttraumatic conditions in veterans of the Vietnam War. The current DSM-IV-TR criteria for PTSD are presented in Table 11–15. As in DSM-III-R, the disorder continues to be classified with the anxiety disorders, and the major criteria of an extreme precipitating stressor, intrusive recollections, emotional numbing, and hyperarousal have been maintained. The DSM-III-R descriptor of the traumatic event as one "outside the range of usual human experience" was considered rather vague and unreliable and was eliminated. New duration criteria were also established, subdividing the disorder into acute or chronic.

Not all investigators agree that PTSD belongs with the anxiety disorders. Although anxiety is a prominent symptom, so are depression and dissociation. The diagnostic criterion of a precipitating stressor or trauma in PTSD makes this disorder different from other anxiety disorders and is more reminiscent of conditions such as brief reactive psychosis, acute stress disorder, patho-logical bereavement, and adjustment disorders. The International Classification of Diseases, Tenth Revision (ICD-10; World Health Organization 1992), for example, classifies all such disorders as stress related. In acknowledgment of the spectrum of disorders stemming from severe stress, DSM-IV added acute stress disorder (ASD) to the anxiety disorders. Acute stress disorder is similar to PTSD with regard to the precipitating traumatic event and to symptomatology but is time limited, occurring up to 1 month after the event. In addition, dissociative symptoms figure prominently in the definition of acute stress disorder, whereas they are not addressed in the PTSD description. It has now been well established by a number of studies, including prospective ones, that ASD is a highly reliable predictor of developing PTSD down the road; it may well be that the two should not be defined as discrete disorders. In a study of people who sustained mild traumatic brain injury in motor vehicle accidents, 82% of those who met ASD criteria were diagnosed with PTSD 6 months later (Bryant and Harvey 1998), as opposed to only 11% of those without ASD, and a steady 80% were diagnosed with PTSD 2 years after the accident (Harvey and Bryant 2000). The DSM-IV-TR diagnostic criteria for ASD are presented in Table 11–16.

Beyond the symptoms of PTSD per se, increasing attention has been drawn to an enduring constellation of traits that frequently develop in individuals subjected to chronic trauma as children or adults. Investigators such as Herman and van der Kolk had originally suggested that a discrete entity of complicated posttraumatic syndromes be recognized, otherwise designated as DESNOS (disorders of extreme stress not otherwise specified), characterized by lasting changes in identity, interpersonal relationships, and the sense of life's meaning (Herman et al. 1989; van der Kolk and Saporta 1991). Similar personality changes are recognized in ICD-10 and are classified as "enduring personality change after catastrophic experience." In the past decade, attention has increasingly been focused on the concept of "trauma-spectrum" disorders, which can include admixtures of posttraumatic stress, dissociative, somatoform, and conversion symptoms, and the classification approach to trauma-related conditions is a subject of ongoing debate.

Clinical Description

A soldier participates in the torture and murder of civilians. A passenger is the sole survivor of a commercial airliner crash. A woman is raped and severely beaten by an unknown assailant. The characteristic features that may develop after a traumatic event such as these include psy-

TABLE 11–15. DSM-IV-TR diagnostic criteria for posttraumatic stress disorder

A. The person has been exposed to a traumatic event in which both of the following were present:
    (1) the person experienced, witnessed, or was confronted with an event or events that involved actual or threatened death or serious injury, or a threat to the physical integrity of self or others
    (2) the person's response involved intense fear, helplessness, or horror.   **Note:** In children, this may be expressed instead by disorganized or agitated behavior
B. The traumatic event is persistently reexperienced in one (or more) of the following ways:
    (1) recurrent and intrusive distressing recollections of the event, including images, thoughts, or perceptions.   **Note:** In young children, repetitive play may occur in which themes or aspects of the trauma are expressed.
    (2) recurrent distressing dreams of the event.   **Note:** In children, there may be frightening dreams without recognizable content.
    (3) acting or feeling as if the traumatic event were recurring (includes a sense of reliving the experience, illusions, hallucinations, and dissociative flashback episodes, including those that occur on awakening or when intoxicated).   **Note:** In young children, trauma-specific reenactment may occur.
    (4) intense psychological distress at exposure to internal or external cues that symbolize or resemble an aspect of the traumatic event
    (5) physiological reactivity on exposure to internal or external cues that symbolize or resemble an aspect of the traumatic event
C. Persistent avoidance of stimuli associated with the trauma and numbing of general responsiveness (not present before the trauma), as indicated by three (or more) of the following:
    (1) efforts to avoid thoughts, feelings, or conversations associated with the trauma
    (2) efforts to avoid activities, places, or people that arouse recollections of the trauma
    (3) inability to recall an important aspect of the trauma
    (4) markedly diminished interest or participation in significant activities
    (5) feeling of detachment or estrangement from others
    (6) restricted range of affect (e.g., unable to have loving feelings)
    (7) sense of a foreshortened future (e.g., does not expect to have a career, marriage, children, or a normal life span)
D. Persistent symptoms of increased arousal (not present before the trauma), as indicated by two (or more) of the following:
    (1) difficulty falling or staying asleep
    (2) irritability or outbursts of anger
    (3) difficulty concentrating
    (4) hypervigilance
    (5) exaggerated startle response
E. Duration of the disturbance (symptoms in Criteria B, C, and D) is more than 1 month.
F. The disturbance causes clinically significant distress or impairment in social, occupational, or other important areas of functioning.
Specify if:
    Acute: if duration of symptoms is less than 3 months
    Chronic: if duration of symptoms is 3 months or more
Specify if:
    With Delayed Onset: if onset of symptoms is at least 6 months after the stressor

chic numbing, reexperiencing of the trauma, and increased autonomic arousal. The trauma is reexperienced in recurrent painful and intrusive recollections, daydreams, or nightmares. Dissociative states may occur, lasting from minutes to days, in which there is a dream-like, unreal state with hazy memory and a distorted sense of time. Psychic numbing or emotional anesthesia is manifested by diminished responsiveness to the external world, with feelings of being detached from other people, loss of interest in usual activities, and inability to feel emotions such as intimacy, tenderness, or sexual interest. Symptoms of excessive autonomic arousal may include hyperactivity and irritability, an exaggerated startle

response, difficulty concentrating, and sleep abnormalities. Rape or mugging victims sometimes become afraid to venture out alone for variable periods of time. Situations reminiscent of the original trauma may be systematically avoided.

Other symptoms may include guilt about having survived, guilt about not having prevented the traumatic experience, depression, anxiety, panic attacks, shame, and rage. There may be prolonged episodes of intense affect; increased irritability; explosive, hostile behavior; and impulsive behavior. Other accompanying or complicating symptoms associated with PTSD may include substance abuse, self-injurious behavior and suicide

---

TABLE 11–16. DSM-IV-TR diagnostic criteria for acute stress disorder

A. The person has been exposed to a traumatic event in which both of the following were present:
   (1) the person experienced, witnessed, or was confronted with an event or events that involved actual or threatened death or serious injury, or a threat to the physical integrity of self or others
   (2) the person's response involved intense fear, helplessness, or horror

B. Either while experiencing or after experiencing the distressing event, the individual has three (or more) of the following dissociative symptoms:
   (1) a subjective sense of numbing, detachment, or absence of emotional responsiveness
   (2) a reduction in awareness of his or her surroundings (e.g., "being in a daze")
   (3) derealization
   (4) depersonalization
   (5) dissociative amnesia (i.e., inability to recall an important aspect of the trauma)

C. The traumatic event is persistently reexperienced in at least one of the following ways: recurrent images, thoughts, dreams, illusions, flashback episodes, or a sense of reliving the experience; or distress on exposure to reminders of the traumatic event.

D. Marked avoidance of stimuli that arouse recollections of the trauma (e.g., thoughts, feelings, conversations, activities, places, people).

E. Marked symptoms of anxiety or increased arousal (e.g., difficulty sleeping, irritability, poor concentration, hypervigilance, exaggerated startle response, motor restlessness).

F. The disturbance causes clinically significant distress or impairment in social, occupational, or other important areas of functioning or impairs the individual's ability to pursue some necessary task, such as obtaining necessary assistance or mobilizing personal resources by telling family members about the traumatic experience.

G. The disturbance lasts for a minimum of 2 days and a maximum of 4 weeks and occurs within 4 weeks of the traumatic event.

H. The disturbance is not due to the direct physiological effects of a substance (e.g., a drug of abuse, a medication) or a general medical condition, is not better accounted for by brief psychotic disorder, and is not merely an exacerbation of a preexisting Axis I or Axis II disorder.

---

attempts, occupational impairment, and interference with interpersonal relationships.

Epidemiology

Although there are marked individual differences in how people react to stress, when stressors become extreme, such as in concentration camp situations or in extended combat, the rate of morbidity rapidly increases (Eitinger 1971; Krystal 1968). Posttraumatic syndromes may be found in up to 30% of victims of disasters (Chapman 1962). Long-term physical health effects have been noted in persons 30 years after their having survived concentration camps (Eitinger 1971).

Although this disorder has been more extensively studied in select groups, such as survivors of combat, concentration camps, and natural disasters, the ECA study investigated the occurrence of PTSD in the general population (Helzer et al. 1987). A 1% lifetime prevalence of PTSD was found (0.5% in men and 1.3% in women). The nature of the precipitating trauma differed between the two sexes. Combat and witnessing someone's injury or death were the two traumas identified in men, whereas physical attack or threat accounted for almost half of the traumas in women. In another large, random community survey of young adults, the lifetime prevalence of PTSD was 9.2%, higher than that found in the ECA study (Breslau et al. 1991). As in the ECA study, the prevalence was higher in women (11.3%) than in men (6%). In the more recent National Comorbidity Survey, the lifetime prevalence of PTSD was similarly found to be 7.8%, much higher than in the ECA study, and was more common in women. The most common stressors were combat exposure in men and sexual assault in women (Kessler et al. 1995).

Symptoms of PTSD, albeit too few in number to meet the full diagnostic criteria, are quite common in the general population. In a Canadian community survey, full PTSD was found in 2.7% of women and 1.2% of men, whereas partial PTSD was found in an additional 3.4% of women and 0.3% of men. Such individuals, seemingly women in particular, may be important to identify, because they experience clinically meaningful distress and functional impairment (M.B. Stein et al. 1997). The gender difference in PTSD prevalence, higher in women, has been consistent across several studies. It appears that women are more likely to develop PTSD than are men with comparable exposure to traumatic events, especially if exposure is before age 15 years (Breslau et al. 1997b). This difference is not well understood and could involve characteristics of both the individuals and the traumatic experiences.

A high rate of comorbid disorders is found in PTSD. In the ECA study, the highest comorbidity was with affective disorders and OCD. Men with PTSD had no increased risk for panic disorder or phobias, whereas women with PTSD had a three- to fourfold increased risk for these disorders (Helzer et al. 1987). In the survey by Breslau et al. (1991), a high comorbidity risk was found for OCD, agoraphobia, panic, and depression, whereas the association with drug or alcohol abuse was weaker. Comorbidity of PTSD with depression is a very consistent finding, although the nature of the relationship between the two conditions is controversial. Epidemiological analyses suggest that in trauma survivors, the vulnerabilities for PTSD and depression are not separate; rather, the risk for depression is highly elevated in just those trauma survivors who manifest PTSD (Breslau et al. 2000). On the other hand, a prospective study of a large sample of trauma survivors found depression and PTSD to be independent sequelae of trauma (Shalev et al. 1998b). Regardless of causality, it is clear that PTSD in women increases the risk for a new onset of both depression and alcohol use disorder (Breslau et al. 1997a). Individuals with PTSD may be more likely to manifest borderline or self-defeating personality disorder, and it appears that the actual PTSD diagnosis rather than the trauma history accounts for this association (Shea et al. 2000).

Etiology

The Role of the Stressor

The severity of the stressor in PTSD differs in magnitude from that found in adjustment disorder, which is usually less severe and within the range of common life experience. However, this relationship between the severity of the stressor and the type of subsequent symptomatology is not always predictable. For example, studies of bereavement and divorce have found that stressors within the range of usual human experience can also produce a distinctive syndrome of reexperiencing the trauma (Horowitz et al. 1980). In effect, it has generally been underemphasized that in the average community setting, events such as sudden loss of a spouse are a much more frequent cause of PTSD than are assault and violence (Breslau et al. 1998).

Nevertheless, events such as sexual assault or armed robbery, which are interpersonal insults to integrity, self-esteem, and security, are particularly likely to lead to PTSD. When stressors become extreme (e.g., rape, extended combat, torture, concentration camp experiences), the rate of morbidity significantly increases. For example, the ECA study found that in men who had served in Vietnam, 4% of those who were in combat but were not wounded had PTSD, whereas 20% of combat veterans who had been wounded developed PTSD. In even more horrendous conditions, such as those endured by U.S. prisoners of war of the Japanese in World War II, extremely high PTSD incidence rates have been

reported: 84% lifetime and 59% decades after (Engdahl et al. 1997). Variable PTSD rates have been found in individuals subjected to major noninterpersonal trauma; for example, reported rates in severely injured accident victims range from a very low 2% (Schnyder et al. 2001) to 32% (Koren et al. 1999). In those sustaining severe traumatic brain injury, a 27% PTSD incidence has been reported (Bryant et al. 2000a). Childhood interpersonal trauma can often result in PTSD, as is widely known clinically and documented by numerous studies. In an inner-city child psychiatry clinic, more than half of the traumatized children had syndromal or subsyndromal PTSD, with experiencing physical abuse or witnessing domestic violence being the strongest contributors (Silva et al. 2000). In a large community sample followed prospectively into young adulthood, about one-third of the children who had suffered substantiated sexual abuse, physical abuse, or neglect had PTSD (Widom 1999). On average, it is estimated that approximately one-fourth of all individuals who experience major trauma develop PTSD (Breslau et al. 1991). In addition, as described by McFarlane, a definite dose–response relationship exists between the impact of the trauma and PTSD. Still, it is rare even for overwhelming trauma to lead to PTSD in more than half of the exposed populations, clearly suggesting that other etiological factors also play a role (McFarlane 1990). A discussion of such predictors follows.

Risk Factors and Predictors

There is general agreement in the literature that a variety of premorbid risk factors predispose to the development of PTSD. Although the disorder can certainly develop in people without significant preexisting psychopathology, a number of biological and psychological variables have been identified that render individuals more vulnerable to the development of PTSD. In one study in a Vietnam veteran outreach center, a prior history of good adolescent friendships was predictive of PTSD, whereas a history of poor adolescent friendships was more likely in those who did not have PTSD. In addition, this study described several patients with good premorbid adjustment, low childhood trauma, and good adolescent relationships who developed severe PTSD after experiencing prolonged trauma in Vietnam (Lindy et al. 1984). In general, however, previous adversity has been associated with a higher likelihood of developing PTSD.

It has been suggested that the greater the amount of previous trauma experienced by an individual, the more likely he or she is to develop symptoms after a stressful life event (Horowitz et al. 1980). In addition, individuals with previous traumatic experiences may be more likely to become exposed to future traumas, because they can be prone to reenact the original trauma behaviorally (van der Kolk 1989). In a study of Vietnam veterans, individuals with PTSD had higher rates of childhood physical abuse than veterans without PTSD, as well as a significantly higher rate of total traumatic events before entrance into the military (Bremner et al. 1993a).

McFarlane (1989) found that the severity of exposure to disaster was the major determinant of early posttraumatic morbidity, whereas preexisting psychological disorders better predicted the persistence of posttraumatic symptoms over time. A number of psychiatric conditions in probands and in their relatives appear to predispose these individuals to develop PTSD. In the ECA sample, a history of childhood conduct problems before age 15 years was predictive of PTSD. Patients with anxious premorbid states and family histories of anxiety may also respond to a trauma with pathological anxiety and develop PTSD (Scrignar 1984). An epidemiological survey identified, albeit retrospectively, different risk factors for becoming exposed to trauma versus developing PTSD after traumatic exposure (Breslau et al. 1991). Risk factors for exposure to trauma were male sex, childhood conduct problems, extraversion, and family history of substance abuse or psychiatric problems. Risk factors for developing PTSD after traumatic exposure were disrupted parental attachments, anxiety, depression, and family history of anxiety. Having an Axis II disorder also increases the risk for chronic PTSD (Ursano et al. 1999). Having a past history of PTSD increases the risk for both acute and chronic PTSD (Ursano et al. 1999). Compared with nonchronic PTSD, chronic PTSD of more than 1 year's duration has been specifically associated with higher rates of comorbid anxiety and depressive disorders and a family history of antisocial behavior (Breslau and Davis 1992).

Interestingly, parental PTSD is a risk factor for PTSD in offspring, even in the absence of elevated trauma (Yehuda et al. 1998b). Findings with regard to gender are conflicting, in that female gender was found to be associated with chronic PTSD in one study (Breslau and Davis 1992) but with only acute PTSD in another (Ursano et al. 1999a). An additional factor that has been associated with a higher likelihood of developing PTSD is lower premorbid intelligence (Macklin et al. 1998). Neurological compromise, with increased neurological soft signs and a childhood history of neurodevelopmental problems and lower intelligence, is associated with PTSD and could possibly be a predisposing risk factor (Gurvits et al. 2000).

Early predictors of PTSD after a traumatic event have also received great attention, and their potential significance for early intervention and prevention is obvious. As previously stated, the occurrence of ASD in the first month after trauma is a very strong predictor of later PTSD. ASD diagnosis combined with a resting heart rate greater than 90 has a surprisingly high sensitivity, 88%, and specificity, 85%, in predicting development of PTSD (Bryant et al. 2000b). Similarly, high heart rate and decreased cortisol in the acute aftermath of trauma strongly correlate with later PTSD (Yehuda et al. 1998a). Even elevated heart rate, on its own, shortly after trauma is a significant predictor of later PTSD (Shalev et al. 1998a). The importance of the very early reaction to a traumatic event in predicting PTSD cannot be underestimated: early PTSD-type symptoms within 1 week of a traffic accident predict PTSD 1 year later (Koren et al. 1999).

In recent years, increased attention has been given to dissociative phenomena and to their relationship with posttraumatic symptoms (Spiegel and Cardena 1990). Greater dissociation around the time of the traumatic event is a strong predictor of subsequent development of PTSD (Marmar et al. 1994; Shalev et al. 1996). Individuals with peritraumatic dissociation are 4–5 times more likely than those without such phenomena to develop both acute and chronic PTSD (Ursano et al. 1999b). It may be that early peritraumatic dissociation can serve as a "marker" to identify individuals who will be at high risk of developing PTSD in the future.

Cognitive and Behavioral Theories

A cognitive model proposed to explain the persistence of PTSD symptoms postulates that PTSD becomes persistent when individuals process their trauma in a way that leads to a sense of serious and current threat. Such threat processing consists of excessively negative appraisals of the trauma or its consequences and a disruption in autobiographical memory involving poor contextualization and strong associative memory (Ehlers and Clark 2000).

Behavioral theory suggests that a disturbance of conditioned responses occurs in PTSD. Autonomic responses to both innocuous and aversive stimuli are elevated, with larger responses to unpaired cues and reduced extinction of conditioned responses (Peri et al. 2000). It is proposed that individuals with PTSD have higher sympathetic system arousal at the time of conditioning and therefore are more conditionable than trauma-exposed individuals without PTSD (Orr et al. 2000). Individuals with PTSD also generalize fear-related conditioned responses across stimuli, having been sensitized by stress (Grillon and Morgan 1999).

Recent studies have also revealed a number of disturbances in cognitive processes associated with PTSD. For example, the high incidence of PTSD after severe traumatic brain injury involving loss of consciousness but few traumatic memories suggests that trauma can mediate PTSD in part at an implicit level (Bryant et al. 2000a). Impairments in explicit memory have been associated with PTSD (Bremner et al. 1993b; Jenkins et al. 1998) and may be related to hippocampal toxicity resulting from stress-mediated elevations in norepinephrine (Bremner et al. 1995). In addition, subjects with PTSD may exhibit recall deficits not for trauma-related words, but rather for positive and neutral words, suggesting that avoidance of the encoding of disturbing information does not occur in PTSD (McNally et al. 1998). This appears consistent with the intrusive nature of traumatic memories clinically encountered in the disorder. Indeed, there appears to be an attentional bias toward traumatic stimuli in PTSD (Bryant and Harvey 1997), whereas generalized attentional disturbances have not been found (Golier et al. 1997).

Biological Theories

More than a century ago, Janet described the breakdown in normal adaptation, information processing, and action that can result from overwhelming trauma and noted the automatic emotional and physical overreaction that occurs with reexposure (van der Kolk and van der Hart 1989). Freud (1919/1955) implicated a biological basis to posttraumatic symptoms, in the form of a physical fixation to the trauma. Pavlov (1927/1960) demonstrated chronic change in autonomic nervous system activity level in response to repeated traumatic exposure. Kardiner (1959) comprehensively described the phenomenology of war traumatic neurosis, identifying five cardinal features: 1) persistence of startle response, 2) fixation on the trauma, 3) atypical dream life, 4) explosive outbursts, and 5) overall constriction of personality. He called this condition a *physioneurosis*, a term implying an interaction of psychological and biological processes, which served as a forerunner of current psychobiological models of PTSD.

Noradrenergic system. The neurobiological response to acute stress and trauma involves the release of various stress hormones that allow the organism to respond adaptively to stress. These releases include heightened secretion of catecholamines and cortisol. When PTSD develops under severe or repeated trauma, the stress response becomes dysregulated and chronic autonomic hyperactivity sets in, manifesting itself in the "positive" symptoms of PTSD—that is, the hyperarousal and intrusive

recollections. A wide range of data support this hypothesis. The noradrenergic system, originating in the locus coeruleus, regulates arousal (Southwick et al. 1999). Animals exposed to inescapable shock initially show evidence of increased turnover of norepinephrine, with subsequent depletion of central norepinephrine (Anisman et al. 1980). Animals that have experienced previous inescapable shock are more sensitive to norepinephrine depletion. In patients with PTSD, heightened physiological responses to stressful stimuli, such as blood pressure, heart rate, respiration, galvanic skin response, and electromyographic activity, have been consistently documented (Kolb 1987; Pitman et al. 1987). Long-standing increases in the urinary catecholamines norepinephrine and epinephrine have been found in patients with PTSD (Kosten et al. 1987; Spivak et al. 1999), as well as elevated plasma norepinephrine (Spivak et al. 1999). Agents that stimulate the arousal system, such as lactate (Rainey et al. 1987) and yohimbine (Southwick et al. 1993, 1997), induce flashbacks and increases in core PTSD symptoms. Clinical improvement in intrusive recollections and hyperarousal during open treatment with adrenergic-blocking agents, such as clonidine or propranolol, also suggests adrenergic hyperactivity (Kolb et al. 1984). A decrease in the number and sensitivity of α_2-adrenergic receptors, possibly as a consequence of chronic noradrenergic hyperactivity, has been reported in PTSD (Perry et al. 1987). Downregulation of the α_2-adrenergic receptor is also supported by one case report of a PTSD patient with a blunted GH response to clonidine, which normalized after behavioral treatment (Hansenne et al. 1991).

Endogenous opioid system. Whereas affective numbing was understood, in the past, primarily as a psychological defense against overwhelming emotional pain, more recent research has suggested a biological component to the "negative" symptoms of PTSD. van der Kolk et al. (1984) proposed that animal models of inescapable shock may parallel the development of PTSD in humans. Animals prevented from escaping from severe stress develop a syndrome of learned helplessness (Maier and Seligman 1976) that resembles the symptoms of constricted affect, withdrawal, amotivation, and decline in functioning associated with PTSD.

Animals exposed to prolonged or repeated inescapable stress develop analgesia, which appears to be mediated by release of endogenous opiates and which is blocked by the opiate antagonist naloxone (Kelly 1982; Maier et al. 1980). Similarly, it is suggested that in humans who have experienced prolonged or repeated trauma, endogenous opiates are readily released with any stimulus that is reminiscent of the original trauma, leading to analgesia and psychic numbing (van der Kolk et al. 1984). Pitman et al. (1990) compared pain intensity in response to thermal stimuli in Vietnam veterans with PTSD and veterans without PTSD who were watching a war videotape. PTSD patients, but not control subjects, had a 30% analgesic effect (i.e., decreased pain intensity) when pretreated with a placebo injection; this analgesia was eliminated with naloxone pretreatment. On the basis of such findings, the concept of trauma addiction has been proposed (van der Kolk et al. 1984). After a transient opioid burst on reexposure to traumatic stimuli, accompanied by a subjective sense of calm and control, opiate withdrawal may set in. This withdrawal may then contribute to the hyperarousal symptoms of PTSD, leading the individual into a vicious cycle of traumatic reexposures to gain transient symptomatic relief.

The noradrenergic and opiatergic systems of the brain interact and may serve reciprocal functions. Clonidine, an α_2-adrenergic agonist, has been shown to suppress opiate withdrawal symptoms in opiate addiction (Gold et al. 1980). Open treatment with clonidine in Vietnam veterans with PTSD demonstrated substantial decreases in hyperreactivity (Kolb et al. 1984).

Serotonergic system. The serotonergic system has also been implicated in the symptomatology of PTSD (van der Kolk and Saporta 1991), although such work is still in its infancy. The septohippocampal brain system contains serotonergic pathways and mediates behavioral inhibition and constraint. The role of serotonergic deficit in impulsive aggression has been studied extensively. In animals, repeated inescapable shock can lead to serotonin depletion. Thus, the irritability and outbursts seen in patients with PTSD may be related to serotonergic deficit. The partial serotonin agonist m-CPP induces an increase in PTSD symptoms suggestive of serotonergic sensitization; interestingly, the PTSD subjects showing this response appear to constitute a separate subgroup from the ones exhibiting noradrenergic sensitization (Southwick et al. 1997). Decreased plasma serotonin levels have been found in PTSD (Spivak et al. 1999). A blunted prolactin response to fenfluramine challenge is similarly supportive of central serotonergic dysregulation in PTSD (Davis et al. 1999). The efficacy of SSRIs in PTSD is indirectly supportive of dysregulated serotonergic modulation in PTSD.

Hypothalamic-pituitary-adrenal axis. A number of findings in PTSD have implicated a chronic dysregulation of HPA axis functioning that is highly characteristic of this disorder and distinct from that seen in other psychiatric disorders such as depression. The findings include elevated CSF corticotropin-releasing hormone (D.G. Baker et al. 1999; Bremner et al. 1997a), low urinary cortisol concentrations (J.W. Mason et al. 1986) and an elevated urinary norepinephrine–cortisol ratio (J.W. Mason et al. 1988), a blunted ACTH response to CRF (Smith et al. 1989), enhanced suppression of cortisol in response to dexamethasone administration, and a decrease in lymphocyte glucocorticoid receptor number. All of these findings are consistent with a model of a highly sensitized HPA axis that is hyperresponsive to stress and the effects of cortisol (Yehuda et al. 1993, 1995a).

Brain circuitry and neuroimaging findings. A number of neuroimaging findings, both structural and functional, in PTSD studies over the past several years have begun to delineate a model suggestive of limbic sensitization and diminished cortical inhibition in PTSD, with specific dysfunction in brain areas involved in memory, emotion, and visuospatial processing (Bremner et al. 1999a). Functional deficits in verbal memory have been correlated with decreased hippocampal volume on MRI in combat-related PTSD (Bremner et al. 1995). Similarly, a decrease in hippocampal volume has been found in adult survivors of childhood abuse (Bremner et al. 1997b). PET imaging with PTSD symptom provocation via audiotaped traumatic scripts revealed activation of the right limbic and paralimbic systems and of the visual cortex (Rauch et al. 1996). PET imaging during auditory exposure to traumatic scripts has shown that abuse memories are associated with decreased blood flow in the medial prefrontal cortex, hippocampus, and visual association cortex (Bremner et al. 1999a). When mental images of combat-related pictures are generated by PTSD veterans, blood flow increases in the amygdala and anterior cingulate and decreases in Broca's area. These patterns may relate to the nonverbal emotional visual imagery involved in the reexperiencing of PTSD symptoms (Shin et al. 1997). Enhanced amygdalar responses to general negative stimuli (not specifically related to trauma) have been found in PTSD and appear to be dissociated from higher cortical influences (Rauch et al. 2000). Indeed, exposure of subjects with PTSD to traumatic stimuli results in decreased blood flow in the medial prefrontal cortex, an area responsible for the regulation of emotional response via inhibition of the amygdala (Bremner et al. 1999b). There is evidence, based on case reports, that successful treatment of PTSD with eye movement desensitization and reprocessing (EMDR) may result not in reduced limbic activity but rather in increased cingulate and prefrontal activity, which enhances the ability to differentiate real threat (Levin et al. 1999).

Genetics. A large study of Vietnam veteran twins found that genetic factors accounted for 13%–34% of the variance in liability to the various PTSD symptom clusters, whereas no etiological role was found for shared environment (True et al. 1993). Molecular genetic studies of PTSD are sparse. An initial study found an association between PTSD and a polymorphism of the dopamine D_2 receptor (Comings et al. 1996); however, this finding was not replicated in a later study (Gelernter et al. 1999).

Course and Prognosis

Scrignar (1984) divided the clinical course of PTSD into three stages. Stage I involves the response to trauma. Nonsusceptible persons may experience an adrenergic surge of symptoms immediately after the trauma but do not dwell on the incident. Predisposed persons have higher levels of anxiety and dissociation at baseline, an exaggerated response to the trauma, and an obsessive preoccupation with the trauma after the trauma has occurred. If symptoms persist beyond 4–6 weeks, the patient enters stage II, or acute PTSD. Feelings of helplessness and loss of control, symptoms of increased autonomic arousal, reliving of the trauma, and somatic symptoms may occur. The patient's life becomes centered around the trauma, with subsequent changes in lifestyle, personality, and social functioning. Phobic avoidance, startle responses, and angry outbursts may occur. In stage III, chronic PTSD develops, with disability, demoralization, and despondency. The patient's emphasis changes from preoccupation with the actual trauma to preoccupation with the physical disability resulting from the trauma. Somatic symptoms, chronic anxiety, and depression are common complications at this time, as are substance abuse, disturbed family relations, and unemployment. Some patients may focus on compensation and lawsuits.

A retrospective study examined patterns of treatment length in PTSD and compared characteristics of short-term patients (i.e., those who were successfully treated within 3 months) with those of long-term patients (i.e., those who received treatment for more than 12 months) (Burstein 1986). All patients were treated with medication and psychotherapy. No difference was found between the two groups with regard to type of stressor, reported symptom distress, possible financial compensation factors, length of time from trauma to intervention, and various demographic features. In this study, the number of patients who were treated successfully in a brief period was almost equal to the number of patients who underwent a prolonged course of treatment. Compared with the patients who were treated over a short period, the patients who required long-term treatment needed higher daily doses of imipramine and may have been more depressed after the first 3 months of treatment. This study did not relate imipramine effects to presence of panic attacks.

In another study, it was found that the rate of full remission from chronic PTSD over a 5-year prospectively studied period was only 18%, highlighting the frequent chronicity of the illness. Histories of alcohol abuse and childhood trauma were associated with less remission (Zlotnick et al. 1999). Even when studies correct for comorbid psychiatric or medical disorders, people with PTSD are found to manifest significant impairment in major domains of living, such as physical limitations, unemployment, poor physical health, and diminished well-being. Thus, in multiply afflicted patients, it may be crucial to specifically target and treat PTSD if present (Zatzick et al. 1997).

Diagnosis

The diagnosis of PTSD is usually not difficult if there is a clear history of exposure to a traumatic event, followed by symptoms of intense anxiety lasting at least 1 month, along with arousal and stimulation of the autonomic nervous system, numbing of responsiveness, and avoidance or reexperiencing of the traumatic event. However, a wide variety of anxiety, depressive, somatic, and behavioral symptoms for which the relationship between their onset and the traumatic event is less clear-cut may easily lead to misdiagnosis.

Differential Diagnosis

Organic Mental Disorders

Following acute physical traumas, head trauma, or concussion, an organic mental disorder must be ruled out, because this diagnosis has important treatment implications. Mild concussions may leave no immediate apparent neurological signs but may have residual long-term effects on mood and concentration. A careful evaluation of the nature of the head trauma, including a review of medical records and witnesses' observations, followed by mental status evaluation and neurological examination, and, if indicated, laboratory examinations, is essential in a diagnostic workup. Malnutrition may occur during prolonged stressful periods and may also lead to organic brain syndromes. Survivors of death camps may have symptoms of an organic mental disorder such as failing memory, difficulty concentrating, emotional lability, headaches, and vertigo. Other causes of organic mental disorder may occasionally mimic PTSD if anxiety, depression, personality changes, or abnormal behaviors are present. Abnormalities of cognition, memory, altered sensorium or level of consciousness, or focal neurological signs would suggest an organic mental disorder.

Organic mental disorders that could mimic PTSD include organic personality syndrome, delirium, amnestic syndrome, organic hallucinosis, and organic intoxication and withdrawal states. In addition, patients with PTSD may cope with their disorder through excessive use of alcohol, drugs, caffeine, or tobacco and thus may present with a combination of organic and psychological factors. In such cases, each concomitant disorder should be diagnosed.

Mood and Anxiety Disorders

Major depression. There is much overlap between PTSD and major mood disorders. Symptoms such as psychic numbing, irritability, sleep disturbance, fatigue, anhedonia, impairments in family and social relationships, anger, concern with physical health, and pessimistic outlook may occur in both disorders. In some veteran outreach populations, 70%–80% of patients meet diagnostic criteria for both disorders. Major depression is a frequent complication of PTSD; when it occurs, major depression must be treated aggressively, because comorbidity carries an increased risk of suicide. If major depression develops secondary to PTSD, both disorders should be diagnosed. Dysthymic symptoms are frequently secondary to PTSD, but if they are of sufficient severity, the additional diagnosis of dysthymic disorder should be made.

Phobic disorders. After a traumatic event, patients may be aversively conditioned to the surroundings of the trauma and may develop a phobia of objects, surroundings, or situations that remind them of the trauma itself. Phobic patients experience anxiety in the feared situation, whereas avoidance is accompanied by anxiety reduction that reinforces the avoidant behavior. In PTSD, the phobia may be symptomatically similar to specific phobia, but the nature of the precipitant and the symptom cluster of PTSD distinguish this condition from simple phobia.

Generalized anxiety disorder. The symptoms of GAD, such as motor tension, autonomic hyperactivity, apprehensive expectation, and vigilance and scanning, are also present in PTSD. However, the onset and course of the illness differ: GAD has an insidious or gradual onset and a course that fluctuates with environmental stressors, whereas PTSD has an acute onset often followed by a chronic course. Phobic symptoms, which are absent in GAD, are often present in PTSD. DSM-IV does not allow for the diagnosis of GAD if PTSD is present.

Panic disorder. Patients with PTSD may also experience panic attacks. In some patients, panic attacks predate the PTSD or do not occur exclusively in the context of stimuli reminiscent of the traumatic event. In other patients, however, panic attacks develop after the PTSD and are cued solely by traumatic stimuli.

Adjustment disorder. Adjustment disorders are maladaptive reactions to identifiable psychosocial pressures. Signs and symptoms may include a wide variety of disturbances and emerge within 3 months of the stressful event. If symptoms are of sufficient severity to meet other Axis I criteria, the diagnosis of adjustment disorder is not made. Adjustment disorder differs from PTSD in that the stressor in adjustment disorder is usually less severe and within the range of common experience and the characteristic symptoms of PTSD, such as reexperiencing the trauma, are absent. The prognosis of full recovery in adjustment disorder is usually excellent.

Compensation neurosis (factitious disorder and malingering). Both factitious disorder and malingering involve conscious deception and feigning of illness, although the motivation for each condition differs. Factitious disorder may present with physical or psychological symptoms, the feigning of symptoms is under voluntary control, and the motivation is to assume the "patient" role. Chronic factitious disorder with physical symptoms (i.e., Munchausen syndrome) involves frequent doctor visits and surgical interventions. PTSD differs from this disorder by absence of fabricated symptoms, acute onset after a trauma, and absence of a bizarre pretraumatic medical history.

Malingering involves the conscious fabrication of an illness for the purpose of achieving a definite goal such as obtaining money or compensation. Malingerers often reveal an inconsistent history, unexpected symptom clusters, a history of antisocial behavior and substance abuse, and a chaotic lifestyle, and there is often a discrepancy between history, claimed distress, and objective data.

Postconcussion syndrome. Mental disorders secondary to head injury are influenced by physiological, psychological, and environmental factors. Psychological symptoms are extremely common after mild closed-head injuries, even when the injuries do not involve loss of consciousness. The so-called postconcussion syndrome encompasses the symptoms of headache, dizziness, irritability, and emotional lability after head injury with concussion. Depression and lethargy are the affective symptoms that occur most commonly. These symptoms bear no relation to the degree of physical injury.

Treatment

Pharmacotherapy

A variety of different psychopharmacological agents have been used in the treatment of PTSD by clinicians and reported in the literature as case reports, open clinical trials, and controlled studies. A summary of the pharmacological treatment of PTSD is presented in Table 11–17. In the past few years, SSRIs and other serotonergic agents have emerged as the first-line pharmacological treatment of PTSD.

TABLE 11–17. Pharmacotherapy of posttraumatic stress disorder (PTSD)

Selective serotonin reuptake inhibitors (SSRIs)

General indications: first-line treatment; well tolerated; once-daily dosing; documented efficacy

Sertraline: U.S. Food and Drug Administration–approved, large controlled trials

Fluoxetine: large controlled trials

Fluvoxamine, paroxetine: open trials, similar efficacy

Nefazodone: next first-line option if poor response to or intolerance of SSRIs; several open trials, one in treatment-refractory patients; no controlled trials

Other antidepressants

Tricyclics: overall modest results when tested in double-blind fashion

Monoamine oxidase inhibitors: may be superior to tricyclics, especially for intrusive symptoms

Augmentation

General indications: when response to first-line options not adequate; additional treatment of specific PTSD symptoms or comorbid disorders

Clonidine: some efficacy in open treatment

Lithium: improvement in intrusive symptoms and irritability in open trial

Carbamazepine: decrease intrusive symptoms, anger, impulsivity in open treatment

Valproate: decreased hyperarousal and intrusion, not numbing, in open treatment

Lamotrigine: very small controlled trial, some efficacy

Buspirone: efficacy in an open trial

Triiodothyronine: improvement in small open trial, possibly antidepressant response

Cyproheptadine: case reports of decreased nightmares

Bupropion: no change in PTSD, improvement in depression

Trazodone, benzodiazepines, diphenhydramine: sleep disturbance

Nefazodone

Adrenergic blockers. Kolb et al. (1984) treated 12 Vietnam veterans with PTSD in an open trial of the β-blocker propranolol over a 6-month period. Dosage ranged from 120 to 160 mg/day. Eleven patients reported a positive change in self-assessment at the end of the 6-month period, with less explosiveness, fewer nightmares, improved sleep, and a decrease in intrusive thoughts, hyperalertness, and startle response. Another open pilot study by this group (Kolb et al. 1984) using clonidine, an noradrenergic α₂ agonist, was conducted in nine Vietnam veterans with PTSD. Daily doses of 0.2–0.4 mg of clonidine were administered over a 6-month period. Eight patients reported reduced explosiveness and improvement in their capacity to control their emotions, and a majority reported improvements in sleep and nightmares; lowered startle response, hyperalertness, and intrusive thinking; and psychosocial improvement. These findings support the role of noradrenergic hyperactivity in the maintenance of autonomic arousal symptoms in PTSD. In a retrospective treatment review of Cambodian patients with PTSD, Kinzie and Leung (1989) found that most benefited from the combination of clonidine and a TCA, as opposed to either medication taken alone. Controlled studies of adrenergic blockers in PTSD are needed.

Tricyclic antidepressants. Until about a decade ago, most reports on the pharmacotherapy of PTSD involved the use of TCAs. A retrospective study by Bleich et al. (1986) of 25 patients with PTSD treated with a variety of different antidepressants, including TCAs and MAOIs, reported good or moderate results in 67% of the patients treated. Response was not clearly related to the presence of somatization symptoms, depression, or panic attacks. Antidepressants appeared to be more useful than major tranquilizers. Although antidepressants improved intrusion-type symptoms, their most prominent impact was decreased insomnia and an overall sedative effect. Antidepressants also were found to have a positive impact on psychotherapy in 70% of cases.

Burstein (1984), in administering imipramine at daily doses of 50–350 mg to 10 patients with recent-onset PTSD, observed significant improvement in intrusive recollections, sleep and dream disturbance, and flashbacks. Similar improvement in intrusive symptomatology was reported with an open trial of desipramine (Kauffman et al. 1987). A positive effect of imipramine on posttraumatic night terrors was reported by J. R. Marshall (1975).

Although controlled studies of TCAs in PTSD were subsequently conducted, they were unable to replicate the earlier trials' success in decreasing posttraumatic symptoms. In a 4-week, double-blind crossover study of desipramine and placebo in 18 veterans with PTSD, only depressive symptoms improved; anxiety, intrusive symptoms, and avoidance did not change with desipramine therapy (Reist et al. 1989). Davidson et al. (1990) conducted a 4- to 8-week double-blind comparison of amitriptyline and placebo in 46 veterans with PTSD. Although depression and anxiety decreased with amitriptyline therapy, the decrease in intrusive and avoidant symptoms was apparent only in the subgroup of patients who completed 8 weeks of amitriptyline therapy and was marginal. At the end of the study, roughly two-thirds of patients in both treatment groups still met the criteria for PTSD.

Monoamine oxidase inhibitors. An early study of MAOIs described five patients with "traumatic war neurosis" in whom phenelzine, at doses of 45–75 mg/day, improved traumatic dreams, flashbacks, startle reactions, and violent outbursts (Hogben and Cornfield 1981). Panic attacks were also described in all of the patients in this study. Positive effects of phenelzine on intrusive posttraumatic symptoms have been reported in subsequent small open trials (Davidson et al. 1987; van der Kolk 1983).

An 8-week randomized double-blind trial subsequently compared phenelzine (71 mg), imipramine (240 mg), and placebo in 34 veterans with PTSD (Frank et al. 1988). Both antidepressants resulted in some overall improvement in patients' posttraumatic symptoms, and phenelzine tended to be superior to imipramine. The most marked improvement was the decrease in intrusive symptoms in patients receiving phenelzine, with an average reduction of 60% on the intrusion scale measure.

Serotonin reuptake inhibitors. Earlier on, multiple open trials with SSRIs suggested that these medications had at least modest efficacy for the treatment of PTSD, and in the past few years SSRIs have become the medications of choice for this disorder. Several initial open trials of fluoxetine reported marked improvement in PTSD symptoms at a wide range of doses (Davidson et al. 1991; McDougle et al. 1991b; Shay 1992). Subsequently, in a double-blind trial comparing fluoxetine and placebo, fluoxetine led to a significant reduction of PTSD symptomatology, especially for arousal and numbing symptoms (van der Kolk et al. 1994). An initial open trial of sertraline (Brady et al. 1995) also claimed benefit for PTSD. Sertraline is now FDA approved for the treatment of PTSD, in the wake of two large controlled trials that recently documented its efficacy. In a 12-week, multicenter, placebo-controlled trial, sertraline at doses of 50–200 mg/day resulted in significant benefits that began to appear by week 2. The response rate was over 50%, and improvement in both numbing and arousal symptoms, although not in reexperiencing, was significantly greater than with placebo (Brady et al. 2000). Comparable results were reported in another large sertraline study with very similar design (Davidson et al. 2001), with a 60% response rate by conservative intent-to-treat analysis. Open trials of other SSRIs, such as fluvoxamine (De Boer et al. 1992) and paroxetine (R.D. Marshall et al. 1998), suggest that these medications have similar efficacy in PTSD, despite the lack of controlled trials.

Mood stabilizers and anticonvulsants. In a small open trial of lithium treatment of PTSD, van der Kolk (1983) reported improvement in intrusive recollections and irritability in more than half of the patients treated. However, there have been no controlled trials. In an open trial of carbamazepine in 10 patients with PTSD, Lipper et al. (1986) reported moderate to great improvement in intrusive symptoms in 7 patients. Wolf et al. (1988) reported decreased impulsivity and angry outbursts in 10 veterans who were also treated with carbamazepine; all patients had normal EEGs. Valproate was initially reported to decrease irritability and angry outbursts in two veterans with PTSD (Szymanski and Olympia 1991). More recently, in an open trial of 16 patients treated with valproate for 8 weeks, a significant decrease in symptoms of hyperarousal and intrusion, but not of numbing, was reported (Clark et al. 1999b). In a very small, placebo-controlled trial of lamotrigine at doses up to 500 mg/day, more patients appeared to respond to lamotrigine than to placebo (Hertzberg et al. 1999), a finding warranting larger studies.

Other medications. Several open trials have described benefits with nefazodone treatment. A 12-week study using a mean dose of 430 mg/day showed improvement in all three symptom clusters in patients with previously treatment-refractory PTSD (Zisook et al. 2000). An 8-week open trial reported similar improvements in patients with chronic PTSD (Davis et al. 2000), whereas another report found a 60% response rate in treatment completers (Davidson et al. 1998), and yet another described improvement in all 10 patients treated (Hertzberg et al. 1998). Thus, nefazodone appears very promising in treating PTSD and a controlled trial is warranted.

A small open trial of buspirone reported that seven out of eight patients experienced a significant reduction in PTSD symptoms; there are no controlled studies (Duffy and Malloy 1994). In a small open trial, triiodothyronine was reported to result in significant clinical improvement in four out of five PTSD patients who had only partial responses to SSRIs; however, it remains unclear whether this was not primarily an antidepressant response (Agid et al. 2001). Cyproheptadine has been reported to greatly decrease the nightmares characteristic of PTSD (Clark et al. 1999a; Gupta et al. 1998). An open trial of bupropion in PTSD reported global improvement secondary to decreased depression, but PTSD symptoms remained mostly unchanged (Canive et al. 1998).

Psychotherapy

It is generally agreed that some form of psychotherapy is necessary in the treatment of posttraumatic pathology. Crisis intervention shortly after the traumatic event is effective in reducing immediate distress, possibly preventing chronic or delayed responses, and, if the pathological response is still tentative, may allow for briefer intervention.

Brief dynamic psychotherapy has been advocated both as an immediate treatment procedure and as a way of preventing chronic disorder. The therapist must establish a working alliance that allows the patient to work through his or her reactions.

The literature has suggested that persons with disrupted early attachments or abuse, who have been traumatized earlier in their lives, are more likely to develop PTSD than are those with stable backgrounds. The occurrence of psychic trauma in a person's past may psychologically and biologically predispose him or her to respond excessively and maladaptively to intense experiences and affects (Herman et al. 1989; Krystal 1968; van der Kolk 1987b). Therefore, attempting to modify preexisting conflicts, developmental difficulties, and defensive styles that render the person especially vulnerable to traumatization by particular experiences is central to the treatment of traumatic syndromes.

The "phase oriented" treatment model suggested by Horowitz (1976) strikes a balance between initial supportive interventions to minimize the traumatic state and increasingly aggressive "working through" at later stages of treatment. Establishment of a safe and communicative relationship, reappraisal of the traumatic event, revision of the patient's inner model of self and world, and planning for termination with a reexperiencing of loss are all important therapeutic issues in the treatment of PTSD. Herman et al. (1989) emphasized the importance of validating the patient's traumatic experiences as a precondition for reparation of damaged self-identity.

Embry (1990) outlined seven major parameters for effective psychotherapy in war veterans with chronic PTSD: 1) initial rapport building, 2) limit setting and supportive confrontation, 3) affective modeling, 4) defocusing on stress and focusing on current life events, 5) sensitivity to transference–countertransference issues, 6) understanding of secondary gain, and 7) therapist's maintenance of a positive treatment attitude.

Group psychotherapy can also serve as an important adjunctive treatment, or as the central treatment mode, in traumatized patients (van der Kolk 1987a). Because of past experiences, such patients are often mistrustful and reluctant to depend on authority figures, whereas the identification, support, and hopefulness of peer settings can facilitate therapeutic change.

Drug treatment has been impressionistically reported to have a beneficial effect on psychotherapy in 70% of cases, with improvements in symptom severity leading to a more positive and motivated approach to psychotherapy and an enhanced accessibility to uncovering and working through (Bleich et al. 1986).

Cognitive and Behavioral Therapies

A variety of cognitive and behavioral techniques have gained increasing popularity and validation in the treatment of PTSD. People involved in traumatic events such as accidents frequently develop phobias or phobic anxiety related to or associated with these situations. When a phobia or phobic anxiety is associated with PTSD, systematic desensitization or graded exposure has been found to be effective. This is based on the principle that when patients are gradually exposed to a phobic or anxiety-provoking stimulus, they will become habituated or deconditioned to the stimulus. Variations of this treatment include using imaginal techniques (i.e., imaginal desensitization) and exposure to real-life situations (i.e., in vivo desensitization). Prolonged exposure (i.e., flooding), if tolerated by a patient, can also be useful and has been reported to be successful in the treatment of Vietnam veterans (Fairbank and Keane 1982).

Relaxation techniques produce the beneficial physiological result of reducing motor tension and lowering the activity of the autonomic nervous system, effects that may be particularly efficacious in PTSD. Progressive muscle relaxation involves contracting and relaxing various muscle groups to induce the relaxation response. This technique is useful for symptoms of autonomic arousal such as somatic symptoms, anxiety, and insomnia. Hypnosis has also been used, with success, to induce the relaxation response in PTSD.

Cognitive therapy and thought stopping, in which a phrase and momentary pain are paired with thoughts or images of the trauma, have been used to treat unwanted mental activity in PTSD. A recent randomized trial compared imaginal exposure and cognitive therapy in 72 patients with chronic PTSD (Tarrier et al. 1999). Both treatments resulted in comparable significant improvement, although not complete remission, of symptoms. Another controlled study in 87 patients with chronic PTSD compared exposure therapy, cognitive restructuring, their combination, and simple relaxation techniques (Marks et al. 1998). Both the behavioral and the cognitive treatment resulted in marked improvement, with gains maintained after 6 months; in contrast, their combination was of no additional benefit, and relaxation yielded only modest improvement. In another study, exposure therapy, stress inoculation training, their combination, and a waiting-list control condition were compared in women with chronic PTSD who had experienced an assault (Foa et al. 1999). The three active treatments produced comparable improvement, and the gains were maintained through 1-year follow-up. In another study that attempted to boost the effects of individual exposure therapy by adding family behavioral interventions, the latter rendered no additional benefit (Glynn et al. 1999).

Another approach, affect management, also appears to be beneficial. In a randomized study of adult women with PTSD and a history of childhood sexual abuse who were already receiving individual psychotherapy and pharmacotherapy, those who underwent a 3-month course of group affect-management treatment demonstrated significantly fewer PTSD and dissociative symptoms after the treatment (Zlotnick et al. 1997).

These psychotherapies appear to be highly beneficial for children and adolescents as well, although they have been less rigorously studied in those populations. In an open trial of CBT in 17 elementary school and junior high school students with PTSD, more than half no longer met disorder criteria after treatment, and were doing even better at 6-month follow-up (March et al. 1998a).

Other Treatments

EMDR is a relatively new technique that has been applied to the treatment of trauma-related pathology in the past decade. There continues to be controversy in the literature regarding EMDR's efficacy as well as the underlying mechanisms of its action. In a 5-year follow-up study of a small group of veterans who had initially been treated with EMDR with modest benefits, all benefit had disappeared at follow-up (Macklin et al. 2000). Although EMDR has been found to be superior to relaxation in treating PTSD (Carlson et al. 1998), relaxation

is not considered one of the first-line treatments for this disorder. A recent randomized study comparing EMDR with CBT found that CBT was significantly more effective and that its superiority was even more apparent at 3-month follow-up (Devilly and Spence 1999).

Transcranial magnetic stimulation was found to have some transient efficacy in decreasing core PTSD symptoms in 10 patients treated openly, and thus may warrant more investigation in PTSD (Grisaru et al. 1998).

Conclusion

In this chapter we endeavored to present a comprehensive discussion of panic disorder, GAD, the phobic disorders, OCD, and PTSD. A review of history, differing theoretical models, and new developments in epidemiology, classification, pathophysiology, and treatment, has been presented. An explosion of research has led to dramatic developments in the understanding and alleviation of various forms of anxiety and has made the anxiety disorders an exciting field of modern psychiatry.

References

Abelson JL, Glitz D, Cameron OG, et al: Blunted growth hormone response to clonidine in patients with generalized anxiety disorder. Arch Gen Psychiatry 48:157–162, 1991

Abelson JL, Weg JG, Nesse RM, et al: Persistent respiratory irregularity in patients with panic disorder. Biol Psychiatry 49:588–595, 2001

Ackerman DL, Greenland S, Bystritsky A, et al: Predictors of treatment response in obsessive-compulsive disorder: multivariate analyses from a multicenter trial of clomipramine. J Clin Psychopharmacol 14:247–254, 1994

Adler CM, McDonough-Ryan P, Sax KW, et al: fMRI of neuronal activation with symptom provocation in unmedicated patients with obsessive compulsive disorder. J Psychiatr Res 34:317–324, 2000

Agid O, Shalev AY, Lerer B: Triiodothyronine augmentation of selective serotonin reuptake inhibitors in posttraumatic stress disorder. J Clin Psychiatry 62:169–173, 2001

Aikins DE, Craske MG: Cognitive theories of generalized anxiety disorder. Psychiatr Clin North Am 24:57–74, 2001

Akhtar S, Wig NN, Varma VK, et al: A phenomenological analysis of symptoms in obsessive-compulsive neurosis. Br J Psychiatry 127:342–348, 1975

Alden LE, Wallace ST: Social phobia and social appraisal in successful and unsuccessful social interactions. Behav Res Ther 33:497–505, 1995

Allgulander C, Lavori PW: Excess mortality among 3302 patients with "pure" anxiety neurosis. Arch Gen Psychiatry 48:599–602, 1991

Brady KT, Sonne SC, Roberts JM: Sertraline treatment of comorbid posttraumatic stress disorder and alcohol dependence. J Clin Psychiatry 56:502–505, 1995

Brady K[T], Pearlstein T, Asnis GM, et al: Efficacy and safety of sertraline treatment of posttraumatic stress disorder: a randomized controlled trial. JAMA 283:1837–1844, 2000

Brambilla F, Bellodi L, Perna G, et al: Dopamine function in obsessive-compulsive disorder: growth hormone response to apomorphine stimulation. Biol Psychiatry 42:889–897, 1997

Brantigan CO, Brantigan TA, Joseph N: Effect of beta blockade and beta stimulation on stage fright. Am J Med 72:88–94, 1982

Brawman MO, Lydiard RB, Emmanuel N, et al: Psychiatric comorbidity in patients with generalized anxiety disorder. Am J Psychiatry 150:1216–1218, 1993

Breiter HC, Rauch SL, Kwong KK, et al: Functional magnetic resonance imaging of symptom provocation in obsessive-compulsive disorder. Arch Gen Psychiatry 53:595–606, 1996

Breitholtz E, Johansson B, Ost LG: Cognitions in generalized anxiety disorder and panic disorder patients: a prospective approach. Behav Res Ther 37:533–544, 1999

Bremner JD, Southwick SM, Johnson DR, et al: Childhood physical abuse and combat-related posttraumatic stress disorder in Vietnam veterans. Am J Psychiatry 150:235–239, 1993a

Bremner JD, Scott TM, Delaney RC, et al: Deficits in short-term memory in posttraumatic stress disorder. Am J Psychiatry 150:1015–1019, 1993b

Bremner JD, Steinberg M, Southwick SM, et al: Use of the Structured Clinical Interview for DSM-IV Dissociative Disorders for systematic assessment of dissociative symptoms in posttraumatic stress disorder. Am J Psychiatry 150:1011–1014, 1993c

Bremner JD, Randall P, Scott TM, et al: MRI-based measurement of hippocampal volume in patients with combat-related posttraumatic stress disorder. Am J Psychiatry 152:973–981, 1995

Bremner JD, Licinio J, Darnell A, et al: Elevated CSF corticotropin-releasing factor concentrations in posttraumatic stress disorder. Am J Psychiatry 154:624–629, 1997a

Bremner JD, Randall P, Vermetten E, et al: Magnetic resonance imaging-based measurement of hippocampal volume in posttraumatic stress disorder related to childhood physical and sexual abuse: a preliminary report. Biol Psychiatry 41:23–32, 1997b

Bremner JD, Staib LH, Kaloupek D, et al: Neural correlates of exposure to traumatic pictures and sound in Vietnam combat veterans with and without posttraumatic stress disorder: a positron emission tomography study. Biol Psychiatry 45:806–816, 1999a

Bremner JD, Narayan M, Staib LH, et al: Neural correlates of memories of childhood sexual abuse in women with and without posttraumatic stress disorder. Am J Psychiatry 156:1787–1795, 1999b

Bremner JD, Innis RB, White T, et al: SPECT [I-123] iomazenil measurement of the benzodiazepine receptor in panic disorder. Biol Psychiatry 47:96–106, 2000

Breslau N, Davis GC: DSM-III generalized anxiety disorder: an empirical investigation of more stringent criteria. Psychiatry Res 15:231–238, 1985

Breslau N, Davis GC: Posttraumatic stress disorder in an urban population of young adults: risk factors for chronicity. Am J Psychiatry 149:671–675, 1992

Breslau N, Davis GC, Andreski P, et al: Traumatic events and posttraumatic stress disorder in an urban population of young adults. Arch Gen Psychiatry 48:216–222, 1991

Breslau N, Davis GC, Peterson EL, et al: Psychiatric sequelae of posttraumatic stress disorder in women. Arch Gen Psychiatry 54:81–87, 1997a

Breslau N, Davis GC, Andreski P, et al: Sex differences in posttraumatic stress disorder. Arch Gen Psychiatry 54:1044–1048, 1997b

Breslau N, Kessler RC, Chilcoat HD, et al: Trauma and posttraumatic stress disorder in the community: the 1996 Detroit Area Survey of Trauma. Arch Gen Psychiatry 55:626–632, 1998

Breslau N, Davis GC, Peterson EL, et al: A second look at comorbidity in victims of trauma: the posttraumatic stress disorder–major depression connection. Biol Psychiatry 48:902–909, 2000

Breuer T, Freud S: Studies on hysteria (1893–1895), in The Standard Edition of the Complete Psychological Works of Sigmund Freud, Vol 2. Edited by Strachey J. London, England, Hogarth Press, 1955, pp 1–319

Bryant RA, Harvey AG: Attentional bias in posttraumatic stress disorder. J Trauma Stress 10:635–644, 1997

Bryant RA, Harvey AG: Relationship between acute stress disorder and posttraumatic stress disorder following mild traumatic brain injury. Am J Psychiatry 155:625–629, 1998

Bryant RA, Marosszeky JE, Crooks J, et al: Posttraumatic stress disorder after severe traumatic brain injury. Am J Psychiatry 157:629–631, 2000a

Bryant RA, Harvey AG, Guthrie RM, et al: A prospective study of psychophysiological arousal, acute stress disorder, and posttraumatic stress disorder. J Abnorm Psychol 109:341–344, 2000b

Buchsbaum MS, Wu J, Haier R, et al: Positron emission tomography assessment of effects of benzodiazepines on regional glucose metabolic rate in patients with anxiety disorder. Life Sci 40:2393–2400, 1987

Burstein A: Treatment of post-traumatic stress disorder with imipramine. Psychosomatics 25:681–687, 1984

Burstein A: Treatment length in post-traumatic stress disorder. Psychosomatics 27:632–637, 1986

Butler G, Fennell M, Robson P, et al: Comparison of behavior therapy and cognitive behavior therapy in the treatment of generalized anxiety disorder. J Consult Clin Psychol 59:167–175, 1991

Caillard V, Rouillon F, Viel JF, et al: Comparative effects of low and high doses of clomipramine and placebo in panic disorder: a double-blind, controlled study. French University Antidepressant Group. Acta Psychiatr Scand 99:51–58, 1999

Calvocoressi L, Lewis B, Harris M, et al: Family accommodation in obsessive-compulsive disorder. Am J Psychiatry 152:441–443, 1995

Canive JM, Clark RD, Calais LA, et al: Bupropion treatment in veterans with posttraumatic stress disorder: an open study. J Clin Psychopharmacol 18:379–383, 1998

Capstick N, Seldrup V: Obsessional states: a study in the relationship between abnormalities occurring at birth and subsequent development of obsessional symptoms. Acta Psychiatr Scand 56:427–439, 1977

Carey G, Gottesman II: Twin and family studies of anxiety, phobic, and obsessive disorders, in Anxiety: New Research and Changing Concepts. Edited by Klein DF, Rabkin J. New York, Raven, 1981, pp 117–136

Carlson JG, Chemtob CM, Rusnak K, et al: Eye movement desensitization and reprocessing (EMDR) treatment for combat-related posttraumatic stress disorder. J Trauma Stress 11:3–24, 1998

Carter RM, Wittchen HU, Pfister H, et al: One-year prevalence of subthreshold and threshold DSM-IV generalized anxiety disorder in a nationally representative sample. Depress Anxiety 13:78–88, 2001

Cassidy J: Attachment and generalized anxiety disorder, in Rochester Symposium on Developmental Psychopathology, Vol 6: Emotion, Cognition and Representation. Edited by Cicchetti D, Toth S. New York, University of Rochester Press, 1995

Cavallini MC, Di-Bella D, Pasquale L, et al: 5HT2C CYS23/SER23 polymorphism is not associated with obsessive-compulsive disorder. Psychiatry Res 77:97–104, 1998

Chambless DL, Gillis MM: Cognitive therapy of anxiety disorders. J Consult Clin Psychol 61:248–260, 1993

Chapman D: A brief introduction to contemporary disaster research, in Man and Society in Disaster. Edited by Boher G, Chapman D. New York, Basic Books, 1962

Charney DS, Heninger GR: Abnormal regulation of noradrenergic function in panic disorders: effects of clonidine in healthy subjects and patients with agoraphobia and panic disorder. Arch Gen Psychiatry 43:1042–1054, 1986

Charney DS, Heninger GR, Breier A: Noradrenergic function in panic anxiety: effects of yohimbine in healthy subjects and patients with agoraphobia and panic disorder. Arch Gen Psychiatry 41:751–763, 1984

Charney DS, Goodman WK, Price LH, et al: Serotonin function in obsessive-compulsive disorder: a comparison of the effects of tryptophan and m-chlorophenylpiperazine in patients and healthy subjects. Arch Gen Psychiatry 45:177–185, 1988

Chartier MJ, Walker JR, Stein MB: Social phobia and potential childhood risk factors in a community sample. Psychol Med 31:307–315, 2001

Chouinard G: Sertraline in the treatment of obsessive compulsive disorder: two double-blind, placebo-controlled studies. Int Clin Psychopharmacol 7(suppl 2):37–41, 1992

Christensen KJ, Kim SW, Dysken MW, et al: Neuropsychological performance in obsessive-compulsive disorder. Biol Psychiatry 31:4–18, 1992

Ciesielski KT, Beech HR, Gordon PK: Some electrophysiological observations in obsessional states. Br J Psychiatry 138:479–484, 1981

Clark DM, Salkovskis PM, Chalkly AJ: Respiratory control as a treatment for panic attacks. J Behav Ther Exp Psychiatry 16:23–30, 1985

Clark DM, Salkovskis PM, Hackmann A, et al: A comparison of cognitive therapy, applied relaxation therapy and imipramine in the treatment of panic disorder. Br J Psychiatry 164:759–769, 1994

Clark RD, Canive JM, Calais LA, et al: Cyproheptadine treatment of nightmares associated with posttraumatic stress disorder. J Clin Psychopharmacol 19:486–487, 1999a

Clark RD, Canive JM, Calais LA, et al: Divalproex in posttraumatic stress disorder: an open-label clinical trial. J Trauma Stress 12:395–401, 1999b

Clayton IC, Richards JC, Edwards CJ: Selective attention in obsessive-compulsive disorder. J Abnorm Psychol 108:171–175, 1999

Clomipramine Collaborative Study Group: Clomipramine in the treatment of patients with obsessive-compulsive disorder. Arch Gen Psychiatry 48:730–738, 1991

Cohen ME, White ID: Life situation, emotions, and neurocirculatory asthenia. Res Nerv Ment Dis Proc 29:832–869, 1950

Comings DE, Muhleman D, Gysin R: Dopamine D2 receptor (DRD2) gene and susceptibility to posttraumatic stress disorder: a study and replication. Biol Psychiatry 40:368–372, 1996

Cooper AM: Will neurobiology influence psychoanalysis? Am J Psychiatry 142:1395–1402, 1985

Cooper PJ, Eke M: Childhood shyness and maternal social phobia: a community study. Br J Psychiatry 174:439–443, 1999

Coplan JD, Lydiard RB: Brain circuits in panic disorder. Biol Psychiatry 44:1264–1276, 1998

Coplan JD, Pine D, Papp L, et al: Uncoupling of the noradrenergic-hypothalamic-pituitary-adrenal axis in panic disorder patients. Neuropsychopharmacology 13:65–73, 1995

Coplan JD, Papp LA, Pine D, et al: Clinical improvement with fluoxetine therapy and noradrenergic function in patients with panic disorder. Arch Gen Psychiatry 54:643–648, 1997

Coryell W, Noyes R, Clancy J: Excess mortality in panic disorder: a comparison with primary unipolar depression. Arch Gen Psychiatry 39:701–703, 1982

Cottraux J, Note I, Albuisson E, et al: Cognitive behavior therapy versus supportive therapy in social phobia: a randomized controlled trial. Psychother Psychosom 69:137–146, 2000

Coupland NJ, Bell C, Potokar J, et al: Flumazenil challenge in social phobia. Anxiety 111:27–30, 2000

Cowley DS, Dager SR, McClellan J, et al: Response to lactate infusion in generalized anxiety disorder. Biol Psychiatry 24:409–414, 1988

Craske MG, Brown TA, Barlow DH: Behavioral treatment of panic disorder: a two-year follow-up. Behav Ther 22:289–304, 1991

Crowe RR, Noyes R, Pauls DL, et al: A family study of panic disorder. Arch Gen Psychiatry 40:1065–1069, 1983

Crowe RR, Wang Z, Noyes R, et al: Candidate gene study of eight GABAA receptor subunits in panic disorder. Am J Psychiatry 154:1096–1100, 1997

Curtis GC, Thyer B: Fainting on exposure to phobic stimuli. Am J Psychiatry 140:771–774, 1983

Curtis GC, Abelson JL, Gold PW: Adrenocorticotropic hormone and cortisol responses to corticotropin-releasing hormone: changes in panic disorder and effects of alprazolam treatment. Biol Psychiatry 41:76–85, 1997

Dadds MR, Barrett PM, Rapee RM, et al: Family process and child anxiety and aggression: an observational analysis. J Abnorm Child Psychol 24:187–203, 1996

Dannon PN, Sasson Y, Hirschmann S, et al: Pindolol augmentation in treatment-resistant obsessive compulsive disorder: a double-blind placebo controlled trial. Eur Neuropsychopharmacol 10:165–169, 2000

Davidson J[R], Walker JI, Kilts C: A pilot study of phenelzine in the treatment of post-traumatic stress disorder. Br J Psychiatry 150:252–255, 1987

Davidson J[R], Kudler H, Smith R, et al: Treatment of posttraumatic stress disorder with amitriptyline and placebo. Arch Gen Psychiatry 47:259–266, 1990

Davidson J[R], Roth S, Newman E: Fluoxetine in post-traumatic stress disorder. Journal of Traumatic Stress 4:419–423, 1991

Davidson JR, Hughes DL, George LK, et al: The epidemiology of social phobia: findings from the Duke Epidemiological Catchment Area Study. Psychol Med 23:709–718, 1993a

Davidson JR, Potts N, Richichi E, et al: Treatment of social phobia with clonazepam and placebo. J Clin Psychopharmacol 13:423–428, 1993b

Davidson JR, Weisler RH, Malik ML, et al: Treatment of posttraumatic stress disorder with nefazodone. Int Clin Psychopharmacol 13:111–113, 1998

Davidson JR, DuPont RL, Hedges D, et al: Efficacy, safety, and tolerability of venlafaxine extended release and buspirone in outpatients with generalized anxiety disorder. J Clin Psychiatry 60:528–535, 1999

Davidson JR, Rothbaum BO, van der Kolk BA, et al: Multicenter, double-blind comparison of sertraline and placebo in the treatment of posttraumatic stress disorder. Arch Gen Psychiatry 58:485–492, 2001

Davis LL, Clark DM, Kramer GL, et al: D-fenfluramine challenge in posttraumatic stress disorder. Biol Psychiatry 45:928–930, 1999

Davis LL, Nugent AL, Murray J, et al: Nefazodone treatment for chronic posttraumatic stress disorder: an open trial. J Clin Psychopharmacol 20:159–164, 2000

DeBellis MD, Casey BJ, Dahl RE, et al: A pilot study of amygdala volumes in pediatric generalized anxiety disorder. Biol Psychiatry 48:51–57, 2000

de Beurs E, van Balkom AJ, Lange A, et al: Treatment of panic disorder with agoraphobia: comparison of fluvoxamine, placebo and psychological panic management combined with exposure and of exposure in vivo alone. Am J Psychiatry 152:683–691, 1995

De Boer M, Op den Velde W, Falger PJ, et al: Fluvoxamine treatment for chronic PTSD: a pilot study. Psychother Psychosom 57:158–163, 1992

Deckert J, Catalano M, Heils A, et al: Functional promoter polymorphism of the human serotonin transporter: lack of association with panic disorder. Psychiatr Genet 7:45–47, 1997

Deckert J, Nothen MM, Franke P, et al: Systematic mutation screening and association study of the A1 and A2a adenosine receptor genes in panic disorder suggest a contribution of the A2a gene to the development of the disease. Mol Psychiatry 3:81–85, 1998

Deckert J, Catalano M, Syagailo YV, et al: Excess of high activity monoamine oxidase A gene promoter alleles in female patients with panic disorder. Hum Mol Genet 81:228–234, 1999

de Haan E, Hoogduin KA, Buitelaar JK, et al: Behavior therapy versus clomipramine for the treatment of obsessive-compulsive disorder in children and adolescents. J Am Acad Child Adolesc Psychiatry 37:1022–1029, 1998

Delle Chiaie R, Pancheri P, Casacchia M, et al: Assessment of the efficacy of buspirone in patients affected by generalized anxiety disorder, shifting to buspirone from prior treatment with lorazepam: a placebo-controlled, double-blind study. J Clin Psychopharmacol 15:12–19, 1995

DeMartinis N, Schweizer E, Rickels K: An open-label trial of nefazodone in high comorbidity panic disorder. J Clin Psychiatry 57:245–248, 1996

DeMartinis N, Rynn M, Rickels K, et al: Prior benzodiazepine use and buspirone response in the treatment of generalized anxiety disorder. J Clin Psychiatry 61:91–94, 2000

Den Boer JA: Serotonergic Mechanisms in Anxiety Disorders: An Inquiry into Serotonin Function in Panic Disorder. The Hague, The Netherlands, Cip-Gegevens Koninklijke Bibliotheek, 1988

Devilly GJ, Spence SH: The relative efficacy and treatment distress of EMDR and a cognitive-behavior trauma treatment protocol in the amelioration of posttraumatic stress disorder. J Anxiety Disord 13:131–157, 1999

DeWit DJ, Ogborne A, Offord DR, et al: Antecedents of the risk of recovery from DSM-III-R social phobia. Psychol Med 29:569–582, 1999

Dimsdale JE, Moss J: Plasma catecholamines in stress and exercise. JAMA 243:340–342, 1980

Dorow R, Horowski R, Paschelke G, et al: Severe anxiety induced by FG-7142, a beta-carboline ligand for benzodiazepine receptors. Lancet 2:98–99, 1983

Duffy JD, Malloy PF: Efficacy of buspirone in the treatment of posttraumatic stress disorder: an open trial. Ann Clin Psychiatry 6:33–37, 1994

Durham RC, Murphy R, Allan T, et al: Cognitive therapy, analytic psychotherapy and anxiety management training for generalized anxiety disorder. Br J Psychiatry 165:315–323, 1994

Dyck IR, Phillips KA, Warshaw MG, et al: Patterns of personality pathology in patients with generalized anxiety disorder, panic disorder with and without agoraphobia, and social phobia. J Personal Disord 15:60–71, 2001

Eaton WW, Keyl PM: Risk factors for the onset of Diagnostic Interview Schedule/DSM-III agoraphobia in a prospective, population-based study. Arch Gen Psychiatry 47:819–824, 1990

Eaton WW, Dryman A, Weissman MM: Panic and phobia, in Psychiatric Disorders in America. Edited by Robins LN, Regier DA. New York, Free Press, 1991, pp 155–179

Ehlers A, Clark DM: A cognitive model of posttraumatic stress disorder. Behav Res Ther 38:319–345, 2000

Eisen JL, Beer DA, Pato MT, et al: Obsessive-compulsive disorder in patients with schizophrenia or schizoaffective disorder. Am J Psychiatry 154:271–273, 1997

Eitinger L: Organic and psychosomatic after effects of concentration camp imprisonment. International Psychiatry Clinics 8:205–215, 1971

Elam M, Yoat TP, Svensson TH: Hypercapnia and hypoxia: chemoreceptor-mediated control of locus coeruleus neurons and splanchnic, sympathetic nerves. Brain Res 222:373–381, 1981

Embry CK: Psychotherapeutic interventions in chronic posttraumatic stress disorder, in Posttraumatic Stress Disorder: Etiology, Phenomenology, and Treatment. Edited by Wolf ME, Mosnaim AD. Washington, DC, American Psychiatric Press, 1990, pp 226–236

Emmanuel NP, Lydiard BR, Ballenger JC: Treatment of social phobia with bupropion. J Clin Psychopharmacol 11:276–277, 1991

Engdahl B, Dikel TN, Eberly R, et al: Posttraumatic stress disorder in a community group of former prisoners of war: a normative response to severe trauma. Am J Psychiatry 154:1576–1581, 1997

Essau CA, Conradt J, Petermann F: Frequency, comorbidity, and psychosocial impairment of specific phobia in adolescents. J Clin Child Psychol 29:221–231, 2000

Fairbank TA, Keane TM: Flooding for combat-related stress disorders: assessment of anxiety reduction across traumatic memories. Behav Ther 13:499–510, 1982

Fallon BA, Campeas R, Schneier FR, et al: Open trial of intravenous clomipramine in five treatment-refractory patients with obsessive-compulsive disorder. J Neuropsychiatry Clin Neurosci 4:70–75, 1992

Fallon BA, Liebowitz MR, Campeas R, et al: Intravenous clomipramine for obsessive-compulsive disorder refractory to oral clomipramine: a placebo-controlled study. Arch Gen Psychiatry 55:918–924, 1998

Faravelli C, Pallanti S: Recent life events and panic disorder. Am J Psychiatry 146:622–626, 1989

Ferrarese C, Appollonio I, Frigo M, et al: Decreased density of benzodiazepine receptors in lymphocytes of anxious patients: reversal after chronic diazepam treatment. Acta Psychiatr Scand 82:169–173, 1990

Fitzgerald KD, Stewart CM, Tawile V, et al: Risperidone augmentation of serotonin reuptake inhibitor treatment of pediatric obsessive compulsive disorder. J Child Adolesc Psychopharmacol 9:115–123, 1999

Flament MF, Rapoport JL, Berg CJ, et al: Clomipramine treatment of childhood obsessive-compulsive disorder: a double-blind controlled study. Arch Gen Psychiatry 42:977–983, 1985

Flament MF, Rapoport JL, Murphy DL, et al: Biochemical changes during clomipramine treatment of childhood obsessive-compulsive disorder. Arch Gen Psychiatry 44:219–225, 1987

Flescher J: A dualistic viewpoint on anxiety. J Am Psychoanal Assoc 3:415–446, 1955

Flint AJ: Epidemiology and comorbidity of anxiety disorders in the elderly. Am J Psychiatry 151:640–649, 1994

Flor-Henry P: The obsessive-compulsive syndrome, in Cerebral Basis of Psychopathology. Edited by Flor-Henry P. Boston, MA, John Coright, 1983, pp 301–311

Foa EB, Steketee G, Grayson JB, et al: Deliberate exposure and blocking of obsessive-compulsive rituals: immediate and long-term effects. Behav Ther 15:450–472, 1984

Foa EB, Kozak MJ, Goodman WK, et al: DSM-IV field trial: obsessive-compulsive disorder. Am J Psychiatry 152:90–96, 1995

Foa EB, Dancu CV, Hembree EA, et al: A comparison of exposure therapy, stress inoculation therapy, and their combination for reducing posttraumatic stress disorder in female assault victims. J Consult Clin Psychol 67:194–200, 1999

Frank JB, Kosten TR, Giller EL Jr, et al: A randomized clinical trial of phenelzine and imipramine for posttraumatic stress disorder. Am J Psychiatry 145:1289–1291, 1988

Franklin ME, Kozak MJ, Cashman L, et al: Cognitive-behavioral treatment of pediatric obsessive-compulsive disorder: an open clinical trial. J Am Acad Child Adolesc Psychiatry 37:412–419, 1998

Franklin ME, Abramowitz JS, Kozak MJ, et al: Effectiveness of exposure and ritual prevention for obsessive-compulsive disorder: randomized compared with nonrandomized samples. J Consult Clin Psychol 68:594–602, 2000

Fredrikson M, Wik G, Greitz T, et al: Regional cerebral blood flow during experimental phobic fear. Psychophysiology 30:126–130, 1993

Freeman CP, Trimble MR, Deakin JF, et al: Fluvoxamine versus clomipramine in the treatment of obsessive compulsive disorder: a multicenter, randomized, double-blinded, parallel group comparison. J Clin Psychiatry 55:301–305, 1994

Freeston MH, Rheaume J, Ladouceur R: Correcting faulty appraisals of obsessional thoughts. Behav Res Ther 34:433–446, 1996

Freud S: Obsessions and phobias (1895[1894]), in The Standard Edition of the Complete Psychological Works of Sigmund Freud, Vol 3. Translated and edited by Strachey J. London, England, Hogarth, 1962a, pp 69–84

Freud S: On the grounds for detaching a particular syndrome from neurasthenia under the description anxiety neurosis (1895[1894]), in The Standard Edition of the Complete Psychological Works of Sigmund Freud, Vol 3. Translated and edited by Strachey J. London, England, Hogarth, 1962b, pp 85–117

Freud S: Analysis of a phobia in a five-year-old boy (1909), in The Standard Edition of the Complete Psychological Works of Sigmund Freud, Vol 10. Translated and edited by Strachey J. London, England, Hogarth, 1955, pp 1–149

Freud S: The disposition to obsessional neurosis: a contribution to the problem of choice of neurosis (1913), in The Standard Edition of the Complete Psychological Works of Sigmund Freud, Vol 12. Translated and edited by Strachey J. London, England, Hogarth, 1958, pp 311–326

Freud S: Introduction to Psychoanalysis and the War Neuroses (1919), in The Standard Edition of the Complete Psychological Works of Sigmund Freud, Vol 17. Translated and edited by Strachey J. London, England, Hogarth, 1955, pp 205–215

Freud S: Inhibitions, symptoms and anxiety (1926), in The Standard Edition of the Complete Psychological Works of Sigmund Freud, Vol 20. Translated and edited by Strachey J. London, England, Hogarth Press, 1959, pp 75–175

Frisch A, Michaelovsky E, Poyurovsky M, et al: Association between obsessive-compulsive disorder and polymorphisms of genes encoding components of the serotonergic and dopaminergic pathways. Eur Neuropsychopharmacol 10:205–209, 2000

Frohlich ED, Tarazi KC, Duston HP: Hyperdynamic beta-adrenergic circulatory state. Arch Intern Med 123:1–7, 1969

Fyer AJ: Current approaches to etiology and pathophysiology of specific phobia. Biol Psychiatry 44:1295–1304, 1998

Fyer AJ, Mannuzza S, Gallops MS, et al: Familial transmission of simple phobias and fears: a preliminary report. Arch Gen Psychiatry 47:252–256, 1990

Gabbard GO: Psychodynamic Psychiatry in Clinical Practice, 3rd Edition. Washington, DC, American Psychiatric Publishing, 2000

Galderisi S, Mucci A, Catapano F, et al: Neuropsychological slowness in obsessive-compulsive patients. Is it confined to tests involving the fronto-subcortical systems? Br J Psychiatry 167:394–398, 1996

Gelenberg AJ, Lydiard RB, Rudolph RL, et al: Efficacy of venlafaxine extended-release capsules in nondepressed outpatients with generalized anxiety disorder: a 6-month randomized controlled trial. JAMA 283:3082–3088, 2000

Gelernter CS, Uhde TW, Cimbolic P, et al: Cognitive-behavioral and pharmacological treatments of social phobia: a controlled study. Arch Gen Psychiatry 48:938–945, 1991

Gelernter J. Southwick S, Goodson S, et al: No association between D2 dopamine receptor (DRD2) "A" system alleles or DRD2 haplotypes and posttraumatic stress disorder. Biol Psychiatry 45:620–625, 1999

Geracioti TD: Venlafaxine treatment of panic disorder: a case series. J Clin Psychiatry 56:408–410, 1995

Germine M, Goddard AW, Woods SW, et al: Anger and anxiety responses to m-chlorophenylpiperazine in generalized anxiety disorder. Biol Psychiatry 32:457–461, 1992

Ghaemi SN, Zarate CA, Popli AP, et al: Is there a relationship between clozapine and obsessive-compulsive disorder? A retrospective chart review. Compr Psychiatry 36:267–270, 1995

Giedd JN, Rapoport JL, Garvey MA, et al: MRI assessment of children with obsessive-compulsive disorder or tics associated with streptococcal infection. Am J Psychiatry 157:281–283, 2000

Gilbert AR, Moore GJ, Keshavan MS, et al: Decrease in thalamic volumes of pediatric patients with obsessive-compulsive disorder who are taking paroxetine. Arch Gen Psychiatry 57:449–456, 2000

Gittelman-Klein R, Klein DF: Controlled imipramine treatment of school phobia. Arch Gen Psychiatry 25:204–207, 1971

Gittleson NL: The effect of obsessions on depressive psychosis. Br J Psychiatry 112:253–259, 1966

Glynn SM, Eth S, Randolph ET, et al: A test of behavioral family therapy to augment exposure for combat-related posttraumatic stress disorder. J Consult Clin Psychol 67:243–251, 1999

Goddard AW, Mason GF, Almai A, et al: Reductions in occipital cortex GABA levels in panic disorder detected with 1H-magnetic resonance spectroscopy. Arch Gen Psychiatry 58:556–561, 2001

Gold M, Pottash AC, Sweeney DR, et al: Opiate withdrawal using clonidine. JAMA 243:343–346, 1980

Goldstein RB, Wickramaratne PJ, Horwath E, et al: Familial aggregation and phenomenology of "early" onset (at or before age 20 years) panic disorder. Arch Gen Psychiatry 54:271–278, 1997

Golier J, Yehuda R, Cornblatt B, et al: Sustained attention in combat-related posttraumatic stress disorder. Integr Physiol Behav Sci 32:52–61, 1997

Goodman WK, Price LH, Rasmussen SA, et al: Efficacy of fluvoxamine in obsessive-compulsive disorder: a double-blind comparison with placebo. Arch Gen Psychiatry 46:36–44, 1989

Goodman WK, McDougle CJ, Price LH, et al: Beyond the serotonin hypothesis: a role for dopamine in some forms of obsessive compulsive disorder? J Clin Psychiatry 51(suppl):36–43, 1990a

Goodman WK, Price LH, Delgado PL, et al: Specificity of serotonin reuptake inhibitors in the treatment of obsessive-compulsive disorder: comparison of fluvoxamine and desipramine. Arch Gen Psychiatry 47:577–585, 1990b

Goodnick PJ, Ruiz A, DeVane CL, et al: Mirtazapine in major depression with comorbid generalized anxiety disorder. J Clin Psychiatry 60:446–448, 1999

Gorman JM, Fyer AF, Gliklich J, et al: Effect of imipramine on prolapsed mitral valves of patients with panic disorder. Am J Psychiatry 138:977–978, 1981

Gorman JM, Levy GF, Liebowitz MR, et al: Effect of acute β-adrenergic blockade on lactate-induced panic. Arch Gen Psychiatry 40:1079–1082, 1983

Gorman JM, Askanazi J, Liebowitz MR, et al: Response to hyperventilation in a group of patients with panic disorder. Am J Psychiatry 141:857–861, 1984

Gorman JM, Liebowitz MR, Fyer AJ, et al: Lactate infusions in obsessive-compulsive disorder. Am J Psychiatry 142:864–866, 1985

Gorman JM, Fyer MR, Goetz R, et al: Ventilatory physiology of patients with panic disorder. Arch Gen Psychiatry 45:31–39, 1988

Gorman JM, Battista D, Goetz RR, et al: A comparison of sodium bicarbonate and sodium lactate infusion in the induction of panic attacks. Arch Gen Psychiatry 46:145–150, 1989a

Gorman JM, Liebowitz MR, Fyer AJ, et al: A neuroanatomical hypothesis for panic disorder. Am J Psychiatry 146:148–161, 1989b

Gorman JM, Kent JM, Sullivan GM, et al: Neuroanatomical hypothesis of panic disorder, revised. Am J Psychiatry 157:493–505, 2000

Grady TA, Pigott TA, L'Heureux F, et al: Double-blind study of adjuvant buspirone for fluoxetine-treated patients with obsessive-compulsive disorder. Am J Psychiatry 150:819–821, 1993

Greenberg BD, George MS, Martin JD, et al: Effect of prefrontal repetitive transcranial magnetic stimulation in obsessive-compulsive disorder: a preliminary study. Am J Psychiatry 154:867–869, 1997

Greist J, Chouinard G, DuBoff E, et al: Double-blind parallel comparison of three dosages of sertraline and placebo in outpatients with obsessive-compulsive disorder. Arch Gen Psychiatry 52:289–295, 1995a

Greist JH, Jefferson JW, Kobak KA, et al: Efficacy and tolerability of serotonin transport inhibitors in obsessive-compulsive disorder. A meta-analysis. Arch Gen Psychiatry 52:53–60, 1995b

Greist JH, Jefferson JW, Kobak KA, et al: A 1 year double-blind placebo-controlled fixed dose study of sertraline in the treatment of obsessive-compulsive disorder. Int Clin Psychopharmacol 10:57–65, 1995c

Grillon C, Morgan CA: Fear-potentiated startle conditioning to explicit and contextual cues in Gulf War veterans with posttraumatic stress disorder. J Abnorm Psychol 108:134–142, 1999

Grimshaw L: Obsessional disorder and neurological illness. J Neurol Neurosurg Psychiatry 27:229–231, 1964

Grisaru N, Amir M, Cohen H, et al: Effect of transcranial magnetic stimulation in posttraumatic stress disorder: a preliminary study. Biol Psychiatry 44:52–55, 1998

Gupta S, Popli A, Bathurst E, et al: Efficacy of cyproheptadine for nightmares associated with posttraumatic stress disorder. Compr Psychiatry 39:160–164, 1998

Gurvits TV, Gilbertson MW, Lasko NB, et al: Neurologic soft signs in chronic posttraumatic stress disorder. Arch Gen Psychiatry 57:181–186, 2000

Han L, Nielsen DA, Rosenthal NE, et al: No coding variant of the tryptophan hydroxylase gene detected in seasonal affective disorder, obsessive-compulsive disorder, anorexia nervosa, and alcoholism. Biol Psychiatry 45:615–619, 1999

Hansenne M, Pitchot W, Ansseau M: The clonidine test in posttraumatic stress disorder (letter). Am J Psychiatry 148:810–811, 1991

Hartley LR, Ungapen S, Davie I, et al: The effect of beta adrenergic blocking drugs on speakers' performance and memory. Br J Psychiatry 142:512–517, 1983

Harvey AG, Bryant RA: Two-year prospective evaluation of the relationship between acute stress disorder and posttraumatic stress disorder following mild traumatic brain injury. Am J Psychiatry 157:626–628, 2000

Hay P, Sachdev P, Cumming S, et al: Treatment of obsessive-compulsive disorder by psychosurgery. Acta Psychiatr Scand 87:197–207, 1993

Hayward C, Killen JD, Draemer HC, et al: Linking self-reported childhood behavioral inhibition to adolescent social phobia. J Am Acad Child Adolesc Psychiatry 37:1308–1316, 1998

Hedges DW, Reimherr FW, Strong RE, et al: An open trial of nefazodone in adult patients with generalized anxiety disorder. Psychopharmacol Bull 32:671–676, 1996

Heimberg RG, Dodge CS, Hope DA, et al: Cognitive behavioral group treatment for social phobia: comparison with a credible placebo control. Cognitive Therapy and Research 14:1–23, 1990a

Heimberg RG, Hope DA, Dodge CS, et al: DSM-III-R subtypes of social phobia: comparison of generalized social phobics and public speaking phobics. J Nerv Ment Dis 178:172–179, 1990b

Heimburg RG, Liebowitz MR, Hope DA, et al: Cognitive behavioral group therapy vs phenelzine therapy for social phobia: a 12-week outcome. Arch Gen Psychiatry 55:1133–1141, 1998

Helzer JE, Robins LN, McEvoy L: Post-traumatic stress disorder in the general population: findings of the Epidemiologic Catchment Area survey. N Engl J Med 317:1630–1634, 1987

Herman JL, Perry JC, van der Kolk BA: Childhood trauma in borderline personality disorder. Am J Psychiatry 146:490–495, 1989

Hertzberg MA, Feldman ME, Beckham JC, et al: Open trial of nefazodone for combat-related posttraumatic stress disorder. J Clin Psychiatry 59:460–464, 1998

Hertzberg MA, Butterfield MI, Feldman ME, et al: A preliminary study of lamotrigine for the treatment of posttraumatic stress disorder. Biol Psychiatry 45:1226–1229, 1999

Hewlett WA, Vinogradov S, Agras WS: Clonazepam treatment of obsessions and compulsions. J Clin Psychiatry 51:158–161, 1990

Hewlett WA, Vinogradov S, Agras WS: Clomipramine, clonazepam, and clonidine treatment of obsessive-compulsive disorder. J Clin Psychopharmacol 12:420–430, 1992a

Hewlett WA, Vinogradov S, Martin K, et al: Fenfluramine stimulation of prolactin in obsessive-compulsive disorder. Psychiatry Res 42:81–92, 1992b

Himle JA, Crystal D, Curtis GC, et al: Mode of onset of simple phobia subtypes: further evidence of heterogeneity. Psychiatry Res 36:37–43, 1991

Hirschmann S, Dannon PN, Iancu I, et al: Pindolol augmentation in patients with treatment-resistant panic disorder: a double-blind, placebo-controlled trial. J Clin Psychopharmacol 20:556–559, 2000

Hoehn-Saric R, Merchant AF, Keyser ML, et al: Effects of clonidine on anxiety disorders. Arch Gen Psychiatry 38:1278–1282, 1981

Hoehn-Saric R, McLeod DR, Zimmerli WD: Differential effects of alprazolam and imipramine in generalized anxiety disorder: somatic versus psychic symptoms. J Clin Psychiatry 49:293–301, 1988

Hoehn-Saric R, McLeod DR, Hipsley PA: Effect of fluvoxamine on panic disorder. J Clin Psychopharmacol 13:321–326, 1993a

Hoehn-Saric R, Hazlett RL, McLeod DR: Generalized anxiety disorder with early and late onset of anxiety symptoms. Compr Psychiatry 34:291–298, 1993b

Hogben GL, Cornfield RB: Treatment of traumatic war neurosis with phenelzine. Arch Gen Psychiatry 38:440–445, 1981

Hollander E, Liebowitz MR, Gorman JM, et al: Cortisol and sodium lactate-induced panic. Arch Gen Psychiatry 46:135–140, 1989

Hollander E, Schiffman E, Cohen B, et al: Signs of central nervous system dysfunction in obsessive-compulsive disorder. Arch Gen Psychiatry 47:27–32, 1990

Hollander E, DeCaria C, Gully R, et al: Effects of chronic fluoxetine treatment on behavioral and neuroendocrine responses to meta-chlorophenylpiperazine in obsessive-compulsive disorder. Psychiatry Res 36:1–17, 1991a

Hollander E, DeCaria C, Nitescu A, et al: Noradrenergic function in obsessive-compulsive disorder: behavioral and neuroendocrine responses to clonidine and comparison to healthy controls. Psychiatry Res 37:161–177, 1991b

Hollander E, DeCaria CM, Nitescu A, et al: Serotonergic function in obsessive-compulsive disorder: behavioral and neuroendocrine responses to oral m-chlorophenylpiperazine and fenfluramine in patients and healthy volunteers. Arch Gen Psychiatry 49:21–28, 1992

Hollander E, Kwon J, Weiller F, et al: Serotonergic function in social phobia: comparison to normal control and obsessive-compulsive disorder subjects. Psychiatry Res 79:213–217, 1998

Hollander E, Bienstock C, Pallanti S, et al: The International Treatment Refractory OCD Consortium: preliminary findings. Presented at the 5th International OCD Conference, Sardinia, Italy, March 29–April 1, 2001

Hollingsworth CE, Tanguay PE, Grossman L, et al: Long-term outcome of obsessive-compulsive disorder in childhood. Journal of the American Academy of Child Psychiatry 19:134–144, 1980

Horesh N, Amir M, Kedem P, et al: Life events in childhood, adolescence and adulthood and the relationship to panic disorder. Acta Psychiatr Scand 96:373–378, 1997

Hornig CD, McNally RJ: Panic disorder and suicide attempt. A reanalysis of data from the Epidemiologic Catchment Area study. Br J Psychiatry 167:76–79, 1995

Horowitz MJ: Stress-Response Syndromes. New York, Jason Aronson, 1976

Horowitz MJ, Wilner N, Kaltreider N, et al: Signs and symptoms of posttraumatic stress disorders. Arch Gen Psychiatry 37:88–92, 1980

Horwath E, Johnson J, Hornig CD: Epidemiology of panic disorder in African-Americans. Am J Psychiatry 150:465–469, 1993

Hudson J, Rapee R: The origins of social phobia. Behav Modif 24:102–129, 2000

Insel TR, Murphy DL, Cohen RM, et al: Obsessive-compulsive disorder: a double-blind trial of clomipramine and clorgyline. Arch Gen Psychiatry 40:605–612, 1983

Insel TR, Mueller EA, Alterman I, et al: Obsessive-compulsive disorder and serotonin: is there a connection? Biol Psychiatry 20:1174–1188, 1985

Ishiguro H, Arinami T, Yamada K, et al: An association study between a transcriptional polymorphism in the serotonin transporter gene and panic disorder in a Japanese population. Psychiatry Clin Neurosci 51:333–335, 1997

James IA, Blackburn IM: Cognitive therapy with obsessive-compulsive disorder. Br J Psychiatry 166:444–450, 1995

James IM, Griffith DNW, Pearson RM, et al: Effect of oxprenolol on stage-fright in musicians. Lancet 2:952–954, 1977

James IM, Borgoyne W, Savage IT: Effect of pindolol on stress-related disturbances of musical performance: preliminary communication. J R Soc Med 76:194–196, 1983

Janet P: Les Obsessions et la Psychasthenie, 2nd Edition. Paris, France, Bailliere, 1908

Jenike MA, Hyman S, Baer L, et al: A controlled trial of fluvoxamine in obsessive-compulsive disorder: implications for a serotonergic theory. Am J Psychiatry 147:1209–1215, 1990a

Jenike MA, Baer L, Summergrad P, et al: Sertraline in obsessive-compulsive disorder: a double-blind comparison with placebo. Am J Psychiatry 147:923–928, 1990b

Jenike MA, Baer L, Buttolph L, et al: Buspirone augmentation of fluoxetine in patients with obsessive-compulsive disorder. J Clin Psychiatry 52:13–14, 1991a

Jenike MA, Baer L, Ballantine HT, et al: Cingulotomy for refractory obsessive-compulsive disorder: a long-term follow-up of 33 patients. Arch Gen Psychiatry 48:548–555, 1991b

Jenike MA, Baer L, Minichiello WE, et al: Placebo-controlled trial of fluoxetine and phenelzine for obsessive-compulsive disorder. Am J Psychiatry 154:1261–1264, 1997

Jenkins MA, Langlasi PJ, Delis D, et al: Learning and memory in rape victims with posttraumatic stress disorder. Am J Psychiatry 155:278–279, 1998

Johnson J, Weissman MM, Klerman GL: Panic disorder, comorbidity, and suicide attempts. Arch Gen Psychiatry 47:805–808, 1990

Johnson MR, Lydiard RB, Zealberg JJ, et al: Plasma and CSF HVA levels in panic patients with comorbid social phobia. Biol Psychiatry 36:425–427, 1994

Johnson MR, Marazziti D, Brawman MO, et al: Abnormal benzodiazepine receptor density associated with generalized social phobia. Biol Psychiatry 43:306–309, 1998

Kagan J, Reznick JS, Snidman N: The physiology and psychology of behavioral inhibition in children. Child Dev 58:1459–1473, 1987

Kahn RJ, McNair DM, Lipman RS, et al: Imipramine and chlordiazepoxide in depressive and anxiety disorders, II: efficacy in anxious outpatients. Arch Gen Psychiatry 43:79–85, 1986

Karayiorgou M, Altemus M, Galke BL, et al: Genotype determining low catechol-O-methyltransferase activity as a risk factor for obsessive-compulsive disorder. Proc Natl Acad Sci USA 94:4572–4575, 1997

Karayiorgou M, Sobin C, Bludell ML, et al: Family based association studies support a sexually dimorphic effect of COMT and MAOA on genetic susceptibility to obsessive-compulsive disorder. Biol Psychiatry 45:1178–1189, 1999

Kardiner A: Traumatic neurosis of war, in American Handbook of Psychiatry, Vol 1. Edited by Arieti S. New York, Basic Books, 1959, pp 245–257

Karno M, Golding JM, Sorenson SB, et al: The epidemiology of obsessive-compulsive disorder in five US communities. Arch Gen Psychiatry 45:1094–1099, 1988

Katerndahl DA: Panic and prolapse. Meta-analysis. J Nerv Ment Dis 181:539–544, 1993

Katschnig H, Amering M, Stolk JM, et al: Long-term follow-up after a drug trial for panic disorder. Br J Psychiatry 167:487–494, 1995

Katzelnick DJ, Kobak KA, Greist JH, et al: Sertraline for social phobia: a double-blind, placebo-controlled crossover study. Am J Psychiatry 152:1368–1371, 1995

Kauffman CD, Reist C, Djenderedjian A, et al: Biological markers of affective disorders and posttraumatic stress disorder: a pilot study with desipramine. J Clin Psychiatry 48:366–367, 1987

Keck PE, Taylor VE, Tugrul KC, et al: Valproate treatment of panic disorder and lactate-induced panic attacks. Biol Psychiatry 33:542–546, 1993

Kehl PA, Marks IM: Neurological factors in obsessive-compulsive disorder: two case reports and a review of the literature. Br J Psychiatry 149:315–319, 1986

Keijsers GP, Hoogduin CA, Schaap CP: Predictors of treatment outcome in the behavioral treatment of obsessive-compulsive disorder. Br J Psychiatry 165:781–786, 1994

Kelly DD: The role of endorphins in stress-induced analgesia. Ann N Y Acad Sci 398:260–271, 1982

Kendler KS, Neale MC, Kessler RC, et al: Generalized anxiety disorder in women: a population-based twin study. Arch Gen Psychiatry 49:267–272, 1992a

Kendler KS, Neale MC, Kessler RC, et al: The genetic epidemiology of phobias in women: the interrelationship of agoraphobia, social phobia, situational phobia, and simple phobia. Arch Gen Psychiatry 49:273–281, 1992b

Kendler KS, Neale MC, Kessler RC, et al: Panic disorder in women: a population-based twin study. Psychol Med 23:397–406, 1993

Kennedy JL, Bradwejn J, Koszycki D, et al: Investigation of cholecystokinin system genes in panic disorder. Mol Psychiatry 4:284–285, 1999

Kessler RC, McGonagle KA, Zhao S, et al: Lifetime and 12-month prevalence of DSM-III-R psychiatric disorders in the United States. Results from the National Comorbidity Survey. Arch Gen Psychiatry 51:8–19, 1994

Kessler RC, Sonnega A, Bromet E, et al: Posttraumatic stress disorder in the National Comorbidity Survey. Arch Gen Psychiatry 52:1048–1060, 1995

Kessler RC, Stein MB, Berglund P: Social phobia subtypes in the National Comorbidity Survey. Am J Psychiatry 155:613–619, 1998

Kessler RC, DuPont RL, Berglund P, et al: Impairment in pure and comorbid generalized anxiety disorder and major depression at 12 months in two national surveys. Am J Psychiatry 156:1915–1923, 1999a

Kessler RC, Stang P, Wittchen HU, et al: Lifetime co-morbidities between social phobia and mood disorders in the US National Comorbidity Survey. Psychol Med 29:555–567, 1999b

Kim SJ, Veenstra-VanderWeele J, Hanna GL, et al: Mutation screening of human 5HT(2B)receptor gene in early onset obsessive-compulsive disorder. Mol Cell Probes 14:47–52, 2000

Kinzie JD, Leung P: Clonidine in Cambodian patients with posttraumatic stress disorder. J Nerv Ment Dis 177:546–550, 1989

Klein DF: Delineation of two drug responsive anxiety syndromes. Psychopharmacologia 5:397–408, 1964

Klein DF: Anxiety reconceptualized, in Anxiety: New Research and Changing Concepts. Edited by Klein DF, Rabkin JG. New York, Raven Press, 1981, pp 235–263

Klein DF: False suffocation alarms, spontaneous panics, and related conditions: an integrative hypothesis. Arch Gen Psychiatry 50:306–317, 1993

Klein DF, Zitrin CM, Woerner MG, et al: Treatment of phobias, II: behavior therapy and supportive psychotherapy: are there any specific ingredients? Arch Gen Psychiatry 40:139–145, 1983

Klein M: A contribution to the theory of anxiety and guilt. Int J Psychoanal 29:114–123, 1948

Knesevich JW: Successful treatment of obsessive-compulsive disorder with clonidine hydrochloride. Am J Psychiatry 139:364–365, 1982

Knowles JA, Fyer AJ, Vieland VJ, et al: Results of a genome-wide genetic screen for panic disorder. Am J Med Genet 28:139–147, 1998

Kobak KA, Greist JH, Jefferson JW, et al: Behavioral versus pharmacological treatments of obsessive compulsive disorder: a meta-analysis. Psychopharmacology (Berl) 136:205–216, 1998

Kolb LC: A neuropsychological hypothesis explaining posttraumatic stress disorders. Am J Psychiatry 144:989–995, 1987

Kolb LC, Burris BC, Griffiths S: Propranolol and clonidine in treatment of the chronic post-traumatic stress disorders of war, in Post-Traumatic Stress Disorder: Psychological and Biological Sequelae. Edited by van der Kolk BA. Washington, DC, American Psychiatric Press, 1984, pp 97–105

Koponen H, Lepola U, Leinonen E, et al: Citalopram in the treatment of obsessive-compulsive disorder: an open pilot study. Acta Psychiatr Scand 96:343–346, 1997

Koran LM, McElroy SL, Davidson JR, et al: Fluvoxamine versus clomipramine for obsessive-compulsive disorder: a double-blind comparison. J Clin Psychopharmacol 16:121–129, 1996

Koran LM, Ringold AL, Elliott MA: Olanzapine augmentation for treatment-resistant obsessive-compulsive disorder. J Clin Psychiatry 61:514–517, 2000

Koren D, Arnon I, Klein E: Acute stress response and posttraumatic stress disorder in traffic accident victims: a one-year prospective, follow-up study. Am J Psychiatry 156:367–373, 1999

Kosten TR, Mason JW, Giller EL, et al: Sustained urine norepinephrine and epinephrine elevation in PTSD. Psychoneuroendocrinology 12:13–20, 1987

Kronig MH, Apter J, Asnis G, et al: Placebo-controlled, multicenter study of sertraline treatment for obsessive-compulsive disorder. J Clin Psychopharmacol 19:172–176, 1999

Krystal H: Massive Psychic Trauma. New York, International Universities Press, 1968

Leckman JF, Goodman WK, North WG, et al: Elevated cerebrospinal fluid levels of oxytocin in obsessive-compulsive disorder. Comparison with Tourette's syndrome and healthy controls. Arch Gen Psychiatry 51:782–792, 1994

Leckman JF, Grice DE, Boardman J, et al: Symptoms of obsessive compulsive disorder. Am J Psychiatry 154:911–917, 1997

Lecrubier Y, Judge R: Long-term evaluation of paroxetine, clomipramine and placebo in panic disorder. Collaborative Paroxetine Panic Study Investigators. Acta Psychiatr Scand 95:153–160, 1997

Lecrubier Y, Bakker A, Dunbar G, et al: A comparison of paroxetine, clomipramine and placebo in the treatment of panic disorder. Collaborative Paroxetine Panic Study Investigators. Acta Psychiatr Scand 95:145–152, 1997

Lelliott P, Marks I, McNamee G, et al: Onset of panic disorder with agoraphobia: toward an integrated model. Arch Gen Psychiatry 46:1000–1004, 1989

Leonard HL, Swedo SE, Rapoport JL, et al: Treatment of obsessive-compulsive disorder with clomipramine and desipramine in children and adolescents: a double-blind crossover comparison. Arch Gen Psychiatry 46:1088–1092, 1989

Leonard HL, Swedo SE, Lenane MC, et al: A double-blind desipramine substitution during long-term clomipramine treatment in children and adolescents with obsessive-compulsive disorder. Arch Gen Psychiatry 48:922–927, 1991

Leonard HL, Swedo SE, Lenane MC, et al: A 2- to 7-year follow-up study of 54 obsessive compulsive children and adolescents. Arch Gen Psychiatry 50:429–439, 1993

Lepine JP, Chignon JM, Teherani M: Suicide attempts in patients with panic disorder. Arch Gen Psychiatry 50:144–149, 1993

Lepola UM, Wade AG, Leinonen EV, et al: A controlled, prospective, 1-year trial of citalopram in the treatment of panic disorder. J Clin Psychiatry 59:528–534, 1998

Lesch KP, Hoh A, Disselkamp-Tietze J, et al: 5-Hydroxytryptamine1A receptor responsivity in obsessive-compulsive disorder: comparison of patients and controls. Arch Gen Psychiatry 48:540–547, 1991

Levin P, Lazrove S, van der Kolk B: What psychological testing and neuroimaging tell us about the treatment of posttraumatic stress disorder by Eye Movement Desensitization and Reprocessing. J Anxiety Disord 13:159–172, 1999

Liden S, Gottfries CG: Beta-blocking agents in the treatment of catecholamine-induced symptoms in musicians (letter). Lancet 2:529, 1974

Lieb R, Wittchen HU, Hofler M, et al: Parental psychopathology, parenting styles, and the risk of social phobia in offspring: a prospective-longitudinal community study. Arch Gen Psychiatry 57:859–866, 2000

Liebowitz MR, Fyer AJ, McGrath P, et al: Clonidine treatment of panic disorder. Psychopharmacol Bull 17:122–123, 1981

Liebowitz MR, Fyer AJ, Gorman JM, et al: Lactate provocation of panic attacks, I: clinical and behavioral findings. Arch Gen Psychiatry 41:764–770, 1984a

Liebowitz MR, Quitkin FM, Stewart JW, et al: Phenelzine versus imipramine in atypical depression: a preliminary report. Arch Gen Psychiatry 41:669–677, 1984b

Liebowitz MR, Gorman JM, Fyer AJ, et al: Lactate provocation of panic attacks, II: biochemical and physiological findings. Arch Gen Psychiatry 42:709–719, 1985a

Liebowitz MR, Gorman JM, Fyer AJ, et al: Social phobia: review of a neglected anxiety disorder. Arch Gen Psychiatry 42:729–736, 1985b

Liebowitz MR, Schneier F, Campeas R, et al: Phenelzine vs atenolol in social phobia: a placebo-controlled comparison. Arch Gen Psychiatry 49:290–300, 1992

Liebowitz MR, Heimberg RG, Schneier FR, et al: Cognitive-behavioral therapy versus phenelzine in social phobia: long-term outcome. Depress Anxiety 10:89–98, 1999

Lindy JD, Grace MC, Green BL: Building a conceptual bridge between civilian trauma and war trauma: preliminary psychological findings from a clinical sample of Vietnam veterans, in Post-Traumatic Stress Disorder: Psychological and Biological Sequelae. Edited by van der Kolk BA. Washington, DC, American Psychiatric Press, 1984, pp 44–57

Lipper S, Davidson JRT, Grady TA, et al: Preliminary study of carbamazepine in post-traumatic stress disorder. Psychosomatics 27:849–854, 1986

Lippitz BE, Mindus P, Meyerson BA, et al: Lesion topography and outcome after thermocapsulotomy or gamma knife capsulotomy for obsessive-compulsive disorder: relevance of the right hemisphere. Neurosurgery 44:452–458, 1999

Lipsitz JD, Markowitz JC, Cherry S, et al: Open trial of interpersonal psychotherapy for the treatment of social phobia. Am J Psychiatry 156:1814–1816, 1999a

Lipsitz JD, Mannuzza S, Klein DF, et al: Specific phobia 10–16 years after treatment. Depress Anxiety 10:105–111, 1999b

Londborg PD, Wolkow R, Smith WT, et al: Sertraline in the treatment of panic disorder: A multi-site, double-blind, placebo-controlled, fixed-dose investigation. Br J Psychiatry 173:54–60, 1998

Lucey JV, Barry S, Webb MG, et al: The desipramine-induced hormone response and the dexamethasone suppression test in obsessive-compulsive disorder. Acta Psychiatr Scand 86:367–370, 1992

Lum LC: Hyperventilation and anxiety states. J R Soc Med 74:1–4, 1981

Lundh LG, Czyzykow S, Ost LG: Explicit and implicit memory bias in panic disorder with agoraphobia. Behav Res Ther 35:1003–1014, 1997

MacDonald PA, Antony MM, Macleod CM, et al: Memory and confidence in memory judgements among individuals with obsessive compulsive disorder and non-clinical controls. Behav Res Ther 35:497–505, 1997

Macklin ML, Metzger LJ, Litz BT, et al: Lower precombat intelligence is a risk factor for posttraumatic stress disorder. J Consult Clin Psychol 66:323–326, 1998

Macklin ML, Metzger LJ, Lasko NB, et al: Five-year follow-up study of eye movement desensitization and reprocessing therapy for combat-related posttraumatic stress disorder. Compr Psychiatry 41:24–27, 2000

MacLeod C, Cohen IL: Anxiety and the interpretation of ambiguity: a text comprehension study. J Abnorm Psychol 102:238–247, 1993

MacLeod C, McLaughlin K: Implicit and explicit memory bias in anxiety: a conceptual replication. Behav Res Ther 33:1–14, 1995

Magee WJ, Eaton WW, Wittchen HU, et al: Agoraphobia, simple phobia, and social phobia in the National Comorbidity Survey. Arch Gen Psychiatry 53:159–168, 1996

Maier SF, Seligman ME: Learned helplessness: theory and evidence. J Exp Psychol 105:3–46, 1976

Maier SF, Dovies S, Gran JW: Opiate antagonists and long-term analgesic reaction induced by inescapable shock in rats. J Comp Physiol Psychol 94:1172–1183, 1980

Maletzky B, McFarland B, Burt A: Refractory obsessive compulsive disorder and ECT. Convuls Ther 10:34–42, 1994

Malizia AL, Cunningham VJ, Bell CJ, et al: Decreased brain GABA(A)-benzodiazepine receptor binding in panic disorder: preliminary results from a quantitative PET study. Arch Gen Psychiatry 55:715–720, 1998

Mannuzza S, Schneier FR, Chapman TF, et al: Generalized social phobia. Reliability and validity. Arch Gen Psychiatry 52:230–237, 1995

Marazziti D, Dell'Osso L, Gemignani A, et al: Citalopram in refractory obsessive-compulsive disorder: an open study. Int Clin Psychopharmacol 16:215–219, 2001

March JS, Amaya-Jackson L, Murray MC, et al: Cognitive-behavioral psychotherapy for children and adolescents with posttraumatic stress disorder after a single-incident stressor. J Am Acad Child Adolesc Psychiatry 37:585–593, 1998a

March JS, Biederman J, Wolkow R, et al: Sertraline in children and adolescents with obsessive-compulsive disorder: a multicenter randomized controlled trial. JAMA 280:1752–1756, 1998b

Markowitz JS, Weissman MM, Ouellette R, et al: Quality of life in panic disorder. Arch Gen Psychiatry 46:984–992, 1989

Marks IM: Fears and Phobias. New York, Academic, 1969

Marks I: Behaviour therapy for obsessive-compulsive disorder: a decade of progress. Can J Psychiatry 42:1021–1027, 1997

Marks IM, Gelder MG: Different ages on onset in varieties of phobia. Am J Psychiatry 123:218–221, 1966

Marks IM, Hodgson R, Rachman S: Treatment of chronic obsessive-compulsive neurosis by in vivo exposure: a two-year follow-up and issues in treatment. Br J Psychiatry 127:349–364, 1975

Marks IM, Stern RS, Mawson D, et al: Clomipramine and exposure for obsessive-compulsive rituals, I. Br J Psychiatry 136:1–25, 1980

Marks IM, Gray S, Cohen D, et al: Imipramine and brief therapist-aided exposure in agoraphobics having self-exposure homework. Arch Gen Psychiatry 40:153–162, 1983

Marks IM, Lelliott P, Basoglu M, et al: Clomipramine, self-exposure and therapist-aided exposure for obsessive-compulsive rituals. Br J Psychiatry 152:522–534, 1988

Marks I, Lovell K, Noshirvani H, et al: Treatment of posttraumatic stress disorder by exposure and/or cognitive restructuring: a controlled study. Arch Gen Psychiatry 55:317–325, 1998

Marmar CR, Weiss DS, Schlenger WE, et al: Peritraumatic dissociation and posttraumatic stress in male Vietnam theater veterans. Am J Psychiatry 151:902–907, 1994

Marshall JR: The treatment of night terrors associated with posttraumatic syndrome. Am J Psychiatry 132:293–295, 1975

Marshall RD, Schneier FR, Fallon BA, et al: An open trial of paroxetine in patients with noncombat-related, chronic posttraumatic stress disorder. J Clin Psychopharmacol 18:10–18, 1998

Marten PA, Brown TA, Barlow DH, et al: Evaluation of the ratings comprising the associated symptom criterion of DSM-III-R generalized anxiety disorder. J Nerv Ment Dis 181:676–682, 1993

Mason JW, Giller EL, Kosten TR, et al: Urinary free-cortisol levels in posttraumatic stress disorder patients. J Nerv Ment Dis 174:145–149, 1986

Mason JW, Giller EL, Kosten TR, et al: Elevation of urinary norepinephrine/cortisol ratio in posttraumatic stress disorder. J Nerv Ment Dis 176:498–502, 1988

Mason ST, Fibiger HC: Anxiety: the locus ceruleus disconnection. Life Sci 25:2141–2147, 1979

Mataix-Cols D, Rauch SL, Manzo PA, et al: Use of factor-analyzed symptom dimensions to predict outcome with serotonin reuptake inhibitors and placebo in the treatment of obsessive-compulsive disorder. Am J Psychiatry 156:1409–1416, 1999

Mathew RJ, Ho BT, Kralik P, et al: Catecholamines and monoamine oxidase activity in anxiety. Acta Psychiatr Scand 63:245–252, 1981

Mattes J: More on panic disorder and mitral valve prolapse (letter). Am J Psychiatry 138:1130, 1981

Mattick RP, Peters L, Clarke JC: Exposure and cognitive restructuring for social phobia: a controlled study. Behav Ther 20:3–23, 1989

Mavissakalian M, Michelson L: Agoraphobia: relative and combined effectiveness of therapist-assisted in vivo exposure and imipramine. J Clin Psychiatry 47:117–122, 1986a

Mavissakalian M, Michelson L: Two-year follow-up of exposure and imipramine treatment of agoraphobia. Am J Psychiatry 143:1106–1112, 1986b

Mavissakalian M, Perel JM: Imipramine dose-response relationship in panic disorder with agoraphobia: preliminary findings. Arch Gen Psychiatry 46:127–131, 1989

Mavissakalian M, Perel JM: Clinical experiments in maintenance and discontinuation of imipramine therapy in panic disorder with agoraphobia. Arch Gen Psychiatry 49:318–323, 1992

Mavissakalian M, Hamann MS, Haidar SA, et al: DSM-III personality disorders in generalized anxiety, panic/agoraphobia, and obsessive-compulsive disorders. Compr Psychiatry 34:243–248, 1993

Mavissakalian M, Perel JM: Imipramine treatment of panic disorder with agoraphobia: dose ranging and plasma level-response relationships. Am J Psychiatry 152:673–682, 1995

McBride PA, DeMeo MD, Sweeney JA, et al: Neuroendocrine and behavioral responses to challenge with the indirect serotonin agonist dl-fenfluramine in adults with obsessive-compulsive disorder. Biol Psychiatry 31:19–34, 1992

McCafferty JP, Bellew KM, Zaninelli RM: Paroxetine treatment of GAD: an analysis of response by dose. Poster presented at the 154th annual meeting of the American Psychiatric Association, New Orleans, LA, May 2001

McDougle CJ, Goodman WK, Price LH, et al: Neuroleptic addition in fluvoxamine-refractory obsessive-compulsive disorder. Am J Psychiatry 147:652–654, 1990

McDougle CJ, Price LH, Goodman WK, et al: A controlled trial of lithium augmentation in fluvoxamine-refractory obsessive-compulsive disorder: lack of efficacy. J Clin Psychopharmacol 11:175–181, 1991a

McDougle CJ, Southwick SM, Charney DS, et al: An open trial of fluoxetine in the treatment of posttraumatic stress disorder. J Clin Psychopharmacol 11:325–327, 1991b

McDougle CJ, Goodman WK, Leckman JF, et al: The efficacy of fluvoxamine in obsessive-compulsive disorder: effects of comorbid chronic tic disorder. J Clin Psychopharmacol 13:354–358, 1993a

McDougle CJ, Goodman WK, Leckman JF, et al: Limited therapeutic effect of addition of buspirone in fluvoxamine-refractory obsessive-compulsive disorder. Am J Psychiatry 150:647–649, 1993b

McDougle CJ, Goodman WK, Leckman JF, et al: Haloperidol addition in fluvoxamine-refractory obsessive-compulsive disorder. A double-blind, placebo-controlled study in patients with and without tics. Arch Gen Psychiatry 51:302–308, 1994

McDougle CJ, Barr LC, Goodman WK, et al: Lack of efficacy of clozapine monotherapy in refractory obsessive-compulsive disorder. Am J Psychiatry 152:1812–1814, 1995

McDougle CJ, Epperson CN, Pelton GH, et al: A double-blind, placebo-controlled study of risperidone addition in serotonin reuptake inhibitor-refractory obsessive-compulsive disorder. Arch Gen Psychiatry 57:794–801, 2000

McFarlane AC: The aetiology of post-traumatic morbidity: predisposing, precipitating and perpetuating factors. Br J Psychiatry 154:221–228, 1989

McFarlane AC: Vulnerability to posttraumatic stress disorder, in Posttraumatic Stress Disorder: Etiology, Phenomenology, and Treatment. Edited by Wolf ME, Mosnaim AD. Washington, DC, American Psychiatric Press, 1990, pp 2–20

McGuire PK, Bench CJ, Frith CD, et al: Functional anatomy of obsessive-compulsive phenomena. Br J Psychiatry 164:459–468, 1994

McKay D: A maintenance program for obsessive-compulsive disorder using exposure with response prevention: 2-year follow-up. Behav Res Ther 35:367–369, 1997

McKeon J, McGuffin P, Robinson P: Obsessive-compulsive neurosis following head injury: a report of four cases. Br J Psychiatry 144:190–192, 1984

McNair DM, Kahn RJ: Imipramine compared with a benzodiazepine for agoraphobia, in Anxiety: New Research and Changing Concepts. Edited by Klein DF, Rabkin JG. New York, Raven, 1981, pp 69–80

McNally RJ, Kohlbeck PA: Reality monitoring in obsessive-compulsive disorder. Behav Res Ther 31:24–53, 1993

McNally RJ, Hornig CD, Otto MW, et al: Selective encoding of threat in panic disorder: application of a dual priming paradigm. Behav Res Ther 35:543–549, 1997

McNally RJ, Metzger LJ, Lasko NB, et al: Directed forgetting of trauma cues in adult survivors of childhood sexual abuse with and without posttraumatic stress disorder. J Abnorm Psychol 107:596–601, 1998

Michels R, Frances A, Shear MK: Psychodynamic models of anxiety, in Anxiety and the Anxiety Disorders. Edited by Tuma AH, Maser JD. Hillsdale, NJ, Lawrence Erlbaum, 1985, pp 595–618

Michelson D, Lydiard RB, Pollack MH, et al: Outcome assessment and clinical improvement in panic disorder: evidence from a randomized controlled trial of fluoxetine and placebo. The Fluoxetine Panic Disorder Study Group. Am J Psychiatry 155:1570–1577, 1998

Michelson D, Pollack M, Lydiard RB, et al: Continuing treatment of panic disorder after acute response: randomized, placebo-controlled trial with fluoxetine. The Fluoxetine Panic Disorder Study Group. Br J Psychiatry 174:213–218, 1999

Michelson L, Marchione K, Greenwald M, et al: Panic disorder: cognitive-behavioral treatment. Behav Res Ther 28:141–151, 1990

Mikkelsen EJ, Detlor J, Cohen DJ: School avoidance and social phobia triggered by haloperidol in patients with Tourette's syndrome. Am J Psychiatry 138:1572–1576, 1981

Miller HE, Deakin JF, Anderson IM: Effect of acute tryptophan depletion on CO2-induced anxiety in patients with panic disorder and normal volunteers. Br J Psychiatry 176:182–188, 2000

Milrod B, Busch F, Leon AC, et al: Open trial of psychodynamic psychotherapy for panic disorder: a pilot study. Am J Psychiatry 157:1878–1880, 2000

Mindus, Jenike MA: Neurosurgical treatment of malignant obsessive-compulsive disorder. Psychiatr Clin North Am 15:921–938, 1992

Mogg K, Mathews A, Weinman J: Selective processing of the threat cues in anxiety states: a replication. Behav Res Ther 27:317–323, 1989

Mogg K, Millar N, Bradley BP: Biases in eye movements to threatening facial expressions in generalized anxiety disorder and depressive disorder. J Abnorm Psychol 109:695–704, 2000

Montgomery SA, McIntyre A, Osterheider M, et al: A double-blind, placebo-controlled study of fluoxetine in patients with DSM-III-R obsessive-compulsive disorder. The Lilly European OCD Study Group. Eur Neuropsychopharmacol 3:143–152, 1993

Montgomery SA, Kasper S, Stein DJ, et al: Citalopram 20 mg, 40 mg, and 60 mg are all effective and well tolerated compared with placebo in obsessive-compulsive disorder. Int Clin Psychopharmacol 16:75–86, 2001

Mountjoy CQ, Roth M, Garside RF, et al: A clinical trial of phenelzine in anxiety depressive and phobic neuroses. Br J Psychiatry 131:486–492, 1977

Mountz JM, Modll JG, Wilson MW, et al: Positron emission tomographic evaluation of cerebral blood flow during state anxiety in simple phobia. Arch Gen Psychiatry 46:501–504, 1989

Mowrer O: A stimulus response analysis of anxiety and its role as a reinforcing agent. Psychol Rev 46:553–565, 1939

Mundo E, Bianchi L, Bellodi L: Efficacy of fluvoxamine, paroxetine, and citalopram in the treatment of obsessive-compulsive disorder: a single-blind study. J Clin Psychopharmacol 17:267–271, 1997

Mundo E, Richter MA, Sam F, et al: Is the 5-HT(1Dbeta) receptor gene implicated in the pathogenesis of obsessive-compulsive disorder? Am J Psychiatry 157:1160–1161, 2000a

Mundo E, Maina G, Uslenghi C: Multicentre, double-blind, comparison of fluvoxamine and clomipramine in the treatment of obsessive-compulsive disorder. Int Clin Psychopharmacol 15:69–76, 2000b

Muris P, Schmidt H, Meckelbach H: Ther structure of specific phobia symptoms among children and adolescents. Behav Res Ther 37:863–868, 1999

Murphy TK, Goodman WK, Fudge MW, et al: B lymphocyte antigen D8/17: a peripheral marker for childhood-onset obsessive-compulsive disorder and Tourette's syndrome? Am J Psychiatry 154:402–407, 1997

Nagy LM, Krystal JH, Woods SW, et al: Clinical and medication outcome after short-term alprazolam and behavioral group treatment in panic disorder: 2.5-year naturalistic follow-up study. Arch Gen Psychiatry 46:993–999, 1989

Nee LE, Caine ED, Polinsky RJ, et al: Gilles de la Tourette syndrome: clinical and family study of 50 cases. Ann Neurol 7:41–49, 1982

Neftel KA, Adler RH, Kappell K, et al: Stage fright in musicians: a model illustrating the effect of beta blockers. Psychosom Med 44:461–469, 1982

Nelson EC, Grant JD, Bucholz KK, et al: Social phobia in a population-based female adolescent twin sample: comorbidity and associated suicide-related symptoms. Psychol Med 30:797–804, 2000

Nemiah JC: A psychoanalytic view of phobias. Am J Psychoanal 41:115–120, 1981

Nemiah JC: The psychodynamic view of anxiety: an historical approach, in Handbook of Anxiety, Vol 1. Edited by Roth M, Noyes R, Burrows GD. Amsterdam, The Netherlands, Elsevier, 1988, pp 277–303

Nestadt G, Lan T, Samuels J, et al: Complex segregation analysis provides compelling evidence for a major gene underlying obsessive-compulsive disorder and for heterogeneity by sex. Am J Hum Genet 67:1611–1616, 2000a

Nestadt G, Samuels J, Riddle M, et al: A family study of obsessive-compulsive disorder. Arch Gen Psychiatry 57:358–363, 2000b

Neziroglu F, Anemone R, Yaryura-Tobias JA: Onset of obsessive-compulsive disorder in pregnancy. Am J Psychiatry 149:947–950, 1992

Nicolson R, Swedo SE, Lenane M, et al: An open trial of plasma exchange in childhood-onset obsessive-compulsive disorder without poststreptococcal exacerbations. J Am Acad Child Adolesc Psychiatry 39:1313–1315, 2000

Noyes R Jr, Clarkson C, Crow RR, et al: A family study of generalized anxiety disorder. Am J Psychiatry 144:1019–1024, 1987

Noyes R Jr, Garvey MJ, Cook BL: Follow-up study of patients with panic disorder and agoraphobia with panic attacks treated with tricyclic antidepressants. J Affect Disord 16:249–257, 1989

Noyes R Jr, Reich JH, Christiansen J, et al: Outcome of panic disorder: relationship to diagnostic subtypes and comorbidity. Arch Gen Psychiatry 47:809–818, 1990

Noyes R Jr, Reich JH, Suelzer M, et al: Personality traits associated with panic disorder: change associated with treatment. Compr Psychiatry 32:283–294, 1991

Noyes R Jr, Clancy J, Woodman C, et al: Environmental factors related to the outcome of panic disorder: a seven-year follow-up study. J Nerv Ment Dis 181:529–538, 1993

Noyes R Jr, Moroz G, Davidson JRT, et al: Moclobemide in social phobia: a controlled dose-response trial. J Clin Psychopharmacol 17:247–254, 1997

Nutt DJ: Altered central a2-adrenoreceptor sensitivity in panic disorder. Arch Gen Psychiatry 46:165–169, 1989

Nutt DJ, Glue P, Lawson C, et al: Flumazenil provocation of panic attacks: evidence for altered benzodiazepine receptor sensitivity in panic disorder. Arch Gen Psychiatry 47:917–925, 1990

O'Connor K, Robillard S: Inference processes in obsessive-compulsive disorder: some clinical observations. Behav Res Ther 33:887–896, 1996

Oehrberg S, Christiansen PE, Behnke K, et al: Paroxetine in the treatment of panic disorder. A randomised, double-blind, placebo-controlled study. Br J Psychiatry 167:374–379, 1995

Ohara K, Suzuki Y, Ochiai M, et al: A variable-number-tandem-repeat of the serotonin transporter gene and anxiety disorders. Prog Neuropsychopharmacol Biol Psychiatry 23:55–65, 1999

Ohman A, Soares JF: "Unconscious anxiety": phobic responses to masked stimuli. J Abnorm Psychol 103:231–240, 1994

O'Rourke D, Fahy TJ, Brophy J, et al: The Galway study of panic disorder, III: outcome at 5 to 6 years. Br J Psychiatry 168:462–469, 1996

Orr SP, Metzger LJ, Lasko NB, et al: De novo conditioning in trauma-exposed individuals with and without posttraumatic stress disorder. J Abnorm Psychol 109:290–298, 2000

Ost LG: Age of onset of different phobias. J Abnorm Psychol 96:223–229, 1987

Ost LG, Breitholtz E: Applied relaxation versus cognitive therapy in the treatment of generalized anxiety disorder. Behav Res Ther 38:777–790, 2000

Ost LG, Westling BE: Applied relaxation vs cognitive behavior therapy in the treatment of panic disorder. Behav Res Ther 33:145–158, 1995

Otto MW: Normal and abnormal information processing: a neuropsychological perspective on obsessive-compulsive disorder. Psychiatr Clin North Am 15:825–848, 1992

Otto MW, Pollack MH, Sachs GS, et al: Discontinuation of benzodiazepine treatment: efficacy of cognitive-behavioral therapy for patients with panic disorder. Am J Psychiatry 150:1485–1490, 1993

Otto MW, Pollack MH, Gould RA, et al: A comparison of the efficacy of clonazepam and cognitive-behavioral group therapy for the treatment of social phobia. J Anxiety Disord 14:345–358, 2000

Pacella BL, Polatin P, Nagler SH: Clinical and EEG studies in obsessive-compulsive states. Am J Psychiatry 100:830–838, 1944

Pallanti S, Quercioli L, Paiva RS, et al: Citalopram for treatment-resistant obsessive-compulsive disorder. Eur Psychiatry 14:101–106, 1999

Pande AC, Davidson JRT, Jefferson JW, et al: Treatment of social phobia with gabapentin: a placebo-controlled study. J Clin Psychopharmacol 19:341–348, 1999

Pande AC, Pollack MH, Crockatt J, et al: Placebo-controlled study of gabapentin treatment of panic disorder. J Clin Psychopharmacol 20:467–471, 2000

Papp LA, Klein DF, Gorman JM: Carbon dioxide hypersensitivity, hyperventilation and panic disorder. Am J Psychiatry 150:1149–1157, 1993

Papp LA, Coplan JD, Marinez JM, et al: Efficacy of open-label nefazodone treatment in patients with panic disorder. J Clin Psychopharmacol 20:544–546, 2000

Pato MT, Zohar-Kadouch R, Zohar J, et al: Return of symptoms after discontinuation of clomipramine in patients with obsessive-compulsive disorder. Am J Psychiatry 145:1521–1525, 1988

Pato MT, Pigott TA, Hill JL, et al: Controlled comparison of buspirone and clomipramine in obsessive-compulsive disorder. Am J Psychiatry 148:127–129, 1991

Pauls DL, Towbin KE, Leckman JF, et al: Gilles de la Tourette's and obsessive-compulsive disorder: evidence supporting a genetic relationship. Arch Gen Psychiatry 43:1180–1182, 1986

Pavlov IP: Conditional Reflexes: An Investigation of the Physiological Activity of the Cerebral Cortex (1927). Edited by Anrep GV. New York, Bover, 1960

Pecknold JC, Swinson RP, Kuch K, et al: Alprazolam in panic disorder and agoraphobia: results from a multicenter trial, III: discontinuation effects. Arch Gen Psychiatry 45:429–436, 1988

Perani D, Colombo C, Bressi S, et al: [18F] FDG PET study in obsessive-compulsive disorder. A clinical/metabolic correlation study after treatment. Br J Psychiatry 166:244–250, 1995

Peri T, Ben Shakhar G, Orr SP, et al: Psychophysiologic assessment of aversive conditioning in posttraumatic stress disorder. Biol Psychiatry 47:512–519, 2000

Perlmutter SJ, Leitman SF, Garvey MA, et al: Therapeutic plasma exchange and intravenous immunoglobulin for obsessive-compulsive disorder and tic disorders in childhood. Lancet 354:1153–1158, 1999

Perna G, Bussi R, Allevi L, et al: Sensitivity to 35% carbon dioxide in patients with generalized anxiety disorder. J Clin Psychiatry 60:379–384, 1999

Peroutka SJ, Price SC, Wilhoit TL, et al: Comorbid migraine with aura, anxiety and depression is associated with dopamine D2 receptor (DRD2) NcoI alleles. Mol Med 4:14–21, 1998

Perry BD, Giller EL Jr, Southwick SM: Altered plasma alpha2-adrenergic binding sites in posttraumatic stress disorder (letter). Am J Psychiatry 144:1511–1512, 1987

Perse TL, Greist JH, Jefferson JW, et al: Fluvoxamine treatment of obsessive-compulsive disorder. Am J Psychiatry 144:1543–1548, 1987

Pfanner C, Marazziti D, Dell'Osso L, et al: Risperidone augmentation in refractory obsessive-compulsive disorder: an open-label study. Int Clin Psychopharmacol 15:297–301, 2000

Piccinelli M, Pini S, Bellantuono C, et al: Efficacy of drug treatment in obsessive-compulsive disorder. A meta-analytic review. Br J Psychiatry 166:424–443, 1995

Pigott TA, Pato MT, Bernstein SE, et al: Controlled comparisons of clomipramine and fluoxetine in the treatment of obsessive-compulsive disorder: behavioral and biological results. Arch Gen Psychiatry 47:926–932, 1990

Pigott TA, Pato MT, L'Heureux F, et al: A controlled comparison of adjuvant lithium carbonate or thyroid hormone in clomipramine-treated patients with obsessive-compulsive disorder. J Clin Psychopharmacol 11:242–248, 1991

Pigott TA, L'Heureux F, Rubenstein CS, et al: A double-blind, placebo controlled study of trazodone in patients with obsessive-compulsive disorder. J Clin Psychopharmacol 12:156–162, 1992a

Pigott TA, L'Heureux F, Hill JL, et al: A double-blind study of adjuvant buspirone hydrochloride in clomipramine-treated patients with obsessive-compulsive disorder. J Clin Psychopharmacol 12:11–18, 1992b

Pigott TA, Hill JL, L'Heureux, et al: A comparison of the behavioral effects of oral versus intravenous m-CPP administration in OCD patients and the effect of metergoline prior to iv m-CPP. Biol Psychiatry 33:3–14, 1993

Pitman RK, Orr SP, Forgue DF, et al: Psychophysiologic assessment of post-traumatic stress disorder imagery in Vietnam combat veterans. Arch Gen Psychiatry 44:970–975, 1987

Pitman RK, van der Kolk BA, Orr SP, et al: Naloxone-reversible analgesic response to combat-related stimuli in posttraumatic stress disorder: a pilot study. Arch Gen Psychiatry 47:541–544, 1990

Pitts FN, McClure JN: Lactate metabolism in anxiety neurosis. N Engl J Med 277:1329–1336, 1967

Pohl RB, Wolkow RM, Clary CM: Sertraline in the treatment of panic disorder: a double-blind multicenter trial. Am J Psychiatry 155:1189–1195, 1998

Pollack MH, Worthington JJ 3rd, Otto MW, et al: Venlafaxine for panic disorder: results of a double-blind, placebo-controlled study. Psychopharmacol Bull 32:667–670, 1996

Pollack MH, Zaninelli R, Goddard A, et al: Paroxetine in the treatment of generalized anxiety disorder: results of a placebo-controlled, flexible-dosage trial. J Clin Psychiatry 62:350–357, 2001

Potts NL, Davidson JR, Krishnan KR, et al: Magnetic resonance imaging in social phobia. Psychiatry Res 52:35–42, 1994

Power KG, Simpson RJ, Swanson V, et al: A controlled comparison of cognitive-behaviour therapy, diazepam, and placebo, alone and in combination, for the treatment of generalized anxiety disorder. J Anxiety Disord 4:267–292, 1990

Purcell R, Maruff P, Kyrios M, et al: Neuropsychological deficits in obsessive-compulsive disorder: a comparison with unipolar depression, panic disorder, and normal controls. Arch Gen Psychiatry 55:415–423, 1998

Quitkin F, Babkin J: Hidden psychiatric diagnosis in the alcoholic, in Alcoholism and Clinical Psychiatry. Edited by Soloman J. New York, Plenum, 1982, pp 129–140

Rachman SJ, Hodgson RJ: Obsessions and Compulsions. Englewood Cliffs, NJ, Prentice-Hall, 1980

Rachman S, Thordarson DS, Shafran R, et al: Perceived responsibility: structure and significance. Behav Res Ther 33:779–784, 1995

Radomsky AS, Rachman S: Memory bias in obsessive-compulsive disorder (OCD). Behav Res Ther 37:605–618, 1999

Rainey JM Jr, Pohl RB, Williams M, et al: A comparison of lactate and isoproterenol anxiety states. Psychopathology 17(suppl 1):74–82, 1984

Rainey JM Jr, Aleem A, Ortiz A, et al: Laboratory procedure for the inducement of flashbacks. Am J Psychiatry 144:1317–1319, 1987

Rapaport MH, Pollack MH, Clary CM, et al: Panic disorder and response to sertraline: the effect of previous treatment with benzodiazepines. J Clin Psychopharmacol 21:104–107, 2001

Rapoport JL, Elkins R, Langer DH, et al: Childhood obsessive-compulsive disorder. Am J Psychiatry 138:1545–1554, 1981

Raskin M, Peeke HVS, Dickman W, et al: Panic and generalized anxiety disorders: developmental antecedents and precipitants. Arch Gen Psychiatry 39:687–689, 1982

Rasmussen SA, Tsuang MT: Clinical characteristics and family history in DSM-III obsessive compulsive disorder. Am J Psychiatry 143:317–322, 1986

Rasmussen S, Hackett E, DuBoff E, et al: A 2-year study of sertraline in the treatment of obsessive-compulsive disorder. Int Clin Psychopharmacol 12:309–316, 1997

Rauch SL, Jenike MA, Alpert NM, et al: Regional cerebral blood flow measured during symptom provocation in obsessive-compulsive disorder using oxygen 15-labeled carbon dioxide and positron emission tomography. Arch Gen Psychiatry 51:62–70, 1994

Rauch SL, Savage CR, Alpert NM, et al: A positron emission tomographic study of simple phobic symptom provocation. Arch Gen Psychiatry 52:20–28, 1995

Rauch SL, van der Kolk BA, Fisler RE, et al: A symptom provocation study of posttraumatic stress disorder using positron emission tomography and script-driven imagery. Arch Gen Psychiatry 53:380–387, 1996

Rauch SL, Whalen PJ, Shin LM, et al: Exaggerated amygdala response to masked facial stimuli in posttraumatic stress disorder: a functional MRI study. Biol Psychiatry 47:769–776, 2000

Ravizza L, Barzega G, Bellino S, et al: Predictors of drug treatment response in obsessive-compulsive disorder. J Clin Psychiatry 56:368–373, 1995

Redmond DE Jr: New and old evidence for the involvement of a brain norepinephrine system in anxiety, in Phenomenology and Treatment of Anxiety. Edited by Fann WE, Karacan I, Pokorny AD, et al. New York, Spectrum, 1979, pp 153–203

Regier DA, Boyd JH, Burke JD Jr, et al: One-month prevalence of mental disorders in the United States, based on five Epidemiologic Catchment Area sites. Arch Gen Psychiatry 45:977–986, 1988

Reich J, Noyes R, Yates W: Anxiety symptoms distinguishing social phobia from panic and generalized anxiety disorders. J Nerv Ment Dis 176:510–513, 1988

Reist C, Kauffmann CD, Haier RJ, et al: A controlled trial of desipramine in 18 men with posttraumatic stress disorder. Am J Psychiatry 146:513–516, 1989

Rettew DC: Avoidant personality disorder, generalized social phobia, and shyness: putting the personality back into personality disorders. Harv Rev Psychiatry 8:283–297, 2000

Rice KM, Blanchard EB, Purcell M: Biofeedback treatments of generalized anxiety disorder: preliminary results. Biofeedback Self Regul 18:93–105, 1993

Rickels K, Csanalosi I, Greisman P, et al: A controlled clinical trial of alprazolam for the treatment of anxiety. Am J Psychiatry 140:82–85, 1983

Rickels K, Schweizer E, Csanalosi I, et al: Long-term treatment of anxiety and risk of withdrawal: prospective comparison of clorazepate and buspirone. Arch Gen Psychiatry 45:444–450, 1988

Rickels K, Downing R, Schweizer E, et al: Antidepressants for the treatment of generalized anxiety disorder: a placebo-controlled comparison of imipramine, trazodone, and diazepam. Arch Gen Psychiatry 50:884–895, 1993a

Rickels K, Schweizer E, Weiss S, et al: Maintenance drug treatment for panic disorder, II: short- and long-term outcome after drug taper. Arch Gen Psychiatry 50:61–68, 1993b

Rickels K, Pollack MH, Sheehan DV, et al: Efficacy of extended-release venlafaxine in nondepressed outpatients with generalized anxiety disorder. Am J Psychiatry 157:968–974, 2000a

Rickels K, DeMartinis N, Garcia-Espana F, et al: Imipramine and buspirone in treatment of patients with generalized anxiety disorder who are discontinuing long-term benzodiazepine therapy. Am J Psychiatry 157:1973–1979, 2000b

Riddle MA, Scahill L, King RA, et al: Double-blind, crossover trial of fluoxetine and placebo in children and adolescents with obsessive-compulsive disorder. J Am Acad Child Adolesc Psychiatry 31:1062–1069, 1992

Riddle MA, Reeve EA, Yaryura-Tobias JA, et al: Fluvoxamine for children and adolescents with obsessive-compulsive disorder: a randomized, controlled, multicenter trial. J Am Acad Child Adolesc Psychiatry 40:222–229, 2001

Rocca P, Fonzo V, Scotta M, et al: Paroxetine efficacy in the treatment of generalized anxiety disorder. Acta Psychiatr Scand 95:444–450, 1997

Rocca P, Beoni AM, Eva C, et al: Peripheral benzodiazepine receptor messenger RNA is decreased in lymphocytes of generalized anxiety disorder patients. Biol Psychiatry 43:767–773, 1998

Romach M, Busto U, Somer G, et al: Clinical aspects of chronic use of alprazolam and lorazepam. Am J Psychiatry 152:1161–1167, 1995

Romano S, Goodman W, Tamura R, et al: Long-term treatment of obsessive-compulsive disorder after an acute response: a comparison of fluoxetine versus placebo. J Clin Psychopharmacol 21:46–52, 2001

Rosenbaum JF, Moroz G, Bowden CL: Clonazepam in the treatment of panic disorder with or without agoraphobia: a dose–response study of efficacy, safety, and discontinuance. Clonazepam Panic Disorder Dose–Response Study Group. J Clin Psychopharmacol 17:390–400, 1997

Rosenberg DR, Keshavan MS, O'Hearn KM, et al: Frontostriatal measurement in treatment-naïve children with obsessive-compulsive disorder. Arch Gen Psychiatry 54:824–830, 1997

Rosenberg DR, Keshavan MS: A.E. Bennett Research Award. Toward a neurodevelopmental model of obsessive-compulsive disorder. Biol Psychiatry 43:623–640, 1998

Rosenberg DR, Stewart CM, Fitzgerald KD, et al: Paroxetine open-label treatment of pediatric outpatients with obsessive-compulsive disorder. J Am Acad Child Adolesc Psychiatry 38:1180–1185, 1999

Rosenberg DR, MacMaster FP, Keshavan MS, et al: Decrease in caudate glutamatergic concentrations in pediatric obsessive-compulsive disorder patients taking paroxetine. J Am Acad Child Adolesc Psychiatry 39:1096–1103, 2000a

Rosenberg DR, Benazon NR, Gilbert A, et al: Thalamic volume in pediatric obsessive-compulsive disorder patients before and after cognitive behavioral therapy. Biol Psychiatry 48:294–300, 2000b

Roth D, Antony MM, Swinson RP: Interpretations for anxiety symptoms in social phobia. Behav Res Ther 39:129–138, 2001

Rowe DC, Stever C, Gard JM, et al: The relation of the dopamine transporter gene (DAT1) to symptoms of internalizing disorders in children. Behav Genetics 28:215–225, 1998

Roy-Byrne PP, Cowley DS, Greenblatt DJ, et al: Reduced benzodiazepine sensitivity in panic disorder. Arch Gen Psychiatry 47:534–538, 1990

Rubenstein CS, Peynircioglu ZF, Chambless DL, et al: Memory in sub-clinical obsessive-compulsive checkers. Behav Res Ther 31:759–765, 1993

Ruiz AT: A double-blind study of alprazolam and lorazepam in the treatment of anxiety. J Clin Psychiatry 44:60–62, 1983

Saletu ZG, Saletu B, Anderer P, et al: Nonorganic insomnia in generalized anxiety disorder, I: controlled studies on sleep, awakening and daytime vigilance utilizing polysomnography and EEG mapping. Neuropsychobiology 36:117–129, 1997

Salkovskis PM, Westbrook D: Behaviour therapy and obsessional ruminations: can failure be turned into success? Behav Res Ther 27:149–160, 1989

Salkovskis PM, Jones DRO, Clark DM: Respiratory control in the treatment of panic attacks: replication and extension with concurrent measurement of behaviour and pCO2. Br J Psychiatry 148:526–532, 1986

Salkovskis PM, Wroe AL, Gledhill A, et al: Responsibility attitudes and interpretations are characteristic of obsessive compulsive disorder. Behav Res Ther 38:347–372, 2000

Salzman L: Comments on the psychological treatment of obsessive-compulsive patients, in Obsessive-Compulsive Disorder: Psychological and Pharmacological Treatment. Edited by Mavissakalian M, Turner SM, Michelson L. New York, Plenum, 1985, pp 155–165

Samuels J, Nestadt G, Bienvenu OJ, et al: Personality disorders and normal personality dimensions in obsessive-compulsive disorder. Br J Psychiatry 177:457–462, 2000

Sanderson WC, Rapee RM, Barlow DH: The influence of an illusion of control on panic attacks induced via inhalation of 5.5% carbon dioxide-enriched air. Arch Gen Psychiatry 46:157–162, 1989

Saxena S, Wang D, Bystritsky A, et al: Risperidone augmentation of SRI treatment for refractory obsessive-compulsive disorder. J Clin Psychiatry 57:303–306, 1996

Schilder P: The organic background of obsessions and compulsions. Am J Psychiatry 94:1397–1416, 1938

Schindler KM, Richter MA, Kennedy JL, et al: Association between homozygosity at the COMT gene locus and obsessive-compulsive disorder. Am J Med Genet 96:721–724, 2000

Schneider F, Weiss U, Kessler C, et al: Subcortical correlates of differential classical conditioning of aversive emotional reactions in social phobia. Biol Psychiatry 45:863–871, 1999

Schneier FR, Johnson J, Hornig CD, et al: Social phobia: comorbidity and morbidity in an epidemiologic sample. Arch Gen Psychiatry 49:282–288, 1992

Schneier FR, Saoud JB, Campeas R, et al: Buspirone in social phobia. J Clin Psychopharmacol 13:251–256, 1993

Schneier FR, Heckelman LR, Garfinkel R, et al: Functional impairment in social phobia. J Clin Psychiatry 55:322–331, 1994

Schneier FR, Goetz D, Campeas R, et al: Placebo-controlled trial of moclobemide in social phobia. Br J Psychiatry 172:70–77, 1998

Schneier F, Liebowitz MR, Abi-Dargham A, et al: Low dopamine D2 binding potential in social phobia. Am J Psychiatry 157:457–459, 2000

Schnyder U, Moergeli H, Klaghofer R, et al: Incidence and prediction of posttraumatic stress disorder symptoms in severely injured accident victims. Am J Psychiatry 158:595–599, 2001

Schwartz C, Snidman N, Kagan J: Adolescent social anxiety as an outcome of inhibited temperament in childhood. J Am Acad Child Adolesc Psychiatry 38:1008–1015, 1999

Schwartz JM, Stoessel PW, Baxter LR, et al: Systematic changes in cerebral glucose metabolic rate after successful behavior modification treatment in obsessive-compulsive disorder. Arch Gen Psychiatry 53:109–113, 1996

Schweizer E, Rickels K, Lucki I: Resistance to the anti-anxiety effect of buspirone in patients with a history of benzodiazepine use. N Engl J Med 314:719–720, 1986

Schweizer E, Rickels K, Weiss S, et al: Maintenance drug treatment of panic disorder, I: results of a prospective, placebo-controlled comparison of alprazolam and imipramine. Arch Gen Psychiatry 50:51–60, 1993

Scott JP: Effects of psychotropic drugs on separation distress in dogs, in Proceedings of the IX Congress of Neuropsychopharmacology. Amsterdam, The Netherlands, Excerpta Medica, 1975, pp 735–745

Scrignar CB: Post-Traumatic Stress Disorder: Diagnosis, Treatment, and Legal Issues. New York, Praeger, 1984

Seedat S, Stein DJ: Inositol augmentation of serotonin reuptake inhibitors in treatment-refractory obsessive-compulsive disorder: an open trial. Int Clin Psychopharmacol 14:353–356, 1999

Sevy S, Papadimitriou GN, Surmont DW, et al: Noradrenergic function in generalized anxiety disorder, major depressive disorder, and healthy subjects. Biol Psychiatry 15:141–152, 1989

Shafran R, Ralph J, Tallis F: Obsessive-compulsive symptoms and the family. Bull Menninger Clin 59:472–479, 1996

Shalev AY, Peri T, Canetti L, et al: Predictors of PTSD in injured trauma survivors: a prospective study. Am J Psychiatry 153:2219–2225, 1996

Shalev AY, Sahar T, Freedman S, et al: A prospective study of heart rate response following trauma and the subsequent development of posttraumatic stress disorder. Arch Gen Psychiatry 55:553–559, 1998a

Shalev AY, Freedman S, Peri T, et al: Prospective study of posttraumatic stress disorder and depression following trauma. Am J Psychiatry 155:630–637, 1998b

Shay J: Fluoxetine reduces explosiveness and elevates mood of Vietnam combat vets with PTSD. J Trauma Stress 5:97–101, 1992

Shea MT, Zlotnick C, Dolan R, et al: Personality disorders, history of trauma, and posttraumatic stress disorder in subjects with anxiety disorders. Compr Psychiatry 41:312–325, 2000

Shear MK, Cooper AM, Klerman GL, et al: A psychodynamic model of panic disorder. Am J Psychiatry 150:859–866, 1993

Sheehan DV, Ballenger J, Jacobsen G: Treatment of endogenous anxiety with phobic, hysterical, and hypochondriacal symptoms. Arch Gen Psychiatry 37:51–59, 1980

Shin LM, Kosslyn SM, McNally RJ, et al: Visual imagery and perception in posttraumatic stress disorder: a positron emission tomographic investigation. Arch Gen Psychiatry 54:233–241, 1997

Silva RR, Alpert M, Munoz DM, et al: Stress and vulnerability to posttraumatic stress disorder in children and adolescents. Am J Psychiatry 157:1229–1235, 2000

Simpson HB, Gorfinkle KS, Liebowitz MR: Cognitive-behavioral therapy as an adjunct to serotonin reuptake inhibitors in obsessive-compulsive disorder: an open trial. J Clin Psychiatry 60:584–590, 1999

Skolnick P, Paul SM: Benzodiazepine receptors in the central nervous system. Int Rev Neurobiol 23:103–140, 1982

Skoog G, Skoog I: A 40-year follow-up of patients with obsessive-compulsive disorder. Arch Gen Psychiatry 56:121–127, 1999

Skre I, Onstad S, Torgensen S, et al: A twin study of DSM-III-R anxiety disorders. Acta Psychiatr Scand 88:85–92, 1993

Smith MA, Davidson J, Ritchie JC, et al: The corticotropin releasing hormone test in patients with posttraumatic stress disorder. Biol Psychiatry 26:349–355, 1989

Solyom C, Solyom K, LaPierre Y, et al: Phenelzine and exposure in the treatment of phobias. Biol Psychiatry 16:239–247, 1981

Solyom L, Heseltine GFD, McClure DJ, et al: Behavior therapy versus drug therapy in the treatment of phobic neurosis. Can J Psychiatry 18:25–32, 1973

Southwick SM, Krystal JH, Morgan CA, et al: Abnormal noradrenergic function in posttraumatic stress disorder. Arch Gen Psychiatry 50:266–274, 1993

Southwick SM, Krystal JH, Bremner JD, et al: Noradrenergic and serotonergic function in posttraumatic stress disorder. Arch Gen Psychiatry 54:749–758, 1997

Southwick SM, Bremner JD, Rasmusson A, et al: Role of norepinephrine in the pathophysiology and treatment of posttraumatic stress disorder. Biol Psychiatry 46:1192–1204, 1999

Spiegel D, Cardena E: Dissociative mechanisms in posttraumatic stress disorder, in Posttraumatic Stress Disorder: Etiology, Phenomenology, and Treatment. Edited by Wolf ME, Mosnaim AD. Washington, DC, American Psychiatric Press, 1990, pp 22–34

Spiegel DA, Bruce TJ, Gregg SF, et al: Does cognitive behavior therapy assist slow-taper alprazolam discontinuation in panic disorder? Am J Psychiatry 151:876–881, 1994

Spence SH, Donovan C, Brechman-Toussant M: Social skills, social outcomes, and cognitive features of childhood social phobia. J Abnorm Psychol 108:211–221, 1999

Spence SH, Donovan C, Brechman TM: The treatment of childhood social phobia: the effectiveness of a social skills training-based, cognitive-behavioural intervention, with and without parental involvement. J Child Psychol Psychiatry 41:713–762, 2000

Spivak B, Vered Y, Graff E, et al: Low platelet-poor plasma concentrations of serotonin in patients with combat-related posttraumatic stress disorder. Biol Psychiatry 45:840–845, 1999

Starcevic V, Fallon S, Uhlenhuth EH: The frequency and severity of generalized anxiety disorder symptoms. Toward a less cumbersome conceptualization. J Nerv Ment Dis 182:80–84, 1994

Starkman MN, Cameron OG, Nesse RM, et al: Peripheral catecholamine levels and the symptoms of anxiety: studies in patients with and without pheochromocytoma. Psychosom Med 52:129–142, 1990

Stein DJ, Spadaccine E, Hollander E: Meta-analysis of pharmacotherapy trials for obsessive-compulsive disorder. Int Clin Psychopharmacol 10:11–18, 1995

Stein DJ, Montgomery SA, Kasper S, et al: Predictors of response to pharmacotherapy with citalopram in obsessive-compulsive disorder. Int Clin Psychopharmacol 16:357–361, 2001

Stein MB, Asmundson GJ: Autonomic function in panic disorder: cardiorespiratory and plasma catecholamine responsivity to multiple challenges of the autonomic nervous system. Biol Psychiatry 36:548–558, 1994

Stein MB, Kean YM: Disability and quality of life in social phobia: epidemiologic findings. Am J Psychiatry 157:1606–1613, 2000

Stein MB, Leslie WD: A brain single photon emission computed tomography (SPECT) study of generalized social phobia. Biol Psychiatry 39:825–828, 1996

Stein MB, Asmundson G, Chartier M: Autonomic responsivity in generalized social phobia. J Affect Disord 31:211–221, 1994

Stein MB, Millar TW, Larsen DK, et al: Irregular breathing during sleep in patients with panic disorder. Am J Psychiatry 152:1168–1173, 1995a

Stein MB, Delaney SM, Chartier M, et al: 3H paroxetine binding to platelets of patients with social phobia: comparison to patients with panic disorder and healthy volunteers. Biol Psychiatry 37:224–228, 1995b

Stein MB, Walker JR, Anderson G, et al: Childhood physical and sexual abuse in patients with anxiety disorders and in a community sample. Am J Psychiatry 153:275–277, 1996

Stein MB, Walker JR, Hazen AL, et al: Full and partial posttraumatic stress disorder: findings from a community survey. Am J Psychiatry 154:1114–1119, 1997

Stein MB, Chartier MJ, Hazen AL, et al: A direct-interview family study of generalized social phobia. Am J Psychiatry 155:90–97, 1998a

Stein MB, Chartier MJ, Kozak MV, et al: Genetic linkage to the serotonin transporter protein and 5HT2A receptor genes excluded in generalized social phobia. Psychiatry Res 81:283–291, 1998b

Stein MB, Liebowitz MR, Lydiard B, et al: Paroxetine treatment of generalized social phobia (social anxiety disorder): a randomized controlled trial. JAMA 280:708–713, 1998c

Stein MB, Fyer AJ, Davidson JRT, et al: Fluvoxamine treatment of social phobia (social anxiety disorder): a double-blind, placebo-controlled study. Am J Psychiatry 156:756–760, 1999

Steketee GS, Foa EB, Grayson JB: Recent advances in the behavioral treatment of obsessive-compulsives. Arch Gen Psychiatry 39:1365–1371, 1982

Stemberger RT, Turner SM, Beidel DC, et al: Social phobia: an analysis of possible developmental factors. J Abnorm Psychol 104:526–531, 1995

Stopa L, Clark DM: Social phobia and interpretation of social events. Behav Res Ther 38:273–283, 2000

Strohle A, Kellner M, Holsboer F, et al: Behavioral, neuroendocrine, and cardiovascular response to flumazenil: no evidence for an altered benzodiazepine receptor sensitivity in panic disorder. Biol Psychiatry 45:321–326, 1999

Suomi SJ, Seaman SF, Lewis JK, et al: Effects of imipramine treatment of separation-induced social disorders in rhesus monkeys. Arch Gen Psychiatry 35:321–325, 1978

Swedo SE: Rituals and releasers: an ethological model of obsessive-compulsive disorder, in Obsessive-Compulsive Disorder in Children and Adolescents. Edited by Rapoport JL. Washington, DC, American Psychiatric Press, 1989, pp 269–288

Swedo SE, Schapiro MB, Grady CL, et al: Cerebral glucose metabolism in childhood-onset obsessive-compulsive disorder. Arch Gen Psychiatry 46:518–523, 1989a

Swedo SE, Rapoport JL, Cheslow DL, et al: Increased incidence of obsessive-compulsive symptoms in patients with Sydenham's chorea. Am J Psychiatry 146:246–249, 1989b

Swedo SE, Rapoport JL, Leonard H, et al: Obsessive-compulsive disorder in children and adolescents: clinical phenomenology of 70 consecutive cases. Arch Gen Psychiatry 46:335–341, 1989c

Swedo SE, Pietrini P, Leonard HL, et al: Cerebral glucose metabolism in childhood-onset obsessive-compulsive disorder: revisualization during pharmacotherapy. Arch Gen Psychiatry 49:690–694, 1992a

Swedo SE, Leonard HL, Kruesi MJP, et al: Cerebrospinal fluid neurochemistry in children and adolescents with obsessive-compulsive disorder. Arch Gen Psychiatry 49:29–36, 1992b

Szegedi A, Wetzel H, Leal M, et al: Combination treatment with clomipramine and fluvoxamine: drug monitoring, safety, and tolerability data. J Clin Psychiatry 57:257–264, 1996

Szeszko PR, Robinson D, Alvir JM, et al: Orbital frontal and amygdala volume reductions in obsessive-compulsive disorder. Arch Gen Psychiatry 56:913–919, 1999

Szymanski HV, Olympia J: Divalproex in posttraumatic stress disorder (letter). Am J Psychiatry 148:1086–1087, 1991

Tancer ME, Stein MB, Uhde TW: Growth hormone response to intravenous clonidine in social phobia: comparison to patients with panic disorder and healthy volunteers. Biol Psychiatry 34:591–595, 1993

Tancer ME, Mailman RB, Stein MB, et al: Neuroendocrine responsivity to monoaminergic system probes in generalized social phobia. Anxiety 1:216–223, 1994

Tarrier N, Pilgrim H, Sommerfield C, et al: A randomized trial of cognitive therapy and imaginal exposure in the treatment of chronic posttraumatic stress disorder. J Consult Clin Psychol 67:13–18, 1999

Telch MJ, Agras WG, Taylor CM, et al: Combined pharmacological and behavioral treatment for agoraphobia. Behav Res Ther 23:325–335, 1985

Telch MJ, Lucas JA, Schmidt NB, et al: Group cognitive-behavioral treatment of panic disorder. Behav Res Ther 31:279–287, 1993

The International Multicenter Clinical Trial Group on Moclobemide in Social Phobia. Moclobemide in social phobia. A double-blind, placebo-controlled study. Eur Arch Psychiatry Clin Neurosci 247:71–80, 1997

Thomsen PH: Child and adolescent obsessive-compulsive disorder treated with citalopram: findings from an open trial of 23 cases. J Child Adolesc Psychopharmacol 7:157–166, 1997

Thomsen PH, Mikkelsen HU: Development of personality disorders in children and adolescents with obsessive-compulsive disorder: a 6- to 22-year follow-up study. Acta Psychiatr Scand 87:456–462, 1993

Thoren P, Asberg M, Cronholm B, et al: Clomipramine treatment of obsessive-compulsive disorder, I: a controlled clinical trial. Arch Gen Psychiatry 37:1281–1285, 1980a

Thoren P, Asberg M, Bertilsson L, et al: Clomipramine treatment of obsessive-compulsive disorder, II: biochemical aspects. Arch Gen Psychiatry 37:1289–1294, 1980b

Tiffon L, Coplan JD, Papp LA, et al: Augmentation strategies with tricyclic or fluoxetine treatment in seven partially responsive panic disorder patients. J Clin Psychiatry 55:66–69, 1994

Tiihonen J, Kuikka J, Rasanen P, et al: Cerebral benzodiazepine receptor binding and distribution in generalized anxiety: a fractal analysis. Molecular Psychiatry 2:463–471, 1997a

Tiihonen J, Kuikka J, Bergstrom K, et al: Dopamine reuptake site densities in patients with social phobia. Am J Psychiatry 154:239–242, 1997b

Tillfors M, Furmark T, Ekselius L, et al: Social phobia and avoidant personality disorder as related to parental history of social anxiety: a general population study. Behav Res Ther 39:289–298, 2001

Tollefson GD, Rampey AH, Potvin JH, et al: A multicenter investigation of fixed-dose fluoxetine in the treatment of obsessive-compulsive disorder. Arch Gen Psychiatry 51:559–567, 1994

Torgersen S: Genetic factors in anxiety disorders. Arch Gen Psychiatry 40:1085–1089, 1983

Towey J, Bruder G, Hollander E, et al: Endogenous event-related potentials in obsessive-compulsive disorder. Biol Psychiatry 28:92–98, 1990

True WR, Rice J, Eisen SA, et al: A twin study of genetic and environmental contributions to liability for posttraumatic stress symptoms. Arch Gen Psychiatry 50:257–264, 1993

Turner SM, Beidel DC, Cooley-Quille MR: Two-year follow-up of social phobias treated with Social Effectiveness Therapy. Behav Res Ther 33:553–555, 1995

Tweed JL, Schoenbach VJ, George LK, et al: The effects of childhood parental death and divorce on six-month history of anxiety disorders. Br J Psychiatry 154:823–828, 1989

Tynes LL, Salins C, Skiba W, et al: A psychoeducational and support group for obsessive-compulsive disorder patients and their significant others. Compr Psychiatry 33:197–201, 1992

Tyrer P, Candy J, Kelly D: A study of the clinical effects of phenelzine and placebo in the treatment of phobic anxiety. Psychopharmacology (Berl) 32:237–254, 1973

Uhde TW, Stein MB, Vittone BJ, et al: Behavioral and physiologic effects of short-term and long-term administration of clonidine in panic disorder. Arch Gen Psychiatry 46:170–177, 1989

Uhde TW, Tancer ME, Gelernter CS, et al: Normal urinary free cortisol and postdexamethasone cortisol in social phobia: comparison to normal volunteers. J Affect Disord 30:155–161, 1994

Ursano RJ, Fullerton CS, Epstein RS, et al: Acute and chronic posttraumatic stress disorder in motor vehicle accident victims. Am J Psychiatry 156:589–595, 1999a

Ursano RJ, Fullerton CS, Epstein RS, et al: Peritraumatic dissociation and posttraumatic stress disorder following motor vehicle accidents. Am J Psychiatry 156:1808–1810, 1999b

Vallejo J, Olivares J, Marcos T, et al: Clomipramine versus phenelzine in obsessive-compulsive disorder: a controlled clinical trial. Br J Psychiatry 161:665–670, 1992

Van Ameringen M, Mancini C, Streiner DL: Fluoxetine efficacy in social phobia. J Clin Psychiatry 54:27–32, 1993

Van Ameringen M, Mancini C, Streiner D: Sertraline in social phobia. J Affect Disord 31:141–145, 1994

Van Ameringen M, Mancini C, Oakman JM: Nefazodone in social phobia. J Clin Psychiatry 60:96–100, 1999

Van Ameringen MA, Lane RM, Walker JR, et al: Sertraline treatment of generalized social phobia: a 20-week, double-blind, placebo-controlled study. Am J Psychiatry 158:275–281, 2001

van Balkom AJ, de Haan E, van Oppen P, et al: Cognitive and behavioral therapies alone versus in combination with fluvoxamine in the treatment of obsessive compulsive disorder. J Nerv Ment Dis 186:492–499, 1998

van den Hout M, Arntz A, Hoekstra R: Exposure reduced agoraphobia but not panic, and cognitive therapy reduced panic but not agoraphobia. Behav Res Ther 32:447–451, 1994

van den Hout M, Tenney N, Huygens K, et al: Preconscious processing bias in specific phobia. Behav Res Ther 35:29–34, 1997

van der Kolk BA: Psychopharmacological issues in posttraumatic stress disorder. Hosp Community Psychiatry 34:683–691, 1983

van der Kolk BA: The role of the group in the origin and resolution of the trauma response, in Psychological Trauma. Edited by van der Kolk BA. Washington, DC, American Psychiatric Press, 1987a, pp 153–171

van der Kolk BA: The separation cry and the trauma response: developmental issues in the psychobiology of attachment and separation, in Psychological Trauma. Edited by van der Kolk BA. Washington, DC, American Psychiatric Press, 1987b, pp 31–62

van der Kolk BA: The compulsion to repeat the trauma: reenactment, revictimization, and masochism. Psychiatr Clin North Am 12:389–411, 1989

van der Kolk BA, Saporta J: The biological response to psychic trauma: mechanisms and treatment of intrusion and numbing. Anxiety Research 4:199–212, 1991

van der Kolk BA, van der Hart O: Pierre Janet and the breakdown of adaptation in psychological trauma. Am J Psychiatry 146:1530–1540, 1989

van der Kolk BA, Boyd H, Krystal J, et al: Post-traumatic stress disorder as a biologically based disorder: implications of the animal model of inescapable shock, in Post-Traumatic Stress Disorder: Psychological and Biological Sequelae. Edited by van der Kolk BA. Washington, DC, American Psychiatric Press, 1984, pp 123–134

van der Kolk BA, Dreyfuss D, Michaels M, et al: Fluoxetine in posttraumatic stress disorder. J Clin Psychiatry 55:517–522, 1994

Van der Linden G, van Heerden B, Warwick J, et al: Functional brain imaging and pharmacotherapy in social phobia: single photon emission computed tomography before and after treatment with the selective serotonin reuptake inhibitor citalopram. Prog Neuropsychopharmacol Biol Psychiatry 24:419–438, 2000

vanOppen P, Arntz A: Cognitive therapy for obsessive-compulsive disorder. Behav Res Ther 32:79–87, 1994

vanOppen P, deHaan E, vanBalkom AJ, et al: Cognitive therapy and exposure in vivo in the treatment of obsessive compulsive disorder. Behav Res Ther 33:379–390, 1995

van Vliet IM, den Boer JA, Westenberg HG: Psychopharmacological treatment of social phobia: a double blind placebo controlled study with fluvoxamine. Psychopharmacology (Berl) 115:128–134, 1994

van Vliet IM, den Boer JA, Westenberg HGM, et al: Clinical effects of buspirone in social phobia: a double-blind placebo-controlled study. J Clin Psychiatry 58:164–168, 1997

Verburg C, Griez C, Meijer J: A 35% carbon dioxide challenge in simple phobias. Acta Psychiatr Scand 90:420–423, 1994

Versiani M, Mundim FD, Nardi AE, et al: Tranylcypromine in social phobia. J Clin Psychopharmacol 8:279–283, 1988

Villareal G, Johnson MR, Rubey R, et al: Treatment of social phobia with the dopamine agonist pergolide. Depress Anxiety 11:45–47, 2000

Wade AG, Lepola U, Koponen HJ, et al: The effect of citalopram in panic disorder. Br J Psychiatry 170:549–553, 1997

Wallace ST, Alden LE: Social phobia and positive social events: the price of success. J Abnorm Psychol 106:416–424, 1997

Wang Z, Valdes J, Noyes R, et al: Possible association of a cholecystokinin promoter polymorphism (CCK-36CT) with panic disorder. Am J Med Genet 81:228–234, 1998

Warneke LB: Intravenous chlorimipramine in the treatment of obsessional disorder in adolescence: case report. J Clin Psychiatry 46:100–103, 1985

Warshaw MG, Dolan RT, Keller MB: Suicidal behavior in patients with current or past panic disorder: five years of prospective data from the Harvard/Brown Anxiety Research Program. Am J Psychiatry 157:1876–1878, 2000

Weiss EL, Potenza MN, McDougle CJ, et al: Olanzapine addition in obsessive-compulsive disorder refractory to selective serotonin reuptake inhibitors: an open-label case series. J Clin Psychiatry 60:524–527, 1999

Weissman MM, Leckman JF, Merikangas KR, et al: Depression and anxiety disorders in parents and children. Arch Gen Psychiatry 41:845–852, 1984

Weissman MM, Markowitz JS, Ouellette R, et al: Panic disorder and cardiovascular/cerebrovascular problems: results from a community survey. Am J Psychiatry 147:1504–1508, 1990

Weissman MM, Wickramaratne P, Adams PB, et al: The relationship between panic disorder and major depression: a new family study. Arch Gen Psychiatry 50:767–780, 1993

Wells A, Carter K: Preliminary tests of a cognitive model of generalized anxiety disorder. Behav Res Ther 37:585–594, 1999

Welner A, Reich T, Robins E, et al: Obsessive-compulsive neurosis: record, family, and follow-up studies. Compr Psychiatry 17:527–539, 1976

Westphal K: Ueber Zwangsverstellungen [obsessional thoughts]. Arch Psychiatr Neurol 8:734–750, 1878

Widom CS: Posttraumatic stress disorder in abused and neglected children grown up. Am J Psychiatry 156:1223–1229, 1999

Wiborg IM, Dahl AA: Does brief dynamic psychotherapy reduce the relapse rate of panic disorder? Arch Gen Psychiatry 53:689–694, 1996

Wilkinson DJ, Thompson JM, Lambert GW, et al: Sympathetic activity in patients with panic disorder at rest, under laboratory mental stress, and during panic attacks. Arch Gen Psychiatry 55:511–520, 1998

Wise SP, Rapoport JL: Obsessive-compulsive disorder: is it a basal ganglia dysfunction?, in Obsessive-Compulsive Disorder in Children and Adolescents. Edited by Rapoport JL. Washington, DC, American Psychiatric Press, 1989, pp 327–344

Wittchen HU, Zhao S, Kessler RC, et al: DSM-III-R generalized anxiety disorder in the National Comorbidity Survey. Arch Gen Psychiatry 51:355–364, 1994

Wittchen HU, Carter RM, Pfister H, et al: Disabilities and quality of life in pure and comorbid generalized anxiety disorder and major depression in a national survey. Int Clin Psychopharmacol 15:319–328, 2000

Wlazlo Z, Schroeder-Hartwig K, Hand I, et al: Exposure in vivo vs social skills training for social phobia: long-term outcome and differential effects. Behav Res Ther 28:181–193, 1990

Wolf ME, Alavi A, Mosnaim AD: Posttraumatic stress disorder in Vietnam veterans, clinical and EEG findings: possible therapeutic effects of carbamazepine. Biol Psychiatry 23:642–644, 1988

Woodman CL, Noyes R: Panic disorder: treatment with valproate. J Clin Psychiatry 55:134–136, 1994

Woodman CL, Noyes R, Black DW, et al: A 5-year follow-up study of generalized anxiety disorder and panic disorder. J Nerv Ment Dis 187:3–9, 1999

Woodruff R, Pitts FN Jr: Monozygotic twins with obsessional illness. Am J Psychiatry 120:1075–1080, 1964

Woody SR, Chambless DL, Glass CR: Self-focused attention in the treatment of social phobia. Behav Res Ther 35:117–129, 1997

World Health Organization: International Statistical Classification of Diseases and Related Health Problems, Tenth Revision (ICD-10). Geneva, Switzerland, World Health Organization, 1992

Wu JC, Buchsbaum MS, Hershey TG, et al: PET in generalized anxiety disorder. Biol Psychiatry 29:1181–1199, 1991

Yehuda R, Southwick SM, Krystal JH, et al: Enhanced suppression of cortisol following dexamethasone administration in posttraumatic stress disorder. Am J Psychiatry 150:83–86, 1993

Yehuda R, Boisoneau D, Lowy MT, et al: Dose-response changes in plasma cortisol and lymphocyte glucocorticoid receptors following dexamethasone administration in combat veterans with and without posttraumatic stress disorder. Arch Gen Psychiatry 52:583–593, 1995a

Yehuda R, Keefe RS, Harvey PD, et al: Learning and memory in combat veterans with posttraumatic stress disorder. Am J Psychiatry 152:137–139, 1995b

Yehuda R, McFarlane AC, Shalev AY: Predicting the development of posttraumatic stress disorder from the acute response to a traumatic event. Biol Psychiatry 44:1305–1313, 1998a

Yehuda R, Schmeidler J, Wainberg M, et al: Vulnerability to posttraumatic stress disorder in adult offspring of Holocaust survivors. Am J Psychiatry 155:1163–1171, 1998b

Yonkers KA, Warshaw MG, Massion AO, et al: Phenomenology and course of generalised anxiety disorder. Br J Psychiatry 168:308–313, 1996

Zatzick DF, Marmar CR, Weiss DS, et al: Posttraumatic stress disorder and functioning and quality of life outcomes in a nationally representative sample of male Vietnam veterans. Am J Psychiatry 154:1690–1695, 1997

Zisook S, Chentsova-Dutton YE, Smith-Vaniz A, et al: Nefazodone in patients with treatment-refractory posttraumatic stress disorder. J Clin Psychiatry 61:203–208, 2000

Zitrin CM, Klein DF, Woerner MG: Treatment of agoraphobia with group exposure in vivo and imipramine. Arch Gen Psychiatry 37:63–72, 1980

Zitrin CM, Klein DF, Woerner MG, et al: Treatment of phobias, I: comparison of imipramine hydrochloride and placebo. Arch Gen Psychiatry 40:125–138, 1983

Zlotnick C, Shea TM, Rosen K, et al: An affect-management group for women with posttraumatic stress disorder and histories of childhood sexual abuse. J Trauma Stress 10:425–436, 1997

Zlotnick C, Warshaw M, Shea MT, et al: Chronicity in posttraumatic stress disorder (PTSD) and predictors of course of comorbid PTSD in patients with anxiety disorders. J Trauma Stress 12:89–100, 1999

Zohar J, Insel TR: Obsessive-compulsive disorder: psychobiological approaches to diagnosis, treatment, and pathophysiology. Biol Psychiatry 22:667–687, 1987

Zohar J, Judge R: Paroxetine versus clomipramine in the treatment of obsessive-compulsive disorder. OCD Paroxetine Study Investigators. Br J Psychiatry 169:468–474, 1996

Zohar J, Mueller EA, Insel TR, et al: Serotonergic responsivity in obsessive-compulsive disorder: comparison of patients and healthy controls. Arch Gen Psychiatry 44:946–951, 1987

Zohar J, Insel TR, Zohar-Kadouch RC, et al: Serotonergic responsivity in obsessive-compulsive disorder: effects of chronic clomipramine treatment. Arch Gen Psychiatry 45:167–172, 1988

CHAPTER 12

Psychological Factors Affecting Medical Conditions

James L. Levenson, M.D.

The fact that psychological factors and psychiatric disorders may affect the clinical course of medical illness is incontrovertible and is no longer the topic of serious debate. For example, psychiatric disorders may adversely affect outcome and length of stay in general hospital patients (Levenson et al. 1990b; Saravay and Lavin 1994), and the presence of major depression increases morbidity and mortality in patients with coronary artery disease (Carney et al. 1988; Frasure-Smith et al. 1993). In some situations, timely psychiatric intervention in medical patients can improve psychosocial adjustment (Evans et al. 1988) and even survival (Spiegel et al. 1989). It should be noted, however, that although most of the consultation-liaison literature has focused on interrelationships between comorbid psychiatric and medical disorders, a wealth of epidemiological research has identified behavioral risk factors for the development of medical illness. Research has documented that behavioral factors such as cigarette smoking, obesity, alcohol and substance dependence, and hazardous sexual practices are major causes of premature death and medical morbidity both in the United States and worldwide (Stoudemire et al. 1987). A description of areas of investigation (Lipowski 1986) for classifying the psychological, behavioral, and social factors that may affect physical health is presented in Table 12–1.

TABLE 12–1. Psychological and behavioral factors affecting medical conditions

I. Psychophysiology
    A. Physiological reactions to psychological and behavioral variables
    B. Biological regulatory mechanisms associated with behavioral and psychological variables
        1. Psychoneurophysiology
        2. Psychoneuroendocrinology
        3. Psychoneuroimmunology
        4. Psychocardiology
II. Effects of concurrent psychiatric illness on the course and outcome of medical disorders
III. Behavioral risk factors for disease and injury
    A. Personality variables
    B. Cigarette smoking
    C. Dietary habits
    D. Alcohol and substance abuse
    E. Hazardous sexual behavior
    F. Risk-taking behaviors (accidents, injury)
    G. Noncompliance with medical treatment
    H. Violence, suicide, homicide
    I. Stressful or disruptive life change

Source. Reprinted with permission from Stoudemire A, Hales RE: "Psychological and Behavioral Factors Affecting Medical Conditions and DSM-IV: An Overview." *Psychosomatics* 32:5–13, 1991. Copyright 1991 Academy of Psychosomatic Medicine.

The author of this chapter would like to thank J. Stephen McDaniel, M.D., Michael G. Moran, M.D., and Alan Stoudemire, M.D., who were coauthors for earlier versions of this chapter, and members of the DSM-IV Workgroup who contributed to earlier reviews of the topic. This chapter is dedicated in memory of Alan Stoudemire.

This chapter builds on the work of the committee that examined the DSM-III-R (American Psychiatric Association 1987) diagnostic category "psychological factors affecting physical condition" for revisions that are reflected in DSM-IV (American Psychiatric Association 1994) (see Table 12–2). Detailed literature reviews were conducted, with emphasis on studies that used systematic methodology to examine the relation among psychiatric, behavioral, and psychological factors and the onset, precipitation, and exacerbation of medical disorders. Expanded versions of those reviews—organized largely by organ system and medical specialty categories—have been published elsewhere (Stoudemire 1995). These reviews were summarized in previous editions of this book and have been updated, with special emphasis on their implications for clinical practice. The diagnosis and treatment of psychiatric disorders are covered in detail elsewhere (Stoudemire et al. 2000).

Role of Psychological Factors in Cancer Onset and Progression

The relation between psychological factors and the onset and course of neoplastic disease serves as a prototype in examining the literature on this topic because many health care professionals and laypersons believe that psychological factors play a major role in cancer onset and progression. This belief has been strengthened, in part, by a rapidly growing literature, both scientific and popular, examining the role of psychological factors in cancer. Enthusiasm for therapeutic interventions based on "psychosomatic" relationships in oncology should be tempered by the recognition that the scientific evidence of such relationships is still in a relatively early stage of development and has many methodological limitations. In this section, I critically summarize the literature on cancer and its potential connections to affective states, coping/defensive style and personality traits, interpersonal relationships, stressful life events, and psychosocial interventions.

Affective States and Cancer

The relation between depression and cancer has been the focus of extensive study from several perspectives. The large epidemiological Western Electric study reported that depressive symptoms were associated with twice as high a risk of death from cancer 17 years later and with a higher-than-normal incidence of cancer for the first 10 years (Shekelle et al. 1981). This finding persisted at

TABLE 12–2. DSM-IV-TR diagnostic criteria for specified psychological factor affecting general medical condition

A. A general medical condition (coded on Axis III) is present.
B. Psychological factors adversely affect the general medical condition in one of the following ways:
   (1) the factors have influenced the course of the general medical condition as shown by a close temporal association between the psychological factors and the development or exacerbation of, or delayed recovery from, the general medical condition
   (2) the factors interfere with the treatment of the general medical condition
   (3) the factors constitute additional health risks for the individual
   (4) stress-related physiological responses precipitate or exacerbate symptoms of the general medical condition

Choose name based on the nature of the psychological factors (if more than one factor is present, indicate the most prominent):
   Mental Disorder Affecting...[Indicate the General Medical Condition] (e.g., an Axis I disorder such as major depressive disorder delaying recovery from a myocardial infarction)
   Psychological Symptoms Affecting...[Indicate the General Medical Condition] (e.g., depressive symptoms delaying recovery from surgery; anxiety exacerbating asthma)
   Personality Traits or Coping Style Affecting...[Indicate the General Medical Condition] (e.g., pathological denial of the need for surgery in a patient with cancer; hostile, pressured behavior contributing to cardiovascular disease)
   Maladaptive Health Behaviors Affecting...[Indicate the General Medical Condition] (e.g., overeating; lack of exercise; unsafe sex)
   Stress-Related Physiological Response Affecting...[Indicate the General Medical Condition] (e.g., stress-related exacerbations of ulcer, hypertension, arrhythmia, or tension headache)
   Other or Unspecified Psychological Factors Affecting...[Indicate the General Medical Condition] (e.g., interpersonal, cultural, or religious factors)

20-year follow-up (Persky et al. 1987). The Western Electric study has been cited for many years as supporting the association between depressive symptoms and increased cancer risk. Other studies, however, have reported negative findings (e.g., see Hahn and Petitti 1988). Dattore et al. (1980) found significantly *lower* depression scores in men who subsequently developed any type of cancer. A study by Zonderman et al. (1989) with a 10-year follow-up from the National Health and

Nutrition Examination Survey found no significant depressive symptoms that could be seen as predictors of cancer morbidity or mortality, as did another study with a 15-year follow-up (Vogt et al. 1994). A meta-analysis of studies relating depression to cancer development reported a small but significant association but of a magnitude of little practical significance (McGee et al. 1994).

Besides epidemiological studies, other studies have examined the effect of depression on outcome in cancer patients, most often examining survival with breast cancer. Breast cancer patients who had a "fighting spirit" or who used denial had a higher survival rate than did those with stoic acceptance or expressed hopelessness and helplessness (Greer et al. 1979). Subsequent studies have provided positive, negative, or mixed associations between depression and mortality in cancer patients (Garssen and Goodkin 1999; Levenson and McDonald, in press). Outcome variables other than mortality are worthy of investigation because depression could be reasonably expected to result in poorer pain control (Glover et al. 1995), less adherence to treatment (Ayres et al. 1994; McDonough et al. 1996), and decreased desire for life-sustaining therapy (Lee and Ganzini 1992).

Other affective states have received much less attention. Emotional distress in general may lead to decreased survival in patients with lung cancer (Faller et al. 1999), as may anger in patients with metastatic melanoma (Butow et al. 1999). Bereavement has been recognized as a significant stressor and often has been assumed to be a risk factor in cancer onset and progression. An early retrospective study showed that the onset of hematological malignancy appeared to be preceded by significant losses in children and young adults (Greene et al. 1956). Subsequent studies have been retrospective or prospective, clinical, or population-based (see Levenson and McDonald, in press). McKenna et al. (1999), in a meta-analysis of 46 studies of breast cancer, found only a modest association between separation or loss experiences and development of cancer. Bereavement has not to date been convincingly shown to influence cancer onset or progression.

Coping Styles, Personality Traits, and Cancer

A large body of literature has described the cancer patient's degree of emotional expressiveness versus repressiveness and its purported effect on prognosis. Temoshok et al. (1985) described a type C behavior pattern (in contrast to the type A studied in coronary disease), typified as a cooperative, unassertive patient who suppresses negative emotions, particularly anger, and

who accepts and complies with external authorities. Type C has been associated with increased melanoma tumor thickness, and its characteristics were found to be more common in melanoma patients than in control subjects (Kneier and Temoshok 1984). The Melbourne Colorectal Cancer Study found that cancer patients were more likely to have certain personality traits (similar to the type C pattern) than were control subjects (Kune et al. 1991). Research over the past two decades has both supported and refuted the belief that cancer development or mortality is influenced by coping, defensive style, or personality traits (Levenson and McDonald, in press).

Cassileth et al. (1988) found that none of the multiple psychosocial factors thought to be predictive of health predicted cancer survival. No differences in coping styles were found between breast cancer patients and control subjects (Buddeberg et al. 1991) or head and neck cancer patients and control subjects (Yamagiwa et al. 1991), and no relation was seen between coping style and breast cancer course (Edwards et al. 1990). Kreitler et al. (1993) found that repression and defensiveness increased in patients *after* the diagnosis of cancer was made, which highlights one of the flaws in retrospective studies. Epidemiological studies have not supported a relation between "emotional repression" and cancer incidence or mortality (Bleiker et al. 1996; Shekelle et al. 1981). The meta-analysis by McKenna et al. (1999) found only a modest association between denial or repression coping and breast cancer onset. In a review, Garssen and Goodkin (1999) concluded that several coping and personality variables are associated with cancer progression.

Relatively less research has examined the effects of interpersonal variables on cancer. One prospective study of former medical students reported that lack of closeness with parents and less satisfactory relationships were associated with later development of cancer (Graves et al. 1991). A prospective study of breast cancer patients found several positive relationship variables that were predictive of increased survival (Waxler-Morrison et al. 1991).

Stressful Life Events and Cancer

Both retrospective clinical and prospective epidemiological human studies have shown an increased incidence of stressful life events preceding the onset of breast, colorectal, cervical, pancreatic, gastric, and lung cancer, but many other studies have failed to find such associations (Levenson and McDonald, in press). Some work has linked stressful life events to progression or recurrence of cancer, but more recent reports have found no effect of stressful life events on relapse or progression (e.g., Giraldi et al. 1997). Most of the studies used aggregate measures of stressful life events rather than examining specific types of stress. Recent research implicated work stress and/or loss of employment as increasing the risk of lung cancer (Jahn et al. 1995; Lynge and Anderson 1997) and colorectal cancer (Courtney et al. 1993). In a review of human and animal studies, Fox (1983) concluded that if stressful events do have an effect on cancer incidence, it is small—a conclusion still appropriate today.

Psychosocial Intervention and Cancer Outcome

In contrast to studies lacking convincing support for an etiological relation between psychological factors and cancer, some studies have shown improvement in the quality of life in cancer patients receiving group therapy (Classen et al. 2001; Fawzy et al. 1990a; Spiegel et al. 1989). Relaxation training (Bindemann et al. 1991; Holland et al. 1991) and cognitive-behavioral therapy (Greer et al. 1991) also have reduced anxiety and depression in cancer patients.

Spiegel and colleagues (Spiegel and Bloom 1983; Spiegel et al. 1981, 1989) performed a small randomized controlled trial of supportive group therapy with training in self-hypnosis for pain control in women with metastatic breast cancer. At 1 year, the psychotherapy treatment group had less mood disturbance and fewer phobic responses (Spiegel et al. 1981) and complained of half as much pain (Spiegel and Bloom 1983). The treatment group also had increased survival compared with the control group (34.8 vs. 18.9 months). Greater longevity was associated with less mood disturbance and greater vigor (Spiegel et al. 1989).

Fawzy et al. (1990a) evaluated the immediate and prolonged effects of a 6-week structured psychiatric group intervention for postsurgical patients with malignant melanoma. Patients who received the intervention had greater vigor than did control subjects at 6 weeks and less depression, fatigue, and total mood disturbance at 6-month follow-up. Experimental subjects showed more active coping than control subjects both at the conclusion of the intervention and at follow-up. This study was the first to examine group psychiatric intervention in patients with early-stage cancer and good prognosis. The investigators also reported that patients who received group therapy had statistically significant increases in immunological function at 6-month follow-up (Fawzy et al. 1990b). Six years later, those who had received group therapy had significantly lower mortality and a trend for less recurrence of melanoma (Fawzy et al. 1993).

Other controlled trials of group psychotherapy showed survival benefit in metastatic cancer (e.g., Cunningham et al. 1998), but others found no beneficial differences in cancer progression or mortality after psychotherapeutic intervention (Gellert et al. 1993).

Mechanisms

The question of *how* psychological factors might influence cancer onset and progression has many potential answers. The immune system is probably important for some, but not all, cancer surveillance, and much research has focused on the influence of psychological factors on immune function relevant to cancer.

Various behavioral explanations that may account for the effects of psychological factors on cancer development and course also have been examined. The effect of some psychological factors (e.g., cynicism) on mortality may be mediated by smoking and alcohol (Almada et al. 1991), although these relations may be interactive rather than simple (Grossarth-Maticek and Eysenck 1990). Psychological factors also affect how patients seek medical attention for their initial cancer symptoms (Vracko-Tusevljak and Kambic 1989) and their self-care and treatment preferences (Greimel et al. 1997; Margolis et al. 1989). Cancer prevention also is influenced by psychological factors, which affect, for example, use of mammography (Schwartz et al. 1999) and genetic testing (Lerman et al. 1999). Some relationships between psychological factors, behavior, and cancer may be cancer-type specific (e.g., sexual behavior and cervical cancer [Lambley 1993]).

In summary, several studies have lent some support to the relationship among a variety of psychological factors and the onset, exacerbation, or outcome of neoplastic disease. Currently, no clear associations (let alone causal relationships) have been proven, both because of methodological limitations in the positive studies and because of the failure of other studies of comparable methodology to find such relationships. Compared with other known risk factors, psychological factors alone (other than cigarette smoking and alcoholism) make a small contribution to cancer onset. However, more recent, more methodologically sound studies have suggested that cancer progression, rather than onset, may be influenced more by psychosocial factors.

Clinical Implications

Depression and anxiety remain common but relatively underdiagnosed and undertreated in cancer patients. Whether mood disorders affect the incidence, course, or clinical outcomes of cancer has not yet been definitively answered by systematic research. Nevertheless, depression and anxiety warrant clinical attention because of their clearly adverse effects on quality of life. Behaviors with obviously harmful effects on patients with cancer (e.g., smoking, alcohol abuse, noncompliance with treatment) also should be targeted for intervention. The current literature on coping and personality style does not support the conclusions that any particular type of coping style is superior for all patients. Popular literature may lead some patients to feel responsible for their disease (or relapse) because they were unable to develop the "right attitude" or personality characteristics to "beat" cancer. Psychiatrists have a responsibility not only to avoid contributing to such simplistic, guilt-generating views but also to help patients (and some other physicians) understand the value of a range of individualized approaches to adaptation.

Psychotherapeutic interventions may be of great benefit to cancer patients. Studies show that psychotherapy can reduce anxiety, depression, and traumatic stress in patients with cancer (Bindemann et al. 1991; Classen et al. 2001; Fawzy et al. 1990a; Greer et al. 1991; Holland et al. 1991; Spiegel and Bloom 1983; Spiegel et al. 1981, 1989). A smaller number of studies appear to show reduced mortality in patients receiving such interventions (Cunningham et al. 1998; Fawzy et al. 1993; Spiegel et al. 1989). If it is suggested, however, in an overly optimistic manner that psychological therapies will actually deliver cure or remission, there is a risk of deeply disappointing patients and their families and distracting from the direct benefits of psychiatric treatment for quality of life. Psychiatrists should keep in mind that psychosocial interventions are more

likely to contribute to *quality* than to *quantity* of life in cancer patients. There is much enthusiasm among many professionals and laypersons for treatments promising to overcome cancer through "mind over body," but current scientific evidence supports a more cautious view. Psychiatric interventions are primarily justified if they reduce distress and dysfunction, such as when depressive or anxiety disorders are diagnosed in the context of oncological illness. Several studies have shown the benefits of antianxiety and antidepressant medications in cancer patients (Costa et al. 1985; Holland et al. 1991). The diagnosis and treatment of psychiatric disorders in these patients are discussed in detail elsewhere (Holland et al. 1998; McDaniel et al. 1995). Several of the most important findings in the relation between psychological factors and cancer, including several sentinel outcome studies, are highlighted in Table 12–3.

Psychoneuroimmunology

The idea that psychosocial variables may affect cancer, with the immune system as a mediating mechanism, belongs to psychoneuroimmunology, a field that has developed around the now well-documented bidirectional interrelation between the brain and the immune system (Greer 2000; McDaniel et al. 1995). There is central nervous system (CNS) innervation of immune system organs, and lymphocyte receptors have been identified for a variety of neurotransmitters, neuropeptides, and CNS hormones. In the other direction of influence, the brain is susceptible to certain lymphokines (i.e., substances produced by lymphocytes).

TABLE 12–3. Illustrative studies supporting the effects of psychological factors on cancer

Psychological factor	Study type	Cancer type	Findings	Reference(s)
Depression	Epidemiological	Mixed	2× risk of death from cancer at 17-year follow-up	Shekelle et al. 1981
Personality traits	Case control	Colorectal	Cancer patients less likely to have expressive personality traits	Kune et al. 1991
Stressful life events	Case control	Breast	Increased stressful life events preceding cancer onset	Geyer 1991
Group therapy with training in self-hypnosis	Randomized controlled trial	Breast	Reductions in distress and pain and increased survival in treatment group	Spiegel and Bloom 1983; Spiegel et al. 1981, 1989
Group therapy	Randomized controlled trial	Melanoma	Less distress, better coping, and increased immune function in treatment group	Fawzy et al. 1990a, 1990b

Several psychological processes have been studied regarding their effects on the immune system. Although a wide variety of effects have been found, findings have not always been replicated. Even when they have, the clinical significance of the findings usually has been uncertain. Nevertheless, the accumulating evidence makes this an exciting frontier. Direct suggestion under hypnosis inhibits the immediate-type hypersensitivity reaction (Black 1963). Psychological stress increases susceptibility to the common cold (S. Cohen et al. 1991). Kiecolt-Glaser and colleagues (Kiecolt-Glaser and Glaser 1995; Kiecolt-Glaser et al. 1984, 1986, 1987a, 1987b, 1988) reported various decreases in humoral and cellular immunity in individuals under stress, including family caregivers of patients with dementia, medical students taking examinations, and persons experiencing marital discord. Convincing evidence indicates that patients with high levels of psychological stress have suppressed secondary (but not primary) antibody responses to immunization (S. Cohen et al. 2001). However, some immune functions may be increased under psychological stress (Schulz and Schulz 1992).

A large amount of research has focused on the effects of depression on the immune system. Cellular immunity is impaired in patients with depression, whereas a variety of antibodies may be increased (Greer 2000). Stein et al. (1991) critically reviewed this literature, noting many methodological problems, and concluded that "alterations in the immune system in [major depression] do not appear to be a specific biological correlate of this disorder" (p. 175). Several studies have detected reduced lymphocyte proliferation in bereaved spouses or partners, but conflicting findings exist regarding effects of bereavement on natural killer (NK) cell activity (Greer 2000). Some studies in patients infected with HIV have documented associations between depression and adverse immunological changes, HIV progression, and HIV-related symptoms and mortality, although other investigators have not found such associations (Ickovics et al. 2001). Coping style, personality, and emotional support also have been associated with changes in immune functions, as have psychological interventions in patients with cancer or HIV/AIDS.

The emergence of the field of psychoneuroimmunology has made it no longer tenable to regard the immune system as autonomous, independent of the nervous system. The implications of this body of research sometimes have generated imaginative conclusions and speculations that go beyond the data. One of many methodological limitations is that most of the demonstrated changes in immune function have been in vitro, and their correlation with actual in vitro immune responses and clinical significance is not clear.

Clinical Implications

The research literature suggests that immune modulation by psychosocial stressors and/or interventions may influence health status. However, the methodological limitations and uncertain clinical implications of the studies to date should lead to the recognition that psychoneuroimmunology's findings are not currently suitable for direct translation into clinical practice (notwithstanding the large and growing popular simplistic literature, much of it by physicians, that attempts to do so). The studies reporting that psychological interventions in patients with cancer might decrease medical morbidity and be associated with positive changes in immunity (e.g., Fawzy et al. 1990b) have generated much excitement, but the major evidence-based justification for providing such therapeutic interventions is the improvement in mental well-being and quality of life they produce.

Psychological Factors and Endocrine Disease

Although there is a considerable amount of literature on psychoneuroendocrinology, particularly regarding the biology of mood disorders, little methodologically sound research exists regarding the clinical aspects of psychological factors and how these factors potentially influence endocrine diseases. Beardsley and Goldstein (1995) critically reviewed empirical findings on these factors and their influences. Of the existing literature, most research is focused primarily on three diseases: diabetes mellitus, Graves' disease, and Cushing's disease. The following discussions explore these three diseases and how psychological factors may influence them. The subject of psychiatric symptoms caused or exacerbated by endocrine disorders is not reviewed.

Diabetes Mellitus

Since the seventeenth century, there has been speculation about the role of psychological factors and the onset of diabetes mellitus. Although early studies aimed to show a relation between stress and the onset of diabetes mellitus, these studies were significantly flawed, yielding inconclusive findings regarding the causal relation between stress and disease onset (Beardsley and Goldstein 1995).

However, later investigations supported a relation between stressful life events and diabetes mellitus. For example, Robinson and Fuller (1985) examined 13 newly diagnosed patients with type 1 diabetes mellitus to ascertain the role of stressful life events as etiological triggering factors. These investigators found a higher frequency of severe life events in the 3 years before diagnosis of type 1 diabetes mellitus in the patients compared with control subjects. In their study of 338 children with type 1 diabetes mellitus, Hagglof et al. (1991) found significant increases in events related to actual or threatened loss within the family of the patients compared with the nondiabetic control subjects. Because these investigators found no difference in the total frequency of life events between the two groups, their findings suggest that qualitative aspects of stress may be a more important cofactor than frequency of life events in understanding the relation between stress and diabetes onset. Studies of this type are subject to recall bias, and other investigators have found no evidence of a causal relation between stressful life events and the onset of diabetes mellitus (Gendel and Benjamin 1946), including one large prospective study of air traffic controllers (Cobb and Rose 1973). One group avoided recall bias by assessing the number of stressful life events in 2,262 community residents ages 50–74 without any history of diabetes before administering a glucose tolerance test. Diabetes was newly diagnosed in 5% and positively associated with the number of stressful life events (Mooy et al. 2000). In one review, Wales (1995) took into account these conflicting data and suggested that, in general, psychological stress may produce a deterioration in glycemic control in the as-yet-undiagnosed, asymptomatic patient, which precipitates symptoms and makes the diagnosis evident.

Other investigators have examined the role of psychological factors in affecting the course of diabetes mellitus. Although early studies were flawed primarily because of difficulties in accurately measuring glucose control, more recent studies measure hemoglobin A_{1c} (HbA1c), a reliable measure of metabolic control.

Studies in clinical samples have generally found an association between perceived stress and poorer metabolic control whether assessed by blood glucose (Garay-Sevilla et al. 2000; Halford et al. 1990) or HbA1c (Herpertz et al. 2000; Lloyd et al. 1999), but such studies are typically cross-sectional, limiting any conclusions about causality. More persuasive are prospective within-subject analyses showing that poorer metabolic control is caused by standardized laboratory stress (Goetsch et al. 1993; Gonder-Frederick et al. 1990) or normal life stress (Kramer et al. 2000), although these studies used relatively small numbers of subjects.

Depression (symptoms or diagnosis) may adversely affect glycemic control and increase the risk for diabetic complications, but study findings have been variable. As assessed by HbA1c, metabolic control has been found to be poorer in depressed children (Lernmark et al. 1999), in depressed men but not women (Lloyd et al. 2000), and in depressed type 1 but not type 2 diabetic persons (de

Groot et al. 1999). It is logical to suspect that poorer compliance might account for depression's effects on diabetic management, and data support this. Ciechanowski et al. (2000) found that depressive symptom severity was associated with poorer adherence to diet and medications as well as more functional impairment and higher health costs. These investigators also found that adherence in diabetes is lacking in patients with a "dismissing attachment" style of relating, who also had poorer doctor–patient communication (Ciechanowski et al. 2001).

As with other medical illnesses, the role of personality characteristics and coping strategies also has been studied with relation to the course of diabetes mellitus in both children and adults, but no clear conclusions have emerged. For example, one study found poorer glycemic control only in patients with a "Cluster B dependent profile" (Orlandini et al. 1997), another found poorer glycemic control only in those who are more altruistic (Lane et al. 2000), and a third found no correlation with any personality variables (Perros et al. 1998). Similarly, studies in children have provided mixed and counterintuitive associations between personality and glucose control.

Although several studies have reported the effects of behavioral or psychosocial interventions on glucose control in diabetic patients, results have not been consistent. However, randomized controlled trials have found that cognitive-behavioral therapy, relaxation training, or coping skills training can improve glucose control in diabetes (Grey et al. 2000; Lammers et al. 1984; Lustman et al. 1998). Antidepressant treatment of depression in diabetes is effective and produces an early trend toward better glycemic control, although some antidepressants can cause moderate hyperglycemia or hypoglycemia (Lustman et al. 1997, 2000).

Deterioration in glucose tolerance in currently treated schizophrenic patients is likely to be caused by most of the newer antipsychotic drugs. However, diabetes was a major problem for schizophrenic patients even before the widespread use of antipsychotic drugs, presumably because of obesity (a side effect of conventional antipsychotics), unhealthy diets, and poorer health care (Dixon et al. 2000). Optimal management of diabetes requires patients to be organized, precise, meticulous, and consistent, making this very difficult to attain for most patients who also have schizophrenia.

Further studies evaluating the role of psychological factors in the onset and course of diabetes mellitus are needed to clarify the current conflicting data regarding stress and this disease. Clarifying this relationship will improve our understanding of the potential role of behavioral interventions as mediators in the effects of stress on diabetic patients. Examples of key findings in the relation between psychological factors and diabetes are shown in Table 12–4.

TABLE 12–4. Illustrative studies supporting the effects of psychological factors on diabetes mellitus

Psychological factor	Study type	Findings	Reference(s)
Stressful life events	Prospective epidemiological	New-onset diabetes associated with number of stressful events	Mooy et al. 2000
Perceived stress	Cross-sectional	Poor metabolic control	Lloyd et al. 1999
Depression	Cross-sectional	Poor adherence, more impairment, higher costs, poor doctor–patient relationships	Ciechanowski et al. 2000, 2001
Cognitive-behavioral therapy	Randomized controlled trial	Improved glucose control	Lustman et al. 1998

Graves' Disease

Graves' disease, sometimes called *exophthalmic goiter*, has been in the differential diagnosis of psychosomatic illness used by clinicians for many years. Weiner (1977) provided the classic review of psychological factors in Graves' disease in his textbook *Psychobiology and Human Disease*. It is apparent from Weiner's review that numerous methodological flaws have made previous studies difficult to interpret. Complicating the studies of Graves' disease are the variable onset and course of the disease itself, making it difficult to measure changes in onset and course related to psychological factors. Furthermore, hyperthyroidism is often characterized by numerous psychological, behavioral, and neuropsychiatric signs and symptoms.

There appears to be minimal evidence to date suggesting that psychological characteristics of patients predispose them to develop Graves' disease or any thyroid disorder for that matter (Weiner 1977). However, more recent studies identified stressful life events as risk factors for Graves' disease (Radosavljevic et al. 1996; Sonino et al. 1993; Winsa et al. 1991). Japanese investigators found that stressful life events and smoking were associated with Graves' disease in women but not men (Yoshiuchi et al. 1998b). However, as with other diseases, such studies of stressful life events preceding disease onset are nonspecific and do not shed light on etiology. A recent study took a more focused approach, examining whether patients with chronic stress due to panic disorder had any differences in thyroid function, antibodies, and echography compared with control subjects. No evidence was found for previous or present Graves' hyperthyroidism occurring more frequently in the patients with panic disorder (Chiovato et al. 1998). One prospective study in patients newly diagnosed with Graves' disease found that after adjusting for confounding variables, psychological stress affected the response to treatment, resulting in less control of hyperthyroidism (Yoshiuchi et al. 1998a). More prospective studies are needed to confirm these results before concluding that psychological factors affect the course of Graves' disease.

Cushing's Disease

Dr. Cushing himself argued that emotional stress contributed to the development of the disease that bears his name. As is the case for Graves' disease, although some evidence suggests that preceding stressful life events are more common than in control subjects (Sonino and Fava 1998), compelling evidence that psychological factors affect Cushing's disease is lacking. Although it is clearly known that stressful stimuli may acutely lead to increased secretion of corticosteroids, hypercortisolism per se cannot be equated with illness and disease (Beardsley and Goldstein 1995). However, there is strong evidence that hypercortisolism of several etiologies, including Cushing's disease, has been associated with the development of a wide range of neuropsychiatric phenomena (Kelly 1996). Controlled human studies are needed to clarify these and other questions pertaining to psychological conditions and effects on endocrine disorders.

Psychocardiology

Coronary Artery Disease

The effects of psychological, social, and behavioral factors on cardiovascular disease have garnered considerable clinical attention and have been a primary focus of epidemiological and psychosomatic medicine research for the past 30 years. Evidence from methodologically rigorous studies of a strong association between coronary artery disease (CAD) and depressive disorders is especially compelling (Glassman and Shapiro 1998; Musselman et al. 1998). The prevalence of major depression in patients with CAD is much higher, especially after myocardial infarction, than in the general population. Depression not only commonly occurs alongside CAD but also negatively affects outcome in CAD. The magnitude of the effects of depression on morbidity and mortality in CAD is on a par with the effects of the recognized medical risk factors.

TABLE 12–5. Illustrative studies supporting the effects of psychological factors on coronary artery disease

Psychological factor	Study type	Findings	Reference(s)
Depression	Prospective	Higher mortality after myocardial infarction	Frasure-Smith et al. 1993, 1995a
Anxiety	Prospective clinical trial	More ischemic events and death after myocardial infarction	Moser and Dracup 1996
Mental stress	Epidemiological studies after disasters	More sudden deaths and more myocardial infarctions	Krantz et al. 2000; Leor et al. 1996
Schizophrenia	Retrospective	Less likely to receive catheterization	Druss et al. 2000

Major depression is a significant predictor of mortality at 6 months and 18 months after an acute myocardial infarction, equal to the effect of predictors such as history of myocardial infarction or indexes of cardiac function (Frasure-Smith et al. 1993, 1995a). In an epidemiological study that followed up a cohort of 3,000 individuals ages 55–85 for 4 years, major depression tripled the relative risk of cardiac mortality in those without heart disease and quadrupled it in those who did have cardiac disease (Penninx et al. 2001). In patients with CAD undergoing cardiac catheterization, major depression was a better predictor of cardiac morbidity and mortality than were physiological measures such as left ventricular function (Carney et al. 1988). Patients hospitalized for unstable angina who also had depressive symptoms were four times more likely to have myocardial infarction or die the following year than were those without depression (after adjusting for other factors) (Lesperance et al. 2000).

In addition to its effects on morbidity and mortality in CAD, depression can profoundly affect patients' quality of life and functioning. The severity of depressive symptoms has a greater effect on functional disability in CAD than does the number of stenosed coronary arteries (Sullivan et al. 1997). Some illustrative studies demonstrating the effects of various psychological factors on CAD are shown in Table 12–5.

There are a number of candidate explanations for the effects of depression on clinical outcome in CAD (Glassman and Shapiro 1998; Musselman et al. 1998). As discussed later in this chapter (see "Lifestyle Risk Factors"), depression is closely associated with nicotine addiction, but depression still adversely affects CAD outcome even after controlling for smoking (Glassman and Shapiro 1998). Depression may interfere with compliance with recommended lifestyle modification, medication, and cardiac rehabilitation (Carney et al. 1988, 1995). Evidence is accumulating that depressed patients may have alterations in platelet aggregation mediated by alterations in plasma serotonin (Musselman et al. 1998). Another potential mechanism contributing to the diminished survival of depressed patients with CAD is reduced heart rate variability (Musselman et al. 1998). It is also possible that some of the adverse effects of depression are mediated through the cardiac effects of stress, as described later in this section. Depression's effects on heart rate variability and resting heart rate may explain the increased risk of ventricular arrhythmias and sudden death in depressed cardiac patients (Glassman and Shapiro 1998).

Anxiety is also extremely common in patients with CAD, and it too adversely affects outcome in CAD. Some evidence indicates that anxiety after myocardial infarction leads to more frequent readmission for unstable angina and more recurrences of myocardial infarction, after controlling for many confounding factors including comorbid depression (Frasure-Smith et al. 1995b). In a large clinical trial, patients who had a high level of anxiety after myocardial infarction had almost five times the risk for serious ischemic events or death compared with those without anxiety, making post–myocardial infarction anxiety one of the strongest predictors of in-hospital complications (Moser and Dracup 1996). Anxiety's adverse effects on outcome in CAD may be mediated via effects on heart rate variability, QT interval prolongation, or other abnormalities in autonomic nervous responses (Januzzi et al. 2000). As with depression, some of anxiety's effects may be related to the effects of stress on the heart (described in the following paragraph).

There are many forms of stress, and many studies report the adverse effects of stress on patients with preexisting heart disease (Krantz et al. 2000). Psychological stress has been considered to play an important role in precipitating cardiac events and sudden death in such patients (Leor et al. 1996). Psychological stress lowers the threshold for life-threatening ventricular arrhythmias. Experimental standardized mental stressors provoke ischemia in many patients with CAD, usually silent (asymptomatic). Such experimental stress-induced silent ischemia is clinically significant. Those who experience it are twice as likely to later have fatal and nonfatal cardiac events compared with those who do not (Jiang et al. 1996). Mental tension, frustration, and sadness double the risk of regular ischemia in CAD (Gullette et al. 1997).

Studies that document increases in myocardial infarction and/or sudden death after missile attacks, earthquakes, and other disasters confirm the effects of stress on heart disease (Krantz et al. 2000; Leor et al. 1996). A recent prospective study of middle-aged women who had been hospitalized for myocardial infarction or unstable angina found that after adjusting for other psychosocial and cardiac variables, women with severe marital stress had triple the risks of recurrent coronary events than did those women without marital stress (Orth-Gomér et al. 2000).

The relation between type A behavior and CAD has been controversial. Type A is a complex construct of multiple traits, including impatience, hostility, intense achievement drive, and time urgency (M. Friedman and Rosenman 1959; Lachar 1993). Many studies have supported type A behavior as a risk factor for the development of CAD and a predictor of worse outcome, but an equal number of studies have been negative. Overall, the majority of the most rigorous studies support the proposition that type A behavior is associated with an increased risk of developing heart disease. However, type A behavior does not appear to cause increased morbidity or mortality in those who have already developed CAD (Lachar 1993; Williams and Littman 1996). Because of the conflicting findings across many studies, investigators have attempted to identify a particular component of the type A syndrome that might be more significantly predictive. Of the type A traits, hostility has been the most consistently associated with increased cardiac events and mortality (Lachar 1993). Anger, which is related but not identical to the concept of hostility, appears to be an especially potent trigger of ischemia (Ironson et al. 1992). How hostility or other elements of type A behavior might lead to CAD, or worsen its outcome, is unknown. Mechanisms considered have included alterations in the balance between sympathetic and parasympathetic nervous system activity (Williams and Littman 1996) and related changes in blood pressure and heart rate control.

Sudden cardiac death after acute psychological stress has long been reported anecdotally but is difficult to study empirically. Evidence suggests that a variety of psychological stressors may sometimes play an important role in precipitating serious ventricular arrhythmias. A systematic review of published cases of ventricular fibril-lation occurring in patients without any known cardiac disease identified preceding psychological distress in 22% (Viskin and Belhassen 1990).

Hypertension

Because about 85% of hypertension cases are classified as primary (essential) hypertension, in which the etiology cannot be specified, psychological factors have been intensively studied as potential contributors to its pathogenesis (Markovitz et al. 1993; Shapiro 1988). The magnitude of blood pressure reactivity to stress has received some support as a factor in the development of hypertension and its progression. Many investigators have examined the relations between personality, coping style, blood pressure reactivity, and hypertension, but conclusions remain controversial. Findings regarding blood pressure reactivity in response to stress in normotensive individuals are not necessarily relevant to clinical hypertension. In some, but not all, studies, a high level of anxiety has been a strong prospective predictor for the development of hypertension, as has job strain. Studies of psychological treatments for hypertension, primarily relaxation techniques and biofeedback, have sometimes found modest but clinically significant sustained reductions in blood pressure. However, such techniques are less effective than drug therapy (De-Ping et al. 1988).

Overall, the evidence for an important role for psychological factors affecting hypertension is equivocal compared with the evidence relating depression and mental stress to CAD (R. Friedman et al. 2001).

Clinical Implications

The role of psychological factors in cardiac disease is one of the most investigated categories of psychosomatic medicine, but as noted earlier, ambiguity and controversy regarding the importance of specific factors remain. Nevertheless, there is sufficient replicated evidence that significant psychiatric disorders, especially major depression, have adverse effects on clinical outcome after myocardial infarction. Patients with mental disorders also may fare poorly because they are less likely to receive definitive interventions such as cardiac catheterization and angioplasty. Druss et al. (2000) found that patients with schizophrenia who had had myocardial infarctions were only 41% as likely to undergo catheterization as those without mental disorders. Because of the weight of the evidence implicating psychological factors, especially depression, in the development and outcome of CAD, there are strong arguments for psychological and psychiatric intervention for prevention of heart disease

(Ketterer 1993; Rozanski et al. 1999). There have been several clinical trials of psychological and psychopharmacological interventions, some of which have been successful in both reducing emotional distress and improving medical outcomes. Two multicenter trials have been under way and will soon be reported: the Sertraline Antidepressant Heart Attack Randomized Trial (SADHART) and a trial of a psychological intervention, the Enhancing Recovery in Coronary Heart Disease (ENRICHD) study (The ENRICHD Investigators 2000). The diagnosis and treatment of psychiatric disorders in patients with heart disease are discussed in detail elsewhere (Levenson and Dwight 2000).

Lifestyle Risk Factors

As emphasized in the introduction to this chapter, it is now well established that lifestyle behaviors are risk factors that significantly contribute to the mortality rate in the United States (see Table 12–1). The most widely studied risk factors are cigarette smoking, obesity, and alcohol consumption, all of which affect the development, perpetuation, and exacerbation of medical illnesses.

Cigarette smoking remains the single most important modifiable risk factor for illness and the greatest single cause of preventable premature deaths (Peto et al. 1992). Cigarette smoking is a powerful independent contributor to the occurrence of myocardial infarction, sudden death, peripheral vascular disease, and stroke. It has been shown to act synergistically with other traditional risk factors such as hypertension and high blood cholesterol to increase the risk of CAD. Smoking accounts for about 80% of the deaths related to chronic obstructive pulmonary disease (COPD). Tobacco's role in causing lung cancer has long been established, but its use increases the risk of many other types of cancer. Psychological factors affect initiation of, continuation of, withdrawal from, and relapse into smoking. For example, girls with lower self-esteem are more likely to smoke than are those with higher self-esteem (Lewis et al. 2001). Overall, persons with mental illness are about twice as likely to smoke as others are, and the increased risk is found with all the major anxiety, mood, and psychotic disorders (Lasser et al. 2000).

Unfortunately, smoking cessation is a difficult intervention. The difficulty is compounded by the physical dependence on nicotine in chronic smokers, which led to a separate category for nicotine dependence in DSM-IV. Effective treatments are now available, especially when behavioral and pharmacological approaches are combined (Agency for Health Care Policy and Research 1996), but abstinence is maintained at 1 year in only about one-third

of the research subjects receiving the most effective intervention (bupropion plus cessation counseling). On the positive side, mentally ill smokers have substantial quit rates (about 37%) with or without smoking cessation treatment (Lasser et al. 2000).

After cigarette smoking, obesity is the second most widely studied risk factor associated with increased morbidity and mortality. A strong association exists between obesity and hypertension, hypercholesterolemia, and diabetes mellitus as risk factors for cardiovascular disease. Obesity also may increase the risk of prostate, colon, and rectal cancer in men and endometrial, cervical, ovarian, breast, and gallbladder cancer in women. For those individuals with morbid obesity (more than 100 pounds overweight), sudden death, lung disease, sleep apnea, cardiomyopathy, congestive heart failure, liver dysfunction, and thromboembolic disease are common complications. Functional limitations and negative psychosocial sequelae also are well-documented outcomes in individuals with morbid obesity.

Because of obesity's medical complications, weight reduction has become an important medical intervention. However, recent evidence has shown that individuals who repeatedly diet are more likely to increase their weight over time when compared with obese individuals who do not repeatedly attempt to lose weight. This finding has led to speculation that repeated dieting may be associated with increases in morbidity.

The concept of weight reduction is complicated by psychological, social, and cultural differences. Evidence indicates that psychological factors such as anxiety, depression, and stress contribute to overeating in some individuals. Several neural and hormonal inputs to the hypothalamus modulate the release of neuropeptides known to affect food intake and energy expenditure (Rosenbaum et al. 1997). However, overall, only modest evidence shows that psychological and behavioral factors play a role in the development of obesity (Power and Parsons 2000). Still, behavioral treatments for obesity have shown efficacy for mild to moderate obesity, especially when they have focused on maintenance of behavior change. Strategies combining exercise, dietary restriction, longitudinal monitoring, and professionally led skills training have produced positive outcomes.

Alcohol consumption is associated with increased morbidity and mortality from accidents, violence, suicide, gastrointestinal ulcers and bleeding, cirrhosis, and several cancers, but regular modest intake is associated with reductions in coronary heart disease and thrombotic stroke (Thun et al. 1997). Other lifestyle factors that have been associated with negative health outcomes include sedentary lifestyle; diet high in cholesterol and fats and low in fiber; sexual practices known to increase the risk of infection with HIV, hepatitis B, and other transmissible organisms; overexposure to sun and other ultraviolet light; lack of use of safety restraints when riding in motor vehicles; and other psychoactive substance use and abuse.

Clinical Implications

With the currently established evidence of the morbidity and mortality associated with lifestyle risk factors, psychiatrists have a responsibility to collaborate with other health care professionals in assisting patients with behavioral changes. This is especially true for patients with psychotic disorders, who have high rates of smoking and obesity (LeFevre 2001). With cigarette smoking being the single most important modifiable risk factor for illness in the United States, treatment of nicotine dependence should play a central role in the treatment plans of those patients who continue to abuse tobacco, with special attention to any comorbid depressive or anxiety disorders. Similarly, interventions for preventing or reducing obesity are of central importance in treating conditions such as heart disease, diabetes, pulmonary disease, and chronic pain. Lifestyle risk factors may be only one part of the explanation of how psychological factors can affect the development and outcome of medical disorders, but they are identifiable and at least potentially modifiable.

Pulmonary Diseases

Asthma

Asthma historically was considered a classic "psychosomatic" illness (Alexander 1950; Dunbar 1947); that is, it was believed that specific personality types and/or particular unconscious conflicts created vulnerability to asthma and could precipitate asthmatic attacks. More systematic research over the ensuing decades has largely discredited this view that asthma can be understood and treated via psychoanalytic theory and treatment but also has documented that psychological factors do affect the course of asthma. The evidence to date indicates that no specific "asthmatic personality" exists and that psychopathology does not account for asthma's etiology. Psychopathology (anxiety, depression, personality disorders) may or may not be more frequent in adult and pediatric patients with asthma (Bauer and Duijsens 1998; Janson et al. 1994; Vila et al. 1999). Patients with more severe asthma do seem to have higher levels of emotional distress, but the latter may be a result of the former (Miles et al. 1997;

Vamos and Kolbe 1999), and some investigators have found no psychological differences between patients with mild and severe asthma (ten Brinke et al. 2001b).

What is clearer is that psychological factors do have profound effects on the symptoms and course of asthma. Rimington et al. (2001) noted that asthma practice guidelines advise assessing changes in symptoms to monitor the effectiveness of treatment. However, their study of 114 general practice patients with asthma found that anxiety and depression helped to explain asthma symptom scores, even after controlling for lung function and treatment. A multicenter European study of 715 community-dwelling young adults found that anxiety and depression scores independently predicted more wheezing, breathlessness, and nocturnal chest tightness but not a diagnosis of asthma (Janson et al. 1994). Rietveld et al. (1999) provided additional support for this relationship in a controlled experiment comparing adolescents with asthma and nonasthmatic control subjects exposed to a standardized stressor (a frustrating computer task). Breathlessness increased in all the patients with asthma after the stressor, but no changes occurred in any objective pulmonary functions. Thus, psychological stress and distress make patients with asthma feel physically worse, despite no actual change in lung function in these studies.

However, the theory that psychological factors might adversely affect pulmonary function in asthma remains quite possible. Le Son and Gershwin (1996) analyzed a retrospective cohort of 550 young adult hospitalized patients with asthma to determine risk factors for intubation. Psychological factors and psychosocial problems were more powerful predictors for intubation (odds ratio = 25.0; 95% confidence interval = 12.4–50.8) than any other examined variable (e.g., smoking, infection, prior hospitalization). Although impressive, this finding does not shed light on how psychological factors' effects on outcome in asthma are mediated, but other studies do. Psychological morbidity is associated with high levels of denial and delays in seeking medical attention in severe asthma, which may be life threatening (Campbell et al. 1995; Miles et al. 1997). Overuse of sympathomimetic drugs, especially over-the-counter agents or herbal remedies containing ephedrine, contributes to asthma mortality, as does underuse of inhaled corticosteroids. Psychological morbidity is associated with less adherence to prescribed inhaled steroids and consequently poorer control of asthma (Cluley and Cochrane 2001). In particular, noncompliant patients with asthma are more depressed than are compliant patients (Bosley et al. 1995). Perhaps as a consequence, psychiatric symptoms in patients with severe asthma are associated with increased health care use (independent of severity of asthma), including more frequent visits to primary care physicians, emergency department visits, exacerbations, and hospitalizations (ten Brinke et al. 2001a).

Chronic Obstructive Pulmonary Disease

COPD encompasses emphysema and chronic bronchitis, which are most often caused by cigarette smoking. Although patients with COPD differ from those with asthma in demographics, pathophysiology, treatment, and prognosis, there are similarities in the effects of psychological factors on each. Depression and anxiety are common in COPD patients (Aydin and Ulusahin 2001; Withers et al. 1999; Yohannes et al. 2000), although this in part reflects the frequency of depression and anxiety disorders in past or current smokers. Psychological distress amplifies perceived dyspnea, or breathlessness, without causing changes in measured pulmonary functions. Depression and anxiety appear to result in lower exercise tolerance (Withers et al. 1999), less adherence to treatment (Bosley et al. 1996), and more disability (Aydin and Ulusahin 2001). One small, prospective, double-blind study found higher mortality in those patients who had higher (more pathological) Minnesota Multiphasic Personality Inventory scores (Ashutosh et al. 1997). Panic and anxiety in patients with COPD may produce significant morbidity through phobic avoidance of activity, excessive anxiolytic use, and more frequent hospitalizations (Smoller et al. 1996). Both pulmonary rehabilitation and cognitive-behavioral psychotherapy may improve exercise tolerance in anxious patients with COPD (Eiser et al. 1997; Withers et al. 1999).

COPD itself, through adverse effects on arterial oxygen and/or carbon dioxide concentrations, can cause cognitive dysfunction that impairs compliance. Chronic hypoxemia may result in irreversible hypoxic brain injury. Memory and concentration disturbances are especially common. Patients on chronic ventilation present some diagnostic and therapeutic problems, and psychological factors can affect weaning.

Clinical Implications

A history that suggests a connection between stressful events and aggravation of asthmatic symptoms should lead to psychiatric consultation. A specific aim of the consultation would include helping the patient develop heightened awareness of the typical stressors that appear to trigger dyspnea so that the patient can develop coping strategies for dealing with them. The psychiatrist also can evaluate the role of anxiolytics or antidepressants in those asthmatic patients for whom pharmacotherapy is indicated. Generally, asthmatic patients do not chronically retain carbon dioxide unless they also have COPD; thus, the judicious use of low-dose benzodiazepines is not necessarily contraindicated. Panic attacks may be difficult to distinguish from acute asthmatic attacks or may occur intertwined with each other. Patients may inappropriately use bronchodilator medications for the treatment of such anxiety, which may then sympathomimetically exacerbate anxiety symptoms. Benzodiazepines are appropriate acutely in such situations, and antidepressants should be considered for prophylactic management.

As noted, adverse effects of psychological morbidity, such as poorer adherence, exacerbation of subjective dyspnea, and more emergency department visits and hospitalizations, are also seen in patients with asthma or COPD. The appropriate treatment of anxiety disorders or major depression thus forms an essential part of the medical management of patients with chronic or recurrent pulmonary disease. Pathological avoidance or denial, whether by the patient or, in the case of pediatric patients with asthma, the family, also calls for intervention. Nothing is more critical in the management of asthma or COPD than smoking cessation. Failure to treat a comorbid mood or anxiety disorder will undermine the success of interventions to help the patient stop smoking. Some of the key findings regarding psychological factors and pulmonary disease are shown in Table 12–6.

TABLE 12–6. Illustrative studies supporting the effects of psychological factors on pulmonary disease

Psychological factor	Study type	Findings	Reference(s)
Stress	Standardized experimental stressor	Increased breathlessness in asthmatic patients	Rietveld et al. 1999
Psychopathology	Clinical cohort	More asthma exacerbations, more health care use	ten Brinke et al. 2001a
Depression and anxiety	Varied	Lower exercise tolerance, less compliance, more disability	Aydin and Ulusahin 2001; Bosley et al. 1996; Withers et al. 1999

Rheumatological Disease

Among patients and physicians, there is widespread anecdotal agreement that emotional factors affect the clinical course of rheumatoid arthritis. Since the work of Alexander and others, there has been interest in the personality profiles of rheumatoid arthritis patients, although the theory that certain neurotic conflicts or personality types were specific to rheumatoid arthritis has been disproven. Patients with rheumatoid arthritis were seen as self-sacrificing, masochistic, inhibited, and perfectionistic (Moos 1964). The loss of mobility, jobs, and relationships contributes to depression and withdrawal, eroding support systems that are so necessary in any chronically ill patient's struggle for rehabilitation. Certain "personality traits" and an increased incidence of psychiatric disturbance should be considered complications of rheumatoid arthritis and not causes of the disease.

Some earlier research suggested that stressful life events play a role in the development or onset of rheumatoid arthritis, but recent studies have not supported any significant relation between the two (Carette et al. 2000; Leymarie et al. 1997). As with other chronic diseases, psychological factors do exert significant effects on symptoms, disability, and treatment in rheumatoid arthritis. Depression is very common in rheumatoid arthritis (Soderlin et al. 2000) and is associated with more pain and greater disability independent of objective indexes of disease severity. Even a history of major depression predicts higher levels of pain in rheumatoid arthritis years later (Fifield et al. 1998). Randomized controlled trials of antidepressants in depressed rheumatoid arthritis patients show both the efficacy of treatment and the improvement in pain, morning stiffness, and disability scores (Ash et al. 1999; Bird and Broggini 2000). However, casual relationships should not be understood simplistically; for example, some antidepressants have analgesic effects independent of their antidepressant effects (Ash et al. 1999). In children with juvenile rheumatoid arthritis, maternal emotional distress as well as the child's emotional distress are associated with higher reported pain after adjusting for disease characteristics (Ross et al. 1993).

The mechanisms by which psychological factors affect the course of rheumatoid arthritis have not been well characterized. Psychoneuroimmunological explanations appear less fitting than psychological effects on pain perception, energy, exercise tolerance, analgesic use, and treatment compliance. Although the early view of rheumatoid arthritis as a classic psychosomatic disorder has been discarded, the consensus in the rheumatological literature is that psychological factors are important, but their relations with illness in rheumatoid arthritis are complex in both adults (Newman and Mulligan 2000; Wolfe 1999) and children (Kroll et al. 1999).

Clinical Implications

Psychological morbidity in rheumatoid arthritis patients, as noted, results in higher levels of pain, but it also leads to poorer quality of life, more work disability, more joint surgery, use of more resources, and lower compliance (Kroll et al. 1999; Newman and Mulligan 2000; Wolfe 1999). Psychiatrists should be especially alert to the existence of mood disorders because depressive symptoms may be falsely attributed to rheumatoid arthritis itself.

Assessment of the support system is an early step in the total evaluation of a patient, and active attempts should be made to maintain the involvement of the patient's family and friends. Depression and demoralization can easily lead to a downward spiral of inactivity, social withdrawal, and nonparticipation in physical therapy, with associated deconditioning, loss of muscle mass, and distancing or even abandonment by the patient's support system. The amplification of pain by depression or other emotional distress often leads to overuse of analgesics and their chronic risks of toxicity.

Gastrointestinal Disorders

Peptic Ulcer Disease

Early investigators of psychosomatic illnesses focused on duodenal ulcer, for which psychological factors were thought to play a larger role than in gastric ulcer. Alexander (1950) suggested that duodenal ulcer occurred after an increase in responsibility or frustration in individuals with unmet wishes to be cared for ("oral dependency"). In a classic study testing this hypothesis, Weiner et al. (1957) combined preexisting individual psychological characteristics and a biological trait (high pepsinogen secretion) to successfully predict when men undergoing the stress of army draft would develop duodenal ulcer.

Understanding the pathogenesis of peptic ulcers has been revolutionized by the discovery of the central role of the bacterium *Helicobacter pylori*. Consequently, many physicians have concluded that peptic ulcer is an infectious disease, except when attributable to nonsteroidal anti-inflammatory drugs (NSAIDs), and that psychological factors are irrelevant. However, only a fraction of the people colonized by *H. pylori* or taking NSAIDs develop peptic ulcers, leaving open the possibility of other contributing factors. A substantial body of research shows that psychosocial factors contribute to 30%–65% of ulcers (Levenstein 2000), summarized in Table 12–7. Psychological factors are most likely to be present in patients with duodenal ulcer who have few conventional medical risk factors (especially *H. pylori*) (Levenstein et al. 1995a). Psychological stress is an independent risk factor for the development (Armstrong et al. 1994) and recurrence (Levenstein et al. 1995b) of duodenal ulcer. It has been repeatedly shown that peptic ulcer has been triggered by stress after a variety of disasters, including bombardment, earthquake, economic crises, being a prisoner of war, or being one of the "boat people" refugees. Job or wage conflicts and family problems also increase the risk of developing peptic ulcer. Depression, maladjustment, and hostility also are prospectively associated with peptic ulcer (Levenstein et al. 1997). Stress, anxiety, and depression retard healing of ulcers and worsen the prognosis.

Whether specific emotions or character traits are pathogenic for peptic disease remains controversial, and some "neurotic" traits may be the consequence rather than the cause of ulcer (Jess and Eldrup 1994). Psychological factors appear to influence peptic ulcer development or course through both health risk behaviors and psychophysiological mechanisms. The former include smoking, alcohol abuse, overuse of NSAIDs, poor diet, and insomnia. The latter include pepsinogen and acid secretion, altered blood flow, impairment of mucosal defenses, and cortisol's slowing of healing (Levenstein 2000).

Irritable Bowel Syndrome

Psychopathology is extremely common in patients with irritable bowel syndrome (IBS), including anxiety (especially panic attacks), depression, and somatization, but there is no unique pattern of psychological characteristics (Walker et al. 1990). Patients with IBS are more likely to have a history of childhood sexual abuse compared with patients who have other gastrointestinal disorders (Walker et al. 1993), but this finding is most characteristic of those patients seeking care at tertiary referral centers. There does not appear to be any increased incidence of childhood sexual abuse in individuals in the community with symptoms of IBS who have not sought treatment. Indeed, almost all of the psychological traits or symptoms that are more common in IBS are differentially increased only in those who have sought medical care for their symptoms (Herschbach et al. 1999). Although both patients with IBS and their doctors observe that their gastrointestinal symptoms seem aggra-

TABLE 12–7. Factors affecting the development and progression of peptic ulcer disease

Primary	Secondary
Helicobacter pylori	Disasters
Nonsteroidal anti-inflammatory drugs	Occupational or family conflict
	Psychological distress (anxiety, depression)
	Smoking
	Alcohol abuse
	Poor diet
	Insomnia

vated by stress, no clear evidence shows that stress causes a gastrointestinal smooth muscle response different from that in control subjects without IBS. Thus, the predominant effect of psychological factors in IBS appears to be on pain and other symptom sensitivity and perception (Whitehead and Palsson 1998) and health-care-seeking behaviors. For example, Gwee et al. (1999) prospectively followed up a cohort of patients who had an episode of infectious gastroenteritis to determine which factors might predict those patients who would go on to develop IBS. They found that those who had more stressful life events and those with higher hypochondriasis scores were more likely to develop IBS, even though there were no differences in intestinal physiological measures between those who did and did not develop IBS.

Inflammatory Bowel Disease

Ulcerative colitis was described in early literature as a psychosomatic disease, but no specific psychological factor has ever been shown to contribute to the cause of ulcerative colitis or Crohn's disease. Psychological distress is common in both types of inflammatory bowel disease (IBD), but it may be a consequence of the chronic disease and its complications or a contributing stressor. Anxiety (state, not trait) and depression are correlated with more physical morbidity and malnutrition in IBD, but the direction of causation is not clear (Addolorato et al. 1997). However, psychological stress does affect symptom complaints and aggravate mucosal disease activity in ulcerative colitis (Levenstein et al. 1994). The presence of a concurrent psychiatric disorder contributes substantially to disability and distress in patients with IBD (Walker et al. 1996). Indeed, depression and a depressive style of coping are better predictors of subjective impairment in IBD than is inflammatory activity (Cuntz et al. 1999).

Clinical Implications

Patients with peptic ulcer of the duodenum whose condition is refractory to treatment should be screened for high state and trait anxiety characteristics. Cognitive-behavioral therapy can help patients feel a greater sense of mastery over feared calamities and less helpless and overwhelmed. One randomized trial found no benefits in preventing recurrence, but other benefits were found (Wilhelmsen et al. 1994). Psychiatrists also can evaluate patients for appropriate use of anxiolytics. Clinicians also should identify depression, overuse of NSAIDs, alcohol abuse, smoking, job stress, and other psychosocial factors that may aggravate peptic ulcer for appropriate therapeutic intervention.

Patients with IBS should be evaluated for the presence of anxiety, mood, and somatoform disorders. Many patients seem to benefit from antianxiety and antidepressant drugs, but the benefits may sometimes be unrelated to psychotropic effects (e.g., tricyclics' anticholinergic effects may reduce some IBS symptoms). Cognitive therapy also may be helpful in treatment of IBS, as demonstrated in controlled trials (Payne and Blanchard 1995).

Psychoanalytic treatment of IBD is no longer common, although some proponents remain (Chessick 1995). However, psychotherapy can significantly aid patients struggling to cope with ulcerative colitis or Crohn's disease. A recent European prospective multi-center controlled trial of psychotherapy in Crohn's disease did not find statistically significant differences, but the trends were toward fewer episodes of IBD and less surgery resulting from failure of drug treatment in patients who received standard treatment plus psychotherapy (Jantschek et al. 1998). The treatment of psychiatric complications of gastroenterological disease is examined in detail elsewhere (Epstein et al. 2000).

Dermatological Disorders

By way of its appearance and sensory capacities, the skin serves as a major interface for emotional expression in the interpersonal world. The range of normal emotions affects the appearance of the skin (e.g., flushing, sweating, and blanching). Psychophysiological reactions are more easily observed in the skin than in any other organ through, for example, changes in skin conductance and blood flow. Although understudied empirically, the effects of psychological factors on skin have long been recognized by clinicians. Angioedema for many years was called angioneurotic edema. Pathological behavioral processes also come into play, including neglect of normal skin care and compulsive scratching and picking. It has long been believed that stressful life events trigger or exacerbate skin diseases. There is some empirical support for this in psoriasis, alopecia areata, atopic dermatitis, and urticaria but less evidence in vitiligo, lichen planus, acne, pemphigus, and seborrheic dermatitis (Picardi and Abeni 2001). Because of the central social and psychological role played by the skin and its appearance, skin diseases in turn can produce a host of psychological reactions, including depressive reactions, shame, social withdrawal, obsessive-compulsive behaviors, and rage (Folks and Kinney 1992). Psychiatric consultation is thus an important part of the treatment approach with many dermatological patients.

Psoriasis

Psoriasis produces hyperproliferative dry patches that require chronic treatment with topical preparations. It is a common illness, affecting up to 3 million individuals in the United States. Psychological factors are stronger determinants of disability in patients with psoriasis than are objective indexes of disease severity (Richards et al. 2001). The anxiety and shame associated with the disorder combine to exact a tremendous psychological toll, with intense anticipation of rejection, a sense of defectiveness, and social withdrawal. Patients with psoriasis (and many other skin diseases) feel very stigmatized because others avoid touching them. Bleeding psoriatic lesions are especially strongly correlated with feelings of stigma. Stigmatization and deprivation of social touching result in depression, despair, isolation, and noncompliance (Gupta et al. 1998; Ramsay and O'Reagan 1988). Stress- and depression-related neuropeptides may have a role in the pathogenesis of psoriasis (Panconesi and Hautmann 1996). More than half of all patients with the disease never enter remission and may be at greatest risk for social isolation. Defensive maneuvers such as social isolation contribute to the lack of potentially helpful relationships that could provide the regulation of painful affects. In a longitudinal study, Scharloo et al. (2000) found that patients with psoriasis who more actively coped, expressed more emotion, and sought more social support had better physical health, were less anxious and depressed, and needed less treatment 1 year later.

Dermatitis

Dermatitis was one of Alexander's (1950) "Holy Seven" psychosomatic illnesses, arising, he believed, from intense conflicts over cravings for physical closeness and exhibitionistic wishes. Now we would be more likely to view these as psychological reactions to the illness. The coexistence of IBS and migraine headaches with dermatitis kindled interest in a common neurophysiological mediator; serotonergic pathways have been implicated (Garvey and Tollefson 1988). Indexes of family stress correlate positively with severity of dermatitis symptoms (Gil et al. 1987). Activation of mast cells by stress, with release of vasoactive, nociceptive, and proinflammatory mediators, may be an intervening mechanism (Singh et al. 1999).

Acne

Many psychological studies of patients with acne show a high prevalence of emotional symptoms, with anxiety and depression, especially poor self-esteem and negative self-image, being the most common (Kilkenney et al. 1997; Rubinow et al. 1987). Successful treatment of severe acne tends to reverse symptoms such as depressive affect and anxiety but produces little change in personality structure (Van der Meeren et al. 1985). Although adherence to treatment regimens constitutes an important variable in outcome, few studies have examined the psychological factors involved. Self-excoriative behavior is an important aggravating factor in acne, and it is more strongly correlated with psychological factors (poor self-concept, perfectionistic and compulsive personality traits) than with dermatological indexes of acne severity (Gupta et al. 1996).

Urticaria and Self-Induced Dermatoses

Urticaria is a common dermatological syndrome, producing wheal and flare "hives" that disappear within 24 hours. Lesions lasting longer should raise the suspicion of a vasculitic process and provoke a focus on etiologies other than the drugs and psychological causes common in transient urticaria. Neurophysiological mechanisms in anxiety-induced urticaria are similar to those in systemic anaphylaxis (Sell 1990). Treatment generally involves antihistamines and reassurance about the transience of the lesions.

Self-induced dermatoses and mutilation occur frequently among psychiatric patients. Occurring in borderline personality disorder, depression, schizophrenia, obsessive-compulsive disorder, malingering, and mental retardation, the lesions vary widely in their appearance and course (Levitz and Tan 1988). Serious lesions may result in tendon and nerve injury, as well as infection.

Clinical Implications

The psychological sequelae of dermatological illnesses may be as important as the antecedents, and as noted earlier, they have erosive effects on support systems and compliance. Active psychiatric intervention in collaboration with dermatologists can interrupt this downward spiral. For many patients with skin diseases characterized by chronic pruritus, psychosocial stressors have a direct exacerbating effect, and psychotherapy, with or without anxiolytics, may help immensely in mitigating the adverse effects of such stressors. Patients with idiopathic urticaria commonly experience flares caused by anxiety. Anxiolytics and antidepressants may be quite helpful. Dermatologists often prescribe doxepin, although its efficacy against pruritus may derive primarily from its potent antihistaminic effects.

End-Stage Renal Disease

As treatment for end-stage renal disease (ESRD) has evolved, there has been extensive interest in the psychiatric and psychosocial aspects of dialysis and transplantation (Kimmel 2000). In the following sections, the literature regarding quality of life and different treatment modalities, the effects of depression and noncompliance on outcome, and the case of patients who wish to withdraw from dialysis are discussed.

Quality of Life and Treatment Modality

Several studies have compared psychosocial quality of life for patients who have dialysis compared with renal transplantation. Of the studies in the United States (Simmons and Abress 1990) and in other countries (Laupacis et al. 1996), most have found better psychosocial functioning in transplant patients. Similar results have been found in children with renal failure (Brownbridge and Fielding 1991). Other studies have shown no difference in the psychological adjustment of patients receiving either of the two treatment modalities (Sayag et al. 1990). Investigators also have compared the quality of life among patients receiving different dialysis modalities. Some have found continuous ambulatory peritoneal dialysis to be associated with better psychological outcome (Brownbridge and Fielding 1991). Others have found mixed results or no differences in psychosocial outcomes (Griffin et al. 1994). Home dialysis is preferred over center dialysis by those patients capable of handling it (Oberley and Schatell 1996). All of these quality-of-life studies must be interpreted cautiously because patients are never randomized to receive a particular form of dialysis or transplantation. Thus, outcome differences may be related to pretreatment differences in medical, psychosocial, or other variables.

Effects of Depression on Outcome in Renal Patients

Depressive symptoms predict overall quality of life more than does adequacy of biochemical dialysis, even after adjusting for other variables (Steele et al. 1996). A Canadian research group (Burton et al. 1986) found that *depression* was a better predictor of shorter survival than was age or a composite physiological index of clinical variables. Several other investigators have noted that depression in patients with ERSD is associated with higher mortality and morbidity (Shulman et al. 1989). Other studies have found no effects of depression on survival (Devins et al. 1990; Kutner et al. 1994). A fundamental weakness of most early studies was that no attempt was made to measure and/or to control for disease severity, a major confounding factor in studies relating psychopathology to outcome in the medically ill (Levenson et al. 1990a). More recent studies have controlled for illness severity and other potential confounds, and depression still predicts higher mortality (Kimmel et al. 2000).

Effects of Compliance on Outcome

From a clinical standpoint, compliance is an important factor in the management of dialysis patients. Noncompliance may appear as skipped or shortened dialysis sessions, excessive interdialytic weight gain, and medication or dietary noncompliance. Psychosocial factors with demonstrated effects on compliance in ESRD include patients' beliefs about their health behaviors (Cummings et al. 1982), "locus of control" and self-efficacy (Schneider et al. 1991), family problems (Cummings et al. 1982), social support (O'Brien 1990), and daily stress (Everett et al. 1995). Compliance also varies between cultures. Bleyer et al. (1999) found rates of missed hemodialysis treatments of 28.1 per 100 patient months in the United States, compared with no missed treatments in any of the Japanese or Swedish patients. Compliance is a complex, multidimensional array of behaviors, and the relation between compliance and health outcomes in dialysis patients is not a simple one. Different forms of compliance usually are intercorrelated but not always (Leggat et al. 1998; Sensky et al. 1996). Cluster analysis was recently used to identify three distinct profiles of noncompliance among renal transplant recipi-

ents: accidental noncompliers, invulnerables, and decisive noncompliers (Greenstein and Siegal 1998). The multiple dimensions and types of noncompliance in dialysis patients, as well as confounding factors such as culture and substance abuse, make it unsurprising that the literature to date does not show noncompliance clearly predicting higher morbidity and mortality. Nevertheless, clinicians' experience that noncompliance leads to worse outcomes, including higher risk of death, is supported by large recent multicenter studies (Leggat et al. 1998). After heart disease, noncompliance is the most common "medical contraindication" excluding patients from renal transplantation (Holley et al. 1998).

Small studies of kidney transplant patients have shown that pretransplant noncompliance predicts posttransplant noncompliance and graft failure (Rodriguez et al. 1991). Noncompliant kidney transplant patients are more likely to be depressed and have other psychosocial problems than are compliant patients (Rodriguez et al. 1991). Overall, although the effects of noncompliance on dialysis and renal transplant patients are well recognized by clinicians, compliance should be regarded as a complex set of behaviors that require more detailed investigation.

Withdrawal From Dialysis

Psychiatric consultation may be requested when long-term dialysis patients wish to discontinue treatment, raising clinical, liaison, and ethical issues (L.M. Cohen et al. 2000). In a large study of dialysis patients (Neu and Kjellstrand 1986), dialysis was discontinued in 9%, accounting for 22% of all deaths. Half of the patients withdrawn were incompetent and required surrogate decision making. Similar studies have been done in other countries (Catalano et al. 1996). Early studies that had pointed to a high rate of suicide in dialysis patients overestimated suicide prevalence by not distinguishing rational treatment withdrawal from suicide. A more recent study points to a suicide rate of 4% of those withdrawing from dialysis (Catalano et al. 1996). The true rate of suicide in dialysis has not been established systematically, nor has there been sufficient empirical characterization of the psychological factors that may affect the decision to withdraw from treatment.

Several of the major studies examining psychological factors and outcome in renal disease are summarized in Table 12–8.

Mechanisms

The current state of research allows for informed speculation on how psychological factors such as depression

TABLE 12–8. Illustrative studies supporting the effects of psychological factors on end-stage renal disease

Psychological factor	Study type	Treatment modality	Findings	Reference(s)
Depression	Cohort	Hemodialysis	Depression predicts shorter survival	Burton et al. 1986; Kimmel et al. 2000
Cultural differences	Survey	Hemodialysis	28.1 missed treatments per 100 patient months in United States versus none in Japan and Sweden	Bleyer et al. 1999
Noncompliance	Cohort	Renal transplantation	Pretransplant noncompliance predicts posttransplant noncompliance and graft failure	Rodriguez et al. 1991

might influence outcome in ESRD. As noted earlier in this chapter (see "Psychoneuroimmunology"), depression may adversely affect immune function. Clinical experience is that depressed ESRD patients are more likely to evidence poor self-care, noncompliance, and poor medical follow-up. Noncompliance may be the key intervening mechanism for the effects of depression and other psychological factors. Depression also has been associated in other populations with increased use of analgesics, which have been shown to have a role in the etiology and exacerbation of chronic renal failure (Sandler et al. 1989). Depression is associated with smoking, alcoholism, and other forms of substance abuse that are highly prevalent in patients with ESRD (Hegde et al. 2000) and are major causes of increased morbidity and mortality themselves. Depression may adversely affect outcome in ESRD by serving as a risk factor for other medical comorbidity—for example, myocardial infarction or malnutrition.

Clinical Implications

Psychiatrists are sometimes asked to participate in decision making about which ESRD treatment modality best suits a particular patient. Current research sheds some light on this question, but it still must be answered based on the preferences and needs of the particular patient. Which modality is most appealing to the patient (i.e., regarding lifestyle, body image, and demands of the treatment)? With which treatment will the patient be most successful in compliance?

Depression is the most common psychiatric disorder in ESRD patients, and the symptoms may be difficult to distinguish from uremia or other comorbid medical conditions (Levenson and Glocheski 1991). Careful differential diagnosis will identify those patients who should

receive treatment for depression, with subsequent expectable improvement in quality of life and functional capacity. Details of the treatment of psychiatric disorders in renal failure and dialysis patients may be found elsewhere (Levy 2000).

Noncompliance remains the reason that psychiatrists are most often consulted by nephrologists. The psychiatrist should help the ESRD treatment team avoid simplistic thinking about noncompliance and be aware of the risk of scapegoating the patient. Noncompliance, as previously noted, represents a complex set of behaviors and interpersonal relationships (patient, family, physician, nurse) with important cultural and ethical considerations. The most extreme form of noncompliance is refusal to accept, or withdrawal from, treatment for ESRD. Some clinicians err in regarding such patients as always depressed and suicidal, whereas others err in the opposite direction, too often accepting such a decision at face value as rational. Psychiatrists have a crucial role in what can be a difficult distinction between autonomous rational decision making and irrational suicidal giving up, symptomatic of a treatable depression (L. M. Cohen et al. 2000).

Conclusion

The DSM-IV-TR diagnostic criteria for psychological factors affecting medical condition are shown in Table 12–2. This chapter has attempted to recognize and illustrate the complexity of the myriad relationships between psychological factors and medical conditions, including onset, course, and outcome of illness. Psychological factors appear to be independent risk factors for some medical diseases, although confounding with other risk factors is typical. Psychological factors may physiologically affect somatic symptoms but more often affect patients' perception of their symptoms. The importance of such "subjective" effects should not be underestimated; as noted in this chapter, cardinal symptoms of many diseases are more closely correlated with psychological factors than with objective indexes of disease severity. The mechanisms by which psychological factors affect medical conditions are still being worked out and require much more research. The range of possible mechanisms is wide, including effects via psychophysiology (e.g., psychoneuroimmunology), the doctor–patient relationship, compliance, and health care use. Although controlled trials now support the value of timely psychiatric and psychotherapeutic interventions in many medical illnesses, much work remains to determine the most effective applications of mental health services in medically ill patients.

References

Addolorato G, Capristo E, Stefanini GF, et al: Inflammatory bowel disease: a study of the association between anxiety and depression, physical morbidity, and nutritional status. Scand J Gastroenterol 32:1013–1021, 1997

Agency for Health Care Policy and Research: Smoking cessation clinical practice guideline. JAMA 275:1270–1280, 1996

Alexander F: Psychosomatic Medicine: Its Principles and Applications. New York, WW Norton, 1950

Almada SJ, Zonderman AB, Shekelle RB, et al: Neuroticism and cynicism and risk of death in middle-aged men: the Western Electric Study. Psychosom Med 53:165–175, 1991

American Psychiatric Association: Diagnostic and Statistical Manual of Mental Disorders, 3rd Edition, Revised. Washington, DC, American Psychiatric Association, 1987

American Psychiatric Association: Diagnostic and Statistical Manual of Mental Disorders, 4th Edition. Washington, DC, American Psychiatric Association, 1994

Armstrong D, Arnold R, Classen M, et al: RUDER—a prospective, two-year, multicenter study of risk factors for duodenal ulcer relapse during maintenance therapy with ranitidine. RUDER Study Group. Dig Dis Sci 39:1425–1433, 1994

Ash G, Dickens CM, Creed FH, et al: The effects if dothiepin on subjects with rheumatoid arthritis and depression. Rheumatology 38:959–967, 1999

Ashutosh K, Haldipur C, Boucher ML: Clinical and personality profiles and survival inpatients with COPD. Chest 111:95–98, 1997

Aydin IO, Ulusahin A: Depression, anxiety comorbidity, and disability in tuberculosis and chronic obstructive pulmonary disease patients: applicability of GHQ-12. Gen Hosp Psychiatry 23:77–83, 2001

Ayres A, Hoon PW, Franzoni JB, et al: Influences of mood and adjustment to cancer on compliance with chemotherapy among breast cancer patients. J Psychosom Res 38:393–402, 1994

Bauer H, Duijsens IJ: Personality disorders in pulmonary patients. Br J Med Psychol 71:165–173, 1998

Beardsley G, Goldstein MG: Endocrine diseases, in Psychological Factors Affecting Medical Conditions. Edited by Stoudemire A. Washington, DC, American Psychiatric Press, 1995, pp 173–186

Bindemann S, Soukop M, Kaye SB: Randomized controlled study of relaxation training. Eur J Cancer 27:170–174, 1991

Bird H, Broggini M: Paroxetine versus amitriptyline for treatment of depression associated with rheumatoid arthritis: a randomized, double blind, parallel group study. J Rheumatol 27:2791–2797, 2000

Black S: Inhibition of immediate-type hypersensitivity response by direct suggestion under hypnosis. BMJ 1:925–929, 1963

Bleiker EM, van der Ploeg HM, Hendriks JH, et al: Personality factors and breast cancer development: a prospective longitudinal study. J Natl Cancer Inst 88:1478–1482, 1996

Bleyer AJ, Hylander B, Sudo H, et al: An international study of patient compliance with hemodialysis. JAMA 281:1211–1213, 1999

Bosley CM, Fosbury JA, Cochrane GM: The psychological factors associated with poor compliance with treatment in asthma. Eur Respir J 8:899–904, 1995

Bosley CM, Corden ZM, Rees PJ, et al: Psychological factors associated with use of home nebulized therapy for COPD. Eur Respir J 9:2346–2350, 1996

Brownbridge G, Fielding DM: Psychosocial adjustment to end-stage renal failure: comparing hemodialysis, continuous ambulatory peritoneal dialysis and transplantation. Pediatr Nephrol 5:612–616, 1991

Buddeberg C, Wolf C, Sieber M, et al: Coping strategies and course of disease of breast cancer patients: results of a 3-year longitudinal study. Psychother Psychosom 55:151–157, 1991

Burton JJ, Kline SA, Lindsay RM, et al: Relationship of depression to survival in chronic renal failure. Psychosom Med 48:261–269, 1986

Butow PN, Coates AS, Dunn SM: Psychosocial predictors of survival in metastatic melanoma. J Clin Oncol 17:2256–2263, 1999

Campbell DA, Yellowlees PM, McLennan G, et al: Psychiatric and medical features of near fatal asthma. Thorax 50:254–259, 1995

Carette S, Surtees PG, Wainwright NW, et al: The role of life events and childhood experiences in the development of rheumatoid arthritis. J Rheumatol 27:2123–2130, 2000

Carney RM, Rich MW, Freedland KE, et al: Major depressive disorder predicts cardiac events in patients with coronary artery disease. Psychosom Med 50:627–633, 1988

Carney RM, Freeland KE, Eisen SA, et al: Major depression and medication adherence in elderly patients with coronary artery disease. Health Psychol 14:88–90, 1995

Cassileth BR, Walsh WP, Lusk EJ: Psychosocial correlates of cancer survival: a subsequent report 3 to 8 years after cancer diagnosis. J Clin Oncol 6:1753–1759, 1988

Catalano C, Goodship TH, Graham KA, et al: Withdrawal of renal replacement therapy in Newcastle Upon Tyne. Nephrol Dial Transplant 11:133–139, 1996

Chessick RD: The psychoanalytic treatment of ulcerative colitis revisited. J Am Acad Psychoanal 23:243–261, 1995

Chiovato L, Marino M, Perugi G, et al: Chronic recurrent stress due to panic disorder does not precipitate Graves' disease. J Endocrinol Invest 21:758–764, 1998

Ciechanowski PS, Katon WJ, Russo JE: Depression and diabetes: impact of depressive symptoms on adherence, function, and costs. Arch Intern Med 160:3278–3285, 2000

Ciechanowski PS, Katon WJ, Russo JE, et al: The patient–provider relationship: attachment theory and adherence to treatment in diabetes. Am J Psychiatry 158:29–35, 2001

Classen C, Butler LD, Koopman C, et al: Supportive-expressive group therapy and distress in patients with metastatic breast cancer. Arch Gen Psychiatry 58:494–501, 2001

Cluley S, Cochrane GM: Psychological disorder in asthma is associated with poor control and poor adherences to inhaled steroids. Respir Med 95:37–39, 2001

Cobb S, Rose RM: Hypertension, peptic ulcer, and diabetes in air traffic controllers. JAMA 224:489–492, 1973

Cohen LM, Steinberg MD, Hails KC, et al: Psychiatric evaluation of death-hastening requests: lessons from dialysis discontinuation. Psychosomatics 41:195–203, 2000

Cohen S, Tyrrell DAJ, Smith AP: Psychological stress and susceptibility to the common cold. N Engl J Med 325:606–612, 1991

Cohen S, Miller GE, Rabin BS: Psychological stress and antibody response to immunization: a critical review of the human literature. Psychosom Med 63:7–18, 2001

Costa D, Mogos I, Toma T: Efficacy and safety of mianserin in the treatment of depression of women with cancer. Acta Psychiatr Scand Suppl 72:85–92, 1985

Courtney JG, Longnecker MP, Theorell T, et al: Stressful life events and the risk of colorectal cancer. Epidemiology 4:407–414, 1993

Cummings K, Becker M, Kirscht J, et al: Psychosocial factors affecting adherence to medical regimens in a group of hemodialysis patients. Med Care 20:567–580, 1982

Cunningham AJ, Edmonds CVI, Jenkins GP, et al: A randomized controlled trial of the effects of group psychological therapy on survival in women with metastatic breast cancer. Psychooncology 7:508–517, 1998

Cuntz U, Welt J, Ruppert E, et al: Determination of subjective burden from chronic inflammatory bowel disease and its psychosocial consequences: results from a study of 200 patients. Psychother Psychosom Med Psychol 49:494–500, 1999

Dattore PJ, Shontz FC, Coyne L: Premorbid personality differentiation of cancer and noncancer groups: a test of the hypothesis of cancer proneness. J Consult Clin Psychol 48:388–394, 1980

de Groot M, Jacobson AM, Samson JA, et al: Glycemic control and major depression in patients with type 1 and type 2 diabetes mellitus. J Psychosom Res 46:425–435, 1999

De-Ping LD, DeQuattro V, Allen J, et al: Behavioral vs. beta-blocker therapy in patients with primary hypertension: effects on blood pressure, left ventricular function and mass, and the pressor surge of social stress anger. Am Heart J 116:637–644, 1988

Devins GM, Mann J, Mandin H, et al: Psychosocial predictors of survival in end-stage renal disease. J Nerv Ment Dis 178:127–133, 1990

Dixon L, Weiden P, Delahanty J, et al: Prevalence and correlates of diabetes in national schizophrenia samples. Schizophr Bull 26:903–912, 2000

Druss BG, Bradford DW, Rosenheck RA, et al: Mental disorders and use of cardiovascular procedures after myocardial infarction. JAMA 283:506–511, 2000

Dunbar F: Mind and Body: Psychosomatic Medicine. New York, Random House, 1947

Edwards JR, Cooper CL, Pearl SS, et al: The relationship between psychosocial factors and breast cancer: some unexpected results. Behav Med 16:5–14, 1990

Eiser N, West C, Evans S, et al: Effects of psychotherapy in moderately severe COPD: a pilot study. Eur Respir J 10:1581–1584, 1997

Epstein SA, Wise TN, Goldberg RL: Gastroenterology, in Psychiatric Care of the Medical Patient, 2nd Edition. Edited by Stoudemire A, Fogel BS, Greenberg DB. New York, Oxford University Press, 2000, pp 775–790

Evans DL, McCartney CF, Haggerty JJ, et al: Treatment of depression in cancer patients is associated with better life adaptation: a pilot study. Psychosom Med 50:72–76, 1988

Everett KD, Brantley PJ, Sletten C, et al: The relation of stress and depression to interdialytic weight gain in hemodialysis patients. Behav Med 21:25–30, 1995

Faller H, Bulzebruck H, Drungs P, et al: Coping, distress, and survival among patients with lung cancer. Arch Gen Psychiatry 56:756–762, 1999

Fawzy FI, Cousins N, Fawzy NW, et al: A structured psychiatric intervention for cancer patients, I: changes over time in methods of coping and affective disturbance. Arch Gen Psychiatry 47:720–725, 1990a

Fawzy FI, Kemeny ME, Fawzy NW, et al: A structured psychiatric intervention for cancer patients, II: changes over time in immunological measures. Arch Gen Psychiatry 47:729–735, 1990b

Fawzy FI, Fawzy NW, Hyun CS, et al: Malignant melanoma: effects of an early structured psychiatric intervention, coping, and affective state on recurrence and survival 6 years later. Arch Gen Psychiatry 50:681–689, 1993

Fifield J, Tennen H, Reisine S, et al: Depression and the long-term risk of pain, fatigue, and disability in patients with rheumatoid arthritis. Arthritis Rheum 41:1851–1857, 1998

Folks DG, Kinney FC: The role of psychological factors in dermatologic conditions. Psychosomatics 33:45–54, 1992

Fox BH: Current theory of psychogenic effects on cancer incidence and prognosis. Journal of Psychosocial Oncology 1:17–31, 1983

Frasure-Smith N, Lesperance F, Talajic M: Depression following myocardial infarction: impact on 6-month survival. JAMA 270:1819–1825, 1993

Frasure-Smith N, Lesperance F, Talajic M: Depression and 18-month prognosis after myocardial infarction. Circulation 91:999–1005, 1995a

Frasure-Smith N, Lesperance F, Talajic M: The impact of negative emotions on prognosis following myocardial infarction: is it more than depression? Health Psychol 14:388–398, 1995b

Friedman M, Rosenman RH: Association of specific overt behavior pattern with blood and cardiovascular findings. JAMA 169:1085–1096, 1959

Friedman R, Schwartz JE, Schnall PL, et al: Psychological variables in hypertension: relationship to casual or ambulatory blood pressure in men. Psychosom Med 63:19–31, 2001

Garay-Sevilla ME, Malacara JM, Gonzalez-Contreras E, et al: Perceived psychological stress in diabetes mellitus type 2. Rev Invest Clin 52:241–245, 2000

Garssen B, Goodkin K: On the role of immunological factors as mediators between psychosocial factors and cancer progression. Psychiatry Res 85:51–61, 1999

Garvey MJ, Tollefson GD: Association of affective disorder with migraine headaches and neurodermatitis. Gen Hosp Psychiatry 10:148–149, 1988

Gellert GA, Maxwell RM, Siegel BS: Survival of breast cancer patients receiving adjunctive psychosocial support therapy: a 10-year follow-up study. J Clin Oncol 11:66–69, 1993

Gendel BR, Benjamin JE: Psychogenic factors in the etiology of diabetes. N Engl J Med 234:556–562, 1946

Gil KM, Keefe FJ, Sampson HA, et al: The relation of stress and family environment to atopic dermatitis symptoms in children. J Psychosom Res 31:673–684, 1987

Giraldi T, Rodani MG, Cartei G, et al: Psychosocial factors and breast cancer: a 6-year Italian follow-up study. Psychother Psychosom 66:229–236, 1997

Glassman AH, Shapiro PA: Depression and the course of coronary artery disease. Am J Psychiatry 155:4–11, 1998

Glover J, Dibble SL, Dood MJ, et al: Mood states of oncology outpatients: does pain make a difference? J Pain Symptom Manage 10:120–128, 1995

Goetsch VL, VanDorsten B, Pbert LA, et al: Acute effects of laboratory stress on blood glucose in non-insulin-dependent diabetes. Psychosom Med 55:492–496, 1993

Gonder-Frederick LA, Carter WR, Cox DJ, et al: Environmental stress and blood glucose change in IDDM. Health Psychol 9:503–515, 1990

Graves PL, Thomas CB, Mead LA: Familial and psychological predictors of cancer. Cancer Detect Prev 15:59–64, 1991

Greene WA, Young LE, Swisher SN: Psychological factors and reticuloendothelial disease. Psychosom Med 18:284–303, 1956

Greenstein S, Siegal B: Compliance and noncompliance in patients with a functioning renal transplant: a multicenter study. Transplantation 66:1718–1726, 1998

Greer S: What's in a name? Neuroimmunomodulation or psychoneuroimmunology? Ann N Y Acad Sci 917:568–574, 2000

Greer S, Morris T, Pettingale KW: Psychological response to breast cancer: effect on outcome. Lancet 2:785–787, 1979

Greer S, Moorey S, Baruch J: Evaluation of adjuvant psychological therapy for clinically referred cancer patients. Br J Cancer 63:257–260, 1991

Greimel ER, Padilla GV, Grant MM: Self-care response to illness of patients with various cancer diagnoses. Acta Oncol 36:141–150, 1997

Grey M, Boland EA, Davidson M, et al: Coping skills training for youth with diabetes mellitus has long-lasting effects on metabolic control and quality of life. J Pediatr 137:107–113, 2000

Griffin KW, Wadhwa NK, Friend R, et al: Comparison of quality of life in hemodialysis and peritoneal dialysis patients. Adv Perit Dial 10:104–108, 1994

Grossarth-Maticek R, Eysenck HJ: Personality, smoking, and alcohol as synergistic risk factors for cancer of the mouth and pharynx. Psychol Rep 67:1024–1026, 1990

Gullette ECD, Blumenthal JA, Babyak M, et al: Effects of mental stress on myocardial ischemia during daily life. JAMA 277:1521–1525, 1997

Gupta MA, Gupta AK, Schork NJ: Psychological factors affecting self-excoriative behavior in women with mild-to-moderate facial acne vulgaris. Psychosomatics 37:127–130, 1996

Gupta MA, Gupta AK, Watteel GN: Perceived deprivation of social touch in psoriasis is associated with greater psychologic morbidity: an index of the stigma experience in dermatologic disorders. Cutis 61:339–342, 1998

Gwee KA, Leong YL, Graham C, et al: The role of psychological and biological factors in postinfective gut dysfunction. Gut 44:400–406, 1999

Hagglof B, Dahlquist G, Lonnbert G, et al: The Swedish childhood diabetes study: indications of severe psychological stress as a risk factor for type 1 (insulin dependent) diabetes mellitus in childhood. Diabetologia 34:579–583, 1991

Hahn RC, Petitti DB: Minnesota Multiphasic Personality Inventory–rated depression and the incidence of breast cancer. Cancer 61:845–848, 1988

Halford WK, Cuddily S, Mortimer RH: Psychological stress and blood glucose regulation in type 1 diabetic patients. Health Psychol 9:516–528, 1990

Hegde A, Veis JH, Seidman A, et al: High prevalence of alcoholism in dialysis patients. Am J Kidney Dis 35:1039–1043, 2000

Herpertz S, Johann B, Lichtblau K, et al: Patients with diabetes mellitus: psychosocial stress and use of psychosocial support: a multicenter study. Med Klin 95:369–377, 2000

Herschbach P, Henrich G, von Rad M: Psychological factors in functional gastrointestinal disorders: characteristics of the disorder or of the illness behavior? Psychosom Med 61:148–153, 1999

Holland JC, Morrow GR, Schmale A, et al: A randomized clinical trial of alprazolam versus progressive muscle relaxation in cancer patients with anxiety and depressive symptoms. J Clin Oncol 9:1004–1011, 1991

Holland JC, Romano SJ, Heiligenstein JH, et al: A controlled trial of fluoxetine and desipramine in depressed women with advanced cancer. Psychooncology 7:291–300, 1998

Holley JL, Monaghan J, Byer B, et al: An examination of the renal transplant evaluation process focusing on cost and the reasons for patient exclusion. Am J Kidney Dis 32:567–574, 1998

Ickovics JR, Hamburger ME, Vlahov D, et al: Mortality, CD4 cell count decline, and depressive symptoms among HIV-seropositive women. JAMA 285:1466–1474, 2001

Ironson G, Taylor CB, Boltwood M, et al: Effects of anger on left ventricular ejection fraction in coronary artery disease. Am J Cardiol 70:281–285, 1992

Jahn I, Becker U, Jockel KH, et al: Occupational life course and lung cancer risk in men: findings from a socio-epidemiological analysis of job-changing histories in a case-control study. Soc Sci Med 40:961–975, 1995

Janson C, Bjornsson E, Hetta J, et al: Anxiety and depression in relation to respiratory symptoms and asthma. Am J Respir Crit Care Med 149:930–934, 1994

Jantschek G, Zeitz M, Pritsch M, et al: Effect of psychotherapy on the course of Crohn's disease: result of the German prospective multicenter psychotherapy treatment study of Crohn's disease. German Study Group on Psychosocial Intervention in Crohn's Disease. Scand J Gastroenterol 33:1289–1296, 1998

Januzzi JL, Stern TA, Pasternak RC, et al: The influence of anxiety and depression on outcomes of patients with coronary artery disease. Arch Intern Med 160:1913–1921, 2000

Jess P, Eldrup J: The personality patterns of inpatients with duodenal ulcer and ulcer-like dyspepsia and their relationship to the course of the diseases—Hvidovre Ulcer Project Group. J Intern Med 235:589–594, 1994

Jiang W, Babyak M, Krantz DS, et al: Mental stress-induced myocardial ischemia and cardiac events. JAMA 275:1651–1656, 1996

Kelly WF: Psychiatric aspects of Cushing's syndrome. QJM 89:543–551, 1996

Ketterer MW: Secondary prevention of ischemic heart disease: the case for aggressive behavioral monitoring and intervention. Psychosomatics 34:78–84, 1993

Kiecolt-Glaser JK, Glaser R: Psychoneuroimmunology and health consequences: data and shared mechanisms. Psychosom Med 57:269–274, 1995

Kiecolt-Glaser JK, Garner W, Speicher C, et al: Psychosocial modifiers of immunocompetence in medical students. Psychosom Med 46:7–14, 1984

Kiecolt-Glaser JK, Glaser R, Strain EC, et al: Modulation of cellular immunity in medical students. J Behav Med 9:5–21, 1986

Kiecolt-Glaser JK, Glaser R, Shuttleworth EC, et al: Chronic stress and immunity in family caregivers of Alzheimer's disease victims. Psychosom Med 49:523–535, 1987a

Kiecolt-Glaser JK, Fisher L, Ogrocki P, et al: Marital quality, marital disruption, and immune function. Psychosom Med 49:13–34, 1987b

Kiecolt-Glaser JK, Kennedy S, Malkoff S, et al: Marital discord and immunity in males. Psychosom Med 50:213–229, 1988

Kilkenney M, Stathakis V, Hibbert ME, et al: Acne in Victorian adolescents: associations with age, gender, puberty and psychiatric symptoms. J Paediatr Child Health 33:430–433, 1997

Kimmel PL: Psychosocial factors in adult end-stage renal disease patients treated with hemodialysis: correlates and outcomes. Am J Kidney Dis 35:S132–S140, 2000

Kimmel PL, Peterson RA, Weihs KL, et al: Multiple measurements of depression predict mortality in a longitudinal study of chronic hemodialysis outpatients. Kidney Int 57:2093–2098, 2000

Kneier AW, Temoshok L: Repressive coping reactions in patients with malignant melanoma as compared to cardiovascular patients. J Psychosom Res 28:145–155, 1984

Kramer JR, Ledolter J, Manos GN, et al: Stress and metabolic control in diabetes mellitus: methodological issues and an illustrative analysis. Ann Behav Med 22:17–28, 2000

Krantz DS, Sheps DS, Carney RM, et al: Effects of mental stress in patients with coronary artery disease: evidence and clinical implications. JAMA 283:1800–1802, 2000

Kreitler S, Chaitchik S, Kreitler H: Repressiveness: cause or result of cancer? Psychooncology 2:43–54, 1993

Kroll T, Barlow JH, Shaw K: Treatment adherence in juvenile rheumatoid arthritis: a review. Scand J Rheumatol 28:10–18, 1999

Kune GA, Kune S, Watson LF, et al: Personality as a risk factor in large bowel cancer: data from the Melbourne Colorectal Cancer Study. Psychol Med 21:29–41, 1991

Kutner NG, Lin LS, Fielding B, et al: Continued survival of older hemodialysis patients: investigation of psychosocial predictors. Am J Kidney Dis 24:42–49, 1994

Lachar BL: Coronary-prone behavior: type A behavior revisited. Tex Heart Inst J 20:143–151, 1993

Lambley P: The role of psychological processes in the aetiology and treatment of cervical cancer: a biopsychological perspective. Br J Med Psychol 66:43–60, 1993

Lammers CA, Naliboff BD, Straatmeyer AJ: The effects of progressive relaxation on stress and diabetic control. Behav Res Ther 22:641–650, 1984

Lane JD, McCaskill CC, Williams PG, et al: Personality correlates of glycemic control in type 2 diabetes. Diabetes Care 23:1321–1325, 2000

Lasser K, Boyd JW, Woolhandler S, et al: Smoking and mental illness: a population-based prevalence study. JAMA 284:2606–2610, 2000

Laupacis A, Keown P, Pus N, et al: A study of the quality of life and cost-utility of renal transplantation. Kidney Int 50:235–242, 1996

Lee MA, Ganzini L: Depression in the elderly: effect on patient attitudes toward life-sustaining therapy. J Am Geriatr Soc 40:983–988, 1992

LeFevre PD: Improving the physical health of patients with schizophrenia: therapeutic nihilism or realism? Scott Med J 46:11–13, 2001

Leggat JE Jr, Orzol SM, Hulbert-Shearin TE, et al: Noncompliance in hemodialysis: predictors and survival analysis. Am J Kidney Dis 32:139–145, 1998

Leor J, Poole WK, Kloner RA: Sudden cardiac death triggered by an earthquake. N Engl J Med 334:413–419, 1996

Lerman C, Hughes C, Trock BJ, et al: Genetic testing in families with heredity nonpolyposis colon cancer. JAMA 281:1618–1622, 1999

Lernmark B, Persson B, Fisher L, et al: Symptoms of depression are important to psychological adaptation and metabolic control in children with diabetes mellitus. Diabet Med 16:14–22, 1999

Le Son S, Gershwin ME: Risk factors for asthmatic patients requiring intubation, III: observations in young adults. J Asthma 33:27–35, 1996

Lesperance F, Frasure-Smith N, Juneau M, et al: Depression and 1-year prognosis in unstable angina. Arch Intern Med 160:1354–1360, 2000

Levenson JL, Dwight M: Cardiovascular disease, in Psychiatric Care of the Medical Patient, 2nd Edition. Edited by Stoudemire A, Fogel BS, Greenberg DB. New York, Oxford University Press, 2000, pp 717–732

Levenson JL, Glocheski S: Psychological factors affecting end-stage renal disease: a review. Psychosomatics 32:382–389, 1991

Levenson JL, McDonald MK: The role of psychological factors in cancer onset and progression: a critical appraisal, in The Psychoimmunology of Cancer, 2nd Edition. Edited by Lewis CE, O'Brien R, Barraclough J. New York, Oxford University Press, in press

Levenson JL, Colenda C, Larson DB, et al: Methodology in consultation-liaison research: a classification of biases. Psychosomatics 31:367–376, 1990a

Levenson JL, Hamer RM, Rossiter LF: Relation of psychopathology in general medical inpatients to use and cost of services. Am J Psychiatry 147:1498–1503, 1990b

Levenstein S: The very model of a modern etiology: a biopsychosocial view of peptic ulcer. Psychosom Med 62:176–185, 2000

Levenstein S, Prantera C, Varvo V, et al: Psychological stress and distress activity in ulcerative colitis: a multidimensional cross-sectional study. Am J Gastroenterol 89:1219–1225, 1994

Levenstein S, Prantera C, Varvo V, et al: Patterns of biologic and psychologic risk factors in duodenal ulcer patients. J Clin Gastroenterol 21:110–117, 1995a

Levenstein S, Kaplan GA, Smith M: Sociodemographic characteristics, life stressors, and peptic ulcer: a prospective study. J Clin Gastroenterol 21:185–192, 1995b

Levenstein S, Kaplan GA, Smith MW: Psychological predictors of peptic ulcer incidence in the Alameda County Study. J Clin Gastroenterol 24:140–146, 1997

Levitz SM, Tan OT: Factitious dermatosis masquerading as recurrent herpes zoster. Am J Med 84:781–783, 1988

Levy NB: End-stage renal disease and its treatment: dialysis and transplantation, in Psychiatric Care of the Medical Patient. Edited by Stoudemire A, Fogel BS, Greenberg DB. New York, Oxford University Press, 2000, pp 791–800

Lewis PC, Harrell JS, Bradley C, et al: Cigarette use in adolescents: the cardiovascular health in children and youth study. Res Nurs Health 24:27–37, 2001

Leymarie F, Jolly D, Sanderman R, et al: Life events and disability in rheumatoid arthritis: a European cohort. Br J Rheumatol 36:1106–1112, 1997

Lipowski ZJ: Psychosomatic medicine: past and present, III: current research. Can J Psychiatry 31:14–21, 1986

Lloyd CE, Dyer PH, Lancashire RJ, et al: Association between stress and glycemic control in adults with type 1 (insulin-dependent) diabetes. Diabetes Care 22:1278–1283, 1999

Lloyd CE, Dyer PH, Barnett AH: Prevalence of symptoms of depression and anxiety in a diabetes clinic population. Diabet Med 17:198–202, 2000

Lustman PJ, Griffith LS, Clouse RE, et al: Effects of nortriptyline on depression and glycemic control in diabetes: results of a double-blind, placebo-controlled trial. Psychosom Med 59:241–250, 1997

Lustman PJ, Freedland KE, Griffith LS, et al: Predicting response to cognitive behavior therapy of depression in type 2 diabetes. Gen Hosp Psychiatry 20:302–306, 1998

Lustman PJ, Freedland KE, Griffith LS, et al: Fluoxetine for depression in diabetes: a randomized double-blind placebo-controlled trial. Diabetes Care 23:618–623, 2000

Lynge E, Anderson O: Unemployment and cancer in Denmark, 1970–1975 and 1986–1990. IARC Sci Publ 138:353–359, 1997

Margolis GJ, Goodman RL, Rubin A, et al: Psychological factors in the choice of treatment for breast cancer. Psychosomatics 30:192–197, 1989

Markovitz JH, Matthews KA, Wing RR, et al: Psychological predictors of hypertension in the Framingham Study: is there tension in hypertension? JAMA 270:2439–2443, 1993

McDaniel JS, Musselman DL, Porter MR, et al: Depression in patients with cancer: diagnosis, biology, and treatment. Arch Gen Psychiatry 52:89–99, 1995

McDonough EM, Boyd JH, Varvares MA, et al: Relationship between psychological status and compliance in a sample of patients treated for cancer of the head and neck. Head Neck 18:267–269, 1996

McGee R, Williams S, Elwood M: Depression and the development of cancer: a meta-analysis. Soc Sci Med 38:187–192, 1994

McKenna MC, Zevon MA, Corn B, et al: Psychosocial factors and the development of breast cancer: a meta-analysis. Health Psychol 18:520–531, 1999

Miles JF, Garden GM, Tunnicliffe WS, et al: Psychological morbidity and coping skills in patients with brittle and non-brittle asthma: a case-control study. Clin Exp Allergy 27:1151–1159, 1997

Moos RH: Personality factors associated with rheumatoid arthritis: a review. Journal of Chronic Diseases 17:41–55, 1964

Mooy JM, deVries H, Grootenhuis PA, et al: Major stressful life events in relation to prevalence of undetected type 2 diabetes: the Hoorn Study. Diabetes Care 23:197–201, 2000

Moser DK, Dracup K: Is anxiety early after myocardial infarction associated with subsequent ischemic and arrhythmic events? Psychosom Med 58:395–401, 1996

Musselman DL, Evans DL, Nemeroff CB: The relationship of depression to cardiovascular disease. Arch Gen Psychiatry 55:580–592, 1998

Neu S, Kjellstrand CM: Stopping long-term dialysis: an empirical study of withdrawal of life-supporting treatment. N Engl J Med 314:14–20, 1986

Newman S, Mulligan K: The psychology of rheumatic diseases. Baillieres Best Pract Res Clin Rheumatol 14:773–786, 2000

Oberley ET, Schatell DR: Home hemodialysis: survival, quality of life, and rehabilitation. Adv Ren Replace Ther 3:147–153, 1996

O'Brien ME: Compliance behavior and long-term maintenance dialysis. Am J Kidney Dis 15:209–214, 1990

Orlandini A, Pastore MR, Fossati A, et al: Personality traits and metabolic control: a study in insulin-dependent diabetes mellitus patients. Psychother Psychosom 66:307–313, 1997

Orth-Gomér K, Wamala SP, Horsten M, et al: Marital stress worsens prognosis in women with coronary heart disease: the Stockholm Female Coronary Risk Study. JAMA 284:3008–3014, 2000

Panconesi E, Hautmann G: Psychophysiology of stress in dermatology: the psychobiologic pattern of psychosomatics. Dermatol Clin 14:399–421, 1996

Payne A, Blanchard EB: A controlled comparison of cognitive therapy and self-help support groups in the treatment of irritable bowel syndrome. J Consult Clin Psychol 63:779–786, 1995

Penninx BWJH, Beekman ATF, Honig A, et al: Depression and cardiac mortality. Arch Gen Psychiatry 58:221–227, 2001

Perros P, Deary IJ, Frier BM: Factors influencing preference of insulin regimen in people with type 1 (insulin-dependent) diabetes. Diabetes Res Clin Pract 39:23–29, 1998

Persky VW, Kempthorne-Rawson J, Shekelle RB: Personality and risk of cancer: 20-year follow-up of the Western Electric Study. Psychosom Med 49:435–449, 1987

Peto R, Lopez AD, Boreham J, et al: Mortality from tobacco in developed countries: indirect estimation from national vital statistics. Lancet 339:1268–1278, 1992

Picardi A, Abeni D: Stressful life events and skin diseases: disentangling evidence from myth. Psychother Psychosom 70:118–136, 2001

Power C, Parsons T: Nutritional and other influences in childhood as predictors of adult obesity. Proc Nutr Soc 59:267–272, 2000

Radosavljevic VR, Jankovic SM, Marinkovic JM: Stressful life events in the pathogenesis of Graves' disease. Eur J Endocrinol 134:699–701, 1996

Ramsay B, O'Reagan M: A survey of the social and psychological effects of psoriasis. Br J Dermatol 118:195–201, 1988

Richards HL, Fortune DG, Griffiths CE, et al: The contribution of perceptions of stigmatization to disability in patients with psoriasis. Psychosom Res 50:11–15, 2001

Rietveld S, van Beest I, Everaerd W: Stress-induced breathlessness in asthma. Psychol Med 29:1359–1366, 1999

Rimington LD, Davies DH, Lowe D, et al: Relationship between anxiety, depression, and morbidity in adult asthma patients. Thorax 56:266–271, 2001

Robinson N, Fuller JH: Role of life events and difficulties in the onset of diabetes mellitus. J Psychosom Res 29:583–591, 1985

Rodriguez A, Diaz M, Colon A, et al: Psychosocial profile of noncompliant transplant patients. Transplant Proc 23:1807–1809, 1991

Rosenbaum M, Leibel RL, Hirsch J: Obesity. N Engl J Med 337:396–406, 1997

Ross CK, Lavigne JV, Hayford JR, et al: Psychological factors affecting reported pain in juvenile rheumatoid arthritis. J Pediatr Psychol 18:561–573, 1993

Rozanski A, Blumenthal JA, Kaplan J: Impact of psychological factors on the pathogenesis of cardiovascular disease and implications for therapy. Circulation 99:2192–2217, 1999

Rubinow DR, Peck GL, Squillace KM, et al: Reduced anxiety and depression in cystic acne patients after successful treatment with oral isotretinoin. J Am Acad Dermatol 17:25–32, 1987

Sandler DP, Smith JC, Weinberg CR, et al: Analgesic use and chronic renal disease. N Engl J Med 320:1238–1243, 1989

Saravay SM, Lavin M: Psychiatric comorbidity and length of stay in the general hospital: a critical review of outcome studies. Psychosomatics 35:233–252, 1994

Sayag R, Kaplan De-Nour A, Shapire Z, et al: Comparison of psychosocial adjustment of male nondiabetic kidney transplant and hospital hemodialysis patients. Nephron 54:214–218, 1990

Scharloo M, Kaptein AA, Weinman J, et al: Patients' illness perceptions and coping as predictors of functional status in psoriasis: a 1-year follow-up. Br J Dermatol 142:899–907, 2000

Schneider MS, Friend R, Whitaker P, et al: Fluid noncompliance and symptomatology in end-stage renal disease: cognitive and emotional variables. Health Psychol 10:209–215, 1991

Schulz K-H, Schulz H: Overview of psychoneuroimmunological stress and intervention studies in humans with emphasis on the uses of immunological parameters. Psychooncology 1:51–70, 1992

Schwartz MD, Taylor KL, Willard KS, et al: Distress, personality, and mammography utilization among women with a family history of breast cancer. Health Psychol 18:327–332, 1999

Sell S: Immunopathology (hypersensitivity diseases), in Anderson's Pathology, 9th Edition. Edited by Kissane JE. St. Louis, MO, CV Mosby, 1990, pp 487–545

Sensky T, Leger C, Gilmour S: Psychosocial and cognitive factors associated with adherence to dietary and fluid restriction regimens by people on chronic hemodialysis. Psychother Psychosom 65:36–42, 1996

Shapiro PA: Psychological factors in hypertension: an overview. Am Heart J 116:632–637, 1988

Shekelle RB, Raynor WJ Jr, Ostfeld AM: Psychological depression and 17-year risk of death from cancer. Psychosom Med 43:117–125, 1981

Shulman R, Price JD, Spinelli J: Biopsychosocial aspects of long-term survival on end-stage renal failure therapy. Psychol Med 19:945–954, 1989

Simmons RG, Abress L: Quality of life issues for end-stage renal disease patients. Am J Kidney Dis 15:201–208, 1990

Singh LK, Pang X, Alexacos N, et al: Acute immobilization stress triggers skin mast cell degranulation via corticotropin releasing hormone, neurotensin, and substance P: a link to neurogenic skin disorders. Brain Behav Immun 13:225–239, 1999

Smoller JW, Pollack MH, Otto M, et al: Panic anxiety, dyspnea, and respiratory disease: theoretical and clinical considerations. Am J Respir Crit Care Med 154:6–17, 1996

Soderlin MK, Hakala M, Nieminen P: Anxiety and depression in a community-based rheumatoid arthritis population. Scand J Rheumatol 29:177–183, 2000

Sonino N, Fava G: Psychosomatic aspects of Cushing's disease. Psychother Psychosom 67:140–146, 1998

Sonino N, Girelli ME, Boscaro M, et al: Life events in the pathogenesis of Graves' disease: a controlled study. Acta Endocrinol 128:293–296, 1993

Spiegel D, Bloom JR: Group therapy and hypnosis reduce metastatic breast carcinoma pain. Psychosom Med 45:333–339, 1983

Spiegel D, Bloom JR, Yalom I: Group support for patients with metastatic cancer: a randomized prospective outcome study. Arch Gen Psychiatry 38:527–533, 1981

Spiegel D, Bloom JR, Kraemer HC, et al: Effect of psychosocial treatment on survival of patients with metastatic breast cancer. Lancet 2:888–891, 1989

Steele TE, Baltimore D, Finkelstein SH, et al: Quality of life in peritoneal dialysis patients. J Nerv Ment Dis 184:368–374, 1996

Stein M, Miller AH, Trestman RL: Depression, the immune system, and health and illness: findings in search of meaning. Arch Gen Psychiatry 48:171–177, 1991

Stoudemire A (ed): Psychological Factors Affecting Medical Conditions. Washington, DC, American Psychiatric Press, 1995

Stoudemire A, Wallack L, Hedemark N: Alcohol dependence and abuse. Am J Prev Med 3(suppl):9–18, 1987

Stoudemire A, Fogel BS, Greenberg DB (eds): Psychiatric Care of the Medical Patient, 2nd Edition. New York, Oxford University Press, 2000

Sullivan MD, La Croix AZ, Baum C, et al: Functional status in coronary artery disease: a one-year prospective study of the role of anxiety and depression. Am J Med 103:348–356, 1997

Temoshok L, Heller BW, Sageviel RW, et al: The relationship of psychological factors of prognostic indicators in cutaneous malignant melanoma. J Psychosom Res 29:139–153, 1985

ten Brinke A, Ouwerkerk ME, Zwinderman AH, et al: Psychopathology in patients with severe asthma is associated with increased health care utilization. Am J Respir Crit Care Med 163:1093–1096, 2001a

ten Brinke A, Ouwerkerk ME, Bel EH, et al: Similar psychological characteristics in mild and severe asthma. J Psychosom Res 50:7–10, 2001b

The ENRICHD Investigators: Enhancing recovery in coronary artery disease patients (ENRICHD): study design and methods. Am Heart J 139:1–9, 2000

Thun MJ, Peto R, Lopez AD, et al: Alcohol consumption and mortality among middle-aged and elderly U.S. adults. N Engl J Med 337:1705–1714, 1997

Vamos M, Kolbe J: Psychological factors in severe chronic asthma. Aust N Z J Psychiatry 33:538–544, 1999

Van der Meeren HLM, Van der Schaar WW, Van den Hurk CMAM: The psychological impact of severe acne. Cutis 36:84–86, 1985

Vila G, Nollet-Clemencon C, Vera M, et al: Prevalence of DSM-IV disorders in children and adolescents with asthma versus diabetes. Can J Psychiatry 44:562–569, 1999

Viskin S, Belhassen B: Idiopathic ventricular fibrillation. Am Heart J 120:661–671, 1990

Vogt T, Pope C, Mullooly J, et al: Mental health status as a predictor of morbidity and mortality: a 15-year follow-up of members of a health maintenance organization. Am J Public Health 84:227–231, 1994

Vracko-Tusevljak M, Kambic V: The significance of psychological factors in the early diagnosis of laryngeal and hypopharyngeal tumors. Laryngorhinootologie 68:118–121, 1989

Wales JK: Does psychological distress cause diabetes? Diabet Med 12:109–112, 1995

Walker EA, Roy-Byrne RP, Katon WJ: Irritable bowel syndrome and psychiatric illness. Am J Psychiatry 174:565–572, 1990

Walker EA, Katon WJ, Roy-Byrne RP, et al: Histories of sexual victimization in patients with irritable bowel syndrome or inflammatory bowel disease. Am J Psychiatry 150:1502–1506, 1993

Walker EA, Gelfand MD, Gelfand AN, et al: The relationship of current psychiatric disorder to functional disability and distress in patients with inflammatory bowel disease. Gen Hosp Psychiatry 18:220–229, 1996

Waxler-Morrison N, Hislop TG, Mears B, et al: Effects of social relationships on survival for women with breast cancer: a prospective study. Soc Sci Med 33:177–183, 1991

Weiner H: Psychobiology and Human Disease. New York, Elsevier, 1977

Weiner H, Thaler M, Reiser MF, et al: Etiology of duodenal ulcer, I: relation of specific psychological characteristics to rate of gastric secretion (serum pepsinogen). Psychosom Med 19:1–10, 1957

Whitehead WE, Palsson OS: Is rectal pain sensitivity a biological marker for irritable bowel syndrome: psychological influences on pain. Gastroenterology 115:1263–1271, 1998

Wilhelmsen I, Haug TT, Ursin H, et al: Effect of short-term cognitive psychotherapy on recurrence of duodenal ulcer: a prospective randomized trial. Psychosom Med 56:440–448, 1994

Williams RB, Littman AB: Psychosocial factors: role in cardiac risk and treatment strategies. Cardiol Clin 14:97–104, 1996

Winsa B, Adami HO, Bergstrom R, et al: Stressful life events and Graves' disease. Lancet 338:1475–1479, 1991

Withers NJ, Rudkin ST, White RJ: Anxiety and depression in severe chronic obstructive pulmonary disease: the effects of pulmonary rehabilitation. J Cardiopulm Rehabil 19:362–365, 1999

Wolfe F: Psychological distress and rheumatic disease. Scand J Rheumatol 28:131–136, 1999

Yamagiwa M, Harada T, Kubo M, et al: Psychological states and personality as factors in the morbidity of head and neck malignant tumors. Nippon Jibiinkoka Gakkai Kaiho 94:67–73, 1991

Yohannes AM, Baldwin RC, Connolly MJ: Depression and anxiety in elderly outpatients with chronic obstructive pulmonary disease: prevalence and validation of the BASDEC screening questionnaire. Int J Geriatr Psychiatry 15:1090–1096, 2000

Yoshiuchi K, Kumano H, Nomura S, et al: Psychological factors influencing the short-term outcome of antithyroid drug therapy in Graves' disease. Psychosom Med 60:592–596, 1998a

Yoshiuchi K, Kumano H, Nomura S, et al: Stressful life events and smoking were associated with Graves' disease in women, but not in men. Psychosom Med 60:182–185, 1998b

Zonderman AB, Costa PT Jr, McCrae RR: Depression as a risk factor for cancer morbidity and mortality in a nationally representative sample. JAMA 262:1191–1195, 1989

Somatoform Disorders

Sean H. Yutzy, M.D.

The somatoform disorders were first delineated as a class of psychiatric disorders in DSM-III (American Psychiatric Association 1980). The class was created to facilitate the differential diagnosis of disorders characterized primarily by "physical symptoms suggesting physical disorder (hence *somatoform*) for which there are no demonstrable organic findings or known physiological mechanisms and for which there is positive evidence, or a strong presumption, that the symptoms are linked to psychological factors or conflicts" (American Psychiatric Association 1980, p. 241). With minor modifications, this grouping and its underlying concept were retained in DSM-III-R (American Psychiatric Association 1987) and, after some debate (Martin 1995), in DSM-IV (American Psychiatric Association 1994) and DSM-IV-TR (American Psychiatric Association 2000). (Noteworthy here was that the explicit diagnostic criteria from DSM-IV remained the same in DSM-IV-TR.) In contrast to factitious disorders and malingering, somatoform disorder symptoms are *not* under voluntary control. The stipulation in DSM-IV-TR that symptoms are *not* fully accounted for by known physiological mechanisms distinguishes somatoform disorders from disorders formerly designated as psychophysiological disorders, some of which are included in DSM-IV-TR under "Psychological Factors Affecting Medical Condition." Beliefs or preoccupations with symptoms are not of delusional intensity, except for body dysmorphic disorder. Symptoms are not better accounted for by other mental disorders.

In DSM-IV-TR, the disorders included under the somatoform rubric are *somatization disorder, undifferentiated somatoform disorder, conversion disorder, pain disorder, hypochondriasis, body dysmorphic disorder*, and the residual category *somatoform disorder not otherwise specified (NOS)*. DSM-IV-TR criteria for these disorders are outlined in Table 13–1. The grouping is based on the clinical utility of a shared diagnostic concern rather than assumptions regarding shared etiology or mechanism: the exclusion of occult "physical" or "organic" pathology underlying the symptoms. In DSM-IV-TR terminology, such etiologies are referred to as "general medical conditions" or the "direct effects of a substance." General medical conditions include all conditions not included in the mental disorders section of ICD-10 (World Health Organization 1992b). As examples, all infectious and parasitic, endocrine, nutritional, metabolic, immunity, and congenital disorders affecting virtually any organ system (including the nervous system) are considered general medical conditions. This terminology was adopted to avoid the implication that *mental* (i.e., psychiatric) conditions do not have *organic* causes and to underscore the view that psychiatric disorders are also *medical* conditions.

The utility of grouping disorders on the basis of a shared clinical concern was endorsed by the symptom-driven *Diagnostic and Statistical Manual of Mental Disorders, Fourth Edition, Primary Care Version* (DSM-IV–PC; American Psychiatric Association 1995), which included "unexplained physical symptoms" as the basis of 1 of its 10 algorithms. Likewise, the ICD-10 *Diagnostic and Management Guidelines for Mental Disorders in Primary Care* (World Health Organization 1996) was organized with a diagnostic category for "unexplained somatic complaint."

Criticisms of the somatoform disorders category were summarized by M.R. Murphy (1990), who contended that the category is "superficial" because it is delineated on the basis of presenting physical symptoms. Furthermore, the individual disorders are not qualitatively distinct, would be better described dimensionally than categorically, are derived from data on hospital- rather than community- or primary care–based populations, give the "spurious impression of understanding" leading to "naive assumptions about disease entities," and

TABLE 13–1. DSM-IV-TR somatoform disorders: a comparison

DSM-IV-TR somatoform disorder	General description	Temporal and other requirements	Exclusions by other psychiatric illness	Other exclusions
Somatization disorder	History of many physical complaints: pain in at least four different sites or functions, two nonpain gastrointestinal, one sexual or reproductive, one pseudoneurological (conversion or dissociative).	Onset before age 30. Occurs over a period of several years. Treatment sought, or significant impairment in social, occupational, or other important areas of functioning.	Not specified.	Not fully explained by a known general medical condition or the direct effect of a substance.
Undifferentiated somatoform disorder	One or more physical complaints.	Duration of at least 6 months. Clinically significant distress or impairment in social, occupational, or other important areas of functioning.	Not better accounted for by another mental disorder.	Not fully explained by a known general medical condition or pathophysiological mechanism (i.e., the effects of injury, medication, drugs, alcohol).
Conversion disorder	Symptoms or deficits affecting voluntary motor or sensory function suggesting a neurological or other general medical condition.	Psychological factors associated. Clinically significant distress or impairment in social, occupational, or other important areas of functioning; or warrants medical evaluation.	Not limited to pain or sexual dysfunction. Not exclusively during course of somatization disorder. Not better accounted for by another mental disorder.	Not intentionally produced or feigned. Not fully explained by a neurological or other general medical condition, or by the direct effect of a substance, or as a culturally sanctioned behavior or experience.
Pain disorder	Pain as predominant focus of clinical presentation. Of sufficient severity to warrant clinical attention.	Clinically significant distress or impairment in social, occupational, or other important areas of functioning. Psychological factors have an important role.	Not better accounted for by a mood, anxiety, or psychotic disorder, and does not meet criteria for dyspareunia.	Not specified.
Hypochondriasis	Preoccupation with fears of having, or the idea that one has, a serious disease based on the misinterpretation of bodily symptoms. Persists despite appropriate medical evaluation and reassurance.	Duration of at least 6 months. Clinically significant distress or impairment in social, occupational, or other important areas of functioning.	Not exclusively during course of a generalized anxiety, obsessive-compulsive, or panic disorder; a major depressive episode; separation anxiety; or another somatoform disorder.	Not of delusional intensity. Not restricted to circumscribed concern about appearance.

TABLE 13–1. DSM-IV-TR somatoform disorders: a comparison (*continued*)

DSM-IV-TR somatoform disorder	General description	Temporal and other requirements	Exclusions by other psychiatric illness	Other exclusions
Body dysmorphic disorder	Preoccupation (may be of delusional intensity) with imagined defect in appearance or markedly excessive concern with slight physical anomaly.	Clinically significant distress or impairment in social, occupational, or other important areas of functioning.	Not better accounted for by another mental disorder (e.g., dissatisfaction with body shape or size in anorexia nervosa).	Not specified.
Somatoform disorder not otherwise specified	Disorders with specified somatoform symptoms. Examples: pseudocyesis; disorders of less than 6 months' duration with fatigue or body weakness, nonpsychotic hypochondriacal symptoms, or other physical complaints.	Can be of less than 6 months' duration.	Does not meet criteria for any specific somatoform disorder.	Not specified.

Source. Adapted with permission from Martin RL: "Somatoform Disorders in the General Hospital Setting," in *Handbook of Studies on General Psychiatry*. Edited by Judd FK, Burrows GD, Lipsitt DR. Amsterdam, The Netherlands, Elsevier, 1991, pp 251–266. Copyright 1991 Elsevier Science Publishers.

morphic disorder), somatoform autonomic dysfunction (a category not included in DSM-IV-TR that corresponds, in part, to the DSM-I and DSM-II psychophysiological disorders), persistent somatoform pain disorder, other somatoform disorders, and somatoform disorder, unspecified. Conversion disorder is not included as a somatoform disorder but is subsumed under a fused dissociative (conversion) disorder. As is discussed in the section on conversion disorder in this chapter, this option was considered carefully in the preparation of DSM-IV, but it was decided to leave conversion disorder in the somatoform grouping on the basis that it met the essential requirement of presentation with physical symptoms suggesting a general medical condition but for which there is no adequate medical or physiological explanation (Martin 1996).

Despite inconsistencies between DSM-IV and ICD-10, sufficient overlap existed to permit generalizations regarding specific somatoform disorders, as long as the differences were kept in mind. The comparability and, by design, compatibility of DSM-IV and ICD-10 provided evidence of expanding international cooperation in developing a common language to foster better communication among clinicians and researchers worldwide.

Given the heterogeneity of the somatoform disorder class, extensive discussion of the class, in general, is not particularly useful. The specific somatoform disorders are best discussed individually. Thus, with the exception of pain disorder, which is reviewed in a separate chapter of this textbook (see Chapter 23 by King), we review the somatoform disorders included in DSM-IV-TR. For convenience, the disorders are discussed in the order in which they appear in DSM-IV-TR.

Somatization Disorder

Definition and Clinical Description

The core features of somatization disorder are recurrent multiple physical complaints that are not fully explained by physical factors and that result in medical attention or significant impairment.

A patient with somatization disorder is typified by the following example:

> An internist referred a married 35-year-old woman to a psychiatrist because of the physician's inability to establish a clear longitudinal history and medical explanation for her numerous physical complaints. Physical examination and laboratory testing had been completely unrevealing. The physician had treated her for anxiety and depressive complaints; however, the pharmaco-

therapy, which was initially apparently effective, subsequently failed.

> On presentation to the psychiatrist, the patient offered a laundry list of physical complaints in a dramatic yet vague manner. The patient often went into elaborate and flamboyant discussions of her marital, social, and occupational problems. Careful review of the presentation identified a long history of chronic physical complaints without medical explanation. Furthermore, the physical problems appeared to be temporally associated with multiple psychosocial stressors.

Somatization disorder is the most pervasive somatoform disorder. By definition, somatization disorder is a polysymptomatic disorder affecting multiple body systems. Symptoms of other specific somatoform disorders (e.g., conversion disorder and pain disorder) are included in the diagnostic criteria for somatization disorder. Undifferentiated somatoform disorder, in essence, represents a syndrome similar to somatization disorder but with a less extensive symptomatology. From a hierarchical perspective, none of these disorders is diagnosed if symptoms occur exclusively during the course of somatization disorder.

Somatization disorder has been the most rigorously studied somatoform disorder and is the best validated in terms of diagnostic reliability, stability over time, prediction of medical utilization, and even heritability. Yet its validity as a discrete syndrome has been challenged (Bass and Murphy 1990). Vaillant (1984), noting that most of the research on this disorder has emanated from four academic centers in the midwestern United States, went so far as to state that the diagnosis "lies in the eyes of the beholder" (p. 543).

Diagnosis

History

The DSM-IV-TR criteria for somatization disorder are the product of a long and inconsistent approach to a syndrome characterized by multiple unexplained physical complaints (Martin 1988). Originally designated as *hysteria*, the syndrome was first described at least 4,000 years ago, with its conceptualization probably originating in Egypt (Goodwin and Guze 1996). In Egyptian medicine, it was believed that physical displacement of the uterus precipitated symptoms (Veith 1965); treatment consisted of attempting to attract the "wandering womb" back to its proper site.

Freud devoted a great deal of attention to the concept of hysteria (Breuer and Freud 1893–1895/1955). In fact, many of the principles of psychoanalysis were developed through observations of hysteria. Dynamic theorists postulated the operation of the ego defense mechanism of conversion in hysteria. This mechanism was conceptualized as the converting of "psychic energy" into physical symptoms. Later, Stekel (1943) coined the term *somatization*, which he regarded as similar to Freud's concept of conversion.

Pierre Briquet (1859) described in his monograph *Traité, Clinique et Thérapeutique Y l'Hystérie* a syndrome corresponding to somatization disorder as it is conceptualized today. He described hysteria as characterized by multiple dramatic and excessive medical complaints in the absence of demonstrable organic pathology. Purtell et al. (1951) resurrected Briquet's concept, adding a quantitative perspective by providing a list of associated symptoms, which was further refined by Perley and Guze (1962).

Hysteria was included as one of the 14 "canonized" psychiatric disorders in the influential criteria described by Feighner et al. (1972). The disorders included were those considered by the authors to have been validated sufficiently. For hysteria, the Feighner criteria required a chronic or recurrent illness beginning before age 30 that includes a dramatic, vague, or complicated medical history. The diagnosis required 25 "positive" medically unexplained symptoms (from a list of 59) in 9 of 10 groups (Table 13–3); 20 symptoms in the same number of groups were necessary for a probable diagnosis. To be counted as positive, a symptom had to 1) have caused the patient to see a physician or other health care provider, 2) have precipitated disability that interfered with the patient's life, 3) have led the patient to take medicine on one or more occasions, 4) have been of "clinical significance" despite not fulfilling one of the three previously mentioned criteria. An example of this fourth criterion would be a brief spell of blindness that the patient minimizes.

As is discussed in this chapter, the syndrome as defined by Feighner et al. (1972) remains the gold standard because it has been the best validated. In particular, clinical, epidemiological, and follow-up studies that used the Feighner criteria support their validity, reliability, and internal consistency (Barsky 1989). The stability of the disorder is supported by the finding that in the 6–8 years after initial diagnosis, there is a 90% probability that the clinical picture will remain essentially unchanged and that no general medical condition or new mental disorder will develop to explain the original symptoms (Barsky 1989).

Despite such validation, the construct was underused by clinicians (Cloninger 1994). This underuse has been attributed to two sources: the pejorative connotation of the term *hysteria* and the complexity of remembering the numerous symptoms divided into various groups not organized according to any obvious logic. The criteria

TABLE 13–3. Feighner symptom list for hysteria (somatization disorder)

Group 1	Group 6
Headaches	Abdominal pain
Sickly most of life	Vomiting
Group 2	**Group 7**
Blindness	Dysmenorrhea
Paralysis	Menstrual irregularity
Anesthesia	Amenorrhea
Aphonia	Excessive bleeding
Fits or convulsions	**Group 8**
Unconsciousness	Sexual indifference
Amnesia	Frigidity
Deafness	Dyspareunia
Hallucinations	Other sexual difficulties
Urinary retention	Vomiting all 9 months of pregnancy at least once, or hospitalization for hyperemesis gravidarum
Trouble walking	
Other unexplained "neurological" symptoms	
Group 3	**Group 9**
Fatigue	Back pain
Lump in throat	Joint pain
Fainting spells	Extremity pain
Visual blurring	Burning pains of the sexual organs, mouth, or rectum
Weakness	Other bodily pains
Dysuria	
Group 4	**Group 10**
Breathing difficulty	Nervousness
Palpitation	Fears
Anxiety attacks	Depressed feelings
Chest pain	Need to quit working, or inability to carry on regular duties because of feeling sick
Dizziness	
Group 5	Crying easily
Anorexia	Feeling life is hopeless
Weight loss	Thinking a good deal about dying
Marked fluctuations in weight	
Nausea	Wanting to die
Abdominal bloating	Thinking of suicide
Food intolerances	Suicide attempts
Diarrhea	
Constipation	

Note. Twenty-five positive symptoms in nine groups required for a diagnosis of definite hysteria; 20 positive symptoms in nine groups required for a diagnosis of probable hysteria.

Source. Adapted from Perley and Guze 1962. Reprinted with permission from Cloninger CR: "Somatoform and Dissociative Disorders," in *The Medical Basis of Psychiatry*, Second Edition. Edited by Winokur G, Clayton P. Philadelphia, PA, WB Saunders, 1994, pp 169–192. Copyright 1994 WB Saunders Company.

were intended principally for a research setting in which the investigator completed his or her systematic assessment with a checklist to evaluate for the presence of the syndrome.

In addition to its definition as a syndrome characterized by many somatic complaints, hysteria was frequently confused with the dramatic and volatile hysterical personality characteristics as described by Chodoff and Lyons (1958). Guze (1970) suggested the more neutral eponym *Briquet's syndrome*. In DSM-III, the syndrome was descriptively renamed *somatization disorder*. The criteria in DSM-III were simplified as follows:

1. The required number of symptoms was lowered to 14 for women and 12 for men, from a list of 37 commonly identified somatic complaints. The 37 symptoms listed were those that best discriminated somatization disorder from other disorders. The number of symptoms required of men was lowered in an attempt to reduce a possible sex bias because of the impossibility of menstrual and pregnancy symptoms in men.
2. The group requirement was eliminated because it seemed to add little information.
3. Depressive and panic attack symptoms were eliminated to avoid overlap with depressive and panic disorders.

The diagnostic criteria for somatization disorder also required a history of physical symptoms of several years' duration beginning before the patient was 30 years old. Conditions similar to those defined by the Feighner criteria were necessary to consider a symptom positive. Exclusion of a medical explanation was determined if the symptoms were not adequately explained by a "physical disorder or physical injury" and were "not side effects of medication, drugs or alcohol" (American Psychiatric Association 1980, p. 243). The clinician did not need to be convinced that the symptom had actually occurred; a patient's report was sufficient.

The criteria for somatization disorder were modified only slightly for DSM-III-R. The changes included shortening the symptom list to 35 and requiring 13 symptoms for the diagnosis in both sexes. A symptom was not counted if it occurred only during a panic attack. Symptoms were to be counted as present if there was no specific pathology or pathophysiological mechanism. In addition, if organic pathology was identified, the complaint or resulting social or occupational impairment must have grossly exceeded what would be expected from the physical findings.

Unfortunately, diagnostic concordance between the simplified DSM-III somatization disorder criteria and the Feighner criteria was less than optimal. As a result, the question was raised whether the types of cases identified by DSM-III criteria constituted a valid disease entity (Cloninger et al. 1986; Guze et al. 1986). The ade-

quacy of the criteria also was questioned when the National Institute of Mental Health (NIMH) Epidemiologic Catchment Area (ECA) studies (L.N. Robins et al. 1984), which used DSM-III criteria, found a much lower lifetime prevalence rate (0.2%–0.3%) of somatization disorder for women in the general population than the 2% estimated by Woodruff et al. (1971), who used Feighner criteria. Furthermore and particularly noteworthy was that many psychiatrists considered both the DSM-III and the DSM-III-R criteria too lengthy and complex for routine clinical use.

DSM-IV Criteria

In an attempt to address these issues for DSM-IV, a comprehensive reassessment of the extant literature and preexisting data sets was coordinated by the American Psychiatric Association. On the basis of this review, Cloninger and Yutzy (1993) suggested a diagnostic strategy that simplified the criteria for somatization disorder and appeared useful in routine practice. Data from a sample of 500 psychiatric outpatients were reanalyzed, leading to the development of an empirically derived algorithm to diagnose somatization disorder. This algorithm required four pain symptoms, two nonpain gastrointestinal symptoms, one nonpain sexual or reproductive symptom, and one pseudoneurological (conversion or dissociative) symptom. This approach was adopted for DSM-IV (Table 13–4). The data reanalysis criteria identified nearly the same patients as did both the original Feighner criteria for hysteria and the DSM-III-R criteria for somatization disorder ($\kappa = .79$; sensitivity = 81%; specificity = 96%) (Yutzy et al. 1992).

The new criteria were tested in a multicenter field trial designed to examine their concordance with previous diagnostic criteria. This study (Yutzy et al. 1995) found excellent agreement with the newly proposed diagnostic strategy and these earlier criteria: DSM-III-R ($\kappa = .84$; sensitivity = 84%; specificity = 98%), DSM-III ($\kappa = .82$; sensitivity = 82%; specificity = 98%), and the original Feighner criteria for hysteria ($\kappa = .79$; sensitivity = 80%; specificity = 97%). These findings supported the DSM-IV diagnostic strategy for somatization disorder.

Differential Diagnosis

The symptom picture encountered in somatization disorder is frequently nonspecific and can overlap with a multitude of medical disorders. According to Cloninger (1994), three features are useful in discriminating between somatization disorder and physical illness: 1) involvement of multiple organ systems, 2) early onset

TABLE 13–4. DSM-IV-TR diagnostic criteria for somatization disorder

A. A history of many physical complaints beginning before age 30 years that occur over a period of several years and result in treatment being sought or significant impairment in social, occupational, or other important areas of functioning.

B. Each of the following criteria must have been met, with individual symptoms occurring at any time during the course of the disturbance:

    (1) *four pain symptoms:* a history of pain related to at least four different sites or functions (e.g., head, abdomen, back, joints, extremities, chest, rectum, during menstruation, during sexual intercourse, or during urination)

    (2) *two gastrointestinal symptoms:* a history of at least two gastrointestinal symptoms other than pain (e.g., nausea, bloating, vomiting other than during pregnancy, diarrhea, or intolerance of several different foods)

    (3) *one sexual symptom:* a history of at least one sexual or reproductive symptom other than pain (e.g., sexual indifference, erectile or ejaculatory dysfunction, irregular menses, excessive menstrual bleeding, vomiting throughout pregnancy)

    (4) *one pseudoneurological symptom:* a history of at least one symptom or deficit suggesting a neurological condition not limited to pain (conversion symptoms such as impaired coordination or balance, paralysis or localized weakness, difficulty swallowing or lump in throat, aphonia, urinary retention, hallucinations, loss of touch or pain sensation, double vision, blindness, deafness, seizures; dissociative symptoms such as amnesia; or loss of consciousness other than fainting)

C. Either (1) or (2):

    (1) after appropriate investigation, each of the symptoms in Criterion B cannot be fully explained by a known general medical condition or the direct effects of a substance (e.g., a drug of abuse, a medication)

    (2) when there is a related general medical condition, the physical complaints or resulting social or occupational impairment are in excess of what would be expected from the history, physical examination, or laboratory findings

D. The symptoms are not intentionally produced or feigned (as in factitious disorder or malingering).

TABLE 13–5. Features useful in discriminating between somatization disorder and general medical conditions

Involvement of multiple organ systems
Early onset and chronic course without development of physical signs of structural abnormalities
Absence of characteristic laboratory abnormalities of the suggested physical disorder

TABLE 13–6. General medical conditions that may be confused with somatization disorder

Multiple sclerosis
Systemic lupus erythematosus
Acute intermittent porphyria
Hemochromatosis

and chronic course without development of physical signs of structural abnormalities, and 3) absence of characteristic laboratory abnormalities of the suggested physical disorder (Table 13–5). These features should be considered in cases for which careful analysis leaves the etiology unclear. The clinician also should be aware that several medical disorders may be confused with somatization disorder (Table 13–6). Patients with multiple sclerosis and systemic lupus erythematosus (SLE) may have vague functional and sensory disturbances with unclear physical signs. Patients with acute intermittent porphyria (AIP) may have a history of episodic pain and various neurological disturbances, and patients with hemochromatosis often have vague and diffuse pains, which may be confused with patients who have somatization disorder.

According to Cloninger (1994), three psychiatric disorders must be carefully considered in the differential diagnosis of somatization disorder: anxiety disorders (in particular, panic disorder), mood disorders, and schizophrenia. The most troublesome distinction is between anxiety disorders and somatization disorder. Individuals with generalized anxiety disorder may have a multitude of physical complaints that are also frequently found in patients with somatization disorder. Individuals with anxiety disorders also may have disease concerns and hypochondriacal complaints common to somatization disorder. Similarly, patients with somatization disorder often report panic (anxiety) attacks. Although the usual parameters of age at onset and course may be helpful in differentiating between an anxiety disorder and somatization disorder, the presence of certain traits, symptoms, and social factors can be of assistance. In particular, the presence of histrionic personality traits, conversion and dissociative symptoms, sexual and menstrual problems, and social impairment supports a diagnosis of somatization disorder (Cloninger 1994). In addition, gender should be considered because men are much more likely to have anxiety disorders than somatization disorder. Precise diagnosis, although difficult, is clinically important because the medical management of somatization disorder differs from that of anxiety disorders.

Patients with mood disorders, especially depression, may have somatic complaints. Commonly, the chief complaint may be headache, gastrointestinal disturbance, or unexplained pain. However, such symptoms resolve with successful treatment of the mood disorder, whereas in somatization disorder, the physical complaints continue. Patients with somatization disorder frequently complain of depression and often fulfill the criteria for major depression (DeSouza et al. 1988). It is not clear, however, whether these complaints truly reflect the clinical state or are simply a reflection of overreporting.

Patients with schizophrenia may have unexplained somatic complaints. Careful evaluation often identifies delusions, hallucinations, and/or a formal thought disorder. Rarely will the somatic symptoms be extensive enough to meet the criteria for somatization disorder. It should be noted that occasionally a patient with extensive somatic symptomatology and no evidence of psychosis subsequently will develop clinical symptoms of schizophrenia (Goodwin and Guze 1996). As described in the section on conversion disorder later in this chapter, reports of hallucinations are common among women with somatization disorder (R.L. Martin, unpublished observations, 1998). Caution must be taken not to equate such reports with a psychotic diagnosis, which can lead to unnecessary long-term treatment with neuroleptics.

Individuals with antisocial, borderline, and/or histrionic personality disorder may have an associated somatization disorder (Cloninger et al. 1997; Hudziak et al. 1996; Stern et al. 1993). Antisocial personality disorder has been shown to cluster both within individuals and within families (Cloninger and Guze 1970; Cloninger et al. 1975) and may have a common etiology in many cases.

Patients with somatization disorder often complain of psychological or interpersonal problems in addition to somatic symptoms. Wetzel et al. (1994) summarized these as "psychoform symptoms." In this study, Minnesota Multiphasic Personality Inventory (MMPI; Hathaway and McKinley 1943) profiles of somatization disorder patients mimicked multiple psychiatric disorders.

Commonly, individuals with somatization disorder are inconsistent historians, and obtaining the medical records often will be necessary to definitively establish the diagnosis.

Natural History

E. Robins and O'Neal (1953) found somatization disorder to be unusual in children younger than 9 years. In most cases, characteristic symptoms begin during adolescence, and the criteria are satisfied by the mid-20s (Guze and Perley 1963; Purtell et al. 1951).

Somatization disorder is a chronic illness with fluctuations in the frequency and diversity of symptoms, but it rarely, if ever, totally remits (Guze and Perley 1963; Guze et al. 1986). The most active symptomatic phase is usually early adulthood, but aging does not lead to total remission (Goodwin and Guze 1996). Pribor et al. (1994) found that patients with somatization disorder age 55 years and older did not differ from younger patients in terms of the number of somatization symptoms or the use of health care services. Longitudinal prospective studies have confirmed that 80%–90% of the patients diagnosed with somatization disorder maintain consistent clinical syndrome and retain the same diagnosis over many years (Cloninger et al. 1986; Guze et al. 1986; Perley and Guze 1962).

According to Goodwin and Guze (1996), the most frequent and important complications of somatization disorder are repeated surgical operations, drug dependence, suicide attempts, and marital separation or divorce. These authors suggested that the first two complications are preventable if the disorder is recognized and the patient's symptoms are managed appropriately. Generally, because of awareness that somatization disorder is an alternative explanation for various pains and other symptoms, invasive techniques can be withheld or postponed when objective indications are absent or equivocal. There is no evidence of excess mortality in patients with somatization disorder.

Avoidance of prescribing habit-forming or addictive substances for persistent or recurrent complaints of pain should be paramount in the mind of the treating physician. Suicide attempts are common, but completed suicide is not (Martin et al. 1985; G.E. Murphy and Wetzel 1982). It is unclear whether marital or occupational dysfunction can be minimized through psychotherapy.

Epidemiology

The lifetime risk, prevalence, and incidence of somatization disorder are unclear. The lifetime risk for somatization disorder was estimated at about 2% in women when age at onset and method of assessment were taken into account (Cloninger et al. 1975). This risk is similar to the previously noted 2% prevalence rate identified by Woodruff et al. (1971). Cloninger et al. (1984), using complete lifetime medical records, found a 3% frequency of somatization disorder in 859 Swedish women in the general population. However, the ECA study (L.N. Robins et al. 1984), using nonphysician interviewers, found a lifetime risk of somatization disorder of only 0.2%–0.3% for women. However, the prevalence of somatization disorder may be underestimated in studies relying on interviews by nonphysicians. In a study by L.N. Robins et al. (1981), nonphysicians, when compared with psychiatrists, showed high (i.e., 97%–99%) diagnostic specificity for somatization disorder. However, diagnostic sensitivity for nonphysicians was low (55% for Feighner-defined hysteria and 41% for DSM-III-defined somatization disorder). The diagnostic criteria for somatization disorder require judgments as to whether symptoms are fully explained medically. Patients with somatization disorder often attribute symptoms to various physical disorders. Nonphysicians rarely have the expertise to evaluate such statements critically and may tend to accept them. To properly assess somatic complaints relative to objective findings and the known course of disease may require that the interviewer have an adequate medical background (Cloninger 1994). Additionally, patients may be less inclined to describe physical complaints to nonphysicians. All of these factors may lead to the underdiagnosis of somatization disorder, which may account for the low prevalence of somatization disorder in large-scale population surveys that use nonphysician interviewers.

Somatization disorder is diagnosed predominantly in women and rarely in men. Some have suggested that this sex difference may be artifactual because somatization disorder criteria are biased against making the diagnosis in men because of the inapplicability of pregnancy and menstrual complaints. Also, men tend to report fewer symptoms than do women. Some investigators have suggested an adjustment for this discrepancy (Temoshok and Attkisson 1977). DSM-III reduced the number of symptoms required to diagnose somatization disorder from 14 (in women) to 12 in men, compensating for the inapplicable gynecological symptoms but not for the response bias in the number of somatic complaints. Diagnosis of somatization disorder remains much less frequent in men than in women unless the number of somatic complaints required for diagnosis in men is reduced to half (i.e., 7) of the 14 required in women (Cloninger 1994). The symptoms of somatization disorder were counted in a study of psychiatric outpatients and their relatives (Cloninger et al. 1986). The frequency counts were identified for probands and for the relatives of nonsomatizing subjects. The prevalence of somatization disorder was 22% in outpatient women when DSM-III criteria of 14 unexplained symptoms in women were used, compared with 2.9% in the female relatives of nonsomatizing subjects. When the DSM-III criterion of 12 unexplained symptoms in men was applied, the prevalence of somatization disorder in the male relatives of nonsomatizing subjects was only 0.3%, making the disorder more than 10 times as prevalent in women as in men. When the symptom count for men was reduced to 7 or 8 symptoms, the prevalences in men and women were about the same. However, according to Cloninger

(1994), men who had from 7 to 11 somatic complaints had a mixed picture of anxiety and personality disorders and did not cluster in families with somatizing subjects of either sex.

Etiology

The etiology of somatization disorder is unknown, but it is clearly a familial disorder. In several studies, approximately 20% of the female first-degree relatives of patients with somatization disorder also met criteria (Cloninger and Guze 1970; Guze et al. 1986; Woerner and Guze 1968). Guze et al. (1986) further demonstrated the familial nature of somatization disorder in a "blind" family study and documented an association between somatization disorder and antisocial personality in male and female relatives. In addition, several studies have suggested that male relatives of female patients with somatization disorder have an increased risk of antisocial personality disorder and alcoholism (Cloninger et al. 1975; Woerner and Guze 1968). Cloninger et al. (1986) found that men with multiple somatic complaints were clinically heterogeneous and did not aggregate in families with either male or female somatizing subjects. Overall, these findings suggest that somatization disorder in women shares a common etiology with antisocial personality disorder, whereas somatization disorder in men may be related more to anxiety disorders (Cloninger et al. 1984, 1986).

A relation between somatization disorder and certain personality disorders has been posited. Hudziak et al. (1996) and Cloninger et al. (1997) identified similarities and even overlap between somatization disorder and borderline personality disorder, as did Stern et al. (1993) with personality disorders broadly. These studies support interpretations that somatization disorder is more of a personality (Axis II) disorder than an Axis I disorder, considering its early onset, nonremitting nature, and pervasiveness, which in some cases results in chronic dysfunctional states.

Familial aggregation in somatization disorder could result from genetic factors, environmental influences, or both. Bohman et al. (1984) used comprehensive lifetime medical records in an adoption study in Sweden and identified two discrete types of somatoform disorders in women. One form, described as "high-frequency somatization," was characterized by frequent headaches, backaches, gastrointestinal disturbances, and gynecological complaints associated with psychiatric disability (Figure 13–1). Review of the psychiatric evaluations showed overlap with somatization disorder. Women who were adopted before age 3 years had a fivefold increase in high-frequency somatization disorder if their biological par-

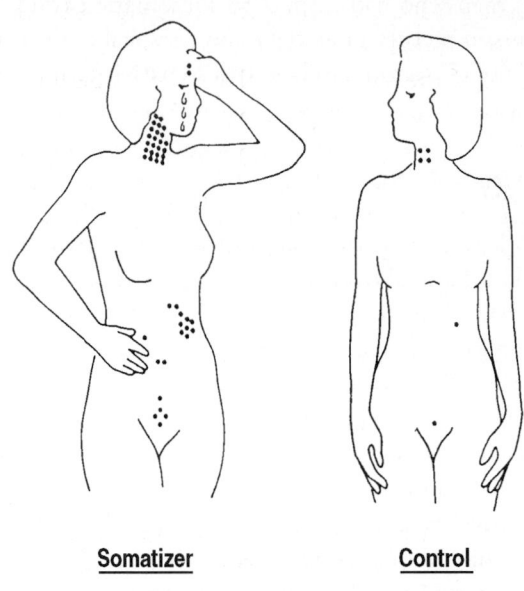

Somatizer   **Control**

- 1 Somatic sick leave/10 person years
- 1 Psychiatric sick leave/10 person years

FIGURE 13–1. Distribution and number of sick leave occasions in Swedish somatizing ("high-frequency") subjects and control nonsomatizing subjects.

Source. Reprinted with permission from Cloninger CR: "Somatoform and Dissociative Disorders," in *The Medical Basis of Psychiatry*, Second Edition. Edited by Winokur G, Clayton PJ. Philadelphia, PA, WB Saunders, 1994, pp 169–192. Copyright 1994 WB Saunders Company.

ents had alcoholism or were antisocial. Risk of somatization disorder in the adopted children varied according to the social status of the adoptive parents. In a cross-fostering analysis that considered the possible combinations of genetic background and postnatal influences, both factors contributed independently to the risk of somatization.

Experimental neuropsychological testing indicates that individuals with somatization disorder have difficulty with information processing related to problems with attention and memory (Almgren et al. 1978; Bendefeldt et al. 1976; Ludwig 1972). Flor-Henry et al. (1981) investigated the neuropsychological functioning of patients with somatization disorder and compared them with control subjects, psychotic depressive patients, and schizophrenic patients. All comparison groups were matched to the patients with somatization disorder for sex, age, handedness, and Wechsler Adult Intelligence Scale—Revised (WAIS-R; Wechsler 1981) full-scale IQ. Compared with the control subjects, patients with somatization disorder had bilateral, symmetrical patterns of frontal lobe dysfunction. The authors also noted nondominant hemisphere dysfunction, with impairment

greater in the anterior as opposed to the posterior regions. Patients with somatization disorder had greater dominant hemisphere impairment than did control subjects and psychotic depressive patients, a finding also reported for persons with antisocial personality disorder. Patients with somatization disorder had less nondominant hemisphere disorganization than did schizophrenic patients. This pattern of neuropsychological impairment permitted identification of patients with somatization disorder from control subjects and patients in the comparison groups.

Other theories attempt to explain the characteristics of patients with somatization disorder. In particular, Shapiro (1965) and Horowitz (1977) suggested that "hysterical" information processing may be responsible for many of the clinical features. The information-processing deficit may be the basis for the somatic complaints, mental status findings of vagueness and circumstantiality, and many social, interpersonal, and occupational problems prominent in these patients and their biological relatives (Cloninger 1978; Flor-Henry et al. 1981; Horowitz 1977). Ford (1983) and Quill (1985) postulated a social communication model based on the theory that individuals with somatization disorder learn to somatize as a means of expressing emotion (i.e., distress) in their family constellation, evoking support and care from significant individuals. Further work needs to be done to evaluate these theories.

Treatment

Somatization disorder is difficult to treat, and there appears to be no single superior treatment approach (G.E. Murphy 1982). Primary care physicians generally can manage patients with somatization disorder adequately, but the expertise of at least a consulting psychiatrist has been shown to be useful. In a prospective, randomized controlled study, Smith et al. (1986) found a reduction in health care costs for patients with somatization disorder who received a psychiatric consultation as opposed to those who did not receive a consultation. Reduced expenditures were largely the result of decreased rates of hospitalization. These gains were accomplished with no decrement in medical status or in patient satisfaction, suggesting that many of the evaluations and treatments otherwise provided to patients with somatization disorder are unnecessary. Smith et al. (1986) suggested that treatment include regularly scheduled visits with an appropriate physician. The frequency of visits should be determined on the basis of support for the patient, not in response to the frequency or severity of complaints.

Scallet et al. (1976) reviewed the earlier psychiatric literature on treatment of hysteria and reported the success rates of various approaches. Although most of the studies were uncontrolled and otherwise methodologically flawed, one study by Luff and Garrod (1935) noted a 51% improvement rate at 3-year follow-up in patients treated with an "eclectic approach." As summarized by Scallet et al. (1976), this treatment involved "reeducation, reassurance and suggestion" (p. 348). These techniques also were described by Carter (1949) as being effective in the treatment of acute conversion.

An eclectic approach comports well with the general principles of treatment recommended by Quill (1985), Cloninger (1994), and Smith et al. (1986). Three important suggestions emerge from review of these reports: 1) establish a firm therapeutic alliance with the patient, 2) educate the patient about the manifestations of somatization disorder, and 3) provide consistent reassurance. Implementation of these principles, as described in more detail in the following paragraphs, may greatly facilitate clinical management of somatization disorder and prevent potentially serious complications, including the effects of unnecessary diagnostic and therapeutic procedures. The superiority of more specific treatment approaches has not been documented by controlled trials (Kellner 1989).

First, a firm therapeutic alliance must be established. The basis of any satisfactory treatment relationship is a firm therapeutic alliance; it is particularly important in the treatment of patients with somatization disorder, but it is often difficult to attain. Generally, multiple physicians already have been consulted in an attempt to discover a physical explanation for the symptoms offered. The patient usually has received the message (overtly or covertly) that the difficulty is "mental," "psychological," or "psychiatric," and the physician is not particularly interested in continuing to provide care to him or her. That message promotes a pattern of "doctor shopping," which may lead to unnecessary diagnostic procedures and treatments. To prevent harm, a therapeutic alliance is essential. The first step in establishing such an alliance is for the physician to acknowledge the patient's pain and suffering. This acknowledgment communicates to the patient that the physician is caring, compassionate, and interested in providing assistance. The physician should then conduct an exhaustive review of the patient's medical history, including careful examination of medical records. Such a review generally will strengthen the incipient therapeutic bond, demonstrating the physician's willingness to take the time and effort to gain an understanding of the patient. In addition, this step is crucial in ruling out medical disorders that can include nonspecific motor and sensory abnormalities or transient or equivocal signs (e.g., multiple sclerosis, SLE, AIP, hemochromatosis) (Table 13–6). Also, a thorough medical knowledge of the patient initially will allow better ongoing assessment of symptomatology. After the diagnosis of somatization disorder is firmly established, elaborate diagnostic evaluations should be conducted based on objective evidence and not just subjective complaints. However, the clinician must always remain cognizant that patients with somatization disorder are not immune to developing physical illness.

Education is the second general principle. Cloninger (1994) favors informing the patient of the diagnosis and describing the various facets of somatization disorder in a positive light. The patient should be advised that he or she is not "crazy" but has a medically recognized illness. The condition will not lead to chronic mental or physical deterioration (or death). The clinician should be careful to strike a balance between painting a positive picture of the disorder and conducting a realistic discussion of prognosis, goals, and treatment.

The third principle is consistent reassurance. Patients with somatization disorder often become concerned that the physician is not performing a sufficiently thorough evaluation and may threaten to seek care from a different physician. Such challenges should be directly addressed with reassurance that the possibility of an undiscovered physical illness is being appropriately assessed on a continuing basis and that changing physicians would place decisions in the hands of someone unaware of the complexities of the patient's case. The patient should be reassured that there is no evidence of a physical cause for the complaint but that there may be a link with "stress." A thorough review of complaints commonly identifies a temporal association of symptoms with interpersonal, social, or occupational problems. Discussion of such associations may help the patient gain insight that the problems may precipitate somatic or psychological symptoms. In patients for whom introspection is difficult, modification of behavior by using simple behavioral management techniques may be useful.

In addition to these general principles, several other issues merit consideration in the treatment of somatization disorder. Because patients with somatization disorder also frequently complain of anxiety and depressive symptoms, prescription medications for these complaints should be held to a minimum and carefully monitored. Wheatley (1962, 1964, 1965) found that low doses of anxiolytic drugs provided some improvement in symptoms in a series of double-blind clinical trials. Although chlordiazepoxide was recommended for reasons of safety, patient preference, and effectiveness in symptom relief, the best results were obtained by optimistic physicians using low doses of anxiolytic medications, regardless of which drug was given (Wheatley 1965). Pharmacotherapy in the management of patients with somatization disorder must be tempered with the knowledge that these patients may take medicines inconsistently and unpredictably, may develop drug dependence, and may overdose in suicide gestures or attempts.

The clinician should develop a relationship with the patient's family. This facilitates attaining a better appreciation of the patient's social structure, which may be crucial to understanding and managing the patient's often chaotic personal lifestyle. When appropriate, the clinician must place firm limits on excessive demands, manipulations, and attention seeking (G.E. Murphy 1982; G.E. Murphy and Guze 1960).

Undifferentiated Somatoform Disorder

Definition and Clinical Description

The essential aspect of undifferentiated somatoform disorder is the presence of one or more clinically significant medically unexplained somatic symptoms with a duration of 6 months or more that are not better accounted for by another mental disorder (Table 13–7; see also Table 13–1 for comparison with other somatoform disorders). In effect, this category serves to capture syndromes that resemble somatization disorder but do not meet the full criteria. Symptoms that may be seen include the same as those that are considered for somatization disorder.

Diagnosis

History

The category of undifferentiated somatoform disorder did not exist prior to DSM-III-R. At that time, it was added to cover those syndromes that in DSM-III simply would have been included under "atypical somatoform disorder." It is not clear whether the category undifferentiated somatoform disorder has been well adopted by clinicians, but several studies support its existence. Alternative terms that have been proposed include subsyndromal, forme fruste, or abridged somatization disorder (Kirmayer and Robbins 1991) and more recently multisomatoform disorder (Kroenke et al. 1997).

DSM-IV Criteria

After some debate, minor changes in the category undifferentiated somatoform disorder were made in DSM-IV.

TABLE 13–7. DSM-IV-TR diagnostic criteria for undifferentiated somatoform disorder

A. One or more physical complaints (e.g., fatigue, loss of appetite, gastrointestinal or urinary complaints).
B. Either (1) or (2):
(1) after appropriate investigation, the symptoms cannot be fully explained by a known general medical condition or the direct effects of a substance (e.g., a drug of abuse, a medication)
(2) when there is a related general medical condition, the physical complaints or resulting social or occupational impairment is in excess of what would be expected from the history, physical examination, or laboratory findings
C. The symptoms cause clinically significant distress or impairment in social, occupational, or other important areas of functioning.
D. The duration of the disturbance is at least 6 months.
E. The disturbance is not better accounted for by another mental disorder (e.g., another somatoform disorder, sexual dysfunction, mood disorder, anxiety disorder, sleep disorder, or psychotic disorder).
F. The symptom is not intentionally produced or feigned (as in factitious disorder or malingering).

Because of perceived low use of the diagnosis undifferentiated somatoform disorder by clinicians, which was attributed to ambiguity of the term undifferentiated disorder, the term multisomatoform disorder was suggested. However, because the few empirical data available seemed to indicate a variable course, with unclear boundaries with normality and other mental disorders (especially anxiety and depressive disorders), this term was not adopted. As a result, the only changes involved substituting the standard "general medical condition" for DSM-III-R's "organic pathology." A threshold for diagnosis also was added, requiring clinically significant distress or impairment. Instead of excluding the diagnosis on the basis of "occurrence exclusively during the course of another mental disorder," exclusion in DSM-IV was on the basis of "not better accounted for by another mental disorder."

Kroenke et al. (1997) used improved diagnostic criteria with inclusion and exclusion criteria and found that the proposed multisomatoform disorder had a large and independent effect on impairment in a study of 1,000 patients from four primary care sites. Still lacking in terms of validity of the proposed disorder is evidence of temporal stability.

Differential Diagnosis

Principal considerations in the differential diagnosis include the question of whether, with follow-up, criteria for somatization disorder will be met. Patients with somatization disorder are typically inconsistent historians. During one evaluation, they may report many symptoms and fulfill criteria for the full syndrome, whereas during another, they may report fewer symptoms, perhaps only fulfilling criteria for an abridged syndrome (Martin et al. 1979). Another consideration is whether the somatic symptoms qualifying a patient for the diagnosis of undifferentiated somatoform disorder are the manifestation of a depressive or an anxiety disorder. Indeed, high rates of major depression and anxiety disorders have been found in somatizing patients attending family medicine clinics (Kirmayer et al. 1993).

Epidemiology

Some investigators have argued that undifferentiated somatoform disorder is the most common somatoform disorder. Escobar et al. (1991) used a construct requiring six somatic symptoms for women and four for men and reported that in the United States 11% of non-Hispanic whites and Hispanics, as well as 15% of blacks, fulfilled the criteria. In Puerto Rico, 20% met the criteria. A preponderance of women was evident in all groups except the Puerto Rican sample.

Etiology

If undifferentiated somatoform disorder is simply an abridged form of somatization disorder, etiological theories reviewed under that diagnosis should also apply to undifferentiated somatoform disorder. Of theoretical interest would be the question of why the syndrome is fully expressed in some and only partially in others. Some investigators postulate theories of etiology involving primarily the concept of somatization, for which there are numerous explanations. As reviewed by Kirmayer and Robbins (1991), somatization can be viewed as a pattern of illness behavior by which bodily idioms of distress may serve as symbolic means of social regulation as well as protest or contestation. As yet, there is little, if any, empirical evidence for such theories.

Treatment

Existing data have been derived from studies fraught with methodological problems, including the use of diverse groups with only a certain number of chronic somatic complaints in common. Several studies suggested that improvement is accelerated with psychotherapy of a supportive, rather than a nondirective, type. However, a substantial proportion of patients improve or recover with no formal psychotherapy. Judicious use of pharmacotherapy appears to be beneficial, with trials of antidepressant medications indicated for patients with depressive symptoms and trials of buspirone, benzodiazepines, and propranolol for patients with anxiety symptoms. Again, definitive recommendations await a more extensive empirical database.

Conversion Disorder

Definition and Clinical Description

The essential features of conversion disorder are the nonintentionally produced symptoms or deficits affecting voluntary motor or sensory function that suggest but are not fully explained by a neurological or general medical condition, by the direct effects of a substance, or by a culturally sanctioned behavior or experience. Specific symptoms mentioned as examples in DSM-IV-TR include motor symptoms such as impaired coordination or balance, paralysis or localized weakness, difficulty swallowing or lump in throat (e.g., "globus hystericus"), aphonia, and urinary retention; sensory symptoms, including hallucinations, loss of touch or pain sensation, double vision, blindness, and deafness; and seizures or convulsions with voluntary motor or sensory components. Single episodes usually involve one symptom, but longitudinally, other conversion symptoms will be evident as well. Psychological factors generally appear to be involved in that symptoms often occur in the context of a conflictual situation that may in some way be resolved with the development of the symptom.

An example of a typical patient with conversion disorder follows:

A woman in her early 20s was brought to the emergency department by female relatives after an argument with her husband that led to his leaving the household. She showed variable impairment in gait, at times appearing quite unstable and needing the support of another person, a piece of furniture, or the walls to ambulate. At other times, her gait was only mildly unsteady. A psychiatry consultation was requested, but before it occurred, the woman was observed to have a "seizure" during which she showed generalized shaking that seemed to wax and wane. No incontinence was noted. Following the episode, she had a questionable Babinski sign on the left side. Her eyes remained closed, and she was variably responsive to questions. When unresponsive, she showed no spontaneous voluntary movement, but she resisted passive movement, such as when attempts were made to open her eyelids to evaluate her pupils.

Internal medicine consultation resulted in routine laboratory work, lumbar puncture, and magnetic resonance imaging (MRI). The patient was admitted to the medical intensive care unit. No abnormalities were noted in any of the laboratory or imaging procedures.

The next day, the patient was fully responsive, showed no impairment in gait, and had no episodes of "seizures." She had a hazy recollection of the preceding day, but when questioned, she did remember the argument with her husband. She reported unhappiness about her marital difficulties, but she did not report enough symptoms to warrant diagnosis of a depressive episode. She was not particularly interested in exploring psychological issues. She denied prior psychiatric problems or treatment, although relatives reported a similar episode 4 years previously, after a disagreement with a boyfriend. The patient had a normal neurological examination except for a questionable Babinski sign on the left side. It was concluded that her apparent neurological presentation was attributable to a mixture of conversion and dissociative symptoms. The patient and her family were cautioned to be vigilant for any symptoms suggesting neurological dysfunction.

She was transferred to the psychiatry service, from which she was discharged 2 days later with a follow-up plan that included marital counseling.

This case illustrates several typical aspects of the presentation and course of conversion disorder to be discussed later in this section.

Diagnosis

History

Some of the major early contributions to the study of conversion disorder were by neurologists, including Charcot (Torack 1978) and Breuer and Freud (1893–1895/1955) in the late nineteenth century and early twentieth century. As shown in Table 13–2, conversion disorder was called "conversion reaction" in DSM-I and "hysterical neurosis, conversion type" in DSM-II. In both DSM-I and DSM-II, the conversion process was restricted to the production of symptoms affecting the voluntary motor and sensory nervous system. Symptoms considered to generally be related to the autonomic nervous system were subsumed under the psychophysiological disorders.

Other terms such as *acute hysteria* also have been used. Unfortunately, conversion disorder or *conversion hysteria* was used by some clinicians synonymously with *hysteria*, a term replaced by somatization disorder in DSM-III. Generally, hysteria was used to describe a more pervasive, chronic, and polysymptomatic disorder. Although conversion symptoms are perhaps the most dramatic symptoms of somatization disorder, the disorder is characterized by multiple unexplained symptoms in many organ systems. In conversion disorder, a single symptom, traditionally of a pseudoneurological type (i.e., suggesting neurological disease), suffices. Such inconsistency in the use of terms has resulted in a great deal of confusion, both in research and in clinical practice.

Adding to this confusion was a change introduced in DSM-III and retained in DSM-III-R, wherein the concept of conversion was expanded to include disorders characterized by symptoms involving any "loss of, or alteration in, physical functioning suggesting a physical disorder" (American Psychiatric Association 1987, p. 259) as long as the mechanism of conversion was evident; that is, the symptom was "an expression of a psychological conflict or need" (American Psychiatric Association 1987, p. 257). Thus, symptoms involving the autonomic or endocrine systems, such as vomiting (supposedly representing revulsion and disgust) and pseudocyesis (as a manifestation of unconscious conflict about, or the need for, pregnancy), were included as examples of conversion symptoms.

DSM-IV Criteria

Several questions about modifications of conversion disorder criteria for DSM-IV were carefully considered. These included, in particular, where in the nosological framework conversion disorder should be placed (i.e., should it remain with the somatoform disorders or be grouped with the dissociative disorders?) and what the syndrome boundaries should be (i.e., what types of symptoms are to be included?) (Martin 1992, 1996). Although the symptomatic, epidemiological, and perhaps pathogenetic similarities of conversion and dissociative symptoms were acknowledged, the review argued for the retention of conversion disorder with the somatoform disorders because of the advantages of facilitating the critical differential diagnosis of patients who have physical symptoms that suggest physical disorders. Review of the literature supported the utility of again restricting conversion disorder to symptoms affecting voluntary motor and sensory functions.

As defined in DSM-IV-TR, nonintentional "symptoms or deficits affecting voluntary motor or sensory function" (American Psychiatric Association 2000, p. 498) are central to conversion disorder (see Table 13–8). The majority of such symptoms will suggest a neurological condition (i.e., are pseudoneurological), but other general medical conditions may be suggested as well. Pseudoneurological symptoms remain the classic symptomatology. By definition, symptoms limited to pain or disturbance in sexual functioning are not included.

In conversion disorder, as in the other somatoform disorders, the symptom cannot be fully explained by a

TABLE 13–8. DSM-IV-TR diagnostic criteria for conversion disorder

A. One or more symptoms or deficits affecting voluntary motor or sensory function that suggest a neurological or other general medical condition.
B. Psychological factors are judged to be associated with the symptom or deficit because the initiation or exacerbation of the symptom or deficit is preceded by conflicts or other stressors.
C. The symptom or deficit is not intentionally produced or feigned (as in factitious disorder or malingering).
D. The symptom or deficit cannot, after appropriate investigation, be fully explained by a general medical condition, or by the direct effects of a substance, or as a culturally sanctioned behavior or experience.
E. The symptom or deficit causes clinically significant distress or impairment in social, occupational, or other important areas of functioning or warrants medical evaluation.
F. The symptom or deficit is not limited to pain or sexual dysfunction, does not occur exclusively during the course of somatization disorder, and is not better accounted for by another mental disorder.

Specify type of symptom or deficit:
With Motor Symptom or Deficit
With Sensory Symptom or Deficit
With Seizures or Convulsions
With Mixed Presentation

known physical disorder. This criterion is perhaps the most imperative diagnostic consideration. In addition, the symptom is defined as not fully explained by a culturally sanctioned behavior or experience. Symptoms such as seizurelike episodes occurring in conjunction with certain religious ceremonies and culturally expected responses, in times past, such as women swooning in response to excitement would qualify as examples.

DSM-IV-TR specifies that the symptoms in conversion disorder are not intentionally produced, thus distinguishing conversion symptoms from those of a factitious disorder or malingering. Although this judgment is difficult to make, it is an important one because the recommended management and expected outcome of factitious disorder and malingering are markedly different.

Clinical judgment also is required in determining whether psychological factors are etiologically related to the symptom. Inclusion of this criterion is perhaps a holdover from the initial conceptualization of conversion symptoms as representing the conversion of unconscious psychic conflict into a physical symptom. As reviewed by Cloninger (1987), such determination is virtually impossible except in cases in which there is a temporal relationship between a psychosocial stressor and the symptom or

in cases in which similar situations led to conversion symptoms in the past.

Differential Diagnosis

Conversion symptoms suggest physical illness, and nonpsychiatrists are generally seen initially. Neurologists are frequently consulted by primary care physicians for such symptoms because most suggest neurological disease. It has been estimated that 1% of the patients admitted to the hospital for neurological problems have conversion symptoms (Marsden 1986).

One major problem with conversion symptoms is that they suggest neurological or general medical conditions, and conversion (mis)diagnosis may be applied when the true illness is present. Some older studies found that significant proportions of patients initially diagnosed with conversion symptoms had neurological illnesses on follow-up. Slater and Glithero (1965) found a misdiagnosis rate of 50% during a 7- to 11-year follow-up; Gatfield and Guze (1962) reported 21%; but more recently, Mace and Trimble (1996) observed a rate of 15%. The trend toward less misdiagnosis may reflect increasing sophistication in neurological diagnosis. Although Slater and Glithero's study often has been used to challenge the validity of hysteria (now somatization disorder), its importance lies in underscoring the need to remain tentative in making a diagnosis of conversion disorder.

Symptoms of various neurological illnesses may seem to be inconsistent with known neurophysiology or neuropathology and may suggest conversion. Diseases to be considered include multiple sclerosis (consider blindness secondary to optic neuritis with initially normal fundi), myasthenia gravis, periodic paralysis, myoglobinuric myopathy, polymyositis, other acquired myopathies (all of which may include marked weakness in the presence of normal deep tendon reflexes), and Guillain-Barré syndrome, in which early weakness of the arms and legs may be inconsistent (Cloninger 1994). As reviewed by Ford and Folks (1985), more than 13% of actual neurological cases are diagnosed as "functional" before the elucidation of a neurological illness. Initial evidence of some neurological disease is predictive of a subsequent neurological explanation (Mace and Trimble 1996).

Complicating diagnosis is the fact that physical illness and conversion (or other apparent psychiatric overlay) are not mutually exclusive. Patients with incapacitating and frightening physical illnesses may appear to exaggerate their symptoms. Patients with actual neurological illness also may have "pseudosymptoms." For example, patients with actual seizures often have pseudoseizures (Desai et al. 1982).

Considering these observations, physicians should resist an incautious diagnosis of conversion disorder when faced with difficult-to-interpret symptoms. The occurrence of apparent conversion symptoms mandates a thorough evaluation for possible underlying physical explanation. This evaluation may include physical and psychiatric examination, X rays, and blood and urine tests as the symptoms and signs would indicate.

Longitudinal studies indicate the most reliable predictor that a patient with apparent conversion symptoms will not later be shown to have a physical disorder is a history of conversion or other unexplained symptoms (Cloninger 1994). Patients with somatization disorder will manifest multiple symptoms in multiple organ systems, including the voluntary motor and sensory nervous systems. Thus, apparent conversion symptoms in the context of somatization disorder should indicate that an underlying physical disorder is unlikely. Although conversion symptoms may occur at any age, vulnerability for conversion symptoms is first manifested most often in late adolescence or early adulthood (Cloninger 1994). Conversion symptoms first occurring in middle age or later should increase suspicion of an occult physical illness.

DSM-IV-TR lists hallucinations among the sensory nervous system examples. Reports of hallucinations suggest psychosis, especially schizophrenia, or a mood disorder with psychotic features. In fact, DSM-III and DSM-III-R virtually forced this interpretation in that the only contexts in which hallucinations were mentioned in conjunction with a nonpsychotic disorder were with the reexperiencing of the traumatic event in posttraumatic stress disorder and with the hearing, by one personality, the voice(s) of one or more of the other personalities in multiple personality disorder (dissociative identity disorder in DSM-IV). Hallucinations as conversion symptoms have long been reported (Andrade and Srinath 1986; Fitzgerald and Wells 1977; Goodwin et al. 1971; Modai and Cygielman 1986). In the DSM-IV's somatization disorder field trial, one-third of a large sample of nonpsychotic women with evidence of unexplained somatic complaints reported a history of hallucinations. Among the 40% who met criteria for somatization disorder, more than one-half reported hallucinations (R.L. Martin, unpublished observations, 1998). Women with other conversion symptoms were more likely to report hallucinations than were those women with no other conversion symptoms, giving further support for including hallucinations as conversion symptoms.

Generally, conversion disorder hallucinations differ in several ways from hallucinations in psychotic conditions and are referred to by some as *pseudohallucinations*. Conversion disorder hallucinations typically occur in the absence of other psychotic symptoms. Insight that the hallucinations are not "real" is generally retained. Conversion hallucinations often involve more than one modality, whereas hallucinations in psychoses generally involve a single sensory modality (especially auditory; secondarily, tactile). They may have a naive, fantastic, or childish content, as in a fairy tale, and are described eagerly as an interesting story (e.g., "A big green frog came in, sat down next to me, and began talking to me"). Conversion hallucinations are often psychologically meaningful (e.g., "I heard my ex-boyfriend's voice telling me that he had made a big mistake"). Because hallucinations as part of psychoses also may share some of these features, vigilance must be maintained for the emergence of other signs of psychosis. A diagnosis of conversion disorder should not be made if the hallucinations are better accounted for by posttraumatic stress disorder or dissociative identity disorder (multiple personality disorder).

An association between conversion symptoms affecting voluntary motor and sensory functioning and dissociative symptoms affecting memory and identity should be noted. Traditionally, such symptoms have been attributed to similar psychological mechanisms. The two types of symptoms often occur in the same individual, sometimes during the same episode of illness (consider the example of the patient with conversion disorder discussed at the beginning of this section). Thus, patients with conversion disorder should be screened for dissociative symptoms, and patients with dissociative disorder should be evaluated for conversion symptoms.

Natural History

Onset is generally from late childhood to early adulthood. Conversion disorder is rare before age 10 years (Maloney 1980) and seldom first presents after age 35 years, but it has been reported to begin as late as the ninth decade (Weddington 1979). When onset is in middle or late age, the possibility of a neurological or other medical condition is increased.

Onset of conversion disorder is generally acute, but it may be characterized by gradually increasing symptomatology. The typical course of individual conversion symptoms is generally short; half (Folks et al. 1984) to nearly all (Carter 1949) patients show a disappearance of symptoms by the time of hospital discharge. However, 20%–25% will relapse within 1 year. Factors traditionally associated with good prognosis include acute onset, presence of clearly identifiable stress at the time of onset, short interval between onset and institution of treatment, and good intelligence (Toone 1990). One recent study noted a better outcome for patients with affective illnesses and a poor prognosis for those with personality disorders (Mace and Trimble 1996). The study also reported that a diagnosis of somatization disorder at follow-up was especially associated with chronicity. Symptoms of blindness, aphonia, and paralysis have been noted to have a relatively good prognosis, whereas seizures and tremor were identified to be more persistent (Toone 1990). However, these findings were not supported in the Mace and Trimble study. When followed up longitudinally, some patients initially diagnosed only with conversion disorder will subsequently meet the criteria for somatization disorder (Kent et al. 1995; Mace and Trimble 1996).

Generally, individual conversion symptoms are self-limited and do not lead to physical changes or disabilities. Occasionally, physical sequelae such as atrophy may occur, but this is rare. Morbidity in terms of marital and occupational impairment appears to be less than that in somatization disorder (Kent et al. 1995; Tomasson et al. 1991). In a long-term follow-up study (up to 44 years) of a small number ($N = 28$) of individuals with conversion disorder, excess mortality by unnatural causes was observed (Coryell and House 1984). None of the deaths in this study was by suicide.

Epidemiology

Conclusions regarding the epidemiology of conversion disorder are compromised by methodological differences in diagnostic boundaries as well as by ascertainment procedures from study to study. Vastly different estimates have been reported. Lifetime prevalence rates of treated conversion symptoms in general populations have ranged from 11/100,000 to 500/100,000 (Ford and Folks 1985; Toone 1990). A marked excess of women compared with men develop conversion symptoms. More than 25% of healthy postpartum and medically ill women report having had conversion symptoms sometime during their lives (Cloninger 1994).

Approximately 5%–24% of psychiatric outpatients, 5%–14% of general hospital patients, and 1%–3% of outpatient psychiatric referrals have a history of conversion symptoms (Cloninger 1994; Ford 1983; Toone 1990). Conversion is associated with lower socioeconomic status, lower education, lack of psychological sophistication, and rural setting (Folks et al. 1984; Guze and Perley 1963; Lazare 1981; Stefansson et al. 1976; Weinstein et al. 1969). Consistent with this finding, much higher rates (nearly 10%) of outpatient psychiatric referrals in developing countries are for conversion symptoms. As countries develop, there may be a declining incidence over time, which may relate to increasing levels of education and sophistication (Stefanis et al. 1976).

Conversion disorder appears to be diagnosed more often in women than in men, with ratios varying from 2:1 (Ljundberg 1957; Stefansson et al. 1976) to 10:1 (Raskin et al. 1966). In part, this variance may relate to referral patterns, but it also appears that indeed a predominance of women compared with men develop conversion symptoms.

Etiology

An etiological hypothesis is implicit in the term *conversion*. The term conversion, in fact, is derived from the hypothesized conversion of psychological conflict into a somatic symptom. Several psychological factors have been implicated in the pathogenesis, or at least pathophysiology, of conversion disorder. However, as the following discussion will show, such etiological relationships are difficult to establish.

In *primary gain*, anxiety is theoretically reduced by keeping an internal conflict or need out of awareness by symbolic expression of an unconscious wish as a conversion symptom. However, individuals with active conversion symptoms often continue to show marked anxiety, especially on psychological tests (Lader and Sartorious 1968; Meares and Horvath 1972). Symbolism is infrequently evident, and its evaluation involves highly inferential and unreliable judgments (Raskin et al. 1966). Interpretation of symbolism in persons with occult medical disorder has been noted to contribute to misdiagnosis. *Secondary gain*, whereby conversion symptoms allow avoidance of noxious activities or the obtaining of otherwise unavailable support, also may occur in persons who have medical conditions, who often take advantage of such benefits (Raskin et al. 1966; Watson and Buranen 1979).

Individuals with conversion disorder may show a lack of concern, in keeping with the nature or implications of the symptom (the so-called *la belle indifférence*). However, such indifference to symptoms is not invariably present in conversion disorder (Lewis and Berman 1965; Sharma and Chaturvedi 1995), and it also can be seen in individuals with general medical conditions (Raskin et al. 1966), sometimes as denial or stoicism (Pincus 1982). Conversion symptoms may be revealed in a dramatic or histrionic fashion. A minority of individuals with conversion disorder fulfill criteria for histrionic personality disorder. A dramatic presentation of conversion disorder can be seen in distressed individuals with medical conditions. Even symptoms based on underlying medical conditions often respond to suggestion, at least temporarily (Gatfield and Guze 1962). Patients with conversion disorder may have a history of disturbed sexuality (Lewis 1974), with many (one-third) reporting a history of sexual abuse, especially incestuous. (Thus, two-thirds do *not* report such a history.) Individuals with conversion disorder are often reported to be the youngest, or else the youngest of a sex, in sibling order, but these are not consistent findings (Stephens and Kamp 1962; Ziegler et al. 1960).

Limited data suggest that conversion symptoms are more frequent in relatives of individuals with conversion disorder (Toone 1990). Rates that were 10 times greater than similarly derived general population estimates in female relatives and approximately 5 times the corresponding rate in male relatives were reported in a nonblind study (Ljundberg 1957). Accumulated data from available twin studies show 9 concordant and 33 discordant monozygotic pairs and 0 concordant and 43 discordant dizygotic pairs (Inouye 1972). Nongenetic familial factors, particularly incestuous childhood sexual abuse, also may be frequent. Nearly one-third of the individuals with medically unexplained seizures reported childhood sexual abuse, as compared with fewer than 10% of those with complex partial epilepsy (Alper et al. 1993). High rates also have been noted in overlapping dissociative conditions. Rates of reported childhood sexual abuse as high as 83% have been noted in individuals with dissociative identity disorder. Women with somatization disorder (many of whom will have conversion or dissociative symptoms) have rates of reported abuse as high as 50% (Martin 1996).

If not directly etiological, many factors have been suggested as predisposing individuals to conversion disorder. In many instances, preexisting personality disorders are diagnosable and may predispose some individuals to conversion disorder. Several psychosocial factors in addition to a history of abuse may be involved. Individuals from rural backgrounds and those who are psychologically and medically unsophisticated appear to be predisposed to conversion disorder, as are those with existing neurological disorders. In the last case, a tendency to conversion symptoms has been attributed to "modeling"; that is, patients with neurological disorders are likely to observe in others, as well as in themselves, various neurological symptoms that they at other times simulate as conversion symptoms.

Treatment

Generally, the initial aim in treating conversion disorder is the removal of the symptom. The pressure behind accomplishing this goal depends on the distress and disability associated with the symptom (Merskey 1989). If the patient is not in particular discomfort and the need to regain function is not great, direct attention may not be necessary. In any situation, direct confrontation is not recommended. Such a communication may cause a patient to feel even more isolated. A conservative approach of reassurance and relaxation is effective. Reassurance need not come from a psychiatrist but can be performed effectively by the primary physician. Once physical illness is excluded, prognosis for conversion symptoms is good. Folks et al. (1984), for example, found that half of 50 general hospital patients with conversion symptoms showed complete remission by the time of discharge.

If symptoms do not resolve with a conservative approach and there is an immediate need for symptom resolution, several techniques, including narcoanalysis (e.g., amobarbital interview), hypnosis, and behavior therapy, may be tried (Merskey 1989). It does appear that prompt resolution of conversion symptoms is important in that the duration of conversion symptoms is associated with greater risk of recurrence and chronic disability (Cloninger 1994).

In narcoanalysis, amobarbital or another sedative-hypnotic medication such as lorazepam is given to the patient intravenously to the point of drowsiness. Sometimes this is followed by administration of a stimulant medication such as methamphetamine. The patient is then encouraged to discuss stressors and conflicts. This technique may be effective in the short term, leading to at least temporary symptom relief and expansion of the information known about the patient. This technique has not been shown to be especially effective with more chronic conversion symptoms. In hypnotic therapy, symptoms may be removed during a hypnotic state, with the suggestion that the symptoms will gradually improve posthypnotically. Information about stressors and conflicts may be explored as well. Behavior therapy, including relaxation training and even aversion therapy, has been proposed and reported by some investigators to be effective.

It is evident that it may not be the particular technique that is associated with symptom relief but the influence of suggestion. Various rituals such as exorcism and other religious ceremonies undoubtedly have led to immediate "cures." Suggestion seems to play a big part in cases of mass hysteria, in which individuals exposed to a "toxin" develop similar symptoms that do not appear to have any organic basis. Often, the epidemic can be contained if affected individuals are segregated. Simple announcements that no toxin was present and that reported "symptomatology" is linked to mass hysteria have been effective.

Anecdotal reports exist of positive response to somatic treatments such as phenothiazines, lithium, and even electroconvulsive therapy (ECT). Of course, in some cases, such a response again may be attributable to suggestion. In others, it may be that symptom removal occurred because of resolution of another psychiatric disorder, especially a mood disorder.

Thus far, the discussion on treatment of conversion disorder has centered on acute treatment primarily for symptom removal. Longer-term approaches would include strategies that were previously discussed for somatization disorder. These involve a pragmatic, conservative approach that entails support for and exploration of various areas of conflict, particularly interpersonal relationships. Ford (1995) suggested a treatment strategy based on "three Ps," whereby predisposing factors, precipitating stressors, and perpetuating factors are identified and addressed. A certain degree of insight may be attained, at least in terms of appreciating relationships between various conflicts and stressors and the development of symptoms. More ambitious goals have been adopted by some in terms of long-term, intensive insight-oriented psychotherapy, especially of a psychodynamic nature. Reports of such approaches date from Freud's work with Anna O. Three studies involving a series of patients treated with psychoanalytic psychotherapy have reported success (Merskey 1989).

Hypochondriasis

Definition and Clinical Description

The essential feature in hypochondriasis is preoccupation not with symptoms themselves but rather with the fear or idea of having a serious disease, based on the misinterpretation of bodily signs and sensations (Table 13–1). The preoccupation persists despite evidence to the contrary and reassurance from physicians. Some degree of preoccupation with disease is apparently quite common. As reviewed by Kellner (1987), 10%–20% of "normal" and 45% of "neurotic" persons have intermittent, unfounded worries about illness, with 9% of patients doubting reassurances given by physicians. In another review, Kellner (1985) estimated that 50% of all patients attending physicians' offices "suffer either from primary hypochondriacal syndromes or have 'minor somatic disorders with hypochondriacal overlay'" (p. 822). How these estimates relate to hypochondriasis as a disorder is difficult to assess because they do not appear to distinguish between preoccupation with symptoms (as is present in somatization disorder) and preoccupation with the implications of the symptoms (as is the case in hypochondriasis).

Diagnosis

History

Clinical descriptions of a syndrome designated *hypochondriasis* and characterized by preoccupation with bodily function can be found in the writings of the Hippocratic era (Stoudemire 1988). The Greeks attributed the syndrome to disturbances of viscera below the xiphoid cartilage, hence the term *hypochondria*. Even into the nineteenth century, the term *hypochondriasis*, unlike the topographically nonspecific concept of more recent usage, was used specifically for somatic complaints below the diaphragm (Cloninger et al. 1984). As reviewed by M. R. Murphy (1990), Gillespie, in 1928, encapsulated a concept of hypochondriasis that is essentially identical to modern concepts, emphasizing preoccupation with a disease conviction "far in excess of what is justified," implying "an indifference to the opinion of the environment, including irresponsiveness to persuasion" (p. 28). Gillespie considered hypochondriasis a discrete disease entity. DSM-I did not include hypochondriasis as a separate illness, only mentioning "hypochondriacal preoccupation" as one of the malignant symptoms observed in psychotic but not reactive depression. As shown in Table 13–2, the syndrome was included in DSM-II as hypochondriacal neurosis and in ICD-9, DSM-III, DSM-III-R, and ICD-10 as hypochondriasis.

Throughout the modern period, there has been controversy over whether hypochondriasis represents an independent, discrete disease entity, as proposed by Gillespie. Kenyon (1976), in an often quoted but perhaps methodologically flawed study (see M. R. Murphy 1990), concluded that hypochondriasis was virtually always secondary to another psychiatric disorder, usually depression. Barsky and various colleagues (Barsky and Klerman 1983; Barsky et al. 1986, 1993) extensively studied patients with hypochondriacal complaints using a set of operational criteria derived from DSM-III. These authors concluded that of the many patients with such complaints, few will meet criteria for the full diagnosis. However, they noted no bimodality, suggesting that hypochondriasis represents a continuum rather than a discrete entity.

DSM-IV Criteria

Specific criteria for the diagnosis of hypochondriasis are included in Table 13–9. As mentioned previously, in hypochondriasis, emphasis is on the patient's preoccupation with the implication that a serious illness is present based on the misinterpretation of bodily symptoms. There was some debate in the development of DSM-IV

TABLE 13–9. DSM-IV-TR diagnostic criteria for hypochondriasis

A. Preoccupation with fears of having, or the idea that one has, a serious disease based on the person's misinterpretation of bodily symptoms.

B. The preoccupation persists despite appropriate medical evaluation and reassurance.

C. The belief in Criterion A is not of delusional intensity (as in delusional disorder, somatic type) and is not restricted to a circumscribed concern about appearance (as in body dysmorphic disorder).

D. The preoccupation causes clinically significant distress or impairment in social, occupational, or other important areas of functioning.

E. The duration of the disturbance is at least 6 months.

F. The preoccupation is not better accounted for by generalized anxiety disorder, obsessive-compulsive disorder, panic disorder, a major depressive episode, separation anxiety, or another somatoform disorder.

Specify if:

With Poor Insight: if, for most of the time during the current episode, the person does not recognize that the concern about having a serious illness is excessive or unreasonable

---

that it was not necessary that a symptom be present. However, on the basis of empirical data, it was determined that this symptom requirement was a valid one and helped to distinguish the "disease conviction" of hypochondriasis from "disease fear" as in a phobic disorder (Cote et al. 1996). "Bodily symptoms" may be interpreted broadly to include misinterpretation of normal bodily functions. The requirement that the preoccupation persist despite medical evaluation and reassurance was included to emphasize the disease conviction aspect of the syndrome. The exclusionary criterion of delusion was debated. Although this criterion was maintained for the purpose of discriminating hypochondriasis from delusional disorders, somatic type, the specifier "with poor insight" was added. To distinguish hypochondriasis from clinically insignificant states, the requirement for distress or impairment is as in the other somatoform disorders. A requirement of 6 months' duration was maintained to distinguish hypochondriasis from transient syndromes that have been shown to have a more variable longitudinal course, suggesting heterogeneity (Barsky et al. 1993).

As is explained in the following discussion, hypochondriasis is not diagnosed if symptoms occur exclusively during the course of generalized anxiety disorder, anxiety disorder, obsessive-compulsive disorder, panic disorder, a major depressive episode, separation anxiety, or another somatoform disorder.

Differential Diagnosis

The first step in evaluating patients with hypochondriasis is to assess the possibility of physical disease. The list of serious diseases associated with the type of complaints seen in hypochondriacal patients is extensive, yet certain general categories emerge (Kellner 1985, 1987). These include neurological diseases, such as myasthenia gravis and multiple sclerosis; endocrine diseases; systemic diseases, such as SLE, that affect several organ systems; and occult malignancies.

If after appropriate assessment the probability of physical illness appears low, the condition should be considered relative to other psychiatric disorders (i.e., whether the hypochondriacal symptoms represent a primary disorder or are secondary to another psychiatric illness). As previously mentioned, one useful criterion is whether the belief is of delusional proportions. Patients with hypochondriasis as a primary disorder, although extremely preoccupied, are generally able to acknowledge the possibility that their concerns are unfounded. Delusional patients, on the other hand, are not. Hypochondriasis, with poor insight, would lie somewhere in between, with the patient not recognizing that the concern is unwarranted for most of the episode. Somatic delusions of serious illness are seen in some cases of major depressive disorder and in schizophrenia. A useful discriminator is the presence of other psychiatric symptoms. A patient with hypochondriacal concerns secondary to depression should show other symptoms of depression such as sleep and appetite disturbance, feelings of worthlessness, and self-reproach, although elderly patients particularly may deny sadness or other expressions of depressed mood. Generally, schizophrenic patients will have bizarre delusions of illness (e.g., "I have congenital Hodgkin's caused by a snail hormone imbalance") and will show other signs of schizophrenia such as looseness of associations, peculiarities of thought and behavior, hallucinations, and other delusions. A confounding feature is the fact that hypochondriacal patients often will develop anxiety or depression in association with their hypochondriacal concerns. In general, characterizing the chronology of the episode will separate such patients from those with hypochondriasis.

Treatment trials also may have diagnostic significance. Depressed patients who are hypochondriacal may respond to antidepressant medication or ECT (often necessary in reversing a depressive state of sufficient severity to lead to such profound symptoms), with resolution of the hypochondriacal as well as the depressive symptoms. In schizophrenic patients, a disease-related delusion may show improvement with neuroleptic treatment.

Although, if questioned carefully, the patient still may report a somatic delusion, preoccupation with the delusion will have diminished.

Natural History

Traditionally, limited data suggested that approximately one-fourth of the patients with a diagnosis of hypochondriasis do poorly, two-thirds show a chronic but fluctuating course, and one-tenth recover. However, such predictions may not reflect advances in psychopharmacology. It also must be remembered that such findings pertain to the full syndrome. A much more variable course is seen in patients with some hypochondriacal concerns.

Epidemiology

Estimates of the frequency of hypochondriacal symptoms warranting a diagnosis are somewhat compromised in that DSM-III-R did not provide threshold criteria, other than requiring a duration of more than 6 months. The ECA study (L. N. Robins et al. 1984) did not assess for hypochondriasis. One study reported prevalence figures ranging from 3% to 13% in different cultures (Kenyon 1965), but it is not clear whether this range represented the full syndrome or just hypochondriacal symptoms. As previously mentioned, many patients have such symptoms as part of other psychiatric disorders, particularly depressive and anxiety disorders, whereas others develop transient hypochondriacal symptoms in response to stress, particularly serious physical illness.

Etiology

In considering hypochondriasis as an aspect of depression or anxiety disorders, it has been posited that these conditions create a state of hypervigilance to insult, including overperception of physical problems (Barsky and Klerman 1983). Hypochondriasis has been discussed extensively in the psychoanalytic literature. Freud hypothesized that it represented "the return of object libido onto the ego with cathexis to the body" (Viederman 1985, p. 10). This theory has formed the basis for a number of psychoanalytic interpretations, including disturbed object relations, repressed hostility displaced to the body so that anger can be communicated indirectly to others, and dynamics involving masochism, guilt, conflicted dependency needs, and a need to suffer and be loved at the same time (Stoudemire 1988). Such "narcissistic" mechanisms have been thought to make patients unanalyzable. Other psychological theories involve defenses against feelings of low self-esteem, inadequacy, percep-

tual and cognitive abnormalities, and reinforcement for assuming the sick role.

More recently, hypochondriasis has been included by some in a posited "obsessive-compulsive spectrum disorder," which includes, in addition to obsessive-compulsive disorder, body dysmorphic disorder, anorexia nervosa, Tourette's disorder, and certain impulsive disorders (e.g., trichotillomania and pathological gambling; Hollander et al. 1992). This clustering is based, in part, on the phenomenological similarity of repetitive thoughts and behaviors that are difficult or impossible to delay or inhibit (Martin and Yutzy 1997).

Treatment

Patients referred early for psychiatric evaluation and treatment of hypochondriasis appear to have a better prognosis than those continuing with only medical evaluations and treatments (Kellner 1983). Psychiatric referral should be performed with sensitivity. Perhaps the best guideline to follow is for the referring physician to stress that the patient's distress is serious and that psychiatric evaluation will be a supplement to, not a replacement for, continued medical care.

Hypochondriacal symptoms secondary to depressive and anxiety disorders may improve with successful treatment of the primary disorder. However, until recently, hypochondriasis as a primary condition was not considered to be responsive to known psychopharmacological medications. Early results of placebo-controlled, double-blind studies are pending, but anecdotal case reports, open-label trials, and review of preliminary data show some promise for the selective serotonin reuptake inhibitors (SSRIs; Fallon et al. 1996). Interestingly, these medications have been shown to be effective in obsessive-compulsive disorder, and preliminary data are promising for their use in other obsessive-compulsive spectrum disorders, including body dysmorphic disorder and anorexia nervosa.

Investigators have tried many psychotherapeutic approaches in treating hyphochondriasis. These may be summarized as supportive, rational, ventilative, and educative (Kellner 1987). However, no evidence shows the superiority of any one of these methods over the others. An approach suggested by Stoudemire (1988)—one that includes consistent treatment, generally by the same primary physician, with supportive, regularly scheduled office visits not based on the evaluation of symptoms—should be considered. Hospitalization, medical tests, and medications with addictive potential are to be avoided if possible. Focus during the office visits gradually should be shifted from symptoms to social or interpersonal problems. Psychotherapeutic approaches may be enhanced greatly by the promising potential of effective pharmacotherapy. Thus, there is increasing hope for attaining the overriding goal in treating hypochondriacal patients: preventing adoption of the sick role and chronic invalidism (Kellner 1987).

Body Dysmorphic Disorder

Definition and Clinical Description

The essential feature of body dysmorphic disorder is a preoccupation with some imagined defect in appearance or markedly excessive concern with a minor physical anomaly (Table 13–10). Such preoccupation persists even after reassurance. Common complaints include a diversity of imagined flaws of the face or head, such as various defects in the hair (too much or too little), skin, shape of the face, or facial features. However, any body part may be the focus, including genitals, breasts, buttocks, extremities, shoulders, and even overall body size. De Leon et al. (1989) stated that the nose, ears, face, and sexual organs are most often involved. It is not surprising, then, that patients with body dysmorphic disorder are found most commonly among persons seeking cosmetic surgery.

The following case example illustrates some of the diagnostic and therapeutic uncertainties involving body dysmorphic disorder, especially regarding overlap with depressive and obsessive-compulsive disorders.

> The patient, a male in his mid-20s, received outpatient psychiatric care after 4 years of preoccupation with facial asymmetry and a blemish, defects not evident to others. He had been treated previously with unsuccessful trials of imipramine, phenelzine, perphenazine, and haloperidol. Seeing his reflection in a mirror or shiny surface resulted in a compulsion (accompanied by "a sick, anxious feeling") to inspect the blemish; thus, the patient avoided viewing all such surfaces. He also experienced what he described as a "sinking feeling" in his chest if he touched his face, particularly in the area of the blemish. He grew a beard so that he would not have to shave himself and then went to a barber weekly for a shave. He retained insight that there was no actual defect but had once made an appointment with a plastic surgeon. He was embarrassed about his preoccupation and concealed it from others. Although diligent in his work and studies and somewhat perfectionistic in general, he had no other evident obsessions or compulsions.
>
> From the start of his current treatment, an educative approach was taken. He did extensive reading on body dysmorphic and obsessive-compulsive disorders and their therapies.

TABLE 13–10. DSM-IV-TR diagnostic criteria for body dysmorphic disorder

A. Preoccupation with an imagined defect in appearance. If a slight physical anomaly is present, the person's concern is markedly excessive.

B. The preoccupation causes clinically significant distress or impairment in social, occupational, or other important areas of functioning.

C. The preoccupation is not better accounted for by another mental disorder (e.g., dissatisfaction with body shape and size in anorexia nervosa).

> The SSRIs fluoxetine, sertraline, paroxetine, and fluvoxamine were not available at the time the patient was treated. While taking clomipramine (100 mg/day—he was not able to tolerate larger doses because of extreme dry mouth), he showed some improvement because he was less dysphoric when ruminating about the blemish, but the preoccupation remained. Similarly, alprazolam "only took the edge off."
>
> The patient became markedly dysphoric and developed suicidal ideation after a breakup with a girlfriend. He received six ECT treatments, and his depressive and body dysmorphic symptoms improved dramatically. Although the "idea" of the blemish remained, it no longer preoccupied him. For the first time in several years, he could actually look at himself in the mirror and touch his face without discomfort. Although the benefit from ECT was transient, it gave him hope that he could be free of his preoccupation. He continued taking clomipramine.
>
> On his own initiative, he obtained bromazepam, a benzodiazepine available in Europe but not the United States. He reported that with this drug, his preoccupation was "more under control." This drug has been found in some, but not all, studies to be effective in treating obsessive-compulsive disorder (Hewlett 1993). After fluvoxamine was introduced, he began taking this drug. He tolerated it much better than clomipramine, and the dose was increased to 300 mg/day. Buspirone was added, and the bromazepam was discontinued. On this regimen, he still has concerns about his face, but "it doesn't rule me the way it used to." He maintains a successful professional practice. He has never married but has had a succession of girlfriends.

Diagnosis

History

As is evident in Table 13–2, body dysmorphic disorder was not even mentioned in the official nomenclatures until DSM-III and then only parenthetically as *dysmorphophobia*. The syndrome, generally under the rubric of dysmorphophobia, has a long history in the European and Japanese literature, with much less attention in the United States literature (Phillips and Hollander 1996).

Because the symptoms are not really of a typical phobic nature with avoidance behavior, the condition was renamed *body dysmorphic disorder* in DSM-III-R. Debate continues as to whether body dysmorphic disorder is a discrete disorder. It is variously argued that it represents a variant of one of the major disorders, including social phobia, mood disorder, obsessive-compulsive disorder, hypochondriasis, and psychosis (particularly delusional disorder), or just the extreme of the continuum of normal concern with appearance. ICD-9 did not include the disorder. ICD-10 lists it as a type of hypochondriacal disorder. Since inclusion of body dysmorphic disorder in DSM-III-R, increased study has occurred so that the disorder is now more clearly characterized.

DSM-IV-TR Criteria

In DSM-IV-TR, the essential feature of body dysmorphic disorder is preoccupation with an imagined defect in appearance or markedly excessive concern for a slight anomaly (Table 13–10). This criterion represents a slight change from that in DSM-III-R, in which the phrase "in a normal-appearing person" was included. Because a person with some defect may have a preoccupation with a different imagined or exaggerated defect, this phrase was dropped.

As in other somatoform disorders, diagnosis requires that the preoccupation causes clinically significant distress or impairment to exclude those individuals with trivial symptoms. As is explained in the following discussion, body dysmorphic disorder is not diagnosed if the preoccupation is better accounted for by another mental disorder. On the other hand, DSM-IV-TR dropped exclusion on the basis of the preoccupation being delusional, which was included in DSM-III-R and in ICD-10.

Differential Diagnosis

By definition, body dysmorphic disorder is not diagnosed when the body preoccupation is better accounted for by another mental disorder. Anorexia nervosa, in which there is dissatisfaction with body shape and size, is specifically mentioned in the criteria as an example of such an exclusion. In DSM-III-R, transsexualism (gender identity disorder in DSM-IV-TR) also was mentioned as such a disorder. Although not specifically mentioned in DSM-IV, if a preoccupation is limited to discomfort or a sense of inappropriateness of one's primary and secondary sex characteristics, coupled with a strong and persistent cross-gender identification, body dysmorphic disorder would not be diagnosed. Diagnostic problems may develop when a patient has the mood-congruent ruminations of major depression (e.g., preoccupation with a per-

ceived unattractive appearance in association with poor self-esteem). However, such concerns generally lack the focus on a particular body part that is seen in body dysmorphic disorder. Somatic obsessions and even grooming or cleaning rituals in obsessive-compulsive disorder may suggest body dysmorphic disorder; however, in such cases, other obsessions and compulsions are seen as well. In body dysmorphic disorder, the preoccupations are limited to concerns with appearance. Preoccupations in body dysmorphic disorder may reach delusional proportions, and patients with this disorder may show ideas of reference regarding defects in their appearance, which may lead to consideration of the diagnosis of schizophrenia. However, bizarre delusions and hallucinations are not seen in patients with body dysmorphic disorder. From the other perspective, schizophrenic patients with somatic delusions generally do not focus on a specific defect in appearance.

Unlike the diagnostic guideline for hypochondriasis, if the preoccupation is of psychotic proportions, a diagnosis of body dysmorphic disorder still can be made. De Leon et al. (1989) point out the difficulties in determining whether a dysmorphophobic concern is delusional or not. They suggest that cases be classified as "primary dysmorphophobia" without attempting to distinguish between delusional and nondelusional concerns, as long as schizophrenia, major depression, and organic mental disorders are excluded. This point of view was adopted in DSM-IV (Phillips and Hollander 1996). In body dysmorphic disorder, it appears that a continuum exists between preoccupations and delusions, and thus it is difficult, if not impossible, to draw a discrete boundary between body dysmorphic disorder and delusional disorder, somatic type. Furthermore, individual patients seem to move along this continuum. Thus, it was decided to allow both diagnoses if a dysmorphic preoccupation was delusional.

Patients with body dysmorphic disorder often isolate themselves, and social phobia may be suspected. However, in social phobia alone the person may feel self-conscious but will not focus on a specific imagined defect. Persons with histrionic personality disorder may be vain and excessively concerned with appearance. However, in this disorder, the focus is on maintaining a good or even an exceptional appearance rather than preoccupation with a defect.

Natural History

Onset of body dysmorphic disorder peaks in adolescence or early adulthood (Phillips 1991). The disorder is generally a chronic condition, with a waxing and waning of intensity but rarely full remission (Phillips et al. 1993). Over a lifetime, multiple preoccupations are typical. (In their study, Phillips et al. 1993 found an average of four.) In some people, the same preoccupation remains unchanged; in others, preoccupations with newly perceived defects are added to the original ones. In some individuals, symptoms remit only to be replaced by others.

Body dysmorphic disorder is highly incapacitating. Almost all persons with this disorder show marked impairment in social and occupational activities. About 75% will never marry, and among those who do, most will divorce (Phillips 1995). Perhaps a third become housebound. Most attribute their limitations to embarrassment concerning their "defect." The extent to which patients with body dysmorphic disorder receive surgery or medical treatments is unknown. Superimposed depressive episodes are common, as are suicidal ideation and suicide attempts. The actual suicide risk is unknown.

Epidemiology

The lifetime risk of body dysmorphic disorder in the general population is unknown. Although body dysmorphic disorder is seldom seen in psychiatric settings, Andreasen and Bardach (1977) estimated that 2% of the patients seeking corrective cosmetic surgery have this disorder. Generally, patients with body dysmorphic disorder are seen psychiatrically only after referral from plastic surgery, dermatology, and otorhinolaryngology clinics (De Leon et al. 1989). The male-to-female ratio is about 1:1 (Phillips 1995).

Etiology

Traditionally, little emphasis was devoted to etiological possibilities other than suggested relationships to underlying mood disorders, schizophrenia, obsessive-compulsive disorder, or social phobia. More recently, body dysmorphic disorder has been included with a posited obsessive-compulsive spectrum disorder and with delusional disorders for which a variety of biological pathologies have been proffered (Phillips et al. 1995). The latter association is reflected in DSM-IV-TR's allowing both disorders to be diagnosed in the same patient for the same symptoms.

Treatment

Simply recognizing that a complaint derives from body dysmorphic disorder may have therapeutic benefit by interrupting an unending procession of repeated evalua-

tions by physicians and eliminating the possibility of needless surgery. Surgery actually has been recommended as a treatment for this disorder, but there is no clear evidence that it is helpful. There is a long history of anecdotal reports suggesting the value of diverse treatments, including behavior therapy, dynamic psychotherapy, and pharmacotherapy. Recommended medications include neuroleptics and antidepressants (De Leon et al. 1989). Response to neuroleptic treatment has been suggested as a diagnostic test to distinguish body dysmorphic disorder from delusional disorder, somatic type (Riding and Munro 1975). Delusional syndromes, in general, may respond to neuroleptics, whereas in body dysmorphic disorder, even when the bodily preoccupations are psychotic, there is less likelihood of success. Pimozide has been singled out as a neuroleptic having specific effectiveness for somatic delusions, but this drug does not appear to be any more effective than other neuroleptics in treating body dysmorphic disorder.

In earlier reports, it was not clear if reported response to antidepressant drugs or ECT was due to amelioration of dysmorphic symptoms per se or to improvement in depressive symptoms. Several studies have suggested that SSRIs, including fluoxetine, fluvoxamine, and clomipramine, have been effective in treating the disorder (Hollander et al. 1993; Phillips et al. 1993). Patients showing a partial response to the SSRI may benefit further from augmentation with buspirone. Improvement with SSRIs seems to be a primary effect in that response was not predicted on the basis of coexisting major depression or obsessive-compulsive disorder. Also of note are observations that patients with somatic delusions may respond to SSRIs.

Somatoform Disorder Not Otherwise Specified

Definition and Clinical Description

Somatoform disorder NOS is the true residual category for the somatoform disorders. By definition, conditions included under this category are characterized by somatoform symptoms that do not meet the criteria for any of the specified somatoform disorders. DSM-IV-TR gives several examples, but syndromes potentially included under this category are not limited to those examples. Unlike undifferentiated somatoform disorder, no minimum duration is required. In fact, some disorders may be relegated to NOS because they do not meet the time requirements for a specified somatoform disorder.

Diagnosis

History

DSM-III included *atypical somatoform disorder*, a minimally defined residual category requiring only that the predominant disturbance of a disorder be characterized by organically or pathophysiologically unexplained physical symptoms or complaints that are apparently linked to psychological factors. The only example given was dysmorphophobia. In DSM-III-R, the atypical category was renamed and redefined, requiring only the presence of "somatoform symptoms" (implying that no organic or pathophysiological mechanism was present) and that criteria for any specific somatoform or other psychiatric disorder with physical symptoms were not present. Examples given included nonpsychotic hypochondriacal symptoms and physical complaints of less than 6 months' duration that are not related to stress.

DSM-IV-TR Criteria

The basic DSM-IV-TR requirement for a diagnosis of somatoform disorder NOS is that a disorder with somatoform symptoms does not meet criteria for a specified somatoform disorder. The first example listed in DSM-IV-TR is pseudocyesis. In DSM-III and DSM-III-R, pseudocyesis was included as a conversion disorder under criteria broadened to include any alteration or loss of physical functioning, suggesting a physical disorder that was an expression of psychological conflict or need. After contraction of conversion disorder to voluntary motor and sensory dysfunction in DSM-IV, pseudocyesis was excluded and relegated to the NOS category. Oddly enough, pseudocyesis lends itself to a quite specific definition (see Table 13–11). The criteria for pseudocyesis were derived from a review of the existing literature. However, given its rarity, pseudocyesis is not listed as a specified somatoform disorder.

Two other examples given are syndromes that resemble specified somatoform syndromes, somatization disorder, undifferentiated somatoform disorder, or hypochondriasis but have a duration less than the required 6 months. An additional example is a condition described as involving complaints such as fatigue or body weakness not due to another mental disorder, again with a duration of less than 6 months. Such a syndrome would resemble neurasthenia, a syndrome with a long historical tradition. Included in DSM-II, ICD-9, and ICD-10, neurasthenia was considered for inclusion as a specified DSM-IV somatoform disorder. After careful review, neurasthenia was not adopted because it was difficult to delineate from depressive, anxiety, and other somatoform disor-

TABLE 13–11. DSM-IV-TR criteria for somatoform disorder not otherwise specified

This category includes disorders with somatoform symptoms that do not meet the criteria for any specific somatoform disorder. Examples include

1. Pseudocyesis: a false belief of being pregnant that is associated with objective signs of pregnancy, which may include abdominal enlargement (although the umbilicus does not become everted), reduced menstrual flow, amenorrhea, subjective sensation of fetal movement, nausea, breast engorgement and secretions, and labor pains at the expected date of delivery. Endocrine changes may be present, but the syndrome cannot be explained by a general medical condition that causes endocrine changes (e.g., a hormone-secreting tumor).
2. A disorder involving nonpsychotic hypochondriacal symptoms of less than 6 months' duration.
3. A disorder involving unexplained physical complaints (e.g., fatigue or body weakness) of less than 6 months' duration that are not due to another mental disorder.

ders, and there was a lack of systematic study supporting it. Finally, there was concern that neurasthenia would become a wastebasket category, the availability of which might promote premature closure of the diagnostic process so that other mental disorders, as well as other general medical disorders, would be overlooked.

Differential Diagnosis

As mentioned in the preceding discussion, DSM-IV-TR lists several syndromes that, if not for their short duration, would qualify for a diagnosis as the specified somatoform disorder that they resemble.

Pseudocyesis deserves further attention. Although not mentioned in DSM-II, it probably would have fit best as a psychophysiological endocrine disorder. In DSM-III and DSM-III-R, pseudocyesis was specifically listed as a conversion symptom. Its presumed mechanism was ambivalence about pregnancy, with the resulting conflict expressed somatically, leading to resolution (primary gain) and unconsciously needed environmental support (secondary gain). Pseudocyesis could have been subsumed under the heading "Psychological Factors Affecting Medical Condition." An argument can be made for its inclusion as a medical condition because, based on a literature review (Martin 1996), in most if not all cases, it appears that a neuroendocrine change accompanies, and at times may antedate, the false belief of pregnancy. However, in most instances, a discrete general medical condition (such as a hormone-secreting tumor) cannot be identified. It might have been included as a specified somatoform disorder except for its rarity; Whelan and Stewart (1990) reported six cases in 20 years of consulting to a unit delivering 2,500 women per year. Yet, pseudocyesis appears as a reasonably discrete syndrome such that specific criteria derived from the literature are included in its listing as a somatoform disorder NOS (see Table 13–11).

Epidemiology, Etiology, and Treatment

Discussion of epidemiology, etiology, and treatment for a residual category such as somatoform disorder NOS would not be meaningful because it represents a grouping of diverse disorders. Conditions that would warrant diagnosis of a specified somatoform disorder except for their insufficient duration (less than 6 months) are probably best considered to be in the spectrum of the resembled disorder. Thus, the epidemiological, etiological, and treatment considerations pertaining to the specified disorder should be reviewed because these may apply, at least in part, to the shorter-duration syndromes.

In a comprehensive review of pseudocyesis, Small (1986) stated: "Of all that has been written on the subject [of pseudocyesis], therapy is least discussed." In another report, Whelan and Stewart (1990) emphasized two principles in treating pseudocyesis. First, the patient is to be clearly, yet "empathically" advised that she (or the rare he) is not pregnant. If such simple advice is not effective, objective procedures such as ultrasound are recommended to demonstrate to the patient that there is no visible evidence of a fetus. Alternatively, menses are to be induced. Remarkably, such straightforward approaches are often effective (Cohen 1982). According to Whelan and Stewart (1990), the second principle, which goes hand in hand with the first, is that the patient's expectations, fears, and fantasies should be explored to discover the reason that the false pregnancy was "needed." They also advised providing a face-saving resolution to the patient's lack of pregnancy, such as allowing the patient to take the position that a "miscarriage" has occurred. However, systematic data on the effectiveness of these and other approaches are lacking. Whatever the therapy, relapses are common. According to Ford (1995), there are limited data on the prognosis for women with pseudocyesis. Concomitant disorders such as major depression should be treated in the usual manner.

Conclusion

Syndromes now subsumed under the rubric "somatoform disorders" have had a tortuous course in the evolution of psychiatric nosology and therapy. Yet, they are extremely important because they are disorders that must be differentiated from conditions with identifiable, and often treatable, physical bases.

Developments in the past decade are encouraging. Coordinated effort has been made to establish a common, globally used nomenclature. Somatoform disorders as delineated in DSM-IV-TR are compatible with, although not identical to, counterparts in ICD-10. A common and more explicitly defined nosology is conducive to empirical research that is truly comparable from one investigation to the next. Initial observations on the pharmacological treatment of several of the disorders, namely hypochondriasis and body dysmorphic disorder, are promising and not only may add to our therapeutic armamentarium but also may suggest avenues for improved pathophysiological as well as etiological understanding of these two somatoform disorders.

Ultimately, it may prove possible to obtain a better understanding of the somatoform disorders, a group of complex, incapacitating disorders. Better understanding should facilitate more effective treatments. Already, there has been some preliminary discussion regarding the development of practice guidelines for somatoform disorders. Consideration of guidelines would have been highly unlikely even a few years ago.

References

Alexander F: Psychosomatic Medicine: Its Principles and Applications. New York, WW Norton, 1950

Almgren P-E, Nordgren L, Skantze H: A retrospective study of operationally defined hysterics. Br J Psychiatry 132:67–73, 1978

Alper K, Devinsky O, Vasquez B, et al: Nonepileptic seizures and childhood sexual and physical abuse. Neurology 43:1950–1953, 1993

American Psychiatric Association: Diagnostic and Statistical Manual: Mental Disorders. Washington, DC, American Psychiatric Association, 1952

American Psychiatric Association: Diagnostic and Statistical Manual of Mental Disorders, 2nd Edition. Washington, DC, American Psychiatric Association, 1968

American Psychiatric Association: Diagnostic and Statistical Manual of Mental Disorders, 3rd Edition. Washington, DC, American Psychiatric Association, 1980

American Psychiatric Association: Diagnostic and Statistical Manual of Mental Disorders, 3rd Edition, Revised. Washington, DC, American Psychiatric Association, 1987

American Psychiatric Association: Diagnostic and Statistical Manual of Mental Disorders, 4th Edition. Washington, DC, American Psychiatric Association, 1994

American Psychiatric Association: Diagnostic and Statistical Manual of Mental Disorders, 4th Edition, Primary Care Version. Washington, DC, American Psychiatric Association, 1995

American Psychiatric Association: Diagnostic and Statistical Manual of Mental Disorders, 4th Edition, Text Revision. Washington, DC, American Psychiatric Association, 2000

Andrade C, Srinath S: True auditory hallucinations as a conversion symptom. Br J Psychiatry 148:100–102, 1986

Andreasen NC, Bardach J: Dysmorphophobia: symptom or disease? Am J Psychiatry 134:673–676, 1977

Bach M, Bach D, de Zwaan M: Independency of alexithymia and somatization. Psychosomatics 37:451–458, 1996

Barsky AJ: Somatoform disorders, in Comprehensive Textbook of Psychiatry, 5th Edition, Vol 1. Edited by Kaplan HI, Sadock BJ. Baltimore, MD, Williams & Wilkins, 1989, pp 1009–1027

Barsky AJ, Klerman GL: Overview: hypochondriasis, bodily complaints, and somatic styles. Am J Psychiatry 140:273–283, 1983

Barsky AJ, Wyshak G, Klerman GL: Hypochondriasis: an evaluation of the DSM-III criteria in medical outpatients. Arch Gen Psychiatry 43:493–500, 1986

Barsky AJ, Cleary PD, Sarnie MK, et al: The course of transient hypochondriasis. Am J Psychiatry 150:484–488, 1993

Bass CM, Murphy MR: Somatization disorder: critique of the concept and suggestions for future research, in Somatization: Physical Symptoms and Psychological Illness. Edited by Bass C. Oxford, England, Blackwell Scientific, 1990, pp 301–332

Bendefeldt F, Miller LL, Ludwig AM: Cognitive performance in conversion hysteria. Arch Gen Psychiatry 33:1250–1254, 1976

Bohman M, Cloninger CR, von Knorring A-L, et al: An adoption study of somatoform disorders, III: cross-fostering analysis and genetic relationship to alcoholism and criminality. Arch Gen Psychiatry 41:872–878, 1984

Breuer J, Freud S: Studies on hysteria (1893–1895), in the Standard Edition of the Complete Psychological Works of Sigmund Freud, Vol 2. Translated and edited by Strachey J. London, England, Hogarth, 1955, pp 1–311

Briquet P: Traité Clinique et Thérapeutique Y l'Hystérie. Paris, France, J-B Balliere & Fils, 1859

Carter AB: The prognosis of certain hysterical symptoms. BMJ 1:1076–1079, 1949

Chodoff P, Lyons H: Hysteria, the hysterical personality and "hysterical" conversion. Am J Psychiatry 114:734–740, 1958

Cloninger CR: The link between hysteria and sociopathy: an integrative model based on clinical, genetic, and neurophysiological observations, in Psychiatric Diagnosis: Explorations of Biological Predictors. Edited by Akiskal HS, Webb WL. New York, Spectrum, 1978, pp 189–218

Cloninger CR: Diagnosis of somatoform disorders: a critique of DSM-III, in Diagnosis and Classification in Psychiatry: A Critical Appraisal of DSM-III. Edited by Tischler GL. New York, Cambridge University Press, 1987, pp 243–259

Cloninger CR: Somatoform and dissociative disorders, in The Medical Basis of Psychiatry, 2nd Edition. Edited by Winokur G, Clayton P. Philadelphia, PA, WB Saunders, 1994, pp 169–192

Cloninger CR, Guze SB: Psychiatric illness and female criminality: the role of sociopathy and hysteria in the antisocial woman. Am J Psychiatry 127:303–311, 1970

Cloninger CR, Yutzy S: Somatoform and dissociative disorders: a summary of changes for DSM-IV, in Current Psychiatric Therapy. Edited by Dunner DL. Philadelphia, PA, WB Saunders, 1993, pp 310–313

Cloninger CR, Reich T, Guze SB: The multifactorial model of disease transmission, III: familial relationship between sociopathy and hysteria (Briquet's syndrome). Br J Psychiatry 127:23–32, 1975

Cloninger CR, Sigvardsson S, von Knorring A-L, et al: An adoption study of somatoform disorders, II: identification of two discrete somatoform disorders. Arch Gen Psychiatry 41:863–871, 1984

Cloninger CR, Martin RL, Guze SB, et al: A prospective follow-up and family study of somatization in men and women. Am J Psychiatry 143:873–878, 1986

Cloninger CR, Bayon C, Przybeck TR: Epidemiology and Axis I comorbidity of antisocial personality, in Handbook of Antisocial Behavior. Edited by Stoff DM, Breiling J, Maser JD. New York, Wiley, 1997, pp 12–21

Cohen LM: A current perspective of pseudocyesis. Am J Psychiatry 139:1140–1144, 1982

Coryell W, House D: The validity of broadly defined hysteria and DSM-III conversion disorder: outcome, family history, and mortality. J Clin Psychiatry 45:252–256, 1984

Cote G, O'Leary T, Barlow DM, et al: Hypochondriasis: integrative review for DSM-IV, in DSM-IV Sourcebook, Vol 2. Edited by Widiger TA, Frances AJ, Pincus HA, et al. Washington, DC, American Psychiatric Press, 1996, pp 933–947

De Leon J, Bott A, Simpson GM: Dysmorphophobia: body dysmorphic disorder or delusional disorder, somatic subtype? Compr Psychiatry 30:457–472, 1989

Desai BT, Porter RJ, Penry K: Psychogenic seizures: a study of 42 attacks in six patients, with intensive monitoring. Arch Neurol 39:202–209, 1982

DeSouza C, Othmer E, Gabrielli W Jr, et al: Major depression and somatization disorder: the overlooked differential diagnosis. Psychiatr Ann 18:340–348, 1988

Escobar JI, Swartz M, Rubio-Stipec M, et al: Medically unexplained symptoms: distribution, risk factors, and comorbidity, in Current Concepts of Somatization: Research and Clinical Perspectives. Edited by Kirmayer LJ, Robbins JM. Washington, DC, American Psychiatric Press, 1991, pp 63–78

Fallon BA, Schneir FR, Narshall R, et al: The pharmacotherapy of hypochondriasis. Psychopharmacol Bull 32:607–611, 1996

Feighner JP, Robins E, Guze SB, et al: Diagnostic criteria for use in psychiatric research. Arch Gen Psychiatry 26:57–63, 1972

Fitzgerald BA, Wells CE: Hallucinations as a conversion reaction. Diseases of the Nervous System 38:381–383, 1977

Flor-Henry P, Fromm-Auch D, Tapper M, et al: A neuropsychological study of the stable syndrome of hysteria. Biol Psychiatry 16:601–626, 1981

Folks DG, Ford CV, Regan WM: Conversion symptoms in a general hospital. Psychosomatics 25:285–295, 1984

Ford CV: The Somatizing Disorders: Illness as a Way of Life. New York, Elsevier, 1983

Ford CV: Conversion disorder and somatoform disorder not otherwise specified, in Treatment of Psychiatric Disorders, 2nd Edition. Edited by Gabbard GO. Washington, DC, American Psychiatric Press, 1995, pp 1737–1753

Ford CV, Folks DG: Conversion disorders: an overview. Psychosomatics 26:371–383, 1985

Gatfield PD, Guze SB: Prognosis and differential diagnosis of conversion reactions (a follow-up study). Diseases of the Nervous System 23:623–631, 1962

Goodwin DW, Guze SB: Psychiatric Diagnosis, 5th Edition. New York, Oxford University Press, 1996

Goodwin DW, Alderson P, Rosenthal R: Clinical significance of hallucinations in psychiatric disorders. Arch Gen Psychiatry 24:76–80, 1971

Guze SB: The role of follow-up studies: their contribution to diagnostic classification as applied to hysteria. Seminars in Psychiatry 2:392–402, 1970

Guze SB, Perley MJ: Observations on the natural history of hysteria. Am J Psychiatry 119:960–965, 1963

Guze SB, Cloninger CR, Martin RL, et al: A follow-up and family study of Briquet's syndrome. Br J Psychiatry 149:17–23, 1986

Hathaway SR, McKinley JC: Minnesota Multiphasic Personality Schedule. Minneapolis, MN, University of Minnesota Press, 1943

Hewlett HA: The use of benzodiazepines in obsessive-compulsive disorder and Tourette's syndrome. Psychiatr Ann 23:309–316, 1993

Hollander E, Neville D, Frenkel M, et al: Body dysmorphic disorder: diagnostic issues and related disorders. Psychosomatics 33:156–165, 1992

Hollander E, Cohen LJ, Simeon D: Body dysmorphic disorder. Psychiatr Ann 23:359–364, 1993

Horowitz MJ: Hysterical Personality. New York, Jason Aronson, 1977

Hudziak JJ, Boffeli TJ, Kreisman JJ, et al: Clinical study of the relation of borderline personality disorder to Briquet's syndrome (hysteria), somatization disorder, antisocial personality disorder, and substance abuse disorders. Am J Psychiatry 153:1598–1606, 1996

Inouye E: Genetic aspects of neurosis. International Journal of Mental Health 1:176–189, 1972

Kellner R: The prognosis of treated hypochondriasis: a clinical study. Acta Psychiatr Scand 67:69–79, 1983

Kellner R: Functional somatic symptoms and hypochondriasis: a survey of empirical studies. Arch Gen Psychiatry 42:821–833, 1985

Kellner R: Hypochondriasis and somatization. JAMA 258:2718–2722, 1987

Kellner R: Somatization disorder, in Treatments of Psychiatric Disorders: A Task Force Report of the American Psychiatric Association, Vol 3. Washington, DC, American Psychiatric Association, 1989, pp 2166–2171

Kellner R: Somatization: theories and research. J Nerv Ment Dis 178:150–160, 1990

Kent D, Tomasson K, Coryell W: Course and outcome of conversion and somatization disorders: a four-year follow-up. Psychosomatics 36:138–144, 1995

Kenyon FE: Hypochondriasis: a survey of some historical, clinical, and social aspects. Br J Psychiatry 138:117–133, 1965

Kenyon FE: Hypochondriacal states. Br J Psychiatry 129:1–14, 1976

Kirmayer LJ, Robbins JM: Introduction: concepts of somatization, in Current Concepts of Somatization: Research and Clinical Perspectives. Edited by Kirmayer LJ, Robbins JM. Washington, DC, American Psychiatric Press, 1991, pp 1–19

Kirmayer LJ, Robbins JM, Dworkind M, et al: Somatization and the recognition of depression and anxiety in primary care. Am J Psychiatry 150:734–741, 1993

Kroenke K, Spitzer RL, de Gruy FV, et al: Multisomatoform disorder: an alternative to undifferentiated somatoform disorder for the somatizing patient in primary care. Arch Gen Psychiatry 54:352–358, 1997

Lader M, Sartorius N: Anxiety in patients with hysterical conversion symptoms. J Neurol Neurosurg Psychiatry 31:490–495, 1968

Lazare A: Conversion symptoms. N Engl J Med 305:745–748, 1981

Lewis WC: Hysteria: the consultant's dilemma: twentieth century demonology, pejorative epithet, or useful diagnosis? Arch Gen Psychiatry 30:145–151, 1974

Lewis WC, Berman M: Studies of conversion hysteria, I: operational study of diagnosis. Arch Gen Psychiatry 13:275–282, 1965

Lipowski ZJ: Somatization: the concept and its clinical application. Am J Psychiatry 145:1358–1368, 1988

Ljundberg L: Hysteria: clinical, prognostic and genetic study. Acta Psychiatr Scand Suppl 32:1–162, 1957

Ludwig AM: Hysteria: a neurobiological theory. Arch Gen Psychiatry 27:771–777, 1972

Luff MC, Garrod M: The after-results of psychotherapy in 500 adult cases. BMJ 2:54–59, 1935

Mace CJ, Trimble MR: Ten-year prognosis of conversion disorder. Br J Psychiatry 169:282–288, 1996

Maloney MJ: Diagnosing hysterical conversion disorders in children. J Pediatr 97:1016–1020, 1980

Marsden CD: Hysteria: a neurologist's view. Psychol Med 16:277–288, 1986

Martin RL: Problems in the diagnosis of somatization disorder: effects on research and clinical practice. Psychiatr Ann 18:357–362, 1988

Martin RL: DSM-IV in progress: diagnostic issues for conversion disorder. Hosp Community Psychiatry 43:771–773, 1992

Martin RL: DSM-IV changes in the somatoform disorders. Psychiatr Ann 25:29–39, 1995

Martin RL: DSM-IV diagnostic options for conversion disorder: proposed autonomic arousal disorder and pseudocyesis, in DSM-IV Sourcebook, Vol 2. Edited by Widiger TA, Frances AJ, Pincus HA, et al. Washington, DC, American Psychiatric Press, 1996, pp 893–914

Martin RL, Yutzy SH: Somatoform disorders, in Psychiatry. Edited by Tasman A, Kay J, Lieberman JA. Philadelphia, PA, WB Saunders, 1997, pp 1119–1155

Martin RL, Cloninger CR, Guze SB: The evaluation of diagnostic concordance in follow-up studies, II: a blind prospective follow-up of female criminals. J Psychiatr Res 15:107–125, 1979

Martin RL, Cloninger CR, Guze SB, et al: Mortality in a follow-up of 500 psychiatric outpatients, II: cause-specific mortality. Arch Gen Psychiatry 42:58–66, 1985

Meares R, Horvath T: "Acute" and "chronic" hysteria. Br J Psychiatry 121:653–657, 1972

Merskey H: Conversion disorder, in Treatments of Psychiatric Disorders: A Task Force Report of the American Psychiatric Association, Vol 3. Washington, DC, American Psychiatric Association, 1989, pp 2152–2159

Modai I, Cygielman G: Conversion hallucinations: a possible mental mechanism. Psychopathology 19:324–326, 1986

Murphy GE: The clinical management of hysteria. JAMA 247:2559–2564, 1982

Murphy GE, Guze SB: Setting limits. Am J Psychother 14:30–47, 1960

Murphy GE, Wetzel RD: Family history of suicidal behavior among suicide attempters. J Nerv Ment Dis 170:86–90, 1982

Murphy MR: Classification of the somatoform disorders, in Somatization: Physical Symptoms and Psychological Illness. Edited by Bass C. Oxford, England, Blackwell Scientific, 1990, pp 10–39

Perley M, Guze SB: Hysteria: the stability and usefulness of clinical criteria: a quantitative study based upon a 6–8 year follow-up of 39 patients. N Engl J Med 266:421–426, 1962

Phillips KA: Body dysmorphic disorder: the distress of imagined ugliness. Am J Psychiatry 148:1138–1149, 1991

Phillips KA: Body dysmorphic disorder: clinical features and drug treatment. CNS Drugs 3:30–40, 1995

Phillips KA, Hollander E: Body dysmorphic disorder, in DSM-IV Sourcebook, Vol 2. Edited by Widiger TA, Frances AJ, Pincus HA, et al. Washington, DC, American Psychiatric Press, 1996, pp 949–960

Phillips KA, McElroy SL, Keck PE Jr, et al: Body dysmorphic disorder: 30 cases of imagined ugliness. Am J Psychiatry 150:302–308, 1993

Phillips KA, Kim JM, Hudson JI: Body image disturbance in body dysmorphic disorder and eating disorders: obsessions or delusions? Psychiatr Clin North Am 18:317–334, 1995

Pincus J: Hysteria presenting to a neurologist, in Hysteria. Edited by Roy A. London, England, Wiley, 1982, pp 131–144

Pribor EF, Smith DS, Yutzy SH: Somatization disorder in the elderly. Am J Geriatr Psychiatry 2:109–117, 1994

Purtell J, Robins E, Cohen M: Observations on clinical aspects of hysteria: a quantitative study of 50 hysteria patients and 156 control subjects. JAMA 146:902–909, 1951

Quill TE: Somatization disorder: one of medicine's blind spots. JAMA 254:3075–3079, 1985

Raskin M, Talbott JA, Meyerson AT: Diagnosis of conversion reactions: predictive value of psychiatric criteria. JAMA 197:530–534, 1966

Riding J, Munro A: Pimozide in the treatment of monosymptomatic hypochondriacal psychosis. Acta Psychiatr Scand 52:23–30, 1975

Robins E, O'Neal P: Clinical features of hysteria in children. The Nervous Child 10:246–271, 1953

Robins LN, Helzer JE, Croughan J, et al: National Institute of Mental Health Diagnostic Interview Schedule: its history, characteristics, and validity. Arch Gen Psychiatry 38:381–389, 1981

Robins LN, Helzer JE, Weissman MM, et al: Lifetime prevalence of specific psychiatric disorders in three sites. Arch Gen Psychiatry 41:949–958, 1984

Scallet A, Cloninger CR, Othmer E: The management of chronic hysteria: a review and double-blind trial of electrosleep and other relaxation methods. Diseases of the Nervous System 37:347–353, 1976

Shapiro D: Neurotic Styles. New York, Basic Books, 1965

Sharma P, Chaturvedi SK: Conversion disorder revisited. Acta Psychiatr Scand 92:301–304, 1995

Slater ETO, Glithero C: A follow-up of patients diagnosed as suffering from "hysteria." J Psychosom Res 9:9–13, 1965

Small GW: Pseudocyesis: an overview. Can J Psychiatry 31:452–457, 1986

Smith GR Jr, Monson RA, Ray DC: Psychiatric consultation in somatization disorder: a randomized controlled study. N Engl J Med 314:1407–1413, 1986

Stefanis C, Markidis M, Christodoulou G: Observations on the evolution of the hysterical symptomatology. Br J Psychiatry 128:269–275, 1976

Stefansson JH, Messina JA, Meyerowitz S: Hysterical neurosis, conversion type: clinical and epidemiological considerations. Acta Psychiatr Scand 59:119–138, 1976

Stekel W: The Interpretation of Dreams: New Developments and Technique, Vols 1 and 2. Translated by Paul E, Paul C. New York, Liveright, 1943

Stephens JH, Kamp M: On some aspects of hysteria: a clinical study. J Nerv Ment Dis 134:305–315, 1962

Stern J, Murphy M, Bass C: Personality disorders in patients with somatization disorder: a controlled study. Br J Psychiatry 163:785–789, 1993

Stoudemire GA: Somatoform disorders, factitious disorders, and malingering, in American Psychiatric Press Textbook of Psychiatry. Edited by Talbott JA, Hales RE, Yudofsky SC. Washington, DC, American Psychiatric Press, 1988, pp 533–556

Temoshok L, Attkisson CC: Epidemiology of hysterical phenomena: evidence for a psychosocial theory, in Hysterical Personality. Edited by Horowitz MJ. New York, Jason Aronson, 1977, pp 143–222

Tomasson K, Kent D, Coryell W: Somatization and conversion disorders: comorbidity and demographics at presentation. Acta Psychiatr Scand 84:288–293, 1991

Toone BK: Disorders of hysterical conversion, in Physical Symptoms and Psychological Illness. Edited by Bass C. London, England, Blackwell Scientific, 1990, pp 207–234

Torack RM: Historical overview of dementia, in The Pathologic Physiology of Dementia. Edited by Torack RA. New York, Springer-Verlag, 1978, pp 1–16

Vaillant GE: The disadvantages of DSM-III outweigh its advantages. Am J Psychiatry 141:542–545, 1984

Veith I: Hysteria: The History of a Disease. Chicago, IL, University of Chicago Press, 1965

Viederman M: Somatoform and factitious disorders, in Psychiatry, Vol 1. Edited by Cavenar JO. Philadelphia, PA, JB Lippincott, 1985, pp 1–20

Watson CG, Buranen C: The frequency and identification of false positive conversion reactions. J Nerv Ment Dis 167:243–247, 1979

Wechsler D: Wechsler Adult Intelligence Scale—Revised. New York, Psychological Corporation, 1981

Weddington WW: Conversion reaction in an 82-year-old man. J Nerv Ment Dis 167:368–369, 1979

Weinstein EA, Eck RA, Lyerly OG: Conversion hysteria in Appalachia. Psychiatry 32:334–341, 1969

Wetzel RD, Guze SB, Cloninger CR, et al: Briquet's syndrome (hysteria) is both a somatoform and a "psychoform" illness: an MMPI study. Psychosom Med 56:564–569, 1994

Wheatley D: Evaluation of psychotherapeutic drugs in general practice. Psychopharmacol Bull 2:25–32, 1962

Wheatley D: General practitioner clinical trials: phenobarbitone compared with an inactive placebo in anxiety states. Practitioner 192:147–151, 1964

Wheatley D: General practitioner clinical trials: chlordiazepoxide in anxiety states, II: long-term study. Practitioner 195:692–695, 1965

Whelan CI, Stewart DE: Pseudocyesis: a review and report of six cases. Int J Psychiatry Med 20:97–108, 1990

Woerner PI, Guze SB: A family and marital study of hysteria. Br J Psychiatry 114:161–168, 1968

Woodruff RA, Clayton PJ, Guze SB: Hysteria: studies of diagnosis, outcome, and prevalence. JAMA 215:425–428, 1971

World Health Organization: The ICD-9 Classification of Mental and Behavioural Disorders, 9th Revision: Clinical Descriptions and Diagnostic Guidelines. Geneva, Switzerland, World Health Organization, 1977

World Health Organization: The ICD-10 Classification of Mental and Behavioural Disorders, 10th Revision: Clinical Descriptions and Diagnostic Guidelines. Geneva, Switzerland, World Health Organization, 1992a

World Health Organization: International Statistical Classification of Diseases and Related Health Problems, 10th Revision. Geneva, Switzerland, World Health Organization, 1992b

World Health Organization: Diagnostic and Management Guidelines for Mental Disorders in Primary Care: ICD-10 Chapter V Primary Care Version. Gottingen, Germany, Hogrefe & Huber, 1996

Yutzy SH, Pribor EF, Cloninger CR, et al: Reconsidering the criteria for somatization disorder. Hosp Community Psychiatry 43:1075–1076, 1149, 1992

Yutzy SH, Cloninger CR, Guze SB, et al: The DSM-IV field trial: somatization disorder: testing a new proposal. Am J Psychiatry 152:97–101, 1995

Ziegler FJ, Imboden JB, Meyer E: Contemporary conversion reactions: a clinical study. Am J Psychiatry 116:901–910, 1960

Factitious Disorders and Malingering

Martin H. Leamon, M.D.

Marc D. Feldman, M.D.

Charles L. Scott, M.D.

Factitious Disorder

Introduction

Factitious disorder is characterized by a person intentionally fabricating or inducing signs or symptoms of other illnesses solely to become identified as "ill" or as a "patient." Such patients have been described in medical writing throughout history (Feldman et al. 1994; Gavin 1843) and throughout the world (Bappal et al. 2001; Cizza et al. 1996; Linde 1996; Mizuta et al. 2000; Seersholm et al. 1991). The concept became firmly established in modern medical thinking in 1951 when Asher (1951) described what has since been classified a subtype of factitious disorders, Munchausen syndrome. In many patients, factitious disorders remain undiagnosed, and even when recognized, they often go untreated (Toth and Baggaley 1991). Yet, factitious disorders cause significant morbidity and mortality (Baker and Major 1994; Folks 1995; Higgins 1990), consume an astonishing amount of medical resources (Feldman 1994a; Frumkin and Victoroff 1990; Higgins 1990; Powell and Boast 1993a; Schwarz et al. 1993), and cause significant emotional distress in the patients themselves, in their caregivers, and in their close relationships (Feldman and Smith 1996). Over the past decade, the medical literature about factitious disorders has continued to expand, with the publication of lay and professional books on the topic (Feldman and Eisendrath 1996; Feldman et al. 1994) and the establishment of a factitious disorders Web site (http://munchausen.com; Feldman 2001).

Classification

DSM-IV-TR (American Psychiatric Association 2000) requires three criteria for the diagnosis of factitious disorder (Table 14–1). The first, the intentional production or feigning of physical or psychological signs or symptoms, distinguishes factitious disorder from the somatoform disorders, in which physical symptoms are viewed as unconsciously produced. The second and third criteria, that the motivation for the behavior is to assume the sick role and that external incentives for the behavior are absent, distinguish factitious disorder from malingering.

DSM-IV-TR classifies the disorder based on the predominant type of factitious symptom presented—physical or psychological. Individual case histories (Bauer and Boegner 1996; Craddock and Brown 1993; Miner and Feldman 1998) suggest that this categorization may be somewhat arbitrary because the same patient may have different presentations across time. Predominantly physical symptoms may be feigned at one time and predominantly psychological or a mixed picture at another. Rogers et al. (1989) also raised epistemological objections to this subtyping, arguing, in part, that factitious disorder with predominantly psychological signs and symptoms confers a psychiatric disorder to someone who, by definition, is merely pretending to have one. The fourth subtype is factitious disorder not otherwise specified (Table 14–2). This code should be used for disorders with factitious symptoms that do not meet criteria for one of the other subtypes. An example is factitious disorder by proxy (discussed in the "Factitious Disorder by Proxy" section later in this chapter).

TABLE 14–1. DSM-IV-TR diagnostic criteria for factitious disorder

A. Intentional production or feigning of physical or psychological signs or symptoms.
B. The motivation for the behavior is to assume the sick role.
C. External incentives for the behavior (such as economic gain, avoiding legal responsibility, or improving physical well-being, as in Malingering) are absent.

Code based on type:

300.16 With Predominantly Psychological Signs and Symptoms: if psychological signs and symptoms predominate in the clinical presentation

300.19 With Predominantly Physical Signs and Symptoms: if physical signs and symptoms predominate in the clinical presentation

300.19 With Combined Psychological and Physical Signs and Symptoms: if both psychological and physical signs and symptoms are present but neither predominates in the clinical presentation

TABLE 14–2. DSM-IV-TR diagnostic criteria for factitious disorder not otherwise specified

This category includes disorders with factitious symptoms that do not meet the criteria for factitious disorder. An example is factitious disorder by proxy: the intentional production or feigning of physical or psychological signs or symptoms in another person who is under the individual's care for the purpose of indirectly assuming the sick role.

ICD-10 (World Health Organization 1992), although slightly different, uses similarly defined operational criteria, emphasizing that the motivation for this behavior is almost always obscure and presumed internal (Freyberger and Schneider 1994). The ICD-10 criteria also highlight the prevalence of comorbid psychiatric disorders.

Other authors have used different typologies. Nadelson (1979) distinguished between factitious disorders of the Munchausen and the non-Munchausen type. This typology may have prognostic and treatment implications. *Munchausen syndrome*, a term coined by Asher (1951), comprises about 10% of patients with factitious disorders (Eisendrath 1994). The eponym remains in wide use and describes a variant of DSM-IV-TR's factitious disorder with predominantly physical signs and symptoms. In this special type of factitious disorder, multiple hospitalizations with dramatic and often life-threatening presentations, wandering from hospital to hospital (peregrination), and pathological lying (*pseudologia fantastica*, the telling of dramatic tales that merge truth and falsehood and that the listener initially finds

intriguing) are prominent. The Munchausen patient shows a pattern of feigning illness at numerous hospital emergency departments, often in different cities; gaining admission and sometimes receiving invasive procedures; becoming quarrelsome with the staff; and often being discharged against medical advice or simply disappearing when the ruse is discovered. Asher, using the anglicized spelling, drew the term from Rudolf Erich Raspe's 1784 book, *Baron Münchhausen's Narrative of His Marvelous Travels and Campaigns in Russia*, which further exaggerated (Carswell 1950) the whimsical accounts of the sporting and military adventures, as well as the peregrinations, of a real-life German cavalry officer in the Russian army, Baron Karl Friedrich Hieronymous von Münchhausen (1720–1797) (Raspe 1787).

Other expressions concerning patients of this type have been quite colorful but often with derogatory overtones: *peregrinating problem patients* (Chapman 1957), *hospital hobos* (Clarke and Melnick 1958), and *hospital addicts* (Barker 1962). Additional terms for the disorder have included *chronic factitious illness* (Spiro 1968), *Kopenickades* or *Ahasuerus syndrome* (Clinical Case Conference 1984), and, for a subset of plastic surgical patients, *the SHAFT syndrome* (Kasdan et al. 1998).

As described, the vast majority of factitious disorder patients are of the non-Munchausen type. Characterized by several authors (Carney 1980; Ford 1986; Freyberger et al. 1994; Guziec et al. 1994; Plassmann 1994b; Reich and Gottfried 1983), these patients are mostly young women with conforming lifestyles and more family support and involvement than Munchausen patients. These patients have been described as passive and immature, and a significant proportion have health-related jobs or training. Most are not wanderers, have single-system complaints, and generate fewer hospitalizations than do Munchausen patients, but the overall severity and morbidity of their illness may be just as great (Sutherland and Rodin 1990).

Others (Eisendrath 1996; Overholser 1990) have classified patients with factitious disorders according to the manner in which illness is simulated and by the type of simulated illness. Patients may simply report invented symptoms and false medical histories—for example, in Internet "chat rooms" (Feldman 2000) or directly to clinicians, as in the case example in the following "Diagnosis" section. They may exaggerate symptoms, for example, by claiming that occasional tension headaches are continual crippling migraines. They may manipulate diagnostic instruments to give false readings, such as manipulating electrocardiogram (ECG) leads to simulate arrhythmia (Ludwigs et al. 1994) or rubbing thermometers to fake fevers (Aduan et al. 1979). They also may tamper with laboratory specimens, adding blood to urine or sputum. Finally, they may purposefully cause actual tissue damage or biochemical abnormalities in their bodies, either inducing new injury or exacerbating existing conditions, by methods such as intentionally traumatic self-catheterization, self-induced infection of wounds or skin with bacteria, injection of unneeded or excessive insulin, or ingestion of thyroid hormones or anticoagulants.

Classification by type of simulated illness is most useful to the clinician who begins to suspect factitious illness and who then looks for evidence to support the suspicion. Wallach (1994) and Nordmeyer (1994) give thorough descriptions of presentations of factitious illness in the different organ systems and some suggestions for their detection. Almost any conceivable condition can be simulated, depending on the knowledge, motivation, creativity, and covert skill of the patient. An exhaustive list of the medical disorders that have been feigned or produced by patients with factitious disorder would approximate the index of a pathology textbook (Feldman et al. 2001).

Diagnosis

Mr. A, a middle-aged, middle-ranking United States military officer, was stationed at what was widely held to be a desirable post in Europe. He was married with no children, by mutual decision with his attentive wife. His superiors described his military career performance as slightly better than average. He was hospitalized for evaluation when a sentry discovered him one evening walking around outside, disorganized and talking disjointedly about Vietnam.

Mr. A was psychiatrically hospitalized at a United States military psychiatric ward in Europe, where he described long-standing symptoms of posttraumatic stress disorder (PTSD) from his experiences as part of an elite covert operations team functioning behind enemy lines. He readily engaged in ward activities and in his treatment program. The historical details he provided were accurate, although he said that he could not reveal some details because of their classified nature. He was evaluated by experienced psychiatrists, psychologists, and nursing staff. His cognitive and affective presentations in ward activities, group psychotherapy, and individual psychotherapy were thought to be consistent with delayed-onset PTSD. When he showed no improvement after 2 weeks of intensive treatment, he was transferred to a military medical center in the United States for further treatment.

Mr. A's presentation remained unchanged, although he seemed to show some improvement. He received much support from the other military patients and was regarded as tragically courageous. The psychiatric resident responsible for Mr. A's direct care (one of the authors of this chapter) spent time reading the litera-

ture on the treatment of PTSD, and Mr. A received extra individual psychotherapy, a valued commodity on a busy inpatient service. A search of his military records detected no history of Vietnam service, and Mr. A carefully explained that his record had been officially manipulated, again because of the classified nature of his activities. Knowledgeable military sources confirmed that although Mr. A's explanation was unusual, it could be correct. In couples psychotherapy sessions, Mr. A gently explained to his wife that he had withheld this important part of his premarital history from her because of the pain it caused him to recall these experiences, as well as the classified nature of his activities. She continued to be emotionally supportive, after gradually accepting that her husband had been so secretive. As time went on, it became clear that Mr. A was facing discharge from military service, which neither he nor his wife wanted. For several reasons, it also seemed unlikely that Mr. A would receive any disability payments once discharged.

After several months of hospitalization, Mr. A's mother was contacted (with his consent). She seemed to be a reliable source but expressed complete bewilderment at her son's predicament. She explained that Mr. A had not been in Vietnam or even in the military during the time he claimed but had been living with her, working in a store.

When Mr. A was presented with his mother's information, he seemed nonplussed, confirmed that his mother was correct, and acknowledged that he had fabricated the Vietnam and PTSD history. He would not engage in further discussion of his hospitalization or his story. The other patients on the ward continued to support Mr. A and were indignant that his doctors questioned the veracity of his story (despite Mr. A's public admission of its invention). His wife was confused. He continued to be superficially pleasant and cooperative on the ward until he was released from the hospital and the military. He received no disability, returned to his wife's hometown, and was lost to follow-up at that time.

Many factors can suggest a diagnosis of factitious disorder (Freyberger et al. 1994; Popli et al. 1992). There can be discrepancies between objective findings, such as pronounced differences between oral and rectal temperatures or involuntary contractions measured in "paralyzed" limbs (Ziv et al. 1998). Objective findings might be inconsistent with clinical history or symptoms, as in the preceding case example or when mixed bowel flora is isolated from "spontaneous" skin lesions. The illness course could be markedly atypical, or the condition can fail to respond as expected to usual therapies, as demonstrated by erratic blood sugars or failure of wounds to heal. A patient may be unusually acquiescent to invasive diagnostic studies or may be unusually quarrelsome and argumentative with staff, particularly when it comes to trying to obtain old records to confirm history. A patient who describes a flamboyant, fascinating life with connections to well-known people may nevertheless have no visitors or callers. Unexplained medical paraphernalia or medications may be found in the patient's hospital room.

These indicators notwithstanding, verification of the DSM-IV-TR diagnostic criteria can be problematic. The first criterion requires that the patient be feigning or intentionally producing illness. The physician becomes a detective, working against the patient's overt desires, trying to discover the ruse. This role shift destabilizes the relationship (Duffy 1993; Paar 1994). The dilemma is especially complex when patients have combinations of feigned and actual illness (Nordmeyer 1994; Sutherland and Rodin 1990) or develop an actual illness in the attempt to simulate one. An example is the ambulance attendant who repeatedly infected her surgical incision with fecal material; with worsening infections and continued antibiotic treatment, she developed kidney failure (Feldman et al. 1994). Similarly, the patient who has had multiple abdominal surgeries for factitious causes may still develop adhesions that may require surgical intervention. Additionally, some general medical conditions may be difficult to diagnose initially, leading to an erroneous clinical impression of fabricated symptoms (Baddley et al. 1998; Koo et al. 1996). Other illnesses, such as multiple sclerosis or systemic lupus erythematosus, may have fluctuating courses, or in themselves produce inconsistent findings suggestive of factitious disorder (Liebson et al. 1996).

The DSM-IV-TR criteria also require that the feigning be intentional. Psychoses (Gielder 1994), mood disorders (Roy and Roy 1995), and dissociative disorders (Goodwin 1988; Toth and Baggaley 1991) need to be ruled out as alternative etiologies. The hunt for intentionality raises ethical and legal issues of informed consent, right to privacy, and malpractice (Frumkin and Victoroff 1990; Houck 1992; Markantonakis and Lee 1988; Powell and Boast 1993a). Almost by definition, patients with factitious disorders deny their simulations. Rather than being proved irrefutably, intentionality is more likely to be inferred through a process of diagnostic and treatment procedures that "confirm the absence" of any naturally occurring disease process that can account for the observed physical problem (Dixon and Abbey 1995; Feldman et al. 2001).

Furthermore, the patient's specific motivation must be "to assume the sick role" (American Psychiatric Association 2000). Yet such patients often are unaware of their motivations, despite being aware of their role in producing their illness (Bhugra 1988; Eisendrath 1996). Patients can be extremely resistant to psychological inquiry or may prematurely leave the hospital (Bauer and Boegner 1996), rendering psychological motivational assessment incomplete (Baker and Major 1994; Churchill et al. 1994; Harrington et al. 1990; Topazian and Binder 1994). Motivations may be multiple and mixed (Rogers et al. 1989), with clear secondary gains coexisting with less conscious or more subtle ones (Khan et al. 2000; Lawrie et al. 1993). Nonetheless, thorough attempts must be made to investigate and clarify the motivational factors operative in the patients (e.g., Feldman and Russell 1991; Feldman et al. 1994).

The notion of the sick role (Parsons 1951) is complex. Some authors see it as a psychological position in which the patient receives overt empathic support and is subject to overtly reduced expectations; that is, the sick role is a nonpathological mode of functioning that the factitious disorder patient adopts for pathological reasons. Others see the sick role of the factitious disorder patient as inherently pathological. Plassmann (1994b) saw it in terms of the patient's "disturbed relationship to his or her own body" combined with a "seriously disturbed doctor–patient relationship." Spivak et al. (1994) similarly described "disturbances in the sense of self and in the sense of reality."

Another factor complicating the diagnosis is the high prevalence of comorbid disorders (Sutherland and Rodin 1990). Substance use disorders (Bauer and Boegner 1996; Burge and Lacey 1993; Kent 1994; McDaniel et al. 1992; Parker 1993; Popli et al. 1992), personality disorders (particularly borderline and antisocial) (Bauer and Boegner 1996; Nadelson 1979; Overholser 1990; Parker 1993), malingering (Gorman and Winograd 1988; Harrington et al. 1990), dissociative disorders (Goodwin 1988; Toth and Baggaley 1991), eating disorders (Burge and Lacey 1993; Mizuta et al. 2000), suicidality, and mood disorders (Gielder 1994; Paar 1994; Roy and Roy 1995; Sutherland and Rodin 1990) may coexist. The comorbidities can overwhelm the diagnostic picture, and the diagnosis can be ignored altogether (Roy and Roy 1995; Toth and Baggaley 1991).

There are no diagnostic tests for factitious disorders. Psychological testing may reflect comorbid conditions (Babe et al. 1992) or, in cases of factitious disorder with predominantly psychological signs and symptoms, may give "fake bad" or invalid results (Zimmerman et al. 1991). Such results are not pathognomonic (Liebson et al. 1996) but of the same order as spurious thermometer readings in cases of factitious fever. Neuroimaging studies are discussed in the "Etiology" section later in this chapter.

Epidemiology

Data on incidence and prevalence rates for the factitious disorders are difficult to gather, vary considerably, and must be viewed with a critical eye. The covert nature of the disorder can lead to missed diagnosis and underestimation of rates or, conversely, to the same case being counted twice (Duffy 1992, 1993; Ifudu and Friedman 1993; Ifudu et al. 1992) and inflating apparent rates. There has even been one "case," humorously invented and "reported" by its physician authors, that was accepted and cited in the literature as genuine (Feldman 1992; Gurwith and Langston 1992). Sutherland and Rodin (1990) diagnosed factitious disorder in 0.8% of all psychiatric consultation-liaison service referrals of medical or surgical inpatients. Bhugra (1988) found 0.5% of psychiatric admissions to have Munchausen syndrome. Ballas (1996) found that 0.9% of the patients in a sickle cell program could have factitious disorder. Bauer and Boegner (1996) diagnosed factitious disorders in 0.3% of neurological admissions. Others (Eisendrath 1996) have reported rates between approximately 2% and 10%, with the higher rates in case series of fevers of unknown origin. Most reported cases have been in patients in their 20s to 40s, but it has been reported in children, adolescents, and geriatric patients (Joseph-Di Caprio and Remafedi 1997; Libow 2000; Pfefferbaum et al. 1999; Zimmerman et al. 1991).

Etiology

Psychodynamic explanations for these paradoxical disorders have been provided by several authors. Many have noted the apparent prevalence of histories of early childhood physical or sexual abuse, with disturbed parental relationships and emotional deprivation. Histories of early illness or extended hospitalizations also have been noted. Nadelson (1979) conceptualized factitious disorder as a manifestation of borderline character pathology rather than as an isolated clinical syndrome. The patient becomes both the "victim and the victimizer" by garnering medical attention from physicians and other health care workers while defying and devaluing them. Projection of hostility and worthlessness onto the caregiver occurs as he or she is both desired and rejected. Plassmann (1994b, 1994c) viewed the disorders as a "symptom of a psychic problem complex." Early traumas are dealt with narcissistically and through dissociation, denial, and a type of projection. The patient's body, or part of the body, becomes perceived as an external object or as a fused, symbiotic combination of self and object, which then comes to represent negative affects (hate, fear, pain), the associated negative object concepts, and negative self-concepts. In the face of early deprivation and assaults, the "body self" is split off to preserve the "psychic self" (Hirsch 1994). When subsequent life events activate these affects or concepts, the result is extreme anxiety and growing derealization. Eventually, the patient acts out or involves the medical system in a type of countertransference identification, which results in manipulations of the body of the patient. The manipulation results in emotional relief, albeit transient and incomplete, in the manner of most repetitious compromises. Other intrapsychic, cognitive, social learning, and behavioral theories have been advanced as well (Barsky et al. 1992; Ford 1996b; Schwartz et al. 1994; Spivak et al. 1994).

Neuropathological bases for the disorders also have been suggested, on the basis of abnormal single photon emission computed tomography (SPECT) scans (Lawrie et al. 1993; Mountz et al. 1996), computed tomography (CT) abnormalities (Babe et al. 1992), magnetic resonance imaging (MRI) abnormalities (Fenelon et al. 1991), and neuropsychological testing (Pankratz and Lezak 1987). No consistent findings have yet been reported. Intriguing, however, is the suggestion that *pseudologia fantastica* may be a syndrome related to, but distinct from, factitious disorders, with its own associated pathology (Abed 1995; Hardie and Reed 1998; Mountz et al. 1996; Newmark et al. 1999).

Although many cases of factitious disorder are chronic (Sutherland and Rodin 1990; Zimmerman et al. 1991), the stressor of recurrent object loss, or fear of loss, occurs over and over in the literature as an antecedent of a factitious episode (Ballard and Stoudemire 1992; Linde 1996; Rothchild 1994; Songer 1995). For example, Carney (1980) found that 74% of his patients with factitious disorder experienced severe sexual or marital stress prior to the development of factitious signs or symptoms.

Treatment

Once the diagnosis is suspected, it is essential to examine the treatment system for countertransference reactions. Plassmann (1994b) saw the patient's ability to induce a countertransference identification in the physician as a core of the disorder, and several authors (Amirault 1995; Freyberger et al. 1994; Kalivas 1996) viewed the physician's countertransference feelings as partially diagnostic for the disorder. In general medical settings, the risk of nontherapeutic countertransference reactions usually calls for obtaining psychiatric consultation (Stotland 1989) that then often involves working with the entire treatment team of physicians, nurses, ethics and risk management committees, and others (Eisendrath and Feder 1996). In psychiatric settings, this step may call for some additional reflection on the case, a treatment planning conference, or a discussion with a clinical consultant or with colleagues. As Feldman and Feldman (1995) described, countertransference can lead to several adverse consequences. "Therapeutic nihilism" on the part of the treatment system may lead to an unexamined assumption that the patient cannot or should not be treated, with subsequent failure to diagnose or refer (Bhugra 1988; Toth and Baggaley 1991). "Anger and aversion" can rupture any therapeutic alliance, undermine the unity of a treatment team, or lead to punitive acting out against the patient. Genuine comorbid or concomitant illness may be ignored (Lewis 1993; Powell and Boast 1993a). Breaches of confidentiality may ensue in the diagnostic hunt or in the supposed effort to "warn" colleagues (Markantonakis and Lee 1988; Powell and Boast 1993a). Overidentification with the patient or activation of rescue fantasies can sabotage treatment efforts and, as Willenberg (1994) warns, can reinforce the patient's internal splitting and actually support continued factitious behaviors.

As discussed previously, the diagnosis must be confirmed. Erroneous diagnosis of a factitious disorder can result in its own trauma and may be perpetuated in medical records (Feldman et al. 1994; Guziec et al. 1994). Teasell and Shapiro (1994), however, argued against the necessity of a completely accurate diagnosis of factitious disorder once the contribution of general medical illness has been factored out. The patient then must be informed of a change in treatment plan, and an attempt must be made to enlist him or her in that plan. The literature generally refers to this process (perhaps alluding to its countertransference aspects) as containing an element of "confrontation." There is now general agreement that treatment begins at this point and that it is best done indirectly, with minimal expectation that the patient "confess" or acknowledge the deception. It is a delicate process, with patients frequently leaving the hospital against medical advice or otherwise leaving treatment (Baile et al. 1992; Baker and Major 1994; Ballas 1996; Songer 1995). Guziec et al. (1994) aptly likened this process to making a psychodynamic interpretation. Eisendrath (1989) described techniques for reducing confrontation, such as using inexact interpretations, therapeutic double binds, and other strategic and face-saving techniques to allow the patient tacitly to relinquish the factitious signs and symptoms.

Some authors recommend inpatient psychiatric hospitalization, often protracted and/or involuntary (Aduan et al. 1979; Plassmann 1994a; Powell and Boast 1993b). However, many (e.g., Ballard and Stoudemire 1992; Guziec et al. 1994; Parker 1993; Rothchild 1994; Spivak et al. 1994; Teasell and Shapiro 1994) describe treat-

ment being initiated in the general medical inpatient setting where the factitious disorder has been diagnosed and continuing in the psychiatric outpatient setting. Whereas the patient with Munchausen syndrome is regarded as less likely to engage in treatment (Eisendrath 1989; Stotland 1989), and the patient with general factitious disorder is seen as more available for intervention, there are case reports of Munchausen patients responding favorably to treatment (Parker 1993; Rothchild 1994; Spivak et al. 1994).

No comparative studies of different therapeutic approaches have been done, but several different techniques have been described. Regardless of modality, treatment must be collaborative and involve some level of communication among all of the patient's treatment providers (Eisendrath and Feder 1996; Feldman and Duval 1997; Higgins 1990). The psychodynamic approach to treatment (Plassmann 1994a; Spivak et al. 1994) generally focuses not on the factitious behaviors themselves but on the underlying dynamic issues, with the therapist taking a neutral stance toward the factitious nature of the behaviors. Strategic-behavioral approaches also have been used (Solyom and Solyom 1990; Teasell and Shapiro 1994), implementing standard behavioral techniques as well as the therapeutic double bind, in which the only way out is to abandon the target factitious behaviors. In one particularly intractable case, Schwarz et al. (1993) used a unique combination strategy, involving weekly psychotherapy provided by the primary care physician and a carefully designed paradoxical unrestricted hospital admission policy to control factitious behavior. Pharmacotherapy, when used, targets specific symptoms, such as depression or transient psychosis, or comorbid disorders. Some patients cease factitious behaviors on their own as a result of unanticipated life change (e.g., marriage or involvement in a church group that provides the requisite attention and support). Perceiving an "addictive" quality to their factitious behaviors, others have creatively evolved personal "12-step" programs that have helped them end the deceptions.

The treatment of factitious disorders is not without its pitfalls. In addition to the challenges of diagnosis and countertransference, significant medicolegal issues must be considered, both in the malpractice and in the workers' compensation arenas. Houck (1992) provided a thorough review, and Janofsky (1994) discussed several forensic cases.

Insufficient studies have been done to address conclusively the prognostic factors in factitious disorder, but children, patients with major depression, and those without personality disorders may have better prognoses (Folks 1995; Libow 2000). The literature on this disorder is certainly ample, and it implies that the factitious disorder patient, although requiring considerable therapeutic skill, may be approached with a cautious hope for improvement (Feldman 1992; Mayo and Haggerty 1984).

Factitious Disorder by Proxy

Introduction

In 1977, the British pediatrician Roy Meadow described another scenario involving factitious illness (R. Meadow 1977). He presented his observations on a number of cases in each of which a mother had intentionally induced illness in her infant, not in herself. Concealing the deception, the mother then presented the child for medical care, resulting in extensive, often invasive, evaluations and examinations of the child. The mother seemed to be very concerned and caring. Despite the outward appearance of being concerned and caring, the mother continued to fabricate illness in her child. Meadow coined the term *Munchausen syndrome by proxy* (MSBP) to describe such scenarios. The children in these situations may be subject to considerable and prolonged morbidity, with a mortality of 6%–10% (Rosenberg 1987; Schreier and Libow 1993b; Sheridan, in press).

As Schreier and Libow wrote, "With the exception perhaps of incest, this simultaneously long-term, close-yet-destructive relationship between perpetrator and victim has no parallel in human psychology" (Schreier and Libow 1993a, p. 53). Over the past decade, there has been a continued expansion of the medical literature about this type of fabricated illness, with the publication of lay and professional books on the topic (Adshead and Brooke 2001; Allison and Roberts 1998; Brownlee 1996; Feldman and Eisendrath 1996; Firstman and Talan 1997; Levin and Sheridan 1995; Schreier and Libow 1993a, 1996).

Classification

DSM-IV-TR provides research criteria for factitious disorder by proxy in the appendix "Criteria Sets and Axes Provided for Further Study" (American Psychiatric Association 2000). The criteria are similar to those for factitious disorder, with the addition of the "by proxy" specification (see Table 14–3). Much of the literature, however, retains the use of the eponym MSBP, and there is considerable debate about how best to use the terms *factitious disorder by proxy* and *MSBP* (Fisher and Mitchell 1995; R. Meadow 1995; Morley 1995).

TABLE 14–3. DSM-IV-TR research criteria for factitious disorder by proxy

A. Intentional production or feigning of physical or psychological signs or symptoms in another person who is under the individual's care.
B. The motivation for the perpetrator's behavior is to assume the sick role by proxy.
C. External incentives for the behavior (such as economic gain) are absent.
D. The behavior is not better accounted for by another mental disorder.

The debate revolves around four questions:

1. Does the syndrome require legally defined child abuse to have occurred?
2. Does the syndrome pertain to the diagnosis of an individual (implying some degree of homogeneous individual psychopathology), or does it pertain to a situation (without homogeneous psychopathology in the fabricator)?
3. Does the syndrome require an attribution or determination of the fabricator's primary motivation, and if so, what is the nature of that motivation?
4. Does the conferring of a psychiatric diagnosis mitigate the fabricator's responsibility for egregious behavior?

DSM-IV-TR uses factitious disorder by proxy to describe *a mental disorder in an individual* who is specifically motivated to attain the sick role through someone else who is under that individual's care. Technically, because factitious disorder by proxy is a research diagnosis, an individual meeting factitious disorder by proxy criteria would actually be given a diagnosis of factitious disorder not otherwise specified. The proxy, if psychiatrically diagnosed, could receive different diagnoses, depending on the circumstances and the proxy's psychiatric symptoms (American Psychiatric Association 2000).

R. Meadow (1995) used MSBP to refer to *a particular form of child abuse* characterized by a particular behavior and attitude on the part of the mother and would reserve factitious disorder by proxy as an individual diagnosis were one needed. MSBP is something a mother commits, not a disorder she has (S.R. Meadow 1995). Bools (1996) viewed the attempt to label the perpetrator of child abuse with any new diagnosis as "(pseudo) psychiatric" and reserved either term to describe a situation of child abuse. Other authors similarly use the terms to refer to situations of abuse (Blix and Brack 1988; Donald and Jureidini 1996; Fisher and

Mitchell 1995; Rosenberg 1996). In contrast to DSM-IV-TR, ICD-10 also classifies factitious disorder by proxy not as a disorder but as a form of child abuse (World Health Organization 1992).

Schreier and Libow (1993a) applied the term *MSBP* to describe a disorder in the fabricator who has a specific and particular primary motivation, which is "the mother's intense need to be in a relationship with doctors and/or hospitals. The child is used to gain and maintain this contact" (p. 13). This motivation is a true perversion in the analytical sense of the term (Schreier 1992). Schreier's (1996) later writing included perpetrators who fabricate with a proxy in order to build "a highly manipulative relationship with a powerful transferential figure," specifically "professionals who occupy positions of power in society," not just physicians.

Another authority, Ford (1996a), argued that the fabricator should receive no syndrome-related diagnosis for the factitious behavior out of concern that diagnosis may provide a legal defense for behavior he views as predominantly criminal. Uniquely, however, he would use the diagnosis of factitious disorder not otherwise specified to apply to the proxy-victim.

DSM-IV-TR criteria allow the proxy to be other than a child and the caregiver other than the mother. Although the overwhelming majority of cases involve mother and child (McClure et al. 1996), instances have been described in which the proxies were able-bodied adults or hospital and nursing home patients and the perpetrators were fathers, other relatives, baby-sitters, partners, health care professionals, or paraprofessionals (Chantada et al. 1994; Repper 1995; Sigal et al. 1986; Yorker 1996a).

The earlier discussion notwithstanding, for the purposes of this chapter, we use DSM-IV-TR terminology. We also use the terms *factitious disorder by proxy* and *MSBP* (Rappaport and Hochstadt 1993) interchangeably, rely primarily on the DSM-IV-TR research criteria, and use the paradigm of the mother perpetrator and the child proxy-victim.

Diagnosis

Certain clusters of warning signs (Table 14–4) can suggest a diagnosis of factitious disorder by proxy.

A proposed diagnostic indicator, described by Szajnberg et al. (1996), is a particular type of countertransference that the clinician experiences (even in cases in which the illness fabrication has been proven): "the clinician has a recurrent, uncanny, ego-dystonic, and uncomfortable sense of *disbelief* that this parent has perpetrated his or her child's symptoms and illness" (p. 230). They recommend that two clinicians be present during a diag-

TABLE 14–4. Warning signs for factitious disorder by proxy

The episodes of illness begin only when the child is, or has recently been, with the parent.

The parent has taken the child to numerous caregivers, resulting in multiple diagnostic evaluations but neither cure nor definitive diagnosis.

The other parent (usually the father) is notably uninvolved despite the ostensive health crises.

The parent is proved to have provided false information to health care professionals or others.

The parent is not reassured by normal test results and continually advocates for painful or risky diagnostic tests for the child.

The child persistently fails to tolerate or respond to usual medical therapies.

Signs and symptoms abate or do not occur when the child is separated from the parent.

Another child in the family has had unexplained illness or childhood death.

The parent has a personal history of factitious disorder.

Source. Data from Bools et al. 1992; Jani et al. 1992; Jureidini 1993; Libow 1995; R. Meadow 1982; Schreier and Libow 1996.

nostic factitious disorder by proxy interview: one to conduct the interview and the other to observe the interpersonal process.

Verification of the DSM-IV-TR diagnosis is a process fraught with the same type of difficulties mentioned in the discussion of factitious disorder earlier in this chapter. The mother's principal motivation must be determined (Kahan and Yorker 1991; Morley 1995; Schreier 1996), and any motivation other than attaining the sick role by proxy must be ruled out (Bools 1996; R. Meadow 1995). Also required is the determination that the mother is intentionally fabricating or inducing the child's illness. Because child abuse is a crime, proving the fabrication becomes a forensic process rather than a clinical medical investigation (Yorker 1996b). Various techniques have been used, including covert video surveillance in the hospital (Byard and Burnell 1994; Lacey et al. 1993; Samuels et al. 1992), searching rooms and belongings (Ford 1996a; Ostfeld and Feldman 1996), and special handling of laboratory specimens (Kahan and Yorker 1991). Some of these techniques raise obvious legal and ethical issues that must be resolved before their implementation (Evans 1995; Ford 1996a; Samuels et al. 1992). Once the deceptions are exposed, the intentionality usually is readily inferred, given the amount of premeditation that is required, for example, to repeatedly suffocate (Samuels et al. 1992), poison (McClure et al. 1996), or inject (Sigal et al. 1990) the proxy-victim.

The ability of the mother with factitious disorder by proxy to deceive and to appear to be a caring, concerned parent can be astounding. In one case in which the mother confessed to repeatedly poisoning two of her children with salt, the mother was "so convincing in her performance that local authorities were reported as digging up pipes in the street looking for contamination," presumably of the water supply (Coombe 1995, p. 195). Video surveillance has clearly shown how the caring presentation is a performance; when the mother thinks she is unobserved, she gives the child minimal attention (Samuels et al. 1992) or is abusive.

The cautions against making a false-positive diagnosis of factitious disorder apply to factitious disorder by proxy as well (R. Meadow 1995; Schreier and Libow 1994). Added to these risks is that of making false criminal accusations with adverse results on the involved family (Rand and Feldman 1999; Schreier and Libow 1993b).

Once factitious disorder by proxy has been diagnosed, it is important to assess the entire family, including the proxy. Other children also may be proxies, other family members may be participating in the factitious behavior, and the proxy himself or herself may be actively cooperating with the fabrications (Alexander et al. 1990; Kosmach et al. 1996; Rand 1996; Smith and Ardern 1989).

Epidemiology

The prevalence of factitious disorder by proxy is unknown, but one study estimated 2.8 cases per 100,000 children age 1 year or younger or 0.5 cases per 100,000 children age 16 years or younger (McClure et al. 1996). Among select populations, such as in cases of fevers of unknown origin (Chantada et al. 1994), discharges against medical advice (Jani et al. 1992), or pediatric specialty registers (Schreier and Libow 1993b), the rates may be substantially higher. The child typically is 2–5 years old at diagnosis (Donald and Jureidini 1996; Sheridan, in press; Yorker and Kahan 1990). Length of time from onset of symptoms in the child to diagnosis can vary widely, averaging 15 months (±14 months) in one series (Rosenberg 1987) to years in another (Libow 1995). Methods are legion, but smothering, poisoning, and fabricated history of seizures or fever are most commonly reported (McClure et al. 1996). In most cases, however, multiple methods have been used to fabricate a variety of illnesses in the child (Bools et al. 1992). Behavioral conditions and psychiatric disorders also may be feigned (Schreier 2000). In a high percentage of cases, other siblings had been proxy-victims as well (Alexander et al. 1990; Sheridan, in press).

A substantial minority (i.e., greater than would be expected in a general population sample but still the minority) of the mothers have connections to the health professions (Ostfeld and Feldman 1996), have received prior psychiatric attention (Alexander et al. 1990; Samuels et al. 1992), or have indications of preexisting factitious disorder in themselves (R. Meadow 1982). Actual psychosis is rare (Bools 1996). No consistent profile on psychological testing has been shown (Rand 1996). In contrast to factitious disorder, the most common comorbid psychiatric disorder in factitious disorder by proxy is a personality disorder (Schreier 1992), and substance use disorders are less commonly reported.

Etiology

Although perpetrators rarely make themselves available for psychiatric or psychological study, most authors postulate that the maternal pathology arises from childhood roots, characterized by "quietly traumatic" emotional neglect and abandonment. Some descriptions of the hypothesized childhood deficits suggest that they occur later than those hypothesized to result in factitious disorder, whereas other authors see the dynamics as more similar (Schreier and Libow 1993a; Sigal et al. 1988). Others have emphasized the role of modern medicine, with its predilection for invasive and aggressive diagnostic testing, in the etiology of the syndrome (Donald and Jureidini 1996). Schreier and Libow (1993a) and Parnell and Day (1998) have written extensively on the etiological hypotheses, and the reader is referred to their texts.

Treatment and Prognosis

Mothers with factitious disorder by proxy are universally regarded as very resistant and difficult to treat (Schreier and Libow 1994). Some of the difficulty stems from the mother's massive use of denial and projective identification (Coombe 1995; Feldman 1994b; Schreier 1992). Another source stems from the process by which treatment is usually initiated. Experience with factitious disorder has shown that an indirect, nonconfrontational approach is most effective and that some continuing of the factitious behavior is to be expected during the course of treatment. In factitious disorder by proxy, because of the necessity to protect the proxy, an indirect approach permitting continued factitious behavior is not possible. The first stage of treatment in factitious disorder by proxy usually begins with the involvement of child protection authorities, the initiation of legal proceedings against the parent, and the removal of the child from the home.

Treatment of factitious disorder by proxy requires coordinated multidisciplinary, multiagency involvement (Coombe 1995; Lyons-Ruth et al. 1991; Parnell and Day 1998; Smith and Ardern 1989). Individual treatment is long-term psychotherapy (group, individual, or combined) and focuses on helping the perpetrator express feelings and needs for support and recognition more directly, with less use of projection and with the development of empathic capacity (Coombe 1995; Lyons-Ruth et al. 1991). As with the treatment of factitious disorder, the factitious behavior is rarely the primary focus. Pharmacotherapy is used only to treat comorbid conditions.

One study (Berg and Jones 1999) followed up 13 mothers who were specifically selected "on the basis of the likelihood of successful intervention" for a mean of 27 months after an inpatient intervention. All of these perpetrators were atypical in that they freely admitted to having engaged in the abuse. Ten (77%) were reunited with their children, with only one recurrence of factitious disorder by proxy illness during the follow-up period. However, the results in more typical, unselected samples have been distinctly unfavorable; thus, the overall prognosis is guarded, with a high likelihood of continued factitious disorder by proxy behavior (Bools et al. 1993, 1994; Davis et al. 1998; Libow 1995; R. Meadow 1993). Management is usually coordinated and directed through the legal system, and protection of the child is the priority (Brady 1994; Kahan and Yorker 1991; Ostfeld and Feldman 1996).

Malingering

Classification

In DSM-IV-TR, malingering is classified under "Other Conditions That May Be a Focus of Clinical Attention" and is not considered to be a mental disorder or a psychiatric illness. Malingering is defined as the "intentional production of false or grossly exaggerated physical or psychological symptoms, motivated by external incentives" (American Psychiatric Association 2000, p. 739). The term *malingering by proxy* also has been suggested (Bools 1996) for those cases in which illness is fabricated in a child for secondary gain; for example, for the purpose of obtaining social assistance benefits money (Cassar et al. 1996). External incentives that may motivate a person to malinger symptoms include avoiding work, evading criminal prosecution, obtaining drugs, receiving financial compensation, avoiding military duty, or escaping other intolerable situations. DSM-IV-TR recommends that malingering be suspected if a combination of the factors listed in Table 14–5 is noted.

TABLE 14–5.   Warning signs for malingering

The individual's evaluation occurs in a medicolegal context, such as referral from an attorney.

A marked discrepancy exists between the person's claims and objective findings.

The individual is uncooperative during the diagnostic evaluation and in complying with the prescribed treatment regimen.

Antisocial personality disorder is present.

Source.   Adapted from American Psychiatric Association 2000.

Other disorders to consider in the differential diagnosis of malingering include factitious disorder, conversion disorder, and somatoform disorders. Although all three of these diagnoses may involve physical symptoms, none involve the production of symptoms for external incentives. In factitious disorder, the individual may intentionally produce symptoms because of an intrapsychic need to maintain the sick role. Individuals with a conversion disorder or somatoform disorder experience symptoms that cannot be fully explained by a medical condition and are often connected to psychological reasons of which the person is unaware. Finally, individuals who confabulate should be distinguished from malingerers because they are unintentionally filling in information that they believed to have happened, when, in fact, it did not happen at all (Newmark et al. 1999; Resnick 2000).

Diagnostic confusion between malingering and other mental disorders, particularly factitious disorders, can be traced to Asher's (1951) original description of Munchausen syndrome. He attributed several possible motives for Munchausen syndrome, including "a desire to escape from the police" and "a desire to get free board and lodgings for the night" (p. 339), motives that would now clearly classify feigned illness behavior as malingering. The tendency to include malingering within the factitious disorders spectrum was further reinforced by Spiro (1968), who recommended that in individuals with Munchausen syndrome, "malingering should only be diagnosed in the absence of psychiatric illness and the presence of behavior appropriately adaptive to a clear-cut long-term goal" (p. 569). There are, however, many examples of patients with factitious disorder who also malinger (see "Diagnosis" subsection of "Factitious Disorder" section earlier in this chapter).

Diagnosis

Malingering is "so easy to define but so difficult to diagnose" (Resnick 1997). When a clinician suspects that a symptom may be fabricated or exaggerated, he or she should be on alert for various inconsistencies that may appear in the individual's evaluation. First, the individual may present inconsistencies in what he or she actually reports. For example, a person may report that he or she is currently unable to talk while speaking eloquently throughout the interview. Second, a malingerer's observed behavior may differ significantly from the symptoms he or she reports. The person who describes active, continuous, disturbing hallucinations during the interview but shows no evidence of distraction illustrates this type of inconsistency suggestive of malingering. Third, malingerers may behave in a dramatically different way depending on who they believe is observing them. This disparity in presentation is illustrated by a person who acts in a confused, disoriented manner in the clinician's office and shortly after leaving is observed by ward staff winning a brilliant game of chess. Fourth, psychological test data may be inconsistent with the history provided by malingerers. Finally, malingerers often report symptoms that are inconsistent with how genuine symptoms normally manifest. The better clinicians understand characteristics of a true illness, the more likely they will be able to detect feigned symptoms (Resnick 2000).

Physicians are trained to assess and treat individuals who actually have medical or mental health symptoms. A care provider's natural inclination is to accept the person's reported symptoms at face value. Rosenhan (2001) conducted a famous study that showed clinicians' tendency to blindly accept reported mental health symptoms. In this study, eight non–mentally ill individuals presented to a psychiatric hospital alleging that they were hearing very atypical voices. Based on this one reported symptom, every person was admitted to the hospital and given schizophrenia diagnoses, even though each person ceased reporting any symptom after admission.

Table 14–6 provides a suggested clinical decision model for the assessment of malingered psychosis (Resnick 1997). In determining whether reported hallucinations or delusions are fabricated or exaggerated, the factors outlined in Table 14–7 also may prove helpful (Resnick 1997). Note that a bona fide diagnosis of a past psychotic disorder does not necessarily exclude a presentation of manufactured psychotic symptoms (Tyrer et al. 2001).

When evaluating possible malingering, the clinician should consider obtaining additional information from collateral sources and psychological testing to verify the person's reported symptoms. In addition to the clinical interview, sources of information that may be useful include interviews with family members, friends, co-workers, employers, clinical staff, other therapists, jail or prison personnel, and probation or parole officers. Records often relevant to the malingering assessment include past medical records, psychiatric records, educa-

---

TABLE 14–6. Clinical decision model for the assessment of malingering

The evaluee's presentation meets the following criteria:

A. Understandable motive to malinger.

B. Marked variability of presentation as observed in at least one of the following:
   1. Marked discrepancies in interview and noninterview behavior.
   2. Gross inconsistencies in reported psychotic symptoms.
   3. Blatant contradictions between reported prior episodes and documented psychiatric history.

C. Improbable psychiatric symptoms as evidenced by one or more of the following:
   1. Reporting elaborate psychotic symptoms that lack common paranoid, grandiose, or religious themes.
   2. Sudden emergence of purported psychotic symptoms to explain antisocial behavior.
   3. Atypical hallucinations or delusions (see Table 14–7).

D. Confirmation of malingered psychosis by either
   1. Admission of malingering following confrontation.
   2. Presence of strong corroborative information, such as psychometric data or history of malingering.

TABLE 14–7. Threshold model for the assessment of hallucinations and delusions

Malingering should be suspected if any combination of the following are observed:

Hallucinations
Continuous rather than intermittent hallucinations
Vague or inaudible hallucinations
Hallucinations not associated with delusions
Stilted language reported in hallucinations
Inability to state strategies to diminish voices
Self-report that all command hallucinations were obeyed
Visual hallucinations in black and white

Delusions
Abrupt onset or termination
Eagerness to call attention to delusions
Conduct markedly inconsistent with delusions
Bizarre content without disordered thinking

---

tional records, work records, rap sheets, court evaluations, and prior disability claims. Psychological testing is often used in malingering assessments and may include structured interviews to evaluate psychotic symptoms (Rogers 1992), various personality inventories, and neuropsychological testing to assess cognitive deficits (Liebson et al. 1996). Witztum et al. (1996) described several military inductees who received erroneous diagnoses of malingering; diagnoses of severe psychiatric disorders were missed because of assessment problems. They also noted, as did

DuAlba and Scott (1993), the important role of cross-cultural issues in the assessment of malingering.

Epidemiology

Malingering of psychiatric symptoms is not a rare event. In a study of malingered mental illness in a metropolitan emergency department, 13% of patients were strongly suspected or considered to be malingering. Reasons identified for malingering included seeking hospitalization for food and shelter, attempting to gain medication, attempting to avoid incarceration, and seeking financial gain (Yates et al. 1996). Rogers et al. (1993) estimated that approximately half of the individuals evaluated for personal injury claims were feigning all or part of their cognitive deficits. In a survey of forensic mental health experts, approximately 17% of the individuals evaluated in forensic settings and nearly 8% of those evaluated in nonforensic settings were assessed as malingering (Rogers 1997). Finally, in a study of individuals referred for evaluation of insanity, more than 20% of the defendants received diagnoses of suspected or definite malingering (Rogers and Shuman 2000).

Treatment

When a determination of malingering is made, the clinician is faced with the dilemma of how to "treat" a non-disorder. Depending on the situation, the clinician may elect to confront the individual with the assessment. Pankratz and Erickson (1990) emphasized the importance of permitting the malingerer to save face. Possible verbal interventions include statements such as "You haven't told me the whole truth" or "The type of symptoms that you are reporting are not consistent with known mental illness" (Inbau and Reid 1967). The clinician should be prepared for some individuals to react defensively and to refuse to accept this diagnosis, even when faced with strong evidence that they are faking symptoms. In contrast, when other individuals are confronted, they admit that their symptoms were faked and give up the charade. Finally, many of Houck's (1992) warnings about the medicolegal pitfalls in the assessment and treatment of a factitious disorder also apply to the assessment and disposition of the malingerer.

References

Abed RT: Voluntary false confessions in a Munchausen patient: a new variant of the syndrome? Irish Journal of Psychological Medicine 12:24–26, 1995

Adshead G, Brooke D (eds): Munchausen's Syndrome By Proxy: Current Issues in Assessment, Treatment and Research. London, England, Imperial College Press, 2001

Aduan RP, Fauci AS, Dale DC, et al: Factitious fever and self-induced infection: a report of 32 cases and review of the literature. Ann Intern Med 90:230–242, 1979

Alexander R, Smith W, Stevenson R: Serial Munchausen syndrome by proxy. Pediatrics 86:581–585, 1990

Allison DB, Roberts MS: Disordered Mother or Disordered Diagnosis? Munchausen By Proxy Syndrome. Hillsdale, NJ, Analytic Press, 1998

American Psychiatric Association: Diagnostic and Statistical Manual of Mental Disorders, 4th Edition, Text Revision. Washington, DC, American Psychiatric Association, 2000

Amirault C: Pseudologica fantastica and other tall tales: the contagious literature of Munchausen syndrome. Lit Med 14:169–190, 1995

Asher R: Munchausen's syndrome. Lancet 1:339–341, 1951

Babe KS Jr, Peterson AM, Loosen PT, et al: The pathogenesis of Munchausen syndrome: a review and case report. Gen Hosp Psychiatry 14:273–276, 1992

Baddley J, Daberkow D, Hilton C: Insulinoma masquerading as factitious hypoglycemia. South Med J 91:1067–1069, 1998

Baile WF Jr, Kuehn CV, Straker D: Factitious cancer. Psychosomatics 33:100–105, 1992

Baker CE, Major E: Munchausen's syndrome: a case presenting as asthma requiring ventilation. Anaesthesia 49:1050–1051, 1994

Ballard RS, Stoudemire A: Factitious apraxia. Int J Psychiatry Med 22:275–280, 1992

Ballas S: Factitious sickle cell acute painful episodes: a secondary type of Munchausen syndrome. Am J Hematol 53:254–258, 1996

Bappal B, George M, Nair R, et al: Factitious hypoglycemia: a tale from the Arab world. Pediatrics 107:180–181, 2001

Barker JC: The syndrome of hospital addiction (Munchausen syndrome): a report on the investigation of seven cases. Journal of Mental Science 108:167–182, 1962

Barsky AJMD, Wyshak G, Klerman GL: Psychiatric comorbidity in DSM-III-R hypochondriasis. Arch Gen Psychiatry 49:101–108, 1992

Bauer M, Boegner F: Neurological syndromes in factitious disorder. J Nerv Ment Dis 184:281–288, 1996

Berg B, Jones D: Outcome of psychiatric intervention in factitious illness by proxy (Munchausen's syndrome by proxy). Arch Dis Child 81:465–472, 1999

Bhugra D: Psychiatric Munchausen's syndrome: literature review with case reports. Acta Psychiatr Scand 77:497–503, 1988

Blix S, Brack G: The effects of a suspected case of Munchausen's syndrome by proxy on a pediatric nursing staff. Gen Hosp Psychiatry 10:402–409, 1988

Bools C: Factitious illness by proxy: Munchausen syndrome by proxy. Br J Psychiatry 169:268–275, 1996

Bools CN, Neale BA, Meadow SR: Co-morbidity associated with fabricated illness (Munchausen syndrome by proxy). Arch Dis Child 67:77–79, 1992

Bools CN, Neale BA, Meadow SR: Follow up of victims of fabricated illness (Munchausen syndrome by proxy). Arch Dis Child 69:625–630, 1993

Bools C, Neale B, Meadow R: Munchausen syndrome by proxy: a study of psychopathology. Child Abuse Negl 18:773–788, 1994

Brady MM: Munchausen syndrome by proxy: how should we weigh our options? Law and Psychology Review 18:361–375, 1994

Brownlee S: Mother love betrayed: children are tools for parents with a rare psychiatric disorder. U.S. News and World Report 120:29, 1996

Burge CK, Lacey JH: A case of Munchausen's syndrome in anorexia nervosa. Int J Eat Disord 14:379–381, 1993

Byard RW, Burnell RH: Covert video surveillance in Munchausen syndrome by proxy: ethical compromise or essential technique? Med J Aust 160:352–356, 1994

Carney MW: Artefactual illness to attract medical attention. Br J Psychiatry 136:542–547, 1980

Carswell J: The Romantic Rogue; Being the Singular Life and Adventures of Rudolph Eric Raspe, Creator of Baron Munchausen. New York, Dutton, 1950

Cassar J, Hales E, Longhurst J, et al: Can disability benefits make children sicker? J Am Acad Child Adolesc Psychiatry 35:700–701, 1996

Chantada G, Casak S, Plata JD, et al: Children with fever of unknown origin in Argentina: an analysis of 113 cases. Pediatr Infect Dis J 13:260–263, 1994

Chapman JS: Peregrinating problem patients; Munchausen's syndrome. JAMA 165:927–933, 1957

Churchill DR, De Cock KM, Miller RF: Feigned HIV infection/AIDS: malingering and Munchausen's syndrome. Genitourinary Medicine 70:314–316, 1994

Cizza G, Nieman L, Doppman J, et al: Factitious Cushing syndrome. J Clin Endocrinol Metab 81:3573–3577, 1996

Clarke E, Melnick SC: The Munchausen syndrome or the problem of hospital hoboes. Am J Med 25:6–12, 1958

Clinical Case Conference: Case records of the Massachusetts General Hospital: Weekly clinicopathological exercises. Case 28-1984: a 39-year-old man with gas in the soft tissues of the left forearm. N Engl J Med 311:108–115, 1984

Coombe P: The inpatient psychotherapy of a mother and child at the Cassel Hospital: a case of Munchausen's syndrome by proxy. British Journal of Psychotherapy 12:195–207, 1995

Craddock N, Brown N: Munchausen syndrome presenting as mental handicap. Mental Handicap Research 6:184–190, 1993

Davis P, McClure R, Rolfe K, et al: Procedures, placement, and risks of further abuse after Munchausen syndrome by proxy, non-accidental poisoning, and non-accidental suffocation. Arch Dis Child 78:217–221, 1998

Dixon D, Abbey S: Cupid's arrow: an unusual presentation of factitious disorder. Psychosomatics 36:502–504, 1995

Donald T, Jureidini J: Munchausen syndrome by proxy: child abuse in the medical system. Arch Pediatr Adolesc Med 150:753–758, 1996

DuAlba L, Scott RL: Somatization and malingering for workers' compensation applicants: a cross-cultural MMPI study. J Clin Psychol 49:913–917, 1993

Duffy TP: The Red Baron. N Engl J Med 327:408–411, 1992

Duffy TP: Kidney-related Munchausen's syndrome and the Red Baron. N Engl J Med 328:61–62, 1993

Eisendrath SJ: Factitious physical disorders: treatment without confrontation. Psychosomatics 30:383–387, 1989

Eisendrath SJ: Factitious physical disorders. West J Med 160:177–179, 1994

Eisendrath SJ: Current overview of factitious physical disorders, in The Spectrum of Factitious Disorders. Edited by Feldman MD, Eisendrath SJ. Washington, DC, American Psychiatric Press, 1996, pp 21–36

Eisendrath SJ, Feder A: Management of factitious disorders, in The Spectrum of Factitious Disorders. Edited by Feldman MD, Eisendrath SJ. Washington, DC, American Psychiatric Press, 1996, pp 195–213

Evans D: The investigation of life-threatening child abuse and Munchausen syndrome by proxy. J Med Ethics 21:9–13, 1995

Feldman MD: Factitious Munchausen's syndrome: a confession. N Engl J Med 327:438–439, 1992

Feldman MD: The costs of factitious disorders. Psychosomatics 35:506–507, 1994a

Feldman MD: Denial in Munchausen syndrome by proxy: the consulting psychiatrist's dilemma. Int J Psychiatry Med 24:121–128, 1994b

Feldman M: Munchausen by Internet: detecting factitious illness and crisis on the Internet. South Med J 93:669–672, 2000

Feldman MD: Factitious Disorders, Munchausen, and Munchausen by Proxy Web page. Available at http://munchausen.com. Accessed July 1, 2001

Feldman M, Duval N: Factitious quadriplegia: a rare new case and literature review. Psychosomatics 38:76–80, 1997

Feldman MD, Eisendrath SJ (eds): The Spectrum of Factitious Disorders. Washington, DC, American Psychiatric Press, 1996

Feldman MD, Feldman JM: Tangled in the web: countertransference in the therapy of factitious disorders. Int J Psychiatry Med 25:389–399, 1995

Feldman MD, Russell JL: Factitious cyclic hypersomnia: a new variant of factitious disorder. South Med J 84:379–381, 1991

Feldman MD, Smith R: Personal and interpersonal toll of factitious disorders, in The Spectrum of Factitious Disorders. Edited by Feldman MD, Eisendrath SJ. Washington, DC, American Psychiatric Press, 1996, pp 175–194

Feldman MD, Ford CV, Reinhold T: Patient or Pretender: Inside the Strange World of Factitious Disorders. New York, Wiley, 1994

Feldman MD, Hamilton JC, Deemer HN: A critical analysis of factitious disorders, in Somatoform and Factitious Disorders. Edited by Phillips KA. Washington, DC, American Psychiatric Publishing, 2001, pp 129–166

Fenelon G, Mahieux F, Roullet E, et al: Munchausen's syndrome and abnormalities on magnetic resonance imaging of the brain. BMJ 302:996–997, 1991

Firstman R, Talan J: The Death of Innocents. New York, Bantam Books, 1997

Fisher GC, Mitchell I: Is Munchausen syndrome by proxy really a syndrome? Arch Dis Child 72:530–534, 1995

Folks DG: Munchausen's syndrome and other factitious disorders. Neurol Clin 13:267–281, 1995

Ford CV: The somatizing disorders. Psychosomatics 27:327–331, 335–337, 1986

Ford CV: Ethical and legal issues in factitious disorders: an overview, in The Spectrum of Factitious Disorders. Edited by Feldman MD, Eisendrath SJ. Washington, DC, American Psychiatric Press, 1996a, pp 51–63

Ford CV: Lies! Lies!! Lies!!! The Psychology of Deceit. Washington, DC, American Psychiatric Press, 1996b

Freyberger HJ, Schneider W: Diagnosis and classification of factitious disorder with operational diagnostic systems. Psychother Psychosom 62:27–29, 1994

Freyberger H, Nordmeyer JP, Freyberger HJ, et al: Patients suffering from factitious disorders in the clinico-psychosomatic consultation liaison service: psychodynamic processes, psychotherapeutic initial care and clinico-interdisciplinary cooperation. Psychother Psychosom 62:108–122, 1994

Frumkin LR, Victoroff JI: Chronic factitious disorder with symptoms of AIDS. Am J Med 88:694–696, 1990

Gavin H: On Feigned and Factitious Diseases, Chiefly of Soldiers and Seamen, on the Means Used to Simulate or Produce Them, and on the Best Mode of Discovering Imposters: Being the Prize Essay in the Class of Military Surgery, in the University of Edinburgh, Session, 1835-6, With Additions. London, England, John Churchill Princes Street Soho, 1843

Gielder U: Factitious disease in the field of dermatology. Psychother Psychosom 62:48–55, 1994

Goodwin J: Munchausen's syndrome as a dissociative disorder. Dissociation: Progress in the Dissociative Disorders 1:54–60, 1988

Gorman WF, Winograd M: Crossing the border from Munchausen to malingering. J Fla Med Assoc 75:147–150, 1988

Gurwith M, Langston C: Factitious Munchausen's syndrome: a confession—reply (letter). N Engl J Med 327:439, 1992

Guziec J, Lazarus A, Harding JJ: Case of a 29-year-old nurse with factitious disorder: the utility of psychiatric intervention on a general medical floor. Gen Hosp Psychiatry 16:47–53, 1994

Hardie T, Reed A: Pseudologia fantastica, factitious disorder and impostership: a deception syndrome. Med Sci Law 38:198–201, 1998

Harrington WZ, Jackimczyk KC, Seligson RA: Thiopental-facilitated interview in respiratory Munchausen's syndrome. Ann Emerg Med 19:941–942, 1990

Higgins PM: Temporary Munchausen syndrome. Br J Psychiatry 157:613–616, 1990

Hirsch M: The body as a transitional object. Psychother Psychosom 62:78–81, 1994

Houck CA: Medicolegal aspects of factitious disorder. Psychiatric Medicine 10:105–116, 1992

Ifudu O, Friedman EA: Kidney-related Munchausen's syndrome and the Red Baron (letter). N Engl J Med 328:61, 1993

Ifudu O, Kolasinski SL, Friedman EA: Brief report: kidney-related Munchausen's syndrome. N Engl J Med 327:388–389, 1992

Inbau FE, Reid JE: Criminal Interrogation and Confessions. Baltimore, MD, Williams & Wilkins, 1967

Jani S, White M, Rosenberg LA, et al: Munchausen syndrome by proxy. Int J Psychiatry Med 22:343–349, 1992

Janofsky JS: The Munchausen syndrome in civil forensic psychiatry. Bulletin of the American Academy of Psychiatry and the Law 22:489–497, 1994

Joseph-Di Caprio J, Remafedi GJ: Adolescents with factitious HIV disease. J Adolesc Health 21:102–106, 1997

Jureidini J: Obstetric factitious disorder and Munchausen syndrome by proxy. J Nerv Ment Dis 181:135–137, 1993

Kahan B, Yorker BC: Munchausen syndrome by proxy: clinical review and legal issues. Behav Sci Law 9:73–83, 1991

Kalivas J: Malingering versus factitious disorder (letter). Am J Psychiatry 153:1108, 1996

Kasdan ML, Soergel TM, Johnson AL, et al: Expanded profile of the SHAFT syndrome. J Hand Surg [Am] 23:26–31, 1998

Kent JD: Munchausen's syndrome and substance abuse. J Subst Abuse Treat 11:247–251, 1994

Khan I, Fayaz I, Ridgley J, et al: Factitious clock drawing and constructional apraxia. J Neurol Neurosurg Psychiatry 68:106–107, 2000

Koo J, Gambla C, Fried R: Pseudopsychodermatologic disease. Dermatol Clin 14:525–530, 1996

Kosmach B, Tarbell S, Reyes J, et al: "Munchausen by proxy" syndrome in a small bowel transplant recipient. Transplant Proc 28:2790–2791, 1996

Lacey SR, Cooper C, Runyan DK, et al: Munchausen syndrome by proxy: patterns of presentation to pediatric surgeons. J Pediatr Surg 28:827–832, 1993

Lawrie SM, Goodwin G, Masterton G: Munchausen's syndrome and organic brain disorder. Br J Psychiatry 162:545–549, 1993

Levin AV, Sheridan MS (eds): Munchausen Syndrome by Proxy: Issues in Diagnosis and Treatment. New York, Lexington Books, 1995

Lewis EJ: Kidney-related Munchausen's syndrome and the Red Baron. N Engl J Med 328:60–61, 1993

Libow JA: Munchausen by proxy victims in adulthood: a first look. Child Abuse Negl 19:1131–1142, 1995

Libow J: Child and adolescent illness falsification. Pediatrics 105:336–342, 2000

Liebson E, White R, Albert M: Cognitive inconsistencies in abnormal illness behavior and neurological disease. J Nerv Ment Dis 184:122–125, 1996

Linde P: A bewitching case of factitious disorder in Zimbabwe. Gen Hosp Psychiatry 18:440–443, 1996

Ludwigs U, Ruiz H, Isaksson H, et al: Factitious disorder presenting with acute cardiovascular symptoms. J Intern Med 236:685–690, 1994

Lyons-Ruth K, Kaufman M, Masters N, et al: Issues in the identification and long-term management of Munchausen by proxy syndrome within a clinical infant service. Infant Mental Health Journal 12:309–320, 1991

Markantonakis A, Lee AS: Psychiatric Munchausen's syndrome: a college register (letter). Br J Psychiatry 152:867, 1988

Mayo JP Jr, Haggerty JJ Jr: Long-term psychotherapy of Munchausen syndrome. Am J Psychother 38:571–578, 1984

McClure RJ, Davis PM, Meadow SR, et al: Epidemiology of Munchausen syndrome by proxy, non-accidental poisoning, and non-accidental suffocation. Arch Dis Child 75:57–61, 1996

McDaniel JS, Desoutter L, Firestone S, et al: Factitious disorder resulting in bilateral mastectomies. Gen Hosp Psychiatry 14:355–356, 1992

Meadow R: Munchausen syndrome by proxy: the hinterland of child abuse. Lancet 2:343–345, 1977

Meadow R: Munchausen syndrome by proxy. Arch Dis Child 57:92–98, 1982

Meadow R: False allegations of abuse and Munchausen syndrome by proxy. Arch Dis Child 68:444–447, 1993

Meadow R: What is, and what is not, 'Munchausen syndrome by proxy'? Arch Dis Child 72:534–538, 1995

Meadow SR: Munchausen syndrome by proxy. Med Leg J 63:89–104, 1995

Miner I, Feldman M: Factitious deafblindness: an imperceptible variant of factitious disorder. Gen Hosp Psychiatry 20:48–51, 1998

Mizuta I, Fukunaga T, Sato H, et al: A case report of comorbid eating disorder and factitious disorder. Psychiatry Clin Neurosci 54:603–606, 2000

Morley CJ: Practical concerns about the diagnosis of Munchausen syndrome by proxy. Arch Dis Child 72:528–529, 1995

Mountz JM, Parker PE, Liu HG, et al: Tc-99m HMPAO brain SPECT scanning in Munchausen syndrome. J Psychiatry Neurosci 21:49–52, 1996

Nadelson T: The Munchausen spectrum: borderline character features. Gen Hosp Psychiatry 1:11–17, 1979

Newmark N, Adityanjee, Kay J: Pseudologia fantastica and factitious disorder: review of the literature and a case report. Compr Psychiatry 40:89–95, 1999

Nordmeyer JP: An internist's view of patients with factitious disorders and factitious clinical symptomatology. Psychother Psychosom 62:30–40, 1994

Ostfeld BM, Feldman MD: Factitious disorder by proxy: clinical features, detection, and management, in The Spectrum of Factitious Disorders. Edited by Feldman MD, Eisendrath SJ. Washington, DC, American Psychiatric Press, 1996, pp 83–108

Overholser JC: Differential diagnosis of malingering and factitious disorder with physical symptoms. Special Issue: Malingering and Deception: An Update. Behav Sci Law 8:55–65, 1990

Paar GH: Factitious disorders in the field of surgery. Psychother Psychosom 62:41–47, 1994

Pankratz L, Erickson RC: Two views of malingering. Clinical Neuropsychologist 4:379–389, 1990

Pankratz L, Lezak MD: Cerebral dysfunction in the Munchausen syndrome. Hillside Journal of Clinical Psychiatry 9:195–206, 1987

Parker PE: A case report of Munchausen syndrome with mixed psychological features. Psychosomatics 34:360–364, 1993

Parnell TF, Day DO: Munchausen by Proxy Syndrome: Misunderstood Child Abuse. Thousand Oaks, CA, Sage Publications, 1998

Parsons T: The Social System. Glencoe, IL, Free Press, 1951

Pfefferbaum B, Allen J, Lindsey E, et al: Fabricated trauma exposure: an analysis of cognitive, behavioral, and emotional factors. Psychiatry 62:293–302, 1999

Plassmann R: Inpatient and outpatient long-term psychotherapy of patients suffering from factitious disorder. Psychother Psychosom 62:96–107, 1994a

Plassmann R: Munchausen syndromes and factitious diseases. Psychother Psychosom 62:7–26, 1994b

Plassmann R: Structural disturbances in the body self. Psychother Psychosom 62:91–95, 1994c

Popli AP, Masand PS, Dewan MJ: Factitious disorders with psychological symptoms. J Clin Psychiatry 53:315–318, 1992

Powell R, Boast N: The million dollar man: resource implications for chronic Munchausen's syndrome. Br J Psychiatry 162:253–256, 1993a

Powell R, Boast N: Resource implications of Munchausen's syndrome (letter). Br J Psychiatry 162:848, 1993b

Rand DC: Comprehensive psychosocial assessment in factitious disorder by proxy, in The Spectrum of Factitious Disorders. Edited by Feldman MD, Eisendrath SJ. Washington, DC, American Psychiatric Press, 1996, pp 109–133

Rand DC, Feldman MD: Misdiagnosis of Munchausen syndrome by proxy: a literature review and four new cases (review). Harv Rev Psychiatry 7:94–101, 1999

Rappaport SR, Hochstadt NJ: Munchausen syndrome by proxy (MSBP): an intergenerational perspective. Journal of Mental Health Counseling 15:278–289, 1993

Raspe RE: Gulliver Revived Containing Singular Travels, Campaigns, Voyages, and Adventures, in Russia, Iceland, Turkey, Egypt, Gibraltar, Up the Mediterranean, and on the Atlantic Ocean: Also, an Account of a Voyage Into the Moon, With Many Extraordinary Particulars Relative to the Cooking Animal, in That Planet, Which Are Here Called the Human Species, 4th Edition. Norfolk, VA, John M'Lean, 1787

Reich P, Gottfried LA: Factitious disorders in a teaching hospital. Ann Intern Med 99:240–247, 1983

Repper J: Munchausen syndrome by proxy in health care workers. J Adv Nurs 21:299–304, 1995

Resnick PJ: Malingered psychosis, in Clinical Assessment of Malingering and Deception, 2nd Edition. Edited by Rogers R. New York, Guilford, 1997, pp 47–67

Resnick PJ: The clinical assessment of malingered mental illness, in Annual Board Review Course Syllabus. Bloomfield, CT, American Academy of Psychiatry and the Law, 2000, pp 842–866

Rogers R: Structured Interview of Reported Symptoms. Odessa, FL, Psychological Assessment Resources, 1992

Rogers R: Introduction, in Clinical Assessment of Malingering and Deception, 2nd Edition. Edited by Rogers R. New York, Guilford, 1997, pp 1–9

Rogers R, Shuman DW: Conducting Insanity Evaluations, 2nd Edition. New York, Guilford, 2000

Rogers R, Bagby RM, Rector N: Diagnostic legitimacy of factitious disorder with psychological symptoms. Am J Psychiatry 146:1312–1314, 1989

Rogers R, Harrell EH, Liff CD: Feigning neuropsychological impairment: a critical review of methodological and clinical considerations. Clin Psychol Rev 13:255–274, 1993

Rosenberg DA: Web of deceit: a literature review of Munchausen syndrome by proxy. Child Abuse Negl 11:547–563, 1987

Rosenberg D: Child neglect and Munchausen syndrome by proxy. Washington, DC, National Criminal Justice Reference Service, 1996

Rosenhan DL: On being sane in insane places, in Down to Earth Sociology: Introductory Readings, 11th Edition. Edited by Henslin JA. New York, Free Press, 2001, pp 278–289

Rothchild E: Fictitious twins, factitious illness. Psychiatry 57:326–332, 1994

Roy M, Roy A: Factitious hypoglycemia: an 11-year follow-up. Psychosomatics 36:64–65, 1995

Samuels MP, McClaughlin W, Jacobson RR, et al: Fourteen cases of imposed upper airway obstruction. Arch Dis Child 67:162–170, 1992

Schreier HA: The perversion of mothering: Munchausen syndrome by proxy. Bull Menninger Clin 56:421–437, 1992

Schreier HA: Repeated false allegations of sexual abuse presenting to sheriffs: when is it Munchausen by proxy? Child Abuse Negl 20:985–991, 1996

Schreier H: Factitious disorder by proxy in which the presenting problem is behavioral or psychiatric. J Am Acad Child Adolesc Psychiatry 39:668–670, 2000

Schreier HA, Libow JA: Hurting for Love: Munchausen by Proxy Syndrome. New York, Guilford, 1993a

Schreier HA, Libow JA: Munchausen syndrome by proxy: diagnosis and prevalence. Am J Orthopsychiatry 63:318–321, 1993b

Schreier HA, Libow JA: Munchausen by proxy syndrome: a clinical fable for our times. J Am Acad Child Adolesc Psychiatry 33:904–905, 1994

Schreier HA, Libow JA: Munchasusen by proxy: the deadly game. Saturday Evening Post 268:40–41, 1996

Schwartz SM, Gramling SE, Mancini T: The influence of life stress, personality, and learning history on illness behavior. J Behav Ther Exp Psychiatry 25:135–142, 1994

Schwarz K, Harding R, Harrington D, et al: Hospital management of a patient with intractable factitious disorder. Psychosomatics 34:265–267, 1993

Seersholm NJ, Frolich S, Jensen NH, et al: Factitious disorder: an iatrogenic disease? Ugeskr Laeger 153:2133–2135, 1991

Sheridan MS: The deceit continues: an updated literature review of Munchausen syndrome by proxy. Child Abuse Negl (in press)

Sigal MD, Altmark D, Carmel I: Munchausen syndrome by adult proxy: a perpetrator abusing two adults. J Nerv Ment Dis 174:696–698, 1986

Sigal M, Carmel I, Altmark D, et al: Munchausen syndrome by proxy: a psychodynamic analysis. Med Law 7:49–56, 1988

Sigal M, Gelkopf M, Levertov G: Medical and legal aspects of the Munchausen by proxy perpetrator. Med Law 9:739–749, 1990

Smith NJ, Ardern MH: "More in sickness than in health": a case study of Munchausen by proxy in the elderly. Journal of Family Therapy 11:321–334, 1989

Solyom C, Solyom L: A treatment program for functional paraplegia/Munchausen syndrome. J Behav Ther Exp Psychiatry 21:225–230, 1990

Songer DA: Factitious AIDS: a case reported and literature review. Psychosomatics 36:406–411, 1995

Spiro HR: Chronic factitious illness: Munchausen's syndrome. Arch Gen Psychiatry 18:569–579, 1968

Spivak H, Rodin G, Sutherland A: The psychology of factitious disorders: a reconsideration. Psychosomatics 35:25–34, 1994

Stotland NL: Munchausen syndrome. JAMA 261:447, 1989

Sutherland AJ, Rodin GM: Factitious disorders in a general hospital setting: clinical features and a review of the literature. Psychosomatics 31:392–399, 1990

Szajnberg NM, Moilanen I, Kanerva A, et al: Munchausen-by-proxy syndrome: countertransference as a diagnostic tool. Bull Menninger Clin 60:229–237, 1996

Teasell RW, Shapiro AP: Strategic-behavioral intervention in the treatment of chronic non-organic motor disorders. Am J Phys Med Rehabil 73:44–50, 1994

Topazian M, Binder HJ: Factitious diarrhea detected by measurement of stool osmolality. N Engl J Med 330:1418–1419, 1994

Toth EL, Baggaley A: Coexistence of Munchausen's syndrome and multiple personality disorder: detailed report of a case and theoretical discussion. Psychiatry 54:176–186, 1991

Tyrer P, Babidge N, Emmanuel J, et al: Instrumental psychosis: the good soldier Svejk syndrome. J R Soc Med 94:22–25, 2001

Wallach J: Laboratory diagnosis of factitious disorders. Arch Intern Med 154:1690–1696, 1994

Willenberg H: Countertransference in factitious disorder. Psychother Psychosom 62:129–134, 1994

Witztum E, Grinshpoon A, Margolin J, et al.: The erroneous diagnosis of malingering in a military setting. Mil Med 161:225–229, 1996

World Health Organization: The ICD-10 Classification of Mental and Behavioral Disorders. Geneva, Switzerland, World Health Organization, 1992

Yates BD, Nordquist CR, Schultz-Ross RA: Feigned psychiatric symptoms in the emergency room. Psychiatr Serv 47:998 1000, 1996

Yorker BC: Hospital epidemics of factitious disorder by proxy, in The Spectrum of Factitious Disorders. Edited by Feldman MD, Eisendrath SJ. Washington, DC, American Psychiatric Press, 1996a, pp 157–174

Yorker BC: Legal issues in factitious disorder by proxy, in The Spectrum of Factitious Disorders. Edited by Feldman MD, Eisendrath SJ. Washington, DC, American Psychiatric Press, 1996b, pp 135–156

Yorker BC, Kahan BB: Munchausen's syndrome by proxy as a form of child abuse. Arch Psychiatr Nurs 4:313–318, 1990

Zimmerman JG, Hussian RA, Tintner R, et al: Factitious disorder in a geriatric patient. Clin Gerontol 11:3–11, 1991

Ziv I, Djaldetti R, Zoldan Y, et al: Diagnosis of "non-organic" limb paresis by a novel objective motor assessment: the quantitative Hoover's test. J Neurol 245:797–802, 1998

Dissociative Disorders

José R. Maldonado, M.D.

David Spiegel, M.D.

The dissociative disorders involve a disturbance in the integrated organization of identity, memory, perception, or consciousness. Events normally experienced on a smooth continuum are isolated from the other mental processes with which they would ordinarily be associated. This isolation results in a variety of dissociative disorders depending on the primary cognitive process affected. When memories are poorly integrated, the resulting disorder is *dissociative amnesia.* Fragmentation of identity results in *dissociative fugue* or *dissociative identity disorder* (DID; formerly multiple personality disorder). Disordered perception yields *depersonalization disorder.* Dissociation of aspects of consciousness produces *acute stress disorder* and various dissociative trance and possession states (see Table 15–1).

These dissociative disorders are a disturbance more in the organization or structure of mental contents than in the contents themselves. Memories in dissociative amnesia are not so much distorted or bizarre as they are segregated from one another. The identity temporarily lost in dissociative fugue, or the aspects of the self that are fragmented in DID, are two-dimensional aspects of an overall personality structure. In this sense, it has been said that patients with DID suffer not from having more than one personality, but rather from having less than one personality. The problem is the failure of integration rather than the contents of the fragments. In summary, all types of dissociative disorders have in common a lack of immediate access to the entire personality structure or mental content in one form or another.

The dissociative disorders have a long history in classical psychopathology but until recently have been largely ignored. Nonetheless, the phenomena are sufficiently persistent and interesting that they have elicited growing attention from both professionals and the public. The dis-

TABLE 15–1. DSM-IV-TR dissociative disorders
Dissociative amnesia (300.12)
Dissociative fugue (300.13)
Dissociative identity disorder (300.14; formerly multiple personality disorder)
Depersonalization disorder (300.6)
Dissociative disorder not otherwise specified (300.15)
Others
Dissociative trance disorder
Acute stress disorder (308.3)

sociative disorders remain an area of psychopathology for which the best treatment is psychotherapy (Maldonado et al. 2000). As mental disorders, they have much to teach us about the way humans adapt to traumatic stress and about information processing in the brain.

The dissociative disorders were included in DSM-III (American Psychiatric Association 1980) and its revised edition, DSM-III-R (American Psychiatric Association 1987), and have been retained with some changes in nomenclature and diagnostic criteria in DSM-IV (American Psychiatric Association 1994) and DSM-IV-TR (American Psychiatric Association 2000). The discussion of each disorder later in this chapter follows the DSM-IV-TR structure.

Development of the Concept

Jean Martin Charcot (1890), a well-known French neurologist, became interested in the dissociated-like features experienced by some of his patients who had unusual neurological-like symptoms. He discovered that hypnosis could reproduce and reverse some of the deficits manifested by his patients. Charcot believed that even a normal process such as hypnosis, which could be used to access desegregated mental contents, was itself evidence of pathology (*un etat nerveux artificiel ou experimentale*, "an artificial or experimental nervous state"). He thought, for example, that once patients were cured of hysteria, they would no longer be hypnotizable. We now know this not to be the case because many "normal" individuals are highly hypnotizable (Hilgard 1965; H. Spiegel and Spiegel 1978/1987).

Nevertheless, the French physician and psychologist Pierre Janet (1920) is credited with the initial description of dissociation as a disorder, a *desagregation mentale*. The term *desagregation* carries with it a slightly different nuance than does the English translation (i.e., dissociation) because it implies a separation of certain mental contents from their general tendency to aggregate or be processed together. Janet (1920) described hysteria as "a malady of the *personal synthesis*" (p. 332). He viewed dissociation as a purely pathological process. Janet's theory on hysteria was based on three psychological models. First, in the hierarchical model, Janet related hysterical symptoms to the activities within the lower strata of mental hierarchy (*automatisms psychologiques*), which were seen during somnambulism. The second model was based on the concept of a psychological system, hypothetically composed of ideas, images, feelings, sensations, and movements. Thus, the dissociation of psychological functions was fundamental to the mechanism of hysteria in which the loss of integration was thought to engender fixed ideas (*ideas fixes*) and to lead to the development of a system totally isolated from the whole personality system. Finally, the third model, the economic model, explained various psychiatric disorders as a loss of equilibration between psychological force and psychological tension. In this model, an unexpected emotional experience causes a consumption of reserved psychological force, which is followed by exhaustion, leading to or associated with hysterical symptoms. Janet was probably the first to study psychological trauma as a principal cause of dissociation.

The dissociative disorders might have been studied more intensively during the twentieth century had not Janet's and Charcot's work been so thoroughly eclipsed by the psychoanalytic approach pioneered by Freud. Freud learned the use of hypnotic techniques from Charcot and applied them in the treatment of some of his first cases. In his early writings with Breuer, Freud began an exploration of dissociative phenomena, similar to those that Janet had described earlier. Cases in the *Studies on Hysteria* (Breuer and Freud 1893–1895/1955), such as that of Anna O., clearly involved dissociative phenomena. Indeed, Anna O. had many symptoms suggestive of DID (Nakdimen 1988). However, Breuer and Freud reformu-

lated the role of the capacity to dissociate through the concept of "hypnoid states, rather than the mechanism of dissociation." Indeed, they thought that dissociative symptoms should be attributed to the capacity to enter these hypnoid states rather than the reverse (Breuer and Freud 1893–1895/1955). However, in an effort to develop a more general theory of human psychopathology, Freud went on to study other kinds of patients, such as those with "obsessive compulsive neurosis" (i.e., obsessive-compulsive disorder) (Freud 1909/1955) and schizophrenia (Freud 1911/1958). This shift in the patient population studied may well account for much of Freud's waning interest in dissociation as a defense and his increasing interest in repression as a more general model for motivated forgetting in unconscious processes. Much has recently been made of the fact that Freud abandoned the seduction theory of the etiology of the neuroses. What may have happened is that he abandoned the study of individuals for whom trauma plausibly could be applied as an etiological factor in their psychiatric disorder.

Discussion about dissociation and its relation to trauma all but disappeared after Janet. However, during World War II and the postwar period, some psychiatrists began to pay attention to two emerging phenomena: 1) a high incidence of dissociative symptoms such as fugue and amnesia among combatants and 2) traumatic neurosis frequently observed among ex-inmates of concentration camps. In the 1970s, interest in dissociation and trauma was revived in different areas: the feminism movement was linked with concerns about child sexual abuse, public curiosity about multiple personalities was heightened by novels and movies, and posttraumatic stress disorder (PTSD) was recognized among Vietnam War veterans. Hilgard (1977) developed a neodissociation theory designed to revive interest in Janetian psychology and psychopathology. He postulated a mental structure with divisions that were horizontal rather than vertical, as in Freud's (1923/1961) archaeological model. Unlike Freud's system, Hilgard's model would allow for immediate access to consciousness of any of a variety of warded-off memories. In the dynamic unconscious model, repressed memories must first go through a process of transformation as they are accessed and lifted from the depths of the unconscious. In Hilgard's model, amnesia is a crucial mediating mechanism that provides the barriers that divide one set of mental contents from another. Thus, the flexible and reversible use of amnesia is a key defensive tool, whereas the reversal of amnesia is an important therapeutic tool.

Repression as a general model for keeping information out of conscious awareness differs from dissociation in six important ways (see Table 15–2):

TABLE 15–2. Differences between dissociation and repression

	Dissociation	**Repression**
Organizational structure	Horizontal	Vertical
Barriers	Amnesia	Dynamic conflict
Etiology	Trauma	Developmental conflict over unacceptable wishes
Contents	Untransformed: traumatic memories	Disguised, primary process: dreams, slips
Means of access	Hypnosis	Interpretation
Psychotherapy	Access, control, and working through traumatic memories	Interpretation, transference

1. The organizational structure of mental contents in dissociation is horizontal, with subunits of information divided from one another but equally available to consciousness (Hilgard 1977). Repressed information, on the other hand, is presumed to be stored in an archeological manner, at various depths, and therefore different parts are not equally accessible (Freud 1923/1961).

2. Subunits of information are presumed to be divided by amnesic barriers in dissociation, whereas dynamic conflict, or motivated forgetting, is the mechanism underlying repression.

3. The information kept out of awareness in dissociation is often for a discrete and sharply delimited time, usually for a traumatic experience, whereas repressed information may be for a variety of experiences, fears, or wishes scattered across time. Dissociation seems to be elicited as a defense, especially after episodes of physical trauma, whereas repression is a response to warded-off fears and wishes or in response to other dynamic conflicts.

4. Dissociated information is stored in a discrete and untransformed manner, whereas repressed information usually is disguised and fragmented. Even when repressed information becomes available to consciousness, its meaning is hidden (e.g., in dreams, slips of the tongue).

5. Retrieval of dissociated information often can be direct. Techniques such as hypnosis can be used to access warded-off memories. In contrast, uncovering of repressed information often requires repeated recall trials through intense questioning, psychotherapy, or psychoanalysis with subsequent interpretation (i.e., of dreams).

6. The focus of psychotherapy for dissociation is integration, via control of access to dissociated states and working through of traumatic memories. The classical psychotherapy for repression involves interpretation, including working through of the transference.

There is debate about whether dissociation is a subtype of repression or vice versa. Such a dispute is probably not resolvable, but what has become clear in recent years is that given the complexity of human information processing, the accomplishment of a sense of mental unity is an achievement, not a given (Kihlstrom and Hoyt 1990; D. Spiegel 1990a). What is remarkable is not that dissociative disorders occur but rather that they do not occur more often, given the fact that information processing comprises a variety of reasonably autonomous subsystems involving perception, memory storage and retrieval, intention, and action (Baars 1988; Cohen and Servan-Schreiber 1992a, 1992b; Rumelhart and McClelland 1986; D. Spiegel 1991c).

Models and Mechanisms of Dissociation

Dissociation and Information Processing

Modern information processing–based theories, including connectionist and parallel distributed processing (PDP) models (Rumelhart and McClelland 1986), take a bottom-up rather than a top-down approach to cognitive organization. Traditional models emphasize a superordinate organization in which broad categories of information structure the processing of specific examples. In the more Aristotelian PDP models, subunits or neural nets process information through computation of co-occurrence of input stimuli. The activation patterns in these neural nets allow for category recognition. For example, the category "kitchen" is built up from the frequent co-occurrence of "appliances of a certain type" rather than being the basis for recognizing its components. The output of one set of nets becomes the input to another, thereby gradually building up integrated and complex patterns of activation and inhibition. Such bottom-up processing models have the advantage of accounting for the processing of vast amounts of information and for the human ability to recognize patterns on the basis of approximate information. However, such models make the classification and integration of information problematic. In PDP models, it is theoretically likely that failures in integration of mental contents will occur. Indeed, attempts have been made to model psychopathology based on difficulties in neural net information processing, for example, in schizophrenia and bipolar disorder (Hoffman 1987), as well as in dissociative disorders (D. Li and Spiegel 1992). The idea is that when a net runs into difficulty in balancing the processing of input information (a model for traumatic input), it is more likely to have difficulty achieving a unified and balanced output. Such neural nets tend to fall into a "dissociated" situation in which they move in one direction or another but cannot reach an optimal balanced solution, and therefore they are unable to process smoothly all of the incoming information.

Such bottom-up information-processing systems have more the problems of a democracy than a monarchy. The difficulty is achieving unity of representation and action. In such models, consciousness is viewed as analogous to the rostrum in a legislature where competing subunits vie for attention and the ability to broadcast their input to the system as a whole (Baars 1988). Indeed, such information-processing models have now become of considerable interest in cognitive psychology (Kihlstrom 1987), and modern memory research, as mentioned earlier in this chapter, provides other examples of structural dissociation of mental elements (Schacter 1996).

Dissociation and Memory Systems

Modern research on memory shows that there are at least two broad categories of memory, variously described as *explicit* and *implicit* (Schacter 1992; Squire 1992) or *episodic* and *semantic* (Tulving 1983). These two memory systems serve different functions. *Explicit* (or *episodic*) *memory* involves recall of personal experience identified with the self (e.g., "I was at the ball game last week"). *Implicit* (or *semantic*) *memory* involves the execution of routine operations, such as riding a bicycle or typing. Such operations may be carried out with a high degree of proficiency with little conscious awareness of either their current execution or the learning episodes on which the skill is based. Indeed, these two types of memory may well have different anatomical localizations: the limbic system, especially the hippocampal formation, and mammillary bodies for episodic memory; and the basal ganglia and cortex for procedural (or semantic) memory (Mishkin 1987; Squire 1992).

Indeed, the distinction between these two types of memory may account for certain dissociative phenomena (D. Spiegel et al. 1993). The automaticity observed in certain dissociative disorders may be a reflection of the separation of self-identification in certain kinds of explicit memory from routine activity in implicit or semantic memory. It is thus not at all foreign to our mental processing to act in an automatic way devoid of explicit self-identification. Were it necessary for us to retrieve explicit memories of how and when we learned all of the activities we are required to perform, it is highly unlikely that we would be able to function with anything like the degree of efficiency we have. Many athletes report focusing on some detail of the event and allowing their bodies to do what they need to, when in fact they are performing extremely well. There is thus a fundamental model in memory research for the dissociation between identity and performance that may well find its pathological reflection in disorders such as dissociative amnesia, fugue, and identity disorder.

Meares (1999) suggested that traumatic memories are represented in a way that is qualitatively different from nontraumatic memories. His argument depends on a concept of self that is double, involving mental life and the individual's own reflection on it. If trauma is seen as causing an uncoupling, or dedoubling, of consciousness, then the traumatic diminishment of the subject–object distinction in psychic life will have several effects. First, it will change the form of conscious awareness to a state that is focused on the present and on immediate stimuli. Second, the memory system in which the traumatic events are recorded will be nonepisodic, thus lacking the reflective component, making it unconscious. Third, the traumatized–traumatizer dyad will be represented not as two persons in a relationship, but more as a nearly fused unit. This fused representation will not be integrated into the system of self as the stream of consciousness but is more likely to remain relatively sequestered. Finally, in an "uncoupled" state, the interpretation of the "meaning" of the traumatic event is impaired, and its construction will be determined by affect.

Dissociation and Trauma

An important development in the modern understanding of dissociative disorders is the exploration of the link between trauma and dissociation (D. Spiegel and Cardeña 1991). Trauma can be understood as the experience of being made into an object or a thing, the victim of someone else's rage or of nature's indifference. It is the ultimate experience of helplessness and loss of control over one's own body. There is growing clinical and some empirical evidence that dissociation may occur especially as a defense during trauma—an attempt to maintain mental control at the very moment when physical control has been lost (Bremner and Brett 1997; Butler et al. 1996; Eriksson and Lundin 1996; Kluft 1984a, 1984c; Koopman et al. 1995, 1996; Putnam 1985; D. Spiegel 1984; D. Spiegel et al. 1988). One patient with DID reported "going to a mountain meadow full of wildflowers" when she was being sexually assaulted by her drunken father. She would concentrate on how pleasant and beautiful this imaginary scene was as a way of detaching herself from the immediate experience of terror, pain, and helplessness. Such individuals often report seeking comfort from imaginary playmates or imagined protectors or absorbing themselves in some perceptual distraction, such as the pattern of the wallpaper. Many rape victims report floating above their bodies, feeling sorry for the persons being assaulted beneath them. Evidence (Putnam 1993; Terr 1991) indicates that children exposed to multiple traumas are more likely to use dissociative defense mechanisms, which include spontaneous trance episodes and amnesia.

As is noted in the discussion on DID later in this chapter, an accumulating literature suggests a connection between a history of physical and sexual abuse in childhood and the development of dissociative symptoms (Anderson et al. 1993; L. Brown et al. 1999; Chu et al. 1999; Coons 1994; Coons and Milstein 1986; Ellason et al. 1996; Farley and Keaney 1997; Irwin 1999; Kaplan et al. 1995; Kluft 1984c, 1985b; Mulder et al. 1998; Roesler and McKenzie 1994; Sar et al. 1996, 2000; Saxe et al. 1993; Scroppo et al. 1998; D. Spiegel 1984). Similarly, evidence is accumulating that dissociative symptoms are more prevalent in patients with Axis II disorders such as borderline personality disorder when there has been a history of childhood abuse (Brenner 1996a, 1996b; Brodsky et al. 1995; Chu and Dill 1990; Darves-Bornoz 1997; Herman et al. 1989; Zweig-Frank et al. 1994). When Mulder et al. (1998) examined the relation between childhood sexual abuse, childhood physical abuse, current psychiatric illness, and measures of dissociation in an adult population, they found that 6.3% of the abused population had three or more frequently occurring dissociative symptoms. Among these individuals, the rate of childhood sexual abuse was two and one-half times as high, the rate of physical abuse was five times as high, and the rate of current psychiatric disorder was four times as high as the respective rates for the other subjects.

However, another way to examine the connection between dissociation and trauma is to look at the link between recent trauma and dissociative symptoms (Carlier et al. 1996; Darves-Bornoz 1997; Darves-Bornoz et al. 1999; Eriksson and Lundin 1996; Koopman et al. 1994, 1995, 1996; Marmar et al. 1996; D. Spiegel 1991a, 1991b; D. Spiegel and Cardeña 1991; van der Kolk et al. 1994). If it is indeed the case that trauma seems to elicit dissociation, this should be observable in the immediate aftermath of natural disasters, combat, and physical assault.

The early literature examining responses to trauma provides hints of dissociative symptoms, but these symptoms often were not systematically assessed. In a classic article on the symptomatology and management of acute grief in the aftermath of the Coconut Grove fire, Lindemann (1944) noted that those individuals who had been injured or had lost loved ones but who acted as though little or nothing had happened had an extremely poor prognosis. Indeed, it was the absence of posttraumatic symptoms in this group compared with the agitation, dysphoria, and restlessness that typified most survivors that led Lindemann to formulate the normal process of acute grief.

Researchers have observed that numbing (i.e., loss of responsiveness in the wake of trauma) is a predictor of later PTSD symptomatology. For example, Z. Solomon et al. (1988, 1989) observed that psychic numbing accounted for 20% of the variance in later PTSD among Israeli combat soldiers. McFarlane (1986) found that numbing in response to the Ash Wednesday bush fires in Australia was a strong predictor of later posttraumatic symptomatology. Similarly, research on hostages and survivors of other life-threatening events indicates that more than half have experienced feelings of unreality, automatic movements, lack of emotion, and a sense of detachment (Madakasira and O'Brien 1987; Noyes and Kletti 1977; Sloan 1988). Symptoms of depersonalization and hyperalertness also frequently occur (Noyes and Slymen 1978–1979). Numbing, loss of interest, and an inability to feel deeply about anything were reported in about a third of the survivors of the Hyatt Regency skywalk collapse (Wilkinson 1983) and in a similar proportion of survivors of the North Sea oil rig collapse (Holen 1993). This finding is consistent with studies of survivors of the Loma Prieta earthquake (Cardeña and Spiegel 1993), in which a quarter of a sample of healthy students reported marked depersonalization during and immediately after the earthquake.

More recently, a study comparing psychiatric patients and a general population sample proposed a model in which alexithymic characteristics contribute to the development of pathological dissociation and stress-related disorders such as PTSD (Grabe et al. 2000).

Such dissociative experiences, especially numbing, have been found to be rather strong predictors of later

PTSD (McFarlane 1986). In fact, Z. Solomon et al. (1989) found numbing to be the single best predictor of a later diagnosis of PTSD. After the Loma Prieta earthquake in 1989, Weiss et al. (1995) found a strong correlation between peritraumatic dissociation and later PTSD among earthquake rescue workers. McFarlane (1992) found that high levels of intrusion, measured 4 months after the trauma, strongly predicted the development of PTSD. Koopman et al. (1994) discovered that a combination of acute dissociative and anxiety symptoms was a significant predictor of PTSD 7 months after the Oakland-Berkeley fires. Shalev et al. (1993, 1996) found that symptoms of intrusion as measured by the Impact of Event Scale (IES; Horowitz et al. 1979) remained elevated in subjects with PTSD, whereas they decreased in subjects who did not develop PTSD. They also found that avoidance symptoms dramatically increased between the first week and the 6-month follow-up examination, although they remained low in subjects without PTSD (Shalev et al. 1996). S. Perry et al. (1992) found similar results following burn trauma.

A recent study by Johnson et al. (2001) confirmed that peritraumatic dissociation was strongly related to later development of PTSD, dissociation, and depression in patients seeking treatment for childhood sexual abuse. Data analysis indicated that women who experienced penile penetration, believed someone or something else would be killed, or were injured as a result of the abuse had more severe peritraumatic dissociation. Regression analyses indicated that peritraumatic dissociation was the only variable to significantly predict symptom severity across symptom type or disorder. This study confirmed previous findings by O'Toole et al. (1999) that having been wounded was not related to lifetime or current PTSD, whereas peritraumatic dissociation was related to all diagnostic components of PTSD.

Draijer and Langeland (1999) administered the Dissociative Experience Scale (DES) and the Structured Trauma Interview to 160 inpatients consecutively admitted to a general psychiatric hospital. They found that 18% of the patients had a DES score greater than 30, which is usually considered the cutoff for dissociative disorders. In their sample, 26.4% of the patients reported early separation, 30.1% had witnessed interparental violence, 23.6% reported physical abuse, 34.6% reported sexual abuse, 11.7% reported rape before age 16, and 42.1% reported sexual and/or physical abuse. In this population, the level of dissociation was primarily related to reported overwhelming childhood experiences (e.g., sexual and physical abuse). Furthermore, when sexual abuse was severe (e.g., involving penetration or several perpetrators, lasting more than 1 year), dissociative symptoms

were even more prominent. The highest dissociation levels were found in patients reporting cumulative sexual trauma (e.g., intrafamilial and extrafamilial) or both sexual and physical abuse. In particular, maternal dysfunction was related to the level of dissociation. With control for gender and age, stepwise multiple regression analysis indicated that the severity of dissociative symptoms was best predicted by reported sexual abuse, physical abuse, and maternal dysfunction. These findings echoed those of Nijenhuis et al. (1998), who reported that patients with dissociative disorder experienced more severe and multifaceted traumatization. In their study, physical and sexual trauma predicted somatoform dissociation, and sexual trauma predicted psychological dissociation as well. These results suggest that pathological dissociation was best predicted by early onset of reported intense, chronic, and multiple traumatization. Thus, physical trauma seems to elicit dissociation or compartmentalization of experience and often may become the matrix for later posttraumatic symptomatology, such as dissociative amnesia for the traumatic episode. Indeed, more extreme dissociative disorders, such as DID, have been conceptualized as chronic PTSD (Kluft 1984b, 1991; D. Spiegel 1984, 1986a). Recollection of trauma tends to have an off–on quality involving either intrusion or avoidance (Horowitz 1976), in which victims either intensively relive the trauma as though it were recurring or have difficulty remembering it (Cardeña and Spiegel 1993; Christianson and Loftus 1987; Madakasira and O'Brien 1987).

Universality and Transcultural Aspects of Dissociation

In the United States, the incidence of dissociative symptoms and dissociative disorders varies depending on the population under study. Dissociative symptoms also have been reported in virtually every major psychiatric disorder and, in less severe forms, even in nonpatient ("normal") populations (Giese et al. 1997). In the general population, 6.3% of adults have reported three to four dissociative symptoms (Mulder et al. 1998). In the acute and subacute psychiatric population of a day hospital, Lussier et al. (1997) found a 9% incidence of dissociative disorder. Coons (1998) reported that dissociative disorders might be present in 5%–10% of psychiatric populations.

Similarly, dissociative disorders have been described in many cultures and settings. An evaluation of a Turkish psychiatric inpatient population found a 10.2% incidence of dissociative disorders and a 5.4% incidence of DID (Tutkun et al. 1998). A more recent study (Sar et al. 2000) suggested that dissociative disorders occurred in

12% of psychiatric outpatient subjects in Turkey. On the other hand, a study of DID in the general (nonpsychiatric) population in Turkey yielded an incidence of 1.7% (Akyuz et al. 1999). Friedl and Draijer (2000) conducted a study of Dutch psychiatric inpatients and found that 8% had dissociative disorders and 2% presented with factitious DID. Similarly, a study of admitted Swiss psychiatric inpatients reported a 5% incidence of dissociative disorders (Mihaescu et al. 1998; Modestin et al. 1996). Middleton and Butler (1998) found that DID was not uncommon among psychiatric Australian patients. In Ethiopia, Awas et al. (1999) described a lifetime prevalence of dissociative disorders of 6.3% among 501 subjects in a rural community. Gast et al. (2001) conducted a study of hospitalized German psychiatric patients and found a 4.4% incidence of dissociative disorders, including a 0.9% incidence of both DID and depersonalization disorder and a 2.6% incidence of DID not otherwise specified. Draijer and Langeland (1999) described an 18% incidence of dissociative disorders in patients admitted to a general psychiatric hospital in the Netherlands.

Acute Stress Disorder

Although acute stress disorder is classified among the anxiety disorders in DSM-IV-TR, mention is made of it in this chapter because half of the symptoms of this disorder are dissociative in nature (Table 15–3). The diagnostic criteria for this disorder would designate as symptomatic approximately one-fourth to one-third of individuals exposed to serious trauma. These symptoms are strongly predictive of later development of PTSD (Butler et al. 1996; Koopman et al. 1994). Similarly, the occurrence of PTSD is predicted by intrusion, avoidance, and hyperarousal symptoms in the immediate aftermath of rape (Rothbaum and Foa 1993) and combat trauma (Blank 1993; Z. Solomon and Mikulincer 1988). Although most individuals experiencing serious trauma are initially symptomatic, most will recover without developing PTSD. Most studies show that 25% or fewer of those who experience serious trauma later become symptomatic. Harvey and Bryant (1999) reported that the occurrence of full and subsyndromal acute stress disorder was approximately 13% and 21%, respectively. They found that most subjects who met criteria for subsyndromal acute stress disorder did not meet the acute stress disorder criteria for dissociation. At least 80% of the individuals who reported derealization also reported reduced awareness and depersonalization.

This diagnostic category should be useful not only for research on the normal and abnormal processes of adjust-

TABLE 15–3. DSM-IV-TR diagnostic criteria for acute stress disorder

A. The person has been exposed to a traumatic event in which both of the following were present:
   (1) the person experienced, witnessed, or was confronted with an event or events that involved actual or threatened death or serious injury, or a threat to the physical integrity of self or others
   (2) the person's response involved intense fear, helplessness, or horror

B. Either while experiencing or after experiencing the distressing event, the individual has three (or more) of the following dissociative symptoms:
   (1) a subjective sense of numbing, detachment, or absence of emotional responsiveness
   (2) a reduction in awareness of his or her surroundings (e.g., "being in a daze")
   (3) derealization
   (4) depersonalization
   (5) dissociative amnesia (i.e., inability to recall an important aspect of the trauma)

C. The traumatic event is persistently reexperienced in at least one of the following ways: recurrent images, thoughts, dreams, illusions, flashback episodes, or a sense of reliving the experience; or distress on exposure to reminders of the traumatic event.

D. Marked avoidance of stimuli that arouse recollections of the trauma (e.g., thoughts, feelings, conversations, activities, places, people).

E. Marked symptoms of anxiety or increased arousal (e.g., difficulty sleeping, irritability, poor concentration, hypervigilance, exaggerated startle response, motor restlessness).

F. The disturbance causes clinically significant distress or impairment in social, occupational, or other important areas of functioning or impairs the individual's ability to pursue some necessary task, such as obtaining necessary assistance or mobilizing personal resources by telling family members about the traumatic experience.

G. The disturbance lasts for a minimum of 2 days and a maximum of 4 weeks and occurs within 4 weeks of the traumatic event.

H. The disturbance is not due to the direct physiological effects of a substance (e.g., a drug of abuse, a medication) or a general medical condition, is not better accounted for by brief psychotic disorder, and is not merely an exacerbation of a preexisting Axis I or Axis II disorder.

ing to trauma but also as a means of providing an important opportunity for early preventive intervention. Dissociation may work well at the time of trauma, but if the defense persists too long, it interferes with the working through (in Lindemann's terms, the "grief work") necessary to put traumatic experience into perspective and reduce the likelihood of later PTSD or other symptomatology. Therefore, psychotherapy aimed at helping individuals acknowledge, bear, and put into perspective traumatic experience shortly after the trauma should be helpful in reducing the incidence of later PTSD.

In the following discussions, we review the diagnosis and treatment of the dissociative disorders as defined in DSM-IV-TR.

Dissociative Amnesia

The hallmark of dissociative amnesia is the inability to recall important personal information, usually of a traumatic or stressful nature, which cannot be explained by ordinary forgetfulness (American Psychiatric Association 2000) (Table 15–4). Dissociative amnesia is considered the most common of all dissociative disorders (Putnam 1985). Amnesia is a symptom commonly found in several other dissociative and anxiety disorders, including acute stress disorder, PTSD, somatization disorder, dissociative fugue, and DID (American Psychiatric Association 2000). A higher incidence of dissociative amnesia has been described in the context of war and natural and other disasters (Maldonado et al. 2000). There appears to be a direct relation between the severity of the exposure to trauma and the incidence of amnesia (G.R. Brown and Anderson 1991; Chu and Dill 1990; Kirshner 1973; Putnam 1985, 1993; Sargant and Slater 1941).

Dissociative amnesia is the classical functional disorder of memory and involves difficulty in retrieving discrete components of episodic memory (see Table 15–2). It does not, however, involve a difficulty in memory storage, as in Wernicke-Korsakoff syndrome. Because the amnesia involves primarily difficulties in retrieval rather than encoding or storage, the memory deficits usually are reversible. Once the amnesia has cleared, normal memory function is resumed (Schacter et al. 1982). Dissociative amnesia has three primary characteristics:

1. The memory loss is episodic. The first-person recollection of certain events is lost, rather than knowledge of procedures.
2. The memory loss is for a discrete period of time, ranging from minutes to years. It is not vagueness or inefficient retrieval of memories, but rather a dense unavailability of memories that had been clearly available. Unlike in the amnestic disorders, for example, from damage to the medial temporal lobe in surgery (Squire and Zola-Morgan 1991) or in Wernicke-Korsakoff syndrome, there is usually no difficulty in learning *new* episodic information. Thus, the amnesia is typically retrograde rather than anterograde (Loew-

---

TABLE 15–4. DSM-IV-TR diagnostic criteria for dissociative amnesia

A. The predominant disturbance is one or more episodes of inability to recall important personal information, usually of a traumatic or stressful nature, that is too extensive to be explained by ordinary forgetfulness.

B. The disturbance does not occur exclusively during the course of dissociative identity disorder, dissociative fugue, posttraumatic stress disorder, acute stress disorder, or somatization disorder and is not due to the direct physiological effects of a substance (e.g., a drug of abuse, a medication) or a neurological or other general medical condition (e.g., amnestic disorder due to head trauma).

C. The symptoms cause clinically significant distress or impairment in social, occupational, or other important areas of functioning.

---

enstein 1991a), with one or more discrete periods of past information becoming unavailable. However, Kluft (1988) observed a syndrome of continuous difficulty in incorporating new information that mimics organic amnestic syndromes.

3. The memory loss is generally for events of a traumatic or stressful nature. In one study (Coons and Milstein 1986), the majority of cases involved child abuse (60%), but disavowed behaviors such as marital problems, sexual activity, suicide attempts, criminal behavior, and the death of a relative also were precipitants.

Dissociative amnesia is most common in the third and fourth decades of life (Abeles and Schilder 1935; Coons and Milstein 1986). It usually involves one episode, but multiple periods of lost memory are not uncommon (Coons and Milstein 1986). Comorbidity with conversion disorder, bulimia, alcohol abuse, and depression is common, and Axis II diagnoses of histrionic, dependent, and borderline personality disorders occur in a substantial minority of such patients (Coons and Milstein 1986). Legal difficulties, such as driving under the influence of alcohol, also accompany dissociative amnesia in a minority of cases. Occasionally, there may be a history of head trauma. If that is the case, usually the trauma is too slight to have physiological consequences.

The typical course of dissociative amnesia is described in the following case:

A 54-year-old man was involved in a motorcycle accident. He was wearing a helmet, which was damaged but did protect him during the accident. He was found to have suffered no significant head trauma. The patient did not lose consciousness, and he talked with a friend after the accident about it. However, he had no memory of the accident or of the 12 hours afterward. His first recollection was of a friend telling him, "You crashed my motorcycle." When he returned the next day to the hospital where he had been treated, he recognized a nurse as someone familiar, and she told him that he had been yelling when they treated his injured left knee. Yet this visit did not stimulate any direct recollection of his time in the hospital. The man had recovered no memory of the accident a month later.

Dissociative amnesia usually involves discrete boundaries around the period of time unavailable to consciousness. Individuals with such a disorder lose the ability to recall what happened during a specific time. They demonstrate not vagueness or spotty memory but rather a loss of any episodic memory for a finite period. Such individuals initially may not be aware of the memory loss—that is, they may not remember that they do not remember. However, they may find, for example, new purchases in their homes but have no memory of having obtained them. They report being told that they have done or said things that they cannot remember.

Dissociative amnesia most frequently occurs after an episode of trauma, and the onset may be sudden or gradual.

A 30-year-old woman was beaten and raped by a man who drove her home from a party. She had refused to let him enter her apartment, but he returned a few minutes later, claiming that he had to make a telephone call. He then sexually assaulted her. She screamed and struggled and called the police immediately afterward. The man was arrested when he returned to retrieve some jewelry she had pulled off his neck during the struggle. Although she had not sustained a concussion, she began to lose memory of the rape in the ensuing week. By the end of the week, she had no memory of the rape but became listless and depressed. In psychotherapy, she used hypnosis to help retrieve her memory, which she was gradually able to do.

Some individuals do experience episodes of selective amnesia, usually for specific traumatic incidents, which may be more interwoven with periods of intact memory. In these cases, the amnesia is for a type of material remembered rather than for a discrete period of time.

Despite the fact that certain information is kept out of consciousness in dissociative amnesia, such information may exert an influence on consciousness. For example, a rape victim with no conscious recollection of the assault will nonetheless behave like someone who has been sexually victimized. Such individuals often show detachment and demoralization, are unable to enjoy intimate relationships, and show hyperarousal to stimuli reminiscent of the trauma. This phenomenon is similar to priming in memory research. Individuals who have read a word in a list will complete a word stem for such a word (e.g., a partial word such as *pre* for *prepare*) minutes or hours later more quickly than they would for a word they have not recently seen. This phenomenon occurs even though they cannot consciously recall having read the word. Similarly, individuals instructed in hypnosis to forget having seen a list of words will nonetheless show priming effects from the hypnotically suppressed list. It is the essence of dissociative amnesia that material being kept out of conscious awareness is nonetheless active and may influence consciousness indirectly: out of sight does not mean out of mind.

Individuals with dissociative amnesia generally do not have disturbances of identity, except to the extent that their identity is influenced by the warded-off memory. It is not uncommon for such individuals to develop depressive symptoms as well, especially when the amnesia is in the wake of a traumatic episode.

Treatment

To date, no controlled studies have addressed the treatment of dissociative amnesia. No established pharmacological treatments are available, except for the use of benzodiazepines or barbiturates for drug-assisted interviews (Maldonado et al. 2000). Most cases of dissociative amnesia revert spontaneously, especially when the individuals are removed from stressful or threatening situations, when they feel physically and psychologically safe, and/or when they are exposed to cues from the past (i.e., family members) (W. Brown 1918; Kardiner and Spiegel 1947; Loewenstein 1991b; Maldonado et al. 2000; Reither and Stoudemire 1988). When a safe environment is not enough to restore normal memory functioning, the amnesia sometimes can be breached using techniques such as pharmacologically mediated interviews (i.e., barbiturates and benzodiazepines) (Baron and Nagy 1988; Naples and Hackett 1978; J.C. Perry and Jacobs 1982; Wettstein and Fauman 1979).

On the other hand, most patients with dissociative disorder are highly hypnotizable on formal testing and therefore are easily able to make use of hypnotic techniques such as age regression (H. Spiegel and Spiegel 1978/1987). Patients are hypnotized and instructed to experience a time before the onset of the amnesia as though it were the present. Then the patients are reoriented in hypnosis to experience events during the amnesic period. Hypnosis can enable such patients to reorient temporally and therefore to achieve access to otherwise dissociated memories.

If the warded-off memory has traumatic content, patients may abreact (i.e., express strong emotion) as these memories are elicited, and they will need psychotherapeutic help in integrating these memories and the associated affect into consciousness.

One technique that can help bring such memories into consciousness while modulating the affective response to them is the screen technique (D. Spiegel 1981). In this approach, patients are taught, by using hypnosis, to relive the traumatic event as if they were watching it on an imaginary movie or television screen. This technique is often helpful for individuals who are unable to relive the event as if it were occurring in the present tense, either because that process is too emotionally taxing or because they are not sufficiently hypnotizable to be able to engage in hypnotic age regression. The screen technique also can be used to provide dissociation between the psychological and the somatic aspects of the memory retrieval. Individuals can be put into self-hypnosis and instructed to get their bodies into a state of floating comfort and safety. They are reminded that no matter what they see on the screen, their bodies will be safe and comfortable.

> A victim of a violent attempted rape had developed a selective amnesia for much of the physical struggle itself. She had sustained a basilar skull fracture, but she had not been rendered unconscious. She also had a generalized seizure shortly after the assault. She initially sought help with hypnosis in an attempt to improve her recollection of the assailant's face.
>
> The woman was instructed in the screen technique and used it to relive the assault. She remembered two things that she had not previously recalled: 1) the assailant was surprised at how hard she was fighting with him, and 2) she recognized that he intended not merely to rape her but to kill her. She became convinced that had she let him drag her into her apartment, she likely would not have survived. She was tearful and frightened as she recalled this aspect of the assault that had been previously unavailable to consciousness.
>
> She was then instructed to divide the imaginary screen in half, picturing on the left side an image of the viciousness and intensity of the assault on her and on the other side recognizing what she had done to protect herself. She was instructed to concentrate on these two aspects of the assault and then, when she was ready, to bring herself out of the state of self-hypnosis. She was told that she could use this as a self-hypnosis exercise several times a day if she wished, as a means of putting her memories of the rape into perspective. This cognitive and emotional restructuring of the traumatic memories made them more bearable in consciousness.
>
> Before this psychotherapy, she had blamed herself for having fought so hard that she was seriously injured. Afterward, she recognized that she may have saved her life by fighting off the assailant so vigorously. This positive therapeutic outcome occurred despite the fact that she was unable to recall any new details about the assailant's physical appearance.

Psychotherapy for dissociative amnesia involves accessing the dissociated memories, working through affectively loaded aspects of these memories, and supporting the patient through the process of integrating these memories into consciousness.

Dissociative Fugue

Dissociative fugue combines failure of integration of certain aspects of personal memory with loss of customary identity and automatisms of motor behavior (Table 15–5). Patients appear "normal," usually showing no signs of psychopathology or cognitive deficit. Fugue involves one or more episodes of sudden, unexpected, purposeful travel away from home, coupled with an inability to recall portions or all of one's past, and a loss of identity or the assumption of a new identity. In contrast to patients who have DID, if patients with dissociative fugue develop a new identity, the old and new identities do not alternate. The onset is usually sudden, and it frequently occurs after a traumatic experience or bereavement. A single episode is not uncommon, and spontaneous remission of symptoms can occur without treatment.

It was thought that the assumption of a new identity, as in the classical case of the Reverend Ansel Bourne (James 1890/1950), was typical of dissociative fugue. However, Reither and Stoudemire (1988), in their review of the literature, documented that in most cases, there is loss of personal identity but no clear assumption of a new identity.

Many cases of dissociative fugue remit spontaneously. But again, hypnosis can be useful in accessing dissociated material. The following case was reported by H. Spiegel and Spiegel (1978/1987):

TABLE 15–5.   DSM-IV-TR diagnostic criteria for dissociative fugue

A. The predominant disturbance is sudden, unexpected travel away from home or one's customary place of work, with inability to recall one's past.

B. Confusion about personal identity or assumption of a new identity (partial or complete).

C. The disturbance does not occur exclusively during the course of dissociative identity disorder and is not due to the direct physiological effects of a substance (e.g., a drug of abuse, a medication) or a general medical condition (e.g., temporal lobe epilepsy).

D. The symptoms cause clinically significant distress or impairment in social, occupational, or other important areas of functioning.

A woman who appeared dazed but physically unharmed was brought into an army hospital emergency department by the base guards because she had been found wandering near the army base. She reported that she did not know who she was, where she lived, or how she happened to be there. Initially, plans were made to admit her to the hospital for a full neurological and psychiatric evaluation. She proved to be highly hypnotizable, and in hypnosis, age regression was used to take her back to an earlier year. She then reported her name and that she lived some 500 miles away. The time was changed again in hypnosis to a period just before this apparent fugue episode. She then reported having received unsigned letters from someone at the army base where her husband was stationed, reporting that her husband was having an affair. This had deeply upset her, and it turned out that her husband was indeed a soldier on the base near which she had been found wandering. They were reunited and reconciled, and the fugue episode ended.

Not infrequently, fugue episodes represent dissociated but purposeful activity, as in the following case:

A businessman found himself on several occasions on transatlantic flights from California to London without recollecting who he was or how he had gotten on the airplane. In psychotherapy exploring these fugue episodes, it was determined that he had had an extremely conflicted relationship with a successful but neglectful father. The father had recently died, leaving the patient financially well off but emotionally ambivalent, with a sense of incompleteness about his relationship with his father. The patient had spent his boyhood years in London, and he recognized in therapy that the travel to London seemed to represent an unconscious attempt to revisit his childhood years and "set his father straight"—something he had never been able to do while his father was alive.

In this case, the dissociative fugue was a form of pathological grief reaction.

Hypnosis can be helpful in accessing otherwise unavailable components of memory and identity. The approach used is similar to that for dissociative amnesia. Hypnotic age regression can be used as the framework for accessing information available at a previous time. Demonstrating to patients that such information can be made available to consciousness enhances their sense of control over the material and facilitates the therapeutic working through of emotionally laden aspects of it.

A woman in a Veterans Administration hospital had lost all memory of the preceding 10 months and insisted that she was in another hospital where she had been during the previous December. She proved on testing with the Hypnotic Induction Profile (H. Spiegel and Spiegel 1978/1987) to be highly hypnotizable. She was then put into hypnosis with a simple, rapid induction technique involving the following instruction: On 1, do one thing: look up. On 2, do two things: slowly close your eyes, and take a deep breath. On 3, do three things: let the breath out, let your eyes relax but keep them closed, and let your body float. Then let one hand or the other float up into the air like a balloon, and that is your signal to yourself that you are ready to concentrate.

When she did this, she was told that we would be changing times, that we would count backward in years, and that when her eyes opened, she would be at an earlier time in her life. We agreed that when I touched her forehead, she would close her eyes and we would change times again. We then began counting several years back. When she opened her eyes, she spoke as though she were in some different place earlier in her life. She was reoriented to the time when she really was in another psychiatric hospital in a different city, and she talked about that experience. She was then instructed to close her eyes again and count forward in months to the present month. She opened her eyes and was then properly oriented and had episodic memory for what had transpired in her life in recent months.

Once reorientation is established and the overt aspects of the fugue have been resolved, it is important to work through interpersonal or intrapsychic issues that underlie the dissociative defenses. Individuals with dissociative fugue are often relatively unaware of their reactions to stress because they so effectively can dissociate them (H. Spiegel 1974). Thus, effective psychotherapy is also anticipatory, helping patients to recognize and modify their tendency to set aside their own feelings in favor of those of others.

Patients with dissociative fugue may be helped with a psychotherapeutic approach that facilitates conscious integration of dissociated memories and motivations for behavior previously experienced as automatic and unwilled. It is often helpful to address current psychosocial stressors, such as marital conflict, with the involved individuals, as in the previously discussed case of the woman found on the army base. To the extent that current psychosocial stress triggers fugue, resolution of that stress can help resolve the fugue state and reduce the likelihood of recurrence. Highly hypnotizable individuals prone to these extreme dissociative symptoms (D. Spiegel et al. 1988; H. Spiegel 1974; H. Spiegel and Spiegel 1978/1987) often have great difficulty in asserting their own point of view in a personal relationship. Rather, they interact with others as though they were undergoing a spontaneous trance experience. One individual described herself as a "disciple in search of a teacher." Psychotherapy can be effective in helping such individuals recognize and modify their tendency toward unthinking compliance with others and toward extreme sensitivity to rejection and disapproval.

In the past, sodium amobarbital or other short-acting sedatives were used to reverse dissociative amnesia or fugue. However, such techniques offer no advantage over hypnosis and are not especially effective (J.C. Perry and Jacobs 1982). Not infrequently, the ceremony of injecting the drug elicits spontaneous hypnotic phenomena before the pharmacological effect is felt, and sedation and other side effects can be troublesome.

There is at least one case report on the use of a locator beacon attached to a patient with dissociative fugue, which has proven effective in the curtailment of dissociative fugue episodes (Macleod 1999).

Depersonalization Disorder

The essential feature of depersonalization disorder is the occurrence of persistent feelings of unreality, detachment, or estrangement from oneself or one's body, usually with the feeling that one is an outside observer of one's own mental processes (Steinberg 1991). Thus, depersonalization disorder is primarily a disturbance in the integration of perceptual experience (Table 15–6). Individuals who have depersonalization disorder are distressed by it. Different from those with delusional disorders and other psychotic processes, those with depersonalization disorder have intact reality testing. Patients are aware of some distortion in their perceptual experience and therefore are not delusional. The symptom is often transient and may co-occur with a variety of other symptoms, especially anxiety, panic, or phobic symptoms. Indeed, the content of the anxiety may involve fears of "going crazy." Derealization frequently co-occurs with depersonalization disorder, in which affected individuals notice an altered perception of their surroundings, resulting in the world seeming unreal or dreamlike. Affected individuals often will ruminate about this alteration and be preoccupied with their own somatic and mental functioning.

Depersonalization as a symptom is seen in several psychiatric and neurological disorders (Pies 1991; Putnam 1985). Unlike other dissociative disorders, the presence of which excludes other mental disorders such as schizophrenia and substance abuse, depersonalization disorder frequently co-occurs with such disorders. It is often a symptom of anxiety disorders and PTSD. In fact, about 69% of patients with panic disorder experience depersonalization or derealization during their panic attacks (Ball et al. 1997). Episodes of depersonalization also may occur as a symptom of alcohol and drug abuse, as a side effect of prescription medication, and during stress and sensory deprivation. Depersonalization is con-

TABLE 15–6. DSM-IV-TR diagnostic criteria for depersonalization disorder

A. Persistent or recurrent experiences of feeling detached from, and as if one is an outside observer of, one's mental processes or body (e.g., feeling like one is in a dream).
B. During the depersonalization experience, reality testing remains intact.
C. The depersonalization causes clinically significant distress or impairment in social, occupational, or other important areas of functioning.
D. The depersonalization experience does not occur exclusively during the course of another mental disorder, such as schizophrenia, panic disorder, acute stress disorder, or another dissociative disorder, and is not due to the direct physiological effects of a substance (e.g., a drug of abuse, a medication) or a general medical condition (e.g., temporal lobe epilepsy).

sidered a disorder when it is a persistent and predominant symptom. The phenomenology of the disorder involves both the initial symptoms themselves and the reactive anxiety caused by them.

Treatment

Depersonalization is most often transient and may remit without formal treatment. Recurrent or persistent depersonalization should be thought of both as a symptom in and of itself and as a component of other syndromes requiring treatment, such as anxiety disorders and schizophrenia.

The symptom itself may respond to self-hypnosis training. Often, hypnotic induction will induce transient depersonalization symptoms in patients. This is a useful exercise because by having a structure for inducing the symptoms, one provides patients with a context for understanding and controlling them. The symptoms are presented as a spontaneous form of hypnotic dissociation that can be modified. Individuals for whom this approach is effective can be taught to induce a pleasant sense of floating lightness or heaviness in place of the anxiety-related somatic detachment. Often, the use of an imaginary screen to picture problems in a way that detaches them from the typical somatic response is also helpful (H. Spiegel and Spiegel 1978/1987).

Other treatment modalities used (Maldonado et al. 2000) include behavioral techniques, such as paradoxical intention (Blue 1979), record keeping, and positive reward (Dollinger 1983); flooding (Sookman and Solyom 1978); psychotherapy, especially psychodynamic (Noyes and Kletti 1977; Schilder 1939; Shilony and Grossman 1993; Torch 1987); and psychoeducation (Fewtrell

1986; Torch 1987). Some have suggested the use of psychotropic medications, including psychostimulants (Cattell and Cattell 1974; Davison 1964; Shorvon 1946), antidepressants (Fichtner et al. 1992; Hollander et al. 1989, 1990; Noyes et al. 1987; Walsh 1975), antipsychotics (Ambrosino 1973; Nuller 1982), anticonvulsants (Stein and Uhde 1989), and benzodiazepines (Ballenger et al. 1988; Nuller 1982; Spier et al. 1986; Stein and Uhde 1989). Finally, others have suggested the use of electroconvulsive therapy (ECT; Ambrosino 1973; Davison 1964; Roth 1959; Shorvon 1946). Appropriate treatment of comorbid disorders is an important part of treatment. Use of antianxiety medications for generalized anxiety or phobic disorders and antipsychotic medications for schizophrenia should help in these conditions.

Dissociative Identity Disorder (Multiple Personality Disorder)

Prevalence

There are no convincing studies of the absolute prevalence of DID. The initial systematic report on the epidemiology of DID estimated a prevalence in the general population of 0.01% (Coons 1984). The estimated prevalence is approximately 3% of psychiatric inpatients (Ross 1991; Ross et al. 1991b). Studies conducted in the general population suggest a prevalence higher than initially reported by Coons (1984) but lower (about 1%) than the one described in psychiatric settings and specialized treatment units (Ross 1991; Vanderlinden et al. 1991). Loewenstein (1994) reported that the prevalence in North America is about 1%, compared with a prevalence of 10% for all dissociative disorders as a group. Loewenstein's findings were replicated by Rifkin et al. (1998), who studied 100 randomly selected women, ages 16–50 years, who had been admitted to an acute psychiatric hospital and found that 1% of the subjects had DID.

The number of reported DID cases has risen considerably in recent years. Factors that account for this increase include a more general awareness of the diagnosis among mental health professionals; the availability, starting with DSM-III, of specific diagnostic criteria (Table 15–7); and reduced misdiagnosis of DID as schizophrenia or borderline personality disorder. Although the increase in reported cases is best documented in North America, a recent study showed similar phenomenology and link to trauma history in Europe (Boon and Draijer 1993a, 1993b; Gast et al. 2001; Nijenhuis et al. 1998). In fact, there are reports of DID in almost all societies and races, making it a true cross-cultural diagnosis

---

TABLE 15–7. DSM-IV-TR diagnostic criteria for dissociative identity disorder

A. The presence of two or more distinct identities or personality states (each with its own relatively enduring pattern of perceiving, relating to, and thinking about the environment and self).

B. At least two of these identities or personality states recurrently take control of the person's behavior.

C. Inability to recall important personal information that is too extensive to be explained by ordinary forgetfulness.

D. The disturbance is not due to the direct physiological effects of a substance (e.g., blackouts or chaotic behavior during alcohol intoxication) or a general medical condition (e.g., complex partial seizures). **Note:** In children, the symptoms are not attributable to imaginary playmates or other fantasy play.

(Coons et al. 1991). Case reports have described DID or related disorders among Asians (Putnam 1989; Yap 1960), blacks (Coons and Milstein 1986; R. Solomon 1983; Stern 1984), Europeans (Boon and Draijer 1993a, 1993b; Freyberger et al. 1998; Nijenhuis et al. 1998; Spitzer et al. 1999; van der Hart 1993), Hispanics (Allison 1974; Ronquillo 1991; R. Solomon 1983), and inhabitants of Australia and New Zealand (L. Brown et al. 1999; Gelb 1993; Middleton and Butler 1998; Price and Hess 1979), Canada (Horen et al. 1995; Ross et al. 1989, 1991a, 1991b; Vincent and Pickering 1988), the Caribbean (Wittkower 1970), India (Adityanjee et al. 1989; Varma et al. 1981), Japan (Berger et al. 1994), the Netherlands (Boon and Draijer 1993b; Draijer and Langeland 1999; Friedl and Draijer 2000; Nijenhuis et al. 1997; Sno and Schalken 1999; van der Hart and Nijenhuis 1993; Vanderlinden et al. 1991; van Dyck 1993), Norway (Boe et al. 1993), Sweden (Eriksson and Lundin 1996), Switzerland (Modestin et al. 1996), and Turkey (Akyuz et al. 1999; Chodoff 1997; Sar et al. 1996, 2000; Tutkun et al. 1998; Yargic et al. 1998).

Other authors attribute the increase in reported cases to hypnotic suggestion and misdiagnosis (Brenner 1994, 1996a; Frankel 1990; Ganaway 1989, 1995; Mayer-Gross et al. 1969; McHugh 1995a, 1995b; Piper 1994; Spanos et al. 1985, 1986). Proponents of this point of view argue that individuals with DID are as a group highly hypnotizable and therefore quite suggestible and that a few specialist clinicians usually make the vast majority of diagnoses. However, it has been observed that the symptomatology of patients diagnosed by specialists in dissociation does not differ from that assessed by psychiatrists, psychologists, and physicians in more general practices, who diagnose one or two cases a year. On the other hand, Akyuz et al. (1999) examined the prevalence of DID in the general population of a rural area in Turkey. They found that 1.7% received a diagnosis of dissociative disorder according to a structured interview, and half of these fulfilled clinical criteria for DID, yielding a minimum prevalence of 0.4% for DID. Thus, their data, derived from a population with no public awareness about DID and no exposure to systematic psychotherapy (thus eliminating the possible "iatrogenic contamination factor"), suggest that DID cannot be considered simply an iatrogenic artifact, a culture-bound syndrome, or a phenomenon induced by media influences.

In a study (Chu et al. 1999) of female patients admitted to a unit specializing in the treatment of trauma-related disorders, participants reporting any type of childhood abuse had elevated levels of dissociative symptoms that were significantly higher than those in subjects not reporting abuse. Higher dissociative symptom levels were correlated with early age at onset of physical and sexual abuse and with more frequent sexual abuse. A substantial proportion of participants with all types of abuse reported partial or complete amnesia for abuse memories. For physical and sexual abuse, early age at onset was correlated with greater levels of amnesia. Participants who reported recovering memories of abuse generally recalled these experiences while at home, alone, or with family or friends. Although some participants were in treatment at the time, very few were in therapy sessions during their first memory recovery. Suggestion was generally denied as a factor in memory recovery, and most participants were able to find strong corroboration of their recovered memories.

If such patients were so suggestible and subject to directive influence by diagnosticians, then it is surprising that their presenting symptoms persisted for an average of 6.5 years before the diagnosis was made (Putnam et al. 1986). Rather, it would seem likely that such patients would accept a suggestion that they have another disorder, such as schizophrenia or borderline personality disorder, because they encounter many clinicians who are unaware of or not familiar with DID. Because these patients are indeed highly hypnotizable and therefore suggestible (Frischholz 1985), care must be taken in the manner in which the illness is presented to them. However, it is unlikely that the increased number of cases currently reported is accounted for by suggestion alone. Rather, a reduction in previous misdiagnoses and an increase in recognition of the prevalence and sequelae of physical and sexual abuse in childhood (Braun 1990; Bryer et al. 1987; Coons et al. 1988; Finkelhor 1984; Frischholz 1985; Goodwin 1982; Herman et al. 1989; Kluft 1984c, 1991; Pribor and Dinwiddie 1992; Putnam

1988; Putnam et al. 1986; Ross 1989; Russell 1986; D. Spiegel 1984; Terr 1991) are also likely explanations. There have been reports of "definite independent confirmation of the histories of abuse" (Coons 1994; Martinez-Taboas 1996) confirming not only the association between dissociative disorders and trauma but also the occurrence of amnesia in response to traumatic experiences. Furthermore, a recent study among Dutch psychiatrists (Sno and Schalken 1999) reported that 40% have made the diagnosis of DID at least once. The diagnosis was made statistically significantly more frequently by female psychiatrists, by psychiatrists age 50 years or younger, and by those certified after 1982. No correlation was observed with primary theoretical orientation or the type or topography of work facility. The mean age of the selected patients was 33.2, and the female-to-male ratio was 9:1. Similar to their American counterparts, most patients were seen once a week in an outpatient setting, and individual psychotherapy and adjunctive anxiolytic or antidepressant medications were the most widely endorsed treatment modalities. Different from more typical American practice, hypnosis was rarely used. This study suggested that the diagnosis of DID should not be dismissed as a local (American) eccentricity and minimized the roles of suggestibility, hypnosis, and culture.

The skepticism regarding the existence of DID is compounded in the case of criminals because of issues of suspected malingering. Lewis et al. (1997) reviewed the clinical records of 12 murderers with a DSM-IV-defined diagnosis of DID. Data were gathered from medical, psychiatric, social service, school, military, and prison records and from records of interviews with subjects' family members. In their sample, they were able to independently corroborate the presence of signs and symptoms of DID in childhood and adulthood from several sources in all 12 cases. Furthermore, objective evidence of severe abuse was obtained in 11 cases. Of interest, most subjects had amnesia for most of the abuse and thus underreported it. Marked changes in writing style and/or signatures were documented in 10 cases.

Course

DID is diagnosed in childhood with increasing frequency (Kluft 1984a; 1984b) but typically emerges between adolescence and the third decade of life; it rarely presents as a new disorder after an individual reaches age 40 years, but there is often considerable delay between initial symptom presentation and diagnosis (American Psychiatric Association 2000; Putnam et al. 1986). The female-to-male sex ratio of DID is 5:4 in children and adolescents and 9:1 in adults (Hocke and Schmidtke 1998; Sno and Schalken 1999).

Untreated, DID is a chronic and recurrent disorder. It rarely remits spontaneously, but the symptoms may not be evident for some time (Kluft 1985c). DID has been called "a pathology of hiddenness" (Gutheil, as quoted in Kluft 1988, p. 575). The dissociation itself hampers self-monitoring and accurate reporting of symptoms. Many patients with the disorder are not fully aware of the extent of the dissociative symptomatology. They may be reluctant to bring up symptoms because of having encountered frequent skepticism. Furthermore, because most patients with DID report histories of sexual and physical abuse (Braun and Sachs 1985; Coons and Milstein 1992; Coons et al. 1988; Kluft 1985b, 1988, 1991; Putnam 1988; Putnam et al. 1986; Ross 1989; Ross et al. 1990; Schultz et al. 1989; D. Spiegel 1984), the shame associated with that experience, as well as fear of retribution, may inhibit reporting of symptoms.

One last consequence of DID is the subjects' inability to be adequate parents, at least while symptomatic. In a qualitative analysis of the experience of parenting of mothers with dissociative disorders, Benjamin et al. (1998) reported that the functioning of DID mothers, as well as their subjective experience of mothering, was poorer than that of either clinical or nonclinical control mothers. All five symptom areas of dissociation (amnesia, depersonalization, derealization, identity confusion, and identity alteration) impeded their parenting efforts. Their findings highlight the need to address parenting in the treatment of mothers with dissociative disorders.

Comorbidity

The major comorbid psychiatric illnesses of DID are the depressive disorders (Putnam et al. 1986; Ross and Norton 1989; Ross et al. 1989; Yargic et al. 1998), substance use disorders (Anderson et al. 1993; Coons 1984; Dunn et al. 1995; Ellason et al. 1996; Putnam et al. 1986; Rivera 1991), and borderline personality disorder (Anderson et al. 1993; Brodsky et al. 1995; Horevitz and Braun 1984; Shearer 1994; Yargic et al. 1998). Sexual (Brenner 1996b; van der Kolk et al. 1994), eating (Berger et al. 1994; Valdiserri and Kihlstrom 1995; van der Kolk et al. 1994), somatoform (Spitzer et al. 1999; Yargic et al. 1998), and sleep disorders (Putnam et al. 1986) occur less commonly. Patients with DID frequently engage in self-mutilative behavior (Bliss 1980, 1984; Coons 1984; Gainer and Torem 1993; Greaves 1980; Putnam et al. 1986; Ross and Norton 1989; Zweig-Frank et al. 1994), impulsiveness, and overvaluing and devaluing of relationships that make approximately a third of DID patients fit

the criteria for borderline personality disorder as well. Such individuals also show higher levels of depression (Horevitz and Braun 1984). Conversely, research shows dissociative symptoms in many patients with borderline personality disorder, especially those who report histories of physical and sexual abuse (Chu and Dill 1990; Ogata et al. 1990).

In a study attempting to identify the risk factors associated with the dissociative symptomatology of borderline personality disorder patients, four risk factors were found to be significantly associated with the level of dissociation reported: 1) inconsistent treatment by a caregiver, 2) sexual abuse by a caregiver, 3) witnessing sexual violence as a child, and 4) adult rape history (Zanarini et al. 2000b). The results of this study suggested that both sexual trauma and something intrinsic to the borderline diagnosis itself are risk factors for dissociative phenomena among borderline patients. Indeed, the impulsiveness, splitting, and hostility frequently seen in some older personality states are similar to the presentations seen in many patients with borderline personality disorder. Wildgoose et al. (2000) suggested that the single factor mediating the main differences between borderline personality disorder and other personality disorders is the presence of dissociation. When compared with control groups, patients with borderline personality disorder have higher levels of dissociation (26% in borderline personality disorder group vs. 3% in control subjects), as measured by the DES (Zanarini et al. 2000a). The researchers also found a wider range of dissociative experiences in this population, including absorption, depersonalization, and amnesia. Golynkina and Ryle (1999) described how in borderline personality disorder partial dissociation provoked by trauma and deprivation in childhood results in the persistence of separate self states, as is the case in DID. The characteristics of these and alternations between them are seen to account for the main features of the condition. As in cases of DID, patients with borderline personality disorder have difficulties in recalling specific autobiographical memories. These difficulties are related to their tendency to dissociate, and it may help patients with borderline personality disorder (as it does patients with DID) to avoid episodic information that would evoke acutely negative affect (Jones et al. 1999). Similarly, a study of patients engaging in deliberate self-injurious behavior (Low et al. 2000) found that the frequency of this behavior was primarily related to increased dissociation, and a secondary component was mediated by low self-esteem, anger, impulsivity, and a history of sexual and physical abuse.

Comorbidity is complex in that patients with concurrent diagnoses of DID and borderline personality disorder (approximately one-third) also are more likely to meet the criteria for major depressive disorder. In addition, they frequently meet the criteria for PTSD, with intrusive flashbacks, recurring dreams of physical and sexual abuse, avoidance and loss of pleasure of usually pleasurable activities, and symptoms of hyperarousal, especially when exposed to reminders of childhood trauma (Kluft 1985a, 1991; Putnam 1993; D. Spiegel 1990b; van der Kolk and Fisler 1995; van der Kolk et al. 1994, 1996). Brenner (1999) postulated that dissociation may be seen as a complex defense and that DID may be thought of as a "lower level dissociative character." Furthermore, Brenner believes that patients with DID have a unique psychic structure—the "dissociative self"—whose function is to create "alter personalities" out of disowned affects, memories, fantasies, and drives. According to his theory, this "dissociative self" must be dissolved to integrate the "alter personalities."

In addition, these patients often receive misdiagnoses of schizophrenia (Coons 1984; Ellason and Ross 1995; Kluft 1987; Putnam et al. 1986; Ross and Norton 1988; Ross et al. 1990; Steinberg et al. 1994). This diagnostic confusion is understandable given that the first-rank criterion for schizophrenia is that the patient has an apparent delusion (e.g., that his or her body is occupied by more than one person). These patients frequently have auditory hallucinations in which one personality state speaks to or comments on the activities of another (Bliss 1986; Bliss et al. 1983; Coons 1984; Kluft 1987; Peterson 1995; Putnam et al. 1986; Ross et al. 1990). When these patients receive misdiagnoses of schizophrenia, they are frequently given neuroleptics, with poor therapeutic response.

Individuals with DID report an average of 15 somatic or conversion symptoms (Anderson et al. 1993; Bowman 1993; Bowman and Markand 1996; Kaplan et al. 1995; Ross et al. 1989, 1990) and other psychosomatic symptoms such as migraine headaches (D. Spiegel 1987). Studies show that approximately one-third of these patients have complex partial seizures (Schenk and Bear 1981), although more recent studies have not found seizure rates to be that high and do not show substantial elevations in DES scores in patients with complex partial seizures compared with those in other neurological patients (Loewenstein and Putnam 1988). There is sufficient comorbidity that patients receiving recent diagnoses of DID should be evaluated for the possibility of a seizure disorder.

Genetics

Jang et al. (1998) conducted a classic twin study to assess the relative influence of genetic and environmental influ-

ences on measures of pathological and nonpathological dissociative experience. Subjects included 177 monozygotic and 152 dizygotic volunteer general population twin pairs who completed two measures of dissociative capacity identified from the items constituting the DES. The genetic correlation between these measures was estimated at 0.91, suggesting common genetic factors underlying pathological and nonpathological dissociative capacity. Genetic and environmental correlations between the DES and measures of personality disorder traits (Dimensional Assessment of Personality Pathology—Basic Questionnaire; DAPP-BQ) also were estimated. Significant genetic correlations (median = 0.38) were found between the DES and the DAPP-BQ measures of cognitive dysregulation, affective lability, and suspiciousness, suggesting that the genetic factors underlying particular aspects of personality disorder also influence dissociative capacity.

Psychological Testing

The diagnosis of DID can be facilitated by psychological testing (Scroppo et al. 1998). Form level on the Rorschach Test usually is within the normal range, but emotionally dramatic responses are common, often involving mutilation, especially on the color cards (such responses are often seen in patients with histrionic personality disorder as well). Good form level is useful in distinguishing DID patients from schizophrenic patients, who have poor form level. Leavitt and Labott (1998) replicated these findings. Their results indicated that Rorschach signs for the Labott, Barach, and Wagner Rorschach markers were significantly better than chance at classifying patients as having DID or as not having DID. The Labott system, which performed the best, was able to accurately classify 92% of the sample. The fact that two relatively rare sets of signs (DID and Rorschach) converged in the same small sector of the psychiatric population represents evidence of linkage that is clinically meaningful and not explainable on the basis of artificial creation. That the Rorschach signs operate independent of external bias, yet correspond to the diagnoses obtained through psychiatric evaluation in an inpatient setting, argues for the validity of the DID diagnosis. Also, unlike individuals with schizophrenia, those with DID score far higher than healthy individuals on standard measures of hypnotizability, whereas schizophrenic patients tend to show lower than normal or the absence of high hypnotizability (Lavoie and Sabourin 1980; Lavoie et al. 1973; Pettinati 1982; Pettinati et al. 1990; D. Spiegel and Fink 1979; D. Spiegel et al. 1982; van der Hart and Spiegel 1993). Thus, there is comparatively little overlap in the hypnotizability scores of schizophrenic patients and those of DID patients.

More recently, scales of trait dissociation have been developed (Bernstein and Putnam 1986; Ross 1989), and patients with DID score extremely high on these scales in contrast to healthy populations and other patient groups (Ross et al. 1990; Steinberg et al. 1990). These include the DES (Bernstein and Putnam 1986; Carlson et al. 1993), the Somatoform Dissociation Questionnaires (SDQ-20 and SDQ-5; Nijenhuis et al. 1996, 1997, respectively), the Clinician-Administered Dissociative States Scale (Bremner et al. 1998), the Structured Clinical Interview for DSM-IV Dissociative Disorders—Revised (Steinberg 2000), and the Adolescent Dissociative Experiences Scale (Armstrong et al. 1997).

The DES is widely used for the screening of dissociative experiences. The scale has been translated and validated in French (Darves-Bornoz et al. 1999), German (the "Fragebogen zu dissoziativen Symptomen"; Freyberger et al. 1998; Gast et al. 2001; Spitzer et al. 1998), Spanish (Icaran et al. 1996; Martinez-Taboas and Bernal 2000), and Turkish (Sar et al. 1996).

Treatment

Psychotherapy

Therapeutic direction. It is possible to help patients with DID gain control in several ways over the dissociative process underlying their symptoms. The fundamental psychotherapeutic stance should involve meeting patients halfway in the sense of acknowledging that they experience themselves as fragmented, yet the reality is that the fundamental problem is a failure of integration of disparate memories and aspects of the self. Therefore, the goal in therapy is to facilitate integration of disparate elements. This can be done in a variety of ways.

Secrets are frequently a problem with DID patients, who attempt to use the therapist to reinforce a dissociative strategy that withholds relevant information from certain personality states. Such patients often like to confide plans or stories to the therapist with the idea that the information is to be kept from other parts of the self, for example, traumatic memories or plans for self-destructive activities. Clear limit setting and commitment on the part of the therapist to helping all portions of a patient's personality structure learn about warded-off information are important. It is wise to clarify explicitly that the therapist will not become involved in secret collusion. Furthermore, when important agreements are negotiated,

such as a commitment on the part of the patient to seek medical help before acting on a thought to harm self or others, it is useful to discuss with the patient that this is an "all-points bulletin," that is, one that requires attention from all the relevant personality states. The excuse that certain personality states were "not aware" of the agreement should not be accepted.

Maldonado (2000) described a series of "Rules of Engagement" (see Table 15 8) to be used in the treatment of DID. These rules were designed to facilitate the therapist–patient contract by establishing clear lines of communication, delineating therapeutic boundaries, eliminating splitting, and enhancing control over dissociative experiences. The rules call for free access to all pertinent old records and permission to discuss all past and current pertinent information with previous therapists; cooperation in the completion of a full organic/neurological workup; a contract for safety; the establishment of a hierarchical pattern of communication and a hierarchical pattern of responsibility; agreement for a limited exploration followed by therapeutic condensation of memories—that is, an "all details are not needed" policy rather than an endless fishing exploration; a "no secrets" policy; an increased level of communication and cooperation between patient and therapist and between alters; detailed rules regarding therapist–patient contact during hospitalization and continued therapy after discharge; need for videotaping; and, finally, clear understanding of the ultimate treatment goal: "full integration."

TABLE 15–8. "Rules of engagement" in the treatment of dissociative identity disorder

1. Free access to all pertinent records
2. Review of all available and pertinent records
3. Freedom to discuss all past and current pertinent information with previous therapists
4. Complete organic/neurological workup
5. Contract for safety
6. Increased communication and cooperation among alters
7. "No secrets" policy
8. Establishment of hierarchical pattern of communication
9. Establishment of hierarchical pattern of responsibility
10. Limited exploration followed by therapeutic condensation of memories
11. "All details are not needed" policy
12. Rules regarding contact during hospitalizations and continued therapy after discharge
13. Videotaping
14. Ultimate goal: "full integration"
15. "One day you will make me obsolete" principle

For example, a patient with DID who had been in treatment for many years demonstrated a new alter who threatened to arrange for an apparently accidental death. The therapist told the alter that he, the therapist, would have to share this information with the other personalities. "You can't do that," the alter replied. "That would violate doctor–patient confidentiality." Suppressing a smile, the therapist explained that confidentiality did not apply between identities.

Hypnosis. Hypnosis can be helpful in therapy as well as in diagnosis (Braun 1984; Kluft 1982, 1985a, 1985c, 1992, 1999; Maldonado and Spiegel 1995, 1998; Maldonado et al. 2000; Smith 1993; H. Spiegel and Spiegel 1978/1987).

First, the simple structure of hypnotic induction may elicit dissociative phenomena. For example, the Hypnotic Induction Profile (H. Spiegel and Spiegel 1978/1987) was administered to a woman who had experienced hysterical pseudoseizures. In the middle of a routine induction, her head suddenly turned to the side and she relived, with considerable affect, as if it were happening in present tense, an episode in which she had been abducted and sexually assaulted. This enabled her and the clinician to reanalyze her symptoms as spontaneous dissociation, similar to the hypnotic state she had been in. The capacity to elicit such symptoms on command provides the first hint of the ability to control these symptoms. Most of these patients have the experience of being unable to stop dissociative symptoms but are often intrigued by the possibility of starting them. This carries with it the potential for changing or stopping the symptoms as well.

Hypnosis can be helpful in facilitating access to dissociated personalities. The personalities may simply occur spontaneously during hypnotic induction. An alternative strategy is to hypnotize the patient and use age regression to help the patient reorient to a time when a different personality state was manifest. An instruction later to change times back to the present tense usually elicits a return to the other personality state. This then becomes an alternative means of teaching the patient control over the dissociation.

Alternatively, entering the state of hypnosis may make it possible to simply "call up" different identities or personality states. Patients can be taught a simple self-hypnosis exercise (as noted earlier in this chapter in the "Dissociative Fugue" section and covered in more detail in Chapter 30). For example, the patient can be told to count to himself or herself from one to three: On 1, do one thing: look up. On 2, do two things: slowly close your eyes, and take a deep breath. On 3, do three things: let

the breath out, let your eyes relax but keep them closed, and let your body float. Then let one hand float up into the air like a balloon. Develop a pleasant sense of floating throughout your body. After some formal exercises such as this, it is often possible to simply ask to speak with a given alter personality, without the formal use of hypnosis. Merely asking to talk with a given identity usually suffices after a while.

Memory retrieval. Because loss of memory in DID is complex and chronic, its retrieval is likewise a more extended and integral part of the psychotherapeutic process. The therapy becomes an integrating experience of information sharing among disparate personality elements. In conceptualizing DID as a chronic PTSD, the psychotherapeutic strategy involves a focus on working through traumatic memories in addition to controlling the dissociation.

Controlled access to memories greatly facilitates psychotherapy. As in the treatment of dissociative amnesia, a variety of strategies can be used to help DID patients break down amnesic barriers. Use of hypnosis to go to that place in imagination and ask one or more such parts of the self to interact can be helpful.

Once these memories of earlier traumatic experience have been brought into consciousness, it is crucial to help the patient work through the painful affect, inappropriate self-blame, and other reactions to these memories. A model of grief work is helpful, enabling the patient to acknowledge and bear the import of such memories (Lindemann 1944; D. Spiegel 1981). It may be useful to have the patient visualize the memories rather than relive them as a way of making their intensity more manageable. It also can be useful to have the patient divide the memories onto two sides of an imaginary screen; for example, on one side, picturing something an abuser did to him or her and on the other side, picturing how the patient tried to protect himself or herself from the abuse.

> A young woman with DID remembered a particularly painful episode in hypnosis. When she was 12 years old, her stepfather smoked a good deal of marijuana and then forced her to have oral sex with him. She recalled being repelled by what he was forcing her to do and then remembered that she had gagged and vomited all over him. "I spoiled his fun. He threw me up against a wall, but it did not bother me a bit because I knew I ruined it for him." She was instructed to picture on one side of the screen what he had done to her and on the other what she had done to him.

Such techniques can help make the traumatic memories more bearable by placing them in a broader perspective, one in which the trauma victim also can identify adaptive aspects of his or her response to the trauma.

This technique and similar approaches can help these individuals work through traumatic memories, enabling them to bear the memories in consciousness and therefore reducing the need for dissociation as a means of keeping such memories out of consciousness. Although these techniques can be helpful and often result in reduced fragmentation and integration (Kluft 1985a, 1985c, 1986, 1992; Maldonado and Spiegel 1995, 1998; D. Spiegel 1984, 1986a), several complications can occur in the psychotherapy of these patients as well.

The information retrieved from memory in these ways should be reviewed, traumatic memories put into perspective, and emotional expression encouraged and worked through, with the goal of sharing the information as widely as possible among various parts of the patient's personality structure. Instructing other alter personalities to "listen" while a given alter is talking, and reviewing previously dissociated material uncovered, can be helpful. The therapist conveys his or her desire to disseminate the information, without accepting responsibility for transmitting it across all personality boundaries.

The "rule of thirds." Psychotherapy with a DID patient can be a time-consuming and emotionally taxing process. The "rule of thirds" (Kluft 1988, 1991) is a helpful guideline. The therapist should spend the first third of the psychotherapy session assessing the patient's current mental state and life problems and defining a problem area that might benefit from retrieval into conscious memory and working through. The therapist should spend the second third of the session accessing and working through this memory. The therapist should allow a final third for helping the patient assimilate the information, regulate and modulate emotional responses, and discuss any responses to the therapist and plans for the immediate future.

It is wise to use this final third of the session for debriefing and helping the patient to reorient, to attempt to integrate the new material, to transmit information across personalities, and to prepare to terminate the session. There may be resistance on the part of the therapist to doing this because the intense abreactive materials are often so compelling and interesting. There also may be resistance on the part of the patient to sharing of information across personalities.

Given the intensity of the material that often emerges involving memories of sexual and physical abuse, and the sudden shifts in mental state accompanied by amnesia, the therapist is called on to take a clear and structured role in managing the psychotherapy. Appropriate limits must be set about self-destructive or threat-

ening behavior and agreements made regarding physical safety and treatment compliance, and other matters must be presented to the patient in such a way that dissociative ignorance is not an acceptable explanation for failure to live up to agreements.

Traumatic transference. Transference applies with special meaning in patients who have been physically and sexually abused. These patients have had presumed caregivers who acted instead in an exploitative and sometimes sadistic fashion. These patients thus expect the same from their therapists. Although their reality testing is good enough that they can perceive genuine caring, they expect therapists either to exploit them, with the patients viewing the working through of traumatic memories as a reinflicting of the trauma and the therapists' taking sadistic pleasure in the patients' suffering, or to be excessively passive, with the patients identifying the therapists with some uncaring family figure who knew abuse was occurring but did little or nothing to stop it. It is important in managing the therapy to keep these issues in mind and make them frequent topics of discussion. Attention to these issues can diffuse, but not eliminate, such traumatic transference distortions of the therapeutic relationship (Maldonado and Spiegel 1995, 1998; D. Spiegel 1988).

Integration. The ultimate goal of psychotherapy for patients with DID is integration of the disparate states. There can be considerable resistance to this process. Early in therapy, the patient views the dissociation as tremendous protection: "I knew my father could get some of me, but he couldn't get all of me." Indeed, he or she may experience efforts of integration as an attempt on the part of the therapist to "kill" personalities. These fears must be worked through and the patient shown how to control the degree of integration, giving the patient a sense of gradually being able to control his or her dissociative processes in the service of working through traumatic memories. The process of the psychotherapy, in emphasizing control, must alter rather than reinforce the content, which involves reexperiencing of helplessness, a symbolic reenactment of trauma (D. Spiegel 1986b).

As previously mentioned, a patient with DID often fears integration as an attempt to kill alter personalities and make the patient more vulnerable to mistreatment by depriving him or her of the dissociative defense. At the same time, this defense represents an internalization of the abusive person or persons in the patient's memory. Setting aside the defense also means acknowledging and bearing the discomfort of helplessness at having been victimized and working through the irrational self-blame that gave the patient a fantasy of control over events that he or she was in fact helpless to control. Yet difficult as it is, ultimately, the goal of psychotherapy is mastery over the dissociative process, controlled access to dissociative states, integration of warded-off painful memories and material, and a more integrated continuum of identity, memory, and consciousness (Maldonado and Spiegel 1995, 1998; D. Spiegel 1988). Although there have been no controlled trials of psychotherapy outcome in patients with this disorder, case series reports indicate a positive outcome in most cases (Kluft 1984c, 1986, 1991).

Cognitive-Behavioral Approaches

Fine (1999) summarized the tactical-integration model for the treatment of dissociative disorders. This consists of structured cognitive-behavioral–based treatments that foster symptom relief, followed by integration of the personalities and/or ego states into one mainstream of consciousness. This approach promotes proficiency in control over posttraumatic and dissociative symptoms, is collaborative and exploratory, and conveys a consistent message of empowerment to the patient.

Psychopharmacology

To date, no good evidence shows that medication of any type has a direct therapeutic effect on the dissociative process manifested by patients with DID (Loewenstein 1991b; Markowitz and Gill 1996; Putnam 1989). In fact, most dissociative symptoms seem relatively resistant to pharmacological intervention (Loewenstein 1991a, 1991b). Thus, pharmacological treatment has been limited to the control of signs and symptoms afflicting patients with DID or comorbid conditions rather than the treatment of dissociation per se.

Whereas in the past, short-acting barbiturates such as sodium amobarbital were used intravenously to reverse functional amnesias, this technique is no longer used, largely because of poor results (J.C. Perry and Jacobs 1982).

Benzodiazepines have at times been used to facilitate recall through controlling secondary anxiety associated with retrieval of traumatic memories. However, these effects may be nonspecific at best. Furthermore, sudden mental state transitions induced by medications may increase rather than decrease amnesic barriers, as the recent concern about triazolam, a short-acting benzodiazepine hypnotic, indicates. Thus, inducing state changes pharmacologically could in theory add to difficulty in retrieval. The only systematic study on the use of benzodiazepines in patients with DID was conducted by Loewenstein et al. (1988). In their study, they used clonaze-

pam successfully to control PTSD-like symptoms in a small sample ($n = 5$) of DID patients, achieving improvement in sleep continuity and a decrease in frequency of flashbacks and nightmares.

Antidepressants are the most useful class of psychotropic agents for patients with DID. Such patients frequently have dysthymic disorder or major depression as well, and when these disorders are present, especially with somatic signs and suicidal ideation, antidepressant medication can be helpful. At least two studies report on the successful use of antidepressant medications (Barkin et al. 1986; Kluft 1984a, 1985b). The use of antidepressants should be limited to the treatment of DID patients who experience symptoms of major depression (Barkin et al. 1986). The newer selective serotonin reuptake inhibitors (SSRIs) are effective at reducing comorbid depressive symptoms and have the advantage of far less lethality in overdose compared with tricyclics and monoamine oxidase inhibitors (MAOIs). Medication compliance is a problem with such patients because dissociated personality states may interfere with the taking of medication by the patients' "hiding" or hoarding of pills, or patients may overdose.

Antipsychotics are rarely useful in reducing dissociative symptoms. They are used occasionally for containing impulsive behavior, with varying effect. More often, they are used with little benefit when DID patients have been given misdiagnoses of schizophrenia (Kluft 1987). In addition to the risks of side effects such as tardive dyskinesia, the neuroleptics may reduce the range of affect, thereby making patients with DID look spuriously as though they were schizophrenic. In fact, most DID researchers have reported an extremely high incidence of adverse side effects with the use of neuroleptic medications (Barkin et al. 1986; Kluft 1984a, 1988; Putnam 1989; Ross 1989).

Anticonvulsants have been used to treat seizure disorders (Mesulam 1981; Schenk and Bear 1981), which have a high rate of comorbidity with DID, mood disorders (Fichtner et al. 1990), and the impulsiveness associated with personality disorders. These agents have been used to reduce impulsive behavior but are rarely definitively helpful. The high incidence of serious side effects (Devinsky et al. 1989) and abuse or overdose potential also should be kept in mind.

Case reports have suggested that β-blockers may be useful in the treatment of hyperarousal, anxiety, poor impulse control, disorganized thinking, and rapid or uncontrolled switching in patients with DID (Braun 1990). However, little information is available about the actual success rate, comorbid diagnoses, or prevalence of adverse drug reactions.

DeBattista et al. (1998) reported on four cases of DID associated with severe self-destructive behavior and comorbid major depression treated with ECT. In three of the patients, ECT appeared to be helpful in treating the comorbid depression without adversely affecting the DID.

Eye Movement Desensitization and Reprocessing

Studies of eye movement desensitization and reprocessing (EMDR) have provided mixed outcomes and little support for any specific effect of the use of structured eye movements during psychotherapy. It may well mobilize therapeutic elements common to various exposure, densensitization, and cathartic methods. In the past few years, it has become a rather popular technique used by therapists dealing with trauma victims who have PTSD and DID. Fine and Berkowitz (2001) described EMDR as a technique that "has come to the forefront of clinical awareness in the last ten years, seems aptly suited for the treatment of trauma, but which can be destabilizing." They proposed a treatment protocol—the "Wreathing Protocol"—that calls for the "imbricated use of EMDR and hypnosis" in the treatment of trauma victims.

Wade and Wade (2001) also suggested combining ego-state therapy, hypnosis, and EMDR in a psychosocial developmental context. They suggested that eye movements and hypnosis may promote corrective developmental experiences leading to resolution of grief and trauma, the acquisition of needed skills and abilities, and the promotion of co-consciousness and negotiation among ego states.

Legal Aspects of Memory Work and Hypnosis Recall

Maldonado (2000) summarized and adapted the guidelines provided by the American Medical Association (AMA; Orne et al. 1985) and the American Society of Clinical Hypnosis (ASCH; Hammond et al. 1985) for the use of hypnosis as a method of memory enhancement. The guidelines suggest that when hypnosis or any other memory enhancement method is being used for forensic purposes or in the context of working out traumatic memories, especially those related to childhood physical and/or sexual abuse, the steps shown in Table 15–9 should be applied. Please refer to Chapter 30, "Hypnosis," for an extensive review of hypnotic technique and the uses, potential side effects, and legal implications of hypnosis.

TABLE 15–9. Guidelines for the use of hypnosis in memory work

1. Before hypnosis use, perform a thorough evaluation of the patient.
2. Explore the patient's expectations about treatment in general and hypnosis use in particular.
3. Obtain the patient's permission to consult with his or her attorney.
4. Clarify your role (i.e., therapist vs. forensic consultant) before initiating any assessment and/or treatment. Make sure the patient clearly understands your role in the case.
5. Obtain written informed consent regarding the nature of hypnotic retrieval (explain to the subject and his or her attorney about the nature of hypnotically retrieved memories) and possible side effects of memory work.
6. Clarify the patient's expectation regarding hypnotically enhanced or recovered memories.
7. Maintain neutrality throughout every interaction with the patient.
8. Make a videotape recording of the interview and hypnotic session.
9. Thoroughly document any and all prehypnosis memories.
10. Objectively measure hypnotizability.
11. Carefully document your discussion of hypnosis and memory, issues of accuracy of memory, informed consent, and the maintenance of a stance of neutrality and nonleading approach.
12. Use an expert as a hypnosis consultant.
13. Conduct the interview in a neutral tone; avoid leading or suggestive questions.
14. Demonstrate a balance between supportiveness and empathy, while assisting the patient to critically evaluate the elicited material.
15. Do not encourage patients to institute litigation or to confront alleged perpetrators based solely on information retrieved under hypnosis.
16. Carefully debrief the subject at the end of each session.
17. Carefully document and produce a report containing
    Detailed prehypnotic memories
    Hypnotizability score
    Hypnotic techniques used
    Any significant behavior
    Any confirmed or new memories and details

Dissociative Trance Disorder

Cultural Context

Dissociative phenomena are ubiquitous around the world, occurring in virtually every culture (Castillo 1994a, 1994b; Kirmayer 1993; Lewis-Fernandez 1993). These phenomena seem to be more prevalent in the less heavily industrialized Second and Third World countries, although they can be found everywhere. For this reason, some scholars have argued against the inclusion of possession or trance disorder as a DSM diagnostic category (Noll 1993). There are descriptions of mediums or possession episodes in different cultures, but they all may serve a similar purpose. There are shamans among Hispanics (Alonso 1988; Pineros et al. 1998) and in Brazil (Shapiro 1992), China (Gaw et al. 1998; Kua et al. 1993), India (Moore 1993; Nuckolls 1991), Iran (Safa 1988), Israel (Bilu and Beit-Hallahmi 1989; Shirali et al. 1986), Japan (Eguchi 1991; Etsuko 1991), Madagascar (Lambek 1988; Sharp 1990, 1994), Malaysia (McLellan 1991; Ong 1988), New Guinea (Schieffelin 1996), Samoa (Mageo 1996), Singapore (Kua et al. 1986), South Africa (Heap and Ramphele 1991), South Asia (Castillo 1994a, 1994b), Thailand (Trangkasombat et al. 1995, 1998), Zambia (Pullela 1986), and Zanzibar (Tantam 1993). Other dissociative syndromes include demonic possession in Brazil (Heap and Ramphele 1991), Chilopa ritual sacrifices in Malawi (Machleidt and Peltzer 1991), and Zar possession in Northern Sudan (Boddy 1988) and Ethiopia (Witztum et al. 1996).

Most scholars agree that the most common clinical features of trance states are amnesia, emotional disturbances, and loss of identity (D. Li and Spiegel 1992). In a study comparing the characteristic features of the possession trance in three different ethnic groups of Chinese, Malayans, and Indians, Kua et al. (1986) found a set of similarities, including alteration in the level of consciousness, amnesia for the period of the trance, stereotyped behavior characteristic of a deity, duration of less than 1 hour, fatigue at the termination of the trance, normal behavior in the interval between trances, onset before age 25 years, low social class status, poor educational level, and prior witnessing of a trance.

Dissociative symptoms are widely understood as an idiom of distress. The major purposes served by possession and trance states include the need to gain power, prestige, and status and the desire to express aggressive and sexual impulses (Shirali et al. 1986), especially given the cultural overdetermination of women's selfhood (Boddy 1988). Spirit-possession rituals may mystify the source of women's suppression and absolve women of any responsibility for an otherwise unacceptable challenge to patriarchal control (Sered 1994). They also may provide the subject with a sense of social association and ultimately attempt to make something socially useful from feelings such as aggression that were previously socially disintegrative (Tantam 1993), may provide a release from normative structural constraints, and may facilitate role reversal and role enhancement (McLellan 1991). Dissociative trance disorders, especially posses-

sion disorder, are probably more common than is usually thought. Ferracuti et al. (1996) reported on 10 patients undergoing exorcisms for devil trance possession state. Subjects were studied with the Dissociative Disorders Diagnostic Schedule and the Rorschach Test. Subjects were found to have many traits in common with patients with DID. Despite claiming possession by a demon and various paranormal phenomena, most of them managed to maintain normal social functioning. Thus, in this sample of subjects reporting demonic possession, dissociative trance disorder appeared to be a distinct clinical manifestation of a dissociative continuum, sharing some features with dissociative disorders in general and DID in particular.

Ataque de nervios is a common, self-labeled Hispanic folk diagnosis that describes episodic, dramatic outbursts of negative emotion in response to a stressor, sometimes involving destructive behavior. A study among 70 Hispanic outpatients conducted by Schechter et al. (2000) found that significantly more subjects with an anxiety or a mood disorder plus ataque de nervios reported a history of physical abuse, sexual abuse, and/or a substance-abusing caregiver than did those with psychiatric disorder but no ataque de nervios. As in the case of dissociative disorders, in some Hispanic individuals, ataque de nervios may represent a culturally sanctioned expression of extreme affect dysregulation associated with antecedent childhood trauma.

In a case-controlled study of 32 girls ages 9–14 years afflicted with an outbreak of spirit possession in the south of Thailand, Trangkasombat and colleagues (1998) found that the children with spirit possession were firstborn and came from small families (e.g., one to three children). Compared with the control subjects, their family life was characterized by more psychosocial stressors, and they had significantly higher rates of psychiatric disorders, anxious and fearful character traits, histrionic character traits, and histories of recurrent trance states. The history of traumatic experiences and exposure to spirit possession ceremonies were more frequent in the spirit-possessed children than in the control children.

Similarly, Gaw et al. (1998) described the clinical characteristics of 20 hospitalized psychiatric patients in the Hebei Province of China who believed that they were possessed. These patients had been given the Chinese diagnosis of *yi-ping* (hysteria) by Chinese physicians before being recruited for the study. The investigators found that among their subjects, the mean age was 37 years; most patients were women from rural areas with little education; and most reported significant events preceding the episode of possession, including interpersonal conflicts, subjectively meaningful circumstances, illness, and death of an individual or dreaming of a deceased individual. Possessing entities were thought to be spirits of deceased individuals, deities, animals, and devils. About one-fifth of their sample reported multiple possessions. In most instances, the initial experience of possession typically came on acutely and often became a chronic relapsing event. Almost all subjects manifested the loss of control over their actions, change in their usual pattern of behavior, loss of awareness of surroundings, loss of personal identity, inability to distinguish reality from fantasy, change in tone of voice, and loss of perceived sensitivity to pain. The authors suggested that their findings indicate that this type of possession syndrome is clinically similar to the DSM-IV-TR diagnosis of dissociative trance disorder under the category of dissociative disorder not otherwise specified.

Some even suggest that possession can be interpreted as historical discourse, usually containing tales of tradition (Mageo 1996), or even as an alternative method of healing—not too different from Western psychotherapy (Li et al. 1992; Machleidt and Peltzer 1991; Mulhern 1991; Tantam 1993)—thus performing a wider social function. In fact, "when the embodiment of an alternative identity is exercised in the cross-cultural complex of spirit possession, it provides a conduit through which subjective suffering can be transcended and through which the past, present, and future can be expressed" (Mulhern 1991).

The trance and possession categories of dissociative trance disorder constitute by far the most common kinds of dissociative disorders around the world. Several studies of dissociative disorders in India, for example, reported that dissociative trance and possession are the most prevalent dissociative disorders (i.e., approximately 3.5% of psychiatric admissions; Adityanjee et al. 1989; Saxena and Prasad 1989). On the other hand, DID, which is relatively more common in the United States, is virtually never diagnosed in India. Cultural and biological factors may account for the different content and form of dissociative symptoms. Nonetheless, the underlying dissociative mechanism inhibiting integration of perception, memory, and identity makes these syndromes an important class of dissociative disorders.

Differences in culture clearly influence almost all mental disorders, and therefore the contents of religious delusions will be different in a Hindu or Muslim person with schizophrenia than in a Christian person with the same disorder. Depression takes a very different form in China, resembling what used to be called *neurasthenia*, with a variety of somatic symptoms predominating more than the guilty ruminations seen in the West (Kleinman 1977). Likewise, the variations in form of the dissociative disorders only serve to underscore the ubiquity of the dissociative mechanism. Nonetheless, the variety of mental content is worthy of attention. The DSM-IV Task Force voted to include dissociative trance disorder in an appendix to DSM-IV to stimulate further research on the question of whether it should be a separate Axis I disorder rather than an example in the category of dissociative disorders not otherwise specified, in which it was placed in DSM-III-R (Table 15–10). Some suggest, and we agree, that the inclusion of trance and possession disorder in DSM-IV intends to develop a sense of cultural sensitivity and internationalization of DSM. On the other hand, designating trance and possession disorder as a formal diagnostic disorder carries with it the risks of attempting to craft a global nosological system, an impossible task. Furthermore, the composite category "dissociative trance disorder," encompassing both trance and possession phenomena, may be misinterpreted as "a single, uniform diagnostic construct and may suggest a greater degree of phenomenological uniformity than exists among indigenous syndromes, creating a hybrid nosological entity without validity" (Lewis-Fernandez 1993, pp. 123–167).

These dissociative episodes usually are understood as an idiom of distress, yet they are not viewed as normal. That is, they are not a generally accepted part of cultural and religious practice that may often involve normal trance phenomena, such as trance dancing in the Balinese Hindu culture. Trance dancers in that culture are remarkable for being the only portion of this socially stable society able to elevate their social status. This elevation of social status is done through developing an ability to enter trance states. They are able within the social ceremony to induce an altered state of consciousness in which they dance over hot coals, hold a sword at their throat, or in other ways show exceptional powers of concentration and physical prowess. They are frequently watched by other dancers to make sure that they retain control and do not hurt themselves. This form of trance is considered socially normal and even exalted. By contrast, trance and possession disorder is viewed by the local community as a common but aberrant form of behavior that requires intervention. Although trance and possession disorder is clearly an idiom of distress (e.g., discomfort in a new family environment), most individuals use an array of alternative strategies for coping with such distress. Thus, cultural informants make it clear that persons with trance and possession trance disorders are acting abnormally, if recognizably.

It is interesting that the most common form of dissociative disorder in the West is DID—that is, the experience of fragmentation of individual identity—whereas in the East, this disorder involves possession by an outside

TABLE 15–10. DSM-IV-TR research criteria for dissociative trance disorder

A. Either (1) or (2):
  (1) trance, i.e., temporary marked alteration in the state of consciousness or loss of customary sense of personal identity without replacement by an alternate identity, associated with at least one of the following:
    (a) narrowing of awareness of immediate surroundings, or unusually narrow and selective focusing on environmental stimuli
    (b) stereotyped behaviors or movements that are experienced as being beyond one's control
  (2) possession trance, a single or episodic alteration in the state of consciousness characterized by the replacement of customary sense of personal identity by a new identity. This is attributed to the influence of a spirit, power, deity, or other person, as evidenced by one (or more) of the following:
    (a) stereotyped and culturally determined behaviors or movements that are experienced as being controlled by the possessing agent
    (b) full or partial amnesia for the event
B. The trance or possession trance state is not accepted as a normal part of a collective cultural or religious practice.
C. The trance or possession trance state causes clinically significant distress or impairment in social, occupational, or other important areas of functioning.
D. The trance or possession trance state does not occur exclusively during the course of a psychotic disorder (including mood disorder with psychotic features and brief psychotic disorder) or dissociative identity disorder and is not due to the direct physiological effects of a substance or a general medical condition.

spirit, deity, or other entity. Given the greater sociocentric organization of culture in the East, it makes sense that the dissociative problem would take the form of an intruding outside identity, whereas in the West, the disorder takes the form of competing internal identities.

Nevertheless, some have proposed that possession trance and multiple personality disorders arose on the basis of similar histories of child abuse and the use of dissociation as a defense mechanism (Bourguignon 1989). Still, different cultures apply their own idiosyncratic etiological theories. The therapeutic approaches and subjects' responses may be rather similar or radically different, depending on the traditional beliefs of the culture in question.

Classification

Dissociative trance disorder has been divided into two broad categories: dissociative trance and possession trance (Table 15–11).

Dissociative Trance

Dissociative trance phenomena are characterized by a sudden alteration in consciousness not accompanied by distinct alternative identities. In this form, the dissociative symptom involves consciousness rather than identity. Also, in dissociative trance, the activities performed are rather simple, usually involving sudden collapse, immobilization, dizziness, shrieking, screaming, or crying. Memory is rarely affected, and amnesia, if any, is fragmented.

Dissociative trance phenomena frequently involve sudden, extreme changes in sensory and motor control. Classic examples include ataque de nervios, which is prevalent throughout Latin America. This condition, for example, is estimated to have a 12% lifetime prevalence rate in Puerto Rico (Lewis-Fernandez 1993). Typically, the individual suddenly starts to shake convulsively, hyperventilate, scream, and show agitation and aggressive movements. These behaviors may be followed by collapse and loss of consciousness. Afterward, such individuals report being exhausted and may have some amnesia for the event (Lewis-Fernandez 1993).

TABLE 15–11. Comparison of Western and Eastern types of dissociative syndromes

Dissociative phenomenon	Western	Eastern
Identity	DID: multiple internal identities	Possession trance: control by external identities
	Dissociative fugue	
Memory	Dissociative amnesia	Secondary in dissociative trance, more common in possession trance
Perception	Depersonalization disorder	Dissociative trance (e.g., *latah*, *ataque de nervios*)
Consciousness	Acute stress disorder	Dissociative trance

Note. DID = dissociative identity disorder.

Falling out occurs frequently among African Americans in the southern United States. Affected individuals may collapse suddenly, unable to see or speak even though they are conscious. These persons may be confused afterward but usually are not amnesic to the episode (Lewis-Fernandez 1993).

In the Malay version of trance disorder, *latah*, affected individuals may have a sudden vision of a spirit that is threatening them. These persons scream or cry, strike out physically, and may need restraints. They may report amnesia, but they do not clearly take on the identity of the offending spirit (Lewis-Fernandez 1993).

Possession Trance

In contrast to dissociative trance, possession trance involves the assumption of a distinct alternate identity, usually that of a deity, an ancestor, or a spirit. The person in this trance often engages in rather complex activities, which may take the form of expressing otherwise forbidden thoughts or needs, negotiating for change in family or social status, or engaging in aggressive behavior. Possession usually involves amnesia for a large portion of the episode during which the alternate identity was in control of the person's behavior.

In Indian possession syndrome, the affected individual suddenly begins speaking in an altered voice with an altered identity, usually that of a deity recognizable to others. Through this voice, a person may refer to himself or herself in the third person. The affected person's "spirit" may negotiate for changes in the family environment or become agitated or aggressive. Possession syndrome typically occurs in a recently married woman who finds herself uncomfortable or unwelcome in her mother-in-law's home. Such individuals usually are unable to directly express their discomfort.

Treatment

Treatment of these disorders varies from culture to culture. Most syndromes occur within the context of acute social stress and thus serve the purpose of recruiting help from the family and other support systems or removing the subject from the immediate danger or threat. Ceremonies to remove or appease the invading spirit are commonly used (Pineros et al. 1998). The role of psychiatry should be focused on ruling out any possible organic cause for the symptoms shown, treating comorbid psychiatric conditions (if any are present), avoiding excess medication, understanding the social context and role of the syndrome, and facilitating a favorable outcome.

Conclusion

The dissociative disorders constitute a challenging component of psychiatric illness. The failure of integration of memory, identity, perception, and consciousness seen in these disorders results in symptomatology that illustrates fundamental problems in the organization of mental processes. Dissociative phenomena often occur during and after physical trauma but also may represent transient or chronic defensive patterns. Dissociative disorders are generally treatable and constitute a domain in which psychotherapy is a primary modality, although pharmacological treatment of comorbid conditions such as depression can be quite helpful. The dissociative disorders are ubiquitous around the world, although they take a variety of forms. They represent a fascinating window into the processing of identity, memory, perception, and consciousness, and they pose a variety of diagnostic, therapeutic, and research challenges.

References

Abeles M, Schilder P: Psychogenic loss of personal identity: amnesia. Archives of Neurology and Psychiatry 34:587–604, 1935

Adityanjee, Raju GSP, Khandelwal SK: Current status of multiple personality disorder in India. Am J Psychiatry 146:1607–1610, 1989

Akyuz G, Dogan O, Sar V, et al: Frequency of dissociative identity disorder in the general population in Turkey. Compr Psychiatry 40:151–159, 1999

Allison RB: A new treatment approach for multiple personalities. Am J Clin Hypn 17:15–32, 1974

Alonso L: Mental illness complicated by the santeria belief in spirit possession. Hosp Community Psychiatry 39:1188–1191, 1988

Ambrosino SV: Phobic anxiety-depersonalization syndrome. New York State Journal of Medicine 73:419–425, 1973

American Psychiatric Association: Diagnostic and Statistical Manual of Mental Disorders, 3rd Edition. Washington, DC, American Psychiatric Association, 1980

American Psychiatric Association: Diagnostic and Statistical Manual of Mental Disorders, 3rd Edition, Revised. Washington, DC, American Psychiatric Association, 1987

American Psychiatric Association: Diagnostic and Statistical Manual of Mental Disorders, 4th Edition. Washington, DC, American Psychiatric Association, 1994

American Psychiatric Association: Diagnostic and Statistical Manual of Mental Disorders, 4th Edition, Text Revision. Washington, DC, American Psychiatric Association, 2000

Anderson G, Yasenik L, Ross CA: Dissociative experiences and disorders among women who identify themselves as sexual abuse survivors. Child Abuse Negl 17:677–686, 1993

Armstrong JG, Putnam FW, Carlson EB, et al: Development and validation of a measure of adolescent dissociation: the Adolescent Dissociative Experiences Scale. J Nerv Ment Dis 185:491–497, 1997

Awas M, Kebede D, Alem A: Major mental disorders in Butajira, southern Ethiopia. Acta Psychiatr Scand Suppl 397:56–64, 1999

Baars BJ: A Cognitive Theory of Consciousness. New York, Cambridge University Press, 1988

Ball S, Robinson A, Shekhar A, et al: Dissociative symptoms in panic disorder. J Nerv Ment Dis 185:755–760, 1997

Ballenger JC, Burrows GD, Dupont RL, et al: Alprazolam in panic disorder and agoraphobia: results from a multicenter trial, I: efficacy in short term treatment. Arch Gen Psychiatry 45:413–422, 1988

Barkin R, Braun BG, Kluft RP: The dilemma of drug therapy for multiple personality disorder, in Treatment of Multiple Personality Disorder. Edited by Braun BG. Washington, DC, American Psychiatric Press, 1986, pp 107–132

Baron DA, Nagy R: The amobarbital interview in a general hospital setting, friend or foe: a case report. Gen Hosp Psychiatry 10:220–222, 1988

Benjamin LR, Benjamin R, Rind B: The parenting experiences of mothers with dissociative disorders. J Marital Fam Ther 24:337–354, 1998

Berger D, Saito S, Ono Y, et al: Dissociation and child abuse histories in an eating disorder cohort in Japan. Acta Psychiatr Scand 90:274–280, 1994

Bernstein EM, Putnam FW: Development, reliability, and validity of a dissociation scale. J Nerv Ment Dis 174:727–735, 1986

Bilu Y, Beit-Hallahmi B: Dybbuk-possession as a hysterical symptom: psychodynamic and socio-cultural factors. Isr J Psychiatry Relat Sci 26:138–149, 1989

Blank AS Jr: The longitudinal course of posttraumatic stress disorder, in Posttraumatic Stress Disorder: DSM-IV and Beyond. Edited by Davidson JRT, Foa EB. Washington, DC, American Psychiatric Press, 1993, pp 3–22

Bliss EL: Multiple personalities: a report of 14 cases with implications for schizophrenia and hysteria. Arch Gen Psychiatry 37:1388–1397, 1980

Bliss EL: A symptom profile of patients with multiple personalities, including MMPI results. J Nerv Ment Dis 172:197–202, 1984

Bliss EL: Multiple Personality, Allied Disorders, and Hypnosis. New York, Oxford University Press, 1986

Bliss EL, Larson EM, Nakashima SR: Auditory hallucinations and schizophrenia. J Nerv Ment Dis 171:30–33, 1983

Blue FR: Use of directive therapy in the treatment of depersonalization neurosis. Psychol Rep 49:904–906, 1979

Boddy J: Spirits and selves in Northern Sudan: the cultural therapeutics of possession and trance. American Ethnologist 15:4–27, 1988

Boe T, Haslerud J, Knudsen H: Multiple personality: a phenomenon also in Norway? Tidsskr Nor Laegeforen 113:3230–3232, 1993

Boon S, Draijer N: Multiple personality disorder in the Netherlands: a clinical investigation of 71 patients. Am J Psychiatry 150:489–494, 1993a

Boon S, Draijer N: Multiple Personality Disorder in the Netherlands: A Study on Reliability and Validity of the Diagnosis. Amsterdam, The Netherlands, Swets & Zeitlinger, 1993b

Bourguignon E: Multiple personality, possession trance, and the psychic unity of mankind. Ethos 17:371–384, 1989

Bowman ES: Etiology and clinical course of pseudoseizures: relationship to trauma, depression, and dissociation. Psychosomatics 34:333–342, 1993

Bowman ES, Markand ON: Psychodynamics and psychiatric diagnoses of pseudoseizure subjects. Am J Psychiatry 153:57–63, 1996

Braun BG: Uses of hypnosis with multiple personality. Psychiatr Ann 14:34–36, 39–40, 1984

Braun BG: Multiple personality disorder: an overview. Am J Occup Ther 44:971–976, 1990

Braun BG, Sachs RG: The development of multiple personality disorder: predisposing, precipitating, and perpetuating factors, in Childhood Antecedents of Multiple Personality Disorder. Edited by Kluft RP. Washington, DC, American Psychiatric Press, 1985, pp 37–64

Bremner JD, Brett E: Trauma-related dissociative states and long-term psychopathology in posttraumatic stress disorder. J Trauma Stress 10:37–49, 1997

Bremner JD, Krystal JH, Putnam FW, et al: Measurement of dissociative states with the Clinician-Administered Dissociative States Scale (CADSS). J Trauma Stress 11:125–136, 1998

Brenner I: The dissociative character: a reconsideration of "multiple personality." J Am Psychoanal Assoc 42:819–846, 1994

Brenner I: The characterological basis of multiple personality. Am J Psychother 50:154–166, 1996a

Brenner I: On trauma, perversion, and "multiple personality." J Am Psychoanal Assoc 44:785–814, 1996b

Brenner I: Deconstructing DID. Am J Psychother 53:344–360, 1999

Breuer J, Freud S: Studies on hysteria (1893–1895), in The Standard Edition of the Complete Psychological Works of Sigmund Freud, Vol 2. Translated and edited by Strachey J. London, England, Hogarth Press, 1955, pp 201–319

Brodsky BS, Cloitre M, Dulit RA: Relationship of dissociation to self-mutilation and childhood abuse in borderline personality disorder. Am J Psychiatry 152:1788–1792, 1995

Brown GR, Anderson B: Psychiatric morbidity in adult inpatients with childhood histories of sexual and physical abuse. Am J Psychiatry 148:55–61, 1991

Brown L, Russell J, Thornton C, et al: Dissociation, abuse and the eating disorders: evidence from an Australian population. Aust N Z J Psychiatry 33:521–528, 1999

Brown W: The treatment of cases of shell shock in an advanced neurological centre. Lancet 2:197–200, 1918

Bryer JB, Nelson BA, Miller JB, et al: Childhood sexual and physical abuse as factors in adult psychiatric illness. Am J Psychiatry 144:1426–1430, 1987

Butler LD, Duran EFD, Jasiukatis P, et al: Hypnotizability and traumatic experience: a diathesis-stress model of dissociative symptomatology. Am J Psychiatry 153:42–63, 1996

Cardeña E, Spiegel D: Dissociative reactions to the San Francisco Bay Area earthquake of 1989. Am J Psychiatry 150:474–478, 1993

Carlier IV, Lamberts RD, Fouwels AJ, et al: PTSD in relation to dissociation in traumatized police officers. Am J Psychiatry 153:1325–1328, 1996

Carlson EB, Putnam FW, Ross CA, et al: Validity of the Dissociative Experiences Scale in screening for multiple personality disorder: a multicenter study. Am J Psychiatry 150:1030–1036, 1993

Castillo RJ: Spirit possession in South Asia, dissociation or hysteria? I: theoretical background. Cult Med Psychiatry 18:1–21, 1994a

Castillo RJ: Spirit possession in South Asia, dissociation or hysteria? II: case histories. Cult Med Psychiatry 18:141–162, 1994b

Cattell JP, Cattell JS: Depersonalization: psychological and social perspectives, in American Handbook of Psychiatry. Edited by Arieti S. New York, Basic Books, 1974, pp 767–799

Charcot JM: Oeuvres Completes de J M Charcot, Tome XI. Paris, France, Lecrosnier et Babe, 1890

Chodoff P: Turkish dissociative identity disorder (letter). Am J Psychiatry 154:1179, 1997

Christianson SA, Loftus EF: Memory for traumatic events. Applied Cognitive Psychology 1:225–239, 1987

Chu JA, Dill DL: Dissociative symptoms in relation to childhood physical and sexual abuse. Am J Psychiatry 147:887–892, 1990

Chu JA, Frey LM, Ganzel BL, et al: Memories of childhood abuse: dissociation, amnesia, and corroboration. Am J Psychiatry 156:749–755, 1999

Cohen JD, Servan-Schreiber D: Introduction to neural network models in psychiatry. Psychiatr Ann 22:113–118, 1992a

Cohen JD, Servan-Schreiber D: A neural network model of disturbances in the processing of context in schizophrenia. Psychiatr Ann 22:131–136, 1992b

Coons PM: The differential diagnosis of multiple personality: a comprehensive review. Psychiatr Clin North Am 7:51–65, 1984

Coons PM: Confirmation of childhood abuse in child and adolescent cases of multiple personality disorder and dissociative disorder not otherwise specified. J Nerv Ment Dis 182:461–464, 1994

Coons PM: The dissociative disorders: rarely considered and underdiagnosed. Psychiatr Clin North Am 21:637–648, 1998

Coons PM, Milstein V: Psychosexual disturbances in multiple personality: characteristics, etiology, and treatment. J Clin Psychiatry 47:106–110, 1986

Coons PM, Milstein V: Psychogenic amnesia: a clinical investigation of 25 cases. Dissociation 5:73–79, 1992

Coons PM, Bowman ES, Milstein V: Multiple personality disorder: a clinical investigation of 50 cases. J Nerv Ment Dis 17:519–527, 1988

Coons PM, Bowman ES, Kluft RP, et al: The cross-cultural occurrence of MPD: additional cases from a recent survey. Dissociation 4:124–128, 1991

Darves-Bornoz JM: Rape-related psychotraumatic syndromes. Eur J Obstet Gynecol Reprod Biol 71:59–65, 1997

Darves-Bornoz JM, Degiovanni A, Gaillard P: Validation of a French version of the Dissociative Experiences Scale in a rape-victim population. Can J Psychiatry 44:271–275, 1999

Davison K: Episodic depersonalization: observations on 7 patients. Br J Psychiatry 110:505–513, 1964

DeBattista C, Solvason HB, Spiegel D: ECT in dissociative identity disorder and comorbid depression. J ECT 14:275–279, 1998

Devinsky O, Putnam F, Grafman J, et al: Dissociative states and epilepsy. Neurology 39:835–840, 1989

Dollinger S: A case report of dissociative neurosis (depersonalization disorder) in an adolescent treated with family therapy and behavior modification. J Consult Clin Psychol 51:479–484, 1983

Draijer N, Langeland W: Childhood trauma and perceived parental dysfunction in the etiology of dissociative symptoms in psychiatric inpatients. Am J Psychiatry 156:379–385, 1999

Dunn GE, Ryan JJ, Paolo AM, et al: Comorbidity of dissociative disorders among patients with substance use disorders. Psychiatr Serv 46:153–156, 1995

Eguchi S: Between folk concepts of illness and psychiatric diagnosis: kitsune-tsuki (fox possession) in a mountain village of western Japan. Cult Med Psychiatry 15:421–451, 1991

Ellason JW, Ross CA: Positive and negative symptoms in dissociative identity disorder and schizophrenia: a comparative analysis. J Nerv Ment Dis 183:236–241, 1995

Ellason JW, Ross CA, Sainton K, et al: Axis I and II comorbidity and childhood trauma history in chemical dependency. Bull Menninger Clin 60:39–51, 1996

Eriksson NG, Lundin T: Early traumatic stress reactions among Swedish survivors of the Estonia disaster. Br J Psychiatry 169:713–716, 1996

Etsuko M: The interpretations of fox possession: illness as metaphor. Cult Med Psychiatry 15:453–477, 1991

Farley M, Keaney JC: Physical symptoms, somatization, and dissociation in women survivors of childhood sexual assault. Women Health 25:33–45, 1997

Ferracuti S, Sacco R, Lazzari R: Dissociative trance disorder: clinical and Rorschach findings in ten persons reporting demon possession and treated by exorcism. J Pers Assess 66:525–539, 1996

Fewtrell W: Depersonalization: a description and suggested strategies. British Journal of Guidance and Counseling 14:263–269, 1986

Fichtner CG, Kuhlman DT, Gruenfeld MJ, et al: Decreased episodic violence and increased control of dissociation in a carbamazepine-treated case of multiple personality. Biol Psychiatry 27:1045–1052, 1990

Fichtner CG, Horevitz RP, Braun BG: Fluoxetine in depersonalization disorder. Am J Psychiatry 149:1750–1751, 1992

Fine CG: The tactical-integration model for the treatment of dissociative identity disorder and allied dissociative disorders. Am J Psychother 53:361–376, 1999

Fine CG, Berkowitz AS: The wreathing protocol: the imbrication of hypnosis and EMDR in the treatment of dissociative identity disorder and other dissociative responses: eye movement desensitization reprocessing. Am J Clin Hypn 43:275–290, 2001

Finkelhor D: Child Sexual Abuse: New Theory and Research. New York, Free Press, 1984

Frankel FH: Hypnotizability and dissociation. Am J Psychiatry 147:823–829, 1990

Freud S: Notes upon a case of obsessional neurosis (1909), in The Standard Edition of the Complete Psychological Works of Sigmund Freud, Vol 10. Translated and edited by Strachey J. London, England, Hogarth Press, 1955, pp 151–320

Freud S: Psycho-analytic notes on an autobiographical account of a case of paranoia (dementia paranoides) (1911), in The Standard Edition of the Complete Psychological Works of Sigmund Freud, Vol 12. Translated and edited by Strachey J. London, England, Hogarth Press, 1958, pp 1–82

Freud S: The ego and the id (1923), in The Standard Edition of the Complete Psychological Works of Sigmund Freud, Vol 19. Translated and edited by Strachey J. London, England, Hogarth Press, 1961, pp 3–66

Freyberger HJ, Spitzer C, Stieglitz RD, et al: Questionnaire on dissociative symptoms: German adaptation, reliability and validity of the American Dissociative Experience Scale (DES). Psychother Psychosom Med Psychol 48:223–229, 1998

Friedl MC, Draijer N: Dissociative disorders in Dutch psychiatric inpatients. Am J Psychiatry 157:1012–1013, 2000

Frischholz EJ: The relationship among dissociation, hypnosis, and child abuse in the development of multiple personality disorder, in Childhood Antecedents of Multiple Personality Disorder. Edited by Kluft RP. Washington, DC, American Psychiatric Press, 1985, pp 99–126

Gainer MJ, Torem MS: Ego-state therapy for self-injurious behavior. Am J Clin Hypn 35:257–266, 1993

Ganaway GK: Historical versus narrative truth: clarifying the role of exogenous trauma in the etiology of MPD and its variants. Dissociation 2:205–220, 1989

Ganaway GK: Hypnosis, childhood trauma, and dissociative identity disorder: toward an integrative theory. Int J Clin Exp Hypn 43:127–144, 1995

Gast U, Rodewald F, Nickel V, et al: Prevalence of dissociative disorders among psychiatric inpatients in a German university clinic. J Nerv Ment Dis 189:249–257, 2001

Gaw AC, Ding Q, Levine RE, et al: The clinical characteristics of possession disorder among 20 Chinese patients in the Hebei province of China. Psychiatr Serv 49:360–365, 1998

Gelb JL: Multiple personality disorder and satanic ritual abuse. Aust N Z J Psychiatry 27:701–708, 1993

Giese AA, Thomas MR, Dubovsky SL: Dissociative symptoms in psychotic mood disorders: an example of symptom nonspecificity. Psychiatry 60:60–66, 1997

Golynkina K, Ryle A: The identification and characteristics of the partially dissociated states of patients with borderline personality disorder. Br J Med Psychol 72:429–445, 1999

Goodwin J: Sexual Abuse: Incest Victims and Their Families. Boston, MA, Wright/PSG, 1982

Grabe HJ, Rainermann S, Spitzer C, et al: The relationship between dimensions of alexithymia and dissociation. Psychother Psychosom 69:128–131, 2000

Greaves GB: Multiple personality: 165 years after Mary Reynolds. J Nerv Ment Dis 168:577–596, 1980

Hammond DC, Garver RB, Mutter CB, et al: Clinical Hypnosis and Memory: Guidelines for Clinicians and for Forensic Hypnosis. Bloomingdale, IL, American Society of Clinical Hypnosis Press, 1995

Harvey AG, Bryant RA: Dissociative symptoms in acute stress disorder. J Trauma Stress 12:673–680, 1999

Heap M, Ramphele M: The quest for wholeness: health care strategies among the residents of council-built hostels in Cape Town. Soc Sci Med 32:117–126, 1991

Herman JL, Perry JC, van der Kolk BA: Childhood trauma in borderline personality disorder. Am J Psychiatry 146:490–495, 1989

Hilgard ER: Hypnotic Susceptibility. New York, Harcourt, Brace & World, 1965

Hilgard ER: Divided Consciousness: Multiple Controls in Human Thought and Action. New York, Wiley-Interscience, 1977

Hocke V, Schmidtke A: "Multiple personality disorder" in childhood and adolescence. Z Kinder Jugendpsychiatr Psychother 26:273–284, 1998

Hoffman RE: Computer simulations of neural information processing and the schizophrenia-mania dichotomy. Arch Gen Psychiatry 44:178–188, 1987

Holen A: Normal and pathological grief: recent views. Tidsskr Nor Laegeforen 113:2089–2091, 1993

Hollander E, Fairbanks J, Decaria C, et al: Pharmacological dissection of panic and depersonalization (letter). Am J Psychiatry 146:402, 1989

Hollander E, Liebowitz MR, Decaria C, et al: Treatment of depersonalization with serotonin reuptake blockers. J Clin Psychopharmacol 10:200–203, 1990

Horen SA, Leichner PP, Lawson JS: Prevalence of dissociative symptoms and disorders in an adult psychiatric inpatient population in Canada. Can J Psychiatry 40:185–191, 1995

Horevitz RP, Braun BG: Are multiple personalities borderline? An analysis of 33 cases. Psychiatr Clin North Am 7:69–87, 1984

Horowitz MJ: Stress Response Syndromes. New York, Jason Aronson, 1976

Horowitz MJ, Wilner NR, Alvarez W: Impact of Event Scale: a measure of objective distress. Psychosom Med 41:208–218, 1979

Icaran E, Colom R, Orengo-Garcia F: Validation study of the Dissociative Experiences Scale in Spanish population sample. Actas Luso Esp Neurol Psiquiatr Cienc Afines 24:7–10, 1996

Irwin HJ: Pathological and nonpathological dissociation: the relevance of childhood trauma. J Psychol 133:157–164, 1999

James W: The Principles of Psychology (1890). New York, Dover, 1950

Janet P: The Major Symptoms of Hysteria: Fifteen Lectures Given in the Medical School of Harvard University, 2nd Edition. New York, Macmillan, 1920

Jang KL, Paris J, Zweig-Frank H, et al: Twin study of dissociative experience. J Nerv Ment Dis 186:345–351, 1998

Johnson DM, Pike JL, Chard KM: Factors predicting PTSD, depression, and dissociative severity in female treatment-seeking childhood sexual abuse survivors. Child Abuse Negl 25:179–198, 2001

Jones B, Heard H, Startup M, et al: Autobiographical memory and dissociation in borderline personality disorder. Psychol Med 29:1397–1404, 1999

Kaplan ML, Asnis GM, Lipschitz DS, et al: Suicidal behavior and abuse in psychiatric outpatients. Compr Psychiatry 36:229–235, 1995

Kardiner A, Spiegel H: War, Stress and Neurotic Illness. New York, Hoeber, 1947

Kihlstrom JF: The cognitive unconscious. Science 237:1445–1452, 1987

Kihlstrom JF, Hoyt IP: Repression, dissociation, and hypnosis, in Repression and Dissociation: Implications for Personality Theory, Psychopathology, and Health. Edited by Singer JL. Chicago, IL, University of Chicago Press, 1990, pp 181–208

Kirmayer LJ: Pacing the void: social and cultural dimensions of dissociation, in Dissociation: Culture, Mind, and Body. Edited by Spiegel D. Washington, DC, American Psychiatric Press, 1993, pp 91–122

Kirshner LA: Dissociative reactions: an historical review and clinical study. Acta Psychiatr Scand 49:698–711, 1973

Kleinman A: Depression, somatization and the "new cross-cultural psychiatry." Soc Sci Med 11:3–10, 1977

Kluft RP: Varieties of hypnotic intervention in the treatment of multiple personality. Am J Clin Hypn 24:230–240, 1982

Kluft RP: An introduction to multiple personality disorder. Psychiatric Annals 14:19–24, 1984a

Kluft RP: Multiple personality in childhood. Psychiatr Clin North Am 7:121–134, 1984b

Kluft RP: Treatment of multiple personality disorder: a study of 33 cases. Psychiatr Clin North Am 7:9–29, 1984c

Kluft RP: Hypnotherapy of childhood multiple personality disorder. Am J Clin Hypn 27:201–210, 1985a

Kluft RP: The natural history of multiple personality disorder, in Childhood Antecedents of Multiple Personality. Edited by Kluft RP. Washington, DC, American Psychiatric Press, 1985b, pp 197–238

Kluft RP: Using hypnotic inquiry protocols to monitor treatment progress and stability in multiple personality disorder. Am J Clin Hypn 28:63–75, 1985c

Kluft RP: Personality unification in multiple personality disorder: a follow-up study, in Treatment of Multiple Personality Disorder. Edited by Braun BG. Washington, DC, American Psychiatric Press, 1986, pp 29–60

Kluft RP: First-rank symptoms as a diagnostic clue to multiple personality disorder. Am J Psychiatry 144:293–298, 1987

Kluft RP: The dissociative disorders, in American Psychiatric Press Textbook of Psychiatry. Edited by Talbott JA, Hales RE, Yudofsky SC. Washington, DC, American Psychiatric Press, 1988, pp 557–585

Kluft RP: Multiple personality disorder, in American Psychiatric Press Review of Psychiatry, Vol 10. Edited by Tasman A, Goldfinger SM. Washington, DC, American Psychiatric Press, 1991, pp 161–188

Kluft RP: The use of hypnosis with dissociative disorders. Psychiatr Med 10:31–46, 1992

Kluft RP: An overview of the psychotherapy of dissociative identity disorder. Am J Psychother 53:289–319, 1999

Koopman C, Classen C, Spiegel D: Predictors of posttraumatic stress symptoms among survivors of the Oakland/Berkeley, Calif., firestorm. Am J Psychiatry 151:888–894, 1994

Koopman C, Classen C, Cardeña E, et al: When disaster strikes, acute stress disorder may follow. J Trauma Stress 8:29–46, 1995

Koopman C, Classen C, Spiegel D: Dissociative responses in the immediate aftermath of the Oakland/Berkeley firestorm. J Trauma Stress 9:521–540, 1996

Kua EH, Sim LP, Chee KT: A cross-cultural study of the possession-trance in Singapore. Aust N Z J Psychiatry 20:361–364, 1986

Kua EH, Chew PH, Ko SM: Spirit possession and healing among Chinese psychiatric patients. Acta Psychiatr Scand 88:447–450, 1993

Lambek M: Spirit possession/spirit succession: aspects of social continuity among Malagasy speakers in Mayotte. American Ethnologist 15:710–731, 1988

Lavoie G, Sabourin M: Hypnosis and schizophrenia: a review of experimental and clinical studies, in Handbook of Hypnosis and Psychosomatic Medicine. Edited by Burrows GD, Dennerstein L. New York, Elsevier, 1980

Lavoie G, Sabourin M, Langlois J: Hypnotic susceptibility, amnesia, and IQ in chronic schizophrenia. Int J Clin Exp Hypn 21:157–168, 1973

Leavitt F, Labott SM: Rorschach indicators of dissociative identity disorders: clinical utility and theoretical implications. J Clin Psychol 54:803–810, 1998

Lewis DO, Yeager CA, Swica Y, et al: Objective documentation of child abuse and dissociation in 12 murderers with dissociative identity disorder. Am J Psychiatry 154:1703–1710, 1997

Lewis-Fernandez R: Culture and dissociation: a comparison of ataque de nervios among Puerto Ricans and "possession syndrome" in India, in Dissociation: Culture, Mind, and Body. Edited by Spiegel D. Washington, DC, American Psychiatric Press, 1993, pp 123–167

Li C, Sun Y, Fang M: Trance states, altered states of consciousness, and related issues. Chinese Mental Health Journal 6:167–170, 1992

Li D, Spiegel D: A neural network model of dissociative disorders. Psychiatr Ann 22:144–147, 1992

Lindemann E: Symptomatology and management of acute grief. Am J Psychiatry 101:141–148, 1944

Loewenstein RJ: An official mental status examination for complex chronic dissociative symptoms and multiple personality disorder. Psychiatr Clin North Am 14:567–604, 1991a

Loewenstein RJ: Psychogenic amnesia and psychogenic fugue: a comprehensive review, in American Psychiatric Press Review of Psychiatry, Vol 10. Edited by Tasman A, Goldfinger SM. Washington, DC, American Psychiatric Press, 1991b, pp 189–222

Loewenstein RJ: Diagnosis, epidemiology, clinical course, treatment, and cost effectiveness of treatment of dissociative disorders and MPD: report submitted to the Clinton Administration Task Force on Health Care Financing Reform. Dissociation 7:3–11, 1994

Loewenstein RJ, Putnam FW: A comparative study of dissociative symptoms in patients with complex partial seizures, multiple personality disorder and posttraumatic stress disorder. Dissociation 1:17–23, 1988

Loewenstein RJ, Hornstein N, Farber B: Open trial of clonazepam in the treatment of posttraumatic stress symptoms in MPD. Dissociation 1:3–12, 1988

Low G, Jones D, MacLeod A, et al: Childhood trauma, dissociation and self-harming behaviour: a pilot study. Br J Med Psychol 73:269–278, 2000

Lussier RG, Steiner J, Grey A, et al: Prevalence of dissociative disorders in an acute care day hospital population. Psychiatr Serv 48:244–246, 1997

Machleidt W, Peltzer K: The Chilopa ceremony: a sacrificial ritual for mentally (spiritually) ill patients in a traditional healing centre in Malawi. Psychiatria Danubina 3:205–227, 1991

Macleod AD: Posttraumatic stress disorder, dissociative fugue and a locator beacon. Aust N Z J Psychiatry 33:102–104, 1999

Madakasira S, O'Brien KF: Acute posttraumatic stress disorder in victims of a natural disaster. J Nerv Ment Dis 175:286–290, 1987

Mageo JM: Spirit girls and marines: possession and ethnopsychiatry as historical discourse in Samoa. American Ethnologist 23:61–82, 1996

Maldonado JR: Diagnosis and treatment of dissociative disorders, in Manual for the Course: Advanced Hypnosis: The Use of Hypnosis in Medicine and Psychiatry. Annual meeting of the American Psychiatric Association, Chicago, IL, May 13–18, 2000

Maldonado JR, Spiegel D: Using hypnosis, in Treating Women Molested in Childhood. Edited by Classen C. San Francisco, CA, Jossey-Bass, 1995, pp 163–186

Maldonado JR, Spiegel D: Trauma, dissociation, and hypnotizability, in Trauma, Memory, and Dissociation. Edited by Marmar CR, Bremner JD. Washington, DC, American Psychiatric Press, 1998, pp 57–106

Maldonado JR, Butler LD, Spiegel D: Treatment of dissociative disorders, in Treatments That Work. Edited by Nathan P, Gorman JM. New York, Oxford University Press, 2000, pp 463–493

Markowitz JS, Gill HS: Pharmacotherapy of dissociative identity disorder. Ann Pharmacother 30:1498–1499, 1996

Marmar CR, Weiss DS, Metzler TJ, et al: Characteristics of emergency services personnel related to peritraumatic dissociation during critical incident exposure. Am J Psychiatry 153(suppl 7):94–102, 1996

Martinez-Taboas A: Repressed memories: some clinical data contributing toward its elucidation. Am J Psychother 50:217–230, 1996

Martinez-Taboas A, Bernal G: Dissociation, psychopathology, and abusive experiences in a nonclinical Latino university student group. Cultural Diversity and Ethnic Minority Psychology 6:32–41, 2000

Mayer-Gross W, Slater E, Roth M: Clinical Psychiatry, 3rd Edition. London, England, Bailliere, Tindal & Cassell, 1969

McFarlane AC: Posttraumatic morbidity of a disaster: a study of cases presenting for psychiatric treatment. J Nerv Ment Dis 174:4–14, 1986

McFarlane AC: Avoidance and intrusion in posttraumatic stress disorder. J Nerv Ment Dis 180:439–445, 1992

McHugh PR: Dissociative identity disorder as a socially constructed artifact. Journal of Practical Psychiatry and Behavioral Health 1:158–166, 1995a

McHugh PR: Witches, multiple personalities, and other psychiatric artifacts. Nat Med 1:110–114, 1995b

McLellan S: Deviant spirits in West Malaysian factories. Anthropologica 33:145–160, 1991

Meares R: The "adualistic" representation of trauma: on malignant internalization. Am J Psychother 53:392–402, 1999

Mesulam MM: Dissociative states with abnormal temporal lobe EEG: multiple personality and the illusion of possession. Arch Neurol 38:178–181, 1981

Middleton W, Butler J: Dissociative identity disorder: an Australian series. Aust N Z J Psychiatry 32:794–804, 1998

Mihaescu G, Vanderlinden J, Sechaud M, et al: The Dissociation Questionnaire DIS-Q: preliminary results with a French-speaking Swiss population. Encephale 24:334–346, 1998

Mishkin M, Appenzeller T: The anatomy of memory. Sci Am 256:80–89, 1987

Modestin J, Ebner G, Junghan M, et al: Dissociative experiences and dissociative disorders in acute psychiatric inpatients. Compr Psychiatry 37:355–361, 1996

Moore EP: Gender, power, and legal pluralism: Rajasthan, India. American Ethnologist 20:522–542, 1993

Mulder RT, Beautrais AL, Joyce PR, et al: Relationship between dissociation, childhood sexual abuse, childhood physical abuse, and mental illness in a general population sample. Am J Psychiatry 155:806–811, 1998

Mulhern S: Patients reporting ritual abuse in childhood (letter and comment). Child Abuse Negl 15:609–613, 1991

Nakdimen KA: Psychoanalysis and multiple personality. Am J Psychiatry 145:896–897, 1988

Naples M, Hackett T: The Amytal interview: history and current uses. Psychosomatics 19:98–105, 1978

Nijenhuis ER, Spinhoven P, van Dyck R, et al: The development and psychometric characteristics of the Somatoform Dissociation Questionnaire (SDQ-20). J Nerv Ment Dis 184:688–694, 1996

Nijenhuis ER, Spinhoven P, van Dyck, et al: The development of the Somatoform Dissociation Questionnaire (SDQ-5) as a screening instrument for dissociative disorders. Acta Psychiatr Scand 96:311–318, 1997

Nijenhuis ER, Spinhoven P, van Dyck R, et al: Degree of somatoform and psychological dissociation in dissociative disorder is correlated with reported trauma. J Trauma Stress 11:711–730, 1998

Noll R: Exorcism and possession: the clash of worldviews and the hubris of psychiatry. Dissociation 6(special issue):250–253, 1993

Noyes R, Kletti R: Depersonalization in response to life-threatening danger. Compr Psychiatry 18:375–384, 1977

Noyes R, Slymen DJ: The subjective response to life-threatening danger. Omega 9:313–321, 1978–1979

Noyes R, Kupperman S, Olson SB: Desipramine: a possible treatment for depersonalization. Can J Psychiatry 32:782–784, 1987

Nuckolls CW: Deciding how to decide: possession-mediumship in Jalari divination. Med Anthropol 13(special issue):57–82, 1991

Nuller YL: Depersonalization: symptoms, meaning, therapy. Acta Psychiatr Scand 66:451–458, 1982

Ogata SN, Silk KR, Goodrich S, et al: Childhood sexual and physical abuse in adult patients with borderline personality disorder. Am J Psychiatry 147:1008–1013, 1990

Ong A: The production of possession: spirits and the multinational corporation in Malaysia. American Ethnologist 15:28–42, 1988

O'Toole BI, Marshall RP, Schureck RJ, et al: Combat, dissociation, and posttraumatic stress disorder in Australian Vietnam veterans. J Trauma Stress 12:625–640, 1999

Orne MT, Axelrad AD, Diamond BL, et al: Scientific status of refreshing recollection by the use of hypnosis. JAMA 253:1918–1923, 1985

Perry JC, Jacobs D: Overview: clinical applications of the Amytal interview in psychiatric emergency settings. Am J Psychiatry 139:552–559, 1982

Perry S, Difede J, Musngi G, et al: Predictors of posttraumatic stress disorder after burn injury. Am J Psychiatry 149:931–935, 1992

Peterson G: Auditory hallucinations and dissociative identity disorder. Am J Psychiatry 152:1403–1404, 1995

Pettinati HM: Measuring hypnotizability in psychotic patients. Int J Clin Exp Hypn 30:404–416, 1982

Pettinati HM, Kogan LG, Evans FJ, et al: Hypnotizability of psychiatric inpatients according to two different scales. Am J Psychiatry 147:69–75, 1990

Pies R: Depersonalization's many faces. Psychiatric Times 8:27–28, 1991

Pineros M, Rosselli D, Calderon C: An epidemic of collective conversion and dissociation disorder in an indigenous group of Colombia: its relation to cultural change. Soc Sci Med 46:1425–1428, 1998

Piper A Jr: Multiple personality disorder. Br J Psychiatry 164:600–612, 1994

Pribor EF, Dinwiddie SH: Psychiatric correlates of incest in childhood. Am J Psychiatry 149:52–56, 1992

Price J, Hess NC: Behaviour therapy as precipitant and treatment in a case of dual personality. Aust N Z J Psychiatry 13:63–66, 1979

Pullela S: An outbreak of epidemic hysteria: an illustrative case study. Irish Journal of Psychiatry 7:9–11, 1986

Putnam FW: Dissociation as a response to extreme trauma, in Childhood Antecedents of Multiple Personality. Edited by Kluft RP. Washington, DC, American Psychiatric Press, 1985, pp 65–97

Putnam FW: The disturbance of "self" in victims of childhood sexual abuse, in Incest-Related Syndromes of Adult Psychopathology. Edited by Kluft RP. Washington, DC, American Psychiatric Press, 1988, pp 113–132

Putnam FW: Diagnosis and Treatment of Multiple Personality Disorder. New York, Guilford, 1989

Putnam FW: Dissociative disorders in children: behavioral profiles and problems. Child Abuse Negl 17:39–45, 1993

Putnam FW, Guroff JJ, Silberman EK, et al: The clinical phenomenology of multiple personality disorder: review of 100 recent cases. J Clin Psychiatry 47:285–293, 1986

Reither AM, Stoudemire A: Psychogenic fugue states: a review. South Med J 81:568–571, 1988

Rifkin A, Ghisalbert D, Dimatou S, et al: Dissociative identity disorder in psychiatric inpatients. Am J Psychiatry 155:844–845, 1998

Rivera M: Multiple personality disorder and the social systems: 185 cases. Dissociation 4:79–82, 1991

Roesler TA, McKenzie N: Effects of childhood trauma on psychological functioning in adults sexually abused as children. J Nerv Ment Dis 182:145–150, 1994

Ronquillo EB: The influence of "espiritismo" on a case of multiple personality disorder. Dissociation 4:39–45, 1991

Ross CA: Multiple Personality Disorder: Diagnosis, Clinical Features, and Treatment. New York, Wiley, 1989

Ross CA: Epidemiology of multiple personality disorder and dissociation. Psychiatr Clin North Am 14:503–518, 1991

Ross CA, Norton GR: Multiple personality disorder patients with a prior diagnosis of schizophrenia. Dissociation 1:39–42, 1988

Ross CA, Norton GR: Suicide and parasuicide in multiple personality disorder. Psychiatry 52:365–371, 1989

Ross CA, Norton GR, Wozney K: Multiple personality disorder: an analysis of 236 cases. Can J Psychiatry 34:413–418, 1989

Ross CA, Miller SD, Reagor P, et al: Structured interview data on 102 cases of multiple personality disorder from four centers. Am J Psychiatry 147:596–601, 1990

Ross CA, Joshi S, Currie R: Dissociative experiences in the general population: a factor analysis. Hosp Community Psychiatry 42:297–301, 1991a

Ross CA, Anderson G, Fleischer WP, et al: The frequency of multiple personality disorder among psychiatric inpatients. Am J Psychiatry 148:1717–1720, 1991b

Roth M: The phobic-anxiety-depersonalization syndrome. Proceedings of the Royal Society of Medicine 52:587–595, 1959

Rothbaum BO, Foa EB: Subtypes of posttraumatic stress disorder and duration of symptoms, in Posttraumatic Stress Disorder: DSM-IV and Beyond. Edited by Davidson JRT, Foa EB. Washington, DC, American Psychiatric Press, 1993, pp 23–35

Rumelhart DE, McClelland JL: Parallel Distributed Processing: Explorations in the Microstructure of Cognition, Vols 1 and 2. Cambridge, MA, MIT Press, 1986

Russell DEH: The Secret Trauma: Incest in the Lives of Girls and Women. New York, Basic Books, 1986

Safa K: Reading Saedi's Ahl-e Hava: pattern and significance in spirit possession beliefs on the southern coasts of Iran. Cult Med Psychiatry 12:85–111, 1988

Sar V, Yargic LI, Tutkun H: Structured interview data on 35 cases of dissociative identity disorder in Turkey. Am J Psychiatry 153:1329–1333, 1996

Sar V, Tutkun H, Alyanak B, et al: Frequency of dissociative disorders among psychiatric outpatients in Turkey. Compr Psychiatry 41:216–222, 2000

Sargant W, Slater E: Amnestic syndromes in war. Proceedings of the Royal Society of Medicine 34:757–764, 1941

Saxe GN, van der Kolk BA, Berkowitz R, et al: Dissociative disorders in psychiatric inpatients. Am J Psychiatry 150:1037–1042, 1993

Saxena S, Prasad KVSR: DSM-III subclassification of dissociative disorders applied to psychiatric outpatients in India. Am J Psychiatry 146:261–262, 1989

Schacter DL: Understanding implicit memory: a cognitive neuroscience approach. Am Psychol 47:559–569, 1992

Schacter DL: In Search of Memory. Cambridge, MA, Harvard University Press, 1996

Schacter DL, Wang PL, Tulving E, et al: Functional retrograde amnesia: a quantitative case study. Neuropsychologia 20:523–532, 1982

Schechter DS, Marshall R, Salman E, et al: Ataque de nervios and history of childhood trauma. J Trauma Stress 13:529–534, 2000

Schenk L, Bear D: Multiple personality and related dissociative phenomena in patients with temporal lobe epilepsy. Am J Psychiatry 138:1311–1316, 1981

Schieffelin EL: Evil spirit sickness, the Christian disease: the innovation of a new syndrome of mental derangement and redemption in Papua, New Guinea. Cult Med Psychiatry 20:1–39, 1996

Schilder P: The treatment of depersonalization. Bulletin of the New York Academy of Science 15:258–272, 1939

Schultz R, Braun BG, Kluft RP: Multiple personality disorder: phenomenology of selected variables in comparison to major depression. Dissociation 2:45–51, 1989

Scroppo JC, Drob SL, Weinberger JL, et al: Identifying dissociative identity disorder: a self-report and projective study. J Abnorm Psychol 107:272–284, 1998

Sered SS: Ideology, autonomy, and sisterhood: an analysis of the secular consequences of women's religions. Gender and Society 8:486–506, 1994

Shalev AY, Schreiber S, Galai T: Early psychiatric responses to traumatic injury. J Trauma Stress 6:441–450, 1993

Shalev AY, Peri T, Canetti L, et al: Predictors of PTSD in injured trauma survivors: a prospective study. Am J Psychiatry 153:219–225, 1996

Shapiro DJ: Symbolic fluids: the world of spirit mediums in Brazilian possession groups. Dissertation Abstracts International 53:867–868, 1992

Sharp LA: Possessed and dispossessed youth: spirit possession of school children in northwest Madagascar. Cult Med Psychiatry 14:339–364, 1990

Sharp LA: Exorcists, psychiatrists, and the problems of possession in northwest Madagascar. Soc Sci Med 38:525–542, 1994

Shearer SL: Dissociative phenomena in women with borderline personality disorder. Am J Psychiatry 151:1324–1328, 1994

Shilony E, Grossman FK: Depersonalization as a defense mechanism in survivors of trauma. J Trauma Stress 6:119–128, 1993

Shirali P, Kishwar A, Bharti SP: Life stress, demographic variables and personality (TAT) in eleven cases of possession (trance-medium) in Shimla Tehsil. Personality Study and Group Behaviour 6:73–81, 1986

Shorvon HJ: The depersonalization syndrome. Proceedings of the Royal Society of Medicine 39:779–785, 1946

Sloan P: Posttraumatic stress in survivors of an airplane crash landing: a clinical and exploratory research intervention. J Trauma Stress 1:211–229, 1988

Smith WH: Incorporating hypnosis into the psychotherapy of patients with multiple personality disorder. Bull Menninger Clin 57:344–354, 1993

Sno HN, Schalken HF: Dissociative identity disorder: diagnosis and treatment in the Netherlands. European Psychiatry: the Journal of the Association of European Psychiatrists 14:270–277, 1999

Solomon R: The use of the MMPI with multiple personality patients. Psychol Rep 53:1004–1006, 1983

Solomon Z, Mikulincer M: Psychological sequelae of war: a 2-year follow-up study of Israeli combat stress reaction casualties. J Nerv Ment Dis 176:264–269, 1988

Solomon Z, Mikulincer M, Bleich A: Characteristic expressions of combat-related posttraumatic stress disorder among Israeli soldiers in the 1982 Lebanon war. Behav Med 14:171–178, 1988

Solomon Z, Mikulincer M, Benbenisty R: Combat stress reaction: clinical manifestations and correlates. Military Psychology 1:17–33, 1989

Sookman D, Solyom L: Severe depersonalization treated with behavior therapy. Am J Psychiatry 135:1543–1545, 1978

Spanos NP, Weekes JR, Bertrand LD: Multiple personality: a social psychological perspective. J Abnorm Psychol 94:362–376, 1985

Spanos NP, Weekes JR, Menary E, et al: Hypnotic interview and age regression procedures in elicitation of multiple personality symptoms: a simulation study. Psychiatry 49:298–311, 1986

Spiegel D: Vietnam grief work using hypnosis. Am J Clin Hypn 24:33–40, 1981

Spiegel D: Multiple personality as a post-traumatic stress disorder. Psychiatr Clin North Am 7:101–110, 1984

Spiegel D: Dissociating damage. Am J Clin Hypn 29:123–131, 1986a

Spiegel D: Dissociation, double binds, and posttraumatic stress in multiple personality disorder, in Treatment of Multiple Personality Disorder. Edited by Braun BG. Washington, DC, American Psychiatric Press, 1986b, pp 61–77

Spiegel D: Chronic pain masks depression, multiple personality disorder. Hosp Community Psychiatry 38:933–935, 1987

Spiegel D: Dissociation and hypnosis in posttraumatic stress disorders. J Trauma Stress 1:17–33, 1988

Spiegel D: Hypnosis, dissociation, and trauma: hidden and overt observers, in Repression and Dissociation: Implications for Personality Theory, Psychopathology, and Health. Edited by Singer JL. Chicago, IL, University of Chicago Press, 1990a, pp 121–142

Spiegel D: Trauma, dissociation, and hypnosis, in Incest-Related Syndromes of Adult Psychopathology. Edited by Kluft RL. Washington, DC, American Psychiatric Press, 1990b, pp 247–261

Spiegel D: Dissociation and trauma, in American Psychiatric Press Review of Psychiatry, Vol 10. Edited by Tasman A, Goldfinger SM. Washington, DC, American Psychiatric Press, 1991a, pp 261–275

Spiegel D: Dissociative disorders: afterword, in American Psychiatric Press Review of Psychiatry, Vol 10. Edited by Tasman A, Goldfinger SM. Washington, DC, American Psychiatric Press, 1991b, p 276

Spiegel D: Dissociative disorders: foreword, in American Psychiatric Press Review of Psychiatry, Vol 10. Edited by Tasman A, Goldfinger SM. Washington, DC, American Psychiatric Press, 1991c, pp 143–144

Spiegel D, Cardeña E: Disintegrated experience: the dissociative disorders revisited. J Abnorm Psychol 100:366–378, 1991

Spiegel D, Fink R: Hysterical psychosis and hypnotizability. Am J Psychiatry 136:777–781, 1979

Spiegel D, Detrick D, Frischholz E: Hypnotizability and psychopathology. Am J Psychiatry 139:431–437, 1982

Spiegel D, Hunt T, Dondershine HE: Dissociation and hypnotizability in posttraumatic stress disorder. Am J Psychiatry 145:301–305, 1988

Spiegel D, Frischholz EJ, Spira J: Functional disorders of memory, in American Psychiatric Press Review of Psychiatry, Vol 12. Edited by Oldham JM, Riba MB, Tasman A. Washington, DC, American Psychiatric Press, 1993, pp 747–782

Spiegel H: The grade 5 syndrome: the highly hypnotizable person. Int J Clin Exp Hypn 22:303–319, 1974

Spiegel H, Spiegel D: Trance and Treatment: Clinical Uses of Hypnosis (1978). Washington, DC, American Psychiatric Press, 1987

Spier SA, Tesar GE, Rosenbaum JF, et al: Treatment of panic disorder and agoraphobia with clonazepam. J Clin Psychiatry 47:238–242, 1986

Spitzer C, Freyberger HJ, Stieglitz RD, et al: Adaptation and psychometric properties of the German version of the Dissociative Experience Scale. J Trauma Stress 11:799–809, 1998

Spitzer C, Spelsberg B, Grabe HJ, et al: Dissociative experiences and psychopathology in conversion disorders. J Psychosom Res 46:291–294, 1999

Squire LR: Memory and the hippocampus: a synthesis from findings with rats, monkeys, and humans. Psychol Rev 99:195–231, 1992

Squire LR, Zola-Morgan S: The medial temporal lobe memory system. Science 253:1380–1386, 1991

Stein MB, Uhde TW: Depersonalization disorder: effects of caffeine and response to pharmacotherapy. Biol Psychiatry 26:315–320, 1989

Steinberg M: The spectrum of depersonalization: assessment and treatment, in American Psychiatric Press Review of Psychiatry, Vol 10. Edited by Tasman A, Goldfinger SM. Washington, DC, American Psychiatric Press, 1991, pp 223–247

Steinberg M, Rounsaville B, Cicchetti DV: The Structured Clinical Interview for DSM-III-R Dissociative Disorders: preliminary report on a new diagnostic instrument. Am J Psychiatry 147:76–82, 1990

Steinberg M, Cicchetti D, Buchanan J, et al: Distinguishing between multiple personality disorder (dissociative identity disorder) and schizophrenia using the Structured Clinical Interview for DSM-IV Dissociative Disorders. J Nerv Ment Dis 182:495–502, 1994

Steinberg M: Advances in the clinical assessment of dissociation: the SCID-D-R. Bull Menninger Clin 64:146–163, 2000

Stern CR: The etiology of multiple personalities. Psychiatr Clin North Am 7:149–160, 1984

Tantam D: An exorcism in Zanzibar: insights into groups from another culture. Group Analysis 26:251–260, 1993

Terr LC: Childhood traumas: an outline and overview. Am J Psychiatry 148:10–20, 1991

Trangkasombat U, Su-Umpan U, Churujikul V, et al: Epidemic dissociation among school children in southern Thailand. Dissociation 8:130–141, 1995

Trangkasombat U, Su-Umpan U, Churujiporn V, et al: Risk factors for spirit possession among school girls in southern Thailand. J Med Assoc Thai 81:541–546, 1998

Torch EM: The psychotherapeutic treatment of depersonalization disorder. Hillside Journal of Clinical Psychiatry 9:133–143, 1987

Tulving E: Elements of Episodic Memory. Oxford, England, Clarendon Press, 1983

Tutkun H, Sar V, Yargic LI, et al: Frequency of dissociative disorders among psychiatric inpatients in a Turkish university clinic. Am J Psychiatry 155:800–805, 1998

Valdiserri S, Kihlstrom JF: Abnormal eating and dissociative experiences. Int J Eat Disord 17:373–380, 1995

van der Hart O: Multiple personality disorder in Europe: impressions. Dissociation 6:102–118, 1993

van der Hart O, Nijenhuis E: Dissociative disorders, especially multiple personality disorder. Ned Tijdschr Geneeskd 137:1865–1868, 1993

van der Hart O, Spiegel D: Hypnotic assessment and treatment of trauma-induced psychoses: the early psychotherapy of Breukink and modern views. Int J Clin Exp Hypn 41:191–209, 1993

van der Kolk BA, Fisler R: Dissociation and the fragmentary nature of traumatic memories: overview and exploratory study. J Trauma Stress 8:505–525, 1995

van der Kolk BA, Hostetler A, Herron N, et al: Trauma and the development of borderline personality disorder. Psychiatr Clin North Am 17:715–730, 1994

van der Kolk BA, Pelcovitz D, Roth S, et al: Dissociation, somatization, and affect dysregulation: the complexity of adaptation of trauma. Am J Psychiatry 153(suppl 7):83–93, 1996

Vanderlinden J, Van Dyck R, Vandereycken W, et al: Dissociative experiences in the general population of the Netherlands and Belgium: a study with the Dissociative Questionnaire (DIS-Q). Dissociation 4:180–184, 1991

van Dyck R: Dissociation, hypnosis and multiple personality disorders. Ned Tijdschr Geneeskd 137:1863–1864, 1993

Varma VK, Bouri M, Wig NN: Multiple personality in India: comparison with hysterical possession state. Am J Psychother 35:113–120, 1981

Vincent M, Pickering MR: Multiple personality disorder in childhood. Can J Psychiatry 33:524–529, 1988

Wade TC, Wade DK: Integrative psychotherapy: combining ego-state therapy, clinical hypnosis, and eye movement desensitization and reprocessing (EMDR) in a psychosocial developmental context. Am J Clin Hypn 43:233–245, 2001

Walsh RN: Depersonalization: definition and treatment (letter). Am J Psychiatry 132:873–874, 1975

Weiss DS, Marmar CR, Metzler TJ, et al: Predicting symptomatic distress in emergency services personnel. J Consult Clin Psychol 63:361–368, 1995

Wettstein RM, Fauman BJ: The amobarbital interview. JACEP 8:272–274, 1979

Wildgoose A, Waller G, Clarke S, et al: Psychiatric symptomatology in borderline and other personality disorders: dissociation and fragmentation as mediators. J Nerv Ment Dis 188:757–763, 2000

Wilkinson CB: Aftermath of a disaster: the collapse of the Hyatt Regency hotel skywalks. Am J Psychiatry 140:1134–1139, 1983

Wittkower ED: Transcultural psychiatry in the Caribbean: past, present and future. Am J Psychiatry 127:162–166, 1970

Witztum E, Grisaru N, Budowski D: The "Zar" possession syndrome among Ethiopian immigrants to Israel: cultural and clinical aspects. Br J Med Psychol 69:207–225, 1996

Yap PM: The possession syndrome: a comparison of Hong Kong and French findings. Journal of Mental Science 106:114–137, 1960

Yargic LI, Sar V, Tutkun H, et al: Comparison of dissociative identity disorder with other diagnostic groups using a structured interview in Turkey. Compr Psychiatry 39:345–351, 1998

Zanarini MC, Ruser T, Frankenburg FR, et al: The dissociative experiences of borderline patients. Compr Psychiatry 41:223–227, 2000a

Zanarini MC, Ruser TF, Frankenburg FR, et al: Risk factors associated with the dissociative experiences of borderline patients. J Nerv Ment Dis 188:26–30, 2000b

Zweig-Frank H, Paris J, Guzder J: Psychological risk factors for dissociation and self-mutilation in female patients with borderline personality disorder. Can J Psychiatry 39:259–264, 1994

Sexual and Gender Identity Disorders

Judith V. Becker, Ph.D.

Bradley R. Johnson, M.D.

Clinicians see patients who have a variety of sexual disorders or dysfunctions. A woman who is sexually assaulted may no longer experience sexual desire. A man who is recently widowed may experience difficulty in achieving erections when he begins to date. A woman with multiple sclerosis may no longer have orgasms. A man who is taking antihypertensive medication may have difficulty obtaining an erection. Recent postmenopausal women may find intercourse painful. Patients given antidepressants or antipsychotic medication may report impairment in sexual functioning. An adolescent may request a consultation because his cross-dressing troubles him. An adult man who has been fantasizing about sex with prepubertal children may seek treatment because he is fearful that he will act on his fantasies. Adolescents or adults may compulsively view pornographic images on the Internet or visit sexual chat rooms to the point that it interferes with life functions. Consequently, it is important for clinicians to become educated about the categories of sexual disorders and become adept at taking sexual histories and using the various modalities and interventions.

In reviewing the literature on the sexual disorders, it is readily apparent that most research conducted to date has been on sexual disorders or dysfunctions experienced by men. Many researchers and clinicians have been concerned about the lack of focus on women and how various theories, models, and interventions have been applied to women without empirical investigation. Recently, an international multidisciplinary consensus development conference on female sexual dysfunction was convened to address problems with current classification systems. The international panel of experts had research and/or clinical expertise in the area of female sexual disorders. The panel issued a consensus report. Their final classification system preserved the four major categories of female sexual dysfunctions listed in DSM-IV-TR (American Psychiatric Association 2000), but some alterations were made. (Interested readers are referred to the *Journal of Sex and Marital Therapy*, Volume 17, Number 2, 2001, for the report and commentaries.)

The criteria for the sexual and gender identity disorders discussed in this chapter are as defined in DSM-IV-TR.

Gender Identity Disorders

Gender and Sexual Differentiation

The genetic sex of an individual is determined at conception, but development from that point on is influenced by many factors. For the first few weeks of gestation, the gonads are undifferentiated. If the Y chromosome is present in the embryo, the gonads will differentiate into testes. A substance referred to as the H-Y antigen is responsible for this transformation. If the Y chromosome or H-Y antigen is not present in the developing embryo, the gonads will develop into ovaries.

Like the gonads, the internal and external genital structures are initially undifferentiated in the fetus. If the gonads differentiate into testes, fetal androgen (i.e., testosterone) is secreted, and these structures develop into male genitalia (epididymis, vas deferens, ejaculatory

Smith et al. (2001) conducted a prospective follow-up study with 20 treated adolescent transsexuals to evaluate early sex reassignment and with 21 nontreated and 6 delayed-treatment adolescents to evaluate the decisions not to allow them to start sex reassignment, especially at an early age. The treated group who received sex-reassignment surgery did not continue to have gender dysphoria, and they were thought to be psychologically and socially functioning quite well 1–4 years postoperatively. None of these individuals expressed regret over their decision to have the surgery. However, although the nontreated group also showed improvement, they had a more dysfunctional psychological profile; therefore, it is important to carefully screen those who are cleared for reassignment and treatment, especially if they are too young or have made their decision to do so too quickly and without careful thought.

Sex reassignment is a long process that must be carefully monitored. Patients with other primary psychiatric diagnoses and secondary transsexuals should be screened out and given other appropriate treatment. If the patient is considered appropriate for sex reassignment, psychotherapy should be started to prepare the patient for the cross-gender role. The patient should then go out into the world and live in the cross-gender role before surgical reassignment. Males should cross-dress, have electrolysis, and practice female behaviors. They can even change their identity to female on official documents and at work. Females should cut their hair, bind or conceal their breasts, and similarly take on the identity of a man. After 1–2 years, if these measures have been successful and the patient still wishes reassignment, hormone treatment is begun. Estrogens are given to the male patient, resulting in redistribution of body fat in a more "feminine" pattern and enlargement of the breasts. This treatment is not without possible medical complications, and patients should be followed up closely by a physician. Side effects of estrogen treatment may include deep vein thrombosis, thromboembolic disorders, increased blood pressure, weight gain, impaired glucose tolerance, liver abnormalities, and depression. Testosterone given to the female patient causes redistribution of fat, growth of facial and body hair, enlargement of the clitoris, and deepening of the voice. Unwanted side effects of testosterone treatment include acne, edema secondary to sodium retention, and impairment of liver function. After 1–2 years of hormone therapy, the patient may be considered for surgical reassignment if such a procedure is still desired. In the male-to-female patient, this consists of bilateral orchiectomy, penile amputation, and creation of an artificial vagina. Female-to-male patients undergo bilateral mastectomy and optional hysterectomy with removal of ovaries. Efforts to create an artificial penis have met with mixed results thus far; at this point, it is better to counsel the patient to downplay the role of the penis in sexual activity. Overall cosmetic and functional results from surgery have been variable in both male and female transsexuals. Postsurgical complications can occur and include the following: for genetic females, chest wall scars and polycystic ovary disease, and for genetic males, urethral stenosis, misdirected urinary streams, vaginal strictures, and rectovaginal fistulas. Psychotherapy after surgery is indicated to help the patient adjust to the surgical changes and discuss sexual functioning and satisfaction.

Gender Identity Disorder of Childhood

Because of the difficulty and turmoil involved in treating late-adolescent and adult patients who have gender identity disorder, researchers and clinicians began to evaluate and treat children with gender identity problems. Strictly speaking, this disorder is seen in a child who perceives himself or herself as being of the opposite sex.

However, it is often difficult to separate gender identity from gender role behavior in children. Boys with normal gender identity may play with "girl" dolls. Many girls in our culture are "tomboys" and like rough and contact games. However, in this gender identity syndrome, there is a repeated pattern of opposite-gender role behavior accompanied by a disturbance in the child's perception of "being" a boy or a girl. The exact incidence of gender identity disorder in children is not known, but, like adult gender dysphoria, it is a rare disorder.

Children with gender identity problems express a desire to become a member of the opposite sex. Boys wish to have a vagina and may play at breast-feeding. Girls wish to have a penis and may simulate a penis with various objects or stand to urinate. Boys cross-dress with dresses, makeup, and jewelry, whereas girls may resist wearing dresses at any cost and wear short hair. Both sexes identify with role models of the opposite sex (e.g., a boy insists that he is Supergirl in a game). In evaluating a child, it is important not to look solely at behavior; there must be a disturbance in the child's sexual identity. As in the evaluation of adults, the child should be evaluated for other psychiatric disorders such as psychosis or adjustment disorder.

Etiology

As with adult gender dysphoria, the etiology of childhood gender identity disorder is unclear. The theories outlined earlier in this chapter for adults who have gender identity disorder also apply to children. Additional factors that have been suggested are parents' indifference to or encouragement of opposite-sex behavior; regular cross-dressing as a young boy by a female; lack of male playmates during a boy's first years of socialization; excessive maternal protection, with inhibition of rough-and-tumble play; or absence of or rejection by an older male early in life (Green 1974). Gender identity disorder in children has been posited as being the result of child and family pathology (Zucker and Bradley 1995).

Physical Appearance

It is interesting to note that several studies have associated gender identity disorder with greater physical attractiveness in boys when compared with the physical attractiveness of clinical control subjects who did not have the disorder (Green 1987; Zucker et al. 1993). Fridell et al. (1996) concluded that girls with gender identity disorder often were seen as less attractive than those in a control group.

Course

Retrospective studies of transsexuals (Green 1974) have shown a high incidence of childhood cross-gender behavior. Follow-up studies of children with gender identity disorder have found a high incidence of continued manifestations in adulthood, with a higher incidence of homosexual or bisexual behavior and fantasies than those in a control group (Green 1985).

Treatment

Treatment of gender identity disorder in the child is offered in an attempt to help the child avoid peer ostracism and humiliation, be comfortable with his or her own sex, and avoid the possible development of adult gender dysphoria. Behavior therapy has been used to modify specific cross-gender behaviors in a manner similar to that described for adults, as well as to enhance contingency management (e.g., reinforcing appropriate behaviors with tokens). Analytically oriented treatment deals with the family dynamics (e.g., a powerful, masculine-devaluing mother; an ineffective, emotionally absent father) and individual dynamics (e.g., castration anxiety following surgery) of the child. An eclectic approach to treatment has been advocated that involves developing a close, trusting relationship between a male therapist and the boy; stopping parental encouragement of feminine behaviors; interrupting the excessively close relationship between mother and son; enhancing the role of father and son; and reinforcing male behaviors (Green 1974).

Sexual Dysfunctions

Male and Female Physiology

Human sexual functioning requires a complex interaction of the nervous, vascular, and endocrine systems to produce arousal and orgasm. Sexual arousal in men occurs in the presence of visual stimuli (e.g., a naked partner), fantasies, or physical stimulation of the genitals or other areas of the body (e.g., the nipples). This stimulation leads to involuntary discharge in the parasympathetic nerves that control the diameter and valves of the penile blood vessels. Blood flow increases into the corpora cavernosa, two cylinders of specialized tissue in the penis that distend with blood to produce an erection. Continued stimulation leads to emission of semen and ejaculation, which are controlled through sympathetic fibers and the pudendal nerve. Dopaminergic systems in the central nervous system facilitate arousal and ejaculation, whereas serotonergic systems inhibit these functions. In addition, androgens must be present to expedite sexual arousal (and to some extent erection and ejaculation).

In women, as in men, arousal depends on fantasies, visual stimuli, and physical stimulation; in general, the latter is more important for women, whereas visual cues are more important for men. Again, this stimulation leads to parasympathetic nervous discharge that increases blood flow to the female genitalia, resulting in lubrication of the vagina and some enlargement of the clitoris. Continued stimulation of the clitoris either directly or through intercourse results in orgasm. Estrogens and progestins play a role in female sexual functioning; however, androgens are important in the maintenance of sexual arousal in women. As in men, dopaminergic systems facilitate female sexual arousal and orgasm, whereas serotonergic systems inhibit these functions.

It is readily apparent that normal sexual functioning and processes require intact neural and vascular connections to the genitals along with normal endocrine functioning. Any illness that interferes with these systems can lead to sexual dysfunction: neurological diseases (e.g., multiple sclerosis, lumbar or sacral spinal cord trauma, herniated disks), thrombosis of the arteries or veins of the penis, diabetes mellitus (which causes both neurological and vascular damage), endocrine disorders (e.g., hyperprolactinemia), liver disease (which leads to a buildup of estrogens), and so forth.

Similarly, drugs that affect these systems also can impair sexual functioning (Table 16–2). Thus, antihypertensives, because of their antiadrenergic effects, can

TABLE 16–2. Some commonly used medications that may interfere with sexual functioning

Abused drugs
- Alcohol
- Opiates
- Cocaine

Antihypertensives
- Diuretics (thiazides, spironolactone)
- Methyldopa
- Clonidine
- β-Blockers
- Reserpine
- Guanethidine

Antipsychotics
- Thioridazine (retarded ejaculation)
- Thiothixine
- Chlorpromazine
- Perphenazine
- Fluphenazine
- Risperidone
- Olanzapine

Antidepressants
- Tricyclics
- Monoamine oxidase inhibitors
- Serotonin reuptake inhibitors
- Trazodone (priapism)
- Nefazodone (rare)
- Venlafaxine
- Mirtazapine (rare)

Others
- Cimetidine
- Steroids
- Estrogens

impair erectile function in men and lubrication in women. Antipsychotics, tricyclic antidepressants, and monoamine oxidase inhibitors can inhibit these same functions through their anticholinergic effects. Antipsychotics can impair arousal and orgasm because of their dopamine-blocking effects, whereas serotonin reuptake inhibitors (e.g., fluoxetine, sertraline, paroxetine, fluvoxamine, and citalopram) can inhibit arousal and orgasm through their serotonergic effects. Spironolactone, steroids, and estrogens can decrease sexual desire through their antiandrogenic effects.

The sexual response cycle of men and women consists of four stages: appetitive, excitement, orgasm, and resolution (Masters and Johnson 1970). The *appetitive stage* is characterized by sexual fantasies or a desire to have sexual activity. The *excitement stage* in both men and women is characterized by erotic feelings that lead to vaginal lubrication in women and penile erection in men.

Also, both heart rate and blood pressure increase. During the male *orgasmic stage*, semen is ejaculated from the penis in spurts. Orgasm for women consists of reflex rhythmic contractions of the circumvaginal muscles. During *resolution*, the final stage, the sex-specific physiological responses return to a resting state. In men, there is a refractory period after orgasm during which it is not possible to have another erection (the length of this period varies between individuals and increases with age). Women are variable: some have a refractory period after orgasm, whereas others do not and can have multiple sequential orgasms.

Sexual dysfunctions (Table 16–3) occur when there are disruptions of any of the four stages of sexual response because of anatomical, physiological, or psychological factors. Sexual orientation is not a determining factor; consequently, heterosexual, homosexual, or bisexual individuals may experience a sexual dysfunction at some point in their lives. Sexual dysfunctions may be lifelong or may develop after a period of normal sexual functioning. For example, a woman who has never achieved an orgasm would be classified as having a primary female orgasmic disorder, whereas a woman who has been orgasmic at one point in her life but is currently unable to achieve orgasm is experiencing a secondary orgasmic disorder. Sexual dysfunctions may be further characterized as to whether they are present in all sexual activities or are situational. For example, a man who has an erection during masturbation but not during sexual interaction with a partner has a situational erectile disorder.

When a sexual dysfunction is diagnosed, the following types should be specified: dysfunction due to psychological factors or dysfunction due to combined psychological factors and a general medical condition. The dysfunction may be recent or lifelong.

TABLE 16–3. Sexual dysfunctions

Hypoactive sexual desire disorder
Sexual aversion disorder
Female sexual arousal disorder
Male erectile disorder
Female orgasmic disorder (i.e., inhibited female orgasm)
Male orgasmic disorder (i.e., inhibited male orgasm)
Premature ejaculation
Dyspareunia (not due to a general medical condition)
Vaginismus (not due to a general medical condition)
Sexual dysfunction due to a general medical condition
Substance-induced sexual dysfunction
Sexual dysfunction not otherwise specified

Epidemiology

The exact prevalence of sexual dysfunctions is difficult to determine. Frank et al. (1978) surveyed 100 well-educated, happily married couples. Forty percent of the men reported erectile or ejaculatory dysfunctions at some point during their lives. Sixty-three percent of the women reported arousal or orgasmic dysfunctions at some point. In addition, 50% of the men and 77% of the women reported other sexual difficulties, including lack of interest or inability to relax. Nathan (1986) analyzed the findings of 22 sex surveys of the general population to estimate prevalence rates for various sexual dysfunctions; Spector and Carey (1990) evaluated 23 community samples to estimate prevalence rates. These studies found a wide range in prevalence estimates for sexual dysfunctions. Studies of clinical samples suggest an increase in the frequency of hypoactive sexual desire disorder, male and female orgasmic disorder, and male erectile disorder as presenting problems and a decrease in premature ejaculation as a presenting problem (Spector and Carey 1990).

Simons and Cary (2001) recently reviewed the published literature since the publication of the Spector and Carey (1990) review. They reported prevalence figures for community samples of 0%–3% for male orgasmic disorder, 0%–5% for male erectile disorder, 0%–3% for male hypoactive sexual desire disorder, and 4%–5% for premature ejaculation. For female orgasmic disorder, the rates were 7%–10%. The authors noted that prevalence estimates were higher when obtained from primary care and sexuality clinic samples.

A comprehensive survey conducted on a representative sample of the United States population between ages 19 and 59 suggested the following prevalence estimates: 3% for male dyspareunia, 15% for female dyspareunia, 10% for male orgasm problems, 25% for female orgasm problems, 33% for female hypoactive sexual desire, 27% for premature ejaculation, 20% for female arousal problems, and 10% for male erectile difficulties (American Psychiatric Association 2000) (Table 16–4). Clearly, a significant percentage of men and women in our society experience sexual problems at some time in their lives.

Etiology

Kaplan (1974) argued for a multicausal theory of sexual dysfunctions on several levels (intrapsychic, interpersonal, and behavioral) and listed four factors as playing a role in the development of these disorders (Table 16–5).

Other factors that may lead to the development of a sexual dysfunction include an unacknowledged homo-

TABLE 16–4. Prevalence estimates of sexual dysfunctions

Sexual disorder	%
Male orgasm	10
Female orgasm	25
Premature ejaculation	27
Female hypoactive sexual desire	33

TABLE 16–5. Multicausal theory of sexual dysfunctions

1. Misinformation or ignorance regarding sexual and social interaction
2. Unconscious guilt and anxiety concerning sex
3. Performance anxiety, as the most common cause of erectile and orgasmic dysfunctions
4. Partners' failure to communicate to each other their sexual feelings and those behaviors in which they want to engage

sexual orientation and attempts to function sexually with a person of the opposite sex. Some sexual dysfunctions lead to secondary sexual problems; for example, an individual who does not have erections or cannot achieve orgasm may develop a lack of sexual desire secondary to not experiencing any positive gratification from the sexual interaction.

Many sexual problems are related to sexual trauma. For example, a history of incest, child sexual abuse, or rape may place an individual at risk for developing sexual problems (Becker et al. 1986).

Many sexual dysfunctions occur secondary to major psychiatric disorders such as schizophrenia, depression, and severe personality disorders (Fagan et al. 1988).

As previously discussed, physical, neurological, and physiological problems can lead to sexual dysfunction. The use of a single medication, or multiple medications, is one of the most common causes of sexual dysfunction.

The side effects of various forms of medications also may cause sexual dysfunctions. A multicenter, prospective, descriptive clinical study was conducted with 344 patients who were taking selective serotonin reuptake inhibitors (SSRIs). The sample consisted of 192 women and 152 men. Of interest is that the incidence of sexual dysfunctions was higher when the patients were directly asked (58%) as opposed to when expected to spontaneously report them (14%). Of the 344 patients, 200 reported some form of sexual dysfunction. The adverse effects varied by type of SSRI. Paroxetine is more likely to interfere with erection than is fluoxetine, fluvoxamine, or sertraline. Sexual dysfunctions included loss of libido, delayed orgasm or ejaculation, anorgasmia, and erectile dysfunction. Although the male patients showed a higher incidence of sexual dysfunction, the women's dysfunctions were more intense. The dysfunction remitted within 6 months in only 5.8% of the patients (Montejo-Gonzalez et al 1997).

Finally, many cases of dysfunction involve both organic and psychogenic factors, especially in the case of an erectile disorder. A man may have a mild degree of organic impairment (e.g., due to diabetes or vascular insufficiency), fail several times at obtaining an erection, and become vulnerable to performance anxiety. In this case, treatment aimed at reducing the psychogenic factors may be sufficient to improve sexual functioning. Conversely, even if a man has evidence of psychological factors contributing to erectile disorder, it is still necessary to evaluate him for organic abnormalities (LoPiccolo and Stock 1986).

Interestingly, no DSM category describes a primary disorder of increased sexual desire, but this has been reported in a few cases with the use of SSRIs (Greil et al. 2001).

Differential Diagnosis

Patients with a sexual dysfunction should be medically evaluated by a gynecologist or urologist to rule out treatable organic etiologies. These organic factors may be local diseases of the genitals, vascular illnesses, neurological diseases, endocrine disorders, or systemic illnesses. Patients always should be asked about medications, including over-the-counter medicines and illegal drugs.

Psychophysiological procedures have been developed to assess patients' erections. During rapid eye movement (REM) sleep, men experience penile erections defined as nocturnal penile tumescence (NPT). Although NPT measures can be equivocal, they help in evaluating a patient with erectile problems for organic factors (e.g., a man with "psychogenic" impotence should have erections while sleeping, whereas a man with "organic" impotence should not have an erection at any time). However, many men have both organic and psychological causes for erectile problems, and thus the results of NPT testing must be interpreted cautiously. Men with a predominance of psychogenic factors may not have nocturnal tumescence, whereas men with an organically based dysfunction actually may have nocturnal erections.

Researchers also have identified the occurrence of vaginal vascular changes in women during REM sleep, and assessment techniques are being explored to evaluate these changes in women who have sexual dysfunctions. Recently, the feasibility of measuring clitoral blood flow with standard color Doppler ultrasonography was

assessed. It was determined that with further refinements, this technique will be useful in clinically assessing female sexual arousal (Khalife et al. 2000). Other assessment procedures include Doppler flow studies and penile blood pressure measurement, arteriography and papaverine injections of the corpora cavernosa to assess vascular competence, and nerve root stimulation to assess neurological impairment.

Descriptions and Treatments of Sexual Dysfunctions

Sexual Desire Disorders

Hypoactive sexual desire disorder. Hypoactive sexual desire disorder (also known as inhibited sexual desire) is characterized by the following DSM-IV-TR criteria:

A. Persistently or recurrently deficient sexual fantasies and desire for sexual activity.
B. The disturbance also causes marked distress or interpersonal difficulty.
C. The diagnosis is made if the dysfunction does not occur exclusively during the course of another Axis I disorder (e.g., major depression) and is not due to the direct effects of a substance (alcohol or illegal drugs or prescription drugs) or a general medical condition.

It is also important to determine whether hypoactive sexual desire is the primary problem or the consequence of another underlying sexual problem. Frequently, a male or female who is experiencing either inhibited sexual excitement or an orgasmic problem may develop hypoactive sexual desire because sexual activity is not found to be reinforcing. It is also important to differentiate this disorder, in which there is an absence of sexual desire and fantasies, from sexual aversion, in which there is avoidance of sexual activity because of extreme anxiety. As with the other dysfunctions, this disorder may be lifelong, may occur after a period of good sexual appetite, or may occur only in a certain context (e.g., with the individual's current partner). It is important to assess whether the desire disorder is substance induced (i.e., drugs or medications). Assessment of individuals with hypoactive sexual desire disorder requires medical workup, psychological evaluation, and assessment of the relationship.

Hypoactive sexual desire disorder has been the most difficult of all the dysfunctions to treat. Testosterone has been used (in both men and women) to treat inhibited sexual desire; however, masculinizing side effects make its use problematic in women. No consistent evidence indicates that it is useful in raising sexual interest in men, even when serum testosterone levels are low (O'Carroll and Bancroft 1984). In addition, a placebo-controlled study in women found no advantage of testosterone over therapy (Dow and Gallagher 1989).

Recently, Segraves et al. (2001) reported on the use of bupropion sustained release in the treatment of hypo-active sexual desire disorder in nondepressed women. Results indicated that 29% of the evaluable participants responded to the treatment.

The most effective treatments involve a combination of cognitive therapy to deal with maladaptive beliefs (e.g., that partners must always want sex at the same time), behavioral treatment (e.g., exercises to enhance sexual pleasure and communication), and marital therapy (e.g., to deal with the individual's use of sex to control the relationship). When the problem is secondary to prescription medication, one could consider waiting for the patient to accommodate to the drug, lowering the dose, giving drug holidays, changing to another drug within the same therapeutic class, changing to a new therapeutic class, or adding a pharmacological antidote (although none is currently approved by the Food and Drug Administration for this purpose) (Finger 2001). These suggestions can apply to drug-induced sexual problems, including those discussed later in this chapter.

Sexual aversion disorder. Sexual aversion disorder is characterized by the following DSM-IV-TR criteria:

A. A persistent or recurrent extreme aversion to, and avoidance of, all (or almost all) genital sexual contact with a partner.
B. The disturbance causes marked distress or interpersonal difficulty.
C. The sexual dysfunction is not better accounted for by another Axis I disorder.

The major goal of treatment is to reduce the patient's fear and avoidance of sex. This goal can be accomplished via systematic desensitization, in which the patient is gradually exposed in imagination and then in vivo to the actual sexual situations that generate anxiety. Kaplan et al. (1982) reported successful treatment of sexual phobias with tricyclic medications and sex therapy.

Sexual Arousal Disorders

Male erectile disorder. Male erectile disorder is characterized by the following DSM-IV-TR criteria:

A. Persistent or recurrent inability to attain, or to maintain until completion of the sexual activity, an adequate erection.
B. The disturbance causes marked distress or interpersonal difficulty.
C. The erectile difficulty is not better accounted for by another Axis I disorder.

The treatment of erectile problems is generally easier if the patient has a willing sexual partner to participate in therapy. However, treatment is possible without a partner's attendance.

Initially, the clinician should inform the patient with male erectile dysfunction that he is not alone in this problem and that, in fact, most men are unable to generate an erection at some time in their lives. Feldman et al. (1994) reported that 35% of men between ages 40 and 70 have severe or complete erectile dysfunction, as do 50% of men older than 70. Until recently, the most frequently used interventions have been behavioral. However, with the introduction of a new pharmacological agent, sildenafil citrate, many patients are opting for a convenient medication form of treatment. Before discussing the research on pharmacological treatments, we review the behavioral interventions.

A successful treatment for arousal and erectile disorders in patients with partners has been the use of behavioral assignments to gradually decrease performance anxiety. Sensate focus exercises (Masters and Johnson 1970) are examples of such techniques in which the patient engages in nongenital, nondemand caressing with a partner and concentrates on pleasurable feelings. Gradually, the patient engages in pleasurable, genital sexual activities (e.g., touch, oral contact) with no penetration permitted until anxiety has been decreased sufficiently to permit full erectile function. Sarwer and Durlak (1997) reported on the effectiveness of behavioral treatment for sexual dysfunctions. Three hundred sixty-five married couples received treatment over a 7-week period. Sessions were once a week for approximately 4 hours. Couples presented with a variety of sexual dysfunctions. The treatment success rate for the total sample was 65%.

Group therapy, hypnotherapy, and systematic desensitization also have been used successfully in cases of erectile difficulties. Again, these treatments act to reduce anxiety associated with being sexual. Although psychoanalysis is not indicated in the treatment of simple erectile dysfunction, psychodynamic interventions may be helpful in alleviating intrapsychic conflicts contributing to performance anxiety. Couples therapy also is often helpful in treating these patients (Leiblum and Rosen 1991).

Various somatic treatments also can be used for erectile disorders, even when these disorders are primarily due to nonorganic factors. Testosterone is often used by nonpsychiatric physicians to treat impotence; however, there is no indication for its use except when erectile problems are due to hypogonadism (O'Carroll and Bancroft 1984).

Vasoactive injections into the corpora cavernosa can be used to treat erectile disorders. These injections can produce erections that last up to several hours. Most injections consist of a combination of papaverine (a smooth-muscle relaxant) and phentolamine (an α-adrenergic blocker), although other agents (e.g., prostaglandin E_1) also can be used (Mahmoud et al. 1992). Side effects of the injections include priapism (i.e., a prolonged, painful erection), fibrotic nodules in the penis, and mild alteration in liver function tests (Levine et al. 1989). Success rates for this treatment are high (about 85%), with improvements in erectile capacity, sexual satisfaction, and frequency of intercourse (Althof et al. 1991). However, the dropout rate is high (about 55%) because of pain of the injection, side effects, and the fact that the injections should not be used more than twice a week (Cooper 1991). The combination of traditional sex therapy techniques and these injections may be helpful even in those men with purely psychogenic erectile dysfunction (Weiss et al. 1991).

Topical medications also may play a role in the treatment of erectile dysfunction by directly relaxing arterial smooth muscle in the penis. Nitroglycerin patches have been found to improve erectile function in about 40% of patients (Meyhoff et al. 1992); the most common side effect is headache. Topical minoxidil also has been found to be helpful in some patients (Cavallini 1991); however, further evaluation of this treatment is required.

Oral medications such as yohimbine, an α-adrenergic antagonist, also have been used to treat erectile dysfunction. Full or partial improvement has been reported in about 34%–38% of patients when compared with those taking a placebo, although the benefits can take several weeks to develop (Sonda et al. 1990; Susset et al. 1989). Dopamine agonists such as bromocriptine also have been found to be effective in preliminary trials (Lal et al. 1991).

Sildenafil is now widely used in the treatment of erectile disorders by releasing nitric oxide into the corpus cavernosum. This activates the enzyme guanylate cyclase, which results in increased levels of cyclic guanosine monophosphate (cGMP), producing smooth-muscle relaxation in the corpus cavernosum and allowing inflow of blood during sexual stimulation. Salerian et al. (2000) recently reported on the treatment of 61 men and 31 women who had psychotropic-induced sexual dysfunction. Ninety-one percent of the men reported improvement in erectile functioning. Seidman et al. (2001) also recently reported not only that sildenafil was efficacious for erectile dysfunction but also that the improvement in erectile dysfunction due to sildenafil was associated with marked improvement in the depressive symptoms often seen in this population.

A major noninvasive, nonpharmacological treatment for erectile dysfunction is an external vacuum device. The device consists of a plastic cylinder with one end open and the other end connected to a vacuum pump. A vacuum is created that draws blood into the penis. A tension ring is then slipped from the cylinder to the base of the penis for up to 30 minutes. This treatment has a high success rate (about 85%) and a low dropout rate (about 20% per year) (Turner et al. 1991). The external vacuum device has the advantages of being noninvasive, being relatively inexpensive, and having few side effects (bruising, physical discomfort, and blocked ejaculation are the most common). Disadvantages are that erections last only 30 minutes and the patient must interrupt sexual activity to use the device (Turner et al. 1992).

For men with pure organic or combination organic–psychogenic impotence who do not respond to other treatment measures, penile prostheses can be implanted. Two types are currently available: a bendable silicone implant and an inflatable implant. However, these should be used only after careful psychiatric, sexual, and urological evaluations. Several drawbacks must be taken into account when considering patients for this form of treatment: the risk of surgery and postoperative infection, the destruction of natural erectile capacity, and mechanical breakdown (about 20%). However, follow-up studies have suggested high patient and partner satisfaction in carefully screened candidates (Pedersen et al. 1988).

Female sexual arousal disorder. Female sexual arousal disorder is characterized by the following DSM-IV-TR criteria:

A. Persistent or recurrent inability to attain, or to maintain until completion of the sexual activity, an adequate lubrication-swelling response of sexual excitement.
B. The disturbance causes marked distress or interpersonal difficulty.
C. The sexual dysfunction is not better accounted for by another Axis I disorder (except another sexual dysfunction) and is not due to the direct physiological effects of a substance (e.g., a drug of abuse, a medication) or a general medical condition.

Treatment of impairment of sexual arousal in women often involves the reduction of anxiety associated with sexual activity. Thus, behavioral techniques such as those involving sensate focus are most often effective (Kaplan 1974). The pharmacological agent sildenafil also has been described as being successful in the treatment of psychotropic-induced sexual dysfunctions in females. Although not yet approved by the Food and Drug Administration for use in women, treatment with sildenafil improved sexual arousal in 77% of the women in one study (Salerian et al. 2000). Similar findings were reported by Berman et al. (2001). Forty-eight women presenting with primary complaints of sexual arousal disorder and secondary complaints consistent with hypoactive sexual desire disorder and orgasmic disorder were administered 100 mg of sildenafil. Both self-report data and physiological measures were taken. Both subjective and physiological responses indicated improvement in sexual functioning. Seventy-one percent of the women reported improved sexual experience and indicated that they would continue taking the medication. The authors recommend that in future clinical studies involving the evaluation of drug therapies for women with sexual dysfunctions, complete medical and psychosocial evaluations should be conducted and the partner or spouse should be included in the treatment whenever possible.

Orgasmic Disorders

Female orgasmic disorder. Female orgasmic disorder is characterized by the following DSM-IV-TR criteria:

A. Persistent or recurrent delay in, or absence of, orgasm following a normal sexual excitement phase. Women exhibit wide variability in the type or intensity of stimulation that triggers orgasm. The diagnosis of female orgasmic disorder should be based on the clinician's judgment that the woman's orgasmic capacity is less than would be reasonable for her age, sexual experience, and the adequacy of sexual stimulation she receives.
B. The disturbance causes marked distress or interpersonal difficulty.
C. The orgasmic dysfunction is not better accounted for by another Axis I disorder and is not due exclusively to the direct physiological effects of a substance or a general medical condition.

The most likely way for a woman with general anorgasmia (i.e., never having had an orgasm) to become orgasmic is through a program of directed masturbation (LoPiccolo and Stock 1986). Any discomfort that the patient may feel about exploring her own body should be discussed. Next, the patient should be instructed in a systematic program for exercising the pubococcygeal muscle, a muscle involved in orgasms. Once the patient has mastered these exercises, she should be placed on a masturbatory program that begins with a gradual visual and tactile exploration of her body and moves toward focused genital touching. Use of sexual fantasies combined with stimulation is also taught. The clinician may recommend use of a vibrator if the woman is unable to have an orgasm when engaging in focused genital touching. Once the woman is able to have an orgasm through self-stimulation, she then teaches her sexual partner (using sensate focus exercises) the type of genital stimulation she requires to have an orgasm.

For a woman with situational anorgasmia, it is imperative to explore the relationship and involve her partner in treatment. Couples therapy, if indicated, and graduated exposure exercises also can be used in treatment. Treatments that focus on communication and relationship skills have been found to have high success rates (Milan et al. 1988).

The most frequent complaint of women experiencing an orgasmic problem is that they are not orgasmic through penile–vaginal intercourse. When becoming orgasmic through intercourse is a patient's treatment goal, the clinician should ensure that she and her partner are aware that adequate stimulation both before and during intercourse is necessary. In addition, the clinician may suggest various sexual positions that allow stimulation of the clitoris by the patient or her partner during intercourse. For women who are fearful of "letting go" during intercourse, systematic desensitization is often helpful. The therapist may wish to explore with the patient psychodynamic reasons, religious concerns, or personal beliefs regarding intercourse and sexual pleasure. Appropriate therapy can be offered to deal with these issues while still working within the parameters of the patient's personal beliefs and morals. Finally, the patient should be told not to expect to have an orgasm every time she has intercourse because only a minority of women are orgasmic regularly during intercourse.

Recently, there have been reports of improved orgasmic responding in women who have been prescribed sildenafil. Berman et al. (2001) reported that 67% of the women in their study reported an increased ability to have an orgasm, as did 67% of the women in the Salerian et al. (2000) study.

Male orgasmic disorder. Male orgasmic disorder is characterized by the following DSM-IV-TR criteria:

A. Persistent or recurrent delay in, or absence of, orgasm following a normal sexual excitement phase during sexual activity that the clinician, taking into account

Assessment for Sexual Interest is an instrument that measures the subject's viewing time of specially designed photographs of clothed models, assuming that the length of viewing time may correlate to the measure of sexual interest. Although this seems like a less invasive and simple method compared with the plethysmograph, the procedure and its reliability, sensitivity, and specificity must be corroborated (Krueger et al. 1998). Abel et al. (1998) reported, however, that data support the use of their instrument. Measuring sexual interest may not be the same as sexual arousal; thus, both the Abel Assessment for Sexual Interest and plethysmography may have their separate uses.

Treatment

Biological treatments traditionally have been reserved for individuals with pedophilia or exhibitionism, although occasionally, individuals with other paraphilias receive treatment with medications. In view of the important role androgens play in maintaining sexual arousal, treatments have focused on blocking or decreasing the level of circulating androgens. Surgical castration has been used widely in Europe with incarcerated sex offenders. However, studies have suggested that surgical castration is not an effective means of eliminating deviant sexual behavior and that almost one-third of castrated men can still engage in intercourse. Many view surgical castration not only as highly intrusive but also as cruel and unusual punishment. The results from this procedure are variable, unpredictable, and irreversible (Heim 1981).

Antiandrogenic medications have been used widely throughout the world since the late 1960s to treat sex offenders. The most extensively used and studied are the progestin derivatives medroxyprogesterone acetate (MPA) and cyproterone acetate (CPA). They have been used less extensively in the United States because of ethical and legal considerations involving the ability of an individual facing a prison term to give informed consent. MPA appears to act by blocking testosterone synthesis, whereas CPA acts primarily by blocking central and peripheral androgen receptors. These medications may be given orally or via long-acting intramuscular depot injection (to improve compliance). They do not appear to influence the direction of sexual drive toward appropriate adult partners; rather, they act to decrease libido and thus break the individual's pattern of compulsive deviant sexual behavior. MPA and CPA thus work best in those paraphilic persons with a high sexual drive and less well in those with a low sexual drive or an antisocial personality (Cooper 1986).

Some researchers have examined the effect that CPA has on sleeping and waking penile erections in pedo-philes. Cooper and Cernovovsky (1992) reported that all measures of NPT decreased while the patients were taking CPA. Results of arousal assessment while patients were awake were somewhat more variable. While the subjects were taking CPA, levels of serum testosterone, follicle-stimulating hormone (FSH), and luteinizing hormone (LH) also decreased, but prolactin levels did not show consistent changes. These medications never should be used as the only form of treatment; the patient must acknowledge his or her responsibility for his or her sexual behavior and participate in individual or group psychotherapy. The most significant long-term side effects are weight gain, increased blood pressure, impaired glucose tolerance, and gallbladder disease (W.J. Meyer et al. 1985). The use of antiandrogenic medications often is referred to as *chemical castration*. Although the legal issues raised concerning surgical castration are similar to those concerning chemical castration, the use of these medications is at least reversible and less invasive.

Another promising focus of research has been on the use of other forms of pharmacological treatment. Fluoxetine has been used successfully in the treatment of patients with voyeurism (Emmanuel et al. 1991), exhibitionism, pedophilia, and frottage (Perilstein et al. 1991) and in persons who have committed rape (Kafka 1991).

Stein et al. (1992) discussed the use of serotonergic medications (i.e., fluoxetine, clomipramine, fluvoxamine, or fenfluramine) in the treatment of sexual obsessions, addictions, and paraphilias. Stein et al. (1992) hypothesized that compulsivity and impulsivity may occur on a neurobiological spectrum on which obsessions and compulsions are at the compulsive end of the spectrum and paraphilias are at the impulsive end.

Kafka (2000) summarized data regarding the current knowledge of using SSRIs in the treatment of both paraphilias and paraphilia-related disorders. The SSRIs can be prescribed in the typical antidepressant doses, although in our experience, higher doses, as often are necessary in the treatment of obsessions, are sometimes necessary. It is important to realize, however, that more research is needed regarding the use of SSRIs for this purpose because the knowledge is based mostly on case reports and open clinical trials. There are no current published double-blind, placebo-controlled studies of their use in the sex offender population or with men or women who have paraphilias.

Kafka and Hennen (2000) described an open trial of psychostimulants added to SSRIs when treating paraphilias in men. They concluded that methylphenidate sustained release can be cautiously and effectively combined with SSRIs in ameliorating paraphilias in some selected cases. Coleman et al. (2000) published results of a retrospective study that concluded that nefazodone may decrease the frequency of sexual obsessions without the undesired sexual side effects sometimes seen with SSRIs.

Krueger and Kaplan (2001) reported on the successful treatment of paraphilias with depot leuprolide. This new class of antiandrogen medication has fewer side effects than MPA does. The authors reported that treatment resulted in a significant suppression of deviant sexual interests and behavior as measured by self-report. Of the 12 patients receiving the therapy, 3 who were receiving long-term treatment developed bone mineralization.

Psychoanalysis and psychodynamic therapy have been used in treating paraphilias. Identification and resolution of early conflicts, trauma, and humiliation are thought to remove the individual's anxiety toward appropriate partners and enable him or her to give up the paraphilic fantasies. Although psychodynamic psychotherapy has been useful in the treatment of some individuals, there has been disappointment with the results of this therapy as the sole form of treatment in cases of deviant sexual arousal (Crawford 1981).

A variety of behavior therapies have been used to treat paraphilias. Various aversive conditioning methods (e.g., noxious odors) and covert sensitization have been used to decrease deviant sexual behavior. (In the latter approach, the individual pairs his or her inappropriate sexual fantasies with aversive, anxiety-provoking scenes, under the guidance of a therapist.) Satiation is a technique in which the individual uses his or her deviant fantasies postorgasm in a repetitive manner to the point of satiating himself or herself with the deviant stimuli, in essence making the fantasies and behavior boring (Marshall and Barbaree 1978).

Skills training and cognitive restructuring to change the individual's maladaptive beliefs are also used in behavioral treatments. Marshall et al. (1991), in an extremely comprehensive review of the literature of treatment outcome studies for a variety of sex offenders, concluded that treatment programs that use comprehensive cognitive-behavioral interventions, as well as those that use antiandrogens in combination with psychological treatment, are the most effective. Recent outcome studies of sex offender programs have yielded generally optimistic results regarding recidivism outcome (Freeman-Longo and Knopp 1992; Marshall and Pithers 1994).

Hanson (in press) conducted a meta-analytic review of the effectiveness of psychological treatment for sex offenders. Forty-two studies were reviewed (combined sample of 9,316 participants). Treatment was associated with a reduction in both sexual and general recidivism.

Risk Assessment of Sex Offenders

Several risk assessment tools have recently emerged to aid in the prediction of recidivism of sexual offenses by individuals, some of whom have a paraphilic disorder. Hanson and Bussiere (1998) published the most well-established predictors of sexual offense recidivism based on meta-analysis. These risk factors include plethysmographic evidence of sexual interest in children, any deviant sexual preference, prior sexual offenses, any stranger victim, early onset of offensive behavior, any unrelated victim, a history of diverse sexual crimes, antisocial personality disorder, being young, being single, and dropping out of treatment. Risk scales have now been developed based on risk factors to aid in this assessment process, including the Rapid Risk Assessment for Sexual Offense Recidivism (Hanson 1997), the Static-99 (Hanson and Thornton 1999), the Violence Risk Appraisal Guide (Quinsey et al. 1998), the Sex Offender Risk Appraisal Guide (Quinsey et al. 1998), the Hare Psychopathy Checklist (Hare 1991), and the Minnesota Sex Offender Screening Tool—Revised (Epperson et al. 1998).

The use of risk assessment tools is considered an actuarial assessment. It has not been established that any single tool can accurately predict the risk of recidivism. In fact, some have been critical of these actuarially derived decisions, arguing that they should not replace a generalized clinical approach to assessment (Sreenivasan et al. 2000). Others question their reliability and validity (Freeman 2001). However, the combination of both actuarial and clinical assessments is considered by most to be the best alternative.

Sexual Dysfunction or Paraphilia Not Otherwise Specified

Several sexual disturbances do not meet criteria for any specific sexual dysfunction or paraphilia. Examples include no (or substantially diminished) subjective erotic feelings despite otherwise normal arousal and orgasm (sexual dysfunction not otherwise specified) and, for the paraphilias, necrophilia (corpses), telephone scatologia (obscene telephone calls), and zoophilia (animals).

References

Abel GG, Becker JV, Cunningham-Rathner J: Complications, consent, and cognitions in sex between children and adults. Int J Law Psychiatry 7:89–103, 1984

Abel GG, Mittelman MS, Becker JV: Sexual offenders: results of assessment and recommendations for treatment, in Clinical Criminology. Edited by Ben-Aron HH, Hucker SI, Webster CD. Toronto, ON, Canada, MM Graphics, 1985, pp 191–205

Abel GG, Osborn CA, Twigg DA: Sexual assault through the life span: adult offenders with juvenile histories, in The Juvenile Sex Offender. Edited by Barbaree HE, Marshall WL, Hudson SM. New York, Guilford, 1993, pp 104–117

Abel GG, Huffman J, Warberg BW, et al: Visual reaction time and plethysmography as measures of sexual interest in child molesters. Sex Abuse 10:81–95, 1998

Althof SE, Turner LA, Levine SB, et al: Sexual, psychological, and marital impact of self-injection of papaverine and phentolamine: a long-term prospective study. J Sex Marital Ther 17:101–112, 1991

American Psychiatric Association: Diagnostic and Statistical Manual of Mental Disorders, 3rd Edition. Washington, DC, American Psychiatric Association, 1980

American Psychiatric Association: Diagnostic and Statistical Manual of Mental Disorders, 3rd Edition, Revised. Washington, DC, American Psychiatric Association, 1987

American Psychiatric Association: Diagnostic and Statistical Manual of Mental Disorders, 4th Edition. Washington, DC, American Psychiatric Association, 1994

American Psychiatric Association: Diagnostic and Statistical Manual of Mental Disorders, 4th Edition, Text Revision. Washington, DC, American Psychiatric Association, 2000

Araji S, Finkelhor D: Explanations of pedophilia: review of empirical research. Bulletin of the American Academy of Psychiatry and the Law 13:17–37, 1985

Bancroft J: Homosexual orientation: the search for a biological basis. Br J Psychiatry 164:437–440, 1994

Barbaree HE, Marshall WL: Erectile responses among heterosexual child molesters, father-daughter incest offenders, and matched non-offenders: five distinct age preference profiles. Canadian Journal of Behavioral Sciences 21:70–82, 1989

Barlow DH, Abel GG, Blanchard EB: Gender identity change in transsexuals: follow-up and replications. Arch Gen Psychiatry 36:1001–1007, 1979

Baum N, Spieler B: Medical management of premature ejaculation. Medical Aspects of Human Sexuality 1:15–25, 2001

Becker JV, Skinner LJ, Abel GG, et al: Level of postassault sexual functioning in rape and incest victims. Arch Sex Behav 15:37–49, 1986

Berman JR, Berman LA, Lin H, et al: Effect of sildenafil on subjective and physiologic parameters of the female sexual response in women with sexual arousal disorder: J Sex Marital Ther 27:411–420, 2001

Bradford JMW, McLean D: Sexual offenders, violence, and testosterone: a clinical study. Can J Psychiatry 29:335–343, 1984

Byne W, Parsons B: Human sexual orientation: the biological theories reappraised. Arch Gen Psychiatry 50:228–239, 1993

Cavallini G: Minoxidil versus nitroglycerin: a prospective double-blind controlled trial in transcutaneous erection facilitation for organic impotence. J Urol 146:50–53, 1991

Cocores JA, Miller NS, Pottash AC, et al: Sexual dysfunction in abusers of cocaine and alcohol. Am J Drug Alcohol Abuse 14:169–173, 1988

Coleman E, Gratzer T, Nesvacil L, et al: Nefazodone and the treatment of nonparaphilic compulsive sexual behavior: a retrospective study (abstract). J Clin Psychiatry 61:282–284, 2000

Collaer ML, Hines M: Human behavioral sex differences: a role for gonadal hormones during early development? Psychol Bull 118:55–107, 1995

Colpi GM, Fanciullacci F, Aydos K, et al: Effectiveness mechanism of clomipramine by neurophysiological tests in subjects with true premature ejaculation. Andrologia 23:45–47, 1991

Cooper AJ: Progestogens in the treatment of male sex offenders: a review. Can J Psychiatry 31:73–79, 1986

Cooper AJ: Evaluation of I-C papaverine in patients with psychogenic and organic impotence. Can J Psychiatry 36:574–578, 1991

Cooper AJ, Cernovovsky Z: The effects of cyproterone acetate on sleeping and waking penile erections in pedophiles: possible implications for treatment. Can J Psychiatry 37:33–39, 1992

Crawford D: Treatment approaches with pedophiles, in Adult Sexual Interest in Children. Edited by Cook M, Howells K. New York, Academic, 1981, pp 181–217

Dougher MJ: Clinical assessment of sex offenders, in The Sex Offender, Vol 1: Corrections, Treatment and Legal Practice. Edited by Schwartz BK, Cellini HR. Kingston, NJ, Civic Research Institute, 1995, pp 11.1–11.13

Dow MGT, Gallagher J: A controlled study of combined hormonal and psychological treatment for sexual unresponsiveness in women. Br J Clin Psychol 28:201–212, 1989

Ehrhardt AA, Meyer-Bahlburg HFL: Effects of prenatal sex hormones on gender-related behavior. Science 211:1312–1318, 1981

Emmanuel NP, Lydiard RB, Ballenger JC: Fluoxetine treatment of voyeurism (letter). Am J Psychiatry 148:950, 1991

Epperson DL, Kaul JD, Hesselton D: Final report on the development of the Minnesota Sex Offender Screening Tool—Revised (MnSOST-R). Presentation at the Association for the Treatment of Sexual Abusers 17th Annual Conference, Vancouver, BC, Canada, November 1998

Fagan PJ, Schmidt CW Jr, Wise TN, et al: Sexual dysfunction and dual psychiatric diagnoses. Compr Psychiatry 29:278–284, 1988

Fallen KC: Characteristics of a clinical sample of sexually abused children: how boy and girl victims differ. Child Abuse Negl 13:281–291, 1989

Fein RL: Intracavernous medication for treatment of premature ejaculation. Urology 35:301–303, 1990

Feldman HA, Goldstein I, Hatzichristou DG, et al: Impotence and its medical and psychosocial correlates: results of the Massachusetts Male Aging Study. J Urol 15:54–61, 1994

Finger WW: Antidepressants and sexual dysfunction: managing common treatment pitfalls. Medical Aspects of Human Sexuality 1:12–18, 2001

Finkelhor D: Source Book on Child Sex Abuse. Beverly Hills, CA, Sage, 1986

Frank E, Anderson C, Rubenstein D: Frequency of sexual dysfunctions in normal couples. N Engl J Med 299:111–115, 1978

Freeman D: False prediction of future dangerousness: error rates and Psychopathy Checklist—Revised. J Am Acad Psychiatry Law 29:89–95, 2001

Freeman-Longo RE, Knopp FH: State-of-the-art sex offender treatment: outcome and issues. Annals of Sex Research 5:141–160, 1992

Freund K, Blanchard R: Phallometric diagnosis of pedophilia. J Consult Clin Psychol 57:100–105, 1989

Freund K, Watson R, Rienzo D: Signs of feigning in the phallometric test. Behav Res Ther 26:105–112, 1988

Fridell SR, Zucker KJ, Bradley SJ, et al: Physical attractiveness of girls with gender identity disorder. Arch Sex Behav 25:17–31, 1996

Gebhard PH, Gagnon JH, Pomeroy WB, et al: Sex Offenders. New York, Harper & Row, 1965

Graziottin A: Clinical approaches to dyspareunia. J Sex Marital Ther 27:489–501, 2001

Green R: Sexual Identity Conflict in Children and Adults. New York, Basic Books, 1974

Green R: Gender identity in childhood and later sexual orientation: follow-up of 78 males. Am J Psychiatry 142:339–341, 1985

Green R: "The Sissy Boys Syndrome" and the Development of Homosexuality. New Haven, CT, Yale University Press, 1987

Green R, Fleming DT: Transsexual surgery follow-up: status in the 1990s, in Annual Review of Sex Research, Vol 1. Edited by Bancroft J, Davis CM, Weinstein D. Lake Mills, IA, Society for the Scientific Study of Sex, 1990, pp 163–174

Greil W, Horvath A, Sassim N, et al: Disinhibition of libido: an adverse effect of SSRI? J Affect Disord 62:225–228, 2001

Hanson RK: The Development of a Brief Actuarial Risk Scale for Sexual Offense Recidivism (User Report 97-04). Ottawa, ON, Canada, Department of the Solicitor General of Canada, 1997

Hanson RK: The 2000 ATSA report on the effectiveness of treatment for sex offenders. Sex Abuse Vol 12, 2000

Hanson RK, Bussiere MT: Predicting relapse: a meta-analysis of sexual offender recidivism studies. J Consult Clin Psychol 66:348–362, 1998

Hanson RK, Thornton D: Static-99: Improving Actuarial Risk Assessments for Sex Offenders. (User Report 99-02), Ottawa, ON, Canada, Department of the Solicitor of Canada, 1999

Hare RD: The Revised Psychopathy Checklist. Toronto, ON, Canada, Multi-Health Systems, 1991

Heim N: Sexual behavior of castrated sex offenders. Arch Sex Behav 10:11–19, 1981

Hoenig J: Etiology of transsexualism, in Gender Dysphoria: Development, Research, Management. Edited by Steiner BW. New York, Plenum, 1985, pp 33–73

Kafka MP: Successful treatment of paraphilic coercive disorder (a rapist) with fluoxetine hydrochloride. Br J Psychiatry 158:844–847, 1991

Kafka MP: Psychopharmacologic treatments for nonparaphilic compulsive sexual behaviors. CNS Spectrums 5:49–59, 2000

Kafka MP, Hennen J: Psychostimulant augmentation during treatment with selective serotonin reuptake inhibitors in men with paraphilias and paraphilia-related disorders: a case series. J Clin Psychiatry 61:664–670, 2000

Kaplan HS: The New Sex Therapy: Active Treatment of Sexual Dysfunctions. New York, Brunner/Mazel, 1974

Kaplan HS, Fyer AJ, Novick A: Sexual phobia. J Sex Marital Ther 8:3–28, 1982

Khalife S, Binik YM, Cohen DR, et al: Evaluation of clitoral blood flow by color Doppler ultrasonography. J Sex Marital Ther 26:187–189, 2000

Krueger RB, Kaplan MS: Depot-leuprolide acetate for treatment of paraphilias: a report of twelve cases: Arch Sex Behav 30:409–422, 2001

Krueger RB, Bradford JW, Glancy GD: Report from the Committee on Sex Offenders: the Abel Assessment for Sexual Interest—a brief description. J Am Acad Psychiatry Law 26:277–280, 1998

Lal S, Kiely ME, Thavundayil JX, et al: Effect of bromocriptine in patients with apomorphine-responsive erectile impotence: an open study. J Psychiatry Neurosci 16:262–266, 1991

Leiblum SR, Rosen RC: Couples therapy for erectile disorders: conceptual and clinical considerations. J Sex Marital Ther 17:147–59, 1991

Levine SB, Althof SE, Turner LA, et al: Side effects of self-administration of intracavernous papaverine and phentolamine for the treatment of impotence. J Urol 141:54–57, 1989

LoPiccolo J, Stock WE: Treatment of sexual dysfunction. J Consult Clin Psychol 54:158–167, 1986

Lothstein L: The postsurgical transsexual: empirical and theoretical considerations. Arch Sex Behav 9:547–564, 1980

Mahmoud KZ, el Dakhli MR, Fahmi IM, et al: Comparative value of prostaglandin E_1 and papaverine in treatment of erectile failure: double-blind crossover study among Egyptian patients. J Urol 147:623–626, 1992

Marshall WL, Barbaree HE: The reduction of deviant arousal: satiation treatment for sexual aggressors. Criminal Justice and Behavior 5:294–303, 1978

Marshall WL, Pithers W: A reconsideration of treatment outcome with sex offenders. Criminal Justice and Behavior 21:6–27, 1994

Marshall WL, Jones R, Ward T, et al: Treatment outcome with sex offenders. Clin Psychol Rev 11:465–485, 1991

Masters WH, Johnson VE: Human Sexual Inadequacy. Boston, MA, Little, Brown, 1970

Metz ME, Pryor JL: Premature ejaculation: a psychophysiological approach for assessment and management. J Sex Marital Ther 26:293–320, 2000

Meyer JK: The theory of gender identity disorders. J Am Psychoanal Assoc 30:381–418, 1982

Meyer WJ, Walker PA, Emory LE, et al: Physical, metabolic, and hormonal effects on men of long-term therapy with medroxyprogesterone acetate. Fertil Steril 43:102–109, 1985

Meyhoff HH, Rosenkilde P, Bodker A: Non-invasive management of impotence with transcutaneous nitroglycerin. Br J Urol 69:88–90, 1992

Milan RJ, Kilmann PR, Boland JP: Treatment outcome of secondary orgasmic dysfunction: a two- to six-year follow-up. Arch Sex Behav 17:463–480, 1988

Money J, Ehrhardt AA: Man and Woman, Boy and Girl: The Differentiation and Dimorphism of Gender Identity From Conception to Maturity. Baltimore, MD, Johns Hopkins University Press, 1974

Montejo-Gonzalez AL, Llorca G, Izquierdo JA, et al: SSRI-induced sexual dysfunction: fluoxetine, paroxetine, sertraline, and fluvoxamine in a prospective, multicenter, and descriptive clinical study of 344 patients. J Sex Marital Ther 23:176–194, 1997

Nathan SG: The epidemiology of the DSM-III psychosexual dysfunctions. J Sex Marital Ther 12:267–281, 1986

O'Carroll R, Bancroft J: Testosterone therapy for low sexual interest and erectile dysfunctions in men: a controlled study. Br J Psychiatry 145:146–151, 1984

Pedersen B, Tiefer L, Ruiz M, et al: Evaluation of patients and partners 1 to 4 years after penile prosthesis surgery. J Urol 139:956–958, 1988

Perilstein RD, Lipper S, Friedman LJ: Three cases of paraphilias responsive to fluoxetine treatment. J Clin Psychiatry 52:169–170, 1991

Person E, Ovesey L: The transsexual syndrome in males, II: secondary transsexualism. Am J Psychother 28:174–193, 1974

Quinsey VL, Harris GT, Rice ME, et al: Violent Offenders: Appraising and Managing Risk. Washington, DC, American Psychological Association, 1998

Risin LI, Koss MP: The sexual abuse of boys: childhood victimizations reported by a national survey, in Rape and Sexual Assault II. Edited by Burgess AW. New York, Garland, 1988, pp 91–104

Salerian AJ, Vittone BJ, Geyer SP, et al: Sildenafil for psychotropic-induced sexual dysfunction in 31 women and 61 men. J Sex Marital Ther 26:133–140, 2000

Sarwer DB, Durlak JA: A field trial of the effectiveness of behavioral treatment for sexual dysfunction. J Sex Marital Ther 23:87–102, 1997

Schiavi RC: Chronic alcoholism and male sexual dysfunction. J Sex Marital Ther 16:23–33, 1990

Scholl GM: Prognostic variables in treating vaginismus. Obstet Gynecol 72:231–235, 1988

Segraves RT, Croft H, Kavoussi R, et al: Bupropion sustained release (SR) for the treatment of hypoactive sexual desire (HSDD) in nondepressed women. J Sex Marital Ther 27:303–316, 2001

Seidman SN, Roose SP, Menza MA, et al: Treatment of erectile dysfunction in men with depressive symptoms: results of a placebo-controlled trial with sildenafil citrate. Am J Psychiatry 158:1623–1630, 2001

Semans JH: Premature ejaculation: a new approach. South Med J 9:353–357, 1956

Simons JS, Carey M: Prevalence of sexual dysfunctions: results from a decade of research. Arch Sex Behav 30:177–219, 2001

Smith Y, Ban Goozen S, Cohen-Kettenis PT: Adolescents with gender identity disorder who were accepted or rejected for sex reassignment surgery: a prospective follow-up study. J Am Acad Child Adolesc Psychiatry 40:472–481, 2001

Sonda LP, Mazo R, Chancellor MB: The role of yohimbine for the treatment of erectile impotence. J Sex Marital Ther 16:15–21, 1990

Spector IP, Carey MP: Incidence and prevalence of the sexual dysfunctions: a critical review of the empirical literature. Arch Sex Behav 19:389–408, 1990

Sreenivasan S, Kirkish P, Garrick T, et al: Actuarial risk assessment models: a review of critical issues related to violence and sex-offender recidivism assessments. J Am Acad Psychiatry Law 28:438–448, 2000

Stein DJ, Hollander E, Anthony DT, et al: Serotonergic medications for sexual obsessions, sexual addictions and paraphilias. J Clin Psychiatry 53:267–271, 1992

Stoller RJ: Sex and Gender, Vol 1: The Development of Masculinity and Femininity. New York, Science House, 1968

Stoller RJ: Perversion: The Erotic Form of Hatred. New York, Pantheon, 1975a

Stoller RJ: Sex and Gender, Vol 2: The Transsexual Experiment. London, England, Hogarth Press, 1975b

Stoller RJ: Fathers of transsexual children. J Am Psychoanal Assoc 27:837–866, 1979

Susset JG, Tessier CD, Wincze J, et al: Effect of yohimbine hydrochloride on erectile impotence: a double-blind study. J Urol 141:1360–1363, 1989

Turner LA, Althof SE, Levine SB, et al: External vacuum devices in the treatment of erectile dysfunction: a one-year study of sexual and psychosocial impact. J Sex Marital Ther 17:81–93, 1991

Turner LA, Althof SE, Levine SB, et al: Twelve-month comparison of two treatments for erectile dysfunction: self-injection versus external vacuum devices. Urology 39:139–144, 1992

Weiss JN, Ravalli R, Badlani GH: Intracavernous pharmacotherapy in psychogenic impotence. Urology 37:441–443, 1991

Zucker KJ, Bradley SJ: Gender Identity Disorder and Psychosexual Problems in Children and Adolescents. New York, Guilford, 1995

Zucker KJ, Green R: Gender identity and psychosexual disorders, in Textbook of Child and Adolescent Psychiatry, 2nd Edition. Edited by Wiener JM. Washington, DC, American Psychiatric Press, 1997, pp 657–676

Zucker KJ, Bradley SJ, Lowry Sullivan CB, et al: A gender identity interview for children. J Pers Assess 61:443–456, 1993

Adjustment Disorders

James J. Strain, M.D.

Jeffrey Newcorn, M.D.

$\mathbf{I}$n the gray area of diagnosis that lies between normal behavior, problem-level issues, and major disorders reside the *subthreshold* disorders, which are often poorly defined, overlap with other diagnostic groupings, have indefinite symptomatology, and consequently present confounds for reliability and validity. DSM-IV-TR (American Psychiatric Association 2000) describes these boundary categories within another conceptual framework:

> A compelling literature documents that there is much "physical" in "mental" disorders and much "mental" in "physical" disorders.... No definition adequately specifies precise boundaries for the concept of "mental disorder." The concept...lacks a consistent operational definition that covers all situations.... Whatever its original cause, it must currently be considered a manifestation of a behavioral, psychological, or biological dysfunction in the individual. (pp. xxx–xxxi)

The issue of defining boundaries is especially problematic in the subthreshold diagnoses (e.g., the adjustment disorders), for which there are no symptom checklists, algorithms, or guidelines for the "quantification of attributes" (p. xxxii).

Adjustment disorder—a subthreshold diagnosis—has undergone a major evolution since DSM-I (American Psychiatric Association 1952) (Table 17–1). DSM-IV-TR has updated the "Associated Features and Disorders" section to clarify comorbidity with other disorders. For example,

> Adjustment Disorders are associated with suicide attempts, suicide, excessive substance use, and somatic complaints. Adjustment Disorder has been reported in individuals with preexisting mental disorders in selected samples, such as children and adolescents and in general medical and surgical patients. The presence of an Adjustment Disorder may complicate the course of illness in individuals who have a general medical condition (e.g., decreased compliance with the recommended medical regimen or increased length of hospital stay). (pp. 680–681)

With regard to specific culture, age, and gender issues, it is necessary to take these attributes into account in making the clinical judgment of whether the individual's response to the stressor is maladaptive or in excess of that which normally would be expected. Women are given the diagnosis of adjustment disorder twice as often as men. However, in children and adolescents, the gender assignment of adjustment disorder is equivalent.

The section on prevalence has been altered to include rates in children, adolescents, and the elderly (2%–8% in community samples). "Adjustment Disorder has been diagnosed in up to 12% of general hospital inpatients who are referred for a mental health consultation, in 10%–30% of those in mental health outpatient settings, and in as many as 50% in special populations that have experienced a specific stressor (e.g., following cardiac surgery)" (p. 681). Those populations with increased stressors (e.g., from poverty) are at higher risk for adjustment disorder.

In the "Course" section, information about progression to other disorders has been added. Adjustment disorder may progress to more severe mental disorders in children and adolescents more frequently than in adults. However, this increased risk may be secondary to the co-

This work was funded by The Malcolm Gibbs Foundation, Inc., New York, New York

TABLE 17–1. Diagnostic categories of adjustment disorder

DSM-I (1952): Transient Situational Personality Disorder
 Gross stress reaction
 Adult situational reaction
 Adjustment reaction of infancy
 Adjustment reaction of childhood
 Adjustment reaction of adolescence
 Adjustment reaction of late life
 Other transient situational personality disturbance

DSM-II (1968): Transient Situational Disturbance
 Adjustment reaction of infancy
 Adjustment reaction of childhood
 Adjustment reaction of adolescence
 Adjustment reaction of adult life
 Adjustment reaction of late life

DSM-III (1980): Adjustment Disorder
 Adjustment disorder with depressed mood
 Adjustment disorder with anxious mood
 Adjustment disorder with mixed emotional features
 Adjustment disorder with disturbance of conduct
 Adjustment disorder with mixed disturbance of emotions
  and conduct
 Adjustment disorder with work (or academic) inhibition
 Adjustment disorder with withdrawal
 Adjustment disorder with atypical features

DSM-III-R (1987): Adjustment Disorder
 Adjustment disorder with depressed mood
 Adjustment disorder with anxious mood
 Adjustment disorder with mixed emotional features
 Adjustment disorder with disturbance of conduct
 Adjustment disorder with mixed disturbance of emotions
  and conduct
 Adjustment disorder with work (or academic) inhibition
 Adjustment disorder with withdrawal
 Adjustment disorder with physical complaints
 Adjustment disorder not otherwise specified

DSM-IV (1994) and DSM-IV-TR (2000): Adjustment Disorder
 Adjustment disorder with depressed mood
 Adjustment disorder with anxiety
 Adjustment disorder with mixed anxiety and depressed
  mood
 Adjustment disorder with disturbance of conduct
 Adjustment disorder with mixed disturbance of emotions
  and conduct
 Adjustment disorder unspecified

occurrence of other mental disorders or the fact that the subthreshold presentation was an early phase of a more pernicious mental disorder.

As a subthreshold diagnosis, the adjustment disorder diagnosis can be used with another Axis I diagnosis if the symptoms of that diagnosis meet criteria for a major diag-nosis (e.g., major depressive disorder) even if a stressor had precipitated that major depressive disorder. The not otherwise specified disorders do not require a stressor. Posttraumatic stress disorder (PTSD) and acute stress disorder require extreme stressors and the presence of a specifically defined array of symptoms. If the symptoms extant are secondary to the direct physiological effects of a general medical condition and/or its treatment, adjust-ment disorder should not be diagnosed.

As with all subthreshold diagnoses, the adjustment disorders present major taxonomic and diagnostic dilem-mas, which present major impediments for the clinician, the educator, and the researcher. Conceptually, the adjustment disorders are positioned between problem-level diagnoses (e.g., phase of life problem, normal bereavement [the V codes]) and the major mental disor-ders. Demoralization has been suggested as another V-code category and should be distinguished from adjust-ment disorder and other pathological conditions (Slavney 1999). At the same time, the "indefiniteness" of the sub-threshold disorders permits the classification of early or transitional states when the clinical picture is vague and indiscrete, and yet the morbid state is more than that expected in a normal reaction. Therefore, adjustment disorder occupies an important place in the psychiatric lexicon spectrum: 1) normal behavior, 2) problem-level diagnoses (V codes), 3) adjustment disorders, 4) catego-ries of disorders classified as not otherwise specified, and 5) major mental disorders. Adjustment disorders would "trump" problem-level disorders but be "trumped" by a specific diagnosis, even if it were in the not otherwise specified category. And, as stated earlier in this section, adjustment disorder may occur comorbidly with other DSM-IV-TR diagnoses.

In the previous edition of this textbook, numerous questions about the diagnosis of adjustment disorder remained unanswered because of the absence of empiri-cal evidence. These questions included those about the role of stressors and the value of specific stressors in the adjustment disorders, the importance of age and medical conditions, the clarity of the diagnostic criteria, the lack of a symptom checklist, and the issues of treatment and prognosis. New research findings have enhanced our understanding of some of these uncertainties.

Adjustment disorder is a stress-related phenomenon in which the stressor has precipitated maladaptation and symptoms (within 3 months of the occurrence of the stressor) that are time limited until the stressor is removed or a new state of adaptation has occurred (Table 17–2). As the diagnosis of adjustment disorder has evolved, the recognition of other stress-related disorders (e.g., PTSD) has occurred. Other acute stress disorders

TABLE 17–2. DSM-IV-TR diagnostic criteria for adjustment disorders

A. The development of emotional or behavioral symptoms in response to an identifiable stressor(s) occurring within 3 months of the onset of the stressor(s).

B. These symptoms or behaviors are clinically significant as evidenced by either of the following:

    (1) marked distress that is in excess of what would be expected from exposure to the stressor

    (2) significant impairment in social or occupational (academic) functioning

C. The stress-related disturbance does not meet the criteria for another specific Axis I disorder and is not merely an exacerbation of a preexisting Axis I or Axis II disorder.

D. The symptoms do not represent bereavement.

E. Once the stressor (or its consequences) has terminated, the symptoms do not persist for more than an additional 6 months.

Specify if:

    Acute: if the disturbance lasts less than 6 months

    Chronic: if the disturbance lasts for 6 months or longer adjustment disorders are coded based on the subtype, which is selected according to the predominant symptoms. The specific stressor(s) can be specified on Axis IV.

    309.0 With Depressed Mood

    309.24 With Anxiety

    309.28 With Mixed Anxiety and Depressed Mood

    309.3 With Disturbance of Conduct

    309.4 With Mixed Disturbance of Emotions and Conduct

    309.9 Unspecified

were described as possible diagnoses during the development of DSM-IV (American Psychiatric Association 1994)—for example, those stress reactions that follow a disaster or cataclysmic personal event (e.g., acute stress disorder) (Spiegel 1994).

The stress disorders are also unique in the psychiatric DSM lexicon in that they are diagnoses with a known etiology (not atheoretical) and in which the etiological agent is essential for the diagnosis. DSM by design was intended to have an atheoretical and phenomenological basis as the cornerstone of its conceptual framework for diagnostic assignment. The stress-induced disorders require the diagnostician to impute etiological significance (individual, cultural, societal) to a life event—a stressor—and relate its effect in clinical terms to the patient. The diagnosis of adjustment disorder also requires a careful assessment of the timing of the stressor to the adverse psychological sequelae, and until DSM-IV, a time limit was imposed on how long this diagnosis could be used. Formerly, adjustment disorder was a transitory diagnosis that could not exceed 6 months, after which if

the patient remained symptomatic, it was necessary to invoke another diagnosis. In DSM-IV-TR, adjustment disorder has an acute form (less than 6 months) and a chronic form (6 months or more).

The etiological and dynamic attributes of adjustment disorder make it an intriguing diagnostic category that constitutes a *linchpin* on the border between normality, problems of living, and pathology. Spitzer has used the term *wild card* for the adjustment disorders because it permits a diagnosis and psychiatric intervention for a condition that may be subthreshold or a "form fruste" of pathology to come (R.L. Spitzer, personal communication, April 1992).

Definition and History

Wise (1988) summarized the historical evolution of the adjustment disorders since 1945. Early on, the diagnostic concept included the notion of a transient situational disturbance, initially codified by developmental epochs (Table 17–1). It evolved to embody a disorder of adjustment characterized by mood, behavior, or work (or academic) inhibition (DSM-III [American Psychiatric Association 1980]). Finally, it was defined to include physical complaints as well as other mood and behavioral disturbances (DSM-III-R [American Psychiatric Association 1987]).

With the opportunity to develop yet another evolutionary step—the DSM-IV initiative—the subthreshold diagnostic category of adjustment disorder was reexamined. From a review of the literature, reanalysis of existing data sets, and observations of the other pertinent diagnoses (e.g., minor depression, PTSD, minor anxiety), modifications for DSM-IV and their rationale were formulated based on empirical evidence.

As a result of the review of the literature and the Western Psychiatric Institute and Clinic data reanalysis supported by a MacArthur grant, the American Psychiatric Association (APA) Task Force on Psychological System Interface Disorders recommended that specific changes be included in DSM-IV and now DSM-IV-TR:

1. Enhance the clarity of the language.

2. Describe the time of the reaction to reflect duration: acute (less than 6 months) or chronic (6 months or longer).

3. Allow for the continuation of the stressor for an indefinite period.

4. Eliminate the subtypes of mixed emotional features, work (or academic) inhibition, withdrawal, and physical complaints.

Finally, the DSM-IV-TR changes regarding associated features; culture, age, and gender; prevalence; course; and differential diagnoses have been described in detail earlier in this chapter.

Although it might be argued that the adjustment disorders could be placed in an innovative category of "stress response syndromes" or, for that matter, in several diverse locations within the DSM classification (Strain et al. 1993), the literature does not offer data to support such an alternative placement. In the extreme, adjustment disorder could be eliminated altogether, with the advantage of maintaining the atheoretical approach of DSM-III-R, DSM-IV, and DSM-IV-TR. This solution, however, did not seem beneficial in view of the findings that show that adjustment disorder is a valid diagnosis (Kovacs et al. 1994, 1995).

Kovacs et al. (1994) examined prospectively the course of adjustment disorder among 30 subjects aged 8–13 years to determine whether long-term negative outcomes of those with adjustment disorder are referable to the disorder itself or to comorbid conditions and compared them with control subjects without adjustment disorder. Those with adjustment disorder recovered rapidly and had similar rates of new psychiatric disorders as those without adjustment disorder.

The criterion and predictive validity of the diagnosis of adjustment disorder in 92 children who had new-onset type 1 diabetes mellitus were examined. DSM-III criteria plus four clinically significant signs or symptoms were used, and the time frame was extended to 6 months after the diagnosis of diabetes. Thirty-three percent of the cohort developed adjustment disorder (mean = 29 days after the medical diagnosis), and the average episode length was 3 months, with a recovery rate of 100%. The 5-year cumulative probability of a new psychiatric disorder was 0.48 in comparison to 0.16 for the non–adjustment disorder subjects. The findings support the criterion validity of the adjustment disorder diagnosis.

Construct validity also was observed in a retrospective data study comparing outpatients with single-episode major depression, recurrent major depression, dysthymia, depression not otherwise specified, and adjustment disorder with depressed mood with or without mixed anxiety (Jones et al. 1999). The Medical Outcomes Study 36-item Short Form Health Status Survey (SF-36) was completed before and 6 months after treatment. Multivariate analysis of variance, multivariate analysis of covariance, and χ^2 test were used to clarify the relations among diagnosis, sociodemographic data, Physical Component Summary scores, and Mental Component Summary scores on the SF-36. The diagnostic categories were significantly different at baseline but did not differ with regard to outcome at follow-up. Females were significantly more likely to be given the diagnosis of major depression or dysthymia than adjustment disorder. Females also were more likely than males to score lower on the Mental Component Summary scales of the SF-36 scales at admission. Patients with adjustment disorder scored higher on all SF-36 scales, as did the other diagnostic groups at baseline and again at follow-up. No significant difference was seen among diagnostic groups with regard to treatment outcome. The authors concluded that the results support the construct validity of the adjustment disorder diagnostic category (Jones et al. 1999).

In following the guidelines for recommending changes for DSM-IV—based on scientifically derived data—no clear evidence exists for selecting a placement alternative to this disorder's independent listing.

In reviewing the diagnosis of adjustment disorder for DSM-IV, two issues emerged as fundamental. First, the effect of the imprecision of this diagnosis on reliability and validity because of the lack of behavioral or operational criteria must be determined. One study (Aoki et al. 1995), however, found three psychological tests— Zung's Self-Rating Anxiety Scale (Zung 1971), Zung's Self-Rating Depression Scale (Zung 1965), and Profile of Mood States (McNair et al. 1971)—to be useful tools for adjustment disorder diagnosis among physical rehabilitation patients. Although Aoki et al. (1995) succeeded in reliably differentiating patients with adjustment disorder from healthy patients, they did not distinguish them from patients with major depression or PTSD.

Second, the classification of syndromes that do not fulfill the criteria for a major mental illness but indicate serious (or incipient) symptomatology that requires intervention and/or treatment, by default, may be viewed as "subthreshold" and afforded a subthreshold interest by health care workers and third-party payers. Thus, the construct of adjustment disorder is designed as a means for classifying psychiatric conditions having a symptom profile that is as yet insufficient to meet the more specifically operationalized criteria for the major syndromes but that is 1) clinically significant and deemed to be in excess of a normal reaction to the stressor in question (taking culture into account), 2) associated with impaired vocational or interpersonal functioning, and 3) not solely the result of a psychosocial problem (V code) requiring medical attention (e.g., noncompliance, phase of life problem).

Attention to minor mental symptomatology (and psychiatric morbidity) may forestall its evolution to more serious disorders and allow remediation before relationships, work, and functioning have been so impaired that they are disrupted or permanently sundered. In the gray area of early diagnosis, enormous salutary effects with modest therapeutic investment may occur. In the era of early diagnosis, guidelines are the most tenuous. It is the professionals at the "front door"—those involved in primary care, triage, and emergency department treatment—who must be assisted to make this most difficult call: Is there sufficient psychiatric morbidity to warrant mental health assessment and/or intervention?

Studies indicate that because of the subthreshold nature of the adjustment disorder diagnosis and an absence of a symptom checklist, nonpsychiatric physicians and nurses find adjustment disorder more difficult to diagnose than a major psychiatric disorder (Fincannon 1995; Margolis 1994; Perez-Jimenez et al. 1994; Silverstone 1996). Without a symptom checklist, the presence of medical symptoms does not confound the diagnosis. For example, in major mood disorders, if seminal symptoms key to the diagnosis (e.g., appetite, sleep, energy, and libido) are attributable to a medical diagnosis, they cannot be used to support a psychiatric diagnosis. Of course, at times the attribution of the symptoms is unclear and impossible to discern. The symptom checklist then itself becomes problematic in the medically or surgically ill patient.

In contrast to other DSM-IV-TR disorders, adjustment disorder includes no specific profile (or checklist) of symptoms that collectively constitutes a psychiatric (medical) syndrome or disorder. Field studies, however, were performed (i.e., Strain et al. 1998a) to ascertain if a reliable checklist from an elaborate list of symptoms associated with adjustment disorder can be created (Table 17–3). (The V codes, a problem level of diagnoses, understandably are devoid of a symptom-based diagnostic schema.) The imprecision of the diagnostic criteria for adjustment disorder is immediately apparent in DSM-IV-TR's description of this disorder as a maladaptive reaction to an identifiable psychosocial or physical stressor, or stressors, that occurs within 3 months after onset of the stressor. It is assumed that the disturbance will remit soon after the stressor ceases or, if the stressor persists, when a new level of adaptation is achieved (American Psychiatric Association 2000). Difficulties are inherent within these diagnostic conceptual elements.

First, with regard to the "maladaptive reaction," it is unclear how this concept can or should be operationalized. The social, vocational, and relationship dysfunctions that are qualitatively or quantitatively unspecified lend

themselves neither to reliability nor to validity—or even to agreement when this clinical situation arises. The concept of maladaptive reaction is further confounded by the elements of culture—that is, the expectable reactions within a specific cultural environment, gender responses, developmental level differences, and the "meaning" of events to an individual and his or her reactions to them. "Average expectable environment" and "patient's explanatory belief" are models in which cultural and subjective differences are taken into account in the assessment of an individual's mental state and reaction (Kleinman 1980). Such individual and cultural considerations are not part of the decision-making algorithm of DSM-IV-TR, which strives for a phenomenological, atheoretical orientation to enhance reliability and validity by describing what can be seen and heard rather than relying on subjective feelings or clinical impressions. Another question is whether the assessment of maladaptation is subjective or objective and who makes the determination—by a third party, by a mental health professional, by the patient, or by an admixture of these. When does an individual cross the threshold into "patienthood," and who will make the decision? As mentioned previously, detection of early states with poorly developed psychiatric prodromes—leading to early warning or prevention—is desired but presents a quandary. Nowhere is this more apparent than in the assessment of "maladaptation."

The patient's functional status evaluation (Axis V) is not linked via an algorithm to the adjustment disorder construct in DSM-IV-TR. Fabrega et al. (1987) contend that both subjective symptoms and decrement in social function can be considered maladaptive and that the severity of either of these is subject to great individual variation. Using data from Axis V and their "Axis VI"—an additional and more specific functional status axis on their Initial Evaluation Form (Mezzich et al. 1981)[1]—these authors could not conclude that the level of psychopathology correlates with impaired functioning. However, Bodlund et al. (1994) found that, according to Axis V, the Global Assessment of Functioning Scale self-report was a poor predictor for an adjustment disorder with depressive symptoms because patients who have this illness tended to score themselves lower.

Second, no criteria or "guidelines" are offered in DSM-IV-TR to quantify stressors for adjustment disorder or to assess their effect or meaning for a particular individual at a given time. Many of the statements regarding maladaptation described previously apply to

[1]The functional status measure, involving seven levels of impairment, is used to assess "current functioning" of patients in three dimensions: "at work or at school, with family, and with other persons or groups" (Fabrega et al. 1987, p. 569).

TABLE 17–3. Symptomatological comparisons among subtypes of adjustment disorder (AD) in 2,224 adult (ages 19–64 years) psychiatric patients

Differential symptoms	AD AII	ADD	ADA	ADE	ADC	ADM
Hyposomnia	1.19	1.33[a]	0.99	1.03	0.63	0.98
Appetite decreased	0.76	0.89[a]	0.41	0.58	0.35	0.66
Weight decreased	0.47	0.53[a]	0.22	0.33	0.23	0.40
Alcohol use	0.60	0.67	0.20	0.35	0.70	1.03[a]
Non-CNS depressant	0.45	0.51	0.10	0.28	0.40	0.66[a]
Violent behavior	0.44	0.30	0.19	0.33	1.14[a]	0.95
Impulsivity	0.72	0.69	0.41	0.57	1.67[a]	1.35
Other antisocial behavior	0.24	0.25	0.09	0.16	0.35	0.46[a]
Self-centered	0.12	0.08	0.15	0.17	0.09	0.28[a]
Undue perfectionism	0.15	0.11	0.31[a]	0.26	0.00	0.04
Decreased motor activity	0.39	0.48[a]	0.09	0.30	0.12	0.28
Increased motor activity	0.44	0.32	0.68[a]	0.58	0.58	0.65
Social withdrawal	0.58	0.67[a]	0.29	0.52	0.16	0.36
Bizarre behavior	0.03	0.03	0.01	0.02	0.21[a]	0.09
Hostility	0.28	0.23	0.11	0.26	0.60	0.71[a]
Generalized anxiety	0.63	0.49	1.52[a]	0.85	0.37	0.55
Panic attacks	0.11	0.08	0.32[a]	0.16	0.00	0.04
Situational anxiety	0.13	0.09	0.37[a]	0.20	0.00	0.09
Depressed mood	1.52	1.78[a]	0.70	1.27	0.65	1.16
Low self-esteem	0.98	1.10[a]	0.82	0.84	0.51	0.77
Elated mood	0.04	0.02	0.03	0.05	0.00	0.13[a]
Suspiciousness	0.21	0.19	0.16	0.22	0.14	0.37[a]
Somatic preoccupation	0.09	0.07	0.24[a]	0.13	0.05	0.05
Suicidal indicators	0.87	1.04[a]	0.14	0.56	0.77	1.04
Homicidal ideation	0.21	0.19	0.02	0.18	0.42	0.48[a]
Homicidal behavior	0.07	0.05	0.02	0.05	0.40[a]	0.23
Developmental intellectual deficit	0.06	0.04	0.07	0.07	0.26[a]	0.11
Lack of insight	0.60	0.56	0.37	0.57	1.42[a]	0.97

Note. AD AII = AD Axis II; ADD = AD with depression; ADA = AD with anxiety; ADE = AD with emotional features; ADC = AD with conduct disorder; ADM = AD with mixed features; CNS = central nervous system.
[a]Group with the highest score, significantly higher than at least one other AD subtype at $P<0.01$.

the assessment of stressors as well (Cohen 1981; Perris et al. 1984; Zilberg et al. 1982). Mezzich et al. (1981) attempted to classify and quantify the psychosocial stressors into 13 domains: health, bereavement, love and marriage, parental, family stressors for children and adolescents, other familial relationships, other relationships outside the family, work, school, financial, legal, housing, and miscellaneous. Another study (Despland et al. 1995) showed that the type of stressor may indeed be of help in diagnosing adjustment disorder. Their work showed that adjustment disorder with depressed mood and mixed mood was associated with more marital problems than were depressive disorders, whereas adjustment disorder with anxiety could be distinguished from other anxiety disorders by the quantity of family and marital problems. The measurement of the severity of the stressor, however, and its temporal and causal relationship to demon-strable symptoms are often uncertain and at times impossible to discern.

Furthermore, the assessment of stress is not linked by an algorithm to Axis IV in DSM-IV-TR—a statement of stress during the previous year—so internal consistency or reinforcement within the diagnostic lexicon is not required (D. Schafer, personal communication, April 1990).

The time course and chronicity of both stressors and symptoms need further exploration. The modifications introduced in DSM-IV, which differentiate between acute and chronic forms of adjustment disorder, solved the problem of a 6-month limitation in DSM-III-R's criteria. This change was validated by Despland et al. (1995), who observed that 16% of the patients with adjustment disorder required treatment for longer than 1 year, with the mean length exceeding the prior limitation of 6 months.

Although the diagnosis of adjustment disorder is not scientifically rigorous, this imprecision makes the diagnosis useful to psychiatry. It is difficult to identify an emerging illness in its early stages, and in such instances, the diagnosis of adjustment disorder serves as a temporary diagnosis that can be modified with information from longitudinal evaluation and treatment. It is a way to "tag" an individual for possible difficulty before the morbidity becomes more apparent.

Even serious symptomatology (e.g., suicidal behavior) that is not regarded as part of a major mental disorder needs treatment and a "diagnosis" under which it can be placed. De Leo et al. (1986a, 1986b) reported on adjustment disorder and suicidality. Recent life events, which would constitute an acute stress, were commonly found to correlate with suicidal behavior in a group that included those with adjustment disorder (Isometsa et al. 1996). Spalletta et al. (1996) observed that assessment of suicidal behavior is an important tool in differentiating major depression, dysthymia, and adjustment disorder. Furthermore, patients with adjustment disorder were observed to be among the most common recipients of a deliberate self-harm diagnosis, with the majority involving self-poisoning (Vlachos et al. 1994). Thus, deliberate self-harm is more common in these patients (Vlachos et al. 1994), whereas the percentage of suicidal behavior was found to be higher in depressed patients (Spalletta et al. 1996).

It had been suggested by the DSM-IV Adjustment Disorder Work Group that suicide and deliberate self-harm could be subtypes of adjustment disorder, but the problem of suicidal symptomatology without another psychiatric diagnosis is placed in the F-code section in DSM-IV-TR, "Other Conditions That May Be a Focus of Clinical Attention." Clearly, what is regarded as a subthreshold diagnosis—adjustment disorder—does not necessarily imply the presence of subthreshold symptomatology.

Finally, the issue of boundaries between depression not otherwise specified, anxiety not otherwise specified, and adjustment disorder remains problematic. How often are the major syndromes associated with a stressor? How different are the symptom profiles of depression and anxiety not otherwise specified from those of adjustment disorder? Studies have been performed to examine these issues in an attempt to further the understanding of the specificity of the diagnosis and the construct of the stressor-related disorders and of those disorders not related to stressors. The MacArthur field trials on the minor depressive and anxiety disorders that have collected data on the presence of stressors immediately preceding the occurrence of symptoms have become important databases to establish whether stress per se is a distinguishing characteristic between adjustment disorder and the other minor mood disorders.

Although some of the findings seem to shed light on these issues, other data are still controversial. The diagnosis of adjustment disorder was consistently associated with shorter length of stay compared with that for major psychiatric diagnoses (Despland et al. 1995; Greenberg et al. 1995). Whereas Despland et al. (1995) found a significantly greater number of Axis II comorbidities in patients with adjustment disorder compared with patients who have other psychiatric diagnoses, Spalletta et al. (1996) observed the prevalence of Axis II personality disorder to occur the least among patients with adjustment disorder with depressed mood relative to patients with major depression or dysthymia.

Mixed anxiety-depressive disorder is another subthreshold diagnosis that only recently was included in DSM-IV. The disorder is similar to adjustment disorder with mixed anxiety and depressed mood, thus making it difficult to draw a boundary between the two disorders, except that less emphasis is placed on a stressor as a precipitating cause. Furthermore, until DSM-IV had been implemented, the main difference between the two diagnoses was the chronicity of the mixed anxiety-depressive disorder, as was noted in the mixed anxiety-depression field trial (Zinbarg et al. 1994). In DSM-III-R, chronic adjustment disorder was not yet described. Now, with the change in criterion C for adjustment disorder, chronic or recurrent disturbance does not eliminate adjustment disorder, and the problem of differentiating the two subthreshold diagnoses remains a gray area. This uncertainty is further complicated by the question of treatment. Is this an anxiety accompanied by depression that should be treated with anxiolytics, such as benzodiazepines, or is this a depression accompanied by anxiety that should be treated with an antidepressant, such as a selective serotonin reuptake inhibitor (SSRI)?

Research is needed to demarcate more carefully the boundaries among the problem-level, subthreshold, minor, and major disorders and, in particular, to establish the role of stressors as etiological precipitants, concomitants, or essentially unrelated factors.

DSM-III-R has been described as "medical illness and age unfair" (i.e., it does not sufficiently take into account the issues of age and/or medical illness) (L. George, personal communication, June 1981; Strain 1981). Eventually, to enhance reliability and validity, there needs to be a psychiatric taxonomy that considers developmental epochs (e.g., children and youth, adults, young elderly, and old elderly) and medical illness with its symptomatology. For example, with regard to the latter issue, Endicott (1984) has described replacing vegetative with ideational symptoms when evaluating depressed patients with medical illness. Rapp and Vrana (1989) confirmed Endicott's proposed changes in the diagnostic criteria for depression in medically ill elderly persons and observed a maintenance of specificity and sensitivity, respectively, when substituting ideational for vegetative symptoms. Recent studies found patients with adjustment disorder to be significantly younger compared with patients who have a major psychiatric diagnosis (Despland et al. 1995; Mok and Walter 1995). Zarb's (1996) study suggested that cognitively impaired elderly, when evaluated with individual items of the Geriatric Depression Scale (Yesavage et al. 1982–1983), had adjustment disorder rather than major depression. In addition, Despland et al. (1995) reported that the patient group with adjustment disorder with depressive or mixed symptoms included more women than men, thus resulting in a sex ratio resembling that for major depression or dysthymia. Therefore, future editions of DSM may be able to take into account the differences encountered in symptom profiles for gender, various developmental epochs, and medical and psychiatric comorbidity. (See Table 17–2 for DSM-IV-TR diagnostic criteria for adjustment disorders.)

Epidemiology

Andreasen and Wasek (1980) reported that 5% of an inpatient and outpatient sample were labeled as having adjustment disorder. Fabrega et al. (1987) observed that 2.3% of a sample of patients at a walk-in clinic (diagnostic and evaluation center) met criteria for adjustment disorder, with no other diagnoses on Axis I or Axis II; 20% had the diagnosis of adjustment disorder when patients with other Axis I diagnoses (i.e., Axis I comorbidities) also were included. In general hospital psychiatric consultation populations, adjustment disorder was diagnosed in 21.5% (Popkin et al. 1990), 18.5% (Foster and Oxman 1994), and 11.5% (Snyder and Strain 1989).

Strain et al. (1998b) examined the consultation-liaison data from seven university teaching hospitals in the United States, Canada, and Australia. The sites had all used a common clinical database to examine 1,039 consecutive referrals. Adjustment disorder was diagnosed in 125 patients (12.0%); it was the sole diagnosis in 81 (7.8%) and comorbid with other Axis I and II diagnoses in 44 (4.2%). It had been considered as a "rule-out" diagnosis in an additional 110 (10.6%). Adjustment disorder with depressed mood, anxious mood, or mixed emotions were the most common subcategories used.

Adjustment disorder was diagnosed comorbidly most frequently with personality disorder and organic mental disorder. Sixty-seven (6.4%) were assigned a V-code diagnosis only. Patients with adjustment disorder were referred significantly more often for problems of anxiety, coping, and depression; had less past psychiatric illness; and were rated as functioning better than those patients with major mental disorders—all consistent with the construct of adjustment disorder as a maladaptation to a psychosocial stressor. Interventions used for this general hospital inpatient cohort were similar to those for other Axis I and II diagnoses, in particular, the prescription of antidepressant medications. Patients with adjustment disorder required a similar amount of clinical time and resident supervision when compared with patients with other Axis I and II disorders.

Oxman et al. (1994) observed that 50.7% of elderly patients (age 55 years or older) receiving elective surgery for coronary artery disease developed adjustment disorder related to the stress of surgery. Thirty percent had symptomatic and functional impairment 6 months after surgery. Kellermann et al. (1999) reported that 27% of elderly patients examined 5–9 days after a cerebrovascular accident fulfilled the criteria for adjustment disorder. Spiegel (1996) observed that half of all cancer patients have a psychiatric disorder, usually an adjustment disorder with depression. Because patients treated for their mental states had longer survival time, treatment of depression in cancer patients should be considered integral to their medical treatment. Adjustment disorder is frequently diagnosed in patients with head and neck surgery (16.8%) (Kugaya et al. 2000), patients with HIV (dementia and adjustment disorder, 73%) (Pozzi et al. 1999), cancer patients from a multicenter survey of consultation-liaison psychiatry in oncology (27%) (Grassi et al. 2000), dermatology patients (29% of the 9% who had psychiatric diagnoses) (Pulimood et al. 1996), and suicide attempters (22%) examined in an emergency department (Schnyder and Valach 1997). Other studies include the diagnosis of adjustment disorder in more than 60% of burned inpatients (Perez-Jimenez et al. 1994), 20% of patients in early stages of multiple sclerosis (Sullivan et al. 1995), and 40% of poststroke patients (Shima et al. 1994).

D. Schafer (personal communication, April 1990) noted that up to 70% of children in the psychiatric setting may be given the diagnosis of adjustment disorder in a variety of mental health care settings. Faulstich et al. (1986) reported the prevalence (12.5%) of DSM-III adjustment disorder and conduct issues for adolescent psychiatric inpatients. Andreasen and Wasek (1980), using a chart review, stated that more adolescents than adults with adjustment disorder experienced acting out and behavioral symptoms, but adults had significantly more depressive symptomatology (87.2% vs. 63.8%). Anxiety symptoms were frequent at all ages.

Fabrega et al. (1987) and Mezzich et al. (1981) evaluated 64 symptoms present in three cohorts: subjects with specific diagnoses, those with adjustment disorder, and those who were not ill. Vegetative, substance use, and characterological symptoms were greatest in the specific-diagnosis group, intermediate in the adjustment disorder group, and least in the group with no illness. The symptoms of mood and affect, general appearance, behavior, disturbance in speech and thought pattern, and cognitive functioning had a similar distribution. The adjustment disorder group was significantly different from the no-illness group with regard to more "depressed mood" and "low self-esteem" ($P<0.0001$). The adjustment disorder and no-illness groups both had minimal pathology of thought content and perception. Twenty-nine percent of the adjustment disorder group, compared with 9% of the no-illness group, had a positive response on the suicide indicators. The three cohorts did not differ on the frequency of Axis III disorders.

An example of associated features in adjustment disorder was provided by Andreasen and Wasek (1980), who observed that in their adjustment disorder cohorts, 21.6% of the adolescents' and 11.8% of the adults' fathers had problems with alcohol. Greenberg et al. (1995) observed more substance abuse in adults with diagnosed adjustment disorder compared with those with other diagnoses. Breslow et al. (1996) examined patients with adjustment disorder and patients with other psychiatric diagnoses and found that alcohol or substance use/abuse did not help to differentiate between diagnostic groups. Thus, a higher rate of substance use at this time does not serve as an incontrovertible prediction factor for the diagnosis of an adjustment disorder.

Runeson et al. (1996) observed from psychological autopsy methods that the median interval between first suicidal communication and suicide was very short in the patients with adjustment disorder (<1 month) compared with patients who have major depression (3 months), borderline personality disorder (30 months), or schizophrenia (47 months).

Family functioning was evaluated by the Family Assessment Device in families who had a member with one of seven mental disorders: schizophrenia, bipolar disorder, major depression, anxiety disorder, eating disorder, substance abuse, and adjustment disorder (Friedmann et al. 1997). Regardless of the specific psychiatric diagnosis, having a family member in an acute phase of any of these psychiatric disorders—even a subthreshold

diagnosis such as adjustment disorder—was a risk factor for poor family functioning. Adjustment disorder in a family member was a significant family stressor.

Etiology

Stress has been described as the etiological agent for adjustment disorder. However, diverse variables and modifiers are involved regarding who will experience an adjustment disorder following stress. Cohen (1981) argued that 1) acute stresses are different from chronic ones in both psychological and physiological terms, 2) the meaning of the stress is affected by "modifiers" (e.g., ego strengths, support systems, prior mastery), and 3) the manifest and latent meanings of the stressor(s) must be differentiated (e.g., loss of job may be a relief or a catastrophe). Adjustment disorder with maladaptive denial of pregnancy, for example, can be a consequence of a stressor such as separation from a partner (Brezinka et al. 1994). An objectively overwhelming stress may have little effect on one individual, whereas a minor one could be regarded as cataclysmic by another. A recent minor stress superimposed on a previous underlying (major) stress that has no observable effect on its own may have a significant additive effect (i.e., concatenation of events) (B. Hamburg, personal communication, April 1990).

The chronological relationship between the stressor and symptoms has been examined less extensively. Depue and Monroe (1986) and Skodol et al. (1990) identified significant methodological problems in evaluating the quality, quantity, and timing of both stressors and symptoms. Depue and Monroe (1986) and Rahe (1990) stated that the model of a single stressor impinging on an undisturbed individual to cause symptoms at a single point in time is insufficient to account for the many presentations of stress and illness in the clinical situation. Limitations of the current construct of stress for research have been described (Cohen 1981). Holmes and Rahe (1967) assigned relative values to specific stressors, but there has been much concern about the methodology used and the results obtained (Cohen 1981).

Other life event scales (Dohrenwend et al. 1978; Paykel and Tanner 1976; Paykel et al. 1971; Tennant 1983) also have been shown to be inconsistent in their ability to link stress and illness. Many authors have cautioned that the vulnerability of the individual (e.g., ego strengths, support system, underlying personality disorders, timing and concatenation of the stressors, control over the stressors, and desirability of the event) needs to be assessed to ascertain the import of the stressor on the individual. Axis IV of DSM-III was included to allow the clinician to assess the presence of stress in the multiaxial diagnoses of psychiatric disorders, but it has been confounded by low reliability (Rey et al. 1988; Spitzer and Forman 1979; Zimmerman et al. 1987). Almost 100% presence of stressors on Axis IV was reported by Despland et al. (1995) for adjustment disorder with depressed mood, whereas 83% was reported for major depression, 80% for dysthymia, and only 67% for nonspecific depression, supporting the importance of stressors in the adjustment disorder diagnosis.

Hirschfeld (1981) and Winokur (1985) discussed both sides of the controversy regarding *neurotic* (i.e., related to a stressor) and *endogenous* (i.e., not related to a stressor) depression. From the examination of several studies, it has been difficult to establish a significant temporal link between the onset of an identified stressor and the occurrence of depressive illness (Akiskal et al. 1978; Andreasen and Winokur 1979; Benjaminsen 1981; Garvey et al. 1984; Hirschfeld 1981; Paykel and Tanner 1976; Winokur 1985).

Andreasen and Wasek (1980) described the differences between the types of stressors found in adolescents and those found in adults: 59% and 35%, respectively, of the precipitants had been present for a year or more and 9% and 39% for 3 months or less. Fabrega et al. (1987) reported that their adjustment disorder group had greater registration of stressors compared with the specific-diagnosis and the nonillness cohorts. There was a significant difference in the amount of stressors reported relevant to the clinical request for evaluation: the group with adjustment disorder, compared with the specific-diagnosis and the nonillness patients, was overrepresented in the "higher stress category." Popkin et al. (1990) reported that in 68.6% of the cases in their consultation cohort, the medical illness itself was judged to be the primary psychosocial stressor. Snyder and Strain (1989) observed that stressors as assessed on Axis IV were significantly higher ($P = 0.0001$) for consultation patients with adjustment disorder than for patients with other diagnostic disorders.

Clinical Features

Nine different types of adjustment disorder are listed in DSM-III-R. As in DSM-III, DSM-III-R adjustment disorder is classified according to the predominant symptoms extant. In DSM-IV-TR, adjustment disorder was reduced to six types that again are classified according to their clinical features: with depressed mood, with anxiety, with mixed anxiety and depressed mood, with disturbance of conduct, with mixed disturbance of emotions and conduct, and unspecified (Table 17–4). In their

TABLE 17–4. Types of DSM-IV-TR adjustment disorder

Adjustment disorder with depressed mood	The predominant symptoms are those of a minor depression. For example, the symptoms might be depressed mood, tearfulness, and hopelessness.
Adjustment disorder with anxiety	This type of adjustment disorder is diagnosed when anxiety symptoms are predominant, such as nervousness, worry, and jitteriness. The differential diagnosis would include anxiety disorders.
Adjustment disorder with mixed anxiety and depressed mood	This category should be used when the predominant symptoms are a combination of depression and anxiety or other emotions. An example would be an adolescent who, after moving away from home and parental supervision, reacts with ambivalence, depression, anger, and signs of increased dependence.
Adjustment disorder with disturbance of conduct	The symptomatic manifestations are those of behavioral misconduct that violated societal norms or the rights of others. Examples are fighting, truancy, vandalism, and reckless driving.
Adjustment disorder with mixed disturbance of emotions and conduct	This diagnosis is made when the disturbance combines affective and behavioral features of adjustment disorder with mixed emotional features and adjustment disorder with disturbance of conduct.
Adjustment disorder unspecified	This is a residual diagnosis within the diagnostic category. This diagnosis can be used when a maladaptive reaction that is not classified under other adjustment disorders occurs in response to stress. An example would be a patient who, when given a diagnosis of cancer, denies the diagnosis of malignancy and is noncompliant with treatment recommendations.

study, Despland et al. (1995) suggested reducing the subtypes even further, demonstrating identical profiles for adjustment disorder with depressed mood and adjustment disorder with mixed anxiety and depressed mood and proposing assimilation of mixed anxiety and depressed mood into the depressed mood category. These two groups represented 57% of their adjustment disorder sample; the remainder was classified as adjustment disorder with anxiety and other categories.

Treatment

Treatment of adjustment disorder rests primarily on psychotherapeutic measures that enable reduction of the stressor, enhanced coping with the stressor that cannot be reduced or removed, and establishment of a support system to maximize adaptation. The first goal is to note significant dysfunction secondary to a stressor and help the patient to moderate this imbalance. Many stressors may be avoided or minimized (e.g., taking on more responsibility than can be managed by the individual or putting oneself at risk by having unprotected sex with an unknown partner). Other stressors may elicit an overreaction on the part of the patient (e.g., abandonment by a lover). The patient may attempt suicide or become reclusive, damaging his or her source of income. In this situation, the therapist would attempt to help the patient put his or her rage and other feelings into words rather than into destructive actions and assist more optimal adaptation and mastery of the trauma-stressor. The role of verbalization cannot be overestimated in an attempt to reduce the pressure of the stressor and enhance coping. The therapist also needs to clarify and interpret the meaning of the stressor for the patient. For example, a mastectomy may have devastated a patient's feelings about her body and herself. It is necessary to clarify that the patient is still a woman, capable of having a fulfilling relationship, including a sexual one, and that the patient can have the cancer removed or treated and not have a recurrence. Otherwise, the patient's pernicious fantasies—"all is lost"—may take over in response to the stressor (i.e., the mastectomy) and make her dysfunctional in work and/or sex and precipitate a painful disturbance of mood that is incapacitating.

Counseling, psychotherapy, crisis intervention, family therapy, and group treatment may be used to encourage the verbalization of fears, anxiety, rage, helplessness, and hopelessness related to the stressors imposed on a patient. The goals of treatment in each case are to expose the concerns and conflicts that the patient is experiencing, identify means to reduce the stressors, enhance the patient's coping skills, and help the patient gain perspective on the adversity and establish relationships (i.e., a support network) to assist in the management of the stressors and the self. Cognitive-behavioral therapy was successfully used in young military recruits (Nardi et al. 1994).

The primary treatment for adjustment disorder is talking. However, in some patients, as in the following case example, small doses of antidepressants and anxiolytics may be appropriate.

> A 35-year-old married woman, mother of three children, was desperate when she learned she had cancer and would need a mastectomy followed by chemotherapy and radiation. She was convinced that she would not recover, that her body would be forever distorted and ugly, that her husband would no longer find her attractive, and that her children would be ashamed of her baldness and the fact that she had cancer. She wondered if anyone would ever want to touch her again. Because her mother and sister also had experienced breast cancer, the patient felt she was fated to an empty future. Despite several sessions to deal with her feelings, the patient's dysphoria remained quite profound. It was decided to add antidepressant chemotherapy (fluoxetine, 20 mg/day) to her psychotherapy sessions to decrease the patient's continuing unpleasant symptoms. Three weeks later, the patient reported that she was feeling less despondent and less concerned about the future and that she had a desire to start resuming her former activities with her family.

Minimal data are available on pharmacological treatment of adjustment disorder, and randomized controlled pharmacological trials are rare. Formal psychotherapy appears to be the current treatment of choice (Uhlenhuth et al. 1995), although psychotherapy combined with benzodiazepines also is used, especially for patients with severe life stress(es) and a significant anxious component (Shaner 2000; Uhlenhuth et al. 1995). Tricyclic antidepressants or buspirone was recommended in place of benzodiazepines for patients with current or past heavy alcohol use because of the greater risk of dependence in these patients (Uhlenhuth et al. 1995). In a 25-week multicenter, randomized, placebo-controlled, double-blind trial, WS 1490 (a special extract from kava-kava) was reported to be effective in adjustment disorder with anxiety and did not have the tolerance issues associated with tricyclics and benzodiazepines (Volz and Kieser 1997). Tianeptine, alprazolam, and mianserin were found to be equally effective in symptom improvement in patients with adjustment disorder with anxiety (Ansseau et al. 1996). In a randomized double-blind study, trazodone was more effective than clorazepate in cancer patients for the relief of anxious and depressed symptoms (Razavi et al. 1999). Similar findings were observed in HIV-positive patients with adjustment disorder (DeWit et al. 1999).

It is important to note that there are no randomized controlled trials employing SSRIs, mixed SSRI atypicals (nefazodone and venlafaxine), buspirone, or mirtazapine. These newer antidepressant medications have fewer side effects and may offer symptom relief of dysphoric moods with minimal adverse reactions and interactions. The difficulty in obtaining an adjustment disorder study cohort with reliable and valid diagnoses may impede the conduct of a controlled clinical trial comparing these newer antidepressant agents against placebo and psychotherapy.

A significant aspect of treatment is for the physician to keep alert to the fact that the diagnosis of adjustment disorder may indicate a patient who is in the early phase of a major mental disorder that has not yet evolved to full-blown symptoms. Therefore, if a patient continues to worsen, becomes more symptomatic, and does not respond to treatment, it is critical to review the patient's symptoms and the diagnosis for the presence of a major mental disorder. The patient in the earlier case example may have been in the early phase of a major depressive disorder, but at the time of assessment, she appeared at a subthreshold level of diagnosis.

Course and Prognosis

With regard to the long-term outcome of adjustment disorder, Andreasen and Hoenk (1982) suggested that the prognosis is good for adults but that in adolescents, many major psychiatric illnesses eventually occur. At 5-year follow-up, 71% of the adults were completely well, 8% had an intervening problem, and 21% developed a major depressive disorder or alcoholism. In adolescents at 5-year follow-up, only 44% were without a psychiatric diagnosis; 13% had an intervening psychiatric illness, and 43% went on to develop major psychiatric morbidity (e.g., schizophrenia, schizoaffective disorder, major depression, bipolar disorder, substance abuse, personality disorders). In contrast to the predictors for major pathology in adults, the chronicity of the illness and the presence of behavioral symptoms in the adolescents were the strongest predictors for major pathology at the 5-year follow-up. The number and type of symptoms were less useful than the length of treatment and chronicity of symptoms as predictors of future outcome.

Mezzich et al. (1981) and Strain et al. (1998a) observed that many of the subtypes of adjustment disorder were infrequently used (e.g., "with mixed emotional features"), whereas "with physical complaints," a DSM-III-R category, had insufficient time to be observed. Both subtypes were deleted in DSM-IV-TR.

As Chess and Thomas (1984) reported, it is important to note that adjustment disorder with disturbance of conduct, regardless of age, has a more guarded outcome. Just as Andreasen and Wasek (1980) observed, Chess and Thomas (1984) underscored that "a significant number [of adjustment disorder patients] did not improve or even grew worse in adolescence and early adult life, and it was not always possible to predict the developmental course of the disorder in the early period after its identification. Hence, we would suggest active appropriate therapeutic intervention in all cases" (p. 58).

Despland et al. (1997) observed 52 patients with adjustment disorder at the end of treatment or after 3 years of treatment. Results showed the occurrence of psychiatric comorbidity (31%), suicide attempts (14%), development of a more serious psychiatric disorder (29%), and an unfavorable clinical state (23%). Adjustment disorder is an important disorder requiring follow-up and observation. The authors concluded that the difficulty in interpreting the importance of stress on the evolution of AD is related to the methodological issues linked to the atheorism of DSM-III-R. Of course, the conceptual framework of atheorism has continued into DSM-IV-TR.

Spalletta et al. (1996) stated that suicidal behavior and deliberate self-harm are important predictors in diagnosis of adjustment disorder. These symptoms can lead to the most distressing consequence—death. However, there was considerable discussion regarding the inclusion of a subtype of adjustment disorder for patients with suicidal thoughts and/or deliberate self-harm in the DSM-IV revision process. Consensus was that such additions to the taxonomy would raise other conflicts. None of the other diagnoses has a subcode for suicidal behavior or deliberate self-harm, although it is commonly encountered in major depression, substance abuse, and borderline personality disorders. In fact, suicidal behavior or deliberate self-harm can accompany any psychiatric diagnosis. There was concern that adjustment disorder with suicidal intent or attempt would be used as a diagnostic assignment rather than the major mental disorder that did not list the opportunity to specify suicide. The desire to specify and highlight the behavior of suicidality could co-opt the obligation for the accurate diagnosis. In effect, a behavior would trump the syndromal diagnosis of a disorder. Consequently, the behavior of suicide or self-mutilation is coded in DSM-IV-TR under an F code: "Other Conditions That May Be a Focus of Clinical Attention." Therefore, there would be two Axis I designations: the primary disorder and the condition indicated by the F code.

Conclusion

The issues of diagnostic rigor and clinical utility seem at odds for the adjustment disorders. Clinicians need a "wild card," and field studies need to use reliable and valid instruments (e.g., depression or anxiety rating scales, stress assessments, length of disability, treatment outcome, family patterns) to determine more exact specification of the parameters of the diagnosis. Identification of the time course, remission or evolution to another diagnosis, and evaluation of stressors (characteristics, duration, and nature of adaptation to stress) would enhance the understanding of the concept of a stress-response illness.

Studies with adequate symptom checklists rated independently from the establishment of the diagnosis would help clarify the threshold between major and minor depression and anxiety, as well as help guide an entry cutoff point for adjustment disorder. Although the upper threshold is established by the criteria for the major syndromes, the lower threshold between an adjustment disorder and problems of living/normality is bereft of operational criteria that would define an entry "boundary." The careful examination of associated demographic and treatment outcome variables also would enable clinicians to describe more specifically the boundaries between diagnoses. Associated features such as family history, biological correlates, treatment response, and long-term course are all critical to establishing the authenticity of a diagnosis—that is, construct and criterion validity. The theory and practice of medicine have documented the need for a comprehensive multidimensional formulation of multiple physiological and functional variables to describe an illness.

Regardless of their position on the diagnostic tree, subthreshold syndromes can encompass significant psychopathology that must be not only recognized but also treated (e.g., suicidal ideation or behavior). Cross-sectionally, adjustment disorder may appear to be the incipient phase of an emerging major syndrome. Consequently, adjustment disorder, despite its problems with reliability and validity, serves an important diagnostic function in the practice of psychiatry. Problem- and subthreshold-level diagnoses are critical to the function of any medical discipline. Because this disorder may be the initial phase, or a mild form, of a dysfunction that is not yet fully developed, the relation between the incipient and the developed and between the subthreshold and the defined must be described. This apparent chaos, lack of specificity, and questionable reliability and validity are the hallmark of interface disorders and subthreshold phenomena, whether they be in diabetes mellitus, hypertension, or depression.

Combined with the remaining problem of the certainty of the diagnosis, the question prevails: Should drugs be used in the treatment of adjustment disorders? The solution to this dilemma demands a caution with regard to pharmacological intervention; the pharmacological studies are currently inconclusive. The diagnostic uncertainty of adjustment disorder presents sufficient difficulty in and of itself, with its mixed features, frequent combination with medical comorbidity, and place-

ment in the gray area of diagnoses (Hosaka et al. 1994; Hugo et al. 1996; Oxman et al. 1994). It is better to be cautious and delay psychotropic drug administration rather than subject the patient to the risk of unfavorable other drug–psychotropic drug interaction(s). The condition may resolve, or it may evolve into a major psychiatric illness that needs to be treated accordingly, which could include pharmacological agents.

The characteristics of a mental disorder vary over the life cycle, and this variation is clearly illustrated by the adjustment disorders. Certain developmental epochs may be associated with a particular symptom profile, as seen with acute myocardial infarction and appendicitis. The effect of the stressor may vary, and the assessment of functioning must be "measured" according to the demands of the developmental stage (e.g., school [youth], work [adults], self-care and maintenance [elderly]). The symptom characteristics and functional assessment of other diagnoses also may vary along the developmental schema from birth to senescence. Illnesses such as major depressive disorders, organic mental disorders, sexual dysfunctions, and eating disorders need to be reformulated in another hierarchy to incorporate the vicissitudes of the stage of the life cycle extant at the time of the assessment. Considering normal variations across developmental epochs would make adjustment disorder and other DSM-IV-TR disorders much more reliable and valid and less vulnerable to being characterized as "unfair" in regard to the aged, children and youth, or the medically ill (L. George, personal communication, May 1981; Strain 1981). The result would be a taxonomy accommodating to the vicissitudes of development, gender, age, and medical illness.

Such an effort also may make adjustment disorder, and DSM-IV-TR and future editions of DSM, more useful to child psychiatrists, pediatricians, geriatricians, geriatric psychiatrists, and primary care specialists, who currently believe that too often their patients' problems do not conform to psychiatry's lexicon. In fact, a significant number of their patients remain at the problem level of diagnoses with their somatic complaints as well. It is common for a fever of unknown origin not to be diagnosed or for chest pain to remain unspecified. It is the *art* of medicine that makes it a profession, and it is a most difficult one at the interface of medicine and psychiatry, or at the interface of normality and pathology. Anna Freud (1968) emphasized the difficulty of understanding normality and pathology in her assessments of childhood. This important advice would prevail across the life cycle and be an important challenge to the developers of the subthreshold diagnoses (e.g., adjustment disorder) and future editions of DSM.

References

Akiskal HS, Bitar AH, Puzantian VR, et al: The nosological status of neurotic depression: a prospective three- to four-year follow-up examination in light of the primary-secondary and unipolar-bipolar dichotomies. Arch Gen Psychiatry 35:756–766, 1978

American Psychiatric Association: Diagnostic and Statistical Manual: Mental Disorders. Washington, DC, American Psychiatric Association, 1952

American Psychiatric Association: Diagnostic and Statistical Manual of Mental Disorders, 3rd Edition. Washington, DC, American Psychiatric Association, 1980

American Psychiatric Association: Diagnostic and Statistical Manual of Mental Disorders, 3rd Edition, Revised. Washington, DC, American Psychiatric Association, 1987

American Psychiatric Association: Diagnostic and Statistical Manual of Mental Disorders, 4th Edition. Washington, DC, American Psychiatric Association, 1994

American Psychiatric Association: Diagnostic and Statistical Manual of Mental Disorders, 4th Edition, Text Revision. Washington, DC, American Psychiatric Association, 2000

Andreasen NC, Hoenk PR: The predictive value of adjustment disorders: a follow-up study. Am J Psychiatry 139:584–590, 1982

Andreasen NC, Wasek P: Adjustment disorders in adolescents and adults. Arch Gen Psychiatry 37:1166–1170, 1980

Andreasen NC, Winokur G: Secondary depression: familial, clinical, and research perspectives. Am J Psychiatry 136:62–66, 1979

Ansseau M, Bataille M, Briole G, et al: Controlled comparison of tianeptine, alprazolam and mianserin in the treatment of adjustment disorders with anxiety and depression. Human Psychopharmacology Clinical and Experimental 11:293–298, 1996

Aoki T, Hosaka T, Ishida A: Psychiatric evaluation of physical rehabilitation patients. Gen Hosp Psychiatry 17:440–443, 1995

Benjaminsen S: Stressful life events preceding the onset of neurotic depression. Psychol Med 11:369–378, 1981

Bodlund O, Kullgren G, Ekselius L, et al: Axis V—Global Assessment of Functioning Scale: evaluation of a self-report version. Acta Psychiatr Scand 90:342–347, 1994

Breslow RE, Klinger BI, Erickson BJ: Acute intoxication and substance abuse among patients presenting to a psychiatric emergency service. Gen Hosp Psychiatry 18:183–191, 1996

Brezinka C, Huter O, Biebl W, et al: Denial of pregnancy: obstetrical aspects. J Psychosom Obstet Gynaecol 15:1–8, 1994

Chess S, Thomas A: Origins and Evolution of Behavior Disorders: From Infancy to Early Adult Life. New York, Brunner/Mazel, 1984

Cohen F: Stress and bodily illness. Psychiatr Clin North Am 4:269–286, 1981

De Leo D, Pellegrini C, Serraiotto L: Adjustment disorders and suicidality. Psychol Rep 59:355–358, 1986a

De Leo D, Pellegrini C, Serraiotto L, et al: Assessment of severity of suicide attempts: a trial with the dexamethasone suppression test and two rating scales. Psychopathology 19:186–191, 1986b

Depue RA, Monroe SM: Conceptualization and measurement of human disorder in life stress research: the problem of chronic disturbance. Psychol Bull 99:36–51, 1986

Despland JN, Monod L, Ferrero F: Clinical relevance of adjustment disorder in DSM-III-R and DSM-IV. Compr Psychiatry 36:456–460, 1995

Despland JN, Monod L, Ferrero F: Etude clinique du trouble de l'adaptation selon le DSM-III-R. Schweizer Archiv fues Neurologie und Psychiatrie 148:19–24, 1997

DeWit S, Cremers L, Hirsch D, et al: Efficacy and safety of trazodone versus clorazepate in the treatment of HIV-positive subjects with adjustment disorders: a pilot study. J Int Med Res 27:223–232, 1999

Dohrenwend BS, Krasnoff L, Askenasy AR, et al: Exemplification of a method for scaling life events: the PERI Life Event Scale. J Health Soc Behav 19:205–229, 1978

Endicott J: Measurement of depression in patients with cancer. Cancer 53:2243–2249, 1984

Fabrega H Jr, Mezzich JE, Mezzich AC: Adjustment disorder as a marginal or transitional illness category in DSM-III. Arch Gen Psychiatry 44:567–572, 1987

Faulstich ME, Moore JR, Carey MP, et al: Prevalence of DSM-III conduct and adjustment disorders for adolescent psychiatric inpatients, in Adolescence, Vol 21, No 82. San Diego, CA, Libra Publishers, 1986, pp 333–337

Fincannon JL: Analysis of psychiatric referrals and interventions in an oncology population. Oncol Nurs Forum 22:87–92, 1995

Foster P, Oxman T: A descriptive study of adjustment disorder diagnoses in general hospital patients. Irish Journal of Psychological Medicine 11:153–157, 1994

Freud A: Normality and Pathology: Assessment of Childhood. New York, International Universities Press, 1968

Friedmann MS, McDermut WH, Solomon DA, et al: Family functioning and mental illness: a comparison of psychiatric and nonclinical families. Fam Process 36:357–367, 1997

Garvey MJ, Tollefson GD, Mungas D, et al: Is the distinction between situational and nonsituational primary depression valid? Compr Psychiatry 25:372–375, 1984

Grassi L, Gritti P, Rigatelli M, et al: Psychosocial problems secondary to cancer: an Italian multicenter survey of consultation-liaison psychiatry in oncology. Italian Consultation-Liaison Group. Eur J Cancer 36:579–585, 2000

Greenberg WM, Rosenfeld DN, Ortega EA: Adjustment disorder as an admission diagnosis. Am J Psychiatry 152:459–461, 1995

Hirschfeld RMA: Situational depression: validity of the concept. Br J Psychiatry 139:297–305, 1981

Holmes TH, Rahe RH: The Social Readjustment Rating Scale. J Psychosom Res 11:213–218, 1967

Hosaka T, Aoki T, Ichikawa Y: Emotional states of patients with hematological malignancies: preliminary study. Jpn J Clin Oncol 24:186–190, 1994

Hugo FJ, Halland AM, Spangenberg JJ, et al: DSM-III-R classification of psychiatric symptoms in systemic lupus erythematosus. Psychosomatics 37:262–269, 1996

Isometsa E, Heikkinen M, Henriksson M, et al: Suicide in non-major depressions. J Affect Disord 36:117–127, 1996

Jones R, Yates WR, Williams S, et al: Outcome for adjustment disorder with depressed mood: comparison with other mood disorders. J Affect Disord 55:55–61, 1999

Kellermann M, Fekete I, Gesztelyi R, et al: Screening for depressive symptoms in the acute phase of stroke. Gen Hosp Psychiatry 21:116–121, 1999

Kleinman A: Patients and Healers in the Context of Culture: An Exploration of the Borderland Between Anthropology, Medicine, and Psychiatry. Berkeley, CA, University of California Press, 1980

Kovacs M, Gatsonis C, Pollock M, et al: A controlled prospective study of DSM-III adjustment disorder in childhood: short term prognosis and long-term predictive validity. Arch Gen Psychiatry 51:535–541, 1994

Kovacs M, Ho V, Pollock MH: Criterion and predictive validity of the diagnosis of adjustment disorder: a prospective study of youths with new-onset insulin-dependent diabetes mellitus. Am J Psychiatry 152:523–528, 1995

Kugaya A, Akechi T, Okuyama T, et al: Prevalence, predictive factors, and screening for psychologic distress in patients with newly diagnosed head and neck cancers. Cancer 88:2817–2823, 2000

Margolis RL: Nonpsychiatrist house staff frequently misdiagnose psychiatric disorders in general hospital inpatients. Psychosomatics 35:485–491, 1994

McNair DM, Lorr M, Doppelman LF (eds): Manual for the Profile of Mood States. San Diego, CA, Educational & Industrial Testing Service, 1971

Mezzich JE, Dow JT, Rich CL, et al: Developing an efficient clinical information system for a comprehensive psychiatric institute, II: initial evaluation form. Behavioral Research Methods and Instrumentation 13:464–478, 1981

Mok H, Walter C: Brief psychiatric hospitalization: preliminary experience with an urban short-stay unit. Can J Psychiatry 40:415–417, 1995

Nardi C, Lichtenberg P, Kaplan Z: Adjustment disorder of conscripts as a military phobia. Mil Med 159:612–616, 1994

Oxman TE, Barrett JE, Freeman DH, et al: Frequency and correlates of adjustment disorder relates to cardiac surgery in older patients. Psychosomatics 35:557–568, 1994

Paykel ES, Tanner J: Life events, depressive relapse and maintenance treatment. Psychol Med 6:481–485, 1976

Paykel ES, Prusoff BA, Uhlenhuth EH: Scaling of life events. Arch Gen Psychiatry 25:340–347, 1971

Perez-Jimenez JP, Gomez-Bajo GJ, Lopez-Catillo JJ, et al: Psychiatric consultation and post-traumatic stress disorder in burned patients. Burns 20:532–536, 1994

Perris H, von Knorring L, Oreland L, et al: Life events and biological vulnerability: a study of life events and platelet MAO activity in depressed patients. Psychiatry Res 12:111–120, 1984

Popkin MK, Callies AL, Colón EA, et al: Adjustment disorders in medically ill patients referred for consultation in a university hospital. Psychosomatics 31:410–414, 1990

Pozzi G, Del Borgo C, Del Forna A, et al: Psychological discomfort and mental illness in patients with AIDS: implications for home care. AIDS Patient Care STDS 13:555–564, 1999

Pulimood S, Rajagopalan B, Rajagopalan M, et al: Psychiatric morbidity among dermatology inpatients. Natl Med J India 9:208–210, 1996

Rahe RH: Psychosocial stressors and adjustment disorder: Van Gogh's life chart illustrates stress and disease. J Clin Psychiatry 51(suppl):13–19, 1990

Rapp SR, Vrana S: Substituting nonsomatic for somatic symptoms in the diagnosis of depression in elderly male medical patients. Am J Psychiatry 146:1197–1200, 1989

Razavi D, Kormoss N, Collard A, et al: Comparative study of the efficacy and safety of trazodone versus clorazepate in the treatment of adjustment disorders in cancer patients: a pilot study. J Int Med Res 27:264–272, 1999

Rey JM, Stewart GW, Plapp JM, et al: DSM-III Axis IV revisited. Am J Psychiatry 145:286–292, 1988

Runeson BS, Beskow J, Waern M: The suicidal process in suicides among young people. Acta Psychiatr Scand 93:35–42, 1996

Schnyder U, Valach L: Suicide attempters in a psychiatric emergency room population. Gen Hosp Psychiatry 19:119–129, 1997

Shaner R: Benzodiazepines in psychiatric emergency settings. Psychiatr Ann 30:268–275, 2000

Shima S, Kitagawa Y, Kitamura T, et al: Poststroke depression. Gen Hosp Psychiatry 16:286–289, 1994

Silverstone PH: Prevalence of psychiatric disorders in medical inpatients. J Nerv Ment Dis 184:43–51, 1996

Skodol AE, Dohrenwend BP, Line BG, et al: The nature of stress: problems of measurement, in Stressors and the Adjustment Disorders. Edited by Noshpitz JD, Coddington RD. New York, Wiley, 1990, pp 3–20

Slavney PR: Diagnosing demoralization in consultation psychiatry. Psychosomatics 40:325–329, 1999

Snyder S, Strain JJ: Differentiation of major depression and adjustment disorder with depressed mood in the medical setting. Gen Hosp Psychiatry 12:159–165, 1989

Spalletta G, Troisi A, Saracco M, et al: Symptom profile: Axis II comorbidity and suicidal behaviour in young males with DSM-III-R depressive illnesses. J Affect Disord 39:141–148, 1996

Spiegel D: DSM-IV Options Book. Washington, DC, American Psychiatric Association, 1994

Spiegel D: Cancer and depression. Br J Psychiatry 168(suppl 30):109–116, 1996

Spitzer RL, Forman JBW: DSM-III field trials, II: initial experience with the multiaxial system. Am J Psychiatry 136:818–820, 1979

Strain JJ: Diagnostic considerations in the medical setting. Psychiatr Clin North Am 4:287–300, 1981

Strain JJ, Newcorn J, Wolf D, et al: Considering changes in adjustment disorder. Hosp Community Psychiatry 44:13–15, 1993

Strain JJ, Newcorn JH, Mezzich JE, et al: Adjustment disorder: the MacArthur reanalysis, in DSM-IV Sourcebook, Vol 4. Washington, DC, American Psychiatric Association, 1998a, pp 403–424

Strain JJ, Smith GC, Hammer JS, et al: Adjustment disorder: a multisite study of its utilization and interventions in the consultation-liaison psychiatry setting. Gen Hosp Psychiatry 20:139–149, 1998b

Sullivan MJ, Winshenker B, Mikail S: Screening for major depression in the early stages of multiple sclerosis. Can J Neurol Sci 22:228–231, 1995

Tennant C: Life events and psychological morbidity: the evidence from prospective studies. Psychol Med 13:483–486, 1983

Uhlenhuth EH, Balter MB, Ban TA, et al: International study of expert judgment on therapeutic use of benzodiazepines and other psychotherapeutic medications, III: clinical features affecting experts' therapeutic recommendations in anxiety disorders. Psychopharmacol Bull 31:289–296, 1995

Vlachos IO, Bouras N, Watson JP, et al: Deliberate self-harm referrals. European Journal of Psychiatry 8:25–28, 1994

Volz HP, Kieser M: Kava-kava extract WS 1490 versus placebo in anxiety disorders: a randomized placebo-controlled 25-week outpatient trial. Pharmacopsychiatry 30:1–5, 1997

Winokur G: The validity of neurotic-reactive depression: new data and reappraisal. Arch Gen Psychiatry 42:1116–1122, 1985

Wise MG: Adjustment disorders and impulse disorders not otherwise classified, in American Psychiatric Press Textbook of Psychiatry. Edited by Talbot JA, Hales RE, Yudofsky SC. Washington, DC, American Psychiatric Press, 1988, pp 605–620

Yesavage JA, Brink TL, Rose TL, et al: Development and validation of geriatric depression screening scale: a preliminary report. J Psychiatry Res 17:37–49, 1982–1983

Zarb J: Correlates of depression in cognitively impaired hospitalized elderly referred for neuropsychological assessment. J Clin Exp Neuropsychol 18:713–723, 1996

Zilberg NJ, Weiss DS, Horowitz MJ: Impact of Event Scale: a cross-validation study and some empirical evidence supporting a conceptual model of stress response syndromes. J Consult Clin Psychol 50:407–414, 1982

Zimmerman M, Pfohl B, Coryell W, et al: The prognostic validity of DSM-III Axis IV in depressed inpatients. Am J Psychiatry 144:102–106, 1987

Zinbarg RE, Barlow DH, Liebowitz M, et al: The DSM-IV field trial for mixed anxiety-depression. Am J Psychiatry 151:1153–1162, 1994

Zung W: A self-rating depression scale. Arch Gen Psychiatry 12:63–70, 1965

Zung W: A rating instrument for anxiety disorders. Psychosomatics 12:371–379, 1971

Impulse-Control Disorders Not Elsewhere Classified

Charles L. Scott, M.D.

Donald M. Hilty, M.D.

Michael Brook, B.S.

The DSM-IV-TR (American Psychiatric Association 2000) category "impulse-control disorders not elsewhere classified" includes five separate diagnoses whose single unifying theme is clinically significant impulsive behavior that is not better accounted for by another DSM-IV-TR diagnosis (Frances et al. 1995). The five diagnoses described in this section are intermittent explosive disorder, kleptomania, pyromania, pathological gambling, and trichotillomania. The diagnosis of impulse-control disorder not otherwise specified describes those individuals who have an impulse-control disorder that does not meet criteria for any of the specific impulse-control disorders or other DSM-IV-TR diagnoses.

When considering a diagnosis of an impulse-control disorder, the clinician must carefully review the established criteria for each of the diagnoses. Numerous other psychiatric disorders have impulsive behavior as one component. The possible diagnostic range for impulsive behavior includes antisocial and borderline personality disorders, conduct disorder, attention-deficit/hyperactivity disorder, oppositional defiant disorder, delirium, dementia, substance-related disorders, schizophrenia and other psychotic disorders, and mood disorders. The clinician should consider alternative motivations such as vengeance or monetary gain that may account for the impulsive-appearing behavior, particularly when considering the diagnoses of intermittent explosive disorder, kleptomania, and pyromania. Even if a person qualifies for an impulse-control disorder, such a diagnosis generally does not excuse criminal behavior in the vast majority of the United States.

Intermittent Explosive Disorder

Definition and Diagnostic Criteria

The classification of individuals who have episodic violent behavior has undergone considerable change in the literature (Table 18–1). In 1956, Menninger and Mayman introduced the term *episodic dyscontrol*, and Menninger (1963), in his book *The Vital Balance*, subdivided dyscontrol into three distinct types: 1) chronic, repetitive aggressive behavior (antisocial personality); 2) episodic, impulsive violence (homicidal assaultiveness, shell shock, hypomania, and delirious syndromes); and 3) disorganized episodic violence (seizure disorders and brain-damage syndromes).

In 1970, Mark and Ervin described a "dyscontrol syndrome," characterized by 1) a history of physical assault, especially spouse and child abuse; 2) the symptom of pathological intoxication; 3) a history of impulsive sexual behavior, at times including sexual assaults; and 4) a history of many traffic violations and serious automobile accidents. This syndrome was thought to represent behavioral manifestations of disordered brain physiology, particularly in the limbic system. That same year, Monroe (1970) reinforced the idea that subtle brain dysfunction could cause episodic violent behavior and also used the term *episodic dyscontrol*.

Eventually, terms began appearing in formal classification systems. The diagnostic term *intermittent explosive disorder* first appeared in ICD-9-CM (World Health Organization 1978). This was the first time that an offi-

TABLE 18–1. Diagnosis of episodic violent behavior: historical perspective

1952	DSM-I	Passive-aggressive personality (aggressive type)
1955	ICD-7	Immature personality (aggressiveness subtype)
1956	Menninger and Mayman	"Episodic dyscontrol"
1963	Menninger	Dyscontrol: chronic, repetitive; episodic, impulsive; disorganized
1968	DSM-II	Explosive personality
1970	Monroe	Episodic behavioral disorders
1970	Mark and Ervin	"Dyscontrol syndrome"
1977	ICD-9	Explosive personality (exclude: dyssocial, hysterical)
1979	ICD-9-CM	Intermittent explosive disorder
		Recurrent, significant outbursts
		Not due to other mental disorder
		Aggression disproportionate to stressors
		Regret, self-reproach (remorse) present
1980	DSM-III	Intermittent explosive disorder
		Several discrete, serious episodes
		Aggression disproportionate to stressors
		No other impulsivity, aggression
		Exclude: schizophrenia, antisocial personality disorder, conduct disorder
1987	DSM-III-R	Intermittent explosive disorder
		Several discrete, serious episodes
		Aggression disproportionate to stressors
		No other impulsivity, aggression
		Exclude: psychosis, organic personality syndrome, antisocial personality disorder, borderline personality disorder, conduct disorder, intoxication
1994	DSM-IV	Intermittent explosive disorder
		Several discrete, serious episodes
		Aggression disproportionate to stressors
		Exclude: antisocial personality disorder, borderline personality disorder, a psychotic disorder, a manic episode, conduct disorder, attention-deficit/hyperactivity disorder, substance intoxication, and a general medical condition that caused the aggression

cial diagnostic nomenclature had categorized episodic violence as a disorder separate from personality. Intermittent explosive disorder with different diagnostic criteria appeared in DSM-III (American Psychiatric Association 1980) and then in DSM-III-R (American Psychiatric Association 1987). In the DSM-IV-TR diagnostic criteria for intermittent explosive disorder (Table 18–2), the requirement that impulsivity be absent between episodes has been eliminated and additional exclusionary diagnoses have been added.

Two DSM-IV-TR diagnoses are currently available to the clinician who wishes to diagnose primarily episodic violent behavior: *intermittent explosive disorder* and *personality change due to a general medical condition, aggressive type*. Intermittent explosive disorder has numerous exclusion criteria, whereas personality change due to a general medical condition requires the presence of a specific organic factor that is judged to be causally related to the violence, including a medication (Shaw and Fletcher 2000). Most individuals with episodic violent

TABLE 18–2. DSM-IV-TR diagnostic criteria for intermittent explosive disorder

A. Several discrete episodes of failure to resist aggressive impulses that result in serious assaultive acts or destruction of property.

B. The degree of aggressiveness expressed during the episodes is grossly out of proportion to any precipitating psychosocial stressors.

C. The aggressive episodes are not better accounted for by another mental disorder (e.g., antisocial personality disorder, borderline personality disorder, a psychotic disorder, a manic episode, conduct disorder, or attention-deficit/hyperactivity disorder) and are not due to the direct physiological effects of a substance (e.g., a drug of abuse, a medication) or a general medical condition (e.g., head trauma, Alzheimer's disease).

behavior do not meet the diagnostic criteria for either disorder but have another psychiatric disorder such as schizophrenia, paranoid disorder, mania, substance abuse, drug withdrawal, delirium, a personality disorder (especially borderline or antisocial), mental retardation, a conduct disorder, or organic brain disease (Tardiff 1992).

Epidemiology

According to a review of the literature published between 1937 and 1991, episodic violent behavior is quite common in the general population, but strictly diagnosed intermittent explosive disorder is quite rare because of the exclusionary criteria (American Psychiatric Association 1994b). However, DSM-IV-TR is more inclusive than past DSM editions. Males account for 80% of the persons who have episodic violence (American Psychiatric Association 1994b). In the introduction to a volume titled *Psychopharmacologic Treatment of Pathologic Aggression* in *The Psychiatric Clinics of North America*, Fava (1997) correctly noted that patients diagnosed with intermittent explosive disorder are complex and heterogeneous in terms of symptoms and etiologies. As important are violent patients with other psychiatric disorders (e.g., bipolar) whose symptoms and etiologies may overlap with intermittent explosive disorder (McElroy et al. 1996, 1998).

The characteristics of 842 individuals who were reported to have episodic violent behavior are summarized in Table 18–3 (American Psychiatric Association 1994b). When all 842 cases were carefully reviewed and compared against DSM-III-R criteria for intermittent explosive disorder, only 17 patients were found to have possible intermittent explosive disorder. Mattes (1990) reported 4 of 51 (8%) patients diagnosed with intermittent explosive disorder who were free of any evidence of organicity.

Patients with episodic violent behavior frequently have abnormal neurological examination results (65%), abnormal neuropsychological test results (58%), abnormal electroencephalogram (EEG) results (55%), a history of attention-deficit/hyperactivity disorder (45%), or a history of learning disability (38%) (Table 18–3). Despite evidence of central nervous system (CNS) dysfunction, it is often impossible to establish a clear cause-and-effect relationship between the CNS dysfunction and episodic violent behavior.

Etiology

Episodic violent behavior occurs in patients because of biological (e.g., neuronal discharges), psychological (e.g., motivational), and social reasons (Lesch and Merschdorf 2000). A continuum exists between "faulty learning" and "faulty equipment" (Monroe 1970). Research has implicated abnormalities in serotonergic and noradrenergic function (Eichelman 1992; Kruesi et al. 1992; Tardiff 1992; Virkkunen et al. 1996), as well as high testosterone levels, increased dopamine levels, and increased arginine vasopressin levels (Kavoussi et al. 1997), in individuals with episodic violence. Reduced γ-aminobutyric acid (GABA) and acetylcholine function also have been associated with agitation (Lindenmayer 2000). Chernasky and Hollander (1997) reviewed the neurobiology and neurophysiology of aggression and impulsivity. It is unclear if all of these findings pertain to those with intermittent explosive disorder. Experimental paradigms of punishment, extinction, and novelty provide a method for studying the neurobiology of behavioral inhibition (Stein et al. 1993). For example, decrease in serotonergic transmission leads to an inability to adopt passive or waiting attitudes or to accept situations that necessitate or create inhibitory tendencies (Soubrie 1986). Animal studies of impulse control typically have used one of three models: delay of reward, differential reinforcement, or autoshaping (behaviors naturally engaged without reinforcement) (Monterosso and Ainslie 1999). Models of self-control also may be of utility, including control of attention, control of emotions, and choice bundling (bundling a current choice with a series of future choices) (Monterosso and Ainslie 1999).

Associated Diagnoses

Because relatively few patients have intermittent explosive disorder, associated diagnoses have not been thoroughly evaluated. By definition (i.e., exclusionary diagnostic criteria), it may not occur with many disorders. In terms of symptoms, as well as etiology, there may be significant overlap with other disorders with agitation (e.g., dementia) or impulse-control dysregulation (e.g., kleptomania). Patients with a medical etiology (e.g., cerebrovascular accident) may be prone to other psychiatric disorders such as depression.

Despite the knowledge that individuals who have episodic violence often have personality disorders, no investigator of intermittent explosive disorder has evaluated personality in a systematic fashion. This is a critical factor because antisocial personality disorder and borderline personality disorder are part of the exclusion criteria for the intermittent explosive disorder diagnosis. Coccaro et al. (1998) evaluated revised intermittent explosive disorder criteria for patients with a known personality disorder in an attempt to better understand the impulsivity of these disorders and the similarities between them and intermittent explosive disorder.

TABLE 18–3. Characteristics of 842 patients with episodic violent behavior

	Patients examined out of total sample, % (N=842)	Number positive/ total examined (%)
History of seizures	87	215/733 (29)
Legal problems	74	216/621 (35)
Head trauma	73	182/617 (29)
History of attention deficit	69	262/582 (45)
Drugs involved	65	82/547 (15)
Neurological abnormality	64	350/539 (65)
History of psychosis	62	33/527 (6)
Antisocial personality	53	15/445 (3)
Alcohol abuse/pathological intoxication	50	238/417 (57)
Electroencephalogram	44	202/368 (55)
Family history of violence	31	109/264 (41)
Prodromal symptoms	24	77/202 (38)
Other personality disorder	20	39/168 (23)
Neuropsychological tests	20	97/167 (58)
Presence of remorse	18	96/153 (63)
Genetic abnormality	18	4/151 (3)
Learning disability	12	38/99 (38)
Computed tomography scan	12	16/98 (16)

Evaluation

The evaluation of the patient with potential intermittent explosive disorder includes a review of the chief complaint, history of the present illness, psychiatric and substance use history, family history, personal and developmental history, medical history (e.g., history of seizures), mental status, and results of physical examination. Information from the patient, relatives, therapist, primary care physician, prior evaluations of violence, and police and criminal records may be of utility. The onset, course, and severity of the violent behavior, as well as other types of reckless behavior (e.g., suicidal behavior, reckless driving, destruction of property, reckless spending, and reckless sexual behavior), are assessed. It may be helpful to quantify the behavior with the Overt Aggression Scale (Yudofsky et al. 1986) or Overt Agitation Severity Scale (Yudofsky et al. 1997). Visual evoked potential studies and special diagnostic techniques (e.g., electroencephalographic activation with chloralose) may prove useful in evaluation of these patients (Bars et al. 2001; Monroe 1970).

Treatment

Although information on the management and treatment of aggressive behavior is available, no information exists on the treatment of rigorously diagnosed intermittent explosive disorder. Studies of aggressive behavior consist primarily of anecdotal case reports or open drug trials; few studies are placebo controlled. Research in this area is also complicated by the ethical dilemma of randomizing potentially violent patients to placebo treatment, although this is critical because the rates of response are most likely lower than those for other disorders (e.g., depression).

The treatment of a patient who becomes acutely violent, regardless of the underlying etiology, commonly involves physical restraint, seclusion, and sedation. Neuroleptics and benzodiazepines, such as haloperidol and lorazepam (or a combination of the two), are often appropriate and effective interventions to control an acutely violent individual (Wise et al., in press). It is more difficult to decide how to treat a patient who has long-standing bouts of aggressive behavior. A task force of professionals from more than 40 disciplines recently reviewed the literature with regard to practice parameters for intravenous sedation for adult patients in the intensive care setting (Shapiro et al. 1995). Evidence for use of haloperidol was convincingly justifiable on scientific evidence alone, whereas use of lorazepam was reasonably justifiable by available scientific evidence and strongly supported by expert critical care opinion. However, intravenous haloperidol may induce arrhythmia such that a pretreatment check of the QTc interval and monitoring are recommended (Lawrence and Nasraway 1997).

The development of a treatment plan for a patient who has long-standing, episodic aggressive behavior is complicated and involves the assessment and amelioration (when possible) of multiple factors: temperament, sensory cues, neuroanatomy, neurochemical and neuroendocrine function, stress, and social conditions (Eichelman 1992). Long-term psychotherapy is effective in diminishing violent behavior in some individuals (Eichelman 1992; Tardiff 1992).

No drug is currently specifically approved by the U.S. Food and Drug Administration (FDA) for the treatment of intermittent explosive disorder or other forms of aggression. However, numerous pharmacological agents have been reported as effective in diminishing violent behavior in some individuals, largely in anecdotal reports: neuroleptics, benzodiazepines, lithium, β-blockers (especially propranolol), anticonvulsants (especially carbamazepine), serotonin-modulating drugs (tryptophan, trazodone, buspirone, clomipramine, selective serotonin reuptake inhibitors [SSRIs]), polycyclic antidepressants, monoamine oxidase inhibitors (MAOIs), and psychostimulants (Eichelman 1992; Tardiff 1992). The task for the clinician is to select the most effective and safest intervention for an individual patient who either is acutely violent or has chronic difficulty controlling violent impulses. Medications with few long-term side effects are advantageous because the duration of the disorder is currently unknown but may be persistent like other aggressive disorders.

Because no universally effective antiaggression medications are available, selection of a pharmacological agent is based on the clinical diagnosis of the patient and associated symptoms. For example, aggressive behavior often can be linked with other psychiatric symptoms or disorders: psychosis (antipsychotic), mania or mood lability (mood stabilizer), anxiety (buspirone, SSRI), or depression (SSRI). In the absence of a treatable psychiatric condition, these drug classes and others (e.g., propranolol) are increasingly being used in the management of chronic aggressive behavior.

Lithium and other mood stabilizers may be useful in the treatment of aggression not associated with a manic episode. Campbell et al. (1984) treated children who had conduct disorder with lithium and reported decreases in aggressive behavior, especially when the behavior contained strong affective components. In a double-blind, placebo-controlled study, Sheard et al. (1976) found that lithium reduced aggression in prisoners who did not have mood disorders. Fava (1997) noted that lithium appears to be effective in the treatment of aggression in prison inmates without epilepsy, mentally retarded and disabled patients, children with conduct disorder, and patients with bipolar disorder. On the basis of the hypothetical relationship between seizures and aggressive behavior,

carbamazepine was used in the early 1970s to treat patients with rage outbursts, especially patients who had seizure foci located in the temporal lobe or limbic structures (Mattes 1986). Carbamazepine reduces aggressive behavior in patients with intermittent explosive disorder and without overt epilepsy (Mattes 1990); the average dose was 860 mg, and the mean serum level was 8.6 μg/mL. Other studies have suggested the benefit of carbamazepine for developmentally disabled persons with agitation (Folks et al. 1982) and those with dementia (Gleason and Schneider 1990), as well as valproate for borderline personality disorder (Stein et al. 1995a) and dementia (Lott et al. 1995; Narayan and Nelson 1997).

Antipsychotic medication has been used for acute and long-term violence, although the side effect risk has prompted reevaluation of that practice. Atypical antipsychotics have a better profile than typical antipsychotics. In a 12-week, double-blind, placebo-controlled trial, risperidone was better than haloperidol and placebo for behavioral disturbance associated with dementia (De Deyn et al. 1999).

Elliott (1977) was among the first to use propranolol to treat the aggressive behavior seen in brain-injured patients. Numerous other studies showed the relative benefit of β-blockers in patients with and without overt brain injury (Mattes 1990; Sheard 1988; Williams et al. 1982; Yudofsky et al. 1981). More recent research has suggested that compounds that modulate serotonin transmission, such as buspirone, serotonin reuptake inhibitors, trazodone, and clomipramine, may benefit some patients. This also appears true in disorders of pathological aggression (Fava 1997).

Course and Prognosis

Few patients are under study for intermittent explosive disorder in terms of its epidemiology, diagnosis, treatment, and course. Accordingly, more data need to be collected in each of these areas.

Kleptomania

Definition and Diagnostic Criteria

The term *kleptomania* derives from the Greek words *kleptein* and *mania*, meaning "stealing madness." By the early 1800s, Matthey coined the term *klopemanie* to define the stealing of useless objects easily obtained by legitimate purposes. In 1838, Marc and Esquirol changed *klopemanie* to *kleptomanie* when describing the behavior of several kings who stole worthless items. *Kleptomanie* was defined as a "conscious urge to steal in an individual in whom there is no ordinary disturbance in consciousness" (Seguier 1966). DSM-I (American Psychiatric Association 1952) did not include kleptomania as a separate diagnosis but considered it as a supplementary term.

Kleptomania first appeared in DSM-II (American Psychiatric Association 1968) and has been included in each subsequent DSM edition (Winer and Pololock 1980). In DSM-IV-TR, kleptomania is defined as the recurrent failure to resist impulses to steal objects that are not needed for personal use or for their monetary gain (Table 18–4). The individual with kleptomania experiences an increasing sense of tension immediately before the theft, followed by a sense of pleasure, gratification, or relief at the time of committing the theft. The stealing is not in response to psychotic symptoms, such as a delusion or hallucination, and is not committed to express anger or vengeance. In addition, the individual is not given the diagnosis of kleptomania if the stealing is better accounted for by conduct disorder, a manic episode, or antisocial personality disorder (American Psychiatric Association 2000).

Kleptomania should be distinguished from other behaviors such as stealing and compulsive buying. Stealing involves the planned taking of objects for secondary gain or profit (Christenson et al. 1994; Yates 1986). In contrast, compulsive buying involves the purchase rather than the theft of items. Although compulsive buying is not a recognized DSM-IV-TR diagnosis, proposed criteria include maladaptive preoccupations or impulses with buying or shopping that cause marked distress; are time-consuming; significantly interfere with social, occupational, or financial functioning; and do not occur exclusively during periods of hypomania or mania (McElroy et al. 1994).

Goldman (1991, p. 986) described the typical person with kleptomania as a 35-year-old married woman "who has been apprehended for the theft of objects she could easily afford and does not need. Her stealing began at age 20 and she has been caught several times." Goldman noted that individuals with kleptomania often keep piles of unopened packages in their homes and sometimes stay indoors to limit opportunities to steal. Although the act of stealing may bring a sense of relief, the individual with kleptomania may keep his or her behavior secret because of associated feelings of shame and guilt. Other characteristics associated with kleptomania described by Goldman include an unhappy marriage with sexual difficulties, long-standing dysphoria, a stressful childhood, and a personality disorder.

TABLE 18–4. DSM-IV-TR diagnostic criteria for kleptomania

A. Recurrent failure to resist impulses to steal objects that are not needed for personal use or for their monetary value.

B. Increasing sense of tension immediately before committing the theft.

C. Pleasure, gratification, or relief at the time of committing the theft.

D. The stealing is not committed to express anger or vengeance and is not in response to a delusion or a hallucination.

E. The stealing is not better accounted for by conduct disorder, a manic episode, or antisocial personality disorder.

In their study of 20 persons with kleptomania, McElroy et al. (1991b) found that some individuals with kleptomania atoned for stealing by donating stolen goods to charity, returning to victimized stores to pay for stolen items or to buy unneeded items, or calling stores to alert clerks of their stealing.

Epidemiology

Kleptomania has been described as a rare diagnosis. Prevalence estimates among identified shoplifters range between 4% (Singer 1978) and 8% (Bradford and Balmaceda 1983). Because many persons with kleptomania are never caught, the actual prevalence may be higher (McElroy et al. 1995). Although some authors have suggested that kleptomania is more common in men (Gibbens 1962), most case reports and studies indicate that kleptomania occurs primarily in women. Patients with bulimia may have a higher prevalence of kleptomania; one study indicated that nearly one-fourth of bulimic patients also met DSM-III-R criteria for kleptomania (Hudson et al. 1983). Some authors have proposed that kleptomania occurs more commonly during menstruation or pregnancy (Benedek 1960). However, this finding has not been duplicated in other studies (Elizur and Jaffe 1968).

Etiology

Numerous theories have been proposed in an effort to understand the stealing behavior of individuals with kleptomania. Explanations have included a need for stimulation to help treat underlying depression (Fishbain 1987) and a desire to emotionally compensate for an actual or anticipated loss (Cupchik and Atcheson 1983). Psychoanalytic theory proposes that stealing gratifies id impulses (Fenichel 1945) and compensates for issues related to childhood neglect (Abraham 1953). Although psychoanalysts have suggested that kleptomania involves sexual conflicts or wishes (Fenichel 1945; Wittels 1942), this proposed linkage has not been confirmed in follow-up research (Bradford and Balmaceda 1983).

Human and animal research suggests that serotonergic neurotransmission is important in the development of impulse-control disorders (Virkkunen et al. 1989) and therefore may play a role in the etiology of kleptomania. Finally, various neurological conditions have been described as precipitating the onset of kleptomania-type behavior. These include dementia (Khan and Martin 1977), intracranial lesions or masses (Chiswick 1976), and normal-pressure hydrocephalus (McIntyre and Emsley 1990).

Associated Diagnoses

Substantial comorbid psychopathology has been described in studies of individuals with kleptomania. Associated disorders that have been reported include mood disorders, anxiety disorders, eating disorders (Wiedemann 1998), other impulse-control disorders, obsessive-compulsive disorder (OCD), and alcohol and substance abuse disorders (Hudson and Pope 1990; McElroy et al. 1991a). Because of a possible relation to mood, anxiety, and eating disorders, Hudson and Pope proposed that kleptomania belongs to a family of "affective spectrum disorders" that may be linked by a common pathophysiological pathway.

In a study of 37 individuals who had a DSM-IV (American Psychiatric Association 1994a) diagnosis of kleptomania, more than 80% reported current psychiatric problems, 54% reported family psychiatric illness, and nearly half were receiving psychiatric treatment at the time of the study. The most common diagnoses were depressive disorders, anxiety disorders, and sleeping disorders. More than 30% had attempted suicide, and more than 20% had a history of alcohol misuse or abuse (Sarasalo et al. 1996).

Several authors have compared kleptomania with OCD because individuals with kleptomania report intrusive, repetitive thoughts combined with urges to steal. Although high rates of obsessive-compulsive symptoms have been described in kleptomania (McElroy et al. 1995), Wiedemann (1998) found no evidence that kleptomania was correlated with OCD in a study examining comorbid psychiatric diagnoses among persons with kleptomania.

Evaluation

When evaluating an individual for possible kleptomania, the clinician should carefully determine whether the per-

son meets the diagnostic criteria for this disorder. The practitioner must consider whether the stealing behavior represents a choice to commit an antisocial act with potential secondary gain rather than the taking of items not needed for personal use. Because many patients with kleptomania do not report their stealing behavior to mental health evaluators, specific questions must be asked. Such questions involve the onset, frequency, duration, and magnitude of stealing behavior as well as any previous treatment. In addition, the clinician should evaluate for a comorbid psychiatric disorder, including depression, mania, alcohol or substance abuse, anxiety disorder, eating disorder, personality disorder, or other impulse-control disorder, as well as a family history of mental illness. The evaluator also should screen for any possible head injury or organic disorder, with particular attention in elderly individuals referred for new-onset stealing behavior (Moak 1988).

Treatment

Various treatment approaches have been described for kleptomania. Nonpharmacological treatments that have been used include systematic desensitization (Marzagao 1972), "assertive training" (Wolpe 1958), aversive conditioning (Keutzer 1972), covert sensitization (Gauthier and Pellerin 1982; Glover 1985), self-imposed banning by shoppers (Goldman 1991), adjunctive sexual counseling for those with disturbed sexual relationships (Turnball 1987), and Shoplifters Anonymous. Pharmacotherapy also has been used to help decrease impulsive urges to steal.

A few published case reports suggest that SSRIs such as paroxetine (Kraus 1999), fluvoxamine (Chong and Low 1996), and fluoxetine (McElroy et al. 1989) may be useful in decreasing the frequency of stealing behavior in individuals with kleptomania. The use of antidepressants may be particularly helpful in individuals with kleptomania with a comorbid depressive disorder. Therapeutic efficacy also has been reported with lithium, valproate, amitriptyline, imipramine, nortriptyline, trazodone, and electroconvulsive therapy (ECT) in adults with kleptomania (McElroy et al. 1995).

Course and Prognosis

Kleptomania appears to be a disorder that has a pattern established early in life (Goldman 1991), with most patients having an onset of symptoms before age 21. In most patients, the symptoms are long-standing, lasting more than 10 years (Sarasalo et al. 1996).

Pyromania

Definition and Diagnostic Criteria

In the United States, Isaac Ray (1844) provided one of the first definitions of pyromania in his book *A Treatise on the Medical Jurisprudence of Insanity*. In this text, Ray quoted European authorities in describing pyromania as a "distinct form of insanity, annulling responsibility for the acts to which it leads" (p. 84). Ray's view of pyromania was not uniformly accepted by other leading psychiatrists, and the concept that fire setting represented a mental disorder was highly controversial. During the latter half of the nineteenth century, most of the medical and psychiatric community rejected the notion that pyromania was a distinct mental disorder. Sigmund Freud's psychodynamic explanations for fire-setting behavior in the 1930s rejuvenated the theory that pyromania stemmed from an irresistible impulse, giving rebirth to this diagnostic controversy (Geller et al. 1986).

The debate over whether pyromania is a mental disorder also has been reflected in the various DSM editions. Although DSM-I classified pyromania as an obsessive-compulsive reaction, DSM-II failed to mention the term. The term *pyromania* reappeared in DSM-III and was defined in part as a "recurrent failure to resist impulses to set fires" (American Psychiatric Association 1980). The diagnosis of pyromania has been retained in all subsequent DSM editions. In DSM-IV-TR, pyromania is defined as deliberate and purposeful fire setting on more than one occasion. The DSM-IV-TR criteria describe a period of tension or arousal preceding the act, fascination with fire and its consequences, followed by pleasure, gratification, or relief (Table 18–5). DSM-IV-TR outlines circumstances in which the diagnosis of pyromania should not be given, including when the individual is intoxicated or is acting under the influence of a hallucination or delusion.

Individuals who commit acts of arson should be distinguished from those who meet diagnostic criteria for pyromania. Arson is commonly defined as the willful and malicious setting of a fire. Numerous motives for fire setting, independent of pyromania, exist and include anger or revenge toward an individual or agency, insurance fraud, vandalism, crime concealment, or a failed suicide attempt.

Epidemiology

Studies indicate that pyromania is diagnosed in 0%–4% of examined arsonists when DSM-III or DSM-IV criteria are used (Koson and Dvoskin 1982; Rasanen et al. 1995;

TABLE 18–5. DSM-IV-TR diagnostic criteria for pyromania

A. Deliberate and purposeful fire setting on more than one occasion.

B. Tension or affective arousal before the act.

C. Fascination with, interest in, curiosity about, or attraction to fire and its situational contexts (e.g., paraphernalia, uses, consequences).

D. Pleasure, gratification, or relief when setting fires, or when witnessing or participating in their aftermath.

E. The fire setting is not done for monetary gain, as an expression of sociopolitical ideology, to conceal criminal activity, to express anger or vengeance, to improve one's living circumstances, in response to a delusion or hallucination, or as a result of impaired judgment (e.g., in dementia, mental retardation, substance intoxication).

F. The fire setting is not better accounted for by conduct disorder, a manic episode, or antisocial personality disorder.

Ritchie and Huff 1999). Although pyromania is rare, acts of arson are common in the United States. In 1997, more than 80,000 acts of arson were reported to the Federal Bureau of Investigation (1998). However, pyromania is rarely diagnosed when established criteria are applied to arsonists. Although Lewis and Yarnell (1951) diagnosed 39% of their sample of 1,500 arsonists with pyromania, this significant percentage was achieved by a poorly defined classification system.

Fire setting is also relatively common among the mentally ill. Geller and Bertsch (1985) found that 26% of nongeriatric state hospital psychiatric inpatients had engaged in some form of fire-setting behavior, and 18% had actually set fires (Geller et al. 1992a, 1992b).

Etiology

The vast majority of the literature related to fire setting addresses factors associated with arsonists, individuals who usually do not qualify for a diagnosis of pyromania. Family backgrounds of fire setters have indicated higher than expected rates of mental illness, antisocial personality disorder, and alcoholism. Common family features noted include absent fathers or fathers with substance abuse or antisocial personality disorder, depressed mothers, distant family relationships, and childhood physical abuse (Smith and Short 1995).

Sigmund Freud (1932[1931]/1964, p.187) theorized that fire setting in males was related to psychosexual conflicts with homosexual features. In particular, he described that "in order to gain control over fire, men had to renounce the homosexually tinged desire to put it out with a stream of urine." However, no empirical research evidence to date supports this analytic theory of causation (Harris and Rice 1984).

Biological factors associated with arson also have been examined. In their study of arsonists, Lewis and Yarnell (1951) found that arsonists had a higher than expected frequency of long-standing physical abnormalities. Case reports of individuals whose fire-setting behavior was assessed as secondary to seizure activity also have been described (Brook et al. 1996; Carpenter and King 1989). In one study, more than 18% of the arsonists were noted to have EEG abnormalities (Hill et al. 1982). Reactive hypoglycemia and decreased cerebrospinal fluid concentrations of 3-methoxy-4-hydroxyphenylglycol (MHPG) and 5-hydroxyindoleacetic acid (5-HIAA) also have been found in arsonists and violent offenders (Virkkunen et al. 1994).

Associated Diagnoses

Although most arsonists will not meet the DSM criteria for pyromania, many will have a psychiatric diagnosis. In his study of 153 adult arsonists, Rix (1994) found that 54% of the arsonists met criteria for a personality disorder. The most common personality disorder was antisocial personality disorder, although borderline, avoidant, dependent, and paranoid types were nearly as common. In addition, intoxication with alcohol, drugs, or both was frequently noted. Research indicates that between one-third and two-thirds of fire setters are intoxicated at the time of their act (Ritchie and Huff 1999; Rix 1994). Other diagnoses overrepresented among fire setters when compared with the general population include schizophrenia (Lewis and Yarnell 1951; Ritchie and Huff 1999), mania (Ritchie and Huff 1999), and mental retardation (Hill et al. 1982; Rix 1994).

Evaluation

When evaluating a fire setter for the diagnosis of pyromania, the clinician must carefully determine whether the individual meets the established diagnostic criteria for this disorder. Additional important areas to review include the person's motive; location of the fire; means of starting the fire; history and progression of fire-setting behavior; age at first offense; aggression toward other inanimate objects; presence or absence of a co-conspirator; intent to harm persons, property, or both; history of violence; history of "watching" other fires or spending time in fire stations; history of setting off fire alarms; actions during the fire; behaviors after setting the fire; self-injurious behavior using fire; history of smoking; access to flammables; and a family history of arson.

The clinician also must determine what role, if any, a comorbid psychiatric diagnosis played in the fire setting. A detailed psychiatric history is important and includes exploration of developmental issues, relationships, social factors, psychosexual adjustments, medical history, legal history, and personality characteristics (Smith and Short 1995). An EEG is appropriate for those individuals with symptoms consistent with a seizure disorder.

In some situations, fire setting represents a suicide attempt, and further inquiry regarding suicidal intent is recommended. Careful attention also must be given to the presence of intoxication, personality disorders, mental retardation, mood disorders, and psychosis. In particular, psychotic arsonists almost always act alone (Molnar et al. 1984), and their targets are frequently outsiders of the community rather than individuals they know (Virkkunen 1974). Virkkunen (1974) also found that hallucinations and delusions were the principal motivation for the fire-setting behavior in one-third of schizophrenic arsonists.

Treatment

Limited studies have been conducted on effective treatment strategies for pyromania. Traditional psychoanalytic approaches have not proven effective, and no research supports the theory that pyromania is caused by unresolved psychosexual conflicts. Other treatment modalities that have been implemented include behavior therapy with aversive conditioning (McGrath and Marshall 1979), positive reinforcement (Bumpass et al. 1983), social skills training (Jackson et al. 1987), and implementation of a relapse prevention plan (Stewart 1993). A relapse prevention plan proposes to assist the person in understanding his or her offense cycle with treatment focused on the development of coping behaviors, avoidance of high-risk situations, relaxation training, and assertiveness and cognitive restructuring (Smith and Short 1995). Because no single approach has been proven effective for all fire setters, treatment should be individualized with a combination of interventions as appropriate. The treatment provider should target treatment interventions to minimize those factors that facilitate fire-setting behavior in the individual examined. Such interventions can include substance abuse treatment for those with a substance abuse diagnosis, mood stabilizers for those with mania, and antipsychotics for individuals whose arson was secondary to psychosis.

Course and Prognosis

Virtually all research examining the course and prognosis of individuals who set fires deals with fire setters whose symptoms do not meet criteria for pyromania. A study of 243 male arsonists found that repeat fire setters differed from those with only one episode by being younger, having more extensive criminal histories, being less likely to set fires for psychotic reasons, and being more likely to have a personality disorder (Rice and Harris 1991). A 20-year follow-up of 67 arsonists found a conviction rate for arson of approximately 4%. Those who reoffended were solitary offenders with chronic problems of social adjustment (Soothill and Pope 1973).

Mentally disordered fire setters have been shown to have a higher rate of recurrence than do non–mentally disordered fire setters (Barnett et al. 1997). Furthermore, Barnett et al. (1999) found that 9% of the arsonists who had been found not guilty by reason of insanity received a conviction of arson in a 10-year follow-up period. When examining a group of 50 patients who had engaged in at least one fire-setting behavior in their lifetime, Geller et al. (1992a, 1992b) determined that 28% of these had fire-setting behavior, and 16% actually set a fire in the 7-year follow-up period.

Pathological Gambling

Definition and Diagnostic Criteria

Access to gambling activities in the United States has increased dramatically since the 1980s as new avenues of gambling such as state lotteries, tribal casinos, and Internet games became available. A 1999 survey indicated that all but three states have some type of legalized gambling, and approximately 80% of Americans engage in a gambling activity on a regular basis. An increase in incidence of problems associated with gambling has paralleled this rise in gambling avenues. According to one estimate, 5.7 million Americans are now classified as having a gambling problem (Committee on the Social and Economic Impact of Pathological Gambling 1999).

The American Psychiatric Association first classified pathological gambling as a disorder of impulse control in 1980, when it was included in DSM-III. DSM-IV-TR criteria for pathological gambling are outlined in Table 18–6. According to DSM-IV-TR, pathological gambling is characterized by a continuous or periodic inability to control gambling behavior, a preoccupation with gambling and with obtaining gambling funds, irrational thinking, and a continuation of the behavior despite adverse consequences and/or desire to quit. Pathological gambling is a disorder that results in a high degree of emotional and physical suffering to gamblers and those around them. Approximately 60% of pathological gamblers engage in

TABLE 18–6. DSM-IV-TR diagnostic criteria for pathological gambling

A. Persistent and recurrent maladaptive gambling behavior as indicated by five (or more) of the following:
   (1) is preoccupied with gambling (e.g., preoccupied with reliving past gambling experiences, handicapping or planning the next venture, or thinking of ways to get money with which to gamble)
   (2) needs to gamble with increasing amounts of money in order to achieve the desired excitement
   (3) has repeated unsuccessful efforts to control, cut back, or stop gambling
   (4) is restless or irritable when attempting to cut down or stop gambling
   (5) gambles as a way of escaping from problems or of relieving a dysphoric mood (e.g., feelings of helplessness, guilt, anxiety, depression)
   (6) after losing money gambling, often returns another day to get even ("chasing" one's losses)
   (7) lies to family members, therapist, or others to conceal the extent of involvement with gambling
   (8) has committed illegal acts such as forgery, fraud, theft, or embezzlement to finance gambling
   (9) has jeopardized or lost a significant relationship, job, or educational or career opportunity because of gambling
   (10) relies on others to provide money to relieve a desperate financial situation caused by gambling
B. The gambling behavior is not better accounted for by a manic episode.

criminal activities, such as forgery and fraud, to maintain their addiction (Blaszczynski and Silove 1996). Stress-related medical conditions such as hypertension, peptic ulcer disease, and migraine headaches are also common among pathological gamblers. Twenty percent of the individuals seeking treatment for pathological gambling have a history of a suicide attempt (American Psychiatric Association 2000).

Studies of pathological gamblers classified two broad subtypes: antisocial-impulsive (also known as action subtype) and obsessive-dependent (escape subtype). Although both subtypes have characteristics common to many pathological gamblers (such as neuroticism, low self-esteem, and manipulativeness), important differences exist. Action gamblers are predominantly male and achieve a euphoric state through gambling. Such individuals tend to be domineering, controlling, and manipulative; have an above-average IQ; and view themselves as friendly, sociable, gregarious, and generous. They are often energetic, assertive, persuasive, and confident in their interpersonal interactions. Action gamblers are reluctant to recognize that they have a gambling problem and generally are resistant to treatment. In contrast, escape gamblers are represented nearly equally by men and women. These individuals tend to be nurturing, responsible, and active in their family life prior to the onset of pathological gambling. In their interpersonal relationships, they are passive-avoidant, unassertive, and in need of empowerment. Escape gamblers often have a history of physical, sexual, or emotional abuse and use gambling as a means to escape their problems. These individuals describe feelings of temporary elation and release from physical and emotional pain while gambling. They may seek professional help for assistance with their gambling, relationship issues, or both. Escape gamblers are more malleable to treatment, with a better prognosis when compared with action gamblers (Blaszczynski et al. 1997; Committee on the Social and Economic Impact of Pathological Gambling 1999). Until recently, most of the research has been done on male pathological gamblers of the antisocial-impulsive subtype; many experimental findings on pathological gambling are specific to action gamblers and therefore may not be generalizable outside this subtype.

Epidemiology

The exact prevalence of pathological gambling is difficult to estimate because of inconsistencies in both screening techniques and diagnostic criteria used in research studies of gamblers. Shaffer et al. (1997) conducted an extensive meta-analysis examining the prevalence rates and lifetime extent of pathological gambling in the United States and Canada. In this study, prevalence of pathological gambling in the adult population was reported as 1.1%. The likelihood that an individual would have a gambling addiction at some point in his or her life was estimated as 1.6%. Groups with a higher prevalence of pathological gambling included adolescents (6.1%) and adults of low socioeconomic status (17.2%). As described in the previous subsection, action gamblers are primarily men, whereas escape gamblers are represented nearly equally by men and women (Committee on the Social and Economic Impact of Pathological Gambling 1999; Lepage et al. 2000).

Etiology

Freud characterized pathological gambling as a neurosis that reflects self-punishment for guilt derived from ambivalence toward the father. Subsequent psychoanalysts interpreted the gambler's behavior as the acting out of a subconscious plea for encouragement and favor to a surrogate parent figure such as Fate or Lady Luck (Bergler 1957; Bolen and Boyd 1968). More recent theories regarding the development of pathological gambling have focused on abnormalities in the autonomic nervous system or certain neurotransmitters. Anderson and Brown (1987) proposed that gamblers have low autonomic arousal that they seek to augment by gambling. Consequently, pathological gamblers become addicted to their own arousal because of its self-reinforcing physical and psychological effects. Follow-up studies suggest that increased arousal and risk taking described in pathological gamblers may be linked to noradrenergic system dysfunction (Roy et al. 1988). Although abnormalities in the endorphin system also have been suggested as a possible contributor to increased arousal in pathological gamblers, studies examining this link have not noted significant differences in plasma β-endorphin levels between pathological gamblers and nongamblers (Blaszczynski et al. 1986). Abnormalities in the dopaminergic reward pathways of pathological gamblers have been shown to account for the addictive symptoms of the disorder (Bergh et al. 1997; Comings 1998), and serotonergic system dysfunction has been linked to the impulsive and compulsive traits (DeCaria et al. 1998). Blanco et al. (1996) reported lower platelet monoamine oxidase activity (a peripheral marker of serotonin function) among pathological gamblers as compared with nongamblers.

An increased prevalence of pathological gambling has been described in family members of individuals diagnosed with the disorder when compared with individuals who gamble recreationally. In their study of 3,359 twins, Eisen et al. (1998) showed that 56% of three or more and 62% of four or more DSM-III-R criteria for pathological gambling endorsed by the participants in their study could be accounted for by familial factors, such as genetic predisposition and environmental influences. Comings et al. (1999) identified a repeat polymorphism of the 48th base pair of the D_4 dopamine receptor gene (*DRD4*) as a potential genetic abnormality in pathological gamblers.

Associated Diagnoses

A significant relationship exists between pathological gambling and substance abuse, with more than 60% of pathological gamblers meeting criteria for a substance abuse disorder at least once in their lifetime. The incidence of pathological gambling is 8–10 times greater among those with alcohol dependence than in the general population (Crockford and el-Guebaly 1998; Lejoyeux et al. 2000). One study examining the overlap of alcoholism and pathological gambling suggested a common genetic vulnerability for these two disorders (Slutske et al. 2000).

Mood disorders have been frequently described in individuals with pathological gambling, with a reported suicide rate between 17% and 24%. According to some estimates, more than 50% of pathological gamblers have a comorbid mood disorder, suggesting that pathological gambling may be an "affective spectrum disorder" (Linden et al. 1986). A more recent analysis, however, indicated that the mood symptoms tend to occur after and as a result of pathological gambling. Revised estimates show that depressive disorders co-occur in approximately 18% of pathological gamblers, a rate similar to that found among substance-dependent populations (Crockford and el-Guebaly 1998).

Personality disorders have been reported to have moderate comorbidity with pathological gambling. In a study of 82 inpatient pathological gamblers, more than 90% met criteria for a personality disorder, primarily narcissistic, histrionic, or borderline (Blaszczynski and Steel 1998; Steel and Blaszczynski 1998). Although possible comorbidity with antisocial personality disorder has been alluded to in the literature, research shows that the antisocial behavior conducted by individuals with pathological gambling typically occurs after their gambling becomes problematic rather than as a result of a separate antisocial personality disorder (Blaszczynski and Silove 1996).

Evaluation

Pathological gamblers often seek help only after they have been pressured to do so by their family, friends, or the legal system. The evaluator's primary task is to carefully determine whether the individual meets the diagnostic criteria for pathological gambling and assess the extent of comorbid conditions. In addition to the DSM-IV-TR criteria, rating scales such as the South Oaks Gambling Screen (Lesieur and Blume 1987) and the Lie/Bet Questionnaire (Johnson et al. 1998) may be useful in assessing the severity of the gambling behavior. Important potential comorbid diagnoses to consider include alcohol and substance abuse, personality disorders, depression, and bipolar mania. Pathological gambling is not diagnosed if the gambling behavior is the result of a manic episode. The examiner's challenge is to distinguish between the elation sometimes induced by gambling behavior and the euphoria secondary to mania.

Because of the high suicide risk among pathological gamblers, a brief inpatient stay may be warranted.

Collateral contacts are helpful in evaluating the extent of the individual's gambling and his or her veracity regarding his or her behavior. Useful sources of information include significant others, family members, credit reports, credit card statements, banking statements, and employers.

Treatment

For many years, psychoanalysis was the most common treatment approach to pathological gambling, although research validating this approach is limited. The goal of psychodynamic therapy is to help the gambler gain insight into, and then confront, the subconscious conflicts that underlie his or her behavior. Bergler (1957) reported having achieved abstinence from gambling in 60 compulsive gamblers through psychodynamic therapy; however, long-term follow-up data on these patients have not been described.

Behavioral and cognitive-behavioral approaches have been identified as highly successful in achieving abstinence from gambling in the short term (i.e., 1 month or less). For example, behavioral models emphasizing desensitization and aversion have been successful in achieving short-term abstinence in 30% of treated patients (Committee on the Social and Economic Impact of Pathological Gambling 1999; Symes and Nicki 1997). Sylvain et al. (1997) described a multimodal cognitive-behavioral approach, which combined cognitive restructuring, problem solving, social skills training, and active relapse prevention and was shown to alleviate pathological symptomology in 86% of participating gamblers, most of whom were able to maintain abstinence as indicated at the 6- and 12-month follow-up assessment.

Several pharmacological agents have been prescribed with varied rates of success, particularly in the presence of a comorbid psychiatric disorder. Lithium carbonate has helped decrease gambling behavior in pathological gamblers with bipolar disorder (Moskowitz 1980). A single case report of clomipramine in a female gambler with social phobia and compulsive personality traits resulted in a cessation of the gambling for approximately 7 months (Hollander et al. 1992). SSRIs have been shown to assist particularly in alleviating impulsive and compulsive aspects of gambling behavior. Hollander et al. (2000) reported complete cessation of gambling for 8 weeks in 7 of 10 pathological gamblers in response to 220 mg/day of fluvoxamine therapy. Studies note that comorbid diagnosis of depression may further warrant treatment with an antidepressant that affects serotonergic activity. Concerns have been raised about the possibility that SSRIs may induce underlying mania in some patients with mood disorders. Screening for comorbid mood disorders should diminish the possibility of a manic episode following SSRI treatment of pathological gambling. Opioid antagonists have been shown to block the excitement or pleasure of addictive behavior and have been suggested as a possible treatment for pathological gambling. In particular, naltrexone has shown promising results for curbing intense cravings that often accompany pathological gambling behavior (Kim 1998).

Relapse prevention strategies such as self-help and group therapies are important in achieving successful and lasting abstinence (Hodgins and el-Guebaly 2000). Gamblers Anonymous is one popular self-help group and is modeled on the 12-Step approach used by Alcoholics Anonymous. Surveys show that people are more likely to turn to Gamblers Anonymous for help than any other form of intervention; however, follow up studies indicate that 82% of "graduates" relapse within 1 year of completing the program (Committee on the Social and Economic Impact of Pathological Gambling 1999).

Course and Prognosis

One suggested course of pathological gambling is illustrated in Figure 18–1 and consists of three progressive stages: 1) the winning phase, 2) the losing phase, and 3) the desperation phase. During the winning stage, pathological gamblers regard gambling as a social activity and are often able to attain substantial profits. This self-reinforcing dynamic facilitates feelings of grandiosity, with the increase in finances directed toward gambling. In the losing stage, gamblers begin to "chase" their losses by placing increasingly larger bets. Gamblers fantasize about winning and attempt to conceal their addiction by lying to family and friends, borrowing money from various resources, and taking out loans. Once the desperation phase is reached, the gambler experiences feelings of hopelessness as losses continue to mount and personal relationships crumble. Gamblers no longer see their gambling as a choice. They often become aloof and emotionally callous and may engage in antisocial behaviors such as stealing, swindling, or forgery to continue gambling. The risk of suicide is highest at this stage (Lesieur and Custer 1984). Compulsive gamblers commonly experience all three phases before seeking help.

The prognosis for pathological gambling appears to be affected by age at onset and type of gambling behavior. In general, the earlier the gambling behavior begins, the bigger the likelihood the individual will develop pathological symptoms. In comparing action with escape gamblers, action gamblers tend to begin gambling at an early age (often in adolescence) and gradually progress through the stages of the disease. In contrast, escape gamblers usually begin gambling later in life (often after 30) but experience the onset of pathological symptoms earlier in the course of their gambling career (Committee on the Social and Economic Impact of Pathological Gambling 1999).

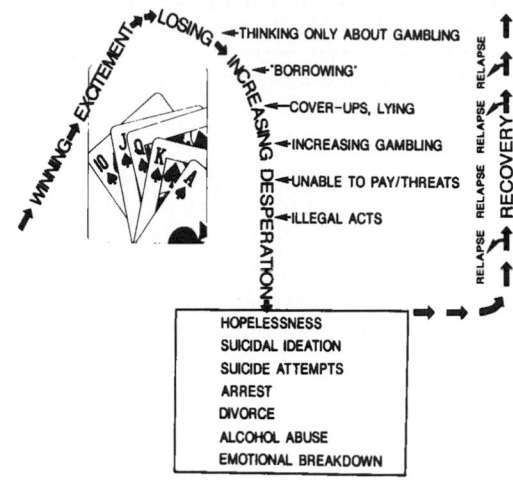

FIGURE 18–1. The clinical course of a pathological gambler.

Trichotillomania

Definition and Diagnostic Criteria

Trichotillomania is a term created by Hallopeau in 1889 to describe a compulsion to pull out one's own hair (Krishnan et al. 1985). DSM-IV-TR diagnostic criteria include recurrent pulling out of one's hair, tension before pulling (Criterion B), and pleasure or gratification when pulling (Criterion C) (Table 18–7). A significant number of individuals considered to have trichotillomania, however, do not fulfill Criteria B and C (Christenson and Crow 1996). Trichotillomania produces irregular, nonscarring focal patches of hair loss that are linear, rectangular, or oval (Figure 18–2). Hair loss usually occurs in the scalp region but can involve eyebrows, eyelashes, or pubic hair. These areas of hair loss are more likely to be found on the opposite side of the body from the dominant hand. Within the area of hair loss, broken hairs of varying lengths are found, and the scalp may have a slight brownish discoloration secondary to rubbing the area. In addition to the current impulse-control disorder classification, trichotillomania has been conceptualized as an affective or anxiety (e.g., OCD) spectrum disorder (Christenson et al. 1991b; Jenike 1989; McElroy et al. 1992; Swedo and Leonard 1992). Krishnan et al. (1985) noted that trichotillomania can be present as a major symptom in OCD, mental retardation, schizophrenia, borderline personality disorder, and depression.

TABLE 18–7. DSM-IV-TR diagnostic criteria for trichotillomania

A. Recurrent pulling out of one's hair resulting in noticeable hair loss.

B. An increasing sense of tension immediately before pulling out the hair or when attempting to resist the behavior.

C. Pleasure, gratification, or relief when pulling out the hair.

D. The disturbance is not better accounted for by another mental disorder and is not due to a general medical condition (e.g., a dermatological condition).

E. The disturbance causes clinically significant distress or impairment in social, occupational, or other important areas of functioning.

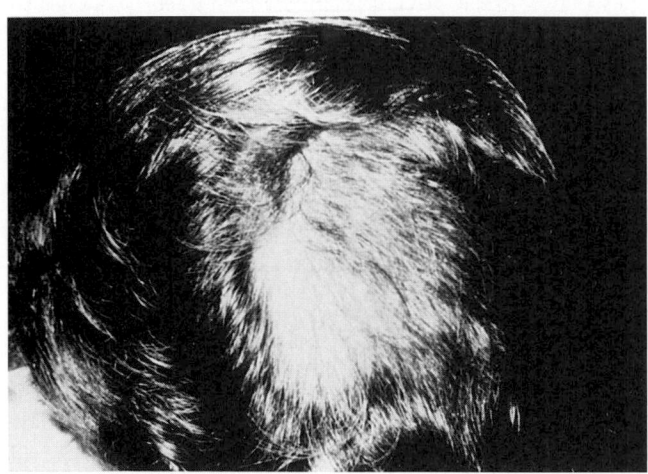

FIGURE 18–2. Trichotillomania.

Note the irregular pattern of hair loss, the hair of varying lengths within the patch of hair loss, and the scalp, which has no evidence of scarring.

Epidemiology

In a questionnaire survey of 2,579 first-year college students, Christenson et al. (1991b) found a prevalence between 0.6% and 1.5% for males and between 0.6% and 3.4% for females. This suggested that trichotillomania may not be as rare as previously suspected and that males may be affected as frequently as females. In another survey of college students, between 10% and 13% reported hair pulling, although only 1% indicated that this behavior resulted in clinically significant hair loss and/or distress (Rothbaum et al. 1993). Most patients seeking treatment are female (Christenson et al. 1991a; Swedo et al. 1989).

The dermatological literature most commonly reports pathological hair pulling in preadolescent children. Stroud (1983), a dermatologist, reported that of 59 patients who came to his office with hair loss in 1982, 31 (53%) had tinea capitis, 12 (20%) had alopecia areata

(i.e., a suspected autoimmune phenomenon), 7 (12%) had traction alopecia (i.e., a disorder associated with hairstyles that apply excessive prolonged tension to the hair), and 6 (10%) had trichotillomania. Oranje et al. (1986) found that the female-to-male ratio was 2.5:1 and also that 25% of the children with trichotillomania had associated onychophagy, trichophagy, or automutilation.

Christenson et al. (1991a) described the phenomenology of trichotillomania in a report of 60 adult hair pullers. The mean age at onset was 13 years, and 93% of the subjects were female. Hair pulling can last from a few minutes to a few hours (Swedo et al. 1991; Winchel et al. 1992a). Hair was pulled primarily from the scalp (67%); however, subjects also pulled eyelashes (22%), eyebrows (8%), facial hair (2%), and pubic hair (2%). Subjects in this study were just as likely to use the nondominant as the dominant hand for hair pulling. All subjects believed that their hair pulling was an excessive or unusual behavior, and 95% reported a diurnal variation, with the worst hair pulling in the evening. Interestingly, it has been reported that symptoms of trichotillomania may worsen the week before menstruation (Keuthen et al. 1997). After pulling, 48% of patients also initiate oral behaviors (e.g., running the hair across their lips, eating the hair) (Christenson et al. 1991a). Accordingly, dental erosion and trichophagy may occur, as well as skin infections.

Etiology

A number of biological etiologies have been proposed for trichotillomania. Christenson et al. (1992) reported that 8% of 161 patients knew a first-degree relative who had pulled hair, and in other family studies, between 4% and 5% of relatives reported current or past hair-pulling behavior (Diefenbach et al. 2000). A neuroethological theory views trichotillomania and OCD as pathology of the neurobiological mechanisms responsible for grooming behavior. Neurotransmitter dysregulation is supported by phenomenological similarities of trichotillomania symptoms to those of other disorders, studies of neurotransmitter and other neuroendocrine function, and treatment studies with SSRIs. Some literature suggests that trichotillomania may be a type of OCD (Jenike 1989; Swedo et al. 1989). Stanley et al. (1992, 1993), however, reported several differences between OCD and trichotillomania, including the facts that hair pulling usually is associated with pleasure, patients with trichotillomania have few associated obsessive-compulsive symptoms, and patients with OCD differ from patients with trichotillomania in terms of anxiety, depression, and personality characteristics. Blunting of neuroendocrine response to *m*-chlorophenylpiperazine (m-CPP), a measure of serotonin responsivity sometimes present in patients with OCD, was not found in 10 patients with trichotillomania (Stein et al. 1995b). In addition, Ninan et al. (1992) did not find abnormalities in cerebrospinal fluid cortisol, 5-HIAA, homovanillic acid, or MHPG levels in patients with trichotillomania but did find that baseline cerebrospinal fluid 5-HIAA levels correlated with response to treatment with SSRI-type antidepressants. Regional cerebral blood flow studies indicate that women with trichotillomania have increased activity of the cerebellar and right superior parietal area, compared with increased frontal cortex activity in women with OCD (Christenson and Crow 1996; Swedo et al. 1991). One way to understand these findings is a dimension from primarily impulsive (i.e., risk seeking) to primarily compulsive (i.e., harm avoidance) (Hollander et al. 1996). Trichotillomania may be closer to the impulsive end, whereas obsessive-compulsive disorder may be closer to the compulsive end. Trichotillomania also appears to share phenomenological and neuropathological overlap with Tourette's disorder.

Many psychosocial theories have been described for trichotillomania. From a psychoanalytic perspective, hair can represent beauty, virility, sexual conflicts, physical prowess, and sexuality; haircutting or plucking can signify castration (Krishnan et al. 1985). Hair pulling may result from poor object relations or a means of working through real or perceived threats of object loss (Greenberg and Sarner 1965; Krishnan et al. 1985). Behavior theories include tension reduction (i.e., negative reinforcement), modeling, and response covariation (e.g., thumb sucking and hair pulling co-occur, and with treatment of the former, the latter resolves). For children, the syndrome usually develops at a time of psychosocial stress (e.g., a disturbed mother–child relationship, hospitalization, or family stress) (Oranje et al. 1986) but may persist even though the stressor(s) may no longer be present.

Associated Diagnoses

Psychiatric disorders are commonly comorbid with trichotillomania (Table 18–8) (Christenson et al. 1991b; Diefenbach et al. 2000; Soriano et al. 1996; Swedo et al. 1992; Winchel et al. 1992a).

Evaluation

The clinical interview requires a substantial collection of historical information, including: quantitative and qualitative pulling of one's hair from the scalp, eyelashes, eyebrows, facial hair, and other regions; tension before pulling; and pleasure or gratification when pulling. A relation,

TABLE 18–8. Lifetime prevalence of psychiatric disorders of chronic hair pullers

Diagnosis	% of sample
Trichotillomania	83[a]
Mood disorders	65
Anxiety disorders	57
Personality disorders	25–55
Body dysmorphic disorder	23
Substance abuse	22
Eating disorders	20
Psychotic disorders	2
No disorder (except trichotillomania)	18

Note. [a]Not all individuals had both an increasing sense of tension before pulling out the hair and gratification or a relief when pulling out the hair (both are required in DSM-IV-TR).

if any, to psychosocial stressors, menstruation, and other triggers should be explored. Collateral report from relatives and friends may be helpful. Family history of hair pulling should be noted. Screening for symptoms of obsessive-compulsive, depressive, other anxiety, and tic disorders may identify comorbid psychiatric conditions. Medical disorders (e.g., dermatological) are prudent to evaluate in collaboration with primary and other specialty physicians as indicated.

Self-monitoring, self-report, and clinical interview instruments are available for use in the diagnosis of trichotillomania. A daily diary of hair pulling and saving pulled hairs may be useful but can be limited by trichophagy, pulling without awareness, and nonadherence for various reasons. The Massachusetts General Hospital Hairpulling Scale is the only self-report questionnaire with established psychometric properties (Keuthen et al. 1995; O'Sullivan et al. 1995). Several clinical rating scales for trichotillomania have been developed, including the Yale-Brown Obsessive-Compulsive Scale modified for trichotillomania (Y-BOCS TM; Stanley et al. 1992) and the Psychiatric Institute Trichotillomania Scale (PITS; Winchel et al. 1992b). The Y-BOCS TM substitutes "thoughts of hair-pulling" for obsessions and "hair-pulling" for compulsions. The PITS is more specific to trichotillomania and can be administered more quickly.

Physical examination and procedures may substantiate the diagnosis of trichotillomania. Adult patients generally do not have changes in fingernails or toenails (except possibly signs of nail biting) usually associated with dermatological conditions. Hair regrowth follows the application of collodion to the area of hair loss for 1 week. In children, careful parental observation of the child, which includes looking for hair among the child's playthings, is often helpful in making the diagnosis. The child also may practice onychophagia (i.e., nail biting). If the child complains of gastrointestinal symptoms such as abdominal pain, diarrhea, and/or constipation, or decreased appetite, examination of the oral cavity for evidence of trichophagy (i.e., eating hair) and X-ray examination of the stomach for a trichobezoar (i.e., hairball) are warranted. In addition, a skin biopsy may provide evidence for the diagnosis by ruling out other conditions. Finally, longitudinal photographs may facilitate changes in the course or responses to treatment.

Treatment

Patients who receive both behavioral and medication treatment show a greater reduction in hair-pulling scores than do those receiving either treatment alone (Keuthen et al. 1998). A review of the literature finds several controlled medication trials, many open case series, and a multitude of case reports for the acute treatment of trichotillomania. Swedo et al. (1989) found that clomipramine was significantly more effective than desipramine in a double-blind crossover treatment of 20 patients with trichotillomania. Rothbaum and Ninan (1992) found that clomipramine was superior to placebo, but in a repeat trial, the difference was not significant (Ninan et al. 2000). Recently, Neudecker et al. (2001) reported that paroxetine was superior to placebo. Christenson et al. (1991d), in another placebo-controlled, double-blind crossover study, reported that fluoxetine was no better than placebo for 21 patients with chronic hair pulling. Streichenwein and Thornby (1995), in a placebo-controlled, double-blind crossover trial, found that fluoxetine was not effective in 23 chronic hair pullers.

Open trials indicate favorable response to fluoxetine (Winchel et al. 1992a), fluvoxamine (Stanley et al. 1997), venlafaxine (Ninan et al. 1998), lithium carbonate (Christenson et al. 1991c), and haloperidol (Van Ameringen et al. 1999). Augmentation of SSRIs also has been successful with haloperidol (Van Ameringen et al. 1999), pimozide (Stein and Hollander 1992), and risperidone (Epperson et al. 1999; Stein et al. 1997). Isolated case reports of successful treatment of trichotillomania in adults have been published regarding the following drugs: buspirone, citalopram, amitriptyline, a monoamine oxidase inhibitor, chlorpromazine in a patient with comorbid schizophrenia, and olanzapine augmentation of an SSRI. For children and adolescents, paroxetine and fluoxetine use has been reported. A steroid topical cream also has been used in combination with clomipramine when hair pulling is cued by itch (Black and Blum 1992). Another topical cream has been used to increase physical sensitivity (Ristvedt and Christenson 1996).

Psychosocial treatments are now beginning to be evaluated in controlled trials. Ninan et al. (2000) showed in a study of 23 patients that cognitive-behavioral treatment had a dramatic effect in reducing symptoms of trichotillomania and was significantly more effective than clomipramine or placebo. Neudecker et al. (2001) reported that multimodal behavior therapy, weekly for 45 treatments, was superior to placebo in a study of 20 patients. Multimodal behavior therapy consisted of behavioral, functional, and motivation analysis and training in symptom-centered techniques. In open trials, a behavioral technique called habit reversal training was reportedly the most effective for trichotillomania and includes increasing awareness, learning alternative behaviors, using alternative coping skills, and maintaining motivation against hair pulling (Baer 1992). Hypnosis (Christenson and Crow 1996) and individual behavior modification techniques (e.g., biofeedback, aversion therapy, extinction, response prevention) (Krishnan et al. 1985) also may be useful. Finally, habit reversal training modified for group therapy has been useful and reduces isolation (Stanley and Mouton 1996).

Course and Prognosis

According to Stroud (1983), most cases of trichotillomania in young children resolve spontaneously because it usually represents a transient behavior in response to a psychosocial stressor or a habit without the presence of an obvious precipitant. If hair loss persists, psychiatric consultation is indicated, and inquiry into areas of parent–child relationships or other areas of potential conflict may illuminate the problem. Oranje et al. (1986), in their study of 21 children younger than 15 years, found that psychiatric consultation was necessary in 11 cases (52%); 4 of these consultees (19%) required psychiatric intervention. Psychiatric evaluation is indicated when trichotillomania occurs in adolescents and adults. Trichotillomania in adults typically follows a chronic course, frequently involves multiple hair sites, and is associated with high rates of psychiatric comorbidity (Christenson et al. 1991a).

The long-term response of symptoms to pharmacotherapy and behavior therapy is variable. At 4-year follow-up, a 40% reduction of symptoms was maintained with clomipramine (Swedo et al. 1993). Keuthen et al. (1998) completed a naturalistic survey study of 63 patients who had received behavioral treatment (90%), medication (73%), or both (41%). At 6-year follow-up, 52% of the subjects rated themselves as treatment responders, and 51% were still in active treatment, with 62% receiving therapy or medication and 25% receiving both; those receiving both showed a greater reduction in hair-pulling scores than did those receiving either treatment alone. In a longitudinal study evaluating hair pulling, sickness impact, and self-esteem in a more structured fashion, Keuthen et al. (2001) noted that responders maintained their symptomatic improvement but did not continue to improve. Interestingly, self-esteem continued to be problematic even with reduced hair-pulling and sickness impact scores.

References

Abraham K: Manifestation of the female castration complex, in Selected Papers on Psychoanalysis, Vol 1. Translated by Bryan D, Strachey A. New York, Basic Books, 1949, pp 338–369

American Psychiatric Association: Diagnostic and Statistical Manual: Mental Disorders. Washington, DC, American Psychiatric Association, 1952

American Psychiatric Association: Diagnostic and Statistical Manual of Mental Disorders, 2nd Edition. Washington, DC, American Psychiatric Association, 1968

American Psychiatric Association: Diagnostic and Statistical Manual of Mental Disorders, 3rd Edition. Washington, DC, American Psychiatric Association, 1980

American Psychiatric Association: Diagnostic and Statistical Manual of Mental Disorders, 3rd Edition, Revised. Washington, DC, American Psychiatric Association, 1987

American Psychiatric Association: Diagnostic and Statistical Manual of Mental Disorders, 4th Edition. Washington, DC, American Psychiatric Association, 1994a

American Psychiatric Association: DSM-IV Sourcebook, Vol 2. Washington, DC, American Psychiatric Association, 1994b

American Psychiatric Association: Diagnostic and Statistical Manual of Mental Disorders, 4th Edition, Text Revision. Washington, DC, American Psychiatric Association, 2000

Anderson G, Brown RIF: Some applications of reversal theory to the explanation of gambling and gambling addictions. Journal of Gambling Behavior 3:179–189, 1987

Baer L: Behavior therapy for obsessive-compulsive disorder and trichotillomania, in Advances in Neurology. Edited by Chase TN, Friedhoff AJ, Cohen DJ. New York, Raven, 1992, pp 333–340

Barnett W, Richter P, Sigmund D, et al: Recidivism and concomitant criminality in pathological firesetters. J Forensic Sci 42:879–883, 1997

Barnett W, Richter P, Renneberg B: Repeated arson: data from criminal records. Forensic Sci Int 101:49–54, 1999

Bars DR, Heyrend FL, Simpson CD, et al: Use of visual evoked-potential studies and EEG data to classify aggressive, explosive behavior of youths. Psychiatr Serv 52:81–86, 2001

Benedek TF: Sexual function in women and their disturbance, in American Handbook of Psychiatry, Vol I. Edited by Arieti S. New York, Basic Books, 1960, pp 727–748

Bergh C, Eklund P, Sodersten P, et al: Altered dopamine action in pathological gambling. Psychol Med 27:473–475, 1997

Bergler E: The Psychology of Gambling. New York, International Universities Press, 1957

Black DW, Blum N: Trichotillomania treated with clomipramine and a topical steroid (letter). Am J Psychiatry 149:842–843, 1992

Blanco C, Orensanz-Munoz L, Blanco-Jerez C, et al: Pathological gambling and platelet MAO activity: a psychobiological study. Am J Psychiatry 153:119–121, 1996

Blaszczynski A, Silove D: Pathological gambling: forensic issues. Aust N Z J Psychiatry 30:358–369, 1996

Blaszczynski A, Steel Z: Personality disorders among pathological gamblers. Journal of Gambling Studies 14:51–71, 1998

Blaszczynski AP, Winter SW, Simon W, et al: Plasma endorphin levels in pathological gambling. Journal of Gambling Behavior 2:3–14, 1986

Blaszczynski A, Steel Z, McConaghy N: Impulsivity in pathological gambling: the antisocial impulsivist. Addiction 92:75–87, 1997

Bolen DW, Boyd WH: Gambling and the gambler: a review and preliminary findings. Arch Gen Psychiatry 18:617–630, 1968

Bradford J, Balmaceda R: Shoplifting: is there a specific psychiatric syndrome? Can J Psychiatry 28:248–253, 1983

Brook R, Dolan M, Coorey P: Arson and epilepsy. Med Sci Law 36:268–271, 1996

Bumpass ER, Fagelman FD, Brix RJ: Intervention with children who set fires. Am J Psychother 37:328–345, 1983

Campbell M, Perry R, Green WH, et al: Use of lithium in children and adolescents. Psychosomatics 25:95–101, 105–106, 1984

Carpenter PK, King AL: Epilepsy and arson. Br J Psychiatry 154:554–556, 1989

Chernasky S, Hollander E: The neuropsychiatric aspects of impulsivity and aggression, in The American Psychiatric Press Textbook of Neuropsychiatry, 3rd edition. Edited by Yudofsky SC, Hales RE. Washington, DC, American Psychiatric Press, 1997, pp 488–492

Chiswick D: Shoplifting, depression and an unusual intracranial lesion (case report). Med Sci Law 16:266–268, 1976

Chong SA, Low BL: Treatment of kleptomania with fluvoxamine. Acta Psychiatr Scand 93:314–315, 1996

Christenson GA, Crow SJ: The characterization and treatment of trichotillomania. J Clin Psychiatry 57:42–49, 1996

Christenson GA, Mackenzie TB, Mitchell JE: Characteristics of 60 adult chronic hair pullers. Am J Psychiatry 148:365–370, 1991a

Christenson GA, Pyle RL, Mitchell JE: Estimated lifetime prevalence of trichotillomania in college students. J Clin Psychiatry 52:415–417, 1991b

Christenson GA, Popkin MK, Mackenzie TB, et al: Lithium treatment of chronic hair pulling. J Clin Psychiatry 52:116–120, 1991c

Christenson GA, Mackenzie TB, Mitchell JE, et al: A placebo-controlled, double-blind crossover study of fluoxetine in trichotillomania. Am J Psychiatry 148:1566–1571, 1991d

Christenson GA, Mackenzie TB, Reeve EA: Familial trichotillomania (letter). Am J Psychiatry 149:283, 1992

Christenson GA, Faber RJ, de Zwaan M, et al: Compulsive buying: descriptive characteristics and psychiatric comorbidity. J Clin Psychiatry 55:5–11, 1994

Coccaro EF, Kavoussi RJ, Berman ME, et al: Intermittent explosive disorder—revised: development, reliability, and validity of research criteria. Compr Psychiatry 39:368–376, 1998

Comings DE: The molecular genetics of pathological gambling. CNS Spectrums 3:20–37, 1998

Comings DE, Gonzalez N, Wu S, et al: Studies of the 48 repeat polymorphism of the DRD4 gene in impulsive, compulsive, addictive behaviors; Tourette syndrome; ADHD; pathological gambling; and substance abuse. Am J Med Genet 88:358–368, 1999

Committee on the Social and Economic Impact of Pathological Gambling (CSEIPG), Committee on Law and Justice, Commission on Behavioral and Social Sciences and Education, National Research Council: Pathological Gambling: A Critical Review. Washington, DC, National Academy Press, 1999

Crockford DN, el-Guebaly N: Psychiatric comorbidity in pathological gambling: a critical review. Can J Psychiatry 43:43–50, 1998

Cupchik W, Atcheson JD: Shoplifting: an occasional crime of the moral majority. Bull Am Acad Psychiatry Law 11:343–352, 1983

DeCaria CM, Begaz T, Hollander E: Serotonergic and noradrenergic function in pathological gambling. CNS Spectrums 3:38–47, 1998

De Deyn PP, Rabheru K, Rasmussen A, et al: A randomized trial of risperidone, placebo, and haloperidol for behavioral symptoms of dementia. Neurology 53:946–955, 1999

Diefenbach GJ, Reitman D, Williamson DA: Trichotillomania: a challenge to research and practice. Clin Psychol Rev 20:289–309, 2000

Eichelman B: Aggressive behavior: from laboratory to clinic. Quo vadit? Arch Gen Psychiatry 49:488–492, 1992

Eisen SA, Lin N, Lyons MJ, et al: Familial influences on gambling behavior: an analysis of 3359 twin pairs. Addiction 93:1375–1384, 1998

Elizur A, Jaffe R: Stealing as a pathological symptom. Isr J Psychiatry Relat Sci 6:52–61, 1968

Elliott FA: Propranolol for the control of belligerent behavior following acute brain damage. Ann Neurol 1:489–491, 1977

Epperson CN, Fasula D, Wasylink S, et al: Risperidone addition in serotonin reuptake inhibitor-resistant trichotillomania: three cases. J Child Adolesc Psychopharmacol 9:43–49, 1999

Fava M: Psychopharmacologic treatment of pathologic aggression, in The Psychiatric Clinics of North America. Edited by Fava M. Philadelphia, PA, WB Saunders, 1997, p 444

Federal Bureau of Investigation: Crime in the United States: Uniform Crime Reports for the United States. Washington, DC, U.S. Department of Justice, 1998

Fenichel O: The Psychoanalytic Theory of Neurosis. New York, WW Norton, 1945

Fishbain DA: Kleptomania as risk-taking behavior in response to depression. Am J Psychother 41:598–603, 1987

Folks DG, King LD, Dowdy SB, et al: Carbamazepine treatment of selected affectively disordered inpatients. Am J Psychiatry 139:115–117, 1982

Frances A, First MB, Pincus HA: Impulse control disorders not elsewhere classified, in DSM-IV Guidebook. Washington, DC, American Psychiatric Press, 1995, pp 343–352

Freud S: The acquisition and control of fire (1932 [1931]), in Standard Edition of the Complete Psychological Works of Sigmund Freud, Figure 22. Translated and edited by Strachey J. London, England, Hogarth Press, 1964, pp 181–193

Gauthier J, Pellerin D: Management of compulsive shoplifting through covert sensitization. J Behav Ther Exp Psychiatry 13:73–75, 1982

Geller JL, Bertsch G: Firesetting behavior in the histories of a state hospital population. Am J Psychiatry 142:464–468, 1985

Geller JL, Erlen J, Pinkus RL: A historical appraisal of America's experience with "pyromania": a diagnosis in search of a disorder. Int J Law Psychiatry 9:201–229, 1986

Geller JL, Fisher WH, Moynihan K: Adult lifetime prevalence of fire setting behaviors in a state hospital population. Psychiatr Q 63:129–142, 1992a

Geller JL, Fisher WH, Bertsch G: Who repeats? A follow-up study of state hospital patients' firesetting behavior. Psychiatr Q 63:143–156, 1992b

Gibbens TCN: Shoplifting. Med Leg J 30:6–19, 1962

Gleason RP, Schneider LS: Carbamazepine treatment of agitation in Alzheimer's outpatients refractory to neuroleptics. J Clin Psychiatry 51:115–118, 1990

Glover J: A case of kleptomania treated by covert sensitization. Br J Clin Psychol 24:213–214, 1985

Goldman MJ: Kleptomania: making sense of the nonsensical. Am J Psychiatry 148:986–996, 1991

Greenberg HR, Sarner CA: Trichotillomania: symptom and syndrome. Arch Gen Psychiatry 12:482–489, 1965

Harris GT, Rice ME: Mentally disordered firesetters: psychodynamic vs. empirical approaches. Int J Law Psychiatry 7:19–34, 1984

Hill RW, Langevin R, Paitich D, et al: Is arson an aggressive act or a property offense? A controlled study of psychiatric referrals. Can J Psychiatry 27:648–654, 1982

Hodgins DC, el-Guebaly N: Natural and treatment-assisted recovery from gambling problems: a comparison of resolved and active gamblers. Addiction 95:777–789, 2000

Hollander E, Frenkel M, DeCaria C, et al: Treatment of pathological gambling with clomipramine. Am J Psychiatry 149:710–711, 1992

Hollander E, Kwon JH, Stein DJ, et al: Obsessive-compulsive spectrum disorders: overview and quality of life issues. J Clin Psychiatry 57(suppl 8):3–6, 1996

Hollander E, DeCaria CM, Finkell JN, et al: A randomized double-blind fluvoxamine/placebo crossover trial in pathologic gambling. Biol Psychiatry 47:813–817, 2000

Hudson JI, Pope HG Jr: Affective spectrum disorder: does antidepressant response identify a family of disorders with a common pathophysiology? Am J Psychiatry 147:552–564, 1990

Hudson JI, Pope HG, Jonas JM, et al: Phenomenologic relationship of eating disorders to major affective disorders. Psychiatry Res 9:345–354, 1983

Jackson HF, Glass C, Hope S: A functional analysis of recidivistic arson. Br J Clin Psychol 26:175–185, 1987

Jenike MA: Obsessive-compulsive and related disorders (editorial). N Engl J Med 321:539–541, 1989

Johnson EE, Hamer RM, Nora RM: The Lie/Bet Questionnaire for screening pathological gamblers: a follow-up study. Psychol Rep 83:1219–1224, 1998

Kavoussi R, Armstead P, Coccaro E: The neurobiology of impulsive aggression, in The Psychiatric Clinics of North America. Edited by Fava M. Philadelphia, PA, WB Saunders, 1997, pp 395–403

Keuthen NJ, O'Sullivan RL, Ricciardi JN, et al: The Massachusetts General Hospital (MGH) Hairpulling Scale, 1: development and factor analyses. Psychother Psychosom 64:141–145, 1995

Keuthen NJ, O'Sullivan RL, Hayday CF, et al: The relationship of menstrual cycle and pregnancy to compulsive hairpulling. Psychother Psychosom 66:33–37, 1997

Keuthen NJ, O'Sullivan RL, Goodchild P, et al: Retrospective review of treatment outcome for 63 patients with trichotillomania. Am J Psychiatry 155:560–561, 1998

Keuthen NJ, Fraim C, Deckersbach T, et al: Longitudinal follow-up of naturalistic treatment outcome in patients with trichotillomania. J Clin Psychiatry 62:101–107, 2001

Keutzer CS: Kleptomania: a direct approach to treatment. Br J Med Psychol 45:159–163, 1972

Khan K, Martin ICA: Kleptomania as a presenting feature of cortical atrophy. Acta Psychiatr Scand 56:168–172, 1977

Kim SW: Opioid antagonists in the treatment of impulse-control disorders. J Clin Psychiatry 59:159–164, 1998

Koson DF, Dvoskin J: Arson: a diagnostic study. Bull Am Acad Psychiatry Law 10:39–49, 1982

Kraus JE: Treatment of kleptomania with paroxetine. J Clin Psychiatry 60:793, 1999

Krishnan KRR, Davidson JRT, Guajardo C: Trichotillomania: a review. Compr Psychiatry 26:123–128, 1985

Kruesi MJP, Hibbs ED, Zahn TP, et al: A 2-year prospective follow-up study of children and adolescents with disruptive behavior disorders: prediction by cerebrospinal fluid 5-hydroxyindoleacetic acid, homovanillic acid, and autonomic measures? Arch Gen Psychiatry 49:429–435, 1992

Lawrence K, Nasraway S: Conduction disturbances associated with administration of butyrophenone antipsychotics in the critically ill: a review of the literature. Pharmacotherapy 17:531–537, 1997

Lejoyeux M, McLoghlin M, Ades J: Epidemiology of behavioral dependence: literature review and results of original studies. European Psychiatry 15:129–134, 2000

Lepage C, Ladouceur R, Jacques C: Prevalence of problem gambling among community service users. Community Ment Health J 36:597–601, 2000

Lesch KP, Merschdorf U: Impulsivity, aggression, and serotonin: a molecular psychobiological perspective. Behav Sci Law 18:581–604, 2000

Lesieur HR, Blume SB: The South Oaks Gambling Screen (SOGS): a new instrument for the identification of pathological gamblers. Am J Psychiatry 144:1184–1188, 1987

Lesieur HR, Custer RL: Pathological gambling: roots, phases and treatments. Annals of the American Academy of Political and Social Science 74:146–156, 1984

Lewis NDC, Yarnell H: Pathological Firesetting (Pyromania) (Nervous and Mental Disease Monogr 82). New York, Coolidge Foundation, 1951

Linden RD, Pope HG Jr, Jonas JM: Pathological gambling and major affective disorder: preliminary findings. J Clin Psychiatry 47:201 203, 1986

Lindenmayer J-P: The pathophysiology of agitation. J Clin Psychiatry 61(suppl 14):5–10, 2000

Lott AD, McElroy SL, Keys MA: Valproate in the treatment of behavioral agitation in elderly patients with dementia. J Neuropsychiatry Clin Neurosci 7:314–319, 1995

Mark V, Ervin F: Violence and the Brain. New York, Harper & Row, 1970

Marzagao LR: Systematic desensitization treatment of kleptomania. J Behav Ther Exp Psychiatry 3:327–328, 1972

Mattes JA: Psychopharmacology of temper outbursts: a review. J Nerv Ment Dis 174:464–470, 1986

Mattes JA: Comparative effectiveness of carbamazepine and propranolol for rage outbursts. J Neuropsychiatry Clin Neurosci 2:159–164, 1990

McElroy SL, Keck PE, Pope HG, et al: Pharmacological treatment of kleptomania and bulimia nervosa. J Clin Psychopharmacol 9:358–360, 1989

McElroy SL, Hudson JI, Pope HG Jr, et al: Kleptomania: clinical characteristics and associated psychopathology. Psychol Med 21:93–108, 1991a

McElroy SL, Harrison G, Hudson JI, et al: Kleptomania: a report of 20 cases. Am J Psychiatry 148:652–657, 1991b

McElroy SL, Hudson JI, Pope HG Jr, et al: The DSM-III-R impulse control disorders not elsewhere classified: clinical characteristics and relationship to other psychiatric disorders. Am J Psychiatry 149:318–327, 1992

McElroy SL, Keck PE Jr, Pope HG Jr, et al: Compulsive buying: a report of 20 cases. J Clin Psychiatry 55:242–248, 1994

McElroy SL, Keck PE, Phillips KA: Kleptomania, compulsive buying, and binge-eating disorder. J Clin Psychiatry 56(suppl 4):14–26, 1995

McElroy SL, Pope HG Jr, Keck PE, et al: Are impulse-control disorders related to bipolar disorder? Compr Psychiatry 37:229–240, 1996

McElroy SL, Soutullo CA, Beckman DA, et al: DSM-IV intermittent explosive disorder: a report of 27 cases. J Clin Psychiatry 59:203–210, 1998

McGrath P, Marshall PG: A comprehensive treatment program for a fire setting child. J Behav Ther Exp Psychiatry 10:69–72, 1979

McIntyre AW, Emsley RA: Shoplifting associated with normal-pressure hydrocephalus: report of a case. J Geriatr Psychiatry Neurol 3:229–230, 1990

Menninger KA: The Vital Balance. New York, Viking, 1963

Menninger KA, Mayman M: Episodic dyscontrol: a third order of stress adaptation. Bull Menninger Clin 20:153–165, 1956

Moak GS: Clinical perspectives on elderly first-offender shoplifters. Hospital and Community Psychiatry 39:648–651, 1988

Molnar G, Keitner L, Harwood BT: A comparison of partner and solo arsonists. J Forensic Sci 29:574–583, 1984

Monroe RR: Episodic Behavioral Disorders. Cambridge, MA, Harvard University Press, 1970

Monterosso J, Ainslie G: Beyond discounting: possible experimental models of impulse control. Psychopharmacology 146:339–347, 1999

Moskowitz JA: Lithium and lady luck: use of lithium carbonate in compulsive gambling. New York State Journal of Medicine 80:785–788, 1980

Narayan M, Nelson JC: Treatment of dementia with behavioral disturbance using divalproex or a combination of divalproex and a neuroleptic. J Clin Psychiatry 58:351–354, 1997

Neudecker A, Rufer M, Hand I, et al: Paroxetine versus multimodal behavioral therapy in the treatment of trichotillomania: a pilot study (NR579), in 2001 New Research Program and Abstracts, American Psychiatric Association 154th Annual Meeting, New Orleans, LA, May 5–10, 2001. Washington, DC, American Psychiatric Association, 2001

Ninan PT, Rothbaum BO, Stipetic M, et al: Assessment update: trichotillomania. CSF 5-HIAA as a predictor of treatment response in trichotillomania. Psychopharmacol Bull 28:451–455, 1992

Ninan PT, Knight B, Kirk L, et al: A controlled trial of venlafaxine in trichotillomania: interim phase I results. Psychopharmacol Bull 34:221–224, 1998

Ninan PT, Rothbaum BO, Marsteller FA, et al: A placebo-controlled trial of cognitive-behavioral therapy and clomipramine in trichotillomania. J Clin Psychiatry 61:47–50, 2000

Oranje AP, Pureboom-Wynia JDR, De Raeymaechec CMJ: Trichotillomania in childhood. J Am Acad Dermatol 16:614–619, 1986

O'Sullivan RL, Keuthen NJ, Hayday CF, et al: The Massachusetts General Hospital (MGH) Hairpulling Scale, 2: reliability and validity. Psychother Psychosom 64:146–148, 1995

Rasanen P, Hakko H, Valsanen E: The mental state of arsonists as determined by forensic psychiatric examinations. Bull Am Acad Psychiatry Law 23:547–553, 1995

Ray I: A Treatise on the Medical Jurisprudence of Insanity, 2nd Edition. Boston, MA, William D Tickner, 1844

Rice ME, Harris GT: Firesetters admitted to a maximum psychiatric institution. Journal of Interpersonal Violence 6:461–475, 1991

Ristvedt SL, Christenson GA: The use of pharmacologic pain sensitization in the treatment of repetitive hair-pulling. Behav Res Ther 34:647–648, 1996

Ritchie EC, Huff T: Psychiatric aspects of arsonists. J Forensic Sci 44:733–740, 1999

Rix KJB: A psychiatric study of adult arsonists. Med Sci Law 34:21–34, 1994

Rothbaum BO, Ninan TA: Treatment of trichotillomania: behavior therapy versus clomipramine. Poster presented at the annual meeting of the Association for Advancement of Behavior Therapy, Boston, MA, November 1992

Rothbaum BO, Shaw L, Morris R, et al: Prevalence of trichotillomania in a college freshman population (letter). J Clin Psychiatry 54:72–73, 1993

Roy A, Custer R, Lorenz V, et al: Depressed pathological gamblers. Acta Psychiatr Scand 77:163–165, 1988

Sarasalo E, Bergman B, Toth J: Personality traits and psychiatric and somatic morbidity among kleptomaniacs. Acta Psychiatr Scand 94:358–364, 1996

Seguier H: Revue historique de la notion de kleptomanie. L'Encephale 55:336–369, 1966

Shaffer HJ, Hall MN, Vander Bilt J: Estimating the Prevalence of Disordered Gambling Behaviour in the United States and Canada: A Meta-Analysis. Boston, MA, Harvard Medical School Division on Addictions, 1997

Shapiro BA, Warren J, Egol AB, et al: Practice parameters for intravenous analgesia and sedation for adult patients in the intensive care unit: an executive summary. Crit Care Med 23:1596–1600, 1995

Shaw SC, Fletcher AP: Aggression as an adverse drug reaction. Adverse Drug React Toxicol Rev 19:35–45, 2000

Sheard MH: Clinical pharmacology of aggressive behavior. Clin Neuropharmacol 11:483–492, 1988

Sheard MH, Marini JL, Bridges CI, et al: The effect of lithium on impulsive aggressive behavior in man. Am J Psychiatry 133:1409–1413, 1976

Singer BA: A case of kleptomania. Bull Am Acad Psychiatry Law 6:414–422, 1978

Slutske WS, Eisen S, True WR, et al: Common genetic vulnerability for pathological gambling and alcohol dependence in men. Arch Gen Psychiatry 57:666–673, 2000

Smith J, Short J: Mentally disordered firesetters. British Journal of Hospital Medicine 53:136–140, 1995

Soothill KL, Pope PJ: Arson: a twenty-year cohort study. Med Sci Law 13:127–138, 1973

Soriano JL, O'Sullivan RL, Baer L, et al: Trichotillomania and self-esteem: a survey of 62 female hair pullers. J Clin Psychiatry 57:77–82, 1996

Soubrie P: Reconciling the role of central serotonin neurones in human and animal behavior. Behav Brain Sci 9:319–364, 1986

Stanley MA, Mouton SG: Trichotillomania treatment manual, in Sourcebook of Psychological Treatment Manuals for Adult Disorders. Edited by Van Hasselt VB, Hersen M. New York, Plenum, 1996, pp 657–687

Stanley MA, Swann AC, Bowers TC, et al: A comparison of clinical features in trichotillomania and obsessive-compulsive disorder. Behav Res Ther 30:39–44, 1992

Stanley MA, Prather RC, Wagner AL, et al: Can the Yale-Brown Obsessive Compulsive Scale be used to assess trichotillomania? A preliminary report. Behav Res Ther 31:171–177, 1993

Stanley MA, Breckenridge JK, Swann AC: Fluvoxamine treatment of trichotillomania. J Clin Psychopharmacol 17:278–283, 1997

Steel Z, Blaszczynski A: Impulsivity, personality disorders and pathological gambling severity. Addiction 93:895–905, 1998

Stein DJ, Hollander E: Low-dose pimozide augmentation of serotonin reuptake blockers in the treatment of trichotillomania. J Clin Psychiatry 53:123–126, 1992

Stein DJ, Hollander E, Liebowitz MR: Neurobiology of impulsivity and the impulse control disorders. J Neuropsychiatry Clin Neurosci 5:9–17, 1993

Stein DJ, Simeon D, Frenkel M, et al. An open trial of valproate in borderline personality disorder. J Clin Psychiatry 56:506–510, 1995a

Stein DJ, Hollander E, Cohen L, et al: Serotonergic responsivity in trichotillomania: neuroendocrine effects of m-chlorophenylpiperazine. Biol Psychiatry 37:414–416, 1995b

Stein DJ, Bouwer C, Hawkridge S, et al: Risperidone augmentation of serotonin reuptake inhibitors in obsessive-compulsive and related disorders. J Clin Psychiatry 58:119–122, 1997

Stewart LA: Profile of female firesetters: implications for treatment. Br J Psychiatry 163:248–256, 1993

Streichenwein SM, Thornby JI: A long-term, double-blind, placebo-controlled crossover trial of the efficacy of fluoxetine for trichotillomania. Am J Psychiatry 152:1192–1196, 1995

Stroud JD: Hair loss in children. Pediatr Clin North Am 30:641–657, 1983

Swedo SE, Leonard HL: Trichotillomania: an obsessive compulsive spectrum disorder? Psychiatr Clin North Am 15:777–790, 1992

Swedo SE, Leonard HL, Rapoport JL, et al: A double-blind comparison of clomipramine and desipramine in the treatment of trichotillomania (hair pulling). N Engl J Med 321:497–501, 1989

Swedo SE, Rapoport JL, Leonard HL, et al: Regional cerebral glucose metabolism of women with trichotillomania. Arch Gen Psychiatry 48:828–833, 1991

Swedo SE, Lenane MC, Leonard HL: Long-term treatment of (hair pulling) (letter). N Engl J Med 329:141–142, 1993

Sylvain C, Ladoceur R, Boisvert JM: Cognitive and behavioral treatment of pathological gambling: a controlled study. J Consult Clin Psychol 65:727–732, 1997

Symes BA, Nicki RM: A preliminary consideration of cue-exposure, response-prevention treatment for pathological gambling behavior: two case studies. Journal of Gambling Studies 13:145–157, 1997

Tardiff K: The current state of psychiatry in the treatment of violent patients. Arch Gen Psychiatry 49:493–499, 1992

Turnbull JM: Sexual relationships of patients with kleptomania. South Med J 80:995–997, 1987

Van Ameringen M, Mancini C, Oakman JM, et al: The potential role of haloperidol in the treatment of trichotillomania. J Affect Disord 56:219–226, 1999

Virkkunen M: On arson committed by schizophrenics. Acta Psychiatr Scand 50:152–160, 1974

Virkkunen M, DeLong J, Bartko J, et al: Relationship of psychobiological variables to recidivism in violent offender and impulsive fire setters. Arch Gen Psychiatry 46:600–603, 1989

Virkkunen M, Rawlings R, Takola R, et al: CSF biochemistries, glucose metabolism, and diurnal activity rhythms in alcoholic, violent offenders, fire setters, and healthy volunteers. Arch Gen Psychiatry 51:20–27, 1994

Virkkunen M, Eggert M, Rawlings R, et al: A prospective follow-up study of alcoholic violent offenders and fire setters. Arch Gen Psychiatry 53:523–529, 1996

Wiedemann G: Kleptomania: characteristics of 12 cases. European Psychiatry 13:67–77, 1998

Williams DT, Mehl R, Yudofsky S, et al: The effect of propranolol on uncontrolled rage outbursts in children and adolescents with organic brain dysfunction. J Am Acad Child Psychiatry 21:129–135, 1982

Winchel RM, Jones JS, Stanley B, et al: Clinical characteristics of trichotillomania and its response to fluoxetine. J Clin Psychiatry 53:304–308, 1992a

Winchel RM, Jones JS, Molcho A, et al: The Psychiatric Institute Trichotillomania Scale (PITS). Psychopharmacol Bull 28:463–476, 1992b

Winer JA, Pollock GH: Adjustment and impulse control disorders, in Comprehensive Textbook of Psychiatry, 3rd Edition, Vol 2. Edited by Kaplan HI, Freedman AM, Saddock BJ. Baltimore, MD, Williams & Wilkins, 1980, pp 1812–1829

Wise MG, Hilty DM, Cerda GM: Delirium (Confusional States), in The American Psychiatric Publishing Textbook of Consultation-Liaison Psychiatry: Psychiatry in the Medically Ill, 2nd Edition. Edited by Wise MG, Rundell JR. Washington, DC, American Psychiatric Publishing, 2002, pp 257–272

Wittels F: Kleptomania and other psychopathic crimes. Journal of Criminal Psychopathology 4:205–216, 1942

Wolpe J: Psychotherapy by Reciprocal Inhibition. Stanford, CA, Stanford University Press, 1958

World Health Organization: International Classification of Diseases, 9th Revision, Clinical Modification. Ann Arbor, MI, Commission on Professional and Hospital Activities, 1978

Yates E: The influence of psycho-social factors on non-sensical shoplifting. International Journal of Offender Therapy and Comparative Criminology 30:203–211, 1986

Yudofsky SC, Williams D, Gorman J: Propranolol in the treatment of rage and violent behavior in patients with chronic brain syndromes. Am J Psychiatry 138:218–220, 1981

Yudofsky SC, Silver JM, Jackson W, et al: The Overt Aggression Scale for objective rating of verbal and physical aggression. Am J Psychiatry 143:35–39; 1986

Yudofsky SC, Kopecky HJ, Kunik M, et al: The Overt Agitation Severity Scale for the objective rating of agitation. J Neuropsychiatry Clin Neurosci 9:541–548, 1997

Personality Disorders

Katharine A. Phillips, M.D.

Shirley Yen, Ph.D.

John G. Gunderson, M.D.

All clinicians frequently encounter patients with personality disorders. These patients are commonly seen in a variety of treatment settings, both inpatient and outpatient. Studies indicate that 30%–50% of outpatients have a personality disorder (Koenigsberg et al. 1985) and that 15% of inpatients are hospitalized primarily for problems caused by a personality disorder; as many as half of the remaining inpatients have a comorbid personality disorder (Loranger 1990) that significantly affects their response to treatment. It has also been estimated that personality disorders are relatively common in the general population, the prevalence being between 10% and 13% (Lenzenweger et al. 1997; Weissman 1993).

Patients with personality disorders present with problems that are among the most complex and challenging that clinicians encounter. Some patients intensely desire relationships but fearfully avoid them because they anticipate rejection; others seek endless admiration and are engrossed with grandiose fantasies of limitless power, brilliance, or ideal love. Still others have a self-concept so disturbed that they feel they embody evil or do not exist. This complexity is amplified by the fact that these and other personality disorder characteristics are not simply a problem the person has but are in fact central to who the person is.

Personality disorders, according to DSM-IV (American Psychiatric Association 1994), are patterns of inflexible and maladaptive personality traits that cause subjective distress, significant impairment in social or occupational functioning, or both. These traits must also deviate markedly from the culturally expected and accepted range, or *norm*, and this deviation must be manifested in more than one of the following areas: cognition,

affectivity, control over impulses and need gratification, and ways of relating to others. In addition, the deviation must have been stably present and enduring since adolescence or early adulthood, and it must be pervasive—that is, it must manifest itself across a broad range of situations, rather than in only one specific triggering situation or in response to a particular stimulus.

Although useful, this definition has ambiguities and limitations. It can be difficult, for example, to determine whether personality traits are inflexible or to differentiate deviance from the norm or sickness from health. Whether dependence on others, compulsive work habits, or passive resistance to demands is considered excessive or problematic depends to some extent on the personal, social, and cultural context in which each occurs. Furthermore, the stability of personality disorders has recently been called into question (Ferro et al. 1998).

Nonetheless, it is important that clinicians attempt to recognize personality disorders in their patients. First, personality disorders do, by definition, cause significant problems for those who have them. Persons with these disorders often suffer, and their relationships with others are problematic. They have difficulty responding flexibly and adaptively to the environment and to the changes and demands of life, and they lack resilience when under stress. Instead, their usual ways of responding tend to perpetuate and intensify their difficulties. However, these individuals are often oblivious to the fact that their personality causes them problems, and they may instead blame others for their difficulties or even deny that they have any problems at all.

Personality disorders also often cause problems for others and are costly to society. Individuals with personality disorders frequently have considerable difficulty in their family, academic, occupational, and other roles. They have elevated rates of separation, divorce, child custody proceedings, unemployment, homelessness (Caton et al. 1994), and perpetration of child abuse (Dinwiddie and Bucholz 1993). They also have increased rates of accidents (McDonald and Davey 1996); police contacts (Gandhi et al. 2001); emergency department visits; medical hospitalization (J.[H.] Reich et al. 1989); violence, including homicide (Miller et al. 1993; Raine 1993); self-injurious behavior (Hillbrand et al. 1994); attempted suicide (Pirkis et al. 1999); and completed suicide (Brent et al. 1994; Hawton et al. 1993). A high percentage of criminals (70%–85% in some studies) (Jordan et al. 1996), 60%–70% of alcoholic individuals, and 70%–90% of persons who abuse drugs have a personality disorder.

Finally, personality disorders need to be identified because of their treatment implications. These disorders often need to be a focus of treatment or, at the very least, need to be taken into account when comorbid Axis I disorders are treated, because their presence often affects an Axis I disorder's prognosis and treatment response. For example, patients with depressive disorders (Black et al. 1988; Nelson et al. 1994), bipolar disorder (Calabrese et al. 1993), panic disorder (J.H. Reich 1988), obsessive-compulsive disorder (Jenike et al. 1986), and substance abuse (Fals-Stewart 1992) often respond less well to pharmacotherapy when they have a comorbid personality disorder. The presence of a comorbid personality disorder is also associated with poor compliance with pharmacotherapy (Colom et al. 2000). Furthermore, personality disorders have been shown to predict the development and relapse of major depression (Alnæs and Torgersen 1997; Lewinsohn et al. 2000), and individuals with a personality disorder are less likely to remit from major depression (O'Leary and Costello 2001), bipolar disorder (Dunayevich et al. 2000), and generalized anxiety disorder (Yonkers et al. 2000).

As most clinicians are well aware, the characteristics of patients with personality disorders are likely to be manifested in the treatment relationship, whether or not the personality disorder is the focus of treatment. For example, some patients may be overly dependent on the clinician, others may not follow treatment recommendations, and still others may experience significant conflict about getting well. Although individuals with personality disorders tend to use psychiatric services extensively, they are more likely to be dissatisfied with the treatment they receive (Kelstrup et al. 1993; Kent et al. 1995).

What follows is a clinically oriented overview of the personality disorders and a description of each disorder.

These descriptions, although based on clinical tradition, have also been informed by the recent explosion of empirical research on the personality disorders—a development facilitated by the placement of these disorders on a separate axis in DSM-III (American Psychiatric Association 1980). This research has focused on many different aspects of these disorders, such as their descriptive features, family history, course, treatment response, and etiology, including their psychodynamic, biogenetic, and sociocultural roots. This ongoing research is greatly enhancing our understanding of these complex disorders.

General Considerations

History of Personality Disorders

Personality types and disorders have been described for thousands of years, as evidenced by Hippocrates' description of four temperaments: the pessimistic melancholic, the overly optimistic sanguine, the irritable choleric, and the apathetic phlegmatic. It is interesting that the early Greeks' theory that these temperaments were determined by the relative proportion of the four bodily humors (black bile, blood, yellow bile, and phlegm, respectively) is reflected in current attempts to discover biogenetic bases of personality.

In the early 1800s, psychiatrists such as Pinel, Esquirol, Rush, and Pritchard described socially maladaptive personality types seen in clinical settings. More specific personality types were then described at the turn of the century, when, for example, Janet (1901) and Freud (Breuer and Freud 1893–1895/1957) described the psychological traits associated with hysteria, the forerunner of histrionic personality disorder. Subsequently, within the framework of early psychoanalytic instinct theory, Abraham proposed that arrests at the three psychosexual stages of childhood development—the oral, anal, and phallic phases—led to the development of the dependent, obsessive-compulsive, and hysterical character types, respectively. However, this view changed as early instinct theory and the subsequent ego-psychological model of psychoanalytic theory were gradually supplanted by object relations theory, which proposes that personality is shaped largely by the child's early parental relationships. In this framework, dependent personality traits derive from parental deprivation, obsessive-compulsive traits from control struggles with parental figures, and hysterical traits, in part, from parental eroticization and competition. The borderline and narcissistic personality disorder concepts also developed out of the object relations framework.

From a quite different perspective, in the 1920s the German phenomenologists Kraepelin (1921) and Kretschmer (1925) described personality types in terms of the spectrum concept—the theory that personality types are biogenetically related variants of the paranoid and affective psychoses (which would now be considered Axis I disorders). These early spectrum personality types were forerunners of the current paranoid, schizotypal, cyclothymic, and depressive personality disorders. In contrast, Schneider (1958), another German phenomenologist, did not subscribe to the spectrum concept but considered personality disorders to represent socially deviant and extreme variants of normally occurring personality traits. He developed the first comprehensive system of personality disorder categories, which provided the template for many of those contained in the *International Statistical Classification of Diseases and Related Health Problems, 10th Revision* (ICD-10; World Health Organization 1992) and DSM-IV.

Personality disorders have been included in every version of DSM, but only paranoid, obsessive-compulsive, and antisocial personality disorders have been consistent DSM "members." Some current categories (e.g., borderline) were added to later editions, whereas others (e.g., inadequate personality) were dropped. The theoretical underpinnings of the DSM personality disorder categories have also changed over the years (Gunderson 1992).

DSM-I, published in 1952 by the American Psychiatric Association, defined personality disorders not as stable and enduring patterns but as traits that malfunction under stressful circumstances, which leads to inflexible and maladaptive behavior. DSM-II (American Psychiatric Association 1968) emphasized that personality disorders involve distress and impairment in functioning, not merely socially deviant behavior.

In DSM-III, several major changes in personality disorder conceptualization and classification were made. There was a shift away from a psychoanalytic orientation toward an atheoretical, descriptive approach. Specific diagnostic criteria were added, and the personality disorders were placed on a separate axis, which highlighted their importance.

The changes made in DSM-III-R (American Psychiatric Association 1987) and DSM-IV attempted to increase the validity of the personality disorder categories by incorporating findings from the growing empirical literature. Although current DSM descriptions attempt to represent an optimal synthesis of clinical tradition and research findings, such descriptions are likely to continue to evolve over time as our understanding of these disorders increases.

Classification Issues

Since DSM-III, the personality disorders have been grouped into three clusters: the *odd or eccentric cluster* (schizotypal, schizoid, and paranoid); the *dramatic, emotional, or erratic cluster* (borderline, histrionic, narcissistic, and antisocial); and the *anxious or fearful cluster* (avoidant, dependent, and obsessive-compulsive) (Table 19–1). Although these clusters were originally based on face validity alone, they have since received some empirical support (Kass et al. 1985; Zimmerman and Coryell 1989). Nonetheless, these clusters are limited because they are based on descriptive similarities rather than on similarities in etiology or external validators such as family history or treatment response.

Another classification issue is whether the personality disorders are best classified as dimensions or categories (Frances 1982; Gunderson et al. 1991b). Do personality disorders exist along dimensions that reflect extreme variants of normal personality, or are they distinct categories that are qualitatively different, and clearly demarcated, from normal personality traits and one another? Each model has its advantages and disadvantages. For example, the *dimensional model*, with its potential use of many personality descriptors and its ability to assess the degree to which traits are present, may more comprehensively cover problematic traits. It does not confine clinicians to the use of a limited number of categories. In addition, most of the traits embodied by Axis II criteria can be found in less extreme form in psychiatrically healthy people. Indeed, one of the frontiers in personality disorder research is the development of types that relate to personality dimensions found in populations that are psychiatrically healthy (Widiger 2000). Of special significance are the widely heralded "Big Five" dimensions of neuroticism, extroversion, openness, agreeableness, and conscientiousness (Table 19–2; Costa and McCrae 1990). Cloninger's seven-dimension psychobiological model of temperament and character, which is theoretically linked to abnormalities in specific neurotransmitter systems, is also of great interest and is receiving increasing investigation (Table 19–3; Cloninger et al. 1993). Both models have received empirical support (O'Connor and Dyce 1998), and dimensional models in general are consistent with the genetic and phenotypic structure of traits delineating personality disorders (Livesley et al. 1998).

The *categorical model*, however, better reflects how clinicians think—that is, in terms of pathological syndromes that a person either has or does not have. The use of categories also makes it possible for clinicians succinctly to summarize patients' difficulties and facilitates communication about them. Although DSM-IV is based

TABLE 19–1. Summary of personality disorder features

Cluster	Model	Key clinical features	Treatment	Course/prognosis
A: Odd, eccentric	Spectrum disorders	Social deficits, absence of close relationships	Structure, rehabilitation, support, medication	Stable/poor
B: Dramatic, emotional, erratic	Self disorders	Social and interpersonal instability	Support, exploration, sociotherapy, individual therapy, medication	Unstable/some remission with age
C: Anxious, fearful	Dimensional disorders	Interpersonal and intrapsychic conflicts	Exploration, individual therapy, group therapy	Modifiable/good

primarily on the categorical model, it also incorporates a dimensional approach to some extent, in that it encourages clinicians to identify problematic personality traits that are subthreshold for any particular diagnosis. Classification models that incorporate both a dimensional and a categorical approach may ultimately prove most useful to clinicians, and several such models have been proposed (Gunderson 1992).

These and other classification issues are currently being debated and researched, and this may lead to changes in the future classification of personality disorders. Whatever system is used, it is important that it be useful to clinicians and, ultimately, reflect what is known about the etiology of these disorders.

Assessment Issues and Methods

The assessment of Axis II disorders is in some ways more complex than that of Axis I disorders. It can be difficult to assess multiple domains of experience and behavior (i.e., cognition, affect, intrapsychic experience, and interpersonal interactions) and to determine that traits are not only distressing, impairing, and of early onset, but also pervasive and enduring. Nonetheless, a personality disorder assessment is essential to the comprehensive evaluation and adequate treatment of all patients. What follows is a discussion of such an assessment and steps that can be taken to avoid commonly encountered problems.

Comprehensiveness of Evaluation

A skilled clinical interview is the mainstay of personality disorder diagnosis and requires the clinician to be familiar with DSM criteria, take a longitudinal view, and use multiple sources of information. A psychodynamic perspective may contribute depth to the assessment through its attention to defenses, attitudes, and development. However, because an open-ended approach may inadequately cover all Axis II disorders, the additional use of a self- report or semistructured (i.e., interviewer-administered) personality disorder assessment instrument can be useful (Table

19–4). Such instruments systematically assess each personality disorder criterion with the use of standard questions or probes. Although self-report instruments have the advantage of saving the interviewer time, they often yield false-positive diagnoses and allow contamination of Axis II traits by Axis I states (Widiger and Frances 1987). Semistructured interviews—which require the interviewer to use certain questions but allow further probing—facilitate accurate diagnosis in several ways: they allow the interviewer to attempt to differentiate Axis II traits from Axis I states, clarify contradictions or ambiguities in the patient's response, and determine that traits are pervasive rather than limited to a specific situation.

Nonetheless, even with the use of a structured interview, the interviewer must often use his or her judgment. For example, is a given trait present in enough situations to be considered pervasive? How much distress or impairment is necessary to consider the criterion present? Is a given characteristic a personality trait or a symptom of an Axis I disorder (i.e., a state)? Another limitation is that agreement among existing instruments is fairly low, and the instruments do not indicate which disorder in any given patient is most severe or should be the focus of treatment.

Syntonicity of Traits

As was noted earlier, because personality disorders to some extent reflect who the person is—and not simply what he or she has—some patients are unaware of the traits that reflect their disorder or may not perceive them as problematic. This limited self-awareness can interfere with personality disorder assessment, especially if the questions asked have negative or unflattering implications. This problem can be minimized by the use of multiple sources of information (e.g., medical records and informants who know the patient well). Still, the fact that studies have shown low concordance rates between patient-based and informant-based interviews (Bernstein et al. 1997; Ferro and Klein 1997) means that interviewers will often need to rely on their personal experience with the patient to reach a conclusion.

TABLE 19–2. Five-factor model of personality

Factor domains	Facets (primary adjective correlates)
Neuroticism	Anxiety (anxious, fearful, worrying)
	Angry hostility (anxious, irritable, impatient)
	Depression (worrying, –contented, –confident)
	Self-consciousness (shy, –self-confident, timid)
	Impulsiveness (moody, irritable, sarcastic)
	Vulnerability (–clear-thinking, –self-confident, –confident)
Extraversion	Warmth (friendly, warm, sociable)
	Gregariousness (sociable, outgoing, pleasure-seeking)
	Assertiveness (aggressive, –shy, assertive)
	Activity (energetic, hurried, quick)
	Excitement-seeking (pleasure-seeking, daring, adventurous)
	Positive emotions (enthusiastic, humorous, praising)
Openness	Fantasy (dreamy, imaginative, humorous)
	Aesthetics (imaginative, artistic, original)
	Feelings (excitable, hurried, quick)
	Actions (interests wide, imaginative, adventurous)
	Ideas (idealistic, interests wide, inventive)
	Values (–conservative, unconventional, –cautious)
Agreeableness	Trust (forgiving, trusting, –suspicious)
	Straightforwardness (–complicated, –demanding, –clever)
	Altruism (warm, soft-hearted, gentle)
	Compliance (–stubborn, –demanding, –headstrong)
	Modesty (–show-off, –clever, –assertive)
	Tender-mindedness (friendly, warm, sympathetic)
Conscientious-ness	Competence (efficient, self-confident, thorough)
	Order (organized, thorough, efficient)
	Dutifulness (–defensive, –distractible, –careless)
	Achievement-striving (thorough, ambitious, industrious)
	Self-disciplined (organized, –lazy, efficient)
	Deliberation (–hasty, –impulsive, –careless)

Note. Minus signs before adjectives indicate negative correlations with the facet scale.
Source. Adapted with permission from McCrae RR, Costa PT Jr: "Discriminant Validity of NEO PI-R Facet Scales," in *Education and Psychological Measurement* 52:229–237, 1992.

State Versus Trait

Another potential problem in personality disorder assessment is that the presence of an Axis I disorder can complicate the assessment of Axis II traits. For example, a person with social withdrawal, low self-esteem, and lack of motivation or energy due to major depression might appear to have avoidant or dependent personality disorder, when in fact these features reflect the Axis I condition. Or a hypomanic person with symptoms of grandiosity or hypersexuality might appear narcissistic or histrionic. In some cases, assessment of Axis II disorders may need to wait until the Axis I condition, such as florid psychosis or mania, has subsided. However, the clinician can often differentiate personality traits from Axis I states during an Axis I episode by asking the patient to describe his or her usual personality outside Axis I episodes; the use of informants who have observed the patient over time and without an Axis I disorder can be helpful. Prior systematic assessment of Axis I conditions is invaluable in terms of alerting the clinician to which Axis II traits will need particularly careful assessment. This task can be very difficult, however, in patients with Axis I conditions that are chronic and of early onset.

Medical Illness Versus Trait

Similarly, the interviewer must ascertain that what appear to be personality traits are not symptoms of a medical illness. For example, aggressive outbursts caused by a seizure disorder should not be attributed to borderline or antisocial personality disorder; nor should the unusual perceptual experiences that can accompany temporal lobe epilepsy be attributed to schizotypal personality disorder. A medical evaluation should be included in a thorough patient assessment.

Situation Versus Trait

The interviewer should also ascertain that personality disorder features are pervasive—that is, not limited to only one situation or occurring in response to only one specific trigger. Similarly, these features should be enduring rather than transient. Asking the patient for behavioral examples of traits can help determine that the trait is indeed present in a wide variety of situations and is expressed in many relationships.

Sex and Cultural Bias

Although most research suggests that existing personality disorder criteria are relatively free of sex bias, interviewers can unknowingly allow such bias to affect their assess-

TABLE 19–3. The seven-factor model of personality: temperament and character inventory

Temperament	Descriptors of extreme variants		Character	Descriptors of extreme variants	
	High	Low		High	Low
Harm avoidance	Pessimistic	Optimistic	Self-directedness	Responsible	Blaming
	Fearful	Daring		Purposeful	Aimless
	Shy	Outgoing		Resourceful	Inept
	Fatigable	Energetic		Self-accepting	Vain
				Disciplined	Undisciplined
Novelty seeking	Exploratory	Reserved	Cooperative	Tender hearted	Intolerant
	Impulsive	Rigid		Empathic	Insensitive
	Extravagant	Frugal		Helpful	Hostile
	Irritable	Stoic		Compassionate	Revengeful
				Principled	Opportunistic
Reward dependence	Sentimental	Critical	Self-transcendent	Self-forgetful	Unimaginative
	Open	Aloof		Transpersonal	Controlling
	Warm	Detached		Spiritual	Materialistic
	Sympathetic	Independent		Enlightened	Possessive
				Idealistic	Practical
Persistence	Industrious	Lazy			
	Determined	Spoiled			
	Ambitious	Underachieving			
	Perfectionistic	Pragmatic			

Source. Adapted with permission from Cloninger CR: "The Genetics and Psychobiology of the Seven-Factor Model of Personality," in *Biology of Personality Disorders.* Edited by Silk KR. Washington, DC, American Psychiatric Press, 1998, pp. 63–92. Copyright 1998 American Psychiatric Press.

ments. It is important, for example, that histrionic, borderline, and dependent personality disorders be assessed as carefully in men as in women and that obsessive-compulsive, antisocial, and narcissistic personality disorders be assessed as carefully in women as in men. Interviewers should also be careful to avoid cultural bias when diagnosing personality disorders, especially when evaluating such traits as promiscuity, suspiciousness, or recklessness, which may have different norms in different cultures.

Diagnosing Personality Disorders in Children and Adolescents

Because the personality of children and adolescents is still developing, personality disorders should be diagnosed with care in this age group. It is in fact often preferable to defer these diagnoses until late adolescence or early adulthood, at which time a personality disorder diagnosis may be appropriate if the features appear to be pervasive, stable, and likely to be enduring. The diagnosis, however, may prove to be wrong as any stage-specific difficulties of adolescence resolve and as the person further matures.

Etiology and Pathogenesis

What causes personality disorders is the most enigmatic and challenging question pertaining to this group of complex disorders. As was described in the section on the history of personality disorders, various hypotheses have been formulated over the years. Psychoanalytic theory has tended to emphasize the contribution of developmental and environmental factors, such as pathological or inadequate parenting, whereas neurobiological perspectives have emphasized genetic, constitutional, or biological factors.

As is the case with other psychiatric disorders, the answer is not likely to be simple. It is unlikely that any personality disorder has a single cause, whether environmental (e.g., childhood abuse) or biological (e.g., a single gene). Rather, available data suggest that personality disorders (as well as normal personality traits) result from a complex combination of, and interaction between, temperament (genetic and other biological factors) and psychological (developmental or environmental) factors (Paris 1993). Although the degree to which genetic and environmental factors contribute to etiology may vary for different personality disorders, the first major twin study

TABLE 19–4. Features of interviews and self-report instruments for the assessment of personality disorders

Interview or instrument	Author	Type	Special features
Structured Interview for DSM-IV Personality Disorders (SIDP)	Pfohl et al. 1994	Interview	Patient and informant questions
Personality Disorders Examination (PDE)	Loranger 1988	Interview	Detailed instruction manual
Structured Clinical Interview for DSM-IV Personality Disorders (SCID-II)	First et al. 1996	Interview	Axis I section; Axis II screening questionnaire
Diagnostic Interview for DSM-IV Personality Disorders (DIPD)	Zanarini et al. 1996	Interview	Good test–retest reliability
Personality Interview Questions—II (PIQ-II)	Widiger 1987	Interview	Nine-point scale for traits and behaviors
Personality Diagnostic Questionnaire—4+ (PDQ-4+)	Hyler et al. 1994	Self-report	Face-valid items
Millon Clinical Multiaxial Inventory—III (MCMI-III)	Millon 1994	Self-report	Dimensions of Axis I and Axis II psychopathology
Wisconsin Personality Inventory (Revised) (WPI-R)	M. Klein 1990	Self-report	Integrates structural analysis of social behavior model[a]
Schedule for Nonadaptive and Adaptive Personality (SNAP)	Clark 1990	Self-report	Normal and abnormal personality measures

Note. All instruments listed assess the full range of personality disorders. Other instruments are available to assess certain individual personality disorders.
[a]See Benjamin 1974.
Source. Adapted from Skodol and Oldham 1991.

indicates that both factors are important in all of these disorders (Torgersen et al. 2000). Of relevance, too, are studies showing that approximately half the observed variance in personality traits such as neuroticism, introversion, and submissiveness can be traced to genetic variation (Carey and DiLalla 1994; Tellegen et al. 1988).

Investigation of the underlying neurobiology of these disorders is rapidly increasing. A growing body of evidence supports the importance of various neurobiological abnormalities in persons with schizotypal personality disorder; alterations in brain structure and function have been shown to be related to deficitlike symptoms, and increased dopaminergic function to psychosislike symptoms. Abnormalities in the serotonin system, which appears to mediate behavioral inhibition, have been found in individuals with borderline and antisocial personality disorders. The finding (which requires replication) that neuroticism is influenced by two alleles of a gene encoding a transporter for serotonin (Lesch et al. 1996) is an example of the groundbreaking work being done in this important area.

Increasing numbers of studies of environmental antecedents of personality disorders, such as family environment and sexual and physical abuse, are substantiating a likely role for such factors in the development of certain disorders, particularly borderline personality disorder

(Zanarini 1997). In addition, defense mechanisms appear to play an important role in the expression of personality disorders, which are characterized by less mature defense mechanisms such as projection and acting out (Vaillant 1994). Research in these areas is expected to continue to increase rapidly. In addition to providing information about the origins of the personality disorders, such findings are expected to open new avenues for treating these often difficult-to-treat patients.

Treatment

Because personality disorders consist of deeply ingrained attitudes and behavior patterns that consolidate during development and have endured since early adulthood, they have always been believed to be very resistant to change. Moreover, as previously noted, treatment efforts are further confounded by the degree to which patients with a personality disorder do not recognize their maladaptive personality traits as undesirable or needing to be changed. Although these reasons have fostered a general wariness about the treatability of patients with personality disorders, there is increasing evidence from longitudinal studies that personality disorders are quite variable in their course and much more malleable than had been thought (Grilo et al. 1999).

Psychoanalysts pioneered the hope that persons with personality disorders could respond to treatment. The original conception of neurosis as a discrete set of symptoms related to a discrete developmental phase or to discrete conflicts was gradually replaced by the idea that more enduring defensive styles and identification processes were the building blocks of character traits. From this perspective, Wilhelm Reich (1949) and others developed the concepts of *character analysis* and *defense analysis*. These processes refer to an analyst's efforts to address the ways in which a person resists learning or the confrontations by which the analyst draws attention to the maladaptive effects of the patient's character traits (i.e., his or her usual interpersonal and behavioral style). A parallel development in technique evolved from group therapy experience. Maxwell Jones (1953) identified the value of confrontations delivered within group settings in which peer pressure made it difficult for patients to ignore feedback or to leave the group. Here, too, a primary goal of treatment was to render more dystonic the ego-syntonic but maladaptive aspects of the patient's interpersonal and behavioral style. This general principle was subsequently adopted by other forms of sociotherapies, notably those within hospital milieus and family therapies.

Families or couples may present complications insofar as the designated patient's disordered interpersonal and behavioral patterns may serve functions for, or be complementary to, the disordered patterns of persons with whom the patient is closely associated. For example, a dependent person is apt to bond with an overly authoritarian partner, or an emotionally constricted obsessional person may find an emotionally expressive, hysterical person particularly compatible. Under these circumstances, treatment is primarily directed not at confronting the maladaptive aspects of one person's character traits but rather at identifying the way in which these aspects may be welcomed and reinforced in one setting but maladaptive and impairing in others.

Significant developments in the treatment of personality disorders involve the use of multiple modalities, the growth of an empirical base, and greater optimism about treatment effectiveness. The overall development of treatment strategies for personality disorders has involved a movement away from therapeutic nihilism to the present widespread but still inconsistent use of a full spectrum of treatment modalities. A review of psychotherapy outcome studies, including psychodynamic/ interpersonal, cognitive-behavioral, mixed, and supportive therapies, found that psychotherapy was associated with a significantly faster rate of recovery compared with the natural course of personality disorders (Perry et al. 1999).

An overview of our knowledge about the potential usefulness of the three major types of psychiatric treatment—psychotherapies, sociotherapies, and pharmacotherapies—is provided in Table 19–5. It is expected that use of these therapies will increasingly be guided by more specific and empirically based information on which modalities, in what sequence, are most effective for treatment of each personality disorder.

One of the most significant developments has been the use of cognitive-behavioral strategies. These strategies generally are more focused and structured than psychodynamic therapies. They typically involve efforts to diminish traits such as impulsivity or to increase assertiveness by using relaxation techniques, role-playing exercises, and other behavioral strategies. Cognitive strategies involve first identifying specific internal mental schemes by which patients typically misunderstand certain situations or misrepresent themselves, and then learning how to modify those internal schemes.

In the past decade, the use of pharmacotherapy for personality disorders has begun to be explored. To the prospect of using specific medications for specific disorders has been added that of identifying biological dimensions of personality psychopathology that may respond to different medication classes (Cloninger 1987; Coccaro and Kavoussi 1997; Siever and Davis 1991). For example, research has increasingly suggested that impulsivity and aggression may respond to serotonergic medications; mood instability and lability may respond to serotonergic medications, other antidepressants, and mood stabilizers; and psychosislike experiences may respond to antipsychotics (Coccaro and Kavoussi 1997; Cornelius et al. 1993; Soloff et al. 1993).

TABLE 19–5. Evidence of treatment effectiveness for personality disorders

	ST	SZ	P	B	AS	H	N	OC	D	AV
Psychotherapies	–	+	–	+	–	++	++	++	++	++
Sociotherapies	±	+	–	++	+	–	–	–	+	+
Pharmacotherapies	+	–	±	+	–	–	–	–	–	±

Note. – = no support; ± = uncertain support; + = modestly helpful; ++ = significantly helpful. ST = schizotypal; SZ = schizoid; P = paranoid; B = borderline; AS = antisocial; H = histrionic; N = narcissistic; OC = obsessive-compulsive; D = dependent; AV = avoidant.

Specific Personality Disorders

Paranoid Personality Disorder

History

Paranoid personality disorder has been richly and consistently represented in this century's descriptive psychiatric literature. It was described by Mayer, Koch, Kraepelin, Bleuler, Kretschmer, and Schneider under such rubrics as the "pseudoquerulent type" and the "fanatic psychopath" (Millon 1981). This disorder has, however, received less attention in the psychoanalytic literature than have many other personality disorders.

Paranoid personality disorder is one of the few personality disorders to have been included in every version of DSM, and its description has consistently focused on the disorder's central feature of a pervasive and unwarranted mistrust of others (Bernstein et al. 1993).

Clinical Features

Persons with paranoid personality disorder have a pervasive, persistent, and inappropriate mistrust of others (Table 19–6). They are suspicious of others' motives and assume that others intend to harm, exploit, or trick them. Thus, they may question, without justification, the loyalty or trustworthiness of friends or sexual partners, and they are reluctant to confide in others for fear the information will be used against them. Persons with paranoid personality disorder appear guarded, tense, and hypervigilant, and they frequently scan their environment for clues of possible attack, deception, or betrayal. They often find "evidence" of such malevolence by misinterpreting benign events (such as a glance in their direction) as demeaning or threatening. In response to perceived or actual insults or betrayals, these individuals overreact, quickly becoming excessively angry and responding with counterattacking behavior. They are unable to forgive or forget such incidents and instead bear long-term grudges against their supposed betrayers; some persons with paranoid personality disorder are litigious. Whereas some individuals with this disorder appear quietly and tensely aloof and hostile, others are overtly angry and combative. Persons with this disorder are usually socially isolated and, because of their paranoia, often have difficulties with co-workers.

Differential Diagnosis

Unlike paranoid personality disorder, the Axis I disorders paranoid schizophrenia and delusional disorder, paranoid type, are both characterized by prominent and persistent

TABLE 19–6. DSM-IV-TR diagnostic criteria for paranoid personality disorder

A. A pervasive distrust and suspiciousness of others such that their motives are interpreted as malevolent, beginning by early adulthood and present in a variety of contexts, as indicated by four (or more) of the following:

(1) suspects, without sufficient basis, that others are exploiting, harming, or deceiving him or her

(2) is preoccupied with unjustified doubts about the loyalty or trustworthiness of friends or associates

(3) is reluctant to confide in others because of unwarranted fear that the information will be used maliciously against him or her

(4) reads hidden demeaning or threatening meanings into benign remarks or events

(5) persistently bears grudges, i.e., is unforgiving of insults, injuries, or slights

(6) perceives attacks on his or her character or reputation that are not apparent to others and is quick to react angrily or to counterattack

(7) has recurrent suspicions, without justification, regarding fidelity of spouse or sexual partner

B. Does not occur exclusively during the course of schizophrenia, a mood disorder with psychotic features, or another psychotic disorder and is not due to the direct physiological effects of a general medical condition.

Note: If criteria are met prior to the onset of schizophrenia, add "premorbid," e.g., "paranoid personality disorder (premorbid)."

paranoid delusions of psychotic proportions; paranoid schizophrenia is also accompanied by hallucinations and other core symptoms of schizophrenia. Although paranoid and schizotypal personality disorders both involve suspiciousness, paranoid personality disorder does not entail perceptual distortions and eccentric behavior.

Etiology

Some theories suggest that paranoid personality disorder originates from having been the object of excessive parental rage or from having been repeatedly humiliated by others. Either type of experience could lead to feelings of inadequacy and vulnerability, followed by projection onto others of hostility and rage, as well as a tendency to blame others for one's shortcomings and problems. The defense mechanism of projection is generally assumed to be involved in the expression of this disorder's features (Vaillant 1992).

It seems likely that paranoid personality disorder has biogenetic contributions. Early in this century, Kraepelin (1921) theorized that this personality disorder was the premorbid character type of persons predisposed to paranoia (now known as Axis I delusional disorder). An association between these two disorders has received some support from family history studies that found a greater morbid risk of paranoid personality disorder in the first-degree relatives of delusional disorder probands than in relatives of probands with schizophrenia or medical illness (Kendler and Gruenberg 1982). Such a link implicates the involvement of both environmental and constitutional factors in the etiology of paranoid personality disorder.

Treatment

Because they mistrust others, persons with paranoid personality disorder usually avoid psychiatric treatment. If they do seek treatment, the therapist immediately encounters the challenge of engaging them and keeping them in treatment. This can best be accomplished by maintaining an unusually respectful, straightforward, and unintrusive style aimed at building trust. If a problem develops in the treatment relationship—for example, the patient accuses the therapist of some fault—it is best simply to offer a straightforward apology, if warranted, rather than to respond evasively or defensively. It is also best to avoid an overly warm style, because excessive warmth and expression of interest can exacerbate the patient's paranoid tendencies. A supportive psychotherapy that incorporates such an approach may be the best treatment for these patients.

Although group treatment or cognitive-behavioral treatment (Turkat and Maisto 1985) aimed at anxiety management and the development of social skills might be of benefit, these patients, because of their suspiciousness and fears of losing control and being criticized, tend to resist such approaches.

Antipsychotic medications are sometimes useful in the treatment of this disorder. Patients may view such treatment with mistrust; however, these medications are particularly indicated in the treatment of the overtly psychotic decompensations that these patients sometimes experience.

Schizoid Personality Disorder

History

Schizoid personality disorder was originally conceptualized as the personality type associated with schizophrenia—a role that is now largely assumed by schizotypal personality disorder. As such, during the early part of this century, schizoid personality disorder as a traitlike variant of schizophrenia was described by Hoch (1910) as the "shut-in personality," by Bleuler (1922) as "schizoidie,"

and by Kraepelin (1919) as "autistic personality." A similar personality type was also described in the psychoanalytic literature by the object relations theorists Fairbairn (1940/1952) and Guntrip (1971), who used the term in a broader fashion to describe socially withdrawn patients who had difficulties with intimacy and some of those behavioral peculiarities now subsumed by schizotypal personality disorder.

Schizoid personality disorder has been included in every version of DSM, but its meaning has varied significantly in the different DSM editions (Kalus et al. 1993). Broadly defined in DSM-I and DSM-II, the category was later divided into the schizoid, avoidant, and schizotypal types of personality disorder.

Clinical Features

Schizoid personality disorder is characterized by a profound defect in the ability to relate to others in a meaningful way (Table 19–7). Persons with this disorder have little or no desire for relationships with others and, as a result, are extremely socially isolated. They prefer to engage in solitary, often intellectual, activities, such as computer games or puzzles, and they often create an elaborate fantasy world into which they retreat and which substitutes for relationships with others. As a result of their lack of interest in relationships, they have few or no close friends or confidants. They date infrequently and seldom marry, and they often work at jobs requiring little interpersonal interaction (e.g., in a laboratory). These individuals are also notable for their lack of affect. They usually appear cold, detached, aloof, and constricted, and they have particular discomfort when experiencing warm feelings. Few, if any, activities or experiences give them pleasure, which is reflected in their chronic anhedonia.

Differential Diagnosis

Schizoid personality disorder shares the features of social isolation and restricted emotional expression with schizotypal personality disorder, but it lacks the latter disorder's characteristics of cognitive and perceptual distortion. Unlike individuals with avoidant personality disorder, who intensely desire relationships but avoid them because of exaggerated fears of rejection, persons with schizoid personality disorder have little or no interest in developing relationships with others.

Etiology

Clinicians have noted that schizoid personality disorder occurs in adults who experienced cold, neglectful, and

TABLE 19–7. DSM-IV-TR criteria for schizoid personality disorder

A. A pervasive pattern of detachment from social relationships and a restricted range of expression of emotions in interpersonal settings, beginning by early adulthood and present in a variety of contexts, as indicated by four (or more) of the following:

  (1) neither desires nor enjoys close relationships, including being part of a family
  (2) almost always chooses solitary activities
  (3) has little, if any, interest in having sexual experiences with another person
  (4) takes pleasure in few, if any, activities
  (5) lacks close friends or confidants other than first-degree relatives
  (6) appears indifferent to the praise or criticism of others
  (7) shows emotional coldness, detachment, or flattened affectivity

B. Does not occur exclusively during the course of schizophrenia, a mood disorder with psychotic features, another psychotic disorder, or a pervasive developmental disorder and is not due to the direct physiological effects of a general medical condition.

Note: If criteria are met prior to the onset of schizophrenia, add "premorbid," e.g., "schizoid personality disorder (premorbid)."

ungratifying relationships in early childhood, which leads these persons to assume that relationships are not valuable or worth pursuing. There is reason to believe that constitutional factors contribute to the childhood pattern of shyness that often precedes the disorder. Introversion, which characterizes schizoid (as well as avoidant and schizotypal) personality disorder, appears to be highly heritable. Although family history studies give stronger support to a link between schizophrenia and schizotypal personality disorder, some studies suggest an association of schizophrenia with schizoid personality disorder, which would implicate the importance of genetic factors in the latter disorder's etiology.

Treatment

Persons with schizoid personality disorder, like those with schizotypal personality disorder, rarely seek treatment. They do not perceive the formation of any relationship—including a therapeutic relationship—as potentially valuable or beneficial. They may, however, occasionally seek treatment for an associated problem, such as depression, or they may be brought for treatment by others. Whereas some patients can tolerate only a supportive therapy or treatment aimed at the resolu-

tion of a crisis or associated Axis I disorder, others do well with insight-oriented psychotherapy aimed at effecting a basic shift in their comfort with intimacy and affects.

Development of a therapeutic alliance may be difficult and can be facilitated by an interested and caring attitude and an avoidance of early interpretation or confrontation. Some authors have suggested the use of so-called inanimate bridges, such as writing and artistic productions, to ease the patient into the therapy relationship. Incorporation of cognitive-behavioral approaches that encourage gradually increasing social involvement may be of value (Liebowitz et al. 1986). Although many patients may be unwilling to participate in a group, group therapy may also facilitate the development of social skills and relationships.

Schizotypal Personality Disorder

History

Early concepts, like current concepts, of schizotypal personality disorder were linked to schizophrenia. Bleuler's (1922) concept of latent schizophrenia, which consisted of mild or attenuated schizophrenia symptoms without deterioration into psychosis, was one of the major clinical forerunners of schizotypal personality disorder. The term *schizotype*, coined by Rado (1956), denoted a nonpsychotic phenotypic variant of the schizophrenia genome. This term was later used as an alternative label for the "borderline schizophrenia" syndrome identified in Danish adoption studies, which was a milder schizophrenia-like disorder present in the biological relatives of schizophrenic probands (Kety et al. 1968).

Schizotypal personality disorder was new to DSM-III and was based on the characteristics of the relatives (i.e., the "schizotypes") identified in the Danish adoption studies. An additional impetus for its addition to DSM-III was the concern that the schizoid and borderline personality disorder constructs were too broadly defined (Siever et al. 1991).

Clinical Features

Persons with schizotypal personality disorder experience cognitive or perceptual distortions, behave in an eccentric manner, and are socially inept and anxious (Table 19–8). Their cognitive and perceptual distortions include ideas of reference, bodily illusions, and unusual telepathic and clairvoyant experiences. These distortions, which are inconsistent with subcultural norms, occur frequently and are an important and pervasive component of the person's experience. They are in keeping with the odd

TABLE 19–8. DSM-IV-TR criteria for schizotypal personality disorder

A. A pervasive pattern of social and interpersonal deficits marked by acute discomfort with, and reduced capacity for, close relationships as well as by cognitive or perceptual distortions and eccentricities of behavior, beginning by early adulthood and present in a variety of contexts, as indicated by five (or more) of the following:

  (1) ideas of reference (excluding delusions of reference)

  (2) odd beliefs or magical thinking that influences behavior and is inconsistent with subcultural norms (e.g., superstitiousness, belief in clairvoyance, telepathy, or "sixth sense"; in children and adolescents, bizarre fantasies or preoccupations)

  (3) unusual perceptual experiences, including bodily illusions

  (4) odd thinking and speech (e.g., vague, circumstantial, metaphorical, overelaborate, or stereotyped)

  (5) suspiciousness or paranoid ideation

  (6) inappropriate or constricted affect

  (7) behavior or appearance that is odd, eccentric, or peculiar

  (8) lack of close friends or confidants other than first-degree relatives

  (9) excessive social anxiety that does not diminish with familiarity and tends to be associated with paranoid fears rather than negative judgments about self

B. Does not occur exclusively during the course of schizophrenia, a mood disorder with psychotic features, another psychotic disorder, or a pervasive developmental disorder.

Note: If criteria are met prior to the onset of schizophrenia, add "premorbid," e.g., "schizotypal personality disorder (premorbid)."

and eccentric behavior characteristic of this disorder. These individuals may, for example, talk to themselves in public, gesture for no apparent reason, or dress in a peculiar or unkempt fashion. Their speech is often odd and idiosyncratic—unusually circumstantial, metaphorical, or vague, for instance—and their affect is constricted or inappropriate. Such a person may, for example, laugh inappropriately when discussing his or her problems.

Persons with schizotypal personality disorder are socially uncomfortable and isolated, and they have few friends. This isolation is often due to their eccentric cognitions and behavior as well as their lack of desire for relationships, which stems in part from their suspiciousness of others. If they develop a relationship, they tend to remain distant or may even terminate it because of their persistent social anxiety and paranoia.

Differential Diagnosis

Schizotypal personality disorder shares the feature of suspiciousness with paranoid personality disorder and that of social isolation with schizoid personality disorder, but these latter two disorders lack the markedly peculiar behavior and significant cognitive and perceptual distortions typically present in schizotypal personality disorder. Schizotypal personality disorder, although on a spectrum with Axis I schizophrenia, lacks enduring overt psychosis.

Etiology

Schizotypal personality disorder is a schizophrenia spectrum disorder—that is, it is related to Axis I schizophrenia. Phenomenological, biological, genetic, treatment response, and outcome data support this link. For example, family history studies show an increased risk for schizophrenia-related disorders in relatives of schizotypal probands and, conversely, an increased risk for schizotypal personality disorder in relatives of schizophrenia probands (Kendler et al. 1993; Torgersen et al. 1993). In addition, at least some forms of schizotypal personality disorder involve biological abnormalities characteristic of schizophrenia—for example, an increased ventricular–brain ratio on computed tomography scan (Wei et al. 1997); increased cerebrospinal fluid volume not attributable to ventricular volume (Dickey et al. 2000); higher cerebrospinal fluid homovanillic acid concentrations (Siever et al. 1993); impaired smooth-pursuit eye movements; and impaired performance on tests of executive function and other tests of visual or auditory attention, such as the Wisconsin Card Sorting Test, the backward masking task, the continuous performance task, and sensory gating tests, suggesting altered precortical functioning (Siever et al. 1991; Trestman et al. 1995). They have also been shown to have deficits on verbal learning and memory tasks (Bergman et al. 1998; Voglmaier et al. 2000), attention-orienting tasks (Raine et al. 1997), and instrumental motor tasks (Cadenhead et al. 2000; Neumann and Walker 1999).

Because of this evidence, schizotypal personality disorder is classified in ICD-10 with schizophrenia rather than with the personality disorders. However, it may be that certain subtypes of this personality disorder are not related to schizophrenia—a reflection of the fact that schizotypal personality disorder's DSM definition has been modified over time to better reflect clinical impressions of a syndrome characterized by cognitive, perceptual, and behavioral eccentricities and to better differentiate it from near-neighbor personality disorders. It is not clear whether those variants of schizotypal personality disorder that are related to schizophrenia represent a milder, traitlike, nonpsychotic variant of schizophrenia or whether they in fact constitute schizophrenia's core features, on which the more florid psychotic episodes of schizophrenia can be superimposed.

Treatment

Because they are socially anxious and somewhat paranoid, persons with schizotypal personality disorder usually avoid psychiatric treatment. They may, however, seek such treatment—or be brought for treatment by concerned family members—when they become depressed or overtly psychotic. As with patients with paranoid personality disorder, it is difficult to establish an alliance with schizotypal patients, and they are unlikely to tolerate exploratory techniques that emphasize interpretation or confrontation. A supportive relationship that counters cognitive distortions and ego-boundary problems may be useful (Stone 1985). This may involve an educational approach that fosters the development of social skills or encourages risk-taking behavior in social situations, or, if these efforts fail, encourages the development of activities with less social involvement. If the patient is willing to participate, cognitive-behavioral therapy and highly structured educational groups with a social skills focus may also be helpful.

Several case series support the usefulness of low-dose antipsychotic medications in the treatment of schizotypal personality disorder (Goldberg et al. 1986; Serban and Siegel 1984). These medications may ameliorate the anxiety and psychosis-like features associated with this disorder, and they are particularly indicated in the treatment of the more overt psychotic decompensations that these patients can experience. In addition, results of an open-label trial suggested that fluoxetine may also diminish features of schizotypal personality disorder (Markovitz et al. 1991).

Antisocial Personality Disorder

History

Pritchard (1835) used the term *moral insanity* to describe people with a pattern of repeated immoral behaviors for which they were not fully responsible. The disorder he characterized has been described by many other psychiatric luminaries under a variety of labels (Millon 1981). Even as psychiatry has decried the use of this diagnosis for excusing antisocial acts, it has been steadfast in recognizing that such persons have significant psychological impairment.

By the late nineteenth century, the term *psychopathic personality* had become a broadly applicable category for persons with socially undesirable character traits. Harvey Cleckley's 1941 definition of the psychopath (Cleckley 1964) heavily influenced the DSM-I and DSM-II definitions of antisocial personality, whereas the definitions of antisocial personality in DSM-III and DSM-III-R rested on the empirical work of Robins (1966). The DSM-III and DSM-III-R definitions consisted of an established pattern of conduct disorder in childhood as well as a set of socially noxious behaviors (e.g., arrests, truancy, and assaultiveness) occurring in adulthood. These definitions had the assets of being explicitly behavioral and of permitting reliable assessment but had the liabilities of being cumbersome and too specific to Western culture. On the basis of empirical evidence, in DSM-IV the Robins behaviorally based version is combined with Cleckley's personologic traits to bring the disorder's definition back in line with clinical observations and with personality trait–based descriptions.

Clinical Features

The central characteristic of antisocial personality disorder is a long-standing pattern of socially irresponsible behaviors that reflects a disregard for the rights of others (Table 19–9). Many persons with this disorder engage in repetitive unlawful acts. The more prevailing personality characteristics include a lack of interest in or concern for the feelings of others, deceitfulness, and, most notably, a lack of remorse over the harm they may cause others. These characteristics generally make these individuals fail in roles requiring fidelity (e.g., as a spouse or a parent), honesty (e.g., as an employee), or reliability in any social role. Some antisocial persons possess a glibness and charm that can be used to seduce, outwit, and exploit others. Although most antisocial persons are indifferent to their effects on others, a notable subgroup takes sadistic pleasure in being harmful. Antisocial personality disorder is associated with high rates of substance abuse (Dinwiddie et al. 1992).

Differential Diagnosis

The primary differential diagnostic issue involves narcissistic personality disorder. Indeed, these two disorders may be variants of the same basic type of psychopathology (Hare et al. 1991). However, the antisocial person, unlike the narcissistic person, is likely to be reckless and impulsive. In addition, narcissistic individuals' exploitiveness and disregard for others are attributable to their sense of uniqueness and superiority rather than to a desire for materialistic gains.

Etiology

Twin and adoptive studies indicate that genetic factors predispose to the development of antisocial personality

TABLE 19–9. DSM-IV-TR criteria for antisocial personality disorder

A. There is a pervasive pattern of disregard for and violation of the rights of others occurring since age 15 years, as indicated by three (or more) of the following:

(1) failure to conform to social norms with respect to lawful behaviors as indicated by repeatedly performing acts that are grounds for arrest

(2) deceitfulness, as indicated by repeated lying, use of aliases, or conning others for personal profit or pleasure

(3) impulsivity or failure to plan ahead

(4) irritability and aggressiveness, as indicated by repeated physical fights or assaults

(5) reckless disregard for safety of self or others

(6) consistent irresponsibility, as indicated by repeated failure to sustain consistent work behavior or honor financial obligations

(7) lack of remorse, as indicated by being indifferent to or rationalizing having hurt, mistreated, or stolen from another

B. The individual is at least age 18 years.

C. There is evidence of conduct disorder with onset before age 15 years.

D. The occurrence of antisocial behavior is not exclusively during the course of schizophrenia or a manic episode.

---

disorder (Grove et al. 1990; Lyons et al. 1995). Nonetheless, it is unclear how much variance is accounted for by genetic factors and whether the nature of the predisposition is relatively specific or is best conceptualized in terms of relatively nonspecific traits such as impulsivity, excitability, or hostility (Widiger et al. 1992). Growing evidence indicates that the impulsive and aggressive behaviors may be mediated by abnormal serotonin transporter functioning in the brain (Coccaro et al. 1996). It is clear that the early family life of these persons often poses severe environmental handicaps in the form of absent, assaultive, or inconsistent parenting. Indeed, many family members also have significant action-oriented psychopathology such as substance abuse or antisocial personality disorder itself. Notably, children who have seen a sibling treated harshly (in ways that might render the sibling likely to engage in antisocial behavior) may learn inhibitions and civility, and thus the exposure may have protective effects on them (Reiss et al. 1995).

Treatment

It is clinically important to recognize antisocial personality disorder because an uncritical acceptance of these individuals' glib or shallow statements of good intentions and collaboration can permit them to have a disruptive influence on treatment teams and other patients. However, there is little evidence to suggest that this disorder can be successfully treated by usual psychiatric interventions. Of interest, nonetheless, are reports suggesting that in confined settings, such as the military or prisons, depressive and introspective concerns may surface (Vaillant 1975). Under these circumstances, confrontation by peers may bring about changes in the antisocial person's social behaviors. It is also notable that some antisocial patients demonstrate an ability to form a therapeutic alliance with psychotherapists, which augurs well for these patients' future course (Woody et al. 1985). These findings contrast with the clinical tradition that emphasizes such persons' inability to learn from harmful consequences. Yet longitudinal follow-up studies have shown that the prevalence of this disorder diminishes with age as these individuals become more aware of the social and interpersonal maladaptiveness of their most noxious social behaviors.

Borderline Personality Disorder

History

The borderline personality disorder construct originated from the observations of psychoanalytic psychotherapists who were impressed by these patients' demanding search for nurturance, their disregard for the usual boundaries of therapy, and their tendency to regress in unstructured situations. Impelled by the clinical importance of foreseeing such problems and by a new wave of psychotherapeutic optimism, empirical work was done to better define this disorder. This work raised the question of whether such patients had an atypical form of mood disorder rather than an atypical form of schizophrenia, as had been previously thought, and, more importantly, led to this disorder's inclusion in DSM-III.

The development of operationalized diagnostic criteria provoked an effusion of further empirical research that has led to revisions of this disorder's construct and informed its treatment (Gunderson et al. 1991a). Borderline personality disorder is the most widely studied personality disorder. It is also common, occurring in approximately 2%–3% of the population and in every culture. Evidence for its validity is growing, and the disorder is now recognized as the most prevalent Axis II disorder in all kinds of clinical settings (Gunderson 2001).

Clinical Features

Borderline personality disorder is characterized by instability and dysfunction in affective, behavioral, and interpersonal domains. Central to the psychopathology of this disorder are a severely impaired capacity for attachment and predictably maladaptive behavior patterns related to separation (Gunderson 1996). When borderline patients feel cared for, held on to, and supported, depressive features (notably loneliness and emptiness) are most evident (Table 19–10). When there is the threat of losing such a sustaining relationship, the idealized image of a beneficent caregiver is replaced by a devalued image of a cruel persecutor. This shift is called *splitting*. An impending separation also evokes intense abandonment fears. To minimize these fears and to prevent the separation, rageful accusations of mistreatment and cruelty and angry self-destructive behaviors may occur. These behaviors often elicit a guilty or fearful protective response from others.

Another central feature of this disorder is extreme affective instability that often leads to impulsive (Herpertz et al. 1997) and self-destructive (Kemperman et al. 1997) behaviors. These episodes are usually brief and reactive and involve extreme alternations between mood states. The experience and expression of anger can be particularly difficult for the borderline patient. During periods of unusual stress, dissociative experiences, ideas of reference, or desperate impulsive acts (including substance abuse and promiscuity) commonly occur.

Differential Diagnosis

Borderline patients' intense feelings of being bad or evil are distinctly different from the idealized self-image of narcissistic persons. Although patients with borderline personality disorder, like persons with antisocial personality disorder, may be reckless and impulsive, their behaviors are primarily interpersonally oriented and aimed toward obtaining support rather than materialistic gains.

Etiology

Psychoanalytic theories have emphasized the importance of early parent–child relationships in the etiology of borderline personality disorder. Such reports have emphasized maternal mismanagement of the 2- to 3-year-old child's efforts to become autonomous (Masterson 1972), exaggerated maternal frustration that aggravates the child's anger (Kernberg 1975), and inattention to the child's emotions and attitudes (Adler 1985). A considerable body of empirical research has embellished these theories by documenting a high frequency of traumatic early abandonment, physical abuse, and sexual abuse. These traumatic experiences appear to occur within a context of sustained neglect from which the pre-borderline child develops an enduring rage and self-hatred. The lack of reliably involved attachment during

TABLE 19–10. DSM-IV-TR criteria for borderline personality disorder

A pervasive pattern of instability of interpersonal relationships, self-image, and affects, and marked impulsivity beginning by early adulthood and present in a variety of contexts, as indicated by five (or more) of the following:

(1) frantic efforts to avoid real or imagined abandonment. **Note:** Do not include suicidal or self-mutilating behavior covered in Criterion 5.

(2) a pattern of unstable and intense interpersonal relationships characterized by alternating between extremes of idealization and devaluation

(3) identity disturbance: markedly and persistently unstable self-image or sense of self

(4) impulsivity in at least two areas that are potentially self-damaging (e.g., spending, sex, substance abuse, reckless driving, binge eating). **Note:** Do not include suicidal or self-mutilating behavior covered in Criterion 5.

(5) recurrent suicidal behavior, gestures, or threats, or self-mutilating behavior

(6) affective instability due to a marked reactivity of mood (e.g., intense episodic dysphoria, irritability, or anxiety usually lasting a few hours and only rarely more than a few days)

(7) chronic feelings of emptiness

(8) inappropriate, intense anger or difficulty controlling anger (e.g., frequent displays of temper, constant anger, recurrent physical fights)

(9) transient, stress-related paranoid ideation or severe dissociative symptoms

development is a source of borderline patients' inability to maintain a stable sense of themselves or of others without ongoing contact (i.e., their defects of object constancy or lack of stable introjects) (Gunderson 1996). Zanarini and Frankenburg (1997) proposed a tripartite causative model consisting of a traumatic childhood, a vulnerable temperament, and triggering events. The biosocial theory of borderline personality disorder suggests that a biological disposition toward emotional vulnerability, exposure to invalidating environments, and deficits in emotion-regulation skills are key etiological factors (Linehan 1993).

Twin study evidence of 69% heritability has mobilized efforts to identify the genetic sources of borderline traits. Siever and Davis (1991) posited that these traits consist of a combination of affective instability and impulsive aggression. There is evidence for serotonergic involvement in borderline traits (Coccaro and Kavoussi 1997; Siever and Davis 1991; Verkes et al. 1998). Although the etiology of borderline personality disorder has yet to be determined, it is likely multifactorial in origin.

Treatment

Borderline patients are high utilizers of psychiatric outpatient, inpatient, and psychopharmacologic treatment (Bender et al. 2001). The extensive literature on the treatment of borderline personality disorder universally notes the extreme difficulties that clinicians encounter with these patients. These problems derive from the patients' appeal to their treaters' nurturing qualities and their rageful accusations in response to their treaters' perceived failures. Often therapists develop intense countertransference reactions that lead them to attempt to re-parent or reject borderline patients. As a consequence, regardless of the treatment approach used, personal maturity and considerable clinical experience are important assets.

As a result of the work of Kernberg (1968) and Masterson (1972), much of the treatment literature has focused on the value of intensive exploratory psychotherapies directed at modifying borderline patients' basic character structure. However, this literature has increasingly suggested that improvement may be related not to the acquisition of insight but to the corrective experience of developing a stable, trusting relationship with a therapist who fails to retaliate in response to these patients' angry and disruptive behaviors. Paralleling this development has been the suggestion that supportive psychotherapies or group therapies may bring about similar changes. Recent evidence has provided support for the effectiveness of an 18-month psychoanalytic treatment program in a partial hospital setting (Bateman and Fonagy 1999). In addition, a long-term, phased model of psychodynamic therapy that combined hospital-based and community-based strategies was reported to be more effective than hospital-based treatment alone (Chiesa and Fonagy 2000).

Treatment of borderline patients has now expanded to include pharmacological and cognitive-behavioral interventions (American Psychiatric Association 2001). Although no one medication has been found to have dramatic or predictable effects, studies indicate that many medications may diminish specific problems such as impulsivity, affective lability, or intermittent cognitive and perceptual disturbances (Table 19–11), as well as irritability and aggressive behavior (Coccaro and Kavoussi 1997; Cornelius et al. 1993; Cowdry and Gardner 1988; Salzman et al. 1995; Soloff 1989; Soloff et al. 1993). Linehan et al. (1991) showed that behavioral treatment consisting of a once-weekly individual and twice-weekly group regimen can effectively diminish the self-destructive behaviors and hospitalization of borderline patients. The success and cost benefits of this treatment, called *dialectical behavior therapy*, have led to its rapid adoption and modification in a variety of settings. In general, the profusion of treatment modalities and the introduction of empiricism point toward the increasing use of more focused treatment strategies.

Histrionic Personality Disorder

History

The forerunner of histrionic personality disorder can be found in turn-of-the-century accounts of hysteria by Pierre Janet and Sigmund Freud. Janet was impressed with the role of actual seduction (or other trauma) in childhood, whereas Freud focused on the unconscious elaboration of the child's sexual drive (i.e., libido). Subsequent psychoanalytic observers noted that hysterical symptoms were often associated with a particular set of character traits, which led to the designation of a hysterical type of personality disorder in DSM-II.

The initial empirical examination of hysterical personality traits used factor-analytic methods, which helped consolidate this syndrome's components but also led to a broad definition (Lazare et al. 1970). Indeed, this disorder's early definitions were so broad that they rendered the diagnosis "meaningless" (Easser and Lesser 1965).

TABLE 19–11. Medication efficacy in borderline personality disorder

Medication	Mood	Suicidality/self-destructiveness	Impulsivity	Psychosislike features
Monoamine oxidase inhibitors	+	+	+	?
Serotonin reuptake inhibitors	++	++	++	+
Tricyclic antidepressants	±	±	±	±
Antipsychotics	+	+	+	++
Mood stabilizers	+	+	+	+
Benzodiazepines	±	−	−	?

Note. The information in this table should be considered tentative; some medications have received relatively little investigation, many medication trials have been small and open, and few of the medications listed have been directly compared with one another. + + = clear improvement; + = modest improvement; ± = variable improvement or worsening; − = some worsening. Most published studies of serotonin reuptake inhibitors have used fluoxetine.

The label *hysterical* was changed to the label *histrionic* in DSM-III in an effort to use a term that was more theoretically neutral and more in line with psychiatry's descriptive tradition. Whereas the term *hysterical personality* still connotes the conflicted eroticization of parental figures, the term *histrionic* that replaced it in DSM-III reflects the diagnostician's concern with the observable features of emotional instability and attention seeking. The DSM-III version of the operationalized criteria of this disorder largely captured its more severe "oral" and manipulative variants and thereby unintentionally magnified its overlap with other categories, such as borderline personality disorder (Pfohl 1991).

The modifications of DSM-III-R and DSM-IV helped distinguish this category from others and placed it within the range of less severe personality disorders that can be conceptualized as maladaptive variants of normally occurring traits. This view was reflected by Chodoff's (1982) suggestion that this disorder represents a caricature of stereotypic femininity.

Clinical Features

Central to histrionic personality disorder is an overconcern with attention and appearance (Table 19–12). Persons with this disorder spend an excessive amount of time seeking attention and making themselves attractive. The desire to be found attractive may lead to inappropriately seductive or provocative dress and flirtatious behavior, and the desire for attention may lead to other flamboyant acts or self-dramatizing behavior. All of these features reflect these persons' underlying insecurity about their value as anything other than a fetching companion. Persons with histrionic personality disorder also display an effusive but labile and suspiciously shallow range of feelings. They are often overly impressionistic and given to hyperbolic descriptions of others (e.g., "She's wonderful" or "She's horrible"). More generally, these persons do not attend to detail or facts, and they are reluctant or unable to make reasoned critical analyses of problems or situations. Persons with this disorder often present with complaints of depression, somatic problems of unclear origin, and a history of disappointing romantic relationships.

Differential Diagnosis

This disorder can be confused with dependent, borderline, and narcissistic personality disorders. Histrionic individuals are often willing, even eager, to have others make decisions and organize their activities for them. However, unlike persons with dependent personality disorder, histrionic persons are uninhibited and lively companions who willfully forgo appearing autonomous because they

TABLE 19–12. DSM-IV-TR criteria for histrionic personality disorder

A pervasive pattern of excessive emotionality and attention seeking, beginning by early adulthood and present in a variety of contexts, as indicated by five (or more) of the following:

(1) is uncomfortable in situations in which he or she is not the center of attention

(2) interaction with others is often characterized by inappropriate sexually seductive or provocative behavior

(3) displays rapidly shifting and shallow expression of emotions

(4) consistently uses physical appearance to draw attention to self

(5) has a style of speech that is excessively impressionistic and lacking in detail

(6) shows self-dramatization, theatricality, and exaggerated expression of emotion

(7) is suggestible, i.e., easily influenced by others or circumstances

(8) considers relationships to be more intimate than they actually are

believe that others desire this. Unlike persons with borderline personality disorder, they do not perceive themselves as bad, and they lack ongoing problems with rage or willful self-destructiveness. Persons with narcissistic personality disorder also seek attention to sustain their self-esteem but differ in that their self-esteem is characterized by grandiosity, and the attention they crave must be admiring—for example, unlike the histrionic person, they would not want to be described as "cute" or "silly."

Etiology

Psychoanalytic theory proposes that histrionic personality disorder originates in the oedipal phase of development (i.e., 3–5 years of age) when an overly eroticized relationship with the opposite-sex parent is unduly encouraged and the child fears that the consequences of this excitement will be the loss of, or retaliation by, the same-sex parent. This conflict results in lasting character formations of exaggerated fantasy and exhibitionistic promise with inhibited factual analysis and diminished actual productivity. Research suggests that qualities such as emotional expressiveness and attention seeking may be characteristics of a biogenetically determined temperament. From this perspective, histrionic personality disorder would be considered an extreme variant of a temperamental disposition, the environmental contributions of which may be less specific than those of the aforementioned theories.

Treatment

Individual psychodynamic psychotherapy, including psychoanalysis, remains the cornerstone of most treatment for persons with histrionic personality disorder. This treatment is directed at increasing patients' awareness of 1) how their self-esteem is maladaptively tied to their ability to attract attention at the expense of developing other skills, and 2) how their shallow relationships and emotional experience reflect unconscious fears of real commitments. Much of this increase in awareness occurs through analysis of the here-and-now doctor–patient relationship rather than through the reconstruction of childhood experiences. Therapists should be aware that the typical idealization and eroticization that such patients bring into treatment are the material for exploration, and thus therapists should be aware of countertransferential gratification.

Narcissistic Personality Disorder

History

Havelock Ellis (1898) introduced the term *narcissism* in 1898 to describe a type of sexual perversion involving treating oneself as a sexual object. Freud then adopted the term to describe a more general attitude of self-absorption and self-love. Later, analysts moved the concept toward excessive self-love and grandiosity that develop in response to injured self-esteem (Morrison 1989; Pulver 1970). The concept of a narcissistic type of personality disorder developed only during the 1980s and was inspired largely by the enormous attention given to pathological narcissism in the psychoanalytic community (Gunderson et al. 1991c). Ironically, this attention was largely an outgrowth of Heinz Kohut's (1971, 1977) theoretical and clinical contributions, many of which focused on nonpathological narcissism.

Clinical Features

Because persons with narcissistic personality disorder have grandiose self-esteem, they are vulnerable to intense reactions when their self-image is damaged (Table 19–13). They respond with strong feelings of hurt or anger to even small slights, rejections, defeats, or criticisms. As a result, persons with narcissistic personality disorder usually go to great lengths to avoid exposure to such experiences and, when that fails, react by becoming devaluative or rageful. Serious depression can ensue, which is the usual precipitant for their seeking clinical help. In relationships, narcissistic persons are often quite distant, try

---

TABLE 19–13. DSM-IV-TR criteria for narcissistic personality disorder

A pervasive pattern of grandiosity (in fantasy or behavior), need for admiration, and lack of empathy, beginning by early adulthood and present in a variety of contexts, as indicated by five (or more) of the following:

(1) has a grandiose sense of self-importance (e.g., exaggerates achievements and talents, expects to be recognized as superior without commensurate achievements)

(2) is preoccupied with fantasies of unlimited success, power, brilliance, beauty, or ideal love

(3) believes that he or she is "special" and unique and can only be understood by, or should associate with, other special or high-status people (or institutions)

(4) requires excessive admiration

(5) has a sense of entitlement, i.e., unreasonable expectations of especially favorable treatment or automatic compliance with his or her expectations

(6) is interpersonally exploitative, i.e., takes advantage of others to achieve his or her own ends

(7) lacks empathy: is unwilling to recognize or identify with the feelings and needs of others

(8) is often envious of others or believes that others are envious of him or her

(9) shows arrogant, haughty behaviors or attitudes

---

to sustain "an illusion of self-sufficiency" (Modell 1975), and may exploit others for self-serving ends. They are likely to feel that those with whom they associate need to be special and unique because they see themselves in these terms; thus, they usually wish to be associated only with persons, institutions, or possessions that will confirm their sense of superiority. The DSM-IV criteria are most accurate in identifying the arrogant, socially conspicuous forms of narcissistic personality disorder; however, there are other forms in which a conviction of personal superiority is hidden behind social withdrawal and a facade of self-sacrifice and even humility (Cooper and Ronningstam 1992).

Differential Diagnosis

Narcissistic personality disorder can be most readily confused with histrionic and antisocial personality disorders. Like persons with antisocial personality disorder, those with narcissistic personality disorder are capable of exploiting others but usually rationalize their behavior on the basis of the specialness of their goals or their personal virtue. In contrast, antisocial persons' goals are materialistic, and their rationalizations, if offered, are based on a view that others would do the same to them. The narcissistic person's excessive pride in achievements, relative constraint in expression of feelings, and disregard for other people's rights and sensitivities help distinguish him or her from persons with histrionic personality disorder. Perhaps the most difficult differential diagnostic problem is whether a person who meets criteria for narcissistic personality disorder has a stable personality disorder or an adjustment reaction. When the emergence of narcissistic traits has been defensively triggered by experiences of failure or rejection, these traits may diminish radically and self-esteem may be restored when new relationships or successes occur.

Etiology

Little scientific evidence is available about the pathogenesis of narcissistic personality disorder. Reconstructions based on developmental history and observations in psychoanalytic treatment indicate that this disorder develops in persons who have had their fears, failures, or dependency responded to with criticism, disdain, or neglect during their childhood years. Such experiences leave them contemptuous of such reactions in themselves and others and inexperienced in viewing others as sources of comfort and support. They develop a veneer of invulnerability and self-sufficiency that masks their underlying emptiness and constricts their capacity to feel deeply.

Treatment

Individual psychodynamic psychotherapy, including psychoanalysis, is the cornerstone of treatment for persons with narcissistic personality disorder. Following Kohut's lead, some therapists believe that the vulnerability to narcissistic injury indicates that intervention should be directed at conveying empathy for the patient's sensitivities and disappointments. This approach, in theory, allows a positive idealized transference to develop that will then be gradually disillusioned by the inevitable frustrations encountered in therapy—disillusionment that will clarify the excessive nature of the patient's reactions to frustrations and disappointments. An alternative view, explicated by Kernberg (1974, 1975), is that the vulnerability should be addressed earlier and more directly by interpretations and confrontations by which these persons will come to recognize their grandiosity and its maladaptive consequences. With either approach, the psychotherapeutic process usually requires a relatively intensive schedule over a period of years in which the narcissistic patient's hypersensitivity to slights is foremost in the therapist's mind and interventions.

Avoidant Personality Disorder

History

Avoidant personality disorder, which was new to DSM-III, was theoretically derived from Millon's (1981) typology of personality disorders (corresponding to his active–detached pattern). Despite its theoretical basis, the disorder does have some historical clinical antecedents, including Kretschmer's (1925) hyperaesthetic type, Schneider's (1959) sensitive type, Horney's (1945) detached type, and Fenichel's (1945) phobic character. In DSM-III-R, in fact, the avoidant personality disorder construct was brought closer to the psychoanalytic construct of the phobic character. The changes of DSM-IV focused on better differentiating this disorder from the Axis I condition of generalized social phobia (Millon 1991).

Clinical Features

Persons with avoidant personality disorder experience excessive and pervasive anxiety and discomfort in social situations and in intimate relationships (Table 19–14). Although strongly desiring relationships, they avoid them because they fear being ridiculed, criticized, rejected, or humiliated. These fears reflect their low self-esteem and hypersensitivity to negative evaluation by others. When they do enter into social situations or relationships, they feel inept and are self-conscious, shy, awkward, and preoccupied with being criticized or rejected. Their lives are constricted in that they tend to avoid not only relationships but also new activities because they fear that they will embarrass or humiliate themselves.

Differential Diagnosis

Schizoid personality disorder also involves social isolation, but the schizoid person does not desire relationships, whereas the avoidant person desires them but avoids them because of anxiety and fears of humiliation and rejection. Whereas avoidant personality disorder is characterized by avoidance of situations and relationships involving possible rejection or disappointment, Axis I social phobia usually consists of specific fears related to social performance (e.g., a fear of saying something inappropriate or of being unable to answer questions in social situations).

Etiology

Millon (1981), from whose work DSM avoidant personality disorder was derived, suggested that the disorder develops from parental rejection and censure, which may be reinforced by rejecting peers. Psychodynamic theory

TABLE 19–14. DSM-IV-TR criteria for avoidant personality disorder

A pervasive pattern of social inhibition, feelings of inadequacy, and hypersensitivity to negative evaluation, beginning by early adulthood and present in a variety of contexts, as indicated by four (or more) of the following:

    (1) avoids occupational activities that involve significant interpersonal contact, because of fears of criticism, disapproval, or rejection

    (2) is unwilling to get involved with people unless certain of being liked

    (3) shows restraint within intimate relationships because of the fear of being shamed or ridiculed

    (4) is preoccupied with being criticized or rejected in social situations

    (5) is inhibited in new interpersonal situations because of feelings of inadequacy

    (6) views self as socially inept, personally unappealing, or inferior to others

    (7) is unusually reluctant to take personal risks or to engage in any new activities because they may prove embarrassing

suggests that avoidant behavior may derive from early life experiences that lead to an exaggerated desire for acceptance or an intolerance of criticism. Research in the biological sphere has implicated the importance of inborn temperament in the development of avoidant behavior. Kagan (1989) found that some children as young as 21 months manifest increased physiological arousal and avoidant traits in social situations (e.g., retreat from the unfamiliar and avoidance of interaction with strangers) and that this social inhibition tends to persist for many years.

Treatment

Because of their excessive fear of rejection and criticism and their reluctance to form relationships, persons with avoidant personality disorder may be difficult to engage in treatment. Engagement in psychotherapy may be facilitated by the therapist's use of supportive techniques, sensitivity to the patient's hypersensitivity, and gentle interpretation of the defensive use of avoidance. Although early in treatment these patients may tolerate only supportive techniques, they may eventually respond well to all kinds of psychotherapy, including short-term, long-term, and psychoanalytic approaches. Clinicians should be aware of the potential for countertransference reactions such as overprotectiveness, hesitancy to adequately challenge the patient, or excessive expectations for change.

Although few data exist, it seems likely that assertiveness and social skills training may increase patients' confidence and willingness to take risks in social situations. Cognitive techniques that gently challenge patients' pathological assumptions about their sense of ineptness may also be useful. Group experiences—perhaps, in particular, homogeneous supportive groups that emphasize the development of social skills—may prove useful for avoidant patients.

Promising preliminary data suggest that avoidant personality disorder may improve with treatment with monoamine oxidase inhibitors or serotonin reuptake inhibitors (Deltito and Stam 1989; Versiani et al. 1992). Anxiolytics sometimes help patients better manage anxiety (especially severe anxiety) caused by facing previously avoided situations or trying new behaviors.

Dependent Personality Disorder

History

Abraham's (1927) "oral" character was the major clinical forerunner of dependent personality disorder. This character type was thought to result from fixation at the first, or oral, stage of psychosexual development—a theory that was reflected in Fenichel's (1945) observation that "certain persons act as nursing mothers in all their object relationships" (p. 489). This personality type was similar to Horney's "compliant" type (Millon 1981).

Dependent personality disorder was a subtype of passive-aggressive personality disorder in DSM-I and did not become a separate disorder until DSM-III. The changes of DSM-IV put greater emphasis on the disorder's central features and attempted to diminish its overlap with other personality disorders (Hirschfeld et al. 1991).

Clinical Features

Dependent personality disorder is characterized by an excessive need to be cared for by others, which leads to submissive and clinging behavior and excessive fears of separation from others (Table 19–15). Although these individuals are able to care for themselves, they so doubt their abilities and judgment, and they view others as so much stronger and more capable than they, that they can be quite disabled. These persons excessively rely on "powerful" others to initiate and do things for them, make their decisions, assume responsibility for their actions, and guide them through life. Low self-esteem and doubt about their effectiveness lead them to avoid positions of responsibility. Because they feel unable to function without excessive guidance, they go to great

---

TABLE 19–15. DSM-IV-TR criteria for dependent personality disorder

---

A pervasive and excessive need to be taken care of that leads to submissive and clinging behavior and fears of separation, beginning by early adulthood and present in a variety of contexts, as indicated by five (or more) of the following:

(1) has difficulty making everyday decisions without an excessive amount of advice and reassurance from others

(2) needs others to assume responsibility for most major areas of his or her life

(3) has difficulty expressing disagreement with others because of fear of loss of support or approval.   **Note:** Do not include realistic fears of retribution.

(4) has difficulty initiating projects or doing things on his or her own (because of a lack of self-confidence in judgment or abilities rather than a lack of motivation or energy)

(5) goes to excessive lengths to obtain nurturance and support from others, to the point of volunteering to do things that are unpleasant

(6) feels uncomfortable or helpless when alone because of exaggerated fears of being unable to care for himself or herself

(7) urgently seeks another relationship as a source of care and support when a close relationship ends

(8) is unrealistically preoccupied with fears of being left to take care of himself or herself

---

lengths to maintain the dependent relationship. They may, for example, always agree with those on whom they depend, and they tend to be excessively clinging, submissive, passive, and self-sacrificing. If the dependent relationship ends, these individuals feel helpless and fearful because they feel incapable of caring for themselves, and they often indiscriminately find another person with whom to have a relationship so that they can be provided with direction and nurturance—an unfulfilling or even an abusive relationship may seem better than being on their own.

Differential Diagnosis

Although persons with borderline personality disorder also dread being alone and need ongoing support, dependent persons want others to assume a controlling function that would frighten the borderline patient. Moreover, persons with dependent personality disorder become appeasing rather than rageful or self-destructive when threatened with separation. Although both avoidant and dependent personality disorders are characterized by low self-esteem, rejection sensitivity, and an excessive need for reassurance, persons with dependent

personality disorder seek out rather than avoid relationships, and they quickly and indiscriminately replace ended relationships instead of further withdrawing from others.

Etiology

Abraham suggested that the dependent character derives from either overindulgence or underindulgence during the oral phase of development (i.e., birth to age 2). Subsequent empirical data have given more support to the underindulgence hypothesis. However, studies of adults have not supported a specific association between feeding or other oral habits in childhood and dependency in adulthood. It may be that ongoing patterns unrelated to the oral phase per se—for example, chronic physical illness or underindulgent parenting that also prohibits independent behavior—are more important to this disorder's development. Genetic or constitutional factors, such as innate submissiveness, may also be a factor in this disorder's etiology; twin studies have found that monozygotic twins score more similarly on scales measuring submissiveness than do dizygotic twins.

Cultural and social factors may also play a role in the development of dependent personality disorder. Dependency is considered not only normative but desirable in certain cultures, and Gilligan (1982) argued that it is encouraged in women in our culture. Thus, dependent personality disorder may represent an exaggerated and maladaptive variant of normal dependency; that is, it may—along with histrionic, obsessive-compulsive, and avoidant personality disorders—best be conceptualized as a "trait" disorder (i.e., occurring on a continuum with normal personality traits). It is important to recognize that to qualify as dependent personality disorder, the dependent traits should be so extreme that they cause significant distress or impairment in functioning.

Treatment

Patients with dependent personality disorder often enter therapy with complaints of depression or anxiety that may be precipitated by the threatened or actual loss of a dependent relationship. They often respond well to various types of individual psychotherapy. Treatment may be particularly helpful if it explores the patients' fears of independence; uses the transference to explore their dependency; and is directed toward increasing patients' self-esteem, sense of effectiveness, assertiveness, and independent functioning. These patients often seek an excessively dependent relationship with the therapist, which can lead to countertransference problems that may actually reinforce their dependence. The therapist may, for example, overprotect or be overly directive with the patient, give inappropriate reassurance and support, or prolong the treatment unnecessarily. He or she may also have excessive expectations for change or withdraw from a patient who is perceived as too needy.

Group therapy and cognitive-behavioral therapy aimed at increasing independent functioning, including assertiveness and social skills training, may be useful for some patients. If the patient is in a relationship that is maintaining and reinforcing his or her excessive dependence, couples or family therapy may be helpful.

Obsessive-Compulsive Personality Disorder

History

In the early 1900s, Freud (1908/1924) made his often-cited observation that persons with obsessive-compulsive personality disorder were characterized by the three "peculiarities" of orderliness (which included cleanliness and conscientiousness), parsimoniousness, and obstinacy. Similarly, in 1918, Ernest Jones (1918/1938) described these individuals as being preoccupied with cleanliness, money, and time. These observations were repeatedly cited and amplified in the subsequent psychoanalytic literature—the disorder often being referred to as *anal character*—and in the descriptive literature (Millon 1981).

This disorder's DSM description has closely mirrored these earlier clinical observations (Pfohl and Blum 1991). In addition, in keeping with its consistent representation in the clinical literature, obsessive-compulsive personality disorder is one of the few personality disorders that has been included in every version of DSM. In European psychiatry, this disorder has been referred to as *anancastic personality disorder*, a term used by Kretschmer and Schneider in the 1920s and still used in ICD-10.

Clinical Features

As Freud noted, and as DSM-IV criteria reflect, persons with obsessive-compulsive personality disorder are excessively orderly (Table 19–16). They are neat, punctual, overly organized, and overconscientious. Although these traits might be considered virtues, especially in cultures that subscribe to the Puritan work ethic, to qualify as obsessive-compulsive personality disorder the traits must be so extreme that they cause significant distress or impairment in functioning. As Abraham (1923) noted, these individuals' perseverance is unproductive. For example, attention to detail is so excessive or time consuming that the point of the activity is lost, conscien-

TABLE 19–16. DSM-IV-TR criteria for obsessive-compulsive personality disorder

A pervasive pattern of preoccupation with orderliness, perfectionism, and mental and interpersonal control, at the expense of flexibility, openness, and efficiency, beginning by early adulthood and present in a variety of contexts, as indicated by four (or more) of the following:

  (1) is preoccupied with details, rules, lists, order, organization, or schedules to the extent that the major point of the activity is lost

  (2) shows perfectionism that interferes with task completion (e.g., is unable to complete a project because his or her own overly strict standards are not met)

  (3) is excessively devoted to work and productivity to the exclusion of leisure activities and friendships (not accounted for by obvious economic necessity)

  (4) is overconscientious, scrupulous, and inflexible about matters of morality, ethics, or values (not accounted for by cultural or religious identification)

  (5) is unable to discard worn-out or worthless objects even when they have no sentimental value

  (6) is reluctant to delegate tasks or to work with others unless they submit to exactly his or her way of doing things

  (7) adopts a miserly spending style toward both self and others; money is viewed as something to be hoarded for future catastrophes

  (8) shows rigidity and stubbornness

tiousness is so extreme that it causes rigidity and inflexibility, and perfectionism interferes with task completion. And although these individuals tend to work extremely hard, they do so at the expense of leisure activities and relationships. As Shapiro (1965) pointed out, the most characteristic thought of obsessive-compulsive persons is "I should"—a phrase that aptly reflects their severe superego and captures their overly high standards, drivenness, and excessive conscientiousness, perfectionism, rigidity, and devotion to work and duties.

These individuals also tend to be overly concerned with control—not only over the details of their own lives but also over their emotions and other people. They have difficulty expressing warm and tender feelings, often using stilted, distant phrasing that reveals little of their inner experience. And they may be obstinate and reluctant to delegate tasks or to work with others unless others submit exactly to their way of doing things, which reflects their need for interpersonal control as well as their fear of making mistakes. Their tendency to doubt and worry also manifests itself in their inability to discard worn-out or worthless objects that might be needed for future catastrophes, and, as Freud and Jones noted, persons with obsessive-compulsive personality are miserly toward themselves and others. A caricatured description of such persons is Rado's (1959) "living machines."

Differential Diagnosis

Obsessive-compulsive personality disorder differs from Axis I obsessive-compulsive disorder in that the latter disorder consists of specific repetitive thoughts and ritualistic behaviors rather than personality traits. In addition, obsessive-compulsive disorder has traditionally been considered ego-dystonic, whereas obsessive-compulsive personality disorder has been considered ego-syntonic. These two disorders are sometimes, but not necessarily, comorbid.

Etiology

Freud's view that obsessive-compulsive personality disorder derives from difficulties occurring during the anal stage of psychosexual development (age 2–4 years) was echoed and elaborated on by subsequent psychoanalytic thinkers, such as Karl Abraham and Wilhelm Reich (1933). According to this theory, children's infantile anal–erotic libidinal impulses conflict with parental attempts to socialize them—in particular, to toilet train them. Although these theories emphasize the importance of children's perception of parental disapproval during toilet training, and of ensuing parent–child control struggles—what Rado (1959) referred to as "the battle of the chamber pot"—these factors are not currently considered central to this disorder's etiology. It may be, however, that conflicts arising during toilet training—such as those characteristic of Erikson's (1950) stage of autonomy versus shame—and continuing during other developmental stages do play a role in this disorder's etiology (Perry and Vaillant 1989). In particular, excessive parental control, criticism, and shaming may result in an insecurity that is defended against with perfectionism, orderliness, and an attempt to maintain excessive control.

Freud believed that constitutional factors also play an important role in the formation of this personality type; similarly, Rado postulated the etiological importance of constitutionally excessive rage that leads to power struggles with others. As is the case with other personality disorders, empirical studies are needed to clarify this disorder's sources.

Treatment

Persons with obsessive-compulsive personality disorder may seem difficult to treat because of their excessive

intellectualization and difficulty expressing emotion. However, these patients often respond well to psychoanalytic psychotherapy or psychoanalysis. Therapists usually need to be relatively active in treatment. They should also avoid being drawn into interesting but affectless discussions that are unlikely to have therapeutic benefit. In other words, rather than intellectualizing with the patient, therapists should focus on the feelings these patients usually avoid. Other defenses common in this disorder, such as rationalization, isolation, undoing, and reaction formation, should also be identified and clarified. Power struggles that may occur in treatment offer opportunities to address the patient's excessive need for control.

Cognitive techniques may also be used to diminish the patient's excessive need for control and perfection. Although patients may resist group treatment because of their need for control, dynamically oriented groups that focus on feelings may provide insight and increase their comfort with exploring and expressing new affects.

Other Personality Disorders

The following three personality disorders were considered for inclusion on DSM-IV Axis II on the basis of their historical tradition, clinical utility, and/or empirical support. However, for various reasons they were thought to require further study. Of note, all three disorders involve chronically morose people who have problems with direct expression of their aggression.

Depressive Personality Disorder

Of all the personality disorders, depressive personality disorder may have the longest clinical tradition, having been recognized 2,000 years ago by Hippocrates in his description of the "black gall," or melancholic, temperament (Phillips et al. 1990). Kraepelin (1921) also described this temperament and, like Hippocrates, considered it a depressive-spectrum disorder—a constitutional traitlike variant of the more severe depressive disorders and one predisposing to them. Schneider's (1959) description of this personality type led to its inclusion in ICD-9 as an affective personality disorder. Kernberg (1988), who drew from the writings of Laughlin, emphasized this personality type's psychodynamic features, which include a severe superego, the inhibited expression of aggression, and an excessive dependence that is defended against with counterdependence. Because of the strength of this disorder's historical tradition, its inclusion in ICD-9, and some empirical evidence in its support, depressive personality disorder was added to the appendix in DSM-IV.

Persons with this disorder are persistently gloomy, burdened, worried, serious, pessimistic, and incapable of enjoyment or relaxation (Table 19–17). They also tend to be guilty, moralistic, self-denying, passive, unassertive, and introverted. They have low self-esteem and are excessively sensitive to criticism and rejection. Although they may be critical of others, they have difficulty directing criticism or any form of aggression toward others and find it easier to criticize themselves. They are also overly dependent on the love and acceptance of others, but they inhibit the expression of this dependency and may instead appear counterdependent.

Although concern has been expressed that this personality disorder may overlap excessively with Axis I depressive disorders—in particular, dysthymia—available data suggest that its overlap with dysthymia, major depression, and other personality disorders is far from complete and that depressive personality disorder appears to be a separate construct (D.N. Klein 1990; D.N. Klein and Shih 1998; Phillips et al. 1998). This disorder should not be diagnosed, however, if it occurs only during major depressive episodes. Although depressive personality disorder appears distinct from Axis I depressive disorders, family history and other data suggest that it may be related to these disorders, giving support to Kraepelin's spectrum concept.

Depressive personality disorder has been noted to respond well to psychoanalytic psychotherapy and psychoanalysis. Although it has been proposed that the major depressive episodes that can co-occur with this personality type may be particularly responsive to antidepressant medications (Akiskal 1983), this hypothesis awaits further empirical validation.

Negativistic Personality Disorder

Negativistic personality disorder entered the appendix in DSM-IV (where it is labeled passive-aggressive [negativistic] personality disorder) as a replacement for the excessively narrow category of passive-aggressive personality disorder, which was thought to represent a single defense mechanism rather than a personality disorder. Other limitations of passive-aggressive personality disorder in previous versions of DSM were its scant empirical support and the fact that passive-aggressive behavior can be normative, even laudable, in certain situations. Negativistic personality disorder is a broader construct that has some historical precedents, including Schneider's (1923) "ill-tempered depressives."

TABLE 19–17. DSM-IV-TR research criteria for depressive personality disorder

A. A pervasive pattern of depressive cognitions and behaviors beginning by early adulthood and present in a variety of contexts, as indicated by five (or more) of the following:

    (1) usual mood is dominated by dejection, gloominess, cheerlessness, joylessness, unhappiness

    (2) self-concept centers around beliefs of inadequacy, worthlessness, and low self-esteem

    (3) is critical, blaming, and derogatory toward self

    (4) is brooding and given to worry

    (5) is negativistic, critical, and judgmental toward others

    (6) is pessimistic

    (7) is prone to feeling guilty or remorseful

B. Does not occur exclusively during major depressive episodes and is not better accounted for by dysthymic disorder.

Negativistic personality disorder, like passive-aggressive personality disorder, describes a pervasive pattern of passive resistance to demands for social and occupational performance (Table 19–18). But it also encompasses a wide range of negativistic attitudes and behaviors, such as anger, pessimism, and cynicism; sullenness and argumentativeness; criticism of others; and envy of those who are perceived as more fortunate. In addition, these individuals tend to alternate between hostile self-assertion and contrite submission. A recent factor-analytic study found that negativistic personality disorder is a unidimensional construct that is associated with narcissistic personality disorder (Fossati et al. 2000). The clinical features of this disorder and its differentiation from other personality disorders remain to be empirically confirmed.

Self-Defeating Personality Disorder

Self-defeating personality disorder has been the subject of much controversy. This personality type has a significant historical and clinical tradition, beginning with Kraft-Ebbing's nineteenth-century description of sexual masochism (which is classified as a paraphilia in DSM) and Freud's subsequent description of moral masochism, a pattern of nonsexual submissive behavior that leads to psychological pain and mistreatment. Nonetheless, concerns have been raised about the misuse of the diagnosis—in particular, that it may be misapplied to women who are actually being abused and thereby be used to blame the victim. In part a reflection of these concerns, self-defeating personality disorder has never been an official psychiatric diagnosis. It was included in the DSM-III-R appendix (Fiester 1991) and is not included in DSM-IV. However, this disorder's proponents argue that its fea-

TABLE 19–18. DSM-IV-TR research criteria for passive-aggressive personality disorder

A. A pervasive pattern of negativistic attitudes and passive resistance to demands for adequate performance, beginning by early adulthood and present in a variety of contexts, as indicated by four (or more) of the following:
   (1) passively resists fulfilling routine social and occupational tasks
   (2) complains of being misunderstood and unappreciated by others
   (3) is sullen and argumentative
   (4) unreasonably criticizes and scorns authority
   (5) expresses envy and resentment toward those apparently more fortunate
   (6) voices exaggerated and persistent complaints of personal misfortune
   (7) alternates between hostile defiance and contrition
B. Does not occur exclusively during major depressive episodes and is not better accounted for by dysthymic disorder.

tures are distinctive, predict the occurrence of impairment and distress, and apply to men as well as to women, and that the disorder is a clinically useful concept with important treatment implications (Cruz et al. 2000).

Self-defeating personality disorder applies to persons who exhibit a pervasive pattern of self-defeating behavior that does not occur only in response to, or in anticipation of, physical, sexual, or psychological abuse. Persons with this disorder feel unworthy of being treated well and, as a result, treat themselves poorly and unwittingly encourage others to make them suffer. They may, for example, reject opportunities for pleasure, choose people or situations that lead to mistreatment or failure, and incite others to become angry with them or reject them. If things do go well for them, they attempt to undermine themselves by, for example, becoming depressed or causing themselves pain.

The treatment of the disorder is complicated by the patient's self-defeating tendencies; patients may unknowingly undermine the treatment and their progress because they feel undeserving of improvement or happiness. Exploring the patient's need to be victimized and making their investment in suffering ego-dystonic may allow a successful outcome with insight-oriented psychotherapy or psychoanalysis.

Conclusions

Clinical interest and research in the personality disorders have grown enormously since 1980, when these disorders were put on a separate axis in DSM-III. The ensuing period has brought to light more specific and effective treatment strategies and a better understanding of these disorders' prognosis and etiology. Even more dramatic than the knowledge gained are the heightened awareness of these disorders and the new and more informed questions that this awareness has generated. Remaining challenges include an explication of the boundaries between personality disorders and both normalcy and Axis I conditions, the discovery of biogenetic bases for personality disorders and their classification, and the development of even more effective treatments. There is good reason to believe that with continued inquiry by clinical and basic-science investigators, the classification system will continue to change so that it becomes even more tightly linked to these disorders' etiology and treatment response.

References

Abraham K: Contributions to the theory of the anal character. Int J Psychoanal 4:400–418, 1923

Abraham K: The influence of oral eroticism on character formation, in Selected Papers on Psychoanalysis. Edited by Jones E. London, England, Hogarth Press, 1927, pp 393–406

Adler G: Borderline Psychopathology and Its Treatment. New York, Jason Aronson, 1985

Akiskal HS: Dysthymic disorder: psychopathology of proposed chronic depressive subtypes. Am J Psychiatry 140:11–20, 1983

Alnæs R, Torgersen S: Personality and personality disorders predict development and relapses of major depression. Acta Psychiatr Scand 95:336–342, 1997

American Psychiatric Association: Diagnostic and Statistical Manual: Mental Disorders. Washington, DC, American Psychiatric Association, 1952

American Psychiatric Association: Diagnostic and Statistical Manual of Mental Disorders, 2nd Edition. Washington, DC, American Psychiatric Association, 1968

American Psychiatric Association: Diagnostic and Statistical Manual of Mental Disorders, 3rd Edition. Washington, DC, American Psychiatric Association, 1980

American Psychiatric Association: Diagnostic and Statistical Manual of Mental Disorders, 3rd Edition, Revised. Washington, DC, American Psychiatric Association, 1987

American Psychiatric Association: Diagnostic and Statistical Manual of Mental Disorders, 4th Edition. Washington, DC, American Psychiatric Association, 1994

American Psychiatric Association: Diagnostic and Statistical Manual of Mental Disorders, 4th Edition, Text Revision. Washington, DC, American Psychiatric Association, 2000

American Psychiatric Association: Practice guideline for the treatment of patients with borderline personality disorder. Am J Psychiatry 158(suppl):1–52, 2001

Bateman A, Fonagy P: Effectiveness of partial hospitalization in the treatment of borderline personality disorder: a randomized controlled trial. Am J Psychiatry 156:1563–1569, 1999

Bender DS, Dolan RT, Skodol AE, et al: Treatment utilization by patients with personality disorders. Am J Psychiatry 158:295–302, 2001

Benjamin LS: Structural analysis of social behavior. Psychol Rev 81:392–425, 1974

Bergman AJ, Harvey PD, Roitman SL, et al: Verbal learning and memory in schizotypal personality disorder. Schizophr Bull 24:635–641, 1998

Bernstein DP, Kasapis C, Bergman A: Assessing Axis II disorders by informant interview. J Personal Disord 11:158–167, 1997

Bernstein DP, Useda D, Siever LJ: Paranoid personality disorder: a review of its current status. J Personal Disord 7:53–62, 1993

Black DW, Bell S, Hulbert J, et al: The importance of Axis II in patients with major depression: a controlled study. J Affect Disord 14:115–122, 1988

Bleuler E: Die Probleme der Schizoidie und der Syntonie. Zeitschrift für die gesamte Neurologie und Psychiatrie 78:373–388, 1922

Brent DA, Johnson BA, Perper J, et al: Personality disorder, personality traits, impulsive violence, and completed suicide in adolescents. J Am Acad Child Adolesc Psychiatry 33:1080–1086, 1994

Breuer J, Freud S: Studies on Hysteria (1893–1895). Translated and edited by Strachey J. New York, Basic Books, 1957

Cadenhead KS, Light GA, Geyer MA, et al: Sensory gating deficits assessed by the P50 event-related potential in subjects with schizotypal personality disorder. Am J Psychiatry 157:55–59, 2000

Calabrese JR, Woyshville MJ, Kimmel SE, et al: Predictors of valproate response in bipolar rapid cycling. J Clin Psychopharmacol 13:280–283, 1993

Carey G, DiLalla DL: Personality and psychopathology: genetic perspectives. J Abnorm Psychol 103:32–43, 1994

Caton CL, Shrout PE, Eagle PF, et al: Risk factors for homelessness among schizophrenic men: a case-control study. Am J Public Health 84:265–270, 1994

Chiesa M, Fonagy P: Cassel personality disorder study. Br J Psychiatry 176:485–491, 2000

Chodoff P: Hysteria and women. Am J Psychiatry 139:545–551, 1982

Clark LA: Schedule for Normal and Abnormal Personality (SNAP). Dallas, TX, Southern Methodist University, 1990

Cleckley H: The Mask of Sanity, 4th Edition. St Louis, MO, CV Mosby, 1964

Cloninger CR: A systematic method for clinical description and classification of personality variants. Arch Gen Psychiatry 44:573–588, 1987

Cloninger CR, Svrakic DM, Przybeck TR: A psychobiological model of temperament and character. Arch Gen Psychiatry 50:975–990, 1993

Coccaro EF, Kavoussi RJ: Fluoxetine and impulsive aggressive behavior in personality-disordered subjects. Arch Gen Psychiatry 54:1081–1088, 1997

Coccaro EF, Kavoussi RJ, Sheline YI, et al: Impulsive aggression in personality disorder correlates with tritiated paroxetine binding in the platelet. Arch Gen Psychiatry 53:531–536, 1996

Colom F, Vieta E, Martínez-Arán A, et al: Clinical factors associated with treatment noncompliance in euthymic bipolar patients. J Clin Psychiatry 61:549–555, 2000

Cooper AM, Ronningstam E: Narcissistic personality disorder, in American Psychiatric Press Review of Psychiatry, Vol 11. Edited by Tasman A, Riba ME. Washington, DC, American Psychiatric Press, 1992, pp 80–97

Cornelius JR, Soloff PH, Perel JM, et al: Continuation pharmacotherapy of borderline personality disorder with haloperidol and phenelzine. Am J Psychiatry 150:1843–1848, 1993

Costa P, McCrae R: Personality disorders and the five-factor model of personality. J Personal Disord 4:362–371, 1990

Cowdry RW, Gardner DL: Pharmacotherapy of borderline personality disorder: alprazolam, carbamazepine, trifluoperazine, and tranylcypromine. Arch Gen Psychiatry 45:111–119, 1988

Cruz J, Joiner TE, Johnson JG, et al: Self-defeating personality disorder reconsidered. J Personal Disord 14:64–71, 2000

Deltito JA, Stam M: Psychopharmacological treatment of avoidant personality disorder. Compr Psychiatry 30:498–504, 1989

Dickey CC, Shenton ME, Hirayasu Y, et al: Large CSF volume not attributable to ventricular volume in schizotypal personality disorder. Am J Psychiatry 157:48–54, 2000

Dinwiddie SH, Bucholz KK: Psychiatric diagnoses of self-reported child abusers. Child Abuse Negl 17:465–476, 1993

Dinwiddie SH, Reich T, Cloninger CR: Psychiatric comorbidity and suicidality among intravenous drug users. J Clin Psychiatry 53:364–369, 1992

Dunayevich E, Sax KW, Keck PE Jr, et al: Twelve-month outcome in bipolar patients with and without personality disorders. J Clin Psychiatry 61:134–139, 2000

Easser BR, Lesser SR: Hysterical personality: a re-evaluation. Psychoanal Q 34:390–405, 1965

Ellis H: Auto-erotism: a psychological study. Alienist and Neurologist 19:260–299, 1898

Erikson EH: Childhood and Society. New York, WW Norton, 1950

Fairbairn WRD: Schizoid factors in the personality (1940), in Psychoanalytic Studies of the Personality. London, England, Tavistock, 1952, pp 3–27

Fals-Stewart W: Personality characteristics of substance abusers: an MCMI cluster typology of recreational drug users treated in a therapeutic community and its relationship to length of stay and outcome. J Pers Assess 59:515–527, 1992

Fenichel O: The Psychoanalytic Theory of the Neurosis. New York, WW Norton, 1945

Ferro T, Klein DN: Family history assessment of personality disorders, I: concordance with direct interview and between pairs of informants. J Personal Disord 11:123–136, 1997

Ferro T, Klein D, Schwartz JE, et al: 30 month stability of personality disorder diagnosis in depressed outpatients. Am J Psychiatry 155:653–659, 1998

Fiester SJ: Self-defeating personality disorder: a review of data and recommendations for DSM-IV. J Personal Disord 5:194–209, 1991

First MB, Gibbon M, Spitzer RL, et al: Structured Clinical Interview for DSM-IV (SCID-IV). New York, Biometrics Research Department, New York State Psychiatric Institute, 1996

Fossati A, Maffei C, Bagnato M, et al: A psychometric study of DSM-IV passive-aggressive (negativistic) personality disorder criteria. J Personal Disord 14:72–83, 2000

Frances A: Categorical and dimensional systems of personality diagnosis: a comparison. Compr Psychiatry 23:516–527, 1982

Freud S: Character and anal erotism (1908), in Collected Papers, Vol 2. London, England, Hogarth Press, 1924, pp 45–50

Gandhi N, Tyrer P, Evans K, et al: A randomized controlled trial of community oriented and hospital-oriented care for discharged psychiatric patients: influence of personality disorder on police contacts. J Personal Disord 15:94–102, 2001

Gilligan C: In a Different Voice: Psychological Theory and Women's Development. Cambridge, MA, Harvard University Press, 1982

Goldberg SC, Schulz C, Schulz PM, et al: Borderline and schizotypal personality disorders treated with low-dose thiothixene vs placebo. Arch Gen Psychiatry 43:680–686, 1986

Grilo CM, McGlashan TH, Oldham JM: Course and stability of personality disorders. J Pract Psychiatry Behav Health 1:61–75, 1999

Grove WM, Eckert ED, Heston L, et al: Heritability of substance abuse and antisocial behavior: a study of monozygotic twins reared apart. Biol Psychiatry 27:1293–1304, 1990

Gunderson JG: Diagnostic controversies, in American Psychiatric Press Review of Psychiatry, Vol 11. Edited by Tasman A, Riba M. Washington, DC, American Psychiatric Press, 1992, pp 9–24

Gunderson JG: The borderline patient's intolerance of aloneness: insecure attachment and therapist availability. Am J Psychiatry 153:752–758, 1996

Gunderson JG: Borderline Personality Disorder: A Clinical Guide. Washington, DC, American Psychiatric Press, 2001

Gunderson JG, Zanarini MC, Kissiel C: Borderline personality disorder: a review of data on DSM-III-R descriptions. J Personal Disord 5:340–352, 1991a

Gunderson JG, Links PS, Reich JH: Competing models of personality disorders. J Personal Disord 5:60–68, 1991b

Gunderson JG, Ronningstam E, Smith LE: Narcissistic personality disorder: a review of data on DSM-III-R descriptions. J Personal Disord 5:167–177, 1991c

Guntrip HJ: The schizoid problem, in Psychoanalytic Theory, Therapy, and the Self. New York, Basic Books, 1971, pp 145–174

Hare RD, Hart SD, Harpur TJ: Psychopathy and the DSM-IV criteria for antisocial personality disorder. J Abnorm Psychol 100:391–398, 1991

Hawton K, Fagg J, Platt S, et al: Factors associated with suicide after parasuicide in young people. BMJ 306:1641–1644, 1993

Herpertz S, Gretzer EM, Steinmeyer V, et al: Affective instability and impulsivity in personality disorder. J Affect Disord 44:31–37, 1997

Hillbrand M, Krystal JH, Sharpe KS, et al: Clinical predictors of self-mutilation in hospitalized forensic patients. J Nerv Ment Dis 182:9–13, 1994

Hirschfeld RMA, Shea MT, Weise R: Dependent personality disorder: perspectives for DSM-IV. J Personal Disord 5:135–149, 1991

Hoch A: Constitutional factors in the dementia praecox group. Review of Neurology and Psychiatry 8:463–475, 1910

Horney K: Our Inner Conflicts: A Constructive Theory of Neurosis. New York, WW Norton, 1945

Hyler SE: Personality Diagnostic Questionnaire—4+ (PDQ-4+). New York, New York State Psychiatric Institute, 1994

Janet P: The Mental State of Hystericals: A Study of Mental Stigmata and Mental Accidents. Translated by Corson CR. New York, GP Putnam's Sons, 1901

Jenike MA, Baer L, Minichiello WE, et al: Coexistent obsessive-compulsive disorder and schizotypal personality disorder: a poor prognostic indicator (letter). Arch Gen Psychiatry 43:296, 1986

Jones E: Anal-erotic character traits (1918), in Papers on Psychoanalysis. London, England, Balliere, Tindall & Cox, 1938, pp 531–555

Jones M: The Therapeutic Community: A New Treatment in Psychiatry. New York, Basic Books, 1953

Jordan BK, Schlenger WE, Fairbank JA, et al: Prevalence of psychiatric disorders among incarcerated women. Arch Gen Psychiatry 53:513–519, 1996

Kagan J: Temperamental influences on the preservation of styles of social behavior. McLean Hospital Journal 14:23–34, 1989

Kalus O, Bernstein DP, Siever LJ: Schizoid personality disorder: a review of its current status. J Personal Disord 7:43–52, 1993

Kass F, Skodol AE, Charles E, et al: Scaled ratings of DSM-III personality disorders. Am J Psychiatry 142:627–630, 1985

Kelstrup A, Lund K, Lauritsen B, et al: Satisfaction with care reported by psychiatric inpatients. Relationship to diagnosis and medical treatment. Acta Psychiatr Scand 87:374–379, 1993

Kemperman I, Russ MJ, Shearin E: Self-injurious behavior and mood regulation in borderline patients. J Personal Disord 11:146–157, 1997

Kendler KS, Gruenberg AM: Genetic relationship between paranoid personality disorder and the "schizophrenic spectrum" disorders. Am J Psychiatry 139:1185–1186, 1982

Kendler KS, McGuire M, Gruenberg AM, et al: The Roscommon family study, III: schizophrenia-related personality disorders in relatives. Arch Gen Psychiatry 50:781–788, 1993

Kent S, Fogarty M, Yellowlees P: A review of studies of heavy users of psychiatric services. Psychiatr Serv 46:1247–1253, 1995

Kernberg OF: Treatment of patients with borderline personality organization. Int J Psychoanal 49:600–619, 1968

Kernberg OF: Further contributions to the treatment of narcissistic personalities. Int J Psychoanal 55:215–240, 1974

Kernberg OF: Borderline Conditions and Pathological Narcissism. New York, Jason Aronson, 1975

Kernberg OF: Clinical dimensions of masochism. J Am Psychoanal Assoc 36:1005–1029, 1988

Kety SS, Rosenthal D, Wender PH, et al: The types and prevalence of mental illness in the biological and adoptive families of adopted schizophrenics, in The Transmission of Schizophrenia. Edited by Rosenthal D, Kety SS. Oxford, England, Pergamon, 1968, pp 345–362

Klein DN: Depressive personality: reliability, validity, and relation to dysthymia. J Abnorm Psychol 99:412–421, 1990

Klein DN, Shih JH: Depressive personality: associations with DSM-III-R mood and personality disorders and negative and positive affectivity, 30-month stability, and prediction of course of Axis I depressive disorders. J Abnorm Psychol 107:319–327, 1998

Klein M: Wisconsin Personality Inventory—Revised. Madison, WI, University of Wisconsin, 1990

Koenigsberg HW, Kaplan RD, Gilmore MM, et al: The relationship between syndrome and personality disorder in DSM-III: experience with 2,462 patients. Am J Psychiatry 142:207–212, 1985

Kohut H: The Analysis of the Self: A Systematic Approach to the Psychoanalytic Treatment of Narcissistic Personality Disorders. New York, International Universities Press, 1971

Kohut H: The Restoration of the Self. New York, International Universities Press, 1977

Kraepelin E: Dementia Praecox and Paraphrenia. Edinburgh, Scotland, E & S Livingstone, 1919

Kraepelin E: Manic-Depressive Insanity and Paranoia. Translated by Barclay RM. Edited by Robertson GM. Edinburgh, Scotland, E & S Livingstone, 1921

Kretschmer E: Physique and Character. New York, Harcourt, Brace, 1925

Lazare A, Klerman G, Armor D: Oral, obsessive and hysterical personality patterns: replication of factor analysis in an independent sample. J Psychiatr Res 7:275–279, 1970

Lenzenweger MF, Loranger AW, Korfine L, et al: Detecting personality disorders in a nonclinical population. Arch Gen Psychiatry 54:345–351, 1997

Lesch KP, Bengel D, Heils A: Association of anxiety-related traits with a polymorphism in the serotonin transporter gene regulatory region. Science 274:1527–1531, 1996

Lewinsohn PM, Rhode P, Seeley JR, et al: Natural course of adolescent major depressive disorder in a community sample: predictors of recurrence in young adults. Am J Psychiatry 157:1584–1591, 2000

Liebowitz MR, Stone MH, Turkat ID: Treatment of personality disorders, in Psychiatry Update: American Psychiatric Association Annual Review, Vol 5. Edited by Frances AJ, Hales RE. Washington, DC, American Psychiatric Press, 1986, pp 356–393

Linehan MM: Cognitive-Behavioral Treatment of Borderline Personality Disorder. New York, Guilford Press, 1993

Linehan MM, Armstrong HE, Suarez A, et al: Cognitive behavioral treatment of chronically parasuicidal borderline patients. Arch Gen Psychiatry 48:1060–1064, 1991

Livesley WJ, Jang KL, Vernon PA: Phenotypic and genetic structure of traits delineating personality disorder. Arch Gen Psychiatry 55:941–948, 1998

Loranger AW: Personality Disorders Examination (PDE) Manual. Yonkers, NY, DV Communications, 1988

Loranger AW: The impact of DSM-III on diagnostic practice in a university hospital. Arch Gen Psychiatry 47:672–675, 1990

Lyons MJ, True WR, Eisen SA, et al: Differential heritability of adult and juvenile antisocial traits. Arch Gen Psychiatry 52:906–915, 1995

Markovitz PJ, Calabrese JR, Schulz SC, et al: Fluoxetine in the treatment of borderline and schizotypal personality disorders. Am J Psychiatry 148:1064–1067, 1991

Masterson JF: Treatment of the Borderline Adolescent: A Developmental Approach. New York, Wiley-Interscience, 1972

McDonald AS, Davey GCL: Psychiatric disorders and accidental injury. Clinical Psychology Review 16:105–127, 1996

Miller RJ, Zadolinnyj K, Hafner RJ: Profiles and predictors of assaultiveness for different psychiatric ward populations. Am J Psychiatry 150:1368–1373, 1993

Millon T: Disorders of Personality—DSM-III: Axis II. New York, Wiley, 1981

Millon T: Avoidant personality disorder: a brief review of issues and data. J Personal Disord 5:353–362, 1991

Millon T: Millon Clinical Multiaxial Inventory—III. Minneapolis, MN, National Computer Systems, 1994

Modell AH: A narcissistic defense against affects and the illusion of self-sufficiency. Int J Psychoanal 56:275–282, 1975

Morrison AP: Introduction, in Essential Papers on Narcissism. Edited by Morrison AP. New York, New York University Press, 1989, pp 1–11

Nelson JC, Mazure CM, Jatlow PI: Characteristics of desipramine-refractory depression. J Clin Psychiatry 55:12–19, 1994

Neumann E, Walker EF: Motor dysfunction in schizotypal personality disorder. Schizophr Res 38:159–168, 1999

O'Connor BP, Dyce JA: A test of models of personality disorder configuration. J Abnorm Psychol 107:3–16, 1998

O'Leary D, Costello F: Personality and outcome in depression: an 18-month prospective follow-up study. J Affect Disord 63:67–78, 2001

Paris J: Personality disorders: a biopsychosocial model. J Personal Disord 7:255–264, 1993

Perry JC, Banon E, Ianni F: Effectiveness of psychotherapy for personality disorders. Am J Psychiatry 156:1312–1321, 1999

Perry JC, Vaillant GE: Personality disorders, in Comprehensive Textbook of Psychiatry/V, 5th Edition, Vol 2. Edited by Kaplan HI, Sadock BJ. Baltimore, MD, Williams & Wilkins, 1989, pp 1352–1387

Pfohl B: Histrionic personality disorder: a review of available data and recommendations for DSM-IV. J Personal Disord 5:150–166, 1991

Pfohl B, Blum N: Obsessive-compulsive personality disorder: a review of available data and recommendations for DSM-IV. J Personal Disord 5:363–375, 1991

Pfohl B, Blum N, Zimmerman M: The Structured Interview for DSM-IV Personality Disorders: SIPD-IV. Iowa City, IA, University of Iowa Press, 1994

Phillips KA, Gunderson JG, Hirschfeld RMA, et al: A review of the depressive personality. Am J Psychiatry 147:830–837, 1990

Phillips KA, Gunderson JG, Triebwasser J, et al: Reliability and validity of depressive personality disorders. Am J Psychiatry 155:1044–1048, 1998

Pirkis J, Burgess P, Jolley D: Suicide attempts by psychiatric patients in acute inpatient, long-stay inpatient and community care. Soc Psychiatry Psychiatr Epidemiol 34:634–644, 1999

Pritchard JC: A Treatise on Insanity. London, England, Sherwood, Gilbert and Piper, 1835

Pulver SE: Narcissism: the term and the concept. J Am Psychoanal Assoc 18:319–341, 1970

Rado S: Schizotypal organization: preliminary report on a clinical study of schizophrenia, in Psychoanalysis and Behavior. New York, Grune & Stratton, 1956, pp 1–10

Rado S: Obsessive behavior, in American Handbook of Psychiatry, Vol 1. Edited by Arieti S. New York, Basic Books, 1959, pp 324–344

Raine A: Features of borderline personality and violence. J Clin Psychology 49:277–281, 1993

Raine A, Benishay D, Lencz T, et al: Abnormal orienting in schizotypal personality disorder. Schizophr Bull 23:75–82, 1997

Reich JH: DSM-III personality disorders and the outcome of treated panic disorder. Am J Psychiatry 145:1149–1152, 1988

Reich J[H], Boerstler H, Yates W, et al: Utilization of medical resources in persons with DSM-III personality disorders in a community sample. Int J Psychiatry Med 19:1–9, 1989

Reich W: Charakteranalyse: Technik und Grundlagen für studierende und praktizierende Analytiker. Leipzig, Germany, IM Selbstverlage des Verfassers, 1933

Reich W: On the technique of character analysis, in Character Analysis, 3rd Edition. New York, Simon & Schuster, 1949, pp 39–113

Reiss D, Hetherington EM, Plomin R, et al: Genetic questions for environmental studies: differential parenting and psychopathology in adolescence. Arch Gen Psychiatry 52:925–936, 1995

Robins LN: Deviant Children Grown Up: A Sociological and Psychiatric Study of Sociopathic Personality. Baltimore, MD, Williams & Wilkins, 1966

Salzman C, Wolfson AN, Schatzberg A, et al: Effect of fluoxetine on anger in symptomatic volunteers with borderline personality disorder. J Clin Psychopharmacol 15:23–29, 1995

Schneider K: Die psychopathischen Personlichkeiten. Vienna, Austria, Deuticke, 1923

Schneider K: Psychopathic Personalities. Springfield, IL, Charles C Thomas, 1958

Schneider K: Clinical Psychopathology. Translated by Hamilton MW. London, England, Grune & Stratton, 1959

Serban G, Siegel S: Response of borderline and schizotypal patients to small doses of thiothixene and haloperidol. Am J Psychiatry 141:1455–1458, 1984

Shapiro D: Neurotic Styles. New York, Basic Books, 1965

Siever LJ, Davis KL: A psychobiological perspective on the personality disorders. Am J Psychiatry 148:1647–1658, 1991

Siever LJ, Bernstein DP, Silverman JM: Schizotypal personality disorder: a review of its current status. J Personal Disord 5:178–193, 1991

Siever LJ, Amin F, Coccaro EF, et al: CSF homovanillic acid in schizotypal personality disorder. Am J Psychiatry 150:149–151, 1993

Skodol AE, Oldham JM: Assessment and diagnosis of borderline personality disorder. Hosp Community Psychiatry 42:1021–1028, 1991

Soloff PH: Psychopharmacologic therapies in borderline personality disorder, in American Psychiatric Press Review of Psychiatry, Vol 8. Edited by Tasman A, Hales RE, Frances AJ. Washington, DC, American Psychiatric Press, 1989, pp 65–83

Soloff PH, Cornelius J, George A, et al: Efficacy of phenelzine and haloperidol in borderline personality disorder. Arch Gen Psychiatry 50:377–385, 1993

Stone M: Schizotypal personality: psychotherapeutic aspects. Schizophr Bull 11:576–589, 1985

Tellegen A, Lykken DT, Bouchard TJ, et al: Personality similarity in twins reared apart and together. J Pers Soc Psychol 54:1031–1039, 1988

Torgersen S, Lygren S, Øien PA, et al: A twin study of personality disorders. Compr Psychiatry 41:416–425, 2000

Torgersen S, Onstad S, Skre I, et al: "True" schizotypal personality disorder: a study of co-twins and relatives of schizophrenic probands. Am J Psychiatry 150:1661–1667, 1993

Trestman RL, Keefe RSE, Mitropoulou V, et al: Cognitive function and biological correlates of cognitive performance in schizotypal personality disorder. Psychiatry Res 59:127–136, 1995

Turkat I, Maisto S: Application of the experimental method to the formulation and modification of personality disorders, in Clinical Handbook of Psychological Disorders. Edited by Barlow D. New York, Guilford, 1985, pp 502–570

Vaillant GE: Sociopathy as a human process: a viewpoint. Arch Gen Psychiatry 32:178–183, 1975

Vaillant GE: Ego Mechanisms of Defense: A Guide for Clinicians and Researchers. Washington, DC, American Psychiatric Press, 1992

Vaillant GE: Ego mechanisms of defense and personality psychopathology. J Abnorm Psychol 103:44–50, 1994

Verkes RJ, Van der Mast RC, Kerkhof AJFM, et al: Platelet serotonin, monoamine oxidase activity, and [3H] paroxetine binding related to impulsive suicide attempts and borderline personality disorder. Biol Psychiatry 43:740–746, 1998

Versiani M, Nardi AE, Mundim FD, et al: Pharmacotherapy of social phobia. A controlled study with moclobemide and phenelzine. Br J Psychiatry 161:353–360, 1992

Voglmaier MM, Seidman LJ, Nizmikiewicz MA, et al: Verbal and nonverbal neuropsychological test performance in subjects with schizotypal personality disorder. Am J Psychiatry 157:787–793, 2000

Wei T, Silverman J, Siever LJ: Ventricular volume and asymmetry in schizotypal personality disorder and schizophrenia assessed with magnetic resonance imaging. Schizophr Res 27:45–53, 1997

Weissman MM: The epidemiology of personality disorders: a 1990 update. J Personal Disord 7:44–62, 1993

Widiger TA: Personality Interview Questions—II. Lexington, KY, University of Kentucky, 1987

Widiger TA: Personality disorders in the 21st century. J Personal Disord 14:3–16, 2000

Widiger TA, Frances AJ: Interviews and inventories for the measurement of personality disorders. Clinical Psychology Review 7:49–75, 1987

Widiger TA, Corbitt EM, Millon T: Antisocial personality disorder, in American Psychiatric Press Review of Psychiatry, Vol 11. Edited by Tasman A, Riba ME. Washington, DC, American Psychiatric Press, 1992, pp 63–79

Woody GE, McLellan AT, Luborsky L, et al: Sociopathy and psychotherapy outcome. Arch Gen Psychiatry 42:1081–1086, 1985

World Health Organization: International Statistical Classification of Diseases and Related Health Problems, 10th Revision. Geneva, Switzerland, World Health Organization, 1992

Yonkers KA, Dyck IR, Warshaw M, et al: Factors predicting the clinical course of generalised anxiety disorder. Br J Psychiatry 176:544–549, 2000

Zanarini M: Role of Sexual Abuse in the Etiology of Borderline Personality Disorder. Washington DC, American Psychiatric Press, 1997

Zanarini M, Frankenburg FR: Pathways to the development of borderline personality disorder. J Personal Disord 11:93–104, 1997

Zanarini MC, Frankenburg FR, Chauncey DL, et al: The Diagnostic Interview for DSM-IV Personality Disorders. Belmont, MA, McLean Hospital, Laboratory for the Study of Adult Development, 1996

Zimmerman M, Coryell W: DSM-III personality disorder diagnoses in a nonpatient sample: demographic correlates and comorbidity. Arch Gen Psychiatry 46:682–689, 1989

Disorders Usually First Diagnosed in Infancy, Childhood, or Adolescence

Charles W. Popper, M.D.

G. Davis Gammon, M.D.

Scott A. West, M.D.

Charles E. Bailey, M.D.

Childhood is recognized in psychiatry as a period of vulnerability and progressive development toward adult personality and character. The psychiatric disorders in children and adolescents are increasingly coming into focus as serious but treatable conditions and as precursors of adult psychopathology.

In this chapter, the discrete psychopathological entities that are usually first diagnosed in youth are discussed. These disorders often emerge in combinations, change in presentation during maturation, interact with one another over time, and can be obscured or amplified by intervening developmental events. As in DSM-IV-TR (American Psychiatric Association 2000), these childhood-onset disorders are described here as crystalline abstract entities, a presentation that does not respect the individuality of their appearance in each child, cradled in a particular family and society, and undergoing continual change.

The primary "work" of children is to change and grow, a task that reflects their push to interact and modify in multiple dimensions. Rigid crystallized descriptions of their disorders do not convey the liveliness and energy of children who are coping and growing in ways that are characteristic of these disorders and in ways quite independent of psychiatric states.

The main message of this chapter concerns the dynamic undercurrent: not the rigidity of diagnostic categories but the flux and change that these abstract entities produce in the lives of children—and of the adults they become.

Multiple psychiatric disorders are typical in a single child psychiatric patient. Each primary psychiatric disorder in childhood can lead to secondary developmental complications, such as conduct disorder or school failure, and more persistently to low self-esteem and disorders of social assertiveness. Primary syndromes quickly expand with secondary complications during development, blurring the boundaries of the "original" psychiatric disorder. Certain disorders move in clusters through families and individuals and interact with one another to produce more virulent forms of the disorders. These interactive effects of multiple concurrent disorders are particularly evident in children and adolescents. Even though personality diagnoses usually are withheld before age 18 years, the typical child psychiatric outpatient carries two separate DSM diagnoses, and the typical inpatient carries four.

This developmental expansion of childhood psychopathology may generate a lifetime of "associated features." In dyslexia, the ectopic neurons and cytoarchitectonic anomalies in the cerebral cortex commonly lead to low frustration tolerance in childhood, rigidity in learning in adolescence, and underachievement in adulthood. The adult outcome of childhood psychopathology depends partly on the ways in which the psychopathology is amplified or contained by individual, family, cultural, and therapeutic forces.

Where were adult psychiatric patients during their childhoods? Part of the answer rests in the ability to observe and diagnose disorders in children. Not long ago, it was believed that mood disorders did not begin until mid- or late adolescence. Now it is known that all "adult" psychiatric disorders in DSM-IV-TR can begin during childhood. Any diagnosis can be used as a primary diagnostic label in a child. Even personality disorders, except for antisocial personality disorder, may be diagnosed in children if the characteristics of the personality disorder appear pervasive and unusually persistent. We also now know that all childhood-onset disorders can have major sequelae in adults or develop into adult disorders.

Medical conditions in children are crucial in evaluating their behavior; even mild or transient Axis III medical problems can cause flagrant behavioral symptoms, especially in young children (Cantwell and Baker 1988). The prevalence of psychiatric disorders is doubled in children with non–central nervous system (CNS) physical disabilities and diseases (Rutter and Yule 1970). On Axis IV, DSM-IV-TR provides a modified version of the Severity of Psychosocial Stressors Scale for children and adolescents. Parental absence or neglect, physical and sexual abuse, psychiatric disorders among caregivers, and even puberty exert age-specific effects on children. The Axis V Global Assessment of Functioning Scale incorporates features of the Children's Global Assessment Scale (Shaffer et al. 1983).

Developmental stage can influence the presentation, significance, and course of a psychiatric disorder. Coping functions and adaptive strengths change with development and are not related in a simple way to chronological age. Under the current DSM system, such developmental characteristics are not classified, and the clinician is left to personal judgment to assess the developmental stage of the individual and the developmental significance of presenting symptoms.

The DSM-IV-TR category "Disorders Usually First Diagnosed in Infancy, Childhood, or Adolescence" includes conditions that not only begin in childhood but also are typically *diagnosed* during childhood (Table 20–1). Some behavioral patterns are normal at certain developmental stages but become pathological at later developmental stages (e.g., separation anxiety disorder, enuresis, encopresis, and oppositional defiant disorder). Most of the behaviors shown in these disorders, however, are not "normal" at any age.

In this chapter, we do not discuss adjustment disorders in children (Newcorn and Strain 1992) or problems of parent–child relationships. Child development and

TABLE 20–1. DSM-IV-TR disorders usually first diagnosed in infancy, childhood, or adolescence

Mental retardation
  Mild mental retardation
  Moderate mental retardation
  Severe mental retardation
  Profound mental retardation
  Mental retardation, severity unspecified
Learning disorders
  Reading disorder
  Mathematics disorder
  Disorder of written expression
  Learning disorder not otherwise specified
Motor skills disorder
  Developmental coordination disorder
Pervasive developmental disorders
  Autistic disorder
  Rett's disorder
  Childhood disintegrative disorder
  Asperger's disorder
  Pervasive developmental disorder not otherwise specified
Attention-deficit and disruptive behavior disorders
  Attention-deficit/hyperactivity disorder
    Predominantly inattentive type
    Predominantly hyperactive-impulsive type
    Combined type
    Not otherwise specified
  Conduct disorder
  Oppositional defiant disorder
  Disruptive behavior disorder not otherwise specified
Feeding and eating disorders of infancy or early childhood
  Pica
  Rumination disorder of infancy
  Feeding disorder of infancy or early childhood
Tic disorders
  Tourette's disorder
  Chronic motor or vocal tic disorder
  Transient tic disorder
  Tic disorder not otherwise specified
Communication disorders
  Expressive language disorder
  Mixed receptive-expressive language disorder
  Phonological disorder
  Stuttering
  Communication disorder not otherwise specified
Elimination disorders
  Encopresis
  Enuresis
Other disorders of infancy, childhood, or adolescence
  Separation anxiety disorder
  Selective mutism
  Reactive attachment disorder of infancy or early childhood
  Stereotypic movement disorder
  Disorder of infancy, childhood, or adolescence not otherwise specified

child psychiatric treatment are discussed in Chapters 2 and 33, respectively. Important psychiatric disorders in youth, including mood and anxiety disorders, substance use disorders, eating disorders, and schizophrenia, also are described elsewhere in this volume. Although these conditions generally present with symptoms during childhood, they are frequently not diagnosed until the individual reaches maturity.

Just as psychopathological influences can undergo developmental expansion during early life, so can early therapeutic interventions. In knowing and treating childhood psychopathology, professionals are serving not only the children and the adults they become but also their parents and caregivers.

Disruptive Behavior Disorders

Attention-Deficit/Hyperactivity Disorder

Children and adults with attention-deficit/hyperactivity disorder (ADHD) show the behavioral characteristics of impulsivity and motor hyperactivity and the cognitive characteristics of inattention. The DSM-IV-TR criteria (Table 20–2) no longer suggest that ADHD is a childhood disorder—a loose mix of scattered attention and annoying behaviors—or a problem that is confined to one setting. It is now understood that ADHD persists into adulthood in many individuals (Biederman 1998; Faraone et al. 2000a; T. Spencer et al. 1998a; Wender 1998), and this body of research characterizing the phenomenology, comorbidity, and treatment of adult populations is growing. Thus far, most findings concerning ADHD in adults have been consistent with previous findings in children and adolescents (Biederman et al. 2000), where most of the available research remains concentrated at this time.

Originally described in antiquity and documented anecdotally throughout the world literature, ADHD was first identified on a large scale in the early twentieth century, when children with von Economo's encephalitis developed symptoms of hyperactivity, impulsivity, and inattention. Impulsive children such as these have been labeled as having "minimal brain damage" (even though there is no direct evidence of brain damage), "minimal brain dysfunction," "hyperkinetic syndrome," and "hyperactivity syndrome." As our understanding of this disorder has grown, the current nomenclature has subclassified ADHD into several discreet clinical entities.

The current ongoing debate is whether ADHD should be conceptualized in dimensional terms, described by a set of numbers quantifying various symptoms and their severity, or in categorical terms, described

as either present or absent—regardless of symptom severity. These two models support different concepts of the illness: ADHD as a diverse group of behavior-management problems or as a disorder with a final, common physiological pathway. Clinically, both models are useful concepts. Indeed, the National Institute of Mental Health Consensus Statement (1998) concluded that although there are differing clinical models for ADHD, substantial evidence supports the validity of the disorder and the adverse long-term effects that may result from lack of appropriate diagnosis and treatment.

Clinical Description

Symptoms of ADHD fall into three primary domains: motor hyperactivity, impulsivity, and inattention. These core symptoms may present in different ways at different ages, but they reflect the shared basic characteristics of the disorder (see Table 20–3).

Measures of activity and attention are weakly correlated, and these symptom clusters appear to reflect independent dimensions of psychopathology. In factor analyses of behavioral ratings on Conners' Hyperactivity Scale and the Achenbach Child Behavioral Checklist (CBCL; Achenbach and Ruffle 1998), the "hyperactivity" factor emerges robustly as a distinct component of general childhood behavior, and "inattention" emerges as a separate factor, not as powerful but consistent in clinical and community samples of children. This separation between the cognitive and the behavioral factors is clinically useful. The DSM-IV-TR subtyping of ADHD into "predominantly inattentive," "predominantly hyperactive-impulsive," and "combined" types allows the diagnostic label of ADHD to designate three of the most pronounced symptom complexes. Each of these three DSM-IV-TR ADHD subtypes appears to have a distinct prognosis and response to treatment; therefore, a separate clinical assessment of inattention and hyperactivity-impulsivity is necessary when evaluating for ADHD.

The DSM-IV-TR diagnosis of ADHD not otherwise specified (NOS) subsumes conditions similar to ADHD that do not fulfill diagnostic criteria. Although this might be expected to be a diagnosis of convenience rather than a biologically distinct disorder, researchers using quantitative electroencephalography and evoked response potentials have found electrophysiological characteristics that distinguish ADHD NOS from the three main forms of ADHD (Kuperman et al. 1996). This finding suggests that an additional subtype of ADHD may indeed exist, currently hidden within the group of patients with ADHD NOS, and that further research on individuals with ADHD NOS may be warranted.

TABLE 20–2. DSM-IV-TR diagnostic criteria for attention-deficit/hyperactivity disorder

A. Either (1) or (2):

    (1) six (or more) of the following symptoms of **inattention** have persisted for at least 6 months to a degree that is maladaptive and inconsistent with developmental level:

       Inattention

       (a) often fails to give close attention to details or makes careless mistakes in schoolwork, work, or other activities

       (b) often has difficulty sustaining attention in tasks or play activities

       (c) often does not seem to listen when spoken to directly

       (d) often does not follow through on instructions and fails to finish schoolwork, chores, or duties in the workplace (not due to oppositional behavior or failure to understand instructions)

       (e) often has difficulty organizing tasks and activities

       (f) often avoids, dislikes, or is reluctant to engage in tasks that require sustained mental effort (such as schoolwork or homework)

       (g) often loses things necessary for tasks or activities (e.g., toys, school assignments, pencils, books, or tools)

       (h) is often easily distracted by extraneous stimuli

       (i) is often forgetful in daily activities

    (2) six (or more) of the following symptoms of **hyperactivity-impulsivity** have persisted for at least 6 months to a degree that is maladaptive and inconsistent with developmental level:

       Hyperactivity

       (a) often fidgets with hands or feet or squirms in seat

       (b) often leaves seat in classroom or in other situations in which remaining seated is expected

       (c) often runs about or climbs excessively in situations in which it is inappropriate (in adolescents or adults, may be limited to subjective feelings of restlessness)

       (d) often has difficulty playing or engaging in leisure activities quietly

       (e) is often "on the go" or often acts as if "driven by a motor"

       (f) often talks excessively

       Impulsivity

       (g) often blurts out answers before questions have been completed

       (h) often has difficulty awaiting turn

       (i) often interrupts or intrudes on others (e.g., butts into conversations or games)

B. Some hyperactive-impulsive or inattentive symptoms that caused impairment were present before age 7 years.

C. Some impairment from the symptoms is present in two or more settings (e.g., at school [or work] and at home).

D. There must be clear evidence of clinically significant impairment in social, academic, or occupational functioning.

E. The symptoms do not occur exclusively during the course of a pervasive developmental disorder, schizophrenia, or other psychotic disorder and are not better accounted for by another mental disorder (e.g., mood disorder, anxiety disorder, dissociative disorder, or a personality disorder).

Code based on type:

    314.01 Attention-Deficit/Hyperactivity Disorder, Combined Type: if both Criteria A1 and A2 are met for the past 6 months

    314.00 Attention-Deficit/Hyperactivity Disorder, Predominantly Inattentive Type: if Criterion A1 is met but Criterion A2 is not met for the past 6 months

    314.01 Attention-Deficit/Hyperactivity Disorder, Predominantly Hyperactive-Impulsive Type: if Criterion A2 is met but Criterion A1 is not met for the past 6 months

Coding note: For individuals (especially adolescents and adults) who currently have symptoms that no longer meet full criteria, "in partial remission" should be specified.

Although people with ADHD tend to be symptomatic in many if not all settings, the intensity of symptoms varies across settings. Symptoms tend to be more pronounced with more environmental structure, such as classrooms and restaurants; during high levels of sensory stimulation; and during high emotional states. Children tend to experience more environmental demands at school, where they are expected to maintain concentration, focus, and inhibit their physical and mental impulses, than at home. Indeed, patients with ADHD may appear quite different to observers in different environments, with symptoms often more apparent in the crowded waiting rooms or clinic hallways than to a physician in a quiet office.

TABLE 20–3. Different presentations of attention-deficit/hyperactivity disorder (ADHD) through the life cycle

Developmental stage	Characteristics of ADHD	Comments
Infancy	Frequent crying; difficult to soothe; sleep disturbances; feeding difficulties	May cry to an extent that interferes with nutritional intake; may be excessively drowsy and unresponsive or sleep poorly because of overreactivity and restlessness.
Preschool	Motor restlessness; insatiable curiosity; vigorous and sometimes destructive play; demanding of parental attention; low-level compliance (especially with boys); excessive temper tantrums; difficulty completing developmental tasks; decreased and/or restless sleep; delays in motor or language development; family difficulties	Often difficult to distinguish from normal behaviors in children at this age; the child seems as if "driven by a motor"; climbs on and gets into things constantly; often accidentally breaks toys and household objects; accidental injuries are also common; severity, frequency, and duration of tantrums far exceed those in children without ADHD.
School-aged children	Easily distracted; engages in off-task activities; unable to sustain attention; impulsive; displays aggression; acts as a "class clown"; social deficits include having difficulty waiting for a turn, following rules, losing gracefully, curbing temper, showing consideration for others; frequently becomes overly excited or may act very silly	May call out in class inappropriately, fidget excessively, have difficulty staying in seat; assignments are frequently messy and disorganized with many mistakes. Symptoms affect academic performance and cause increasing difficulty in peer relationships and social interactions as the child grows older; failures in these areas may lead to poor self-esteem and depression.
Adolescents	Excessive motor activity (e.g., excessive running and climbing, not staying in seat) tends to decrease, although fidgetiness and inner restlessness may continue; problem behaviors include discipline problems, family conflict, anger and emotional lability, difficulty with authority, significant lags in academic performance; poor peer relationships; poor self-esteem; hopelessness; lethargy and lack of motivation; driving mishaps, speeding, accidents.	Impulsive symptoms may lead adolescents to break rules and get into conflict with authority figures.
Adults	Difficulty with concentration and performing sedentary tasks; disorganization; forgetfulness; losing things; failure to plan; depending on others to maintain order; difficulty keeping track of several things at once; trouble both getting started on and finishing tasks; changing plans or jobs in midstream; misjudging time; restlessness; impulsivity; being "absentminded"	May have employment difficulties, especially in desk jobs, which may lead to short durations of employment; higher incidence of antisocial acts and arrests than in the general population.

Source. Reprinted with permission from Conners CK, March JS, Frances A, et al (eds): "Treatment of Attention-Deficit/Hyperactivity Disorder: Expert Consensus Guidelines." *Journal of Attention Disorders* 4(suppl 1):7–128, 2001.

Although DSM-IV-TR emphasizes the three core symptoms, pathological functioning is also seen in motivation, emotionality, anger control, and aggression. Motivational problems in ADHD can include variability, unpredictability, difficulty in sustaining interest and completing projects, and simple frustration and discouragement. Although these characteristics are considered in DSM-IV-TR to be associated features of ADHD, lack of motivation and difficulty in self-organization may produce more functional interference than do the core symptoms of

ADHD. Emotional impulsivity is most obvious in anger and aggressive behavior, symptoms that can be regularly triggered in response to only minor provocation. Exploratory behavior can seem aggressive, involving an energetic foraging into new places and things. On entering a room, a child with ADHD may immediately begin to touch and climb. These inclinations can lead to rough handling of objects, accidental breakage, intrusive entry into unsafe areas, physical injuries, and even accidental ingestions. Property damage may result without malicious intent.

However, it is important to remember that many children with ADHD do not have behavior problems, hyperactivity, or excessive aggression. The predominantly inattentive type of ADHD is very common and often is found in settings such as primary care offices and learning disorder clinics, where the threshold for evaluation does not require high levels of hyperactivity and/or aggression. In contrast to children with the predominantly hyperactive-impulsive type of ADHD, predominantly inattentive children show more manageable behavior, mild anxiety and shyness, more sluggishness and drowsiness, less impulsivity, less conduct disorder and problem behavior, and more mood and anxiety disorders (Gaub and Carlson 1997; Lahey et al. 1987).

Girls and women with ADHD have received more attention in recent years, as attempts have been made to closely examine populations other than preadolescent boys with ADHD. Historically, girls have been reported to have less impulsivity, hyperactivity, and comorbid conduct disorder than boys (Berry et al. 1985). However, factor analysis of behavioral data in adults with ADHD suggests that certain inattention and impulsivity items load on different factors in men than in women; that is, gender affects factor composition (M.A. Stein et al. 1995). Recent studies indicate that there are far more similarities than differences in core ADHD symptoms between boys and girls (Biederman et al. 1999a; Rucklidge and Tannock 2001). Moreover, these studies have found that girls are at higher risk for more psychological impairment, with more fear, depression, mood swings, cognitive difficulties, and language problems than boys with ADHD. These recent data seem to dispel the myth that females suffer silently with minimal symptoms, because their outcome is often worse than that of males (Faraone et al. 2000b).

Although inattention and hyperactivity-impulsivity are currently the two defining dimensions of ADHD in DSM-IV-TR, the organizational deficits, motivational problems, and impaired time sense in ADHD deserve considerably more clinical attention and warrant further research because they might constitute additional dimensions of ADHD. Currently, the three-dimensional concept of ADHD has a high degree of clinical usefulness and scientific validity, but the construct of ADHD will likely become more differentiated and multidimensional as research continues.

Epidemiology

In the United States, approximately 6% of school-age children have ADHD (range=3%–10%). ADHD is present in 30%–50% of children in child psychiatric outpatient clinics and inpatient treatment centers. The strong male predominance in ADHD (3–10 to 1) may be partly the result of diagnostic expectations rather than true predominance. Despite this potential bias, girls are generally reported to constitute up to 25% of children with ADHD and may constitute a higher proportion of the predominantly inattentive subtype.

The prevalence of childhood ADHD has been traditionally higher in the United States than in other countries, a difference that may be a result of diagnostic practices. In the past, about 2% of child psychiatric outpatients in Great Britain had a diagnosis of ADHD compared with 40% in the United States. Prevalence rates have become more uniform among countries as different internationally used diagnostic systems have come into greater concordance.

Pharmacoepidemiological studies have estimated that 2%–4% of the United States school population is receiving psychostimulant medications, with recent trends indicating an increase in the number of prescriptions each year. Between 1990 and 1995, there was a 2.5-fold rise in the use of psychostimulants in the United States (Safer et al. 1996), and significant increases also have been noted in Australia (Valentine et al. 1997). Factors that have been proposed to explain these continual increases in psychostimulant use include the growing recognition and treatment of ADHD in adolescents and adults, increasing drug treatment of predominantly inattentive ADHD, more extensive treatment of young females, lengthier treatments, physician familiarity and comfort in prescribing psychostimulants, increased visibility of ADHD and its treatment in the public media, and the growth of national organizations such as Children and Adults With ADD (ChADD) that provide grassroots support and information to individuals and families affected by ADHD.

Etiology

No evidence indicates that there is only one attention deficit or that a single brain mechanism is responsible for all manifestations of ADHD. Similarly, there is no evidence of a single gene defect or a specific mechanism of genetic transmission in ADHD, and the hereditary component is likely to be polygenic (S.G. Vandenberg et al. 1986). Different etiologies and different sites of pharmacological action may be relevant for different individuals or subpopulations with ADHD.

Genetics. Although family studies have suggested strong genetic and nongenetic contributions (Pauls 1991), the genetic factors appear to predominate (Faraone and Doyle 2001; Sherman et al. 1997). The prevalence of psychopathology is two to three times higher in the relatives of children with ADHD, even after controlling for socioeconomic class and family intactness. In adopted children with ADHD, biological parents have been found to have more psychopathology than adopting parents (Deutsch et al. 1982). Family members of children with ADHD show an increased prevalence of ADHD, conduct disorder and antisocial personality disorder, mood disorders, anxiety disorders, and substance abuse.

A strong genetic influence is consistent with findings that ADHD appears to form clusters with certain comorbid psychiatric conditions that are transmitted together in particular families. Such findings suggest that genetic factors related to comorbidity might be relevant to an etiologically based subtyping of ADHD. For example, ADHD is often diagnosed in some children who would be more accurately diagnosed as having bipolar disorder or anxiety disorder, so that the presence of ADHD symptoms might reflect other genetically transmitted disorders. As a result, the early literature on familial patterns of ADHD is full of inconsistencies, and some controversies regarding comorbidity persist. Furthermore, separate genetic factors may be involved in the etiology of different features of ADHD or of associated features of ADHD.

Although the extent of genetic influence appears to vary, several specific genes have been implicated in the development of ADHD (Sprich et al. 2000). Indeed, ADHD is most likely a polygenic disorder involving dopamine, norepinephrine, serotonin, γ-aminobutyric acid (GABA), and other neurotransmitters (Comings 2001; Comings et al. 2000a).

Genes for components of the dopamine neurotransmitter system have received the most attention. In particular, linkage studies have associated ADHD with allelic variants of the D_4 dopamine receptor gene (*DRD4*) (Faraone et al. 2001; LaHoste et al. 1996; McCracken et al. 2000; Roman et al. 2001; Sunohara et al. 2000; Swanson et al. 1998; Todd et al. 2001) and of the *DAT1* gene that codes for the dopamine transporter 1 protein involved in presynaptic reuptake of dopamine (Barr et al. 2001; Cook et al. 1995; Gill et al. 1997; Rowe et al. 2001; D.J. Vandenbergh et al. 2000). The 7-repeat allele of *DRD4*, the variant that has been associated with ADHD, codes for a form of the receptor that appears to transduce a diminished intracellular response to dopamine. This finding suggests that decreased postreceptor response to postsynaptic dopamine might be a plausible pathophysiological mechanism underlying at least some forms of ADHD. It also has been proposed that the "defective gene" might be a marker for nonresponsiveness to psychostimulants (Seeger et al. 2001b). Interestingly, the *DRD4* gene, distributed in cortical and limbic regions, has been associated in some studies (but not all) with novelty-seeking behavior (Benjamin et al. 1996; Ebstein et al. 1996). In a similar manner, the 10-repeat allelic variant of the dopamine transporter gene (*DAT1*) may be associated with hyperefficient reuptake of dopamine from the synaptic cleft (Swanson et al. 2000), suggesting that reduced intrasynaptic dopamine might represent another potential mechanism underlying ADHD. Although the association of ADHD with these allelic variants of the *DRD4* and *DAT1* genes has been supported in most studies, other studies have failed to confirm these associations. Also, some limited evidence indicates linkage of ADHD with the *DRD5* gene that encodes the D_5 dopamine receptor (Comings 2001) and with the *DRD2* gene that encodes the D_2 dopamine receptor (Blum et al. 1996).

Genes for the norepinephrine receptor α_{1C} (*ADRA1C*), dopamine β-hydroxylase (*DBH*), epinephrine-synthesizing enzyme phenylethanolamine *N*-methyltransferase (*PNMT*), catecholamine-breakdown enzymes catechol-*O*-methyltransferase (*COMT*) and monoamine oxidase A (*MAOA*), and the norepinephrine transporter also have been postulated to play a significant role in ADHD (Comings et al. 2000b). This preliminary genetic evidence is consistent with the efficacy of noradrenergic reuptake inhibitors in ADHD (Michelson et al. 2001).

An association with a polymorphism of the promotor region for the serotonin transporter (5-HTTLPR) also has been proposed (Manor et al. 2001; Seeger et al. 2001a) and may show significant interaction with *DRD4* (Auerbach et al. 2001). The *HTR1A* gene for the serotonin 1A receptor and other serotonin genes (including *TD02* and *HTR1DA*) also are being investigated.

Taken together, these genetic findings suggest that multiple genetic or polygenic mechanisms may contribute and that gene variants coding for dopamine (and possibly also other) neurotransmitter system structures may underlie the pathophysiology of ADHD. Although these data are congruent with the family studies examining the phenomenology, comorbidity, and familial patterns of ADHD, many of these data require confirmation through further investigation and replication to increase the reliability of the findings on specific genetic contributions. Indeed, not all investigations have confirmed the current genetic findings, even for the *DRD4* and *DAT1* genes (Barr et al. 2000; Castellanos et al. 1998; Payton et al. 2001).

General medical factors. Various medical factors can lead to the appearance of ADHD or ADHD-like symptoms, including streptococcal infection, generalized resistance to thyroid hormone, hyperthyroidism, ordinary hunger, and even occasionally constipation. Certain psychiatric medications also may mimic ADHD by inducing anxiety, agitation, mood swings, behavioral activation, or disinhibition. These medications include psychostimulants, antidepressants, anticonvulsants, benzodiazepines, and substances such as caffeine and theophylline.

Pediatric autoimmune neuropsychiatric disorders associated with streptococcal infections (PANDAS), such as obsessive-compulsive disorder (OCD) and Tourette's disorder, also may present with ADHD symptoms. Indeed, about half of the preadolescent children diagnosed with PANDAS have symptoms of ADHD (Peterson et al. 2000; Swedo et al. 1998).

Generalized resistance to thyroid hormone results from an autosomal dominant mutation in human thyroid hormone receptors (chromosome 3) that makes them underresponsive to the action of thyroid hormone, and 50% of the cases present with ADHD (Hauser et al. 1993). It is interesting that generalized resistance to thyroid hormone in males is associated with brain abnormalities accrued during early fetal development, including multiple appearances of Heschl's gyrus bilaterally and Sylvian fissure anomalies in the left hemisphere (C.M. Leonard et al. 1995). Although generalized resistance to thyroid hormone is often associated with ADHD, the reverse is not true: the prevalence of generalized resistance to thyroid hormone among patients with ADHD is too low to warrant routine thyroid screening. Apart from the uncommon disorder of generalized resistance to thyroid hormone, thyroid disorders are diagnosed in about 2%–3% of the children with ADHD, which is within the 1%–4% prevalence rate for a general pediatric population (Valentine et al. 1997). However, the association of generalized resistance to thyroid hormone with low intelligence might be stronger than its association with ADHD (R.E. Weiss et al. 1994), and the apparent association of generalized resistance to thyroid hormone and ADHD might be mediated by intelligence.

Because nutrition is a critical factor in the development of the CNS, severe early malnutrition may be a common cause of ADHD worldwide. In children who experience severe malnutrition during the first year of life, 60% show inattention, impulsivity, and hyperactivity persisting at least into adolescence (Galler et al. 1983). In addition, pyloric stenosis is associated with the subsequent appearance of ADHD, even when corrected by age 2 months. At this time, the specific nutritional deficiencies that contribute to the etiology of ADHD are unknown.

Neuromedical factors. Neuromedical etiologies of ADHD include brain damage (often frontal cortex), neurological disorders, low birth weight, extreme perinatal anoxia, and exposure to neurotoxins. Intrauterine exposure to toxic substances, including alcohol, lead, cigarette smoke, and probably cocaine, can produce teratological effects on behavior. For example, fetal alcohol syndrome includes hyperactivity, impulsivity, and inattention as well as physical anomalies and diminished intelligence.

Children with ADHD have higher mean blood lead levels than do their siblings. A large-scale study in Ottawa, Ontario, showed a topological distribution of ADHD children living in public housing, perhaps reflecting the lead-containing paints in residential buildings. However, far higher Conners' Teacher Rating Scale scores were observed among children who lived near a major roadway, apparently showing the strong effect of lead-containing gasolines. In first-grade students generally, a dose–response relation has been found between lead concentrations in hair and teachers' ratings of disruptive behavior, regardless of socioeconomic class (Tuthill 1996). Lead can produce a broad range of toxic effects, especially during development, and these effects are more common and more persistent than generally realized. Both prenatal and postnatal toxic lead exposure can precede ADHD and other cognitive deficits (Bellinger et al. 1987). Transient lead exposure during childhood produces neurocognitive and neurobehavioral abnormalities that may persist for 10 or more years (Needleman et al. 1990). Although its physical toxicity rises in a dose-dependent manner, there appears to be no minimal level below which lead ceases to have toxic effects on the development of cognition (Winneke and Krämer 1997).

Intrauterine exposure to cigarette smoke also may be associated with ADHD. In one study, 22% of the mothers of children with ADHD smoked during pregnancy, compared with 8% of the mothers of children without ADHD (Milberger et al. 1996).

Obstetrical complications during late pregnancy or delivery occasionally may result in ADHD. Generally, obstetrical difficulties and perinatal asphyxia are not highly correlated with the appearance of neurological disorders such as cerebral palsy (Nelson and Ellenberg 1986), and such events probably do not account for more than a small percentage of cases of ADHD (Nichols and Chen 1981). Furthermore, correlations between perinatal distress and ADHD may not reflect a causal link.

Overt neurological disorders, most commonly seizures and cerebral palsy, are present in approximately 5% of the children with ADHD, although they do not correlate with the severity of ADHD symptoms. Like children with other psychiatric disorders, children with ADHD may have multiple minor physical and neurological anomalies. Nonlocalizing neurological soft signs (such as clumsiness, left-right confusion, perceptual-motor dyscoordination, and dysgraphia) are common in children with ADHD. However, approximately 15% of the children without ADHD have up to five neurological soft signs, so the clinical relevance usually is presumed to be insignificant.

ADHD with onset after toddlerhood may indicate the presence of acquired neuropathological changes, such as traumatic brain injury, encephalitis, or CNS infection. Frontal lobe injury often results in ADHD symptoms, but brain lesions in a variety of other locations can lead to a clinical picture that resembles ADHD and responds to medication in a similar manner.

Right hemisphere syndrome. ADHD-like symptoms are present in 93% of the patients with right hemisphere syndrome (Voeller 1986). Typically evident from birth, right hemisphere syndrome is not a medical disorder, a result of injury or disease, or a learning disorder in the usual sense that involves a particular skill, such as reading or arithmetic. Instead, it consists of a series of right cortical deficits that can appear in healthy individuals who have difficulties with learning, memory, concentration, and organization (García-Sánchez et al. 1997). The entire right hemisphere appears to be involved, with no specific localization.

Right hemisphere syndrome is readily identifiable in routine intelligence testing by a Verbal IQ score that is significantly higher than the Performance IQ score. Usually, a 20-point IQ difference can generate noticeable characteristics, and 20- to 50-point differences account for most cases. Extreme cases can involve differences of 100 points or more, with the level of intelligence of individuals with right hemisphere syndrome ranging from retarded to brilliant.

The crucial feature in right hemisphere syndrome is not poor right hemisphere functioning but a marked mismatch between the intelligence of each hemisphere. Because neither hemisphere is usually defective, right hemisphere syndrome is typically conceptualized as a difference in functioning rather than as a medical disorder. In addition to the expected right-sided characteristics classically seen in patients with right hemisphere neurological damage, individuals with right hemisphere syndrome have what might be called "social dyslexia": difficulty in perceiving and reacting to social cues; incomplete comprehension of other people's sense of humor, even though they may be quite witty themselves; slow acquisition of social skills; being viewed by others as strange or odd; and a tendency to become angry or aggressive because of these social misunderstandings. Depressive disorders seem to be very common, perhaps because of the diminished social functioning and demoralization that may occur. As children and adults, individuals with right hemisphere syndrome are frequently far more verbally gifted than their other achievements might suggest.

Unlike ADHD, the ADHD-like symptoms of right hemisphere syndrome typically respond poorly to medications, but cognitive-behavioral treatment appears helpful. An ambitious approach is developmentally guided cognitive therapy, similar in some ways to the neuropsychological rehabilitative treatments offered to people who have sustained major brain trauma. This constructional treatment involves step-by-step learning, starting with simple mental tasks, progressively building on newly acquired skills, with the progression of specific steps determined by cognitive and developmental principles.

Misdiagnosis. Misidentification does not normally function as an etiological factor, but ADHD can be viewed as a special case because many psychiatric disorders may, on the surface, look similar to ADHD in their clinical presentation. Disorders that look like ADHD include oppositional defiant disorder, conduct disorder, bipolar disorder, Tourette's disorder, posttraumatic stress disorder (PTSD), abuse or neglect, and even major depressive disorder (Table 20–4). For example, about 25% of the patients who traditionally might have been given diagnoses of ADHD are now given diagnoses of bipolar disorder—and vice versa.

Comorbidity

Often misdiagnosed for other disorders (Table 20–4), ADHD represents a true challenge in many individuals because of the valid and extensive comorbidity often present. Unfortunately, these comorbid conditions are often the only diagnosis made, causing particular concern when these diagnoses are the result of a primary diagnosis of ADHD, such as substance abuse and depression. Indeed, the high prevalence of comorbidity in ADHD poses a variety of problems for both diagnostic practice and the understanding of the etiology of the disorder. ADHD is unique, at least in psychiatry, in being a highly prevalent disorder that may frequently be misdiagnosed in a large proportion of cases. Although misdiagnosis can distort the understanding and treatment of any medical condition, ADHD is a special case because of the high frequency of diagnostic error. To minimize this possibility, structured assessments may be a critical tool to adequately tease apart complicated and at times overlapping

TABLE 20–4. Psychiatric disorders often associated with attention-deficit/hyperactivity disorder

Conduct disorder
Oppositional defiant disorder
Anxiety disorders
Learning disorders
Motor skills disorder
Substance use disorders
Communication disorders
Bipolar disorder
Major depression
Posttraumatic stress disorder
Obsessive-compulsive disorder
Tourette's disorder
Schizophrenia
Mental retardation
Pervasive developmental disorders, including autistic disorder

Note. Various psychiatric states should be assessed clinically in individuals with attention-deficit/hyperactivity disorder, even though strong statistical associations have not been shown for each of these conditions.

symptom clusters. To accurately diagnose ADHD, all confounding and potentially comorbid diagnoses should be considered.

Conduct disorder and oppositional defiant disorder. Conduct disorder (not merely conduct problems or symptoms) is seen in 40%–70% of the children with ADHD, and about the same percentage of children with conduct disorder have ADHD (Kadesjo and Gillberg 2001; Soussignan and Tremblay 1996). Children whose conduct disorder is diagnosed before age 12 years nearly always meet criteria for ADHD, whereas about one-third of children with adolescent-onset conduct disorder meet ADHD criteria.

Children and adolescents with comorbid ADHD and conduct disorder differ sufficiently from those with ADHD alone that comorbid ADHD and conduct disorder is increasingly recognized as a separate subtype (Jensen 2001). Although laboratory measures of attention, activity, and impulsivity generally have failed to show differences between these groups (Werry et al. 1987), teachers consistently rate children with comorbid ADHD and conduct disorder as more hyperactive-impulsive and less attentive than those with ADHD alone (Reeves et al. 1987; S.K. Shapiro and Garfinkel 1986). Similarly, in a recent subanalysis of the Multimodal Treatment Study of Children With ADHD (MTA), children with comorbid ADHD and conduct disorder were rated as more impulsive than inattentive on continuous performance testing (Newcorn et al. 2001). Children with

ADHD and delinquency were more likely (36%) than children with ADHD alone (19%) or control subjects (7%) to have reading disorder (McGee et al. 1984), and they were more likely to have impaired language skills, visual-motor integration, and visuospatial skills (Moffitt 1990; Moffitt and Silva 1988). Children with the predominantly hyperactive-impulsive subtype of ADHD plus conduct disorder have been found to have high levels of family psychopathology, whereas the predominantly inattentive type of ADHD has been linked to neurological disorders, lower IQ, and additional cognitive deficits (August et al. 1983; Lahey et al. 1988b). The relatives of children with ADHD and comorbid ADHD and conduct disorder have been reported to have an approximately similar prevalence of ADHD, but the relatives of children with comorbid ADHD and conduct disorder appeared to have a higher prevalence of conduct disorder (26% vs. 13%), and comorbid ADHD and conduct disorder appeared to cosegregate in the families (Biederman et al. 1992).

Anxiety disorders. About one-third of the children with ADHD have an anxiety disorder (MTA Cooperative Group 1999a), reflecting a two- to fourfold increase in prevalence compared with children in the general population (Bird et al. 1993; P. Cohen et al. 1993). Family genetic studies have suggested that the risk for anxiety disorders may be transmitted separately from the risk for ADHD (Biederman et al. 1991, 1992; Perrin and Last 1996).

A child's self-report of anxiety is considered more reliable than the parents' (Pliszka 1992), as is often the case with internalizing disorders. However, their perceptions of their other problems might be distorted by anxiety. Children with comorbid ADHD and anxiety disorders report more school problems than do their peers with ADHD alone, although they were not found to have higher frequencies of learning disorders or impaired school performance (Biederman et al. 1991). They also report a range of social difficulties more frequently, such as stressful life events (Jensen et al. 1993), and divorce was found to be more frequent in their families (Biederman et al. 1991).

Some reports suggest that children with ADHD and comorbid anxiety may be less likely to respond to psychostimulants (Pliszka 1989; Taylor et al. 1987), although this finding remains controversial. For example, in the large-scale MTA study, comorbid anxiety did not predict nonresponse to psychostimulants. Interestingly, children with comorbid ADHD and anxiety disorders appeared more likely than children with ADHD alone to benefit from combined psychostimulant and psychosocial treatment (MTA Cooperative Group 1999b).

Mood disorders. Children with ADHD may have an increased prevalence of major depressive disorder, although these findings have been mixed. Nonetheless, whether minimal or robust, the connection is likely in part biological. Both ADHD and major depressive disorder are associated with decreased rapid eye movement (REM) latency, responsiveness to noradrenergic antidepressants, genetic interrelationships, anxiety disorders, and bipolar disorder. More than half of the children with bipolar disorder also fulfill criteria for ADHD (Butler et al. 1995; West et al. 1995, 1996), and about 20%–25% of the children with ADHD also fulfill criteria for bipolar disorder (Biederman et al. 1996a; Butler et al. 1995). Thus, certain children with ADHD may have precursor conditions of bipolar disorder or they may have true comorbid conditions that significantly affect the course of treatment (T. Spencer et al. 2001a; West et al. 1995; Wozniak et al. 2001a).

Tic disorders. Tourette's disorder is overrepresented in patients with ADHD, and at least 25% of males with Tourette's disorder have ADHD. OCD in children also appears to be linked to ADHD, often in association with Tourette's disorder. More recently, children who have comorbid tic disorder with ADHD as well as those who have comorbid OCD with ADHD have been found to have PANDAS antistreptococcal/antineuronal antibodies. About half of these cases also fulfill criteria for ADHD (Peterson et al. 2000; Swedo et al. 1998).

The comorbid appearance of ADHD, Tourette's disorder, and OCD has emerged as a clinically significant cluster of diagnoses, with each of these three disorders apparently sharing a common genetic etiology. Their shared genetic characteristics suggest that ADHD associated with Tourette's disorder and/or OCD might be different from other forms of ADHD in terms of physiological, phenomenological, or pharmacological features (T. Spencer et al. 2001b). For example, certain genes might increase vulnerability to streptococcal infections, leading to the autoimmune forms of ADHD symptoms. Alternatively, aggressive behavior in some patients with ADHD may result partially from the anxiety associated with OCD or from the complex tics associated with Tourette's disorder.

Pervasive developmental disorders. Autism presents so commonly with ADHD that the DSM-III-R criteria (American Psychiatric Association 1987) for ADHD excluded its diagnosis in the presence of autism. That exclusion was removed in DSM-IV (American Psychiatric Association 1994), so patients with autistic disorder and ADHD can legitimately be treated with psychostim-

ulants without the necessity of declaring autism to be a new indication for psychostimulants.

Psychotic agitation. Although relatively uncommon, accurate differential diagnosis of psychotic agitation is essential because psychostimulant or antidepressant treatment can exacerbate psychotic symptoms. Typically, patients with ADHD have absolutely no hallucinations, delusional thinking, or breakthroughs of primary process thinking. However, similar to patients with psychotic disorders, ADHD patients may have loose thought patterns, engage in self-endangering behavior, and show little awareness of their environment. The motor activity in ADHD appears continuous and endless, and the tempo of the impulsivity is roughly constant, in contrast to the irregular and less predictable body and affective tempo of psychotic children. Psychotic children may show anger and emotional overreactions that are primarily derived from cognitive distortions and can have a long duration (30 minutes to 5 hours). In contrast, emotional overreactions in patients with ADHD usually are based on misunderstandings and accidents, and tantrums in these patients usually resolve within 30 minutes. Generally, the long-term course of ADHD is gradual improvement (Biederman et al. 2000), in contrast to psychotic disorders, which typically worsen with time. Also of interest, though, is that some children of mothers with schizophrenia have motor and attention deficits and, according to follow-up studies, often grow up to become adults with schizophrenia; and their non-ADHD siblings have a low incidence of adult schizophrenia (Marcus et al. 1985).

Learning disorders. ADHD is associated with a high prevalence of all learning and communication disorders. Similarly, ADHD has a relatively high prevalence in samples of individuals with mental retardation. Language disorders and reading disorders (Purvis and Tannock 2000) may occur in patients with ADHD and are often not reflected in routine IQ testing and scores (Tirosh and Cohen 1998), suggesting a need for specific testing when clinically appropriate.

Psychosocial factors. Psychosocial factors such as situational anxiety, child abuse and neglect, and simple boredom can clinically manifest in symptoms that mimic ADHD. Examination of the course of illness distinguishes these conditions from ADHD.

Pathogenesis

Elucidating the pathophysiology of ADHD is a complex and ongoing task that is complicated by the remaining diagnostic and conceptual ambiguities. The large array of etiological factors, mechanisms, symptom overlap, comorbid disorders, developmental changes, and complications of illness—and especially their interactions—explain why it has been difficult to identify the core symptoms of ADHD as distinct from those of other disorders. The task of cleaning up the blur of diagnostic boundaries is an essential step in the formation of a definition of ADHD. Research on the etiology and pathophysiology is complicated by the incompleteness of this effort.

Although both biological and psychosocial factors are involved in shaping the appearance of ADHD in individuals, it appears that most cases of ADHD have a pronounced biological origin. A wide variety of biological findings in ADHD may contribute to the descriptive and etiological understanding of this disorder. Although current findings remain largely incomplete, scattered, and discrepant, some emerging trends can be noted. Diverse studies provide glimpses of potentially significant correlations among abnormal functional (behavioral, neuropsychological), anatomical, biochemical (neurochemical, pharmacological), and developmental findings.

Neuropsychological studies. Many methodological and conceptual issues remain to be worked out, but the neuropsychological literature implicates disturbances in response inhibition and various executive functions in the pathogenesis of ADHD (see Tannock 1998 and Barkley 2000 for reviews).

Deficits in response inhibition have been long recognized as a component of ADHD, and this feature has been increasingly recognized as a central element in the disorder (Barkley 1990; Quay 1997; Schachar et al. 2000). Response inhibition can be assessed on simple well-established neuropsychological tasks that assess the capacity for withholding or suppressing a physical or mental response that otherwise might be expected (Schachar et al. 2000). The effect of response inhibition is to hold impulsive reactions in check. The delay of such reactions, which are often semiautomatic responses, may permit more effective participation of various higher-level frontal cortical executive functions (Barkley 1997a, 1997b) and lead to more adaptive behavioral outcomes—or, more simply stated, allow more time for thought before acting.

The neuropsychological literature also has provided evidence for impairments in working memory (Barkley et al. 2001; Levy and Farrow 2001), semantic processing (Tannock et al. 2000), and executive functions (Barkley et al. 2001; Biederman 1998; Denckla and Reader 1993) in the pathogenesis of ADHD. These functional deficits

contribute to a range of difficulties in structuring a narrative (Purvis and Tannock 1997), in accurately appraising the moment-to-moment consequences of actions and interactions with others (self-monitoring), and in coordinating complex intertwined activities (multitasking and multiprocessing).

An integrated model of ADHD ties these observations together (Barkley 1997a, 1997b), positing that deficient response inhibition is the core feature of the disorder and is central to the development and proper working of four executive neuropsychological functions: 1) working memory; 2) self-regulation of affect, motivation, and arousal; 3) internalization of speech; and 4) reconstitution (behavioral analysis and synthesis). The difficulty in response inhibition leads to reduced reliance on (and use of) these critical functions in organizing and guiding responses to various tasks and demands. The various deficits and problem behaviors characteristic of ADHD are viewed as consequences of disturbances in executive functions that arise secondary to impaired response inhibition.

Specific defects in the four executive functions and other neuropsychological functions also may be present in conduct disorder and in learning and language disorders, exacerbating the neuropsychological difficulties of ADHD (Seidman et al. 2001).

Neurochemical and pharmacological studies. Neurochemical studies of ADHD were initially organized around the catecholamine hypothesis, beginning with norepinephrine as the crucial neurotransmitter (Wender 1971). Although this hypothesis has undergone numerous revisions over the years, a strong emphasis remains on dopamine and norepinephrine (Biederman and Spencer 1999). It has been suggested that norepinephrine neuronal projections are involved in alerting (i.e., signaling) the posterior attention system of the cortex to receive incoming stimuli and that the dopamine system might influence the cortical anterior attention system, which subserves executive functions that are linked to behavioral responses (Pliszka et al. 1996). These findings are consistent with a norepinephrine/attention and dopamine/activity model of ADHD—with "activity" encompassing hyperactivity, impulsivity, and behavioral self-control. Another chemical model suggests an association of norepinephrine with hyperactivity, dopamine with impulsivity, and serotonin with aggression (Castellanos et al. 1994a). Numerous such models are possible. Peripheral and possibly central epinephrine might be involved in the mechanism of psychostimulant action on attention and impulsivity, and roles of GABA (Pliszka et al. 1996), glutamate (Carlsson 2000), and acetylcholine are also being investigated.

The early "monotransmitter theories" of ADHD have been replaced by more sophisticated models that reflect the heterogeneous neurochemical mechanisms that are likely to be etiological in ADHD (Zametkin and Rapoport 1987). Neuronal circuitry models of ADHD now routinely synthesize findings concerning multiple neurotransmitter systems. Conceptualizations linking specific brain functions with neurotransmitter systems in ADHD are being synthesized with emerging findings in human neurochemical anatomy and cognitive neuroscience. Although these rough neurochemical models do not account for a considerable amount of discrepant data, they provide simple heuristic models for further exploration.

Neuroanatomical studies. Quantitative magnetic resonance imaging (MRI) studies have identified several anatomical characteristics of ADHD, with consistent findings implicating abnormal structural changes in the frontal lobes, basal ganglia, and cerebellar vermis (Giedd et al. 2001). Total brain volume appears to be reduced by about 4%–5% in boys and girls with ADHD (Castellanos et al. 1994b, 2001); the lack of progressive change with age suggests an early and global disruption of brain growth, possibly implicating neurotrophic growth factors (Rapoport et al. 2001). The possibility of disrupted brain development in early gestation is consistent with findings of abnormal neuronal migration in some individuals with ADHD (Nopoulos et al. 2000). The anterior frontal cortex has been reported to be smaller on the right side (Castellanos et al. 1996; Filipek et al. 1997), a finding corroborated with decreased blood flow in the frontal regions compared with normal control subjects (Lou et al. 1998) and consistent with a defect in cortical-striatal-thalamic-cortical (CSTC) circuits in the right hemisphere. The caudate region shows abnormal structural asymmetry; this finding suggests that the caudate does not have its normal extent of developmental reduction in size and is consistent with a disruption of the normal developmental transfer of functions from the basal ganglia to the frontal cortex (Castellanos et al. 1994b; Filipek et al. 1997; Mataro et al. 1997; Pueyo et al. 2000). The putamen, which is involved in regulation of motoric behavior, also has been implicated in ADHD (Teicher et al. 2000). Another consistent finding is reduced cerebellar volume, particularly the posterior inferior lobe of the vermis, in both boys and girls with ADHD (Berquin et al. 1998; Castellanos et al. 2001). Cerebellar involvement in cognitive processes, possibly including executive functions, as well as in motor control and inhibition suggests that a prefrontal-thalamic-cerebellar network may be involved in core symptoms of ADHD.

Findings on the corpus callosum in ADHD have been less consistent (Giedd et al. 1994; Overmeyer et al. 2000; Semrud-Clikeman et al. 1994). The corpus callosum, presumably involved in the transfer of information between hemispheres, may be more relevant to understanding the symptoms reflecting the imbalance in hemispheric functioning observed in right hemisphere syndrome rather than ADHD. Some initial data suggest the possibility of predicting psychostimulant efficacy based on anatomical characteristics (Filipek et al. 1997).

Neurophysiological studies. Although routine clinical electroencephalograms (EEGs) are interpreted as normal in most patients with ADHD, quantitative EEG data have shown that 93% of children with ADHD could be categorized as having either hyperarousal or hypoarousal relative to control subjects without ADHD (Chabot and Serfontein 1996). Studies of evoked potentials (event-related electrical waves in the brain) also have reported numerous findings in ADHD suggestive of abnormal arousal and attention. Some of these evoked potential characteristics have been found to change with age, correlate to specific ADHD symptoms or associated features (such as aggressive behavior), and be corrected by psychostimulants. An abnormality in the right frontal cortex associated with impaired attention and information processing (small P300 amplitude) may correlate with diminished effectiveness of psychostimulants in some patients.

These neurophysiological findings suggest that ADHD involves a disorder of arousal in addition to defects in attention, response inhibition, and executive functioning. The disorder of arousal may present as either hyperarousal or hypoarousal in different patients, and both may be linked to high or low autonomic reactivity. Both hyperarousal and hypoarousal appear associated with abnormalities in the function of frontal circuits. The data on arousal seem to imply that there are different forms of dysregulation of the frontal cortex in ADHD rather than a simple decrease in frontal activity, and such differences in arousal characteristics might be significant to ADHD subtyping.

Neuroimaging studies. An early positron emission tomography (PET) scan study of adults with ADHD found an overall reduction in global cerebral glucose metabolism of 8%, with the largest decreases observed in the premotor cortex and superior prefrontal cortex. More recent PET scan evidence of redistribution of blood flow, some following successful treatment with psychostimulants, further supports relative hypofrontality and compensatory redistribution of blood flow in patients with ADHD (Bush et al. 1999; Lou 1996; Lou et al. 1989; Matochik et al. 1994; Schweitzer et al. 2000). The newer generation of studies that examine structure–function correlations suggest significant roles of the right prefrontal and caudate areas in specific cognitive functions. For example, changes in performance on neuropsychological tasks that require response inhibition have been correlated with anatomical changes in the right frontostriatal neuronal circuits (Casey et al. 1997; Teicher et al. 2000).

Current studies have increasingly used a combination of sophisticated neuropsychological testing methods (i.e., task performance) with neuroimaging techniques. Such studies have permitted more refined structure–function correlations and promise to eventually allow a more fine anatomical dissection of the neuronal network dysregulations involved in the pathogenesis of ADHD. Especially as neurotransmitter-specific neuroimaging methods promote a biochemical characterization of the circuit dysfunctions in ADHD, the pharmacological effects in the frontal cortex, basal ganglia, thalamus, and cerebellum on neuropsychological dysfunctions that contribute to ADHD are likely to be clarified.

Course and Prognosis

Although generalizations about the course and prognosis of ADHD are difficult, it is now recognized that most cases of ADHD are both congenital and lifelong. The symptoms of inattention, impulsivity, and hyperactivity are manifest in different ways as an individual develops, reflecting the developmental tasks and normal activities at different points in the life cycle (see Table 20–3). However, an adult with pronounced inattention, impulsivity, and hyperactivity does not necessarily have ADHD because the DSM-IV-TR diagnosis of ADHD in adults requires a history of ADHD during childhood. ADHD can be diagnosed by age 3 years, but it is usually difficult to recognize the disorder before age 5 years because a normal developmental stage of increased activity begins at about age 2 years. Identification is often delayed until elementary school, when demands for physical stillness and focus are greater, comparison to peers is easier, and more group stimulation is involved. Individuals with ADHD often experience their most challenging adjustments during the regimented school years. This is in part because they are not yet free to select areas of learning and schoolwork that are least affected by their cognitive and behavioral symptoms. In addition to academic challenges and behavioral infractions, school-age children with ADHD may be significantly compromised in social skills and self-esteem.

The hyperactivity of ADHD often improves during childhood and early adolescence (Biederman 1998). In general, the symptoms of hyperactivity improve notably, impulsivity improves to a lesser degree, but the inattention does not seem to improve (Hart et al. 1995). Despite the improvement in some symptoms over time, social skills and general adaptive abilities appear to fall progressively further behind with age (Roizen et al. 1994). The prevalence of ADHD is estimated to decline by 50% about every 5 years until the mid-20s (J.C. Hill and Schoener 1996), regardless of the type and duration of treatment (Hart et al. 1995). Features of impulsivity persist into adolescence in 70% and into adulthood in 30%–50% of cases of childhood ADHD (Barkley 1990; Gittelman et al. 1985; G. Weiss and Hechtman 1986). These compelling data highlight the need for aggressive treatment in adolescents and adults who might have a reduction in symptoms but remain at high risk for poor functional outcomes.

Clearly, ADHD is not a benign or self-limited childhood disorder. By young adulthood, ADHD is associated with fewer completed years of schooling, more changes of residence, more cigarette smoking, more marijuana use, more alcohol use, more traffic violations, more speeding, more car accidents and crashes, more court appearances, and more felony convictions (T. Spencer et al. 1999; Wilens et al. 1998). In terms of psychiatric symptoms, young adults with ADHD have more mood disorders, suicide attempts, phobic anxiety, somatization symptoms, and psychosexual traumas.

Substance use disorders emerge in children with ADHD earlier and more often than in children without ADHD, and substance use continues into adulthood in about half of the patients with ADHD (Pomerleau et al. 1995). ADHD may be an independent risk factor for the development of substance abuse, including alcohol and nicotine (Biederman et al. 1997b; Sullivan and Rudnik-Levin 2001; Wilens et al. 1998). These findings contrast with earlier data that suggested that, in the absence of conduct disorder, ADHD does not appear to be associated with subsequent substance abuse (Disney et al. 1999; Lynskey and Fergusson 1995). The links between ADHD and substance abuse probably can be explained in some patients by psychiatric comorbidity, such as bipolar disorder or conduct disorder in children and antisocial personality or personality disorder in adults. Alternatively, characteristics such as risk-taking behavior, difficulty in anticipating or planning for consequences, or aggressive behavior may play a role. Despite these conflicting data, it appears that treatment of ADHD may lead to significant reductions in substance abuse and dependence (Biederman et al. 1998; Greene et al. 1999; Wilens et al. 1998).

Other comorbid psychiatric disorders also may have a significant effect on the course and prognosis of ADHD. Indeed, ADHD symptoms tend to improve gradually over time if they are not complicated by other comorbidities. Disorders that present episodically, such as mood disorders, tend to yield periodic exacerbations of the ADHD symptoms. More chronic or deteriorative psychiatric disorders, such as conduct or personality disorders, anxiety disorders, and substance abuse, tend to intensify ADHD symptoms over time. Subsequently, at times it is difficult to distinguish the natural course of ADHD from comorbid disorders so that appropriate clinical decisions can be made.

Although historically overemphasized, antisocial personality disorder in adulthood is one of the most common serious outcomes of ADHD. The high risk of antisocial outcome is likely to be concentrated in children with ADHD who have comorbid conduct disorder. Follow-up studies examining some of the populations with more severe ADHD and comorbid conduct disorder have reported that 25%–30% of these children eventually develop antisocial personality disorder. Although this is not likely generalizable to the entire ADHD population, when it occurs, it seems to be mediated by the interaction of hyperactivity-impulsivity symptoms with conduct disorder. Inattention does not appear to play a significant role in development of symptoms of criminality (August et al. 1983; Babinski et al. 1999).

As an individual with ADHD enters parenthood, problems of impulsivity in caregiving, inattentiveness to child-rearing details, disorganization, identification with the child's ADHD, projection of the parent's ADHD tendencies, and guilt regarding genetic transmission to the child often become evident. It is not reasonable to assume that parents with ADHD know how to manage a child with ADHD because of their familiarity with the symptoms of ADHD. The parent's own ability to overcome the obstacles of his or her own disorder, or failure to initiate pharmacological treatment of his or her disorder, can have a major effect on the child's treatment, course of illness, and prognosis. Psychostimulant treatment of a parent with ADHD can produce clinically significant improvement in the child's ADHD symptoms. When both parent and child have ADHD, treatment of either the parent or the child can improve the condition of the other. Alternatively, failure to treat parent or child can be a rate-limiting step in the clinical improvement of both. As in many disorders, the concurrent treatment of child and family usually is a major advantage in managing ADHD in a child. In general, the interpersonal and social complications of ADHD can be complex, even in relatively mild cases (Whalen et al.

1989). Subsequently, complications in family functioning are virtually inevitable (Hechtman 1996). A child's ADHD is likely to influence parental satisfaction, marital harmony, and sibling development. Behavioral observation studies indicate that parents tend to have a more anxious, controlling, and directive structure setting and give more negative responses to their children with ADHD. At least a part of the parents' behavior appears to be elicited by the difficult behavior of the child (Barkley 1990). Similar effects on peer relationships and behavior are also worthy of clinical monitoring because of their effect on the child's socialization.

Diagnostic Evaluation

Clinical evaluation includes assessing the specific symptoms of ADHD, considering similarly presenting disorders, and delineating concomitant psychiatric and neurological disorders (Table 20–5). In addition to a routine and thorough psychiatric evaluation of the individual and a general family assessment, special emphasis is warranted in several areas. These include school reports of grades and behavior (including behavior on the bus and in the cafeteria) or work history, concomitant learning disorders and other common comorbid psychiatric disorders, social functioning and social skills, obstetrical history (maternal alcohol use, fetal overactivity, prenatal or perinatal injury), family residence (lead exposure in paints and car exhaust fumes), family psychiatric history (including ADHD in males), family medical history (thyroid disorder), medication use (barbiturates, benzodiazepines, psychostimulants, carbamazepine), history of child abuse or neglect, and potential risks of medication abuse by the patient or family members. Essential sources of information include the patient, parents, teachers, significant others, and treating physicians.

Physical examination and laboratory testing can identify physical anomalies and thyroid disorders. Neurological evaluation can uncover possible localizing symptoms, neuromaturational signs such as choreiform movements, overflow and mirror movements, tremor, gross and fine motor function, cerebral laterality, and baseline (premedication) frequency of tics or dystonias. Lead screening is appropriate when excessive lead exposure is suspected; the screening test is a plasma level of zinc protoporphyrin, which has replaced the free erythrocyte protoporphyrin because it has fewer false-positive results and is an indicator of long-term lead exposure. A plasma lead level is optional at initial screening because it reflects lead exposure over the previous 4 weeks only. A baseline sample of handwriting permits visual documentation of clinical change in the medical record. In the absence of

TABLE 20–5.　Differential diagnosis of attention-deficit/hyperactivity disorder (ADHD)

Psychiatric
　Conduct disorder
　Oppositional defiant disorder
　Major depression
　Anxiety (situational, developmental)
　Separation anxiety disorder
　Posttraumatic stress disorder
　Panic disorder
　Phobic disorder
　Dissociative disorders
　Bipolar disorder
　Early schizophrenia
　Psychotic agitation
　Substance use disorders (intoxication or withdrawal)
　Attention-seeking or manipulative behavior
Psychosocial
　Physical or sexual abuse
　Neglect
　Boredom
　Overstimulation
　Sociocultural deprivation
Medical
　Thyroid disorders
　Drug-induced agitation
　Recreational stimulants
　Medical stimulants: pseudoephedrine
　Barbiturates, benzodiazepines
　Carbamazepine
　Theophylline
Extreme prenatal or perinatal problem (rare)
　Brain damage (following trauma or infection)
　Lead poisoning (postnatal toxicity)
　Teratogenic effect of exposure to alcohol, cocaine, lead, probably cigarette smoke
Dietary
　Excessive caffeine
Hunger
Constipation
Minor persistent pain
Normal behavior

Note. Various etiological factors give rise to ADHD or to conditions that look like ADHD. ADHD look-alike disorders may be more clinically appropriate diagnoses for individual patients than ADHD, and some look-alikes may be better diagnosed as comorbid conditions with ADHD. Because of the common co-occurrence of ADHD and ADHD look-alike conditions, all of these disorders and some etiological conditions that give rise to them must be considered in the differential diagnosis of ADHD. In clinical practice, all of the factors listed in the table (disorders, symptoms, situations, and states) should be considered—either identified or ruled out—before a firm diagnosis of ADHD is made. In effect, ADHD is a "diagnosis of exclusion"—a diagnosis that is made by the exclusion of other factors.

suggestive symptoms, baseline (premedication) EEG, electrocardiogram, and thyroid evaluation are not essential and probably not cost-effective. Laboratory tests, other than for the routine management of medications, are not routinely necessary.

Educational testing and, often, neuropsychological evaluation are useful to assess academic achievement, intelligence, cortical functioning, attention, impulsivity, and developmental skills; including symptoms of learning, motor skills, and communication disorders.

Comorbidity rates are sufficiently high that evaluations of ADHD should be initially based on the expectation that concurrent psychiatric disorders will be identified. ADHD is often diagnosed in association with conduct disorder, oppositional defiant disorder, bipolar disorder, depression, and learning disorders (Table 20–4). The differential diagnosis of ADHD is also challenging at times because of a high rate of comorbidity of neurological disorders and the extensive phenomenological similarity to other psychiatric disorders and to normal behavior.

Many of the defining criteria of ADHD are shared with numerous psychiatric disorders. Notable progress has been made in eliminating diagnostic criteria of ADHD that are common behaviors of "normal" people, but several of the 18 symptoms of ADHD listed in DSM-IV-TR are still problematic. Fidgeting, acting driven or "on the go," talking excessively, interrupting or intruding, making careless mistakes, glossing over errors, and engaging reluctantly in effortful thinking are hardly overt signs of significant psychopathology. However, taken together, these symptoms help to create a clinical picture that reliably distinguishes ADHD from normal behavior and other differential diagnoses, such as oppositional defiant disorder and conduct disorder. Indeed, the primary clinical challenge is no longer differentiating ADHD from normal behavior but differentiating ADHD from other psychiatric disorders. Some of the earlier diagnostic criteria for ADHD were discarded after the field trials for DSM-IV because they lacked the power to differentiate DSM-IV ADHD from other DSM-IV disorders, including anxiety and bipolar disorder. For example, the symptom of thoughtless self-endangering behavior was found to be too nonspecific to warrant its continued use.

Bipolar disorder and ADHD have many symptoms in common—and some overlapping diagnostic criteria—two disorders mimicking each other enough to lead to diagnostic error. All conditions with ADHD-like symptoms need to be considered in the evaluation of ADHD and viewed as part of the differential diagnosis to reduce the risk of overdiagnosing ADHD. Moreover, the comorbidity of similarly appearing disorders presents additional problems that complicate the differential diagnosis.

Although they resemble and mimic each other, both ADHD and bipolar disorder can appear comorbidly as distinct disorders. They may present simultaneously in any one individual, even if their symptom overlap can make them difficult to differentiate. As noted earlier in this chapter, about 20%–25% of the youths with ADHD also have bipolar disorder by DSM-IV criteria (Butler et al. 1995), and between 50% and 100% of youths with bipolar disorder fulfill criteria for ADHD (Butler et al. 1995; West et al. 1996). Therefore, caution must be taken to avoid oversimplifying by diagnosing a single disorder because this can significantly impair treatment and prognosis (Sachs et al. 2000; T. Spencer et al. 2001a).

In addition to the comorbidity, ADHD is typically accompanied by certain associated features, as described in DSM-IV-TR. For instance, when compared with adolescents with bipolar disorder, adolescents who have both bipolar disorder and ADHD are more likely to have mixed mania, irritability, higher scores on mania rating scales, and sometimes lower serum thyroxine concentrations (West et al. 1996). Such findings highlight the fact that clinically relevant features of ADHD are difficult to conceptualize but nonetheless can be helpful in clinical diagnosis.

Often in psychiatry, diagnostic confidence cannot be achieved, and a working diagnosis is used as a basis for treatment. With ADHD, this approach can lead to an empirical trial of psychostimulants. However, a positive treatment response to a psychostimulant does not necessarily imply a diagnosis of ADHD because patients with several other disorders also may show a therapeutic response to psychostimulants. On the other hand, a negative response to a psychostimulant does not rule out ADHD because patients with ADHD may respond only to certain psychostimulants or to another class of medications altogether. At times it may be helpful to keep the diagnostic process open ended and to expect that emerging clinical data will confirm or refute initial diagnostic impressions.

At present, clinical diagnosis of ADHD rests to a large degree on clinical judgment. The looseness of this approach is unsatisfactory for the diagnosis of a significant psychiatric disorder in children. Furthermore, the use of purely behavioral features, cognitive performance, and affective symptoms is particularly frustrating in distinguishing ADHD from the many ADHD look-alike conditions. The eventual identification of specific and sensitive criteria for ADHD will create a major advantage in diagnosing ADHD and differentiating it from other conditions and from normalcy. An easy and objective method to assess both attention and hyperactivity-impulsivity is solely needed, and some progress is being made in this direction (Teicher et al. 1996).

Currently, making a diagnosis of ADHD is much more complicated than in past decades. It is difficult to make a firm diagnosis of ADHD without assessing the presence or absence of many disorders (Table 20–4). It is no longer easy to make this diagnosis in many patients in a single office visit because the accumulation of adequate clinical data to address each of these possibilities requires careful evaluation and observation over time. In effect, ADHD may appear to be a diagnosis of exclusion. The continual refinement of specific and sensitive diagnostic criteria for ADHD across the life span will create a major advantage in diagnosing ADHD and differentiating it from other conditions in the future.

Treatment

Various treatment methods are useful; both multimodal and sequential approaches are generally needed. Certain interventions are specific to particular etiologies, but some treatments are helpful regardless of etiology. A major study of the multimodal treatment of ADHD (the MTA study) has solidified knowledge and provided important new insights into the roles and contributions of psychopharmacological and psychosocial treatments in the management of ADHD.

Psychostimulants remain the primary treatment for ADHD because they are more effective than alternative medications and modalities for improving inattention and other cognitive symptoms. The use of psychostimulants in ADHD is one the oldest and most established psychopharmacological treatments. There have been more than 200 double-blind demonstrations of its efficacy and safety in children, with additional trials confirming its benefits in adult populations. The effect of psychostimulants in treating core symptoms of ADHD is as effective in girls as in boys. The effectiveness of these drugs has been shown to persist for at least 15 months (Gillberg et al. 1997; Sharp et al. 1999) and, in clinical use, appears to endure for many years.

A small percentage of patients may develop tolerance to psychostimulants after several months of treatment; the psychostimulants appear to become ineffective despite dose increases. If a therapeutic effect diminishes over time and is not due to intercurrent (including psychiatric) illness or stress, this problem generally can be clinically managed by alternating between two different psychostimulants every few weeks or months.

The "quieting" effects of psychostimulants on the impulsivity, hyperactivity, inattention, and emotional lability of ADHD are distinct from caffeine-induced focusing of attention, the antianxiety effect of benzodiazepines, or the tranquilization of antipsychotic agents.

These agents act by different neurochemical and neurophysiological mechanisms, and they produce chemically different forms of "sedation." Children with ADHD can show a calming response to other medical psychostimulants (pseudoephedrine) and behavioral excitation to sedatives (benzodiazepines and barbiturates). Such "paradoxical" clinical effects may not be specific to hyperactive children. Under laboratory conditions, boys and men without ADHD show a qualitatively similar psychostimulant-induced reduction of motor behavior, but the quantitative effect in hyperactive boys is significantly larger (Rapoport et al. 1980). The explanation of this apparent difference in the human laboratory, and of the clinical finding that not all people with ADHD respond "therapeutically" to psychostimulants, is uncertain. It appears that psychostimulant responsiveness is not specifically tied to diagnostic state but reflects more basic biological mechanisms.

In addition to reducing the core symptoms of inattention, impulsivity, and hyperactivity, psychostimulant treatment often appears to lead to enduring improvement in social skills and self-esteem. Improvements in academic performance, socialization, and school or work productivity are further enhanced by concurrent changes in external structure and support (Barkley and Cunningham 1978; Jensen et al. 2001b). Controlled follow-up studies examining physical growth also have found that most deficits are temporary and tend to normalize by late adolescence, even with continued treatment. This has been hypothesized to suggest that the growth deficits may be mediated by ADHD itself and not psychostimulants (T. Spencer et al. 1998c).

Some patients do not experience therapeutic effects from psychostimulants. Several factors can be considered in these cases. Some comorbid psychiatric disorders, including anxiety disorders or symptoms, bipolar disorder, and schizophrenia, are aggravated by psychostimulants. Most psychotic disorders or symptoms can be aggravated by psychostimulants. Any neurological condition or neurodevelopmental idiosyncrasy that occurs concomitantly with ADHD might lead to drug-induced neurotoxic symptoms, often at unexpectedly low doses of psychotropic medications. The presence of anxiety (and perhaps other internalizing symptoms) has been reported by numerous research groups to be associated with a weaker and less prevalent therapeutic effect of psychostimulants. Patients with internalizing disorders tend to be overly inhibited, whereas ADHD patients typically have deficits in inhibitory self-control (Oosterlaan and Sergeant 1996). It may be hypothesized that the changing balance between these characteristics and the intermittent nature of anxiety contribute to the unevenness of psychostimulant effects in patients with ADHD and anxiety. In some cases, the dosage of the psychostimulant may need to be altered when ADHD with comorbid anxiety is treated in order to obtain stable therapeutic effects (Livingston et al. 1992).

Current concepts of the mechanism or mechanisms of psychostimulant action in ADHD are undergoing continual revision. The largely dopaminergic, lesser adrenergic, still lesser serotonergic, possibly some cholinergic, and probably other pharmacological effects of the psychostimulants are consistent with many different (and conflicting) models of ADHD. Simple single neurotransmitter explanations are viewed as unlikely. Newer theories, incorporating nonpharmacological and neurophysiological findings, can become quite elaborate and interesting. For instance, the unexpected finding that methylphenidate slows right hemisphere processing (i.e., slower reaction time on neuropsychological tasks without a change in accuracy) seems to imply that the therapeutic effects of psychostimulants must be strong enough to outweigh their seemingly negative effects on right-sided functioning (Campbell et al. 1996).

In healthy individuals, the most serious risks of psychostimulants include tics and psychosis. Seizures are not induced by psychostimulants, and cardiac and cardiovascular effects are generally not clinically significant. Common side effects include delayed sleep onset, minor increase in blood pressure and heart rate, decreased appetite, reduced (or slowed) height and weight gain, tremor or adventitious movements, cognitive overfocusing, anxiety, dysphoria, irritability, nightmares, and social withdrawal.

In general, nonpsychostimulant medications are notably less effective in treating ADHD, especially in treating symptoms of inattention. Tricyclic antidepressants (TCAs) are also able to treat the core symptoms of ADHD but are typically less effective than psychostimulants for symptoms of inattention. Their efficacy has been shown in double-blind, placebo-controlled studies conducted by 11 separate research groups over the past 30 years. Low dosages of TCAs (e.g., nortriptyline 0.3–2.0 mg/kg/day) provide therapeutic effects that last 24 hours, allowing for convenient once-daily dosing.

Reports of sudden death during routine desipramine treatment in five children and adolescents (Popper and Elliott 1990; Riddle et al. 1991, 1995) have led to general concern about the use of TCAs in youths, particularly for treating nonlethal disorders such as ADHD. The problem appears to be specific to desipramine; even imipramine has not been implicated, probably because its anticholinergic side effects are cardioprotective. Most of these cases of sudden death involved treatments for ADHD rather than mood disorders or enuresis, which is the most common pediatric use of TCAs. Some of the patients who died had significant preexisting cardiovascular risks, including one patient whose coronary artery anomaly could not have been identified before death unless invasive arteriography had been obtained. Desipramine treatment of ADHD is easy to avoid because so many other TCAs are readily available, and all appear to be equally effective in treating ADHD. Therefore, TCAs may be reasonably considered if rebound effects of psychostimulants are disruptive, if tics emerge specifically during rebound, if once-a-day administration is needed for treatment adherence, if the child or family is potentially drug abusing, if a comorbid mood disorder is present, if sleep disturbance is prominent, and perhaps if a strong family psychiatric history of mood disorder exists.

Selective noradrenergic reuptake inhibitors, such as atomoxetine or reboxetine, also appear to have anti-ADHD properties. Atomoxetine has been more adequately examined and appears effective for both children and adults with ADHD (Michelson et al. 2001).

Bupropion has been successfully used in adults with ADHD (Wender and Reimherr 1990), and findings in children are mixed (Casat et al. 1989; Clay et al. 1988; Conners et al. 1996). The anti-ADHD effects of bupropion appear smaller than those of standard psychostimulant drugs. In a controlled drug comparison study with methylphenidate, bupropion produced comparable but consistently weaker therapeutic effects (Barrickman et al. 1995). An unexpectedly high incidence of severe skin rash has been associated with bupropion treatment in children (Conners et al. 1996).

Monoamine oxidase inhibitor (MAOI) antidepressants usually are clinically effective, but they are not typically used for treating ADHD because of the dietary restrictions and potential risks. The newer MAOIs, such as L-deprenyl (selegiline) and moclobemide (available in Canada), are more isoenzyme specific than traditional MAOIs. Early findings suggested that moclobemide is effective in ADHD (Trott et al. 1992) and that L-deprenyl is not (Ernst et al. 1996; Feigin et al. 1996).

α_2-Agonists such as clonidine have become widely used to treat ADHD (Hunt et al. 1990), but the two randomized double-blind, placebo-controlled studies of clonidine in children with ADHD found only minor effects on ADHD (Jaselskis et al. 1992; Singer et al. 1995). A meta-analysis estimated that clonidine has some value (mean effect size = 0.58) for treating ADHD but less than that of psychostimulants (Connor et al. 1999). In general, clonidine appears to treat behavioral hyperactivity and impulsivity, as well as associated aggressive behavior and insomnia, but not the attentional

symptoms (van der Meere et al. 1999). Its potentially serious adverse cardiovascular effects, including hypotension and bradycardia, are typically benign, but either one can result in syncope. Abrupt discontinuation (including running out of pills) can induce significant tachycardia and hypertension but also has been associated with severe ventricular tachyarrhythmias in adults (Jain and Misra 1991) and children (Coumel et al. 1978). Clinicians are advised to monitor blood pressure and heart rate before and during any treatment involving clonidine, alone or in combination with other drugs. Guanfacine is a similar agent with some pharmacological advantages (Hunt et al. 1995; Scahill et al. 2001)

Other medications for consideration include venlafaxine, β-adrenergic blockers, donepezil, and possibly modafinil or nicotine. Antipsychotic medications may be appropriate for treating ADHD in the context of significant comorbidity, including tic disorders, bipolar disorder, or other psychotic conditions.

Despite the medications used, dose optimization in patients with ADHD is complicated by the variations in the level of ambient environmental stimulation, changes in emotionality and excitement, and diurnal patterns of hunger and arousal. These factors produce shifts in attentional and neurophysiological reactivity, as well as shifts in psychostimulant-induced effects. Clinically significant differences often exist between home and school (or job) environments. Dose selection becomes an artful task in which one attempts to optimize the balance of behaviors in different settings and physical maturation and growth. Periodic dose adjustments may be needed for changes in body weight, varying environmental or developmental stress, or changes in drug metabolism, especially because approximately 50% of the individuals with ADHD will continue to need treatment into adulthood (Barkley 1990; Gittelman et al. 1985; G. Weiss and Hechtman 1986).

In the nonpharmacological management of ADHD, various psychosocial interventions appear helpful in supporting the patient and family and in relieving some of the predictable problems associated with ADHD. Education of the family members about ADHD, its treatment, and its management is necessary as well. Family members usually can be "coached" in behavioral management techniques that can be applied at home. For children, the psychological effect of the parents can be pivotal in exacerbating or diminishing symptoms; therefore, focused parent counseling is sensible in many cases.

Education and support for parents and family members are crucial, and they can be provided through programmed group training sessions (Barkley 1990). National organizations for parents, such as ChADD, have many local chapters throughout the United States that can provide crucial support, education, and advocacy for families and patients.

Environmental management of sensory stimulation can reduce overstimulation from external sources, keep impulsivity and aggressivity in better control, and provide a sense of control and basis for self-esteem. Environmental measures can involve arranging the patient's home and job or school setting to reduce stimuli and distractions. For children at home, parents can be advised to establish quiet spaces, decorate with simple furniture and subdued colors, keep toys in the closet, permit only one friend to visit at a time, avoid supermarkets and parties, and encourage fine motor exercises (e.g., jigsaw puzzles). At work, adolescents and adults should be encouraged to make arrangements to use a quiet, small office space with no officemates; to have a minimum of visitors; to avoid chatting or visual contact with passersby; and to have few telephone interruptions. The work environment should be uncluttered and undistracting, containing few windows and no nearby refrigerator, radio or television, or sound-making machinery. These recommendations have not been evaluated in controlled studies, but they are commonly offered and appear clinically valuable.

Special education is generally required because children with ADHD are typically below achievement levels expected for school grade, even after accounting for IQ (Cantwell and Baker 1988). At school, beneficial accommodations include a small and self-contained classroom, small-group activities, thoughtful selection of seating location to minimize distractions, high teacher-to-student ratio, quiet ambience, routine and predictable structure, one-to-one tutoring, and use of a resource room. Arrangements for supervision or modifications at recess, in physical education class, on the bus, and in the cafeteria are sometimes helpful. Careful management of transitions to new schools and between programs requires administrative foresight and detail-oriented planning. It is essential to inform school officials about the child's strengths and problems, self-esteem, social skills, and useful environmental measures as well as to receive regular reports from school personnel about behavior and academic performance. An individualized educational plan (IEP) can be developed with the school to facilitate classroom arrangements, perhaps with concomitant interventions to accommodate specific learning disorders.

Contingent rewards, response-cost management, and time-outs can help build impulse control in children. Behavioral methods can be as effective as psychostimulants in modifying classroom behavior, but generalization beyond the treatment setting may be limited. Cognitive-behavioral therapy is used for teaching problem-solving strategies, self-monitoring, verbal mediation (using internal speech) for self-praise and self-instruction, and seeing rather than glossing over errors.

Group treatments can be helpful for children and adolescents with ADHD who need training in social skills. Deficits in the development of social skills are commonly found in individuals with ADHD, including those without aggressive behavior, oppositional behavior, impulsivity, or hyperactivity. Other areas of adaptive functioning are also compromised, even in patients with predominantly inattentive ADHD. Children of normal intelligence (Full-Scale IQ of 101 ± 14) who have ADHD may have low-to-borderline scores on the Vineland Adaptive Behavior Scale (73 ± 14), and this discrepancy increases with age (Roizen et al. 1994). Social and adaptive dysfunctions only recently have been viewed as standard components of ADHD, and they may justify incorporation into the routine management of ADHD (M.A. Stein et al. 1995).

Reinforcement of smoking prevention attitudes is also very important in this population, along with the acquisition of alternative means of dealing with peer pressure, self-image, anxiety, and peers' opinions. Children with ADHD tend to be less future-oriented and less concerned about future health problems (and other delayed risks). Their novelty-seeking behavior also may interfere with subsequent smoking cessation efforts (Downey et al. 1997). Early intervention is particularly valuable for youths with ADHD, who generally start smoking earlier than their peers who do not have ADHD (Biederman et al. 1999b; Downey et al. 1997). Among youths with ADHD, appropriate treatment with psychiatric medications may result in up to an 85% reduction in subsequent substance abuse disorder (Biederman et al. 1999b). However, in view of the possible therapeutic effects of nicotine on ADHD symptoms (Levin et al. 1996), symptoms may worsen during smoking cessation, making it even more difficult for persons with ADHD to stop smoking. In a similar manner, preventive measures to stem alcohol and other substance use disorders are useful.

Nutritional therapy of ADHD has a murky history, involving a string of cures too good to be true and "new" treatments that have been used for years. Perhaps frustrated by behavioral methods and frightened by "mind drugs," parents are often interested in hearing physicians' views on nutritional and other unproven treatments of ADHD. Some of these parents seem willing to accept that their child has a "physical problem" but are not ready to acknowledge a "medical disorder." It is also striking that ADHD has attracted more medical and professional advocates of nutritional treatment than any other psychiatric and most other medical disorders. Possibly reflecting acute clinical intuition, numerous forms of elimination diets have been enthusiastically promulgated and enforced for years on the basis of anecdotes and repeated assertions, without the benefit of adequate testing or even attempts at controlled trials.

Although no dietary treatment of ADHD has been consistently shown to have clinical value, some studies cannot be readily dismissed. Several reasonable reports are consistent with a possible role of dietary factors in the etiology and treatment of ADHD. In a controlled trial that used dye washout periods and high-dose dye challenges, specific restriction of a set of food dyes (with no other restrictions) was found to be effective for treating a subgroup (5%–10%) of children with ADHD. In another controlled rechallenge study, a diet that minimized the intake of certain "reactive" foods, preservatives, and artificial food dyes was found to produce a clinically and statistically significant improvement in children with ADHD (M. Boris and Mandel 1994); in this study, atopic children with ADHD appeared to be more likely to respond than other children with ADHD. In an EEG study examining children whose ADHD appeared to be aggravated by specific foods (as determined by previous deprivation and challenge), an increase was found in beta activity in the frontotemporal cortex during rechallenge with the sensitizing food (Uhlig et al. 1997). A controlled study of a low-antigen diet found no changes on attention or activity measures, but the children with ADHD reported significant subjective improvement (Schulte-Körne et al. 1996).

Other dietary treatments of ADHD have been examined but without convincing evidence of clinical value. The well-publicized Feingold diet, involving reduced dietary intake of salicylates and food dyes, has yielded contradictory findings in controlled trials. Data on salicylate elimination and challenge have indicated minimal effects (Perry et al. 1996). Sugar toxicity, sugar withdrawal, and reactive hypoglycemia have been reported to induce ADHD symptoms, but these claims do not appear to be valid unless perhaps there were preexisting nutritional deficiencies. It has been well documented that aspartame has no clinical effects on ADHD. Dietary treatments based on trace mineral content in hair analysis, particularly zinc deficiency and cadmium excess, have not been rigorously evaluated. Megavitamin treatments appear ineffective and can cause toxic effects.

Despite prevailing skepticism of dietary treatments of ADHD, some studies of dietary treatments of ADHD have produced enough suggestive evidence to warrant a measure of respect and to justify further disciplined

research. Reasonably good evidence suggests that some foods or food dyes induce hyperactive behavior or other ADHD symptoms in a very small percentage of children (Arnold 2002). Some data seem to confirm the folklore that mood and sleep are influenced by a broad range of foods in children (Breakey 1997). Based on the involvement of iron in mechanisms affecting dopaminergic activity, a well-conducted open-label study suggested that boys with ADHD may respond to 30-day iron supplementation (Sever et al. 1997). Reduced blood levels of omega-3 and omega-6 fatty acids have been reported in children with ADHD (Arnold et al. 1994; Mitchell et al. 1987; Stevens et al. 1995, 1996), with these reductions possibly correlating to severity of symptoms. Double-blind, placebo-controlled studies in youths have suggested some effect of omega-6 γ-linolenic acid in treating ADHD (Arnold 2001), and recent data have suggested that relative zinc deficiency may explain why some patients with ADHD do not show a more robust response to psychostimulants (Arnold et al. 2000).

To monitor treatment effects in research and clinical practice, a variety of standardized scales have been developed. The best available instrument for adults is the Wender Utah Rating Scale, which is also useful in assessing ADHD symptoms in children (M.A. Stein et al. 1995). Other options are available for children as well. The Child Attention/Activity Profile (CAP) assesses both the inattention and the hyperactivity-impulsivity factors and is sensitive to psychostimulant effects (Edelbrock 1987). Early versions of the Conners' Parent Rating Scale and the Conners' Teacher Rating Scale (Rapoport et al. 1985) were widely used, but they functioned as nonspecific measures of "misbehavior" and conduct problems; they were not as useful for monitoring specific ADHD symptoms or for the predominantly inattentive type of ADHD. However, Conners updated these scales to keep pace, and the current versions appear to function quite well (Conners et al. 1996). The Home Situations Questionnaire can be used by parents or residential caregivers (Barkley 1990); it assesses behaviors in a variety of different settings and also can measure drug effects. All these instruments, although developed for drug research, can be applied to outcome assessment of ADHD for any treatment method. An additional method of assessment, which is one of the best but not as systematic or reproducible as the scales, is an arrangement for clinicians to receive reports on behavior and cognition from teachers as well as parents.

Certain performance tests, mostly variations on the Continuous Performance Test (CPT), have been used clinically to measure attentiveness and responsiveness to changing sensory cues. Although these tests, computerized or otherwise, have been used to monitor treatment and to adjust medication dosages, their usefulness is open to question. Attentional performance in a laboratory is not necessarily related to naturalistic behavior or cognitive functioning in different life spaces.

Multimodal treatment of ADHD is currently the standard of care for children, especially those with major psychiatric or neurological comorbidity, behavior disorders, aggression, disruptiveness, learning disorders, developmental disorders, or poor prognosis. However, appropriate pharmacological treatment remains the cornerstone of all effective treatment regimens. Indeed, numerous large- and small-scale studies have found that in the absence of appropriate pharmacotherapy, outcomes are very poor; but there is a lot to be gained by supporting medication treatment with appropriate educational, psychosocial, and family interventions (Ialongo et al. 1993; Jensen et al. 2001b; Pelham et al. 1993; Vitiello et al. 2001).

Clinical Comment

ADHD provides an example of a congenital or early-onset disorder, often with a genetic or neurological etiology, that can be modified by life experiences. Untoward genetic and biological processes that are prominent during early childhood can be washed over in time by social and environmental factors. Socioeconomic opportunities, family variables, education, and the ability to seek and use medical treatment exert prominent influences on the development of behavior and behavior disorders, regardless of cause. In this way, ADHD characteristics can be amplified into psychopathology or channeled into useful energetic activity, depending on a series of psychosocial factors.

A large variety of etiologies, environmental circumstances, developmental processes, and psychiatric disorders can result in behavioral hyperactivity, impulsivity, and inattention. Whether a final common pathway, similar among all subtypes of ADHD, exists remains to be determined. Although genetic and some potentially toxin-induced forms of ADHD appear to share virtually identical clinical features and possibly common pathways, a single physiological explanation of ADHD is doubtful in view of the apparent differences in medication responsiveness of ADHD.

Continued ADHD research has provided some unexpected findings, challenging the ability to rethink conceptual organization of this disorder. The traditional view of ADHD as a benign, self-limited, and perhaps amusing or irritating childhood condition has been discarded. Longitudinal studies have provided convincing evidence that many children with ADHD grow up to have significant adult psychopathology. Although multimodal treatment is the long-established norm in patients with ADHD, this approach has been challenged by findings that the addition of psychosocial treatments may provide relatively less added benefit compared with the use of psychostimulants alone in uncomplicated cases. If simple psychostimulant treatment is the optimal single treatment, and if additional psychosocial interventions do not yield as much as generally believed, it is conceivable that long-term developmentally oriented early intervention might be less powerful than assumed. The advantage of early intervention is a bedrock concept in child psychiatric treatment, but recent findings concerning ADHD suggest that even bedrock should be examined and tested. The experience with ADHD serves as a reminder that, even with the oldest and most established diseases and treatments, empirical study is needed to define the scope and limits of knowledge.

Conduct Disorder

Conduct disorder is the most common diagnosis of child and adolescent patients in both clinic and hospital settings. This disorder entails repeated violations of personal rights or societal rules, including violent and nonviolent behaviors. The syndrome is not a single medical entity but consists of various forms of misbehavior—some more extreme than others but all with the core feature of basic disregard for people and property. The diagnostic criteria include offenses ranging from frequent lying, cheating, and truancy to vandalism, running away, car theft, arson, and rape (Table 20–6). The validity of a single categorical grouping has been questioned by proponents of more symptomatic or dimensional approaches to conduct problems. Conduct disorders can present with or derive from comorbid psychiatric disorder, such as mood disorders, psychosis, ADHD, substance abuse, organic impairment, mental retardation, psychodevelopmental (or personality) disorders, and learning disorders. However, in most cases, family, socioeconomic, and environmental factors appear to contribute heavily to the genesis of conduct disorder (Loeber et al. 2000).

Conduct disorder encompasses some of the most severe behavior disorders of childhood (Frick 1998). Only a fraction of the children with this disorder receive treatment. Many can be rehabilitated or habilitated, but some lead lives of delinquency or undergo long-term incarceration. Early onset has been found to be the strongest predictor of poor outcome in a variety of studies, forming the basis for the DSM-IV-TR subtyping of conduct disorder into early and late onset (Lahey et al.

TABLE 20–6. DSM-IV-TR diagnostic criteria for conduct disorder

A. A repetitive and persistent pattern of behavior in which the basic rights of others or major age-appropriate societal norms or rules are violated, as manifested by the presence of three (or more) of the following criteria in the past 12 months, with at least one criterion present in the past 6 months:

Aggression to people and animals
   (1) often bullies, threatens, or intimidates others
   (2) often initiates physical fights
   (3) has used a weapon that can cause serious physical harm to others (e.g., a bat, brick, broken bottle, knife, gun)
   (4) has been physically cruel to people
   (5) has been physically cruel to animals
   (6) has stolen while confronting a victim (e.g., mugging, purse snatching, extortion, armed robbery)
   (7) has forced someone into sexual activity

Destruction of property
   (8) has deliberately engaged in fire setting with the intention of causing serious damage
   (9) has deliberately destroyed others' property (other than by fire setting)

Deceitfulness or theft
   (10) has broken into someone else's house, building, or car
   (11) often lies to obtain goods or favors or to avoid obligations (i.e., "cons" others)
   (12) has stolen items of nontrivial value without confronting a victim (e.g., shoplifting, but without breaking and entering; forgery)

Serious violations of rules
   (13) often stays out at night despite parental prohibitions, beginning before age 13 years
   (14) has run away from home overnight at least twice while living in parental or parental surrogate home (or once without returning for a lengthy period)
   (15) is often truant from school, beginning before age 13 years

B. The disturbance in behavior causes clinically significant impairment in social, academic, or occupational functioning.

C. If the individual is age 18 years or older, criteria are not met for antisocial personality disorder.

Code based on age at onset:

   312.81 Conduct Disorder, Childhood-Onset Type: onset of at least one criterion characteristic of conduct disorder prior to age 10 years

   312.82 Conduct Disorder, Adolescent-Onset Type: absence of any criteria characteristic of conduct disorder prior to age 10 years

   312.89 Conduct Disorder, Unspecified Onset: age at onset is not known

Specify severity:

   Mild: few if any conduct problems in excess of those required to make the diagnosis **and** conduct problems cause only minor harm to others

   Moderate: number of conduct problems and effect on others intermediate between "mild" and "severe"

   Severe: many conduct problems in excess of those required to make the diagnosis **or** conduct problems cause considerable harm to others

1998c; Tolan 1987). Compared with adolescent-onset conduct disorder, childhood-onset conduct disorder is more predominantly seen in males and is more likely to be associated with physical aggression, ADHD, an early history of oppositional defiant disorder, and antisocial personality disorder in adulthood.

Clinical Description

Conduct disorder accounts for 50% of convicted juvenile delinquents and a higher proportion of incarcerated youths. These youths are often products of low socioeconomic status, unstable homes with family discord, mater-

nal rejection, and absent or alcoholic fathers (DeKlyen et al. 1998; Farrington and Loeber 2000; Lahey et al. 1999), but some youths with conduct disorder come from more favorable environments. As a group, youths with conduct disorder have measurably lower cognitive and moral development, more behavioral impulsivity, greater susceptibility to boredom and stimulus-seeking behavior, and in some cases lower nutritional status. Many of these patients tend to be overtly aggressive, even to the point of being homicidal, particularly toward parents but more generally toward authority figures (Fergusson et al. 1994; Vitiello and Stoff 1997). Outcome and course depend partially on involvement in a delinquency group, the nature of the delinquency group, the availability of alternative social supports, concurrent psychiatric disorders, and the age at onset.

Not all delinquent behavior is conduct disorder. Youths with *adaptive delinquency* or *subcultural delinquency* are conceptualized to have made an "adaptive" response to social and cultural disadvantage, parental neglect, and delinquent peers. Viewed as social victims rather than as mentally ill, these youths are commonly seen in juvenile delinquency centers and inner-city clinics and less commonly in prisons. Adaptive delinquency has a wide range of severity, and the condition is not always apparent. The diagnosis of conduct disorder was developed to identify more serious and chronic cases that may have psychiatric dimensions. Misconduct (especially severe delinquency) is more frequent in boys, but the symptom profile is similar in both sexes (Zoccolillo et al. 1996).

A crucial feature of conduct disorder is the absence of impulsivity (Halperin et al. 1995). Impulsive anger in patients with conduct disorder typically derives from comorbid disorders, especially ADHD. Both impulsive and nonimpulsive anger can play a role in the conduct of illegal behavior. Dealing (selling) drugs requires much more thoughtful planning and effective action than does abusing drugs. The strong association between conduct disorder and impulsivity is most likely an artifact of the frequent comorbid presentation of ADHD and conduct disorder. In fact, many of the characteristics attributed to conduct disorder result from comorbid psychiatric disorders. The high rate of comorbidity has complicated delineation of the features specific to conduct disorder, of which impulsivity is just one example.

Across a diversity of presentations, children and adolescents with conduct disorder show alterations of mood (sullenness, anger) and cognition, including attention and learning disorders. Cognitive problems include a faulty sense of size and time, a distorted view of the consequences of previous events, difficulty in imagining the expectable outcome of future events, underestimation of risks, disrupted awareness of cause and effect (particularly regarding their own behavior), reduced problem-solving ability, blocks in logical thinking, and impaired moral reasoning. Pathological defenses include minimizing, avoiding, lying, externalizing, unconscious manipulation, and denial. Interpersonal impairments appear as suspiciousness or paranoia (with cognitive distortions sometimes triggering fights and resentments), a minimum of guilt and empathy, and difficulty in relating to professionals.

Although symptoms such as driving recklessly, carrying weapons, and showing impulsive and nonimpulsive violence may be observed, wanton dangerousness to the public is not typical of all youths with conduct disorder. However, dangerousness may be significant in the small subgroup of children whose aggressive or suicidal behavior is a direct response to hallucinations.

Typically, comorbid psychiatric or neurological pathology is observed in association with the more severe cases of conduct disorder (Biederman et al. 1997a). At least some children with oppositional defiant disorder later develop conduct disorder (Biederman et al. 1996b; Langbehn et al. 1998), and it appears that most children with conduct disorder had an early history consistent with oppositional defiant disorder (August et al. 1999). In general, the antecedent oppositional defiant disorder is associated with childhood-onset rather than adolescent-onset conduct disorder. Adolescents in prisons, especially those slated for execution, show an exceedingly high prevalence of conduct disorder, comorbid neuropsychiatric disorders, and brain injury (D.O. Lewis et al. 1982). Substance use disorders contribute to both the severity and the duration of symptoms. Alcohol and substance use for self-stimulation or self-medication (of anxiety, depression, boredom, pathological excitement, temper, or psychosis) can become a complicating (and mediating) factor that aggravates the impulsivity, rage, and passivity associated with comorbid disorders. Low self-esteem and passivity are common but might be disguised by an exterior of bravado or "toughness." Academic underachievement is typical and may be related to the commonly comorbid learning and communication disorders, especially reading disorder and expressive language disorders. If behavioral impulsivity and hyperactivity are present, they can be a result of ADHD. In general, concomitant psychopathology is often present and can contribute to the chronicity, severity, and social spread of conduct disorder (Loeber et al. 2000).

Embedded within the concept of conduct disorder is the stereotype of the young "hardened criminal" who is dangerous and sociopathic but has not yet been imprisoned. DSM-IV-TR makes no attempt to designate such youths. In attempts at a more precise description of these youths, researchers have considered various attributes hypothesized to be more specific to these individuals, including callousness, low emotional reactivity, and family history of antisocial personality disorder, illegal behavior, and career criminality (Barry et al. 2000).

Epidemiology

Although abundant epidemiological information about crime is available, the data about conduct disorder are very limited and contaminated by comorbidity. Delinquency is a legal concept and refers to behavior that violates criminal law, whereas behavioral criteria for conduct disorder include behaviors that do not necessarily involve legal violations. The prevalence of delinquency in the general child and adolescent population in the United States is approximately 10% (range = 5%–15%), and there is a male predominance for property crimes (4:1) and violent crimes (8:1) among youths. The distribution of violent crimes in the United States among urban, suburban, and rural areas is 10:2:1. After adjustment for population density, however, violent crime is found to be highest in rural areas. Minors (younger than 18 years) are responsible for 40% of arrests for property crimes and 20% of arrests for violent crimes. Children younger than 15 years account for 5.5% of all arrests for violent crimes (Federal Bureau of Investigation 2001). When self-report data are used instead of official statistics, the prevalence of misconduct and delinquent behaviors becomes much greater, and the male predominance declines to about 2:1. These prevalence statistics probably overestimate the general worldwide problem because violent crime appears to be more prevalent in the United States than in other countries.

The prevalence estimates for conduct disorder range from 1% to 10%. Conduct disorder has been found to be more prevalent in youths residing in large cities, although adjustments for population size diminish this disparity (Wichstrøm et al. 1996). The prevalence of conduct disorders has been increasing in females in recent years, so that the traditional male predominance is decreasing over time (Zoccolillo et al. 1996). Conduct disorder is more prevalent in areas of low income, high crime, and social disorganization (Lahey et al. 1999; Sampson et al. 1997). The epidemiology of conduct disorder will continue to vary, depending on diagnostic criteria used, population size and distribution, family and community structure, socioeconomic conditions, and information source.

Etiology

A wide variety of etiological factors have been described, reflecting the full range of explanatory models of behavioral causation and the importance of delinquency as a central societal concern. Early speculation centered on intrapsychic structures, such as "superego defects" (Aichhorn 1925/1955), and on parental influences on unconscious motivation (A.M. Johnson et al. 1941), such as "superego lacunae" and the "acting out" of parents' unverbalized antisocial wishes or impulses. These inferences were never subjected to large-scale or epidemiological studies in children or adults.

Sociological theories focus on the effects of social deprivation, substance abuse, local variations in behav-

ioral norms, gang formation, status seeking, escape from social entrapment, early rejection by peers, and school failure. Researchers in the field of sociology use sophisticated mathematical modeling to determine the role of specific socialization experiences in the path that leads to delinquent behavior and drug use (Elliott et al. 1985).

Parent, caregiver, and home microenvironment characteristics are believed to be particularly important in the presentation of conduct disorder. Proposed factors in the etiology of conduct disorder include fathers with antisocial personality disorder, absent or alcoholic fathers, large families, shifting caregivers, parental rejection, parental abandonment, parental role modeling of impulsive or injurious behaviors, inadequate limit setting, harsh discipline, inconsistent or unpredictable discipline, parental overstimulation or understimulation, parental manipulative behavior, separation from parents, institutional care, early onset of unsanctioned use of alcohol, proximity of a delinquent peer group, and chronic poverty. Empirical evidence for the validity of these factors (and their interactions) varies in strength. Each factor most likely contributes significantly in some cases.

Some counterintuitive findings are clinically instructive. Coming from a single-parent home does not appear to be a major risk factor. Family discord rather than separation appears to mediate the risk for conduct disorder (Rutter and Giller 1984), although other factors associated with single-parent homes also appear to be mediating factors (Lahey et al. 1988a, 1999). This suggests that keeping families together may, in some cases, have disastrous developmental consequences.

Certain microenvironmental factors can also statistically protect a child. Intelligence and small family size repeatedly have been found to be protective factors against both the development and the persistence of conduct disorder. Adequate supervision at home, especially when parents are away, has been shown to reduce the risk of conduct disorder. After-school activities, involvement of neighbors and relatives, community centers, and extended school hours can provide this type of supervision.

Neurophysiological characteristics of conduct disorder, such as decreased resting heart rate, have been reported in numerous studies. The combination of decreased heart rate, lowered skin conductance, and increased slow-wave activity on EEG at age 15 was found to be an independent predictor of criminality at age 24. This suggests that autonomic underarousal, presumably associated with low levels of anxiety, may be a biological mediator of the tendency toward the development of conduct disorder (Raine et al. 1990). And more recently, P300 decrements (Bauer and Hesselbrock 1999) and left hemispheric focal abnormalities (Pillmann et al. 1999) have been reported in patients with conduct disorder and criminal behavior, further evidence supporting biological underpinnings.

Neurological factors appear significant in some individuals with conduct disorder, especially in more aggressive and violent children. Conduct disorder is associated with an increased prevalence of neurological symptoms, both hard and soft signs; neuropsychological deficits, especially inattention; and seizures. The degree of aggression correlates with a history of physical abuse, head and face injuries, neurological findings, and ADHD. Elevated bone lead levels are associated with aggression and conduct symptoms (Needleman et al. 1996). In extremely violent youths, severe learning and communication problems appear to be common. Psychomotor seizures occur in 20% of these individuals, compared with less than 1% in a general population of youths (D.O. Lewis et al. 1982). Furthermore, psychotic symptoms appear in up to 60% of severely violent youths with conduct disorder (D.O. Lewis et al. 1988).

Family history studies show an overrepresentation of antisocial personality, substance abuse, addictive behaviors, mood disorders, ADHD, learning disorders, and schizophrenia (Lahey et al. 1999). The incidence of antisocial behavior and conduct disorder is increased in fathers and other male relatives of children with conduct disorder. Although these findings can be explained by familial or genetic transmission, it is apparent that both environmental and genetic factors influence the development of conduct disorder (Goldstein et al. 2001; Holmes et al. 2001; Jacobson et al. 2000).

Family studies suggest some inheritable predisposing factors. Elevated rates of conduct disorder in adopted-away children complicate the use of adoption studies, but both adoption and twin studies suggest that genetic and environmental factors are operational. For example, one twin study found that a family history of antisocial personality disorder increased a child's risk of having aggressive behavior and conduct disorder in adolescence and antisocial features in adulthood. An adverse home environment was found to predispose a child to the development of conduct disorder but only if antisocial personality disorder was present in the biological family history. That is, a problematic home in the absence of the genetic loading does not necessarily lead to conduct disorder (Cadoret et al. 1995).

The conduct disorders likely will be shown to have polygenic transmission that interacts etiologically with environmental and other biological mechanisms. Studies have implicated the dopamine transporter gene (*DAT1*; Rowe et al. 2001), the D_5 dopamine receptor gene (*DRD5*; Vanyukov et al. 2000), the serotonin transporter gene (Seeger et al. 2001a), and the androgen receptor gene (Comings et al. 1999). An interaction of dopamine, serotonin, and norepinephrine also has been proposed (Comings et al. 2000a), as well as involvement of the hypothalamic-pituitary-cortisol axis (McBurnett et al. 2000).

Indeed, any dysfunction in the neuronal circuitry regulating conduct is certain to be highly complex. Although such biochemical findings provide direction for further research, they should be viewed as very preliminary (R.J. Davidson et al. 2000). Moreover, more fruitful findings may come from studies that take the more dimensional approach of seeking biological markers for individual symptoms of conduct disorder rather than for the entire diagnostic category of conduct disorder, especially considering the potential contaminating influences of comorbidity (Zubieta and Alessi 1993).

One might conclude that many of the etiological factors for conduct disorder could be predicted with the use of common sense alone; indeed, there are few surprises. However, as noted, there are counterintuitive findings and interactions among multiple factors, and these easily overload any rigorous etiological explanation about the individuality of each case. Although common sense and basic psychiatric knowledge can make a large proportion of these cases understandable in a general way, the appearance of conduct disorder is not readily predictable. No single factor mentioned is able to account for more than 50% of the variance in the occurrence of childhood disorders. When factors are grouped together, no combination of factors can account for more than 70% of the variance in the occurrence of conduct disorder (Elliott et al. 1985). Given this variety of factors operating at the population level, it is a daunting—if not impossible—task to accumulate predictive knowledge about the development of individual cases of conduct disorder.

Course and Prognosis

The major outcome risk of conduct disorder in childhood is antisocial personality disorder in adulthood. In a 30-year follow-up study of 500 child guidance clinic patients (Robins 1966), antisocial behavior in childhood was found to predict maladjustment and a high prevalence (37%) of severe psychopathology in adulthood: antisocial behavior, alcohol abuse, psychiatric hospitalization, child neglect, nonsupport, financial dependency, and poor employment and military records. The children of these patients showed a high prevalence of truancy, running away, theft, and dropping out of high school. Of particular interest was the finding that the natural course of conduct disorder did not appear to be influenced by psychiatric treatment, lengthy incarceration, job or military experiences, or degree of religious involvement (Robins 1966). In contrast, marriage to a stable spouse, support from siblings and parents, and brief incarceration were found to be helpful in promoting stability.

In a separate follow-up study of 9,945 Philadelphia, Pennsylvania, boys with conduct disorder, 35% were arrested by their eighteenth birthday, and 6% became chronic offenders accounting for more than 50% of delinquencies. Recidivists in this sample were more likely to have early onset, poor school grades, and low socioeconomic status (Wolfgang et al. 1972). Another study found that about 50% of youths (median age = 15) with conduct disorder had no Axis I diagnosis at follow-up 18–21 months later, but 33% had antisocial personality disorder; about 25% of these adults had anxiety disorders, and 25% had substance use disorders (Storm-Mathisen and Vaglum 1994).

Among youths with conduct disorder, childhood predictors of chronicity and unfavorable outcome in adulthood include early onset, attentional problems, school failure, anxiety disorders (two or more in childhood), substance abuse, antisocial behavior, arson, socialization deficits, family discord, family history of antisocial personality disorder, and low socioeconomic status. Family risk factors appear to be more prognostically significant for the development of conduct disorder than for any other child psychiatric diagnosis (Fendrich et al. 1990).

Better socialization, positive social experiences, and adequate social skills—especially assertiveness and effective problem-solving—are useful in predicting a better long-term outcome (Jenkins 1973; Rutter and Giller 1984). The nature of involvement with peers is also a predictor of course and severity. Peer ratings of misbehavior and low popularity in first grade were found to predict delinquent behavior during adolescence (Tremblay et al. 1988). Furthermore, ratings of aggressivity made by a child's peers at age 8 years may predict certain features of the person's psychiatric, marital, and legal status at age 28–30 (Huesmann et al. 1984).

Complications of conduct disorder are numerous: school failure, school suspension, legal problems, injuries due to fighting or retaliation, accidents, sexually transmitted disease, teenage pregnancy, prostitution, being raped or murdered, criminal activity, imprisonment, fugitive status, abandonment of family, drug addiction, suicide, and homicide. Consequences of comorbid attention deficits and learning disorders can include low frustration tolerance, educational failure, loss of interest in school, underdevelopment of verbal skills, school dropout, and subsequent unemployment. Children with conduct dis-

order have a high rate of physical injuries, accidents, and illnesses, as well as emergency department visits and hospitalizations. At follow-up, the most common causes of mortality in conduct disorder were found to be suicide, motor vehicle accidents, and death from uncertain causes (Rydelius 1988).

When compared with children with conduct disorder alone, children with comorbid ADHD and conduct disorder tend to have an earlier onset of symptoms, more aggressive behavior, more severe and diverse conduct problems, and a more troubled course and outcome. The fathers of children presenting with comorbid ADHD and conduct disorder tend to be more aggressive and to be imprisoned more often (Walker et al. 1987). Both conduct disorder and ADHD appear to contribute separately to the development of illegal behavior (Foley et al. 1996).

As age increases, up to about 26 years old, there is a tendency toward progressively more serious crime and a higher incidence of incarceration or, alternatively, toward general improvement in overall self-management and outcome. Over time, interactions among etiological factors become accumulative. These tendencies to "spiral down" and "spiral up" are viewed as the result of cumulative interactions among disadvantages and advantages.

The prevalence of conduct disorder among incarcerated youths is 85%. About 20% have ADHD or a learning disorder; and about 50% have an IQ below 85. Therefore, although conduct disorder is highly linked to family factors, incarceration status is more strongly associated with psychiatric diagnosis (or intelligence) than with family or economic variables (Hollander and Turner 1985).

Despite the extremely high incidence of major psychopathology, maladjustment, and incarceration, about half of the children with conduct disorder achieve a favorable adult adjustment (Lahey et al. 1999; Loeber 1982; Rutter and Giller 1984). There is a tendency toward a reduction in antisocial symptoms after age 40 (Hare et al. 1988; Robins 1966). Although later onset, adequate supervision at home, and good socialization skills are predictors of better course and adult outcome, it is unknown to what degree the good outcomes are associated with the natural course of illness, life experiences, therapeutic intervention, comorbidity, or preexisting characteristics.

Diagnostic Evaluation

For youths with conduct disorder who have impaired verbal skills, use manipulative defenses, or become uncomfortable when talking with professionals, interactive diagnostic interviews can be difficult. Specific verbal inquiries or repetitive questioning can elicit inconsistent or hostile responses. For these individuals, standard interviews can be ineffective or even counterproductive. Assessments based on highly verbal and structured interviews may overestimate psychopathology and underestimate the interpersonal or intellectual strengths of these individuals.

Child self-reports of conduct symptoms are often unreliable. Although parents' reports are generally more trustworthy, there are good reasons to question the accuracy of these data. Because some of the behaviors of conduct disorder appear infrequently, historical rather than observational data are often preferred. However, the secrecy of the behaviors, the fears of or wishes for punishment, and the amplifying or diminishing influences of extraneous feelings and biases confound the reliability of all reporters, including child, parents, teachers, and police. Correlations between the behavioral reports of different types of reporters are quite low (Achenbach and McConaughy 1996), leading to unresolved clinical dilemmas concerning how to combine the data derived from different informants.

Virtually any child psychiatric disorder can present with behavior problems or with comorbid conduct disorder. In assessing an individual with conduct disorder, it is essential to evaluate the full range of psychiatric diagnoses, neurological status, intelligence and neuropsychological features, educational skills and deficits, social adaptation and assertiveness, and family functioning.

A search for comorbid psychiatric diagnoses, especially bipolar disorder, is critical (Biederman et al. 1997a; McGee and Williams 1988). It appears that up to 25% of adolescents with conduct disorder also may have bipolar disorder (Arredondo and Butler 1994), and much higher lifetime rates have been reported. This common comorbidity may be explained in a variety of ways (Jensen et al. 2001a; T. Spencer et al. 2001a; Wozniak et al. 2001b), including the possibility that conduct symptoms and substance abuse are increased during affective episodes involving elevated or expansive mood. Interestingly, conduct disorder does not appear to have similarly high rates of comorbidity with other mood disorders, such as major depressive disorder or dysthymic disorder (Arredondo and Butler 1994; Rey 1994). Adolescents with conduct disorder have major depressive disorder at the rate that would be expected if there were no association between the two disorders. Anxiety disorders may present in children with comorbid conduct and major depressive disorders but not generally in children with conduct disorder only (Meller and Borchardt 1996).

The finding that up to 25% of children with conduct disorder also have bipolar disorder, but that there is no overrepresentation of conduct disorder with major depressive disorder, challenges the common clinical belief that a diagnosis of conduct disorder is a signal that the child might be depressed. Instead, conduct disorder can be more appropriately interpreted as a signal that the child might have bipolar disorder. Conduct disorder can appear before or after the apparent onset of bipolar disorder, and the conduct disorder may persist or remit after the resolution of the bipolar symptoms (Kovacs et al. 1988; T. Spencer et al. 2001a).

Substance abuse, although very common among patients with conduct disorder, is commonly underdiagnosed. It is not unusual for the substance abuse to remain undiagnosed until these patients present for treatment as adults (Schubiner et al. 2000; Whitmore et al. 1997).

In addition to bipolar disorder and substance abuse, it is clinically helpful to emphasize that learning and communication disorders are common concomitants of conduct disorder and can contribute to a chronic course. Developmental deficits in social skills and other adaptive functions are often apparent, even in individuals who have predominantly inattentive ADHD. Mild mental retardation is often overlooked. Prepsychotic children and intermittently psychotic children may have or appear to have conduct disorder.

The understanding of conduct disorder has progressed dramatically from the days when delinquency was viewed largely in terms of personality development or family functioning. At present, it would be a significant error to assume that a child with conduct disorder should be conceptualized as having merely a "personality disorder" or a "prepersonality disorder." The differential diagnosis of conduct disorder has become more complex, responding to increasing awareness of the multiple paths that lead to conduct and behavior problems. Children with conduct disorders challenge the capacity to think and respond in a multidimensional manner.

Treatment

Psychiatric treatment of conduct disorder depends more on individual variables than on diagnosis. Given the diversity of presentations and severities of conduct disorder, it is not surprising that treatment can move in several directions: legal sanctions, family interventions, social support, psychotherapeutic treatment of individual or family psychopathology, or pharmacological treatment (Kazdin 1987). The biopsychosocial treatment of conduct disorder can involve a large multidisciplinary team, conceivably including a psychiatrist, a psychologist, a pediatrician, a neurologist, an educational consultant, a speech and language specialist, an occupational and recreational supervisor, a social worker, a legal adviser, a parole officer, a school liaison person, and a case manager. The treatment site can be a home, school, hospital, residential school, or specialized delinquency program.

From the very start to the end of treatment, the quick establishment of a containment structure and an expectation of effective limit setting—to provide both safety and a holding environment for treatment—are essential. Limit setting at home may be compromised by parental conflict, parental absence, inconsistent discipline, vague or low behavioral expectations, or parental depression or other psychiatric illness. Creating or reinforcing limits can involve parent counseling, psychiatric treatment of parents, increased supervision at home, surveillance at school, or use of legal mechanisms. Guardianship, hearings before judges, counseling by parole officers, and brief incarceration may be essential for effective limit setting and for communicating the significance of behavioral violations. Treatment of conduct disorder typically requires the involved management of multiple systems (Kazdin 1997).

The possible primary and sustaining roles of comorbid mental disorders in most cases of conduct disorder require that mental health professionals evaluate and follow up psychiatric factors in essentially all cases. The minimum required would be a consultative role in a multimodal treatment program. A single treatment method can be decisive for some individuals with conduct disorder, but the vast majority of patients require multimodal treatment.

Pharmacological research on conduct disorder is quite limited, and most therapeutic effects have appeared to be more closely related to the comorbidity than to the conduct disorder itself. Indeed, the range of medications used in treatment reflects the range of comorbidity presenting with conduct disorder, and it appears to have little to do with specific treatment of conduct disorder per se. Pharmacotherapy can involve virtually any psychotropic drug, depending on the concomitant neuropsychiatric findings in the individual: psychostimulants for ADHD, lithium or anticonvulsants for bipolar disorders, antidepressants for depressive disorders, neuroleptics for psychotic features or impulsive behavior (Findling et al. 2000), and β-adrenergic blocking agents for severe aggression.

Lithium treatment has been examined in several controlled trials, but the exclusive focus has been on conduct disorder with prominent aggressive features, and findings have been mixed (Campbell et al. 1995a, 1995b; Malone et al. 2000; Rifkin et al. 1997). Lithium may be exerting a substantial effect in the subgroup of patients with true bipolarity, which may be why clinicians widely report that it appears to be effective in many cases.

Similarly, limited controlled data suggest that anticonvulsants may be helpful for conduct disorder and associated aggression. In a small trial, valproate improved both explosive tempers and mood lability (Donovan et al. 2000). Trials of carbamazepine have yielded mixed results, with one controlled study reporting no difference between carbamazepine and placebo (Cueva et al. 1996; Kafantaris et al. 1992).

For treating comorbid ADHD and conduct disorder, a wide variety of medications could be useful, including psychostimulants, but the risks of comorbid substance abuse and drug dealing need to be considered. In a 4-year prospective study, 58% of the youths with comorbid conduct disorder and ADHD had their conduct symptoms remit with adequate treatment of their ADHD (Biederman et al. 2001b), a significant finding that emphasizes the importance of early and aggressive treatment of ADHD. Open trials of pemoline (Shah et al. 1994) also have indicated some therapeutic effects, but there is no evidence of the value of this drug in treating conduct disorder in the absence of ADHD. When using pemoline, the risks of drug-induced chemical hepatitis (potentially fulminant), substance abuse (although less than with short-acting psychostimulants), and drug dealing must be considered. Open-label clonidine also has been reported helpful in treating comorbid conduct disorder and ADHD (Schvehla et al. 1994).

The value of nonpharmacological treatments often can be seen when pharmacological therapies are not initiated immediately in treatment. Especially with psychiatric hospitalization, the cost-cutting method of starting pharmacotherapy on admission increases the risk of misattributing clinical stabilization to medications rather than to hospitalization, the milieu, and other treatments (Malone et al. 1997). Unnecessary drug treatments and excessive dosing can potentially be avoided by delaying pharmacotherapy long enough to make a specific diagnosis of a comorbid medication-responsive disorder rather than quickly starting a nonspecific drug treatment.

A variety of psychotherapeutic treatments may be helpful, including cognitive-behavioral therapy for anger and impulse-control management (Faulstich et al. 1988) and individual psychotherapy for problem-solving skills (Kazdin et al. 1989; Kernberg and Chazan 1991). Group therapy, particularly in residential treatment or group-oriented facilities, often permits the "gang orientation" of these youths to be used in promoting positive change and improving socialization skills.

Youths with conduct disorder often have family members with externalizing behaviors and psychiatric disorders. Psychiatric treatment is often needed for the psychiatric disorders of the parents or siblings. A major focus of working with family members may involve maintaining effective limits and a focused orientation toward treatment (rather than punishment). Functional family therapy can be useful in some cases for reducing interpersonal manipulation (Patterson 1982) and for limiting projective identification between family members (Tolan et al. 1986).

School interventions can include individualized educational programming, vocational training, and remediation of language and learning disorders. Evidence indicates that the early treatment of learning disorders may help prevent the development of conduct disorder.

Because of the complexity of individual cases, most youths with conduct disorder need lengthy therapeutic interventions. Because treatment may "terminate" by graduation into another treatment or facility, a therapist may not see the long-term effects of a particular intervention. Management of a case often entails repeated setbacks that can frustrate caregivers.

For treatment-resistant patients, effortful attention and purposeful persistence may be needed to establish empathic understanding of the child's view of life and to develop a motivation for change. Failure to diagnose additional concomitant psychiatric disorders (in child or family) is a common source of poor outcome in conduct disorder. When necessary, parent counseling involves helping parents learn to secure psychiatric hospitalization, use the legal system, avoid inappropriate attempts at defending or excusing the child's actions, or, in extreme cases, accept the "loss" of the child to a life of imprisonment, crime, or fugitive status. The treatment of conduct disorder, with or without concurrent psychiatric disorders, often requires a chronic regimen that can be quite taxing.

Clinical Comment

There has been a debate regarding whether the diagnosis of conduct disorder should be constructed to be independent of gender and social class: should criteria be selected to remove gender and class bias so that all children are viewed democratically as equally likely to have conduct disorder? Or should the definition of conduct disorder be constructed by using criteria that make no attempt to diminish or hide differences in the prevalence of conduct disorder that might appear among cultural, socioeconomic, ethnic, or gender subgroups? Even if the definitional criteria for conduct disorder were selected to be class-independent, it is not surprising that patterns of referral, availability of treatments, and course of illness would remain class-dependent.

Governmental planning for a full and balanced range of treatment services for conduct disorder requires a mandated sense of priority at the national and state levels. Outpatient clinics, hospital units, residential treatment facilities, aftercare (posthospitalization) services, emergency and short-term care facilities, specialized delinquency programs and correctional services, and juvenile courts are essential services to permit a child with conduct disorder to move through an appropriate sequence of treatments.

Controlled comparisons of the psychiatric and legal models for the management of the conduct disorders are not currently available, despite the widespread use of both models. In practice, both models are blended in many treatments. The evaluation of such complicated large-scale, multiyear, multimodal treatments would be exceedingly costly. In the meantime, the treatment of these children remains subject to judgments made in numerous locales and based on a variety of child-rearing and psychiatric treatment philosophies.

Conduct disorder is an umbrella term that unifies tremendously diverse forms of misbehavior that derive from biological, psychodynamic, familial, and social factors. Attempts to subcategorize conduct disorder need to become more sophisticated, allowing for multiple dimensions and their interactions (e.g., aggressive vs. nonaggressive, socialized vs. unsocialized, impulsive vs. nonimpulsive, early vs. late onset, with vs. without family history of antisocial personality disorder). Until psychiatry can delineate specific criteria for clinically useful subgroups, treatment will continue to be offered in individualized but nonspecific psychiatric plans for this mixture of children with "major misbehavior."

Oppositional Defiant Disorder

Children with oppositional defiant disorder show argumentative and disobedient behavior but, unlike children with conduct disorder, respect the personal "rights" of other people. Similar provocative and antiauthority behavior is common in children with conduct disorders and ADHD, but oppositional defiant disorder is a separate diagnosis in its own right. In addition, children may show oppositional or defiant behavior during major affective episodes (depression or hypomania) or more enduringly in chronic mood disorder. However, the term *oppositional defiant disorder* describes children whose provocative, antiauthority, or angry behavior occurs apart from psychosis or symptomatic periods of mood disorders (Table 20–7). Oppositional defiant disorder often presents in association with ADHD, conduct disorder, bipolar disorder, and other psychiatric diagnoses (Greene and Doyle 1999).

TABLE 20–7. DSM-IV-TR diagnostic criteria for oppositional defiant disorder

A. A pattern of negativistic, hostile, and defiant behavior lasting at least 6 months, during which four (or more) of the following are present:
(1) often loses temper
(2) often argues with adults
(3) often actively defies or refuses to comply with adults' requests or rules
(4) often deliberately annoys people
(5) often blames others for his or her mistakes or misbehavior
(6) is often touchy or easily annoyed by others
(7) is often angry and resentful
(8) is often spiteful or vindictive
Note: Consider a criterion met only if the behavior occurs more frequently than is typically observed in individuals of comparable age and developmental level.
B. The disturbance in behavior causes clinically significant impairment in social, academic, or occupational functioning.
C. The behaviors do not occur exclusively during the course of a psychotic or mood disorder.
D. Criteria are not met for conduct disorder, and, if the individual is age 18 years or older, criteria are not met for antisocial personality disorder.

This diagnostic designation permits the study and treatment of "difficult" behavior that is not as severe as conduct disorder and that presumably does not have the same genetic transmission, psychodynamics, family features, or drug responsiveness as the psychotic and mood disorders.

Clinical Description

Oppositional and defiant features can be normal for young children ages 18–36 months and for adolescents; the 6-month minimum duration criterion for oppositional defiant disorder is used to exclude ordinary developmental phenomena.

Anger-related symptoms are the presenting behavior problems, but management of anger appears to be a circumscribed problem. Unlike children with ADHD, the oppositional and angry behavior of these children does not lead to impulsivity throughout their behavior, affect, and cognition (Halperin et al. 1995). The anger is typically directed at parents and teachers, and a lesser degree of anger dyscontrol may be seen in peer relationships. Temper tantrums typically subside in minutes, at most in 30 minutes. Children with mood disorders can require considerably longer to reorganize after an angry outburst.

A crucial feature of oppositional struggling is the self-defeating stand that these children take in arguments. They may be willing to lose something they want (a privilege or toy) rather than lose a struggle. The oppositional struggle takes on a life of its own in the child's mind and becomes more important than the reality of the situation. This "holding onto" or "winning" the struggle may feel paramount to the child. "Rational" objections voiced to the child become counterproductive, and the child may experience these interventions as the adult continuing the argument.

Passive-aggressive and "sneaky" behavior also can be seen, but it does not have the self-centered manipulative quality or the persistent continuity of the coping style seen in children with conduct disorder. Alternatively, oppositional children can show excessive compliance, passivity, and "goody-goody" or perfectionistic behavior. At times, these children seem to live by their own sense of justice, without regard for the realities or circumstances of other people.

The oppositional and defiant symptoms are generally reported by parents and caregivers; the children typically are not able to provide reliable information pertaining to this diagnosis. The children often do not view themselves as oppositional or argumentative, and they externalize blame onto parents, authority figures, and peers. More generally, children with oppositional defiant disorder may have abnormal social cognitions and be inclined to misperceive social information (Coy et al. 2001). In addition to the oppositional behavior, intentional defiance is a hallmark of this disorder. Behavior problems may include verbal fighting and bullying.

In a follow-up study of children with oppositional defiant disorder and conduct disorder, there was little crossover between these two diagnostic categories in the course of 18 months. The distinction between the disruptive behavior disorders, on the basis of the criterion of "violation of personal rights and societal rules," appears to be useful and stable.

Epidemiology

Approximately 6% of children have oppositional defiant disorder, with estimates ranging from 1% to 10%. Along with ADHD, it is the most prevalent psychiatric disorder in 5- to 9-year-old children (August et al. 1996). A male predominance of 2–3:1 was reported in a nonreferred epidemiological sample (Anderson et al. 1987). Oppositional defiant disorder is commonly seen in classrooms for emotionally disturbed and learning-disabled children.

Etiology

The etiology of oppositional defiant disorder is not well understood. The influences of comorbid diagnoses, especially comorbid mood disorders and ADHD, will be important to sort out in studies that attempt to establish etiology. Oppositional defiant disorder often appears to be a characteristic of a family rather than of a child (K.E. Fletcher et al. 1996). In the absence of direct studies of the etiology of oppositional defiant disorder, several psychosocial mechanisms have been hypothesized: 1) parental problems (too harsh or inadequate) in disciplining, structuring, and limit-setting; 2) identification by the child with an impulse-disordered or aggressive parent, who sets a role model for oppositional and defiant interactions with other people; 3) attachment deficits caused by parents' emotional or physical unavailability (e.g., depression, separation, evening work hours); and 4) impairments in the development of affect regulation and social cognition. For example, the persistence of the diagnosis has been associated with both adverse parenting practices and the presence of psychiatric disorders in parents (August et al. 1999). Evidence also indicates that a history of victimization, but not trauma that is unassociated with personal victimization, may be associated with oppositional defiant disorder (Ford et al. 1999).

Neurological, neurobiological, and temperamental factors also may contribute. Traumatic brain injury has been associated with oppositional and defiant symptoms that appear approximately 2 years after injury (Max et al. 1998). Elevated dehydroepiandrosterone sulfate levels in children were found to be highly specific to a diagnosis of oppositional defiant disorder, suggesting a potential role of adrenal androgen functioning (van Goozen et al. 2000). Reduced plasma levels of serotonin (5-hydroxy-indoleacetic acid [5-HIAA]) and dopamine (homovanillic acid [HVA]) metabolites were found in boys with oppositional defiant disorder, with degree of reduction correlating to aggressive and delinquent behaviors (van Goozen et al. 1999). Reduced circulating cortisol levels suggest changes in the hypothalamic-pituitary-adrenal axis, and altered baseline and stressed heart rate levels suggest changes in sympathetic autonomic functioning (van Goozen et al. 1998). Preliminary results suggest a familial aggregation of oppositional defiant disorder, but mechanisms of transmission are undetermined.

Course and Prognosis

Oppositional defiant disorder can be diagnosed after age 3 years but usually appears in late childhood. Follow-up studies suggest that 40% of the children with oppositional defiant disorder retain the diagnosis for at least 4 years, and 93% retain psychiatric symptoms (Cantwell and Baker 1989). Some evidence suggests a developmental progression for some individuals with oppositional defiant disorder to conduct disorder in adolescence and antisocial personality disorder in adulthood (Biederman et al. 1996b; Langbehn et al. 1998). However, even though conduct disorder is often preceded by oppositional defiant disorder, oppositional defiant disorder does not generally develop into conduct disorder (August et al. 1999; Speltz et al. 1999). Parental use of physical discipline appears to be associated with a less favorable outcome at 2-year follow-up (Speltz et al. 1998).

Diagnostic Evaluation

Behavioral evidence of oppositional defiant disorder often can be obtained within 30 minutes by observing peer interactions (Matthys et al. 1995). Psychiatric evaluation of the child and family is needed to investigate family and psychosocial factors as well as to identify comorbid presentations with conduct disorder, ADHD, mood disorders, or psychotic disorders. It is also worthwhile to evaluate for a learning disorder, language disorder, or low intelligence; the persistence of these conditions can contribute to a child's oppositional behavior.

Treatment

Several studies in the psychology literature have reported that behavioral techniques can modify oppositional behavior. Different presentations of oppositional defiant disorder and different comorbidity may justify different behavioral approaches to treatment (Greene and Doyle 1999). Parent training has been particularly useful in ameliorating oppositional behavior in children (Danforth 1998). One large-scale study reported that psychoanalytic psychotherapy had greater effectiveness in treating oppositional defiant disorder (56%) than in treating conduct disorder (23%), especially if the patient and family did not drop out during the first year of treatment (Fonagy and Target 1994). No controlled studies support the typical practice of treating these children with individual or family psychotherapy.

Clinical Comment

Although oppositional defiant disorder is a distinct disruptive behavior disorder, considerable research is needed to define its clinical characteristics, epidemiology, etiology, course, relation to other disorders, and treatment.

Although the oppositional behavior and defiance are distressing to families, these symptoms are not necessarily more pathological than excessive compliance in a child. Pathological compliance can be a significant developmental liability and reason for treatment, but it is not recognized as a psychopathological entity in a culture that places a high social value on harmonious conformity.

Learning, Motor Skills, and Communication Disorders

Developmental problems and barriers to the acquisition or performance of specific skills are usually first diagnosed in childhood and can have major consequences for lifetime functioning. Three major domains of skills are addressed by DSM-IV-TR. The learning disorders involve a series of impairments in the learning of academic skills, particularly reading, mathematics, and expressive writing. Motor skills disorder entails difficulty with physical coordination. The communication disorders involve developmental problems with language and speech, specifically deficits of expressive language, receptive (plus expressive) language, stuttering, and articulation.

These disorders often occur in combination and often with other psychiatric comorbidity in individuals and families. In practice, these children commonly present with psychiatric or behavior problems, and the learning and communication disorders are uncovered secondarily.

Most of these disorders are defined by a particular skill or area of functioning that is impaired relative to general intelligence. DSM-IV-TR criteria specify that these diagnoses should be based on more than simple clinical observation; when possible, standardized test protocols are important for documenting the presence of a specific deficit. Depending on the disorder, formal measurements of both intelligence and specific skills may be required for diagnosis.

As a group, these disorders are present in 10%–15% of the school-age population. Most of these disorders have a male predominance of 3:1–4:1. Equal sex ratios are reported for reading disorder, mathematics disorder, and mixed receptive-expressive language disorder. All of these disorders run in families.

The etiology is unknown but is generally believed to be related to dysmaturation or early damage to the brain areas related to these specific processing functions. The strength of the direct evidence for genetic or biological abnormalities varies with each disorder, and nonbiological factors also are clearly involved in shaping outcome. There is no reason to assume that each disorder is due to a single pathological mechanism, and subtyping may become possible as the brain mechanisms involved become better understood. The clustering of these disorders in the same individuals suggests that these neuropsychological impairments reflect an early disruption in developmental processes, can involve wide-ranging but potentially related cerebral dysfunctions, and are likely to require multimodal educational remediation and subsequent educational accommodations.

These learning, motor skills, and communication disorders are commonly associated with high rates of comorbid psychiatric disorders and various psychological complications, including low self-esteem ("feeling stupid"), poor frustration tolerance, passivity, rigidity in new learning situations, truancy, and dropping out of school. Disruptive behavior disorder can be a complication of these disorders, but signs of developmental dysfunction may appear before school failure, in the preschool years. Although there has been considerable emphasis on the "emotional overlay" resulting from learning and communication disorders, there is an increasing awareness of the neuropsychiatric and sociofamilial antecedents of these disorders.

Over time, mild cases may "resolve" through persistent education and practice. Certain individuals may compensate by "overlearning," but others retain specific deficits in adulthood. Often, the associated behavioral symptoms and intrapsychic complications persist beyond the duration of the developmental deficits, and they may remain problematic during adult life (J. Cohen 1985).

Psychoeducational evaluation includes intelligence testing, a battery of specific achievement tests (of the full range of academic skills, language, speech, and motor coordination), and observation of the child's behavior in the classroom. A general determination of the quality of teaching available at the school is needed before a diagnosis is made. It is also essential to evaluate for possible mental retardation, ADHD, mood disorder (causing low motivation), and other psychiatric and neurological disorders. Sensory perception tests are given to assess possible impairments of vision or hearing, which can aggravate or mimic features of these disorders.

Two federal laws, Section 504 of the Rehabilitation Act of 1973 (whose regulatory explanation was set forth in 1997) and the Individuals With Disabilities Educational Act of 1990/1997 (IDEA, successor to Public Law 94-142, the Education for Handicapped Children Act of 1978), entitle individuals with these disorders to treatment and accommodation as part of their guarantee to a "free and appropriate public education" in the "least restrictive setting."

Section 504 prohibits ostensibly discriminatory acts that, by omission or commission, exclude "handicapped" students from a free and appropriate public education in the least restrictive setting, and it provides broad legal remedy when special educational and remedial services (accommodations) have been withheld through a mandated "accommodation plan." The IDEA entitles "disabled" students to special educational services determined by an IEP, and it provides a funding mechanism for federal and state assistance to local school districts in financing such services.

New laws, changes in the regulatory explanations of these laws, and legal precedents have generally broadened the range of disorders covered and the services provided in recent years. In addition to mental retardation and the learning, communication, and pervasive developmental disorders, various neurological and medical disorders, other health impairments (ADHD included), and serious emotional disturbances, such as depression, are now recognized as disabilities under the IDEA. Under Section 504, the definition of handicapping conditions has been construed even more broadly.

Part-time resource rooms, full-time self-contained classrooms, and mainstream classrooms (with special education consultants) provide the major part of special educational services. Sometimes, specialized schools and residential treatment programs are used. Multidisciplinary communication is essential because many specialists and teachers may be involved in the education of a single child. Careful communication, particularly during transitions, is vital to maintain developmental and educational progress.

Parents of children with learning and communication disorders often fear the irreversibility of these conditions and may contribute to a climate of negativity and criticism. These parents may be responsive to supportive interventions such as involvement in educational planning and adjustment of expectations to anticipate slower-than-standard learning with no clear "ceiling" on educational outcome.

In practice, the provision of "mandated" special education is often inequitable. Although an IEP is designed for each child, in school systems with lower socioeconomic status student populations, in particular, restrictive budgets and limited advocacy may constrain the availability of services. Frequently, remediation of only the more basic skills in the most severe cases is funded. On the other hand, well-informed parents in some school districts have begun to enlist the services of lawyers specializing in this area to force schools under Section 504 to finance extraordinarily expensive residential mental health accommodation plans. Such arrangements have too often been poor proxies for the intermediate and longer-term inpatient treatments that have become otherwise unavailable since managed care has defaulted on their provision. These costly settlements have sometimes threatened the quality of services available to other students.

Although children with these underdiagnosed and undertreated disorders have begun to receive remediation during childhood, the many types of psychoeducational and educational techniques in use nationwide have been too infrequently evaluated in comparative studies.

Psychopharmacological therapy is not helpful in treating learning, communication, or motor skills disorders. Aggressive management is required for psychological effects on self-esteem, patience, assertiveness, and flexibility. The evaluation and treatment of concurrent psychiatric disorders, as well as the management of secondary psychological complications, require more than a purely educational or neuropsychiatric perspective.

These neurodevelopmental disorders appear to be predominantly genetic or neuromaturational in origin; however, socioenvironmental factors are critical in the appearance of the complications of these disorders, so that psychosocial and interpersonal factors are central in treatment and prognosis.

Learning Disorders

The learning disorders involve deficits in the acquisition and performance of reading, writing (not handwriting but expressive writing), or arithmetic. These conditions are meant to designate individuals who have specific deficits in acquiring skills and neurointegrative processing, and so are qualitatively different from other slow learners.

Learning disorders are defined to exclude individuals whose slow learning is explainable by weak educational opportunities, low intelligence, motor or sensory (visual or auditory) handicaps, or neurological problems. In understanding the effect of these disorders, it is helpful to hold a broad psychiatric and neurological view of development in childhood and functioning in adulthood because the estimated 5%–10% of the population with learning disorders is at increased risk for other psychiatric disorders. People with learning disorders commonly have a comorbid communication or motor skills disorder, low self-esteem, motivational problems, and symptoms of anxiety.

The diagnosis of a learning disorder is often made initially during grade school. During the early school years, basic skills, attention, and motivation are building blocks for subsequent learning. Major impairments in these fundamental abilities require identification and remediation to avoid developmental derailment in multiple spheres of functioning. In later school years, organizational skills become increasingly significant: problems with note taking, time management, and book and paper arrangements may be signs of cortical deficits, even for individuals whose basic skills are well remedied. In high school and college, these students may have difficulty in learning foreign languages, writing efficiently, reading for fun, enjoying sports, pursuing scientific studies, setting high personal goals, and striving to achieve their goals (J. Cohen 1985).

At a certain point in the remediation process, a limit is reached in what remediation can accomplish to facilitate automatic and skillful performance, and some residual skills deficits may remain. Thereafter, usually during high school or college, a greater emphasis is placed on accommodation rather than remediation. The goal of intervention then becomes more focused on learning ways to optimize performance in view of the residual learning disability.

Depending on the type of disorder, a child can be encouraged to make use of a calculator or word processor, take "time-extended" tests, receive tutoring individually or in a small group, or use self-paced programmed texts or computerized self-instruction. Cognitive-behavioral techniques are used to emphasize success, develop pride and self-esteem, foster enjoyment of mastering a skill, give opportunities to experiment with less defensive rigidity, enhance learning by confronting established patterns ("do something new"), and promote interests in new situations and new experiences.

Reading Disorder

Learning to read can be compromised in many ways, but reading disorder is a specific neuropsychiatric form of reading disability. Commonly called developmental dyslexia, this learning disorder is characterized by a slow acquisition of reading skills resulting from demonstrable cognitive deficits, primarily in cortical function, in the presence of normal intelligence, educational opportunity, motivation, and emotional control. Slow reading speed, impaired comprehension, word omissions or distortions, and letter reversals result in functioning below the expected performance levels based on age and intelligence (Table 20–8).

TABLE 20–8. DSM-IV-TR diagnostic criteria for reading disorder

A. Reading achievement, as measured by individually administered standardized tests of reading accuracy or comprehension, is substantially below that expected given the person's chronological age, measured intelligence, and age-appropriate education.

B. The disturbance in Criterion A significantly interferes with academic achievement or activities of daily living that require reading skills.

C. If a sensory deficit is present, the reading difficulties are in excess of those usually associated with it.

Coding note: If a general medical (e.g., neurological) condition or sensory deficit is present, code the condition on Axis III.

Although the distinctiveness of this disorder was once questioned, reading disorder has been validated as a specific disorder. The historically influential Isle of Wight study (Rutter and Yule 1975) showed a hump at the "slow" end of the curve for reading acquisition and no analog of "fast" learners at the high end of the curve; these findings were taken for many years to support reading disorder as an entity distinct from simple learning slowness or other causes of difficulty learning to read. In retrospect, these findings appear to result from an artifact of the reading test used in the study (Van der Wissel and Zegers 1985). However, subsequent data suggested that reading ability follows a normal distribution in the population, similar to blood pressure. Reading disability is determined by a cutoff score, just as is hypertension. Like many other medical conditions, reading disorder is now viewed as a lifelong condition with familial genetic transmission, heterogeneous etiology, and important environmental determinants of outcome.

Clinical description. The "core" specific dysfunction in most dyslexic patients involves a defect in phonological processing. In phonological processing, words are decomposed (decoded) into their constituent units of sound (phonemes) and then mapped onto the appropriate groups of letters (graphemes). Impairment in the accuracy and speed of reading single words is the "gold standard" difficulty in reading disorder, and it arises specifically from the difficulty with phonological processing. Slow and inaccurate reading of phonetically "legal" nonsense words is the most accurate predictor of reading problems (Grigorenko 2001). Reading disorder seems to involve dysfunction of a largely "posterior" cortical system specialized for reading (Shaywitz et al. 1998). Contrary to earlier belief, support for specific visuospatial processing problems is currently rather limited.

The symptoms of word omissions or distortions may imply the existence of a much less common subtype of reading disorder. In this hypothesized dyseidetic dyslexia (in contrast to dysphonic dyslexia), problems in the orthographic processing subsystem of the posterior cortical reading system result in impairments in recognizing letters, in letter grouping, and in matching letters and sounds (i.e., in mapping graphemes onto phonemes). This subtype is generally less disabling because bright, motivated individuals can master rapid automatic contextual reading with excellent comprehension.

Other factors are important for reading to develop normally. In addition to the posterior cortical reading system, a wide variety of neurological and psychiatric functions must be intact, including vision, receptive and expressive language capacities, global intelligence, motivation, and attention. Comorbid psychiatric disorders (especially if associated with symptoms of anxiety, agitation, or inattention), sensory deficits, cultural deprivation, inadequate schooling, brain damage, and mental retardation can further impair reading development and academic and social-emotional success. Other maturational ("reading readiness") skills are necessary, including the ability to take instruction, remain seated, and avoid disrupting other individuals in the classroom.

The prominent features of reading disorder may present differently at different ages. Children with reading disorder frequently manifest early or preclinical signs of the disorder. Difficulties in learning the letters of the alphabet and the names of numbers, in learning to associate sounds with letters, and in rhyming words or being confused by words that sound alike are common. Additionally, mild language delays and mild expressive language difficulties, such as difficulties with word finding, mispronunciation, and breaks in speech, may be early indicators of risk for reading disorder. They may be early indicators of more general language difficulties as well.

With increasing age, delays in reading acquisition, slow oral reading, and poor comprehension are appreciated. In the elementary school years, problems associating letters with sounds evolve into problems sounding out written words (particularly "legal" nonsense words) and translating spoken words into properly spelled (orthographically correct) words. Syllables may be elided or their letters reversed, as may letters of similar phonology or morphology, such as *b* and *d*. In oral reading or dictation, words may be left out, unfamiliar words creatively spelled, and familiar words substituted for unfamiliar words with similar general appearance. Difficulty with the reading of single words and especially difficulty in reading phonetically "legal" nonsense words are the strongest predictors of poor reading comprehension in elementary school.

Reading disorder is a lifelong disability. Of the children with reading disorder identified in the first grade, 74% have significantly impaired reading in the tenth grade. The spelling problems typically associated with reading disorder usually are lifelong and may be more severe and long lasting than the reading problem. Because reading disorder persists, strategies for accommodation will eventually supplant remediation because reading will be slower and laborious in most dyslexic patients.

Comorbid learning, communicational, and coordination difficulties are common. Virtually all individuals with reading disorder have spelling problems. About 80% of the individuals with reading disorder have other verbal language deficits. Many have the DSM-IV-TR disorder of written expression, phonological disorder,

motor skills disorder, or poor handwriting. Some have seizures or symptoms of nondominant hemisphere injury. Attentional difficulties are common, even on tasks that are unrelated to reading and language. Anxiety, mood, and disruptive behavior disorders are also frequently associated with reading disorder. Conduct disorder, usually beginning before adolescence and sometimes before the school years, may be present in 25% of the patients; and about one-third of the children with conduct disorder have reading disorder. Disturbances in self-esteem, social adjustment, and academic performance are common.

Epidemiology. Reading disorder is by far the most prevalent of the learning disorders, involving 80% of all individuals with learning disorders. Prevalence estimates for reading disorder vary widely; DSM-IV-TR cites a prevalence of 4% in the United States, but figures up to 17.5% of the general population have been reported. Reading disorder was believed to show the 3:1–4:1 male predominance observed in most learning disorders, but more recent data suggest an equal prevalence in males and females (Shaywitz et al. 1990; Wadsworth et al. 1992). Reading disorder is familial, and current data suggest that from 23% to 65% of the affected children have an affected parent. Increased prevalence of reading disorder is associated with low socioeconomic class, large family size, and social disadvantage. Prevalence has been reported to vary with geographic region, but this may reflect different standards for classification or other differences in ascertainment. The prevalence of reading disorder may differ across countries, where demands for high-quality reading may vary and where reading may involve different linguistic structures or pictographic symbols.

Etiology. Several lines of evidence lend support for the central role of the phonological processing deficits in reading disorder (Grigorenko 2001; Swank 1999). Measures of phonological processing are predictive of later reading success (Torgesen et al. 1994). Deficits in phonological awareness distinguish normal readers from dyslexic patients (Stanovitch and Siegel 1994). These deficits persist into adult life and continue to be associated with the degree of reading impairment (Bruck 1992). Interventions to improve phonological awareness have been found to promote reading acquisition (Foorman et al. 1997; Wise and Olson 1995).

The phonological processing system is conceptualized as a lower-level "module" within complex (and still generally poorly understood) language and reading systems. Models of the phonological module posit hierarchical processing and analysis. Phonological awareness (the capacity to recognize and to rapidly code and decode abstract representations of the sound attributes of written and spoken words into phonemes) represents the lower end, and metaphonology (the knowledge of rules for combining and blending phonemes) represents the higher end of the hierarchical phonological system. A possibly separate module for orthographic analysis may be involved in the representation and ordering of graphemes and the direct rapid mapping of graphemes onto phonemes.

Reading disorder appears to be related to dysfunction principally in the superior temporal gyrus, the posterior superior temporal gyrus (Wernicke's area), the angular gyrus, the striate cortex, the inferior frontal gyrus (Broca's area), and the inferior lateral extrastriate cortex. These neurological structures appear to be involved in the rapid sequencing of spoken language into phonemes and in subsequent phonological and metaphonological processing.

Various imaging and neuroanatomical studies, for example, have suggested abnormalities in the development of lateralization in the brain hemispheres and abnormalities in interhemispheric information transfer. Anomalous cerebral morphology in the bilateral frontal and left temporoparietal regions has been described in numerous imaging studies of reading disorder. A recent large-scale study showed that reading disorder was associated with enlargement of the retrocallosal cortex and smaller insula and anterior superior neocortical regions (Pennington et al. 1999), consistent with subtle differences in cortical development.

Developmental abnormalities of the cerebral cortex in reading disorder are also suggested by neuroanatomical anomalies that have been shown in neuropathological studies. These neuronal ectopias and dysplasias are widespread throughout the cortex but are primarily concentrated in the left hemisphere, especially in the perisylvian region. In the inferior frontal and superior temporal regions, these neuronal anomalies include micropolygyria, neuronal ectopia in layer 1, nodules (brain warts), and architectonic dysplasias.

Also, the usual cerebral pattern of a larger language-dominant region (Broca's area) in the left hemisphere is absent (Haslam et al. 1981). Instead, the planum temporale is symmetrical in these brains, indicating that the usual asymmetry in this part of the brain is absent and suggesting that the normal development of a differentiated language center does not occur in reading disorder.

These studies provide evidence of a relatively underdeveloped Broca's area (left planum temporale) as well as more widespread cortical anomalies. The neuronal ectopias and anomalous symmetry imply a relative failure in brain development that is not restricted to language-dominant regions. More generalized dysfunction is implied by findings that cerebral blood flow is more left-asymmetrical (i.e., predominates on the left side of the brain) during a semantics task in individuals with reading disorder (Rumsey et al. 1985b). These anomalous brain structures are associated with a broad range of cerebral functions, including spatial and verbal abilities, motor dominance (i.e., handedness), and left–right sense. The wide distribution of anomalous structures and function may be consistent with the other comorbid learning disorders that frequently accompany reading disorder, suggesting that the developmental defects that underlie reading disorder are often part of a larger neurodevelopmental, dysmaturational process that may produce disturbances in other areas of psychological functioning.

MRI data show subtle variations in the morphology of the corpus callosum. The reduction in the anterior (genu) volume of the corpus callosum suggests potential difficulties with interhemispheric transfer (Hynd et al. 1995). These studies also found a significant correlation between corpus callosum volume and reading achievement. A recent functional MRI (fMRI) study suggested abnormalities in activation in the left prefrontal cortex and in the right cerebellum (Temple et al. 2000). Together, these findings suggest that structural changes in the anterior corpus callosum that interfere with interhemispheric transfer or coordination of information might play a role in reading disorder.

The cytoarchitectural anomalies probably were acquired during the midgestational period of massive neuronal migration in the topographic formation of the cerebral cortex. Because early acquired lesions can cause a reorganization of the structure and interconnections of the cortex (even at distant points, remote from the original lesions), brain architectural and connectional features may lead to a "cerebral reorganization" and deliver unusual functioning in people with reading disorder. Such alterations in organization suggest that older theories based on "loss-of-function" models of reading disorder significantly underestimate these individuals' potentials and special talents.

Numerous findings and theories regarding hemisphere function and specialization during development have been proposed. A study comparing strongly left-handed and strongly right-handed people found that left-handers (and their relatives) had more reading disorder, stuttering, and immune disorders (Geschwind and Behan 1982). Geschwind and Galaburda (1985) speculated that a prenatal testosterone spurt may lead to slowed cortical lateralization (reduced left hemisphere function), reading disorder, left-handedness, and autoimmune disease (thymus suppression). Although many of the predictions based on this hypothesis have been shown to be incorrect, some biological interconnections among these conditions (Galaburda 1993) underscore the medical basis of reading disorder.

It has been suggested that the fluent word identification necessary for accurate and rapid reading is mediated through two consolidated systems within the left hemispheric posterior cortical reading system (Pugh et al. 2000): a dorsal (temporoparietal) circuit and a ventral (occipitotemporal) circuit. In contrast to normal readers, individuals with reading disorder had heightened reliance on both inferior frontal and right hemispheric posterior regions to compensate for difficulties in the posterior left hemispheric system. For normal readers, the dorsal circuit appears to predominate at first in development and is associated with analytic processing necessary for learning to integrate orthographic features with phonological and lexical-semantic features of printed words. The ventral circuit constitutes a later-developing and faster word identification system that underlies fluent word recognition in skilled readers.

Family psychiatric histories show an overrepresentation of reading, speech, and language disorders in siblings and parents of patients with reading disorder. A concordance rate approaching 100% in identical twins has been found in several studies of reading disorder (S.G. Vandenberg et al. 1986), although DeFries and Alarcon (1996) reported "unbiased" concordances of 68% for identical twins and 38% for fraternal twins. The lower concordance in fraternal twins supports a genetic factor. When the heritability of various components of the reading process has been examined, evidence for the heritability of phonological processing is strong, and some support exists for the heritability of orthographic processing. Family pedigrees generally are not consistent with a single mode of transmission, suggesting that the disorder is genetically heterogeneous. Gene linkage analysis has implicated chromosome 15 in the autosomal dominant transmission of certain cases of reading disorder (S. Smith et al. 1983). Chromosome 6 is also involved in some cases (Cardon et al. 1994; Grigorenko et al. 1997), and other linkages have been established as well.

Despite the neurogenetic factors in the etiology of reading disorder, environmental factors exert a strong influence on its expression and clinical presentation. Although the main etiological factors appear to be neurological, symptom severity and duration may be affected by learning and experience. The phonological and orthographic demands of one's language, educational opportunity, and self-expectations may affect outcome. Reading disorder can be negatively influenced by maternal smoking, low birth weight, and prenatal and perinatal mishaps. In the positive direction, reading disorder can be beneficially influenced by educational opportunities; family support; and individual personality, drive, and ambition. In this sense, none of the neurological abnormalities can be assumed to be causes of reading disorder because educational and environmental factors interact to alter the expression of these neuronal lesions.

Course and prognosis. For reading disorder and slow reading acquisition, adequate reading skills eventually may be acquired with sufficient time and effort. Educational interventions appear to accelerate this process, especially if family support and personal motivation are strong. The extent of residual symptoms in reading disorder and its associated features is quite variable.

Delayed acquisition of reading skills usually is identified in grade school. Typically, by third grade, the child with reading disorder is 1–2 years behind expectations and may fall farther behind unless remediation is received. Adolescents may become frustrated with learning, lose interest in school, and drop out of school; in addition, there may be an exacerbation (or clinical recognition) of conduct disorder or other concomitant psychiatric disorders. Although reading usually improves over time, spelling problems and delinquency may persist. In adulthood, the rate of unemployment and placement in unskilled jobs is elevated.

Some adults never attain substantial reading skills and may adapt by hiding the disability from their children, friends, and employers. They may not seek remedial education or may continue to resist remediation in adulthood, because of either embarrassment, pride, or the required effort. The associated feature of rejection of help may be both a cause and a complication of persistent reading problems. Mismanagement of this major problem in early learning can become a model for the child's subsequent approach to problem solving. Alternatively, proper management can teach the child how to persevere in the face of a seemingly hopeless personal problem.

Diagnostic evaluation. It can be useful to obtain neurological and psychiatric assessment (especially regarding disruptive behavior, ADHD, other learning and communication disorders, and social deprivation); hearing and vision tests; and IQ, psychological, neuropsychological, and educational measurements (including reading speed, comprehension, and spelling). The new neuroimaging techniques are expected to contribute significantly to diagnostic assessment in the future.

The evaluation of students with reading disorder often includes an assessment that determines whether they will receive extra training or accommodations through a special education program at school. Among students whose reading achievement scores are substantially below their intelligence measures, most would be classified as qualifying for special education services because their reading achievement scores are below the cutoff scores. However, bright students with reading disorder might have substantial reading underachievement relative to their intelligence but not "qualify" for special education services because their reading achievement scores exceed the cutoff scores. To allow such students to receive intervention, the evaluation process that determines which students receive special education requires thoughtfulness and flexibility.

Treatment. Early educational intervention may involve one of several remedial programs. Comparative studies of the different educational approaches to reading disorder are still limited, but growing evidence supports the use of phonologically based interventions. In an interesting approach to outcome measurement, an intensive 3-week program that emphasized phonological segmentation and comprehension was found to normalize lactate metabolism in the inferior frontal gyrus in dyslexic children at the end of treatment (Richards et al. 2000).

In addition to remediating the phonological and reading deficits, treatment should be directed at comorbid learning or communication disorders, disruptive behavior disorders (i.e., conduct disorder or ADHD), or mood or anxiety disorder. Self-esteem may need to be bolstered to help the child (or adult) tolerate the remedial efforts. Parental involvement is crucial in providing support for the educational program and for the child's persistent efforts in a criticism-free learning environment. Some parents may advocate alternative vitamin or dietary approaches, but no data support these options for treating learning disorders (Arnold 2002). Parents can be advised that it is beneficial for them to listen to their children read at home daily (Tizard et al. 1982).

The standard psychotropic medications are not useful in treating reading disorder. Somewhat unexpectedly, piracetam has been reported in double-blind, placebo-controlled studies, with standardized reading tests among the outcome measures, to improve reading in children with developmental reading disorder. Such studies have shown that the improvements in children are modest but consistent and statistically significant, and the longer studies (5–9 months) showed more pronounced improvements in reading. Furthermore, five double-blind, placebo-controlled studies in adults with reading disorder confirmed the findings in children. Piracetam, a derivative of GABA, has been used outside the United States to treat cognitive changes in the elderly. It is not a psychostimulant and does not alter levels of alertness or arousal. With accumulating evidence that piracetam can modestly improve reading in children and adults with reading disorder, further investigation of noötropic agents (memory or learning enhancer) should be entertained.

Mathematics Disorder

The capacity for making simple mathematical calculations is critical in a consumer economy and high-technology culture. Arithmetic, calculation (fractions, decimals, percentages), measurement (space, time, weight), and logical reasoning are basic skills.

Clinical description. Mathematics disorder can present with circumscribed deficits associated with fact retrieval or with more globalized deficits associated with problem conceptualization. Arithmetic facts may be deficient despite preserved mathematical conceptual knowledge (Hittmair-Delazer et al. 1995). Individuals with mathematics disorder (Table 20–9) have difficulty in learning to count, doing simple mathematical calculations, conceptualizing sets of objects, and thinking spatially (right/left, up/down, east/west). Deficits may be seen in copying shapes, mathematical memory, number and procedure sequencing, and the naming of mathematical concepts and operations. Also, reading and spelling problems may be seen in association with mathematics disorder.

TABLE 20–9. DSM-IV-TR diagnostic criteria for mathematics disorder

---

A. Mathematical ability, as measured by individually administered standardized tests, is substantially below that expected given the person's chronological age, measured intelligence, and age-appropriate education.

B. The disturbance in Criterion A significantly interferes with academic achievement or activities of daily living that require mathematical ability.

C. If a sensory deficit is present, the difficulties in mathematical ability are in excess of those usually associated with it.

Coding note: If a general medical (e.g., neurological) condition or sensory deficit is present, code the condition on Axis III.

Factors that produce slow academic development of mathematical abilities include neurological, genetic, psychological, and socioeconomic conditions as well as learning experiences. Typically, arithmetic ability correlates with IQ and classroom training. However, mathematics disorder is not defined to designate individuals who are merely slow learners or who have poor educational opportunities; instead, it labels individuals whose mathematical abilities are low for their IQ. In addition, these individuals often have comorbid psychiatric disorders or symptoms, although descriptions of the psychiatric concomitants of this disorder are limited.

Epidemiology. Approximately 3%–6% of the population is affected by mathematics disorder, and the sex distribution appears to be equal (Gross-Tsur et al. 1996; C. Lewis et al. 1994; Shalev et al. 2000). As in other learning disabilities, psychiatric comorbidities are common, especially conduct disorder. Also, about 20% of the patients have dyslexia, and about 25% have ADHD; children comorbid for dyslexia were more profoundly impaired on math skills and other neuropsychological measures than were children with mathematics disorder alone or with mathematics disorder and comorbid ADHD (Shalev et al. 1997). Attentional problems may lead to arithmetic difficulties (Ehlers et al. 1997) in children who do not have mathematics disorder, but children with such difficulties need to be evaluated for this disorder. Lower socioeconomic classes show an overrepresentation of mathematics disorder as well as other learning disorders. Studies of genetic contributions are sparse. In a large study of patients with developmental dyscalculia, about half of the siblings (Shalev et al. 2001) and 42% of the first-degree relatives of the index child (Gross-Tsur et al. 1996) were reported to have learning disabilities; the risks of dyscalculia in the first-degree relatives of affected children exceeded the risks to first-degree relatives of control children by 5- to 10-fold.

Etiology. Etiological factors are not well defined. Individuals with mathematics disorder appear to have a type of neurocortical abnormality that is linked to a deficit in processing speed in some areas of mathematics (Bull and Johnston 1997). Neuropsychological deficits in number manipulation, spatial relationships, and mathematical reasoning may be present. Both verbal (sequencing) and visuospatial deficits can contribute to mathematics disorder, suggesting that bilateral hemisphere dysfunction may be involved (Rourke 1993; Rourke and Strang 1983), although gross neurological deficit in the language-dominant hemisphere is not typically demonstra-

ble. Nonetheless, evidence indicates that the left hemisphere may play a relatively more important role, at least in certain functional deficits (Shalev et al. 1995). For example, the left prefrontal region has been implicated in mathematics disorder (Tohgi et al. 1995). Subcortical mechanisms also have been proposed.

Course and prognosis. During the school years, the course of mathematics disorder usually entails a progressive increase in disability because the learning of mathematical skills is based on the developmental completion of earlier steps. Some children perform well on rote arithmetic and fail later in trigonometry and geometry, which require more abstract and spatial thinking. Over time, most individuals show gradual improvement. As in other learning disorders, complications include low self-esteem, truancy, dropping out of school, symptoms of disruptive behavior disorders, and avoidance (or poor performance) of jobs that require mathematical skills.

Diagnostic evaluation. Evaluation for mathematics disorder includes psychiatric (i.e., disruptive behavior disorders, other learning disorders, and mental retardation), neurological, cognitive (i.e., intelligence, psychological, neuropsychological, and educational achievement testing), and social assessments. Standardized tests of arithmetic skills may need to be individually adjusted for the child's educational experience with an older (rote calculation) or newer (logical concept) mathematics curriculum.

Treatment. Treatment of mathematics disorder involves special education, with initial evaluation and subsequent monitoring of the possible need for psychiatric and neurological intervention. It is interesting that when mathematics disorder is accompanied by ADHD, salient auditory stimulation has been found to improve mathematical performance (et al. 1996).

The mathematical skills of a fifth- or sixth-grader without mathematics disorder are quite sufficient for the practical requirements of most adults, although concomitant social and nonverbal deficits that accompany mathematics disorder may be more significant and enduring (Semrud-Clikeman and Hynd 1990). After the school years (and even during them), weakness in arithmetic skills is not socially stigmatic and may not be a direct source of personal distress. It is likely that this disorder is quietly present in many adults, who make accommodations in their lives and choice of work to manage a residue of dysfunctions that were more evident during school years.

Disorder of Written Expression

Disorder of written expression is not well characterized in the psychiatric literature, and its assessment and treatment are not well developed. Spelling, grammar, sentence and paragraph formation, organizational structure, and punctuation are the areas of difficulty (Table 20–10).

Clinical description. Symptoms include slow writing speed, low written yield, illegibility, letter reversals, word-finding and syntax errors, erasures, rewritings, spacing errors, and punctuation and spelling problems. A more generalized "developmental output failure" may be suggested by low productivity, refusal to complete work or submit assignments, and chronic underachievement (Levine et al. 1981). Ideational content and intellectual abstraction may be limited, although not necessarily. The "sense of audience," a social cognition of the interests and needs of the reader, may be impaired (Gregg and McAlexander 1989).

Epidemiology and etiology. The prevalence of disorder of written expression is not well delineated. There is a standard 3:1–4:1 male predominance. These deficits in written expression may result from underlying problems with graphomotor (hand and pencil control), fine motor, and visuomotor function; attention; memory; concept formation and organization (prioritizing and flow); and expressive language function. Other motor dysfunctions may be present. Like other learning disorders, disorder of written expression is presumed to result from neurocortical dysfunctions, which may be modified by environmental experiences.

Diagnostic evaluation. Formal methods for assessment and measurement of expressive writing have been developed (Brown et al. 2000), but adequate clinical screening can be obtained from samples of copied, dictated, and spontaneous writing. In evaluating disorder of written expression, it is worthwhile to screen for developmental coordination disorders and other motor abnormalities.

Treatment. Genuine remedial therapy is possible. Educational interventions traditionally have consisted of alternative writing formats and skill building. The wide availability of computers has promoted new methods in remediation. Pending more specific research, the psychiatric evaluation and intervention for the disorder of written expression resemble the approach to the other learning disorders.

TABLE 20–10. DSM-IV-TR diagnostic criteria for disorder of written expression

A. Writing skills, as measured by individually administered standardized tests (or functional assessments of writing skills), are substantially below those expected given the person's chronological age, measured intelligence, and age-appropriate education.

B. The disturbance in Criterion A significantly interferes with academic achievement or activities of daily living that require the composition of written texts (e.g., writing grammatically correct sentences and organized paragraphs).

C. If a sensory deficit is present, the difficulties in writing skills are in excess of those usually associated with it.

Coding note: If a general medical (e.g., neurological) condition or sensory deficit is present, code the condition on Axis III.

Motor Skills Disorder

Developmental Coordination Disorder

Developmental coordination disorder, the only motor skills disorder recognized in DSM-IV-TR, involves deficits in the learning and performance of motor skills (Table 20–11). Integration of motor functions and memory of motor tasks also are impaired. Overall, about 5%–6% of children have significant impairments of gross or fine motor functions, which are apparent in running, throwing a ball, buttoning, holding a pencil, and moving with grace; the disorder also may manifest as generalized physical awkwardness. Although the learning of new motor skills may be slow or delayed, some already-learned motor skills may be performed very well, whereas other learned movements are performed poorly. Movements that require coordinated symmetrical or bilateral actions (such as jumping or swimming), good balance (ice skating), or continuous positional changes (running, tennis) may be particularly difficult. Most of these children have difficulties with handwriting (Miller et al. 2001a). Perceptual problems are common, especially visuospatial processing (P.H. Wilson and McKenzie 1998). None of the motor impairments in developmental coordination disorder can be explained by fixed or localizable neurological abnormalities or by mechanical interference. It was previously assumed that these children would "outgrow" their motor learning problems, but long-term data suggest that the impairments commonly persist into adulthood (Cantell and Kooistra 2002; Fox and Lent 1996).

Although this disorder is rarely the primary complaint leading to psychiatric evaluation, it is commonly found in association with many psychiatric disorders, especially

dren with communication disorders (70%) are placed in special education or repeat a grade within the first 10 years of schooling (Aram et al. 1984).

As in the learning disorders, recent research in communication disorders is moving away from an emphasis on deficits in audioperceptual processing and toward a conceptualization based on language and symbolic functions. Sensory, perceptual, motor, and cognitive processes are closely connected in cerebral development. During the course of early development of the cerebral cortex, there is a progressive leftward lateralization of language functions, including speech (sound production), phonetic and syntactic analysis, and verbal (as well as nonverbal) sequence analysis. The right hemisphere appears to be more involved in sound recognition than the left. Lesion data and neurobiological theory have implicated the left perisylvian regions in the processing of phonemes and auditory information. These findings have been confirmed by MRI, single photon emission spectroscopy, and PET. The areas of the planum temporale and angular gyrus appear compromised in both children and adults with language impairments (Semrud-Clikeman 1997). Also, evidence is emerging of familial transmission of these precise deficits (Tallal et al. 2001).

Socioeconomic and cultural factors are associated with speech and language impairments (Tomblin et al. 1997a) and may contribute to their risk. Prematurity, CNS infections, and other pre- and perinatal risk factors may increase the severity of or account for speech and language impairments (Tomblin et al. 1997b).

Hearing loss plays a significant role in the etiology of the communication disorders (Bennett and Haggard 1999). Hearing is crucial in the development of speech and language, and impairments of hearing operate etiologically alongside genetic, neurological, environmental, and educational factors. Deafness is associated with clear reduction in communication skills, but milder hearing decrements also may be developmentally significant. A mild hearing loss (25–40 decibels) resulting from chronic otitis media or perforation of the tympanic membrane may delay development of articulation, expressive and receptive language, and spelling. During the formative period for language development, fluctuating hearing capacity can diminish verbal intelligence and academic performance in a persistent way (Howie 1980).

Early middle-ear pathology may cause language or speech symptoms, particularly if the hearing impairment is chronic. Otitis media, a common infectious disease in children, may leave a residual hearing decrement in 20% of the American population. The degree of language and speech delay may correlate to the number of otitis epi-sodes. Determinants of otitis media include socioeconomic class, allergies, and oropharyngeal (palate) or craniofacial malformations. Hearing loss also may result from genetic and metabolic disorders, chromosomal anomalies, low birth weight, perinatal anoxic damage, CNS infections, ototoxic medications (e.g., antibiotics, diuretics), and toxin exposures (e.g., alcohol, anticonvulsants). Sociofamilial as well as medical factors can contribute, via otitis media, to the appearance of communication disorders.

It appears that impairment in cognitive and educational development may occur at levels of hearing loss that are considered medically insignificant (Howie 1980). It may be speculated that early fluctuations in conductive hearing lead to anomalies in brain development, perhaps leading to enduring changes in auditory attention or signal/noise discrimination. However, not all children who have had episodes of otitis media have developmental delays. Sensory stimulation is crucial in organizing the visual cortex (Wiesel 1982), but there is less clarity regarding the effect of early auditory experience on the acquisition of language, speech, and central auditory-processing mechanisms.

An interesting line of research has led to the proposal that the neurophysiological problem in language disorders may be a deficit in processing rapidly presented stimuli (Stark and Tallal 1988; Temple et al. 2000). This problem in the perception and memory of rapidly appearing stimuli may involve not only linguistic tasks but also a variety of sensory and motor functions and integrative processing. Laboratory tests to identify these neuropsychological deficits might be helpful in the direct diagnosis of language disorders, without the use of standard neuropsychological testing batteries, at least in certain children. These sensory and motor deficits in response to rapid stimuli are also found in children with reading disorder (although not phonological disorder), again supporting the notion of a continuity between language and learning disorders.

It has been speculated that the mechanisms involved in early influences on the development of the cerebral cortex may be useful in understanding the pathogenesis of learning disorders as well as communication disorders, and they may apply to a broader range of mental functions.

Speech and language skills are eventually acquired in virtually all children with communication disorders, but lower IQ and concomitant psychopathology appear to predict less favorable outcome. Complications include progressive academic impairments, psychological distress, low self-esteem, rigidity regarding learning, and dropping out of school.

Evaluation includes a medical, psychiatric, social, and developmental workup as well as language and speech assessment (Cantwell and Baker 1987). Because 20% of children have hearing deficits caused by otitis media, it is helpful to test for hearing acuity with methods such as audiometry or auditory evoked response (which does not require a young child's cooperation). Parents may give a history of few startle reactions, lack of sound imitation (at 6 months) or reactiveness (at 12 months), unintelligibility (at 2.5 years), loud speech, frequent misunderstandings ("Huh?"), speech avoidance, or communication-associated embarrassment or tension (e.g., blinking). Assessing family characteristics (e.g., family size, birth order, socioeconomic status, parental verbal skills, familial speech patterns, interpersonal stimulation), as well as observing free speech between parents and child, may be useful. The child's speech may be studied for language comprehension (linguistic structures), expression (structure and length of utterances), and logical reasoning. Auditory attention (e.g., keeping up with the flow of conversation, ability to hear in a crowd, lack of distractibility), discrimination (e.g., distinguishing similar sounds), and memory (e.g., the ability to repeat sequences of words or digits) can be assessed informally or formally. In neuropsychological tests, nonverbal measures of IQ (e.g., Leiter International Performance Scale, Columbia Scale of Mental Maturity) are used. Also, a neurological evaluation may be indicated for children with a communication disorder in whom a motor abnormality is suspected.

Treatment of communication disorders includes educational and behavioral interventions, as well as treatment of concomitant medical (e.g., hearing), neurological (e.g., seizures), and psychiatric problems. Aggressive treatment of otitis media is particularly indicated in these children, despite the uncertainty about the relation of this disease to language and speech development. It is particularly helpful to encourage social involvement, imitation, and imaginative play as a means of increasing verbal, communicative, and symbolic exercise. There is no evidence that use of nonverbal communication by child or parents inhibits the development of language skills, and it might even enhance such skills.

Advances in linguistics, psychology, the neurosciences, and genetics hold increasing promise for correlating the neurobiology of speech and language to its functional components. A sense of the future direction of this field may be gleaned from one result of the applied integration of these fields, the recent characterization of an autosomal dominant gene that accounts for a severe rare developmental communication disorder (Lai et al. 2001). Psycholinguistic studies (Vargha-Khadem et al. 1995) characterized the complex phenotype of the disorder.

Symptoms include problems with articulation (impaired selection and sequencing of orofacial movements), problems with phonemic awareness and processing (coding and decoding speech into its constituent sounds), disordered use of grammar and syntax, and difficulties with semantics and understanding. The responsible genetic locus was mapped to chromosome 7 at site 7q31 (S.E. Fisher et al. 1998) and the *FOXP2* gene. The forkhead/winged-helix (*FOX*) genes regulate transcription and play important roles in early development. Extrapolation from other FOX autosomal disorders suggests that *FOXP2* plays a critical regulatory role in the cascade of developmental processes mediated by gene–environment interactions that form the language system of the brain. Although few specifics underlying disturbances in neurological functioning that produce the distinctive phenotype are understood, neuroimaging studies have reported bilateral dysfunction of the basal ganglia (Vargha-Khadem et al. 1998) consistent with the role subcortical systems may play in speech and language (Crosson 1999).

Expressive Language Disorder

In expressive language disorder, a linguistic "encoding" problem, the symbolic production and communicative use of language are impaired. The individual cannot put the idea into words ("I can't get the words out") and also has problems in nonverbal expression. These individuals have similar difficulties with repeating, imitating, pointing to named objects, or acting on commands. Unlike autistic and pervasive developmental disorders, comprehension is typically normal in verbal and nonverbal communication. In verbal language, both semantic and syntactic errors occur so that word selection and sentence construction may be impaired; paraphrasing, narrating, and explaining are weak in intelligibility or coherence. The child with expressive language disorder may use developmentally earlier forms of language expression and may rely more on nonverbal communication for requests and comments. Short sentences and simple verbal structures may be used, even with nonverbal communications such as sign language (Paul et al. 1994). This feature implies a problem in symbolic development across language modalities, leading to a diverse group of delays in articulation, vocabulary, and grammar (Table 20–12).

Individuals with expressive language disorder generally learn language in a normal sequence but slowly. These children can adjust their speech to talk appropriately to young children (Fey et al. 1981), suggesting some facility and flexibility in the use of their language skills. There may be associated learning disorders, phonological disorder, inattentiveness, impulsivity, or aggressivity.

TABLE 20–12. DSM-IV-TR diagnostic criteria for expressive language disorder

A. The scores obtained from standardized individually administered measures of expressive language development are substantially below those obtained from standardized measures of both nonverbal intellectual capacity and receptive language development. The disturbance may be manifest clinically by symptoms that include having a markedly limited vocabulary, making errors in tense, or having difficulty recalling words or producing sentences with developmentally appropriate length or complexity.

B. The difficulties with expressive language interfere with academic or occupational achievement or with social communication.

C. Criteria are not met for mixed receptive-expressive language disorder or a pervasive developmental disorder.

D. If mental retardation, a speech-motor or sensory deficit, or environmental deprivation is present, the language difficulties are in excess of those usually associated with these problems.

Coding note: If a speech-motor or sensory deficit or a neurological condition is present, code the condition on Axis III.

When frustrated, the child may have tantrums during the early years or may briefly refuse to speak when older. Problems in social interactions may lead to peer problems and overdependence on family members.

Approximately 1 in 1,000 children have a severe form of expressive language disorder, but mild forms may be 10 times more common. The standard 3:1–4:1 male predominance of some of the other developmental disorders is seen in this disorder.

DSM-IV-TR recognizes both congenital and acquired forms of expressive language disorder. Diverse etiologies involving neurological, genetic, environmental, and familial factors have been described. Teratogenic, perinatal, toxic, and metabolic influences are linked to certain cases. When hearing loss is present, the degree to which hearing is lost strongly correlates with the amount of language impairment (J.A.M. Martin 1980). Children with expressive language disorder are reported to have low cerebral blood flow to the left hemisphere (Raynaud et al. 1989).

Although expressive language disorder is often associated with seemingly secondary behavioral and attentional problems, a high incidence of various psychiatric problems is also observed in relatives, suggesting that concomitant psychiatric disorders may be present in children with difficulties in expressive language.

This condition usually causes parental concern by the time the child reaches age 2–3 years, when the child may appear to be bright but is not yet talking, has acquired only a small vocabulary, or is difficult to comprehend. The period from age 4 to age 7 years is crucial. By age 8, one of two developmental courses is usually established. The child may be progressing toward nearly normal speech, retaining only subtle defects and perhaps symptoms of other learning disorders. Alternatively, the child may remain disabled, show slow progress, and subsequently lose some previously achieved capacities. There appears to be a decrease in nonverbal IQ, possibly because of the failure of development of sequencing, categorization, and related higher cortical functions. The child may lose some of his or her earlier brightness and come to resemble a mentally retarded adolescent. In both courses, complications of expressive language disorder include shyness, withdrawal, and emotional lability.

Evaluation includes psychiatric (attentional and behavior problems), neurological, cognitive, and educational assessments. Intelligence is determined by a nonverbal measure of IQ. A test of hearing acuity is sensible, and workup for concomitant learning disorders is essential.

Few studies of language disorders in recent years have examined DSM-IV-TR expressive language disorder as a discrete entity. Instead, psychiatric research on language problems has focused on receptive or mixed receptive-expressive language disorder.

Mixed Receptive-Expressive Language Disorder

Mixed receptive-expressive language disorder is the impaired development of language comprehension that entails impairments in both decoding (i.e., comprehension) and encoding (i.e., expression). Multiple cortical and subcortical deficits usually are observed, including sensory, integrative, recall, and sequencing functions (Table 20–13). Although receptive aphasia in adults leaves expression intact, a similar condition during development generally leaves a child impaired in the learning of a first verbal language, so that the learning of both receptive and expressive functions are disrupted. Depending on the nature of the deficits, nonverbal comprehension may be preserved or disrupted. Involving receptive and expressive language deficits, mixed receptive-expressive language disorder is considerably more severe and socially disruptive than simple expressive or receptive language disorders (Beitchman et al. 2001; D. Cohen et al. 1976; C.J. Johnson et al. 1999).

Psychiatric comorbidity is often extensive, and mild presentations of mixed receptive-expressive language disorder are frequently overlooked or eclipsed by more evident social-emotional and learning difficulties, resulting in a lost opportunity for early intervention.

TABLE 20–13.   DSM-IV-TR diagnostic criteria for mixed receptive-expressive language disorder

A. The scores obtained from a battery of standardized individually administered measures of both receptive and expressive language development are substantially below those obtained from standardized measures of nonverbal intellectual capacity. Symptoms include those for expressive language disorder as well as difficulty understanding words, sentences, or specific types of words, such as spatial terms.

B. The difficulties with receptive and expressive language significantly interfere with academic or occupational achievement or with social communication.

C. Criteria are not met for a pervasive developmental disorder.

D. If mental retardation, a speech-motor or sensory deficit, or environmental deprivation is present, the language difficulties are in excess of those usually associated with these problems.

Coding note: If a speech-motor or sensory deficit or a neurological condition is present, code the condition on Axis III.

In mild cases, there may be slow "processing" of certain linguistic forms (e.g., unusual, uncommon, or abstract words; spatial or visual language) or slow comprehension of complicated sentences. There also may be difficulty in understanding humor and idioms and in "reading" situational cues. In severe cases, these difficulties may extend to simpler phrases or words, reflecting slow auditory processing. Muteness, echolalia, or neologisms may be observed. During the developmental period, the learning of expressive language skills becomes impaired by the slowness in receptive language processing.

The developmental type of mixed receptive-expressive language disorder may be distinguished from aphasia (which is not a developmental disorder but a loss of pre-existing language functions), other acquired deficits (usually caused by neurological trauma or disease), or the absence of language (a rare condition usually associated with profound mental retardation). Although DSM-IV-TR considers the developmental and the acquired forms to be subtypes of mixed receptive-expressive language disorder, the developmental subtype corresponds more closely to the learning disorders.

Psychiatric comorbidity often includes learning and motor skills disorders, in addition to emotional and disruptive behavior disorders (Beitchman et al. 2001; C.J. Johnson et al. 1999). Mixed receptive and expressive language impairments at age 5 years are associated with aggressiveness and ADHD, and their presence predicts academic failure and antisocial outcome. A strong association with low socioeconomic status, unmarried parents,

impaired hearing, and visual motor deficits has been noted.

Mixed receptive-expressive language disorder may approach the severity of autistic disorder during adolescence because of social awkwardness, stereotypies, resistance to change, and low frustration tolerance (D. Cohen et al. 1976). However, these individuals typically have better social skills, environmental awareness, abstraction, and nonverbal communication than do those with autism.

About 3%–6% of school-age children have mixed receptive-expressive language disorder, but severe cases have a prevalence of 1 in 2,000. Unlike the male predominance of expressive language disorder and many of the learning disorders, an equal sex ratio is found in mixed receptive-expressive language disorder, although sex may influence the range and expression of concomitant social and behavioral difficulties.

The main etiology of mixed receptive-expressive language disorder appears to be neurobiological, usually genetic factors or cerebral damage. Neurological examination detects abnormalities in about two-thirds of cases. Electroencephalographic findings include a slight increase in nondiagnostic abnormalities, especially in the language-dominant hemisphere. Computed tomography (CT) scans may show abnormalities, but these are not uniform or diagnostic. Similarly, dichotic listening may be abnormal but without specific or lateralizing findings.

Evaluation includes assessment of nonverbal IQ, social skills, hearing acuity, articulation, receptive skills (understanding single words, word combinations, and sentences), nonverbal communication (vocalizations, gestures, and gazes), and expressive language skills. Expressive language skills can be measured in terms of the mean length of utterances, which is compared with developmental norms. Syntactic structures should be assessed and also compared with developmental norms. Standardized instruments are available to assess comprehension, with norms starting at age 18 months. Concomitant medical, neurological, and psychiatric (e.g., learning disorders, mood disorders, disruptive behavior disorders, autistic disorder and other pervasive developmental disorders, mental retardation, and selective mutism) diagnoses should be considered.

For treatment of expressive and receptive language problems, special education should be maintained until the symptoms improve. After a child is "mainstreamed," supplemental academic and language supports may be helpful. Psychiatric treatment for attention deficits, behavior problems, and other comorbidity, as well as speech therapy for phonological disorder, may be needed.

Some stuttering is associated with mental retardation, specifically trisomy 21 (Down syndrome) and Hunter-Hurler syndrome (a mucopolysaccharide disorder). In rare cases, stutterlike dysfluency can be caused by psychotropic medications (TCAs, neuroleptics, lithium, alprazolam).

Stuttering often starts at age 2–4 years or, less commonly, at age 5–7 years. For toddlers, stuttering is usually a transient developmental symptom lasting less than 6 months, but about 25% of early-onset patients have persistent stuttering beyond age 12 years. For onset during latency, symptoms are usually stress related, and a benign course of 6 months' to 6 years' duration is typical.

At the onset, the child usually is unaware of the symptom. Symptoms usually appear gradually and then take on a waxing and waning course. The disorder may gradually improve during childhood and essentially resolve by mid-adolescence, or it may worsen and lead to a chronic course. Males tend to have more chronic forms of the disorder. Persons with persistent stuttering have greater phonological and articulation deficits (Paden et al. 1999).

If the condition progresses, word blocking and involuntary tension of the jaw and face muscles may become conspicuous. In persistent cases, people who stutter become painfully aware of the problem. These individuals find that anxiety further aggravates their dysfluency and that they cannot improve their speech by slowing their speech rate or by focusing attention on their speech.

Neurological and acquired stuttering tend to be more constant and fixed, in contrast to a greater variability of the genetic, constitutional, and psychodynamic forms. For nonneurogenic stuttering, the symptoms are often absent during singing, reading aloud, talking in unison, or talking to pets or inanimate objects.

Complications include fearful anticipation, eye blinking, tics, and avoidance of problematic words and situations. The child may experience negative emotional reactions of family and peers (embarrassment, guilt, anger), teasing, and social ostracism. Speech avoidance and poor self-image may affect language and social development and may lead to academic and occupational problems.

Evaluation of stuttering includes a workup for possible neurological causes (cortical, basal ganglial, cerebellar). A full developmental history and general evaluation of speech, language, and hearing are needed. Behavioral assessment includes delineating any restrictions in social interactions and activities. Referral for evaluation to a speech and language pathologist is indicated in all cases of stuttering. It is helpful to assess the dysfluency in monologue, conversation, play, and anxiety; to test the effects of slowed speech and focused attention on the dysflu-ency; and to observe parent–child interactions for communicative stress placed on the child (e.g., rapid questioning, interruptions, repeated corrections, frequent topic shifts).

Speech therapy involves some elements of behavior therapy, including modifying environmental and conversational factors that trigger stuttering, relaxation, rhythm control, feedback, and dealing with accessory body movements, as well as fostering self-esteem and social assertiveness. Specific therapies for stuttering include intensive smooth speech, intensive electromyography feedback, and home-based smooth speech; all have been reported to reduce stuttering frequency by 85%–90%, and these gains have persisted 6 years after treatment (Craig et al. 1996; Hancock et al. 1998). Other methods include imitation, role-playing, practice in speaking (while reading, choral reading, conversing), and talking in different settings (alone, in a group, in front of a classroom, on a telephone) and with different people (parents, relatives, friends, strangers).

Education and counseling of family members are advised. Psychotherapy is generally not indicated, but it might be considered if stuttering persists or begins in adolescence. Antianxiety drugs are generally of minimal value. Neuroleptics may be useful in some cases, but there are no controlled studies. Some studies have suggested the possible effectiveness of serotonin reuptake inhibitors for stuttering. A controlled trial found that clonidine did not improve stuttering (Althaus et al. 1995). Therefore, the role of pharmacotherapy seems limited at best, especially in view of the effectiveness of speech therapy.

Clinical Comment

The preceding neurodevelopmental disorders highlight the potential for underachievement in specific domains. Despite educational opportunities, adequate intelligence, and emotional stability, they emerge in both clinical populations and "normal" samples.

Anomalous strengths and special talents can be associated with these "disorders." Mental age and IQ do not set an upper level for achievement for individuals with any of these disorders. In theory and in practice (Rutter and Yule 1975), many children and adults attain personal goals that are far beyond predicted capacity.

For learning and language disorders that are defined as a weakness relative to general intelligence, no formal standards exist yet for selecting which instruments should be used to assess the specific developmental skills or for determining what degree of test score discrepancies should count for diagnosis. Clinically, it is also difficult to be precise about distinguishing "ordinary statistical slowness" (i.e., at the low end of the normal curve for learning rate) from genuine neurodevelopmental slowness, especially in individuals who have other signs of delays.

In some areas of this overarching diagnostic category, such as reading disorder, important research developments are already holding the promise to revolutionize clinical treatment. In other areas, such as phonological disorder, psychiatric and neuropsychological findings are quite thin—especially in view of the broad effect of these disorders on the education of children and opportunities for adults. Wide-reaching recommendations are still too often made for educational programs and legally mandated treatments on the basis of little rigorous research and relatively simple theories of cognitive functioning.

Although spelling problems are commonly seen in association with these disorders, they are not classified as a separate disorder. In the general population, spelling problems are typically a result of weak instruction or concentration problems rather than cognitive processing deficits. In some cases, however, a "spelling disorder" can be labeled as a "learning disorder not otherwise specified," as can certain types of spatial processing difficulties, handwriting problems, social skills deficits, or (in a slightly different world) lack of musicality. The focus on learning, motor skills, and communication is based on culturally defined notions of essential skills as well as the psychiatric comorbidity that accompanies deficits in these functions.

In view of suggestions that learning problems may be increased through prenatal exposure by maternal use of cigarettes (Nichols and Chen 1981) or alcohol (S.E. Shaywitz et al. 1980), some cases of these disorders may be preventable.

Mental Retardation

Intelligence (e.g., as measured by IQ) might be considered an independent dimension that deserves its own separate DSM-IV-TR axis. However, the diagnosis of mental retardation encompasses more than low intelligence; it also requires deficits in adaptive functioning. The diagnostic concept of mental retardation as constituting low IQ plus adaptive deficits was developed by the American Association on Mental Retardation (1992) and essentially adopted by DSM-IV. It emphasizes that mental retardation is not an innate characteristic of an individual but the result of an interaction between personal intellectual capacities and the environment.

At least 90% of the individuals with low intelligence are identified by age 18 years, but the diagnosis of mental retardation requires onset during the developmental period. Furthermore, developmental understanding is basic to the treatment of mental retardation, although psychiatric treatment of mental retardation is typically provided by general and child psychiatrists.

The definition of mental retardation encompasses three features: 1) subaverage intelligence (e.g., IQ of 70 or below), 2) impaired adaptive functioning, and 3) childhood onset (Table 20–16). The system for subclassifying the severity of mental retardation in DSM-IV-TR is based on IQ scores, but the American Association on Mental Retardation (1992) instead subclassifies by the required "intensity and pattern of support systems" (intermittent, limited, extensive, and pervasive).

TABLE 20–16. DSM-IV-TR diagnostic criteria for mental retardation

A. Significantly subaverage intellectual functioning: an IQ of approximately 70 or below on an individually administered IQ test (for infants, a clinical judgment of significantly subaverage intellectual functioning).

B. Concurrent deficits or impairments in present adaptive functioning (i.e., the person's effectiveness in meeting the standards expected for his or her age by his or her cultural group) in at least two of the following areas: communication, self-care, home living, social/interpersonal skills, use of community resources, self-direction, functional academic skills, work, leisure, health, and safety.

C. The onset is before age 18 years.

Code based on degree of severity reflecting level of intellectual impairment:

317   **Mild Mental Retardation:** IQ level 50–55 to approximately 70

318.0   **Moderate Mental Retardation:** IQ level 35–40 to 50–55

318.1   **Severe Mental Retardation:** IQ level 20–25 to 35–40

318.2   **Profound Mental Retardation:** IQ level below 20 or 25

319   **Mental Retardation, Severity Unspecified:** when there is strong presumption of Mental Retardation but the person's intelligence is untestable by standard tests

---

Intelligence is routinely measured by standardized tests, such as the Wechsler Adult Intelligence Scale—Revised (WAIS-R), the Wechsler Intelligence Scale for Children—Third Edition (WISC-III) for 6- to 16-year-olds, the Stanford-Binet Intelligence Scale, 4th Edition, for 2- to 18-year-olds, or sections of the Bayley Scales of

culty in "reading" facial expressions. With delays in speech and language development, limitations in communication may inhibit expression of negative affect, leading to instances of apparent affective hyperreactivity including impulsive anger, low frustration tolerance, and reactive agitation. In extreme cases, impulse dyscontrol may lead to violence and destructiveness. These behavioral manifestations may show only modest improvement over time, especially in patients with severe or profound mental retardation (Reid and Ballinger 1995). Interestingly, the usual signals of distress may not be evident in patients with severe or profound mental retardation, leading to an underestimation of their discomfort and subjective stress in a variety of circumstances, including medical evaluation and procedures (Cavaliere et al. 1999).

The ordinary complexities of daily human interactions may test an individual's cognitive limits (Sigman 1985). Cognitive capacities may be taxed in the parallel processing of speech production; thought communication; listening; and the understanding of situational context, social cues, and emotional signals. Changes in daily situation may stretch cognitive capacities and coping abilities, sometimes leading to frustration. Resistance to novelty and environmental change may be viewed as an associated finding or a developmental consequence of mental retardation.

Defensive style can include rigidity or withdrawal. Primitive reactions to frustration and tension may involve not only aggressive responses but also self-injurious, self-stimulatory, or habitual behaviors. SIB is commonly observed in this population, although visual and auditory deficits can induce or aggravate such behavior (P.W. Davidson et al. 1996; Wieseler et al. 1995). Psychosocial opportunities, both within and outside of treatment programs, may be severely limited by defensive withdrawal and by societal rejection. An inclination to be less persistent in dealing with challenges (Kozub et al. 2000) has important implications for adaptive functioning.

Habilitation may be inhibited by the individual's difficulty in recognizing the historical and interpersonal dimensions of his or her behavioral and affective problems, limitations in memory, cognitive processing, abstract thinking, sense of time, and perspective taking.

Medical comorbidity is approximately twice as frequent as in the general population (Ryan and Sunada 1997). Such medical problems (including associated neurological or metabolic disorders, physical disabilities, and sensory deficits) often are undertreated. When motor deficits are present, their specific characteristics should be identified and targeted for treatment. However, receiving adequate medical care may require organizational and social skills that exceed the easy grasp of mentally retarded people.

Generalizations about mental retardation are increasingly coming into question as research permits the understanding and differentiation of specific mental retardation syndromes. Contrasting with the old notion that mental retardation is a nonspecific form of slow development, newer phenomenological data indicate that these syndromes share many commonalities but are not the same. For example, persons with trisomy 21 (Down syndrome) and fragile X syndrome tend to have quite different characteristics of language, cognition, social behavior, and adaptive skills (Bregman and Hodapp 1991; Lachiewicz et al. 1994) as well as different psychiatric comorbidity (Bregman 1991). "Theory of mind" abilities may be impaired, but the etiology of the mental retardation is a major factor in determining "theory of mind" abilities and deficits (Yirmiya et al. 1998). Such findings suggest that individuals with mental retardation of different etiologies, not just of different severities, have distinct profiles of strengths and weaknesses that may be expected to influence their development.

Epidemiology

Prevalence figures in the United States range from 1% to 3%, depending mainly on the definition of adaptive functioning (Larson et al. 2001). Approximately 85%–90% of patients are mildly retarded (IQ = 55–70). There appears to be a male predominance at all levels of mental retardation of about 1.5:1, although ratios as high as 6:1 have been reported; there may be a female predominance in severe mental retardation (Katusic et al. 1996).

Diagnostic labeling is low before age 5 years, rises sharply in the early school years, peaks in the later school years (about age 15), and then declines during adulthood toward 1%. High prevalence rates during the school years usually are attributed to the adaptive and intellectual demands of school (especially social and abstract thinking) and the high degree of supervision in classrooms (increased recognition of the child's difficulties). The decline during adulthood usually is attributed to improving social and economic skills, less supervision at work, and possibly (in some cases) delayed intellectual development. Typically, more severe levels of mental retardation have an earlier age at diagnosis.

Socioeconomic class is a crucial variable. Severe and profound mental retardation are distributed uniformly across all socioeconomic classes, but mild mental retardation is more common in low socioeconomic classes (Stromme and Magnus 2000) (Figure 20–2). In the lowest socioeconomic class, the prevalence of mental retardation in the American school-age population is 10%–30%. This "multiply disadvantaged" poverty class consists of inhabitants of city slums and poor rural areas, migrant workers, and economically oppressed groups. This fact highlights the etiological role of genetic–environmental interactions in mental retardation, especially in cases for which there is no obvious cause (Croen et al. 2001; Thapar et al. 1994).

In underdeveloped countries, the quality of nutrition, hygiene, sanitation, prenatal care, and mass immunization influences the incidence of mental retardation, but prevalence is reduced by infant mortality. In technologically advanced countries, medical and social supports enhance survival and longevity, although the effect on quality of life is less clear.

Etiology

There are almost 1,000 recognized biological syndromes involving mental retardation, entailing disruptions in virtually any sector of brain biochemical or physiological functioning (Castellvi-Bel and Mila 2001; Grossman 1983; Johnston et al. 2001). Disruption of neurogenesis, neuronal migration, cellular differentiation, intercellular communication, cytoskeleton organization, synaptic vesicle transport, and other cellular functions are typical arenas of pathological change. The most common anatomical features of mental retardation are dendritic abnormalities, which may range from generalized dysgenesis to highly syndrome-specific abnormalities or from multiform changes resulting from neuronal damage and reorganization to particular cytoarchitectural formations and changes over time (Kaufmann and Moser 2000).

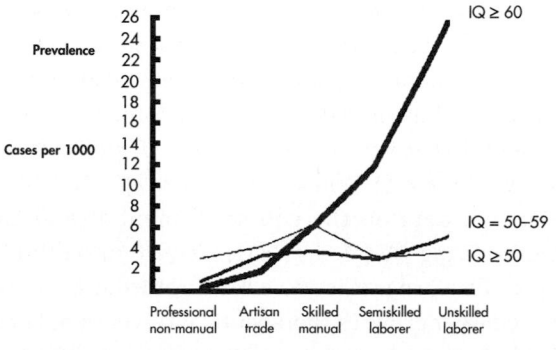

FIGURE 20–2. Prevalence of mental retardation in children from various socioeconomic classes.

The more serious forms of mental retardation show an even distribution across socioeconomic class, but mild mental retardation is more prevalent in lower socioeconomic groups. Social class is indicated by occupation of the child's father.

Source. Adapted from Birch et al. 1970.

Mild retardation is generally idiopathic and familial, but severe and profound retardation are typically genetic or related to brain damage. Specific syndromes of mental retardation, such as Down syndrome or fragile X syndrome, can be identified on the basis of consistent clinical features. Even in cases of nonspecific mental retardation, in which no consistent and distinctive features are present, specific causes might be identified; for example, eight gene sites have so far been linked with nonspecific X-linked mental retardation (Castellvi-Bel and Mila 2001).

The most common form is idiopathic mental retardation, a "nonspecific" form that is associated with sociocultural or psychosocial disadvantage and typically is seen in the offspring of retarded parents ("familial"). The degree of retardation in this form is generally mild and sometimes moderate. Intellectual and adaptive deficits are presumed to be determined by a polygenic mechanism, although emphasis is currently placed on the role of intervening social factors. These individuals live in low socioeconomic circumstances, and their functioning is influenced by poverty, disease, deficiencies in health care, and impaired help seeking. Family size may exceed parental capacities for attention and positive stimulation of the children, inducing marked effects on several dimensions of development. Social disadvantage contributes heavily to the etiology of some forms of mild mental retardation. Nonetheless, the overrepresentation of various genetic, physical, and neurological abnormalities in people with mild mental retardation is a reminder that social forces may not be the predominant etiological factors.

Both inherited (presumably polygenic) factors and environmental mechanisms may contribute to the familial transmission of mild mental retardation across generations (Castellvi-Bel and Mila 2001). This common form of mental retardation is associated with a high prevalence of conduct, attention, and language disorders.

Moderate and severe forms of mental retardation are less likely to be idiopathic. Specific biomedical etiologies may be identified in 60%–70% of all cases of mental retardation and in a higher proportion of cases of severe or profound mental retardation. These moderate and severe cases usually are first diagnosed in infancy or early childhood, and 90% have prenatal causes. Major mechanisms include genetic and neurodevelopmental damage. When biological causes are identifiable, there are more severe disabilities, physical limitations, and dependency.

In cases of idiopathic mental retardation, there is substantial evidence for a biological basis of brain abnormalities. Enlarged ventricles, similar to findings in schizophrenia, have been reported in 75% of the children with mental retardation of unknown cause (Prassopoulos et al. 1996). Infants with mental retardation show an abnormal thickening of the corpus callosum during development in the first year of life (Fujii et al. 1994).

Neurodevelopmental damage or dysmorphogenesis may be produced by a variety of mechanisms. Physical insults that are typically damaging to the brain are catastrophic in early development. Because the fetus has no demonstrable immunological response in early gestation, maternal infections (e.g., congenital AIDS or toxoplasmosis) may cause major damage. If rubella is contracted during the first month of pregnancy, there is a 50% rate of fetal abnormalities. Intrauterine exposure to toxins (e.g., lead), medications, and radiation may result in intrauterine growth retardation and other toxic effects on brain development (Herskowitz 1987). Similarly, intrauterine exposures to nicotine, alcohol, and cocaine are preventable causes of mental retardation (Drews et al. 1996). Intrauterine seizures can be a prenatal cause of brain damage and impaired brain development (Volpe 1987). Certain forms of maternal illness (toxemia or diabetes) also may be dangerous to the developing nervous system in utero.

At birth, obstetrical trauma and Rh isoimmunization may cause brain injury. Birth asphyxia is probably not a significant source of mental retardation; there has been a deemphasis on the role of perinatal hypoxia in the etiology of neuropsychiatric problems (Nelson 1991). Hypoxic changes typically result in maturational delays that are no longer diagnosed by age 7 years, except perhaps in severe and profound mental retardation. Prematurity (or low birth weight) is not typically causal, but it may be in extreme cases (e.g., <28 weeks' gestation or birth weight<1,500 g) (Vexler and Ferriero 2001). Taken together, low birth weight, low gestational age, and low Apgar scores contribute significantly to only about 4% of the children with mental retardation (Stromme 2000).

Several forms of neurodevelopmental damage may occur postnatally. Environmental factors are particularly crucial in underdeveloped countries, where distribution of medical care may be limited. Neurological infections and disease, including seizures, may contribute. Neurological trauma may result from falls, accidents, athletic injury, extreme fever, child abuse, and severe malnutrition.

Chromosomal factors can be identified in 10% of institutionalized individuals with mental retardation. Apart from polygenetic inheritance, the major chromosomal mechanisms include dominantly inherited single-gene defects, recessively inherited inborn errors of metabolism, recessive chromosomal aberrations, and early developmental (embryonic) gene alterations.

As mental retardation in general and the specific disorders are more intensively studied, there is an emerging picture of the extraordinary complexity of genetic and neurodevelopmental processes, as well as of sociodevelopmental processes, that contribute to the different presentations. Specific genetic mechanisms, molecular events, developmental courses, cognitive features, language abilities, and adaptive strengths and weaknesses are being identified for the various mental retardation syndromes (Bregman and Hodapp 1991). Two examples, trisomy 21 and fragile X syndrome, provide an interesting contrast to illustrate the distinctive qualities among different syndromes of mental retardation.

Course and Prognosis

Although biological factors of each mental retardation syndrome in each individual may determine certain aspects of development, the course and outcome of mental retardation generally depend largely on social, economic, health/medical, educational, and developmental circumstances. Whether the disorder is a mild familial form or the result of a severe inborn metabolic error, the course of mental retardation is influenced by interactions with environmental opportunities and barriers. Parental characteristics may entail advantages that are compensatory or disadvantages that are compounding. Such features of the microenvironment operate as intervening factors and may have a stronger influence on adult psychiatric outcome than the causative factors, except in extreme cases. The course and prognosis of mental retardation is much less predictable than originally believed.

Neurodevelopmental evaluation during the first year can predict intellectual outcome and neurological status in later childhood in nearly 90% of premature children (Largo et al. 1990). Premature infants with intracranial hemorrhage (demonstrated on ultrasound) are especially likely to have impaired cognitive and motor abilities later, especially if there are persistent signs of periventricular abnormalities (M.L. Williams et al. 1987).

Current data on the course of mental retardation reflect varying degrees of aggressivity in habilitative efforts. The prognosis in mental retardation may be expected to improve as therapeutic interventions become available to more members of the general public and as adaptive behavior improves over the course of a lifetime.

The period between ages 18 and 26 has been identified as a particularly critical interval in development for people with mental retardation (Blacher 2001). During this time, most individuals experience a completion of their state-supported formal education and the transition toward personal independence. Vocational training and placement, setting up residential arrangements, and the establishment of a social matrix and self-expectations are prominent during this time. This time also coincides with a withdrawal of organized community supports.

At present, about two-thirds of mentally retarded individuals shed their diagnoses in adulthood, as adaptive skills increase (Grossman 1983). Typically, the global level of adaptive functioning is found to change over the course of months or years in response to changes in economic and social supports, living arrangements, work opportunities, and parental support.

For mental retardation at all levels of severity, and for cases of both idiopathic and known etiologies, the developmental course is slow but not "deviant." The normal sequence of cognitive developmental stages is observed. The speed of developmental change is slow, and there appears to be a "ceiling" on ultimate achievement. In addition, secondary emotional and social "complications" may influence the clinical presentation and outcome.

Excessively low or high expectations maintained by family, therapeutic team, or patient constitute significant obstacles to therapeutic improvement. The habitual resignation to low expectation of achievement has a chilling effect on self-esteem, hope, and outcome.

Common psychological complications include frequent experiencing of failure, low self-esteem, frustration in fulfillment of dependency needs and wishes for love, wavering parental support, regressive wishes for institutionalization, anticipation of failure (leading to avoidance of problem solving and challenges, reduced curiosity and exploration, and impaired mastery seeking and pride), defensive rigidity, and excessive caution (e.g., resistance to dealing with new people and places, including helping professionals). Additional psychosocial complications are impaired interactions and communications, inappropriate social assertiveness, and vulnerability to being exploited. Financial complications (poverty) entail further medical complications, including impaired care seeking (delayed treatment, excessive use of emergency facilities), rarity of preventive treatment (prenatal and well-baby care, periodic checkups), accidents and trauma, malnutrition, lead exposure, child abuse, prematurity, and teenage pregnancy. It is apparent that complications of mental retardation are numerous. A lack of aggressivity, integration, or continuity in the provision of care can hinder basic medical treatment. Institutionalization may promote passivity and excessive compliance. Societal ignorance and stigmatization may lead to avoidance by potential social companions and professionals.

Family complications may include parental disappointment, anger, guilt, overprotectiveness, infantilization, overinvolvement, or detachment. Siblings may experience annoyance at sharing in sibling care, loss of parents' attention, parents' compensatory overexpectations, and realistic fears concerning genetic risks for their own children. The effect on parents of having a child with mental retardation is, however, positive in many cases (Taanila et al. 1996).

Death is often sudden and unexpected among individuals with mental retardation, especially among patients with seizure disorders (Chaney and Eyman 2000; McKee and Bodfish 2000). Prenatal etiology of mental retardation and low IQ are also risk factors for early mortality (Chaney and Eyman 2000).

A major part of the care of mentally retarded individuals includes prevention and management of the numerous medical, psychological, and family complications. Another major component of care is the monitoring of overall speed of progress: a lack of developmental improvement raises the possibility of concomitant psychiatric diagnoses.

Diagnostic Evaluation

It cannot be overemphasized that all psychiatric diagnoses may co-occur with mental retardation and that all personality types may occur in mental retardation. Up to one-half of these patients may have ADHD. Mentally retarded individuals also may have unipolar and bipolar mood disorders, anxiety disorders, psychotic reactions, autistic disorder, and learning disorders (G. Masi et al. 2000a; Menolascino et al. 1986). Some psychiatric rating scales have been formally tested (Aman 1991), but some standard evaluation instruments might perform differently in this population (Borthwick-Duffy et al. 1997; Embregts et al. 2000). Many patients with mental retardation never receive psychiatric evaluation and endure their comorbid mental disorders without treatment (Stromme and Diseth 2000).

Sadness, depression, lack of enthusiasm, excessive anxiety, and "primary process" associations are not primary features of mental retardation; these symptoms should be evaluated as complications or as signs of concomitant disorders.

Medical evaluation should include physical examination (seeking physical stigmata) and laboratory tests, including thyroid function, lead testing, chromosomal analysis, and molecular screening for amino and organic acids and mucopolysaccharides, among others. However, specialized studies are best ordered by a clinical geneticist or other specialist in mental retardation because the rates of positive findings are dramatically higher for these expensive tests if they have been ordered on the basis of specifically leading physical and clinical findings (Hunter

2000). X-ray studies of long bones and wrists should be obtained. Neurological evaluation should be performed to discover possible treatable causes of mental retardation, seizure disorders, and possibly deafness and blindness. Head and face size and symmetries, head shape (including hair patterns), eye and ear position, and asymmetries of motor and sensory function should be examined. A history of maternal miscarriage, toxic exposures, infections, and fetal size and activity should be elicited. Neuroimaging, such as MRI and perhaps EEG, may be appropriate for patients with neurological symptoms, abnormal cranial size (microcephaly or macrocephaly), or unusual cranial contour (Curry et al. 1997). Psychological testing, including neuropsychological evaluation, is commonly required. Adaptive skills of the individual should be measured (e.g., the Vineland Adaptive Behavior Scale) to target areas of remediation and strength.

Families of individuals with mental retardation experience considerable challenge. The burden of management can tax the efforts of any family (Cooper 1981), especially the parents (Figure 20–3). Because intensive intervention is required to minimize developmental complications, this burden can continue for many years. The growth-promoting characteristics of the family can be assessed (through interviews and home visit) by investigating the level of stimulation, emotional support, help seeking, decision making, future orientation, and financial planning for the mentally retarded individual.

Evaluation of these patients should be continued, sometimes over several years, to allow sequential assessments to fully characterize behavioral and physical features (Curry et al. 1997). It is not unusual for the etiological diagnosis to be changed during the course of such extended evaluations (Stromme 2000).

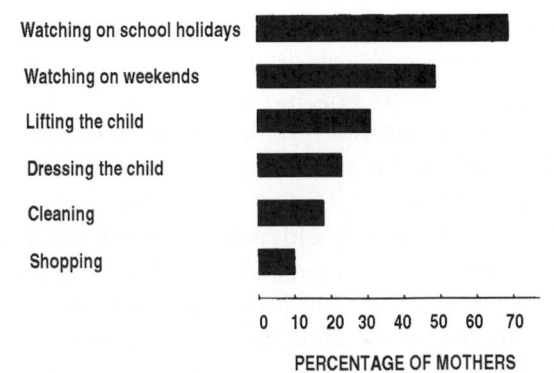

FIGURE 20–3. Caregiving burdens described by mothers of children with mental retardation.

The care of a child with mental retardation places practical responsibilities as well as emotional strains on the families.

Source. Adapted from Birch et al. 1970.

Treatment

Treatment of the multiple handicaps and complications commonly associated with mental retardation is typically multimodal, with a developmental orientation (Szymanski and King 1999). Long-term habilitative programs involve many specialists and agencies working collaboratively over time and across agency boundaries.

The vast majority of children and a sizable proportion of adults with mental retardation are able to live at home with their parents (Braddock et al. 2001). Out-of-home placements become more common as the child matures and continue to increase as the individual ages. Actual accommodations and opportunities are often highly dependent on the local availability of resources and the choices made by responsible authorities in government or private agencies. The progressive trend away from the use of large centralized institutions has led to increased community-based placement in group homes. The group of residents is typically larger than the average family, requiring the homes to undergo special architectural and zoning accommodations. The transition from living with parents to living in a residential facility can be managed in a manner that promotes the satisfaction and well-being of all concerned, even when the aging of the patient's parents requires a late-life transition (Seltzer et al. 2001).

Psychiatric hospitalization may be needed in certain cases, usually for the same reasons that justify inpatient management in the nonretarded population. Outreach programs may be an alternative to hospitalization for some patients with mental retardation and major psychiatric disorders (van Minnen et al. 1997).

Large state-operated psychiatric hospitals providing custodial care are still used in certain cases. Although many specialized chronic inpatient programs are well managed, some institutions have problems with neglect and physical abuse. In these settings, staff perpetrators tend to be new male employees with a history of perpetration, and the likelihood of such abuse being uncovered is increased by recent in-service training on abuse prevention (McCartney and Campbell 1998). Also, some custodial inpatient placements are clinically inappropriate, a problem that can be successfully challenged by class action lawsuit, resulting in improved patient adaptation (Dudley et al. 1997).

The specific psychiatric component includes the coordination of the primary diagnostic evaluation of medical and psychiatric conditions, parental guidance (behavioral management, educational and environmental planning, long-term monitoring, and advocacy), and the usual variety of psychiatric therapies for specific concomitant psychiatric disorders (Szymanski 1987; Szymanski and Tanguay 1980). Substance abuse treatment and prevention may be necessary, although research available to guide interventions is minimal (Christian and Poling 1997).

Behavior modification can be useful for treating symptoms of aggressivity, defiance, overactivity, asocial behavior, self-injury, stereotypies, and pica; in some cases, toilet training, dressing and grooming, and eating skills may be taught. Response-contingent procedures appear particularly effective (Didden et al. 1997). Educational and developmental training to enhance speech and language, motor, cognitive, occupational, social, recreational, sexual, and adaptive skills are commonly provided by specialized professionals (Felce and Emerson 2001). Cognitive training may be enhanced by methods that bring information from the periphery of attention ("out of focus") that is then faded into focus (Carlin et al. 2001). The individual may be trained to initiate task simplifications, request communicational clarifications, and perform environmental improvements. Parent counseling and education, as well as family support, are standard. Even within structured and protective residential programs, the average size of the social network of adults with mental retardation, excluding staff members, is two people (J. Robertson et al. 2001); thus, psychosocial skills training is useful, including concrete assistance in making and sustaining friendships. Cognitive-behavioral approaches to prevention of potential sexual and verbal abuse are appropriate (Khemka and Hickson 2000). Special attention is needed for managing the conflicts regarding standard of living (economic) and behavioral expectations between home and treatment settings.

Although treatments based on abstract thinking may not be helpful, developmentally oriented psychotherapeutic interventions may be effective for crisis management or for achieving long-term psychosocial goals. For some adolescent or adult patients with mild mental retardation, verbal psychotherapy may be used to promote self–other differentiation, self-esteem, identity formation, interpersonal development, emotional and behavioral control, management of power, and expression of love and sexuality. Technical modifications include the use of briefer and clearer verbalizations, focus on current events and feelings, reinforcement of reality–fantasy differentiations, management of projections, teaching about the nature of emotional life, and free use of positive reinforcement. Brief frequent sessions may be more useful than standard formats. For children, play therapy may be used.

Pharmacotherapy may be helpful in the management of some symptoms associated with mental retardation as well as in the treatment of comorbid psychiatric disorders. Unfortunately, there is a paucity of controlled research in mental retardation, necessitating extrapolation from small open-label adult trials and studies conducted on other diagnostic groups (Aman et al. 2000). Behavioral manifestations may show only modest improvement over time, especially in patients with severe or profound mental retardation (Reid and Ballinger 1995). Treatment is primarily symptom-oriented or targets comorbid psychiatric conditions (Matson et al. 2000). Although controlled studies are still relatively few, atypical neuroleptics may be useful for treating aggressive and agitated behavior (Antonacci and de Groot 2000; Buitelaar 2000; Buitelaar et al. 2001; H. Williams et al. 2000). Less well-established treatments include use of β-adrenergic blockers, clonidine for agitation (Agarwal et al. 2001), psychostimulants for hyperactivity, TCAs for depressive disorders, serotonin reuptake inhibitors for mood and perseverative symptoms, anticonvulsants for seizures, mood stabilizers for bipolar disorders (Carta et al. 2001), and naltrexone for SIBs. Although published reports are few, electroconvulsive therapy may be used, and there does not appear to be an increased vulnerability to its adverse effects (Thuppal and Fink 1999).

Clinical Comment

The development of treatment resources for mentally retarded individuals requires the collaboration of professionals in the fields of medicine, psychology, education, law, and ethics, as well as representatives of private agencies and government. The ethical issues involved in the treatment of mentally retarded patients may inhibit some physicians and other professionals from taking an aggressive therapeutic stance. The tremendous dependency needs and the lifelong duration of treatment also may operate to scare physicians away.

In schools, the ongoing controversy about the merits of "mainstream" classroom versus specialized "resource room" placements remains to be resolved by psychological and educational outcome assessment; the debate will interact with public and political processes.

In underdeveloped countries, improved nutrition, hygiene, sanitation, and prenatal care, as well as mass immunizations, are crucial to the prevention and treatment of mental retardation. Within the United States, large variations in the regional distribution of mental retardation treatment programs, in addition to the high needs of inner cities and some rural areas, limit the effectiveness of governmental service and planning.

Advances in medicine are fostering the survival of very premature and low-weight infants, whose persistent neurological and intellectual deficits are a new source of mental retardation. There is also an increasing number of known causes of mental retardation and an expanding awareness of the effectiveness of aggressive treatment. In research, mental retardation offers the opportunity for investigating the interrelationships of intellectual and emotional functioning in human development. The revolution in molecular medicine and neuroscience will undoubtedly lead to further identification of genetic, morphogenetic, and physiological (including neuronal plasticity and brain "reorganization") processes that underlie or remediate many presentations of mental retardation.

This ancient disorder, described in classical Thebes, has been viewed with tolerance and respect in many historical cultures, although the Christian concept of the "feeble-minded" established a curious mix of sensitivities. In the eighteenth century, John Locke made the pivotal distinction between mental retardation and emotional disorders. In the nineteenth century, a period of habilitative optimism was followed by subsequent disillusionment at slow therapeutic progress. In the twentieth century, some states enacted laws that required sterilization of mentally retarded individuals. By mid-century, medical research had challenged the ancient notion of untreatability. In 1975, federal law P.L. 94-142 mandated special educational services for all mentally retarded children. Currently, some legal anachronisms and funding limitations remain that obstruct opportunities for contributory work, dignified living, and personal growth. Interest in this disorder is unfashionable in this age, which is oriented toward productivity and efficiency. However, within professional circles, it is believed that aggressive treatment works and that the implementation of a humane public policy entails funding of the required services.

Medical professionals will continue to investigate causes, psychiatric concomitants, psychological complications, and psychosocial treatment interventions. The ongoing revolutions in molecular medicine and neuroscience will undoubtedly lead to further identification of genetic, morphogenetic, and physiological processes that underlie the many presentations of mental retardation. Management of the family's "postdiagnosis crisis," the siblings' psychological burdens, and the family's financial planning is the most immediate way to improve the mentally retarded child's microenvironment. Family support also can be provided by local chapters of the Association for Retarded Citizens. Research on adaptive skills, education, and development remains the focus of long-term efforts. A particular contribution of psychiatrists is in aiding patients with comorbid psychiatric diagnoses (Patja et al. 2001).

There are numerous aspects of prevention, including public education, destigmatization, alleviation of poverty, wider medical care, genetic counseling, advocacy in law and government for development of treatment resources and special education, and advocacy for research. Significant obstacles to research in mental retardation include individuals' barriers in the decision-making process, lack of information and support, limited experience in exercising their own choice, and cognitive limitations (Freedman 2001). These obstacles must be overcome to further define effective pharmacological and psychosocial clinical treatment.

Aggressive management can improve the quality of life and longevity of mentally retarded persons, and aggressive research efforts are needed as well. At least some future cases of mental retardation may be prevented or treated through genetic alteration, possibly involving prenatal intervention through intrauterine gene transfer (Ye et al. 2001).

Pervasive Developmental Disorders

The pervasive developmental disorders make up a neurobiologically diverse group of conditions characterized by deficits across many areas of functioning that lead to a remarkably pervasive but diffuse disruption of developmental processes. These multiply handicapped individuals typically have a developmental process that is not merely slow or limited but is "atypical" or "deviant." Anomalous strengths can emerge from this developmental process in some cases, but many of these individuals have mental retardation. Comorbidity may include any of the psychiatric disorders, and there may be an increased prevalence of OCD (often identified as "perseveration"), stereotypic movement disorder, tic disorders, ADHD, and mood disorders among individuals with a pervasive developmental disorder.

DSM-IV-TR recognizes several pervasive developmental disorders that differ in course of illness, symptoms, and severity. *Autistic disorder* involves an early onset of impairments in social interaction, communication deficits, and restricted activities and interests; there is some tendency toward partial improvement over time, but unpredictable periods of rapid improvement appear between extended periods of minimal change. *Childhood disintegrative disorder* entails symptoms that are largely similar, but the symptoms follow at least 2 years of seemingly normal development; the child then loses early developmental gains and reaches a stable level of autistic-like functioning. *Rett's disorder*, an early-onset progressive disorder of females, is associated with mental retardation, generalized growth retardation, and multiple neurological symptoms (including stereotyped movements of the hands); this disorder appears similar to autistic disorder during early childhood, but it progressively takes on characteristics of a neurodegenerative or neurodevelopmental disorder. *Asperger's disorder* is largely similar to "high-functioning" autistic disorder in its relative preservation of language skills and intellect; despite some remaining skepticism about its validity as a distinct DSM-IV-TR disorder, several features of Asperger's disorder have been found that distinguish it from autism and other developmental disorders.

Early intervention and multiyear treatment of the pervasive developmental disorders emphasize communication and occupational functions. The treatment can be effective, although the benefits accrue slowly, and its value has not been well documented in controlled studies. General management requires a long-term, multimodal, developmentally oriented clinical program. Medical treatments are aimed at symptom relief and management of any comorbid neurological or psychiatric disorders.

Autistic Disorder

Autistic disorder, an early-onset pervasive developmental disorder, entails disabilities in virtually all psychological and behavioral sectors. In view of the severity of extreme cases of autistic disorder, it is remarkable that this condition was not documented until the late nineteenth century and not described until the mid twentieth century. However, most individuals with autistic disorder do not have the massive, severe developmental impairments seen in the classically described cases. Although it was initially conceptualized as a deprivation syndrome, later evidence of neuropsychiatric dysfunction led to a more biological construct of the affective, cognitive, social, communicative, motor, neurovegetative, integrative, and adaptive abnormalities of autistic disorder (D. Cohen et al. 1987). The current view of the phenomenology is remarkably similar to the early description, but there have been major shifts in the understanding of prevalence, severity, etiology, and especially treatment.

Clinical Description

The DSM-IV-TR definition of autistic disorder puts particular emphasis on the impairments in social interaction and reciprocity, the difficulties with verbal and nonverbal communication (and related capacities such as symbolization), and the stereotyped pattern of behaviors and interests (Table 20–18).

Autistic disorder presents in a wide spectrum of severities. The classic form of "early infantile autism," described by Kanner (1943), was a severe infancy-onset disorder with profoundly disturbed social relationships (e.g., detachment, aloofness), communication disruption, motor abnormalities, affective atypicality, massive cognitive impairments, multiple behavioral oddities, distorted perception, and bizarre thoughts. These symptoms led to conceptualizations based on failed ego development or severe regression, and the bizarre thoughts and behaviors were viewed as suggestive of psychotic development. The notion of autistic disorder as a variant of schizophrenia or of any psychotic disorder is no longer considered heuristically useful.

Despite the extremely disrupted integration of brain functions, an almost chaotic form of disorganization, and cognitive and emotional confusion, autistic disorder is not associated with delusions, hallucinations, or loose associations. It is no longer viewed as a psychotic disorder, and emphasis is placed on the neurointegrative features of the disorganization and the idiosyncratic traits of the individual. In the relatively mild forms of autistic disorder, the social, communicative, and behavioral abnormalities are so subtle that they merge into the range of character pathology.

Children with autistic disorder may show limited social interactiveness, a seeming indifference to human warmth, little imitation or sharing, and rare smiling. Socially, these children appear passive and aloof, initially avoiding social contact, but they can come to enjoy and seek interpersonal experiences. Autistic children often have difficulty in comprehending verbal and nonverbal language and are often misinterpreted; typically, these issues need to be a focus of treatment. They often show persistent deficits in sensing or appreciating the feelings of other people and in understanding the process and nuances of social communication. Communicative speech and gesturing are limited and may be difficult to understand because of echolalia, pronoun reversals, and idiosyncratic meanings. Speech is typically late and unusual, and it sometimes fails to develop altogether. Phonological (i.e., sound production) and syntactic (i.e., grammar) functions may be relatively spared, with more significant impairments of semantics (i.e., sociocultural meanings) and pragmatics (i.e., rules of interpersonal exchange), as well as other aspects of communication. Imaginative and symbolic functions (e.g., use of toys in play) may be deeply affected. Rituals, stereotypies (e.g., rocking, whirling), self-stimulation, SIB, and unusual mannerisms are common. Autistic children often have an obsessive attachment to certain people or objects (resistance to change) and a lack of ordinary spontaneity.

TABLE 20–18. DSM-IV-TR diagnostic criteria for autistic disorder

A. A total of six (or more) items from (1), (2), and (3), with at least two from (1), and one each from (2) and (3):

  (1) qualitative impairment in social interaction, as manifested by at least two of the following:
   (a) marked impairment in the use of multiple non-verbal behaviors such as eye-to-eye gaze, facial expression, body postures, and gestures to regulate social interaction
   (b) failure to develop peer relationships appropriate to developmental level
   (c) a lack of spontaneous seeking to share enjoyment, interests, or achievements with other people (e.g., by a lack of showing, bringing, or pointing out objects of interest)
   (d) lack of social or emotional reciprocity

  (2) qualitative impairments in communication as manifested by at least one of the following:
   (a) delay in, or total lack of, the development of spoken language (not accompanied by an attempt to compensate through alternative modes of communication such as gesture or mime)
   (b) in individuals with adequate speech, marked impairment in the ability to initiate or sustain a conversation with others
   (c) stereotyped and repetitive use of language or idiosyncratic language
   (d) lack of varied, spontaneous make-believe play or social imitative play appropriate to developmental level

  (3) restricted repetitive and stereotyped patterns of behavior, interests, and activities, as manifested by at least one of the following:
   (a) encompassing preoccupation with one or more stereotyped and restricted patterns of interest that is abnormal either in intensity or focus
   (b) apparently inflexible adherence to specific, nonfunctional routines or rituals
   (c) stereotyped and repetitive motor mannerisms (e.g., hand or finger flapping or twisting, or complex whole-body movements)
   (d) persistent preoccupation with parts of objects

B. Delays or abnormal functioning in at least one of the following areas, with onset prior to age 3 years: (1) social interaction, (2) language as used in social communication, or (3) symbolic or imaginative play.

C. The disturbance is not better accounted for by Rett's disorder or childhood disintegrative disorder.

Affect may be "shallow," overly responsive to small changes, oblivious to large changes in the environment, and unpredictably labile and odd. Fear responses may be exaggerated or may be absent even when appropriate.

Impulsivity, agitation, and tantrum behavior is common, especially in the early years. Cognitive deficits include impairments in abstraction, sequencing, and integration. There may be distorted perception for smell, taste, or touch and underdevelopment of visual and auditory processing. Eating patterns may be restricted ("picky eating") or indiscriminate (pica).

Most individuals with autistic disorder show subnormal intelligence, but some show significant "increases" in measured IQ during the course of treatment or development. There are often dramatic inconsistencies, with extraordinary "scatter" of capabilities among different IQ subtests and over time. Unusual or special capacities ("savant" skills) may be present in particular areas, such as music, drawing, arithmetic, or calendar calculation.

Epidemiology

The available prevalence estimates for autistic disorder are based on criteria that emphasize the more severe forms of this disorder. When these criteria are used, prevalence is estimated at approximately 1 in 2,000. The less severe forms are more common, with estimates as high as 1 in 250. There is a male predominance of approximately 4:1–5:1, but females often have more severe symptoms. Contrary to early belief, increased prevalence is not associated with higher socioeconomic class or higher intelligence.

Etiology

Contrary to popular opinion, there is no significant evidence that psychosocial factors or parenting abnormalities cause autistic disorder or that exposure to mumps-measles-rubella vaccination increases the risk of autistic disorder.

Genetic and biological factors appear to play a significant role in autistic disorder (Folstein and Piven 1991), but what is inherited appears to be a spectrum of cognitive and social deficits rather than autism per se. The higher concordance in monozygotic than dizygotic twins (60%–91% vs. 0%) supports a genetic factor (Bailey et al. 1995). Family genetic studies establish higher rates of autism, social and communication deficits, and stereotyped behaviors (i.e., broader autism phenotype) in the relatives of autistic patients (Piven et al. 1997b). The reports of chromosome 15 abnormalities and the 2%–5% incidence of autism in individuals with fragile X syndrome initially led to optimism that genetic linkage studies might define genes for autistic disorder, but early attempts failed. A two-stage genomewide scan by the International Molecular Genetic Study of Autism Consortium (S. Barrett et al. 1999; Philippe et al. 1999) failed to identify candidate genes, probably because the power of current techniques is challenged by the large number of genes that contribute to the liability to autistic disorder. Identification of candidate genetic loci might be assisted by accidents of nature, such as deletions or translocations, that permit the association of a small chromosomal region with either autism or some of its traits (M. Smith et al. 2001). Despite the difficulties, recent findings provide strong evidence of linkage with chromosome arms 2q, 7q, and 16p (International Molecular Genetic Study of Autism Consortium 2001).

The probable overrepresentation of ADHD, obsessive-compulsive symptoms, and Tourette's disorder also may suggest that autistic disorder involves genetic factors that are related to the transmission of these disorders and, perhaps, the transmission of the syndrome entailing all three conditions (J.S. Stern and Robertson 1997). The first-degree (parents) and second-degree (aunts, uncles, and grandparents) relatives of individuals with autistic disorder have been reported to have significantly higher rates of major depressive disorder and social phobia, in comparison to relatives of patients with Down syndrome (Piven and Palmer 1999). Shared genetic mechanisms may account for this overrepresentation.

Siblings of autistic children show a prevalence of autistic disorder of 2%–5% (more than 50 times the expected prevalence), and about 5%–25% of the siblings have delays in learning (usually language or speech disorder), mental retardation, or physical defects. Family studies have suggested autosomal recessive inheritance for certain cases of autistic disorder. Neuropathological studies have suggested that neurodevelopmental changes begin early in gestation, probably in the second trimester (Bauman 1991). Decreased numbers of Purkinje's cells and fetal cerebellar circuitry also have been reported.

Early neuroimaging studies have yielded findings that are inconsistent, nonspecific, nondiagnostic, or suggestive of general neuromaturational delays, adding little to the understanding of the pathogenesis of the pervasive developmental disorders. Failure to appreciate and properly correct for the effects of important covariates such as gender, age, performance IQ, and total brain volume in sample construction appears to have accounted for much of the inconsistency, but underlying etiological heterogeneity may play an important role as well. The most consistent neuroimaging findings implicate abnormalities in the temporal and parietal lobes of patients with autistic disorder.

The most common changes noted in MRI studies have been reductions in the volume of the hippocampus and amygdala (Aylward et al. 1999; DeLong and Heinz 1997; Saitoh et al. 2001) and the posterior corpus callo-

sum (Manes et al. 1999; Piven et al. 1997a; Rimland and Baker 1996). Hypoplasia of the cerebellar vermis of the cerebellum often has been reported (Courchesne et al. 1988; Levitt et al. 1999; Peterson 1995; Pierce and Courchesne 2001) but not replicated in other studies (Hardan et al. 2001; Manes et al. 1999; Piven et al. 1997c, 1998; Schaefer et al. 1996). Vermal hypoplasia has been correlated with reductions in environmental exploration and repetitive behavior (Pierce and Courchesne 2001) and with spatial attentional tasks (Townsend et al. 1999). An inverse correlation has been found between vermal hypoplasia and frontal lobe size (Carper and Courchesne 2000). Data on evoked response potentials have implicated impaired cerebello-frontal spatial attention networks in the attentional dysfunction in autistic disorder (Townsend et al. 2001).

PET studies have shown reductions in the volume and metabolic activity of the anterior cingulate gyrus as well as bitemporal glucose hypometabolism (Haznedar et al. 1997; Zilbovicius et al. 2000). High-resolution single photon emission computed tomography (SPECT) scanning also has identified abnormalities in the temporal and parietal lobes (Mountz et al. 1995). Alterations of serotonin synthesis in the dentatothalamocortical pathway, which is relevant to language production and sensory integration, have been reported in children (Chugani et al. 1997) and adults (R.A. Muller et al. 1998) with autistic disorder. The serotonin system in autistic disorder shows evidence of developmental abnormalities as well (Chugani et al. 1999).

A specific medical cause may be identified in some individuals. An elevated prevalence of early developmental problems, such as postnatal neurological infections, congenital rubella, and phenylketonuria, has been reported. About 2%–5% of autistic individuals appear to have fragile X syndrome. Seizure disorders are also common in autism, including both major motor seizures and complex partial seizures. Seizure onset typically is either during early childhood or during adolescence, and clinical seizures can be observed in up to 50% of autistic persons by age 20 years. Children with an early onset of seizures may show an increase in seizure symptoms during adolescence. Adolescence-onset seizures are observed more commonly in autistic disorder than in mental retardation.

Neurochemical assays suggest a decrease in urinary catecholamines (and related metabolites) and perhaps an increase in the dopamine metabolite HVA in cerebrospinal fluid. Elevated blood serotonin concentration appears to be a stable trait that remains for decades in one-third of patients with autism, but it does not appear to correlate with specific clinical features. Regional studies have suggested asymmetries of serotonin synthesis in the frontal cortex, thalamus, and dentate nucleus of the cerebellum (Chugani et al. 1997). Acute tryptophan depletion markedly exacerbated symptoms of autism, again suggesting a role for serotonin (McDougle et al. 1996). Elevated plasma levels of the excitatory amino acids glutamine and asparagine have been found (Moreno-Fuenmayor et al. 1996). Oxytocin and vasopressin may be involved in social attachment, which might be relevant to the symptoms of autistic disorder (Insel 1997). Other studies support the possible involvement of opiate peptides in autistic disorder (Sandman 1991; Willemsen-Swinkels et al. 1996).

Various immunological abnormalities have been proposed to contribute to the development of autism. Several reports have suggested an overrepresentation of several different autoimmune disorders in autistic patients. Preliminary reports have suggested the possible role of various autoantibodies and of interleukin, but these findings have not been replicated.

Neuropsychological testing typically shows global dysfunctions, but no discrete pathways or regions are consistently identified. Low IQ is associated with a higher prevalence of seizures, social impairment, bizarre behavior, self-mutilation, and poor prognosis. The increase in seizures during adolescence is observed particularly often in autistic individuals with low IQ. There is delayed development of cerebral dominance and an excess of non-right-handedness, primitive neurological reflexes, soft neurological signs, and physical anomalies.

Together, these findings suggest that autistic disorder entails 1) neuromaturational abnormalities that affect the development of brain structure and cerebral asymmetry, 2) pervasive and diffuse changes in widely disparate parts of the brain, 3) diffuse but pervasive symptoms in a variety of dimensions, and 4) serotonergic abnormalities in at least a subgroup of patients. The etiology of the neuromaturational problem is unknown, but such atypical brain development might be induced by genetic predisposition, infection or immunological reaction in the second trimester, or a metabolic disturbance in brain chemistry during early or mid-gestation. It may be speculated that the serotonergic abnormalities are related to comorbid obsessive-compulsive features, mood or anxiety disorder, or immunological changes. In summary, the neurobiological dysfunction appears to be quite diffuse, and no clear "primary" deficit is found in most autistic individuals.

Course and Prognosis

Autistic disorder is often apparent at birth or early infancy, and parents may seek a medical evaluation during the child's first year (often for deafness). Some symptoms are usually recognized, at least in retrospect, in more than 80% of children with autistic disorder by age 2 years. The DSM-IV-TR definition of autistic disorder requires an apparent onset before age 3 years.

The general course of autistic disorder is gradual improvement, but there is a high degree of irregularity and unpredictability in the speed of improvement. Periods of rapid developmental growth alternate with periods of slow, stable growth. The changes in maturational tempo occur abruptly or gradually. Developmental progress can be slow or rapid, and the periods of improvement may last for a couple of weeks or many months. Developmental change may be made in particular skills without improvement in other areas of functioning, or it may occur pervasively across many areas of functioning. Episodes of overt regression may occur during concurrent medical illness, situational stress, or puberty and even during periods of otherwise rapid developmental progress unexplained by environmental factors. Overall, predictors of good adaptive outcome include later onset, higher IQ, better language skills (especially vocabulary), and greater social and communicative skills.

The availability of educational and supportive services has a marked beneficial effect, just as in mental retardation. In the severe, classic forms, some adaptive skills can be learned. In the less severe forms, the acquired social skills and adaptations eventually may permit performance in an ordinary occupation. Even a relatively interactive and pleasant social life can be attained.

Over the years, the time course of change remains unpredictable. As adults, autistic individuals continue to show a gradual clearing of symptoms but retain clinical evidence of residual deficits (Rumsey et al. 1985a). Depending on the severity of the autistic disorder, perhaps 2%–15% achieve a nonretarded level of cognitive and adaptive functioning. Obsessive-compulsive features remain predominant in adulthood and may include stereotyped pacing, rocking, perseveration, and stuttering. Adults with autistic disorder remain socially aloof and often retain an oppositional streak. Expressive and receptive language often become normal, although speech may continue to have a singsong or monotonous sound. No delusions or hallucinations are evident. Autistic adults may achieve employment (generally in simple rote jobs) and the capacity for independent residence, but they rarely marry. The few outcome studies currently available describe the follow-up of severe and largely untreated cases; adult outcome may be better in less severe and more aggressively treated cases. It is unclear whether the features that persist into adulthood are core symptoms or developmental complications of autistic disorder, but these persistent features are not typically shared by individuals with mental retardation. Many other complications of autistic disorder, even in the nonretarded subgroup, are similar to the complications typically seen in mental retardation.

Diagnostic Evaluation

In addition to the standard psychiatric and behavioral evaluation, a workup of autistic disorder includes assessment of language skills, cognition, social skills, and adaptive functioning. Standardized scales and interviews have been developed to assess these areas of functioning (Tanguay 2000). Psychological and neuropsychological testing for mental retardation and mixed receptive-expressive language disorder are valuable, but it can be difficult to obtain reliable and consistent findings. Evaluation for communication disorders may be particularly formidable if the child's nonverbal skills are also impaired. An assessment of the home environment and emotional supportiveness of the family is essential.

Neurological examination includes consideration of possible inborn metabolic and degenerative diseases. Screening for phenylketonuria is probably cost-effective. MRI studies may be helpful in some cases as a part of the general neurological evaluation, but they cannot be used for diagnosis of autistic disorder at this time. It is typically worthwhile to obtain an EEG in view of the high prevalence of seizure disorders in this population, although the EEG patterns are often nonspecifically abnormal in the absence of seizures. Chromosomal analysis also should be considered to evaluate for relatively frequent genetic abnormalities, such as fragile X syndrome. In some cases, audiological examination for possible deafness and examinations for other sensory deficits may be considered.

Patients with autistic disorder also must be evaluated for psychiatric comorbidity, especially OCD, ADHD, tic disorders, mood disorders (particularly major depressive or dysthymic disorder), and psychotic disorders. Although ADHD may be functionally present and fulfill diagnostic criteria, it is not designated as a separate DSM-IV-TR disorder when it occurs in the context of a pervasive developmental disorder.

Differential diagnosis includes congenital deafness (although deaf children typically learn an alternate lip or sign language, lose their isolative behaviors, and develop sensitive expressive communication), congenital blindness (although blind children relate more socially), mental retardation (although mentally retarded children do not show the islands of special capacity that autistic children sometimes have), expressive and mixed receptive-expressive language disorder (although children with these disorders typically are more interactive and can communicate well in gestures), schizophreniform disorder, schizotypal personality disorder, and juvenile-onset schizophrenia (although children with schizophrenia typically have hallucinations, delusions, or thought disorder).

In many cases, particularly those involving less severe forms, it is difficult to make a definitive diagnosis of autistic disorder. The appearance of hallucinations, delusions, or clear thought disorder should lead to the consideration of a primary psychotic disorder rather than autism. However, children and adults with autistic disorder may have concomitant psychotic disorders, comorbid mood disorders, or anxiety disorders.

Treatment

Historically, treatment neglect resulted in a generation of individuals with autistic disorders who had a relatively poor outcome. More recently, several studies have shown that rigorous multimodal treatment may be useful and sometimes has dramatic effects, although controlled and systematic studies are needed.

Behavior therapy has been helpful in controlling unwanted symptoms, promoting social interactions, increasing self-reliance, and facilitating exploration (i.e., novelty-seeking behavior). Specialized assertiveness training may be helpful in enhancing adaptive skills. Special education, vocational training, the teaching of adaptive skills, and support in managing major life events are basic. Environmental management, especially predictable or programmed structure, has a particularly powerful effect.

Providing guidance to parents is critical, especially for those who are making the chronically afflicted child the emotional center of their lives. Although this attentiveness may have beneficial effects for the child, it is often driven by unjustified guilt, unrealistic pessimism, or narcissism. Parents can contribute to the child's learning of self-care and adaptive skills, arrange for special education and management with schools and other public agencies, and make long-term plans for the child's future. Because long-term treatment is essential, periodic medical reassessment is needed to monitor for the possible appearance of seizures or concomitant psychiatric disorders that may be masked by the autistic disorder.

A long-term program involving high levels of supervision and structure is generally required. Specialized day-care and group settings, incorporating elements of behavioral treatment in a naturalistic setting with a stable interpersonal network, are helpful in some cases (Landesman and Vietze 1987). At times, residential care is needed to provide a more enveloping structure of protection and supervision.

Most of the pharmacological studies of autistic disorder have been conducted in children, with little research concerning adults. No drug treatment of autistic disorder itself is available, but psychotropic medications can be used to target particular symptoms, symptom clusters, and comorbid disorders in individual patients. No psychotropic medications provide generally useful treatment for most cases of autistic disorder.

The symptoms most amenable to pharmacotherapy include perseverative behaviors (comparable to obsessive-compulsive symptoms), depressive disorders, aggressivity, impulsivity, destructiveness, bipolar disorders, anxiety, hyperactivity, hypoactivity, pica, and SIBs. Management of seizures is also approached medically. In general, the risk of overmedication requires continual attentiveness.

Although no single medication is generally indicated, different agents can provide symptomatic benefit. Low doses of nonsedating conventional neuroleptics (such as haloperidol) have been found helpful for promoting learning, controlling behavioral symptoms, reducing excessive activity levels, controlling aggressive and disruptive behavior, and enhancing the effects of behavior therapy and other interventions. The newer atypical antipsychotics, such as risperidone, appear to be more beneficial in some patients (McDougle et al. 1998), better tolerated, and less risky. Olanzapine is generally less satisfactory because of its tendency to aggravate obsessive-compulsive symptoms. Psychostimulants, anticonvulsants, and neuroleptics may be useful for symptoms of impulsivity. Psychostimulants are used for children who either are underactive or have concurrent ADHD. β-Blocking agents and perhaps clonidine might have some value in managing symptoms of impulsivity and aggression. Early reports on naltrexone, an opiate receptor blocking agent, suggested that this drug could improve affective availability, promote social reciprocity, and reduce stereotyped motor behavior and SIBs; however, more recent data suggest that it has little or no clinically significant effects. Several preliminary reports have suggested that fluoxetine can be helpful in treating obsessional and depressive symptoms in patients with autistic disorder. Serotonin reuptake inhibitors also have been found to reduce anxiety symptoms in some children (Steingard et al. 1997). In a controlled study of adults with autism, fluvoxamine was significantly more beneficial than placebo (McDougle et al. 1997), and lithium has been found to be helpful as an adjunctive treatment, particularly when supplementing serotonin reuptake inhibitors. Other researchers have suggested possible benefits of H_1 (niaprazine) and H_2 (famotidine) blockers, corticotropin analogues, and inositol. Secretin has been reported to be helpful in this disorder, but controlled studies (Owley et al. 2001; W. Roberts et al. 2001) have not confirmed its utility. Some popularly touted treatments, including dimethylglycine (Bolman and Richmond 1999) and high-dose magnesium-pyridoxine (Findling et al. 1997), have not been supported in controlled studies.

The controlled clinical studies of intervention in autistic disorder have been almost exclusively restricted to behavioral and pharmacological treatments. Reports on family, individual, group, and program interventions are generally based on impressionistic evaluations.

Working closely with autistic children may present a challenge to a therapist's empathic capacities. These individuals learn about reality in slow steps and may take considerable time to learn about human beings and the nature of feelings. Children with less severe cases of autistic disorder may present more subtle empathic challenges. Over time, many of these children are capable of deeply joyous and genuine interpersonal interactions, albeit unusual ones that may be lacking in the more transcendental aspects of human interaction.

Childhood Disintegrative Disorder

Clinical Description

Childhood disintegrative disorder, as defined in DSM-IV-TR, differs from autistic disorder in time of onset, clinical course, and prevalence. In contrast to autistic disorder, this disorder involves an early period of normal development until age 3–4 years. This is followed by a period of marked deterioration of adaptive, communicative, and social functioning (Table 20–19), usually occurring rapidly over the course of 6–9 months. Childhood disintegrative disorder may begin with behavioral symptoms, such as anxiety, anger, or outbursts, but the general loss of functions becomes pervasive and severe. The deterioration leads to a syndrome that is symptomatically similar to autistic disorder, except that mental retardation (typically in the moderate-to-profound range) tends to be more frequent and pronounced (Volkmar and Rutter 1995), and significantly more children appear to develop seizures (Mouridsen et al. 1998). Over time, the deterioration remains stable, although some capacities may be regained to a limited degree. About 20% regain the ability to speak in sentences, but their communication skills remain impaired (A.E. Hill and Rosenbloom 1986). Most adults are completely dependent and require institutional care, and some have a shortened life span.

TABLE 20–19. DSM-IV-TR diagnostic criteria for childhood disintegrative disorder

A. Apparently normal development for at least the first 2 years after birth as manifested by the presence of age-appropriate verbal and nonverbal communication, social relationships, play, and adaptive behavior.

B. Clinically significant loss of previously acquired skills (before age 10 years) in at least two of the following areas:
   (1) expressive or receptive language
   (2) social skills or adaptive behavior
   (3) bowel or bladder control
   (4) play
   (5) motor skills

C. Abnormalities of functioning in at least two of the following areas:
   (1) qualitative impairment in social interaction (e.g., impairment in nonverbal behaviors, failure to develop peer relationships, lack of social or emotional reciprocity)
   (2) qualitative impairments in communication (e.g., delay or lack of spoken language, inability to initiate or sustain a conversation, stereotyped and repetitive use of language, lack of varied make-believe play)
   (3) restricted, repetitive, and stereotyped patterns of behavior, interests, and activities, including motor stereotypies and mannerisms

D. The disturbance is not better accounted for by another specific pervasive developmental disorder or by schizophrenia.

The syndromal validity of childhood disintegrative disorder has remained controversial (Mouridsen et al. 2000). Attempts to validate a distinction between autism and childhood disintegrative disorder have not been decisive. Comparisons of lifetime psychopathology in parents, neuroimaging studies, and genetic findings in childhood disintegrative disorder and childhood autistic disorder have uncovered mostly minor differences, except for a significantly higher rate of electroencephalographic abnormalities in childhood disintegrative disorder (Mouridsen et al. 1998, 1999a, 1999b, 2000).

Epidemiology

Childhood disintegrative disorder is rare, with prevalence estimates ranging from 1 to 4 in 100,000, which is about 1/100th the frequency of autistic disorder. There appears to be a male predominance of greater than 4:1.

Etiology

No specific neurobiological deficit or cause of childhood disintegrative disorder has been identified (Volkmar and Cohen 1989). Early associations of childhood disintegra-

tive disorder with specific neurological and medical disorders have not been supported. Significant psychosocial or medical stressors have been reported in association with the onset or worsening of the disorder, but their etiological significance is unclear.

Diagnostic Evaluation and Treatment

The evaluation and treatment of childhood disintegrative disorder are essentially comparable to the approach to autistic disorder, although much more active support, behavioral treatment, neurological care, and medical monitoring are needed. Studies attempting to characterize this very rare disorder have been difficult to conduct, and research on the pathophysiology and treatment of this disorder has lagged behind research on the other specific pervasive developmental disorders. A change in the disease label is also needed because of the crudity of the term *disintegrative*, especially when used in speaking with parents about their child.

Rett's Disorder

Clinical Description

Rett's disorder is a progressive neurodevelopmental disorder and one of the most common causes of mental retardation in females.

Epidemiology

Its estimated prevalence ranges from 4 to 22 in 100,000 girls (Kozinetz et al. 1993; Skjeldal et al. 1997). Because Rett's disorder occurs almost exclusively in females, it had been proposed that Rett's disorder is caused by an X-linked dominant mutation with lethality in hemizygous males. This proposal has been confirmed with the discovery that Rett's disorder results from mutations in the X-linked methyl-CpG-binding protein 2 (*MECP2*) gene (Amir et al. 1999).

Etiology

Once considered a clearly neurodegenerative process, serial neurodevelopmental evaluations have provided support for an arrest of developmental functions at various stages, particularly during periods of rapid neuronal growth, pruning, and maturation (Naidu et al. 1995), and increasing support exists for Rett's disorder as a neurodevelopmental disorder that arises from a poorly understood failure in the epigenesis of neural systems (Johnston et al. 2001). Debate continues about the neurodevelopmental versus neurodegenerative nature of the disease process and course, but it is clear that the onset of Rett's disorder can be observed in very young girls and that progressive clinical decline is the hallmark.

Recent identification of nonlethal mutations in the *MECP2* gene in males with classic and variant presentations of Rett's disorder (Clayton-Smith et al. 2000; Laccone et al. 2001) suggests that a range of variation in phenotype may arise from mutations at this site, and screening of the *MECP2* gene should be considered also in males with severe mental retardation in whom the most common forms of mental retardation have been excluded (Couvert et al. 2001; Hoffbuhr et al. 2001). Recent reports of three males (two males with Klinefelter's syndrome with classic Rett's disorder and a hemizygous male infant with an Xq27–28 inversion novel 32 base pair frameshift deletion) suggested that other novel mechanisms may produce Rett's disorder in males as well (Hoffbuhr et al. 2001; Schwartzman et al. 2001), although the probability of such cases is low (if Rett's disorder and Klinefelter's syndrome occur independently, for example, the probability of a joint presentation approximates 1 in 10–15 million births).

The progressive clinical decline is not initially apparent. Typically, after 6–18 months of relatively normal development, the first social, language, neurological, and motor deficiencies become apparent. Initially, the clinical decline is gradual, but it becomes quite evident by age 4 years (Table 20–20). Head and body growth retardation, along with other developmental delays, can be seen during this phase. Then, starting during the early school years, there is a period of more rapid functional deterioration in which intellectual and communicative capacities diminish, and purposeful control of hand movements is replaced with apraxia, wringing, and washing motions. Following this rapid deterioration, these girls appear to have a pervasive developmental disorder, which usually is identified as autistic disorder or childhood disintegrative disorder (Moeschler et al. 1988). This rapid decline in functioning usually reaches an apparent plateau that may last for months or years. However, this plateau is eventually seen to be a gradual decline that is much slower than that of the previous stage. Gait and truncal ataxia, respiratory symptoms involving dysregulation of breathing functions, and scoliosis typically begin to emerge during this slow decline.

By age 3–5 years, girls with Rett's disorder are less likely to be viewed as having either autistic or childhood disintegrative disorder because of the progressive appearance of increasingly severe neurological symptoms. Mental retardation is generally apparent, and most patients have intelligence scores in the severely retarded range. Seizures, decreasing physical mobility, spasticity, muscle weakness, severe scoliosis, wasting, dystonia, and choreoathetosis may emerge. Typically, these girls are eventually

TABLE 20–20. DSM-IV-TR diagnostic criteria for Rett's disorder

A. All of the following:
(1) apparently normal prenatal and perinatal development
(2) apparently normal psychomotor development through the first 5 months after birth
(3) normal head circumference at birth
B. Onset of all of the following after the period of normal development:
(1) deceleration of head growth between ages 5 and 48 months
(2) loss of previously acquired purposeful hand skills between ages 5 and 30 months with the subsequent development of stereotyped hand movements (e.g., hand-wringing or hand washing)
(3) loss of social engagement early in the course (although often social interaction develops later)
(4) appearance of poorly coordinated gait or trunk movements
(5) severely impaired expressive and receptive language development with severe psychomotor retardation

confined to wheelchairs, often before adolescence. Feeding can become quite difficult because of compromised motor functioning (swallowing). Caregivers need to be aware of the high risk of aspiration, which may be compounded by the dysregulation of breathing. Seizures occur in 80% of these patients and add to the management problems. Some girls with Rett's disorder die suddenly of unexplained causes; some patients have a normal life span despite the severe symptoms and disabilities, but life expectancy is generally reduced.

The discovery of the gene for Rett's disorder is the result of a decade-long search. Extensive "exclusion" mapping studies of families with Rett's disorder mapped the locus of the putative gene(s) to Xq28. A systematic gene screening approach identified mutations in the *MECP2* gene as the cause of Rett's disorder (Amir et al. 1999). Subsequent studies confirmed the finding, and they have begun to better characterize the range of mutations and of their expression. In classic Rett's disorder, studies suggest that patterns of X chromosome inactivation may play a greater role in determining the clinical severity than the type of mutation; in variant presentations, however, the mutation may more strongly affect disease severity. Familial cases of Rett's disorder are rare and are due to X chromosomal inheritance from a carrier mother, who is often mildly affected. In sporadic cases of Rett's disorder, de novo mutations of the gene in the paternally derived X chromosome appear common (Trappe et al. 2001).

The immediate activity of the X-linked *MECP2* gene's nuclear protein product is understood: it selectively binds CpG dinucleotides in the mammalian genome and mediates transcriptional repression through interaction with chromatin-remodeling complexes associated with histone deacetylase and the corepressor SIN3A, and it appears to have a central role in methylation-dependent regulation of gene expression. *MECP2* is expressed at high levels in the postnatal brain, indicating that methylation-dependent regulation of gene expression may have a crucial role in the mammalian CNS. How disturbances in its functioning account for the "classical" and "variant" Rett's disorder and non–Rett's disorder phenotypes, ranging from mild learning disability in females to severe mental retardation, seizures, ataxia, and sometimes neonatal encephalopathy in males, remains uncertain, although effects on gene expression and possibly on translation or transcription are involved. The discovery of the cause of the disorder, however, has begun to drive research in this area in a more concerted fashion.

MECP2-deficient mice have phenotypes that resemble some of the symptoms of patients with Rett's disorder (Chen et al. 2001; Guy et al. 2001). *MECP2*-null mice are normal until age 5 weeks, when they began to develop manifestations of the disease. Mutant brains showed substantial reduction in both weight and neuronal cell size but no obvious structural defects or signs of neurodegeneration. Brain-specific deletion of *MECP2* at embryonic day (E) 12, when rapid development gets under way, moreover, results in a phenotype identical to that of the null mutation, indicating that the phenotype is caused by *MECP2* deficiency in the CNS rather than in peripheral tissues. Deletion of *MECP2* in postnatal CNS neurons led to a similar neuronal phenotype, although at a later age. The later finding implies that the role of *MECP2* is not restricted to the immature brain but becomes critical in mature neurons. *MECP2* deficiency in these neurons is sufficient to cause neuronal dysfunction with symptomatic manifestation similar to Rett's disorder. Murine models promise to advance research in this area (Chen et al. 2001).

An atypical glycolipid has been described in most of these patients. Investigators evaluating the cerebrospinal fluid of patients with Rett's disorder have reported reduced concentrations of substance P (Matsuishi et al. 1997) and nerve growth factor and elevated concentrations of β-endorphin and glutamate. Abnormalities of monoamine levels have been reported. Two studies showed underpigmentation in the zona compacta. Neuropathological studies found a generalized atrophy involving both the cerebrum and the cerebellum, a generalized decrease in neuronal cell size and an increase in cell density, a reduction in the number of basal forebrain cholinergic neurons, and a reduction in the number of melanin-containing neurons in the substantia nigra (Wong et al. 1998). The impoverished patterns of branching of dendrites of pyramidal neurons in premotor frontal, motor, and limbic cortex have been reported less in Rett's disorder than in control (trisomy 21) brains (Armstrong et al. 1998).

Diagnostic Evaluation

Data from neuroimaging studies are preliminary, but SPECT studies have suggested that bifrontal hypoperfusion correlates with severity of Rett's disorder. Diffuse atrophy (most notably in the prefrontal, posterior frontal, and anterior temporal regions) was noted in an MRI study. Abnormal EEG results are typically found after age 2 years; despite the high prevalence of seizures, the EEG findings are typically nonspecific. Taken together, the neurobiological abnormalities suggest an X-linked generalized atrophy with global dysfunction that correlates with severity of the symptoms.

Treatment

Treatment of Rett's disorder is supportive. Generally, these multiply handicapped patients require intensive care (Lindberg 1992). The role of psychopharmacotherapy is limited, but several reports have found carbamazepine to be more effective than other anticonvulsants for seizure control in girls with Rett's disorder. Lamotrigine might also be useful.

In contrast to childhood disintegrative disorder, Rett's disorder is an excellent example of rapid progress in recent research in the pervasive developmental disorders. Older findings will need to be reconsidered in light of the revolution that molecular genetics is catalyzing in this area.

Asperger's Disorder

Asperger's disorder is another pervasive developmental disorder that is similar to autistic disorder, except that language acquisition, cognitive development, learning skills, and even most adaptive behaviors are largely preserved (Table 20–21). The autistic features of impaired social interactions and stereotyped behaviors and interests are present but are generally more subtle (Klin et al. 2000). Rather than a relative lack of interest in other people or a general weakness in communication, conversational interactions may be merely impaired. These

TABLE 20–21. DSM-IV-TR diagnostic criteria for Asperger's disorder

A. Qualitative impairment in social interaction, as manifested by at least two of the following:
 (1) marked impairment in the use of multiple nonverbal behaviors such as eye-to-eye gaze, facial expression, body postures, and gestures to regulate social interaction
 (2) failure to develop peer relationships appropriate to developmental level
 (3) a lack of spontaneous seeking to share enjoyment, interests, or achievements with other people (e.g., by a lack of showing, bringing, or pointing out objects of interest to other people)
 (4) lack of social or emotional reciprocity
B. Restricted repetitive and stereotyped patterns of behavior, interests, and activities, as manifested by at least one of the following:
 (1) encompassing preoccupation with one or more stereotyped and restricted patterns of interest that is abnormal either in intensity or focus
 (2) apparently inflexible adherence to specific, nonfunctional routines or rituals
 (3) stereotyped and repetitive motor mannerisms (e.g., hand or finger flapping or twisting, or complex whole-body movements)
 (4) persistent preoccupation with parts of objects
C. The disturbance causes clinically significant impairment in social, occupational, or other important areas of functioning.
D. There is no clinically significant general delay in language (e.g., single words used by age 2 years, communicative phrases used by age 3 years).
E. There is no clinically significant delay in cognitive development or in the development of age-appropriate self-help skills, adaptive behavior (other than in social interaction), and curiosity about the environment in childhood.
F. Criteria are not met for another specific pervasive developmental disorder or schizophrenia.

individuals may "interact" through seemingly endless monologues on a topic of extreme interest to themselves, without reading nonverbal and even verbal cues, continuing on without apparent awareness that the other person views the topic as eccentric or idiosyncratic. They may become quite knowledgeable, or at least collect large numbers of facts, about a topic. Even social communications might be learned as a set of rules and scripts. Such a child's "precocious" interest in particular topics can fascinate adults but may not engage peers or draw emotional responsiveness.

Because of its similarities to autism, the status of Asperger's disorder as a distinct form of pervasive devel-

opmental disorder is often questioned, and many specialists believe that it is a mild version of autistic disorder (i.e., high-functioning autism) rather than a separate and distinct disorder (Gillberg 1989; Rapin 1991; Szatmari 2000). Analysis of speech and communication patterns, cognitive batteries, and WISC findings (Ehlers et al. 1997) have supported the DSM-IV-TR interpretation that Asperger's and autistic disorders are distinct entities. However, the distinction is challenged by evidence suggesting that a spectrum of cognitive and social deficits (i.e., the "broad" autistic phenotype) may be inherited rather than autism per se (Bailey et al. 1995). The view of Asperger's and autistic disorders as representing "parallel but potentially overlapping developmental trajectories" (Szatmari et al. 2000) is consistent with the concept of Asperger's disorder as a part of an autistic spectrum.

With the relative sparing of intelligence, language, and cognition, Asperger's disorder differs from autism in having a low prevalence of mental retardation. Also unlike in autism, verbal functioning is stronger than nonverbal functioning. Only 12% of the children with Asperger's disorder have IQ scores below 70. It is characteristic of these patients to misread nonverbal cues, have marked difficulties with peer interactions (especially in groups), focus repetitively in conversation on topics of interest only to themselves, appear not particularly empathic, and speak without normal inflection and tone variation; they may be relatively unexpressive affectively, and they tend to have few friends (Wing 1981). Even with these limitations, persons with Asperger's disorder are often quite sociable and talkative, and they may form affectionate bonds with family members (Frith 1991). Symptoms of right hemisphere syndrome, ADHD, or developmental coordination disorder may be observed.

The course tends to be stable over time, often with some gradual gains (Szatmari et al. 1989, 2000). The verbal strengths may hide social deficits, especially from adults, who are often inclined to misinterpret behavioral abnormalities as laziness or stubbornness. Although social skills may improve with age, relative weakness in interpersonal interactions and lack of social spontaneity may become more limiting in later childhood and adolescence, leading to increasing isolation, anxiety, and depression. Nonetheless, long-term educational and occupational adjustment are markedly better than in autistic disorder, and financial and social independence are generally achieved.

Epidemiological data are limited, but the prevalence of the more severe presentations of Asperger's disorder is estimated at 5–15 in 100,000. The male predominance is 3:1–4:1.

The etiology of Asperger's disorder remains unknown. In some cases, it follows a familial pattern, consistent with genetic, psychosocial, or environmental transmission. A possible role of fetal exposure to alcohol has been raised (Aronson et al. 1997).

Neurobiological studies are extremely limited. About 30% of the patients with Asperger's disorder have non-specific EEG abnormalities, and 15% show evidence of brain atrophy. In a recent SPECT study, abnormal right hemisphere metabolism was reported; although the significance of this finding is not entirely known, it lends some support to the concept of "right-hemisphere-only autistic disorder" (McKelvey et al. 1995; Szatmari et al. 1995).

Treatment includes social and motor skills training, remedial educational interventions when indicated, and vocational training (Attwood and Wing 1998). The relative sparing of language and intelligence allows individuals with Asperger's disorder to have a better outcome than do most persons with autistic disorder. Temple Grandin is a productive member of society with good verbal skills who has Asperger's disorder (formerly diagnosed as autism). Her self-report (Grandin and Scariano 1986) shows that a high-functioning individual with a pervasive developmental disorder can vividly describe personal experiences and complex cognitions. Persons with Asperger's disorder, despite their relative handicaps in social functioning, can become quite expert and effective in their chosen activities, and perhaps they are even helped in these accomplishments by the highly focused nature of their interests.

Clinical Comment on the Pervasive Developmental Disorders

A sensible subtyping of pervasive developmental disorders has long been awaited (Table 20–22), and recent research and the clinical awareness of the diversity of pervasive developmental disorders can be expected to lead to improved understanding and eventually to improved treatments. At this time, however, treatments remain largely supportive and symptomatic.

TABLE 20–22. Characteristics and differential diagnosis of the pervasive developmental disorders

Characteristics	Autistic disorder	Childhood disintegrative disorder	Rett's disorder	Asperger's disorder	PDD NOS
Feature	Standard autism	Delayed-onset but severe autism	"Mid childhood" autism	High-functioning autism	Atypical and sub-threshold
Intelligence	Severe MR to normal	Severe MR	Severe MR	Mild MR to normal	Mild MR to normal
Age at recognition (years)	0–3	>2	0.5–2.5	Usually >2	Variable
Communication skills	Usually limited	Poor	Poor	Limited to fair	Limited to fair
Social skills	Very limited	Very limited	Vary with age	Limited	Variable
Loss of skills	Usually not	Marked	Marked	Usually not	Usually not
Restricted interests	Variable	Not applicable	Not applicable	Marked	Variable
Seizure disorder	Uncommon	Frequent	Uncommon	Common	Common
Head growth deceleration	No	No	Yes	No	No
Prevalence per 100,000 estimated	20–200	1–4	4–20	5–15	>15
Family history of similar problems	Uncommon	No	No	Frequent	Unknown
Sex ratio	M>F	M>F	F	M>F	M>F
Course in adulthood	Stable	Declining	Declining	Stable	Usually stable
Outcome	Poor	Very poor	Very poor	Fair to poor	Fair to good

Note. MR = mental retardation; PDD NOS = pervasive developmental disorder not otherwise specified.
Source. Modified with permission from Volkmar FR, Cohen DJ: "Nonautistic Pervasive Developmental Disorders," in *Psychiatry.* Edited by Michels R, Cooper AM, Guze SB, et al. Philadelphia, PA, JB Lippincott, 1991.

These disorders, relatively rare and still of unknown etiology, are receiving intensive study. Because maternal factors are no longer considered primary or in any way etiological, research has focused on biological description and evaluation of psychosocial treatment interventions. The critical role of aggressive treatment and the need for a variety of community resources have been generally accepted, although the development of appropriate community supports is limited by funding. Effective public advocacy has provided some genuine opportunities for individuals with pervasive developmental disorders. With improving treatment, increasingly more adults with pervasive developmental disorder have overcome the disease label.

Tic Disorders

Tics are sudden, rapid, nonrhythmic, stereotyped movements (motor tics) or vocalizations (vocal tics). Their form may be simple (motor: jerking movements, shrugging, eye blinking; vocal: grunting, sniffing, throat clearing) or complex (motor: grimacing, bending, banging; vocal: echolalia, odd inflections and accents). Tic movements are often preceded by a "premonitory urge" (Leckman et al. 1993); these uncomfortable and irresistible somatosensory experiences, sometimes termed *sensory tics* (Kurlan et al. 1989; A.K. Shapiro et al. 1998), seem to motivate or compel about 30% of the movements and vocalizations.

Although tics are experienced as irresistible, they may be temporarily delayed or suppressed. The fact that tics may be consciously suppressed distinguishes them from choreiform movements (i.e., disruptions of normal synergistic movement by coordinated muscle groups, such as blinks or grimaces), athetosis (i.e., slow writhing), dystonias (i.e., abnormal muscle tone), other dyskinesias (i.e., disruptions of voluntary and involuntary motions), and other neurological movement disorders with which they may be confused. Instead, tics are brief and repetitive (but not rhythmic) motor or vocal responses. They are purposeless but may resemble purposeful acts. Although they involve recurrent movements of the same muscle groups, their location can change gradually over time.

Distinguishing tics from compulsive or impulsive symptoms can be challenging, particularly because OCD and ADHD often present comorbidly with Tourette's or chronic tic disorders. For example, patients with tics may be driven to recurrently touch surfaces, touch other people, touch their own genitals inappropriately, engage in SIBs such as head-banging or self-mutilating behaviors such as scratching a patch of skin to rawness (M.M. Robertson et al. 1989), or have aggressive or obscene verbal (coprolalic) or motoric (copropraxic) outbursts.

Individual tics or ticlike movements may be seen occasionally in children and adults without tic disorders, but such "twitches" (e.g., blinks, grimaces) and habits are not diagnosed as disorders unless they persist for at least 2 weeks.

DSM-IV-TR recognizes three discrete tic disorders: transient tic, chronic tic, and Tourette's disorders (Table 20–23). These conditions are closely related in descriptive, etiological, genetic, pathophysiological, and developmental characteristics.

Tic disorders are believed to arise from abnormal functioning of CSTC neural circuitry involved in motor control and sensorimotor integration. Genetic studies show that 50% of male (and 30% of female) first-degree relatives of patients with Tourette's disorder have transient tic disorder, chronic tic disorder, OCD (Hebebrand et al. 1997), and often ADHD. This overrepresentation suggests a genetic interrelationship among the three tic disorders, OCD, and perhaps ADHD. Environmental factors, including infections triggering autoimmune reactions against key portions of the brain, are also important in the developmental pathogenesis of these disorders. Because the symptoms of these disorders are subject to moment-to-moment influences from environmental and internal stimuli, tic disorders have been seen as prototypic illnesses for the study of interacting biopsychosocial influences (Chase et al. 1992; D. Cohen et al. 1988; Kurlan 1993).

Because the etiologies of the three tic disorders seem closely interrelated, it is appropriate that tic disorders are subtyped by clinical description and course rather than by etiology. Tourette's disorder is generally the most serious of these disorders and has been the best studied. Transient and chronic tic disorders are less well characterized.

Transient Tic Disorder

Transient tic disorder is diagnosed if daily tics persist for 4 weeks to 1 year, the threshold for the diagnosis of chronic tic disorder. Although a single symptomatic period may be observed in some patients, recurrent episodes may come and go for years.

Transient tics are usually motoric, but they are otherwise similar in appearance to chronic and Tourette's tics. Transient tic disorder may be relabeled later in its course if tics persist. These tics do not appear to be consistently associated with other symptoms, but situational or developmental anxiety may be prominent during episodes. Studies of comorbidity are sparse.

TABLE 20–23. DSM-IV-TR diagnostic criteria for tic disorders

Diagnostic criteria for transient tic disorder

A. Single or multiple motor and/or vocal tics (i.e., sudden, rapid, recurrent, nonrhythmic, stereotyped motor movements or vocalizations)

B. The tics occur many times a day, nearly every day for at least 4 weeks, but for no longer than 12 consecutive months.

C. The onset is before age 18 years.

D. The disturbance is not due to the direct physiological effects of a substance (e.g., stimulants) or a general medical condition (e.g., Huntington's disease or postviral encephalitis).

E. Criteria have never been met for Tourette's disorder or chronic motor or vocal tic disorder.

Specify if:

Single Episode or **Recurrent**

Diagnostic criteria for chronic motor or vocal tic disorder

A. Single or multiple motor or vocal tics (i.e., sudden, rapid, recurrent, nonrhythmic, stereotyped motor movements or vocalizations), but not both, have been present at some time during the illness.

B. The tics occur many times a day nearly every day or intermittently throughout a period of more than 1 year, and during this period there was never a tic-free period of more than 3 consecutive months.

C. The onset is before age 18 years.

D. The disturbance is not due to the direct physiological effects of a substance (e.g., stimulants) or a general medical condition (e.g., Huntington's disease or postviral encephalitis).

E. Criteria have never been met for Tourette's disorder.

Diagnostic criteria for Tourette's disorder

A. Both multiple motor and one or more vocal tics have been present at some time during the illness, although not necessarily concurrently. (A *tic* is a sudden, rapid, recurrent, nonrhythmic, stereotyped motor movement or vocalization.)

B. The tics occur many times a day (usually in bouts) nearly every day or intermittently throughout a period of more than 1 year, and during this period there was never a tic-free period of more than 3 consecutive months.

C. The onset is before age 18 years.

D. The disturbance is not due to the direct physiological effects of a substance (e.g., stimulants) or a general medical condition (e.g., Huntington's disease or postviral encephalitis).

Up to 12% of children have tic symptoms, but the prevalence of transient tic disorder is undetermined.

Both genetic and psychosocial factors influence the appearance of transient tic disorder. Episodes are typically seen during periods of increased stress or excitement, which contribute to the transient presentation and the variability of symptom intensity. When tics present in apparent response to physical or emotional trauma, the individual generally has an underlying genetic vulnerability (Alegre et al. 1996).

The onset of single or recurrent episodes of transient tic disorder usually is during middle childhood (ages 5–10 years) or early adolescence. If episodes recur, the frequency and severity of symptoms typically diminish over the course of years. The tics usually do not interfere with functioning, although they may interact with anxiety and social stressors to produce interpersonal and self-esteem complications.

For mild presentations of transient tic disorder, medical workup is often omitted in actual practice. For more significant or persistent presentations, psychiatric, neurological, and medical evaluations should assess possible concomitant disorders such as mood and anxiety disorders (particularly OCD), ADHD, neurological comorbidity (including other movement disorders), and general pediatric illnesses, including virus-induced tics (usually herpetic), autoimmune conditions, and posttraumatic tics from head trauma. Psychosocial sources of anxiety that might aggravate tic severity, developmental details, and family genetic history should be ascertained.

Transient tic disorder typically does not require treatment. It is usually helpful to advise the family to reduce attention to the symptom and criticism of the child. Behavioral techniques (e.g., relaxation), medications (e.g., minor tranquilizers), or brief psychotherapy may be helpful in certain cases for anxiety management and tic control. In the absence of significant comorbidity or psychosocial stressors, the patient and family may be provided with education and reassurance, and they may be encouraged to return for reevaluation if symptoms persist.

Chronic Motor or Vocal Tic Disorder

Chronic motor or vocal tic disorder is diagnosed if either a motor or a vocal tic persists for more than 1 year. Tourette's disorder is diagnosed if both motor and vocal tics are chronic.

Chronic tics usually are motoric and similar in form to those in other motor tic disorders. Chronic vocal tics are rare, are usually mild, and generally consist of grunts (e.g., diaphragmatic contractions) rather than true vocal or verbal tics. The persistence of chronic tics can be associated with anxiety or depressive disorders, both of which may aggravate tic disorders.

Prevalence data are not available for chronic tic disorders because the durational characteristics of tics have not been studied epidemiologically. Chronic tic disorder is probably less common than Tourette's disorder in clinical populations, but it is unclear whether this reflects general prevalence or referral bias (such as help seeking).

The intensity of chronic tics typically varies little over the course of weeks, although changes may be noted over the course of months or years. The onset is usually during early childhood (ages 5–10 years). In about two-thirds of patients, the disorder ends during adolescence, but some cases may persist in mild form for years or even decades. A subtype of chronic tic disorder also can appear in adulthood, typically after age 40.

Pediatric, neurological, and psychiatric evaluations, similar to the workup for transient tic disorder, are indicated. A child whose transient tics have persisted should be reevaluated after 6–12 months, so that comorbidity and psychosocial stressors can be reassessed and so that treatment can be considered.

Similar to transient tic disorder, both behavioral and pharmacological treatments are effective. Psychosocial interventions may be used to target symptoms of anxiety. Minor tranquilizers, or low doses of major tranquilizers, may be considered. Serotonin reuptake inhibitors may be appropriate to treat comorbid anxiety, especially comorbid OCD. Although systematic data are lacking, anecdotal information suggests that these medications are quite useful.

Tourette's Disorder

Tourette's disorder entails the presence of both vocal tics and multiple motor tics. Transient tic disorder is diagnosed during the first 12 months that both motor and verbal tics are observed, and the diagnosis is converted to Tourette's disorder beyond 1 year. The DSM-IV-TR definition of Tourette's disorder is considerably looser than the classic criteria and permits inclusion of a wider range of patients.

Although Tourette's disorder is often considered a lifelong disease, prevalence is 10-fold higher among children than adults, and longitudinal studies indicate that symptoms decline or fully resolve in 50% of affected individuals by age 18 years (Leckman et al. 1998), suggesting a more benign and less chronic outcome for many individuals.

Clinical Description

Both the motor and the vocal tics may be simple or complex. The behavioral component can be suppressed voluntarily, but then a premonitory sensory urge builds, usually with a subjective sense of tension. This sensation of craving before a tic is relieved temporarily when patients allow themselves to express their tics in action. Many patients experience their tics as a voluntary response to these premonitory urges, and they may feel more troubled by the continual pre-tic tension than by the tics themselves (Leckman et al. 1993). They also may engage in self-reproach, faulting themselves for not controlling their "voluntary" behaviors.

Some patients find that they can control their tics during the day at school or work and then "let off the tension" later, when alone in their bedrooms. For these individuals, the use of the home as a haven for the release of symptoms can be an effective way to reduce the effect of their symptoms on their social and occupational life. However, some patients with severe Tourette's disorder feel that "saving" their tics in this manner is even more problematic because it interferes with the comfort of family members.

The symptoms of chronic tic and Tourette's disorders typically wax and wane over time. Anxiety and excitement typically lead to increased symptoms, relaxation and focused attention can reduce symptoms, and symptoms are typically minimal or absent during sleep. Severity varies widely. Mild cases may go undiagnosed (even in television personalities), whereas severe cases may be disabling and socially disfiguring. Increased symptom severity may be evident for several minutes during stressful situations, may last for months during periods of developmental anxiety and stress, or may last for years—particularly when associated with concomitant anxiety or mood disorders (Coffey et al. 2000; Elstner et al. 2001), ADHD, or other comorbidity.

Vocal tics may be disguised, for example, in feigned coughing. Complex motor tics may appear to be purposeless, or they may be camouflaged by being blended into other purposeful movements.

Sometimes complex motor tics are self-destructive, such as scratching or cutting oneself, or violent, with temper tantrums and assaults.

Obsessive-compulsive features appear in about 20%–40% of patients, and full OCD presents in 7%–10%. Although the diagnostic criteria are clearly defined, the clinical boundaries between Tourette's disorder, ADHD, and OCD are blurred in the many patients who have combined features of these three disorders (Cath et al. 2001a, 2001b; Miguel et al. 2000).

Comorbid conduct, mood, and anxiety disorders are also common. Although disruptive behavior, mood, and anxiety disorders as well as cognitive dysfunctions may be accounted for by comorbidity with ADHD, the comorbid presentation of ADHD and Tourette's disorder appears to be a more severe condition than ADHD alone (J. Spencer et al. 2000).

There is no evidence of increased risk of psychosis, impaired reality sense, or cognitive deterioration in Tourette's disorder, but aggressive (Stefl 1983) or sexual

(Jagger et al. 1982) behaviors are seen in up to one-third of patients with Tourette's disorder.

Specific cognitive deficits that have been reported in Tourette's disorder consist of visual-motor integration problems, impaired fine motor skill, and executive dysfunction (Como 2001). The presence of comorbid conditions, notably ADHD and OCD, appears to significantly increase the likelihood that an individual with Tourette's disorder also will have learning problems or some demonstrable cognitive impairment, and they may, in fact, account for most such problems.

Structured diagnostic assessments in adults with Tourette's disorder have found a significantly elevated rate of personality disorders in comparison to the general population (64% vs. 6%). In adulthood, it is common for patients with Tourette's disorder to meet criteria for more than one personality disorder. Moreover, depressive and anxiety disorders are significantly more prevalent in patients with Tourette's disorder than in control samples (M.M. Robertson et al. 1997).

Neurological symptoms are typically observed in patients with Tourette's disorder, including soft signs in 50% of patients and choreiform movements in 30% of patients. Approximately 50% of patients show abnormal EEG findings, particularly immature patterns consisting of excess slow waves and posterior sharp waves. CT scans usually are normal.

Some patients have a form of Tourette's disorder that is an autoimmune reaction to a streptococcal infection; that is, PANDAS. Choreiform "piano-playing" movements are present in many patients. About 80% of the patients with PANDAS also have OCD, and about 50% have ADHD. Other neuropsychiatric symptoms associated with PANDAS include emotional lability, oppositional behavior, separation anxiety, bedtime rituals, phobias, and deterioration in math skills and handwriting (Swedo et al. 1998).

Epidemiology

Up to 12% of children may have tic symptoms, which usually are transient. The general prevalence of tic disorders is currently estimated at 1%–2%, but it is probably higher in children and adolescents. Prevalence estimates for Tourette's disorder range from 1 in 350 to 1 in 2,000. A male predominance of 3:1–10:1 has been reported, but the actual ratio may be closer to 2:1. No socioeconomic skewing is apparent. Cross-cultural studies have suggested that Tourette's disorder presents similarly across cultures in its clinical features, comorbidity, family history, and treatment outcomes, consistent with a strong neurobiological etiology (Freeman et al. 2000; Staley et al. 1997).

Etiology

Genetic, biological, and psychosocial factors appear operative in Tourette's disorder and other tic disorders. Tics are noted in two-thirds of the relatives of patients with Tourette's disorder, and tic disorders are found in 5%–10% of their siblings. The higher concordance of Tourette's disorder in monozygotic (50%–56%) than dizygotic (10%) twins suggests a heritable component; when chronic tics are included in the ascertainment, the concordance between monozygotic twins is nearly 100%. Genetic studies show a link between Tourette's disorder, chronic tics, and OCD. There also may be a link between Tourette's disorder and ADHD, even in the absence of OCD (Sheppard et al. 1999).

Several segregation analyses of families of Tourette's patients have provided support for autosomal dominant transmission, with partial penetrance and gender threshold effects, of Tourette's disorder (Curtis et al. 1992; Pauls and Leckman 1986). Two studies have suggested more complex transmission (Walkup et al. 1996), perhaps even nonmendelian (Seuchter et al. 2000).

A gender threshold effect (Pauls and Leckman 1986), specifically involving a lower penetrance of Tourette's disorder in girls at a given level of genetic loading, could account for the higher prevalence in boys than in girls. A gender threshold effect also could explain findings that girls show a higher prevalence of Tourette's and chronic tic disorders in their families. When all presumed forms of the disorder were considered in the segregation analysis, the penetrance was estimated as essentially complete (100%) in males and 71% for females. Consistent with a gender threshold effect, males within affected families were more likely to have tic disorders, and females were more likely to have OCD (Pauls and Leckman 1986). In this model, about 10% of the individuals with Tourette's disorder were estimated to have a nonheritable form of the disorder, perhaps the result of an environmental exposure.

The search for candidate genes, while promising, has been inconclusive to date. Possible associations of Tourette's disorder with dopamine-related genes have been mixed (Rowe et al. 1998; Thompson et al. 1998; D.J. Vandenberg et al. 2000). Examination of serotonin receptor genes suggests that this neurotransmitter system plays a minor role, if any (Brett et al. 1995).

A distinct environmentally triggered etiology has been proposed for genetically predisposed individuals. An autoimmune mechanism following streptococcal infection may lead to some cases of Tourette's disorder, chronic tic disorder, and comorbid obsessive-compulsive phenomena and inattention or hyperactivity. The prevalence of these entities as autoimmune phenomena is not well established, but 10%–20% of tic disorders may have an autoimmune basis. These PANDAS are diagnosed if five criteria are met: 1) presence of tic disorder and/or OCD, 2) prepubertal onset, 3) sudden onset or episodic course, 4) temporal association between streptococcal infections and neuropsychiatric symptom exacerbations, and 5) associated neurological abnormalities (H.L. Leonard and Swedo 2001).

PANDAS-associated episodes are caused or triggered by group A β-hemolytic streptococcal infections, such as pharyngitis, upper respiratory infections, or subclinical streptococcal infections (Singer et al. 2000). Antibodies directed against group A β-hemolytic streptococcus also recognize and cross-react with neuronal antigens (epitopes) in the basal ganglia (Singer et al. 1998; Swedo 1994; Swedo et al. 1998) and are believed to produce Syndenham's chorea, tic disorders, and OCD. They also might cause or contribute to some cases of anorexia nervosa (Sokol and Gray 1997). Consistent with this mechanism, MRI studies found enlargement of the basal ganglia in patients with streptococcal-related Tourette's disorder and OCD (Giedd et al. 2000).

A monoclonal antibody (D8/17) identifies a B lymphocyte antigen with expanded expression in nearly all patients with rheumatic fever as well as in most patients with childhood-onset Tourette's disorder or OCD (Hoekstra et al. 2001; T.K. Murphy et al. 1997). The antigen is believed to be a trait marker for susceptibility to this complication of group A β-hemolytic streptococcal infections, although it is also overexpressed in patients with autistic disorder. This finding provides further support for a role for group A β-hemolytic streptococcal infections in the pathogenesis of some cases of tic disorders and OCD.

A leading hypothesis suggests that Tourette's disorder is associated with a supersensitivity of postsynaptic D_2 dopaminergic receptors in the basal ganglia. The upregulation of dopa-decarboxylase, an enzyme critical in presynaptic dopamine turnover, has been suggested to play a potential role in this phenomenon (Ernst et al. 1999). However, abnormalities of serotonin, dynorphin, GABA, acetylcholine, and norepinephrine neurotransmitters, which participate in the CSTC system, also have been described.

The metabolites of dopamine and sometimes serotonin are reduced in the cerebrospinal fluid of patients with Tourette's disorder. Decreased levels of the endogenous opiate dynorphin A1-17 have been found in striatal pathways projecting to the globus pallidus (Haber and Wolfer 1992), and dynorphin A1-8 is increased in the cerebrospinal fluid of Tourette's patients (Leckman et al.

1988), which is consistent with the involvement of opioid mechanisms. Autopsy studies have described abnormalities of dopamine in the striatum, of serotonin in the basal ganglia, of dynorphin in the globus pallidus, and of glutamic acid in the subthalamic region.

Imaging studies are generally consistent in finding involvement of the basal ganglia, although specific findings vary. The globus pallidus is reported to be small and the caudate enlarged, perhaps with greater changes on the left side (Peterson et al. 1993). A quantitative MRI study of monozygotic twins concordant for tics found significantly reduced right caudate volumes in the more severely affected twins (Hyde et al. 1995). Also, the more severely affected twins did not have the normal asymmetry of the lateral ventricles observed in the less affected twins and in control groups in previous studies. SPECT studies have shown decreased cerebral blood flow in the left lenticular nucleus (Riddle et al. 1992) and a significant decrease in right basal ganglia activity; these findings are suggestive of functional asymmetry (Klieger et al. 1997; Peterson et al. 1998). A PET study quantifying dopamine receptors in Tourette's disorder found an elevated number of D_2 dopamine receptors (Wong et al. 1997). Taken together, these older data implicate the basal ganglia, both anatomically and functionally, in the pathophysiology of Tourette's disorder.

A simplistic model could relate motor tics to abnormalities in the functioning of neurons in nigrostriatal pathways and the other symptoms of Tourette's disorder to disturbances of limbic and cortical connections. However, interactions between the basal ganglia and the limbic system are complex and incompletely understood (Haber and Lynd-Balta 1993). More recent studies have suggested thalamic and cortical involvement, especially the prefrontal cortex (Hendren et al. 2000; Peterson et al. 2001b; E. Stern et al. 2000). Relevant pathways may include dopaminergic nigrostriatal projections, mesopontine nuclei, and ventral tegmental cortical and limbic projections. In addition, corticothalamic pathways, which are involved in motor and sensorimotor functions, use the basal ganglia as a relay site. Tics observed in Tourette's disorder may originate from a primary subcortical disorder and influence the motor and prefrontal cortex through disinhibited afferent signals or through impaired inhibition directly at the cortical level (Ziemann et al. 1997). This type of prefrontal-CSTC mechanism is consistent with neuropsychological evidence of subtle disturbances in the inhibition of voluntary movements and eye tracking (antisaccade).

The usual absence of motor developmental delays in Tourette's disorder (Bruun 1988) suggests that a relatively specific effect is exerted on the involved neural pathways rather than a generalized neurodevelopmental effect on neuromotor functions. Additional etiological factors are suggested by retrospective findings of increased prenatal and perinatal complications, lower birth weight (in affected monozygotic rather than dizygotic twins), greater emotional stress during pregnancy, more nausea and vomiting during the first trimester, and poorer prenatal care (Burd et al. 1999; Leckman et al. 1990). It may be speculated that such environmental factors modulate the expression of the genetic predisposition to Tourette's disorder, perhaps operating through stress- or gender-related hormonal mechanisms.

Thus, converging evidence suggests variant or disturbed functioning of CSTC circuitry in Tourette's disorder, as well as in OCD and ADHD, with developmental, genetic, immunological, and perhaps hormonal influences. The system is complicated and still little understood, but it appears involved in voluntary motor control and sensorimotor integration.

Course and Prognosis

Tics usually appear first in middle childhood or early adolescence, although they may begin later in adult life or as early as 2 years. Tics typically wax and wane in intensity over time. They often worsen during times of psychosocial stress (including teasing and social ostracism), intrapsychic conflict, and positive or negative emotional excitement. Psychosocial stress may be particularly symptom inducing at the start of the school year, at times of parental separation and divorce, and during physical fatigue.

As many as 50% of affected individuals experience significant improvement or complete remission of their symptoms by age 18 years, consistent with a 10-fold higher prevalence of Tourette's disorder in children than in adults.

The clinical presentation of Tourette's disorder may change during the course of development (Leckman et al. 1998). The mean age at onset of tics (usually motor) is 5–7 years; earlier age at onset is associated with a stronger family history of tics (Freeman et al. 2000). Symptoms typically worsen with time but in a waxing and waning pattern. The progression in severity of the tics is sufficient to seriously jeopardize functioning in school in up to 22% of these children. Severity typically peaks at about age 10 years, but the onset of puberty is not associated with the timing or severity of tics.

Motor tics typically show a rostral-caudal progression with age, with symptoms involving head before trunk and limbs. Phonic and vocal tics become evident at about age 10 or 11 years. Vocal tics may start as a single syllable,

progress to longer exclamations, and occasionally progress to complex verbal structures and gestures.

Sensory tics appear to lag behind the first appearance of tics by 3 years on the average and typically present in a rostral-caudal distribution (Chee and Sachdev 1997). Speculatively, this delay may result from maturation in the cognitive processing of sensory information that permits these "subtle and elusive" phenomena access to consciousness (Leckman et al. 1993). Alternatively, the apparent delay may reflect the later presentation of tics in the shoulders and hands, where sensory tics are typically experienced; that is, motor tics usually first appear around age 7 but do not reach the shoulders and hands until about age 10–11 years (A.K. Shapiro et al. 1998).

Classic coprolalia, observed in 30%–60% of the patients with Tourette's disorder, usually first emerges in early adolescence. Copropraxia (complex obscene gestures) may appear later as coprolalia resolves.

Early in development, before the initial appearance of tics, 25%–50% of the children with Tourette's disorder show symptoms of impulsivity, hyperactivity, and inattention similar to ADHD. Obsessive-compulsive symptoms often follow the onset of simple tics by 5–10 years (Bruun 1988; Peterson et al. 2001a) and subsequently may elaborate extensively.

Comorbidity is an important determinant of outcome. Patients with only tic symptoms tend to have a relatively benign course, whereas patients with ADHD and/or OCD have courses complicated by aggressive and disruptive symptoms and social and academic failure (Budman et al. 2000; Coffey et al. 2000; T. Spencer et al. 1998b; Stephens and Sandor 1999). Concurrent mood and anxiety disorders often aggravate the course of tic disorders (Coffey et al. 2000).

In the autoimmune form of Tourette's disorder (PANDAS), tic symptoms usually begin with an acute and even dramatic onset at around age 7–8 years (Swedo et al. 1998). Exacerbations may occur days to months after the onset of the streptococcal infection. The interval between first infection and initial appearance of tics may be weeks or months, but subsequently the interval between recurrent infections and symptom exacerbation typically decreases over time to a few days or weeks. Tic symptoms can be worsened by a "strep throat" or an "ordinary" upper respiratory infection. PANDAS can even be triggered by simple exposure to people with streptococcal infections, without any apparent clinical symptoms until the appearance or exacerbation of the neuropsychiatric syndrome.

Complications of severe Tourette's disorder may include impaired academic and social functioning and impaired self-esteem, interacting with the symptoms and complications that typically attend the comorbid disorders. Teasing, shame, self-consciousness, and social ostracism are common features in patients with predominantly internalizing comorbidities, whereas antisocial or criminal outcomes may be the manifestations with prominent externalizing comorbidity. Some patients may show a reluctance to involve themselves in socially demanding situations, particularly if their symptoms are severely socially disfiguring. Others may adopt an aggressive stance toward the world. Patients may avoid entering intimate relationships, marriage, and other interpersonally gratifying activities. The rate of unemployment is reportedly as high as 50% in adults with Tourette's disorder.

Diagnostic Evaluation

A complete psychiatric evaluation of the child and parents is indicated, including the assessment of possible ADHD, conduct disorder, OCD, learning disorders, pervasive developmental disorders, and mental retardation. A family genetic history should specifically include tic disorders, ADHD, OCD, and streptococcus-related illnesses. Neurological examination is appropriate to rule out other movement disorders, including Wilson's disease. An EEG is helpful in ruling out myoclonic seizures and other neurological disorders. An assessment of baseline dyskinesias is necessary before neuroleptic drug treatments are started. School reports, including those addressing academic performance, general behavior, severity of tics, and social skills, are useful. The child's self-consciousness, management of teasing and social ostracism, and assertiveness may be assessed. The possibility of concurrent mood or anxiety disorder should be evaluated. Along with assessment of family psychopathology and stressors, direct evaluation of tic and related disorders in siblings and parents may be considered.

A careful history of potential poststreptococcal neuropsychiatric sequelae should be obtained. Antibodies to streptococcal enzymes streptolysin O and DNase B increase during infection, and elevated titers may persist for some months thereafter. Measurement of these titers can be obtained as evidence of a possible association between an infection and the appearance or exacerbation of tic symptoms. Throat or nasopharyngeal swabs may be cultured to confirm acute infection. However, the clinical utility of these studies in documenting or tracking PANDAS has not been established. Nonetheless, evaluation for antistreptococcal antibodies should be considered in children with tic disorders, possibly with measurement of the stable B-cell antigen identified by the monoclonal antibody D8/17; this antigen, when overexpressed, appears to be a trait marker for susceptibility to the complications of group A β-hemolytic streptococcal infection, including rheumatic fever and the neuropsychiatric syndromes (PANDAS).

The clinician's task in following up the course of patients with Tourette's disorder is complicated by the great variability in the severity and appearance of tics. Symptom lists are idiosyncratic to individuals, and the specific form of the tics will change over time. It is helpful to obtain periodic individual evaluations of tic severity, symptom shifting, and functional interference because these symptoms interact with comorbidity, developmental stage, and circumstance.

Treatment

Pharmacotherapy, behavior therapy, and sometimes psychotherapy and special education may be used, although longitudinal studies of complex interventions have yet to be conducted. Although medications may play a vital role in the management of Tourette's disorder, a child's adaptive capacities, comorbid diagnoses, coping mechanisms, interpersonal skills, and social support play a significant role in outcome. Also, in view of the studies suggesting a frequently benign resolution of Tourette's symptoms toward the end of adolescence, the presumption of extended or lifelong psychopharmacological treatment should be questioned or at least clinically tested in individual cases.

Neuroleptic drugs have been the cornerstone of pharmacotherapy. Although largely replaced by the newer atypical antipsychotic agents, studies of conventional neuroleptics have reported that approximately 60%–80% of Tourette's patients show clinically significant improvement. Low dosages of high-potency neuroleptics, such as haloperidol and pimozide, have been prescribed most commonly, but low-potency neuroleptics appear to be approximately as effective. The neuroleptic dosages are typically low in comparison to antipsychotic doses; dose elevations may be required gradually over time, but decreases in dosage also may be possible because of the waxing and waning of symptoms. Atypical antipsychotics, including olanzapine, risperidone, and ziprasidone, have been effective in controlled trials of Tourette's disorder (Bruggeman et al. 2001; Onofrj et al. 2000; Sallee et al. 2000). Despite the reduced incidence of adverse motor effects with the atypical antipsychotics, it is important to keep in mind that all neuroleptics carry a risk of inducing neuroleptic malignant syndrome (Latz and McCracken 1992; Steingard et al. 1992) and tardive tourettism (Bharucha and Sethi 1995).

Clonidine is an alternative treatment that has been reported to be helpful in about 50% of patients with Tourette's disorder, particularly for children with behavior disorders whose ADHD might be improved by clonidine. At low dosages, clonidine stimulates α_2-adrenergic presynaptic receptors, leading acutely to decreased norepinephrine neurotransmission and, with chronic treatment, to increased dopamine use through an unknown indirect mechanism possibly involving serotonin. The clinical effect of clonidine might increase over the course of 2–3 months of treatment. Guanfacine, a similar α_2-adrenergic receptor agonist, has been found in controlled studies to be effective and safe in this population (Chappell et al. 1995; Scahill et al. 2001). The effects of long-term clonidine and guanfacine treatment are not well defined.

The use of stimulants and TCAs in treating Tourette's disorder remains controversial because of past findings that these agents may exacerbate or trigger tic disorders. Although some controlled findings suggest that these agents exacerbate tics in many children (Gadow et al. 1995; Riddle et al. 1995), many physicians have returned to using these agents with only occasional complaints of tic induction. With or without the use of stimulants and TCAs, continued vigilance regarding tic induction is advisable if over-the-counter sympathomimetic drugs are used by patients with Tourette's disorder. Similarly, special warnings are needed concerning the recreational use of cocaine and related drugs. At this time, it is acceptable practice to prescribe psychostimulants in treating chronic tic disorders with comorbid ADHD, and TCAs may be considered for patients with comorbid anxiety or depressive disorders.

Controlled trials support the use of various other agents in Tourette's disorder, including the selective MAOI selegiline (Feigin et al. 1996), mixed dopamine agonist pergolide (Gilbert et al. 2000), nicotinic receptor antagonist mecamylamine (Silver et al. 2001), GABA receptor agonist baclofen (Singer et al. 2001), and opioid agonist propoxyphene (Kurlan et al. 1991). Interestingly, botulinum toxin A, the neuromuscular blocking agent, was found in an open-label study to reduce motor tics and also to diminish the premonitory sensations (Kwak et al. 2000). Also, some evidence indicates that androgens and the opiate receptor antagonist naltrexone may worsen tics and associated obsessive-compulsive symptoms and therefore should be avoided.

If comorbid psychiatric disorders are present in patients with Tourette's disorder, treatment of the comorbidity may improve the symptoms of Tourette's disorder. This parallel improvement can be seen with most comorbid psychiatric disorders, including mood and anxiety disorders, ADHD, and other behavior disorders. Although there remains debate about the possible risk of tic induction or aggravation by use of psychostimulants, a growing body of literature supports their chronic use in treating ADHD with comorbid Tourette's disorder with little evidence of stimulant-induced tic exacerbation (Gadow et al. 1999; T. Spencer et al. 2001b).

For children with tic disorders associated with streptococcal infection, several immunological treatments are under investigation, including plasmapheresis, intravenous immunoglobulins, antibiotic prophylaxis, and prednisone (Allen et al. 1995; H.L. Leonard and Swedo 2001; Matarrazo 1992). A multiyear follow-up study suggested that antibiotic prophylaxis of PANDAS symptoms may be helpful in patients for whom the treatment is effective in suppressing recurrence of streptococcal infection (H.L. Leonard and Swedo 2001).

Neuropsychologically based educational interventions can be helpful in dealing with some of the "frontal" symptoms of ADHD (Denckla and Reader 1993). Various behavioral techniques have been used, but they are not uniformly effective. Standard procedures have not been established.

Although psychotherapy is not a specific treatment of Tourette's disorder, it may be useful to help an individual deal with the stigma of illness and with self-esteem problems, promote interpersonal comfort and social skills, improve the opportunities for and the odds of successful marriage, and enhance functioning and satisfaction at work. In addition to enhancing adaptive skills, psychotherapy may reduce the anxiety that aggravates tic severity (K.P. O'Connor et al. 2001).

The family response to this disfiguring disorder is often significant, and its management is important for the welfare of both the family and the patient (D. Cohen et al. 1988). The Tourette Syndrome Association is a national organization that provides support and education to families and patients, funds and helps locate subjects for research, and advocates with public agencies.

Clinical Comment

The high incidence of social ostracism and self-consciousness, as well as the high rates of adult unemployment, among patients with Tourette's disorder requires special attention to the psychosocial consequences of this disorder. Control of the tics does not constitute the end point of treatment. This classic "neurological" disorder is no longer considered rare, is a common comorbid disorder with other psychiatric disorders, and has a firm place in the psychiatric nosology.

Feeding and Eating Disorders of Infancy or Early Childhood

Anorexia nervosa and bulimia nervosa, usually first diagnosed in adolescence, are discussed in Chapter 22. Three additional eating disorders usually first diagnosed in childhood are pica, rumination disorder of infancy, and feeding disorder of infancy or early childhood.

Pica and rumination disorder are rarely treated as isolated entities by psychiatrists, but these disorders are significant medical conditions with definite psychiatric dimensions. Feeding disorder of infancy or early childhood corresponds to a subcategory of the pediatric diagnosis of nonorganic failure to thrive.

Pica

A pattern of eating nonfood materials can be seen in young children, individuals with severe or profound mental retardation, and pregnant women. Pica has been extensively documented in the pediatric literature but minimally documented in the psychiatric literature—despite its presumed biopsychosocial etiology and its potential for major behavioral, cognitive, neurological, and developmental complications.

Pica appears to be quite common in children, particularly young children, but is frequently underdiagnosed. When pica occurs in mentally retarded persons or in pregnant women, it can require a physician's vigilant inquiry to uncover. The psychiatric significance of pica is very different in these distinct populations.

Geophagia (the eating of clay or soil) is a similar phenomenon that is an ordinary and sanctioned activity in many cultures worldwide, especially in indigenous populations that live close to the soil. Even in some American locations, including the central Piedmont region of Georgia, chalk eating is a cultural norm (Grigsby et al. 1999). Such culturally determined forms of pica are not considered a mental disorder (Table 20–24). Whatever the basis for the pica, the risk of accidental poisoning is significant.

Clinical Description

Children and people with mental retardation may eat paper, paint, coins, string, rags, hair, feces, vomitus, leaves, bugs, worms, and cloth. Pica in children is typically observed in association with behavior and other medical problems, but such children are rarely brought for psychiatric treatment of the isolated problem of pica. Pica behavior can vary considerably across days, but some

---

TABLE 20–24. DSM-IV-TR diagnostic criteria for pica

A. Persistent eating of nonnutritive substances for a period of at least 1 month.
B. The eating of nonnutritive substances is inappropriate to the developmental level.
C. The eating behavior is not part of a culturally sanctioned practice.
D. If the eating behavior occurs exclusively during the course of another mental disorder (e.g., mental retardation, pervasive developmental disorder, schizophrenia), it is sufficiently severe to warrant independent clinical attention.

---

children have been documented to ingest 25–60 g of soil in a single day (Calabrese et al. 1997).

Pregnant women, apart from their common craving for fruit and sharp-tasting foods, have been reported at times to seek and eat starchy materials, refrigerator frost, or substances containing minerals. Cultural geophagia commonly involves the eating of earth, clay, sand, and pebbles. Geophagia is also common in children and in pregnant women.

Epidemiology

Few epidemiological data are available on DSM-defined pica, but picalike behaviors are common. About 10%–20% of children in the United States exhibit picalike behavior at some point in their lives, and up to 50%–70% of children living in the inner cities have pica between ages 1 and 6 years. Boys and girls are equally involved. Epidemiological studies show that children with pica typically come from a low socioeconomic class, have pets at home, and show various behavioral abnormalities. Typically, they are not referred for treatment unless complications, such as lead poisoning, or concomitant disorders are identified. More than 50% of the children hospitalized for accidental ingestions have been found to have pica (Millican et al. 1968).

Mental retardation is associated with a high prevalence of pica. Approximately 20%–40% of institutionalized people with severe or profound mental retardation have pica. Gender prevalence is equal.

The prevalence of pica among pregnant women has been reported to vary geographically from 0% to 70%. In the lower socioeconomic classes of the United States, persistent nonnutritive eating is seen in about 60% of pregnant women. The specific eating of ice and freezer frost was reported by 8% of the pregnant women in the inner city of Washington, DC (Edwards et al. 1994). Most children with pica have mothers or siblings who also have pica.

Pica increases the risk of exposure to environmental toxins. Lead poisoning has been reported in as many as 92% of children living near a lead smelter in Brazil (Silvany-Neto et al. 1996). Households may become contaminated by toxins inadvertently brought home from job sites despite precautions to avoid occupational exposure and transportation of potentially toxic materials (Chiaradia et al. 1997). Even in affluent locations, pica is a major route of exposure to lead, pesticides, and organic toxins through the ingestion of house dust in carpets, mattresses, and sofas (J.W. Roberts and Dickey 1995).

Culturally based pica is seen in some families of Third World origins (Vermeer and Frate 1979). For example, geophagia is observed in the general population (nonclinical samples) in many parts of Africa, South America, Asia, and aboriginal Australia. In different regions, earth eating is used as a simple "pacifier" for infants, a routine pastime (like smoking), or a culturally based method for respecting or incorporating magical spirits; it also is used for presumed medicinal value (e.g., to suppress nausea). The practice is not indiscriminate but involves careful selection of certain types of clay and specific preparations (such as cooking). When culturally proper soil or clay is not available to Americans of African descent in inner cities, laundry starch is used as a common substitute because of its claylike texture and consistency. The risks of pica remain potentially serious, even when culturally sanctioned. Among children, the prevalence of lead intoxication has been reported as high as 73% in Kenya and 90% in Pakistan (Hafeez and Malik 1996).

Etiology

Childhood pica is sometimes interpreted as an ordinary part of exploratory learning or as a reflection of a young child's inability to differentiate food from inedible objects. The findings of increased childhood pica in households with pets and of the eating of pet food by children suggest that imitation can be an etiological factor. Most children with pica have parents with a history of pica; the disorder may be passed along by a variety of mechanisms, including cultural ones. Psychoanalytic hypotheses have emphasized impairments in aggressivity or orality. Disorders of parent–child nurturance and of psychosocial deprivation (disruptive feeding, traumatic weaning, unmet "oral" needs) may contribute in certain cases. The overrepresentation of pica in lower socioeconomic classes may be a partial marker for psychosocial stress or family pathology, which can be involved in the etiology. Parental depression, neglect, and inadequate supervision are clearly related to the risk of toxic inges-

tions in children (Bithoney et al. 1985) and are presumed to be tangible behavioral factors that contribute to the appearance of pica. Mothers of children with pica have been described as immature, emotionally unavailable, and overwhelmed by parenting tasks. In general, the cultural and environmental origins of pica need to be considered because they may explain some aspects of the family transmission of pica.

In individuals with severe or profound mental retardation, the primary mechanism is believed to be self-stimulation rather than impaired judgment. Children and adults with mental retardation and pica tend to engage in pica with a favorite object.

A nutritional etiology has been proposed for some adults, who are believed to have an instinctive craving for vitamins and minerals, especially iron and perhaps zinc or calcium. The eating is hypothesized to be an attempt to correct a nutritional deficiency. Evidence indicates that this mechanism operates in animals, but few data support this notion in humans. Eating of ice (or refrigerator frost) has been reported in pregnant women in association with iron deficiency, and prescription of iron supplements has been found to improve the anemia and reduce the ice eating (Danford 1982). Pica can instead be a cause of malnutrition because the consumed objects or substances may interfere with the absorption of nutrients. Because anemia does not regularly induce pica in adults, it is more likely that pica causes nutritional imbalances in adults. The relevance of the nutritional deficiency theory of pica to children is undetermined.

Certain medical factors can contribute to the appearance of pica in adults, including brain disorders, gastrointestinal disease, parasitic infestations, and inflammations. Family psychiatric history and biological concomitants of pica have not been systematically studied. However, some data have suggested that mood disorders may be overrepresented in families with pica.

Course and Prognosis

In children, pica usually starts at age 12–24 months and resolves by age 6 years. However, in mentally retarded persons, pica can endure and persist into adulthood. In pregnant women, geophagia usually resolves at the end of pregnancy, although it may recur in subsequent pregnancies.

Complications of pica are numerous and potentially severe. Constipation and gastrointestinal malabsorption are common. Fecal impaction may occur repetitively. Ingestion of foreign bodies or hair balls can lead to intestinal obstruction, potentially leading to intestinal perforation or biliary obstruction, which sometimes requires colostomy. Anemias can be produced by nutritional deficiencies and sometimes traumatic intestinal bleeding. Mineral toxicity, salt imbalances, parasitic infections, vomiting, poisoning, and dental injury may be seen. Ingestion of radioactively contaminated soil is also a public health concern (Simon 1998).

Ingestion of lead-containing paint, plaster, and earth can lead to toxic encephalopathy in severe cases, fatigue and weight loss (with constipation) in moderate cases, and learning impairments in mild cases. Approximately 80% of the children with severe lead poisoning have pica, and at least 30% of the children with pica show lead-related symptoms.

Lead intake by pregnant women can cause congenital plumbism. However, pica has developmental significance even without toxin ingestions: pregnant women who eat ice give birth to infants with smaller head circumferences than do women without pica (Edwards et al. 1994). Children with pica can have slow motor and mental development, growth retardation, seizures, and neurological deficits, as well as behavioral abnormalities both before and after the period of pica. A long-term follow-up study suggested that young children with pica are at increased risk for the subsequent development of bulimia nervosa, with an odds ratio of 6.7 (Marchi and Cohen 1990).

Diagnostic Evaluation

Evaluation of children with pica involves behavioral and psychiatric evaluation of the child and parents, psychosocial evaluation of the home (including caregiver availability and presence of pets), nutritional status, feeding history, lead exposure, and cultural values. The possibility of inadequate supervision of children or parental neglect needs assessment.

The diagnosis is often missed because children are typically brought for evaluation of other problems. Adults may not have directly observed the pica behavior in children or may volunteer such observations about their family only reluctantly.

Pica should be actively considered in children and adults (not only persons with mental retardation) with anemia, chronic constipation, fecal impaction, or accidental ingestions. Lead poisoning may be present in children with ADHD, unexplained fatigue or weight loss, learning impairments, mental retardation, or gingival "lead lines."

In view of the high risk of lead intoxication, it is reasonable to assess children with pica by obtaining both a zinc protoporphyrin and a plasma lead level. Although debate remains about whether there is a developmentally "safe" minimal blood level of lead, there is general agreement about the upper limits of acceptable plasma levels of lead (10 µg/dL) and zinc protoporphyrin (30 µg/dL). When identifying a child with pica, it is advisable to examine siblings and parents for pica as well.

Treatment

Behavior therapy has been used for children and mentally retarded individuals with pica. Rewarding appropriate eating, teaching the differentiation of edible foods, overcorrection (immediate enforcement of oral hygiene), and negative reinforcement (time-outs, physical restraint) have been successful, especially for mentally retarded people. Psychosocial interventions include promotion of maternal supervision and stimulation, improvement of play opportunities (new toys), and placement in day care.

Concomitant medical treatments may be required. Management of lead poisoning may be handled in the routine manner. It has been suggested that nutritional iron and zinc treatments produce short-term improvements in some individuals. Nutritional treatments have not been systematically assessed, although some preliminary evidence suggests that multivitamins might be able to reduce pica in some cases (Pace and Toyer 2000).

Psychosocial interventions also have not been evaluated, but improvements in personal and household hygiene appear to be beneficial. Removal of old or synthetic carpets and furniture, elimination of sources of dust and particulates, or even a family move away from a problematic home may be required in some cases.

Public health measures for reducing environmental lead levels have been shown to be dramatically effective in reducing plasma lead levels of children on a national level. Although the mean plasma lead level has been reduced by more than 80% in the United States since the 1970s, minority groups living in urban poverty remain at high risk for elevated lead levels; this is especially true for immigrants (Rothenberg et al. 1999).

Effective correction of lead intoxication may not induce lasting improvements. For example, even after comprehensive management of lead poisoning in children with pervasive developmental disorder, 75% became reexposed to lead during the course of their medical management. In many cases of childhood pica, ongoing reassessments of lead and zinc protoporphyrin levels are advisable beyond the course of acute medical treatment.

Clinical Comment

Pica in children and mentally retarded individuals is a significant disorder that generally has not received systematic psychiatric attention. Nonnutritive eating in pregnant women and among some socioeconomic groups may represent a related or dissimilar condition. Increased clinical surveillance and research studies are needed to delineate possible differences in the forms of pica that appear in different populations, including the normative forms of pica that are prevalent in certain regions of the world.

The basic psychiatric dimensions of childhood pica are yet to be described, but the routine evaluation of the siblings and parents of American children with pica is clinically advisable. The increased risk for bulimia nervosa among children with pica highlights the psychiatric significance of this behavior. Beyond studies on lead exposure, no long-term follow-up studies of pica or its treatment have been done.

Rumination Disorder of Infancy

Certain infants show a pleasurable relaxation as they regurgitate, rechew, drool, and reswallow their food, usually in the absence of caregivers and other sources of stimulation. Their continuing self-stimulation, apparent satisfaction, and languorous obliviousness highlight their full engrossment in rumination. Their obvious enjoyment and enthusiasm occur despite malnourishment and diminished weight gain and are in marked contrast to their parents' disgust at this activity.

This potentially fatal disorder of infants may reflect abnormal development of early self-stimulation and physiological regulation, and it is particularly apparent when infants are alone (Table 20–25). Rumination (merycism) may be a cause or result of disrupted parent–child attachments, and it can be associated with major developmental delays and mental retardation. It is recognized by gastroenterologists as a functional disorder of infancy (Rasquin-Weber et al. 1999).

The symptom of rumination is relatively common in adults with mental retardation; it has been reported in up to 10% of institutionalized adults with severe or profound mental retardation (Fredericks et al. 1998). In addition, patients with eating disorders are occasionally observed to ruminate (Eckern et al. 1999; Weakley et al. 1997). Rumination also may present in developmentally normal children (Reis 1994), adolescents (Khan et al. 2000), and adults (Parry-Jones 1994), seemingly as a transient response to situational stressors. The relation of these forms of rumination to the pathological condition of rumination disorder in infants is unclear.

Clinical Description

Rumination involves the continued eating of partially digested stomach contents that are regurgitated into the esophagus or mouth. It is different from vomiting, in

TABLE 20–25. DSM-IV-TR diagnostic criteria for rumination disorder

A. Repeated regurgitation and rechewing of food for a period of at least 1 month following a period of normal functioning.

B. The behavior is not due to an associated gastrointestinal or other general medical condition (e.g., esophageal reflux).

C. The behavior does not occur exclusively during the course of anorexia nervosa or bulimia nervosa. If the symptoms occur exclusively during the course of mental retardation or a pervasive developmental disorder, they are sufficiently severe to warrant independent clinical attention.

which the stomach contents are expelled through the mouth.

Rumination may start with the infant's placing fingers or clothes in the mouth to induce regurgitation, with rhythmic body or neck motions, or it may begin without any apparent initiating action. During rumination, the infant generally lies quietly, may look happy or "spacey," and may hold body and head in a characteristic arching position while sucking. No nausea, discomfort, or disgust is apparent. If observed, the infant usually stops and fixes visual attention on the intruder; when the infant is no longer aware of being observed, sucking and tongue movements restart in seconds. When he or she is not ruminating, the infant may appear apathetic and withdrawn, irritable and fussy, or seemingly normal.

Self-stimulatory behaviors are commonly seen in association with rumination disorder. Often, thumb sucking, cloth sucking, head banging, and body rocking are observed, lending support to the hypothesis that rumination can be an infantile form of self-stimulation.

Epidemiology

No prevalence figures are available, but rumination disorder is rare and decreasing in prevalence in the general population, perhaps because of improving infant and child care. The disorder has almost disappeared in some countries (Guedeney 1995). However, rumination disorder is not rare in infants with mental retardation. About 10% of institutionalized mentally retarded adults show similar medically unexplained symptoms. About 93% of the adults with rumination have severe or profound mental retardation. The few available studies consist of small samples and report contradictory findings on sex ratio. Both male predominance and equal sex prevalence have been reported.

Etiology

There is strong evidence of both organic and environmental contributions to the etiology of rumination. Rumina-

Feeding Disorder of Infancy or Early Childhood

In pediatrics, the diagnosis of failure to thrive indicates a retardation of body growth or milestone attainment as a result of inadequate nutritional intake. The "organic" forms of failure to thrive can result from chronic physical illness (congenital AIDS), neurological disease, sensory deficit, or virtually any serious pediatric disease. The "nonorganic" forms, constituting at least 80% of cases of failure to thrive, encompass 1) homeostatic disorders of infancy (sleep and feeding dysregulation), 2) pathological food refusal, 3) protein-calorie malnutrition, and 4) social and emotional factors interfering with adequate nutritional care (including reactive attachment disorder, which is discussed later in the chapter).

The DSM-IV-TR diagnosis of feeding disorder of infancy or early childhood does not include all forms of nonorganic failure to thrive but only the types of eating failure that occur in the context of adequate provision of food (Table 20–26). This disorder does not include cases of child neglect or cases of inadequate eating due to obviously defective parenting or feeding.

Clinical Description

Infants may gag when fed or refuse to open their mouths. Young children might decline to eat, or they may eat so slowly that their intake is drastically reduced. In infants, the retardation in weight gain is typically accompanied by motor, social, and linguistic delays as well as a problematic relationship with the feeder or caregiver (as a result if not a cause of the disorder). In early childhood, symptoms may include impaired interpersonal relationships and interactions, mood symptoms, behavior problems, developmental delays, unusual food preferences, excessively rigid or narrow food choices, and perhaps bizarre eating and foraging behaviors.

TABLE 20–26. DSM-IV-TR diagnostic criteria for feeding disorder of infancy or early childhood

A. Feeding disturbance as manifested by persistent failure to eat adequately with significant failure to gain weight or significant loss of weight over at least 1 month.

B. The disturbance is not due to an associated gastrointestinal or other general medical condition (e.g., esophageal reflux).

C. The disturbance is not better accounted for by another mental disorder (e.g., rumination disorder) or by lack of available food.

D. The onset is before age 6 years.

Epidemiology

About 25% of the infants in the general population are reported to have some type of feeding problem, but a prevalence of 80% is described in children with developmental delays (Manikam and Perman 2000). Approximately 1%–5% of pediatric hospital admissions are for nonorganic failure to thrive, and community-based estimates of the prevalence of nonorganic failure to thrive are approximately 1%–4%. Epidemiological data concerning the DSM-IV-TR diagnosis of feeding disorder of infancy or early childhood are not available.

Etiology

The relative loss of weight is due to malnutrition, but the malnutrition may have various causes (Woolston 1983). Both physical and psychosocial etiologies may be involved, although the definition of the disorder excludes cases that clearly result from overt medical problems or other psychiatric disorders.

Various mechanisms (and potential subtypes) include difficulties with physiological homeostasis, attachment to the caregiver, and autonomy from the caregiver, as well as posttraumatic responses (Chatoor et al. 1985).

Homeostatic control of sleep and feeding is an early developmental accomplishment that is generally easy to achieve. The lability of the autonomic nervous system, presumably seen in colicky infants, needs the calming and soothing responses of the caregiver to promote development of self-regulation. Even the physical requirements of eating may induce fatigue and interfere with feeding in some infants, especially those with medical conditions unrelated to feeding.

Attachment problems, reflected in impaired relatedness and reciprocal interactions with the caregiver, may operate to inhibit adequate feeding. The ordinary signals, including eye contact, smiling, vocal contact, visual stimulation, and physical touching, may not be provided (or responded to) by child or parent, undermining the reciprocal signaling that underlies effective feeding. Apathy might replace the enjoyment of feeding experienced by child and caregiver.

Autonomy struggles, reflecting the negotiation of separation from the feeder, may be manifest by the child's food refusal, "pickiness" about food choices, or undereating. Between ages 6 months and 3 years (the developmental period of separation and individuation), the child's agenda may effectively become "I will decide who puts food in my mouth." If the parent interprets the child's actions as rebellion or personal insult, a power struggle may become evident in feeding (before it becomes clear in other developmental arenas). Food refusal is often accompanied by other displays of autonomy and power, including temper tantrums and aggressivity (Chatoor 1989). The result is that the child's eating patterns become determined by the interpersonal and emotional struggle with the parent rather than nutritional needs or internal physiological hunger signals (Chatoor et al. 2000).

Additional socioemotional factors that might reduce nutritional intake and body growth include posttraumatic responses to medical procedures involving the mouth, child abuse, emotional deprivation, or family pathology. Maternal psychopathology appears to increase the risk of feeding problems, such as food refusal or pickiness, in infants.

Feeding disorder is distinct from general problems in feeding, but some findings on infants with feeding problems may be relevant. Although mood and anxiety disorders do not appear to be overrepresented in the mothers of children with feeding problems (Whelan and Cooper 2000), almost one-third of the children with a feeding disorder have mothers with current or past DSM-IV eating disorders (Whelan and Cooper 2000). Such mothers appeared to have difficulty in tolerating normal child feeding behavior and appeared to react to it in a manner that reflected the mother's concerns about food and eating rather than the child's developmental needs (A. Stein et al. 1999). These mothers appear to show excessive concern about the weight, shape, and consistency of the food; concern about the shape and weight of the child; attitudes toward dieting and food restriction; uneasiness with child's use of food for nonnutritive purposes such as play; and discomfort with vomiting and mess.

A category of "posttraumatic feeding disorder" has been proposed to describe infants whose feeding problems appeared to result from a traumatic event involving the esophagus or oropharynx, such as an actual incident of choking or gagging, postsurgical retching, or a surgical procedure. Only a small percentage of children with such physical trauma develop these symptoms, so it is inferred that the temperamental, physiological, experiential, or comorbidity factors are crucial in its development (Chatoor et al. 2001). Phenomenologically, the child shows resistant behaviors suggestive of intense distress (crying, arching, refusing to open mouth, spitting) even when being positioned, similar to anticipatory anxiety. Whereas other types of feeding disorder may suggest a child's lack of appetite, this posttraumatic form is more suggestive of a fear of eating or swallowing.

Another type of feeding disorder is the pediatric syndrome called *psychosocial dwarfism*. This disorder has a later age at onset (or later age at recognition) and usually is based on a failure to gain height (whereas weight is the criterion in the DSM-IV-TR definition of feeding disorder). This form of nonorganic failure to thrive involves developmental and behavioral features similar to those of feeding disorder, as well as enuresis or encopresis, irritability, or apathy. These children typically also have a clinically apparent sleep problem and a reduced secretion of growth hormone at night. The reduced growth hormone secretion may result from the disturbed sleep and may serve as a biological marker for psychosocial dwarfism. Other forms of nonorganic failure to thrive and reactive attachment disorder (discussed later in the chapter) do not appear to have the sleep or growth hormone abnormality of psychosocial dwarfism.

Course and Prognosis

The untreated course of these disorders may depend on the specific subtype or mechanisms involved, but the expected outcome ranges from spontaneous remission to malnutrition, infection, susceptibility to chronic illness, and death. Both nutritional and psychosocial deprivation may result in long-term behavioral changes, hyperactivity, short stature, and lowered IQ. In some cases of prolonged food refusal, such as seen in the posttraumatic form, the lack of practice in chewing or eating may lead to oromotor delays (Chatoor et al. 2001). The relation of these feeding disorders to other psychiatric disorders in adulthood is undetermined, but some evidence indicates increased risk for later eating disorders (Jacobs and Isaacs 1986; Marchi and Cohen 1990).

Evaluation and Treatment

It is not clear from the DSM-IV-TR definition whether feeding disorder of infancy or early childhood includes cases in which food is available but the caregiver is simply an inept feeder. It is also unclear whether the reversal of the symptoms with appropriate care is characteristic.

In some cases, disturbed eating patterns based on power struggling may be approached by a behavioral-cognitive approach with the mother. However, in some cases, a more extensive psychotherapeutic approach is needed to address the mother's dependency and control issues (Chatoor 1989). Support for the mother of a temperamentally challenging infant might include modeling, direct coaching on how to read the infant's cues, teaching how to allow appropriate autonomy during meals, reducing the mother's distractions during feeding, fostering of self-feeding, tolerating mess, and using contingency management and praise. In contrast, for a child's posttraumatic feeding disturbances, gradual and graded desensitization to fear objects, such as the high chair and feeding utensils, can be useful (Chatoor et al. 2000).

In most cases of feeding disorder of infancy, however, the services of a multidisciplinary team, preferably in a hospital setting, are appropriate for evaluating and initiating treatment. Specialists in gastroenterology, nutrition, behavior, and development can be helpful. Many potential specialized procedures are available for evaluating feeding and swallowing disorders in children (Lefton-Greif and Loughlin 1996), but the medical workup of such children will depend on a variety of factors. Evaluation includes assessment of body growth as well as observations of the mother–child interactions in general and in feeding in particular. (A more detailed description of the multidisciplinary treatment is found in the section "Reactive Attachment Disorder of Infancy or Early Childhood" later in this chapter.)

Clinical Comment

Although feeding disorder of infancy or early childhood is described in DSM-IV-TR as a unitary entity, attempts have been made to parse this condition into a set of subtypes. This new classification distinguishes four subtypes based on their developmental characteristics, reflecting the age at their initial presentation and the developmental struggles that they represent. Three subtypes are defined in terms of medical factors that precipitate them, including anatomical defects, neurological impairment, and general medical disease. A posttraumatic subtype is described. Two other eating disorders, pica and rumination disorder, are already recognized in DSM-IV-TR. This refined subtyping reflects new knowledge regarding the specific forms and presentations of the feeding and eating disorders that present in early childhood, and each subtype is associated with a distinctive approach to treatment.

TABLE 20–27. DSM-IV-TR diagnostic criteria for encopresis

A. Repeated passage of feces into inappropriate places (e.g., clothing or floor) whether involuntary or intentional.

B. At least one such event a month for at least 3 months.

C. Chronological age is at least 4 years (or equivalent developmental level).

D. The behavior is not due exclusively to the direct physiological effects of a substance (e.g., laxatives) or a general medical condition except through a mechanism involving constipation.

Code as follows:
787.6   With Constipation and Overflow Incontinence
307.7   Without Constipation and Overflow Incontinence

Elimination Disorders

Encopresis

Encopresis includes fecal soiling of clothes, voiding in bed, and excretion onto the floor, occurring after age 4 years when full bowel control is developmentally expected. Because "organic" causes of encopresis need to be excluded, medical examination for structural and other nonfunctional abnormalities must be obtained before the diagnosis is made (Table 20–27). Although the term *encopresis* is used loosely to denote both types of soiling, the medically explained cases are technically *fecal incontinence*, and the idiopathic ones are *encopresis* (Loening-Baucke 1996). Both biopsychiatric and psychodynamic theories have been proposed to explain the etiology of encopresis. However, if a specific neurobiological explanation were identified, the condition would no longer be idiopathic. *Idiopathic encopresis* would be a clearer term for this psychiatric disorder.

Behavior problems are found in one-third of the children with encopresis (van der Plas et al. 1996). Some of the psychological and behavioral difficulties appear to resolve when the encopresis improves. In such cases, encopresis appears to function as an etiological factor for the development of behavioral symptoms. In other cases, major psychiatric disorders appear comorbidly with encopresis and require concurrent treatment.

Most cases of encopresis result from chronic constipation that leads to overflow. The stool may be formed, semiformed, or liquid. At least some children have encopresis without constipation. Children who have encopresis with constipation have a longer colonic transit time (slower movement) than encopretic children without constipation (Benninga et al. 1994), suggesting that some additional mechanisms might be involved. Children with soiling showed a general increase in behavioral symptoms, as measured on the Child Behavior Checklist, which were comparable in magnitude for both the constipated and the nonconstipated children (Benninga et al. 1994).

Clinical Description

Encopresis is usually a result of chronic constipation and is generally accompanied by pain during defecation, smell, and embarrassment. Parents usually repeatedly ask the child to try to relieve the symptoms in the toilet. Encopresis during the daytime is much more common than nocturnal encopresis. Half of these patients have primary encopresis: these individuals have never established fecal continence. The other half have secondary encopresis: these children initially learned bowel control, were continent for at least 1 year, and then regressed, typically by age 8 years.

Primary encopresis may be viewed as reflecting slow development or an early developmental fixation. In fact, it is associated in boys with a high rate of developmental delays (and enuresis) compared with secondary encopresis. Secondary encopresis, in which control was learned and then lost, is associated more strongly with conduct disorder and psychosocial stressors than is primary encopresis (Foreman and Thambirajah 1996).

About 75%–90% of the children with encopresis have the DSM-IV-TR subtype designated as "with constipation and overflow incontinence." These "retentive" cases involve a low frequency of bowel movements, impaction, overflow of liquid around a partially hardened stool, and leakage of liquid into the clothing. The cause may be chronic constipation, inadequate bowel training (e.g., overly coercive), pain (e.g., from an anal fissure), or phobic avoidance of toilets. These retentive episodes usually extend for several days and are followed by painful defecation.

Encopresis without constipation and overflow incontinence can involve a variety of causes, including a lack of sphincter awareness or weak sphincter control. In cases of postbath soiling, physical stimulation may be causative. If soiling is deliberate and the child is typically impulsive or hostile, antisocial or major psychiatric disorders may be associated. Smearing may be accidental (the child who tries to hide the accident) or purposeful (defiant or vindictive).

Behavior problems such as conduct disorder are common in the psychiatrically referred population of youths with encopresis (Friman et al. 1988), but there is comparatively little behavioral disturbance in samples seen by pediatricians (Gabel et al. 1988). In the psychiatric population, 25% of the children with encopresis also have functional enuresis; in the pediatric population, this diagnostic overlap is less common. Some children withhold both urine and feces; they may develop megabladder and megacolon.

Chronic constipation, even without overflow incontinence, tends to be severe and is commonly associated with large stools and pain. In girls, urinary tract infection and chronic pyelonephritis are frequent.

Typically, children with encopresis experience shame and embarrassment, feel dirty, and have low self-esteem. They may endure accusations from their parents and siblings, fear discovery by their peers, and hide physically and emotionally.

Epidemiology

Encopresis is less common than enuresis. Prevalence is approximately 1.5% after age 5 years; the disorder diminishes with age and is rare in adolescents. There is a 4:1 male predominance. Slightly higher prevalence rates are associated with the lower socioeconomic classes and with mental retardation, particularly in moderate and severe cases. However, most cases of encopresis are not associated with low intelligence. Overall, neither social class nor intelligence appears to correlate with the presence of encopresis.

Etiology

Medical causes of fecal incontinence include hypothyroidism, hypercalcemia, anal fissure or malformation, rectal stenosis, lactase deficiency, overeating of fried and fatty foods, trauma or surgery, congenital aganglionic megacolon (although Hirschsprung's disease is usually associated with large feces rather than incontinence), meningomyelocele (tissue protrusion through a defect in the vertebral column), and other neuromedical disorders. Pathophysiological mechanisms include altered colon motility and contraction patterns, stretching and thinning of colon walls (megacolon), and decreased sensation or perception (usually appearing early in development). During infancy, fecal soiling may result from severe diaper rash: fecal withholding might help the infant avoid rectal pain. These medical causes of fecal soiling exclude the diagnosis of encopresis.

Abnormal secretion of gastrointestinal hormones or altered motility in the gastrointestinal tract could lead to constipation and overflow incontinence. Children with encopresis were reported to have normal secretion of gastrin and cholecystokinin; however, their levels of pancreatic polypeptide were found to reach their peak and remain abnormally high following meals, whereas postprandial motilin levels were diminished (H.P. Stern et al. 1995). These differences in hormone secretion and motility might explain the unusually chronic constipation associated with fecal overflow, although their association with encopresis also might be a result of the constipation.

Some encopretic children show neurodevelopmental symptoms, such as inattention, hyperactivity, impulsivity, low frustration tolerance, and dyscoordination. Neurodevelopmental theories of encopresis have been proposed, although most children with neurodevelopmental delays or disorders do not have encopresis, and most children with encopresis do not appear to have significant neurodevelopmental symptoms. Children with primary encopresis appear to have comorbid developmental delays and enuresis, whereas secondary enuresis is more likely to present with conduct disorder and psychosocial stressors (Foreman and Thambirajah 1996). This clustering supports a neurodevelopmental factor in the etiology of primary encopresis.

A familial occurrence of encopresis is well documented. About 15% of the children with encopresis have fathers who had encopresis during childhood. Unlike the findings in enuresis, psychosocial factors appear to be stronger than genetic factors in the familial transmission of encopresis.

Psychosocial stressors (suggestive of adverse circumstances) and conduct disorder (suggestive of family psychopathology) are associated with encopresis, specifically secondary enuresis (Foreman and Thambirajah 1996). Presumably, the loss of previously established sphincter control is secondary to intercurrent life events, such as disorder in the family and environment. In general, family psychopathology is overrepresented in encopresis and, in some cases, intrudes on the development of self-control and disrupts its consolidation.

Inadequate or punitive toilet training appears to be a cause of encopresis in some cases. Pathogenic approaches are those that usually are considered coercive, aggressive, perfectionistic, inconsistent, or neglectful. Some cases of encopresis reflect developmental complications. For example, encopresis can result from toilet-related fears that are not properly managed or from physical discomfort associated with inadequate physical support during toilet training (e.g., feet do not touch the ground). Stress-related factors appear causative in one-half of the cases of secondary encopresis, for example, frenetic rushing before school or during television commercials.

Course and Prognosis

Prevalence typically decreases over time throughout childhood, for both medically untreated and treated children. In children with chronic constipation and encopresis who also have concurrent psychiatric or medical disorders (unrelated to the encopresis), the disorder appearing comorbidly with encopresis can be the primary determinant of prognosis. For example, a more protracted course of encopresis is associated with the presence of conduct disorder, the use of soiling as a direct expression of anger, and parental disinterest in dealing with the problem.

Diagnostic Evaluation

Initial medical evaluation is required to evaluate possible structural abnormalities (e.g., anal fissure) and may involve barium enema. Psychiatric evaluation includes assessment of comorbid psychopathology, which is found in 35% of the children with encopresis. Typical comorbidity with encopresis includes conduct disorder, oppositional defiant disorder, psychotic disorders, mood disorders, and mental retardation.

Treatment

Many cases can be treated in a pediatric model by decompaction and behavioral treatment, but resistant cases may require psychiatric intervention. Pediatric management of cases may include bowel cleansing (laxatives, enemas), daily maintenance on mineral oil and high-fiber diets, counseling (education, reducing interpersonal struggles and negative affects, and rewards), and follow-up. Planned toilet sitting times can be helpful because bowel habits can be very susceptible to changes in daily routine in children (Youssef and Di Lorenzo 2001). Psychiatric comorbidity is higher among children who do not respond to these measures (Buttross 1999).

Although various behavioral treatments have been studied, relatively few have been well controlled (Brooks et al. 2000); none of these interventions are well established (McGrath et al. 2000). Anal sphincter biofeedback also appears effective for children when used in combination with conventional treatment (Cox et al. 1996), although its value may be time-limited. When used in association with conventional pediatric management, biofeedback can increase the response rate after 6 weeks of treatment from 20% to about 40% of children. However, both types of treatment produced improvement in about 50% of the children after 1 year of treatment (van der Plas et al. 1996).

Cisapride, a serotonin type 4 (5-HT$_4$) receptor agonist used to treat gastroesophageal influx, increases gastric motility and has been found helpful in a controlled trial for treating chronic constipation in children (Nurko et al. 2000); however, its tendency to induce QT prolongation makes this an undesirable treatment in routine cases.

In pediatric practice, approximately 50%–75% of the cases improve during the initial months of treatment (Levine 1982). Only 7% of the children with pediatrically treated encopresis and chronic constipation were encopretic at 7-year follow-up, and those patients had significant behavioral symptoms. In contrast, children whose chronic constipation (without encopresis) was pediatrically treated usually become asymptomatic. At 7-year follow-up, 70% of such children had a complete resolution of symptoms, and 25% had mild constipation occasionally; only 5% required occasional laxatives (Sutphen et al. 1995). Thus, a small but significant fraction of children with encopresis remain encopretic despite extended medical treatment (Rockney et al. 1996). In adults with encopresis, the effectiveness of medical treatment is not well delineated. Generally, residual encopresis in adolescence and adulthood is associated with psychopathology.

In resistant cases, or if aggressive pediatric treatment becomes counterproductive, individual and family psychiatric interventions are indicated. The focus of treatment then shifts from the encopresis to a more general treatment of associated psychopathological disorders.

Clinical Comment

Encopresis may be successfully approached with a pediatric model in most cases, but treatment-resistant cases may need psychiatric intervention. Even if major psychopathology can be immediately identified, medical evaluation is required in all cases to rule out possible organic causes.

Encopresis is commonly experienced by clinicians as "unattractive" because of both personal meanings and odor. This symptom and the patients who have it may be unconsciously but systematically avoided, and this avoidance constitutes a complication in psychiatric treatment as well as in the child's development.

Enuresis (Not Due to a General Medical Condition)

Urinary incontinence in young children, and occasionally in older children after the completion of toilet training, is a normal developmental phenomenon. Enuresis (not due to a general medical condition) is diagnosed when medically unexplained urinary incontinence is frequent, distressing, or interfering with activities (Table 20–28). Urinary bladder control is typically attained by age 3 or 4; therefore, DSM-IV-TR diagnosis requires a minimal age of 5 years. Before these presentations are designated as psychiatric disorders, a medical assessment of physical causes of enuresis (such as bladder infection or seizures) is required.

The DSM-IV-TR term *enuresis (not due to a general medical condition)* is inconvenient for efficient communication, but it avoids the problems connected with the DSM-III-R term *functional enuresis*. "Functional" disorders were originally distinguished from "organic" disorders to refer separately to the physical/medical and the mental/psychiatric realms. As the concepts of those realms have progressively merged, the terms have become outdated. Because the terms are convenient, however, they are used in the following discussion: *functional enuresis* refers here to enuresis not due to a general

TABLE 20–28. DSM-IV-TR diagnostic criteria for enuresis

A. Repeated voiding of urine into bed or clothes (whether involuntary or intentional).
B. The behavior is clinically significant as manifested by either a frequency of twice a week for at least 3 consecutive months or the presence of clinically significant distress or impairment in social, academic (occupational), or other important areas of functioning.
C. Chronological age is at least 5 years (or equivalent developmental level).
D. The behavior is not due exclusively to the direct physiological effect of a substance (e.g., a diuretic) or a general medical condition (e.g., diabetes, spina bifida, a seizure disorder).

Specify type:
 Nocturnal Only
 Diurnal Only
 Nocturnal and Diurnal

medical condition, and *enuresis* refers to enuresis regardless of cause.

Clinical Description

Bed-wetting is more common than daytime urinary incontinence. In the large majority of school-aged children, nocturnal enuresis is monosymptomatic (Varan et al. 1996), that is, not accompanied by daytime wetting or other urological conditions. Bed-wetting typically occurs 30 minutes to 3 hours after sleep onset, with the child either sleeping through the episode or being awakened by the moisture; however, for some children, enuresis may occur at any time during the night. Children with daytime (diurnal) enuresis usually have nocturnal enuresis too. About 30% of the children with nocturnal enuresis also have enuresis during the daytime (Kalo and Bella 1996).

In 80% of enuretic children, bladder control has not yet been attained, and the enuresis is primary (caused either by a uromedical disorder or by delayed learning of bladder control). In 20%, urinary incontinence is secondary (reappearing after competent functioning is attained, apparently caused by an intercurrent process). Several studies have suggested that primary (dysfunctional) enuresis is associated with less emotional disturbance or with mental retardation and that secondary (regressive) enuresis implies more serious psychopathology or stress (von Gontard et al. 1997). However, the distinction between primary and secondary enuresis has not been supported by other empirical studies. Most studies have found that stressors (concerning family stability, stressful life events before age 6 years, current psychosocial difficulties) are significant in both primary and secondary enuresis. Stronger evidence is available in youths to associate more comorbid psychopathology with older age at onset. Thus, the labels of *primary* and *secondary* enuresis may be used for descriptive rather than explanatory or mechanistic purposes. For some purposes, a more useful categorization is based on the distinction between patients with enuresis at night only, in the daytime only (rare), and in both the night and the day.

Epidemiology

Enuresis is common, but prevalence figures vary widely, depending partially on quantitative aspects of the definitional criteria. Nocturnal enuresis may occur occasionally in 25% of boys, but more problematic enuresis persists beyond age 5 in 7%–10% of boys and 3% of girls. The male predominance persists but decreases with age. At age 10 years, 3%–5% of boys and 2%–3% of girls are still diagnosable. In adulthood, general prevalence is 1%. A correlation with socioeconomic status has been suggested but not established.

Etiology

The mechanisms involved in developing and maintaining bladder control are not well described, and multiple etiologies are believed to produce enuresis. Three major mechanisms include 1) low nocturnal release of vasopressin, which may lead to increased urine volume, associated with a possible circadian abnormality; 2) bladder abnormalities, such as small functional volume and/or detrusor hyperactivity; and 3) inability to achieve adequate arousal during sleep to experience bladder fullness sensations. These different mechanisms are not necessarily independent.

Some children with nocturnal enuresis do not have a normal nighttime release of vasopressin (antidiuretic hormone) and so may not have the usual reduction in the formation of urine at night (Rittig et al. 1989). The low overnight plasma levels of vasopressin (from 11:00 P.M. to 4:00 A.M.) are associated with increased urination volume and decreased osmolality (Aikawa et al. 1999). No pituitary abnormalities were found on MRI to explain the defective control of the circadian rhythm of vasopressin (Hunsballe et al. 1996). Among the 1% of adults with nocturnal enuresis, nocturnal vasopressin release appears to be normal, but instead the mechanism appears to involve a reduced sensitivity of the kidneys to the antidiuretic effects of vasopressin (G. Robertson et al. 1999). In both children with decreased nocturnal vasopressin secretion and adults with decreased nocturnal vaso

pressin sensitivity, the lack of antidiuretic function is the basis for pharmacological treatment with desmopressin, an analogue of vasopressin.

Nocturnal polyuria has become recognized as a major factor in the etiology of many cases of "functional" enuresis. In fact, nocturnal bed-wetting sometimes can be induced in healthy children with ingestion of a water load at bedtime. In these cases, the wetting is elicited by a threshold volume that is specific to each individual and bears no correlation to bladder filling rate (Kirk et al. 1996).

Enuresis also can be caused by urological (urinary tract infection, especially in secondary enuresis in girls, or obstruction), anatomical (spinal disease, weak bladder or supporting musculature), physiological (abnormally low bladder pressure threshold or detrusor hyperactivity, leading to early emptying), metabolic (diabetes), and neurological (seizure disorder) mechanisms.

Disorders of sleep or diurnal rhythm may be etiological in some cases of functional enuresis. Although the nocturnal vasopressin changes can be interpreted in terms of a failure in diurnal regulation, some cases of enuresis are hypothesized to involve a failure of the reticular activating system to produce an adequate level of arousal during sleep to regulate bladder control (Neveus et al. 2000). The EEG findings are still debated; enuretic episodes can occur during any EEG stage, but there seems to be a concentration of episodes during delta (Stages III and IV, non-REM) sleep or postdelta arousal (transition from delta into REM sleep). One subtyping of enuresis involves the coupling of sleep EEG with sleep cystometry (Watanabe and Azuma 1989). In addition, some children with enuresis are described by their parents as "deep" sleepers, and "at-home" studies have confirmed that they were more difficult to awaken (arouse) in the morning.

A "maturational" disorder is suggested in certain cases by findings of short stature, low mean bone age for chronological age, delayed sexual maturation, and small volume of voidings (suggestive of small bladder capacity); however, bladder capacity is typically normal. More generally, enuresis is associated with an overrepresentation of developmental delays (Steinhausen and Gobel 1989). Also, children who have behavior problems and enuresis have more developmental delays and smaller voiding volumes than do enuretic children who do not have behavior problems; this finding suggests that at least some forms of enuresis with behavior problems are reflections of a developmental delay (Shaffer et al. 1984).

Approximately 50% of the children with functional enuresis have emotional or behavioral symptoms, but it is unclear whether this result represents cause, effect, or an associated finding (e.g., poor parental limit setting).

Functional enuresis also may be related to stress, trauma, or psychosocial crisis, such as the birth of a sibling, start of school, a move, hospitalization, a loss, parental absence, car accident, or developmental crisis. In contrast to other types of enuresis, stress-induced cases are equally prevalent in boys and girls. However, the roles of environmental stress, family support, and socioeconomic status have been questioned (Fergusson et al. 1986).

A higher prevalence of functional enuresis is associated with moderate and severe mental retardation. Voluntary enuresis may imply psychopathology, but it is often difficult to identify such psychopathology in individual cases or events, particularly if voluntary episodes are used to camouflage or cover for unintentional events.

Some forms of functional enuresis may run in families, particularly in males. Approximately 65%–70% of the children with this disorder have a first-degree relative with functional enuresis. The chances of a child having enuresis are 77% if both parents have history of enuresis and 44% if one parent has such a history (Bakwin 1973). A genetic linkage study of nocturnal enuresis in children suggested that up to 40% of families may be linked to loci on chromosome 22, but there was also evidence of broader genetic heterogeneity involving chromosomes 8, 12, and 13 among several others (von Gontard et al. 1999). A recessive mode of inheritance was observed in 9% of the families (Arnell et al. 1997; Eiberg et al. 1995).

Course and Prognosis

Enuresis remits spontaneously at a rate of approximately 15% per year (Forsythe and Butler 1989). Approximately 1% of boys (and fewer girls) still have this condition at age 18 years, generally with little associated psychopathology. The adolescent-onset form of enuresis, however, appears to have more associated psychopathology and a less favorable outcome. In adults, the onset of nocturnal enuresis, without daytime symptoms, often signifies serious urological pathology (Sakamoto and Blaivas 2001).

The symptoms of functional enuresis, at any age, can lead to embarrassment, anger and punishment from caregivers, teasing by peers, avoidance of overnight visiting and camp, social withdrawal, and angry outbursts. These complications, if not properly managed, can have a greater effect on long-term outcome than the enuresis itself.

Diagnostic Evaluation

An initial medical assessment is required to rule out the various nonfunctional forms of enuresis. With extensive urological evaluation, about 20% of youths with nocturnal enuresis are found to have a urological abnormality. In certain cases, a sleep evaluation may be useful, but an EEG is not routinely required. Measurement of certain maturational indexes may be useful for identifying simple developmental variance.

A specific form of enuresis, *giggle incontinence*, appears to result from altered muscle tone during laughter or emotionally intense moments. Although this form was traditionally resistant to treatment, psychostimulants appear to be effective. Giggle incontinence should be routinely considered during diagnostic evaluation because of its distinctive treatment.

Psychiatric evaluation of the child and parents includes assessment of associated psychopathology, recent psychosocial stressors, family concern about the symptom, and previous management of the symptoms. Inquiry about possible enuresis in the siblings is appropriate in view of their threefold increased risk. The proposed specific association of enuresis and depressive disorders has not been consistently supported in well-designed studies, but a stronger link has been found with ADHD. Children with ADHD are three times more likely to have nocturnal enuresis and five times more likely to have daytime enuresis than are children without ADHD (Robson et al. 1997); therefore, evaluation for ADHD is advisable in children with enuresis.

Treatment

Most cases of functional enuresis are treated by pediatricians, who strongly prefer behavioral to pharmacological interventions for enuresis (Skoog et al. 1997). Behavioral methods for treating nocturnal enuresis include restriction of prebedtime fluid intake, planned midsleep awakenings for voiding in toilet, and rewards for successful nights.

Since the 1930s, nocturnal enuresis has been commonly treated by a simple device: a moisture-sensitive blanket that, during an enuretic episode, sounds a bell that arouses the patient from sleep. The "bell and pad" method has a high success rate (80%–90%), but it also has a high relapse rate (up to 15%–40%). A lower relapse rate usually can be achieved if the bell is set up to awaken the parents, who themselves then awaken the child. If relapse occurs, reinitiation of the bell system is often effective (Forsythe and Butler 1989). There is sometimes considerable resistance to the consistent use of the alarm system by either parent or child. One recent innovation has been the use of a noninvasive ultrasound device that detects bladder size and gives feedback when bladder volume reaches a critical size (Pretlow 1999). Other behavioral methods are in widespread use, but they have not been as systematically tested.

Desmopressin, an analogue of the antidiuretic hormone vasopressin, has been successful in several double-blind trials in treating nocturnal enuresis (Glazener and Evans 2000a) and is now popularly prescribed by family practitioners and pediatricians. Its efficacy in 50%–80% of cases (Bonde et al. 1994; Caione et al. 1997; Wille 1986) is not as high as that of bell alarms, and the extent of improvement appears more limited. Only 60%–65% of patients with primary nocturnal enuresis have a marked reduction in wet nights (Skoog et al. 1997; Uygur et al. 1997). Some evidence indicates that desmopressin might be more effective in older children. Desmopressin also appears to be more effective for patients with a demonstrable excess of nocturnal vasopressin release (Rittig et al. 1997). Relapse is common when desmopressin treatment is discontinued. Adverse effects are usually minimal, with only 4% of patients experiencing significant side effects (nasal irritation, nose bleeds); however, 0.8% of the patients had hyponatremic seizures resulting from desmopressin-induced water intoxication. Because the seizures usually appear following excessive fluid intake, they might be significantly reduced if patients avoid excessive fluid ingestion, especially in the evening and near bedtime. Another major disadvantage is cost: a daily dosage of desmopressin costs more than $5 (average wholesale price in 2001), which is considerably higher than treatment with TCAs or the bell system.

TCAs can be helpful if a patient does not respond well to behavioral interventions, if daytime and nighttime enuresis are present, or if mood or anxiety disorder is associated. TCAs have been shown to be effective in many double-blind studies (Glazener and Evans 2000b), typically in low dosages (e.g., imipramine 25–125 mg or about 2 mg/kg nightly; EEG monitoring is absolutely mandatory; a daily dosage of 5 mg/kg is not to be exceeded). Some reports have suggested that the success rate is only 15% after discontinuation of antidepressants, but the success rate is probably higher if the dosage is tapered gradually. In view of the high rate of remission with placebo, it is sensible to attempt to lower the medication dosage every 4–6 months. In view of the high lethality of TCAs in overdose (particularly desipramine) and the reported sudden deaths during desipramine treatment (see "Treatment" subsection in the "Attention-Deficit/Hyperactivity Disorder" section earlier in this chapter), treatment of enuresis with desipramine should be avoided. Imipramine is much safer and is effective in treating enuresis. Carbamazepine is also efficacious in treating nocturnal enuresis (Al-Waili 2000). Also, access to pill bottles at home should be carefully controlled to minimize risks of overdose, which might result from the

child's attempt to make treatment go faster, a suicide attempt, or accidental ingestion by younger siblings.

The mechanism for the effect of TCAs on enuresis is unknown, but it is not the anticholinergic properties (anticholinergic agents are not effective); it may be related to the antidepressant property (MAOIs are also effective). Consistent with a catecholamine/alertness hypothesis, pseudoephedrine was reported to provide statistically significant improvement in primary nocturnal enuresis (Varan et al. 1996). Selective serotonin reuptake inhibitors have not been examined for antienuretic properties. In patients with nocturnal polyuria (without enuresis), imipramine may produce reductions in urine osmolality as well as volume, suggesting that imipramine may have an antidiuretic effect that is independent of its antienuretic effect (Hunsballe et al. 1997).

For daytime enuresis, oxybutynin has been reported to produce significant improvement in 54% of cases (Caione et al. 1997). Oxybutynin treats enuresis mainly by acting as a smooth muscle relaxant through its effect of blocking cholinergic receptors on the detrusor muscle. By diminishing bladder muscle contraction, oxybutynin increases bladder capacity, allows delay of the need to urinate, and thereby reduces the urgency and frequency of involuntary voiding (and voluntary urination). Oxybutynin may be used in combination with desmopressin or even with tricyclics (Kaneko et al. 2001) but may be less useful in patients with normal bladder function (Kosar et al. 1999).

For treating nocturnal enuresis in general, the alarm interventions, desmopressin, and TCAs are about equally effective during the treatment period (Glazener and Evans 2001). Desmopressin produces a more rapid therapeutic effect than the alarm system, but the alarm bell has a slightly higher rate of improvement and is slightly more likely to maintain effective symptom control after treatment discontinuation. In addition, on the basis of a cost-effectiveness analysis, researchers in Denmark concluded that the use of the alarm system would produce substantial net savings to society, whereas use of desmopressin would produce net losses (Ankjaer-Jensen and Sejr 1994). Overall, probably the most effective treatment for nocturnal enuresis is the bell alarm combined with desmopressin (Mellon and McGrath 2000), although imipramine might be used instead of desmopressin if cost is a concern and immediate symptom control is not essential.

Other interventions usually are not necessary in most cases of functional enuresis, although the presence of secondary enuresis might suggest possible benefits from counseling. Psychotherapy may be useful for the uncommon case in which the symptom of enuresis is interpersonally cathected (e.g., into an oppositional struggle or into expression of rage) or for patients with significant comorbid psychopathology.

Management of the embarrassment, low self-esteem, and behavioral avoidance that often accompany this disorder is usually a critical part of the treatment for children and adults in the United States. In contrast, enuresis does not cause as much concern in Australia, either for the child or for the family (Bower et al. 1996). When dealing with the emotional complications of enuresis, it is usually helpful to deemphasize the conscious or unconscious explanations that might engender shame or guilt and instead to focus more specifically on the symptom alleviation.

Clinical Comment

Like encopresis, enuresis (not due to a general medical condition) may be managed successfully in most cases by pediatricians who use behavioral interventions. Even when secondary functional enuresis appears to signal significant psychosocial or developmental stress, pediatric interventions may be sufficient to restore adequate developmental progress. Psychiatric intervention is crucial in certain cases of functional enuresis, particularly when psychopathology, late-onset enuresis without medical explanation, or interpersonal cathexis of the symptoms is associated. The high success rate in treating nocturnal enuresis with a vasopressin analogue, coupled with findings of diminished nocturnal release of the antidiuretic hormone, has added a new dimension to the understanding of this medical disorder. The hormonal and/or circadian abnormalities, coupled with the apparent genetic and pathophysiological heterogeneity, show that even "functional" disorders may not be as "psychological" as previously believed.

Other Disorders of Infancy, Childhood, or Adolescence

Separation Anxiety Disorder

In addition to normal situational and developmental anxiety, children can show genuine anxiety disorders. These pathological states are common but are frequently dismissed by parents, pediatricians, and psychiatrists as mere "anxiety." Children are commonly imagined to be innately fearful, and adolescence is seen as naturally anxiety provoking. Anxiety is viewed as so ordinary in children that often due consideration is not given to the possibility of an anxiety disorder.

Separation anxiety, a normal developmental phenomenon at age 18–30 months, has been traditionally described in terms of attachment and separation theory (see Chapter 2). A nonpathological form of separation anxiety is sometimes observed in adults or children who have been geographically displaced and are feeling homesick; examples include students, soldiers, immigrants, refugees, and hospitalized patients (Van Tilburg et al. 1996).

In separation anxiety disorder, cognitive, affective, somatic, and behavioral symptoms appear in response to genuine or fantasied separation from attachment figures (Table 20–29). Separation anxiety disorder can present clinically in a variety of ways, including difficulty in falling asleep (prebedtime agitation) and school absenteeism (Bernstein and Borchardt 1991).

Separation anxiety disorder is the only anxiety disorder listed in DSM-IV-TR as a disorder usually first diagnosed infancy, childhood, or adolescence. Like other anxiety disorders in children, separation anxiety disorder can lead to social problems, academic underachievement, and interference with developing assertiveness skills and personal autonomy, often resulting in social awkwardness (or "immaturity") and sometimes a reluctance to date. Unlike many child psychiatric disorders, the anxiety disorders often cause more distress to the children than to the parents (although the parents may themselves be quite anxious because of their own anxiety disorders).

As in adults, anxiety disorders tend to present in clusters, and most children with separation anxiety disorder have other comorbid anxiety disorders. In fact, the comorbidity of separation anxiety disorder with other anxiety disorders is so extensive that it is difficult to examine separation anxiety disorder in isolation from social phobia, generalized anxiety disorder, and panic disorder. At present, much of the medical literature on separation anxiety disorder is actually about separation anxiety disorder in the context of other anxiety disorders, and one of the major research challenges remains to distinguish what is distinct about separation anxiety disorder itself.

Clinical Description

The usual focus of the anxiety is fear of separation from a major attachment object, typically a parent or caregiver, but it can be a favorite toy or familiar place. Generally, even a young child can specify the attachment object that gives a sense of protection or safety (from anxiety). Common presentations include preoccupying or morbid fear of parents' death, clinging to parents, school avoidance, sleep refusal, resistance to being alone, nightmares, antic-

TABLE 20–29. DSM-IV-TR diagnostic criteria for separation anxiety disorder

A. Developmentally inappropriate and excessive anxiety concerning separation from home or from those to whom the individual is attached, as evidenced by three (or more) of the following:
   (1) recurrent excessive distress when separation from home or major attachment figures occurs or is anticipated
   (2) persistent and excessive worry about losing, or about possible harm befalling, major attachment figures
   (3) persistent and excessive worry that an untoward event will lead to separation from a major attachment figure (e.g., getting lost or being kidnapped)
   (4) persistent reluctance or refusal to go to school or elsewhere because of fear of separation
   (5) persistently and excessively fearful or reluctant to be alone or without major attachment figures at home or without significant adults in other settings
   (6) persistent reluctance or refusal to go to sleep without being near a major attachment figure or to sleep away from home
   (7) repeated nightmares involving the theme of separation
   (8) repeated complaints of physical symptoms (such as headaches, stomachaches, nausea, or vomiting) when separation from major attachment figures occurs or is anticipated
B. The duration of the disturbance is at least 4 weeks.
C. The onset is before age 18 years.
D. The disturbance causes clinically significant distress or impairment in social, academic (occupational), or other important areas of functioning.
E. The disturbance does not occur exclusively during the course of a pervasive developmental disorder, schizophrenia, or other psychotic disorder and, in adolescents and adults, is not better accounted for by panic disorder with agoraphobia.

Specify if:
   Early Onset: if onset occurs before age 6 years

ipatory worrying, cognitive disruption, or somatization. Although the anxiety is usually centered around separation from a parent, the fear can instead manifest as an anticipatory fear of being injured, kidnapped, or killed. Interference with autonomous functioning can extend to inability to sleep in one's own bed, visit friends, go on errands, or stay at camp.

Homesickness, a manifestation of separation anxiety, appears to be a distinct phenomenon from separation anxiety disorder. Homesickness was reported by 18% of 8- to 16-year-old boys at a 2-week summer camp. Although it appeared to be associated with depressive and anxiety symptoms, it decreased with age and separation experiences (Thurber 1999). Homesickness may be freely described by young children ("I want my mommy") but can be difficult to admit for adolescents, especially boys. In contrast, the symptoms of separation anxiety disorder are often quite evident and freely admitted to parents by children. Separation anxiety disorder usually is relieved temporarily by physical proximity to the attachment object, but children whose actual life circumstances involve separation are not necessarily at increased risk for separation anxiety disorder (Federer et al. 2000).

Children with separation anxiety may sense a clear "line of demarcation" that separates safe from unsafe: they may be able to enter the school hallways but not the classroom, or they may be able to play in the school yard but not be able to walk into the school building; they may be able to leave the house but not cross a particular street.

More than 92% of the children with separation anxiety disorder have other DSM-IV-TR disorders, typically anxiety or mood disorders (Table 20–30). Many children with major depressive disorder also fulfill criteria for separation anxiety disorder.

These children typically have internalizing behaviors and psychological mechanisms. Pathological compliance, perfectionism, and "nicey-nice" presentation of self may be seen. The children can show somatizations (stomachaches, headaches) in the morning on school days, a fear of teachers ("They're mean"), or passive-aggressive traits. In some cases, however, anxiety disorders in children can become the basis for disruptive behavior symptoms.

The prominence of somatization with separation anxiety is similar to that of panic, phobic, generalized anxiety, and depressive disorders of adulthood. Children with separation anxiety disorder commonly experience stomachaches and palpitations, and they generally have more somatic complaints than do children with any other psychiatric disorder (Livingston et al. 1988). Separation anxiety disorder has many characteristics of phobic disorders, which often appear comorbidly. Separation anxiety disorder differs from other anxiety disorders in its focus on separation and its early appearance (usually first diagnosed in childhood). It differs from phobic disorders in that the latter may be directed toward myriad potential sources of fear.

School absenteeism is reported in about 75% of the children with separation anxiety disorder, and separation anxiety disorder is reported in up to 50%–80% of school absentees (Klein and Last 1989); however, these conditions are quite distinct. The terms *school phobia*, *school avoidance*, and *school refusal* are misnomers: most school "phobics" are not in fact phobic, and the terms *avoidance*

TABLE 20–30. Comparison of children with separation anxiety disorder and children with school-related phobic disorders

	Children with separation anxiety disorder	Children with phobic disorders
Age at referral (mean)	9 years	14 years
Sex ratio (M:F)	1:2	2:1
Low socioeconomic class (Hollingshead IV or V)	32%	68%
Concurrent DSM-III disorder	92%	63%
Concurrent anxiety disorder	50%	53%
Concurrent mood disorder	33%	32%
Maternal anxiety disorder	83%	57%
Maternal mood disorder	63%	14%

Note. These children were referred to an outpatient psychiatric clinic and were diagnosed with separation anxiety disorder or a phobic disorder (simple or social) regarding school. Although concomitant mood and anxiety disorders are common in both disorders, the children and mothers showed more psychopathology associated with separation anxiety disorder than with phobic disorders.
Source. Data from Last et al. 1987.

and *refusal* imply psychological mechanisms that may not apply. A more descriptively neutral and accurate label is *school absenteeism*, a term that has the advantage of highlighting a possible connection with job absenteeism. School absenteeism has a variety of etiologies (Table 20–31). Not all children with school absenteeism have separation anxiety, and not all children with separation anxiety disorder have school absenteeism (Last et al. 1987).

In some cases of school absenteeism, the parent and child are bound to each other by psychodynamically based fears of separation. The classical psychoanalytic description (A.M. Johnson et al. 1941) is consistent with recent findings of mood disorders and separation anxiety in both parent and child associated with school absenteeism. A more modern construct showed that the presence of separation anxiety disorder in children was associated with excessive criticism and emotional overinvolvement by parents in an "expressed emotion" paradigm (Hirshfeld et al. 1997).

Epidemiology

Separation anxiety disorder is common and tends to run in families. Epidemiological studies report a prevalence of 2%–5% among children (B. Masi et al. 2001) and a decrease with age. The sex ratio is equal or female predominant (2:1). Unlike other anxiety disorders, 50%–75% of these children's families live in low socioeconomic status (Last et al. 1992; Velez et al. 1989).

School absenteeism is common, with 75% of adults admitting to this behavior during childhood. At some inner-city schools, absenteeism may be observed in more than 90% of students. Large-scale studies of school absenteeism have not been pursued from a psychiatric

TABLE 20–31. Sources of school absenteeism

Separation anxiety disorder
Truancy (often associated with conduct disorder)
Psychiatric disorders usually first diagnosed in adulthood
  Mood disorders
    Major depressive disorder
    Bipolar disorder
  Other anxiety disorders
    Overanxious disorder
    Phobic disorder
    Panic disorder
    Obsessive-compulsive disorder
  Overt psychotic disorders (rare)
Sociocultural conformity
  Permission granted by family (e.g., overt or covert support to stay at home to take care of siblings, to earn money, or to avoid tests)
  Normative peer behavior in certain locales (spending time with peers rather than going to school)
Realistic fear of bodily harm in dangerous school setting
Drug-induced absenteeism (e.g., propranolol, haloperidol)

point of view. The extent of school absenteeism that is specifically due to separation anxiety disorder, and not to comorbidity, is undetermined.

Etiology

Developmental theorists have speculated about mechanisms contributing to separation anxiety disorder. A temperamental factor is suggested by the findings that children who are shy, fearful, or "behaviorally inhibited" before age 3 years (Kagan et al. 1987) have an increased prevalence of anxiety disorders at follow-up. Insecure (resistant) attachment during infancy, as assessed on the Strange Situation test (Ainsworth et al. 1978), was found to be associated with the presence of anxiety disorders in 28% of the patients followed up to age 17 years (Warren et al. 1997).

The relation of separation anxiety disorder and school absenteeism to mood and other anxiety disorders has been an area of active research. There remains some debate about whether separation anxiety disorder in children exists entirely independently of associated major depressive disorder or other anxiety disorders. The comorbidity and familial and developmental relationships are extremely involved. Biological markers suggest that separation anxiety disorder is related to both depressive and panic disorders.

Cross-sectionally, separation anxiety disorder is commonly seen in association with major depressive disorder in children. Children with dysthymic disorder who did not have concurrent major depression had a high prevalence of anxiety disorder, especially separation anxiety disorder (33%) (G. Masi et al. 2001). Among children and adolescents with panic disorder, separation anxiety disorder was comorbid in 73% (G. Masi et al. 2000b). However, youths do not appear to show a cross-sectional association between separation anxiety disorder and agoraphobia (Federer et al. 2000).

Separation anxiety disorder occurs at higher frequency in children whose family histories include alcoholism, panic disorder with agoraphobia, or depression. More than half of the children with separation anxiety disorder have parents with mood or anxiety disorders (Table 20–30). The risk of separation anxiety in a child is increased by the presence of panic disorder or major depression in a parent, for both individual and comorbid presentations of these disorders (Biederman et al. 2001a; Unnewehr et al. 1998).

Similar to children with separation anxiety disorder, many children with school absenteeism have mood disorders or one of several anxiety disorders, and their parents also may have these disorders (Figure 20–4). When children with school absenteeism are divided into those with phobic disorder and those with separation anxiety disorder, it appears that the parents of the school absentees with phobic disorder have an increased prevalence of simple or social phobia, whereas the parents of school absentees with separation anxiety disorder have an increased prevalence of panic disorder (C. Martin et al. 1999).

Another proposed etiological factor for separation anxiety disorder is PTSD. Separation anxiety disorder was the most common comorbid diagnosis in the 50% of sexually and/or physically abused boys who developed

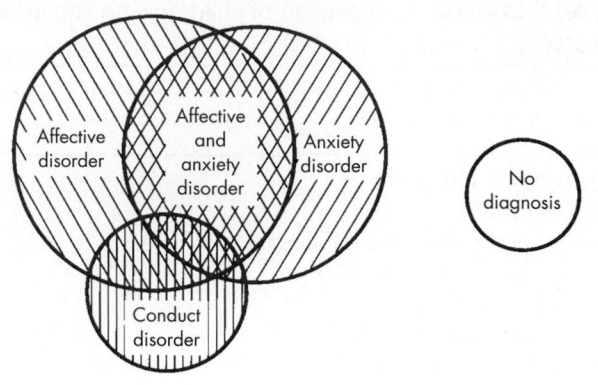

FIGURE 20–4. School absenteeism: overlap with affective, anxiety, and conduct disorders.
Source. Reprinted with permission from Bernstein GA, Garfinkel BD: "School Phobia: The Overlap of Affective and Anxiety Disorders." *Journal of the American Academy of Child Psychiatry* 25:235–241, 1986. Copyright 1986, American Academy of Child Psychiatry.

PTSD (Dykman et al. 1997). Also, children living with parental violence are at increased risk for separation anxiety disorder (Pelcovitz et al. 2000). It is unclear whether the appearance of separation anxiety disorder in this group is a result of traumatic abuse, PTSD, psychological grief, or concurrent depressive disorders or whether it is a marker for family chaos and abuse.

Biological markers suggest possible connections of separation anxiety disorder to depressive and panic disorders. A study of dexamethasone suppression testing in children with separation anxiety disorder suggested that positive test results (nonsuppression) are seen nearly as often as in children with major depressive disorder (Livingston et al. 1984), possibly reflecting the high rate of comorbidity or a physiological similarity between separation anxiety disorder and major depressive disorder. In addition, children with separation anxiety disorder have been found to show an increased physiological sensitivity to inhaled carbon dioxide (Pine et al. 2000), similar to adults with panic disorder. Children with other anxiety disorders also showed this increased sensitivity, including somatic symptoms and respiratory changes, but the most pronounced changes were seen in separation anxiety disorder.

Course and Prognosis

Separation anxiety disorder may be diagnosed after the normative period of separation anxiety, but it is typically not observed before age 4 years. It is usually first recognized in early or mid childhood. Separation anxiety disorder is typically a chronic disorder, but exacerbations may occur at times of actual separations, deaths, illness, family moves, or natural disasters. Symptoms might be aggravated during episodes of comorbid psychiatric disorders. Symptoms also may worsen during or after medical illness, particularly chronic medical conditions with acute exacerbations. Multiple medical examinations are commonly sought by the child or parents.

School absentees often show academic underachievement and social avoidance, and they can be at risk for chronic unemployment in adulthood. Just as they have difficulty getting to school, they have difficulty getting to their jobs. A long-term follow-up study of school absentees after age 30 (Flakierska-Praquin et al. 1997) found that, compared with psychiatric and nonclinical control subjects, they were more likely to live with their parents and had fewer children. When compared with child psychiatric control subjects, the former school absentees had better general psychosocial adjustment but had received more psychiatric treatment.

Just as the biological markers of separation anxiety suggested relations to both panic and depressive disorder, similar suggestions are seen in longitudinal studies. Long-term follow-up studies have suggested an increased risk for the development of other anxiety disorders, especially panic disorder with agoraphobia, and possibly depressive disorder (Klein and Last 1989). A follow-up study of children with separation anxiety disorder (who also had a communication disorder) found that 44% no longer had an anxiety disorder after 4 years; however, 11% still had separation anxiety disorder, and 33% had a different diagnosis, typically another anxiety disorder (Cantwell and Baker 1989). Also, separation anxiety disorder in childhood appears associated with early-onset panic disorder (Battaglia et al. 1995) but not in all studies (Hayward et al. 2000). Adults with panic disorder, especially those with agoraphobia, reported childhood symptoms of separation anxiety disorder even more often than did adults with generalized anxiety disorder or phobic disorder (Silove et al. 1995). The developmental link with childhood separation anxiety disorder does not appear to be specific to adult panic disorder because separation anxiety disorder appears to function as a risk factor for the comorbid appearance of multiple anxiety disorders in adults (Lipsitz et al. 1994). However, one study found that panic disorder with agoraphobia was the only anxiety disorder in adults that was associated with retrospectively recalled childhood separation anxiety (Manicavasagar et al. 1998).

The majority (68%) of children of adults with agoraphobia were found to have diagnosable psychiatric disorders, especially anxiety disorders in general and separation anxiety disorder in particular (Capps et al. 1996; Unnewehr et al. 1998). One-half of the children of parents with social phobia were found to have an anxiety disorder, and 19% of the total had separation anxiety disorder (Mancini et al. 1996). Agoraphobic mothers reported a high incidence of stomachaches during their own childhoods, and their reports indicated that their children had a high incidence of school absenteeism (14%) and stomachaches (Berg 1976). It may be speculated that childhood separation anxiety develops into adult panic disorder or, at least, that childhood separation anxiety is one of several possible antecedents of panic disorder in adults (Ollendick et al. 1994).

A much simpler connection between childhood and adult anxiety disorders has more recently been examined. Perhaps because of the prominence of panic and other anxiety disorders in adults, the presence of separation anxiety disorder in adults has been relatively underdiagnosed, and the developmental connection between childhood and adult separation anxiety disorder has not been emphasized. In fact, 63% of the children with separation anxiety disorder have at least one parent who fulfills the criteria for the disorder (Manicavasagar et al. 2001). The symptoms appeared to persist from childhood, typically preceding the appearance of other anxiety disorders, and severity of childhood symptoms accounted for 33% of the variance in separation anxiety scores in adulthood (Manicavasagar et al. 2000). These children may later develop panic disorder and find that their separation anxiety disorder becomes neglected (Manicavasagar and Silove 1997).

The link between separation anxiety disorder and suicidality is complex. Independently of depressive disorders, separation anxiety is strongly associated with suicidality in adolescents (Feldman and Wilson 1997). However, in children younger than 16 years, separation anxiety was present in a lower percentage of actual attempters than among children with suicidal ideation or nonsuicidal youth (Strauss et al. 2000), perhaps suggesting that the presence of separation anxiety disorder might reduce the risk of a suicidal youth actually attempting a suicidal act.

Diagnostic Evaluation

The workup includes assessment of possible mood disorder or anxiety (phobic, panic) disorder. These disorders, as well as separation anxiety disorder, also should be evaluated in the parents.

Clinically, it is sometimes difficult to distinguish the presenting symptoms of separation anxiety disorder from ordinary acute anxiety. Both conditions can involve distractibility, distorted cognition, depersonalization, transient impairment in reality sense, motoric overactivity, and angry outbursts. However, the presence of separation anxiety disorder implies that separation-related psychodynamics are the primary trigger of the acute anxiety.

Some severe disorders may present with separation anxiety and exclude a separate diagnosis of separation anxiety disorder. Children with autistic disorder or other pervasive developmental disorders often have separation anxiety, but evidence of neurological and psychiatric dysfunction usually can be identified across a wide area of functions. Schizophrenia can initially present in children as separation anxiety, with impaired early object relations (e.g., being viewed as "weird" by peers, living as a "loner") appearing before more overt psychotic symptoms emerge.

Occasionally, separation anxiety disorder, school absenteeism, and panic attacks are drug-induced. Propranolol (used for treating headache) or haloperidol (for associated Tourette's disorder or psychosis) may induce transient periods of separation anxiety disorder or school absenteeism that resolve on discontinuation of medication (Popper 1993). Risperidone might be more likely than olanzapine to induce separation anxiety (Hanna et al. 1999). Therefore, it is worth evaluating current medication regimens for agents that might aggravate "depression."

Differential diagnosis may be complicated by an unexpected form of separation anxiety. Developmentally normal children who had low birth weights and neonatal ultrasound evidence of ventricular enlargement or brain parenchymal lesions were found to have an increased likelihood of separation anxiety at age 6 years (Whitaker et al. 1997). In contrast, separation anxiety was not identified in similar children with neonatal intraventricular hemorrhage or brain matrix disorders, suggesting some degree of neuropathological specificity. This finding implies that early brain injury could be an etiology of some forms of separation anxiety in children.

Treatment

The traditional treatment of separation anxiety disorder entails psychosocial interventions (individual psychotherapy combined with family therapy or parental guidance), often with antianxiety or antidepressant medication.

Antidepressants are commonly used for treating separation anxiety disorder. Fluoxetine has been reported in uncontrolled case series to be useful for treating separation anxiety disorder (Birmaher et al. 1994; Fairbanks et al. 1997; Manassis and Bradley 1994). In a controlled study, fluvoxamine was effective for children with anxiety disorders such as separation anxiety disor-

der (Research Unit on Pediatric Psychopharmacology Anxiety Study Group 2001), but selective serotonin reuptake inhibitors have not been rigorously examined for treating separation anxiety per se or for treating school absenteeism. TCAs have been studied mainly in children with school absenteeism and separation anxiety disorder, and a substantial literature questions their usefulness for this indication (Klein et al. 1992; Popper 1993). Newer antidepressants, such as bupropion or venlafaxine, have not been systematically examined.

Antidepressant treatments may be considered for children whose school absenteeism exceeds 2 weeks and is not explained by a medical problem, truancy, overt psychosis, sociocultural conformity, or realistic fear of physical danger. An open-label study of fluoxetine reported clinical improvement in all 10 children and adolescents with separation anxiety disorder and 8 of 10 youths with social phobia but only 1 of 7 with generalized anxiety disorder (Fairbanks et al. 1997). Antidepressants are probably effective in the many cases of school absenteeism in which the underlying etiology is separation anxiety disorder, mood disorder, phobic disorder, or panic disorder. However, the value of these treatments remains in question because the available studies are small; no large-scale investigations of antidepressants for treating either separation anxiety disorder or school absenteeism have been done.

Benzodiazepines (mainly alprazolam and clonazepam) and buspirone also have been used for children and parents with separation anxiety disorder, although with mixed success (Bernstein et al. 1990; Graae et al. 1994; Kranzler 1988; Simeon et al. 1992). Clinically, these agents appear to be helpful for the "anticipatory" anxiety that can develop secondarily around "primary" anxiety symptoms, but adequate studies are needed.

If a parent has an anxiety or a mood disorder causing difficulty in separating from the child, the parent should receive direct psychiatric treatment as well as behavioral guidance for parenting. Antidepressant treatment of mood or anxiety disorders in a parent is commonly a part of the treatment of separation anxiety disorder in a child.

Separation anxiety disorder also can be partially alleviated by the use of a "high-tech" method: the attachment figure is given an electronic beeper, and the child is given a coin, allowing a telephone call to the parent in the event of a surge of anxiety. Typically, the child will use the beeper to contact the parent once or twice and then uses the coin as a symbol of the capacity to reach the attachment figure if needed. The parent tends to relax once it is clear that the child feels less anxious when separated. This technique also can be useful in facilitating school attendance.

Cognitive-behavioral therapy and family management appear to be useful in controlled studies for treating separation anxiety disorder (P.M. Barrett 1998; P.M. Barrett et al. 1996; Kendall 1994; Kendall et al. 2001; Muris et al. 2001; Southam-Gerow et al. 2001) and school absenteeism (N.J. King et al. 1998). Goals of cognitive-behavioral treatment may include positive self-instruction and self-talk, cognitive restructuring, emotive imagery, graded exposure and desensitization, reduction in social anxiety, social problem solving, social skills training, and increasing levels of social participation. Parent involvement is also useful (Mendelowitz et al. 1999) to reinforce the child's successes, promote the child's social participation, and model appropriate behaviors. Forced school attendance appears to be highly effective for cases of school "refusal" (Blagg and Yule 1984), but it may be judged inappropriate in individual cases.

Psychodynamic aspects of individual and family psychotherapies have more regularly appearing characteristics for this disorder than for most childhood disorders. For children with separation anxiety disorder, the child's experience of psychotherapy is organized around the actual "separations within the therapy." It is advisable to pay special attention to planned and unplanned absences (vacations by the patient or therapist, school transitions, therapist or teacher pregnancy, parental unavailability, therapist illness, deaths) and to the termination of treatment. It is often useful to give the child a concrete object or souvenir, or a clearly verbalized image of the therapist's future activity, at the time of interruption or termination. Preventive verbal anticipation, preparation of the parents as well as the child, and active discussion of the practicalities surrounding expected separations are useful in the management of these cases.

It is advised that strong emphasis be placed on termination work with the parents as well as with the child. The parents' own separation issues and psychopathology may lead them to be intolerant of the "loss" affects, to push for an abrupt finish, or to undervalue the importance of psychodynamic issues elicited at termination. Both child and parents may be observed to "rehearse" different aspects of the treatment termination before its completion. Much like their children, parents with separation anxiety disorder may have distorted cognitions regarding terminations ("I was not sure that you would allow us to come back"); therefore, explicit articulation of this point before termination is useful. Particularly for parents with mood or anxiety disorders, who may themselves be vulnerable at times of psychological loss or stress, it is useful to be specific about the mechanism for return to treatment.

More generally, there is extensive dynamic interaction between the separation anxiety of the child and the anxiety of the parent or parents, even if the family conceals their more overt wishes to encourage the child's dependency and their worry about the child's independent action. The treatments of the child and the parent will interact extensively as well, giving a clinician opportunities to intervene at two points in the self-stimulating system. Children with anxiety disorders tend to have dysfunctional cognitions that lead them to underestimate their ability to cope with dangerous or ambiguous situations (Bogels and Zigterman 2000), and parents often share and reinforce these viewpoints; thus, a cognitive-behavioral approach that involves child and parents may be useful for enhancing their attitudes to self-management. In the event that hospitalization of the child is needed, the parent's own separation fears might make it difficult for him or her to tolerate having the child away from home. This may appear to be a lack of cooperation with treatment, but it is more helpful to understand that the parent can only view the measure as too extreme. Management of the parent's separation anxiety at this juncture is crucial and a major part of the treatment because it allows the successful initiation of genuine psychotherapy for the separation anxiety disorder in the child. Occasionally, this situation can lead to joint hospitalization of the child and the parent (Chabrol et al. 1995).

A common pitfall in the treatment of this disorder is an overemphasis by the parents and professionals on the presenting symptoms (e.g., poor school attendance) rather than on the child's broader problems and long-term development. A child's ability to attend school consistently or to manage anxiety quietly signifies behavioral improvement, but the child may be left with psychodevelopmental liabilities. It is essential to maintain a wide perspective on the psychopathology and the risk for adult impairment to prevent premature closure of therapeutic work.

Another pitfall in the treatment of this disorder in children and parents involves pathological compliance. Some parents and children have an overly "good" or "nice" presentation of self, and their perfectionistic manner of managing themselves can prevent them from exposing their deeper thoughts and feelings. "Pathological pleasantness" in a child or parents needs to be monitored during the course of treatment and not mistaken for substantial understanding, support, or change.

Limit setting in the treatment of separation anxiety disorder can be useful or disruptive. If the child has a panic disorder or major depressive episode, limit setting can be counterproductive and aggravate the symptoms. Forcing a child with panic disorder to attend school can result in a temper tantrum or physical assault. However, "therapeutic coercion," sensitively applied, can be helpful in some cases of true separation anxiety disorder, particularly if the intervention is appropriately timed after drug treatment. For treating truancy (a far more common cause of school absenteeism), limit setting is certainly a useful and often necessary measure for establishing a routine daily structure in the child's life.

Psychosocial measures are also appropriate for managing school absenteeism based on fear of physical danger, family "permission," or subcultural "hanging out" with peers.

Clinical Comment

The emerging view is that children with separation anxiety disorder tend to become separation-anxious adults with panic disorder, but the long-term diagnostic outcome of children with school absenteeism is less clear. School absenteeism appears to be a more heterogeneous category, deriving from a variety of etiologies.

Comorbidity, family, longitudinal, biological marker, and pharmacological data suggest that separation anxiety disorder is related to panic disorder and, less clearly, depressive disorders. Indeed, a debate remains about whether separation anxiety disorder exists in the absence of mood or anxiety disorders, raising questions about the validity of this diagnosis. It is interesting to note that there are parallel debates about whether separation anxiety disorder exists as a distinct disorder in adults and whether panic disorder exists in children.

Research is needed regarding the relation of separation anxiety disorder to other child and adult psychiatric disorders, especially in view of the high prevalence of school absenteeism and adult unemployment. Treatment in these children requires a serious focus beyond their prominent presenting symptoms. The high prevalence of concurrent psychopathology and long-term developmental liabilities requires anticipatory clinical attention. Helping parents and school personnel to recognize the broader psychopathology and psychodevelopmental risks of separation anxiety disorder requires ongoing collaborative work, consultation, and advocacy at schools.

Selective Mutism

Children with selective mutism do not use speech in specific settings and show abnormalities of interpersonal behavior and social assertiveness. This uncommon disorder was initially described more than 100 years ago, but the medical literature on selective mutism consisted mainly of individual case reports until quite recently. The paucity of large-scale controlled studies impeded the accumulation of systematic and statistical descriptions, which are only now becoming available. This disorder, formerly viewed in almost exclusively psychodynamic terms, is now reconceptualized in view of findings of the prominent role of anxiety disorders and developmental delays.

Clinical Description

In selective mutism, children do not speak in one or several of the major environments in which they live. Even though they can talk without difficulty in certain places (usually at home), partial or total muteness appears selectively in unfamiliar places or particular social situations (Table 20–32). Typically, speech is normal at home when the child is alone with parents and siblings, and communication is constricted in the presence of teachers, peers, and strangers. When separated from a familiar or comfortable environment, these children might freely or hesitantly use gestural speech, nods, monosyllabic responses, written notes, or whispers, but they avoid full vocalization and verbal speech.

Although many children with selective mutism have normal language capabilities, developmental disorders or delays appear to be present in most of these children (Kristensen 2000). Approximately one-third of these children have a language disorder, and about one-half have a speech disorder or delayed speech development (Kolvin and Fundudis 1981). In addition, children with selective mutism have an increased prevalence of neurological disorders and mental retardation. The traditional assumption that children with selective mutism have normal speech, language, and biological development is not true in most cases.

TABLE 20–32. DSM-IV-TR diagnostic criteria for selective mutism

A. Consistent failure to speak in specific social situations (in which there is an expectation for speaking, e.g., at school) despite speaking in other situations.

B. The disturbance interferes with educational or occupational achievement or with social communication.

C. The duration of the disturbance is at least 1 month (not limited to the first month of school).

D. The failure to speak is not due to a lack of knowledge of, or comfort with, the spoken language required in the social situation.

E. The disturbance is not better accounted for by a communication disorder (e.g., stuttering) and does not occur exclusively during the course of a pervasive developmental disorder, schizophrenia, or other psychotic disorder.

Anxiety disorders are highly prevalent among these children (Black and Uhde 1995; Dummit et al. 1997; Kristensen 2000). Many children with selective mutism have school absenteeism, problems with separation, anxiety, and obsessive-compulsive features. Most children had behavioral abnormalities that were observed before age 6 years.

Usually, widespread impairments of social behavior and, sometimes, behavioral control are seen. Many of these children show early and persistent shyness, submissiveness, excessive dependency, timidity in activities involving personal assertiveness, clinging to parents, sulky behavior with strangers, temper tantrums, and regressive behaviors. At times, these children may show streaks of oppositionality, demanding and controlling behavior, passive-aggressiveness, and defiance.

In many of the published case reports, overly strong emotional ties to the mother and maternal overprotectiveness were emphasized. Parental fear, anxiety, agoraphobia, and shyness, but also parental aggressivity and violence, were often described. The parents' use of silence as a weapon of anger and a means of coercion also was repeatedly highlighted.

Early facial injury, mouth trauma (dental surgery), or oral punishment (washing out the mouth, slapping the face) were commonly described, especially during the period of speech development. Children with selective mutism are sometimes compared with children who, after the developmental period of normal stranger anxiety, are hesitant to speak in new situations. Many psychiatrically normal children have major difficulty in speaking on initially entering kindergarten, but this hesitancy resolves as the people and environment become familiar.

In a large study of 68 children with selective mutism (Hayden 1980), four subtypes of this disorder were distinguished on the basis of psychodynamic and behavioral features. The *symbiotic* form of selective mutism involves a dominant mother who is openly jealous of the child's relationships with other people, a father who is passive or speaks minimally, and a child who seems submissive but can be intensely manipulative. This subgroup is the largest, and its description closely parallels the usual clinical descriptions. *Passive-aggressive* children with selective mutism use silence in a defiant and hostile manner, show antisocial and often aggressive behaviors, and generally have parents with overt antisocial features. *Reactive* (or perhaps depressed) children commonly show depressive features and social withdrawal, have a parent with a mood disorder, and often have a family history of shyness. The *speech-phobic* children appear literally afraid to hear their own voices, show autonomic excitatory reactions in response to hearing themselves talk

(even on audiotape), show obvious ritualistic and compulsive behaviors, and show a strong motivation to overcome their symptoms.

In the same study, Hayden (1980) also reported a high prevalence of physical and sexual abuse in children with all forms of selective mutism; the cases of physical and sexual abuse were documented by independent social welfare agencies. A similarly high rate of child abuse was found in an independent study (MacGregor et al. 1994) but not in all studies (Black and Uhde 1995). These findings suggest that, in some cases, selective mutism might be a posttraumatic phenomenon, which would have implications for the clinical management of these children and their families.

Epidemiology

An estimated prevalence of 180 per 100,000 children has recently been reported (Kopp and Gillberg 1997), indicating a higher prevalence than generally was reported in the past (when more stringent definitional criteria were used). Teachers describe up to 2% prevalence of mute behavior in class (Kumpulainen et al. 1998). There is a slight female predominance, with a sex ratio of 1:1–1:2. An increased prevalence of selective mutism in children from immigrant families is also reported.

Etiology

Although traditional views of the etiology of selective mutism have been predominantly psychodynamic in nature, more recent findings suggest a variety of biological factors. The association of selective mutism with a history of early-onset shyness or a family history of shyness is consistent with a psychodynamic model, but it is also consistent with a constitutional or temperamental contribution to childhood shyness (Kagan et al. 1987), anxiety disorders, or mood disorders.

Virtually all children with selective mutism in two studies fulfilled criteria for social phobia or avoidant personality disorder (Black and Uhde 1995; Dummit et al. 1997), with another report describing the prevalence at 74% (Kristensen 2000). About one-half had additional anxiety disorders (Dummit et al. 1997), with about 30% having simple phobia (Black and Uhde 1995). Although anxiety disorders are highly represented, the prevalence of ADHD or oppositional defiant disorder is very low.

In addition to the well-established association of selective mutism with anxiety disorders, comorbidity studies have indicated that most children with selective mutism also have a developmental disorder or delay (Kristensen 2000). The association of selective mutism with communication disorders, mental retardation, pervasive developmental disorder, and neurological disorder suggests a neurodevelopmental etiological factor. These conditions can potentially aggravate the speech of a child with selective mutism. Interestingly, more than 30% of the children with selective mutism also have a comorbid elimination disorder (Kristensen 2000). The co-occurrence of an anxiety disorder and a developmental disorder or delay was reported in 46% of the children with selective mutism and 1% of the control subjects (Kristensen 2000).

Various descriptive observations are consistent with psychodynamic factors, including the selective appearance of symptoms in specific environments. Selective mutism is often conceptualized in psychodynamic terms as a coping behavior and as a reflection of primitively asserted autonomy. Muteness also can be interpreted as a defense against emotional distress, pain, fear of punishment, and interpersonal interaction, occurring in families with a tendency toward family enmeshment and overprotectiveness. Separation anxiety and abandonment fears are common, which appear to be caused by both biological and psychodynamic forces.

A posttraumatic etiology is supported by the data suggesting a high prevalence of physical and sexual abuse, parental violence, and early mouth trauma. An etiology related to separation anxiety is consistent with some overt behavioral symptoms, as well as strong maternal ties, family history of mood disorder, and history of loss (e.g., through geographic move or sociopolitical change). In family studies, relatives of children with selective mutism are found to be taciturn and also to have an elevated prevalence of speech and language disorders (Steinhausen and Adamek 1997). Immigrant status and parents' use of foreign language also have been frequently cited in these families. A lack of confidence and personal autonomy in managing the external world appears to be a contributing factor.

At the other end of the etiological spectrum, brain lesions, especially cerebellar damage, have been implicated in rare cases of selective mutism (Gordon 2001). Specific gene involvement has been suggested (Grosso et al. 1999; Hagerman et al. 1999; Simons et al. 1997) but not systematically explored.

Course and Prognosis

Selective mutism typically starts at ages 3–5, when developmentally normal children may still show brief periods of mutism on meeting strangers or in new settings. Although the gradual emergence of early "shyness" may be identified retrospectively (Kolvin and Fundudis 1981), selective mutism is typically diagnosed at ages 5–8, when symptoms become obvious at school. If school attendance is adequate and social behavior is compliant, recognition and referral for treatment may be delayed or avoided.

Symptoms may last for several weeks, months, or years. Some children improve without therapy. About 50% of children are no longer selectively mute by age 10, but the prognosis appears less encouraging if speech behaviors do not improve by then (Kolvin and Fundudis 1981).

Certain cases of selective mutism do not emerge until adolescence. These individuals typically do not speak to family members or outsiders, often show prominent passive-aggressive or antisocial features, and tend to have a less favorable prognosis (Hayden 1980).

Complications include academic underachievement, scapegoating, and satisfaction with the secondary gains of illness. The disadvantages of inappropriate special class and school placements are incurred, as teachers become helpless in dealing with the socially disruptive silence. Many children experience teasing and humiliation, but some children are apparently protected by peers, who may speak on their behalf or who bestow special services and personal attention. Excessive protection and tolerance by peers or parents usually reinforce the mute behavior.

The long-term outcome is not known. The abnormal social behavior, interpersonal manipulations, shyness, and aggressivity appear to persist beyond the period of symptomatic muteness. Further information about the natural course of illness may be derived from studies on comorbidity. Selective mutism may be related to mood, separation anxiety, and phobic disorders. The finding that 97% of the children with selective mutism fulfill criteria for social phobia has led to the proposal that selective mutism may be a symptom or form of social phobia (Black and Uhde 1992).

Diagnostic Evaluation

A full psychiatric evaluation of the child and parents is warranted, with special attention to mood and anxiety disorders (Anstendig 1999). Neurological assessment is helpful to consider possible brain damage, mental retardation, pervasive developmental disorder, expressive language disorder, receptive aphasia, and deafness. Speech and language evaluation is needed, including examination of familial patterns of communication, silence, and anger. The child and family should be assessed for physical and sexual abuse, antisocial behavior, shyness, psychosocial deprivation, and mental retardation. At times, a home visit is helpful to evaluate the communication environment; in some cases, it may be essential to evaluate the child's speech because home may be the only place where the child is willing to talk (Cleator and Hand 2001). Differential diagnosis includes anxiety disorders such as social phobia, disuse of speech in schizophrenia (alogia) or schizotypal personality, deafness, aphasia, and hysteria.

Treatment

Selective mutism was notoriously difficult to treat until serotonin reuptake inhibitors were shown to produce substantial improvement in both mutism and global functioning of these children, as rated by parents (Black and Uhde 1994; J.S. Carlson et al. 1999). This finding was particularly striking in view of the inability of TCAs to treat this condition. However, most fluoxetine-treated children were still quite symptomatic after 12 weeks of treatment (Black and Uhde 1994), and the therapeutic effect appeared to decrease with increasing age (Dummit et al. 1996); therefore, the use of other methods is necessary. Anxiolytics or atypical neuroleptics might be helpful as adjuvants, and MAOIs might be considered in treatment-resistant cases (Golwyn and Sevlie 1999).

After pharmacotherapy, behavior therapy appears to have the next best outcome (Krohn et al. 1992; Labbe and Williamson 1984). Contingency management, positive reinforcement, desensitization, and assertiveness training generally have been used. At present, behavior therapy probably should be used in combination with a selective serotonin reuptake inhibitor. Speech and language therapy are often indicated for children with selective mutism, especially in view of their communication disorders and neurodevelopmental problems.

Parent counseling can be effective. Parents and teachers often make accommodations to the child's muteness; however, it is generally useful to maintain a clear expectation that the child talk and communicate, at least for a structured period each day at home, at each school period, and at each treatment session. It is important for the parents, especially the symbiotic parent, to be explicit with the child about the expectation of talking at school and in therapy. Most parents and teachers need to be supported and repeatedly reminded to refrain from reinforcing the child's passivity or contributing to the secondary gain.

Therapists have anecdotally described a variety of practical techniques aimed at reducing the child's muteness. Minimizing the "directness" of verbal interaction can reduce the subjective feelings of threat or aggressivity that the child may experience in communicating. Clinicians have used approaches such as covering their own mouths during speech, reducing eye contact with the child, using averted body positions, speaking in gestures

(pantomime), silent mouthing of words, or using electronic devices to mediate communication. Often, simple questions to the child are asked that require writing a response, tapping the therapist's hand, or making a one-word utterance. For children whose anxiety results from speech phobia, the production of a single word may be preceded by increased tension and rigidity and followed by a sense of relief and pride, which a therapist can positively reinforce. It is unclear whether such methods are therapeutic or counterproductive.

Once the mute speech is improving, it may be anticipated that the child and parents will continue to require treatment for associated psychiatric disorders. Initial symptomatic improvement of the mutism may be followed by resistance to further pursuit of treatment by both child and parents, with the risk of leaving comorbidity, causal factors, and social and academic complications inadequately managed. Both individual and family psychotherapy aimed at reducing the mutism usually are found to be slow, difficult, and disappointing. It may be helpful to focus the psychotherapies on issues related to fear, including self-esteem, separation and autonomy, and assertiveness. During the course of treatment, particularly of children with significant separation issues, missed appointments and illness may be followed by regressive behavior and speech.

Use of short-term therapy (Wright et al. 1985) or hospitalization have been suggested but not pursued. In general, psychosocial treatment should include consideration of social skills training, possibly including help for the family in constructing structured daily activities.

Clinical Comment

There is a clear need for systematic studies of virtually all aspects of selective mutism, including the largely uncharted territory of its natural course, epidemiology, genetics and biological features, etiological role of abuse and neglect, and treatment outcomes. Investigation of selective mutism, which was dormant for years, has now been enlivened by the growing interest in its comorbidity with other psychiatric disorders (especially anxiety and mood disorders), the role of developmental disorders and delays, the controversial effects of abuse and neglect, the possible etiological role of (developmental) stranger anxiety, and the "serotonergic view" of the disorder. Just as separation anxiety disorder in children appears to share some important links with panic disorder in adults, emerging evidence is strengthening the conceptual links between selective mutism and social phobia. At the level of clinical care, however, each case of this uncommon disorder teaches its own lessons.

Reactive Attachment Disorder of Infancy or Early Childhood

Following exposure to severe and prolonged neglect or physical or emotional abuse, infants and young children may show a variety of disturbances in interpersonal relatedness, social behavior, emotional reactivity and excitability, and cognition. Such disturbances are inferred to arise from disordered development of early interpersonal attachment (Table 20–33). Reactive attachment disorder encompasses both increased and decreased social interactiveness after trauma in infancy or early childhood.

The grossly pathological care that may lead to this posttraumatic syndrome includes physical or sexual abuse, neglect, the absence of stable attachment figures (such as in some institutional or foster care settings), the failure of an emotionally disturbed caregiver to read or respond to a child's emotional or physical needs, or the failure of caregivers to become attached to the child (Tibbits-Kleber and Howell 1985). According to DSM-IV-TR, any failure of normal development may be labeled as reactive attachment disorder if preceded by gross failures in child care.

The hallmark of reactive attachment disorder is the appearance of profoundly disturbed interpersonal relationships following grossly inadequate early care in childhood (with or without evidence of their linkage). The pediatric label of nonorganic failure to thrive is a broader diagnostic category that encompasses 1) cases of reactive attachment disorder that involve physical growth retardation, 2) the DSM-IV-TR category of feeding and eating disorders of infancy or early childhood, and 3) some cases of retarded physical growth without prominent social abnormalities.

In normal development, an infant is expected to show overt behavioral signs of attachment and bonding to a parent by age 8 months. Attachment behavior, defined by Bowlby as an innate biological system that motivates behavior whose evolutionary advantage is the elicitation of protection and comfort for the infant, entails the seeking and engagement of selected adults to care for the child (N.W. Boris and Zeanah 1998).

Attachment behavior in children has been empirically examined with the Strange Situation test (Ainsworth et al. 1978), which is based on observations of an infant or a child following separation and reunion with a caregiver. The resulting classification of attachment behavior (Ainsworth et al. 1978; Main and Solomon 1990) is useful in describing clear differences between populations of low-risk and maltreated infants (V. Carlson et al. 1989; Van Ijzendoorn et al. 1999), but not all children showing abnormal attachment behavior on the Ainsworth para-

TABLE 20–33. DSM-IV-TR diagnostic criteria for reactive attachment disorder of infancy or early childhood

A. Markedly disturbed and developmentally inappropriate social relatedness in most contexts, beginning before age 5 years, as evidenced by either (1) or (2):
  (1) persistent failure to initiate or respond in a developmentally appropriate fashion to most social interactions, as manifest by excessively inhibited, hypervigilant, or highly ambivalent and contradictory responses (e.g., the child may respond to caregivers with a mixture of approach, avoidance, and resistance to comforting, or may exhibit frozen watchfulness)
  (2) diffuse attachments as manifest by indiscriminate sociability with marked inability to exhibit appropriate selective attachments (e.g., excessive familiarity with relative strangers or lack of selectivity in choice of attachment figures)

B. The disturbance in Criterion A is not accounted for solely by developmental delay (as in mental retardation) and does not meet criteria for a pervasive developmental disorder.

C. Pathogenic care as evidenced by at least one of the following:
  (1) persistent disregard of the child's basic emotional needs for comfort, stimulation, and affection
  (2) persistent disregard of the child's basic physical needs
  (3) repeated changes of primary caregiver that prevent formation of stable attachments (e.g., frequent changes in foster care)

D. There is a presumption that the care in Criterion C is responsible for the disturbed behavior in Criterion A (e.g., the disturbances in Criterion A began following the pathogenic care in Criterion C).

Specify type:
  Inhibited Type: if Criterion A1 predominates in the clinical presentation
  Disinhibited Type: if Criterion A2 predominates in the clinical presentation

digm have attachment disorders. Other types of behavior that may be more clinically significant to attachment disorders include affectionate or comfort-seeking behavior, cooperation with caregiver, exploratory behavior, and tendency to maintain contact with caregiver during exploration (N.W. Boris et al. 1997). In general, the relation of attachment behavior to psychiatric diagnosis has received only limited research attention, but there are suggestions that attachment behavior may be predictive of borderline personality traits (Fonagy et al. 1996) and anxiety disorder (Warren et al. 1997).

Clinical Description

In attachment disorders, a variety of behavioral, cognitive, and affective presentations may be seen at different ages. In children, odd social responsiveness, weak interpersonal attachment, apathy or inappropriate excitability, and mood abnormalities are common. In early infancy, diagnosis is based on the failure to achieve developmental expectations: lack of eye tracking or responsive smiling by age 2 months and failure to play simple games or reach out to be picked up by 5 months.

Children with reactive attachment disorder may present with inhibited or disinhibited subtypes, which are recognized by DSM-IV-TR. *Inhibited* infants with reactive attachment disorder may appear lethargic or show little activity. Their body movements are weak. Sleep is excessive and disrupted, and weight gain is slow. They may seem spacey and unengaged or, alternatively, hypervigilant and avoidant. The infants have little interactive interest in the environment and often resist being held. As young children, individuals with reactive attachment disorder may appear withdrawn, passive, or disinterested in people, or they may respond to interpersonal stimuli in odd or inconsistent ways. Children who have the inhibited subtype of reactive attachment disorder seem to have closed down on incoming stimulation, interpersonal and otherwise, as if their general responsiveness were diminished and their reactivity were inhibited.

Children with the *disinhibited* form of reactive attachment disorder may show overly rapid familiarity. They may show inappropriate touching or clinging, excessive interest, and a sort of unmodulated "enthusiasm" with people, even in a first-time meeting. They readily switch their intense "attachment" from one person to another, acting as though people are interchangeable parts ("indiscriminate sociability") and repetitively reenacting a few rigid "scripts" in their interactions ("I love you. Take me home"). Their behavior appears to convey the message "You can take care of me forever." Their immediate emotional involvement may seem initially gratifying to a stranger, but it is also experienced as weird or unusual.

In older children, reactive attachment disorder typically presents with socialization defects. In the absence of socialization problems, such a child might be labeled with a V code (parent–child relational problem) or given a diagnosis of PTSD. At present, the DSM designation of this disorder has led to relatively little further research on reactive attachment disorder, either biological or psychosocial. The extent and nature of cognitive changes in these children have not been extensively examined. Although relations between attachment and cognitive function have been hypothesized, the apparent correlations might be due to covarying factors (T.G. O'Connor et al. 2000).

Epidemiology

Adequate epidemiological data are unavailable. The prevalence of reactive attachment disorder is estimated at about 1% (Zeanah and Embe 1995), largely based on the approximately 1%–5% of pediatric hospital admissions that are due to nonorganic failure to thrive.

Etiology

The etiology of reactive attachment disorder is written into its DSM-IV-TR definition. Previous abuse, neglect, or grossly impaired caregiving is definitionally required, and the disease label suggests that a disruption of caregiver–child bonding is the crucial mechanism. Although it emphasizes the interpersonal or social effects on the child, the definition implies that the parenting is the cause of the child's problem.

Many factors can potentially interfere with attachment behavior. The failure to offer normal instinctive parenting, or even minimally adequate parenting, is typically the result of an overt emotional or psychiatric problem afflicting parent or caregiver: major depressive disorder, psychosis, substance abuse, or mental retardation; child phobia or fear of committing infanticide; frustration with a "difficult" child; active hostility; preoccupation; insensitivity; or indifference. Other factors that might serve as obstacles to parenting include medical illness, parental isolation (lack of social support), poverty, poor education, or grossly disturbed family life. Infant characteristics include being handicapped, unwanted, lethargic, or chronically ill.

Children who are adopted from institutional care are at increased risk for reactive attachment disorder. Although the large majority of children adopted from such facilities do not have behavior problems (Zeanah 2000), it appears that both earlier age and longer duration of deprivation can increase the risk of subsequent insecure attachment, socialization disturbances, disruptive behaviors, and autistic-like changes (L. Fisher et al. 1997; T.G. O'Connor et al. 2000; Rutter et al. 1999).

The foster care system is another source of children with reactive attachment disorder. Entry into the foster care system begins with a disruption of the primary attachment relationships, and the system itself often contributes to the problem by supplying a sequence of multiple caregivers with multiple relationship disruptions. Thus, the system designed to manage the problem is, at times, another factor contributing to the maintenance of this psychopathology.

Biological factors also appear to play an etiological role. A specific suppression of growth hormone release has been described in infants with reactive attachment disorder, and it has been interpreted as closely resembling the growth hormone hyposecretion in rat pups during maternal separation (Katz et al. 1996). Whether growth hormone suppression is a cause, a result, or neither (perhaps related instead to separation anxiety or hyperexploratory behavior) is unclear, and the clinical relevance of this putative animal model remains speculative. More extensive research has been conducted on the pediatric disorder of failure to thrive, but that disorder is sufficiently different from reactive attachment disorder to prevent meaningful comparison. Nonetheless, these studies might suggest directions for further research on reactive attachment disorder, including a correlation of biological markers and temperamental factors.

Course and Prognosis

If this disorder is untreated, the course may vary from spontaneous remission to malnutrition, infection, or death. Both nutritional and psychosocial deprivation may result in long-term behavioral changes, hyperactivity, short stature, and lowered IQ. If emotional deprivation continues but enforced feeding is provided, children may show improved weight gain. However, even when body growth is preserved, ongoing emotional deprivation can cause depressive-type changes and developmental delays in infants. This consequence appears to be illustrated in the historical entity of *hospitalism* (Provence and Lipton 1962). Specific predictors of behavioral, cognitive, and physical sequelae have not been identified. However, among children adopted from institutional care, the postinstitutional environment has been shown to be a significant factor in mitigating the expression of behavior and emotional problems (Zeanah 2000).

For those children with the disinhibited type of reactive attachment disorder, the feature of indiscriminate sociability may persist in these children, even after subsequent environmental improvement and return to developmental trajectories have been achieved. Adopting parents are not generally concerned about this behavior, suggesting that it is accepted as a personality trait rather than viewed as maladaptive psychopathology.

As longitudinal studies of reactive attachment disorder become available, more specific phenomenological and developmental details will be known about this disorder. The relation of reactive attachment disorder to the subsequent appearance of mood disorders, anxiety disorders, eating disorders, and personality disorders has not been determined.

Diagnostic Evaluation

A diagnosis of reactive attachment disorder should be considered whenever a child shows socially unusual behavior, including disruptive behavior (such as conduct disorder or oppositional defiant disorder). Early history and sociability factors might, in some cases, be submerged under a complex history of behavior problems (S.L. Wilson 2001).

In infants and younger children, professional observation of mother–child interactions in the medical setting and at home might be required. A home visit is central to evaluation and diagnosis. Psychiatric evaluation of the parents is essential. When possible, siblings should be assessed regarding their psychosocial experiences, social functioning, and possible psychiatric disorders. Medical assessment of the child patient is required to rule out chronic physical illness (organic failure to thrive), homeostatic sleep and feeding disorders, food refusal, malnutrition, neurological disease, and sensory deficit.

The diagnosis is essentially confirmed by the child's symptomatic improvement following the provision of adequate care. The evaluation of the child's response can be most readily conducted in a hospital, which permits direct evaluation of the child and the parent–child interactions. Hospitalization also allows a multidisciplinary team to make the observations necessary for diagnosis. An alternative to hospitalization is a planned parent–child separation, which involves removal of the child to a different environment in which the caregiver has the capacity for care and observation.

Assessment of caregiver–child interactions can involve a high degree of sophistication and technical skill. Minimally, it involves observation of the caregiver's simple capacity for physical holding, physical and interpersonal stimulation, empathy, attentiveness to the child's behavior, fear of the child, anger, or indifference.

With or without hospitalization, home visits are generally indicated for evaluation of the adequacy of housing, safety, nutrition, stability, regularity of actions during the day and over time, use of space, supervision, other home dwellers, behavioral standards, and parental involvement with the child. Multiple shifts of routine, caregiver, home, and environment may undermine the consistency of the child's life and contribute to the development of reactive attachment disorder.

Although home visits can contribute to the evaluation of any psychiatric patient (including adults), reactive attachment disorder is the only psychiatric disorder for which a home visit is virtually required. In practice, however, parents may be reluctant to allow even one home visit. Parents may be defensive, angry, and ashamed concerning the professional's interest in home visits. The handling of privacy and personal concerns presents a challenge to the clinician to maintain empathy for the caregivers, especially if a child's suffering is at stake.

Issues of privacy often generate sharp limitations on the evaluation of these children.

Many parents of children with this disorder are aware that their child is not receiving what is needed. They may wish to give care but find themselves incapable of providing it. It is a clinical error to presume that parents of children with reactive attachment disorder are not interested in what is best for the child. Parents often are gratified to receive outside assistance, help for the child (despite the sense of humiliation at "failing" to provide), and support and treatment for themselves.

Psychiatric evaluation of the parents is an essential component of the overall assessment. Particularly for the primary caregiver, the evaluation must be thorough, including the full range of debilitating psychiatric disorders and psychosocial stressors. The therapist must assess the extent or lack of supports, the onset of the psychiatric disorder in relation to the period of neglect, the possibility of physical or sexual abuse, and the causes of any previous treatment failures. Child abuse and, at times, neglect may not be readily identifiable during the initial weeks or months of the treatment; they may not be detected until months later, when the parents become more comfortable and trusting.

Treatment

Basic medical care, provision of adequate caregiving, parental education, and parental psychiatric treatment are generally needed to treat reactive attachment disorder of infancy or early childhood. Medical hospitalization, which is useful in evaluation, is generally justified also for performing this massive intervention.

The use of hospitalization is much preferable to parent–child separation for infants or very young children, but it can be useful for children at any age. Both removal from the home environment and hospitalization permit the establishment of normal feeding and physiological patterns as well as the opportunity for evaluating and expanding the parents' caregiving capacities.

Given the complexity of medical and psychiatric problems, the need for proficiency in baby care and nurturance, the required sensitivity in managing the parents, and the frequent need for social services and legal procedures, it is a major advantage for treatment to be delivered by a specialized team working in a hospital. This multidisciplinary team typically provides care on a pediatric inpatient unit and in an outpatient clinic, with a determined emphasis on coordination and continuity.

Hospitalization or treatment intervention typically leads to a major improvement in the clinical status of the child. This improvement in response to treatment is considered confirmation of the diagnosis of reactive attachment disorder. Clinical nonresponsiveness implies the presence of a different disorder, an additional disorder, or persistent physical damage resulting from extreme medical complications that occurred before treatment was begun.

If treatment is initiated long after the period of abuse and neglect, when early attachment problems are already a part of the history and abnormal social behavior is prominent, standard psychiatric evaluation and treatment of child and parents are indicated. Hospitalization is not crucial if the child is no longer in the abusive phase. Although no controlled studies of treatment outcome are available, current medical and psychiatric practice involves multimodal therapy with child and parents.

Standard psychotherapeutic approaches to children with reactive attachment disorder need to be adjusted (S.L. Wilson 2001). Trust and reciprocity cannot be assumed as a basis for the treatment relationship. Many of these children have difficulty in learning from social experiences, may not have the usual level of insight or desire for change, and may not value authority figures in the usual manner. Nonetheless, the goals of treatment remain the traditional ones of self-understanding and self-control, acceptance of reality and its limitations, and the development of meaningful relationships.

Clinical Comment

The creation of a diagnostic category that entails a reasonable but hypothetical mechanism is an unusual occurrence in the DSM-IV-TR system. Confusion may arise in individual cases if socialization defects are not preceded by clear antecedent abuse or neglect or if demonstrably disordered early attachment results in behavioral or affective symptoms without sociability deficits. The linkage between an early traumatic experience and subsequent symptoms may be speculative in individual cases, but repeated clinical observations of this coupling in many children allows the diagnosis to be defined by its apparent etiology. Nonetheless, in clinical care, this is a conceptually cumbersome diagnosis.

In individual cases of reactive attachment disorder, the value of an etiology-based definition can appear questionable (Richters and Volkmar 1994). The limitations often placed on the availability of accurate historical and social information may preclude fulfillment of the etiological criterion, forcing clinicians to improvise. The etiological criterion is also questionable because of the possibility, for example, that this condition is a developmental disorder such as atypical development (pervasive developmental disorder) and that the attachment deficits are not essential to this disorder.

TABLE 20–34. An alternative classification of attachment disorder subtypes

Nonattachment disorders

Nonattachment with emotional withdrawal	No evidence of attachment to caregiver; no pattern of comfort seeking; constricted affect; little social pleasure or exploration
Nonattachment with indiscriminate sociability	Lack of age-appropriate cautiousness about approaching, being held by, or engaging with relative strangers; will seek comfort from strangers; shallow, perhaps brittle affect

Disordered attachment disorders

Disordered attachment with inhibition	Has focused attachment figure but either clings anxiously around unfamiliar people when caregiver present (less so when caregiver absent) with constricted affect or has inhibition characterized by fear and hypervigilance with exaggerated compliance and lack of pleasure
Disordered attachment with self-endangerment	Has focused attachment figure but does not use this person to monitor cues about danger; is reckless, is accident-prone, and shows aggressive behaviors in the context of the relationship
Disordered attachment with role reversal	Has focused attachment figure but has heightened or precocious concern for that caregiver's well-being; caretaking of self or otherwise may alternate with bossy and punitive behavior

Disrupted attachment disorder

	Prolonged separation from caregiver before onset of search behaviors; refusal to accept comfort from others; emotional withdrawal; sleep and eating disturbance and regression

Source. Reprinted with permission from Boris NW, Zeanah CH, Larrieu JA, et al: "Attachment Disorders in Infancy and Early Childhood: A Preliminary Investigation of Diagnostic Criteria." *American Journal of Psychiatry* 155:295–297, 1998.

The focus in the DSM-IV-TR definition on pathogenic care and social abnormalities rather than abnormal attachment behaviors highlights the blending of concepts and dimensions that can be confusing at a clinical level (Zeanah 1996). An alternative classification (Table 20–34) has been proposed that is based on the nature of the attachment behaviors rather than on presence or absence of pathogenic care. This alternative definition and subtyping of reactive attachment disorder was found to have better reliability than the DSM-IV classification (N.W. Boris et al. 1998). This approach raises the possibility that this disorder can be conceptualized without reliance on historical information or the arbitrary hypothesized linkage between history and current symptoms.

"Disorganized" attachment, one of the types of pathological attachment that can be identified with the Ainsworth paradigm (Main and Solomon 1990), has been associated with a *DRD4* gene polymorphism (Lakatos et al. 2000). This is the same 48–base pair 7-repeat allele that has been associated with the human personality trait of novelty seeking (Benjamin et al. 1996; Ebstein et al. 1996) and with ADHD (LaHoste et al. 1996; Swanson et al. 1998). The possible association of the *DRD4* gene with neonatal temperament (Auerbach et al. 1999; Ebstein et al. 1998) raises the possibility that the genetics of temperament and attachment may be a critical factor, perhaps more than life circumstances and parenting experiences, in the development of pathological attachment and attachment disorders.

Stereotypic Movement Disorder

Certain repetitive and purposeless motor behaviors may be seen in young children, sensory-deprived (deaf or blind) people, or individuals with mental retardation, pervasive developmental disorders, and some psychotic disorders (e.g., schizophrenia, mood disorders with psychomotor changes). Many stereotypies appear to have a self-stimulatory component, but the diagnosis of stereotypic movement disorder is made only if these repetitive behaviors cause functional interference or physical injury (Table 20–35). SIB is a common and clinically important form of stereotypic behavior.

Clinical Description

Examples of stereotypies include head banging, body rocking, hand flapping, whirling, stereotyped laughter, thumb sucking, hair fingering, facial touching, eye poking, object biting, self-biting, self-scratching, self-hitting, teeth grinding, and breath holding. Although one behavioral stereotypy may predominate, it is typical for several stereotypies to co-occur. Different stereotypies may become prominent at different times. The rhythm of the

---

TABLE 20–35. DSM-IV-TR diagnostic criteria for stereotypic movement disorder

A. Repetitive, seemingly driven, and nonfunctional motor behavior (e.g., hand shaking or waving, body rocking, head banging, mouthing of objects, self-biting, hitting own body).

B. The behavior markedly interferes with normal activities or results in self-inflicted bodily injury that requires medical treatment (or would result in an injury if preventive measures were not used).

C. If mental retardation is present, the stereotypic or self-injurious behavior is of sufficient severity to become a focus of treatment.

D. The behavior is not better accounted for by a compulsion (as in obsessive-compulsive disorder), a tic (as in tic disorder), a stereotypy that is part of a pervasive developmental disorder, or hair pulling (as in trichotillomania).

E. The behavior is not due to the direct physiological effects of a substance or a general medical condition.

F. The behavior persists for 4 weeks or longer.

Specify if:

With Self-Injurious Behavior: if the behavior results in bodily damage that requires specific treatment (or that would result in bodily damage if protective measures were not used)

---

repetitive behavior may be slow and gentle, fast and energetic, or even violently energized. Sometimes waves of increasing and decreasing energy may be seen over the course of several minutes. Frequency may increase during periods of tension, frustration, boredom, and isolation, as well as just before bedtime.

Two of the most common presentations are head banging and body rocking. Head banging may last for hours, particularly at bedtime or on morning awakening. The head banging can be soft and quiet, occurring during periods of isolation or boredom, and appear to have a self-stimulatory and pleasurable quality. Alternatively, head banging may occur during a clearly unpleasurable state. During a temper tantrum, a child may thrash on the floor, with limbs flailing and head banging vigorously against the floor or wall.

Body rocking may be slow swaying, with quiet murmuring or singing, or it may be violent enough to move a child's bed across the room. Whether pleasurable or unpleasurable, there is typically a self-absorbed quality of mentation.

Among individuals with serious developmental disabilities, the severity of the symptoms of stereotypic movement disorder may be associated with the severity of mental retardation or pervasive developmental disorder (Bodfish et al. 2000).

Epidemiology

Approximately 15%–20% of a normal pediatric population may have a history of transient stereotypies, but no data are available regarding the prevalence of stereotypic movement disorder with physical injury or functional interference in the general population. Stereotypic behaviors appear to show equal sex prevalence. There are no data regarding socioeconomic influences. The prevalence is higher in individuals with mental retardation. Among institutionalized people with severe and profound mental retardation, about 60% have stereotypic movement disorder, and 15% engage in SIBs (Schroeder et al. 1979).

Etiology

Stereotypic movement disorder has no clear etiology, but several theories have been advanced, and multiple contributing or interacting factors are probably involved.

Organic influences are supported by the increased incidence of stereotypic movement disorder in individuals with abnormal brain structure or function, such as mental retardation, auditory or visual sensory deficit (blindness, deafness), brain disease (seizures, postinfection, metabolic abnormality), psychotic disorder, and drug-induced psychosis (amphetamines). A presumed final common pathway might involve disruption of the balance among elements of basal ganglia motor circuitry (Canales and Graybiel 2000). Neurochemical mechanisms involving serotonin (regarding impulse control) and opioids (controlling pain) have been proposed (Villalba and Harrington 2000), and purinergic systems (regulating aggression) also have been suggested (Lara et al. 2000).

An etiological role of self-stimulation (or autoerotic stimulation) is suggested by the characteristic self-absorbed and apparently pleasurable appearance and by the occurrence of this behavior during periods of boredom or physical isolation. Self-stimulation through repetitive physical activity may be satisfying if normal forms of stimulation are unavailable or ineffective. For example, patients with extreme impairments in cognition may body rock if the ordinary array of sights and sounds is not as interpretable or pleasurable as the physical activity. Alternatively, a tension-relieving purpose is plausible because these behaviors increase during periods of anxiety, tension, and frustration. An arousal factor also has been proposed because the behaviors sometimes are more evident at bedtime or on arising in the morning. Thus, head banging during temper tantrums may be viewed in terms of self-stimulation, tension discharge, or arousal. However, functional analyses of various "typologies" of stereotypic movement disorder suggest that the aberrant behaviors serve multiple functions and are maintained by a variety of different forms of reinforcement in different individuals (Kennedy et al. 2000).

SIBs are particularly difficult to explain etiologically. Theories are easy to generate, but they are often shaped by counterintuitive clinical observations. For example, protective physical restraints that inhibit SIB are welcomed and found to be relaxing by some people, yet removal of the restraints may lead promptly to a marked return or increase in stereotyped behavior. These patients can experience pain (in response to a pinch or an electric shock) and, at times, seem to try to protect themselves from self-injury. These observations are difficult to integrate in terms of a general capacity to feel or avoid discomfort. It has been theorized that such observations concerning SIB suggest a form of pain sensitivity that can be drastically altered by emotion, situation, or physiology in some unusual manner in patients with specific psychiatric disorders (e.g., autistic disorder).

Although stereotypic movement disorder is overrepresented among individuals with a history of neglect, understimulation, and mental retardation, these behaviors can be seen in patients with normal intelligence and normal caregiving experiences. Body rocking, for example, has been observed in 3%–25% of college students, although the movements appear to be more associated with situational factors and smaller in physical amplitude than similar stereotypies seen in people with mental retardation (Berkson et al. 1999). Thumb sucking and body rocking in persons of normal intelligence appear to be associated with a lifetime diagnosis of mood or anxiety disorders (Castellanos et al. 1997) and with obsessive-compulsive, perfectionistic, or impulsive-aggressive traits (Niehaus et al. 2000; Wilhelm et al. 1999).

Certain types of stereotypies occur in normal development, particularly during the period of learning of motor patterns and rhythms (Kravitz and Boehm 1971). These behaviors appear to function as motoric exercises, aiding the child in feeling and acting within his or her neuromuscular and motoric system. Biological markers and physiological studies of stereotypic movement disorder are unavailable.

Course and Prognosis

Certain stereotypies, such as head banging and body rocking, begin as early as 6–12 months. These behaviors typically resolve in 80% of children without mental disorders by age 4 years, although more subtle habits may persist, such as finger tapping or teeth grinding (DeLissovoy 1962). In people with mental retardation or pervasive developmental disorders, such early-onset stereotypies may persist for years. Later-onset stereotypies may be

descriptively similar, but they appear episodically and only during periods of anxiety or stress.

A complication of stereotypic movement disorder results from the attention that the behaviors (especially SIBs) invoke from caregivers. These various forms of attention and care may unwittingly become sustaining behavioral reinforcers, leading to more intense or enduring symptoms.

Diagnostic Evaluation

When the disorder begins during infancy or in very early childhood, evaluation for concurrent mental retardation and other developmental disabilities is appropriate. For disorders with later onset, it is necessary to evaluate for agitation or anxiety associated with psychosis or mood disorders as well as for mental retardation and pervasive developmental disorders. In some cases, the use of psychostimulant medications and other dopamine agonists may aggravate or produce stereotypic behaviors; therefore, evaluation of current medication use is appropriate.

Stereotypic movement disorder is not diagnosed if the symptoms can be explained by concomitant tic disorder or OCD. Stereotypies may be distinguished from tics or compulsions when they have a self-stimulatory or pleasurable component. Although tics or compulsions may carry a tension-discharging function, they are not experienced as pleasurable.

Treatment

The symptoms of stereotypic movement disorder are often treatment resistant. Behavioral techniques, especially overcorrection, have been found most effective. Interventions involving anxiety reduction, sensory stimulation, and the offering of alternatives to self-stimulation are also helpful.

Although behavioral methods usually rely on reward systems when possible, positive reinforcement in treating stereotypic movement disorder is generally not effective when used alone. Overcorrection has the best empirical support, but it is a coercive treatment that may invoke anger, oppositionalism, and symptom substitution.

Blocking pleasurable feedback from self-stimulation can be useful. The particular technique depends on the sensory mode of predominant self-stimulation. For self-stimulation based on sound, white noise or tape-recorded music may be considered. For rocking, a vibrator taped to the hand may distract from other kinesthetic self-stimulation. For finger waving, beads on a string may provide alternative proprioceptive stimulation. For visual stimulation, ambient lighting may be altered or a bubble-blower may be provided. Such distraction from self-stimulation and use of stimuli substitution can be helpful in some individuals (Baroff 1986).

In cases of noninjurious behaviors, extinction (ignoring the symptom rather than giving attention) is sometimes suggested. In treating significant SIB, mildly aversive stimuli might be needed, such as facial puffs of air, sharp (Tabasco) or sour (lemon) tastes, or scratchy skin contact (burlap). Physical restraints also may be used protectively or as a reward for increasing periods of abstaining from self-injury.

Pharmacological treatment has been extensively explored, but no single approached has emerged as consistently helpful. Case reports suggest that serotonin reuptake inhibitors, atypical neuroleptics, and the opiate blocker naltrexone have some value in certain patients with mental retardation (C. Turner et al. 1999). Serotonin reuptake inhibitors have been reported to be helpful (Hellings et al. 1996) but may aggravate symptoms for some individuals. The effectiveness of naltrexone, presumably mediated by blocking endorphin-mediated pleasure sensations, might be predicted by elevated levels of certain pro-opiomelanocortin peptide fragments (Sandman et al. 2000). Case reports also have described some use for anticonvulsants, clonidine, diphenhydramine, and even allupurinol. Psychostimulants and other dopamine agonists may aggravate or induce the appearance of stereotypic behaviors.

Increased parental attention and involvement during performance of the stereotypies may be therapeutic, similar to treatment of apparent self-stimulation in rumination disorder. For example, during head banging, parents are advised to hold or sit with the child, holding and protecting the head until banging stops. Although this process can reduce the overall duration, it may take a long time, and parents often have difficulty in following through on suggestions to provide additional time with or attention to a child.

When stereotypies originate from a psychotic disorder, increased attention may be unhelpful or counterproductive. Treatment with antipsychotic or other sedative medications may be needed.

Some clinicians use simple and practical management techniques, such as directing a child to bang his or her head on a soft surface, combined with interventions for stress reduction. Controlled studies of most treatments of stereotypic movement disorder are lacking.

Clinical Comment

Stereotypic movement disorder, encompassing a variety of behavioral stereotypies, allows the diagnostic labeling of certain behavior problems at any age. Although it may be found to represent a distinct diagnostic category in its own right, it might represent a stress-related behavioral condition that reaches clinical significance under certain conditions, especially the restrictive environmental circumstances often encountered by those with developmental disabilities (Verhoeven et al. 1999). In all patients with stereotypic movement disorder, it is advisable at present to evaluate aggressively for possible concurrent mental retardation, developmental disorders, psychotic disorders, and agitation associated with mood or anxiety disorders (or related incipient or precursor conditions).

Standardized Assessment Instruments for Children and Adolescents

Structured and semistructured interview protocols, checklists, questionnaires, and rating scales have been developed for the evaluation and follow-up of many child psychiatric disorders (American Psychiatric Association Task Force for the Handbook of Psychiatric Measures 2000; Corcoran and Fischer 2000; Rapoport et al. 1985). Similar to instruments developed for evaluating the major diagnoses in adults, these instruments are useful in clinical practice as well as research protocols (Rutter et al. 1987). Available instruments can provide a systematic review of general behaviors, psychiatric symptoms, and all DSM-IV-TR diagnoses of childhood, as well as a global assessment of general functioning (Achenbach and Rescorla 2001; Achenbach and Ruffle 1998).

Standardized instruments can yield findings that differ from those of clinical evaluations. The sources of these differences are numerous, and neither approach can be rigidly interpreted as correct. Clinicians tend to underreport substance abuse and related disorders in adolescents, and standardized instruments are typically more systematic and complete than clinicians in scanning across all of the DSM-IV-TR diagnoses.

Children and parents each contribute useful but different observations. In general, children are more effective in reporting mood symptoms, and parents are more effective in reporting behavioral symptoms. However, features of conduct disorder may be reported at higher rates either by children or by parents, depending on the clinical situation. Children likely report more when the information will not be self-indicting but less if punishment or treatment is being considered.

It is clear that no single informant can give a full description of a child. Children, teachers, parents, relatives, community members, and clinicians all view the child from different settings and with different biases. The sex, age, and psychiatric diagnosis of the child and the parents might influence the nature of observations. However, the differences between parents' and teachers' observations, and between two parents' observations, often relate to genuine variations in the behavior of children in different settings and with different people. Studies comparing the data of different reporters, evaluation techniques, and diagnostic subgroups are clarifying the sources of complexity that have long been inherent in the clinical process.

The standardized diagnostic instruments will facilitate epidemiological studies of the major psychiatric disorders in the general child and adolescent population. The classic work of Rutter, on the Isle of Wight and in inner-city London, has provided the first major comprehensive set of epidemiological data on psychiatric disorders in children (Rutter 1989; Rutter et al. 1970, 1976). Current estimates for prevalence and sex ratio for many childhood-onset disorders are still preliminary and sometimes vague (Table 20–36). These data are expected to improve as more information becomes available based on current diagnostic criteria and standardized assessments of childhood psychopathology.

TABLE 20–36. Estimates of epidemiological characteristics of disorders usually first diagnosed in infancy, childhood, or adolescence

Diagnosis	Sex ratio (male:female)	Lifetime prevalence (per 100,000)
Reading disorder	2:1–4:1	4,000–17,000
Developmental coordination disorder	2:1–4:1	5,000–6,000
Attention-deficit/hyperactivity disorder	3:1–10:1	3,000–10,000
Conduct disorder	2:1–5:1	1,000–15,000
Oppositional defiant disorder	2:1–3:1	1,000–10,000
Expressive language disorder	3:1–4:1	3,000–10,000 (1,000 for severe cases)
Mixed receptive-expressive language disorder	1:1	3,000–6,000 (500 for severe cases)
Mathematics disorder	1:1–2:1	3,000–6,000
Phonological disorder	2:1–3:1	2,000–6,000
Separation anxiety disorder	1:1–2:1	2,000–5,000
Feeding disorder of infancy	1:1–2:1	1,000–4,000
Mental retardation	1.5:1–3:1	1,000–3,000
Tic disorders other than Tourette's	2:1–5:1	1,000–2,000
Stuttering	3:1–4:1	1,000–2,000
Enuresis	2:1–3:1	1,000 (males at age 18)
Encopresis	4:1	1,000–1,500 (at age 5)
Pica	1:1	500–1,000 (estimate)
Stereotypy/habit disorder	1:1–3:1	100–1,000
Reactive attachment disorder	?	100–1,000
Rumination disorder	1:1	100–200 (estimate)
Tourette's disorder	3:1–9:1	50–300 among children, 10–20 among adults
Autistic disorder	4:1–5:1	20–200
Selective mutism	1:1–1:2	180
Asperger's disorder	3:1–4:1	5–15
Rett's disorder	All female	4–20
Childhood disintegrative disorder	>4:1	1–4
Disorder of written expression	3:1–4:1	?

Note. These estimates are based on current and often preliminary data from a variety of sources using different methods and diagnostic criteria. Thus, they are likely to be revised substantially as more studies become available. It is particularly important to note that the order of descending prevalence listed here is only approximate (and in some places arbitrary) because of the wide range of uncertainty and unknowns in the current prevalence estimates.

Complexity and the Capacity for Change

Rarely can a child psychiatric disorder be viewed as a single or simple disturbance. Although each DSM-IV-TR disorder has been discussed here in isolation, multiple concurrent diagnoses are typical in children and adolescents. Moreover, early-onset psychiatric disorders typically induce developmental complications that manifest across multiple domains of functioning, producing cumulative and enduring impairments in adaptation. These disorders and their multiply interacting complications tend to organize and snowball into final common pathways of child psychopathology, including academic impairment (declining school grades, progressive learning delays, school failure, dropout), compromised peer and family relationships (aggressive behavior, isolation, ostracism, retaliation), damaged self-concept (disturbed self-esteem, disordered social assertiveness, identity diffusion), demoralization, societal marginalization or criminal outcome, and chronic dissatisfaction and underachievement.

Even more than in adult psychiatry, the developmental complications of child psychiatric illness make it difficult to place a precise definitional boundary around the core features of a psychiatric disorder in a child. The delineation of a child psychiatric disorder—whose core features can be distinguished from its developmental complications and comorbidity—is a task that is best approached in successive approximations. DSM-IV-TR provides a snapshot in the progressive elaboration and scientific clarification of psychopathology in youth.

Current developmental theories presume intricate and enmeshed interactions among biological, environmental, and psychosocial forces in normal and pathological development. Biological deficits render children more vulnerable to socioenvironmental hazards and, similarly, unsupportive formative environments amplify the consequences of biological liabilities. Complex deficits in multiple functional dimensions and developmental lines are not generally amenable to monotherapies. As a result, multimodal intervention is the standard of care for nearly all serious childhood psychiatric disorders.

It is axiomatic in child psychiatry that early intervention can reduce the developmental consequences of early-onset psychiatric disorders. By intervening before the appearance or accrual of secondary complications (primary intervention), there is often greater potential for treatment gains during the developmental period than during adulthood. In practice, however, the powerful effects of early intervention are often obscured by the heightened biological severity and more pathogenic environment commonly associated with early-onset biopsychiatric disorders. Nonetheless, early intervention is strongly advantageous for virtually all child and adolescent psychiatric disorders.

The Child and the Family

Focusing on the child can itself be an oversimplification. Psychiatric disorders and developmental disturbances in a child affect parents, siblings, extended families, schools, and communities. A child's parents may overfocus on symptoms or be overprotective, over- or underestimate a child's psychopathology, over- or underestimate the child's strengths, shower excessive criticism or compensatory solicitousness on the child, avoid the parental role, show their own inappropriate behavioral responses to stressors, or act on their own psychopathology.

Siblings may experience the direct effects of a patient's behavior and mood, resent the patient's freedom to misbehave while getting away with lessened parental discipline, feel jealous of the patient for being the recipient of special parental concern and efforts, or act on the anger at their parents for the parents' reduced availability and divided attention. Often, these siblings' concerns are based in reality.

Clinicians are sometimes too ready to accept a parent's statement that a child patient's siblings are receiving sufficient support or are adjusting adequately to the extra burdens, when in fact professional intervention might be sorely needed. Even seasoned clinicians may collude with a parent's feeling of "having enough to do without worrying about" a sibling, unintentionally fostering the growth of complications of a child's psychiatric disorders and enlarging the family burden.

The transmission of psychiatric disorders across generations usually is the result of genetic mechanisms and family culture. Effective treatment has the potential to reduce the generational transmission of some of these disorders. Overly focused treatments that do not address the complex and multidimensional scope of these disorders often fail to use this opportunity, especially in this era of managed care. Generally, whenever a child with a psychiatric disorder is identified, clinicians should evaluate the family system and consider the direct evaluation of siblings and parents for specific psychopathology. This surveillance of family members should continue throughout a child's treatment and, in some cases, beyond.

Instilling Hope

Even in children with genetically severe psychiatric disorders or extreme psychosocial circumstances, a supportive set of environmental modifiers (including pharmaco-therapy and psychosocial treatment) may be the dominant influence on long-term outcome. Children and parents find it difficult to believe that many pathogenic forces and problematic symptoms in a child can be "washed over" by later developmental experiences and opportunities.

It is often difficult for the clinician to accurately estimate the inner personal strengths of a child and the supportive capacities of a family or to reasonably gauge a child's prognosis during a crisis or its aftermath. Failure by the clinician to gain this perspective can undermine a child's sense of confidence in the future.

Timely treatment can dramatically improve prognosis, although this may depend critically on the family's and the child's ability to seek and use treatment. A child with a psychiatric disorder—even severe—who is brought into treatment promptly and responds well to therapy may experience minimal interference with functioning and perhaps little detriment in personal development, family life, education, work achievement, initiative, or lifetime satisfaction. On the other hand, a child who does not or cannot make use of treatment is more likely to have a life of chronic dissatisfaction, underachievement, and lower income, even if the psychiatric disorder is relatively mild. The ability to seek treatment can, in many cases, play a more decisive role in determining the prognosis than either the diagnosis or the severity of illness.

Treatment seeking can be taught. Learning to seek treatment is often a gradual process, for both the child and the family. It may take place over several years, especially when psychotherapeutic methods are needed for children and families with "resistance" to help seeking. This process often requires reiteration, perhaps needing several cycles of relapse and treatment-induced remission before an understanding begins to take hold.

Understanding the disorder is a key element for succeeding in treatment and no less for children than for adults. For a child to be effectively involved in treatment, he or she must understand his or her illness in terms that are age- and intellect-appropriate. During the course of treatment, the child enters progressively higher levels of cognitive functioning and self-awareness. Over the years, the child will be required to repeatedly revise and reformulate his or her understanding of the disorder, of the treatment, and of himself or herself.

As a child's caregivers seek medical treatment for him or her, they model and teach help-seeking activity. The child gradually internalizes these functions in stages. The clinician can help both the parents and the child with this developmental process. Children and adolescents can begin to take certain help-seeking steps on their own, and some older adolescents can begin to assume primary responsibility for managing the illness. The teaching of treatment-seeking behavior can begin when the child is young. Early intervention allows the physician and family to collaborate in helping the child conceptualize the disorder in a way that promotes coping with the illness and to foster the child's self-image.

A child's recognition of personal strengths, including treatment-seeking and help-using abilities, is an essential part of coming to terms with a psychiatric illness.

For better and for worse, the psychiatric disorders of children and adolescents are traditionally described from the point of view of the medical model of disease. In psychiatry, we have come to define "disorders" on the basis of functional interference, pathological causes, and long-term developmental consequences.

If we are imbedded in a medical model of the psychiatric disorders usually first diagnosed in youth, young patients will see that we do not perceive an important side of their beings and the promise of their realistic hopes. They will come to feel, correctly, that we do not understand them. If, instead, we view these individuals as having medical conditions that are part of "the human condition" that they can struggle against and use their abilities to overcome, we will be able to understand these children—and the adults they become—in a more accurate, balanced, and complete way.

References

Abikoff H, Courtney ME, Szeibel PJ, et al: The effects of auditory stimulation on the arithmetic performance of children with ADIID and nondisabled children. J Learn Disabil 29:238–246, 1996

Achenbach TM, McConaughy SH: Empirically Based Assessment of Child and Adolescent Psychopathology: Practical Applications, 2nd Edition. Thousand Oaks, CA, Sage, 1996

Achenbach TM, Rescorla LA: Manual for the ASEBA School-Age Forms and Profiles. Burlington, VT, University of Vermont, Research Center for Children, Youth, and Families, 2001

Achenbach TM, Ruffle T: Medical Practitioners' Guide for the Child Behavior Checklist and Related Forms. Burlington, VT, University of Vermont College of Medicine, Department of Psychiatry, 1998

Agarwal V, Sitholey P, Kumar S, et al: Double-blind, placebo-controlled trial of clonidine in hyperactive children with mental retardation. Ment Retard 39:259–267, 2001

Aichhorn A: Wayward Youth (1925). New York, Meridian Books, 1955

Aikawa T, Kasahara T, Uchiyama M: Circadian variation of plasma arginine vasopressin concentration, or arginine vasopressin in enuresis. Scand J Urol Nephrol Suppl 202:47–49, 1999

Ainsworth MD, Blehar MC, Waters E, et al: Patterns of Attachment: A Psychological Study of the Strange Situation. Hillsdale, NJ, Erlbaum, 1978

Airaksinen EM, Matilainen R, Mononen T, et al: A population-based study on epilepsy in mentally retarded children. Epilepsia 41:1214–1220, 2000

Al-Waili NS: Carbamazepine to treat primary nocturnal enuresis: double-blind study. Eur J Med Res 5:40–44, 2000

Alegre S, Chacon J, Redondo L, et al: Post-traumatic tics. Rev Neurol 24:1280–1282, 1996

Allen AJ, Leonard HL, Swedo SE: Case study: a new infection-triggered, autoimmune subtype of pediatric OCD and Tourette's syndrome. J Am Acad Child Adolesc Psychiatry 34:307–311, 1995

Almost D, Rosenbaum P: Effectiveness of speech intervention for phonological disorders: a randomized controlled trial. Dev Med Child Neurol 40:319–325, 1998

Althaus M, Vink HJ, Minderaa RB, et al: Lack of effect of clonidine on stuttering in children. Am J Psychiatry 152:1087–1089, 1995

Aman MG, Kern RA: The efficacy of folic acid in fragile X syndrome and other developmental disabilities. J Child Adolesc Psychopharmacol 1:285–295, 1991

Aman MG, Collier-Crespin A, Lindsay RL: Pharmacotherapy of disorders in mental retardation. Eur Child Adolesc Psychiatry 9(suppl 1):98–107, 2000

American Association on Mental Retardation: Mental Retardation: Definition, Classification, and Systems of Supports, 9th Edition. Washington, DC, American Association on Mental Retardation, 1992

American Psychiatric Association Task Force for the Handbook of Psychiatric Measures: Handbook of Psychiatric Measures. Washington, DC, American Psychiatric Association, 2000

American Psychiatric Association: Diagnostic and Statistical Manual of Mental Disorders, 3rd Edition, Revised. Washington, DC, American Psychiatric Association, 1987

American Psychiatric Association: Diagnostic and Statistical Manual of Mental Disorders, 4th Edition. Washington, DC, American Psychiatric Association, 1994

American Psychiatric Association: Diagnostic and Statistical Manual of Mental Disorders, 4th Edition, Text Revision. Washington, DC, American Psychiatric Association, 2000

Amir RE, Van den Veyver IB, Wan M, et al: Rett syndrome is caused by mutations in X-linked MECP2, encoding methyl-CpG-binding protein 2. Nat Genet 23:127–128, 1999

Anderson JC, Williams S, McGee R, et al: DSM-III disorders in preadolescent children: prevalence in a large sample from the general population. Arch Gen Psychiatry 44:69–76, 1987

Ankjaer-Jensen A, Sejr TE: Costs of the treatment of enuresis nocturna: health economic consequences of alternative methods in the treatment of enuresis nocturna. Ugeskr Laeger 156:4355–4360, 1994

Anstendig KD: Is selective mutism an anxiety disorder? Rethinking its DSM-IV classification. J Anxiety Disord 13:417–434, 1999

Antonacci DJ, de Groot CM: Clozapine treatment in a population of adults with mental retardation. J Clin Psychiatry 61:22–25, 2000

Aram DM, Ekelman BL, Nation JE: Preschoolers with language disorder: 10 years later. Journal of Speech and Hearing Research 27:232–244, 1984

Armstrong DD, Dunn K, Antalffy B: Decreased dendritic branching in frontal, motor and limbic cortex in Rett syndrome compared with trisomy 21. J Neuropathol Exp Neurol 57:1013–1017, 1998

Arnell H, Hjälmas K, Jägervall M, et al: The genetics of primary nocturnal enuresis: inheritance and suggestion of a second major gene on chromosome 12q. J Med Genet 34:360–365, 1997

Arnold LE: Alternative treatments for adults with attention-deficit hyperactivity disorder (ADHD), in Adult Attention Deficit Disorders: Brain Mechanisms and Life Outcomes. Edited by Wasserstein J, Wolfe LE, Lefever FF. New York, New York Academy of Sciences, 2001, pp 310–341

Arnold LE: Treatment alternatives for attention-deficit/hyperactivity disorder, in Attention Deficit Hyperactivity Disorder: State of the Science; Best Practices. Edited by Jensen PS, Cooper J. Kingston, NJ, Civic Research Institute, 2002

Arnold LE, Kleykamp D, Votolato N, et al: Potential link between dietary intake of fatty acids and behavior: pilot exploration of serum lipids in attention-deficit hyperactivity disorder. J Child Adolesc Psychopharmacol 4:171–182, 1994

Arnold LE, Pinkham SM, Votolato N: Does zinc moderate essential fatty acid and amphetamine treatment of attention-deficit/hyperactivity disorder? J Child Adolesc Psychopharmacol 10:111–117, 2000

Aronson M, Hagberg B, Gillberg C: Attention deficits and autistic spectrum problems in children exposed to alcohol during gestation: a follow-up study. Dev Med Child Neurol 39:583–587, 1997

Arredondo DE, Butler SF: Affective comorbidity in psychiatrically hospitalized adolescents with conduct disorder or oppositional defiant disorder: should conduct disorder be treated with mood stabilizers? J Child Adolesc Psychopharmacol 4:151–158, 1994

Attwood T, Wing L: Asperger's Syndrome: A Guide for Parents and Professionals. London, England, Jessica Kingsley Publishers, 1998

Auerbach J, Geller V, Lezer S, et al: Dopamine D4 receptor (DRD4) and serotonin transporter promoter (5-HTTLPR) polymorphisms in the determination of temperament in 2-month-old infants. Mol Psychiatry 4:369–373, 1999

Auerbach JG, Benjamin J, Faroy M, et al: DRD4 related to infant attention and information processing: a developmental link to ADHD? Psychiatr Genet 11:31–35, 2001

August GJ, Stewart MA, Holmes CS: A four-year follow-up of boys with and without conduct disorder. Br J Psychiatry 143:192–198, 1983

August GJ, Realmuto GM, MacDonald AW, et al: Prevalence of ADHD and comorbid disorders among elementary school children screened for disruptive behavior. J Abnorm Child Psychol 24:571–595, 1996

August GJ, Realmuto GM, Joyce T, et al: Persistence and desistance of oppositional defiant disorder in a community sample of children with ADHD. J Am Acad Child Adolesc Psychiatry 38:1262–1270, 1999

Aylward EH, Minshew NJ, Goldstein G, et al: MRI volumes of amygdala and hippocampus in non-mentally retarded autistic adolescents and adults. Neurology 53:2145–2150, 1999

Babinski LM, Hartsough CS, Lambert NM: Childhood conduct problems, hyperactivity-impulsivity, and inattention as predictors of adult criminal activity. J Child Psychol Psychiatry 40:347–355, 1999

Bailey A, Le Couteur A, Gottesman I, et al: Autism as a strongly genetic disorder: evidence from a British twin study. Psychol Med 25:63–77, 1995

Bakwin H: The genetics of enuresis, in Bladder Control and Enuresis. Edited by Kolvin RC, MacKeith RC, Meadow SR. London, England, W Heinemann Medical Books, 1973, pp 73–78

Balboni G, Pedrabissi L, Molteni M, et al: Discriminant validity of the Vineland Scales: score profiles of individuals with mental retardation and a specific disorder. Am J Ment Retard 106:162–172, 2001

Barkley RA (ed): Attention Deficit Hyperactivity Disorder: A Handbook for Diagnosis and Treatment. New York, Guilford, 1990

Barkley RA: Attention-deficit/hyperactivity disorder, self-regulation, and time: toward a more comprehensive theory. J Dev Behav Pediatr 18:271–279, 1997a

Barkley RA: Behavioral inhibition, sustained attention, and executive functions: constructing a unifying theory of ADHD. Psychol Bull 121:65–94, 1997b

Barkley RA: Genetics of childhood disorders, XVII: ADHD, part 1: the executive functions and ADHD. J Am Acad Child Adolesc Psychiatry 39:1064–1068, 2000

Barkley RA, Cunningham CE: Do stimulant drugs improve the academic performance of hyperkinetic children? A review of outcome studies. Clin Pediatr 17:85–92, 1978

Barkley RA, Edwards G, Laneri M, et al: Executive functioning, temporal discounting, and sense of time in adolescents with attention deficit hyperactivity disorder (ADHD) and oppositional defiant disorder (ODD). J Abnorm Child Psychol 29:541–556, 2001

Baroff GS: Mental Retardation: Nature, Cause and Management. New York, Hemisphere, 1986

Barr CL, Wigg KG, Feng Y, et al: Attention-deficit hyperactivity disorder and the gene for the dopamine D5 receptor. Mol Psychiatry 5:548–551, 2000

Barr CL, Xu C, Kroft J, et al: Haplotype study of three polymorphisms at the dopamine transporter locus confirm linkage to attention-deficit/hyperactivity disorder. Biol Psychiatry 49:333–339, 2001

Barrett PM: Evaluation of cognitive-behavioral group treatments for childhood anxiety disorders. J Clin Child Psychol 27:459–468, 1998

Barrett PM, Dadds MR, Rapee RM: Family treatment of childhood anxiety: a controlled trial. J Consult Clin Psychol 64:333–342, 1996

Barrett S, Beck JC, Bernier R, et al: An autosomal genomic screen for autism: collaborative linkage study of autism. Am J Med Genet 88:609–615, 1999

Barrickman LL, Perry PJ, Allen AJ, et al: Bupropion versus methylphenidate in the treatment of attention-deficit hyperactivity disorder. J Am Acad Child Adolesc Psychiatry 34:649–657, 1995

Barry CT, Frick PJ, DeShazo TM, et al: The importance of callous-unemotional traits for extending the concept of psychopathy to children. J Abnorm Psychol 109:335–340, 2000

Battaglia M, Bertella S, Politi E, et al: Age at onset of panic disorder: influence of familial liability to the disease and of childhood separation anxiety disorder. Am J Psychiatry 152:1362–1364, 1995

Bauer LO, Hesselbrock VM: P300 decrements in teenagers with conduct problems: implications for substance abuse risk and brain development. Biol Psychiatry 46:263–272, 1999

Bauman ML: Microscopic neuroanatomical abnormalities in autism. Pediatrics 87(suppl):791–796, 1991

Beitchman JH, Nair R, Clegg M, et al: Prevalence of psychiatric disorders in children with speech and language disorders. Journal of the American Academy of Child Psychiatry 25:528–535, 1986

Beitchman JH, Wilson B, Johnson CJ, et al: Fourteen-year follow-up of speech/language-impaired and control children: psychiatric outcome. J Am Acad Child Adolesc Psychiatry 40:75–82, 2001

Bellinger D, Leviton C, Waternaux H, et al: Longitudinal analyses of prenatal and postnatal lead exposure and early cognitive development. N Engl J Med 316:1037–1043, 1987

Benjamin J, Li L, Patterson C, et al: Population and familial association between the D4 dopamine receptor gene and measures of novelty seeking. Nat Genet 12:81–84, 1996

Bennett KE, Haggard MP: Behaviour and cognitive outcomes from middle ear disease. Arch Dis Child 80:28–35, 1999

Benninga MA, Buller HA, Heymans HS, et al: Is encopresis always the result of constipation? Arch Dis Child 71:186–193, 1994

Berg I: School phobia in the children of agoraphobic women. Br J Psychiatry 128:86–89, 1976

Berkson G, Rafaeli-Mor N, Tarnovsky S: Body-rocking and other habits of college students and persons with mental retardation. Am J Ment Retard 104:107–116, 1999

Bernstein GA, Borchardt CM: Anxiety disorders of childhood and adolescence: a critical review. J Am Acad Child Adolesc Psychiatry 30:519–532, 1991

Bernstein GA, Garfinkel BD, Borchardt CM: Comparative studies of pharmacotherapy for school refusal. J Am Acad Child Adolesc Psychiatry 29:773–781, 1990

Berquin PC, Giedd JN, Jacobsen LK, et al: Cerebellum in attention-deficit hyperactivity disorder: a morphometric MRI study. Neurology 50:1087–1093, 1998

Berry CA, Shaywitz SE, Shaywitz BA: Girls with attention deficit disorder: a silent minority? A report on behavioral and cognitive characteristics. Pediatrics 76:801–809, 1985

Bharucha KJ, Sethi KD: Tardive tourettism after exposure to neuroleptic therapy. Mov Disord 10:791–793, 1995

Biederman J: Attention-deficit/hyperactivity disorder: a life-span perspective. J Clin Psychiatry 59(suppl 7):4–16, 1998

Biederman J, Spencer T: Attention-deficit/hyperactivity disorder (ADHD) as a noradrenergic disorder. Biol Psychiatry 46:1234–1242, 1999

Biederman J, Faraone SV, Keenan K, et al: Familial association between attention deficit disorder and anxiety disorders. Am J Psychiatry 148:251–256, 1991

Biederman J, Faraone SV, Keenan K, et al: Further evidence for family genetic risk factors in attention deficit hyperactivity disorder: patterns of comorbidity in probands and relatives psychiatrically and pediatrically referred samples. Arch Gen Psychiatry 49:728–738, 1992

Biederman J, Faraone S, Mick E, et al: Attention-deficit hyperactivity disorder and juvenile mania: an overlooked comorbidity? J Am Acad Child Adolesc Psychiatry 35:997–1008, 1996a

Biederman J, Faraone SV, Milberger S, et al: Is childhood oppositional defiant disorder a precursor to adolescent conduct disorder? Findings from a four-year follow-up study of children with ADHD. J Am Acad Child Adolesc Psychiatry 35:1193–1204, 1996b

Biederman J, Faraone SV, Hatch M, et al: Conduct disorder with and without mania in a referred sample of ADHD children. J Affect Disord 44:177–188, 1997a

Biederman J, Wilens T, Mick E, et al: Is ADHD a risk factor for psychoactive substance use disorders? Findings from a four-year prospective follow-up study. J Am Acad Child Adolesc Psychiatry 36:21–29, 1997b

Biederman J, Wilens TE, Mick E, et al: Does attention-deficit hyperactivity disorder impact the developmental course of drug and alcohol abuse and dependence? Biol Psychiatry 44:269–273, 1998

Biederman J, Faraone SV, Mick E, et al: Clinical correlates of ADHD in females: findings from a large group of girls ascertained from pediatric and psychiatric referral sources. J Am Acad Child Adolesc Psychiatry 38:966–975, 1999a

Biederman J, Wilens T, Mick E, et al: Pharmacotherapy of attention-deficit/hyperactivity disorder reduces risk for substance use disorder (abstract). Pediatrics 104:e20, 1999b

Biederman J, Mick E, Faraone SV: Age-dependent decline of symptoms of attention deficit hyperactivity disorder: impact of remission definition and symptom type. Am J Psychiatry 157:816–818, 2000

Biederman J, Faraone SV, Hirshfeld-Becker DR, et al: Patterns of psychopathology and dysfunction in high-risk children of parents with panic disorder and major depression. Am J Psychiatry 158:49–57, 2001a

Biederman J, Mick E, Faraone SV, et al: Patterns of remission and symptom decline in conduct disorder: a four-year prospective study of an ADHD sample. J Am Acad Child Adolesc Psychiatry 40:290–298, 2001b

Birch HG, Richardson SA, Baird D, et al: Mental Subnormality in the Community: A Clinical and Epidemiological Study. Baltimore, MD, Williams & Wilkins, 1970

Bird HR, Gould MS, Staghezza BM: Patterns of diagnostic comorbidity in a community sample of children aged 9 through 16 years. J Am Acad Child Adolesc Psychiatry 32:361–368, 1993

Birmaher B, Waterman GS, Ryan N, et al: Fluoxetine for childhood anxiety disorders. J Am Acad Child Adolesc Psychiatry 33:993–999, 1994

Bithoney WG, Snyder J, Michalek J, et al: Childhood ingestions as symptoms of family distress. Am J Dis Child 139:456–459, 1985

Blacher J: Transition to adulthood: mental retardation, families, and culture. Am J Ment Retard 106:173–188, 2001

Black B, Uhde TW: Elective mutism as a variant of social phobia. J Am Acad Child Adolesc Psychiatry 31:1090–1094, 1992

Black B, Uhde TW: Treatment of elective mutism with fluoxetine: a double-blind, placebo-controlled study. J Am Acad Child Adolesc Psychiatry 33:1000–1006, 1994

Black B, Uhde TW: Psychiatric characteristics of children with selective mutism: a pilot study. J Am Acad Child Adolesc Psychiatry 34:847–856, 1995

Blagg N, Yule W: The behavioral treatment of school refusal: a comparative study. Behav Res Ther 22:119–127, 1984

Blum K, Sheridan PJ, Wood RC, et al: The D_2 dopamine receptor gene as a determinant of reward deficiency syndrome. J R Soc Med 89:396–400, 1996

Bodfish JW, Symons FJ, Parker DE, et al: Varieties of repetitive behavior in autism: comparisons to mental retardation. J Autism Dev Disord 30:237–243, 2000

Bogels SM, Zigterman D: Dysfunctional cognitions in children with social phobia, separation anxiety disorder, and generalized anxiety disorder. J Abnorm Child Psychol 28:205–211, 2000

Bolman WM, Richmond JA: A double-blind, placebo-controlled, crossover pilot trial of low dose dimethylglycine in patients with autistic disorder. J Autism Dev Disord 29:191–194, 1999

Bonde HV, Andersen JP, Rosenkilde P: Nocturnal enuresis: change of nocturnal voiding pattern during alarm treatment. Scand J Urol Nephrol 28:349–352, 1994

Boris M, Mandel FS: Foods and additives are common causes of the attention deficit hyperactive disorder in children. Ann Allergy 72:462–468, 1994

Boris NW, Zeanah CH: Clinical disturbances of attachment in infancy and early childhood. Curr Opin Pediatr 10:365–368, 1998

Boris NW, Fueyo M, Zeanah CH: The clinical assessment of attachment in children under 5. J Am Acad Child Adolesc Psychiatry 36:291–310, 1997

Boris NW, Zeanah CH, Larrieu JA, et al: Attachment disorders in infancy and early childhood: a preliminary investigation of diagnostic criteria. Am J Psychiatry 155:295–297, 1998

Borthwick-Duffy SA, Lane KL, Widaman KF: Measuring problem behaviors in children with mental retardation: dimensions and predictors. Res Dev Disabil 18:415–433, 1997

Bouffard M, Watkinson EJ, Thompson LP, et al: A test of the activity deficit hypothesis with children with movement difficulties. Adapted Physical Activity Quarterly 13:61–73, 1996

Bower WF, Moore KH, Shepherd RB, et al: The epidemiology of childhood enuresis in Australia. Br J Urol 78:602–606, 1996

Braddock D, Emerson E, Felce D, et al: Living circumstances of children and adults with mental retardation or developmental disabilities in the United States, Canada, England and Wales, and Australia. Mental Retardation and Developmental Disabilities Research Reviews 7:115–121, 2001

Breakey J: The role of diet and behaviour in childhood. J Paediatr Child Health 33:190–194, 1997

Bregman JD: Current developments in the understanding of mental retardation, part 2: psychopathology. J Am Acad Child Adolesc Psychiatry 30:861–872, 1991

Bregman JD, Hodapp RM: Current developments in the understanding of mental retardation, part 1: biological and phenomenological perspectives. J Am Acad Child Adolesc Psychiatry 30:707–719, 1991

Brett PM, Curtis D, Robertson MM, et al: Exclusion of the 5-HT1A serotonin neuroreceptor and tryptophan oxygenase genes in a large British kindred multiply affected with Tourette's syndrome, chronic motor tics, and obsessive-compulsive behavior. Am J Psychiatry 152:437–440, 1995

Brooks RC, Copen RM, Cox DJ, et al: Review of the treatment literature for encopresis, functional constipation, and stool-toileting refusal. Ann Behav Med 22:260–267, 2000

Brosch S, Haege A, Kalehne P, et al: Stuttering children and the probability of remission: the role of cerebral dominance and speech production. Int J Pediatr Otorhinolaryngol 47:71–76, 1999

Brown MB, Giandenoto MJ, Bolen LM: Diagnosing written language disabilities using the Woodcock-Johnson Tests of Educational Achievement—Revised and the Wechsler Individual Achievement Test. Psychol Rep 87:197–204, 2000

Bruck M: Persistence of dyslexics' phonologic awareness deficits. Dev Psychol 28:874–886, 1992

Bruggeman R, van der Linden C, Buitelaar JK, et al: Risperidone versus pimozide, I: Tourette's disorder: a comparative double-blind parallel-group study. J Clin Psychiatry 62:50–56, 2001

Bruun RD: The natural history of Tourette's syndrome, in Tourette's Syndrome and Tic Disorders: Clinical Understanding and Treatment. Edited by Cohen D, Bruun R, Leckman J. New York, Wiley, 1988

Budman CL, Bruun RD, Park KS, et al: Explosive outbursts in children with Tourette's disorder. J Am Acad Child Adolesc Psychiatry 39:1270–1276, 2000

Buitelaar JK: Open-label treatment with risperidone of 26 psychiatrically hospitalized children and adolescents with mixed diagnoses and aggressive behavior. J Child Adolesc Psychopharmacol 10:19–26, 2000

Buitelaar JK, van der Gaag RJ, Cohen-Kettenis P, et al: A randomized controlled trial of risperidone in the treatment of aggression in hospitalized adolescents with subaverage cognitive abilities. J Clin Psychiatry 62:239–248, 2001

Bull R, Johnston RS: Children's arithmetical difficulties: contributions from processing speed, item identification, and short-term memory. J Exp Child Psychol 65:1–24, 1997

Burd L, Severud R, Klug MG, et al: Prenatal and perinatal risk factors for Tourette disorder. J Perinat Med 27:295–302, 1999

Burgard JF, Donohue B, Azrin NH, et al: Prevalence and treatment of substance abuse in the mentally retarded population: an empirical review. J Psychoactive Drugs 32:293–298, 2000

Bush G, Frazier JA, Rauch SL, et al: Anterior cingulated cortex dysfunction in attention-deficit/hyperactivity disorder revealed by fMRI and the Counting Stroop. Biol Psychiatry 45:1542–1552, 1999

Butler SF, Arredondo DE, McCloskey V: Affective comorbidity in children and adolescents with attention deficit hyperactivity disorder. Ann Clin Psychiatry 7:51–55, 1995

Buttross S: Encopresis in the child with a behavioral disorder: when the initial treatment does not work. Pediatr Ann 28:317–321, 1999

Cadoret RJ, Yates WR, Troughton E, et al: Genetic-environmental interaction in the genesis of aggressivity and conduct disorders. Arch Gen Psychiatry 52:916–924, 1995

Caione P, Arena F, Biraghi M, et al: Nocturnal enuresis and daytime wetting: a multicentric trial with oxybutynin and desmopressin. Eur Urol 31:459–463, 1997

Calabrese EJ, Stanek EJ, James RC, et al: Soil ingestion: a concern for acute toxicity in children. Environ Health Perspect 105:1354–1358, 1997

Campbell M, Adams PB, Small AM, et al: Lithium in hospitalized aggressive children with conduct disorder: a double-blind and placebo-controlled study. J Am Acad Child Adolesc Psychiatry 34:445–453, 1995a

Campbell M, Kafantaris V, Cueva JE: An update on the use of lithium carbonate in aggressive children and adolescents with conduct disorder. Psychopharmacol Bull 31:93–102, 1995b

Campbell L, Malone MA, Kershner JR, et al: Methylphenidate slows right hemisphere processing in children with attention-deficit/hyperactivity disorder. J Child Adolesc Psychopharmacol 6:229–239, 1996

Canales JJ, Graybiel AM: A measure of striatal function predicts motor stereotypy. Nature Neuroscience 3:377–383, 2000

Cantell M, Kooistra L: Long-term outcomes of developmental coordination disorder, in Developmental Coordination Disorder. Edited by Cermak SA, Larkin D. Albany, NY, Singular Publishing Group, 2002

Cantwell DP, Baker L: Developmental Speech and Language Disorders. New York, Guilford, 1987

Cantwell DP, Baker L: Issues in classification of child and adolescent psychopathology. J Am Acad Child Adolesc Psychiatry 27:521–533, 1988

Cantwell DP, Baker L: Stability and natural history of DSM-III childhood diagnoses. J Am Acad Child Adolesc Psychiatry 28:691–700, 1989

Capps L, Sigman M, Sena R, et al: Fear, anxiety and perceived control in children of agoraphobic parents. J Child Psychol Psychiatry 37:445–452, 1996

Cardon LR, Smith SD, Fulker DW, et al: Quantitative trait locus for reading disability on chromosome 6. Science 266:276–279, 1994

Carlin MT, Soraci SA, Dennis NA, et al: Enhancing free-recall rates of individuals with mental retardation. Am J Ment Retard 106:314–326, 2001

Carlson JS, Kratochwill TR, Johnston HF: Sertraline treatment of 5 children diagnosed with selective mutism: a single-case research trial. J Child Adolesc Psychopharmacol 9:293–306, 1999

Carlson V, Cicchetti D, Barnett D, et al: Disorganized/disoriented attachment relationships in maltreated infants. Dev Psychol 25:525–531, 1989

Carlsson ML: On the role of cortical glutamate in obsessive-compulsive disorder and attention-deficit hyperactivity disorder, two phenomenologically antithetical conditions. Acta Psychiatr Scand 102:401–413, 2000

Carper RA, Courchesne E: Inverse correlation between frontal lobe and cerebellum sizes in children with autism. Brain 123:836–844, 2000

Carta MG, Hardoy MC, Dessi I, et al: Adjunctive gabapentin in patients with intellectual disability and bipolar spectrum disorders. J Intellect Disabil Res 45:139–145, 2001

Casat CD, Pleasants DZ, Schroeder DH, et al: Bupropion in children with attention deficit disorder. Psychopharmacol Bull 25:187–201, 1989

Casey BJ, Castellanos FX, Giedd JN, et al: Implication of right frontostriatal circuitry in response inhibition and attention-deficit/hyperactivity disorder. J Am Acad Child Adolesc Psychiatry 36:374–383, 1997

Castellanos FX, Elia J, Kruesi MJ, et al: Cerebrospinal fluid monoamine metabolites in boys with attention deficit hyperactivity disorder. Psychiatry Res 52:305–316, 1994a

Castellanos FX, Giedd JN, Eckburg P, et al: Quantitative morphology of the caudate nucleus in attention deficit hyperactivity disorder. Am J Psychiatry 151:1791–1796, 1994b

Castellanos FX, Giedd JN, Marsh WL, et al: Quantitative brain magnetic resonance imaging in attention-deficit hyperactivity disorder. Arch Gen Psychiatry 53:607–616, 1996

Castellanos FX, Ritchie GF, Marsh WL, et al: DSM-IV stereotypic movement disorder: persistence of stereotypies of infancy in intellectually normal adolescents and adults. J Clin Psychiatry 58:177–178, 1997

Castellanos FX, Lau E, Tayebi N, et al: Lack of an association between a dopamine-4 receptor polymorphism and attention-deficit/hyperactivity disorder: genetic and brain morphometric analyses. Mol Psychiatry 3:431–434, 1998

Castellanos FX, Giedd JN, Berquin PC, et al: Quantitative brain magnetic resonance imaging in girls with attention-deficit/hyperactivity disorder. Arch Gen Psychiatry 58:289–295, 2001

Castellvi-Bel S, Mila M: Genes responsible for nonspecific mental retardation. Mol Genet Metab 72:104–108, 2001

Cath DC, Spinhoven P, van Woerkom TC, et al: Gilles de la Tourette's syndrome with and without obsessive-compulsive disorder compared with obsessive-compulsive disorder without tics: which symptoms discriminate? J Nerv Ment Dis 189:219–228, 2001a

Cath DC, Spinhoven P, Hoogduin CA, et al: Repetitive behaviors in Tourette's syndrome and OCD with and without tics: what are the differences? Psychiatry Res 101:171–185, 2001b

Cavaliere F, Cormaci S, Cormaci M, et al: Clinical and hormonal response to general anaesthesia in patients affected by different degrees of mental retardation. Minerva Anestesiol 65:499–505, 1999

Cermak SA, Gubbay SS, Larkin D: What is developmental coordination disorder? in Developmental Coordination Disorder: Theory and Practice. Edited by Cermak SA, Larkin D. Albany, NY, Delmar Thompson Learning, 2001

Chabot RJ, Serfontein G: Quantitative electroencephalographic profiles of children with attention deficit disorder. Biol Psychiatry 40:951–963, 1996

Chabrol H, Fouraste R, Morón P, et al: Father-child hospitalization in separation anxiety [in Spanish]. Actas Luso Esp Neurol Psiquiatr Cienc Afines 23:223–226, 1995

Chaney RH, Eyman RK: Patterns in mortality over 60 years among persons with mental retardation in a residential facility. Ment Retard 38:289–293, 2000

Chappell PB, Riddle MA, Scahill L, et al: Guanfacine treatment of comorbid attention deficit hyperactivity disorder and Tourette's syndrome: preliminary clinical experience. J Am Acad Child Adolesc Psychiatry 34:1140–1146, 1995

Chase TN, Friedhoff AJ, Cohen DJ (eds): Tourette Syndrome: Genetics, Neurobiology, and Treatment (Advances in Neurology Series, Vol 58). New York, Raven, 1992

Chatoor I: Infantile anorexia nervosa: a developmental disorder or separation and individuation. J Am Acad Psychoanal 17:43–64, 1989

Chatoor I, Dickson L, Einhorn A: Rumination: etiology and treatment. Pediatr Ann 13:924–929, 1984

Chatoor I, Dickson L, Schaefer S, et al: A developmental classification of feeding disorders associated with failure to thrive: diagnosis and treatment, in New Directions in Failure to Thrive: Research and Clinical Practice. Edited by Drotar D. New York, Plenum, 1985

Chatoor I, Ganiban J, Hirsch R, et al: Maternal characteristics and toddler temperament in infantile anorexia. J Am Acad Child Adolesc Psychiatry 39:743–751, 2000

Elliott DS, Huizinga D, Ageton SS: Explaining Delinquency and Drug Use. Beverly Hills, CA, Sage, 1985

Elstner K, Selai CE, Trimble MR, et al: Quality of life (QOL) of patients with Gilles de la Tourette's syndrome. Acta Psychiatr Scand 103:52–59, 2001

Embregts PJ: Reliability of the Child Behavior Checklist for the assessment of behavioral problems of children and youth with mild mental retardation. Res Dev Disabil 21:31–41, 2000

Ernst M, Liebenauer LL, Jons PH, et al: Selegiline in adults with attention deficit hyperactivity disorder: clinical efficacy and safety. Psychopharmacol Bull 32:327–334, 1996

Ernst M, Zametkin AJ, Jons PH, et al: High presynaptic dopaminergic activity in children with Tourette's disorder. J Am Acad Child Adolesc Psychiatry 38:86–94, 1999

Fairbanks JM, Pine DS, Tancer NK, et al: Open fluoxetine treatment of mixed anxiety disorders in children and adolescents. J Child Adolesc Psychopharmacol 7:17–29, 1997

Faraone SV, Doyle AE: The nature and heritability of attention-deficit/hyperactivity disorder. Child Adolesc Psychiatr Clin North Am 10:299–316, 2001

Faraone SV, Biederman J, Spencer T, et al: Attention-deficit/hyperactivity disorder in adults: an overview. Biol Psychiatry 48:9–20, 2000a

Faraone SV, Biederman J, Mick E, et al: Family study of girls with attention deficit hyperactivity disorder. Am J Psychiatry 157:1077–1083, 2000b

Faraone SV, Doyle AE, Mick E, et al: Meta-analysis of the association between the 7-repeat allele of the dopamine D(4) receptor gene and attention deficit hyperactivity disorder. Am J Psychiatry 158:1052–1057, 2001

Farrington DP, Loeber R: Epidemiology of juvenile violence. Child Adolesc Psychiatr Clin N Am 9:733–748, 2000

Faulstich ME, Moore JR, Roberts RW, et al: A behavioral perspective on conduct disorders. Psychiatry 51:116–130, 1988

Federal Bureau of Investigation: Crime in the United States 2000: Uniform Crime Reports. Washington, DC, U.S. Department of Justice, 2001

Federer M, Herrle J, Margraf J, et al: [Separation anxiety and agoraphobia in 8-year-old children.] Prax Kinderpsychol Kinderpsychiatr 49:83–96, 2000

Feigin A, Kurlan R, McDermott MP, et al: A controlled trial of deprenyl in children with Tourette's syndrome and attention deficit hyperactivity disorder. Neurology 46:965–968, 1996

Felce D, Emerson E: Living with support in a home in the community: predictors of behavioral development and household and community activity. Mental Retardation and Developmental Disabilities Research Reviews 7:75–83, 2001

Feldman M, Wilson A: Adolescent suicidality in urban minorities and its relationship to conduct disorders, depression, and separation anxiety. J Am Acad Child Adolesc Psychiatry 36:75–84, 1997

Felsenfeld S, Kirk KM, Zhu G, et al: A study of the genetic and environmental etiology of stuttering in a selected twin sample. Behav Genet 30:359–366, 2000

Fendrich M, Warner V, Weissman MM: Family risk factors, parental depression, and psychopathology in offspring. Dev Psychol 26:40–50, 1990

Fergusson DM, Horwood LJ, Shannon FT: Factors related to the age of attainment of nocturnal bladder control. Pediatrics 78:884–890, 1986

Fergusson DM, Horwood LJ, Lynskey MT: Structure of DSM-III-R criteria for disruptive childhood behaviors: confirmatory factor models. J Am Acad Child Adolesc Psychiatry 33:1145–1157, 1994

Fey M, Leonard L, Wilcox K: Speech style modification in language-impaired children. Journal of Speech and Hearing Disorders 46:91–96, 1981

Filipek PA, Semrud-Clikeman M, Steingard RJ, et al: Volumetric MRI analysis comparing subjects having attention-deficit hyperactivity disorder with normal controls. Neurology 48:589–601, 1997

Findling RL, Maxwell K, Scotese-Wojtila L, et al: High-dose pyridoxine and magnesium administration in children with autistic disorder: an absence of salutary effects in a double-blind, placebo-controlled study. J Autism Dev Disord 27:467–478, 1997

Findling RL, McNamara NK, Branicky LA, et al: A double-blind pilot study of risperidone in the treatment of conduct disorder. J Am Acad Child Adolesc Psychiatry 39:509–516, 2000

Fisher L, Ames EW, Chisholm K, et al: Problems reported by parents of Romanian orphans adopted to British Columbia. International Journal of Behavioral Development 20:67–82, 1997

Fisher SE, Vargha-Khadem F, Watkins KE, et al: Localization of a gene implicated in a severe speech and language disorder. Nat Genet 18:168–170, 1998

Flakierska-Praquin N, Lindstrom M, Gillberg C: School phobia with separation anxiety disorder: a comparative 20- to 29-year follow-up study of 35 school refusers. Compr Psychiatry 38:17–22, 1997

Fletcher KE, Fischer M, Barkley RA, et al: A sequential analysis of the mother-adolescent interactions of ADHD, ADHD+ODD, and normal teenagers during neutral and conflict discussions. J Abnorm Child Psychol 24:271–297, 1996

Foley HA, Carlton CO, Howell RJ: The relationship of attention deficit hyperactivity disorder and conduct disorder to juvenile delinquency: legal implications. Bull Am Acad Psychiatry Law 24:333–345, 1996

Folstein SE, Piven J: Etiology of autism: genetic influences. Pediatrics 87(suppl):767–773, 1991

Fonagy P, Target M: The efficacy of psychoanalysis for children with disruptive disorders. J Am Acad Child Adolesc Psychiatry 33:45–55, 1994

Fonagy P, Steele M, Steele H, et al: The relation of attachment status, psychiatric classification, and response to psychotherapy. J Consult Clin Psychol 64:22–31, 1996

Foorman BR, Francis DJ, Beeler T, et al: Early interventions for children with problems: study designs and preliminary findings. Learning Disabilities 8:63–71, 1997

Ford JD, Racusin R, Daviss WB, et al: Trauma exposure among children with oppositional defiant disorder and attention deficit-hyperactivity disorder. J Consult Clin Psychol 67:786–789, 1999

Foreman DM, Thambirajah MS: Conduct disorder, enuresis and specific developmental delays in two types of encopresis: a case-note study of 63 boys. Eur Child Adolesc Psychiatry 5:33–37, 1996

Forsythe WI, Butler RJ: Fifty years of enuretic alarms. Arch Dis Child 64:879–885, 1989

Fox AM, Lent B: Clumsy children: primer on developmental coordination disorder. Can Fam Physician 42:1965–1971, 1996

Fredericks DW, Carr JE, Williams WL: Overview of the treatment of rumination disorder for adults in a residential setting. J Behav Ther Exp Psychiatry 29:31–40, 1998

Freedman RI: Ethical challenges in the conduct of research involving persons with mental retardation. Ment Retard 39:130–141, 2001

Freeman RD, Fast DK, Burd L, et al: An international perspective on Tourette syndrome: selected findings from 3,500 individuals in 22 countries. Dev Med Child Neurol 42:436–447, 2000

Frick PJ: Conduct Disorders and Severe Antisocial Behavior. New York, Plenum, 1998

Friman PC, Mathew JR, Finney JW, et al: Do encopretic children have clinically significant behavior problems? Pediatrics 82:407–409, 1988

Frith U (ed): Autism and Asperger Syndrome. Cambridge, England, University of Cambridge, 1991

Fujii Y, Konishi Y, Kuriyama M, et al: Corpus callosum in developmentally retarded infants. Pediatr Neurol 11:219–223, 1994

Gabel S, Chandra R, Shindledecker R: Behavior ratings and outcome of medical treatment for encopresis. J Dev Behav Pediatr 9:129–133, 1988

Gadow KD, Sverd J, Sprafkin J, et al: Efficacy of methylphenidate for attention deficit hyperactivity disorder in children with tic disorder. Arch Gen Psychiatry 52:444–455, 1995

Gadow KD, Sverd J, Sprafkin J, et al: Long-term methylphenidate therapy in children with comorbid attention-deficit hyperactivity disorder and chronic multiple tic disorder. Arch Gen Psychiatry 56:330–336, 1999

Galaburda AM (ed): Dyslexia and Development: Neurobiological Aspects of Extra-Ordinary Brains. Cambridge, MA, Harvard University Press, 1993

Galler JR, Ramsey F, Solimano G, et al: The influence of early malnutrition on subsequent behavioral development, II: classroom behavior. Journal of the American Academy of Child Psychiatry 22:16–22, 1983

García-Sánchez C, Estévez-González A, Suárez-Romero E, et al: Right hemisphere dysfunction in subjects with attention-deficit disorder with and without hyperactivity. J Child Neurol 12:107–115, 1997

Gaub M, Carlson CL: Behavioral characteristics of DSM-IV ADHD subtypes in a school-based population. J Abnorm Child Psychol 25:103–111, 1997

Geschwind N, Behan P: Left-handedness: association with immune disease, migraine, and developmental learning disorder. Proc Natl Acad Sci U S A 79:5097–5100, 1982

Geschwind N, Galaburda AM: Cerebral lateralization: biological mechanisms, associations, and pathology. Arch Neurol 42:428–459, 521–552, 634–654, 1985

Getting P: Emerging principles governing the operations of neural networks. Annu Rev Neurosci 12:185–204, 1989

Giedd JN, Castellanos FX, Casey BJ, et al: Quantitative morphology of the corpus callosum in attention deficit hyperactivity disorder. Am J Psychiatry 151:665–669, 1994

Giedd JN, Rapoport JL, Garvey MA, et al: MRI assessment of children with obsessive-compulsive disorder or tics associated with streptococcal infection. Am J Psychiatry 157:281–283, 2000

Giedd JN, Blumenthal J, Molloy E: Brain imaging of attention deficit/hyperactivity disorder. Ann N Y Acad Sci 931:33–49, 2001

Gierut JA: Treatment efficacy: functional phonological disorders in children. J Speech Lang Hear Res 41:S85–100, 1998

Gilbert DL, Sethuraman G, Sine L, et al: Tourette's syndrome improvement with pergolide in a randomized, double-blind, crossover trial. Neurology 54:1310–1315, 2000

Gill M, Daly G, Heron S, et al: Confirmation of association between attention deficit hyperactivity disorder and a dopamine transporter polymorphism. Mol Psychiatry 2:311–313, 1997

Gillberg C: Asperger syndrome in 23 Swedish children. Dev Med Child Neurol 31:520–531, 1989

Gillberg C, Persson E, Grufman M, et al: Psychiatric disorders in mildly and severely mentally retarded urban children and adolescents: epidemiological aspects. Br J Psychiatry 149:68–74, 1986

Gillberg C, Melander H, von Knorring AL, et al: Long-term stimulant treatment of children with attention-deficit hyperactivity disorder symptoms: a randomized, double-blind, placebo controlled trial. Arch Gen Psychiatry 54:857–864, 1997

Gittelman R, Mannuzza S, Shenker R, et al: Hyperactive boys almost grown up, I: psychiatric status. Arch Gen Psychiatry 42:937–947, 1985

Glazener CM, Evans JH: Desmopressin for nocturnal enuresis in children. Cochrane Database Syst Rev 2:CD002112, 2000a

Glazener CM, Evans JH: Tricyclic and related drugs for nocturnal enuresis in children. Cochrane Database Syst Rev 3:CD002117, 2000b

Glazener CM, Evans JH: Alarm interventions for nocturnal enuresis in children. Cochrane Database System Review 1:CD002911, 2001

Goldstein RD, Prescott CA, Kendler KS: Genetic and environmental factors in conduct problems and adult antisocial behavior among adult female twins. J Nerv Ment Dis 189:201–209, 2001

Golwyn DH, Sevlie CP: Phenelzine treatment of selective mutism in four prepubertal children. J Child Adolesc Psychopharmacol 9:109–113, 1999

Gordon N: Mutism: elective or selective, and acquired. Brain Dev 23:83–87, 2001

Gostason R: Psychiatric illness among the mentally retarded: a Swedish population study. Acta Psychiatr Scand 318(suppl):1–117, 1985

Graae F, Milner J, Rizzotto L, et al: Clonazepam in childhood anxiety disorders. J Am Acad Child Adolesc Psychiatry 33:372–376, 1994

Grandin T, Scariano MM: Emergence Labeled Autistic. Novato, CA, Arena Press, 1986

Greene RW, Doyle AE: Toward a transactional conceptualization of oppositional defiant disorder: implications for assessment and treatment. Clinical Child and Family Psychology Review 2:129–148, 1999

Greene RW, Biederman J, Faraone SV, et al: Further validation of social impairment as a predictor of substance use disorders: findings from a sample of siblings of boys with and without ADHD. J Clin Child Psychol 28:349–354, 1999

Gregg N, McAlexander PA: The relation between sense of audience and specific learning disabilities: an exploration. Annals of Dyslexia 39:206–226, 1989

Grigorenko EL: Developmental dyslexia: an update on genes, brains, and environments. J Child Psychol Psychiatry 42:91–125, 2001

Grigorenko EL, Wood FB, Meyer MS, et al: Susceptibility loci for distinct components of developmental dyslexia on chromosomes 6 and 15. Am J Hum Genet 60:27–39, 1997

Grigorenko EL, Sternberg RJ, Ehrman ME: A theory-based approach to the measurement of foreign language learning ability: the canal-F theory and test. Modern Language Journal 84:390–405, 2000

Grigorenko EL, Wood FB, Meyer MS, et al: Linkage studies suggest a possible locus for developmental dyslexia on chromosome 1p. Am J Med Genet 105:120–129, 2001

Grigsby RK, Thyer BA, Waller RJ, et al: Chalk eating in middle Georgia: a culture-bound syndrome of pica? South Med J 92:190–192, 1999

Gross-Tsur V, Manor O, Shalev RS: Developmental dyscalculia: prevalence and demographic features. Dev Med Child Neurol 38:25–33, 1996

Grossman HJ (ed): Classification in Mental Retardation. Washington, DC, American Association on Mental Deficiency, 1983

Grosso S, Cioni M, Pucci L, et al: Selective mutism, speech delay, dysmorphisms, and deletion of the short arm of chromosome 18: a distinct entity? J Neurol Neurosurg Psychiatry 67:830–831, 1999

Guedeney A: An update on merycism and early depression: a critical review of the literature and a psychopathological hypothesis [in French]. Psychiatr Enfant (Paris) 38:345–363, 1995

Guy J, Hendrich B, Holmes M, et al: A mouse Mecp2-null mutation causes neurological symptoms that mimic Rett syndrome. Nat Genet 27:322–326, 2001

Haber SN, Lynd-Balta E: Basal ganglia-limbic system interactions, in Handbook of Tourette's Syndrome and Related Tic and Behavioral Disorders. Edited by Kurlan R. New York, Marcel Dekker, 1993

Haber SN, Wolfer D: Basal ganglia peptidergic staining in Tourette syndrome, in Tourette Syndrome: Genetics, Neurobiology, and Treatment (Advances in Neurology Series, Vol 58). Edited by Chase TN, Friedhoff AJ, Cohen DJ. New York, Raven, 1992

Hafeez A, Malik QU: Blood lead levels in preschool children in Rawalpindi. JPMA J Pak Med Assoc 46:272–274, 1996

Hagerman RJ, Hills J, Scharfenaker S, et al: Fragile X syndrome and selective mutism. Am J Med Genet 83:313–317, 1999

Halperin JM, Newcorn JH, Matier K, et al: Impulsivity and the initiation of fights in children with disruptive behavior disorders. J Child Psychol Psychiatry 36:1199–1211, 1995

Hancock K, Craig A, McCready C, et al: Two- to six-year controlled-trial stuttering outcomes for children and adolescents. J Speech Lang Hear Res 41:1242–1252, 1998

Hanna GL, Fluent TE, Fischer DJ: Separation anxiety in children and adolescents treated with risperidone. J Child Adolesc Psychopharmacol 9:277–283, 1999

Hardan AY, Minshew NJ, Harenski K, et al: Posterior fossa magnetic resonance imaging in autism. J Am Acad Child Adolesc Psychiatry 40:666–672, 2001

Hare RD, McPherson LM, Forth AE: Male psychopaths and their criminal careers. J Consult Clin Psychol 56:710–714, 1988

Harris EC, Barraclough B: Suicide as an outcome for mental disorders: a meta-analysis. Br J Psychiatry 170:205–228, 1997

Hart EL, Lahey BB, Loeber R, et al: Developmental change in attention-deficit hyperactivity disorder in boys: a four-year longitudinal study. J Abnorm Child Psychol 23:729–749, 1995

Haslam RH, Dalby JT, Johns RD, et al: Cerebral asymmetry in developmental dyslexia. Arch Neurol 38:679–682, 1981

Hauser P, Zametkin AJ, Martinez P, et al: Attention deficit-hyperactivity disorder in people with generalized resistance to thyroid hormone. N Engl J Med 328:997–1001, 1993

Hayden TL: Classification of elective mutism. Journal of the American Academy of Child Psychiatry 19:118–133, 1980

Hayward C, Killen JD, Kraemer HC, et al: Predictors of panic attacks in adolescents. J Am Acad Child Adolesc Psychiatry 39:207–214, 2000

Haznedar MM, Buchsbaum MS, Metzger M, et al: Anterior cingulate gyrus volume and glucose metabolism in autistic disorder. Am J Psychiatry 154:1047–1050, 1997

Hebebrand J, Klug B, Fimmers R, et al: Rates for tic disorders and obsessive compulsive symptomatology in families of children and adolescents with Gilles de la Tourette syndrome. J Psychiatr Res 31:519–530, 1997

Hechtman L: Families of children with attention deficit hyperactivity disorder: a review. Can J Psychiatry 41:350–360, 1996

Hellings JA, Kelley LA, Gabrielli WF, et al: Sertraline response in adults with mental retardation and autistic disorder. J Clin Psychiatry 57:333–336, 1996

Hendren RL, De Backer I, Pandina GJ: Review of neuroimaging studies of child and adolescent psychiatric disorders from the past 10 years. J Am Acad Child Adolesc Psychiatry 39:815–828, 2000

Herskowitz J: Developmental neurotoxicology, in Psychiatric Pharmacosciences of Children and Adolescents. Edited by Popper C. Washington, DC, American Psychiatric Press, 1987, pp 81–124

Hill AE, Rosenbloom L: Disintegrative psychosis of childhood: teenage follow-up. Dev Med Child Neurol 28:34–40, 1986

Hill EL: A dyspraxic deficit in specific language impairment and developmental coordination disorder? Evidence from hand and arm movements. Dev Med Child Neurol 40:388–395, 1998

Hill JC, Schoener EP: Age-dependent decline of attention deficit hyperactivity disorder. Am J Psychiatry 153:1143–1146, 1996

Hirshfeld DR, Biederman J, Brody L, et al: Associations between expressed emotion and child behavioral inhibition and psychopathology: a pilot study. J Am Acad Child Adolesc Psychiatry 36:205–213, 1997

Hittmair-Delazer M, Sailer U, Benke T: Impaired arithmetic facts but intact conceptual knowledge: a single case study of dyscalculia. Cortex 31:139–147, 1995

Hoekstra PJ, Bijzet J, Limburg PC, et al: Elevated D8/17 expression on B lymphocytes, a marker of rheumatic fever, measured with flow cytometry in tic disorder patients. Am J Psychiatry 158:605–610, 2001

Hoffbuhr K, Devaney JM, LaFleur B, et al: MeCP2 mutations in children with and without the phenotype of Rett syndrome. Neurology 56:1486–1495, 2001

Hollander HE, Turner FD: Characteristics of incarcerated delinquents: relationship between development disorders, environmental and family factors, and patterns of offense and recidivism. Journal of the American Academy of Child Psychiatry 24:221–226, 1985

Holmes SE, Slaughter JR, Kashani J: Risk factors in childhood that lead to the development of conduct disorder and antisocial personality disorder. Child Psychiatry Hum Dev 31:183–193, 2001

Howie VM: Developmental sequelae of chronic otitis media: a review. J Dev Behav Pediatr 1:34–38, 1980

Huesmann LR, Eron LD, Lefkowitz MM, et al: The stability of aggression over time and generations. Dev Psychol 20:1120–1134, 1984

Humphries T, Wright M, Snider L, et al: A comparison of the effectiveness of sensory integrative therapy and perceptual-motor training in treating children with learning disabilities. J Dev Behav Pediatr 13:31–40, 1992

Hunsballe JM, Lundorf E, Norgaard JP: The pituitary gland in nocturnal enuresis: MR findings. Scand J Urol Nephrol 30:85–87, 1996

Hunsballe JM, Rittig S, Pedersen EB, et al: Single dose imipramine reduces nocturnal urine output in patients with nocturnal enuresis and nocturnal polyuria. J Urol 158:830–836, 1997

Hunt RD, Capper L, O'Connell P: Clonidine in child and adolescent psychiatry. J Child Adolesc Psychopharmacol 1:87–102, 1990

Hunt RD, Arnsten AF, Asbell MD: An open trial of guanfacine in the treatment of attention-deficit hyperactivity disorder. J Am Acad Child Adolesc Psychiatry 34:50–54, 1995

Hunter AG: Outcome of the routine assessment of patients with mental retardation in a genetics clinic. Am J Med Genet 90:60–68, 2000

Hyde TM, Stacey ME, Coppola R, et al: Cerebral morphometric abnormalities in Tourette's syndrome: a quantitative MRI study of monozygotic twins. Neurology 45:1176–1182, 1995

Hynd GW, Hall J, Novey ES: Dyslexia and corpus callosum morphology. Arch Neurol 52:32–38, 1995

Ialongo NS, Horn WF, Pascoe JM, et al: The effects of multimodal intervention with ADHD children: a 9-month follow-up. J Am Acad Child Adolesc Psychiatry 32:182–189, 1993

Individuals With Disabilities Education Act 20 U.S.C. Chapter 33 As last amended by The Individuals with Disabilities Education Act Amendments of 1997 Pub.L. 105–17 (June 4, 1997)

Insel TR: A neurobiological base of social attachment. Am J Psychiatry 154:726–735, 1997

International Molecular Genetic Study of Autism Consortium (IMGSAC): A genome-wide screen for autism: strong evidence for linkage to chromosomes 2q, 7q, and 16p. Am J Hum Genet 69:570–581, 2001

Jacobs BW, Isaacs S: Pre-pubertal anorexia nervosa. J Child Psychol Psychiatry 27:237–250, 1986

Jacobson KC, Prescott CA, Kendler KS: Genetic and environmental influences on juvenile antisocial behavior assessed on two occasions. Psychol Med 30:1315–1325, 2000

Jagger J, Proshoff BA, Cohen DJ, et al: The epidemiology of Tourette syndrome: a pilot study. Schizophr Bull 8:267–279, 1982

Jain P, Misra A: Nonsustained ventricular tachycardia following clonidine withdrawal (letter). Postgrad Med J 33:403–404, 1991

Jaselskis CA, Cook EH, Fletcher K, et al: Clonidine treatment of hyperactive and impulsive children with autistic disorder. J Clin Psychopharmacol 12:322–327, 1992

Jenkins RL: Behavior Disorders of Childhood and Adolescence. Springfield, IL, Charles C Thomas, 1973

Jensen PS: Introduction: ADHD comorbidity and treatment outcomes in the MTA. J Am Acad Child Adolesc Psychiatry 40:134–136, 2001

Jensen PS, Shervette RE, Xenakis SN, et al: Anxiety and depressive disorders in attention deficit disorder with hyperactivity: new findings. Am J Psychiatry 150:1203–1209, 1993

Jensen PS, Hinshaw SP, Kraemer HC, et al: ADHD comorbidity findings from the MTA study: comparing comorbid subgroups. J Am Acad Child Adolesc Psychiatry 40:147–158, 2001a

Jensen PS, Hinshaw SP, Swanson JM, et al: Findings from the NIMH Multimodal Treatment Study of ADHD (MTA): implications and applications for primary care providers. J Dev Behav Pediatr 22:60–73, 2001b

Johnson AM, Falstein EI, Szurek SA, et al: School phobia. Am J Orthopsychiatry 11:702–711, 1941

Johnson CJ, Beitchman JH, Young A, et al: Fourteen-year follow-up of children with and without speech/language impairments: speech/language stability and outcomes. J Speech Lang Hear Res 42:744–760, 1999

Johnston MV, Nishimura A, Harum K, et al: Sculpting the developing brain. Adv Pediatr 48:1–38, 2001

Kadesjo B, Gillberg C: The comorbidity of ADHD in the general population of Swedish school-age children. J Child Psychol Psychiatry 42:487–492, 2001

Kafantaris V, Campbell M, Padron-Gayol MV, et al: Carbamazepine in hospitalized aggressive conduct disorder children: an open pilot study. Psychopharmacol Bull 28:193–199, 1992

Kagan J, Reznick JS, Snidman N: The physiology and psychology of behavioral inhibition in children. Child Dev 58:1459–1473, 1987

Kalo BB, Bella H: Enuresis: prevalence and associated factors among primary school children in Saudi Arabia. Acta Paediatr 85:1217–1222, 1996

Kaneko K, Fujinaga S, Ohtomo Y, et al: Combined pharmacotherapy for nocturnal enuresis. Pediatr Nephrol 16:662–664, 2001

Kanner L: Autistic disturbances of affective contact. Nervous Child 2:217–250, 1943

Kaplan BJ, Polatajko HJ, Wilson BN, et al: Reexamination of sensory integration treatment: a combination of two efficacy studies. J Learn Disabil 26:342–347, 1993

Katusic SJ, Colligan RC, Beard CM, et al: Mental retardation in a birth cohort, 1976–1980, Rochester, Minnesota. Am J Ment Retard 100:335–344, 1996

Katz LM, Nathan L, Kuhn CM, et al: Inhibition of GH in maternal separation may be mediated through altered serotonergic activity at 5-HT2A and 5-HT2C receptors. Psychoneuroendocrinology 21:219–235, 1996

Kaufmann WE, Moser HW: Dendritic anomalies in disorders associated with mental retardation. Cereb Cortex 10:981–991, 2000

Kazdin AE: Conduct Disorders in Childhood and Adolescence. Newbury Park, CA, Sage, 1987

Kazdin AE: Practitioner review: psychosocial treatments for conduct disorder in children. J Child Psychol Psychiatry 38:161–178, 1997

Kazdin AE, Bass D, Siegel T, et al: Cognitive-behavioral therapy and relationship therapy in the treatment of children referred for antisocial behavior. J Consult Clin Psychol 57:522–535, 1989

Kendall PC: Treating anxiety disorders in children: results of a randomized clinical trial. J Consult Clin Psychol 62:100–110, 1994

Kendall PC, Brady EU, Verduin TL: Comorbidity in childhood anxiety disorders and treatment outcome. J Am Acad Child Adolesc Psychiatry 40:787–794, 2001

Kennedy CH, Meyer KA, Knowles T, et al: Analyzing the multiple functions of stereotypical behavior for students with autism: implications for assessment and treatment. J Appl Behav Anal 33:559–571, 2000

Kent RD: Research on speech motor control and its disorders: a review and prospective. J Commun Disord 33:391–427, 2000

Kernberg PF, Chazan SE: Children With Conduct Disorders: A Psychotherapy Manual. New York, Basic Books, 1991

Khan S, Hyman PE, Cocjin J, et al: Rumination syndrome in adolescents. J Pediatr 136:528–531, 2000

Khemka I, Hickson L: Decision-making by adults with mental retardation in simulated situations of abuse. Ment Retard 38:15–26, 2000

Kidd KK: Genetic models of stuttering. Journal of Fluency Disorders 5:187–201, 1980

King BH, DeAntonio C, McCracken JT, et al: Psychiatric consultation in severe and profound mental retardation. Am J Psychiatry 151:1802–1808, 1994

King NJ, Tonge BJ, Heyne D, et al: Cognitive-behavioral treatment of school-refusing children: a controlled evaluation. J Am Acad Child Adolesc Psychiatry 37:395–403, 1998

Kirk J, Rasmussen PV, Rittig S, et al: Provoked enuresis-like episodes in healthy children 7 to 12 years old. J Urol 156:210–213, 1996

Klein RG, Last CG: Anxiety Disorders in Children. Newbury Park, CA, Sage, 1989

Klein RG, Koplewicz HS, Kanner A: Imipramine treatment of children with separation anxiety disorder. J Am Acad Child Adolesc Psychiatry 31:21–28, 1992

Klieger PS, Fett KA, Dimitsopulos T, et al: Asymmetry of basal ganglia perfusion in Tourette's syndrome shown by technetium-99m-HMPAO SPECT. J Nucl Med 38:2188–2191, 1997

Klin A, Volkmar FR, Sparrow SS (eds): Asperger Syndrome. New York, Guilford, 2000

Kolvin I, Fundudis T: Elective mute children: psychological development and background factors. J Child Psychol Psychiatry 22:219–232, 1981

Kopp S, Gillberg C: Selective mutism: a population-based study: a research note. J Child Psychol Psychiatry 38:257–262, 1997

Kosar A, Arikan N, Dincel C: Effectiveness of oxybutynin hydrochloride in the treatment of enuresis nocturna: a clinical and urodynamic study. Scand J Urol Nephrol 33:115–118, 1999

Kovacs M, Paulauskas S, Gatsonis C, et al: Depressive disorders in childhood, III: a longitudinal study of comorbidity with and risk for conduct disorders. J Affect Disord 15:205–217, 1988

Kozinetz CA, Skender ML, MacNaughton N, et al: Epidemiology of Rett syndrome: a population-based registry. Pediatrics 91:445–450, 1993

Kozub FM, Porretta DL, Hodge SR: Motor task persistence of children with and without mental retardation. Ment Retard 38:42–49, 2000

Kranzler HR: Use of buspirone in an adolescent with overanxious disorder. J Am Acad Child Adolesc Psychiatry 27:789–790, 1988

Kravitz H, Boehm JJ: Rhythmic habit patterns in infancy: their sequence, age of onset, and frequency. Child Dev 42:399–413, 1971

Kristensen H: Selective mutism and comorbidity with developmental disorder/delay, anxiety disorder, and elimination disorder. J Am Acad Child Adolesc Psychiatry 39:249–256, 2000

Krohn DD, Weckstein SM, Wright HL: A study of the effectiveness of a specific treatment for elective mutism. J Am Acad Child Adolesc Psychiatry 31:711–718, 1992

Kumpulainen K, Rasanen E, Raaska H, et al: Selective mutism among second-graders in elementary school. Eur Child Adolesc Psychiatry 7:24–29, 1998

Kuperman S, Johnson B, Arndt S, et al: Quantitative EEG differences in a nonclinical sample of children with ADHD and undifferentiated ADD. J Am Acad Child Adolesc Psychiatry 35:1009–1017, 1996

Kurlan R (ed): Handbook of Tourette's Syndrome and Related Tic and Behavioral Disorders. New York, Marcel Dekker, 1993

Kurlan R, Lichter D, Hewitt D: Sensory tics in Tourette's syndrome. Neurology 39:731–734, 1989

Kurlan R, Majumdar L, Deeley C, et al: A controlled trial of propoxyphene and naltrexone in patients with Tourette's syndrome. Ann Neurol 30:19–23, 1991

Kwak CH, Hanna PA, Jankovic J: Botulinum toxin in the treatment of tics. Arch Neurol 57:1190–1193, 2000

Labbe EE, Williamson DA: Behavioral treatment of elective mutism: a review of the literature. Clin Psychol Rev 4:273–294, 1984

Laccone F, Huppke P, Hanefeld F, et al: Mutation spectrum in patients with Rett syndrome in the German population: evidence of hot spot regions. Hum Mutat 17:183–190, 2001

Lachiewicz AM, Spiridigliozzi GA, Gullion CM, et al: Aberrant behaviors of young boys with fragile X syndrome. Am J Ment Retard 98:567–579, 1994

Lahey BB, Schaughency EA, Hynd GW, et al: Attention deficit disorder with and without hyperactivity: comparison of behavioral characteristics of clinic-referred children. J Am Acad Child Adolesc Psychiatry 26:718–723, 1987

Lahey BB, Hartdagen S, Frick PJ, et al: Conduct disorder: parsing the confounded relation to parental divorce and antisocial personality. J Abnorm Psychol 97:334–337, 1988a

Lahey BB, Piacentini JC, McBurnett K, et al: Psychopathology in the parents of children with conduct disorder and hyperactivity. J Am Acad Child Adolesc Psychiatry 27:163–170, 1988b

Lahey BB, Loeber R, Quay HC, et al: Validity of DSM-IV subtypes of conduct disorder based on age of onset. J Am Acad Child Adolesc Psychiatry 37:435–442, 1998c

Lahey BB, Miller TL, Gordon RA, et al: Developmental epidemiology of the disruptive behavior disorders, in Handbook of the Disruptive Behavior Disorders. Edited by Quay HC, Hogan A. New York, Plenum, 1999, pp 23–48

LaHoste GJ, Swanson JM, Wigal SB, et al: Dopamine D4 receptor gene polymorphism is associated with attention deficit hyperactivity disorder. Mol Psychiatry 1:121–124, 1996

Lai CSL, Fisher SE, Hurst JA, et al: A fork-head domain gene is mutated in a severe speech and language disorder. Nature 431:519–523, 2001

Lakatos K, Toth I, Nemoda Z, et al: Dopamine D4 receptor (DRD4) gene polymorphism is associated with attachment disorganization in infants. Mol Psychiatry 5:633–637, 2000

Landesman S, Vietze P: Living Environments and Mental Retardation. Washington, DC, American Association on Mental Deficiency, 1987

Langbehn DR, Cadoret RJ, Yates WR, et al: Distinct contributions of conduct and appositional defiant symptoms to adult antisocial behavior: evidence from an adoption study. Arch Gen Psychiatry 55:821–829, 1998

Lara DR, Belmonte-de-Abreu P, Souza DO: Allopurinol for refractory aggression and self-inflicted behaviour. J Psychopharmacol 14:81–83, 2000

Largo RH, Graf S, Kundu S, et al: Predicting developmental outcome at school age from infant tests of normal, at-risk, and retarded infants. Dev Med Child Neurol 32:30–45, 1990

Larson SA, Lakin KC, Anderson L, et al: Prevalence of mental retardation and developmental disabilities: estimates from the 1994/1995 National Health Interview Survey Disability Supplements. Am J Ment Retard 106:231–252, 2001

Last CG, Francis G, Hersen M, et al: Separation anxiety and school phobia: a comparison using DSM III criteria. Am J Psychiatry 144:653–657, 1987

Last CG, Perrin S, Hersen M, et al: DSM-III-R anxiety disorders in children: sociodemographic and clinical characteristics. J Am Acad Child Adolesc Psychiatry 31:1070–1076, 1992

Latz SR, McCracken JT: Neuroleptic malignant syndrome in children and adolescents: two case reports and a warning. J Child Adolesc Psychopharmacol 2:123–129, 1992

Lavigne JV, Burns WJ, Cotter PD: Rumination in infancy: recent behavioral approaches. Int J Eat Disord 1:70–82, 1981

Leckman JF, Riddle MA, Berrettini WH, et al: Elevated CSF dynorphin A [1–8] in Tourette's syndrome. Life Sci 43:2015–2023, 1988

Leckman JF, Dolnansky ES, Hardin MT, et al: Perinatal factors in the expression of Tourette's syndrome: an exploratory study. J Am Acad Child Adolesc Psychiatry 29:220–226, 1990

Leckman JF, Walker DE, Cohen DJ: Premonitory urges in Tourette's syndrome. Am J Psychiatry 150:98–102, 1993

Leckman JF, Zhang H, Vitale A, et al: Course of tic severity in Tourette syndrome: the first two decades. Pediatrics 102:14–19, 1998

Lefton-Greif MA, Loughlin GM: Specialized studies in pediatric dysphagia. Semin Speech Lang 17:311–329, 1996

Leonard CM, Martinez P, Weintraub BD, et al: Magnetic resonance imaging of cerebral anomalies in subjects with resistance to thyroid hormone. Am J Med Genet 60:238–243, 1995

Leonard HL, Swedo SE: Paediatric autoimmune neuropsychiatric disorders associated with streptococcal infection (PANDAS). Int J Neuropsychopharmacol 4:191–198, 2001

Levin ED, Conners CK, Sparrow E, et al: Nicotine effects on adults with attention-deficit/hyperactivity disorder. Psychopharmacology (Berl) 123:55–63, 1996

Levine MD: Encopresis: its potentiation, evaluation, and alleviation. Pediatr Clin North Am 29:315–330, 1982

Levine MD, Oberklaid F, Meltzer LJ: Developmental output failure: a study of low productivity in school-aged children. Pediatrics 67:18–25, 1981

Levitt JG, Blanton R, Capetillo-Cunliffe L, et al: Cerebellar vermis lobules VIII-X in autism. Prog Neuropsychopharmacol Biol Psychiatry 23:625–633, 1999

Levy F, Farrow M: Working memory in ADHD: prefrontal/parietal connections. Current Drug Targets 2:347–352, 2001

Lewis C, Hitch GJ, Walker P: The prevalence of specific arithmetic difficulties and specific reading difficulties in 9 to 10 year old and girls. J Child Psychol Psychiatry 35:283–292, 1994

Lewis DO, Pincus JH, Shanok SS, et al: Psychomotor epilepsy and violence in a group of incarcerated adolescent boys. Am J Psychiatry 139:882–887, 1982

Lewis DO, Pincus JH, Bard B, et al: Neuropsychiatric, psychoeducational and family characteristics of 14 juveniles condemned to death in the United States. Am J Psychiatry 145:584–589, 1988

Lindberg B: Understanding Rett Syndrome: A Practical Guide for Parents, Teachers, and Therapists. Göttingen, Germany, Hogrefe & Huber, 1992

Lipsitz JD, Martin LY, Mannuzza S, et al: Childhood separation anxiety disorder in patients with adult anxiety disorders. Am J Psychiatry 151:927–929, 1994

Livingston R, Reis CJ, Ringdahl IC: Abnormal dexamethasone suppression test results in depressed and nondepressed children. Am J Psychiatry 141:106–108, 1984

Livingston R, Taylor JL, Crawford SL: A study of somatic complaints and psychiatric diagnosis in children. J Am Acad Child Adolesc Psychiatry 27:185–187, 1988

Livingston RL, Dykman RA, Ackerman PT: Psychiatric comorbidity and response to two doses of methylphenidate in children with attention deficit disorder. J Child Adolesc Psychopharmacol 2:115–122, 1992

Loeber R: The stability of antisocial and delinquent childhood behavior. Child Dev 53:1431–1446, 1982

Loeber R, Green SM, Lahey BB, et al: Findings on disruptive behavior disorders from the first decade of the developmental trends study. Clinical Child and Family Psychology Review Vol 3, 2000

Loening-Baucke V: Encopresis and soiling. Pediatr Clin North Am 43:279–298, 1996

Lou HC: Etiology and pathogenesis of attention-deficit hyperactivity disorder (ADHD): significance of prematurity and perinatal hypoxic-haemodynamic encephalopathy. Acta Paediatr 85:1266–1271, 1996

Lou HC, Henriksen L, Bruhn P, et al: Striatal dysfunction in attention deficit and hyperkinetic disorder. Arch Neurol 46:48–52, 1989

Lou HC, Andresen J, Steinberg B, et al: The striatum in a putative cerebral network activated by verbal awareness in normals and in ADHD children. Eur J Neurol 5:67–74, 1998

Lynskey MT, Fergusson DM: Childhood conduct problems, attention deficit behaviors, and adolescent alcohol, tobacco, and illicit drug use. J Abnorm Child Psychol 23:281–302, 1995

MacGregor R, Pullar A, Cundall D: Silent at school: elective mutism and abuse. Arch Dis Child 70:540–541, 1994

Main M, Solomon J: Procedures for identifying infants as disorganized/disoriented during the Ainsworth Strange Situation, in Attachment in the Preschool Years. Edited by Greenberg MT, Cicchetti D, Cummings EM. Chicago, IL, University of Chicago Press, 1990, pp 121–160

Malcolm A, Thumshirn MB, Camilleri M, et al: Rumination syndrome. Mayo Clin Proc 72:646–652, 1997

Malone RP, Luebbert JF, Delaney MA, et al: Nonpharmacological response in hospitalized children with conduct disorder. J Am Acad Child Adolesc Psychiatry 36:242–247, 1997

Malone RP, Delaney MA, Luebbert JF, et al: A double-blind placebo-controlled study of lithium in hospitalized aggressive children and adolescent with conduct disorder. Arch Gen Psychiatry 57:649–654, 2000

Manassis K, Bradley S: Fluoxetine in anxiety disorders. J Am Acad Child Adolesc Psychiatry 33:761–762, 1994

Mancini C, van Ameringen M, Szatmari P, et al: A high-risk pilot study of the children of adults with social phobia. J Am Acad Child Adolesc Psychiatry 35:1511–1517, 1996

Mandich AD, Polatajko HJ, Macnab JJ, et al: Treatment of children with developmental coordination disorder: what is the evidence? Physical and Occupational Therapy in Pediatrics 20:51–68, 2001

Manes F, Piven J, Vrancic D, et al: An MRI study of the corpus callosum and cerebellum in mentally retarded autistic individuals. J Neuropsychiatry Clin Neurosci 11:470–474, 1999

Manicavasagar V, Silove D: Is there an adult form of separation anxiety disorder? A brief clinical report. Aust N Z J Psychiatry 31:299–303, 1997

Manicavasagar V, Silove D, Hadzi-Pavlovic D: Subpopulations of early separation anxiety: relevance to risk of adult anxiety disorders. J Affect Disord 48:181–190, 1998

Manicavasagar V, Silove D, Curtis J, et al: Continuities of separation anxiety from early life into adulthood. J Anxiety Disord 14:1–18, 2000

Manicavasagar V, Silove D, Rapee R, et al: Parent-child concordance for separation anxiety: a clinical study. J Affect Disord 65:81–84, 2001

Manikam R, Perman JA: Pediatric feeding disorders. J Clin Gastroenterol 30:34–46, 2000

Manor I, Eisenberg J, Tyano S, et al: Family based association study of the serotonin transporter promoter region polymorphism (5-HTTLPR) in attention deficit hyperactivity disorder. Am J Med Genet 105:91–95, 2001

Marchi M, Cohen P: Early childhood eating behaviors and adolescent eating disorders. J Am Acad Child Adolesc Psychiatry 29:112–117, 1990

Marcus J, Hans SL, Mednick SA, et al: Neurological dysfunctioning in offspring of schizophrenics in Israel and Denmark. Arch Gen Psychiatry 42:753–761, 1985

Martin C, Cabrol S, Bouvard MP, et al: Anxiety and depressive disorders in fathers and mothers of anxious school-refusing children. J Am Acad Child Adolesc Psychiatry 38:916–922, 1999

Martin JAM: Syndrome delineation in communication disorders, in Language and Language Disorders in Children. Edited by Hersov LA, Berger M. Oxford, England, Pergamon, 1980

Masi B, Mucci M, Millepiedi S: Separation anxiety disorder in children and adolescents: epidemiology, diagnosis, and management. CNS Drugs 15:93–104, 2001

Masi G, Favilla L, Mucci M: Generalized anxiety disorder in adolescents and young adults with mild mental retardation. Psychiatry 63:54–64, 2000a

Masi G, Favilla L, Mucci M, et al: Panic disorder in clinically referred children and adolescents. Child Psychiatry Hum Dev 31:139–151, 2000b

Masi G, Favilla L, Mucci M, et al: Depressive symptoms in children and adolescents with dysthymic disorder. Psychopathology 34:29–35, 2001

Mataro M, Garcia-Sanchez C, Junque C, et al: Magnetic resonance imaging measurement of the caudate nucleus in adolescents with attention-deficit hyperactivity disorder and its relationship with neuropsychological and behavioral measures. Arch Neurol 54:963–968, 1997

Matochik JA, Liebenauer LL, King AC, et al: Cerebral glucose metabolism in adults with attention deficit hyperactivity disorder after chronic stimulant treatment. Am J Psychiatry 151:658–664, 1994

Matson JL, Bamburg JW, Mayville EA, et al: Psychopharmacology and mental retardation: a 10 year review (1990–1999). Res Dev Disabil 21:263–296, 2000

Matsuishi T, Nagamitsu S, Yamashita Y, et al: Decreased cerebrospinal fluid levels of substance P in patients with Rett syndrome. Ann Neurol 42:978–981, 1997

Matthys W, Van Loo P, Pachen V, et al: Behavior of conduct disordered children in interaction with each other and with normal peers. Child Psychiatry Hum Dev 25:183–195, 1995

Max JE, Castillo CS, Bokura H, et al: Oppositional defiant disorder symptomatology after traumatic brain injury: a prospective study. J Nerv Ment Dis 186:325–332, 1998

Mayes SD, Humphrey FJ 2d, Handford HA, et al: Rumination disorder: differential diagnosis. J Am Acad Child Adolesc Psychiatry 27:300–302, 1988

McBurnett K, Lahey BB, Rathouz PJ, et al: Low salivary cortisol and persistent aggression in boys referred for disruptive behavior. Arch Gen Psychiatry 57:38–43, 2000

McCartney JR, Campbell VA: Confirmed abuse cases in public residential facilities for persons with mental retardation: a multi-state study. Ment Retard 36:465–473, 1998

McCracken JT, Smalley SL, McGough JJ, et al: Evidence for linkage of a tandem duplication polymorphism upstream of the dopamine D4 receptor gene (DRD4) with attention deficit hyperactivity disorder (ADHD). Mol Psychiatry 5:531–536, 2000

McDougle CJ, Naylor ST, Cohen DJ, et al: Effects of tryptophan depletion in drug-free adults with autistic disorder. Arch Gen Psychiatry 53:980–983, 1996

McDougle CJ, Holmes JP, Bronson MR, et al: Risperidone treatment of children and adolescents with pervasive developmental disorders: a prospective open-label study. J Am Acad Child Adolesc Psychiatry 36:685–693, 1997

McDougle CJ, Holmes JP, Carlson DC, et al: A double-blind, placebo-controlled study of risperidone in adults with autistic disorder and other pervasive developmental disorders. Arch Gen Psychiatry 55:633–641, 1998

McGee R, Williams S: A longitudinal study of depression in nine-year-old children. J Am Acad Child Adolesc Psychiatry 27:342–348, 1988

McGee R, Williams S, Silva PA: Behavioral and developmental characteristics of aggressive, hyperactive, and aggressive-hyperactive boys. J Am Acad Child Adolesc Psychiatry 23:280–284, 1984

McGillicuddy NB, Blane HT: Substance use in individuals with mental retardation. Addict Behav 24:869–878, 1999

McGrath ML, Mellon MW, Murphy L: Empirically supported treatments in pediatric psychology: constipation and encopresis. J Pediatr Psychol 25:225–254, 2000

McKee JR, Bodfish JW: Sudden unexpected death in epilepsy in adults with mental retardation. Am J Ment Retard 105:229–235, 2000

McKelvey JR, Lambert R, Mottron L, et al: Right-hemisphere dysfunction in Asperger's syndrome. J Child Neurol 10:310–314, 1995

Meller WH, Borchardt CM: Comorbidity of major depression and conduct disorder. J Affect Disord 39:123–126, 1996

Mellon MW, McGrath ML: Empirically supported treatments in pediatric psychology: nocturnal enuresis. J Pediatr Psychol 25:193–214, 2000

Mendelowitz SL, Manassis K, Bradley S, et al: Cognitive-behavioral group treatments in childhood anxiety disorder: the role of parental involvement. J Am Acad Child Adolesc Psychiatry 38:1223–1229, 1999

Menolascino FJ, Levitas A, Greiner C: The nature and types of mental illness in the mentally retarded. Psychopharmacol Bull 22:1060–1071, 1986

Michelson D, Faries D, Wernicke J, et al: Atomoxetine in the treatment of children and adolescents with attention-deficit/hyperactivity disorder: a randomized, placebo-controlled, dose-response study (abstract). Pediatrics 108:E83, 2001

Miguel EC, do Rosario-Campos MC, Prado HS, et al: Sensory phenomena in obsessive-compulsive disorder and Tourette's disorder. J Clin Psychiatry 61:150–156, 2000

Milberger S, Biederman J, Faraone SV, et al: Is maternal smoking during pregnancy a risk factor for attention deficit hyperactivity disorder in children? Am J Psychiatry 153:1138–1142, 1996

Miller LT, Missiuna CA, Macnab JJ, et al: Clinical description of children with developmental coordination disorder. Canadian Journal of Occupational Therapy 68:5–15, 2001a

Miller LT, Polatajko HJ, Missiuna C, et al: A pilot trial of a cognitive treatment for children with developmental coordination disorder. Human Movement Science 20:183–210, 2001b

Millican FK, Layman EM, Lourie RS, et al: Study of an oral fixation: pica. Journal of the American Academy of Child Psychiatry 7:79–107, 1968

Missiuna C (ed): Children With Developmental Coordination Disorder: Strategies for Success. New York, Haworth, 2001

Mitchell EA, Aman MG, Turbott SH, et al: Clinical characteristics and serum essential fatty acid levels in hyperactive children. Clin Pediatr 26:406–411, 1987

Miyahara M, Mobs I: Developmental dyspraxia and developmental coordination disorder. Neuropsychol Rev 5:245–268, 1995

Moeschler JB, Charman CD, Berg SZ, et al.: Rett syndrome: natural history and management. Pediatrics 82:1–10, 1988

Moffitt TE: Juvenile delinquency and attention deficit disorder: boys' developmental trajectories from age 3 to age 15. Child Dev 61:893–910, 1990

Moffitt TE, Silva PA: Self-reported delinquency, neuropsychological deficit, and history of attention deficit disorder. J Abnorm Child Psychol 16:553–569, 1988

Molteni M, Moretti G: Minor psychiatric disorders as possible complication of mental retardation. Psychopathology 32:107–112, 1999

Moreno-Fuenmayor H, Borjas L, Arrieta A, et al: Plasma excitatory amino acids in autism. Invest Clin 37:113–128, 1996

Mountz JM, Tolbert LC, Lill DW, et al: Functional deficits in autistic disorder: characterization by technetium-99m-HMPAO and SPECT. J Nucl Med 36:1156–1162, 1995

Mouridsen SE, Rich B, Isager T: Validity of childhood disintegrative psychosis: general findings of a long-term follow-up study. Br J Psychiatry 172:263–267, 1998

Mouridsen SE, Rich B, Isager T: Epilepsy in disintegrative psychosis and infantile autism: a long-term validation study. Dev Med Child Neurol 41:110–114, 1999a

Mouridsen SE, Rich B, Isager T: The natural history of somatic morbidity in disintegrative psychosis and infantile autism: a validation study. Brain Dev 21:447–452, 1999b

Mouridsen SE, Rich B, Isager T: A comparative study of genetic and neurobiological findings in disintegrative psychosis and infantile autism. Psychiatry Clin Neurosci 54:441–446, 2000

MTA Cooperative Group: A 14-month randomized clinical trial of treatment strategies for attention-deficit/hyperactivity disorder. The MTA Cooperative Group: Multimodal Treatment Study of Children With ADHD. Arch Gen Psychiatry 56:1073–1086, 1999a

MTA Cooperative Group: Moderators and mediators of treatment response for children with attention-deficit/hyperactivity disorder: the Multimodal Treatment Study of Children With Attention-Deficit/Hyperactivity Disorder. Arch Gen Psychiatry 56:1088–1096, 1999b

Muller RA, Chugani DC, Behen ME, et al: Impairment of dentato-thalamo-cortical pathway in autistic men: language activation data from positron emission tomography. Neurosci Lett 245:1–4, 1998

Muris P, Mayer B, Bartelds E, et al: The revised version of the Screen for Child Anxiety Related Emotional Disorders (SCARED-R): treatment sensitivity in an early intervention trial for childhood anxiety disorders. Br J Clin Psychol 40:323–336, 2001

Murphy TK, Goodman WK, Fudge MW, et al: B lymphocyte antigen D8/17: a peripheral marker for childhood-onset obsessive-compulsive disorder and Tourette's syndrome? Am J Psychiatry 154:402–407, 1997

Naidu S, Hyman S, Harris EL, et al: Rett syndrome studies of natural history and search for a genetic marker. Neuropediatrics 26:63–66, 1995

National Institute of Mental Health (NIMH) Consensus Statement: Diagnosis and treatment of attention deficit hyperactivity disorder (ADHD). NIH Consens Statement 16:1–37, 1998

Needleman HL, Schell A, Bellinger D, et al: The long-term effects of exposure to low doses of lead in childhood: an 11-year follow-up report. N Engl J Med 322:83–88, 1990

Needleman HL, Riess JA, Tobin MJ, et al: Bone lead levels and delinquent behavior. JAMA 275:363–369, 1996

Nelson KB: Prenatal and perinatal factors in the etiology of autism. Pediatrics 87(suppl):761–766, 1991

Nelson KB, Ellenberg JH: Antecedents of cerebral palsy: multivariate analysis of risk. N Engl J Med 315:81–86, 1986

Neveus T, Lackgren G, Tuvemo T, et al: Enuresis: background and treatment. Scand J Urol Nephrol Suppl 206:1–44, 2000

Newcorn JH, Strain J: Adjustment disorder in children and adolescents. J Am Acad Child Adolesc Psychiatry 31:318–327, 1992

Newcorn JH, Halperin JM, Jensen PS, et al: Symptom profiles in children with ADHD: effects of comorbidity and gender. J Am Acad Child Adolesc Psychiatry 40:137–146, 2001

Nichols PL, Chen T-C: Minimal Brain Dysfunction: A Prospective Study. Hillsdale, NJ, Erlbaum, 1981

Niehaus DJ, Emsley RA, Brink P, et al: Stereotypies: prevalence and association with compulsive and impulsive symptoms in college students. Psychopathology 33:31–35, 2000

Nopoulos P, Berg S, Castellenos FX, et al: Developmental brain anomalies in children with attention-deficit hyperactivity disorder. J Child Neurol 15:102–108, 2000

Nurko S, Garcia-Aranda JA, Worona LB, et al: Cisapride for the treatment of constipation in children: a double-blind study. J Pediatr 136:35–40, 2000

O'Connor KP, Brault M, Robillard S, et al: Evaluation of a cognitive-behavioural program for the management of chronic tic and habit disorders. Behav Res Ther 39:667–681, 2001

O'Connor TG, Rutter M, English and Romanian Adoptees Study Team: Attachment disorder behavior following early severe deprivation: extension and longitudinal follow-up. J Am Acad Child Adolesc Psychiatry 39:703–712, 2000

Ollendick TH, Mattis SG, King NJ: Panic in children and adolescents: a review. J Child Psychol Psychiatry 35:113–134, 1994

Onofrj M, Paci C, D'Andreamatteo G, et al: Olanzapine in severe Gilles de la Tourette syndrome: a 52-week double-blind cross-over study vs. low-dose pimozide. J Neurol 247:443–446, 2000

Oosterlaan J, Sergeant JA: Inhibition in ADHD, aggressive, and anxious children: a biologically based model of child psychopathology. J Abnorm Child Psychol 24:19–36, 1996

Overmeyer S, Simmons A, Santosh J, et al: Corpus callosum may be similar in children with ADHD and siblings of children with ADHD. Dev Med Child Neurol 42:8–13, 2000

Owen SE, McKinlay IA: Motor difficulties in children with developmental disorders of speech and language. Child Care Health Dev 23:315–325, 1997

Owley T, McMahon W, Cook EH, et al: Multisite, double-blind, placebo-controlled trial of porcine secretin in autism. J Am Acad Child Adolesc Psychiatry 40:1293–1299, 2001

Pace GM, Toyer EA: The effects of a vitamin supplement on the pica of a child with severe mental retardation. J Appl Behav Anal 33:619–622, 2000

Paden EP, Yairi E: Phonological characteristics of children whose stuttering persisted or recovered. J Speech Hear Res 39:981–990, 1996

Paden EP, Yairi E, Ambrose NG: Early childhood stuttering, II: initial status of phonological abilities. J Speech Lang Hear Res 42:1113–1124, 1999

Parry-Jones B: Merycism or rumination disorder: a historical investigation and current assessment. Br J Psychiatry 165:303–314, 1994

Patja K, Iivanainen M, Raitasuo S, et al: Suicide mortality in mental retardation: a 35-year follow-up study. Acta Psychiatr Scand 103:307–311, 2001

Patterson GR: Coercive Family Processes. Eugene, OR, Castalia, 1982

Paul R, Cohen D, Caparulo B: A longitudinal study of patients with severe, specific developmental language disorders. Journal of the American Academy of Child Psychiatry 22:525–534, 1994

Pauls DL: Genetic factors in the expression of attention-deficit hyperactivity disorder. J Child Adolesc Psychopharmacol 1:353–360, 1991

Pauls DL, Leckman JF: The inheritance of Gilles de la Tourette's syndrome and associated behaviors. N Engl J Med 315:993–997, 1986

Payton A, Holmes J, Barrett JH, et al: Examining for association between candidate gene polymorphisms in the dopamine pathway and attention-deficit hyperactivity disorder: a family based study. Am J Med Genet 105:464–470, 2001

Pearson DA, Lachar D, Loveland KA, et al: Patterns of behavioral adjustment and maladjustment in mental retardation: comparison of children with and without ADHD. Am J Ment Retard 105:236–251, 2000

Pelcovitz D, Kaplan SJ, DeRosa RR, et al: Psychiatric disorders in adolescents exposed to domestic violence and physical abuse. Am J Orthopsychiatry 70:360–369, 2000

Pelham WE, Carlson C, Sams SE, et al: Separate and combined effects of methylphenidate and behavior modification of boys with attention deficit hyperactivity disorder in the classroom. J Consult Clin Psychol 61:506–515, 1993

Pennington BF, Filipek PA, Lefly D, et al: Brain morphometry in reading-disabled twins. Neurology 53:723–729, 1999

Perrin S, Last CG: Relationship between ADHD and anxiety in boys: results from a family study. J Am Acad Child Adolesc Psychiatry 35:988–996, 1996

Perry CA, Dwyer J, Gelfand JA, et al: Health effects of salicylates in foods and drugs. Nutr Rev 54:225–240, 1996

Peterson BS: Neuroimaging in child and adolescent neuropsychiatric disorders. J Am Acad Child Adolesc Psychiatry 12:1560–1576, 1995

Peterson B, Riddle MA, Cohen DJ, et al: Reduced basal ganglia volumes in Tourette's syndrome using three-dimensional reconstruction techniques from magnetic resonance images. Neurology 43:941–949, 1993

Peterson BS, Skudlarski P, Anderson AW, et al: A functional magnetic resonance imaging study of tic suppression in Tourette syndrome. Arch Gen Psychiatry 55:326–333, 1998

Peterson BS, Leckman JF, Tucker D, et al: Preliminary findings of antistreptococcal antibody titers and basal ganglia volumes in tic, obsessive-compulsive, and attention deficit/hyperactivity disorders. Arch Gen Psychiatry 57:364–372, 2000

Peterson BS, Pine DS, Cohen P, et al: Prospective, longitudinal study of tic, obsessive-compulsive, and attention-deficit/hyperactivity disorders in an epidemiological sample. J Am Acad Child Adolesc Psychiatry 40:685–695, 2001a

Peterson BS, Staib L, Scahill L, et al: Regional brain and ventricular volumes in Tourette syndrome. Arch Gen Psychiatry 58:427–440, 2001b

Petryshen TL, Kaplan BJ, Liu MF, et al: Absence of significant linkage between phonological coding dyslexia and chromosome 6p23–21.3, as determined by use of quantitative-trait methods: confirmation of qualitative analyses. Am J Hum Genet 66:708–714, 2000

Petryshen TL, Kaplan BJ, Fu Liu M, et al: Evidence for a susceptibility locus on chromosome 6q influencing phonological coding dyslexia. Am J Med Genet 105:507–517, 2001

Philippe A, Martinez M, Guilloud-Bataille M, et al: Genome-wide scan for autism susceptibility genes. Paris Autism Research International Sibpair Study. Hum Mol Genet 8:805–812, 1999

Pierce K, Courchesne E: Evidence for a cerebellar role in reduced exploration and stereotyped behavior in autism. Biol Psychiatry 49:655–664, 2001

Pillmann F, Rohde A, Ullrich S, et al: Violence, criminal behavior, and the EEG: significance of left hemispheric focal abnormalities. J Neuropsychiatry Clin Neurosci 11:454–457, 1999

Pine DS, Klein RG, Coplan JD, et al: Differential carbon dioxide sensitivity in childhood anxiety disorders and nonill comparison group. Arch Gen Psychiatry 57:960–967, 2000

Piven J, Palmer P: Psychiatric disorder and the broad autism phenotype: evidence from a family study of multiple-incidence autism families. Am J Psychiatry 156:557–563, 1999

Piven J, Bailey J, Ranson BJ, et al: An MRI study of the corpus callosum in autism. Am J Psychiatry 154:1051–1056, 1997a

Piven J, Palmer P, Jacobi D, et al: Broader autism phenotype: evidence from a family history study of multiple-incidence autism families. Am J Psychiatry 154:185–190, 1997b

Piven J, Saliba K, Bailey J, et al: An MRI study of autism: the cerebellum revisited. Neurology 49:546–551, 1997c

Piven J, Bailey J, Ranson BJ, et al: No difference in hippocampus volume detected on magnetic resonance imaging in autistic individuals. J Autism Dev Disord 28:105–110, 1998

Pliszka SR: Effect of anxiety on cognition, behavior, and stimulant response in ADHD. J Am Acad Child Adolesc Psychiatry 28:882–887, 1989

Pliszka SR: Comorbidity of attention-deficit hyperactivity disorder and overanxious disorder. J Am Acad Child Adolesc Psychiatry 31:197–203, 1992

Pliszka SR, McCracken JT, Maas JW: Catecholamines in attention-deficit hyperactivity disorder: current perspectives. J Am Acad Child Adolesc Psychiatry 35:264–272, 1996

Polatajko HJ, Macnab JJ, Anstett B, et al: A clinical trial of the process-oriented treatment approach for children with developmental co-ordination disorder. Dev Med Child Neurol 37:310–319, 1995

Pomerleau OF, Downey KK, Stelson FW, et al: Cigarette smoking in adult patients diagnosed with attention deficit hyperactivity disorder. J Subst Abuse 7:373–378, 1995

Popper C: Psychopharmacological treatment of anxiety disorders in adolescents and children. J Clin Psychiatry 54(suppl):52–63, 1993

Popper CW, Elliott GR: Sudden death and tricyclic antidepressants: clinical considerations for children. J Child Adolesc Psychopharmacol 1:125–132, 1990

Prassopoulos P, Cavouras D, Ioannidou M, et al: Study of subarachnoid spaces in children with idiopathic mental retardation. J Child Neurol 11:197–200, 1996

Pretlow RA: Treatment of nocturnal enuresis with an ultrasound bladder volume controlled alarm device. J Urol 162:1224–1228, 1999

Provence S, Lipton RC: Infants and Institutions. New York, International Universities Press, 1962

Pueyo R, Maneru C, Vendrell P, et al: Attention deficit hyperactivity disorder: cerebral asymmetry observed on magnetic resonance. Rev Neurol 30:920–925, 2000

Pugh KR, Mencl WE, Jenner AR, et al: Functional neuroimaging studies of reading and reading disability (developmental dyslexia). Mental Retardation and Developmental Disabilities Research Reviews 6:207–213, 2000

Purvis KL, Tannock R: Language abilities in children with attention deficit hyperactivity disorder, reading abilities, and normal controls. J Abnorm Child Psychol 25:133–144, 1997

Purvis KL, Tannock R: Phonological processing, not inhibitory control, differentiates ADHD and reading disability. J Am Acad Child Adolesc Psychiatry 39:485–494, 2000

Quay HC: Inhibition and attention deficit hyperactivity disorder. J Abnorm Child Psychol 25:7–13, 1997

Raine A, Venables PH, Williams M: Relationships between central and autonomic measures of arousal at age 15 years and criminality at age 24 years. Arch Gen Psychiatry 47:1003–1007, 1990

Rapin I: Autistic children: diagnosis and clinical features. Pediatrics 87(suppl):751–760, 1991

Rapoport JL, Buchsbaum MS, Weingartner H, et al: Dextroamphetamine: its cognitive and behavioral effects in normal and hyperactive boys and normal men. Arch Gen Psychiatry 37:933–943, 1980

Rapoport JL, Conners CK, Reatig N: Rating scales and assessment instruments for use in pediatric psychopharmacology research. Psychopharmacol Bull 21:713–1125, 1985

Rapoport JL, Castellanos FX, Gogate N, et al: Imaging normal and abnormal brain development: new perspectives for child psychiatry. Aust N Z J Psychiatry 35:272–281, 2001

Rasmussen P, Gillberg C: Natural outcome of ADHD with developmental coordination disorder at age 22 years: a controlled, longitudinal, community-based study. J Am Acad Child Adolesc Psychiatry 39:1424–1431, 2000

Rasquin-Weber A, Hyman PE, Cucchiara S, et al: Childhood functional gastrointestinal disorders. Gut 45:II60–II68, 1999

Raynaud C, Billard C, Tzongrig H, et al: Study of rCBF developmental dysphasia children at rest and during verbal stimulation. J Cereb Blood Flow Metab 1(suppl):S323, 1989

Reeves JC, Werry JS, Elkind GS, et al: Attention deficit, conduct, oppositional, and anxiety disorders in children, II: clinical characteristics. J Am Acad Child Adolesc Psychiatry 26:144–155, 1987

Rehabilitation Act of 1973, Pub.L. 93-112, as amended by the Rehabilitation Act Amendments of 1974, Pub.L. 93-516, 29 U.S.C. 794

Reid AH, Ballinger BR: Behaviour symptoms among severely and profoundly mentally retarded patients: a 16–18 year follow-up study. Br J Psychiatry 167:452–455, 1995

Reis S: Rumination in two developmentally normal children: case report and review of the literature. J Fam Pract 38:521–523, 1994

Research Unit on Pediatric Psychopharmacology Anxiety Study Group: Fluvoxamine for the treatment of anxiety disorders in children and adolescents. N Engl J Med 344:1279–1285, 2001

Rey JM: Comorbidity between disruptive disorders and depression in referred adolescents. Aust N Z J Psychiatry 28:106–113, 1994

Richards TL, Corina D, Serafini S, et al: The effects of phonologically driven treatment for dyslexia on lactate levels as measured by proton MSRI. Am J Neuroradiol 25:40–47, 2000

Richters MM, Volkmar FR: Reactive attachment disorder of infancy or early childhood. J Am Acad Child Adolesc Psychiatry 33:328–332, 1994

Riddle MA, Nelson JC, Kleinman CS, et al: Sudden death in children receiving Norpramin: a review of three reported cases and commentary. J Am Acad Child Adolesc Psychiatry 30:104–108, 1991

Riddle MA, Rasmussen AM, Woods SW, et al: SPECT imaging of cerebral blood flow in Tourette syndrome, in Tourette Syndrome: Genetics, Neurobiology, and Treatment (Advances in Neurology Series, Vol 58). Edited by Chase TN, Friedhoff AJ, Cohen DJ. New York, Raven, 1992, pp 207–211

Riddle MA, Lynch KA, Scahill L, et al: Methylphenidate discontinuation and reinitiation during long-term treatment of children with Tourette's disorder and attention-deficit/hyperactivity disorder: a pilot study. J Child Adolesc Psychopharmacol 5:205–214, 1995

Rifkin A, Karajgi B, Dicker R, et al: Lithium treatment of conduct disorders in adolescents. Am J Psychiatry 154:554–555, 1997

Rimland B, Baker SM: Brief report: alternative approaches to the development of effective treatments for autism. J Autism Dev Disord 26:237–241, 1996

Rittig S, Knudsen UB, Norgaard JP, et al: Abnormal diurnal rhythm of plasma vasopressin and urinary output in patients with enuresis. Am J Physiol 256:F664–F671, 1989

Rittig S, Schaumburg H, Schmidt F, et al: Long-term home studies of water balance in patients with nocturnal enuresis. Scand J Urol Nephrol Suppl 183:25–56, 1997

Roberts JW, Dickey P: Exposure of children to pollutants in house dust and indoor air. Rev Environ Contam Toxicol 143:59–78, 1995

Roberts W, Weaver L, Brian J, et al: Repeated doses of porcine secretin in the treatment of autism: a randomized, placebo-controlled trial. Pediatrics 107:E71, 2001

Robertson G, Rittig S, Kovacs L, et al: Pathophysiology and treatment of enuresis in adults. Scand J Urol Nephrol Suppl 202:36–38, 1999

Robertson J, Emerson E, Gregory N, et al: Social networks of people with mental retardation in residential settings. Ment Retard 39:201–214, 2001

Robertson MM, Trimble MR, Lees AJ: Self-injurious behaviour and the Gilles de la Tourette syndrome: a clinical study and review of the literature. Psychol Med 19:611–625, 1989

Robertson MM, Banerjee S, Hiley PJ, et al: Personality disorder and psychopathology in Tourette's syndrome: a controlled study. Br J Psychiatry 171:283–286, 1997

Robins LN: Deviant Children Grown Up. Baltimore, MD, Williams & Wilkins, 1966

Robson WL, Jackson HP, Blackhurst D, et al: Enuresis in children with attention-deficit hyperactivity disorder. South Med J 90:503–505, 1997

Rockney RM, McQuade WH, Days AL, et al: Encopresis treatment outcome: long-term follow-up of 45 cases. J Dev Behav Pediatr 17:380–385, 1996

Roizen NJ, Blondis TA, Irwin M, et al: Adaptive functioning in children with attention-deficit hyperactivity disorder. Arch Pediatr Adolesc Med 148:1137–1142, 1994

Roman T, Schmitz M, Polanczyk G, et al: Attention-deficit hyperactivity disorder: a study of association with both the dopamine transporter gene and the dopamine D4 receptor gene. Am J Med Genet 105:471–478, 2001

Rothenberg SJ, Manalo M, Jiang J, et al: Maternal blood lead level during pregnancy in South Central Los Angeles. Arch Environ Health 54:151–157, 1999

Rourke BP: Arithmetic disabilities, specific and otherwise: a neuropsychological perspective. J Learn Disabil 26:214–226, 1993

Rourke BP, Strang JD: Subtypes of reading and arithmetic disabilities: a neuropsychological analysis, in Developmental Neuropsychiatry. Edited by Rutter M. New York, Guilford, 1983

Rowe DC, Stever C, Gard JM, et al: The relation of the dopamine transporter gene (DAT1) to symptoms of internalizing disorders in children. Behav Genet 28:215–225, 1998

Rowe DC, Stever C, Chase D, et al: Two dopamine genes related to reports of childhood retrospective inattention and conduct disorder symptoms. Mol Psychiatry 6:429–433, 2001

Rucklidge JJ, Tannock R: Psychiatric, psychosocial, and cognitive functioning of female adolescents with ADHD. J Am Acad Child Adolesc Psychiatry 40:530–540, 2001

Rumsey JM, Rapoport JL, Sceery WR: Autistic children as adults: psychiatric, social, and behavioral outcomes. Journal of the American Academy of Child Psychiatry 24:465–473, 1985a

Rumsey JM, Duara R, Grady C, et al: Brain metabolism in autism: resting cerebral glucose utilization rates as measured with positron emission tomography. Arch Gen Psychiatry 42:448–455, 1985b

Rutter M: Isle of Wight revisited: twenty-five years of child psychiatric epidemiology. J Am Acad Child Adolesc Psychiatry 28:633–653, 1989

Rutter M, Giller H: Juvenile Delinquency: Trends and Perspectives. New York, Guilford, 1984

Rutter M, Yule W: A Neuropsychiatric Study in Childhood. Suffolk, England, Lavenhan Press, 1970

Rutter M, Yule W: The concept of specific reading retardation. J Child Psychol Psychiatry 16:181–197, 1975

Rutter M, Tizard J, Whitmore K: Education, Health and Behaviour: Psychological and Medical Study of Childhood Development. Harlow, England, Longman, 1970

Rutter M, Tizard J, Yule W, et al: Isle of Wight studies, 1964–1974. Psychol Med 6:313–332, 1976

Rutter M, Tuma A, Lann I: Assessment and Diagnosis in Child Psychopathology. New York, Guilford, 1987

Rutter M, Anderson-Wood L, Beckett C, et al: Quasi-autistic patterns following severe early global privation. J Child Psychol Psychiatry 40:537–550, 1999

Ryan R, Sunada K: Medical evaluation of persons with mental retardation referred for psychiatric assessment. Gen Hosp Psychiatry 19:274–280, 1997

Rydelius A: The development of antisocial behavior and sudden violent death. Acta Psychiatr Scand 77:398–403, 1988

Sachs GS, Baldassano CF, Truman CJ, et al: Comorbidity of attention deficit hyperactivity disorder with early and late-onset bipolar disorder. Am J Psychiatry 157:466–468, 2000

Safer DJ, Zito JM, Fine EM: Increased methylphenidate usage for attention deficit disorder in the 1990s. Pediatrics 98:1084–1088, 1996

Saitoh O, Karns CM, Courchesne E: Development of the hippocampal formation from 2 to 42 years: MRI evidence of smaller area dentata in autism. Brain 124:1317–1324, 2001

Sakamoto K, Blaivas JG: Adult onset nocturnal enuresis. J Urol 165:1914–1917, 2001

Sallee FR, Kurlan R, Goetz CG, et al: Ziprasidone treatment of children and adolescents with Tourette's syndrome: a pilot study. J Am Acad Child Adolesc Psychiatry 39:292–299, 2000

Sampson RJ, Raudenbusch SW, Earls F: Neighborhoods and violent crime: a multilevel study of collective efficacy. Science 277:918–924, 1997

Sandman CA: The opiate hypothesis in autism and self-injury. J Child Adolesc Psychopharmacol 1:237–248, 1991

Sandman CA, Hetrick W, Talyor D, et al: Uncoupling of proopiomelanocortin (POMC) fragments is related to self-injury. Peptides 21:785–791, 2000

Sauvage D, Leddet I, Hameury L, et al: Infantile rumination: diagnosis and follow-up of twenty cases. Journal of the American Academy of Child Psychiatry 24:197–203, 1985

Scahill L, Chappell PB, Kim YS, et al: A placebo-controlled study of guanfacine in the treatment of children with tic disorders and attention deficit hyperactivity disorder. Am J Psychiatry 158:1067–1074, 2001

Schachar R, Mota VL, Logan GD, et al: Confirmation of an inhibitory control deficit in attention-deficit/hyperactivity disorder. J Abnorm Child Psychol 28:227–235, 2000

Schaefer GB, Thompson JN, Bodensteiner JB, et al: Hypoplasia of the cerebellar vermis in neurogenetic syndromes. Ann Neurol 39:382–385, 1996

Schroeder S, Schroeder C, Smith B, et al: Prevalence of self-injurious behaviors in a large state facility for the retarded: a three-year follow-up study. Journal of Autism and Childhood Schizophrenia 8:261–269, 1979

Schubiner H, Tzelepis A, Milberger S, et al: Prevalence of attention-deficit/hyperactivity disorder and conduct disorder among substance abusers. J Clin Psychiatry 61:244–251, 2000

Schulte-Körne G, Deimel W, Gutenbrunner C, et al: Effect of an oligo-antigen diet on the behavior of hyperkinetic children [in German]. Zeitschrift Fur Kinder Und Jugendpsychiatrie 24:176–183, 1996

Schvehla TJ, Mandoki MW, Sumner GS: Clonidine therapy for comorbid attention deficit hyperactivity disorder and conduct disorder: preliminary findings in a children's inpatient unit. South Med J 87:692–695, 1994

Schwartzman JS, Bernardino A, Nishimura A, et al: Rett syndrome in a boy with a 47,XXY karyotype confirmed by a rare mutation in the MECP2 gene. Neuropediatrics 32:162–164, 2001

Schweitzer JB, Faber TL, Grafton ST, et al: Alterations in the functional anatomy of working memory in adult attention deficit hyperactivity disorder. Am J Psychiatry 157:278–280, 2000

Seeger G, Schloss P, Schmidt MH: Functional polymorphism within the promotor of the serotonin transporter gene is associated with severe hyperkinetic disorders. Mol Psychiatry 6:235–238, 2001a

Seeger G, Schloss P, Schmidt MH: Marker gene polymorphisms in hyperkinetic disorder—predictors of clinical response to treatment with methylphenidate? Neurosci Lett 313:45–48, 2001b

Seidman LJ, Biederman J, Monuteaux MC, et al: Learning disabilities and executive dysfunction in boys with attention-deficit/hyperactivity disorder. Neuropsychology 15:544–556, 2001

Seltzer MM, Krauss MW, Hong J, et al: Continuity or discontinuity of family involvement following residential transitions of adults who have mental retardation. Ment Retard 39:181–194, 2001

Semrud-Clikeman M: Evidence from imaging on the relationship between brain structure and developmental language disorders. Semin Pediatr Neurol 4:117–124, 1997

Semrud-Clikeman M, Hynd GW: Right hemispheric dysfunction in nonverbal learning disabilities: social, academic, and adaptive functioning in adults and children. Psychol Bull 107:196–209, 1990

Semrud-Clikeman M, Filipek PA, Biederman J, et al: Attention deficit hyperactivity disorder: magnetic resonance imaging morphometric analyses of the corpus callosum. J Am Acad Child Adolesc Psychiatry 33:875–881, 1994

Seuchter SA, Hebebrand J, Klug B, et al: Complex segregation analysis of families ascertained through Gilles de la Tourette syndrome. Genet Epidemiol 18:33–47, 2000

Sever Y, Ashkenazi A, Tyano S, et al: Iron treatment in children with attention deficit hyperactivity disorder: a preliminary report. Neuropsychobiology 35:178–180, 1997

Shaffer D, Gardner A, Hedge B: Behavior and bladder disturbance of enuretic children: a common disorder. Dev Med Child Neurol 26:781–792, 1984

Shaffer D, Gould MS, Brasic J, et al: A Children's Global Assessment Scale (CGAS). Arch Gen Psychiatry 40:1228–1231, 1983

Shah MR, Seese LM, Abikoff H, et al: Pemoline for children and adolescents with conduct disorder: a pilot investigation. J Child Adolesc Psychopharmacol 4:255–261, 1994

Shalev RS, Manor O, Amir N, et al: Developmental dyscalculia and brain laterality. Cortex 31:357–365, 1995

Shalev RS, Manor O, Gross-Tsur V: Neuropsychological aspects of developmental dyscalculia. Math Cognition 33:105–120, 1997

Shalev RS, Auerbach J, Manor O, et al: Developmental dyscalculia: prevalence and prognosis. Eur Child Adolesc Psychiatry 9(suppl 2):58–64, 2000

Shalev RS, Manor O, Kerem B, et al: Developmental dyscalculia is a familial learning disability. J Learn Disabil 34:59–65, 2001

Shapiro AK, Shapiro ES, Young JG, et al: Gilles de la Tourette Syndrome. New York, Raven, 1998

Shapiro SK, Garfinkel HD: The occurrence of behavior disorders in children: the interdependence of attention deficit disorder and conduct disorder. Journal of the American Academy of Child Psychiatry 25:809–819, 1986

Sharp WS, Walter JM, Marsh WL, et al: ADHD in girls: clinical comparability of a research sample. J Am Acad Child Adolesc Psychiatry 38:40–47, 1999

Shaywitz SE, Cohen DJ, Shaywitz BA: Behavior and learning difficulties in children of normal intelligence born to alcoholic mothers. J Pediatr 96:978–982, 1980

Shaywitz SE, Shaywitz BA, Fletcher JM, et al: Prevalence of reading disability in boys and girls: results of the Connecticut Longitudinal Study. JAMA 264:998–1002, 1990

Shaywitz SE, Shaywitz BA, Pugh KR, et al: Functional disruption in the organization of the brain for reading in dyslexia. Proc Natl Acad Sci U S A 95:2636–2641, 1998

Sheppard DM, Bradshaw JL, Purcell R, et al: Tourette's and comorbid syndromes: obsessive compulsive and attention deficit hyperactivity disorder: a common etiology? Clin Psychol Rev 19:531–552, 1999

Sherman DK, Iacono WG, McGue MK: Attention-deficit hyperactivity disorder dimensions: a twin study of inattention and impulsivity-hyperactivity. J Am Acad Child Adolesc Psychiatry 36:745–753, 1997

Sigman M (ed): Children With Emotional Disorders and Developmental Disabilities: Assessment and Treatment. Orlando, FL, Grune & Stratton, 1985

Silove D, Harris M, Morgan A, et al: Is early separation anxiety a specific precursor of panic disorder-agoraphobia? A community study. Psychol Med 25:405–411, 1995

Silvany-Neto AM, Carvalho FM, Tavares TM, et al: Lead poisoning among children of Santo Amaro, Bahia, Brazil in 1980, 1985, and 1992. Bulletin of the Pan American Health Organization 30.51–62, 1996

Silver AA, Shytle RD, Sheehan KH, et al: Multicenter, double-blind, placebo-controlled study of mecamylamine monotherapy for Tourette's disorder. J Am Acad Child Adolesc Psychiatry 40:1103–1110, 2001

Simeon JG, Ferguson HB, Knott V, et al: Clinical, cognitive, and neurophysiological effects of alprazolam in children and adolescents with overanxious and avoidant disorder. J Am Acad Child Adolesc Psychiatry 31:29–33, 1992

Simon SL: Soil ingestion by humans: a review of history, data, and etiology with application to risk assessment of radioactively contaminated soil. Health Phys 74:647–672, 1998

Simons D, Goode S, Fombonne E: Elective mutism and chromosome 18 abnormality. Eur Child Adolesc Psychiatry 6:112–124, 1997

Singer HS, Brown J, Quaskey S, et al: The treatment of attention-deficit hyperactivity disorder in Tourette's syndrome: a double-blind placebo-controlled study with clonidine and desipramine. Pediatrics 95:74–81, 1995

Singer HS, Giuliano JD, Hansen BH, et al: Antibodies against human putamen in children with Tourette syndrome. Neurology 50:1618–1624, 1998

Singer HS, Giuliano JD, Zimmerman AM, et al: Infection: a stimulus for tic disorders. Pediatr Neurol 22:380–383, 2000

Singer HS, Wendlandt J, Krieger M, et al: Baclofen treatment in Tourette syndrome: a double-blind, placebo-controlled, crossover trial. Neurology 56:599–604, 2001

Skinner RA, Piek JP: Psychosocial implications of poor motor coordination in children and adolescents. Human Movement Science 20:73–94, 2001

Skjeldal OH, von Tetzchner S, Aspelund F, et al: Rett syndrome: geographic variation in prevalence in Norway. Brain Dev 19:258–261, 1997

Skoog SJ, Stokes A, Turner KL: Oral desmopressin: a randomized double-blind placebo controlled study of effectiveness in children with primary nocturnal enuresis. J Urol 158:1035–1040, 1997

Smith M, Escamilla JR, Filipek P, et al: Molecular genetic delineation of 2q37.3 deletion in autism and osteodystrophy: report of a case and of new markers for deletion screening by PCR. Cytogenet Cell Genet 94:15–22, 2001

Smith S, Kimberling W, Pennington B, et al: Specific reading disability: identification of an inherited form through linkage analysis. Science 219:1345–1347, 1983

Snowling M, Bishop DV, Stothard SE: Is preschool language impairment a risk factor for dyslexia in adolescence? J Child Psychol Psychiatry 41:587–600, 2000

Sokol MS, Gray NS: An infection-triggered, autoimmune subtype of anorexia nervosa. J Am Acad Child Adolesc Psychiatry 36:1128–1133, 1997

Soussignan R, Tremblay R: Other disorders of conduct, in Hyperactivity Disorders of Childhood. Edited by Sandberg S. Cambridge, England, Cambridge University Press, 1996

Southam-Gerow MA, Kendall PC, Weersing VR: Examining outcome variability: correlates of treatment response in a child and adolescent anxiety clinic. J Clin Child Psychol 30:422–436, 2001

Sparrow SS, Balla DA, Cicchetti DV: Vineland Adaptive Behavior Scales. Circle Pines, MN, American Guidance Service, 1984

Speltz ML, Coy K, DeKlyen M, et al: Early onset oppositional defiant disorder: what factors predict its course? Seminars in Clinical Neuropsychiatry 3:302–319, 1998

Speltz ML, McClellan J, DeKlyen M, et al: Preschool boys with oppositional defiant disorder: clinical presentation and diagnostic change. J Am Acad Child Adolesc Psychiatry 38:838–845, 1999

Spencer J, O'Brien J, Riggs K, et al: Motion processing in autism: evidence for a dorsal stream deficiency. Neuroreport 11:2765–2767, 2000

Spencer T, Biederman J, Wilens TE, et al: Adults with attention-deficit/hyperactivity disorder: a controversial diagnosis. J Clin Psychiatry 59(suppl 7):59–68, 1998a

Spencer T, Biederman J, Harding M, et al: Disentangling the overlap between Tourette's disorder and ADHD. J Child Psychol Psychiatry 39:1037–1044, 1998b

Spencer T, Biederman J, Wilens T: Growth deficits in children with attention deficit hyperactivity disorder. Pediatrics 102:501–506, 1998c

Spencer T, Biederman J, Wilens T: Attention-deficit hyperactivity disorder and comorbidity. Pediatr Clin North Am 46:915–927, 1999

Spencer TJ, Biederman J, Wozniak J, et al: Parsing pediatric bipolar disorder from its associated comorbidity with the disruptive behavior disorders. Biol Psychiatry 49:1062–1070, 2001a

Spencer T, Biederman J, Coffey B, et al: Tourette disorder and ADHD. Adv Neurol 85:57–77, 2001b

Sprich S, Biederman J, Crawford MH: Adoptive and biological families of children and adolescents with ADHD. J Am Acad Child Adolesc Psychiatry 39:1432–1437, 2000

Staley D, Wand R, Shady G: Tourette disorder: a cross-cultural review. Compr Psychiatry 38:6–19, 1997

Stanovich KE, Siegel LS: Phenotypic performance profile of children with reading disabilities: a regression-based test of the phonological-core-variable-difference model. Journal of Educational Psychology 86:24–53, 1994

Stark R, Tallal P: Language, Speech, and Reading Disorders in Children: Neuropsychological Studies. Boston, MA, College-Hill Press, 1988

Stefl ME: The Ohio Tourette's Study. Cincinnati, OH, University of Cincinnati School of Planning, 1983

Stein A, Woolley H, McPherson K: Conflict between mothers with eating disorders and their infants during mealtimes. Br J Psychiatry 175:455–461, 1999

Stein MA, Sandoval R, Szumowski E, et al: Psychometric characteristics of the Wender Utah Rating Scale (WURS): reliability and factor structure for men and women. Psychopharmacol Bull 31:425–433, 1995

Steingard R, Khan A, Gonzalez A, et al: Neuroleptic malignant syndrome: review of experience with children and adolescents. J Child Adolesc Psychopharmacol 2:183–198, 1992

Steingard RJ, Zimnitzky B, DeMaso DR, et al: Sertraline treatment of transition-associated anxiety and agitation in children with autistic disorder. J Child Adolesc Psychopharmacol 7:9–15, 1997

Steinhausen HC, Adamek R: The family history of children with elective mutism: a research report. Eur Child Adolesc Psychiatry 6:107–111, 1997

Steinhausen HC, Gobel D: Enuresis in child psychiatric clinic patients. J Am Acad Child Adolesc Psychiatry 28:279–281, 1989

Stephens RJ, Sandor P: Aggressive behaviour in children with Tourette syndrome and comorbid attention-deficit hyperactivity disorder and obsessive-compulsive disorder. Can J Psychiatry 44:1036–1042, 1999

Stern E, Silbersweig DA, Chee KY, et al: A functional neuroanatomy of tics in Tourette syndrome. Arch Gen Psychiatry 57:741–748, 2000

Stern HP, Stroh SE, Fiedorek SC, et al: Increased plasma levels of pancreatic polypeptide and decreased plasma levels of motilin in encopretic children. Pediatrics 96:111–117, 1995

Stern JS, Robertson MM: Tics associated with autistic and pervasive developmental disorders. Neurol Clin 15:345–355, 1997

Stevens LJ, Zentall SS, Deck JL, et al: Essential fatty acid metabolism in boys with attention-deficit hyperactivity disorder. Am J Clin Nutr 62:761–768, 1995

Stevens LJ, Zentall SS, Abate ML, et al: Omega-3 fatty acids in boys with behavior, learning, and health problems. Physiol Behav 59:915–920, 1996

Storm-Mathisen A, Vaglum P: Conduct disorder patients 20 years later: a personal follow-up study. Acta Psychiatr Scand 89:416–420, 1994

Strauss J, Birmaher B, Bridge J, et al: Anxiety disorders in suicidal youth. Can J Psychiatry 45:739–745, 2000

Stromme P: Aetiology in severe and mild mental retardation: a population-based study of Norwegian children. Dev Med Child Neurol 42:76–86, 2000

Stromme P, Diseth TH: Prevalence of psychiatric diagnoses in children with mental retardation: data from a population-based study. Dev Med Child Neurol 42:266–270, 2000

Stromme P, Magnus P: Correlations between socioeconomic status, IQ and aetiology in mental retardation: a population-based study of Norwegian children. Soc Psychiatry Psychiatr Epidemiol 35:12–18, 2000

Sullivan MA, Rudnik-Levin F: Attention deficit/hyperactivity disorder and substance abuse: diagnostic and therapeutic considerations. Ann N Y Acad Sci 931:251–270, 2001

Sunohara GA, Roberts W, Malone M, et al: Linkage of the dopamine D4 receptor gene and attention-deficit/hyperactivity disorder. J Am Acad Child Adolesc Psychiatry 39:1537–1542, 2000

Sutphen JL, Borowitz SM, Hutchison RL, et al: Long-term follow-up of medically treated childhood constipation. Clin Pediatr (Phila) 34:576–580, 1995

Swank LK: Specific developmental disorders: the language-learning continuum. Child Adolesc Psychiatr Clin North Am 8:89–112, 1999

Swanson JM, Sunohara GA, Kennedy JL, et al: Association of the dopamine receptor D4 (DRD4) gene with a refined phenotype of attention deficit hyperactivity disorder (ADHD): a family based approach. Mol Psychiatry 3:38–41, 1998

Swanson JM, Flodman P, Kennedy J, et al: Dopamine genes and ADHD. Neurosci Biobehav Rev 24:21–25, 2000

Swedo SE: Sydenham's chorea: a model for childhood autoimmune neuropsychiatric disorders. JAMA 272:1788–1791, 1994

Swedo SE, Leonard HL, Garvey M, et al: Pediatric autoimmune neuropsychiatric disorders associated with streptococcal infections: clinical description of the first 50 cases. Am J Psychiatry 154:264–271, 1998

Szatmari P: The classification of autism, Asperger's syndrome, and pervasive developmental disorder. Can J Psychiatry 45:731–738, 2000

Szatmari P, Bremner R, Nagy J: Asperger's syndrome: a review of clinical features. Can J Psychiatry 34:554–560, 1989

Szatmari P, Archer L, Fisman S, et al: Asperger's syndrome and autism: differences in behavior, cognition, and adaptive functioning. J Am Acad Child Adolesc Psychiatry 34:1662–1671, 1995

Szatmari P, Bryson SE, Streiner DL, et al: Two-year outcome of preschool children with autism or Asperger's syndrome. Am J Psychiatry 157:1980–1987, 2000

Szymanski LS: Prevention of psychosocial dysfunction in persons with mental retardation. Ment Retard 25:215–218, 1987

Szymanski L, King BH: Summary of the Practice Parameters for the Assessment and Treatment of Children, Adolescents, and Adults With Mental Retardation and Comorbid Mental Disorders. American Academy of Child and Adolescent Psychiatry. J Am Acad Child Adolesc Psychiatry 38:1606–1610, 1999

Szymanski LS, Tanguay LS (eds): Emotional Disorders of Mentally Retarded Persons. Baltimore, MD, University Park Press, 1980

Taanila A, Kokkonen J, Järvelin MR: The long-term effects of children's early onset disability on marital relationships. Dev Med Child Neurol 38:567–577, 1996

Tallal P: Developmental language disorders, in Learning Disabilities: Proceedings of the National Conference. Edited by Kavanagh JF, Truss TJ. Parkton, MD, York, 1988, pp 181–272

Tallal P, Hirsch LS, Realpe-Bonilla T, et al: Familial aggregation in specific language impairment. J Speech Lang Hear Res 44:1172–1182, 2001

Taminiau JA: Gastro-oesophageal reflux in children. Scand J Gastroenterol Suppl 223:18–20, 1997

Tanaka Y, Yoshida A, Kawahata N, et al: Diagnostic dyspraxia: clinical characteristics, responsible lesion and possible underlying mechanism. Brain 119:859–873, 1996

Tanguay PE: Pervasive developmental disorders: a 10-year review. J Am Acad Child Adolesc Psychiatry 39:1079–1095, 2000

Tannock R: Attention deficit hyperactivity disorder: advances in cognitive, neurobiological, and genetic research. J Child Psychol Psychiatry 39:65–99, 1998

Tannock R, Martinussen R, Frijters J: Naming speed performance and stimulant effects indicate effortful, semantic processing deficits in attention-deficit/hyperactivity disorder. J Abnorm Child Psychol 28:237–252, 2000

Taylor E, Schachar R, Thorley G, et al: Which boys respond to stimulant medication? A controlled trial of methylphenidate in boys with disruptive behavior. Psychol Med 17:121–143, 1987

Teicher MH, Ito Y, Glod CA, et al: Objective measurement of hyperactivity and attentional problems in ADHD. J Am Acad Child Adolesc Psychiatry 35:334–342, 1996

Teicher MH, Anderson CM, Polcari A, et al: Functional deficits in basal ganglia of children with attention-deficit/hyperactivity disorder shown with functional magnetic resonance imaging relaxometry. Nat Med 6:470–473, 2000

Temple E, Poldrack RA, Protopapas A, et al: Disruption of the neural response to rapid acoustic stimuli in dyslexia: evidence from functional MRI. Proc Natl Acad Sci U S A 97:13907–13912, 2000

Thapar A, Gottesman II, Owen MJ, et al: The genetics of mental retardation. Br J Psychiatry 164:747–758, 1994

Thompson M, Comings DE, Feder L, et al: Mutation screening of the dopamine D1 receptor gene in Tourette's syndrome and alcohol dependent patients. Am J Med Genet 81:241–244, 1998

Thuppal M, Fink M: Electroconvulsive therapy and mental retardation. J ECT 15:140–149, 1999

Thurber CA: The phenomenology of homesickness in boys. J Abnorm Child Psychol 27:125–139, 1999

Tibbits-Kleber AL, Howell RJ: Reactive attachment disorder of infancy (RAD). J Clin Child Psychol 14:304–310, 1985

Tirosh E, Cohen A: Language deficit with attention-deficit disorder: a prevalent comorbidity. J Child Neurol 13:493–497, 1998

Tizard J, Schofield WN, Hewison J: Collaboration between teachers and parents in assisting children's reading. Br J Educ Psychol 52:1–15, 1982

Todd RD, Neuman RJ, Lobos EA, et al: Lack of association of dopamine D4 receptor gene polymorphisms with ADHD subtypes in a population sample of twins. Am J Med Genet 105:432–438, 2001

Wiesel TN: Postnatal development of the visual cortex and the influence of environment. Nature 299:583–592, 1982

Wieseler NA, Hanson RH, Nord G: Investigation of mortality and morbidity associated with severe self-injurious behavior. Am J Ment Retard 100:1–5, 1995

Wilens T, Spencer T, Frazier J, et al: Psychopharmacology in children and adolescents, in Handbook of Child Psychopathology. Edited by Ollendick T, Hersen M. New York, Plenum Publishing, 1998, pp 603–636

Wilhelm K, Parker G, Dewhurst-Savellis J, et al: Psychological predictors of single and recurrent major depressive episodes. J Affect Disord 54:139–147, 1999

Wille S: Comparison of desmopressin and enuresis alarm for nocturnal enuresis. Arch Dis Child 61:30–33, 1986

Willemsen-Swinkels SH, Buitelaar JK, Weijnen FG, et al: Plasma beta-endorphin concentrations in people with learning disability and self-injurious and/or autistic behavior. Br J Psychiatry 168:105–109, 1996

Williams H, Clarke R, Bouras N, et al: Use of the atypical antipsychotics olanzapine and risperidone in adults with intellectual disability. J Intellect Disabil Res 44:164–169, 2000

Williams ML, Lewandowski LJ, Coplan J, et al: Neurodevelopmental outcome of preschool children both preterm with and without intracranial hemorrhage. Dev Med Child Neurol 29:243–249, 1987

Wilson PH, McKenzie BE: Information processing deficits associated with developmental coordination disorder: a meta-analysis of research findings. J Child Psychol Psychiatry 39:829–840, 1998

Wilson SL: Attachment disorders: review and current status. J Psychol 135:37–51, 2001

Wing L: Asperger's syndrome: a clinical account. Psychol Med 11:115–130, 1981

Winneke G, Krämer U: Neurobehavioral aspects of lead neurotoxicity in children. Cent Eur J Public Health 5:65–69, 1997

Wise BW, Olson RK: Computer-based phonologic awareness and reading instruction. Annals of Dyslexia 45:99–122, 1995

Wolfgang ME, Figlio RM, Cellin T: Delinquency in a Birth Cohort. Chicago, IL, University of Chicago Press, 1972

Wong DF, Singer HS, Brandt J, et al: D_2-like dopamine receptor density in Tourette syndrome measured by PET. J Nucl Med 38:1243–1247, 1997

Wong DF, Ricaurte G, Grunder G, et al: Dopamine transporter changes in neuropsychiatric disorders. Adv Pharmacol 42:219–223, 1998

Woolston JL: Eating disorders in infancy and early childhood. Journal of the American Academy of Child Psychiatry 22:114–121, 1983

Wozniak J, Biederman J, Richards JA: Diagnostic and therapeutic dilemmas in the management of pediatric bipolar disorder. J Clin Psychiatry 14:10–15, 2001a

Wozniak J, Biederman J, Faraone SV, et al: Heterogeneity of childhood conduct disorder: further evidence of a subtype of conduct disorder linked to bipolar disorder. J Affect Disord 64:121–131, 2001b

Wright HH, Miller MD, Cook MA, et al: Early identification and intervention with children who refuse to speak. Journal of the American Academy of Child Psychiatry 24:739–746, 1985

Ye X, Mitchell M, Newman K, et al: Prospects for prenatal gene therapy in disorders causing mental retardation. Mental Retardation and Developmental Disabilities Research Reviews 7:65–72, 2001

Yirmiya N, Erel O, Shaked M, et al: Meta-analyses comparing theory of mind abilities of individuals with autism, individuals with mental retardation, and normally developing individuals. Psychol Bull 124:283–307, 1998

Youssef NN, Di Lorenzo C: Childhood constipation: evaluation and treatment. J Clin Gastroenterol 33:199–205, 2001

Zametkin AJ, Rapoport JL: Neurobiology of attention deficit disorder with hyperactivity: where have we come in 50 years? J Am Acad Child Adolesc Psychiatry 26:676–686, 1987

Zeanah CH: Beyond insecurity: a reconceptualization of attachment disorders in infancy. J Consult Clin Psychol 64:42–52, 1996

Zeanah CH: Disturbances of attachment in young children adopted from institutions. J Dev Behav Pediatr 21:230–236, 2000

Zeanah CH, Embe RN: Attachment disorders in infancy and childhood, in Child and Adolescent Psychiatry, 3rd Edition. Edited by Rutter M, Hersov L, Taylor E. London, England, Blackwell, 1995

Ziemann U, Paulus W, Rothenberger A: Decreased motor inhibition in Tourette's disorder: evidence from transcranial magnetic stimulation. Am J Psychiatry 154:1277–1284, 1997

Zilbovicius M, Boddaert N, Belin P, et al: Temporal lobe dysfunction in childhood autism: a PET study: positron emission tomography. Am J Psychiatry 157:1988–1993, 2000

Zoccolillo M, Tremblay R, Vitaro F: DSM-III-R and DSM-III criteria for conduct disorder in preadolescent girls: specific but insensitive. J Am Acad Child Adolesc Psychiatry 35:461–470, 1996

Zubieta JK, Alessi NE: Is there a role of serotonin in the disruptive behavior disorders? A literature review. J Child Adolesc Psychopharmacol 3:11–35, 1993

Sleep Disorders

Thomas C. Neylan, M.D.

Charles F. Reynolds III, M.D.

David J. Kupfer, M.D.

The 2001 Sleep in America Poll showed that 69% of adult Americans experience frequent sleep problems. Approximately two-thirds of adults average less than 8 hours of sleep per night, and a full one-third habitually sleep less than 7 hours (National Sleep Foundation 2001). Furthermore, this survey showed that Americans are working more and spending less time sleeping or in recreation than 5 years before. Despite increased attention to the health consequences of disturbed sleep and the phenomenal growth of organized sleep medicine, sleep disturbances remain pandemic and mostly undertreated. In this chapter we provide a broad overview of sleep disorders and summarize current treatment guidelines for each disorder.

Normal Human Sleep

The brain has three major states of activity and function: wakefulness, rapid eye movement (REM) sleep, and non-REM sleep. REM sleep, identified in 1953 by Aserinsky and Kleitman, is a dramatic physiologic state in that the brain becomes electrically and metabolically activated with frequencies approaching those of wakefulness. Perhaps as a defense to preserve sleep, there is a generalized muscle atonia that is detected polysomnographically by the disappearance of electromyographic activity. REMs occur in phasic bursts and are accompanied by fluctua-

tions in respiratory and cardiac rate. Finally, dreaming in REM sleep is frequently vivid and affectively charged and is associated with activation of the amygdala (L.D. Sanford et al. 2001), which is thought to regulate emotionally influenced memory (Macquet et al. 1996).

Healthy sleep in humans consists of recurring 70- to 120-minute cycles of non-REM and REM sleep characterized polysomnographically by the electroencephalogram (EEG), the electrooculogram (EOG), and the electromyogram (EMG) (Rechtschaffen and Kales 1968). The conventional EEG lead used for sleep staging is either C3 or C4 (Jasper 1958). Eye movements are detected by the EOG because of the presence of an electrical dipole between the cornea and retina. Typically, sleep progresses from wakefulness through the four stages of non-REM sleep until the onset of the first REM period. In the healthy adult, the deepest stages of sleep, non-REM Stages III and IV (collectively referred to as *slow-wave sleep*), occur in the first two non-REM periods. In contrast, the REM periods in the first half of the sleep period are brief and lengthen in successive cycles.

During wakefulness, the EEG is characterized by low-voltage fast activity consisting of a mix of alpha (8–13 Hz) and beta (>13 Hz) frequencies. *Stage I* of non-REM sleep is a transitional stage between wakefulness and sleep during which the predominant alpha rhythm disappears, giving way to the slower theta (4–7 Hz) frequencies. Tonic electromyographic activity decreases,

Supported in part by the General Clinical Research Center (UCSF: 5M01RR-00079) and National Institutes of Mental Health Grants MH57157 (TCN); M01RR00056, P30MH05247, MH37869, MH43832 (CFR); P30MH30915, MH59769 (DJK).

and the eyes move in a slow, rolling pattern. *Stage II* is characterized by a background theta rhythm and the episodic appearance of sleep spindles (i.e., brief bursts of 12- to 14-Hz activity) and K complexes (i.e., a high-amplitude, slow-frequency electronegative wave followed by an electropositive wave). Muscle tone remains diminished, and eye movements are rare. *Stages III* and *IV* are defined as epochs of sleep consisting of greater than 20% and 50%, respectively, of high-amplitude activity in the delta band (0.5–3.0 Hz). Muscle tone is nearly atonic, and eye movements are absent.

Neuroanatomy of Sleep

Several discrete areas in the pontine brain stem are involved in the regulation of REM sleep. REM sleep onset is driven by ascending cholinergic cells of both the pedunculopontine tegmental nucleus (PPT) and the lateral dorsal tegmental nucleus (LDT). These cells receive inhibitory projections from the serotonergic cells of the dorsal raphe nuclei and the noradrenergic cells of the locus coeruleus. The oscillation between the pro-REM cholinergic cells and the inhibitory serotonergic and noradenergic cells accounts for the ultradian cycling of REM sleep. In addition, areas of the limbic forebrain become activated during REM sleep (Figure 21–1). Descending inputs from limbic areas, particularly the amygdala, can affect phasic REM activity (e.g., the frequency of eye movements in each epoch of REM sleep). These inputs may account for the observed associations of acute stress, posttraumatic stress disorder (PTSD), and major depression with increased phasic REM activity (Mellman et al. 1997). Pontine lesions below the cholinergic REM on cells eliminate the muscle atonia that normally characterizes REM sleep. Incomplete muscle atonia can lead to pathological motor activity during sleep (described in "REM Sleep Behavior Disorder" subsection later in this chapter).

Non-REM sleep is less focally regulated than REM sleep. Non-REM sleep is driven in part by cells in the preoptic/anterior hypothalamic area (POAH). These cells send γ-aminobutyric acid (GABA)–mediated projections to the posterior hypothalamus ending at the tuberomammillary nucleus (TM), resulting in inhibition of the tonic histamine-mediated activity involved in regulating arousal. In addition, the cholinergic cells of the ascending reticular activating system (ARAS) are also inhibited by an unknown mechanism. Elimination of arousal activity from the ARAS and TM allows for emergence of slower-frequency thalamocortical rhythms characteristic of non-REM sleep (Steriade et al. 2001).

Recent advances in molecular biology have led to the discovery of another neurotransmitter system that appears to regulate the sleep cycle. Hypocretins are neuropeptides regulating neurons that are located in the posterior hypothalamus and have projections to monoaminergic cell groups throughout the entire brain (De Lecea et al. 1998; Sakurai et al. 1998). The hypocretins are excitatory in nature and promote wakefulness and suppress REM sleep (Bourgin et al. 2000). Hypocretin deficiency is implicated in both canine and human narcolepsy as discussed further ahead.

Sleep and Circadian Rhythms

The timing of our daily sleep–wake cycle is mainly under the control of the suprachiasmatic nucleus (SCN) in the hypothalamus, which establishes a daily, or circadian, rhythm. Destruction of the SCN eliminates circadian rhythmicity (Moore and Eichler 1972; Rusak and Zucker 1979), although sleep cycles persist. Hence, sleep is also regulated by a homeostatic drive that causes us to feel sleepy after sustained wakefulness. The circadian oscillator promotes sleepiness both in the afternoon and at night in those with a typical sleep–wake schedule. Thus, the interaction of circadian and homeostatic regulation explains the observation that a person may feel subjectively more alert at 7:00 P.M. than at 4:00 P.M. despite having had a longer period of sustained wakefulness. The circadian oscillator reacts and entrains to environmental cues (e.g., the light–dark cycle) that are called *zeitgebers* (literally, "time-givers"). The discovery of several genes responsible for familial forms of circadian rhythm disorders, including the "Clock" gene, has provided new insight into the mechanism of genetic regulation of circadian rhythms (Toh et al. 2001). These circadian pacemaker genes may control the oscillations of various systems, such as neuroendocrine activity and thermoregulation. Exposure to bright light may affect the regulation of these genes, thus allowing a shift in the circadian timing of multiple systems.

Ontogeny of Sleep Stages

During the first 3 years of life, the sleep–wake rhythm develops from an ultradian to a circadian pattern, with the principal sleep phase occurring at night. Sleep in prepubertal children is characterized by large percentages of REM and high-amplitude slow-wave sleep. During adolescence, a precipitous decrease in slow-wave sleep (Feinberg 1974) occurs during a period of rapid neuronal

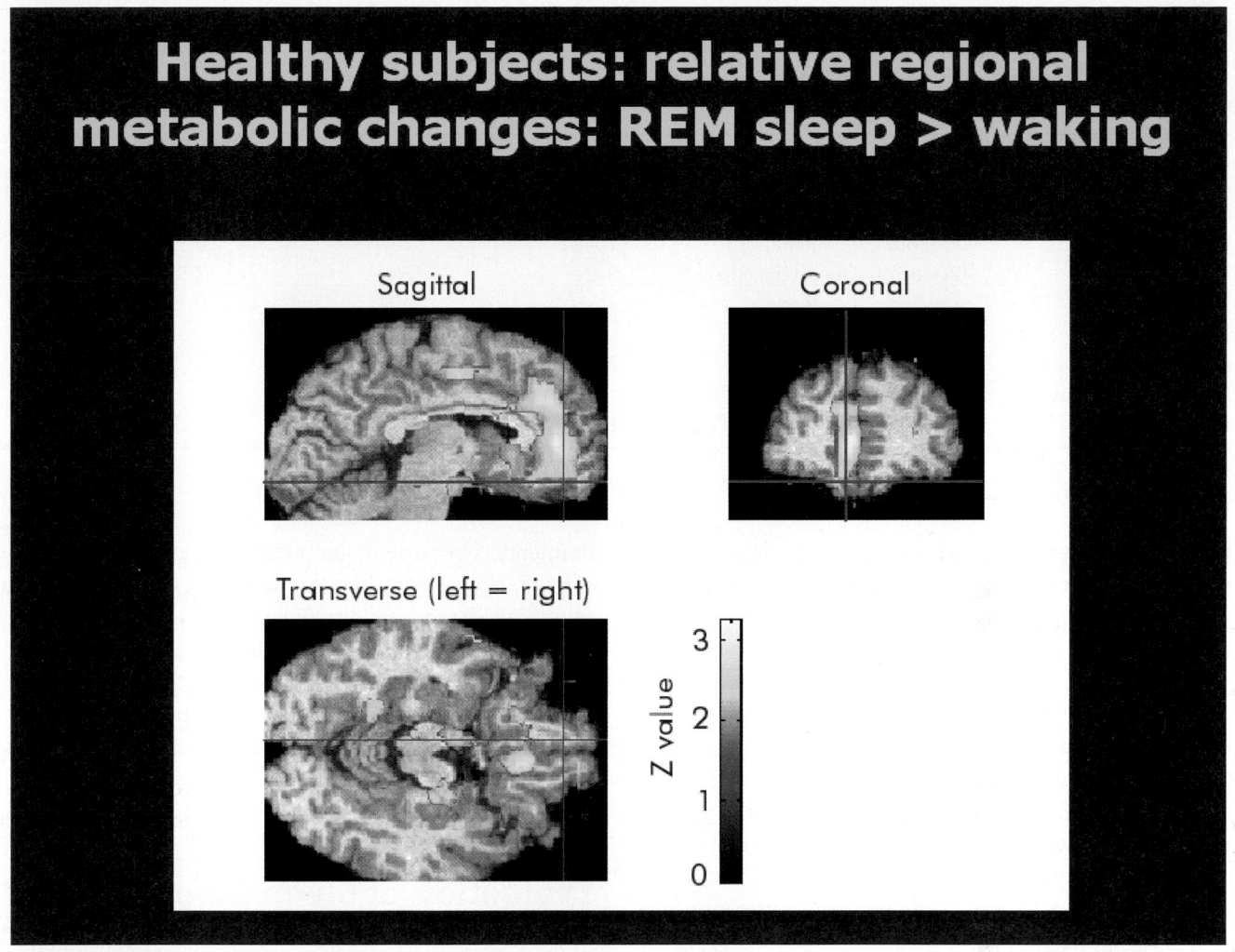

FIGURE 21–1. Relative regional metabolic changes between rapid eye movement (REM) sleep and waking in healthy subjects.

Figure shows all of the regions in the brain that have statistically greater relative cerebral metabolism during REM sleep than during wakefulness.

Source. Nofzinger et al. 1997.

senescence and synaptic pruning (Feinberg 1982; Huttenlocher 1979). In the third through sixth decades, there is a gradual and slight decline in sleep efficiency and total sleep time. With advancing age, sleep becomes more fragmented and lighter in depth. There are more transient arousals, as well as sleep stage shifts, and there is also a gradual disappearance of slow-wave sleep (Gillin and Ancoli-Israel 1992). In addition, the diurnal sleep–wake pattern decays as sleep is redistributed into the light phase in the form of frequent naps (Buysse et al. 1992).

Sleep Pharmacology

Prior to the 1960s, when benzodiazepines were introduced, barbiturates were the most commonly prescribed sedative-hypnotic medications. Because of their superior tolerability and safety, benzodiazepines quickly supplanted the barbiturates. Currently, benzodiazepines and atypical sedative-hypnotics are used to induce sleep onset and to improve overall sleep continuity (Table 21–1). Within the class of benzodiazepines, the duration of action and the presence of active metabolites are the main variables to consider when using these agents. Long-acting benzodiazepines such as flurazepam, which have active metabolites with half-lives in excess of 200 hours, often cause problems with daytime alertness and are associated with more errors while driving an automobile as compared with short-acting agents. Short-half-life benzodiazepines such as triazolam are useful for sleep-onset insomnia but will not benefit those with sleep maintenance difficulties in the latter half of the night. Furthermore, short-half-life agents produce more pro-

TABLE 21–1. Hypnotic agents

Generic	Trade	Onset	Half-life (h)[a]	Active metabolites	Dose (mg)
Benzodiazepines					
Flurazepam	Dalmane	Rapid	40–250	Yes	15, 30
Quazepam	Doral	Rapid	40–250	Yes	7.5, 15
Estazolam	ProSom	Rapid	10–24	Yes	0.5, 1, 2
Temazepam	Restoril	Intermediate	8–22	No	7.5, 15
Triazolam	Halcion	Rapid	<6	No	0.125, 0.25, 0.50
Imidazopyridine					
Zolpidem	Ambien	Rapid	2.5	No	5, 10
Pyrazolopyrimidine					
Zaleplon	Sonata	Rapid	1	No	5, 10, 20

Note. [a]Parent compound and active metabolites.

nounced and rapid rebound anxiety and insomnia. However, slow tapering of these agents can prevent the discontinuation syndrome. In general, it is thought that sedative-hypnotic therapy should be limited to agents with short and intermediate half-lives. The adverse effects of using long-duration sedative-hypnotics for periods of insomnia include impaired memory and psychomotor performance and an increased risk of motor vehicle accidents (Menzin et al. 2001). For example, the use of benzodiazepines and other sedatives increases the risk of hip fracture in elderly patients.

Zolpidem is a short-half-life nonbenzodiazepine drug that binds selectively to the type 1 benzodiazepine receptor (Langer et al. 1987). It has no effect on nocturnal respiratory function in patients with obstructive lung disease (Girault et al. 1996). In therapeutic doses, it has minimal effects on sleep architecture and does not cause rebound insomnia after discontinuation (Kryger et al. 1991; Merlotti et al. 1989). Like triazolam, zolpidem causes short-term impairment of memory that is reversible with flumazenil (Wesensten et al. 1995). Zaleplon has a mechanism of action similar to that of zolpidem. The primary difference is its very short duration of action, which makes it potentially useful for the management of sleep-onset insomnia and early-morning awakening (Weitzel et al. 2000).

A number of medications used in the treatment of insomnia are not approved by the U.S. Food and Drug Administration (FDA) for the treatment of insomnia (Table 21–2). Antihistamines are frequently used despite having poorer efficacy relative to the benzodiazepines and more adverse daytime effects. Trazodone is a sedating antidepressant that is frequently used as a sedative. It has been found to improve sleep continuity and subjective sleep quality. Although trazodone is frequently rec-

ommended because of its putative absence of tolerance effects, data on its long-term efficacy have not been obtained. Trazodone's major side effects include priapism, hypotension, and morning hangover. Melatonin has been used to treat insomnia despite warnings from multiple experts in sleep medicine. The safety of over-the-counter melatonin is unknown, given the lack of regulatory oversight by the FDA.

Clinical Manifestations and Evaluation of Sleep Disorders

In community and clinical studies, insomnia has been associated with poor job performance, fatigue, accidents, impaired physical well-being, and increased use of alcohol (Ford and Kamerow 1989; Gallup Organization 1995; Kales et al. 1984; Mellinger et al. 1985; National Commission on Sleep Disorders Research 1993). Studies of insomnia subjects suggest that sleep loss per se is a biological stressor that results in an increase in aggressive behavior in animals and human subjects (Hicks et al. 1979; Hipolide et al. 1995; O'Reilly 1995; Peder et al. 1986) and a worsening of anxiety in anxiety disorder subjects (Roy-Byrne et al. 1986). Conservative estimates of the total annual cost of insomnia in the United States range from $92.5 to $107.5 billion (Stoller 1994). The chief complaint usually is related to disrupted or too little sleep, excessive sleepiness, or adverse events associated with the sleep period.

A thorough medical and psychiatric history is essential for diagnosing conditions that have an impact on sleep–wake function. The entire 24-hour period should be explored with respect to sleep–wake habits. Patients with insomnia should be questioned about their views on

TABLE 21–2. Unapproved agents used in the treatment of insomnia

Agent	Advantages	Disadvantages
Antidepressants		
Amitriptyline	No tolerance	Anticholinergic delirium, increased risk of falls, daytime sedation
Doxepin	No tolerance	Increased risk of falls, daytime sedation
Trazodone	No tolerance, no anticholinergic effects	Increased risk of falls, daytime sedation
Antipsychotics		
Haloperidol	No tolerance, few anticholinergic effects	Extrapyramidal effects, increased risk of falls, not very sedating
Thioridazine	No tolerance	Extrapyramidal effects, increased risk of falls, anticholinergic delirium
Barbiturates	No pertinent advantages over benzodiazepines	High risk of addiction, dangerous withdrawal syndrome, overdose potential, daytime sedation
Miscellaneous		
Chloral hydrate	Less addictive than benzodiazepines	Overdose potential, tolerance to hypnotic effects over time, nausea
Diphenhydramine	No tolerance	Anticholinergic delirium, increased risk of falls, daytime sedation, memory impairment

what constitutes healthy sleep. Very often patients who by virtue of their constitution are short sleepers are subjectively distressed by their inability to sleep for the popular standard of 8 hours. The severity of insomnia can be understood only in terms of its impact on daytime function such as mood, fatigue, muscle aches, attention, and concentration. Asking patients about the total number of hours of sleep typically obtained has limited value, given the overlap between good and poor sleepers. Self-rating instruments such as the Pittsburgh Sleep Quality Index (Buysse et al. 1989) are useful for measuring subjective sleep quality. A 2-week sleep–wake log is invaluable for obtaining a history of irregular sleep–wake patterns; napping; use of stimulants, hypnotics, or alcohol; diet; activity during the day; number of arousals; and perceived length of sleep time and its relationship to daytime mood and alertness.

Approximately 4%–5% of the general population complains of excessive sleepiness (Bixler et al. 1979). Sleepiness relates to the propensity to sleep, such as after sleep deprivation. Clinically, it is more alarming than insomnia because of the higher degree of psychosocial impairment as well as the high rate of automobile and occupational accidents (Guilleminault and Carskadon 1977; Mitler et al. 1988; Roth et al. 1994). Patients should be asked about symptoms of morning headaches, cataplexy, hypnagogic or hypnopompic hallucinations, sleep paralysis, automatic behavior, or sleep drunkenness (Table 21–3). In addition, they should be questioned carefully about falling asleep while driving or

while performing any other potentially dangerous activity. Additional history should be obtained from bed partners for events that are usually not perceived by the patients, such as snoring, respiratory pauses longer than 10 seconds, unusual body movements, or somnambulism.

Patients who complain of disturbances associated with the sleep period should be questioned about nocturnal incontinence or polyuria, orthopnea, paroxysmal nocturnal dyspnea, headaches that interrupt sleep, jaw clenching or bruxism, sleeptalking, somnambulism, and, in the case of males, painful nocturnal erections (Aldrich 1994).

Polysomnography remains the principal diagnostic tool in the field of sleep medicine. A thorough polysomnographic study provides data on sleep continuity, sleep architecture, REM physiology, sleep-related respiratory impairment, oxygen desaturation, cardiac arrhythmias, and periodic movements. Additional measures may include nocturnal penile tumescence, temperature, and infrared video monitoring. The routine use of polysomnography in the evaluation of hypersomnolent patients is well justified given the high incidence of sleep apnea and narcolepsy in this group. Polysomnography should be used in any patient with a parasomnia in which there is clinical suspicion of sleep apnea or nocturnal seizure disorder. Practice guidelines for the use of polysomnography in the evaluation of chronic insomnia have been developed by the American Academy of Sleep Medicine (Chesson et al. 2000; Table 21–4).

TABLE 21–3. Sleep definitions

Apnea	Cessation of airflow for at least 10 seconds.
Cataplexy	Sudden loss in muscle tone, usually precipitated by a sudden emotional response such as fear or laughter.
Chronobiology	The study of natural physiological rhythms.
Circadian rhythm	A regular pattern of fluctuation in physiology or behavior that is usually linked to the 24-hour light–dark cycle.
Diurnal	A behavior or physiological variable that is tied to daytime.
Hypersomnia	Excessive sleepiness. Pertains to the propensity to fall asleep.
Hypnagogic or hypno-pompic hallucinations	Hallucinations occurring at the beginning or end of sleep that are usually a manifestation of REM sleep.
Hypopnea	Reduction in airflow by at least 50% for at least 10 seconds.
Insomnia	Difficulty with initiating or maintaining sleep.
Myoclonus	Abrupt contraction of a group of muscles, usually in the lower extremity.
Paradoxical sleep	Synonym for REM sleep.
Parasomnia	Adverse physiological or behavioral event occurring during sleep.
Phase advance or delay	Shift of the sleep or wake cycle to an earlier or later position in the 24-hour day.
Polysomnography	The electrophysiological recording of multiple biological parameters during sleep.
Zeitgeber	An environmental factor, such as the light–dark cycle, that helps entrain biological rhythms to a 24-hour time period.

Note. REM = rapid eye movement.
Source. Data from American Sleep Disorders Association Diagnostic Classification Steering Committee 1990.

The Multiple Sleep Latency Test (MSLT; Carskadon et al. 1986) is the most objective and valid measure of excessive sleepiness. Other measures such as the Stanford Sleepiness Scale (Hoddes et al. 1973) and the Maintenance of Wakefulness Test (Mitler et al. 1982) are less reliable, although they are easy and inexpensive to use. The Epworth Sleepiness Scale measures daytime sleepiness in eight common real-life situations (Johns 1991). In the MSLT, the patient is given the opportunity to fall

TABLE 21–4. Practice guidelines for the use of polysomnography in the evaluation of insomnia

Polysomnography is not routinely indicated for transient or chronic insomnia.

Polysomnography is indicated when sleep apnea or myoclonus is suspected, particularly in older patients.

Polysomnography should be considered if the diagnosis is uncertain *and* behavior or drug therapy is ineffective.

Polysomnography is indicated for patients with confusional or violent arousals, particularly if the clinical diagnosis is uncertain.

Polysomnography should be considered for circadian rhythm disorders if the clinical diagnosis is uncertain.

Source. Data from Chesson et al. 2000.

asleep in a darkened room for five 20-minute periods in 2-hour intervals across the patient's usual period of wakefulness. The average latency to sleep onset, measured polysomnographically, is a direct measure of the propensity to fall asleep. Multiple studies have shown that an average sleep latency of less than 5 minutes indicates a pathological degree of sleepiness associated with a high rate of intrusive sleep episodes during the wake period and decrements in work performance (Carskadon et al. 1981; Dement et al. 1978; Nicholson and Stone 1986). The detection of sleep-onset REM periods in the MSLT has become a cornerstone in the diagnosis of narcolepsy (Mitler 1982).

Classification of Sleep Disorders

DSM-IV-TR (American Psychiatric Association 2000) divides sleep disorders into four major categories: primary sleep disorders, sleep disorders related to another mental disorder, sleep disorder due to a general medical condition, and substance-induced sleep disorder.

Primary Sleep Disorders

Dyssomnias

Primary Insomnia

Primary insomnia is the term used to describe difficulty initiating or maintaining sleep, or nonrestorative sleep, lasting at least a month in duration. By definition, primary insomnia results in significant daytime impairment and is not secondary to another sleep disorder. Sleep fragmentation can usually be validated by polysomnography, which shows prolonged sleep latencies, decreased sleep efficiency, and a predominance of the lighter stages of non-REM sleep (Hauri and Fisher 1986; Hauri and Olmstead 1980). An overview of the evaluation of chronic insomnia is provided in Table 21–5.

For some patients, primary insomnia represents a lifetime disorder or trait characteristic in which the patient has a constitutional predisposition for fragmented sleep (Hauri and Olmstead 1980). The pathophysiology, although unknown, is presumed to be secondary to a neurochemical or structural disorder involving neural networks governing sleep–wake states. Patients with this pattern of primary insomnia are extremely light sleepers and are easily perturbed by environmental noise, temperature fluctuations, and situational anxiety. Several studies suggest that primary insomnia can be conceptualized as a disorder of hyperarousal (Regestein et al. 1993). For example, patients with insomnia have a greater 24-hour metabolic rate than do age- and weight-matched normal sleepers (Bonnet and Arand 1995). Patients with insomnia have longer average sleep latencies on the MSLT (Stepanski et al. 1988).

Some patients develop primary insomnia following a period of severe stress. In these patients, the symptoms of insomnia do not remit with the resolution of the stressful event, either because new behaviors that disrupt sleep have been adapted or because environmental cues in the sleeping area have become paired with conditioned arousal. In addition, patients with chronic insomnia will sometimes develop a form of performance anxiety associated with going to sleep. Their struggles to fall asleep and their anxiety about possible daytime fatigue set up a conditioned association between bedtime behavior and anxious arousal. The disorder can become chronic, persisting over many years, and can cause chronic fatigue, muscle aches, and mood disturbance (Hauri and Fisher 1986).

There are several effective treatment approaches to chronic insomnia that do not involve the use of hypnotics (Chesson et al. 1999a). Education about normal sleep and counseling around habits for promoting good sleep hygiene are a good but insufficient intervention when used alone (Hauri 1989; Morin et al. 1994). Various relaxation therapies such as hypnosis, meditation, deep breathing, and progressive muscle relaxation can be helpful. These techniques, in contrast to the use of hypnotics, are not immediately beneficial but require several weeks of practice to improve sleep (McClusky et al. 1991). Success is dependent on a high degree of motivation in patients, who must devote considerable time to practicing these techniques. Those who succeed in learning these techniques have a greater satisfaction with maintenance treatment than do patients chronically using hyp-

TABLE 21–5. Evaluation of chronic insomnia

Step 1	Evaluate for a general medical condition that may adversely affect sleep.
Step 2	Evaluate whether medications or substance use is disrupting sleep.
Step 3	Evaluate whether another mental disorder such as depression, schizophrenia, or anxiety disorder is causing sleep disruption.
Step 4	Consider a breathing-related sleep disorder, particularly if the patient snores or is obese.
Step 5	Consider a sleep–wake schedule disorder if the patient has an irregular schedule or is involved in shift work.
Step 6	Consider a parasomnia diagnosis if the patient complains of behavioral or mental events that occur during sleep.
Step 7	If insomnia has persisted for more than a month and is not related to the above disorders, then the diagnosis is primary insomnia.
Step 8	If insomnia is not described by the above criteria, then the diagnosis of dyssomnia not otherwise specified is used.

Source. Data from Reynolds et al. 1995.

notics (Bootzin and Perlis 1992; Morin et al. 1992, 1999). Furthermore, responders to behavioral interventions have sustained benefits after 6 months (G.D. Jacobs et al. 1996). Biofeedback can be helpful in those patients who are not sensitive to their internal state of arousal (Hauri and Esther 1990). Patients are provided an external measure of a biological variable such as an EMG or EEG that allows them a means to influence their own level of arousal.

Stimulus control behavior modification focuses on eliminating environmental cues associated with arousal (Bootzin 1972). This technique is similar to implementing rules for sleep hygiene in that patients are instructed to use their bed only for sleep and intimacy, to go to bed only when sleepy, to remove clocks from sight, and to adhere to a stable sleep–wake schedule. The goal is to limit the amount of wake time spent in bed, thereby reestablishing the association between the bed and sleep.

Sleep restriction therapy is similarly aimed at reducing the amount of wake time spent in bed (Spielman et al. 1987). Patients are asked to record in a sleep diary the amount of time they estimate they are asleep. They are then instructed to restrict their time in bed to a degree commensurate to their estimate of their total sleep time. Patients often have their usual difficulties with sleep fragmentation during the first few nights and become sleep deprived. Sleep deprivation helps consolidate sleep on subsequent nights, thereby improving sleep efficiency. Increases in length of time in bed can subsequently be titrated to the presence of daytime fatigue.

Hypnotics should be considered only after a thorough diagnostic assessment of secondary causes of insomnia, after sleep hygiene has been improved, and after behavioral treatments have been attempted. If these approaches are unsuccessful, then hypnotics can be used, starting with very low doses and limiting use to short periods. Long-term efficacy studies of behavioral and pharmacological interventions in insomnia are clearly needed.

Primary Hypersomnia

The diagnosis of primary hypersomnia subsumes two previous categories: idiopathic hypersomnia and recurrent hypersomnia (Kleine-Levin syndrome). Both variants are characterized by prolonged nocturnal sleep and severe daytime sleepiness that can be objectively documented by a short mean sleep latency on the MSLT. Primary hypersomnia is a diagnosis of exclusion, made when other disorders causing excessive sleepiness have been ruled out. A recurrent form of primary hypersomnia is characterized by intermittent attacks of hypersomnolence and hyperphagia, often associated with indiscrete hypersexuality, poor social judgment, mood disturbance, and hallucinations. Between episodes there can be a complete remission of symptoms. This pattern of primary hypersomnia occurs most frequently in males in their late adolescence and early 20s, after which time there is a gradual decline in the frequency and duration of the episodes (Critchley 1962). The pathophysiology of primary hypersomnia is postulated to involve an underlying disturbance of limbic and hypothalamic function. Several abnormal laboratory findings have been documented, including slowing of background rhythm on the EEG, altered secretory pattern of growth hormone and thyroid-stimulating hormone, and elevated cerebrospinal-fluid serotonin and dopamine metabolites (Billiard 1989; Chesson et al. 1991). Treatment usually involves the use of psychostimulants to reduce daytime hypersomnolence.

Narcolepsy

Narcolepsy is a common cause of daytime hypersomnolence in which REM sleep repeatedly and suddenly intrudes into wakefulness. It represents an impairment in the ability to maintain a stable neural state; REM is no longer segregated in its usual ultradian rhythm during sleep. The clinical phenomenology of narcolepsy is best understood through a consideration of normal REM physiology (e.g., activated EEG, generalized atonia, dream cognition). Both cataplexy and sleep paralysis involve muscle atonia occurring at a time when the patient is cognizant of the environment and subjectively feels awake. Hypnagogic hallucinations are not well understood but are thought to be related to the dreamlike perceptual phenomenon of REM sleep. Nocturnal sleep is characterized by short REM latency and frequent arousals and shifts from non-REM sleep to REM sleep to wakefulness (Rechtschaffen et al. 1963).

Recent advances in molecular biology have clarified the pathophysiology of narcolepsy. Canine narcolepsy is caused by a mutation in the hypocretin gene (Lin et al. 1999). Preprohypocretin knockout mice have symptoms suggestive of narcolepsy. Finally, human narcolepsy has been found to be associated with generalized deficiency of hypocretin (Nishino et al. 2000; Peyron et al. 2000; Thannickal et al. 2000). It is possible that decreased tone of monoaminergic cells and increased cholinergic sensitivity, characteristic of narcolepsy (Nishino and Mignot 1997), are caused by the absence of excitatory inputs from hypocretin cells in the hypothalamus (Hungs and Mignot 2001). Low hypocretin levels in cerebrospinal fluid, which have been reported in studies of narcolepsy, may be an additional diagnostic tool in the evaluation of hypersomnolence (Nishino et al. 2000).

Studies have shown that narcolepsy affects psychological state as well as cognition. Patients have been found to have more job-related injuries, problems with occupational or academic performance, and a higher prevalence of anxiety and mood disorders (Richardson et al. 1990). Several studies of patients with narcolepsy have shown impaired performance in tasks requiring sustained attention, as a result of intrusive microsleeps. However, not all performance decrements can be attributed to impaired arousal, because attention deficits have been found in narcoleptic patients during EEG-verified wakefulness (for a review, see Mendelson 1987). In one study (Reynolds et al. 1983a), 20% of 25 patients with narcolepsy met criteria for major depression, 8% for generalized anxiety disorder, and 12% for alcohol abuse. An unresolved issue is whether the higher prevalence of psychiatric symptomatology is a response to the psychosocial consequences of having a chronic disorder in which existing treatments are often inadequate or whether the mood and affective disturbance are driven by a common pathophysiology.

The treatment of narcolepsy primarily involves the use of dopaminomimetic stimulants such as dextroamphetamine, methamphetamine, methylphenidate, or pemoline. These agents can release presynaptic pools of monoamines, block their reuptake, or inhibit monoamine oxidase metabolism of norepinephrine and dopamine. Discontinuation of agents that release dopamine appears to result in rebound insomnia. Additional agents used to treat narcolepsy include γ-hydroxybutyrate and modafinil. Modafinil, an atypical psychostimulant that affects postsynaptic α_1-adrenergic receptors, promotes wakefulness and is rarely associated with substance dependence (Besset et al. 1996). Modafinil is less effective than amphetamine in controlling cataplexy (Shelton et al. 1995). REM-suppressing agents such as tricyclic antidepressants and γ-hydroxybutyrate have been found to control cataplexy. An important nonpharmacological approach is the use of scheduled naps throughout the wake period (Helmus et al. 1997). Practice guidelines for the use of stimulants in the treatment of narcolepsy have been recommended by the American Academy of Sleep Medicine (Table 21–6).

Sleep Apnea

If evolution had led to the development of a stiff upper airway, the problems of snoring and obstructive apnea would never have occurred. Because it must be flexible for purposes of swallowing and production of speech, the upper airway has an inherent potential for collapse during respiration. To compensate for this vulnerability, there is a complex set of muscles that dilate the upper airway during inspiration. In addition, anatomic factors that affect lumen size (e.g., obesity) and exogenous factors that reduce phasic muscle activity of the upper airway (e.g., sedative-hypnotics [Bonora et al. 1984]) can independently lead to an increased potential for airway collapse. Genetic factors, independent of obesity, contribute to the heritability of sleep apnea, through the influence of craniofacial traits (Mathur and Douglas 1995; Nelson and Hans 1997).

Sleep-disordered breathing is an age-related disorder affecting approximately 24% of community-dwelling individuals over age 65 years (Ancoli-Israel et al. 1991) and 42% of elderly persons living in nursing homes (Ancoli-Israel 1989). In contrast, in a large sample of college freshman in Hong Kong, the prevalence was found to be approximately 0.1% (Hui et al. 1999). The estimated prevalence of apnea in a random sample of employed middle-aged subjects is 9% for women and 24% for men (Young et al. 1993). Although occasionally causing insomnia, sleep apnea is typically an occult disorder that causes daytime somnolence, impaired concentration and intellectual functioning, and morning headaches. It is associated with obesity, loud snoring, systemic and pulmonary hypertension, cardiac arrhythmias, nocturnal cardiac ischemia, myocardial infarction, and excessive

TABLE 21–6. Practice guidelines for the use of stimulants in the treatment of narcolepsy

The diagnosis of narcolepsy should be established by a polysomnogram and the Multiple Sleep Latency Test.

Stimulants should be used to alleviate daytime sleepiness, not to maximize performance.

Pemoline, methylphenidate, dextroamphetamine, methamphetamine, and modafinil have proven efficacy.

The recommended maximum daily doses for some of the stimulants used to treat narcolepsy are as follows:

  Pemoline 150 mg

  Methylphenidate 100 mg

  Dextroamphetamine 100 mg

  Methamphetamine 80 mg

Combining short- and long-acting stimulants may be indicated in some patients.

Tolerance is most likely to occur in treatment with high-dose amphetamines.

Amphetamines have the highest potential for illicit use.

Most female patients should discontinue taking stimulants during pregnancy if this does not present intolerable risk to the woman.

Caution is urged in prescribing stimulants to nursing mothers.

Source. Data from American Sleep Disorders Association Standards of Practice Committee 1995.

mortality (H. Schafer et al. 1997; Strollo and Rogers 1996; Yamashiro and Kryger 1994). It can be caused by an impairment in central respiratory drive (central apnea), intermittent upper airway obstruction (obstructive apnea), or a combination of the two (mixed apnea). Patients with this disorder experience frequent respiratory pauses during sleep that are associated with oxygen desaturation. The apneic events are terminated by loud gasping, thrashing movements, and arousal on EEG. Patients, who usually have no awareness of these events, are often brought to clinical attention by alarmed bed partners (Guilleminault 1982).

Sleep apnea is quantified polysomnographically by measuring oral and nasal airflow with thermistors, which are warmed by exhaled air; respiratory effort with either thoracic and abdominal strain gauges, diaphragmatic or intercostal EMG, or an esophageal pressure gauge; oxygen saturation with an oximeter; and sleep architecture with a standard sleep montage (i.e., EEG, EOG, EMG). Patients with severe sleep apnea typically have evidence of pathological sleepiness as measured by latencies to sleep onset of less than 5 minutes on the MSLT. Ball et al. (1997) found that an effort by sleep specialists to increase awareness of obstructive sleep apnea among primary care physicians succeeded in dramatically increasing case recognition and treatment of the disorder.

The clinical impact of sleep apnea is related to two phenomena: hypoxia and sleep fragmentation. Cerebral hypoxia can lead to intellectual deterioration, impaired attention and memory, and personality changes. Successful treatment improves neurocognitive performance on most, but not all, measures, which suggests that permanent anoxic injury occurs in some patients (Bedard et al. 1993). Several investigators have attempted to discern whether hypersomnolence is related to sleep hypoxia or to sleep fragmentation. Roehrs et al. (1989) reported a study of 466 patients with obstructive sleep apnea in which multiple polysomnographic variables, including arousals on EEG and oxygen desaturations, were independently analyzed for prediction of excessive daytime somnolence. Although the number of arousals and hypoxic events covaried significantly, it was the arousal index that best predicted short latencies on the MSLT. This finding suggests that hypersomnolence is secondary to the disruption in quantity and quality of sleep. A study of older insomnia patients with and without mild to moderate sleep apnea showed that when sleep fragmentation is controlled, apneas and hypoxic events do not predict additional psychomotor impairment (Stone et al. 1994).

There are a variety of behavioral, medical, pharmacological, and surgical treatments for sleep apnea. Behavioral approaches include weight loss, abstinence from sedative-hypnotics, and sleep-position training (which helps the patient avoid the supine position during sleep). Mechanical approaches include use of tongue-retaining devices, orthodontic appliances that advance the mandible (Loube and Strauss 1997; Nakazawa et al. 1992), and nasal continuous positive airway pressure (CPAP). Surgical techniques aim to increase the lumen size of the oropharynx and include uvulopalatopharyngoplasty (UPPP), maxillomandibular and hyoid advancement, and chronic tracheostomy (Powell et al. 1994). Follow-up studies of patients who have undergone UPPP show that approximately half of the subjects benefit from surgery, and some who do benefit relapse after several years (Janson et al. 1997). Preliminary data suggest that laser-assisted UPPP is inferior to conventional UPPP in enhancing oropharyngeal air space; however, the clinical significance of this finding has not been established (Finkelstein et al. 1997).

To date, nasal CPAP remains the initial treatment of choice for moderate to severe sleep apnea. CPAP acts as a pneumatic splint that maintains the patency of the oropharynx during respiration (Sullivan and Grunstein 1994). The air pressure required to maintain airway patency should be directly titrated in the sleep laboratory. Reports of long-term compliance are variable, ranging from 25% to 70% (Guilleminault et al. 1992).

Nightly compliance is required for optimal benefit. One night of discontinuation of nasal CPAP results in complete reversal of the gains made in daytime alertness (Kribbs et al. 1993).

Circadian Rhythm Sleep Disorder

The sleep–wake cycle, under the circadian control of endogenous regulators or oscillators, can be disrupted by a misalignment between biological rhythms and external demands on waking behavior. Circadian rhythm sleep disorders present with either insomnia or hypersomnolence, depending on the juxtaposition of performance demands and the underlying circadian cycle.

Circadian rhythm sleep disorders are associated with significant medical comorbidity and impairment in psychosocial functioning. Rotating-shift workers have been found to have an injury rate two to three times that of their co-workers who work stable day, evening, or night shifts (M. Smith and Colligan 1982). *Shift work type disorder* is associated with high rates of gastrointestinal, cardiac, and reproductive disorders (Czeisler and Allan 1988). Workers who rotate onto different shifts experience an acute misalignment in their underlying biological rhythms: 65% of workers on rotating shifts complain of poor sleep as compared with 20% of workers on stable shifts (Czeisler et al. 1982). Night shift workers are usually in a state of permanent circadian misalignment because of their tendency to revert to conventional schedules on their days off. Air traffic controllers and attending emergency physicians make more cognitive errors while working night shifts (Luna et al. 1997; Smith-Coggins et al. 1994). Shift workers have higher rates of on-the-job sleepiness, as well as higher rates of drug use and divorce (Regestein and Monk 1991). The *jet lag type* is one of the most common of these disorders. Travelers flying across multiple time zones must re-entrain their circadian sleep–wake rhythms with respect to both social schedule and the acquired light–dark cycle (Spitzer et al. 1999). Patients with *delayed sleep phase type disorder* are described as night owls, with an innate preference for beginning sleeping in the late hours of night and sleeping until the late morning or early afternoon. They experience sleep-onset insomnia and morning hypersomnolence when forced to comply with a conventional sleep–wake schedule. There are reports of patients with a phase advance in their sleep–wake schedule who experience hypersomnolence in the early evening hours, as well as midnight arousal. Typically these are older patients, because with age there is a tendency for the sleep–wake cycle to advance relative to clock time. The general treatment approach is to promote good sleep hygiene, with the goal of properly aligning patients' circadian systems with their sleep–wake schedules. Treatment may also involve manipulation or augmentation of external zeitgebers, such as with the use of bright-light therapy.

Phototherapy.   Multiple studies have shown that exposure to light at 2,000 lux or more can shift circadian rhythms (Terman 1994). Bright light entrains multiple biological rhythms by means of a direct retinohypothalamic tract and excitatory amino acids transducing information to the suprachiasmatic nuclei (Dijk et al. 1995). One hypothesis concerning the therapeutic value of morning bright light is related to its ability to phase-advance or realign these rhythms to a healthy baseline (Lewy et al. 1987; Terman et al. 1988). Recent studies have shown that rapid tryptophan depletion under double-blind conditions reverses the therapeutic gains of bright light, which suggests that serotonergic mechanisms are involved in phototherapy (Lam et al. 1996; Neumeister et al. 1997).

With respect to sleep disorders, bright light has been found to be effective in treating delayed sleep phase type disorder (Rosenthal et al. 1990) and jet lag (Daan and Lewy 1984). Furthermore, it has been found to improve alertness and cognitive performance in night shift workers (Campbell et al. 1995a). Bright-light therapy improves sleep–wake patterns in institutionalized elderly persons. For example, evening light exposure improves sleep maintenance insomnia in the elderly (Campbell et al. 1995b; Mishima et al. 1994; Yamadera et al. 2000). Bright-light exposure in the evening reduces sundowning behavior in hospitalized patients with Alzheimer's disease (Satlin et al. 1992).

In one method of therapy, patients are instructed to sit 3 feet in front of a bright-light source of at least 2,500-lux intensity (Terman 1994). Typically, patients require between 30 minutes and 2 hours of exposure, depending on therapeutic response. Side effects include eyestrain, headache, and mild psychomotor agitation. At present, there is no evidence that long-term use of bright-light therapy results in any ocular damage (Gallin et al. 1995). The timing of exposure depends on the direction in which patients wish to shift their sleep–wake schedule. Morning or evening exposure will phase-advance or phase-delay the sleep–wake schedule, respectively.

Melatonin.   The rationale for the clinical use of melatonin is its ability to re-entrain the underlying circadian sleep–wake rhythm (Sack et al. 2000). Endogenous melatonin increases after the onset of the dark cycle and is inhibited by photic stimuli transduced by the retinohy-

pothalamic tract to the suprachiasmatic nucleus to the pineal gland. Exogenously administered melatonin in the early evening causes the endogenous melatonin release to occur earlier and produces an enhanced propensity for an earlier sleep onset (Lewy et al. 1995). Exogenous melatonin has been proposed as a potential alternative to bright-light therapy for manipulating sleep–wake rhythms to manage jet lag and facilitate adaptation to rotating work shifts. However, controlled trials of this strategy have not demonstrated its efficacy in either alleviating jet lag (Spitzer et al. 1999) or facilitating adaptation to night shift work (Wright et al. 1998).

Dyssomnia Not Otherwise Specified

The category of dyssomnia not otherwise specified (NOS) includes the phenomenon of *nocturnal myoclonus*, which is characterized by periodic leg movements of sufficient severity to cause sleep continuity disturbance, leading to complaints of either insomnia or daytime sleepiness. Nocturnal myoclonus consists of repetitive, brief leg jerks that occur in regular 20- to 40-second intervals. These movements are frequently associated with transient arousals that lead to sleep fragmentation and a predominance of the lighter stages of non-REM sleep (Karadeniz et al. 2000). Patients are usually unaware of this disorder, except that they may have the experience of morning leg cramps and a sense of insufficient sleep. Periodic leg movements are frequently found on polysomnographic record and are not correlated with subjective measures of sleep quality (Mendelson 1996).

Nocturnal myoclonus is seen frequently in association with sleep apnea, narcolepsy, uremia, diabetes, and a variety of disorders affecting the cortex, brain stem, and spinal cord (Coleman et al. 1980). Typically, nocturnal myoclonus is idiopathic, with no evidence of gross central nervous system pathology. It is a normal phenomenon at birth, disappears in childhood, and frequently reemerges in old age. The emergence of myoclonus is thought to be secondary to the loss of inhibition of a naturally occurring pacemaker operating at the level of the spinal cord (Lugaresi et al. 1972; R.C. Smith 1985).

Restless legs syndrome is a syndrome that causes sleep-onset insomnia. It is typically characterized by deep paresthesias in the calf muscles, prompting the urge to keep the legs in motion. However, it also can involve the arms in approximately half of those with the syndrome (Montplaisir et al. 1997). Restless legs syndrome can be extremely distressing and has been linked to suicide. It is associated with anemia, pregnancy, and nocturnal myoclonus. It is also associated with uremia and has been diagnosed in 20% of patients with end-stage renal disease

(Winkelman et al. 1996). There is a familial form of this disorder with an autosomal dominant pattern of transmission with complete penetrance (Trenkwalder et al. 1996).

The most common treatments involve the use of benzodiazepines or dopaminomimetics such as L-dopa or bromocriptine (Montplaisir et al. 1992; Trenkwalder et al. 1995). Other agents currently under investigation for use in treatment of restless legs syndrome include opioids, carbamazepine, clonidine, and baclofen (Wagner et al. 1996). Practice parameters for the treatment of nocturnal myoclonus and restless legs syndrome have been developed by the American Academy of Sleep Medicine and are presented in Table 21–7.

Parasomnias

Parasomnias are adverse events that occur during sleep. Many of these disorders have been described as disorders of partial arousal from various sleep stages. There has been much debate regarding whether these disorders emerge from specific sleep stages such as delta and REM. Mahowald and Schenck (1992) argued that parasomnias and narcolepsy represent dissociated states with mixed features of REM sleep, non-REM sleep, and wakefulness. *Sleepwalking disorder* and *sleep terror disorder* involve intrusions of wake behavior into non-REM sleep. Similarly, *REM sleep behavior disorder*, in which patients are motorically active during dreams, represents an intrusion of wake behavior into a sleep state. This model is also helpful in understanding how some antidepressant medications cause sleep dissociation, as in the case of intrusion of REMs during non-REM sleep with fluoxetine treatment (Schenck et al. 1992).

Sleepwalking and Night Terrors

Sleepwalking and *night terrors* are found normally in young children and are associated with psychopathology only if persisting into adulthood. Typically, they involve a partial arousal from sleep during the first third of the night, a period characterized by a predominance of slow-wave sleep (Gaudreau et al. 2000). In sleepwalking, subjects become partially aroused and ambulatory; they are typically difficult to awaken and have amnesia for the events. Data from the Finnish Twin Cohort show that concordance for sleepwalking in childhood is 0.55 in monozygotic and 0.35 in dizygotic pairs (Hublin et al. 1997). Nocturnal violent behavior, seen predominantly in men, can be associated with sleepwalking (Alkassar et al. 2000; Moldofsky et al. 1995). Several forensic cases have involved the argument that sleep-related violence was defensible on the basis of its being a noninsane

TABLE 21–7. Practice guidelines for the treatment of nocturnal myoclonus (NM) and restless legs syndrome (RLS)

The diagnosis of nocturnal myoclonus or restless legs syndrome should be established by the patient's history, bed partner report, and possible polysomnogram.

Secondary causes of NM and RLS should be evaluated and treated.

Levodopa/carbidopa, oxycodone, propoxyphene, carbamazepine, and clonazepam have proven efficacy. Gabapentin and clonidine have possible efficacy.

Close physician monitoring of adverse effects is required.

Iron supplementation is useful for RLS patients with iron deficiency.

Most female patients should discontinue taking medication during pregnancy.

No information is known about the use of medications in children with NM or RLS.

Source. Data from Chesson et al. 1999b.

automatism (Broughton et al. 1994; Schenck and Mahowald 1995). In one survey of 170 adults with injurious parasomnias, long-term nightly use of benzodiazepines was found to be safe and effective (Schenck and Mahowald 1996). Night terrors involve an emergence of intense fear associated with autonomic arousal in which patients are inconsolable, difficult to awaken fully, and unable to assign specific cognitions associated with the anxiety. Treatment is directed toward reducing stress, anxiety, and sleep deprivation, all of which are known to exacerbate these disorders. In extreme cases, low-dose benzodiazepines are indicated and effective.

Nightmare Disorder

Nightmare disorder, formerly known as *dream anxiety disorder*, occurs in 10%–50% of children (American Psychiatric Association 1994). The incidence of the disorder peaks between the ages of 3 and 6 (Leung and Robson 1993) and declines with age (Hartmann 1984). In a survey of 1,006 adults (ages 18–80 years) in Los Angeles, 5.3% of respondents reported that "frightening dreams" were a current problem (Bixler et al. 1979). Results of this survey and others (Coren 1994) have indicated that there is a higher prevalence of frightening dreams in women. Unfortunately, there is no reliable information about nightmare disorder in adults because nightmares are rarely captured in the sleep laboratory and because subjects are often confused about the difference between night terrors and nightmares, which can obscure survey data (Hartmann 1984). Individuals with nightmare disorder, unlike those with night terrors, have anxiety-provoking dreams characterized by vivid, detailed imagery that is associated with good recall. Furthermore, in none of the aforementioned studies were attempts made to adjust or control for exposure to traumatic stress.

Nightmares have been postulated to be a hallmark of traumatic stress responses (Ross et al. 1989). DSM-IV (American Psychiatric Association 1994) acknowledges that the prevalence of nightmare disorder is unknown. Given that this diagnosis is excluded when PTSD is present, the validity of nightmare disorder as a separate nosological entity has not been well established.

REM Sleep Behavior Disorder

REM sleep behavior disorder, which is listed as a parasomnia NOS in DSM-IV, occurs when there is incomplete or absent muscle atonia during REM sleep. The disorder is characterized by prominent motor activity during dreaming. Several dramatic cases have involved patients who suddenly assaulted their bed partners in response to frightening dreams. REM sleep behavior disorder can emerge transiently during drug intoxication or withdrawal or exist as a chronic condition, most typically in patients with demonstrable neurological disease (Mahowald and Schenck 1992; Nofzinger and Reynolds 1994), particularly Parkinson's disease (Olson et al. 2000). REM sleep behavior disorder has also been reported in patients with lesions of the pons, where normal muscle atonia of REM sleep is regulated (Kimura et al. 2000). Benzodiazepines, particularly clonazepam, and carbamazepine have been found to be useful in reducing these events (Bamford 1993; Mahowald and Schenck 1994). Treatment with the acetylcholinesterase inhibitor donepezil has also been found to be effective (Ringman and Simmons 2000).

Nocturnal Paroxysmal Dystonia

Nocturnal paroxysmal dystonia, another disorder subsumed under parasomnia NOS in DSM-IV, is characterized by stereotypical and violent movements of the trunk and limbs of short duration. These movements can resemble seizure activity and respond to treatment with carbamazepine (Provini et al. 2000). They can occur multiple times during the night and are associated with non-REM sleep.

Some parasomnias occur during sleep–wake transitions. Head banging, formerly known as *jactatio capitis nocturnus*, is a rhythmic movement disorder that is thought to be a self-soothing behavior in children during the transition from wakefulness to sleep. Sleep starts, or hypnic jerks, are sudden muscle contractions that often occur during sleep onset and are thought to be clinically insignificant.

Sleep Disorders Related to Another Mental Disorder

Mood Disorders

Sleep disturbance is verifiable in 90% of patients with major depression and is characterized by sleep fragmentation, decreased quantity and altered distribution of delta sleep, reduced duration of the first non-REM period (i.e., REM latency), redistribution of REM sleep into the first half of the night, and increased number of REMs per minute of REM sleep (Kupfer and Foster 1972; Kupfer and Reynolds 1992; Reynolds and Kupfer 1987). Multiple studies have shown that disturbed sleep antedates the development of major depression (Breslau et al. 1996; Chang et al. 1997; Ford and Kamerow 1989; Roberts et al. 2000).

A review of findings from sleep studies in depressed patients leads to the conclusion that no single variable, such as REM latency, has diagnostic specificity (Benca et al. 1992). However, REM latency has been found to be a reliable marker for particular state and trait variables and to have value in predicting clinical course and treatment outcome. For example, first-degree relatives of depressed patients with short REM latency have been found to be at increased risk for major depression (Giles et al. 1988). In addition, first-degree relatives concordant for depression have been found also to be concordant for REM latency (Giles et al. 1987b). Kupfer et al. (1976) showed that the degree of REM latency prolongation and total REM suppression seen during initiation of treatment with amitriptyline predicted clinical response. Similarly, REM suppression by clomipramine has been found to predict response to treatment (Höchli et al. 1986). Short REM latency during an index episode of depression confers a higher risk of relapse after clinical remission (Giles et al. 1987a).

Multiple studies have shown that REM latency is related to state-dependent factors in major depression. For example, Giles et al. (1986) found that REM latency helped distinguish endogenous depression from nonendogenous depression. Short REM latency was related to appetite loss, terminal insomnia, anhedonia, and unreactive mood. In contrast, sleep electroencephalography does not support the biological validity of the diagnoses of primary versus secondary depression, in that the polysomnographic characteristics of each are similar (Thase et al. 1984). Reynolds et al. (1992) showed that subjects with bereavement-related depression had more sleep continuity disturbance and shorter REM latencies than did bereaved subjects without depression. Kupfer et al.

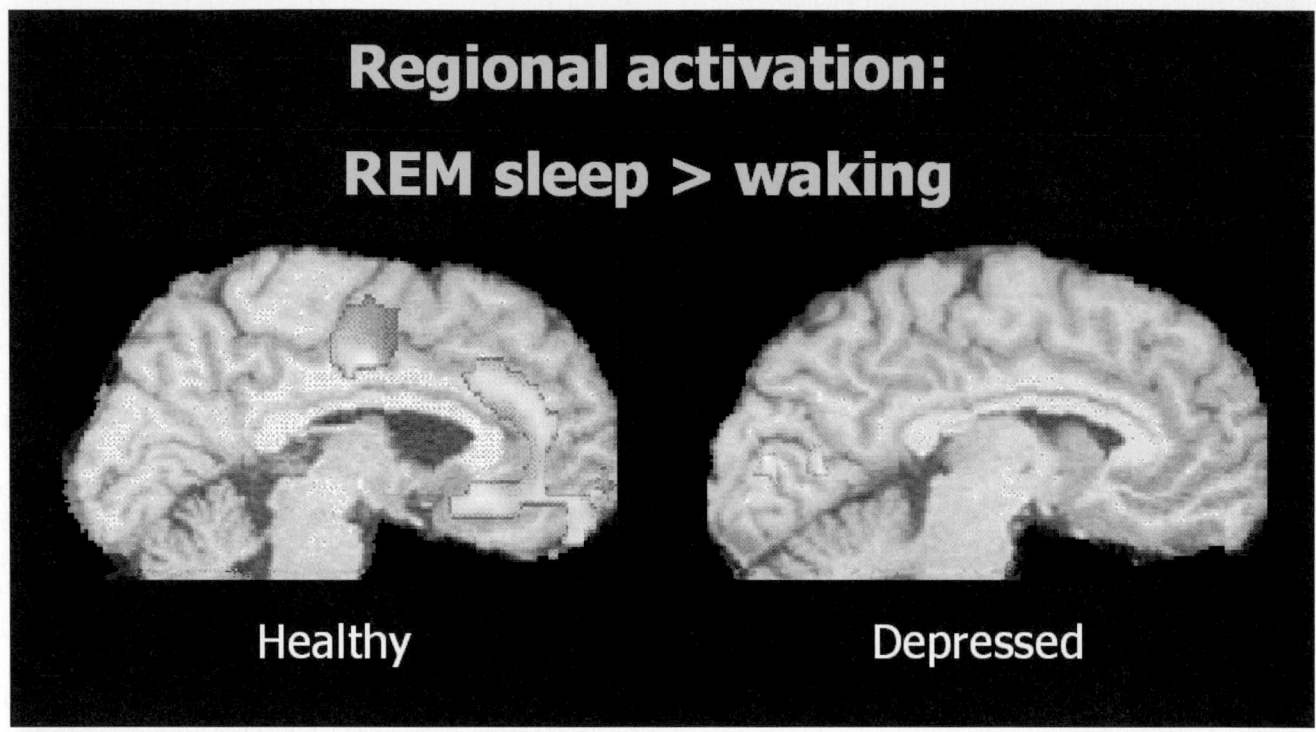

FIGURE 21–2. Regional activation during rapid eye movement (REM) sleep and wakefulness in healthy and depressed subjects.

Source. Nofzinger et al. 1999.

(1988) demonstrated, in one of the first longitudinal studies of sleep in depression, that REM latency is shorter during the earlier phases of relapse in recurrent major depression. This finding was replicated in a study of elderly patients with depression (Dew et al. 1996). Short REM latency is more prevalent among inpatients with depression than among outpatients with depression, suggesting a relationship with the severity of the index episode (Spiker et al. 1978). Disturbed sleep, as measured by REM latency, REM density, and sleep efficiency, predicts a poorer response to cognitive-behavioral therapy (Thase et al. 1996, 1998).

Recent studies of functional imaging in depressed subjects have helped guide efforts to describe the functional neuroanatomy of depression. Positron emission tomography (PET) imaging has been used to examine specific brain regions during REM and non-REM sleep. Nofzinger et al. (1999) found that depressed patients are distinguished from control subjects by the lack of activation of anterior paralimbic structures during REM sleep compared with waking (Figure 21–2). Ho et al. (1996) found that whole-brain metabolic rates were increased in depressed versus control subjects during non-REM sleep, which suggests that depression is associated with brain hyperarousal. Depressed subjects who respond to sleep deprivation with improvement in mood have elevated

brain metabolism in the cingulate and medial frontal lobe as documented by PET imaging (Wu et al. 1999). Improvements in depression ratings following sleep deprivation were shown to be associated with decreases in glucose metabolism in the anterior cingulate and medial frontal cortex in a study that used serial PET images (G.S. Smith et al. 1999).

There have been several attempts to integrate the aforementioned findings into a model that explains the association of sleep physiology with both state and trait characteristics in depression. A subgroup of patients may have as a heritable characteristic an inherently weak slow-wave sleep process that allows REM to be expressed earlier (Kupfer and Ehlers 1989; Giles et al. 1998). Patients with short REM latency may have a lifelong vulnerability for major depression. For example, Lauer et al. (1995) showed that subjects with no lifetime psychiatric disorder and a family history of depression have reduced slow-wave sleep and increased REM density in the first sleep cycle. In other patients, state-dependent phenomena such as arousal or stress temporarily affect sleep architecture. In this group, a short REM sleep measure serves as a state marker that is related to the severity of the episode. For example, unmedicated subjects with depression who are successfully treated with cognitive or interpersonal psychotherapy show a reduction in REM density (Buysse et al. 1997; Thase et al. 1994). Similarly, depressed patients with central nervous system hyperarousal, as indicated by decreased sleep efficiency, and increased REM density are less likely to respond well to interpersonal or cognitive-behavioral therapy (Thase et al. 1996, 1997). Current research in sleep and depression is aimed at clarifying the influence of age, gender, and family history on sleep physiology.

Antidepressant medications vary in their effects on sleep continuity and architecture. Tricyclic antidepressants have different effects on sleep latency and stage I and stage II sleep, but all increase slow-wave sleep, suppress REM sleep, and prolong REM latency. Most tricyclics produce daytime sedation, which limits their tolerability; this is particularly true of amitriptyline and doxepin. The sedative effect may explain why tricyclics enhance sleep continuity (Benca 1994; Kupfer et al. 1991; Shipley et al. 1985). Monoamine oxidase inhibitors prolong sleep latency, decrease sleep continuity, greatly suppress REM sleep, and prolong REM latency (Benca 1994; Minot et al. 1993). Selective serotonin reuptake inhibitors decrease sleep continuity, increase REM latency, and usually decrease REM time (Hendrickse et al. 1994; Mahowald and Schenck 1992; Nicholson and Pascoe 1988; Saletu et al. 1991). Trazodone increases slow-wave sleep, increases REM latency, decreases REM time, and improves sleep continuity (Muratorio et al. 1974; Scharf and Sachais 1990). Nefazodone produces no change in slow-wave sleep and improves sleep continuity but, in contrast to most other antidepressants, modestly increases REM sleep (Armitage et al. 1994; Rickels et al. 1994; Sharpley et al. 1992; Ware et al. 1994). Bupropion decreases sleep continuity and slow-wave sleep and, like nefazodone, increases REM sleep (Nofzinger et al. 1995). No data are available about the effects of venlafaxine on polysomnographic measures of sleep.

Schizophrenia

Two years after the discovery of REM sleep, the first of many reports on REM sleep and schizophrenia was published (Dement 1955). The early studies were driven, in part, by the exciting prospect of finding a link between dream cognition and perception, and psychosis. In the latter half of the 1960s, approximately 50% of all studies of sleep and psychiatric disorders involved patients with schizophrenia (Nofzinger et al. 1993b). Although a specific link between REM sleep and psychosis was never found, most studies clearly show that patients with schizophrenia have disrupted sleep. Many studies are difficult to interpret because of the lack of suitable control subjects for confounding variables such as age, presence

of centrally active medication, proximity to drug withdrawal, clinical features (e.g., negative and positive symptoms), and state-dependent characteristics such as acute relapse. Nevertheless, patients with schizophrenia have been found to have prolonged sleep latencies, sleep fragmentation with multiple arousals, decreased slow-wave sleep, variability in REM latency, and decreased REM rebound after REM sleep deprivation (Benson and Zarcone 1993; Ganguli et al. 1987; Keshavan et al. 1990b; Martin et al. 2001; Zarcone et al. 1987).

Several investigators have attempted to find correlations between clinical features of schizophrenia and specific sleep variables. For example, the variability in REM latency in schizophrenia has been found to be linked to family history of affective disorder (Keshavan et al. 1990a), presence of negative symptoms (Maggini et al. 1987; Tandon et al. 1989), tardive dyskinesia (Thaker et al. 1989), neuroleptic withdrawal (Neylan et al. 1992; Nofzinger et al. 1993a; Tandon et al. 1992), and nonsuppression of cortisol by dexamethasone (Tandon et al. 1996). Increased REM sleep time and increased REM activity in subjects with schizophrenia are associated with suicidal behavior (Lewis et al. 1996). Diminished slow-wave sleep is one of the most replicated and stable findings in schizophrenia (Feinberg and Hiatt 1978; Keshavan et al. 1996, 1998; Maixner et al. 1998), although it has not been observed in all studies (Lauer et al. 1997). It has been found to be associated with poor performance on neuropsychological tests of attention (Orzack et al. 1977) and with negative symptoms (Ganguli et al. 1987; Keshavan et al. 1995b; Tandon et al. 1992; van Kammen et al. 1988). Three studies have shown an inverse relationship between slow-wave sleep and cerebral atrophy as measured by the ventricular brain ratio on computed tomography scans (Benson and Zarcone 1992; Benson et al. 1996; van Kammen et al. 1988). A recent study of 31-P magnetic resonance spectroscopy found an inverse relationship between slow-wave sleep and brain anabolic processes (Keshavan et al. 1995a). Slow-wave sleep has also been found to be correlated with the serotonin metabolite 5-hydroxyindoleacetic acid (Benson et al. 1991) and delta sleep–inducing peptide-like immunoreactivity (van Kammen et al. 1992) in the cerebrospinal fluid of volunteers with schizophrenia.

Anxiety Disorders

Sleep in patients with generalized anxiety disorder is similar to that in patients with primary insomnia in that there are prolonged sleep latencies and increased sleep fragmentation. Subjective sleep quality is significantly impaired in subjects with social phobia (Stein et al.

1993). Sleep in patients with anxiety disorders differs from that seen in patients with major depression: patients with anxiety disorders exhibit normal REM latencies and decreased REM percentage (Reynolds et al. 1983b). It has been suggested that patients with symptoms of both depression and anxiety may be segregated with respect to sleep variables on the basis of the presence or absence of a family history of depression (Sitaram et al. 1984). Furthermore, sleep deprivation does not result in symptomatic improvement in patients with anxiety disorders (Labbate et al. 1998; Roy-Byrne et al. 1986), in contrast to the case in depressive patients.

A study on sleep and panic disorder by Mellman and Uhde (1989) confirmed that panic attacks can arise during sleep. Six of 13 patients with panic disorder were observed to have panic symptoms during sleep when they were being studied electrographically. Of interest, all panic attacks occurred during non-REM sleep, particularly during transitions from stage II to delta sleep. This finding adds further data to support the theory that panic attacks can be physiologically provoked. The mild hypercapnia normally found in sleep may predispose patients to sleep panic, although this hypothesis needs further testing (Mellman and Uhde 1989). Patients with panic disorder who are experiencing sleep panic do have more irregularities in tidal volume and increased numbers of microapneas than do control subjects (Stein et al. 1995). Patients with sleep panic attacks have an earlier onset of illness and greater occurrence of comorbid mood and other anxiety disorders (Labbate et al. 1994).

Multiple studies have demonstrated that patients with PTSD have significant sleep continuity disturbance and increased REM phasic activity such as eye movements (Mellman et al. 1995a, 1995b; Ross et al. 1994; Woodward et al. 1996); these symptoms are directly correlated with PTSD symptom severity. Several studies suggest that nightmares may be uniquely related to exposure to traumatic stress. A survey of Holocaust survivors by Rosen et al. (1991) showed that the number of complaints of nightmares was higher in survivors with longer periods of imprisonment in the concentration camps. True et al. (1993) obtained self-report data about sleep in 4,042 monozygotic and dizygotic Vietnam era–veteran twins with varying degrees of combat exposure. Combat exposure was highly correlated with reports of dreams and nightmares but was only weakly associated with sleep-onset and sleep-maintenance insomnia. Neylan et al. (1998) conducted a secondary data analysis of the questionnaire items that address complaints about sleep from the National Vietnam Veterans Readjustment Study (Kulka et al. 1990), a major population-based study that sampled to represent the entire group of 3.1 million men and women who served in the Vietnam War. The results show that complaints of frequent nightmares are relatively rare and are found exclusively in subjects with PTSD (Neylan et al. 1998). These results support the hypothesis published by Ross et al. (1989), who stated that nightmares and disturbances of REM sleep are a hallmark of PTSD.

Dementia

Patients with dementia of the Alzheimer's type have more sleep fragmentation (Grace et al. 2000), less delta and REM sleep (Vitiello and Prinz 1988), and little to no spindle and K-complex activity (Reynolds et al. 1985a; Smirne et al. 1977) in comparison with age-matched control subjects. Vitiello et al. (1992) suggested that the poor sleep of these patients results from the loss of neurons from areas that participate in the regulation of sleep such as the nucleus basalis of Meynert (McKinney et al. 1982; Sterman and Clemente 1974) and the brain-stem reticular formation (Hirano and Zimmerman 1962). Patients with dementia have more sleep-related phenomena, such as sundowning and nocturnal wanderings, that provoke attempts to consolidate nocturnal sleep with hypnotics as well as prompt families to institutionalize their elderly relatives (J.R.A. Sanford 1975). Patients with Alzheimer's dementia spend as much as half of the 24-hour day in bed, often experiencing a polyphasic sleep–wake pattern (D. Jacobs et al. 1989; Witting et al. 1990). Perhaps aggravating this pattern is the fact that institutionalized elderly patients spend less than 2 minutes per day exposed to bright light (Ancoli-Israel and Kripke 1989).

Studies examining the relationship between sleep, aging, and dementia suggest an important relationship between normal sleep–wake function and cognition. The severity of dementia has been found to correlate with severity of sleep disturbances (Bliwise et al. 1995). Feinberg et al. (1967) suggested that the sleep EEG is an indicator of the functional integrity of the cerebral cortex. An important unanswered question is whether sleep loss in aging is related to cognitive impairment or whether the two emerge secondary to some underlying, independent biological process.

There is evidence that the prevalence of sleep apnea is higher in patients with probable Alzheimer's dementia than in age- and sex-matched control subjects. Further, the severity of dementia is correlated with the severity of apnea (Hoch et al. 1986; Reynolds et al. 1985b). One study has shown that demented patients with sleep apnea have a higher rate of mortality at 2-year follow-up (Hoch et al. 1989).

Sleep Disorder Due to a General Medical Condition

Sleep can be adversely affected by multiple medical disorders, particularly those that compromise cardiopulmonary function or cause chronic pain. Endocrine disorders such as diabetes and hyperthyroidism can cause significant sleep continuity disturbance. Hot flashes associated with normal menopause can occur in sleep and cause arousals. Patients may complain of insomnia, hypersomnia, parasomnia, or a combination of symptoms.

Sleep and Seizures

Non-REM sleep has a well-known activating effect on seizure activity. This is in contrast to REM sleep, during which epileptic discharges usually are suppressed. EEG synchronization may explain the higher prevalence of seizures and interictal discharges seen in non-REM sleep (Shouse 1994). Many patients with epilepsy have their seizures predominantly during sleep or on arousal from sleep (Janz 1962). The clinical course depends on the type and severity of the seizure disorder. Although complaints of insomnia are unusual, sleep can be sufficiently fragmented to cause daytime fatigue and hypersomnolence (Bazil et al. 2000).

Unusual nocturnal motor behavior, sleep-related incontinence, or nocturnal tongue biting warrants an evaluation for sleep seizures. Often seizure-related behavior is difficult to distinguish from parasomnias such as enuresis and somnambulism. Family history of either parasomnias or seizure disorder is useful collaborative evidence. Persons who exhibit somnambulism usually have more purposeful motor behavior and are easier to redirect. Finally, an all-night EEG may be needed to screen for epileptiform activity.

Sleep and Parkinson's Disease

Sleep disturbance is reported in approximately 50% of patients with Parkinson's disease (Shulman et al. 2001). Sleep in this disease is characterized by an increased number of awakenings, decreased delta and REM sleep, and a scarcity of sleep spindles. The resting tremor usually subsides with the onset of stage I sleep, but, depending on the severity of the disorder, it can persist into stage II or reemerge during sleep stage changes (April 1966). The pathophysiology of the sleep disturbance is unclear. Patients with Parkinson's disease have been shown to have a higher prevalence of sleep-disordered breathing (Hardie et al. 1986). Nigrostriatal degeneration may have a direct or indirect impact on the neural substrate regulating sleep. Dopaminomimetic drugs such as L-dopa have dose-dependent effects on sleep and promote daytime somnolence (D. Schäfer and Greulich 2000).

Substance-Induced Sleep Disorder

Substance-induced sleep disorder is related to both direct and indirect toxic effects on sleep. Both alcohol- and hypnotic-induced sleep disorders involve the development of tolerance to the sleep-inducing effects of the agent, as well as increased arousals during withdrawal periods. Many studies have shown that acute alcohol administration causes REM sleep suppression in the first half of the night followed by a rebound increase of REM sleep and arousals in the second half (Mendelson 1987). Acute alcohol use in high doses suppresses REM sleep for the entire night (Knowles et al. 1968). During acute withdrawal, there is marked sleep continuity disturbance and prominent REM sleep rebound (Johnson et al. 1970). Alcoholic individuals admitted to a treatment unit who have evidence of increased REM pressure have a higher rate of relapse at 3 months (Gillin et al. 1994). Abstinent alcoholic subjects have been shown to have decreased slow-wave sleep and increased sleep stage changes for many months after alcohol withdrawal (Adamson and Burdick 1973).

Stimulants cause sleep-onset insomnia during usage and rebound hypersomnia during withdrawal. Food allergy– and toxin-induced sleep disorders presumably involve indirect toxic effects on the physiological substrate regulating sleep. In all of these disorders, careful removal of the offending agent either eliminates the problem or exposes an additional sleep disorder.

Conclusions

Careful assessment and treatment of sleep disorders can dramatically improve the quality of psychiatric care. Disordered sleep has protean effects on mood, attention, memory, and general sense of vigor. Further, disturbance in sleep has clear prognostic value and must be addressed to optimize clinical care. The search for the core function of sleep remains an exciting area for scientific research, with clear implications for our understanding of basic brain homeostatic mechanisms.

References

Adamson J, Burdick JA: Sleep of dry alcoholics. Arch Gen Psychiatry 28:146–149, 1973

Aldrich MS: Cardinal manifestations of sleep disorders, in Principles and Practice of Sleep Medicine, 2nd Edition. Edited by Kryger MH, Roth T, Dement WC. Philadelphia, PA, WB Saunders, 1994, pp 413–425

Alkassar Z, Couvez A, Guieu JD: [Fratricide occurring during a nocturnal episode of somnambulism: a case report]. Encephale 26:27–32, 2000

American Psychiatric Association: Diagnostic and Statistical Manual of Mental Disorders, 4th Edition. Washington, DC, American Psychiatric Association, 1994

American Psychiatric Association: Diagnostic and Statistical Manual of Mental Disorders, 4th Edition, Text Revision. Washington, DC, American Psychiatric Association, 2000

American Sleep Disorders Association Diagnostic Classification Steering Committee: International Classification of Sleep Disorders: Diagnostic and Coding Manual. Rochester, MN, American Sleep Disorders Association, 1990

American Sleep Disorders Association Standards of Practice Committee: Practice parameters for the use of polysomnography in the evaluation of insomnia. Sleep 18:55–57, 1995

Ancoli-Israel S: Epidemiology of sleep disorders. Clin Geriatr Med 5:347–362, 1989

Ancoli-Israel S, Kripke DF: Now I lay me down to sleep: the problem of sleep fragmentation in elderly and demented residents of nursing homes. Bulletin of Clinical Neurosciences 54:127–132, 1989

Ancoli-Israel S, Kripke DF, Klauber MR, et al: Sleep disordered breathing in community dwelling elderly. Sleep 14:486–495, 1991

April RS: Observations on parkinsonian tremor in all-night sleep. Neurology (New York) 16:720–724, 1966

Armitage R, Rush AJ, Trivedi M, et al: The effects of nefazodone on sleep architecture in depression. Neuropsychopharmacology 10:123–127, 1994

Aserinsky E, Kleitman N: Regularly occurring periods of eye motility and concomitant phenomena during sleep. Science 118:273–274, 1953

Ball EM, Simon RD Jr, Tall AA, et al: Diagnosis and treatment of sleep apnea within the community: the Walla Walla Project. Arch Intern Med 157:419–424, 1997

Bamford CR: Carbamazepine in REM sleep behavior disorder. Sleep 16:33–34, 1993

Bazil CW, Castro LH, Walczak TS: Reduction of rapid eye movement sleep by diurnal and nocturnal seizures in temporal lobe epilepsy. Arch Neurol 57:363–368, 2000

Bedard MA, Montplaisir J, Malo J, et al: Persistent neuropsychological deficits and vigilance impairment in sleep apnea syndrome after treatment with continuous positive airway pressure (CPAP). J Clin Exp Neuropsychol 15:330–341, 1993

Benca RM: Mood disorders, in Principles and Practice of Sleep Medicine, 2nd Edition. Edited by Kryger MH, Roth T, Dement WC. Philadelphia, PA, WB Saunders, 1994, pp 899–913

Benca RM, Obermeyer WH, Thisted RA, et al: Sleep and psychiatric disorders: a meta-analysis. Arch Gen Psychiatry 49:651–668, 1992

Benson KL, Zarcone VP: Slow wave sleep and brain structural imaging in schizophrenia (abstract). Sleep Research 21:250, 1992

Benson KL, Zarcone VP Jr: Rapid eye movement sleep eye movements in schizophrenia and depression. Arch Gen Psychiatry 50:474–482, 1993

Benson KL, Faull KF, Zarcone VP: Evidence for the role of serotonin in the regulation of slow wave sleep in schizophrenia. Sleep 14:133–139, 1991

Benson KL, Sullivan EV, Lim KO, et al: Slow wave sleep and computed tomographic measures of brain morphology in schizophrenia. Psychiatry Res 60:125–134, 1996

Besset A, Chetrit M, Carlander B, et al: Use of modafinil in the treatment of narcolepsy: a long term follow-up study. Neurophysiol Clin 26:60–66, 1996

Billiard M: The Kleine-Levin syndrome, in Principles and Practice of Sleep Medicine. Edited by Kryger MH, Roth T, Dement WC. Philadelphia, PA, WB Saunders, 1989, pp 377–378

Bixler EO, Kales A, Soldatos CR, et al: Prevalence of sleep disorders in the Los Angeles metropolitan area. Am J Psychiatry 136:1257–1262, 1979

Bliwise DL, Hughes M, McMahon PM, et al: Observed sleep/wakefulness and severity of dementia in an Alzheimer's disease special care unit. J Gerontol A Biol Sci Med Sci 50:M303–M306, 1995

Bonnet MH, Arand DL: 24-hour metabolic rate in insomniacs and matched normal sleepers. Sleep 18:581–588, 1995

Bonora M, Shields G, Knuths S, et al: Selective depression by ethanol of upper airway respiratory motor activity in cats. American Review of Respiratory Disease 130:156–161, 1984

Bootzin RR: A stimulus control treatment for insomnia (abstract), in Proceedings of the Annual Meeting of the American Psychological Association. Washington, DC, American Psychological Association, 1972, pp 395–396

Bootzin RR, Perlis ML: Nonpharmacologic treatments of insomnia. J Clin Psychiatry 53(suppl):37–41, 1992

Bourgin P, Huitrón-Résendiz S, Spier AD, et al: Hypocretin-1 modulates rapid eye movement sleep through activation of locus coeruleus neurons. J Neurosci 20:7760–7765, 2000

Breslau N, Roth T, Rosenthal L, et al: Sleep disturbance and psychiatric disorders: a longitudinal epidemiological study of young adults. Biol Psychiatry 39:411–418, 1996

Broughton R, Billings R, Cartwright R, et al: Homicidal somnambulism: a case report. Sleep 17:253–264, 1994

Buysse DJ, Reynolds CF, Monk TH, et al: The Pittsburgh Sleep Quality Index: a new instrument for psychiatric practice and research. Psychiatry Res 28:193–213, 1989

Buysse DJ, Browman KE, Monk TH, et al: Napping and 24-hour sleep/wake patterns in healthy elderly and young adults. J Am Geriatr Soc 40:779–786, 1992

Buysse DJ, Frank E, Lowe KK, et al: Electroencephalographic sleep correlates of episode and vulnerability to recurrence in depression. Biol Psychiatry 41:406–418, 1997

Campbell SS, Dijk DJ, Boulos Z, et al: Light treatment for sleep disorders: consensus report, III: alerting and activating effects. J Biol Rhythms 10:129–132, 1995a

Campbell SS, Terman M, Lewy AJ, et al: Light treatment for sleep disorders: consensus report, V: age-related disturbances. J Biol Rhythms 10:151–154, 1995b

Carskadon MA, Harvey K, Dement WC: Sleep loss in young adolescents. Sleep 4:299–312, 1981

Carskadon MA, Dement WC, Mitler MM, et al: Guidelines for the Multiple Sleep Latency Test (MSLT): a standard measure of sleepiness. Sleep 9:519–524, 1986

Chang PP, Ford DE, Mead LA, et al: Insomnia in young men and subsequent depression: the Johns Hopkins Precursors Study. Am J Epidemiol 146:105–114, 1997

Chesson AL, Anderson WM, Littner M, et al: Practice parameters for the nonpharmacologic treatment of chronic insomnia: an American Academy of Sleep Medicine report. Standards of Practice Committee of the American Academy of Sleep Medicine. Sleep 22:1128–1133, 1999a

Chesson AL, Wise M, Davila D, et al: Practice parameters for the treatment of restless legs syndrome and periodic limb movement disorder: an American Academy of Sleep Medicine Report. Standards of Practice Committee of the American Academy of Sleep Medicine. Sleep 22:961–968, 1999b

Chesson A , Hartse K, Anderson WM, et al: Practice parameters for the evaluation of chronic insomnia. An American Academy of Sleep Medicine report. Standards of Practice Committee of the American Academy of Sleep Medicine. Sleep 23:237–241, 2000

Coleman RM, Pollack CP, Weitzman ED: Periodic movements in sleep (nocturnal myoclonus): relationship to sleep disorders. Ann Neurol 8:416–421, 1980

Coren S: The prevalence of self-reported sleep disturbances in young adults. Int J Neurosci 79:67–73, 1994

Critchley M: Periodic hypersomnia and megaphagia in adolescent males. Brain 59:494–515, 1962

Czeisler CA, Allan JS: Pathologies of the sleep–wake schedule, in Sleep Disorders: Diagnosis and Treatment, 2nd Edition. Edited by Williams RL, Karacan I, Moore CA. New York, Wiley, 1988, pp 109–129

Czeisler CA, Moore-Ede MC, Coleman RM: Rotating shift work schedules that disrupt sleep are improved by applying circadian principles. Science 217:460–463, 1982

Daan S, Lewy AJ: Scheduled exposure to daylight: a potential strategy to reduce "jet lag" following transmeridian flight. Psychopharmacol Bull 20:566–568, 1984

de Lecea L, Kilduff TS, Peyron C, et al: The hypocretins: hypothalamus-specific peptides with neuroexcitatory activity. Proc Natl Acad Sci U S A 95:322–327, 1998

Dement W[C]: Dream recall and eye movements during sleep in schizophrenics and normals. J Nerv Ment Dis 122:263–269, 1955

Dement WC, Carskadon MA, Richardson GS: Excessive daytime sleepiness in the sleep apnea syndrome, in Sleep Apnea Syndromes. Edited by Guilleminault C, Dement WC. New York, Alan R Liss, 1978, pp 23–46

Dew MA, Reynolds CF, Buysse DJ, et al: Electroencephalographic sleep profiles during depression: effects of episode duration and other clinical and psychosocial factors in older adults. Arch Gen Psychiatry 53:148–156, 1996

Dijk DJ, Boulos Z, Eastman CI, et al: Light treatment for sleep disorders: consensus report, II: basic properties of circadian physiology and sleep regulation. J Biol Rhythms 10:113–125, 1995

Feinberg I: Changes in sleep cycle patterns with age. J Psychiatr Res 10:283–306, 1974

Feinberg I: Schizophrenia: caused by a fault in programmed synaptic elimination during adolescence? J Psychiatr Res 17:319–334, 1982

Feinberg I, Hiatt JF: Sleep patterns in schizophrenia: a selective review, in Sleep Disorders: Diagnosis and Treatment. Edited by Williams RC, Karacan I. New York, Wiley, 1978, pp 205–231

Feinberg I, Koresko RL, Heller N: EEG sleep patterns as a function of normal and pathological aging in man. J Psychiatr Res 5:107–144, 1967

Finkelstein Y, Shapiro-Feinberg M, Stein G, et al: Uvulopalatopharyngoplasty vs laser-assisted uvulopalatoplasty: anatomical considerations. Arch Otolaryngol Head Neck Surg 123:265–276, 1997

Ford DE, Kamerow DB: Epidemiologic study of sleep disturbances and psychiatric disorders: an opportunity for prevention? JAMA 262:1479–1484, 1989

Gallin PF, Terman M, Reme CE, et al: Ophthalmologic examination of patients with seasonal affective disorder, before and after bright light therapy. Am J Ophthalmol 119:202–210, 1995

Gallup Organization: Sleep in America. Princeton, NJ, Gallup, 1995

Ganguli R, Reynolds CF, Kupfer DJ: Electroencephalographic sleep in young, never-medicated schizophrenics: a comparison with delusional and nondelusional depressives and with healthy controls. Arch Gen Psychiatry 44:36–44, 1987

Gaudreau H, Joncas S, Zadra A, et al: Dynamics of slow-wave activity during the NREM sleep of sleepwalkers and control subjects. Sleep 23:755–760, 2000

Giles DE, Roffwarg HP, Schlesser MA, et al: Which endogenous depressive symptoms relate to REM latency reduction? Biol Psychiatry 21:473–482, 1986

Giles DE, Jarrett RB, Roffwarg HP, et al: Reduced rapid eye movement latency: a predictor of recurrence in depression. Neuropsychopharmacology 1:33–39, 1987a

Giles DE, Roffwarg HP, Rush AJ: REM latency concordance in depressed family members. Biol Psychiatry 22:910–914, 1987b

Giles DE, Biggs MM, Rush AJ, et al: Risk factors in families of unipolar depression, I: psychiatric illness and reduced REM latency. J Affect Disord 14:51–59, 1988

Giles DE, Kupfer DJ, Rush AJ, et al: Controlled comparison of electrophysiological sleep in families of probands with unipolar depression. Am J Psychiatry 155:192–199, 1998

Gillin JC, Ancoli-Israel S: The impact of age on sleep and sleep disorders, in Clinical Geriatric Psychopharmacology, 2nd Edition. Edited by Salzman C. Baltimore, MD, Williams & Wilkins, 1992, pp 213–234

Gillin JC, Smith TL, Irwin M, et al: Increased pressure of REM sleep at admission predicts relapse in non-depressed patients with primary alcoholism at 3 month follow-up. Arch Gen Psychiatry 51:189–197, 1994

Girault C, Muir JF, Mihaltan F, et al: Effects of repeated administration of zolpidem on sleep, diurnal and nocturnal respiratory function, vigilance, and physical performance in patients with COPD. Chest 110:1203–1211, 1996

Grace JB, Walker MP, McKeith IG: A comparison of sleep profiles in patients with dementia with Lewy bodies and Alzheimer's disease. Int J Geriatr Psychiatry 15:1028–1033, 2000

Guilleminault C: Sleep and breathing, in Sleep and Waking Disorders: Indications and Techniques. Edited by Guilleminault C. Menlo Park, CA, Addison-Wesley, 1982, pp 155–182

Guilleminault C, Carskadon M: Relationship between sleep disorders and daytime complaints, in Sleep 1976. Edited by Koeller WP, Oevin PW. Basel, Switzerland, S Karger, 1977, pp 95–100

Guilleminault C, Stoohs R, Quera-Salva MA: Sleep-related obstructive and nonobstructive apneas and neurologic disorders. Neurology 42(suppl 6):53–60, 1992

Hardie RJ, Efthimiou J, Stern GM: Respiration and sleep in Parkinson's disease. J Neurol Neurosurg Psychiatry 49:1326, 1986

Hartmann E: The Nightmare: The Psychology and Biology of Terrifying Dreams. New York, Basic Books, 1984

Hauri P: Primary insomnia, in Treatment of Psychiatric Disorders, Vol 3. Washington, DC, American Psychiatric Association, 1989, pp 2424–2433

Hauri PJ, Esther MS: Insomnia. Mayo Clin Proc 65:869–882, 1990

Hauri P, Fisher J: Persistent psychophysiologic (learned) insomnia. Sleep 9:38–53, 1986

Hauri P, Olmstead P: Childhood-onset insomnia. Sleep 3:59–65, 1980

Helmus T, Rosenthal L, Bishop C, et al: The alerting effects of short and long naps in narcoleptic, sleep deprived, and alert individuals. Sleep 20:251–257, 1997

Hendrickse WA, Roffwarg HP, Grannemann BD, et al: The effects of fluoxetine on the polysomnogram of depressed outpatients: a pilot study. Neuropsychopharmacology 10:85–91, 1994

Hicks RA, Moore JD, Hayes C, et al: REM sleep deprivation increases aggressiveness in male rats. Physiol Behav 22:1097–1100, 1979

Hipolide DC, Tufik S: Paradoxical sleep deprivation in female rats alters drug-induced behaviors. Physiol Behav 57:1139–1143, 1995

Hirano A, Zimmerman H: Alzheimer's neurofibrillary changes: a topographic study. Arch Neurol 7:227, 1962

Ho AP, Gillin JC, Buchsbaum MS, et al: Brain glucose metabolism during non-rapid eye movement sleep in major depression: a positron emission tomography study. Arch Gen Psychiatry 53:645–652, 1996

Hoch CC, Reynolds CF, Kupfer DJ, et al: Sleep-disordered breathing in normal and pathologic aging. J Clin Psychiatry 47:499–503, 1986

Hoch CC, Reynolds CF, Houck PR, et al: Predicting mortality in mixed depression and dementia using EEG sleep variables. J Neuropsychiatry Clin Neurosci 1:366–371, 1989

Höchli D, Riemann D, Zulley J, et al: Initial REM sleep suppression by clomipramine: a prognostic tool for treatment response in patients with a major depressive disorder. Biol Psychiatry 21:1217–1220, 1986

Hoddes E, Zarcone VP, Smythe H, et al: Quantification of sleepiness: a new approach. Psychophysiology 10:431–436, 1973

Hublin C, Kaprio J, Partinen M, et al: Prevalence and genetics of sleepwalking: a population-based twin study. Neurology 48:177–181, 1997

Hui DS, Chan JK, Ho AS, et al: Prevalence of snoring and sleep-disordered breathing in a student population. Chest 116:1530–1536, 1999

Hungs M, Mignot E: Hypocretin/orexin, sleep and narcolepsy. Bioessays 23:397–408, 2001

Huttenlocher PR: Synaptic density in human frontal cortex: developmental changes and effects of aging. Brain Res 163:195–205, 1979

Jacobs D, Ancoli-Israel S, Parker L, et al: 24-hour sleep/wake patterns in a nursing home population. Psychol Aging 4:352–356, 1989

Jacobs GD, Benson H, Friedman R: Perceived benefits in a behavioral-medicine insomnia program: a clinical report. Am J Med 100:212–216, 1996

Janson C, Gislason T, Bengtsson H, et al: Long-term follow-up of patients with obstructive sleep apnea treated with uvulopalatopharyngoplasty. Arch Otolaryngol Head Neck Surg 123:257–262, 1997

Janz D: The grand mal epilepsies and the sleeping–waking cycle. Epilepsia 3:69–109, 1962

Jasper NH: The ten-twenty electrode system of the International Federation. Electroencephalogr Clin Neurophysiol 10:371–375, 1958

Johns MW: A new method for measuring daytime sleepiness: the Epworth sleepiness scale. Sleep 14:540–555, 1991

Johnson LC, Burdick JA, Smith J: Sleep during alcohol intake and withdrawal in the chronic alcoholic. Arch Gen Psychiatry 22:406–418, 1970

Kales JD, Kales A, Bixler EO, et al: Biopsychobehavioral correlates of insomnia, V: clinical characteristics and behavioral correlates. Am J Psychiatry 141:1371–1376, 1984

Karadeniz D, Ondze B, Besset A, et al: EEG arousals and awakenings in relation with periodic leg movements during sleep. J Sleep Res 9:273–277, 2000

Keshavan MS, Reynolds CF, Ganguli R, et al: EEG sleep in familial subgroups of schizophrenia. Sleep Research 19:330, 1990a

Keshavan MS, Reynolds CF, Kupfer KJ: Electroencephalographic sleep in schizophrenia: a critical review. Compr Psychiatry 31:34–47, 1990b

Keshavan MS, Pettegrew JW, Reynolds CF III, et al: Biological correlates of slow wave sleep deficits in functional psychoses: 31P-magnetic resonance spectroscopy. Psychiatry Res 57:91–100, 1995a

Keshavan MS, Miewald J, Haas G, et al: Slow-wave sleep and symptomatology in schizophrenia and related psychotic disorders. J Psychiatr Res 29:303–314, 1995b

Keshavan MS, Reynolds CF III, Miewald JM, et al: A longitudinal study of EEG sleep in schizophrenia. Psychiatry Res 59:203–211, 1996

Keshavan MS, Reynolds CF III, Miewald MJ, et al: Delta sleep deficits in schizophrenia: evidence from automated analyses of sleep data. Arch Gen Psychiatry 55:443–448, 1998

Kimura K, Tachibana N, Kohyama J, et al: A discrete pontine ischemic lesion could cause REM sleep behavior disorder. Neurology 55:894–895, 2000

Knowles JB, Laverty SG, Kuechler HA: The effects of alcohol on REM sleep. Quarterly Journal of Studies on Alcohol 29:342–349, 1968

Kribbs NB, Pack AI, Kline LR, et al: Effects of one night without nasal CPAP treatment on sleep and sleepiness in patients with obstructive sleep apnea. American Review of Respiratory Disease 147:1162–1168, 1993

Kryger MH, Steljes D, Pouliot Z, et al: Subjective versus objective evaluation of hypnotic efficacy: experience with zolpidem. Sleep 14:399–407, 1991

Kulka RA, Schlenger WE, Fairbank JA, et al: The National Vietnam Veterans Readjustment Study: Tables and Findings and Technical Appendices. New York, Brunner/Mazel, 1990

Kupfer DJ, Ehlers CL: Two roads to rapid eye movement latency. Arch Gen Psychiatry 46:945–948, 1989

Kupfer DJ, Foster FG: Interval between onset of sleep and rapid-eye-movement sleep as an indicator of depression. Lancet 2:684–686, 1972

Kupfer DJ, Reynolds CF: Sleep and affective disorders, in Handbook of Affective Disorders, 2nd Edition. Edited by Paykel ES. New York, Guilford, 1992, pp 311–323

Kupfer DJ, Foster FG, Reich L, et al: EEG sleep changes as predictors in depression. Am J Psychiatry 133:622–626, 1976

Kupfer DJ, Frank E, Grochocinski VJ, et al: Electroencephalographic sleep profiles in recurrent depression: a longitudinal investigation. Arch Gen Psychiatry 45:678–681, 1988

Kupfer DJ, Perel JM, Pollock BG, et al: Fluvoxamine versus desipramine: comparative polysomnographic effects. Biol Psychiatry 29:23–40, 1991

Labbate LA, Pollack MH, Otto MW, et al: Sleep panic attacks: an association with childhood anxiety and adult psychopathology. Biol Psychiatry 36:57–60, 1994

Labbate LA, Johnson MR, Lydiard RB, et al: Sleep deprivation in social phobia and generalized anxiety disorder. Biol Psychiatry 43:840–842, 1998

Lam RW, Zis AP, Grewal A, et al: Effects of rapid tryptophan depletion in patients with seasonal affective disorder in remission after light therapy. Arch Gen Psychiatry 53:41–44, 1996

Langer SZ, Arbilla S, Scatton B, et al: Receptors involved in the mechanism of action of zolpidem, in Imidazopyridines in Sleep Disorders: A Novel Experimental and Therapeutic Approach. Edited by Sauvanet JP, Langer SZ, Morselli PL. New York, Raven, 1987, pp 55–72

Lauer CJ, Schreiber W, Holsboer F, et al: In quest of identifying vulnerability markers for psychiatric disorders by all-night polysomnography. Arch Gen Psychiatry 52:145–153, 1995

Lauer CJ, Schreiber W, Pollmacher T, et al: Sleep in schizophrenia: a polysomnographic study on drug-naive patients. Neuropsychopharmacology 16:51–60, 1997

Leung AK, Robson WL: Nightmares. J Natl Med Assoc 85:233–235, 1993

Lewis CF, Tandon R, Shipley JE, et al: Biological predictors of suicidality in schizophrenia. Acta Psychiatr Scand 94:416–420, 1996

Lewy AJ, Sack RA, Miller S, et al: Antidepressant and circadian phase-shifting effects of light. Science 235:352–354, 1987

Lewy AJ, Sack RL, Blood ML, et al: Melatonin marks circadian phase position and resets the endogenous circadian pacemaker in humans. Ciba Found Symp 183:303–317, 1995

Lin L, Faraco J, Li R, et al: The sleep disorder canine narcolepsy is caused by a mutation in the hypocretin (orexin) receptor 2 gene. Cell 98:365–376, 1999

Loube MD, Strauss AM: Survey of oral appliance practice among dentists treating obstructive sleep apnea patients. Chest 111:382–386, 1997

Lugaresi E, Coccagna G, Mantovani M, et al: Some periodic phenomenon arising during drowsiness and sleep in man. Electroencephalogr Clin Neurophysiol 32:701–705, 1972

Luna TD, French J, Mitcha JL: A study of USAF air traffic controller shiftwork: sleep, fatigue, activity, and mood analyses. Aviat Space Environ Med 68:18–23, 1997

Macquet P, Peters J, Aerts J, et al: Functional neuroanatomy of human rapid-eye-movement sleep and dreaming. Nature 383:163–166, 1996

Maggini C, Guazzeli M, Ciapparelli A: All-night sleep abnormalities in schizophrenia, in Schizophrenia: A Psychobiological View. Edited by Casacchia M, Rossi A. Dordrecht, The Netherlands, Kluwer Academic Publishers, 1987, pp 125–136

Mahowald MW, Schenck CH: Dissociated states of wakefulness and sleep. Neurology 42(suppl 6):44–52, 1992

Mahowald MW, Schenck CH: REM sleep behavior disorder, in Principles and Practice of Sleep Medicine, 2nd Edition. Edited by Kryger MH, Roth T, Dement WC. Philadelphia, PA, WB Saunders, 1994, pp 574–588

Maixner S, Tandon R, Eiser A, et al: Effects of antipsychotic treatment on polysomnographic measures in schizophrenia: a replication and extension. Am J Psychiatry 155:1600–1602, 1998

Martin J, Jeste DV, Caliguiri MP, et al: Actigraphic estimates of circadian rhythms and sleep/wake in older schizophrenia patients. Schizophr Res 47:77–86, 2001

Mathur R, Douglas NJ: Family studies in patients with sleep apnea-hypopnea syndrome. Ann Intern Med 122:174–178, 1995

McClusky HY, Milby JB, Switzer PK, et al: Efficacy of behavioral versus triazolam treatment in persistent sleep-onset insomnia. Am J Psychiatry 148:121–126, 1991

McKinney M, Hedreen C, Coyle JT: Cortical cholinergic innervation: implications for the pathophysiology and treatment of Alzheimer's disease, in Alzheimer's Disease: A Report of Progress in Research. Edited by Corkin S, Davis K, Crowden J, et al. New York, Raven, 1982, pp 259–265

Mellinger GD, Balter MB, Uhlenhuth EH: Insomnia and its treatment: prevalence and correlates. Arch Gen Psychiatry 42:225–232, 1985

Mellman TA, Uhde TW: Electroencephalographic sleep in panic disorder: a focus on sleep-related panic attacks. Arch Gen Psychiatry 46:178–184, 1989

Mellman TA, David D, Kulick-Bell R, et al: Sleep disturbance and its relationship to psychiatric morbidity after Hurricane Andrew. Am J Psychiatry 152:1659–1663, 1995a

Mellman TA, Kulick-Bell R, Ashlock LE, et al: Sleep events among veterans with combat-related posttraumatic stress disorder. Am J Psychiatry 152:110–115, 1995b

Mellman TA, Nolan B, Hebding J, et al: A polysomnographic comparison of veterans with combat-related PTSD, depressed men, and non-ill controls. Sleep 20:46–51, 1997

Mendelson WB: Human Sleep: Research and Clinical Care. New York, Plenum, 1987

Mendelson WB: Are periodic leg movements associated with clinical sleep disturbance? Sleep 19:219–223, 1996

Menzin J, Lang KM, Levy P, et al: A general model of the effects of sleep medications on the risk and cost of motor vehicle accidents and its application to France. Pharmacoeconomics 19:69–78, 2001

Merlotti L, Roehrs T, Koshorek G, et al: The dose effects of zolpidem on the sleep of healthy normals. J Clin Psychopharmacol 9:9–14, 1989

Minot R, Luthringer R, Macher JP: Effect of moclobemide on the psychophysiology of sleep/wake cycles: a neuroelectrophysiological study of depressed patients administered moclobemide. Int Clin Psychopharmacol 7:181–189, 1993

Mishima K, Okawa M, Hishikawa Y, et al: Morning bright light therapy for sleep and behavior disorders in elderly patients with dementia. Acta Psychiatr Scand 89:1–7, 1994

Mitler MM: The Multiple Sleep Latency Test as an evaluation for excessive somnolence, in Disorders of Sleeping and Waking: Indications and Techniques. Edited by Guilleminault C. Menlo Park, CA, Addison-Wesley, 1982, pp 145–153

Mitler MM, Gujavarty KS, Browman CP: Maintenance of wakefulness test: a polysomnographic technique for evaluating treatment efficacy in patients with excessive somnolence. Electroencephalogr Clin Neurophysiol 53:658–661, 1982

Mitler MM, Carskadon MA, Czeisler CA, et al: Catastrophes, sleep, and public policy: consensus report. Sleep 11:100–109, 1988

Moldofsky H, Gilbert R, Lue FA, et al: Sleep-related violence. Sleep 18:731–739, 1995

Montplaisir J, Lapierre O, Warnes H, et al: The treatment of the restless legs syndrome with or without periodic leg movements in sleep. Sleep 15:391–395, 1992

Montplaisir J, Boucher S, Poirier G, et al: Clinical, polysomnographic, and genetic characteristics of restless legs syndrome: a study of 133 patients diagnosed with new standard criteria. Mov Disord 12:61–65, 1997

Moore RY, Eichler VB: Loss of a circadian adrenal corticosterone rhythm following suprachiasmatic lesions in the rat. Brain Res 42:210–216, 1972

Morin CM, Gaulier B, Barry T, et al: Patients' acceptance of psychological and pharmacological therapies for insomnia. Sleep 15:302–305, 1992

Morin CM, Culbert JP, Schwartz SM: Nonpharmacological interventions for insomnia: a meta-analysis of treatment efficacy. Am J Psychiatry 151:1172–1180, 1994

Morin CM, Colecchi C, Stone J, et al: Behavioral and pharmacological therapies for late-life insomnia: a randomized controlled trial. JAMA 281:991–999, 1999

Muratorio A, Maggini C, Coccagna G, et al: Polygraphic study of the all-night sleep pattern in neurotic and depressed patients treated with trazodone. Mod Probl Pharmacopsychiatry 9:182–189, 1974

Nakazawa Y, Sakamoto T, Yasutake R, et al: Treatment of sleep apnea with prosthetic mandibular advancement (PMA). Sleep 15:499–504, 1992

National Commission on Sleep Disorders Research: Wake Up, America: A National Sleep Alert. Submitted to the United States Congress, January 1993

National Sleep Foundation: 2001 Sleep in America Poll. Washington, DC, National Sleep Foundation, 2001

Nelson S, Hans M: Contribution of craniofacial risk factors in increasing apneic activity among obese and nonobese habitual snorers. Chest 111:154–162, 1997

Neumeister A, Praschak-Rieder N, Besselmann B, et al: Effects of tryptophan depletion on drug-free patients with seasonal affective disorder during a stable response to bright light therapy. Arch Gen Psychiatry 54:133–138, 1997

Neylan TC, van Kammen DP, Kelley ME, et al: Sleep in schizophrenic patients on and off haloperidol therapy: clinically stable vs relapsed patients. Arch Gen Psychiatry 49:643–649, 1992

Neylan TC, Marmar CR, Metzler TJ, et al: Sleep disturbances in the Vietnam generation: an analysis of sleep measures from the National Vietnam Veteran Readjustment Study. Am J Psychiatry 155:929–933, 1998

Nicholson AN, Pascoe PA: Studies on the modulation of the sleep-wakefulness continuum in man by fluoxetine, a 5-HT uptake inhibitor. Neuropharmacology 27:597–602, 1988

Nicholson AN, Stone BM: Impaired performance and the tendency to sleep. Eur J Clin Pharmacol 30:27–32, 1986

Nishino S, Mignot E: Pharmacological aspects of human and canine narcolepsy. Progress in Neurobiology 52:27–78, 1997

Nishino S, Ripley B, Overeem S, et al: Hypocretin (orexin) deficiency in human narcolepsy. Lancet 355:39–40, 2000

Nofzinger EA, Reynolds CF III: REM sleep behavior disorder. JAMA 271:820, 1994

Nofzinger EA, van Kammen DP, Gilbertson MW, et al: Electroencephalographic sleep in clinically stable schizophrenic patients: two-weeks versus six-weeks neuroleptic-free. Biol Psychiatry 33:829–835, 1993a

Nofzinger EA, Buysse DJ, Reynolds CF, et al: Sleep disorders related to another mental disorder (nonsubstance/primary): a DSM-IV literature review. J Clin Psychiatry 54:244–255, 1993b

Nofzinger EA, Reynolds CF III, Thase ME, et al: REM sleep enhancement by bupropion in depressed men. Am J Psychiatry 152:274–276, 1995

Nofzinger EA, Mintun MA, Wiseman M, et al: Forebrain activation in REM sleep: an FDG PET study. Brain Res 770:192–201, 1997

Nofzinger EA, Nichols TE, Meltzer CC, et al: Changes in forebrain function from waking to REM sleep in depression: preliminary analyses of [18F]FDG PET studies. Psychiatry Res 91:59–78, 1999

Olson EJ, Boeve BF, Silber MH: Rapid eye movement sleep behaviour disorder: demographic, clinical and laboratory findings in 93 cases. Brain 123(pt 2):331–339, 2000

O'Reilly MF: Functional analysis and treatment of escape-maintained aggression correlated with sleep deprivation. J Appl Behav Anal 28:225–226, 1995

Orzack MH, Hartmann EL, Kornetsky C: The relationship between attention and slow-wave sleep in chronic schizophrenia. Psychopharmacol Bull 13:59–61, 1977

Peder M, Elomaa E, Johansson G: Increased aggression after rapid eye movement sleep deprivation in Wistar rats is not influenced by reduction of dimensions of enclosure. Behav Neural Biol 45:287–291, 1986

Peyron C, Faraco J, Rogers W, et al: A mutation in a case of early onset narcolepsy and a generalized absence of hypocretin peptides in human narcoleptic brains. Nat Med 6:991–997, 2000

Powell NB, Guilleminault C, Riley RW: Surgical therapy for obstructive sleep apnea, in Principles and Practice of Sleep Medicine, 2nd Edition. Edited by Kryger MH, Roth T, Dement WC. Philadelphia, PA, WB Saunders, 1994, pp 706–771

Provini F, Plazzi G, Lugaresi E: From nocturnal paroxysmal dystonia to nocturnal frontal lobe epilepsy. Clinical Neurophysiology 111(suppl 2):S2–S8, 2000

Rechtschaffen A, Kales A: A Manual of Standardized Terminology, Techniques, and Scoring System for Sleep Stages of Human Subjects. Bethesda, MD, U.S. Department of Health, Education and Welfare, Public Health Service, 1968, pp 1–60

Rechtschaffen A, Wolpert EA, Dement WC, et al: Nocturnal sleep of narcoleptics. Electroencephalogr Clin Neurophysiol 15:599–609, 1963

Regestein QR, Monk TH: Is the poor sleep of shift workers a disorder? Am J Psychiatry 148:1487–1493, 1991

Regestein QR, Dambrosia J, Hallett M, et al: Daytime alertness in patients with primary insomnia. Am J Psychiatry 150:1529–1534, 1993

Reynolds CF III, Kupfer DJ: Sleep research in affective illness: state of the art circa 1987. Sleep 10:199–215, 1987

Reynolds CF III, Shaw DH, Newton TF, et al: EEG sleep in outpatients with generalized anxiety: a preliminary comparison with depressed outpatients. Psychiatry Res 8:81–89, 1983a

Reynolds CF III, Christiansen CL, Taska LS, et al: Sleep in narcolepsy and depression: does it all look alike? J Nerv Ment Dis 171:290–295, 1983b

Reynolds CF III, Kupfer DJ, Taska LS, et al: EEG sleep in elderly depressed, demented, and healthy subjects. Biol Psychiatry 20:431–442, 1985a

Reynolds CF III, Kupfer DJ, Taska LS, et al: Sleep apnea in Alzheimer's dementia: correlation with mental deterioration. J Clin Psychiatry 46:257–261, 1985b

Reynolds CF III, Hoch CC, Buysse DJ, et al: Electroencephalographic sleep in spousal bereavement and bereavement-related depression of late life. Biol Psychiatry 31:69–82, 1992

Reynolds CF III, Buysse DJ, Kupfer DJ: Disordered sleep: developmental and biopsychosocial perspectives on the diagnosis and treatment of persistent insomnia, in Psychopharmacology: The Fourth Generation of Progress. Edited by Bloom FE, Kupfer DJ. New York, Raven, 1995, pp 1617–1629

Richardson JW, Fredrickson PA, Siong-Chi L: Narcolepsy update. Mayo Clin Proc 65:991–998, 1990

Rickels K, Schweizer E, Clary C, et al: Nefazodone and imipramine in major depression: a placebo-controlled trial. Br J Psychiatry 164:802–805, 1994

Ringman JM, Simmons JH: Treatment of REM sleep behavior disorder with donepezil: a report of three cases. Neurology 55:870–871, 2000

Roberts RE, Shema SJ, Kaplan GA, et al: Sleep complaints and depression in an aging cohort: a prospective perspective. Am J Psychiatry 157:81–88, 2000

Roehrs T, Zorick F, Wittig R, et al: Predictors of objective level of daytime sleepiness in patients with sleep-related breathing disorders. Chest 95:1202–1206, 1989

Rosen J, Reynolds CF, Yeager AL, et al: Sleep disturbances in survivors of the Nazi Holocaust. Am J Psychiatry 148:62–66, 1991

Rosenthal NE, Joseph-Vanderpool JR, Levendosky AA, et al: Phase-shifting effects of bright morning light as treatment for delayed sleep phase syndrome. Sleep 13:354–361, 1990

Ross RJ, Ball WA, Sullivan KA, et al: Sleep disturbance as the hallmark of posttraumatic stress disorder. Am J Psychiatry 146:697–707, 1989

Ross RJ, Ball WA, Dinges DF, et al: Rapid eye movement sleep disturbance in posttraumatic stress disorder. Biol Psychiatry 35:195–202, 1994

Roth T, Roehrs T, Carskadon M, et al: Daytime sleepiness and alertness, in Principles and Practice of Sleep Medicine, 2nd Edition. Edited by Kryger MH, Roth T, Dement WC. Philadelphia, PA, WB Saunders, 1994, pp 40–49

Roy-Byrne PP, Uhde TW, Post RM: Effects of one night's sleep deprivation on mood and behavior in panic disorder: patients with panic disorder compared with depressed patients and normal controls. Arch Gen Psychiatry 43:895–899, 1986

Rusak B, Zucker I: Neural regulation of circadian rhythms. Physiol Rev 59:449–526, 1979

Sack RL, Brandes RW, Kendall AR, et al: Entrainment of free-running circadian rhythms by melatonin in blind people. N Engl J Med 343:1070–1077, 2000

Sakurai T, Amemiya A, Ishii M, et al: Orexins and orexin receptors: a family of hypothalamic neuropeptides and G protein-coupled receptors that regulate feeding behavior. Cell 92:573–585, 1998

Saletu B, Frey R, Krupka M, et al: Sleep laboratory studies on the single-dose effects of serotonin reuptake inhibitors paroxetine and fluoxetine on human sleep and awakening qualities. Sleep 14:439–447, 1991

Sanford JRA: Tolerance of debility in elderly dependants by supporters at home: its significance for hospital practice. BMJ 3:471–473, 1975

Sanford LD, Silvestri AJ, Ross RJ, et al: Influence of fear conditioning on elicited ponto-geniculo-occipital waves and rapid eye movement sleep. Archives Italiennes de Biologie 139:169–183, 2001

Satlin A, Volicer L, Ross V, et al: Bright light treatment of behavioral and sleep disturbances in patients with Alzheimer's disease. Am J Psychiatry 149:1028–1032, 1992

Schäfer D, Greulich W: Effects of parkinsonian medication on sleep. Journal of Neurology 247(suppl 4):IV/24–IV/7, 2000

Schafer H, Koehler U, Ploch T, et al: Sleep-related myocardial ischemia and sleep structure in patients with obstructive sleep apnea and coronary heart disease. Chest 111:387–393, 1997

Scharf MB, Sachais BA: Sleep laboratory evaluation of the effects and efficacy of trazodone in depressed insomniac patients. J Clin Psychiatry 51:13–17, 1990

Schenck CH, Mahowald MW: A polysomnographically documented case of adult somnambulism with long-distance automobile driving and frequent nocturnal violence: parasomnia with continuing danger as a noninsane automatism? Sleep 18:765–772, 1995

Schenck CH, Mahowald MW: Long-term, nightly benzodiazepine treatment of injurious parasomnias and other disorders of disrupted nocturnal sleep in 170 adults. Am J Med 100:333–337, 1996

Schenck C, Mahowald M, Won Kim S, et al: Prominent eye movements during non-REM sleep and REM sleep behavior disorder associated with fluoxetine treatment of depression and obsessive-compulsive disorder. Sleep 15:226–235, 1992

Sharpley AL, Walsh AES, Cowen PJ: Nefazodone—a novel antidepressant—may increase REM sleep. Biol Psychiatry 31:1070–1073, 1992

Shelton J, Nishino S, Vaught J, et al: Comparative effects of modafinil and amphetamine on daytime sleepiness and cataplexy of narcoleptic dogs. Sleep 18:817–826, 1995

Shipley JE, Kupfer DJ, Griffin SJ, et al: Comparison of effects of desipramine and amitriptyline on EEG sleep of depressed patients. Psychopharmacology 85:14–22, 1985

Shouse MN: Epileptic seizure manifestations during sleep, in Principles and Practice of Sleep Medicine, 2nd Edition. Edited by Kryger MH, Roth T, Dement WC. Philadelphia, PA, WB Saunders, 1994, pp 801–814

Shulman LM, Taback RL, Bean J, et al: Comorbidity of the nonmotor symptoms of Parkinson's disease. Mov Disord 16:507–510, 2001

Sitaram N, Gillin JC, Bunney WE Jr: Cholinergic and catecholaminergic receptor sensitivity in affective illness: strategy and theory, in Neurobiology of Mood Disorders. Edited by Post RM, Ballenger JC. Baltimore, MD, Williams & Wilkins, 1984, pp 629–651

Smirne S, Come G, Franceschi M, et al: Sleep in presenile dementia, in Communications in EEG. International Federation of Societies for Electroencephalography and Clinical Neurophysiology, 9th Congress. 1977, pp 521–522

Smith GS, Reynolds CF III, Pollock B, et al: Cerebral glucose metabolic response to combined total sleep deprivation and antidepressant treatment in geriatric depression. Am J Psychiatry 156:683–689, 1999

Smith M, Colligan M: Health and safety consequences of shift work in the food processing industry. Ergonomics 25:133–144, 1982

Smith RC: Relationship of periodic movements in sleep (nocturnal myoclonus) and the Babinski sign. Sleep 8:239–243, 1985

Smith-Coggins R, Rosekind MR, Hurd S, et al: Relationship of day versus night sleep to physician performance and mood. Ann Emerg Med 24:928–934, 1994

Spielman A, Saskin P, Thorpy M: Treatment of chronic insomnia by restriction of time in bed. Sleep 10:45–56, 1987

Spiker DG, Coble P, Cofsky J, et al: EEG sleep and severity of depression. Biol Psychiatry 13:485–488, 1978

Spitzer RL, Terman M, Williams JB, et al: Jet lag: clinical features, validation of a new syndrome-specific scale, and lack of response to melatonin in a randomized, double-blind trial. Am J Psychiatry 156:1392–1396, 1999

Stein MB, Kroft CD, Walker JR: Sleep impairment in patients with social phobia. Psychiatry Res 49:251–256, 1993

Stein MB, Millar TW, Larsen DK, et al: Irregular breathing during sleep in patients with panic disorder. Am J Psychiatry 152:1168–1173, 1995

Stepanski E, Zorick F, Roehrs T, et al: Daytime alertness in patients with chronic insomnia compared with asymptomatic control subjects. Sleep 11:54–60, 1988

Steriade M, Timofeev I, Grenier F: Natural waking and sleep states: a view from inside neocortical neurons. Journal of Neurophysiology 85:1969–1985, 2001

Sterman MB, Clemente CD: Forebrain mechanisms for the onset of sleep, in Basic Sleep Mechanisms. Edited by Petre-Quadens O, Schlag JD. New York, Academic Press, 1974, pp 83–97

Stoller MK: Economic effects of insomnia. Clin Ther 16:873–897, 1994

Stone J, Morin CM, Hart RP, et al: Neuropsychological functioning in older insomniacs with or without obstructive sleep apnea. Psychol Aging 9:231–236, 1994

Strollo PJ Jr, Rogers RM: Obstructive sleep apnea. N Engl J Med 334:99–104, 1996

Sullivan CE, Grunstein RR: Continuous positive airway pressure in sleep-disordered breathing, in Principles and Practice of Sleep Medicine, 2nd Edition. Edited by Kryger MH, Roth T, Dement WC. Philadelphia, PA, WB Saunders, 1994, pp 694–705

Tandon R, Shipley JE, Eiser AS, et al: Association between abnormal REM sleep and negative symptoms in schizophrenia. Psychiatry Res 27:359–361, 1989

Tandon R, Shipley JE, Taylor S, et al: Electroencephalographic sleep abnormalities in schizophrenia: relationship to positive/negative symptoms and prior neuroleptic treatment. Arch Gen Psychiatry 49:185–194, 1992

Tandon R, Lewis C, Taylor SF, et al: Relationship between DST nonsuppression and shortened REM latency in schizophrenia. Biol Psychiatry 40:660–663, 1996

Terman M: Light therapy, in Principles and Practice of Sleep Medicine, 2nd Edition. Edited by Kryger MH, Roth T, Dement WC. Philadelphia, PA, WB Saunders, 1994, pp 1012–1029

Terman M, Terman JS, Quitkin FM, et al: Response of the melatonin cycle to phototherapy for seasonal affective disorder. J Neural Transm 72:147–165, 1988

Thaker GK, Wagman AM, Kirkpatrick B, et al: Alterations in sleep polygraphy after neuroleptic withdrawal: a putative supersensitive dopaminergic mechanism. Biol Psychiatry 25:75–86, 1989

Thannickal TC, Moore RY, Nienhuis R, et al: Reduced number of hypocretin neurons in human narcolepsy. Neuron 27:469–474, 2000

Thase ME, Kupfer DJ, Spiker DG: Electroencephalographic sleep in secondary depression: a revisit. Biol Psychiatry 19:805–814, 1984

Thase ME, Reynolds CF III, Frank E, et al: Polysomnographic studies of unmedicated depressed men before and after cognitive behavioral therapy. Am J Psychiatry 151:1615–1622, 1994

Thase ME, Simons AD, Reynolds CF: Abnormal electroencephalographic sleep profiles in major depression: association with response to cognitive behavior therapy. Arch Gen Psychiatry 53:99–108, 1996

Thase ME, Buysse DJ, Frank E, et al: Which depressed patients will respond to interpersonal psychotherapy? The role of abnormal EEG sleep profiles. Am J Psychiatry 154:502–509, 1997

Thase ME, Fasiczka AL, Berman SR, et al: Electroencephalographic sleep profiles before and after cognitive behavior therapy of depression. Arch Gen Psychiatry 55:138–144, 1998

Toh KL, Jones CR, He Y, et al: An hPer2 phosphorylation site mutation in familial advanced sleep phase syndrome. Science 291:1040–1043, 2001

Trenkwalder C, Stiasny K, Pollmacher T, et al: L-dopa therapy of uremic and idiopathic restless legs syndrome: a double-blind, crossover trial. Sleep 18:681–688, 1995

Trenkwalder C, Seidel VC, Gasser T, et al: Clinical symptoms and possible anticipation in a large kindred of familial restless legs syndrome. Mov Disord 11:389–394, 1996

True WR, Rice J, Eisen SA, et al: A twin study of genetic and environmental contributions to liability for posttraumatic stress symptoms. Arch Gen Psychiatry 50:257–264, 1993

van Kammen DP, van Kammen WB, Peters J, et al: Decreased slow-wave sleep and enlarged lateral ventricles in schizophrenia. Neuropsychopharmacology 1:265–271, 1988

van Kammen DP, Widerlov E, Neylan TC, et al: Delta sleep–inducing peptide-like immunoreactivity (DSIP-LI) and delta sleep in schizophrenic volunteers. Sleep 15:519–525, 1992

Vitiello MV, Prinz PN: Aging and sleep disorders, in Sleep Disorders: Diagnosis and Treatment, 2nd Edition. Edited by Williams RL, Karacan I, Moore CA. New York, Wiley, 1988, pp 293–312

Vitiello MV, Bliwise DL, Prinz PN: Sleep in Alzheimer's disease and the sundown syndrome. Neurology 42(suppl 6):83–94, 1992

Wagner ML, Walters AS, Coleman RG, et al: Randomized, double-blind, placebo-controlled study of clonidine in restless legs syndrome. Sleep 19:52–58, 1996

Ware JC, Rose FV, McBrayer RH: The acute effects of nefazodone, trazodone and buspirone on sleep and sleep-related penile tumescence in normal subjects. Sleep 17:544–550, 1994

Weitzel KW, Wickman JM, Augustin SG, et al: Zaleplon: a pyrazolopyrimidine sedative-hypnotic agent for the treatment of insomnia. Clin Ther 22:1254–1267, 2000

Wesensten NJ, Balkin TJ, Davis HQ, et al: Reversal of triazolam- and zolpidem-induced memory impairment by flumazenil. Psychopharmacology 121:242–249, 1995

Winkelman JW, Chertow GM, Lazarus JM: Restless legs syndrome in end-stage renal disease. Am J Kidney Dis 28:372–378, 1996

Witting W, Kwa IH, Eikelenboom P, et al: Alterations in the circadian rest–activity rhythm in aging and Alzheimer's disease. Biol Psychiatry 27:563–572, 1990

Woodward SH, Friedman MJ, Bliwise DL: Sleep and depression in combat-related PTSD inpatients. Biol Psychiatry 39:182–192, 1996

Wright SW, Lawrence LM, Wrenn KD, et al: Randomized clinical trial of melatonin after night-shift work: efficacy and neuropsychologic effects. Ann Emerg Med 32(pt 1):334–340, 1998

Wu J, Buchsbaum MS, Gillin JC, et al: Prediction of antidepressant effects of sleep deprivation by metabolic rates in the ventral anterior cingulate and medial prefrontal cortex. Am J Psychiatry 156:1149–1158, 1999

Yamadera H, Ito T, Suzuki H, et al: Effects of bright light on cognitive and sleep–wake (circadian) rhythm disturbances in Alzheimer-type dementia. Psychiatry Clin Neurosci 54:352–353, 2000

Yamashiro Y, Kryger MH: Why should sleep apnea be diagnosed and treated? Clinical Pulmonary Medicine 1:250–259, 1994

Young T, Palta M, Dempsey J, et al: The occurrence of sleep-disordered breathing among middle-aged adults. N Engl J Med 328:1230–1235, 1993

Zarcone VP Jr, Benson KL, Berger PA: Abnormal rapid eye movement latencies in schizophrenia. Arch Gen Psychiatry 44:45–48, 1987

Eating Disorders

Anorexia Nervosa, Bulimia Nervosa, and Obesity

Katherine A. Halmi, M.D.

The eating disorders *anorexia nervosa* and *bulimia nervosa* and the condition of *obesity* have been known since earliest times in Western civilization. Well-documented case reports of anorexia nervosa are found in literature describing early Christian saints. Bell (1985) reported the severe starving behavior and bingeing episodes of Saint Catherine of Siena, described the kind of reed she used to induce vomiting, and listed the herbal cathartics that she used for purging. Although binge eating and purging behavior are certainly described in Roman civilization, the disorder bulimia nervosa as we define it today has not been so well documented.

The eating disorders are entities or syndromes and not specific diseases with a common cause, common course, and common pathology. They are best conceptualized as syndromes and are therefore classified on the basis of the clusters of symptoms they present.

Because an important interaction exists between psychology and physiology in the eating disorders, this chapter begins with a brief section on the physiology of eating. Following this, the characteristics of anorexia nervosa, bulimia nervosa, and obesity are reviewed, with emphasis on the distinctive clinical features, medical complications, epidemiology, course, prognosis, pathogenic development, treatment, and theories of etiology.

Physiology and Behavioral Pharmacology of Eating

A Systems Conceptualization

A major conceptual revision for understanding the physiology and behavior of eating has expanded the dual-center theory of hypothalamic facilitatory and inhibitory centers for eating. The sensitive hypothalamic eating centers are part of a broad complex of neuroregulator interactions that includes a peripheral satiety system (gastrointestinal and pancreatic hormones released by food passing through the gastrointestinal tract) and a broad neural network affecting feeding, within the brain. Eating behavior is now known to reflect an interaction between an organism's physiological state and environmental conditions. Salient physiological variables include the balance of various neuropeptides and neurotransmitters, metabolic state, metabolic rate, condition of the gastrointestinal tract, amount of storage tissue, and sensory receptors for taste and smell. Environmental conditions include features of the food such as taste, texture, novelty, accessibility, and nutritional composition, as well as other external conditions such as ambient temperature, presence of other people, and stress (Blundell and Hill 1986).

To understand eating behavior, it is also important to recognize the role of conditioned (learned) components in the initiation and termination of nutrient ingestion. Because of methodological complexities, this area has received little study. Booth (1985) provided the best discussion of conditioned appetites and satieties because he focused attention on the interaction between psychological and physiological phenomena.

It is important to remember that when an exogenous agent such as a drug or peptide is given to an animal or a human, it does not simply activate a specific set of receptors that induce specific responses; it intervenes in a complex transactional fabric as well (Blundell and Hill 1986).

Neurotransmitters

Biogenic Amines

The study of catecholaminergic pathways in the hypothalamus by Leibowitz (1980) led to the discovery of the role of α_2-adrenergic receptors in the paraventricular nucleus (PVN) and the β_2-adrenergic receptors in the perifornical hypothalamus (PFH) in feeding. Microinjection of α_2 agonists to the PVN produces hyperphagia and causes a preferential ingestion of carbohydrate. This adrenergic β_2-responsive circuit in the PFH inhibits feeding. Underweight anorexia nervosa patients and persons without eating disorders in times of dieting have reduced central and peripheral norepinephrine activity (Pirke 1996). This is confirmed by hypothermia, bradycardia, and hypotension.

Serotonin, an indoleamine, has been shown to facilitate satiety (Hoebel 1977) and may at least in part control the intake of carbohydrate (Wurtman and Wurtman 1979). Serotonin injected peripherally and centrally into the PVN suppresses deprivation-induced and norepinephrine-induced eating (Leibowitz 1980).

The serotonin type 2A (5-HT_{2A}) receptor is a G protein–coupled receptor that controls signal transduction by activating phospholipase C (Eison and Mullins 1996). Properties of the 5-HT_{2A} receptor such as ligand affinity receptor downregulation or signal transduction could be affected by any disturbance or alteration in a genetic coding variant for this receptor. Such an aberration may contribute to the disturbed and disordered eating behavior in anorexia nervosa and bulimia nervosa.

Some evidence indicates that serotonin neuronal activity is involved in behavioral inhibition (Soubrie 1986), obsessive-compulsive disorder (OCD) (Barr et al. 1992), anxiety and fear (Charney et al. 1990), and depression (Grahame-Smith 1992); serotonin neuronal activity also has well-established involvement with satiety for food intake. Anorexia nervosa has comorbid or coexisting disturbances of behavioral inhibition, obsessive-compulsive problems, excessive anxiety and fear, and depression. Bulimia nervosa is frequently characterized by behavioral disinhibition and depression.

Dopamine seems to play a more complicated role in eating behavior. Low doses of dopamine and dopamine agonist stimulate feeding, whereas higher doses inhibit feeding (Leibowitz 1980). Glucose administration suppresses firing in substantia nigra dopamine neurons. There is evidence of increased hypothalamic dopamine turnover during feeding. This finding suggests that central dopamine mechanisms mediate the rewarding effects of food as they mediate the rewarding effects of intracranial self-stimulation and the self-stimulation of psychoactive drugs. The dopamine antagonist pimozide suppresses sham feeding intake of sucrose. This may be due to the inhibition of the rewarding effect of glucose (Gibbs and Smith 1984). In free-feeding rats, however, pimozide causes an increase in meal size.

Peptides and Opioids

Corticotropin-releasing factor (CRF) acts within the PVN to inhibit feeding. Norepinephrine seems to inhibit the CRF inhibitory feeding effect. The pancreatic polypeptide neuropeptide Y increases both food and water intake when injected into the PVN. Another pancreatic polypeptide, peptide YY, is a more potent stimulator of feeding than neuropeptide Y (Morley and Levine 1985).

Opioid antagonism decreases feeding in many species but has no effect in reducing food intake in other species. Under some physiological conditions, such as starving or insulin-induced hypoglycemia, naloxone fails to inhibit feeding. Stress-induced eating is probably driven by activation of the opioid system. Dynorphin, an endogenous κ opioid receptor ligand, enhances feeding. Again, the major site of action for dynorphin appears to be the PVN (Morley and Levine 1985).

Vasopressin and oxytocin are neuropeptides distributed in the brain and function as long-acting neuromodulators with complex behavioral effects that are often reciprocal. Oxytocin antagonizes vasopressin's consolidation of learning acquired during aversive conditioning (Bohus et al. 1978). The dysregulation of secretion of these hormones in anorexia nervosa (Demitrek et al. 1992) may enhance the retention of cognitive distortions of the aversive consequences of eating.

Peripheral Satiety Network

Several peptides are released by ingested food from the gastrointestinal tract. Some of these inhibit feeding by activating ascending vagal fibers. Cholecystokinin (CCK) is the most extensively studied of these peptides. Its effects, mediated by vagal fibers, have been traced to the PVN of the hypothalamus, where lesions will abolish CCK's effect on feeding. Low doses of CCK infused into the PVN attenuate feeding, and central infusions of CCK antibodies enhance feeding. The potency of the satiety effect of CCK varies across animal species. Other peptides that appear to inhibit feeding via vagal fibers are glucagon, somatostatin, and thyrotropin-releasing hormone.

Bombesin is a gastric peptide that inhibits feeding, independent of vagal fibers. Gastrin-releasing peptide and calcitonin also inhibit feeding (Gibbs and Smith 1984). Some of these peptides, such as CCK, bombesin, and glucagon, when administered parenterally to humans, have produced satiety. However, their usefulness as therapeutic agents at present is limited because of their restricted absorption from the gut and because the high doses required induce adverse effects such as nausea.

Leptin is a protein hormone secreted by adipose tissue cells and believed to act as an afferent signal and regulator of body fat stores (Zhang et al. 1994). Leptin activates receptors and is coded by the *DB* gene in the hypothalamus and OB receptors in the choroid plexus (Tartaglia et al. 1995). Defects in the leptin coding sequence in rodents result in leptin deficiency and defects in leptin receptors, which are associated with obesity (Chen et al. 1996). Leptin is positively correlated with fat mass in humans in all weight ranges (Considine et al. 1996). Underweight patients with anorexia nervosa have significantly reduced plasma and cerebrospinal fluid (CSF) leptin concentrations compared with normal-weight control subjects (Mantzoros et al. 1997). These levels reach normal values with weight restoration. Because acute fasting-induced weight loss provokes a decline in leptin concentration that is disproportionate to the amount of fat loss (Boden et al. 1996), it has been hypothesized that leptin is a protecting regulator against starvation. Reduced leptin concentrations induce a variety of neuroendocrine responses, including decreased thyroid thermogenesis, increased secretion of stress steroid, and decreased procreation (Ahima et al. 1996).

Anorexia Nervosa

Definition

Anorexia nervosa is a disorder characterized by preoccupation with body weight and food, behavior directed toward losing weight, peculiar patterns of handling food, weight loss, intense fear of gaining weight, disturbance of body image, and amenorrhea. DSM-IV-TR (American Psychiatric Association 2000a) criteria for anorexia nervosa are included in Table 22–1.

Clinical Features

Individuals with anorexia nervosa typically express an intense fear of gaining weight, tend to be preoccupied with thoughts of food, and worry irrationally about fatness. Denial of their own clearly observable symptoms is characteristic of anorexic patients. They frequently look in mirrors to make sure they are thin, and they inces-

TABLE 22–1. DSM-IV-TR diagnostic criteria for anorexia nervosa

A. Refusal to maintain body weight at or above a minimally normal weight for age and height (e.g., weight loss leading to maintenance of body weight less than 85% of that expected; or failure to make expected weight gain during period of growth, leading to body weight less than 85% of that expected).

B. Intense fear of gaining weight or becoming fat, even though underweight.

C. Disturbance in the way in which one's body weight or shape is experienced, undue influence of body weight or shape on self-evaluation, or denial of the seriousness of the current low body weight.

D. In postmenarcheal females, amenorrhea, i.e., the absence of at least three consecutive menstrual cycles. (A woman is considered to have amenorrhea if her periods occur only following hormone, e.g., estrogen, administration.)

Specify type:

Restricting Type: during the current episode of anorexia nervosa, the person has not regularly engaged in binge-eating or purging behavior (i.e., self-induced vomiting or the misuse of laxatives, diuretics, or enemas)

Binge-Eating/Purging Type: during the current episode of anorexia nervosa, the person has regularly engaged in binge-eating or purging behavior (i.e., self-induced vomiting or the misuse of laxatives, diuretics, or enemas)

santly express concern about looking fat and feeling flabby. Collecting recipes and preparing elaborate meals for their families are other behaviors that reflect their preoccupation with food. Peculiar handling of food is frequent in individuals with anorexia. They will hide carbohydrate-rich foods and hoard large quantities of candies, carrying them in their pockets and purses. Often they will try to dispose of their food surreptitiously to avoid eating. Anorexic persons will spend a great deal of time cutting food into small pieces and rearranging the food on their plates.

Anorexic patients' fear that they are gaining weight exists even in the face of increasing cachexia, and they characteristically show disinterest in and even resistance to treatment. Persons with this disorder lose weight by drastically reducing their total food intake and disproportionately decreasing the intake of high-carbohydrate and fatty foods. Some individuals with anorexia will develop rigorous exercise programs, and others simply will be as active as possible at all times. Self-induced vomiting and laxative and diuretic abuse are other purging behaviors by which anorexic persons attempt to lose weight. Weight loss and a refusal to maintain body weight over a minimal normal weight for age and height are the most characteristic features of this disorder. Anorexic individuals have a disturbance in the way in which they experience their body weight and shape. They often fail to recognize that their degree of emaciation is dangerous. Their cognition is so distorted that they judge their self-worth predominantly by body shape and weight.

Obsessive-compulsive behavior often develops after the onset of anorexia nervosa. An obsession with cleanliness, an increase in housecleaning activities, and a more compulsive approach to studying are not uncommonly observed in these patients.

Amenorrhea can appear before noticeable weight loss has occurred. Poor sexual adjustment is frequently present in patients with anorexia. Many adolescent patients with anorexia have delayed psychosocial sexual development, and adults often have a markedly decreased interest in sex with the onset of anorexia nervosa.

Patients with anorexia nervosa can be divided into two groups: those who binge eat and purge and those who merely restrict food intake to lose weight. There is a relatively frequent association with impulsive behavior such as suicide attempts, self-mutilation, stealing, and substance abuse (including alcohol abuse) among bulimic anorexic individuals, who are also less likely to be regressed in their sexual activity and may in fact be promiscuous. Bulimic anorexic patients are more likely to have discrete personality disorder diagnoses (Halmi 1987).

Medical Complications

Most of the physiological and metabolic changes in anorexia nervosa are secondary to the starvation state or purging behavior and are reversed with nutritional rehabilitation. We often find abnormalities in hematopoiesis, such as leukopenia and relative lymphocytosis, in acutely emaciated anorexic patients. Individuals with anorexia nervosa who engage in self-induced vomiting or who abuse laxatives and diuretics are liable to develop hypokalemic alkalosis. These patients often have elevated serum bicarbonate levels, hypochloremia, and hypokalemia. Patients with electrolyte disturbances have physical symptoms of weakness and lethargy and, at times, have cardiac arrhythmias. The latter condition may threaten sudden cardiac arrest, a frequent cause of death in patients who purge. Other complications of bingeing and purging are discussed in the section on bulimia nervosa.

Elevation of serum enzymes reflects fatty degeneration of the liver and is observed both in the emaciated anorexic phase and during refeeding. Elevated serum cholesterol levels tend to occur more frequently in younger patients. Carotenemia is often observed in malnourished anorexic patients. All of these physiological changes reverse themselves with nutritional rehabilitation (Halmi and Falk 1981). Amenorrhea, which is a major diagnostic criterion for anorexia nervosa, is not related simply to weight loss and is discussed in the section "Etiology and Pathogenesis" later in this chapter.

Epidemiology, Course, and Prognosis

The incidence of anorexia nervosa has increased in the past 30 years both in the United States and in Western Europe. In Monroe County, New York, the average annual incidence rate of 0.35 per 100,000 population in the 1960s increased to 0.64 per 100,000 in the 1970s (Jones et al. 1980). In London, the prevalence of anorexia nervosa was one severe case in approximately 200 girls ages 12–18 years in the 1970s (Crisp et al. 1976). An incidence study in northeastern Scotland in the 1980s found four cases of anorexia nervosa per 100,000 population per annum (Szmukler 1985). A more recent incidence study conducted in northeastern Scotland (Eagles et al. 1995), reported that between 1965 and 1991, the incidence of anorexia nervosa increased nearly sixfold (from 3 per 100,000 to 17 per 100,000 cases). These studies probably underestimate the true incidence because not all cases come to the attention of health care providers. Hoek (1991) found the incidence of anorexia nervosa at the primary care level in Holland to be 6.3 per 100,000 population per year during the period 1985–1986 and 8.1 during the period 1987–1989. Rooney et al. (1995) surveyed patients recruited for study from the level of primary care in England. The prevalence of anorexia nervosa was 20.2 cases per 100,000 population (0.02% of the total population). The prevalence among female patients ages 15–29 years was 115.4 cases per 100,000 (0.1%). In Rochester, Minnesota, Lucas et al. (1991) recorded a point prevalence of anorexia nervosa of 0.2% for females and 0.02% for males on January 1, 1980. Five years later, their survey showed that the point prevalence of anorexia nervosa had increased to 0.48% among female adolescents ages 15–19 years. A more recent survey that followed up high school students to age 24 found the incidence of eating disorders to be 2.8% by age 18 and 1.3% for ages 19–23. The lifetime prevalence of anorexia nervosa was 0.6% (Lewinsohn et al. 2000). Only 4%–6% of the anorexic population is male (Halmi 1974).

In a community epidemiological survey in Canada, Woodside et al. (2001) found that men with eating disorders were very similar to women with the same diagnoses. The pattern of familial aggregation of eating disorders in males with anorexia nervosa was found to be highly similar to that observed in recent family studies of affected females (Strober et al. 2001).

The course of anorexia nervosa varies from a single episode with weight and psychological recovery to nutritional rehabilitation with relapses to an unremitting course resulting in death. Two of the most methodologically satisfying long-term follow-up studies have shown a mortality rate of 6.6% at 10 years after a well-defined treatment program (Halmi et al. 1991) and a mortality rate of 18% at 30-year follow-up (Theander 1985).

These studies, in addition to a follow-up study by Hsu and Crisp (1979), found that many patients with anorexia may show considerable improvement in their medical condition, but most still had the characteristic psychological set of the illness. Fewer than one-fourth of these patients could be considered to have made a good psychological adjustment when they were followed up to ages 20 through 50 years. In his 30-year follow-up study, Theander (1985) found that 75% of his patients could be classified as being in a psychologically stable state. This was not true at the time of earlier follow-up examinations. Generally speaking, poor outcome in the studies mentioned earlier was associated with longer duration of illness, older age at onset, previous admissions to psychiatric hospitals, poor childhood social adjustment, premorbid personality difficulties, and disturbed relationships between patients and other family members.

A prospective 5-year study of 95 patients with anorexia nervosa in Australia found that 3 had died, 56 patients had no eating disorder diagnosis, and the remainder had a continuation of their illness with psychosocial difficulties (Ben-Tovin et al. 2001). All of these outcome studies indicate that anorexia nervosa is a serious, chronic disorder.

Etiology and Pathogenesis

A specific etiology and pathogenesis leading to the development of anorexia nervosa are unknown. Anorexia nervosa begins after a period of severe food deprivation, which may be due to any of the following:

- Willful dieting for the purpose of being more attractive
- Willful dieting for the purpose of being more professionally competent (e.g., ballet dancers, gymnasts, jockeys)
- Food restriction secondary to severe stress
- Food restriction secondary to severe illness and/or surgery
- Involuntary starvation

Previous periods of severe food restriction are often reported, and a history of earlier dieting is not unusual. The question is, what is unique about the individual who goes on to develop anorexia nervosa?

The psychological theories concerning the causes of anorexia have centered mostly on phobic mechanisms and psychodynamic formulations. Crisp (1976) postulated that anorexia nervosa constitutes a phobic avoidance response to food resulting from the sexual and social tension generated by the physical changes associated with puberty.

Psychodynamic theories have focused on fantasies of oral impregnation and dependent seductive relationships with warm, passive fathers and guilt over aggression toward ambivalently regarded mothers.

A cognitive and perceptual developmental defect was postulated by Bruch (1962) as the cause of anorexia nervosa. She described the disturbances of body image (denial of emaciation), disturbances in perception (lack of recognition or denial of fatigue, weakness, hunger), and a sense of ineffectiveness as being caused by untoward learning experiences.

Russell (1969) suggested that the amenorrhea may be caused by a primary disturbance of hypothalamic function and that the full expression of this disturbance is induced by psychological stress. He thought that the malnutrition of anorexia nervosa perpetuates the amenorrhea but is not primarily responsible for the endocrine disorder. This hypothesis is supported by the fact that the return of normal menstrual cycles lags behind the return to a normal body weight; the resumption of menses in anorexia nervosa is associated with marked psychological improvement (Falk and Halmi 1982).

Further support for the theory of disturbed hypothalamic function in anorexia nervosa comes from neurotransmitter studies. The increased cortisol production present in anorexia nervosa has been traced to the hypothalamus. Two groups of investigators (Gold et al. 1986; Hotta et al. 1986) showed that patients with anorexia have increased CRF in their CSF, which probably means that increased CRF production from the hypothalamus is causing the cortisol changes observed in anorexia. Because central neurotransmitters such as dopamine, serotonin, and norepinephrine all influence appetite, satiety, and eating behavior, it is reasonable to study these neurotransmitters in patients with anorexia.

Although assessment of neurotransmitter function in the brain in humans has serious methodological problems, preliminary indirect studies indicate that a dysregulation of all three of these neurotransmitters probably occurs. Kaye et al. (1984b) showed a decreased serotonin turnover in bulimic anorexic patients compared with restricting anorexic patients. In addition, Kaye et al. (1984a) showed low CSF norepinephrine levels in long-term anorexic patients who have attained a weight within at least 15% of their normal weight range. Owen et al. (1983) showed that individuals with anorexia have a blunted growth hormone response to L-dopa, indicating a defect at the postsynaptic dopamine receptor sites. More recently, Brambilla et al. (2001) reported a blunted growth hormone response to the postsynaptic D_2 receptor stimulation with apomorphine in underweight anorexic patients. They suggested that the postsynaptic D_2 receptors are downregulated in anorexia nervosa because of a peripheral negative feedback linked to a hyperfunctioning somatotropic axis or to a hypothalamic presynaptic dopamine hypersecretion and/or reduced dopamine reuptake. In this study, growth hormone responses did not correlate with body mass index (BMI) but did correlate negatively with scores on the Eating Disorder Inventory Scale. Thus, dopamine alteration in anorexia nervosa may be linked to psychopathological parameters.

Neuropeptide Y, a powerful endogenous stimulant of eating behavior in the central nervous system, was found to be significantly elevated in the CSF of emaciated patients with anorexia (Kaye et al. 1990). The neuropeptide Y levels generally returned to a normal range with long-term weight restoration. A reduction of food intake may produce a homeostatic increase in neuropeptide Y secretion that should serve to stimulate feeding, but this mechanism seems to be ineffective in the patient with anorexia nervosa. The relation between neuropeptide Y and CRF and luteinizing hormone secretion in anorexia nervosa is an area that needs further investigation (see Table 22–2).

There is increasing evidence for genetic influences in the development of anorexia nervosa. Strober et al. (1985) found increased rates of anorexia nervosa, bulimia nervosa, and subclinical anorexia nervosa in first- and second-degree relatives of anorexic probands compared with the relatives of nonanorexic psychiatrically ill control probands. They proposed that the pattern of familial clustering of these disorders represents variable expressions of a common underlying psychopathology.

Another study providing evidence that both anorexia nervosa and bulimia nervosa are familial and that clustering of the disorder in families may arise partly from genetic transmission of risk was done by Lilenfeld et al. (1998). In a large epidemiological sample of twins obtained from the Virginia Twin Registry, a strong association between anorexia nervosa and bulimia nervosa was found; the co-twin of a twin affected with anorexia nervosa was 2.6 times more likely to have a lifetime diagnosis of bulimia nervosa compared with co-twins of unaffected twins. This evidence suggested some sharing of familial risk and liability factors between anorexia nervosa and bulimia nervosa (Kendler et al. 1991; Walters and Kendler 1995).

Family studies of anorexia nervosa have shown a tendency toward familial occurrence of this disorder and a high association with mood disorder. Theander (1970) calculated the morbidity risk for a sister of a patient with anorexia to be 6.6%, much higher than would be expected. In a study of 30 female twin pairs in London, 9 of 16 of the monozygotic and 1 of 14 of the dizygotic pairs were concordant for anorexia nervosa (Holland et al. 1984). In a later expansion of this study, Holland et al. (1988) concluded that their data indicated a genetic predisposition that could become manifest under adverse conditions, such as inappropriate dieting or emotional stress. The authors proposed that this genetic vulnerability might implicate a particular personality type or a general susceptibility to psychiatric instability (in particular, mood disorder) or might directly involve a hypothalamic dysfunction. A monozygotic twin carrying one or more vulnerability factors would have both the potential for developing anorexia nervosa under conditions of stress and some less specific genetic loading for this disorder. Family studies of anorexia nervosa have shown an increased frequency of mood disorder in the first-degree relatives of the probands with anorexia compared with the first-degree relatives of subjects without anorexia. In two controlled studies, the prevalence of eating disorder was not higher in the first-degree relatives of probands with mood disorder. This suggests that an independent predisposition to anorexia must be superimposed on a predisposition to mood disorder for anorexia nervosa to be manifest. More recent family and twin studies examining comorbidity between eating disorders and other psychiatric diagnoses were reviewed in detail by Lilenfeld et al. (1997). Studies of major affective illness in anorexia nervosa probands reported familial risk estimates in the range of 7%–25%, with relative estimates in the range of 2.1–3.4. Family studies show relatively low rates of substance abuse among relatives of restricting anorexia nervosa probands and independent familial transmission of OCD and anorexia nervosa (Lilenfeld et al. 1998). In another study, the morbidity risk for obsessive-compulsive spectrum disorders was significantly higher among 436 relatives of eating disorder probands than among 358 relatives of comparison subjects (9.69% vs. 0%). The eating disorder probands and comparison subjects did not differ in familial risk for eating disorders (Bellodi et al. 2001).

TABLE 22–2. Neurotransmitters and neuropeptides in anorexia nervosa

Hormone	Effect on eating behavior	Functional status in anorexia nervosa	Clinical manifestations
Norepinephrine	Inhibits the CRF-inhibiting feeding effect	↓	Decreased food intake
Serotonin	Facilitates satiety	↑	Feeling full after a minimal intake of food
Dopamine	Mediates rewarding effects of food	↓	?
Corticotropin-releasing factor (CRF)	Inhibits feeding; stimulates motor activity	↑	Decreased food intake; increased motor activity
Neuropeptide Y	Increases food intake	↑	Should stimulate feeding, but ineffective in anorexia nervosa
Cholecystokinin	Attenuates feeding	↑	Decreased meal size

Note. This table is, of course, oversimplified; actual phenomena are more complex.

In a study comparing the mothers of 57 anorexic patients with those of age- and sex-matched control subjects, Halmi et al. (1991) found a significantly greater prevalence of OCD in the mothers of the anorexic patients. Serotonin dysregulation may be a link between the OCD of the mothers and the anorexia nervosa in their daughters.

Treatment

A multifaceted treatment endeavor with medical management and behavioral, individual, cognitive, and family therapy is necessary to treat anorexia nervosa (Table 22–3). The first step in treatment is to obtain the anorexic patient's cooperation in a treatment program. Most patients with anorexia nervosa are disinterested and even resistant to treatment and are brought to the therapist's office unwillingly by relatives or friends. For these patients, it is important to emphasize the benefits of treatment and to reassure them that treatment can bring about a relief of insomnia and depressive symptoms, a decrease in the obsessive thoughts about food and body weight that interfere with the ability to concentrate on other matters, an increase in physical well-being and energy, and an improvement in peer relationships.

The immediate aim of treatment should be to restore the patient's nutritional state to normal. Mere emaciation or the state of being mildly underweight (15%–25%) can cause irritability, depression, preoccupation with food, and sleep disturbance. It is exceedingly difficult to achieve behavioral change with psychotherapy in a patient who is experiencing the psychological effects of emaciation. Outpatient therapy as an initial approach has the best chance for success in patients with anorexia who 1) have had the illness for less than 6 months, 2) are not

bingeing and vomiting, and 3) have parents who are likely to cooperate and effectively participate in family therapy.

The more severely ill patient with anorexia may present an extremely difficult medical-management challenge and should be hospitalized and undergo daily monitoring of weight, food and calorie intake, and urine output. In the patient who is vomiting, frequent assessment of serum electrolytes is necessary. Behavior therapy is most effective in the medical management and nutritional rehabilitation of the patient with anorexia, although there are times when other target behaviors can be changed with this approach. Behavior therapy can be used in both outpatient and inpatient settings.

The operant conditioning paradigm has been the most effective form of behavior therapy for the treatment of anorexia nervosa. This can be used both in the context of a structured ward setting and in an individualized treatment program set up after a behavioral analysis of the patient has been completed. Positive reinforcements are used and consist of increased physical activity, visiting privileges, and social activities contingent on weight gain. An individual behavioral analysis may show other positive reinforcements to be more clinically relevant in the particular cases. The timing of reinforcement is important in behavior therapy. An adolescent patient needs at least a daily reinforcement for weight increase, which should be approximately 0.5 lb or 0.1 kg per day. Making positive reinforcements contingent only on weight gain is helpful in reducing the staff–patient arguments and stressful interactions concerning how and what the patient is eating because weight is an objective measure. In addition to being used to induce weight gain, behavior therapy can be used to stop vomiting. A response-prevention technique is used when bingeing and purging patients are required to stay in an observed dayroom area for 2–3 hours after

TABLE 22–3. Treatment of anorexia nervosa

Type of treatment	Key elements	Measurements	Indications
Medical management	Weight restoration	Weight (outpatient—weekly; inpatient—daily)	Below normal weight for age and height by ≥10%
	Rehydration and correction of serum electrolytes	Serum electrolytes	History of vomiting, laxative abuse, severe restriction of food and fluids
Behavior therapy	Positive reinforcements for weight gain	Weight (outpatient—weekly; inpatient—daily)	Underweight
	Response prevention for binge eating and purging	Serum electrolytes and serum amylase	Weakness, puffy cheeks–parotid enlargement, scars on dorsum of hands, fainting spells
Cognitive therapy	Operationalizing beliefs, evaluating automatic thoughts, prospective hypothesis testing, examination of underlying assumptions	Assessment of distorted cognitions (e.g., all-or-none/black-or-white thinking), feeling fat, self-worth measured solely by body image, pervasive sense of ineffectiveness except in losing weight	Disturbance in way one's body weight or shape is experienced; denial of seriousness of low body weight; relentless pursuit of thinness for control of environment
Family therapy	Family counseling or therapy format based on needs of specific family	Analysis of family functioning, roles, and interactions	If patient is living with family, some type of family counseling or therapy is essential
Pharmacotherapy			
Chlorpromazine	Liquid form, start low doses, such as 10 mg tid, and gradually increase	Complete blood count, lying and standing blood pressure	Severely delusional, overactive, hospitalized patients
Cyproheptadine	Liquid form, start 4 mg bid and increase to 8 mg tid if necessary	Complete blood count with platelets	Severely overactive anorexic patient who does not binge and purge
Fluoxetine	Preferable to use after weight restoration because of tendency to induce arousal	Complete blood count, observation of total sleep and activity	Severely obsessive-compulsive behaviors related or unrelated to eating disorders, severe depression
Clomipramine	Necessary to start in very low doses because of hypotension side effects; preferable to use after weight restoration	Complete blood count, lying and standing blood pressure, electrocardiogram	Severely obsessive-compulsive behaviors
Tricyclic antidepressants	Necessary to start in very low doses because of hypotension side effects; preferable to use after weight restoration	Complete blood count, lying and standing blood pressure, electrocardiogram	Severe depression

every meal. Very few patients vomit in front of other people, and thus the emesis response is prevented and, eventually, stopped completely.

Cognitive therapy techniques for treating anorexia nervosa were developed by Garner and Bemis (1982). The assessment of cognition is a first step in cognitive therapy. Patients are asked to write down their thoughts on an assessment form so that cognitions can be examined for systematic distortions in the processing and interpretation of events. Cognitive techniques include operationalizing beliefs, decentering, using the "what if" technique, evaluating autonomic thoughts, testing prospective hypotheses, reinterpreting body image misperception, examining underlying assumptions, and modifying basic assumptions.

Cognitive-behavioral treatment for prevention of relapse of anorexia nervosa was further developed by Kleifield et al. (1996), who created an easy-to-use treatment manual. The cognitive-behavioral treatment is based on two core assumptions about the disorder. The first assumption is that anorexia nervosa has a significant positive functioning in the patient's life and develops as a way of coping with adverse experiences often associated with developmental transitions and distressing life events. The anorexic patient's deficient coping abilities produce anxiety and fear, and the patient is distracted from these anxieties by an overwhelming preoccupation with food and weight. The anorexic condition is also a reinforcing one, in that the patient experiences a surge of confidence and a sense of competence and control after being successful in dieting. The second assumption is that food restriction and ritualistic food avoidance behaviors become independent of the events or issues provoking them. The anorexic patient's extreme anxiety about gaining weight and becoming fat is alleviated by not eating. The relief of anxiety about gaining weight—the anxiety being alleviated through avoidance of food—is another strong reinforcement and thus a key factor in the persistence with which these patients pursue food restriction.

On the basis of the aforementioned assumptions, two separate pathways are taken in treatment. First, the dietary restriction is regarded as a food phobia, and change in eating behavior is a primary objective. Behavioral methods such as monitoring food intake and the details surrounding food intake, along with techniques such as increasing exposure, are used to increase the patient's food intake gradually. Cognitive-behavioral methods are used to reduce the anxiety associated with behavioral change. Cognitive techniques such as cognitive restructuring and problem solving help the patient deal with distorted and overvalued beliefs about food and thinness and cope with life's stresses.

A family analysis should be done on all patients with anorexia who are living with their families. On the basis of this analysis, a clinical judgment should be made regarding what type of family therapy or counseling is clinically advisable. In some cases, family therapy will not be possible. However, in those cases, issues of family relationships must be dealt with in individual therapy and, in some cases, in brief counseling sessions with immediate family members. A controlled family therapy study by Russell et al. (1987) showed that patients with anorexia younger than 18 benefited from family therapy and patients older than 18 did worse in family therapy compared with the control therapy. There are no controlled studies of the combination of individual and family therapy. In actual practice, many clinicians provide individual therapy and some sort of family counseling in managing anorexia nervosa.

Drugs can be useful adjuncts in the treatment of anorexia nervosa. The first drug used in treating anorexia was chlorpromazine. This medication is especially effective in patients with anorexia who are severely obsessive-compulsive. No controlled double-blind study has been done to prove definitely the efficacy of chlorpromazine in inducing weight gain in persons with anorexia. This is surprising, given that it was the first drug used and that it is the preferred drug for most severely ill anorexic patients. Another category of drugs frequently used in the treatment of anorexia nervosa is the antidepressants. A double-blind study in which 72 patients with anorexia were randomly assigned to amitriptyline, cyproheptadine (an antihistaminic drug), and placebo therapy showed that both cyproheptadine and amitriptyline had a marginal effect in decreasing the number of days necessary to achieve a normal weight. Cyproheptadine had an unexpected antidepressant effect, demonstrated by a significant decrease in scores on the Hamilton Rating Scale for Depression (Halmi et al. 1986). In the bulimic subgroups of patients with anorexia, cyproheptadine had a negative effect compared with both placebo and amitriptyline. This differential effect within the bulimic anorexic subgroups indicates a real medical distinction and appears to justify this subgrouping. Cyproheptadine has the advantage of not having the tricyclic antidepressant side effects of reducing blood pressure and increasing heart rate. This makes it especially attractive for use in emaciated individuals with anorexia.

Other drugs have been tested in patients with anorexia but have not had much of an effect. The results of small studies exploring the efficacy of fluoxetine and clomipramine suggest that both of these medications warrant further study (Crisp et al. 1987; Gwirtsman et al. 1990). Both fluoxetine and clomipramine are potent inhibitors of serotonin reuptake, and both have proven effective in OCD as well as depression. These medications may be effective in preventing relapse in anorexia nervosa. Because of certain side effects (anorexia and hyperactivity in fluoxetine therapy; hypotension and tachycardia in clomipramine therapy), special caution is necessary when these medications are given to underweight anorexic patients. At a 6- to 18-month follow-up of 31 patients who had been taking fluoxetine after inpatient weight restoration, 29 patients were found to have maintained their weight at or above 85% of average body weight (Kaye et al. 1991). In this study, restricting anorexic patients responded significantly better than did bulimic and purging-type anorexic patients. The authors judged the overall response to be good in 10 patients, partial in 17, and poor in 4 patients.

A multifaceted treatment approach is necessary for effective care of patients with anorexia nervosa. As medical rehabilitation proceeds, an associated improvement in psychological state occurs. Behavioral contingencies are useful for inducing weight gain and changing the medical condition of the patient. Cyproheptadine may be helpful in facilitating weight gain and decreasing depressive symptomatology in the restricting anorexic patient. If an anorexic patient has a predominance of depressive symptoms and is within 80% of a normal weight range, fluoxetine should be useful for treating the depression.

Severely obsessive-compulsive, anxious, and agitated anorexic patients are likely to require chlorpromazine or an atypical antipsychotic medication such as risperidone or olanzapine. All patients need cognitive individual psychotherapy. The more severely ill patients need hospitalization initially, followed by a well-planned continued outpatient treatment program (Garner and Garfinkel 1985). Prevention of relapse is a major part of the treatment of anorexia nervosa. Multicenter controlled treatment studies are being conducted to test the efficacy of a specific cognitive-behavioral therapy (CBT) and serotonin reuptake inhibitors in the prevention of relapse in this disorder.

Bulimia

Definition

Bulimia is a term that means "binge eating." This behavior has become a common practice among female students in universities and, more recently, in high schools. Not all persons who engage in binge eating require a psychiatric diagnosis. Bulimia can occur in anorexia nervosa; when this happens, the patient, under the DSM-IV-TR system, should have a diagnosis of *anorexia nervosa, binge-eating/purging type*. Bulimia also can occur in a normal-weight condition associated with psychological symptomatology. In that case, a diagnosis of *bulimia nervosa* applies (Table 22–4). Normal-weight bingeing and purging patients can fall into two categories: 1) normal-weight bulimic patients who have never had a history of anorexia nervosa and 2) those who have had a history of anorexia nervosa. Unfortunately, the DSM-IV-TR classification system does not separate these two subgroups of bulimic patients. The term *bulimia nervosa* implies a psychiatric impairment and therefore is a better label than simply *bulimia*.

Bulimia nervosa is a disorder in which the behavior of bulimia or binge eating is the predominant behavior. Binge eating is defined as an episodic, uncontrolled, rapid ingestion of large quantities of food over a short period. Abdominal pain or discomfort, self-induced vomiting,

TABLE 22–4. DSM-IV-TR diagnostic criteria for bulimia nervosa

A. Recurrent episodes of binge eating. An episode of binge eating is characterized by both of the following:
   (1) eating, in a discrete period of time (e.g., within any 2-hour period), an amount of food that is definitely larger than most people would eat during a similar period of time and under similar circumstances
   (2) a sense of lack of control over eating during the episode (e.g., a feeling that one cannot stop eating or control what or how much one is eating)
B. Recurrent inappropriate compensatory behavior in order to prevent weight gain, such as self-induced vomiting; misuse of laxatives, diuretics, enemas, or other medications; fasting; or excessive exercise.
C. The binge eating and inappropriate compensatory behaviors both occur, on average, at least twice a week for 3 months.
D. Self-evaluation is unduly influenced by body shape and weight.
E. The disturbance does not occur exclusively during episodes of anorexia nervosa.
Specify type:
   Purging Type: during the current episode of bulimia nervosa, the person has regularly engaged in self-induced vomiting or the misuse of laxatives, diuretics, or enemas
   Nonpurging Type: during the current episode of bulimia nervosa, the person has used other inappropriate compensatory behaviors, such as fasting or excessive exercise, but has not regularly engaged in self-induced vomiting or the misuse of laxatives, diuretics, or enemas

sleep, or social interruption terminates the bulimic episode. Feelings of guilt, depression, or self-disgust follow. Bulimic patients often use cathartics for weight control and have an eating pattern of alternate binges and fasts. Bulimic patients have a fear of not being able to stop eating voluntarily. The food consumed during a binge usually has a highly dense calorie content and a texture that facilitates rapid eating. Frequent weight fluctuations occur but without the severity of weight loss present in anorexia nervosa.

Bulimia is also encountered in DSM-IV-TR *binge-eating disorder* (BED), which did not exist in DSM-III-R (American Psychiatric Association 1987). This disorder is listed as an example under the category "eating disorder not otherwise specified" (Tables 22–5 and 22–6). Insufficient data are currently available to make BED a distinct Axis I diagnosis. Preliminary field studies show that most persons who meet criteria for BED are obese. In the next 5 years, epidemiological studies will determine whether BED is a distinct disorder or merely the nonpurging type of bulimia.

TABLE 22–5. DSM-IV-TR criteria for eating disorder not otherwise specified

The eating disorder not otherwise specified category is for disorders of eating that do not meet the criteria for any specific eating disorder. Examples include

1. For females, all of the criteria for anorexia nervosa are met except that the individual has regular menses.
2. All of the criteria for anorexia nervosa are met except that, despite significant weight loss, the individual's current weight is in the normal range.
3. All of the criteria for bulimia nervosa are met except that the binge eating and inappropriate compensatory mechanisms occur at a frequency of less than twice a week or for a duration of less than 3 months.
4. The regular use of inappropriate compensatory behavior by an individual of normal body weight after eating small amounts of food (e.g., self-induced vomiting after the consumption of two cookies).
5. Repeatedly chewing and spitting out, but not swallowing, large amounts of food.
6. Binge-eating disorder: recurrent episodes of binge eating in the absence of the regular use of inappropriate compensatory behaviors characteristic of bulimia nervosa.

Clinical Features

Bulimia nervosa usually begins after a period of dieting of a few weeks to a year or longer. The dieting may or may not have been successful in achieving weight loss. Most binge-eating episodes are followed by self-induced vomiting. Episodes are less frequently followed by use of laxatives. A minority of bulimic patients use diuretics for weight control. The average length of a bingeing episode is about 1 hour. Most patients learn to vomit by sticking their fingers down their throat, and after a short time they learn to vomit on a reflex basis. Some patients have abrasions and scars on the backs of their hands (called *Russell's sign*) from their persistent efforts to induce vomiting. Most bulimic patients do not eat regular meals and have difficulty feeling satiety at the end of a normal meal. Bulimic patients usually prefer to eat alone and at their homes. Approximately one-third to one-fifth of bulimic patients will choose a weight within a normal weight range as their ideal body weight. About one-fourth to one-third of the patients with bulimia nervosa have had a history of anorexia nervosa.

Most bulimic patients have depressive signs and symptoms. They have problems with interpersonal relationships, self-concept, and impulsive behaviors and show high levels of anxiety and compulsivity. Chemical dependency is not unusual in this disorder, alcohol abuse being the most common. Bulimic persons will abuse

TABLE 22–6. DSM-IV-TR research criteria for binge-eating disorder

A. Recurrent episodes of binge eating. An episode of binge eating is characterized by both of the following:
   (1) eating, in a discrete period of time (e.g., within any 2-hour period), an amount of food that is definitely larger than most people would eat in a similar period of time under similar circumstances
   (2) a sense of lack of control over eating during the episode (e.g., a feeling that one cannot stop eating or control what or how much one is eating)
B. The binge-eating episodes are associated with three (or more) of the following:
   (1) eating much more rapidly than normal
   (2) eating until feeling uncomfortably full
   (3) eating large amounts of food when not feeling physically hungry
   (4) eating alone because of being embarrassed by how much one is eating
   (5) feeling disgusted with oneself, depressed, or very guilty after overeating
C. Marked distress regarding binge eating is present.
D. The binge eating occurs, on average, at least 2 days a week for 6 months.
   Note: The method of determining frequency differs from that used for bulimia nervosa; future research should address whether the preferred method of setting a frequency threshold is counting the number of days on which binges occur or counting the number of episodes of binge eating.
E. The binge eating is not associated with the regular use of inappropriate compensatory behaviors (e.g., purging, fasting, excessive exercise) and does not occur exclusively during the course of anorexia nervosa or bulimia nervosa.

amphetamines to reduce their appetite and to lose weight. Impulsive stealing usually occurs after the onset of binge eating; however, about one-fourth of patients actually begin stealing before the onset of bulimia. Food, clothing, and jewelry are the items most commonly stolen.

Medical Complications

Patients with bulimia nervosa who engage in self-induced vomiting and abuse purgatives or diuretics are susceptible to hypokalemic alkalosis. These patients have electrolyte abnormalities, including elevated serum bicarbonate levels, hypochloremia, hypokalemia, and, in a few cases, low serum bicarbonate levels, indicating a metabolic acidosis. The latter is particularly true among individuals who abuse laxatives. It is important to remember that fasting can promote dehydration, which results in volume depletion. This can promote generation of aldosterone, which promotes further potassium excretion from the kidneys.

Thus, there can be an indirect renal loss of potassium as well as a direct loss through self-induced vomiting. Patients with electrolyte disturbances have physical symptoms of weakness and lethargy and at times have cardiac arrhythmias. The latter, of course, can lead to a sudden cardiac arrest. Patients with bulimia nervosa can have severe attrition and erosion of the teeth, causing an irritating sensitivity, pathological pulp exposures, loss of integrity of the dental arches, diminished masticatory ability, and an unaesthetic appearance.

Parotid gland enlargement associated with elevated serum amylase levels is commonly observed in patients who binge and vomit. In fact, the serum amylase level is an excellent way to follow reduction of vomiting in patients with eating disorders who deny purging episodes. Acute dilatation of the stomach is a rare emergency condition for patients who binge. Esophageal tears also can occur through the process of self-induced vomiting. A complication of shock can result subsequent to the esophageal tear and should be treated by experienced medical and surgical personnel. Severe abdominal pain in the patient with bulimia nervosa should alert the physician to a diagnosis of gastric dilatation and the need for nasogastric suction, X rays, and surgical consultation.

Cardiac failure caused by cardiomyopathy from ipecac intoxication is a medical emergency that is being reported more frequently and that usually results in death. Symptoms of precardial pain, dyspnea, and generalized muscle weakness associated with hypotension, tachycardia, and abnormalities on the electrocardiogram should alert one to possible ipecac intoxication. Other laboratory findings may include elevated liver enzymes and an increased erythrocyte sedimentation rate. Obviously, at this point the patient should be under a cardiologist's care. An echocardiogram will show a cardiomyopathy contraction pattern associated with congestive heart failure.

Other mechanisms for cardiac arrhythmias and sudden death in bulimic patients probably exist. The arrhythmias noted here are associated with electrolyte disturbances and ipecac intoxication. More recent studies have shown arrhythmias associated with bingeing behavior even when serum electrolytes are within normal limits.

A summary of medical complications is presented in Table 22–7.

Epidemiology, Course, and Prognosis

No satisfactory incidence studies on bulimia nervosa have been reported. This is not surprising, given the fact that this disorder emerged only in 1980 as the distinct diagnostic entity presented in DSM-III (American Psychiatric Association 1980). In DSM-III, bulimia nervosa was referred to as "bulimia," and the criteria did not allow one to distinguish between occasional binge eating episodes and the truly incapacitating disorder of bulimia nervosa. The bulimia nervosa diagnostic criteria have been revised every few years, and this may account for the disparity in reported prevalence rates for this disorder. Studies that used strict criteria found prevalence rates between 1 and 3.8 per 100 females (Hart and Ollendick 1985; Schotte and Stunkard 1987). In a study combining surveys and interviews of women in the first year of college, Kurth et al. (1995) found the prevalence of bulimia nervosa to be 2%. In a Canadian community sample, in a study in which a structured interview was used, prevalence rates of this disorder were 1% (Garfinkel et al. 1995). Hoek (1991) found a 1-year prevalence rate of bulimia nervosa of 0.17% among adolescent girls and young women ages 15–29 years in a primary care health delivery system. The prevalence of males in the bulimia nervosa population varies between 10% and 15%. In most studies, the average age at onset of bulimia nervosa is 18 years (range = 12–35 years). These studies have shown a much higher representation of the social classes IV and V in patients with bulimia nervosa compared with patients with anorexia nervosa.

Intervention studies on the prevention of eating disorders to date have not produced impressive results. Most studies have been designed to target and measure

TABLE 22–7. Medical complications of bulimia nervosa

Behavioral and physical aberrations	Physiological disturbances
Binge eating	Acute dilatation of stomach—shock
Self-induced vomiting	Esophageal tears—shock; dehydration
	Metabolic alkalosis—hypochloremia, hypokalemia, weakness, lethargy
	Cardiac arrhythmias—cardiac arrest
	Erosion of dental enamel—caries, exposure of pulp
Parotid gland enlargement (self-induced vomiting or excessive gum chewing)	Elevated serum amylase
Ipecac use	Hypotension, tachycardia, electrocardiographic abnormalities, elevated liver enzymes

change on the individual level. Austin (2000) suggested that expecting children to develop resilience to unhealthy pressures may be a less successful strategy than making significant changes in the social environment. An example would be "a model of proactive primary prevention targeted at environmental change and cross-disciplinary collaboration with coronary heart disease, cancer and obesity prevention intervention research" (Austin 2000, p. 1253).

There are virtually no long-term follow-up studies on patients with bulimia nervosa. Thus, little information is available on the natural course of this disorder and on outcome predictors.

Etiology and Pathogenesis

Fairburn and Cooper (1984) found that a rigid diet was the most commonly reported precipitant of binge-eating behavior and that a gross bingeing bout was the most common precipitant for vomiting behavior. This finding may shed some light on the physiological mechanisms involved in binge eating and purging. For example, the period of strict dieting may influence peptide and neurotransmitter secretion, which may in turn affect appetite and satiety mechanisms. Studies of satiety responses in patients with eating disorders have shown that the perceptions of hunger and of satiety are disturbed in patients who binge and purge (Halmi and Sunday 1991). Another study showed distinct differences in taste preferences for sweetness and "fattiness" in restricting anorexic patients, bulimic anorexic patients, normal-weight bulimic patients, and control subjects (Sunday and Halmi 1990). Further identification of disturbances in the psychological processes of hunger, satiety, and taste could provide important clues concerning impaired central mechanisms. Evidence for dysregulation of serotonergic neurotransmission in bulimia nervosa consists of blunted prolactin response to the serotonin receptor agonist m-chlorophenylpiperazine (m-CPP), 5-hydroxytryptophan, and dl-fenfluramine and enhanced migrainelike headache response to m-CPP challenge. Low levels of CSF 5-hydroxyindoleacetic acid are associated with impulsive and aggressive behaviors and are also present in bulimia nervosa patients (Jimerson et al. 1997; Levitan et al. 1997). In a large interview study by Braun et al. (1994), 31% of the bulimic subgroups had a Cluster B (impulsive) disorder. Borderline personality disorder was present in 25% of the bulimic subgroups and was the most common Cluster B condition.

In a study of clinical features, Hatsukami et al. (1984) found that 43.5% of a sample of 108 women with bulimia nervosa had an affective disorder at some time in their lives and 18.5% had a history of alcohol or drug abuse. Although there is a high association of mood disorder with bulimia nervosa, insufficient current evidence is available to support describing bulimia nervosa as a mere forme fruste of mood disorder. Bulimia nervosa theoretically fits well into an addictive model (Szmukler and Tantam 1984).

A study that used the Minnesota Multiphasic Personality Inventory to compare women with bulimia nervosa with women who abused alcohol and drugs found that the two groups had similar profiles. They had elevations on the scales denoting depression, impulsivity, anger, rebelliousness, anxiety, rumination, social withdrawal, and idiosyncratic thinking (Hatsukami et al. 1982). Two studies that used the Social Adjustment Scale found that women with bulimia nervosa were significantly worse in all areas of adjustment (work, social, and leisure activities; relationship with extended family; role as spouse; role as parent, and membership in a family unit) than were women in a control sample (Johnson and Berndt 1983; Norman and Herzog 1984). These findings remained stable after a year. These latter studies indicate that one might expect to find a higher prevalence of Axis II DSM-IV-TR diagnoses in the patients with bulimia nervosa than in a normal population.

The percentage of individuals with DSM-III-R bulimia (including anorexic bulimic individuals) who have at least one personality disorder has been reported to be 77% (Powers et al. 1988), 69% (Wonderlich et al. 1990), 62% (Gartner et al. 1989), 61% (Schmidt and Telch 1990), 33% (Ames-Frankel et al. 1992), and 23% (Herzog et al. 1992). All of these studies used established diagnostic interviews, but the findings are not in agreement. This is probably a result of several factors: 1) some of the studies with very small numbers of patients may represent a biased sample; 2) studies used different criteria, ranging from DSM-III to DSM-III-R, for both eating disorders and personality disorders; and 3) some of the Axis II interviewers lacked information about the patients' Axis I diagnosis, which may have led to false-positive personality disorder diagnoses. Nonetheless, substantial evidence indicates that personality disorders are commonly associated with bulimia nervosa.

A study determining coherent groupings of personality profiles of bulimia and anorexia patients was conducted by psychiatrists and psychologists who used a Q-sort procedure. With a cluster-analytic procedure, three categories of patients emerged: 1) a high functioning–perfectionistic group, 2) a constricted-overcontrolled group, and 3) an emotionally dysregulated–undercontrolled group. These categorizations were significantly effective in predicting eating disorder symptoms (Westen and

TABLE 22–8. Treatment of bulimia nervosa

Type of treatment	Indications	Measurements	Key elements
Cognitive-behavioral therapy (CBT)			
Group	Outpatients—young adults	Psychiatric and medical evaluations before entering therapy	Psychoeducational component on all aspects of the bulimic disorder
Individual	Inpatients; outpatients—adolescents and adults with severe character disorders	Self-recording of medical consultations available throughout treatment	Self-monitoring, cognitive restructuring
Behavior therapy	Usually used in conjunction with computed tomography	Same as for CBT	Restricting exposure to cues, developing alternative behaviors, response prevention to stop vomiting
Interpersonal therapy	Outpatients—young adults	Psychiatric and medical evaluations before entering therapy and consultation available during treatment	Focuses on interpersonal relationships
Pharmacotherapy Antidepressants Desipramine Imipramine Nortriptyline Phenelzine Fluoxetine	Binge-eating behavior, depression, unwillingness to enter CBT	Initial evaluation: complete blood count, serum electrolytes and amylase electrocardiogram, blood pressure. Repeat above after 1 week and as often as clinically indicated	The antidepressant drugs affect catecholamine and indoleamine function, which modulates eating behavior.

Harden-Fischer 2001). Thus, personality patterns may account for meaningful variations within eating disorder diagnoses.

Treatment

Treatment studies of bulimia nervosa have proliferated in the past 15 years, in contrast to the relatively few treatment studies of anorexia nervosa. This is probably because of the greater prevalence of bulimia nervosa and the fact that this disorder usually can be treated on an outpatient basis. Specific therapy techniques such as behavior therapy, cognitive therapy, psychodynamic therapy, and "psychoeducation therapy" have been conducted in both individual and group therapies (Table 22–8). There are no controlled studies in which patients were randomly assigned to individual or group therapy for any of these techniques. Multiple controlled drug treatment studies also have been conducted in the past decade. Often a variety of therapy techniques such as cognitive therapy, behavior therapy, and drug treatment may be used together in either individual or group therapy. Unfortunately, there is no way to predict at present what bulimic patient will respond to what type of therapy or treatment. "The Practice Guideline for the Treatment of

Patients With Eating Disorders" (Revision) (American Psychiatric Association 2000b) has a helpful section on developing a treatment plan for the individual patient. Factors that need to be considered are level of care (outpatient, intensive outpatient, partial hospitalization, residential treatment center, or inpatient hospitalization), site of treatment (availability of medical care), and family assessment and treatment.

Psychodynamic Therapy

Lacey (1983) described the use of psychodynamic therapy with cognitive and behavioral techniques in both the individual and the group therapy formats. Common themes that need to be dealt with are poor self-esteem, dependency problems, and a sense of ineffectiveness.

Cognitive-Behavioral Therapy

Fourteen published controlled studies have examined the efficacy of CBT in bulimia nervosa. One of the first and best descriptions of CBT was by Fairburn (1981). All of the subjects in these 14 studies were outpatients, with the exception of one study of the effectiveness of CBT in individual therapy, involving inpatients. Nearly all of the studies used a psychoeducational component that included information on the social-cultural emphasis on thinness; set point theory; the physical effects and medical complications of bingeing, purging, and abuse of laxatives and diuretics; and how dieting and fasting precipitate binge–purge cycles. Self-monitoring was an important part of all of these studies and usually consists of a daily record of the times and durations of meals and a record of binge-eating and purging episodes, as well as descriptions of moods and circumstances surrounding binge–purge episodes. The studies stressed the importance of eating regular meals.

Cognitive restructuring is the basis of all the CBT programs. The first step in cognitive therapy is the assessment of cognition. Patients are asked to write their thoughts on an assessment form so that cognitions can be examined for systematic distortions in the processing and interpretation of events. Two reviews of controlled studies of CBT for bulimia nervosa concluded that CBT benefits most patients (Fairburn et al. 1992a; Gotestam and Agras 1989). CBT was more effective than treatment with antidepressants alone, self-monitoring plus supportive psychotherapy, and behavioral treatment without the cognitive treatment component. One-year follow-up studies with CBT have shown a good maintenance of change, superior to that following treatment with antidepressants.

Behavior therapy is used specifically to stop the binge-eating/purging behaviors. Behavioral approaches include restricting exposure to cues that trigger a binge-purge episode, developing a strategy of alternative behaviors, and delaying the vomiting response to eating. Response prevention is a technique used specifically to prevent vomiting. After eating, a patient is placed in a situation in which it is very difficult for him or her comfortably to vomit. Adding exposure (i.e., requiring the patient to binge) did not seem to enhance the effects of response prevention (Rosen 1982).

The combined effects of CBT and antidepressant medication for bulimia nervosa were examined in three studies. Mitchell et al. (1990) found that group CBT was superior to imipramine therapy for decreasing binge eating and purging, and the combined treatment showed no additive effects for those treated with group CBT alone. Agras et al. (1992) had similar results comparing individual CBT, desipramine therapy, and the combination at 16 weeks. However, at 32 weeks, only the combined treatment given for 24 weeks was superior to medication given for 16 weeks. In a third study, CBT plus medication (desipramine, followed by fluoxetine in nonresponders) was superior to medication alone, but supportive psychotherapy plus medication was not. CBT plus medication was superior to CBT alone.

A study of interpersonal therapy (IPT), which targets interpersonal functioning, showed that IPT was equivalent to CBT in reducing bulimic symptoms and psychopathology; at follow-up, it was actually superior to CBT (Fairburn et al. 1992b). This was the first study to show that bulimia nervosa may be treated successfully without focusing directly on the patient's eating habits and attitudes toward shape and weight. In another study comparing CBT with IPT, bulimic patients had 19 sessions of treatment over a 20-week period and were evaluated for 1 year after treatment in a multisite study. CBT was significantly superior to IPT at the end of treatment for the number of participants recovered (29% vs. 6%). At a 1-year follow-up, no significant difference was found between the two treatments. However, CBT was significantly more rapid in initiating improvement in patients with bulimia nervosa compared with IPT. Therefore, the authors suggested that CBT should be considered the preferred psychotherapeutic treatment for bulimia nervosa (Agras et al. 2000).

Currently, multicenter treatment studies that use a sequential design are under way, which more realistically represents the practice of treating bulimia nervosa by primary care physicians. In these studies, usually one form of treatment such as CBT or a serotonin reuptake inhibitor is administered for a period of 4 months. If the patients have not completely ceased bingeing and purging behavior at the end of that time, they are then assigned to another treatment modality. One study showed that individuals with bulimia nervosa who did not respond to or had relapsed following CBT or IPT had a significantly better response to fluoxetine compared with placebo (Walsh et al. 2000). In the next 3–4 years, these studies will yield some very useful data to aid in the decisions about what kind of therapy should be given to which patients.

Drug Therapy

Studies of antidepressant medications have consistently shown some efficacy in the treatment of bulimia nervosa. These studies were prompted by observations that patients with bulimia nervosa also had significant mood disturbances. Since 1980, more than a dozen double-blind, placebo-controlled trials of various antidepressants were conducted in normal-weight outpatients with bulimia nervosa. (For a review of these studies, see Fairburn et al. 1992a.) All of these trials found a significantly greater reduction in binge eating when antidepressant medication was administered than when placebo was given. Antidepressants improved mood and reduced psychopathological symptoms such as preoccupation with shape and weight. These studies provide evidence for the short-term efficacy of antidepressant medication, but long-term efficacy remains unknown. The average rate of abstinence from bingeing and purging in these studies was 22%, indicating that most patients remain symptomatic at the end of treatment with antidepressants. Both of the systematic studies conducted to evaluate maintenance of change in bulimic symptomatology yielded disappointing results: most subjects did not maintain improvement (Pyle et al. 1990; Walsh et al. 1991). The dosage of antidepressant medication to treat bulimia nervosa was similar to that used in the treatment of depression. The antidepressants used in the controlled treatment studies of bulimia nervosa included desipramine, imipramine, amitriptyline, nortriptyline, phenelzine, and fluoxetine.

The current data suggest that the treatment of choice for bulimia nervosa should be CBT and that a single antidepressant administered in the absence of psychotherapy cannot be considered an adequate treatment.

Obesity

Definition

In contrast to anorexia nervosa and bulimia nervosa, obesity is classified not as a psychiatric disorder but as a medical disorder. Obesity is an excessive accumulation of body fat and operationally is defined as being overweight. The BMI, which is weight (kg)/height (m^2), has the highest correlation, 0.8, with body fat measured by other, more precise laboratory methods. *Mildly overweight* is defined as having a BMI of 25–30, or body weight between the upper limit of normal and 20% above that limit on standard height-weight charts. *Obesity* is defined as a BMI greater than 30, or body weight greater than 20% above the upper limit for height (Bray 1978).

Clinical Features

The most obvious clinical features of obesity are physical; these features are discussed in the following section on medical complications. The psychological and behavioral aspects of obesity are best considered grouped in two categories: *eating behavior* and *emotional disturbance*. There is considerable heterogeneity in eating patterns. Most commonly, obese persons complain that they cannot restrain their eating and that they have difficulty achieving satiety. Some obese persons cannot distinguish hunger from other dysphoric states and will eat when they are emotionally upset.

The most methodologically satisfying studies have shown that there is no distinct or excess psychopathology in obesity. In one study of severely obese patients who had gastric bypass surgery, the most prevalent psychiatric diagnosis was major depressive disorder. However, this diagnosis was no more prevalent in the obese patients than in the general population. Self-disparagement of body image is especially present in those who have been obese since childhood. This may be due to the continual bombardment of social prejudice against obese people. The stigmatization and prejudice against obese types is well documented in studies of educational disadvantages and of employment prejudices against obese persons. Many obese individuals develop anxiety and depression when they attempt to diet (Halmi et al. 1980). Because health risks and mortality vary with degree of adiposity, Bray (1986) proposed a classification into low-risk (BMI=25–30), moderate-risk (BMI=31–40), and high-risk (BMI>40) individuals.

Medical Complications

Obesity affects a great variety of physiological functions. Blood circulation may be overtaxed as body weight increases, and congestive heart failure may occur in grossly obese individuals. Hypertension is strongly associated with obesity, and the prevalence of carbohydrate intolerance in grossly obese subjects is approximately 50%. Increased body fat in the upper region of the body as opposed to the lower region is more likely to be associated with the onset of diabetes mellitus. The impairment of pulmonary function becomes extreme in severe obesity and involves hypoventilation, hypercapnia, hypoxia, and somnolence (i.e., pickwickian syndrome). The latter has a high mortality rate. Obesity may accelerate the development of osteoarthritis and of dermatological problems from stretching of the skin, intertrigo, and acanthosis nigricans. Obese women are an obstetrical risk, being susceptible to toxemia and hypertension.

Obesity has been associated with several types of cancer. Obese males have a higher rate of prostate and colorectal cancer, and obese females have increased incidences of gallbladder, breast, cervical, endometrial, uterine, and ovarian cancer. Most studies on the topic suggest that obesity influences the development and progression of both endometrial and breast cancer through influences on estrogen production. Low-density lipoprotein levels are increased in obesity, and levels of high-density lipoproteins (HDL cholesterol) are reduced. The low levels of HDL may be one mechanism by which obesity is associated with an increased risk for cardiovascular disease.

Epidemiology, Course, and Prognosis

If obesity is defined as the state of being 20% above ideal weight, then nearly a quarter of the United States population would be considered obese (VanItallie 1985). Socioeconomic status is highly correlated with obesity: the condition is much more common among women (less so among men) of low status. This relationship is also present in obese children. Increasing age and obesity are associated until age 50. The prevalence of obesity is higher in women compared with men; in those older than 50 years, this may be due to the increased mortality rate among obese men with advancing age.

Unfortunately, life expectancy and obesity studies are restricted to life insurance studies and therefore do not represent a random American population. Despite these limitations, studies have shown a progressive increase in "excess mortality" as BMI increased (Society of Actuaries 1992). Another study of grossly obese persons showed that excess mortality was greatly increased in younger men (aged 25–34 years) and gradually declined with age (Stevens et al. 1998).

Etiology and Pathogenesis

It is unlikely that obesity has a single etiology. In the first section of this chapter, the complex neural mechanisms involved in the control of feeding behavior were discussed. Lipid, amino acid, and glucose metabolism all seem to affect, in some way, central neural regulatory mechanisms that influence eating behavior. Obesity is regarded today by most investigators as a disorder of energy balance, a disorder with a strong genetic component that is modulated by cultural and environmental influences.

Obesity has a definite familial aspect. Eighty percent of the offspring of two obese parents are obese, compared with 40% of the offspring of one obese parent and only 10% of the offspring of lean parents. Findings of twin studies and adoption studies suggest that genetic factors play a strong role in the development of obesity.

The cloning and sequencing of the mouse obese (*Ob*) gene and its human homologue in 1994 (Zhang et al. 1994) provided the basis for further research into the pathways that regulate adiposity and body weight. Leptin, the gene product of the *Ob* gene, was shown to be a 16-kd protein that is present in mouse and human plasma (Halaas et al. 1995). Intraperitoneal injections of recombinant leptin decrease food intake and increase energy expenditure in wild-type mice. Leptin reduces body fat in mice, and its absence in mice with the *Ob* gene leads to a massive increase in body fat. In both humans and rodents, leptin is highly correlated with BMI and amount of body fat (Maffei et al. 1995). Weight loss due to food restriction was associated with a decrease in plasma leptin concentrations in mice and obese humans. These data suggest that leptin serves an endocrine function, regulating body weight and stores of body fat.

Obese persons have larger and more numerous fat cells. Cellular proliferation tends to occur early in life but also will occur in adult life when the existing fat cells are greatly enlarged. The regulation of fat cell proliferation and size is not well understood. The relation of physical activity to obesity is complex. It is known that obese people are less active than people of normal weight. The increase in caloric expenditure by physical activity is small. Animal studies show that physical activity actually decreases food intake and may actually prevent the decline in metabolic rate that usually accompanies dieting.

Treatment

For mild obesity (20%–40% overweight), the most efficient treatment to date is behavioral modification in groups, a balanced diet, and exercise. This is usually done by both commercial and nonprofit large organizations. For moderate obesity (41%–100% overweight), a medically supervised protein-sparing modified fast (400–700 calories per day) is often necessary. This diet may or may not be combined with behavioral modification techniques. A behavior analysis is necessary to set up a sensible behavioral modification program. Antecedents of eating behavior, the eating behavior itself, the consequences of the behavior, and the acceptable rewards for carrying out various prescribed behaviors are all analyzed. Behavioral treatment programs include self-monitoring, nutrition education, physical activity, and cognitive restructuring.

The use of medication such as phenylpropanolamine or fenfluramine was popular in the past. The problem with these drugs is that on withdrawal, a rebound ballooning up of weight occurs; some patients have concomitant lethargy and depression. In 1997, fenfluramine was removed by the U.S. Food and Drug Administration from the market and for approved use for treatment of obesity because of the adverse effects of pulmonary hypertension and mitral valve impairment.

Only one long-term (5 years) controlled study has documented the safety and efficacy of the fenfluramine-phentermine combination (Weintraub 1992). The National Task Force on the Prevention and Treatment of Obesity (1996) reviewed all English-language reports of studies in which human obesity was treated with medication that was given for at least 24 weeks. The task force found that the net weight loss attributable to medication use was modest, ranging from 2 kg to 10 kg. The weight loss tends to reach a plateau by 6 months. Most adverse effects are mild and self-limited, but rare serious outcomes such as pulmonary hypertension have been reported. The task force's conclusion was that pharmacotherapy for obesity, when combined with appropriate behavioral approaches to change diet and amount of physical activity, helps some obese patients lose weight and maintain weight loss for at least 1 year (National Task Force on the Prevention and Treatment of Obesity 1996). The task force also stated that until more data are available, pharmacotherapy cannot be recommended for routine use in obese individuals. They did acknowledge that it may be helpful in carefully selected patients.

Severe obesity (greater than 100% over a normal weight) is the least common form of obesity and is most effectively treated by surgical procedures that reduce the size of the stomach. These procedures produce a large weight loss and show a good record of weight loss maintenance.

Behavioral modification is the treatment of choice for overweight children and should include involvement of the parents and the schools. Psychotherapy is not recommended as a treatment per se for obesity, although some patients may have particular problems that may be effectively treated or helped with psychotherapy. For excellent discussions on the treatment of obesity, see Stunkard (1984), Brownell (1984), and Lasagna (1987).

Conclusion

The eating disorders are complex syndromes in which the interactions among environmental, psychological, and physiological factors both create and maintain the disturbed eating behavior. The more precise an understanding we obtain of the connectedness of basic physiological changes, psychological changes, and eating behavior, the better we will be able to design effective treatment interventions.

Many questions remain to be asked about our current treatment interventions. For example, how long should the bulimic patient be treated with antidepressants? Would periodic follow-up behavioral sessions prevent relapse in bulimic patients treated with behavior therapy? How can we identify the most likely effective treatment for a patient?

Continued prospective longitudinal studies are necessary for bulimia nervosa because no information is avail-

able on what happens to this addictive-like bingeing–purging behavior over the course of a lifetime. Although disturbed eating behavior has been present throughout the history of humankind, it has been systematically studied with scientific methodology only in the past few decades. There is a continued need for further study of eating disorders.

References

Agras WS, Rossiter EM, Arnow B, et al: Pharmacologic and cognitive-behavioral treatment for bulimia nervosa: a controlled comparison. Am J Psychiatry 149:82–87, 1992

Agras WS, Walsh BT, Fairburn CG: A multicenter comparison of cognitive-behavioral therapy and interpersonal psychotherapy for bulimia nervosa. Arch Gen Psychiatry 57:459–466, 2000

Ahima RS, Prabakarn D, Mantzoros C, et al: Role of leptin in the neuroendocrine response to fasting. Nature 382:250–252, 1996

American Psychiatric Association: Diagnostic and Statistical Manual of Mental Disorders, 3rd Edition. Washington, DC, American Psychiatric Association, 1980

American Psychiatric Association: Diagnostic and Statistical Manual of Mental Disorders, 3rd Edition, Revised. Washington, DC, American Psychiatric Association, 1987

American Psychiatric Association: Diagnostic and Statistical Manual of Mental Disorders, 4th Edition, Text Revision. Washington, DC, American Psychiatric Association, 2000a

American Psychiatric Association: Practice guideline for the treatment of patients with eating disorders (revision). Am J Psychiatry 157(suppl):1–39, 2000b

Ames-Frankel J, Devlin MJ, Walsh BT, et al: Personality disorders and eating disorders. J Clin Psychiatry 53:90–96, 1992

Austin B: Prevention research in eating disorders: theory and new directions. Psychol Med 30:1249–1262, 2000

Barr LC, Goodman WK, Price LH, et al: The serotonin hypothesis of obsessive compulsive disorder: implications of pharmacological challenge studies. Clin Psychiatry 53:17–28, 1992

Bell RM: Holy Anorexia. Chicago, IL, University of Chicago Press, 1985

Bellodi L, Cavallini MC, Bertelli S: Morbidity risk for obsessive-compulsive spectrum disorders in first-degree relatives of patients with eating disorders. Am J Psychiatry 158:563–569, 2001

Ben-Tovin D, Walker K, Gilchrist P: Outcome in patients with eating disorders: a 5 year study. Lancet 357:1254–1257, 2001

Blundell JE, Hill A: Behavioral pharmacology of feeding: relevance of animal experiments for studies in man, in Pharmacology of Eating Disorders. Edited by Carruba M, Blundell J. New York, Raven, 1986, pp 51–70

Boden G, Chen X, Mazzoli M, et al: Effect of fasting on serum leptin in normal subjects. J Clin Endocrinol Metab 81:3419–3423, 1996

Bohus B, Kovacs GL, de Wied D: Oxytocin, vasopressin and memory: opposite effects on consolidation and retrieval processes. Brain Res 157:414–417, 1978

Booth DA: Food-conditioned eating preferences and aversions with interceptive elements: conditioned appetite and satieties. Ann N Y Acad Sci 443:22–41, 1985

Brambilla F, Bellodi L, Arancio C, et al: Central dopaminergic function in anorexia and bulimia nervosa: a psychoneuroendocrine approach. Psychoneuroendocrinology 26:393–409, 2001

Braun DL, Sunday SR, Halmi KA: Psychiatric comorbidity in patients with eating disorders. Psychol Med 24:859–867, 1994

Bray GA: Definitions, measurements and classification of the syndromes of obesity. Int J Obesity 2:99–112, 1978

Bray GA: Effects of obesity on health and happiness, in Handbook of Eating Disorders: Physiology, Psychology, and Treatment. Edited by Brownell KD, Foreyt JP. New York, Basic Books, 1986, pp 3–44

Brownell KD: New developments in the treatment of obese children and adolescents, in Eating and Its Disorders. Edited by Stunkard AJ, Stellar E. New York, Raven, 1984, pp 175–184

Bruch H: Perceptual and conceptual disturbance in anorexia nervosa. Psychosom Med 24:187–195, 1962

Charney DS, Wood SW, Krystal JH, et al: Serotonin function and human anxiety disorders. Ann N Y Acad Sci 600:558–573, 1990

Chen H, Charlat O, Tartaglia LA, et al: Evidence that the diabetes gene encodes the leptin receptor: identification of a mutation in the leptin receptor gene in the DB/DB mice. Cell 84:491–495, 1996

Considine RV, Sinha MK, Heiman ML, et al: Serum immunoreactive-leptin concentrations in normal-weight and obese humans. N Engl J Med 334:292–295, 1996

Crisp AH: The possible significance of some behavioral correlates of weight and carbohydrate intake. J Psychosom Res 11:117–123, 1976

Crisp AH, Palmer RL, Kalucy RS, et al: How common is anorexia nervosa? A prevalence study. Br J Psychiatry 128:549–552, 1976

Crisp AH, Lacey JH, Crutchfield M: Clomipramine and 'drive' in people with anorexia nervosa: an inpatient study. Br J Psychiatry 150:355–358, 1987

Demitrack MA, Kalogeras KT, Altemus M, et al: Plasma and cerebrospinal fluid measures of arginine vasopressin secretion in patients with bulimia nervosa and in healthy subjects. J Clin Endocrinol Metab 74:1277–1283, 1992

Eagles T, Johnston M, Hunter D, et al: Increasing incidence of anorexia nervosa in the female population of northeast Scotland. Am J Psychiatry 152:1266–1271, 1995

Eison AS, Mullins UL: Regulation of central 5-HT$_{2A}$ receptors: a review of in vivo studies. Behav Brain Res 73:177–181, 1996

Fairburn C: A cognitive behavioral approach to the treatment of bulimia. Psychol Med 11:707–711, 1981

Fairburn CG, Cooper PJ: The clinical features of bulimia nervosa. Br J Psychiatry 144:238–246, 1984

Fairburn CG, Agra WS, Wilson GT: The research on the treatment of bulimia nervosa: practical and theoretical implications, in Biology of Feast and Famine: Relevance to Eating Disorders. Edited by Anderson GH, Kennedy SH. New York, Academic Press, 1992a, pp 318–340

Fairburn CG, Jones R, Pevelar RC, et al: Three psychological treatments for bulimia nervosa: a comparative trial. Arch Gen Psychiatry 48:463–469, 1992b

Falk JR, Halmi KA: Amenorrhea in anorexia nervosa: examination of the critical body hypothesis. Biol Psychiatry 17:799–806, 1982

Garfinkel P, Goering L, Spegg C, et al: Bulimia nervosa in a Canadian community sample: prevalence and comparison of subgroups. Am J Psychiatry 52:1052–1058, 1995

Garner DM, Bemis KM: A cognitive-behavioral approach to anorexia nervosa. Cognitive Therapy and Research 6:1223–1250, 1982

Garner DM, Garfinkel PE: Handbook of Psychotherapy for Anorexia Nervosa. New York, Guilford, 1985

Gartner AF, Marcus RN, Halmi KA, et al: DSM-III-R personality disorders in patients with eating disorders. Am J Psychiatry 146:1585–1591, 1989

Gibbs J, Smith GP: Satiety hormones, in Frontiers in Neuroendocrinology, Vol 8. Edited by Martini L, Gonong W. New York, Raven, 1984, pp 98–132

Gold PW, Gwirtsman H, Kaye W, et al: Pathophysiologic mechanisms in underweight and weight corrected patients. N Engl J Med 314:335–342, 1986

Gotestam KA, Agras WS: Bulimia nervosa: pharmacologic and psychologic approaches to treatment. Nordisk Psykiatrisk Tidsskrift 43:543–551, 1989

Grahame-Smith DG: Serotonin in affective disorders. Int Clin Psychopharmacol 6(suppl 4):5–13, 1992

Gwirtsman HE, Guze BH, Yager J, et al: Fluoxetine treatment of anorexia nervosa: an open trial. J Clin Psychiatry 51:378–382, 1990

Halaas J, Gajiwala K, Maffei M, et al: Weight-reducing effects of the protein encoded by the obese gene. Science 269:543–546, 1995

Halmi KA: Anorexia nervosa: demographic and clinical features in 94 cases. Psychosom Med 36:18–26, 1974

Halmi KA: Anorexia nervosa and bulimia, in Handbook of Adolescent Psychology. Edited by Hersen M, Van Hasselt T. New York, Pergamon, 1987, pp 265–287

Halmi KA, Falk JR: Common physiological changes in anorexia nervosa. Int J Eat Disord 1:16–27, 1981

Halmi KA, Sunday SR: Temporal patterns of hunger and satiety ratings and related cognitions in anorexia and bulimia. Appetite 16:219–237, 1991

Halmi KA, Stunkard AJ, Mason EE: Emotional responses to weight reduction by three methods: gastric bypass, jejunoileal bypass, diet. Am J Clin Nutr 33:446–451, 1980

Halmi KA, Eckert E, LaDu T, et al: Anorexia nervosa: treatment efficacy of cyproheptadine and amitriptyline. Arch Gen Psychiatry 43:177–181, 1986

Halmi KA, Eckert E, Marchi P, et al: Comorbidity of psychiatric diagnoses in anorexia nervosa. Arch Gen Psychiatry 48:712–718, 1991

Hart K, Ollendick TH: Prevalence of bulimia in working and university women. Am J Psychiatry 142:851–854, 1985

Hatsukami J, Mitchell J, Eckert E: Similarities and differences on the MMPI between women with bulimia and women with alcohol and drug abuse problems. Addict Behav 7:435–439, 1982

Hatsukami J, Mitchell J, Eckert E, et al: Affective disorder and substance abuse in women with bulimia. Psychol Med 14:704–710, 1984

Herzog DB, Keller MB, Lavori PW, et al: The prevalence of personality disorders in 210 women with eating disorders. J Clin Psychiatry 53:147–152, 1992

Hoebel BG: Pharmacological control of feeding. Annu Rev Pharmacol Toxicol 17:605–621, 1977

Hoek H: The incidence and prevalence of anorexia nervosa and bulimia nervosa in primary care. Psychol Med 21:455–460, 1991

Holland AJ, Crisp A, Russell GFM, et al: Anorexia nervosa: a study of 34 twin pairs and one set of triplets. Br J Psychiatry 145:414–419, 1984

Holland AJ, Sicotte N, Tresure J: Anorexia nervosa: evidence for a genetic basis. J Psychosom Res 32:561–571, 1988

Hotta M, Chibasaki T, Masuda A, et al: The responses of plasma adrenal corticotropin and cortisol to corticotropin-releasing hormone and cerebral spinal fluid immunoreactive CRH in anorexia nervosa patients. J Clin Endocrinol Metab 62:319–321, 1986

Hsu G, Crisp A: Outcome of anorexia nervosa. Lancet 1:61–65, 1979

Jimerson DC, Wolfe BE, Metzger ED, et al: Decrease serotonin function in bulimia nervosa. Arch Gen Psychiatry 54:529–534, 1997

Johnson C, Berndt DJ: Preliminary investigation of bulimia and life adjustment. Am J Psychiatry 140:774–777, 1983

Jones D, Fox MM, Babigian HM, et al: Epidemiology of anorexia nervosa in Monroe County, N.Y., 1960–1976. Psychosom Med 42:551–558, 1980

Kaye WH, Ebert MH, Raleigh M, et al: Abnormalities in CNS monoamine metabolism in anorexia nervosa. Arch Gen Psychiatry 41:350–355, 1984a

Kaye WH, Ebert M, Gwirtsman H, et al: Differences in brain serotonergic metabolism between nonbulimic and bulimic patients with anorexia nervosa. Am J Psychiatry 141:1598–1601, 1984b

Kaye WH, Berrettini W, Gwirtsman HE, et al: Altered cerebral spinal fluid neuropeptide Y and peptide YY immunoreactivity in anorexia and bulimia nervosa. Arch Gen Psychiatry 47:548–556, 1990

Kaye WH, Welzin T, Hsu J: An open trial of fluoxetine in patients with anorexia nervosa. J Clin Psychiatry 52:464–471, 1991

Kendler SK, MacLean C, Neale M, et al: The genetic epidemiology of bulimia nervosa. Am J Psychiatry 148:1627–1637, 1991

Kleifield E, Wagner S, Halmi K: Cognitive-behavioral treatment of anorexia nervosa. Psychiatr Clin North Am 19:715–734, 1996

Kurth C, Krahn D, Nairn K, et al: The severity of dieting and bingeing behaviors in college women: interview validation of survey data. J Psychiatry Res 29:211–225, 1995

Lacey JH: An outpatient treatment program for bulimia nervosa. Int J Eat Disord 2:209–241, 1983

Lasagna L: The pharmacotherapy of obesity, in Psychopharmacology: The Third Generation of Progress. Edited by Meltzer HY. New York, Raven, 1987, pp 1281–1284

Leibowitz SF: Neurochemical systems of the hypothalamus: control of feeding and drinking behavior and water electrolyte excretion, in Handbook of the Hypothalamus, Vol 3. Edited by Morgane PJ, Panksepp J. New York, Raven, 1980, pp 299–347

Levitan RD, Kaplan AS, Joffe RT, et al: Hormonal and subjective responses to intravenous meta-chlorophenylpiperazine in bulimia nervosa. Arch Gen Psychiatry 54:521–527, 1997

Lewinsohn PM, Striegel-Moore RH, Seeley JR: Epidemiology and natural course of eating disorders in young women from adolescence to young adulthood. J Am Acad Child Adolesc Psychiatry 39:1284–1292, 2000

Lilenfeld LR, Kaye WH, Greeno CG, et al: Psychiatric disorders in women with bulimia nervosa and their first degree relatives: effects of comorbid substance dependence. Int J Eat Disord 22:253–264, 1997

Lilenfeld LR, Kaye WH, Greeno CG, et al: A controlled family study of anorexia nervosa and bulimia nervosa: psychiatric disorders in first-degree relatives and effects of proband comorbidity. Arch Gen Psychiatry 55:603–610, 1998

Lucas A, Beard C, O'Fallon W, et al: Fifty year trends in the incidence of anorexia nervosa in Rochester, Minnesota: a population-based study. Am J Psychiatry 148:917–922, 1991

Maffei M, Halaas J, Ravussin E, et al: Leptin levels in human and rodent: measurement of plasma leptin and OB RNA in obese and weight-reduced subjects. Nat Med 1:1155–1161, 1995

Mantzoros C, Flier JS, Lesem MD, et al: Cerebrospinal fluid leptin in anorexia nervosa: correlation with nutritional status and potential role in resistance to weight gain. J Clin Endocrinol Metab 82:1845–1851, 1997

Mitchell JE, Pyle RL, Eckert ED, et al: A comparison study of antidepressants and structured intensive group therapy in the treatment of bulimia nervosa. Arch Gen Psychiatry 47:149–157, 1990

Morley J, Levine AS: Pharmacology of eating behavior. Annu Rev Pharmacol Toxicol 25:127–146, 1985

National Task Force on the Prevention and Treatment of Obesity: Long-term pharmacotherapy in the management of obesity. JAMA 276:1907–1915, 1996

Norman KA, Herzog DB: Persistent social maladjustment in bulimia: one year follow-up. Am J Psychiatry 141:444–446, 1984

Owen WP, Halmi KA, Lasley E, et al: Dopamine regulation in anorexia nervosa. Psychopharmacol Bull 19:578–580, 1983

Pirke KM: Central and peripheral noradrenalin regulation in eating disorders. Psychiatry Res 62:43–49, 1996

Powers PS, Covert DL, Brightwell DR, et al: Other psychiatric disorders among bulimic patients. Compr Psychiatry 29:503–508, 1988

Pyle RL, Mitchell JE, Eckert ED, et al: Maintenance treatment and 6 month outcome for bulimia patients who respond to initial treatment. Am J Psychiatry 147:871–875, 1990

Rooney B, McClelland L, Crisp AH, et al: The incidence and prevalence of anorexia nervosa in three suburban health districts in southwest London, UK. Int J Eat Disord 18:299–307, 1995

Rosen J: Bulimia nervosa: treatment with exposure and response prevention. Behavior Therapy 13:117–124, 1982

Russell GFM: Metabolic, endocrine and psychiatric aspects of anorexia nervosa. Scientific Basis of Medicine Annual Review 14:236–255, 1969

Russell GFM, Szmukler JI, Dare C, et al: An evaluation of family therapy in anorexia nervosa and bulimia nervosa. Arch Gen Psychiatry 44:1047–1056, 1987

Schmidt ND, Telch MJ: Prevalence of personality disorders among bulimics, non-bulimic binge eaters and normal controls. Journal of Psychopathology and Behavioral Assessment 12:170–185, 1990

Schotte D, Stunkard A: Bulimia vs. bulimic behaviors on a college campus. JAMA 9:1213–1215, 1987

Society of Actuaries: Life tables for the United States Social Security Area 1900–2080: Actuarial Study No 107, August 1992 (SSA Publ No 11-11536). Washington, DC, U.S. Department of Health and Human Services, 1992

Soubrie P: Reconciling the role of central serotonin neurosis in human and animal behavior. Behav Brain Sci 9:319–363, 1986

Stevens J, Ooi J, Pamuk E, et al: The effect of age on the association between body mass index and mortality. N Engl J Med 338:1–7, 1998

Strober M, Morell W, Burroughs J, et al: A controlled family study of anorexia nervosa. Psychiatry Res 19:329–346, 1985

Strober M, Freeman R, Lampert C, et al: Males with anorexia nervosa: a controlled study of eating disorders in first-degree relatives. Int J Eat Disord 29:263–269, 2001

Stunkard AJ: The current status of treatment for obesity in adults, in Eating and Its Disorders. Edited by Stunkard AJ, Stellar E. New York, Raven, 1984, pp 157–174

Sunday SR, Halmi KA: Taste perceptions and hedonics in eating disorders. Physiol Behav 48:587–594, 1990

Szmukler JI: The epidemiology of anorexia nervosa and bulimia. J Psychiatry Res 19:1243–1253, 1985

Szmukler JI, Tantam D: Anorexia nervosa: starvation dependence. Br J Med Psychol 57:305–310, 1984

Tartaglia LA, Dembski M, Weng X, et al: Identification and expression cloning of a leptin receptor, OB-R. Cell 83:1263–1271, 1995

Theander S: Anorexia nervosa. Acta Psychiatr Scand 214:1–300, 1970

Theander S: Outcome and prognosis in anorexia nervosa and bulimia, in Anorexia Nervosa and Bulimic Disorders. Edited by Szmukler GI, Slade PD, Harris P, et al: London, Pergamon, 1985, pp 493–508

VanItallie TB: Health implications of overweight and obesity in the United States. Ann Intern Med 103:983–988, 1985

Walsh BT, Hadigan CM, Devlin MJ, et al: Long-term outcome of antidepressant treatment for bulimia nervosa. Am J Psychiatry 148:1206–1212, 1991

Walsh BT, Agras WS, Devlin MJ, et al: Fluoxetine in bulimia nervosa following poor response to psychotherapy. Am J Psychiatry 157:1332–1334, 2000

Walters EE, Kendler KS: Anorexia nervosa an anorectic-like syndromes in a population-based twin sample. Am J Psychiatry 152:64–71, 1995

Weintraub M: Long-term weight control: the National Heart, Lung and Blood Institute funded multi-modal intervention study. Clin Pharmacol Ther 51:581–585, 1992

Westen D, Harden-Fischer J: Personality profiles in eating disorders: rethinking the distinction between Axis I and Axis II. Am J Psychiatry 158:547–562, 2001

Wonderlich SA, Swift WJ, Slotnick HB, et al: DSM-III-R personality disorders and eating disorder subtypes. Int J Eat Disord 9:607–616, 1990

Woodside DB, Garfinkel PE, Lin E, et al: Comparisons of men with full or partial eating disorders, men without eating disorders, and women with eating disorders in the community. Am J Psychiatry 158:570–574, 2001

Wurtman JJ, Wurtman RJ: Drugs that enhance central serotonergic transmission diminished elective carbohydrate consumption by rats. Life Sci 24:895–904, 1979

Zhang Y, Prenca R, Maffei M, et al: Positional cloning of the mouse obese gene and its human homologue. Nature 372:425–432, 1994

Pain Disorders

Steven A. King, M.D., M.S.

Of all the problems faced by physicians, pain is among the most pervasive and difficult to diagnose and treat. It is not only one of the most frequently encountered complaints in medicine in general but also a common symptom of other mental disorders. The scope of the problem is illustrated by a recent survey that reported that 43% of American households have at least one family member with chronic pain (Partners Against Pain 2001). The increasing recognition of pain as an important health issue is demonstrated by the decision of the Joint Commission on the Accreditation of Health Care Organizations (JCAHO) to require that hospitals and other health care organizations implement procedures for ensuring that all patients are assessed for pain and, if necessary, provided treatment for it (Joint Commission on Accreditation of Health Care Organizations 2000).

This chapter presents an overview of current concepts regarding the diagnosis and treatment of pain, with special emphasis on the role of the psychiatrist.

Definition of Pain

One of the difficulties encountered by clinicians and researchers is defining pain. Although pain has not traditionally been considered a mental disorder, the current definitions of pain accept the primacy of psychological factors in the pain experience. The most commonly accepted definition is that presented by the Committee on Taxonomy of the International Association for the Study of Pain: "An unpleasant sensory and emotional experience associated with actual or potential tissue damage, or described in terms of such damage.... Activity induced in the nociceptor and nociceptive pathways by a noxious stimulus is not pain, *which is always a psychological state*, even though we may well appreciate that

pain most often has a proximate physical cause" (Merskey and Bogduk 1994, p. 210; emphasis added). The Institute of Medicine Committee on Pain, Disability, and Chronic Illness Behavior reported that "the experience of pain is more than a simple sensory process. It is a complex perception involving higher levels of the central nervous system, emotional states, and higher order mental processes" (Osterweis et al. 1987, p. 13).

These definitions indicate the necessity of terminating the dualistic concept that pain should be divided into that associated with identifiable organic pathology and that considered secondary to psychological factors. This outdated view has many drawbacks, most notably its often leading to the belief that the former is "real pain," whereas the latter is "imaginary," even though when the etiological factors involved in the pain are psychological, the patient's perception of the pain is the same and his or her suffering is just as real.

Diagnostic Classification of Pain

Problems were encountered in employing the pain-related diagnoses included in the previous editions of the *Diagnostic and Statistical Manual of Mental Disorders* (DSM) (King and Strain 1996). Therefore, a new pain-related category—*pain disorder*—was introduced in the fourth edition, DSM-IV (American Psychiatric Association 1994), and retained in the text revision of this edition (American Psychiatric Association 2000; Table 23–1). This is the first DSM category to address the issues of and provide for diagnoses in which acute pain is the primary problem and for conditions in which both psychological factors and general medical conditions are involved in the development or maintenance of the pain.

TABLE 23–1. DSM-IV-TR diagnostic criteria for pain disorder

A. Pain in one or more anatomical sites is the predominant focus of the clinical presentation and is of sufficient severity to warrant clinical attention.

B. The pain causes clinically significant distress or impairment in social, occupational, or other important areas of functioning.

C. Psychological factors are judged to have an important role in the onset, severity, exacerbation, or maintenance of the pain.

D. The symptom or deficit is not intentionally produced or feigned (as in factitious disorder or malingering).

E. The pain is not better accounted for by a mood, anxiety, or psychotic disorder and does not meet criteria for dyspareunia.

Code as follows:

307.80 Pain Disorder Associated With Psychological Factors: psychological factors are judged to have the major role in the onset, severity, exacerbation, or maintenance of the pain. (If a general medical condition is present, it does not have a major role in the onset, severity, exacerbation, or maintenance of the pain.) This type of pain disorder is not diagnosed if criteria are also met for somatization disorder.

Specify if:

Acute: duration of less than 6 months

Chronic: duration of 6 months or longer

307.89 Pain Disorder Associated With Both Psychological Factors and a General Medical Condition: both psychological factors and a general medical condition are judged to have important roles in the onset, severity, exacerbation, or maintenance of the pain. The associated general medical condition or anatomical site of the pain (see below) is coded on Axis III.

Specify if:

Acute: duration of less than 6 months

Chronic: duration of 6 months or longer

Note: The following is not considered to be a mental disorder and is included here to facilitate differential diagnosis.

Pain Disorder Associated With a General Medical Condition: a general medical condition has a major role in the onset, severity, exacerbation, or maintenance of the pain. (If psychological factors are present, they are not judged to have a major role in the onset, severity, exacerbation, or maintenance of the pain.) The diagnostic code for the pain is selected based on the associated general medical condition if one has been established or on the anatomical location of the pain if the underlying general medical condition is not yet clearly established—for example, low back (724.2), sciatic (724.3), pelvic (625.9), headache (784.0), facial (784.0), chest (786.50), joint (719.40), bone (733.90), abdominal (789.0), breast (611.71), renal (788.0), ear (388.70), eye (379.91), throat (784.1), tooth (525.9), and urinary (788.0).

As yet, the extent of the use of this new diagnostic category has been the subject of limited research. King (1996) reported that 51% of patients with pain who were evaluated by a psychiatric consultation-liaison service fulfilled the diagnostic criteria for pain disorder, whereas fewer than 2% met the criteria for *somatoform pain disorder,* its predecessor in DSM-III-R (American Psychiatric Association 1987). Anooshian et al. (1999) found that 88% of patients treated at a psychiatric pain clinic met the criteria for pain disorder.

Other diagnostic classification systems for pain have been proposed, but none has yet been widely employed (King 2000). The most extensive of these was developed by the Task Force on Taxonomy of the International Association for the Study of Pain (Merskey and Bogduk 1994). This five-axis classification system for categorizing pain is displayed in Table 23–2. The schema provides for comments on psychological factors on both the second axis, where psychiatric illness can be coded under the nervous system, and on the fifth axis, where possible etiologies include "psychophysiological" and "psychological." However, the diagnosis of the psychiatric illness is based on other classification systems for mental disorders, such as DSM.

Although it is not contained in any formal diagnostic classification systems for pain, the term *chronic pain syndrome* is frequently applied to extended pain. There are different views concerning what should be subsumed under this syndrome, but most clinicians employ Black's (1975) criteria:

TABLE 23–2. International Association for the Study of Pain classification of chronic pain

Axis I	Regions (head, face, and mouth; abdominal region; lower back, etc.)
Axis II	Systems (musculoskeletal system and connective tissue; nervous system; gastrointestinal system, etc.)
Axis III	Temporal characteristics of pain: pattern of occurrence (single episode, limited duration; continuous or nearly continuous, nonfluctuating; recurring irregularly, etc.)
Axis IV	Patient's statement of intensity: time since onset of pain (mild, medium, or severe with appropriate duration)
Axis V	Etiology (inflammatory; neoplasm; degenerative; dysfunctional, including psychophysiological; psychological origin, etc.)

Source.   Adapted from Merskey and Bogduk 1994.

intractable, often multiple pain complaints, which are usually inappropriate to existing somatogenic problems; multiple physician contacts and many nonproductive diagnostic procedures; excessive preoccupation with the pain problem; [and] an altered behavior pattern with some of the features of depression, anxiety, and neuroticism. (p. 1000)

Because of the extremely subjective nature of many of the criteria, the validity of this diagnosis is questionable. Furthermore, some of the factors described, such as the overuse of diagnostic procedures, may be related as much to limitations in training and knowledge about pain among medical professionals as to patient behavior. Because of these limitations and the pejorative connotations that have surrounded its use, the diagnostic category *chronic pain syndrome* is best avoided.

Gate Control Theory of Pain

Over the years, a variety of theories have been promulgated to explain pain. Although there is no universal acceptance of any one concept, the *gate control theory* developed by Melzack and Wall (1965) has received much attention. These authors believe that the transmission of nerve impulses from the periphery to the spinal cord is modified by a gatelike mechanism in the dorsal horn. The position of the gate and the amount of information subsequently conveyed to the brain are determined by several factors. Large A-beta fibers as well as small A-delta and C fibers carry impulses from the periphery to the substantia gelatinosa and spinal cord transmission (T) cells. Activation of the large fibers inhibits transmission to the T cells, thus closing the gate, whereas activation of the small fibers increases transmissions, thus opening the gate. The impact of the large and small fibers on the T cells is mediated by the substantia gelatinosa.

In addition to the impulses from the periphery, the gating mechanism is also influenced by descending messages from the brain and by a "central control" mechanism that is activated by the large-diameter fibers and involves certain cognitive processes. Thus, according to this theory, pain is determined not only by peripheral stimulation, but also by information traveling from the brain to the spinal cord. This reaffirms the role of the mind–body interaction.

Although more recent research indicates that the gating system is more complicated than first conceived and that there may be more than one such mechanism involved, the basic concept remains intact (Melzack 1996; Wall 1996).

Pain Disorders and Other Mental Disorders

Although there is unquestionably a relationship between pain and other mental disorders, the exact nature of this relationship is unclear. Most research on this issue has focused on the frequency of psychiatric disorders among patients whose primary complaint is pain, but the few studies that addressed pain among psychiatric patients reported it to be a common problem. Delaplaine et al. (1978) reported that 38% of patients admitted to a psychiatric hospital complained of pain. King et al. (1998) found that on interview, 87% of psychiatric inpatients reported having pain, with 58% of these patients stating that their pain had been present for 2 years or longer. King and Timko (1999) reported that 59% of patients referred to a psychiatric consultation-liaison service complained of pain on initial evaluation, although only 6% of all patients were referred for this problem. Chaturvedi (1987b) identified pain in 18% of patients attending a psychiatric clinic. In both this study and that by Delaplaine et al. (1978), pain was noted to be much more frequent among the patients whose diagnosis was neurosis than among those with schizophrenia or other psychoses.

Chronic pain appears to be frequently associated with both anxiety disorders and various forms of depressive disorders, including major depression, dysthymic disorder, and adjustment disorder with depressed mood. In the current literature, the range of prevalence of depression in patients with chronic pain is 10%–100% (Gureje et al. 1998; King 1997; Romano and Turner 1985). Although the variability of these results may reflect difficulties in applying these diagnoses in patients with pain, it may also be due to differences in the patient populations studied. These disorders have been identified both in patients in whom there is clear evidence of an organic etiology for the pain and in patients in whom there is not, although it appears that the depressive disorders may be more common among the latter group (Magni 1987).

Although much research on pain has focused on the importance of psychological factors in the development and perpetuation of chronic pain, there is substantial evidence to support the role of these factors in acute pain and the role of psychologically based treatment modalities in its management. The decision to include a diagnostic category for acute pain in DSM-IV reflects this. Research demonstrates that pain ranging from traumatic to postoperative is strongly influenced by the mental state of the patient (Acute Pain Management Guideline Panel 1992; Chapman and Turner 1986).

It is often conceived that patients develop depression as a response to pain, but other opinions regarding this have been voiced. Blumer and Heilbronn (1982) suggested that the associated mental disorder may precede the pain and possibly predispose one to it, and they described the pain-prone individual whose pain is a form of masked depression. Research indicates that depressive disorders may be more common in the first-degree relatives of people with chronic pain, which suggests a possible environmental or genetic predisposition for developing pain (Chaturvedi 1987a; Hudson et al. 1985; Katon et al. 1985; Magni 1987; Violon and Giurgea 1984). Other studies suggest that depression is secondary to the pain (Atkinson et al. 1991; Brown 1990) or that these two problems may coexist either independently or as the result of a common psychological or neurochemical pathway (Feinmann 1985; Gamsa 1990; Magni 1987; von Knorring and Ekselius 1994). Pain is also a very common presenting symptom of depression and in fact may often be the only symptom (Simon et al. 1999). The relationship between pain and depression may be affected by variables such as age (Turk et al. 1995). As Magni et al. (1994) noted, all of the theories appear to have some validity, and currently the best conclusion seems to be that "depression promotes pain and pain promotes depression" (Magni et al. 1994, p. 289).

Certain forms of acute pain also appear to be frequently associated with other mental disorders. Beitman et al. (1988, 1989) observed that more than 30% of patients with chest pain and normal coronary arteries by cardiac catheterization met the criteria for panic disorder.

Assessment of Pain

Although physicians and health care professionals often seek to obtain evidence of the presence and severity of pain, in fact pain is a subjective experience for which there are no objective measures. The literature indicates that there is little correlation between the level of pain and physical findings. For example, Gore et al. (1987) reported that there was no relationship between radiological findings and the severity of neck pain experienced. In a study in which magnetic resonance imaging of the lumbar spine was performed on asymptomatic subjects, Jensen et al. (1994) found that 64% had at least one abnormal lumbar disk and 38% had two or more. It is estimated that a clear physiological etiology cannot be identified for as many as 85% of patients with isolated low-back pain (Deyo and Weinstein 2001).

Determining how much pain an individual patient should have requires the evaluation of multiple psychosocial factors that appear to influence the pain experience, including past pain, cultural factors, and family history of pain and mental disorders. Studies also suggest that the failure to identify underlying physical conditions etiologically related to the pain may result from these conditions' not having reached the threshold of clinical detection or may reflect deficiencies in the training of physicians in the diagnosis of pain-related conditions (Gunn and Sola 1989; Hendler et al. 1982; Rosomoff et al. 1989). Furthermore, many of the therapies used for pain—for example, medications, surgery, and extended periods of inactivity—can themselves cause or exacerbate pain, further obscuring the original etiology of the pain (Kouyanou 1997). Because mental health professionals usually do not evaluate patients with pain until long after its onset, if they evaluate such patients at all, these professionals are further handicapped in their attempts to assess the factors involved in the development of the pain.

Given that pain is a complex, subjective experience, its is not surprising that many different methods for assessing and measuring it have been developed (Acute Pain Management Guideline Panel 1992; Jacox et al. 1994; King 2000; Williams 1988; Table 23–3). The JCAHO guidelines on pain (Joint Commission on Accreditation of Health Care Organizations 2000) do not specify which assessment tools should be used in fulfilling its requirements. Although no single method has been found to be universally valid or reliable, the approaches described in the following paragraphs are among the most commonly used.

The simplest pain measurement is the Numerical Rating Scale (Scott and Huskisson 1976), in which the patient is asked to assign a numerical score to the pain. A typical scale ranges from 0 to 10, where "0" represents no pain and "10" represents the worst pain imaginable. A similar scale, the Visual Analog Scale (Scott and Huskisson 1976), requires the patient to mark a place on a 10-cm line, the ends of which are similarly labeled.

The McGill Pain Questionnaire permits a more in-depth analysis of the pain the patient is experiencing (Melzack 1975). The test lists 20 sets of words describing pain. These words are assigned to sensory, affective, and evaluative scales. The test can be scored based on the total number of words chosen or by the rank order of the words. Research indicates that patterns of response vary according to the type of pain experienced (Reading et al. 1982). The McGill Pain Questionnaire has been criticized for its reliance on language skills; results may reflect the patient's intelligence level, education, or cultural background.

TABLE 23–3. Commonly used instruments for assessing pain

Instrument	Description	Comments
Numerical Rating Scale	Patient rates pain on 0–10 scale	Simple to administer
Visual Analog Scale	Patient marks point on 10-cm line to identify level of pain	Simple to administer
McGill Pain Questionnaire	Patient identifies terms describing pain from 20 sets of words	Results may be affected by language skills
West Haven–Yale Multidimensional Pain Inventory	52-question instrument assessing various aspects of pain and its impact on patient's life	More complex to score and interpret
Faces Scale	Pictures of faces ranging from smiling to crying indicating level of discomfort	Simple to administer; useful for patients with limited language skills due to age (young children) or illness (older patients)
Psychological instruments (Minnesota Multiphasic Personality Inventory, Beck Depression Inventory)	Inquire about various aspects of patient's psychological and physical functioning	Results may be difficult to interpret in patients with physical illness

An alternative is the West Haven–Yale Multidimensional Pain Inventory, a 52-question instrument that measures the patient's perception of how others respond to his or her pain; participation in daily activities; and the effect of pain on the patient's overall lifestyle (Kerns et al. 1985).

Other, more traditional psychological testing instruments have also been used with pain patients, most notably the Minnesota Multiphasic Personality Inventory (MMPI; Hathaway and McKinley 1989). However, the validity of this and similar psychological instruments is controversial when these tests are applied to patients with physical ailments such as pain. For example, it was reported more than 40 years ago that patients whose back pain did not have an organic etiology were more likely to demonstrate a certain configuration on the MMPI, the so-called Conversion V or neurotic triad, in which elevations on the hypochondriasis and hysteria scales were believed to reflect the patient's concerns about his or her health (Hanvik 1951). A lower depression score suggested that the patient was indifferent to these concerns. Although some support for this view still remains, other research indicates that this configuration may actually reflect adjustment to chronic illness and can be found among patients with chronic health problems, whether or not there is an identifiable organic etiology (Naliboff et al. 1982; Watson 1982). Similarly, instruments to detect depression, such as the Beck Depression Inventory, may be overinclusive, because many items such as problems with sleep, appetite, and health are as likely to be related to the pain as to depression (Novy et al. 1995). The MMPI and other psychological instruments have at times also been used to determine whether patients who develop chronic pain are characterologically

prone to this problem, but studies have failed to reveal any marked evidence for this (Main et al. 1991).

To aid physicians in determining whether a patient's pain is of organic or psychological origin, Waddell et al. (1980) described five signs that they believed indicated that low-back pain was of nonorganic origin:

- Tenderness that is superficial or nonanatomic in distribution
- Pain brought on by movements that should not cause pain but are simulations of those that do
- The disappearance of positive physical findings when the patient is distracted
- Regional disturbances involving weakness or sensory deficits that are nonanatomic in origin
- Overreaction by the patient during the examination

However, the authors noted that these signs are subject to a range of interpretation on the part of the clinicians and may be invalid for certain connective-tissue disorders. Main and Waddell (1998) recommended that these signs be taken as "yellow flags" signaling the possible involvement of psychological issues and not as final determinants as to the presence or absence of physical disorders.

Because pain can be influenced by such a wide variety of factors, the concept of *illness behavior* has been found by some to be useful (Mechanic 1962; Pilowsky 1968). Criteria included in illness behavior are

- Pain perception
- Decision making regarding whether to seek treatment and from whom to seek such treatment

- The meaning of the pain to the patient
- The manner in which the patient communicates about pain
- The effect pain has on the patient's functioning

Among the factors that affect illness behavior are cultural background, socioeconomic status, psychological functioning, experiences, memory, and learning.

Although the concept of illness behavior has been more frequently applied to chronic pain, extensive evidence indicates that some of these factors also play a major role in acute pain. In a pioneering study, Beecher (1946) observed that soldiers severely wounded in battle often did not complain of pain or described pain of a level far below that which would be expected. He postulated that this may have reflected the relief felt by the soldiers, who realized that they would be removed from the battlefield and their lives would no longer be endangered. Conversely, stressful life events may contribute to the development of chronic pain (Atkinson et al. 1988).

A person's knowledge of and expectations regarding a potentially painful insult to the body have also been demonstrated to alter patient response. Egbert et al. (1964) found that preoperative psychological preparation of the patient can have a profound influence on postsurgical recovery, including the degree of pain experienced.

The Problem of Pain in Special Populations

Because pain is a subjective problem, physicians must rely on patient self-report. However, in groups in which verbal skills may be diminished, most notably very young and elderly populations, this does not suffice. Unfortunately, failure to recognize this has resulted in the undertreatment of pain for both these groups. Furthermore, because these patients are often unable to complain of pain, myths have developed that they feel less pain than do nongeriatric adults (Acute Pain Management Guideline Panel 1992). Physicians who are caring for these patients must be especially vigilant for signs that the patients are in pain, and they must use their experience to identify conditions and procedures that are likely to cause pain and treat it appropriately (American Geriatrics Society Panel on Chronic Pain in Older Persons 1998; Cummings et al. 1996; Sengstaken and King 1993). Assessment of pain may at times require the use of different tools—for example, the substitution of non-verbal scales of pain measurement, such as one employing faces ranging from happy to sad, developed for small children in place of the Numerical Rating and Visual Analog Scales (Hunter et al. 2000). The recommendations for pain management in these two groups are similar to those for nongeriatric adults, although extra caution must be taken when providing medications to children and geriatric patients.

The care of the terminally ill is an issue that has received increasing attention as a result of the recent ongoing debate over physician-assisted suicide. Although there is a tendency for psychiatrists to focus on depression experienced by many terminally ill patients, it is important to remember that a large number of these patients also experience severe pain, which is often poorly managed (Jacox et al. 1994). The presence of depression and pain appear to increase the likelihood that a patient will request physician-assisted suicide, and both problems need to be addressed (Foley 1997). Unfortunately, although psychiatrists accept the importance of their role in evaluating and treating depression among the terminally ill, they may consider pain management to be better handled by other physicians, whom they believe undergo more extensive training in this field. However, it is important to note that physicians in general, including those in primary care, also tend to receive limited training in pain during their postgraduate education (Sengstaken and King 1994).

Effect of Litigation

Because many patients with chronic pain have developed the problem as the result of an injury, and because we live in an increasingly litigious society, psychiatrists who evaluate and treat such patients must be aware of the potential effects that involvement in the judicial system may have on the patient and his or her pain. When there is financial gain from having pain, the possibility of malingering is often paramount; however, concerns about this possibility are overstated. Patients may exaggerate symptoms and the extent of disability to attain secondary gains, but such exaggerations usually occur after the presence of the illness that initiated the pain is established. Actual falsification of pain and injury appears to be infrequent. The Report of the Commission on the Evaluation of Pain (1987) found that malingering was a rare problem in the Social Security Administration's disability system. Leavitt and Sweet (1986) similarly found malingering to be rare in individuals complaining of low-back pain.

Studies have both supported and rejected the detrimental effects of litigation and involvement in workers' compensation systems on chronic pain. In their review,

Osterweis et al. (1987) reported that the only consistent finding among these patients was that those who were employed at the outset of treatment appeared to do better. Unfortunately, involvement in the legal system may promote inactivity, which in turn can exacerbate pain and make it even more difficult for patients to return to their preinjury lifestyles. For example, in some situations, patients may find it more financially lucrative not to return to work. Even when patients desire to increase their activity levels, they may be fearful that this will demonstrate that they are not in pain and they will therefore lose benefits that are needed and are due. Patients in this situation often feel torn with regard to which of the possibly conflicting recommendations of physicians, friends, relatives, and lawyers to accept. Physicians who treat patients with chronic pain must be cognizant of this potential conflict and must make their patients aware that it is the individual's well-being that is of utmost importance.

Management of Pain

Although acute and chronic pain are often managed with similar therapeutic modalities, there are important differences in how these two types are approached and in the goals that the treating clinician should try to accomplish.

No method of differentiating acute pain from chronic pain has yet received universal acceptance. In its classification system, the Task Force on Taxonomy of the International Association for the Study of Pain recommends a criterion of 3 months' duration for chronic pain (Merskey and Bogduk 1994). Others suggest that the term *chronic pain* not be defined by any specific time limit but rather be used when the pain lasts beyond the expected period for its resolution (Brena et al. 1984). However, in the literature, the criterion most frequently employed is pain with a duration of 6 months or longer, and this is the criterion included in DSM-IV-TR.

Approaches to Management

Acute Pain

The goal of treatment for acute pain is primarily to relieve the pain. Although the methods for effectively treating most cases of this form of pain appear to be available, it is often undertreated. Marks and Sachar (1973) found that of 37 medical inpatients being treated for pain with narcotic analgesics, 32% were continuing to experience severe distress and another 41% experienced moderate distress, despite the medication regimen. The

authors observed that misconceptions among physicians about the pharmacokinetics of these medications and concern about the potential for addiction were major factors in the physicians' failing to address adequately their patients' pain. Unfortunately, other studies indicate that problems with undertreatment have continued (Abbott et al. 1992; Choiniere et al. 1990; Melzack et al. 1987; Owen et al. 1990). Notwithstanding physicians' concerns about starting a patient on the road to addiction by treating acute pain with opioid analgesics, the potential for developing iatrogenic opioid dependence after being prescribed one of these medications for acute pain appears to be quite low.

Although the management of postoperative and other forms of acute pain will usually be provided by surgeons, anesthesiologists, and other physicians directly involved in the care of the patient, psychiatrists should be aware that there is much they can contribute to the care of patients with pain. The Acute Pain Management Guideline Panel (1992) highlighted the importance of employing cognitive and behaviorally based interventions such as relaxation, imagery, biofeedback, and education and instruction in the management of postoperative and other acute pain. However, many nonpsychiatric physicians involved in caring for patients with these forms of pain may lack the training and experience psychiatrists have that are needed to provide these therapeutic modalities.

Guidelines for the psychiatric approach to acute pain are presented in Table 23–4.

TABLE 23–4. Guidelines for the psychiatric approach to acute pain

1. In acute pain, the primary goal is to alleviate the pain as much as possible.
2. Although the appropriate use of analgesic medications is the mainstay of the effective management of acute pain, psychologically based interventions are also efficacious and should be employed.
3. The pain and the effectiveness of the therapeutic modalities being used to treat it should be frequently assessed.
4. Problems for which psychiatric consultations are often obtained on patients with acute pain, such as anxiety, depression, and problems coping with the illness, may reflect poor pain management.
5. When acute pain is accompanied by other mental disorders, relief of the pain may improve the mental state of the patient.
6. Be aware of the special issues that may be encountered in the management of acute pain. For example, patients with cancer pain may develop suicidal ideation.
7. Opioid analgesics may be safely used for the management of acute pain with minimal risk of abuse or dependence.

Chronic Pain

In treating chronic pain, it is important to address functioning as well as the pain. The goal of treatment should be to manage the pain as opposed to curing it. In many cases, this requires refocusing the patient away from the pain. In essence, patients with chronic pain must wrest control of their lives back from the pain. Much of the benefit from the use of the psychologically based treatment modalities may relate more to their effect on the patient as a whole than to directly reducing the pain itself. In a meta-analysis of 109 studies of psychological treatments for pain, Malone and Strube (1988) found that these therapies had a greater effect on mood and the number of subjective symptoms than on the frequency, intensity, and duration of pain.

Although only a small percentage of patients with acute pain develop chronic pain, it is still unclear who these individuals are and whether there is any way to predict long-term disability. The literature supports the importance of psychosocial factors rather than organic variables in determining whether a person will recover from his or her pain (Dworkin et al. 1985; Osterweis et al. 1987).

In approaching the patient with chronic pain, the psychiatrist faces a number of obstacles. Unfortunately, many patients with this problem tend to view referrals to psychiatrists and other mental health practitioners negatively. They fear that such referrals may indicate that their treating physicians do not believe that the pain is "real." Furthermore, many patients with this problem believe that the physicians, in making such referrals, are giving up and that acceptance of the referrals forces patients to acquiesce to this condition. As Blumer and Heilbronn (1987) noted, "The chronic pain sufferer argues that he or she has no mental problem and needs no psychiatric intervention, that the only real problem is the pain and that the doctors better find out what is wrong where it hurts" (p. 216). To help these patients, psychiatrists must recognize and address these concerns.

Many colleagues of psychiatrists may also mistakenly assume that psychiatrists have a role to play only when there is no organic pathology and may ask them to help determine whether the pain is real. Psychiatrists who are called on to settle this question might consider the following reply: "Pain occurring in unicorns, griffins and jabberwockies is always imaginary pain, since these are imaginary animals; patients, on the other hand are real, and so they always have real pain" (Sapira 1976, p. 116).

By the time patients with chronic pain are referred to psychiatrists, they often feel frustrated and abused by the health care system. Furthermore, if the pain is the result of an accident involving litigation, the patient has the additional problem of coping with the judicial system. In many cases, the specific form of therapy chosen may be less important than the therapist's willingness to display empathy and understanding and to set realistic goals for treatment. Unfortunately, modern Western medicine has, to a great degree, emphasized therapies that are performed on patients—rather than recognized that for many problems it is what patients do for themselves, not what is done to them, that is the most effective. This is especially true for chronic pain.

One of the obstacles that must frequently be overcome in cases of chronic pain is the common fears that the pain indicates the presence of a severe underlying condition that must be detected and that an increase in activity will exacerbate rather than improve the pain. Patients who manage to avoid or conquer these concerns tend to do better than those who retain them (Jensen et al. 1991).

Guidelines for the psychiatric approach to chronic pain are presented in Table 23–5.

Psychologically Based Modalities

Psychologically based treatment approaches are considered to be a vital part of pain management programs (Fordyce et al. 1985). A wide variety of psychotherapies have been reported to be beneficial for pain, including many forms of individual, group, and family therapy. The most commonly used approaches fall into two major categories: 1) operant conditioning and 2) cognitive-behavioral therapies, including biofeedback, relaxation training, and hypnosis (Table 23–6). Each of these is more fully described elsewhere in this book; the following is a brief overview of their specific application to pain.

Operant conditioning is based on the concept that certain operant or learned behaviors develop in response to environmental cues. Common examples among pain patients include complaints of pain and reluctance to indulge in certain activities. The anticipated response to pain is often receipt of medication and being excused from work or normal daily tasks. The goal of operant conditioning is to reinforce the positive or "healthy" behaviors and to diminish the destructive behaviors that maintain the patient's pain.

Cognitive-behavioral therapy involves identifying and correcting the patient's distorted attitudes, beliefs, and expectations. The goal of this therapy is, first, to make the patient more aware of factors that exacerbate and diminish the pain and, second, to cause the patient therefore to modify behavior accordingly. A variety of thera-

TABLE 23–5. Guidelines for the psychiatric approach to chronic pain

1. The focus of the management of chronic pain should be on improving function rather than on alleviating pain.
2. Unless there is clear evidence that the patient is malingering, accept that the reported pain is present.
3. When evaluating patients with chronic pain, explain that psychiatrists' involvement in their care in no way suggests that they do not have "real" pain or that the pain is "all in their head."
4. To determine an appropriate treatment plan, attempt to discern the roles that psychological factors and a general medical condition are playing in the onset and maintenance of the pain. Be aware that even when a general medical condition is playing a major role in the pain, psychologically based therapeutic approaches are often efficacious.
5. Because psychosocial factors often determine the responses of patients with chronic pain to many therapeutic modalities, psychiatrists should endeavor to assist their nonpsychiatric physician colleagues in evaluating these patients before treatment plans are created.
6. Recognize that pain is often comorbid with other mental disorders. The pain may be a symptom of these mental disorders, lead to them, or coexist with them.
7. Be aware that the effective management of chronic pain often depends on the willingness and ability of patients with this problem to learn and practice strategies that will assist them in coping with their pain.
8. Be supportive. Patients with chronic pain often feel angry and frustrated about many issues, including interactions with the health care and legal systems.
9. Avoid therapeutic modalities such as the extended use of benzodiazepines or opioid analgesics that may worsen the patient's problems.

peutic modalities may be used to achieve this. In biofeedback, electronic equipment is employed to measure certain physiological functions of which the patient is usually unaware and to convey this information to the patient. One example of such physiological parameters is muscle tension. The patient may be instructed in specific relaxation techniques or be encouraged to achieve certain goals involving the biofeedback equipment, such as lowering the pitch of a tone.

A wide variety of relaxation techniques can be taught to patients. Among the most common methods is progressive muscle relaxation, in which the patient learns to relax different muscle groups by contracting and then relaxing each one (Jacobson 1970).

Although the exact nature of hypnosis and the associated trance remains the subject of debate, a British Medical Association (1955) report offered the following apt description:

A temporary condition of altered attention in the subject which may be induced by another person and in which a variety of phenomena may appear spontaneously or in response to verbal or other stimuli. These phenomena included alterations in consciousness and memory, increased susceptibility to suggestion, and the production in the subject of responses and ideas unfamiliar to him in his usual state of mind. Further, phenomena such as anesthesia, paralysis and rigidity of muscles, and vasomotor changes can be produced and removed in the hypnotic state. (p. 191)

Although hypnosis involves relaxation, its efficacy in the treatment of pain extends beyond this. Patients can be taught to reduce pain through hypnotic suggestions such as forming a visual image of the pain and changing it or dissociating the painful part from the rest of the body. The benefits of hypnosis for acute pain are well documented, but, unfortunately, support for its efficacy in chronic pain is based primarily on anecdotal evidence (Hilgard and Hilgard 1983).

The application of each of these techniques to the management of pain has been studied to varying degrees, and controversy still remains concerning which approach is most efficacious. However, research suggests certain general guidelines regarding how each is best used. Through reviews of the literature, Turner and Chapman (1982a, 1982b) and Linton (1986) found that operant therapy is especially useful in decreasing patients' medication use and increasing their activity levels. In contrast, cognitive-behavioral therapy was observed to be helpful in reducing pain complaints. Biofeedback was found to be of benefit in certain pain conditions, especially tension and migraine headaches, but was discovered overall to be inferior or at best equal to relaxation therapy, which appears to be efficacious in the treatment of a wide variety of both acute and chronic pain conditions.

Each of these therapies may be employed when pain is the primary problem. However, when pain is the symptom of a mental disorder, that disorder should be addressed: appropriate treatment with psychotherapy and/or psychotropic medications must be initiated.

One additional method of treatment, the efficacy and actions of which are controversial, is the use of placebo. Research indicates that placebos can have a definite analgesic effect on a variety of painful conditions, including those in which there is an identifiable organic etiology (Turner et al. 1994).

Pharmacological Management of Pain

Opioid Analgesics

Although opioid analgesics play a primary role in the management of acute pain and the pain associated with

TABLE 23–6. Psychologically based treatments of pain

Type of treatment	Description	Comments
Operant conditioning	Based on reinforcing positive behaviors and diminishing destructive behaviors that are formed in response to environmental cues	May be helpful for reducing medication use and improving activity level
Cognitive-behavioral therapy	Based on identifying and correcting distorted attitudes, beliefs, and expectations	May be helpful for reducing level of pain complaints and coping with pain
Relaxation techniques	Various techniques for helping patients cope with stress	Easy to learn and employ
Biofeedback	Patient learns to affect physiological parameters through use of electronic instrumentation	Some patients may find the techniques difficult to employ when not using the instrumentation; may result in patient overfocusing on physiological parameters
Hypnosis	Involves relaxation, increased suggestibility, and dissociation	Can provide significant pain relief; some patients may resist receiving this therapy out of invalid fears that they will lose control of their behavior

cancer, the prescribing of opioid analgesics for patients with chronic noncancer pain continues to be the subject of controversy.

There still appears to be widespread concern among physicians that prescribing opioids to patients with chronic pain will result in the institution of sanctions by state and federal authorities, although scant evidence exists to support this view. In an attempt to allay physicians' fears in this regard, the Federation of State Medical Boards of the United States in 1998 issued model guidelines on the use of controlled substances for the management of pain. A majority of state medical boards in the United States have adopted these guidelines either totally or in part. The guidelines highlight the importance of offering patients appropriate treatment for pain: "Physicians should not fear disciplinary action from the Board or other state regulatory or enforcement agency for prescribing, dispensing, or administering controlled substances, including opioid analgesics for a legitimate medical purpose and in the usual course of professional practice" (Federation of State Medical Boards of the United States 1998, p. 2). The concern held by many physicians that an investigation will automatically be instituted if they administer or prescribe high doses of opioids for chronic pain is also addressed in the guidelines' statement that judgment regarding "the validity of prescribing [will be] based on the physician's treatment of the patient and on available documentation, rather than on the quantity and chronicity of prescribing" (p. 2). It is recommended that physicians who prescribe opioids should become familiar with their own state regulations.

Studies have shown that these medications can be safely prescribed and are effective for chronic nonmalignant pain (Portenoy 1994; Zenz et al. 1992). Furthermore, there is evidence that many painful conditions are undertreated and mismanaged because of physicians' concerns about the use of these drugs. However, physicians must also be aware that these medications are subject to abuse and can have potentially life-shattering side effects, the most notable being the development of psychological dependence. Other potential problems must also be considered. Because patients can obtain medications from multiple sources, it may be difficult to determine whether they are being honest about their drug use.

The number of chronic patients who will abuse or develop psychological dependence on opioids prescribed for pain remains unclear. One of the most-cited references on the limited risk of the development of opioid abuse and addiction continues to be a letter published by Porter and Jick in 1980. The authors reported that of 11,882 patients who received at least one dose of an opioid analgesic during hospitalization, only 4 who did not have previous history of addiction developed this problem. However, no breakdown was provided to as to the types of pain experienced by the patients described, and one might assume that many, if not most, of the patients studied suffered postoperative or other posttraumatic pain or pain related to a terminal illness, rather than chronic pain. In contrast, a study by Bouckoms et al. (1992) of 59 patients with chronic pain and no detectable history of substance abuse or dependence disorder who were followed for an average of 36 months found that 27% abused these medications and 24% developed addiction. The authors were unable to identify any predictive factors for those who developed these problems. Hoffman et al. (1995), in a study of 414 chronic pain patients, reported that 12.6% had current psychological dependence on opioid analgesics and 2.9% were in remission for this problem. The results of these studies should in no way be interpreted as supporting a restriction of opioid use. Rather, they should make health care professionals aware that a substantial number of patients may develop problems with these medications when they are prescribed for pain and that vigilance in watching for such problems is therefore essential.

The best recommendation is to consider the prescription of opioid analgesics for chronic pain on a case-by-case basis, with close monitoring of patients and continuous scrutiny for signs of abuse. Clearly, the use of these medications for chronic pain should be limited to patients for whom objective benefits of treatment, such as an increase in activity levels or a return to or continuation of employment, can be observed. Physicians should be hesitant to prescribe these medications when the only sign of improvement is a reduction in pain without any other concurrent changes that would support the validity of this self-report.

Psychiatrists may at times be asked by their physician colleagues for help in assessing whether a patient is abusing an opioid analgesic. Because most physicians receive scant training in the problems of drug abuse and dependence and their management, it falls to psychiatrists to possess the appropriate knowledge. Perhaps of most importance is understanding what is meant by the DSM-IV-TR terms *dependence* and *abuse* and by the commonly employed term *addiction*. It is vital to recognize that these words refer to psychological states that differ from physical dependence and tolerance. The latter two are the result of the pharmacological properties of medications and appear to occur in any patient who takes an opioid at a high enough dose for a long enough period. *Physical dependence* reflects the withdrawal states that will occur if these medications are discontinued or their dosage is markedly reduced without tapering. *Tolerance* refers to the requirement for increasing doses of an opioid over time in order to receive the same degree of analgesia (American Society of Addiction Medicine 1998). Unfortunately, failure to understand these terms may result in unnecessary suffering. Patients who are undertreated for their pain and who express desire for more effective pain management may be mislabeled as being drug dependent, a problem that has been termed *pseudoaddiction* (Weissman and Haddox 1989).

In the treatment of patients who are receiving opioid analgesics, the recognition of withdrawal syndromes is vital. The DSM-IV-TR criteria for opioid withdrawal are shown in Table 23–7.

When opioid analgesics are being considered, the following guidelines should be employed (Table 23–8).

TABLE 23–7. DSM-IV-TR diagnostic criteria for opioid withdrawal.

A. Either of the following:
   (1) cessation of (or reduction in) opioid use that has been heavy and prolonged (several weeks or longer)
   (2) administration of an opioid antagonist after a period of opioid use
B. Three (or more) of the following, developing within minutes to several days after Criterion A:
   (1) dysphoric mood
   (2) nausea or vomiting
   (3) muscle aches
   (4) lacrimation or rhinorrhea
   (5) pupillary dilation, piloerection, or sweating
   (6) diarrhea
   (7) yawning
   (8) fever
   (9) insomnia
C. The symptoms in Criterion B cause clinically significant distress or impairment in social, occupational, or other important areas of functioning.
D. The symptoms are not due to a general medical condition and are not better accounted for by another mental disorder.

Guideline 1. In the case of mild to moderate postoperative and other acute pain, a nonsteroidal anti-inflammatory drug (NSAID) or acetaminophen should be used. More severe acute pain should be treated with an opioid analgesic. Treatment for cancer-related and chronic noncancer pain should begin with nonopioid analgesics, such as the NSAIDs and tricyclic antidepressants (TCAs), and other forms of pain management. The World Health Organization Expert Committee (1990) recommends a stepwise approach starting with nonopioid analgesics, with the addition of opioid analgesics if pain is not controlled. Even if the nonopioid analgesics are insufficient for pain relief, they should be continued after the introduction of an opioid. By providing analgesia via mechanisms different from the opioids, they may enable analgesia to be attained at a lower dosage of the opioid than would be required if it were used alone. Furthermore, it appears that both NSAIDs and TCAs may bolster the analgesic effects of opioids, thus allowing them to be administered at a lower dosage that will result in a reduction in frequency and severity of opioid-related side effects.

Guideline 2. Acute pain may initially require treatment with a stronger opioid analgesic such as morphine or hydromorphone. When treatment with opioid analgesics is initiated for cancer-related and chronic noncancer

TABLE 23–8. Guidelines for the use of opioid analgesics

1. Opioid analgesics may be used as the initial treatment for more severe acute pain conditions. In the case of cancer-related and chronic noncancer pain, initiate treatment with nonopioid analgesics (e.g., nonsteroidal anti-inflammatory drugs and tricyclic antidepressants) and other forms of pain management before employing opioid analgesics. Even if the addition of opioids is required, these other therapeutic modalities should be continued if they are providing analgesia.
2. In the case of acute pain, a stronger opioid may be initially required. Treatment for cancer-related and chronic noncancer pain should begin with the milder opioid analgesics such as codeine, oxycodone, and hydrocodone rather than the more potent ones.
3. Prescribe on a fixed schedule rather than on an "as needed" (prn) basis.
4. Unless a patient is unable to take medications in oral form, administer medications orally rather than parenterally.
5. Be aware of the available routes of administration and the potential side effects associated with these medications.

pain, the milder medications, such as codeine, oxycodone, and hydrocodone, should be tried first. If these are insufficient, the stronger narcotics, including morphine, methadone, fentanyl, and hydromorphone, should be considered. All of the opioids just mentioned are μ opioid receptor agonists. The other basic class of opioid analgesics consists of the mixed agonist–antagonists, which bind at the κ opioid receptors and block μ opioid receptors, and the partial agonists, which bind selectively at the μ receptors. Although it has been reported that this second group of medications may have less potential for abuse than do the μ receptor agonists, they do not appear to offer any marked benefit and they have the potential to create additional problems. Patients who take a mixed agonist–antagonist after receiving pure agonists may develop withdrawal. Furthermore, pentazocine, a commonly used mixed agonist–antagonist, can cause psychotomimetic effects, including hallucinations. The use of mixed agonist–antagonists is therefore not generally recommended. However, the mixed agonist–antagonist butorphanol is available in a nasal spray and thus is suitable for patients who require an opioid but are temporarily unable to take one by mouth because of nausea and vomiting (e.g., patients with severe migraine headaches).

μ Opioid analgesics also have individual properties that affect their efficacy. Several commonly used opioids are metabolized to their analgesic forms by the hepatic cytochrome P450 (CYP) 2D6 enzyme system (Virani et al. 1997). Codeine is metabolized to morphine by this system, as are oxycodone to oxymorphone and hydrocodone to hydromorphone. In the case of a patient who is prescribed a medication that may inhibit this system, such as some of the selective serotonin reuptake inhibitor (SSRI) antidepressants, the analgesic effects of these medications may be markedly reduced. The opioid in tramadol also is metabolized to its active form by this system.

Codeine, oxycodone, and hydrocodone are usually given in combination with acetaminophen. Over time, patients may develop tolerance to the analgesic effects of the opioids but not to the potential hepatic toxic effects of acetaminophen. Thus, if patients will require one of these medications for an extended period, providing codeine or oxycodone alone (hydrocodone is only available in combination with other medications) should be considered. This allows for separate prescription and dose titration of acetaminophen or an NSAID.

When methadone is used, it must be given three or four times a day to be effective, because its duration of analgesia is shorter than its half-life. Also because of its long half-life, methadone may take 2–3 days before it provides effective analgesia. Therefore, another opioid analgesic should be provided for breakthrough pain during this period. The clinician should also be aware that because in the United States methadone is strongly associated with drug addiction, it is imperative that when the drug is prescribed for pain, the patient be made aware that it is being employed for its analgesic effects.

Meperidine is a strong opioid analgesic that is used in a variety of pain settings. Although the drug is an effective treatment for acute pain, the Acute Pain Management Guideline Panel (1992) stated that it is overused even for this indication and that other opioid analgesics are more effective. The extended use of meperidine (i.e., for more than 2–3 days) is contraindicated because repeated dosing may result in the accumulation of the toxic metabolite normeperidine, a cerebral irritant that can cause problems ranging from marked anxiety to convulsions. The oral bioavailability of meperidine is also poor, necessitating the switch to an alternative analgesic when parenteral administration is no longer required. Psychiatrists should know that, apparently alone among the opioid analgesics, meperidine can have a lethal interaction with monoamine oxidase inhibitors (MAOIs) (Browne and Lintner 1987) and increase the risk of postoperative delirium (Marcantonio et al. 1994).

Tramadol (Ultram) is a unique medication that combines a weak μ opioid receptor agonist (1/6,000 the potency of morphine) with a weak inhibitor of norepinephrine and serotonin (5-hydroxytryptamine [5-HT]) reuptake ("Tramadol" 1995). The analgesic effect of this medication appears to be primarily related to this latter effect (i.e., inhibition of norepinephrine and 5-HT) rather than to its opioid actions. This is why the analgesic effect of tramadol is only minimally reduced if a CYP 2D6 inhibitor is prescribed with it. Tramadol has been reported to be beneficial for both acute and chronic pain, although in the United States it is currently available only in oral form, which somewhat limits its usefulness in certain cases of acute pain. Because of tramadol's weak μ opioid receptor affinity, it has been suggested that tolerance for, dependence on, and abuse of this agent are less likely than for other opioids. The recommended oral dose is 50–100 mg every 4–6 hours up to 200 mg/day.

Recommended starting and equianalgesic doses of the opioid analgesics are listed in Table 23–9. However, when switching from one opioid to another, it is important to remember that because of the presence of multiple opioid receptors, there is only partial cross-tolerance between these medications (Bruera et al. 1996). Thus, the table should be considered a general guide; the exact dosages administered should be determined on a case-by-case basis according to the status of the individual patient.

TABLE 23–9. Opioid analgesics: recommended starting and equianalgesic doses

Drug (trade name)	Approximate equianalgesic oral dose	Approximate equianalgesic parenteral dose	Recommended starting dose	
			Oral	Parenteral
μ Opioid agonist				
Morphine	30 mg q 3–4 hr (around-the-clock dosing); 60 mg q 3–4 hr (single dose or intermittent dosing)	10 mg q 3–4 hr	30 mg q 3–4 hr	10 mg q 3–4 hr
Sustained-release morphine (MS Contin, Oramorph, Kadian)	60 mg q 12 hr	Not available	30 mg q 12 hr	Not available
Methadone	20 mg q 6–8 hr	10 mg q 6–8 hr	20 mg q 6–8 hr	10 mg q 6–8 hr
Transdermal fentanyl (Duragesic)		25 μg q hr		25 μg q hr (via transdermal patch)
Transmucosal fentanyl (Actiq)	200 μg q hr		200 μg q hr (via transmucosal absorption)	
Hydromorphone (Dilaudid)	7.5 mg q 3–4 hr	1.5 mg q 3–4 hr	6 mg q 3–4 hr	1.5 mg q 3–4 hr
Meperidine (Demerol)	300 mg q 2–3 hr	100 mg q 3 hr	Not recommended	100 mg q 3 hr
Codeine	130 mg q 3–4 hr	75 mg q 3–4 hr	60 mg q 3–4 hr	60 mg q 2 hr (intramuscular/subcutaneous)
Oxycodone (Percodan, Percocet, Tylox) and hydrocodone (Vicodin, Lortab)	30 mg q 3–4 hr	Not available	10 mg q 3–4 hr	Not available
Sustained-release oxycodone (OxyContin)	30 mg q 12 hr	Not available	10 mg q 12 hr	Not available
Propoxyphene (Darvon-N, Darvocet-N)	250 mg q 3–4 hr	Not available	200 mg q 3–4 hr	Not available
Opioid agonist–antagonist and partial agonist				
Buprenorphine (Buprenex)	Not available	0.3–0.4 mg q 6–8 hr	Not available	0.4 mg q 6–8 hr
Butorphanol (Stadol)	Not available	2 mg q 3–4 hr	Not available	2 mg q 3–4 hr
Nalbuphine (Nubain)	Not available	10 mg q 3–4 hr	Not available	10 mg q 3–4 hr
Pentazocine (Talwin)	150 mg q 3–4 hr	60 mg q 3–4 hr	50 mg q 3–4 hr	Not recommended

Source. Adapted from Jacox et al. 1994.

Guideline 3. The medications should be given on a fixed schedule rather than as needed (prn). When a fixed schedule is employed, better analgesia is often provided. Also, the patient is freed from the multitude of decisions that prn dosing engenders. The patient does not have to decide whether the pain is sufficient to warrant taking the medication, whether to take it as the pain is beginning or to wait until it becomes unbearable, or whether to delay taking it so that it will remain available. Unfortunately, these decisions tend to focus the patient's mind on the pain rather than away from it—the opposite of what is desired in the management of most cases of pain.

In patients requiring more than two doses a day of a short-acting opioid who will need to be on an opioid for more than a few days, the use of a long-acting opioid—such as slow-release forms of oxycodone (OxyContin) and morphine (MS Contin, Kadian, Oramorph), methadone, or transdermal fentanyl (Duragesic)—should be considered. These medications need to be taken less often and provide more stable analgesia than do the shorter-acting forms.

Patient-controlled analgesic (PCA) devices commonly combine a baseline fixed-schedule infusion of opioids with prn dosing. These devices have received widespread acceptance for the management of postoperative pain. However, there is currently no substantial evidence that this method provides better analgesia than fixed-schedule dosing alone.

Guideline 4. Physicians who prescribe opioid analgesics should be aware of the various ways they can be administered and of the potential side effects associated with them. Routes of administration for these medications include orally; intramuscularly; intravenously, either by bolus, continuous infusion, or pumps such as PCA devices; rectally; by epidural or intrathecal infusion; transdermally; and by nasal spray.

Fentanyl is available in two forms not currently available for other opioids: transdermal and transmucosal. Fentanyl administered by a transdermal patch (Duragesic) may provide a useful alternative to other forms of parenteral administration in patients who are unable to ingest oral medications. Because the patches need be changed only at 72-hour intervals and are easily applied, this method of opioid administration may be especially beneficial for outpatients. However, in general, because oral administration is the simplest and usually the least expensive, oral preparations are preferred unless the patient is unable to tolerate them or this method of administration has ceased to be effective. Transmucosal fentanyl citrate is provided as a lozenge on a stick (Actiq). At present, the transmucosal preparation is indicated only in the management of breakthrough pain in cancer patients who are using moderate to high doses of a strong opioid such as morphine or transdermal fentanyl.

A major advantage of parenteral administration of an opioid is more rapid onset of peak analgesia. For most of the opioids, the peak is reached at 30 minutes to 1 hour when the medication is given parenterally, compared with 1 to 2 hours when provided orally. However, this becomes a less important factor when the medication is provided on a fixed schedule. Furthermore, parenteral administration often results in a 1- to 2-hour reduction in the duration of analgesia when compared with oral administration (4–6 hours versus 4–7 hours).

Guideline 5. The side effects most commonly associated with the opioid analgesics are constipation, nausea and vomiting, and sedation. Treatment with stool softeners (e.g., docusate) and a large-bowel stimulant laxative (e.g., senna) should be initiated prophylactically to prevent constipation. Nausea and vomiting can be treated with hydroxyzine or a phenothiazine antiemetic. Transdermal fentanyl has been associated with a lower incidence of marked gastrointestinal problems than other opioids. In patients with cancer who require high doses of opioids to control their pain, excessive sedation may be managed with a psychostimulant medication. Respiratory depression may develop with the administration of opioids and is the most frequent cause of mortality associated with this class of drugs. It may occur acutely as the result of an overdose, but in clinical situations it more commonly results from the gradual accumulation of the opioid.

Multiple protocols for detoxifying patients from opioid analgesics are available. The simplest method is a gradual tapering of the opioid being used. This is usually accomplished by placing the patient on a fixed schedule and then reducing the dose. Several factors should be considered in determining the appropriate schedule: the length of time the patient has been using the medication, the dose, the patient's desire for detoxification and willingness to cooperate with the process, and the degree of pain still being experienced. Generally, the dose of the opioids can be safely reduced by 10%–20% each day with minimal risk of withdrawal.

An alternative schedule, one that is especially useful when the patient is taking large doses of an opioid, is a substitution/detoxification schedule employing methadone. In this case, the equianalgesic dose of methadone is determined (see Table 23–9). The methadone is then provided on a four-times-a-day schedule. To avoid the necessity of waking the patient during the night, a schedule of 8:00 A.M., 12:00 P.M., 5:00 P.M., and 9:00 P.M. is often followed. The methadone dose is then reduced by 10%–20%

each day. Patient compliance may be improved by providing the methadone in a "pain cocktail" mixed with cherry syrup so that the patient is unaware of the amount of medication being taken. This method is commonly provided by inpatient pain management programs and, with the help of cooperative pharmacies, in outpatient settings. The methadone withdrawal protocol should not be employed for patients using mixed agonist–antagonist opioids.

Although detoxification can be performed quickly and safely, most patients with chronic pain require the institution of other forms of pain management to prevent relapse. Simply detoxifying such patients without addressing the reasons why they required an opioid analgesic in the first place may make physicians feel they have accomplished something but offers little long-term benefit for the patients.

Nonsteroidal Anti-Inflammatory Drugs

The NSAIDs and acetaminophen (Table 23–10) are effective analgesics for a wide range of pain conditions. NSAIDs are especially effective for the pain associated with bone metastases, one of the most common cancer-related pains.

The NSAIDs appear to exert their analgesic actions primarily through the inhibition of cyclooxygenase (COX) and, in turn, the synthesis of prostaglandins, although recent research indicates that NSAIDs may have also have a central nervous system effect. The mechanism by which acetaminophen provides analgesia is still unknown.

The process of deciding which NSAID to employ has changed substantially with the introduction of the COX-2 inhibitors. The rationale for use of these drugs lies in the separate functions of the two major COX systems. The COX-1 system is primarily involved in what are often called the body's "housekeeping chores"—for example, protection of the stomach lining and of renal and platelet function. The COX-2 system plays the major role in inflammation and (it is conjectured) in pain; it is this system that is specifically targeted by the COX-2 inhibitors. At the time of this writing, three COX-2 inhibitors were available in the United States: celecoxib (Celebrex), rofecoxib (Vioxx), and valdecoxib (Bextra). However, a number of others are currently in development and will no doubt be available in the near future. Although the primary advantage of the COX-2 inhibitors is that they appear less likely to cause gastrointestinal problems than the older NSAIDs, gastrointestinal complaints, including bleeding, are also the leading side effects related to the use of the COX-2 inhibitors (Hawkins and Hanks 2000). These medications have the additional advantages of not

TABLE 23–10. Nonsteroidal anti-inflammatory drugs and acetaminophen

Drug (trade name)	Usual adult dose
Oral	
Acetaminophen	650–975 mg q 4 hr
Aspirin	650–975 mg q 4 hr
Choline magnesium trisalicylate (Trilisate)	1,000–1,500 mg bid
Celecoxib (Celebrex)	100–200 mg q 12 hr
Diflunisal (Dolobid)	500 mg q 12 hr
Diclofenac sodium (Voltaren)	50 mg tid
Etodolac (Lodine)	200–400 mg q 4–6 hr
Fenoprofen calcium (Nalfon)	200 mg q 4–6 hr
Flurbiprofen (Ansaid)	50 mg q 4–6 hr
Ibuprofen (Motrin, Advil)	400 mg q 4–6 hr
Indomethacin (Indocin)	25–50 mg q 8 hr
Ketoprofen (Orudis)	25–75 mg q 6–8 hr
Magnesium salicylate	650 mg q 4 hr
Meclofenamate sodium (Meclomen)	50 mg q 4–6 hr
Mefenamic acid (Ponstel)	250 mg q 6 hr
Nabumetone (Relafen)	1,000 mg q 24 hr
Naproxen (Naprosyn)	250 mg q 6–8 hr
Naproxen sodium (Anaprox, Naprelan)	275 mg q 6–8 hr
Oxaprozin (Daypro)	1,200 mg q 24 hr
Piroxicam (Feldene)	20 mg q 24 hr
Rofecoxib (Vioxx)	25–50 mg q 24 hr
Salsalate (Disalcid)	500 mg q 4 hr
Sodium salicylate	325–650 mg q 3–4 hr
Sulindac (Clinoril)	200 mg q 12 hr
Valdecoxib (Bextra)	10 mg q 24 hr
Parenteral	
Ketorolac (Toradol)	30 or 60 mg im initial dose followed by 15 or 30 mg q 6 hr Oral dose following im dosage: 10 mg q 6–8 hr

Source. Adapted from Jacox et al. 1994.

affecting platelet functioning and of being less likely to precipitate renal toxicity in comparison with the older NSAIDs; however, COX-2 inhibitors are no more efficacious than the older agents. Many patients do not require a COX-2 inhibitor and can be safely treated with NSAIDs such as ibuprofen and naproxen, which, because they are available in over-the-counter preparations, are much less expensive than the COX-2 inhibitors (Peterson and Cryer 1999). If one NSAID is not beneficial after a 1- to 2-week period at a sufficient dose, an alternative should be considered.

Ketorolac, the first NSAID to be available in parenteral form in the United States, can be prescribed to patients who are unable to tolerate oral medications. In many cases, it also provides an effective alternative to opioid analgesics for the management of postoperative pain. However, because of its possible gastrointestinal side effects and its cost, ketorolac should be used for no more than 5 days parenterally and 14 days orally, and the oral form should be used only in patients being switched from the parenteral form. Acetaminophen has not traditionally been considered an NSAID, but it is an effective analgesic, and there is evidence to suggest that it may have an anti-inflammatory effect (Bradley et al. 1991).

Antidepressants

During the past 35 years, there has been an increase in evidence supporting the analgesic properties of antidepressant medications, most notably the TCAs, for both cancer pain and chronic nonmalignant pain. Although this effect was initially thought to be related to the antidepressant properties of these medications, substantial research indicates that they have separate analgesic effects unrelated to the emotional state of the patient.

The antidepressants appear to be efficacious for a wide range of painful conditions, including neuropathic pain, tension and migraine headaches (for which the drugs are used prophylactically), fibromyalgia, osteoarthritis and rheumatoid arthritis, and irritable bowel syndrome (Clouse 1994; King 1995; Max 1994; Saper 1997). The TCAs are considered first-line drugs for the treatment of pain related to neuropathies, including postherpetic neuralgia and diabetic neuropathy (Sindrup and Jensen 1999; Wiffen et al. 2000). It should be noted that although many physicians still consider opioids the most potent analgesics available, painful conditions involving injury to the nerves often respond poorly to these drugs.

How antidepressants exert their analgesic effect is unclear. The primary focus has been on their effects on serotonin and norepinephrine reuptake; and it appears that the medications that act on both neurotransmitters, such as the TCAs, are more effective than those that act only on serotonin (Max 1994). Other mechanisms of action that have been suggested include enhancement of endorphin secretion; effects on sodium channels; antihistaminic and anticholinergic effects; inhibition of substance P, a neuropeptide involved in pain transmission; and antagonism of N-methyl-D-aspartate (NMDA) receptors. It should be noted that these mechanisms are not mutually exclusive and may have varying importance depending on the specific pain conditions.

Although amitriptyline is still widely believed to be the TCA with the strongest analgesic effect, there is little literature to support this. All of the TCAs appear to be equally analgesic. The only advantage of amitriptyline appears to be its strong sedative effect, which may be beneficial for patients with chronic pain whose sleep is significantly impaired by the pain.

The few studies that have examined the analgesic effects of the SSRIs indicate that their analgesic properties are inferior to those of the TCAs and may not be markedly better than placebo (Smith 1998). Of the newer antidepressants, venlafaxine appears to be more promising as an analgesic than nefazodone, mirtazapine, or bupropion (Ansari 2000). The author considers extended-release venlafaxine (Effexor XR) to be the second-line antidepressant for analgesia for patients who are unable to tolerate TCAs or for whom these medications are contraindicated because of the presence of other medical conditions, such as cardiac disease.

Although the TCAs may exert their analgesic effects at lower dosage levels than are required for their antidepressant actions, analgesia appears to be dose related. A commonly repeated myth is that the ceiling dose for analgesia is 75 mg/day of amitriptyline or the equivalent. In fact, the literature indicates that the optimal analgesic dose is usually in the 100- to 150-mg range. The best way to initiate treatment for analgesia with a TCA is to start at a dose smaller than the usual initial dose for depression and then to increase the dose gradually until side effects, most commonly daytime sedation, develop. For example, for analgesia the initial dose of amitriptyline is 25 mg 1–2 hours before bedtime. The dose can be increased by 25 mg every third day until side effects develop. Because the duration of analgesia appears to be similar to that of the antidepressant effect, once-a-day dosing is often sufficient. However, some patients may obtain a better analgesic effect with divided doses. Although patients often show improvement after only a few days of treatment, as in the case of depression, the analgesic effects of the TCAs may take several weeks to develop. The optimal analgesic dose of extended-release venlafaxine has yet to be determined, but the author recommends trying to attain a dosage between 225 and 375 mg/day.

As in the treatment of depression, the recommended length of maintenance therapy with antidepressants for chronic pain varies from patient to patient. These medications carry a lower risk of side effects than other medications that are commonly used for chronic pain. Therefore, if a patient is doing well, these should be the last medications that are discontinued. Physicians should reassess the continuing need for an antidepressant every few months and should consider tapering and discontinuing the medication after the patient's condition has stabilized.

Anticonvulsants

The analgesic effects of anticonvulsants for neuropathic pain have long been known. The older anticonvulsants—phenytoin, carbamazepine, and sodium valproate—were reported to provide pain relief (McQuay et al. 1995). Of the newer anticonvulsants, gabapentin (Neurontin) has been the one most studied as an analgesic (Backonja 2000) and has the advantage of a more benign side effect profile than the older ones. Although gabapentin appears be efficacious for neuropathic pain, there is no evidence that it is better than or even as good as the TCAs for this problem. Gabapentin may exert its analgesic effects through calcium or sodium channel blockade or through enhancement of γ-aminobutyric acid (GABA) levels in the brain produced by increasing GABA synthesis and release (Ross 2000). The usual starting dose is 100 mg three times a day with eventual increase up to 3,600 mg/day. Other newer anticonvulsants—most notably topiramate (Topamax), oxcarbazepine (Trileptal), and lamotrigine (Lamictal)—also appear to provide analgesia for neuropathic pain. With regard to other specific pain syndromes, carbamazepine continues to be considered the most effective medication in the treatment of trigeminal neuralgia, and sodium valproate is beneficial in prophylactic treatment of migraine headaches.

Benzodiazepines

The use of benzodiazepines for patients with chronic pain is controversial. Benzodiazepines appear to provide little benefit for patients with chronic pain or cancer-related pain, and it is generally recommended that benzodiazepines be avoided when these conditions are present. Because of their GABAergic effects, benzodiazepines may actually exacerbate pain rather than reduce it (Dellemijn and Fields 1994), and they can interfere with the analgesic effects of opioids (Gear et al. 1997). Despite this, King and Strain (1990) found that benzodiazepines are often employed in the management of chronic pain. They also observed that patients' most frequently cited reason for taking these medications was that they improve sleep. Because of the additional analgesic effects provided by the TCAs, it is recommended that they be used to treat the insomnia that may accompany pain. When pain is accompanied by anxiety, the use of a benzodiazepine alternative, such as one of the antidepressants or buspirone, should be considered.

Selected Other Medications Used as Analgesics

Because so many different medications have been employed for pain, it is impossible to provide a comprehensive list here. The following selected medications are included because of their special interest to psychiatrists.

In addition to the antidepressants, other psychotropic medications also appear to have analgesic effects. Several of the neuroleptics, including haloperidol and chlorpromazine, have been reported to provide analgesia, most notably for neuropathic pain. However, methotrimeprazine, a phenothiazine, is the only neuroleptic that has been found in controlled studies to have analgesic effects (Monks 1990).

Lithium has been shown to be beneficial in cases of acute and cluster headaches. Therapeutic dosage is usually similar to that required when this medication is used to treat bipolar disorder.

The triptans are a new class of compounds that act on various 5-HT receptors. These agents, which include sumatriptan (Imitrex), zolmitriptan (Zomig), rizatriptan (Maxalt), and naratriptan (Amerge), are used for abortive treatment of migraine headaches.

Other Treatment Modalities

It is beyond the scope of this chapter to present a comprehensive review of the many therapies available for the treatment of acute and chronic pain. Readers who are interested in a more detailed discussion are referred to textbooks on pain (Loesser et al. 2000; Wall and Melzack 1999).

Among the other therapies found to be beneficial are various surgical interventions, nerve blocks, trigger point injections, acupuncture, physical therapy, and transcutaneous electrical nerve stimulation (TENS). The provision of each of these therapies requires clinicians with specific training and experience. As with the psychologically based modalities, support in the literature for the efficacy of each of these therapies is variable. The best recommendation is that in the absence of a medical emergency, conservative therapies be tried before more invasive ones such as nerve blocks and surgery. Therapeutic interventions such as physical therapy, acupuncture, and TENS carry little risk of side effects or of worsening the patient's pain. It has often been noted that there is a dearth of well-performed research supporting the efficacy of these treatments. However, this statement can be applied to most of the therapies used for chronic pain, including surgery. When any of the organic therapies are employed, they should be used in addition to, not in place of, the interventions that address the psychosocial aspects of the pain.

As the interest in pain has grown during the past quarter century, various forms of pain services, clinics, and treatment centers have been created. These vary from true multidisciplinary establishments to those offering single forms of treatment provided by one or more clinicians. Unfortunately, the type of therapy provided often is based less on what the patient needs than on what the clinician offers. Even when a truly multidisciplinary treatment team is present, the team may fail to recognize the differences between patients, and the clinicians may attempt a "one size fits all" treatment approach (Turk 1990). Patients appear to be much better served when a variety of modalities are available.

Because of the importance of improving the functioning of patients with chronic pain, the best multidisciplinary pain programs offer services that focus on this goal. Central to such programs are physical therapy, occupational therapy, and behaviorally oriented therapies. Although patients may prefer programs in which treatment is done *on* them, lasting improvement appears to depend on health care professionals' teaching patients how to cope with and manage their pain and patients' willingness to do this. Linton (1998) summarized characteristics of successful pain programs as follows:

> Firstly, they appear to take a multidimensional view of the problem. A major emphasis is placed on psychosocial aspects of the problem, e.g. the fear and worry involved. Secondly, a thorough, but "low-tech" examination is provided. Thirdly, after the examination, time is taken to communicate the results, e.g. why it hurts, and provide advice as to how the problem may be best managed. Fourthly, there is an emphasis on self-care, i.e. that the patient's behavior is an integral part in the recovery process. Pain management is a vital aspect, as pharmacological and nonpharmacological methods may be useful. Reducing the pain would also appear to lessen fear and other psychological factors that may fuel long-term problems. Fifthly, there is an attempt to reduce any unfounded fear or anxiety concerning the pain. Sixthly, the programs provide crystal clear recommendations concerning activities and in some cases help patients regain function by providing graded exercises. Lastly, what the programs do not [do] is medicalize the pain, e.g. by the indiscriminant use of high tech exams, referrals as a starting point, sick certificates of more than a few days, providing extensive prescriptions, or advising the patient to "take it easy" or go on bed rest. (pp. 166–167)

Conclusions

Both acute and chronic pain are major health problems. Although the methods for effectively treating most cases of pain are currently available, misconceptions about pain and ignorance of the principles of its management have resulted in needless suffering. Psychiatrists have much to contribute to the care of patients with pain, and it is hoped that they will take a leading role in this important field.

References

Abbott FV, Gray-Donald K, Sewitch MJ, et al: The prevalence of pain in hospitalized patients and resolution over six months. Pain 50:15–28, 1992

Acute Pain Management Guideline Panel: Acute Pain Management: Operative or Medical Procedures and Trauma. Clinical Practice Guideline, AHCPR Publ No 92-0032. Rockville, MD, Agency for Health Care Policy and Research, Public Health Service, U.S. Department of Health and Human Services, February 1992

American Geriatrics Society Panel on Chronic Pain in Older Persons: The management of chronic pain in older persons. American Geriatrics Society. J Am Geriatr Soc 46:635–651, 1998

American Psychiatric Association: Diagnostic and Statistical Manual of Mental Disorders, 3rd Edition, Revised. Washington, DC, American Psychiatric Association, 1987

American Psychiatric Association: Diagnostic and Statistical Manual of Mental Disorders, 4th Edition. Washington, DC, American Psychiatric Association, 1994

American Psychiatric Association: Diagnostic and Statistical Manual of Mental Disorders, 4th Edition, Text Revision. Washington, DC, American Psychiatric Association, 2000

American Society of Addiction Medicine: Public policy statement on definitions related to the use of opioids in pain treatment. J Addict Disord 17:129–131, 1998

Ansari A: The efficacy of newer antidepressants in the treatment of chronic pain: a review of current literature. Harv Rev Psychiatry 7:257–277, 2000

Anooshian J, Streltzer, J, Goebert D: Effectiveness of a psychiatric pain clinic. Psychosomatics 40:226–232, 1999

Atkinson JH, Slater MA, Grant I, et al: Depressed mood in chronic low back pain: relationship with stressful life events. Pain 35:47–55, 1988

Atkinson JH, Slater MA, Patterson TL, et al: Prevalence, onset and risk of psychiatric disorders in men with chronic low back pain: a controlled study. Pain 45:111–122, 1991

Backonja MM: Anticonvulsants (antineuropathics) for neuropathic pain syndromes. Clin J Pain 16:S67–S72, 2000

Beecher HK: Pain in men wounded in battle. Ann Surg 123:98–105, 1946

Beitman BD, Mukerji V, Flaker G, et al: Panic disorder, cardiology patients, and atypical chest pain. Psychiatr Clin North Am 11:387–397, 1988

Beitman BD, Mukerji V, Lamberti JW, et al: Panic disorder in patients with chest pain and angiographically normal coronary arteries. Am J Cardiol 63:1399–1403, 1989

Black RG: The chronic pain syndrome. Surg Clin North Am 55:999–1011, 1975

Blumer D, Heilbronn M: Chronic pain as a variant of depressive disease: the pain-prone disorder. J Nerv Ment Dis 170:381–394, 1982

Blumer D, Heilbronn M: Depression and chronic pain, in Presentations of Depression. Edited by Cameron OG. New York, Wiley, 1987, pp 215–235

Bouckoms AJ, Masand P, Murray GB, et al: Chronic nonmalignant pain treated with long-term oral narcotic analgesics. Ann Clin Psychiatry 4:185–192, 1992

Bradley JD, Brandt KD, Katz BP, et al: Comparison of an anti-inflammatory dose of ibuprofen and acetaminophen in the treatment of patients with osteoarthritis of the knee. N Engl J Med 325:87–91, 1991

Brena SF, Crue BL, Stieg RL: Comments on the classification of chronic pain: its clinical significance. Bull Clin Neurosci 49:67–81, 1984

British Medical Association: Report: medical use of hypnotism. BMJ I(suppl):190–193, 1955

Brown GK: A causal analysis of chronic pain and depression. J Abnorm Psychol 99:127–137, 1990

Browne B, Lintner S: Monoamine oxidase inhibitors and narcotic analgesics: a critical review of the implications for treatment. Br J Psychiatry 151:210–212, 1987

Bruera E, Pereira J, Watanabe S, et al: Opioid rotation in patients with cancer pain. Cancer 78:852–857, 1996

Chapman CR, Turner JA: Psychological control of acute pain in medical settings. J Pain Symptom Manage 1:9–20, 1986

Chaturvedi SK: A comparison of depressed and anxious chronic pain patients. Gen Hosp Psychiatry 9:383–386, 1987a

Chaturvedi SK: Prevalence of chronic pain in psychiatric patients. Pain 19:231–237, 1987b

Choiniere M, Melzack R, Girard N, et al: Comparisons between patients' and nurses' assessment of pain and medication efficacy in severe burn injuries. Pain 40:143–152, 1990

Clouse RE: Antidepressants for functional gastrointestinal syndromes. Dig Dis Sci 39:2352–2363, 1994

Cummings EA, Reid GJ, Finley GA, et al: Prevalence and source of pain in pediatric inpatients. Pain 68:25–31, 1996

Delaplaine R, Ifabumuyi OI, Merskey H, et al: Significance of pain in psychiatric hospital patients. Pain 4:361–366, 1978

Dellemijn PLI, Fields HL: Do benzodiazepines have a role in chronic pain management? Pain 57:137–152, 1994

Deyo RA, Weinstein JN: Low back pain. N Engl J Med 344:363–370, 2001

Dworkin RH, Handlin DS, Richlin DM, et al: Unraveling the effects of compensation, litigation, and employment on treatment response in chronic pain. Pain 23:49–59, 1985

Egbert LD, Battit GE, Welch CD, et al: Reduction of postoperative pain by encouragement and instruction of patients. N Engl J Med 270:825–827, 1964

Feinmann C: Pain relief by antidepressants: possible modes of action. Pain 23:1–8, 1985

Federation of State Medical Boards of the United States: Model Guidelines for the Use of Controlled Substances for the Treatment of Pain. Euless, TX, Federation of State Medical Boards, 1998

Foley KM: Competent care for the dying instead of physician-assisted suicide. N Engl J Med 336:54–57, 1997

Fordyce WE, Roberts AH, Sternbach RA: The behavioral management of chronic pain: a response to critics. Pain 22:113–125, 1985

Gamsa A: Is emotional disturbance a precipitator or a consequence of chronic pain? Pain 42:183–195, 1990

Gear RW, Miaskowki C, Heller PH, et al: Benzodiazepine mediated antagonism of opioid analgesia. Pain 71:25–29, 1997

Gore DR, Scpic SB, Gardner GM, et al: Neck pain: a long-term follow-up of 205 patients. Spine 12:1–5, 1987

Gunn CC, Sola AE: Chronic intractable benign pain (CIBP) (letter). Pain 39:364–365, 1989

Gureje O, Von Korff M, Simon GE: Persistent pain and well-being. JAMA 280:147–151, 1998

Hanvik LJ: MMPI profiles in patients with low-back pain. J Consult Clin Psychol 5:350–353, 1951

Hathaway SR, McKinley JC: Minnesota Multiphasic Personality Inventory–2. Minneapolis, MN, University of Minnesota, 1989

Hawkins C, Hanks GW: The gastroduodendal toxicity of nonsteroidal anti-inflammatory drugs: a review of the literature. J Pain Symptom Manage 20:140–151, 2000

Hendler N, Uematesu S, Long D: Thermographic validation of physical complaints in "psychogenic pain" patients. Psychosomatics 23:283–287, 1982

Hilgard ER, Hilgard JR: Hypnosis in the Relief of Pain, Revised Edition. Los Altos, CA, William Kaufman, 1983

Hoffman NG, Olofsson O, Salen B, et al: Prevalence of abuse and dependency in chronic pain patients. Int J Addict 30:919–927, 1995

Hudson JI, Hudson MS, Pliner LF, et al: Fibromyalgia and major affective disorder: a controlled phenomenology and family history study. Am J Psychiatry 142:441–446, 1985

Hunter M, McDowell L, Hennessy R, et al: An evaluation of the faces pain scale with young children. J Pain Symptom Manage 20:122–129, 2000

Jacobson E: Modern Treatment of Tense Patients. Springfield, IL, Charles C Thomas, 1970

Jacox A, Carr DB, Payne R, et al: Management of Cancer Pain. Clinical Practice Guideline, AHCPR Publ No 94-0592. Rockville, MD, Agency for Health Care Policy and Research, Public Health Service, U.S. Department of Health and Human Services, March 1994

Jensen MP, Turner JA, Romano JM, et al: Coping with chronic pain: a critical review. Pain 47:249–283, 1991

Jensen MC, Bran-Zawadzki MN, Obuchowski N, et al: Magnetic resonance imaging of the lumbar spine in people without back pain. N Engl J Med 331:69–73, 1994

Joint Commission on Accreditation of Health Care Organizations: Implementing the new pain management standards. Oakbrook Terrace, IL, Joint Commission on Accreditation of Health Care Organizations, 2000

Katon W, Egan K, Miller D: Chronic pain: lifetime psychiatric diagnoses and family history. Am J Psychiatry 142:1156–1160, 1985

Kerns RD, Turk DC, Rudy TE: The West Haven–Yale Multidimensional Pain Inventory (WHYMPI). Pain 23:345–356, 1985

King SA: Antidepressants: a valuable adjunct for musculoskeletal pain. Journal of Musculoskeletal Medicine 12:51–57, 1995

King SA: The clinical application of DSM-IV for patients with pain, in Proceedings of the 8th World Congress on Pain. Vancouver, BC, IASP Press, 1996

King SA: Depression and pain: assessment and therapeutic strategies. J Back Musculoskel Rehab 9:223–231, 1997

King SA: The classification and assessment of pain. Int Rev Psychiatry 12:86–90, 2000

King SA, Strain JJ: Benzodiazepine use by chronic pain patients. Clin J Pain 6:143–147, 1990

King SA, Strain JJ: Somatoform pain disorder, in DSM-IV Sourcebook, Vol 2. Edited by Widiger TA, Frances AJ, Pincus HA, et al. Washington, DC, American Psychiatric Press, 1996, pp 915–931

King SA, Roy P, Lawser A: The problem of pain among psychiatric inpatients. Paper presented at the annual meeting of the American Pain Society, San Diego, CA, November 1998

King SA, Timko JV: The problem of pain among patients referred to a psychiatric consultation/liaison service. Paper presented at the 9th World Congress on Pain, Vienna, Austria, August 1999

Kouyanou K, Pither CE, Wesseley S: Iatrogenic factors and chronic pain. Psychosom Med 59:597–604, 1997

Leavitt F, Sweet JJ: Characteristics and frequency of malingering among patients with low back pain. Pain 25:357–374, 1986

Linton SJ: Behavioral remediation of chronic pain: a status report. Pain 24:125–141, 1986

Linton SJ: The socioeconomic impact of chronic back pain: is anyone benefiting? Pain 75:163–168, 1998

Loesser JD, Butler SH, Chapman CR, et al: Bonica's Management of Pain. Philadelphia, PA, Lippincott Williams & Wilkins, 2000

Magni G: On the relationship between chronic pain and depression when there is no organic lesion. Pain 31:1–21, 1987

Magni G, Moreschi C, Rigatti-Luchini S, et al: Prospective study on the relationship between depressive symptoms and chronic musculoskeletal pain. Pain 56:289–297, 1994

Main CJ, Evans PJD, Whitehead RC: An investigation of personality structure and other psychological features in patients presenting with low-back pain: a critique of the MMPI, in Proceedings of the VIth World Congress on Pain. Edited by Bond MR, Charlton JE, Woolf CJ. Amsterdam, The Netherlands, Elsevier, 1991, pp 207–218

Main CJ, Waddell G: Behavioral responses to examination. Spine 23:2367–2371, 1998

Malone MD, Strube MJ: Meta-analysis of non-medical treatments for chronic pain. Pain 34:231–244, 1988

Marcantonio ER, Juarez G, Goldman L, et al: The relationship of postoperative delirium with psychoactive medications. JAMA 272:1518–1522, 1994

Marks RM, Sachar EJ: Undertreatment of medical inpatients with narcotic analgesics. Ann Intern Med 78:173–181, 1973

Max MB: Antidepressants as analgesics, in Progress in Pain Research and Management, Vol 1. Edited by Fields HL, Liebeskind JC. Seattle, WA, IASP Press, 1994, pp 229–246

McQuay H, Carroll D, Jadad AR, et al: Anticonvulsant drugs for management of pain: a systematic review. BMJ 311:1047–1052, 1995

Mechanic D: The concept of illness behavior. Journal of Chronic Disease 15:189–194, 1962

Melzack R: The McGill Pain Questionnaire: major properties and scoring methods. Pain 1:277–299, 1975

Melzack R: Gate control theory. Pain Forum 5:128–138, 1996

Melzack R, Wall PD: Pain mechanisms: a new theory. Science 150:971–979, 1965

Melzack R, Abbott FV, Zackon W, et al: Pain on a surgical ward: a survey of the duration and intensity of pain and the effectiveness of medication. Pain 29:67–72, 1987

Merskey H, Bogduk N (eds): International Association for the Study of Pain Classification of Chronic Pain, 2nd Edition. Seattle, WA, IASP Press, 1994

Monks R: Psychotropic drugs, in The Management of Pain. Edited by Bonica JJ. Philadelphia, PA, Lea & Febiger, 1990, pp 1676–1689

Naliboff BD, Cohen MJ, Yellen AN: Does the MMPI differentiate chronic illness from chronic pain? Pain 13:333–341, 1982

Novy DM, Nelson DV, Berry LA: What does the Beck Depression Inventory measure in chronic pain? A reappraisal. Pain 61:261–270, 1995

Osterweis M, Kleinman A, Mechanic D (eds): Pain and Disability. Washington, DC, National Academy Press, 1987

Owen H, McMillan V, Rogowski D: Postoperative pain therapy: a survey of patients' expectations and their experiences. Pain 41:303–307, 1990

Partners Against Pain: A survey of pain in America. http://www.partnersagainstpain.com/html/survey, 2001

Peterson WL, Cryer B: Cox-1-sparing NSAIDs: is the enthusiasm justified? JAMA 282:1961–1963, 1999

Pilowsky I: Abnormal illness behavior. Br J Med Psychol 42:347–351, 1968

Portenoy RK: Opioid therapy for chronic nonmalignant pain: current status, in Progress in Pain Research and Management, Vol 1. Edited by Fields HL, Liebeskind JC. Seattle, WA, IASP Press, 1994, pp 247–264

Porter J, Jick H: Addiction rare in patients treated with narcotics (letter). N Engl J Med 302:123, 1980

Reading AE, Everitt BS, Sledmere CM: The McGill Pain Questionnaire: a replication of its construction. Br J Clin Psychol 21:339–349, 1982

Report of the Commission on the Evaluation of Pain. U.S. Department of Health and Human Services, Social Security Administration, Office of Disability, Publ No 64-031, 1987

Romano JM, Turner JA: Chronic pain and depression: does the literature support a relationship? Psychol Bull 97:18–34, 1985

Rosomoff HL, Fishbain DA, Goldberg M, et al: Physical findings in patients with chronic intractable benign pain of the neck and/or back. Pain 37:279–287, 1989

Ross EL: The evolving role of antiepileptic drugs in treating neuropathic pain. Neurology 55(suppl 1):S41–S46, 2000

Saper JR: Diagnosis and symptomatic treatment of migraine. Headache 37(suppl 1):S1–S14, 1997

Sapira J: Real pain (letter). N Engl J Med 295:116, 1976

Scott J, Huskisson EC: Graphic representation of pain. Pain 2:175–184, 1976

Sengstaken EA, King SA: The problems of pain and its detection among geriatric nursing home residents. J Am Geriatr Soc 41:541–544, 1993

Sengstaken EA, King SA: Primary care physicians and pain: education during residency. Clin J Pain 10:303–309, 1994

Simon GE, Von Korff M, Piccinelli M, et al: An international study of the relation between somatic symptoms and depression. N Engl J Med 341:1329–1335, 1999

Sindrup, SH, Jensen TS: Efficacy of pharmacological treatments of neuropathic pain: an update and effect related to mechanism of drug action. Pain 83, 389–400, 1999

Smith AJ: The analgesic effects of selective serotonin reuptake inhibitors. J Psychopharmacol 12:407–413, 1998

Tramadol: a new oral analgesic. Med Lett Drugs Ther 37:59–60, 1995

Turk DC: Customizing treatment for chronic pain patients: who, what, and why. Clin J Pain 6:255–270, 1990

Turk DC, Okifuji A, Scharff L: Chronic pain and depression: role of perceived impact and perceived control in different age cohorts. Pain 61:93–101, 1995

Turner JA, Chapman CR: Psychological interventions for chronic pain: a critical review, I: relaxation training and biofeedback. Pain 12:1–21, 1982a

Turner JA, Chapman CR: Psychological interventions for chronic pain: a critical review, II: operant conditioning, hypnosis, and cognitive-behavioral therapy. Pain 12:23–46, 1982b

Turner JA, Deyo RA, Loeser JD, et al: The importance of placebo effects in pain treatment and research. JAMA 271:1609–1614, 1994

Violon A, Giurgea D: Familial models for chronic pain. Pain 18:199–203, 1984

Virani A, Mailis A, Shapiro LE, et al: Drug interactions in human neuropathic pain pharmacotherapy. Pain 73:3–13, 1997

von Knorring L, Ekselius L: Idiopathic pain and depression. Qual Life Res 3(suppl 1):S57–S68, 1994

Waddell G, McCulloch JA, Kummel E, et al: Nonorganic physical signs in low back pain. Spine 5:117–125, 1980

Wall PD: Comments after 30 years of the gate control theory. Pain Forum 5:12–22, 1996

Wall PD, Melzack R: Textbook of Pain, 4th Edition. Philadelphia, PA, WB Saunders, 1999

Watson D: Neurotic tendencies among chronic pain patients: an MMPI item analysis. Pain 14:365–385, 1982

Weissman DE, Haddox JD: Opioid pseudoaddiction: an iatrogenic syndrome. Pain 36:363–366, 1989

Wiffen P, Collins S, McQuay H, et al: Anticonvulsant drugs for acute and chronic pain (Cochrane Review), in The Cochrane Library, Issue 4, 2000. Oxford: Update Software

Williams RC: Toward a set of reliable and valid measures for chronic pain assessment and outcome research. Pain 35:239–251, 1988

World Health Organization Expert Committee on Cancer Pain Relief and Active Supportive Care: Cancer Pain Relief and Palliative Care: Report of a WHO Expert Committee (WHO Technical Series 804). Geneva, Switzerland, World Health Organization, 1990

Zenz M, Strumpf M, Tryba M: Long-term oral opioid therapy in patients with chronic nonmalignant pain. J Pain Symptom Manage 7:69–77, 1992

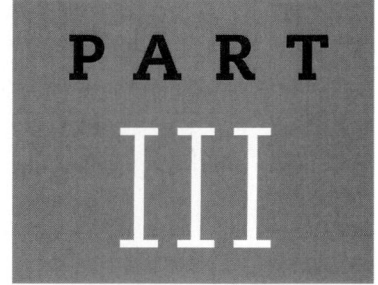

PART

III

Psychiatric Treatments

Psychopharmacology and Electroconvulsive Therapy

Lauren B. Marangell, M.D.

Jonathan M. Silver, M.D.

Donald C. Goff, M.D.

Stuart C. Yudofsky, M.D.

The skillful practice of psychopharmacology requires a broad knowledge of psychiatry, pharmacology, and medicine. We begin this chapter with an overview of general principles relevant to the safe and effective use of psychotropic medications. Subsequent sections cover the major classes of psychotropic medications—antidepressants, antipsychotics, anxiolytics, and mood stabilizers—and the disorders for which they are prescribed. The reader should be aware that this nomenclature is somewhat artificial; for example, many antidepressant medications are also used to treat anxiety disorders.

General Principles

Initial Evaluation

Like all areas of medicine, the art of psychopharmacology rests on proper diagnosis and delineation of medication-responsive target symptoms. Additional considerations include ruling out nonpsychiatric causes, such as endocrine or neurological disorders and substance abuse; noting the presence of other medical problems that will influence drug selection, such as cardiac or hepatic disease; evaluating other medications that the patient is taking that might cause a drug–drug interaction; and evaluating personal and family history of medication responses.

Target Symptoms

A key component of a well-considered decision to use a medication is the delineation of target symptoms. The physician should determine and list the specific symptoms that are designated for treatment and monitor the response of these symptoms to treatment. Standard rating scales, such as the Hamilton Rating Scale for Depression (Hamilton 1960) and the Overt Aggression Scale (OAS; Silver and Yudofsky 1991; Yudofsky et al. 1986), provide specific methods for assessing symptoms and target behaviors and are useful for monitoring change with treatment. In the absence of formal rating scales, target symptoms can be rated on a 1–10 scale. In addition, the clinician should monitor functional status. The goal of treatment is not just to alleviate symptoms but also to restore normal functioning to the extent possible.

Multiple Medications

A frequent and dangerous clinical error is the treatment of specific symptoms of a disorder with multiple drugs,

The authors would like to thank Holly Zboyan for her invaluable assistance in the preparation of this chapter.

The "Drug Interactions" section contains material developed over many years for other purposes in collaboration with Ann Callahan, M.D., and Terence Ketter, M.D.

rather than treating, more specifically, the underlying disorder. For example, it is not uncommon for a psychiatrist to receive a referral for a patient who is taking one type of benzodiazepine for anxiety, a different type of benzodiazepine for insomnia, an analgesic for nonspecific somatic complaints, and a subtherapeutic dosage of an antidepressant (e.g., 50 mg/day of imipramine) for feelings of sadness. Often, the somatic complaints, insomnia, and anxiety are components of an underlying depression, which may be aggravated by the polypharmaceutical approach inherent in symptomatic treatment.

However, many patients have psychiatric conditions that require the concomitant use of several psychotropic agents. The carefully considered, rational use of several psychiatric medications must be distinguished from ill-considered polypharmacy. An example of useful combined treatment is augmentation of an antidepressant agent with lithium for patients who have experienced only a partial therapeutic response to an antidepressant alone.

Choice of Drug

Selection of a drug for a given diagnosis or symptom is made on the basis of both patient-specific and drug-specific considerations. Patient-specific factors include comorbid medical and psychiatric disorders, other medications being taken, history of response to medication, family history of medication responses, and life circumstances that will likely be affected by the specific side effects of the chosen agent. For example, for an elderly man with depression and prostatic hypertrophy, an antidepressant drug with minimal anticholinergic properties should be chosen to avoid urinary retention. For a patient with both panic disorder and major depression, an antidepressant medication that also treats panic disorder should be chosen. For an architect with bipolar disorder, medications that cause a hand tremor might be problematic. For a woman taking oral birth control pills, carbamazepine may increase the hepatic metabolism of the contraceptive agent, thereby lowering the contraceptive efficacy. Patients often, but not always (Post et al. 1992), respond positively to medications that were helpful in the past. For example, a patient with severe depression that was previously responsive to phenelzine but is now unresponsive to a variety of newer antidepressants might respond again to phenelzine.

The clinician also must consider the physical, intellectual, and psychological capacities of the patient and of his or her caregivers when selecting a new medication. For example, in patients with dementia, it may not be safe to use a monoamine oxidase inhibitor (MAOI), for which it is important to remember dietary restrictions and potential drug interactions. An elderly patient with mild memory impairment may have difficulty following instructions about increasing the dosage of an antidepressant medication. In general, the more complicated the instructions or the more medications that are prescribed, the more difficulty the patient will have in complying with the therapeutic regimen.

Drug-specific factors include available preparations and cost. In most cases, once-a-day dosing is preferred for patient convenience and compliance. The choice of a particular medication also may depend on whether that drug is available in injectable and liquid forms in addition to tablet, pill, or capsule forms.

Generic Substitution

Generic substitution, when available, may provide a less expensive alternative to the original proprietary (brand-name) formulation; however, some caution is warranted because generic "equivalents" may not be truly equivalent in all circumstances. After patent expiration, information relevant to producing a medication is in the public domain. At that point, other pharmaceutical companies may produce the medication, provided the drug is formulated according to U.S. Food and Drug Administration (FDA) requirements. The current FDA requirements center around the concept of *bioequivalence;* products are bioequivalent if there is no significant difference in the rate at which or extent to which the active ingredient becomes available to the site of action, given the same dose and conditions (Food and Drug Administration 1992). However, in some cases, even small differences in bioavailability, or other differences in preparations such as type of preservatives or excipients, may become clinically meaningful. For example, a patient may have an allergic reaction to one generic preparation but not another of the same drug because of differences in the dye used to color the pill.

Initial generic product selection is of less clinical significance than is switching between formulations. For example, if a patient is in remission and without side effects while taking one formulation of generic amitriptyline, pharmacy substitution risks both loss of efficacy and toxicity if the new preparation has a slightly lower or higher bioavailability. This type of substitution generally occurs when the patient changes pharmacies or when the pharmacy buys a different, often less expensive, generic preparation. This risk of an adverse clinical outcome is highest when switching between two generic preparations (Hauck and Anderson 1992). In many circumstances, generic substitution is a safe and effective cost-saving tool, but the clinician should be aware of potential problems and, in the event of an unexpected reaction, should ask the patient if the medication has changed in appearance. The change in appearance, such as in size, shape, or color, should alert the clinician to a probable change in generic formulations.

Patient Information and Patient–Physician Communication

A general principle is that the more the patient and his or her family understand about the illness and the reason that medications have been chosen to treat the illness, the more compliant the patient and the more supportive the family will be. Failure to devote adequate time to discussion and instruction before recommending a medication may result in poor therapeutic response, poor compliance by the patient, areas of mistrust and miscommunication, and the requirement at a later time of extensive professional time and effort. We believe that excellent communication among the physician, the patient, and the family before the selection of a medication will increase the likelihood of a positive outcome.

Therapeutic skill and creativity on the part of a clinician are essential for effective treatment with medications. For example, the clinician must expect a patient with major depression associated with significant anxiety and somatic complaints to be concerned about and fearful of drug side effects. The way in which the clinician discusses such side effects with the patient will ultimately affect the patient's confidence in the treatment plan and his or her compliance. It is often useful to emphasize that common early side effects, such as nausea, are not dangerous and will likely improve with time. Situations that require immediate intervention to ensure patient safety must be clearly communicated. For example, it is essential that patients be aware of the signs of lithium toxicity.

Compliance

Only a minority of patients who require subacute or chronic treatment continue to take their medications as prescribed. As discussed earlier, we believe that communication and patient education are the most important interventions to improve patient compliance. In addition to oral communication, written instructions are often helpful, particularly if the patient is to remember more complicated information, such as dose titration or instructions for multiple medications. Whenever possible, medication regimens should be simplified. For example, once-a-day dosing should be used when possible, and any medication that requires more than twice-a-day dosing usually should be avoided if a suitable alternative exists. To assist patients who have difficulty remembering to take their medication, the physician should help to identify cues from the daily routine that can be used as reminders (Cramer 1995). Often it is easiest to incorporate medication times with morning or evening toiletry routines; patients may be instructed to leave their medication by their toothbrush or razor. Midday doses are the most difficult to incorporate reliably into most people's daily activities and should be avoided if possible, unless the patient is extremely well motivated.

Patients value medication not only in terms of absolute efficacy but also in terms of how the medication affects all areas of their lives (Morris and Shulz 1993). As such, the patient must be an active part of the treatment, and the medication decisions must be tailored to conform to the patient's lifestyle and values. For example, a benzodiazepine may be an appropriate medication for a patient with acute anxiety, but if the patient believes it to be a dangerous and addictive medication, despite physician reassurance, noncompliance is more likely. When multiple medications cannot be avoided, a pillbox with sections for each day of the week can be purchased at most pharmacies. Use of a pillbox is also helpful for patients who do not remember whether they have taken their medication each day. When applicable, blood levels of medications can be used to monitor compliance.

Evaluation of Response

The treatment plan should include a predetermined dose and duration that will provide an adequate trial of the medication. Far too frequently, medications are discontinued with the assumption of failure of response without the benefit of an adequate drug trial (e.g., inadequate dosage or duration of treatment). A patient's treatment plan should be revised if the patient has an unusual sensitivity to the medication, if dangerous or disabling side effects emerge, or if the patient does not respond to an adequate drug trial. In such cases, a diagnostic reevaluation of the patient may be indicated, with further tests to detect any underlying nonpsychiatric illness that did not appear during the initial assessment and consideration of alternative treatments.

For patients who do respond, an end point for treatment must be determined. Far too often, medication regimens are continued beyond the point at which therapeutic benefit is derived. A common example is the use of benzodiazepines for the treatment of anxiety in which patients may be maintained for years without the assessment of the therapeutic benefit of the drug by gradual discontinuation.

Antidepressant Drugs

Overview

The modern era of the treatment of depression with medication began in the 1950s when iproniazid, an MAOI used for the treatment of tuberculosis, was noted to elevate mood (Selikoff et al. 1952). Unfortunately, hepatic necrosis was a side effect of iproniazid, and this led to its withdrawal from clinical use. In addition, dangerous hypertensive reactions associated with the MAOIs initially were poorly understood, and most psychiatrists were reluctant to use these drugs. Imipramine, the first of the tricyclic antidepressants (TCAs), was developed as a derivative of chlorpromazine; it was hoped that imipramine would be more effective than chlorpromazine as an antipsychotic agent. Although imipramine did not show antipsychotic efficacy, it was shown to be effective in the treatment of depression (Kuhn 1958). Subsequently, many other antidepressants have been approved for use in the United States. To date, all antidepressants appear to be equally effective for treating major depression, but individual patients may respond preferentially to one agent or another. In addition, these medications are significantly different from one another with regard to side effects, lethality in overdose, pharmacokinetics, and the ability to treat comorbid psychiatric disorders.

Mechanisms of Action

All current antidepressant drugs affect the serotonergic and/or catecholaminergic systems in the central nervous system (CNS), by either presynaptic reuptake inhibition, blocking catabolism, or receptor agonist or antagonist effects (for a review, see Charney 1998; Frazer 1997; W.K. Goodman and Charney 1985). The effects of antidepressants on monoamine availability are immediate, but the clinical response is typically delayed for several weeks. Downregulation of presynaptic autoreceptors, α- and β-noradrenergic receptors, and the serotonin type 1 (5-HT$_1$) receptors more closely parallels the time course of clinical response. This downregulation can be conceptualized as a marker of antidepressant-induced neuronal adaptation. More important, most of the receptors that are immediately affected by antidepressants are linked to G proteins. A defective linkage between the receptor and the G protein may result in abnormal intracellular transduction mechanisms (Bourin and Baker 1996). In actuality, antidepressants most likely act via modulating G proteins, second messenger systems, and gene expression (for a review of molecular mechanisms, see Duman 1998).

Indications

Although the antidepressants have many potential therapeutic uses, the primary approved indication for these drugs is the treatment of major depression, as defined by DSM-IV-TR (American Psychiatric Association 2000). Overall, approximately 70% of the patients with depression respond to an adequate trial of antidepressant medication, although far fewer achieve full remission of symptoms. In addition, antidepressants are effective for patients with obsessive-compulsive disorder (OCD) (selective serotonin reuptake inhibitors [SSRIs] and clomipramine), panic disorder (TCAs and SSRIs), bulimia (TCAs, SSRIs, and MAOIs), dysthymia (SSRIs), bipolar depression (after treatment with a mood stabilizer), social phobia (MAOIs and SSRIs), posttraumatic stress disorder (PTSD) (SSRIs), irritable bowel syndrome (TCAs), enuresis (TCAs), neuropathic pain (TCAs), migraine headache (TCAs), attention-deficit/hyperactivity disorder (bupropion), smoking cessation (bupropion), autism (SSRIs), and late luteal phase dysphoric disorder (SSRIs); however, the FDA has not evaluated or approved the use of antidepressants to treat many of these conditions.

Clinical Use

Each of the commonly used classes of antidepressants is discussed in the following sections and summarized in Table 24–1. The antidepressant classes are based on similarity of receptor effects and side effects. All are effective for depression when administered in therapeutic doses. The choice of antidepressant medication is based on the patient's psychiatric symptoms, his or her history of previous treatment response, family members' history of previous response, medication side effect profile, comorbid psychiatric or medical disorders, and risk of suicide by overdose (Tables 24–2 and 24–3). In general, the SSRIs and the other newer antidepressants are better tolerated and safer than either the TCAs or the MAOIs, although many patients still benefit from these older drugs. In the following sections, clinically relevant information is presented for each of the antidepressant medication classes individually, followed by a discussion of the pharmacological treatment of depression. Principles germane to the use of antidepressants to treat anxiety disorders can be found at the end of the section on anxiety later in this chapter.

TABLE 24–1. Commonly used antidepressant drugs

Generic (trade) name	Starting dosage (mg)[a]	Usual daily dosage (mg)	Available oral dosages (mg)	Mean drug [active metabolite] half-life (hours)
Tricyclics and tetracyclics				
Tertiary amine tricyclics				
Amitriptyline (Elavil, Endep)	25–50	100–300	10, 25, 50, 75, 100, 150	15.6 [26.6]
Clomipramine (Anafranil)	25	100–250	25, 50, 75	32 [69]
Doxepin (Sinequan)	25–50	100–300	10, 25, 50, 75, 100, 150	16.8
Imipramine (Tofranil, Tofranil PM)	25–50	100–300	10, 25, 50, 75, 100, 125, 150	7.6 [17.1]
Trimipramine (Surmontil)	25–50	100–300	25, 50, 100	24
Secondary amine tricyclics				
Desipramine (Norpramin)	25–50	100–300	25, 50, 75, 100, 150	17.1
Nortriptyline (Pamelor, Aventyl)	25	50–200	10, 25, 50, 75	26.6
Protriptyline (Vivactil)	10	15–60	5, 10	78.4
Tetracyclics				
Amoxapine (Asendin)	50	100–400	25, 50, 100, 150	8
Maprotiline (Ludiomil)	50	100–225	25, 50, 75	43
Selective serotonin reuptake inhibitors				
Citalopram (Celexa)	20	20–60[b]	20, 40	35
Fluoxetine (Prozac, Sarafem)	20	20–60[b]	10, 20, liq, 90 (weekly)	72 [144]
Fluvoxamine (Luvox)	50	50–300[b]	50, 100	15
Paroxetine (Paxil)	20	20–60[b]	10, 20, 30, 40	20
Sertraline (Zoloft)	50	50–200[b]	50, 100	26 [66]
Dopamine-norepinephrine reuptake inhibitors				
Bupropion (Wellbutrin)	150	300	75, 100	14
Bupropion SR (Wellbutrin SR, Zyban)	150	300	100, 150	21
Serotonin-norepinephrine reuptake inhibitors				
Venlafaxine (Effexor)	37.5	75–225	25, 37.5, 50, 75, 100	5 [11]
Venlafaxine (XR) (Effexor XR)	37.5	75–225	37.5, 75, 150	5 [11]
Serotonin modulators				
Nefazodone (Serzone)	50	150–300	100, 150, 200, 250	4
Trazodone (Desyrel)	50	75–300	50, 100, 150, 300	7
Norepinephrine-serotonin modulator				
Mirtazapine (Remeron)	15	15–45	15, 30	20
Monoamine oxidase inhibitors				
Irreversible, nonselective				
Phenelzine (Nardil)	15	15–90	15	2
Tranylcypromine (Parnate)	10	30–60	10	2
Reversible MAOI-A				
Moclobemide (Aurorix, Manerex)	150	300–600	100, 150	2

Note. [a]Lower starting dosages are recommended for elderly patients and for those with panic disorder, significant anxiety, or hepatic disease.
[b]Dosage varies with diagnosis. See text for specific guidelines.

Source. Dosing information is from American Psychiatric Association 1993. Half-life information is compiled from Amsterdam et al. 1980 and *Physicians' Desk Reference* 2001, 55th Edition. Montvale, NJ, Medical Economics, 2001.

Tricyclic and Heterocyclic Antidepressants

Receptor Effects

Most TCAs inhibit the reuptake of norepinephrine, serotonin, and, to a lesser extent, dopamine. These mechanisms are thought to be responsible for the therapeutic action of TCAs. In addition, TCAs block muscarinic cholinergic receptors, H_1 histamine receptors, and α_1-adrenergic receptors. These mechanisms are thought to account for the side effects of the TCAs.

TABLE 24–2. Guidelines for choosing an antidepressant medication

Unipolar depression	All antidepressants are equally effective. Choose on the basis of previous response, side effects, comorbid medical and psychotic disorders.
Depression with melancholia features	TCA[a]
Depression with atypical features	SSRI, MAOI[b]
Depression with psychotic features	Antidepressant plus antipsychotic, or ECT; avoid bupropion
Bipolar depression[c]	Lithium, lamotrigine
Depression + OCD	SSRI, clomipramine
Depression + panic disorder	SSRI, TCA, MAOI[b]
Depression + seizures	Avoid bupropion and TCAs
Depression + Parkinson's disease	Bupropion
Depression + sexual dysfunction	Bupropion, nefazodone, mirtazapine

Note. ECT = electroconvulsive therapy; MAOI = monoamine oxidase inhibitor; OCD = obsessive-compulsive disorder; SSRI = selective serotonin reuptake inhibitor; TCA = tricyclic antidepressant.

[a]Although some data suggest that TCAs are superior in melancholic depression, many clinicians choose the newer agents, even in melancholia, on the basis of improved tolerability and safety.

[b]Although MAOIs are highly effective, they are not used as first-line agents because of their increased risk relative to the newer agents.

[c]Mood stabilizers are first-line treatment for all phases of bipolar disorder (see text section on mood stabilizers).

Background

The name *tricyclic* is based on the chemical structure; all tricyclics have a three-ring nucleus. Currently, most clinicians are moving away from use of TCAs as first-line drugs; relative to the newer antidepressants, they tend to have more side effects, to require gradual titration to achieve an adequate antidepressant dose, and to be lethal in overdose. Some data suggest that TCAs may be more effective than SSRIs in the treatment of major depression with melancholic features (Danish University Antidepressant Group 1990; Perry 1996); however, many skilled clinicians and researchers continue to prefer the newer antidepressants, even in melancholia, for the aforementioned reasons. Newer medications that affect both norepinephrine and serotonin (e.g., venlafaxine and mirtazapine) also may have superior efficacy in severely ill depressed patients or when remission is defined as the outcome (Thase et al. 2001).

Imipramine, amitriptyline, clomipramine, trimipramine, and doxepin are tertiary amines. Desipramine, nortriptyline, and protriptyline are secondary amines.

The tertiary amines have more potent serotonin reuptake inhibition, and the secondary amines have more potent noradrenergic reuptake inhibition. The tertiary amines tend to have more side effects than do the secondary amines; in our opinion, the tertiary amines usually do not offer any additional therapeutic benefits. Desipramine and protriptyline tend to be activating. Among the TCAs, nortriptyline is the least likely to produce orthostatic hypotension. Amoxapine has an active metabolite that antagonizes D_2 dopamine receptors and can therefore cause treatment-emergent extrapyramidal side effects (EPS; Coupet et al. 1979; see section on antipsychotic drugs later in this chapter). Maprotiline is characterized as a heterocyclic agent. The receptor effects of maprotiline are most similar to those of protriptyline.

Clinical Use

Before initiation of treatment with TCAs, the physician must obtain a comprehensive cardiovascular history and review of symptoms. Because TCAs often cause orthostasis, other potential risk factors for hypotension should be considered, and patients should be instructed to change from sitting or lying to the standing position slowly. For patients with preexisting heart disease and for all patients older than 40, an electrocardiogram (ECG) should be obtained before TCA treatment is initiated. If the initial ECG shows clinically significant abnormalities, another ECG must be taken after the patient's medication has reached a steady-state level. For patients with bundle branch block, TCAs should not be used unless all other options have failed.

The following dosage guidelines are for healthy adults with minimal anxiety. Patients with significant anxiety, panic, or a tendency to be sensitive to side effects should receive initial dosages that are 50% lower. Similarly, elderly patients and those with cardiovascular or hepatic disease should receive lower initial dosages.

Imipramine, amitriptyline, doxepin, desipramine, clomipramine, and trimipramine can be initiated at 25–50 mg/day. Divided dosing may be used initially to minimize side effects, but eventually the entire dosage can be given at bedtime. The dosage can be increased to 150 mg/day the second week, 225 mg/day the third week, and 300 mg/day the fourth week. The dosage of clomipramine should not exceed 250 mg/day because of an increased risk of seizures at higher dosages.

Nortriptyline should be initiated at 25 mg/day and increased to 75 mg/day over 1–2 weeks depending on tolerability and clinical response. Some patients require dosages up to 150 mg/day. Amoxapine should be started at 50 mg/day and titrated up to 400 mg/day; it has a short

TABLE 24–3. Summary of key features and side effects of antidepressant medications

Medication	Proposed mechanism/ receptor effects	Dosing	Titration required	Sedation	Weight gain	Sexual dysfunction	Other key side effects
TCAs	5-HT + NE reuptake inhibition	Once daily	Yes	Most, yes	Yes	Yes	Anticholinergic,[a] orthostasis, quinidine-like effects on cardiac condition, lethal in overdose
SSRIs	5-HT reuptake inhibition	Once daily	Minimal	Minimal	Rare	Yes	Initial: nausea, loose bowel movements, headache, insomnia
Bupropion SR	DA + NE reuptake inhibition	Multiple, if dose > 200 mg	Some	Rare	Rare	Rare	Initial: nausea, headache, insomnia, anxiety/agitation; seizure risk
Venlafaxine XR	5-HT + NE > DA reuptake inhibition	Once daily	Some	Minimal	Rare	Yes	Similar to SSRIs; dose-dependent hypertension
Nefazodone	5-HT₂ antagonist + weak 5-HT + NE reuptake inhibition	Twice daily	Yes	Yes	Rare	Rare	Initial: nausea, dizziness, confusion, visual changes, sedation
Trazodone	5-HT₂ antagonist + weak 5-HT₂ reuptake inhibition	Twice daily	Yes	Yes	Rare	Rare	Initial sedation, priapism, dizziness, orthostasis
Mirtazapine	α₂-Adrenergic + 5-HT₂ antagonism	Once daily	Minimal	Yes	Yes	Rare	Anticholinergic[a]; may increase serum lipids; rare: orthostasis, hypertension, peripheral edema, agranulocytosis
MAOIs	Inhibit monoamine oxidase	Two or three times a day	Yes	Rare	Yes	Yes	Orthostatic hypotension, insomnia, peripheral edema; avoid in patients with CHF, avoid phenelzine in patients with hepatic impairment; potentially life-threatening drug interactions; dietary restrictions

Note. CHF = congestive heart failure; DA = dopamine; 5-HT = serotonin; NE = norepinephrine; MAOIs = monoamine oxidase inhibitors;. SSRIs = selective serotonin reuptake inhibitors; TCAs = tricyclic antidepressants.
[a]Anticholinergic side effects include dry mouth, blurred vision, constipation, urinary retention, tachycardia, and possible confusion.

half-life and should be given in divided doses. Protriptyline can be started at 10 mg/day and increased to 60 mg/day. Maprotiline should be started at 50 mg/day and maintained at that dosage for 2 weeks because of an increased risk of seizure if the dosage is raised too quickly. The dosage can be increased over 4 weeks to 225 mg/day.

Plasma Levels and Therapeutic Monitoring

Clinically meaningful plasma levels are available for imipramine, desipramine, and nortriptyline. For imipramine, the combined sum of the plasma levels of imipramine and the desmethyl metabolite (desipramine) should be greater than 200 ng/mL. Desipramine levels should be greater than 125 ng/mL. A therapeutic window has been observed for nortriptyline, with optimal response between 50 and 150 ng/mL. These therapeutic levels are based on steady-state concentrations, which are reached after 5–7 days for these medications. Blood should be drawn approximately 10–14 hours after the last dose of medication.

Most patients respond to usual dosages of antidepressants and do not require monitoring of plasma levels. For example, in two-thirds of physically healthy adult patients with depression, a dosage of 75 mg/day of nortriptyline results in an optimal therapeutic plasma level of this drug (Åsberg 1974). Therefore, this dosage is used as a general guideline for initiating treatment and, in most cases, will lead to a satisfactory treatment response. Nonetheless, there are times when a plasma level determination can be useful (Table 24–4).

Risks, Side Effects, and Their Management

Anticholinergic effects. Anticholinergic side effects result from antagonism of muscarinic receptors. The most common anticholinergic side effects are dry mouth, constipation, urinary retention, blurred vision, and tachycardia. In predisposed patients, such as elderly persons, anticholinergic medications may cause cognitive impairment and confusion. Because the tertiary amines and protriptyline have a particularly high affinity for the muscarinic receptors, these medications are more likely than others to cause anticholinergic side effects.

Cholinergic medications have been reported to relieve some of the anticholinergic side effects (Everett 1976; Yager 1986). Bethanechol chloride may alleviate dry mouth, constipation, urinary hesitancy and retention, and erectile and ejaculatory dysfunction. The addition of a medication to treat side effects should be considered only after dosage reduction and alternative antidepressants with fewer anticholinergic side effects have been attempted. One must proceed with great caution when using antidepressants with anticholinergic side effects in treating patients with prostatic hypertrophy, narrow-angle glaucoma, or cognitive impairment. The newer antidepressant drugs may be preferable for patients with these disorders.

Sedation. The relative sedating properties of the TCAs appear to parallel their respective histamine receptor binding affinities. Trimipramine, amitriptyline, and doxepin are the most sedating TCAs. Desipramine and protriptyline are less sedating.

Cardiac effects. Many of the TCAs have cardiovascular effects, including orthostatic hypotension and cardiac conduction delays. For many patients, especially those with preexisting heart disease, TCAs have clinically relevant effects on blood pressure, heart rate, cardiac conduction, and cardiac rhythm (Glassman 1984; L. S. Goodman et al. 1986; Roose 1992).

Orthostatic hypotension is the cardiovascular side effect that most commonly results in serious morbidity,

TABLE 24–4. Indications for use of antidepressant levels

1. Patient has not responded to an adequate trial of nortriptyline, desipramine, or imipramine.
2. Patient is at high risk because of age or medical illness and requires treatment with the lowest possible effective dose.
3. Patient requires rapid increases in dosage because of extraordinary suicide risk.
4. Concern about patient compliance with medication regimen.
5. Documentation is needed of plasma level to which the patient responded for use in future treatment.
6. Potential of drug interactions that may lead to an increase or a decrease in plasma levels.

Source. Reprinted with permission from Charney DS, Berman RM, Miller HL: "Treatment of Depression," in *The American Psychiatric Press Textbook of Psychopharmacology*, 2nd Edition. Edited by Schatzberg AF, Nemeroff CB. Washington, DC, American Psychiatric Press, 1998, pp. 716–717. Copyright 1998 American Psychiatric Press, Inc.

especially in elderly patients and in patients with congestive heart failure (Glassman and Bigger 1981; Glassman et al. 1983). Glassman et al. (1979) reported an injury rate of 4% for patients with an average age of 60 years who were treated with imipramine. These injuries included fractures and lacerations requiring sutures. Although orthostatic hypotension may occur with any TCA, nortriptyline is the TCA least likely to cause this side effect (Roose et al. 1981). Orthostatic hypotension from TCAs may not be dose dependent; therefore, lowering the dosage of the antidepressant may not lessen the dizziness or the changes in blood pressure.

Increases in heart rate that occur with TCAs rarely result in morbidity or mortality (Glassman and Bigger 1981); however, patients often find tachycardia frightening or distracting. Antidepressants with greater anticholinergic properties are associated with a higher incidence of this side effect, which may be quite troublesome to patients with panic disorder.

Because TCAs at toxic levels (as occur in overdose) can cause life-threatening arrhythmias, many clinicians believe that these drugs can cause dangerous arrhythmias at treatment doses. In fact, TCAs are potent antiarrhythmic agents, possessing quinidine-like properties (Glassman and Bigger 1981). Because prolongation of the P-R and QRS intervals can occur with TCA use, these drugs should not be used in patients with preexisting heart block (especially right bundle branch block and left bundle branch block). In such patients, TCAs often lead to second- or third-degree heart block, both of which are life-threatening conditions (Roose et al. 1987).

Weight gain. Patients treated with TCAs may experience undesirable weight gain. This side effect appears to be unrelated to improvement in the patient's mood (Fernstrom et al. 1986; Kupfer et al. 1979).

Neurological effects. A dose-related risk of seizures has been found with clomipramine, which has led to the recommendation that the daily dosage of this drug should not exceed 250 mg (Clomipramine Collaborative Study Group 1991; see also Anafranil package insert). Overdoses of TCAs, particularly amoxapine and desipramine, are associated with seizures (Wedin et al. 1986). Whether therapeutic dosages of TCAs lower the seizure threshold is controversial (Dailey and Naritoku 1996). Nonetheless, other classes may be safer options for individuals with epilepsy (Rosenstein et al. 1993).

Amoxapine, which has a mild neuroleptic effect, can cause EPS, akathisia, and even tardive dyskinesia (Gammon and Hansen 1984; Ross et al. 1983; Thornton and Stahl 1984). For this reason, we do not recommend that amoxapine be prescribed as a first-line treatment for depression.

Overdose. The major complications from overdose with TCAs include those that arise from neuropsychiatric impairment, hypotension, cardiac arrhythmias, and seizures. Because the TCAs have significant anticholinergic activity, anticholinergic delirium may occur. This is particularly true for elderly patients and for patients with neuropsychiatric conditions. Other complications of anticholinergic overdose include agitation, supraventricular arrhythmias, hallucinations, severe hypertension, and seizures (Goldfrank et al. 1986). Patients with anticholinergic delirium manifest hot dry skin, dry mucous membranes, dilated pupils, absent bowel sounds, and tachycardia. Anticholinergic delirium constitutes a medical emergency and requires full supportive medical care. Physostigmine, a centrally and peripherally acting reversible anticholinesterase, may be used as a diagnostic agent in cases of suspected anticholinergic toxicity. This agent is administered at a dose of 1–2 mg intramuscularly or intravenously at a slow, controlled rate of no more than 1 mg/minute. Physostigmine should not be used to maintain reversal of the toxicity, however, because a cholinergic crisis may result. A cholinergic crisis is characterized by nausea, vomiting, bradycardia, and seizures. This reaction can be reversed by the administration of a potent anticholinergic drug such as atropine. A more detailed explanation of the treatment of these complications can be found elsewhere (Goldfrank et al. 1986).

Hypotension, which may result from norepinephrine depletion and from other causes related to the peripheral

and central effects of TCAs, should be treated with vigorous fluid replacement. Seizures and cardiac complications also may occur with antidepressant overdose (Boehnert and Lovejoy 1985). When the QRS interval is below 0.10, the likelihood of seizures or ventricular arrhythmias decreases (Boehnert and Lovejoy 1985). Ventricular arrhythmias that occur secondary to overdose are typical of the arrhythmias that occur with high doses of quinidine-like agents, and these begin within the first 24 hours after hospital admission (Goldberg et al. 1985). Ventricular arrhythmias should be treated with lidocaine, propranolol, or phenytoin. Prophylactic treatment with phenytoin and insertion of a temporary pacemaker should be considered in patients with prolonged QRS intervals (i.e., >120 msec; Goldfrank et al. 1986).

Seizures associated with TCA overdose should be managed with standard emergency procedures (i.e., airway maintenance, proper ventilation, and treatment of the seizures with agents such as intravenous diazepam). Because many overdose situations involve combinations of drugs, the clinician should be alert to the possibility that alcohol or benzodiazepines also may have been ingested.

Allergic reactions. Allergic and hypersensitivity reactions may occur with TCAs, as they may with most drugs. If a mild rash develops, the drug may be continued and symptomatic treatment instituted. For more serious skin eruptions, the drug should be discontinued, preferably over several days to reduce the possibility of cholinergic rebound symptoms. If further antidepressant treatment is necessary, it is preferable to avoid drugs that are metabolites of the offending drug (i.e., one should not use nortriptyline if a reaction develops to amitriptyline or desipramine if a reaction develops to imipramine). Elevated temperature or signs of infection associated with the rash necessitate a complete medical evaluation, including complete blood count and liver function tests.

Drug interactions. Because the liver metabolizes the TCAs, drugs that inhibit or induce hepatic microsomal enzymes may alter plasma tricyclic levels. This is particularly true for 2D6 inhibitors. In some individuals, this interaction may cause dangerously high levels of the TCA (Vaughan 1988; see section on drug interactions later in this chapter).

Although several agents affect tricyclic levels, the effect is usually not reciprocal: the TCAs rarely affect the metabolism of other drugs. A notable exception to this general rule is the drug sodium valproate, levels of which may decrease when a TCA is administered concurrently (Preskorn and Burke 1992). By a different mode of action, the TCAs also may interfere with the mechanism of action of two antihypertensive drugs. Both guanethidine and clonidine lose effectiveness if administered concomitantly with drugs, such as TCAs, that block reuptake of catecholamines into adrenergic neurons.

Selective Serotonin Reuptake Inhibitors

Mechanism of Action

SSRIs inhibit the presynaptic serotonin reuptake pump. This reuptake inhibition initially increases serotonin in the synaptic cleft, which then causes presynaptic autoreceptors to downregulate and ultimately increases net serotonin transmission (De Montigny et al. 1981). As discussed earlier in this chapter, the ultimate mechanism of action is likely to be related to secondary effects on signal transduction and gene transcription.

Background

SSRIs were developed in an attempt to formulate reuptake-blocking drugs that lacked the troublesome side effects of the TCAs. SSRIs largely lack four of the five pharmacological properties characteristic of TCAs— blockade of muscarinic receptors, of H_1-histaminergic receptors, and of α_1-adrenergic receptors, and norepinephrine reuptake-blocking properties—leaving only the serotonin reuptake inhibitor property intact. This selectivity has several advantages, including a reduction in dangerous side effects. The SSRIs are much safer in overdose than the TCAs because they do not have life-threatening effects at high plasma concentrations. A 15-day supply of TCAs is lethal in most patients. In addition, SSRIs are unlikely to affect the seizure threshold or cardiac conduction, making these drugs an excellent choice for patients for who have epilepsy or cardiac disease.

Because of the more tolerable side effects and once-a-day dosing, patients are more likely to comply with SSRI than with TCA treatment. Compliance is particularly important when considering first-line treatment and overall health care costs. In addition, SSRIs have an unusually broad spectrum of action. They are efficacious in the treatment not only of depression but also of many other psychiatric disorders, as listed earlier in this chapter. This broad spectrum of efficacy is advantageous when treating patients who have more than one disorder. For example, only the SSRIs and clomipramine have been shown to be effective for the treatment of OCD in randomized controlled trials.

The SSRIs are started at or near their therapeutic antidepressant doses, without the long titration period required with most TCAs. The most significant disadvan-

tage of these medications is a high incidence of treatment-emergent sexual dysfunction (discussed later), which often persists for as long as the patient continues taking the medication.

All of the SSRIs have a similar spectrum of efficacy and a similar side effect profile. However, they are structurally and, in some instances, clinically distinct. For example, allergy to one SSRI does not predict allergy to another. Similarly, response or nonresponse to one does not ensure a similar reaction to another medication in the class. The SSRIs also have distinct pharmacokinetic properties, the most important of which are differences in half-life and the propensity to inhibit cytochrome P450 (CYP) enzymes.

Fluvoxamine has an average half-life of 12–15 hours after a single oral dose, but this is prolonged by 30%–50% at steady state (van Harten 1995). Fluvoxamine requires twice-a-day administration at dosages greater than 50 mg/day. Sertraline and paroxetine both have an elimination half-life of approximately 24 hours. Sertraline has an active metabolite, desmethylsertraline, that has a half-life of 62–104 hours. Citalopram has a half-life of 35 hours and no clinically significant metabolites. The moderate half-life of these drugs warrants once-daily dosing and allows for washout within about a week. Fluoxetine has a half-life of 2–4 days, and its active metabolite, norfluoxetine, has a half-life of 7–15 days. Although this long half-life results in a longer time to reach steady-state concentrations, the onset of therapeutic effects is not delayed beyond the 2–4 weeks required of all current antidepressant medications. A long half-life may be advantageous for patients who forget to take their medication.

Although drug–drug interactions are significantly less common with SSRIs than with either TCAs or MAOIs, most SSRIs inhibit various hepatic cytochrome P450 enzymes, which may increase levels of other drugs. The individual drugs in the class have different profiles of cytochrome P450 inhibition, as discussed later in this chapter.

Clinical Use

Although all patients with depression should receive a thorough medical evaluation, no specific tests are required before treatment is initiated with an SSRI. The usual starting dosages for the SSRIs are summarized in Table 24–1. These standard dosages should be decreased by 50% for patients with hepatic disease and for elderly persons. In addition, patients with panic disorder or significant anxiety symptoms are often intolerant of the initial stimulating side effects that commonly occur with

SSRIs. In these cases, the initial dosage also should be decreased by 50% (or more) and then increased as tolerated to the usual therapeutic dosage. It is often advantageous to apply this approach to patients who generally tend to be sensitive to side effects. A liquid preparation of fluoxetine is available for patients who require doses of less than 10 mg or who have difficulty swallowing pills. The other SSRIs are available in scored tablets.

The usual therapeutic dosages for the treatment of depression are citalopram 20 mg, fluoxetine 20 mg, paroxetine 20 mg, and sertraline 50–150 mg. Although the manufacturer of fluvoxamine has not pursued FDA approval for the treatment of depression in the United States (fluvoxamine is approved only for the treatment of OCD), this medication is an effective antidepressant at 50–150 mg/day (Claghorn et al. 1996; Walczak et al. 1996). For the treatment of depression, the SSRIs have a flat dose–response curve, meaning that higher dosages tend not to be more effective than standard dosages, although isolated patients respond better to higher dosages. Premature escalation of the SSRI dosage when treating a patient with depression is most likely to add side effects without improved antidepressant efficacy. Therefore, we recommend maintaining the usual therapeutic dosage for 4 weeks. If there is no improvement at that time, a trial of a higher dose may be warranted. If a partial response is evident at 4 weeks, the dosage should remain constant for an additional 2 weeks because improvement to the initial dosage may continue.

The treatment of OCD requires a longer duration and often higher dosages to assess efficacy. A therapeutic trial for OCD is 8–12 weeks. In fixed-dose studies, fluoxetine and sertraline have appeared to be effective at dosages similar to those used to treat depression (Greist et al. 1995; Tollefson et al. 1994). However, some patients clearly benefit from higher doses. To avoid unnecessary side effects, the best course of action often is to treat first with modest dosages of medication and then increase the dosage if needed. The most common reason for nonresponse in patients with OCD is failure to increase the dose adequately.

In the treatment of panic disorder, data indicate that 40–60 mg/day of paroxetine is more efficacious than lower dosages (Ballenger et al. 1998; Oehrberg et al. 1995). However, available data indicate that the other SSRIs are effective for the treatment of panic disorder at their typical antidepressant dosages (Tiller et al. 1999; van Vliet et al. 1996). Use of fluoxetine in panic disorder has been studied only in small, open studies, but the drug appears to show antipanic effects at low dosages (Louie et al. 1993). Fluoxetine should be initiated at 5 mg/day and gradually increased to 20 mg/day because patients with panic disorder tend to be exquisitely sensitive to side effects (see subsection on the treatment of panic disorder in the section on anxiolytics in this chapter).

Late luteal phase dysphoric disorder appears to respond to doses similar to those used to treat depression. Interestingly, late luteal phase dysphoric disorder can be treated with medication administered only during the symptomatic period before menses (Gelenberg 1997; Wikander et al. 1998). Fluoxetine is effective in the treatment of bulimia at a dosage of 60 mg/day (Mitchell et al. 1993). Although the other SSRIs also may be effective for the treatment of bulimia, dosing guidelines are not available. The use of SSRIs to attenuate symptoms associated with borderline personality disorder and PTSD may require relatively higher dosages.

Risks, Side Effects, and Their Management

Common side effects. Mild nausea, loose bowel movements, anxiety, headache, insomnia, and increased sweating are frequent initial side effects of SSRI treatment. They are usually dosage related and may be minimized with low initial dosing and gradual titration. These early adverse effects almost always attenuate after the first few weeks of treatment. Sexual dysfunction, discussed later, is the most common longer-term side effect of the SSRIs.

Neurological effects. Tension headaches are common early in treatment. These usually can be managed with over-the-counter pain relief preparations. SSRIs may initially worsen migraine headaches, but if the patient can tolerate the first few weeks of treatment with symptomatic relief, SSRIs are often effective in reducing the severity and frequency of migraines (Doughty and Lyle 1995; Hamilton and Halbreich 1993; Manna et al. 1994).

Tremor and akathisia are less common and can be managed with dosage reduction or the addition of a β-blocker. There are isolated case reports of SSRI-related dystonia and increasing reports of SSRI-related exacerbation of Parkinson's disease (Leo 1996; Lipinski et al. 1989; Tate 1989). However, in a review of case reports of movement disorders associated with SSRIs, Leo (1996) found that more than half were confounded by the concomitant use of other medications that can contribute to EPS. The advisability of SSRI use in depressed patients with Parkinson's disease remains to be determined. Bupropion and electroconvulsive therapy (ECT) may be reasonable alternatives for patients with both Parkinson's disease and depression.

Stimulation/insomnia. Some patients complain of jitteriness, restlessness, muscle tension, and disturbed sleep. These side effects typically occur early in treatment, before the antidepressant effect. All patients should be informed of the possibility of these side effects and reassured that if they develop, they tend to be transient. Patients with preexisting anxiety should be started at low dosages with subsequent titration as tolerated. In this way, if overstimulation occurs, it will be less likely to be severe enough to result in a lack of compliance with medication. The short-term use of a benzodiazepine also may help the patient cope with overstimulation in the early stages of treatment, until tolerance to this side effect occurs. Despite these common transient stimulating effects, SSRIs are clearly effective for patients with anxiety or agitated depression. Similarly, insomnia that commonly occurs early in treatment may be tolerable if the patient is reassured that the side effect will be transient. Symptomatic treatment with short-term use of benzodiazepines or low-dose trazodone (e.g., 50–150 mg) at bedtime is reasonable (Jacobsen 1990; Nierenberg and Keck 1989).

Sedation. Despite occasional stimulating effects, SSRIs may induce sedation in some patients. In our experience, patients who experience significant treatment-emergent sedation with these medications often require lower dosages of the medication. Altering the time of administration (e.g., moving the time the medication is taken from morning to evening) often is not successful.

Weight gain or loss. All the SSRIs have the potential to cause weight gain in some individuals (Bouwer and Harvey 1996; Fisher et al. 1995). In a recent controlled study, Fava et al. (2000) found that paroxetine was associated with greater weight gain than fluoxetine or sertraline. However, most commonly, the SSRIs are weight neutral.

Gastrointestinal symptoms. Nausea and diarrhea may occur after treatment with an SSRI. This side effect is dose dependent and often transient.

Sexual dysfunction. Decreased libido, anorgasmia, and delayed ejaculation are common side effects of SSRIs. When possible, the management of sexual side effects should be postponed until the patient has completed an adequate trial of the antidepressant. In some cases, tolerance to sexual side effects develops.

When significant sexual dysfunction persists for more than 1 month despite a positive response to treatment, a reduction in the dosage should be considered. In some cases, this results in a diminution of the symptoms without loss of therapeutic benefit. Unfortunately, in other instances, there is no therapeutic dosage that does not

cause the sexual side effect. In such cases, two strategies are available: the antidepressant can be replaced with an alternative, or other drugs may be prescribed to counteract the side effect. The decision to try a different antidepressant is potentially problematic because an equivalent therapeutic response is not guaranteed. In our experience, switching from one SSRI to another does not tend to decrease sexual side effects. Antidepressants that do not commonly cause sexual dysfunction are bupropion, nefazodone, and mirtazapine.

Several medications have been suggested as antidotes for the sexual side effects associated with antidepressants. Bupropion, 75 or 150 mg/day, has been added to an SSRI regimen with some success for improving libido (Labbate and Pollack 1994). Sildenafil has been used on an as-needed basis prior to sexual activity with some success with improved erectile and ejaculatory function (Ashton and Bennett 1999).

Because the sexual side effects of SSRIs reverse rapidly when the medication is stopped, it is sometimes feasible for patients to skip 1 or 2 days of medication each week and experience unimpaired sexual function the next day (Rothschild 1995). This "drug holiday" or "sex holiday," as it is sometimes referred to, is most easily accomplished with the shorter half-life agents. However, there is some concern regarding relapse and fostering noncompliance with this strategy.

The syndrome of inappropriate secretion of antidiuretic hormone. Case reports have identified an association between SSRIs and the development of the syndrome of inappropriate secretion of antidiuretic hormone (SIADH). However, the actual incidence remains unclear, and a causative relation has yet to be established (Woo and Smythe 1997). Published reports have indicated that elderly persons may be at a higher risk (Liu et al. 1996). Symptoms include lethargy, headache, hyponatremia, elevated urinary sodium excretion, and hyperosmolar urine. Acute treatment of SIADH should consist of discontinuation of the drug as well as restriction of fluid intake. Patients experiencing severe confusion, convulsions, or coma should receive intravenous sodium chloride. Physicians should be aware of this potentially serious but reversible side effect, especially when treating elderly patients.

Vivid dreams. Reports of vivid dreams, distinct from nightmares, are common with SSRIs. The mechanism is unknown.

Rash. If a mild rash develops, the drug may be continued and symptomatic treatment instituted. Severe rashes require discontinuation of medication. Because the SSRIs share a similar mechanism but not similar structures, an allergy to one agent does not predict an allergy to another.

Serotonin syndrome. There have been several reports of a medication-induced syndrome that has been attributed to excessive stimulation of the serotonergic system. This condition arises more commonly among patients treated concurrently with two or more serotonergic drugs (e.g., fluoxetine and an MAOI). However, it also may occur in patients receiving SSRI monotherapy. Affected individuals have the constellation of lethargy, restlessness, confusion, flushing, diaphoresis, tremor, and myoclonic jerks. As the condition progresses, hyperthermia, hypertonicity, rhabdomyolysis, renal failure, and death may occur (Metz and Shader 1990). The syndrome must be identified as rapidly as possible because discontinuation of the serotonergic medications is the first step in treatment, followed by emergency medical treatment, as required. Life-threatening serotonin syndrome is fortunately rare and most often occurs with medication combinations that involve MAOIs.

Discontinuation syndromes. Several reports have described a series of symptoms following discontinuation or dose reduction of serotonergic antidepressant medications. The most common symptoms include dizziness, headache, paresthesia, nausea, diarrhea, insomnia, and irritability. Of note, these symptoms are also seen when a patient misses doses. A prospective double-blind, placebo substitution study confirmed that discontinuation symptoms are most common with short-half-life antidepressants, such as paroxetine (Rosenbaum et al. 1998).

Apathy syndromes. We and others have noted an apathy syndrome in some patients after months or years of successful treatment with SSRIs. Patients often confuse this syndrome with a recurrence of depression, but the two conditions are quite distinct. The syndrome is characterized by a loss of motivation, increased passivity, and often feelings of lethargy and "flatness." However, there is no associated sadness, tearfulness, emotional angst, decreased concentration, or thoughts of hopelessness, worthlessness, or suicide. If specifically asked, patients often remark that the symptoms are not experientially similar to their original depressive symptoms. This syndrome has, to date, not been adequately studied, and the pathophysiology is not known. However, there is speculation that subchronic stimulation of central serotonin may attenuate dopamine functioning in several areas of the brain, including the frontal cortex. In this respect, it

is notable that the clinical presentation mirrors that of a frontal lobe syndrome.

The syndrome appears to be dose dependent and reversible. Mistakenly interpreting the apathy and lethargy for a relapse of depression, and hence increasing the dose of medication, will worsen the symptoms. If dosage reduction is not effective, patients may benefit from the addition of a stimulant. Other agents that increase dopamine also may be effective. Other treatments, such as the use of adjunctive olanzapine, are under study based on the ability of this compound to increase frontal lobe dopamine.

Drug interactions. Several deaths have been reported in patients taking a combination of SSRIs and MAOIs, presumably resulting from the serotonin syndrome (Francois et al. 1997; Hodgman et al. 1997; Kolecki 1997). Because of the potential lethality of this interaction, when it is necessary to switch from an SSRI to an MAOI, the patient must remain off the SSRI for a long enough time to ensure that it has been fully eliminated from the body. This time frame is the equivalent of five times the half-life of the SSRI. Therefore, at least 5 weeks are required between the discontinuation of fluoxetine and the institution of an MAOI (Beasley 1993) and about 1 week between other SSRIs and an MAOI. A 2-week waiting period is required when switching from an MAOI to an SSRI to allow resynthesis of the enzyme.

SSRIs vary with regard to inhibition of cytochrome P450 isozymes. Enzyme inhibition may result in increased blood levels of concomitantly administered medications (see section on drug interactions later in this chapter).

Bupropion

Mechanism of Action

Bupropion's mechanism of antidepressant activity remains unclear. Bupropion is metabolized to hydroxybupropion, which appears to be the active entity. Hydroxybupropion inhibits the reuptake of norepinephrine and dopamine, hence the designation dopamine-norepinephrine reuptake inhibitor (DNRI).

Background

Bupropion's unique spectrum of putative receptor effects provides a useful addition to the therapeutic armamentarium. The most significant advantage of bupropion is its relative lack of sexual side effects. Indeed, the addition of low doses of bupropion may attenuate the sexual dysfunction caused by other medications. There has been some suggestion, on the basis of small clinical trials and case reports, that bupropion may be less likely than other antidepressants to precipitate mania or rapid cycling in patients with bipolar disorder (Ketter et al. 1995; Sachs et al. 1994; Stoll et al. 1994; Zarate et al. 1995). Because bupropion facilitates dopamine transmission, many clinicians preferentially use this agent for patients with Parkinson's disease. The fact that dopamine is integrally related to the brain's reward mechanisms, which are stimulated by nicotine and other addictive substances, has provided the theoretical underpinning for recent research indicating that bupropion is an effective aid to smoking cessation. Two placebo-controlled trials with nondepressed chronic cigarette smokers reported a dose-dependent increase in the percentage of patients able to achieve abstinence. Individuals receiving 300 mg/day were able to sustain abstinence longer than those receiving 150 mg/day, and both groups were superior to placebo groups (Zyban package insert). Bupropion is being marketed under the name Zyban for smoking cessation.

Several small clinical trials have indicated that bupropion may be beneficial in the treatment of attention-deficit/hyperactivity disorder (Conners et al. 1996; Cook et al. 1995; Greenhill 1992). Unfortunately, bupropion does not treat panic disorder or OCD, and clinical experience suggests that it has less ability than the SSRIs to attenuate symptoms of general anxiety.

Overall, bupropion has a favorable side effect profile with little or no weight gain, few effects on cardiac conduction (Roose et al. 1991), and minimal sexual side effects (Kiev et al. 1994). Disadvantages include an increased risk of medication-induced seizures at higher than recommended dosages and the requirement for twice-daily dosing in most patients.

Clinical Use

We recommend using the sustained-release preparation rather than the original preparation because of increased tolerability and decreased seizure risk. The sustained-release preparation is initiated at 150 mg, preferably taken in the morning. After 4 days, the dosage may be increased to 150 mg twice a day. For the short-acting preparation, bupropion is initiated at 75 mg twice a day and increased as tolerated to a total daily dosage of 300 mg. Patients who do not respond after 4 weeks may warrant a trial of 450 mg/day. No single dose should exceed 200 mg. Gradual dose titration helps to minimize initial anxiety and insomnia. The temporary use of anxiolytic or hypnotic agents is reasonable in some patients but generally should be limited to the first few weeks of treatment.

Contraindications

Patients with seizure disorders should not use bupropion. Similarly, consideration of an alternative treatment is advised for patients with a history of significant head trauma, CNS tumor, or an active eating disorder.

Risks, Side Effects, and Their Management

The most common side effects of bupropion are initial headache, anxiety, insomnia, increased sweating, and gastrointestinal upset. Tremor and akathisia also may occur. Management is the same as previously discussed concerning the SSRIs. Bupropion is not associated with anticholinergic side effects, orthostatic hypotension, weight gain, or cardiac conduction changes.

The incidence of seizures is 0.4% with dosages less than 450 mg/day, provided no single dose of the short-acting preparation exceeds 150 mg. The incidence increases to 5% with dosages between 450 and 600 mg/day. The sustained-release preparation has a seizure incidence of 0.1% in dosages less than 300 mg/day and 0.4% in dosages between 300 and 400 mg/day. Higher dosages of the sustained-release preparation have not been evaluated. Patients who have a history of seizures or who are taking concomitant medications that lower the seizure threshold should be given bupropion with caution.

Psychosis. Reports of delusions, hallucinations, and paranoia are consistent with bupropion-mediated increases in central dopamine. Bupropion should be used with caution in patients with psychotic disorder.

Overdose. Much more is known about overdose with the immediate-release formulation of bupropion than with the newer, sustained-release formulation. Reported reactions with the immediate-release form include seizures, hallucinations, loss of consciousness, and sinus tachycardia. Treatment of overdose should include induction of vomiting, administration of activated charcoal, and ECG and electroencephalographic (EEG) monitoring. For seizures, an intravenous benzodiazepine preparation is recommended.

The danger of bupropion overdose is, for the most part, limited to the risk of seizures. However, seizures are seldom a life-threatening event, unless they result in motor vehicle accidents, falls, or other trauma-related events. On the other hand, bupropion's lack of significant cardiovascular or respiratory toxicity means that it is rarely lethal in overdose.

Drug interactions. Combination with an MAOI is potentially dangerous, but less so than the combination of serotonergic drugs and MAOIs. Although the practice is not recommended, there are reports of combining MAOIs and bupropion in patients with refractory depression.

In vitro data suggest that bupropion is metabolized by CYP2B6. Bupropion is now known to inhibit CYP2D6. Because of the risk of dose-dependent seizures, caution is warranted when bupropion is combined with other medications that might inhibit its metabolism.

Venlafaxine

Mechanism of Action

Venlafaxine hydrochloride is a potent inhibitor of norepinephrine and serotonin reuptake. At lower dosages, serotonin reuptake inhibition is prominent. At higher dosages, inhibition of norepinephrine reuptake becomes more significant. Inhibition of dopamine reuptake is manifest at the higher end of the dosage range (Ellingrod and Perry 1994).

Background

Venlafaxine is a phenylethylamine antidepressant released in the United States in 1994. Venlafaxine is approved by the FDA for the treatment of both major depression and generalized anxiety disorder. Preliminary data suggest that it might also have a role in the treatment of chronic pain conditions and perhaps other disorders for which SSRIs are effective. In addition, venlafaxine may be effective for patients who have not responded to other antidepressants; a 33% response rate to venlafaxine was reported in patients who failed to improve during adequate trials of other antidepressant treatments, including MAOIs and ECT (Nierenberg et al. 1994). Venlafaxine is 27% protein bound, which is substantially lower than all the other antidepressants. This property is advantageous when it is necessary to minimize the likelihood of protein-binding interactions. Venlafaxine is unlikely to inhibit cytochrome P450 enzymes, which further decreases the likelihood of drug interactions. Venlafaxine extended-release allows for once-a-day dosing. Blood pressure elevation may occur at higher doses, as discussed in the section on side effects.

Clinical Use

The recommended dosage range of venlafaxine is 75–225 mg/day. The extended-release preparation, which allows for once-daily dosing, is preferred. The usual starting dosage is 37.5–75 mg/day. Doses up to 375 mg/day have been used for patients who are otherwise nonresponsive to treatment. Blood pressure monitoring is recommended because of dose-dependent increases in mean diastolic blood pressure in some patients.

Unlike the SSRIs, venlafaxine shows a positive dose–response relationship; patients with mild depression may respond to lower doses, whereas patients with more severe or recurrent depression may respond better to higher doses. Kelsey (1996) hypothesized that this difference exists because the mechanism of action involves mixed reuptake, with differential effects at higher dosages.

Risks, Side Effects, and Their Management

The side effect profile of venlafaxine is similar to that of the SSRIs, including gastrointestinal symptoms, sexual dysfunction, and transient discontinuation symptoms. Like the SSRIs, venlafaxine does not affect cardiac conduction or lower the seizure threshold. For most patients, venlafaxine is not associated with sedation or weight gain. Side effects that differ from those of the SSRIs are hypothesized to be related to the increased noradrenergic activity of this drug at higher doses, specifically dose-dependent anxiety in some patients and hypertension.

Hypertension. Modest dose-dependent increases in blood pressure may occur with venlafaxine treatment. A large meta-analysis found that the magnitude of change in blood pressure with venlafaxine is statistically significant but is unlikely to be of clinical significance at doses less than 300 mg/day (Thase 1998). For clinically significant treatment-emergent hypertension, dosage reduction or treatment discontinuation should be considered.

Overdose. Few data are available regarding venlafaxine in overdose, but its pharmacological profile suggests that it is safer than the TCAs. Of the reported cases to date, most patients did not have symptoms. For others, somnolence, mild sinus tachycardia, and generalized convulsions were reported. Recommended treatment includes general supportive and symptomatic measures; in severe cases, dialysis should be considered.

Drug interactions. Venlafaxine does not appear to significantly inhibit cytochrome P450 enzymes, and it is the antidepressant least likely to contribute to protein-binding interactions. Venlafaxine should not be combined with MAOIs because of the risk of serotonin syndrome.

Nefazodone

Mechanism of Action

Nefazodone is a 5-HT$_2$ receptor antagonist and a weak inhibitor of neuronal serotonin and norepinephrine reuptake. Together these properties are believed to enhance 5-HT$_{1A}$-mediated neuronal transmission.

Background

Nefazodone entered the United States market in 1995. The advantages of nefazodone are a low incidence of sexual dysfunction (Goldberg 1995) and early attenuation of symptoms of anxiety and insomnia (Armitage et al. 1994; Fawcett et al. 1995). The disadvantages are prominent early sedation, twice-a-day dosing, slow dosage titration, and inhibition of CYP3A3/4.

Clinical Use

The clinically effective dosage range has been determined to be between 300 and 600 mg/day. Because of prominent early side effects, we recommend an initial dosage of 50 mg twice a day or at bedtime, with subsequent increases every 5–7 days, as tolerated, until the total daily dosage reaches 600 mg/day in divided doses or a therapeutic response emerges. The therapeutic range for elderly patients is slightly lower (i.e., between 200 and 400 mg/day in divided doses). As with other antidepressants, an adequate trial of at least 4 weeks is necessary to evaluate efficacy.

Risks, Side Effects, and Their Management

Common side effects are sedation, nausea, dizziness, confusion, and blurred vision. Nefazodone does not appear to cause weight gain or sexual dysfunction.

Visual effects. Visual symptoms, such as blurred or abnormal vision, may accompany nefazodone treatment. Nefazodone does not have significant anticholinergic effects, and the mechanism for visual changes is not known. Treatment-emergent visual symptoms are generally mild and transient.

Overdose. Few data on nefazodone overdose exist. No deaths have been reported. Treatment should consist of supportive measures with specific attention to hypotension and excessive sedation. Gastric lavage is encouraged.

Contraindications and drug interactions. Coadministration with most medications that are metabolized by CYP3A3/4 should be undertaken with caution, and the dosages of the other medications that are 3A3/4 substrates should be reduced (see the section on drug interactions later in this chapter). The interaction of nefazodone with MAOIs has not yet been evaluated, but it may be as dangerous as that of the SSRIs. Therefore, this combination should be avoided.

Trazodone

Mechanism of Action

Trazodone, like nefazodone, is a postsynaptic 5-HT$_2$ antagonist and a weak inhibitor of serotonin reuptake.

Background

Trazodone is an older antidepressant associated with significant sedative activity. Currently, trazodone is not recommended as a first-line antidepressant because of an increased risk of orthostatic hypotension, arrhythmias, and priapism. Also, when compared with other available antidepressants, trazodone does not offer an advantage in terms of therapeutic efficacy (Haria et al. 1994). However, trazodone may be useful in patients with insomnia. It is currently common practice to use low dosages of trazodone, such as 50–100 mg, to assist with initial insomnia while starting one of the newer antidepressants to treat the underlying depression. If this strategy is used, we recommend tapering the dosage and discontinuing treatment with trazodone after 4–6 weeks.

Clinical Use

Trazodone is prescribed in much the same manner as the TCAs, although there is less danger of toxicity at higher doses. The recommended therapeutic dosage range for the treatment of depression is 200–400 mg/day in divided doses. Initial dosing should begin with 50 mg/day, with subsequent increases as tolerated. Most of the daily dosage should be administered in the evening to minimize daytime sedation.

Risks, Side Effects, and Their Management

Excessive sedation is the most commonly encountered side effect of trazodone. Although trazodone has virtually no anticholinergic effects, dry mouth and blurred vision occur more frequently with trazodone treatment than with placebo.

Priapism. Trazodone is the only antidepressant that has been associated with priapism (Scher et al. 1983), which may be irreversible and require surgical intervention (Mitchell and Popkin 1983). This risk must always be considered before trazodone is chosen to treat male patients.

Cardiovascular effects. Trazodone can cause orthostatic hypotension and dizziness (Glassman 1984; Spivak et al. 1987), although these side effects do not appear to correlate with trazodone's binding to the α$_2$-adrenergic receptor. Because trazodone does not cause a significant change in cardiac conduction, for some time it was thought to be the antidepressant of choice among patients with cardiac conduction defects. However, there are now several reports of increased ventricular irritability among patients with conduction defects and preexisting ventricular arrhythmias (Aronson and Hafez 1986; Jankowsky et al. 1983; Vitullo et al. 1990), and multiple newer agents exist that do not appear to affect cardiac conduction.

Overdose. There is a risk in overdose of myocardial irritation in patients with preexisting ventricular conduction abnormalities.

Mirtazapine

Mechanism of Action and Receptor Effects

Mirtazapine facilitates central serotonergic and noradrenergic transmission by antagonizing α_2-noradrenergic autoreceptors and heteroreceptors (De Boer 1996). In addition, mirtazapine antagonizes postsynaptic 5-HT$_{2A}$, 5-HT$_3$, and H$_1$ receptors. 5-HT$_{2A}$ antagonism may be related to the antidepressant properties of this drug and is likely to account for the low occurrence of drug-induced sexual dysfunction. 5-HT$_3$ antagonism is thought to prevent nausea. Antagonism of H$_1$ receptors may account for the side effects of sedation and weight gain. Mirtazapine has moderate activity at α_1 receptors and muscarinic receptors.

Background

Mirtazapine entered the United States market in 1996. It has been shown to reduce anxiety symptoms and sleep disturbances associated with depression as early as 1 week after the start of treatment (Bremmer 1995; Smith et al. 1990). Other advantages are minimal sexual dysfunction, minimal nausea, and once-daily dosing. In addition, mirtazapine is unlikely to be associated with cytochrome P450–mediated drug interactions. The disadvantages of mirtazapine are weight gain and prominent early sedation.

Clinical Use

Mirtazapine treatment is initiated with 15 mg at bedtime. Depending on clinical response and side effects, the dosage can be increased to a maximum of 45 mg at bedtime, although higher dosages are sometimes used in patients with treatment-resistant illness. Elderly patients and those with renal or hepatic disease may require lower dosages.

Risks, Side Effects, and Their Management

As noted previously, sexual dysfunction and nausea are not commonly associated with mirtazapine treatment. The most common side effects are sedation, weight gain, and dizziness.

Somnolence. Somnolence occurs in more than 50% of the patients treated with mirtazapine (Bremmer 1995; Smith et al. 1990). Tolerance to this side effect develops after the first few weeks of treatment.

Weight gain. The weight gain associated with mirtazapine use may be partially a result of an increased appetite. A mean increase of 8.2 lb over the first 28 weeks of treatment has been reported in several controlled studies (Bremmer 1995; Smith et al. 1990).

Agranulocytosis. In preliminary clinical trials, 2 of 2,796 mirtazapine-treated patients developed agranulocytosis, and 1 developed severe neutropenia. All 3 patients recovered after medication discontinuation, and other possible etiologies were present in at least 1 of these individuals. Thirteen patients with pretreatment neutropenia did not progress to more severe neutropenia or agranulocytosis. Postmarketing evaluation to date has not established a causal relation between mirtazapine and agranulocytosis. Routine laboratory monitoring is not currently recommended.

Anticholinergic effects. Mirtazapine is associated with modest anticholinergic side effects, including dry mouth and constipation. Anticholinergic side effects and their management are discussed in the earlier section of this chapter concerning TCAs.

Increased serum lipid levels. Nonfasting serum cholesterol levels increased by 20% or more in 15% of patients and to levels greater than or equal to 500 mg/dL in 6% of patients who participated in the United States clinical trials. These rates are twice those of patients taking either placebo or an active comparison drug. The clinical significance of mirtazapine-induced increases in serum lipid levels is not known.

Cardiac effects. Hypertension, orthostatic hypotension, dizziness, and vasodilation with peripheral edema may occur with mirtazapine treatment.

Overdose. Little is known about mirtazapine overdose. To date, patients who have overdosed have fully recovered. Warning signs include drowsiness, impaired memory, and tachycardia. Recommended treatment includes gastric lavage, cardiac monitoring, and supportive measures.

Drug interactions. Mirtazapine does not significantly inhibit hepatic cytochrome P450 enzymes. Additive effects may occur when mirtazapine is combined with other drugs with sedative or vascular effects. Mirtazapine should not be used in combination with an MAOI or within 14 days of discontinuing therapy with an MAOI.

Monoamine Oxidase Inhibitors

Mechanism of Action

The enzyme monoamine oxidase (MAO) inactivates biogenic amines such as norepinephrine, serotonin, dopamine, and tyramine through oxidative deamination. MAOIs block this inactivation and thereby increase the amount of these transmitters available for synaptic release. There are two types of MAO: A and B. Type A (MAO-A) acts selectively on the substrates norepinephrine and serotonin, whereas type B (MAO-B) preferentially affects phenylethylamine. Both MAO types oxidize dopamine and tyramine. MAO-A inhibition appears to be most relevant to the antidepressant effects of these drugs. Drugs that contain both MAO-A and MAO-B are called *nonselective*. The MAOI antidepressants currently available in the United States are nonselective inhibitors. Because tyramine can be metabolized by either MAO-A or MAO-B, drugs that selectively inhibit either one of these enzymes, but not the other, do not require dietary restrictions. MAO-A–selective drugs, such as moclobemide, are available in other countries for the treatment of depression. MAO-B–selective drugs, such as pargyline and L-deprenyl, are marketed for other indications and do not appear to treat depression in their usual dosages. At higher dosages, both of these drugs become nonselective.

Another important characteristic of MAOIs is the production of reversible versus irreversible enzyme inhibition. An irreversible inhibitor permanently disables the enzyme. This means that MAO must be resynthesized, in the absence of the drug, before the activity of the enzyme can be reestablished. Resynthesis of the enzyme may take up to 2 weeks. For this reason, 10–14 days are required after discontinuation of irreversible inhibitors before instituting other antidepressants or before permitting the use of the drugs or foods that are known to be contraindicated (see the following subsection on clinical use of MAOIs). On the other hand, a reversible inhibitor can move away from the active site of the enzyme, enabling the enzyme to be available to metabolize other substances. The reversibility and selectivity of the currently available MAOIs are summarized in Table 24–5.

Clinical Use

The MAOIs are not currently used as first-line agents because of the improved tolerability and safety of the newer antidepressants. However, the MAOIs continue to be excellent medications for a subset of patients who do not respond to the newer antidepressants. Patients with a depressive syndrome characterized by mood reactivity (i.e., mood that is responsive acutely to favorable and unfavorable life experiences), oversleeping, overeating, extreme lethargy, and extreme sensitivity to rejection—the so-called atypical subtype—may show a preferential response to MAOI therapy (Liebowitz et al. 1984; Quitkin et al. 1979; Ravaris et al. 1980; Zisook 1985). These atypical symptoms may, in fact, provide a marker for patients who are likely to respond to MAOIs.

More so than with other medications, it is imperative to review the patient's medical status and current medications before prescribing an MAOI. The importance of following the dietary and medication restrictions, as outlined later, should be discussed with the patient; the discussion should be supplemented with written instructions, as presented in Table 24–6. Patients also should be warned against gaining a false sense of confidence if dietary guidelines are broken without consequences. We often recommend that our patients who take MAOIs read chapters on antidepressants in books written specifically for patients and their families (e.g., Gorman 1990; Kass et al. 1992; Yudofsky et al. 1991). Because the current use of MAOIs is predominantly in patients with refractory depression—patients who are often suicidal—too often clinicians are hesitant to use these medications for fear that patients will intentionally not comply with dietary restrictions in order to harm themselves. This is a difficult paradox: if the medication is effective, the patient will no longer want to commit suicide. Furthermore, withholding of effective treatment, with the likely continuation of the depressed state, is associated with a higher risk for suicide. In these cases, we often emphasize to the patient that failure to adhere to the instructions is more likely to cause cerebral hemorrhage and disability than to cause death.

Phenelzine is initiated with 15 mg in the morning and increased by 15 mg every other day until a total daily dosage of 60 mg is reached. If no response occurs within 2 weeks, the dosage may be increased in 15-mg increments to a usual maximum of 90 mg/day. Higher dosages are sometimes used, if tolerated, in patients with severe and refractory depression. Tranylcypromine is initiated at 10 mg and then increased every other day to 30 mg/day. As with phenelzine, higher doses may be necessary when the condition is refractory to treatment (Amsterdam and

TABLE 24–5. Summary of monoamine oxidase (MAO) inhibitor reversibility and selectivity

Drug	Reversible inhibition	Enzyme selectivity	Indication
Phenelzine	No	MAO-A + B	Depression
Tranylcypromine	No	MAO-A + B	Depression
L-Deprenyl	No	MAO-B[a]	Parkinson's disease
Pargyline	No	MAO-B[a]	Hypertension
Moclobemide[b]	Yes	MAO-A	Depression

[a]MAO-B is selective at lower doses, nonselective at higher doses.
[b]Not available in the United States.

Berwish 1989). After tolerance to the hypotensive side effects has developed, usually after 1 or 2 weeks, the patient may take the medication as a single daily dose in the morning. Morning dosing is preferred because these medications tend to be activating, especially tranylcypromine, which is related to amphetamine. Some data suggest that once-daily dosing of the MAOIs may be therapeutically superior to multiple dosing (Weise et al. 1980).

Risks, Side Effects, and Their Management

The following risks and side effects apply to the irreversible, nonselective MAOI antidepressants (phenelzine and tranylcypromine). The most common side effects are orthostatic hypotension, headache, insomnia, weight gain, sexual dysfunction, peripheral edema, and afternoon somnolence. Although the MAOIs do not have significant affinity for muscarinic receptors, anticholinergic-like side effects are present at the start of treatment. Dry mouth is common but not as marked as with the TCAs. Fortunately, the more serious risks, such as hypertensive crisis and serotonin syndrome, are not common.

Hypertensive crisis. The inactivation of intestinal MAO impairs the metabolism of tyramine. Tyramine can act as a false transmitter and displace norepinephrine from presynaptic storage granules. Thus, large amounts of dietary tyramine can result in a hypertensive crisis in patients taking MAOIs because increased amounts of norepinephrine result in profound α-adrenergic activation. This reaction also has been called the "cheese reaction" because tyramine is present in relatively high concentrations in aged cheese.

Tyramine is formed in foods by the decarboxylation of tyrosine during the aging, ripening, and decay process of foods. Patients receiving MAOI treatment should be instructed to avoid eating the foods listed in Table 24–7. The key foods to avoid are aged cheeses, fermented sausage, sauerkraut, soy sauce, yeast extracts such as

Marmite, fava beans and broad beans (which contain dopamine), and any food that is overripe or spoiled. Fresh, unaged cheeses, such as cottage cheese, ricotta, and cream cheese, are safe. Several foods that were formerly considered dangerous are no longer included on the list of prohibited substances. For example, domestic bottled or canned beer is now considered safe when consumed in moderation (Gardner et al. 1996). Most wines and liquors are also considered safe when taken in moderation. Liver, if fresh, is also probably safe, and caffeine and chocolate are of concern only when consumed in large amounts.

Some drugs with sympathomimetic activity, including certain decongestants and cough syrups, should be avoided because of the risk of precipitating a hypertensive crisis (Table 24–7). However, pure antihistamine drugs, such as diphenhydramine, and pure expectorants without dextromethorphan (e.g., guaifenesin) are permissible.

Unfortunately, even perfect compliance with the dietary and other restrictions does not guarantee complete protection from MAOI-induced hypertensive crises. Rare reports of spontaneous hypertension associated with MAOI use have come from several independent sources. Most of these reports involve the use of tranylcypromine, but phenelzine also has been implicated (Fallon et al. 1988; Kahn 1988; Krause 1989; Linet 1986).

These reactions can range from mild to severe. In the mildest form, the patient may complain of sweating, palpitations, and a mild headache. The most severe form manifests as a hypertensive crisis, with severe headache, increased blood pressure, and possible intracerebral hemorrhage. If a patient experiences a severely painful or unremitting occipital headache when taking an MAOI, he or she should immediately seek medical assessment and monitoring.

If the blood pressure is severely elevated, pharmacological treatment should be instituted. We often recommend that patients purchase a home blood pressure cuff to help distinguish a true hypertensive crisis from more

TABLE 24–6.   Instructions for patients taking monoamine oxidase inhibitors

While taking this medication

1. Avoid all the foods and drugs indicated on the list (see Table 24–7).
2. In general, all the foods you should avoid are decayed, fermented, or aged in some way. Avoid any spoiled food even if it is not on the list.
3. If you get a cold or flu, you may use aspirin or Tylenol. For a cough, glycerin cough drops or cough syrup without dextromethorphan may be used.
4. All laxatives or stool softeners for constipation may be used.
5. For infections, all antibiotics may be safely prescribed, such as penicillin, tetracycline, or erythromycin.
6. Do not take any other medications without first checking with me. These include any over-the-counter medicines bought without prescription, such as cold tablets, nose drops, cough medicine, and diet pills.
7. Eating one of the restricted foods may cause a sudden elevation of your blood pressure. If this occurs, you will get an explosive headache, particularly in the back of your head and in your temples. Your head and face will feel flushed and full, your heart may pound, and you may perspire heavily and feel nauseated. If this rare reaction occurs, do not lie down because this elevates your blood pressure further. If your blood pressure is high, go to the nearest emergency center for evaluation and treatment. Do not wait for a telephone call from our office.
8. If you need medical or dental care while taking this medication, show these restrictions and instructions to the doctor or dentist. Have the doctor or dentist call my office if he or she has any questions or needs further clarification or information.
9. Side effects such as postural light-headedness, constipation, delay in urination, delay in ejaculation and orgasm, muscle twitching, sedation, fluid retention, insomnia, and excess sweating are quite common. Many of these side effects lessen after the third week.
10. Light-headedness may occur after sudden changes in position. This can be avoided by getting up slowly. If tablets are taken with meals, this and the other side effects are lessened.
11. The medication is rarely effective in less than 3 weeks.
12. Care should be taken while operating any machinery or driving; some patients have episodes of sleepiness in the early phase of treatment.
13. Take the medication precisely as directed. Do not regulate the number of pills without first consulting me.
14. In spite of the side effects and special dietary restrictions, your medication (an MAO inhibitor) is safe and effective when taken as directed.
15. If any special problems arise, call me at my office.

Source.   Adapted from Jenike 1987.

common, and benign, headaches of other etiologies. Currently, the most common treatment for MAOI-induced hypertension is the calcium channel blocker nifedipine. An oral dose of 10 mg of nifedipine often normalizes blood pressure in 1–5 minutes with little risk of overshoot hypotension (Schenk and Remick 1989). If patients are supplied with a prescription for nifedipine in advance, they may administer the medication immediately and then proceed to a hospital for further monitoring and treatment. A drug with α-adrenergic-blocking properties, such as intravenous phentolamine (5 mg) or intramuscular chlorpromazine (25–50 mg), also may be administered. Because treatment with phentolamine may be associated with cardiac arrhythmias or severe hypotension, this approach should be carried out only in an emergency department setting (Tollefson 1983).

It is advisable to have patients taking MAOIs carry an identification card as notification to emergency medical personnel that they are currently taking an MAOI. Patients should always carry the list of prohibited foods and medications, and they should be told to notify physicians that they are taking an MAOI before accepting any medication or anesthetic (Tables 24–6 and 24–7). When patients have dental procedures performed, local anesthetics without vasoconstrictors (e.g., epinephrine) must be used.

Serotonin syndrome.   The combination of serotonergic drugs, such as the SSRIs, with MAOIs can result in serotonin syndrome, which may be fatal. As the condition progresses, hyperthermia, hypertonicity, myoclonus, and death may occur. The syndrome must be identified as rapidly as possible. Discontinuation of the serotonergic medications is the first step in treatment, followed by emergency medical treatment, as required.

The combination of MAOIs with meperidine, and perhaps with other phenylpiperidine analgesics, also has been implicated in the fatal reactions that were attributed to the serotonin syndrome. Aspirin, nonsteroidal anti-inflammatory drugs, and acetaminophen should be used for mild to moderate pain. Among narcotic agents, codeine and morphine are safe in combination with MAOIs, although doses may need to be lower than usual.

Cardiovascular effects.   The MAOIs cause significant hypotension, which is often the dosage-limiting side effect of these drugs. Expansion of the intravascular volume by using salt tablets or fludrocortisone may be an effective treatment. However, some patients manifest peripheral edema, which may mandate a reduction in salt intake. The addition in low dosage of a psychostimulant medication has been shown to alleviate this side effect as well.

TABLE 24–7.　Dietary and medication restrictions for patients taking monoamine oxidase inhibitors (MAOIs)

Foods that must be avoided while taking an MAOI and for 2 weeks after stopping the medication[a]	Aged cheeses (fresh cheese such as cream cheese, cottage cheese, ricotta cheese, American cheese, and moderate amounts of mozzarella are currently considered safe)
	Aged or fermented meats, such as sausages, salami, and pepperoni (smoked salmon and whitefish are currently considered safe)
	Sauerkraut
	Soy sauce
	Fava beans and broad bean pods
	All food that may be spoiled
	Alcohol may be consumed in moderation, but tap beer should be avoided, including nonalcoholic tap beer
	Yeast or meat extracts such as Marmite and Bovril (yeast and baked goods containing yeast are safe)
	Yogurt, if fresh, is safe

Drugs that must be avoided while taking an MAOI and for 2 weeks after stopping the medication[b]

All sympathomimetics and stimulant drugs, including

Amphetamines	Local anesthetic drugs containing ephedrine or cocaine
Diet medications	Demerol
Ephedrine	Levodopa and dopamine
Isoproterenol	Fenfluramine and dexfenfluramine
Methylphenidate	Other antidepressant medications
Phenylpropanolamine	Buspirone
Phenylephrine	

Over-the-counter nasal decongestants and cold, sinus, and allergy medications containing pseudoephedrine, phenylephrine, or phenylpropanolamine

Actifed	Robitussin PE, DM, CF, Night Relief
Alka-Seltzer Plus	Sine-Aid
Allerest	Sine-Off
Contact	Sinex
Coricidin D	Triaminic
CoTylenol	Tylenol
Dristan	Vicks Formula 44M, 44D, Nyquil
Neo-Synephrine	

Safe cold/allergy medications	Tylenol (plain)
	Robitussin (plain)
	Alka-Seltzer (plain)
	Chlor-Trimeton Allergy (without decongestant)
	Steroid inhalers
Other safe medications	Nonsteroidal anti-inflammatory drugs
	Codeine
	Morphine
	Antibiotics
	Laxatives and stool softeners
	Local anesthetics without epinephrine or cocaine

Note.　[a]Food restrictions are based on tyramine contact data from Walker et al. 1996.
[b]It is advisable to check the current *Physicians' Desk Reference* for any drug that is not known to be safe before prescribing it in combination with an MAOI.
Source.　Feinburg and Holzer 1997, 2000; Schulman and Walker 1999, 2000; Walker et al. 1997; Wing and Chen 1997.

Weight gain. MAOIs are associated with a risk of significant weight gain during treatment. It appears that this side effect occurs less frequently with tranylcypromine than it does with phenelzine (Rabkin et al. 1985).

Sexual dysfunction. MAOIs are commonly associated with treatment-emergent sexual dysfunction, including decreased libido, delayed ejaculation, anorgasmia, and impotence. Some patients become tolerant to this side effect over time, but more often the problem persists unless the dose is reduced or another medication is used to counter the sexual side effects. The treatment of sexual side effects is discussed in the section on SSRIs.

CNS effects. Headache and insomnia are common initial side effects that usually dissipate after the first few weeks of treatment. Patients taking MAOIs commonly experience somnolence in the afternoon, which is often described as an irresistible urge to take a nap. Even a brief nap (e.g., 20 minutes) will effectively restore alertness. This interesting effect is not related to insomnia or the timing of medication administration, but rather is a more direct chronobiological effect.

Overdose. The MAOIs fall between the TCAs and the SSRIs in terms of lethality in overdose. Most complications related to MAOI overdose arise from its stimulation of the sympathetic nervous system. MAOIs are most dangerous when patients have hypertensive crises as the result of ingesting foods with high tyramine content.

Drug interactions. The inhibition of MAO can cause severe interactions with other drugs, as detailed in the earlier subsections on hypertensive crisis and the serotonin syndrome. A list of MAOI drug interactions is provided in Table 24–7. In addition, MAOIs may prolong and amplify the sedative effects of medications and alcohol.

Moclobemide

Moclobemide is a reversible inhibitor of MAO-A (RIMA). This drug is not available in the United States, but it is available in many other countries, including Mexico and Canada. As discussed earlier in this section, because the RIMAs are reversible and selective, dietary restrictions are not necessary. Moclobemide is initiated at 150 mg twice a day. Although the suggested therapeutic range is 300–600 mg/day, we and others have found that dosages of 900 mg/day are often required to obtain optimal antidepressant effects.

Issues of Treatment

Treatment of Acute Major Depression

The choice of an antidepressant medication is based on factors discussed earlier in this section and outlined in Table 24–2. The initial therapeutic response of the depressed patient to medications may be detected as early as the first week, but it is often delayed by several weeks. Neurovegetative symptoms usually improve before mood improves. The clinician must inform the patient of this latency in therapeutic response because many patients expect antidepressants to be effective with the first dose. For patients with severe anxiety or insomnia, the concurrent use of a benzodiazepine may be considered. However, we restrict this practice solely to the treatment of depressed patients with marked anxiety, and we discontinue it by tapering the benzodiazepine dosage as the antidepressant begins to exert its therapeutic effect. A patient may experience a return of energy and motivation while still experiencing the subjective symptoms of hopelessness and excessive guilt. For such patients, there may be an increased risk of suicide because a return of energy in an extremely dysphoric individual may provide the impetus and wherewithal for an act of self-destruction.

A clinical challenge in the evaluation of side effects of antidepressant drugs is to distinguish symptoms of the illness from complaints that are secondary to side effects. Nelson et al. (1984) carefully studied patient complaints before and during treatment with desipramine. Many symptoms that the patients attributed to antidepressant treatment, such as constipation, poor memory or concentration, nausea or vomiting, diarrhea, difficulty sitting still, drowsiness, difficulty with urination, palpitations, urinary frequency, and tremors, were attributable to the illness rather than to medication side effects. A great deal of the skill required to treat patients with major depression involves encouraging them to continue treatment despite their perception of early medication side effects. It is important to inform patients that the more serious antidepressant side effects subside after the first 2 weeks of treatment.

An adequate trial of antidepressant medication traditionally has been defined as treatment with therapeutic dosages of a drug for a total of 6–8 weeks. On the basis of more recent data, Quitkin et al. (1996) suggested that 4 weeks may be a more clinically meaningful point for reevaluation of treatment. After 4 weeks of antidepressant treatment, the patient can be conceptualized as falling into one of three groups, depending on whether there has been 1) a full response, 2) a partial response, or 3) no response at all. For the fortunate patients who achieve full remission, treatment should continue for a minimum of 4–6 months, or longer when there is a history of a recurrent course (see the subsection "Maintenance Treatment of Major Depression" later in this chapter). If a partial response has been achieved by 4 weeks, a full response may be evident within an additional 2 weeks without further intervention. If there is no response at all, the dosage should be increased, the medication should be changed to another antidepressant, or the therapy should be augmented with another medication (see the subsection "Treatment-Resistant Depression" later in this chapter). These guidelines are summarized in Figure 24–1.

Treatment of Depression With Psychotic Features

Patients with psychotic depression have been reported to respond to combined treatment with antidepressants and antipsychotics (Nelson and Bowers 1978); they also show a dramatic response to ECT, which is often the treatment of choice in this disorder (Yudofsky 1981). Long-term antipsychotic medications are generally not warranted, but prophylactic antidepressant medication must be continued as in nonpsychotic depression.

Treatment of Bipolar Depression

A history of previous episodes of mania or hypomania should alert the clinician to the diagnosis of bipolar disorder. Because antidepressants can precipitate manic episodes and increase cycling in bipolar patients (Wehr and Goodwin 1979), mood stabilizers (e.g., lithium, valproate) are the appropriate first step in the treatment of bipolar depression (see section "Mood Stabilizers" later in this chapter).

Maintenance Treatment of Major Depression

Antidepressant therapy should not be discontinued before there have been 4–5 symptom-free months (Prien and Kupfer 1986). Most clinicians treat single episodes of depression for a minimum of 6 months. Antidepressants should be continued at the same dosage that resulted in remission of the acute episode. Strong evidence indicates that relapse is more likely when the antidepressant dosage is lowered from acute treatment levels (Frank et al. 1990).

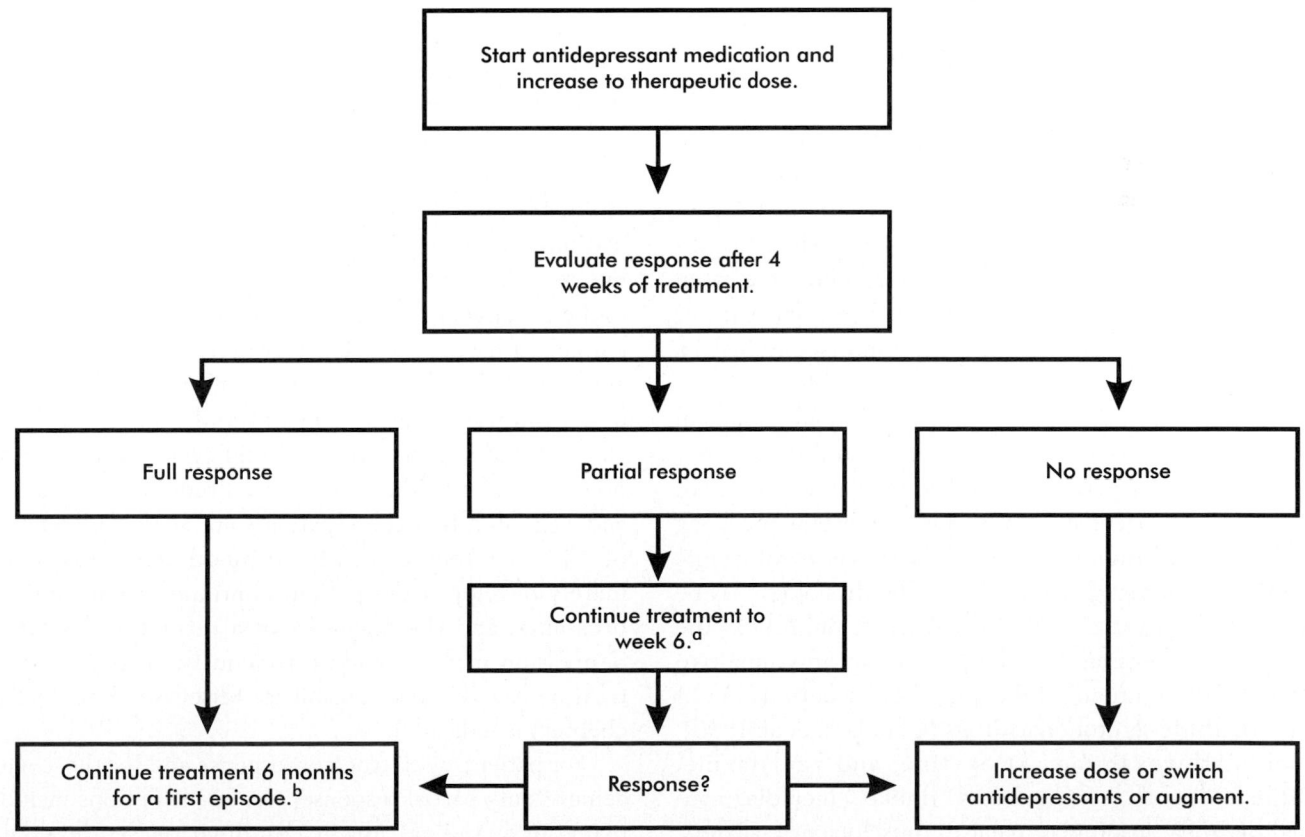

FIGURE 24–1. Algorithm for the acute treatment of major depression.

[a]If no further response is seen at week 5, it is not necessary to wait until week 6. [b]See text for maintenance treatment guidelines for patients with recurrent depression.

Unfortunately, depression is often a recurrent disorder. After one episode of depression, there is a 50% chance that the patient will have a second episode; after three episodes, there is a 90% chance of recurrence (Angst 1990). Therefore, longer periods of antidepressant treatment, often called *maintenance treatment*, are warranted to protect against recurrence (NIMH Consensus Development Conference Statement 1985). The value of maintenance antidepressant treatment, with and without psychotherapy, for patients with recurrent depression has been established by Frank et al. (1990) in an elegant four-arm, double-blind, placebo-controlled trial. Current World Health Organization guidelines recommend maintenance treatment for patients who have had two or more episodes of major depression within a 5-year period (Coppen et al. 1986). In patients with more than three episodes of depression, long-term prophylaxis is strongly recommended. The duration of treatment is individualized on the basis of the severity and effect of past episodes, and the time between episodes. Some patients may require lifelong antidepressant maintenance treatment. There is no evidence of increased risk associated with long-term use of antidepressants.

Antidepressant Discontinuation

Discontinuation of antidepressant medication should be concordant with the guidelines for treatment duration, as outlined earlier. It is advisable to taper the medication while monitoring for signs and symptoms of relapse. Abrupt discontinuation is also more likely to lead to antidepressant discontinuation symptoms, which are often referred to as *withdrawal* symptoms. The occurrence of these symptoms following medication discontinuation does not imply that antidepressants are "addictive."

Abrupt discontinuation of TCAs commonly results in diarrhea, increased sweating, anxiety, and dizziness—symptoms previously attributed to cholinergic rebound. However, the occurrence of similar symptoms following the discontinuation of many of the newer serotonergic antidepressants suggests that the pathophysiology may be more closely related to changes in serotonin. Among the newer antidepressants, withdrawal symptoms appear to occur most commonly following the discontinuation of short-half-life serotonergic drugs (Coupland et al. 1996), such as fluvoxamine, paroxetine, and venlafaxine. Patients describe symptoms as "flulike," including nausea, diarrhea, insomnia, malaise, muscle aches, anxiety, irritability, dizziness, vertigo, and vivid dreams (Coupland et al. 1996). Often and for unknown reasons, patients who experience this constellation of symptoms

have transient "electric shock" sensations. This unique symptom is diagnostically useful and strongly suggests to the clinician that the patient is in fact experiencing withdrawal because the symptom rarely occurs in other conditions such as viral infections or as a side effect of a new medication.

Symptoms usually occur for 1–2 days following the abrupt discontinuation of the medication and subside within 7–10 days. However, in some instances symptoms also may occur during tapering and dose reduction, and they may persist for up to 3 weeks. Restarting the medication with a slower taper may be necessary, although it is often possible to attenuate withdrawal symptoms produced by short-half-life SSRIs by administering one dose of fluoxetine (which has a more prolonged half-life). In our experience, the short-term addition of a benzodiazepine is often helpful.

Treatment-Resistant Depression

Careful review of the clinical history and response to previous treatment often reveals that patients in whom depression has been resistant to standard antidepressant treatment have had an inadequate therapeutic trial with the antidepressant (Lydiard 1985) or have been noncompliant with the medication. Failure to complete an adequate therapeutic trial with an antidepressant drug does not constitute a depression that is resistant to pharmacotherapy. In another presentation, patients report a history of robust but short-lived responses to several antidepressants. This patient may be manifesting a medication-induced rapid-cycling course. Mild episodes of hypomania during the course of treatment may be overlooked, especially in a high-functioning, productive patient with a premorbid history of hyperthymic personality, which is defined as a chronic state of mild hypomania. Kukopoulos et al. (1983) and Akiskal (1992) claimed that hyperthymia and mild cyclothymia may be predictors of a medication-induced rapid-cycling course and suggested that these patients are at the milder end of a bipolar spectrum. Mixed mood states may ultimately develop if the patient continues taking antidepressants, and the diagnosis of a refractory, agitated depression may be made erroneously. In these cases, treatment with a mood stabilizer (discussed later in this chapter) is indicated.

For patients with true nonresponse and for those who achieve only partial response, treatment options include using an augmentation or combination strategy and switching to another antidepressant. Augmentation involves adding another agent that is not an antidepressant, such as lithium, thyroid hormone, or a psychostimulant. Combination treatment refers to combining two antidepressants with different mechanisms of action to produce synergistic effects. Whether to switch, augment, or combine depends on many factors, including the severity of illness, side effects of the current medication, and the patient's willingness to take more than one medication. For example, if a patient's illness is significantly interfering with daily function, augmentation or combination should be considered if the current antidepressant is well tolerated because this may result in a quicker response. On the other hand, a patient with a milder illness, significant side effects of the current medication, and a general uneasiness about taking medication will probably be better off if the current medication is switched to a different, single antidepressant.

Of the augmentation strategies, lithium augmentation has the best evidence from randomized controlled trials; however, almost all of these data are with the TCAs. Since De Montigny and colleagues first reported successful antidepressant treatment with adjunctive lithium in 1981, there have been many reports of patients who failed to respond to TCA or SSRI treatment alone but whose depressions improved when the antidepressant was combined with lithium (Dinan and Barry 1989; Ontiveros et al. 1991; Thase et al. 1989). Although some of these patients manifested a rapid and dramatic response when lithium was added to their antidepressant regimen, improvement may require several weeks. Patients often respond to dosages of lithium lower than are used for the treatment of bipolar disorder. We typically start with 600 mg at bedtime. If there is no response after 2 weeks, the dosage should be increased as tolerated.

Thyroid supplementation has received a more mixed endorsement in the scientific literature. Goodwin et al. (1982) performed the first double-blind study that found triiodothyronine (T_3) to be a useful adjunct in former nonresponders. However, Gitlin et al. (1987), in a follow-up study, found no benefit to this approach. A study by Joffe (1988) reported that patients who did respond to the addition of T_3 were less likely to benefit from adjunctive lithium, and vice versa. This double-blind, placebo-controlled trial found a 50% response rate for both lithium and T_3 augmentation. For unclear reasons, it appears that T_3 is more effective than thyroxine (T_4) as an augmenting agent in unipolar depression (Joffe and Singer 1990).

Stimulants such as amphetamine and methylphenidate have been used to treat depression for many years. Stimulants should not be used as monotherapy, except perhaps in geriatric patients with prominent apathy, medically ill patients with depression, or patients with poststroke depression (Lingam et al. 1988). However, psychostimulants are useful for augmentation of antidepressants in the treatment of refractory depression and are generally safe, even for most patients with cardiac disorders. Fawcett et al. (1991) reported the successful use of stimulant-MAOI combinations among a group of patients who were nonresponders to various other treatments, including ECT. Only 1 of their 32 patients could not tolerate the combination because of hypertensive side effects. The nonamphetamine stimulant modafinil has been reported to be useful in a recent uncontrolled report of seven subjects (Menza et al. 2000).

The use of more than one antidepressant for patients with treatment-resistant depression is potentially beneficial. SSRI-TCA combinations have been reported to be effective for patients who do not respond to monotherapy and, perhaps, to cause a more rapid antidepressant effect (Nelson et al. 1991; Weilburg et al. 1989). Some SSRIs can cause tricyclic levels in the blood to rise (Aranow et al. 1989; Downs et al. 1989), but this effect is not likely to account for the synergism between the two antidepressants. However, because of this pharmacokinetic interaction, augmentation of the TCA dose should be reduced to achieve the same blood levels. Although there are few systematic data, other antidepressant combinations are commonly used in clinical practice to treat refractory depression. The principle of combining two antidepressants is to choose agents that have different mechanisms of action. For example, it makes little sense to combine two different SSRIs. However, the combination of an SSRI with mirtazapine or bupropion may provide mechanistic synergy. When combining antidepressants, it is important first to ensure that the patient has had an adequate trial of a single agent and to be aware of possible drug interactions or additive side effects.

Despite concerns about severe reactions that may occur with concomitant treatment with TCAs and MAOIs, the combination may be safely prescribed, provided specific precautions are taken. It has been firmly established that it is hazardous to add a TCA to ongoing MAOI therapy. However, there are reports of the safe addition of an MAOI to ongoing treatment with a TCA (Kahn et al. 1989; for a review, see Pande et al. 1991). Some evidence indicates that such a combination may prove effective in depressed patients who have failed monotherapy with a TCA and an SSRI (Schmauss et al. 1988; White and Simpson 1981). There are two general strategies for combined therapy with MAOIs: 1) the MAOI is added to the TCA, or 2) the two drugs are begun concurrently. If the MAOI is to be added, the TCA should be raised, as usual, to a therapeutic level. The MAOI should be added in small increments over protracted periods of time until a therapeutic response occurs or until side effects intervene. Because of the risk of the serotonin syndrome, TCAs with strong serotonin reuptake inhibition, especially clomipramine, should be avoided in combination with MAOIs (Marley and Wozniak 1984). This caveat must be extended to the entire class of SSRIs and venlafaxine, all of which must never be administered together with an MAOI.

Particular care must be exercised in switching patients from an MAOI to other antidepressant classes. For patients who have completed an MAOI trial without therapeutic response, other antidepressants should not be started until 14 days after the original MAOI has been discontinued. Equal care is required when switching from most other antidepressants to an MAOI. A time period equal to five times the half-life of the drug, including active metabolites, is required between stopping other antidepressant medications and starting an MAOI. A 2-week interval is also recommended when switching from phenelzine to tranylcypromine because tranylcypromine is an amphetamine derivative. Theoretically, switching from tranylcypromine, which has a short half-life, to phenelzine should not require as prolonged a waiting period. A recent case series published by Szuba et al. (1997) suggested that some patients could be switched from one MAOI to another without a 14-day washout. The authors emphasized that this strategy should be used only when clinically essential and with close monitoring.

Switching between other antidepressants is less problematic. Current practice is to discontinue the first medication before starting the second one. There is no need for a medication-free period if neither medication is an MAOI. However, some patients report increased side effects and anxiety when switching from fluoxetine to nefazodone. This reaction is most likely because fluoxetine and its active metabolite norfluoxetine inhibit CYP2D6, which metabolizes a metabolite of nefazodone, which is known to be anxiogenic. Therefore, it may be prudent to wait 1–2 weeks between the discontinuation of fluoxetine and the start of nefazodone.

Nonpharmacological options also should be considered in patients who have not adequately responded to treatment. As discussed later in this chapter, ECT is a highly effective treatment. In addition, several novel treatment options, including vagus nerve stimulation, are showing promising results for moderately treatment-resistant patients (also discussed later in this chapter). In addition, psychotherapy has an important role in the treatment of depression (as is discussed in various chapters throughout this volume).

Anxiolytics, Sedatives, and Hypnotics

Overview

Anxiety and insomnia are prevalent symptoms with multiple etiologies. Effective treatments are available, but they vary by diagnosis. In most instances, the best course of action is to treat the underlying disorder rather than reflexively instituting treatment with a nonspecific anxiolytic. For example, a patient who has anxiety symptoms related to paranoid delusions should be given an antipsychotic medication not an anxiolytic. Likewise, patients with panic disorder, OCD, or major depression should receive medications indicated for those disorders. In these cases, anxiety may be a target symptom, one of the group of target symptoms of the underlying disorder.

In some cases, anxiolytics serve a transitional purpose. Consider a patient with acute-onset panic disorder, severe anticipatory anxiety, and a family history of depression. An antidepressant medication that also has antipanic effects may be the optimal treatment, but it will not help the patient for several weeks, during which time there is a risk of progression to agoraphobia. For this patient, we recommend starting the antidepressant and also targeting acute symptom relief with a benzodiazepine. After 4 weeks, the benzodiazepine should be slowly tapered so that the patient's symptoms are controlled with the antidepressant alone.

In this section, we discuss the pharmacology of medications classified as anxiolytic, sedative, or hypnotic, primarily the benzodiazepines, buspirone, zolpidem, and zaleplon. Subsequently, we present diagnosis-specific treatment guidelines as outlined in Table 24–8. The commonly used anxiolytics and hypnotics, together with their usual dosages, are shown in Table 24–9. In addition, many antidepressant medications are effective in the treatment of anxiety disorders. The pharmacology of the antidepressants was discussed in the previous section; their clinical use in anxiety disorders is included in the diagnosis-specific subsections that follow.

Benzodiazepines

Mechanisms of Action

Benzodiazepines facilitate the inhibitory properties of γ-aminobutyric acid (GABA), the major inhibitory neurotransmitter in the brain (reviewed by Tallman et al. 1980). The benzodiazepine receptor is a subtype of the GABA$_A$ receptor. Activation of the benzodiazepine

TABLE 24–8. Medications of choice for specific anxiety disorders

Generalized anxiety disorder	Buspirone, benzodiazepines, venlafaxine, SSRIs[a]
Obsessive-compulsive disorder	Clomipramine, SSRIs
Panic disorder	SSRIs, TCAs, MAOIs, benzodiazepines
Performance anxiety	β Blockers, benzodiazepines
Social phobia	SSRIs, MAOIs, benzodiazepines, buspirone

Note. MAOI = monoamine oxidase inhibitor; SSRI = selective serotonin reuptake inhibitor; TCA = tricyclic antidepressant.

[a]Paroxetine was recently approved for the treatment of generalized anxiety disorder, but other SSRIs are probably also effective.

receptor facilitates the action of endogenous GABA, which results in the opening of chloride ion channels and a decrease in neuronal excitability. Benzodiazepines act rapidly because ion channels can open and close relatively quickly, in contrast to the slower onset of action that occurs when a drug acts via a metabotropic receptor and the resultant cascade of G proteins, second messengers, and subsequent intracellular effects.

Indications and Efficacy

Benzodiazepines are highly effective anxiolytics and sedatives; they also possess muscle relaxant and anticonvulsant properties. Benzodiazepines effectively treat both acute and chronic generalized anxiety (Elie and Lamontagne 1985; Greenblatt et al. 1983; Rickels 1986; Rickels et al. 1983) and panic disorder. The high-potency benzodiazepines alprazolam and clonazepam have received more attention as antipanic agents (Tesar 1990; Tesar et al. 1991), but double-blind studies also have confirmed the efficacy of diazepam (Dunner et al. 1986) and lorazepam (Charney and Woods 1989) in the treatment of panic disorder. Although only a few benzodiazepines have specific, FDA-approved indications for the treatment of insomnia, almost all benzodiazepines may be used for this purpose. Benzodiazepines are most clearly valuable as hypnotics in the general hospital setting, where high levels of sensory stimulation, pain, and acute stress may interfere with sleep. The safe, effective, and time-limited use of benzodiazepine hypnotics may, in fact, prevent chronic sleep difficulties from taking hold (NIMH Consensus Development Conference 1984). Benzodiazepines are also used to treat akathisia and catatonia and as an adjunct in the treatment of acute mania.

TABLE 24–9. Commonly used anxiolytic and hypnotic medications

Generic (trade) name	Single dose (mg)	Usual therapeutic dosage (mg/day)	Approximate dose equivalent (mg)	Methods of administration and supplied form	Approximate elimination half-life, including metabolites[a]
Benzodiazepines					
Alprazolam (Xanax and generics)	0.25–1	1–4	0.5	po: 0.25/0.5 mg	12 hours
Chlordiazepoxide (Librium and generics)	5–25	15–100	10	po: 5/10/25 mg; iv, im[b]	1–4 days
Clonazepam (Klonopin)	0.5–2	1–4	0.25	po: 0.5/2 mg	1–2 days
Clorazepate (Tranxene and generics)	3.75–22.5	15–60	7.5	po: 3.75/7.5/30 mg	2–4 days
Diazepam (Valium and generics)	2–10	4–40	5	po: 2/5/10 mg; iv, im[b]	2–4 days
Lorazepam (Ativan and generics)	0.5–2	1–6	1	po, s/l: 0.5/1/2 mg; iv, im[b]	12 hours
Oxazepam (Serax and generics)	10–30	30–120	15	po: 10/15/30 mg	12 hours
Nonbenzodiazepines					
Buspirone (BuSpar)	10–30	30–60	NA	po: 5/10/15 mg	2–3 hours

Note. NA = not applicable.

[a]The clinical duration of action for the benzodiazepines does not correlate with the elimination half-life. See text for discussion.

[b]Lorazepam im is well absorbed. We do not recommend chlordiazepoxide or diazepam im.

Source. Adapted from Teboul and Chouinard 1990 and *Physicians' Desk Reference* 2001.

Because alcohol and barbiturates also act, in part, via the GABA$_A$ receptor–mediated chloride ion channel, benzodiazepines show cross-tolerance with these substances. As such, benzodiazepines are used frequently for the treatment of alcohol or barbiturate withdrawal and detoxification. Alcohol and barbiturates are more dangerous than benzodiazepines because at high doses they can act directly at the chloride ion channel. In contrast, benzodiazepines have no direct effect on the ion channel; the effects of benzodiazepines are limited by the amount of endogenous GABA.

Three of the benzodiazepines are indicated for use in the control of seizure disorders. Diazepam is rapidly effective in the control of status epilepticus when administered intravenously. Clonazepam, either alone or in addition to other anticonvulsants, is indicated for control of absence, myoclonic, and atonic seizures. Clorazepate is indicated as adjunctive therapy for the control of grand mal and other seizure disorders. Intravenous lorazepam has gained acceptance as the treatment of choice for status epilepticus; its pharmacokinetic and pharmacodynamic properties result in a more prolonged anticonvulsant effect than is found with intravenous diazepam, which was formerly the standard treatment (Leppik et al. 1983).

Choice of Benzodiazepine

In equipotent doses, all benzodiazepines have similar effects. The choice among benzodiazepines is generally based on differences in half-life, rapidity of onset, metabolism, and potency. One frequently misunderstood issue is the relation between pharmacokinetic half-life and pharmacodynamic effect. The pharmacodynamics (i.e., the effects of the drug on the CNS) depend on several factors, including pharmacokinetic half-life, affinity of the drug for the benzodiazepine receptor, and lipid solubility of the drug. For example, lorazepam has a higher binding affinity for the benzodiazepine receptor than does diazepam (Jack et al. 1982); therefore, lorazepam binds to the receptor for a longer time. Lipid solubility is another important factor in determining pharmacodynamic effects of benzodiazepines. A drug that is highly lipid soluble will rapidly distribute to fat tissues, including those within the brain, whereas a drug with lower lipid solubility will reach the brain more slowly but maintain brain levels longer. Therefore, although diazepam (with high lipid solubility) has a more rapid onset of action than lorazepam (with moderate lipid solubility), the acute therapeutic effects will not last as long as those of lorazepam. When compared with diazepam, a single dose of lorazepam takes longer to produce sedation, but

this sedation persists longer (Ellinwood et al. 1985). This occurs despite the fact that lorazepam has a markedly briefer pharmacokinetic half-life than does diazepam and its metabolites (8 hours vs. 48 hours, respectively).

The metabolism of benzodiazepines also is important in the choice of the specific therapeutic agent. For example, diazepam is metabolized in the liver to desmethyldiazepam, a metabolite with a long half-life. Lorazepam and oxazepam are not converted to active metabolites by the liver. Therefore, for patients with hepatic dysfunction, lorazepam and oxazepam are clinically indicated for relief of anxiety because their elimination from the body will not be significantly affected (Abernethy et al. 1984).

Sedative effects of diazepam have been shown to persist for up to 2 weeks following discontinuation, after only 14 days of administration of diazepam 3 mg three times a day (Salzman et al. 1983). For patients with brain disorders and for elderly patients, benzodiazepines that are brief acting and devoid of active metabolites are usually indicated (e.g., lorazepam). As with all psychotropic medications, the most critical issue is that the lowest effective doses should be used in elderly patients, with careful and continuous monitoring of side effects.

Risks, Side Effects, and Their Management

Sedation and impairment of performance. Benzodiazepine-induced sedation may be considered either a therapeutic action or a side effect. Residual daytime somnolence is a function of two variables: drug half-life and dosage (Roth and Roehrs 1992). With longer-acting agents, such as flurazepam and quazepam, a morning-after hangover is common, although some tolerance to this effect may develop with time. On the other hand, any benzodiazepine, short or long acting, can cause daytime drowsiness if the nighttime dose is too great. In general, it is clinically unclear and theoretically uncertain whether sedation is a desirable component of anxiolytic activity. Many patients both expect and desire some degree of sedation when they are intensely anxious. Anxious patients who have received chronic treatment with benzodiazepines rarely complain about daytime sedation, even when compared with drug-free anxious subjects (Lucki et al. 1986).

Impairment of performance on sensitive psychomotor tests has been well documented after the administration of benzodiazepines. Diazepam, administered in a dosage of 10 mg three times a day, impaired driving skills in anxious patients during the first weeks of treatment (Linnoila et al. 1983). Lucki et al. (1986) found no impairment in a series of cognitive tasks in a group of anxious patients who had been taking benzodiazepines for an average of 5 years. Whether or not sedation is desired, patients must be warned that driving, engaging in dangerous physical activities, and using hazardous machinery should be avoided during the acute stages, and possibly during the later stages, of treatment with benzodiazepines.

Dependence, withdrawal, and rebound effects. Concerns about physical and psychological dependence on benzodiazepines are frequently raised by patients and often affect a clinician's choice of treatment. On the basis of the criterion of self-reinforcement, however, most of the benzodiazepines, with the possible exception of diazepam, have low abuse potential when properly prescribed and supervised (American Psychiatric Association 1990; Sellers et al. 1992). Illicit street traffic in potent agents such as alprazolam and triazolam has remained low, possibly because the rapidly developing sedation produced by these drugs interferes with the desired euphoriant effects (Mendelson 1992). Physical dependence often occurs when benzodiazepines are taken in higher than usual dosages or for prolonged periods of time (Busto et al. 1986; Schopf 1983; Tyrer et al. 1983).

If benzodiazepines are discontinued precipitously, withdrawal effects that include hyperpyrexia, seizures, psychosis, and even death may occur. Despite various methodological shortcomings, several studies also suggest that physical dependence may occur even when benzodiazepines are taken in usual clinical doses for prolonged periods beyond several weeks and that the symptoms of withdrawal may arise even when drug discontinuation is not abrupt (Ashton 1991; Noyes et al. 1988). The signs and symptoms of withdrawal may include tachycardia, increased blood pressure, muscle cramps, anxiety, insomnia, panic attacks, impairment of memory and concentration, and perceptual disturbances. In addition, withdrawal-related derealization, hallucinations, and other psychotic symptoms have been reported. These withdrawal symptoms may begin as soon as the day after discontinuation of benzodiazepines and may continue for weeks to months. Evidence indicates that withdrawal reactions peak more rapidly and more intensely with the benzodiazepines that have a briefer half-life (Busto et al. 1986). These withdrawal effects are rapidly reversed with the readministration of benzodiazepines. Although it is generally believed that there is cross-tolerance for all benzodiazepines, there has been a report of withdrawal symptoms from alprazolam that were not reversed with diazepam (Zipursky et al. 1985).

Rebound anxiety is defined as the return, on discontinuation of a benzodiazepine, of the anxiety signs and symptoms with greater intensity than existed before treatment. For this diagnosis, accurate documentation of specific symptoms and operationalized measures of the severity of preexisting anxiety are required. Fontaine et al. (1984) treated patients with generalized anxiety disorder for 4 weeks either with diazepam (a benzodiazepine with a long half-life) in a dosage of 15 mg/day or with placebo. After this time, both the drug and the placebo were withdrawn either abruptly or gradually. The patients who experienced abrupt withdrawal from diazepam had a 10% increase in anxiety, whereas no patient on the gradual withdrawal schedule or with placebo treatment had increased anxiety. Muscle spasms, insomnia, gastric symptoms, and agitation were documented in the benzodiazepine withdrawal group compared with the placebo group. Fewer cases of rebound anxiety were seen with diazepam than with bromazepam (which has a briefer half-life than diazepam).

Kales and Kales (1983) described rebound insomnia occurring after abrupt withdrawal of benzodiazepine drugs with relatively rapid elimination rates, such as triazolam. For patients with panic disorder treated with alprazolam, tapering and discontinuation of the medication may be associated with significant rebound anxiety and panic (Pecknold and Swinson 1986). Fyer et al. (1987) reported that significant withdrawal effects may occur when alprazolam, administered in a dosage of 2.5–8.0 mg/day for 12–47 weeks, is tapered at a rate of 10% every 3 days. In addition, there have been several reports of seizures occurring after the sudden discontinuation of alprazolam (Breier et al. 1984; Levy 1984). Kales et al. (1986) found no rebound effects with the discontinuation of the long-acting benzodiazepines flurazepam and quazepam. However, the patients were observed for only 15 days, which may be an insufficient length of time. In another study, the discontinuation of flurazepam led to rebound insomnia that occurred only during the second week of observation, whereas the rebound after triazolam discontinuation came within 2 days (Mitler et al. 1984).

A general principle for most psychoactive medications is that discontinuation should be accomplished gradually. For patients taking benzodiazepines for longer than 2–3 months, we suggest that the dosage be decreased by approximately 10% per week. Therefore, for a patient receiving 4 mg/day of alprazolam, the dosage should be tapered by 0.5 mg/week for 8 weeks. The last few dosage levels may be the most difficult to discontinue, and the patient will require increased attention and support from the physician during this time.

Memory impairment. Intravenous use of the benzodiazepines is associated with significant anterograde amnesia (Dixon et al. 1984; Reitan et al. 1986). For midazolam, diazepam, and lorazepam, this phenomenon may have clinical benefits because amnesia for surgical or other invasive therapeutic procedures is often desired. Amnesia appears to be mediated through the central benzodiazepine receptor; therefore, it may occur with any benzodiazepine (Lister 1985). In contrast to use in anesthesia, when benzodiazepines are used to treat insomnia or anxiety, amnesia may be a serious liability. Several studies have documented the deleterious effects on memory of oral benzodiazepines (Angus and Romney 1984; Mac et al. 1985). Tolerance to these amnestic effects may not develop. The degree of anterograde amnesia appears to be related to dosage, and the amnesia may occur in the first several hours after each dose of benzodiazepine is taken, even after repeated use (Lucki et al. 1986). There is some evidence, however, that the disruption of memory may be, at least in part, a retrograde effect produced by the onset of sleep itself (Roth et al. 1980); for example, benzodiazepine doses too low to induce sleep are less likely to cause amnestic effects (Roth et al. 1984).

The newer, briefer-acting benzodiazepines have been associated in some reports with a greater tendency to produce memory impairments (Roth et al. 1980), although a review of controlled studies did not seem to bear this out (Rothschild 1992). Following a 0.5-mg dose of triazolam, several individuals were unable to recall a whole series of complex, but routine, daily activities (Ewing et al. 1988; Morris and Estes 1987).

Disinhibition and dyscontrol. An area of controversy is the allegation that benzodiazepines may, in some instances, cause behavioral disinhibition, leading to acts of aggression (Medawarn and Rassaby 1991; Regestein and Reich 1985). Greenblatt et al. (1984), in their review of double-blind, controlled studies of triazolam and flurazepam that included more than 5,400 patients, found no reports of bizarre, disinhibitory reactions. However, there is a long history of anecdotal reports suggesting that many of the benzodiazepines can cause paradoxical anger and behavioral disinhibition that is dose related (see review by Rothschild 1992). A history of hostility, impulsivity, or borderline or antisocial personality disorder has been implicated as a potential predictor of this reaction. In light of the heightened attention focused on triazolam and the resulting potential for a significant reporting bias, the increase in anecdotal reports citing this particular agent is difficult to interpret. At present, some caution should be exercised when benzodiazepines are prescribed to patients with a history of poor impulse control and aggression (see section on the treatment of aggression later in this chapter); this possibility should be communicated to patients and documented in the medical record.

Overdose. Benzodiazepines are remarkably safe when taken in overdose. Dangerous effects occur when the overdose includes several sedative drugs, especially when alcohol is included, because of synergistic effects at the chloride ion site and resultant membrane hyperpolarization. In an extensive review by Greenblatt et al. (1977a), no patient who took an overdose of benzodiazepines alone became seriously ill or had serious complications. When the overdose occurred in combination with other drugs, however, the complications depended on the type and quantity of the nonbenzodiazepines. Finkle et al. (1979) essentially confirmed these results by finding that in only 2 of 1,239 overdoses with benzodiazepines were the deaths associated with the benzodiazepine alone.

The diagnosis of benzodiazepine overdose usually is made on the basis of questioning by the clinician of the patient, family, or friends about what drugs were ingested. The result is confirmed by physical examination finding signs and symptoms of toxicity with a CNS depressant (e.g., sedation, mental confusion, reduced respiration) and by either urine or blood drug screens. Because the standard urine drug screen assay may not detect the presence of many commonly prescribed benzodiazepines, including lorazepam, alprazolam, clonazepam, temazepam, and triazolam, the clinician should actively research the presence and accuracy of these tests in the laboratory that he or she uses. A safe and effective benzodiazepine antagonist, flumazenil, now exists that may be used via intravenous injection in an emergency setting to reverse the effects of any potential overdose with a benzodiazepine (Votey et al. 1991). However, medical management of a patient who has had an overdose often still requires physical supportive measures, such as ensuring proper respiratory function.

Drug interactions. Most sedative drugs, including narcotics and alcohol, potentiate the sedative effects of benzodiazepines. In addition, medications that inhibit hepatic CYP3A3/4, as discussed later in this chapter, increase blood levels and hence side effects of clonazepam, alprazolam, midazolam, and triazolam. Lorazepam, oxazepam, and temazepam are not dependent on hepatic enzymes for metabolism and therefore are not affected by hepatic disease or the inhibition of hepatic enzymes.

Use in pregnancy. Anxiolytics, like most medications, should be avoided during pregnancy and breast-feeding when possible. Although there have been concerns that benzodiazepines, when ingested during the first trimester of pregnancy, may increase the risk of the development of cleft palate, this has not been substantiated in controlled studies (Rosenberg et al. 1983; Shiono and Mills 1983).

Buspirone

The azapirones are agonists at the 5-HT$_{1A}$ receptors. Unlike benzodiazepines and barbiturates, they do not interact with the GABA receptor or directly with chloride ion channels. As such, these medications do not produce sedation, interact with alcohol, impair psychomotor performance, or pose a risk of abuse. There is no cross-tolerance between benzodiazepines and azapirones. As such, it is important to bear in mind that these classes of medication are not interchangeable. Like the antidepressants, azapirones have a relatively slow onset of action. Buspirone is the only azapirone currently available in the United States.

Mechanism of Action

The anxiolytic effect of the azapirones is the result of a selective stimulation of the 5-HT$_{1A}$ receptor. Acute administration suppresses neuronal firing in the dorsal raphe through autoreceptor stimulation. Chronic administration desensitizes presynaptic, but not postsynaptic, 5-HT$_{1A}$ receptors (Suranyi-Cadotte et al. 1990).

Indications and Efficacy

Buspirone is effective in the treatment of generalized anxiety. Although it has a longer onset of action, its efficacy is not statistically different from that of the benzodiazepines (Cohn and Wilcox 1986; Goldberg and Finnerty 1979). Despite its successes in the treatment of generalized anxiety disorder, buspirone does not appear to be effective in the treatment of panic disorder (Sheehan et al. 1990), except perhaps in an auxiliary role for the treatment of anticipatory anxiety (Gastfried and Rosenbaum 1989). Buspirone is also used as an augmenting agent in the treatment of OCD (Harvey and Balon 1995; Laird 1996) and depression (Rickels et al. 1988; Sramek et al. 1996), and some evidence suggests that buspirone may be an effective treatment for social phobia (Munjack et al. 1991; Schneier et al. 1992).

Buspirone is available for oral administration in a variety of dosage forms, including the 15-mg and 30-mg "dividose" tablets. These tablets are scored for division into bisections or trisections. We recommend an initial dosage of 7.5 mg twice a day, increased after 1 week to 15 mg twice a day. The dosage may then be increased as needed to achieve optimal therapeutic response. The usual recommended maximum daily dosage is 60 mg, but many patients safely tolerate and benefit from 90 mg/day. Because buspirone is metabolized by the liver and excreted by the kidneys, it should not be administered to patients with severe hepatic or renal impairment. Buspirone is metabolized by CYP3A3/4. Therefore, the initial dose should be lower in patients who are also taking medications that are known to inhibit this enzyme system, such as nefazodone.

Side Effects

The side effects that are more common with buspirone than with the benzodiazepines are nausea, headache, nervousness, insomnia, dizziness, and light-headedness (Rakel 1990). Restlessness also has been reported, which theoretically may be related to the activity of this drug at the dopamine receptor. Buspirone does not appear to interact with alcohol or other CNS depressants to increase sedation and motor impairment (Moskowitz and Smiley 1982). When administered to subjects who had histories of recreational sedative abuse, buspirone showed no abuse potential (Cole et al. 1982), a finding confirmed by subsequent studies (Sellers et al. 1992). As mentioned previously, buspirone is not sedating and does not impair mechanical performance, such as driving (Moskowitz and Smiley 1982). However, because side effects in any individual patient cannot be predicted, these activities should be avoided during the initial stages of buspirone therapy.

Drug Interactions

Buspirone should not be administered in combination with an MAOI.

Overdose

No fatal outcomes of buspirone overdose have been reported. However, overdose of buspirone with other drugs may result in more serious outcomes.

Zolpidem and Zaleplon

Zolpidem (Ambien) and Zaleplon (Sonata) are hypnotics that act at the omega-1 subtype of the central benzodiazepine receptor. This selectivity is hypothesized to be associated with a lower risk of dependence. Unlike the benzodiazepines, zolpidem and zaleplon do not appear to have significant anxiolytic, muscle relaxant, or anticonvulsant properties. However, amnestic effects may occur.

Indications

Zolpidem is a short-acting hypnotic with established efficacy in inducing and maintaining sleep. Because of the short half-life of this drug, most patients report minimal daytime sedation. Zaleplon is an ultra short-acting hypnotic, which allows this drug to be administered in the middle of the night with minimal residual sedative effects after 4 hours.

Clinical Use

Both zolpidem and zaleplon are available in 5- and 10-mg tablets for oral administration. The maximum recommended dosage for adults is 10 mg/day, administered at night. The initial dosage for elderly persons should not exceed 5 mg. Caution is advised in patients with hepatic dysfunction. In general, hypnotics should be limited to short-term use, with re-evaluation for more extended therapy (see discussion of the treatment of insomnia later in this chapter).

Risks, Side Effects, and Their Management

In general, the side effects of zolpidem and zaleplon are similar to those of the short-acting benzodiazepines. These agents should not be considered free of abuse potential.

Overdose

Both zolpidem and zaleplon appear to be nonfatal in overdose. However, overdoses in combination with other CNS-depressant agents pose a greater risk. Recommended treatment consists of general symptomatic and supportive measures including gastric lavage. Use of flumazenil may be helpful.

Drug Interactions

Research on drug interactions is limited for these agents, but any drug with CNS-depressant effects could potentially enhance the CNS-depressant effects of zolpidem and zaleplon via pharmacodynamic interactions. In addition, zolpidem is primarily metabolized by cytochrome P450 3A3/4 and zaleplon is partially metabolized by 3A3/4. As such, inhibitors of this enzyme may increase zolpidem blood levels and toxicity.

Pharmacotherapy for Generalized Anxiety Disorder

Generalized anxiety disorder can be treated with benzodiazepines, buspirone, and certain of the antidepressants (e.g., venlafaxine). Some of these agents are compared in Table 24–10.

Benzodiazepines have the advantage of being rapidly effective and the obvious disadvantages of abuse potential and sedation. Although benzodiazepines are indicated for relatively short-term use only (i.e., 1–2 months), they are, in general, safe and effective for long-term use for the minority of patients who require such medication (Greenblatt et al. 1983; Rickels et al. 1983). Whereas tolerance to sedation often develops, the same is not true of the anxiolytic effects of these agents.

All benzodiazepines indicated for the treatment of anxiety are equally efficacious. The choice of a specific agent usually depends on the pharmacokinetics and pharmacodynamics of the drug. Some patients respond to extremely low dosages, such as 0.125 mg of alprazolam twice a day, although mean dosages are higher. When using benzodiazepines to treat anxiety, we advocate starting with 0.25 mg of alprazolam two or three times a day or an equivalent dosage of another benzodiazepine (Table 24–9) and then titrating according to anxiolysis versus sedation. Benzodiazepines should be avoided in patients with a history of recent and/or significant substance abuse, and all patients should be advised to take their first dose at home in a situation that would not be dangerous in the event of greater than expected sedation.

Buspirone does not cause the sedative or abuse problems of the benzodiazepines, but some clinicians have observed that the anxiolytic properties do not appear to be as potent as those of the benzodiazepines, particularly in patients who have previously received a benzodiazepine (Schweizer et al. 1986). Because buspirone is not sedating (Seidel et al. 1985) and has no psychomotor effects, it has a distinct advantage over the benzodiazepines when optimal alertness and motor performance are necessary. Buspirone has been assessed in subjects with histories of recreational sedative abuse (Cole et al. 1982) and in recently detoxified alcoholic patients (Griffith et al. 1986); in these groups, it showed no abuse potential. Response to buspirone occurs in approximately 2–4 weeks. There is also evidence that the azapirones have modest antidepressant effects, perhaps at high doses (Jenkins et al. 1990; Lucki 1991).

Buspirone does not show cross-tolerance with benzodiazepines and other sedative-hypnotic drugs such as alcohol, barbiturates, and chloral hydrate. Therefore, buspirone does not suppress benzodiazepine withdrawal symptoms (Lader and Olajide 1987). For anxious patients taking a benzodiazepine who require a switch to buspirone, the benzodiazepine must be tapered gradually to avoid withdrawal symptoms, despite the fact that the patient is receiving buspirone.

TABLE 24–10. Comparison of benzodiazepines, buspirone, and selective serotonin reuptake inhibitors (SSRIs)

Characteristic	Benzodiazepines	Buspirone	SSRIs
Therapeutic effect of single dose	Yes	No	No
Time to full therapeutic action	Days	Weeks	Weeks
Sedation	Yes	No	Unlikely
Dependence liability	Yes	No	No
Impairs performance	Yes	No	No
Suppresses sedative withdrawal symptoms	Yes	No	No
Once-a-day dosing	No	No	Yes
Treats comorbid depression	No	No	Yes
Side effects	Sedation, memory impairment	Dizziness	Gastrointestinal, sexual dysfunction

Patients with generalized anxiety disorder also respond to antidepressant treatment (Hoehn-Saric et al. 1988; Kahn et al. 1986). In studies comparing benzodiazepines, MAOIs, SSRIs, and TCAs in the treatment of concurrent anxiety and depression, all had some measure of success depending on the degree of depression and the type of anxiety disorder (Keller and Hanks 1995). Kahn et al. (1986) reported success comparable with that found with chlordiazepoxide in treating patients with generalized anxiety disorder with 75–150 mg/day of imipramine. Like the effect reported with buspirone, this anxiolytic effect was noted to have a delayed onset of approximately 2–3 weeks. Another research group, comparing imipramine with alprazolam in patients with generalized anxiety disorder, found imipramine to be more effective in treating the psychic symptoms, such as dysphoria and negative anticipatory thinking, and alprazolam more effective in treating the somatic symptoms (Hoehn-Saric et al. 1988). In a controlled study comparing imipramine, trazodone, diazepam, and placebo in 230 patients with generalized anxiety disorder not complicated by depression or panic disorder, moderate-to-marked improvement was reported by 73% of those treated with imipramine, 69% of those treated with trazodone, 66% of those treated with diazepam, and only 47% of those treated with placebo (Rickels et al. 1993). SSRIs also appear to be effective, but controlled studies are lacking. Venlafaxine has been reported in controlled clinical trials to be effective in the treatment of generalized anxiety disorder (Davidson et al. 1999; Rickels et al. 2000) and has received FDA approval for this indication.

The duration of pharmacotherapy for generalized anxiety disorder is controversial. Psychotherapy is recommended for most patients with this disorder, and it may facilitate the tapering of medication. However, generalized anxiety is often a chronic condition, and some patients require long-term pharmacotherapy. As in other anxiety disorders, the need for ongoing treatment should be reassessed every 6–12 months.

Pharmacotherapy for Panic Disorder

Benzodiazepines, TCAs, MAOIs, and SSRIs are all effective in the treatment of panic disorder. Among the benzodiazepines, the higher-potency agents alprazolam and clonazepam are preferred because they are well tolerated in the higher dose ranges often required to treat panic disorder (Spier et al. 1986; Tesar 1990). Clonazepam has the advantage of a longer elimination half-life, which provides more stable plasma drug levels and allows twice-a-day dosing, whereas the shorter half-life of alprazolam is better suited for acute dosage titration. For the treatment of panic disorder, clonazepam is started at 0.5 mg twice a day and increased to a total of 1–2 mg/day in two divided doses. Higher dosage levels may be necessary for complete relief of symptoms. The starting dosage of alprazolam is usually 0.25 or 0.5 mg three times a day (Tesar 1990).

Because long-term exposure to high-dose benzodiazepines may place some patients at risk for physical and/or psychological dependence, we recommend the use of antidepressants for the treatment of panic disorder. Many antidepressants have been shown to be effective in this setting, including TCAs (Klein et al. 1987; Zitrin et al. 1983), MAOIs (Sheehan et al. 1980; van Vliet et al. 1993), and SSRIs (den Boer et al. 1995; Oehrberg et al. 1995; Schneier et al. 1990; Westenberg and den Boer 1988). For most patients, the SSRIs should be considered first-line agents. The choice should be based on the same factors discussed in the section on antidepressant drugs. MAOIs usually are reserved for patients who have not responded to SSRIs and TCAs. A major caveat is that patients with panic disorder initially may be highly sensitive to the stimulant effects of small doses of antidepressants. For highly anxious patients with panic disorder, we often initiate treatment with clonazepam or alprazolam and add a low-dose antidepressant, which is then increased slowly. The rapid onset of action of the benzodiazepine is helpful to the patient until the antidepressant becomes effective. When panic symptoms have not been present for several weeks, the benzodiazepine is slowly tapered. In patients with marked residual anticipatory anxiety, longer-term use of a benzodiazepine or buspirone should be considered as an adjunct to the antidepressant. Although some patients respond to lower doses, standard to high-standard antidepressant doses generally are used for the treatment of panic disorder.

For most patients, pharmacotherapy combined with time-limited cognitive-behavioral therapy is highly effective in reducing panic attacks but possibly less effective in attenuating avoidance behavior. Unfortunately, there are no guidelines for the duration of pharmacotherapy. We recommend attempting to taper medication every 6–12 months if the patient has been relatively symptom-free. However, many patients require longer-term pharmacotherapy.

Pharmacotherapy for Social Phobia

Social phobia responds to a variety of medications, including SSRIs (Black et al. 1992; den Boer et al. 1995; Van Ameringen et al. 1993; Westenberg and den Boer 1993), MAOIs (Liebowitz et al. 1988; Marshall et al. 1994), benzodiazepines (Davidson et al. 1991; Gelernter et al. 1991; Jefferson 1995), and buspirone (Munjack et al. 1991; Schneier et al. 1992). TCAs, although highly effective in the treatment of panic disorder, appear to be ineffective for most patients with social phobia. Similarly, β-blockers, although effective in treating performance anxiety, are not effective in treating generalized social phobia (Jefferson 1995).

The risks and side effects of the SSRIs, MAOIs, and benzodiazepines are discussed extensively elsewhere in the chapter. Dosages for the treatment of social phobia are similar to dosages of these medications for other disorders.

The high-potency agents alprazolam (Gelernter et al. 1991) and clonazepam (Davidson et al. 1991; Jefferson 1995) appear to be the most effective benzodiazepines for treating social phobia. Preliminary studies have shown that patients with generalized and specific social phobia benefited from treatment with the reversible MAOIs (moclobemide), but the irreversible MAOI phenelzine remains the best studied (Jefferson 1995). Although the MAOIs are highly effective in reducing both social anxiety and social avoidance, these drugs are not first-line

agents, as they are not in the treatment of depression, because of their increased risks compared with other available agents.

Pharmacotherapy for Performance Anxiety

Several studies have shown the efficacy of β-blockers in the treatment of performance anxiety. Taken within 2 hours of the stressor, propranolol, in doses ranging from 20 to 80 mg, may improve performance on examinations (Drew et al. 1985), in public speaking (Hertley et al. 1983), and in musical performances (Brantigan et al. 1982). A trial dose of 40 mg of propranolol (e.g., during a vacation day) should be administered before the specific performance situation in which the patient anticipates anxiety. This initial dose should not be taken in a high-risk or critical situation in which any unexpected side effect could result in serious consequences. Subsequently, doses of propranolol should be administered approximately 2 hours before the situation in which disabling performance anxiety is expected. The dose may be increased gradually by 20-mg increments during successive performances until adequate relief of performance distress is achieved (Yudofsky and Silver 1987). The risks and side effects of β-blockers are discussed extensively later in this chapter, in the section "Antiaggression Drugs."

Pharmacotherapy for Obsessive-Compulsive Disorder

The discovery of the SSRIs brought about a revolution in the treatment of OCD. As a consequence of the development of these drugs, the understanding of OCD and related conditions multiplied manyfold. Clomipramine, a tricyclic with potent serotonin reuptake inhibition, was the first medication with established efficacy for treatment of OCD (Clomipramine Collaborative Study Group 1991). Currently, clomipramine and the SSRIs provide the foundation of pharmacological treatment of OCD. In contrast to the experience of patients treated with pharmacotherapy for many other Axis I disorders, most patients with OCD experience only a 35%–60% improvement in symptoms (Jenike 1990). In addition, medication responses may not be apparent until treatment has been given for 10 weeks. Cognitive-behavioral therapy should be combined with pharmacological approaches.

Before initiating clomipramine treatment, the clinician must heed all the precautions associated with the use of any TCA (see discussion of TCAs earlier in this chapter). Initial dosing and titration of clomipramine also must follow the guidelines for TCAs, with the additional caveat that 250 mg is the maximum recommended dosage because of an increased risk of seizures above this level. Plasma levels are available but are only weakly correlated with therapeutic effect (Mavissakalian et al. 1990). Most patients with OCD respond to dosages of clomipramine between 150 and 200 mg/day. Because side effects associated with the anticholinergic, antihistaminic, and α_2-adrenergic actions of clomipramine may occur, patients must be monitored for and made aware of the potential for symptoms such as constipation, dry mouth, urinary hesitancy, sedation, and orthostatic hypotension.

As in the treatment of depression, the SSRIs tend to be better tolerated than the TCAs. Fluoxetine has been compared with clomipramine under double-blind conditions and found to have an approximately equivalent antiobsessional effect (Pigott et al. 1990). It has been suggested that an effective antiobsessional dosage of fluoxetine may be higher than its usual antidepressant dosage. Many clinicians seek to establish a daily dose of 60–80 mg in treating OCD. No systematic study of this issue has confirmed this common impression and widely used practice. In fact, a report by Wheadon (1991) found no greater antiobsessional effect of fluoxetine at 40 or 60 mg/day compared with 20 mg/day. Nonetheless, on the basis of the current knowledge of the treatment of OCD, a trial of fluoxetine should not be considered complete until the patient has failed to respond to 80 mg/day after 8 weeks (Jenike 1990). In an open-label study, 198 patients with OCD who were previously nonresponsive to fixed doses of fluoxetine benefited from dosage titration up to 80 mg, with two-thirds achieving an optimal response within 24 weeks (Tollefson et al. 1994).

The other SSRIs are also effective treatments for OCD. Therapeutic dosages of fluvoxamine range from 100 to 300 mg/day in divided doses (Freeman et al. 1994; Goodman et al. 1990, 1996; Perse et al. 1988). In a double-blind comparison of flexible doses of paroxetine, clomipramine, and placebo, paroxetine was found to be as effective as clomipramine and significantly more effective than placebo in the treatment of OCD (Zohar and Judge 1996). The recommended dosage range for paroxetine in the treatment of OCD is 40–60 mg/day. In a double-blind comparison of three dosages of sertraline (50, 100, and 200 mg/day) and placebo in patients with OCD, all three sertraline groups showed significantly greater improvement than the placebo group after 12 weeks (Greist et al. 1995).

Several augmentation strategies have been suggested, none with uniformly positive results in controlled trials but with possible effectiveness in selected patients. OCD augmentation strategies include use of fenfluramine (Hollander et al. 1990), lithium (Feder 1988), antipsychotics (McDougle et al. 1990, 1995), clonazepam (Hewlett et al. 1990), and buspirone (Jenike et al. 1991; Markovitz et al. 1990), typically added to a serotonergic antidepressant.

As in the other anxiety disorders, relatively few data are available to address longer-term treatment of OCD. OCD is often a lifelong disorder with a waxing and waning course, for which many patients require prolonged pharmacotherapy. Although relatively high dosages of SSRIs are recommended for the acute treatment, lower dosages may be effective for maintenance treatment (Mundo et al. 1997). In a 2-year follow-up study comparing 130 obsessive-compulsive patients who were responders to treatment with clomipramine (150 mg/day), fluoxetine (40 mg/day), or fluvoxamine (300 mg/day) for 6 months, those who continued treatment with the same daily dosage or half dosage had significantly superior outcomes when compared with those who discontinued treatment. No differences in efficacy between the full and half doses were found (Ravizza et al. 1996).

Pharmacotherapy for Insomnia

Although the benzodiazepines, zolpidem, and zaleplon are the mainstay of pharmacotherapy for insomnia, other sedating drugs, such as trazodone or chloral hydrate, also may be used. As discussed previously, insomnia should first be addressed diagnostically, and in most cases nonpharmacological interventions should be tried before treatment with a hypnotic is instituted. Hypnotic agents should be administered in the lowest effective dose. Medications commonly prescribed to treat insomnia, their recommended dosages, time of onset, and half-lives are shown in Table 24–11. General principles for using medications to treat insomnia are outlined in Table 24–12.

Each hypnotic benzodiazepine has a distinct pharmacodynamic and pharmacokinetic profile that has an important influence on its use in clinical practice. Whereas all the currently available benzodiazepine hypnotics are absorbed relatively rapidly from the gastrointestinal tract and achieve peak plasma levels in approximately 1.5 hours (Greenblatt 1992), affinity for the benzodiazepine receptor and elimination half-life both affect the clinical use of these agents. For example, flurazepam and quazepam are both ultimately metabolized into a clinically active compound, desalkylflurazepam, which has an elimination half-life of 40–50 hours (Greenblatt 1992; Greenblatt et al. 1981). With successive days of treatment, the accumulation of this

TABLE 24–11. Medications commonly prescribed to treat insomnia

Medication (trade name)	Usual therapeutic dosage (mg/day)		Time until onset of action (minutes)	Half-life (including metabolites; hours)
	Adult	Geriatric		
Clonazepam (Klonopin)[a]	0.5–2	0.25–1	20–60	19–60
Clorazepate (Tranxene)	3.75–15	3.75–7.5	30–60	48–96
Estazolam (ProSom)	1–2	0.5–1	15–30	8–24
Lorazepam (Ativan)[a]	1–4	0.25–1	30–60	8–24
Oxazepam (Serax)	15–30	10–15	30–60	2.8–5.7
Quazepam (Doral)	7.5–15	7.5	20–45	39–120
Temazepam (Restoril)	15–30	7.5–15	45–60	3–25
Triazolam (Halcion)	0.125–0.25	0.125	15–30	1.5–5
Chloral hydrate[b]	500–2,000	500–2,000	30–60	4–8
Trazodone (Desyrel)[a,b]	50–150	25–100	30–60	5–9
Zaleplon (Sonata)[b]	5–10	5	30	1.0
Zolpidem (Ambien)[b]	5–10	5	30	1.5–4.5

Note. [a]Use of this drug as a hypnotic agent is not an indication approved by the Food and Drug Administration.
[b]These drugs are not benzodiazepines.
Source. Adapted with permission from Kupfer KJ, Reynolds CF: "Management of Insomnia." *New England Journal of Medicine* 336:341–346, 1997. Also adapted from *Physicians' Desk Reference* 2001.

TABLE 24–12. Guidelines for pharmacotherapy for insomnia

1. Use the lowest effective dose.
2. Use agents with short or intermediate half-lives to avoid daytime sedation.
3. Use intermittent dosing (two to four times a week).
4. Use for no more than 3–4 weeks.
5. Discontinue medication gradually.
6. Be alert for rebound insomnia.

Source. Adapted with permission from Kupfer KJ, Reynolds CF: "Management of Insomnia." *New England Journal of Medicine* 336:341–346, 1997. Also adapted from *Physicians' Desk Reference* 2001.

compound in the body may adversely affect motor performance and cause daytime drowsiness, a so-called hangover effect. Although tolerance to the daytime sedation may develop with time (Greenblatt et al. 1977b), we believe that for elderly patients and many others, the risks of CNS side effects are too great with flurazepam and quazepam. On the other hand, a long elimination half-life reduces the risk of early-morning awakening and rebound insomnia after drug discontinuation, so that these agents may be appropriate for brief treatment. With a half-life of just 1.5–5 hours, triazolam is at the opposite end of the spectrum among the benzodiazepines (Greenblatt et al. 1983). The risks of accumulation of triazolam in the body are avoided in healthy patients, but the risk of rebound insomnia makes triazolam less useful

for patients with early-morning awakening. Temazepam and estazolam have intermediate half-life values (Greenblatt 1992), and, as a result, day-after and rebound insomnia are less likely with these agents. Quazepam is unique among the benzodiazepines in that it is selective for the type 1 benzodiazepine receptor (Wamsley and Hunt 1991); however, desalkylflurazepam, a metabolite of quazepam, is a long-acting and nonselective benzodiazepine receptor agonist, which accounts for at least some of the clinical effects of this drug.

The nonbenzodiazepine hypnotic agents zolpidem and zaleplon act at the type 1 benzodiazepine receptor. As discussed previously, the clinical characteristics of zolpidem and zaleplon are similar to those of triazolam, but zolpidem appears to be less likely to produce rebound insomnia. Sedating antidepressants such as trazodone are often effective and do not carry the risk of abuse associated with more traditional hypnotics.

Pharmacotherapy for Alcohol Withdrawal

A relatively simple procedure for treating alcohol withdrawal is the benzodiazepine loading dose technique (Sellers et al. 1983). This technique takes advantage of the long half-lives of benzodiazepines such as diazepam and chlordiazepoxide. Doses of 20 mg of diazepam (or 100 mg of chlordiazepoxide) are administered hourly to patients until they have no signs or symptoms of alcohol withdrawal. This state is usually accompanied by mild to moderate sedation. Thereafter, no further doses of benzodiazepine are administered. Because of the long half-life of diazepam and other long-acting benzodiazepines, the therapeutic plasma level of the benzodiazepine is maintained during the period of risk for alcohol withdrawal symptoms. Sullivan and Sellers (1986) recommended that healthy patients receive at least 60 mg of diazepam or 300 mg of chlordiazepoxide in the initial loading dose regimen. This technique has advantages over the method of repeat dosing with benzodiazepines in that the accumulation of benzodiazepines may lead to prolonged sedation and the development of benzodiazepine dependence in a population at high risk for chemical dependence.

Antipsychotic Drugs

Antipsychotic medications, previously referred to as *major tranquilizers* or *neuroleptics*, are effective for the treatment of a variety of psychotic symptoms, such as hallucinations, delusions, and thought disorders, regardless of etiology (other indications are discussed later). The term *major tranquilizer* is a misnomer because sedation is generally a side effect, not the principal treatment effect. Similarly, the term *neuroleptic* is based on the neurological side effects characteristic of the older antipsychotic drugs, such as catalepsy in animals and EPS in humans.

Antipsychotic drugs can be classified in several ways. One classification is based on chemical structure; for example, phenothiazines and butyrophenones constitute two chemical classes. We use the term *conventional* to signify the older antipsychotic drugs, to differentiate them from the newer, *atypical* or "second generation" antipsychotics. All conventional antipsychotics are equally effective when given in equivalent doses (Table 24–13). Among the conventional antipsychotics, we commonly distinguish between high- and low-potency agents; as we discuss later, this characteristic predicts side effects. Although the term *atypical antipsychotic* lacks a single consistent definition, it generally implies fewer EPS and superior efficacy, particularly for the negative symptoms of schizophrenia. Atypical antipsychotics are also less likely to produce hyperprolactinemia. Currently, the atypical antipsychotics include clozapine, risperidone, olanzapine, quetiapine, and ziprasidone.

The favorable efficacy and neurological side effect profiles of atypical antipsychotics have led some authorities to recommend that they be used uniformly as first-line agents, with the exception of clozapine, which is restricted in its use because of the risk of agranulocytosis (Lieberman 1996). The therapeutic advantages of atypical antipsychotics over conventional agents may be greater in first-episode patients than in chronically ill patients, further arguing against second-line status (Sanger et al. 1999). On the other hand, atypical antipsychotics are markedly more expensive and may place some patients at risk for medical morbidity resulting from weight gain (particularly clozapine and olanzapine), hyperprolactinemia (risperidone), and cardiac conduction delay (ziprasidone). Whereas most pharmacoeconomic studies have indicated that increased costs of the atypical antipsychotics are offset by reduced rates of hospitalization, the long-term safety of these drugs remains to be fully characterized. Discussion of the properties common to most of the antipsychotic medications follows, with specific comments on each of the atypical antipsychotics at the end of this section.

Mechanisms of Action

For many years, the prevailing theory regarding the mechanism of action of antipsychotic drugs was based on the observation that all the available antipsychotics antagonize D_2 dopamine receptors in vitro and that the relative affinities of the typical antipsychotic drugs for striatal D_2 receptors correlate with the dosage required to treat psychotic symptoms (Creese et al. 1976; Seeman et al. 1976). Yet the theory that psychosis results from hyperdopaminergia is overly simplistic. Underactivity of dopamine in mesocortical pathways, specifically those projecting to the frontal lobes, may account for the negative symptoms of schizophrenia (e.g., anergia, apathy, aspontaneity; (K. Davis et al. 1991; Goff and Evins 1998). At the same time, this underactivity in the frontal lobe may serve to disinhibit mesolimbic dopamine activity via a corticolimbic feedback loop (Pycock et al. 1980). An overactivity of mesolimbic dopamine is the result, manifested by the positive symptoms of schizophrenia (e.g., hallucinations, delusions; K. Davis et al. 1991). This revised dopamine hypothesis is concordant with the clinical observation that conventional antipsychotic drugs are more effective in treating positive symptoms than negative symptoms (Breier et al. 1987).

Antagonism of the 5-HT$_2$ receptor may modify dopamine activity in a regionally specific manner. When combined with conventional antipsychotics, 5-HT$_2$ blockade preserves firing of nigrostriatal (A9) dopamine neurons (Svensson et al. 1989; Ugedo et al. 1989). Early studies reported that addition of 5-HT$_2$ antagonism to conventional antipsychotics decreased EPS in rats and improved negative symptoms in patients with schizo-

TABLE 24–13. Commonly used antipsychotic drugs

Generic (trade) name	Usual daily dosage (mg)	Methods of administration	Available oral doses (mg)	Approximate oral dose equivalents (mg)[a]
Conventional antipsychotics				
Phenothiazines				
Chlorpromazine (Thorazine)	300–600	po, im	10, 25, 50, 100, 200	100
Piperidines				
Thioridazine (Mellaril)	300–600	po, im	10, 15, 25, 50, 100, 150, 200	100
Mesoridazine (Serentil)	150–300	po	10, 25, 50, 100	50
Pimozide (Orap)	2–6	po	2	1–2
Piperazines				
Trifluoperazine (Stelazine)	15–30	po	1, 2, 5, 10	5
Fluphenazine (Prolixin)	5–15	po, L, im, D	1, 2.5, 5, 10	2
Perphenazine (Trilafon)	32–64	po	2, 4, 8, 16	10
Thioxanthenes				
Thiothixene (Navane)	15–30	po, L, im	1, 2, 5, 10, 20	5
Butyrophenones				
Haloperidol (Haldol)	5–15	po, im, D	0.5, 1, 2, 5, 10, 20	2
Dibenzoxazepines				
Loxapine (Loxitane)	45–90	po	5, 10, 25, 50	15
Molindone (Moban)	30–60	po	5, 10, 25, 50, 100	10
Atypical antipsychotics				
Clozapine (Clozaril)	250–500	po	25, 100	50
Risperidone (Risperdal)	4–6	po	1, 2, 3, 4	1
Olanzapine (Zyprexa)	10–20	po	2.5, 5, 7.5, 10	2–3
Quetiapine (Seroquel)	300–600	po	25, 100, 200, 300	100
Ziprasidone (Geodon)	80–160	po	20, 40, 60, 80	

Note.   D = long-acting decanoate preparation; im = short-acting intramuscular; L = liquid; po = oral tablets or capsules.
[a]Equivalent doses from American Psychiatric Association 1997.

phrenia (Duinkerke et al. 1993; Gelders 1989). This dual 5-HT$_2$/D$_2$ antagonism is believed to account, at least in part, for the superior efficacy and side effect profile of the atypical antipsychotics (Meltzer et al. 1989), although this model has recently been challenged (Kapur and Seeman 2001). On the basis of this dual antagonism, atypical antipsychotics are often referred to as *serotonin-dopamine antagonists*. Other investigators have suggested that noradrenergic (Baldessarini et al. 1992) and glutaminergic (Goff and Coyle 2001) effects may contribute to the efficacy of atypical antipsychotics. A recent view holds that reduced liability for EPS, lower prolactin levels, and preservation of certain physiological dopaminergic functions with atypical agents may reflect in part the dissociation constant, or degree of "loose binding" to the D$_2$ receptor (Kapur and Seeman 2001). In addition, the GABAergic system (Reynolds and Stroud 1993) and neuropeptides, specifically cholecystokinin (Garver et al. 1990), neurotensin (Bisette and Nemeroff 1988; Garver et al. 1991), and vasopressin (Beckman et al. 1985; Sorensen et al. 1985), may be involved in the pathophys-

iology of schizophrenia and may serve as targets for future therapeutic approaches.

Indications and Efficacy

The most common indications for the use of antipsychotic drugs are in the treatment of acute psychosis and the maintenance of a remission of psychotic symptoms in patients with schizophrenia. All conventional antipsychotics have comparable efficacy but differing side effect profiles. Clozapine, risperidone, and olanzapine appear to be at least as effective as the older medications for the treatment of positive symptoms and more efficacious for the treatment of negative symptoms of schizophrenia; the other atypical agents are less well studied. Ziprasidone and quetiapine have shown antipsychotic efficacy comparable to conventional agents, but their comparative effects on negative symptoms remain to be clarified (Arvanitis and Miller 1997; Goff et al. 1998). Clozapine is effective in approximately 30% of patients who were nonresponsive to several trials of conventional antipsychotics (Kane 1996). Risperidone and olanzapine also may be advantageous for this difficult patient population, but adequate controlled trials are lacking, and results are not fully consistent (Chakos et al. 2001).

Antipsychotic drugs are also effective in ameliorating psychotic symptoms that result from many diverse etiologies, such as mood disorders with psychotic features, drug toxicities, psychosis secondary to other brain disorders, and delusional disorders. Low dosages of antipsychotics may be effective in some patients with borderline or schizotypal personality disorders, particularly when used to target psychotic ideation (Gunderson 1986). In the treatment of severe OCD, antipsychotics have been used to augment antiobsessional agents (McDougle et al. 1990). Antipsychotics and other drugs with dopamine receptor–blocking action (e.g., metoclopramide) are also used for their antiemetic effect. Gilles de la Tourette's syndrome may be controlled with antipsychotic agents; haloperidol and pimozide are the most frequently used drugs for this disorder.

The sedative side effect of antipsychotic medications may lead to the misuse of these drugs in several clinical situations. Antipsychotics frequently are improperly prescribed as hypnotic or anxiolytic agents. In addition, antipsychotic drugs are administered to patients who are chronically agitated and violent. Because of the potential long-term risks of these drugs (see subsection "Tardive Disorders" later in this section), antipsychotics are not recommended for the treatment of uncomplicated anxiety or insomnia.

Clinical Use

Medication Selection

The choice of antipsychotic medication is often determined, in large part, by anticipated side effects. When appropriate, involvement of the patient and family members in this process can enhance the alliance and minimize distress when side effects develop. A patient who has selected a particular drug, taking into account possible side effects, is generally less upset when the anticipated side effect develops, especially if the patient understands that other treatment options are available. In most circumstances, the atypical antipsychotics (except for clozapine) are best tolerated and are preferred as first-line agents. Although atypical antipsychotics generally appear to have modest advantages for negative symptoms over the conventional agents, differences in efficacy among atypical agents are not well established. Head-to-head comparisons of atypical agents have been few, and findings of differential efficacy between agents

generally have been inconsistent and contested (Conley and Mahmoud 2001; Tran et al. 1997). Depot preparations of conventional agents continue to play an important clinical role in the absence of delayed-release formulations of atypical agents. Clozapine is generally reserved for refractory patients because of the risk of agranulocytosis.

A useful construct for conceptualizing differences in side-effect profiles for the conventional antipsychotics is the concept of "high potency" versus "low potency." Drug potency refers to the milligram equivalence of drugs, not to the relative efficacy. For example, although haloperidol is more potent than chlorpromazine (haloperidol 2 mg = chlorpromazine 100 mg), therapeutically equivalent doses are equally effective (haloperidol 12 mg = chlorpromazine 600 mg). Potency of the antipsychotic drugs has generally been determined in two ways: 1) by ascertaining dosages that are efficacious in clinical trials and clinical practice and 2) by comparing affinities of the drug for the D_2 receptor. Typically, the potency of antipsychotic drugs is compared with a standard 100-mg dose of chlorpromazine. As a rule, for conventional antipsychotics only, the high-potency antipsychotic drugs have an equivalent dose of less than 5 mg (Table 24–13). These medications have a high degree of EPS but less sedation, fewer anticholinergic side effects, and less hypotension. Low-potency conventional antipsychotic drugs have an equivalent dose of greater than 40 mg. These drugs have a high level of sedation, anticholinergic side effects, and hypotension but a lower degree of acute EPS. Tardive dyskinesia rates do not differ between high- and low-potency conventional antipsychotics. Antipsychotic drugs with intermediate potency (i.e., equivalent dose between 5 and 40 mg) have a side effect profile that lies between the profiles of these two groups. In most circumstances, high-potency drugs are preferred among the conventional antipsychotics because EPS usually can be minimized by using the lowest effective dosage or by symptomatic treatment, whereas anticholinergic and autonomic side effects are potentially more dangerous and difficult to manage. Intermediate-potency conventional antipsychotic drugs are sometimes useful for patients who cannot tolerate either high- or low-potency drugs.

The atypical antipsychotics produce fewer EPS than even the low-potency conventional antipsychotics. Distress related to EPS may compromise compliance; in addition, akathisia may be confused with agitation, and drug-induced parkinsonism may be misinterpreted as negative symptoms of schizophrenia. Clozapine and quetiapine have the least EPS liability and so are recommended for treatment of psychosis in patients with Parkinson's disease. Growing evidence suggests that the atypical agents are associated with substantially lower rates of tardive dyskinesia than are conventional agents. With the notable exception of risperidone, the atypical antipsychotics produce substantially less hyperprolactinemia than do conventional agents. Because of associated medical morbidity, as well as the potential effect on self-esteem and compliance, weight gain is also an important side effect associated to varying degrees with all atypical agents except ziprasidone. Concerns about cardiac conduction delay with ziprasidone require careful consideration, as do concerns about cataract formation with quetiapine. Cataracts have been linked to quetiapine in beagle dogs but not in humans or in nonhuman primates. Finally, sedation may be problematic with atypical agents, particularly with clozapine and quetiapine, and the risk of orthostatic hypotension necessitates early dose titration with clozapine, quetiapine, and risperidone.

Optimal Dosages

An optimal dosage or therapeutic range of blood levels has not been identified for most of the antipsychotics. Older high-dosage strategies and "rapid tranquilization," which involved rapidly escalating intramuscular doses of high-potency agents for the control of acute psychosis, are no longer recommended. Antipsychotic drugs, with the exception of clozapine, have a high therapeutic index, and they can be administered at dosages substantially above the optimal therapeutic dosage without immediate and obvious adverse events. However, carefully controlled studies have confirmed that more modest dosages of conventional antipsychotic drugs have equal efficacy and are better tolerated. Several reviews of controlled trials of conventional antipsychotics concluded that the optimal dosage for most patients is between 300 and 600 mg/day of chlorpromazine-equivalents, with some patients responding to lower dosages and with little benefit at doses greater than 700 mg/day (Appleton and Davis 1980; Baldessarini et al. 1988; J.M. Davis 1985).

The concept of a "therapeutic window" has been proposed for haloperidol, with optimal efficacy associated with serum concentrations between 5 and 15 ng/mL, typically achieved by daily doses of about 5–10 mg. Higher levels of D_2 receptor blockade increase the risk for EPS and secondary negative symptoms. Because EPS also are dose-related with risperidone, careful titration is required to avoid adverse effects at higher doses. Clozapine and quetiapine do not appear to have dose-limiting neurological side effects, but safety data are not available for doses greater than 900 mg/day of clozapine and 750 mg/day of quetiapine. Although olanzapine was studied at doses of 10–15 mg/day in premarketing trials, recent evidence suggests that efficacy may be enhanced in some refractory patients with an increase in dose to 20–30 mg/day.

In the initial stages of treatment with antipsychotic medication, sedation may predominate over the specific antipsychotic effects. Many psychiatrists incorrectly believe that if psychosis does not rapidly respond with the use of antipsychotics, higher dosages are necessary. In fact, as in antidepressant therapy, reversal of psychosis is often gradual and may occur over several weeks to several months. Guidelines for the acute use of antipsychotic drugs are summarized in Table 24–14; usual dosages for each of the commonly used antipsychotic drugs are summarized in Table 24–13.

Long-Acting Injectable Antipsychotics

For patients with chronic psychotic symptoms who do not comply with a daily medication regimen, a long-acting depot preparation should be considered after stabilization with oral medication. Fluphenazine decanoate and haloperidol decanoate are the only long-acting injectables currently available in the United States.

Conversion to a decanoate preparation is complicated by the highly variable individual pharmacokinetics of the oral and long-term depot agents. Most patients respond to a fluphenazine decanoate dosage of between 10 and 30 mg every 2 weeks (Baldessarini et al. 1988). A loading dose strategy has been established for haloperidol decanoate, in which patients receive an initial dose that is 20 times the oral maintenance dosage (Ereshefsky et al. 1993). The maximum volume per injection of haloperidol decanoate should not exceed 3 cc, and the maximum dose per injection should not exceed 100 mg. If 20 times the oral dose is greater than 100 mg, the dose is given in divided injections spaced 3–7 days apart. Subsequent doses are decreased monthly to about 10 times the oral dose by the third or fourth month. Ten times the oral dose, administered every 4 weeks, is a typical maintenance dose with haloperidol decanoate. For patients who are elderly or debilitated, the initial dose is 10–15 times the previous oral daily dosage. Many clinicians prefer to continue oral medication at approximately half the previous maintenance dose during the first few months of depot neuroleptic administration rather than administer a loading dose of depot medication. This approach allows greater flexibility of initial dose titration. In either approach, breakthrough psychotic symptoms are treated with supplemental oral medication, and the dose of the next scheduled depot injection can be increased accord-

TABLE 24–14. Guidelines for the acute use of antipsychotic drugs

1. Before the initiation of treatment, obtain a medical history and perform a complete physical and neurological examination. The history and physical examination are necessary not only to ensure accurate diagnosis of the etiology of the psychosis but also to ensure safe administration of the antipsychotic drugs. Because each antipsychotic drug has a slightly different side effect profile, the examination may be tailored as appropriate. Among the elements of the examination that have particular importance are pulse rate and blood pressure, ophthalmological examination, and neurological examination with emphasis on extrapyramidal signs and symptoms and tardive dyskinesia.

2. After discussion with the patient and family about the risks and benefits of treatment, select the appropriate antipsychotic agent on the basis of the patient's physical status, the side effect profile of the drug, and the history of response to medication, if available.

3. Inform and educate the patient and family about the risks of development of tardive dyskinesia. Document this discussion in the patient's chart.

4. Initiate antipsychotic medications in moderate doses (e.g., 4–10 mg haloperidol, 4–6 mg risperidone [titrate from lower dose], or 10 mg olanzapine for healthy adults).

5. Consider anticholinergic medication for the prophylaxis of extrapyramidal symptoms when prescribing high-potency conventional antipsychotic drugs to patients at high risk for dystonia. Avoid anticholinergic medication in patients with confusion or urinary retention and in patients who are at low risk for dystonia, such as the elderly.

6. Maintain the treatment dosage for 2–4 weeks because the response to antipsychotics is gradual.

7. When medication is necessary to control acute agitation, a sedative such as lorazepam 2 mg may be effective.

8. If possible, give all the antipsychotic medication at bedtime to increase compliance and minimize daytime side effects.

9. If there is no response, side effects are minimal, and you believe poor compliance is not the reason, increase the dosage gradually until mild side effects are seen (e.g., sedation, hypotension, extrapyramidal effects).

10. If no further improvement is seen after an additional 2–4 weeks at this dosage, substitute another antipsychotic drug from another class. Consider the use of another atypical antipsychotic drug.

ingly. Steady-state serum concentrations are achieved after approximately 10 weeks (five injection intervals) with fluphenazine decanoate and after approximately 20 weeks with haloperidol decanoate. Note that side effects may take months to subside, and withdrawal dyskinesia may not appear for months after discontinuation of the decanoate formulation.

Risks, Side Effects, and Their Management

Many of the side effects of antipsychotic drugs can be understood on the basis of their receptor-blocking properties. When antipsychotics reduce dopamine activity in the nigrostriatum (via dopamine receptor blockade), extrapyramidal signs and symptoms result, similar to those of Parkinson's disease. Another locus of dopamine receptors resides in the pituitary and hypothalamus (the tuberoinfundibular system), where dopamine is synonymous with prolactin-inhibiting factor. Blockade of dopamine in this system results in hyperprolactinemia. Similarly, antagonism of acetylcholine receptors produces symptoms such as dry mouth, blurred vision, and constipation. Antagonism of α_1-adrenergic receptors results in hypotension, and antagonism of histamine receptors is associated with sedation.

Extrapyramidal Effects

Extrapyramidal symptoms include acute dystonic reactions, parkinsonian syndrome, akathisia, neuroleptic malignant syndrome (NMS), and tardive dyskinesia. Although high-potency antipsychotics are more likely to produce extrapyramidal symptoms, all conventional antipsychotic drugs are equally likely to produce tardive dyskinesia. The atypical antipsychotics produce substantially fewer EPS, although careful titration of risperidone is necessary to avoid neurological side effects. Although use of anticholinergic agents or amantadine may prevent or ameliorate most occurrences of EPS, use of atypical agents is increasingly recommended to avoid these side effects without introducing additional medications. Long-term use of anticholinergics should be minimized because these agents can produce significant side effects, including impairments of memory and attention. Clozapine appears to be the only agent that does not cause tardive dyskinesia, although preliminary data suggest a reduced risk with olanzapine and risperidone (Jeste et al. 1999; Tollefson et al. 1997); relative tardive dyskinesia rates with quetiapine and ziprasidone have not been reported.

Acute dystonic reactions are among the most disturbing and acutely disabling adverse drug reactions that can occur with the administration of antipsychotic drugs. This reaction most frequently occurs within hours or days of the initiation of a high-potency conventional antipsychotic medication. The uncontrollable tightening of muscles typically involves spasms of the neck, back (opisthotonos), tongue, or muscles that control lateral eye movement (oculogyric crisis). Laryngeal involvement

TABLE 24–15. Drugs commonly used for the treatment of acute extrapyramidal side effects

Generic (trade) name	Mechanism	Usual dosage	Indications
Benztropine (Cogentin)	Anticholinergic	1–2 mg po bid	D, P
		2 mg iv[a]	Acute dystonia
Diphenhydramine (Benadryl)	Anticholinergic	25–50 mg po tid	D, P
		25 mg im/iv[a]	Acute dystonia
Trihexyphenidyl (Artane)	Anticholinergic	5–10 mg po bid	D, P
Amantadine (Symmetrel)	Dopaminergic	100 mg po bid	P
Propranolol (Inderal)	β-Blocker	20 mg po tid	A
		1 mg iv	

Note. Rabbit syndrome and akinesia respond to the medications used to treat parkinsonian syndrome.
A = akathisia; D = dystonia; im = intramuscularly; iv = intravenously; P = parkinsonian syndrome.
[a]Follow with po medication.

may compromise the airway and result in ventilatory difficulties (stridor). These reactions are often terrifying to the patient and may seriously jeopardize compliance with medications. Intravenous or intramuscular administration of anticholinergic medication is a rapid and effective treatment of acute dystonia. The drugs and dosages used to treat dystonic reactions are listed in Table 24–15. The anticholinergic drug given to reverse the dystonia will wear off after several hours. Because antipsychotic drugs have long half-lives and durations of action, additional oral anticholinergic drugs should be prescribed for several days after an acute dystonic reaction or longer if the antipsychotic drug is continued unchanged. Amantadine should be considered for treatment of EPS in elderly patients who are highly sensitive to anticholinergic activity, particularly if a switch to an atypical agent is not appropriate.

Acute dystonic reactions may be treated prophylactically with anticholinergic medications; for example, benztropine 1–2 mg twice a day may be initiated at the same time as the antipsychotic agent haloperidol (Goff et al. 1991). Young patients taking high-potency antipsychotic drugs are at particularly high risk for the development of acute dystonia. We suggest that prophylactic treatment be considered for patients for whom the risk of developing extrapyramidal reactions is high, especially patients younger than 40 years starting high-potency conventional agents (Arana et al. 1988). Anticholinergic medication can be tapered and stopped after 10 days.

Parkinsonian syndrome (or pseudoparkinsonism) has many of the features of classic idiopathic Parkinson's disease: diminished range of facial expression (masked facies), cogwheel rigidity, slowed movements (bradykinesia), drooling, small handwriting (micrographia), and pill-rolling tremor. As in Parkinson's disease, the pathophysiology involves disproportionally less dopamine than

acetylcholine in the basal ganglia. The onset of this side effect is gradual, and it may not appear for weeks after antipsychotics have been administered. The most common treatments for idiopathic Parkinson's disease restore the dopamine:acetylcholine balance by increasing dopamine. Because dopamine antagonism is putatively involved in the therapeutic effects of antipsychotics, treatment of parkinsonism most often involves decreasing the level of acetylcholine (although amantadine, a dopaminergic drug, often effectively attenuates parkinsonian side effects without exacerbating the underlying psychotic illness). Drugs used in the treatment of the parkinsonian side effects of antipsychotic agents are listed in Table 24–15.

The rabbit syndrome, consisting of fine, rapid movements of the lips that resemble the chewing movements of a rabbit, is often considered a subset of parkinsonian side effects. This side effect occurs after more prolonged treatment and may be confused with buccolingual tardive dyskinesia (Baldessarini 1988; Deshmukh et al. 1990). It has been found in approximately 4% of patients receiving antipsychotics without concomitant anticholinergics (Yassa and Lal 1986). Like parkinsonian side effects, the rabbit syndrome is treated effectively with anticholinergic drugs.

Akinesia is defined as a behavioral state of diminished spontaneity characterized by decreased gestures, unspontaneous speech, apathy, and difficulty with initiating usual activities (Rifkin et al. 1975). Akinesia may appear after several weeks of therapy and is often an element of the parkinsonism syndrome. This drug-induced syndrome may be mistaken for depression or for negative symptoms of schizophrenia. The drugs listed in Table 24–15 provide effective treatment.

Akathisia is an extrapyramidal disorder consisting of a subjective feeling of restlessness in the lower extremities, often manifested in an inability to sit still. It is a common reaction that most often occurs shortly after the initiation of conventional antipsychotic medication. After a single oral dose of 5 mg of haloperidol, 40% of the patients in one study experienced akathisia; after 1 week of receiving a 10-mg nighttime dose, this rate increased to 75% (van Putten et al. 1984). Akathisia is frequently mistaken for an exacerbation of psychotic symptoms, anxiety, and/or depression. If the dosage of antipsychotic medication is increased, the restlessness continues and eventually worsens. Lowering the dosage may improve the symptoms. Akathisia is among the most treatment resistant of the acute EPS, although it generally resolves if the patient is switched to an atypical agent. In the past, anticholinergic drugs were suggested as the first line of therapy, but they are often ineffective, helping only occasionally when akathisia occurs in combination with other extrapyramidal symptoms, such as rigidity. Benzodiazepines are helpful in some cases.

The treatment of choice for akathisia is either a switch to an atypical agent or the addition of a β-adrenergic-blocking drug, particularly propranolol. Several well-controlled studies have documented that propranolol, in dosages up to 120 mg/day, is an effective treatment for akathisia (Adler et al. 1985, 1989; Lipinski et al. 1984). In general, the lipophilic β-blockers are more effective in treating akathisia than the hydrophilic ones (Dupuis et al. 1987; Reiter et al. 1987; Zubenko et al. 1984). At present, controversy remains as to whether β-selective drugs effectively treat akathisia, with some negative findings (Zubenko et al. 1984) and some positive reports (Dumon et al. 1992; Dupuis et al. 1987). These drugs avoid the risk of bronchospasm in susceptible patients and, therefore, would be a welcome treatment alternative (Adler et al. 1991; Dumon et al. 1992; Lewis and Lofthouse 1993). Although akathisia is uncommon with atypical agents, it may occur, particularly with high-dose administration of risperidone, olanzapine, or ziprasidone.

Tardive Disorders

Tardive dyskinesia is a disorder characterized by involuntary choreoathetoid movements of the face, trunk, or extremities. The syndrome is usually associated with prolonged exposure to dopamine receptor–blocking agents, most frequently, antipsychotic drugs. However, the antidepressant amoxapine and the antiemetic agents metoclopramide and prochlorperazine can also cause tardive dyskinesia. Spontaneous dyskinesias also occur relatively frequently in nonmedicated elderly. The American Psychiatric Association (APA) Task Force on Tardive Dyskinesia estimated a cumulative incidence of 5% per year of exposure among young adults and a prevalence of 30% after 1 year of treatment among elderly patients (American Psychiatric Association 1992). Clozapine seems to carry little or no risk of inducing tardive dyskinesia. The incidence of tardive dyskinesia in association with the other atypical antipsychotics has not yet been adequately determined. Preliminary evidence suggests a level of risk for olanzapine and risperidone between the conventional antipsychotics and clozapine (Jeste et al. 1999; Tollefson et al. 1997).

The diagnostic features of tardive dyskinesia are listed in Table 24–16. These features have been adapted from the Abnormal Involuntary Movement Scale (AIMS). Although this scale is primarily for research use, physicians who prescribe antipsychotic drugs should be familiar with its contents in order to perform a thorough examination for the presence of tardive dyskinesia (Munetz and Benjamin 1988). A procedure for examining a patient for tardive dyskinesia can be found in Table 24–17.

TABLE 24–16. Clinical features of tardive dyskinesia

1. Facial and oral movements
   a. Muscles of facial expression: involuntary movement of forehead, eyebrows, periorbital area, cheeks; involuntary frowning, blinking, smiling, grimacing.
   b. Lips and perioral area: involuntary puckering, pouting, smacking.
   c. Jaw: involuntary biting, clenching, chewing, mouth opening, lateral movements.
   d. Tongue: involuntary protrusion, tremor, choreoathetoid movements (i.e., rolling, worm-like movement without displacement from the mouth).
2. Extremity movements
   a. Involuntary movement of upper arms, wrists, hands, fingers: choreic movements (i.e., rapid, objectively purposeless, irregular, spontaneous), athetoid movements (i.e., slow, irregular, complex, serpentine), tremor (i.e., repetitive, regular, rhythmic).
   b. Involuntary movement of lower legs, knees, ankles, toes: lateral knee movement, foot tapping, foot squirming, inversion and eversion of foot.
3. Trunk movements: Involuntary movement of neck, shoulders, hips: rocking, twisting, squirming, pelvic gyrations.

Source. Adapted from the Abnormal Involuntary Movement Scale (AIMS), National Institute of Mental Health 1988 ("AIMS: Abnormal Involuntary Movement Scale" 1988).

An evaluation for abnormal movements should be conducted before treatment begins and every 6 or 12 months thereafter. In typical cases, the patient often is not aware of mild involuntary movements. Less common

TABLE 24–17. Examination procedure for tardive dyskinesia

Either before or after completing the examination procedure, unobtrusively observe the patient at rest (e.g., in the waiting room). The chair to be used in this examination should be a hard, firm one without arms.

Examination procedure:

1. Ask patient whether there is anything in his or her mouth (e.g., gum, candy), and if there is, ask him or her to remove it.
2. Ask patient about the current condition of his or her teeth. Ask patient if he or she wears dentures. Do teeth or dentures bother patient now?
3. Ask patient whether he or she notices any movements in mouth, face, hands, or feet. If yes, ask him or her to describe them and to assess to what extent they currently bother the patient or interfere with his or her activities.
4. Have patient sit in chair with hands on knees, legs slightly apart, and feet flat on floor. (Look at entire body for movements while patient is in this position.)
5. Ask patient to sit with hands hanging unsupported (if male) between legs or (if female and wearing a dress) hanging over knees. (Observe hands and other body areas.)
6. Ask patient to open mouth. (Observe tongue at rest within mouth.) Do this twice.
7. Ask patient to protrude tongue. (Observe abnormalities of tongue movement.) Do this twice.
8. Ask patient to tap thumb, with each finger, as rapidly as possible for 10–15 seconds, separately with right hand, then with left hand. (Observe facial and leg movements.)
9. Flex and extend patient's left and right arms one at a time. (Note any rigidity.)
10. Ask patient to stand up. (Observe in profile. Observe all body areas again, hips included.)
11. Ask patient to extend both arms outstretched in front with palms down. (Observe trunk, legs, and mouth.)
12. Have patient walk a few paces, turn, and walk back to chair. (Observe hands and gait.) Do this twice.

Source. Adapted from the Abnormal Involuntary Movement Scale (AIMS), National Institute of Mental Health 1988 ("AIMS: Abnormal Involuntary Movement Scale" 1988).

are severe dyskinetic movements, which can be disfiguring or even disabling as a result of involvement of speech or swallowing. Although the most common form of tardive disorder is the dyskinetic variety (nonrhythmic, quick, choreiform movements), other types have been identified. These include tardive akathisia, tardive dystonia, and tardive tics (Fahn 1985).

The most commonly accepted hypothesis of the mechanism for the development of tardive dyskinesia is that postsynaptic dopamine receptors develop supersensitivity to dopamine after prolonged dopamine receptor blockade. This model does not account for the time course of tardive dyskinesia onset nor does it account for the persistence of tardive dyskinesia after medication is discontinued (Jenner and Marsden 1986). Other hypotheses have been proposed, including the generation of free radicals by dopamine blockade (Cadet et al. 1986). Recent research has implicated an interaction between oxidative load (free radicals) and glutamatergic neurotoxicity (Tsai et al. 1998).

The most significant and consistently documented risk factor for the development of tardive dyskinesia is increasing age of the patient (Branchey and Branchey 1984; Jeste and Wyatt 1982; Kane and Smith 1982). The duration of exposure to a conventional antipsychotic is also an important factor, as the cumulative incidence has been shown to remain constant at about 5% for the first 8 years in nonelderly patients. Women have been found to be at a greater risk for severe tardive dyskinesia, although the evidence suggests that this finding is limited to geriatric populations (Kennedy et al. 1971; Seide and Muller 1967). Other risk factors may include EPS early in the course of treatment, a history of drug holidays (a greater number of drug-free periods is associated with an increased risk), the presence of brain damage, diabetes mellitus, and a diagnosis of mood disorder.

The issue of informed consent with respect to the risk of tardive dyskinesia has been extensively reviewed (Munetz and Roth 1985; Roth 1983). It is usually difficult to obtain informed consent from a patient with acute psychosis. In many circumstances, full informed consent may not be obtainable from a patient with acute psychosis for several weeks. A general guideline is to inform and educate the family of the patient about the risks of tardive dyskinesia before starting the antipsychotic and to educate the patient about this disorder as soon as possible. Although the evidence for reduced risk of tardive dyskinesia with atypical agents is not yet conclusive, patients and families should be informed that treatment with a conventional agent may increase the likelihood of irreversible movements compared with treatment with an atypical agent. The psychiatrist also needs to be aware that some states (e.g., California and New Jersey) legally mandate that informed consent be obtained from patients before the initiation of antipsychotic treatment. All such discussions with patients and their families should be documented in the patients' records. Informed consent that is exclusively in the written form has been shown to be less effective in communicating information to the patient than verbal communication combined with written information (Munetz and Roth 1985). The psychiatrist must allocate adequate time to the provision of informed consent consistent with the confusional state and cognitive capabilities of the patient. Further discussion of this area may be found in Chapter 40 of this textbook.

Because antipsychotic medications are the most effective treatment for most patients with schizophrenia, the situation often arises in which a patient develops tardive dyskinesia but still requires the medication to function. If discontinuation of the antipsychotic drug is clinically possible, gradual improvement in tardive dyskinesia may occur, although involuntary movements often worsen initially with tapering of the antipsychotic, a phenomenon referred to as *withdrawal dyskinesia* (Glazer et al. 1984). Withdrawal dyskinesias also may appear when a patient is switched from a conventional agent to an atypical antipsychotic. Withdrawal dyskinesias typically resolve within 6 weeks; however, suppressed or latent tardive dyskinesia that has been suppressed by D_2 receptor blockade, once it appears, may not resolve. Conversely, movements may be masked temporarily by increasing the dosage of the antipsychotic medication, but the symptoms eventually reemerge, often in a more severe form. Anticholinergic drugs may reversibly worsen dyskinetic movements (Reunanen et al. 1982; Yassa 1985), whereas anticholinergic drugs in high doses may improve tardive dystonia (Burke et al. 1982; Fahn 1985).

No definitive treatment exists for tardive dyskinesia. In several small studies, α-tocopherol (vitamin E) was shown to be of some benefit, most often for patients who had tardive dyskinesia for less than 5 years (Adler et al. 1993; Akhtar et al. 1993; Dabiri et al. 1994; Egan et al. 1992; Elkashef et al. 1990; Lohr and Caligiuri 1996; Lohr et al. 1987), but no benefit was discerned with vitamin E in a recent Veterans Affairs trial (Adler et al. 1998). Vitamin E is a relatively benign antioxidant that may protect neurons from the damaging effects of free radicals, which have been implicated in the etiology of tardive dyskinesia. The typical dosage of vitamin E is 1,600 IU/day. Despite inconsistent evidence for efficacy, prophylaxis with vitamin E has been recommended.

For patients with tardive dyskinesia who cannot discontinue their antipsychotic, a switch to an atypical agent may be prudent. In an open trial, Lieberman et al. (1991) reported a 50% or greater improvement in the severity of tardive dyskinesia among 43% of the patients switched from a conventional antipsychotic to clozapine. Severe tardive dyskinesia, and especially tardive dystonia, was most likely to respond. The efficacy of the other atypical antipsychotics has not been systematically evaluated in this regard, but it is reasonable to attempt to use these agents prior to a clozapine trial.

Neuroleptic Malignant Syndrome

In rare instances, patients taking antipsychotic medications may develop a potentially life-threatening disorder known as *NMS*. Although it occurs most frequently with the use of high-potency conventional antipsychotic drugs, this condition may accompany treatment with any antipsychotic agent, including the atypical antipsychotics. Patients with NMS typically have marked muscle rigidity, although this feature may be absent with the atypical antipsychotics. Other salient features include fever, autonomic instability, elevated white blood cell count (>15,000/mm^3), elevated creatinine phosphokinase (CPK) levels (>300 U/mL), and delirium. The elevated CPK is due to muscle breakdown, which can lead to myoglobinuria and acute renal failure.

In a large prospective study, Rosebush and Stewart (1989) found that NMS was associated most often with the initiation or increase of antipsychotic medication, and in every case it occurred within 1 month of admission to a psychiatric unit. Episodes that occurred in patients taking stable dosages of antipsychotic medications were almost always associated with antecedent dehydration. Lithium use increases the risk appreciably, as does the presence of a mood disorder. Higher dosages, rapid escalation of dosage, and intramuscular injections of antipsychotics are all associated with the development of NMS (Keck et al. 1989). The keys to treatment after recognition of the syndrome are discontinuation of all medications, thorough medical evaluation, intravenous fluids, antipyretic agents, and cooling blankets. Dantrolene and bromocriptine have been reported in uncontrolled trials to improve symptoms of NMS, but their efficacy over supportive care has not been proved and is controversial (Rosebush et al. 1991). Rosebush et al. (1989) reviewed 20 cases of patients who developed NMS while taking conventional agents and found that delaying reinitiation of an antipsychotic by at least 2 weeks after resolution of symptoms was associated with a markedly decreased risk of relapse.

Bromocriptine is a centrally active dopamine agonist that has been used successfully in some cases of NMS (Guze and Baxter 1985). The symptoms of rigidity may respond rapidly, although the temperature elevation, blood pressure instability, and creatinine kinase level may normalize only after several days. This drug should be administered in an initial dosage of 1.25–2.5 mg twice a day, and it may be increased to 10 mg three times a day (Guze and Baxter 1985).

Dantrolene sodium, also used in the treatment of malignant hyperthermia (a rare reaction to anesthetic drugs), is a direct-acting muscle relaxant that may reduce the thermogenesis of NMS caused by the tonic contraction of skeletal muscles (Guze and Baxter 1985). The manufacturer's recommendation for administration of dantrolene for acute malignant hyperthermia is 1 mg/kg by rapid intravenous push. The drug should be continued until the symptoms are reversed or until a maximum dose of 10 mg/kg is given. The oral dosage of dantrolene after a malignant hyperthermic crisis is 4–8 mg/kg/day in four divided doses. This regimen should be continued until all symptoms resolve. The clinician should be aware that dantrolene has a significant potential for hepatotoxicity and thus should not be administered to patients with liver dysfunction.

Anticholinergic Side Effects

In general, the anticholinergic potency of the antipsychotic drugs is less than that of the anticholinergic antiparkinsonian drugs. However, when low-potency antipsychotic drugs (including clozapine) are given in high dosages, anticholinergic side effects often become pronounced. Anticholinergic effects are categorized as peripheral or central. The most common peripheral side effects are dry mouth, decreased sweating, decreased bronchial secretions, blurred vision (due to inhibition of accommodation), difficulty in urination, constipation, and tachycardia. Bethanechol chloride, a cholinergic drug that does not cross the blood–brain barrier, may effectively treat these side effects at a dosage of 25–50 mg three times a day; it may be required for the duration of therapy with the antipsychotic medication.

Central side effects of anticholinergic drugs include impairment in concentration, attention, and memory, and these side effects must be differentiated from symptoms caused by the patient's psychosis. Some patients are subject to these symptoms at relatively low dosages of medication. In cases of toxicity, anticholinergic delirium, which includes hot dry skin, dry mucous membranes, dilated pupils, absent bowel sounds, and tachycardia, may appear. Anticholinergic delirium constitutes a medical emergency and requires full supportive medical care. Physostigmine, a centrally and peripherally acting reversible anticholinesterase, may be used as a diagnostic agent in cases of suspected anticholinergic toxicity. This agent is administered intramuscularly at a dose of 1.0–2.0 mg or intravenously at a slow controlled rate of no more than 1 mg/minute. Physostigmine should not be used to maintain reversal of the toxicity, however, because a cholinergic crisis may result, which is characterized by nausea, vomiting, bradycardia, and seizures. This reaction can be reversed by the administration of a potent anticholinergic drug such as atropine.

Adrenergic Side Effects

Antipsychotics also block α-adrenergic receptors, which can result in orthostatic hypotension and dizziness. Orthostatic hypotension is quite commonly associated with low-potency conventional agents, and among the atypical agents, clozapine, risperidone, and ziprasidone require initial dose titration, particularly in the elderly, to avoid orthostatic hypotension. The administration of epinephrine, which stimulates both α- and β-adrenergic receptors, will result in a paradoxical drop in blood pressure as a result of the stimulation of β receptors in the presence of α-receptor blockade. In asthmatic patients who require treatment with antipsychotics as well as episodic treatment with α-adrenergic drugs, specific warnings are necessary regarding the dangers inherent in the use of epinephrine in the treatment of an acute asthmatic attack.

Endocrine and Sexual Side Effects

All the conventional antipsychotic medications and risperidone may produce hyperprolactinemia. Side effects mediated, at least in part, by hyperprolactinemia include gynecomastia, galactorrhea, amenorrhea, and decreased libido. Although such side effects were frequently associated with hyperprolactinemia resulting from conventional antipsychotics (Ghadirian et al. 1982; A.I. Green and Brown 1988), a review of clinical experience with risperidone found relatively low rates of side effects despite markedly elevated prolactin levels (Kleinberg et al. 1997). Because ascertainment of these side effects can be problematic, the true incidence and relation to prolactin levels remain controversial. Hyperprolactinemia secondarily can lower estrogen levels, resulting in amenorrhea and theoretically placing patients at risk for osteoporosis and pathological fractures (Klibanski et al. 1981).

A combination of anticholinergic effects, α-adrenergic-receptor blockade, and hormonal effects may lead to several types of sexual difficulty. In men, inability to achieve or maintain erections, decreased ability to achieve orgasm, and changes in the pleasurable quality of orgasm have been reported with conventional agents (Ghadirian et al. 1982). Thioridazine may cause painful retrograde ejaculation, in which semen is ejected into the bladder (Shader 1964). Priapism, which necessitates immediate urological consultation, has been reported, especially with thioridazine and chlorpromazine (Mitchell and Popkin 1982), although atypical agents also have been linked to priapism (Deirmenjian et al. 1998; Emes and Millson 1994; Rosen and Hanno 1992). Women may experience changes in the quality of orgasm as well as decreased ability to achieve orgasm with use of antipsychotics. Sexual side effects are usually very troubling to patients and often interfere with treatment compliance. Therefore, regular assessment by the clinician of sexual side effects is important. Reducing the dosage or changing the type of agent may reverse these symptoms, although this important topic remains poorly studied. (Other treatment strategies are discussed in the subsection on sexual side effects of antidepressant drugs earlier in this chapter.)

Weight Gain

Many patients experience weight gain while taking antipsychotic medication. Allison et al. (1999) analyzed results from all published controlled trials of antipsychotic agents and estimated the mean weight change after 10 weeks of treatment for each agent. The effect of conventional antipsychotics ranged from a mean loss of 0.4 kg with molindone to a mean gain of 3.2 kg with thioridazine. Haloperidol produced a mean 1.1-kg weight gain. Among atypical agents, only ziprasidone produced no change in weight; the other atypical agents were associated with the following estimates of weight gain at 10 weeks: risperidone 2.1 kg, olanzapine 4.15 kg, and clozapine 4.45 kg. Insufficient data were available to calculate mean weight gain with quetiapine. Weight gain with atypical agents is quite variable; approximately 20% of the patients treated with olanzapine gain no weight, whereas morbid obesity can occur in about 10% of patients. Weight gain with olanzapine appears to plateau within the first 6 months and is not dose dependent.

Ocular Effects

Antipsychotics may cause pigmentary changes in the lens and retina, especially with long-term treatment. Pigment deposition in the lens of the eye does not affect vision; however, pigmentary retinopathy, which can lead to irreversible blindness, has been associated specifically with the use of thioridazine. Although pigmentary retinopathy has most often been reported with dosages above the recommended ceiling (i.e., 800 mg/day) of thioridazine, this condition also has occurred at usual clinical doses (Ball and Caroff 1986; Hamilton 1985). The clinician should be aware that drug interactions may increase plasma levels of thioridazine, which may increase the risk of development of this dangerous side effect (Silver et al. 1986).

Quetiapine was associated with cataracts in preclinical safety studies conducted in beagles. Subsequent studies performed in nonhuman primates did not detect an elevated risk of cataracts; postmarketing surveys have not detected an increased risk of cataracts with quetiapine compared with other antipsychotics. However, the incidence of cataracts is elevated in schizophrenia patients in general. Patients starting quetiapine should be informed of the potential risk of cataracts and the recommendation in the package insert that appropriate eye examinations be performed every 6 months. This precaution may be scientifically unsupported at present but remains an issue of liability.

Dermatological Effects

Patients taking antipsychotics, especially the aliphatic phenothiazines (e.g., chlorpromazine), may become more sensitive to sunlight, which can lead to severe sunburn. Especially in the summer months, patients should avoid excessive sun exposure and use ultraviolet-blocking agents such as sunscreens that contain fully protective levels of para-aminobenzoic acid (PABA). As with many other medications, allergic maculopapular skin eruptions may occur. These are best treated by discontinuation of the agent, accompanied by symptomatic treatment with antihistamines such as diphenhydramine. For subsequent treatment of psychosis, the patient should be given a drug from another family of antipsychotics. Photosensitivity reactions have not been reported with the atypical agents.

Cardiac Effects

Several reports of sudden death have been attributed to thioridazine or chlorpromazine therapy in young, healthy patients (Aherwadker et al. 1964; Giles and Modlin 1968). Thioridazine slows atrial and ventricular conduction and prolongs refractory periods (Descotes et al. 1979; Hartigan-Go et al. 1996; Yoon et al. 1979). Because the effect is concentration dependent, thioridazine can be quite dangerous if taken in overdose or in combination with quinidine-like drugs (Risch et al. 1981). Chlorpromazine also prolongs QT intervals and atrioventricular conduction, even at relatively low doses (150 mg/day) (Ban and St. Jean 1964). Pimozide also may produce significant changes in cardiac conduction as a result of its calcium channel blocking properties (Opler and Feinberg 1991). It is recommended that serial ECGs be performed when treatment with pimozide is started, and the drug should be stopped if the QT interval exceeds 520 msec in adults or 470 msec in children (Baldessarini 1985). Extremely high doses of intravenous haloperidol (up to 1,000 mg in 24 hours) have been administered safely in patients with cardiac disease, although rare cases of torsade de pointes have been reported at these doses (Metzger and Friedman 1993).

In materials submitted to the Psychopharmacological Drugs Advisory Committee of the FDA, Pfizer, Inc., reported results from a trial designed to examine the ECG effects of atypical agents and thioridazine at maximum therapeutic serum concentrations and at the potentially higher concentrations that might occur in clinical practice if these agents were co-prescribed with metabolic inhibitors. After correcting the QT interval for heart rate, thioridazine produced the greatest mean delay in QTc (35.6 msec), followed by ziprasidone (20.6 msec), quetiapine (9.1 msec), olanzapine (6.8 msec), and haloperidol (4.7 msec). Quetiapine produced the greatest increase in heart rate (11 beats/minute). Addition of metabolic inhibitors only produced further increases in QTc when added to quetiapine (19.7 msec) and haloperidol (8.9 msec). Although the mean 39% increase in serum ziprasidone concentrations produced by ketoconazole coadministration did not result in an increase in the mean QTc duration, ziprasidone serum concentrations weakly correlate with QTc duration. In eight cases of overdose reported by the manufacturer and one published case (Burton et al. 2000), ziprasidone did not produce significant cardiac toxicity. Only 2 of 3,095 subjects (0.06%) in premarketing trials developed QTc intervals longer than 500 msec; however, participants in these trials were screened to exclude cardiac disease. In two reports of overdose with quetiapine, prolongation of the QT interval has been observed (Gajwani et al. 2000; Hustey 1999), whereas most reported cases of overdose with risperidone and olanzapine have described relatively benign ECG findings (Acri and Henretig 1998; L.G. Cohen et al. 1999). The cardiac effect of atypical agents in patients with underlying heart disease has not been adequately studied.

Hepatic Effects

Increased levels on liver function tests have been associated with antipsychotic treatment. Many cases of this reaction were linked to impurities in the original formulation of chlorpromazine, and the incidence has decreased over the years. These abnormalities usually suggest obstructive liver disease, with increases in bilirubin and alkaline phosphatase. In such circumstances, the drug must be immediately discontinued and a different antipsychotic drug initiated. This reaction appears to be more common with low-potency conventional antipsychotics. Transient elevations in hepatic enzymes have been observed with olanzapine and quetiapine, but these laboratory findings have not been linked to liver injury.

Hematological Effects

Transient leukopenia and, in rare cases, agranulocytosis have been associated with neuroleptic treatment (Balon and Berchou 1986). Although agranulocytosis is strictly defined as a complete absence of all granulocytes in the blood, it also may refer to severe neutropenia, with a neutrophil count of less than 500/mL. This is an idiosyncratic reaction that usually occurs within the first 3–4 weeks after the initiation of treatment with an antipsychotic drug. However, the period of risk for agranulocytosis and leukopenia continues for 2–3 months of treatment. A higher risk for agranulocytosis is associated with low-potency conventional antipsychotic drugs and, most significantly, clozapine (Balon and Berchou 1986). (For discussion of clozapine-induced agranulocytosis, see subsection on the side effects of clozapine later in the chapter.)

Signs and symptoms of this reaction include high fever, stomatitis, severe pharyngitis, lymphadenopathy, and malaise. Treatment of this reaction requires immediate discontinuation of all medications and immediate medical evaluation and treatment. Agranulocytosis usually resolves after discontinuation of the causative agent. There must be vigorous treatment of any infections that develop. Further treatment of psychosis must be with an agent of a completely different chemical class.

Effects on Seizure Threshold

Chlorpromazine had been marketed for less than 1 year before a case of seizure was associated with its use (Anton-Stephens 1953). Data from the Boston Collaborative Drug Surveillance Program indicated a 0.22% frequency of seizures in patients treated with chlorpromazine (Jick et al. 1970). Other surveys have supported the relation between seizures and higher doses of phenothiazines (Messing et al. 1984; Schlichther et al. 1956), although the incidence of seizures with most antipsychotics is quite low (Devinsky et al. 1991). Of all the conventional antipsychotics, molindone and fluphenazine have most consistently been shown to have the lowest potential for this side effect (Itil and Soldatos 1980; Oliver et al. 1982). In a study of patients with epilepsy, the addition of psychotropic medication, including antipsychotics, was generally associated with improved seizure control (Ojemann et al. 1987). Clozapine is an exception among the antipsychotics because it dose-dependently lowers the seizure threshold and has been estimated to produce seizures in as many 10% of the patients receiving the drug for 3.8 years.

The mechanism by which antipsychotic agents affect seizure threshold remains unclear. Animal models and in vitro methods for assessing relative drug effects on seizure threshold have produced complex and often conflicting results (Chen et al. 1968; Oliver et al. 1982; Tedeschi et al. 1958). Effects on seizure threshold may follow curvilinear relationships with respect to brain concentrations for some conventional neuroleptics (Oliver et al. 1982). Olanzapine is reported to increase slowing on the EEG but is not associated with epileptiform activity or seizures (Beasley et al. 2000; Pillmann et al. 2000).

Effects on Temperature Regulation

Antipsychotic drugs directly affect the hypothalamus and suppress temperature regulation. In combination with the α-adrenergic receptor– and cholinergic receptor–blocking effects of antipsychotics, this effect becomes particularly serious in hot, humid weather. Severe hyperthermia, rhabdomyolysis, renal failure, and death may result. This potentially life-threatening condition requires immediate medical intervention and supportive treatment. It is mandatory that a cool environment and adequate amounts of fluids be provided for patients taking antipsychotic agents. Also, care must be taken that patients do not overexert themselves in warm weather or hot environments. Special monitoring is also required for acutely agitated or manic patients and for patients in restraints because they are prone to this dangerous condition.

Use in Pregnancy

Like most other drugs, antipsychotic agents should be avoided, if possible, during pregnancy and during lactation periods for mothers who breast-feed their infants. There is a possible increase in birth defects among infants born to mothers who were first exposed to antipsychotic drugs during the sixth to tenth week of gestation (Edlund and Craig 1984). Edlund and Craig (1984) pointed out that because there is an increased risk of fetal death in psychotic mothers, the small risk of neuroleptic-induced teratogenesis must be assessed carefully and balanced against the risks involved in withholding treatment. These important issues have been reviewed in detail elsewhere (Altshuler et al. 1996).

In addition, antipsychotic agents should be prescribed with great caution in the peripartum period. Extrapyramidal symptoms (Hill et al. 1966; Levy and Wisniewski 1974; Tamer et al. 1969) and neonatal jaundice (Scokel and Jones 1962) have been reported in infants following in utero exposure to conventional antipsychotic drugs. Also, neonates may be exposed to small amounts of antipsychotics in breast milk (Stewart et al. 1980). It is therefore necessary to reassess the potential risks and benefits of antipsychotic treatment as the pregnancy comes to term. As a general guideline, antipsychotic drugs should be used in pregnant patients only if absolutely necessary, at the minimal dose required, and for the briefest possible time. Documentation of informed consent from both the mother and the father is necessary. Use of ECT to treat acute psychosis in pregnant mothers should be considered.

Drug Interactions

Antipsychotic drugs have profound effects on multiple CNS receptors, and these effects are compounded when other medications are added. For example, the α-adrenergic-receptor blockade of antipsychotics may interfere with the efficacy of the antihypertensive drug guanethidine. The sedative and anticholinergic effects of antipsychotic drugs are increased with the addition of other sedating or anticholinergic drugs. As mentioned previously, patients taking drugs with potentially serious adverse effects (such as the risk of retinopathy with thioridazine) should be monitored through plasma level determinations when other medications are used concurrently.

Pharmacokinetic interactions with antipsychotic drugs are common and have been reviewed elsewhere (Goff and Baldessarini 1995). Most conventional antipsychotic agents are metabolized by the hepatic CYP2D6 isoenzyme. The activity of this enzyme varies greatly between individuals based on genetic polymorphisms and can be inhibited by certain drugs, such as SSRIs. For example, addition of fluoxetine raised haloperidol serum concentrations by 20% and fluphenazine concentrations by 65% in one study (Goff et al. 1995). Two categories of potential drug–drug interactions are of particular concern. The first includes interactions that can elevate clozapine serum concentrations to toxic levels. This has been described with addition of inhibitors of CYP3A4 and CYP1A2 isoenzymes, such as erythromycin and fluvoxamine (L.G. Cohen et al. 1996; Wetzel et al. 1998). The other category of potentially serious interactions includes those that induce metabolism of antipsychotic agents, thereby lowering serum concentrations below a therapeutic threshold. Large reductions in clozapine and haloperidol serum concentrations have been reported with the addition of carbamazepine, phenobarbital, and phenytoin (Arana et al. 1986; Byerly and DeVane 1996). Of note, cigarette smoking can affect antipsychotic metabolism; serum concentrations of clozapine in particular are reduced with smoking and increased after smoking cessation (Byerly and DeVane 1996; Haring et al. 1989).

Atypical Antipsychotic Drugs

Clozapine, the first of the class of atypical antipsychotic drugs, was a landmark in the treatment of schizophrenia for several reasons. It was the first medication shown to be efficacious in otherwise nonresponsive patients, many of whom seemed destined to live out their lives in state psychiatric hospitals. Although it was not uniformly effective, clozapine was a "miracle" for many of these individuals. In addition, clozapine was the first agent to attenuate significantly the negative symptoms of schizophrenia, such as marked social withdrawal and apathy, thereby helping many patients return to meaningful and productive lives. Also, clozapine rarely produces EPS, and to date it is the only antipsychotic drug that is not associated with treatment-emergent tardive dyskinesia. This important clinical property is concordant with the observation that chronic administration of clozapine results in selective inhibition of dopamine neurons in the mesolimbic pathways, with little functional effect on striatal dopamine tracts. Finally, clozapine has minimal effects on the tuboinfundibular system, and therefore it does not cause hyperprolactinemia.

Clozapine has a wide range of physiological actions, and although several hypotheses are available to explain its unique spectrum of effects, the definitive answer awaits further research. A great deal of research has focused on clozapine's relatively greater 5-HT_2 than D_2 antagonism, and this property has been the predominant focus of new drug development in the class of drugs currently referred to as atypical antipsychotics. Risperidone, olanzapine, quetiapine, and ziprasidone have subsequently been approved for use in the United States. In general, the atypical antipsychotic drugs provide superior efficacy for the treatment of negative symptoms, produce fewer acute motor side effects, and may reduce the risk of tardive dyskinesia compared with conventional antipsychotic drugs. These drugs may also improve cognitive function in patients with schizophrenia (M.F. Green et al. 1997; Hagger et al. 1993; Purdon et al. 2000; Rossi et al. 1997). Although the use of these agents, as opposed to the less expensive, conventional drugs, is currently the subject of debate, it is hoped that the atypical antipsychotics may substantially improve the quality of life for individuals with chronic psychotic disorders by improving compliance, negative symptoms, and cognitive functioning (M. Green 1996).

Clozapine

Clozapine, a dibenzodiazepine, is the prototypical atypical antipsychotic. Because of the approximately 1% risk of producing a potentially fatal agranulocytosis, the use of clozapine is restricted to patients who have not responded to or cannot tolerate other antipsychotic drugs. Kane et al. (1988) studied patients with chronic schizophrenia who had failed to improve after at least three adequate trials of conventional antipsychotics. Data from this large, multicenter, double-blind prospective study indicated a significant improvement in 30% of the patients taking clozapine, compared with only 4% of those taking chlorpromazine. Clozapine produced significant improvement, compared with chlorpromazine, in positive and negative symptoms, as well as tension and hostility (Kane et al. 1988). Less rigorous data suggest that clozapine also may be effective in refractory schizoaffective disorder, psychotic mood disorders, and rapid-cycling bipolar disorder, even in the absence of psychosis (Calabrese et al. 1996; Keck et al. 1996; McElroy et al. 1991; Suppes et al. 1992; Zarate et al. 1995). Because clozapine appears to be devoid of parkinsonian side effects, it is also useful in low dosages (25 mg/day) for patients with Parkinson's disease and psychosis induced by dopamine agonists (Ostergaard and Dupont 1988). Other indications require higher dosages, as discussed later, and an extended period of titration to achieve therapeutic dosages and clinical response.

Clozapine is a difficult drug for both patient and physician, but when other treatments have failed, there is no doubt that the potential benefits of this remarkable medication are worth the risks for many patients with severe psychotic illnesses.

Mechanism of action. Clozapine shows high in vitro receptor affinities for the D_4, 5-HT_2, α_1-adrenergic, muscarinic, and histamine H_1 receptors, and a relatively weak affinity for D_1, D_2, and D_3 receptors (Brunello et al. 1995; Meltzer et al. 1989). The high 5-HT_2:D_2 ratio is hypothesized to be responsible for many of clozapine's advantages over typical antipsychotic drugs, either directly or indirectly (Meltzer 1991). Other investigators have suggested that clozapine's superior efficacy may be related to the drug's ability to increase norepinephrine outflow (Breier et al. 1994) or may be due to indirect effects on glutamatergic systems (Goff and Coyle 2001). Unlike conventional agents, clozapine reverses several effects produced by blockade of glutamatergic N-methyl-D-aspartate (NMDA) receptors in animal models thought to be predictive of therapeutic response in schizophrenia (Goff and Coyle 2001).

Clinical use. Because of prominent sedation and orthostatic hypotension, clozapine is initiated at a dosage of 12.5 mg/day and quickly increased to 12.5 mg twice a day. The dosage is then increased as tolerated, generally by 25- or 50-mg increments every day or every other day. Clozapine is usually added to the previous antipsychotic agent in a cross-titration in which the previous drug is tapered once a clozapine dose of approximately 100 mg/day has been achieved. This strategy should be used with caution if the existing medication is a low-potency conventional antipsychotic because of additive α-adrenergic and anticholinergic side effects. Initiation of clozapine in an inpatient setting with monitoring of vital signs can be much more rapid than in an outpatient setting. The typical target dosage is 300–500 mg/day in divided doses, with a greater amount given in the evening to minimize daytime sedation. Although routine blood level monitoring is not recommended, it should be noted that a serum level of greater than 350 ng/mL is associated with a higher response rate (Perry et al. 1991). Serum levels should be ascertained in nonresponders. The duration of treatment required to assess the medication response is longer than for most medications: typically, 3–6 months (Meltzer 1994). It is important that both the patient and the family understand this time frame before initiating treatment with clozapine. If patients are nonresponsive after 6 months of continuous clozapine treatment, the dosage may be gradually increased to a maximum of 900 mg/day. Not uncommonly, patients may not show a significant reduction in symptoms with clozapine, but review of their course over a 6-month or 1-year period indicates a dramatic reduction in rates of relapse and hospitalization.

Risks, side effects, and their management. *Agranulocytosis.* Agranulocytosis occurs in 0.8% of the patients taking clozapine during the first year of treatment, with a peak incidence at 3 months (Alvir and Lieberman 1994; Alvir et al. 1993). The dispensing of clozapine in the United States is linked to weekly white blood cell monitoring during the first 6 months, then biweekly thereafter. On the basis of the patient's white blood cell and absolute neutrophil count, strict guidelines have been set (Table 24–18). The system of white blood cell monitoring has successfully reduced fatalities from agranulocytosis to extremely low levels (Honigfeld et al. 1998).

There may be a genetic susceptibility to clozapine-induced agranulocytosis. Although it was first reported in patients of Ashkenazi Jewish descent (Lieberman et al. 1990), the finding has been extended to non-Jewish populations and appears to be related to genetic variations in the major histocompatibility complex (Corzo et al. 1995; Turbay et al. 1997; Yunis et al. 1995). Although there are some promising leads for genetic markers, at this time

---

TABLE 24–18. Guidelines for hematological monitoring of patients taking clozapine

1. Initial white blood cell (WBC) count must be greater than 3,500/mm³.
2. A weekly WBC count is required throughout treatment and for 4 weeks after discontinuation of clozapine.[a]
3. If WBC count is 2,000–3,000/mm³ *or* granulocyte count is 1,000–1,500/mm³, interrupt therapy and monitor for signs of infection. Check WBC count and differential daily. If there are no symptoms of infection, WBC count returns to greater than 3,000/mm³, and granulocyte level is greater than 1,500/mm³, resume clozapine with twice-weekly WBC and differential counts until the total WBC count returns to above 3,500/mm³.
4. If WBC count is less than 2,000/mm³ *or* granulocyte count is less than 1,000/mm³, discontinue clozapine and do not rechallenge. Check WBC count and differential daily. Treat infection with antibiotics. Consider bone marrow aspiration to ascertain granulopoietic status. If granulopoiesis is deficient, consider protective isolation.

Note. [a]Monitoring every 14 days has recently been recommended for patients who have been taking clozapine for 6 months or longer.

---

genetic testing is not of clinical benefit, and these findings do not preclude the use of clozapine in any ethnic group. For unknown reasons, women and elderly persons also may be at greater risk for clozapine-induced agranulocytosis.

If agranulocytosis develops, prompt consultation with a hematologist is indicated. Reverse isolation and prophylactic antibiotics may be used to prevent infection. Granulocyte-stimulating factors may be used to shorten the duration and reduce the morbidity of agranulocytosis (Barnas et al. 1992; Chengappa et al. 1996; Gerson et al. 1992; Nielsen 1993). Although lithium often causes leukocytosis, it does not appear to treat or prevent clozapine-induced agranulocytosis. Once a patient has developed agranulocytosis while taking clozapine, he or she should not be rechallenged with this medication.

Clozapine is contraindicated in patients with myeloproliferative disorders or who are immunocompromised as a result of diseases such as tuberculosis or human immunodeficiency virus (HIV) infection because of their increased risk of developing agranulocytosis. Concomitant medications that are associated with bone marrow suppression, such as carbamazepine, are also contraindicated.

Extrapyramidal effects. EPS are uncommon with clozapine at any dosage, although some patients experience akathisia or hand tremors.

Neuroleptic malignant syndrome. Despite the absence of EPS in clozapine-treated patients, there have been reports of NMS in patients taking clozapine alone (Anderson and Powers 1991; Das Gupta and Young 1991; Miller et al. 1991).

Sedation. Sedation is the most common side effect of clozapine, and it is particularly prominent early in treatment. Sedation generally attenuates with dosage reduction, when tolerance to this side effect develops, or when a disproportionate amount is given at bedtime.

Cardiovascular effects. Hypotension and tachycardia occur in most patients taking clozapine. Rare cases of myocarditis of uncertain etiology also have been reported in patients taking clozapine.

Weight gain. Weight gain occurs in most patients; many patients gain 10% or more of their original body weight (Umbricht et al. 1994). One naturalistic study found that weight gain did not plateau with clozapine until year 4 and was not dose related (Henderson et al. 2000). In addition, new-onset diabetes mellitus was reported at a rate of about 7% of patients per year but was not statistically associated with weight gain (Henderson et al. 2000). Patients should receive nutritional counseling at the initiation of treatment with clozapine, and fasting blood sugar levels should be monitored every 6 months.

Hypersalivation. Hypersalivation occurs in one-third of the patients taking clozapine, particularly at night. Although the basis for this side effect is unknown, the symptom is not related to drug-induced parkinsonism. Because clozapine has potent anticholinergic properties, addition of an anticholinergic agent is not recommended for control of drooling.

Fever. For unclear reasons, clozapine treatment is associated with benign, transient temperature elevations, generally within the first 3 weeks of treatment. Patients taking clozapine who develop fevers should be evaluated for infectious etiologies, agranulocytosis, and NMS.

Seizures. Clozapine treatment is associated with a dose-dependent risk of seizures. The vast majority of clozapine-induced seizures are tonic-clonic, but myoclonic seizures also occur. Dosages of less than 300 mg/day are associated with a 1%–3% seizure risk. Dosages of 300–600 mg/day carry a 3%–4% risk, and dosages greater than 600 mg/day are associated with a 5% risk of seizures. Because of this risk, clozapine dosages greater than 600 mg/day are not recommended unless the patient has failed to respond at lower dosages. Many clinicians avoid using clozapine for patients who have abnormal EEG findings. Our clinical impression is that EEG abnormalities associated with clozapine use are much more common than clozapine-induced seizures. Once a seizure has occurred, the question of whether to continue using clozapine requires clinical judgment. Because only those patients with fairly serious and otherwise refractory illnesses receive clozapine, the medication is usually continued, with the addition of an anticonvulsant. Carbamazepine must be avoided because of the additive risk of bone marrow suppression. At present, valproate appears to be the safest anticonvulsant for patients taking clozapine.

Anticholinergic effects. Anticholinergic side effects, such as dry mouth, blurred vision, constipation, and urinary retention, are common early side effects.

Obsessive-compulsive symptoms. Treatment with clozapine has been reported to exacerbate symptoms of OCD, probably because of 5-HT$_2$ antagonism (Ghaemi et al. 1995). If this effect occurs, symptoms are usually controlled with the addition of an SSRI.

Drug interactions. Clozapine should not be combined with any drugs that have the potential to suppress bone marrow function, such as carbamazepine. There have been isolated reports of respiratory arrest in patients who were taking both clozapine and a high-potency benzodiazepine. Because of these reports, benzodiazepines should be avoided, particularly at high doses, in patients who are taking clozapine.

Clozapine is metabolized by hepatic CYP1A2 and, to a lesser degree, CYP3A3/4; therefore, it is subject to changes in serum concentration when combined with medications that inhibit or induce these enzymes (see section on drug interactions later in this chapter). Clozapine serum levels are increased by coadministration of fluvoxamine and erythromycin and decreased by phenobarbital, phenytoin, and cigarette smoking (Byerly and DeVane 1996). These pharmacokinetic interactions are particularly important because of the dose-dependent risk of seizures.

Risperidone

Risperidone, a novel benzisoxazole derivative, is an atypical antipsychotic medication that combines D$_2$-receptor antagonism with potent 5-HT$_2$ receptor antagonism. Risperidone has a higher affinity for D$_2$ receptors than does clozapine. Risperidone also antagonizes D_1, D_4, α_1, α_2, and H_1 histaminic receptors. Risperidone was more effective than haloperidol 20 mg/day against both the positive and the negative symptoms of chronic schizophrenia (Chouinard et al. 1993; Marder and Meibach 1994). The optimal dosage of risperidone in the North American trials was 6 mg/day, but subsequent clinical experience has indicated that most patients do well on lower doses of 3–6 mg/day, and the elderly may require doses as low as 0.5 mg/day. Clinicians should titrate the dose of risperidone to avoid EPS. Unlike the other atypical agents, risperidone elevates prolactin levels, often higher than levels associated with conventional agents.

Bondolfi et al. (1996) reported that risperidone was comparable to clozapine in treatment-refractory schizophrenia; however, the patients in their study were not as highly refractory as were the patients in the earlier studies of clozapine in refractory schizophrenia, and the dose of clozapine administered to the comparison group was quite low (Kane et al. 1988). Although clinical experience suggests that risperidone is unlikely to be as effective as clozapine in highly refractory cases, Marder and Meibach (1994) found that schizophrenia patients presumed to be treatment resistant on the basis of having been hospitalized for 6 months or longer at the time of study entry did not respond to haloperidol 20 mg/day but significantly improved with risperidone 6 mg/day or 16 mg/day compared with placebo.

Clinical use. Risperidone is most effective in the 4- to 6-mg range. For initial treatment, we recommend using divided doses, starting at 1 mg twice a day and quickly increasing to 2 mg twice a day. For elderly persons, the initial dosage should be much lower (0.25–0.5 mg/day). After the first week of treatment, the entire dosage can be given at bedtime. This usually helps the patient to sleep and reduces daytime side effects. However, we do not suggest this practice for elderly persons because of an increased risk of falling. In addition, some patients feel an activating effect from risperidone; in these individuals, the medication should be administered in the morning.

Risks, side effects, and their management. Insomnia, hypotension, agitation, headache, and rhinitis are the most common side effects of risperidone. These tend to lessen with time. Risperidone produces weight gain, which is intermediate in magnitude compared with other atypical agents. Overall, the drug tends to be well tolerated. Risperidone is not associated with significant anticholinergic side effects. Whereas hyperprolactinemia is a common finding with risperidone, the incidence of clinical manifestations is less clear.

Extrapyramidal effects. In comparison to relatively high doses of haloperidol (20 mg/day), risperidone is associated with a lower prevalence of acute extrapyramidal effects and akathisia (Owens 1996). EPS occurs in a dose-dependent manner, with more frequent occurrence when the dosage is greater than 6 mg/day.

Cardiovascular effects. Brief hypotension may occur, as expected with α blockade (Owens 1994). Tachycardia is also common.

Tardive dyskinesia. Risperidone at low doses produces few parkinsonian side effects (Gwinn and Caviness 1997; Umbricht and Kane 1996). The incidence of risperidone-induced tardive dyskinesia is not known, but it is assumed to be between that of clozapine and the conventional antipsychotics. In one 9-month study of elderly patients, risperidone produced very low rates of tardive dyskinesia compared with haloperidol (Jeste et al. 1999).

Weight gain. Weight gain associated with risperidone treatment is quite variable and is less than weight gain associated with olanzapine and clozapine (Allison et al. 1999). The mean weight gain after 10 weeks of exposure to risperidone is approximately 2.1 kg.

Drug interactions. Risperidone is metabolized primarily by the CYP2D6 enzyme (Byerly and DeVane 1996). Medications that inhibit this enzyme, such as many of the SSRIs, cause increased risperidone plasma levels. However, several studies have not found an increase in side effects resulting from such an interaction, possibly because the primary metabolite of risperidone, 9-OH risperidone, is fully active and is excreted unchanged by the kidneys. Inhibition of the 2D6 enzyme may merely alter the balance between parent drug and metabolite without significantly altering total D_2 occupancy. Pharmacodynamic interactions may occur when risperidone is combined with other medications that share a similar physiological effect, such as orthostatic hypotension.

Olanzapine

Olanzapine, a thienobenzodiazepine, represents a modification of the clozapine molecule. Compared with clozapine, olanzapine has greater D_2 and weaker D_4 and α-adrenergic affinity. Despite the structural similarity of these two drugs, olanzapine is not associated with higher than expected rates of agranulocytosis. Although in vitro binding studies have indicated a high affinity for M_1 receptors, anticholinergic side effects are not as prominent as these data would predict.

Olanzapine has dose-dependent therapeutic effects on both positive and negative symptoms and a favorable side effect profile (Beasley et al. 1996). Acute dystonia is uncommon. Akathisia is more common but significantly less common than with the conventional antipsychotic drugs. In prospective double-blind studies, treatment-emergent tardive dyskinesia was reported to occur in 1% of the olanzapine group compared with 4.6% of the haloperidol group (Tollefson et al. 1997). Olanzapine is associated with modest dose-dependent elevations in serum prolactin levels, but most often these elevations are transient and within the normal reference range (Tollefson et al. 1997).

Olanzapine has shown superior efficacy for negative symptoms, depressive symptoms, and cognitive impairments compared with haloperidol (Beasley Jr et al. 1997; Purdon et al. 2000; Tollefson and Sanger 1997; Tollefson et al. 1998). Studies of olanzapine in refractory patients have produced inconsistent results, although recent data suggest that olanzapine may be more effective in some refractory patients at doses up to 40 mg/day (Breier and Hamilton 1999; Conley et al. 1998).

Clinical use. The recommended starting dosage of olanzapine is 10 mg at bedtime, subsequently titrated on the basis of tolerability and therapeutic effect. The clinically effective range is 7.5–20 mg/day, administered as a single daily dose at bedtime. Higher dosages may be more effective but result in increased side effects. Clinically meaningful improvement may not be evident for the first several weeks after initiating treatment, but improvement usually continues through week 6 and perhaps longer.

Although there are no systematic data regarding switching from other antipsychotic drugs to olanzapine, early clinical experience favors a gradual cross-titration. Commonly, olanzapine is added to the existing antipsychotic medication, which is then tapered after 1–2 weeks. This strategy is applicable when switching from clozapine to olanzapine, but a word of caution is warranted. For patients who are stable while taking clozapine, it is tempting to consider substituting olanzapine to avoid the risk of clozapine-induced agranulocytosis; however, it cannot be assumed that patients will do equally well on another atypical antipsychotic. There have been many instances of poor patient outcomes after attempts to switch from clozapine to another atypical antipsychotic (Henderson et al. 1998). However, before initiating a trial of clozapine, it is reasonable to try olanzapine or risperidone in patients whose illness is refractory to conventional antipsychotic drugs.

Risks, side effects, and their management. *Somnolence.* As one would predict on the basis of the histamine H_1 antagonism, somnolence is a common side effect of olanzapine. Somnolence and psychomotor slowing are dose dependent, and patients often become tolerant to this side effect over time.

Anticholinergic side effects. Anticholinergic side effects are clinically less significant than would be predicted on the basis of in vitro muscarinic receptor-binding affinity. However, dry mouth has been reported in association with olanzapine treatment (Beasley et al. 1996).

Seizures. Premarketing studies reported a 0.9% incidence of seizures, some of which were attributed to concomitant medical disorders. Olanzapine should be used with caution in patients with a history of seizures and in those with conditions that may lower the seizure threshold, such as dementia.

Hepatic effects. Increased transaminase levels were reported in 2% of the patients taking olanzapine in premarketing evaluation. In many cases, these levels normalized without medication discontinuation, and all cases to date have been clinically benign. Routine laboratory monitoring is not recommended, but olanzapine should be used with caution in patients with hepatic disease or with additional risk factors for hepatic toxicity. In this group of patients, serum transaminase levels must be monitored.

Weight gain. Treatment-emergent weight gain is common with olanzapine and averages about 7 kg (15 lb). However, approximately 20% of patients may not gain weight. Nutritional education should be provided to patients, along with monitoring of caloric intake by diet diaries, and exercise should be strongly encouraged. Weight reduction groups are often helpful in providing instructional materials and offering support.

Drug interactions. Olanzapine is metabolized by several pathways and is therefore unlikely to be affected by concurrent administration with other medications. Because olanzapine does not appear to inhibit any of the cytochrome P450 enzymes, it should not increase the availability of other medications through this mechanism. Additive pharmacodynamic effects are expected if olanzapine is combined with medications that also have anticholinergic, antihistaminic, or α-adrenergic side effects.

Quetiapine

Quetiapine is a dibenzothiazapine derivative with weak affinity for 5-HT$_{1A}$, 5-HT$_2$, D$_1$, D$_2$, H$_1$, α_1, and α_2 receptors. Quetiapine has very "loose" binding to D_2 receptors. For example, D_2 receptor occupancy may drop from approximately 57% when measured 3 hours after an oral quetiapine dose of 400 mg to 20% after 9 hours. In a fixed-dose comparison of quetiapine to haloperidol (12 mg/day) and placebo, quetiapine was superior to placebo at doses of 150–750 mg on most measures but superior to placebo for the treatment of negative symptoms only at the 300-mg dose (Arvanitis and Miller 1997). Quetiapine was not statistically superior to haloperidol in efficacy measures but was comparable to placebo with regard to treatment-emergent EPS (Arvanitis et al. 1997). A comparison of high-dose quetiapine (approximately 500 mg/day) and low-dose quetiapine (approximately 250 mg/day) found significantly greater efficacy with the higher dose (Small et al. 1997). Quetiapine's relatively high 5-HT_2:D_2 ratio is consistent with the hypothesized advantageous properties of the atypical antipsychotics, antagonism of H_1 receptors is associated with sedative side effects, and α_1 antagonism is associated with orthostatic hypotension.

Clinical use.   Quetiapine is initiated at a dose of 25 mg twice a day and then increased on day 2 to 50 mg twice a day, on day 3 to 100 mg twice a day, and on day 4 to 100 mg in the morning and 200 mg in the evening. The optimal dose for most patients appears to range between 400 mg/day and 600 mg/day, although the drug is safe and efficacious for some patients within a dose range of 150–750 mg. A slower titration and lower daily doses may be warranted for patients with hepatic disease and for elderly patients. Because of a relatively short half-life of 8 hours, quetiapine is usually administered twice daily.

Risks, side effects, and their management.   Quetiapine was no different from placebo in doses to 750 mg/day regarding EPS and changes in serum prolactin levels (Arvanitis and Miller 1997).

Somnolence.   Somnolence is one of the most common side effects of quetiapine. Somnolence and psychomotor slowing are dose dependent, and patients often become tolerant to this side effect over time.

Ocular changes.   The development of cataracts was observed in association with quetiapine treatment in preclinical studies of dogs, but a causal relation has not been established in humans. Postmarketing experience has not detected an increase in incidence of cataracts with quetiapine compared with other antipsychotics; however, cataracts are more common in schizophrenic patients in general compared with the general population. Even though concerns raised by safety studies in dogs have not been substantiated in clinical practice, it is currently recommended that patients receive an ocular examination of sufficient sensitivity to detect cataract formation, such as a slit-lamp examination, at the initiation of treatment and at 6-month intervals. Because this is not an acute change, if the clinical situation dictates, quetiapine may be begun shortly before the ocular examination.

Cardiovascular effects.   As predicted with α_1 antagonism, quetiapine may induce orthostatic hypotension and concomitant symptoms of dizziness, tachycardia, and syncope. The risk of symptomatic hypotension is particularly pronounced during initial dose titration. Quetiapine should be used with caution in patients with cardiovascular disease, cerebral vascular disease, or other illnesses predisposing to hypotension.

Hepatic effects.   Increased transaminase levels were reported in 6% of the patients taking quetiapine in premarketing evaluation. These changes usually occur in the first weeks of treatment and to date have been benign. Routine laboratory monitoring is not recommended, but quetiapine should be used with caution in patients with hepatic disease or with additional risk factors for hepatic toxicity.

Weight gain.   Quetiapine may induce weight gain. In premarketing placebo-controlled studies, a weight gain of 7% or more of body weight was observed in 23% of quetiapine-treated patients, compared with 6% of placebo-control subjects. Early clinical experience suggests that weight gain associated with quetiapine treatment is not generally as marked as has been observed with olanzapine, although insufficient data are available to compare it directly with other agents (Allison et al. 1999).

Drug interactions.   Quetiapine is metabolized by the hepatic CYP3A3/4 enzyme. Concurrent administration of cytochrome P450–inducing drugs, such as carbamazepine, decreases quetiapine blood levels. In such circumstances, increased doses of quetiapine are appropriate. Quetiapine does not appreciably affect the pharmacokinetics of other medications. Pharmacodynamic effects are expected if quetiapine is combined with medications that also have antihistaminic or α-adrenergic side effects. Because of its potential for producing hypotension, quetiapine also may enhance the effects of certain antihypertensive agents.

Ziprasidone

Ziprasidone is the most recent atypical agent to become available in the United States. Ziprasidone combines a high affinity for 5-HT$_2$ receptors with intermediate affinity for D$_2$, resulting in a very high 5-HT$_2$:D$_2$ affinity ratio. Ziprasidone also has substantial agonist activity at 5-HT$_{1a}$ receptors and moderately inhibits reuptake of serotonin and norepinephrine—suggesting possible antidepressant activity. Ziprasidone appears to be similar to other atypical agents in efficacy, although no head-to-head comparisons have been reported between ziprasidone and other atypical agents. The FDA delayed approval of ziprasidone until additional safety data could be obtained regarding effects on cardiac conduction. Ziprasidone delays the QTc interval at maximum therapeutic blood levels by approximately 20 msec, on average, which is a larger effect than with other atypical agents but less than with thioridazine. Although monitoring of ECGs is not routinely required, clinicians should consider the relative risk of cardiac conduction delay compared with the benefits of ziprasidone (which include tolerability and minimal weight gain) when selecting a medication.

Clinical use. Ziprasidone is usually started at a dosage of 20–40 mg twice a day and can be rapidly titrated over 2–4 days to a typical therapeutic dosage of 60–80 mg twice a day in medically healthy, nonelderly patients. In one study, a starting dosage of 60 mg twice a day was well tolerated without significant orthostatic hypotension. Dosing in the elderly and in patients with cardiovascular disease has not been well studied to date. Ziprasidone has a half-life of 5–10 hours and is usually administered twice daily with meals. Food increases absorption by approximately 100%. Ziprasidone at a dosage of 80 mg twice a day was comparable to haloperidol 15 mg/day in overall efficacy, and substantially fewer patients receiving ziprasidone required antiparkinsonian medication compared with those receiving haloperidol (10% vs. 53%) (Goff et al. 1998).

Ziprasidone has shown efficacy for negative symptoms in placebo-controlled trials (Daniel et al. 1999; Keck 1998). Because safety data with ziprasidone are largely derived from studies that excluded subjects with cardiac disease, clinicians should screen patients for cardiac risk factors, preferably with a baseline ECG and serum electrolytes, before initiating ziprasidone. Patients with QTc prolongation at baseline must be monitored very closely; consultation from a cardiologist is recommended. However, ziprasidone may improve cardiovascular risk factors related to obesity and hyperlipidemia.

Risks, side effects, and their management. In the few studies that have been published to date, ziprasidone has been well tolerated. The most common side effects have included headache, dyspepsia, nausea, constipation, abdominal pain, somnolence, and EPS. Ratings of parkinsonism and akathisia with ziprasidone 120 mg/day did not differ from those with placebo. Although dizziness has been reported, rates of orthostatic hypotension have not differed from those with placebo in controlled clinical trials. Ziprasidone produces transient hyperprolactinemia, which returns to predrug baseline levels after 12 hours; prolactin levels are significantly lower with ziprasidone than with haloperidol (Goff et al. 1998).

Cardiovascular side effects. Ziprasidone produced a mean QTc prolongation of 21 msec at maximal blood levels achieved during exposure to typical therapeutic doses. Twenty-one percent of the subjects had QTc prolongation of 60 msec or greater, and 3% developed QTc prolongation of 75 msec or greater. However, in all clinical trials, the rate of QTc intervals greater than 500 msec (considered a threshold for arrhythmia risk) did not differ from that with placebo (<0.1%). Ziprasidone blood levels were increased by about 40% by coadministration of ketoconazole (a metabolic inhibitor) without any change in QTc duration detected. Consistent with the weak relation between drug levels and QTc effect, the 10 published cases of overdose with ziprasidone have been relatively benign.

Weight gain. Ziprasidone produces less weight gain than do other atypical antipsychotic agents. Allison et al. (1999) calculated a mean weight gain of less than 1 kg after 10 weeks of ziprasidone treatment.

Drug interactions. Drugs that inhibit the CYP3A4 isoenzyme reduce metabolism of ziprasidone: concurrent treatment with ketoconazole increased ziprasidone blood levels by approximately 40%. Carbamazepine (and possibly other enzyme inducers) may lower ziprasidone levels by about 35%. Effects of ziprasidone on metabolism of other drugs have not been reported.

Pharmacological Treatment of Schizophrenia

General Principles

Evidence shows that the long-term outcome for a patient with schizophrenia is better when treatment of the acute episode is initiated rapidly. After a patient's first episode of schizophrenia, the antipsychotic medication should be continued for at least 1 year after a full remission of psychotic symptoms. After that time, a trial period without medication may be considered, except for patients with a history of serious suicide attempts or violent aggressive behavior (American Psychiatric Association 1997). The patient and his or her family should be informed of the early signs and symptoms of relapse, such as suspiciousness, difficulty sleeping, and argumentativeness and should be warned that relapse is highly likely. The patient should be carefully monitored during this period.

For patients with a chronic, relapsing form of schizophrenia, antipsychotic medication should be continued for up to 5 symptom-free years before discontinuation (Johnson 1985) and probably indefinitely. Kane et al. (1983) performed careful studies of patients maintained with high-dose (12.5–50.0 mg every 2 weeks) and low-dose (1.25–5.0 mg every 2 weeks) treatment with fluphenazine decanoate. Although the high-dose medication prevented relapse better than the low-dose treatment, patients who were given low-dose medication had fewer EPS. In addition, the mild exacerbations of the psychoses were successfully treated with periodic increases in medication, without the necessity of hospitalization. Marder et al. (1984) compared the clinical course in patients with schizophrenia treated with 5 or 25 mg of fluphenazine decanoate administered every 2 weeks. They found no difference in relapse rates between the two groups, although the higher-dose group had evidence of more side effects. Subsequent studies have further documented the advantage of dose reduction in the maintenance of schizophrenia (Johnson et al. 1987; Marder et al. 1987; Schooler et al. 1997); however, intermittent treatment is associated with a greater relapse rate and is not recommended (Herz et al. 1991; Schooler et al. 1997).

Recently, Herz et al. (2000) reported that a relatively simple program of weekly monitoring of patients in medication groups combined with rapid response to early signs of destabilization markedly reduced relapse rates. The atypical antipsychotics have generally shown superior efficacy in preventing relapse—it is unclear if this reflects improved compliance or whether these agents additionally provide greater stabilization, perhaps by modulating the effect of environmental stress.

In light of these important studies, we recommend that patients be maintained on the lowest dosage of antipsychotic drugs possible. In addition, patients should be monitored closely for symptoms of relapse. If the patient is compliant with treatment, oral medications are usually sufficient. However, if there is concern, on the basis of the previous treatment history, that the patient may not reliably take daily oral medication, a long-acting depot preparation may be indicated.

Treatment-Resistant Schizophrenia

If the symptoms do not respond to the indicated treatment, minimal side effects (e.g., EPS, hypotension, sedation) occur, and poor compliance is not the cause, the physician can gradually increase the dosage until mild side effects are seen. If no further improvement is seen after an additional 2–4 weeks at this dosage, another antipsychotic drug from another class should be substituted. Atypical antipsychotics should be considered in patients who have not responded to conventional antipsychotic medication. At this time, adequate data do not exist to suggest greater efficacy of one atypical antipsychotic, other than clozapine. A trial of clozapine should be considered for patients who continue to have positive symptoms, frequent relapses, or aggression despite an adequate trial of at least one other antipsychotic medication and for patients with intolerable side effects to at least two different antipsychotic medications from different classes (American Psychiatric Association 1997). At least one of these drugs should be an atypical antipsychotic.

An additional strategy to use with nonresponsive patients is to add another medication to augment the therapeutic effects of the antipsychotic. The most common agents used to augment antipsychotic medications in the treatment of schizophrenia are lithium (Cole et al. 1984; Delva and Letemednia 1982), valproate (Linnoila et al. 1976), and benzodiazepines (Csernansky et al. 1988; Douyon et al. 1989; Nestoros et al. 1982). These medications are often quite helpful when there is a need to target specific symptoms, such as affective lability, aggression, or anxiety, in a patient with schizophrenia. However, with the current availability of the atypical antipsychotics, particularly clozapine, the use of these augmenting strategies in patients with antipsychotic-resistant schizophrenia should be reserved for patients who cannot take clozapine or who have not fully responded to clozapine (American Psychiatric Association 1997). Augmentation with SSRIs may be helpful for depression and for negative symptoms, although clinicians should monitor carefully for pharmacokinetic interactions (Evins and Goff 1996). Although there are no systematic data to guide the treatment of patients who have not responded to clozapine, some patients may benefit from the combination of clozapine and one of the other atypical antipsychotics (Henderson and Goff 1996). Because of the potential side effects and added cost, combination therapy should be attempted only after an adequate trial of monotherapy has been completed. If clear benefit is not apparent after 6 weeks of combination therapy, the augmenting agent should be discontinued. Recent work with cognitive-behavioral therapy has shown considerable promise when combined with medication in refractory patients (Gould et al. 2001).

Other Uses of Antipsychotic Medications

The use of antipsychotic medications to treat other disorders is addressed elsewhere in this chapter (e.g., in the "Treatment of Mania" section and "Antipsychotic Drugs" subsection in the "Acute Aggression and Agitation" section later in this chapter).

Mood Stabilizers

Overview

After an initial observation by Cade (1949) that the calming effect of lithium in animals could be extended to humans with manic-depressive illness, Baastrup and Schou (1967) conclusively demonstrated that lithium was effective in the prophylaxis of recurrence of affective disorders. Although lithium continues to be an invaluable primary treatment for acute mania and maintenance therapy in bipolar disorder, it is ineffective or suboptimal for many patients. Fortunately, clinical trials are under way to evaluate a variety of other compounds, most prominently medications that are typically classified as anticonvulsants or mood stabilizers. The anticonvulsant valproate and the atypical antipsychotic olanzapine are approved by the FDA for the treatment of mania. These medications are collectively referred to as *mood stabilizers* because of their ability to stabilize mood oscillations regardless of etiology. In this section, we review the clinical use of lithium and the anticonvulsants that are definite or probable mood stabilizers. The general properties of the antipsychotics, including olanzapine, were reviewed in the preceding section. In this section, we expand on the use of these compounds for the treatment of bipolar disorder.

Lithium

Mechanism of Action

Lithium is a monovalent cation that is believed to affect intracellular second messenger systems. According to a review by Jope and Williams (1994), lithium inhibits several steps in phosphoinositide metabolism as well as G-protein functioning (Manji et al. 1995). Lithium has been reported to inhibit the stimulation of adenylate cyclase by several different neurotransmitters without suppressing basal adenylate cyclase activity (Belmaker et al. 1983; Ebstein et al. 1980; Zohar et al. 1982) and to inhibit protein kinase C (PKC) after subchronic administration (Bitran et al. 1995; Lenox et al. 1992; Manji et al. 1993). These effects on signal transduction have broad effects on neuronal function and gene expression (for an excellent review, see Manji et al. 1999).

Indications and Efficacy

Lithium has been proved effective for acute and prophylactic treatment of both manic and depressive episodes in patients with bipolar illness (Consensus Development Panel 1985; Prien et al. 1984) and cyclothymia (Akiskal et al. 1979). However, patients with rapid-cycling bipolar disorder (i.e., four or more mood disorder episodes per year) have been reported to respond less well to lithium treatment (Dunner and Fieve 1974; Prien et al. 1984; Wehr et al. 1988). Lithium is also effective in the prevention of future depressive episodes in patients with recurrent unipolar depressive disorder (Consensus Development Panel 1985) and as an adjunct to antidepressants in depressed patients whose illness is partially refractory to treatment with antidepressants alone (discussed earlier in this chapter in the section on antidepressant drugs). Furthermore, lithium may be useful in the maintenance of remission of depressive disorder after ECT (Coopen et al. 1981; Sackeim et al. 2001) and in the maintenance of the antidepressant effect of sleep deprivation (Baxter et al. 1986). Lithium also has been used effectively in some cases of aggression and behavioral dyscontrol (see section on the treatment of aggression later in this chapter).

Clinical Use

Before they begin treatment with lithium, patients should be told that they might experience nausea, diarrhea, polyuria, increased thirst, and fine hand tremor. These are often transient, but in some patients they persist with therapeutic lithium levels. Because of a narrow range between the therapeutic and toxic doses of lithium and the wide variability of lithium pharmacokinetics among different individuals, the optimal dosage for an individual patient cannot be based on the dosage administered. Rather, lithium dosing should be based on the concentration of lithium in the plasma. Lithium carbonate is completely absorbed by the gastrointestinal tract and reaches peak plasma levels in 1–2 hours. The elimination half-life is approximately 24 hours. Steady-state lithium levels are obtained in approximately 5 days.

Therapeutic plasma levels for patients undergoing lithium therapy range from 0.5 to 1.5 mEq/L. Although lower plasma levels are associated with less troubling side effects, most clinicians seek to establish levels of at least 0.8 mEq/L in treating acute manic episodes. Therefore, when intolerable side effects have not intervened, treatment of acute mania with lithium should not be considered a failure until plasma levels of 1.2–1.5 mEq/L have been reached and maintained for 2 weeks. However, when levels this high are necessary for acute treatment, the dosage often may be reduced to the range of 0.8–1.0 mEq/L for maintenance therapy. Although Gelenberg et al. (1989) initially reported that levels in the range of 0.8–1.0 mEq/L provide better prophylaxis against relapse, this finding may be applicable only to patients who require relatively high levels for initial stabilization. Patients who are stabilized with blood levels in the range of 0.4–0.8 mEq/L may do well remaining at these relatively low levels, often with a reduced side effect burden. Therapeutic lithium levels have not been established for other disorders.

Lithium is dosed to achieve therapeutic blood levels and clinical response. Lithium levels should be obtained 12 hours after the last lithium dose. After therapeutic lithium levels have been established, levels should be monitored every month for the first 3 months and every 3 months thereafter. For patients who have remained stable and who are aware of early signs of both relapse and lithium toxicity, lithium levels may be obtained less frequently.

Because lithium has a serum half-life of approximately 24 hours, it may be administered as a single daily dose. The results of several investigations favor such a dosing schedule. Divided daily doses with the usual carbonate salt result in several peak levels throughout the day, with a relatively rapid decrease between doses. The multiple-dose regimen exposes the kidney to multiple peak levels of intermediate concentration, whereas single daily dosing exposes the kidney to a single peak of higher absolute concentration. It has been suggested that nephrotoxicity is related to the duration of exposure to peak lithium levels and not to the absolute level of any particular peak (Bowen et al. 1991; Hetmar et al. 1987; Plenge et al. 1982). It is for this reason that single daily dosing is recommended. Although slow-release preparations of lithium are available, these are not necessary for obtaining adequate 24-hour levels. The main advantage of sustained release is that less lithium ion is released in the stomach, where it can act as an irritant, and more is released in the small intestine (Schatzberg and Cole

1991). For patients who experience nausea and gastric irritation, the slow-release formulations may provide protection from this unpleasant side effect. Patients with diarrhea may prefer the standard-release formulations. The patient and appropriate family members must be informed of the potential acute side effects and long-term consequences of lithium therapy. Side effects are described in detail in the subsection "Risks, Side Effects, and Their Management" later in this section. General guidelines for lithium treatment are listed in Table 24–19.

Contraindications and Pretreatment Medical Evaluation

Lithium should not be administered to patients with fluctuating or unstable renal function. In patients with statically impaired renal function, another mood stabilizer, such as valproate, is preferred. For patients who are unresponsive to alternative treatments, lithium may be administered if the dosage and dose frequency are suitably reduced to avoid toxic blood levels. Because lithium may affect functioning of the cardiac sinus node, patients with sinus node dysfunction (e.g., sick sinus syndrome) should not receive lithium. Although lithium also has acute and chronic effects on the thyroid, patients with hypothyroidism may receive lithium if the thyroid disease is adequately treated and monitored. Laboratory tests that should be performed before the initiation of lithium or valproate are outlined in Table 24–20.

TABLE 24–19. Guidelines for lithium treatment

1. Review medical history and review of systems with particular attention to renal, thyroid, and cardiac status.
2. Order pretreatment pregnancy test and levels of BUN, creatinine, electrolytes, and thyrotropin. If the patient is older than 40 years or has evidence of cardiac disease, order ECG.
3. Inform patient and family of proper use of lithium. Include a discussion of common side effects, the importance of monitoring of lithium levels, early signs and symptoms of toxicity, and potential long-term side effects. If patient is female, include warnings about pregnancy during treatment.
4. Initiate therapy at 300 mg bid, and increase by 300 mg every 3–4 days.
5. Obtain lithium levels (12 hours after last dose) twice a week, until there is a clinical response or the lithium level reaches approximately 1.0 mEq/L.
6. Monitor BUN and creatinine.
7. Monitor thyrotropin every 6–12 months if symptoms of hypothyroidism develop.

Note. BUN = blood urea nitrogen; ECG = electrocardiogram.

TABLE 24–20. Characteristics of commonly used mood stabilizers

	Lithium	Valproate	Carbamazepine
Available preparations	Lithium carbonate (Eskalith, Lithonate, Lithotabs, generics; 300-mg tabs, caps) Lithium citrate liquid (8 mEq/ 5 mL) Extended release (Eskalith CR 450 mg; Lithobid 300 mg)	Divalproex sodium (Depakote 125-, 250-, 500-mg tabs, 125-mg sprinkle caps) Depacon iv Valproic acid (Depakene, generics, 250-mg caps; Depakene 250 mg/5 mL syrup) Divalproex ER 500 mg	Tegretol, generics (200-mg tabs, 100-mg chewable tabs, 100 mg/5 mL suspension) Tegretol-XR sustained release (100-, 200-, 400-mg tabs)
Half-life	24 hours	9–16 hours	24/12 hours[a]
Starting dosage	300 mg bid	250 mg tid or 20 mg/kg	200 mg bid
Blood level	0.8–1.2 mEq/L	45–125 µg/mL	4–12[b] µg/mL
Metabolism	Renal	Hepatic	Hepatic
Contraindications[c]	Unstable renal function	Hepatic dysfunction	Hepatic dysfunction
Pretreatment laboratory evaluation	Chem 20,[d] CBC, thyrotropin, ECG if ≥40 years old or cardiac disease; pregnancy test	Aspartate aminotransferase, alanine aminotransferase, pregnancy test	CBC, aspartate aminotransferase, alanine aminotransferase, pregnancy test

Note. CBC = complete blood count; ECG = electrocardiogram.
[a]24 hours before hepatic autoinduction; 12 hours after autoinduction. [b]Not correlated with clinical response. [c]All current mood stabilizers should be avoided in pregnancy. See text for discussion. [d]Especially blood urea nitrogen, creatinine, sodium, and calcium.

Although initial uncontrolled reports suggested a markedly increased risk of Ebstein's anomaly of the heart in infants who were exposed to lithium in utero (Nora et al. 1974), subsequent controlled data predicted a 0.1%–0.7% absolute risk (Edmonds and Oakley 1990; Jacobson et al. 1992; Kallen and Tandberg 1983; Zalzstein et al. 1990) compared with 0.01% in the general population. The overall risk of major congenital anomalies in association with lithium exposure is 4%–12%, compared with 2%–4% in comparison groups (L.S. Cohen et al. 1994). The increased risk of malformations must be weighed against the risk for both mother and fetus if lithium discontinuation results in a manic relapse. Guidelines for lithium use in pregnancy are outlined in Table 24–21.

Risks, Side Effects, and Their Management

Renal effects. For all patients taking lithium, a measure of serum blood urea nitrogen (BUN) and creatinine should be obtained at baseline and every 3–6 months after lithium therapy has commenced, with more frequent testing if there are specific complaints or signs of renal dysfunction. Most of the effects of lithium on the kidney are reversible after discontinuation of the drug. Although permanent morphological changes in renal structure have been reported, the clinical implications of these changes have yet to be established, and to date there have been no published reports of irreversible renal failure as a result of chronic, nontoxic lithium therapy (Hetmar et al. 1991).

However, lithium inhibits vasopressin with resultant impairment in renal concentrating ability. Termed *nephrogenic diabetes insipidus* (NDI), this condition results in polyuria for up to 60% of patients taking lithium (Lokkegaard et al. 1985). This side effect is associated with higher plasma lithium levels, a longer duration of treatment (DePaulo et al. 1986), and a multiple daily dosing schedule (Hetmar et al. 1991). NDI may result in serious complications, including dehydration, lithium toxicity, and electrolyte imbalance. Although clinically significant polyuria usually reverses itself after discontinuation of lithium therapy, it may persist for many months (Ramsey and Cox 1982; Simon et al. 1977). However, less serious increases in urine volume may persist indefinitely, an effect that some investigators believe is a consequence of renal tubular atrophy (Hetmar et al. 1991).

Preventive and management strategies for NDI include increasing the patient's fluid intake and decreasing the amount of lithium given to the lowest effective dosage. Once-a-day dosing also results in lower urinary output than the multiple-dosing schedule (Hetmar et al. 1991; Plenge et al. 1982). If these simpler management strategies fail to correct the polyuria, potassium supplementation, 10–20 mEq/day, may be effective (Klemfuss 1992; Martin 1993). Diuretics also may be used in the treatment of lithium-induced NDI. By causing sodium depletion, diuretics ultimately create in the kidney a compensatory conservation of sodium. The osmotic effect of this sodium conservation constrains the kidney's

TABLE 24–21. Treatment recommendations for lithium use in women with bipolar disorder

I. Encourage careful contraceptive practices for all women of childbearing age.

II. Evaluate the need for lithium prophylaxis.

   A. In women with single episodes of affective instability and long intervening periods of well-being:

      1. Attempt gradual tapering and discontinuation of lithium prophylaxis before pregnancy.

      2. Maintain lithium-free well-being for the entire pregnancy if possible; reintroduce lithium during the second and third trimesters if necessary.

   B. In women with severe bipolar disorder in whom discontinuation of lithium prophylaxis poses a *substantial* risk of increased morbidity:

      1. Temporarily discontinue lithium therapy for a period coinciding as closely as possible with that of embryogenesis.

      2. Consider reintroduction of lithium and/or treatment with antipsychotic agents if clinical deterioration occurs.

   C. In women with severe bipolar disorder in whom discontinuation of lithium prophylaxis poses an *unacceptable* risk of increased morbidity, maintain lithium therapy throughout pregnancy.

III. Other considerations for women who take lithium during all or part of the first trimester of pregnancy:

   A. Provide reproductive risk counseling as early in pregnancy as possible.

   B. Offer prenatal diagnosis by fetal echocardiography and high-resolution ultrasound examination at 16–18 weeks of gestation.

Source. Reprinted with permission from Cohen LS, Friedman JM, Jefferson JW, et al: A reevaluation of risk of in utero exposure to lithium. *Journal of the American Medical Association* 271:146–150, 1994. Copyright 1994, American Medical Association.

ability to dilute urine, thereby alleviating the polyuria. However, thiazide diuretics can raise lithium levels into the toxic range, an effect that is particularly dangerous in a patient who is already at risk for dehydration from polyuria. For this reason, the nonthiazide diuretic amiloride is now the preferred treatment for lithium-induced NDI because it does not appear to increase plasma lithium levels (Battle et al. 1985). Amiloride apparently acts by blocking the absorption of lithium in the renal tubules, where the lithium would otherwise interfere with the action of vasopressin (Billings 1985). For lithium-induced NDI, amiloride is prescribed in a dosage of 5 mg twice a day and increased to 10 mg twice a day if necessary. Despite the claim that amiloride does not raise lithium levels, we believe it is prudent to continue to monitor serum lithium levels with greater frequency (at least every 2 months) when amiloride is combined with lithium.

Interstitial nephritis has been reported to be a consequence of long-term lithium therapy. Hetmar et al. (1987) performed renal biopsies on 46 bipolar patients with a mean of 8 years of lithium therapy and found that the proportion of sclerotic glomeruli, atrophic tubules, and interstitial fibrosis was significantly greater in patients who had received a multiple daily dosing schedule, compared with patients with a history of once-daily dosing and with a control group with no history of lithium exposure. Lokkegaard et al. (1985) reported that decreases in the glomerular filtration rate (GFR) are detectable only after many years of lithium therapy; however, most investigators have found no clinically significant effect on the GFR (Hetmar et al. 1991; Schou 1989; Waller and Edwards 1989). Proteinuria has been reported as a rare side effect and is thought to be the consequence of either glomerular leakage or the inhibition of tubular resorption (Waller and Edwards 1989; Wood et al. 1989).

Thyroid dysfunction. Reversible hypothyroidism may occur in as many as 20% of the patients treated with lithium (Lindstedt et al. 1977; Myers et al. 1985). Although this occurrence is hypothesized to be related to the effect of lithium on thyrotropin adenylate cyclase, lithium may have important effects on other key areas of thyroid function (Waller 1985). Lithium-induced hypothyroidism occurs more frequently in women, in patients with thyroid antibodies, and in patients with an exaggerated thyrotropin response to thyrotropin-releasing hormone (TRH; Calabrese et al. 1985; Myers et al. 1985). Because the development of hypothyroidism in bipolar patients is associated with intractable depression (Yassa et al. 1988) and with the development of a rapid-cycling course (Bauer et al. 1990), thyroid function must be monitored every 6–12 months during lithium treatment or if symptoms develop that might be attributable to thyroid dysfunction. The thyrotropin level is the most sensitive test for detecting hypothyroidism, especially with recent refinements in the assay. If laboratory tests indicate the development of hypothyroidism, the patient should be evaluated clinically for signs and symptoms of hypothyroidism and be referred to an endocrinologist for any further tests. In collaboration with the endocrinologist, the psychiatrist should decide on the appropriate treatment—in most cases, thyroid hormone replacement and continuation of lithium therapy.

Parathyroid dysfunction. The effects of lithium on calcium metabolism may be related to lithium-induced hyperparathyroidism (Anath and Dubin 1983; Mallette and Eichhorn 1986). Clinically significant effects of hypercalcemia associated with lithium have been reported, including back pain, kyphoscoliosis, osteoporosis, hypertension, cardiomegaly, and impaired renal function (Clur 1989). Potential neuropsychiatric sequelae include affective changes, anxiety, aggressiveness, sleep disturbance, apathy, psychosis, delirium, dementia, and seizures (Borer and Bhanot 1985). Although they are rare, symptoms of hyperparathyroidism may be misdiagnosed as lithium toxicity or the effects of the underlying mood disorder. When signs or symptoms that might be related to hyperparathyroidism develop, serum calcium ion levels should be checked, and if they are abnormal, parathyroid hormone levels should be obtained and an endocrinologist consulted.

Neurotoxicity. Lithium therapy may be associated with several types of neurological dysfunction. Fine resting tremor is a neurological side effect that may be detected in as many as one-half of the patients taking lithium (Vestergaard et al. 1980). β-Adrenergic-blocking drugs, such as propranolol in divided daily doses below 80 mg/day, are effective in treating this tremor (Zubenko et al. 1984). Subjective memory impairment occurs in approximately 28% of the patients taking lithium and is among the most frequent reasons for noncompliance (Goodwin and Jamison 1990). ECT-induced confusion is likely to be worsened by concurrent lithium administration; therefore, lithium is relatively contraindicated for patients who are receiving a course of ECT (Consensus Conference 1985; Penney et al. 1990).

Cardiac effects. Mitchell and Mackenzie (1982) reported changes in T-wave morphology on the ECG (flattening or inversion) in 20%–30% of patients taking lithium, changes that are most likely benign. Lithium also may suppress the function of the sinus node and result in sinoatrial block. Patients with sinus disease or conduction defects, therefore, should not be given lithium. Cases have also been reported of aggravation of preexisting ventricular arrhythmias with lithium therapy. An ECG should be checked before treatment with lithium is started in patients older than 40 years or in those with a history or symptoms of cardiac disease.

Weight gain. Weight gain is a frequent side effect of lithium treatment (Peselow et al. 1980; Vendsborg et al. 1976; Vestergaard et al. 1980). Vendsborg et al. (1976) found a correlation between liquid intake and weight gain. Patients with polydipsia may drink fluids with a high caloric content, such as carbonated soft drinks, and

thereby gain weight. These patients should be instructed to drink low-calorie liquids. Peselow et al. (1980) reviewed several hypotheses indicating that weight gain also may be a direct effect of lithium therapy. Possible mechanisms include influences on carbohydrate metabolism, changes in glucose tolerance, or changes in lipid metabolism. Dieting and exercise should be recommended early in treatment.

Dermatological reactions. Dermatological reactions to lithium include acne, follicular eruptions, and psoriasis (Bakris et al. 1980–1981; Deandrea et al. 1982). The most frequent of these reactions is skin rash, which is reported in up to 7% of lithium-treated patients (Bone et al. 1980). Changes in hair, including hair loss, hair thinning, and loss of wave, also have been reported. Except for cases of exacerbation of psoriasis, these reactions are usually benign and may not warrant discontinuation of lithium treatment. Lithium-induced acne responds to topical treatment with steroidal agents, such as tretinoin (Retin-A).

Gastrointestinal side effects. Gastrointestinal difficulties occur frequently with lithium treatment, especially nausea and diarrhea. Although these side effects may be manifestations of toxicity, they also occur at lithium levels within the therapeutic range. Gastrointestinal symptoms may improve with reduction of dosage or ingestion of lithium with meals. Slow-release formulations are more often associated with nausea, whereas sustained-release preparations are more commonly associated with diarrhea.

Hematological side effects. The most frequent hematological change detected in patients taking lithium is leukocytosis (approximately 15,000 white blood cells/mm^3). As reviewed by Brewerton (1986), this change is generally benign; lithium may, in fact, be used to treat several conditions associated with granulocytopenia. (The use of lithium to treat carbamazepine-induced granulocytopenia is discussed later in this section.) Lithium-induced leukocytosis is readily reversible with discontinuation of lithium therapy.

Overdose and toxicity. Because of the narrow range between therapeutic and toxic plasma lithium levels, the physician must devote sufficient time to informing the patient and the family about the signs and symptoms of early lithium toxicity and the circumstances that may increase the chances of toxicity, such as drinking insufficient amounts of fluids, becoming overheated with increased perspiration, or ingesting too much medication.

The physician must emphasize the prevention of lithium toxicity through the maintenance of adequate salt and water intake, especially during hot weather and exercise. Toxic lithium levels can produce severe neurotoxic reactions, with symptoms such as dysarthria, ataxia, and intention tremor. The signs and symptoms of lithium toxicity may be divided into those that usually occur at lithium levels between 1.5 and 2.0 mEq/L, those that occur between 2.0 and 2.5 mEq/L, and those that occur above 2.5 mEq/L (Table 24–22), although some patients may become clinically toxic with lithium levels in the standard therapeutic range. The recommended management of lithium toxicity is reviewed in Table 24–23.

TABLE 24–22. Signs and symptoms of lithium toxicity

**Mild-to-moderate intoxication
(lithium level = 1.5–2.0 mEq/L)**

Gastrointestinal	Vomiting
	Abdominal pain
	Dryness of mouth
Neurological	Ataxia
	Dizziness
	Slurred speech
	Nystagmus
	Lethargy or excitement
	Muscle weakness

**Moderate-to-severe intoxication
(lithium level = 2.0–2.5 mEq/L)**

Gastrointestinal	Anorexia
	Persistent nausea and vomiting
Neurological	Blurred vision
	Muscle fasciculations
	Clonic limb movements
	Hyperactive deep tendon reflexes
	Choreoathetoid movements
	Convulsions
	Delirium
	Syncope
	Electroencephalographic changes
	Stupor
	Coma
	Circulatory failure (lowered blood pressure, cardiac arrhythmias, and conduction abnormalities)

**Severe lithium intoxication
(lithium level > 2.5 mEq/L)**

Generalized convulsions
Oliguria and renal failure
Death

TABLE 24–23. Management of lithium toxicity

1. The patient should immediately contact his or her personal physician or go to a hospital emergency department.
2. Lithium should be discontinued and the patient instructed to ingest fluids, if possible.
3. Physical examination should be completed, including vital signs and a neurological examination with complete formal mental status examination.
4. Lithium level, serum electrolytes, renal function tests, and electrocardiogram should be obtained as soon as possible.
5. For significant acute ingestion, residual gastric contents should be removed by induction of emesis, gastric lavage, and absorption with activated charcoal.[a]
6. Vigorous hydration and maintenance of electrolyte balance are essential.
7. For any patient with a serum lithium level greater than 4.0 mEq/L or with serious manifestations of lithium toxicity, hemodialysis should be initiated.[a]
8. Repeat dialysis may be required every 6–10 hours, until the lithium level is within nontoxic range and the patient has no signs or symptoms of lithium toxicity.

Note. [a]Information from Goldfrank et al. 1986.

Drug interactions. Because of the narrow therapeutic range of lithium, knowledge of its drug–drug interactions is of paramount importance. Because of the narrow therapeutic range of lithium, knowledge of its drug-drug interactions is of paramount importance. Because the kidney excretes lithium, any medication that alters renal function can affect lithium levels. Thiazide diuretics reduce lithium clearance and hence may increase lithium levels. Loop diuretics (e.g., furosemide) do not have this effect. Nonsteroidal anti-inflammatory drugs may also increase lithium levels by decreasing clearance. It is particularly important to inform patients of this effect because these medications are often self-prescribed. Other medications that may increase lithium levels include angiotensin-converting enzyme inhibitors and COX-2 inhibitors (e.g., celecoxib, rofecoxib). Drugs that may decrease lithium levels include theophylline and aminophylline. Lithium may potentiate the effects of succinylcholine-like muscle relaxants. Concerns about increased risk of delirium, NMS, and irreversible brain damage have been raised for the combination of lithium and neuroleptic drugs on the basis of case reports (W.J. Cohen and Cohen 1974). However, a controlled investigation found no difference in side effects or complications between a group of patients with mania treated with antipsychotic medications alone and a group of patients with mania treated with antipsychotic drugs and lithium (Goldney and Spence 1986); this result is concordant with clinical experience. The preponderance of evidence indicates that lithium and antipsychotic medications, including haloperidol, can be safely and effectively combined, with appropriate monitoring.

Valproate

Lambert et al. (1966) were the first to report success in treating bipolar disorder with valproate. Since that time, numerous uncontrolled studies have supported this initial claim. After the early 1980s, several controlled studies established that valproate is effective in acute mania (Gerner and Stanton 1992; Keck et al. 1992; Pope et al. 1991). More recently, a collaborative study by Bowden et al. (1994) directly compared valproate with lithium and placebo in patients with mania. This study found valproate to be as effective as lithium in patients with euphoric mania. It is concordant with previous observations (Calabrese et al. 1992; McElroy et al. 1992; Post et al. 1987) that valproate was found to be more effective than lithium in patients with rapid-cycling and dysphoric mania. Valproate also has been reported to be especially effective for mania occurring in patients with a history of closed-head trauma (McElroy et al. 1989) and in patients with EEG abnormalities (Pope et al. 1988). Although several open-trial studies have suggested that valproate is also effective for prophylaxis in bipolar disorder, no controlled studies have confirmed this finding to date (Keck et al. 1992). The efficacy of valproate in the treatment of acute bipolar depression has yet to be studied systematically. Divalproex sodium is approved by the FDA for the treatment of mania.

Mechanism of Action

Although many putative mechanisms have been proposed, the basis for the mood-stabilizing effects of valproate is most likely concordant with the mechanism of lithium, specifically by attenuating the activity of PKC and other steps in the signal transduction pathway leading to neuronal adaptation and changes in gene expression (Chen et al. 1994; Manji et al. 1999).

Clinical Use

Before beginning treatment with valproate, patients should be told that they might experience nausea, sedation, and a fine hand tremor. These are often transient, but in some patients they persist. Several valproate preparations are available in the United States, including valproic acid, sodium valproate, divalproex sodium, and an extended-release preparation of divalproex sodium. Divalproex sodium is a dimer of sodium valproate and valproic acid with an enteric coating, and

it is much better tolerated than other oral valproate preparations. An intravenous preparation also has become available, but it has not yet been well studied in psychiatric disorders. The half-life of valproate is 10 hours.

Valproate may be initiated gradually with subsequent dosage titration or with a more rapid "loading" strategy. Most commonly, valproate is initiated at a dosage of 250 mg three times a day and subsequently increased by 250 mg every 3 days. Most patients require a dosage of 1,250–2,500 mg/day. Although valproate has a relatively short half-life, moderate doses may be given once a day at bedtime to reduce daytime sedation, often without compromising clinical efficacy. This strategy should not be used when valproate is administered to treat seizure disorders, for which more constant serum levels are required.

In situations for which rapid stabilization is of paramount importance, valproate treatment can be initiated at a dose of 20 mg per kilogram of body weight (Keck et al. 1993). Some patients require relatively high dosages of valproate, sometimes greater than 4,000 mg/day, to achieve a sufficient plasma level and clinical response, and some patients do not respond until plasma valproate levels are greater than 100 mg/mL. As with all psychotropic medications, the final dosage is more dependent on the balance between clinical response and side effects than on absolute blood level. However, plasma levels of 45–100 mg/mL are recommended for the treatment of acute mania (Bowden et al. 1996). Patients with less severe symptoms, such as bipolar II disorder or cyclothymia, often respond at lower dosages and blood levels (Jacobsen 1993). Blood levels in other phases of bipolar disorder, such as bipolar depression, or in other indications, such as aggression, have not been established. The extended-release preparation of divalproex sodium has 80%–90% of the bioavailability of the initial divalproex sodium, so doses may need to be slightly higher when using this preparation.

Contraindications

Valproate is relatively contraindicated for patients with hepatitis or liver disease; it may be pursued as treatment for such patients only as a last resort and with the approval and continuous involvement of a gastroenterologist. Valproate has been linked to spina bifida and other neural tube defects in the offspring of patients exposed to this medication in the first trimester of pregnancy (Lammer et al. 1987; Robert and Guibaud 1982). As such, the risks of continuing valproate during pregnancy must be balanced against the risk of relapse.

Risks, Side Effects, and Their Management

Hepatic toxicity.   Although there have been reports of rare, non-dose-related hepatic failure with fatalities—estimated to occur in 1 in 118,000 patients—no cases have occurred in patients older than 10 years who were receiving valproate monotherapy (Dreifuss et al. 1987, 1989). Nonetheless, baseline liver function tests are indicated. If baseline test results are normal, monitoring for clinical signs of hepatotoxicity is more important than routine monitoring of liver enzymes, which has little predictive value and may be less effective than clinical monitoring (Pellock and Willmore 1991).

Transient, mild elevations in the liver enzymes, up to three times the upper limit of normal, do not require the discontinuation of valproate. Although γ-glutamyl transferase (GGT) levels are often checked by clinicians, this test is often elevated without clinical significance in patients receiving valproate and carbamazepine (Dean and Penry 1992). Likewise, plasma ammonia levels are often elevated transiently with valproate treatment, but this finding does not require that the treatment be interrupted (Jaeken et al. 1980). Because increases in transaminase levels are often dose dependent, if there is no suitable alternative treatment, dosage reduction and careful monitoring may be attempted.

Hematological effects.   Valproate has been associated with changes in platelet count, but clinically significant thrombocytopenia has rarely been documented (Dean and Penry 1992). Coagulation defects also have been reported. Overall, the risk of inducing a coagulation disturbance in an otherwise healthy adult is extremely low. However, in patients for whom anticoagulation is strictly contraindicated and in patients who already are receiving anticoagulation therapy, monitoring of the coagulation profile is required at baseline, at 1 month, and then every 3 months.

Gastrointestinal side effects.   Indigestion, heartburn, and nausea are common side effects of valproate therapy. We recommend the divalproex sodium preparation to help mitigate these effects. Patients also may be encouraged to take their doses with food. The symptomatic use of histamine$_2$ blockers or famotidine is sometimes warranted. In most cases, however, dyspepsia is transient and not severe. Pancreatitis has been reported as a rare occurrence among some patients receiving relatively high doses of valproate (M.J. Murphy et al. 1981). If vomiting and severe abdominal pain develop in the context of valproate therapy, a serum amylase level should be obtained immediately.

Weight gain.   Weight gain is a common side effect of valproate treatment. Isojarvi et al. (1996) reported significant weight gain with associated hyperinsulinemia in approximately 50% of a cohort of women taking valproate. This side effect does not appear to be dose dependent. Dieting and exercise should be recommended early in treatment.

Neurological effects.   One of the most common side effects associated with valproate use is benign essential tremor. This tremor is apparently not dose related and may first occur as late as 1 year after the initiation of therapy (Hyman et al. 1979). Drowsiness is another common side effect of valproate treatment, but tolerance often develops once a steady-state level of the drug is reached. A more gradual initial titration of valproate may be indicated for patients who complain of marked daytime sleepiness. In addition, once-a-day bedtime dosing often achieves symptomatic remission with less daytime sedation. Rarely, persistent somnolence, ataxia, or even delirium may occur, but these effects are more likely when other potentially sedating medications are being prescribed concurrently.

Alopecia.   Both transient and persistent hair loss have been associated with valproate use. When hair loss occurs, it often begins 3 months or longer after the initiation of treatment and is probably not dose related. Regrowth may result in hair that is wavier or curlier than before (Jeavons et al. 1977). It is our observation that patients with thyroid abnormalities who receive valproate are more likely to experience hair loss, even when ongoing thyroid replacement treatment has normalized their thyroid function. Patients with valproate-induced alopecia may benefit from zinc supplementation, at a dosage of 22.5 mg/day (Hurd et al. 1984). We routinely recommend supplementation with a multivitamin preparation containing zinc and selenium at the onset of valproate treatment.

Overdose.   Valproate overdose results in increasing sedation, confusion, and ultimately coma. The patient also may manifest hyperreflexia or hyporeflexia, seizures, respiratory suppression, and superventricular tachycardia (Labar 1992). Treatment should include gastric lavage, ECG monitoring, treatment of emergent seizures, and respiratory support as indicated.

Drug interactions.   Because valproate may inhibit hepatic enzymes, there is the potential for increases in the levels of other medications (Dean and Penry 1992). Valproate is also highly bound to plasma proteins and may displace other highly bound drugs from protein-binding sites. Therefore, coadministered drugs that are either highly protein bound or reliant on hepatic metabolism may require dose adjustment.

Carbamazepine

Takezaki and Hanaoka (1971) reported that carbamazepine was effective in controlling manic behavior; the first report from the United States of its efficacy for mania was by Ballenger and Post (1980). Subsequently, evidence from controlled studies has indicated that carbamazepine is effective in both the acute and the prophylactic treatment of mania, with overall response rates comparable to those of lithium treatment (Gerner and Stanton 1992; Keck et al. 1992). There is less evidence, however, to support the efficacy of carbamazepine in the acute treatment of depression and in the prophylactic treatment of unipolar depression. In two controlled studies, carbamazepine treatment was found to be effective in a subgroup of patients with refractory depression, with response rates greater among the patients with bipolar depression than among those with unipolar depression (Post et al. 1986; Small 1990). A systematic, controlled study of the antidepressant effects of carbamazepine in a more typical group of patients with depression remains to be conducted.

Clinical Use

Carbamazepine should be initiated at a dosage of 200 mg twice a day with increments of 200 mg/day every 3–5 days. Plasma levels of 8–12 µg/mL are based on clinical use in patients with seizure disorders and do not correlate with clinical response in psychiatric disorders. We recommend dosage titration to clinical response and side effects, rather than targeting of a particular dosage or blood level. During the titration phase, patients may be particularly prone to side effects such as sedation, dizziness, and ataxia, which indicate that a more gradual titration, such as 100 mg twice a day, should be instituted. Although the maximum dosage of carbamazepine recommended by the manufacturer is 1,200 mg/day, higher dosages are frequently required on the basis of plasma level determinations and clinical response (Placidi et al. 1986; Post et al. 1984). Tegretol-XR is a sustained-release preparation that is less likely to cause gastrointestinal side effects. Generic preparations of carbamazepine are often poorly tolerated. Because carbamazepine induces its own metabolism (autoinduction), dose adjustments may be required for weeks or months after the initiation of treatment to maintain therapeutic plasma levels (Eichelbaum et al. 1985). Some investigators have

suggested that the carbamazepine metabolite carbamazepine-10,11-epoxide has a major role in the therapeutic activity of carbamazepine in affective illness, especially in the treatment of depression (Post et al. 1983).

Contraindications

Because of the potential for hematological and hepatic toxicity, carbamazepine should not be administered to patients with liver disease or thrombocytopenia or those who are at risk for agranulocytosis. For this reason, carbamazepine is strictly contraindicated in patients receiving clozapine. Because of reports of teratogenicity, including increased risks of spina bifida (Rosa 1991), microcephaly (Bertollini et al. 1987), and craniofacial defects (Jones et al. 1989), carbamazepine is relatively contraindicated for use in pregnant women. Pretreatment evaluation should include a complete blood count, an aspartate aminotransferase level, and an alanine aminotransferase level. Because carbamazepine has a tricyclic structure, theoretical concerns have been raised about coadministration with MAOIs, but Ketter et al. (1995a) described a case series in which this combination was well tolerated.

Risks, Side Effects, and Their Management

Hematological disorders. The most serious toxic hematological side effects of carbamazepine are agranulocytosis and aplastic anemia, which can be fatal. Whereas carbamazepine-induced agranulocytosis or aplastic anemia is extremely rare, now estimated to occur at the rate of 1 in 125,000 patients (Pellock 1987), leukopenia (total white blood cell count <3,000 cells/mm^3) is more common, with a prevalence of approximately 10%. Persistent leukopenia with thrombocytopenia occurs in approximately 2% of patients, and mild anemia occurs in fewer than 5% of patients. Although it is important to assess hematological function and risk factors before initiating treatment, there appears to be no benefit to ongoing monitoring in the absence of clinical indicators. When carbamazepine-induced agranulocytosis occurs, the onset is rapid, so that a normal complete blood count one day does not provide reassurance that agranulocytosis will not develop the next day. Therefore, as opposed to routine monitoring, we advise patients to call if they develop fever, sore throat, infection, petechiae, or extreme weakness and pallor.

Carbamazepine should be discontinued if the absolute neutrophil count is less than 1,000. Consultation with a hematologist is also required at this point. It is interesting that the use of lithium to counteract leukopenia induced by carbamazepine has been suggested (Brewerton 1986). However, lithium does not reverse the underlying pathophysiological effects of carbamazepine; therefore, the clinician should monitor patients taking carbamazepine as they are being withdrawn from lithium because clinically significant leukopenia may be unmasked.

Hepatic toxicity. Carbamazepine occasionally causes hepatic toxicity (Gram and Bentsen 1983), usually a hypersensitivity hepatitis that appears after a latency period of several weeks and is associated with elevations in aspartate aminotransferase, alanine aminotransferase, and lactic dehydrogenase (LDH). Cholestasis is also possible, with increases in bilirubin and alkaline phosphatase. Mild, transient elevations in transaminase levels generally can be monitored without discontinuation of carbamazepine. If aspartate aminotransferase or alanine aminotransferase levels increase above three times the upper limit of normal, carbamazepine should be discontinued.

Dermatological conditions. An exanthematous rash is one of the more common side effects associated with carbamazepine, occurring in 3%–17% of patients (Warnock and Knesevich 1988). This reaction typically begins within 2–20 weeks after the start of treatment. Carbamazepine is generally discontinued if a rash develops because of the risk of progression to an exfoliative dermatitis or Stevens-Johnson syndrome, a severe bullous form of erythema multiforme (Patterson 1985). In patients who are nonresponsive to all other mood stabilizers, carbamazepine may be reinstituted along with initial prednisone coverage (J.M. Murphy et al. 1991; Vick 1983).

Endocrinological disorders. Carbamazepine may cause a reduction in the circulating levels of T_3 and T_4, possibly by inducing their hepatic metabolism (Bentsen et al. 1983; Yeo et al. 1978); this effect rarely has clinical significance. However, when carbamazepine is used in combination with other agents that antagonize thyroid function, such as lithium, a clinically significant synergistic effect may emerge (Kramingler and Post 1990). Carbamazepine may simultaneously reduce thyrotropin levels because it appears to diminish the pituitary response to TRH (Joffe et al. 1984).

SIADH with resultant hyponatremia may be induced by carbamazepine treatment. Alcoholic patients may be at greater risk for developing hyponatremia. If a patient taking carbamazepine develops confusion, the serum sodium level should be checked. When hyponatremia develops, it is often transient; however, even more severe cases of this condition can often be managed by fluid restriction, the addition of lithium, or use of the antibiotic demeclocycline (Brewerton and Jackson 1994).

Weight gain does not appear to be a side effect of carbamazepine therapy (Joffe et al. 1986).

Gastrointestinal disorders. Nausea and occasional vomiting are common side effects of carbamazepine, as they are with other mood stabilizers. Dosage reduction and institution of a slower titration rate help to minimize these effects.

Neurological effects. Patients may develop dizziness, drowsiness, and ataxia. These symptoms often occur at therapeutic plasma levels, especially in the early phases of treatment, and in such cases the dosage should be reduced and a slower titration schedule implemented.

Drug interactions. Carbamazepine induces hepatic cytochrome P450 enzymes, which may reduce the levels of other medications. Through the mechanism of hepatic enzyme induction, carbamazepine has been implicated in oral contraceptive failure (Coulam and Annegers 1979); therefore, women should be advised to consider alternative forms of birth control while taking carbamazepine. Similarly, medications or substances that inhibit CYP3A3/4 (discussed in the section on drug interactions later in this chapter) may result in significant elevations of plasma carbamazepine levels (Brodie and MacPhee 1986; Ketter et al. 1995b).

Overdose. Carbamazepine overdose is first manifested by neuromuscular disturbances, such as nystagmus, myoclonus, and hyperreflexia, with later progression to seizures and coma. Cardiac conduction changes are possible at higher dosages. Nausea, vomiting, and urinary retention also may occur. Treatment should include induction of vomiting, gastric lavage, and supportive care. Monitoring of blood pressure and respiratory and kidney functioning should follow for several days after a serious overdose.

Lamotrigine

Lamotrigine is an anticonvulsant medication that decreases sustained high-frequency repetitive firing of the voltage-dependent sodium channel, which may then decrease glutamate release (Leach et al. 1991; Mac-Donald and Kelly 1995). The efficacy of lamotrigine in treating bipolar depression has been established in a double-blind, placebo controlled trial (Calabrese et al. 1999). This multicenter study included patients with bipolar I disorder who were experiencing a major depressive episode. Participants received lamotrigine monotherapy (50 or 200 mg) or placebo for 7 weeks. The response rate was 51% in the group that received 200 mg, 41% in the group that received 50 mg, and 26% in the control group. A separate 6-month study in patients with rapid-cycling bipolar disorder reported that lamotrigine monotherapy was more effective in preventing relapse than placebo, especially in bipolar II disorder. Although further data are required, particularly regarding the ability of lamotrigine to prevent or treat the manic phase of bipolar disorder, lamotrigine is already a valuable addition to the current therapeutic armamentarium, particularly for the depressed phase of bipolar disorder. Lamotrigine is well tolerated and to date is not associated with hepatotoxicity, weight gain, or significant sedation.

Lamotrigine treatment is usually initiated at 25 mg once a day and increased in 25-mg increments every week. This dosage should be reduced by half for patients who are also taking valproate and increased for those taking carbamazepine because of hepatic enzyme inhibition and induction, respectively. Lamotrigine requires slow dosage titration to minimize the risk to the patient of developing a skin rash. A maculopapular rash develops in 5% of the patients taking lamotrigine, usually in the first 4 weeks of treatment. Stevens-Johnson syndrome may occur, with an estimated risk of 1 in 1,000 patient years (Richens 1994). Stevens-Johnson syndrome is potentially fatal. It is essential to advise patients of this risk and to emphasize that they should call the office immediately if they develop a rash. Development of a rash with concomitant systemic symptoms is a particularly ominous sign and should be evaluated immediately.

Although lamotrigine is generally well tolerated, common early side effects include headache, dizziness, gastrointestinal distress, and blurred or double vision.

Treatment of Mania

The first step in treating mania is to initiate treatment with a mood stabilizer. Currently lithium, valproate, and olanzapine are indicated as monotherapy agents for the treatment of mania. Valproate appears to be particularly effective for patients with mixed mania and depression (Swann et al. 1997). The efficacy of olanzapine in the treatment of mania is independent of the presence or absence of psychotic symptoms.

Other factors to consider in selecting a mood stabilizer include previous response to treatment, family history of response to a particular agent, side effects, concomitant medical problems, and concurrent medications. Lithium and valproate both cause gastrointestinal side effects, weight gain, and tremor. Olanzapine is also associated with weight gain and rarely with impaired glucose metabolism (as discussed earlier in this chapter). Starting

dosages and rapidity of titration depend on balancing the clinical need for rapid control of symptoms, which dictates faster titration, with the improved tolerability of slower dose escalations. For example, after the clinician diagnoses acute mania and decides to use valproate as the primary mood stabilizer, the initial dose depends on the urgency of the clinical situation. If the patient is highly agitated on an inpatient hospital unit, use of the "loading" strategy may be indicated, in which the patient is started with 20 mg/kg of divalproex. On the other hand, a patient with hypomania may do well at a substantially lower dose. Often patients with bipolar II disorder do well taking smaller doses of mood stabilizers, such as lithium 600 mg at bedtime or valproate 500 mg at bedtime. Olanzapine is started at a dose of 15 mg in acute mania, but lower doses may be effective for the treatment of hypomania in outpatients. Olanzapine does not require monitoring of blood levels, which may be advantageous in some clinical situations. Although the mood stabilizers provide definitive treatment, they often require 1–2 weeks, and occasionally longer, before their efficacy is apparent. Because agitation and behavioral dyscontrol are often prominent in mania, additional agents are frequently used in the acute setting. The benzodiazepines lorazepam (Lenox et al. 1992) and clonazepam (Chouinard et al. 1983, 1993), even in high doses, can be used to treat agitation and insomnia until the primary antimanic medication takes effect. Alprazolam is not recommended for patients with mania because, like all agents with antidepressant effects, it may precipitate mania (Arana et al. 1988).

In general, antipsychotic medication should be tapered after the acute episode, with continuation of the mood stabilizer as prophylaxis against recurrent episodes. Conventional antipsychotics should be avoided because they are associated with a greater degree of EPS and tardive dyskinesia compared with the atypical antipsychotics.

When patients fail to respond to a single agent, the next step is to combine medications. Adding a second agent is preferred to substituting one mood stabilizer for another, unless there was a toxic or allergic reaction to the first drug. This strategy provides synergy and avoids the risk of exacerbating the patient's symptoms by withdrawing the first agent, which although seemingly ineffective may have been providing some therapeutic benefit. After the patient is stabilized, it may be reasonable to consider tapering the first agent, although it is not unusual for patients with bipolar disorder to require long-term treatment with a combination of medications. Lithium in combination with carbamazepine (Lipinski and Pope 1982; Moss and James 1983) or with valproate

(McElroy et al. 1989) has produced remission for some patients who were unresponsive to lithium alone. In addition, some patients respond to a combination of two anticonvulsants even if they have previously failed to respond to each agent individually (Ketter et al. 1992).

Lithium with valproate is the most common and least complicated combination. Combinations of lithium or valproate with atypical antipsychotics are also effective. Valproate and carbamazepine can be combined, but the pharmacokinetics are complicated. To compensate for the bimodal pharmacokinetic interactions, valproate dosages need to be higher and carbamazepine dosages lower than when these agents are used singly. Valproate shifts the metabolism of carbamazepine toward its active metabolite, which is not reflected in the serum carbamazepine levels. Therefore, carbamazepine levels appear artificially low.

If these combinations prove ineffective, preliminary data suggest that clozapine is an effective mood stabilizer, even in nonpsychotic patients (Suppes et al. 1992). ECT is an effective treatment for acute mania and is especially useful for patients who cannot safely wait until medication becomes effective (Hirschfeld et al. 1994). In addition, myriad other medications are being studied for the treatment of bipolar disorder, most often for the manic phase of the illness. Studies are under way to evaluate other anticonvulsants and atypical antipsychotic medications. To date, there are case reports regarding the use of these other agents but not peer-reviewed controlled clinical trial data. The importance of not assuming that all anticonvulsants are effective is illustrated by two negative controlled trials of gabapentin in the treatment of bipolar disorder (Frye et al. 2000), despite numerous positive case reports.

Bipolar Depression

Treatment

A common mistake is to treat bipolar depression in the same manner as unipolar depression, overlooking the need for a mood stabilizer. In bipolar depression, the first pharmacological intervention should be to start or optimize treatment with a mood stabilizer rather than to start an antidepressant medication. In addition, thyroid function should be evaluated, particularly if the patient is taking lithium. Subclinical hypothyroidism, diagnosed by an elevated thyrotropin level and normal T_3 and T_4 levels, may present as depression in affectively predisposed individuals. In such cases, the addition of thyroid hormones may be beneficial, even if there is no other evidence of hypothyroidism.

Unless treatment history or comorbid medical problems dictate otherwise, lithium continues to be a first-line treatment for bipolar depression. The response rate to lithium in bipolar depression is 79% (Zornberg and Pope 1993). The efficacy of lamotrigine in treating bipolar depression has been shown in a double-blind, placebo-controlled trial (Calabrese et al. 1999). Although the Calabrese study used lamotrigine as a monotherapy for bipolar depression, we are hesitant to do this in patients with bipolar I disorder because to date no compelling data indicate that lamotrigine prevents mania. Lamotrigine can be combined with lithium, valproate, or carbamazepine. As noted earlier in this chapter, lower doses of lamotrigine are started, and the dose titration is more gradual when this medication is added to valproate.

If treatment with a single mood stabilizer is ineffective, some experts recommend adding a second mood stabilizer, whereas others recommend careful addition of an antidepressant (Sachs et al. 2000). Although the switch rate into mania or induction of rapid cycling by antidepressants is controversial (Peet 1994; Wehr and Goodwin 1987), these agents do appear to present a risk for some patients, often with devastating consequences. Controlled comparative data on the use of specific antidepressant drugs in the treatment of bipolar depression are sparse. Current treatment guidelines extrapolate from these few studies and rely heavily on anecdotal clinical experience. MAOIs appear to be more effective than TCAs in bipolar depression (Himmelhoch et al. 1991). Some data suggest that bupropion also may be less likely to induce mania or cycle acceleration (Sachs et al. 1994; Shopsin 1983) compared with the TCAs. The serotonin reuptake inhibitors also appear to be relatively safe for many patients (Cohn et al. 1989). Overall, TCAs should be avoided when other viable treatment options exist. ECT, as discussed later in this chapter, should be considered in severe cases.

Prophylaxis

Patients with bipolar disorder require lifelong prophylaxis with a mood stabilizer, both to prevent new episodes and to decrease the likelihood that the illness will progress to a more malignant course. Ninety percent of bipolar patients relapse on stopping lithium, most within 6 months (Suppes et al. 1991). In addition to the single episode that may occur, each episode may further kindle the illness, thereby inducing a more malignant course of illness with decreased treatment responsiveness. The more episodes a patient has had, the less likely he or she is to respond to treatment (Gelenberg et al. 1989).

An additional rationale for continuing effective prophylactic treatment is the phenomenon of discontinuation-induced refractoriness (Post et al. 1992). It appears that some patients whose symptoms were previously successfully treated with lithium and then have another episode after lithium has been discontinued fail to respond to the reinstitution of lithium. Moreover, these individuals tend to be poorly responsive to other treatments. Although to date discontinuation-induced refractoriness has been reported only with lithium, it is feasible that the phenomenon may occur with other agents. However, if tolerance develops, a period of time off the ineffective medication, combined with the institution of a different agent, is indicated. In most situations in which it is necessary to discontinue a mood stabilizer, it should be done with as slow a taper as possible. Abruptly stopping lithium is associated with a substantially higher rate of relapse than is tapering the drug (Faedda et al. 1994). Again, although most currently available data are for lithium, there is no reason to suspect that the principles differ for other mood stabilizers.

Finally, prophylaxis is best achieved when patients understand their illness, including the importance of treatment and the consequences of discontinuing medication. Referral to local support groups, such as the National Depressive and Manic-Depressive Association, can be invaluable. It is also helpful to simplify medication schedules, such as using at-bedtime lithium dosing as opposed to divided doses. Minimizing side effects is also important.

Drug Interactions

A drug interaction occurs when the pharmacological action of a medication is altered by a concurrently administered drug (or exogenous substance). With the increased use of psychotropic medications, the importance of drug interactions in psychopharmacology is increasingly apparent. Simultaneously, the characterization of specific cytochrome P450 isozymes facilitates the use of a more clinically meaningful and simpler conceptual framework to understand and predict many of the drug–drug interactions.

There are three types of drug interactions. *Pharmacokinetic interactions* involve an alteration by a second agent in the absorption, distribution, metabolism, or excretion of a drug, which changes the plasma concentration of the drug. *Pharmacodynamic interactions* involve a change in the action of a drug at a receptor or biologically active site, which alters the pharmacological effect of a given plasma concentration of the drug. *Idiosyncratic interactions* occur unpredictably in a small number of patients; they are unexpected, given the known pharmacological actions of the individual drugs.

Pharmacokinetic Interactions

Cytochrome P450 Enzymes

Clinically significant drug interactions are most commonly caused by changes in drug metabolism. Cytochrome P450 enzymes metabolize all psychotropic drugs, except lithium. These enzymes are a heterogeneous group of mixed-function oxidases found predominantly in the liver and, to varying degrees, in the gut and brain. These enzymes catalyze the oxidative metabolism of a large number of drugs as well as many other endogenous and exogenous substances. The cytochrome P450 enzymes are classified by families and subfamilies on the basis of similarities in amino acid sequence (Nelson et al. 1993). Enzymes within subfamilies have relatively specific affinities for various drugs and other substances. The enzymes that are primarily involved in drug metabolism are CYP1A2, CYP2C, CYP2D6, and CYP3A3/4.

If one of these enzymes is inhibited by another drug, the result is an increase in the plasma level of concurrently administered drugs that rely on the enzyme for metabolism. A common analogy is blocking a drain, which results in a buildup of water. The drain is the metabolic pathway, the block is the enzyme inhibitor, and the water is the medications that are substrates for the enzyme. For example, the 2D6 enzyme is essential for the usual metabolism of TCAs (they are substrates for this enzyme). Fluoxetine inhibits the 2D6 enzyme. If a patient is taking a TCA and fluoxetine is added, or vice versa, TCA plasma levels increase, which may result in increased side effects or toxicity. Anticipating the potential for this reaction, the clinician can use a lower dosage of the TCA. This example illustrates the key clinical principle of prescribing enzyme inhibitors: in most cases, the combination of an enzyme inhibitor and a medication that is a substrate for that enzyme is not contraindicated, but the patient should be monitored for signs and symptoms related to increased substrate levels, with appropriate lowering of the substrate dose if necessary. The specific P450 enzymes that metabolize many medications are not yet known, but information about the role of the cytochrome P450 enzymes in drug metabolism is rapidly evolving. Table 24–24 provides a list of the better-recognized and clinically important substrates and inhibitors for each of the cytochrome P450 enzymes. In most cases, enzyme inhibitors and substrates can be safely combined, provided the dosage of the substrate is lowered if needed.

TABLE 24–24. Partial list of clinically relevant cytochrome P450 (CYP) substrates and inhibitors

Enzyme	CYP1A2	CYP2C9/10	CYP2C19	CYP2D6	CYP3A3/4/5	
Substrates[a]	Aminophylline	Phenytoin	Barbiturates	Most antipsychotics	Acetaminophen	Lidocaine
	Amitriptyline	Warfarin	Diazepam	Codeine	Alprazolam	Midazolam
	Caffeine		Divalproex	Donepezil	Amiodarone	Oral contraceptives
	Clozapine (in part)			Encainide	Antiarrhythmics	Oxcarbazine
	Imipramine			Flecainide	Buspirone	Pimozide
	Methadone			Galanthamine	Calcium channel	Propafenone
	Olanzapine			Lipophilic β-blockers	blockers	Protease inhibitors
	Propranolol			Mexiletine	Carbamazepine	Quinidine
	Tacrine			TCAs[c]	Cyclosporine	Statins
	Theophylline			Tromodol	Donepezil	Steroids
	Verapamil			Trazodone	Ethosuximide	Tamoxifen
				Type IC antiarrhythmics	Galanthamine	Triazolam
				Venlafaxine	Lamotrigine	
Inhibitors[b]	Cimetidine	Cimetidine	Fluoxetine	Bupropion	Diltiazem	
	Ciprofloxacin	Fluoxetine	Fluvoxamine	Cimetidine	Fluvoxamine	
	Enoxacin	Fluvoxamine		Fluoxetine	Grapefruit juice	
	Fluvoxamine	Modafinil		Paroxetine	Imidazole antifungal	
	Grapefruit juice	Ritonavir		Phenothiazines	agents (e.g., keto-	
	Ketoconazole			Quinidine	conazole)	
	Norfloxacin			Ritonavir	Some macrolides	
				Sertraline	antibiotics	
					Nefazodone	
					Protease inhibitors	
					Verapamil	

Note.   TCA = tricyclic antidepressant.
[a]Medications and substances metabolized by a given enzyme. [b]May increase levels of substrates. [c]The 2D6 enzyme is the final common pathway for the metabolism of TCAs.
Source.   Adapted from Callahan et al. 1996.

In general, enzyme inhibition is competitive and depends on both the relative concentration of the inhibitor and its affinity for the enzyme. The effects of inhibitors are relatively rapid (minutes to hours) and are reversible within a time frame that depends on the half-life of the inhibitor. There is a large amount of interindividual variation in drug metabolism and the propensity for enzyme inhibition to alter metabolism. Part of this variation is the result of genetic polymorphism (Shimada et al. 1994), which is a heritable alteration in the enzyme. The 2C19 and 2D6 enzymes are known to exhibit polymorphism. Persons who have a genetic polymorphism causing a large reduction in the amount of active enzyme are referred to as "poor metabolizers" and are at risk for increased drug levels, which may lead to toxicity. Approximately 15%–20% of Asians and 1% of Caucasians have reduced amounts of the CYP2C19 enzyme (Nakamura et al. 1985; Xie et al. 1996), whereas 7%–10% of Caucasians lack the CYP2D6 enzyme (Dahl et al. 1995). In contrast, some persons have increased amounts of the CYP2D6 enzyme (Johansson et al. 1993). These individuals are referred to as "ultrarapid metabolizers" and may have reduced levels of drugs that are metabolized by this enzyme, resulting in decreased efficacy. Polymorphism accounts for much of the well-known interindividual differences in drug metabolism and the occurrence of drug-drug interactions mediated by cytochrome P450.

In addition, the cytochrome P450 enzymes can be induced (Watkins et al. 1985). Cytochrome P450 enzyme induction causes the liver to produce a greater amount of the enzyme, which can increase elimination and reduce plasma levels of a second drug or its metabolites. When clinically relevant, the drug dosage should be increased to achieve the same serum concentration. The effects of inducers tend to be delayed days to weeks because this process involves enzyme synthesis. Barbiturates, carbamazepine, phenytoin, rifampin, dexamethasone, smoking, and chronic alcohol use induce cytochrome P450 enzymes.

Protein Binding

Medications are distributed to their sites of action through the circulatory system. In the bloodstream, all the psychotropic medications except lithium are bound to plasma proteins to varying degrees. A drug is considered highly protein bound if more than 90% is bound to plasma proteins. A reversible equilibrium exists between the bound and unbound drug; the unbound fraction is pharmacologically active, whereas the bound fraction is inactive and therefore cannot be metabolized or excreted. When two drugs exist simultaneously in the plasma, competition for protein-binding sites occurs. This can cause displacement of the previously protein-bound drug, which in the free state becomes pharmacologically active. Interactions that occur by this mechanism are called *protein-binding interactions*. They are transient because, although the plasma concentration of free drug initially increases, the drug then becomes subject to redistribution, metabolism, and excretion, producing a new steady-state concentration. This type of interaction is generally not clinically significant unless the drugs involved are highly protein bound (which results in a large change in plasma concentration of free drug from a small amount of drug displacement) and have a low therapeutic index or narrow therapeutic window (in which case small changes in plasma levels can result in toxicity or loss of efficacy (Callahan et al. 1996).

Absorption and Excretion

Changes in plasma level as a result of alterations in absorption or excretion are less common with psychiatric medications. Drugs with anticholinergic effects, such as TCAs, tend to decrease gastrointestinal motility, which allows for longer periods of absorption of other medications (Greiff and Rowbotham 1994). Prolonged absorption may result in increased plasma levels of concomitantly administered medications. Changes in drug plasma concentration as a result of changes in excretion are most germane to lithium, which is dependent on renal excretion. Any medication that alters the kidney's excretion of lithium may result in clinically significant changes in the serum lithium level (as reviewed by Goodwin and Jamison 1990). These medications are listed in Table 24–24.

Pharmacodynamic Interactions

Pharmacodynamic interactions involve a change in the pharmacological effect of a drug resulting from the action of a second drug at a common receptor or bioactive site. These interactions can be mediated directly or indirectly. Direct pharmacodynamic interactions involve agonist or antagonist actions of two drugs at a common site, which produces increased (additive) or decreased pharmacological effects. Such interactions generally result from known pharmacological actions of a drug, and for this reason agents with a multiplicity of pharmacological effects are more likely to be involved. For example, low-potency antipsychotics and tertiary amine TCAs have anticholinergic, antihistaminic, α-adrenergic antagonist, and quinidine-like effects. In light of this, it can be predicted that the concurrent administration of chlorpromazine and imipramine will result in additive sedation, constipation, postural hypotension, and depression of cardiac conduction.

Indirect interactions involve changes in physiological functions caused by the combined action of two drugs at a common site. These interactions cannot be predicted on the basis of known pharmacological effects, and their mechanisms are poorly understood. Many indirect pharmacodynamic interactions have clinically significant consequences. For example, the adjunctive use of lithium with various antidepressant agents can potentiate antidepressant effects (synergism). On the other hand, the concurrent administration of a serotonin reuptake inhibitor or meperidine with an MAOI can produce a potentially lethal hypermetabolic reaction.

Summary

Remembering the myriad of psychotropic drug interactions is extremely difficult. Nevertheless, by applying a systematic approach, the clinician can often predict the occurrence and time course of such interactions. Several factors must be considered when assessing the potential consequences of drug interactions. Drug-related factors that increase the risk for clinically significant interactions include a low therapeutic index or narrow therapeutic window, a multiplicity of pharmacological actions, and inhibition or inducement of cytochrome P450 enzymes. Next, patient-related factors that can increase the risk for significant drug interactions should be considered. These include genetically based variations in drug-metabolizing capacity, as well as advanced age, underlying medical illness, and comorbid substance abuse. Finally, the literature should be carefully reviewed to ascertain the potential clinical relevance of available data. If a clinically significant drug interaction appears likely to occur, the patient's clinical status should be followed up closely; therapeutic drug monitoring should be used, if applicable, and dosage adjustments should be made accordingly. Rational polypharmacy requires an understanding of the pharmacological principles governing drug interactions and a knowledge of the factors that increase the likelihood of clinically significant variations in drug action. This understanding will allow the clinician to maximize beneficial effects while minimizing the risk of adverse events.

Antiaggression Drugs

Overview

Aggressive and violent behaviors are frequently encountered in patients with underlying disorders as diverse as traumatic brain injury; brain tumor; hereditary or metabolic brain disease; mental retardation; dementia; seizure disorders; sequelae of CNS infections; sequelae of substance abuse; DSM-IV (American Psychiatric Association 1994) Axis I psychiatric disorders such as schizophrenia, bipolar disorder, and conduct disorder; and Axis II personality disorders such as antisocial and borderline personality disorders (Anderson and Silver 1999; Silver and Yudofsky 1987). Dyscontrol of aggression in many of these conditions is often the most significant source of disability and dysfunction among all the symptoms and signs associated with the underlying illness. These episodes range in severity from irritability to outbursts that result in damage to property or assaults on others. In severe cases, affected individuals cannot remain in the community or with their families and often are referred to the most restrictive long-term psychiatric or neurobehavioral facilities.

In establishing a treatment plan for patients with agitation or aggression, the overarching principle is that diagnosis comes before treatment. The history of the development of symptoms in a biopsychosocial context is usually the most critical part of the evaluation. It is essential to determine the mental status of the patient before the agitated or aggressive event, the nature of the precipitant, the physical and social environment in which the behavior occurs, the ways in which the event is mitigated, and the primary and secondary gains related to agitation and aggression (Corrigan et al. 1993; Silver and Yudofsky 1994; Yudofsky et al. 1998). We suggest using the consensus guidelines for the treatment of agitation in the elderly with dementia as a framework for the assessment and management of agitation and aggression (Alexopolous et al. 1998). After appropriate assessment of possible etiologies of these behaviors, treatment is focused on the occurrence of comorbid neuropsychiatric conditions (depression, psychosis, insomnia, anxiety, delirium). Evaluation and documentation of aggressive behaviors and agitation with objective measures such as the Overt Aggression Scale (Silver and Yudofsky 1991;

Yudofsky et al. 1986) and the Overt Agitation and Severity Scale (Yudofsky et al. 1997) are often helpful. Other factors that influence the choice of medication include whether the treatment is in the acute (hours to days) or chronic (weeks to months) phase and the severity of the behavior (mild to severe).

Although no medication has been approved by the FDA specifically for the treatment of aggression, medications are widely used (and commonly misused) in the management of acute or chronic aggression. We divide the use of pharmacological interventions for aggression into two major categories: 1) the use of the sedating effects of medications, as required in acute or severe situations, so that the patient does not harm himself or herself or others, and 2) the use of nonsedating medications for the treatment of chronic aggression (Corrigan et al. 1993; Silver and Yudofsky 1994; Yudofsky et al. 1998).

Acute Aggression and Agitation

Medications that are sedating may be indicated for the treatment of agitation and for treating severe episodes of aggressive behavior. Because these drugs are not specific in their ability to inhibit aggressive behaviors, however, there may be detrimental effects on arousal and cognitive function. Therefore, the use of sedation-producing medications must be time-limited to avoid the emergence of seriously disabling side effects ranging from oversedation to tardive dyskinesia. Unless aggressive behavior is clearly related to psychotic ideation that is responding to treatment with antipsychotic agents, we prefer to limit the use of both antipsychotic agents and benzodiazepines for "sedating" aggression to a maximum period of 4 weeks. Beyond this time, the clinician must consider whether the aggression is chronic and alter the treatment plan accordingly to use medications recommended to treat chronic behaviors (see the following section).

Antipsychotic Drugs

Antipsychotics are the most commonly used medications in the treatment of aggression. Although these agents are appropriate and effective when aggression is derivative of active psychosis, the use of antipsychotic agents to treat chronic aggression, especially secondary to organic brain injury, is often ineffective and entails risks that the patient will develop serious complications. Usually, it is the sedative side effects rather than the antipsychotic properties of antipsychotics that are used (i.e., misused) to "treat" (i.e., mask) the aggression. Often, patients develop tolerance to the sedative effects of the medication and, therefore, require increasing doses. As a result, especially with the older conventional antipsychotic medications, extrapyramidal and anticholinergic-related side effects occur. Paradoxically (and frequently), because of the development of akathisia, the patient may become more agitated and restless as the dose of neuroleptic is increased, especially when a high-potency antipsychotic such as haloperidol is administered. The akathisia is often mistaken for increased irritability and agitation, and a vicious cycle of increasing neuroleptic doses and worsening akathisia occurs.

There is some evidence from studies of injury to motor neurons in animals that haloperidol retards recovery. This effect was seen only when animals actively participated in a behavioral task and not when the animals were restrained after drug administration (Feeney et al. 1982). It is possible that the effect on decreasing dopamine and inhibiting neuronal function, which may be the mechanism of action to treat aggression, has other detrimental effects on recovery. Whether this finding is generalizable to recovery in brain injury remains unclear. However, the finding raises important potential risk–benefit issues that must be considered before antipsychotic drugs are used to treat aggressive behavior in patients with neuronal damage.

In patients with acute aggression, we recommend starting a high-potency antipsychotic such as risperidone at low dosages of 0.5 mg orally with repeated administration every hour until control of aggression is achieved. If intramuscular medication were required, haloperidol would be used. If after several administrations of risperidone the patient's aggressive behavior does not improve, the hourly dose may be increased until the patient is sedated sufficiently that he or she no longer shows agitation or violence. Once the patient is not aggressive for 48 hours, the daily dosage should be decreased gradually (i.e., by 25% each day) to ascertain whether aggressive behavior reemerges. In this case, the clinician must decide whether it is best to increase the dose of risperidone or to initiate treatment with a more specific antiaggressive drug.

Sedatives and Hypnotics

The literature is inconsistent on the effects of the benzodiazepines in the treatment of aggression. The sedative properties of benzodiazepines are especially helpful in the management of acute agitation and aggression. Most likely, this is due to the effect of benzodiazepines on increasing the inhibitory neurotransmitter GABA. Paradoxically, several studies reported increased hostility, aggression, and the induction of rage in patients receiving benzodiazepines. However, these reports are balanced by the observation that this phenomenon is rare (Dietch and Jennings 1988). Benzodiazepines can produce amnesia, and preexisting memory dysfunction can be exacerbated by the use of benzodiazepines. Brain-injured patients also may experience increased problems with coordination and balance with benzodiazepine use.

For treatment of acute aggression, lorazepam 1–2 mg may be administered every hour by either oral or intramuscular route until sedation is achieved (Silver and Yudofsky 1994). Intramuscular lorazepam has been suggested as an effective medication in the emergency treatment of the violent patient (Bick and Hannah 1986). Intravenous lorazepam is also effective, although the onset of action is similar when administered intramuscularly. Caution must be taken with intravenous administration, and it should be injected in doses less than 1 cc (1 mg) per minute to avoid laryngospasm. As is done with neuroleptics, gradual tapering of lorazepam may be attempted when the patient has been in control for 48 hours. If aggressive behavior recurs, medications for the treatment of chronic aggression may be initiated. Lorazepam in 1- or 2-mg doses, administered either orally or by injection, may be given, if necessary, in combination with an antipsychotic medication (risperidone 1–2 mg). Other sedating medications such as paraldehyde, chloral hydrate, or diphenhydramine may be preferable to sedative antipsychotic agents.

Chronic Aggression

If periods of agitation or aggression continue beyond several weeks, the use of specific antiaggressive medications should be initiated to prevent these episodes from occurring. Because no medication has been approved by the FDA for treatment of aggression, the clinician uses medications that may be antiaggressive but have been approved for other uses (e.g., seizure disorders, depression, anxiety, hypertension) (Silver and Yudofsky 1994; Yudofsky et al. 1998).

Antipsychotic Medications

If, after thorough clinical evaluation, it is determined that the aggressive episodes result from psychosis, such as paranoid delusions or command hallucinations, then antipsychotic medications will be the treatment of choice. Risperidone has been used to treat agitation in elderly patients with dementia with good results (Goldberg and Goldberg 1995). Olanzapine and quetiapine also may be used. The differential side effects of these medications are discussed earlier in this chapter. Clozapine may have greater antiaggressive effects than other antipsychotic medications (Michals et al. 1993; Ratey et al. 1993). However, the increased risk of seizures and agranulocytosis must be carefully assessed.

Antianxiety Medications

Serotonin appears to be a key neurotransmitter in the modulation of aggressive behavior. In preliminary reports, buspirone, a 5-HT$_{1A}$ agonist, has been reported to be effective in the management of aggression and agitation for patients with head injury, dementia, and developmental disabilities and autism (Silver and Yudofsky 1994). In rare instances, some patients become more aggressive when treated with buspirone. We usually initiate buspirone at 7.5 mg twice a day for 1 week and then increase the dosage to 15 mg twice a day. Dosages of 45–60 mg/day may be required before there is improvement in aggressive behavior, although we have noted dramatic improvement within 1 week.

Clonazepam may be effective in the long-term management of aggression, although controlled, double-blind studies have not yet been conducted. Freinhar and Alvarez (1986) found that clonazepam decreased agitation in three elderly patients with organic brain syndromes. Keats and Mukherjee (1988) reported antiaggressive effects of clonazepam in a patient with schizophrenia and seizures. We use clonazepam when pronounced aggression and anxiety occur together or when aggression occurs in association with neurologically induced tics and similarly disinhibited motor behaviors. Doses should be initiated at 0.5 mg twice a day and may be increased to as high as 2–4 mg twice a day, as tolerated. Sedation and ataxia are frequent side effects.

Anticonvulsants

The anticonvulsant carbamazepine, commonly used for the treatment of bipolar disorders, also has been advocated for the control of aggression in both epileptic and nonepileptic populations. Several open studies have indicated that carbamazepine may be effective in decreasing aggressive behavior associated with traumatic brain injury dementia (Chatham-Showalter 1996), developmental disabilities, schizophrenia, and a variety of other organic brain disorders (Silver and Yudofsky 1994; Yudofsky et al. 1998). Carbamazepine can be a highly effective medication to treat aggression in the brain-injured patient. Reports also indicate that the antiaggressive response of carbamazepine can be found in patients with and without EEG abnormalities (Silver and Yudofsky 1994).

In our experience and that of others, the anticonvulsant valproic acid also may be helpful to some patients with organically induced aggression (Geracioti 1994;

Giakas et al. 1990; Mattes 1992; Wroblewski et al. 1997). For patients with aggression and epilepsy whose seizures are being treated with anticonvulsant drugs such as phenytoin and phenobarbital, switching to carbamazepine or to valproic acid may treat both conditions.

Gabapentin has been used effectively for the treatment of agitation in patients with dementia (Herrmann et al. 2000; Roane et al. 2000). Doses have ranged from 200 to 2,400 mg/day.

Lithium

Although lithium is known to be effective in controlling aggression related to manic excitement, many studies suggest that it also may have a role in the treatment of aggression in selected, nonbipolar patient populations. Included are patients with traumatic brain injury (Bellus et al. 1996), patients with mental retardation who have self-injurious or aggressive behavior, children and adolescents with behavior disorders, prison inmates, and patients with other organic brain syndromes.

Patients with brain injury have increased sensitivity to the neurotoxic effects of lithium (Hornstein and Seliger 1989; Moskowitz and Altshuler 1991). Because of lithium's potential for neurotoxicity and its relative lack of efficacy in many patients with aggression secondary to brain injury, we limit the use of lithium in those patients whose aggression is related to manic effects or recurrent irritability related to cyclic mood disorders.

Antidepressants

The antidepressants that have been reported to control aggressive behaviors are those that act preferentially (amitriptyline) or specifically (trazodone and fluoxetine) on serotonin. In open studies, Mysiw et al. (1988) and Jackson et al. (1985) reported that amitriptyline (maximum dose 150 mg/day) was effective in the treatment of patients with recent severe brain injury whose agitation had not responded to behavioral techniques. Szlabowicz and Stewart (1990) successfully treated a 43-year-old man with aggressive behavior subsequent to anoxic encephalopathy with amitriptyline 75 mg at bedtime. Trazodone also has been reported to be effective in the treatment of aggression that occurs with organic mental disorders (Silver and Yudofsky 1994; Yudofsky et al. 1998). Gedye (1991) reported a case in which a 17-year-old mentally handicapped and autistic male with aggressive and self-injurious behavior had a favorable response following treatment with trazodone. Two individuals with Huntington's disease and aggressiveness were treated effectively with sertraline (Ranen et al. 1996). Fluoxetine, a potent serotonergic antidepressant, has been reported to be effective in the treatment of aggressive behavior in a patient who had brain injury as well as in patients with personality disorders and depression and adolescents with mental retardation and self-injurious behavior (Silver and Yudofsky 1994; Yudofsky et al. 1998). We have used SSRIs with considerable success in aggressive patients with brain lesions. The dosages used are similar to those for the treatment of mood lability and depression.

We have evaluated and treated many patients with emotional lability that is characterized by frequent episodes of tearfulness and irritability and the full symptomatic picture of neuroaggressive syndrome (Silver and Yudofsky 1994). These patients, who would be diagnosed according to DSM-IV-TR as having "personality change, labile type, due to traumatic brain injury," have responded well to antidepressants.

There have been several reports of the beneficial effects of fluoxetine for "emotional incontinence" secondary to several neurological disorders (Brown et al. 1998; Nahas et al. 1998; Panzer and Mellow 1992; Seliger et al. 1992; Sloan et al. 1992). In our experience, all SSRIs can be effective, and the dosage guidelines are similar to those used in the treatment of depression. In addition, other antidepressants, such as nortriptyline, can be effective for emotional lability. We emphasize that for many patients it may be necessary to administer these medications at standard antidepressant dosages to obtain full therapeutic effects, although response may occur for others within days of initiating treatment at relatively low doses.

Antihypertensive Medications: β-Blockers

Since the first report of the use of β-adrenergic receptor blockers in the treatment of acute aggression in 1977, more than 25 articles have appeared in the neurological and psychiatric literature reporting experience in using β-blockers with more than 200 patients with aggression (Yudofsky et al. 1987). Most of these patients had been unsuccessfully treated with antipsychotics, minor tranquilizers, lithium, and/or anticonvulsants before treatment with β-blockers. The β-blockers that have been investigated in controlled prospective studies include propranolol (a lipid-soluble, nonselective receptor antagonist), nadolol (a water-soluble, nonselective receptor antagonist), and pindolol (a lipid-soluble, nonselective β-receptor antagonist with partial sympathomimetic activity). A growing body of preliminary evidence suggests that β-adrenergic receptor blockers are effective agents for the treatment of aggressive and violent behaviors, particularly those related to organic brain syndrome. The effectiveness of propranolol in reducing agitation has been confirmed during the initial hospitalization after traumatic brain injury (Brooke et al. 1992). When a patient requires the use of a once-a-day medication because of compliance difficulties, long-acting propranolol (i.e., Inderal LA) or nadolol can be used. When patients develop bradycardia that prevents prescribing of therapeutic dosages of propranolol, pindolol can be substituted, using one-tenth the dosage of propranolol. Pindolol's intrinsic sympathomimetic activity stimulates the β receptor and restricts the development of bradycardia.

The major side effects of β-blockers when used to treat aggression are a lowering of blood pressure and pulse rate. Because peripheral β receptors are fully blocked in doses of 300–400 mg/day, further decreases in these vital signs usually do not occur even when doses are increased to much higher levels. Despite reports of depression with the use of β-blockers, controlled trials and our experience indicate that it is a rare occurrence. Because the use of propranolol is associated with significant increases in plasma levels of thioridazine, which has an absolute dosage ceiling of 800 mg/day, the combination of these two medications should be avoided whenever possible.

Conclusion

Table 24–25 summarizes our recommendations for the use of various classes of medication in the treatment of chronic aggressive disorders associated with traumatic brain injury. Acute aggression may be treated by using the sedative properties of neuroleptics or benzodiazepines. In treating aggression, the clinician, when possible, should diagnose and treat underlying disorders and use, when possible, antiaggressive agents specific to those disorders. When there is partial response after a therapeutic trial with a specific medication, adjunctive treatment with a medication that has a different mechanism of action should be instituted. For example, a patient with partial response to β-blockers can have additional improvement with the addition of an anticonvulsant.

Electroconvulsive Therapy

Overview

ECT is the use of electrically induced repetitive firings of the neurons in the CNS (i.e., grand mal seizures) to treat psychiatric illnesses such as depression or mania and psychiatric symptoms such as psychosis or catatonia. Although ECT was first used in the late 1930s, before the era of potent psychopharmacological treatment of major mood disorders, the treatment today remains clinically

TABLE 24–25. Pharmacotherapy for agitation

	Drug	Primary indication
Acute agitation/severe aggression	High-potency antipsychotic drugs (haloperidol, risperidone)	
	Benzodiazepines (lorazepam)	
Chronic agitation	Atypical antipsychotics (risperidone, olanzapine, quetiapine, clozapine)	Psychosis
	Valproic acid, carbamazepine, ?gabapentin	Seizure disorder, severe aggression
	Serotonergic antidepressants (SSRIs, trazodone)	Depression, mood lability
	Buspirone	Anxiety
	β-Blockers	Aggression without concomitant neuro-psychiatric sequelae

Note. SSRI = selective serotonin reuptake inhibitor.

relevant because of its high degree of efficacy, safety, and usefulness. Despite the extraordinary practical difficulties involved, scientific efforts to define its clinical efficacy and diagnostic indications have resulted in six published controlled trials since 1968 in which ECT has been shown to be superior to simulated treatment (Lerer and Belmaker 1986). For many patients, ECT is the safest and most effective form of treatment (American Psychiatric Association 1990). Many years ago, ECT was used primarily in large state hospitals for the treatment of chronic psychiatric disorders, including schizophrenia. Currently, in the United States, ECT is used primarily in the private sector for patients who do not receive prolonged inpatient care (Asnis et al. 1978).

Mechanisms of Action

The mechanisms of action of ECT are complex and not completely understood. ECT has been found to affect many of the neurotransmitters and receptors that have been implicated in depression and its treatment. In studies involving both humans and animals, ECT has been found to affect serotonin, GABA, endogenous opiates and their receptors, and catecholamines (including dopamine, norepinephrine, and epinephrine and their receptors). It also affects a wide variety of other neurotransmitters, neuropeptides, and neuroendocrine pathways (Kapur and Mann 1993; Nutt and Glue 1993). In addition, neurophysiological hypotheses regarding a range of effects of ECT (e.g., on kindling and on regional cerebral blood flow) are under investigation.

Indications

The principal diagnostic indication for ECT is major depression, especially when a rapid response is needed

for either medical or psychiatric reasons (American Psychiatric Association 2001). Depressed patients adequately treated with either drugs or ECT have significantly lower mortality rates, not only related to suicide but also from natural causes, than patients with depression who do not receive treatment with one of these methods (Avery and Winokur 1976). According to an analysis of rigorously controlled studies that compared the efficacy of ECT with that of simulated ECT, placebo, and antidepressants, ECT was clearly superior for severe depression (Janicak et al. 1985). However, more recent studies indicate that the likelihood of response to ECT is reduced in patients who have previously failed one or more adequate antidepressant trials (Prudic et al. 1996). In a study by Prudic et al. (1996), which included 100 patients, the acute response rate in patients who had previous antidepressant trials that were considered inadequate (i.e., they were not treatment-resistant) was 91.4% immediately after ECT, but the response rate decreased to 74.3% after 1 week. In contrast, patients who were medication-resistant (i.e., they had failed one or more adequate antidepressant trials before ECT) had an immediate response rate of 63.1%, which decreased to 47.7% a week after cessation of ECT.

ECT also may be of benefit in the treatment of mania that is not responsive to medications (Small et al. 1986). Patients with schizophrenia who have affective and catatonic symptoms may have a beneficial response to ECT; however, there is no indication that ECT alters the fundamental psychopathology of schizophrenia (Small et al. 1986).

Yudofsky (1981) outlined clinical situations in which ECT may be advantageous over other treatment approaches. Among these situations, which are by no means all-inclusive, are the following:

1. Patients whose severe mood disorders have not responded to adequate psychopharmacological treatment (i.e., with appropriate dosage and duration of treatment).

2. Patients with delusional depression (Avery and Lubrano 1979; Glassman and Roose 1981; Paul et al. 1977).

3. Patients—particularly elderly patients—who cannot tolerate the cardiovascular, genitourinary, or CNS side effects of antidepressant or antipsychotic agents.

4. Patients whose acute symptoms are so severe (i.e., manic excitement, active suicidal behavior, psychomotor retardation, or catatonia) that a rapid and dramatic response is required.

5. Patients with histories of depressive episodes that have responded successfully to previous electroconvulsive treatments.

Contraindications

There are relatively few contraindications to ECT (American Psychiatric Association 2001). First, patients with clinically significant space-occupying cerebral lesions or conditions with increased intracranial pressure must not receive this treatment because of the risk of brain stem herniation (Maltbie et al. 1980). Second, patients with significant cardiovascular problems, such as recent myocardial infarction, severe cardiac ischemia, and moderate to severe hypertension (including pheochromocytoma), are more prone to the transient fluctuations in the cardiovascular system that occur during and shortly after ECT. Such patients may or may not safely be given ECT, and they must be evaluated before treatment by a cardiologist familiar with the potential side effects of ECT. Patients with recent intracerebral hemorrhage are at increased risk, as are those with bleeding or unstable vascular aneurysm or abnormalities, or with retinal detachment. Before the use of muscle relaxants in ECT, degenerative diseases of the spine and other bones constituted a significant risk from ECT. Today, however, adequate anesthetic and muscle relaxant techniques render ECT generally safe in patients with these disorders. Although it has been suggested that patients should discontinue taking MAOIs at least 2 weeks before the initiation of ECT to prevent dangerous increases in blood pressure during treatment, ECT has been administered to patients currently treated with MAOIs without adverse effects (Wells and Bjorkstein 1989).

Medical Evaluation Before Treatment

Before receiving ECT, patients should have a complete medical and neurological examination, a complete blood count, a serum electrolyte analysis, and an ECG. An X ray of the lumbosacral region should be obtained if spinal orthopedic problems are suspected. A chest X ray must be obtained because of the use of positive pressure respiration during general anesthesia. Evaluation by an anesthesiologist to determine risk of anesthesia is recommended. In specific clinical situations, such as when there is clinical evidence of a brain tumor or intracerebral bleeding or if there are CNS symptoms of uncertain etiology, electroencephalography and brain computed tomography or magnetic resonance imaging are also required.

Informed consent of a competent patient is essential. Because of the high degree of fear and misinformation related to ECT, we encourage that ample time be devoted to the discussion of the risks, benefits, and techniques of ECT and of all treatment alternatives with patients and their families. This includes meeting with patients and family members to provide an ample opportunity for the exchange of ideas, feelings, and information related to electroconvulsive treatment. We consider this process an integral part of the overall ECT procedure. The clinician may wish to have the patient and his or her family read specially prepared information about the risks and benefits of ECT (Yudofsky et al. 1991).

Technique

Anesthesia and Muscle Relaxation

ECT is used primarily for psychiatric inpatients, and it is common for an anesthetist or anesthesiologist to assist the psychiatrist in administering the treatment. The APA Task Force on Electroconvulsive Therapy (American Psychiatric Association 2001) recommended pretreatment with an anticholinergic drug such as atropine (0.4–1.0 mg iv) or glycopyrrolate (0.2–0.4 mg intravenously) to decrease the morbidity of cardiac bradyarrhythmias and aspiration. General anesthesia is induced only to the degree that a light coma is produced, using a fast-acting anesthetic such as methohexital, which has fewer cardiac side effects than slower-acting barbiturates such as thiopental. A starting dose of approximately 0.75–1.0 mg/kg of intravenous methohexital is recommended, but the amount required to induce safe and brief anesthesia may vary from considerably lower to considerably higher amounts depending on the patient's metabolism of the drug. Once the patient is anesthetized, intravenous succinylcholine is used for muscular relaxation. In general, approximately 0.5–1 mg/kg of intravenous succinylcholine is administered rapidly, immediately after the onset of general anesthesia. If there are preexisting skeletal

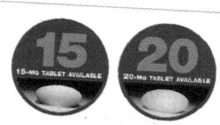
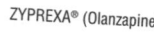
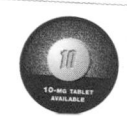

the seizure threshold). Unfortunately, higher electrical dosages also were equated with greater cognitive problems.

Course of Treatment

In the United States, ECT treatments are generally given on an every-other-day basis for 2–3 weeks, usually Monday, Wednesday, and Friday. Twice-weekly treatments may be equally effective with fewer cognitive side effects but with a slower onset of action (Lerer et al. 1995). Duration of seizure for longer than 20 seconds per treatment (as assessed by motor activity, not EEG seizure activity) is considered adequate for therapeutic purposes. The number of treatments administered is generally determined by a patient's clinical response; the therapy is discontinued when successive treatm55ents do not elicit further beneficial effects (Weiner 1979). With depressed patients, a typical course of ECT consists of 6–10 treatments, but sometimes more are required. We do not recommend more than 20 treatments in a single course of ECT.

After a course of treatment, ample time and permission must be given for the patient to discuss with the professional his or her feelings about having been depressed and having received ECT. Occasionally, a patient will erroneously attribute his or her inability to recall a name to permanent side effects of the procedure. In this situation, the normal forgetting process to which most people are subject can become a frightening and unwarranted symbol of depression and ECT. In addition, there must be the recognition that ECT is a specific therapeutic tool that should be used as a component of a larger therapeutic strategy (Yudofsky 1982; Yudofsky et al. 1991). Because the beneficial response to ECT is often so rapid and dramatic, insufficient emphasis may be placed on sociological and intrapsychic stresses that have contributed to the initial depression. It is only after the patient's affective illness has been improved by ECT that he or she is able to use psychotherapy, family therapy, and behavior therapy effectively to address the conditions that contributed to the depression.

Risks and Side Effects

In general, ECT is an unusually safe procedure, with morbidity and mortality not significantly greater than that associated with general anesthesia. The mortality rate of patients with ECT is 2 per 100,000 treatments (Fink 1978). The most frequent complaints of patients are memory impairment, headaches, and muscle aches (Gomez 1975); the most significant risks associated with ECT are cardiovascular and intracerebral (Abrams 1992).

unilateral electrode placement is related to fewer cognitive side effects compared with bilateral stimulus, studies also have suggested that unilateral placement is less efficacious if comparable stimulus doses are used (Abrams 1986; American Psychiatric Association 1990; Malitz and Sackeim 1986; Sackeim et al. 1993). Recent studies that used higher-dose unilateral ECT reported improved efficacy. Sackeim and co-workers (2000) randomized 80 depressed patients to right unilateral ECT, with an electrical dosage 50%, 150%, or 500% above the seizure threshold, or bilateral ECT, with an electrical dosage 150% above the threshold. In this study, high-dose right unilateral ECT and bilateral ECT were equally effective (response rate = 65%), and both were approximately twice as effective as low- or moderate-dose ECT. High-dose right unilateral ECT produced less severe cognitive side effects than bilateral ECT. A separate study by McCall et al. (2000) produced very similar results; specifically, fixed-dose right unilateral ECT produced a higher antidepressant response rate than lower stimulus parameters. Increased stimulation resulted in an increased response rate (stimulations up to 8–12 times

Medical Risks

Ictal and postictal fluctuations in autonomic tone can elicit cardiac arrhythmias of many varieties, including premature ventricular contractions during the immediate postictal period. Increase in vagal tone may result in sinus bradycardia or sinus arrest, whereas increases in sympathetic tone can elicit ventricular ectopy and increases in blood pressure and heart rate (Abrams 1992). To evaluate the safety of ECT in the cardiovascular realm, Dec et al. (1985) assessed serial ECGs and serum cardiac enzyme values of 29 patients who received a course of this therapy. The investigators could not find persistent electrocardiographic changes, elevations in CPK, or elevations in aspartate aminotransferase levels after 85 treatments in these patients. It is important to note that 24% of these patients had stable, preexisting cardiovascular disease, which included conduction system disease, recent myocardial infarction, and depressed ventricular function. The authors concluded that with careful cardiac monitoring before and after the procedure, with frequent checks of electrolyte values, and with careful tailoring of the anesthetic regimen to the individual patient, cardiovascular morbidity and mortality could be minimized, even for patients with known cardiovascular disease. As we noted earlier, patients who have preexisting disorders that increase intracranial pressure (e.g., space-occupying brain lesions), other CNS dysfunctions, hypertension, degenerative bone disease, or severe cardiac disease are at increased risk for serious side effects related to ECT. Such patients may receive ECT only after thorough evaluation and carefully documented approval by the relevant nonpsychiatric medical specialists.

Memory Impairment

The initial confusion and cognitive deficits associated with ECT treatment are usually temporary, lasting approximately 30 minutes. Whereas many patients report no problems with their memory, aside from the time immediately surrounding the ECT treatments, others report that their memory is not as good as it was before receiving ECT (Squire and Slater 1983). However, the controversy surrounding the effect of ECT on memory results primarily from public misinformation (Reid 1993).

To date, no reliable data have shown permanent memory loss caused by modern ECT. Prospective computed tomography and magnetic resonance imaging studies of the brain show no evidence of ECT-induced structural changes (Coffey et al. 1991; Devanand et al. 1994). A comparison of eight patients who received more than 100 ECT treatments with matched control subjects who had never received ECT found no significant differences

in cognitive function (Devanand et al. 1991). Ninety-two depressed patients receiving either unilateral or bilateral ECT were interviewed regarding side effects both before and after the course of treatment. There was no change in cognitive complaints from pre-ECT to immediately after the ECT course (Devanand et al. 1995). In considering the possible effects of ECT on memory and cognition, it is important to keep in mind that depression itself commonly results in both memory and cognitive deficits. For patients with cognitive impairment secondary to depression, the therapeutic effect of ECT may contribute to improved cognitive functioning over time (Stoudemire et al. 1995).

The use of brief-pulse stimulation instead of sine wave stimulation can reduce the memory impairment (Squire et al. 1975). Unilateral stimulation results in fewer cognitive problems. Other cognitive deficits include memory deficits for nonverbal information and transient disorientation. Patients with pretreatment global cognitive impairment and prolonged disorientation in the acute postictal periods were the most vulnerable to persistent retrograde amnesia (Sobin et al. 1995). Memory loss is greatest for public events, with less impairment in memory for autobiographical information (Lisanby et al. 2000).

Post-ECT Prophylactic Treatment

Despite the acute efficacy of ECT, appropriate prophylactic treatment must be instituted after ECT to prevent relapse. Most commonly, antidepressant medications are used for this purpose. Unfortunately, many patients who receive ECT have been previously nonresponsive to standard antidepressant medications, and the efficacy of these treatments post-ECT is not clear (Sackeim et al. 1990). In such patients, lithium carbonate may be a useful agent for continuation therapy (Coppen et al. 1981; Perry and Tsuang 1979; Shapira et al. 1995). In a recent controlled study, the combination of nortriptyline and lithium resulted in a 39% relapse rate after 24 weeks, compared with 60% for nortriptyline alone and 84% for those who received placebo following response to ECT (Sackeim et al. 2001a). For patients who fail to respond to other prophylactic therapies, maintenance ECT (i.e., an outpatient treatment every week to every several weeks) may be effective (Schwarz et al. 1995).

Conclusion

After more than 50 years of use, ECT remains a safe, specific, and effective treatment regimen in psychiatry. The treatment is particularly effective in patients with severe depressions, including those that have delusional, suicidal, or psychomotor components. It is important, as it is concerning all somatic interventions in psychiatry, that ECT be recognized as a specific therapeutic tool that is only one component of a larger treatment plan and that includes psychosocial and other biological interventions. Adequate time must be allocated to discuss the risks, benefits, side effects, and overall experience of the procedure with patients and their families and to answer their questions.

Other Nonpharmacological Somatic Treatments

Several other nondrug methods have been investigated for the treatment of depression.

Light

Some patients with mood disorder have recurrent annual depressions, a condition termed *seasonal affective disorder* (SAD). The most common form of this condition involves regularly occurring winter depressions, characterized by the reverse neurovegetative pattern found in atypical depressions (e.g., hypersomnia, hyperphagia with carbohydrate craving, weight gain; Wehr and Rosenthal 1989). Summer depressions also have been reported; these seem to present with a clinical picture consistent with typical depression. Although many patients with SAD have bipolar disorder (usually type II or cyclothymic), some debate remains among investigators as to whether patients with SAD have exclusively bipolar disorders (Blehar and Rosenthal 1989). Strong evidence now indicates that patients with SAD who have winter depressions respond to phototherapy. Morning exposure to bright light appears to be the most efficacious (Terman et al. 1989), with current recommendations for a minimum of 2,500 lux for 2 hours each day for 1 week. Doses as high as 10,000 lux for briefer daily periods of exposure may be even more effective. Patients with milder depressions respond best to this form of treatment (Terman et al. 1989). Partial sleep deprivation also may induce remission in depressed patients (Post et al. 1976). This antidepressant effect is usually transient, but it may be prolonged by concomitant administration of lithium (Baxter et al. 1986).

Vagus Nerve Stimulation

Vagus nerve stimulation delivered by an implantable, programmable pulse generator is effective in reducing the frequency, duration, and/or intensity of seizures in patients with treatment-resistant, partial-onset epilepsy. The extension of vagus nerve stimulation from a treatment for epilepsy to possible treatment of depression parallels the use of anticonvulsants for treatment of mood disorders. The exact mechanisms of vagus nerve stimulation are still under investigation but are probably related to the neuroanatomical pathways of the vagus nerve (cranial nerve X), which included prominent connections to multiple areas of the brain that are implicated in mood disorders (for a review of the proposed mechanisms of action of vagus nerve stimulation, see George et al. 2000b). Vagus nerve stimulation is known to affect a variety of neurotransmitters, including norepinephrine, serotonin, GABA, and glutamate.

A recent pilot study of 30 patients with treatment-resistant depression reported a 40% response rate after 10 weeks of vagus nerve stimulation (Rush et al. 2000). Several tests of neuropsychological function showed improvements in this group (Sackeim et al. 2001b). After an additional 9 months of vagus nerve stimulation, the response rate was sustained and the remission rate significantly increased (Marangell et al. 2001). Vagus nerve stimulation treatment was well tolerated. Based on these data, vagus nerve stimulation was approved by the European Union and Canada in 2001 as a treatment for depression (unipolar or bipolar) in patients who are unresponsive to or intolerant of medications. Consideration of vagus nerve stimulation for FDA approval is pending the results of a larger controlled trial, which is currently under way.

Transcranial Magnetic Stimulation

Transcranial magnetic stimulation (TMS) uses a magnetic field to stimulate or inhibit cortical neurons. As opposed to electrical stimulation, the TMS device generates a focal magnetic field that easily moves through the skull. In current applications, TMS is not intended to produce a seizure, so anesthesia is not required. The area of cortex stimulated is related to placement of the coil on the skull—for example, placing the coil over motor cortex results in motor movement. For depression, the coil is most often placed over the left dorsolateral prefrontal cortex. In a 2-week study, 30 participants with major depressive episodes (unipolar or bipolar) received TMS (20 minutes every weekday to left prefrontal cortex) or a sham procedure. Nine of 20 participants in the TMS group responded, compared with none in the sham group (George et al. 2000a). Positive results also have been reported by other investigators (Berman et al. 2000; Grunhaus et al. 2000; Klein et al. 1999; Pascual-Leone et al. 1996). However, as noted in an editorial by Sackeim (2000), the TMS research to date has not shown that a substantial number of patients receive marked symptomatic relief for any meaningful period. Longer-term data and further refinement of this technique are needed before TMS becomes a clinically viable treatment option.

General Principles

Amsterdam JD, Brunswick DJ, Mendels J: The clinical application of tricyclic antidepressant pharmacokinetics and plasma levels. Am J Psychiatry 137:653–662, 1980

Cramer JA: Optimizing long-term patient compliance. Neurology 45:S25–S28, 1995

Food and Drug Administration: Bioavailability and bioequivalence requirements. Federal Register 57:17997–18001, 1992

Hamilton M: Rating depressive patients. J Clin Psychiatry 41:21–24, 1960

Hauck WW, Anderson S: Types of bioequivalence and related statistical considerations. International Journal of Clinical Pharmacology, Therapy, and Toxicology 30:181–187, 1992

Morris LS, Schulz RM: Medication compliance: the patient's perspective. Clin Ther 15:593–606, 1993

Physicians' Desk Reference, 51st Edition. Montvale, NJ, Medical Economics, 2001

Post RM, Leverich GS, Altshuler L, et al: Lithium-discontinuation-induced refractoriness: preliminary observations. Am J Psychiatry 149:1727–1729, 1992

Silver JM, Yudofsky SC: The Overt Aggression Scale: overview and clinical guidelines. J Neuropsychiatry Clin Neurosci 3:S22–S29, 1991

Yudofsky SC, Silver JM, Jackson W, et al: The Overt Aggression Scale for the objective rating of verbal and physical aggression. Am J Psychiatry 143:35–39, 1986

Antidepressant Drugs

Akiskal HS: Depression in cyclothymic and related temperaments: clinical and pharmacologic considerations (monograph). J Clin Psychiatry 10:37–43, 1992

American Psychiatric Association: Practice Guidelines for Major Depressive Disorder in Adults. Washington, DC, American Psychiatric Association, 1993

American Psychiatric Association: Diagnostic and Statistical Manual of Mental Disorders, 4th Edition, Text Revision. Washington, DC, American Psychiatric Association, 2000

Amsterdam J, Berwish NJ: High dose tranylcypromine therapy for refractory depression. Pharmacopsychiatry 22:21–25, 1989

Angst J: Natural history and epidemiology of depression, in Results of Community Studies in Prediction and Treatment of Recurrent Depression. Edited by Cobb J, Goeting N. Southampton, England, Duphar Medical Relations, 1990

Aranow A, Hudson J, Pope HG Jr, et al: Elevated antidepressant plasma levels after addition of fluoxetine. Am J Psychiatry 148:911–913, 1989

Armitage R, Rush AJ, Trivedi M, et al: The effects of nefazodone on sleep architecture in depression. Neuropsychopharmacology 10:123–127, 1994

Aronson MD, Hafez H: A case of trazodone-induced ventricular tachycardia. J Clin Psychiatry 47:388–389, 1986

Åsberg M: Individualization of treatment with tricyclic compounds. Med Clin North Am 58:1084–1091, 1974

Ashton AK, Bennett RG: Sildenafil treatment of serotonin reuptake inhibitor–induced sexual dysfunction. J Clin Psychiatry 60:194–195, 1999

Ballenger JC, Wheadon DE, Steiner M, et al: Double-blind, fixed-dose, placebo-controlled study of paroxetine in the treatment of panic disorder. Am J Psychiatry 155:36–42, 1998

Beasley CM Jr, Masica DN, Heiligenstein JH, et al: Possible monoamine oxidase inhibitor-serotonin uptake inhibitor interaction: fluoxetine clinical data and preclinical findings. J Clin Psychopharmacol 13:312–320, 1993

Boehnert MT, Lovejoy FH: Value of the QRS duration versus the serum drug level in predicting seizures and ventricular arrhythmias after an acute overdose of tricyclic antidepressants. N Engl J Med 313:474–479, 1985

Bourin M, Baker GB: The future of antidepressants. Biomed Pharmacother 50:7–12, 1996

Bouwer CD, Harvey BH: Phasic craving for carbohydrate observed with citalopram. Int Clin Psychopharmacol 11:273–278, 1996

Bremmer JD: A double blind comparison of mirtazapine, amitriptyline, and placebo in major depression. J Clin Psychiatry 56:519–525, 1995

Charney DS: Monoamine dysfunction and the pathophysiology and treatment of depression. J Clin Psychiatry 59(suppl 14):11–14, 1998

Claghorn JL, Earl CQ, Walczak DD, et al: Fluvoxamine maleate in the treatment of depression: a single-center, double-blind, placebo-controlled comparison with imipramine in outpatients. J Clin Psychopharmacol 16:113–120, 1996

Clomipramine Collaborative Study Group: Clomipramine in the treatment of patients with obsessive-compulsive disorder. Arch Gen Psychiatry 48:730–738, 1991

Conners CK, Casat CD, Gualtieri CT, et al: Bupropion hydrochloride in attention deficit disorder with hyperactivity. J Am Acad Child Adolesc Psychiatry 35:1314–1321, 1996

Cook EH Jr, Stein MA, Krasowski MD, et al: Association of attention-deficit disorder and the dopamine transporter gene. Am J Hum Genet 56:993–998, 1995

Coppen A, Mendelwicz J, Kielholz P: Pharmacotherapy of Depressive Disorders: A Consensus Statement. Geneva, Switzerland, World Health Organization, 1986

Coupet J, Rauh CE, Szues-Myers VA, et al: 2-Chloro-11-(1-piperazinyl) dibenz [b, f] [1, 4] oxazepine (amoxapine), an antidepressant with antipsychotic properties: a possible role for 7-hydroxyamoxapine. Biochem Pharmacol 28:2514–2515, 1979

Coupland NJ, Bell CJ, Potokar JP: Serotonin reuptake inhibitor withdrawal. J Clin Psychopharmacol 16:356–362, 1996

Dailey JW, Naritoku DK: Antidepressants and seizures: clinical anecdotes overshadow neuroscience. Biochem Pharmacol 52:1323–1329, 1996

Danish University Antidepressant Group: Paroxetine: a selective serotonin reuptake inhibitor showing better tolerance, but weaker antidepressant effect than clomipramine in a controlled multicenter study. J Affect Disord 18:289–299, 1990

De Boer T: The pharmacologic profile of mirtazapine. J Clin Psychiatry 57(suppl 4):19–25, 1996

De Montigny C, Gunberg S, Mayer A, et al: Lithium induces rapid relief of depression in tricyclic antidepressant nonresponders. Br J Psychiatry 138:252–256, 1981

Dinan TG, Barry S: A comparison of electroconvulsive therapy with a combined lithium and tricyclic combination among depressed tricyclic nonresponders. Acta Psychiatr Scand 80:97–100, 1989

Doughty MJ, Lyle WM: Medications used to prevent migraine headaches and their potential ocular adverse effects. Optometry and Vision Science 72:879–891, 1995

Downs JM, Downs AD, Rosenthal TL, et al: Increased plasma tricyclic antidepressant concentrations in two patients currently treated with fluoxetine. J Clin Psychiatry 50:226–227, 1989

Duman RS: Novel therapeutic approaches beyond the serotonin receptor. Biol Psychiatry 44:324–335, 1998

Ellingrod VL, Perry PJ: Venlafaxine: a heterocyclic antidepressant. American Journal of Hospital Pharmacy 51:3033–3046, 1994

Everett HC: The use of bethanechol chloride with tricyclic antidepressants. Am J Psychiatry 132:1202–1204, 1976

Fallon B, Foote B, Walsh T, et al: Spontaneous hypertensive episodes with monoamine oxidase inhibitors. J Clin Psychiatry 49:163–165, 1988

Fava M, Judge R, Hoog SL, et al: Fluoxetine versus sertraline and paroxetine in major depressive disorder: changes in weight with long-term treatment. J Clin Psychiatry 61:863–867, 2000

Fawcett J, Kravitz HM, Zajecka JM, et al: CNS stimulant potentiation of monoamine oxidase inhibitors in treatment-refractory depression. J Clin Psychopharmacol 11:127–132, 1991

Fawcett J, Marcus RN, Anton SF, et al: Response of anxiety and agitation symptoms during nefazodone treatment of major depression. J Clin Psychiatry 56(suppl 6):37–42, 1995

Fernstrom MH, Krowinski RL, Kupfer DJ: Chronic imipramine treatment and weight gain. Psychiatry Res 17:269–273, 1986

Fisher S, Kent TA, Bryant SG: Postmarketing surveillance by patient self-monitoring: preliminary data for sertraline versus fluoxetine. J Clin Psychiatry 56:288–296, 1995

Francois B, Marquet P, Roustan J, et al: Serotonin syndrome due to an overdose of moclobemide and clomipramine: a potentially life-threatening association. Intensive Care Med 23:122–124, 1997

Frank E, Kupfer DJ, Perel JM, et al: Three-year outcomes for maintenance therapies in recurrent depression. Arch Gen Psychiatry 47:1093–1099, 1990

Frazer A: Antidepressants. J Clin Psychiatry 58(suppl 6):9–25, 1997

Gammon GD, Hansen C: A case of akinesia induced by amoxapine. Am J Psychiatry 141:283–284, 1984

Gardner DM, Shulman KI, Walker SE, et al: The making of a user friendly MAOI diet. J Clin Psychiatry 57:99–104, 1996

Gelenberg AJ: Treating PMS. Biological Therapies in Psychiatry Newsletter 20:1, 1997

Gitlin MJ, Weiner H, Fairbanks L: Failure of T3 to potentiate tricyclic antidepressant response. J Affect Disord 13:267–272, 1987

Glassman AH: The newer antidepressant drugs and their cardiovascular effects. Psychopharmacol Bull 20:272–279, 1984

Glassman AH, Bigger JT: Cardiovascular effects of therapeutic doses of tricyclic antidepressants: a review. Arch Gen Psychiatry 39:815–820, 1981

Glassman AH, Bigger JT, Giardina EGV, et al: Clinical characteristics of imipramine-induced orthostatic hypotension. Lancet 1:468–472, 1979

Glassman AH, Johnson LL, Giardina EGV, et al: Psychotropic drug use in depressed patients with congestive heart failure. JAMA 250:1997–2001, 1983

Goldberg RJ: Nefazodone and venlafaxine: two new agents for the treatment of depression. J Fam Pract 41:591–594, 1995

Goldberg RJ, Capone RJ, Hunt JD: Cardiac complications following tricyclic antidepressant overdose: issues for monitoring policy. JAMA 254:1772–1775, 1985

Goldfrank LR, Lewin NA, Flomenbaum NE, et al: Antidepressants: tricyclics, tetracyclics, monoamine oxidase inhibitors, and others, in Goldfrank's Toxicologic Emergencies, 3rd Edition. Edited by Goldfrank LR, Flomenbaum ME, Lewis NA, et al. Norwalk, CT, Appleton-Century-Crofts, 1986, pp 351–363

Goodman LS, Alexander RD, Laciness DJ: Monoamine oxidase inhibitors and tricyclic antidepressants: comparison of their cardiovascular effects. J Clin Psychiatry 47:225–229, 1986

Goodman WK, Charney DS: Therapeutic applications and mechanisms of action of monoamine oxidase inhibitor and heterocyclic antidepressant drugs. J Clin Psychiatry 46(suppl 12):6–22, 1985

Goodwin FK, Prange AJ, Post RM, et al: Potentiation of antidepressant effects by L-triiodothyronine in tricyclic nonresponders. Am J Psychiatry 139:34–38, 1982

Gorman JM: The Essential Guide to Psychiatric Drugs. New York, St Martin's Press, 1990

Greenhill LL: Pharmacologic treatment of attention deficit hyperactivity disorder. Psychiatr Clin North Am 15:1–27, 1992

Greist JH, Jefferson JW, Kobak KA, et al: A 1 year double-blind placebo-controlled fixed dose study of sertraline in the treatment of obsessive-compulsive disorder. Int Clin Psychopharmacol 10:57–65, 1995

Hamilton JA, Halbreich U: Special aspects of neuropsychiatric illness in women: with a focus on depression. Annu Rev Med 44:355–364, 1993

Haria M, Fitton A, McTavish D: Trazodone: a review of its pharmacology, therapeutic use in depression and therapeutic potential in other disorders. Drugs Aging 4:331–355, 1994

Hodgman MJ, Martin TG, Krenzelok EP: Serotonin syndrome due to venlafaxine and maintenance tranylcypromine therapy. Hum Exp Toxicol 16:14–17, 1997

Jacobsen FM: Low-dose trazodone as a hypnotic in patients treated with MAOIs and other psychotropics: a pilot study. J Clin Psychiatry 51:298–302, 1990

Jankowsky D, Curtis G, Zisook S, et al: Trazodone-aggravated ventricular arrhythmias. J Clin Psychopharmacol 3:372–376, 1983

Jenike MA: Affective illness in elderly patients, part 2. Psychiatric Times 4:1, 1987

Joffe RT: T3 and lithium potentiation of tricyclic antidepressants. Am J Psychiatry 145:1317–1318, 1988

Joffe RT, Singer W: A comparison of triiodothyronine and thyroxine in the potentiation of tricyclic antidepressants. Psychiatry Res 32:241–251, 1990

Kahn D: Mysterious MAOI hypertensive episodes (letter). J Clin Psychiatry 49:38–39, 1988

Kahn D, Silver JM, Opler LA: The safety of switching rapidly from tricyclic antidepressants to monoamine oxidase inhibitors. J Clin Psychopharmacol 9:198–202, 1989

Kass FI, Oldham JM, Pardes H: The Columbia University College of Physicians and Surgeons Complete Home Guide to Mental Health. New York, Henry Holt, 1992

Kelsey JE: Dose-response relationship with venlafaxine. J Clin Psychopharmacol 16(suppl 2):21S–28S, 1996

Ketter TA, Jenkins JB, Schroeder DH, et al: Carbamazepine but not valproate induces bupropion metabolism. J Clin Psychopharmacol 15:327–333, 1995

Kiev A, Masco HL, Wenger TL, et al: The cardiovascular effects of bupropion and nortriptyline in depressed outpatients. Ann Clin Psychiatry 6:107–115, 1994

Kolecki P: Venlafaxine induced serotonin syndrome occurring after abstinence from phenelzine for more than two weeks (letter). J Toxicol Clin Toxicol 35:211–212, 1997

Krause R: Hypertensive episodes with tranylcypromine treatment. J Clin Psychopharmacol 9:232–233, 1989

Kuhn R: The treatment of depressive states with G 22355 (imipramine hydrochloride). Am J Psychiatry 115:459–464, 1958

Kukopoulos A, Caliari B, Tundo A, et al: Rapid cyclers, temperament, and antidepressants. Compr Psychiatry 24:249–258, 1983

Kupfer DJ, Coble PA, Rubinstein MS: Changes in weight during treatment for depression. Psychosom Med 41:535–544, 1979

Labbate LA, Pollack MH: Treatment of fluoxetine-induced sexual dysfunction with bupropion: a case report. Ann Clin Psychiatry 6:13–15, 1994

Leo RJ: Movement disorders associated with the serotonin selective reuptake inhibitors. J Clin Psychiatry 57:449–454, 1996

Liebowitz MR, Quitkin FM, Stewart JW, et al: Phenelzine vs imipramine in atypical depression: a preliminary report. Arch Gen Psychiatry 41:669–677, 1984

Linet LS: Mysterious MAOI hypertensive episodes. J Clin Psychiatry 47:563–565, 1986

Lingam VR, Lazarus LW, Groves L, et al: Methylphenidate in treating post-stroke depression. J Clin Psychiatry 49:151–153, 1988

Lipinski JF, Mallya G, Zimmerman P, et al: Fluoxetine-induced akathisia: clinical and theoretical implications. J Clin Psychiatry 50:339–342, 1989

Liu BA, Mittmann N, Knowles SR, et al: Hyponatremia and the syndrome of inappropriate secretion of antidiuretic hormone associated with the use of selective serotonin reuptake inhibitors: a review of spontaneous reports. Can Med Assoc J 155:519–527, 1996

Louie AK, Lewis TB, Lannon RA: Use of low-dose fluoxetine in major depression and panic disorder. J Clin Psychiatry 54:435–438, 1993

Lydiard RB: Tricyclic-resistant depression: treatment resistance or inadequate treatment? J Clin Psychiatry 46:412–417, 1985

Manna V, Bolino F, Di Cicco L: Chronic tension-type headache, mood depression and serotonin: therapeutic effects of fluvoxamine and mianserine. Headache 34:44–49, 1994

Marley E, Wozniak KM: Interactions of non-selective monoamine oxidase inhibitor, phenelzine, with inhibitors of 5-hydroxytryptamine, dopamine, or noradrenaline re-uptake inhibitors. J Psychiatr Res 18:191–203, 1984

Menza MA, Kaufman KR, Castellanos A: Modafinil augmentation of antidepressant treatment in depression. J Clin Psychiatry 61:378–381, 2000

Metz A, Shader RI: Adverse interactions encountered when using trazodone to treat insomnia associated with fluoxetine. Int Clin Psychopharmacol 5:191–194, 1990

Mitchell JE, Popkin JE: Antidepressant drug therapy and sexual dysfunction in men: a review. J Clin Psychopharmacol 3:76–79, 1983

Mitchell JE, Raymond N, Specker S: A review of the controlled trials of pharmacotherapy and psychotherapy in the treatment of bulimia nervosa. Int J Eat Disord 14:229–247, 1993

Nelson JC, Bowers MB: Delusional unipolar depression: description and drug response. Arch Gen Psychiatry 35:1321–1328, 1978

Nelson JC, Jatlow PI, Quinlan DM: Subjective complaints during desipramine treatment: relative importance of plasma drug concentrations and the severity of depression. Arch Gen Psychiatry 41:55–59, 1984

Nelson JC, Mazure CM, Bowers MB: A preliminary, open study of the combination of fluoxetine and desipramine. Arch Gen Psychiatry 48:303–307, 1991

Nierenberg AA, Keck PE Jr: Management of monoamine oxidase inhibitor-associated insomnia with trazodone. J Clin Psychopharmacol 9:42–45, 1989

Nierenberg AA, Feighner JP, Rudolph R, et al: Venlafaxine for treatment resistant unipolar depression. J Clin Psychopharmacol 14:419–423, 1994

NIMH Consensus Development Conference Statement: Mood disorders: pharmacologic prevention of recurrences. Am J Psychiatry 142:469–476, 1985

Oehrberg S, Christiansen PE, Behnke K, et al: Paroxetine in the treatment of panic disorder: a randomized, double-blind, placebo-controlled study. Br J Psychiatry 167:374–379, 1995

Ontiveros A, Fontaine R, Elie PL, et al: Refractory depression: the addition of lithium to fluoxetine or desipramine. Acta Psychiatr Scand 83:188–192, 1991

Pande AC, Calarco MM, Grunhaus LJ: Combined MAOI-TCA treatment in refractory depression, in Refractory Depression. Edited by Amsterdam J. New York, Raven, 1991, pp 115–121

Perry PJ: Pharmacotherapy for major depression with melancholic features: relative efficacy of tricyclic versus selective serotonin reuptake inhibitor antidepressants. J Affect Disord 39:1–6, 1996

Preskorn SH, Burke M: Somatic therapy for major depressive disorder: selection of an antidepressant. J Clin Psychiatry 53(suppl):5–18, 1992

Prien RF, Kupfer DJ: Continuation drug therapy for major depression episodes: how long should it be maintained? Am J Psychiatry 143:18–23, 1986

Quitkin F, Rifkin A, Klein DF: Monoamine oxidase inhibitors: a review of antidepressant effectiveness. Arch Gen Psychiatry 35:749–760, 1979

Quitkin FM, McGrath PJ, Stewart JW, et al: Chronological milestones to guide drug change: when should clinicians switch antidepressants? Arch Gen Psychiatry 53:785–792, 1996

Rabkin JG, Quitkin FM, McGrath P, et al: Adverse reactions to monoamine oxidase inhibitors, part II: treatment correlates and clinical management. J Clin Psychopharmacol 5:2–9, 1985

Ravaris CL, Robinson DS, Ives JO, et al: Phenelzine and amitriptyline in the treatment of depression: a comparison of present and past studies. Arch Gen Psychiatry 37:1075–1080, 1980

Roose SP: Modern cardiovascular standards for psychotropic drugs. Psychopharmacol Bull 28:35–43, 1992

Roose SP, Glassman AH, Siris SG, et al: Comparison of imipramine- and nortriptyline-induced orthostatic hypotension: a meaningful difference. J Clin Psychopharmacol 1:316–319, 1981

Roose SP, Glassman AH, Giardina EGV, et al: Tricyclic antidepressants in depressed patients with cardiac conduction disease. Arch Gen Psychiatry 44:273–275, 1987

Roose SP, Dalack GW, Glassman AH, et al: Cardiovascular effects of bupropion in depressed patients with heart disease. Am J Psychiatry 148:512–516, 1991

Rosenbaum JF, Fava M, Hoog SL, et al: Selective serotonin reuptake inhibitor discontinuation syndrome: a randomized clinical trial. Biol Psychiatry 44:75–76, 1998

Rosenstein DL, Nelson JC, Jacobs SC: Seizures associated with antidepressants: a review. J Clin Psychiatry 54:289–299, 1993

Ross DR, Walker JI, Paterson J: Akathisia induced by amoxapine. Am J Psychiatry 140:115–116, 1983

Rothschild AJ: Selective serotonin reuptake inhibitor-induced sexual dysfunction: efficacy of a drug holiday. Am J Psychiatry 152:1514–1516, 1995

Sachs GS, Later B, Stol AL, et al: A double-blind trial of bupropion versus desipramine for bipolar depression. J Clin Psychiatry 55:391–393, 1994

Schenk CH, Remick RA: Sublingual nifedipine in the treatment of hypertensive crisis associated with monoamine oxidase inhibitors (letter). Ann Emerg Med 18:114–115, 1989

Scher M, Krieger JN, Juergens S: Trazodone and priapism. Am J Psychiatry 140:1362–1363, 1983

Schmauss M, Kapfhammer HP, Meyr P, et al: Combined MAO-inhibitor and tri-(tetra)cyclic antidepressant treatment in therapy resistant depression. Prog Neuropsychopharmacol Biol Psychiatry 12:523–532, 1988

Selikoff IJ, Robitzek EH, Ornstein GG: Toxicity of hydrazine derivatives of isonicotinic acid in the chemotherapy of human tuberculosis. Quarterly Bulletin of SeaView Hospital 13:17–26, 1952

Smith WT, Glaudin V, Panagides J, et al: Mirtazapine versus amitriptyline versus placebo in the treatment of major depressive disorder. Psychopharmacol Bull 20:191–196, 1990

Spivak B, Ravdan M, Shine M: Postural hypotension with syncope possibly precipitated by trazodone. Am J Psychiatry 144:1512–1513, 1987

Stoll AL, Mayer PV, Kolbrener M, et al: Antidepressant-associated mania: a controlled comparison with spontaneous mania. Am J Psychiatry 151:1642–1645, 1994

Szuba MP, Hornig-Rohan M, Amsterdam J: Rapid conversion from one monoamine oxidase inhibitor to another. J Clin Psychiatry 58:307–310, 1997

Tate JL: Extrapyramidal symptoms in a patient taking haloperidol and fluoxetine (letter). Am J Psychiatry 148:339–340, 1989

Thase ME: Effects of venlafaxine on blood pressure: a meta-analysis of original data from 3744 depressed patients. J Clin Psychiatry 59:502–508, 1998

Thase ME, Kupfer DJ, Frank E, et al: Treatment of imipramine-resistant depressant, II: an open clinical trial of lithium augmentation. J Clin Psychiatry 50:413–417, 1989

Thase ME, Entsuah AR, Rudolph RL: Remission rates during treatment with venlafaxine or selective serotonin reuptake inhibitors. Br J Psychiatry 178:234–241, 2001

Thornton JE, Stahl SM: Case report of tardive dyskinesia and parkinsonism associated with amoxapine therapy. Am J Psychiatry 141:704–705, 1984

Tiller JW, Bouwer C, Behnke K: Moclobemide and fluoxetine for panic disorder. International Panic Disorder Study Group. Eur Arch Psychiatry Clin Neurosci 249(suppl):S7–S10, 1999

Tollefson GD: Monoamine oxidase inhibitors: a review. J Clin Psychiatry 44:280–288, 1983

Tollefson GD, Birkett M, Koran L, et al: Continuation treatment of OCD: double-blind and open-label experience with fluoxetine. J Clin Psychiatry 55:69–76, 1994

van Harten J: Overview of the pharmacokinetics of fluvoxamine. Clin Pharmacokinet 29(suppl 1):1–9, 1995

van Vliet IM, den Boer JA, Westenberg HG, et al: A double-blind comparative study of brofaromine and fluvoxamine in outpatients with panic disorder. J Clin Psychopharmacol 16:299–306, 1996

Vaughan DA: Interaction of fluoxetine with tricyclic antidepressants (letter). Am J Psychiatry 145:1478, 1988

Vitullo RN, Wharton JM, Allen NB, et al: Trazodone-related exercise-induced nonsustained ventricular tachycardia. Chest 98:247–248, 1990

Walczak DD, Apter JT, Halikas JA, et al: The oral dose-effect relationship for fluvoxamine: a fixed-dose comparison against placebo in depressed outpatients. Ann Clin Psychiatry 8:139–151, 1996

Walker SE, Shulman KI, Tailor SA, et al: Tyramine content of previously restricted foods in monoamine oxidase inhibitor diets. J Clin Psychopharmacol 16:383–388, 1996

Wedin GP, Oderda GM, Klein-Schwartz W, et al: Relative toxicity of cyclic antidepressants. Ann Emerg Med 15:797–804, 1986

Wehr TA, Goodwin FK: Rapid cycling in manic-depressives induced by tricyclic antidepressants. Arch Gen Psychiatry 36:555–559, 1979

Weilburg JB, Rosenbaum JF, Biederman J, et al: Fluoxetine added to non-MAOI antidepressant converts non-responders to responders: a preliminary report. J Clin Psychiatry 50:447–449, 1989

Weise CC, Stein MK, Pereira-Ogan J, et al: Amitriptyline once daily versus three times daily in depressed outpatients. Arch Gen Psychiatry 37:555–560, 1980

White K, Simpson G: Combined MAOI-tricyclic antidepressant treatment: a reevaluation. J Clin Psychopharmacol 1:264–282, 1981

Wikander I, Sundblad C, Andersch B, et al: Citalopram in premenstrual dysphoria: is intermittent treatment during luteal phases more effective than continuous medication throughout the menstrual cycle? J Clin Psychopharmacol 18:390–398, 1998

Woo MH, Smythe MA: Association of SIADH with selective serotonin reuptake inhibitors. Ann Pharmacother 31:108–110, 1997

Yager J: Bethanecol chloride can reverse erectile and ejaculatory dysfunction induced by tricyclic antidepressants and mazindol: case report. J Clin Psychiatry 47:210–211, 1986

Yudofsky SC: Electroconvulsive therapy in general hospital psychiatry: a focus of new indications and technologies. Gen Hosp Psychiatry 3:292–296, 1981

Yudofsky SC, Hales RE, Ferguson T: What You Need to Know About Psychiatric Drugs. New York, Grove Weidenfeld, 1991

Zarate CA Jr, Tohen M, Baraibar G, et al: Prescribing trends of antidepressants in bipolar depression. J Clin Psychiatry 56:260–264, 1995

Zisook S: A clinical overview of monoamine oxidase inhibitors. Psychosomatics 26:240–246, 1985

Anxiolytics, Sedatives, and Hypnotics

Abernethy DR, Greenblatt DJ, Ochs HR, et al: Benzodiazepine drug-drug interactions commonly occurring in clinical practice. Curr Med Res Opin 8(suppl 4):80–93, 1984

American Psychiatric Association: Benzodiazepine Dependence, Toxicity, and Abuse: A Task Force Report of the American Psychiatric Association. Washington, DC, American Psychiatric Association, 1990

Angus WR, Romney DM: The effect of diazepam on patients' memory. J Clin Psychopharmacol 4:203–206, 1984

Ashton H: Protracted withdrawal syndromes from benzodiazepines. J Subst Abuse Treat 8:19–28, 1991

Black B, Uhde TW, Tancer ME: Fluoxetine for the treatment of social phobia (letter). J Clin Psychopharmacol 12:293–295, 1992

Brantigan CO, Brantigan TA, Joseph N: Effect of beta blockade and beta stimulation on stage fright. Am J Med 72:88–94, 1982

Breier A, Charney DS, Nelson JC: Seizures induced by abrupt discontinuation of alprazolam. Am J Psychiatry 141:1606–1607, 1984

Busto U, Sellers EM, Naranjo CA, et al: Withdrawal reactions after long-term therapeutic use of benzodiazepines. N Engl J Med 315:854–857, 1986

Charney DS, Woods SW: Benzodiazepine treatment of panic disorder: a comparison of alprazolam and lorazepam. J Clin Psychiatry 50:418–423, 1989

Clomipramine Collaborative Study Group: Clomipramine in the treatment of patients with obsessive-compulsive disorder. Arch Gen Psychiatry 48:730–738, 1991

Cohn J, Wilcox CS: Low-sedation potential of buspirone compared with alprazolam and lorazepam in the treatment of anxious patients: a double-blind study. J Clin Psychiatry 47:409–412, 1986

Cole JO, Orzak MG, Beake B, et al: Assessment of the abuse liability of buspirone in recreational sedative users. J Clin Psychiatry 43:69–74, 1982

Davidson JRT, Ford SM, Smith RD, et al: Long-term treatment of social phobia with clonazepam. J Clin Psychiatry 52(suppl):16–20, 1991

Davidson JR, DuPont RL, Hedges D, et al: Efficacy, safety, and tolerability of venlafaxine extended release and buspirone in outpatients with generalized anxiety disorder. J Clin Psychiatry 60:528–535, 1999

den Boer JA, van Vliet IM, Westenberg HG: Recent developments in the psychopharmacology of social phobia. Eur Arch Psychiatry Clin Neurosci 244:309–316, 1995

Dixon J, Power SJ, Grundy EM, et al: Sedation for local anaesthesia: comparison of intravenous midazolam and diazepam. Anaesthesia 39:372–378, 1984

Drew PJ, Barnes JN, Evans SJ: The effect of acute beta-adrenoceptor blockade on examination performance. Br J Clin Pharmacol 19:783–786, 1985

Dunner DL, Ishiki D, Avery DH, et al: Effect of alprazolam and diazepam on anxiety and panic attacks in panic disorder: a controlled study. J Clin Psychiatry 47:458–460, 1986

Elie R, Lamontagne Y: Alprazolam and diazepam in the treatment of generalized anxiety. J Clin Psychopharmacol 4:125–129, 1985

Ellinwood EH Jr, Heatherly DG, Nikaido MA, et al: Comparative pharmacokinetics and pharmacodynamics of lorazepam, alprazolam and diazepam. Psychopharmacology (Berl) 86:393–451, 1985

Ewing JA, Elliot WJ, Maio LD, et al: You don't have to be a neuroscientist to forget everything with triazolam but it helps. JAMA 259:350–352, 1988

Feder R: Lithium augmentation of clomipramine (letter). J Clin Psychiatry 49:458, 1988

Finkle BS, McCloskey KL, Goodman LS: Diazepam and drug-associated deaths: a survey in the United States and Canada. JAMA 242:429–434, 1979

Fontaine R, Chouinard G, Annable L: Rebound anxiety in anxious patients after abrupt withdrawal of benzodiazepine treatment. Am J Psychiatry 141:848–852, 1984

Freeman CP, Trimble MR, Deakin JF, et al: Fluvoxamine versus clomipramine in the treatment of obsessive-compulsive disorder: a multicenter, randomized, double-blind parallel group. J Clin Psychiatry 55:301–305, 1994

Fyer AJ, Liebowitz JR, Gorman JM, et al: Discontinuation of alprazolam treatment in panic patients. Am J Psychiatry 144:303–308, 1987

Gastfried DR, Rosenbaum JF: Adjunctive buspirone in benzodiazepine treatment of four patient with panic disorder. Am J Psychiatry 146:914–916, 1989

Gelernter CS, Uhde TW, Cimbolic P, et al: Cognitive-behavioral and pharmacologic treatments for social phobia: a preliminary study. Arch Gen Psychiatry 48:938–945, 1991

Goldberg HL, Finnerty RJ: The comparative efficacy of buspirone and diazepam in the treatment of anxiety. Am J Psychiatry 136:1184–1187, 1979

Goodman WK, Price LH, Delgado PL, et al: Specificity of serotonin reuptake inhibitors in the treatment of obsessive-compulsive disorder: comparison of fluvoxamine and desipramine. Arch Gen Psychiatry 47:577–585, 1990

Goodman WK, Kozak MJ, Liebowitz M, et al: Treatment of obsessive-compulsive disorder with fluvoxamine: a multicentre, double-blind, placebo-controlled trial. Int Clin Psychopharmacol 11:21–29, 1996

Greenblatt DJ: Pharmacology of benzodiazepine hypnotics. J Clin Psychiatry 53(suppl):7–13, 1992

Greenblatt DJ, Allen MD, Noel BJ, et al: Acute overdosage with benzodiazepine derivatives. Clin Pharmacol Ther 21:497–514, 1977a

Greenblatt DJ, Allen MD, Shader RI: Toxicity of high dose flurazepam in the elderly. Clin Pharmacol Ther 21:355–361, 1977b

Greenblatt DJ, Divoll M, Harmatz JS, et al: Kinetics and clinical effects of flurazepam in young and elderly noninsomniacs. Clin Pharmacol Ther 30:475–486, 1981

Greenblatt DJ, Shader RI, Abernethy DR: Drug therapy: current status of benzodiazepines. N Engl J Med 309:410–416, 1983

Greenblatt DJ, Shader RI, Divol M, et al: Adverse reactions to triazolam, flurazepam, and placebo in controlled clinical trials. J Clin Psychiatry 45:192–195, 1984

Greist J, Chouinard G, DuBoff E, et al: Double-blind parallel comparison of three dosages of sertraline and placebo in outpatients with obsessive-compulsive disorder. Arch Gen Psychiatry 52:289–295, 1995

Griffith JD, Jasinski DR, Casten GP, et al: Investigation of the abuse liability of buspirone in alcohol-dependent patients. Am J Med 80(suppl 3B):30–35, 1986

Harvey KV, Balon R: Augmentation with buspirone: a review. Ann Clin Psychiatry 7:143–147, 1995

Hertley LR, Ungapen S, Davie I, et al: The effect of beta-adrenergic blocking drugs on speakers' performance and memory. Br J Psychiatry 142:512–517, 1983

Hewlett WA, Vinogradov S, Agras WS: Clonazepam treatment of obsessions and compulsions. J Clin Psychiatry 51:158–161, 1990

Hoehn-Saric R, McLeod DR, Zimmerli WD: Differential effects of alprazolam and imipramine in generalized anxiety disorder: somatic vs psychic symptoms. J Clin Psychiatry 49:293–301, 1988

Hollander E, DeCaria CM, Schneier FR, et al: Fenfluramine augmentation of serotonin reuptake blockade antiobsessional treatment. J Clin Psychiatry 51:119–123, 1990

Jack ML, Colburn WA, Spirt NM, et al: A pharmacokinetic/pharmacodynamic/receptor binding model to predict the onset and duration of pharmacological activity of the benzodiazepines. Prog Neuropsychopharmacol Biol Psychiatry 7:629–635, 1982

Jefferson JW: Social phobia: a pharmacologic treatment overview. J Clin Psychiatry 56(suppl):18–24, 1995

Jenike MA: Approaches to the patient with treatment-refractory obsessive-compulsive disorder. J Clin Psychiatry 51(suppl):15–21, 1990

Jenike MA, Baer L, Buttolph L: Buspirone augmentation of fluoxetine in patients with obsessive-compulsive disorder. J Clin Psychopharmacol 12:13–14, 1991

Jenkins SW, Ruegg R, Moeller FG: Gepirone in the treatment of major depression. J Clin Psychopharmacol 10(suppl):77S–85S, 1990

Kahn RJ, Menair D, Lipman RS, et al: Imipramine and chlordiazepoxide in depressive and anxiety disorders: efficacy in anxious outpatients. Arch Gen Psychiatry 43:79–85, 1986

Kales A, Kales JD: Sleep laboratory studies of hypnotic drugs: efficacy and withdrawal effects. J Clin Psychopharmacol 3:140–150, 1983

Kales A, Bixler EO, Vela-Bueno A, et al: Comparison of short and long half-life benzodiazepine hypnotics: triazolam and guazepam. Clin Pharmacol Ther 40:378–386, 1986

Keller MB, Hanks DL: Anxiety symptom relief in depression treatment outcomes. J Clin Psychiatry 56(suppl):22–29, 1995

Klein DF, Ross DC, Cohen P: Panic and avoidance in agoraphobia; application of path analysis to treatment studies. Arch Gen Psychiatry 44:377–385, 1987

Kupfer KJ, Reynolds CF: Management of insomnia. N Engl J Med 336:341–346, 1997

Lader M, Olajide D: A comparison of buspirone and placebo in relieving benzodiazepine withdrawal symptoms. J Clin Psychopharmacol 7:11–15, 1987

Laird LK: Issues in the monopharmacotherapy and polypharmacotherapy of obsessive-compulsive disorder. Psychopharmacol Bull 32:569–578, 1996

Leppik IE, Derivan AT, Homan RW, et al: Double-blind study of lorazepam and diazepam in status epilepticus. JAMA 249:1452–1454, 1983

Levy AB: Delirium and seizures due to abrupt alprazolam withdrawal: case report. J Clin Psychiatry 45:38–39, 1984

Liebowitz MA, Gorman JM, Fyer AJ, et al: Pharmacotherapy of social phobia: an interim report of a placebo-controlled comparison of phenelzine and atenolol. J Clin Psychiatry 49:252–257, 1988

Linnoila M, Erwin CW, Brendle A, et al: Psychomotor effects of diazepam in anxious patients and healthy volunteers. J Clin Psychopharmacol 3:88 96, 1983

Lister RG: The amnestic action of benzodiazepines in man. Neurosci Biobehav Rev 9:87–94, 1985

Lucki I: Behavioral studies of serotonin receptor antagonists as antidepressant drugs. J Clin Psychiatry 52(suppl):24–31, 1991

Lucki I, Rickels K, Geller AM: Chronic use of benzodiazepines and psychomotor and cognitive test performance. Psychopharmacology (Berl) 88:426–433, 1986

Mac DS, Kumar R, Goodwin DW: Anterograde amnesia with oral lorazepam. J Clin Psychiatry 46:137–138, 1985

Markovitz PJ, Stagro SJ, Calabrese JR: Buspirone augmentation of fluoxetine in obsessive-compulsive disorder. Am J Psychiatry 147:798–800, 1990

Marshall RD, Schneier FR, Fallon BA, et al: Medication therapy for social phobia. J Clin Psychiatry 55:33–37, 1994

Mavissakalian MR, Jones B, Olson S, et al: Clomipramine in obsessive-compulsive disorder: clinical response and plasma levels. J Clin Psychopharmacol 10:261–268, 1990

McDougle CJ, Goodman WK, Price LH, et al: Neuroleptic addition in fluvoxamine-refractory obsessive-compulsive disorder. Am J Psychiatry 147:652–654, 1990

McDougle CJ, Fleischmann RL, Epperson CN, et al: Risperidone addition in fluvoxamine-refractory obsessive-compulsive disorder: three cases. J Clin Psychiatry 56:526–528, 1995

Medawarn C, Rassaby E: Triazolam overdose, alcohol, and manslaughter. Lancet 338:1515–1516, 1991

Mendelson WB: Clinical distinction between long-acting and short-acting benzodiazepines. J Clin Psychiatry 53(suppl):4–7, 1992

Mitler MM, Seidel WF, Van Den Hoel J, et al: Comparative hypnotic effects of flurazepam, triazolam, and placebo: a long-term simultaneous nighttime and daytime study. J Clin Psychopharmacol 4:2–13, 1984

Morris HH, Estes ML: Traveler's amnesia: transient global amnesia secondary to triazolam. JAMA 258:945–946, 1987

Moskowitz H, Smiley A: Effects of chronically administered buspirone and diazepam on driving-related skills and performance. J Clin Psychiatry 43:45–55, 1982

Mundo E, Bareggi SR, Pirola R, et al: Long-term pharmacotherapy of obsessive-compulsive disorder: a double-blind controlled study. J Clin Psychopharmacol 17:4–10, 1997

Munjack DJ, Bruns J, Baltazar PL, et al: A pilot study of buspirone in the treatment of social phobia. J Anxiety Disord 5:87–98, 1991

NIMH [National Institute of Mental Health] Consensus Development Conference: Drugs and insomnia: the use of medication to promote sleep. JAMA 251:2410–2414, 1984

Noyes R Jr, Garvey MJ, Cook BL, et al: Benzodiazepine withdrawal: a review of evidence. J Clin Psychiatry 49:382–389, 1988

Oehrberg S, Christiansen PE, Behnke K, et al: Paroxetine in the treatment of panic disorder: a randomised, double-blind, placebo-controlled study. Br J Psychiatry 167:374–379, 1995

Pecknold JC, Swinson RP: Taper withdrawal studies with alprazolam in patients with panic disorder and agoraphobia. Psychopharmacol Bull 22:173–176, 1986

Perse TL, Greist JH, Jefferson JW, et al: Fluvoxamine treatment of obsessive-compulsive disorder. Am J Psychiatry 144:1543–1548, 1988

Physicians' Desk Reference, 51st Edition. Montvale, NJ, Medical Economics, 2001

Pigott TA, Pato MT, Bernstein SE, et al: Controlled comparisons of clomipramine and fluoxetine in the treatment of obsessive-compulsive disorders: behavioral and biological results. Arch Gen Psychiatry 47:926–932, 1990

Rakel RE: Long-term buspirone therapy for chronic anxiety: a multicenter international study to determine safety. South Med J 83:194–198, 1990

Ravizza L, Barzega G, Bellino S, et al: Drug treatment of obsessive-compulsive disorder (OCD): long-term trial with clomipramine and selective serotonin reuptake inhibitors (SSRIs). Psychopharmacol Bull 32:167–173, 1996

Regestein QR, Reich P: Agitation observed during treatment with newer hypnotic drugs. J Clin Psychiatry 46:280–283, 1985

Reitan JA, Porter W, Braunstein M: Comparison of psychomotor skills and amnesia after induction of anesthesia with midazolam or thiopental. Anesth Analg 65:933–937, 1986

Rickels K: The clinical use of hypnotics: indications for use and the need for a variety of hypnotics. Acta Psychiatr 332(suppl):132–141, 1986

Rickels K, Case WG, Downing RW, et al: Long-term diazepam therapy and clinical outcome. JAMA 250:767–771, 1983

Rickels K, Schweizer E, Csanelosi I, et al: Long-term treatment of anxiety and risk of withdrawal: prospective comparison of clonazepam and buspirone. Arch Gen Psychiatry 45:444–450, 1988

Rickels K, Downing R, Schweizer E, et al: Antidepressants for the treatment of generalized anxiety disorder: a placebo-controlled comparison of imipramine, trazodone, and diazepam. Arch Gen Psychiatry 50:884–895, 1993

Rickles K, Pollack MH, Sheehan DV, et al: Efficacy of extended-release venlafaxine in nondepressed outpatients with generalized anxiety disorder. Am J Psychiatry 157:968–974, 2000

Rosenberg L, Mitchell AA, Parsells JL, et al: Lack of relation of oral clefts to diazepam use during pregnancy. N Engl J Med 309:1282–1285, 1983

Roth T, Roehrs TA: Issues in the use of benzodiazepine therapy. J Clin Psychiatry 53(suppl):14–18, 1992

Roth T, Hartse KM, Saab PG, et al: The effects of flurazepam, lorazepam, and triazolam on sleep and memory. Psychopharmacology (Berl) 70:231–237, 1980

Roth T, Roehr T, Wittig R, et al: Benzodiazepines and memory. Br J Clin Pharmacol 18(suppl):45S–49S, 1984

Rothschild AJ: Disinhibition, amnestic reactions, and other adverse reactions secondary to triazolam: a review of the literature. J Clin Psychiatry 53(suppl):69–79, 1992

Salzman C, Shader RI, Greenblatt DJ, et al: Long vs short half-life benzodiazepines in the elderly: kinetics and clinical effects of diazepam and oxazepam. Arch Gen Psychiatry 40:293–297, 1983

Schneier FR, Liebowitz MR, Davies SO, et al: Fluoxetine in panic disorder. J Clin Psychopharmacol 10:119–121, 1990

Schneier FR, Saoud JB, Campeas RC, et al: Buspirone in social phobia. J Clin Psychopharmacol 13:251–256, 1992

Schopf J: Withdrawal phenomena after long-term administration of benzodiazepines: a review of recent investigations. Pharmacopsychiatrie Neuro-Psychopharmakologie 16:1–8, 1983

Schweizer E, Rickels K, Lucki I: Resistance to anti-anxiety effects of buspirone in patients with a history of benzodiazepine use. N Engl J Med 314:719–720, 1986

Seidel WF, Cohen SA, Bliwise NG, et al: Buspirone: an anxiolytic without sedative effect. Psychopharmacology (Berl) 87:371–373, 1985

Sellers EM, Naranjo CA, Harrison M, et al: Oral diazepam loading: simplified treatment of alcohol withdrawal. Clin Pharmacol Ther 34:822–826, 1983

Sellers EM, Schneiderman JF, Romach MK, et al: Comparative drug effects and abuse liability of lorazepam, buspirone, and secobarbital in nondependent subjects. J Clin Psychopharmacol 12:79–85, 1992

Sheehan DV, Ballenger J, Jacobsen G: Treatment of endogenous anxiety with phobic, hysterical, and hypochondriacal symptoms. Arch Gen Psychiatry 39:51–59, 1980

Sheehan DV, Raj AB, Sheehan KH, et al: Is buspirone effective for panic disorder? J Clin Psychopharmacol 10:3–11, 1990

Shiono PH, Mills JL: Oral clefts and diazepam use during pregnancy (letter). N Engl J Med 311:919–920, 1983

Spier SA, Tesar GE, Rosenbaum JF, et al: Treatment of panic disorder and agoraphobia with clonazepam. J Clin Psychiatry 47:238–242, 1986

Sramek JJ, Tansman M, Suri A, et al: Efficacy of buspirone in generalized anxiety disorder with coexisting mild depressive symptoms. J Clin Psychiatry 57:287–291, 1996

Sullivan JT, Sellers EM: Treating alcohol, barbiturate, and benzodiazepine withdrawal. Rational Drug Therapy 20:1–8, 1986

Suranyi-Cadotte BE, Bodnoff SR, Welner SA: Antidepressant-anxiolytic interactions: involvement of the benzodiazepine-GABA and serotonin systems. Prog Neuropsychopharmacol Biol Psychiatry 14:633–654, 1990

Tallman JF, Paul SM, Skolnick P, et al: Receptors for the age of anxiety: pharmacology of the benzodiazepines. Science 207:274–281, 1980

Teboul E, Chouinard G: A guide to benzodiazepine selection, part 1: pharmacological aspects. Can J Psychiatry 35:700–710, 1990

Tesar GE: High-potency benzodiazepines for short-term management of panic disorder: the U.S. evidence. J Clin Psychiatry 15(suppl):4–10, 1990

Tesar GE, Rosenbaum JF, Pollack MH, et al: Double-blind, placebo-controlled comparison of clonazepam and alprazolam for panic disorder. J Clin Psychiatry 52:69–76, 1991

Tollefson GD, Birkett M, Koran L, et al: Continuation treatment of OCD: double-blind and open-label experience with fluoxetine. J Clin Psychiatry 55(suppl):69–76, 1994

Tyrer PJ, Owen R, Dawling S: Gradual withdrawal of diazepam after long-term therapy. Lancet 1:1402–1406, 1983

Van Ameringen M, Mancini C, Streiner DL: Fluoxetine efficacy in social phobia. J Clin Psychiatry 54:27–32, 1993

van Vliet IM, Westenberg HG, Den Boer JA: MAO inhibitors in panic disorder: clinical effects of treatment with brofaromine: a double blind placebo controlled study. Psychopharmacology 112:483–489, 1993

Votey SR, Bosse GM, Bayer MJ, et al: Flumazenil: a new benzodiazepine antagonist. Ann Emerg Med 20:181–188, 1991

Wamsley JK, Hunt MA: Relative affinity of quazepam for type-1 benzodiazepine receptors in brain. J Clin Psychiatry 52(suppl):15–20, 1991

Westenberg HGM, den Boer JA: Clinical and biochemical effects of selective serotonin-uptake inhibitors in anxiety disorders, in Selective Serotonin Reuptake Inhibitors: Novel or Commonplace Agents? Edited by Gastpar M, Wakelin JS. Basel, Switzerland, S Karger, 1988, pp 84–99

Westenberg HG, den Boer JA: New findings in the treatment of panic disorder. Pharmacopsychiatry 26(suppl):30–33, 1993

Wheadon DE: Placebo controlled multi-center trial of fluoxetine in OCD. Paper presented at the Fifth World Congress of Biological Psychiatry, Florence, Italy, June 1991

Yudofsky SC, Silver JM: Beta-blockers in the treatment of performance anxiety. Harvard Mental Health Letter 4:8, 1987

Zipursky RB, Baker RW, Zimmer B: Alprazolam withdrawal delirium unresponsive to diazepam: case report. J Clin Psychiatry 46:344–345, 1985

Zitrin CM, Klein DF, Woerner MG, et al: Treatment of phobias: comparison of imipramine and placebo. Arch Gen Psychiatry 40:125–138, 1983

Zohar J, Judge R: Paroxetine versus clomipramine in the treatment of obsessive-compulsive disorder. Br J Psychiatry 169:468–474, 1996

Antipsychotic Drugs

Acri AA, Henretig FM: Effects of risperidone in overdose. Am J Emerg Med 16:498–501, 1998

Adler LA, Angrist B, Peselow E, et al: Efficacy of propranolol in neuroleptic-induced akathisia. J Clin Psychopharmacol 5:164–166, 1985

Adler LA, Angrist B, Reiter S, et al: Neuroleptic-induced akathisia: a review. Psychopharmacology (Berl) 97:1–11, 1989

Adler LA, Angrist B, Weinreb H, et al: Studies on the time course and efficacy of β-blockers in neuroleptic-induced akathisia and the akathisia of idiopathic Parkinson's disease. Psychopharmacol Bull 27:107–111, 1991

Adler LA, Peselow E, Rotrosen J, et al: Vitamin E in the treatment of tardive dyskinesia. Am J Psychiatry 150:1405–1407, 1993

Adler LA, Edson R, Lavori P, et al: Long-term treatment effects of vitamin E for tardive dyskinesia. Biol Psychiatry 43:868–872, 1998

Aherwadker SJ, Eferdigil MC, Coulshed N: Chlorpromazine therapy and associated acute disturbances of cardiac rhythm. Br Heart J 36:1251–1252, 1964

AIMS: Abnormal Involuntary Movement Scale. Psychopharmacol Bull 24:781–783, 1988

Akhtar S, Jajor TR, Kumar S: Vitamin E in the treatment of tardive dyskinesia. J Postgrad Med 39:124–126, 1993

Allison DB, Mentore JL, Heo M, et al: Antipsychotic-induced weight gain: a comprehensive research synthesis. Am J Psychiatry 156:1686–1696, 1999

Altshuler LL, Cohen L, Szuba MP, et al: Pharmacologic management of psychiatric illness during pregnancy: dilemmas and guidelines. Am J Psychiatry 153:592–606, 1996

Alvir JMJ, Lieberman JA: Agranulocytosis: incidence and risk factors. J Clin Psychiatry 55(suppl B):137–138, 1994

Alvir JMJ, Lieberman JA, Safferman AZ: Clozapine-induced agranulocytosis: incidence and risk factors in the United States. N Engl J Med 329:162–167, 1993

American Psychiatric Association: Tardive Dyskinesia: A Task Force Report of the American Psychiatric Association. Washington, DC, American Psychiatric Association, 1992

American Psychiatric Association: Practice guideline for the treatment of patients with schizophrenia. Am J Psychiatry 154(suppl):1–63, 1997

Anderson ES, Powers PS: Neuroleptic malignant syndrome associated with clozapine use. J Clin Psychiatry 52:102–104, 1991

Anton-Stephens D: Preliminary observations on the psychiatric use of chlorpromazine. Journal of Mental Science 100:543–547, 1953

Appleton WS, Davis JM: Practical Clinical Psychopharmacology, 2nd Edition. Baltimore, MD, Williams & Wilkins, 1980

Arana GW, Goff DC, Friedman H, et al: Does carbamazepine-induced reduction of plasma haloperidol levels worsen psychotic symptoms? Am J Psychiatry 143:650–651, 1986

Arana GW, Goff DC, Baldessarini RJ, et al: Efficacy of anticholinergic prophylaxis for neuroleptic-induced acute dystonia. Am J Psychiatry 145:993–996, 1988

Arvanitis LA, Miller BG: Multiple fixed doses of "Seroquel" (quetiapine) in patients with acute exacerbation of schizophrenia: a comparison with haloperidol and placebo. (The Seroquel Trial 13 Study Group.) Biol Psychiatry 42:233–246, 1997

Baldessarini R: Chemotherapy in Psychiatry: Principles and Practice. Cambridge, MA, Harvard University Press, 1985

Baldessarini RJ: A summary of current knowledge of tardive dyskinesia. Encephale 14:263–268, 1988

Baldessarini RJ, Cohen BM, Teicher MH: Significance of neuroleptic dose and plasma level in the pharmacological treatment of psychoses. Arch Gen Psychiatry 45:79–91, 1988

Baldessarini R, Huston-Lyons D, Campbell A, et al: Do central antiadrenergic actions contribute to the atypical properties of clozapine? Br J Psychiatry 160(suppl 17):12–16, 1992

Ball WA, Caroff SN: Retinopathy, tardive dyskinesia, and low-dose thioridazine (letter). Am J Psychiatry 143:256–257, 1986

Balon R, Berchou R: Hematologic side effects of psychotropic drugs. Psychosomatics 27:119–127, 1986

Ban TA, St. Jean A: The effects of phenothiazines on the electrocardiogram. Canadian Medical Association Journal 91:537–540, 1964

Barnas C, Zwierzina H, Hummer M, et al: Granulocyte-macrophage colony-stimulating factor (GM-CSF) treatment of clozapine-induced agranulocytosis: a case report. J Clin Psychiatry 53:245–247, 1992

Beasley CM, Tollefson G, Tran P, et al: Olanzapine versus placebo and haloperidol: acute phase results of the Northern American double-blind olanzapine trial. Neuropsychopharmacology 14:111–123, 1996

Beasley C Jr, Tollefson G, Tran P: Efficacy of olanzapine: an overview of pivotal clinical trials. J Clin Psychiatry 58(suppl 10):7–12, 1997

Beckman H, Lang R, Gattoz WF: Vasopressin-oxytocin in cerebrospinal fluid of schizophrenic patients and normal controls. Psychoneuroendocrinology 10:187–191, 1985

Bisette G, Nemeroff CB: Neurotensin and the mesocorticolimbic dopamine system. Ann N Y Acad Sci 537:397–404, 1988

Bondolfi G, Baumann P, Dufour H: Treatment-resistant schizophrenia: clinical experience with new antipsychotics. Eur Neuropsychopharmacol 6(suppl):S21–S25, 1996

Branchey M, Branchey L: Patterns of psychotropic drug use and tardive dyskinesia. J Clin Psychopharmacol 4:41–45, 1984

Breier A, Hamilton SH: Comparative efficacy of olanzapine and haloperidol for patients with treatment-resistant schizophrenia. Biol Psychiatry 45:403–411, 1999

Breier A, Wolkowitz OM, Doran AR, et al: Neuroleptic responsivity of negative and positive symptoms in schizophrenia. Am J Psychiatry 144:1549–1555, 1987

Breier A, Buchanan RW, Waltrip RW II, et al: The effect of clozapine on plasma norepinephrine: relationship to clinical efficacy. Neuropsychopharmacology 10:1–7, 1994

Brunello N, Masotto C, Steardo L, et al: New insights into the biology of schizophrenia through the mechanism of action of clozapine. Neuropsychopharmacology 13:177–213, 1995

Burke RE, Fahn S, Jankovic J, et al: Tardive dyskinesia: late-onset and persistent dystonia caused by antipsychotic drugs. Neurology 32:1335–1346, 1982

Burton S, Heslop K, Harrison K, et al: Ziprasidone overdose (letter). Am J Psychiatry 157:835, 2000

Byerly M, DeVane L: Pharmacokinetics of clozapine and risperidone: a review of the literature. J Clin Psychopharmacol 16:177–187, 1996

Cadet JL, Lohr JB, Jeste DV: Free radicals and tardive dyskinesia (letter). Trends Neurosci 9:107–108, 1986

Calabrese JR, Kimmel SE, Woyshville MJ, et al: Clozapine for treatment-refractory mania. Am J Psychiatry 153:759–764, 1996

Chakos M, Lieberman J, Hoffman E, et al: Effectiveness of second-generation antipsychotics in patients with treatment-resistant schizophrenia: a review and meta-analysis of randomized trials. Am J Psychiatry 158:518–526, 2001

Chen G, Ensor CR, Bohner B: Studies of drug effects on electrically induced extensor seizures and clinical implications. Archives Internationales de Pharmacodynamie et de Therapie 172:183–218, 1968

Chengappa KN, Gopalani A, Haught MK, et al: The treatment of clozapine-associated agranulocytosis with granulocyte colony-stimulating factor (G-CSF). Psychopharmacol Bull 32:111–121, 1996

Chouinard G, Jones BD, Remington G, et al: A Canadian multicenter, placebo-controlled study of fixed doses of risperidone and haloperidol in the treatment of chronic schizophrenic patients. J Clin Psychopharmacol 13:25–40, 1993

Cohen LG, Chessley S, Eugenio L, et al: Erythromycin-induced clozapine toxic reaction. Arch Intern Med 156:675–677, 1996

Cohen LG, Fatalo A, Thompson BT, et al: Olanzapine overdose with serum concentrations. Ann Emerg Med 34:275–278, 1999

Cole JO, Gardos G, Rapkin R, et al: Lithium carbonate in tardive dyskinesia and schizophrenia, in Tardive Dyskinesia and Affective Disorders. Edited by Gardos G, Casey D. Washington, DC, American Psychiatric Press, 1984, pp 50–73

Conley R, Tamminga C, Bartko J, et al: Olanzapine compared with chlorpromazine in treatment-resistant schizophrenia. Am J Psychiatry 155:914–920, 1998

Conley RR, Mahmoud RA: Randomized double-blind study of risperidone and olanzapine in the treatment of schizophrenia or schizoaffective disorder. Am J Psychiatry 158:765–774, 2001

Corzo D, Yunis JJ, Salazar M, et al: The major histocompatibility complex region marked by HSP70-1 and HSP70-2 variants is associated with clozapine-induced agranulocytosis in two different ethnic groups. Blood 86:3835–3840, 1995

Creese I, Burt DR, Snyder SH: Dopamine receptor binding predicts clinical and pharmacological potencies of antischizophrenic drugs. Science 192:481–483, 1976

Csernansky JC, Riney SJ, Lombrozo L: Double-blind comparison of alprazolam, diazepam, and placebo for the treatment of negative schizophrenic symptoms. Arch Gen Psychiatry 45:655–659, 1988

Dabiri LM, Pasta D, Darby JK, et al: Effectiveness of vitamin E for the treatment of long-term tardive dyskinesia. Am J Psychiatry 151:925–926, 1994

Daniel DG, Zimbroff DL, Potkin SG, et al: Ziprasidone 80 mg/day and 160 mg/day in the acute exacerbation of schizophrenia and schizoaffective disorder: a 6-week placebo-controlled trial. Neuropsychopharmacology 20:491–505, 1999

Das Gupta K, Young A: Clozapine-induced neuroleptic malignant syndrome. J Clin Psychiatry 52:105–107, 1991

Davis JM: Maintenance therapy and the natural course of schizophrenia. J Clin Psychiatry 46:18–21, 1985

Davis K, Kahn R, Ko G, et al: Dopamine in schizophrenia: a review and reconceptualization. Am J Psychiatry 148:1474–1486, 1991

Deirmenjian JM, Erhart SM, Wirshing DA, et al: Olanzapine-induced reversible priapism: a case report. J Clin Psychopharmacol 18:351–353, 1998

Delva NJ, Letemednia FJJ: Lithium treatment in schizophrenia and schizoaffective disorders. Br J Psychiatry 141:387–400, 1982

Descotes J, Lievre M, Ollagnier M, et al: Study of thioridazine cardiotoxic effects by means of his bundle activity recording. Acta Pharmacologica Toxicologica 44:370–376, 1979

Deshmukh DK, Joshi VS, Agarwal MR: Rabbit syndrome: a rare complication of long-term neuroleptic medication (case example). Br J Psychiatry 157:293, 1990

Devinsky O, Honigfeld G, Patin J: Clozapine-related seizures. Neurology 41:369–371, 1991

Douyon R, Angrist B, Peselow E, et al: Neuroleptic augmentation with alprazolam: clinical effects and pharmacokinetic correlates (comment). Am J Psychiatry 146:1087–1088, 1989

Duinkerke SJ, Botter PA, Jansen AAI, et al: Ritanserin, a selective 5HT2/1c antagonist, and negative symptoms in schizophrenia: a placebo-controlled double blind trial. Br J Psychiatry 163:451–455, 1993

Dumon J-P, Catteau J, Lanvin F, et al: Randomized, double-blind, crossover, placebo-controlled comparison of propranolol and betaxolol in the treatment of neuroleptic-induced akathisia. Am J Psychiatry 149:647–650, 1992

Dupuis B, Catteau J, Dumon J-P, et al: Comparison of propranolol, sotalol, and betaxolol in the treatment of neuroleptic-induced akathisia. Am J Psychiatry 144:802–805, 1987

Edlund MJ, Craig TJ: Antipsychotic drug use and birth defects: an epidemiologic reassessment. Compr Psychiatry 25:32–37, 1984

Egan MF, Hyde TM, Albers GW, et al: Treatment of tardive dyskinesia with vitamin E. Am J Psychiatry 149:773–777, 1992

Elkashef AM, Ruskin PE, Bacher N, et al: Vitamin E in the treatment of tardive dyskinesia. Am J Psychiatry 147:505–506, 1990

Emes CE, Millson RC: Risperidone-induced priapism. Can J Psychiatry 39:315–316, 1994

Ereshefsky L, Toney G, Saklad SR, et al: A loading-dose strategy for converting from oral to depot haloperidol. Hosp Community Psychiatry 44:1155–1161, 1993

Evins A, Goff D: Adjunctive antidepressant drug therapies in the treatment of negative symptoms of schizophrenia. CNS Drugs 6:130–147, 1996

Fahn S: A therapeutic approach to tardive dyskinesia. J Clin Psychiatry 46:19–24, 1985

Feinberg SS, Holzer B: The monoamine oxidase inhibitor (MAOI) diet and kosher pizza (letter, comment). J Clin Psychopharmacol 17:226–227, 1997

Feinberg SS, Holzer B: Clarifying the safety of the MAOI diet and pizza (letter, comment). J Clin Psychiatry 61:145, 2000

Gajwani P, Pozuelo L, Tesar GE: QT interval prolongation with quetiapine (Seroquel) overdose. Psychosomatics 41:63–65, 2000

Garver DL, Beinfeld MC, Yao JK: Cholecystokinin, dopamine and schizophrenia. Psychopharmacol Bull 26:377–380, 1990

Garver DL, Bisette G, Yao JK, et al: Relation of CSF neurotensin concentrations to symptoms and drug response of psychotic patients. Am J Psychiatry 148:484–488, 1991

Gelders YG: Thymosthenic agents, a novel approach in the treatment of schizophrenia. Br J Psychiatry 155(suppl 5):33–36, 1989

Gerson SL, Gullion G, Yeh HS, et al: Granulocyte colony-stimulating factor for clozapine-induced agranulocytosis (letter). Lancet 340:1097, 1992

Ghadirian AM, Chouinard G, Annable L: Sexual dysfunction and plasma prolactin levels in neuroleptic-treated schizophrenic outpatients. J Nerv Ment Dis 170:463–467, 1982

Ghaemi SN, Zarate CA Jr, Popli AP, et al: Is there a relationship between clozapine and obsessive-compulsive disorder? A retrospective chart review. Compr Psychiatry 36:267–270, 1995

Giles TO, Modlin RK: Death associated with ventricular arrhythmias and thioridazine hydrochloride. JAMA 205:108–110, 1968

Glazer WM, Moore DC, Schooler NR, et al: Tardive dyskinesia: a discontinuation study. Arch Gen Psychiatry 41:623–627, 1984

Goff D, Baldessarini R: Antipsychotics, in Drug Interactions in Psychiatry. Edited by Ciraulo D, Shader R, Greenblatt D, et al. Baltimore, MD, Williams & Wilkins, 1995, pp 129–174

Goff DC, Coyle JT: The emerging role of glutamate in the pathophysiology and treatment of schizophrenia. Am J Psychiatry 158:1366–1377, 2001

Goff D, Evins A: Negative symptoms in schizophrenia: neurobiological models and treatment response. Harv Rev Psychiatry 6:59–77, 1998

Goff D, Arana G, Greenblatt D, et al: The effect of benztropine on haloperidol-induced dystonia, clinical efficacy and pharmacokinetics: a prospective, double-blind trial. J Clin Psychopharmacol 11:106–112, 1991

Goff D, Midha K, Sarid-Segal O, et al: A placebo-controlled trial of fluoxetine added to neuroleptic in patients with schizophrenia. Psychopharmacology 117:417–423, 1995

Goff D, Posever T, Herz L, et al: An exploratory haloperidol-controlled dose-finding study of ziprasidone in hospitalized patients with schizophrenia or schizoaffective disorder. J Clin Psychopharmacol 18:296–304, 1998

Gould RA, Mueser KT, Bolton E, et al: Cognitive therapy for psychosis in schizophrenia: an effect size analysis. Schizophr Res 48:335–342, 2001

Green AI, Brown WA: Prolactin and neuroleptic drugs. Endocrinol Metab Clin North Am 17:213–223, 1988

Green M: What are the functional consequences of neurocognitive deficits in schizophrenia? Am J Psychiatry 153:321–330, 1996

Green MF, Marshall BD Jr, Wirshing WC, et al: Does risperidone improve verbal working memory in treatment-resistant schizophrenia? Am J Psychiatry 154:799–804, 1997

Gunderson JG: Pharmacotherapy for patients with borderline personality disorder. Arch Gen Psychiatry 43:698–700, 1986

Guze BH, Baxter LR: Current concepts: neuroleptic malignant syndrome. N Engl J Med 313:163–166, 1985

Gwinn KA, Caviness JN: Risperidone-induced tardive dyskinesia and parkinsonism. Mov Disord 12:119–121, 1997

Hagger C, Buckley P, Kenny JT, et al: Improvement in cognitive functions and psychiatric symptoms in treatment-refractory schizophrenic patients receiving clozapine. Biol Psychiatry 34:702–712, 1993

Hamilton JD: Thioridazine retinopathy within the upper dosage limit. Psychosomatics 26:823–824, 1985

Haring C, Barnas C, Saria A, et al: Dose-related plasma levels of clozapine. J Clin Psychopharmacol 9:71–72, 1989

Hartigan-Go K, Bateman N, Nyberg G, et al: Concentration-related pharmacodynamic effects of thiordazine and its metabolites in humans. Clin Pharmacol Ther 60:543–553, 1996

Henderson D, Goff D: Risperidone as an adjunct to clozapine therapy in chronic schizophrenics. J Clin Psychiatry 57:395–397, 1996

Henderson DC, Nasrallah RA, Goff DC: Switching from clozapine to olanzapine in treatment-refractory schizophrenia: safety, clinical efficacy, and predictors of response. J Clin Psychiatry 59:585–588, 1998

Henderson D, Cagliero E, Gray C, et al: Clozapine, diabetes mellitus, weight gain, and lipid abnormalities: a five year naturalistic study. Am J Psychiatry 157:975–981, 2000

Herz MI, Glazer WM, Mostert MA, et al: Intermittent versus maintenance medication in schizophrenia: two-year results. Arch Gen Psychiatry 48:333–339, 1991

Herz MI, Lamberti JS, Mintz J, et al: A program for relapse prevention in schizophrenia: a controlled study. Arch Gen Psychiatry 57:277–283, 2000

Hill RM, Desmond NM, Kay JL: Extrapyramidal dysfunction in an infant of a schizophrenic mother. J Pediatr 69:589–595, 1966

Honigfeld G, Arellano F, Sethi J, et al: Reducing clozapine-related morbidity and mortality: 5 years of experience with the Clozaril National Registry. J Clin Psychiatry 59(suppl 3):3–7, 1998

Hustey FM: Acute quetiapine poisoning. J Emerg Med 17:995–997, 1999

Itil TM, Soldatos CL: Epileptogenic side effects of psychotropic drugs: practical recommendations. JAMA 244:1460–1463, 1980

Jenner P, Marsden CD: Is the dopamine hypothesis of tardive dyskinesia completely wrong? Trends Neurosci June:259, 1986

Jeste DV, Wyatt RJ: Understanding and Treating Tardive Dyskinesia. New York, Guilford, 1982

Jeste DV, Lacro JP, Bailey A, et al: Lower incidence of tardive dyskinesia with risperidone compared to haloperidol in older patients. J Am Geriatr Soc 47:716–719, 1999

Jick O, Miettinen OS, Shapiro S, et al: Comprehensive drug surveillance. JAMA 213:1455–1460, 1970

Johnson DAW: Antipsychotic medication: clinical guidelines for maintenance therapy. J Clin Psychiatry 46:6–15, 1985

Johnson DA, Ludlow JM, Street K, et al: Double-blind comparison of half-dose and standard-dose flupenthixol decanoate in the maintenance treatment of stabilized out-patients with schizophrenia. Br J Psychiatry 151:634–638, 1987

Kane JM: Treatment-resistant schizophrenic patients. J Clin Psychiatry 57:35–40, 1996

Kane JM, Smith JM: Tardive dyskinesia: prevalence and risk factors, 1959 to 1979. Arch Gen Psychiatry 39:473–481, 1982

Kane JM, Rifkin A, Woerner M, et al: Low-dose neuroleptic treatment of outpatient schizophrenics, I: preliminary results for relapse rates. Arch Gen Psychiatry 40:893–896, 1983

Kane JM, Honigfeld G, Singer J, et al: Clozapine for the treatment-resistant schizophrenic: a double-blind comparison vs chlorpromazine/benztropine. Arch Gen Psychiatry 45:789–796, 1988

Kapur S, Seeman P: Does fast dissociation from the dopamine D2 receptor explain the action of atypical antipsychotics? A new hypothesis. Am J Psychiatry 158:360–369, 2001

Keck PEA Jr: Ziprasidone 40 and 120 mg/day in the acute exacerbation of schizophrenia and schizoaffective disorder: a 4-week placebo-controlled trial. Psychopharmacology 140:173–184, 1998

Keck PE Jr, Pope HG Jr, Cohen BM, et al: Risk factor for neuroleptic malignant syndrome. Arch Gen Psychiatry 46:914–918, 1989

Keck PE Jr, McElroy SL, Strakowski SM: New developments in the pharmacologic treatment of schizoaffective disorder. J Clin Psychiatry 57(suppl 9):41–48, 1996

Kennedy PF, Hershon HI, McGuire RJ: Extrapyramidal disorders after prolonged phenothiazine therapy. Br J Psychiatry 118:509–518, 1971

Kleinberg D, Brecher M, Davis J: Prolactin levels and adverse events in patients treated with risperidone. Paper presented at the 150th annual meeting of the American Psychiatric Association, San Diego, CA, May 17–22, 1997

Klibanski A, Neer R, Beitins I: Decreased bone density in hyperprolactinemic women. N Engl J Med 303:1511–1514, 1981

Levy W, Wisniewski K: Chlorpromazine causing extrapyramidal dysfunction in newborn infants of psychotic mothers. New York State Journal of Medicine 74:684–685, 1974

Lewis RV, Lofthouse C: Adverse reactions with β-adrenoceptor blocking drugs: an update. Drug Saf 9:272–279, 1993

Lieberman JA: Atypical antipsychotic drugs as a first-line treatment of schizophrenia: a rationale and hypothesis. J Clin Psychiatry 57(suppl 11):68–71, 1996

Lieberman JA, Yunis J, Egea E, et al: HLA-B38, DR4, DQw3 and clozapine induced agranulocytosis in Jewish patients with schizophrenia. Arch Gen Psychiatry 47:945–948, 1990

Lieberman JA, Saltz BL, Johns CA, et al: The effects of clozapine on tardive dyskinesia. Br J Psychiatry 158:503–510, 1991

Linnoila M, Vinkar M, Hiertala O: Effect of sodium valproate on tardive dyskinesia. Br J Psychiatry 129:114–119, 1976

Lipinski JF, Zubenko GS, Cohen BM, et al: Propranolol in the treatment of neuroleptic induced akathisia. Am J Psychiatry 141:412–415, 1984

Lohr JB, Caligiuri MP: A double-blind placebo-controlled study of vitamin E treatment of tardive dyskinesia. J Clin Psychiatry 57:167–173, 1996

Lohr JB, Cadet JL, Lohr MA, et al: L-Alpha-tocopherol in tardive dyskinesia. Lancet 1:913–914, 1987

Marder SR, Meibach RC: Risperidone in the treatment of schizophrenia. Am J Psychiatry 151:825–835, 1994

Marder SR, van Putten T, Mintz J, et al: Costs and benefits of two doses of fluphenazine. Arch Gen Psychiatry 41:1025–1029, 1984

Marder SR, van Putten T, Mintz J, et al: Low and conventional dose maintenance therapy with fluphenazine decanoate: two-year outcome. Arch Gen Psychiatry 44:518–521, 1987

McDougle CJ, Goodman WK, Price LH, et al: Neuroleptic addition in fluvoxamine-refractory obsessive-compulsive disorder. Am J Psychiatry 147:652–654, 1990

McElroy SL, Dessain EC, Pope HG Jr, et al: Clozapine in the treatment of psychotic mood disorders, schizoaffective disorder, and schizophrenia. J Clin Psychiatry 52:411–414, 1991

Meltzer HY: The mechanism of action of novel antipsychotic drugs. Schizophr Bull 17:265–287, 1991

Meltzer HY: An overview of the mechanism of action of clozapine. J Clin Psychiatry 55(suppl B):47–52, 1994

Meltzer HY, Matsubara S, Lee J-C: Classification of typical and atypical antipsychotic drugs on the basis of dopamine D_1, D_2, and serotonin$_2$ pKi values. J Pharmacol Exp Ther 251:238–246, 1989

Messing RO, Closson RG, Simon RP: Drug-induced seizures: a 10 year experience. Neurology 17:869–877, 1984

Metzger E, Friedman R: Prolongation of the corrected QT and torsades de pointes cardiac arrhythmia associated with intravenous haloperidol in the medically ill. J Clin Psychopharmacol 13:128–132, 1993

Miller DD, Sharafuddin MJA, Kathol RG: A case of clozapine-induced neuroleptic malignant syndrome. J Clin Psychiatry 52:99–101, 1991

Mitchell JE, Popkin MK: Antipsychotic drug therapy and sexual dysfunction in men. Am J Psychiatry 139:633–637, 1982

Munetz MR, Benjamin S: How to examine patients using the Abnormal Involuntary Movement Scale. Hosp Community Psychiatry 39:1172–1177, 1988

Munetz MR, Roth LH: Informing patients about tardive dyskinesia. Arch Gen Psychiatry 42:866–871, 1985

Nestoros J, Suranyi B, Spees R, et al: Diazepam in high doses is effective in schizophrenia. Prog Neuropsychopharmacol Biol Psychiatry 6:513–518, 1982

Nielsen H: Recombinant human granulocyte colony-stimulating factor (rhG-CSF; filgrastim) treatment of clozapine-induced agranulocytosis. J Intern Med 34:529–531, 1993

Ojemann LM, Baugh-Bookman C, Dudley DL: Effect of psychotropic medications on seizure control in patients with epilepsy. Neurology 37:1525–1527, 1987

Oliver AP, Luchins DJ, Wyatt RJ: Neuroleptic-induced seizures: an in vitro technique for assessing relative risk. Arch Gen Psychiatry 39:206–209, 1982

Opler LA, Feinberg SS: The role of pimozide in clinical psychiatry: a review. J Clin Psychiatry 52:221–233, 1991

Ostergaard K, Dupont E: Clozapine treatment of drug-induced psychotic symptoms in late stages of Parkinson's disease (letter). Acta Neurol Scand 78:349–350, 1988

Owens DG: Extrapyramidal side effects and tolerability of risperidone: a review. J Clin Psychiatry 55(suppl):29–35, 1994

Owens DG: Adverse effects of antipsychotic agents: do newer agents offer advantages? Drugs 51:895–930, 1996

Perry PJ, Miller DD, Arndt SV, et al: Clozapine and norclozapine plasma concentrations and clinical response of treatment-refractory schizophrenic patients. Am J Psychiatry 148:231–235, 1991

Pillmann F, Schlote K, Broich K, et al: Electroencephalogram alterations during treatment with olanzapine. Psychopharmacology (Berl) 150:216–219, 2000

Purdon SE, Jones BDW, Stip E, et al: Neuropsychological change in early phase schizophrenia during 12 months of treatment with olanzapine, risperidone, or haloperidol. Arch Gen Psychiatry 57:249–258, 2000

Pycock CJ, Carter CJ, Kerwin RW: Effect of 6-hydroxydopamine lesions of the medial prefrontal cortex on neurotransmitter systems in subcortical sites in the rat. J Neurochem 34:91–99, 1980

Reiter S, Adler L, Angrist B, et al: Atenolol and propranolol in neuroleptic-induced akathisia (letter). J Clin Psychopharmacol 7:279–280, 1987

Reunanen M, Kaarnen P, Vaisanen E: The influence of anticholinergic treatment on tardive dyskinesia caused by neuroleptic drugs. Acta Neurol Scand 65(suppl 90):278–279, 1982

Reynolds GP, Stroud D: Hippocampal benzodiazepine receptors in schizophrenia. J Neural Transm 93:151–155, 1993

Rifkin A, Quitkin F, Klein DF: Akinesia: a poorly recognized drug-induced extrapyramidal behavioral disorder. Arch Gen Psychiatry 32:672–674, 1975

Risch SC, Groom GP, Janowsky DS: Interfaces of psychopharmacology and cardiology—part two. J Clin Psychiatry 42:47–57, 1981

Rosebush P, Stewart T: A prospective analysis of 24 episodes of neuroleptic malignant syndrome. Am J Psychiatry 146:717–725, 1989

Rosebush PI, Stewart TD, Gelenberg AJ: Twenty neuroleptic rechallenges after neuroleptic malignant syndrome in 15 patients. J Clin Psychiatry 50:295–298, 1989

Rosebush PI, Stewart T, Mazurek MF: The treatment of neuroleptic malignant syndrome: are dantrolene and bromocriptine useful adjuncts to supportive care? Br J Psychiatry 159:709–712, 1991

Rosen SI, Hanno PM: Clozapine-induced priapism. J Urol 148:876–877, 1992

Rossi A, Mancini F, Stratta P, et al: Risperidone, negative symptoms, and cognitive deficit in schizophrenia: an open study. Acta Psychiatr Scand 95:40–43, 1997

Roth LH: Question the experts. J Clin Psychopharmacol 3:206–207, 1983

Sanger T, Lieberman J, Tohen M, et al: Olanzapine versus haloperidol treatment in first-episode psychosis. Am J Psychiatry 156:79–87, 1999

Schlichther W, Bristow ME, Schultz S, et al: Seizures occurring during intensive chlorpromazine therapy. Can Med Assoc J 74:364–366, 1956

Schooler NR, Keith SJ, Severe JB, et al: Relapse and rehospitalization during maintenance treatment of schizophrenia: the effects of dose reduction and family treatment. Arch Gen Psychiatry 54:453–463, 1997

Scokel PW, Jones WD: Infant jaundice after phenothiazine drugs for labour: an enigma. Obstet Gynecol 20:124–127, 1962

Seeman P, Lee T, Chau-Wong M, et al: Antipsychotic drug doses and neuroleptic/dopamine receptors. Nature 261:717–719, 1976

Seide H, Muller HR: Choreiform movements as side effects of phenothiazine medication in elderly patients. J Am Geriatr Soc 15:517–522, 1967

Shader RI: Sexual dysfunction associated with thioridazine hydrochloride. JAMA 188:1007–1009, 1964

Silver JM, Yudofsky SC, Kogan M, et al: Elevation of thioridazine plasma levels by propranolol. Am J Psychiatry 143:1290–1292, 1986

Small J, Hirsch S, Arvanitis L, et al: Quetiapine in patients with schizophrenia. Arch Gen Psychiatry 54:549–557, 1997

Sorensen SC, Gjerris A, Hammer M: Cerebrospinal fluid vasopressin in neurological and psychiatric disorders. J Neurol Neurosurg Psychiatry 48:50–57, 1985

Stewart RB, Karas B, Springer PK: Haloperidol excretion in human milk. Am J Psychiatry 137:849–850, 1980

Suppes T, McElroy SL, Gilbert J, et al: Clozapine in the treatment of dysphoric mania. Biol Psychiatry 32:270–280, 1992

Svensson TH, Tung CS, Grenhoff J: The 5-HT2 antagonist ritanserin blocks the effect of pre-frontal cortex inactivation on rat A10 dopamine neurons in vivo. Acta Physiol Scand 136:497–498, 1989

Tamer A, McKay R, Arias D, et al: Phenothiazine-induced extrapyramidal dysfunction in the neonate. J Pediatr 75:479–480, 1969

Tedeschi DH, Benigni JP, Elder CJ, et al: Effects of various phenothiazines on minimal electroshock seizure threshold and spontaneous motor activity of mice. J Pharmacol Exp Ther 123:35–38, 1958

Tollefson G, Sanger T: Negative symptoms: a path analytic approach to a double-blind, placebo- and haloperidol-controlled clinical trial with olanzapine. Am J Psychiatry 154:466–474, 1997

Tollefson G, Beasley C, Tamura R, et al: Blind, controlled, long-term study of the comparative incidence of treatment-emergent tardive dyskinesia with olanzapine or haloperidol. Am J Psychiatry 154:1248–1254, 1997

Tollefson GD, Sanger TM, Lu Y, et al: Depressive signs and symptoms in schizophrenia: a prospective blinded trial of olanzapine and haloperidol. Arch Gen Psychiatry 55:250–258, 1998

Tran P, Hamilton S, Kuntz A, et al: Double-blind comparison of olanzapine versus risperidone in the treatment of schizophrenia and other psychotic disorders. J Clin Psychopharmacol 17:407–418, 1997

Tsai G, Goff D, Chang R, et al: Markers of glutamatergic neurotransmission and oxidative stress associated with tardive dyskinesia. Am J Psychiatry 9:1207–1213, 1998

Turbay D, Lieberman J, Alper CA, et al: Tumor necrosis factor constellation polymorphism and clozapine-induced agranulocytosis in two different ethnic groups. Blood 89:4167–4174, 1997

Ugedo L, Grenhoff J, Svenssson TH: Ritanserin, a 5-HT2 receptor antagonist, activates midbrain dopamine neurons by blocking serotonergic inhibition. Psychopharmacology 98:45–50, 1989

Umbricht D, Kane JM: Medical complications of new antipsychotic drugs. Schizophr Bull 22:475–483, 1996

Umbricht D, Pollack S, Kane JM: Clozapine and weight gain. J Clin Psychiatry 55(suppl B):157–160, 1994

van Putten T, May PRA, Marder SR: Akathisia with haloperidol and thiothixene. Arch Gen Psychiatry 31:67–72, 1984

Wetzel H, Anghelescu I, Szegedi A, et al: Pharmacokinetic interactions of clozapine with selective serotonin reuptake inhibitors: differential effects of fluvoxamine and paroxetine in a prospective study. J Clin Psychopharmacol 18:2–9, 1998

Yassa R: Antiparkinsonian medication withdrawal in the treatment of tardive dyskinesia: a report of three cases. Can J Psychiatry 30:440–442, 1985

Yassa R, Lal S: Prevalence of the rabbit syndrome. Am J Psychiatry 143:656–657, 1986

Yoon MS, Han J, Dersham GH, et al: Effects of thioridazine (Mellaril) on ventricular electrophysiologic properties. Am J Cardiol 43:1155–1158, 1979

Yunis JJ, Corzo D, Salazar M, et al: HLA associations in clozapine-induced agranulocytosis. Blood 86:1177–1183, 1995

Zarate CA Jr, Tohen M, Baldessarini RJ: Clozapine in severe mood disorders. J Clin Psychiatry 56:411–417, 1995

Zubenko GS, Lipinski JF, Cohen M, et al: Comparison of metoprolol and propranolol in the treatment of akathisia. Psychiatry Res 11:143–149, 1984

Mood Stabilizers

Akiskal HS, Khani MK, Scott-Strauss A: Cyclothymic temperamental disorders. Psychiatr Clin North Am 2:527–554, 1979

Anath J, Dubin SE: Lithium and symptomatic hyperparathyroidism. J R Soc Med 96:1026–1029, 1983

Arana GW, Epstein S, Molloy M, et al: Carbamazepine-induced reduction of plasma alprazolam concentrations: a clinical case report. J Clin Psychiatry 49:448–449, 1988

Baastrup PC, Schou M: Lithium as a prophylactic agent: its effect against recurrent depressions and manic-depressive psychosis. Arch Gen Psychiatry 16:162–172, 1967

Bakris GL, Smith DW, Tiwari S: Dermatologic manifestations of lithium: a review. Int J Psychiatry Med 10:327–331, 1980–1981

Ballenger JC, Post RM: Carbamazepine in manic-depressive illness: a new treatment. Am J Psychiatry 137:782–790, 1980

Battle DC, von Riotte AB, Gaviria M, et al: Amelioration of polyuria by amiloride in patients receiving long-term lithium therapy. N Engl J Med 312:408–414, 1985

Bauer MS, Whybrow PC, Winokur A: Rapid cycling bipolar affective disorder, I: association with grade I hypothyroidism. Arch Gen Psychiatry 47:427–432, 1990

Baxter LR Jr, Liston EH, Schwartz JM, et al: Prolongation of the antidepressant response to partial sleep deprivation by lithium. Psychiatry Res 19:17–23, 1986

Belmaker RH, Lerer B, Klein E, et al: Clinical implications of research on the mechanism of action of lithium. Prog Neuropsychopharmacol Biol Psychiatry 7:287–296, 1983

Bentsen KD, Gram L, Veje A: Serum thyroid hormones and blood folic acid during monotherapy with carbamazepine or valproate: a controlled study. Acta Neurol Scand 67:235–241, 1983

Bertollini R, Kallen B, Mastroiacovo P, et al: Anticonvulsant drugs in monotherapy: effect on the fetus. Eur J Epidemiol 3:164–171, 1987

Billings PR: Amiloride in the treatment of lithium-induced diabetes insipidus (letter). N Engl J Med 312:1575–1576, 1985

Bitran JA, Manji HK, Potter WZ, et al: Down-regulation of PKC alpha by lithium in vitro. Psychopharmacol Bull 31:449–452, 1995

Bone S, Roose SP, Dunner DL, et al: Incidence of side effects in patients on long-term lithium therapy. Am J Psychiatry 137:103–104, 1980

Borer MS, Bhanot VK: Hyperparathyroidism: neuropsychiatric manifestations. Psychosomatics 26:597–601, 1985

Bowden CL, Brugger AM, Swann AC, et al: Efficacy of divalproex vs lithium and placebo in the treatment of mania. The Depakote Mania Study Group. JAMA 271:918–924, 1994

Bowden CL, Janicak PG, Orsulak P, et al: Relation of serum valproate concentration to response in mania. Am J Psychiatry 153:765–770, 1996

Bowen RC, Grof P, Grof E: Less frequent lithium administration and lower urine volume. Am J Psychiatry 148:189–192, 1991

Brewerton TD: Lithium counteracts carbamazepine-induced leukopenia while increasing its therapeutic effect. Biol Psychiatry 21:677–685, 1986

Brewerton TD, Jackson CW: Prophylaxis of carbamazepine-induced hyponatremia by demeclocycline in six patients. J Clin Psychiatry 55:249–251, 1994

Brodie MJ, MacPhee GJ: Carbamazepine neurotoxicity precipitated by diltiazem. BMJ 292:1170–1171, 1986

Cade JFJ: Lithium salts in the treatment of psychotic excitement. Med J Aust 36:349–352, 1949

Calabrese JR, Gulledge AD, Hahn K, et al: Autoimmune thyroiditis in manic-depressive patients treated with lithium. Am J Psychiatry 142:1318–1321, 1985

Calabrese JR, Markowitz PJ, Kimmel SE, et al: Spectrum of efficacy of valproate in 78 rapid-cycling bipolar patients. J Clin Psychopharmacol 12:53S–56S, 1992

Calabrese JR, Bowden CL, Sach GS, et al: A double-blind placebo-controlled study of lamotrigine monotherapy in outpatients with bipolar I depression. Lamictal 602 Study Group. J Clin Psychiatry 60:79–88, 1999

Chen G, Manji HK, Hawver DB, et al: Chronic sodium valproate selectively decreases protein kinase C alpha and epsilon in vitro. J Neurochem 63:2361–2364, 1994

Chouinard G, Young SN, Annable L: Antimanic effect of clonazepam. Biol Psychiatry 18:451–466, 1983

Chouinard G, Annable L, Turnier L, et al: A double-blind randomized clinical trial of rapid tranquilization with I.M. clonazepam and I.M. haloperidol in agitated psychotic patients with manic symptoms. Can J Psychiatry 38:S114–S121, 1993

Clur AWB: Hypothyroidism and hyperparathyroidism associated with lithium toxicity (letter). S Afr Med J 76:124, 1989

Cohen LS, Friedman JM, Jefferson MD, et al: A reevaluation of risk of in utero exposure to lithium. JAMA 271:146–150, 1994

Cohen WJ, Cohen NH: Lithium carbonate, haloperidol and irreversible brain damage. JAMA 230:1283–1287, 1974

Cohn JB, Collins G, Ashbrook E, et al: A comparison of fluoxetine, imipramine, and placebo in patients with bipolar depressive disorder. Int Clin Psychopharmacol 4:313–322, 1989

Consensus Conference: Electroconvulsant therapy. JAMA 254:2103–2108, 1985

Consensus Development Panel: Mood disorders: pharmacologic prevention of recurrences. Am J Psychiatry 142:469–476, 1985

Coopen A, Abou-Saleh MT, Miller P, et al: Lithium continuation therapy following electroconvulsive therapy. Br J Psychiatry 139:284–287, 1981

Coulam CB, Annegers JF: Do anticonvulsants reduce the efficacy of oral contraceptives? Epilepsia 20:519–525, 1979

Dean JC, Penry JK: Valproate, in The Medical Treatment of Epilepsy. Edited by Resor SR, Kutt H. New York, Marcel Dekker, 1992, pp 265–278

Deandrea D, Walker N, Mehlmauer M, et al: Dermatologic reactions to lithium: a critical review of the literature. J Clin Psychopharmacol 2:199–204, 1982

DePaulo JR, Correa EI, Sapir DG: Renal function and lithium: a longitudinal study. Am J Psychiatry 143:892–895, 1986

Dreifuss FE, Santilli N, Langer DH, et al: Valproic acid hepatic fatalities: a retrospective review. Neurology 37:379–385, 1987

Dreifuss FE, Langer DH, Moline KA, et al: Valproic acid hepatic fatalities, II: US experience since 1994. Neurology 39:201–207, 1989

Dunner DL, Fieve RR: Clinical factors in lithium carbonate prophylaxis failure. Arch Gen Psychiatry 30:229–233, 1974

Ebstein RP, Hermoni M, Belmaker RH: The effect of lithium on noradrenaline-induced cyclic AMP accumulation in rat brain: inhibition after chronic treatment and absence of supersensitivity. J Pharmacol Exp Ther 213:161–167, 1980

Edmonds LD, Oakley GP: Ebstein's anomaly and maternal lithium exposure during pregnancy. Teratology 41:551–552, 1990

Eichelbaum M, Tomson T, Tybring G, et al: Carbamazepine metabolism in man: induction and pharmacogenetic aspects. Clin Pharmacokinet 10:80–90, 1985

Faedda GL, Tondo L, Baldessarini RJ, et al: Outcome after rapid vs. gradual discontinuation of lithium treatment in bipolar disorders. Arch Gen Psychiatry 50:448–455, 1994

Fankhauser MP, Lindon JL, Connolly B, et al: Evaluation of lithium-tetracycline interaction. Clin Pharm 7:314–317, 1988

Frye MA, Ketter TA, Kimbrell TA, et al: A placebo-controlled study of lamotrigine and gabapentin monotherapy in refractory mood disorders. J Clin Psychopharmacol 20:607–614, 2000

Gelenberg AJ, Kane JM, Keller MB, et al: Comparison of standard and low blood levels of lithium for maintenance treatment of bipolar disorder. N Engl J Med 321:1489–1493, 1989

Gerner RH, Stanton A: Algorithm for patient management of acute manic states: lithium, valproate, or carbamazepine? J Clin Psychopharmacol 12(suppl):57S–63S, 1992

Goldney RD, Spence ND: Safety of the combination of lithium and neuroleptic drugs. Am J Psychiatry 143:882–884, 1986

Goodwin FK, Jamison R: Manic-Depressive Illness. New York, Oxford University Press, 1990

Gram LM, Bentsen KD: Hepatic toxicity of antiepileptic drugs: a review. Acta Neurol Scand Suppl 97:81–90, 1983

Hetmar O, Bren C, Clemmesen L, et al: Lithium: long-term effects on the kidney, II: structural changes. J Psychiatr Res 21:279–288, 1987

Hetmar O, Poulsen UJ, Ladefoged J, et al: Lithium: long-term effects on the kidney: a prospective follow-up study ten years after kidney biopsy. Br J Psychiatry 158:53–58, 1991

Himmelhoch JM, Thase ME, Mallinger AG, et al: Tranylcypromine versus imipramine in anergic bipolar depression. Am J Psychiatry 148:910–916, 1991

Hirschfeld RMA, Clayton P, Cohen I, et al: Practice guideline for the treatment of patients with bipolar disorder. Am J Psychiatry 151:1–36, 1994

Hurd RW, Rinsvelt V, Karas WB, et al: Selenium, zinc, and copper changes with valproic acid: possible relation to drug side effects. Neurology 34:1393–1395, 1984

Hyman NM, Dennis PD, Sinclair KG: Tremor due to sodium valproate. Neurology 29:1172–1180, 1979

Isojarvi JI, Laatikainen TJ, Knip M, et al: Obesity and endocrine disorders in women taking valproate for epilepsy. Ann Neurol 39:579–584, 1996

Jacobsen FM: Low-dose valproate: a new treatment for cyclothymia, mild rapid cycling disorders, and premenstrual syndrome. J Clin Psychiatry 54:229–234, 1993

Jacobson SJ, Jones K, Johnson K, et al: Prospective multicentre study of pregnancy outcome after lithium exposure during first trimester. Lancet 339:530–533, 1992

Jaeken J, Casaer P, Corbeel L: Valproate, hyperammonaemia and hyperglycinaemia (letter). Lancet 2:260, 1980

Jeavons PM, Clark JE, Harding GFA: Valproate and curly hair (letter). Lancet 1:359, 1977

Joffe RT, Gold PW, Uhde TW, et al: The effects of carbamazepine on the thyrotropin response to thyrotropin releasing hormone. Psychiatry Res 12:161–166, 1984

Joffe RT, Post RM, Uhde TW: Effect of carbamazepine on body weight in affectively ill patients. J Clin Psychiatry 47:313–314, 1986

Jones KL, Lacro RV, Johnson KA, et al: Pattern of malformations in the children of women treated with carbamazepine during pregnancy. N Engl J Med 320:1661–1666, 1989

Jope RS, Williams MB: Lithium and brain signal transduction systems. Biochem Pharmacol 47:429–441, 1994

Kallen B, Tandberg A: Lithium and pregnancy: a cohort study in manic-depressive women. Acta Psychiatr Scand 68:134–139, 1983

Keck PE Jr, McElroy SL, Nemeroff CB: Anticonvulsants in the treatment of bipolar disorder. J Neuropsychiatry Clin Neurosci 4:395–405, 1992

Keck PE Jr, McElroy SL, Tugrul KC, et al: Valproate oral loading in the treatment of acute mania. J Clin Psychiatry 54:305–308, 1993

Ketter TA, Pazzaglia PJ, Post RM: Synergy of carbamazepine and valproic acid in affective disorders. J Clin Psychopharmacol 12:276–281, 1992

Ketter TA, Post RM, Parekh PI, et al: Addition of monoamine oxidase inhibitors to carbamazepine: preliminary evidence of safety and antidepressant efficacy in treatment-resistant depression. J Clin Psychiatry 56:471–475, 1995a

Ketter TA, Flockhart DA, Post RM, et al: The emerging role of cytochrome P450 3A in psychopharmacology. J Clin Psychopharmacol 15:387–398, 1995b

Klemfuss H: Diminishing toxic effects of lithium administration (letter). Am J Psychiatry 149:846, 1992

Kramlinger KG, Post RM: Addition of lithium carbonate to carbamazepine: hematological and thyroid effects. Am J Psychiatry 147:615–620, 1990

Labar DR: Antiepileptic drug toxic emergencies, in The Medical Treatment of Epilepsy. Edited by Resor SR, Kutt H. New York, Marcel Dekker, 1992, pp 573–588

Lambert P-A, Cavaz G, Borselli S, et al: Action neuropsychotrop diun nouvel anti-epileptique: le Depamide. Ann Med Psychol (Paris) 1:707–710, 1966

Lammer EJ, Sever LE, Oakley GP: Teratogen update: valproic acid. Teratology 35:465–473, 1987

Leach MJ, Baxter MG, Critchley MA: Neurochemical and behavioral aspects of lamotrigine. Epilepsia 32:S4–S8, 1991

Lenox RH, Newhouse PA, Creelman WL, et al: Adjunctive treatment of manic agitation with lorazepam versus haloperidol: a double blind study. J Clin Psychiatry 53:47–52, 1992

Lenox RH, Watson DG, Patel J, et al: Chronic lithium administration alters a prominent PKC substrate in rat hippocampus. Brain Res 570:333–340, 1992

Lindstedt G, Nilsson L, Walinder J, et al: On the prevalence, diagnosis and management of lithium-induced hypothyroidism in psychiatric patients. Br J Psychiatry 130:452–458, 1977

Lipinski JF, Pope HG: Possible synergistic action between carbamazepine and lithium carbonate in the treatment of three acutely manic patients. Am J Psychiatry 139:948–949, 1982

Lokkegaard H, Andersen NF, Henriksen E: Renal function in 153 manic-depressive patients treated with lithium for more than five years. Acta Psychiatr Scand 71:347–355, 1985

MacDonald RL, Kelly KM: Antiepileptic drug mechanisms of action (review). Epilepsia 36:S2–S12, 1995

Mallette LE, Eichhorn E: Effects of lithium carbonate on human calcium metabolism. Arch Intern Med 146:770–776, 1986

Manji HK, Bebchuk JM, Moore GJ, et al: Modulation of CNS signal transduction pathways and gene expression by mood-stabilizing agents: therapeutic implications. J Clin Psychiatry 60(suppl 2):27–39, 1993

Manji HK, Chen G, Shimon H, et al: Guanine nucleotide-binding proteins in bipolar affective disorder: effects of long-term lithium treatment. Arch Gen Psychiatry 52:135–144, 1995

Manji HK, Chen G, Hsiso JK, et al: Regulation of signal transduction pathways by mood-stabilizing agents: implications for the delayed onset of therapeutic efficacy. J Clin Psychiatry 57:34–46, 1999

Martin A: Clinical management of lithium-induced polyuria. Hosp Community Psychiatry 44:427–428, 1993

McElroy SL, Keck PE Jr, Pope HG Jr, et al: Valproate in psychiatric disorders: literature review and clinical guidelines. J Clin Psychiatry 50(suppl):23–29, 1989

McElroy SL, Keck PE Jr, Pope HG Jr, et al: Valproate in the treatment of bipolar disorder: literature review and clinical guidelines. J Clin Psychopharmacol 12(suppl):42S–52S, 1992

McGennis AJ: Lithium carbonate and tetracycline interaction. BMJ 1:1183, 1978

Mitchell JE, Mackenzie TB: Cardiac effects of lithium therapy in man: a review. J Clin Psychiatry 43:47–51, 1982

Moss GR, James CR: Carbamazepine and lithium synergism in mania. Arch Gen Psychiatry 40:588–589, 1983

Murphy JM, Mashman J, Miller JD, et al: Suppression of carbamazepine-induced rash with prednisone. Neurology 41:144–145, 1991

Murphy MJ, Lyon IW, Taylor JW, et al: Valproic acid associated with pancreatitis in an adult (letter). Lancet 1:41–42, 1981

Myers DH, Carter RA, Burns BH, et al: A prospective study of the effects of lithium on thyroid function and on the prevalence of antithyroid antibodies. Psychol Med 15:55–61, 1985

Nora JJ, Nora AH, Toews WH: Lithium, Ebstein's anomaly and other congenital heart defects. Lancet 1:594–595, 1974

Patterson JF: Stevens-Johnson syndrome associated with carbamazepine therapy. J Clin Psychopharmacol 5:185, 1985

Peet M: Induction of mania with selective serotonin re-uptake inhibitors and tricyclic antidepressants. Br J Psychiatry 164:549–550, 1994

Pellock JM: Carbamazepine side effects in children and adults. Epilepsia 28:S64–S70, 1987

Pellock JM, Willmore LJ: A rational guide to routine blood monitoring in patients receiving antiepileptic drugs. Neurology 41:961–964, 1991

Penney JF, Dimwiddie SH, Zarumski CF, et al: Concurrent and close temporal administration of lithium and ECT. Convuls Ther 6:139–145, 1990

Peselow ED, Dunner DL, Fieve RR, et al: Lithium carbonate and weight gain. J Affect Disord 2:303–310, 1980

Placidi GF, Lenzi A, Lazzerini F, et al: The comparative efficacy and safety of carbamazepine versus lithium: a randomized double-blind 3-year trial in 83 patients. J Clin Psychiatry 47:490–494, 1986

Plenge P, Mellerup ET, Bolwig C, et al: Lithium treatment: does the kidney prefer one daily dose instead of two? Acta Psychiatr Scand 66:121–128, 1982

Pope HG Jr, McElroy SL, Sathin A, et al: Head injury, bipolar disorder, and response to valproate. Compr Psychiatry 29:34–38, 1988

Pope HG Jr, McElroy SL, Keck PE Jr, et al: Valproate in the treatment of acute mania: a placebo-controlled study. Arch Gen Psychiatry 48:62–68, 1991

Post RM, Uhde TW, Ballenger JC, et al: Carbamazepine and its 10-11-epoxide metabolite in plasma and CSF: relationship to antidepressant response. Arch Gen Psychiatry 40:673–676, 1983

Post RM, Uhde TW, Ballenger JC: Efficacy of carbamazepine in affective disorders: implications for underlying physiological and biochemical substrates, in Anticonvulsants in Affective Disorders. Edited by Emrich HM, Okuma T, Muller AS. Amsterdam, The Netherlands, Elsevier, 1984, pp 93–115

Post RM, Uhde TW, Roy-Byrne PP, et al: Antidepressant effects of carbamazepine. Am J Psychiatry 143:29–34, 1986

Post RM, Uhde TW, Roy-Byrne PP, et al: Correlates of antimanic response to carbamazepine. Psychiatry Res 21:71–83, 1987

Post RM, Leverich GS, Altshuler L, et al: Lithium-discontinuation-induced refractoriness: preliminary observations. Am J Psychiatry 149:1727–1729, 1992

Prien RF, Kupfer DJ, Mansky PA, et al: Drug therapy in the prevention of recurrences in unipolar and bipolar affective disorders: report of the NIMH Collaborative Study Group comparing lithium carbonate, imipramine, and a lithium carbonate-imipramine combination. Arch Gen Psychiatry 41:1096–1104, 1984

Ramsey TA, Cox M: Lithium and the kidney: a review. Am J Psychiatry 139:443–449, 1982

Richens A: Safety of lamotrigine. Epilepsia 35(suppl 5):S37–S40, 1994

Robert E, Guibaud P: Maternal valproic acid and congenital neural tube defects (letter). Lancet 2:937, 1982

Rosa FW: Spina bifida in infants of women treated with carbamazepine during pregnancy. N Engl J Med 324:674–677, 1991

Sachs GS, Lafer B, Stoll AL, et al: A double-blind trial of bupropion versus desipramine for bipolar depression. J Clin Psychiatry 55:391–393, 1994

Sachs GS, Printz DJ, Kahn DA, et al: The Expert Consensus Guideline Series: medication treatment of bipolar disorder. Postgrad Med Spec No:1–104, 2000

Sackeim HA, Haskett RF, Mulsant BH, et al: Continuation pharmacotherapy in the prevention of relapse following electroconvulsive therapy: a randomized controlled trial. JAMA 285:1299–1307, 2001

Schatzberg AF, Cole JO: Manual of Clinical Psychopharmacology, 2nd Edition. Washington, DC, American Psychiatric Press, 1991

Schou M: Lithium prophylaxis: myths and realities. Am J Psychiatry 146:573–576, 1989

Shopsin B: Bupropion's prophylactic efficacy in bipolar affective illness. J Clin Psychiatry 44:163–169, 1983

Simon MN, Garber E, Arieff AJ: Persistent nephrogenic diabetes insipidus after lithium carbonate. Ann Intern Med 86:446–447, 1977

Small JG: Anticonvulsants in affective disorders. Psychopharmacol Bull 26:25–36, 1990

Suppes T, Baldessarini RJ, Faedda GI, et al: Risk of recurrence following discontinuation of lithium treatment in bipolar disorder. Arch Gen Psychiatry 48:1082–1088, 1991

Suppes T, McElroy SL, Gilbert J, et al: Clozapine in the treatment of dysphoric mania. Biol Psychiatry 32:270–280, 1992

Swann AC, Bowden CL, Morris D, et al: Depression during mania: treatment response to lithium or divalproex. Arch Gen Psychiatry 54:37–42, 1997

Takezaki H, Hanaoka M: The use of carbamazepine (Tegretol) in the control of manic-depressive psychosis and other manic-depressive states. J Clin Psychiatry 13:173–183, 1971

Vendsborg PB, Bech P, Rafaelson OJ: Lithium treatment and weight gain. Acta Psychiatr Scand 53:139–147, 1976

Vestergaard P, Amdisen A, Schou M: Clinically significant side effects of lithium treatment. Acta Psychiatr Scand 62:193–200, 1980

Vick NA: Suppression of carbamazepine-induced skin rash with prednisone. N Engl J Med 309:1193–1194, 1983

Waller DG: Thyroid function and urine-concentrating ability during lithium treatment. J Psychiatr Res 19:569–571, 1985

Waller DG, Edwards JG: Lithium and the kidney: an update. Psychol Med 19:825–831, 1989

Warnock JK, Knesevich J: Adverse cutaneous reactions to antidepressants. Am J Psychiatry 145:425–430, 1988

Wehr TA, Goodwin FK: Do antidepressants cause mania? Psychopharmacol Bull 23:61–65, 1987

Wehr TA, Sack DA, Rosenthal NE, et al: Rapid cycling affective disorder: contributing factors and treatment responses in 51 patients. Am J Psychiatry 145:179–184, 1988

Wood IK, Parmalee DX, Foreman JW: Lithium-induced nephrotic syndrome. Am J Psychiatry 146:84–87, 1989

Yassa R, Saunders A, Nastase C, et al: Lithium-induced thyroid disorders: a prevalence study. J Clin Psychiatry 48:14–16, 1988

Yeo PP, Bates D, Howe JG, et al: Anticonvulsants and thyroid function. BMJ 1:1581–1583, 1978

Zalzstein E, Koren G, Einarson T, et al: A case-control study on the association between first trimester exposure to lithium and Ebstein's anomaly. Am J Cardiol 41:551–552, 1990

Zohar J, Ebstein RP, Belmaker RH: Adenylate cyclase as the therapeutic target site of lithium, in Basic Mechanisms in the Action of Lithium. Edited by Emrich HM, Aldenhoff JB, Lux HD. Amsterdam, The Netherlands, Elsevier, 1982, pp 154–166

Zornberg GL, Pope HGJ: Treatment of depression in bipolar disorder: new directions for research. J Clin Psychopharmacol 13:397–408, 1993

Zubenko GS, Cohen BM, Lipinski JF: Comparison of metoprolol and propranolol in the treatment of lithium tremor. Psychiatry Res 11:163–164, 1984

Drug Interactions

Callahan AM, Marangell LB, Ketter TA: Evaluating the clinical significance of drug interaction: a systematic approach. Harv Rev Psychiatry 4:153–158, 1996

Dahl ML, Johansson I, Bertilsson L, et al: Ultrarapid hydroxylation of debrisoquine in a Swedish population: analysis of the molecular genetic basis. J Pharmacol Exp Ther 274:516–520, 1995

Goodwin FK, Jamison R: Manic-Depressive Illness. New York, Oxford University Press, 1990

Greiff JM, Rowbotham D: Pharmacokinetic drug interactions with gastrointestinal motility modifying agents. Clin Pharmacokinet 27:447–461, 1994

Johansson I, Lundqvist E, Bertilsson L, et al: Inherited amplification of an active gene in the cytochrome P450 CYP2D locus as a cause of ultrarapid metabolism of debrisoquine. Proc Natl Acad Sci U S A 90:11825–11829, 1993

Nakamura K, Goto F, Ray WA, et al: Interethnic differences in genetic polymorphism of debrisoquine and mephenytoin hydroxylation between Japanese and Caucasian populations. Clin Pharmacol Ther 38:402–408, 1985

Nelson DR, Kamataki T, Waxman DJ, et al: The P450 superfamily: update on new sequences, gene mapping, accession numbers, early trivial names of enzymes, and nomenclature. DNA Cell Biol 12:1–51, 1993

Shimada T, Yamazaki H, Mimura M, et al: Interindividual variations in human liver cytochrome P-450 enzymes involved in the oxidation of drugs, carcinogens and toxic chemicals: studies with liver microsomes of 30 Japanese and 30 Caucasians. J Pharmacol Exp Ther 270:414–423, 1994

Watkins PB, Wrighton SA, Maurel P, et al: Identification of an inducible form of cytochrome P-450 in human liver. Proc Natl Acad Sci U S A 82:6310–6314, 1985

Wing YK, Chen CN: Tyramine content in Chinese food (letter, comment). J Clin Psychopharmacol 17:227, 1997

Xie HG, Xu ZH, Luo X, et al: Genetic polymorphism of debrisoquine and S-mephenytoin oxidation metabolism in Chinese populations: a meta-analysis. Pharmacogenetics 6:235–238, 1996

Antiaggression Drugs

Alexopoulos GS, Silver JM, Kahn DA, et al: The Expert Consensus Guideline Series: treatment agitation in older persons with dementia. Postgrad Med: A Special Report, April 1998

American Psychiatric Association: Diagnostic and Statistical Manual of Mental Disorders, 4th Edition. Washington, DC, American Psychiatric Association, 1994

Anderson KA, Silver JM: Neurological diseases and medical diseases, in Medical Management of the Violent Patient: Clinical Assessment and Therapy. Edited by Tardiff K. New York, Marcel Dekker, 1999, pp 87–124

Bellus SB, Stewart D, Vergo JG, et al: The use of lithium in the treatment of aggressive behaviors with two brain-injured individuals in a state psychiatric hospital. Brain Injury 10:849–860, 1996

Bick PA, Hannah AL: Intramuscular lorazepam to restrain violent patients (letter). Lancet 1:206, 1986

Brooke MM, Patterson DR, Questad KA, et al: Agitation and restlessness after closed head injury: a prospective study of 100 consecutive admissions. Arch Phys Med Rehabil 73:917–921, 1992

Brown KW, Sloan RL, Pentland B: Fluoxetine as a treatment for post-stroke emotionalism. Acta Psychiatr Scand 98:455–458, 1998

Chatham-Showalter PE: Carbamazepine for combativeness in acute traumatic brain injury. J Neuropsychiatry Clin Neurosci 8:96–99, 1996

Corrigan PW, Yudofsky SC, Silver JM: Pharmacological and behavioral treatments for aggressive psychiatric inpatients. Hosp Community Psychiatry 44:125–133, 1993

Dietch JT, Jennings RK: Aggressive dyscontrol in patients treated with benzodiazepines. J Clin Psychiatry 49:184–189, 1988

Feeney DM, Gonzalez A, Lewin A: Amphetamine, haloperidol, and experience interact to affect rate of recovery after motor cortex injury. Science 217:855–857, 1982

Freinhar JP, Alvarez WA: Clonazepam treatment of organic brain syndromes in three elderly patients. J Clin Psychiatry 47:525–526, 1986

Gedye A: Trazodone reduced aggressive and self-injurious movements in a mentally handicapped male patient with autism. J Clin Psychopharmacol 11:275–276, 1991

Geracioti TD Jr: Valproic acid treatment of episodic explosiveness related to brain injury. J Clin Psychiatry 55:416–417, 1994

Giakas WJ, Seibyl JP, Mazure CM: Valproate in the treatment of temper outbursts (letter). J Clin Psychiatry 51:525, 1990

Goldberg RJ, Goldberg JS: Low-dose risperidone for dementia related disturbed behavior in nursing home. Paper presented at the 148th annual meeting of the American Psychiatric Association, Miami, FL, May 20–25, 1995

Herrmann N, Lanctot K, Myszak M: Effectiveness of gabapentin for the treatment of behavioral disorders in dementia. J Clin Psychopharmacol 20:90–93, 2000

Hornstein A, Seliger G: Cognitive side effects of lithium in closed head injury (letter). J Neuropsychiatry Clin Neurosci 1:446–447, 1989

Jackson RD, Corrigan JD, Arnett JA: Amitriptyline for agitation in head injury. Arch Phys Med Rehabil 66:180–181, 1985

Keats MM, Mukherjee S: Antiaggressive effect of adjunctive clonazepam in schizophrenia associated with seizure disorder. J Clin Psychiatry 49:117–118, 1988

Mattes JA: Valproic acid for nonaffective aggression in the mentally retarded. J Nerv Ment Dis 180:601–602, 1992

Michals ML, Crismon ML, Roberts S, et al: Clozapine response and adverse effects in nine brain-injured patients. J Clin Psychopharmacol 13:198–203, 1993

Moskowitz AS, Altshuler L: Increased sensitivity to lithium-induced neurotoxicity after stroke: a case report. J Clin Psychopharmacol 11:272–273, 1991

Mysiw WJ, Jackson RD, Corrigan JD: Amitriptyline for post-traumatic agitation. Am J Phys Med Rehabil 67:29–30, 1988

Nahas Z, Arlinghaus KA, Kotrla KJ, et al: Rapid response of emotional incontinence to selective serotonin reuptake inhibitors. J Neuropsychiatry Clin Neurosci 10:453–455, 1998

Panzer MJ, Mellow AM: Antidepressant treatment of pathologic laughing or crying in elderly stroke patients. J Geriatr Psychiatry Neurol 4:195–199, 1992

Ranen NG, Lipsey JR, Treisman G, et al: Sertraline in the treatment of severe aggressiveness in Huntington's disease. J Neuropsychiatry Clin Neurosci 8:338–340, 1996

Raty JJ, Leveroni C, Kilmer D, et al: The effects of clozapine on severely aggressive psychiatric inpatients in a state hospital. J Clin Psychiatry 54:219–223, 1993

Roane DM, Feinbert TE, Meckler L, et al: Treatment dementia-associated agitation with gabapentin. J Neuropsychiatry Clin Neurosci 12:40–43, 2000

Schulman KI, Walker SE: Clarifying the safety of the MAOI diet and pizza (letter, reply). J Clin Psychiatry 61:145–146, 2000

Seliger GM, Hornstein A, Flax J, et al: Fluoxetine improves emotional incontinence. Brain Inj 6:267–270, 1992

Silver JM, Yudofsky SC: Neuropsychiatric aspects of traumatic brain injury, in Textbook of Neuropsychiatry. Edited by Hales RE, Yudofsky SC. Washington, DC, American Psychiatric Press, 1987, pp 179–190

Silver JM, Yudofsky SC: The Overt Aggression Scale: overview and clinical guidelines. J Neuropsychiatry Clin Neurosci 3:S22–S29, 1991

Silver JM, Yudofsky SC: Aggressive disorders, in Neuropsychiatry of Traumatic Brain Injury. Edited by Silver JM, Yudofsky SC, Hales RE. Washington, DC, American Psychiatric Press, 1994, pp 313–354

Sloan RL, Brown KW, Pentland B: Fluoxetine as a treatment for emotional lability after brain injury. Brain Inj 6:315–319, 1992

Szlabowicz JW, Stewart JT: Amitriptyline treatment of agitation associated with anoxic encephalopathy. Arch Phys Med Rehabil 71:612–613, 1990

Wroblewski BA, Joseph AB, Kupfer J, et al: Effectiveness of valproic acid on destructive and aggressive behaviors in patients with acquired brain injury. Brain Inj 11:37–47, 1997

Yudofsky SC, Silver JM, Jackson W, et al: The Overt Aggression Scale for the objective rating of verbal and physical aggression. Am J Psychiatry 143:35–39, 1986

Yudofsky SC, Silver JM, Schneider SE: Pharmacologic treatment of aggression. Psychiatr Ann 17:397–407, 1987

Yudofsky SC, Kopecky HJ, Kunik M, et al: The Overt Agitation Severity Scale for the objective rating of agitation. J Neuropsychiatry Clin Neurosci 9:541–548, 1997

Yudofsky SC, Silver JM, Hales RE: Treatment of agitation and aggression, in The American Psychiatric Press Textbook of Psychopharmacology, 2nd Edition. Edited by Schatzberg AF, Nemeroff CB. Washington, DC, American Psychiatric Press, 1998, pp 881–900

Electroconvulsive Therapy and Other Somatic Treatments

Abrams R: Is unilateral electroconvulsive therapy really the treatment of choice in endogenous depression? Ann N Y Acad Sci 462:50–55, 1986

Abrams R: Electroconvulsive Therapy, 2nd Edition. New York, Oxford University Press, 1992

American Psychiatric Association: The Practice of Electroconvulsive Therapy: Recommendations for Treatment, Training, and Privileging. A Task Force Report of the American Psychiatric Association, 2nd Edition. Edited by Weiner RD. Washington, DC, American Psychiatric Association, 2001

Asnis GM, Fink M, Saferstein S: ECT in metropolitan New York hospitals: a survey of practice, 1975–76. Am J Psychiatry 135:479–482, 1978

Avery D, Lubrano A: Depressions treated with imipramine and ECT: the DeCarolis study reconsidered. Am J Psychiatry 136:559–569, 1979

Avery D, Winokur G: Mortality in depressed patients treated with ECT and antidepressants. Arch Gen Psychiatry 33:1029–1037, 1976

Baxter LR Jr, Liston EH, Schwartz JM, et al: Prolongation of the antidepressant response to partial sleep deprivation by lithium. Psychiatry Res 19:17–23, 1986

Berman RM, Narasimhan M, Sanacora G, et al: A randomized clinical trial of repetitive transcranial magnetic stimulation in the treatment of major depression. Biol Psychiatry 47:332–337, 2000

Blehar MC, Rosenthal NE: Seasonal affective disorders and phototherapy: report of a National Institute of Mental Health-sponsored workshop. Arch Gen Psychiatry 46:469–474, 1989

Coffey CE, Weiner RD, Djang WT, et al: Brain anatomic effects of electroconvulsive therapy: a prospective magnetic resonance imaging study. Arch Gen Psychiatry 48:1013–1021, 1991

Coppen A, Abou-Saleb MT, Miller P, et al: Lithium continuation therapy following electroconvulsive therapy. Br J Psychiatry 139:284–287, 1981

Dec GW, Stern TA, Welsch C: The effects of electroconvulsive therapy on serial electrocardiograms and serum cardiac enzyme values: a prospective study of depressed hospitalized inpatients. JAMA 253:2525–2529, 1985

Devanand DP, Verma AK, Tirumalasetti F, et al: Absence of cognitive impairment after more than 100 lifetime ECT treatments. Am J Psychiatry 148:929–932, 1991

Devanand DP, Dwork AJ, Hutchinson ER, et al: Does ECT alter brain structure? Am J Psychiatry 151:957–970, 1994

Devanand DP, Fitzsimons L, Prudic J, et al: Subjective side effects during electroconvulsive therapy. Convuls Ther 11:232–240, 1995

Fink M: Efficacy and safety of induced seizures (ECT) in man. Compr Psychiatry 19:1–18, 1978

George MS, Nahas Z, Molloy M, et al: A controlled trial of daily left prefrontal cortex TMS for treating depression. Biol Psychiatry 48:962–970, 2000a

George MS, Sackeim HA, Marangell LB, et al: Vagus nerve stimulation: a potential therapy for resistant depression? Psychiatr Clin North Am 23:757–783, 2000b

Glassman AH, Roose SP: Delusional depression: a distinct clinical entity. Arch Gen Psychiatry 38:424–427, 1981

Gomez J: Subjective side effects of ECT. Br J Psychiatry 127:609–611, 1975

Grunhaus L, Dannon PN, Schreiber S, et al: Repetitive transcranial magnetic stimulation is as effective as electroconvulsive therapy in the treatment of nondelusional major depressive disorder: an open study. Biol Psychiatry 47:314–324, 2000

Janicak PG, Davis JM, Gibbons RD, et al: Efficacy of ECT: a meta-analysis. Am J Psychiatry 132:297–302, 1985

Kapur S, Mann JJ: Antidepressant action and the neurobiologic effects of ECT: human studies, in The Clinical Science of Electroconvulsive Therapy. Edited by Coffey CE. Washington, DC, American Psychiatric Press, 1993, pp 236–250

Klein E. Kreinin I, Chistyakov A, et al: Therapeutic efficacy of right prefrontal slow repetitive transcranial magnetic stimulation in major depression: a double-blind controlled study. Arch Gen Psychiatry 56:315–320, 1999

Lerer B, Belmaker RH: ECT and lithium: basic mechanisms, parallels, and controls in receptor mechanisms, in ECT: Basic Mechanisms. Edited by Lerer B, Weiner D, Belmaker R. Washington, DC, American Psychiatric Press, 1986

Lerer B, Shapira B, Calev A, et al: Antidepressant and cognitive effects of twice- versus three-times-weekly ECT. Am J Psychiatry 152:4, 564–570, 1995

Lisanby SH, Maddox JH, Prudic J, et al: The effects of electroconvulsive therapy on memory of autobiographical and public events. Arch Gen Psychiatry 57:581–590, 2000

Malitz S, Sackeim HA, Decina P, et al: The efficacy of electroconvulsive therapy: dose-response interactions with modality. Ann N Y Acad Sci 462:56–64, 1986

Maltbie AA, Wingfield MS, Volow MR, et al: Electroconvulsive therapy in the presence of brain tumor: case reports and an evaluation of risk. J Nerv Ment Dis 168:400–405, 1980

Marangell LB, Rush AJ, George MS, et al: Long-term experience with vagus nerve stimulation (VNS) for treatment resistant depression. Paper presented at annual meeting of the Society of Biological Psychiatry, New Orleans, LA, May 3–5, 2001

McCall WV, Reboussin DM, Weiner RD, et al: Titrated moderately suprathreshold vs fixed high-dose right unilateral electroconvulsive therapy: acute antidepressant and cognitive effects. Arch Gen Psychiatry 57:438–444, 2000

Nutt DJ, Glue P: The neurobiology of ECT: animal studies, in The Clinical Science of Electroconvulsive Therapy. Edited by Coffey CE. Washington, DC, American Psychiatric Press, 1993, pp 213–235

Pascual-Leone A, Rubio B, Pallardo F, et al: Rapid rate transcranial magnetic stimulation of left dorsolateral prefrontal cortex in drug-resistant depression. Lancet 348:233–237, 1996

Paul SM, Extein I, Calih H, et al: The use of ECT with treatment resistant depressed patients at the National Institute of Mental Health. Am J Psychiatry 138:486–489, 1977

Perry P, Tsuang MT: Treatment of unipolar depression following electroconvulsive therapy: relapse rate comparison between lithium and tricyclic therapies following ECT. J Affect Disord 1:123–129, 1979

Post RM, Kotin J, Goodwin FK: Effects of sleep deprivation on mood and central amine metabolism in depressed patients. Arch Gen Psychiatry 33:627–632, 1976

Prudic J, Haskett RF, Mulsant B, et al: Resistance to antidepressant medications and short-term clinical response to ECT. Am J Psychiatry 153:985–992, 1996

Reid WH: Electroconvulsive therapy. Tex Med 89:58–62, 1993

Rush AJ, George MS, Sackeim HA, et al: Vagus nerve stimulation (VNS) for treatment-resistant depression: a multicenter study. Biol Psychiatry 47:276–286, 2000

Sackeim HA: Repetitive transcranial magnetic stimulation: what are the next steps? Biol Psychiatry 48:959–961, 2000

Sackeim HA, Prudic J, Devanand DP, et al: The impact of medication resistance and continuation pharmacotherapy on relapse following response to electroconvulsive therapy in major depression. J Clin Psychopharmacol 10:96–104, 1990

Sackeim HA, Prudic J, Devanand DP, et al: Effects of stimulus intensity and electrode placement on the efficacy and cognitive effects of electroconvulsive therapy. N Engl J Med 328:839–846, 1993

Sackeim HA, Prudic J, Devanand DP, et al: A prospective, randomized, double-blind comparison of bilateral and right unilateral electroconvulsive therapy at different stimulus intensities. Arch Gen Psychiatry 57:425–434, 2000

Sackeim HA, Haskett RF, Mulsant BH, et al: Continuation pharmacotherapy in the prevention of relapse following electroconvulsive therapy: a randomized controlled trial. JAMA 285:1299–1307, 2001a

Sackeim HA, Keilp JG, Rush AJ, et al: The effects of vagus nerve stimulation on cognitive performance in patients with treatment-resistant depression. Neuropsychiatry Neuropsychol Behav Neurol 14:53–62, 2001b

Schulman KI, Walker SE: Refining the MAOI diet: tyramine content of pizzas and soy products. J Clin Psychiatry 60:191–193, 1999

Schwarz T, Loenwenstein J, Isenberg KE: Maintenance ECT: indications and outcome. Convuls Ther 11:14–23, 1995

Shapira B, Gorfine M, Lerer B: A prospective study of lithium continuation therapy in depressed patients who have responded to electroconvulsive therapy. Convuls Ther 11:80–85, 1995

Small JG, Milstein V, Klapper MH, et al: Electroconvulsive therapy in the treatment of manic episodes. Ann N Y Acad Sci 462:37–49, 1986

Sobin C, Sackeim HA, Prudic J, et al: Predictors of retrograde amnesia following ECT. Am J Psychiatry 152:995–1001, 1995

Squire LR, Slater PC: Electroconvulsive therapy and complaints of memory dysfunction: a prospective three-year follow-up study. Br J Psychiatry 142:1–8, 1983

Squire LR, Slater PC, Chance PM: Retrograde amnesia: temporal gradient in very long-term memory following electroconvulsive therapy. Science 187:77–79, 1975

Stoudemire A, Hill CD, Morris R, et al: Improvement in depression-related cognitive dysfunction following ECT. J Neuropsychiatry Clin Neurosci 7:31–34, 1995

Terman M, Terman JS, Quitkin FM, et al: Light therapy for seasonal affective disorder: a review of efficacy. Neuropsychopharmacology 2:1–22, 1989

Walker SE, Shulman KI, Tailor SA: The monoamine oxidase inhibitor (MAOI) diet and kosher pizza (letter, reply). J Clin Psychopharmacol 17:227–228, 1997

Wehr TA, Rosenthal NE: Seasonality and affective illness. Am J Psychiatry 146:829–839, 1989

Weiner RD: The psychiatric use of electrically induced seizures. Am J Psychiatry 136:1507–1516, 1979

Wells DG, Bjorkstein AR: Monoamine oxidase inhibitors revisited. Can J Anaesth 36:64–74, 1989

Yudofsky SC: ECT in general hospital psychiatry: focus on new indications and technologies. Gen Hosp Psychiatry 3:292–296, 1981

Yudofsky SC: Electroconvulsive therapy in the eighties: technique and technologies. Am J Psychother 36:391–398, 1982

Yudofsky SC, Hales RE, Ferguson T: What You Need to Know About Psychiatric Drugs. New York, Grove Weidenfeld, 1991

Brief Dynamic Individual Psychotherapy

Hanna Levenson, Ph.D.

Stephen F. Butler, Ph.D.

Edward Bein, Ph.D.

It has now been established in a number of studies with a variety of patients—across a range of settings with diverse agendas—that regardless of the type of outpatient treatment patients begin (e.g., long-term psychotherapy, short-term therapy), the great majority are seen only for 6–12 sessions (Garfield 1986; Goldman and Taube 1988; Olfson and Pincus 1994; Phillips 1987). In fact, it has been estimated that 50% of all outpatients drop out of treatment before the eighth session (Phillips 1987). These findings hold even when the treatments are specifically psychodynamic in nature.

Although there is evidence that the majority of therapy is brief, most of these therapies have been unplanned brief treatments (e.g., premature terminations, dropouts, no-shows). Levenson and colleagues, however, attempted to assess the prevalence of intentional short-term treatments. In a comprehensive national survey of 3,600 psychologists, psychiatrists, and social workers (response rate=57%), almost all respondents in the three disciplines (89% of psychologists, 77% of psychiatrists, and 84% of social workers) reported conducting some planned brief therapy (i.e., therapy designed to be limited in duration and/or focus) (Davidovitz and Levenson 1995; Levenson and Davidovitz 2000). As expected, cognitive-behavioral therapists conducted brief therapy for the greatest number of hours per week, and psychodynamic therapists spent the least amount of time conducting brief therapy. Overall, the psychodynamically oriented psychiatrists, psychologists, and social workers were responsible for one-quarter of all brief therapy conducted nationally. The type of location in which the therapy was conducted (rural, nonmetropolitan, or metropolitan) had no effect on the proportion of therapists conducting brief therapy or the amount of time spent conducting such therapy. Therefore, most mental health professionals are conducting treatments that are short term, whether by default or by design.

In our first section we examine the past and present practice of short-term dynamic psychotherapy. We then elucidate those qualities that we believe describe contemporary brief dynamic psychotherapy. In subsequent sections we examine clinically relevant research and factors influencing the practice of brief dynamic psychotherapy, such as training and therapist reluctance to use briefer treatment modes. We conclude with our recommendations for improving the challenging arena of brief dynamic psychotherapy.

Historical Perspective and Contemporary Approaches

We provide a history of short-term therapy to emphasize the fact that brief therapy is not new. As pointed out by

The authors gratefully acknowledge the contributions of Drs. Joanna S. Burg, Robert Weisman, and David Overstreet to various sections.

Miller (1996), "to a large extent, the implementation of brief therapy innovations occurred before managed care came to dominate mental health services" (p. 355). From a historical and conceptual viewpoint, short-term dynamic psychotherapies may be conveniently grouped into "generations" (Crits-Christoph et al. 1991). We briefly mention four such generations as a way of tracing the evolution in the thinking and practice of brief dynamic psychotherapy. For further information on the early history of brief dynamic psychotherapy, the reader is referred to Marmor's (1979) overview as well as to the original works.

First Generation: Freud and Psychoanalysis

Contemporary brief dynamic psychotherapy is anchored in the work of Freud. Several of Freud's early treatments were short-term therapies. As described by Marmor (1979), Bruno Walter, the conductor, was treated successfully by Freud in six sessions in 1906, and in 1908 Freud cured Gustav Mahler, the composer, of impotency problems in a single 4-hour session. Even training analyses were conducted in less than 1 year. As psychoanalytic theory became more complex and elaborate, and the goals of analysis became more ambitious, the length of treatments increased. Freud's focus on free association was what Davanloo (1986) called a "fateful step," from which the early advocates of brief psychotherapy began to diverge. Davanloo noted: "Almost all attempts to reverse this trend and develop an effective technique of short-term psychotherapy have been based on taking back some of the control and putting more of the motive power [for the treatment] into the hands of the therapist" (p. 108).

In 1925, Sandor Ferenczi and Otto Rank published *The Development of Psychoanalysis*, in which they advocated time limits, a focus for the treatment, and a frequently active stance for the therapist. Even by today's standards, these authors' contributions to brief dynamic psychotherapy remain innovative and central to modern dynamic approaches. Ferenczi and Rank wished to increase the therapist's activity to counter the patient's passivity. Presaging many aspects both of object relations and of the interpersonal brief therapies was Ferenczi's emphasis on the frankness, empathy, and democracy of the patient–therapist relationship (Rachman 1988). Rank introduced precursors of two additional tenets of modern brief psychotherapy: 1) the issue of separation activated by setting a time limit in advance (Rank's concept of the *birth trauma*) and 2) assessment of the patient's motivation to change (Rank's concept of the *will*). For these rea-

sons, Marmor (1979) wrote that Rank "may well be the most important historical forerunner of the brief dynamic psychotherapy movement" (p. 150).

Several years after Freud's death in 1939, another serious challenge to classical psychoanalysis unfolded. In their seminal book *Psychoanalytic Therapy: Principles and Applications*, Alexander and French (1946) questioned the presumed relationship between therapeutic outcome and length of therapy. Their book has been recognized by some current practitioners as the first brief therapy manual. Alexander and French's best-known recommendation is that psychotherapists should actively adjust their conduct or manner so that patients are provided with a "corrective emotional experience." Alexander and French advocated therapist flexibility and adjustment of the length and frequency of sessions. These maneuvers were intended to prevent the patient's passive dependency and the development of a transference neurosis. Intense controversy occurred within the psychoanalytic community in reaction to the ideas of Ferenczi, Rank, and Alexander and French, and, thus, the contributions of these investigators were ignored for many years.

Second Generation: Short-Term Dynamic Psychotherapies

In this phase, from 1960 to 1980, brief dynamic therapy began to emerge as a legitimate therapeutic method. David Malan of the Tavistock Clinic in London, James Mann of Boston University School of Medicine, Peter Sifneos of Massachusetts General Hospital in Boston, and Habib Davanloo of Montreal General Hospital in Canada are usually seen as the main representatives of this generation.

Malan's brief therapy techniques derive from psychoanalytic principles—an "applied psychoanalysis" (Ursano and Hales 1986). Malan believed that "far reaching changes could be brought about in relatively severe and chronic illnesses by a technique of active interpretation containing all the essential elements of full scale analysis" (Malan 1976, p. 20). Malan concentrated on identification of a focal problem—a "nuclear" or childhood conflict that is manifested in some form in the current presenting problem. He would frame the focal problem in terms of the patient's characteristic defense-anxiety-impulse configurations; that is, the characteristic defensive behaviors the patient employed to protect himself or herself from experiencing anxiety-provoking conflictual impulses or feelings. Malan referred to the defense-anxiety-impulse framework as the *triangle of conflict*, and interpretations would be used to articulate the three components. He would also draw the patient's attention to parallels among the defense-anxiety-impulse configurations the patient had enacted in relationship with the therapist, with others in the patient's current life, and with important figures from the past. The parallels among the three kinds of relationships are referred to as the *triangle of person.* For example, the therapist might point out that a patient's deferential and dependent manner toward the therapist seems characteristic of childhood interactions that the patient had with his or her parents and might explore why the aforementioned patient needed to adopt an acquiescent attitude with the parents.

Mann is credited with deriving a generic theoretical orientation that focuses on the difficulties in dealing with separation and loss (Levenson et al. 1997; Mann 1973). His *time-limited treatment* consists of 12 sessions. It is asserted that the fixed duration forces the patient to face unconscious issues related to the passage of time. In the relationship with the therapist, the patient is thought to relive (in a healthier way) reunion with and separation from that parent who has failed the patient and who is regarded with ambivalence and guilt.

Sifneos (1987) developed techniques and a rationale for his *short-term anxiety-provoking psychotherapy* (STAPP). He contributed greater specificity to selection and exclusion criteria, focus of inquiry, and anxiety-provoking intervention techniques. His work focuses on the efficacy of brief dynamic therapy with relatively high-functioning patients experiencing conflicts associated with oedipal issues. No number of sessions is agreed on at the outset, but a length between 6 and 20 sessions is determined as the therapy proceeds. Sifneos assumes a role that is part therapist and part teacher (Bloom 1992). Burke et al. (1979) more descriptively noted that Sifneos "is like a schoolmaster seeing through the excuses and alibis of his recalcitrant pupils" (p. 178). For example, a STAPP therapist, after hearing "I don't know" from the patient in response to a question about the patient's emotional ties to her father, says, "Oh, come on, of course you know! Just tell me!" (Nielsen and Barth 1991, p. 66).

Davanloo, after training under Malan, developed his *intensive short-term dynamic psychotherapy* (ISTDP) approach. ISTDP was designed to break through the patient's defensive barrier using confrontational techniques similar to those of Sifneos. Vagueness, tentativeness, detachment, evasiveness, diversionary tactics, intellectualization, rationalization, rumination, projection, introjection, and weepiness are dramatically pointed out to patients to intensify feelings and crystallize the patients' resistance. The crisis of being confronted by the therapist "produces intense affects which tap into a res-

ervoir of unconscious thoughts, memories and feelings, and activate the unconscious therapeutic alliance. This dynamic flow speeds and compresses the psychoanalytic process" (Laiken et al. 1991, p. 93). Davanloo (1978) sees himself as "the relentless healer." He is particularly interested in working with patients who have chronic, serious psychopathology; consequently, he offers treatment to a wider range of patients than do many other brief dynamic therapists.

Third Generation: Research-Based Interpersonal Therapies

The approaches of the second generation furthered the practice of brief dynamic psychotherapy, but empirical support was sparse. Selection criteria and interventions were formulated primarily by ideology, clinical judgment, and theoretical inference, rather than by systematic application of research findings (Perry et al. 1983).

The third generation of brief therapies has done much to provide empirical support for the efficacy of brief dynamic therapy, as well as to elucidate its active therapeutic ingredients. However, these therapies have tended to exclude particularly difficult patients from their research for methodological reasons. In addition to an empirical emphasis, the third-generation therapies herald a move away from *intra*psychic (one-person) models of theory and practice to more *inter*personal (two-person) ones. Representatives of this wave are *time-limited dynamic psychotherapy* (TLDP), developed by Hans Strupp and Jeffrey Binder at Vanderbilt University (Strupp and Binder 1984); *short-term supportive-expressive psychotherapy*, formulated by Lester Luborsky at the University of Pennsylvania (Luborsky and Crits-Christoph 1990); and *control mastery theory*, created by Joseph Weiss and Harold Sampson at Mount Zion Hospital in San Francisco (Weiss et al. 1986).

As an example of this research-based interpersonal approach, Strupp and Binder's TLDP will be briefly reviewed. A manual for the practice of TLDP, *Psychotherapy in a New Key* (Strupp and Binder 1984), was developed as part of efforts of the Vanderbilt Psychotherapy Research Team. This manual, which was designed to standardize the application of TLDP technique, represents an attempt to make the model more learnable. (Some of the drawbacks of "manualized" therapies will be discussed later.)

TLDP has a psychoanalytic foundation; however, personality development and functioning are viewed from an interpersonal and object relations perspective. The major objective of TLDP is to examine recurrent maladaptive themes from the patient's range of object relations that are activated in relation to the therapist. Consistent focus is directed to the patient's manner of construing and relating to the therapist both as a significant person in the present and as the personification of past relationships. The patient–therapist relationship is conceived of as a dyadic system in which the behavior of both participants is continually scrutinized and modified (Strupp and Binder 1984). The rationale for this approach stems from the view that regardless of the severity of psychopathology, interpersonal relations are the arena in which intrapsychic conflict is expressed. Very much in the tradition of Alexander and French, the goal of TLDP is to provide patients with corrective interpersonal experiences by helping them "discover, identify, and understand the meanings of the beliefs, feelings, and action patterns that interfere with their current living, built on erroneous and obsolescent assumptions carried forward automatically from earlier phases" (Strupp and Binder 1984, p. 137). The duration of treatment is approximately 25 sessions and is established very early in treatment.

Fourth Generation: Experiential/Integrative Treatments

Contemporary approaches constituting the fourth generation are characterized by two main features. First, they incorporate concepts and/or techniques from various sources external to psychoanalysis (e.g., cognitive-behavioral therapy, child development, neuroscience) into the more traditional psychodynamic perspectives and strategies. Second, they emphasize in-session experiential factors as critical components of the therapeutic process. In addition to theoretical and clinical advances, the fourth-generation approaches were also influenced in the direction of pragmatism and efficiency by powerful economic and sociopolitical forces (Levenson and Burg 2000; also see "Managed Care, Consumerism, and the Zeitgeist" subsection later in this chapter).

Three such experiential/integrative approaches will illustrate. One of them, from McCullough Vaillant (1997), builds on the second-generation approaches of Malan and Davanloo. Accordingly, it attempts to facilitate rapid change by creating opportunities for intense in-session affective experience in relation to the therapist (see also Magnavita 1997 and Fosha 2000). The other two, from Levenson (1995) and Safran and Muran (2000), extend the relational thinking of the third generation and seek to promote experiential learning emanating from in-session transactions between therapist and patient.

McCullough Vaillant's (1997) *short-term anxiety-regulating psychotherapy* (STARP) attempts to heal char-

acter pathology. In essence, it enhances Malan's treatment approach by incorporating perspectives and techniques from outside psychoanalysis. Its theory of personality functioning and psychopathology updates Malan's triangle of conflict with Silvan Tomkins' (1984) affect theory. Its theory of technique applies principles of learning theory to the pursuit of psychoanalytic goals:

> The deepest level of integration in this model occurs in the application of learning theory principles not only to external behavior but also to the *psychodynamic experience and meanings* of the two [Malan] triangles. Behavioral principles (reinforcement, extinction, desensitization, and so on) provide the general mechanisms by which the intrapsychic workings of the mind are altered. (McCullough Vaillant 1997, p. 50)

For example, part of the value of the psychoanalytic analysis of the transference is its activation of anxiety in the patient, which with enough repetitions allows the patient to become desensitized to it and better able to experience the conflictual affects that elicited it. Psychodynamic, experiential (e.g., guided imagery), and behavioral (e.g., desensitization) interventions are all appropriate means for implementing these general mechanisms in order to help patients relinquish defenses and experience disowned affects. McCullough Vaillant, partly due to the influence of self psychology, espouses a less confrontational approach than that of Davanloo. For example, in response to a patient who avoids answering a question about her feelings, the STARP therapist might say, "As I ask you about your feelings, you often look away and become silent. Are you aware that this is happening? Is this topic painful for you to look at? Is there some way that I can help you make it more bearable to face?" (McCullough Vaillant 1997, p. 13). For more impaired patients, McCullough Vaillant will sometimes structure a STARP treatment as a series of blocks of sessions, with the time in between blocks seen as allowing the patient to enhance in-session progress on his or her own.

Levenson's (1995, in press) approach to TLDP is based on Strupp and Binder's (1984) third-generation model for treating chronic and pervasive dysfunctional interpersonal patterns, but it differs from that model in its greater use of concepts and techniques from other theoretical orientations (e.g., schema-focused cognitive, behavioral, systems) and in its greater emphasis on experiential learning (rather than focusing on insight through interpretation). On the basis of the patient's unique way of interacting, particular recursive loops of affective and behavioral changes that signify a new manner of interacting are encouraged so that the patient gains a different appreciation of him- or herself, of the therapist, and of their interaction. These changes provide the patient with experiential learning so that old patterns may be relinquished and new (i.e., healthier) patterns may evolve. For example, the therapist of a subservient, anxiety-ridden patient might try to create situations that encourage the patient to act more assertively in-session, thereby promoting feelings of independence (previously defended against), which in turn would further enable the patient to behave more boldly—thus facilitating a recursive loop of behavior promoting affect promoting behavior.

Safran and Muran's (2000) *brief relational therapy* (BRT) was designed to help therapists recognize and resolve problems in the therapeutic alliance. It is based on contemporary relational perspectives that integrate ideas from object relations theory, self psychology, interpersonal theory, and postmodern theory (Aron 1996; Mitchell and Aron 1999). It also draws on the Buddhist notion of "mindfulness," the goal of which is to "become aware of and then deautomate our habitual ways of structuring our experience through automatic psychological activities and actions" (Safran and Muran 2000, p. 57). Central to the relational perspectives is the notion of a "two-person psychology," according to which "the impact of the analyst [therapist] needs to be examined systematically as an intrinsic part of the transference, which is thought to be based on the mutual contributions of both participants to the interaction" (Aron 1996, p. 50). BRT embraces a "two-person" perspective more comprehensively than did third-generation therapies, emphasizing the therapist's subjectivity and seeing countertransference as more the rule than the exception. It gives intense focus to the "here and now" of treatment, paying special attention to the recognition and repair of ruptures in the therapeutic alliance (Safran and Muran 1996). Such repair requires an ongoing collaboration between patient and therapist in which the contributions of both are examined.

Safran and Muran (2000) stressed the value of therapist "metacommunication" over traditional transference interpretations; although both comment on patient–therapist interactions, the former is less inferential about patient motives and more grounded in the therapist's immediate experience. For example, a therapist who was feeling confused about the lack of emotional depth in recent sessions said to his patient, "You know, I've been trying to figure out what's been going on between us. It feels to me like there's been a quality of flatness to our last few sessions. I think I've been kind of hesitant to bring it up, because of a reluctance to spoil things between us, and because I've had a sense of things going well between us, and of enjoying our time together" (Saf-

ran and Muran 2000, pp. 110–111). During the ensuing discussion, the patient was able to acknowledge the sense of flatness, to recognize that it was due in part to her discomfort with discord, and later to voice her disappointment in the helpfulness of the treatment. BRT also sanctions the use of experiential techniques such as "awareness experiments" as alternative approaches to help promote patient ownership of disowned feelings.

Qualities That Define Brief Dynamic Psychotherapy

What are the essential features that distinguish brief dynamic psychotherapy from other types of therapy? A review of the literature of the past 20 years reveals numerous publications addressing this topic (e.g., Bauer and Kobos 1987; Burlingame and Fuhriman 1987; Crits-Christoph and Barber 1991; Flegenheimer 1982; Gustafson 1984; Koss and Shiang 1994; Koss et al. 1986; Levenson 1995; Levenson et al. 2000; MacKenzie 1991; Magnavita 1993; Marmor 1979; Mendelsohn 1978; Messer and Warren 1995; Small 1979; Wolberg 1980). A content analysis of these papers reveals several fundamental qualities. Some of these qualities have been mentioned repeatedly in the literature and, therefore, appear to be quite essential in defining brief dynamic psychotherapy; others are less frequently reported and seem more peripheral.

The qualities of brief dynamic psychotherapy can, in general, be organized into two main categories: those qualities pertaining to the *brief features* per se and those germane to the *psychodynamic aspects* (Table 25–1). Within each category the qualities are rank-ordered in terms of the number of times they are mentioned in these various publications. These characteristics may be conceptualized as a consensual, operational definition of short-term dynamic psychotherapy. The first four brief qualities—limited focus and goals, limited time, selection criteria, and increased therapist activity—will be examined in some detail, followed by a discussion of brief therapy modifications in psychoanalytic concepts and techniques.

Limited Therapeutic Focus

A major concept distinguishing the brief dynamic psychotherapy approaches from long-term psychotherapy or psychoanalysis is the idea of a limited focus of treatment. Probably the earliest attempt to provide a focus for analytically oriented treatment was when Rank (1929/1936) set a predetermined termination date and concentrated

TABLE 25–1. Qualities that define brief psychodynamic psychotherapy

Brief qualities
Limited focus (and limited goals)
Limited time
Selection criteria
Therapist activity
Therapeutic alliance
Rapid assessment/prompt intervention
Termination
Optimism
Contract
Psychodynamic qualities
Analytic concepts
Analytic techniques

Note. Qualities based on the frequency with which they are mentioned in the literature.

TABLE 25–2. Focus of treatment

Theorist(s)	Focus
Malan	Wish–threat–defense (triangle of conflict)
	Therapist–current relationships–past relationships (triangle of person)
Sifneos	
Short-term anxiety-provoking psychotherapy	Unresolved conflict defined during evaluation—typically oedipal issues
Mann	
Time-limited psychotherapy	Conflict over time limits and loss—especially the pain and limitations imposed by dealing with loss defensively
Davanloo	
Intensive short-term dynamic psychotherapy	Triangle of person; triangle of conflict
Luborsky and Mark[a]	
Short-term supportive-expressive psychotherapy	Core conflictual relationship theme (CCRT)—wish–response from other–response from self
Strupp and Binder	
Time-limited dynamic psychotherapy	Cyclical maladaptive patterns/dynamic focus—acts of self-expectations of others—acts of others—introject
Weiss and Sampson— Mount Zion Group	
Control-mastery theory	Unconscious pathogenic beliefs and intention to get better
McCullough Vaillant	
Short-term anxiety-regulating psychotherapy	Triangle of conflict (revised)
Levenson	
Experiential time-limited dynamic psychotherapy	Corrective interpersonal experiences to change cyclical maladaptive patterns
Safran and Muran	
Brief relational therapy	Moment-to-moment awareness

Note. [a]See Luborsky and Mark 1991.
Source. Some material adapted from Barber and Crits-Christoph 1991, p. 337.

on the separation issues stimulated by this date. Ferenczi and Rank (1925) argued against attempting a complete analysis for every patient when they noted that "in the correctly executed analysis the whole development of the individual is not repeated, but only those phases of development of the infantile libido on which the ego… has remained fixed" (p. 19). Alexander and French (1946) likewise argued that it is not necessary to analyze all aspects of every patient's mental life. Rather, the analysis need extend back only to the point at which the trauma causing the patient difficulty occurred (Flegenheimer 1982). Furthermore, Alexander and French (1946) advocated limiting the patient's regression by using such modifications as reducing the frequency of sessions and using a chair instead of a couch.

Brief therapists need a central theme, topic, or problem to serve as a guide so that they will be able to stay on target—a necessity when time is of the essence. Brief therapists cannot pay attention to all clinical data; even fascinating material must sometimes be ignored. Practitioners working with short-term models must learn to use *selective attention* (Malan 1963) and *benign neglect* (Pumpian-Mindlin 1953) or they run the risk of being overwhelmed by the patient's rich intrapsychic and interpersonal life.

A detailed presentation of the different foci represented by the various brief dynamic theorists is beyond the scope of this chapter. However, in Table 25–2 we summarize the focus of treatment for several of the main brief dynamic theorists. The reader is referred to the original sources or to the excellent volume edited by Crits-Christoph and Barber (1991) for more information.

Examination of the different brief dynamic psychotherapies reveals some general trends in the development of focal methods. As previously stated, the theoretical emphasis of third-generation brief dynamic therapies shifted from an intrapsychic to an interpersonal focus, deemphasizing wishes and impulses in favor of efforts to define recurrent interpersonal patterns that create and maintain dysfunctional relationships in the patient's life. This interpersonal focus is typically identified early in the treatment and communicated to the patient, and digressions away from the focus are discouraged. In general, vignettes of interpersonal interactions with significant others are scrutinized by the therapist to extract repetitive maladaptive efforts to deal with interpersonal conflict. The patient's transference reaction to the therapist is presumed to be an expression of the same basic relationship problems that create difficulty for the patient in his or her daily life. The different theorists proffer different explanations for the link between the patient's core conflicts and the presenting symptomatology, but all agree that these relationship themes must be addressed in the therapy.

A particularly important development in the field is reflected in the efforts of Luborsky and Crits-Christoph (1990), Strupp and Binder (1984), the Mount Zion Psychotherapy Research Group (Weiss et al. 1986), and Horowitz et al. (1984), who offered explicit methodologies for generating a therapeutic focus. Prior to these efforts, a focal theme was left to be intuited based on clinical experience. The development of formalized, systematic methods for defining the focal theme promises more effective means of training therapists (Strupp et al. 1988) and greater accessibility to research protocols for investigating the role actually played by the dynamic focus.

Early research on therapeutic focus was conducted by Malan (1976), who reported that undirected interpretations (i.e., interpretations not associated with a central issue) were negatively associated with outcome. This work, however, has been criticized for its methodology (e.g., no control group, use of case notes rather than audio- or videotapes). Malan's pioneering effort, however, was followed by a study conducted by the Mount Zion group (Silberschatz et al. 1986), which demonstrated that interpretations compatible with the patient's unconscious "plan" to get better were more effective than other interpretations. Similarly, accuracy of interpretations has been found to be predictive of positive outcome (Joyce et al. 1995). A convergence of findings appears to support the efficacy of establishing a focus and maintaining that focus throughout the treatment. However, a caveat is warranted here—namely, that the meager evidence available also supports the notion that the therapist should be *flexible*. Rounsaville et al. (1988) investigated therapists trained to adhere to an interpersonal focus with depressed patients and found that therapists were judged by supervisors to be more skillful when they deviated from the prescribed protocol with difficult patients. Clearly, rigid efforts to adhere to a focus and

discourage deviations are likely to damage the therapeutic alliance and result in poor outcome.

Thus, paying attention to material directly related to the focus does not mean coercing patients or ignoring what is important to them. Schacht et al. (1984) emphasized that disregard for what a patient says or does could weaken the therapeutic alliance and be perceived as unempathic by the patient. The therapist should repeatedly attempt to enable the patient to work on the focal issue: "The therapist's patterning of questions, the timing and shaping of the context for questions, the choices of what to name and what to leave nameless, should all create an associative atmosphere in which focally relevant material predominates because it seems most narratively natural" (Schacht et al. 1984, p. 108). Some general guidelines for developing a psychodynamic focus are given in Table 25–3. These guidelines underscore the importance of sensitive and simultaneous attention to patterns of past and present functioning. As Wolberg (1980) stated,

> Little time is available in short-term therapy to explore the past. Much better use can be made of the treatment hour by dealing with pertinent elements in the here and now. However, where the therapist can determine important past events and contingencies that have molded the personality organization, this will facilitate a better understanding of the patient's illness and help select an appropriate dynamic focus. (p. 101)

TABLE 25–3. General principles for developing a psychodynamic focus

1. Gather historical material and other data, but let the patient tell his or her own story.
2. Study the patient's characteristic defensive pattern.
3. Be sensitive to how present patterns have roots in the past.
4. Watch for transference patterns; deal with negative transference reactions rapidly and supportively.
5. Examine possible countertransference feelings and behavior for clues as to repetitive dysfunctional patterns.
6. Constantly look for resistances that threaten to block progress.

Source. Adapted from Wolberg 1980.

Bauer and Kobos (1987) contend that "the focus of treatment should be clear, specific, and manageable" (p. 157). Related to, but separate from, therapeutic focus is "manageability" of the focus within the allotted time, sometimes referred to as having "limited goals." The aim of brief dynamic psychotherapy is not "cure" once and for all. Rather, the therapy should provide an opportunity to foster some changes in behavior and thinking, permitting more adaptive coping and a better sense of one's self. Brief dynamic therapy is seen as an opportunity to begin a process of change that continues long after the therapy is over. Additionally, brief therapy is also viewed as rendering appropriate help for brief periods throughout the life cycle. This outlook has resulted in a more general-practice framework for brief psychotherapy (Budman and Gurman 1988) in which therapists (like internists or family practitioners) have discontinuous but enduring relationships with patients as the patients deal with developmental stresses and the intermittent strains of life.

Time Limits and Time Management

Naturally, time is the critical variable that defines an approach as *short-term*, *brief*, or *time-limited*. The issue of time is the second most frequently mentioned brief therapy criterion. Although most clinicians set 25 sessions as the upper limit of brief therapy (Koss and Shiang 1994), the number of sessions may range from one session (e.g., Bloom 1992; Hoyt et al. 1992) to as many as 40 (Sifneos 1979).

Time, like focus, can be conceptualized in a variety of ways. Burlingame and Fuhriman (1987) divided considerations of duration into three categories: *specific time limits*, *variable time limits*, and *time-attentive considerations* (MacKenzie 1991). Usually the *limiting* or *rationing* of time is used conceptually to accelerate the therapeutic work, either by raising the patient's awareness of the existential issues of finite time and mortality (e.g., Mann 1973) or by encouraging therapist activity and adherence to a focus (e.g., Horowitz et al. 1984).

Although it is most customary for psychodynamically oriented short-term therapists to use the traditional weekly 50-minute "hour," many are experimenting with the frequency of sessions (e.g., frequent initial sessions with more intermittent later sessions), the duration of each therapy session (e.g., the 20-minute "hour"), and even the number of successive brief therapies (e.g., intermittent brief therapy throughout the life cycle). Marmor (1979) pointed out that setting time limits has three clinical consequences. First, it emphasizes individuation-separation issues, which commonly underlie presenting problems. Second, it acknowledges the autonomy of the patient. Third, it encourages the patient's independence and self-confidence.

Unfortunately, time limits are being used increasingly for administrative and economic reasons instead of therapeutic ones. In the worst of situations, there may be no therapeutic basis for the number of sessions patients receive, such decisions being determined only by the financial bottom line. In the best of situations, managed care programs monitor the quality of care and promote patients' resourcefulness (Levenson and Burg 2000).

The brief dynamic psychotherapies largely have been developed for and researched with highly selected, and usually highly functioning, patients (see "Selection Criteria" subsection below). It may be dangerous to make the assumption that brief (especially very brief) courses of treatment can be readily extended to severely disturbed patients with chaotic lifestyles. The amount of therapy that is appropriate for the treatment of severe conditions remains an important empirical question. *Variable time limits* are used by some therapeutic models that propose altering the time allotted based on various factors such as therapist experience (Malan 1976) or type and severity of presenting complaint (Davanloo 1978). Strupp and Binder (1984) suggested using 25-session "blocks" of therapy, with sharply defined goals for each block, and McCullough Vaillant (1997) has offered similar suggestions.

More recently, however, brief dynamic therapists are moving away from conceptualizing therapy merely in terms of a specific amount of time and are instead addressing ways to make every session count regardless of length of treatment. These models are categorized as *time attentive*. Examples of this approach include the idea of the therapist's *time-limited attitude* (regardless of the actual length of therapy) (Binder et al. 1987) and the notion of brief therapy as a "state of mind of the therapist and of the patient" (Budman and Gurman 1988, p. 10).

Selection Criteria

The importance of selection criteria is a controversial subject in the brief dynamic psychotherapy field. Early in the history of psychoanalysis, as psychoanalytic treatments became progressively longer, Freud (1904/1953) put forth the possibility that treatment might be shortened with healthier patients. Largely based on this comment, rigorous patient selection to identify the healthiest patients became an early and integral part of virtually all brief dynamic psychotherapies.

The problem then arose of how to determine which patients were the "healthiest" and which ones would respond well to a brief course of treatment. Rank (1929/1936) introduced the role of the patient's "will" or motivation for therapeutic change. That patients motivated for change are more likely than others to benefit from brief psychotherapy remains an important idea for modern short-term psychodynamic theorists. Later, Alexander and French (1946) proposed that brief treatment was suitable for patients with mild, chronic, and acute neurosis (Flegenheimer 1982). Good motivation, ego strength, and response to trial interpretations were also mentioned, along with the patient's willingness and ability to take an active role in the treatment. Although Alexander held that severity of symptoms bore no relationship to length of treatment, he reserved standard psychoanalysis for severe chronic neurosis.

Following these early pioneers, modern short-term theorists extended the applications of traditional psychoanalytic concepts to patient selection. In their reviews of the psychoanalytic literature on analyzability, Bachrach and Leaff (1978) noted that a patient's suitability for treatment is typically judged from reports of the patient's history and general level of functioning. Such concepts as high ego strength and a history of good object relations are considered prognostic indicators of significant therapeutic gains. Thus, those credited with bringing brief dynamic psychotherapy into the modern therapeutic arena (Davanloo 1978, 1980; Malan 1963, 1976, 1979; Mann 1973; Sifneos 1972, 1979) specified fairly stringent suitability characteristics:

- Appropriate ego strength
- Ability to become rapidly involved in and contribute to treatment
- Adequate motivation
- A history of meaningful relationships
- Adequate intelligence or psychological sophistication
- A relatively circumscribed problem or symptom presentation (as opposed to wide-ranging difficulties in many aspects of the patient's life)

In addition, these authors specified relatively consistent exclusion criteria, such as psychosis, major affective disorders (especially bipolar disorder), drug use, suicidal tendencies (and other acting out) or impulsive tendencies, organic disorders, and some personality disorders (borderline personality disorder, especially in those patients with histories of acting out, and schizoid personality disorder, when interpersonal unresponsiveness on the part of the patient is noted). Finally, following Malan's (1976) notion of a "trial interpretation," short-term theorists generally suggest an interview or trial session to evaluate the patient's ability to engage in the therapeutic tasks. The inclusion and exclusion criteria for the major short-term dynamic approaches are given in Table 25–4.

How do these selection criteria hold up? Attempts to evaluate patients' suitability for brief dynamic psychotherapy generally recognize that there are two basic approaches. One involves an assessment of the patient's general state of psychological health and tends to focus on psychoanalytic formulations of *patient characteristics* antedating the psychotherapy (such as ego functioning and quality of object relations). However, such concepts are typically highly abstract and difficult to translate into specific clinical and empirical observations. Binder et al. (1987) pointed out that "it is much easier to agree about the importance of 'ego strength' than to specify its manifestations" (p. 156). Similarly, it has proven to be difficult to establish clear, concrete evidence of Sifneos' (1979) requirement of one "meaningful" relationship in the patient's history.

The other approach to evaluate patients' suitability for brief dynamic psychotherapy involves using *performance criteria*, that is, a patient's performance during early interviews. This approach echoes early attempts to gauge the willingness and ability of patients to become actively involved in treatment and their response to trial interpretations. Such trial interpretations were hoped to provide a stimulus from which to assess the patient's insightfulness and manner of dealing with psychological issues, sometimes referred to as *psychological mindedness*. Thus, this in vivo evaluation was thought to provide a direct assessment of the patient's ability to engage in the actual behavior demanded in the therapeutic situation.

Despite its promise, however, performance-based assessment has only minimally enhanced the ability to forecast outcome in brief dynamic psychotherapy. Thackrey and colleagues (1993; Butler et al. 1987) tested a scale that was intended to assess a patient's willingness and ability to engage in psychotherapy and that used low inference judgments made by independent raters and interviewing clinicians. These ratings yielded significant correlations with outcome ($r = .30–.52$), accounting for 9%–25% of the variance in process and outcome measures. Although correlations of this magnitude are not small by the standards of psychotherapy research, nonetheless 75%–91% of the variance was *not accounted for* by ratings of the patient's performance in an early interview.

Several possibilities might explain these modest results. First, as in most controlled psychotherapy studies, this study's inclusion criteria eliminated the most severe psychopathology. Thus, patients with psychosis, patients currently requiring hospitalization, actively suicidal or homicidal patients, and patients with active, severe comorbid substance abuse were excluded. Restricting the range of studied patients in this way would be expected to reduce the chances of obtaining strong correlations. The correlations observed in this study would undoubtedly have been higher had a broader range of patients been included.

Patients with severe personality disorder, for example, would seem less likely to benefit from brief dynamic

TABLE 25–4. Criteria for patient selection for brief dynamic psychotherapy

Theorist(s)	Inclusion criteria	Exclusion criteria
Malan	Capacity to form good relationships Good response to trial interpretations	Addictions, serious suicide attempts, ECT Severe major depression, acting out
Sifneos Short-term anxiety-provoking psychotherapy	Intelligence, psychological mindedness History of meaningful relationships Motivation for change beyond symptom relief Appropriate affect during interview One major and specific complaint	Psychosis, major affective syndrome, addiction Suicidal tendencies and acting out Severe personality disorder
Mann Time-limited psychotherapy	Good ego strength, capacity for rapid affective connection and disconnection Definable focus Mild neurosis and personality disorders	Psychosis, schizoid, and severe obsessional personality disorders Severe psychosomatic disorders
Davanloo Intensive short-term dynamic psychotherapy	Wide range Pass trial therapy	Psychosis, severe major depression, brain damage, suicidal tendencies and acting out, addictions "Decompensation" during or following trial therapy
Luborsky and Mark Short-term supportive-expressive psychotherapy		Psychosis, borderline personality disorder, suicidal acting out, antisocial personality without depression
Strupp and Binder Time-limited dynamic psychotherapy	Coherent, identifiable interpersonal theme Distinction between self and others Capacity for human relationships Ability to form collaborative relationship with therapist	Use Malan's criteria as "red flags," but rely chiefly on the patient's inability to engage in the therapeutic tasks demanded
Weiss and Sampson—Mount Zion Group Control-mastery theory	History of positive interpersonal relationships	Psychosis Organic brain syndrome Mental deficiency Serious substance abuse Suicide potential
McCullough Vaillant Short-term anxiety-regulating psychotherapy	Global Assessment of Functioning rating above 50 Low Axis IV stress score Motivation for treatment Psychological mindedness Positive initial response to treatment	Substance abuse disorders Eating disorders Poor impulse control
Levenson Experiential time-limited dynamic psychotherapy	Therapist can discern a recurrent interpersonal theme	Not able to attend to therapeutic interchange (e.g., psychosis, dementia) Problems can be treated more effectively by other means Cannot tolerate the active–interactive therapeutic process (e.g., impulse-control problems)

TABLE 25–4. Criteria for patient selection for brief dynamic psychotherapy *(continued)*

Theorist(s)	Inclusion criteria	Exclusion criteria
Safran and Muran Brief relational therapy	Not specified, but designed for (but not limited to) those with Depression and anxiety disorders Concomitant personality disorders Difficulty establishing therapeutic alliances	Not specified

Note. ECT = electroconvulsive therapy.
Source. Some material adapted from Barber and Crits-Christoph 1991, pp. 328–330.

psychotherapy. Horowitz et al. (1986) reported that brief (i.e., 12-session) focused dynamic therapy was insufficient to improve the functioning of patients with more severe personality disorders. Likewise, Shea et al. (1990) found that depressed patients with personality disorders had worse outcomes than did patients without personality disorders after 16 sessions of treatment. On the other hand, Winston et al. (1994) reported good outcomes for patients with Cluster C or histrionic personality disorders who received 40-session dynamic treatments, and Levenson and Overstreet (1993) found significant changes in some patients with personality disorders after 15 sessions of dynamic therapy. Also, some patients with personality disorders in the study by Thackrey and colleagues (Butler et al. 1987; Thackrey et al. 1993) were deemed suitable for outpatient brief therapy.

Kopta et al. (1994) found that it took half of the patients with acute distress symptoms (e.g., crying easily) an average of 5 sessions to return to normal functioning, whereas it took the same proportion of patients with chronic distress symptoms (e.g., feelings of guilt) an average of 14 sessions to achieve the same result. Patients with character symptoms (e.g., inability to trust others) required more than 52 sessions.

Hoglend (1993) found that patients with personality disorders did more poorly 2 years after brief dynamic therapy (9–53 sessions) than did patients without personality disorders. These groups, however, were not significantly different at the 4-year follow-up. Furthermore, there was some evidence that patients with personality disorders who received more therapy were the ones who did better in the long run. Perhaps the most interesting point made by this study is a methodological one—namely, that the effects of additional sessions on patients with personality disorders may not be evident at termination or even at the 1-year follow-up, the time point typically used in psychotherapy research designs.

One compounding problem in using such constructs in personality diagnosis to determine suitability was highlighted by Binder et al. (1987). These authors pointed to the fact that certain patients appeared bright, articulate, and seemingly insightful during the trial therapy interview, yet their "insights" tended to be superficial. The intellectual formulations of these patients camouflaged subtle, automatic maneuvers aimed at resisting true collaboration with the therapist. Furthermore, some patients who evidenced verbal fluency and intelligence in an initial interview appeared to use these qualities in therapy to divert attention away from painful emotional concerns. Finally, these evaluations did not take into account the contribution of the therapist. In several cases, the patient's problems in relating interpersonally were exacerbated in therapy by the therapist's counterresponse (i.e., countertransference) to the patient's style.

All of this suggests that prediction of a given patient's response to brief psychotherapy is risky. The kinds of scientific investigations just described are important in terms of identifying and defining explicitly relevant therapist and patient variables and for generating research hypotheses regarding how these variables interact. Clinically, however, such selection criteria can be used only to make very qualified predictions of how an individual patient will respond to therapy. As clinicians, we must also recognize that patients are not mere passive vessels whose conditions we diagnose and offer prognoses for. Rather, patients are responsive to our predictions and may respond to a judgment that they are "too sick" for brief therapy or "not sick enough" for long-term therapy in ways that confound our notions of how psychotherapy is supposed to work.

The present authors' position on the use of selection criteria is that, given the present state of knowledge, virtually any psychotherapy with virtually any patient can benefit from a time-limited attitude on the part of the therapist. This involves the promotion of a consistent, active engagement of both patient and therapist in the therapeutic relationship. Impediments on the part of the patient to becoming so engaged become an important issue to be addressed in the therapy.

Therapist Activity

Flegenheimer (1982) noted that

> it is striking to compare pages of written transcripts of long-term and brief therapy. While the former will show long productions by the patient interspersed with brief comments by the therapist, the brief therapy transcripts show almost equal productions by patient and therapist.... The activity of the therapist also brings a special tone to the therapeutic situation. By his or her activity the therapist shows an interest in the work at hand, and the properly selected patient will respond to this by an increase in motivation and interest in the treatment. (pp. 7–8)

Brief dynamic psychotherapy emphasizes the need for increased amounts of therapist activity. However, *activity* is only necessary to the extent that one needs to maintain the *focus* and make progress within a certain amount of *time*. Thus, activity is integrally related to the aforementioned aspects of focus and time. It is only through the interventions of the therapist that the focus can be achieved within a specified period. Mendelsohn (1978), writing on critical factors in short-term psychotherapy, viewed focusing as a type of therapist activity.

Many clinicians, when learning brief therapy techniques, become confused that therapist activity means confrontation, advice giving, or directive support. What it more appropriately entails is an awareness of the goals of the work and a plan of how to get there while being sensitive to the patient's presentation and the context of the clinical material. Therapist activity should aid the patient in increasing focally relevant thoughts and behaviors. As Schacht et al. (1984) noted, "If [therapy is] carried out in a crude, mechanical, or unempathic manner the patient may reject the therapist's efforts as tedious carping and the therapy may reach an impasse" (p. 108). Similarly, MacKenzie (1991) acknowledged that "clinical skill is required to be active, yet not controlling; stimulating, but not taking over" (p. 403).

That there can be detrimental results from therapist activity has been empirically demonstrated. Henry et al. (1993a) found that training therapists to become more active as they learn how to do TLDP may actually give them more opportunities to make clinical errors (see "Training" subsection later in this chapter). As Strupp (1982) poetically observed, "Therapy without guidance

results in chaos; forcible therapy has its own built-in defeats; the therapist's task is to find the optimum balance. The therapist, like the good parent, needs to know how to love without spoiling and to discipline without hurting" (p. 68). Several writers (e.g., Flegenheimer 1982; MacKenzie 1991) elaborated on how the focusing activity of the therapist not only keeps the therapy on target but also lessens patient regression and the development of a transference neurosis (i.e., the acting out of the patient's conflicts in the therapy), both of which could inhibit therapeutic progress in the abbreviated length of time. Typically the activity of the psychodynamic brief therapist refers to an increase in and earlier timing of interpretations, usually involving transference issues. This brings us to a discussion of brief therapy modifications of analytic concepts and techniques.

Modifications of Psychoanalytic Concepts and Techniques

Brief psychodynamic therapists adhere to many of the psychoanalytically inspired concepts familiar to the various forms of psychotherapy such as Freudian, ego analytic, object relations, interpersonal, and self psychology therapy. Specifically, brief dynamic therapeutic work relies on major psychoanalytic and psychodynamic concepts such as the importance of childhood experiences and developmental history, unconscious determinants of behavior, the role of conflicts, the transference relationship between therapist and patient, the patient's resistance to the therapeutic work, and repetitive behavior. Many brief therapists, however, do not feel obliged to adopt elaborate metapsychological models that incorporate highly inferential constructs. Instead, they prefer to stick close to the observable data. Such an inclination may stem from the need to do pragmatic clinical work and from the interest many brief theorists have in conducting research, for which variables must be precisely defined.

Similarly, the techniques used in brief dynamic psychotherapy have been inspired by those used in psychoanalysis and long-term dynamic therapy:

> That is, the therapist makes use of clarifications and interpretations, pays attention to the transference and countertransference, and addresses other repetitive, often maladaptive, patterns of behavior, especially in the interpersonal domain. In general, no direct advice is given. Unlike formal psychoanalysis, brief dynamic psychotherapies use free association for specific issues and not as a general rule of treatment. (Crits-Christoph and Barber 1991, pp. 2–3)

As Crits-Christoph and Barber's description suggests, some classical techniques have been modified to be more compatible with a limited focus and limited time. Perhaps the most notable of these modifications is that of the *early transference interpretation*. Flegenheimer (1982) saw early interpretation of transference as preventing the occurrence of a transference neurosis: "The early interpretation of transference manifestations brings these phenomena under the scrutiny of the observing portion of the patient's ego, putting the patient on guard, so to speak, against the dangers of dependency and regression which lie ahead" (p. 9). Still others see value in demonstrating to the patient his or her characteristic style of relating. An example from a second hour of a brief psychotherapy will illustrate:

> A 45-year-old patient had been talking about how her parents always found fault with her and tried to make her feel inferior. The therapist pursued a series of questions in an attempt to understand the patient's parental experiences and dynamics better. The patient responded in an angry tone, "Your questions! I just don't know what you want or how to answer." To which the therapist replied, "Do you get the feeling that I want to make you feel stupid like your parents did?"

This early transference interpretation highlighted for the patient how the same interpersonal dynamic evident with her parents might also be occurring with her therapist. In addition, it also served to bring into awareness the negative feelings the patient was having in this early phase of treatment. Making such negative feelings obvious serves to limit their being acted on by the patient (e.g., prematurely ending therapy), a situation that often cannot be dealt with effectively within the brief format.

Another major modification of psychoanalytic technique involves the gathering of psychosocial and historical information. Clearly, in a brief therapy, the amount of time devoted to obtaining background material must be curtailed. Many brief therapists employ the concept of a *focused history*, in which the patient begins to tell his or her own story and the therapist asks clarifying questions designed to obtain information relevant to a particular theme that is emerging in the therapy. For example, a patient might enter therapy saying he is afraid his girlfriend might leave him. The therapist could ask whether he has had similar fears with other persons in the past. Or the therapist could pursue losses the patient has experienced in his life. Both of these lines of inquiry would be different from having a fixed set of intake questions covering such topics as family history and school history.

Also with regard to acquiring information, many brief dynamic therapists put less emphasis on knowing factual genetic material. They are more likely to base their focus and interventions on an assessment of patients in the here and now. How are the patients presenting themselves? Why now? What is the nature of the interaction between patient and therapist? What seem to be the characteristic defenses used? What is the therapist's own countertransference?

Furthermore, as discussed earlier, a number of recently developed brief dynamic therapies have incorporated techniques from experiential and cognitive-behavioral therapy (Fosha 2000; Levenson 1995; Magnavita 1997; McCullough Vaillant 1997; Safran and Muran 2000). In these treatments, the understanding of patients in terms of psychodynamic notions is decoupled from the exclusive use of dynamic techniques.

In summary, short-term psychodynamic psychotherapies can be described as treatments of limited duration in which therapists are active in maintaining a circumscribed focus with limited goals using a framework of psychoanalytically derived concepts and techniques.

Factors Related to the Practice of Brief Dynamic Psychotherapy

Managed Care, Consumerism, and the Zeitgeist

That managed behavioral health care has had an enormous influence on the practice of psychotherapy since its inception in the 1980s is axiomatic by now. The growth of managed care in the 1990s has been nothing short of phenomenal. For instance, whereas only 29% of employees in the United States were covered by managed care plans in 1988, this figure had grown to 81% by 1997 (Newman 1999). More than one-half of the respondents to a national survey (Davidovitz and Levenson 1995) and a California survey (Levenson et al. 1995) reported providing services for a preferred provider organization (PPO) or a health maintenance organization (HMO). Another survey of therapists from several disciplines revealed that two-thirds had adopted time-limited therapy techniques or had shortened the length of therapy because of the restraints of managed care. And 60% reported that their incomes had declined (Fee, Practice and Managed Care Survey 1995).

Managed care systems had been established for the ostensible purpose of controlling costs while promoting efficient and effective (but usually limited-access) treatments. However, Bennett (1988) summarized that "over the past 15 years the health maintenance organization...

movement has abandoned its social objectives in favor of economic ones" (p. 1544). Some writers (e.g., Ackley 1993) have suggested that the managed care industry, now so monetarily driven, be renamed the "managed cost industry," or even worse, "mangled care" because of the poor quality of service (Franko and Erb 1998). These developments have had a major impact not only on mental health care providers and their clients (see, e.g., Barron and Sands 1996; Benedict and Phelps 1998; Fraser 1996) but also on the way that psychotherapy is being conceptualized.

Psychological health care that is provided by HMOs or financed by third-party payers tends to be severely limited in duration by required practice styles, utilization review, or capitation (absolute dollar limits). The maximum number of sessions covered by HMOs or third-party payers is almost always 20 or fewer and in practice is considerably lower; an average of 2.5, 4.7, or 6.6 sessions is not uncommon (Miller 1996). Some authors have distinguished between brief therapy and that practiced in managed care settings by giving the latter a different label (e.g., "HMO-therapy" [Austad and Berman 1991] or "ultrabrief therapy" [Miller 1996]). Most of the models for short-term dynamic psychotherapy specify a treatment duration longer than an HMO would find desirable. Thus, there can be critical differences between brief therapy as practiced traditionally and brief therapy as practiced in many managed care settings.

Aside from an emphasis on brevity of treatment, managed care companies typically favor specific types of approaches. For instance, behavioral descriptions of patient symptoms are favored over interpersonal or intrapsychic formulations, and preference is shown for treatment formulations focused on symptom relief, psychotropic medication, and directive interventions within a radically short-term format (Cushman and Gilford 2000; Levenson and Strupp 1999). This bias has resulted in economic support for approaches that are more congruent with this worldview than is dynamic therapy. For example, approaches such as cognitive-behavioral therapy, solution-focused therapy, and brief strategic therapy have been identified as ideal from the perspective of managed care, in that such modalities are often viewed as having predetermined, structured practices that are precisely tied to behavioral manifestations of symptoms and can be managed through regulation (Gould 1996). These approaches tend to view patients as largely rational, collaborative individuals who wish to return to a premorbid state of feeling and functioning (as one typically does following a bout of strep throat). Patients who do not fit this ideal can be perceived as uncooperative, perhaps even personality disordered (i.e., having an Axis II disorder),

and thus not eligible for treatment coverage by managed care companies. Some authors report that this lack of funding (or coverage) for Axis II personality problems has resulted in limited discussions of such disorders among clinicians (Cushman and Gilford 2000).

Such developments have indeed had a massive impact on dynamic therapy in both its long-term and its brief incarnations. Dynamic therapy has traditionally emphasized underlying, sometimes unobservable "dynamics" that are the focus of treatment. In many cases, these underlying dynamics are viewed as relatively independent of a particular patient's symptomatic presentation. Thus, dynamic therapy techniques have traditionally not been directed at specific symptom constellations. In a sense, the integrative therapies described above can be seen as an effort on the part of dynamic theorists and therapists to incorporate some of the techniques of behavioral approaches. An additional response is a recent trend for some dynamic therapy approaches to target specific symptom presentations or populations, such as posttraumatic stress syndrome, depression, addiction, lower-functioning patients, and so forth. For a review and presentation of some of these targeted brief dynamic therapies, see Levenson et al. (2002).

Recently, there has been a heated debate concerning the clinical, ethical, and practical effects of managed care practices on the delivery of mental health services (e.g., Austad 1996; Chipman 1995; Cummings 1995; Karon 1995; Stern 1993. Each side in this "psychobattle" (Hymowitz and Pollock 1995) has accused the other of bad practices, as is evident in the titles of some of the two sides' publications (e.g., "Is Long-Term Psychotherapy Unethical?" [Austad 1996] and "Managed Care Is Harmful to Outpatient Mental Health Services" [Miller 1996]). Iglehart (1996) made the point that at present little is known about the efficacy and effectiveness of these ultrabrief treatments.

The push for briefer treatments, however, is not based solely on economic considerations. Professionals in the mental health care system are concerned about providing more rapid relief of suffering and making services available to more people. Those persons seeking help are demanding the most for their time and money in an age of consumer awareness. Potential patients (more likely called *clients* or *consumers*) are questioning therapists (*providers*) regarding what results can be expected in what amount of time. Messer and Warren (1995) commented on other factors leading to an increase in short-term interventions: improved access to treatment by the Community Mental Health Centers Act of 1963; increased attention to the benefits of therapy through the popular media; decreased length of hospitalization; and development of brief, empirically based treatments.

Some commentators have also considered that the push toward brief therapies stems from American society's fascination with quick solutions. Cartoons in the popular press depict therapy drive-up windows ("Brief Therapy" 1990), and an article in *U.S. News and World Report* ("Therapy for the '90s" 1992) noted the following:

> Fast food, it is now clear, was only the beginning. Society has moved on to express checkout lines and automated teller machines, to plain-paper faxes and microwaved dinners. Value, in the 1990s, cleaves to what is quick. So it was perhaps inevitable that someone would come up with the idea of "single-session psychotherapy," an expedited approach to dealing with the ills of the psyche. If an hour is too long to wait for baked chicken, who can spend months or years on the analytic couch? (p. 55)

Nearly two decades of managed care and the relentless push toward brief, cheap treatments has resulted in a waning of the popularity of psychodynamic thinking and training opportunities (Rouff 2000). However, despite managed care's general hostility to psychodynamic theory and practice, many authors continue to underscore the benefits that dynamic thinking and therapeutic approaches have to offer (Wheelock 2000). Complex issues such as transference, countertransference (even countertransference related to managed care restrictions!), and difficult, resistive patients will not go away simply because they are not economically profitable or in vogue (Waska 1999). The key may be to develop education and supervision methods that will reliably train psychodynamic therapists to deal effectively with such complex issues.

Training

From the growing mass of clinical and empirical work, it can be stated emphatically that brief dynamic psychotherapy is not simply a shorter version of long-term therapy. The research literature is clear that brief therapy is a different treatment modality requiring specialized training in its own theories and techniques (e.g., Bauer and Kobos 1987; Budman and Stone 1983; Ursano and Hales 1986). However,

> students are instructed in the long-term model (usually psychoanalysis) whereas most patients are, in fact, seen on a short-term basis. The result is that most therapists struggle to develop bootstrap forms of the knowledge they have acquired in formal training to the realities of practice. (Strupp and Binder 1984, p. 6)

Despite its importance, training in brief therapy is far less researched and understood than brief therapy techniques and outcome. Levenson and her colleagues have conducted studies to document the extent, type, and long-term effects of training in brief dynamic psychotherapy. Levenson et al. (1995) found that of those clinicians who regularly offered brief therapy, more than one-third reported having little or no training in it. This is a distressing statistic, particularly because it is now widely accepted that brief therapy is not "dehydrated" long-term therapy (Cummings 1986) or "just less of the same" (Peake et al. 1988). However, the survey data (Davidovitz and Levenson 1995) also revealed that professionals with extensive training were conducting considerably more brief therapy than were those who received no training. In addition, there is a significant positive relationship between the amount of training and attitudes about and skill in conducting brief therapy. The most common type of brief therapy training experience for the practicing professional is reading, followed by workshops, conferences, and supervision. Supervision, not unexpectedly, was considered to be the most useful experience. Psychiatrists (90% of whom identified themselves as having a psychodynamic or eclectic orientation) reported taking significantly more academic courses than psychologists or social workers. Furthermore, over time there appears to have been an increase in the psychiatric brief therapy course offerings, with 90% of current psychiatrists in practice less than 6 years reporting taking a brief therapy course (compared with 64% of new psychiatrists 20 years ago). The findings of a long-term follow-up study of trainees (now therapists) revealed that they were using the TLDP strategies they learned an average of 9 years earlier and were finding these strategies helpful in doing both short- and long-term therapies (LaRue-Yalom and Levenson 2001).

Levenson and Evans (2000) conducted a survey of psychology graduate schools and internships. They found that 60% of institutions with a psychodynamic orientation offered some form of brief therapy training. When the teachers and supervisors in these settings were asked to identify the topics that were most difficult for trainees to grasp, they indicated the following: setting of limited goals, adherence to a focus, making a paradigm shift, rapid development of an alliance, and attitudinal bias toward long-term therapy.

The parallel processes of supervision and treatment have been observed for years (e.g., Ekstein and Wallerstein 1972). Frances and Clarkin (1981) noted that the brief therapy

> treatment context requires a relatively high level of therapist activity and planning, the setting of clear and

limited goals, the focus on a single problem or dynamic conflict, and a quick attachment to and then separation from the therapist. These same conditions are characteristic of the work of brief therapy supervision. (p. 244)

Dasberg and Winokur (1984) also discussed parallels between short-term dynamic treatment and training. Specifically, they mentioned similarities in structure and experiences (e.g., changing attitudes over time) and in attributes and actions (e.g., high motivation, commitment to change) between the learner and the patient in brief therapy. Hoyt (1991) pointed out congruences in phase-specific behaviors between supervisor and trainee. For example, early on, problems of focusing and establishing a working alliance may affect both therapy and supervision. Similarly, the supervisor may unrealistically try to "cram unassimilable amounts of clinical lore and wisdom into the last supervision meetings. The trainee, not feeling 'totally educated' and competent, may invite and welcome these eleventh-hour desperations" (Hoyt 1991, p. 105). This is a process that may be paralleled in the ending trainee–patient relationship. Levenson detailed 10 similarities between supervision in TLDP and TLDP itself (Table 25–5).

Burlingame et al. (1989) randomly exposed trainee and senior staff of a counseling center to one of three training conditions: no training, self-instructional training, and intensive training (i.e., 10 hours of instruction, demonstration, role-playing, and discussion). All therapists then conducted an eight-session time-limited therapy. Although the more experienced therapists had superior outcomes in general, there were indications that greater amounts of training for *both* the inexperienced and the experienced therapists led to greater patient improvements. In other words, even experienced therapists gained significantly from the brief therapy training program. The investigators concluded that "if a mental health agency is moving to a time-limited treatment policy in an attempt to be more cost effective, minimal training of [even experienced] therapists may be a more effective way to proceed than merely putting a limit on the number of sessions" (Burlingame et al. 1989, p. 312).

Training manuals have been one approach to provide more specific descriptions of treatment techniques. Butler and Strupp (1993) reviewed some of the best-known "manualized" psychodynamic/interpersonal therapies. One of these is TLDP (Strupp and Binder 1984; Levenson 1995). At the Vanderbilt Center for Psychotherapy Research, Strupp and colleagues completed a study on the effects of specialized training in TLDP (the Vanderbilt II study). This 5-year Vanderbilt II study examined the effect of manualized training in TLDP on 16 experi-

TABLE 25–5. Parallels between brief therapy supervision and brief therapy treatment

1. Almost same number of meetings (21 vs. 20).
2. Generate hypotheses on relatively little information.
3. Model desirable therapist qualities in supervision (e.g., patience, activity, staying focused, awareness of time constraints, supportive yet confrontative and collaborative).
4. Work actively with trainee resistance.
5. Trainees not only have an educative, intellectual learning experience but also have a new affective experience (e.g., sense of competency).
6. Trainees take responsibility for choosing what they bring up in supervision.
7. Emphasize collaboration between supervisee and supervisor (e.g., supervisor shows own work and is open to feedback from trainees).
8. Create a safe environment in supervision.
9. Concerning termination, trainees are simultaneously dealing with issues about leaving supervision (e.g., have they learned enough) and leaving their patients (e.g., will they be okay).
10. Expectation that trainees will continue to incorporate and integrate what they have learned after the conclusion of the training rotation.

enced therapists (8 psychiatrists and 8 psychologists) and 80 patients. For the first phase of the study, therapists were assigned two patients and asked to treat them in up to 25 weekly sessions, as "they ordinarily would treat such patients" (Strupp 1990). In the second year of the study, therapists went through a training program to learn TLDP. The training program consisted of didactic presentations on TLDP principles and techniques, illustrated with clinical examples, and small-group supervision of each therapist's single training case, including discussion of audio- and videotaped sessions of training cases.

In the third phase, therapists again treated two patients, this time according to the tenets of TLDP. The main Vanderbilt II results indicated that the training program was successful in changing therapists' interventions to be congruent with the manual (Henry et al. 1993a). In comparing the outcomes of the patients who received the therapists' usual treatment and the outcomes of those who received TLDP, at termination the former were superior on several measures, but at 1-year follow-up the TLDP patients showed superior outcomes on TLDP-relevant interpersonal variables (Bein et al. 2000). It is difficult to interpret this finding, however, in large part because a review of the third-phase session tapes suggested that few of the therapists had learned to conduct TLDP with even minimal skill.

The Vanderbilt II findings pertinent to the changes in therapists' behavior and their responses to training are quite complex. Although there were positive changes in adherence to *general* psychodynamic techniques after training (this was not the focus of the training, however), there were also indications of negative changes. For example, the greater activity level of therapists after training resulted in the therapists' having more opportunities to make "mistakes." In addition, after training, therapists appeared less approving and less supportive in their therapies. Because the therapists were not trained to mastery, it may be that there was a decrement in therapists' performance because they were still attempting to adapt their customary style to accommodate new strategies. Based on these and other observations of therapist training, the following should be considered when offering manual-based training: 1) Choose competent but relatively less experienced therapists; 2) Select therapists who are less vulnerable to negative training effects (e.g., less hostile and controlling); 3) Assume that even experienced therapists are novices in the approach to be learned; 4) Provide close, directive, and specific feedback to therapists and focus on therapists' own thought processes; 5) Assign therapists several training cases; and 6) Assess therapist skill based on review of taped sessions (Bein et al. 2000; Henry et al. 1993b).

Some of these suggestions have been followed in subsequent research. A recently completed clinical trial (the National Institute on Drug Abuse [NIDA] Collaborative Cocaine Treatment Study; Crits-Christoph et al. 1999) compared three manualized psychosocial treatments for cocaine abuse. One of these treatments was a brief, dynamic approach (Mark and Faude 1995) based on supportive-expressive therapy as developed by Luborsky (1984). The participating therapists in this study underwent a rigorous selection process involving submission of audiotapes of one of their own ongoing cases (prior to the study). Training consisted of four 2-day workshops and at least four audiotaped training cases with individual supervision (Crits-Christoph et al. 1998). Therapists' adherence to the manual and competence were assessed by their supervisors in up to eight sessions per training case. Even under these exceedingly rigorous training conditions, it appears to be difficult to demonstrate marked training effects; on average, supportive-expressive therapists' adherence and competence did not improve from their first case to their last. Crits-Christoph and colleagues suggest that this lack of a learning effect may be due to the fact that the selected therapists were already generally competent and thus had little room for improvement. This "ceiling effect" explanation is similar to the one offered by Rounsaville et al. (1986) to explain

a lack of training effects for therapists who learned interpersonal therapy for depression. In absolute terms, however, the therapists in the NIDA Cocaine Treatment Study were rated as only adequate (average rating of 3.7 on a scale ranging from 1 to 7). Furthermore, the supervisors of these therapists did not consider the trainees to be outstanding, although some were rated as more competent than the others. Rather, these supervisors concluded that supportive-expressive dynamic therapy is difficult to implement skillfully. These findings are congruent with those of Strupp and colleagues in the Vanderbilt II study. However, Crits-Christoph et al. (1998) did not find the apparent negative effects of training observed in the Vanderbilt II study and described above. Perhaps the extremely rigorous selection process used in the cocaine treatment study resulted in therapists who, although not initially expert in the delivery of this particular form of brief dynamic therapy, were more skilled psychodynamically than those in the Vanderbilt II study.

The difficulties encountered by these studies in attempting to demonstrate training effects in manualized brief dynamic therapy underscore the complexity of what is being asked of therapists. For example, brief dynamic therapy requires therapists to quickly develop a coherent therapeutic focus, tactfully and rapidly elicit possibly difficult material, and provide interpretations (including transference interpretations) to anxious patients who have not been in therapy for very long. In addition, all of this must be done without harming the therapeutic alliance. These results also highlight the need to examine the methods by which dynamic therapy is taught. Perhaps supervisors must more systematically take into account therapists' experience and skill level, as well as therapists' (and, perhaps, supervisors') personality styles.

In addition to manuals, training in brief psychotherapy has emphasized the use of clinical material obtained directly from therapy sessions, including live supervision and use of audio- and videotaping (Levenson and Evans 2000). Most brief dynamic therapy training programs routinely use videotape recordings for supervision and research and usually will not accept patients for treatment who, for whatever reason, cannot consent to videotaping. In addition, videotaping has been widely used in workshops on short-term dynamic psychotherapy given by experts in the field. Supervisors have found few negative effects from such procedures but have encountered resistance from therapists in training who either consciously or unconsciously fear having their work exposed to such close scrutiny. Sifneos (1987) called videotape technology the "microscope" of psychiatry, a label that underscores both its usefulness and its feared inhibiting effect. Therapists who had received TLDP training as part of their clinical education felt that the opportunity to videotape their own cases and to watch their supervisors conduct therapy on videotape was invaluable (LaRue-Yalom and Levenson 2001).

Safran and Muran (2000) noted the value of experiential exercises for trainees in their approach to brief dynamic therapy. Because their therapeutic approach highlights the importance of the therapist's nonjudgmental awareness of his or her subjective reactions during sessions, the exercises are intended to enhance trainee awareness of bodily and emotional experience. For example, in one exercise, trainees are instructed to focus on their breathing; when they notice that their attention has wandered, they are to note what is occupying them and then return focus to their breathing. Over time, trainees become more aware of and tolerant of a wide range of internal experience.

Experience

Experience appears to be another factor that greatly influences the practice of brief dynamic psychotherapy. But how it exerts such influence is somewhat of a paradox. It is widely accepted that brief therapy is a very demanding endeavor—one best suited to be learned after one has already become facile with the basics. As Mann (1973) noted,

> Knowledge of the psychoanalytic theories of mental functioning heavily buttressed by experience in the long-term treatment of patients is the best preparation for this [brief] treatment plan. *Short treatment in no way suggests easy treatment.* In many ways, short treatment is more difficult than longer treatment, even for the experienced therapist. (p. 82; emphasis added)

Mario Andolphi, an Italian family therapist and trainer, is quoted as saying: "To make shorter the therapy, make longer the training" (Ecker and Hulley 1996, p. ix). However, the paradox is that although knowledge and skills gained over the years in conducting long-term therapy seem to be a prerequisite for learning brief therapy, one may need to set aside many of the assumptions of long-term therapy to make full use of the techniques and rationale of brief therapy (Flegenheimer 1982). Sifneos (1987), writing on learning to use STAPP, stated the following:

> From my own observations of the supervision of 70 therapists representing such disciplines as psychiatry, psychology, social work, and nursing during the last 25 years, I can state categorically that the main difficulty in learning to use STAPP has more to do with certain misconceptions about the superiority of long-term psychotherapy which were rigidly embedded in the minds of our trainees, and which they were reluctant to give up, than with anything else, including their relative inexperience. This problem was resolved when we decided…to offer [instruction in STAPP] early so as to avoid their being thoroughly indoctrinated in dogmatic points of view and in preconceived and narrow-minded ideas which tended to obscure their ability to make meaningful observations which interfered with their learning. (p. 189)

Because these inexperienced therapists were presumably open-minded (i.e., not indoctrinated), Sifneos found them easier to train than experienced therapists, and these therapists-in-training, therefore, "more often obtained successful results than did their more experienced counterparts" (Sifneos 1978, p. 493).

The issue of when to train in brief dynamic psychotherapy remains somewhat controversial. However, it seems that the enthusiasm and positive expectation of the neophyte learner may be as valuable as the knowledge and skill of the seasoned clinician. Winokur and Dasberg (1983) found that experienced therapists might suffer from a sense of loss of competence as they experiment with shorter-term treatments. These authors suggested allowing seasoned therapists time to work through negative attitudes they might have toward briefer methods. The diminished self-esteem or narcissistic injury that may occur while therapists are practicing new skills may, in part, account for the posttraining decrements in performance evidenced by the experienced therapists in the Vanderbilt II study described earlier in this section.

Regardless of when brief therapy skills are learned, experience in brief therapy seems to be reliably related to greater skill (Anderson and Lambert 1995; Levenson and Davidovitz 2000). Levenson et al. (1995) found that for those therapists who were conducting brief therapy but who had little experience in that modality, formal training and the amount of brief therapy they were presently conducting were the most potent predictors of skill. However, for more experienced brief therapists, attitude toward brief therapy played a greater role in predicting skill. Levenson et al. (1995) concluded that novice therapists would do well to continue to increase their experience while receiving more training; experienced clinicians, however, might require training that focuses on values and attitudes as well as techniques. Experience alone does not appear to be a sufficient teacher.

Resistances, Attitudes, Expectations

Despite advances in the theory and technique of brief dynamic psychotherapy, as well as the existence of a number of research studies demonstrating its overall effectiveness, many therapists are still reluctant to learn these methods and apply them in their clinical practice (e.g., Bolter et al. 1990; Budman and Gurman 1988; Hoyt 1985; Levenson and Evans 2000; Levenson et al. 1995; Winokur and Dasberg 1983). Important variables in understanding this reluctance are therapists' values and assumptions regarding the nature and practice of brief psychotherapy.

Budman and Gurman (1988) proposed that the value systems of the long-term therapist are different from those of the short-term therapist. These authors identified eight dominant values pertaining to the ideal manner in which long-term therapy is practiced and contrasted these with the corresponding ideal values pertinent to the practice of short-term therapy. For example, Budman and Gurman postulated that one of the ideal value differences between long-term and short-term therapists involves the idea of "cure." Whereas the long-term therapist seeks a change in basic character or "therapeutic perfectionism" (Malan 1963), the short-term therapist does not believe in the notion of "cure" and prefers pragmatism, parsimony, and the least radical intervention.

Bolter et al. (1990) sought to assess empirically whether there were such value differences between short-term and long-term practicing therapists. Two hundred twenty-two psychologists were sent a questionnaire in order that relevant values and preferred therapeutic approaches (short-term vs. long-term) might be measured. The study provided partial support for Budman and Gurman's (1988) proposal: in two of the eight areas, long-term and short-term therapists' responses differed significantly. Short-term therapists believed more strongly that psychological change could occur outside therapy and that setting time limits would intensify the therapeutic work. Furthermore, results indicated that clinicians with a psychodynamic orientation, in contrast to those having a cognitive-behavioral orientation, were more likely to believe that therapy was necessary for change, that the focus of therapy should be on pathology, that therapy should be open-ended, and that ambitious goals were desirable. Thus, although the findings from the study by Bolter et al. (1990) suggest that a short-term orientation is related to therapeutic values, it is important to note that the theoretical orientation of the therapist also plays a significant role in determining values. Similarly, some writers, on the basis of both personal experience (Edbril 1994) and empirical data (Levenson and Davidovitz 2000), have commented that female psychodynamic therapists may experience particular difficulties in making the paradigm shift to briefer interventions because of their preference for continuing therapeutic relationships.

Most of the literature addressing therapists' reluctance to use brief therapy focuses on psychoanalytic or psychodynamic therapists. Bolter (1987) found that 91% of the psychodynamic therapists who responded to an attitude questionnaire favored long-term approaches. Speed (1992) similarly found that 87% of those therapists most comfortable with very long-term therapy were psychodynamic in orientation. In a national survey, psychodynamic brief therapists reported less skill, experience, and training in, and less of a positive attitude concerning the effectiveness of, brief therapy than did their cognitive-behavior therapy colleagues (Davidovitz and Levenson 1995). Yet, these dynamically trained practitioners were conducting a large amount of brief therapy. This fact has tremendous implications for training. Are graduate school curricula, residency training programs, and continuing education experiences geared toward meeting the needs of these dynamic clinicians? The survey data indicate that residency training programs may be doing an excellent job in providing brief therapy courses; 90% of recent graduates have taken at least one such course.

Hoyt (1985) proposed that dynamically trained therapists have resistances toward short-term psychotherapy. When trying to determine why many therapists are not learning and applying short-term dynamic methods as a treatment of choice, Hoyt rejected the idea that the situation is due chiefly to lack of awareness regarding recent clinical and research developments: "Rather, I would suggest, there are a number of myths, erroneous beliefs, and (perhaps unconscious) 'problems about learning' (Ekstein and Wallerstein 1972) that may make clinicians reluctant or resistant to using short-term dynamic methods" (Hoyt 1985, p. 95). Hoyt organized these resistances into six broad categories, as shown in Table 25–6.

TABLE 25–6. Sources of resistance against short-term dynamic psychotherapy

The belief that more is better (e.g., treatment must take a long time to be effective)

Myth of the "pure gold" of analysis

Confusion of patient's interests (in the most efficient, effective help) with the therapist's interests (in uncovering all aspects of the patient's personality)

Demanding hard work (to be active and intensely alert)

Economic and other pressures (desire to hold on to that which is profitable and dependable)

Countertransference and related therapist reactions to termination

---

Source. Adapted from Hoyt 1985.

Negative attitudes toward briefer modes of intervention could adversely affect therapists' willingness and ability to use brief therapy methods effectively. Flegenheimer (1982) warned that problems could arise during a brief psychotherapy if the therapist's values are "inconsistent with the optimism and confidence that the brief therapist must have in the method and which must be brought to the treatment situation" (p. 13).

Similarly, Winokur and Dasberg (1983) suggested that

> when teaching professionals a new approach, it is not enough to rely on lectures, reading materials, or even live demonstrations and individual supervision.... In order to integrate a new approach into their professional identity, particularly if this identity is molded already, they need also to work through the intellectual, quasi-intellectual, and emotional difficulties encountered in the learning process. (p. 51)

Ursano and Dressler (1977) made the point that

> clinicians' attitudes toward various therapeutic approaches strongly influence the use of a particular treatment modality and the effectiveness with which it is conducted. These values are determined by the type of professional training, the amount of clinical experience, and the particular work setting of the clinician, as well as by individual personality characteristics. *A positive attitude toward brief psychotherapy* and a skill in practicing it are extremely important if the trend toward shorter term treatment continues. (p. 55, emphasis added)

Levenson and Bolter (1988) examined the values and attitudes of psychiatry residents and psychology interns before and after a 6-month seminar/supervision in brief dynamic psychotherapy. Findings revealed that after training, trainees were more willing to consider brief therapy for more than minor disorders, more positive about achieving significant insight, more expectant that the benefits would be long-lasting, and less likely to think that an extended "working through" was necessary. Also, they were more willing to be active, more likely to see that a time limit was helpful, and more prepared to believe that patients would change significantly after the therapy was over. An extension of this study (Neff et al. 1996), involving three experienced trainers with three different brief therapy models, indicated that intensive 1-day workshops can lead to more positive and optimistic attitudes toward brief therapy. These studies support the view that attending to values and attitudes associated with short-term versus long-term therapy may be a necessary component of the success of any teaching or training program in brief psychotherapy.

The prevailing evidence suggests that those clinicians who may be naturally drawn to brief treatment models may express values and attitudes different from those whose preference is to conduct long-term therapy. This is not surprising, nor is it surprising that an individual's training greatly influences those values and attitudes. It is crucial, however, to ensure that the current economic climate is not used politically to elevate one set of values and attitudes at the expense of another. Indeed, earlier in this century, those therapists who sought to shorten therapy regularly found those efforts devalued by their peers. Clearly, brief treatment is not a panacea and should not be oversold. Neither should the important observations made by long-term therapists of patients over time be summarily rejected. There is much yet to be learned about the treatment of psychopathology, and it is unlikely that one set of values and attitudes is unquestionably superior.

Research on the Efficacy and Long-Term Outcome of Short-Term Therapy

Several *meta-analyses* have been conducted to evaluate whether brief dynamic psychotherapy is efficacious (i.e., works under experimental conditions). In these studies, statistical procedures were employed to combine the results from a number of outcome studies to determine the relative value of brief dynamic therapy in comparison with no treatment and with alternative brief psychotherapies such as cognitive-behavioral treatment. The first meta-analysis, by Svartberg and Stiles (1991), concluded that brief dynamic therapy was superior to no treatment but inferior to alternative therapies, both at posttreatment and at 1-year follow-up. In contrast, subsequent meta-analyses by Crits-Christoph (1992), Anderson and Lambert (1995), and Leichsenring (2001) concluded that brief dynamic therapy was equivalent in effectiveness to alternative therapies. Anderson and Lambert also found some evidence that more experienced therapists or therapists specifically trained in brief dynamic approaches tended to be more helpful to patients. Empirical studies have failed to demonstrate that long-term (or open-ended) approaches achieve better outcomes than short-term (or time-limited) therapies (Barber 1994; Koss and Shiang 1994). Findings of some studies even indicate that briefer interventions are more effective. For example, Piper et al. (1984) found that short-term (6 months) individual dynamic psychotherapy and long-term (24 months) group therapy produced better outcomes than did long-term individual therapy or short-term group therapy. In sum, then, the best evidence to date suggests that the efficacy of brief dynamic therapy is in general neither superior nor inferior to that of other brief treatment approaches.

Howard et al. (1986) plotted improvement rates for a large number of studies as a function of time; most but not all of the therapists studied offered psychodynamic or interpersonal therapy. They concluded that 50% of patients show significant improvement by the eighth session and 75% by the 26th session. These improvement rates occur within the 10- to 25-session limit typical of many brief dynamic therapies. Moreover, these 50% and 75% effectiveness marks were derived almost exclusively from studies of long-term or open-ended therapies, rather than of ones specifically intended to be brief or time-limited (Hoyt and Austad 1992). However, one must be cautious in interpolating these empirical data. As pointed out by Barber and Ellman (1996), "The lack of studies comparing brief with long-term therapy has led to the unfounded 'verdict' that long-term dynamic psychotherapy is not effective or not worthwhile" (p. 189). When evaluating such findings, one must consider the inherent limitations of research with long-term psychotherapies. For pragmatic reasons, research on long-term therapies usually involves observations of therapies in naturalistic studies, resulting in a loss of the experimental control that is possible in studies of shorter duration.

In assessing long-term outcome, research indicates that patients in brief dynamic therapy tend to maintain their therapeutic gains (Messer and Warren 1995), but there is some indication that treatments of fewer than 16 sessions may not be as effective for depressed patients (Shapiro et al. 1995).

Conclusions and Recommendations

Although there are now many types of brief dynamic individual psychotherapies, these therapies have several qualities in common. We have defined brief psychodynamic psychotherapy as treatment of limited duration in which therapists are active in maintaining a circumscribed focus with limited goals using a basic framework of psychoanalytically derived concepts and techniques. We strongly believe that there is an important and major role for short-term *dynamically informed* therapy in the future. The dynamic brief therapist of the twenty-first century will need to be trained to be able to use appropriately and flexibly a variety of intervention techniques and to work collaboratively with other health care providers. What we envision is an emphasis on a psychodynamic understanding of the patient to provide a guide for these appropriate interventions. As stated by Gabbard (1990) in his book on psychodynamic psychiatry in clinical practice, "Dynamic psychiatry simply provides a coherent conceptual framework within which all treatments are prescribed. Regardless of whether the treatment is dynamic psychotherapy or pharmacotherapy, it is *dynamically informed*" (p. 204). If brief dynamic therapists of the future emphasize the psychodynamic understanding of patients and their situations, they will have a basis for using any one of a number of specialized techniques, such as cognitive restructuring, hypnosis, psychopharmacology, or more traditionally recognizable psychodynamic interventions.

Table 25–7 contains our specific recommendations for the future.

We close with our admonition that brief treatments (psychodynamic or otherwise) must not be oversold. Clearly, brief treatment is not a panacea. There is a danger in this age of limited resources, consumerism, and quick fixes that brief therapy (and especially the ultra-brief treatments) will be touted and then expected to do the impossible. However, brief dynamic psychotherapy that is used in a realistic and informed fashion should continue to help many of our patients.

TABLE 25–7. Specific recommendations for brief dynamic therapies of the future

---

1. Abandon unrealistic, perfectionistic treatment goals and notions of cure. Instead, focus on reasonable yet meaningful change with the expectation that patients will return to therapy several times over their life span.
2. Continue the liberating movement toward integrative stances with an increased focus on clinical phenomena and descriptive formulations to guide effective and efficient treatment.
3. With regard to elaborate selection criteria, assume that patients can be treated briefly until proven otherwise in the course of treatment. Recognize that there will be patients who are not well suited to short-term interventions.
4. Initially use manuals to teach those with little brief therapy experience.
5. Education in brief dynamic psychotherapy is best when there is close, directive, and specific feedback concerning formulation and intervention strategies. Videotape is an invaluable tool in this regard.
6. Focus on those skills that are relevant for the competent practice of brief therapy (e.g., rapid alliance building).
7. The tension between efficiency–effectiveness, quality–quantity, and costs–benefits must be dealt with in an ongoing dialectic between patients–therapists, teachers–students–administrators, and professionals–patients–third-party payers.

Source. Some material adapted from Levenson and Burg 2000; Levenson and Davidovitz 2000; Levenson and Strupp 1999.

References

Ackley DC: Employee health insurance benefits: a comparison of managed care in traditional mental health care: costs and results. The Independent Practitioner 13:49–53, 1993

Alexander F, French T: Psychoanalytic Therapy: Principles and Applications. New York, Ronald Press, 1946

Anderson EM, Lambert MJ: Short-term dynamically oriented psychotherapy: a review and meta-analysis. Clin Psychol Rev 15:503–514, 1995

Aron L: A Meeting of Minds: Mutuality in Psychoanalysis. Hillsdale, NJ, Analytic Press, 1996

Austad CS: Is Long-Term Psychotherapy Unethical? Toward a Social Ethic in an Era of Managed Care. San Francisco, CA, Jossey-Bass, 1996

Austad CS, Berman WH: Managed health care and the evolution of psychotherapy, in Psychotherapy in Managed Health Care: The Optimal Use of Time and Resources. Edited by Austad CS, Berman WH. Washington, DC, American Psychological Association, 1991, pp 3–18

Bachrach HM, Leaff LA: "Analyzability": a systematic review of the clinical and quantitative literature. J Am Psychoanal Assoc 26:881–920, 1978

Barber JP: Efficacy of short-term dynamic psychotherapy: past, present, and future. J Psychother Pract Res 3:108–121, 1994

Barber JP, Crits-Christoph P: Comparison of the brief dynamic therapies, in Handbook of Short-Term Dynamic Psychotherapy. Edited by Crits-Christoph P, Barber JP. New York, Basic Books, 1991, pp 323–356

Barber JP, Ellman J: Advances in short-term dynamic psychotherapy. Current Opinion in Psychiatry 9:188–192, 1996

Barron JW, Sands H (eds): Impact of Managed Care on Psychodynamic Treatment. Madison, CT, International Universities Press, 1996

Bauer GP, Kobos JC: Brief Therapy: Short-Term Psychodynamic Intervention. Northdale, NJ, Jason Aronson, 1987

Bein E, Anderson T, Strupp HH, et al: The effects of training in time-limited dynamic psychotherapy: changes in therapeutic outcome. Psychotherapy Research 10:119–132, 2000

Benedict JG, Phelps R: Introduction: psychology's view of managed care. Professional Psychology: Research and Practice 29:29–30, 1998

Bennett MJ: The greening of the HMO: implications for prepaid psychiatry. Am J Psychiatry 145:1544–1549, 1988

Binder JL, Henry WP, Strupp HH: An appraisal of selection criteria for dynamic psychotherapies and implications for setting time limits. Psychiatry 50:154–166, 1987

Bloom BL: Planned Short-Term Psychotherapy. Boston, MA, Allyn & Bacon, 1992

Bolter K: Differences in therapy-related values and attitudes between short-term and long-term therapists. Unpublished doctoral dissertation, California School of Professional Psychology, Berkeley, CA, 1987

Bolter K, Levenson H, Alvarez W: Differences in values between short-term and long-term therapists. Professional Psychology: Research and Practice 21:285–290, 1990

Brief therapy: fast relief for troubled people. Better Homes and Gardens, September 1990, pp 53–54

Budman SH, Gurman AS: Theory and Practice of Brief Psychotherapy. New York, Guilford, 1988

Budman SH, Stone J: Advances in brief psychotherapy: a review of recent literature. Hosp Community Psychiatry 34:939–946, 1983

Burke JD Jr, White HS, Havens LL: Which short-term therapy? Matching patient and method. Arch Gen Psychiatry 36:177–186, 1979

Burlingame GM, Fuhriman JA: Clinician attitudes toward time-limited and time-unlimited therapy. Professional Psychology: Research and Practice 18:61–65, 1987

Burlingame GM, Fuhriman A, Paul S, et al: Implementing a time-limited therapy program: differential effects of training and experience. Psychotherapy: Theory, Research and Practice 26:303–312, 1989

Butler SF, Strupp HH: Effects of training psychoanalytically oriented therapists to use a manual, in Psychodynamic Treatment Research: A Handbook for Clinical Practice. Edited by Miller NE, Luborsky L, Barber JP, et al. New York, Basic Books, 1993, pp 191–210

Butler SF, Thackrey M, Strupp HH: Capacity for Dynamic Process Scale (CDPS): relation to patient variables, process and outcome. Paper presented at the annual meeting of Society for Psychotherapy Research, Ulm, West Germany, June 1987

Chipman A: Meeting managed care: an identity and value crisis for therapists. Am J Psychother 49:550–567, 1995

Crits-Christoph P: The efficacy of brief dynamic psychotherapy: a meta-analysis. Am J Psychiatry 149:151–158, 1992

Crits-Christoph P, Barber JP (eds): Handbook of Short-Term Dynamic Psychotherapy. New York, Basic Books, 1991

Crits-Christoph P, Barber JP, Kurcias JS: Introduction and historical background, in Handbook of Short-Term Dynamic Psychotherapy. Edited by Crits-Christoph P, Barber JP. New York, Basic Books, 1991, pp 1–12

Crits-Christoph P, Siqueland L, Chittams J, et al: Training in cognitive, supportive-expressive, and drug counseling therapies for cocaine dependence. J Consult Clin Psychol 66:484–492, 1998

Crits-Christoph P, Siqueland L, Blaine J, et al: Psychosocial treatments for cocaine dependence: National Institute on Drug Abuse Collaborative Cocaine Treatment Study. Arch Gen Psychiatry 57:493–502, 1999

Cummings NA: The dismantling of our health system: strategies for the survival of psychological practice. Am Psychol 41:426–431, 1986

Cummings NA: Unconscious fiscal convenience. Psychotherapy in Private Practice 14:23–28, 1995

Cushman P, Gilford P: Will managed care change our way of being? Am Psychol 55:985–996, 2000

Dasberg H, Winokur M: Teaching and learning short-term dynamic psychotherapy: parallel processes. Psychotherapy: Theory, Research and Practice 21:184–188, 1984

Davanloo H (ed): Basic Principles and Techniques in Short-Term Dynamic Psychotherapy. New York, Spectrum, 1978

Davanloo H: A method of short-term dynamic psychotherapy, in Short-Term Dynamic Psychotherapy, Vol 1. Edited by Davanloo H. New York, Jason Aronson, 1980, pp 43–71

Davanloo H: Intensive short-term psychotherapy with highly resistant patients, I: handling resistance. International Journal of Short-Term Psychotherapy 1:107–133, 1986

Davidovitz D, Levenson H: A national survey on practice and training in brief therapy. Paper presented at the annual meeting of the American Psychological Association, New York, NY, August 1995

Ecker B, Hulley L: Depth-Oriented Brief Therapy. San Francisco, CA, Jossey-Bass, 1996

Edbril SD: Gender bias in short-term therapy: toward a new model for working with women patients in managed care settings. Psychotherapy 31:601–609, 1994

Ekstein R, Wallerstein RS: The Teaching and Learning of Psychotherapy. New York, International Universities Press, 1972

Fee, practice and managed care survey. Psychotherapy Finances 21:1–8, 1995

Ferenczi S, Rank O: The Development of Psychoanalysis. New York, Nervous and Mental Disease Publication Company, 1925

Flegenheimer WV: Techniques of Brief Psychotherapy. New York, Jason Aronson, 1982

Fosha D: The Transforming Power of Affect: A Model for Accelerated Change. New York, Basic Books, 2000

Frances A, Clarkin J: Parallel techniques in supervision and treatment. Psychiatr Q 53:242–248, 1981

Franko DL, Erb J: Managed care or mangled care? Psychotherapy: Theory, Research and Practice 35:43–53, 1998

Fraser JS: All that glitters is not gold: medical offset effects and managed behavioral health care. Professional Psychology: Research and Practice 27:335–344, 1996

Freud S: Psycho-analytic method (1904), in Collected Papers: Early Papers, Vol 1. Translated by Riviere J. Edited by Jones E. London, England, Hogarth Press, 1953, pp 264–271

Gabbard GO: Psychodynamic Psychiatry in Clinical Practice. Washington, DC, American Psychiatric Press, 1990

Garfield SL: Research on client variables in psychotherapy, in Handbook of Psychotherapy and Behavior Change, 3rd Edition. Edited by Garfield SL, Bergin AE. New York, Wiley, 1986, pp 213–256

Goldman HH, Taube CA: High users of outpatient mental health services, II: implications for practice and policy. Am J Psychiatry 145:24–28, 1988

Gould RL: The use of computers in therapy, in The Computerization of Behavioral Healthcare. Edited by Trabin T. San Francisco, CA, Jossey-Bass, 1996, pp 39–62

Gustafson JP: An integration of brief dynamic psychotherapy. Am J Psychiatry 141:935–944, 1984

Henry WP, Strupp HH, Butler SF, et al: Effects of training in time-limited dynamic psychotherapy: changes in therapist behavior. J Consult Clin Psychol 61:434–440, 1993a

Henry WP, Schacht TE, Strupp HH, et al: Effects of training in time-limited dynamic psychotherapy: mediators of therapists' responses to training. J Consult Clin Psychol 61:441–447, 1993b

Hoglend P: Personality disorders and long-term outcome after brief dynamic psychotherapy. J Personal Disord 7:168–181, 1993

Horowitz M[J], Marmar CR, Krupnick J, et al: Personality Styles and Brief Psychotherapy. New York, Basic Books, 1984

Horowitz MJ, Marmar CR, Weiss DS, et al: Comprehensive analysis of change after brief dynamic psychotherapy. Am J Psychiatry 143:582–589, 1986

Howard KI, Kopta SM, Krause MS, et al: The dose-effect relationship in psychotherapy. Am Psychol 41:159–164, 1986

Hoyt MF: Therapist resistances to short-term dynamic psychotherapy. J Am Acad Psychoanal 13:93–112, 1985

Hoyt MF: Teaching and learning short-term psychotherapy, in Psychotherapy in Managed Health Care: The Optimal Use of Time and Resources. Edited by Austad CS, Berman WH. Washington, DC, American Psychological Association, 1991, pp 98–107

Hoyt MF, Austad CS: Psychotherapy in a staff model health maintenance organization: providing and assuring quality care in the future. Psychotherapy: Theory, Research and Practice 29:119–129, 1992

Hoyt MF, Rosenbaum R, Talmon M: Planned single-session psychotherapy, in The First Session in Brief Therapy. Edited by Budman S, Hoyt MF, Friedman S. New York, Guilford, 1992, pp 59–86

Hymowitz C, Pollock EJ: Psychobattle: cost-cutting firms monitor couch time as therapists fret. Wall Street Journal, July 13, 1995, p 1

Iglehart JK: Managed care and mental health. N Engl J Med 334:131–135, 1996

Joyce AS, Duncan SC, Piper WE: Task analysis of "working" responses to dynamic interpretation in short-term individual psychotherapy. Psychotherapy Research 5:49–62, 1995

Karon BP: Provision of psychotherapy under managed health care: a growing crisis and national nightmare. Professional Psychology: Research and Practice 26:5–9, 1995

Kopta SM, Howard KI, Lowry JL, et al: Patterns of symptomatic recovery in psychotherapy. J Consult Clin Psychol 62:1009–1016, 1994

Koss MP, Shiang J: Research on brief psychotherapy, in Handbook of Psychotherapy and Behavior Change, 4th Edition. Edited by Bergin AE, Garfield SL. New York, Wiley, 1994

Koss MP, Butcher JN, Strupp HH: Brief psychotherapy methods in clinical research. J Consult Clin Psychol 54:60–67, 1986

Laiken M, Winston A, McCullough L: Intensive short-term dynamic psychotherapy, in Handbook of Short-Term Dynamic Psychotherapy. Edited by Crits-Christoph P, Barber JP. New York, Basic Books, 1991, pp 80–109

LaRue-Yalom T, Levenson H: Long-term outcome of training in time-limited dynamic psychotherapy. Paper presented at the American Psychological Association Convention, San Francisco, CA, August 2001

Leichsenring F: Comparative effects of short-term psychodynamic psychotherapy and cognitive-behavioral therapy in depression: a meta-analytic approach. Clin Psychol Rev 21:401–419, 2001

Levenson H: Time Limited Dynamic Psychotherapy: A Guide to Clinical Practice. New York, Basic Books, 1995

Levenson H: Time-limited dynamic psychotherapy: an integrationist perspective. Journal of Psychotherapy Integration (in press)

Levenson H, Bolter K: Short-term psychotherapy values and attitudes: changes with training. Paper presented at the American Psychological Association Convention, Atlanta, GA, August 1988

Levenson H, Burg J: Training psychologists in the era of managed care, in A Psychologist's Proactive Guide to Managed Mental Health Care. Edited by Kent A, Hersen M. Hillsdale, NJ, Lawrence Erlbaum, 2000, pp 113–140

Levenson H, Davidovitz D: Brief therapy prevalence and training: a national survey of psychologists. Psychotherapy 37:335–340, 2000

Levenson H, Evans SA: The current state of brief therapy training in American Psychological Association accredited graduate and internship programs. Professional Psychology: Research and Practice 31:446–452, 2000

Levenson H, Overstreet D: Long-term outcome with brief psychotherapy. Paper presented at the annual meeting of the Society for Psychotherapy Research, Pittsburgh, PA, June 1993

Levenson H, Strupp HH: Recommendations for the future of training in brief dynamic psychotherapy. J Clin Psychol 55:385–391, 1999

Levenson H, Speed J, Budman S: Therapists' experience, training, and skill in brief therapy: a bicoastal survey. Am J Psychother 49:95–117, 1995

Levenson H, Servis M, Hales RE: Brief psychodynamically informed therapy for medically ill patients, in Medical-Psychiatric Practice, 2nd Edition, Vol 2. Edited by Stoudemire A, Fogel BS. Washington DC, American Psychiatric Press, 2000, pp 3–37

Levenson H, Butler S, Powers T, et al: Concise Guide to Brief Dynamic Psychotherapy. Washington, DC, American Psychiatric Publishing, 2002

Luborsky L: Principles of Psychoanalytic Psychotherapy: A Manual for Supportive-Expressive Treatment. New York, Basic Books, 1984

Luborsky L, Crits-Christoph P: Understanding transference: the CCRT method. New York, Basic Books, 1990

Luborsky L, Mark D: Short-term supportive-expressive psychoanalytic psychotherapy, in Handbook of Short-Term Dynamic Psychotherapy. Edited by Crits-Christoph P, Barber JP. New York, Basic Books, 1991

MacKenzie KR: Principles of brief intensive psychotherapy. Psychiatr Ann 21:398–404, 1991

Magnavita JJ: The evolution of short-term dynamic psychotherapy: treatment of the future? Professional Psychology: Research and Practice 24:360–365, 1993

Magnavita JJ: Restructuring Personality Disorders: A Short-term Dynamic Approach. New York, Guilford, 1997

Malan DH: A Study of Brief Psychotherapy. London, England, Tavistock, 1963

Malan DH: The Frontier of Brief Psychotherapy. New York, Plenum, 1976

Malan DH: Individual Psychotherapy and the Science of Psychodynamics. London, England, Butterworth, 1979

Mann J: Time-Limited Psychotherapy. Cambridge, MA, Harvard University Press, 1973

Mark D, Faude J: Supportive-expressive therapy for cocaine abuse, in Dynamic Therapies for Psychiatric Disorders. Edited by Barber JP, Crits-Christoph P. New York, Basic Books, 1995, pp 294–331

Marmor J: Short-term dynamic psychotherapy. Am J Psychiatry 136:149–155, 1979

McCullough Vaillant L: Changing Character: Short-Term Anxiety-Regulating Psychotherapy for Restructuring Defenses, Affects, and Attachment. New York, Basic Books, 1997

Mendelsohn R: Critical factors in short-term psychotherapy: a summary. Bull Menninger Clin 42:133–149, 1978

Messer SB, Warren CS: Models of Brief Psychodynamic Therapy: A Comparative Approach. New York, Guilford, 1995

Miller IJ: Managed care is harmful to outpatient mental health services: a call for accountability. Professional Psychology: Research and Practice 27:349–363, 1996

Mitchell SA, Aron L (eds): Relational Psychoanalysis: The Emergence of a Tradition. Hillsdale, NJ, Analytic Press, 1999

Neff WL, Lambert MJ, Kirk ML, et al: Therapists' attitudes toward short-term therapy: changes with training. Employee Assistance Quarterly 11:67–77, 1996

Newman R: A tumultuous 10 years. APA Monitor: Available online at http://www.apa.org/monitor/feb99.html (accessed 5/14/01)

Nielsen G, Barth, K: Short-term anxiety-provoking psychotherapy, in Handbook of Short-Term Dynamic Psychotherapy. Edited by Crits-Christoph P, Barber JP. New York, Basic Books, 1991

Olfson M, Pincus HA: Outpatient psychotherapy in the United States, I: volume, costs, and other user characteristics. Am J Psychiatry 151:1281–1288, 1994

Peake TH, Bordin CM, Archer RP: Brief Psychotherapies: Changing Frames of Mind. Beverly Hills, CA, Sage, 1988

Perry S, Frances A, Klar H, et al: Selection criteria for individual dynamic psychotherapies. Psychiatr Q 55:3–16, 1983

Phillips LE: The ubiquitous decay curve: delivery similarities in psychotherapy, medicine and addiction. Professional Psychology: Research and Practice 18:650–652, 1987

Piper WE, Debbane EG, Bienvenu JP, et al: A comparative study of four forms of psychotherapy. J Consult Clin Psychol 52:268–279, 1984

Pumpian-Mindlin E: Consideration in the selection of patients for short-term therapy. Am J Psychother 7:641–652, 1953

Rachman AW: Rule of empathy: Sandor Ferenczi's pioneering contribution to the empathic method in psychoanalysis. J Am Acad Psychoanal 16:1–27, 1988

Rank O: Will Therapy (1929). Translated by Taft J. New York, Knopf, 1936

Rouff LC: Clouds and silver linings: Training experiences of psychodynamically oriented mental health trainees. Am J Psychother 54:549–559, 2000

Rounsaville BJ, Chevron ES, Weissman MM, et al: Training therapists to perform interpersonal therapy in clinical trials. Compr Psychiatry 27:364–371, 1986

Rounsaville BJ, O'Malley S, Foley S, et al: Role of manual-guided training in the conduct and efficacy of interpersonal psychotherapy for depression. J Consult Clin Psychol 56:681–688, 1988

Safran JD, Muran JC: The resolution of ruptures in the therapeutic alliance. J Consult Clin Psychol 64:447–458, 1996

Safran JD, Muran JC: Negotiating the Therapeutic Alliance: A Relational Treatment Guide. New York, Guilford, 2000

Schacht TE, Binder JL, Strupp HH: The dynamic focus, in Psychotherapy in a New Key: A Guide to Time-Limited Dynamic Psychotherapy. Edited by Strupp HH, Binder JL. New York, Basic Books, 1984, pp 65–109

Shapiro D, Rees A, Barkham M, et al: Effects of treatment duration and severity of depression on the maintenance of gains after cognitive-behavioral and psychodynamic-interpersonal psychotherapy. J Consult Clin Psychology 63:378–387, 1995

Shea MT, Pilkonis PA, Beckham E, et al: Personality disorders and treatment outcome in the NIMH Treatment of Depression Collaborative Research Program. Am J Psychiatry 147:711–718, 1990

Sifneos PE: Short-Term Psychotherapy and Emotional Crisis. Cambridge, MA, Harvard University Press, 1972

Sifneos PE: The teaching and supervision of STAPP, in Basic Principles and Techniques of Short-Term Dynamic Psychotherapy. Edited by Davanloo H. New York, Jason Aronson, 1978, pp 491–499

Sifneos PE: Short-Term Dynamic Psychotherapy: Evaluation and Technique. New York, Plenum, 1979

Sifneos PE: Short-Term Dynamic Psychotherapy: Evaluation and Technique, 2nd Edition. New York, Plenum, 1987

Silberschatz G, Fretter PB, Curtis JT: How do interpretations influence the process of psychotherapy? J Consult Clin Psychol 54:646–652, 1986

Small L: The Briefer Psychotherapies. New York, Brunner/Mazel, 1979

Speed JL: Therapists' practice, training, and skill in brief therapy: a survey of California and Massachusetts psychologists. Unpublished doctoral dissertation, Wright Institute Graduate School of Psychology, Berkeley, CA, 1992

Stern S: Managed care, brief therapy, and therapeutic integrity. Psychotherapy 30:162–175, 1993

Strupp HH: The outcome problem in psychotherapy: contemporary perspectives, in Psychotherapy Research and Behavior Change. Edited by Harvey TH, Parks MM. Washington, DC, American Psychological Association, 1982, pp 39–71

Strupp HH: Time-limited dynamic psychotherapy: development and implementation of a training program, in Brief Therapy: Myths, Methods, and Metaphors. Edited by Zeig JK, Gillian SG. New York, Brunner/Mazel, 1990, pp 327–341

Strupp HH, Binder JL (eds): Psychotherapy in a New Key: A Guide to Time-Limited Dynamic Psychotherapy. New York, Basic Books, 1984

Strupp HH, Butler SF, Rosser CL: Training in psychodynamic therapy. J Consult Clin Psychol 56:689–695, 1988

Svartberg M, Stiles TC: Comparative effects of short-term psychodynamic psychotherapy: a meta-analysis. J Consult Clin Psychol 59:704–714, 1991

Thackrey M, Butler SF, Strupp HH: The Capacity for Dynamic Process Scale (CDPS), in A Collection of Psychological Scales. Edited by Canfield ML, Canfield JE. New York, Basic Books, 1993, pp 191–210

Therapy for the '90s. U.S. News and World Report, January 13, 1992, pp 55–56

Tomkins SS: Affect theory, in Approaches to Emotion. Edited by Scherer KR, Ekman P. Hillsdale, NJ, Lawrence Erlbaum, 1984, pp 163–195

Ursano RJ, Dressler DM: Brief versus long-term psychotherapy: clinician attitudes and organizational design. Compr Psychiatry 18:55–60, 1977

Ursano RJ, Hales RE: A review of brief individual psychotherapies. Am J Psychiatry 143:1507–1517, 1986

Waska RT: Psychoanalytic perspectives concerning the impact of managed care on psychotherapy. Psychoanalytic Social Work 6:61–77, 1999

Weiss J, Sampson H, Mount Zion Psychotherapy Research Group: The Psychoanalytic Process: Theory, Clinical Observations, and Empirical Research. New York, Guilford, 1986

Wheelock I: The value of a psychodynamic approach in a managed care setting. Am J Psychother 54:204–215, 2000

Winokur M, Dasberg H: Teaching and learning short-term dynamic psychotherapy: techniques and resistances. Bull Menninger Clin 47:36–52, 1983

Winston A, Laikin M, Pollack J, et al: Short-term psychotherapy of personality disorders. Am J Psychiatry 151:190–194, 1994

Wolberg LR: Handbook of Short-Term Psychotherapy. New York, Thieme-Stratton, 1980

Psychoanalysis, Psychoanalytic Psychotherapy, and Supportive Psychotherapy

Robert J. Ursano, M.D.

Edward K. Silberman, M.D.

Our health is directly and indirectly affected by our behavior: our thoughts, feelings, fantasies, and actions. Because of this effect, both increased morbidity and mortality can result from psychiatric illness. Frequently, psychopathology limits our ability to see options and exercise choices, leading to feelings, thoughts, fantasies, and actions that may be painful, restricted, and repetitive. Psychotherapy is directed toward changing these learned forms of behavior that affect health and performance. Personality is, in fact, a cluster of probable behaviors that each individual characteristically has in a given context (Ursano et al. 2001). Changing these response patterns can change the risk of disease, illness, and negative health behaviors, as well as interpersonal strategies that may decrease productivity and success.

Originally called the *talking cure*, psychotherapy is the generic term for a large number of treatment techniques that are directed toward changing behavior through verbal interchange. In the context of talking, psychotherapy provides understanding, support, new experiences, and new knowledge that can 1) result in learning, 2) increase the range of behaviors available to the patient, 3) relieve symptoms, and 4) alter maladaptive and unhealthy patterns of behavior. In the process of this reorganization, both perception and behavior change.

The target organ of psychotherapy is the brain. Feelings, thoughts, fantasies, and actions are brain functions. If behavior is to change, brain function and activity must alter at some basic level (Kandell 1979, 1989, 1999, 2000). If neuron A used to fire to neuron B, it must now fire to neuron C. Just as past life experience affects the development and maturation of the brain, and therefore brain activity, so too does present life experience, including the experience of psychotherapy.

Our social connectedness, a major focus of psychotherapeutic work, mediates both morbidity and mortality (House et al. 1988) and serves to regulate bodily function (Hofer 1984). The common observation that a phobic individual will approach the phobic object when accompanied by a supportive other illustrates the profound biological activities that accompany interpersonal relations and of which we know very little. How the "outside" (i.e., life experience) changes what is inside (i.e., our biology) is fundamental to an understanding of brain function and to the effectiveness of all psychotherapies. Our understanding of these processes, the science of behavior change, is now emerging (Kandell 1999, 2000; Ursano and Fullerton 1991). For example, Baxter et al. (1992) showed that after psychotherapy, changes in the brain evident through positron emission tomography are similar to those following treatment with fluoxetine, and preclinical studies are now well focused on the close relationship of brain structure, genes, and experience (Meaney 2001; Sapolsky 2000). Psychotherapy is a life experience that affects brain function. The neuroscience of psychotherapy is in its infancy.

Psychotherapy was defined by Harry Stack Sullivan (1954) as primarily a verbal interchange between two individuals in which one of these individuals is designated an expert and the other a help seeker. These two persons work together to identify the patient's characteristic problems in living, with the hope of achieving behavioral change (Table 26–1). This definition of psychotherapy excludes a substantial number of activities that are inaccurately considered psychotherapy. First, psychotherapy by this definition is verbal. Certainly more than 90% of the interchange in psychotherapy is verbal. Although nonverbal communication can be important, it is never the primary activity of psychotherapy. Second, the requirement that one person be the help seeker and the other an expert sets the roles, activities, and boundaries of this interchange. Two friends sharing a drink at a bar or restaurant do not fit this picture. In fact, in the bar or restaurant the social setting and rules are very different. In these settings, the rules of interaction dictate an equal sharing of one's problems. If one person is always the listener, the other begins to feel uncomfortable, because this is not the expected interchange. Rather, at the bar or restaurant, one person talks and then the other often says, "Oh yes, me too," or something similar. Not so in psychotherapy. Here the patient reveals his or her problems, but the physician-therapist provides help, not a reciprocal revelation of problems. The two settings have different rules governing the relationship (Epstein 1995).

TABLE 26–1. Individual psychotherapy

Consists of an interaction between two persons.
Interaction is primarily verbal.
One person is the help seeker and the other an expert.
Goal of the interaction is to identify the characteristic patterns of behavior of the patient that are causing symptoms and problems in living.
Patient has the expectation of help and change.

TABLE 26–2. Nonspecific curative factors of medical intervention

Developing a confiding relationship
Maintaining the expectation of help and benefit
Providing opportunities for abreaction
Providing new information
Providing a rationale/organization/meaning (diagnosis) to seemingly unrelated symptoms and events
Maximizing the probability that the patient will experience a success

---

All medical treatments, including psychotherapy, also show the effects of nonspecific curative factors in their outcomes (Table 26–2). These factors, also called *placebo effects*, include the presence of a confiding relationship,

abreaction (i.e., the expression of intense feelings), the provision of new information, and the provision of a rationale or meaning (i.e., diagnosis) that organizes seemingly unrelated symptoms and events and maximizes the patient's probability of success experiences (J.D. Frank 1971). Clinicians use these principles as part of the art and science of medical treatment to increase their patients' relief of pain and suffering.

In addition to these nonspecific factors, most medical treatments also have specific curative factors. Similarly, the psychotherapies identify specific technical interventions and procedures directed toward behavioral change.

As in other medical treatments, there are contraindications to and dangers in the use of psychotherapy (Crown 1983; Hadley and Strupp 1976). It is not sufficient to take the position that "the operation was a success but the patient died"—or that psychotherapy was a success but no change occurred. Although the therapist in individual psychotherapy does not "require" behavioral change and, depending on the type of psychotherapy, may or may not directly use technical procedures focused on behavioral change per se (e.g., practice, desensitization), the final result of the therapist's technical expertise is behavioral change. Such change includes alterations in the patient's well-being, physical health, social supports, and societal productivity, as well as symptomatic relief. What is dealt with in treatment is what the patient is able to bring into focus, what the patient can tolerate talking about, and what he or she can tolerate the therapist talking about (Coleman 1968).

Psychotherapy is both efficacious and cost-effective (Crits-Christoph 1991, 1992; Lazar 1997; Perry et al. 1999). The effectiveness of psychotherapy is no longer a matter of debate (Luborsky et al. 1975; Parloff 1982; Parloff et al. 1986; Shapiro and Shapiro 1982; Smith et al. 1980; Spiegel and Lazar 1997). However, the answer to the question of which psychotherapy for which patient and by which therapist is still unclear (Parloff 1982).

The cost-effectiveness of psychotherapeutic treatment is a focus of substantial research (Krupnick and Pincus 1992; Lazar 1997). Individual psychotherapy has been shown to result in reduced health care costs for high utilizers of psychiatric services (Guthrie et al. 1999) and fewer days of hospitalization for patients on medical and surgical services of a general hospital. In health clinics and health maintenance organizations, brief psychotherapy decreases the number of visits to primary health care providers, reduces the number of laboratory and X-ray studies, decreases the number of prescriptions given, and, overall, reduces direct health care costs (Longobardi

1981; Sharfstein et al. 1984). Mumford et al. (1984) summarized their meta-analysis of the cost-offset effects of outpatient mental health treatments, most of which were short term. They found that outpatient psychotherapy resulted in an average reduction of 33% in use of medical care. Furthermore, these reductions occurred predominantly in the more expensive inpatient medical services.

In another study (Meyer et al. 1981), 72 patients with major emotional problems who had been treated only by internists in a general medical clinic were compared with 62 patients who, in addition to being treated by internists for medical problems, received 10 weekly psychotherapy visits. Both groups had approximately an equal degree of emotional disturbance. At 4-month and 1-year follow-ups, the brief psychotherapy group reported many more global improvements than did the nonpsychotherapy group. Also, more patients in the brief psychotherapy group than in the nonpsychotherapy group were employed at 1-year follow-up. This study suggests that there are specific beneficial effects of brief psychotherapy when it is used in a medical setting by skilled psychotherapists.

Combining psychotherapy with antidepressant medication has also been shown to produce the best outcome at 1-year follow-up when compared with either treatment alone (DiMascio et al. 1979; Weissman et al. 1981). Smith and colleagues (Smith and Glass 1977; Smith et al. 1980) showed an effect size of psychotherapy of 0.68, a level equivalent to that of several clinical trials that were stopped early because it would have been unethical to withhold such a clearly effective treatment from patients. Crits-Christoph (1992; Crits-Christoph and Barben 1991) demonstrated somewhat larger effect sizes in a review of well-designed studies of brief psychodynamic psychotherapy. This review also found that after brief psychodynamic psychotherapy, patients were better off than 79% of those on a waiting list in terms of psychiatric symptom levels and social adjustment. Howard et al. (1986) found that 74% of patients in psychotherapy were improved after 26 sessions. For a comparison group with only general medical support, this degree of recovery required 2 years (McNeilly and Howard 1991).

Although at times we speak of psychotherapy as beginning as soon as the physician sees the patient, this hyperbole is used primarily to underscore the importance of interpersonal and transferential elements in the initial meeting with the patient. In fact, it is extremely important to distinguish the diagnostic interviews from the ongoing treatment. The evaluation process is distinct from, although related to, the psychotherapy itself. The interventions and technical procedures performed during the evaluation phase are substantially different from the technical procedures of psychotherapy itself. During the evaluation phase, the physician must assess the diagnosis and the patient's ego strength and physical health. In addition, the clinician must closely consider the selection criteria and the different treatment options, including "no treatment indicated" (Frances and Clarkin 1981). This phase constitutes, in Levinson's terminology, the *candidacy stage* (Levinson et al. 1967). Through negotiation with the patient, a treatment decision is reached and the psychotherapy begins.

Many patients do not make it through the evaluation phase of seeking help. Repeatedly, it has been shown that more than 50% of patients drop out by five sessions. It is inappropriate to consider those who drop out as having been in psychotherapy. Clearly, some of these patients experience benefit during their short contact with mental health professionals (Malan et al. 1975)—some through the nonspecific curative factors of help seeking and others through guidance and crisis intervention. In addition, many may drop out because they did not receive what they were looking for.

Psychotherapies can be distinguished by their overall goals, the techniques used, and the diagnostic categories to which the techniques can be applied. In this chapter we review psychoanalytically oriented treatments—psychoanalysis and psychoanalytically oriented (psychodynamic) psychotherapy, interpersonal psychotherapy, (IPT) which has many psychodynamic elements (Markowitz et al. 1998), and finally, supportive psychotherapy. The psychoanalytically oriented and supportive psychotherapies remain the most commonly used psychotherapies. Many of the principles of the psychodynamic/psychoanalytic treatments have been incorporated into other treatment modalities and into the clinical assessment process, medication management, and ward milieu work. Understanding the principles and phenomena observed in psychodynamic treatment, therefore, is often critical to success with other treatments and evaluation techniques (Gabbard 2000). In addition, skill in the briefer forms of psychotherapy is related to skill in the longer-term treatments, although these treatment approaches are not the same.

The psychoanalytically oriented treatments and supportive psychotherapy are applied to a wide array of diagnostic problems. Understanding the techniques and the phases of these therapies can also provide important knowledge and skills for assessment and management of medication, compliance, interpersonal stressors, and past and present family problems, all of which can greatly affect outcome, relapse, rehabilitation, and social function.

Psychoanalytically Oriented Psychotherapies

Primary to the psychodynamic (psychoanalytically oriented) treatments is the importance of the patient feeling engaged and involved in the work. Through the exploration of the patient's conflicts evidenced in symptoms, metaphors, and symbols, both defensive patterns and disturbances in present interpersonal relationships can be identified in the treatment setting as well as in the patient's life. The therapist's ability to hear what the patient has to say and to understand its meaning is central to all psychoanalytically oriented treatments (Solnit 2000). This facet of treatment demands skill in neutral listening and the ability to identify with the patient's perspective and worldview while not losing one's own.

The therapist is always listening for the continuity present, but hidden, between sessions (Coleman 1968). The therapist operates on the hypothesis that each session is related to the previous one. The psychoanalyst and the psychodynamic psychotherapist listen to the patient's subjective experience of the world, interpersonal and internal conflicts, and cognitive defenses that result in the day-to-day changes in moods, thoughts, and behaviors (Mohl and McLaughlin 1997; Silberman and Certa 1997).

In the initial phase of treatment, the therapeutic alliance (i.e., the working alliance) is developed (Greenson 1965; Zetzel 1956). The therapeutic alliance is the reality-based relationship between the analyst (or the therapist) and the patient that forms the basis of working together in a cooperative manner (Sonnenberg et al. 1997). The therapeutic alliance is nurtured through the identification of the patient's initial anxieties about beginning treatment. Fostering the therapeutic alliance is a part of the therapist's establishment of the conditions under which the patient can favorably hear and deal with the interpretations that the therapist will give later in the treatment (Ponsi 2000).

Few empirical studies of psychoanalytic treatment have been done (Bachrach et al. 1985; Galatzer-Levy et al. 2000; Kantrowitz et al. 1986, 1987, 1990; Kernberg et al. 1972; Sandell et al. 2000; Vaughan et al. 2000; Wallerstein 1992). The brief psychodynamic treatments have a somewhat greater empirical database, but much further research is needed here as well (Crits-Christoph 1992; Gomes-Schwartz et al. 1978; Horowitz et al. 1986; Luborsky et al. 1975, 1988; Malan 1980; Milrod et al. 2000; Strupp 1980a, 1980b, 1980c). In general, the studies that have been conducted support the efficacy of psychoanalytically oriented treatment approaches. How-

ever, methodological issues are prominent in most of the research in this area. Moreover, the difficulties of long-term studies are substantial. Handbooks for treatment will go far in improving research in the psychoanalytically oriented treatments (Luborsky 1984; Milrod et al. 1997; Strupp and Binder 1984).

Psychoanalysis

Psychoanalysis was developed by Sigmund Freud beginning in the late nineteenth century. Originally, Freud used hypnosis to recover forgotten memories related to traumas of early childhood. Historically, he progressed from hypnosis to the "pressure technique" and finally to the modern approach of using free association. Perhaps Freud's most important and lasting discovery was the contribution of psychic reality to development and conflict formation. Freud found that it was the subjective experience of events in childhood—that is, the psychic reality of the events—rather than the presence or absence of the actual events, that affected development and conflict formation. This discovery led Freud to identify the role of the unconscious and unremembered experiences of childhood and to develop a mechanism, psychoanalysis, to discover and bring these memories into awareness.

The dangers of neglecting the actuality of traumatic events have been highlighted in recent years and must always be considered by the therapist. In the treatment of children this is particularly important because of the need to intervene to protect the child. Often a neglect of the reality of trauma results if the therapist does not understand that the patient's recall is a mixture of both subjective factors and objective fact, neither of which can be ignored.

Freud identified dreams, slips of the tongue, and free association as important windows on the influence of childhood and the present conflicts of the patient. From the psychoanalytic view, an understanding of the conflicts experienced in childhood is important to gaining knowledge of and changing present behavior (Brenner 1976). The conflicts of childhood are called the *childhood neurosis*.

Conflicts are patterns of feelings, thoughts, and behavior that were "learned" (i.e., incorporated into brain function and patterning) during childhood. "Neurotic" conflicts result in the patient's feelings of anxiety and depression; somatic symptoms; work, social, or sexual inhibition; and maladaptive interpersonal relations. Typically, such conflicts are between libidinal (i.e., sexual/bodily) and aggressive wishes. Libidinal wishes can be thought of as longings for sexual and emotional gratification or more generally as positive feelings and affects (Kernberg 2001). Aggressive wishes are destructive desires (or, as they are more often conceptualized today, negative feelings and affects) that either are primary or result from frustration and deprivation.

The concept of sexual wishes is quite broad in psychoanalysis and is not limited to only genital feelings. Sexual wishes include wishes to be held and touched, to control, to eat, and many others. This concept of sexuality was another of Freud's major contributions: his discovery, and the subsequent confirmation through child observation, of the intimate relationship between children and their bodies. It is through their bodies that children come to know mother, father, and the world. It is hard to overemphasize the radical change in thinking that resulted from beginning to think of the child as having thoughts, feelings, and fantasies and as not being a "tabula rasa" or a "small adult."

The goal of psychoanalysis is the elucidation of the childhood neurosis (i.e., conflicts) as it presents in the transference neurosis (Table 26–3). This is a major undertaking that requires a reasonably psychiatrically healthy individual who can sustain the treatment. Psychoanalysis is frequently criticized for being used to treat reasonably psychiatrically healthy people. In fact, however, this is the tradition of medicine. For example, one may ask who receives triple bypass surgery: the individual with a single left main descending artery occlusion or the individual who is having a myocardial infarction and in the end stage of congestive heart failure? Clearly, the answer is the former. This underscores the frequently forgotten point that medical treatments are given to patients rather than to diseases. All medical treatments, including psychoanalysis, make certain requirements of the patient. These requirements must be considered when the treatment is prescribed. Psychoanalysis is very demanding of patients. It requires an individual who is able to access his or her fantasy life in an active, experiencing manner and is able to leave it behind at the end of a session.

Psychoanalysis focuses on the recovery of childhood experiences as they appear in the relationship with the analyst (Chessick 2000; Coltrera 1980; Freud 1912a/1958; Gill 1982; Greenson 1967). This re-creation in the doctor–patient relationship of a conflicted relationship with a childhood figure is the *transference neurosis*. Frequently, the transference is paternal or maternal, but it need not be. Sibling, aunt, uncle, and grandparent transferences are all important parts of psychoanalytic work. The transference neurosis (in contrast to transference phenomena) is the sustained appearance of the transference over time. When the transference neurosis is present, the patient experiences the analyst in a similar

TABLE 26–3. Psychoanalysis

Goal	Resolution of the childhood neurosis as it presents itself in the transference neurosis
Selection criteria	Experiences conflict that is primarily oedipal
	Experiences conflict as internal
	Is psychologically minded
	Is able to obtain symptom relief through understanding
	Is able to experience and observe strong affects without acting out
	Has supportive relationships available in both the present and the past
Duration	Four to five sessions per week; 3–6 years, average duration
Techniques	Free association
	Therapeutic alliance
	Neutrality
	Abstinence
	Defense analysis
	Interpretation of transference

manner as he or she once did the significant figure from the past. Frequently, this experience is accompanied by other elements of the past being experienced in the patient's life.

Transference is a ubiquitous phenomenon that is increasingly able to be studied empirically (Fried et al. 1992; Luborsky and Crits-Christoph 1990). Several empirical studies support the importance of addressing the transference for a successful outcome of psychodynamic treatment (Brodaty 1983; Donovan 1984; Frances and Perry 1983; Luborsky and Crits-Christoph 1990; Malan 1975, 1976, 1980; Marziali 1984; Marziali and Sullivan 1980). Transference is the result of our tendency to see the past in the present, to exclude new information, and to see what is familiar to us (Table 26–4). This "looking for the familiar" results in our reacting and responding in ways that are characteristic of our relationships with significant figures from our past. The analyst's relative abstinence (i.e., avoiding gratifying wishes) and neutrality (i.e., not encouraging one side or another of the patient's conflict—either the wishes or the defenses and prohibitions) help create a setting in which the transference can emerge and, more important, in which it can be observed and understood by the analyst and the patient. It is the contrast between the patient's experience of the analyst in the transference and his or her experience in the therapeutic alliance that facilitates the recognition that the transference thoughts and feelings are self-generated.

TABLE 26–4. Transference and countertransference

Transference	Seeing the past in the present
	Seeing the familiar
	Excluding new information
Countertransference	
Concordant	Identifying with the patient's feelings (the therapist feels as though he or she were the patient)
Complementary	Reacting to the patient's feelings (the therapist feels as though he or she were the transference figure)

The transference is not a total distortion of the doctor–patient relationship. Rather, it is often an elaboration (without confirming information) of an observation the patient has made about the analyst or his or her office. Reality serves as the foundation on which the transference is constructed. The patient's understanding of the transference aids in the recall of the past and the recovery of lost feelings.

Countertransference is the analyst's transference response to the patient. At times, *countertransference* is also used to describe the analyst's specific neurotic responses to the patient's transference (Table 26–4). However, this is not clearly different from the first, more general, definition (Blum 1986; Sandler et al. 1973). Countertransference is also ubiquitous and it is not limited to the psychoanalytic setting. In fact, it can be an important part of any relationship, particularly the doctor–patient relationship; when present, it may be intense and enduring. Countertransference is increased by life stress and unresolved conflicts in the analyst. It can appear as either an identification with or a reaction to the patient's conscious and unconscious fantasies, feelings, and behaviors (Racker 1957). Through analysis of his or her own countertransference reactions, the analyst recognizes subtle aspects of the transference relationship and is better able to understand the patient's experience (Searles 1965). Skill in recognizing countertransference and transference is an important part of the psychiatrist's armamentarium in all treatment settings, particularly those involving consultation-liaison psychiatry, in which the doctor–patient or nurse–patient relationships can be the major reason a consultation was requested.

The design of the psychoanalytic treatment situation fosters the patient's observing capacity so that the transference neurosis can be analyzed (Stone 1961). Transference is not unique to the psychoanalytic situation. It occurs throughout life in all areas and is a frequent accompaniment to hospitalization of any kind. Entering a hospital, having one's clothes removed, having one's name forgotten, being required to eat when told, and having to submit to medical procedures constitute a highly regressive experience that facilitates the appearance of transferences. The ability to recognize transference phenomena as they appear in all doctor–patient relationships is very important. Psychoanalysis is unique in its efforts to establish a setting in which the transference, when it appears, can be used as a vehicle for understanding.

Modern psychoanalysis continues to require frequent meetings of the analyst and analysand—usually, four to five sessions per week. (Freud originally met with his patients six times per week.) This frequency of sessions is continued, on the average, for 3–6 years. This intensity of meetings is necessary for the patient to develop sufficient trust to explore his or her inner fantasy life. In addition, given the number of events that occur daily in a life, the frequent meetings enable the patient to explore fantasies rather than only the reality-based perceptions of life events (Freud 1912b/1958). Individuals who are in crisis and who therefore are very concerned and focused on the real events in their life are not good candidates to enter psychoanalysis. Psychoanalysis focuses on the patient's experience and fantasies of his or her life rather than on the real events. A crisis does not allow the patient the opportunity to explore fantasies. In general, the patient in psychoanalysis is encouraged to use the couch so that the patient's focus on fantasies rather than on reality will be further facilitated. In addition, the analyst usually sits out of view, allowing the patient better to elaborate his or her fantasies about the analyst.

Free association is a major element in the technique of psychoanalysis. Freud described free association through an analogy of a train ride (Freud 1913/1958). He suggested that if the analyst and analysand were riding together on a train and the analyst were blind, the analysand would not forget to describe the beautiful mountains or the ugly coal slags. This analogy is meant to convey the sense of the patient's reporting of all thoughts that come to mind without censorship and without dismissing them as too trivial. In point of fact, free association is difficult to attain, and much of the work of psychoanalysis is based on identifying those places where free association breaks down (i.e., the occurrence of a defense, clinically experienced by the analyst as resistance). When the patient is able to achieve the highest level of free association, the neurotic conflicts have been removed and termination is near.

Early in treatment, the analyst establishes a therapeutic alliance with the patient that allows for a reality-based consideration of the demands of the treatment and for a working collaboration between analyst and analysand toward the patient's understanding himself or herself (Greenson 1965; Meissner 1998; Zetzel 1956). The analyst focuses on analyzing the defenses the patient uses to minimize conflict and disturbing affects (Freud 1912b/1958, 1913/1958, 1914/1958) (Table 26–5). Defenses such as intellectualization, reaction formation, denial, repression, and other neurotic cognitive mechanisms are identified and repeatedly interpreted to the patient. Through the analysis of defense, the working alliance strengthens and the patient's ability to observe internal fantasies increases. In addition, the patient's comfort with talking about his or her feelings with the analyst increases. In this way, the transference grows more available and can be analyzed.

The analysis of the patient's dreams is an important element of psychoanalytic treatment (Freud 1911/1958; Reiser 2001; Sharpe 1961; Ursano et al. 1998). Dreams, as well as slips of the tongue and symptoms, express the conflicts of the patient in "metaphor," evidencing the out-of-awareness (i.e., unconscious) elements of the conflict. The building blocks of dreams are recent life events. Dreams express both a present and a childhood conflict in much the same way that a rebus expresses a story. The grammar of the dream process is different from that of conscious thought. Rather than following logic and time sequence, dreams are constructed by condensation of multiple meanings and the use of symbols. There are no universal symbols. The symbols, perhaps better thought of as symbolic vehicles available to any given person, are from the "dictionary" of meanings developed as part of the individual's life experience, both in childhood and in adulthood. Thus, dreams (and slips of the tongue and symptoms) are a means for the patient to understand the feelings and thoughts that influence his or her life, that are out of awareness, and that often are derived from childhood experiences, beliefs, and views of the interpersonal world and familial behavior (Weiss and Sampson 1986).

The primary goal of psychoanalysis is the establishment of the transference relationship and the subsequent analysis of this relationship. It is this primary focus that distinguishes psychoanalysis from psychodynamic psychotherapy. The specific treatment effects of psychoanalysis grow from the experience and analysis of the transference, reawakened affects, cognitions, and behaviors linked with significant individuals in the patient's past. In the context of the arousal associated with these figures and the simultaneous understanding of the experience, behavioral change occurs (Loewald 1980).

TABLE 26–5. Defense mechanisms

Repression
Intellectualization
Reaction formation
Regression
Displacement
Sublimation
Reversal
Splitting
Denial
Projection
Inhibition
Projective identification
Asceticism
Omnipotence
Isolation of affect
Devaluing
Identification with the aggressor
Primitive idealization

The analyst uses a number of techniques in his or her interventions, including interpretation and clarification (Bibring 1954; Glover 1968; Sandler et al. 1973). Classically, an interpretation is the linking together of the patient's experience of an event in the present with the transference experience of the analyst and the childhood-significant figure. Rarely are interpretations actually given in one sentence in one session. More frequently, interpretations occur over a period during which the past, the present, and the transference experiences are linked together.

Medications are infrequently used in psychoanalysis, although some analysts are attempting to use psychoanalysis with medication in the treatment of persons with affective disorders. Psychoanalysis is actually a highly supportive treatment for the individual who experiences frequent contact, quiet inquiry, and intellectual understanding as a supportive environment (de Jonghe et al. 1992; Wallerstein 1986, 1989). The supportive elements and their contribution to the treatment process have been less discussed in psychoanalysis than in other treatments. The need for medication may indicate the patient's need for greater support than can be provided in the psychoanalytic treatment.

The analyst operates under several guiding principles that facilitate the analysis of the transference. These principles include 1) neutrality, by which the analyst favors neither the patient's wishes (i.e., id) nor the condemnations of these wishes (i.e., superego); and 2) abstinence, whereby the analyst does not provide gratification to the patient similar to that of the wished-for object (Freud 1915 [1914]/1958) (Table 26–6). It is helpful in understanding

TABLE 26–6. Principles of psychoanalytic technique

Neutrality	The analyst maintains a neutral stance favoring neither the patient's wishes (i.e., id) nor the patient's condemnations of these wishes (i.e., superego).
Abstinence	The analyst does not gratify the patient's desire or expectation that the analyst act like the person from the past. Rather, the analyst helps the patient see and understand this process.

the rule of abstinence to recognize a definition of transference used by Joseph Sandler. Sandler et al. (1973) described transference as the role pressure placed on the analyst to conform to the behaviors of the significant individual from the past. Therefore, transference is experienced by the analyst as an expectation from the patient that the analyst will behave in a certain manner. Abstinence is the avoidance of becoming this figure *in reality* and gratifying these wishes or beliefs. The therapist's abstinence leads to his or her being somewhat silent but not withholding, in order better to observe how the patient organizes his or her psychic world. This stance must be explained and the patient educated about the reason for this stance.

The assessment of a patient for psychoanalysis must include diagnostic considerations as well as an assessment of the patient's ability to make use of the psychoanalytic situation for behavioral change. These considerations include the patient's psychological mindedness; the availability of supports in his or her real environment to sustain the psychoanalysis, which can be felt as quite depriving; and the patient's ability to experience and simultaneously to observe highly charged affective states.

Because of the frequency of the sessions and the duration of the treatment, the cost of psychoanalysis can be prohibitive. Low-fee clinics frequently make available a substantial amount of treatment to some patients who could not otherwise afford it.

Psychoanalysis has been useful in the treatment of obsessional disorders, anxiety disorders, dysthymic disorders, and moderately severe personality disorders. Individuals with substantial preoedipal pathology, usually indicated by chaotic life settings and an inability to establish a supportive dyadic relationship, as is often seen in patients with narcissistic, borderline, schizoid, paranoid, and schizotypal personality disorders, are usually not thought to be candidates for traditional psychoanalysis. In the present climate of emphasis on cost-effectiveness, psychoanalysis is more frequently recommended after a course of brief psychotherapy has proved to be either ineffective or insufficient.

Psychoanalytic Psychotherapy

Psychoanalytically oriented psychotherapy—also known as *psychoanalytic psychotherapy, psychodynamic psychotherapy*, and *explorative psychotherapy*—is a psychotherapeutic procedure that recognizes the development of transference and resistance in the psychotherapy setting (Bruch 1974; Fromm-Reichmann 1950). Both long-term and brief psychodynamic psychotherapy are possible. In the past, the terms *brief psychotherapy* and *long-term psychotherapy* were frequently used synonymously with *supportive psychotherapy* and *explorative psychotherapy*, respectively. However, brief and long-term more accurately describe the duration rather than the technique, focus, or goal of psychoanalytically oriented psychotherapy (Budman and Gurman 1983; Errera et al. 1967; Ursano and Dressler 1977). In addition, newer methods of delivering psychotherapy—including intermittent psychotherapy, which is provided in episodes over an extended period of time, and sequential brief psychotherapy, in which medication is continued after termination of the psychotherapy—are becoming more common than classical long-term psychotherapy.

Brief psychotherapy, in particular, requires the therapist to confront his or her own ambitiousness and perfectionism as well as any exaggerated ideal of personality structure and function. The time limits of brief psychotherapy give the therapy its unique characteristics and distinguish it from long-term psychotherapy and psychoanalysis (Ursano and Dressler 1974). Stierlin (1968) identified two treatment factors that are important to understanding the effectiveness of psychotherapy: the "propitious moment" and the "shared past." Brief psychotherapy uses the propitious moment to create personality change, whereas long-term treatment uses the shared past that develops between therapist and patient. Both the propitious moment and the shared past carry psychotherapeutic advantages and disadvantages, emphasizing certain technical possibilities and limiting others.

Following World War II, the interest in psychoanalysis resulted in a rapid growth in the demand for psychotherapy. This growing demand considerably increased the resultant pressure on psychiatrists to develop briefer and less intense forms of psychotherapy than psychoanalysis. In addition, the community mental health movement, and, more recently, the increasing cost of mental health care, have stimulated efforts to find briefer forms of psychotherapy (Milrod et al. 1997). At present, brief psychotherapy is an important part of the psychiatrist's armamentarium (Kay 1997). (See Chapter 25 for a detailed discussion of brief psychodynamic psychotherapy.)

Psychoanalytic psychotherapy is usually more focused than the extensive reworking of personality undertaken in psychoanalysis (Dewald 1978). In addition, psychoanalytic psychotherapy is oriented somewhat more to the here and now and there is less of an attempt to reconstruct the developmental origins of conflicts. Psychoanalytically oriented psychotherapy may take as its entire goal the analysis of a set of defenses that are interfering with the patient's development. The accomplishment of this task may substantially open up the patient's life and development.

Psychoanalytic psychotherapy recognizes and interprets transference when it occurs (Table 26–7). However, the entire treatment is not directed toward the establishment and analysis of the transference in the thorough manner of a psychoanalysis. Long-term psychodynamic psychotherapy includes more transference work than do the brief psychodynamic psychotherapies. Psychoanalytic psychotherapy also makes use of techniques that are not available in psychoanalysis. This allows for its application to a broader range of patients, including those with psychotic regressive potentials such as borderline personality disorder.

Usually, patients in long-term psychoanalytic psychotherapy are seen one, two, or three times per week; twice per week is desirable in that this frequency allows for sufficient intensity for the transference to unfold and to be interpreted. Patient and therapist meet in face-to-face encounters and free association is encouraged. Psychoanalytic psychotherapy may extend from several months to several years, at times taking as long as a psychoanalysis. The length of treatment is determined by the number of focal problem areas undertaken in the treatment. Medications can be used in psychoanalytic psychotherapy and provide another means of titrating the level of regression a patient may experience. The therapist uses interpretations and clarifications as in psychoanalysis. In addition, however, the therapist may use other interpretative techniques such as suggestion, practice of new behavior patterns and experiences, and confrontation (Bibring 1954). *Practice* in this context (classically called manipulation) refers to learning from experience, such as pointing out that the therapist does not respond in the expected transferential manner. Confrontation is not "fighting" but rather pointing out to the patient when something is being denied or avoided.

The same patients who are treated in psychoanalysis can be treated in psychoanalytic psychotherapy. However, the focus of the treatment is much narrower and the expected outcome less comprehensive. At times, the supportive elements of a psychoanalytic psychotherapy can interfere with the patient's full experience of his or

TABLE 26–7. Psychoanalytic psychotherapy

Goal	Defense and transference analysis with limited reconstruction of the past
Selection criteria	When a narrower focus and less comprehensive outcome is acceptable
	The same selection criteria as in psychoanalysis are used, but they can include more seriously disturbed patients who can use understanding to resolve symptoms when supportive elements are available in the treatment
Duration	One to three sessions per week for 1–6 years on average
Techniques	Therapeutic alliance
	Face to face
	Free association
	Defense and transference interpretation
	More use of clarification, suggestion, and learning through experience than in psychoanalysis
	Medication

her conflicts, which can be more evident to the patient in a psychoanalysis. The psychosocial problems and internal conflicts of patients who could not be treated in psychoanalysis, such as those with major depression, schizophrenia, and borderline personality disorder, can be addressed in a long-term psychoanalytic psychotherapy. The long-term contributions of psychoanalytic psychotherapy to the treatment of major depression and schizophrenia, for which biological treatments have proved efficacious for some of the major symptoms, require further study. Patients with these diagnoses use psychotherapy to modify illness-onset conditions and facilitate readjustment, recovery, and integration into family and community. In long-term psychoanalytic psychotherapy, the regressive tendencies of such patients can be titrated with greater elements of support, the use of medication as needed, and greater reality feedback through the face-to-face encounter with the therapist.

Strupp's studies of college students and Luborsky's work on the helping alliance confirm the importance of interactional variables and support to the outcome in psychotherapy (Butler and Strupp 1993; Horvath et al. 1993; Luborsky et al. 1988; Strupp 1980a, 1980b; Strupp and Binder 1984). Both investigators also found that the quality of the therapeutic interaction and the handling of the transference and countertransference are critical to success or failure in treatment. Strupp's studies indicate that patients treated by nonprofessionally trained therapists are as much improved, on average, as patients treated by professional therapists. However, they also show that such nonexperienced therapists run out of relevant material and soon become unwilling to continue to treat patients over an extended period (Strupp 1980c; Strupp and Hadley 1979). One of the important tasks of training in psychotherapy may be the development of the ability to "endure" with the patient and, over time, with numbers of patients. Technical training and a theoretical framework may allow the therapist to maintain a sense of competence, direction, and interest in the work that the nonprofessional therapist cannot. The dosage and duration of treatment may also relate to the outcome (Freedman et al. 1999; Sandell et al. 2000).

The opening phase of psychodynamic psychotherapy is often marked by the activation of the magical expectations of the patient and the belief that past pains will now be resolved. During the initial phase, the therapist may make few comments and usually accepts the positive transference of the patient. Important aspects of the current problems, the patient's characteristic defense mechanisms and coping styles, and the developmental roots of the central issue become clearer during this phase. In the middle phase of treatment, resistance is likely to appear, as well as the negative transference. The patient experiences the frustration that not all the wished-for changes are occurring. Defenses are identified and analyzed, and usually the transference is sufficiently evident to be worked with.

The patient must be educated about transference phenomena and develop sufficient observing ego to participate with the therapist in wondering about this aspect of his or her internal life. The transference is not suddenly interpreted to the patient, nor should one assume that the patient knows that it is expected or desirable to talk about feelings toward the therapist. It is the skill of the therapist that allows him or her to know when to introduce this topic to the patient and how to help the patient increasingly to explore this area of feelings and thoughts. In the end phase of treatment, termination and the patient's resistances to termination are prominent. Termination is based on having reached a series of life goals that allows the patient to continue on a normal developmental path. Ideal treatment goals are not the end point. Rather, the reestablishment of normal development and the removal of obstacles to the normal recovery processes are the goals of treatment. The patient's increased capacity to understand his or her conflicts and to analyze conflicts independently indicates that the end of treatment will occur shortly.

Interpersonal Psychotherapy

IPT is a psychotherapy developed by Klerman and colleagues (Klerman et al. 1984a, 1984b; Markowitz 1998; Rounsaville et al. 1985b). Whether conducted briefly or longer term, IPT focuses on current interpersonal problems in outpatient nonbipolar, nonpsychotic depressed individuals. IPT has been the major psychotherapeutic modality used in combined psychotherapy and pharmacological treatment studies. This psychotherapy has also been used for the treatment of drug abuse. It did not, however, have a notable impact on outcome when patients were already participating in a well-run treatment program that included weekly group psychotherapy (Rounsaville et al. 1983, 1985a). IPT derives from the interpersonal school of psychiatry that originated with Adolf Meyer and Harry Stack Sullivan. The understanding of social supports and of attachment provides further theoretical underpinning for this form of psychotherapy. IPT focuses on reassurance, clarification of feeling states, improvement in interpersonal communication, testing of perception, and interpersonal skills rather than on personality reconstruction.

In IPT the therapist focuses on the patient's current social functioning (Table 26–8). A complete inventory of current and past significant interpersonal relationships, including the family of origin, friendships, and relations in the community, is a part of the evaluation phase. Patterns of authority, dominance and submission, dependency and autonomy, intimacy, affection, and activities are observed. Cognitions are generally seen as beliefs and attitudes about norms, expectations and roles, and role performance. Defense mechanisms may be recognized, but they are explored in terms of interpersonal relations. Similarly, dreams may be examined as a reflection of current interpersonal problems. In IPT, the therapist may explore distorted thinking by comparing what the patient says with what he or she does or by identifying the patient's view of an interpersonal relationship (Klerman et al. 1984b).

IPT has been primarily used in the treatment of depressed patients (A. F. Frank et al. 1991; O'Hara et al. 2000). In the opening phase of IPT, a detailed symptom history is taken, usually using a structured interview. The symptoms are reviewed with the patient, and the patient receives explicit information about the natural course of depression as a clinical condition. There is an emphasis on legitimizing the patient in the sick role. A second major task of this phase is the assessment of the patient's interpersonal problem areas. There is an attempt to identify

TABLE 26–8. Interpersonal psychotherapy

Goal	Improvement in current interpersonal skills
Selection criteria	Outpatient, nonbipolar, nonpsychotic depression
Duration	Short- and long-term
	Usually once-weekly meetings
Techniques	Reassurance
	Clarification of feeling states
	Improvement of interpersonal communication
	Testing perceptions
	Development of interpersonal skills
	Medication

one or more of four problem areas: grief reaction, interpersonal disputes, role transition, and interpersonal deficits. Each of these areas is thought to be related to depression.

The middle phase of treatment is directed toward resolving the problem area or areas. Clarifying positive and negative feeling states, identifying past models for relationships, and guiding and encouraging the patient in examining and choosing alternative courses of action constitute the basic techniques for handling each problem area (Weissman and Markowitz 1994). The focus is kept on current dilemmas and not past interpersonal relationships. Interpersonal events, rather than intrapsychic or cognitive events, are the focus of IPT.

Much of IPT is based on psychodynamic theory (Markowitz et al. 1998). The therapist's attitude is one of exploration, similar to the attitude in other insight-oriented psychotherapies when applied in a medical model. Applying the dictum of working "from the surface to the depths" results in much of the resemblance of IPT to psychodynamic psychotherapy. However, Klerman and colleagues found it useful to highlight the differences between these approaches to standardize a psychotherapeutic technique. Collaborative clinical trials have demonstrated the advantage of maintenance IPT in enhancing social functioning during recovery from depression and in reducing symptoms and improving functioning during the acute phase of a depressive episode. These effects require 6–8 months to become apparent. Depressed patients undergoing combined pharmacotherapy and IPT have the best outcomes (DiMascio et al. 1979; Weissman et al. 1981). IPT has also been effective in the treatment of postpartum depression, improving depressive symptoms and social adjustment (O'Hara et al. 2000; see also Chapter 27 in this volume).

Comparison of Psychodynamic, Interpersonal, and Cognitive Psychotherapies

Because interpersonal and cognitive (see Chapter 29) psychotherapies are related to the psychodynamic model, there is a high degree of overlap in the problem areas identified in any given patient in these treatments. The conceptualization of the problem, however, is different. In many ways it is complementary rather than mutually exclusive. The psychoanalytic, interpersonal, and cognitive psychotherapies share explorative and change-oriented goals. Cognitive psychotherapy focuses on the patient's thinking; IPT on the patient's interpersonal relations and social supports; and psychoanalytically oriented treatments on the internal experience of the patient and its relationship to past experience. Cognitive and interpersonal psychotherapies are most frequently used to treat depression rather than to treat an entire range of psychopathology. No studies using well-defined psychodynamic psychotherapies and medication have been performed. In this area, IPT and cognitive psychotherapy have been more closely studied.

IPT, cognitive psychotherapy, and the more traditional psychodynamic psychotherapies can be compared (Table 26–9). All three modalities are complex methods of treatment that must be tailored to the individual patient. All demand a high degree of clinical judgment, and the therapist requires a considerable amount of time to acquire competency in administering these treatments (Beck et al. 1979).

The relationship between therapist and patient and the establishment of a therapeutic alliance are essential in IPT, cognitive psychotherapy, and the psychoanalytically oriented treatments. Extensive exploration of the patient's thoughts and feelings, including those involving the therapist, is a major portion of the work. In addition, in all three, the therapist attempts to maintain an investigative, collaborative, and nonjudgmental stance.

In practice, cognitive psychotherapy is similar to the analysis of defense in the psychodynamic approaches. Understanding defenses focuses the patient and therapist on the hidden cognitive distortions that result in the patient's faulty perception of both the internal and the external world. In the dynamic model, defense mechanisms are directed toward the control of anxiety resulting from conflict. The defenses, however, distort perception and cognition—resulting in distortions that are similar to those that are the focus of cognitive psychotherapy. In cognitive psychotherapy, cognitions are seen as the caus-

TABLE 26–9. Comparison of psychoanalytic, interpersonal, and cognitive psychotherapies

	Psychoanalytic/ psychodynamic psychotherapy	Interpersonal psychotherapy	Cognitive psychotherapy
Treatment focus	Internal experience	Interpersonal relationships and social supports	Thoughts/cognitions
Primary diagnoses treated	Anxiety Depression Personality disorders	Depression Anxiety	Depression Anxiety
Skill needed by therapist	++++	++++	++++
Therapeutic alliance	++++	++++	++++
Nonjudgmental stance	++++	++++	++++
Focus			
Cognitive	+++ (defense mechanisms)	+	++++ (cognitive distortions)
Interpersonal	++++ (transference and past relationships)	++++ (interpersonal withdrawal, attachment and models)	+
Technique			
Nondirective	++++	+	+
Directive/behavioral interventions	+	++++	++++

Note. Plus signs indicate degree, from small (+) to great (++++).

ative agent of the patient's distress. Much of the work in identifying these cognitions and alerting the patient to them is similar to the understanding and interpretation of defenses in the psychodynamic psychotherapies. The schemata underlying the faulty cognitions of cognitive psychotherapy are unconscious assumptions, which in the psychodynamic model are viewed as being derived from earlier experience. Both treatments share the importance of identifying these unconscious patterns of behavior and of making them known to the patient. To the extent that a psychodynamic psychotherapy focuses on the here-and-now experience of the patient rather than on the reconstruction of past experience, its similarity to cognitive psychotherapy increases. Frequently, the understanding of a defensive pattern used by a patient to handle an ongoing conflict can be the end point of a well-conducted psychodynamic psychotherapy. In such a case, the outcomes for cognitive and psychodynamic individual psychotherapy might be quite similar.

With regard to the degree of structure and directiveness, however, the two types of psychotherapy are different. In psychodynamic psychotherapy, the structure of the session is largely determined by the flow of the patient's thoughts and the interaction of these thoughts with the therapist's interpretive comments. In contrast, cognitive psychotherapy sessions are structured by an agenda that serves to focus the patient's thoughts and activities. In psychodynamic psychotherapy the role of

the therapist is limited to that of an empathic interpreter and sharer of the patient's experiences, whereas in cognitive psychotherapy the therapist may direct, prescribe, enjoin, educate, train, or role-play as well. Furthermore, in cognitive psychotherapy more emphasis is placed on directly altering psychopathology rather than on facilitating its alleviation through insight and resolution of inferred underlying conflicts.

IPT is most closely related to the psychodynamic object relations perspective. Understanding internal objects rests on understanding the actual interpersonal relationships of the patient, including his or her relationship with the physician. Both interpersonal and psychodynamic psychotherapy share a focus on identifications and transference, which in IPT is defined as "past models for relationships." In addition, in IPT particular attention is paid to withdrawal and detachment, areas related to defenses in the psychodynamic model and to faulty cognitions in the cognitive model. Interpersonal rather than intrapsychic or cognitive events are identified in IPT. This frequently means that the interpersonal psychotherapist's attention is directed toward the same area of disturbance as is the cognitive or psychodynamic psychotherapist's. However, the identified "problem"—interpersonal deficits, faulty cognitions, or intrapsychic conflict—is different.

The differences in the interventions used by these psychotherapies are more striking than the differences in their goals or in the problems they target for treatment (DeRubeis et al. 1982). To what extent it is the differences in psychotherapeutic treatments, not the similarities, that produce behavioral change is not clear. Both cognitive and interpersonal psychotherapy use more directive and behavioral interventions than do psychodynamic approaches. IPT and cognitive psychotherapy make more use of teaching new behavioral skills. More than the cognitive and interpersonal treatments, the psychodynamic psychotherapies rely on the patient to activate and practice new behaviors without direction. The briefer psychotherapies (i.e., IPT, cognitive psychotherapy, and brief psychodynamic psychotherapy) lack the extended working-through and application period of psychoanalysis and of intensive (i.e., long-term) psychodynamic psychotherapy.

Empirical studies comparing well-defined psychodynamic psychotherapy with cognitive and interpersonal psychotherapies have not been undertaken. Future research must address which form of psychotherapy may be most helpful for which patient. To develop research strategies, it would be helpful to conceptualize this question as related to the mode or modes through which any particular patient can most effectively learn new behaviors. An individual's available learning path (e.g., through the study of cognitions, interpersonal relations, and/or subjective experience) is influenced by state, trait, and contextual variables. The process of learning in the psychotherapies and psychoanalysis, a process of altering neuronal organization through behavioral (primarily verbal) means, may be influenced by the patient's diagnosis, medications, history, cognitive style, developmental stage, and affective availability, as well as the doctor–patient match and other variables. The effectiveness of the therapist in any given modality is certainly a critical variable. The differences and similarities in the outcomes of cognitive, interpersonal, and psychodynamic treatments also require study.

Supportive Psychotherapy

The term *supportive* is generally used to distinguish a type of psychotherapy that is less ambitious, less intensive, and less anxiety-provoking than those designated psychoanalytic, insight-oriented, exploratory, or expressive. Universally, supportive psychotherapy is ranked as the most important type of psychotherapy to learn during residency training (Langsley and Yager 1988). Despite its centrality, supportive therapy has traditionally been described only vaguely, as a residual category of treatment for patients not suitable for other forms of

therapy—a modality defined more by what it is not than by what it is. More recently, there has been a growing interest in supportive therapy as a worthy subject in its own right, and increasing numbers of articles and books have been devoted to describing or studying it (Novalis et al. 1997; Pinsker 1997; Rockland 1989b; Werman 1984).

The concept of supportiveness tends to be defined from diverse, often conflicting theoretical, technical, or practical perspectives, and proposed differences between supportive and other psychoanalytically derived therapies do not necessarily hold true in practice. Twice-weekly psychotherapy, for example, has been labeled "supportive" by authors distinguishing it from psychoanalysis, but "psychoanalytic" by others comparing it with less intensive treatments (Holmes 1995). Techniques theoretically specific to supportive therapy may also be integral to psychoanalysis (de Jonghe et al. 1994; Wallerstein 1986). Outcomes in patients randomly assigned to "supportive" versus "expressive" therapies may be surprisingly similar (Hellerstein et al. 1998).

In current thought, supportiveness is seen as an essential element in all forms of psychotherapy, which differ in degree rather than presence of supportive techniques (Ornstein 1986; Rockland 1993). Supportive psychotherapy may best be viewed as one pole on a continuum of therapies with only relative differences in goals, indications, theoretical bases, strategies, and techniques.

Goals

The goals of psychoanalysis and psychoanalytic psychotherapy encompass so broad an array of intrapsychic, interpersonal, adaptive, behavioral, and symptomatic changes that they cannot be distinguished definitively from those of supportive psychotherapy (Table 26–10). However, most authors emphasize amelioration of symptoms, maintenance or restoration of function, improved self-esteem, and improved adaptation to internal and external stresses as the distinctive goals of supportive therapy (Dewald 1994; Freyberger and Freyberger 1994; Holmes 1995; Kernberg 1999; Munich 1997). These stand in contrast to the goals of psychoanalysis and psychoanalytic therapy, which center on reversing underlying pathology and restructuring personality.

This dichotomy is clearest in cases where supportive therapy aims to *maintain* or *restore* function (Table 26–11). It is uncertain whether long-term *improvement* in symptoms, self-esteem, or life functioning can occur without concomitant changes in ego structure—at least in the absence of a continuing relationship with the therapist as an "auxiliary ego." Therefore, whereas separation of patient and therapist ("resolution of the transference") is

TABLE 26–10. Supportive psychotherapy

Goal	Support of reality testing
	Provision of ego support
	Maintenance or reestablishment of usual level of functioning
Selection criteria	Very healthy individual faced with overwhelming crises
	Patient with ego deficits
Duration	Days, months, or years—as needed
Techniques	Predictable availability of therapist
	Use of interpretation to strengthen defenses
	Maintenance of reality-based working relationship grounded in support, concern, and problem solving
	Suggestion, reinforcement, advice, reality testing, cognitive restructuring, reassurance, limit setting, and environmental interventions
	Medication
	Psychodynamic life narrative

TABLE 26–11. Goals

Supportive therapy	Psychoanalytic therapy
Maintenance of function	Reversal of pathology
Restoration of function	Restructuring of personality
Coping with pathology	Resolution of unconscious conflict
Alleviation of symptoms	Understanding of symptoms

an implicit goal of psychoanalytic therapies, it is less important in supportive therapy, where decreased intensity rather than termination of treatment may be more appropriate in the long term (Dewald 1994). When the patient in supportive therapy is able to sustain improvement autonomously, the outcome becomes more similar to that sought by psychoanalytic therapies.

Indications

Because there are relatively few data to support the assignment of patients to one or another therapy type, personal predilection of the therapist often plays a prominent role in the prescription of supportive versus psychoanalytic psychotherapy. Most often, insight-oriented therapy is automatically considered the treatment of first choice and supportive therapy is assigned to those patients who are not considered amenable to change. Some authors, however, have suggested that the two types of treatment should be considered on a more equal

basis, because a briefer or less intense treatment may be in many patients' best interest as a treatment of first choice (Pinsker 1997; Rockland 1989b). Furthermore, research has recently demonstrated that supportive therapy, as defined by *technique*, may be used to attain the same *goals* as expressive or insight-oriented therapy (Hellerstein et al. 1998). Such considerations become especially relevant as economic pressures force clinicians to prescribe the most efficient among potentially effective treatments.

In common clinical practice, patients at both ends of the health–sickness continuum receive supportive psychotherapy: those who are generally very psychiatrically healthy and well adapted but who have become impaired in response to stressful life circumstances and those who have severe pathology that cannot be cured (Table 26–12). The healthy individual, when faced with overwhelming stress or crises—particularly those which include traumas or disasters—may seek help and be a candidate for supportive psychotherapy. The relatively psychiatrically healthy candidate for supportive psychotherapy is a well-adapted individual with good social support and interpersonal relations, flexible defenses, and good reality testing who is experiencing an acute crisis, making use of social supports, not withdrawing, and anticipating resolution of crisis. Although functioning below his or her usual level, this patient remains hopeful about the future and makes use of resources available for problem solving, respite, and growth. This patient uses supportive psychotherapy to reconstitute more rapidly, to avoid errors in judgment by "thinking out loud," to relieve minor symptomatology, and to grow as an individual by learning about the world.

The more typical candidate for supportive psychotherapy has significant deficits in ego functioning, including the following:

- *Poor reality testing*. These patients show an inability to separate fact from fantasy and to recognize boundaries between self and others. They may become psychotic under the stress of psychodynamic psychotherapy and develop psychotic transferences.
- *Poor impulse control*. Such patients need promptly to discharge affects through actions that are often destructive to themselves or others. They are not able to contain and examine feelings as is required by more explorative, insight-oriented psychotherapies.
- *Poor interpersonal relations*. Patients who are unable to form and maintain stable relationships that include reasonable levels of trust and intimacy are limited in their capacity to maintain therapeutic relationships as well, especially those that arouse powerful feelings.

TABLE 26–12. Characteristics of candidates for supportive psychotherapy

Type I: *Patient impaired by overwhelming crisis, trauma, or disaster and functioning below usual level in response to a crisis.*

    Generally very psychiatrically healthy
    Well adapted
    Good social supports
    Good interpersonal relations
    Flexible defenses
    Good reality testing
    Hopeful about future
    Uses resources

Type II: *Patient has chronic ego deficits and impaired functioning.*

    Impaired reality testing
    Difficulty with impulse control
    Limited ability to sublimate
    Limited interpersonal relations
    Frequently high levels of aggression
    Limited ability to self-soothe/refuel
    Low verbal ability and capacity for introspection

- *Poor balance of affects.* This category includes patients who are overwhelmed by anger or anxiety and those who experience little or no affect of any sort.
- *Lack of ability to sublimate.* These patients are unable to channel energy into creative and socially useful activities, reflecting their low ability to master affects and impulses pleasurably.
- *Low capacity for introspection.* Because self-observation is a necessary step toward the attainment of insight, these patients do poorly in psychotherapies that require self-reflection and curiosity about themselves and their interpersonal relations.
- *Low verbal ability.* Most clinicians do not include high intelligence as a prerequisite for insight-oriented psychotherapy. However, patients for psychodynamic psychotherapies do need to be able to identify and communicate their thoughts and feelings intelligibly to the therapist and to derive relief from doing so.

A variety of other factors have been proposed as exclusion criteria for insight-oriented psychotherapy and as possible indications for supportive psychotherapy. Motivation has been stressed by many authors. However, it has yet to be determined whether motivation for symptom change, for behavioral change, for a relationship with the therapist, or for insight (among others) is crucial in assigning patients to explorative/change-oriented versus supportive psychotherapy (Bloch 1979). Alexithymic patients are generally referred for supportive rather than insight psychotherapy. Such patients are characterized by an inability to find words to describe their emotions; they tend to describe situational details and symptoms rather than feelings (Sifneos 1975). These patients are thought to be prone to psychosomatic illnesses and likely unsuited for insight-oriented psychotherapy (Sifneos 1972, 1972–1973, 1975). However, studies of patients with the traditional psychosomatic illnesses have found them to be quite variable in their responses to psychotherapy (Kellner 1975). Patients who are very passive and who lack the conviction that their own efforts are effective may be candidates for supportive rather than insight-oriented psychotherapy (Werman 1981). Some have suggested that a certain level of dependency may be necessary for patients to do well in supportive therapy, and that those with a high need for autonomy are poorly suited for this treatment (Freyberger and Freyberger 1994). Patients who derive substantial practical benefit from their illness, such as financial or emotional support (i.e., secondary gain), may also be appropriate candidates for supportive psychotherapy rather than an insight-oriented approach (Persson and Alström 1983). However, severe antisocial traits generally predict poor response to supportive therapy, as they do to insight-oriented therapy.

Ego strength and the ability to form relationships may be more important than diagnosis in the selection of patients for supportive psychotherapy (Werman 1984). Patients with lower ego strength and lower motivation for therapy have been found to benefit more from supportive techniques than from those specific to exploratory therapy (Horowitz et al. 1984). More attention needs to be paid to which characteristics of the patient may best predict a good response to supportive psychotherapy as opposed to merely a poor response to psychoanalytic psychotherapies. Delineation of the personal qualities needed to benefit from supportive psychotherapy remains an important task for future research.

Theoretical Basis

Psychoanalytic theory is generally viewed as the basis for supportive therapy, although certain aspects are especially emphasized (Werman 1988). Theories of unconscious motivation and defense, internalized objects, and ego psychology inform supportive as well as psychoanalytic therapies (Holmes 1995; Kernberg 1999). However, practice of supportive therapy draws more heavily on the work of Kohut and the British Object Relations School than on Freudian metapsychology (Buckley 1994) (Table 26–13). Thus, the emphasis is less on conflict resolution, as achieved by analysis of transference, than on

TABLE 26–13. Theoretical emphasis	
Supportive therapy	**Psychoanalytic therapy**
Self psychology	Conflict theory
Ego psychology	Object relations theory
Behavioral psychology	Ego psychology
Cognitive psychology	

TABLE 26–14. Strategies	
Supportive therapy	**Psychoanalytic therapy**
Fostering of positive transference	Analysis of transference
Containing the unconscious	Revealing the unconscious
Strengthening defenses	Loosening defenses
Regulation of affects	Mobilization of affects
Clarifying the present	Reconstructing the past
Minimizing regression	Facilitating "regression in the service of the ego"

establishment of a positive and coherent sense of self, mediated by the relationship between patient and therapist.

From this theoretical perspective, the therapist provides a "holding environment" in which patients feel secure, understood, and valued and a relationship through which they can develop a more realistic, less negatively biased view of themselves and others (Winston et al. 1986). Therapeutic gain stems from gradual internalization of aspects of the therapist and the therapeutic relationship, which replace internalized "bad" objects (i.e., critical, punitive, rejecting) to form a stable core of positive identity. From the point of view of attachment theory, the patient forms a secure attachment to the therapist as a necessary precursor to developing increased autonomy.

Theoretical frameworks from outside psychoanalysis have been increasingly used to expand the techniques of supportive therapy. The theory of social constructionism has suggested a strategy of working with patients to derive positive meanings from adverse life experiences (Holmes 1995). Religiously based concepts of mindfulness and self-acceptance have provided the foundation for techniques to support self-destructive patients through change-oriented therapy (Shearin and Linehan 1994). Cognitive and behavioral theories, with their emphasis on conscious thought, behavioral change, learning, and problem solving, inform many of the techniques of supportive therapy. In general, supportive therapy derives from a broader theoretical base than psychoanalytic theory alone.

Strategies

The basic strategy of psychoanalytic therapy is to uncover and resolve unconscious conflicts underlying the difficulties that the patient brings to treatment. This implies understanding the genesis of such conflicts in early relationships and reworking the defensive structure that has evolved to manage them (Table 26–14). By contrast, the basic strategy of supportive therapy is to map out the patient's major areas of life difficulty and ameliorate them in whatever way possible, rather than to discover causes (Kernberg 1999; Rosenthal et al. 1999).

Central to this strategy is helping the patient to strengthen adaptive defenses, diminish use of maladaptive defenses, and improve the balance of impulse and defense—for example, by avoiding overwhelming stress, reducing excessively harsh self-criticism, or containing overly intense impulses (Dewald 1994; Holmes 1995; Kernberg 1999). This strategy entails a focus on the conscious thoughts and feelings of the patient rather than on the unconscious, and on strengthening rather than loosening defenses. Similarly, the attempt is to minimize rather than foster regression, and to help the patient contain rather than mobilize affects.

As in psychoanalytic treatment, the relationship between patient and therapist forms the basis of supportive therapy. However, whereas in the former the relationship serves as a means for clarifying and correcting the patients' projections and distortions (i.e., transference), in the latter it provides an object of identification and a source of security and reassurance (Dewald 1994; Pinsker 1994). In psychoanalytic therapy, the neutrality and abstinence of the therapist mobilize anxiety; in supportive therapy, the transparency and spontaneity of the therapist diminish it.

Improved self-esteem may be a goal of both psychoanalytic and supportive therapies, but the strategies for attaining that goal differ. In psychoanalytic treatment, self-esteem is enhanced by fostering the patient's understanding of the unconscious mental content that undermines it. In supportive therapy, self-esteem is enhanced by helping the patient to improve adaptive functioning and minimize emotional discomfort and by fostering the patient's introjection of the therapist's acceptance and positive regard.

Techniques

Although supportive therapy is often dismissed as mere "hand holding" or "paid friendship," skillful practice of supportive psychotherapy may actually be more difficult than that of change-oriented psychotherapy because the patient may have less capacity to engage beneficially with a therapist (Wallace 1983). Understanding unconscious motivation, psychic conflict, the patient–therapist relationship, and the patient's use of defense mechanisms is essential to comprehending the patient's strengths and vulnerabilities. This knowledge is critical to providing support as well as insight (Bellak and Siegel 1983; Karen Horney Clinic Medical Board 1981; Rockland 1989a).

The basic stance of the therapist in supportive therapy is quite different from that of the therapist conducting psychoanalytic psychotherapy. Rather than being abstinent and neutral, the therapist is both active and reactive, more readily taking positions, answering questions, giving advice, reassuring, praising, and educating the patient. The therapeutic style tends to be more conversational than that in insight-oriented therapy and less one of silent listening (Pinsker 1994) (Table 26–15). By his or her activity, judicious sharing of personal factual information, planned use of verbal and nonverbal reinforcement, and willingness to intervene with practical help when necessary, the supportive therapist presents as more of a real person and less of a "blank screen" than the psychoanalytic therapist.

The structure of supportive therapy is less intensive and more flexible than that of psychoanalytic therapy (Stafford-Clark 1970). Typical frequency of meetings ranges from weekly to monthly, and sessions may be brief or full-length. More-frequent meetings may be appropriate in times of crisis, and unscheduled telephone calls may be viewed as central to the treatment rather than as deviations to be understood and interpreted.

A particular technical challenge in supportive treatment is the therapist's need to maintain spontaneity without acting impulsively or out of countertransference. For example, the therapist must use reinforcement without becoming coercive, give advice or information without presenting as omnipotent (Nurnberg 1984), and respond flexibly to the patient's needs without becoming anxiously protective or overindulgent.

The therapist who is predictably available and safe (i.e., who accepts the patient and puts aside his or her own needs in the service of the treatment) assumes some of the holding functions of the good parent. In such a therapeutic situation, the patient is able to identify with and incorporate the well-functioning aspects of the therapist—such as the capacity for self-observation and the ability to tolerate ambivalence (Adler 1982; Pine 1976). Similarly, permitting the patient to see himself or herself "mirrored" in the therapist as part of an idealized parental figure over long periods may stabilize new internal structures and behaviors. This approach is in contrast to

TABLE 26–15. Techniques

Supportive therapy	Psychoanalytic therapy
Activity; spontaneity	Abstinence
Advice; direction	Neutrality
Reinforcement of defenses	Interpretation of defenses
Clarification of conscious processes	Interpretation of unconscious processes
Acknowledgement of needs	Frustration of wishes
Enhancement of reality testing	Facilitation of fantasy
Benign neglect of process	Attention to process
Reassurance	Confrontation
Therapist as participant ally	Therapist as participant observer
Empathic listening	Empathic listening
Tact	Tact

psychoanalytically oriented psychotherapy, in which such attitudes are generally interpreted rather than accepted.

Patients in supportive psychotherapy frequently develop intensely dependent and ambivalent relationships with the therapist. These relationships often parallel the separation-individuation process of normal child development (Adler 1982). Patients may recapitulate with the therapist the alternating autonomy and rapprochement experienced with the parent. The therapist's respect for the patient's autonomy and need for "refueling" may be important in strengthening the patient's independence and facilitating return to health. The containment of affect is also an important supportive function (Adler 1982; Kernberg 1975, 1984). Patients in need of supportive psychotherapy typically fear the destructive power of their rage and envy. They may be helped to modulate their emotional reactions by the reliable presence of the therapist and a therapeutic relationship that remains unchanged in the face of emotional onslaughts.

The therapist attempts to strengthen defenses and foster the supportive relationship by refraining from interpreting positive transference feelings and waiting until the intensity of feelings has abated before commenting about negative transference feelings (Buckley 1986). Interpretations of the negative transference are limited to those needed to ensure that the treatment is not disrupted. While maintaining a friendly stance toward the patient, the therapist must respect the patient's need to establish a comfortable degree of distance. The therapist must not push for a more intimate or emotion-laden relationship than the patient can tolerate (Robinson and Flaherty 1982). The rapport with the patient that the supportive psychotherapist tries to establish differs from the therapeutic alliance of insight-oriented therapy. The doctor–patient relationship in supportive psychotherapy does not require the patient to observe and report on his or her own feelings and behavior to the same extent as in the change-oriented, explorative psychotherapies. In addition, the therapist acts more as a guide and a mentor. There is unanimous agreement among writers on supportive psychotherapy that fostering a good working relationship with the patient is the first priority. Studies indicate that in the case of more severely ill patients, this may take many months, in contrast to work with psychiatrically healthier patients, in which the therapeutic alliance tends to develop early or not at all (Docherty 1989; A.F. Frank and Gunderson 1990).

Many of the active interventions of supportive psychotherapy are based on the principle of "substitutive psychotherapy" (Werman 1984), in which the psychotherapy substitutes for capacities that the patient lacks. This is sometimes stated as the therapist acting as an "auxiliary ego" for the patient. The deficient ego capacities for which substitution is needed may include basic elements of self-perception, such as attainment of a stable sense of self over time and a clear recognition of boundaries between self and others. Techniques that may support the patients' deficient ego functions include suggestion, reinforcement, clarification, limit setting, environmental interventions, and concurrent use of medication (Dewald 1994; Rockland 1989b; Werman 1984).

Patients may be encouraged to discuss alternative behaviors, goals, and interpretations of events (Castelnuovo-Tedesco 1986). The therapist tries to reinforce the most adaptive defenses of which the patient is capable while discouraging use of more primitive defenses. To do so effectively, the therapist must judge the capacities of the patient and the degree to which a primitive defense might be necessary for the patient's equilibrium. This judgment is particularly important when assessing the primitive defenses of patients with schizophrenia (McGlashan 1982) or limited self-mutilation in those with severe personality pathology (Holmes 1995).

Reassurance takes a variety of forms in supportive psychotherapy, including supporting an adaptive level of denial (such as that employed by a patient in coping with a terminal illness), the patient's experience of the therapist's empathic attitude, or the therapist's reality testing of the patient's negatively biased evaluations (Werman 1984). Reassuring a patient is not easy (Peteet 1982). Reassurance requires a clear understanding of what the patient fears. Overt expression of interest and concern may be reassuring to a patient who fears rejection but threatening to one who fears intrusion. In a similar vein,

Rockland (1989a, 1989b) stressed the need to tailor interventions to fit the character traits and unconscious transference of the patient. Thus, the therapist may stress independence in the case of a patient who fears passivity or loss of control and may give advice and direction to a clinging, dependent patient. Intellectualized language may be more effective with obsessional patients and emotionally toned language with histrionic patients.

Communication of the therapist's knowledge of the patient and his or her circumstances is a pedagogical aspect of supportive psychotherapy (Werman 1981). The therapist uses simple, concrete language that has personal meaning for the patient. The therapist may discuss with the highly inhibited patient the advantages of being more assertive or spontaneous, or may point out to the patient with poorly developed social controls the dangers of impulsive behavior. In this manner, the therapist functions as an "auxiliary superego." In both the very constricted patient and the very impulsive patient, the therapist's recognition and accurate naming of the patient's affects may aid the patient in recognizing and differentiating emotional states, a necessary prerequisite to tolerating and modulating affect (Pine 1976).

Interpretive comments may be used by the supportive therapist, although the form and content of interpretations usually differ from those in psychoanalytically oriented psychotherapy. Interpretations in supportive psychotherapy are given in a manner consistent with the principle of decreasing (rather than increasing) anxiety and strengthening (rather than loosening) defenses. Thus, they deal with material close to the patient's awareness rather than with unconscious material that might be distressing or frightening to the patient, and they can often serve to strengthen the defenses of intellectualization and rationalization (Werman 1984). Interpretations are used not to open up new material to consciousness but rather to diminish anxiety and provide plausible explanations based on what is already conscious. Interpretations are framed in terms of current issues and situations through use of formulations that the patient can readily accept. Such interventions are sometimes referred to as *interpreting upward*. The therapeutic efficacy of this technique was first described by Glover (1931), who pointed out that incomplete or inexact interpretations often alleviate symptoms.

The psychodynamic life narrative can be used as a supportive interpretation (Viederman 1983). The narrative is a formulation of the patient's current difficulties (often a life crisis) as the inevitable product of previous life experiences. The life narrative uses only facts of which the patient is already aware and explanations that do not threaten self-esteem. It serves to provide the patient with a sense of control through understanding, to help him or her accept emotional responses as justifiable and inevitable, and to strengthen the alliance with the therapist, who is seen as giving something valuable. Such a narrative may be contraindicated in patients who can benefit from psychoanalytically oriented psychotherapy because it will strengthen defensive intellectualization, close off avenues to greater understanding, and possibly stir powerful expectations of gratification from the therapist.

Intellectualized interpretations may also be useful in discussing dreams in supportive psychotherapy (Werman 1978). In addition, these interpretations may foster an increased capacity for self-observation (Ermutlu 1977). A technique that has been used for the latter purpose consists of suggesting that pathological behavior is the product of a "sick part" of the patient that is distinct from the patient as a whole. This "induced dichotomy of personality" helps the patient recognize both the pathological behaviors and the better-functioning aspects of himself or herself and fosters the patient's identification with the more mature, adaptive traits.

The suitability of an interpretation may depend more on the manner in which it is given than on its content (Pine 1986). In supportive psychotherapy, interpretations are phrased to relieve the patient of the pressure to make an immediate response. The therapist tries to communicate that although the interpretation may be painful, he or she will stick by the patient through the patient's discomfort. Interpretations can best be made at times of low emotional intensity. The patient can also be given advance warning that a potentially painful comment is going to be made. Such techniques are directed toward sufficiently modulating the patient's emotional response so that the interpretation can be tolerated and processed.

The therapist's expressions of interest, advice giving, and facilitation of ventilation reinforce desired behaviors (P.R. Sullivan 1971). Expressions of interest and solicitude are positively reinforcing. Advice can lead to behavioral change if it is specific and applies to frequently occurring behaviors. Desired behaviors can be rewarded by the therapist's approval and by social reinforcement. Ventilation of emotions may be useful if the therapist can help the patient to safely contain and limit these emotions, thus extinguishing the anxiety response to emotional expression. Cognitive and behavioral psychotherapeutic interventions that strengthen the adaptive and defensive functioning of the ego (e.g., realistic and logical thinking, social skills, containment of affects such as anxiety) can contribute to the supportive aspects of psychotherapy (Novalis et al. 1997).

Except in the case of brief treatment aimed at supporting the patient through a life crisis or traumatic event, termination is not a goal in supportive psychotherapy in the same sense as it is in change-oriented therapies (Dewald 1994). In the most usual situation, the patient's functional deficits necessitate ongoing, long-term support. In such a case, keeping the patient in treatment might be a more appropriate goal than terminating treatment. Over time the treatment may gradually diminish in intensity or, alternatively, may evolve into a more change-oriented treatment. When the latter occurs, it may be appropriate to reevaluate goals and consider possible criteria for termination.

Supportive psychotherapy with special patient populations may require special techniques. Kates and Rockland (1994) described supportive therapy with schizophrenic patients as occurring in three phases: stabilization, maintenance, and working through/termination. Although applying techniques common to most supportive therapies, they particularly stressed the need for a collaborative (versus an authoritarian) patient–therapist relationship, in which goals and parameters of treatment are negotiated bilaterally. Use of the therapeutic interaction as a means of reality testing is also especially important in work with schizophrenic patients.

With somatizing patients who may habitually express feelings through physical symptoms, the first step may be to get the patient talking about him- or herself, while supplying information and advice relevant to the problem (Freyberger and Freyberger 1994). As the therapeutic alliance develops, the patient is encouraged to express more feelings in recounting his or her life story to the therapist. This supportive phase of treatment may prepare some patients to understand emotional cause and effect in their lives and help them begin to appreciate the workings of unconscious processes.

Supportive therapy with medically ill patients may entail providing the patient with a safe place to ventilate anger and grief over illness-related loss and disability (Freyberger and Freyberger 1994). A specific therapeutic task is to help the patient maintain optimism and a problem-solving approach and avoid becoming entirely preoccupied with the illness. Assisting patients in modulating their expressions of anger and dependency may be crucial in maintaining their interpersonal support networks.

Efficacy

Relatively few studies have assessed the efficacy of supportive therapy. Most data come from studies in which supportive psychotherapy was used as a control in testing the efficacy of other treatments (Conte and Plutchik 1986). In such studies, the procedures used in supportive psychotherapy tend to be poorly specified, and no attempts are made to correlate individual supportive techniques with outcome (Conte 1994). There are no studies in which supportive psychotherapy has been compared with no treatment or minimal treatment.

Despite its limitations, the research literature offers some evidence that supportive psychotherapy is an effective treatment. The Menninger Psychotherapy Project assessed long-term (i.e., up to 10 years) explorative and supportive psychotherapy in a group of patients with mixed symptomatic and personality pathology (Wallerstein 1986). A major result of the study was that psychoanalytic therapy was less effective, and supportive therapy was more effective, then expected. In general, the techniques of supportive therapy produced improvement in functioning and ego strength comparable to those of expressive and insight-oriented techniques. This result is consistent with the idea that sophisticated support itself promotes structural change in some patients.

More recently, this result was confirmed in a group of patients with Axis II Cluster C disorders who were treated with either supportive or confrontational dynamic psychotherapy (Hellerstein et al. 1998). Outcomes were comparable in the two groups. At 6 months, the patients who received supportive therapy remained improved in interpersonal functioning, especially in increased assertiveness (Rosenthal et al. 1999). The cases of supportive therapy patients who experienced good outcomes were characterized by highly positive therapeutic alliances throughout treatment, a finding that confirms the importance of the patient–therapist relationship in this type of treatment.

Studies of patients with anxiety disorders have also demonstrated the efficacy of supportive therapy. The effects of imipramine therapy plus behavior therapy have been compared with those of imipramine therapy plus supportive psychotherapy in a group of patients with agoraphobia, mixed phobia, or simple phobia (Klein et al. 1983; Zitrin et al. 1978). The expected benefit of adding behavioral techniques to supportive psychotherapy was not found; patients in both groups fared equally well. Similar results were reported by Alström et al. (1984a, 1984b), who found that psychodynamically oriented supportive psychotherapy was as effective as behavior therapy in the treatment of patients with agoraphobia and social phobia. These results may indicate that the active ingredient in both supportive psychotherapy and behavioral treatments is the encouragement of the patient to expose him- or herself to the feared situation (Klein et al. 1983). A study of supportive psychotherapy

in combination with antidepressants has also shown the combined-treatment group to do best (de Jonghe et al. 2001).

Research in the psychotherapy of schizophrenia has failed to demonstrate the benefit of explorative, expressive techniques (Gomes-Schwartz 1984). By contrast, the use of supportive techniques appears more promising (Hogarty et al. 1974; Munich 1997). May (1968) found that inpatients with nonchronic schizophrenia had somewhat better outcomes when treated with supportive psychotherapy and antipsychotic medication than when treated with medication alone. When these approaches were used singly, however, medication was more effective than psychotherapy. A later study compared medication plus explorative, insight-oriented psychotherapy with reality-adaptive supportive psychotherapy in patients with schizophrenia (Gunderson et al. 1984; Stanton et al. 1984). Patients receiving supportive therapy spent less time in the hospital and performed better in major life roles than did patients receiving insight therapy, a finding seemingly at variance with the lower intensity and cost of supportive treatment. Furthermore, a good therapeutic alliance was associated with decreased symptoms, lower doses of neuroleptics, and better compliance with medication (A.F. Frank and Gunderson 1990). Falloon et al. (1986) found that family behavioral and problem-solving therapy was more effective than individual therapy in decreasing symptom intensity and relapse rates in schizophrenia patients. However, Rea et al. (1991) found that individual supportive therapy produced more improvement than family therapy in coping and interpersonal style. Differences in therapeutic methods may account for these discrepant results.

A larger body of research exists indicating that supportive psychotherapy is an effective component of treatment for patients with a variety of medical illnesses. Karush et al. (1969) reported that ulcerative colitis patients with high dependency and low ego strength improved both somatically and emotionally after supportive psychotherapy, but not after insight-oriented treatment. The best results were found in cases in which the therapist was viewed as warm, understanding, and optimistic and a positive working relationship was formed. Forester et al. (1985) assessed the effects of supportive psychotherapy on patients undergoing radiation treatment. The psychotherapy, which consisted of educational clarification of emotional issues and ventilation of feelings, resulted in less emotional distress and fewer complaints of side effects in treated patients compared with those in the control group, who received no psychotherapy. Mumford et al. (1982) reviewed controlled studies of psychotherapy treatment of patients recovering from myocardial infarction and surgery and found positive effects on experience of pain, cooperation with treatment, incidence of complications, speed of recovery, and number of days in the hospital. The psychotherapies focused on educating the patients about their illnesses and treatments, but also included varying amounts of cognitive and behavioral techniques, ventilation, and reassurance in the context of a supportive relationship. Schindler et al. (1989) demonstrated that supportive therapy reduced medical complications, use of pain medication, and length of hospital stay in patients undergoing coronary artery bypass surgery. Studies of patients with gastrointestinal disease suggest that those who receive supportive therapy fare better and maintain their improvement compared with those receiving medical treatment alone (Conte 1994; Freyberger and Freyberger 1994). A dramatic study by Spiegel et al. (1989) showed that women with metastatic breast cancer who received supportive group therapy had less depression, anxiety, and pain and survived 19 months longer than control patients.

The evidence to date, although preliminary, suggests that supportive psychotherapy can be effective in both psychiatric and medical illnesses and may be more cost-effective than more intense psychotherapies. More research is needed regarding the indications, contraindications, and techniques of supportive psychotherapy.

Education

The importance of individual psychotherapy to the practicing clinician makes mandatory the inclusion of instruction on psychotherapy in psychiatric residency training. The skills learned in psychotherapy—both the ability to intervene and the ability to recognize transference, countertransference, and defense—are important in many other treatment modalities. The clinician skilled in recognizing these phenomena is better able to perform a wide array of treatments, including medication management, family therapy, inpatient psychiatric treatment, and consultation-liaison.

The fundamental skills of establishing the therapeutic alliance, understanding the relationship of transference to anxiety and regression, and providing support are central to psychiatric care. Learning psychodynamic psychotherapy provides the opportunity to work with a specific treatment modality as well as to become skilled in a wide array of areas central to clinical care. Learning long-term psychodynamic psychotherapy is not the equivalent of learning the brief psychotherapies or supportive psychotherapy (Levenson and Strupp 1999; Vaughan et al. 2000);

however, it may be true that the long-term psychotherapist is best prepared for using the briefer psychotherapy, in which there are fewer opportunities to make mistakes and to correct them. In this era of managed care, it is even more likely that the psychiatrist will be called on to supervise others conducting psychotherapy. For this reason also, skills in psychotherapy are necessary.

Psychiatric residents must develop skills to apply all psychotherapeutic treatment modalities and to understand their indications and contraindications. Psychoanalysis, with its extended intensive training requirements, is essentially a subspecialty area and is now generally pursued postresidency. It offers the opportunity for specific patients to gain broad-based understanding in a generally supportive environment. Supportive psychotherapy, the mainstay of psychiatric treatment, is much more complicated than is often recognized. The understanding of which patient for which treatment at which time is as critical for the prescription of psychotherapy as it is for the prescription of psychopharmacological agents (Frances et al. 1984). Given the decrease in the number of psychoanalysts in medical school education, learning the indications for referral for psychoanalysis may be increasingly difficult for future psychiatrists.

The brief psychotherapies (see Chapter 25) are best taught in conjunction with the discussion of the principles of long-term psychotherapy and in the context of learning psychodynamic formulations of pathology and the ways in which defenses, transferences, and countertransferences appear in the psychotherapeutic dyad. The resident can then begin to learn the unique constraints and advantages that accrue within a brief period as well as the unique advantages of long-term psychotherapeutic work. The resident must also learn the advantages and disadvantages of intermittent psychotherapy and sequential psychotherapy with continued medication treatment. Through contrasting the psychotherapies, the trainee learns appropriate patient selection and technical procedures to accomplish psychotherapy. Such training requires both familiarity with the psychotherapy literature and supervised clinical experiences in the various psychotherapies. All physicians should be versed in brief supportive psychotherapy as a technique distinct from pure "counseling" and education.

The evaluation of the patient is an important part of initiating any psychotherapy. Seeing psychotherapy as a modality that must be prescribed in duration, focus, and intensity and with a plan similar to pharmacological treatment of a patient enhances the resident's sense of mastery, accomplishment, and competence in dealing psychotherapeutically with a broad range of patients (Luborsky and Auerbach 1985).

The teaching of supportive psychotherapy requires further development of the knowledge base in supportive psychotherapy and the description of the technical procedures. At present, supportive psychotherapy remains a neglected area of teaching despite its complexity. A clearer delineation of the technical procedures used in psychotherapy and their assessment on a supportive versus change-oriented/explorative continuum should be part of psychotherapy supervision. In addition, such clarification will facilitate comparison among the psychotherapies and foster appropriate research questions, including those concerning the use of supportive psychotherapy as part of medication management.

Conclusions

Individual psychoanalytically oriented and supportive psychotherapies are an effective treatment for a wide range of symptoms and disorders. These treatment modalities require accurate diagnosis, treatment planning, and consistent application of principles and technique. Various types of psychotherapy are now well described. Further research is needed to identify which psychotherapy is most effective for which patient. The identification of specific types of change associated with different psychotherapies may aid this process.

The psychoanalytic treatments—psychoanalysis and psychoanalytic psychotherapy—now span the range of approaches—from brief to long-term and focal to broad based (Kernberg 1999). Interpersonal psychotherapy has primarily been used in research, but highlighted in this form of therapy is the importance of focusing on the social relationships as an aspect of understanding the psychoanalytic components of personality and mind–brain interaction. Interpersonal psychotherapy, cognitive psychotherapy, and supportive psychotherapy have more of an empirical research base than do the more specific psychoanalytic treatments. Research studies with more rigorous designs and conducted over longer periods are needed. Supportive psychotherapy, probably the most widely practiced of the psychotherapies, continues to be lacking in specific research. Better delineation of the specific technique in supportive psychotherapy will aid this development.

Clinicians require training in each of the psychotherapy modalities and in their application in stand-alone treatment plans and used intermittently or in combination or sequence with medication. Such training will enable them to better recognize the relationship of the psychotherapies to each other and the potential therapeutic benefits and costs associated with each.

References

Adler E: Supportive psychotherapy revisited. Hillside Journal of Clinical Psychiatry 4:3–13, 1982

Alström JE, Nordlund CL, Persson G, et al: Effects of four treatment methods on agoraphobic women not suitable for insight-oriented psychotherapy. Acta Psychiatr Scand 70:1–17, 1984a

Alström JE, Nordlund CL, Persson G, et al: Effects of four treatment methods on social phobic patients not suitable for insight-oriented psychotherapy. Acta Psychiatr Scand 70:97–110, 1984b

Bachrach HM, Weber JJ, Solomon M: Factors associated with the outcome of psychoanalysis (IV). International Review of Psycho-Analysis 12:379–389, 1985

Baxter C, Schwartz S, Berman K, et al: Caudate glucose metabolic rate changes with both drug and behavior therapy for obsessive-compulsive disorder. Arch Gen Psychiatry 49:681–689, 1992

Beck AT, Rush AJ, Shaw BF, et al: Cognitive Therapy of Depression. New York, Guilford, 1979

Bellak L, Siegel H: Handbook of Intensive, Brief, and Emergency Psychotherapy. Larchmont, NY, CPS, 1983

Bibring E: Psychoanalysis and the dynamic psychotherapies. J Am Psychoanal Assoc 2:745–770, 1954

Bloch S: Assessment of patients for psychotherapy. Br J Psychiatry 135:193–208, 1979

Blum HP: Countertransference and the theory of technique: discussion. J Am Psychoanal Assoc 34:309–328, 1986

Brenner C: Psychoanalytic Technique and Psychic Conflict. New York, International Universities Press, 1976

Brodaty JH: Techniques in brief psychotherapy. Aust N Z J Psychiatry 17:109–115, 1983

Bruch H: Learning Psychotherapy: Rationale and Ground Rules. Cambridge, MA, Harvard University Press, 1974

Buckley P: [Supportive psychotherapy] A neglected treatment. Psychiatr Ann 16:515–517, 521, 1986

Buckley P: Self psychology, object relations theory and supportive psychotherapy. Am J Psychother 48:519–529, 1994

Budman SH, Gurman AS: The practice of brief therapy. Professional Psychology 14:277–292, 1983

Butler SF, Strupp HH: Effects of training experienced dynamic therapists to use a psychotherapy manual, in Psychodynamic Treatment Research. Edited by Miller NE, Luborsky L, Barber JP, et al. New York, Basic Books, 1993, pp 191–210

Castelnuovo-Tedesco P: The Twenty-Minute Hour: A Guide to Brief Psychotherapy for the Physician. Washington, DC, American Psychiatric Press, 1986

Chessick RD: Psychoanalysis: clinical and theoretical. Am J Psychiatry 157:846–848, 2000

Coleman JV: Aims and conduct of psychotherapy. Arch Gen Psychiatry 18:1–6, 1968

Coltrera JT: Truth from genetic illusion: the transference and the fate of the infantile neurosis, in Psychoanalytic Explorations of Technique: Discourse on the Theory of Therapy. Edited by Blum HP. New York, International Universities Press, 1980, pp 284–313

Conte HR: Review of research in supportive psychotherapy: an update. (Review) (29 refs) Am J Psychiatry 48:494–504, 1994

Conte HR, Plutchik R: Controlled research in supportive psychotherapy. Psychiatr Ann 16:530–533, 1986

Crits-Christoph P: The efficacy of brief dynamic psychotherapy: a meta-analysis. Am J Psychiatry 149:151–158, 1992

Crits-Christoph P, Barben JP (eds): Handbook of Short-Term Dynamic Psychotherapy. New York, Basic Books, 1991

Crown S: Contraindications and dangers of psychotherapy. Br J Psychiatry 143:436–441, 1983

de Jonghe F, Rijnierse P, Janssen R: The role of support in psychoanalysis. J Am Psychoanal Assoc 40:475–499, 1992

de Jonghe F, Rijnierse P, Janssen R: Psychoanalytic supportive psychotherapy. J Am Psychoanal Assoc 42:421–446, 1994

de Jonghe F, Kool S, van Aalst G, et al: Combining psychotherapy and antidepressants in the treatment of depression. J Affect Disord 64:217–229, 2001

DeRubeis RJ, Hollon SD, Evans MD, et al: Can psychotherapies for depression be discriminated? A systematic investigation of cognitive therapy and interpersonal therapy. J Consult Clin Psychol 50:744–756, 1982

Dewald P: The process of change in psychoanalytic psychotherapy. Arch Gen Psychiatry 35:535–542, 1978

Dewald PA: Principles of supportive psychotherapy. Am J Psychother 48:505–518, 1994

DiMascio A, Weissman MM, Prusoff BA, et al: Differential symptom reduction by drugs and psychotherapy in acute depression. Arch Gen Psychiatry 36:1450–1456, 1979

Docherty JP: The individual psychotherapies: efficacy, syndrome-based treatments, and the therapeutic alliance, in Outpatient Psychiatry: Diagnosis and Treatment, 2nd Edition. Edited by Lazare A. Baltimore, MD, Williams & Wilkins, 1989, pp 624–644

Donovan JM: More on transference interpretations (letter). Am J Psychiatry 141:142, 1984

Epstein RS: Keeping Boundaries: Maintaining Safety and Integrity in the Psychotherapeutic Process. Washington, DC, American Psychiatric Press, 1995

Ermutlu I: Induced dichotomy of personality as a technique in supportive psychotherapy. Psychiatric Forum 7:19–22, 1977

Errera P, McKee B, Smith DC, et al: Length of psychotherapy: studies done in a university community psychiatric clinic. Arch Gen Psychiatry 17:454–458, 1967

Falloon I, Pederson J, Al-Khayyal M: Enhancement of health-giving family support versus treatment of faculty pathology. Journal of Family Therapy 8:339–350, 1986

Forester B, Kornfeld DS, Fleiss JL: Psychotherapy during radiotherapy: effects on emotional and physical distress. Am J Psychiatry 142:22–27, 1985

Frances A[J], Clarkin JF: No treatment as the prescription of choice. Arch Gen Psychiatry 38:542–545, 1981

Frances A[J], Perry S: Transference interpretations in focal therapy. Am J Psychiatry 140:405–409, 1983

Frances AJ, Clarkin J, Perry S: Differential Therapeutics in Psychiatry: The Art and Science of Treatment Selection. New York, Brunner/Mazel, 1984

Frank AF, Gunderson JG: The role of the therapeutic alliance in the treatment of schizophrenia: relationship to course and outcome. Arch Gen Psychiatry 47:228–236, 1990

Frank AF, Kupfer DJ, Wagner EF, et al: Efficacy of interpersonal psychotherapy as a maintenance treatment of recurrent depression. Arch Gen Psychiatry 48:1053–1059, 1991

Frank JD: Therapeutic factors in psychotherapy. Am J Psychother 25:350–361, 1971

Freedman N, Hoffenberg JD, Corus N, et al: The effectiveness of psychoanalytic psychotherapy: the role of treatment duration, frequency of sessions, and the therapeutic relationship. J Am Psychoanal Assoc 47:741–742, 1999

Freud S: The handling of dream-interpretation in psychoanalysis (1911), in Standard Edition of the Complete Psychological Works of Sigmund Freud, Vol 12. Translated and edited by Strachey J. London, England, Hogarth Press, 1958, pp 89–96

Freud S: The dynamics of transference (1912a), in Standard Edition of the Complete Psychological Works of Sigmund Freud, Vol 12. Translated and edited by Strachey J. London, England, Hogarth Press, 1958, pp 97–108

Freud S: Recommendations to physicians practising psychoanalysis (1912b), in Standard Edition of the Complete Psychological Works of Sigmund Freud, Vol 12. Translated and edited by Strachey J. London, England, Hogarth Press, 1958, pp 109–120

Freud S: On beginning the treatment (further recommendations on the technique of psycho-analysis I) (1913), in Standard Edition of the Complete Psychological Works of Sigmund Freud, Vol 12. Translated and edited by Strachey J. London, England, Hogarth Press, 1958, pp 121–144

Freud S: Remembering, repeating and working-through (further recommendations on the technique of psycho-analysis II) (1914), in Standard Edition of the Complete Psychological Works of Sigmund Freud, Vol 12. Translated and edited by Strachey J. London, England, Hogarth Press, 1958, pp 145–156

Freud S: Observations on transference-love (further recommendations on the technique of psycho-analysis III) (1915[1914]), in Standard Edition of the Complete Psychological Works of Sigmund Freud, Vol 12. Translated and edited by Strachey J. London, England, Hogarth Press, 1958, pp 157–173

Freyberger H, Freyberger HJ: Supportive psychotherapy. Psychother Psychosom 61:132–142, 1994

Fried D, Crits-Christoph P, Luborsky L: The first empirical demonstration of transference in psychotherapy. J Nerv Ment Dis 180:326–331, 1992

Fromm-Reichmann F: Principles of Intensive Psychotherapy. Chicago, IL, University of Chicago Press, 1950

Gabbard GO: Psychodynamic Psychiatry in Clinical Practice, 3rd Edition. Washington, DC, American Psychiatric Press, 2000

Galatzer-Levy RM, Bachrach H, Skolnikoff A, et al: Does Psychoanalysis Work? New Haven, CT, Yale University Press, 2000

Gill M: The Analysis of Transference, I: Theory and Technique. New York, International Universities Press, 1982

Glover E: The therapeutic effect of inexact interpretation: a contribution to the theory of suggestion. Int J Psychoanal 12:397–411, 1931

Glover E: The Technique of Psychoanalysis. New York, International Universities Press, 1968

Gomes-Schwartz B: Individual psychotherapy of schizophrenia, in Schizophrenia: Treatment, Management, and Rehabilitation. Edited by Bellack AS. Orlando, FL, Grune & Stratton, 1984, pp 307–345

Gomes-Schwartz B, Hadley S, Strupp H: Individual psychotherapy and behavior therapy. Annu Rev Psychol 29:435–447, 1978

Greenson RR: The working alliance and the transference neurosis. Psychoanal Q 34:155–181, 1965

Greenson RR: The Technique and Practice of Psychoanalysis. New York, International Universities Press, 1967

Gunderson JE, Frank AF, Katz HM, et al: Effects of psychotherapy in schizophrenia, II: comparative outcome of two forms of treatment. Schizophr Bull 10:564–598, 1984

Guthrie E, Moorey J, Margison F, et al: Cost effectiveness of brief psychodynamic-interpersonal therapy in high utilizers of psychiatric services. Arch Gen Psychiatry 56:519–526, 1999

Hadley SW, Strupp HH: Contemporary views of negative effects in psychotherapy: an integrated account. Arch Gen Psychiatry 33:1291–1302, 1976

Hellerstein DJ, Rosenthal RN, Pinsker H, et al: A randomized prospective study comparing supportive and dynamic therapies. Outcome and alliance. J Psychother Pract Res 7:261–171, 1998

Hofer MA: Relationships as regulators: a psychobiologic perspective on bereavement. Psychosom Med 46:183–197, 1984

Hogarty GE, Goldberg SC, Schooler NR, et al: Drug and sociotherapy in the aftercare of schizophrenic patients, III: adjustment of nonrelapsed patients. Arch Gen Psychiatry 31:609–618, 1974

Holmes J: Supportive psychotherapy. The search for positive meanings. Br J Psychiatry 167:439–447, 1995

Horowitz MJ, Marmar C, Weiss DS, et al: Brief psychotherapy of bereavement reactions: the relationship of process to outcome. Arch Gen Psychiatry 41:438–448, 1984

Horowitz MJ, Marmar CR, Weiss DS, et al: Comprehensive analysis of change after brief dynamic psychotherapy. Am J Psychiatry 143:582–589, 1986

Horvath A, Gaston L, Luborsky L: The therapeutic alliance and its measures, in Psychodynamic Treatment Research. Edited by Miller NE, Luborsky L, Barber JP, et al. New York, Basic Books, 1993, pp 247–273

House JS, Landis KR, Umberson D: Social relationships and health. Science 241:540–545, 1988

Howard KI, Kopta SM, Krause MS, et al: The dose-effect relationship in psychotherapy. Am Psychol 41:159–164, 1986

Kandell ER: Psychotherapy and the single synapse: the impact of psychiatric thought on neurobiologic research. N Engl J Med 301:1028–1037, 1979

Kandell ER: Genes, nerve cells, and the remembrance of things past. J Neuropsychiatry Clin Neurosci 1:103–125, 1989

Kandell ER: Biology and the future of psychoanalysis: a new intellectual framework for psychiatry revisited. Am J Psychiatry 156:505–524, 1999

Kandell ER: Comment on "Biology and the future of psychoanalysis: a new intellectual framework for psychiatry revisited." Am J Psychiatry 157:839–840, 2000

Kantrowitz JL, Paolitto F, Sashin J, et al: Affect availability, tolerance, complexity, and modulation in psychoanalysis: follow up of a longitudinal, prospective study. J Am Psychoanal Assoc 34:529–559, 1986

Kantrowitz JL, Katz AL, Paolitto F, et al: Changes in the level and quantity of object relations in psychoanalysis: follow up of a longitudinal, prospective study. J Am Psychoanal Assoc 35:23–46, 1987

Kantrowitz JL, Katz AL, Paolitto F: Followup of psychoanalysis five to ten years after termination, I: stability of change. J Am Psychoanal Assoc 38:471–496, 1990

Karen Horney Clinic Medical Board: Guidelines for identifying therapeutic modalities. Am J Psychoanal 41:195–202, 1981

Karush A, Daniels GE, O'Connor JF, et al: The response to psychotherapy in chronic ulcerative colitis, II: factors arising from the therapeutic situation. Psychosom Med 31:201–226, 1969

Kates J, Rockland LH: Supportive psychotherapy of the schizophrenia patient. Am J Psychother 48:543–561, 1994

Kay J: Brief psychodynamic psychotherapies. Past, present, and future challenges. J Psychother Pract Res 6:330–337, 1997

Kellner R: Psychotherapy in psychosomatic disorders: a survey of controlled studies. Arch Gen Psychiatry 32:1021–1028, 1975

Kernberg OF: Borderline Conditions and Pathological Narcissism. New York, Jason Aronson, 1975

Kernberg OF: Severe Personality Disorders: Psychotherapeutic Strategies. New Haven, CT, Yale University Press, 1984

Kernberg OF: Psychoanalysis, psychoanalytic psychotherapy and supportive psychotherapy: contemporary controversies. Int J Psychoanal 80:1075–1091, 1999

Kernberg OF: Affect theory. Paper presented at the annual meeting of the American Psychiatric Association, New Orleans, LA, May 2001

Kernberg OF, Burstein ED, Coyne L, et al: Psychotherapy and psychoanalysis: final report of the Menninger Foundation's Psychotherapy Research Project. Bull Menninger Clin 36:1–275, 1972

Klein DF, Zitrin CM, Woerner MG, et al: Treatment of phobias, II: behavior therapy and supportive psychotherapy: are there any specific ingredients? Arch Gen Psychiatry 40:139–145, 1983

Klerman GL, Weissman MM, Rounsaville BJ, et al: Interpersonal psychotherapy for depression, in Psychiatry Update: The American Psychiatric Association Annual Review, Vol 3. Edited by Grinspoon L. Washington, DC, American Psychiatric Press, 1984a, pp 56–67

Klerman GL, Weissman MM, Rounsaville BJ, et al: Interpersonal Psychotherapy of Depression. New York, Basic Books, 1984b

Krupnick JL, Pincus HA: The cost-effectiveness of psychotherapy: a plan for research. Am J Psychiatry 149:1295–1305, 1992

Langsley D, Yager J: The definition of a psychiatrist: eight years later. Am J Psychiatry 145:469–475, 1988

Lazar SG (ed): Extended dynamic psychotherapy: making the case in an era of managed care. Psychoanalytic Inquiry 17(special supplement), 1997

Levenson H, Strupp HH: Recommendations for future of training in brief dynamic psychotherapy. J Clin Psychol 55:385–391, 1999

Levinson DJ, Merrifield J, Berg K: Becoming a patient. Arch Gen Psychiatry 17:385–406, 1967

Loewald HW: On the therapeutic action of psychoanalysis, in Papers on Psychoanalysis. New Haven, CT, Yale University Press, 1980, pp 221–256

Longobardi PG: The impact of a brief psychological intervention on medical care utilization in an army health care setting. Med Care 19:655–671, 1981

Luborsky L: Principles of Psychoanalytic Psychotherapy: A Manual for Supportive Expressive Treatment. New York, Basic Books, 1984

Luborsky L, Auerbach AH: The therapeutic relationship in psychodynamic psychotherapy: the research evidence and its meaning for practice, in Psychiatry Update: The American Psychiatric Association Annual Review, Vol 4. Edited by Hales RE, Frances AJ. Washington, DC, American Psychiatric Press, 1985, pp 550–561

Luborsky L, Crits-Christoph P: Understanding Transference. New York, Basic Books, 1990

Luborsky L, Singer B, Luborsky L: Comparative studies of psychotherapies: is it true that "everyone has won and all must have prizes"? Arch Gen Psychiatry 32:995–1008, 1975

Luborsky L, Crits-Christoph P, Mintz J, et al: Who Will Benefit From Psychotherapy? New York, Basic Books, 1988

Malan DH: A Study of Brief Psychotherapy. New York, Plenum, 1975

Malan DH: The Frontier of Brief Psychotherapy. New York, Plenum, 1976

Malan DH: Toward the Validation of Dynamic Psychotherapy. New York, Plenum, 1980

Malan DH, Heath ES, Bacal HA, et al: Psychodynamic changes in untreated neurotic patients, II: apparently genuine improvements. Arch Gen Psychiatry 32:110–126, 1975

Markowitz J (ed): Interpersonal Psychotherapy. Washington, DC, American Psychiatric Press, 1998

Markowitz JC, Svartberg M, Swartz HA: Is IPT time-limited psychodynamic psychotherapy? J Psychother Pract Res 7:185–195 1998

Marziali EA: Prediction of outcome of brief psychotherapy from therapist interpretive interventions. Arch Gen Psychiatry 41:301–304, 1984

Marziali EA, Sullivan JM: Methodological issues in the content analysis of brief psychotherapy. Br J Med Psychol 53:19–27, 1980

May PRA: Treatment of Schizophrenia: A Comparative Study of Five Treatment Methods. New York, Science House, 1968

McGlashan TH: DSM-III schizophrenia and individual psychotherapy. J Nerv Ment Dis 170:752–757, 1982

McNeilly CL, Howard KJ: The effects of psychotherapy: a re-evaluation based on dosage. Psychotherapy Research 1:74–78, 1991

Meany MJ: Nature, nurture, and disunity of knowledge. Ann N Y Acad Sci 935:50–61, 2001

Meissner WW: Neutrality, abstinence and the therapeutic alliance. J Am Psychoanal Assoc 46:1089–1128, 1998

Meyer E, Derogatis LR, Miller MJ, et al: Addition of time-limited psychotherapy to medical treatment in a general medical clinic: results at one-year follow-up. J Nerv Ment Dis 169:780–790, 1981

Milrod B, Busch F, Cooper A, et al. (eds): Manual of Panic-Focused Psychodynamic Psychotherapy. Washington, DC, American Psychiatric Press, 1997

Milrod B, Busch F, Leon AC, et al: Open trial of psychodynamic psychotherapy for panic disorder: a pilot study. Am J Psychiatry 157:1878–1880, 2000

Mohl PC, McLaughlin GDW: Listening to the patient, in Psychiatry. Edited by Tasman A, Kay J, Lieberman J. Philadelphia, PA, WB Saunders, 1997, pp 3–18

Mumford E, Schlesinger HJ, Glass CV: The effects of psychological intervention on recovery from surgery and heart attacks: an analysis of the literature. Am J Public Health 72:141–151, 1982

Mumford E, Schlesinger HJ, Glass GV, et al: A new look at evidence about reduced cost of medical utilization following mental health treatment. Am J Psychiatry 141:1145–1158, 1984

Munich RL: Contemporary treatment of schizophrenia. Bull Menninger Clin 61:189–221, 1997

Novalis PN, Rojceicz SJ Jr, Peele R: Clinical Manual of Supportive Psychotherapy. Washington, DC American Psychiatric Press, 1997

Nurnberg HG: Survey of psychotherapeutic approaches to narcissistic personality disorder. Hillside Journal of Clinical Psychiatry 6:204–220, 1984

O'Hara MW, Stuart S, Gorman LL, et al: Efficacy of interpersonal psychotherapy for postpartum depression. Arch Gen Psychiatry 57:1039–1045, 2000

Ornstein A: Supportive psychotherapy: a contemporary view. Clinical Social Work Journal 14:14–30, 1986

Parloff MB: Psychotherapy research evidence and reimbursement decisions: Bambi meets Godzilla. Am J Psychiatry 139:718–727, 1982

Parloff MB, Lond P, Wolfe B: Individual psychotherapy and behavior change. Annu Rev Psychol 37:321–349, 1986

Perry JC, Banon E, Ianni F: Effectiveness of psychotherapy for personality disorders. Am J Psychiatry 156:1312–1321, 1999

Persson G, Alström JE: A scale for rating suitability for insight-oriented psychotherapy. Acta Psychiatr Scand 68:117–125, 1983

Peteet JR: A closer look at the concept of support: some applications to the care of patients with cancer. Gen Hosp Psychiatry 4:19–23, 1982

Pine F: On therapeutic change: perspective from a parent–child model. Psychoanalysis and Contemporary Science 5:537–569, 1976

Pine F: [Supportive psychotherapy] A psychoanalytic perspective. Psychiatr Ann 16:526–529, 1986

Pinkser H: The role of theory in teaching supportive psychotherapy. Am J Psychother 48:530–542, 1994

Pinsker H: A Primer of Supportive Psychotherapy. Hillsdale, NJ, Analytic Press, 1997

Ponsi M: Therapeutic alliance and collaborative interactions. Int J Psychoanal 81:687–704, 2000

Racker H: Meanings and uses of countertransference. Psychoanal Q 26:303–357, 1957

Rea M, Strachan A, Goldstein MJ: Changes in coping style following individual and family treatment for schizophrenia. Gen Hosp Psychiatry 11:358–364, 1991

Reiser MF: The dream in contemporary psychiatry. Am J Psychiatry 158:351–359, 2001

Robinson MV, Flaherty JA: Self-regulation of distance in supportive psychotherapy. Clinical Social Work Journal 10:209–217, 1982

Rockland LH: Psychoanalytically oriented supportive therapy: literature review and techniques. J Am Acad Psychoanal 17:451–462, 1989a

Rockland LH: Supportive Therapy: A Psychodynamic Approach. New York, Basic Books, 1989b

Rockland LH: A review of supportive psychotherapy, 1986–1992. Hosp Community Psychiatry 44:1053–1060, 1993

Rosenthal RN, Muran JC, Pinsker H, et al: Interpersonal change in brief supportive psychotherapy. J Psychother Pract Res 8:55–63, 1999

Rounsaville BJ, Glazer W, Wilber CH, et al: Short-term interpersonal psychotherapy in methadone-maintained opiate addicts. Arch Gen Psychiatry 40:629–636, 1983

Rounsaville BJ, Gawin F, Kleber H: Interpersonal psychotherapy adapted for ambulatory cocaine abusers. Am J Drug Alcohol Abuse 11:171–191, 1985a

Rounsaville BJ, Klerman GL, Weissman MM, et al: Short-term interpersonal psychotherapy (IPT) for depression, in Handbook of Depression: Treatment, Assessment and Research. Edited by Beckham EE, Leber WB. Homewood, IL, Dorsey Press, 1985b, pp 125–150

Sandell R, Blomberg J, Lazar A, et al: Varieties of long-term outcome among patients in psychoanalysis and long-term psychotherapy: a review of findings in the Stockholm Outcome of Psychoanalysis and Psychotherapy Project (STOPP). Int J Psychoanal 81:921–942, 2000

Sandler J, Dare C, Holder A: The Patient and the Analyst: The Basis of the Psychoanalytic Process. New York, International Universities Press, 1973

Sapolsky RM: Glucocorticoids and hippocampal atrophy in neuropsychiatric disorders, Arch Gen Psychiatry 57:925–935, 2000

Schindler B, Shook J, Schwartz G: Beneficial effects of psychiatric intervention on recovery after coronary artery bypass graft surgery. Gen Hosp Psychiatry 11:358–364, 1989

Searles HF: Collected Papers on Schizophrenia and Related Subjects. New York, International Universities Press, 1965

Shapiro DA, Shapiro D: Meta-analysis of comparative therapy outcome studies: a replication and refinement. Psychol Bull 92:581–604, 1982

Sharfstein SS, Muszynski S, Myers E: Health Insurance and Psychiatric Care: Update and Appraisal. Washington, DC, American Psychiatric Press, 1984

Sharpe EF: Dream Analysis. London, England, Hogarth Press, 1961

Shearin E, Linehan M: Dialectical behavior therapy for borderline personality disorder: theoretical and empirical foundations. Acta Psychiatr Scand Suppl 379:61–68, 1994

Sifneos PE: Short-Term Psychotherapy and Emotional Crisis. Cambridge, MA, Harvard University Press, 1972

Sifneos PE: Is dynamic psychotherapy contraindicated for a large number of patients with psychosomatic diseases? Psychother Psychosom 21:133–156, 1972–1973

Sifneos PE: Problems of psychotherapy of patients with alexithymic characteristics and physical disease. Psychother Psychosom 26:65–70, 1975

Silberman EK, Certa K: Psychiatric interview: settings and techniques, in Psychiatry. Edited by Tasman A, Kay J, Lieberman J. Philadelphia, PA, WB Saunders, 1997, pp 19–39

Smith ML, Glass GV: Meta-analysis of psychotherapy outcome studies. Am Psychol 32:752–760, 1977

Smith ML, Glass GV, Miller TI: The Benefits of Psychotherapy. Baltimore, MD, Johns Hopkins University Press, 1980

Solnit AJ: Recovery and adaptation. Psychoanal Study Child 55:252–274, 2000

Sonnenberg SM, Sutton L, Ursano RJ: Physician–patient relationship, in Psychiatry. Edited by Tasman A, Kay J, Lieberman JA. Philadelphia, PA, WB Saunders, 1997, pp 40–50

Spiegel D, Lazar SG: The need for psychotherapy in the medically ill. Psychoanalytic Inquiry 17(suppl):45–50, 1997

Spiegel D, Kraemer H, Bloom J: Effect of psychosocial treatment on survival of patients with metastatic breast cancer. Lancet 2:888–891, 1989

Stafford-Clark D: Supportive psychotherapy, in Modern Trends in Psychological Medicine II. Edited by Price JH. New York, Appleton-Century-Crofts, 1970, pp 277–295

Stanton AH, Gunderson JG, Knapp P, et al: Effects of psychotherapy in schizophrenia, I: design and implementation of a controlled study. Schizophr Bull 10:520–563, 1984

Stierlin H: Short-term versus long-term psychotherapy in the light of a general theory of human relationships. Br J Med Psychol 41:357–367, 1968

Stone L: The Psychoanalytic Situation: An Examination of Its Development and Essential Nature. New York, International Universities Press, 1961

Strupp HH: Success and failure in time-limited psychotherapy: a systematic comparison of two cases: comparison 1. Arch Gen Psychiatry 37:595–603, 1980a

Strupp HH: Success and failure in time-limited psychotherapy. Further evidence (comparison 4). Arch Gen Psychiatry 37:947–954, 1980b

Strupp HH: Success and failure in time-limited psychotherapy. With special reference to the performance of a lay counselor. Arch Gen Psychiatry 37:831–841, 1980c

Strupp HH, Binder J: Psychotherapy in a New Key: Time-Limited Dynamic Psychotherapy. New York, Basic Books, 1984

Strupp HH, Hadley SW: Specific vs nonspecific factors in psychotherapy: a controlled study of outcome. Arch Gen Psychiatry 36:1125–1136, 1979

Sullivan HS: The Psychiatric Interview. Edited by Perry HS, Gawel ML. New York, WW Norton, 1954

Sullivan PR: Learning theories and supportive psychotherapy. Am J Psychiatry 128:763–766, 1971

Ursano RJ, Dressler DM: Brief vs long term psychotherapy: a treatment decision. J Nerv Ment Dis 159:164–171, 1974

Ursano RJ, Dressler DM: Brief versus long-term psychotherapy: clinician attitudes and organizational design. Compr Psychiatry 18:55–60, 1977

Ursano RJ, Fullerton CS: Psychotherapy: medical intervention and the concept of normality, in The Diversity of Normal Behavior: Further Contributions to Normatology. Edited by Offer D, Sabshin M. New York, Basic Books, 1991, pp 39–59

Ursano RJ, Sonnenberg SM, Lazar SG: Concise Guide to Psychodynamic Psychotherapy: Principles and Techniques in the Era of Managed Care. Washington, DC, American Psychiatric Press, 1998

Ursano RJ, Epstein RS, Lazar SG: Behavioral responses to illness: personality and personality disorders, in Textbook of Medical Surgical Psychiatry: Psychiatry in the Medically Ill. Edited by Rundell JR, Wise MG. Washington, DC, American Psychiatric Publishing, 2001, pp 125–146

Vaughan SC, Marshall RD, Mackinnon RA, et al: Can we do psychoanalytic outcome research? A feasibility study. Int J Psychoanal 81:513–527, 2000

Viederman M: The psychodynamic life narrative: a psychotherapeutic intervention useful in crisis situations. Psychiatry 46(3):236–246, 1983

Wallace ER: Dynamic Psychiatry in Theory and Practice. Philadelphia, PA, Lea & Febiger, 1983

Wallerstein RS: Forty-Two Lives in Treatment: A Study of Psychoanalysis and Psychotherapy. New York, Guilford, 1986

Wallerstein RS: Psychoanalysis and psychotherapy: an historical perspective. Int J Psychoanal 70:563–591, 1989

Wallerstein RS: Follow up in psychoanalysis: what happens to treatment gains. J Am Psychoanal Assoc 40:665–690, 1992

Weiss J, Sampson H: The Psychoanalytic Process: Theory, Clinical Observation and Empirical Research. New York, Guilford, 1986

Weissman MM, Markowitz JC: Interpersonal psychotherapy. Arch Gen Psychiatry 51:599–606, 1994

Weissman MM, Klerman GL, Prusoff BA, et al: Depressed outpatients: results one year after treatment with drugs and/or interpersonal psychotherapy. Arch Gen Psychiatry 38:51–55, 1981

Werman DS: The use of dreams in psychotherapy: practical guidelines. Canadian Psychiatric Association Journal 23:153–158, 1978

Werman DS: Technical aspects of supportive psychotherapy. Psychiatric Journal of the University of Ottawa 6:153–160, 1981

Werman DS: The Practice of Supportive Psychotherapy. New York, Brunner/Mazel, 1984

Werman DS: On the mode of therapeutic action of psychoanalytic supportive psychotherapy, in How Does Treatment Help? On the Modes of Action of Psychoanalytic Psychotherapy. Edited by Rothstein A. Madison, CT, International Universities Press, 1988, pp 157–167

Winston A, Pinsker H, McCullough L: A review of supportive psychotherapy. Hosp Community Psychiatry 37:1105–1114, 1986

Zetzel ER: Current concepts of transference. Int J Psychoanal 37:369–376, 1956

Zitrin CM, Klein DF, Woerner MG: Behavior therapy, supportive psychotherapy, imipramine, and phobias. Arch Gen Psychiatry 35:307–316, 1978

Glossary

Abstinence   Therapist's technical stance of being somewhat silent, although not withholding, in order better to observe how the patient organizes his or her psychic world. Requires explanation for and education of the patient.

Acting out   Expressing unconscious conflict in action rather than in words.

Asceticism   Denial of pleasure, including food, sleep, exercise, and sexual gratification, usually with an air of superiority or of doing good for someone else. Typical of adolescence.

Behavior   Thoughts (i.e., cognitions), feelings (i.e., affects), fantasies, and actions.

Brief psychodynamic psychotherapy   Psychodynamic psychotherapy that is focal and of limited duration, usually 12–20 sessions.

Cognitive psychotherapy   Psychotherapy that focuses on inappropriate and inaccurate cognitions and beliefs. Includes homework and behavioral interventions.

Complementary countertransference   Therapist's identification with a significant figure from the patient's past whom the patient is experiencing in the transference.

Concordant countertransference   Therapist's identification with the patient's emotional experience.

Countertransference   Psychotherapist's emotional experience of the patient. May be a help or an impediment to treatment. May be experienced by the therapist as pressure to act in a certain way with the patient.

Defense (see Mechanisms of defense)

Denial   Act of ignoring painful realities as though they were not present—for example, a man in an intensive care unit after a myocardial infarction refuses to believe he has had a heart attack and continues to run his business from his bed as though nothing had happened.

Devaluing   Minimizing and dismissing with an air of contempt.

Displacement   Act of focusing one's anxiety or feelings on a different object or person from the one to which or to whom these feelings are truly related—for example, kicking the dog when being angry with one's spouse.

Ego (see also Superego)   Portion of the personality that mediates between the real world and the internal world. Includes autonomous functions such as thinking.

End phase of treatment (see also Termination)   Last phase of a psychotherapy, which includes consolidation, recapitulation of symptoms and defenses, practice, and end setting.

Evaluation phase   Initial two to four sessions that are used to assess the patient and reach a treatment decision.

Free association   Technical procedure of encouraging the patient to speak as freely as possible, to suspend judgment, and to say whatever comes to mind. Always only a relative term. Requires education of the patient.

Id   Wishful portion of the tripartite psychoanalytic personality model.

Identification with the aggressor   Act of behaving like a significant person in one's life who has been aggressive or violent toward oneself.

Inhibition   Constriction of thoughts, feelings, and/or behaviors to avoid internal conflict.

Insight-oriented psychotherapy (see Psychodynamic psychotherapy)

Intellectualization   Use of excessively intellectual, factual, and cognitive mechanisms to decrease anxiety.

Intermittent psychotherapy   Psychotherapy provided intermittently over a long-term treatment plan. This psychotherapy may be episodic brief psychotherapy or widely spaced individual sessions of psychodynamic, interpersonal, or cognitive psychotherapy.

Interpersonal psychotherapy   Psychotherapy focused on interpersonal relations and social functioning.

Interpretation   Technical procedure of making what is unconscious (i.e., out of the patient's awareness) conscious. May include linking the transference with a present experience and also with a past significant figure.

Isolation of affect   Separation of feelings from awareness. Related to intellectualization.

Long-term psychotherapy (see Psychodynamic psychotherapy)

Mechanisms of defense   Ways of thinking (i.e., cognitions) directed toward decreasing unpleasant affective states (anxiety) and maintaining unconscious conflicts out of awareness. Examples include intellectualization, repression, externalization, somatization, splitting, denial, and acting out.

Neurosis   Older term used in psychoanalytic writings to mean internal conflict.

Object relationships   Internal representational world of "people" as distinguished from the "real" persons; the experiential world of the patient, populated with meanings and perceptions rather than real events.

Objects (see Object relationships)

Omnipotence   Primitive defense in which one exaggerates one's own sense of power and ability.

Primitive idealization   Act of exaggerating the power, ability, and prestige of another person to relieve one's own anxiety.

Projection   Primitive defense in which one attributes one's own conflicted feelings and wishes to another person.

Projective identification   Primitive defense in which one projects one's own feelings onto another and then attempts to control those feelings in that person.

Psychic reality   The "internal world," that is, unconscious perceptions based on the meanings of events rather than on the actual events. Derives from biological givens and developmental experience.

Psychoanalysis   Psychotherapeutic treatment of great intensity, usually several years in length, directed at the elaboration of the patient's psychic reality and world of meaning through examination of the transference. Focuses on how these areas affect behavior. Term also used to describe the theory of mental functioning derived from this technique.

Psychodynamic psychotherapy (also called Explorative psychotherapy; Insight-oriented psychotherapy; Long-term psychotherapy; Psychoanalytic psychotherapy)   The "talking cure" based on the principles of a psychoanalytic understanding of mental functioning (e.g., presence of defenses, transference, and psychic reality) as aspects of mental life. Primary goal is to make what is out of awareness available for conscious processing through identifying patterns of behavior derived from childhood.

Psychoanalytic psychotherapy (see Psychodynamic psychotherapy)

Psychotherapy   The generic term for all "talking cures." Verbal interchange between an expert and a help seeker, the goal of which is to alter characteristic patterns of behavior that are causing the help-seeker difficulties. Includes cognitive psychotherapy, interpersonal psychotherapy, and psychoanalysis, among others.

Reaction formation   Act of doing the opposite of what one feels (e.g., being overly ingratiating to people with whom one is angry).

Reality testing   An ego function. The capacity to distinguish reality from fantasy, and internal wishes and thoughts from external events.

Regression   Return to an earlier mode of functioning to avoid experiences of conflict in the present.

Repression   Act of removing conflicted thoughts and feelings from awareness; act of forgetting.

Resistance   Clinical term used to describe the therapist's experience of the patient's unconscious reluctance to experience disturbing affects related to childhood conflicts. Includes defense mechanisms, secondary gain, reinforcing nature of acting out, need to punish oneself, and need to thwart progress.

Reversal   Act of changing an impulse or wish from active to passive.

Sequential psychotherapy and medication treatment   Psychotherapy with medication treatment followed by termination of the ongoing psychotherapy and continuation of medication management.

Splitting   Primitive defense that separates positive and negative self and object images so that individuals tend to be seen as all good or all bad.

Sublimation   Mature defense mechanism resulting in the application of the energy from previous conflicts in appropriate feelings, thought, and behaviors in the present.

Superego (see also Ego)   That part of the personality that includes one's conscience and one's goals.

Supportive psychotherapy   Psychotherapy directed toward helping the patient reestablish his or her previous best level of functioning. The most common form of psychotherapy, requiring thoughtful and skilled application of psychodynamic principles and techniques.

Termination (see also End phase of treatment)   Act of ending psychotherapy. This phase of treatment is demanding for the therapist as well as for the patient.

Therapeutic alliance   Reality-based relationship of the therapist and the patient who are working together.

Transference   Experience of acting toward, feeling, and/or perceiving another person to be like a significant figure from one's past. Important area of learning in the psychoanalytic psychotherapies but not limited to therapy settings.

Transference neurosis   Prominent, substantial transference typical of psychoanalysis.

Working alliance (see Therapeutic alliance)

CHAPTER 27

Interpersonal Psychotherapy

John C. Markowitz, M.D.

Interpersonal psychotherapy (IPT) is a time-limited treatment that the late Gerald L. Klerman, M.D., and Myrna M. Weissman, Ph.D., developed in the 1970s for adult outpatients with major depression. IPT is well known as a research intervention on the basis of numerous successful randomized controlled clinical trials. In recent years it has begun to spread in clinical practice. This chapter reviews the research-defined indications and outlines the general conduct of this relatively simple yet potent psychotherapy.

IPT is a straightforward, manual-based, focused, pragmatic, and optimistic time-limited treatment that targets particular psychiatric disorders. It was first devised and has been best tested as a treatment of major depressive episodes. IPT has two basic premises: first, that depression is a medical illness that is treatable and not the patient's fault. Second, the disorder does not occur in a vacuum, but rather is influenced by and itself affects the patient's psychosocial environment. The goal of treatment is to help the patient solve a difficulty in his or her role functioning or social environment. Doing so helps the patient gain a sense of mastery over his or her functioning and relieves depressive symptoms.

IPT was defined in a manual (Klerman et al. 1984; updated by Weissman et al. 2000) and tested in randomized clinical trials. Evidence for efficacy in research trials for patients with major depressive disorder led to its adaptation and testing for other mood and nonmood disorders and its modification for adolescent and geriatric depressed patients, for patients with bipolar and dysthymic disorders, for depressed HIV-positive and depressed pregnant patients, and for depressed primary care patients. Nonmood targets have included bulimia, substance abuse, and increasingly the anxiety disorders. IPT has also been adapted for use as a maintenance treatment, for couples and group formats, as a telephone intervention, and in a patient self-help guide.

Begun as a research intervention, IPT has only fairly recently been disseminated among clinicians and in residency training programs. In the wake of publication of efficacy data for IPT, promulgation of practice guidelines that embrace IPT among antidepressant treatments, and endorsement of IPT by *Consumer Reports* ("Mental Health: Does Therapy Work?" 1995; Seligman 1995), there have been increasing requests for training in IPT. Managed care and economic pressures have also aroused growing interest in defined, time-limited, empirically supported treatments such as IPT.

Practice guidelines for treatment of depression appeared in 1993 for mental health professionals (Karasu et al. 1993) and for primary care practitioners (Agency for Health Care Policy and Research 1993a, 1993b, 1993c, 1993d). Each of these discussed IPT as an acute and maintenance treatment for depression, used alone and in combination with medication.

The American Psychiatric Association practice guideline for adults with major depression (Karasu et al. 1993) included IPT among the few recommended psychotherapies. The guideline did not require efficacy data from controlled clinical trials as an inclusion criterion. IPT was deemed useful for patients "in the midst of recent conflicts with significant others and for those having difficulty adjusting to an altered career or social role or other life transition" (p. 6)—that is, for depression associated with life events or interpersonal conflicts. Although many patients do present with such recent life changes, the empirical support for IPT's efficacy in depressed patients—some of which is documented below—makes these indications appear minimal and conservative.

The Agency for Health Care Policy and Research primary care guidelines for depression comprised four volumes (Agency for Health Care Policy and Research 1993a, 1993b, 1993c, 1993d). Both the physician and the patient guidelines listed IPT; cognitive-behavioral therapy

(CBT; Beck et al. 1979); and behavioral, brief dynamic, and marital therapy as treatments for depression. IPT was recommended as an acute treatment for nonpsychotic depression to alleviate symptoms, prevent relapse and recurrence, correct distressing psychological problems with secondary symptom resolution, and address secondary consequences of depression. The guidelines stated that medication alone may suffice as continuation treatment to prevent relapse or recurrence and as maintenance treatment for remitted patients with recurrent depression (Frank et al. 1990, 1991). The panel considered IPT, CBT, and behavioral treatments to be "effective in most cases of mild-to-moderate depression" (Agency for Health Care Policy and Research 1993b, p. 12) but added that indications "for continuation phase psychotherapy are unclear" (p. 18), although "two studies are suggestive that continuation psychotherapy may reduce the relapse rate" (p. 18). The patient guidelines listed behavioral therapy, cognitive therapy, and IPT as the "most well-studied [sic] for their effectiveness in reducing symptoms of major depressive disorder" (Agency for Health Care Policy and Research 1993d, p. 23).

IPT's use is spreading from its initial research base in the United States. The IPT manual has been translated into Italian, German, Japanese, and Spanish and is being used more widely around the world. Descriptions of IPT have appeared in Spanish (Puig 1995) and Dutch journals (Blom et al. 1996). An International Society for Interpersonal Psychotherapy was formed at the American Psychiatric Association annual meeting in May 2000 in Chicago, Illinois. (For a complete description of the IPT method, see Weissman et al. 2000; for the patient guide, see Weissman 1995; for the group adaptation, see Wilfley et al. 2000; for the adaptation for depressed adolescents, see Mufson et al. 1993; and for the dysthymic disorder adaptation, see Markowitz 1998.)

Theoretical and Empirical Foundations

IPT is based on interpersonal theory deriving from the post–World War II work of Adolf Meyer, Harry Stack Sullivan (1953), and later John Bowlby and others (Table 27–1). The main principle abstracted from these theories is that life events occurring after the early childhood years influence psychopathology. IPT uses this principle for practical, not etiological, purposes. It does not presume to discern the *cause* of a depressive episode—the etiology of depression being multifactorial—but pragmatically uses the connection between current life events

TABLE 27–1. Theoretical and empirical foundations of interpersonal psychotherapy (IPT)

I. **Interpersonal theory**
   A. Importance of current life events to psychopathology
      Meyer, Sullivan, and others
   B. Attachment theory
      Bowlby

II. **Empirical support: association of depressive episodes with**
   A. Complicated bereavement (grief)
   B. Marital and other interpersonal disputes (role disputes)
   C. Life events (role transitions)
   D. Isolation and lack of social support (interpersonal deficits)

and the onset of depressive symptoms to help the patient understand and combat his or her episode of illness. IPT is also based on psychosocial and life events research of depression, which bolstered these theories by demonstrating relationships between depression and complicated bereavement, role disputes (e.g., bad marriages), role transitions (and meaningful life changes), and interpersonal deficits.

Conducting IPT

General Principles

IPT therapists define depression as a *medical illness*, a treatable condition that is not the patient's fault. This definition tends to displace the burdensome guilt of the depressed patient from the patient him- or herself to the illness, making the symptoms ego-dystonic and discrete; it also provides hope for a response to treatment. The therapist uses DSM-IV (American Psychiatric Association 1994) to make a diagnosis and employs rating scales such as the Hamilton Rating Scale for Depression (HRSD; Hamilton 1960) or the Beck Depression Inventory (BDI; Beck 1978) to assess and explain the depressive symptoms. This assessment helps the patient to recognize that he or she is dealing with a common mood disorder with a predictable set of symptoms—not the personal failure, weakness, or character flaw that the depressed patient often believes to be the problem. To underscore this idea, IPT therapists give depressed patients the "sick role" (Parsons 1951), excusing them from blame for what their illness prevents them from doing, but also obliging them as patients to work to recover the healthy role they have lost.

By solving an interpersonal problem—dealing with complicated bereavement, a role dispute or transition, or an interpersonal deficit—the IPT patient has an opportunity to improve his or her life situation and simultaneously relieve the symptoms of the depressive episode. This coupled formula has been validated by randomized controlled trials in which IPT has been tested, and hence can be offered with confidence and optimism. Such therapeutic optimism, although hardly specific to IPT, very likely provides part of its power in "remoralizing" the patient.

An eclectic therapy, IPT uses techniques found in other treatment approaches. For example, IPT employs a medical model of depressive illness consistent with pharmacotherapy (which makes it highly compatible in combination with medication). It shares role playing and a "here and now" focus with cognitive therapy, and addresses interpersonal issues in a manner familiar to marital therapists. It is not its specific techniques but rather its overall strategies that make IPT a unique and coherent approach. IPT overlaps to some degree with psychodynamic psychotherapies, and many of its early research therapists came from psychodynamic backgrounds; however, IPT also meaningfully differs from them in its emphasis on the present, not the past; its focus on real-life change rather than self-understanding; its medical model; and its avoidance of the transference and of genetic and dream interpretations (Markowitz et al. 1998a). Although, like CBT, it constitutes a time-limited treatment targeting a syndromal constellation (e.g., major depression), IPT is considerably less structured, assigns no explicit homework, and focuses on interpersonal problem areas rather than automatic thoughts (Table 27–2). Each of the four IPT interpersonal problem areas has discrete—if to some degree overlapping—goals for therapist and patient to pursue.

IPT techniques aid the patient's pursuit of these interpersonal goals. The therapist repeatedly helps the patient relate life events to mood and other symptoms. Techniques include an *opening question* that elicits an interval history of mood and events; *communication analysis*, a reconstruction and evaluation of recent, affectively charged life circumstances; *exploration of the patient's wishes and options*, to pursue those wishes in particular interpersonal situations; *decision analysis*, to help the patient choose which options to employ; and *role playing*, to help patients prepare tactics for real life.

IPT deals with current rather than past interpersonal relationships, focusing on the patient's immediate social context. The IPT therapist attempts to intervene in the areas of symptom formation and social dysfunction asso-

TABLE 27–2. Comparison of interpersonal psychotherapy (IPT) and cognitive-behavioral therapy (CBT)

I. **Points in common**
   A. Common factors of psychotherapy
      1. Helping patient feel understood (Relationship)
      2. Framework for understanding (Rationale)
      3. Providing hope and optimism
      4. Psychoeducation
      5. Technique for getting better (Ritual)
      6. Success experiences
   B. Common features of brief psychotherapies for depression
      1. Manualized
      2. Active
      3. Time limited (with comparable time courses)
      4. Structured (CBT > IPT)
      5. "Here and now" current focus
      6. Can be combined with antidepressant medication
      7. Goals of self-assertion, mastery
      8. Ultimate goal of new skills for prophylaxis
   C. Technical similarities
      1. Mobilizing patient to greater activity
      2. Linking mood to activities and reactions to events, albeit with different emphases
      3. Problem solving: "Exploring options" versus "Empirical hypothesis testing"
      4. Addressing "expectations" versus "assumptions" about others
      5. Role playing
II. **Differences**
   A. IPT: medical model
   B. CBT: homework
   C. Focus on affect (IPT) versus thoughts (→ affect) (CBT)—hence more external versus more intrapsychic approach
III. **Differential therapeutics of major depression: Which works better for whom?**

ciated with depression rather than addressing enduring aspects of personality. Personality is in any case difficult to accurately assess during an episode of an Axis I disorder such as depression (Hirschfeld et al. 1983). IPT does build new social skills (Weissman et al. 1981), a benefit that may be as valuable as changing personality traits.

Phases of Treatment

As an acute treatment, IPT has three phases (Table 27–3). The *first phase*, usually consisting of one to three sessions, includes diagnostic evaluation, psychiatric anamnesis, and setting the framework for the treatment. The therapist reviews symptoms, uses standard criteria

(American Psychiatric Association 1994) to assign a diagnosis of depression, and gives the patient the sick role (Parsons 1951). The psychiatric history includes the "interpersonal inventory," a careful review of the patient's past and current social functioning and close relationships, as well as the patterns of and reciprocal expectations in these relationships. (The interpersonal inventory is not a structured instrument.) Changes in relationships proximal to the onset of symptoms are elucidated—for example, death of a loved one, children leaving home, worsening marital strife, or isolation from a confidant. This review provides a framework for understanding the social and interpersonal context of the onset of depressive symptoms and establishes the basis for a treatment focus.

Having assessed the need for medication on the basis of the patient's symptom severity, past history and response to treatment, and treatment preference, the therapist educates the patient about depression by discussing the constellation of symptoms that define major depression, their psychosocial concomitants, and what the patient may expect from treatment. The therapist next links the depressive syndrome to the patient's interpersonal situation in a formulation (Markowitz and Swartz 1997) centered on one of four interpersonal problem areas (Table 27–4): 1) *grief*, 2) interpersonal *role disputes*, 3) *role transitions*, or 4) *interpersonal deficits*. If the patient explicitly accepts this formulation as a focus for subsequent treatment, therapy enters the middle phase.

It is important to keep treatment focused on a simple theme that even a highly distractible depressed patient can grasp. Any formulation necessarily simplifies a patient's complex situation. Although some patients may present with multiple interpersonal problems, the goal of the formulation is to isolate one or at most two salient problems related to the patient's mood disorder (whether as precipitant or consequence). More than two foci would mean no focus at all. The choice of focal problem area depends on the therapist's clinical acumen, although research has shown that IPT therapists do agree in choosing such areas (Markowitz et al. 2000) and that patients seem to find the foci credible.

In the *middle phase*, the IPT therapist pursues strategies specific to the chosen interpersonal problem area. For *grief*—complicated bereavement following the death of a loved one—the therapist facilitates the catharsis of mourning and helps the patient find new activities and relationships to compensate for the loss. *Role disputes* are conflicts with significant others: a spouse, another family member, a co-worker, or a close friend. The therapist

TABLE 27–3. Phases of interpersonal psychotherapy (IPT)

I. **Early phase**
  A. Deal with the depression
    1. Review depressive symptoms
    2. Name the syndrome: formal diagnosis
    3. Psychoeducation about depression and its treatment
    4. Give patient the "sick role"
    5. Evaluate need for medication
  B. Relate depression to interpersonal context: interpersonal inventory
    1. Nature of interaction with significant persons
    2. Reciprocal expectations of patient and significant others, and whether these were fulfilled
    3. Satisfying and unsatisfying aspects of relationships
    4. Recent changes in key relationships
    5. Changes patient desires in relationships
  C. Identify the major problem area
    1. Determine problem area related to current episode and set treatment goals.
    2. Which relationship is related to the episode? What might change in it?
  D. Explain IPT concepts and contract
    1. Outline understanding of the problem: formulation
    2. Agree on treatment goals (focal problem area)
      a. brief treatment (time limit)
      b. target is depression (not character)
    3. Describe IPT procedures: "here and now" focus, need to discuss important concerns; review of current interpersonal relations; discussion of practical aspects of treatment

II. **Middle phase**
Specific strategies for treating grief, role dispute, role transition, or interpersonal deficits

III. **Termination phase**
  A. Consolidate gains
  B. Foster independence
  C. Address guilt (and blame therapy) if nonresponder
  D. Review risk of relapse and recurrence
  E. Recontract for continuation and maintenance treatment if appropriate

TABLE 27–4. Interpersonal psychotherapy problem areas

Grief (complicated bereavement)
Role dispute
Role transition
Interpersonal deficits (only if none of above appropriate)

helps the patient explore the relationship, the nature of the dispute, whether it has reached an impasse, and available options for resolving it. If these options fail, therapist and patient may conclude that the relationship has reached an impasse and consider ways to change the impasse or to end the relationship. *Role transition* includes change in life status—for example, beginning or ending a relationship or career, moving, promotion, retirement, graduation, or being diagnosed with a medical illness. The patient learns to manage the change by mourning the loss of the old role while recognizing positive and negative aspects of the new role he or she is assuming and by taking steps to gain mastery over the new role. *Interpersonal deficits*, better thought of as "no acute life events," is the residual fourth IPT problem area and is used for patients who lack one of the first three problem areas—that is, patients who report no recent life events that could have precipitated their symptoms. This focus defines the patient as having deficits in social skills, including problems in initiating or sustaining relationships, and helps the patient to develop new relationships and skills. Some patients who might seem to fall into this category may in fact have dysthymic disorder, for which separate strategies have been developed (Markowitz 1998).

IPT sessions address present here-and-now problems rather than childhood or developmental issues. Sessions open with the question: "How have things been since we last met?" This focuses the patient on recent interpersonal events and recent mood, which the therapist helps the patient to link. Therapists take an active, nonneutral, supportive, and hopeful stance to counter the depressed patient's pessimism. They elicit and emphasize the options that exist for change in the patient's life, options that the depressive episode may have prevented the patient from seeing or exploring fully. Nor does understanding the situation suffice: therapists stress the need for patients to test these options in order to improve their lives and simultaneously treat their depressive episodes.

The *final phase* of IPT, which occupies the last few sessions of acute treatment or the last few months of maintenance treatment, strengthens the patient's newly regained sense of independence and competence by recognizing and consolidating therapeutic gains. The therapist secures self-esteem by underscoring that the patient's depressive episode has improved because of his or her actions in changing a life situation—and this at a time when the patient had felt weak and impotent. The therapist also helps the patient to anticipate triggers for and responses to depressive symptoms that might arise in the future. Compared with psychodynamic psychother-

apy, IPT deemphasizes termination: it is a graduation from successful treatment. The sadness of parting is distinguished from depressive feelings. If the patient has not improved, the therapist emphasizes that the treatment has failed, not the patient, and that alternative effective treatment options exist. Patients with multiple prior major depressive episodes who successfully complete acute treatment but remain at high risk for recurrence may contract for maintenance therapy as acute treatment draws to a close.

Case Example

Ms. A, a 37-year-old married Roman Catholic Latina businesswoman, presented with a 4-month history of major depression and a 24-item HRSD score of 28. Symptoms included a depressed and anxious mood with diurnal variation, exhaustion due to insomnia, difficulty concentrating at work, and moments of passive suicidal ideation. Although she initially felt that her symptoms had arisen out of the blue, her therapist's history taking led to the conclusion that it was connected to recent life events. She had recently been promoted at work, an achievement that pleased her but also meant greater work responsibilities and more time spent away from home. Her 4-year-old daughter complained about this, and her husband intensified pressure on her to have a second child. She felt that her husband misunderstood her difficult role as a "modern mother."

Ms. A had had one prior episode of depression 14 years before, shortly after her college graduation and on the brink of marrying Mr. A. That episode had been milder and had resolved with a brief course of antidepressant medication. She had no history of substance abuse, suicide attempts, or previous psychotherapy. Her family history was notable for maternal depression and for a brother's alcohol abuse. Her interpersonal inventory revealed that she had a few close friends, in whom she was more likely to confide than her husband. She also counted on her family of origin for support. Her marriage had many positive aspects but was limited by her lawyer husband's "macho," authoritarian attitude. She felt that she was supposed to defer to him and resentfully complied.

Ms. A was reluctant to take antidepressant medication. Her therapist diagnosed her as having a recurrent major depressive episode, told her her HRSD score, and suggested that the episode was related to an ongoing role dispute with her husband, which had been exacerbated by her promotion. (Because work was going well and she felt less conflicted about this aspect of her life, the therapist focused on the role dispute rather than a role transition.) Ms. A agreed to a 12-week course of IPT and was given the sick role.

Sessions focused on marital communication. Ms. A explained to her husband how important her new job was to her and asked him for support in building her career and in caring for their daughter. They discussed compromises about work hours. She was initially discouraged when her husband reacted angrily in one of these discussions. Ms. A and her therapist then reviewed the encounter and explored options for how she could broach the topic at a calmer time of the week than previously. They role-played this interaction, with the patient testing out different expressions of her feeling and different tones of voice. The next encounter, after the fourth week, was more successful, and in the following week, they had two more productive talks and planned their first family vacation in some time. Ms. A was already feeling much better (HRSD score = 10) and was on better terms with her husband. Their daughter was happier as the result of more attention from both parents. On the subsequent vacation they agreed that it would probably make more sense for them not to have another child.

By week 9 Ms. A was euthymic, functioning well both at work and at home. Her HRSD score was 5. During the termination phase, the IPT therapist emphasized that Ms. A's improvement was due to her own actions—that is, to her finding more effective ways to communicate with her husband in resolving their role dispute. Although they were terminating acute treatment, the therapist pointed out that Ms. A had now experienced two episodes of major depression and was at significant risk for a third. Accordingly, they agreed to continuation treatment with monthly sessions of IPT.

Interpersonal Psychotherapy for Mood Disorders: Efficacy and Adaptations

IPT has been tested for a variety of mood and, increasingly, non–mood disorders (see Table 27–5).

Acute Treatment of Major Depression

IPT was first tested as an acute antidepressant treatment in a four-cell, 16-week randomized trial that compared IPT, amitriptyline, their combination, and a nonscheduled control treatment for 81 outpatients with major depression (DiMascio et al. 1979; Weissman et al. 1979). Of the two active monotherapies, amitriptyline alleviated symptoms more quickly than did IPT, but no significant differences were apparent between IPT and amitriptyline in symptom reduction at the end of treatment. Each active treatment reduced symptoms more efficaciously than the nonscheduled control, and combined amitriptyline–IPT was more efficacious than either active monotherapy. Patients with psychotic depression did poorly on IPT alone. Naturalistic follow-up at 1 year found that many patients sustained improvement from the brief IPT intervention and that IPT patients had developed significantly better psychosocial functioning regardless of whether they received medication. This

TABLE 27–5. Empirically based indications for interpersonal psychotherapy (IPT)

Major depression
    Acute
    Recurrent (prophylaxis)
    Geriatric patients
    Adolescent patients
    HIV-positive patients
    Primary care patients
    Conjoint therapy for depressed married women
    Postpartum and antepartum women
Dysthymic disorder[a]
Bipolar disorder (adjunctive treatment)[a]
Interpersonal counseling for subsyndromal depression
Bulimia (individual or group format)[a]
Social phobia[a]

Note. [a]Preliminary results are encouraging.

effect on social function was not found for amitriptyline alone, nor had it been evident for IPT immediately after the 16-week trial (Weissman et al. 1981).

In the multisite National Institute of Mental Health (NIMH) Treatment of Depression Collaborative Research Program (Elkin et al. 1989), the most ambitious acute treatment study to date, investigators randomly assigned 250 outpatients with major depression to 16 weeks of IPT, CBT, or either imipramine pharmacotherapy or placebo plus clinical management. Most subjects completed at least 15 weeks or 12 treatment sessions. Patients with milder depression (17-item HRSD score <20) improved equally in all four treatments. Among more severely depressed patients (HRSD score ≥ 20), imipramine worked fastest and most consistently outperformed placebo. IPT was comparable to imipramine on several outcome measures, including HRSD improvement, and superior to placebo for more severely depressed patients. CBT was not superior to placebo among the more depressed patients.

Klein and Ross (1993), reanalyzing the NIMH Treatment of Depression Collaborative Research Program data using the Johnson–Neyman statistical technique, found an ordering for treatment efficacy with "medication superior to psychotherapy, [and] the psychotherapies somewhat superior to placebo...particularly among the symptomatic and impaired patients" (p. 241). The authors reported that CBT was "relatively inferior to IPT for patients with BDI scores greater than approximately 30, generally considered the boundary between moderate and severe depression" (p. 247). The reanalysis does not contradict the report of Elkin et al. (1989), but rather sharpens differences among treatments.

In an 18-month naturalistic follow-up study of the NIMH Treatment of Depression Collaborative Research Program subjects, Shea et al. (1992) found no significant differences among the four treatment groups in the percentage of remitters (i.e., those who had minimal or no symptoms after the end of treatment and sustained that state during follow-up). Thirty percent of CBT, 26% of IPT, 19% of imipramine, and 20% of placebo subjects who had acutely remitted remained in remission throughout the follow-up period. Among acute remitters, relapse over the 18-month follow-up was 36% for CBT, 33% for IPT, 50% for imipramine (medication having been stopped at 16 weeks), and 33% for placebo. The authors concluded that for many patients, 16 weeks of specific treatments were insufficient to achieve full and lasting recovery.

Erik Hoencamp and colleagues (personal communications, 1996, 2002) in The Hague, The Netherlands, are completing a study of IPT versus nefazodone, alone and in combination, for acute treatment of major depression.

Maintenance Treatment

IPT was initially developed for and tested in an 8-month, six-cell trial (Klerman et al. 1974; Paykel et al. 1975). Today this study would be considered a "continuation" treatment, as the concept of long-term maintenance antidepressant treatment has lengthened. Acutely depressed outpatient women ($n = 150$) who had responded ($\geq 50\%$ symptom reduction rated by a clinical interviewer) to a 4- to 6-week acute phase of amitriptyline were randomly assigned to receive 8 months of weekly IPT alone, amitriptyline alone, placebo alone, combined IPT–amitriptyline, combined IPT–placebo, or no pill. Randomization to IPT or a low-contact psychotherapy condition occurred at entry into the continuation phase, whereas randomization to medication, placebo, or no pill occurred at the end of the second month of continuation. Maintenance pharmacotherapy was found to prevent relapse and symptom exacerbation, whereas IPT improved social functioning (Weissman et al. 1974). The effects of IPT on social functioning did not appear for 6–8 months. The best outcomes were seen for combined psychotherapy–pharmacotherapy.

Two longer antidepressant maintenance trials of IPT have been conducted. Frank et al. (1990, 1991), studied 128 outpatients with multiply and rapidly recurrent depression. Patients were initially treated with combined high-dose (>200 mg/day) imipramine and weekly IPT. Responders remained on high-dose medication while IPT was tapered to a monthly frequency during a 4-month continuation phase. Patients who remained in remission

were then randomly assigned to 3 years of 1) ongoing high-dose imipramine plus clinical management, 2) high-dose imipramine plus monthly IPT, 3) monthly IPT alone, 4) monthly IPT plus placebo, or 5) placebo plus clinical management. The investigators found high-dose imipramine to be the most efficacious treatment, preventing relapse in more than 80% of patients over 3 years. In contrast, most patients on placebo relapsed within the first few months. Once-monthly IPT, although less efficacious than medication, was statistically and clinically superior to the placebo condition in this high-risk patient population. Reynolds et al. (1999) essentially replicated these maintenance findings in a study of geriatric patients with major depression.

Women of childbearing age are the modal patients with depression. The study finding of an 82-week survival time without recurrence with IPT alone would suffice to protect many women with recurrent depression through pregnancy and nursing without medication. Further study is required to determine the efficacy of IPT relative to newer medications (e.g., selective serotonin reuptake inhibitors), and the efficacy of more-frequent-than-monthly doses of maintenance IPT. A study of differing doses of maintenance IPT for depressed patients is currently under way in Pittsburgh.

Geriatric Depressed Patients

IPT was first used with geriatric depressed patients as an addition to a 6-week pharmacotherapy trial to enhance compliance and to provide some treatment for the placebo control group (Rothblum et al. 1982; Sholomskas et al. 1983). The investigators noted that grief and role transition specific to life changes were the prime focus of treatment. They suggested modifications of IPT, including more flexible duration of sessions and greater use of practical advice and support (e.g., arranging transportation, calling the physician) and recognizing that major role changes may be impractical and detrimental (e.g., divorce at age 75 years). The 6-week trial compared standard IPT with nortriptyline in 30 geriatric depressed patients. Results showed some advantages for IPT, largely because of higher attrition in the medication group due to nortriptyline side effects (Sloane et al. 1985).

Reynolds et al. (1999) at the University of Pittsburgh conducted a 3-year maintenance study of geriatric patients with recurrent depression, using IPT and nortriptyline in a design similar to the Frank et al. (1990) study. The IPT manual was modified to allow more flexibility with session length, on the assumption that some elderly patients might not tolerate 50-minute sessions. The authors found that older patients needed to address early life relationships in their psychotherapy, a departure from the typical here-and-now focus of IPT. Like Sholomskas et al. (1983), they thought that therapists needed to help patients solve practical problems and to acknowledge that some problems may not be amenable to resolutions, such as existential late life issues or lifelong psychopathology (Rothblum et al. 1982). Elderly depressed patients whose sleep quality normalized by the early continuation phase had an 80% chance of remaining well during the first year of maintenance treatment. The response rate was similar for patients who subsequently received either nortriptyline or IPT.

Reynolds et al. (1999) acutely treated 187 geriatric patients (age 60 years and older) with recurrent major depression with the combination of IPT and nortriptyline. One hundred seven remitted and subsequently achieved recovery after continuation therapy. These 107 were then randomly assigned to one of four 3-year maintenance conditions: 1) medication clinic with nortriptyline alone, with steady-state nortriptyline plasma levels maintained in a therapeutic window of 80–120 ng/mL; 2) medication clinic with placebo; 3) monthly maintenance IPT with placebo; or 4) monthly maintenance IPT plus nortriptyline. Recurrence rates were 43% for nortriptyline alone, 90% for placebo, 64% for IPT with placebo, and 20% for combined treatment. Each monotherapy was statistically superior to placebo, whereas combined therapy showed superiority to IPT alone and a trend for superiority over medication alone. Compared with patients in their 60s, those age 70 and older were more likely to suffer recurrence and did so more quickly. This study corroborates the maintenance findings of Frank et al. (1990, 1991), with the difference that combined treatment had advantages over pharmacotherapy alone for the geriatric population.

The comparison of high-dose tricyclic antidepressants with low-dose maintenance IPT, in both the Frank et al. (1990, 1991) study and the Reynolds et al. (1999) study, is easy to misinterpret. Had the tricyclic dosage been lowered comparably to the reduced psychotherapy dosage, recurrence in the medication groups might well have been greater. Nonetheless, because there were no precedents for this research, the monthly dosing interval chosen for maintenance IPT was reasonable and indeed resulted in some benefit. This research raises the issue of dose-finding studies for psychotherapy—for example, what might biweekly maintenance IPT do?

Depressed Adolescents (IPT-A)

Mufson et al. (1993) modified IPT to incorporate adolescent developmental issues, adding as a fifth problem area the single-parent family, an interpersonal situation found frequently among adolescent treatment populations. Mufson and colleagues conducted an open feasibility and follow-up trial and then a controlled 12-week clinical trial comparing IPT for depressed adolescents (IPT-A) and clinical monitoring in 48 clinic-referred adolescents (ages 12–18 years) who met DSM-III-R (American Psychiatric Association 1987) criteria for major depressive disorder. Patients were seen biweekly by an independent evaluator blind to their treatment status for assessment of symptomatology, social functioning, and social problem-solving skills. Thirty-two of the 48 patients completed the protocol (21 assigned to IPT-A, 11 in control [clinical monitoring] group).

Patients who received IPT-A reported significantly greater improvement in depressive symptoms and overall social functioning, including functioning with friends and problem-solving skills. In the intent-to-treat sample, 75% of IPT-A patients met the criterion for recovery (HRSD score ≤ 6), compared with 46% of control patients. The findings support the feasibility, patient acceptance, and efficacy of 12 weeks of IPT-A with acutely depressed adolescents in reducing depressive symptomatology and improving social functioning and interpersonal problem-solving skills (Mufson et al. 1999). Mufson is currently completing an effectiveness study of IPT-A in school-based clinics and pilot-testing it in a group format for depressed adolescents.

Rosello, Bernal, and Rivera at the University of Puerto Rico compared 12 weeks of randomly assigned IPT ($n = 22$), CBT ($n = 25$), and a waiting-list control condition ($n = 24$) for adolescents ages 13–18 years who met DSM-III-R criteria for major depression, dysthymia, or both. The investigators did not use Mufson's IPT-A modification. They found both IPT and CBT to be more efficacious than the control condition in reducing adolescents' self-ratings of depressive symptoms. IPT was more effective than CBT in increasing self-esteem and social adaptation. The effect size for IPT was .73, and for CBT, .43 (Rossello and Bernal 1999).

Depressed HIV-Positive Patients (IPT-HIV)

Markowitz et al. (1992) modified IPT for depressed HIV patients (IPT-HIV), emphasizing common issues among this population, such as concerns about illness and death, grief, and role transitions. In a pilot open trial, 21 of the 24 depressed patients responded with symptom reduction. A 16-week study randomized 101 subjects to IPT-HIV, CBT, supportive psychotherapy, and imipramine plus supportive psychotherapy (Markowitz et al. 1998b).

Echoing the results seen with the more severely depressed subjects in the NIMH Treatment of Depression Collaborative Research Program study (Elkin et al. 1989), all treatments were associated with symptom reduction, but IPT and imipramine–supportive psychotherapy produced symptomatic and functional improvement significantly greater than that seen with CBT or supportive psychotherapy. Many patients reported improvement in depressive physical symptoms that they had mistakenly attributed to HIV infection.

Depressed Primary Care Patients

Schulberg and colleagues compared IPT and pharmacotherapy for depressed ambulatory medical patients in a primary care setting (Schulberg and Scott 1991; Schulberg et al. 1993). Although they did not modify the IPT manual, IPT was integrated into the routine of the primary care center (e.g., nurses took vital signs before each session). If patients were medically hospitalized, IPT was continued in the hospital when possible. Patients with current major depression ($n = 276$) were randomly assigned to IPT, nortriptyline, or primary care physicians' usual care. Patients receiving IPT were seen weekly for 16 weeks and monthly thereafter for 4 months (Schulberg et al. 1996). Depressive symptom severity declined more rapidly with either nortriptyline or IPT than with usual care. Approximately 70% of treatment completers receiving nortriptyline or IPT, but only 20% in usual care, had recovered after 8 months. Brown et al. (1996) found that subjects with a lifetime history of comorbid panic disorder had a poor response across treatments compared with those with major depression alone. These pilot findings on comorbid panic disorder have been corroborated by Frank et al. (2000a).

Conjoint IPT for Depressed Patients With Marital Disputes (IPT-CM)

Marital conflict, separation, and divorce can precipitate or complicate depressive episodes (Rounsaville et al. 1979). Some clinicians believe that individual psychotherapy for depressed patients in marital disputes may lead to premature rupture of marriages (Gurman and Kniskern 1978). Hence, a manual was developed for conjoint therapy of depressed patients with marital disputes (IPT-CM; Klerman and Weissman 1993). IPT-CM includes both spouses in all sessions and focuses on the current marital dispute. Eighteen patients with major depression linked to the onset or exacerbation of marital disputes were randomly assigned to 16 weeks of either individual IPT or IPT-CM. Patients in both treatments showed similar reductions in depressive symptoms, but patients receiving IPT-CM reported significantly better marital adjustment, marital affection, and sexual relations than did patients receiving individual IPT (Foley et al. 1989). These pilot findings require replication with a larger sample and other control groups.

Antepartum/Postpartum Depression

Spinelli at Columbia University is using IPT to treat women with antepartum depression. Examination of this role transition addresses the depressed pregnant woman's self-evaluation as a parent, the physiological changes of pregnancy, and altered relationships with the spouse or significant other and with other children. Spinelli added "complicated pregnancy" as a fifth interpersonal problem area. Timing and duration of sessions are adjusted in response to bed rest, delivery, obstetrical complications, and child care. Postpartum mothers may bring children to sessions. As with depressed HIV-positive patients, telephone sessions and hospital visits are sometimes necessary (Spinelli 1997). A controlled clinical trial comparing IPT with a didactic parent education group intervention in depressed pregnant women over 16 weeks of acute treatment and 6 monthly follow-up sessions is under way.

O'Hara et al. (2000) conducted a comparison of IPT and a waiting-list control condition in 120 women with postpartum depression. The 12-week trial had an 18-month follow-up. The investigators assessed both the mothers' symptom states and their interactions with their infants (Stuart and O'Hara 1995). Of the IPT group, 38% met HRSD and 44% met BDI remission criteria, compared with 14% on each of these measures for the waiting-list group. Sixty percent of IPT patients, versus 16% of control subjects, reported a greater than 50% reduction on the BDI. Women receiving IPT also showed significant improvement in social adjustment relative to the control group.

Klier et al. (2001) treated 17 women with postpartum depression in nine weekly 90-minute group sessions plus an hour-long individual termination session. Scores on the 21-item HRSD fell from 19.7 to 8.0, suggesting the efficacy of this approach. Zlotnick et al. (2001) treated 37 women at risk for postpartum depression with either four 60-minute sessions of a group based on IPT principles or usual treatment. Six of 18 women in the control condition (versus 0 of 17 in the interpersonal group) developed depression 3 months postpartum. This preventive application of what sounds like a group form of interpersonal counseling (Klerman et al. 1987) requires replication but is exciting.

Dysthymic Disorder (IPT-D)

A modification of IPT for dysthymic disorder (IPT-D) encourages patients to reconceptualize what they have considered their lifelong character flaws as ego-dystonic, chronic, mood-dependent symptoms—that is, as chronic but treatable state rather than immutable trait. Therapy itself was defined as an "iatrogenic role transition" from believing oneself flawed in personality to recognizing and obtaining treatment for one's mood disorder. Markowitz (1994, 1998) openly treated 17 pilot subjects with 16 sessions of IPT-D: none worsened, and 11 remitted. Medication benefits roughly half of dysthymic patients (Kocsis et al. 1988; Thase et al. 1996), but nonresponders may need psychotherapy, and even medication responders may benefit from combined treatment (Markowitz 1994). On the basis of these pilot results, a comparative study of 16 weeks of IPT-D alone, supportive psychotherapy, sertraline plus clinical management, and a combined IPT–sertraline cell is approaching completion at Weill Medical College of Cornell University.

Browne, Steiner and others at McMaster University in Hamilton, Ontario, treated more than 700 dysthymic patients in the community with either 12 sessions of standard IPT over 4 months, sertraline for 2 years, or their combination. Patients were followed for 2 years. Although results have not yet been published, preliminary findings have been presented at several conferences (e.g., World Psychiatric Association, Jerusalem, Israel, 1997; American Psychiatric Association Annual Meeting, Chicago, IL, May 2000). Using the criterion of a 40% reduction in score of the Montgomery–Åsberg Depression Rating Scale (MADRS) at 1-year follow-up, 51% of IPT-alone subjects improved, significantly fewer than the 63% taking sertraline and the 62% in combined treatment. On follow-up, however, IPT was associated with significant economic savings in use of health care and social services. Thus, combined treatment was as efficacious as but less expensive than sertraline alone.

Feijò de Mello et al. (2001) randomly assigned 35 dysthymic outpatients to receive moclobemide with or without 16 weekly sessions of IPT. Both groups improved, but there was a nonsignificant trend for greater improvement on the HRSD and MADRS in the combined-treatment group.

Bipolar Disorder

Frank and colleagues are assessing the benefits for bipolar patients of adjunctive IPT modified by social zeitgeber theory—behavioral scheduling of daily and sleep patterns (Ehlers et al. 1988; Malkoff-Schwartz et al. 2000)—as maintenance treatment of lithium-stabilized bipolar patients, comparing interpersonal social rhythms therapy (IPSRT) with medication alone (Frank 1991; Frank et al. 2000b). Acutely ill bipolar patients are treated with medication and are randomly assigned to either IPSRT or clinical management. After achieving 4 weeks of stabilization, they are again randomized to either IPSRT or clinical management for 3 years of maintenance treatment while continuing pharmacotherapy.

A preliminary report comparing adjunctive IPSRT and conventional medication-clinic treatment found no statistically significant differences between the two in the acute phase, although median time to remission was 21 weeks with IPSRT versus 40 weeks with clinical management ($n = 22$). Of the first 82 subjects to enter the maintenance phase, patients who received the same treatment (i.e., IPSRT or clinical management) in both phases had lower recurrence rates and symptom scores over the following 52 weeks than did those reassigned from one treatment to the other (Frank et al. 1999). Yet in subsequent analyses it appeared that the switch from acute IPSRT to maintenance clinical management increased the risk of depressive recurrence (Frank et al. 2000b). Furthermore, patients who received maintenance IPSRT had fewer depressive symptoms but a similar rate of manic episodes compared with patients receiving clinical management (Frank et al. 1999).

Subsyndromally Depressed Hospitalized Elderly Patients

Mossey et al. (1996) noted that even depressive symptoms that did not reach the threshold for major depression impeded recovery of hospitalized elderly patients. They conducted a 10-session trial of a modification of IPT, administered by nonpsychiatric nurses, called interpersonal counseling (IPC; Klerman et al. 1987) for elderly hospitalized medical patients with minor depressive symptoms. Patients were seen for 1-hour sessions on a flexible schedule that accommodated the patient's medical status. Seventy-six hospitalized patients over age 60 years who did not meet criteria for major depression but who had depressive symptoms on two consecutive assessments were randomly assigned to either IPC or usual care. Researchers also followed a euthymic, untreated control group. Patients found IPC tolerable. Assessment after 3 months showed nonsignificantly greater improvement in depressive symptoms and on all outcome variables for IPC relative to usual care, whereas control subjects showed a slight symptomatic worsening. Rehospitalization rates in the IPC and euthymic control groups were virtually identical (11%–15%) and were significantly less than those in the subsyndromally depressed group receiving usual care (50%). Differences between IPC and usual-care groups reached statistical significance at 6 months on depressive symptom reduction and self-rated health, but not on physical or social functioning. The investigators felt that 10 sessions were insufficient for some patients and that a maintenance phase might have been useful.

IPT for Nonmood Disorders

The efficacy of IPT as a treatment for depression has led to its adaptation as a treatment for other psychiatric disorders. Life events are ubiquitous, but when is it useful to focus treatment on them? Research is beginning to answer such questions.

Substance Abuse

IPT failed to demonstrate efficacy in two clinical trials for patients with substance abuse. Rounsaville et al. (1983) at Yale studied 72 methadone-maintained opiate abusers and found that adding adjunctive IPT to standard substance abuse care had no additional benefit in reducing psychopathology. Both treatment groups improved. The same researchers found that IPT was ineffective and marginally inferior to a behavioral control intervention in helping 42 subjects with cocaine abuse to achieve abstinence (Carroll et al. 1991). Although these two negative studies suggest limits to IPT's range of utility, they do not necessarily preclude its use for substance abuse. IPT might be useful, for example, as a treatment for newly abstinent alcohol-dependent patients, who face psychosocial stressors that have been shown to precipitate relapse.

Bulimia

Fairburn et al. (1993) adapted IPT for use with bulimia patients, eliminating the sick-role and role-playing components so that relatively distinct strategies could be contrasted in a comparison of IPT and CBT. Initial trials showed that although CBT achieved results more quickly, IPT had longer-term benefits that were comparable to those of CBT and superior to those of a behavioral control condition (Fairburn et al. 1995). In a subsequent multisite trial, however, CBT was superior to IPT (Agras et al. 2000). A research group in Christchurch, New Zealand, is currently studying the application of IPT to anorexia nervosa.

Wilfley et al. (1993, 2000) developed a modified version of IPT for use in a 16-week, 90-minute-session group format (IPT-G). They compared this intervention with group CBT and a waiting-list control condition for 56 women with nonpurging bulimia. At termination, binge eating had decreased in the IPT-G and CBT groups but not in the waiting-list condition. Results persisted at 1-year follow-up. A randomized clinical trial is now comparing group IPT and CBT for 20 sessions over 20 weeks among 162 women. The initial IPT phase—in which the therapist identifies problem areas, presents IPT concepts, and offers a treatment contract—is conducted individually.

Social Phobia

Although it has not yet been tested in controlled studies as a treatment for anxiety disorders, IPT has been modified for social phobia independently by two research groups. Lipsitz et al. (1999) at Columbia University treated nine IPT pilot cases and found promising results for social phobia. They noted that such standard IPT ingredients as the medical model, provision of the sick role, and the supportive therapeutic stance appear to benefit most patients. A controlled trial is now under way. Stuart and O'Hara at the University of Iowa are also testing IPT for social phobia. Weissman and Jacobson at Columbia University have adapted IPT in a 10-session group intervention for shy patients who experience social phobia in unstructured interpersonal situations (i.e., at parties, in intimate discussions with significant others, but not in defined work situations).

Panic Disorder

Arzt and van Rijsoort in Maastricht, The Netherlands, are studying IPT as a treatment for panic disorder.

Posttraumatic Stress Disorder

Posttraumatic stress disorder (PTSD) is an anxiety disorder defined by a life event, which might suggest the utility of IPT in its treatment. Krupnick and colleagues are assessing a group form of IPT for multiply victimized women in public-sector gynecology clinics in Virginia. Markowitz and colleagues at Cornell University are testing an individual form of IPT for PTSD.

Other Applications

Research groups are testing the applicability of IPT to body dysmorphic disorder, chronic somatization in primary care patients, depression in post–myocardial infarction patients (Stuart and Cole 1996), depression in cancer patients, borderline personality disorder, insomnia, and other disorders (Weissman et al. 2000). IPT's focus on life events suggests its potential applicability to patients with medical illness.

Interpersonal Counseling

Many patients presenting to primary care physicians report psychiatric symptoms yet do not meet full criteria for a psychiatric disorder. Their symptoms can be debilitating and may result in high utilization of medical procedures (Wells et al. 1989). Based on IPT, IPC was designed to treat distressed primary care patients who do not meet full syndromal criteria for psychiatric disorders. IPC is administered for a maximum of six sessions by health care professionals without formal psychiatric training, usually nurse practitioners. The first session can last up to 30 minutes, with subsequent sessions shorter in duration.

In IPC, therapists assess patients' current functioning, recent life events, occupational and familial stressors, and changes in interpersonal relationships. They assume that such events provide the context in which emotional and bodily symptoms occur. Klerman et al. (1987) conducted a study with 128 patients in a primary care clinic who scored 6 or higher on the Goldberg General Health Questionnaire (GHQ), randomizing them either to IPC or to usual care without psychological treatment (Klerman et al. 1987). Over an average of 3 months, often receiving only one or two IPC sessions, patients receiving IPC showed significantly greater symptom relief (especially mood improvement) on the GHQ than did control subjects. IPC subjects were more likely to subsequently make use of mental health services, suggesting a new awareness of the psychological aspect of their symptoms.

IPC and IPT by Telephone

Because many patients avoid or have difficulty traveling to an office for face-to-face treatment, IPC is being tested as a telephone treatment. Weissman and Miller at Columbia University are conducting a pilot feasibility trial comparing IPT by telephone with no treatment in 30 patients with recurrent major depression who have not received regular treatment. Another study, by Neugebauer and colleagues at Columbia University College of Physicians and Surgeons/New York State Psychiatric Institute, is testing telephone IPC as an intervention for women with minor depression postmiscarriage.

IPT Patient Guide

Weissman (1995) developed a user-friendly IPT patient guide with worksheets for depressed readers who want information about or are receiving IPT. The worksheets can be used to facilitate sessions or to monitor problem areas after treatment. The utility of this patient guide in enhancing treatment has not been studied.

Summary

IPT has demonstrated efficacy as an acute and maintenance monotherapy and as a component of combined treatment for major depressive disorder. It also appears to have utility for other mood and nonmood syndromes, although the evidence for these is sparser. Because monotherapy with either IPT or pharmacotherapy is likely to suffice for most depressed patients, combined treatment is probably best reserved for severely or chronically ill patients (Rush and Thase 1999). How best to combine time-limited psychotherapy with pharmacotherapy—for which patients, in what sequence, and so forth—is an exciting area for future research.

When is one treatment likely to have a better outcome than another? Comparative trials are beginning to reveal moderating factors or predictors of treatment outcome. Studies such as the NIMH Treatment of Depression Collaborative Research Program, which compared IPT and CBT, have suggested factors that might predict better outcome with either IPT or CBT (Table 27–6). Sotsky et al. (1991) found that depressed patients with a low baseline level of social dysfunction responded well to IPT, whereas those with severe social deficits (probably equivalent to the "interpersonal deficits" problem area) responded less well. Patients with greater symptom severity and difficulty in concentrating responded poorly to CBT. Initial severity of major depression and of impaired functioning predicted superior response to IPT and to imipramine. Imipramine also worked most efficaciously for patients with difficulty functioning at work, a result that likely reflects its quicker onset of action. Patients with atypical depression responded better to either IPT or CBT than to imipramine or placebo (Shea et al. 1999).

Barber and Muenz (1996), examining only Treatment of Depression Collaborative Research Program completers, found IPT to be more efficacious than CBT for patients with obsessive-compulsive personality disorder, whereas those with avoidant personality disorder fared better with CBT. An abnormal sleep profile on electroencephalogram predicted significantly poorer response to

TABLE 27–6. Choosing between interpersonal psychotherapy (IPT) and cognitive-behavioral therapy (CBT)

Predictor	IPT	CBT
Life events	Present	Absent
Social dysfunction (baseline)	Low	Very high ("interpersonal deficits")
Symptom severity (baseline)	Higher	Lower
Personality disorder	Obsessive	Avoidant

IPT in comparison with normal sleep parameters (Thase et al. 1997). Frank et al. (1991) found that psychotherapist adherence to a focused IPT approach may enhance outcome. The replication and further elaboration of these predictive factors deserve ongoing study.

IPT Training

Until recently, IPT practitioners were few in number and almost exclusively limited to therapists in research studies. In response to clinical demand for this empirically supported treatment, IPT training is now increasingly included in professional workshops and conferences, with training courses conducted at university centers in Canada, the United Kingdom, continental Europe, Asia, New Zealand, and Australia. IPT is taught in a small but growing number of psychiatric residency training programs in the United States (Markowitz 1995) and has been included in family practice and primary care training (L.A. Gillies, personal communication, 1996).

Although the principles and practices of IPT are straightforward, any psychotherapy requires some innate therapeutic ability, and IPT training requires more than reading the manual (Rounsaville et al. 1988; Weissman et al. 1982). Psychotherapy is learned by doing. Most IPT training programs are designed to help experienced therapists refocus their treatment by learning new techniques, not to teach novices how to conduct psychotherapy. Candidates should have a graduate clinical degree (M.D., Ph.D., M.S.W., R.N.), several years of experience conducting psychotherapy, and clinical familiarity with the diagnosis of patients they plan to treat.

The IPT training used in the Treatment of Depression Collaborative Research Program (Elkin et al. 1989) became the model for subsequent research studies. It includes a brief didactic program, review of the manual, and a longer practicum in which the therapist treats two to three patients under close supervision monitored by videotapes of the sessions (Chevron and Rounsaville 1983). Rounsaville et al. (1986) found that psychotherapists who performed well on an initial supervised IPT case often did not require further intensive supervision,

and that experienced therapists committed to the approach required less supervision than others (Rounsaville et al. 1988). Some clinicians have taught themselves IPT by using as guides the IPT manual (Klerman et al. 1984) and peer supervision. For research certification, we continue to recommend at least two or three successfully treated cases with hour-for-hour supervision of taped sessions (Markowitz 2001).

There is no formal certificate for IPT proficiency and no accrediting board. When the practice of IPT was restricted to research settings, this was not a problem: one research group taught another in the manner described above. With the spread of IPT into clinical practice, however, issues have arisen about standards for clinical training, and questions of competence and accreditation have gained greater urgency. As was noted in the surgeon general's recent report (Satcher 1999), IPT training programs are still not widely available. Many psychiatry residency and psychology training programs still focus on long-term psychodynamic psychotherapy or on cognitive therapy; in these programs, too, the lack of exposure to time-limited treatment has been noted (Weissman and Sanderson, in press). Psychiatric residency and other mental health care treatment training programs should include clinical instruction in the time-limited psychotherapies described in manuals, in addition to providing exposure to long-term psychotherapy. To our knowledge, no accepted model psychotherapy curriculum is available.

The educational process for IPT in clinical practice requires further study. We do not know, for example, what levels of education and experience are required to learn IPT, or how much supervision an already experienced psychotherapist is likely to require.

The Future

The history of IPT consists of its testing in a succession of outcome trials that have helped to define its diagnostic indications. Because psychotherapy is underfunded relative to pharmacotherapy, we know far less about the indications for and optimal dosages of IPT than about antidepressant medication. Future outcome trials may continue to define the territory of IPT's utility. These should include trials for different diagnoses (e.g., the anxiety disorders), testing of dosages (i.e., optimal frequency and duration of IPT sessions), and studies of the sequencing of IPT with other treatments. Questions to be answered include the following: When, and for whom, is IPT best combined with pharmacotherapy? Is it best to start with pharmacotherapy and then add IPT? If so, at what interval, and with what frequency? When should IPT be used as augmentation for pharmacotherapy, and vice versa? Other research may help to determine the cost-effectiveness and potential cost-offset of IPT as a treatment that improves both symptoms and social functioning.

IPT is also anomalous among psychotherapies in its nearly pure focus to date on outcome studies. Until recent decades, almost all psychotherapy research consisted of process research—an analysis of what occurred between patient and therapist in sessions. The late Gerald L. Klerman affirmed the primacy of outcome research, emphasizing that if the therapy had no actual clinical benefit, its mechanism would hold little interest. Now that it is clear that IPT helps many patients, process research seems warranted to try to identify its active, mediating factors. Little is known about the specific value of many IPT interventions. It is even unclear, for example, whether focusing on a role transition rather than a role dispute makes a difference for patients, or whether particular sorts of life events are helpful or unhelpful foci. Patient and therapist characteristics may also potentially influence treatment outcome.

Clinical training in IPT is likely to increase. How it spreads will be a function of training programs. Training will probably need to be formalized and accredited, both to ensure clinical competence and to satisfy managed care organizations. Research is needed on how best to teach and disseminate IPT.

In summary, IPT is a time-limited, forward-looking, pragmatically focused psychotherapy that defines psychiatric disorders as treatable medical illnesses and links them to the patient's current social situation. This strategy has proved efficacious for patients with major depression and bulimia, and it shows promise for other mood and nonmood disorders as well.

References

Agency for Health Care Policy and Research: Depression in Primary Care, Vol 1: Detection and Diagnosis (Clinical Guideline Number 5; AHCPR Publ No 93-0550). Rockville, MD, Agency for Health Care Policy and Research, 1993a

Agency for Health Care Policy and Research: Depression in Primary Care, Vol 2: Treatment of Major Depression (Clinical Practice Guideline Number 5; AHCPR Publ No 93-0551). Rockville, MD, Agency for Health Care Policy and Research, 1993b

Agency for Health Care Policy and Research: Depression in Primary Care, Vol 3: Detection, Diagnosis, and Treatment (Quick Reference Guideline Number 5; AHCPR Publ No 93-0552). Rockville, MD, Agency for Health Care Policy and Research, 1993c

Agency for Health Care Policy and Research: Depression in Primary Care, Vol 4. Depression Is a Treatable Illness: A Patient's Guide (Consumer Guideline Number 5; AHCPR Publ No 93-0553). Rockville, MD, Agency for Health Care Policy and Research, 1993d

Agras WS, Walsh BT, Fairburn CG, et al: A multicenter comparison of cognitive-behavioral therapy and interpersonal psychotherapy for bulimia nervosa. Arch Gen Psychiatry 57:459–466, 2000

American Psychiatric Association: Diagnostic and Statistical Manual of Mental Disorders, 3rd Edition, Revised. Washington, DC, American Psychiatric Association, 1987

American Psychiatric Association: Diagnostic and Statistical Manual of Mental Disorders, 4th Edition. Washington, DC, American Psychiatric Association, 1994

Barber JP, Muenz LR: The role of avoidance and obsessiveness in matching patients to cognitive and interpersonal psychotherapy: empirical findings from the Treatment for Depression Collaborative Research Program. J Consult Clin Psychol 64:951–958, 1996

Beck AT: Depression Inventory. Philadelphia, PA, Center for Cognitive Therapy, 1978

Beck AT, Rush AJ, Shaw BF, et al: Cognitive Therapy of Depression. New York, Guilford, 1979

Blom MBJ, Hoencamp E, Zwaan T: Interpersoonlijke psychotherapie voor depressie: een pilot-onderzoek. Tijdschrift voor Psychiatr 38:398–402, 1996

Brown C, Schulberg HC, Madonia MJ, et al: Treatment outcomes for primary care patients with major depression and lifetime anxiety disorders. Am J Psychiatry 153:1293–1300, 1996

Carroll KM, Rounsaville BJ, Gawin FH: A comparative trial of psychotherapies for ambulatory cocaine abusers: relapse prevention and interpersonal psychotherapy. Am J Drug Alcohol Abuse 17:229–247, 1991

Chevron ES, Rounsavillle BJ: Evaluating the clinical skills of psychotherapists: a comparison of techniques. Arch Gen Psychiatry 40:1129–1132, 1983

DiMascio A, Weissman MM, Prusoff BA, et al: Differential symptom reduction by drugs and psychotherapy in acute depression. Arch Gen Psychiatry 36:1450–1456, 1979

Ehlers CL, Frank E, Kupfer DJ: Social zeitgebers and biological rhythms: a unified approach to understanding the etiology of depression. Arch Gen Psychiatry 45:948–952, 1988

Elkin I, Shea MT, Watkins JT, et al: National Institute of Mental Health Treatment of Depression Collaborative Research Program: general effectiveness of treatments. Arch Gen Psychiatry 46:971–982, 1989

Fairburn CG, Jones R, Peveler RC, et al: Psychotherapy and bulimia nervosa: longer-term effects of interpersonal psychotherapy, behavior therapy, and cognitive behavior therapy. Arch Gen Psychiatry 50:419–428, 1993

Fairburn CG, Norman PA, Welch SL, et al: A prospective study of outcome in bulimia nervosa and the long-term effects of three psychological treatments. Arch Gen Psychiatry 52:304–312, 1995

Feijò de Mello M, Myczowisk LM, Menezes PR: A randomized controlled trial comparing moclobemide and moclobemide plus interpersonal psychotherapy in the treatment of dysthymic disorder. J Psychother Pract Res 10:117–123, 2001

Foley SH, Rounsaville BJ, Weissman MM, et al: Individual versus conjoint interpersonal psychotherapy for depressed patients with marital disputes. Int J Fam Psychiatry 10:29–42, 1989

Frank E: Biological order and bipolar disorder. Paper presented at the meeting of the American Psychosomatic Society, Santa Fe, NM, March 1991

Frank E, Kupfer DJ, Perel JM, et al: Three-year outcomes for maintenance therapies in recurrent depression. Arch Gen Psychiatry 47:1093–1099, 1990

Frank E, Kupfer DJ, Wagner EF, et al: Efficacy of interpersonal psychotherapy as a maintenance treatment of recurrent depression. Arch Gen Psychiatry 48:1053–1059, 1991

Frank E, Swartz HA, Mallinger AG, et al: Adjunctive psychotherapy for bipolar disorder: effects of changing treatment modality. J Abnorm Psychol 108:579–587, 1999

Frank E, Shear MK, Rucci P, et al: Influence of panic-agoraphobic spectrum symptoms on treatment response in patients with recurrent major depression. Am J Psychiatry 157:1101–1107, 2000a

Frank E, Swartz HA, Kupfer DJ: Interpersonal and social rhythm therapy: managing the chaos of bipolar disorder. Biol Psychiatry 48:593–604, 2000b

Gurman AS, Kniskern DP: Research on marital and family therapy: progress, perspective, and prospect, in Handbook of Psychotherapy and Behavior Change. Edited by Garfield SB, Bergen AB. New York, Wiley, 1978, pp 817–902

Hamilton M: A rating scale for depression. J Neurol Neurosurg Psychiatry 25:56–62, 1960

Hirschfeld RMA, Klerman GL, Clayton PJ, et al: Assessing personality: effects of the depressive state on trait measurement. Am J Psychiatry 140:695–699, 1983

Karasu TB, Docherty JP, Gelenberg A, et al: Practice guideline for major depressive disorder in adults. Am J Psychiatry 150(suppl):1–26, 1993

Klein DF, Ross DC: Reanalysis of the National Institute of Mental Health Treatment of Depression Collaborative Research Program general effectiveness report. Neuropsychopharmacology 8:241–251, 1993

Klerman GL, Weissman MM: New Applications of Interpersonal Psychotherapy. Washington, DC, American Psychiatric Press, 1993

Klerman GL, DiMascio A, Weissman MM, et al: Treatment of depression by drugs and psychotherapy. Am J Psychiatry 131:186–191, 1974

Klerman GL, Weissman MM, Rounsaville BJ, et al: Interpersonal Psychotherapy of Depression. New York, Basic Books, 1984

Klerman GL, Budman S, Berwick D, et al: Efficacy of a brief psychosocial intervention for symptoms of stress and distress among patients in primary care. Med Care 25:1078–1088, 1987

Klier CM, Muzik M, Rosenblum KL, et al: Interpersonal psychotherapy adapted for the group setting in the treatment of postpartum depression. J Psychother Pract Res 10:124–131, 2001

Kocsis JH, Frances AJ, Voss C, et al: Imipramine treatment for chronic depression. Arch Gen Psychiatry 45:253–257, 1988

Lipsitz JD, Fyer AJ, Markowitz JC, et al: An open trial of interpersonal psychotherapy for social phobia. Am J Psychiatry 156:1814–1816, 1999

Malkoff-Schwartz S, Frank E, Anderson BP, et al: Social rhythm disruption and stressful life events in the onset of bipolar and unipolar episodes. Psychol Med 30:1005–1016, 2000

Markowitz JC: Psychotherapy of dysthymia. Am J Psychiatry 151:1114–1121, 1994

Markowitz JC: Teaching interpersonal psychotherapy to psychiatric residents. Academic Psychiatry 19:167–173, 1995

Markowitz JC: Interpersonal Psychotherapy for Dysthymic Disorder. Washington, DC, American Psychiatric Press, 1998

Markowitz JC: Learning the new psychotherapies, in Treatment of Depression: Bridging the 21st Century. Edited by Weissman MM. Washington, DC, American Psychiatric Publishing, 2001, pp 281–300

Markowitz JC, Swartz HA: Case formulation in interpersonal psychotherapy of depression, in Handbook of Psychotherapy Case Formulation. Edited by Eels TD. New York, Guilford, 1997, pp 192–222

Markowitz JC, Klerman GL, Perry SW, et al: Interpersonal therapy of depressed HIV-seropositive patients. Hosp Community Psychiatry 43:885–890, 1992

Markowitz JC, Svartberg M, Swartz HA: Is IPT time-limited psychodynamic psychotherapy? J Psychother Pract Res 7:185–195, 1998a

Markowitz JC, Kocsis JH, Fishman B, et al: Treatment of HIV-positive patients with depressive symptoms. Arch Gen Psychiatry 55:452–457, 1998b

Markowitz JC, Leon AC, Miller NL, et al: Rater agreement on interpersonal psychotherapy problem areas. J Psychother Pract Res 9:131–135, 2000

Mental health: does therapy help? Consumer Reports, November 1995, pp 734–739

Mossey JM, Knott KA, Higgins M, et al: Effectiveness of a psychosocial intervention, interpersonal counseling, for subdysthymic depression in medically ill elderly. J Gerontol 51A:M172–M178, 1996

Mufson L, Moreau D, Weissman MM: Interpersonal Therapy for Depressed Adolescents. New York, Guilford, 1993

Mufson L, Weissman MM, Moreau D, et al: Efficacy of interpersonal psychotherapy for depressed adolescents. Arch Gen Psychiatry 56:573–579, 1999

O'Hara MW, Stuart S, Gorman LL, et al: Efficacy of interpersonal psychotherapy for postpartum depression. Arch Gen Psychiatry 57:1039–1045, 2000

Parsons T: Illness and the role of the physician: a sociological perspective. Am J Orthopsychiatry 21:452–460, 1951

Paykel ES, DiMascio A, Haskell D, et al: Effects of maintenance amitriptyline and psychotherapy on symptoms of depression. Psychol Med 5:67–77, 1975

Puig JS: Psicoterapia interpersonal (1). Rev Psiquiatría Fac Med Barna 22:91–99, 1995

Reynolds CF III, Frank E, Perel JM, et al: Nortriptyline and interpersonal psychotherapy as maintenance therapies for recurrent major depression: a randomized controlled trial in patients older than 59 years. JAMA 281:39–45, 1999

Rossello J, Bernal G: The efficacy of cognitive-behavioral and interpersonal treatments for depression in Puerto Rican adolescents. J Consult Clin Psychol 67:734–745, 1999

Rothblum ED, Sholomskas AJ, Berry C, et al: Issues in clinical trials with the depressed elderly. J Am Geriatr Soc 30:694–699, 1982

Rounsaville BJ, Weissman MM, Prusoff BA, et al: Marital disputes and treatment outcome in depressed women. Compr Psychiatry 20:483–490, 1979

Rounsaville BJ, Glazer W, Wilber CH, et al: Short-term interpersonal psychotherapy in methadone-maintained opiate addicts. Arch Gen Psychiatry 40:629–636, 1983

Rounsaville BJ, Chevron ES, Weissman MM, et al: Training therapists to perform interpersonal psychotherapy in clinical trials. Compr Psychiatry 27:364–371, 1986

Rounsaville BJ, O'Malley SS, Foley SH, et al: The role of manual-guided training in the conduct and efficacy of interpersonal psychotherapy for depression. J Consult Clin Psychol 56:681–688, 1988

Rush AJ, Thase ME: Psychotherapies for depressive disorders: a review, in Depressive Disorders: WPA Series Evidence and Experience in Psychiatry. Edited by Maj M, Sartorius N. Chichester, UK, Wiley, 1999, pp 161–206

Satcher D: Surgeon General's Reference: Mental Health: A Report of the Surgeon General. Rockville, MD, U.S. Department of Health and Human Services, 1999

Schulberg HC, Scott CP: Depression in primary care: treating depression with interpersonal psychotherapy, in Psychotherapy in Managed Health Care: The Optimal Use of Time and Resources. Edited by Austad CS, Berman WH. Washington, DC, American Psychological Association, 1991, pp 153–170

Schulberg HC, Scott CP, Madonia MJ, et al: Applications of interpersonal psychotherapy to depression in primary care practice, in New Applications of Interpersonal Psychotherapy. Edited by Klerman GL, Weissman MM. Washington, DC, American Psychiatric Press, 1993, pp 265–291

Schulberg HC, Block MR, Madonia MJ, et al: Treating major depression in primary care practice. Arch Gen Psychiatry 53:913–919, 1996

Seligman MEP: The effectiveness of psychotherapy: the Consumer Reports study. Am Psychol 12:965–974, 1995

Shea MT, Elkin I, Imber SD, et al: Course of depressive symptoms over follow-up: findings from the National Institute of Mental Health Treatment for Depression Collaborative Research Program. Arch Gen Psychiatry 49:782–787, 1992

Shea MT, Elkin I, Sotsky SM: Patient characteristics associated with successful treatment: outcome findings from the NIMH Treatment of Depression Collaborative Research Program, in Psychotherapy Indications and Outcomes. Edited by Janowsky DS. Washington, DC, American Psychiatric Press, 1999, pp 71–90

Sholomskas AJ, Chevron ES, Prusoff BA, et al: Short-term interpersonal therapy (IPT) with the depressed elderly: case reports and discussion. Am J Psychother 36:552–566, 1983

Sloane RB, Stapes FR, Schneider LS: Interpersonal therapy versus nortriptyline for depression in the elderly, in Clinical and Pharmacological Studies in Psychiatric Disorders. Edited by Burrows GD, Norman TR, Dennerstein L. London, England, John Libbey, 1985, pp 344–346

Sotsky SM, Glass DR, Shea MT, et al: Patient predictors of response to psychotherapy and pharmacotherapy: findings in the NIMH treatment of depression collaborative research program. Am J Psychiatry 148:997–1008, 1991

Spinelli M: Manual of interpersonal psychotherapy for antepartum depressed women (IPT-P), 1997 (Available through Dr. Spinelli, Columbia University College of Physicians and Surgeons, New York, NY)

Stuart S, Cole V: Treatment of depression following myocardial infarction with interpersonal psychotherapy. Ann Clin Psychiatry 8:203–206, 1996

Stuart S, O'Hara MW: IPT for postpartum depression. J Psychother Pract Res 4:18–29, 1995

Sullivan HS (ed): The Interpersonal Theory of Psychiatry. New York, WW Norton, 1953

Thase ME, Fava M, Halbreich U, et al: A placebo-controlled, randomized clinical trial comparing sertraline and imipramine for the treatment of dysthymia. Arch Gen Psychiatry 53:777–784, 1996

Thase ME, Buysse DJ, Frank E, et al: Which depressed patients will respond to interpersonal psychotherapy? The role of abnormal EEG profiles. Am J Psychiatry 154:502–509, 1997

Weissman MM: Mastering Depression: A Patient Guide to Interpersonal Psychotherapy. Albany, NY, Graywind Publications, 1995 (Currently available through The Psychological Corporation, Order Service Center, P.O. Box 839954, San Antonio, TX 78283-3954, Tel 1-800-228-0752, Fax 1-800-232-1223)

Weissman MM, Sanderson WC: Problems and promises in modern psychotherapy: the need for increased training in evidence-based treatments, in Modern Psychiatry: Challenges in Educating Health Professionals to Meet New Needs. Edited by Hamburg B. New York, Josia Macy Foundation, in press

Weissman MM, Klerman GL, Paykel ES, et al: Treatment effects on the social adjustment of depressed patients. Arch Gen Psychiatry. 30:771–778, 1974

Weissman MM, Prusoff BA, DiMascio A, et al: The efficacy of drugs and psychotherapy in the treatment of acute depressive episodes. Am J Psychiatry 136:555–558, 1979

Weissman MM, Klerman GL, Prusoff BA, et al: Depressed outpatients: results one year after treatment with drugs and/or interpersonal psychotherapy. Arch Gen Psychiatry 38:52–55, 1981

Weissman MM, Rounsaville BJ, Chevron ES: Training psychotherapists to participate in psychotherapy outcome studies: Identifying and dealing with the research requirement. Am J Psychiatry 139:1442–1446, 1982

Weissman MM, Markowitz JC, Klerman GL: Comprehensive Guide to Interpersonal Psychotherapy. New York, Basic Books, 2000

Wells KB, Stewart A, Hayes RD, et al: The functioning and well-being of depressed patients: results of the medical outcomes study. JAMA 262:914–919, 1989

Wilfley DE, Agras WS, Telch CF, et al: Group cognitive-behavioral therapy and group interpersonal psychotherapy for the nonpurging bulimic individual: a controlled comparison. J Consult Clin Psychol 61:296–305, 1993

Wilfley DE, MacKenzie RK, Welch RR, et al: Interpersonal Psychotherapy for Group. New York, Basic Books, 2000

Zlotnick C, Johnson SL, Miller IW, et al: Postpartum depression in women receiving public assistance: pilot study of an interpersonal-therapy-oriented group intervention. Am J Psychiatry 158:638–640, 2001

Behavior Therapies

Robert I. Berkowitz, M.D.

Behavior therapy developed as a scientific approach to human behavior change. The search for an understanding of the process of learning moved from the field of philosophy to the newly developing field of psychology late in the nineteenth century. Association theory had already been developed by the British school of philosophical empiricism, but it was Pavlov and his co-workers who demonstrated the basic principles of learning by contiguity and the way in which new connections could be acquired, generalized, and extinguished. In the United States, first Thorndike and then Skinner and his colleagues demonstrated how the environment alters behavior and introduced principles such as reinforcement, punishment, and stimulus control. In broad terms, Skinner postulated that the environmental consequences of behavior determined which actions would be strengthened and which would be weakened over time.

These developments were contemporary with the development of psychoanalytic theory and practice, and beginning in the 1950s numerous attempts were made to integrate the more recently developed learning theories and psychoanalytic theory. These attempts failed to gain acceptance from either psychoanalytic theorists or learning theorists, perhaps because they did not lead to new testable propositions. Thus, behavior therapy developed as an alternative way of understanding and treating disordered behavior, being sparked by the failure to demonstrate the efficacy of psychoanalysis. Among the basic principles underlying the conceptual basis for behavior therapy are the following:

1. Both normal and abnormal behaviors are assumed to be learned and maintained in the same way; thus, procedures that alter normal behaviors will also be useful in altering deviant behaviors. An example of this is positive reinforcement, which affects a wide range of behaviors across a variety of different species and which has proven useful in modifying many problem behaviors.

2. The social environment plays a key role in the development and maintenance of both normal and abnormal behaviors. A consequence of this view is that the patient's environment may need to be altered to maintain newly acquired behaviors and prevent relapse.

3. The major focus of treatment is on the behavior problem itself, and, thus, specification of both the behaviors to be changed and the circumstances presently maintaining those behaviors is an important facet of assessment and treatment. Behaviors requiring treatment will usually be broken up into discrete components, each of which will be treated using individually tailored procedures depending on the behavior and its antecedents and consequences.

4. Behavior therapy is based on a scientific approach to treatment. Treatment procedures must be well specified so that they can be replicated by others; this involves the development of detailed treatment manuals. Treatment procedures must be evaluated in controlled experiments and the active components of treatment separated from inactive components by additive clinical experimental designs.

Social-cognitive learning theory (Bandura 1986) has now become the most widely accepted theoretical underpinning of behavior therapy. This theory incorporates elements of both Pavlovian and Skinnerian theories but goes beyond these in postulating an interaction between environment, behavior, and cognitive processes. Not only does the environment affect the person, but the person can alter his or her personal environment, thus affecting future behavior. Reinforcement is viewed not as the automatic effect of reward but rather as a source of information about the potential effects of future behavior. Similarly, classical conditioning is no longer viewed as an automatic result of the occurrence of two stimuli occurring closely in time. Experimental work has demonstrated that prior experience and recognition of the relatedness of events are often crucial to this type of learning. Hence, cognitive processes are recognized as important modulators of behavior.

Basic research is beginning to unravel the biology of learning. It is now clear that learning leads to neurochemical changes in the central nervous system. Work with the simple organism *Aplysia*, a sea mollusk, has revealed that when this animal learns avoidance behavior, the chemical structure of cells in the nervous system is altered. When the avoidance behavior disappears—for example, through repeated exposure—the chemical changes are reversed (Kandel 1989). Hence, there is a reciprocal interaction between biological processes in the central nervous system and behavior changes resulting from environmental influences. Because psychotherapy involves learning new ways of behaving, and learning produces neurochemical changes, the behavior changes associated with therapy should be detectable by imaging methods. In a study of patients with obsessive-compulsive disorder (OCD), positron emission tomography was used to investigate changes in rates of glucose metabolism in the cerebrum before and after treatment with behavior therapy (Baxter et al. 1992). Rates of glucose metabolism in the right head of the caudate nucleus changed when the OCD was successfully treated but did not change in patients who did not respond to treatment. Moreover, these changes were similar to those produced by antidepressant treatment.

In addition to developments in theory and practice, behavior therapy has reached into new areas of endeavor. These include the development of behavioral pediatrics and behavioral medicine, which have in turn taken behavior therapy into preventive medicine. Another active area of research involves investigations of the interaction between behavior therapy and pharmacological treatments. Finally, the development of effective manualized therapies derived from perspectives other than behavior therapy not only allows comparisons of behavior therapy with these procedures but also allows the testing of differing hypotheses regarding the processes by which therapeutic behavior change occurs.

It should be recognized that behavior therapy is not a monolithic procedure; rather, it involves the application of a variety of well-specified therapeutic procedures that have been packaged to treat or prevent a variety of disorders. The large number of applications of behavior therapy to the wide variety of psychiatric problems and the extensive research literature preclude a comprehensive account in this chapter. Thus, the focus will be on applications in a few common disorders.

Therapeutic Procedures

In the following paragraphs, some therapeutic procedures commonly used in behavior therapy are detailed. Many of these procedures form one component of a more complex therapeutic package that has been designed for a particular psychiatric disorder and tested in controlled outcome studies. It should be recognized that certain procedures common to all therapies are employed in such therapeutic packages—including a therapeutic rationale and therapeutic instructions—and that a satisfactory therapeutic relationship is as essential to behavior therapy as it is to other psychotherapies.

Systematic Desensitization

Systematic desensitization, a procedure introduced by Wolpe (1958), is most often used in the treatment of phobias (see "Anxiety Disorders" section later in this chapter). After a thorough exploration of the patient's phobia, a hierarchy of feared situations along one dimension is created—for example, for a patient with height phobia, looking down from the second floor of a building to looking down from a skyscraper, with many gradual steps in between. The patient is then taught deep muscle relaxation (see "Relaxation Training" subsection below) and next visualizes the first item in the hierarchy for some 20–30 seconds, signaling if any anxiety has been aroused. When the visualization of the first scene has produced no anxiety on two repetitions, the therapist moves on to the next item in the hierarchy. Because there may be some recrudescence of anxiety between sessions, it is usually wise to drop back a couple of items and to proceed forward from there.

Some patients have difficulty visualizing feared scenes and may need coaching (e.g., to imagine colors and specific details of a particular scene). Systematic desensitization is little used today, having been largely superseded by the use of direct exposure to the feared situation, as will be described in the next subsection. The procedure is useful, however, in extremely fearful patients who will not venture into the feared situation, when it is used before exposure to the feared situation.

Exposure Therapy (Programmed Practice)

Exposure therapy, sometimes known as *programmed practice*, is one of the most investigated and frequently used therapies in the treatment of phobias, including agoraphobia. There are several variants of this therapeutic procedure, although all begin with the construction of a hierarchy of feared situations along a particular dimension. The simplest variant of exposure therapy is known as *exposure instructions*. The therapist helps the patient construct the first few steps in a hierarchy of the feared situation. For example, for the patient with agoraphobia who is housebound, this involves walking a few yards from the front door, then walking half a block, then walking a block, and so on. With the use of the hierarchy, a course is laid out along which the patient is instructed to walk alone. The instructions are to walk as far as possible until mild anxiety is evident. At least one session, lasting approximately 30 minutes, should be held each day. The patient repeats each walk until the anxiety has dissipated and then he or she begins to walk farther. A diary is kept for each trial. At the next session the diary is reviewed, progress is attended to and praised, and any stumbling blocks are discussed and a solution for them is found. Progress is usually slow at first, with occasional setbacks, but as the patient gains experience with the method, he or she is able to make faster progress and eventually can proceed on his or her own.

In *therapist-assisted exposure*, the therapist accompanies the patient to the feared situation and provides direct coaching on facing it. In such cases the therapist may challenge the patient to experience maximal anxiety levels. In addition, the therapist may explore the thoughts of the patient during the exposure experience so that distorted cognitions can be directly challenged.

Group exposure therapy combines individualized exposure instructions and practice with group education concerning the phobia (usually panic disorder with agoraphobia) and with a discussion of the participants' experiences during exposure to the feared situation. Such group sessions are usually 3 hours in duration, comprising a 30-minute educational session, an exposure session with individual practice, and a 45-minute debriefing session. Group sessions are often held daily for 10–14 days.

Flooding is a form of exposure therapy in which patients are exposed to the maximal phobic situation and kept in that situation until their fear dissipates. Although this form of treatment produces positive results more rapidly than does graduated exposure, it may be associated with much discomfort and therefore is rarely used today.

Cognitive Therapy

Although behavior therapy, as its name implies, tends to focus on the current behavior of the patient, from the earliest days of behavior therapy there was at least some focus on the specific cognitions accompanying a particular disorder. The importance of distorted cognitions has

been particularly recognized in the treatment of the anxiety disorders, depression, and the eating disorders. The typical approach to cognitive therapy involves a thorough exploration of the thoughts and feelings preceding, during, and following a particular behavior (e.g., binge eating or purging). For patients who have difficulty recalling such thoughts, self-monitoring is often useful. Once the cognitions have been clearly identified, the reality of such thoughts is considered in detail. When the patient recognizes the unrealistic nature of the thoughts, such thinking can be challenged in vivo by the patient or behavioral experiments designed further to test the reality of such thinking can be devised.

The following case history is an example of the use of cognitive therapy:

> A philosophy student in her late 20s had a sudden panic attack while presenting a paper in her class. She then had several further attacks (apparently precipitated by thoughts of failure), lost her appetite, and began to lose weight. In addition, she began to avoid leaving home unless accompanied by her husband. She was evaluated within a month of the start of her symptoms. During the initial interview, it became clear that this ambitious young woman thought that her life was out of control, that she was a failure, that she could not continue with her projected career as a philosopher, and that her life was essentially over. She was particularly afraid that her wealthy and successful husband would divorce her and find a more suitable companion. Because she was a philosopher and supposedly a logical individual, the therapist asked her to examine the reality of her beliefs. Within the first session she was able to see that her beliefs were unrealistic. She immediately began practicing leaving home alone, challenging her unrealistic thinking when it recurred. Within a few sessions she no longer felt anxious, was able to resume her studies, had no phobic limitation, and once more felt secure in her marriage. At 1-year follow-up she remained, by her assessment, symptom free.

It should be noted that cognitive procedures are usually combined with behavior change procedures, and that many behavior therapies are now referred to as *cognitive-behavioral* therapies.

Reinforcement

Reinforcement consists of making an event contingent on the performance of a behavior that one wishes to change. *Positive reinforcement* is said to occur when the contingent application of the event strengthens the behavior. Positive reinforcers are usually viewed as pleasant (e.g., food, attention, praise, money). All therapists use verbal attention to reinforce particular themes during therapy sessions. Behavior therapists tend to use such reinforcement in a more precise manner, making attention or praise contingent on the occurrence of the behavior that is being strengthened. Although positive reinforcement is an aspect of all therapeutic encounters, it is most often used to strengthen prosocial behaviors in children with conduct disorder or in persons with schizophrenia (discussed later in this chapter). *Negative reinforcement* refers to a process by which a particular behavior removes the reinforcing event, thus strengthening the behavior. The events used in a negative reinforcement paradigm are usually regarded as unpleasant. For example, in the treatment of anorexia nervosa the often-used threat of tube feeding serves as a negative reinforcer, because the patient can avoid the negative occurrence (i.e., tube feeding) by eating and gaining weight.

In addition to using reinforcement within a therapeutic package of some kind, the psychiatrist must review patients' current behavior to identify reinforcers that might be maintaining the pathological behavior. It is also clear that staff attention to problem behaviors increases the frequency of such behaviors. Therefore, nursing and medical staff at all levels should be trained in the application of social reinforcement and extinction procedures. Research has shown that untrained nursing staff attend to problem behaviors more frequently than they attend to prosocial behaviors of patients. Such an approach causes an increase in the frequency of problem behaviors.

Extinction

Removal of positive reinforcement weakens behavior and may lead to its total disappearance. This procedure is known as *extinction*. From a clinical viewpoint, extinction can be used only in environments such as an inpatient unit or a classroom in which reinforcement can be controlled, although relatives of patients can be taught to use extinction in the home. The withdrawal of positive reinforcement may lead to an *extinction burst*, in which the unwanted behavior briefly increases in frequency or strength. If the procedure is being applied by relatives in the home setting, it is important to warn them that an increase in the problem behavior may occur at first, so that they do not abandon the attempt to control the behavior through extinction.

Punishment

The punishment paradigm consists of the application of an aversive stimulus contingent on the unwanted behavior, with the aim of rapidly bringing the behavior under control. Punishment is used infrequently in behavior therapy and only in situations in which the behavior in question threatens physical harm and in which more benign procedures such as positive reinforcement or extinction have failed. An example of the application of punishment is given in the subsection on ruminative vomiting, a life-threatening condition in infancy. The use of punishment, because it raises difficult ethical issues, is usually supervised by a committee that should include an informed layperson. In addition, if the use of punishment does not bring the unwanted behavior rapidly under control, the punishment paradigm should be reviewed for the accuracy of its use and/or stopped.

Aversion Therapy

Aversion therapy, which should not be confused with punishment, is based on the principle of classical conditioning and involves pairing an aversive stimulus with the unwanted behavior. An example of such a paradigm is the pairing of nausea (induced with emetine) with the drinking of alcohol in the treatment of alcoholism. It has been shown that such classical conditioning is more powerful if it involves the same physiological system as the one involved in the unwanted behavior. Thus, drinking is paired with nausea in the case of alcoholism because both involve the gastrointestinal system. One of the problems with aversive therapy is that exposure to the original stimulus (in this case, drinking alcohol) tends to weaken the classically conditioned response and lead to relapse. Therefore, in the original application of such conditioning, booster sessions were found to delay relapse. Nonetheless, the tendency toward relapse after aversion therapy has led to a decrease in enthusiasm for the use of aversion therapy in general.

Biofeedback

The principal aim of biofeedback procedures is to magnify a response that is not accessible to a patient and to provide feedback regarding changes in that response over time. For example, small muscle contractions are not usually discriminable by patients. Such responses can be amplified through the use of electronic monitoring, and a signal can be displayed, either visually or in the form of a continuous tone, that is proportional to the muscle contraction being measured. In this way, the patient can be informed about the degree of contraction and can potentially learn either to increase or to decrease the contractions, depending on the aim of therapy. Thus, in the case of nerve or muscle damage the aim would be to increase contractions in selected muscles, whereas in the case of tension headache the aim would be to reduce tension in the affected muscles. Biofeedback has many potential applications—for example, in fecal incontinence, through training of the anal sphincter; in hypertension, through displaying blood pressure values and allowing patients to discover methods to control their blood pressure; and in Raynaud's disease, through enhancing temperature control. Using small portable biofeedback units, patients can practice in their own homes, and thus learning can be transferred from the office to the patients' own environment.

Relaxation Training

Relaxation training is a relatively simple therapeutic technique that is useful in a variety of conditions (discussed later in this chapter) and often forms a component of a behavior therapy treatment package. Patients are first presented with a rationale. For example, a patient who has tension headaches would be told that muscles tense up as a result of anxiety and this can lead to pain; if the patient were to learn to relax his or her muscles, such pain could be lessened. Patients are then seated comfortably in a chair and are taught to tense and then relax each muscle group systematically. Soon they are able to induce relaxation fairly quickly simply by relaxing all their muscles. Patients are encouraged at the same time to visualize a pleasant, relaxing scene or to use a simple mantra to control distracting thoughts. Patients are given a tape recording of relaxation instructions and are encouraged to use the tape for some 20 minutes each day at home. After several treatment sessions with intervening home practice, patients are taught rapid relaxation techniques. In this procedure, patients are taught to scan their bodies intermittently for tense muscles and to bring on the relaxation response rapidly using the word *relax*, which they have previously paired with a deeply relaxed state. This procedure can then be used during the course of their everyday lives.

Modeling

Modeling refers to a procedure in which a desired behavior is performed by a therapist with the aim of having his or her patient copy that performance. It may be necessary to break a complex behavior pattern into its component parts and model each segment of that behavior sequentially until the entire sequence can be performed by the patient. Reinforcement such as praise is used as the patient gradually masters the desired behavior. The patient is then encouraged to try out the behavior at home. Modeling has been used to treat children's phobias through encouragement to expose themselves to the feared situation; in social skills training in disorders such

as schizophrenia; in marital counseling; and in training in better parenting skills.

Social Skills Training

Social skills training is used in the rehabilitation of patients with schizophrenia (discussed later in this chapter); in the treatment of social phobia, particularly when the phobia is combined with avoidant personality disorder; and in any patient in whom a particular social skills deficit is apparent. The first step is to analyze the social skills deficit in concrete behavioral terms—for example, avoiding eye contact, a slumped body posture that is not conducive to interpersonal communication, or speaking too softly. More appropriate behavior is then gradually developed by means of modeling and social reinforcement, together with opportunities for the patient to practice the new behaviors (e.g., in a group setting). The patient is next encouraged to practice the new behaviors in his or her own environment. Videotapes of the patient performing the desired behavior may also be employed so that the therapist can give detailed feedback on progress.

Anxiety Disorders

Panic Disorder With or Without Agoraphobia

Agoraphobia (and the simple phobias) has been a central focus of behavior therapy since Wolpe's description of systematic desensitization first appeared (Wolpe 1958). The work in this area is an excellent example of the continual refinement of therapeutic hypotheses and procedures based on the results of clinical trials. On the basis of his findings from animal experiments in which fear responses were induced and then treated, Wolpe formulated the hypothesis that if a response that inhibits anxiety occurs in an anxiety-provoking situation, then the anxiety response will be weakened—an example of the principle of *reciprocal inhibition*. In his animal experiments, Wolpe used food to inhibit fear while the animal was exposed to gradually intensifying fear-arousing situations. In humans, relaxation was used to inhibit anxiety; hence, in the clinical application of systematic desensitization, deep muscle relaxation is paired with the imagination of feared scenes presented in a graded hierarchy, beginning with those provoking the least fear and gradually progressing to more fear-arousing scenes. Research in the field was catalyzed by the development of an analog model of phobia, namely, snake fears (Lazovik and Lang 1960). This model allowed for a more rapid delineation of the active and inactive components of systematic desensitization than would have been possible if research had been limited to clinical populations.

Findings from analog research challenged the theory on which systematic desensitization was based. Therapeutic instructions were found to be an essential component of desensitization, and removal of such instructions from the therapeutic package weakened the efficacy of treatment. This finding was not entirely surprising, given that therapeutic instructions have been found to be a major component of all psychotherapies. Such instructions comprise information concerning the therapeutic rationale, a description of the therapeutic procedures to be used, and, perhaps most important, an assessment of the outcome that might be expected from treatment. More surprising was the finding that pairing relaxation with feared scenes was not essential for successful outcome, nor was a gradual approach to the feared situation in imagination. This finding challenged the central notion of reciprocal inhibition. Ultimately, exposure to the feared situation itself was found to be the critical ingredient for successful treatment.

Many controlled clinical trials have demonstrated the effectiveness of graded exposure therapy in the treatment of agoraphobia (Taylor and Arnow 1988). Long-term studies have shown that improvement is well maintained for periods of up to 7 years (Fava et al. 1995). Involving a spouse (or friend) in the treatment process adds to the effectiveness of exposure therapy, probably because the patient's practice in the feared situation is better supported. The addition of couples training in communication skills enhances maintenance of the effects of exposure therapy. Such enhanced communication may allow the couple to adjust better to the agoraphobic individual's newfound freedom of movement, a change that may be stressful for some couples. Overall, exposure therapy is associated with dropout rates of approximately 10%, and more than 80% of patients demonstrate marked improvement. However, exposure therapy may be less effective in reducing panic attacks than in reducing or eliminating phobic behavior.

Behavior Therapy for Panic Disorder

Several studies suggest that the catastrophic interpretation of panic symptoms rather than the frequency of panic attacks is the critical element associated with the severity of agoraphobia. Catastrophic cognitions fall into three categories: 1) fear of illness, 2) fear of loss of control, and 3) fear of embarrassment while having a panic attack. It is hypothesized that persons susceptible to such cognitions misinterpret either mild symptoms of anxiety or other body changes (e.g., dizziness on standing up suddenly) in a catastrophic manner, leading to spiraling anxiety that culminates in a panic attack. It follows that therapy aimed at correcting such misinterpretations should lead to a reduction in panic. Such therapy consists, first, in identifying the type of cognitions experienced by the patient and, second, having the patient expose himself or herself to situations in which the catastrophic cognitions occur, essentially demonstrating to himself or herself that the feared consequences do not occur in reality (e.g., despite a fear of having a heart attack because of an accelerating heart rate, no heart attack occurs). In addition, some physical symptoms leading to the catastrophic thinking patterns can be induced in the therapy situation (e.g., in the case of dizziness, spinning the patient in a chair) and the reality of the frightening thoughts can thus be directly disconfirmed.

Controlled studies have demonstrated the effectiveness of this treatment in reducing panic attacks; between 50% and 90% of patients achieved remission of their symptoms in the various studies (e.g., Barlow et al. 1989; Clark et al. 1994; Craske et al. 1995). Follow-up studies reveal some relapse in symptoms of panic, although, for the most part, maintenance of treatment effects is good. In a study by Fava et al. (1995) in which panic disorder patients with agoraphobia received 12 sessions of behavioral therapy with in vivo exposure, 67% remained in remission for at least 7 years.

Combination Therapy

In general, it appears that the most effective treatment for agoraphobia with panic is a combination of pharmacological treatment and exposure therapy. For example, in a study comparing exposure therapy with and without treatment with fluvoxamine, the addition of medication was found to enhance the outcome of exposure therapy (de Beurs et al. 1995). For patients with agoraphobia who have not experienced panic attacks, exposure therapy alone should suffice. Behavior therapy may also be useful in the discontinuation of treatment with alprazolam, as demonstrated in a study comparing a slow tapering of medication with and without behavior therapy. Patients receiving the combined treatment were more successful in discontinuing alprazolam therapy and were significantly less anxious and depressed after medication discontinuation than those not receiving behavior therapy (Bruce et al. 1995).

Simple Phobia

Because medication appears to have little place in the treatment of simple phobia, the approach to this problem that is most often used is graded exposure therapy. Such treatment is usually fairly easy to arrange and involves the patient's gradually approaching the feared object or situation. Therapist-aided exposure may be used in which the therapist accompanies the patient into the phobic situation and directly arranges exposure trials, or the therapist may simply use instructions regarding the practice of exposure and request that the patient keep a record of such practice. This record is examined at subsequent treatment sessions, and solutions to problems encountered by the patient are worked out. Most patients with simple phobia respond rapidly to such treatment, and follow-up studies suggest that gains are well maintained.

Social Phobia

The number of studies of the treatment of social phobia, once a rather neglected area of research, is now increasing (Heimberg and Barlow 1991; Heimberg et al. 1993). Findings of controlled studies suggest that the behavioral treatment of choice is a combination of exposure therapy and cognitive restructuring. One study found that the addition of cognitive restructuring to exposure therapy prevented relapse. The principal area of focus for cognitive change is in eliciting the details of the social phobic patient's fears of negative evaluation by others and challenging the reality of these ideas. Exposure therapy in social phobia is more difficult to arrange than in the case of simple phobia or agoraphobia because social situations are less controllable by the patient than other phobic situations and may become more intense than expected. Moreover, many social interchanges are of short duration and therefore do not provide the more prolonged exposure characteristic of the therapy for other phobias. Hence, careful planning of exposure situations, ensuring a sufficient number of opportunities for exposure, and providing support for failure experiences when the social situation is more intense than was planned are all important aspects of the treatment of social phobia.

Obsessive-Compulsive Disorder

There have been remarkable advances in the treatment of OCD with behavior therapy, although the results of treatment are not completely satisfactory. Deriving from basic work concerning the relationship between anxiety and avoidance behaviors such as compulsions, *response prevention* of compulsive rituals has become one of the cornerstones of behavior therapy in this condition (Stanley and Turner 1995). The thesis is that the compulsive behavior does not allow for reality testing of the fear. Thus, patients' fear of contamination leading to illness

and death is reinforced by the fact that they do not become sick or die as long as they engage in hand washing.

The main therapeutic procedure is to prevent the patient from engaging in compulsive acts such as hand washing after exposure to "contaminating" situations. This may be accomplished by means of a gradual approach on an outpatient basis in which the patient, perhaps aided by a relative, abstains from engaging in compulsive behavior after exposure to the feared situation. A hierarchical approach is taken, in which the patient begins with the easiest situation and gradually moves toward more difficult tasks. On an inpatient basis, a more intensive approach can be taken—for example, preventing the patient from engaging in hand washing for a period of several days while providing a supportive relationship. The efficacy of this approach was first demonstrated in controlled single-case studies and since then has been examined in a number of controlled clinical trials.

Although response prevention results in marked diminution in compulsive behavior, it does not usually eliminate the fear of contamination. Controlled studies have demonstrated that exposure to contaminating situations results in marked diminution in contamination fears but relatively little change in rituals (Steketee et al. 1982). The combination of the two treatments (exposure plus response prevention) is clearly superior to either one alone. Finally, it has been shown that the addition of desensitization in imagination—focusing on the imagined catastrophic consequences of contamination—results in superior maintenance of recovery. Thus, a three-part behavior therapy dealing with separate components of the disorder appears to be most effective: response prevention for rituals, exposure therapy for phobic anxiety, and imaginal desensitization for obsessive worry.

Relatively little is known about the efficacy of combinations of behavior therapy and pharmacological treatment. A review of the literature suggests that patients in medication studies drop out at higher rates and experience somewhat less positive results than do patients in studies involving behavior therapies. Kozak et al. (2000) studied patients with OCD who were treated with exposure plus response prevention (ERP) alone, clomipramine alone, or the combination. ERP monotherapy produced a response rate similar to that for the combination condition, and both of these conditions resulted in greater improvement than did the clomipramine-alone condition. Furthermore, at follow-up 3 months after the end of treatment, the ERP-alone and combination groups continued to experience greater improvement than did the clomipramine-alone group.

Mood Disorders

Major Depression

The effectiveness of a cognitive-behavioral approach to treating unipolar nonpsychotic depression has been studied extensively in controlled clinical trials. In this treatment, the contingencies maintaining the depressed mood, often conceptualized as a relative lack of environmental reinforcement, are examined. Among the therapeutic procedures used are 1) problem solving combined with the teaching of coping skills to enhance the reinforcement deficit and 2) an examination of self-defeating cognitions, followed by the psychiatrist's teaching the patient to recognize such thoughts, to challenge them, and to substitute more adaptive thinking. Because antidepressant therapy can be viewed as the standard treatment for major depression, much recent research has been aimed at clarifying the relative effectiveness of pharmacological therapy and cognitive-behavioral therapy (CBT) and the effectiveness of the combined treatments (Clarkin et al. 1996).

In one of the first studies to examine this issue systematically, Kovacs et al. (1981) found that both imipramine therapy and CBT produced improvement in depressive symptomatology in a 12-week treatment period and that CBT was marginally superior. At 1-year follow-up, both groups of patients maintained their improvement; however, there was a suggestion that those receiving CBT showed less relapse than those receiving imipramine. In the large-scale National Institute of Mental Health Treatment of Depression Collaborative Research Program (Elkin et al. 1989), CBT, interpersonal therapy (IPT), and antidepressant medication were compared in a multicenter trial. The results suggested that all three therapies were effective but that medication was more effective in cases of severe depression.

Other studies have found that of patients who respond to therapy, those receiving CBT in combination with a tricyclic antidepressant show less tendency to relapse than those receiving antidepressants alone (Simons et al. 1986). Given that patients receiving antidepressants tend to improve more quickly than those receiving CBT, the preferred treatment for major depression would seem to be a combination of CBT and an antidepressant.

Patients with chronic major depression often have serious and unremitting courses. Some studies have reported that responses to CBT are similar to those observed for other forms of psychotherapy or for antidepressant medication. A multicenter trial (Keller et al. 2000) evaluated 662 patients with chronic, nonpsychotic major depression who were randomly assigned to receive 12 weeks of treatment with antidepressant medication (nefazodone), a cognitive-behavioral approach specifically designed to treat chronic depression, or a combination of both treatments. The combination of CBT with nefazodone resulted in significantly greater response (73%) than did either CBT or nefazodone alone (both 48%). Thus, this study supports the clinical notion that a combination of psychotherapy with CBT plus medication may be very useful to patients with chronic depression.

Social skills training has also been used to treat major depression. Such training involves the teaching of more assertive behavior that would be expected to increase social interaction and strengthen environmental reinforcement. Controlled studies have shown that this approach is as effective as CBT. Indeed, one must conclude from a survey of the literature that behavior therapy, IPT, and time-limited focused psychotherapy are all equally effective in the treatment of major depression, although superior maintenance has been demonstrated only in the case of CBT and IPT at this time. This raises the theoretical issue regarding what procedures might be shared by these different approaches to treatment and whether they affect depressed mood through the same or different psychological processes.

Other Depressive Disorders

The place of behavior therapy in more severe depression (e.g., cases meeting research criteria for endogenous depression) is less certain, due to a relative lack of controlled treatment studies in this area. Early work suggests, however, that CBT may be quite effective in both outpatient and inpatient populations and may be a useful alternative to treatment with medication. This modality may perhaps be helpful in patients who are not able to tolerate adequate dosage of antidepressant medication or as an adjunctive treatment combined with medication. CBT has also appeared to be useful in the treatment of dysthymia in initial uncontrolled studies.

Disorders of Eating

The three major disorders of eating are *anorexia nervosa*, *bulimia nervosa*, and *binge-eating disorder* (BED), the latter often associated with obesity. The development of behavior therapy differs significantly between these three disorders for different reasons. In the case of anorexia nervosa, the relative rarity of the disorder has militated against the conducting of controlled trials, and very little is known about the comparative effectiveness of different approaches to treatment over the long term. Bulimia nervosa, although common, markedly increased in prevalence toward the end of the 1970s, and clinical research is now in a state of relative maturity. BED has only recently attracted research attention, and therefore much less is known about the treatment of this disorder, although it would appear that treatments effective in bulimia nervosa are also effective in BED.

Anorexia Nervosa

The behavioral approach to the treatment of anorexia nervosa is aimed at the restoration of normal body weight, usually within an inpatient setting. It is widely agreed that weight restoration in the severely emaciated patient is the first objective of treatment. Next, there should be an attempt to deal with whatever problems appear to have precipitated and are maintaining the eating disorder. Crisp et al. (1991) viewed anorexia nervosa as an avoidance of maturation (a weight and shape phobia); thus, weight restoration is viewed as exposing the patient to problems that are being avoided through starvation (i.e., an exposure therapy).

Single-case controlled research, a useful approach when dealing with a relatively rare disorder, has revealed three procedures that promote increased caloric intake: reinforcement of weight gain in small increments, feedback of information regarding progress (usually accomplished by daily weight and caloric consumption feedback), and the serving of large meals even though the patient will at first leave most of the food untouched. These procedures are used in the context of a carefully negotiated therapeutic contract and a well-designed ward milieu (Agras 1987). Such programs lead to steady weight gain, and studies suggest that behavior therapy is more efficient than other treatment approaches, resulting in shorter hospital stays for equal amounts of weight gain. The only large-scale controlled study of an inpatient behavioral approach to weight restoration suggested that behavior therapy may be relatively more effective in the less severe case of anorexia nervosa.

Research has also been directed toward evaluating outpatient treatments for anorexia nervosa. One study compared inpatient and outpatient care for anorexia nervosa in a randomized controlled trial (Crisp et al. 1991). Surprisingly, the results of outpatient care equaled those of inpatient care, in that weight gains in the patients receiving outpatient care were equivalent to those in the patients receiving inpatient care, and weight gains in the patients in these groups were superior to those in patients

who received no treatment. This study requires replication by other investigators because of methodological problems, including a high rate of dropout from the study. Nonetheless, in an era in which the duration of hospitalization for the anorexic patient is becoming ever shorter, this study may point the way to the future of treatment of anorexia.

Bulimia Nervosa

The upsurge in the number of young women seeking treatment for bulimic symptoms in the late 1970s presented clinicians with a difficult problem because no effective treatment methods had been described for this condition. The work of Fairburn (1981), who first described a CBT for bulimia, has led to the appearance of a large number of controlled trials in the last decade. It is generally agreed that the social pressure for women to remain thin has increased during the past 15 years. This pressure leads a subgroup of young women to restrict their caloric intake markedly and to form rigid rules relating to food, leading to an increased probability of binge eating and eventually, because of threatened weight increase, to purging. It is also probable that the most susceptible young women are those who markedly restrict their food intake despite being genetically programmed for having a fuller figure. Research has shown that some bulimic individuals have a markedly increased energy efficiency, maintaining normal body weight in the absence of purging on a mean daily caloric intake of approximately 1,400 calories. They also tend to eat very little early in the day, which sets the scene for binge eating later in the day.

CBT is aimed at overcoming the dietary restriction and distorted thinking patterns that are believed to maintain bulimia nervosa. The basic components of CBT include self-disclosure to significant others, thus increasing social control over the secretive bulimic behaviors; gradual reintroduction of the consumption of three adequate meals each day; slow introduction of "feared" binge foods to the diet; challenge of distorted cognitions regarding food intake; and a relapse prevention program (Agras 1987; Fairburn 1981). Controlled studies have demonstrated that CBT is more effective in reducing binge eating and purging than are a waiting-list control condition; a pill placebo; psychoeducational treatment; nondirective psychotherapy combined with self-monitoring of eating behavior; stress management; and, in some studies, behavior therapy (i.e., a treatment omitting the procedures aimed at correcting distorted thinking patterns). In other studies, CBT and behavior therapy have been found to be equivalent in effectiveness in reducing binge eating and purging, although patients receiving CBT almost always have psychiatrically healthier attitudes toward weight and shape, attitudes that are specifically targeted by CBT. Overall, some 55% of patients with bulimia recover with the use of CBT, and the majority maintain their gains over follow-up periods of up to 5 years (Fairburn et al. 1993). A substantial proportion of those not fully recovering have a subclinical eating disorder at follow-up.

Combination Therapy

Because both CBT and antidepressant medication have been used in the treatment of bulimia nervosa, the relative effectiveness of these different approaches to treatment and their combination has been investigated. Studies have shown that CBT is superior to antidepressant medication in reducing binge eating and purging and that the combined treatment is no more effective than CBT alone. It appears, however, that the combined treatment more effectively reduces depression and emotionally induced eating, and there is tentative evidence that, as in depression, the combined treatment leads to better maintenance of improvement (Agras et al. 1992; Mitchell et al. 1990). More recently, Walsh et al. (1997) conducted a study in which two antidepressants, desipramine and fluoxetine, were used. These investigators substituted fluoxetine when desipramine was ineffective; such a model is more similar to that used by practitioners. Walsh and colleagues found that the sequential use of these medications was as effective as CBT and that there was a marginally improved effectiveness when medication was combined with CBT.

Other Approaches to Treatment

It has been shown that an adaptation of IPT—an approach that was first demonstrated to be effective in the treatment of depression—to eating disorders is as effective as CBT (Fairburn et al. 1991). This is an interesting finding, given that no attention was paid to eating disturbances in the interpersonal treatment. This suggests that IPT and CBT may work by different processes. There is much evidence that negative affect, frequently arising from interpersonal conflicts, triggers binge eating. It may be that IPT works by reducing negative affect, whereas CBT works by reducing dietary restraint.

Binge-Eating Disorder

The research in bulimia nervosa has resulted in the rediscovery of a subset of obese individuals who binge eat but do not purge. The proportion of overweight individuals who binge eat increases with increasing levels of adiposity, from 10% in mildly obese persons to more than 40% in severely obese persons. Moreover, it appears that these individuals are less successful in their weight loss attempts than are their non-binge-eating counterparts. The similarity of this disorder to bulimia nervosa suggests that treatments effective in that condition should be effective in BED. Initial research has shown this hypothesis to be true: both CBT and IPT have been demonstrated to be equally effective in reducing binge eating in controlled studies (Agras et al. 1994; Wilfley et al. 1993). As is the case with bulimia nervosa, although antidepressant medication appears effective, adding therapy with such medication to CBT does not result in a significant additional reduction in binge eating. However, those receiving antidepressant treatment lose more weight than those not receiving medication.

The optimal approach for treating the obese binge-eating patient is to begin treatment with CBT and follow this with weight loss treatment that does not demand overly restrictive dieting. Patients with BED who stop binge eating and who maintain abstinence also maintain their weight losses.

Psychotic Disorders

The behavioral approach to the treatment of psychotic disorders may be viewed as being adjunctive to pharmacological treatment and directed toward amelioration of specific problem behaviors or, more broadly, toward the social rehabilitation of the disturbed individual. These aims are accomplished using methods deriving from operant conditioning. Thus, precise definition of the problem behavior, combined with the use of reinforcement in various forms, is the core of the approach for patients with either disturbed behavior that does not improve with the use of medication or limitations in social and vocational skills secondary to the psychotic process.

Some of the first applications of behavior therapy were to severely disturbed individuals with chronic psychoses. The early successes of reinforcement therapy, demonstrated largely in single-case experiments, led to many applications in the mental hospital, in which a large number of problems, including aggressive and disruptive behavior, delusional behavior, depression, and apathy, were found susceptible to change (Kazdin 1977). Ayllon and Azrin (1965) demonstrated the effectiveness of using tokens with chronic psychotic patients, thus broadening the range of backup reinforcers that could be used to motivate individuals. One of the most sophisticated applications and testings of a token economy system was the experiment conducted by Paul and Lentz (1977) comparing a social-learning program with a more traditional milieu therapy program. This experiment had many noteworthy features, including the use of multiple outcome measures, continuous monitoring of staff behavior to ensure proper operation of programs, collection of long-term follow-up data, and computation of the cost-effectiveness of the two programs. Patients in both treatment programs showed progress, but those in the social-learning program showed significantly greater improvement across a range of prosocial behaviors, required less medication, and maintained their gains more successfully during the 18-month follow-up. Moreover, the social-learning program was the most cost-efficient of the two programs.

Whereas the token economy focused on generating skills useful to most patients, social skills training, delivered within complex and sophisticated rehabilitation programs and based on a detailed analysis of each patient's interpersonal deficits, now forms a more individualized approach to the patient with schizophrenia. Among the skills taught are maintaining eye contact, reacting more quickly to interpersonal communication, varying intonation, and reinforcing prosocial responses from others. Techniques such as modeling prosocial behaviors are often used. In addition, the patient and family members may be taught more effective conflict resolution through the use of role playing, video feedback, and practice. A number of controlled studies have demonstrated that clinically meaningful changes in behavior occur as a result of social skills training, improvements of up to 70% in social functioning are made, and hospital stays are shortened.

In recognition of the fact that environmental stress is a factor affecting the outcome of treatment in schizophrenic patients, the effectiveness of a behavioral family-based treatment has been studied intensively (Falloon et al. 1985). The main focus of such treatment has been problem solving at the family level. When families are unable to use the problem-solving approach successfully, training in communication skills is added to the program. Specific behavior problems impeding the process of therapy are dealt with using appropriate behavior change techniques. Compared with patients undergoing individual treatment, those receiving behavioral family therapy showed a 10-fold decrease in the number of days spent in the hospital or in jail during follow-up. In addition, the number of days spent in residential facilities decreased 30-fold. Thus, we may conclude that behavioral family treatment is an effective adjunct to the treatment of chronic schizophrenia. Fewer exacerbations are observed

with family behavioral approaches compared with individual approaches or routine care. In addition, family behavioral treatment resulted in lower levels of rejecting attitudes by family members and reduced levels of tension in the patients (Mueser et al. 2001) as compared with a supportive family therapy approach.

Behavioral Medicine

Behavior therapy has been applied to a number of medical disorders, including essential hypertension, hypercholesterolemia, and obesity; headache; sleep disturbance; gastrointestinal problems; and asthma. In addition, therapeutic procedures have been developed for problems common to many medical disorders such as compliance with medication taking and the response to stress.

Obesity

Behavioral treatment for mild to moderate obesity contains the following elements: 1) self-monitoring; 2) reinforcement of an increase in activity levels; 3) slowing of the eating rate; 4) narrowing of the stimuli associated with eating; 5) adherence to a low-fat, high-fiber, heart-healthy diet; and 6) use of reinforcement and self-reinforcement to attain short-term goals. This treatment package has been shown to be more effective than more traditional dietary approaches to weight control, psychotherapy, and even pharmacological treatment in a large number of controlled studies. The degree of weight loss achieved by the average patient is modest, usually averaging approximately 0.5 kg per week of treatment. Treatment programs of 16 weeks' duration result in a mean weight reduction of 8–10 kg. Weight loss is enhanced when reinforcement procedures, such as refund of a monetary deposit depending on weekly weight loss, are used. There is, however, marked variability in weight loss between individuals: some patients do not lose weight, whereas others lose more than 15 kg over the same period. The reasons for such variability are unclear, although there is evidence that poor adherence to the treatment regimen and particularly to self-monitoring is associated with a poorer outcome. In addition, biological factors—for example, adaptation of basal metabolic rate to dietary restriction—may vary between individuals. Finally, as discussed earlier in this chapter, the obese binge-eating patient appears to have more difficulty in losing weight than does the obese non-binge-eating patient.

Group therapy is the most usual behavioral approach to the treatment of obesity and may have advantages over individual treatment in that a wide variety of problem situations and their solutions are presented in a group context. Maintenance of weight loss appears to depend on the continued practice of behaviors learned during treatment. The most crucial of these are adherence to a healthy diet and eating style and continued exercise. Patients who continue to practice these behaviors have been shown to maintain or even increase their initial weight losses up to 5 years after treatment. Those who do not continue such behaviors tend to regain all of the weight that they lost, and some regain even more weight.

Behavior therapy has also been used to enhance the maintenance of weight loss with a very-low-calorie diet (VLCD), a treatment regimen used in moderately to severely obese patients. VLCDs were initially associated with a series of deaths in obese patients undergoing such treatment. These deaths were caused by inadequate protein in the diet accompanied by potassium deficiency, which in susceptible individuals led to ventricular fibrillation. Modern variants of the diet with adequate protein, minerals, and vitamins have proved safe when used with careful medical supervision. One controlled study demonstrated that weight regain after completion of a 12-week VLCD was less in a group of patients who were also receiving behavior therapy than in a group of patients who were not receiving this adjunctive treatment. Clinical studies suggest that mean weight losses of 20 kg or more might be expected with this combination of treatments, as well as marked improvement in cardiovascular risk factors including blood pressure, serum cholesterol levels, and even sleep apnea.

Relapse Prevention and Longer-Term Treatment

Longer-term follow-up studies have demonstrated difficulty with weight regain after acute weight loss (Brownell and Wadden 1986; Stunkard and Penick 1979). The theory of relapse proposed for the addictions but applicable to the treatment of obesity suggests that relapse (i.e., a return to previous behaviors) occurs when a patient who has insufficient ways to cope is confronted by a high-risk situation, problem, or emotional state. Precipitants to overeating often include negative affective states while alone or positive affective states in social situations. Cognitive-behavioral approaches have begun to address the relapse issue.

In a study addressing long-term treatment, Perri et al. (1988) treated a group of obese patients using behavioral techniques. Participants were then randomized to a no-treatment control group and to four other groups, each of which used a variety of behavioral approaches. All of the behavioral groups had continued therapist contact biweekly for an additional year. Problem situations were discussed and new strategies developed to help patients cope without resorting to eating at high-risk times. The participants in the no-treatment control group regained approximately one-half the weight they had lost during the year, whereas the participants in all of the behavioral groups maintained weight losses. In sum, continued therapist contact, longer treatment, and cognitive-behavioral approaches appear necessary for greater weight loss maintenance.

Combined Treatments

As is the case with other disorders, the question arises with regard to whether the effects of behavior therapy and medication might be synergistic. Several studies involving the combination of appetite-suppressant drugs, such as fenfluramine, and behavior therapy have been reported. The most impressive of these found an advantage in terms of weight loss for the group receiving fenfluramine at the end of treatment (Craighead et al. 1981). However, at 1-year follow-up this result was reversed, with those receiving medication regaining more weight than those receiving behavior therapy. The combined-treatment group lost less weight at this time than did those who were treated with behavior therapy alone. It may have been the case that patients receiving medication attributed their weight losses to the medication and thus did not practice the behavior changes needed to maintain the weight losses. The withdrawal of fenfluramine and dexfenfluramine from the market because of their linkage with cardiac valvular damage in a substantial number of cases has reduced the number of available appetite suppressant agents. Sibutramine has been approved for use in the treatment of obesity, and phentermine remains on the market because there is no evidence of a relationship between cardiac damage and the latter medication.

Wadden et al. (2001) found that the addition of a behavioral approach and a portion-controlled diet to pharmacological management of obesity significantly improved weight loss and patients' satisfaction with treatment outcome. At 12 months, obese patients had lost 4.1% of their initial body weight with sibutramine treatment alone, 10.8% when behavioral treatment was added to sibutramine, and 16.5% when behavioral treatment plus a meal-replacement approach using prepackaged food was added to sibutramine treatment.

Headache

The research literature on the treatment of both tension and migraine headache suggests that relaxation and biofeedback procedures are equally effective. Relaxation training is simpler to apply and should thus be the preferred treatment. Both relaxation training and biofeedback are more effective in reducing the number and intensity of tension or migraine headaches than either no treatment or treatment with various types of placebos. One study, however, suggests that patients who do not respond to relaxation training may benefit from biofeedback. Follow-up studies show good maintenance for patients who improved with treatment; however, a fairly large percentage of individuals, perhaps 40%, are nonresponders. For the responder, studies have suggested that booster sessions may lead to lowered relapse rates. The mechanism of action of relaxation training and related procedures in the treatment of headache is uncertain, although it seems likely that lowering of sympathetic nervous system activity is the basis for the effect.

Primary Insomnia

Sleep disturbance uncomplicated by other psychiatric or physical disorders is a common problem in medical practice. Given the potential deleterious effects of long-term use of hypnotic agents, it should not be treated for longer than a few days with medication. Thus, the discovery and testing of nonpharmacological approaches to the treatment of sleep-onset insomnia are important.

Two behavior therapy approaches to sleep disturbance have been shown to be effective in controlled studies. Both of these approaches decrease the amount of time before sleep onset as measured by self-report and polysomnography. The first of these treatments, relaxation training, is based on the rationale that anxiety and other distractions preventing sleep onset can be controlled with such training. The second treatment, stimulus control, is based on the theory that sleep onset should be signaled by a narrow range of stimuli—that is, being in bed in a dark room and feeling drowsy—and that for many patients with sleep-onset disturbance the connection between these stimuli and sleep has broken down. Thus, stimulus control treatment consists of removing distractions such as books, television, and radio from the bedroom. In addition, patients are instructed to get up if they do not fall asleep within 10 minutes and are further instructed not to go back to bed until they are drowsy. It has been shown that this treatment is more effective than relaxation training (Lacks et al. 1983). The preferred treatment approach to uncomplicated sleep-onset disturbance should now be stimulus control training combined with discontinuance of hypnotic medication.

Stress Management

Relaxation training is useful in ameliorating many symptoms of stress, including anxiety, tension headache, and sleep disturbance. In addition, relaxation training appears to modify the Type A behavior pattern, an independent risk factor for cardiovascular disease. Type A behavior, which may represent a maladaptive response to life stress, consists of aggressive striving, time urgency, irritability, and impatience. A long-term controlled study involving patients who had had myocardial infarction demonstrated that it was possible to modify this pattern of behavior with an educational treatment regimen based on relaxation training and that reduction in Type A behavior was associated with fewer recurrent myocardial infarctions (Friedman et al. 1984).

Adherence to a Medical Regimen

A number of controlled studies have demonstrated that behavior change approaches can improve adherence to the medical regimen, particularly medication taking. Appointment keeping, one of the first steps in adherence, has been shown to improve with the use of simple reminder strategies (e.g., a telephone call or a reminder card). Controlled studies suggest that appointment keeping can be improved from levels of approximately 70% to levels of more than 90% with the use of these simple strategies, thereby improving the cost-effectiveness of medical care (Gates and Colborn 1976).

Compliance with medication taking has also been shown to be poor: approximately half of all patients take medication as prescribed, a further 20% take medication approximately 80% of the time, and the remainder take either no medication or very little medication. Behavior change strategies are aimed at several aspects of the problem (Agras 1989). First, the patient's expectations about the effectiveness of the proposed treatment are explored. If the patient does not expect the treatment to work, he or she will be unlikely to adhere to the prescribed regimen. For example, a negative experience of a relative or friend with the prescribed treatment may affect the expectations of a patient regarding outcome. Education regarding the short- and long-term benefits of the medical regimen is important in helping to promote a positive expectation regarding treatment. Second, the complexity of the regimen should be examined, because it has been shown that the more complex the regimen, the poorer the compliance. This includes an examination of all the medications that the patient is currently taking and an attempt to fit the new medication into the current regimen. Third, it has been demonstrated that patients quickly forget instructions given by their physicians; this underlines the need for written instructions. Fourth, it appears important to tie medication taking to other regularly scheduled behaviors (e.g., mealtimes, bedtime) and to have the pills stored in such a way that they are easily accessible at such times. Finally, the early handling of side effects to medication appears critical in maintaining adequate adherence. Patients with preexisting symptoms similar to the side effects of a medication appear particularly likely to prematurely discontinue taking medication. Identification of such symptoms before beginning medication is therefore important.

Cancer

One important role of behavior therapy in the treatment of patients with cancer is the reduction of anxiety and nausea associated with cancer chemotherapy, an example of classical conditioning. Relaxation training can be used for patients who do not respond to modern antiemetic agents. Controlled studies demonstrate that such treatment is effective in reducing anxiety, nausea, and vomiting. Unfortunately, little is known about the comparative effects of medication and relaxation training in reducing nausea and vomiting or whether these two treatment modalities augment each other. A second role of behavior therapy is to enhance coping with cancer. In a randomized controlled study involving patients in whom malignant melanoma had been newly diagnosed, Fawzy et al. (1993) used a structured 6-week group intervention with components including health education, stress management, coping skills, and supportive group psychotherapy. There were several interesting findings. First, the group receiving the intervention used significantly more active-coping methods than did the control (usual care) group. Second, the active-treatment group experienced notable immunological changes. Third, at 6-year follow-up there was a strong trend for recurrence to be lower, and survival to be longer, in the active-treatment group. These results are similar to those of Spiegel et al. (1989), who employed a 1-year program of supportive–expressive group psychotherapy in women with breast cancer. After 1 year of treatment, the group receiving active treatment showed markedly less anxiety and pain than did the control group. In addition, at 10-year follow-up, length of survival time was superior for the group receiving the active treatment. Because the two treatments differed from one another, it is possible that some common mechanism was responsible for the observed results.

Disorders of Childhood

Behavior therapy for children's disorders has been based on the use of operant conditioning, particularly the application of reinforcement procedures. This model emphasizes that behavior is a function of its consequences. Maladaptive behaviors are hypothesized to be learned as a result of complex reinforcement and punishment schedules in specific social environments. By analyzing the contingencies surrounding a behavior, one may change it by altering those contingencies. More recently, therapeutic procedures found to be useful in adults (e.g., in the treatment of anxiety disorder, depression, and OCD) have been successfully applied to children. Selected areas in the treatment of children's disorders are reviewed in the following subsections.

Autism

Autism, a pervasive developmental disorder, is no longer considered to be psychogenic in origin and is now viewed as a central nervous system disorder (Cohen and Shaywitz 1982). Lovaas et al. (1971, 1979) made an important contribution to our understanding of autism by identifying the perceptual problem of *stimulus overselectivity*. When a variety of stimuli are presented to autistic children, as is the case in almost every social contact, only one portion is attended to, and there is a lack of response to the complex stimulus and its meaning. In one study, normal children were able to respond to each component (auditory, visual, and tactile) of a complex cue, while the autistic child responded selectively to only one cue and not the others. Thus, the autistic child's response to situations often appears bizarre. No evidence of sensory deficits is found. When simple cues are presented to autistic children, behavioral responding is more consistent. When well-defined cues are used, along with immediate and tangible reinforcers, desired behaviors can gradually be shaped. Behavioral excesses (e.g., tantrums, aggression, self-stimulatory behaviors) may be either punished (using, for example, time-out from reinforcement, in which a child might be put in a room alone for a few minutes contingent on disruptive behavior) or, if mild, ignored with the aim of weakening them (an example of the removal of reinforcement, i.e., extinction). Therapists and parents can be trained to teach autistic children in this way, and environments can be designed to reinforce desired behaviors systematically. Lovaas (1977) also developed methods to teach language skills to autistic children. Such children are able to learn but require very specific programming. Verbal skills are taught progressively, first with the use of reinforcement for attending to the teacher, then by the use of imitation, then by labeling objects, followed by stating simple sentences. Autistic children are able to improve their language skills substantially with this method; however, improvement is correlated with IQ, and maintenance depends on continued reinforcement. Increasing language skills can also facilitate socialization in children with severe language deficiencies.

In a controlled study, Lovaas (1977) provided intensive treatment to young autistic children and their parents. Parents, along with children, applied a home-based program using operant procedures over a 2-year period. The children received reinforcement for learning, communication, and social behaviors. After the trial, 47% of the children in the intervention group had been placed in a regular first-grade classroom (and IQ levels had markedly increased compared with pretreatment levels), whereas none from the no-treatment control group were able to be placed in such a classroom setting. These results suggest that such early, intensive, and comprehensive treatment may be very useful in autism. Improvements in language and social functioning have also been reported in other studies using intensive behavioral programming, as summarized by Rogers (1998).

Combination Treatment

In a controlled study, Campbell et al. (1978) investigated the use of haloperidol or placebo versus contingent or noncontingent reinforcement in a language training program for hospitalized autistic children. Medication reduced stereotypical and withdrawn behavior in older, but not younger, children, whereas contingency management improved ward behaviors and compliance and imitation in the language training program. The group receiving haloperidol and contingent reinforcement showed the greatest improvement.

Conduct Disorder

Parents often seek help for their children's behavior problems, including aggressiveness, destructiveness, oppositional behavior, temper tantrums, and other negative behaviors (e.g., whining, screaming, threatening). Numerous studies have described a high rate of what Patterson (1976) described as *coercive interactions* in families of these children. Parents of these children respond with coercive behaviors when attempting to control their children's misbehavior. Patterson described a negative reinforcement model in which the coercive behavior of the parent may be reinforced by the reduc-

tion of the aversive behavior of the child. Unfortunately, the parent also models punitive behaviors to the child, who is then trained to behave similarly. In addition, parents may, without intending to, positively reinforce the deviant behaviors, either by attending to them or by fulfilling a demand accompanied by the deviant behavior (Wahler 1976). Often a parent will spend considerable effort and time with a child in attempting to abort a temper tantrum, and this approach may in fact reinforce the behavior.

To address such problems, the primary research effort has been in training parents to use social learning techniques to shape more adaptive and prosocial behaviors in their children. Such programs (Patterson 1976) have taught parents to monitor both prosocial and deviant behaviors, develop positive reinforcement systems (e.g., contingent point systems for obtaining rewards), use extinction (i.e., "ignoring") for minor misbehaviors, and use punishment (e.g., time-out) for serious infractions. Christophersen et al. (1972) examined the use of a home reinforcement system (i.e., token economy) with observations by parents and reliability checks by the experimenters. The token economy is a systematic use of contingent reinforcement using tokens (often points or stars) earned by the child for prosocial behaviors and later used to purchase privileges or desired items. This approach led to a marked reduction in deviant behaviors and increase in prosocial behaviors.

Christophersen et al. (1976) also compared the parent training and home token economy system with conventional outpatient treatment for children with conduct disorder. Parents using the token economy reported a 67% reduction in deviant behavior, whereas those using traditional treatment reported only a 34% reduction. Similar systems have been designed and have been found useful in the classroom, psychiatric inpatient programs, and residential treatment programs for children with behavioral disturbances.

There are, however, limits to the efficacy of such programs. It has been shown, for example, that marital discord is associated with conduct disorder in children. In such cases, improvement is unlikely until the marital discord has been addressed. Other complicating parental factors may include depression, substance abuse, or other psychopathology that will require therapeutic attention for the child to improve using behavioral techniques.

Kazdin and colleagues (Kazdin 1987; Kazdin et al. 1987) reviewed in great detail the behavioral treatments for conduct and oppositional disorders and suggested that the more severe the conduct disorder, the more guarded the outcome. They studied the combined effects of parent management training (using behavioral techniques described earlier in this chapter) and a cognitive-behavioral problem-solving skills training approach for the children, the latter approach aimed at improving maladaptive thinking patterns. Such patterns seen in aggressive children, they noted, include the lack of problem-solving skills and the tendency to believe that others are antagonistic toward them. Those children receiving the combined treatment exhibited less aggressive behavior at home and in school, along with greater overall prosocial behaviors, than did the contact-control group, both following treatment and at 1-year follow-up. Further controlled work is much needed so that more powerful therapies for this important disorder can be developed.

Kazdin (1987) and others advocated earlier treatment for children and their families, that is, treatment before the children became heavily involved in antisocial behaviors and involved in the juvenile justice system. Such research should focus on early intervention to minimize the severity of the conduct disorder and the frequency of antisocial behaviors.

One study (Dumas and Wahler 1985) evaluated mother–child dyads participating in a parent-training program for children with conduct disorder. Mothers who had a low level of community contact (i.e., insular mothers) used more aversive control toward their children than did mothers with a higher level of community contacts. Children of the insular mothers were more aggressive than those of noninsular mothers in general, and in particular when responding to negative maternal behavior. Increasing contacts with friends and social supports in the community may help reduce negative interpersonal interactions.

A number of studies now report that behavioral techniques and parent management training for the treatment of childhood conduct problems can produce significant improvement in child behavior (reviewed by Kazdin 1998). Maintenance of these gains has been found in follow-ups of 1–3 years; one program has even reported maintenance of gains for 10–14 years (Long et al. 1994).

Attention-Deficit/Hyperactivity Disorder

Attention-deficit/hyperactivity disorder (ADHD) and associated learning disabilities may occur in more than 5% of children in the United States. Hyperactive children demonstrate excessive motor activity, distractibility, and impulsivity, which cause adjustment difficulties both at home and in school. These children often have difficulty when concentration is required for task completion. Behavioral studies using contingent reinforcement of desired behaviors in this population demonstrated that when teachers differentially attended to and reinforced

appropriate classroom behavior, deviant behavior was reduced (Becker et al. 1967). Children who were rewarded for increasing academic work through use of free time or through participation in preferred classroom activities made considerable academic gains that were well maintained. Maintenance in school-related gains has been enhanced by the addition of parental reinforcement (Ayllon et al. 1975). When children brought home a good-behavior letter, one indicating cooperation and a reduced level of deviant behavior, they could select home-based rewards (e.g., praise, more allowance money); failure to bring home the letter resulted in an earlier bedtime or withholding of allowance.

Ayllon et al. (1975) evaluated academic performance in children who had been taking methylphenidate and who continued to do poorly academically. When methylphenidate therapy was discontinued, their hyperactivity increased. A token program was instituted whereby first work in math and then work in both math and reading were reinforced. Not only did academic performance improve, but the hyperactivity decreased. The behaviors incompatible with learning were reduced if the child was successful academically. A number of studies have begun to evaluate whether interactive effects exist when both behavioral and pharmacological interventions are used. Controlled studies suggest that medication reduces hyperactive behaviors but does little for either the learning deficits or the impulsive and aggressive behaviors associated with this disorder (Gadow 1985). Thus, a combination of behavior therapy and medication is most commonly used in the treatment of ADHD.

Combination Treatment

Pelham et al. (1993) compared an intensive behavioral intervention with pharmacological treatment (methylphenidate) for children with ADHD. Although both the behavioral and the pharmacological interventions resulted in significant improvements in hyperactive and impulsive behaviors, the effect sizes were greater with the pharmacological treatment. A major clinical trial, the Multimodal Treatment Study of Children with ADHD (1999), examined whether intensive behavioral treatment, when combined with pharmacological treatment, provided added benefits. The subjects who received the combination of behavior therapy plus medication did not differ in measures of hyperactivity from those receiving medication alone. However, those receiving behavior therapy plus medication showed greater improvements than did the medication-alone group in a number of areas—oppositional and aggressive symptoms, social skills, parent–child relations, and achievement in reading—compared with those children who received only the behavioral intervention without medication or the community intervention. These findings suggest that the combination of behavioral and pharmacological treatment may be useful to maximize treatment response in children with ADHD.

Ruminative Vomiting

Ruminative vomiting is seen in infants and in mentally retarded individuals of all ages. Milk, or food in the case of the older child, is regurgitated and spat out. Because in infancy this condition is often life threatening, the principal approach to treatment has been within a punishment paradigm. Punishment is much less useful as a therapeutic procedure than positive reinforcement, because there are unwanted side effects such as aggressive behavior and there is always the possibility of inflicting physical harm. For the most part, punishment is used only in situations in which the behavior to be changed threatens injury to the patient and only when procedures using positive reinforcement have been found not to lead to improvement. In institutions where punishment procedures are frequently used, it is essential that an oversight committee be appointed to monitor the use of punishment.

Infants with ruminative vomiting regurgitate their food mouthful by mouthful, which leads to malnutrition and dehydration and thus poses a threat to life. One approach to treatment is to use the principle of punishment, whereby an unpleasant event is made contingent on each episode of regurgitation. In one controlled study, a drop of lemon juice on the tongue was used as the unpleasant event. During baseline measurement, before treatment was begun, the infant ruminated between 40% and 70% of the time the infant was awake (Sajwaj et al. 1974). Once lemon juice was presented contingent on spitting up food, the rate of ruminative vomiting decreased steadily. Punishment was then briefly removed, and rumination quickly returned to original baseline levels, confirming the effectiveness of lemon juice as a punishing event. Reintroduction of punishment led to disappearance of the behavior and a return to normal weight, with no relapse at 1-year follow-up. Similar procedures have been used successfully in mentally retarded ruminating individuals.

Childhood Depression

Behavioral treatment of childhood depression has been modeled on the demonstrably successful treatment of adult depression using either social skills training or a more comprehensive CBT package. The treatment package used with depressed children is similar to that used with adults and is aimed at decreasing depressive thinking, enhancing social skills, and increasing pleasant activities. Several controlled single-case studies have shown the effectiveness of either the whole cognitive-behavioral package or an element of the package (e.g., social skills training). However, many of these studies focused their assessment of improvement on the specific skills taught, rather than on depression. In one controlled study, it was found that some 50% of adolescents no longer met criteria for depression after treatment, whereas little change was observed in the waiting-list control group. There was continued improvement over a 2-year follow-up: fewer than 10% met criteria for depression at 1 year, and fewer than 20% met criteria at 2 years. This finding suggests that although not everyone improves, the effects of treatment are long lasting. Interestingly, adding therapy for the parents of these children produced no added benefits. Other studies suggest that younger children respond equally well to treatment, but, as with adults, there tends to be no difference between different types of active treatment.

In a randomized controlled trial of adolescents with major depression, Brent et al. (1997) found that CBT resulted in a higher rate of remission (65% achieved absence of depression) compared with individual supportive therapy (39%) or systemic family therapy (38%). The rate of remission was also greater with CBT compared with the other treatments.

Behavioral Pediatrics

As in the case of adults, behavioral approaches have been used increasingly in pediatric populations with medical problems. Chronic diseases in childhood often require complex behavior changes for optimal treatment. Such is the case, for example, for the child with insulin-dependent diabetes mellitus who must comply with medications, diet, and exercise. Epstein et al. (1981) developed an educational intervention aimed at increasing knowledge and skills, using instruction, feedback concerning performance, and reinforcement. The content included insulin dosage, diet, exercise, self-administration of insulin, and the signs and symptoms of hypoglycemia. Parents participated, encouraging child adherence. Substantial improvements were made: urine samples were negative for glucose in 27% of cases during treatment, 39% after treatment, and 45% at 2-month follow-up.

Reinforcement systems have also been used to help children adhere to the demands of hemodialysis (Magrab and Papadopoulou 1977). Children were encouraged to adhere to diet and were rewarded with prizes for improvements in weight and in potassium and blood urea nitrogen levels. Similar reinforcement approaches have been helpful in larger populations, such as for the encouragement of attendance at dental facilities by low-income families (Reiss et al. 1976).

Modeling has proved useful in reducing children's fears before medical procedures. Melamed and Siegel (1975), in a randomized, controlled study, studied children who were about to have surgery. One group of children in the study viewed a film about a child coping with hospitalization and medical procedures, whereas the control group saw a film on another topic. Directly after this film, the experimental group demonstrated more physiological arousal. However, before surgery and a month later, both self-report of fear and physiological arousal were notably less in the experimental group. Fewer children in the experimental group required pain medication after surgery or complained of side effects, and more returned to eating solid foods sooner. This procedure is an excellent example of the use of modeling to aid in adaptive coping with a stressful life event.

References

Agras WS: Eating Disorders: Management of Obesity, Bulimia, and Anorexia Nervosa. New York, Pergamon, 1987

Agras WS: Understanding compliance with the medical regimen: the scope of the problem and a theoretical perspective. Arthritis Care and Research 2(suppl):8–16, 1989

Agras WS, Rossiter EM, Arnow B, et al: Pharmacologic and cognitive-behavioral treatment for bulimia nervosa: a controlled comparison. Am J Psychiatry 149:82–87, 1992

Agras WS, Telch CF, Arnow B, et al: Weight loss, cognitive-behavioral, and desipramine treatments in binge eating disorder: an additive design. Behav Ther 25:209–238, 1994

Ayllon T, Azrin NH: The measurement and reinforcement of behavior of psychotics. J Exp Anal Behav 8:357–383, 1965

Ayllon T, Layman D, Kandel HJ: A behavioral-educational alternative to drug control of hyperactive children. J Appl Behav Anal 8:137–146, 1975

Bandura A: Social Foundations of Thought and Action: A Social Cognitive Theory. Englewood Cliffs, NJ, Prentice-Hall, 1986

Barlow DH, Craske MG, Cerny JA, et al: Behavioral treatment of panic disorder. Behav Ther 20:261–282, 1989

Baxter LB, Schwartz JM, Bergman K, et al: Caudate glucose metabolic rate changes with both drug and behavior therapy for obsessive-compulsive disorder. Arch Gen Psychiatry 49:681–689, 1992

Becker WC, Madsen CH, Arnold CR, et al: The contingent use of teacher attention and praising in reducing classroom behavior problems. Journal of Special Education 1:287–307, 1967

Brent DA, Holder D, Kolko D, et al. A clinical psychotherapy trial for adolescent depression comparing cognitive, family, and supportive therapy. Arch Gen Psychiatry 54:877–885, 1997

Brownell KD, Wadden TA: Behavior therapy for obesity: modern approaches and better results, in Handbook of Eating Disorders: Physiology, Psychology and Treatment of Obesity, Anorexia, and Bulimia. Edited by Brownell KD, Foreyt JP. New York, Basic Books, 1986, pp 180–197

Bruce TJ, Spiegel DA, Gregg SF, et al: Predictors of alprazolam discontinuation with and without cognitive behavior therapy in panic disorder. Am J Psychiatry 152:1156–1160, 1995

Campbell M, Anderson L, Meier M, et al: A comparison of haloperidol and behavior therapy and their interaction in autistic children. Journal of the American Academy of Child Psychiatry 17:640–655, 1978

Christophersen ER, Arnold CM, Hill DW, et al: The home point system: token reinforcement procedures for application by parents of children with behavior problems. J Appl Behav Anal 5:485–497, 1972

Christophersen ER, Barnard JD, Ford D, et al: The family training program: improving parent-child interaction patterns, in Behavior Modification Approaches to Parenting. Edited by Mash EJ, Handy LC, Hamerlynck LA. New York, Brunner/Mazel, 1976, pp 137–155

Clark DM, Salkovskis PM, Hackmann A, et al: A comparison of cognitive therapy, applied relaxation and imipramine in the treatment of panic disorder. Br J Psychiatry 164:759–769, 1994

Clarkin JF, Pilkonis PA, Magruder K: Psychotherapy of depression: implications for reform of the health care system. Arch Gen Psychiatry 53:717–723, 1996

Cohen DJ, Shaywitz BA: Preface to special issue on neurobiological research in autism. J Autism Dev Disord 12:103–109, 1982

Craighead LW, Stunkard AJ, O'Brien R: Behavior therapy and pharmacotherapy of obesity. Arch Gen Psychiatry 38:763–768, 1981

Craske MG, Maidenberg E, Bystritsky A: Brief cognitive-behavioral versus non-directive therapy for panic disorder. J Behav Ther Exp Psychiatry 26:113–120, 1995

Crisp AH, Norton K, Gowers S, et al: A controlled study of the effects of therapies aimed at adolescent and family psychopathology in anorexia nervosa. Br J Psychiatry 159:325–333, 1991

de Beurs E, van Balkom AJ, Lange A, et al: Treatment of panic disorder with agoraphobia: comparison of fluvoxamine, placebo, and psychological panic management combined with exposure and of exposure in vivo alone. Am J Psychiatry 152:683–691, 1995

Dumas JE, Wahler RG: Indiscriminate mothering as a contextual factor in aggressive-oppositional child behavior: "Damned if you do and damned if you don't." J Abnorm Child Psychol 13:1–17, 1985

Elkin E, Shea T, Watkins J, et al: National Institute of Mental Health Treatment of Depression Collaborative Research Program: general effectiveness of treatment. Arch Gen Psychiatry 46:971–982, 1989

Epstein LH, Beck S, Figuera J, et al: The effects of targeting improvements in urine glucose on metabolic control in children with insulin dependent diabetes. J Appl Behav Anal 14:365–376, 1981

Fairburn CG: A cognitive-behavioral approach to the treatment of bulimia. Psychol Med 11:707–711, 1981

Fairburn CG, Jones R, Peveler RC, et al: Three psychological treatments for bulimia nervosa: a comparative trial. Arch Gen Psychiatry 48:463–469, 1991

Fairburn CG, Jones R, Peveler RC, et al: Psychotherapy and bulimia nervosa: longer-term effects of interpersonal psychotherapy, behavior therapy, and cognitive-behavior therapy. Arch Gen Psychiatry 50:419–428, 1993

Falloon IRH, Boyd JL, McGill CW, et al: Family management in the prevention of morbidity of schizophrenia. Arch Gen Psychiatry 42:887–896, 1985

Fava GA, Zielezny M, Savron G, et al: Long-term effects of behavioural treatment for panic disorder with agoraphobia. Br J Psychiatry 166:87–92, 1995

Fawzy FI, Fawzy NW, Hyun CS, et al: Malignant melanoma: effects of an early structured psychiatric intervention, coping, and affective state on recurrence and survival 6 years later. Arch Gen Psychiatry 50:681–689, 1993

Friedman M, Thoresen CE, Gill JJ, et al: Alteration of Type A behavior and reduction in cardiac recurrences in postmyocardial infarction patients. Am Heart J 108:237–248, 1984

Gadow KD: Relative efficacy of pharmacological, behavioral, and combination treatments for enhancing academic performance. Clin Psychol Rev 5:513–533, 1985

Gates SJ, Colborn DK: Lowering appointment failures in a neighborhood health center. Med Care 14:263–267, 1976

Heimberg RG, Barlow DH: New developments in cognitive-behavioral therapy for social phobia. J Clin Psychiatry 52:21–30, 1991

Heimberg RG, Salzman DG, Holt CS, et al: Cognitive-behavioral group treatment for social phobia. Cognitive Therapy Research 14:1–23, 1993

Kandel ER: Genes, nerve cells, and the remembrance of things past. J Neuropsychiatry Clin Neurosci 1:103–107, 1989

Kazdin AE: The Token Economy: A Review and Evaluation. New York, Plenum, 1977

Kazdin AE: Conduct Disorder in Childhood and Adolescence. Newbury Park, CA, Sage, 1987

Kazdin AE: Psychosocial treatments for conduct disorder in children, in A Guide to Treatments That Work. Edited by Nathan PE, Gorman JM. New York, Oxford University Press, 1998, pp 65–89

Kazdin AE, Esveldt-Dawson K, French NH, et al: Effects of parent management and problem solving skills training combined in a treatment of antisocial child behavior. J Am Acad Child Adolesc Psychiatry 26:416–424, 1987

Keller M, McCullough JP, Klein DN, et al: A comparison of nefazodone, the cognitive behavioral-analysis system of psychotherapy, and their combination for the treatment of chronic depression. N Engl J Med 342:1462–1470, 2000

Kovacs M, Rush AJ, Beck AT, et al: Depressed outpatients treated with cognitive therapy or pharmacotherapy: a one-year follow-up. Arch Gen Psychiatry 38:33–39, 1981

Kozak MJ, Liebowitz MR, Foa EB: Cognitive behavior therapy and pharmacotherapy for OCD: the NIMH-sponsored collaborative study, in Treatment Challenges in Obsessive-Compulsive Disorder. Edited by Goodman WK, Rudorfer M, Maser J. Mahwah, NJ, Lawrence Erlbaum, 2000, pp 501–530

Lacks P, Bertelson AD, Gans L, et al: The effectiveness of three behavioral treatments for different degrees of sleep onset insomnia. Behav Ther 14:593–605, 1983

Lazovik AD, Lang PJ: A laboratory demonstration of systematic desensitization psychotherapy. Journal of Psychological Studies 11:238–247, 1960

Long P, Forehand R, Wierson M, et al: Does parent training with young noncompliant children have long-term effects? Behav Res Ther 32:101–107, 1994

Lovaas OI: Language Development Through Behavior Modification. New York, Wiley, 1977

Lovaas OI, Schreibman L, Koegel RI, et al: Selective responding by autistic children to multiple sensory input. J Abnorm Psychol 77:211–222, 1971

Lovaas OI, Koegel RL, Schreibman L: Stimulus overselectivity in autism: a review of research. Psychol Bull 86:1236–1254, 1979

Magrab PR, Papadopoulou ZL: The effect of a token economy on dietary compliance for children on hemodialysis. J Appl Behav Anal 10:573–578, 1977

Melamed BG, Siegel LJ: Reduction of anxiety in children facing hospitalization and surgery by use of filmed modeling. J Consult Clin Psychol 43:511–521, 1975

Mitchell JE, Pyle RL, Eckert ED, et al: A comparison study of antidepressants and structured intensive group psychotherapy in the treatment of bulimia nervosa. Arch Gen Psychiatry 47:149–157, 1990

Mueser KT, Sengupta A, School NR, et al: Family treatment and medication dosage reduction in schizophrenia: effects on patient social functioning, family attitudes, and burden. J Consult Clin Psychol 69:3–12, 2001

Multimodal Treatment Study of Children with ADHD (MTA) Cooperative Group: A 14-month randomized clinical trial of treatment strategies for attention-deficit/hyperactivity disorder. Arch Gen Psychiatry 56:1073–1083, 1999

Patterson GR: The aggressive child: victim and architect of a coercive system, in Behavior Modification and Families. Edited by Mash EJ, Hamerlynck LA, Handy LC. New York, Brunner/Mazel, 1976, pp 93–127

Paul GL, Lentz RG: Psychosocial Treatment of Chronic Mental Patients: Milieu Versus Social Learning Programs. Cambridge, MA, Harvard University Press, 1977

Pelham WE, Carlson CL, Sams SE, et al: Separate and combined effects of methylphenidate and behavior modification on boys with attention-deficit hyperactivity disorder in the classroom. J Consult Clin Psychol 61:506–515, 1993

Perri MG, McAllister DA, Gange JJ, et al: Effects of four maintenance programs on the long-term management of obesity. J Consult Clin Psychol 56:529–534, 1988

Reiss M, Plotrowski WD, Bailey JS: Behavioral community psychology: encouraging low-income parents to seek dental care for their children. J Appl Behav Anal 9:387–398, 1976

Rogers SJ: Empirically supported comprehensive treatments for young children with autism. J Clin Child Psychol 27:167–178, 1998

Sajwaj T, Libet J, Agras WS: Lemon juice therapy: the control of life-threatening rumination in a six-month-old infant. J Appl Behav Anal 7:557–563, 1974

Simons AD, Murphy GE, Levine RD, et al: Cognitive therapy and pharmacotherapy for depression. Arch Gen Psychiatry 43:43–50, 1986

Spiegel D, Bloom JR, Kraemer HC, et al: Effect of psychosocial treatment on survival of patients with metastatic breast cancer. Lancet 2:888–891, 1989

Stanley MA, Turner SM: Current status of pharmacological and behavioral treatment of obsessive-compulsive disorder. Behav Ther 26:163–186, 1995

Steketee G, Foa EB, Grayson FB: Recent advances in the behavioral treatment of obsessive-compulsives. Arch Gen Psychiatry 39:1365–1371, 1982

Stunkard AF, Penick SB: Behavior modification in the treatment of obesity: the problem of maintaining weight loss. Arch Gen Psychiatry 36:801–806, 1979

Taylor CB, Arnow B: The Nature and Treatment of Anxiety Disorders. New York, Free Press, 1988

Wadden TA, Berkowitz RI, Sarwer DB, et al: Benefits of lifestyle modification in the pharmacological treatment of obesity: a randomized trial. Arch Intern Med 161:218–227, 2001

Wahler RG: Deviant child behavior within the family: developmental speculations and behavior change strategies, in Handbook of Behavior Modifications and Behavior Therapy. Edited by Leitenberg H. Englewood Cliffs, NJ, Prentice-Hall, 1976, pp 516–543

Walsh BT, Wilson GT, Loeb KL, et al: Medication and psychotherapy in the treatment of bulimia nervosa: preliminary findings. Am J Psychiatry 154:523–531, 1997

Wilfley DE, Agras WS, Telch CF, et al: Group cognitive-behavioral therapy and group interpersonal therapy for the nonpurging bulimic: a controlled comparison. J Consult Clin Psychol 61:296–305, 1993

Wolpe J: Psychotherapy by Reciprocal Inhibition. Stanford, CA, Stanford University Press, 1958

Cognitive Therapy

Jesse H. Wright, M.D., Ph.D.

Aaron T. Beck, M.D.

Michael E. Thase, M.D.

Cognitive therapy (CT) is a system of psychotherapy based on theories of pathological information processing in mental disorders. Treatment is directed primarily at modifying distorted or maladaptive cognitions and related behavioral dysfunction. Therapeutic interventions are usually focused and problem oriented. Although the use of specific techniques is a major feature of this approach, there can be considerable flexibility and creativity in the clinical application of CT.

In this chapter we trace the historical origins of CT, explain basic cognitive theories, discuss experimental findings on cognitive pathology, and detail commonly used CT techniques. The main focus is on the treatment of depression and anxiety disorders. CT procedures for eating disorders, psychosis, characterological problems, and other psychiatric conditions also are described. Finally, the extensive research on the effectiveness of CT is reviewed and summarized.

Historical Background

The CT approach to depression was first proposed by Beck in the early 1960s (A.T. Beck 1963, 1964). He had begun to study depression from a psychoanalytical perspective several years earlier but had been struck by incongruities between the "retroflexed hostility" concept of psychoanalysis and his observations that depressed individuals usually hold negatively biased constructions of themselves and their environment (A.T. Beck 1963, 1964). Subsequently, a comprehensive CT for depression was articulated, and the treatment model was extended to a variety of other conditions, including anxiety disor-

ders (A.T. Beck 1967, 1976). CT was described in a fully developed form in *Cognitive Therapy of Depression* (A.T. Beck et al. 1979). This volume was the culmination of a series of treatment manuals developed at the Center for Cognitive Therapy at the University of Pennsylvania. The therapy interventions were designed to be compatible with the cognitive model of depression and were drawn from several sources including the clinical experiences of Beck and colleagues and the writings of behaviorists and post-Freudian analysts (A.T. Beck et al. 1979; Thase and Beck 1992).

CT is linked philosophically to the concepts of the Greek Stoic philosophers and eastern schools of thought such as Taoism and Buddhism (A.T. Beck et al. 1979). The writing of Epictetus in the *Enchiridion* ("Men are disturbed not by things, but by the views which they take of them.") captures the essence of the perspective that our ideas or thoughts are a controlling factor in our emotional lives. Modern philosophers also have endorsed the concept that conscious ideas are at the center of human experience and that the meanings attached to events are a primary source of our actions. The phenomenological approach to philosophy, as exemplified in the writings of Kant, Jaspers, Binswanger, and others has significantly influenced the development of CT (A.T. Beck et al. 1979). Frankl's (1985) logotherapy and Mahoney's (1985) and Guidano and Liotti's (1983) theories on constructivism also have played a role in formulating cognitively oriented treatment models. These authors have emphasized the importance of cognitive factors in finding meaning in life and in promoting personal growth.

There have been a number of developments in the field of psychotherapy during the twentieth century that have contributed to the formulation of the CT approach. The neo-Freudians, such as Adler (1936), Horney (1950), Alexander (1950), and Sullivan (1953) focused on the importance of perceptions of the self and on the salience of conscious experience (Raimy 1975). Other contributions came from the field of developmental psychology (Bowlby 1985; Piaget 1954) and from Kelly's (1955) theory of personal constructs. These writers stressed the significance of schemas (cognitive templates) in perceiving, assimilating, and acting on information from the environment.

CT also incorporates theories and treatment methods of behavior therapy. Procedures such as activity scheduling, graded task assignments, exposure, and social skills training play a fundamental role in CT (A.T. Beck et al. 1979; Lewinsohn et al. 1982; Meichenbaum 1977). In addition, Ellis' rational emotive therapy (Ellis 1962, 1973) has helped promulgate CT and related treatments.

Investigations in the field of cognitive psychology have solidified the concepts originally proposed by Beck and have led to a refinement of the CT approach (e.g., Alford and Beck 1997; D.A. Clark et al. 1999; Dobson and Shaw 1986; Hollon and Kendall 1980; LeFebvre 1981; Nelson and Craighead 1977; Rizley 1978). Also, the utility of the cognitive model has been demonstrated in a number of outcome trials reviewed later in this chapter. Recent developments have included the description of cognitive and behavioral techniques for personality disorders (A.T. Beck and Freeman 1990; J. Beck 1997; Perris 1994; Shearin and Linehan 1994), substance abuse (Barrett and Meyer 1993; A.T. Beck et al. 1992a; Carroll et al. 1994a, 1994b; Fisher and Bentley 1996), geriatric patients (Beutler et al. 1987; Steuer et al. 1984; K.C.M. Wilson et al. 1995), eating disorders (Agras et al. 1992; P.J. Cooper and Steere 1995; Fairburn et al. 1991), and bipolar disorder (Basco and Rush 1996). Also, theories and procedures have been developed for combining CT and pharmacotherapy (Rush 1988; J.H. Wright and Schrodt 1989; J.H. Wright and Thase 1992), applying CT principles in the treatment of psychotic patients (Alford and Correia 1994; Garety et al. 1994; Kingdon and Turkington 1991; Perris and Skagerlind 1994), implementing cognitively oriented inpatient treatment (Bowers 1989; Stuart et al. 1997; J.H. Wright et al. 1993b), using CT in behavioral medicine (Bergdahl et al. 1995; Dworkin et al. 1994; Payne and Blanchard 1995; Sensky and Wright 1993; Speckens et al. 1995; White and Neilson 1995), and employing computer-assisted cognitive therapy (CCT) to improve the efficiency of treatment (Selmi et al. 1990; J.H. Wright and Wright 1997; J.H. Wright et al. 2002a, 2002b).

In a review of the evolution of CT over the past 30 years, Beck (A.T. Beck 1993) observed that intensive efforts have been made to have CT fulfill the criteria for a system of psychotherapy (Table 29–1). These criteria include: 1) a comprehensive theory, 2) empirical data to support this theory, 3) an operationalized therapy that interlocks with theoretical concepts, and 4) demonstrated efficacy of the treatment (A.T. Beck 1993). The remainder of this chapter is devoted to describing basic cognitive theories and their experimental basis, the translation of theoretical constructs into clinical practice, and the validation of CT in controlled research.

Basic Concepts

The Cognitive Model

The cognitive model for psychotherapy is grounded on the theory that there are characteristic errors in information processing in depression, anxiety disorders, personality disturbances, and other psychiatric conditions (A.T. Beck 1976; A.T. Beck and Rush 1992). For example, Beck (A.T. Beck 1976; A.T. Beck and Rush 1992) has proposed that there are three major areas of cognitive distortion in depression (the negative cognitive triad of self, world, and future) and that patients with anxiety disorders habitually overestimate the danger or risk in situations. Cognitive distortions such as misperceptions, errors in logic, or misattributions are thought to lead to dysphoric affect and maladaptive behavior. Furthermore, a "vicious cycle" is perpetuated when the behavioral response confirms and amplifies negatively distorted cognitions (J.H. Wright 1988).

This point is illustrated by the case of Mr. S, a 45-year-old recently divorced, depressed man. After being rebuffed on his first attempt to ask a woman for a date, Mr. S had a series of dysfunctional cognitions such as, "You should have known better…. You're a loser… There's no use trying." His subsequent behavioral pattern was consistent with these cognitions—he made no further social contacts and became more lonely and isolated. The negative behavior led to additional maladaptive cognitions (e.g., "No one will want me…. I'll be alone the rest of my life…. What's the use of going on?").

TABLE 29–1. Criteria for a system of psychotherapy

A comprehensive theory
Empirical support for the theory
An operationalized therapy based on theoretical principles
Empirical evidence for effectiveness of the psychotherapy

The CT perspective can be summarized in a working model (Figure 29–1) that expands on the well-known stimulus–response paradigm (J.H. Wright 1988). Cognitive mediation is given the central role in this model. However, an interactive relationship between environmental influences, cognition, emotion, and behavior is also recognized. It should be emphasized that this working model does not presume that cognitive pathology is the cause of specific syndromes or that other factors such as genetic predisposition, biochemical alterations, or interpersonal conflicts are not involved in the etiology of psychiatric illnesses. Instead, the model is used simply as a guide for the actions of the cognitive therapist in clinical practice. It is assumed that most forms of psychopathology have complex etiologies involving cognitive, biological, social, and interpersonal influences, and that there are multiple, potentially useful, approaches to treatment (see, for example, Akiskal and McKinney 1975; Engel 1977; J.H. Wright and Thase 1992; J.H. Wright et al. 1993a). In addition, it is assumed that cognitive changes are accomplished through biological processes and that psychopharmacological treatments can alter cognitions (J.H. Wright and Thase 1992). This position is consistent with outcome research on CT and pharmacotherapy (Blackburn et al. 1981; Imber et al. 1990; Peselow et al. 1990; Simons et al. 1984) and with other studies that have documented neurobiological changes associated with conditioning in animals (Kandel 1979; Kandel and Schwarz 1982; Mohl 1987) or psychotherapy in humans (Baxter et al. 1992; Brody et al. 2001; Martin et al. 2001; J.M. Schwartz et al. 1996; Thase et al. 1998).

The working model in Figure 29–1 posits a close relationship between cognition and emotion. The general thrust of CT is that emotional responses are largely dependent upon cognitive appraisals of the significance of environmental cues. For example, sadness is likely when an event (or memory of an event) is perceived in a negative way (such as a loss, a defeat, or a rejection), and anger is common when it is judged that there are threats to one's self or loved ones (A.T. Beck and Rush 1992). The cognitive model also incorporates the effects of emotion on cognitive processing. Heightened emotion can stimulate and intensify cognitive distortion (Bower 1981; Greenburg and Safran 1984). Therapeutic procedures in CT involve interventions at all points in the working model diagrammed in Figure 29–1. However, most of the effort is directed at stimulating either cognitive or behavioral change.

Levels of Dysfunctional Cognitions

Beck and colleagues (A.T. Beck 1976; A.T. Beck et al. 1979; Dobson and Shaw 1986) have suggested that there

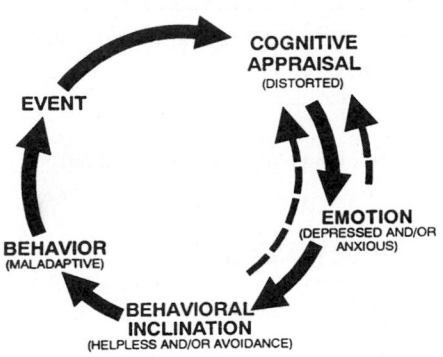

FIGURE 29–1. A working model for cognitive therapy.
Source. Adapted from J.H. Wright 1988.

are two major levels of dysfunctional information processing: 1) automatic thoughts, and 2) basic beliefs incorporated in schemas. Automatic thoughts are the cognitions that occur rapidly while a person is in a situation (or is recalling an event). These automatic thoughts usually are not subjected to rational analysis and often are based on erroneous logic. Although the individual may be only subliminally aware of these cognitions, automatic thoughts are accessible through questioning techniques used in CT (A.T. Beck et al. 1979; J.H. Wright and Beck 1983). The different types of faulty logic in automatic thinking have been termed *cognitive errors* (A.T. Beck et al. 1979). Descriptions of typical cognitive errors such as selective abstraction, arbitrary inference, and absolutistic thinking are found in Table 29–2.

Schemas are deeper cognitive structures that contain the basic rules for screening, filtering, and coding information from the environment (A.T. Beck et al. 1979; D.A. Clark et al. 1999; J.H. Wright and Beck 1983). These organizing constructs are developed through early childhood experiences and subsequent formative influences. Schemas can play a highly adaptive role in allowing rapid assimilation of data and appropriate decision making (Bowlby 1985). However, in psychiatric disorders there are clusters of maladaptive schemas that perpetuate dysphoric mood and ineffective or self-defeating behavior (A.T. Beck 1976; A.T. Beck and Freeman 1990). Examples of adaptive and maladaptive schemas are included in Table 29–3.

D.A. Clark et al. (1999) have suggested that group schemas can be divided into three levels: 1) simple schemas (e.g., rules about objects in the environment) that may have little or no influence on psychopathology; 2) intermediary beliefs, rules, and assumptions (e.g., conditional rules, "if–then" statements such as "to be

TABLE 29–2. Cognitive errors

Selective abstraction (sometimes termed "mental filter")	Drawing a conclusion based on only a small portion of the available data
Arbitrary inference	Coming to a conclusion without adequate supporting evidence or despite contradictory evidence
Absolutistic thinking ("all or none" thinking)	Categorizing oneself or personal experiences into rigid dichotomies (e.g., all good or all bad, perfect or completely flawed, success or total failure)
Magnification and minimization	Over- or undervaluing the significance of a personal attribute, a life event, or a future possibility
Personalization	Linking external occurrences to oneself (e.g., taking blame, assuming responsibility, criticizing oneself) when there is little or no basis for making these associations
Catastrophic thinking	Predicting the worst possible outcome while ignoring more likely eventualities

Source. Adapted with permission from Beck AT, Rush AJ, Shaw BF, et al.: *Cognitive Therapy of Depression.* New York, Guilford, 1979.

TABLE 29–3. Adaptive and maladaptive schemas

Adaptive	Maladaptive
No matter what happens, I can manage somehow.	I must be perfect to be accepted.
If I work at something, I can master it.	If I choose to do something, I must succeed.
I'm a survivor.	I'm a fake.
Others can trust me.	Without a woman [man], I'm nothing.
I'm lovable.	
People respect me.	I'm stupid.
I can figure things out.	No matter what I do, I won't succeed.
If I prepare in advance, I usually do better.	Others can't be trusted.
I like to be challenged.	I can never be comfortable around others.
There's not much that can scare me.	If I make one mistake, I'll lose everything.
	The world is too frightening for me.

accepted, I must always please others"); and 3) core beliefs about the self (e.g., fundamental rules such "I am unlovable") that often have an global and absolute quality. Schemas can vary in their degree of flexibility, permeability (i.e., the degree to which they can be modified by contradictory information), concreteness, valence, and breadth (D.A. Clark et al. 1999). It has been suggested that clusters of interrelated schemas (termed *modes*) help humans to organize and deal with the demands that are placed upon them (D.A. Clark et al. 1999).

One of the basic tenets of CT is that maladaptive schemas often lie dormant until they are triggered by stressful life events (A.T. Beck et al. 1979; D.A. Clark et al. 1999; Miranda 1992). The newly emerged schema(s) then influences the more superficial level of cognitive processing so that automatic thoughts are consistent with the rules of the schema. This theory applies primarily to episodic disorders such as depression. In chronic conditions (e.g., personality disturbances and eating disorders), schemas that pertain to the self may be present consistently and may be more resistant to change than in depression or anxiety disorders (A.T. Beck and Freeman 1990; A.T. Beck and Rush 1992).

> An example of the relationship between schemas and automatic thoughts can be found in the case of Mrs. C, a 39-year-old schoolteacher, married for the second time, who was functioning well until her husband made an unwise financial investment. When the family's economic situation changed, Mrs. C became depressed and started to have crying spells in her classroom. During the course of CT, several important schemas were uncovered. One of these was the maladaptive belief: "You'll fail, no matter how hard you try." This schema was associated with a host of negative automatic thoughts (e.g., "I messed up again.... We'll lose everything.... It's not worth the effort"). Although there had been a significant financial loss, and the marriage was stressed because of the situation, the emergence of Mrs. C's underlying schema led to an overgeneralization of the significance of the problem and a perpetuation of dysfunctional automatic thoughts.

Cognitive Pathology in Depression and Anxiety Disorders

The role of cognitive functioning in depression and anxiety disorders has been studied extensively. Information processing also has been examined in eating disorders, characterological problems, and other psychiatric conditions. In general, the results of this investigative effort have confirmed Beck's hypotheses (A.T. Beck 1963, 1964, 1976; A.T. Beck and Rush 1992; A.T. Beck et al. 1979; D.A. Clark et al. 1999; Rush 1983; J.H. Wright 1988; J.H. Wright and Beck 1983). A full review of this research is not attempted here. However, a synthesis of results of significant studies on depression and anxiety is provided. These findings have played an important role in both confirming and shaping the treatment procedures used in CT. Cognitive pathology in eating disturbances, personality disorders, and psychoses is described in the section on CT applications.

Reviews of the voluminous research on cognitive processes in depression have found strong evidence for a negative cognitive bias in this disorder (D.A. Clark et al. 1999; Haaga 1991). For example, distorted automatic thoughts and cognitive errors have been found to be much more frequent in depressed persons than in control subjects (Blackburn et al. 1986a; Dobson and Shaw 1986; Hollon et al. 1986; LeFebvre 1981; Watkins and Rush 1983). A selective recall bias also has been described. Depressed individuals are more likely to remember negative than positive self-referent information (D.M. Clark and Teasdale 1982; Gotlib 1981; Lloyd and Lishman 1975; Nelson and Craighead 1977; Teasdale and Fogarty 1979).

Substantial evidence has been collected to support the concept of the negative cognitive triad (D.A. Clark et al. 1999). A particularly well designed study in this area of research was performed by Blackburn et al. (1986a) who used the Cognitive Bias Questionnaire to test distortions in the three areas of the negative cognitive triad (self, world, and future). Depressed individuals scored more than twice as high on this scale as nondepressed control subjects. A large group of investigations has established that one of the elements of the negative cognitive triad, hopelessness, is highly associated with suicide risk (A.T. Beck et al. 1975, 1985b; Fawcett et al. 1987; Minkoff et al. 1973; Nekanda-Trepka et al. 1983; Prezant and Neimeyer 1988). A.T. Beck et al. (1985b) found that hopelessness was the strongest predictor of ultimate suicide in a sample of depressed inpatients followed 10 years after discharge. Also, in a related study with outpatients, hopelessness was shown to predict ultimate suicides with a high degree of sensitivity (A.T. Beck et al. 1990).

Research on schemas has been limited by problems in measuring these underlying cognitive structures (see, for example, Bradley and Mathews 1982; D.A. Clark et al. 1999; H. Davis and Unruh 1981; Derry and Kuiper 1981). The most commonly used instrument, the Dysfunctional Attitude Scale (DAS; Weissman 1979) has

been criticized because it appears to tap a general tendency for negatively biased thinking and may not directly assess schemas (D.A. Clark et al. 1999; Hollon et al. 1986). Furthermore, Beck's theories indicate that schemas become dormant during remissions: therefore, these core beliefs would not be expected to be readily accessible with a self-rating instrument such as the DAS. Nevertheless, several investigations have found high DAS scores during periods of depression and marked reductions with symptomatic improvement (e.g., Blackburn et al. 1986a; DeRubeis et al. 1990; Simons et al. 1984). It has been suggested that small residual elevations in DAS scores after recovery from depression may indicate that this scale detects underlying schemas that are a marker for vulnerability to relapse (Blackburn et al. 1986a; D.E. Giles et al. 1989; Riskind and Steer 1984).

Abramson et al. (1978) have proposed that attributions to life events are negatively distorted in depression and that misattributions can play a role in the development of this disorder. The relevance of early research on attributions has been questioned because most investigations were performed with nonclinical experimental subjects (D.A. Clark et al. 1999; Peterson et al. 1985). Also, some studies of carefully diagnosed depressed patients found little or no evidence for attributional distortions (Hargreaves 1985; Miller et al. 1982). Nevertheless, the overall results of research on attributions indicate that clinically depressed individuals are prone to blame themselves for adverse life events, give global meaning to circumscribed occurrences, and believe that negative situations will last indefinitely. In contrast, individuals that do not have depression commonly view noxious events as being due to external forces (e.g., fate, bad luck), as having isolated significance (limited only to the specific events), and being transient situations (Deutscher and Cimbolic 1990; Hammon et al. 1981; Raps et al. 1982; Zautra et al. 1985; Zimmerman et al. 1986).

Studies of responses to feedback have provided another perspective on dysfunctional information processing. Depressed individuals usually underestimate the amount of positive feedback that they receive (D.A. Clark et al. 1999; DeMonbreun and Craighead 1977; Gotlib 1983; Loeb et al. 1964; Nelson and Craighead 1977; Rizley 1978; Wenzloff and Grozier 1988). In analogue experiments, depressed subjects have expended decreased effort on subsequent trials after concluding that they have performed poorly on a task (Klein et al. 1976; Loeb et al. 1971). Interestingly, several studies have found a "positive self-serving bias" in nondepressed control subjects (Alloy and Ahrens 1987; Gotlib and Olson 1983; Rizley 1978). The tendency for nondepressed individuals to hear more positive and/or less negative feedback than they actually receive and to expend extra effort after being told they have not done well, may be an adaptive trait (Rizley 1978).

Studies of information processing in anxiety disorders have provided additional confirmation for the cognitive model of psychopathology. Anxious patients have been found to have an attentional bias in responding to potentially threatening stimuli (Mathews and MacLeod 1987). Individuals with significant levels of anxiety are more likely than nonanxious persons to have a facilitated intake of information about potential threat; and furthermore, those with anxiety disorders are prone to interpret environmental situations as being unrealistically dangerous or risky (Fitzgerald and Phillips 1991; Mathews and MacLeod 1987). Anxious patients also have been shown to have an enhanced recall for memories associated with threatening situations or past anxiety states (Cloitre and Liebowitz 1991; Ingram and Kendall 1987). Thus, dysfunctional thinking in anxiety disorders spans over several phases of information processing, including attention, elaboration and inference, and retrieval from memory.

Automatic thoughts associated with themes of danger, threat, uncontrollability, or anticipated incompetence have been observed at much higher rates in patients with elevated levels of anxiety than those with low anxiety (Ingram and Kendall 1987; Kendall and Hollon 1989). In other studies of cognitive biasing in anxiety disorders, investigators have noted high frequencies of negative self-statements (C.R. Glass and Furlong 1990), beliefs that social behavior is inadequate or standards of others cannot be met (Wallace and Alden 1991), misinterpretations of bodily stimuli (McNally and Foa 1987), and overestimates of future misfortune (Mizes et al. 1987).

Comparisons of depressed and anxious patients have revealed differences between the two groups and common features of the disorders (D.A. Clark et al. 1990; Ingram et al. 1987). In depression, cognitions about hopelessness, low self-worth, and failure are more frequent, whereas in anxiety, cognitive themes are usually related to anticipated harm or danger (D.A. Clark et al. 1990). Also, depressed patients are more likely to have absolute thoughts about negative themes, whereas those with anxiety disorders tend to have questioning thoughts concerning the uncertainty of future events (D.A. Clark et al. 1990; Ingram and Kendall 1987; Kendall and Hollon 1989). Although the content of thoughts may be different, depressed and anxious patients both have demoralization, self-absorption, a predominance of automatic information processing, and a reduction in the cognitive capacity needed for problem solving and task perfor-

mance (D.A. Clark et al. 1990; Ingram and Kendall 1987; Ingram et al. 1987). Findings of studies on cognitive pathology in depression and anxiety disorders are summarized in Table 29–4.

Therapeutic Principles

General Procedures

CT is usually a short-term treatment, lasting from 4 to 20 sessions (J. Beck 1995). In some instances, very brief treatment courses are used for patients with mild or circumscribed problems, or longer series of CT sessions are used for those with chronic or especially severe conditions. However, the typical patient with major depression or an anxiety disorder can be treated successfully within the short-term format. After completion of the initial course of treatment, intermittent booster sessions may be useful in some cases, particularly for individuals with a history of recurrent illness. Booster sessions can help maintain gains, solidify what has been learned in CT, and decrease the chances of relapse (Thase 1992).

Although CT is primarily directed at the "here and now," knowledge of the patient's family background, developmental experiences, social network, and medical history helps guide the course of therapy. Collecting a thorough history is an essential component of the early phase of treatment. History taking can be augmented in CT by asking the patient to write a brief "autobiography" as one of the early homework assignments. This material is then reviewed during a subsequent therapy session.

The bulk of the therapeutic effort in CT is devoted to working on specific problems or issues in the patient's present life. The problem-oriented approach is emphasized for several reasons. First, directing the patient's attention to current problems stimulates the development of action plans that can help reverse helplessness, hopelessness, avoidance, or other dysfunctional symptoms. Second, data on cognitive responses to recent life events are more readily accessible and verifiable than for events that happened years in the past. Third, practical work on present problems helps to prevent the development of excessive dependency or regression in the therapeutic relationship. Finally, current problems usually provide ample opportunity to understand and explore the impact of past experiences (J.H. Wright 1988).

The Therapeutic Relationship

The therapeutic relationship in CT is characterized by a high degree of collaboration between patient and thera-

TABLE 29–4. Pathological information processing in depression and anxiety disorders

Predominant in depression	Predominant in anxiety disorders	Common to both depression and anxiety disorders
Hopelessness	Fears of harm or danger	Demoralization
Low self-esteem	High sensitivity to information about potential threat	Self-absorption
Negative view of environment		Heightened automatic information processing
Automatic thoughts with negative themes	Automatic thoughts associated with danger, risk, uncontrollability, incapacity	Maladaptive schemas
Misattributions		Reduced cognitive capacity for problem solving
Overestimates of negative feedback	Overestimates of risk in situations	
Enhanced recall of negative memories	Enhanced recall of memories for threatening situations	
Impaired performance on cognitive tasks requiring effort, abstract thinking		

pist and an empirical tone to the work of therapy. The therapist and patient function much like an investigative team. They develop hypotheses about the validity of automatic thoughts and schemas or alternately about the effectiveness of patterns of behavior. A series of exercises or experiments is then designed to test the validity of the hypotheses and, subsequently, to modify cognitions or behavior. A.T. Beck et al. (1979) have termed this form of therapeutic relationship *collaborative empiricism.* Methods of building a collaborative and empirical relationship are listed in Table 29–5.

The therapist usually is more active in CT than in most other psychotherapies. The degree of therapist activity varies with the stage of treatment and the severity of the illness. Generally, a more directive and structured approach is emphasized early in treatment, when symptoms are severe. For example, a markedly depressed patient who is beginning treatment may benefit from considerable direction and structure because of symptoms such as helplessness, hopelessness, low energy, and impaired concentration (J.H. Wright and Salmon 1990). As the patient improves and understands more about the methods of CT, the therapist can become somewhat less active. By the end of treatment, the patient should be able to use self-monitoring and self-help techniques with little reinforcement from the therapist.

Collaborative empiricism is fostered throughout the therapy, even when directive work is required. Although the therapist may suggest specific strategies or give homework assignments designed to combat severe depression or anxiety, the patient's input is always solicited and the self-help component of CT is emphasized from the outset of treatment. Also, it is made clear that CT is not an attempt to convert all negative thoughts to positive ones. In fact, bad things do occur to people, and some individuals have behaviors that are ineffective or self-defeating (Krantz 1985). It is emphasized that in CT

TABLE 29–5. Methods of enhancing collaborative empiricism

Work together as an investigative team.
Adjust therapist activity level to match the severity of illness and phase of treatment.
Encourage self-monitoring and self-help.
Obtain accurate assessment of validity of cognitions and efficacy of behavior.
Develop coping strategies for real losses and actual deficits.
Promote essential "nonspecific" therapist variables (e.g., kindness, empathy, equanimity, positive general attitude).
Provide and request feedback on regular basis.
Recognize and manage transference.
Customize therapy interventions.
Use gentle humor.

one seeks to obtain an accurate assessment of 1) the validity of cognitions, and 2) the adaptive versus maladaptive nature of behavior. If cognitive distortions have occurred, then the patient and therapist will work together to develop a more rational perspective. On the other hand, if actual negative experiences or characteristics are identified, they will attempt to find ways to cope or to change.

The development of a collaborative working relationship is dependent on a number of therapist and patient characteristics. The "nonspecific" therapist variables that are important components of all effective psychotherapies (Barrett and Wright 1984; D. Davis and Wright 1994; Traux and Mitchell 1971) are equally significant in CT (Table 29–6). Professionals who are kind, understanding, and can convey appropriate empathy make good cognitive therapists. Other factors of significance are the ability of the therapist to generate trust, to demonstrate a high level of competence, and to exhibit equanimity under pressure (A.T. Beck et al. 1979; Thase and

TABLE 29–6. Structuring procedures for cognitive therapy

Set agenda for therapy sessions.
Give constructive feedback to direct the course of therapy.
Employ common cognitive therapy techniques on a regular basis.
Assign homework to link sessions together.

Beck 1992; J.H. Wright and Davis 1992). Cognitive therapists also must be able to maintain an energetic pace and to sustain their concentration throughout the treatment sessions.

Another characteristic that can influence the therapeutic relationship is the therapist's general attitude. Clinicians with a reasonably positive outlook on life and a belief that individual efforts can lead to significant change are likely to form more adaptive therapeutic relationships than those who may be overly discouraged or pessimistic. If the latter features are present, the therapist may require personal therapy to be able to forge the collaborative and empirical relationships that are necessary for effective CT.

Additional procedures that cognitive therapists use to encourage collaborative empiricism are 1) providing feedback throughout sessions, 2) recognizing and managing transference, 3) customizing therapy interventions, and 4) using gentle humor. The therapist gives feedback to keep the therapeutic relationship anchored in the "here and now," and to reinforce the working aspect of the therapy process. Comments are made frequently throughout the session to summarize major points, to give direction, and to keep the session on target. Also, questions are asked at several intervals in each session to determine how well the patient has understood a concept or has grasped the essence of a therapeutic intervention. Because CT is highly psychoeducational, the therapist functions to some degree as a teacher. Thus, discreet positive feedback is given to help stimulate and reward the patient's efforts to learn. On a cautionary note, however, the cognitive therapist needs to avoid overzealous coaching or providing inaccurate or overdone positive feedback. Such actions will usually undermine the development of a good collaborative relationship.

Patients also are encouraged to give feedback throughout the sessions. In the beginning of treatment, patients are told that the therapist will want to hear from them regularly about how the sessions are going. What are the patient's reactions to the therapist? What things are going well? What would the patient like to change? What points are clear and make sense? What seems confusing?

A collaborative therapeutic relationship with frequent opportunities for two-way feedback generally discourages the formation of a transference neurosis. CT methodology and the short-term nature of treatment promote pragmatic working relationships as opposed to recapitulations of dysfunctional early relationships. Nevertheless, significant transference reactions can occur. These are more likely with patients who have personality disorders or other chronic illnesses that require longer term treatment. The formation of negative or problematic transference reactions is rare in conventional, short-term CT of persons with uncomplicated depression or anxiety disorders. When transference reactions occur, the cognitive therapist applies CT procedures to understand the phenomenon and to intervene. Typically, automatic thoughts and schemas that pertain to the therapeutic relationship are identified, explored, and modified if possible.

Another feature of CT that increases the collaborative nature of the therapeutic relationship is the customization of therapy interventions to meet the level of the patient's cognitive and social functioning. A profoundly depressed or anxious individual of low average intelligence may require a primarily behavioral approach, with limited efforts at understanding concepts such as automatic thoughts and schemas, especially in the beginning of treatment. Conversely, a less symptomatic patient with higher intelligence and ability to grasp abstract concepts may be able to profit from schema assessment early in therapy. If treatment procedures are pitched at a proper level, the patient is more likely to understand the material of therapy and to form a collaborative relationship with the therapist who is directing the treatment.

The therapeutic relationship also can be enhanced by using gentle humor during CT sessions. For example, the therapist may encourage the patient's sense of humor by providing opportunities to laugh together at some improbable situation or humorously distorted cognition. On occasion, the therapist may use hyperbole in a discreet manner to point out an inconsistency or an illogical conclusion. Humor needs to be injected carefully into the therapeutic relationship. Some patients respond quite well to humor. Others may be limited in their ability to use this feature of therapy. However, appropriate use of humor can strengthen the therapeutic relationship in CT if patient and therapist are able to laugh with one another and to use humor to deflate exaggerated or distorted cognitions.

Structuring Therapy

Several of the structuring procedures commonly employed in CT are listed in Table 29–6. One of the most important techniques for CT is the use of a therapy agenda. At the beginning of each session, the therapist and patient work together to derive a short list of topics, usually consisting of two to four items. Generally, it is advisable to shape an agenda that 1) can be managed within the time frame of an individual session, 2) follows up on material from earlier sessions, 3) reviews any homework from the previous session and provides an opportunity for new homework assignments, and 4) contains specific items that are highly relevant to the patient but are not too global or abstract.

Agenda setting helps to counteract hopelessness and helplessness by reducing seemingly overwhelming problems down into workable segments. The agenda setting process also encourages patients to take a problem-oriented approach to their difficulties. Simply articulating a problem in a specific manner often can initiate the process of change. In addition, the agenda keeps the patient focused on salient issues and encourages efficient use of the therapy time.

The agenda is set in a collaborative manner, and decisions to depart from the agenda are made jointly between therapist and patient. When work on an agenda item generates important information on a topic that was not foreseen at the beginning of the session, the therapist and patient discuss the merits of diverting or modifying the agenda. An excessively rigid approach to using a therapy agenda is not advocated. There must be sufficient flexibility to investigate promising new leads or to allow the patient to express significant thoughts or feelings that were unexpected at the beginning of the session. However, an overall commitment to setting and following the therapy agenda gives needed structure to patients who are unable to define problems clearly or think of ways to cope with them.

Feedback procedures described earlier are also used in structuring CT sessions. For example, the therapist may observe that the patient is drifting from the established agenda or is spending time discussing a topic of questionable relevance. In situations such as these, constructive feedback is given to direct the patient back to a more profitable area of inquiry. Heavy-handed, negatively oriented feedback is avoided. Instead, the therapist tends to give encouraging remarks that point the patient to issues that provide significant opportunities for change.

Commonly used CT techniques add an additional structural element to the therapy. Examples include activity scheduling, thought recording, and graded task assignments. These interventions, and others of similar nature, provide a clear and understandable method for reducing symptoms. Repeated use of procedures such as recording, labeling, and modifying automatic thoughts helps to link sessions together, especially if they are introduced in therapy and then assigned as homework.

Psychoeducation

Psychoeducational procedures are a routine component of CT. One of the major goals of the treatment approach is to teach patients a new way of thinking that can be applied in resolving current symptoms and in managing problems that will be encountered in the future. The psychoeducational effort usually begins with the process of socializing the patient to therapy. In the opening phase of treatment, the therapist explains the basic concepts of CT and introduces the patient to the format of CT sessions. The therapist also devotes time early in treatment to discussing the therapeutic relationship in CT and the expectations for both patient and therapist. Psychoeducational work during a course of CT often involves brief explanations or illustrations coupled with homework assignments. These activities are woven into treatment sessions in a manner that emphasizes a collaborative, active learning approach. Some cognitive therapists have described the use of "mini-lectures" (Epstein et al. 1988), but a heavily didactic approach is generally avoided.

Psychoeducation can be facilitated with reading assignments and computer programs that reinforce learning, deepen the patient's understanding of CT principles, and promote the use of self-help methods. Table 29–7 contains a list of useful psychoeducational tools, including a pamphlet, books, and a computer program, that teach the CT model and encourage self-help. Most cognitive therapists liberally use psychoeducational tools as a basic part of the therapy process.

Cognitive Techniques

Identifying Automatic Thoughts

Much of the work of CT is devoted to recognizing and then modifying negatively distorted or illogical automatic thoughts (Table 29–8). The most powerful way of introducing the patient to the effects of automatic thoughts is to find an in vivo example of how automatic thoughts can influence emotional responses. Mood shifts during the therapy session are almost always good places to pause to identify automatic thoughts. The therapist observes that a strong emotion such as sadness, anxiety, or anger has appeared and then asks the patient to describe the thoughts that "went through your head" just prior to the mood shift. This technique is illustrated in the example

TABLE 29–7. Psychoeducational materials and programs for cognitive therapy

Title	Authors	Description
"Coping With Anxiety"	A.T. Beck et al. 1985a	Appendix to book
"Coping With Depression"	A.T. Beck et al. 1995	Brief pamphlet
Feeling Good	Burns 1980, 1999	Book with self-help program
Getting Your Life Back: The Complete Guide to Recovery From Depression	Wright and Basco 2001	Book with self-help program; integrates cognitive therapy and biological approaches
"Good Days Ahead: The Multimedia Program for Cognitive Therapy"	J.H. Wright et al. 2002b	Computer-assisted therapy and self-help program
Mind Over Mood	Greenberger and Padesky 1995	Self-help workbook
Never Good Enough	Basco 1999	Book on perfectionism

TABLE 29–8. Methods for identifying and modifying automatic thoughts

Socratic questioning (guided discovery)
Use of mood shifts to demonstrate automatic thoughts in vivo
Imagery exercises
Role play
Thought recording
Generating alternatives
Examining the evidence
Decatastrophizing
Reattribution
Cognitive rehearsal

of Mr. B, a 50-year-old depressed man who had suffered several recent losses and had developed extremely low self-esteem.

Therapist: "How did you react to your wife's criticism?"

Mr. B: (Suddenly appears much more sad and anxious) "It was just too much to take."

Therapist: "I can see this really upsets you. Can you think back to what went through your mind right after I asked you the last question? Just try to tell me all the thoughts that popped into your head."

Mr. B: (Pause, then recounts) "I'm always making mistakes. I can't do anything right. There's no way to please her. I might as well give up."

Therapist: "I can see why you felt so sad. When these kinds of thoughts just automatically pop into your mind, you don't stop to think if they are accurate or not. That's why we call them automatic thoughts."

Mr. B: "I guess you're right. I hardly realized I was having those thoughts until you asked me to say them out loud."

Therapist: "Recognizing that you're having automatic thoughts is one of the first steps in therapy. Now let's see what we can do to help you with your thinking and with the situation with your wife."

Beck has described emotion as the "royal road to cognition" (A.T. Beck 1989). The patient usually is most accessible during periods of affective arousal, and cognitions such as automatic thoughts and schemas generally are more potent when they are associated with strong emotional responses. Hence, the cognitive therapist capitalizes on spontaneously occurring affective states during the interview and also pursues lines of questioning that are likely to produce intense affect. One of the myths about CT is that it is an overly intellectualized form of therapy. In fact, CT, as formulated by A.T. Beck et al. (1979) involves efforts to increase affect and to use emotional responses as a core ingredient of therapy (J.H. Wright 1988).

One of the most frequently used procedures in CT is Socratic questioning (also termed *guided discovery*). There is no set format or protocol for this technique. Instead, the therapist must rely on his or her experience and ingenuity to formulate questions that will help patients move from having a "closed mind" to a state of inquisitiveness and curiosity. Socratic questioning stimulates recognition of dysfunctional cognitions and development of a sense of dissonance about the validity of strongly held assumptions.

Socratic questioning usually involves a series of inductive questions that are likely to reveal dysfunctional thought patterns. The use of this technique to identify automatic thoughts is illustrated in the case of Ms. W, a 42-year-old woman with an anxiety disorder.

Therapist: "What things seem to trigger your anxiety?"

Ms. W: "Everything. It seems like no matter what I do I'm nervous all the time."

Therapist: "I suppose that 'everything' could trigger your anxiety and that you have no control over it. But, let's stop for a moment and see if there are any other possibilities. Is that okay?"

Ms. W: "Sure."

Therapist: "Then try to think of a situation where your anxiety is very high and one where it's much lower."

Ms. W: "Well, a high anxiety time would be whenever I try to go out in public, like to go shopping or to a party. And a low anxiety time would be sitting at home watching TV."

Therapist: "So there's some variation depending on what you are doing at the time."

Ms. W: "I guess that's right."

Therapist: "Would you like to find out what's behind the variation?"

Ms. W: "I guess. But I suppose it's just because being out with people makes me nervous and being at home feels safe."

Therapist: "That's one explanation. I wonder if there might be any others—ones that would give you some clues on how to get over the problem?"

Ms. W: "I'm willing to look."

Therapist: "Well then, let's try to find out something about the different thoughts that you have about these two situations. When you think of going out to a party, what comes to mind?"

Ms. W: "I'll be embarrassed. I won't have any idea what to say or do. I'll probably panic and run out the door."

This example depicts the typical use of Socratic questions early in the therapy process. Further questioning would be required to help the patient fully understand how dysfunctional cognitions are involved in her anxiety responses and how changing these cognitions could dampen her anxiety and promote a higher level of functioning.

Imagery and role play are used as alternate methods of uncovering cognitions when direct questions are unsuccessful in generating suspected automatic thinking (A.T. Beck et al. 1979). These techniques also are selected when only a limited amount of automatic thoughts can be brought out through Socratic questioning, and the therapist expects that more important automatic thoughts are present. Some patients may be able to use imagery procedures with few prompts or directions. In this case, the clinician only may need to ask the patient to imagine himself or herself back in a particularly troubling or emotion-provoking situation and then to describe the thoughts that occurred. However, most patients, particularly in the early phases of therapy, can benefit from "setting the scene" for the use of imagery (J.H. Wright 1988). The patient is asked to describe the details of the setting. When and where did it take place? What happened immediately before the incident? How did the characters in the scene appear? What were the main physical features of the setting? Questions such as these help bring the scene alive in the patient's mind and facilitate recall of cognitive responses to the situation.

Role play is a related technique for evoking automatic thoughts. When this procedure is used, the therapist first asks a series of questions to try to understand a vignette involving an interpersonal relationship or other social interchange that is likely to stimulate dysfunctional automatic thinking. Then, with the permission of the patient, the therapist briefly steps into the role of the individual in the scene and facilitates the playing out of a typical response set. Role play is used less frequently than Socratic questioning or imagery and is best suited to therapeutic situations in which there is an excellent collaborative relationship and the patient is unlikely to respond to the role play exercise with a negative or distorted transference reaction.

Thought recording is one of the most frequently used CT procedures for identifying automatic thoughts (J. Beck 1995). Patients can be asked to log their thoughts in a number of different ways. The simplest method is the two-column technique—a procedure that often is used when the patient is just beginning to learn how to recognize automatic thoughts. The two-column technique is illustrated in Table 29–9. In this case, the patient was asked to write down automatic thoughts that occurred in stressful or upsetting situations. Alternately, the patient could try to identify emotional reactions in one column and automatic thoughts in the other. A three-column exercise could include a description of the situation, a list of automatic thoughts, and a notation of the emotional response. Thought recording helps the patient to recognize the effects of underlying automatic thoughts and to understand how the basic cognitive model (i.e., relationship between situations, thoughts, feelings, and behaviors) applies to his or her own experiences. This procedure also initiates the process of modifying dysfunctional cognitions.

TABLE 29–9. Two-column thought recording

Situation	Automatic thoughts
Call from boss to submit a report	I can't do this. I don't know what to do. It won't be acceptable.
My wife asks me to help more around the house	Nothing I do is ever enough. She thinks I don't try.
Car won't start	I was stupid to buy this car. Nothing works right anymore. This is the last straw.

Thought recording is usually explained and illustrated in a therapy session and then additional exercises are assigned for homework. Depending on the case conceptualization, the therapist may suggest that the patient pay special attention to certain situations or issues (e.g., panic-inducing environmental cues, recurrent interpersonal problems, or dysfunctional behavioral responses). Also, specific assignments may be made to set up an in vivo experience that is likely to generate automatic thoughts. Examples might include discussing a troubling situation with a family member or attempting to engage in an anxiety provoking situation or behavior that is usually avoided. Automatic thoughts that are recorded during these homework assignments are brought to the next session for review and discussion.

Modifying Automatic Thoughts

There usually is no sharp division in CT between the phases of eliciting and modifying automatic thoughts. In fact, the processes involved in identifying automatic thoughts often are enough to initiate substantive change. As the patient begins to recognize the nature of his or her dysfunctional thinking, there typically is an increased degree of skepticism regarding the validity of automatic thoughts. Although patients can start to revise their cognitive distortions without specific additional therapeutic interventions, modification of automatic thoughts can be accelerated if the therapist applies Socratic questioning and other basic CT procedures to the change process (see Table 29–8).

Techniques used for revising automatic thoughts include 1) generating alternatives, 2) examining the evidence, 3) decatastrophizing, 4) reattribution, 5) thought recording, and 6) cognitive rehearsal (A.T. Beck et al. 1979; J. Beck 1995; J.H. Wright 1988). Socratic questioning is used in all of these procedures. *Generating alternatives* is illustrated in the case of Ms. D, a 32-year-old woman with major depression. The therapist's questions were pointed toward helping Ms. D to see a broader range of possibilities than she had originally considered.

Ms. D: "Every time I think of going back to school, I panic."
Therapist: "And when you start to think of going to school, what thoughts come to mind?"
Ms. D: "I'll botch it up. I won't be able to make it. I'll feel so ashamed when I have to drop out."
Therapist: "What else could happen? Anything even worse, or are there any better possibilities?"
Ms. D: "Well it couldn't get much worse unless I never even tried at all."
Therapist: "How would that be so bad?"
Ms. D: "Then I'd just be the same—stuck in a rut, not going anywhere."
Therapist: "We can take a look at that conclusion later—that not going to school would mean that you would stay in a rut; but for now let's look at the other possibilities if you do try to go to school again."

Ms. D: "Okay. I guess there's some chance that it would go pretty well, but it'll be hard for me to manage school, the house, and all my family responsibilities."
Therapist: "When you try to step back from the situation and not listen to your automatic thoughts, what's the most likely outcome of your going back to school?"
Ms. D: "It will be a difficult adjustment, but it's something I want to do. I have the intelligence to do it if I apply myself."

Examining the evidence is a major component of the collaborative empirical experience in CT. Specific automatic thoughts or clusters of related automatic thoughts are set forth as hypotheses, and the patient and therapist then search for evidence both for and against the hypothesis. In the case of Ms. D, the thought "If I don't go to school, I'd just be the same—stuck in a rut, not going anywhere" was selected for an examining the evidence exercise. The therapist believed that returning to school was probably an adaptive action for the patient to take. However, it also was thought that seeing further education as the only route to change would excessively load this activity with a "make or break" mentality and would promote a disregard for other modifications that might increase self-esteem and self-efficacy.

Decatastrophizing involves efforts to reconceptualize feared outcomes in a manner that encourages coping and problem solving. This technique can be effective even if there is a reasonably high likelihood that a negative prediction will actually occur. For example, a man might correctly judge his marriage to be so troubled that his wife may ask for a divorce. In this instance, the therapist would help the patient to recognize distorted cognitions about his ability to manage a possible breakup of the marriage. The patient might think, "I couldn't make it without her" or "I'd lose everything." The decatastrophizing procedure would involve examining negative automatic thoughts for their validity; looking for previously unrecognized attributes, interests, or coping mechanisms; reviewing the ways that the patient had managed losses in the past; and stimulating the patient to think beyond the immediate situation. The use of *reattribution techniques* is based on findings of studies on the attributional process in depression explained earlier in this chapter. Depressed individuals have been found to have negatively biased attributions in three dimensions: global versus specific, internal versus external, and fixed versus variable (Abramson et al. 1978). Several different types of reattribution procedures are employed, including psychoeducation about the attributional process, Socratic questioning to stimulate reattribution, written exercises to recognize and reinforce alternate attributions, and homework assignments to test out the accuracy of attributions.

Five-column Thought Change Records (TCRs; A.T. Beck et al. 1979) or other similar thought-recording devices are standard tools used in modification of automatic thoughts. The five-column TCR is used to encourage both identification and change of dysfunctional cognitions. A fourth (rational thoughts) and fifth (outcome) column are added to the three-column thought record described earlier. The patient is instructed to use this form to capture and change automatic thoughts. Either a stressful event or a memory of an event or situation is noted in the first column. Automatic thoughts are recorded in the second column and are rated for degree of belief (how much the patient believes them to be true at the moment they occur) on a 0–100 scale. The third column is used to observe the emotional response to the automatic thoughts. The intensity of emotion is rated on a 1–100 scale. The fourth column, rational thoughts, is the most critical part of the TCR. The patient is asked to stand back from the automatic thoughts, assess their validity, and then write out a more rational or realistic set of cognitions. There are a wide variety of procedures that can be used to facilitate the development of rational thoughts for the TCR.

Most patients can learn about cognitive errors and can start to label specific instances of erroneous logic in their automatic thoughts. This is often the first step in generating a more rational pattern of cognitive responses to life events. This process is illustrated in the case of Mr. E, a 58-year-old man with major depression, who completed a TCR during the middle phase of CT (Table 29–10). He had learned how to use the TCR during prior therapy sessions and had been acquainted with the concept of cognitive errors through therapy experiences and from reading self-help materials (see Table 29–7). Mr. E noted the particular cognitive errors involved with each of his automatic thoughts and wrote out a more rational set of cognitions.

Previously described techniques such as generating alternatives, examining the evidence, and reattribution also are used by the patient in a self-help format when the TCR is assigned for homework. In addition, the therapist often is able to help the patient refine or add to the list of rational thoughts when the TCR is reviewed at a subsequent therapy session. Repeated attention to generating rational thoughts on the TCR is very helpful in breaking maladaptive patterns of automatic and negatively distorted thinking.

The fifth column of the TCR, outcome, is used to record any changes that have occurred as a result of revising and modifying automatic thoughts. In the case of Mr.

E, there was a significant decrease in dysphoric affect. Although the use of the TCR will usually lead to the development of a more adaptive set of cognitions and a reduction in painful affect, on some occasions the initial automatic thoughts will prove to be accurate. In such situations, the therapist helps the patient take a problem solving approach, including the development of an action plan, to manage the stressful or upsetting event.

Cognitive rehearsal is used to help uncover potential negative automatic thoughts in advance and to coach the patient in ways of developing more adaptive cognitions. First, the patient is asked to use imagery or role play to identify possible distorted cognitions that could occur in a stressful situation. Second, the patient and therapist work together to modify the dysfunctional cognitions. Third, imagery or role play is used again, this time to practice the more adaptive pattern of thinking. Finally, for a homework assignment, the patient is asked to try out the newly acquired cognitive patterns in vivo.

Identifying and Modifying Schemas

The process of identifying and modifying schemas is somewhat more difficult than changing negative automatic thoughts because these core beliefs are more deeply embedded, may be largely out of the patient's awareness, and usually have been reinforced through years of life experience. However, many of the same techniques described for automatic thoughts are employed successfully in therapeutic work at the schema level (A.T. Beck et al. 1979; Thase and Beck 1992; J.H. Wright 1988). Procedures such as Socratic questioning, imagery, role play, and thought recording are used to uncover maladaptive schemas (Table 29–11).

As the patient gains experience in recognizing automatic thoughts, repetitive patterns begin to emerge that may suggest the presence of underlying schemas. Therapists have several options at this point. A psychoeducational approach can be used to explain the concept of schemas (may be alternately termed *core beliefs* or *basic assumptions*) and their linkage to more superficial, automatic thoughts (Dobson and Shaw 1986). Patients may then start to recognize schemas on their own. However, when the patient first starts to learn about basic assumptions, the therapist may need to suggest that certain schemas might be operative and then engage the patient in collaborative exercises that test these hypotheses.

Modification of schemas may require repeated attention, both in and out of therapy sessions. One commonly used procedure is to ask the patient to keep a list in a therapy notebook of all the schemas that have been identified to date. The schema list can be reviewed before

TABLE 29–10. Thought Change Record—an example

Situation	Automatic thought(s)	Emotion(s)	Rational response	Outcome
Describe: a. Actual event leading to unpleasant emotion; or b. Stream of thoughts, daydream, or recollection leading to unpleasant emotion; or c. Unpleasant physiological sensations	a. Write automatic thought(s) that preceded emotion(s). b. Rate belief in automatic thought(s), 0%–100%.	a. Specify sad, anxious, angry, etc. b. Rate degree of emotion, 1%–100%.	a. Identify cognitive errors. b. Write rational response to automatic thought(s). c. Rate belief in rational response, 0%–100%.	a. Once again, rate belief in automatic thought(s), 0%–100%. b. Specify and rate subsequent emotion(s), 0%–100%.
Date: 4/15/98				
I wake up and I'm immediately troubled. I start to worry about work.	1. I can't face another day. (90%)	Sad: 90% Anxious: 80%	1. Magnification. Even though it has been rough, I have been able to get to work every day. Get a shower and make breakfast—that will get things started. (80%)	Sad: 30% Anxious: 40%
	2. The big project is due in 2 weeks; I'll never get it done. (100%)		2. Catastrophizing, all-or-none thinking. About half of the work is done. Don't panic. Break it down into pieces. Taking one step at a time helps. (95%)	
	3. Everybody knows I'm ready to fall apart. (90%)		3. Overgeneralization, magnification. Some people know I've been in trouble, but they haven't gotten down on me. I'm the one who puts me down. (95%)	
	4. It's hopeless. (85%)		4. Magnification. I know my job well and have a good track record. If I stick with this, I can probably make it. (90%)	

Source. Adapted with permission from Beck AT, Rush AJ, Shaw BF, et al.: *Cognitive Therapy of Depression.* New York, Guilford, 1979.

each session. This technique promotes a high level of awareness of schemas and usually encourages the patient to place issues pertaining to schemas on the agenda for therapy.

CT interventions that are particularly helpful in modifying schemas include examining the evidence, listing advantages and disadvantages, generating alternatives, and using cognitive rehearsal. After a schema has been identified, the therapist may ask the patient to do a pro/con analysis (examining the evidence) using a double-column procedure. This technique usually induces the patient to doubt the validity of the schema and to start to think of

TABLE 29–11. Methods for identifying and modifying schemas

Socratic questioning
Imagery and role play
Thought recording
Identifying repetitive patterns of automatic thoughts
Psychoeducation
Listing schemas in therapy notebook
Examining the evidence
Listing advantages and disadvantages
Generating alternatives
Cognitive rehearsal

TABLE 29–12. Schema modification through examining the evidence

Schema: "I must be perfect to be accepted."

Evidence for	Evidence against
The better I do, the more people seem to like me.	Others who aren't "perfect" seem to be to be loved and accepted. Why should I be different?
Women who have a perfect figure are most attractive to men.	You don't have to have a perfect figure. Hardly anybody has one—just the models on television.
My parents have the highest standards; they are always pushing me to do better.	My parents want me to do well. But they'll probably accept me as long as I try to do my best, even if I don't meet all of their expectations. This statement is absolute and sets me up for failure because no one can be perfect all the time.

alternate explanations. An examining-the-evidence intervention is illustrated in the case of Ms. R, a 24-year-old woman with depression and bulimia (Table 29–12). During the course of her CT, Ms. R identified an important schema that was affecting both the depression and the eating disorder ("I must be perfect to be accepted."). By examining the evidence, she was able to see that her schema was based at least in part on faulty logic.

Ms. R also used the listing advantages and disadvantages technique as part of the strategy to modify this maladaptive schema (Table 29–13). Some schemas appear to have few, if any, advantages (e.g., "I'm stupid"; "I'll always lose in the end"), but many schemas have both positive and negative features (e.g., "If I decide to do something, I must succeed"; "I always have to work harder than others or I'll fail"). The latter group of schemas may be maintained even in the face of their dysfunctional aspects because they encourage hard work, perseverance, or other behaviors that are adaptive. Yet, the absolute and demanding nature of the schemas ultimately leads to excessive stress, failed expectations, low self-esteem, or other deleterious results. Listing advantages and disadvantages helps the patient to examine the full range of effects of the schema and often encourages modifications that can make the schema both more adaptive and less damaging. In Ms. R's case, this exercise set the stage for another step of schema modification, generating alternatives (Table 29–14).

The list of alternative schemas will usually include several different options, ranging from rather minor adjustments to extensive revisions in the schema. The therapist uses Socratic questioning and other CT techniques such as imagery and role play to help the patient recognize potential alternative schemas. A "brainstorming" attitude is encouraged. Instead of trying to be sure that a revised schema is entirely accurate at first glance, the therapist usually suggests that they try to generate a variety of modified schemas without initially considering

TABLE 29–13. Schema modification through listing advantages and disadvantages

Schema: "I must be perfect to be accepted."

Advantages	Disadvantages
I've tried very hard to be the best.	I never really feel accepted because I've never reached perfection.
I've received top marks in school.	I'm always down on myself. I've developed bulimia. I'm obsessed with my body size.
I'm in lots of activities, and I've won dancing competitions.	I have trouble accepting my successes. I drive myself too hard and can't enjoy ordinary things.

their validity or practicality. This stimulates creativity and gives the patient further encouragement to step aside from rigid long-standing schemas.

After alternatives are generated and discussed, the therapy turns toward examining the potential consequences of changing basic attitudes. Cognitive rehearsal can be used in the therapy session to test a schema modification. This may be followed by a homework assignment to try out the revised schema in vivo. Therapist and patient work together to choose the most reasonable modifications for underlying schemas and to reinforce

TABLE 29–14. Schema modification though generating alternatives

Schema: "I must be perfect to be accepted."
Possible alternatives
People that are successful are more likely to be accepted.
If I try to do my best (even if it's not perfect), others are likely to accept me.
I would like to be perfect, but that's an impossible goal. I'll choose certain areas to try to excel (school, work, career) and not demand perfection everywhere.
You don't need to be perfect to be accepted.
I'm worthy of love and acceptance without trying to be perfect.

TABLE 29–15. Behavioral procedures used in cognitive therapy

Questioning to identify behavioral patterns
Activity scheduling with mastery and pleasure recording
Self-monitoring
Graded task assignments
Behavioral rehearsal
Response prevention
Distraction
Relaxation exercises
Respiratory control
Assertiveness training
Modeling
Social skills training

learning these new constructs through multiple practice sessions in therapy sessions and in real-life experiences.

Behavioral Procedures

Behavioral interventions are used in CT to 1) change dysfunctional patterns of behavior (e.g., helplessness, isolation, phobic avoidance, inertia, bingeing and purging); 2) reduce troubling symptoms (e.g., tension, somatic and psychic anxiety, intrusive thoughts); and 3) assist in identifying and modifying maladaptive cognitions (Table 29–15 presents a listing of behavioral techniques). As discussed earlier in this chapter, the cognitive model for therapy (see Figure 29–1) suggests that there is an interactive relationship between cognition and behavior. Thus, behavioral initiatives should influence cognition, and cognitive interventions should have an impact on behavior.

The Socratic questions used in cognitively oriented procedures have a direct parallel when the emphasis is on behavioral change. The therapist asks a series of questions that help differentiate actual behavioral deficits from negatively distorted accounts of behavior (J.H. Wright 1988). Depressed and anxious patients usually overreport their symptomatic distress or the difficulties they have in managing situations. Often, well framed questions can reveal cognitive distortions and also stimulate change as the patient considers the negative impact of dysfunctional behavior. Three specific behavioral techniques—activity scheduling, graded task assignments, and exposure—are explained below.

Activity scheduling is a structured method of learning about the patient's behavioral patterns, encouraging self-monitoring, increasing positive mood, and designing strategies for change (A.T. Beck et al. 1979; Thase and Beck 1992; J.H. Wright and Beck 1983). A daily or weekly activity log is employed in which the patient is asked to record what he or she does during each hour of

the day and then to rate each activity for mastery and pleasure on a 0–10 scale. When the activity record is first introduced, the patient usually is asked to make a record of baseline activities without attempting to make any changes. The data are then reviewed in the next therapy session.

Almost invariably, the patient rates some activities higher than others on mastery and/or pleasure. For example, Mr. G, a 48-year-old depressed man who had told his therapist that "I don't enjoy anything anymore," described several activities on his daily activity log that contradicted this statement. Reading while sitting alone was rated as a 6 on mastery and 8 on pleasure, and attending his son's choir concert was rated as 7 on mastery and 10 on pleasure. Conversely, attempting to work in his home office was rated as a 1 on mastery and a 0 on pleasure. Discussion of the activity scheduling assignment with Mr. G helped him to see that he was still capable of performing reasonably well in certain activities and also that he was able to derive considerable enjoyment from some of his actions. In addition, the schedule was used to target problem areas (e.g., working in his home office) that would require further work in therapy. Finally, the activity schedule provided data that could be used in adjusting Mr. G's daily routine to promote a heightened sense of mastery and greater enjoyment.

Another behavioral procedure, the graded task assignment, can be used when the patient is facing a situation that seems excessively difficult or overwhelming. A challenging behavioral goal is broken down into small steps that can be taken one at a time. The graded task assignment is quite similar to the systematic desensitization protocols that are used in traditional behavior therapy (Wolpe 1969). However, a cognitive component is added to the methodology. There is an added emphasis placed on improving self-esteem and self-efficacy, countering hopelessness and helplessness, and using the graded task assignment to disprove maladaptive thoughts and schemas. With depressed individuals, the graded task assignment typically is used as a problem-solving technique. This stepwise approach, coupled with cognitive techniques such as Socratic questioning and thought recording, can reactivate the patient and focus his or her energy in a productive manner.

An example of the use of a graded task assignment can be found in the case of Mr. G, the 48-year-old man described in the section on activity scheduling. One of the particularly troublesome items uncovered with activity scheduling was the patient's difficulty in getting to work at his home office. Socratic questioning revealed that Mr. G had been unable to work in his home office for over 6 weeks. Mail, bills, and correspondence with friends were piled up to the point that he saw the situation as impossible. Cognitions related to this problem included automatic thoughts such as "It's too much.... I've procrastinated too long this time.... I'm totally swamped.... I can't handle it."

The therapist and patient constructed a series of steps that encouraged Mr. G to approach the task and eventually master the problem. The graded task assignment included the following steps: 1) walk into the office and sit down at the desk for at least 15 minutes; 2) spend at least 20 minutes sorting mail into categories; 3) open and discard any junk mail; 4) open and read any personal letters and write list of responses required; 5) open and stack all bills; 6) clean office; 7) respond in writing to at least one letter; 8) balance checkbook; 9) pay all current or overdue bills; 10) respond to additional letters if necessary. Reasonable goals for specific time intervals were discussed, and the therapist used coaching, Socratic questioning, and other cognitive techniques to help Mr. G accomplish the task.

Exposure techniques are a central part of cognitive-behavioral approaches to anxiety disorders. For example, a phobia can be conceptualized as an unrealistic fear of an object or a situation coupled with a conditioned pattern of avoidance. Treatment can proceed along two complementary lines: cognitive restructuring to modify the dysfunctional thoughts and exposure therapy to break the pattern of avoidance. Typically, a hierarchy of feared stimuli is developed with the patient. The hierarchy should contain a number of different stimuli that cause varying degrees of distress. Usually the items are ranked by degree of distress. One commonly used system involves rating each item on a scale from 0 to 100, with 100 representing the maximum distress possible. After the hierarchy is established, the therapist and patient work collaboratively to set goals for gradual exposure, starting with the items that are ranked lower on the distress scale. Breathing training, relaxation exercises, and other behavioral methods (see Table 29–15) may be used to enhance the patient's ability to carry out the exposure protocol.

Exposure can be done with imagery in treatment sessions or in vivo. Also, innovative virtual-reality methods have been developed for exposure therapy (Rothbaum et al. 1995). Virtual-reality exposure techniques have been shown to be effective in empirical trials, but they are expensive and are not yet widely available. Clinician-administered exposure therapy is frequently used as part of the cognitive-behavioral approach to simple phobias, panic disorder with agoraphobia, social phobia, and obsessive-compulsive disorder (OCD).

Other behavioral techniques used in CT include behavioral rehearsal (a procedure that is usually combined with cognitive rehearsal described earlier), response prevention (a collaborative exercise in which the patient agrees to stop a dysfunctional behavior, such as prolonged crying spells, and to monitor cognitive responses), distraction (alternate activities that can temporarily divert a patient from intrusive thoughts, depressive ruminations, or other dysfunctional cognitions), relaxation exercises, respiratory control, assertiveness training, modeling, and social skills training (D.M. Clark et al. 1985; Meichenbaum 1977; Thase and Wright 1991; J.H. Wright 1988; J.H. Wright and Beck 1983; Young and Beck 1982).

Computer-Assisted Cognitive Therapy

Newer forms of computer-assisted therapy may offer significant potential for increasing the efficiency of cognitive-behavioral interventions and improving access to treatment (Greist 1998; Marks 1999; J.H. Wright and Wright 1997). An early prototype for computerized therapy was developed by Selmi et al. (1982, 1990). Their text-based program teaches patients how to use CT to cope with depression. An outcome study demonstrated that patients with mild to moderate depression responded well to the computer program (Selmi et al. 1990). Subjects who received the computerized therapy improved as much as those who were treated with standard CT, and both active treatments were superior to a wait list control.

Colby and Colby (1990) have produced a computer program that incorporates some of the principles of CT but does not cover the major CT interventions in depth. One of the interesting features of the Colby and Colby program is a dialogue mode in which the computer attempts to carry on a therapeutic conversation with the patient using "natural language." Although this dialogue is highly inventive, it does not simulate the typical therapeutic interview in CT. Also, problems in understanding the patient's typed responses and in giving accurate feedback were observed in an empirical study of this software (Stuart and LaRue 1996). One research group (Bowers et al. 1993) found that the Colby and Colby program was ineffective in treating severely ill inpatients, but Colby (1995) has reported very high patient satisfaction among a large number of users of this program.

Both the Selmi et al. and the Colby and Colby forms of computer-assisted therapy have the disadvantage of being text based. These programs require the patient to type responses and to read large amounts of written material. J.H. Wright et al. (1995a, 1995b, 2002a, 2002b) have introduced a multimedia form of CCT that is designed to be "user friendly" and to be suitable for a wide range of patients, including those with no previous computer or keyboard experience. This program ("Good Days Ahead: The Multimedia Program for Cognitive Therapy") uses a DVD-ROM format and features large amounts of video and audio, along with interactive self-help exercises.

A randomized, controlled trial of CCT for depression conducted with a prototype of the Wright et al. program found that CCT was equivalent to standard CT, even though the total therapist time in CCT was reduced to about 4 hours (J.H. Wright et al. 2001, 2002a). Subjects in this study were drug-free. CCT and standard CT were both highly effective in relieving symptoms of depression, and both were superior to a delayed-treatment control condition.

Possible contributions of CCT may include decreased cost of treatment, increased access to therapy, more rapid socialization to treatment procedures and techniques, and a reduced burden on therapists to teach basic CT concepts (Colby 1995; J.H. Wright and Wright 1997). Opportunities for improved efficiency of treatment, advances in the design of computer programs, and the proliferation of computers in society may promote greater use of computer tools for CT.

Selecting Patients for Cognitive Therapy

CT procedures have been described for a large number of diagnostic categories (A.T. Beck 1993; Freeman and Dattilio 1992; Freeman et al. 1989; F.D. Wright et al. 1993). Although there are no contraindications to using this treatment approach, CT is usually not attempted with patients who have a substantial degree of organic brain disease (e.g., mental retardation, dementia, or delirium). Ludgate et al. (1992) have suggested that CT should be

considered a primary treatment for 1) disorders where it has been proven to be effective in controlled research (e.g., unipolar depression [nonpsychotic], anxiety disorders, eating disorders, and psychophysiological disorders), and 2) other conditions for which a clearly detailed treatment method has been developed (e.g., personality disorders, substance abuse), there is some evidence for effectiveness, and there is no substantive research data to support the superiority of other treatment approaches. CT should be considered an adjunctive therapy for disorders such as major depression with psychotic features, bipolar illness, and schizophrenia in which there is clear evidence for the effectiveness of biological treatments, and the effects of CT alone compared with pharmacotherapy have not been studied.

Several studies have examined possible predictors for outcome in CT. Simons et al. (1985) observed that high scores on a test of self-control predicted an enhanced response to CT compared with a tricyclic antidepressant. Although several later studies (Jarrett et al. 1991; Wetzel et al. 1992) failed to replicate this finding, one other study (Burns et al. 1994) partially replicated it. Miller et al. (1989) found that high levels of cognitive dysfunction in depressed inpatients were associated with a superior response to combined treatment with CT and pharmacotherapy as compared with pharmacotherapy alone. Another group of investigators has reported that patients with chronic or especially severe depression may respond somewhat less well to CT than individuals with lower levels of symptoms. (Thase et al. 1993, 1994b). However, the research of Thase et al. (1993, 1994b) did not include control groups. When CT has been compared directly with pharmacotherapy, most studies have found no relationship between severity or endogenous subtype and treatment outcome (see "Effectiveness of Cognitive Therapy" section later in this chapter).

Investigations of biological predictors have yielded conflicting results. Dexamethasone nonsuppression was associated with a poorer response to both CT and pharmacotherapy in one study (McKnight et al. 1992). Thase et al. (1996) found that the dexamethasone suppression test did not reliably discriminate between responders and nonresponders to CT in group of severely ill inpatients, but high urinary free cortisol levels were associated with a diminished response to CT. Electroencephalographic (EEG) sleep studies usually have not differentiated CT responders and nonresponders (Corbishley et al. 1990; Jarrett et al. 1990; Simons and Thase 1992; Thase et al. 1994a). One large study of 90 outpatients treated with CT found that a profile of multiple EEG sleep abnormalities was associated with a lower recovery rate and higher risk for relapse (Thase et al. 1996). Although studies of biological markers suggest that cortisol levels or EEG findings may help predict treatment response in some cases, the overall findings of research in this area do not support the use of laboratory tests to select patients for CT.

Clinical experience has suggested that patients who are free of severe character pathology (especially borderline or antisocial features) have previously formed strong, trusting relationships with significant others, have a belief in the importance of self-reliance, and have a curious or inquisitive nature are especially suitable for CT (Thase and Beck 1992). Average or above-average intelligence also can be helpful, but CT procedures can be simplified for those with subnormal intellectual skills or impaired learning and memory functioning (Casey and Grant 1992; Thompson 1996; J.H. Wright and Salmon 1990). Of course, most patients do not have a full combination of the ideal features noted above. A flexible approach can be employed in which CT procedures are customized to match the special characteristics of the patient's social background, intellectual level, personality structure, and clinical disorder (Freeman and Dattilio 1992).

Cognitive Therapy Applications

The basic procedures described in this chapter are used in all CT applications. However, the targets for change, selection of techniques, and timing of interventions may vary depending on the condition being treated and the format for therapy. A full discussion of the multiple applications and formats for CT is beyond the scope of this chapter. The reader is referred to comprehensive books on CT for a more detailed accounting of the modifications of this treatment approach for different clinical disorders (Freeman and Dattilio 1992; Freeman et al. 1989; Salkovskis 1996; J.H. Wright et al. 1993a, 1993b). CT methods have been outlined for a number of clinical problems not covered here, including conditions such as substance abuse (Carroll et al. 1994a, 1994b; Fisher and Bentley 1996; Oei et al. 1991; Thase 1997; F.D. Wright et al. 1993), chronic depression (McCullogh 2000; Scott 1992; Scott et al. 1992), hypochondriasis (Warwick and Salkovskis 1990), body dysmorphic disorder (N.B. Schmidt and Harrington 1995), gambling addiction (Bujold et al. 1994; Sharpe and Tarrier 1993), and psychophysiological disorders (Bergdahl et al. 1995; Dworkin et al. 1994; Payne and Blanchard 1995; White and Neilson 1995). Group CT techniques have been described by Covi and Primakoff (1988) and Freeman et al. (1992); and procedures for marital and family CT have been set forth by Beck (A.T. Beck 1988), Epstein et al. (1988), and Wright and Beck (J.H. Wright and Beck 1993). Also, strategies have been developed for using CT as a comprehensive model for inpatient treatment (J.H. Wright et al. 1993a, 1993b). In this portion of the chapter, we briefly examine the distinctive features of CT for five common psychiatric illnesses—depression, anxiety disorders, eating disturbances, personality disorders, and psychosis.

Depression

In the opening phase of treatment of depression, the cognitive therapist focuses on establishing a collaborative relationship and introduces the patient to the cognitive model. Agendas, feedback, and psychoeducational procedures are used to structure sessions. The emphasis is placed on two major forms of cognitive dysfunction: negatively distorted thinking and deficits in learning and memory functioning (Thase and Beck 1992). Early in therapy, a special effort may be placed on relieving hopelessness because of the close link between this element of the negative cognitive triad and suicide risk. Also, reduction in hopelessness can be an important step in reactivating and reenergizing the depressed patient.

Problems with learning and memory functioning are countered with the aforementioned structuring procedures and with learning reinforcement techniques such as written therapy notes, diagrams, and homework assignments (Thase and Wright 1991; J.H. Wright 1988). The clinician carefully matches the therapeutic work to the patient's level of cognitive functioning so that learning is encouraged and the patient is not overwhelmed with the material of therapy. Behavioral techniques, such as activity scheduling and graded task assignments, often are a major component of the opening phase of CT of depression (Thase and Wright 1991).

The middle portion of treatment is usually devoted to eliciting and modifying negatively distorted automatic thoughts. Behavioral techniques continue to be used in most cases. By this point in the therapy, patients should understand the cognitive model and be able to employ thought monitoring techniques to reverse all three elements of the negative cognitive triad (self, world, and future). Typically, the patient is taught to identify cognitive errors (e.g., selective abstraction, arbitrary inference, absolutistic thinking) and to use procedures such as generating alternatives and examining the evidence to alter negatively distorted thinking.

Work on eliciting and testing automatic thoughts continues during the latter portion of treatment. However, if there have been gains in functioning and the patient has grasped the basic principles of CT, therapy can turn primarily to identifying and altering maladaptive schemas.

The concept of schemas usually has been introduced earlier in therapy, but the principal efforts at changing these underlying structures are reserved for the late phase of treatment when the patient is more likely to grasp and retain complex therapeutic initiatives. Before therapy concludes, the therapist helps the patient review what has been learned during the course of treatment and also suggests thinking ahead to possible circumstances that could trigger a return of depression. The potential for relapse is recognized, and problem-solving strategies are developed that can be employed in future stressful situations (Thase 1992).

Anxiety Disorders

Although the techniques used in CT for anxiety disorders are similar to those employed in the treatment of depression, treatment efforts are directed toward altering four major types of dysfunctional anxiety-producing cognitions: 1) overestimates of the likelihood of a feared event, 2) exaggerated estimates of the severity of a feared event, 3) underestimation of personal coping abilities, and 4) unrealistically low estimates of the help that others can offer (D.M. Clark and Beck 1988). Most authors have recommended that a mixture of cognitive and behavioral measures be used in patients who have anxiety disorders (Alford et al. 1990; Barlow and Cerney 1988; A.T. Beck et al. 1985a; D.M. Clark and Beck 1988).

In panic disorder, the emphasis is placed on helping the patient to recognize and change grossly exaggerated estimates of the significance of physiological responses or fears of imminent psychological disaster (A.T. Beck et al. 1985a, 1992b; D.M. Clark 1986). For example, an individual with panic disorder may begin to perspire or breathe more rapidly, after which cognitions such as "I can't catch my breath.... I'll pass out.... I'll have a stroke," increase the intensity of the autonomic nervous system activity. The vicious cycle interaction between catastrophic cognitions and physiological arousal can be broken in two complimentary ways: 1) altering the dysfunctional cognitions and 2) interrupting the cascading autonomic hyperactivity. Commonly used cognitive interventions include Socratic questioning, imagery, thought recording, generating alternatives, and examining the evidence. Behavioral measures such as relaxation training and respiratory control are used to dampen the physiological arousal associated with panic (D.M. Clark et al. 1985). Also, when panic attacks are stimulated by specific situations (e.g., driving, public speaking, crowds), graded exposure may be particularly useful in helping patients to both master a feared task and overcome their panic symptoms.

CT of phobic disorders centers on modifying unrealistic estimates of risk or danger in situations and engaging the patient in a series of graded exposure assignments. Generally, cognitive and behavioral procedures are used simultaneously. For example, a graded task assignment for an individual with agoraphobia might include a stepwise increase in experiences in a social setting accompanied by use of the Daily Record of Dysfunctional Thoughts to record and revise maladaptive automatic thinking. Patients with generalized anxiety disorder (GAD) usually have diffuse cognitive distortions about many circumstances in their lives (e.g., physical health, finances, loss of control, family issues) coupled with persistent autonomic overarousal (A.T. Beck et al. 1985a; J.H. Wright and Borden 1992). The CT approach to GAD is closely related to methods used for panic disorder and phobias. However, special attention is paid to defining the stimuli that are associated with increased anxiety. Breaking down the generalized state of anxiety into workable segments can help the patient gain mastery over what initially appears to be an uncontrollable situation.

Behavioral techniques such as exposure and response prevention are used together with cognitive restructuring for patients with OCD (Emmelkamp and Beens 1991; James and Blackburn 1995; Salkovskis 1985). Cognitive interventions include thought stopping, challenging the validity of obsessional thoughts, attempting to replace dysfunctional cognitions with positive self-statements, and modifying negative automatic thoughts (James and Blackburn 1995). Salkovskis and Warwick (1985) have noted that cognitive procedures may be needed in some cases to help the patient engage in exposure and response prevention.

Eating Disorders

Individuals with eating disorders may have many of the same cognitive distortions that are seen in depression. However, they have an additional cluster of cognitive biases about body image, eating behavior, and weight (D.A. Clark et al. 1989; Schlesier-Carter et al. 1989; Zotter and Crowther 1991). Patients with eating disorders usually place inordinate value on body shape as a measure of self-worth and as a condition for acceptance (e.g., "I must be thin to be accepted"; "If I'm overweight, nobody will want me"; "Fat people are weak"). They also may believe that any variance from their excessive standards means a total loss of control.

CT interventions are used to subject these maladaptive cognitions to empirical testing (Agras et al. 1992; P.J. Cooper and Steere 1995; Fairburn 1985; Garner 1992; Garner and Bemis 1985). Commonly used procedures include eliciting and testing automatic thoughts, examining the evidence, reattribution, and in vivo homework assignments (Bowers 1992). In addition, behavioral techniques are used to stimulate more adaptive eating behavior and to uncover significant cognitions related to eating (Bowers 1992; Garner 1992). As in treatment of other disorders, the relative emphasis on cognitive procedures compared with behavioral measures is dictated by the severity of the illness and the phase of treatment. An individual with anorexia nervosa who is malnourished and has an electrolyte imbalance may require hospitalization during the initial part of treatment for a contingency management program (Bowers 1992). Patients with this level of illness may have a significant impairment in learning and memory functioning and therefore have limited capacity to understand thought recording or other cognitive interventions. In contrast, a patient with uncomplicated bulimia nervosa may be able to benefit from relatively demanding cognitively oriented procedures early in treatment.

One of the critical factors in treating patients with eating disorders is the development of an effective working relationship. Compared with individuals with depression or anxiety disorders, those with eating disturbances often are reluctant to fully engage in therapy. Frequently, they have long-standing patterns of hiding their behavior from others and have developed elaborate methods of maintaining their dysfunctional approach to meals, body weight, and exercise. Thus, the patient with an eating disorder poses a special problem for the cognitive therapist. A thorough psychoeducational effort and considerable patience are usually required for the formation of a collaborative empirical relationship. Also, if the therapist focuses in the beginning on problem areas that the patient clearly wants to change (e.g., low self-esteem, hopelessness, loss of interest), struggles over control of eating disorders can be avoided until there have been successful experiences in working together in therapy.

Personality Disorders

A.T. Beck and Freeman (1990) articulated a CT approach to personality disorders that is based on a cognitive conceptualization of characterological disturbances. They suggest that the different personality types have idiosyncratic cognitions in four main areas: basic beliefs, view of self, view of others, and strategies for social interaction. For example, an individual with a narcissistic personality might believe, "I'm special.... I'm better than the rest.... Ordinary rules don't apply to me." This cognitive set leads to behavioral strategies such as manipulativeness, breaking rules, and exploiting others

(A.T. Beck and Freeman 1990). In contrast, a person with a dependent personality disorder might have core beliefs such as, "I need others to survive.... I can't manage on my own.... I can't be happy if I'm alone." The interpersonal strategies associated with these beliefs would include efforts to cling to or entrap others (A.T. Beck and Freeman 1990).

CT methods typically employed in treatment of affective disorders may not be successful with characterological problems (A.T. Beck and Freeman 1990; Persons et al. 1988; Pretzer and Beck 1996). Recommendations that have been made for modifying CT for treatment of personality disorders are summarized in Table 29–16 (A.T. Beck and Freeman 1990; J. Beck 1997; Linehan 1987, 1993; Shearin and Linehan 1994). The problem-oriented, structured, and collaborative empirical characteristics of CT are retained in therapeutic work with patients who have personality disturbances, but there is an added emphasis on the therapeutic relationship. Persons with characterological disorders often recapitulate in the therapy encounter the impaired relationships that they have had with significant others in the past.

Treatment of personality disorders with CT may take considerably longer than therapy of more circumscribed problems such as depression or anxiety. Patients with personality disturbances have deeply ingrained schemas that are unlikely to change within the short-term format used for other disorders (J. Beck 1997; Perris 1994; Young and Lindemann 1992). When the course of therapy lengthens, there is a greater chance for development of transference and countertransference reactions. In CT, transference is viewed as a manifestation of underlying schemas. Therefore, transferential phenomena are recognized as opportunities for examining and modifying core beliefs.

TABLE 29–16. Modifications of cognitive therapy for personality disorders

Pay special attention to the therapeutic relationship.

Attend to one's own (the therapist's) cognitive responses and emotional reactions.

Develop an individualized case conceptualization (including an assessment of the impact of developmental experiences, significant traumas, and environmental stresses).

Place an initial focus on increasing self-efficacy.

Use behavioral techniques, such as rehearsal and social skills training, to reverse actual deficits in interpersonal functioning.

Set firm, reasonable limits.

Set realistic goals.

Anticipate compliance problems.

Review and repeat treatment interventions.

An individualized case conceptualization is used. This formulation includes hypotheses on the role of maladaptive schemas in symptom production. Consideration also is given to the influences of parent–child conflicts, traumatic experiences, and the current social network on cognitive and behavioral pathology. Patients with personality disorders often have significant real-life problems, including severely disturbed interpersonal relationships and pronounced social skills deficits.

Although an ultimate goal of treatment is to modulate ineffective or maladaptive schemas, initial efforts (using procedures such as behavioral techniques or thought recording) may be directed at more readily accessible targets such as increasing self-efficacy or decreasing dysphoric mood. Self-monitoring, self-help exercises, and the structuring procedures used in CT help prevent excessive dependency. However, patients with character disorders (especially those with borderline, narcissistic, or dependent personalities) are prone to have excessive expectations, to be overly demanding, or to exhibit manipulative behavior. Thus, the cognitive therapist needs to set firm but reasonable limits and to help the patient articulate realistic treatment goals (A.T. Beck and Freeman 1990).

Adherence to treatment recommendations can be another problem in CT of personality disorders. The therapist can use procedures such as Socratic questioning or schema identification to uncover the reasons for noncompliance and help the patient follow through with homework assignments or other therapeutic work. Reviewing and repeating treatment interventions is another important component of CT for personality disorders. Considerable patience and persistence is required from the therapist as efforts are made to help the patient reverse chronic, deeply imbedded psychopathology.

Dialectical behavior therapy (DBT) is a specialized form of cognitive-behavioral therapy (CBT) developed by Marsha Linehan for treatment of borderline personality disorder (Linehan 1993, 1987). DBT employs cognitive and behavioral methods in addition to acceptance strategies derived from Zen teaching and practice. Therapy with DBT is long-term and involves repeated behavioral analysis, behavioral skills instruction, contingency management, cognitive restructuring, exposure interventions to reduce avoidance and dysfunctional emotions, and mindfulness training (Linehan et al. 1999). DBT has been used successfully in borderline patients with suicidal behavior and substance abuse (Linehan et al. 1991, 1993, 1994).

Psychosis

Psychotic illnesses are one of the indications for adjunctive CT (Ludgate et al. 1992). Although biological treatments are the accepted form of therapy for psychotic patients, several randomized, controlled trials have demonstrated that CT can reduce positive symptoms in patients who have residual symptomatology after stabilization on medication. It has also been observed that cognitive psychotherapy can help psychotic individuals understand their disorders, adhere to treatment recommendations, and develop more effective psychosocial functioning (Cochran 1986; Eckman et al. 1992; Fowler and Morley 1989; Kingdon and Turkington 1991; Lecompte 1995; Perris 1989; Perris and Skagerlind 1994; J.H. Wright and Schrodt 1989).

In CT of patients who have psychotic symptoms, the therapist conveys that maladaptive cognitions and reactions to life stress may interact with biological factors in the expression of the illness (Scott et al. 1992). Therefore, attempts to develop more adaptive cognitions or to learn how to cope better with environmental pressures can assist with efforts toward managing the disorder. During the early part of therapy with a psychotic patient, there is a strong emphasis on building a therapeutic alliance (Alford and Beck 1994; Scott et al. 1992). The rationale for antipsychotic medication is explained, and the therapist tries to stimulate hope by modifying intensely negative cognitions about the illness or its treatment (e.g., "I'm to blame…. Nothing will help…. Drugs don't work.") Usually, attempts to challenge hallucinations or delusions directly are delayed until a solid therapeutic relationship has been established. However, efforts are made to reverse delusional self-destructive cognitions as early as possible in the treatment process (Ludgate et al. 1992).

Reality testing is performed in a gentle, nonconfrontational manner (Kingdon and Turkington 1991; Ludgate et al. 1992). Usually delusions with lowest level of conviction are targeted first (Alford and Beck 1994). The therapist uses guided discovery as the major intervention, but also may help the patient to record and change distorted automatic thoughts (Scott et al. 1992). Behavioral techniques such as activity scheduling, graded task assignments, and social skills training also are used with psychotic patients. These procedures can be used to provide needed structure or to teach adaptive behaviors. Initiatives that can reduce the risk of relapse are another component of the CT approach to psychotic disorders. Recommended interventions include 1) use of CT techniques that enhance medication compliance (see, for example, Lecompte 1995; J.H. Wright and Thase 1992), 2) identification of potential triggers for symptom exacerbation, 3) development of cognitive and behavioral strategies to manage stressful life events, and 4) extension of CT to the entire family unit (Scott et al. 1992).

Effectiveness of Cognitive Therapy

CT has been investigated in many carefully designed outcome trials that have documented the effectiveness of this treatment approach. The most intensive research has been directed at CT of depression and anxiety disorders.

Depression

Acute Treatment Phase Studies

Meta-analyses of the numerous outcome studies of CT for depression have found that this form of therapy compares well with other treatments for depression (Dobson 1989; Gaffan et al. 1995; Robinson et al. 1990). For example, Dobson (1989) concluded that CT was at least as effective as pharmacotherapy for depression and that there was some evidence for superiority of CT when all studies were considered together. In a subsequent review, Hollon et al. (1991) argued that some studies have been biased either toward CT or pharmacotherapy and thus suggested that firm conclusions on the relative efficacy of these treatments were still premature. A recent meta-analysis of 65 studies of CT for depression attempted to control for potential bias of the investigator by rating all studies on a researcher allegiance scale (Gaffan et al. 1995). Although researcher allegiance significantly predicted study outcomes, the results of Dobson's (1989) original meta-analysis were upheld.

Studies of CT for depression have been the subject of a detailed review by Thase (2001). Several of the more important investigations are noted here. The first major comparison of CT and pharmacotherapy was performed at the Center for Cognitive Therapy at the University of Pennsylvania (Rush et al. 1977). In this study, CT was found to be superior to imipramine in the treatment of depressed outpatients. However, results of this study have been questioned because of the "Lourdes effect" and because imipramine was tapered and stopped before the end of the trial (Rush et al. 1977). Two later studies, both performed in the United Kingdom, also found CT to be an effective treatment for depression (Blackburn et al. 1981; Teasdale et al. 1984). Blackburn et al. (1981) performed the first outcome trial at a facility other than the center where CT was developed. Patients from one of two settings, hospital outpatient or general practice clinics, were randomly assigned to CT, pharmacotherapy with amitriptyline or clomipramine, or a combination of CT and pharmacotherapy. CT was more effective than pharmacotherapy in the general practice patients, but doubts have been raised about the adequacy of the drug treatment in this sample (Hollon et al. 1991). Patients treated in the hospital outpatient setting responded equally well to all three treatments. There was a trend for the combined treatment to provide greater symptom reduction. Teasdale et al. (1984) compared "treatment as usual" (most, but not all patients treated with antidepressants) in a family practice setting to the same form of treatment plus CT. Patients who received the added CT component were significantly less depressed at the end of the trial.

Two major investigations in the United States replicated the original Rush et al. (1977) study. Murphy et al. (1984) at Washington University in St. Louis randomly assigned depressed outpatients to treatment with CT alone, nortriptyline alone, CT plus placebo, or combined CT and nortriptyline. The results of this study indicated that all treatments were effective for short-term symptom reduction. Similar findings were obtained in an outcome trial completed at the University of Minnesota. Hollon et al. (1992a) assessed the relative efficacy of CT alone, imipramine, and combined treatment with CT and imipramine. As in the Murphy et al. (1984) study, there were no significant differences found between the treatments in the acute phase of the research. Nonsignificant trends were observed for the combined treatment to be superior to either condition alone.

The National Institute of Mental Health (NIMH) Treatment of Depression Collaborative Research Project (Elkin et al. 1989, 1995) also examined the relative efficacies of CT and pharmacotherapy. Additional comparisons were made with another focused psychotherapy for depression, interpersonal therapy (IPT), and with placebo plus clinical management. All four treatments, including placebo plus clinical management, were associated with significant improvement in this trial. In the primary statistical analysis, there were no differences found between either of the psychotherapies and imipramine (plus clinical management). However, when patients were stratified by level of initial severity, CT was less effective (in the more severely affected patients) than the other active treatments (Elkin et al. 1995). This finding is inconsistent with results of other trials that compared CT with pharmacotherapy (DeRubeis et al. 1999) and may be explained by differences in application of CT across sites (Jacobson and Hollon 1996).

In a more recent study, two forms of psychotherapy, CT and applied relaxation, were both superior to desipramine (Murphy et al. 1995). The psychotherapies were conducted over 16 weeks and consisted of up to 20 sessions. Desipramine was given at therapeutic doses, and plasma levels were monitored. The percentages of patients in each treatment group who experienced a remission of depression were 82% for CT, 73% for applied relaxation, and 29% for desipramine. The authors suggested that a possible explanation for the low rate of treatment response in patients who received desipramine was the lack of psychotherapy in the medication group. Although patients on desipramine saw a pharmacotherapist for 20-minute sessions on a weekly or biweekly basis, the physician was specifically instructed not to engage in psychotherapy (Murphy et al. 1995). One possible explanation for the results of the Murphy et al. (1995) study is that some element of psychotherapy may be required for optimal response to antidepressant medication and that pharmacotherapy may be disadvantaged in comparison to CT if psychotherapy is not provided. Blackburn et al. (1981) reported a similar poor outcome for pharmacotherapy alone in subjects treated in a primary care setting.

Another possible reason for the poor showing of the pharmacotherapy group in the Murphy et al. study is that the investigators may have inadvertently sampled a subgroup of depressed patients who were nonresponsive to tricyclics. A parallel finding was observed by Stewart et al. (1998) in a reanalysis of the NIMH Treatment of Depression Collaborative Research Project study. Although CT was not particularly effective in this study overall (e.g., Elkin et al. 1989, 1995), Stewart et al. found that CT was superior to imipramine among the subset of patients with reverse neurovegetative features and preserved mood reactivity. Because such patients may be more responsive to monoamine oxidase inhibitors (MAOIs) or several of the newer antidepressants, comparisons of CT with other forms of pharmacotherapy have been needed. The recent study of Jarrett et al. (1999) found that CT was as effective as an MAOI for atypical depression. In a 10-week study of 108 outpatients with atypical depression, both CT and the MAOI phenelzine were superior to a pill placebo condition.

Further evidence for the effectiveness of CT for depression has come in studies of group CT (Covi and Lipman 1987; Free et al. 1991; Zettle and Rains 1989), geriatric depressed patients (Beutler et al. 1987; Riskind et al. 1985; Steuer et al. 1984; K.C.M. Wilson et al. 1995), and hospitalized depressed patients (Bowers 1990; Miller et al. 1989; Stuart and Bowers 1995; Thase et al. 1991; Whisman et al. 1991). The overall results of CT outcome studies indicate that CT is an effective treatment for depression and is comparable to antidepressants in producing acute symptomatic relief. Studies in which CT was found to be more effective than antidepressants have been questioned because of possible inadequacies in the pharmacotherapy regimens. Conversely, the single controlled study that suggested the possibility that CT might be less effective than medication for severe depression (Elkin et al. 1989) has been criticized because of questions about supervision of cognitive therapists and varied responses at different treatment sites (Jacobson and Hollon 1996; Thase and Beck 1992).

Long-Term Outcome Studies

Several of the investigations reviewed above measured the effects of the short-term therapies 1 and 2 years after treatment was completed. Results of these studies have generally favored CT in preventing relapse. For example, Kovacs et al. (1981) found that patients treated with CT in the Rush et al. (1977) study had a 31% relapse rate at 1 year, compared with a 65% relapse rate for those who had been treated with imipramine. An even higher differential relapse rate was described by Blackburn et al. (1986b). A 2-year naturalistic follow-up investigation of patients treated in the Blackburn et al. (1981) study found a substantially lower relapse rate in patients treated with CT alone (23%) or with combined therapy (21%), as compared with those who had received pharmacotherapy alone (78%).

Simons et al. (1986), who followed patients 1 year after their study, found the lowest relapse rates in patients who received CT alone (20%) or CT plus placebo (18%). Combined treatment was associated with a 43% rate of relapse after pharmacotherapy was withdrawn. The group treated with pharmacotherapy alone had the highest rate of relapse (67%). Patients in the Hollon et al. (1992a) study showed the same pattern of long-term response to treatment (Evans et al. 1992). The relapse rate for those treated with pharmacotherapy (without continuation-phase pharmacotherapy) was over twice the rate for patients who received CT or combined treatment.

The only investigation that did not find superiority for CT in preventing relapse was the NIMH Treatment of Depression Collaborative Research Project (Elkin et al. 1989; Shea et al. 1992). The failure of CT to significantly protect against depressive relapse in that study may be attributable to the relatively poor showing of CT in the acute phase of the study. Specifically, a treatment that is no more effective than a pill placebo in the acute phase may not be expected to have a durable effect posttreatment (Thase 2001). Nevertheless, patients treated with CT were less likely to require treatment in the follow-up period than were those treated with any of the other therapies, and the relapse rate following CT (36%) was somewhat lower than that observed with imipramine plus clinical management (50%) 18 months after the study was completed.

Two more recent studies examined the usefulness of CT in treating residual symptoms of depression in patients who did not respond fully to antidepressants

(Fava et al. 1996; Paykel et al. 1999). In the study by Fava et al. (1996), the relapse rate was 35% for CT and 70% for routine clinical management across a 4-year follow-up. Paykel et al. (1999) similarly observed a significant relapse-prevention effect in a two-center study of incompletely remitted patients receiving continuation pharmacotherapy. Treatment with CT reduced the hazard of relapse from 47% to 29% across 68 weeks of follow-up. Taken together, results of these investigations of the long-term effects of CT support the use of this modality to help reduce relapse and recurrence.

Perhaps the most intriguing results pertaining to longer-term outcomes come from the studies of Fava et al. (1998) and Jarrett et al. (2001). Fava et al. (1998) randomly assigned 45 remitted patients with recurrent depression to receive either 10 every-other-week sessions of CT (in addition to pharmacotherapy) or pharmacotherapy alone prior to medication discontinuation. Whereas 80% of the control group had recurrent depressive episodes across the next 24 months, 75% of the CT-treated group remained well after withdrawal of medication.

Jarrett et al. (2001) examined the role of ongoing continuation-phase CT sessions after response to acute-phase therapy. Previously, Thase et al. (1992) had suggested that CT could be terminated after 12–16 weeks of treatment *if* the initial response was brisk and complete. By contrast, incompletely remitted patients were at high (50%) risk of relapse following discontinuation of acute-phase therapy. Jarrett et al. (2001) confirmed this "at risk" assessment and demonstrated that incompletely remitted patients were "protected" from relapse by continuation-phase CT. By contrast, patients in the lower-risk (fully remitted) stratum gained no benefit from additional CT sessions. The durable relapse-prevention effects of CT may be linked to changes in affectively primed information processing (Teasdale et al. 2000).

Anxiety Disorders

CT also has been found to be an effective therapy for anxiety disorders. Especially strong evidence has been collected to support the utility of CT and related therapies in treatment of panic disorder. Two major forms of therapy have been developed: *panic control treatment* (PCT)—a combination of relaxation training, cognitive restructuring, and exposure (Barlow and Cerney 1988), and *focused cognitive therapy*—a more cognitively oriented treatment that uses exposure but places less emphasis on behavioral interventions than PCT (A.T. Beck et al. 1985a).

Barlow et al. (1989) reported that 87% of patients who completed a course of PCT were panic free after treatment and that PCT was significantly more effective than either relaxation training alone or a waiting list control condition. In a related investigation that compared PCT and alprazolam for panic disorder, this research group observed that PCT was superior to a waiting list control or placebo (Klosko et al. 1990). Of those completing the study, 87% who received PCT were free of panic attacks compared with 50% for alprazolam, 33% for the waiting list control, and 36% for placebo. The treatment protocol designed by Barlow and Cerney (1988) also was efficacious in an open trial of therapy administered by pharmacologically oriented clinicians who received training in this approach (Welkowitz et al. 1991). Shear et al. (1991a) noted that a cognitive and behavioral treatment package closely related to PCT was highly effective in clinical practice and, in addition, was capable of reversing vulnerability to sodium lactate–induced panic (Shear et al. 1991b).

In the largest study of PCT conducted to date, Barlow et al. (2000) found its short-term effects comparable to those of imipramine; both active interventions were significantly more effective than a double-blind pill placebo–clinical management condition. The combination of CT and imipramine demonstrated a modest advantage over the monotherapies. Following termination of treatment, patients treated with PCT had more durable responses than those withdrawn from imipramine.

Focused CT, as described by A.T. Beck et al. (1985a), also has fared well in outcome studies. Sokol et al. (1989) reported dramatic reductions in panic frequency (mean of 4.5 panic attacks a week before treatment to zero attacks per week after treatment) in an uncontrolled study of patients treated at the Center for Cognitive Therapy, University of Pennsylvania. Subsequently, Beck and colleagues (A.T. Beck et al. 1992b) studied panic disorder patients who were randomly assigned to CT or supportive psychotherapy. Results strongly favored CT. After 8 weeks, almost three times as many patients who received CT (versus those who received supportive therapy) were panic free. An additional study compared focused CT, relaxation training, imipramine, and a waiting list control in the treatment of panic disorder (D.M. Clark et al. 1994). All three active treatments were superior to the control condition, but CT led to greater reductions in anxiety levels, catastrophic cognitions, and frequency of panic attacks.

Other investigators also have documented the effectiveness of cognitive and behavioral treatment programs for panic disorder with or without agoraphobia (Arntz and Van Den Hout 1996; J.G. Beck et al. 1994; Bouchard et al. 1996; Craske et al. 1995; Laberge et al. 1993; Ost et al. 1993; Otto et al. 1993; Pollack et al. 1994; Westling and Ost 1995). Otto et al. (1993) have demonstrated that CT is more effective than standard clinical management in helping panic disorder patients discontinue benzodiazepines. Also, studies that have examined the long-term effects of treatment for panic disorder have found significant relapse prevention effects for CT (Otto and Whittal 1995).

Only one investigation found any evidence that CT may be less effective than other treatments. Black et al. (1993) compared a shortened form of CT (eight sessions) with fluvoxamine and placebo in patients with panic disorder. CT subjects were significantly improved compared with placebo on some (e.g., Clinical Global Impression [CGI] scores, panic attack severity scores) but not all ratings. Evidence was found for superiority of fluvoxamine on several clinical measures; however, the panic attack severity score was lowest for CT subjects at the end point analysis (CT = 6.8, fluvoxamine = 8.1, placebo = 15.3).

Although early trials of CT for GAD reported evidence for treatment effectiveness (e.g., Blowers et al. 1987; Durham and Turvey 1987), differences were not always found between CT and supportive or more traditional behavioral approaches (Hollon and Beck 1994). Initial studies of CT for generalized anxiety were marred by design problems such as lack of specificity in the treatment approaches, use of unsophisticated or truncated forms of CT, and selection of cognitive therapists with limited training or experience. Nevertheless, most studies of CT (or combined CT and behavior therapy) for GADs have found CT to be efficacious (Hollon and Beck 1994).

Later trials of CT for generalized anxiety used more precise research designs. Power et al. (1990) randomly assigned patients with GAD to diazepam, placebo, CT, diazepam plus CT, or placebo plus CT. Individuals treated in any of the three CT conditions were substantially improved by the end of the study. Diazepam alone also showed significant treatment effects as compared with placebo, but this was less marked than for CT.

Butler et al. (1991) performed a carefully designed study of CT for generalized anxiety. This research group had extensive previous experience in behavior therapy practice and research. In addition, they received intensive training in CT (including supervision at the Center for Cognitive Therapy, University of Pennsylvania). Adherence to the treatment models (both CT and behavior therapy) was monitored by independent raters. Results of this study indicated that CT was clearly superior to behavior therapy or a waiting list control. Furthermore, patients treated with CT had significantly more change in measures of dysfunctional cognition, including anxious thoughts and maladaptive beliefs. Another well-designed study compared CT with analytic psychotherapy and anxiety management training (a psychoeducation-based therapy that teaches anxiety coping strategies) for treatment of 110 patients with GAD (Durham et al. 1994). CT was clearly superior to the other treatments. The differential response between CT and analytic psychotherapy was so dramatic that the authors questioned whether analytic therapy was suitable for persons with GAD.

Several well executed studies have found evidence for the effectiveness of CT for social phobia (Gelernter et al. 1991; Heimberg et al. 1990; Hope et al. 1995). Heimberg's group cognitive and behavioral method has been the most widely studied (Juster and Heimberg 1995). Overall results of multiple studies indicate that treatment response is best when cognitive and exposure procedures are combined in therapy of social phobia (Juster and Heimberg 1995; Taylor 1996).

Although behavioral treatments have been shown to be effective for OCD (James and Blackburn 1995; Salkovskis and Westbrook 1989), only one outcome trial has been completed in which CT was compared directly with behavioral therapy (Van Oppen et al. 1995). Seventy-one patients with OCD who were not taking antidepressants were randomly assigned to Beck's form of CT or exposure plus response prevention (ERP). Both treatments led to statistically significant improvement, but CT was superior to ERP in reducing symptoms of OCD. Cognitive restructuring and behavioral methods are often combined in treating obsessive-compulsive patients (James and Blackburn 1995; J.M. Schwartz et al. 1996). It is still unclear whether a full package of cognitive and behavioral techniques offers significant advantages over either treatment alone.

Eating Disorders

A large number of experimental trials have found that CT significantly improves the symptoms of bulimia nervosa (Agras et al. 1992a, 1992b, 1994, 2000; P.J. Cooper and Steere 1995; P.J. Cooper et al. 1996; Fairburn et al. 1991, 1993, 1995; Garner 1992; Goldbloom et al. 1997; Leitenberg et al. 1994; Thackwray et al. 1993; Walsh et al. 1997). Reviews of controlled studies of CT for bulimia nervosa have concluded that there is convincing evidence for the efficacy of cognitive-behavioral treatment (Mitchell et al. 1996; Ricca et al. 2000; G.T. Wilson 1999). Typically, CT reduces the frequency of binge behaviors from 73% to 93% (Fairburn et al. 1992) and leads to a complete remission of bulimic symptoms in 51%–71% of cases (Ricca et al. 2000).

Agras et al. (1992) found that CBT and CT combined with desipramine were superior to desipramine alone in treatment of bulimia nervosa. In another study, Fairburn et al. (1991, 1993) compared CT with behavioral treatment and IPT. Although all three psychological treatments used by Fairburn and colleagues led to improvement in bulimic symptoms, CT and IPT were superior to behavior therapy, and CT was the most effective in modifying extreme dieting, emesis, and dysfunctional attitudes (Fairburn et al. 1991, 1993).

Thackwray et al. (1993) noted that bulimic patients who were treated with a full package of cognitive and behavior therapy fared much better over time than did those who received behavioral therapy alone. Six months after treatment, 69% of the subjects who were treated with CBT were abstinent from binge eating and purging. The abstinence rate for those receiving behavior therapy and an attention placebo group were 38% and 15%, respectively. Thus, combined cognitive and behavior therapy appears to offer advantages over a purely behavioral approach to bulimia.

Reviews of studies of combined CT and pharmacotherapy for bulimia have concluded that CT has a significant positive effect when added to antidepressant therapy (Ricca et al. 2000; G.T. Wilson 1999). However, adding medication to CT appears to offer little benefit over treatment with CT alone.

The most recent major investigation of psychological therapies for bulimia nervosa (Agras et al. 2000) involved 220 patients who were randomly assigned to either CT or IPT. CT was found to be significantly superior to IPT at the end of treatment. A 48% remission and a 29% recovery rate were observed for CT, whereas the remission rate (28%) and recovery rate (6%) were much lower for IPT.

Two studies have investigated the utility of CT self-help manuals in the treatment of bulimia. U. Schmidt et al. (1993) gave 28 bulimic patients a CT handbook and no other treatment. Twenty of the subjects were judged to be much improved ($n = 12$) or somewhat improved ($n = 8$) after using the workbook for 4–6 weeks. Another research group reported that a CT program of eight sessions of 20–30 minutes with a social worker plus use of a self-help manual led to an 80% reduction in the frequency of bulimic episodes (P.J. Cooper et al. 1996). Although these studies were uncontrolled, the results suggest that it may be possible to lower the cost of CT and increase access to treatment for bulimia by using self-help methods.

Binge-eating disorder (BED) has been studied less intensively than bulimia nervosa. Nevertheless, there is growing evidence that CT is also effective for this form of eating disorder (Agras et al. 1994b; Ricca et al. 2000; Wilfley 1993; G.T. Wilson 1999). In reviews of studies of CT for BED, G.T. Wilson (1999) and Ricca et al. (2000) noted that CT has been shown to be beneficial in reducing bingeing, but has not been consistently helpful in promoting weight loss in persons with BED. Traditional behavioral weight control programs have been shown to promote weight loss, at least in the short term, in patients with BED (G.T. Wilson 1999).

Psychosis

There has been a growing interest in studying the use of CT and related therapies for psychotic disorders. In several uncontrolled studies, CT has been reported to reduce schizophrenic symptoms (Chadwick and Birchwood 1994; Chadwick and Lowe 1994; Fowler and Morley 1989; Kingdon and Turkington 1991; Perris and Skagerlind 1994). Two groups of investigators have compared CT with a waiting list control; however, randomized assignment was not used (Garety et al. 1994; Tarrier et al. 1993).

Several randomized controlled investigations of CT for psychosis have been completed since 1996. Drury et al. (1996a, 1996b) found substantial improvement in positive symptoms and reduced time required for recovery in a group of inpatients treated with CT. Forty patients with nonaffective psychosis were randomly assigned to CT plus standard clinical management or treatment as usual. CT was more effective than standard therapy in reducing positive symptoms and delusional conviction. The percentages of patients who had moderate to severe residual symptoms after treatment were 5% for those who received the added CT compared with 56% for subjects who were treated with standard therapy.

In another randomized, controlled trial, Kuipers et al. (1997) found superior reduction in Brief Psychiatric Rating Scale scores in patients with nonaffective psychosis treated with CT compared with routine care. However, there were no significant differences observed between the treatment groups for other measures of change. Tarrier et al. (1998) studied 87 persons with schizophrenia who had persistent symptoms despite adequate medication. Subjects were randomly assigned to CT plus routine care, supportive therapy plus routine care, or routine care alone. After completion of treatment, patients who received CT had significantly lower scores on measures of positive symptoms than those treated with supportive therapy or routine care alone. Changes in negative symptoms were equivalent in all three treatment groups.

The most carefully controlled study of CT for psychosis reported to date was conducted by Sensky et al. (2000). Ninety persons who met DSM-IV (American Psychiatric Association 1994) criteria for schizophrenia who had persistent, drug-resistant symptoms were randomly assigned to CT or "befriending" (supportive therapy) plus routine care. Treatment manuals and taped sessions were used to insure fidelity to the treatment method. Medication was equivalent in both treatment groups. At the end of the 9-month course of therapy, there were no differences found between the treatments. Therapy with CT and befriending were both associated with substantial improvements in positive and negative symptoms. However, at the 9-month follow-up examination, patients treated with CT had significantly lower scores on measures of both positive and negative symptoms. For example, the change in Scale for Assessment of Negative Symptoms mean scores from baseline to 9-month follow-up was 49.3% for CT and 19.0% for befriending. Depressive symptoms were also reduced to a greater extent in patients who received CT.

Taken together, studies of CT for nonaffective psychosis suggest that CT can add to the effects of medication and routine care in the treatment of individuals who have persistent symptoms. Treatment protocols in most studies have focused primarily on methods of reducing delusions and hallucinations. Further research on the application of CT for positive symptoms is clearly needed. However, development and testing of specific methods for negative symptoms would be especially welcome because of the frequent resistance of these problems to pharmacotherapy.

One of the important potential targets for CT of severe and chronic mental disorders is treatment adherence (Scott and Wright 1997). CT has been shown to improve adherence to lithium carbonate regimens in patients with bipolar disorder (Cochran 1986), and CT appeared to enhance medication compliance in an uncontrolled study of schizophrenic patients treated in small group homes (Perris and Skagerlind 1994). Additional research is clearly needed on the use of CT for treatment adherence. CT methods have been described as particularly well suited for helping clinicians and patients to collaborate effectively in promoting adherence to treatment recommendations (Lecompte 1995; Rush 1988; Scott and Wright 1997).

Outcome Research for Other Disorders

The majority of CT outcome research has been concerned with depression, anxiety disorders, and eating disorders. However, a substantial amount of investigative work has been completed on the efficacy of CT for other conditions such as psychophysiological disorders, substance abuse, and personality disorders. A broad range of studies have examined the utility of CT in behavioral medicine (Sensky et al. 1993). For example, multiple sclerosis patients treated with CT have been found to have significantly improved psychological and physical functioning (Larcombe and Wilson 1984; Rodgers et al. 1996). In another study, CT was shown to be significantly better than routine care in reducing depression and improving glucose control in persons with type 2 diabetes (Lustman et al. 1998). CT has also been demonstrated to be effective in reducing medication requirements in persons with hypertension (Shapiro et al. 1997).

Several groups have reported that CT can be a helpful approach in the management of chronic pain (Linton and Ryberg 2001; Moore et al. 2000; Phillips 1987; Skinner et al. 1990; Turner and Clancy 1986). A meta-analysis of 25 studies of CT for pain (excluding headache) found that this approach was effective when compared to a waiting list control group and to alternative active treatments (Morley et al. 1999). The cognitive treatment model for chronic pain has been described in detail by Turk et al. (1983).

Other investigators have observed that CT can be useful in the treatment of skin disorders (Horne et al. 1989), epilepsy (Goldstein 1990), asthma (Maes and Schlosser 1988), inflammatory and irritable bowel syndromes (Payne and Blanchard 1995; S.P. Schwartz and Blanchard 1991), myocardial infarction (Friedman et al. 1986), temporomandibular disorders (Dworkin et al. 1994; Mishra et al. 2000), fibromyalgia (White and Nielson 1995), and medically unexplained physical symptoms (Kroenke and Swindle 2000; Speckens et al. 1995). CT also has been shown to be effective in reducing the risk of disability from medical illness. In a randomized study of programs for prevention of disability from spine pain, Linton and Andersson (2000) found that a six-session cognitive-behavioral group intervention led to a ninefold lowering of the risk for long-term work absence.

Attempts to use CT to help patients with rheumatoid arthritis have met with mixed results (Keefe and Van Horn 1993; Kraaimaat et al. 1995; Sharpe et al. 2001). In a study of CT treatment in patients with recent-onset rheumatoid arthritis, Sharpe et al. (2001) observed significant reductions in both psychological and physical morbidity. Leibing et al. (1999) noted that CT helped with coping behaviors, emotional stabilization, and degree of impairment in patients with multiple sclerosis. In other studies, however, the progressive course of this illness tended to reduce gains over time. Generally, results of studies in behavioral medicine indicate that CT can improve psychophysiological functioning, subjective well-being, and/or coping with illness.

In another study, breast cancer patients who had received mastectomies experienced reductions in psychological distress after a course of cognitively oriented therapy (Tarrier and Maguire 1984).

Applications of CT for substance abuse and characterological disturbances have not yet been studied extensively under controlled conditions. However, several important findings have been reported, and a significant amount of research is currently under way. An early investigation for substance abuse suggested that CT (plus paraprofessional drug counseling) may be superior to drug counseling alone in treatment of heroin addicts (Woody et al. 1983). In a large study of treatment for cocaine abuse, Wells et al. (1994) found that a relapse prevention program based in part on cognitive-behavioral methods and a 12-Step approach were equally effective in decreasing both cocaine and alcohol use. The patients who received relapse prevention had a lower use of alcohol than those treated with the 12-Step approach at the follow-up assessment.

Another study of CT-based relapse prevention programs found CBT to be more effective than desipramine or clinical management in reducing cocaine behaviors and fostering abstinence (Carroll et al. 1995). Carroll et al. (1994a, 1994b) observed no differences immediately after treatment in subjects with cocaine dependence who received CT (relapse prevention), desipramine, or placebo. However, the CT subjects had a significantly improved response at the 1-year follow-up. The authors concluded that this effect was likely due to "implementation of the generalizable coping skills conveyed through that treatment."

In contrast, the National Institute on Drug Abuse–sponsored trial comparing CT, supportive-expressive psychotherapy, and individual and group drug counseling failed to demonstrate the effectiveness of CT as a treatment for cocaine-dependent patients (Crits-Christoph et al. 1999). Results strongly favored the combination of group and individual drug counseling; neither psychotherapy benefited patients any more than did group counseling alone, despite 8–10 additional hours of one-to-one intervention.

Limited research has been completed on CT for alcohol abuse, but preliminary studies have shown that alcoholic individuals, even those with significant Axis II pathology, can respond well to a CT approach (Fisher and Bentley 1996; Longabaugh et al. 1994; Schonfeld and Dupree 1995; Sitharthan et al. 1996).

Outcome research on CT for personality disorders is the beginning stage of development. Results of early studies indicate that the presence of an Axis II disorder may complicate the treatment of depression, anxiety disorders, or eating disorders with CT (T.R. Giles et al. 1985; Mavissakalian and Hammon 1987; Persons et al. 1988; Rush and Shaw 1983). Personality disorders did not, however, predict poorer CT response in the multicenter NIMH Treatment of Depression Collaborative Research Project (Shea et al. 1990) or in a single-center study conducted by the Pittsburgh group (Stuart et al. 1992). A large randomized trial of CT for treatment of alcohol abuse similarly found that patients who had antisocial personality disorder responded well to treatment, and in some cases actually did better than subjects without personality disorder (Longabaugh et al. 1994). Also, patients with body dysmorphic disorder and comorbid Axis II disorders were observed to have highly significant and substantial improvement after treatment with CT (Neziroglu et al. 1996).

The most notable research on a cognitive-behavioral approach to personality disorders has been conducted by Linehan and colleagues (Bohus et al. 2000; Linehan 1993; Linehan et al. 1991, 1993, 1994, 1999; Shearin and Linehan 1994). In a randomized trial of 44 borderline patients treated with DBT or treatment as usual, significant reductions in suicidal acts and the medical risk for suicide were observed in those who received DBT (Linehan et al. 1991). At the 6-month posttreatment assessment, DBT was still superior to treatment as usual, but these differences had disappeared by the time of the 12-month assessment (Linehan et al. 1993). Subjects treated with DBT had fewer days of inpatient hospitalization than control subjects during the year after completion of therapy.

Another analysis of data from Linehan's studies indicated that DBT had mixed effects on social and interpersonal functioning (Linehan et al. 1994). In a group of 26 patients with borderline personality and chronic suicidal activities treated with DBT or treatment as usual, DBT was found to significantly improve measures of anger and interviewer-rated social adjustment. Global life satisfaction was not different in the two experimental groups. In a review of Linehan's work, Perris (1994) observed that DBT emphasizes behavioral change more than revision of dysfunctional schemas. He suggested that improvements in interpersonal skills are more likely to be long lasting if patients learn functional "personal rules of living."

A limited number of other studies of CT for personality disorders have been conducted. Two groups investigated the usefulness of group therapy based on DBT

(Shearin and Linehan 1994; Springer et al. 1996). In a study of inpatients with a variety of Axis II diagnoses, DBT was no more effective than supportive group therapy (Springer et al. 1996). The treatment program was quite short compared with the DBT described by Linehan, and a variety of other treatments were used for this inpatient sample. Thus, the study by Springer et al. (1996) does not appear to be an adequate test of DBT. In a later, uncontrolled study, Bohus et al. (2000) reported significant improvements in depression, dissociation, anxiety, and global stress after a 3-month inpatient DBT program.

Shearin and Linehan (1994) have described a small study in which they attempted to teach the skills training component of DBT in a group format. They concluded that DBT cannot be effectively delivered in an abbreviated package of skills training only. In the most recent randomized controlled trial, Linehan et al. (1999) found that DBT was more effective than treatment as usual in reducing drug abuse and improving social adjustment in patients with comorbid borderline personality disorder and substance abuse.

Beck's model for CT of personality disorders has not been tested in controlled trials. Two case series have been reported in which CT appeared to be useful for treatment of people with personality disorders (Davidson and Tyer 1996; Nelson-Gray et al. 1996). Outcome research has been extremely limited for any type of psychotherapy of personality disorders. These conditions are notoriously difficult to treat under controlled conditions because of pervasive interpersonal and skills deficits and a frequent need for long-term therapy. Linehan's groundbreaking research has stimulated hope that additional studies will help elucidate the most effective methods of treating this challenging group of patients.

Conclusions

CT is a recently developed system of psychotherapy that is linked philosophically with a long tradition of viewing cognition as a primary determinant of emotion and behavior. The theoretical constructs of CT are supported by a large body of experimental findings regarding dysfunctional information processing in psychiatric disorders. In clinical practice, CT is usually short-term, problem oriented, and highly collaborative. Therapists and patients work together in an empirical style, seeking to identify and modify maladaptive patterns of thinking. Behavioral techniques are used to uncover distorted cognitions and to promote more effective functioning. Also, psychoeducational procedures and homework assign-

ments help reinforce concepts learned in therapy sessions. The goals of CT include both immediate symptom relief and the acquisition of cognitive and behavioral skills that will decrease the risk for relapse.

The efficacy of CT for depression, generalized anxiety, panic disorder, eating disorders, and other conditions has been established in a wide range of outcome studies. Newer applications for CT, such as personality disorders, substance abuse, and psychosis are beginning to receive attention from investigators. Detailed treatment manuals or other guidelines for therapy have been described for most psychiatric illnesses.

CT has rapidly evolved into one of the major psychotherapeutic orientations in modern psychiatric treatment. Future challenges for this therapy model include study of the relative importance of treatment components, detailed examination of predictors for outcome, elucidation of the interface between biological and cognitive processes, and incorporation of new developments in computer-assisted learning. The empirical nature of CT should promote further exploration of the potential uses for this treatment approach.

References

Abramson LY, Seligman MEP, Teasdale J: Learned helplessness in humans: critique and reformulation. J Abnorm Psychol 87:49–74, 1978

Adler A: The neurotic's picture of the world. International Journal of Individual Psychology 2:3–10, 1936

Agras WS, Rossiter EM, Arnow B, et al: Pharmacologic and cognitive-behavioral treatment for bulimia nervosa: a controlled comparison. Am J Psychiatry 149:82–87, 1992

Agras WS, Rossiter EM, Arnow B, et al: One-year follow-up of psychosocial and pharmacologic treatments for bulimia nervosa. J Clin Psychiatry 55:179–183, 1994a

Agras WS, Telch CF, Arnow B, et al: Weight loss, cognitive-behavioral, and desipramine treatments in binge eating disorder: an additive design. Behav Ther 25:225–238, 1994b

Agras WS, Walsh BT, Fairburn CG, et al: A multicenter comparison of cognitive-behavioral therapy and interpersonal psychotherapy for bulimia nervosa. Arch Gen Psychiatry 57:459–466, 2000

Akiskal HS, McKinney WT: Overview of recent research in depression: integration of ten conceptual models into a comprehensive clinical frame. Arch Gen Psychiatry 32:285–305, 1975

Alexander F: Psychosomatic Medicine: Its Principles and Applications. New York, WW Norton, 1950

Alford BA, Beck AT: Cognitive therapy of delusional beliefs. Behav Res Ther 32:369–380, 1994

Alford BA, Beck AT: The Integrative Power of Cognitive Therapy. New York, Guilford, 1997

Alford BA, Correia CJ: Cognitive therapy of schizophrenia: theory and empirical status. Behav Ther 25:17–33, 1994

Alford BA, Freeman A, Beck AT, et al: Brief focused cognitive therapy of panic disorder. Psychotherapy 27:230–234, 1990

Alloy LB, Ahrens AH: Depression and pessimism for the future: biased use of statistically relevant information in predictions for self versus others. J Pers Soc Psychol 52:366–378, 1987

American Psychiatric Association: Diagnostic and Statistical Manual of Mental Disorders, 4th Edition. Washington, DC, American Psychiatric Association, 1994

Arntz A, Van Den Hout M: Psychological treatments of panic disorder without agoraphobia: cognitive therapy versus applied relaxation. Behav Res Ther 34:113–121, 1996

Barlow DH, Cerney JA: Psychological Treatment of Panic. New York, Guilford, 1988

Barlow DH, Craske MG, Cerney JA, et al: Behavioral treatment of panic disorder. Behav Ther 20:261–268, 1989

Barlow DH, Gorman JM, Shear MK, et al: Cognitive-behavioral therapy, imipramine, or their combination for panic disorder: a randomized controlled trial. JAMA 283:2529–2536, 2000

Barrett CL, Meyer RG: Cognitive therapy with alcoholism, in Cognitive Therapy With Inpatients: Developing a Cognitive Milieu. Edited by Wright JH, Thase ME, Beck AT, et al. New York, Guilford, 1993, pp 315–336

Barrett CL, Wright JH: Therapist variables, in Issues in Psychotherapy Research. Edited by Hersen M, Nichelson L, Bellack AS. New York, Plenum, 1984, pp 361–391

Basco MR: Never Good Enough. New York, Free Press, 1999

Basco MR, Rush AJ: Cognitive-Behavioral Therapy for Bipolar Disorder. New York, Guilford, 1996

Baxter LR Jr, Schwartz JM, Bergman KS, et al: Caudate glucose metabolic rate changes with both drug and behavior therapy for obsessive-compulsive disorder. Arch Gen Psychiatry 49:681–689, 1992

Beck AT: Thinking and depression. Arch Gen Psychiatry 9:324–333, 1963

Beck AT: Thinking and depression, II: theory and therapy. Arch Gen Psychiatry 10:561–571, 1964

Beck AT: Depression: Clinical, Experimental, and Theoretical Aspects. New York, Harper & Row, 1967

Beck AT: Cognitive Therapy and the Emotional Disorders. New York, International Universities Press, 1976

Beck AT: Love is Never Enough. New York, Harper & Row, 1988

Beck AT: Cognitive therapy and research: a 25-year retrospective. Presented at the World Congress of Cognitive Therapy. Oxford, England, 1989

Beck AT: Cognitive therapy: past, present, and future. J Consult Clin Psychol 61:194–198, 1993

Beck AT: Cognitive therapy: a status report. Journal of Clinical Psychology and Psychopathology, in press

Beck AT, Freeman A: Cognitive Therapy of Personality Disorders. New York, Guilford, 1990

Beck AT, Rush AJ: Cognitive therapy, in Comprehensive Textbook of Psychiatry, 6th Edition. Edited by Kaplan HI, Sadock BJ: Baltimore, MD, Williams & Wilkins, 1992, pp 1847–1857

Beck AT, Kovacs M, Weissman A: Hopelessness and suicidal behavior—an overview. JAMA 234:1146–1149, 1975

Beck AT, Rush AJ, Shaw BF, et al: Cognitive Therapy of Depression. New York, Guilford, 1979

Beck AT, Emery GD, Greenberg RL: Anxiety Disorders and Phobias: A Cognitive Perspective. New York, Basic Books, 1985a

Beck AT, Steer RA, Kovacs M, et al: Hopelessness and eventual suicide: a 10-year prospective study of patients hospitalized with suicidal ideation. Am J Psychiatry 142:559–562, 1985b

Beck AT, Brown G, Berchick RJ, et al: Relationship between hopelessness and ultimate suicide: a replication with psychiatric outpatients. Am J Psychiatry 147:190–195, 1990

Beck AT, Wright JH, Neuman C: Cocaine abuse, in Comprehensive Casebook of Cognitive Therapy. Edited by Freeman A, Dattilio FM. New York, Plenum, 1992a, pp 185–192

Beck AT, Sokol L, Clark DA, et al: A cross-over study of focused cognitive therapy for panic disorder. Am J Psychiatry 149:778–783, 1992b

Beck AT, Greenberg RL, Beck J: Coping with depression (a booklet). Bala Cynwyd, PA, The Beck Institute, 1995

Beck J: Cognitive Therapy: Basics and Beyond. New York, Guilford, 1995

Beck J: Cognitive approaches to personality disorders, in The American Psychiatric Press Review of Psychiatry, Vol 16. Edited by Dickstein LJ, Riba MB, Oldham JM. Washington, DC, American Psychiatric Press, 1997, pp 73–106

Beck JG, Stanley MA, Baldwin LE, et al: Comparison of cognitive therapy and relaxation training for panic disorder. J Consult Clin Psychol 62:818–826, 1994

Bergdahl J, Anneroth G, Perris H: Cognitive therapy in the treatment of patients with resistant burning mouth syndrome: a controlled study. J Oral Pathol Med 24:213–215, 1995

Beutler LE, Scogin F, Kinkish P, et al: Group cognitive therapy and alprazolam in the treatment of depression in older adults. J Consult Clin Psychol 55:550–556, 1987

Black DW, Wesner R, Bowers W, et al: A comparison of fluvoxamine, cognitive therapy, and placebo in the treatment of panic disorder. Arch Gen Psychiatry 50:44–50, 1993

Blackburn IM, Bishop S, Glen AIM, et al: The efficacy of cognitive therapy in depression: a treatment trial using cognitive therapy and pharmacotherapy, each alone and in combination. Br J Psychiatry 139:181–189, 1981

Blackburn IM, Jones S, Lewin RJP: Cognitive style in depression. Br J Clin Psychol 25:241–251, 1986a

Blackburn IM, Eunson KM, Bishop S: A two-year naturalistic follow-up of depressed patients treated with cognitive therapy, pharmacotherapy, and a combination of both. J Affect Disord 10:67–75, 1986b

Blowers C, Cobb J, Mathews A: Generalized anxiety: a controlled treatment study. Behav Res Ther 25:493–502, 1987

Bohus M, Haaf B, Stiglmayr C, et al: Evaluation of inpatient dialectical-behavior therapy for borderline personality disorder—a prospective study. Behav Res Ther 38:875–887, 2000

Bouchard S, Gauthier J, Laberge B, et al: Exposure versus cognitive restructuring in the treatment of panic disorder with agoraphobia. Behav Res Ther 34:213–224, 1996

Bower GH: Mood and memory. Am Psychol 36:129–148, 1981

Bowers WA: Cognitive therapy with inpatients, in Handbook of Cognitive Therapy. Edited by Freeman A, Simon KM, Arkowitz H, et al. New York, Plenum, 1989, pp 583–596

Bowers WA: Treatment of depressed inpatients: cognitive therapy plus medication, relaxation plus medication, and medication alone. Br J Psychiatry 156:73–78, 1990

Bowers WA: Inpatient cognitive therapy for eating disorders, in Cognitive Therapy with Inpatients: Developing a Cognitive Milieu. Edited by Wright JH, Thase ME, Beck AT, et al. New York, Guilford, 1992, pp 337–356

Bowers W, Stuart S, MacFarlane R, et al: Use of computer-administered cognitive-behavior therapy with depressed inpatients. Depression 1:294–299, 1993

Bowlby J: The role of childhood experience in cognitive disturbance, in Cognition and Psychotherapy. Edited by Mahoney MJ, Freeman A. New York, Plenum, 1985, pp 181–200

Bradley B, Mathews A: Negative self-schemata in clinical depression. Br J Clin Psychol 22:173–181, 1982

Brody AL, Saxena S, Stoessel P, et al: Regional brain metabolic changes in patients with major depression treated with either paroxetine or interpersonal therapy: preliminary findings. Arch Gen Psychiatry 58:631–640, 2001

Bujold A, Ladouceur R, Sylvain C, et al: Treatment of pathological gamblers: an experimental study. J Behav Ther Exp Psychiatry 25:275–282, 1994

Burns DD: Feeling Good. New York, William Morrow, 1980, 1999

Burns DD, Rude S, Simons AD, et al: Does learned resourcefulness predict the response to cognitive behavioral therapy for depression? Cognitive Therapy and Research 18:277–291, 1994

Butler G, Fennell M, Robson P, et al: Comparison of behavior therapy and cognitive behavior therapy in the treatment of generalized anxiety disorder. J Consult Clin Psychol 59:167–175, 1991

Carroll KM, Rounsaville BJ, Nich C, et al: One-year follow-up of psychotherapy and pharmacotherapy for cocaine dependence. Arch Gen Psychiatry 51:989–997, 1994a

Carroll KM, Rounsaville BJ, Gordon LT, et al: Psychotherapy and pharmacotherapy for ambulatory cocaine abusers. Arch Gen Psychiatry 51:177–187, 1994b

Carroll KM, Nich C, Rounsaville BJ: Differential symptom reduction in depressed cocaine abusers treated with psychotherapy and pharmacotherapy. J Nerv Ment Dis 183:251–259, 1995

Casey DA, Grant RW: Cognitive therapy with depressed elderly inpatients, in Cognitive Therapy with Inpatients: Developing a Cognitive Milieu. Edited by Wright JH, Thase ME, Beck AT, et al. New York, Guilford, 1992, pp 295–314

Chadwick P, Birchwood M: The omnipotence of voices: a cognitive approach to auditory hallucinations. Br J Psychiatry 164:190–201, 1994

Chadwick PDJ, Lowe CF: A cognitive approach to measuring and modifying delusions. Behav Res Ther 32:355–367, 1994

Clark DA, Feldman J, Channon S: Dysfunctional thinking in anorexia and bulimia nervosa. Cognitive Therapy and Research 13:377–387, 1989

Clark DA, Beck AT, Stewart B: Cognitive specificity and positive-negative affectivity: complementary or contradictory views on anxiety and depression? J Abnorm Psychol 99:148–155, 1990

Clark DA, Beck AT, Alford BA: Scientific Foundations of Cognitive Theory and Therapy of Depression. New York, John Wiley & Sons, 1999

Clark DM: A cognitive approach to panic. Behav Res Ther 24:461–470, 1986

Clark DM, Beck AT: Cognitive approaches, in Handbook of Anxiety Disorders. Edited by Last CG, Hersen M. New York, Pergamon, 1988, pp 362–385

Clark DM, Teasdale JD: Diurnal variation in clinical depression and the accessibility of memories of positive and negative experiences. J Abnorm Psychol 91:87–95, 1982

Clark DM, Salkovskis PM, Chalkley AJ: Respiratory control as a treatment for panic attacks. J Behav Ther Exp Psychiatry 16:23–30, 1985

Clark DM, Salkovskis PM, Hackmann A, et al: A comparison of cognitive therapy, applied relaxation and imipramine in the treatment of panic disorder. Br J Psychiatry 164:759–769, 1994

Cloitre M, Liebowitz MR: Memory bias in panic disorder: an investigation of the cognitive avoidance hypothesis. Cognitive Therapy and Research 15:371–386, 1991

Cochran SD: Compliance with lithium regimens in the outpatient treatment of bipolar affective disorders. Journal of Compliance in Health Care 1:151–169, 1986

Colby KM: A computer program using cognitive therapy to treat depressed patients. Psychiatr Serv 46:1223–1225, 1995

Colby KM, Colby PM: Overcoming Depression. Malibu, CA, Artifactual Intelligence Works, 1990

Cooper PJ, Steere J: A comparison of two psychological treatments for bulimia nervosa: implications for models of maintenance. Behav Res Ther 33:875-885, 1995

Cooper PJ, Coker S, Fleming C: An evaluation of the efficacy of supervised cognitive behavioral self-help for bulimia nervosa. J Psychosom Res 40:281–287, 1996

Corbishley M, Beutler L, Quan S, et al: Rapid eye movement density and latency and dexamethasone suppression as predictors of treatment response in depressed older adults. Current Therapeutic Research 47:846–859, 1990

Covi L, Lipman RS: Cognitive behavioral group psychotherapy combined with imipramine in major depression. Psychopharmacol Bull 23:173–176, 1987

Covi L, Primakoff L: Cognitive group therapy, in The American Psychiatric Press Review of Psychiatry. Edited by Frances AJ, Hales RE. Washington, DC, American Psychiatric Press, 1988, pp 608–616

Craske MG, Maidenberg E, Bystritsky A: Brief cognitive-behavioral versus nondirective therapy for panic disorder. J Behav Ther Exp Psychiatry 26:113–120, 1995

Crits-Christoph P, Siqueland L, Blaine J, et al: Psychosocial treatments for cocaine dependence. National Institute on Drug Abuse Collaborative Cocaine Treatment Study. Arch Gen Psychiatry 56:493–502, 1999

Davidson KM, Tyrer P: Cognitive therapy for antisocial and borderline personality disorders: single case study series. Br J Clin Psychol 35:413–429, 1996

Davis D, Wright JH: The therapeutic relationship in cognitive-behavioral therapy: patient perceptions and therapist responses. Cognitive and Behavioral Practice 1:25–45, 1994

Davis H, Unruh WR: The development of the self-schema in adult depression. J Abnorm Psychol 90:125–133, 1981

DeMonbreun BG, Craighead WE: Distortion of perception and recall of positive and neutral feedback in depression. Cognitive Therapy and Research 1:311–329, 1977

Derry PA, Kuiper NA: Schematic processing and self-reference in clinical depression. J Abnorm Psychol 90:286–297, 1981

DeRubeis RJ, Evans MD, Hollon SD, et al: How does cognitive therapy work? Cognitive change and symptom change in cognitive therapy and pharmacotherapy for depression. J Consult Clin Psychol 58:862–869, 1990

DeRubeis RJ, Gelfand LA, Tang TZ, et al: Medication versus cognitive behavior therapy for severely depressed outpatients: mega-analysis of four randomized comparisons. Am J Psychiatry 156:1007–1013, 1999

Deutscher S, Cimbolic P: Cognitive process and their relationship to endogenous and reactive components of depression. J Nerv Ment Dis 178:351–359, 1990

Dobson KS: A meta-analysis of the efficacy of cognitive therapy for depression. J Consult Clin Psychol 57:414–419, 1989

Dobson KS, Shaw BF: Cognitive assessment with major depressive disorders. Cognitive Therapy and Research 10:13–29, 1986

Drury V, Birchwood M, Cochrane R, et al: Cognitive therapy and recovery from acute psychosis: a controlled trial, I: impact on psychotic symptoms. Br J Psychiatry 169:593–601, 1996a

Drury V, Birchwood M, Cochrane R, et al: Cognitive therapy and recovery from acute psychosis: a controlled trial, II: impact on recovery time. Br J Psychiatry 169:602–607, 1996b

Durham RC, Turvey AA: Cognitive therapy vs. behavior therapy in the treatment of chronic general anxiety. Behav Res Ther 25:229–234, 1987

Durham RC, Murphy T, Allan T, et al: Cognitive therapy, analytic psychotherapy and anxiety management training for generalised anxiety disorder. Br J Psychiatry 165:315–323, 1994

Dworkin SF, Turner JA, Wilson L, et al: Brief group cognitive-behavioral intervention for temporomandibular disorders. Pain 59:175–187, 1994

Eckman TA, Wirshing WC, Marder SR, et al: Technique for training schizophrenic patients in illness self-management: a controlled trial. Am J Psychiatry 149:1549–1555, 1992

Elkin I, Shea MT, Watkins JT, et al: NIMH Treatment of Depression Collaborative Research Program, I: general effectiveness of treatments. Arch Gen Psychiatry 46:971–982, 1989

Elkin I, Gibbons RD, Shea MT, et al: Initial severity and differential treatment outcome in the National Institute of Mental Health Treatment of Depression Collaborative Research Program. J Consult Clin Psychol 63:841–847, 1995

Ellis A: Reason and Emotion in Psychotherapy. New York, Lyle Stuart, 1962

Ellis A: Humanistic Psychotherapy: The Rational-Emotive Psychotherapy. New York, McGraw-Hill, 1973

Emmelkamp PMG, Beens H: Cognitive therapy with obsessive-compulsive disorder: a comparative evaluation. Behav Res Ther 29:293–300, 1991

Engel GL: The need for a new medical model: a challenge for biomedicine. Science 196:129–136, 1977

Epstein N, Schlesinger SE, Dryden W: Cognitive-Behavioral Therapy With Families. New York, Brunner/Mazel, 1988

Evans MD, Hollon SD, DeRubeis RJ, et al: Differential relapse following cognitive therapy and pharmacotherapy for depression. Arch Gen Psychiatry 49:802–808, 1992

Fairburn CG: Cognitive-behavioral treatment for bulimia, in Handbook of Psychotherapy for Anorexia Nervosa and Bulimia. Edited by Garner DM, Garfinkel PE. New York, Guilford, 1985, pp 160–169

Fairburn CG, Jones R, Peveler RC, et al: Three psychological treatments for bulimia nervosa. Arch Gen Psychiatry 48:463–469, 1991

Fairburn CG, Agras WS, Wilson GT: The research on treatment of bulimia nervosa: practical and theoretical implications, in The Biology of Feast and Famine: Relevance to Eating Disorders. Edited by Anderson GH, Kennedy SH. San Diego, CA, Academic Press, 1992, pp 318–340

Fairburn CG, Jones R, Peveler RC, et al: Psychotherapy and bulimia nervosa. Arch Gen Psychiatry 50:419–428, 1993

Fairburn CG, Norman PA, Welch SL, et al: A prospective study of outcome in bulimia nervosa and the long-term effects of three psychological treatments. Arch Gen Psychiatry 52:304–312, 1995

Fava GA, Grandi S, Zielezny M, et al: Four-year outcome for cognitive behavioral treatment of residual symptoms in major depression. Am J Psychiatry 153:945–947, 1996

Fava GA, Rafanelli C, Grandi S, et al: Prevention of recurrent depression with cognitive behavioral therapy. Arch Gen Psychiatry 55:816–820, 1998

Fawcett J, Scheftner W, Clark D, et al: Clinical predictors of suicide in patients with major affective disorders: a controlled prospective study. Am J Psychiatry 144:35–40, 1987

Fisher MS, Bentley KJ: Two group therapy models for clients with a dual diagnosis of substance abuse and personality disorder. Psychiatr Serv 47:1244–1250, 1996

Fitzgerald TE, Phillips W: Attentional bias and agoraphobic avoidance: the role of cognitive style. J Anxiety Disord 5:333–341, 1991

Fowler D, Morley S: The cognitive-behavioral treatment of hallucinations and delusions: a preliminary study. Behavioral Psychotherapy 17:262–282, 1989

Frankl VE: Logos, paradox, and the search for meaning, in Cognition and Psychotherapy. Edited by Mahoney MJ, Freeman A. New York, Plenum, 1985, pp 3–49

Free ML, Oei TPS, Sanders MR: Treatment outcome of a group cognitive therapy program for depression. Int J Group Psychother 41:533–547, 1991

Freeman A, Dattilio FM: Comprehensive Casebook of Cognitive Therapy. New York, Plenum, 1992

Freeman A, Simon KM, Beutler LE, et al. (eds): Comprehensive Handbook of Cognitive Therapy. New York, Plenum, 1989

Freeman A, Schrodt GR, Gilson M, et al: Cognitive group therapy with inpatients, in Cognitive Therapy With Inpatients: Developing a Cognitive Milieu. Edited by Wright JH, Thase ME, Beck AT, et al. New York, Guilford, 1992, pp 121–153

Friedman M, Thorensen CD, Gill JJ, et al: Alteration of type A behavior and its effect on cardiac recurrences in post myocardial infarct patients: summary results of the recurrent coronary prevention project. Am Heart J 112:653–665, 1986

Gaffan EA, Tsaousis I, Kemp-Wheeler SM: Researcher allegiance and meta-analysis: the case of cognitive therapy for depression. J Consult Clin Psychol 63:966–980, 1995

Garety PA, Kuipers L, Fowler D, et al: Cognitive behavioral therapy for drug-resistant psychosis. Br J Med Psychol 67:259–271, 1994

Garner DM: Psychotherapy for eating disorders. Current Opinion in Psychiatry 5:391–395, 1992

Garner DM, Bemis KM: A cognitive-behavioral approach to anorexia nervosa. Cognitive Therapy and Research 6:123–150, 1985

Gelernter CS, Uhde TW, Cimbolic P, et al: Cognitive-behavioral and pharmacological treatments of social phobia: a controlled study. Arch Gen Psychiatry 48:938–945, 1991

Giles DE, Etzel BA, Biggs MM: Long-term effects of unipolar depression on cognitions. Compr Psychiatry 30:225–230, 1989

Giles TR, Young RR, Young DE: Behavioral treatment of severe bulimia. Behav Ther 16:393–405, 1985

Glass CR, Furlong M: Cognitive assessment of social anxiety: affective and behavioral correlates. Cognitive Therapy and Research 14:365–384, 1990

Goldbloom DS, Olmsted M, Davis R, et al: A randomized controlled trial of fluoxetine and cognitive behavioral therapy for bulimia nervosa: short-term outcome. Behav Res Ther 35:803–811, 1997

Goldstein LH: Behavioral and cognitive-behavioral treatments for epilepsy: a progress review. Br J Clin Psychol 29:257–269, 1990

Gotlib IH: Self-reinforcement and recall: differential deficits in depressed and nondepressed psychiatric inpatients. J Abnorm Psychol 90:521–530, 1981

Gotlib IH: Perception and recall of interpersonal feedback: negative bias in depression. Cognitive Therapy and Research 7:399–412, 1983

Gotlib IH, Olson JM: Depression, psychopathology, and self-serving attributions. Br J Clin Psychol 22:309–310, 1983

Greenberg LS, Safran JD: Integrating affect and cognition: a perspective on the process of therapeutic change. Cognitive Therapy and Research 8:559–578, 1984

Greenberger D, Padesky CA: Mind Over Mood. New York, Guilford, 1995

Greist JH: Clinical computing: treatment for all: the computer as a patient assistant. Psychiatr Serv 49:887–889, 1998

Guidano VF, Liotti G: Cognitive Processes and Emotional Disorders: A Structural Approach to Psychotherapy. New York, Guilford, 1983

Haaga DA, Dyck MJ, Ernst D: Empirical status of cognitive theory of depression. Psychol Bull 110:215–236, 1991

Hammon C, Krantz SE, Cochran SD: Relationships between depression and causal attributions about stressful life events. Cognitive Therapy and Research 5:351–358, 1981

Hargreaves IR: Attributional style and depression. Br J Clin Psychol 24:65–66, 1985

Heimberg RG, Dodge CS, Hope DA, et al: Cognitive behavioral group treatment for social phobia: comparison with a credible placebo control. Cognitive Therapy and Research 14:1–23, 1990

Hollon SD, Beck AT: Cognitive and cognitive-behavioral therapies, in Handbook of Psychotherapy and Behavior Change: An Empirical Analysis, 4th Edition. Edited by Garfield SL, Bergin AE. New York, Wiley, 1994, pp 428–466

Hollon SD, Kendall PC: Cognitive self-statements in depression: development of an automatic thought questionnaire. Cognitive Therapy and Research 4:383–395, 1980

Hollon SD, Kendall PC, Lumry A: Specificity of depressotypic cognitions in clinical depression. J Abnorm Psychol 95:52–59, 1986

Hollon SD, Shelton RC, Loosen PT: Cognitive therapy and pharmacotherapy for depression. J Consult Clin Psychol 59:88–99, 1991

Hollon SD, DeRubeis RJ, Evans MD, et al: Cognitive therapy and pharmacotherapy for depression: singly and in combination. Arch Gen Psychiatry 49:774–782, 1992a

Hollon SD, DeRubeis RJ, Seligman MEP: Cognitive therapy and the prevention of depression. Applied and Preventive Psychology 1:89–95, 1992b

Hope DA, Heimberg RG, Bruch MA: Dismantling cognitive-behavioral group therapy for social phobia. Behav Res Ther 33:637–650, 1995

Horne DJ, White AW, Varigos GA: A preliminary study of psychological therapy in the management of atopic eczema. Br J Med Psychol 62:241–248, 1989

Horney K: Neurosis and Human Growth: The Struggle Toward Self-Realization. New York, WW Norton, 1950

Imber SD, Pilkonis PA, Sotsky SM, et al: Mode-specific effects among three treatments for depression. J Consult Clin Psychol 58:353–359, 1990

Ingram RE, Kendall PC: The cognitive side of anxiety. Cognitive Therapy and Research 11:523–536, 1987

Ingram RE, Kendall PC, Smith TW, et al: Cognitive specificity in emotional distress. J Pers Soc Psychol 53:734–742, 1987

Jacobson NS, Hollon SD. Prospects for future comparisons between drugs and psychotherapy: lessons from the CBT-versus-pharmacotherapy exchange. J Consult Clin Psychol 64:104–108, 1996

James IA, Blackburn IM: Cognitive therapy with obsessive-compulsive disorder. Br J Psychiatry 166:444–450, 1995

Jarrett R, Rush AJ, Khatami M, et al: Does the pretreatment of polysomnogram predict response to cognitive therapy in depression outpatients? A preliminary report. Psychiatry Res 33:285–299, 1990

Jarrett R, Giles D, Gullion C, et al: Does learned resourcefulness predict response to cognitive therapy in depressed outpatient? J Affect Disord 23:223–229, 1991

Jarrett RB, Schaffer M, McIntire D, et al: Treatment of atypical depression with cognitive therapy or phenelzine: a double-blind, placebo-controlled trial. Arch Gen Psychiatry 56:431–437, 1999

Jarrett RB, Kraft D, Doyle J, et al: Preventing recurrent depression using cognitive therapy with and without a continuation phase: a randomized clinical trial. Arch Gen Psychiatry 58:381–388, 2001

Juster HR, Heimberg RG: Social phobia: longitudinal course and long-term outcome of cognitive-behavioral treatment. Psychiatr Clin North Am 18:821–842, 1995

Kandel ER: Psychotherapy and the single synapse: the impact of psychiatric thought on neurobiologic research. N Engl J Med 301:1028–1037, 1979

Kandel ER, Schwartz JH: Molecular biology of learning: modulation of transmitter release. Science 218:433–443, 1982

Keefe FJ, Van Horn Y: Cognitive-behavioral treatment of rheumatoid arthritis pain. Arthritis Care and Research 6:213–222, 1993

Kelly G: The Psychology of Personal Constructs. New York, WW Norton, 1955

Kendall PC, Hollon SD: Anxious self-talk: development of the Anxious Self-Statements Questionnaire (ASSQ). Cognitive Therapy and Research 13:81–93, 1989

Kingdon D, Turkington D: The use of cognitive behavior therapy with a normalizing rationale in schizophrenia. J Nerv Ment Dis 179:207–211, 1991

Klein DC, Fencil-Morse E, Seligman MEP: Learned helplessness, depression, and the attribution of failure. J Pers Soc Psychol 33:508–516, 1976

Klosko JS, Barlow DH, Tassinari R, et al: A comparison of alprazolam and behavior therapy in treatment of panic disorder. J Consult Clin Psychol 58:77–84, 1990

Kovacs M, Rush AJ, Beck AT, et al: Depressed outpatients treated with cognitive therapy or pharmacotherapy. Arch Gen Psychiatry 38:33–39, 1981

Kraaimaat FW, Brons MR, Geenen R, et al: The effect of cognitive behavior therapy in patients with rheumatoid arthritis. Behav Res Ther 33:487–495, 1995

Krantz SE: When depressive cognitions reflect negative realities. Cognitive Therapy and Research 9:595–610, 1985

Kroenke K, Swindle R: Cognitive-behavioral therapy for somatization and symptom syndromes: a critical review of controlled clinical trials. Psychother Psychosom 69:205–215, 2000

Kuipers E, Garety P, Fowler D: London–East Anglia randomized controlled trial of cognitive-behavioral therapy for psychosis, I: effects of the treatment phase. Br J Psychiatry 171:319–327, 1997

Laberge B, Gauthier JG, Cote G, et al: Cognitive-behavioral therapy of panic disorder with secondary major depression: a preliminary investigation. J Consult Clin Psychol 61:1028–1037, 1993

Larcombe NA, Wilson PH: An evaluation of cognitive-behavior therapy for depression in patients with multiple sclerosis. Br J Psychiatry 145:366–371, 1984

Lecompte D: Drug compliance and cognitive-behavioral therapy in schizophrenia. Acta Psychiatrica Belgica 95:91–100, 1995

LeFebvre MF: Cognitive distortion and cognitive errors in depressed psychiatric and low back pain patients. J Consult Clin Psychol 49:517–525, 1981

Leibing E, Pfingsten M, Bartmann U, et al: Cognitive-behavioral treatment in unselected rheumatoid arthritis outpatients. Clinical J Pain 15:58–66, 1999

Leitenberg H, Rosen J, Wolf R, et al: Comparison of cognitive-behavioral therapy and desipramine in the treatment of bulimia nervosa. Behav Res Ther 32:37–45, 1994

Lewinsohn PM, Sullivan JM, Grosscup SJ: Behavioral therapy: clinical applications, in Short-Term Psychotherapies for Depression. Edited by Rush AJ. New York, Guilford, 1982, pp 50–87

Linehan MM: Dialectical behavior therapy for borderline personality disorder: theory and method. Bull Menninger Clin 51:261–276, 1987

Linehan MM: Cognitive-Behavioral Treatment of Borderline Personality Disorder. New York, Guilford, 1993

Linehan MM, Armstrong HE, Suarez A, et al: Cognitive-behavioral treatment of chronically parasuicidal borderline patients. Arch Gen Psychiatry 48:1060–1064, 1991

Linehan MM, Heard HL, Armstrong HE: Naturalistic follow-up of a behavioral treatment for chronically parasuicidal borderline patients. Arch Gen Psychiatry 50:971–974, 1993

Linehan MM, Tutek DA, Heard HL, et al: Interpersonal outcome of cognitive behavioral treatment for chronically suicidal borderline patients. Am J Psychiatry 151:1771–1776, 1994

Linehan MM, Schmidt H, Dimeff, L, et al: Dialectical behavior therapy for patients with borderline personality disorder and drug-dependence. Am J Addict 8:279–292, 1999

Linton SJ, Andersson T: Can chronic disability be prevented? A randomized trial of cognitive-behavior intervention and two forms of information for patients with spinal pain. Spine 25:2825–2831, 2000

Linton SJ, Ryberg M: A cognitive-behavioral group intervention as prevention for persistent neck and back pain in a non-patient population: a randomized controlled trial. Pain 90:83–90, 2001

Lloyd GG, Lishman WA: Effect of depression on the speed of recall of pleasant and unpleasant experiences. Psychol Med 5:173–180, 1975

Loeb A, Beck AT, Feshbach S, et al: Some effects of reward on the social perception and motivation of psychiatric patients varying in depression. Journal of Abnormal Social Psychology 68:609–616, 1964

Loeb A, Beck AT, Diggory J: Differential effects of success and failure on depressed and nondepressed patients. J Nerv Ment Dis 152:106–114, 1971

Longabaugh R, Rubin A, Malloy P, et al: Drinking outcomes of alcohol abusers diagnosed as antisocial personality disorder. Alcohol Clin Exp Res 18:778–785, 1994

Ludgate JW, Wright JH, Bowers W, et al: Individual cognitive therapy with inpatients, in Cognitive Therapy With Inpatients: Developing a Cognitive Milieu. Edited by Wright JH, Thase ME, Beck AT, et al. New York, Guilford, 1992, pp 91–120

Lustman PJ, Griffith LS, Freedland KE, et al: Cognitive behavior therapy for depression in type 2 diabetes mellitus: a randomized, controlled trial. Ann Intern Med 129:613–621, 1998

Maes S, Schlosser M: Changing health behavior outcomes in asthmatic patients: a pilot study. Soc Sci Med 26:359–364, 1988

Mahoney MJ: Psychotherapy and human change processes, in Cognition and Psychotherapy. Edited by Mahoney MJ, Freeman A. New York, Plenum, 1985

Marks I: Computer aids to mental health care. Can J Psychiatry 44:548–555, 1999

Martin SD, Martin E, Rai SS, et al: Blood flow changes in depressed patients treated with interpersonal psychotherapy or venlafaxine hydrochloride: preliminary findings. Arch Gen Psychiatry 58:641–648, 2001

Mathews A, MacLeod C: An information-processing approach to anxiety. Journal of Cognitive Psychotherapy: An International Quarterly 1:105–115, 1987

Mavissakalian M, Hamman MS: DSM-III personality disorder in agoraphobia, II: changes with treatment. Compr Psychiatry 28:356–361, 1987

McCullough JP Jr: Treatment for Chronic Depression. Cognitive Behavioral Analysis System of Psychotherapy. New York, Guilford, 2000

McKnight DL, Nelson-Gray RO, Barnhill J: Dexamethasone suppression test and response to cognitive therapy and antidepressant medication. Behav Ther 1:99–111, 1992

McNally RJ, Foa EB: Cognition and agoraphobia: bias in the interpretation of threat. Cognitive Therapy and Research 11:567–581, 1987

Meichenbaum DB: Cognitive-Behavior Modification: An Integrative Approach. New York, Plenum, 1977

Miller IW, Klee SH, Norman WH: Depressed and nondepressed inpatients' cognitions of hypothetical events, experimental tasks, and stressful life events. J Abnorm Psychol 91:78–81, 1982

Miller IW, Norman WH, Keitner GI, et al: Cognitive-behavioral treatment of depressed inpatients. Behav Ther 20:25–47, 1989

Minkoff K, Bergman E, Beck AT, et al: Hopelessness, depression, and attempted suicide. Am J Psychiatry 130:455–459, 1973

Miranda J: Dysfunctional thinking is activated by stressful life events. Cognitive Therapy and Research 16:473–483, 1992

Mishra KD, Gatchel RJ, Gardea MA: The relative efficacy of three cognitive-behavioral treatment approaches to temporomandibular disorders. J Behav Med 23:293–309, 2000

Mitchell JE, Hoberman HN, Peterson CB, et al: Research on the psychotherapy of bulimia nervosa: half empty or half full. Int J Eat Disord 20:219–229, 1996

Mizes JS, Landolf-Fritsche B, Grossman-McKee D: Patterns of distorted cognitions in phobic disorders: an investigation of clinically severe simple phobics, social phobics, and agoraphobics. Cognitive Therapy and Research 11:583–592, 1987

Mohl PC: Should psychotherapy be considered a biological treatment? Psychosomatics 28:320–326, 1987

Moore JE, Von Korff M, Cherkin D, et al: A randomized trial of a cognitive-behavioral program for enhancing back pain self care in a primary care setting. Pain 88:145–153, 2000

Morley S, Eccleston C, Williams A: Systematic review and meta-analysis of randomized controlled trials of cognitive behaviour therapy and behaviour therapy for chronic pain in adults, excluding headache. Pain 80:1–13, 1999

Murphy GE, Simons AD, Wetzel RD, et al: Cognitive therapy and pharmacotherapy, singly and together in the treatment of depression. Arch Gen Psychiatry 41:33–41, 1984

Murphy GE, Carney RM, Knesevich MA, et al: Cognitive behavior therapy, relaxation training, and tricyclic antidepressant medication in the treatment of depression. Psychol Rep 77:403–420, 1995

Nekanda-Trepka CJS, Bishop S, Blackburn IM: Hopelessness and depression. Br J Clin Psychol 22:49–60, 1983

Nelson RE, Craighead WE: Selective recall of positive and negative feedback, self-control behaviors and depression. J Abnorm Psychol 86:379–388, 1977

Nelson-Gray RO, Johnson D, Foyle LW, et al: The effectiveness of cognitive therapy tailored to depressives with personality disorders. J Personal Disord 10:132–152, 1996

Neziroglu F, McKay D, Todaro J, et al: Effect of cognitive behavior therapy on persons with body dysmorphic disorder and comorbid Axis II diagnoses. Behav Ther 27:67–77, 1996

Oei TPS, Lim B, Young RM: Cognitive processes and cognitive behavior therapy in the treatment of problem drinking. J Addict Dis 10:63–80, 1991

Ost LG, Westling BE, Hellstrom K: Applied relaxation, exposure in vivo and cognitive methods in the treatment of panic disorder with agoraphobia. Behav Res Ther 31:383–394, 1993

Otto MW, Pollack MH, Sachs GS, et al: Discontinuation of benzodiazepine treatment: efficacy of cognitive-behavioral therapy for patients with panic disorder. Am J Psychiatry 150:1485–1490, 1993

Otto MW, Whittal ML: Cognitive-behavior therapy and the longitudinal course of panic disorder. Psychiatr Clin North Am 18:803–820, 1995

Paykel ES, Scott J, Teasdale JD, et al: Prevention of relapse in residual depression by cognitive therapy. Arch Gen Psychiatry 56:829–835, 1999

Payne A, Blanchard EB: A controlled comparison of cognitive therapy and self-help support groups in the treatment of irritable bowel syndrome. J Consult Clin Psychol 63:779–786, 1995

Perris C: Cognitive Therapy With Schizophrenic Patients. New York, Guilford, 1989

Perris C: Cognitive therapy in the treatment of patients with borderline personality disorders. Acta Psychiatr Scand 89(suppl 379):69–72, 1994

Perris C, Skagerlind L: Cognitive therapy with schizophrenic patients. Acta Psychiatr Scand 89(suppl 382):65–70, 1994

Persons JB, Burns BD, Perhoff JM: Predictors of drop-out and outcome in cognitive therapy for depression in a private practice setting. Cognitive Therapy and Research 12:557–575, 1988

Peselow ED, Robins C, Block P, et al: Dysfunctional attitudes in depressed patients before and after clinical treatment and in normal control subjects. Am J Psychiatry 147:439–444, 1990

Peterson C, Villanova P, Raps CS: Depression and attributions: factors responsible for inconsistent results in the published literature. J Abnorm Psychol 94:165–168, 1985

Phillips HC: The effects of behavioral treatment on chronic pain. Behav Res Ther 25:365–377, 1987

Piaget J: The Construction of Reality in the Child. New York, Basic Books, 1954

Pollack MH, Otto MW, Kaspi SP, et al: Cognitive behavior therapy for treatment-refractory panic disorder. J Clin Psychiatry 55:200–205, 1994

Power KG, Simpson RJ, Swanson V, et al: Controlled comparison of pharmacological and psychological treatment of generalized anxiety disorder in primary care. Br J Gen Pract 40:289–294, 1990

Pretzer J, Beck AT: A cognitive theory of personality disorders, in Major Theories of Personality Disorder. Edited by Clarkin J. New York, Guilford, 1996, pp 36–105

Prezant DW, Neimeyer RA: Cognitive predictors of depression and suicide ideation. Suicide Life Threat Behav 18:259–264, 1988

Raimy V: Misunderstandings of the Self. San Francisco, CA, Jossey Bass, 1975

Raps CS, Peterson C, Reinhard KE, et al: Attributional style among depressed patients. J Abnorm Psychol 91:102–108, 1982

Ricca V, Mannucci E, Zucchi T, et al: Cognitive-behavioural therapy for bulimia nervosa and binge eating disorder: a review. Psychother Psychosom 69:287–295, 2000

Riskind JH, Steer R: Do maladaptive attitudes "cause" depression? Misconception of cognitive theory. Arch Gen Psychiatry 41:1111–1112, 1984

Riskind JH, Beck AT, Steer RA: Cognitive-behavioral therapy in geriatric depression: comment on Steuer et al. J Consult Clin Psychol 53:944–947, 1985

Rizley R: Depression and distortion in the attribution of causality. J Abnorm Psychol 87:32–48, 1978

Robinson LA, Berman JS, Neimeyer RA: Psychotherapy for the treatment of depression: a comprehensive review of controlled outcome research. Psychol Bull 108:30–49, 1990

Rodgers D, Khoo K, MacEachen M, et al: Cognitive therapy for multiple sclerosis: a preliminary study. Alternative Therapies in Health and Medicine 2:70–74, 1996

Rothbaum BO, Hodges LF, Kooper R, et al: Effectiveness of computer-generated (virtual reality) graded exposure in the treatment of acrophobia. Am J Psychiatry 152:626–628, 1995

Rush AJ: Cognitive therapy of depression: rationale, techniques, and efficacy. Psychiatr Clin North Am 6:105–127, 1983

Rush AJ: Cognitive approaches to adherence, in The American Psychiatric Press Review of Psychiatry, Vol 8. Edited by Francis AJ, Hales RE. Washington, DC, American Psychiatric Press, 1988, pp 627–642

Rush AJ, Shaw BF: Failure in treating depression by cognitive therapy, in Failures in Behavior Therapy. Edited by Foa EB, Emmelkamp PGM. New York, Wiley, 1983, pp 213–224

Rush AJ, Beck AT, Kovacs M, et al: Comparative efficacy of cognitive therapy and pharmacotherapy in the treatment of depressed outpatients. Cognitive Therapy and Research 1:17–37, 1977

Salkovskis PM: Obsessional-compulsive problems: a cognitive-behavioral analysis. Behav Res Ther 25:571–583, 1985

Salkovskis PM (ed): Frontiers of Cognitive Therapy. New York, Guilford, 1996

Salkovskis PM, Warwick HM: Cognitive therapy of obsessive-compulsive disorder: treating treatment failures. Behavioural Psychotherapy 13:243–255, 1985

Salkovskis PM, Westbrook D: Behavior therapy and obsessional ruminations: can failure be turned into success? Behav Res Ther 27:149–160, 1989

Schlesier-Carter B, Hamilton SA, O'Neil PM, et al: Depression and bulimia: the link between depression and bulimic cognitions. J Abnorm Psychol 98:322–325, 1989

Schmidt NB, Harrington P: Cognitive-behavioral treatment of body dysmorphic disorder: a case report. J Behav Ther Exp Psychiatry 26:161–167, 1995

Schmidt U, Tiller J, Treasure J: Self-treatment of bulimia nervosa: a pilot study. Int J Eat Disord 13:273–277, 1993

Schonfeld L, Dupree LW: Treatment approaches for older problem drinkers. Int J Addict 30:1819–1842, 1995

Schwartz JM, Stoessel PW, Baxter LR Jr, et al: Systematic changes in cerebral glucose metabolic rate after successful behavior modification treatment of obsessive-compulsive disorder. Arch Gen Psychiatry 53:109–113, 1996

Schwartz SP, Blanchard EB: Evaluation of psychological treatment for inflammatory bowel disease. Behav Res Ther 29:167–177, 1991

Scott J: Chronic depression: can cognitive therapy succeed when other treatments fail? Behavioural Psychotherapy 20:25–36, 1992

Scott J, Wright JH: Cognitive therapy for chronic and severe mental disorders, in American Psychiatric Press Review of Psychiatry, Vol 16. Edited by Dickstein LJ, Riba MB, Oldham JM. Washington, DC, American Psychiatric Press, 1997, pp 135–170

Scott J, Byers S, Turkington D: The chronic patient, in Cognitive Therapy With Inpatients: Developing a Cognitive Milieu. Edited by Wright JH, Thase ME, Beck AT, et al. New York, Guilford, 1992, pp 357–390

Selmi PM, Klein MH, Greist JH, et al: An investigation of computer-assisted cognitive-behavior therapy in the treatment of depression. Behavior Research Methods 14:181–185, 1982

Selmi PM, Klein MH, Greist JH, et al: Computer-administered therapy for depression. Am J Psychiatry 147:51–56, 1990

Sensky T, Wright JH: Cognitive therapy with medical patients, in Cognitive Therapy With Inpatients. Edited by Wright JH, Thase ME, Beck AT, et al. New York, Guilford, 1993, pp 219–246

Sensky T, Turkington D, Kingdon D, et al: A randomized controlled trial of cognitive-behavioral therapy for persistent symptoms in schizophrenia resistant to medication. Arch Gen Psychiatry 57:165–172, 2000

Shapiro D, Hui KK, Oakley ME, et al: Reduction in drug requirements for hypertension by means of a cognitive-behavioral intervention. Am J Hypertens 10:9–17, 1997

Sharpe L, Tarrier N: Towards a cognitive-behavioural theory or problem gambling. Br J Psychiatry 162:407–412, 1993

Sharpe L, Sensky T, Timberlake N, et al: A blind, randomized, controlled trial of cognitive-behavioural intervention for patients with recent onset rheumatoid arthritis: preventing psychological and physical morbidity. Pain 89:275–283, 2001

Shea MT, Pilkonis PA, Beckham E, et al: Personality disorders and treatment outcome in the NIMH treatment of depression collaborative research program. Am J Psychiatry 147:711–718, 1990

Shea MT, Elkin I, Imber SD, et al: Course of depressive symptoms over follow-up: findings from the NIMH treatment of depression collaborative research program. Arch Gen Psychiatry 49:782–787, 1992

Shear MK, Ball G, Fitzpatrick M, et al: Cognitive-behavioral therapy for panic: an open study. J Nerv Ment Dis 179:468–472, 1991a

Shear MK, Fyer AJ, Ball G, et al: Vulnerability to sodium lactate in panic disorder patients given cognitive-behavioral therapy. Am J Psychiatry 148:195–197, 1991b

Shearin EN, Linehan MM: Dialectical behavior therapy for borderline personality disorder: theoretical and empirical foundations. Acta Psychiatr Scand 89(suppl 379):61–68, 1994

Simons AD, Thase ME: Biological markers, treatment outcome, and 1 year follow-up in endogenous depression: electroencephalographic sleep studies and cognitive therapy. J Consult Clin Psychol 60:392–401, 1992

Simons AD, Garfield SL, Murphy CE: The process of change in cognitive therapy and pharmacotherapy for depression. Arch Gen Psychiatry 41:45–51, 1984

Simons AD, Lustman PJ, Wetzel RD, et al: Predicting response to cognitive therapy of depression: the role of learned resourcefulness. Cognitive Therapy and Research 9:79–89, 1985

Simons AD, Murphy GE, Levine JE, et al: Cognitive therapy and pharmacotherapy for depression: sustained improvement over one year. Arch Gen Psychiatry 43:43–49, 1986

Sitharthan T, Kavanagh DJ, Sayer G: Moderating drinking by correspondence: an evaluation of a new method of intervention. Addiction 91:345–355, 1996

Skinner JB, Erskine A, Pearce S, et al: The evaluation of a cognitive-behavioral treatment program in outpatients with chronic pain. J Psychosom Res 34:13–19, 1990

Sokol L, Beck AT, Greenberg RL, et al: Cognitive therapy of panic disorder: a nonpharmacological alternative. J Nerv Ment Dis 177:711–716, 1989

Speckens AEM, van Hemert AM, Spinhoven P, et al: Cognitive behavioural therapy for medically unexplained physical symptoms: a randomised controlled trial. BMJ 311:1328–1332, 1995

Springer T, Lohr NE, Buchtel HA, et al: A preliminary report of short-term cognitive-behavioral group therapy for inpatients with personality disorders. J Psychother Pract Res 5:57–71, 1996

Steuer JL, Mintz J, Hammen CL, et al: Cognitive-behavioral and psychodynamic group psychotherapy in treatment of geriatric depression. J Consult Clin Psychol 52:180–189, 1984

Stewart JW, Garfinkel R, Nunes EV, et al: Atypical features and treatment response in the National Institute of Mental Health Treatment of Depression Collaborative Research Program. J Clin Psychopharmacol 18:429–434, 1998

Stuart S, Bowers WA: Cognitive therapy with inpatients: review and meta-analysis. Journal of Cognitive Psychotherapy: An International Quarterly 9:85–92, 1995

Stuart S, LaRue S: Computerized cognitive therapy: the interface between man and machine. Journal of Cognitive Psychotherapy: An International Quarterly 10:181–191, 1996

Stuart S, Simons AD, Thase ME, et al: Are personality assessments valid in acute major depression? J Affect Disord 24:281–290, 1992

Stuart S, Wright JH, Thase ME, et al: Cognitive therapy with inpatients. Gen Hosp Psychiatry 19:42–50, 1997

Sullivan HS: Interpersonal Theory of Psychiatry. New York, WW Norton, 1953

Tarrier N, Maguire P: Treatment of psychological distress following mastectomy: an initial report. Behav Res Ther 22:81–84, 1984

Tarrier N, Beckett R, Harwoods S, et al: A trial of two cognitive-behavioral methods of treating drug-resistant residual psychotic symptoms in schizophrenic patients, I: outcome. Br J Psychiatry 162:524–532, 1993

Tarrier N, Yusupoff L, Kinney C, et al: Randomized controlled trial of intensive cognitive behavior therapy for patients with chronic schizophrenia. BMJ 317:303–307, 1998

Taylor S: Meta-analysis of cognitive-behavioral treatments for social phobia. J Behav Ther Exp Psychiatry 27:1–9, 1996

Teasdale JD, Fogarty SJ: Differential effects of induced mood on retrieval of pleasant and unpleasant events from episodic memory. J Abnorm Psychol 88:248–257, 1979

Teasdale JD, Fennell MJV, Hibbert GA, et al: Cognitive therapy for major depressive disorder in primary care. Br J Psychiatry 144:400–406, 1984

Teasdale JD, Segal ZV, Williams JM, et al: Prevention of relapse/recurrence in major depression by mindfulness-based cognitive therapy. J Consult Clin Psychol 68:615–623, 2000

Thackwray DE, Smith MC, Bodfish JW, et al: A comparison of behavioral and cognitive-behavioral interventions for bulimia nervosa. J Consult Clin Psychol 61:639–645, 1993

Thase ME: Transition and aftercare, in Cognitive Therapy With Inpatients: Developing a Cognitive Milieu. Edited by Wright JH, Thase ME, Beck AT, et al. New York, Guilford, 1992, pp 414–435

Thase ME: Cognitive-behavioral therapy for substance abuse disorders, in Review of Psychiatry, Vol 16. Edited by Dickstein LJ, Riba MB, Oldham JM. Washington, DC, American Psychiatric Press, 1997, pp 45–71

Thase ME: Depression-focused psychotherapies, in Treatments of Psychiatric Disorders, 3rd Edition, Vol 2. Edited by Gabbard GO. Washington, DC, American Psychiatric Publishing, 2001, pp 1181–1227

Thase ME, Beck AT: An overview of cognitive therapy, in Cognitive Therapy With Inpatients: Developing a Cognitive Milieu. Edited by Wright JH, Thase ME, Beck AT, et al. New York, Guilford, 1992, pp 3–35

Thase ME, Wright JH: Cognitive behavioral therapy with depressed inpatients: an abridged treatment manual. Behav Ther 22:579–595, 1991

Thase ME, Bowler K, Harden T: Cognitive behavior therapy of endogenous depression, part 2: preliminary findings in 16 unmedicated inpatients. Behav Ther 22:469–477, 1991

Thase ME, Simmons AD, McGreary J, et al: Relapse after cognitive behavior therapy of depression: potential implications for longer courses of treatment? Am J Psychiatry 149:1046–1052, 1992

Thase ME, Simons AD, Reynolds III CF: Psychobiological correlates of poor response to cognitive behavior therapy: potential indications for antidepressant pharmacotherapy. Psychopharmacol Bull 29:293–301, 1993

Thase ME, Reynolds III CF, Frank E, et al: Polysomnographic studies of unmedicated depressed men before and after cognitive behavioral therapy. Am J Psychiatry 151:1615–1622, 1994a

Thase ME, Reynolds CF III, Frank E, et al: Response to cognitive-behavioral therapy in chronic depression. J Psychother Pract Res 3:204–214, 1994b

Thase ME, Simons AD, Reynolds CF III: Abnormal electroencephalographic sleep profiles in major depression. Arch Gen Psychiatry 53:99–108, 1996

Thase ME, Fasiczka AL, Berman SR, et al: Electroencephalographic sleep profiles before and after cognitive behavior therapy of depression. Arch Gen Psychiatry 55:138–144, 1998

Thompson LW: Cognitive-behavioral therapy and treatment for late-life depression. J Clin Psychiatry 57(suppl 5):29–37, 1996

Traux CB, Mitchell KM: Research on certain therapist interpersonal skills in relation to process and outcome, in Handbook of Psychotherapy and Behavior Change: An Empirical Analysis. Edited by Bergin AE, Garfield SL. New York, Wiley, 1971, pp 299–344

Turk DC, Meichenbaum D, Genest M: Pain and Behavioral Medicine: A Cognitive-Behavioral Perspective. New York, Guilford, 1983

Turner JA, Clancy S: Strategies for coping with chronic low back pain: relationship to pain and disability. Pain 24:355–364, 1986

Van Oppen P, De Haan E, Van Balkom AJLM, et al: Cognitive therapy and exposure in vivo in the treatment of obsessive compulsive disorder. Behav Res Ther 33:379–390, 1995

Wallace ST, Alden LE: A comparison of social standards and perceived ability in anxious and nonanxious men. Cognitive Therapy and Research 15:237–254, 1991

Walsh BT, Wilson GT, Loeb KL, et al: Medication and psychotherapy in the treatment of bulimia nervosa. Am J Psychiatry 154:523–531, 1997

Warwick HM, Salkovskis PM: Hypochondriasis. Behav Res Ther 28:105–117, 1990

Watkins JT, Rush AJ: Cognitive response test. Cognitive Therapy and Research 7:125–126, 1983

Weissman AN: The dysfunctional attitude scale: a validation study. Dissertation Abstracts International 40:1389B–1390B, 1979

Welkowitz LA, Papp LA, Cloitre M, et al: Cognitive-behavior therapy for panic disorder delivered by psychopharmacologically oriented clinicians. J Nerv Ment Dis 179:473–477, 1991

Wells EA, Peterson PL, Gainey RR, et al: Outpatient treatment for cocaine abuse: a controlled comparison of relapse prevention and twelve-step approaches. Am J Drug Alcohol Abuse 20:1–17, 1994

Wenzloff RM, Grozier SA: Depression and the magnification of failure. J Abnorm Psychol 97:90–93, 1988

Westling BE, Ost L: Cognitive bias in panic disorder patients and changes after cognitive-behavioral treatments. Behav Res Ther 33:585–588, 1995

Wetzel R, Murphy G, Carney R, et al: Prescribing therapy for depression: the role of learned resourcefulness, a failure to replicate. Psychol Rep 70:803–807, 1992

Whisman MA, Miller IW, Norman WH, et al: Cognitive therapy with depressed inpatients: specific effects on dysfunctional cognitions. J Consult Clin Psychol 59:282–288, 1991

White KP, Nielson WR: Cognitive behavioral treatment of fibromyalgia syndrome: a follow-up assessment. J Rheumatol 22:717–721, 1995

Wilfley DE, Agras WS, Telch CF, et al: Group cognitive-behavioral therapy and group interpersonal psychotherapy for the nonpurging bulimic individual: a controlled comparison. J Consult Clin Psychol 61:296–305, 1993

Wilson GT: Cognitive behavior therapy for eating disorders: progress and problems. Behav Res Ther 37:S79–S95, 1999

Wilson KCM, Scott M, Abou-Saleh M, et al: Long-term effects of cognitive-behavioural therapy and lithium therapy on depression in the elderly. Br J Psychiatry 167:653–658, 1995

Wolpe J: The Practice of Behavior Therapy. New York, Pergamon, 1969

Woody GE, Luborsky L, McLellan AT, et al: Psychotherapy for opiate addicts: does it help? Arch Gen Psychiatry 40:639–645, 1983

Wright FD, Beck AT, Newman CF, et al: Cognitive therapy of substance abuse: theoretical rationale. NIDA Res Monogr 137:123–146, 1993

Wright JH: Cognitive therapy of depression, in The American Psychiatric Press Review of Psychiatry, Vol 7. Edited by Frances AJ, Hales RE. Washington, DC, American Psychiatric Press, 1988, pp 554–590

Wright JH, Basco MR: Getting Your Life Back: The Complete Guide to Recovery from Depression. New York, Free Press, 2001

Wright JH, Beck AT: Cognitive therapy of depression: theory and practice. Hosp Community Psychiatry 34:1119–1127, 1983

Wright JH, Beck AT: Family cognitive therapy with inpatients, in Cognitive Therapy With Inpatients: Developing a Cognitive Milieu. Edited by Wright JH, Thase ME, Beck AT, et al. New York, Guilford, 1993, pp 176–191

Wright JH, Borden J: Cognitive therapy of depression and anxiety. Psychiatr Ann 21:424–428, 1992

Wright JH, Davis MH: Hospital psychiatry in transition, in Cognitive Therapy With Inpatients: Developing a Cognitive Milieu. Edited by Wright JH, Thase ME, Beck AT, et al. New York, Guilford, 1992, pp 193–218

Wright JH, Salmon PG: Learning and memory in depression, in Depression: New Directions in Theory, Research, and Practice. Edited by McCann CD, Endler NS. Toronto, ON, Canada, Wall & Thompson, 1990, pp 211–236

Wright JH, Schrodt GR Jr: Combined cognitive therapy and pharmacotherapy, in Handbook of Cognitive Therapy. Edited by Freeman A, Simon MK, Arkowitz H, et al. New York, Plenum, 1989, pp 267–283

Wright JH, Thase ME: Cognitive and biological therapies: a synthesis. Psychiatr Ann 22:451–458, 1992

Wright JH, Wright AS: Computer-assisted psychotherapy. J Psychother Pract Res 6:315–329, 1997

Wright JH, Thase ME, Sensky T: Cognitive and biological therapies: a combined approach, in Cognitive Therapy With Inpatients: Developing a Cognitive Milieu. Edited by Wright JH, Thase ME, Beck AT, et al. New York, Guilford, 1993a, pp 193–218

Wright JH, Thase ME, Beck AT, et al (eds): Cognitive Therapy With Inpatients: Developing a Cognitive Milieu. New York, Guilford, 1993b

Wright JH, Salmon P, Wright AS, et al: Cognitive Therapy: A Multimedia Learning Program. Louisville, KY, MindStreet, 1995a

Wright JH, Salmon P, Wright AS, et al: Cognitive therapy: a multimedia learning program. Paper presented at the 148th annual meeting of the American Psychiatric Association, Miami Beach, FL, May 1995b

Wright JH, Wright AS, Basco MR, et al: Controlled trial of computer-assisted cognitive therapy for depression. World Congress of Cognitive Therapy, Vancouver, BC, Canada, July 2001

Wright JH, Wright AS, Salmon P, et al: Development and initial testing of a multimedia program for computer-assisted cognitive therapy. Am J Psychother 56:76–86, 2002a

Wright JH, Wright AS, Beck AT: Good Days Ahead: The Multimedia Program for Cognitive Therapy. Louisville, KY, MindStreet, 2002b

Young JE, Beck AT: Cognitive therapy: clinical applications, in Short-Term Psychotherapies for Depression. Edited by Rush AJ. New York, Guilford, 1982, pp 182–214

Young JE, Lindemann MD: An integrative schema-focused model for personality disorders. Journal of Cognitive Psychotherapy: An International Quarterly 6:11–23, 1992

Zautra JH, Guenther RT, Chartier GM: Attributions for real and hypothetical events: their relation to self-esteem and depression. J Abnorm Psychol 94:530–540, 1985

Zettle RD, Rains JC: Group cognitive and contextual therapies in treatment of depression. J Clin Psychol 45:436–445, 1989

Zimmerman M, Coryell W, Corenthal C, et al: Dysfunctional attitudes and attribution style in healthy controls and patients with schizophrenia, psychotic depression, and nonpsychotic depression. J Abnorm Psychol 95:403–405, 1986

Zotter DL, Crowther JH: The role of cognitions in bulimia nervosa. Cognitive Therapy and Research 15:413–426, 1991

Hypnosis

José R. Maldonado, M.D.

David Spiegel, M.D.

Hypnosis is a natural state of aroused, attentive focal concentration coupled with a relative suspension of peripheral awareness. It involves an intensity of focus that allows the hypnotized person to make maximal use of innate abilities to control perception, memory, and somatic function. Hypnotic capacity represents both a potential vulnerability to certain kinds of psychiatric illness, such as posttraumatic stress, conversion, and dissociative disorders, and an asset, in that it can facilitate various psychotherapeutic strategies. Because hypnotic capacity is a normal and widely distributed trait, and because entry into hypnotic states occurs spontaneously, hypnotic phenomena occur frequently. Even psychiatrists who make no formal use of hypnosis can enhance their effectiveness by learning to recognize and take advantage of hypnotic mental states.

History

Trance experiences have been described at least as far back as the time of the ancient Greeks, often as vehicles for treatment of mental or physical illness. In non-Western cultures, such experiences tended to be in the domain of the healer, who entered a dissociative state as part of the healing ceremony. Frequently, however, these ceremonies were public and invited both patient and observers to enter the trance state as well.

Hypnosis was identified as a formal phenomenon of psychotherapeutic interest in the eighteenth century. Franz Anton Mesmer employed it as an alternative treatment for many ills that we would now label as stress related or psychosomatic (Lopez 1993). His work is credited with being the first Western conceptualization of a psychotherapy (Ellenberger 1970), a therapeutic talking interaction between doctor and patient. Shortly thereafter, Louis XVI in 1784 appointed two commissions to investigate the phenomenon (known as "animal magnetism") and Mesmer's claims of medical efficacy. The infamous Dr. Guillotin headed one commission; the other, made up of five members of the Academy of Sciences, was headed by Benjamin Franklin, American ambassador to France. Both commissions concluded that the success of mesmerism was due to the manipulation of "heated" imagination. Nevertheless, the panel acknowledged that the phenomenon of suggestion, the influence of one individual on another, was at the root of social order as well as personal change.

In the nineteenth century, interest in hypnosis persisted in this country, as evidenced by the writings of William James (1902), Boris Sidis (1905), and Morton Prince (1906; founder of the *Journal of Abnormal Psychology*), all of whom were fascinated by the extreme symptoms observed in patients with dissociative syndromes such as multiple personality disorder (renamed *dissociative identity disorder* in DSM-IV [American Psychiatric Association 1994]). On the Continent, serious practitioners such as Braid (1843) and Esdaile (Ernst 1995; Esdaile 1846/1957) used hypnosis to treat symptoms, including pain and anxiety. Janet (1907) built a theory of the unconscious involving compartmentalization of memory that differed from Freud's model in that it was horizontal and compartmental rather than vertical and archaeological (E.R. Hilgard 1977). Information kept out of awareness was relatively untransformed and could be accessed directly, using techniques such as hypnosis, which Janet also utilized as evidence of experimentally induced pathology. Breuer and Freud (1893–1895/1955) used hypnotic age regression to treat hysterical symptoms and began to develop their theory linking unconscious determinants to conscious symptoms. They considered "hypnoid" states to be the building blocks of hysterical symptomatology and accurately observed that although hypnotic processes could be normal, they were often mobilized in the service of resolving an unconscious conflict. Hypnoid states were seen as the vehicle for expressing conflicts rather than as the cause of such conflicts or as pathological in themselves. Later, attributing the phenomenon to transference, Freud (1925[1924]/1959) abandoned hypnosis as a technique in favor of free association after a patient emerging from a hypnotic session threw her arms around him. At that moment, he discovered transference and decided to analyze rather than mobilize it, retaining, however, the couch he had used for hypnotic inductions.

In the early part of the twentieth century, there was relatively little clinical use of hypnosis, although new treatment techniques were developed and promulgated (Erickson 1967). Interest revived during World War II, when army psychiatrists found the technique helpful in treating what was then called "traumatic neurosis" (Kardiner and Spiegel 1947). An era of serious laboratory investigation of the phenomenon began in the 1950s with the development of several hypnotizability scales (Stanford Hypnotic Susceptibility Scales [E.R. Hilgard 1965; Weitzenhoffer and Hilgard 1959, 1962]). By the 1970s, several shorter hypnotizability scales were in use in clinical settings (Stanford Hypnotic Clinical Scale [E.R. Hilgard and Hilgard 1975], Hypnotic Induction Profile [H. Spiegel and Spiegel 1987]). Investigations ranged from studies of the relationships among hypnotizability, placebo response, and acupuncture to studies of the differential hypnotizability of patients with psychosis and other psychiatric disorders to investigations used in determining neurophysiological correlates of the hypnotic state and hypnotic capacity, all with varying success.

Thus, hypnosis has persisted in one form or another for more than two centuries. In the mid-1950s, the American Medical Association and the American Psychiatric Association officially recognized hypnosis as a legitimate therapeutic tool. Two professional hypnosis societies have emerged—the Society for Clinical and Experimental Hypnosis, which emphasizes research in the field, and the American Society for Clinical Hypnosis—each of which publishes a journal. Hypnosis is now taught in many major medical schools. A division of the American Psychological Association (Division 30) is devoted to the study of hypnosis, and the use of hypnosis in clinical and investigational areas is increasing.

Definition

Alterations in consciousness occur frequently in the course of ordinary life: at moments of physical or psycho-

logical stress, as a result of formal instruction or direction, in the diurnal sleep–wake cycle, and with the use of a variety of psychoactive substances (H. Spiegel 1963). Indeed, such cyclic variation is the norm, not the exception. Sleep is requisite for normal attention, and it may also be that alterations within wakefulness optimize attention-related processes. Certain variations in consciousness may change the relationship between mental and physical states and alter the degree to which concentration can be focused. One of these alterations in consciousness is *hypnosis*, a naturally occurring phenomenon in which focal concentration is intensified at the expense of peripheral awareness.

Hypnosis is a state of attentive, receptive concentration with a relative suspension of peripheral awareness. Hypnotic phenomena occur spontaneously, and the alteration of consciousness that hypnotized individuals experience has a variety of therapeutic applications. Hypnotic experience involves three main factors: absorption, dissociation, and suggestibility. Each of these factors is discussed here (Figure 30–1).

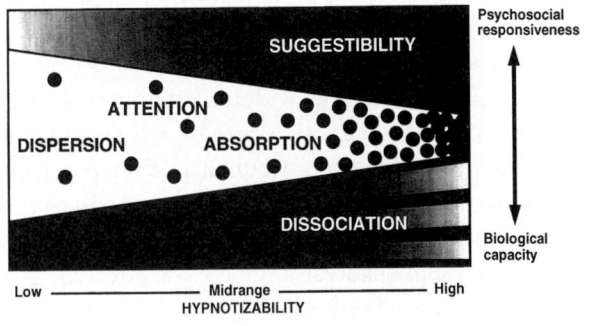

FIGURE 30–1. Continuum of attention and dissociation. This diagram depicts the spectrum of normal attentional focus. Hypnotic phenomena are characterized by intense absorption, with accompanying enhanced dissociation and suggestibility.

Absorption

Absorption is immersion in a central experience at the expense of contextual orientation (J.R. Hilgard 1970; Tellegen 1981; Tellegen and Atkinson 1974). When one is intensely involved in a central object of consciousness, one tends to ignore perceptions, thoughts, memories, or motor activities at the periphery. Hypnotized individuals are intensely absorbed in their trance experience. In a hypnotic age regression, subjects act as though they were younger, suspending awareness that they really are decades older than the assumed age. The subjects are aware of the incongruity of the situation or suggestion, yet they easily ignore it. This makes the experience of acting like a 3-year-old more vivid, because it is not plagued by disbelief and critical evaluation.

Research has shown a correlation between hypnotizability and a spontaneous tendency for people to undergo absorbing experiences (Tellegen and Atkinson 1974). Thus, those who tend to get so caught up in a movie that they lose awareness of being in a theater are in a trance-like state and are relatively more hypnotizable. Whatever a person in a hypnotic trance concentrates on is attended to relatively completely.

Dissociation

This intense absorption means that many routine experiences that would ordinarily be conscious occur out of ordinary conscious awareness. Even complex emotional states or sensory experiences may be dissociated. These experiences may range from the simple, such as a feeling that the hand is not as much a part of the body as usual, to the complex. Some involve memory alterations, such as dissociative amnesia for a traumatic event, whereas others pertain to identity and motor function, as in a fugue episode in which for a period of hours to months an individual functions as though he or she had a different name and residence. Such experiences can be both induced and reversed with the structured use of hypnosis.

Dissociated information is temporarily and reversibly unavailable to consciousness but may nonetheless influence conscious (or other unconscious) experience. A rape victim may have no conscious memory of the crime but may become anxious when exposed to stimuli reminiscent of the event. Absorption and dissociation are complementary constructs. Intense focal attention facilitates putting other information outside conscious awareness.

Suggestibility

Suggestibility is enhanced in hypnosis. Because of their intense absorption in the trance experience, hypnotized individuals usually accept instructions relatively uncritically (hence the term *suggestibility*). Although hypnotized individuals are not deprived of their will, they do have a tendency to accept suggestions or instructions, suspending the usual conscious editing function that raises the question "Why?" when an instruction is given. Thus, hypnotized individuals are more prone to accept directions, no matter how irrational. They are also less prone to distinguish an instruction as coming from another rather than from themselves (i.e., hypnotic source amnesia) and so will tend to act on another person's ideas as though they were their own. Thus, a hyp-

notized individual is especially vulnerable to the nature of the therapeutic intervention; the trance state can enhance responsiveness, either for good or for ill.

Myths Dispelled

There are a variety of common "mythunderstandings" about hypnosis (Table 30–1).

TABLE 30–1. Corrections of common myths about hypnosis

Hypnosis is not sleep.
Hypnotizability is a trait: not everyone is hypnotizable.
Hypnosis is not something *done to* a subject or patient.
Hypnotizability is *not* a susceptibility or a sign of weak-mindedness.
There is nothing intrinsically dangerous about hypnosis.
There is nothing intrinsically therapeutic about hypnosis.

---

1. **Hypnosis is not sleep.** The most prevalent misunderstanding derives from the name itself: the Greek root *hypnos* means "sleep." The hypnotized individual is not asleep but rather is awake and alert. Like a sleeping person, a hypnotized individual has suspended peripheral awareness but, in contrast with what occurs in sleep, his or her focal attention is intense and carefully controlled. The power spectral electroencephalogram (EEG) of hypnotized individuals shows a pattern consistent with resting alertness rather than sleep.

2. **Hypnotizability is a trait: not everyone is hypnotizable.** Hypnotizability is a capacity that varies considerably from one individual to another. Indeed, hypnotizability is a stable and measurable trait, as consistent over a 25-year interval in adulthood as is intelligence (Piccione et al. 1989). Hypnotizability is greatest in late childhood and decreases gradually through adolescence. About 1 of 4 adults is not hypnotizable, and 1 of 10 is highly hypnotizable (H. Spiegel and Spiegel 1987).

3. **Hypnosis is not something *done to* a subject or patient.** Recognition of this fact is helpful for demystifying hypnosis and reducing anxiety on the part of both the doctor inducing hypnosis and the patient. The doctor is not doing something to the patient. Rather, a doctor inducing hypnosis is in the position of the Socratic teacher, one who helps students discover what they already know. A correctly performed hypnotic induction allows the patient and doctor to assess

and explore the patient's hypnotic capacity or lack thereof. This approach tends to minimize power struggles between doctor and patient. For example, there is less chance of misinterpreting a patient's inability to experience a hypnotic trance as resistance. On the other hand, some therapists become frightened when working with a highly hypnotizable patient, because they think that they have imposed an extreme transformation of consciousness on the patient, when in fact they have merely identified and mobilized it.

4. **Hypnotizability is *not* a susceptibility or a sign of weak-mindedness.** Rather, it is an intact capacity for focused concentration that is often associated with, if anything, the absence of serious psychotic and neurological disorders. There are no apparent gender differences in hypnotizability—men and women are equally hypnotizable (Stern et al. 1979).

5. **There is nothing intrinsically dangerous about hypnosis.** Hypnosis is a benign procedure that is tolerated well by patients. The same cognitive flexibility that allows patients to enter the trance facilitates their exit from it with clear structure and support from the therapist. There are few serious contraindications for the use of hypnosis. It is not in itself a dangerous procedure. Indeed, most patients find it relaxing. An occasional patient is slow in exiting from the hypnotic state. Calm reassurance never fails to complete the termination of the trance procedure. Rarely, a paranoid patient may incorporate the attempted hypnotic induction into a delusional system, although careful explanation of the procedures in advance and the use of a hypnotizability test as an initial encounter tend to minimize the likelihood of this occurring. A depressed, suicidal patient may view the use of hypnosis as a last resort and become dangerously disappointed if he or she perceives it as a failure. As with any intervention, careful basic clinical screening is required and appropriate management is necessary, but the procedure itself is, in general, benign and well accepted by patients.

6. **There is nothing intrinsically therapeutic about hypnosis.** Hypnosis is not in and of itself a therapy. Many patients find it a relaxing and comfortable state and may be reassured by the fact that they can produce in a formal state of hypnosis some or all of the symptoms they have experienced spontaneously, such as conversion symptoms, hysterical seizures, or fugue episodes. The use to which the trance state is put, however, is the crucial issue in determining treatment outcome.

Measuring Hypnotizability

Rationale

Because hypnotizability is a stable and measurable trait, a clinical assessment of hypnotizability can be a helpful starting point for the use of hypnosis in treatment (H. Spiegel and Spiegel 1987). This approach combines a hypnotic induction with a procedure that provides the psychiatrist with a deduction of the patient's hypnotic ability. It has several advantages:

1. Hypnotizability testing helps to clarify the hypnotic interaction. It is the therapist's role to systematically assess patients' ability to respond rather than to push them to respond in a certain manner. Such a dispassionate hypnotic induction reduces pressure on therapists to prove their ability to put a patient into a hypnotic state. Likewise, it reduces the sense of pressure on the patient to either comply or resist. Rather, the testing setting creates an atmosphere of scientific exploration that encourages rather than coerces involvement.

2. The use of such a standardized interaction with a large number of patients allows the psychiatrist to make informed inferences about variations in patient response. Patients' relative ability (or inability) to allow the therapist to restructure their inner experience via hypnosis also provides helpful information about their general interpersonal style. For example, highly hypnotizable individuals generally rate themselves as more trusting than do those who are not hypnotizable (Roberts and Tellegen 1973). In addition, hypnotizability testing provides information of relevance to differential diagnosis, as is discussed later in this chapter.

3. Hypnotizability testing provides data about the patient's ability to respond to a treatment that employs hypnosis. Highly hypnotizable individuals can be rationally encouraged. Nonhypnotizable individuals can be offered an alternative approach that is likely to be more efficacious, such as one of the behavioral therapies, biofeedback, or relevant psychoactive medication.

Hypnotizability Scales

Hypnotizability scales have existed since the early part of the century and have been widely used in research—for example, the Stanford Hypnotic Susceptibility Scales, Forms A and B (SHSS: A) and Form C (SHSS: C) (E. R. Hilgard 1965; Weitzenhoffer and Hilgard 1959, 1962) and the Harvard Group Scale of Hypnotic Susceptibility (HGSHS: A; Shor and Orne 1962). These scales involve a structured hypnotic induction and an assessment of the subject's response to a variety of instructions, including alterations in control over movement, sensation, temporal orientation, and perception, such as hallucinatory experiences. Some of these scales have been translated into and validated in other languages; for example, the SHSS: C has been translated into Italian (De Pascalis et al. 2000), and the HGSHS: A has been translated into Danish (Zachariae et al. 2000).

More recently, hypnotizability scales have been developed for clinical use (Hypnotic Induction Profile [HIP; H. Spiegel and Spiegel 1987], Stanford Hypnotic Clinical Scale [SHCS; E.R. Hilgard and Hilgard 1975]). These scales are briefer (5–10 minutes for the HIP and 20 minutes for the SHCS, compared with 1 hour for the Stanford research scales) and are designed for use even with patients who have severe psychiatric disturbances.

The HIP calls for rapid induction commencing with upward gaze and lowering of the eyelids, followed by a series of instructions to the subject to elevate the left hand and keep it in the air, even if the examiner pulls the hand down. Subjects are rated on five items assessing cognitive and behavioral aspects of the hypnotic experience (Table 30–2): 1) their ability to experience a sense of *dissociation* of the left hand from the body; 2) *movement* of the hand, its floating back up in the air after being pulled down, accompanied by 3) a sense of *involuntariness* during elevation of the hand; 4) response to the *cut-off signal* ending the hypnotic experience; and 5) a *sensory alteration* in the hand or elsewhere in the body. The entire procedure can be administered and the scoring done in less than 10 minutes. It predicts responsiveness to a variety of treatments and facilitates differential diagnosis (Figure 30–2) (D. Spiegel et al. 1982, 1988; H. Spiegel and Spiegel 1987).

TABLE 30–2. Responses measured in the Hypnotic Induction Profile

Dissociation
Movement
Involuntariness
Cut-off signal ending hypnotic instruction
Sensory alteration

Prediction of Treatment Responsiveness

Because hypnotic trance involves an intensification of concentration and an increase in receptiveness, it would make sense that the capacity to experience hypnosis

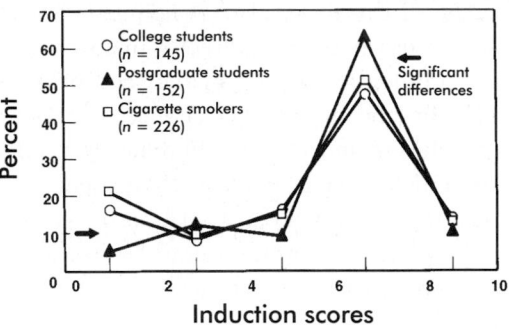

FIGURE 30–2. Hypnotizability as measured by the Hypnotic Induction Profile in three populations.
The variance accounted for by motivational differences may be reflected in the slightly higher scores of postdoctoral students enrolled in a hypnosis course.
Source. D. Spiegel, E. Frischholz, unpublished data, 1980.

should be correlated with responsiveness to treatment. Indeed, this has been found to be the case in treatment with hypnosis of problems such as pain (E.R. Hilgard and Hilgard 1975), smoking cessation (D. Spiegel et al. 1993a; H. Spiegel and Spiegel 1987), and asthma (Collison 1975). Hypnotizability is also correlated with the increased likelihood of responding even to treatments that do not explicitly employ hypnosis, such as acupuncture (Katz et al. 1974).

Outcome studies have generally shown that hypnosis is efficacious and that, in most cases, hypnotizability predicts treatment responsiveness (D. Spiegel et al. 1981). Relatively few well-controlled studies have compared the use of hypnosis as an adjunct with other techniques. Studies conducted among anxiety disorder patient populations have generally found hypnosis to be beneficial, especially when patients request it (Glick 1970; Lazarus 1973). Studies involving student volunteers who are symptomatic tend to show no clear advantage for hypnosis versus desensitization, whereas studies in which stress is induced in nonsymptomatic volunteers demonstrate some advantage for relaxation training over hypnosis (Marks et al. 1968).

M.E. Johnson and Hauck (1999) conducted a study to evaluate the general public's beliefs and opinions about hypnosis as well as to ascertain the sources of those beliefs. The study included samples representing different ages, socioeconomic backgrounds, interests, and geographical locations who completed a 27-item questionnaire. They found that although the various sample groups obtained their information about hypnosis from different sources, their beliefs about hypnosis were remarkably consistent. In general, all groups had an interesting mix of ideas about hypnosis, with most people expressing a positive view of the potential therapeutic benefits. The vast majority of respondents believed that hypnosis reduces the time required to uncover causes of a person's problems and that hypnotized persons can undergo dental and medical procedures without pain. However, Johnson and Hauck's findings also indicated that an extremely large proportion of the general public views hypnosis as a powerful tool for recovering past memories, including accurate memories as far back as birth or even past lives.

Can Hypnotizability Be Enhanced?

A number of articles and studies have addressed the issue of enhancement of hypnotic capacity. All of the published articles consist of case reports, small samples, or anecdotal cases, making it difficult to generalize from the results. Nevertheless, sensory deprivation (Sanders and Reyher 1969) and the use of psychotomimetic drugs (Sjoberg and Hollister 1965) have been associated with enhanced hypnotic responsiveness.

Interestingly, hypnosis seems to have a positive effect on other forms of alternative healing. Lu and Lu's (1999) research combining acupuncture and hypnosis revealed that synergy does exist between the two modalities. In their study, hypnosis augmented the effect of acupuncture, resulting in better treatment outcomes. In addition, hypnosis can be used in the management of needle phobias—for example, in the case of acupuncture patients whose fears prevent them from returning for further treatment despite the fact that acupuncture has rendered good therapeutic results.

Hypnotizability and Psychiatric Disorders

One of the most interesting theoretical areas of research in hypnosis is the relationship between hypnotizability and psychopathology (Figure 30–3). There is accumulating evidence that high hypnotizability is associated with several serious psychiatric disorders. In addition, some authors have associated hypnotizability with personality styles (Rhoades and Edmonston 1969; H. Spiegel and Spiegel 1987).

Hypnotizability in Dissociative and Posttraumatic Stress Disorders

Clinicians have long observed that it is unusual to find a patient with a severe dissociative disorder—such as fugue, amnesia, or dissociative identity disorder (i.e.,

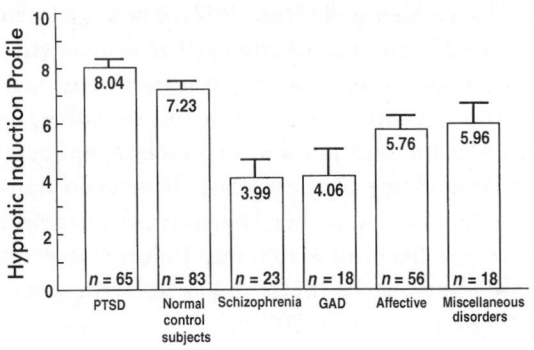

FIGURE 30–3. Psychopathology and hypnotizability.
Hypnotic Induction Profile scores indicate higher than normal responsiveness among patients with posttraumatic stress disorder but lower responsiveness among other psychiatric patient groups. GAD = generalized anxiety disorder; PTSD = posttraumatic stress disorder.
Source. Reprinted with permission from Spiegel D, Hunt T, Dondershine HE: "Dissociation and Hypnotizability in Posttraumatic Stress Disorder." *American Journal of Psychiatry* 145:301–305, 1988. Copyright 1988 American Psychiatric Association.

multiple personality disorder)—who is not highly hypnotizable (see also Chapter 15 in this textbook; Frischholz 1985; Maldonado and Spiegel 1998). The recent literature on dissociative identity disorder indicates that most patients with this disorder are highly hypnotizable and report a history of severe physical and sexual abuse in childhood (Braun and Sachs 1985; Kluft 1985; Maldonado and Spiegel 1998; Maldonado et al. 2000; D. Spiegel 1984). This observation has led to the recognition that the capacity to dissociate—to separate, for example, psychological from physical experience—is mobilized both during and after periods of extreme physical duress such as assault (Bremner and Brett 1997; Butler et al. 1996; Eriksson and Lundin 1996; Kluft 1984a, 1984b; Koopman et al. 1995; Putnam 1985; D. Spiegel 1984, 1986, 1988, 1990a, 1990b; D. Spiegel et al. 1988; van der Kolk and van der Hart 1989; D.P. Wood and Sexton 1997). In two studies, the hypnotizability of combat veterans with posttraumatic stress disorder (PTSD) was found to be significantly higher in comparison with that of other patient groups and of healthy control subjects (Stutman and Bliss 1985; D. Spiegel et al. 1988).

In an attempt to determine the relationship between hypnotizability and acute dissociative reactions to trauma, Bryant et al. (2001) administered the SHCS to acutely traumatized patients ($n=61$) with acute stress disorder, subclinical acute stress disorder (i.e., no dissociative symptoms), and no acute stress disorder within 4 weeks of their traumatic experience. They found that even though patients with acute stress disorder and patients with subclinical acute stress disorder manifested comparable levels of nondissociative psychopathology, acute stress disorder patients had higher levels of hypnotizability and were more likely to display reversible posthypnotic amnesia than were both patients with subclinical acute stress disorder and patients with no acute stress disorder. The authors interpreted these findings in light of a diathesis–stress process mediating trauma-related dissociation and concluded that people who develop acute stress disorder in response to traumatic experiences may have a stronger ability to experience dissociative phenomena compared with people who develop subclinical acute stress disorder or no acute stress disorder.

In some cases, especially cases of repeated, severe assault in childhood, a temporary dissociation that allows the child to tolerate overwhelming fear and pain becomes an ongoing part of the personality structure, and thus the PTSD takes the form of dissociated selves, one of whom suffered and, indeed, in the unconscious, "deserved" the pain and humiliation, others of whom take the stance of protecting the patient from further injury. Because the hypnotic state can be induced in a matter of seconds, and hypnotizability is associated with a higher frequency of spontaneously occurring hypnotic-like experiences, it makes sense that individuals who are highly hypnotizable will have spontaneously mobilized this capacity, especially in the face of serious environmental stress, as in the following example:

> A 16-year-old girl had been beaten by her father during a dispute with her mother when the patient was 4 years old. The girl began developing dissociative episodes in which she would suddenly act and talk like a 4-year-old child. She had no memories of these episodes after they occurred, and they could last for several hours.

[The dissociation between her normal and dissociated mental state is illustrated in Figure 30–4. Both drawings of the same theme, the patient standing next to a tree with her mother, were drawn within a 10-minute period—the former during hypnotically induced dissociation, the latter afterward. The difference in drawing style is clear, as is the disturbed nature of the "4-year-old's" drawing. *Faceless people are floating in air, and the sky merges with the tree.* The other drawing is more age appropriate, and the figures have a kind of stiff placidity (D. Spiegel and Rosenfeld 1984).]

> The patient had dissociated memories and affects associated with this assault by her father. They reemerged much later when she was sexually exploited by an employer. After months of hospitalization, she learned to use self-hypnosis not only to face past traumatic experiences but also in an effort to protect herself. She came to experience the dissociated state as a "protective light" that surrounded her.

Hypnosis is useful early in the treatment of such patients, first, in determining whether they have a dissociative disorder, and, second, in providing rapid access to these dissociated states. This process can be used to demonstrate for these patients how to control dissociation and to begin a process of communication that in the context of well-structured psychotherapy can eventually lead to a reduction in such spontaneous dissociative symptoms. It is important that the impact of whatever physical trauma occurred be recognized and taken into account in the therapy and that the therapy help such patients work through their reactions to that impact. Recognizing and teaching patients with dissociative disorders how to master this capacity is an important psychotherapeutic task (see Chapter 15).

The capacity for hypnotic dissociation has been found to be relevant to a milder but pronounced cluster of symptoms labeled the "Grade 5 syndrome" (H. Spiegel 1974). This cluster has many similarities to the DSM Axis II histrionic personality disorder diagnosis. Patients with these symptoms, who are highly hypnotizable, repeatedly establish naive and dependent relationships, often express symptoms in dramatic ways, are sluggish in reorienting to internal rather than external cues, and form intense affiliations with new ideas and persons, affiliations that tend not to last over time. These patients require a tightly structured, supportive psychotherapy that recognizes their tendency unwittingly to build relationships in which they are vulnerable to control by others. One such patient described herself as a "disciple in search of a teacher." Individuals who in the setting of hypnotizability testing are less able to allow the therapist to restructure their internal world may, in general, be more defended against the influence of other people, whereas those who are highly hypnotizable on formal testing may in less formal circumstances likewise allow other people to reorient them in a hypnotic-like way. In this sense, the hypnotic encounter can be seen as a kind of crystallized transference, a sample of the patient's general style of relating to others.

Hypnotizability in Phobic and Anxiety Disorders

Several studies have proffered evidence that phobic individuals are more highly hypnotizable than are control populations (Frankel and Orne 1976; Gerschman et al. 1979), although other studies have failed to replicate this finding (Frischholz et al. 1982). It is possible that some kinds of phobic symptoms mobilize dissociative capacity, with the symptom representing absorp-

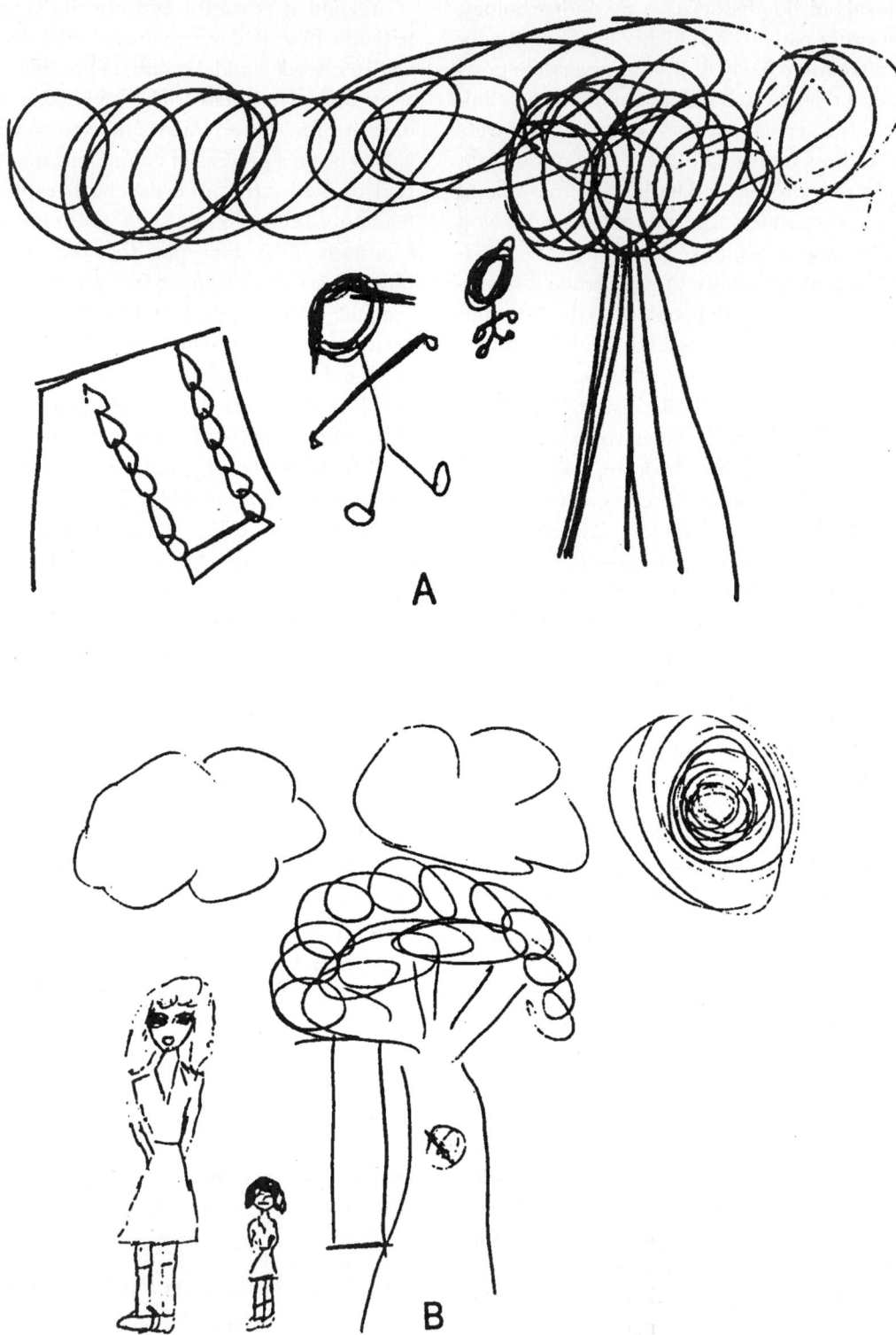

FIGURE 30–4. Hypnotic age regression.

Drawings made during (A) and after (B) hypnotically induced dissociation during which this 16-year-old patient experienced herself as 4 years old.

tion in the fear of the situation and suspension of critical judgment about it. However, patients with generalized anxiety disorder (GAD) have markedly lower scores than do subjects without the disorder (D.

Spiegel et al. 1982). Those patients with GAD who take benzodiazepines tend to have higher hypnotizability scores than do those who are untreated (D. Spiegel 1980).

Hypnotizability in Eating Disorders

Pettinati et al. (1990) administered both the SHSS: C and the HIP to patients with bulimia and anorexia nervosa. The authors observed higher hypnotizability in the bulimic patients than in the restricting patients. These researchers noted that many of the bulimic patients reported that they were in a trancelike state when they engaged in their compulsive bingeing and purging behavior. Vanderlinden et al. (1995) found that compared with control subjects, eating disorder patients scored significantly higher on the Dissociation Questionnaire (DIS-Q) and the SHCS. Covino et al. (1994) examined the levels of hypnotizability and dissociation in an outpatient sample of bulimic women of normal weight and compared these levels with those of healthy control subjects. They found that bulimic patients were significantly more hypnotizable than were control subjects and that they scored higher on self-report scales of dissociative experiences. These findings suggest a possible opportunity for intervention employing hypnosis in controlling this form of eating disorder (Gross 1984).

Hypnotizability in Schizophrenia and Affective Disorders

As far back as 1937, Copeland and Kitching observed that presumably psychotic patients who were hypnotizable were not genuinely psychotic. Given the complex cognitive tasks involved in tests of hypnotic responsiveness, it makes sense theoretically that patients experiencing delusions, loose associations, and hallucinations might score more poorly on tests of hypnotizability, as they do on most other psychological tests. On the other hand, because hallucinations can be produced artificially in hypnotic states, some investigators have predicted that schizophrenic individuals should be equally or even more hypnotizable than subjects without schizophrenia. More than 20 studies have been conducted on the issue, and the findings have generally shown somewhat lower, and the absence of very high, hypnotizability among schizophrenic patients (Lavoie and Sabourin 1980; Pettinati 1982). Schizophrenic patients show a more restricted range of scores, and those who do better on psychological tests such as the Rorschach are more hypnotizable than those who display more thought disorganization.

Thus, psychotic patients, especially those with schizophrenia, score differently on hypnotizability scales than do nonpsychotic individuals. Their scores on the HIP are substantially lower than those of control samples (Pettinati 1982; Pettinati et al. 1990; D. Spiegel et al.

1982). However, mean scores of schizophrenic patients have not been found to be lower than those of psychiatrically healthy individuals in studies employing the SHSS (Lavoie and Elie 1985; Lavoie and Sabourin 1980; Pettinati 1982; Pettinati et al. 1990). These studies do show lower variance in scores, which means there is a relative absence of very high hypnotizability among schizophrenic patients. Furthermore, Lavoie and Elie (1985) found significantly fewer autistic forms of primary process on the Rorschach tests of the more hypnotizable schizophrenic patients. Thus, schizophrenic patients show impairment that interferes with hypnotic concentration: scores on some scales indicate that these individuals are substantially less hypnotizable, and scores on all measures show very few of them to be highly hypnotizable.

Studies using the HIP have in particular shown substantially lower hypnotizability scores for schizophrenic individuals compared with psychiatrically healthy subjects (Pettinati 1982; D. Spiegel et al. 1982), whereas those employing the Stanford scales (SHSS: A and SHSS: C; Weitzenhoffer and Hilgard 1959, 1962) have tended to show a restricted range of scores among schizophrenic patients but mean scores that are not significantly lower than those of comparison groups (Lavoie and Sabourin 1980; Pettinati 1982). In addition, patients with major affective disorders have been found to score higher than schizophrenic patients but lower than subjects without schizophrenia (D. Spiegel et al. 1982) (Figure 30–3). These findings were independent of psychoactive medication use (D. Spiegel 1980). Thus, several psychiatric syndromes—schizophrenia, GAD, and, to a lesser extent, major affective disorder—have been found to be associated with generally lower hypnotic responsiveness. The symptoms of the illness apparently impair expression of a patient's native capacity for hypnotic concentration.

Given these findings, the possibility exists that hypnotizability testing can be used in certain cases to clarify differential diagnosis. For example, it has been increasingly recognized, in part on the basis of genetic data, that an acute psychotic episode is a manifestation of an illness other than chronic and borderline schizophrenia. There is considerable phenomenological overlap among acute psychoses. However, patients with hysterical psychosis or a dissociative disorder should be extremely hypnotizable (D. Spiegel and Fink 1979; Steingard and Frankel 1985; van der Hart and Spiegel 1993). On the other hand, patients with chronic or borderline schizophrenia score at the other end of the hypnotizability spectrum (Lavoie and Sabourin 1980; Pettinati 1982; Pettinati et al. 1990; D. Spiegel and Fink 1979; D. Spiegel et al. 1982; van der Hart and Spiegel 1993).

Hypnosis in Treatment

Brief Treatment: Symptom Restructuring With Hypnosis

Hypnosis has been used as an adjunctive tool in the treatment of a variety of common psychiatric and medical problems, including habit disorders, anxiety and phobic states, psychosomatic problems, and pain. Because the hypnotic state involves an enhanced and altered state of concentration with an ability to produce changes in perception and certain body functions, it makes sense that it would be an effective tool in managing these psychosomatic problems. A variety of techniques have been employed in symptom-oriented treatment using hypnosis. One is the so-called ego-strengthening approach, in which hypnosis is used to provide positive reinforcement for behavior change (Crasilneck and Hall 1985). Erickson (1967) made use of a "therapeutic bind," mobilizing the patient's resistance to treatment by intensifying, or "prescribing," symptoms. The patient would then construe eliminating the symptom as a victory over the therapist. This approach, although not necessary among patients who are well motivated and who have resolved their ambivalence about symptom reduction, has the virtue of demonstrating to patients their ability to modulate symptoms, bypassing defensiveness by worsening rather than lessening them (Erickson 1967). Other therapists employ simple instructions that a symptom will disappear. This authoritarian approach often puts both therapist and patient in an awkward situation—it is unwise to tell a patient something one is not certain is true, whether or not the patient is in a trance. No one can be certain that a symptom will disappear, even in the case of a highly hypnotizable patient.

More recent approaches to the use of hypnosis have emphasized the educational aspects of the experience. In particular, it is most efficient to structure the intervention as a lesson in self-hypnosis that the patient can learn to employ in the service of symptom reduction. Also, it is useful to teach patients a cognitive strategy that alters their perspective on the problem, reinforced by the self-hypnosis. One such approach is *restructuring* (H. Spiegel and Spiegel 1987). Restructuring in hypnosis involves using the intense concentration characteristic of the trance state to help patients develop a strategy for change that amounts to an affirmation experience rather than a struggle, focusing on what they are for rather than what they are against. For example, instead of telling themselves not to smoke or that cigarettes taste bad, patients use the self-hypnosis exercise to focus on a broader commitment to protect their body in the same way that they would protect a child from poison, viewing their bodies as trusting, innocent creatures that depend on them for their protection. In this approach, mind and body are viewed as distinct but interdependent, and the goal is to change the relationship to the body rather than to prevent smoking (Figure 30–5). Thus, these patients' perspective on the problem is enlarged, which makes the resolution of the problem itself an example of a broader pattern of relating to one's body. This therapeutic focus avoids the trap of increasing attention to the problem, in this case smoking, which can actually increase one's desire to engage in the activity (e.g., to smoke) (similar to telling oneself, "Don't think about purple elephants").

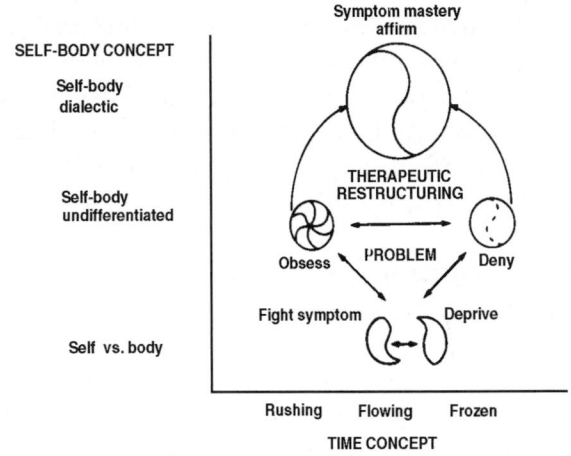

FIGURE 30–5. Model for constructing a restructuring treatment strategy using hypnosis.

This model emphasizes a commitment to affirm a restructured relationship of respect for one's body rather than fight against the symptom, which only amplifies it.

This kind of restructuring strategy can be applied to other problems as well, such as mild to moderate overeating (Barabasz and Spiegel 1989) and pain (Brose et al. 1997; E.R. Hilgard and Hilgard 1975; D. Spiegel 1985). In the latter case, patients are taught to transform the pain signal by making the affected body area colder or warmer, or numb, or to focus on a sensation in some other part of the body. The management of anxiety or panic attacks is not taught by an instruction to relax or not be anxious; rather, patients learn to affiliate with a physical metaphor that connotes relaxation, such as floating in water. In this way, patients can overcome urges or symptoms not by struggling against them, but rather by subsuming them under a commitment to a new way of relating to the body, or through a hypnotically developed capacity to transform sensation (H. Spiegel and Spiegel 1987).

Indications and Contraindications

Hypnosis has been shown to be an effective adjunct to the treatment of a variety of symptoms and problems (Table 30–3). As noted earlier, hypnosis has an important place in the treatment of dissociative disorders—for example, in identifying and controlling dissociative fugue, amnesia, and identity disorder—and in treating PTSD and conversion disorder. Hypnosis also has been widely used in the treatment of anxiety disorders and phobias. A number of studies have demonstrated the efficacy of hypnosis in the treatment of pain. Recent research indicates its utility during medical procedures to help control pain and anxiety (Lang et al. 1996, 2000). Hypnosis has been useful in the control of such psychosomatic problems as asthma and psoriasis. It has been extensively used in habit control, especially for smoking, and to a lesser extent for weight control.

Use of hypnosis should be considered if the patient has the requisite hypnotizability, indicates he or she will be cooperative during the procedure, and has a problem for which hypnosis has been shown to be of adjunctive utility. The first criterion is measured by hypnotizability testing as discussed above. The second criterion can be met by a brief but frank discussion with the patient about the nature of hypnosis, with clarification of the fact that in hypnosis the doctor does not control the patient but rather explores the patient's capacity to focus and intensify concentration. The therapist should be no more interested in using hypnosis than the patient is, and the extremely rare problems arising from the use of hypnosis can generally be avoided if the procedure is never forced on an unwilling or ambivalent patient.

Although transference and other relationship factors must be taken into account when hypnosis is used in psychotherapy, artificial enhancement of transference distortions can be avoided by this dispassionate approach to hypnotic induction and assessment.

Applications of Hypnosis in Psychiatry

Although some psychoanalysts view hypnosis as a contaminant of therapy, Freud himself speculated toward the end of his career that the pure gold of analysis might well have to be alloyed with the baser metal of suggestion. Indeed, the early influence of Charcot as Freud's hypnosis teacher (von Plessen 1996) had a lasting effect; Freud placed a drawing of Charcot inducing hypnosis over the psychoanalytic couch in his last office in London. Psychotherapies employing hypnosis can use, rather than merely analyze, transference. Hypnosis has been used in intensive psychotherapy as a means of gaining access to repressed memories that have not emerged through use of other techniques—for example, when both the patient and the psychotherapist have worked on resistance issues and believe that some additional leverage is necessary. Such a use of hypnosis comes up particularly in regard to traumatic events that may have occurred during childhood and have been dissociated.

Anxiety Disorders and Phobias

The Epidemiologic Catchment Area study sponsored by the National Institute of Mental Health demonstrated that anxiety disorders are among the most widely prevalent psychiatric disturbances, affecting as much as 15% of the population (Myers et al. 1984). Anxiety is a state of psychosomatic discomfort experienced by patients largely in physical terms, with increases in heart rate, gastrointestinal and thoracic discomfort, diaphoresis, and motor restlessness. Panic attacks (i.e., sudden and intense states involving this kind of discomfort) may be associated with irrational avoidance behavior (i.e., phobias). On the other hand, a more chronic state may inhibit psychological comfort and social functioning, as in GAD.

Hypnosis has also been reported to be useful in the treatment of anxiety and phobias (J.C. Clarke and Jackson 1983; Erickson 1967; J.R. Hilgard and LeBaron 1982; Maldonado and Spiegel 1996; McGuinness 1984; Somer 1995; D. Spiegel et al. 1981; Stanton 1993). In fact, a 7-year follow-up of 178 patients treated with a single session of self-hypnosis for flying phobia indicated that 52% were either improved or cured (D. Spiegel et al. 1981).

Whereas, as noted earlier, the hypnotizability of patients with GAD is low, studies show that phobic patients are at least normally and perhaps highly hypnotizable (Frankel and Orne 1976). A variety of treatment strategies employing hypnosis have in common a restructuring of cognition by combining imagery with physical relaxation. Anxious patients are instructed to maintain such a sense of floating relaxation while picturing feared situations on an imaginary screen in the trance state. This approach clearly has elements in common with systematic desensitization (Marks et al. 1968), the difference being that in the former the induction of physical relaxation coupled with a noxious stimulus can be included very quickly without the development and working through of a hierarchy.

Specific phobias call for variation in cognitive strategy. Patients with flying phobia, for example, can be taught to combine the hypnotically induced physical sense of floating with the concept of floating with the airplane. They can then focus on the idea of the plane as an

TABLE 30–3. Uses of hypnosis in psychiatric disorders

Psychiatric disorder	Hypnotic technique(s)	Goal(s)
Bulimia nervosa	Restructuring relationship to body and eating	Control spontaneous dissociative aspects of impulsive behavior
Conversion disorder	Hypnotizability testing, symptom enhancement, symptom alteration	Help make differential diagnosis and to identify, control, and reduce symptoms
Dissociative disorder	Hypnotizability testing, symptom elicitation, regression, restructuring	Clarify diagnosis, enhance symptom control, facilitate access to dissociative states, and facilitate working through
Phobic and anxiety disorders	Dissociating psychological from somatic distress, screen technique, desensitization	Reduce somatic amplification of anxiety, restructure anxiety-inducing stimuli, and separate stimuli from conditioned response
Posttraumatic stress disorder	Regression, abreaction, restructuring	Enhance control over access to traumatic memories, reduce spontaneous "flashbacks," and facilitate working through
Schizophrenia	Hypnotizability testing	Help make differential diagnosis

extension of the body, instead of feeling trapped inside the plane, and can also concentrate on the difference between a possibility and a probability. The mere fact that a crash is possible does not make it likely. This is a technique that can be employed by patients before and during the airplane flight.

Individuals with acrophobia can be taught in the trance state to view gravity not as something likely to pull them off a cliff or building but rather as something that roots them to the ground. Agoraphobic patients may find it useful to imagine a plastic bubble surrounding them that they can take with them even when they leave their protective environment. Thus, whatever sense of safety they feel at home can sometimes be carried with them. Patients with animal phobias can be taught to feel more in control of a situation with an animal by first learning to control their own somatic response to it. Cognitively, they can concentrate on the difference between dangerous and tame animals (D. Spiegel and Spiegel 1988; H. Spiegel and Spiegel 1987). Other approaches using hypnosis have included instructing patients in a trance to imagine that they are literally somewhere else, away from the fearful stimulus (Erickson 1967), or that their capacity to master the situation and their response to it will improve (Crasilneck and Hall 1985). There is generally less attention paid to uncovering techniques that seek to link the complaint of anxiety to some early traumatic experience, although this is most applicable, as noted earlier, to clear cases of PTSD, as opposed to phobic and anxiety disorders.

Nishith et al. (1999) set up an experiment to test whether a simple hypnotic induction following an alprazolam experience could recreate the subjective effects of alprazolam (Xanax). Subjects were initially given 1 mg of

alprazolam. Four days later, the subjects were exposed to the hypnosis-only condition and the hypnosis plus alprazolam experience–based suggestion condition in counterbalanced order. Nishith et al. found that exposure to the hypnosis-plus-suggestion condition produced greater levels of relaxation, as measured by the tension–anxiety scale of the Profile of Mood States (POMS), than did either the alprazolam condition or the hypnosis-only condition. In each of the three conditions, patients with high hypnotizability showed significantly greater levels of relaxation than did those with low hypnotizability. EEG data revealed that frontal and occipital sites were specifically involved in both the alprazolam and the hypnotic-suggestion conditions, a finding suggesting a neurobiological basis for the use of hypnosis as a substitute for sedative drug use.

Dissociative Disorders

Hypnosis can be a helpful tool in the psychotherapy of dissociative disorders. Patients with these disorders experience their fugue states, dissociated identities, and conversion symptoms as occurring suddenly and beyond their control. Hypnosis used formally can serve therapeutic as well as diagnostic purposes (Kluft 1993; see also Chapter 15). The controlled access to the hypnotic state often spontaneously triggers the dissociative symptom (e.g., hysterical pseudoseizures). It is possible to induce the symptom—for example, by using age regression and having the patient reexperience the last time the dissociative symptom was present. In this structured manner, the patient can be taught to practice bringing on the symptom and thereby learn to control it, as in the following example:

A 16-year-old boy was brought to the emergency department writhing and screaming that he was possessed by "demons of Satan." He was initially diagnosed as having schizophrenia and was given antipsychotic medication, to which he did not respond. His history indicated that he had been well until several months earlier, when his girlfriend had left him and he had made a suicide gesture in front of her home. She took him to the local pastor, who referred to the suicide attempt as "Satan's work." The boy then began having possession episodes in which he growled in a strange voice that threatened to put a curse on the patient and to transfer the curse to anyone who tried to interfere. The patient was amnesic for each episode afterward.

The patient was examined with the HIP and scored 10 of 10 points, indicating high hypnotizability. He was then age-regressed to the last possession episode, and he changed abruptly from being polite and subdued to harboring the delusional belief that he was possessed by a demon, laughing in a bizarre manner, sniffling, and growling. The regression was ended and he reassumed his more restrained demeanor. He was congratulated for having been able to bring on the possession episode. His parents were encouraged not to panic as they had previously when these episodes occurred and also to change the bedroom arrangement in the home. He had been sharing a room with an older sister, who it turned out had been sexually active with her boyfriend. Within a few weeks the possession episodes stopped, and the patient maintained his improvement for years afterward without the use of antipsychotic medications.

This patient would have met DSM-IV criteria for dissociative identity disorder, although the presentation was atypical in that the symptoms did not begin in early childhood and were circumscribed and resolved fairly rapidly. This assessment and intervention prevented an incorrect diagnosis from being made and the patient's being treated for schizophrenia (D. Spiegel and Fink 1979).

Posttraumatic Stress Disorder

The use of hypnosis in the psychotherapy of trauma was initially thought to be limited to abreaction, based on Freud's cathartic method. The idea was that some intense affect associated with the traumatic event needed to be released and that simply repeating the event with its associated emotion in the trance state would suffice to resolve the symptoms. However, it became clear to Freud (1914/1958) that conscious, cognitive work must be done on the material for it to be successfully worked through. Hypnotic techniques for the treatment of posttraumatic conditions were often used by the clinical pioneers of the end of the nineteenth century and by military therapists treating soldiers during the twentieth century's conflagrations. More recently, hypnosis has also been used with survivors of sexual assault, accidents, and

other traumas. Nonetheless, there have been almost no systematic studies on the efficacy of hypnosis for posttraumatic disorders (Cardeña 2000). A number of individuals with PTSD have shown high hypnotizability in various studies (D. Spiegel et al. 1988; Stutman and Bliss 1985). Similarly, available reports suggest high hypnotizability in individuals who were victims of severe punishment during childhood (Nash and Lynn 1986; D. Spiegel and Cardeña 1991). If, as proposed by some (Kluft 1984a, 1992; D. Spiegel et al. 1982), the impact of the stress suffered during trauma encouraged a more effective use of self-hypnosis abilities, thus enhancing or mediating symptomatology, hypnosis might be used to help modulate and control symptoms associated with PTSD and to help integrate memories of trauma.

For therapy to be effective, cognitive restructuring, emotional expression, and relationship management must accompany the patient's reexperiencing of the traumatic events. The therapy should provide an enhanced sense of control over the memories of the experience. This may take the form of a symbolic restructuring of the traumatic experiences in hypnosis (H. Spiegel and Spiegel 1987), with the use of a grief work model (D. Spiegel 1981). Hypnosis can be used to provide controlled access to the dissociated or repressed memories of the traumatic experience and then to help patients restructure their memories of the events.

Given the growing evidence that many people enter a dissociated state during physical trauma (Butler et al. 1996; Cardeña and Spiegel 1993; D. Spiegel and Cardeña 1991; van der Kolk and Fisler 1995; van der Kolk et al. 1994), it makes sense that enabling them to enter a structured dissociative state in therapy would facilitate their access to memories of the traumatic experience, memories that can be worked through to resolve the posttraumatic symptomatology. Hypnosis can be helpful in allowing the victim to review aspects of the trauma in a controlled manner. The memories can be experienced for a time with the assurance that they can be put aside afterward. In a trance, patients can be quickly taught how to produce a state of physical relaxation despite whatever psychological stress they experience, thus dissociating the somatic reaction from the psychological preoccupation and allowing for modulation of the traumatic memory and an enhanced sense of control over the experience. Patient and therapist can then find a condensation image that symbolizes some aspect of the trauma.

It is often helpful to have patients do this on an imaginary screen, which gives them some sense of distance from the event. It is also useful to divide the screen in half, having the patient picture on one side some aspect of the event (e.g., a rape victim's image of the assailant) and on the other side of the screen something he or she did to protect himself or herself (e.g., struggling with the assailant, talking with him, running away). This enables the patient to restructure his or her view of the assault, facing it, but not simply in the familiar terms of the humiliation, pain, and fear with which it was initially associated. Victims can better bear their helplessness when they also acknowledge their efforts to protect themselves. Bereaved individuals can picture themselves at the graveside on one side of the screen and at an earlier moment of joy with the deceased on the other side of the screen. They can then be taught a self-hypnosis exercise in which they grieve and work through traumatic memories while enhancing their sense of control over the process (D. Spiegel 1981).

The most distressing thing about a traumatic event is the sense of absolute helplessness that it engenders. This helplessness is reenacted in PTSD through loss of control over state of mind, with spontaneous dissociative states, startle reactions, or intrusive recollections of the event. Furthermore, such patients may tend to identify the therapist with the assailant and feel that the therapy amounts to a reinflicting of the trauma. It is crucial that the therapy, especially when a technique such as hypnosis is used, be structured so that the process enhances patients' sense of control. This approach can allow patients to integrate the image of themselves as victims with the ongoing, more global image of themselves as persons coping effectively with severe stress, making the repressed material conscious and therefore less powerful and enabling them to establish a new, more congruent self-image and absorb the loss into the ongoing flow of their lives.

The principles of this kind of psychotherapy (Table 30–4) can be summarized with the following eight Cs:

TABLE 30–4. Principles of psychotherapy for trauma victims: the eight *C*s

---

Confrontation

Confession

Consolation

Condensation

Consciousness

Concentration

Control

Congruence

---

1. **Confrontation.** It is important to confront the traumatic events directly rather than attribute the symptoms to some long-standing personality problem.

2. **Confession.** It is often necessary to allow such patients to confess deeds or emotions that are embarrassing to them and at times repugnant to the therapist. It is important to help these patients distinguish between misplaced guilt and real remorse. There is always a retrospective wish to change traumatic circumstances through a fantasy that such circumstances could have been controlled. The price is irrational guilt: "I should have known."

3. **Consolation.** The intensity of these experiences requires an actively consoling approach from the therapist, lest he or she be perceived as being judgmental or as collaborating in the pain inflicted on the patient. A kind of traumatic transference can develop in which, for example, rape victims may believe that their therapists are reinflicting the trauma during the "working through" phase. Appropriate expressions of sympathy and concern can be helpful in acknowledging and diffusing this common reaction.

4. **Condensation.** It is important to find an image that condenses a crucial aspect of the traumatic experience. This representation can make the overwhelming aspects of the trauma more manageable by giving them concrete, symbolic form. Furthermore, this approach can be used to facilitate a restructuring of the experience by joining previously disparate images—for example, linking the pain associated with the death of a buddy in combat with the happiness experienced during some earlier shared time. This allows patients to alter the pain of the loss by attending to positive aspects of the lost relationship that remain in memory.

5. **Consciousness.** In a gradual manner, so that the patient is not overwhelmed, the therapist must make conscious previously dissociated traumatic memories.

6. **Concentration.** Use of the intense concentration characteristic of the hypnotic state is helpful in reinforcing the boundaries of the traumatic experience and of the painful affect associated with it. Through sharply focusing attention on the loss, the inference is made that when the hypnotic state is ended, attention can be shifted away from the traumatic experience.

7. **Control.** Because the most painful aspect of severe trauma is the sense of absolute helplessness, the loss of control over one's body and the course of events, it is especially important that the process of the therapeutic intervention enhance the patient's sense of control over the memories. The experience should be structured so that patients are given the opportunity to terminate the working through when they feel they have had enough, can remember as much from the hypnosis as they care to, and feel they are in charge of

the self-hypnosis experience. They should learn to use it on their own as a self-hypnosis exercise as well as with the therapist. Such procedures help patients to deal with traumatic memories with a greater sense of control and mastery.

8. **Congruence.** The goal of the therapy is to help patients integrate dissociated or repressed traumatic material into conscious awareness in such a way that they can tolerate experiencing the memories as part of themselves, so that the traumatic past is not disjunctive and incompatible with the present. Patients should emerge from therapy having reviewed not only what was done to them but what they did to protect themselves, not only what they lost but what they had had that made the loss so painful.

Conversion Disorders

Years ago, Charcot correctly reported an association between conversion disorder and high hypnotic capacity (Charcot 1890). As suggested by Janet, it is our belief that the symptoms of conversion disorder can be understood in part as reflecting the presence of uncontrolled hypnotic states. Bliss (1984) has already reported that conversion patients are very hypnotizable (an average of 9.7 on the HIP 12-point scale). Other studies have corroborated that conversion patients are more highly hypnotizable relative to the general population (Maldonado 1996a, 1996b). For example, studies suggest that the percentage of the general population that is highly hypnotizable is between 20% and 30%, as compared with about 69% in patients suffering from psychogenic seizures (Peterson et al. 1950). Maldonado and colleagues have hypothesized that patients with a conversion disorder may indeed be using their own capacity to dissociate in order to displace the uncomfortable feelings or affects onto a chosen part of the body, which then becomes dysfunctional (Maldonado 1996a, 1996b; Maldonado and Jasiukaitis 1997).

Because highly hypnotizable individuals show an unusual capacity for psychological control over somatic function, it makes sense that hypnotic phenomena may be involved both in the etiology of some somatoform symptoms and in their control (D. Spiegel and Vermetten 1994). Certain classic conversion disorders, such as hysterical paralysis, may well represent dissociative phenomena, because profound alterations in sensation and experience of control over motor function are standard hypnotic phenomena (D. Spiegel and Vermetten 1994). Indeed, hypnosis may be useful in both the diagnosis and the treatment of many psychosomatic illnesses and conversion symptoms (Bowman 1993; Bush et al.

1992; Maldonado 1996a, 1996b; Maldonado and Jasiukaitis 1997).

In the case of conversion disorders, hypnosis should always be used as an adjuvant to, rather than in lieu of, medical treatment. Hypnosis can be used not to remove the process or to restore function, but rather to allow patients to control the effects of their emotional stress and mind states over their body. It is not advisable to force a cure in a patient, as doing so may lead to other complications (e.g., symptom substitution). Rather, patients should be trained in the use of self-hypnotic techniques and then allowed to improve at a pace that feels comfortable to them, while the clinician provides suggestions for improved control and mastery and explores the unconscious psychological reasons behind the presence of symptoms, including the possibility of secondary gain.

In the treatment of conversion disorders, hypnosis may be useful in two ways (Maldonado 1996b; Maldonado and Spiegel 2000a; 2000b). First, it may be diagnostic. In fact, during a hypnotic induction, the clinician may bring on, worsen, or ameliorate symptoms. Second, hypnosis may be therapeutic. Changes in the symptom during or after a trial of hypnosis can be used constructively to teach the patient to use self-hypnosis as a means of enhancing his or her control over the severity of the symptom. This hypnotic modulation makes the symptom seem less alien and threatening. Hypnosis can be appropriately used as part of a rehabilitation strategy, particularly insofar as it can help patients master the reactive anxiety that is associated with real physical dysfunction as well as conversion symptoms. A patient can be taught to use a state of self-hypnosis to develop a sense of floating relaxation while picturing bothersome problems on an imaginary screen. The patient can then work on, for example, improving use of a dysfunctional hand by developing tremors that gradually build up strength and circulation. An interesting case report described a patient with persistent contractures of the entire hand secondary to a compound fracture of the index finger. After having been treated with a variety of techniques for 3 years with no improvement, he chose to try self-hypnosis exercises of this type to focus on rehabilitation rather than seek further information about causation. At the end of a year of daily self-hypnosis exercises, the patient had regained full function of the hand and returned to work (D. Spiegel and Chase 1980; Figure 30–6).

The clinical use of hypnosis in the context of conversion disorder encompasses three phases (Maldonado 1996b, 2001; Maldonado and Spiegel 2000). The first phase involves *exploration of the meaning* that the symptoms have to the patient. By engaging in this process, the

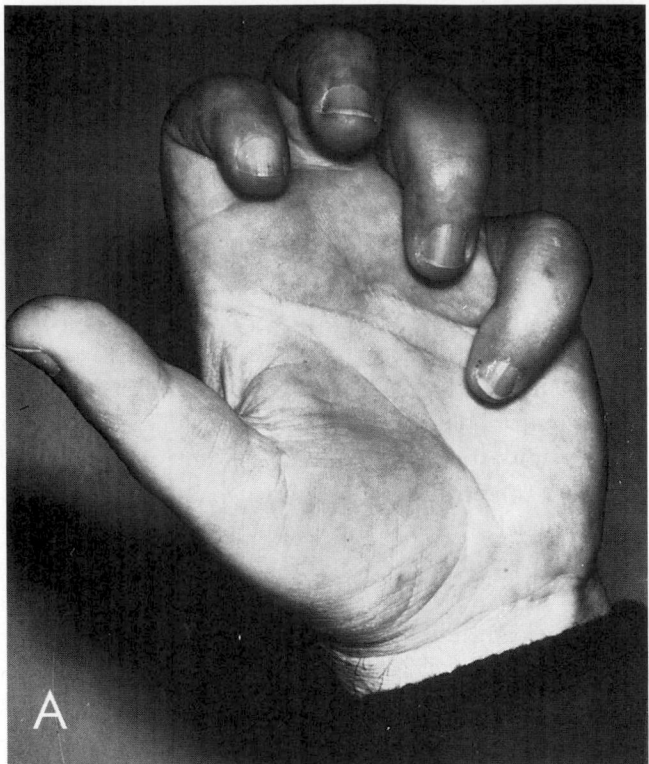

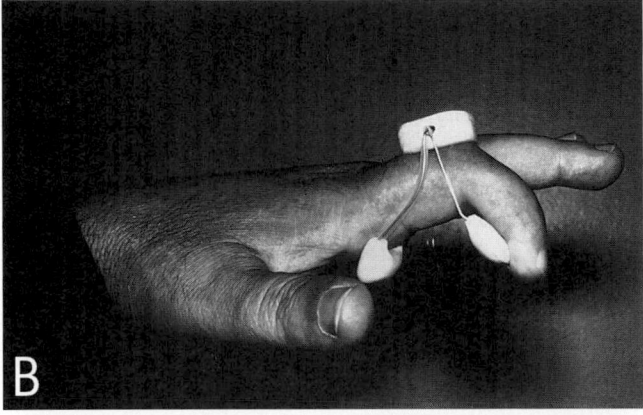

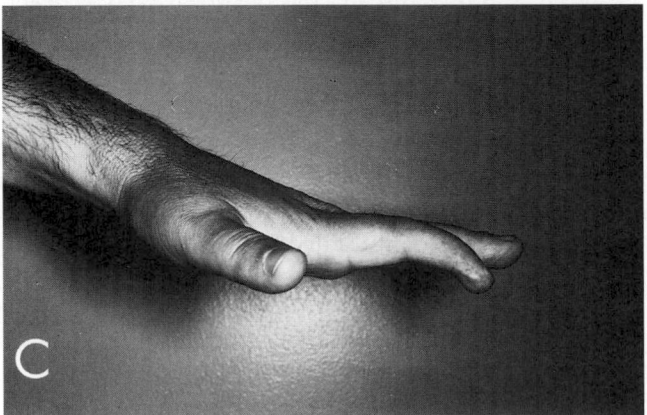

FIGURE 30–6. Treatment of contractures of the hand using self-hypnosis.

Hand in maximal extension before *(A)*, during *(B)*, and after *(C)* treatment using self-hypnosis exercises and dynamic splinting.

therapist will gain a better understanding of the underlying purpose(s) served by the symptom(s). Two golden rules apply to hypnotic exploration of unconscious symptoms: 1) never eliminate a symptom without first understanding its value and purpose, and 2) never take away a symptom without giving the patient a better defense and obtaining the patient's agreement. The second phase involves *symptom alteration*. The best form of symptom alteration is one that takes the patient's mind away from the presenting symptoms while simultaneously allowing the patient to discover more appropriate ways to cope with his or her anxiety. This may be accomplished through either of two symptom-alteration techniques: 1) *symptom substitution*, in which a given symptom is exchanged for another symptom that is less impairing or pathological until the patient is ready to do away with the symptom entirely (i.e., exchanging the perception of intense pain for a numbing, tingling sensation in the same area); or 2) *symptom extinction*, in which the patient agrees to "give up" the symptom after working through the problem in psychotherapy. The third phase in the hypnotic treatment of conversion symptoms involves *maximizing the patient's level of functioning*. Posthypnotic suggestions may be quite useful when the patient is very concrete (i.e., not psychologically sophisticated) and in need of continual support or reassurance. Hypnotic techniques can be used as a *transitional object* while the patient gets on the road of total physical and psychological health (i.e., free of impairing physical symptoms and psychological conflicts). Similarly, the use of *projective techniques* can be quite valuable in helping the patient to envision him- or herself doing better and living without the illness. At this phase, hypnosis may be used to increase the level of motivation, enhance the patient's sense of mastery, and strengthen his or her (ego) defenses.

Maldonado (2001) described a "reverse symptom identification technique" in which the therapist, using the positive transference/countertransference in the therapeutic relationship, may mobilize a patient's healthy defense mechanisms and accelerate the rate of recovery while facilitating a more meaningful exploration of the patients' symptoms, their significance, and the true etiological reason beneath the symptoms (i.e., the psychological conflict being covered or displaced/converted by the presenting symptoms). Patients are taught how to achieve a state of self-hypnosis and are then hypnotized by the therapist. Following trance induction, the therapist proceeds to produce—in a nonaffected body part, preferably a nonaffected contralateral part—a symptom similar in nature and magnitude to the patient's presenting symptom. The therapist discusses with the patient the mechanisms involved in the production of that phenomenon. By stressing the fact that all hypnosis is self-hypnosis, the therapist teaches patients that if they can cause a deficit, they will also be able to effect the cure "whenever they are ready to do so, and not before." Toward the end of the session, the therapist models for the patient what is expected of him or her by providing suggestions for normalization in sensation and function of the "hypnotized" extremity being used as an example. Patients are then encouraged to use these newly learned skills to restore sensation and/or function—as they did in the office—either in the office with the therapist or "at any time in the future when they feel safe and ready."

The above-described phases and techniques are designed to help the patient understand that all hypnosis is self-hypnosis; thus, at the end, patients are taught that their hypnotic ability—which they perceived as a sign of weakness because it caused their symptoms—can be harnessed and used constructively (i.e., turned into a strength) not only to resolve the current problem (i.e., conversion symptom) but also as a tool for mastery and self-control to prevent future deficits and symptoms. This treatment involves a collaborative approach rather than the old suggestion methods used by Bernheim, Janet, and Freud. The therapist adopts the role of a coach guiding the patient through the process rather than doing things for the patient. The patient is helped through the process of understanding the nature, meaning, and usefulness of the conversion symptoms. The patient is then given all the necessary tools to cope with the deficits and to "give up the symptoms when ready." Table 30–5 presents a summary of principles and techniques for the use of hypnosis in the treatment of conversion disorders.

TABLE 30–5. Steps used in the treatment of conversion disorder

1. Symptom exploration
2. Symptom alteration
   a. Symptom substitution
   b. Symptom extinction
3. Maximizing level of functioning
4. Reverse symptom identification

Hypnosis is similarly useful in the treatment of pseudoseizures (Kuyk et al. 1995) and other pseudoneurological deficits. In a study comparing levels of dissociation between patients with pseudoseizures (*n*=20) and a control group, the authors (L.H. Goldstein et al. 2000) found that pseudoseizure patients demonstrated higher levels of dissociation and escape–avoidance coping strategies. They also expressed a greater belief in external control over health and had higher depression scores, in comparison with the control subjects.

In a recent study, Barry et al. (2000) found that hypnotizability scores for epileptic patients were lower than those for pseudoseizure patients. They used hypnosis, while patients were undergoing video-EEG monitoring, to induce an "ictal" event. In their sample, hypnotic seizure induction used as a diagnostic technique of nonepileptic event (NEE) had a sensitivity of 77% and a specificity of 95%. Nevertheless, as already reported by others (Krumholz and Niedermeyer 1983; Ramchandani and Schindler 1993), between 37% and 42% of patients with true epilepsy have coexistence pseudoseizures. We must also consider that even though studies have suggested that only 20%–30% of the general population is hypnotizable to a somnambulistic level (i.e., highest level of hypnotizability), nearly 70% of patients with psychogenic seizures are capable of reaching the same hypnotic level (Peterson et al. 1950). Given this context, it may be dangerous to assume that a hypnotically induced NEE is equivalent to a diagnosis of pseudoseizures (i.e., conversion disorder).

A different use for hypnosis in the diagnosis of pseudoseizures was suggested by Sumner et al. (1952). They proposed the use of hypnosis to elicit memories associated with the time of the seizure itself. In their study, none of the subjects suffering from true epilepsy had any recollection of the events associated with the ictal episode. In contrast, 100% of the patients suffering from pseudoseizures recalled the events. This test had a very high correlation with the EEG data obtained at the time of the ictal activity. Ninety-three percent of those diagnosed as epileptic had abnormal EEG recordings, whereas only 7% of those diagnosed as psychogenic had an abnormal EEG.

Years later, Kuyk et al. (1999) obtained similar results. They studied patients with epileptic seizures and patients with pseudoepileptic seizures and, under hypnosis, which was performed by an investigator who was blind to other data, attempted to recover patients' memories of events that had occurred during the ictal episode. If recall was obtained, the experimental diagnosis of pseudoepilepsy was given; if not, epilepsy was diagnosed. These results were then compared with the clinical EEG-confirmed diagnoses. Hypnotizability was measured in all subjects. The authors found that recall for the ictus was obtained in 85% of the patients diagnosed with pseudoepilepsy. None of the patients with the clinical diagnosis of epilepsy recovered any memories. Fifteen of the patients with pseudoepileptic seizures reported no memories for the ictal event. This result yields a specificity of 100% and a sensitivity of 85% for the recall technique.

Kuyk et al. also found that hypnotizability was significantly higher in patients with pseudoepileptic seizures than in patients with epileptic seizures. They suggested that a positive recall test indicates pseudoepileptic seizures. As is the case with EEGs, however, a positive test is positive, but a negative test is inconclusive.

Insomnia

The use of hypnosis to treat insomnia overlaps considerably with the treatment of anxiety disorders. Because hypnosis is not sleep but a form of concentration, it might seem paradoxical to use hypnosis to help people fall asleep. However, hypnosis can be helpful for inducing a state of physical relaxation that is at least compatible with sleep, diminishing the sympathetic arousal usually associated with anxious preoccupation. Thus, patients can be instructed to go into a state of self-hypnosis and induce a sense of floating relaxation physically; then, if preoccupied with arousing or uncomfortable thoughts, they can project these thoughts onto an imaginary screen in the trance state. Patients are instructed to become "traffic directors" for their own thoughts, or to deal with them on the screen, thereby dissociating them from the evoked physical response (H. Spiegel and Spiegel 1987). Such approaches can be helpful in conjunction with standard sleep laboratory approaches, which include keeping the bedroom as a place where work and other anxiety-arousing activities do not occur and avoiding constantly looking at the clock when awakened. It is also important to distinguish routine insomnia due to situational reactions and anxiety from the more severe early-morning awakening associated with depression and from the repeated arousals from sleep that are associated with sleep apnea syndrome. Few results of formal studies have been reported, but most case reports suggest that hypnosis is useful in the treatment of not only primary insomnia but other sleep disturbances as well (Bauer and McCanne 1980; Becker 1993; Schenck and Mahowald 1995).

Applications of Hypnosis in General Medicine

Anxiety With Dental and Medical Procedures

A number of articles have been published concerning the use of hypnosis as an adjunct to dental procedures and in the treatment of dental phobia (Hammarstrand et al. 1995; Lu 1994; Moore et al. 1996; Peretz 1996; Robb and Crothers 1996; Rustvold 1994; Shaw and Niven 1996; Shaw and Welbury 1996; Wilks 1994) and other dental problems, including periodontal disease (G.J. Wood and Zadeh 1999) and temporomandibular joint disease (Simon and Lewis 2000). The success of use of hypnotic techniques in dental work has created a new interest in teaching these techniques in American dental schools (J.H. Clarke 1996; Herod 1995).

Hypnosis has been successfully used to help patients with phobic states tolerate a number of both invasive and noninvasive procedures such as needle injections (Bell et al. 1983), phlebotomy (Dash 1981; Morse and Cohen 1983; Nugent et al. 1984), needle biopsy (Adams and Stenn 1992), lumbar punctures (Kellerman et al. 1983), and bone marrow aspiration (Liossi and Hatira 1999); tolerate the rigors of hemodialysis (Dy and Fabbri 1972); moderate the symptoms of trichotillomania (Fabbri and Dy 1974); manage sexual disorders (Fabbri 1976); and minimize the claustrophobia in cancer patients undergoing external beam radiation therapy (Steggles 1999).

Similarly, hypnotic techniques have been successfully used to assist phobic patients undergoing a number of medical/surgical and diagnostic procedures, thus diminishing the need for excessive anesthesia or antianxiety medication, improving compliance, and eliminating trauma to patients (Cadranel et al. 1994; Chandler 1996; Covino and Frankel 1993; Deyoub 1980; Ellis and Spanos 1994; J.R. Hilgard and LeBaron 1982; Kessler and Dane 1996; Lambert 1996; Lang et al. 1996, 2000; Mize 1996; Rape and Bush 1994).

Hypnosis may be especially helpful as an adjunctive tool for treating these anxiety states because of the ability of the hypnotized person to control somatic response. For example, Cadranel et al. (1994) described the successful use of hypnosis for patients undergoing colonoscopic examination. They were able to use hypnosis in 50% of patients for whom other forms of anesthesia were not available. These patients reported less intense pain than did patients in whom hypnosis was unsuccessful. Cadranel et al. also reported a much better rate of successfully completed colonoscopies (100% versus 50% in the nonhypnotized group). Patients in the hypnosis group were more compliant with further testing later on, compared with only 2% in the nonhypnosis group. Similarly, Zimmerman (1998) reported on the use of relaxation, imagery, and hypnotic suggestions in patients undergoing upper gastrointestinal endoscopy. He found that the use of hypnosis spares the need for pharmacological sedation, thus eliminating the possible hazards of sedation and the need for postsurgical monitoring after the completion of the examination.

In a recent randomized trial of self-hypnosis analgesia plus patient-controlled (pharmacological) analgesia (PCA) versus PCA alone among patients undergoing invasive radiological procedures, those in the hypnosis-plus-PCA condition used one-ninth the amount of medication, experienced less pain and anxiety, and had fewer medical complications compared with patients in the PCA-alone group (Lang et al. 1996). In a larger and more recent randomized trial involving 241 patients, Lang et al. (2000) found that similar patients who were taught self-hypnosis used half the intravenous medication, had half the pain and anxiety, and experienced fewer episodes of autonomic instability in comparison with control patients; in addition, the procedures required, on average, 20 minutes less time to complete for the self-hypnosis patients. Thus, the addition of self-hypnosis training to medical procedures can effectively reduce pain, anxiety, and utilization of medical resources as well.

The hypnotic session may be used initially to demonstrate to patients that they have a greater degree of control over somatic responsiveness than they imagine. It may also be useful to teach these patients to picture on the screen a place that they find intrinsically relaxing so that they can use their memory of, for example, a mountain lake or the beach as a means of providing a respite from anxious preoccupation. They may use the same trance state as a means of facing their concerns, placing an image of an upcoming performance, for example, on one side of the screen while on the other side testing out various strategies for mastering the situation. The pleasant image may be especially useful for medical patients having to undergo procedures. Phobic responses to magnetic resonance imaging (MRI) tests and computed tomography (CT) scans are among the most common types of phobias we encounter. Again, hypnosis has been highly successful in facilitating the performance of imaging procedures, such as MRI and CT (Chandler 1996; Friday and Kubal 1990; Lang et al. 1996; Simon 1999b). Both in preparation and while in the clinic or hospital, patients can enter a state of self-hypnosis and imagine being somewhere they enjoy, thereby dissociating their psychological experience from the physical aspects of the procedure, as in the following case:

> A 39-year-old woman with a brain tumor found herself unable to tolerate the MRI scanner. She felt a sense of panic when she was enclosed in the scanner, and the noise added to her discomfort. She admitted that she was anxious about the result, a possible recurrence of the tumor, but said she was prepared for that and knew she needed to have the scan. She proved to be moderately hypnotizable (6 of 10 on the HIP) and was taught to enter a state of self-hypnosis in which she imagined that she was waterskiing, her favorite sport. She practiced this several times a day and went into that state in the scanner. Imagining that the clanking sound of the scanner was the boat engine, she tolerated the procedure well.

Pain Syndromes and Anesthesia

Pain is the ultimate psychosomatic phenomenon, always representing both tissue injury and the psychological reaction to such injury. The first formal study of the use of hypnosis in pain was performed more than a century ago in India, when a Scottish surgeon named Esdaile (1846/1957) reported 80% surgical anesthesia for amputations using hypnosis. He was immediately censured by his colleagues and 10 years later withdrew the findings when a report came out from Massachusetts General Hospital that ether anesthesia had been 90% effective. Indeed, one of the surgeons strode to the front of the amphitheater and announced, "Gentlemen, this is no humbug!" to distinguish the use of ether from hypnosis.

Nonetheless, it is clear that psychological factors are major variables in the intensity of the pain experience. A century later, at the same hospital, Beecher (1956) demonstrated that the intensity of pain was directly associated with its meaning. To the extent that pain represented threat and the possibility of future disability, it was more intense among civilian surgical patients than it was among a group of combat soldiers to whom the pain of injury meant that they were likely to get out of combat alive.

Behavioral approaches to pain control emphasize changing patterns of social reinforcement that are contingent on pain-related behavior (Fordyce et al. 1973). Pain is classified as primarily operant (i.e., influenced by secondary gain) or respondent (i.e., driven by a noxious physical stimulus). Respondent pain may gradually be transformed into operant pain as attention and sympathy reinforce pain behavior. This process can be reversed through use of positive reinforcement for nonpain behavior. For example, nurses and family members can be trained to pay a great deal of attention to such patients when they increase their activity level or converse about subjects other than their pain. Social contacts involving the pain itself, such as demands for medication, are best kept brief and formal. This approach can be helpful, especially in chronic pain syndromes, in increasing levels of physical activity and diminishing excessive analgesic medication use.

Hypnosis facilitates alteration of the subjective experience of pain (Brose et al. 1997). The techniques most often employed involve physical relaxation coupled with imagery that provides a substitute focus of attention for the painful sensation (Table 30–6). Patients can be taught to develop a comfortable, floating sensation, and highly hypnotizable individuals may simply imagine receiving an injection of novocaine in the affected area, producing a sense of tingling numbness. Some patients prefer to imagine moving the pain to another part of their body or to develop a sensation of floating above their own bodies, creating distance between themselves and the painful sensation. More moderately hypnotizable patients often prefer to focus on a change in temperature, either warmth or coolness, imagining that they are floating in a warm bath or a mountain stream or immersing a painful hand in a bucket of ice chips. That temperature metaphors are usually effective may be related to the fact that pain and temperature fibers run together in the lateral spinothalamic tract, separate from other sensory fibers. Less hypnotizable patients may benefit from distraction techniques in which they concentrate hard on sensations in other parts of their bodies.

TABLE 30–6. Steps used in hypnotic analgesia

---

1. Induce physical relaxation through use of a metaphor such as floating.
2. Alter perception of the pain by
    Inducing dissociation from current sensory experience.
    Imagining a sense of warmth, coolness, tingling, or numbness.
    Focusing attention on sensation in a nonpainful part of the body.
3. Transform the pain.
4. Provide positive reinforcement for symptom improvement.
5. Use a rehabilitation model for treatment.
6. Reduce secondary gain for symptom maintenance.
7. Treat amplifying comorbid conditions:
    Anxiety related to disease progression
    Depression

Regardless of the metaphor selected, certain general principles can be employed with all uses of hypnosis for pain control. The first principle is to teach patients to filter the hurt out of the pain. Patients learn to transform the pain experience by acknowledging that even though it may exist, there is a distinction between the signal itself and the discomfort the signal causes. The hypnotic metaphor helps them transform the signal into one that is less uncomfortable. The second principle is to expand the perceptual options available to patients by having them change from an experience in which either the pain is there or it is not, to one in which they see a third option, which is that the pain is there but it is transformed by the presence of such competing sensations as tingling, numbness, warmth, or coolness. The third principle is to teach patients not to fight the pain. Fighting pain only enhances the pain by focusing attention on it, by enhancing related anxiety and depression, and by

increasing physical tension that can literally put traction on painful parts of the body and increase the pain signals generated peripherally:

> A world-class competition swimmer had collapsed in an alley as a result of hemorrhaging of an undiagnosed lymphoma in his abdomen. During his chemotherapy the patient lay writhing in his bed, screaming with pain and demanding increasing amounts of analgesic medication, even while he was receiving high doses of opiates. The nursing staff reported him to be exceedingly difficult to manage. Found to be moderately hypnotizable, he was taught a self-hypnosis exercise that involved his imagining that he was somewhere he preferred to be.
> "I'm a great swimmer, but I've never surfed," he said.
> "Good, let's go to Hawaii," the physician suggested. The patient continued to wince, but there was a different tone in his voice.
> "What happened?" the physician asked.
> "I fell off the surfboard," he responded.
> "This time, do it right," the physician replied.
> The patient did this self-hypnosis exercise regularly, and 48 hours later he was no longer taking any pain medications and was joking with the nurses in the hallway. A subsequent notation in the medical record stated: "Patient off of pain medication: tumor must be regressing."

Many have already described the usefulness of hypnotic intervention as an adjunct to analgesia (Moskowitz 1996). When Weinstein and Au (1991) used hypnosis in angioplasty patients, they found that it increased patients' tolerance of the procedure. Faymonville et al. (1995) compared the patients' experience of anxiety, pain, and amount of medication required during plastic surgery. Patients in the hypnosis group reported lower levels of intraoperative anxiety and pain during surgery compared with patients receiving conscious intravenous sedation (control group). Both studies found that hypnotized patients required less narcotic pain medication during the procedure in comparison with control subjects.

Meurisse et al. (1996) reported on 108 patients undergoing thyroidectomies (97 partial or unilateral lobectomies; 11 bilateral lobectomies) and 13 undergoing cervical explorations for hyperparathyroidism performed under a hypnosedation technique combining hypnosis and light conscious sedation. Informed consent was obtained from each patient. Despite the fact that none of the patients was screened for hypnotic capacity preoperatively or underwent a preparatory hypnotic session, no patient required conversion to general anesthesia. When the data from the hypnosedation cases were compared with operative data and postoperative courses from a well-matched population ($n = 70$) of patients operated on for thyroid diseases under general anesthesia, the results were extremely positive. Under hypnosedation, mortality was zero and surgical management was complicated only by unilateral definitive recurrent laryngeal nerve paralysis in one case (0.8%) and the need for neck reexploration for severe hematoma after parathyroidectomy in another case. Hyperparathyroidism was cured in all cases. The surgeons all reported better operating conditions for cervicotomy with hypnosedation ($P < 0.01$). Compared with patients who underwent neck surgery under general anesthesia, the hypnosedation group reported greater satisfaction with the surgical procedure, required less analgesics postoperatively, and had a shorter hospital stay, providing a substantial reduction in medical care cost. Patients in the hypnosedative group also experienced less postoperative fatigue syndrome and had a shorter surgical convalescence and thus were able return sooner to full social or professional activity.

A study comparing the effectiveness of hypnosis versus stress-reducing strategies (control) in patients ($n = 60$) undergoing elective plastic surgery under conscious sedation was conducted by Faymonville et al. (1997). Subjects were randomly allocated to one of the two treatments for the entire surgical procedure. Patients' behavior was monitored during surgery by a psychologist, and patients were asked to score their levels of anxiety; pain; perceived control before, during, and after surgery; postoperative nausea and vomiting; and overall level of satisfaction with intraoperative pain control and surgical conditions. The researchers found that peri- and postoperative levels of anxiety and pain were significantly lower in the hypnosis group. The reductions in the levels of anxiety and pain were achieved despite a significant reduction in intraoperative requirements for midazolam and opiates in the hypnosis group. Also, patients in the hypnosis group reported greater feelings of intraoperative control than did those in the control group ($P < 0.01$). Postoperative nausea and vomiting were also significantly reduced in the hypnosis group (6.5% vs. 30.8%, $P < 0.001$). Similarly, vital signs were more stable, overall surgical conditions were better, and fewer signs of patient discomfort and pain were observed by the psychologist in the hypnosis group ($P < 0.001$). As expected, the patient satisfaction score was significantly higher in the hypnosis group ($P < 0.004$).

Recently, Mauer et al. (1999) conducted a study ($n = 60$) in orthopedic patients who had undergone hand surgery. Patients received either usual treatment or usual treatment plus hypnosis. After controlling for gender, race, and pretreatment scores, the group receiving hypnosis showed significant decreases in measures of perceived pain intensity, perceived pain affect, and state anxiety. In addition, the experimental group experienced

significantly fewer medical complications and demonstrated enhanced postsurgical recovery and rehabilitation in comparison with the control group. Similarly, physicians' ratings of progress were significantly higher for the experimental subjects than for the control subjects.

Similarly, Meurisse et al. (1999) subjected a group of patients ($n = 31$) to a conventional bilateral neck exploration procedure under local anesthesia and hypnosedation (i.e., hypnosis-induced analgesia). A hypnotic state (immobility, subjective well-being, and increased pain thresholds) was induced within 10 minutes; restoration of a fully conscious state was obtained within several seconds after termination of the trance. The researchers found that no patients who had the surgery while under hypnoanalgesia required conversion to general anesthesia. No complications were observed. Despite minimal use of anesthesia, hypnosedation was so effective that it allowed for extensive neck exploration, with up to four glands identified in 84% of cases. The mean operating time was less than 1 hour. All patients rated their level of comfort, recovery, and surgical condition as excellent. Postoperative analgesic consumption was minimal, with a mean length of hospital stay of 1.5 days (± 0.5 days).

Other types of pain syndromes reported to be responsive to hypnotic manipulation include those associated with burns (Ohrbach et al. 1998; Patterson et al. 1997), limb fracture reduction (Iserson 1999), chronic tension-type headache (Gysin 1999; Spinhoven and ter Kuile 2000), and migraine headache (Matthews and Flatt 1999). Andreychuk and Skriver (1975) found that hypnotizability not only was a predictor of treatment response for migraine headaches, but also was a correlate of pretreatment symptom severity. That is, more highly hypnotizable individuals complained of more severe migraine symptoms before treatment but responded better to intervention.

A recent meta-analysis of 18 published studies (Montgomery et al. 2000) examined the effectiveness of hypnosis in pain management by comparing studies that evaluated hypnotic pain reduction in healthy volunteers against studies that used patient samples. Comparison of the effectiveness of hypnoanalgesic effects and participants' degree of hypnotic suggestibility revealed a moderate to large hypnoanalgesic effect. These results suggest that the greater the subject's hypnotic capacity (i.e., suggestibility), the more effective the analgesic effect produced by hypnotic suggestion, supporting the efficacy of hypnotic techniques for pain management. The results also indicated that hypnotic suggestion was equally effective in reducing both clinical and experimental pain.

In 1996, a nonfederal, nonadvocate, 12-member panel representing the fields of family medicine, social medicine, psychiatry, psychology, public health, nursing, and epidemiology met for the purpose of providing physicians with a responsible assessment of the integration of behavioral and relaxation approaches into the treatment of chronic pain. Twenty-three experts in behavioral medicine, pain medicine, sleep medicine, psychiatry, nursing, psychology, neurology, and the behavioral and neurosciences presented data to the panel during a 1½-day public session. The panel concluded that a number of well-defined behavioral and relaxation interventions are effective in the treatment of chronic pain and insomnia, and that strong evidence exists for the use of relaxation techniques and hypnosis for pain resulting from a variety of medical conditions, including cancer. The evidence was moderate for the effectiveness of cognitive-behavioral techniques and biofeedback in relieving chronic pain. The panel's results and recommendations were published in the *Journal of the American Medical Association* (National Institutes of Health [NIH] Technology Assessment Panel 1996).

Consistent with these findings, Faymonville et al. (1998) described their experiences using hypnosis (over a period of 6 years) in more than 1,400 patients undergoing surgery. These authors reported that when hypnosis was used as an adjunct to conscious sedation and local anesthesia, patients reported improved intraoperative comfort; reduced anxiety, pain, and intraoperative requirements for anxiolytic and analgesic drugs; optimal surgical conditions; and a faster postsurgical recovery time.

For children undergoing painful procedures, the main focus is on imagery rather than relaxation, because they are highly hypnotizable and are easily absorbed in images. Some find it helpful to play in an imaginary baseball game, to picture themselves going to another room in the house, or to imagine themselves watching a favorite television show. Another useful technique is for them to imagine that they are visiting their favorite amusement part, playground, or friend's house. This enables them to restructure their experience of what is going on and dissociate themselves psychologically from pain and fear of the procedure. It is helpful to have parents assisting and to go through several rehearsals of the procedure so that the children do not encounter anything unfamiliar. This helps parents as well to feel more effective in comforting their children. Hypnosis has successfully been used in children to significantly reduce the pain associated with invasive procedures (J.R. Hilgard and LeBaron 1982; Iserson 1999; Liossi and Hatira 1999; Zeltzer and LeBaron 1982). The use of imagery techniques with suggestions for a favorable postoperative course has been associated with markedly lower postoperative pain rat-

ings and shorter hospital stays (Lambert 1996). Many recently published articles have addressed the use of hypnosis for pain control in children; thus, these specific techniques will not be discussed here (Celestin-L'hopiteau 2000; Kuttner 1991, 1993; Maldonado and Spiegel 2000b).

The neurophysiological mechanisms of hypnotic analgesia are still under debate. Notwithstanding, hypnotic analgesia seems to work through two mechanisms: *physical relaxation* and *attention control*. Patients in pain tend to splint the painful area instinctively, and yet this enhanced muscle tension around a painful area often increases pain. Most patients find that they can enhance their physical response by focusing on a variety of images that connote physical relaxation, such as a sense of floating. Second, because hypnosis involves an intensification and narrowing of the focus of attention, it allows individuals to place pain at the periphery of their awareness by putting some competing metaphor or sensation at the center of their attention. Thus, by focusing on a memory of dental anesthesia and spreading that numbness to the affected area, making the area warmer or cooler, substituting a sense of tingling or lightness, or focusing on sensation in some nonpainful part of the body, hypnotized individuals can diminish the amount of attention they pay to painful stimuli.

Miller and Bowers (1993) challenged the notion of pure social compliance as the mechanism of action of hypnotic analgesia. They compared the extent of pain reduction produced by hypnotic analgesia with that produced by a stress-inoculation procedure, in a group of highly and poorly hypnotizable subjects. They found that stress inoculation but not hypnotic analgesia impaired performance of a cognitively demanding task that competed with pain reduction for cognitive resources. This finding suggests that hypnotic analgesia occurs with little or no cognitive effort to reduce pain. The results do support the notion of dissociated control, which proposes that suggestions for analgesic relief during hypnosis directly activate pain reduction and thereby avert the need for cognitive strategies to reduce pain. That this hypnotic analgesia is not merely social compliance but involves neurophysiological changes in information processing is suggested by cortical event-related potential (ERP) studies. In these studies, highly hypnotizable individuals could diminish the P100 and P300 components of their event-related response to a somatosensory stimulus by focusing on a hallucinated image that would block their perception of the stimulus (D. Spiegel et al. 1989; Figure 30–7). This cortical attention deployment mechanism is at the moment the most plausible explanation, although a number of studies have tested the idea that

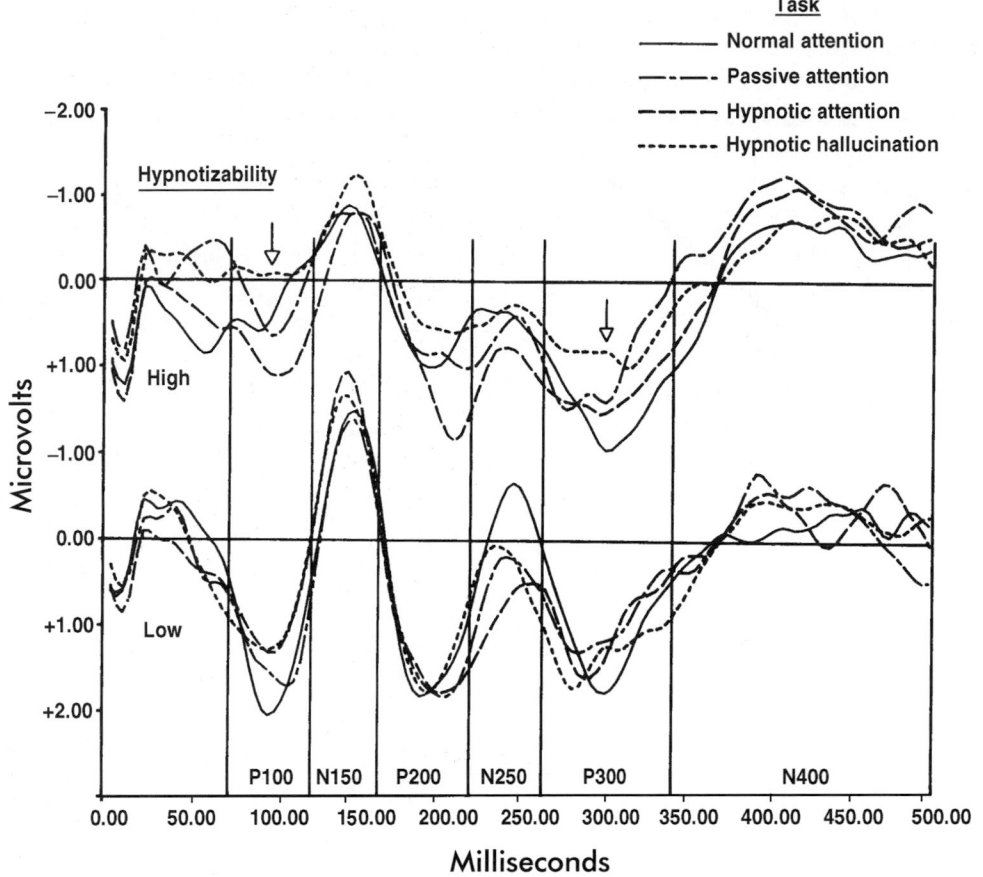

FIGURE 30–7. Somatosensory event-related potentials among 10 highly hypnotizable and 10 poorly hypnotizable individuals.

Hypnotic obstructive hallucination results in reduction of P100 and P300 amplitudes, whereas hypnotic attention is associated with an increase in P100 amplitude.

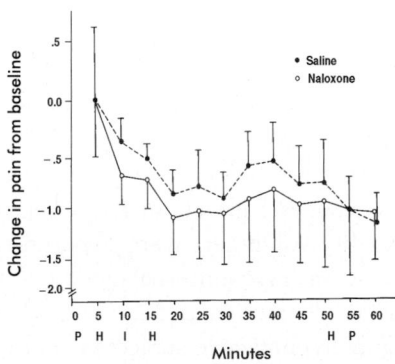

FIGURE 30–8. Effect of naloxone on the hypnotic reduction in clinical pain.

Hypnotic reduction in physical pain is not blocked by naloxone: 10 mg of naloxone, given in a double-blind, crossover design, does not block and reverse hypnotic analgesia. H = hypnotic analgesia exercise; I = injection of naloxone or saline; P = mood assessment.

endogenous opiates are involved in hypnotic analgesia. With one partial exception (Frid and Singer 1979), studies with both volunteers (E. Goldstein and Hilgard 1975) and patients in chronic pain (D. Spiegel and Albert 1983) have shown that hypnotic analgesia is not blocked or reversed by a substantial dose of naloxone given in double-blind, crossover fashion (Figure 30–8).

Kiernan et al. (1995) reported that hypnotic analgesia may act through one of two neurological mechanisms: a reduction of RIII nociceptive reflex, which is related to spinal cord antinociceptive mechanisms; or reductions in pain sensation over and beyond reductions in RIII, which may be related to brain mechanisms that serve to prevent awareness of pain signals once nociception has reached higher centers. Whatever the mechanism, hypnotic analgesia is efficacious (Dahlgren et al. 1995; Faymonville et al. 1995; Genuis 1995; Hargadon et al. 1995). Systematic studies have demonstrated that hypnosis is superior to an attentional control condition for analgesia among

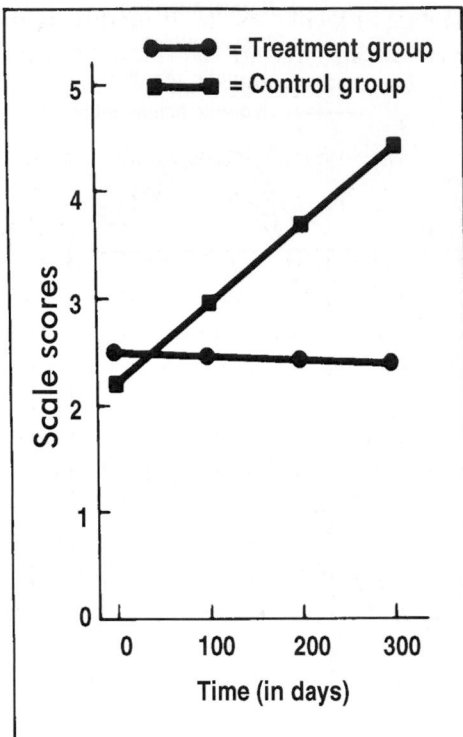 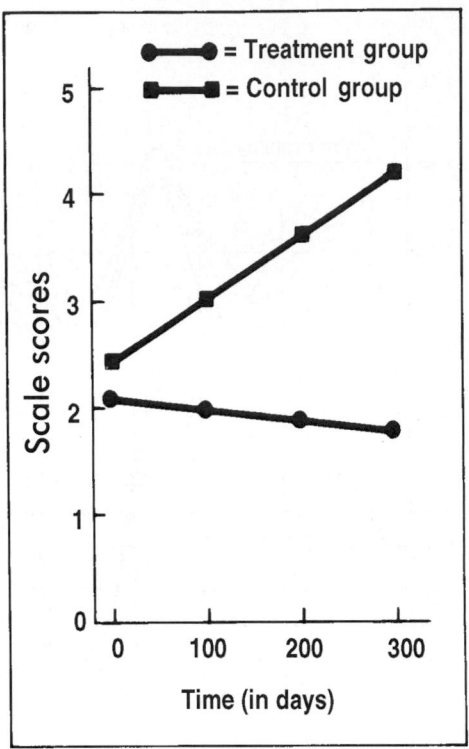

FIGURE 30–9.   Reduction of cancer pain with hypnosis.

Changes in pain sensation *(left)* and suffering *(right)* among 54 women with metastatic breast cancer randomized to weekly treatment with group support and training in self-hypnosis or to a control condition. Note doubling of pain in the control group but reduction of pain in the treatment group.

Source.   Reprinted with permission from Spiegel D: "The Use of Hypnosis in Controlling Cancer Pain." *CA: A Cancer Journal for Clinicians* 35:221–231, 1985.

children undergoing painful procedures (Zeltzer and LeBaron 1982). Furthermore, in a randomized prospective study, a combination of hypnosis and group psychotherapy was shown to result in a 50% reduction in pain among metastatic breast cancer patients (D. Spiegel and Bloom 1983; Figure 30–9), and there was a corresponding reduction in mood disturbance (D. Spiegel et al. 1981). Hypnotic analgesia has also been shown to be more potent than either placebo analgesia (McGlashan et al. 1969) or acupuncture analgesia (Knox and Shum 1977), although there is a correlation between hypnotizability and responsiveness to acupuncture (Katz et al. 1974). Thus, hypnotic mechanisms of pain control may be mobilized by other treatment techniques, but the explicit use of hypnosis with hypnotizable patients has proved to be a more powerful means of controlling pain.

In a review of studies, E.R. Hilgard and Hilgard (1975) estimated a 0.5 correlation between hypnotizability and treatment responsiveness for pain control. The ability of hypnotizable individuals to focus their attention

and to alter their responses to perceptions while at the same time producing a physical state of relaxation allows them to restructure their experience of pain and thereby develop a sense of mastery over it. Because the pain experience is both psychological and physical, this technique mobilizes and focuses cognitive experience while producing a sense of physical relaxation.

In a study that attempted to test the mechanism underlying the analgesic effects of hypnosis, high- and low-hypnotizability volunteers were exposed to a cold-pressor pain test during counterbalanced conditions of waking relaxation, distraction, and hypnosis (Freeman et al. 2000). Highly hypnotizable subjects experienced significantly greater pain relief during hypnosis than during the distraction or waking-relaxation conditions; they also demonstrated significantly greater pain relief in response to hypnosis than did poorly hypnotizable subjects. Quantitative EEG findings revealed significantly greater high-theta (5.5–7.5 Hz) activity for high-hypnotizability subjects than for low-hypnotizability subjects at parietal

(P3) and occipital (O1) sites during both hypnosis and waking-relaxation conditions. These findings provide additional support for the neodissociation theory and for state-based theories of hypnosis.

Crawford et al. (1998) studied adults ($n = 15$) with chronic (mean 4 years) low-back pain, all of whom were moderately to highly hypnotizable. All of the patients achieved significant reduction in perceived pain after receiving instructions for inducing hypnotic analgesia during cold-pressor pain training. In the first part of the study, somatosensory event-related potential (SERP) correlates of noxious electrical stimulation were evaluated during attend and hypnotic analgesia conditions at anterior frontal (Fp1, Fp2), midfrontal (F3, F4), central (C3, C4), and parietal (P3, P4) regions. During hypnotic analgesia, hypothesized inhibitory processing was evidenced by enhanced N140 in the anterior frontal region and by a prestimulus positive-ongoing contingent cortical potential at Fp1; decreased spatiotemporal perception was evidenced by reduced P200 (bilateral midfrontal and central, and left parietal) and P300 (right midfrontal and central) amplitudes. Hypnotic analgesia led to highly significant mean reductions in perceived sensory pain and distress. These results suggest that hypnotic analgesia is an active process that requires inhibitory effort, dissociated from conscious awareness, in which the anterior frontal cortex participates in a topographically specific inhibitory feedback circuit that cooperates in the allocation of thalamocortical activities. In the second part of the study, subjects were evaluated on their ability to successfully apply newly learned skills in experimental pain reduction to reduction of their own chronic pain. Subjects reported diminished chronic pain, enhanced psychological well-being, and improved sleep quality.

In an effort to explore the effects of hypnosis on both pain perception and heterotopic nociceptive stimulation, high- and low-hypnotizability subjects were first randomly assigned to either a control session or a session of hypnotic analgesia while the nociceptive flexion reflex (RIII) was recorded from the biceps femoris muscle in response to stimulation of the sural nerve (Sandrini et al. 2000). The subjective pain threshold, the RIII reflex threshold, and the mean area with suprathreshold stimulation were measured. Heterotopic nociceptive stimulation was examined with the cold-pressor test. During and immediately after the test, the subjective pain threshold, pain tolerance, and mean RIII area were again measured. The same examinations were then repeated during hypnosis. The authors found that in highly hypnotizable subjects, hypnosis significantly reduced subjective pain perception and the nociceptive flexion reflex; it also increased pain tolerance and reduced pain perception

and the nociceptive reflex during the cold-pressor test. Both hypnosis and diffuse noxious inhibitory controls (DNICs) were capable of modifying the perception of pain. In fact, it seems likely that DNICs and hypnosis use the same descending inhibitory pathways for the control of pain.

In a recent study, Benhaiem et al. (2001) obtained thermal detection thresholds for warm and cool stimuli and then measured heat pain thresholds at both the upper and lower left limbs before, during, and after a hypnotic session during which subjects ($n = 32$) were given standardized suggestions of analgesia limited to the left foot. The researchers found that heat pain thresholds were significantly increased at both the lower and upper limbs, suggesting that hypnotic suggestions may selectively and somatotopically alter pain sensation in highly susceptible subjects.

Hypnosis has long been used as the sole anesthetic agent or as an adjunct to conventional anesthesia during minor surgical procedures. In fact, some researchers have proposed that positive suggestion and hypnotic techniques can unequivocally benefit all patients who undergo surgical and obstetrical procedures with modern general or regional anesthesia. Such proposals have in turn prompted others to stipulate that "rather than regarding hypnotic suggestion as a mere adjunct to anesthesia, it should be regarded as an integral part of surgical and obstetrical care" (Erickson 1994).

Gastrointestinal Disorders

Many published articles have addressed the use of hypnosis in the treatment of gastrointestinal disorders. Hypnosis has been reported as successful in ulcerative colitis and related conditions (Schafer 1997), irritable bowel syndrome (IBS) (Francis and Houghton 1996; Houghton et al. 1996; Snape 1994; Whorwell et al. 1984, 1987), dysphagia (Kopel and Quinn 1996), uncontrolled belching (S.B. Spiegel 1996), and peptic ulcer disease (Colgan et al. 1988; Francis and Houghton 1996; Klein and Spiegel 1989). Hypnosis has been repeatedly used with great success in the treatment of emesis, of all causes and in both children (Keller 1995) and adults (Covino and Frankel 1993; Faymonville et al. 1995; Renouf 1998). Zeltzer et al. (1984) reported significant reduction in chemotherapy-induced nausea and vomiting among 19 patients who had been taught hypnosis. Hypnosis has been reported not only to help in the treatment of acute emesis associated with chemotherapy treatment (Genuis 1995; J.R. Hilgard and LeBaron 1982; Jacknow et al. 1994) but also to prevent anticipatory anxiety and emesis associated with cancer therapy (Marchioro et al. 2000; Redd et al. 1982). Even hyperemesis gravidarum and morning sickness have been reported to respond well to hypnotic intervention (Baram 1995; Fuchs et al. 1980; Iancu et al. 1994; Simon 1999a; Simon and Schwartz 1999; Torem 1994).

Relaxation instructions have been helpful for some patients with stress-related bowel disease, such as ulcerative colitis and regional enteritis. Patients have found it helpful to imagine in trance something soothing in the gut; such imagining giving them a sense of control over a symptom that makes them feel especially helpless, thereby diminishing the cycle of reactive anxiety. In a well-conducted randomized trial (Whorwell et al. 1984, 1987) 15 patients with IBS who were treated with hypnosis reported significant improvement in pain, abdominal distension, and diarrhea, as well as emotional well-being, compared with a control group of 15 patients. An 18-month follow-up of 15 of these patients revealed continued remission, and the authors reported similar improvement in 35 additional patients (Houghton et al. 1996).

Six matched pairs of IBS patients were randomly assigned to either a "gut-directed" hypnotherapy or a symptom-monitoring wait-list control condition in a multiple baseline–across–subjects design wherein those assigned to the control condition were later crossed over to the treatment condition (Barabasz et al. 1999). After concurrent psychiatric diagnoses, susceptibility to hypnosis, and various demographic features were controlled, hypnosis treatment was found to be superior ($P < 0.016$) to symptom monitoring. Patients treated with hypnosis reported that symptoms of abdominal pain, constipation, and flatulence were all significantly improved. Similarly, state and trait anxiety scores were seen to decrease significantly after treatment. Treatment gains continued throughout the 2-month follow-up.

In another study in treatment-resistant IBS patients ($n = 27$) (Vidakovic-Vukic 1999), 89% of those treated with "gut-oriented" hypnosis therapy experienced clear improvement—that is, pain and flatulence were reduced or disappeared completely, and bowel habits normalized. More recently, Forbes et al. (2000) compared the effectiveness of "gut-directed hypnotherapy" (six sessions) and a specially devised audiotape intervention in a randomized controlled trial ($n = 52$) of IBS patients during a 12-week study. All patients had previously failed to respond to dietary and pharmacological therapy, and their median symptom duration was 60 months. Successful trance was induced in all hypnotherapy patients. Forbes et al. found that symptom scores improved in 76% of the hypnotherapy patients compared with 59% of the audiotape patients. In addition, a reduction in median symptom score, from 14.0 to 8.5, was seen in hypnother-

apy patients, compared with an unchanged score of 13 in audiotape patients ($P < 0.05$).

Klein and Spiegel (1989) observed significant hypnotic control of gastric acid secretion among 28 highly hypnotizable subjects. When these patients were hypnotized and instructed to eat an imaginary meal, basal acid output increased 89%. In another trial designed to test reduction in acid output, subjects were instructed to use hypnosis to experience deep relaxation. There was a notable 39% decrease in basal acid output. In a third trial, subjects were given an injection of pentagastrin, which stimulates maximal parietal cell output. There was still a marked 11% reduction in pentagastrin-stimulated peak acid output during hypnosis. This study further emphasizes the fact that high hypnotizability is a two-edged sword, in that it may increase or decrease a given physiological parameter, depending on the mental content during the hypnotic state. That these observations may have clinical relevance is illustrated by the findings of a controlled trial of hypnosis in relapse prevention of duodenal ulcers (Colgan et al. 1988). Thirty patients with rapidly relapsing ulcer disease were randomly assigned, after administration of ranitidine, to hypnosis treatment or no treatment. All of the control subjects but only 53% of the hypnosis patients relapsed. More recently, several articles reported the benefits of hypnosis in the treatment of ulcer disease (Francis and Houghton 1996). Thus, hypnosis seems to be an effective adjunct to the management of some gastrointestinal disorders.

Respiratory Disorders

Several articles have reported on the usefulness of hypnosis for a variety of respiratory and pulmonary problems. A number of these have addressed the efficacy of hypnosis in helping asthmatic patients (Aronoff et al. 1975; P.S. Clarke 1970; Collison 1975; Ewer and Stewart 1986; Hackman et al. 2000; Inoue et al. 1995; Kelly and Zeller 1969; Kohen 1986; Kohen and Wynne 1997; Luparello et al. 1968; Maher-Loughnan 1970; McFadden et al. 1969; Moorefield 1971; Morrison 1988; Mun 1969; Smith et al. 1970). Patients can learn to use self-hypnotic techniques rather than medication when they begin to feel an anxiety-precipitated asthmatic attack coming on. This may help interrupt the vicious cycle of anxiety and bronchoconstriction. A common technique is to have asthmatic patients enter a state of self-hypnosis and imagine that they are somewhere where they naturally breathe easily, such as on a beach breathing cool ocean spray (H. Spiegel and Spiegel 1987).

Studies have shown that there is a correlation between hypnotizability and treatment response in asthmatic patients (Collison 1975). In his sample, Collison

(1975) found that one-fifth of his asthma patients experienced "complete symptom resolution" and that one-third had "considerable improvement in symptoms" after hypnotic treatment and training. In a randomized, controlled trial, Ewer and Stewart (1986) studied 39 adults with mild to moderate asthma. After brief treatment with hypnosis, patients with a high hypnotizability score showed marked improvement (74.9%) in the degree of bronchial hyperresponsiveness to a standardized methacholine challenge test. The use of bronchodilators decreased by 26.2%.

Morrison (1988) described dramatic improvements in treatment-resistant chronic asthma patients. After hypnotic treatment and training, patients reported a two-thirds decline in the number of hospital admissions due to complications of asthma. In addition, they reported a decreased need for steroid medications, reduced lengths of hospital stays, and overall improvement in their perception of illness. Similar responses have been described in pediatric asthma patients (Aronoff et al. 1975; Gluzman and Zisel'son 1989; Kohen 1987).

Anbar (2000) reported on the utility of teaching self-hypnosis to patients with cystic fibrosis. In his sample ($n = 49$), patients successfully used self-hypnosis for symptom control 86% of the time. No patients reported worsening of symptoms due to the use of hypnosis (i.e., there were no adverse effects). More than 30% of the patients continued to practice hypnosis on their own for 6 months or longer. Many of the patients used hypnosis for more than one purpose, such as for relaxation (61% of patients), relief of pain associated with medical procedures (31%), headache relief (16%), changing the taste of medications to make them more palatable (10%), and control of other symptoms associated with cystic fibrosis (18%), thus demonstrating that patients can learn to use hypnosis to enhance their control over discomforts associated with cystic fibrosis and its therapy.

In a separate study, Anbar (2001) used self-hypnosis training to help children and adolescents ($n = 16$) to deal with chronic dyspnea (mean duration 2 years) that had been determined to be of psychogenic (i.e., not organic) origin. Patients were taught self-hypnosis in one or two 30-minute sessions and were encouraged to practice at home. After 1 month of hypnosis training, 82% of the subjects reported that their dyspnea and associated symptoms had resolved. The remaining patients reported that their symptoms had improved. At a follow-up 9 months after hypnosis training, the authors found that there was no recurrence of dyspnea, associated symptoms, or onset of new symptoms in patients in whom the dyspnea resolved.

Jacavone and Young (1998) reported on the use of hypnosis, guided imagery, and biofeedback to help "difficult-to-wean" patients discontinue use of ventilators in the critical care setting. Anbar and Hehir (2000) described the use of hypnosis for diagnosis and treatment of psychogenic vocal cord dysfunction.

Dermatological Disorders

Psychogenic factors have been implicated in essentially all skin diseases (Arone di Bertolino 1983; Elitzur and Brenner 1986; Gherardi et al. 1993; R.F. Johnson 1980; Tobia 1982; Tsushima 1988). As reported by Bellini (1998) and Shenefelt (2000), a wide spectrum of dermatological disorders may be improved or cured with hypnosis, including acne excoriee, alopecia areata, atopic dermatitis, congenital ichthyosiform erythroderma, dyshidrotic dermatitis, erythromelalgia, furuncles, glossodynia, herpes simplex, hyperhidrosis, ichthyosis vulgaris, lichen planus, neurodermatitis, nummular dermatitis, postherpetic neuralgia, pruritus, psoriasis, rosacea, trichotillomania, urticaria, verruca vulgaris, and vitiligo. More specifically, hypnosis has been shown to be helpful in the treatment of multiple dermatological conditions, in particular pruritus (Arone di Bertolino 1983), eczema (Hájek et al. 1990), scleroderma (Seikowski et al. 1995), warts (Arone di Bertolino 1983; Ewin 1992; Spanos et al. 1988, 1990; Steele and Irwin 1988), and psoriasis (Kantor 1990; Winchell and Watts 1988).

Shertzer and Lookingbill (1987) studied the effects of hypnosis in patients with chronic urticaria (i.e., of over 7 years' duration) and found that hypnosis sessions produced relief of pruritus as measured by self-report parameters. All subjects were treated with hypnosis, regardless of their level of hypnotizability, but highly hypnotizable subjects had fewer hives and more frequently reported stress as a causative factor of their outbreaks.

Warts have been treated with hypnosis (Ewin 1992), and one carefully controlled study demonstrated that simple hypnotic instructions to the effect that the warts would tingle and disappear resulted in a rate of improvement that was substantially better than the spontaneous remission rate for warts (Surman et al. 1973). Studies employing hypnosis in the treatment of warts have reported success rates ranging from 27% (R.F. Johnson and Barber 1978) to 80% (Ewin 1992). Other studies have shown specific benefits of hypnosis over simple task-motivating instructions in the elimination of warts (Spanos et al. 1988, 1990). Stewart and Thomas (1995) described statistically significant subjective and objective benefits after hypnosis treatment ($P < 0.01$) for 18 adults with extensive atopic dermatitis previously resistant to conventional treatment. Equally important, treatment gains were maintained during a 2-year follow-up.

Tausk and Whitmore (1999) conducted a 3-month randomized, single-blind, controlled trial to evaluate the effects of hypnosis on adults with stable, chronic, plaque-type psoriasis. Subjects were selected for high or moderate hypnotizability and were randomized to receive either hypnosis with active suggestions of improvement or neutral hypnosis with no mention of their disease process, followed by an additional 3 months of hypnosis treatment with active suggestions of improvement for all patients. The highly hypnotizable subjects experienced significantly greater improvement than did than the moderately hypnotizable subjects, independent of the treatment group assignment (active suggestion or neutral hypnosis).

Smoking Cessation

Hypnosis has been employed as an adjunctive tool with a variety of habit-control strategies, primarily for smoking cessation (Table 30–7). It has been used to 1) provide a kind of substitute physical relaxation for the momentary respite that accompanies inhaling a cigarette, 2) enhance self-observation and self-monitoring, 3) provide positive reinforcement for behavior change, 4) diminish the positive reinforcement provided by smoking itself, and 5) facilitate cognitive restructuring of the smoking habit. Hypnosis has been employed in both group and individual settings. More recently, the emphasis has been on teaching patients self-hypnosis rather than having multiple sessions with a therapist. Although some dramatic, immediate results can occur when the patient is being instructed that he or she will find the cigarette distasteful or feel physically uncomfortable while inhaling, such approaches can create unnecessary dependency on the therapist. It is helpful to find a strategy that is intrinsically self-reinforcing and meaningful to the patient and that can be practiced whenever the urge to smoke comes on the patient. One cognitive restructuring model involves emphasizing that smoking is destructive specifically to the patient's body and thereby limits what the patient can do with his or her life. The focus in hypnosis is then on protecting the patient's body from poison in the same way that the patient would protect an infant or a pet from ingesting noxious food. This approach enables the patient to balance the urge to smoke against the urge to protect his or her body from damage—in other words, the focus is on what the patient is *for* rather than what he or she is *against* (H. Spiegel 1970).

No single psychological approach to smoking cessation has been proven to be superior to others. Nevertheless, psychological interventions have been found to contribute significantly to successful treatment outcome in smoking cessation. The available data from clinical and

TABLE 30–7. Objectives of the use of hypnosis in smoking cessation treatment

1. Provide an alternative means of inducing physical relaxation.
2. Enhance self-observation and self-monitoring.
3. Provide positive reinforcement for behavior change.
4. Diminish the positive reinforcement provided by smoking itself.
5. Facilitate cognitive restructuring of the smoking habit.

experimental research studies have been discussed and summarized elsewhere (Covino and Bottari 2001). Factors that account for the utility of hypnosis as an adjunct to smoking cessation treatment include 1) enhanced responsiveness to suggestion (Rabkin et al. 1984; H. Spiegel and Spiegel 1987); 2) alteration of unconscious motivation to smoke (Rabkin et al. 1984); 3) immediate symptom relief (Orne 1977); 4) nonspecific ceremonial, expectational, and placebo factors (Orne 1977); 5) enhanced ability to focus attention on the treatment strategy (Frischholz and Spiegel 1986); and 6) facilitation of ongoing self-administration through self-hypnosis (H. Spiegel and Spiegel 1987).

The generally accepted criterion for evaluating treatment interventions for smoking is complete abstinence at 6 months rather than reduction in smoking. Results of various trials of hypnosis in treatment indicate quit rates ranging from 13% to 64% with individual interventions and a follow-up time of at least 6 months (Crasilneck and Hall 1968; Holroyd 1980, 1991; Hyman et al. 1986; Schwartz 1987, 1991; H. Spiegel 1970; Williams and Hall 1988). The single-session approach developed by H. Spiegel (1970) is widely used (Schwartz 1987, 1991) and produces long-term complete abstinence rates of 20%–35% when undertaken by him (H. Spiegel 1970; H. Spiegel and Spiegel 1987) and others (Ahijevych et al. 2000; Barabasz et al. 1986; Berkowitz et al. 1979; Frank et al. 1986; see Figure 30–10). Abstinence rates as high as 40% at 6 months have been reported (Hyman et al. 1986; Williams and Hall 1988).

These abstinence rates are superior to the rates of unassisted quitting (Gritz and Bloom 1987). In addition, hypnotizability has been shown to predict better outcome (Barabasz et al. 1986; D. Spiegel et al. 1993a; H. Spiegel and Spiegel 1987). Thus, although in general there is no evidence that treatments employing hypnosis are more effective than other interventions for smoking, they may well be more efficient in that they enable patients to employ self-hypnosis to reinforce a cognitive restructuring strategy while at the same time they provide an episode of physical relaxation.

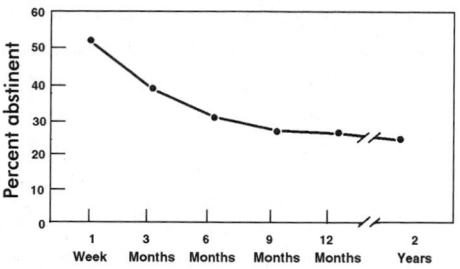

FIGURE 30–10. Percentage of patients taught a single-session, self-hypnosis restructuring strategy to stop smoking who remained continuously abstinent up to follow-up at 2 years.

Weight Control

Hypnosis has been employed as an adjunct to a comprehensive dietary and exercise control program for weight reduction and management. The same restructuring principles discussed previously can be applied to overeating: experiencing an excess of food as damaging to the body, and learning to eat with respect for one's body. Again, this involves focusing on what the patient is *for*—rather than being *against* food. Indeed, an important component of such an approach can be to teach the patient to use self-hypnosis training to control the urge to overeat by preparing a list of foods that constitute eating with respect and then comparing an urge with the foods on the list. If the desired food is on the list, the patient is encouraged to eat it like a gourmet, focusing intently on all aspects of the eating experience. If the food is not on the list, rather than fight the urge, the patient is encouraged to use self-hypnosis to compare it with his or her overall commitment to treat the body with respect and therefore to eat with respect. Patients can thus deal with the desire to eat not as an occasion to feel deprivation but rather as one in which they are enhancing their mastery of the urge by focusing on protecting their body. In addition, hypnosis can be used to help patients provide positive self-reinforcement for compliance with a revised eating regimen (Crasilneck and Hall 1985). It is also useful to have patients concentrate on heightening their responsiveness to internal signals of hunger and satiety: "Eat when you are hungry, and stop eating when you are full."

Clinical experience suggests that persons within 20% of their ideal body weight may obtain some benefit from such restructuring techniques with self-hypnosis in addition to careful attention to diet and exercise. There is evidence that treatment employing hypnosis is effective (Barabasz and Spiegel 1989; Stradling et al. 1998). In a

meta-analysis of studies on the effect of adding hypnosis to cognitive-behavioral treatments for weight reduction, Kirsch (1996) and colleagues (1995) found that the mean weight loss in the hypnosis group was twice that of the group treated without hypnosis. His findings further indicated that the benefits of hypnosis increase substantially over time. Furthermore, hypnotizability has been shown to be correlated with weight reduction in some studies (Anderson 1985).

In general, outcome studies show some overlap between behavioral techniques and hypnosis in both structure and outcome. For example, Kirsch and colleagues (Kirsch 1996; Kirsch et al. 1995) conducted a meta-analysis of 18 studies in which a cognitive-behavioral therapy was compared with the same therapy supplemented with hypnosis. Results indicated that the addition of hypnosis substantially enhanced treatment outcome. The average patient receiving cognitive-behavioral therapy with hypnosis showed greater improvement—about twice the weight loss—than at least 70% of the patients receiving nonhypnotic treatment (mean weight loss was 11.83 lb [5.37 kg] for the hypnosis group and 6.00 lb [2.72 kg] for the group receiving cognitive treatment without hypnosis). The effects of hypnotic intervention seemed especially pronounced at long-term follow-up, which indicates that unlike those in nonhypnotic treatment, patients in whom the hypnotic state had been induced continued to lose weight after the treatment ended ($r = 0.74$). Both approaches—behavioral techniques and hypnosis—involve the use of imagery and restructuring of cognition about the feared stimulus coupled with a means of producing physical relaxation. Hypnosis can be most effective when it is used to enhance patients' sense of mastery and control over psychological experience as well as their somatic response to such experience.

Neurophysiological Aspects of Hypnosis

Efforts to identify neurobiological correlates of the hypnotic state and trait have been frustrating but not unrewarding. The belief that hypnotizability is biologically based dates at least as far back as 1880, to Rudolf Heidenhain, who explained hypnosis physiologically in terms of cortical inhibition. Between 1877 and 1884, Pavlov studied, under Heidenhain, hypnotic phenomena during conditioned reflex experiments. Later, in 1910, Pavlov described hypnotic states and explained them in terms of partial inhibition of the cortex (Windholz

1996). Subsequently, the debate regarding the mechanisms mediating the hypnotic phenomenon continued between Charcot (1890; Wildocher and Dantchev 1994) and Bernheim (1889/1964).

Brain Electrical Activity

Power spectral analysis, the study of resting patterns of electrical activity in the brain, has been relatively unenlightening with regard to hypnosis. There has been some indication of more alpha activity among highly hypnotizable persons, whether or not they are in a trance, and of an alpha laterality difference favoring the left hemisphere among this population (Edmonston and Grotevant 1975; Morgan et al. 1974). This difference suggests that hypnosis may differentially involve the right cerebral hemisphere; alpha is the noise the brain makes when resting but alert, so relatively less alpha on the right suggests more activity. This hypothesis is supported by observations that highly hypnotizable persons tend to be "left-lookers," preferring to activate their right hemispheres (Bakan 1969; Gur and Reyher 1973).

Nevertheless, bilateral EEG measures obtained in highly hypnotizable subjects ($n = 16$) while performing hemisphere-specific tasks during a hypnosis and a no-hypnosis control condition call into question the right-hemisphere-activation interpretation of lateralized brain function during hypnosis (Edmonston and Moscovitz 1990). Instead, these data suggest a lack of task-appropriate activity during hypnosis. Edmonston and Moscovitz contend that failure to attend to baseline activity measurements and use of ratios to evaluate interhemispheric lateralization may potentially contribute to misinterpretation of previously obtained data. In fact, Jasiukaitis et al. (1997) raised new questions and suggested new hypotheses regarding the old theory of right-cerebral-hemisphere dominance of brain activity during hypnosis. Their review of the literature, including evidence from electrodermal responding, visual ERPs, and Stroop interference, suggested that some hypnotic phenomena may be associated with the left hemisphere. They hypothesized that although hemispheric activation on hypnotic challenge may depend in large part on the kind of task the challenge involves, several general aspects of hypnosis might be more appropriately seen as left- rather than right-hemisphere brain functions, including concentrated attentional focus and the role of language in the establishment of hypnotic reality.

More recent studies of power spectral analysis suggest that theta power, especially in the frontal region, best differentiates highly hypnotizable from poorly hypnotizable individuals (Sabourin et al. 1990). Graffin

et al. (1995) obtained EEG measures in both highly and poorly hypnotizable subjects under three separate conditions: an initial baseline period; just preceding and following a standard hypnotic induction; and during the induction. They found a differential pattern of EEG activity between highly hypnotizable subjects and poorly hypnotizable subjects during the baseline period, characterized by greater theta power in the more frontal areas of the cortex for the former group. They also observed that in the period just preceding and following the hypnotic induction, poorly hypnotizable subjects displayed an increase in theta activity, whereas highly hypnotizable subjects displayed a decrease. Furthermore, during the actual hypnotic induction, theta power increased markedly for both groups in the more posterior areas of the cortex, whereas alpha activity increased across all sites. These findings suggest that anterior/posterior cortical differences may be more important than hemispheric laterality for understanding the hypnotic processes.

Crawford et al. (1996) studied the effect of hypnotic susceptibility levels on auditory ERPs measured in subjects instructed to ignore tones while reading a novel or counting their pulse. Subjects were divided into high- and low-hypnotizability groups on the basis of their HGSHS: A and SHSS: C scores. Auditory ERPs were recorded at C3, C4, and Cz to 50 msec 1.961 tone pips 50-, 60-, 70-, and 80-dB intensities, randomly presented at 1.5-second intervals. As predicted, high-hypnotizability subjects evidenced significantly smaller N1 and P2 amplitudes than did low-hypnotizability subjects when ignoring tones. As stimulus intensities increased, N1 latencies decreased for lows but increased for highs. N1 latency slopes across the 50- to 80-dB intensities were significantly more negative for low- than for high-hypnotizability subjects. These findings suggest that the highly hypnotizable individuals diverted greater attentional processing to the tasks at hand, particularly as the tones increased in intensity. They were also slower to respond to not-to-be-attended stimuli, confirming that hypnotic susceptibility is associated with efficient attentional processing such that high-hypnotizability persons can more effectively partition their attention toward relevant stimuli and away from irrelevant stimuli in comparison with low-hypnotizability persons.

Brain electrical activity research has confirmed that some cortical regions show characteristic modification of spontaneous brain electrical activity as a function of hypnotic responsiveness. Using FFT (fast Fourier transform) spectrum of 16-channel EEG recording, Meszaros and Szabo (1999) demonstrated that in highly hypnotizable subjects, the right parietotemporal region showed more electric power than the left one, whereas the low-hypnotizability subjects had left-side predominance or equilibrated power in all derivations. When indirect hypnosis induction was administered, the same right-side preponderance was obtained in low-hypnotizability subjects, suggesting the importance of the right parietotemporal associative area in the alteration of consciousness that characterizes hypnotic states.

Although early results were mixed, studies of the effects of hypnotic hallucination on ERPs have since yielded more promising results. The basic premise of these experiments is that because hypnotized individuals can experience perceptual alterations, including hallucinations, these changes might be reflected in corresponding alterations in the amplitude of the cortical evoked response to stimuli. Whereas some early studies showed no such effects (e.g., Amadeo and Yanovski 1975; Halliday and Mason 1964), others did (e.g., Clynes et al. 1964; Wilson 1968) but were hampered by small sample sizes, nonquantitative analysis of EEGs, limited use of hypnotizability testing, and use of subjects with neurological or psychiatric impairments. However, there is accumulating evidence that highly hypnotizable individuals experiencing a hypnotic hallucination that alters their perception of a stimulus have corresponding amplitude changes in the response evoked by that stimulus. For example, D. Spiegel et al. (1985) found that six highly hypnotizable subjects who experienced a hallucination of a cardboard box obstructing their view of a stimulus generator had significant reductions in P300 amplitude throughout the scalp and in N200 amplitude in the occipital region as well. These alterations occurred in no other hypnotic condition and did not occur among a group of individuals with low hypnotizability who were attempting to experience the same perceptual alteration. Furthermore, the reduction in P300 amplitude was significantly greater in the right than in the left occipital region, a finding that again implicates the right cerebral hemisphere in hypnotic experience. However, more recent visual ERP research (Jasiukaitis et al. 1996) has in fact implicated the left cerebral hemisphere in hypnotic perceptual alteration. These studies indicated greater reduction of occipital P200 amplitude during hypnotic obstructive hallucination when visual stimuli were presented to the right visual field than when they were presented to the left visual field, which demonstrates a stronger hypnotic effect of imagery in the left than the right occipital cortex.

Allen et al. (1995) studied the effect of posthypnotic amnesia using ERPs between simulators and hypnotized subjects. All participants demonstrated larger late positive component (LPC) amplitudes (compared with baseline) when confronted with learned words than when confronted with unlearned words, regardless of whether amnesia was reported. Nevertheless, the highly hypnotizable participants who reported recognition amnesia had significant changes in attention-related (P1 and N1) and recognition-related (N400 and LPC) ERP component amplitudes as a function of whether amnesia was reported, which suggests that posthypnotic amnesia may involve alterations in the processes of attention, selection, and accessibility.

Similar alteration in ERP amplitude congruent with hypnotic perceptual alteration has also been found when somatosensory stimuli are used (D. Spiegel et al. 1989; Figure 30–7). The hypnotic instruction is analogous to that used clinically for pain control. Each subject was told that his or her hand would be cool and numb and that this numbness would filter out any other sensations in the affected area. There was a significant reduction in P300 amplitude and also in P100 amplitude, suggesting earlier filtering of this somatosensory signal in the hypnotic hallucination condition. Thus, these subjects responded cortically as though the stimulus were less intense as well as less relevant. In another condition, subjects were told that the stimuli were pleasant and interesting and they should pay full attention to them. This yielded a significant increase in P100 amplitude but not P300 amplitude in hypnosis. Thus, highly hypnotizable subjects were capable of producing bidirectional changes in ERP amplitude to sensory stimuli, depending on the cognitive task employed during hypnosis. Poorly hypnotizable subjects showed no such changes, even though they were given an identical set of instructions by an experimenter blind to their hypnotizability.

Women with high- ($n = 10$) and low- ($n = 10$) hypnotizability were tested by De Pascalis and Carboni (1997) in a somatosensory target-detection task to evaluate the effects of hypnotic alterations of somatosensory perception on P3 peak amplitude and evoked cardiac response. The stimulus-detection task consisted of standard and target electric stimuli delivered within a fixed foreperiod. The P3 peak amplitude of ERPs recorded from frontal, central, and temporo-parieto-occipital (posterior) scalp sites and phasic heart rate deceleration response were compared in four conditions: 1) normal attention in waking state, 2) hypnotic obstructive hallucination, 3) hypnotic attention, and 4) hypnotic passive attention. The highly hypnotizable subjects demonstrated significant suppression of P3 peak amplitudes to target stimuli in the left frontal and posterior scalp sites during the hypnotic obstructive hallucination condition as compared with the normal attention condition. In the normal attention condition, P3 suppression was paralleled by a smaller anticipatory heart rate deceleration in response to probe stimulus onset. Regardless of condition, the P3 peak response to standard stimuli was found to be significantly greater for subjects with low hypnotizability than for those with high hypnotizability. The authors concluded that hypnotically induced obstructive hallucinations to somatosensory stimuli involve alterations in neural and autonomic responses that are consistent with a trait conception of hypnotizability.

Results similar to those observed in somatosensory studies have been obtained in studies of the auditory system. Sigalowitz et al. (1991) found P300 amplitude differences among highly hypnotizable individuals who were hallucinating a reduction or increase in tones, whereas poorly hypnotizable persons did not show such a change. The amplitude reduction did not reach statistical significance, but the increase during positive hallucination did. Lamas and Valle-Inclan (1998) combined two experimental effects—the noise-compatibility effect and the Simon effect—in a task designed to test negative auditory hallucinations. In the choice reaction task, targets appearing at either side of a screen are defined by color and are accompanied by irrelevant noise, and a negative hallucination suggestion is given for noise stimuli. Highly hypnotizable subjects ($n = 4$) performed the task on two separate occasions, with and without suggestion. The results indicated increases in reaction times and P300 latencies as a function of noise and spatial stimulus–response incompatibility (i.e., Simon effect). Whereas hypnotic suggestion decreased the response times for all types of trials nonsignificantly, it decreased those of left-hand responses significantly. In contrast, suggestion reduced the increase in P300 latencies in noise-incompatible trials but did not influence the Simon effect. These results indicate that hypnotic suggestion specifically affects the processing of hallucinated stimuli, which is consistent with the hallucinatory experience reported by the subjects.

A more recent study (Barabasz et al. 1999) examined the effects of positive obstructive and negative obliterating instructions on visual and auditory ERPs–P300 signals. The two groups of subjects ($n = 20$), selected on the basis of high and low hypnotizability, were requested to perform identical tasks during two conditions: waking state and alert hypnosis state (i.e., eyes open under hypnosis). High hypnotizability subjects showed greater ERP amplitudes while experiencing negative hallucinations and lower ERP amplitudes while experiencing positive obstructive hallucinations, in contrast with low-hypnotizability subjects and their own waking imagination-only conditions. This study demonstrates that when participants are carefully selected for hypnotizability and responses are time-locked to events, rather robust physi-

ological markers of hypnosis emerge. These reflect alterations in consciousness that correspond to participants' subjective experiences of perceptual alteration.

Examination of the SERP literature reveals that a clearly defined electrophysiological response to selective attention was described by Naatanen and Michie (1979). The characteristic response (signature) to somatosensory stimuli consisted of a negative deflection 140 milliseconds after the stimulus was administered, known as the N_{140}. This negative deflection is consistently seen as a response to selective attention to somatic stimulation (Allison 1982; Michie 1984; Naatanen and Michie 1979). Maldonado and colleagues (Maldonado 1996a, 1996b, 2001; Maldonado and Jasiukaitis 1997) postulated that conversion symptoms may represent a form of selective attention needed to create and perpetuate the symptoms or deficits. They examined SERPs in a group of patients presenting with lateralized (i.e., unilateral) deficits and found that subjects exhibited a "normal N_{140}" on the unaffected side (as expected in all "normal" control subjects) but an *enhanced* N_{140} on the affected side (Maldonado 2001). Even more remarkably, when the researchers provided hypnotic suggestions for time regression (e.g., to weeks prior to the onset of symptoms), subjects experienced complete normalization of the SERP's response, showing only the "classic" N_{140} bilaterally. At the end of the hypnosis session, the SERP's tracing returned to the previous pattern—that is, a classic N_{140} on the unaffected side and an enhanced N_{140} in the affected side. All subjects' hypnotizability scores were in the "high" range (i.e., equal to or greater than 8). Maldonado (2001) suggested that a hypnotic-like process facilitating selective hyperattention may mediate motor conversion phenomena.

Brain Imaging

There has been little study of hypnosis using newer brain-imaging techniques such as positron emission tomography (PET), single photon emission computed tomography (SPECT), and MRI. However, a recent PET study indicates that hypnotic reduction of the perceived unpleasantness of a stimulus was associated with significant changes in pain-evoked activity within anterior cingulate but not somatosensory cortex (Rainville et al. 1997). In addition, Szechtman et al. (1998) measured regional cerebral blood flow (rCBF) using PET. Highly hypnotizable subjects were hypnotized and asked to produce vivid auditory hallucinations. Subjects who could produce the hallucinations (8 of the 14 tested) had increased rCBF in the right anterior cingulate gyrus, and the "externality" and "clarity" of the hallucinations were highly correlated with blood flow in this region (Szecht-man et al. 1998). Thus there is evidence of effects of hypnotic perceptual alteration on cerebral blood flow, which may involve activity of frontal attentional regions. Evidence of involvement of primary sensory (temporal) cortex was found in the Szechtman et al. study as well.

Finally, Rainville et al. (1999) investigated the effects of hypnosis and suggestions in highly hypnotizable sub-jects attempting to alter pain perception. The study used PET measures of rCBF and EEG measures of brain elec-trical activity. Subjects were studied under three experi-mental conditions: 1) a (baseline) restful state, followed by 2) hypnotic relaxation alone (hypnosis), and then by 3) hypnotic relaxation with suggestions for altered pain perception (hypnosis with suggestion). During each scan, the left hand was immersed in neutral (35°C) or painfully hot (47°C) water for the first two conditions and in pain-fully hot water for the last condition. The researchers found that hypnosis was accompanied by significant increases in both occipital rCBF and delta EEG activity, which were highly correlated with each other (r = 0.70, $P < 0.0001$). Peak increases in rCBF were also observed in the caudal part of the right anterior cingulate sulcus and bilaterally in the inferior frontal gyri. Hypnosis-related decreases in rCBF were found in the right inferior parietal lobule, the left precuneus, and the posterior cin-gulate gyrus. The hypnosis-with-suggestion condition resulted in additional widespread increases in rCBF in the frontal cortices predominantly on the left side. More-over, the medial and lateral posterior parietal cortices showed suggestion-related increases partially overlapping with regions of hypnosis-related decreases. These results support a state theory of hypnosis in which occipital increases in rCBF and delta activity reflect the alteration of consciousness associated with decreased arousal and possible facilitation of visual imagery. Frontal increases in rCBF associated with suggestions for altered perception might reflect the verbal mediation of the suggestions, working memory, and top-down processes involved in the reinterpretation of the perceptual experience.

These techniques have proven useful in identifying subsystems within the brain devoted to specific types of perceptual and cognitive processing—for example, acti-vation of the left inferior frontal cortex and anterior cingulate gyrus in response to visual and auditory presen-tation of words (Volkow and Tancredi 1991). This brain-imaging work has led to the parsing of attentional processes into a series of components with different neu-roanatomic localizations, using PET imaging of brain responses to various attentional tasks (Posner and Peter-son 1990). The posterior attentional system involves ori-enting, with activation of the posterior or prestriate cor-

tex. Focusing of attention—for example, detecting a faint blip on a radar screen—is associated with activity in the anterior cingulate gyrus. Arousal involves activity in the right frontal cortex. These new theories and the data that support them offer the possibility of greater specificity in identifying the neurophysiological basis of hypnotic pro-cesses. For example, the majority of observations of a connection between hypnosis and alteration in ERP amplitude have involved changes in the P300 amplitude, which is maximal over the frontal and central cortex. This would suggest some specific involvement of the anterior attentional systems in hypnotic concentration. These systems include focusing (anterior cingulate) and arousal (frontal, especially on the right), phenomena that are consistent with the fact that hypnosis involves intense absorption, or focal attention, and a state of resting alert-ness or arousal.

However, hypnotic alteration of perception involves changes in primary sensory association cortex as well (Kosslyn et al. 2000; Figure 30–11). Highly hypnotizable subjects were asked to see a colored pattern in color, a similar gray-scale pattern in color, the color pattern as gray scale, and the gray-scale pattern as gray scale during PET scanning with $^{15}O–CO_2$. First, the classic "color area" in the fusiform/lingual region was identified by ana-lyzing the results when subjects were asked simply to perceive color as color versus when they were asked to perceive gray as gray. During hypnosis, both the left- and the right-hemisphere color areas showed activation when subjects were asked to perceive color, regardless of whether they were actually shown the color or the gray-scale stimulus; moreover, these brain regions exhibited decreased activation when subjects were told to see gray scale, regardless of whether they were actually shown the color or the gray-scale stimulus. Thus, the observed changes in subjective experience achieved during the hypnotic state are reflected by changes in brain function similar to those that occur in perception. Thus hypnotic alteration of perception is more than mere compliance with suggestion—it involves alteration in sensory experi-ence. These findings support the claim that hypnosis is a psychological state with distinct neural correlates and not just the result of adopting a role.

A more recent study (Faymonville et al. 2000) using PET attempted to identify the brain areas in which hyp-nosis modulates cerebral responses to a noxious stimulus. The protocol involved two states, a hypnotic resting state with mental imagery, and a hypnotic state with stimula-tion (warm nonnoxious vs. hot noxious stimuli applied to right thenar eminence). Cerebral blood flow scans were obtained with the $^{15}O–H_2O$ technique during each con-dition, and the subject was asked to rate pain sensation

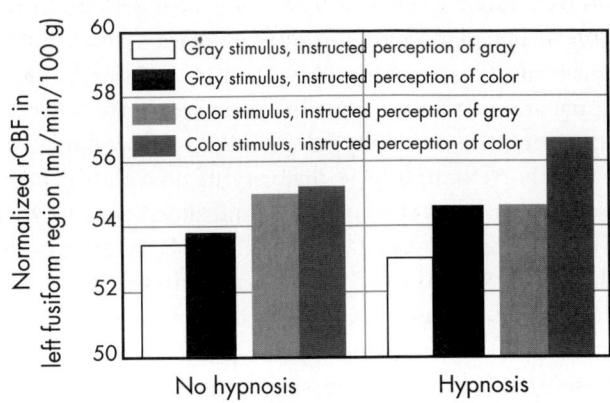

FIGURE 30–11. Effects of hypnotic alteration of color perception on blood flow in the lingual and fusiform gyri measured by positron emission tomography scanning using ^{15}O–CO_2.

Source. Reprinted with permission from Kosslyn SM, Thompson WL, Constantini-Ferrando MF, et al: "Hypnotic Visual Illusion Alters Color Processing in the Brain." *American Journal of Psychiatry* 157:1279–1284, 2000. Copyright 2000 American Psychiatric Publishing, Inc.

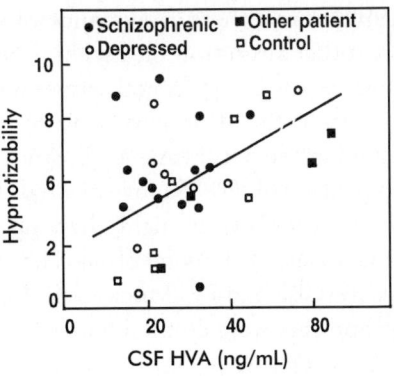

FIGURE 30–12. Hypnotizability as a function of homovanillic acid (HVA) in the cerebrospinal fluid (CSF), with regression line.

and unpleasantness. Statistical parametric mapping demonstrated that noxious stimulation caused an increase in rCBF in the thalamic nuclei and anterior cingulate and insular cortices. The hypnotic state induced significant activation of a right-sided extrastriate area and the anterior cingulate cortex. The interaction analysis revealed that the activity in the anterior (mid-)cingulate cortex showed a different relation to pain perception and unpleasantness in the hypnotic state than in control situations. Results also showed that hypnosis decreased both the sensation of pain and the unpleasantness of noxious stimuli, suggesting that hypnotic modulation of pain is mediated by the anterior cingulate cortex.

Neurotransmitters

Further indirect evidence for the involvement of the frontal cortex in hypnotic phenomena derives from a finding that hypnotizability is significantly correlated with cerebrospinal fluid (CSF) levels of homovanillic acid (HVA), a metabolite of dopamine (D. Spiegel and King 1992; Figure 30–12). High levels of HVA in the CSF primarily reflect activity in the frontal cortex and basal ganglia, regions rich in dopaminergic synapses. Administration of amphetamine, which stimulates the release of dopamine, has been shown to enhance hypnotizability (Sjoberg and Hollister 1965). Although at first the basal ganglia might seem irrelevant to such attention-deployment mechanisms, the automaticity observed in

hypnotic motor behavior could represent an activation of this region (D. Spiegel et al. 1993b), which is involved in both implicit memory (Mishkin 1991; Schacter 1987) and routine motor activity, especially of large muscle groups.

Other Physiological Correlates

Efforts have been made to correlate the hypnotic experience with actual physiological or cerebral physiology changes. Even though a "seat of hypnosis" has not been found in the brain, there is ample clinical and research experience indicating that the hypnotic process affects both brain electrical and metabolic processes, as well as causing more peripheral changes. Williamson et al. (2001) conducted a study attempting to demonstrate the effects of hypnotic manipulation in the subject's effort sense during dynamic exercise by measuring cardiovascular responses and brain activation. Using healthy, highly hypnotizable volunteers, they had subjects exercise under three hypnotic conditions: cycling on a perceived level grade, a perceived downhill grade, and a perceived uphill grade. They found that suggestion of downhill cycling decreased both the ratings of perceived exertion (from 13 ± 2 to 11 ± 2 [SD] units; $P < 0.05$) and the rCBF in the left insular cortex and anterior cingulate cortex, but it did not alter exercise heart rate or blood pressure responses. Perceived uphill cycling elicited significant increases in ratings of perceived exertion (from 13 ± 2 to 14 ± 1 units), heart rate (+16 beats/minute), mean blood pressure (+7 mm Hg), right insular activation ($+7.7 \pm 4\%$), and right thalamus activation ($+9.2 \pm 5\%$). Nevertheless, the decreases in perceived effort do not reduce cardiovascular responses below the level required to sustain metabolic needs.

A study of the autonomic and EEG responses to aversive stimuli presented by means of hypnotic suggestion in highly hypnotizable volunteers suffering from simple phobia revealed significant increases in heart rate and respiratory rate with a shift of the sympathovagal indexes toward a sympathetic predominance during hypnotic exposure to the phobic object (Gemignani et al. 2000). Concomitant with peripheral physiological changes, there was a significant increase in the EEG gamma band with a left frontocentral prevalence.

Other physiological changes include plethysmographic changes caused by rapid vasodilation mediated by direct suggestion, in the case of Raynaud's disease treated by hypnosis (Conn and Mott 1984). Highly hypnotizable individuals have been shown to have the capacity to control peripheral skin temperature and blood flow (Grabowska 1971; Kistler et al. 1999; Zimbardo et al. 1970) and to be able to suppress cortical evoked response to a perceptual stimulus while hallucinating an obstruction to that stimulus (D. Spiegel et al. 1985, 1989). Hypnosis has been implicated in changes in immune function, but there is little in the way of controlled studies. A recent study (Fox et al. 1999) examined psychological and immunological parameters 6 weeks before and 6 weeks after hypnosis treatment in patients suffering from frequently recurrent genital herpes simplex virus (rgHSV). After the hypnosis intervention, the authors observed a significant overall reduction in the number of reported episodes of rgHSV, accompanied by an increase in the numbers of CD3 and CD8 lymphocytes. Patients experiencing symptom improvement also showed significant increases in natural killer (NK) cell counts and in herpes simplex virus–specific lymphokine-activated killer (LAK) activity and reduced levels of anxiety in comparison with nonimprovers.

Forensic and Legal Issues

A major application of hypnosis in the legal setting has been for the purpose of refreshing recollection of witnesses and victims of crimes (Gravitz 1995). There have been some positive results with this technique—for example, the case involving the driver of a hijacked school bus in Chowchilla, California (*People v. Schoenfeld* 1980). Under hypnosis, and not previously, the driver was able to recall the numbers and letters on the license plate of the car that overtook the bus. This led to the arrest and conviction of the kidnappers.

Nonetheless, there has been serious criticism of the use of hypnosis with witnesses and victims. Two charges are leveled at the technique. One is *confabulation*—that

a hypnotized witness will make up material (Laurence and Perry 1983) and become what has been called an "honest liar" (H. Spiegel 1980), someone who believes his or her misstatement out of a desire to please the hypnotist or simply as a result of being in the nonrational hypnotic state itself. The other is *concreting*—that having gone through the process of hypnosis, even if new information is not made up, the subject will emerge with an enhanced conviction that his or her memories are correct and that the subject will therefore be more convincing to a jury than he or she should be (Diamond 1980; Dywan 1995; McConkey 1992; Orne 1979; D. Spiegel and Scheflin 1994; D. Spiegel and Spiegel 1987). There is evidence that under hypnosis people are more likely to make confident errors—the accuracy of the memories they produce is no better than usual but their confidence in the accuracy of their memories increases (McConkey 1992).

Courts have been uniformly unwilling to admit the testimony of a person hypnotized while testifying. More recently, however, courts have also begun to exclude testimony of witnesses who have previously been hypnotized about the event in question. The case law has provided some examples of egregious misuses of hypnosis. For example, in *People v. Shirley* (1982), a woman whose memory of the details of a questionable sexual assault was obscured because of her having ingested a substantial amount of alcohol was hypnotized by a member of the prosecution team the night before she was to testify. Her testimony improved dramatically. The conviction was overturned by the California Supreme Court, which ruled that any witness or victim who had been hypnotized about the facts of a crime could not subsequently testify. In other words, the use of hypnosis created an issue of admissibility rather than weight given to testimony. The court excluded defendants from this prohibition. In a subsequent case, *People v. Guerra* (1984), the conviction of a rapist was likewise overturned, because critical details regarding the nature of the attack were provided by the witness only during a hypnosis session in which considerable pressure was applied for her to remember penetration by the assailant. However, in this case the California Supreme Court left open the possibility that the testimony of a witness whose story had not changed despite a hypnotic interrogation might be salvaged. The Arizona Supreme Court (*State ex rel. Collins v. Superior Court* 1982) retreated from its extreme position and adopted a standard that holds in New York (*People v. Hughes* 1983) and New Jersey (*People v. Hurd* 1980), among other states, which is that such witnesses may testify about their prehypnotic recollection of events. The U.S. Supreme Court, in *Rock v. Arkansas*

(1987), ruled that a defendant could testify about his or her prehypnotic recollection of events, thereby rejecting a per se exclusion of testimony that could have been influenced by hypnosis.

From a practical point of view, it is wise to caution attorneys and witnesses that the use of hypnosis might leave open the possibility of challenge to witnesses' credibility or even to the inadmissibility of their testimony (Scheflin and Shapiro 1989; D. Spiegel and Scheflin 1994). Taking note of this problem, the California Legislature (1985) passed a law stating that witnesses would be allowed to testify after hypnotic interrogation if certain guidelines were followed. These guidelines include the use of an independent expert psychiatrist or psychologist as a hypnosis consultant, careful documentation of the witness's memory before hypnosis, and electronic recording of all interaction preceding, during, and after hypnosis sessions (Maldonado and Spiegel 1998; D. Spiegel and Spiegel 1987). The kind of situation in which hypnosis is most likely to be worth the risk is one in which there is a traumatic amnesia for the events of a crime or in which all other avenues of exploration have been exhausted. Hypnosis should not be used as a replacement for routine police work. The "FBI Guidelines for Use of Hypnosis" (Ault 1979) details the parameters and rules to be followed to maximize the yield of hypnotic recollection while preserving the integrity of the process.

The Council on Scientific Affairs of the American Medical Association convened a panel of experts to examine the research evidence relevant to this problem. The report issued by the panel (Orne et al. 1985) concluded that existing evidence indicated that the use of hypnosis tended to increase the productivity of witnesses, resulting in new memories, some of which were true and some of which were incorrect. Furthermore, some studies showed an increase in the confidence assigned by hypnotized subjects to their memories despite the fact that the percentage of correct responses had not improved. The panel noted that the analogy between the laboratory setting in which most of the studies were done and the real-life situation in the courtroom must be drawn with great caution and that situations in which extreme emotional and physical trauma have occurred differ markedly. The panel recommended that careful guidelines similar to the ones outlined in the California law be followed when hypnosis is used in the forensic setting (Bloom 1994; Maldonado and Spiegel 1997; D. Spiegel and Spiegel 1987).

Certainly, it is clear that hypnosis is no truth serum and that the courts must weigh the effects of any hypnotic induction on a witness. At the same time, hypnosis may in certain cases help a traumatized and amnesic witness to recall details not brought forward through conventional interrogation methods (Brown et al. 1998). Despite the former popularity of hypnosis as a way of "improving" eyewitness memory, many courts almost always regard the use of this testimony as inadmissible, whereas others allow it only when strict procedural guidelines have been followed. Although the U.S. Supreme Court recognized a defendant's constitutional right to admit his own hypnotically elicited testimony, others have recognized a constitutional basis for excluding hypnotically elicited testimony in most other circumstances (Newman and Thompson 1999).

Maldonado (2001) summarized and adapted the guidelines provided by the American Medical Association (1985) and the American Society of Clinical Hypnosis (Hammond 1995) for the use of hypnosis as a method of memory enhancement. These guidelines suggest that when hypnosis or any other memory-enhancement method is employed for forensic purposes or in the context of working out traumatic memories, especially those related to childhood physical and/or sexual abuse, the following steps should be applied:

- Prior to hypnosis use, perform a thorough evaluation of the patient.
- Explore the patient's expectations regarding treatment in general and hypnosis use in particular.
- Obtain the patient's permission to consult with his or her attorney.
- Explain to the subject and his or her attorney (if one is involved) about the nature of hypnotically retrieved memories.
- Clarify your role (i.e., therapist versus forensic consultant) before initiating any assessment and/or treatment. Make sure the patient clearly understands your role in the case.
- After full disclosure, obtain written informed consent:
  - Regarding the nature of hypnotic retrieval
  - Regarding possible side effects of memory work
- Clarify patient's expectation regarding hypnotically enhanced/recovered memories.
- Maintain neutrality throughout every interaction with the patient.
- Making a videotape recording of the interview/hypnotic session is mandatory.
- Thoroughly document any and all prehypnosis memories.
- Objectively measure hypnotizability.
- Carefully document your discussion of hypnosis and memory, issues of accuracy of memory, informed con-

sent, and the maintenance of a stance of neutrality and nonleading approach.

- Use an expert as a hypnosis consultant.
- Conduct the interview in a neutral tone, avoid leading or suggestive questions.
- Demonstrate a balance between supportiveness and empathy while assisting the patient to critically evaluate the elicited material.
- It is inappropriate to encourage patients to institute litigation or to confront alleged perpetrators solely on the basis of information retrieved under hypnosis.
- Carefully debrief the subject at the end of each session.
- Carefully document and produce a report containing the following:
  - Detailed prehypnotic memories
  - Hypnotizability score
  - Hypnotic techniques used
  - Any significant behavior
  - Any confirmed or new memories or details

Conclusions

Hypnotizability is a stable and measurable trait, one that connotes the presence of an intact ability to concentrate intensely, a receptivity to new information, and a flexibility in changing behavior. Thus, the capacity to experience hypnosis constitutes a therapeutic resource in the patient that can be mobilized by formal hypnosis during the therapy session and by self-hypnosis exercises afterward. It is this cognitive flexibility that makes hypnotizable individuals adept at employing strategies such as restructuring that can help them alter their perspective on their symptoms by experiencing symptom resolution as an occasion to enhance their sense of mastery, rather than as submission to the will of the therapist.

Many therapeutic approaches using hypnosis involve patients' changing perspectives on the relationship between their psychological and physical state, dissociating mental from physical stress, adopting a stance of protectiveness toward their body rather than fighting destructive urges, or learning to see sudden discontinuities in consciousness as understandable and controllable hypnotic phenomena. This alteration in consciousness that has long been associated with a myth about losing control can actually be mobilized as a powerful therapeutic tool in enhancing patients' control over their behavior, perceptions, somatic functions, and cognition.

References

Adams PC, Stenn PG: Liver biopsy under hypnosis. J Clin Gastroenterol 15:122–124, 1992

Ahijevych K, Yerardi R, Nedilsky N: Descriptive outcomes of the American Lung Association of Ohio hypnotherapy smoking cessation program. Int J Clin Exp Hypn 48:374–87, 2000

Allen JJ, Iacono WG, Laravuso JJ, et al: An event-related potential investigation of posthypnotic recognition amnesia. J Abnorm Psychol 104:421–430, 1995

Allison T: Scalp and cortical recordings of initial somatosensory cortex to median nerve stimulation in man. Ann N Y Acad Sci 388:671–678, 1982

Amadeo M, Yanovski A: Evoked potentials and selective attention in subjects capable of hypnotic analgesia. Int J Clin Exp Hypn 23:200–210, 1975

American Medical Association: Scientific status of refreshing recollections by the use of hypnosis. Council on Scientific Affairs. JAMA 253:1918-1923, 1985

American Psychiatric Association: Diagnostic and Statistical Manual of Mental Disorders, 4th Edition. Washington, DC, American Psychiatric Association, 1994

Anbar RD: Self-hypnosis for patients with cystic fibrosis. Pediatr Pulmonol 30:461–465, 2000

Anbar RD: Self-hypnosis for management of chronic dyspnea in pediatric patients. Pediatrics 107:E21, 2001

Anbar RD, Hehir DA: Hypnosis as a diagnostic modality for vocal cord dysfunction. Pediatrics 106:E81, 2000

Anderson MS: Hypnotizability as a factor in the treatment of obesity. Int J Clin Exp Hypn 33:150–159, 1985

Andreychuk T, Skriver C: Hypnosis and biofeedback in the treatment of migraine headache. Int J Clin Exp Hypn 23:172–183, 1975

Arone di Bertolino R: Hypnosis in dermatology [in Italian]. Minerva Med 74:2969–2973, 1983

Aronoff GM, Aronoff S, Peck LW: Hypnotherapy in the treatment of bronchial asthma. Ann Allergy 42:356–362, 1975

Ault RL Jr: FBI guidelines for use of hypnosis. Int J Clin Exp Hypn 27:449–451, 1979

Bakan P: Hypnotizability, laterality of eye movements, and functional brain asymmetry. Percept Mot Skills 28:927–932, 1969

Barabasz AF, Baer L, Sheehan DV, et al: A three-year follow-up of hypnosis and restricted environmental stimulation therapy for smoking. Int J Clin Exp Hypn 34:169–181, 1986

Barabasz M, Spiegel D: Hypnotizability and weight loss in obese subjects. Int J Eat Disord 8:335–341, 1989

Barabasz A, Barabasz M, Jensen S, et al: Cortical event-related potentials show the structure of hypnotic suggestions is crucial. Int J Clin Exp Hypn 47:5–22, 1999

Baram DA: Hypnosis in reproductive health care: a review and case reports. Birth 22:37–42,1995

Barry JJ, Atzman O, Morrell MJ: Discriminating between epileptic and nonepileptic events: the utility of hypnotic seizure induction. Epilepsia 41:81–84, 2000

Bauer KE, McCanne TR: An hypnotic technique for treating insomnia. Int J Clin Exp Hypn 28:1–5, 1980

Becker PM: Chronic insomnia: outcome of hypnotherapeutic intervention in six cases. Am J Clin Hypn 36:98–105, 1993

Beecher HK: Relationship of significance of wound to pain experienced. JAMA 161:1609–1616, 1956

Bell DS, Christian ST, Clements RS Jr: Acuphobia in a longstanding insulin-dependent diabetic patient cured by hypnosis (letter). Diabetes Care 6:622, 1983

Bellini MA: Hypnosis in dermatology. Clin Dermatol 16:725–726, 1998

Benhaiem JM, Attal N, Chauvin M, et al: Local and remote effects of hypnotic suggestions of analgesia. Pain 89:167–173, 2001

Berkowitz B, Ross-Townsend A, Kohberger R: Hypnotic treatment of smoking: the single-treatment method revisited. Am J Psychiatry 136:83–85, 1979

Bernheim H: Hypnosis and Suggestion in Psychotherapy: A Treatise on the Nature of Hypnotism (1889). Translated by Herter CA. New Hyde Park, NY, University Books, 1964

Bliss EL: Hysteria and hypnosis. J Nerv Ment Dis 172:203–206, 1984

Bloom PB: Clinical guidelines in using hypnosis in uncovering memories of sexual abuse: a master class commentary. Int J Clin Exp Hypn 42:173–178, 1994

Bowman ES: Etiology and clinical course of pseudoseizures, relationship to trauma, depression and dissociation. Psychosomatics 34:333–342, 1993

Braid J: Neurohypnology, or the Rationale of Nervous Sleep Considered in Relation With Animal Magnetism, Illustrated by Numerous Cases of Its Successful Application in the Relief and Cure of Disease. London, England, John Churchill, 1843

Braun BG, Sachs RG: The development of multiple personality disorder: predisposing, precipitating, and perpetuating factors, in Childhood Antecedents of Multiple Personality Disorder. Edited by Kluft RP. Washington, DC, American Psychiatric Press, 1985, pp 37–64

Bremner JD, Brett E: Trauma-related dissociative states and long-term psychopathology in posttraumatic stress disorder. J Trauma Stress 10:37–49, 1997

Breuer J, Freud S: Studies on hysteria (1893–1895), in The Standard Edition of the Complete Psychological Works of Sigmund Freud, Vol 2. Translated and edited by Strachey J. London, England, Hogarth, 1955, pp 1–319

Brose WG, Gaeta R, Spiegel D: Neuropsychiatric aspects of pain management, in American Psychiatric Press Textbook of Neuropsychiatry, 3rd Edition. Edited by Yudofsky SC, Hales RE. Washington, DC, American Psychiatric Press, 1997, pp 245–275

Brown DP, Scheflin AW, Hammond DC: Memory, Trauma Treatment, and the Law. New York, WW Norton, 1998

Bryant RA, Guthrie RM, Moulds ML: Hypnotizability in acute stress disorder. Am J Psychiatry 158:600–604, 2001

Bush E, Barry JJ, Spiegel D, et al: The successful treatment of pseudoseizures with hypnosis. Epilepsia 33:135, 1992

Butler LD, Duran RE, Jasiukaitis P, et al: Hypnotizability and traumatic experience: a diathesis-stress model of dissociative symptomatology. Am J Psychiatry 153(suppl 7):42–63, 1996

Cadranel JF, Benhamou Y, Zylberberg P, et al: Hypnotic relaxation: a new sedative tool for colonoscopy? J Clin Gastroenterol 18:127–129, 1994

California Legislature: AB 2669 Chapter 7, Hypnosis of Witnesses, added to Chapter 7, Division 6, of the Evidence Code, Enacted January 1, 1985

Cardeña E: Hypnosis in the treatment of trauma: a promising, but not fully supported, efficacious intervention. Int J Clin Exp Hypn 48:225–238, 2000

Cardeña E, Spiegel D: Dissociative reactions to the San Francisco Bay Area earthquake of 1989. Am J Psychiatry 150:474–478, 1993

Celestin-L'hopiteau I: Relaxation and hypnosis for pain in children. Revue de l'Infirmiere 65:34–35, 2000

Chandler T: Techniques for optimizing MRI relaxation and visualization. Administrative Radiology Journal 15:16–18, 1996

Charcot JM: Oeuvres complètes de JM Charcot, Tome IX. Paris, France, Lecrosnier et Babe, 1890

Clarke JC, Jackson JA: Hypnosis and Behavior Therapy: The Treatment of Anxiety and Phobias. New York, Springer, 1983

Clarke JH: Teaching clinical hypnosis in U.S. and Canadian dental schools. Am J Clin Hypn 39:89–92, 1996

Clarke PS: Effects of emotion and cough on airways obstruction in asthma. Med J Aust 1:535–537, 1970

Clynes M, Kohn M, Lifshitz K: Dynamics and spatial behavior of light-evoked potentials, their modification under hypnosis, and on-line correlation in relation to rhythmic components. Ann N Y Acad Sci 112:468–509, 1964

Conn L, Mott T Jr: Plethysmographic demonstration of rapid vasodilation by direct suggestion: a case of Raynaud's disease treated by hypnosis. Am J Clin Hypn 26:166–170, 1984

Colgan SM, Faragher EB, Whorwell PJ: Controlled trial of hypnotherapy in relapse prevention of duodenal ulceration. Lancet 1:1299–1300, 1988

Collison DR: Which asthmatic patients should be treated by hypnotherapy? Med J Aust 1:776–781, 1975

Copeland MD, Kitching EH: Hypnosis in mental hospital practice. Journal of Mental Science 83:316–329, 1937

Covino NA, Bottari M: Hypnosis, behavioral theory, and smoking cessation. J Dent Educ 65:340–347, 2001

Covino NA, Frankel FH: Hypnosis and relaxation in the medically ill. Psychother Psychosom 60:75–90, 1993

Covino NA, Jimerson DC, Wolfe BE, et al: Hypnotizability, dissociation, and bulimia nervosa. J Abnorm Psychol 103:455–459, 1994

Crasilneck HD, Hall JA: Clinical Hypnosis: Principles and Applications, 2nd Edition. New York, Grune & Stratton, 1985

Crasilneck HB, Hall JA: The use of hypnosis in controlling cigarette smoking. South Med J 61:999–1002, 1968

Crawford HJ, Corby JC, Kopell BS: Auditory event-related potentials while ignoring tone stimuli: attentional differences reflected in stimulus intensity and latency responses in low and highly hypnotizable persons. Int J Neurosci 85:57–69, 1996

Crawford HJ, Knebel T, Kaplan L, et al: Hypnotic analgesia: 1. Somatosensory event-related potential changes to noxious stimuli and 2. Transfer learning to reduce chronic low back pain. Int J Clin Exp Hypn 46:92–132, 1998

Dahlgren LA, Kurtz RM, Strube MJ, et al: Differential effects of hypnotic suggestion on multiple dimensions of pain. J Pain Symptom Manage 10:464–470, 1995

Dash J: Rapid hypno-behavioral treatment of a needle phobia in a five-year-old cardiac patient. J Pediatr Psychol 6:37–42, 1981

De Pascalis V, Carboni G: P300 event-related-potential amplitudes and evoked cardiac responses during hypnotic alteration of somatosensory perception. Int J Neurosci 92:187–207, 1997

De Pascalis V, Bellusci A, Russo PM: Italian norms for the Stanford Hypnotic Susceptibility Scale, Form C. Int J Clin Exp Hypn 48:315–323, 2000

Deyoub PL: Hypnosis for the relief of hospital-induced stress. Journal of the American Society of Psychosomatic Dentistry and Medicine 27:105–109, 1980

Diamond BL: Inherent problems in the use of pretrial hypnosis on a prospective witness. California Law Review 68:313–349, 1980

Dy AJ, Fabbri R Jr: The use of hypnosis with the hemodialysis patient. Am J Clin Hypn 14:173–177, 1972

Dywan J: The illusion of familiarity: an alternative to the report-criterion account of hypnotic recall. Int J Clin Exp Hypn 43:194–211, 1995

Edmonston WE Jr, Grotevant WR: Hypnosis and alpha density. Am J Clin Hypn 17:221–232, 1975

Edmonston WE Jr, Moscovitz HC: Hypnosis and lateralized brain functions. Int J Clin Exp Hypn 38:70–84, 1990

Elitzur B, Brenner S: Treatment of infectious skin diseases by hypnosis. Harefuah 110:73–74, 1986

Ellenberger H: The Discovery of the Unconscious: The History and Evolution of Dynamic Psychiatry. New York, Basic Books, 1970

Ellis JA, Spanos NP: Cognitive-behavioral interventions for children's distress during bone marrow aspirations and lumbar punctures: a critical review. J Pain Symptom Manage 9:96–108, 1994

Erickson JC III: The use of hypnosis in anesthesia: a master class commentary. Int J Clin Exp Hypn 42:8–12, 1994

Erickson MH: Advanced Techniques of Hypnosis and Therapy: Selected Papers of Milton H. Erickson, M.D. Edited by Haley J. New York, Grune and Stratton, 1967

Eriksson NG, Lundin T: Early traumatic stress reactions among Swedish survivors of the *Estonia* disaster. Br J Psychiatry 169:713–716, 1996

Ernst W: "Under the influence" in British India: James Esdaile's Mesmeric Hospital in Calcutta, and its critics. Psychol Med 25:1113–1123, 1995

Esdaile J: Hypnosis in Medicine and Surgery (1846). New York, Julian Press, 1957

Ewer TC, Stewart DE: Improvement in bronchial hyper-responsiveness in patients with moderate asthma after treatment with a hypnotic technique: a randomized controlled trial. British Medical Journal of Clinical Research and Education 293:1129–1132, 1986

Ewin DM: Hypnotherapy for warts (verruca vulgaris): 41 consecutive cases with 33 cures. Am J Clin Hypn 35:1–10, 1992

Fabbri R Jr: Hypnosis and behavior therapy: a coordinated approach to the treatment of sexual disorders. Am J Clin Hypn 19:4–8, 1976

Fabbri R Jr, Dy AJ: Hypnotic treatment of trichotillomania: two cases. Int J Clin Exp Hypn 22:210–215, 1974

Faymonville ME, Fissette J, Mambourg PH, et al: Hypnosis as adjunct therapy in conscious sedation for plastic surgery. Reg Anesth 20:145–151, 1995

Faymonville ME, Defechereux T, Joris J, et al: Hypnosis and its application in surgery. Revue Medicale de Liege 53:414–418, 1998

Faymonville ME, Mambourg PH, Joris J, et al: Psychological approaches during conscious sedation. Hypnosis versus stress reducing strategies: a prospective randomized study. Pain 73:361–367, 1997

Faymonville ME, Laureys S, Degueldre C, et al: Neural mechanisms of antinociceptive effects of hypnosis. Anesthesiology 92:1257–1267, 2000

Forbes A, MacAuley S, Chiotakakou-Faliakou E: Hypnotherapy and therapeutic audiotape: effective in previously unsuccessfully treated irritable bowel syndrome? International Journal of Colorectal Disease 15:328–334, 2000

Fordyce WE, Fowler RS, Lehmann JR: Operant conditioning in the treatment of chronic pain. Arch Phys Med Rehabil 54:399–408, 1973

Fox PA, Henderson DC, Barton SE, et al: Immunological markers of frequently recurrent genital herpes simplex virus and their response to hypnotherapy: a pilot study. Int J STD AIDS 10:730–734, 1999

Francis CY, Houghton LA: Use of hypnotherapy in gastrointestinal disorders. Eur J Gastroenterol Hepatol 8:525–529, 1996

Frank RG, Umlauf RL, Wonderlich SA, et al: Hypnosis and behavioral treatment in a worksite smoking cessation program. Addict Behav 11:59–62, 1986

Frankel FH, Orne MT: Hypnotizability and phobic behavior. Arch Gen Psychiatry 33:1259–1261, 1976

Freeman R, Barabasz A, Barabasz M, et al: Hypnosis and distraction differ in their effects on cold pressor pain. Am J Clin Hypn 43:137–148, 2000

Freud S: An autobiographical study (1925[1924]), in The Standard Edition of the Complete Psychological Works of Sigmund Freud, Vol 20. Translated and edited by Strachey J. London, England, Hogarth, 1959, pp 1–74

Freud S: Remembering, repeating and working-through (further recommendations on the technique of psycho-analysis II) (1914), in The Standard Edition of the Complete Psychological Works of Sigmund Freud, Vol 12. Translated and edited by Strachey J. London, England, Hogarth, 1958, pp 145–156

Frid M, Singer G: Hypnotic analgesia in conditions of stress is partially reversed by naloxone. Psychopharmacology (Berl) 63:211–215, 1979

Friday PJ, Kubal WS: Magnetic resonance imaging: improved patient tolerance utilizing medical hypnosis. Am J Clin Hypn 33:80–84, 1990

Frischholz EJ, Spiegel D, Spiegel H, et al: Differential hypnotic responsivity of smokers, phobics, and chronic-pain control patients: a failure to confirm. J Abnorm Psychol 91:269–272, 1982

Frischholz EJ, Spiegel D: Adjunctive uses of hypnosis in the treatment of smoking. Psychiatric Annals 16:87–90, 1986

Frischholz EJ: The relationship among dissociation, hypnosis, and child abuse in the development of multiple personality disorder, in Childhood Antecedents of Multiple Personality Disorder. Edited by Kluft RP. Washington, DC, American Psychiatric Press, 1985, pp 99–126

Fuchs K, Paldi E, Abramovici H, et al: Treatment of hyperemesis gravidarum by hypnosis. Int J Clin Exp Hypn 28:313–323, 1980

Gemignani A, Santarcangelo E, Sebastiani L, et al: Changes in autonomic and EEG patterns induced by hypnotic imagination of aversive stimuli in man. Brain Res Bull 53:105–111, 2000

Genuis ML: The use of hypnosis in helping cancer patients control anxiety, pain, and emesis: a review of recent empirical studies. Am J Clin Hypn 37:316–325, 1995

Gerschman J, Burrows GD, Reade P, et al: Hypnotizability and the treatment of dental phobic illness, in Hypnosis. Edited by Burrows GD, Collison DR, Dennerstein L. Amsterdam, The Netherlands, Elsevier North-Holland Biomedical, 1979, pp 33–39

Gherardi D, Fabrizio E, Chirillo S, et al: Psychiatric aspects in dermatology. Clinical contribution [in Italian]. Minerva Psichiatr 34:19–23, 1993

Glick BS: Conditioning therapy with phobic patients: success and failure. Am J Psychother 24:92–101, 1970

Gluzman SA, Zisel'son AD: Psychotherapy of bronchial asthma in children. Pediatriia 5:107–108, 1989

Goldstein E, Hilgard E: Failure of opiate antagonist naloxone to modify hypnotic analgesia. Proc Natl Acad Sci U S A 71:1041–1043, 1975

Goldstein LH, Drew C, Mellers J, et al: Dissociation, hypnotizability, coping styles and health locus of control: characteristics of pseudoseizure patients. Seizure 9:314–322, 2000

Grabowska MJ: The effect of hypnosis and hypnotic suggestions on the blood flow in the extremities. Pol Med J 10:1044–1051, 1971

Graffin NF, Ray WJ, Lundy R: EEG concomitants of hypnosis and hypnotic susceptibility. J Abnorm Psychol 104:123–131, 1995

Gravitz MA: First admission (1846) of hypnotic testimony in court. Am J Clin Hypn 37:326–330, 1995

Gritz E, Bloom J: Psychosocial sequelae of cancer in long-term survivors and their families. Paper presented at the Western Regional Conference of the American Cancer Society, Los Angeles, CA, January 1987

Gross M: Hypnosis in the therapy of anorexia nervosa. Am J Clin Hypn 26:175–181, 1984

Gur R, Reyher J: Relationship between style of hypnotic induction and direction of lateral eye movements. J Abnorm Psychol 82:499–505, 1973

Gysin T: Clinical hypnotherapy/self-hypnosis for unspecified, chronic and episodic headache without migraine and other defined headaches in children and adolescents. Forschende Komplementarmedizin 6(suppl 1):44–46, 1999

Hackman RM, Stern JS, Gershwin ME: Hypnosis and asthma: a critical review. J Asthma 37:1–15, 2000

Hájek P, Jakoubek B, Radil T: Gradual increase in cutaneous threshold induced by repeated hypnosis of healthy individuals and patients with atopic eczema. Percept Mot Skills 70:549–550, 1990

Halliday AM, Mason AA: Cortical evoked potentials during hypnotic anaesthesia. Electroencephalogr Clin Neurophysiol 16:312–314, 1964

Hammarstrand G, Berggren U, Hakeberg M: Psychophysiological therapy vs. hypnotherapy in the treatment of patients with dental phobia. Eur J Oral Sci 103:399–404, 1995

Hammond DC, Garver RB, Mutter CB, et al: Clinical Hypnosis and Memory: Guidelines For Clinicians and for Forensic Hypnosis. Bloomingdale, IL, American Society of Clinical Hypnosis Press, 1995

Hargadon R, Bowers KS, Woody F.Z: Does counterpain imagery mediate hypnotic analgesia? J Abnorm Psychol 104:508–516, 1995

Herod EL: Psychophysical pain control during tooth extraction. General Dentistry 43:267–269, 1995

Hilgard ER, Hilgard JR: Hypnosis in the Relief of Pain. Los Altos, CA, William Kaufmann, 1975

Hilgard ER: Hypnotic Susceptibility. New York, Harcourt, Brace & World, 1965

Hilgard ER: Divided Consciousness: Multiple Controls in Human Thought and Action. New York, Wiley, 1977

Hilgard JR, LeBaron S: Relief of anxiety and pain in children and adolescents with cancer: quantitative measures and clinical observations. Int J Clin Exp Hypn 30:417–442, 1982

Hilgard JR: Personality and Hypnosis: A Study of Imaginative Involvement. Chicago, IL, University of Chicago Press, 1970

Holroyd J: Hypnosis treatment for smoking: an evaluative review. Int J Clin Exp Hypn 28:341–357, 1980

Holroyd J: The uncertain relationship between hypnotizability and smoking treatment outcome. Int J Clin Exp Hypn 39:93–102, 1991

Houghton LA, Heyman DJ, Whorwell PJ: Symptomatology, quality of life and economic features of irritable bowel syndrome—the effect of hypnotherapy. Aliment Pharmacol Ther 10:91–95, 1996

Hyman GJ, Stanley RO, Burrows GD, et al: Treatment effectiveness of hypnosis and behaviour therapy in smoking cessation: a methodological refinement. Addict Behav 11:355–365, 1986

Iancu I, Kotler M, Spivak B, et al: Psychiatric aspects of hyperemesis gravidarum. Psychother Psychosom 61:143–149, 1994

Inoue H, Kobayashi H, Chiba T: Classification for bronchial asthma from the viewpoint of autonomic nerve function and airway hyperreactivity [in Japanese]. Nippon Kyobu Shikkan Gakkai Zasshi 33(suppl):104–105, 1995

Iserson KV: Hypnosis for pediatric fracture reduction. J Emerg Med 17:53–56, 1999

Jacavone J, Young I: Use of pulmonary rehabilitation strategies to wean a difficult-to-wean patient: case study. Crit Care Nurse 18:29–37, 1998

Jacknow DS, Tschann JM, Link MP, et al: Hypnosis in the prevention of chemotherapy-related nausea and vomiting in children: a prospective study. J Dev Behav Pediatr 15:258–264, 1994

James W: Varieties of Religious Experiences. New York, Random House, 1902

Janet P: The Major Symptoms of Hysteria: Fifteen Lectures Given in the Medical School of Harvard University. New York, Macmillan, 1907

Jasiukaitis P, Nouriani B, Spiegel D: Left hemisphere superiority for event-related potential effects of hypnotic obstruction. Neuropsychologia 34:661–668, 1996

Jasiukaitis P, Nouriani B, Hugdahl K, et al: Relateralizing hypnosis: or, have we been barking up the wrong hemisphere? Int J Clin Exp Hypn 45:158–177, 1997

Johnson ME, Hauck C: Beliefs and opinions about hypnosis held by the general public: a systematic evaluation. Am J Clin Hypn 42:10–20, 1999

Johnson RF: Warts, blisters, and stigmata: role of suggestions in some unusual skin changes. J Am Soc Psychosom Dent Med 27:72–86, 1980

Johnson RF, Barber TX: Hypnosis, suggestions, and warts: an experimental investigation implicating the importance of "believed-in efficacy." Am J Clin Hypn 20:165–174, 1978

Kantor SD: Stress and psoriasis. Cutis 46:321–322, 1990

Kardiner A, Spiegel H: War Stress and Neurotic Illness. New York, Paul Hoeber, 1947

Katz RL, Kao CY, Spiegel H, et al: Pain, acupuncture, and hypnosis. Adv Neurol 4:819–825, 1974

Keller VE: Management of nausea and vomiting in children. J Pediatr Nurs 10:280–286, 1995

Kellerman J, Zeltzer L, Ellenberg L, et al: Adolescents with cancer: hypnosis for the reduction of the acute pain and anxiety associated with medical procedures. Adolesc Health Care 4:85–90, 1983

Kelly E, Zeller B: Asthma and the psychiatrist. J Psychosom Res 13:377–395, 1969

Kessler R, Dane JR: Psychological and hypnotic preparation for anesthesia and surgery: an individual differences perspective. Int J Clin Exp Hypn 44:189–207, 1996

Kiernan BD, Dane JR, Phillips LH, et al: Hypnotic analgesia reduces R-III nociceptive reflex: further evidence concerning the multifactorial nature of hypnotic analgesia. Pain 60:39–47, 1995

Kirsch I: Hypnotic enhancement of cognitive-behavioral weight loss treatments—another meta-reanalysis. J Consult Clin Psychol 64:517–519, 1996

Kirsch I, Montgomery G, Sapirstein G: Hypnosis as an adjunct to cognitive-behavioral psychotherapy: a meta-analysis. J Consult Clin Psychol 63:214–220, 1995

Kistler A, Mariauzouls C, Wyler F, et al: Autonomic responses to suggestions for cold and warmth in hypnosis. Forschende Komplementarmedizin 6:10–14, 1999

Klein KB, Spiegel D: Modulation of gastric acid secretion by hypnosis. Gastroenterology 96:1383–1387, 1989

Kluft RP: An introduction to multiple personality disorder. Psychiatr Ann 14:19–24, 1984a

Kluft RP: Treatment of multiple personality disorder: a study of 33 cases. Psychiatr Clin North Am 7:9–29, 1984b

Kluft RP: Childhood multiple personality disorder: predictors, clinical findings, and treatment results, in Childhood Antecedents of Multiple Personality Disorder. Edited by Kluft RP. Washington, DC, American Psychiatric Press, 1985, pp 167–196

Kluft RP: The use of hypnosis with dissociative disorders. Psychiatric Medicine 10:31–46, 1992

Kluft RP: The treatment of dissociative disorder patients: an overview of discoveries, successes and failures. Dissociation 7:135–137, 1993

Knox VJ, Shum K: Reduction of cold-pressor pain with acupuncture analgesia in high- and low-hypnotic subjects. J Abnorm Psychol 86:639–643, 1977

Kohen DP, Wynne E: Applying hypnosis in a preschool family asthma education program: uses of storytelling, imagery, and relaxation. Am J Clin Hypn 39:169–181, 1997

Kohen DP: Application of relaxation/mental imagery (self-hypnosis) to the management of asthma: report of behavioral outcomes of a two-year, prospective controlled study. Am J Clin Hypn 34:283–294, 1986

Kohen DP: A biobehavioral approach to managing childhood asthma. Children Today 16:6–10, 1987

Koopman C, Classen C, Cardeña E, et al: When disaster strikes, acute stress disorder may follow. J Trauma Stress 8:29–46, 1995

Kopel KF, Quinn M: Hypnotherapy treatment for dysphagia. Int J Clin Exp Hypn 44:101–105, 1996

Kosslyn SM, Thompson WL, Costantini-Ferrando MF, et al: Hypnotic visual illusion alters color processing in the brain. Am J Psychiatry 157:1279–1284, 2000

Krumholz A, Niedermeyer E: Psychogenic seizures: a clinical study with follow up data. Neurology 33:498–502, 1983

Kuttner L: Helpful strategies in working with preschool children in pediatric practice. Pediatr Ann 20:120–122, 1991

Kuyk J, Spinhoven P, van Dyck R: Hypnotic recall: a positive criterion in the differential diagnosis between epileptic and pseudoepileptic seizures. Epilepsia 40:485–491, 1999

Kuyk J, Jacobs LD, Aldenkamp AP, et al: Pseudo-epileptic seizures: hypnosis as a diagnostic tool. Seizure 4:123–128, 1995

Lamas JR, Valle-Inclan F: Effects of a negative visual hypnotic hallucination on ERPs and reaction times. Int J Psychophysiol 29:77–82, 1998

Lambert SA: The effects of hypnosis/guided imagery on the postoperative course of children. J Dev Behav Pediatr 17:307–310, 1996

Lang EV, Joyce JS, Spiegel D, et al: Self-hypnotic relaxation during interventional radiological procedures: effects on pain perception and intravenous drug use. Int J Clin Exp Hypn 44:106–119, 1996

Lang EV, Benotsch EG, Fick LJ, et al: Adjunctive non-pharmacological analgesia for invasive medical procedures: a randomised trial. Lancet 355:1486–1490, 2000

Laurence JR, Perry C: Hypnotically created memory among highly hypnotizable subjects. Science 222:523–524, 1983

Lavoie G, Elie R: The clinical relevance of hypnotizability in psychosis, with reference to thinking processes and sample variances, in Modern Trends in Hypnosis. Edited by Waxman D, Misra P, Gibson M, et al. New York, Plenum, 1985, pp 41–66

Lavoie G, Sabourin M: Hypnosis and schizophrenia: a review of experimental and clinical studies, in Handbook of Hypnosis and Psychosomatic Medicine. Edited by Burrows GD, Dennerstein L. Amsterdam, The Netherlands, Elsevier North-Holland Biomedical, 1980, pp 377–420

Lazarus AA: "Hypnosis" as a facilitator in behavior therapy. Int J Clin Exp Hypn 21:25–31, 1973

Liossi C, Hatira P: Clinical hypnosis versus cognitive behavioral training for pain management with pediatric cancer patients undergoing bone marrow aspirations. Int J Clin Exp Hypn 47:104–116, 1999

Lopez CA: Franklin and Mesmer: an encounter. Yale J Biol Med 66:325–331, 1993

Lu DP: The use of hypnosis for smooth sedation induction and reduction of postoperative violent emergencies from anesthesia in pediatric dental patients. ASDC J Dent Child 61:182–185, 1994

Lu DP, Lu GP: Clinical management of needle-phobia patients requiring acupuncture therapy. Acupuncture and Electro-Therapeutics Research 24:189–201, 1999

Luparello T, Lyons HA, Bleecker ER, et al: Influences of suggestion on airway reactivity in asthmatic subjects. Psychosom Med 30:819–825, 1968

Maher-Loughan GP: Hypnosis and autohypnosis for the treatment of asthma. Int J Clin Exp Hypn 18:1–14, 1970

Maldonado JR: Physiological correlates of conversion disorders. Paper presented at the 149th annual meeting of the American Psychiatric Association, New York, May 1996a

Maldonado JR: Psychological and physiological factors in the production of conversion disorder. Paper presented at the Society for Clinical and Experimental Hypnosis annual meeting, Tampa, FL, November 1996b

Maldonado JR: Reviews in psychiatry: conversion disorder. Paper presented at the 154th annual meeting of the American Psychiatric Association, New Orleans, LA, May 2001

Maldonado JR, Jasiukaitis P: Somatosensory-related potential evidence of selective attention to the affected side in conversion disorders, Psycho-Neurophysiology of Conversion Disorders, 1997 (resubmitted for publication)

Maldonado JR, Spiegel D: Hypnosis, in Psychiatry. Edited by Tashman A, Kay J, Lieberman J. Philadelphia, PA, WB Saunders, 1996, pp 1475–1499

Maldonado JR, Spiegel D: Trauma, dissociation and hypnotizability, in Trauma: Memory and Dissociation. Edited by Marmar R, Bremmer D. Washington, DC, American Psychiatric Press, 1998, pp 57–106

Maldonado JR, Spiegel D: Conversion disorder, in Review of Psychiatry, Vol 20: Somatoform and Factitious Disorders. Edited by Phillips KA. Washington, DC, American Psychiatric Press, 2000a, pp 95–128

Maldonado JR, Spiegel D: Medical hypnosis, in Psychiatric Care of the Medical Patient, 2nd Edition. Edited by Stoudemire A, Fogel BS, Greenberg D, New York, Oxford University Press, 2000b, pp 73–90

Maldonado JR, Butler L, Spiegel D: Treatment of dissociative disorders, in A Guide to Treatments That Work. Edited by Nathan PE, Gorman JM. New York, Oxford University Press, 1997, pp 423–446

Maldonado JR, Butler L, Spiegel D: Treatment of dissociative disorders, in A Guide to Treatments That Work, 2nd Edition. Edited by Nathan PE, Gorman JM. New York, Oxford Press, 2000, pp 463–496

Marchioro G, Azzarello G, Viviani F, et al: Hypnosis in the treatment of anticipatory nausea and vomiting in patients receiving cancer chemotherapy. Oncology 59:100–104, 2000

Marks IM, Gelder MG, Edwards G: Hypnosis and desensitization for phobias: a controlled prospective trial. Br J Psychiatry 114:1263–1274, 1968

Matthews M, Flatt S: The efficacy of hypnotherapy in the treatment of migraine. Nursing Standard 14:33–36, 1999

Mauer MH, Burnett KF, Ouellette EA, et al: Medical hypnosis and orthopedic hand surgery: pain perception, postoperative recovery, and therapeutic comfort. Int J Clin Exp Hypn 47:144–161, 1999

McConkey KM: The effects of hypnotic procedures on remembering, in Contemporary Hypnosis Research. Edited by Fromm E, Nash MR. New York, Guilford, 1992, pp 405–426

McFadden ER Jr, Luparello T, Lyons HA, et al: The mechanism of action of suggestion in the induction of acute asthma attacks. Psychosom Med 31:134–143, 1969

McGlashan TH, Evans FJ, Orne MT: The nature of hypnotic analgesia and the placebo response to experimental pain. Psychosom Med 31:227–246, 1969

McGuinness TP: Hypnosis in the treatment of phobias: a review of the literature. Am J Clin Hypn 26:261–272, 1984

Meszaros I, Szabo C: Correlation of EEG asymmetry and hypnotic susceptibility. Acta Physiologica Hungarica 86:259–263, 1999

Meurisse M, Faymonville ME, Joris J, et al: Endocrine surgery by hypnosis. From fiction to daily clinical application. Annales d Endocrinologie 57:494–501, 1996

Meurisse M, Hamoir E, Defechereux T, et al: Bilateral neck exploration under hypnosedation: a new standard of care in primary hyperparathyroidism? Ann Surg 229:401–408, 1999

Michie P: Selective attention effects on somatosensory event-related potentials. Ann N Y Acad Sci 425:250–255, 1984

Miller ME, Bowers KS: Hypnotic analgesia: dissociated experience or dissociated control? J Abnorm Psychol 102:29–38, 1993

Mishkin M: Cerebral memory circuits, in Perception, Cognition and Brain, 1990 Yakult International Symposium, Yakult Honsha Co, Tokyo, Japan, August 1991

Mize WL: Clinical training in self-regulation and practical pediatric hypnosis: what pediatricians want pediatricians to know. J Dev Behav Pediatr 17:317–322, 1996

Montgomery GH, DuHamel KN, Redd WH: A meta-analysis of hypnotically induced analgesia: how effective is hypnosis? Int J Clin Exp Hypn 48:138–153, 2000

Moore R, Abrahamsen R, Brodsgaard I: Hypnosis compared with group therapy and individual desensitization for dental anxiety. Eur J Oral Sci 104:612–618, 1996

Moorefield CW: The use of hypnosis and behavior therapy in asthma. Am J Clin Hypn 13:162–168, 1971

Morgan AH, MacDonald H, Hilgard ER: EEG alpha: lateral asymmetry related to task and hypnotizability. Psychophysiology 11:275–282, 1974

Morrison JB: Chronic asthma and improvement with relaxation induced by hypnotherapy. J R Soc Med 81:701–704, 1988

Morse DR, Cohen BB: Desensitization using meditation-hypnosis to control "needle" phobia in two dental patients. Anesth Prog 30:83–85, 1983

Moskowitz L: Psychological management of postsurgical pain and patient adherence. Hand Clinics 12:129–137, 1996

Mun CT: The value of hypnotherapy as an adjunct in the treatment of bronchial asthma. Singapore Medical Journal 10:182–186, 1969

Myers JK, Weissman MM, Tischler GL, et al: Six-month prevalence of psychiatric disorders in three communities: 1980 to 1982. Arch Gen Psychiatry 41:959–967, 1984

Naatanen R, Michie PT: Early selective-attention effects on the evoked potential: a critical review and reinterpretation. Biol Psychol 8:81–136, 1979

Nash MR, Lynn SJ: Child abuse and hypnotic ability. Imagination, Cognition and Personality 5:211–218, 1986

National Institutes of Health (NIH) Technology Assessment Panel: Integration of behavioral and relaxation approaches into the treatment of chronic pain and insomnia. NIH Technology Assessment Panel on Integration of Behavioral and Relaxation Approaches into the Treatment of Chronic Pain and Insomnia. JAMA 276:313–318, 1996

Newman AW, Thompson JW Jr: Constitutional rights and hypnotically elicited testimony. J Am Acad Psychiatry Law 27:149–154, 1999

Nishith P, Barabasz A, Barabasz M, et al: Brief hypnosis substitutes for alprazolam use in college students: transient experiences and quantitative EEG responses. Am J Clin Hypn 41:262–268, 1999

Nugent WR, Carden NA, Montgomery DJ: Utilizing the creative unconscious in the treatment of hypodermic phobias and sleep disturbance. Am J Clin Hypn 26:201–205, 1984

Ohrbach R, Patterson DR, Carrougher G, et al: Hypnosis after an adverse response to opioids in an ICU burn patient. Clinical Journal of Pain 14:167–175, 1998

Orne MT, Axelrad AD, Diamond BL, et al: Scientific status of refreshing recollection by the use of hypnosis. JAMA 253:1918–1923, 1985

Orne MT: Hypnosis in the treatment of smoking, in Proceedings of the 3rd World Conference on Smoking and Health, Vol 2 (DHEW NIH 77-1413). Washington, DC, Department of Health, Education and Welfare, 1977, pp 489–507

Orne MT: The use and misuse of hypnosis in court. Int J Clin Exp Hypn 27:311–341, 1979

Patterson DR, Adcock RJ, Bombardier CH: Factors predicting hypnotic analgesia in clinical burn pain. Int J Clin Exp Hypn 45:377–395, 1997

People v Guerra, C-41916 Supreme Court, CA, Orange Co (1984)

People v Hughes, 59 NY2d 523, 466 NYS2d 255, 543 NE2d, 484 (1983)

People v Hurd, Supreme Court, NJ, Somerset Co, April 2, 1980

People v Schoenfeld, 168 Cal Rptr 762, 111 CA3d 671 (1980)

People v Shirley, 31 Cal 3d 18, 641 P2d 775 (1982), modified 918a (1982)

Peretz B: Relaxation and hypnosis in pediatric dental patients. Journal of Clinical Pediatric Dentistry 20:205–207, 1996

Peterson DB, Sumner JW, Jones GA: Role of hypnosis in differentiation of epileptic from convulsive-like seizures. Am J Psychiatry 107:428–433, 1950

Pettinati HM, Kogan LG, Evans FJ, et al: Hypnotizability of psychiatric inpatients according to two different scales. Am J Psychiatry 147:69–75, 1990

Pettinati HM: Measuring hypnotizability in psychotic patients. Int J Clin Exp Hypn 30:404–416, 1982

Piccione C, Hilgard ER, Zimbardo PG: On the degree of stability of measured hypnotizability over a 25-year period. J Pers Soc Psychol 56:289–295, 1989

Posner MI, Peterson SE: The attention system of the human brain. Annu Rev Neurosci 13:25–42, 1990

Prince M: The Dissociation of a Personality. New York, Longmans-Green, 1906

Putnam FW Jr: Dissociation as a response to extreme trauma, in Childhood Antecedents of Multiple Personality Disorder. Edited by Kluft RP. Washington, DC, American Psychiatric Press, 1985, pp 65–97

Rabkin SW, Boyko E, Shane F, et al: A randomized trial comparing smoking cessation programs utilizing behaviour modification, health education or hypnosis. Addict Behav 9:157–173, 1984

Rainville P, Duncan GH, Price DD, et al: Pain affect encoded in human anterior cingulate but not somatosensory cortex. Science 277:968–971, 1997

Rainville P, Hofbauer RK, Paus T, et al: Cerebral mechanisms of hypnotic induction and suggestion. J Cogn Neurosci 11:110–125, 1999

Ramchandani D, Schindler B.: Evaluation of pseudoseizures: a psychiatric perspective. Psychosomatics 34:70–79, 1993

Rape RN, Bush JP: Psychological preparation for pediatric oncology patients undergoing painful procedures: a methodological critique of the research. Children's Health Care 23:51–67, 1994

Redd WH, Andresen GV, Minagawa RY: Hypnotic control of anticipatory emesis in patients receiving cancer chemotherapy. J Consult Clin Psychol 50:14–19, 1982

Renouf D: Hypnotically induced control of nausea: a preliminary report. J Psychosom Res 45:295–296, 1998

Rhoades CD, Edmonston WE Jr: Personality correlates of hypnotizability: a study using the Harvard Group Scale of Hypnotic Susceptibility, the 16-PF and the IPAT. Am J Clin Hypn 11:227–233, 1969

Robb ND, Crothers AJ: Sedation in dentistry, part 2: management of the gagging patient. Dental Update 23:182–186, 1996

Roberts AH, Tellegen A: Ratings of "trust" and hypnotic susceptibility. Int J Clin Exp Hypn 21:289–297, 1973

Rock v Arkansas, 107 S Ct 2704, 97 LEd 2d 37 (1987)

Rustvold SR: Hypnotherapy for treatment of dental phobia in children. General Dentistry 42:346–348, 1994

Sabourin ME, Cutcomb SD, Crawford HJ, et al: EEG correlates of hypnotic susceptibility and hypnotic trance: spectral analysis and coherence. Int J Psychophysiol 10:125–142, 1990

Sanders RS Jr, Reyher J: Sensory deprivation and the enhancement of hypnotic susceptibility. J Abnorm Psychol 74:375–381, 1969

Sandrini G, Milanov I, Malaguti S, et al: Effects of hypnosis on diffuse noxious inhibitory controls. Physiol Behav 69:295–300, 2000

Schacter DL: Implicit memory: history and current status. J Exp Psychol Learn Mem Cogn 13:501–518, 1987

Schafer DW: Hypnosis and the treatment of ulcerative colitis and Crohn's disease. Am J Clin Hypn 40:111–117, 1997

Scheflin AW, Shapiro JL: Trance on Trial. New York, Guilford, 1989

Schenck CH, Mahowald MW: Two cases of premenstrual sleep terrors and injurious sleep-walking. J Psychosom Obstet Gynaecol 16:79–84, 1995

Schwartz JL: Smoking Cessation Methods: United States and Canada, 1978–85 (USPHS NIH 87-2940). Washington, DC, Division of Cancer Prevention and Control, National Cancer Institute, 1987

Schwartz JL: Methods for smoking cessation. Clin Chest Med 12:737–753, 1991

Seikowski K, Weber B, Haustein UF: Effect of hypnosis and autogenic training on acral circulation and coping with the illness in patients with progressive scleroderma. Hautarzt 46:94–101, 1995

Shaw AJ, Niven N: Theoretical concepts and practical applications of hypnosis in the treatment of children and adolescents with dental fear and anxiety. Br Dent J 180:11–16, 1996

Shaw AJ, Welbury RR: The use of hypnosis in a sedation clinic for dental extractions in children: report of 20 cases. ASDC J Dent Child 63:418–420, 1996

Shenefelt PD: Hypnosis in dermatology. Arch Dermatol 136:393–399, 2000

Shertzer CL, Lookingbill DP: Effects of relaxation therapy and hypnotizability in chronic urticaria. Arch Dermatol 123:913–916, 1987

Shor RE, Orne EC: Harvard Group Scale of Hypnotic Susceptibility. Palo Alto, CA: Consulting Psychologists Press, 1962

Sidis B, Goodhart SP: Multiple Personality. New York, Appleton-Century-Crofts, 1905

Sigalowitz SJ, Dywan J, Ismailos L: Electrocortical evidence that hypnotically induced hallucinations are experienced. Paper presented at the Society for Clinical and Experimental Hypnosis Meeting, New Orleans, LA, October 1991

Simon EP: Hypnosis in the treatment of hyperemesis gravidarum. American Family Physician 60:56, 61, 1999a

Simon EP: Improving tolerance of MR imaging with medical hypnosis. Am J Roentgenol 172:1694–1695, 1999b

Simon EP, Lewis DM: Medical hypnosis for temporomandibular disorders: treatment efficacy and medical utilization outcome. Oral Surg Oral Med Oral Pathol Oral Radiol Endod 90:54–63, 2000

Simon EP, Schwartz J: Medical hypnosis for hyperemesis gravidarum. Birth 26:248–254, 1999

Sjoberg BM, Hollister LE: The effects of psychotomimetic drugs on primary suggestibility. Psychopharmacologia 8:251–262, 1965

Smith MM, Colebatch HJ, Clarke PS: Increase and decrease in pulmonary resistance with hypnotic suggestion in asthma. Am Rev Respir Dis 102:236–242, 1970

Somer E: Biofeedback-aided hypnotherapy for intractable phobic anxiety. Am J Clin Hypn 37:54–64, 1995

Snape WJ Jr: Current concepts in the management of the irritable bowel syndrome. Rev Gastroenterologica de Mexico 59:127–132, 1994

Spanos NP, Stenstrom RJ, Johnston JC: Hypnosis, placebo and suggestion in the treatment of warts. Psychosom Med 50:245–260, 1988

Spanos NP, Williams V, Gwynn MI: Effects of hypnotic, placebo, and salicylic acid treatments on wart regression. Psychosom Med 52:109–114, 1990

Spiegel D: Hypnotizability and psychoactive medication. Am J Clin Hypn 22:217–222, 1980

Spiegel D: Vietnam grief work using hypnosis. Am J Clin Hypn 24:33–40, 1981

Spiegel D: Multiple personality as a post-traumatic stress disorder. Psychiatr Clin North Am 7:101–110, 1984

Spiegel D: The use of hypnosis in controlling cancer pain. CA Cancer J Clin 35:221–231, 1985

Spiegel D: Dissociating damage. Am J Clin Hypn 29:123–131, 1986a

Spiegel D: Dissociation, double binds, and posttraumatic stress in multiple personality disorder, in Treatment of Multiple Personality Disorder. Edited by Braun BG. Washington, DC, American Psychiatric Press, 1986b, pp 61–77

Spiegel D: Dissociation and hypnosis in posttraumatic stress disorders. Journal of Traumatic Stress 1:17–33, 1988

Spiegel D: Hypnosis, dissociation, and trauma: hidden and overt observers, in Repression and Dissociation: Implications for Personality Theory, Psychopathology, and Health. Edited by Singer JL. Chicago, IL, University of Chicago Press, 1990a, pp 121–142

Spiegel D: Trauma, dissociation, and hypnosis, in Incest-Related Syndromes of Adult Psychopathology. Edited by Kluft RL. Washington, DC, American Psychiatric Press, 1990b, pp 247–261

Spiegel D, Albert L: Naloxone fails to reverse hypnotic alleviation of chronic pain. Psychopharmacology (Berl) 81:140–143, 1983

Spiegel D, Bloom JR: Group therapy and hypnosis reduce metastatic breast carcinoma pain. Psychosom Med 45:333–339, 1983

Spiegel D, Cardeña E: Disintegrated experience: the dissociative disorders revisited. J Abnorm Psychol 100:366–378, 1991

Spiegel D, Chase RA: The treatment of contractures of the hand using self-hypnosis. J Hand Surg [Am] 5:428–432, 1980

Spiegel D, Fink R: Hysterical psychosis and hypnotizability. Am J Psychiatry 136:777–781, 1979

Spiegel D, King R: Hypnotizability and CSF HVA levels among psychiatric patients. Biol Psychiatry 31:95–98, 1992

Spiegel D, Rosenfeld A: Spontaneous hypnotic age regression: case report. J Clin Psychiatry 45:522–524, 1984

Spiegel D, Scheflin AW: Dissociated or fabricated? Psychiatric aspects of repressed memory in criminal and civil cases. Int J Clin Exp Hyp 42:411–432, 1994

Spiegel D, Spiegel H: Forensic uses of hypnosis, in Handbook of Forensic Psychology. Edited by Weiner IB, Hess AK. New York, Wiley, 1987, pp 490–507

Spiegel D, Spiegel H: Assessment and treatment using hypnosis, in Handbook of Anxiety Disorders. Edited by Last CG, Hersen M. New York, Pergamon, 1988, pp 401–412

Spiegel D, Vermetten E: Effects of hypnosis on somatic functions, in Dissociation: Culture, Mind, and Body. Edited by Spiegel D. Washington, DC, American Psychiatric Press, 1994, pp 185–209

Spiegel D, Frischholz EJ, Maruffi B, et al: Hypnotic responsivity and the treatment of flying phobia. Am J Clin Hypn 23:239–247, 1981

Spiegel D, Detrick D, Frischholz E[J]: Hypnotizability and psychopathology. Am J Psychiatry 139:431–437, 1982

Spiegel D, Cutcomb S, Ren C, et al: Hypnotic hallucination alters evoked potentials. J Abnorm Psychol 94:249–255, 1985

Spiegel D, Hunt T, Dondershine HE: Dissociation and hypnotizability in posttraumatic stress disorder. Am J Psychiatry 145:301–305, 1988

Spiegel D, Bierre P, Rootenberg J: Hypnotic alteration of somatosensory perception. Am J Psychiatry 146:749–754, 1989

Spiegel D, Frischholz EJ, Fleiss JL, et al: Predictors of smoking abstinence following a single-session restructuring intervention with self-hypnosis. Am J Psychiatry 150:1090–1097, 1993a

Spiegel D, Frischholz EJ, Spira J: Functional disorders of memory, in American Psychiatric Press Review of Psychiatry, Vol 12. Edited by Oldham JM, Riba MB, Tasman A. Washington, DC, American Psychiatric Press, 1993b, pp 747–782

Spiegel H: The dissociation-association continuum. J Nerv Ment Dis 136:374–378, 1963

Spiegel H: Termination of smoking by a single treatment. Arch Environ Health 20:736–742, 1970

Spiegel H: The Grade 5 syndrome: the highly hypnotizable person. Int J Clin Exp Hypn 22:303–319, 1974

Spiegel H: Hypnosis and evidence: help or hindrance? Ann N Y Acad Sci 347:73–85, 1980

Spiegel H, Spiegel D: Trance and Treatment: Clinical Uses of Hypnosis. Washington, DC, American Psychiatric Press, 1987

Spiegel SB: Uses of hypnosis in the treatment of uncontrollable belching: a case report. Am J Clin Hypn 38:263–270, 1996

Spinhoven P, ter Kuile MM: Treatment outcome expectancies and hypnotic susceptibility as moderators of pain reduction in patients with chronic tension-type headache. Int J Clin Exp Hypn 48:290–305, 2000

Stanton HE: Using hypnotherapy to overcome examination anxiety. Am J Clin Hypn 35:198–204, 1993

State ex rel Collins v Superior Court, 132 Ariz 180, 644 P2d 1266 (1982), supplemental opinion filed May 4, 1982

Steggles S: The use of cognitive-behavioral treatment including hypnosis for claustrophobia in cancer patients. Am J Clin Hypn 41:319–326, 1999

Steingard S, Frankel FH: Dissociation and psychotic symptoms. Am J Psychiatry 142:953–955, 1985

Steele K, Irwin WG: Treatment options for cutaneous warts in family practice. Fam Pract 5:314–319, 1988

Stewart AC; Thomas SE: Hypnotherapy as a treatment for atopic dermatitis in adults and children. Br J Dermatol 132:778–783, 1995

Stern DL, Spiegel H, Nee JCM: The Hypnotic Induction Profile: normative observations, reliability, and validity. Am J Clin Hypn 21:109–132, 1979

Stradling J, Roberts D, Wilson A, et al: Controlled trial of hypnotherapy for weight loss in patients with obstructive sleep apnoea. Int J Obes Relat Metab Disord 22:278–281, 1998

Stutman RK, Bliss EL: Posttraumatic stress disorder, hypnotizability, and imagery. Am J Psychiatry 142:741–743, 1985

Sumner JW, Cameron RR, Peterson DB: Hypnosis in differentiation of epileptic from convulsive-like seizures. Neurology 27:395–402, 1952

Surman OS, Gottlieb SK, Hackett TP, et al: Hypnosis in the treatment of warts. Arch Gen Psychiatry 28:439–441, 1973

Szechtman H, Woody E, Bowers KS, et al: Where the imaginal appears real: a positron emission tomography study of auditory hallucinations. Proc Natl Acad Sci U S A 95:1956–1960, 1998

Tausk F, Whitmore SE: A pilot study of hypnosis in the treatment of patients with psoriasis. Psychother Psychosom 68:221–225, 1999

Tellegen A, Atkinson G: Openness to absorbing and self-altering experiences ("absorption"), a trait related to hypnotic susceptibility. J Abnorm Psychol 83:268–277, 1974

Tellegen A: Practicing the two disciplines for relaxation and enlightenment: comment on "Role of the Feedback Signal in Electromyograph Biofeedback: The Relevance of Attention," by Qualls and Sheegan. J Exp Psychol Gen 110:217–226, 1981

Tobia L: Hypnosis in dermatology [in Italian]. Minerva Med 73:531–537, 1982

Torem MS: Hypnotherapeutic techniques in the treatment of hyperemesis gravidarum. Am J Clin Hypn 37:1–11, 1994

Tsushima WT: Current psychological treatments for stress-related skin disorders. Cutis 42:402–404, 1988

van der Hart O, Spiegel D: Hypnotic assessment and treatment of trauma-induced psychoses: the early psychotherapy of H. Breukink and modern views. Int J Clin Exp Hypn 41:191–209, 1993

van der Kolk BA, Fisler R: Dissociation and the fragmentary nature of traumatic memories: overview and exploratory study. J Trauma Stress 8:505–525, 1995

van der Kolk BA, Hostetler A, Herron N, et al: Trauma and the development of borderline personality disorder. Psychiatr Clin North Am 17:715–730, 1994

van der Kolk BA, van der Hart O: Pierre Janet and the breakdown of adaptation in psychological trauma. Am J Psychiatry 146:1530–1540, 1989

Vanderlinden J, Spinhoven P, Vandereycken W, et al: Dissociative and hypnotic experiences in eating disorder patients: an exploratory study. Am J Clin Hypn 38:97–108, 1995

Vidakovic-Vukic M. Hypnotherapy in the treatment of irritable bowel syndrome: methods and results in Amsterdam. Scand J Gastroenterol Suppl 230:49–51, 1999

Volkow ND, Tancredi LR: Biological correlates of mental activity studied with PET. Am J Psychiatry 148:439–443, 1991

von Plessen K: Jean Martin Charcot and his controversial research on hysteria. Tidsskr Nor Laegeforen 116:3633–3635, 1996

Weinstein EJ, Au PK: Use of hypnosis before and during angioplasty. Am J Clin Hypn 34:29–37, 1991

Weitzenhoffer AM, Hilgard ER: Stanford Hypnotic Susceptibility Scale, Forms A and B. Palo Alto, CA, Consulting Psychologists Press, 1959

Weitzenhoffer AM, Hilgard ER: Stanford Hypnotic Susceptibility Scale, Form C. Palo Alto, CA, Consulting Psychologists Press, 1962

Whorwell PJ, Prior A, Colgan SM: Hypnotherapy in severe irritable bowel syndrome: further experience. Gut 28:423–425, 1987

Whorwell PJ, Prior A, Faragher EB: Controlled trial of hypnotherapy in the treatment of severe refractory irritable-bowel syndrome. Lancet 1:1232–1234, 1984

Widlocher D, Dantchev N: Charcot and hysteria. Rev Neurol (Paris) 150:490–497, 1994

Wilks CG: The use of hypnosis in the management of gagging and intolerance to dentures (letter). Br Dent J 176:332, 1994

Williams JM, Hall DW: Use of single session hypnosis for smoking cessation. Addict Behav 13:205–208, 1988

Williamson JW, McColl R, Mathews D, et al: Hypnotic manipulation of effort sense during dynamic exercise: cardiovascular responses and brain activation. J Appl Physiol 90:1392–1399, 2001

Wilson NJ: Neurophysiologic alterations with hypnosis. Diseases of the Nervous System 29:618–620, 1968

Winchell SA, Watts RA: Relaxation therapies in the treatment of psoriasis and possible pathophysiologic mechanisms. J Am Acad Dermatol 18(1 Pt 1):101–104, 1988

Windholz G: Hypnosis and inhibition as viewed by Heidenhain and Pavlov. Integr Physiol Behav Sci 31:155–162, 1996

Wood DP, Sexton JL: Self-hypnosis training and captivity survival. Am J Clin Hypn 39:201–211, 1997

Wood GJ, Zadeh HH: Potential adjunctive applications of hypnosis in the management of periodontal diseases. Am J Clin Hypn 41:212–225, 1999

Zachariae R, Jorgensen MM, Christensen S: Hypnotizability and absorption in a Danish sample: testing the influence of context. Int J Clin Exp Hypn 48:306–314, 2000

Zeltzer L, LeBaron S, Zeltzer PM: The effectiveness of behavioral intervention for reduction of nausea and vomiting in children and adolescents receiving chemotherapy. J Clin Oncol 2:683–690, 1984

Zeltzer L, LeBaron S: Hypnosis and nonhypnotic techniques for reduction of pain and anxiety during painful procedures in children and adolescents with cancer. J Pediatr 101:1032–1035, 1982

Zimbardo PG, Maslach C, Marshall G: Hypnosis and the Psychology of Cognitive and Behavioral Control. Stanford, CA, Department of Psychology, Stanford University, 1970

Zimmerman J: Hypnotic technique for sedation of patients during upper gastrointestinal endoscopy. Am J Clin Hypn 40:284–287, 1998

CHAPTER 31

Group Therapy

Sophia Vinogradov, M.D.

Paul D. Cox, M.D.

Irvin D. Yalom, M.D.

Interpersonal relationships are of crucial importance to human psychological development. There are many psychiatric and therapeutic implications to this simple premise. Personality and patterns of behavior can be seen as the result of early interactions with other significant human beings. Modern schools of dynamic psychotherapy underscore the link between psychopathology and distorted interpersonal relationships and emphasize that psychiatric treatment must be directed toward understanding and correcting these distortions. Although this can of course take place in the context of the therapist–patient dyad, it is self-evident that a group of people can serve as an immensely specific therapeutic tool. In such a group setting, patients are provided with a varied array of interpersonal relationships that, with proper guidance, will permit them to identify, explore, and alter maladaptive interpersonal behavior.

Furthermore, the group setting is at once a ubiquitous and elusive phenomenon in our society. After all, groups are everywhere around us throughout our lives, from our early family units to the classroom and our classmates to the persons we surround ourselves with at work, at play, and at home. At the same time, we hear complaints about increasing interpersonal alienation in modern life—a sense of isolation, anonymity, and even social fragmentation. Perhaps because of this, and because it can provide such a powerful and unique therapeutic experience, the group setting is being used more and more not only by mental health professionals but by laypersons. Alcoholics Anonymous, Parents Without Partners, Recovery, Inc., Overeaters Anonymous, Mended Hearts, and Compassionate Friends are but a few of the current specialized and self-help groups available in the lay setting.

A number of specialized groups have been developed to function in a supportive and occasionally highly therapeutic mode in nonpsychiatric medical settings as well. The groundbreaking work of Spiegel et al. (1989) demonstrated a twofold increase in survival rate for patients with metastatic breast carcinoma who participated in a long-term psychodynamically oriented support group. Fawzy et al. (1993) found an improvement both in use of coping strategies and in immune function in patients with malignant melanoma who participated in a short-term group intervention. Group therapy enhances the quality of life of cancer patients (Blake-Mortimer 1999; Greenstein and Breitbart 2000).

Clinical Relevance of Group Therapy

Although the general principles of group therapy are increasingly being employed by the self-help group movement and by other mental health professions, mainstream psychiatric education has deemphasized the teaching and practice of group therapy. Perhaps the remedicalization of psychiatry, with its emphasis on biological modes of treatment for mental illness, accounts for this trend. Also, some psychiatrists may be alienated by the fact that the group treatment modality is being used so often by laypersons in settings that are, strictly speaking, nonpsychiatric. However, a meta-analysis by Barlow et al. (2000) suggested that many self-help groups involve professionals. These authors also noted that the effectiveness of self-help groups is an important new area of research.

Nonetheless, the estrangement of psychiatrists from group work is of some concern; after all, group therapy is a widely practiced mode of psychotherapy that is employed in a vast number of clinical settings with a proven degree of clinical effectiveness. The advent of widespread managed care and population-based care systems will probably necessitate increased use of groups and therefore the teaching of groups.

Efficacy

First and foremost, group therapy is effective treatment. Multiple outcome studies of varying sophistication and methodological design have been performed since the early 1960s. Considerable clinical consensus and research evidence have accumulated indicating that various forms of group therapy are beneficial to their participants (Dies 1979, 1993; Hoag and Burlingame 1997; Kaul and Bednar 1986; MacKenzie 1997a; Orlinsky and Howard 1986; Piper et al. 1992; Smith et al. 1980; Yalom 1983, 1985). Investigators over the years have concluded that group treatment is as effective as individual therapy in treating psychological disorders (D.A. Shapiro and Shapiro 1982; Smith et al. 1980). Thirty-two studies that directly contrasted individual and group treatments were analyzed (Tillitski 1990; Toseland and Siporin 1986); in 24 of the studies, no major differences were found between the two modalities. In the remaining 8 studies, group therapy was found to be more effective than individual therapy.

Numbers of Group Therapy Patients

Enormous numbers of psychiatric patients receive their sole or primary treatment in groups. This is particularly true in institutional settings and for chronically mentally ill persons. At least one-half of all psychiatric hospitals and one-quarter of all correctional institutions, not to mention the vast majority of community mental health centers, use group treatments (J. L. Shapiro 1978). Many health maintenance organizations make substantial use of group therapy as well (Cheifetz and Salloway 1984; MacKenzie 1997b, 2001a; Spitz 1997; Taylor 2001). Altogether, hundreds of thousands of patients undergo group therapy. Furthermore, patients most often found in institutional settings—the chronically ill—represent one of the greatest current challenges to the psychiatric profession and to social policy regarding the mentally ill. When compared with these populations, patients receiving routine individual therapy are a relatively insignificant subset, in terms of both large-scale mental health policy and sheer numbers.

Nonpsychiatric Groups

New orders of magnitude occur when we consider the staggering number of nonpsychiatric clients who receive treatment in specialized therapy groups or in one of the vast number of self-help groups. For example, the use of groups for patients with particular medical conditions—such as cancer support groups, post–myocardial infarction groups, and diabetes education groups—is burgeoning in the health care setting (Fawzy et al. 1995; Stern 1993). In 1983, perhaps 12 million to 14 million individuals attended some form of self-help group (e.g., Alcoholics Anonymous, Compassionate Friends, Recovery, Inc.) (Lieberman 1990). Goodman and Jacobs (1994) suggested that self-help groups may become the treatment of choice for many psychopathologies and nonpsychiatric life predicaments by the year 2010 or 2020. Inevitably, the practicing therapist of nearly every persuasion will encounter clients who have had contact with some form of group experience.

Practical Aspects of Group Therapy: Cost-Effectiveness and Efficiency

At its inception, group therapy was grounded in practical aspects. To facilitate the treatment of large numbers of tuberculosis patients at the turn of the century, a Boston internist named Joseph Pratt developed a workable, efficient treatment format: group meetings. Many of Dr. Pratt's patients were indigent and could not afford private care; many were debilitated, despondent, and ostracized in the healthy community. Needing to work with many different individuals in a highly efficient manner, Dr. Pratt began organizing groups of 20 or 30 patients and lecturing them once or twice a week (Pratt 1922). Even today, of course, group therapy retains this advantageous feature of expediency. Large numbers of patients can be treated and efficient use can be made of time and other resources.

Cost-effectiveness played an important role in the early development of group therapy as well. As noted in the previous paragraph, Pratt himself worked with indigent patients, and several other early pioneers in the group-lecture approach treated psychotic individuals who could afford only institutional care. Alfred Adler, an Austrian psychiatrist who became interested in theories of group behavior and of social interest, also spoke of "bringing psychology to the people" (Ansbacher 1980, p. 733). In England during and after World War II, the overwhelming number of psychiatric casualties and the limited hospital staff available made group treatment the most practical modality and led to an explosion in group therapy practice and research, which included the work of Wilfred Bion and the Tavistock model of group behavior and of S.H. Foulkes and group analysis (Pines and Hutchinson 1993). The same situation holds true today in many understaffed community agencies or institutional settings: treatment groups permit more efficient use of limited staff. Leadership in managed care supports the use of groups in large part for reasons of expediency.

Fortunately, the rationale for group therapy goes well beyond economics and savings in staff time. In examining nine studies comparing the differential efficiency of individual and group therapy, Toseland and Siporin (1986) concluded that group treatment is more consistently efficient and/or cost-effective. As efforts to maintain or improve outcomes while containing costs continue, these practical considerations of expediency and cost and staff efficiency will undoubtedly take on more weight. In fact, more than one group therapist has suggested that clinicians soon may need to justify individual therapy and defend their decision not to use the more cost-effective group therapy (Dies 1986; MacKenzie 1997b). However, although group therapy is more cost-efficient, its advantages transcend simple economic considerations: it is a form of treatment that makes use of unique therapeutic properties not shared by other psychotherapies.

Scope of Current Group Therapy Practice

Current group therapy practice encompasses a wide spectrum, ranging from the long-term interactional outpatient group and the medication–support group to the time-limited psychoeducational group to the acute crisis drop-in group (MacKenzie 1997a; Vinogradov and Yalom 1989). Therapy groups can be categorized by means of four interrelated characteristics (Table 31–1): the setting of the group, its duration, its goals, and its techniques.

Setting

One distinguishing feature among groups is their clinical setting. A particularly clear distinction can be made between psychiatric inpatient and outpatient groups. Inpatient groups on a psychiatric ward tend to meet daily, are usually composed of individuals with acute psychiatric problems, and often involve mandatory participation; turnover is great, with membership fluctuating widely because of the short duration of hospitalization. Psychiatric outpatient groups, in contrast, meet once weekly, consist of individuals who show more similar and more stable levels of functioning, and involve voluntary participation; membership tends to be more stable. There can be exceptions, of course. Some inpatient wards attempt to form more homogeneous groups that are based on level of functioning, although their membership will still vary widely. And psychiatric outpatient groups encompass many variations, ranging from the monthly drop-in group for chronically ill patients in a medication clinic to the twice-weekly interactional group run in a private practitioner's office.

Inpatient versus outpatient is but one distinction. Group therapy is also practiced in myriad other clinical settings, extending from the daily small groups in a psychiatric day hospital to weekly probation groups to staff retreats or support groups. Specialized groups for medical syndromes (e.g., diabetes education groups or lupus support groups) often meet in a hospital or clinic setting, whereas other types of specialized groups (e.g., rape crisis groups, Vietnam veterans' groups) may be associated with a center that offers counseling services (e.g., rape trauma center, veterans' outreach center).

Duration

A second consideration for any therapy group is its duration. Most inpatient groups are an integral part of the treatment program and are thus indefinitely self-sustaining; the ward census may change and different kinds of patients may be hospitalized, but the group meets every day. Outpatient groups have more latitude with regard to duration. They can exist for one session only (e.g., a drop-in crisis group that meets as needed at a student health center), or they can be open-ended and long-term in nature and periodically renew their membership over the years. In an interactionally oriented outpatient group, members will usually stay in therapy for 1–3 years, and "graduating" members are replaced as they leave, so that the size of the group remains approximately constant. A substantial number of groups in the outpatient setting, however, choose a time-limited format, especially if they are focusing on a specific problem. For example, an educational–behavioral group for patients with eating disorders may be designed to meet for six sessions.

Goals

A third factor that can be used to characterize the different kinds of group therapy pertains to the goals of the group, which may be conceptualized as existing along a spectrum. At one end of this spectrum are the ambitious goals of long-term interactional groups: symptom relief

TABLE 31–1. Scope of current group therapy practice

Type of group	Life of group	Attendance	Average length of stay in group	Goals	Major therapeutic factors/techniques	Membership criteria
Prototypical interactionally oriented groups	Indefinite; as permitted by professional schedule of group leaders	Voluntary, but regular attendance essential	1 to 2 years	Character change; symptom relief	Interpersonal learning; corrective recapitulation of primary family group	Higher-functioning patients; interpersonal pathology; desire to change, able to tolerate interpersonal focus; able to attend all sessions
Acute inpatient groups	Indefinite; usually an integral part of ward program	Generally mandatory during hospitalization; will show higher turnover	1 to 2 days up to several weeks, depending on the length of hospitalization	Restoration of function	Instillation of hope; socialization techniques; altruism; existential factors	Patients may be placed in different groups by level of functioning; membership will fluctuate widely
Follow-up or aftercare groups; discharge planning groups; day hospital groups; probation groups	Indefinite; usually associated with a specific program	Often mandatory	Usually a fixed number of sessions	Deinstitutionalization	Instillation of hope; imparting of information; imitative behavior; socializing techniques	Patients require follow-up care or aftercare; able to tolerate group setting and attend required sessions
Medication or clinic groups	Indefinite; usually part of clinic program	Voluntary; often occurring on a drop-in basis	Indefinite; depends on the patient's enrollment in clinic	Support; education; maintaining functions	Universality; imparting of information; socializing techniques; altruism	Patients on long-term psychiatric medication; able to tolerate group setting
Behaviorally oriented groups (e.g., eating disorders group)	Time limited, often 6 to 12 sessions; some are ongoing	Voluntary, but regular attendance generally prerequisite for participation	Life of group	Discrete behavior change	Techniques of behavior modification; universality; imitative behavior	Patients with a specific behavioral problem; desire to change
Specialized groups for medical disorders (e.g., diabetes, heart disease)	Time limited, often 6 to 12 sessions; some are ongoing	Voluntary; often drop-in basis	Life of group or fixed number of sessions	Education; support; socialization	Universality; cohesiveness; imparting of information; imitative behavior; altruism; existential factors	Patients with specific medical problems; desire for further education and support
Specialized groups for life events (e.g., bereavement, divorce)	Tend to be time limited, 8 to 12 sessions	Voluntary; often flexible	Life of group	Support; catharsis; socialization	Cohesiveness; altruism; existential factors	Patients who have undergone a life event; desire for group experience

TABLE 31–1.   Scope of current group therapy practice *(continued)*

Type of group	Life of group	Attendance	Average length of stay in group	Goals	Major therapeutic factors/techniques	Membership criteria
Specialized support groups (e.g., Vietnam veterans outreach, rape crisis, student center drop-in, professional support or professional retreats)	Indefinite; ongoing for professional retreats, which usually last 1 to 3 days	Usually drop-in basis; for staff support groups, especially during retreats, all members of the staff should attend	Variable	Support; catharsis	Cohesiveness; altruism; occasional interpersonal learning	Patients/clients who belong to specialized situation; desire for support

and character change. At the other end, there is the more limited but crucial goal of restoration of function: the deinstitutionalizing role of acute inpatient therapy groups. Between these two extremes lie the goals of the large majority of therapy groups. For some, such as medication clinic groups or inpatient and outpatient groups for chronically mentally ill persons, the most important goal will be maintenance of appropriate psychosocial functioning. Numerous others, including social skills training groups and specialized and self-help groups, attempt to provide education, socialization, and support. Many symptom-oriented short-term groups that are behaviorally focused (e.g., groups centered on bulimia, agoraphobia, or smoking cessation) have the goal of discrete behavior change.

Theoretical Orientation and Techniques

A fourth aspect of any therapy group is its theoretical orientation and the techniques employed by the therapist. This aspect is closely entwined with the goals of the group. An eating disorders group with the goal of discrete behavior change, for example, may have a cognitive-behavioral orientation and may focus on identifying cognitive distortions and triggers to behavioral responses. An analytic therapy group that has the goal of improving patients' ego functioning, on the other hand, may focus on the analysis of transference and resistance.

A wide range of theories and techniques inform the current practice of group therapy (Alonso and Swiller 1993). In this chapter, we will for the most part describe an understanding and an application of group therapy that are based on an interpersonal model of psychological functioning. This interpersonal orientation has a sound clinical and empirical foundation and translates into a set of clear and coherent tasks and techniques for the group therapist.

Membership Criteria

As can be seen from Table 31–1, the specific membership criteria for a given therapy group can vary widely from one type of group to another and are intimately linked to the goals of the group. In a behaviorally oriented group for patients with obsessive-compulsive disorder, for example, inclusion criteria are obsessive-compulsive symptomatology and a desire to change. The exclusion criterion is simply an inability to partake in a group experience (an extremely paranoid and obsessive individual would be excluded, for example). In contrast, a prototypical interactionally oriented group has much more stringent inclusion criteria: a member must admit to some interpersonal pathology, must have the ego strength and functioning necessary to tolerate an interpersonal focus, and must commit to regular attendance.

From these examples, the underlying principle for membership is made clear: whatever the specific nature of the group, a member must be able to perform the group task as the group works toward its goals. A member must therefore have problem areas that are compatible with the goals of the group and must have some motivation to change. Exclusion criteria include any factors that may interfere with the group task, such as marked incompatibility with group norms or with one or more group members, inability to tolerate the group setting, or a tendency to assume a deviant role in the group. These general criteria are outlined in Table 31–2 and are discussed further in the section on selecting patients and composing a therapy group.

In sum, the scope of current group therapy practice is wide indeed; those persons receiving treatment range from

TABLE 31–2. General membership criteria for group therapy

Inclusion criteria
Ability to perform group task
Problem areas compatible with group goals
Motivation to change
Exclusion criteria
Marked incompatibility with group norms for acceptable behavior
Inability to tolerate group setting
Severe incompatibility with one or more members
Tendency to assume deviant role

severely ill hospitalized psychiatric patients to high-functioning outpatients to persons with specific nonpsychiatric problems. Group therapy is a highly flexible psychotherapeutic modality, one that can be adapted to a variety of settings, time constraints, goals, and techniques.

Therapeutic Factors in Group Therapy: The Interpersonal Focus

Consider for a moment a hypothetical therapy group—let us say an outpatient group with eight members. Psychotherapy with one individual patient is a complex enough undertaking, but a group of patients is a potential Tower of Babel! Eight individuals intensively interact together, each with a different presenting complaint, varying psychological needs, unique problems in living, and, of course, a distinct character structure. Certain theorists would even argue that a new entity, with its own personality and characteristics, has been formed: the group itself.

The complexity of understanding and making sense of this enterprise often seems overwhelming to the neophyte therapist. What is needed is some simplifying principle, some mode of distinguishing between the truly essential, mutative aspects of the therapy group experience and those elements that represent the accessory characteristics of conscious and unconscious interaction in the group. We need to ask this question: Of all the dizzying, complex events in a group's transactions, which truly help the patient to change? We must identify the actual mechanisms of change in group therapy.

Identifying the Therapeutic Factors in Group Therapy

Group therapy was practiced for nearly half a century before researchers took steps to determine which factors actually help patients to change. Since the 1950s, a variety of research approaches have been used, including the interview and testing of group therapy patients with successful outcomes, as well as questionnaires directed at experienced group therapists and trained observers. Using these methods, researchers have identified a number of mechanisms of change in group therapy, that is, the curative or therapeutic factors.

There is usually a high degree of overlap among the various classification systems proposed by different investigators (Bloch 1986; Bloch and Crouch 1985; Butler and Fuhriman 1983; Corsini and Rosenberg 1955; Dies 1993; Fuhriman and Burlingame 1990; Yalom 1970). Yalom (1995) derived an atheoretical, 11-factor inventory of the therapeutic mechanisms operating in group therapy (Table 31–3): 1) instillation of hope, 2) universality, 3) imparting of information, 4) altruism, 5) development of socializing techniques, 6) imitative behavior, 7) catharsis, 8) corrective recapitulation of the primary family group, 9) existential factors, 10) group cohesiveness, and 11) interpersonal learning. Yalom suggested that these primary factors, derived from extensive clinical and research evidence, serve as provisional guidelines for determining how group therapy helps patients to change. Furthermore, these factors can constitute the basis for an effective technical approach to therapy. In his comprehensive text on group therapy, *The Theory and Practice of Group Psychotherapy*, Yalom (1995) utilized these therapeutic factors as a central organizing principle.

TABLE 31–3. Yalom's inventory of the therapeutic factors in group therapy

Instillation of hope
Universality
Imparting of information
Altruism
Development of socializing techniques
Imitative behavior
Catharsis
Corrective recapitulation of the primary family group
Existential factors
Group cohesiveness
Interpersonal learning

Let us define and briefly discuss each of these factors. The last factor—the powerful but often misunderstood mechanism of interpersonal learning—will be discussed in greater detail.

Instillation of Hope

Instilling and maintaining hope is crucial in all psychotherapies and plays a unique role in group therapy. Clinical sentiment and research evidence alike indicate that faith in the treatment mode can in itself be therapeutically effective, both when the patient has a high expectation of help and when the therapist believes in the efficacy of the treatment (Bloch and Crouch 1985). In therapy groups of every ilk, there will be patients who have improved as well as members who are at a low ebb; patients will often remark at the end of therapy how important it was for them to observe the improvement of others and thus to hope for their own improvement. Many of the self-help groups that emerged in the 1970s and 1980s, such as Compassionate Friends for bereaved parents or Mended Hearts for cardiac surgery patients, also place a heavy emphasis on the instillation of hope. Groups such as Alcoholics Anonymous that are aimed at substance abuse often use the testimonials of former alcoholic or recovered addicted persons to inspire hope in new members.

Universality

Many patients go through life with a sense of isolation. Secretly convinced that they are unique in their loneliness or their wretchedness, that they alone have certain unacceptable problems or impulses, these persons remain socially isolated and have few opportunities for frank and candid consensual validation. In a therapy group, especially in its early stages, the disconfirmation of a patient's sense of uniqueness comes as a powerful sense of relief. Some specialized groups, in fact, are focused on helping individuals for whom secrecy has been an especially important and isolating part of life. For example, short-term structured groups for bulimic patients require open disclosure about attitudes toward body image and detailed accounts about bingeing and purging behavior. As a rule, patients experience a great sense of relief when they discover that they are not alone, that some of their problems are "universal," and that other group members share the same dilemmas. Often, the degree of relief is directly related to the degree of reluctance to disclose.

Imparting of Information

The imparting of information occurs in a group whenever a therapist gives didactic instruction to patients about mental functioning or whenever advice or direct guidance about life problems is offered either by the leader or by other group members. Although long-term interactional groups generally do not value the use of didactic education or advice, other types of groups rely more or less heavily on these two manners of imparting information. Let us briefly examine each of them in turn.

Many self-help groups such as Recovery, Inc. (for psychological problems), Make Today Count (for cancer patients), and Gamblers Anonymous emphasize *didactic instruction*. Experts are often invited to address the group, and members are strongly encouraged to exchange information among themselves. Most, if not all, specialized groups led by professionals rely heavily on this procedure as well; groups aimed at patients with a specific disorder or facing a specific life crisis (e.g., obesity, trauma such as rape, epilepsy, chronic pain) build in a teaching component and offer explicit instruction about the nature of the patient's illness or life situation. Many day-treatment groups or social skills training groups for chronically mentally ill persons also use teaching and instruction.

Unlike explicit didactic instruction from the therapist, *direct advice* from other members occurs without exception in every kind of therapy group. In dynamic interactional therapy groups, it is invariably part of the early life of the group but is generally of limited value to members. Later, when the group has moved beyond an initial "problem solving" stage and has begun to engage in true interactional work, the reappearance of advice seeking or advice giving around a given issue is an important clue to resistance in the group. In contrast, noninteractionally focused groups often make explicit and effective use of direct suggestions and guidance. For example, members of behavior-shaping groups, discharge groups (those that prepare patients for discharge from the hospital), Recovery, Inc., and Alcoholics Anonymous offer one another considerable direct advice. Discharge groups may discuss the events of a patient's trial home visit and offer suggestions for alternative behavior, whereas Alcoholics Anonymous and Recovery, Inc., use guidance and directive slogans. Research on a behavior-shaping group of male sex offenders found that the most effective form of guidance was either systematic operationalized instructions or alternative suggestions from peers about how to reach a desired goal (Flowers 1979).

Altruism

In a therapy group, patients become enormously helpful to one another: they share similar problems and offer one another support, reassurance, suggestions, and insight. To the patient starting therapy who is demoralized and who feels that he or she has nothing of value to offer anyone, the experience of being helpful to other members of the group can be surprisingly rewarding. Not only does the altruistic act boost self-esteem, it also distracts patients who spend much of their psychic energy immersed in morbid self-absorption. By its very structure, the therapy group fosters the act of being helpful to others and counters overly solipsistic preoccupation.

Development of Socializing Techniques

Social learning—the development of basic social skills—is a therapeutic factor that operates in all therapy groups, although the nature of the skills taught and the explicitness of the process vary greatly according to the type of group therapy. In some groups, such as those preparing long-term hospitalized patients for discharge or those for adolescents with behavioral problems, there may be explicit emphasis on the development of social skills. Role-playing is often employed, in which patients learn to approach prospective employers for a job or adolescent boys learn to invite a girl to a dance. In groups that are more interactionally oriented, patients often learn about maladaptive social behavior from the open feedback they offer one another. A patient may, for example, learn about a disconcerting tendency to avoid eye contact during conversation, or about the effect that his or her whispery voice and constantly folded arms have on others, or about a host of other social habits that, unbeknownst to the patient, have been undermining his or her social relationships.

Imitative Behavior

The importance of imitative behavior as a therapeutic factor in groups is difficult to gauge, but there is some evidence from social psychological research that therapists may underestimate its importance. Bandura et al. (1969), for example, experimentally demonstrated nearly 30 years ago that imitation of healthy behavior is an effective therapeutic force in the treatment of certain phobias. In group therapy we often observe patients who benefit by observing the therapy of another patient with a similar problem constellation, a phenomenon of "vicarious learning." (Bandura 1986) A timid, somewhat repressed female member might observe another woman in the group begin to improve as the woman experiments with more engaging behavior and perhaps a more attractive appearance; the timid patient may then try new ways of presenting herself as well.

Catharsis

Catharsis, or the ventilation of emotions, is a complex therapeutic factor that is linked to other processes in the group, particularly universality and cohesiveness. The sheer act of ventilation, by itself, although often accompanied by a sense of emotional arousal and relief, rarely promotes lasting change for a patient. It is the affective sharing of one's inner world, and then the acceptance by others, that is of paramount importance. Being accepted by others after expressing strong emotions brings into question one's belief that one is basically repugnant, unacceptable, or unlovable. Therapy is both an emotional and a corrective experience; for change to take place, a patient must experience something strongly in the group setting and then understand the implications of that emotional experience. We will return to this fundamental premise later when we discuss the here-and-now focus of group therapy.

Corrective Recapitulation of the Primary Family Group

Patients often enter group therapy with a history of unsatisfactory experiences in their first and most important group experience, the primary family. Because group therapy offers such a vast array of recapitulative possibilities, patients may begin to interact with leaders or other members as they once interacted with parents and siblings (Baker and Baker 1993). A helplessly dependent patient may ascribe unrealistic knowledge and power to the leader. A rebellious and defiant individual may see the therapist as someone who blocks autonomy in the group or who strips members of their individuality. The "primitive" or chaotic patient might attempt to split the co-therapists or even the entire group, igniting fires of bitter disagreement and rivalry. The competitive patient will compete with other members for the therapist's attention or perhaps seek allies in an effort to topple the therapist(s). And a self-effacing individual or one with poor self-esteem may neglect his or her own interests in a seemingly selfless effort to placate or provide for other members. All of these patterns of behavior can represent a recapitulation of early family experiences.

What is of capital importance in interactional group therapy (and to a lesser degree in other group settings that make use of psychological insight) is not only that these kinds of early familial conflicts are reenacted but that they are understood and corrected. The group leader must not permit these growth-inhibiting relationships to freeze into the rigid, impenetrable system that characterizes many family structures. Instead, the leader must constantly explore and challenge fixed roles in the group and must constantly encourage members to test new behaviors. By exploring and altering ingrained patterns of behavior with leaders and other group members, the patient is liberated from the yoke of unfinished business from the past.

Existential Factors

An existential approach to the understanding of patients' concerns posits that the human being's paramount struggle is with the givens of existence: death, isolation, freedom, and meaninglessness (Yalom 1980). In certain kinds of therapy groups, particularly those centered around patients with cancer or chronic and life-threatening medical illnesses, or in bereavement groups, members will often begin to confront some of these existential issues. They will realize that there is a limit to the guidance and support they can receive from others. They may find that the ultimate responsibility for the conduct of their lives is their own. They will often learn that although one can be close to others, there is nonetheless a basic aloneness to existence that cannot be avoided. As they accept some of these issues, many patients who are confronting death learn to face their limitations and their mortality with greater candor and courage. In group therapy, the sound and trusting relationship among members—the basic, intimate encounter—has an intrinsic value in that it provides presence and a "being with" in the face of these harsh existential realities (Benioff and Vinogradov 1993; Yalom and Vinogradov 1988).

Group Cohesiveness

Although it is discussed near the end of this brief description of therapeutic factors, group cohesiveness is one of the more complex and absolutely integral features of a successful therapy group (Dies 1993). Cohesiveness in a group context refers to the affinity that members have for their group and for the other members. The members of a cohesive group are accepting of one another, supportive, and inclined to form meaningful relationships in the group; they are ready to perform the group task. As such, cohesiveness can be conceptualized as a necessary precondition for change rather than a true mechanism of change. And yet, many if not most psychiatric patients have had an impoverished history of belonging; never before have they been a valuable, integral, participating member of any kind of group, and the successful negotiation of a group therapy experience may in itself be curative. For these patients, group cohesiveness appears to be a true therapeutic factor. Furthermore, the social behavior required for members to be esteemed by a cohesive group tends also to be adaptive for the individual in his or her social life outside the group.

How else does group cohesiveness set the stage for change? Quite simply, by providing conditions of acceptance and understanding. Under cohesive conditions, patients are more inclined to express and explore themselves, to become aware of and integrate hitherto unacceptable aspects of themselves, and to relate more deeply to others. Cohesiveness in a group thus favors self-disclosure, risk taking, and the constructive expression of confrontation and conflict—all phenomena that facilitate successful therapy.

Highly cohesive groups are stable groups with better attendance, more active patient commitment and participation, and less membership turnover than groups that have not cohered. Some groups in certain settings, such as those specializing in a particular problem or disorder (e.g., a cancer support group or a group for women law students that is run by a university health center), will by their very nature develop a great deal of cohesiveness. In other kinds of groups, especially those in which membership changes frequently, the leader may need actively to facilitate the development of this important therapeutic factor. We will discuss means of fostering cohesiveness in the sections exploring the group therapist's tasks and techniques.

Interpersonal Learning

Group therapy may make use of any number of the therapeutic factors described here, but its cardinal feature is that it draws together a number of different individuals who wish to change something about themselves or their situations. This provides each member in the group with a unique ensemble of interpersonal interactions to explore. R.D. Laing (1967) suggested, "My experience and my action occur in a social field of reciprocal influence and interaction. I experience myself...as experienced by and acted upon by others..." (p. 9). Surprisingly, this potent mechanism for change in group therapy—interpersonal learning—is often overlooked, misapplied, or misunderstood by leaders, perhaps because the encouragement of interpersonal exploration requires considerable therapist skill and experience. To place the use of interpersonal learning into its full context, we will examine three underlying concepts: the importance of interpersonal relationships, the group as a social microcosm, and learning from behavioral patterns in the social microcosm.

Importance of interpersonal relationships. Humans are gregarious creatures committed for life to a social existence based on interpersonal communication through language. Harry Stack Sullivan (1953) contended that the need for interpersonal acceptance and security is basic and, given the prolonged period of helplessness during infancy, may be as crucial to survival as any biological need. To ensure and promote this interpersonal acceptance, a developing child will accentuate those aspects of behavior that meet with approval or obtain desired ends and will suppress those aspects that engender punishment or disapproval. The human personality can thus be seen as shaped almost entirely by interaction with other significant beings. Goffman (1961) noted: "There seems to be no agent more effective than another person in bringing a world for oneself alive, or, by a glance, a gesture, or a remark, shriveling up the reality in which one is lodged" (p. 41). Psychopathology arises when these interactions have resulted in distortions in how one perceives others and in how one reacts to them.

Psychotherapists who use an interpersonal frame of reference—and what psychotherapist does not do so at one time or another?—concentrate on the interpersonal pathology that underlies or arises from a particular symptom complex. The therapist translates symptoms into interpersonal language. For example, the psychotherapist rarely addresses "depression" per se. The typical symptom cluster of dysphoric mood and neurovegetative signs does not in and of itself offer a handhold for beginning the process of psychotherapeutic change. Instead, the clinician forms a relationship with the person who is depressed and ascertains the underlying interpersonal problems that arise from the depression and that most certainly also exacerbate it (problems such as dependency, obsequiousness, inability to express rage, and hypersensitivity to rejection). Once these maladaptive interpersonal themes have been identified, the therapist and the patient can undertake the work of understanding and altering them.

The group as a social microcosm.   Sooner or later, given enough time and freedom, each person in the group will begin to interact with other group members in the same way that he or she interacts with persons outside the group. In other words, participants create in the group the same type of interpersonal world they inhabit on the outside. The group becomes a laboratory experiment in which interpersonal strengths and weaknesses unfold "in miniature." Slowly but predictably, each individual's interpersonal pathology comes to be displayed in the group. Arrogance, impatience, narcissism, grandiosity, sexualization—all such traits eventually surface. There is hardly any need for members to describe their past or to report present difficulties with relationships in their outside life. Group behavior provides far more accurate and immediate data. Members act out their interpersonal problems before the eyes of everyone in the group, and a freely interacting group will, in time, develop into a social microcosm of each of the members of that group. The following vignettes illustrate this principle:

John, a busy and successful dentist, had serious marital problems and was "coerced" into group therapy by his wife and marriage counselor. His wife complained that he was detached and uninvolved and that she had to throw a "tantrum" to get him to respond. John believed that his wife was always angry and critical toward him for no reason. Although John was polite and ingratiating, his participation in the group remained at a superficial level even after several months. He felt distant and a bit disdainful of the group that he was "forced" to attend. Soon the female members were prodding him, complaining that he wasn't engaged in the group work, asking, "Where is John really at?" They grew angry and more shrill in their interactions with John (just like his wife) in order to elicit a response, any response, from him—a reflection in miniature of the problems in his marriage.

Elizabeth was a very attractive woman who, after her husband's job promotion and transfer, had left a high-powered career and had a baby; she soon entered a severe depression and felt overwhelmed by pain she could not express. She found her life lacking in intimacy, and her outside relationships, as well as her marriage, felt superficial and inauthentic to her. In the group, Elizabeth was very popular. She was charming, sensitive, and concerned about everyone. However, she rarely let the group glimpse behind her composed facade and into the depths of her pain and despair. Her great shame about her depression (after all, she "had it so good") and even deeper shame about the childhood of poverty and abuse from which she had risen resulted in her recreating in the group the same type of cordial but distant and unnourishing relationships she had established in her social life and marriage.

Mark joined the group after his divorce and a string of unsuccessful romantic encounters. He had no close friends, male or female. He was sexually compulsive and competitive, and although he dated frequently, the thrill of the initial sexual conquest would inevitably pall, leaving him with a feeling of emptiness. Mark soon recreated this behavior in the therapy group. Although an active and involved member, he devoted himself almost exclusively to courting the attractive women in the group, including the female co-therapist. The female members began to feel sexualized and withdrew from him. Because he had also adopted an exceedingly competitive stance with the men in the group (especially powerful men, such as the male co-therapist), Mark quickly succeeded in isolating himself from all fulfilling relationships in the social microcosm of the group.

Learning from behavioral patterns in the social microcosm.   These preceding concepts interrelate in the process of group therapy to provide the therapist with an extremely powerful tool for change: interpersonal learning. In this process, psychopathology emerges from and is embodied in distorted interpersonal interactions, in which the group becomes a social microcosm as each member displays his or her interpersonal pathology, and in which feedback allows members to identify and change their interpersonal behavior. This process is described here and is schematically outlined in Figure 31–1 (Yalom 1985, 1986, 1995):

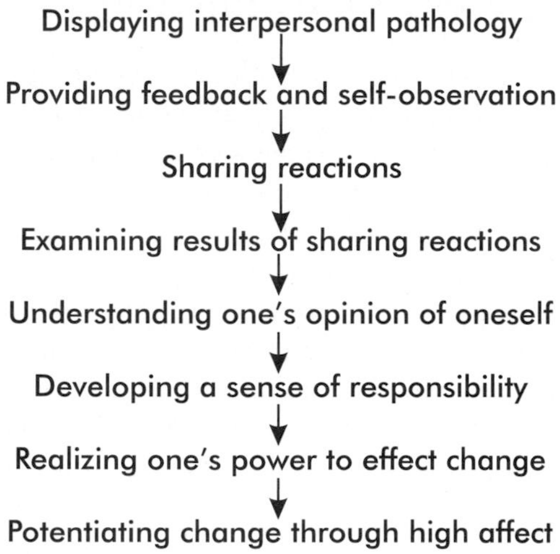

Displaying interpersonal pathology
↓
Providing feedback and self-observation
↓
Sharing reactions
↓
Examining results of sharing reactions
↓
Understanding one's opinion of oneself
↓
Developing a sense of responsibility
↓
Realizing one's power to effect change
↓
Potentiating change through high affect

FIGURE 31–1. Learning from behavioral patterns in the social microcosm of the therapy.

1. *Displaying interpersonal pathology:* Members display their characteristic interpersonally distorted behavior.
2. *Providing feedback and self-observation:* Members share observations of each other and discover some of their own blind spots.
3. *Sharing reactions:* Members point out one another's blind spots and point out how each member's behavior makes them feel.
4. *Examining results of sharing reactions:* Each member begins to have a more objective picture of his or her own behavior and of the impact it has on others.
5. *Understanding one's opinion of oneself:* Each member becomes aware of how one's own behavior influences the opinions of others and, hence, one's opinions of oneself.
6. *Developing a sense of responsibility:* As a result of understanding how one's behavior influences one's sense of self-worth, one becomes more fully aware of responsibility for one's interpersonal life.
7. *Realizing one's power to effect change:* With the acceptance of responsibility for life's interpersonal dilemmas, each member begins to realize that one can change what one has created.
8. *Potentiating change through high affect:* The more emotionally laden are the events of this sequence, the greater is the potential for change.

Interpersonal learning is the primary mechanism for change in unstructured, longer-term, high-functioning interaction groups; in these settings, in fact, the elements of interpersonal learning are typically ranked by members as being the most helpful aspect of the group therapy experience (Butler and Fuhriman 1980; Freedman and Hurley 1980; Lieberman et al. 1973; Yalom 1995). Of course, not all therapy groups concentrate in an explicit manner on interpersonal learning. However, interpersonal interaction, with its rich potential for learning and change, does occur any time a group assembles.

Forces That Modify the Therapeutic Factors in Group Therapy

We have applied a simplifying principle to the group therapeutic process and have identified a comprehensive set of therapeutic factors that operate in group therapy. And yet, group therapy is obviously a forum for change whose form, content, and process vary considerably both across groups and within the same group at any given time. In other words, different types of groups will make use of different clusters of therapeutic factors (see Table 31–1), and, furthermore, as a group evolves, different sets of factors come into play (Dies 1993). Thus, we need to be aware that three modifying forces can influence the therapeutic mechanisms at work in any given group: the type of group, the stage of therapy, and individual differences among patients.

Type of Group

Research on long-term interactional outpatient group therapy indicates that group members consistently select a constellation of three factors—interpersonal learning, catharsis, and self-understanding—as those elements of group therapy most helpful to them (Yalom 1995). Inpatients, in contrast, tend to identify other mechanisms: the instillation of hope and the existential factor of assumption of responsibility (Leszcz et al. 1985; Yalom 1983). This difference in emphasis is due to the fact that inpatient groups have high member turnover and are heterogeneous in clinical composition (i.e., patients with greatly differing ego strength, motivation, goals, and psychopathology meet in the same group for varying lengths of time). Furthermore, psychiatric patients usually enter the hospital in a state of despair, after they have exhausted other available resources. Groups that are centered around self-help concepts, such as Alcoholics Anonymous, Recovery, Inc., and support groups for bereaved parents, rely on the mechanisms of universality, guidance, altruism, and cohesiveness (Lieberman and Borman 1979).

Stage of Therapy

Patients' needs and goals change during the course of therapy and so, too, do the therapeutic factors that are most helpful to them. In its early stages, an outpatient group is most concerned with establishing boundaries and maintaining membership, and factors such as instillation of hope, guidance, and universality loom most important. Other factors, such as altruism and group cohesiveness, will operate throughout the duration of therapy, but their nature changes with the stage of the group. In the case of altruism, for example, early in the group, patients will offer suggestions to each other, ask appropriate questions, and show concern and attention. Later, they will be able to express a deeper caring and greater support for each other and exhibit a true sharing of emotion.

Initially, group cohesiveness occurs through group support and acceptance, whereas later in the life of the group it facilitates self-disclosure. Ultimately, group cohesiveness makes it possible for members to explore issues of confrontation and conflict, issues so essential to interpersonal learning. The longer patients participate in a group, the more they value the therapeutic factors of cohesiveness, self-understanding, and interpersonal interaction (Butler and Fuhriman 1983).

Differences Among Patients

As mentioned at the beginning of this section, each patient in group therapy is different, and patients with different levels of functioning will find different therapeutic factors beneficial. Higher-functioning patients tend to value interpersonal learning more than do lower-functioning patients in the same group. In one study of inpatient groups, both types of patients chose awareness of responsibility and catharsis as helpful elements of group therapy; however, the lower-functioning patients also valued the instillation of hope, and higher-functioning patients selected universality, vicarious learning, and interpersonal learning as additional useful experiences (Leszcz et al. 1985). A group experience is something of a therapeutic cafeteria: many different mechanisms of change are available, but each individual patient will make the most use out of those particular factors that are most suited to his or her needs and problems. A passive, repressed individual may benefit from experiencing and expressing strong affect, through catharsis, for example; whereas someone with impulse dyscontrol may profit from self-restraint and an intellectual structuring of the affective experience through imitative behavior. Some patients need to develop very basic social skills through the development of socializing techniques, whereas others benefit from the identification and exploration of much subtler interpersonal issues—for example, the patient who exaggerates helplessness and irrationality as a means of controlling other persons.

Therapeutic Factors: Summary

In sum, the comparative usefulness and potency of these simplified therapeutic factors are complex and change across groups, across members of the same group, and across time. Research indicates that different types of groups make use of different therapeutic factors, and therapists who are leading groups must have a firm grasp of those factors that are most compatible with the needs and capacities of their group members. An emphasis on interpersonal learning is not appropriate for a behaviorally oriented group for persons with bulimia nervosa, just as time taken for didactic education would frustrate the members of a long-term, intensive interactional group. The therapist thus has the basic task not only of understanding the appropriate mechanisms and goals for change in any given group, but also—as we shall explore in the next section—of establishing and maintaining the group within the setting of those goals.

The Therapist's Basic Tasks in Group Therapy

When a therapist begins individual psychotherapy with a new client, the therapist–patient dyad exists ipso facto, and the initial work of therapy unfolds from this point. But when a therapist starts a therapy group, the process is quite different. Long before the first meeting, the leader will have been hard at work, for the group therapist's initial task is to create a physical entity where none existed. The leader assembles a group and offers the professional help that is the initial raison d'être for the group. The leader selects the members and sets the time, place, and tone for the meetings. In sum, the therapist has the basic tasks of establishing and maintaining the group and resolving the problems typically encountered in the group setting (Table 31–4).

Let us explore some of these general principles of group format, composition, and maintenance, keeping in mind that these basic tasks can be modified to suit the needs of particular kinds of therapy groups.

TABLE 31–4. Therapist's basic tasks in group therapy

1. The decision to establish a therapy group:
   a. Determine setting and size of the group.
   b. Choose frequency and length of group sessions.
   c. Decide on open versus closed group.
   d. Select a co-therapist for the group.
2. The act of creating a therapy group:
   a. Formulate appropriate goals.
   b. Select patients who can perform the group task.
   c. Prepare patients for group therapy.
3. The construction and maintenance of a therapeutic environment:
   a. Build the culture of the group explicitly and implicitly.
   b. Identify and resolve common problems (membership turnover, subgrouping, conflict).
   c. Use procedural aids as appropriate.

Establishing a Therapy Group

Setting and Size

Before the first group meeting takes place, the therapist makes certain decisions about its circumstances. The most pragmatic of these involves choosing an appropriate meeting place. A setting that provides privacy and freedom from distraction is essential, of course, but a group meeting room should also be consistently available and of adequate size and have comfortable seating. A circular seating arrangement is necessary: all of the members must be able to see one another. The use of inpatient wards with long sofas does not permit good interaction. If three or four members sit in a row, they cannot see one another, and consequently most remarks in such groups are directed to the therapist, the one person visible to all. Furniture in the center of the room may hide nuances of body behavior; a table, for example, might mask the clenched fists of a member with a stoic facial expression. Some therapists provide coffee and tea at the meeting place; one effect of this is to increase the sociability of the setting, at least before the actual session.

The optimal size of a group is a function of its therapeutic goals. Organizations such as Alcoholics Anonymous and Recovery, Inc., that operate with group settings of up to 80 members rely heavily on inspiration, guidance, and suppression to change members' behavior. However, leaders working in a large therapeutic community (e.g., in a residential halfway house) might wish to make use of a different set of factors, such as group pressure and interdependence to foster reality testing or to instill a sense of individual responsibility to the social community. In this setting, groups of 15 or so members may be more appropriate.

The ideal size for a prototypical interactional group is 7 or 8 members, and certainly no more than 10. Too few members will not provide the critical mass necessary for interpersonal interactions. In a group that is too small, there will not be enough opportunities for broad consensual validation, and patients will tend to interact one at a time with the therapist rather than with one another. Anyone who has ever tried to conduct a group with only two or three patients knows the frustration of this enterprise. In a group with more than 10 members, however, there may be ample fruitful interaction, but some members will be left out. There will simply be insufficient time to examine and understand all of the interactions.

When the therapist is working with inpatients or leading specialized outpatient groups, his or her focus may not be as explicitly interpersonally oriented as in the prototypical interaction group, but the therapist will still want to aim for a lively and engaging group, one that encourages active participation by as many members as possible. In our clinical experience, the optimal group size that allows members to share experiences with one another ranges from a minimum of 4 or 5 to a maximum of 12; groups of 6–8 members seem to offer the greatest opportunity for verbal exchange among all patients.

Time Constraints and Use of Open Versus Closed Groups

The late 1960s and early 1970s saw a great deal of experimentation with the time variable in group therapy. Weekly 4- to 8-hour groups were not unheard of, and marathon weekend sessions were common. Research has failed to demonstrate any superiority of the time-extended meeting, and today there is a clinical consensus that the optimal duration for a session in ongoing group therapy is between 60 and 120 minutes (Yalom 1995). Usually 20–30 minutes are required for the group to warm up, and at least 60 minutes are needed to work through the major themes of the session. After about 2 hours, most therapists find they begin to fatigue and the group becomes weary and repetitious. Groups that meet frequently, such as daily inpatient groups, or groups that consist of lower-functioning patients who can tolerate only limited social stimuli, do well with briefer sessions. Groups that meet less often or that are centered on higher-functioning interactional work require at least 90 minutes per session in order to be fruitful.

The frequency of meetings can vary from once a day—typically in the inpatient setting, where therapy groups meet from three to six times a week—to once every 3–12 weeks, as in clinic medication–support groups. A once-weekly schedule is most common in outpatient group work and seems well suited to supportive or specialized groups. Long-term interactional groups also tend to meet once per week, although clinical experience suggests that twice-weekly sessions, when feasible, increase the intensity and productivity of this kind of group.

The decision to make a group open or closed is related to the goals of the group and its identified life span. A closed group meets for a predetermined number of sessions, begins with a fixed number of members, and, as of the first session, closes its doors and accepts no new members. For example, therapists working with a specialized group of bereaved spouses or of patients with eating disorders may take in a fixed number of patients for a preset number of sessions, usually 8–12 meetings. In such time-limited groups, each session may follow a predetermined protocol. External time constraints can also influence the format of a group. For example, in a university health center, a support group for graduate students having trouble with their dissertations may be set up to run the length of an academic semester.

In contrast, open groups either are more flexible about size—consider the ongoing inpatient group on a psychiatric ward, which reflects ward census—or may maintain a consistent size by replacing members as they leave the group. Open groups usually have a broader set of therapeutic goals and generally meet indefinitely; although members come and go, the group has a life of its own. Such ongoing outpatient groups at psychiatric teaching centers have been known to continue for more than 20 years and to have been the training ground for generations of residents!

Use of a Co-therapist

Most group therapists prefer to work with a co-therapist. Co-therapists complement and support each other. As the therapists share points of view and examine hunches together, each therapist's observational range is broadened. There is much agreement among clinicians that a male–female co-therapist team has unique advantages. It recreates the parental configuration of the primary family, which for many members increases the affective charge of the group. Many patients can benefit from observing a male therapist and a female therapist working together with mutual respect and without the derogation, exploitation, or sexualizing that the patients too often take for granted in male–female relationships. Moreover, the group is provided with a wider array of transferential possibilities, for patients will differ in their reactions to each of the co-therapists and to the co-therapists' relationship. In a group led by a male–female

co-therapist team, for example, a somewhat histrionic female member may pander to the male leader and ignore his female counterpart, a pattern that would not emerge as clearly in a group led by one therapist. Other members may have fantasies about the relationship between the two co-therapists.

The co-therapy format seems particularly helpful for beginning therapists and for experienced therapists working with an especially difficult patient population. In addition to clarifying transference distortions of each other's presentation in the group, co-therapists can support each other in maintaining objectivity in the face of massive group pressure. We had occasion to work at one point with a lonely female member of a group, a hospital volunteer who became romantically involved with one of her psychiatric patients; she discussed this in a group session and then verbally flagellated herself. In an effort to be supportive, the other members unanimously and vociferously condoned her behavior and attempted to pressure the leaders into a noncritical stance as well. As co-therapists, we were better able to resist the powerful group pressure and maintain our professional objectivity about this woman's behavior.

Similarly, co-therapists are invaluable in helping each other constructively weather an attack from group members. A therapist under the gun may be too threatened either to clarify the attack or to encourage further exploration without appearing defensive or condescending. There is nothing more squelching than when a leader under fire says, "It's really great that you're expressing your feelings and attacking me. Keep it going!" It is usually the co-therapist who can best help members channel and express their anger in an appropriate manner and who can then lead members to examine the source and the meaning of that anger.

There is some question whether co-therapists should openly reveal their differences of opinion during the group session. Two factors to consider are the level of functioning of the group and the maturity of the group. Patients who are lower functioning and who are more fragile or unstable overall should generally not be exposed to conflict between the co-therapists, no matter how gently it is expressed. Likewise, co-therapist disagreement is not helpful early in the work with even higher-functioning patients, for a beginning group usually is not stable or cohesive enough to tolerate divisiveness in leadership. Later in such a group, however, the therapists' honesty about disagreement can contribute substantially to the potency and honesty of the group. Members observe the leaders they respect disagreeing openly and resolving their differences with honesty and tact. Members also experience the therapists not as infallible authority figures but as humans with imperfections, and they thus learn to differentiate others according to individual attributes rather than stereotyped roles.

The major disadvantages of the co-therapy format flow from problems in the co-therapy relationship itself. If coleaders are uncomfortable with each other, closed and competitive, or in wide disagreement about style and strategy, there is little chance that their group will be able to work effectively. Research has demonstrated that the major causes of failure are co-therapists' embracing vastly different ideological positions (Paulson et al. 1976) and failing to address the developmental tasks of the co-therapy relationship as these reflect the developmental tasks of the group (Dugo and Beck 1997). Therefore, when choosing a coleader, it is important to select someone who is different enough in personal style to be complementary but who is similar in theoretical orientation and with whom you can discuss your relationship especially as it pertains to the group's development.

Whenever two therapists of vastly different levels of experience lead a group together, it is important that they be open-minded and mature, comfortable with each other, and comfortable in their roles as co-workers or as teacher and apprentice. Splitting is a phenomenon that often occurs in groups led by co-therapists, and some patients are very perceptive about tensions in the co-therapists' relationship. For example, if a neophyte therapist feels jealous of a senior co-therapist's clinical experience and wisdom, a member might marvel at everything the older therapist says and denigrate the younger therapist's interventions. Occasionally the entire group can become split into two factions, with each co-therapist having a "team" of patients aligned with him or her; this may occur because the patients believe they have a special relationship with one or the other of the therapists or because they believe that one of the therapists is more intelligent, more senior, or more attractive or has a similar ethnic background. Splitting, like the problem of subgrouping that we will discuss later, should always be noted and openly interpreted in the group.

Combining Group Therapy With Other Therapeutic Modalities

The standard group therapy format, in which one therapist meets with six to eight patients, is often combined with other therapeutic modalities. For example, some or all of the patients in a given group may also be involved in concurrent individual psychotherapy with other therapists; this is often described as *conjoint therapy* and is one of the more preferable means for combining psychotherapies. Occasionally, all or some of the members in a group are in concurrent individual therapy with the group therapist in what is known as *combined therapy*. This latter therapy usually arises when a psychotherapist in solo private practice forms a group from the ranks of his or her individual patients. Both conjoint and combined therapies are frequently encountered by therapists who run groups in clinics or on inpatient wards. Amaranto and Benden (1990) are developing models to incorporate the advantages of both.

When is it useful to combine psychotherapeutic modalities? Some patients may go through a life crisis so severe that they require temporary individual support in addition to group therapy. Others may be so chronically disabled by fear, anxiety, or aggression that they require individual therapy to participate effectively in the group and avoid becoming locked into a stereotyped role. At times, active individual intervention is necessary simply to explore the patient's conflicts in group therapy and thus prevent him or her from having an unprofitable experience or from dropping out of the group. Individual or group therapy approaches complement each other most effectively when the individual and group therapists support each other and are in frequent contact and when the individual therapy is interpersonally oriented and explores feelings and incidents related to current group meetings.

Concurrent individual therapy can hinder group therapy in several ways. When there is a marked difference in approach between the individual therapist and the group therapist, patients may become confused and the two therapies may work at cross-purposes. The patient who is used to the support and narcissistic gratification of individual therapy—who is accustomed to exploring fantasies, dreams, associations, and memories and to being the exclusive center of attention of a therapist—may become frustrated by initial group meetings. Early sessions usually offer less personal support and may be dedicated more to building a cohesive unit and to examining here-and-now interactions than to deep exploration of each member's life. Individual therapy and group therapy can also interfere with each other if patients use their individual therapy to drain off affect from the group, reacting to emotionally laden events in the group only later in the sanctum of their individual therapy hour.

Another combination is the use of group therapy with medication clinics, a practical and humane combination of modalities most often, but not exclusively, used with chronic psychiatric patients (Brook 1993, 2001; Cox 2001). In this approach, patients who attend biweekly or monthly medication clinics, usually to receive prescriptions for antipsychotic medication or for mood stabilizers, also participate in a group meeting associated with the clinic. Sessions are generally highly structured and focus on educating patients about their medications, on solving practical problems, and on sharing a difficult plight. A chronically psychotic patient who lives in relative social isolation can use these groups to practice some basic social skills and to receive support for his or her efforts. Group therapy is used to personalize, enhance, and reinforce the patient's experience in a medication clinic.

Creating a Therapy Group

Formulating Goals

As a first step to creating a therapy group, the therapist must carefully examine all of the clinical facts of life that will bear on the group. The *intrinsic* factors (e.g., mandatory attendance for patients on legal probation, duration of treatment in a ward group of hospitalized patients with cancer) are built into the clinical situation and cannot be changed; the group leader must adapt to them. The *extrinsic* factors are those that have become tradition or policy in a given setting—an example might be an inpatient ward's fixed program of daily community meetings. Extrinsic factors are arbitrary and within the power of the therapist to change.

Once a clear view of the clinical facts of life has been obtained, the leader's second step is to construct a reasonable set of clinical goals for the group. This is the most important step in creating a therapy group, for the selection of inappropriate or vaguely defined goals is sure to result in failure. The goals of a long-term outpatient group are ambitious: to offer symptomatic relief and to change character structure. An attempt to apply these same goals to an aftercare group of patients with chronic schizophrenia would result in therapeutic nihilism.

Goals must be shaped that are appropriate to the clinical situation and achievable in the amount of time available. In time-limited, specialized groups, the goals must be focused, achievable, and tailored to the capacity and potential of the group members. It is important that the therapy group be a success experience; patients enter therapy feeling defeated and demoralized, and the last thing they need is another failure.

Selecting Patients and Composing a Therapy Group

Once the therapist has a clear idea of the goals of the group—in other words, a clear idea of the group task—he or she must select members who can achieve these goals and perform the group task. The leader's expertise in the selection and preparation of members will greatly affect the group's fate. The therapist must create a group that coheres, and, because nothing threatens a group's cohesiveness more than the presence of a grossly deviant member, the selection of members must be guided by the notion of group integrity and the avoidance of deviancy. A group of board-and-care-home residents with chronic schizophrenia cannot cohere effectively in the presence of an exploitative and manipulative member with a personality disorder; nor can a high-functioning group of outpatients function well together in the presence of a patient who frequently goes into dissociative states.

The single most important criterion for member selection, no matter what the group, is an ability to perform the group task. Study of group failures reveals that deviancy (i.e., an inability or refusal to engage in the group task) is negatively related to outcome. An individual who considers himself or herself (or is considered by other members) to be "out of the group" or a deviant or mascot has little likelihood of profiting from the group and there is a fair chance of negative outcome for that person (Lieberman et al. 1973). Therefore, selection for group therapy is, in practice, conducted by the process of elimination. Group therapists exclude certain patients from consideration (most often because the therapist predicts the patient will assume a deviant role or because the patient lacks motivation for change) and accept remaining patients.

Once a leader determines that a patient could benefit from group therapy, how does he or she go about actually composing a group? How is it decided which patients will work well together? Above all, the therapist must be concerned about the group's *integrity*. Members selected must be committed to the task of therapy and to regular attendance in the group. To attempt to refine the process of composition even more—to form a group ideally composed to interact therapeutically—is every group therapist's dream, yet we lack the knowledge and instruments necessary to permit us to realize this dream. Perhaps the key concept is group cohesiveness. An effective rule of thumb for longer-term outpatient groups is "homogeneity in ego strength, heterogeneity in problem areas" (Whitaker and Lieberman 1964). In other words, patients profit from a mixture of personality styles, ages, and problem areas—all factors that enrich the broth of the ensuing group interaction—but the group coheres best if all members possess the ego strength necessary to participate equally in the group task.

The situation is different in specialized or symptom-oriented groups; in these cases, members always share at least one major problem area (e.g., an eating disorder, bereavement, chronic pain), but they may be heterogeneous in terms of ego strength. Whenever possible, the therapist aims for similar levels of motivation and psychological-mindedness in the composition of the group. Having one or two members who are fragile, brittle, or work avoidant impedes the work of a fast-paced, highly motivated group. Likewise, a stolid group of more concrete chronically ill psychiatric patients can become destabilized if pushed too hard too fast by a confrontational, agitated, or manic individual (Kahn 1984; Kanas 1985, 1986). Beyond this, leaders may wish to try to balance the group composition along various parameters, such as by composing a group with an equal number of men and women, a wide age range, or varied interpersonal activity levels.

Often (as in, for example, mandatory inpatient groups or a group in a correctional institution) the therapist has minimal influence over group membership. At the very least, he or she must exercise the group therapist's prerogative and exclude those patients who are markedly incompatible with the prevailing group norms for acceptable behavior. Examples might include the physically agitated patient or the manic patient. Patients who cannot tolerate the stress of a group setting, such as extremely paranoid individuals, and patients who are absolutely incompatible with at least one other member also should not be included in the group. Group member screening is even more complicated in managed care settings. On the one hand, therapists often feel pressure from administration to fit patients into a group, and a higher risk of poor fit is tolerated. On the other hand, large institutional settings with large group programs are more likely to have a group that is suitable for any given patient. Unfortunately, the former situation is more common early in group program development.

One reason it is so difficult to compose an ideal group is that it is extremely difficult to predict subsequent group behavior from information available at the time of the screening procedure. An important source of information is the candidate's previous experience in groups. Another important source is the screening procedure itself. In the one or two intake interviews, the therapist should focus on the candidate's interpersonal functioning: past, present, and in the interview itself. The therapist must assess the individual's ability to tolerate interpersonal interactions and to reflect on them. Suitable questions might include the following: "How has the interview been for you so far today?" "Were there any parts that made you uncomfortable?" "What is it like for you to reveal things about yourself to a relative stranger?"

Preparing Patients for Group Therapy

Preparation of the patient for group therapy is another one of the therapist's essential tasks. A great deal of powerful research evidence has demonstrated that pregroup preparation decreases the number of dropouts, increases cohesiveness, and accelerates the work of therapy (Piper and Perrault 1989; Piper et al. 1982; Yalom 1966, 1995). In some settings, such as an inpatient ward or a medication support group, this preparation will of necessity be minimal and will consist mainly of orienting the patient to the time, location, composition, procedure, and goals of the group. But even this brief preparation helps to orient patients to the group experience and provides guidelines about how to benefit from the group.

For most outpatient groups, preparation is best accomplished during one or two individual sessions with each patient before he or she begins group therapy. After deciding during an intake interview that the patient is a suitable candidate for group therapy, the therapist may then proceed to prepare the patient for the group. Patients have ample amounts of primary anxiety, and therapists must avoid adding yet more—the secondary anxiety that arises from being thrown into an ambiguous, intrinsically threatening situation. Therefore, providing clarity is the chief aim of the pregroup preparatory procedure. The therapist provides patients with a cognitive structure that enables them to participate more effectively in the group from the start.

Many patients hold misconceptions about the worth and efficacy of group therapy; they believe that it is cheaper or diluted therapy and therefore not as worthwhile as individual therapy. These negative expectations must be addressed openly and corrected so that the patient will engage fully in treatment. Other patients express concerns about procedure and process: the size of the group, the type of members, the amount of negative confrontation, confidentiality. One of the most pervasive fears is the fear of having to reveal oneself and confess shameful transgressions to an audience of hostile strangers. Another common worry is a fear of mental contagion, of being made sicker through association with other psychiatric patients. Often this fear is a preoccupation of schizophrenic or borderline patients, although the fear may also be observed in patients who project their own feelings of self-contempt or hostility onto others.

A cognitive approach to group therapy preparation has several goals (Table 31–5).

Underlying everything the therapist says is a process of demystification and the establishment of a therapeutic alliance. This comprehensive preparation enables the patient to make an informed decision to enter the therapy group and enhances commitment to the group from the beginning.

TABLE 31–5. Rationales behind group therapy preparation

Provide a rational explanation to the patient about the group therapy process.

Describe the behavior expected of patients in the group.

Establish a treatment contract.

Raise expectations about the effects of the group.

Predict some of the common problems and discouragement that may be encountered in early meetings.

Constructing and Maintaining a Therapeutic Environment

Building the Culture of the Group

Once the group is a physical reality and the first meeting is under way, the leader must establish behavioral norms that will guide the interactions of the newly formed group. In individual therapy the therapist is the sole designated agent of direct change, but in group therapy the situation is more complex. Ideally, *all* of the members of the group will provide support, a sense of universality, and interpersonal feedback—in other words, the members themselves will be important agents of change. Any time a group of people assembles, be it in a professional, social, or even family setting, it will develop a "culture," a set of unwritten rules or norms that determine the acceptable behavioral procedure of the group. In group therapy, it is the leader's task to create a group culture maximally conducive to effective group interaction and to the development of the various therapeutic factors.

Norms constructed early in the group are important. They are shaped both by the expectations of the members as they start the group and by the behavior of the therapist during the early sessions. The therapist influences this process of norm setting in two different ways. First, the leader, in the role of technical expert, can *explicitly* shape the group norms. During early preparation of patients for group therapy, for example, patients can be given explicit instructions about the rules for appropriate behavior in the group, such as sharing concerns about body image in an eating disorders group. Once a group gets under way, the leader may reward desirable behavior through social reinforcement. If a usually shy member begins to participate, or if members start to offer one another spontaneous and honest feedback, this new behavior may be shaped and rewarded verbally or nonverbally through changes in the therapist's body language, eye contact, and facial expression.

The second way the therapist shapes therapeutic norms in the group is through model setting. In an acute inpatient therapy group, for example, leaders offer a model of nonjudgmental acceptance and appreciation of members' strengths as well as problem areas, helping to shape a group that is health oriented. In a social skills training group for schizophrenic patients, the leader might choose to model simple, direct, socially rewarding conversation. No matter what the level and functioning of the group, the effective leader sets a model of interpersonal honesty and spontaneity for his or her group members. But the therapist's honesty must take place in the service of his or her background responsibility; nothing takes precedence over the goal of being helpful to the patient.

There are several basic therapeutic group norms that should be encouraged in any group setting, regardless of its orientation. The first of these is the norm of the *self-monitoring group*, in which the group itself learns to assume responsibility for its own functioning. Any therapist who has ever worked in a group in which the members are completely dependent on the leader for direction knows firsthand the signs of the passive group. The patients seem to be an audience at a play; they appear to be waiting for the leader to make the curtain rise and the action begin. The group begins to feel stilted, heavy, and forced. After every meeting, the leader feels fatigued, powerless, and irritated by the burden of making it all work.

How can the therapist build a culture that encourages the development of a self-monitoring group? This can be accomplished by keeping in mind that initially, only the leader knows when a group has been productive. The therapist must start to share this knowledge with the patients at the very inception of a group and slowly educate them to recognize a good session. The therapist might say, "This was an exciting meeting today and everyone shared a lot. I hate to see it end." The evaluative function can then be shifted to the patients by the therapist's saying, "How is the group going so far today? What's been the most satisfying part?" And, finally, members can be taught that they have the ability to influence the course of a session; the therapist could say, "Things have been slow today. What could we do to make it different?"

There are several other basic norms that influence the therapy. *General procedural norms* must always be actively shaped by the leader. Ideally, the most therapeutic procedural format of a group is one that is unstructured, unrehearsed, and freely flowing. The therapist must intervene actively to preclude the development of a nontherapeutic procedure, for example, a "taking turns" format in which members figuratively line up to discuss specific problems or life crises one after another by rote. In such an instance, the therapist might interrupt and ask how the practice got started or what effect it has on the group. The leader could also indicate that the group has many other procedural options from which to choose.

When *members consider the group important*, group therapy becomes more effective, and the leader who reinforces this norm increases the therapeutic potency of his or her group. Likewise, the therapist augments the power of the group by increasing *the continuity between meetings*. It is the task of the therapist, as the group "time-binder," to call attention to behavioral patterns developing over several meetings. Finally, a group functions best when it sees its *members as agents of help and support;* a truly therapeutic culture implies, both explicitly and implicitly, that members will learn the most and receive the most help from one another.

Identifying and Resolving Common Problems in Group Therapy

Membership problems. The early developmental sequence and potency of a therapy group are strongly affected by *membership problems*. Turnover in membership, tardiness, and absence are facts of life in all groups, yet these events will threaten a group's stability and integrity. Considerable absenteeism will redirect an outpatient group's attention and energy from its developmental tasks to the problem of maintaining membership, whereas continual turnover in inpatient groups powerfully affects group cohesiveness. Tardiness and irregular attendance must be discouraged in all group settings and should be regarded in the same way in which one regards these phenomena in individual therapy.

Leaders of long-term outpatient therapy groups should keep in mind that in the normal course of such groups, 10%–35% of the members will drop out in the first 12–20 meetings (Yalom 1966, 1995). In an open group it is the therapist's task to replace dropouts by adding new members. Dropouts are threatening to the group's stability for two reasons: they impede the development of cohesiveness, and they implicitly (and sometimes explicitly) devalue the group. Dropouts are also threatening to the leader, especially to the neophyte, and the therapist may unwittingly adopt a seductive posture in an effort to keep a patient in the group. The dropout rate can be reduced through vigorous pretherapy selection and preparation (Connelly et al. 1986; McCallum et al. 1992; Orlinsky and Howard 1986; Piper and Perrault 1989). If predictions of the general problems and frustrations that can arise early in a group are made to new members ahead of time, there is less likelihood that dropping out will occur.

Subgrouping. A second problem commonly encountered in group therapy is *subgrouping*—the splitting off of smaller units. A subgroup usually arises from the belief by two or more members that these members can derive more gratification from a relationship with one another than from one with the entire group. Extragroup socializing, which often occurs in outpatient groups (and almost invariably in inpatient groups), is often the first stage of subgrouping. A clique of three or four members will begin to have telephone conversations, to have coffee or dinner, and to share separate observations and interactions with one another. Occasionally, two members will become sexually involved. A subgroup may also coalesce completely within the confines of the group therapy room, as members who perceive themselves to be similar form coalitions based on age, similar values, comparable education, and the like. Remaining group members, excluded from the clique, generally do not possess effective social skills and do not usually coalesce into a second subgroup. This phenomenon of "ingroup" versus "outgroup" can often be strikingly observed in inpatient settings.

The members of a subgroup can be recognized by a code of behavior: they agree with one another regardless of the issue and they avoid confrontations among their own membership; they exchange knowing glances when a member who is not in the clique speaks; they arrive and depart from the meeting together. Complications arise for all members of the therapy group, whether they belong to the subgroup or not. If a member belongs, loyalty to the subgroup is a major issue, secrets begin to be kept, and the free and honest discussion of feelings becomes inhibited. If a member has been excluded from the subgroup, complex feelings of envy, competition, and inferiority are aroused. Unfortunately, as these emotions and the anxiety associated with earlier exclusion experiences are evoked, it becomes exceptionally difficult for members to comment on their feelings of exclusion.

It is not the extragroup socializing that is crippling to a group per se; rather, it is the conspiracy of silence around it that becomes dangerous. The primary task in the group is to examine in depth the interpersonal relationships among all of the members, and extragroup socializing inhibits this examination. Important material—the relationship between members who are interacting outside the group, feelings of exclusion in patients who are not part of this interaction—remains covert, and the task of the group is sabotaged. Patients who violate group norms through the pursuit of subgrouping or through secret extragroup liaisons are opting for immediate need gratification rather than for involvement in interpersonal learning and change. Subgrouping or extragroup behavior that remains covert—that is not examined in the group session—becomes a potent form of resistance. It hobbles the therapist and makes a travesty of other members' efforts to be revealing, to give honest feedback, and to participate fully and authentically in the group process.

Subgrouping represents a situation that contains both high risk and high gain. In pregroup preparation, the therapist attempts to prevent its occurrence by actively encouraging the development of group norms whereby all extragroup behavior is subsequently brought back into the group for discussion. When it does take place, subgrouping must be explicitly identified—usually by the leader—and explored in the light of the group task, which is the in-depth examination of the interpersonal relationships among all members. When the powerful issues that give rise to subgrouping are confronted by the group, discussed openly, and worked through, they can prove to be of considerable therapeutic import in the very group they were hampering.

In fact, deliberate use of subgrouping is part of the conceptual heart of systems-centered therapy. Agazarian (1997) utilized systems theory and directed therapeutic efforts mostly toward subgroups. The group-as-a-whole is a supra-entity (it contains the subgroup) and the individual members are part of subgroups (subgroups of the subgroup). Changes occurring at the level of the subgroup influence the nature of the group-as-a-whole as well as the participating individuals. Such parsimony of effort is further enhanced by the deliberate addressing of details of subgrouping. Noting changes in the "boundaries" between subgroups (e.g., splits, containing and integrating differences) and the direction of the systems or subsystem's energy (vectors) can be the basis for interventions. These interventions, placed in a framework that Agazarian (1997) called "defense modification," appear to quickly move forward the work of the group-as-a-whole as well as that of the individuals. Subgrouping, like any powerful phenomenon, can be destructive if unaddressed. However, it is also potentially instructive and productive. Agazarian enhanced group therapists' ability to use subgrouping effectively.

Conflict. *Conflict*, a third common problem, is inevitable in the course of a group's development. The task of the therapist is to identify conflict as it arises and to harness it in the service of the group task. Conflict resolution is virtually impossible in the presence of off-target or oblique hostility, and, once again, it is the therapist's task to identify and render overt that which has been covert. For example, he or she might say, "Bob, I've noticed that you've cut off Mary a couple of times today. I wonder if

you're feeling a little angry because of the feedback the women in the group gave you last week."

How can the therapist harness conflict in the group and use it in the service of interpersonal growth? One important step is finding the right level for the group at hand. Too much conflict is threatening and counterproductive for just about any group of individuals, but too little conflict—especially with higher-functioning patients—leaves the group stagnant, excessively cautious, and superficial. Here, a judicious amount of confrontation, anger, and conflict resolution can provide an affectively charged learning experience for the group members.

Group cohesiveness is the prime prerequisite for the successful management of conflict. Members must have developed a feeling of mutual respect and trust and must value the group sufficiently to be able to tolerate confrontational or uncomfortable interactions. The leader will need to emphasize that open communication must be maintained if the group is to survive; all members must continue to deal directly with one another, no matter how angry they become. Norms must be established in which it is made clear that group members are there to understand themselves, not to outdo, defeat, or ridicule one another. Furthermore, every member is to be taken seriously. When a group begins to treat one person as someone whose opinions and anger are to be lightly regarded, the hope of effective treatment for that patient has all but officially been abandoned.

Not all groups tolerate the same level of conflict. The open, conflictual confrontation that might take place between two members of a long-term outpatient group would be devastating in a group for schizophrenic patients (Kanas 1985, 1996). Gentle, cautious disagreement would be appropriate in a time-limited group for patients with panic disorder, whereas such disagreement would be seen as an avoidance of the real issues in a long-term outpatient group. Furthermore, even the same group may not tolerate the same level of conflict at different points in its development. Early on, a prototypical group needs to invest its energy in the development of cohesiveness, trust, and support. In its middle phases, such a group will begin the constructive exploration of disagreement and confrontation. Much later, as members are terminating therapy, they may wish to focus again on the positive, more intimate aspects of the group experience rather than the divisive ones.

Finally, therapists should remember that conflict easily gets out of hand, no matter what the group setting. Leaders will often have to intervene vigorously to keep conflict within constructive bounds. Most often, this will include helping patients to express anger more directly and more fairly and ensuring that everyone gets a turn to respond to the anger. As with any affectively charged experience in the group, the therapist will need to encourage active feedback and consensual validation from all of the group members and, more than ever, will need to help patients process the meaning of that experience within the context of the group.

Techniques of the Group Therapist

Although individual and group therapists often use similar psychotherapeutic techniques, a number of interventions are unique to group therapy. These interventions include working in the here and now, using therapist transparency, and employing various procedural aids that can enhance the group work. We shall briefly examine each of these group therapy techniques and then describe how fundamental group therapy technology can be modified to suit a specialized group setting.

Working in the Here and Now

Even in the absence of direct leadership—for example, in a self-help group with no designated leader—an environment can develop in which nearly all of the therapeutic factors, from universality to altruism, will operate. The one important exception is the factor of interpersonal learning. In group therapy, interpersonal learning requires the presence of a leader, one who is well versed in the specific therapeutic techniques of working in the here and now. The principles of working in the here and now and the use of interpersonal learning are of most consequence in prototypic interactional groups, but these fundamental concepts can be modified to suit the needs of other kinds of groups and form an essential part of any group therapist's armamentarium (Dies 1993; Kahn 1984; Rothke 1986).

Goals

The primary goal of the long-term outpatient therapy group, and, to a lesser extent, of many other kinds of groups, is to help each individual understand as much as possible about his or her interactions with the other members of the group, therapists included. To accomplish this, members must learn to focus on the immediate interpersonal transactions occurring in the group. For the therapist, this means that the most fundamental principle of technique is to focus on the present, on what takes place in the therapy room in the here and now of the group interaction. By directly focusing on the here and now, the leader solicits and engages the active participation of all the members and maximizes the power and efficiency of the group. In other words, the therapy group focus is most powerful if it is basically ahistoric—that is, if it deemphasizes the historical past and even the current outside life of the individual members in favor of the here-and-now events in the group. Deemphasis does not imply that history is unimportant; rather, it implies that groups work most efficiently on the interactions occurring in the immediate present.

If it is to be therapeutically effective, a group experience must contain both an affective and a cognitive component. That is, the group members must be involved with one another in an affective matrix: they must interact freely, they must reveal a great deal of themselves, and they must experience and express important emotions. But they must also step outside that experience and examine, understand, and integrate the meaning of the emotional experience they have just undergone (Yalom and Vinogradov 1993). Thus, a here-and-now focus consists of a rotating sequence of affect evocation and affect examination (Figure 31–2).

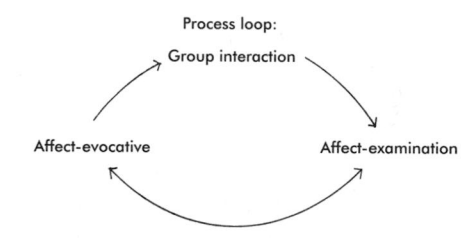

FIGURE 31–2. Schematic representation of the here-and-now technique in group therapy.

The absence of either the affective or the cognitive components of the here-and-now experience jeopardizes therapy. Encounter groups were often powerful and exciting events in the 1960s and 1970s, but many participants found that a strong emotional occurrence without subsequent examination promoted little real learning. No real therapeutic change occurs unless group members can integrate what they have learned in the here and now and then transfer that learning to their real-life situation. Likewise, leaders who focus exclusively on explanations and intellectual integration can end up squelching all expression of spontaneous affect and create a lifeless, sterile group.

Techniques

These two stages of the here-and-now focus—affect evocation followed by affect examination—are different in character and demand two very distinct sets of techniques. For the first stage, the stage of emotional experience, the therapist needs a set of techniques that will plunge the group into the immediate interpersonal interactions. For the second stage, clarification and understanding of the emotional experience, the therapist needs a set of techniques that will help the group transcend itself to examine and interpret its own experience. Let us consider each of these stages in turn.

Plunging the group into the here and now. The starting place for shaping a group focused on the here and now is the pregroup preparation. The leader can offer the patient a rationale of the here-and-now approach through a brief, simplified discussion of the interpersonal approach to therapy. Patients benefit from an explicit description of how various kinds of psychological problems arise from (and are manifested in) patients' relationships with others and how group therapy is an ideal setting to take a close look at interpersonal relationships. Without this preparation, patients may be confused by the here-and-now focus of the group. After all, they sought therapy to deal with painful feelings such as anxiety, anger, or depression; how can they not be puzzled to find themselves in a group in which the therapist is asking them to reveal their feelings toward seven strangers? To alleviate this kind of confusion and to ensure that patients participate fully, the therapist must provide a cognitive bridge for incoming members.

After laying these foundations for the here-and-now focus in the pregroup preparation, the leader continues to reinforce this focus throughout therapy. Experienced group therapists think "here and now" at all times and consider themselves as shepherds keeping the group at work grazing on current interactions. All strays into the past, into outside life, or into intellectualization must be headed off or gently nudged back into the present. Whenever the group engages in some "there and then" discussion, for example, the group leader must think, "How can I bring this back into the here and now?"

The therapist must begin to steer the group into the here and now in its very first session. Consider for a moment the beginning of any therapy group. Typically, some member will get things started by sharing with the group a major life problem or concern and the reasons why he or she is now in this therapy group. Usually this disclosure begets both some support and some similar disclosure from others, and in a short period the group members have begun to share a great deal.

To plunge the group into the here and now, the interactionally oriented therapist may intervene with a comment such as "This group has made a good start, and many of you have shared some important things about yourselves. However, I have a hunch that something else has been happening here today as well. [It is of course more than a hunch. The therapist knows perfectly well that what he or she is about to say has occurred.] Each of you has found himself or herself thrown together with a group of strangers. No doubt you've been observing and sizing up one another and making first impressions." By this time, some persons in the group will be nodding in agreement, and the therapist may then set the task of the group: "Perhaps we could spend the rest of the meeting today discussing what each of you has come up with so far." Or, in a more fragile, lower-functioning group in which members might find this open-ended task threatening, an alternative suggestion could be, "Perhaps we could share what we liked the most about each other's participation so far." Now, this is no subtle intervention. It is a heavy-handed, explicit instruction to begin the process of here-and-now interaction. And yet the vast majority of groups, no matter what their composition or orientation, respond favorably to this intervention. Even groups of hospitalized patients, if proper boundaries are placed, accomplish this task with considerable ease and reward.

Group therapists must be active and continue diligently from session to session to bring the group discussion into the here and now. They must shift the content of the material from outside the group to inside the group, from abstract reflections on problems to specific revelations, from generic statements to personal disclosure. When a patient states that he or she is embarrassed to talk about certain things in the group, the therapist might ask what the patient anticipates happening if he or she were to take the risk and talk about something "embarrassing." If the patient supposes that people might laugh or be judgmental, the leader could then ask, "Who here in the group do you feel would laugh at you?" Once the group member reveals his or her guesses about others' reactions, the door is open to good interactional work. Other group members can confirm or, as is more often the case, disconfirm those guesses.

A useful technique for activating the here and now is to identify an in-group analogue for some outgroup problem and then to work on the in-group analogue rather than the out-group situation. If, for example, a male patient brings in an account of an argument he had with his wife in which she accused him of being unfeeling, it is incumbent on the group leader to search for some type of here-and-now manifestation of that conflict. The therapist might reflect on recent interactions in the group in which members wondered whether this patient was really empathic to their problems. Or the therapist might ask some of the female members of the group to picture being married to this patient. To what degree of close emotional contact could they imagine being in with him? Without an intervention of this sort, the group will spend its energies on helping the patient solve the problems that led to the argument with his wife—an inefficient use of a group's time. Generally presented with incomplete or biased data, groups are almost always destined to fail to solve outside problems, and members end up feeling frustrated or discouraged.

The therapist who is experienced in working in the here and now is able to use almost every incident as a springboard for interactional exploration. If a patient monopolizes the group with a long 20-minute convoluted account of some painful period that occurred earlier in his life, the leader should start to reflect, "What are the interactional aspects of this behavior?" The leader may recall that in the first session, this patient said he often feels others don't listen to him. "Is it possible," the therapist could ask aloud, "that this is one of those times?" Another tack might be to ask why the patient chose to deliver this monologue today in the group. "What do the rest of you think? Could it be related to a feeling of being misunderstood in last week's meeting?" Or the patient could be encouraged to guess how the rest of the group is reacting to what he has been saying. Any one of these approaches has the same effect: it moves the group members away from a content-oriented monologue in which they cannot participate to a discussion of the relationships among members.

Individuals do not engage naturally and easily in the here and now. The experience is new and frightening, especially for the many patients who have not previously had close and honest relationships or who have spent their lives keeping certain thoughts and feelings—anger, pain, intimacy—covert. The therapist must offer much support, reinforcement, and explicit training. A first step is to help patients understand that the here-and-now focus is not synonymous with confrontation and conflict. In fact, many patients have problems not with anger or rage but with closeness and the honest and nondemanding or nonmanipulative expression of positive sentiments. Accordingly, it is important early in the group to encourage the expression of positive feelings as well as critical ones (Yalom and Vinogradov 1993).

The leader must teach group members how to request and how to offer feedback that is centered within the group's interactions and that is specific and personal. Observations or requests that have to do with there-and-

then problems or that are global and abstract—such as "What should I do about my fights with my boyfriend?" or "You're really nice" or "Am I a boring person?"—are always unhelpful. The more specific the question or feedback, the more useful and potent it is. Much more fruitful are requests such as "I'd like to explore why I keep locking horns with the men in this group," and feedback such as "I feel closest to you when you share your pain with me, but I get turned off when you present yourself as having it all together and needing very little from the group."

Understanding the here and now.   The second stage of the here-and-now focus requires an entirely different set of functions and techniques from the therapist. If the first stage demands activation and plunging of the group into the present affective experience, the second stage demands reflection, explanation, and interpretation. Often this latter phase of the group work is referred to as *group process*. If several individuals engage in a discussion, the content of their discussion is obvious; the discussion consists of the actual words spoken and the substantive issues addressed. But the process of the discussion is entirely different. The process refers to how this content was expressed and what it reveals about the nature of the relationship of the individuals holding the discussion.

The group therapist must always attend to the process of the communication in the group—that is, he or she must examine how the words exchanged shed light on the relationships among the participants. Consider, for example, the patient who suddenly reveals in a meeting that as a child she was sexually molested by her stepfather. The group members will probably probe for more "vertical disclosure," for more details such as how long the abuse lasted, what role her mother played, and whether the abuse affected the patient's relationship with men. A process-oriented therapist is more concerned about "horizontal disclosure" (i.e., disclosure about the disclosure) and, accordingly, will attend to the relational aspects of the patient's disclosure (Vinogradov and Yalom 1989). The leader may then pose questions such as "Why is Betty revealing this to us today rather than some other day?" or "What has permitted her to take this risk today?" or "What prevented her from telling us this earlier?" or "How does she anticipate the group will respond?"

The recognition of process is part of the art of psychotherapy and often requires a long apprenticeship. To understand process, one needs to register continually all of the available data. Who chooses which seat? Who is always late? At whom do members look when talking with each other? Who meets with whom at the end of the group? How does the group change when a particular member is absent? Some of the most valuable data are the therapist's own reactions. Feelings of impatience, frustration, or boredom in a group session represent valuable information and should be put to use. Likewise, when the leader feels engaged or excited by the group interactions, this is often the sign of a potent, hard-working meeting.

To recognize and understand the process in the here and now, it is helpful to keep in mind that certain tensions and processes will be present to some degree in every therapy group. One of the most fundamental of these is the struggle for dominance. Others include basic group conflicts faced by each member: the conflicts between sibling rivalry and the need for mutual support, between self-interest and the desire to help another person, and between the wish to immerse oneself in the comforting body of the group on the one hand and the fear of losing one's precious autonomy on the other. Certain theoretical models of group behavior have been developed, by Bion (1959) and others, to describe and explain these basic conflicts.

The therapist who recognizes and identifies these fundamental tensions when they manifest themselves in the group will have illuminated an important part of the here-and-now process. As an example, we once had occasion to work with an articulate and provocative young man who had long enjoyed the role of dominant member of a group. When an older, very successful and aggressive man joined as a new member, the younger man gradually became withdrawn and depressed and soon announced his intention of leaving the group. It was not until the therapist called attention to the struggle for dominance that the patient began to explore some of his feelings about competition and envy.

Use of Transference and Therapist Transparency

Transference

Group members regard group therapists in an unrealistic light for many reasons. True transference or displacement of affect from some prior object, such as an early parental figure, is one reason. Conflicted attitudes toward authority as represented by the leader (e.g., dependency, autonomy, rebellion) are another. And still another reason is the patient's tendency to ascribe superhuman features to therapists so that the patient can use the therapists as a shield against existential anxiety. One realistic source of strong feelings lies in the members' explicit or intuitive appreciation of the great power that group therapists wield. The therapists' consistent presence and impartial-

ity are essential for group survival and stability. Group therapists cannot be exposed; they can add new members, expel old members, and mobilize enormous group pressure around any issue they wish.

True transference does, of course, occur in therapy groups; indeed, it is powerful and radically influences the nature of the group discourse. But just as there will be, in any group, patients whose therapy hinges on the resolution of transference distortion, so there will also be many others whose improvement depends on interpersonal learning stemming not from transferential work with the therapist but from peer-oriented work with another member around such issues as competition, exploitation, or sexual and intimacy conflicts. Thus, if leaders ignore transference considerations, they may seriously misunderstand some important transactions; if, on the other hand, they see only the transference aspects of the group, they will fail to encourage the exploration of many other important interactions and may also fail to relate authentically to many of the group members. The cardinal rule is to maintain flexibility. Group therapists have a variety of tasks: they must make good use of any irrational attitudes toward them without at the same time neglecting a leader's many other functions in the group.

To work effectively with transference in the therapy group, leaders must help patients recognize, understand, and change their distorted attitudes. Two major approaches or techniques facilitate transference resolution in the therapy group. The first of these involves consensual validation (or, as is more often the case, consensual invalidation) by other group members of the patient's distorted views. The second, which shall be discussed separately, makes use of increased therapist transparency.

In consensual validation, a group leader encourages a patient to validate his or her impressions against those of other members. If many or all of the group members concur in the patient's view of and feelings toward the leader (say, that the leader is "too autocratic"), it can be concluded either that the patient's reaction to the therapist stems from global group forces related to the leader's role or that the reaction is not an unrealistic one at all and the patient is perceiving the leader accurately. Therapists, too, have blind spots. If, on the other hand, one member alone possesses a particular view of the therapist, then this member may be helped to examine the possibility that he or she sees the group leader, and perhaps other persons too, through an internal distorting prism.

Therapist Transparency

Group therapists can also allow a patient to confirm or disconfirm irrational impressions by gradually revealing more of themselves, reacting to the patient as a real person in the here and now. Leaders can thus respond to their patients authentically, share their feelings in a judicious and responsible manner, and acknowledge or refute motives and feelings attributed to them. In this approach, they look at their own blind spots and demonstrate respect for the feedback members offer them. In the face of mounting reality-based data about the therapist, it becomes increasingly difficult for members to maintain their fictitious beliefs about the group leader (Vinogradov and Yalom 1990).

One fear that therapists sometimes have concerning personal self-disclosure is the fear of escalation—the fear that once they reveal themselves, the insatiable group will demand even more. But strong forces in the group oppose this trend. Although members are enormously curious about their group leader, they also wish the therapist to remain unknown and all-powerful. Although they appreciate the responsible and growth-promoting use of interpersonal feedback from their leader, few want the therapist to discuss his or her personal problems.

There are many different approaches to therapist transparency, depending on the therapist's personal style and the goals in the group at a particular time. It is helpful to ask oneself what the purpose of self-disclosure is at any given point in the group: "Am I trying to facilitate transference resolution? Am I providing a model in an effort to create therapeutic norms? Am I attempting to assist the interpersonal learning of members by working on their relationship with me? Am I attempting to support and demonstrate my acceptance of members by saying, in effect, 'I value and respect you and demonstrate this by giving of myself'?" At all times, the therapist must consider whether transparency is consonant with other group therapy tasks (Vinogradov and Yalom 1990).

Although therapist self-disclosure generally facilitates group interaction, it is important to keep in mind that the group therapist's primary raison d'être is not to be fully self-disclosing. Furthermore, leader self-revelation must be guided by the different needs of each group member. Not all patients need the same thing, either from the therapist or from the group. Some patients need to relax controls and to learn how to express their emotions in an honest and responsible manner, whether they be anger, love, tenderness, envy, or other emotions. Other patients need the opposite, in that they need to gain impulse control and to accept limits to the expression of their emotions; their lifestyles may already be characterized by labile and immediately acted-on affect. Even the transparent and authentically self-disclosing therapist must provide some cognitive structuring—some intellectual integration to the group experience. Only in this manner can patients learn to generalize their experiences to outside life.

The leader's role undergoes a gradual metamorphosis during the life of any relatively stable interactional group. In the beginning, therapists busy themselves with the many functions necessary for the creation of the group, the development of a social system in which the many therapeutic factors may operate, and the activation and illumination of the here and now. Gradually, the leader begins to interact with each of the members, and the members' early stereotypes of the therapist become more difficult to maintain. This process between the therapist and each of the members is not qualitatively different from the interpersonal learning that ensues as a result of each member's relationship with other members. After all, therapists have no monopoly on authority, dominance, sagacity, or aloofness, and many members work out their conflicts in these areas not only with the leader but also with other members who have these attributes.

Procedural Aids

A group leader's therapeutic armamentarium can be expanded through the use of procedural aids—specialized techniques that are not essential but may facilitate the course of therapy. We discuss three such approaches: written summaries, videotaping, and structured exercises.

Written Summaries

The course of most outpatient therapy groups, especially interactionally oriented groups, is facilitated by the use of written summaries (Yalom 1995; Yalom et al. 1975). The most useful procedure is for the group leader to dictate a candid, concise description of the group session after each meeting and to have a transcription (of approximately two to three single-spaced pages) sent out to the group members the following day. These summaries serve to extend the effect of the group's here-and-now interactions during the week between meetings. Patients have been unanimous in their positive evaluation of this technique. Most await the arrival of the weekly summary with anticipation and read and consider it seriously. Many members reread the summaries several times, and almost all file them for future review. The patients' therapeutic perspectives and commitment are deepened, and the patient–therapist relationship is strengthened. No serious transference complications, breaks in confidentiality, or other adverse consequences have been noted to occur by practitioners of this method.

Weekly summaries are most valuable if they are honest and straightforward about the process of therapy in the group. They are virtually identical to the summaries therapists make for their own files and are based on the assumption that each patient is a full collaborator in the therapeutic process—that psychotherapy is strengthened and not weakened by demystification. The orientation of the material in the summary reflects the therapeutic orientation of the group. In a long-term interaction group, the summary focuses on the interpersonal transactions that occurred in the meeting and the therapist's reflections on some of the dynamics and implications of those transactions. In a time-limited outpatient group for bereaved spouses, the summaries are more descriptive in nature and underline some of the members' modes of coping with bereavement: loneliness, change in social role, disposition of the effects of the dead spouse, and confrontation with existential issues such as death, aloneness, meaning in life, and regret (Yalom and Vinogradov 1988).

The summary serves several functions (Table 31–6). It provides an understanding of the here-and-now events of the session and facilitates the integration of powerful affective experiences. It labels sessions as good or resistive, notes and rewards patient gains in the group, and predicts undesirable developments in the group, thus minimizing their impact. It increases group cohesiveness by emphasizing similarities among members, by underscoring the expressing of caring or other positive emotions, and by providing continuity from one meeting to another. The summary is also an ideal forum for interpretations, either for interpretations made during the session (which may have fallen on deaf ears if delivered in the midst of a heated discussion) or for new interpretations that have occurred to the therapist after the meeting. Finally, the summary provides hope to the patients by helping them realize that the group is an orderly process and that the therapist has some coherent sense of the group's long-term development.

Videotaping

Modern scientific technology has no doubt contributed to the dehumanization of present-day society; to the deconstitution of stable, support-giving social, work, and kinship groups; and, consequently, to the necessity for group therapy. However, it has also created an instrument, the videotape recorder, that has considerable potential benefit for the teaching, practice, and understanding of group therapy. Some therapists make the videotape recording a central feature of therapy; they may arrange for immediate playback of certain segments during a meeting or set up regularly scheduled playback ses-

TABLE 31–6. Benefits of weekly written summary of group therapy session

1. Provides a further understanding of the here-and-now events of the session.
2. Helps integrate powerful affective experiences.
3. Labels the session as good or resistive.
4. Notes and rewards patient gains.
5. Predicts undesirable developments.
6. Increases group cohesiveness by emphasizing similarities among members.
7. Underscores caring or positive emotions.
8. Provides continuity from meeting to meeting.
9. Allows interpretations.
10. Provides a view of the group's long-term development.

Note. Weekly written summaries are sent to all members between sessions.

sions. Other therapists, ourselves included, find the technique of value but prefer to use it as a teaching device or occasionally as an auxiliary aid in the therapeutic process.

Although feedback from others about one's behavior is important, it is never as convincing as information one discovers for oneself, and videotape provides feedback that is not mediated through a second person. Often a patient's cherished self-image is radically challenged by a videotape playback. It is not unusual for a patient suddenly to recall and to accept previous feedback he or she has received from other members. The patient realizes that the group has been honest and, if anything, overprotective in previous confrontations.

Often profound realizations occur: for the first time, patients observe with their own eyes their full behavior and its impact on others. Many initial playback reactions are concerned with physical attractiveness and mannerisms, whereas in subsequent playback sessions patients begin to make more careful note of their interactions with others, their withdrawal or timidity, and their self-preoccupation or aloofness or their hostility.

Patients who will be able to view the playback are usually receptive to the suggestion of videotaping. Often, however, they are concerned about confidentiality and need reassurance on this issue. If the videotape is to be viewed by anyone other than group members (e.g., students, researchers, supervisors), the therapist must be explicit about the purpose of the viewing and the identity of the viewers and must obtain written permission from all of the members.

Structured Exercises

The term *structured exercises* refers to the many group activities in which members follow some specific set of orders, generally prescribed by the leader. These kinds of exercises play an important role in many specialized therapy groups but may be counterproductive in long-term general outpatient groups (Lieberman et al. 1973; McKay and Paleg 1992; Yalom 1985; Yalom et al. 1975). The precise rationale of the procedures varies, but in general, structured exercises are meant to modify the pace of the group and direct group members' attention to factors deemed relevant to the group's goals. In brief interpersonal group therapy, structured exercises (warm-up procedures) permit a bypassing of hesitant, uneasy first steps of the group; others speed up interaction through assignment to individuals of interactional tasks that circumvent cautious, ritualized social behavior; still others speed up individual work by helping members get in touch with suppressed emotions, with unknown or hidden parts of themselves, and with their physical bodies. In a medication support group or cognitive-behavioral group, a structured check-in procedure focuses attention on specific therapeutic issues and aspects of treatment.

A structured exercise may require only a few minutes, or it may consume an entire meeting. Although the exercise may be predominantly nonverbal in nature, there is always a verbal component in that the exercise generates data that subsequently can be discussed by the group. The exercise can involve the group as a whole; for example, a group of chronically mentally ill day-treatment patients may be asked to plan an outing. Or it can involve one member vis-à-vis the group: in a trust exercise, used in an encounter-type group, one member stands, with eyes closed, in the center of the group circle and then falls, allowing the group to support him or her. Exercises can include each individual within the group, such as a "go around," in which each member is asked to give initial impressions of everyone else. In another type of go around that is useful in the early life of a group, each member shares some background history. In working with bereaved spouses, we ask members during an early session to bring in a wedding photograph to share with the rest of the group.

Many of the therapist tasks and techniques for interactive, interpersonal group therapy—norm setting, here-and-now activation, understanding the here and now—involve approaches that have a prescriptive quality (approaches in the form of questions such as "Whose opinion in the group especially matters to you?" or "Can you look at Mary as you talk to her?" or "What has it been like for you to share that with us?" or "On a risk-taking scale of 1 to 10, how much have you risked with us today?"). Every experienced group leader uses some structured exercises, at times in a subtle and spontaneous manner. For example, if a group is tense and blocked and

experiences a silence of a minute or two (a minute's silence feels very long in a group!), the leader might ask for a quick go around in which each member says briefly what he or she had been feeling or had thought of saying, but did not, in that silence. Such an exercise usually generates much valuable data.

Although the judicious use of structured exercises can facilitate the course of group therapy, excessive use of such exercises may be counterproductive, depending on the goals of the group. In long-term interpersonal or psychodynamic group therapy, members make more therapeutic headway if the leaders encourage them to experience their timidity or suspiciousness and to understand the underlying dynamics rather than if the leaders prescribe an exercise that plunges members willy-nilly into deep disclosure or expression (Flowers and Booraem 1990). In acute or short-term settings such as inpatient groups and certain specialized outpatient groups, the situation is more complex. Faced with a limited amount of time in which to be helpful to many different patients, therapists may find that structured exercises are extremely useful: the exercises increase patient participation, provide a discrete, appropriate group task, and increase group efficiency. But there is a pitfall to be avoided. Whenever therapists prescribe structured tasks for a group, even during a single meeting, they run the risk of infantilizing members and establishing norms that block the group from developing into a potent therapeutic force. Members of a highly structured, leader-centered group begin to feel that all help emanates from the leader. They passively await their turn to work with the therapist. They de-skill themselves from an interpersonal point of view and cease to avail themselves of the help and resources that other group members can provide. Therapists leading such groups should deliberately and directly address this dynamic by encouraging task-focused member interactions. For example, in a medication support group, the therapist might encourage discussion among members on managing medication side effects. Although it is useful to impose structure judiciously when working with certain groups, it is essential to use that structure in a way that furthers the group's goals and enhances each member's functioning.

Modification of Basic Techniques for a Specialized Clinical Setting: The Acute Inpatient Therapy Group

The therapist faced with the task of organizing a therapy group in a specialized clinical situation must learn to modify fundamental group principles and techniques. We suggest these three basic steps:

1. *Assessment of the clinical setting:* Determine the immutable clinical restraints surrounding the group.
2. *Formulation of goals:* Develop goals that are appropriate and achievable within the existing clinical restraints.
3. *Modification of traditional technique:* Retain the basic principles of group therapy but alter techniques to adapt them to the clinical setting and to achieve the specified goals.

We shall illustrate these steps by discussing two highly specialized group settings: the acute inpatient therapy group and the outpatient medication support group. We have chosen the first setting for two reasons. First, the *clinical challenge* of inpatient group therapy is severe, and radical modifications of technique and strategy are required in order to lead effective groups in this setting (Kibel 1993). Second, the inpatient group is the most commonly encountered specialized group and is found on virtually every acute psychiatric ward in the country. Medication support groups, on the other hand, are used with less acutely ill patients and are examples of attempts to face the *fiscal challenges* of today's managed care environment. In general, specialized groups provide added value in resource-sensitive environments but require modification of group therapy technique.

Assessment of the Clinical Setting

The clinical setting facing the inpatient therapist appears highly inhospitable to the practice of traditional group therapy. Intrinsic limitations over which the therapist has no control include the rapid turnover of patients (patients will often be present for only a single group meeting) and the severity and heterogeneity of psychopathology among hospitalized patients. Extrinsic constraints that affect the formation of an inpatient group are represented by such matters as ward policy, staffing, and administrative support (or lack thereof) for group therapy.

The therapist must carefully delineate both the intrinsic and extrinsic limitations of the clinical setting and then take steps to change those extrinsic factors that might hinder the group. On an inpatient ward, for example, the therapist can enlist the support of administrative and clinical staff to ensure that group therapy is a part of the ward program, that group time is set aside and protected for all patients, and that there are adequate group meeting facilities.

Formulation of Goals

Taking into account the clinical facts of life or constraints of the inpatient setting, the therapist must proceed to formulate appropriate goals for an inpatient therapy group (Table 31–7). Six achievable goals for the inpatient setting have been highlighted (Yalom 1983):

TABLE 31–7. Goals for acute inpatient therapy groups

Engage patients in the therapeutic process.
Teach patients that talking helps.
Spot problems.
Decrease isolation.
Allow patients to be helpful.
Alleviate hospital-related anxiety.

---

1. *Engage patients in the therapeutic process:* Patients are helped to become involved in a process that they find constructive and supportive and will wish to continue after discharge from the hospital.
2. *Teach patients that talking helps:* Patients are exposed to the benefits of psychotherapy and of improved communication skills.
3. *Spot problems:* Patients are helped to learn to identify their maladaptive interpersonal behavior.
4. *Decrease patients' sense of isolation:* Patients are encouraged to develop satisfying social contacts.
5. *Allow patients to be helpful to others:* Patients are allowed to see that they can contribute to the lives of people around them.
6. *Alleviate hospital-related anxiety:* Patients are encouraged to share concerns about the stigma of psychiatric hospitalization, to discuss distressing events on the ward (e.g., bizarre behavior of other patients, staff tensions, acutely disturbed patients), and to achieve reassurance from other group members.

Modification of Traditional Technique

Once appropriate goals have been established, therapists must modify their standard group therapy techniques in order to lead effective groups on the acute psychiatric inpatient ward (Table 31–8). Four essential modifications that we will discuss are 1) the shortening of the time frame, 2) the use of direct support, 3) emphasis on the here and now, and 4) the provision of structure.

TABLE 31–8. Modifications of basic techniques for acute inpatient therapy groups

Shortening of the time frame
Use of direct support
Emphasis on the here and now
Provision of structure

Shortening of time frame.   The first and most fundamental modification the inpatient group leader makes is to shorten the time frame radically. The therapist in an acute inpatient group must consider the life of the group to be only a single session and must strive to offer something useful for as many patients as possible during that session. Naturally, a single-session time frame demands efficiency. There is no time to waste: the leader has only a single opportunity to engage each patient and must not squander that opportunity. This need for efficiency demands heightened therapist activity. The therapist must be prepared to activate the group, to call on members, to support them, and to interact personally with them.

Use of direct support.   Inpatient group therapists must also learn to offer support quickly and directly. The most direct manner of offering support is simply to acknowledge openly each patient's efforts, intentions, strengths, positive contributions, and risks. If, for example, a member states that he finds a woman in the group very attractive, the leader must judiciously support this patient for the risk he has taken. The leader may wonder whether the group member has previously been able to express his admiration of another person so openly or may note that his openness encourages other members to take risks and reveal important feelings. Inpatient group therapists must try to emphasize the positive rather than the negative aspects of a person's behavior or defense. For example, rather than confront the patient who insists on playing "assistant therapist," the therapist may instead make positive comments on how helpful this patient has been to others. The stage is then set for a gentle remark on the patient's selflessness and reluctance to ask for something personal from the group.

The supportive therapist also makes it a point to help patients—especially objectionable or irritating patients—obtain support from the group. A self-centered patient who incessantly complains about a health condition or an insoluble situational problem will quickly alienate any group. When the therapist identifies such behavior, he or she must intervene quickly to circumvent the development of group animosity and rejection. The therapist may, for example, assign the patient the task of introducing new members into the group, giving positive feedback to other members, or attempting to guess and express what each member's evaluation of the group is that day. Or the leader may reframe the patient's irritating behavior: "Perhaps you have needs, too, but have trouble expressing them. I wonder if your preoccupation with your health [finances, spouse] isn't a way of asking for something from the group." Helping the patient to formulate a specific request for attention from the group often generates a positive response from the other members.

Another approach is to focus on making the group safe. Whereas some conflict and tension are necessary to the therapeutic work in a long-term outpatient group, inpatients are much too vulnerable to tolerate the additional anxiety of group conflict. The group therapist must anticipate and avoid confrontation and conflict whenever possible. If patients are irritable or critical, the leader can channel that work onto himself or herself. If two patients are locked into an adversarial position, the leader can remind them that sparks often fly between two persons who have similarities or who have envious feelings toward each other. Then each of the patients can be invited to talk about those aspects of the other that he or she admires or envies or to discuss the ways that he or she resembles the other.

When the therapist leads a group of severely regressed patients, he or she must provide even more support, in an even more direct fashion. The patients' behavior must be examined and then reframed in some positive way. The therapist can, for example, support the mute patient for staying the whole session, compliment the patient who leaves early for having stayed 20 minutes, or support inactive patients for having paid attention throughout the meeting. At times the therapist must even label inappropriate or bizarre statements as attempts to communicate with the group.

Emphasis on the here and now.   These foregoing considerations of therapist efficiency, activity, and support in the inpatient setting do not make the here-and-now focus any less important than in outpatient therapy. Such a focus helps inpatients learn many important interpersonal skills: those of communicating more clearly, getting closer to others, expressing positive feelings, noticing personal mannerisms that push people away, listening, offering support, revealing oneself, and forming friendships. However, the clinical conditions of extremely brief treatment duration and more severe pathology demand modifications in basic technique. There is insufficient time to work through interpersonal issues. Instead, the therapist simply helps patients to spot major interpersonal problems and to reinforce interpersonal strengths. Explicit instruction must be provided about the relevance of the here and now by, for example, explaining that group therapy focuses on the way people relate to one another because that is what group therapy does best; and that, furthermore, groups do this most effectively by examining the relationships between members of the group. The group leader must emphasize that even though patients may enter the hospital for many different reasons, everyone can benefit from learning how to get more out of their relationships with others.

Provision of structure. Finally, work with the acute inpatient group requires structure, and just as there is no place in acute inpatient group work for the inactive therapist, there is also no place for the nondirective therapist. Group leaders provide structure for the inpatient group in several ways: by instructing patients about and orienting them to the nature and purpose of the meeting, by establishing clear spatial and temporal boundaries for the group, and by using a lucid and confident personal style that reassures confused or anxious patients and contributes to a sense of structure. One of the most potent ways of providing structure is to build into each session a consistent, explicit sequence. Although different group sessions will have different sequences depending on the composition and task of the group, the following are natural lines of division:

1. *The first few minutes:* The therapist provides explicit structure for the group. If there are new members (and there usually are in the acute inpatient group), this is the time to orient them to therapy.
2. *Definition of the task:* The therapist determines the most profitable direction for the group to take in a particular session. The leader may, for example, listen to get a sense of the urgent issues on the ward that day. Or the leader may provide a structured exercise, such as having each patient formulate (with the leader's help) an agenda to follow during that session (Yalom 1983). For example, an agenda of a shy and inhibited young depressed woman might be to try to express some positive feelings in the group.
3. *Accomplishing the task:* The therapist helps the group to address the broad issues raised at the start of the session and, in the process, attempts to have as many patients participate as possible. If the group uses an agenda format, this is the "agenda filling" stage: the shy patient is helped to identify the members toward whom she feels positively and to express those feelings.
4. *The final few minutes:* The leader indicates that the work phase is over and the remaining time is devoted to review and analysis of the meeting. This is the summing-up period and the self-reflective loop of the here-and-now process, in which the therapist attempts to clarify the group interaction that occurred in the session. How, for example, did the group respond when a usually shy and inhibited member openly expressed some positive sentiments?

Modification of Basic Techniques for a Specialized Clinical Setting: The Medication Support Group

Assessment of the Clinical Setting

Therapists often work in clinical settings with significant fiscal limitations. Clinic directors often expect psychiatrists to rely on medication alone and to limit psychotherapy referrals. Insurance plans may reimburse psychiatrists only for medication visits. Patients needing prolonged medication management are often referred back to their primary care doctor. In summary, many psychiatrists face fiscal constraints that preclude leading traditional therapy groups.

Nevertheless, psychiatrists and therapists strive to provide the best treatment with the resources available. Many patients benefit from medication support groups. Here they can access the expertise of psychiatrists and therapists and the support of their peers. However, as in the case of any specialized medical treatment, some patients may need additional services. Specialized groups work best when they are part of a comprehensive treatment program.

Formulation of Goals

The goals of the medication support group are modest but important. Some are similar to those for inpatient groups. Five achievable goals for medication support groups can be pursued:

1. *Provide a flexible treatment setting:* Patients can attend groups more frequently when in crisis and can easily schedule early appointments with their providers.
2. *Teach patients that talking in therapy groups helps:* Patients are exposed to some of the benefits of group psychotherapy.
3. *Spot problems:* Group leaders can observe patients in a more complex and challenging interpersonal environment and can identify undertreated conditions and maladaptive interpersonal behavior.
4. *Decrease patients' sense of isolation:* For example, each patient finds out that he or she is not the only person taking psychiatric medications.
5. *Allow patients to be helpful to others:* Patients share their stories about taking medications and recovering from mental illness and thereby contribute to the lives of people around them.

Modification of Traditional Technique

Three essential modifications that we will discuss are 1) the flexibility of the treatment frame, 2) the management of anxiety, and 3) the provision of structure.

Flexibility of treatment frame. In contrast to attendance at psychotherapy groups, members attend medication support groups irregularly. Similar to the inpatient unit, each meeting has a different membership, and the life of the group lasts only a single session. Therapists are active and structure meetings to achieve the group's goals and to maximize group time. Group membership changes even more than that of inpatient groups. People managing minor crises may attend weekly, although multiple meetings per week are extremely rare. Those undergoing changes in medication may attend every 2–4 weeks. Those who are stable may attend every 4–12 weeks.

There are many benefits to this flexibility. Over the course of a long treatment, patients can use the group in different ways and can participate as members of different subgroups. Patients whose illnesses are acute, resolving, or in remission form three different subgroups. Each has something to offer the others. The stable patient can offer support to the patient undergoing medication changes and can feel justifiably proud and relieved to be stable. Members undergoing medication changes offer those in crisis a model of working with the doctor to optimize treatment. A great deal can be accomplished in medication support groups, but working in the here-and-now is neither possible nor appropriate.

Management of anxiety. Despite their treatment setting and relatively high-functioning membership, medication support groups are more like inpatient than outpatient groups. Therapists must offer support quickly and directly help objectionable or irritating patients. Unlike therapists who work in settings that provide a framework for interpersonal work, medication support group therapists must intervene quickly to maintain group cohesion in the service of the group's modest goals. Work in the here and now is extraordinarily powerful, and like any potent tool, it must be wielded thoughtfully and in the appropriate setting and circumstance. Most members do not attend the group frequently enough to make use of anxiety-inducing here-and-now work. Those attending more frequently are usually in crisis and even less likely to benefit from a here-and-now focus. Although members are not as ill as those on an inpatient unit, the group's leaders do not have the luxury of returning group members to the inpatient unit, where they can be observed after the session. Anxiety management in medication support groups is paramount.

Provision of structure. Similar to the acute inpatient group, medication support groups require structure. Group leaders should introduce every meeting with a brief statement on the purposes and structure of the meeting. To provide appropriate medication management, medication support groups must cover specific content areas for each patient. A comprehensive check-in procedure for each patient is one way to provide a predictable structure. Although the sequential check-in process consumes most of the group time and cannot be characterized as encouraging intermember interaction, check-ins can represent opportunities for tapping therapeutic factors such as instillation of hope, universality, imparting information, and altruism. Catharsis and existential factors are also occasionally addressed. Most patients find written check-in instructions helpful because they attend so infrequently and such procedures help to provide structure. The following instructions exemplify those often used in a check-in process:

- Please tell us your name, medications, dosages, and how you take them (compliance).
- Tell us how the medications help you (What are your target symptoms?).
- Tell us any problems that the medications cause for you (What are the side effects?).
- Tell us about recent or upcoming "big events" (What are the current stresses around which you might need support?).

Group Therapy Programs and Managed Care Systems

> It is the larger work that defines practice and establishes the parameters within which change and adaptation occur. That being the case, we find it puzzling that physicians pay so little attention to how changes in the larger work world affect their lives. (Tischler and Astrachan 1996, p. 959)

The importance of group therapy is growing in today's managed care environment. Community mental health programs, the military, and the Department of Veterans Affairs use systematic approaches to the delivery of mental health care. Group therapy is moving beyond the public sector and the private office to the private sector institution. Health care companies are increasingly careful about allocating resources and tracking outcomes. As health care delivery systems grow, group therapy programs must become more sophisticated.

The most obvious economic reason for increased utilization of group therapy is efficient use of staff time (number of patients per staff hour). However, group therapy as a labor-saving strategy is prone to being misused. Leaders in managed care face significant challenges to expand the use of group therapy to better serve large populations. Therapists, administrators, and staff must change the institutional culture and develop protocols to implement group therapy programs. Developing such programs is similar to applying any other new strategic approach (e.g., preauthorization and concurrent utilization review). New requirements and policies may feel heavy-handed at first, but eventually the techniques useful for initiating change will be refined (Bennett 1993) and become routine. Starting a group therapy program and shifting utilization patterns are huge changes. Despite the obvious economic advantages of group therapy, institutions still face substantial internal resistance and an extraordinarily complicated evolving marketplace.

Managed care brings clinical and business activities together in complex ways. Economic risk threatens to replace clinical scope of practice as the primary paradigm for dividing up responsibility. The importance of being able to predict one's costs necessitates the use of actuarial assessments. Covering large populations enables managed care companies to predict and plan for infrequent but costly illnesses. Many costly illnesses can be prevented, and a large group therapy program can facilitate provision of preventive care for large populations, thus decreasing morbidity through secondary prevention.

Starting a Group Program

Group therapy coordination is an essential function. Someone must oversee a new program's development. Each stage entails different challenges and requires its own blend of strategies. However, facilitating and reinforcing behavior change are always important. Initial attempts may even be awkward. The group program coordinator should carefully plan which groups to start first in order to maximize usefulness to patients and clinicians. There are two basic strategies: One can start several groups that will have heterogeneous memberships (i.e., demographics, diagnoses, and problems)—for example, cycles of brief interpersonal therapy groups and ongoing medication support groups. Alternatively, one can start focused groups for problems, illnesses, or stage-related difficulties that are common in one's treatment setting—for example, cognitive-behavioral group therapy for posttraumatic stress disorder or a relapse prevention group for alcoholism. Not everyone can be effectively treated in the same type of group therapy, and the process of deciding which patient belongs in which group is still being refined (Harwood 1996). Nevertheless, the group program coordinator should start groups that are likely to be used per discussions with the referring staff.

Starting a group program is challenging. The coordinator must maintain the support of the referring staff and attend to numerous practical matters. With each early referral, there are risks of refusal by the patient, the receiving clinician or group therapist, or the group, and a delicate balancing of priorities is required. Referral failures and dropouts discourage both the referring clinician and the group therapist. Initially, the effort put into making decisions such as those concerning which groups to start, when to start them, and how to match patients and groups will be out of proportion to the savings that a small group program produces. As a group program enlarges, fit-and-matching issues become less problematic but still require a coherent, thoughtful approach. Group program coordinators perform or oversee the many essential executive, clerical, and educational tasks necessary to develop, enlarge, and maintain a group program.

The group program should fit as seamlessly as possible with other clinical functions such as intake, crisis stabilization, individual treatment, and referral to extraclinic resources. Evaluations and crisis stabilization are almost always performed individually. After that, group or individual approaches may be used for secondary prevention—either time-limited or maintenance treatments. Preventive efforts, although historically underemphasized, are gaining in esteem as their value in capitated systems becomes apparent. Given the absence of a litmus test for likelihood to fail in group therapy, one could argue that referral to a group should always be a part of the initial treatment plan. Rather than "Who will fail in group treatment?" the question may be, "How can we prepare everyone to benefit from some form of group treatment?"

Long-term groups with highly impaired populations often provide the greatest savings because of their prolonged nature and because they obviate the need for more expensive levels of care (Gabbard et al. 1997; MacKenzie 1997a). Time-limited groups focus on less impaired patients and therefore draw from a larger population. They offer increased flexibility by allowing providers additional treatment options with little impact on clinician time. Clinical benefit is essentially equivalent in a five-person versus an eight-person group, and therapist time is equal.

In settings where the shift to using group therapy is well under way, clinicians and administrators must continue their efforts. Wherever group therapy is not being used, staff members should encourage each other to ask the question "Why not group therapy?" rather than "Why group therapy?" This is an important shift in perspective and lays the basis for changes in the institutional culture.

Delivery Systems and Group Therapy

The penetration of group psychotherapy into clinical services has always been dependent on social and political trends related to access (MacKenzie 1997a, p. 102).

As noted earlier, the first therapy group is credited to the internist Joseph Pratt. At a time when tuberculosis was common, Pratt brought his sanitarium patients together for classes. Soon other practitioners, including early psychoanalysts, began seeing patients in group settings. Over the course of the next several decades, changes in the need for mental health care led to creative work and change in group therapy practice. During World War II, Wilfred Bion, a British psychoanalyst, used group process to care for patients with psychiatric problems brought about by the war. His ideas as described earlier in this chapter continue to influence understanding of institutional dynamics, basic group therapy, and organizational change.

During the 1970s, there was a shift from care in locked institutions to community mental health care, and T-groups and encounter groups were created. Although this was a productive period in many ways, many programs were inadequately funded. Poorly formulated systems often used group gatherings as a panacea. Thus, the psychotic symptoms of some patients suffering from schizophrenia became worse with the use of overly stimulating and anxiety-producing forms of group therapy. Poorly trained group leaders led risky endeavors that resulted in boundary violations and other negative outcomes. During this period, Yalom's empirical research (described earlier in this chapter) led to the creation of a list of therapeutic factors as well as interpersonal group psychotherapy. Group therapy, popularized and overextended during the free-love 1960s, reentered the health care arena in the 1970s.

Since the 1990s, the incentive for developing groups has been increasing. As in the past, we face the challenge of applying group therapy in thoughtful new ways and run the risk of inappropriately using group therapy as a panacea. What can we expect to be different from the past?

Changes inside and outside the field of group therapy will stimulate further development. Bion and Yalom were able to outline truths of group behavior in institutional and small group settings. Their theories are valid for patient treatment groups but are not enough in the case of group program development for primary and secondary prevention. Furthermore, treating brain disease requires integration of group behavior theory and the latest treatments (e.g., therapy with new medication, cog-nitive therapy for drug abuse, interpersonal therapy for eating disorders) (Verhulst 1996). Changes in the health care delivery system will likely stimulate new inquiries into overlooked or underdeveloped applications of group behavior (e.g., psychoeducational groups, medication support groups).

Health services researchers use improved information systems to analyze treatments in real clinical settings rather than just research settings. Even the modest systems currently in place will allow thoughtful planning while protecting against the most egregious misuses and overuses of group therapy. For instance, in larger populations, infrequently occurring illnesses turn up at predictable rates. Knowing this allows large managed care organizations to develop more detailed plans for systems of care, including the formation of specialized therapy groups.

There are many different ways to use group process to enhance patients' treatment. Group analysis focuses on treatment through the group. This approach continues to influence other forms of group therapy. Yalom's therapeutic factors provide a framework for therapists to enhance the efficacy of cognitive, behavioral, and psychoeducational approaches. In group therapy, universality, altruism, increased opportunity for positive modeling, and lending of hope all can amplify the impact that other approaches rely on to help patients. Increasing pressure to provide efficient care changes the direction of development and innovation. For example, homogenous groups cohere more rapidly. This contributed to the development of symptom-specific, illness-specific, and developmental stage–specific groups. The need for resource-sensitive methods has led to the development of different types of time-limited groups. The need for a new way to incorporate group therapy will undoubtedly influence what aspects of group therapy receive the most attention in research and development circles.

Group Programs

Despite the advantage of having multiple groups from which to choose, rarely do group therapists combine forces. However, a few systems such as the Tavistock Clinic (in London) and the New York Group Psychoanalytic Society have increased the number of options available for referral by the evaluating clinician. With adequate communication, a better match between patient and group is possible. However, these two organizations offer a narrow array of group therapies, and the potential members probably self-select. On the other hand, group programs at health maintenance organizations (HMOs) offer a broader array of group therapies but still do not provide a full spectrum. One of the challenges inherent in having many patients and many groups is matching patients to groups.

Unfortunately, there is still no widely applied triage system for such matching. Attaining the best match possible depends on good communication between referring clinicians and group therapists. Every effort should be made to convey to all clinicians and staff information on the type and nature of the groups available (Crosby and Sabin 1995). Patient–treatment matching is an important research topic. Collecting outcome data and improving information systems are two important pieces of the groundwork needed to provide feedback for group therapy programs.

New information systems are allowing and patterns of reimbursement are encouraging more thoughtful utilization of group therapists. Administrative staff use larger, more sophisticated information systems to track the clinical needs of larger and larger populations. Managed care payers reward clinicians for keeping people healthy and intervening more quickly in chronic illnesses by maintaining a framework of regular contact. Although developments in group theory have been substantial and influential, the recent changes outside the field are at least as important.

The Current Response

In 1996, the American Group Psychotherapy Association (AGPA) established the National Registry of Certified Group Psychotherapists. The certification process requires high levels of training including formal didactics with specified content as well as extensive clinical experience and supervision. AGPA proactively addressed the excesses and misapplications that plagued earlier periods of group therapy expansion. Nevertheless, there is still a great deal of work to do.

Treatment–patient matching, pregroup preparation, and group program development are still in their infancy. Many clinicians and academicians focus on developing manualized treatments for specific illness (Spitz 1996). Others study "group process," or how the manner in which group members relate to each other changes as a function of time. Basic scientific research on group therapy is essential. However, developing systems of care based on group therapies is a different type of challenge. Managed care should be eager to meet the challenge of figuring out how best to deploy research-tested, clinically effective, an resource-sensitive treatments. Ironically, the dynamic marketplace encourages group therapy but is changing so quickly that many businesses do not have time to develop and refine innovative group therapy programs.

Established staff-model HMOs lead the effort to identify which types of groups are most useful in providing care for large capitated populations. Group coordinators focus on time-limited groups, especially psychoeducational groups, that help prevent the development of full-blown illness. In the past, groups for chronically, persistently, and severely mentally ill patients were almost exclusively the province of public mental health programs. In the 1990s, several books were written on treating such patients in groups. Bauer and McBride (1996) and Stone (1996) wrote on group therapy for severely mentally ill patients (bipolar affective disorder and chronic mental illness, respectively). Development of group therapy models for psychotic disorders has been even more robust, with books by Kanas (1996), Schermer and Pines (1999), and Martindale et al. (2000). Linehan (1993), MacKenzie (2001b), and Budman et al. (1996), among others, developed or wrote about models for treating severe personality disorders in groups and empirically tested these models for efficacy.

Several approaches to time-limited group treatment for common nonpsychotic disorders are well developed and have been published in both book and workbook form. Many utilize tenets of cognitive or behavioral group therapy (e.g., Padesky on depression, Zueker-White on panic disorder). The theoretical basis and layout of the books lend themselves to a structured, focused approach. Many books provide the reader with pretreatment and posttreatment assessments. Adding tests to assess parameters such as locus of control, motivation, social competence, learned resourcefulness, ego strength, coping style (Piper and Joyce 1996), psychological mindedness (McCallum and Piper 1996), and psychological defenses (Tasca et al. 1994) to the pretest may facilitate the matching of patients and groups. Paleg and Jongsma (2000) made an important contribution to comprehensive approaches to program development by compiling a book on group therapy formats for 28 different presenting problems.

Unlike time-limited cognitive or behavioral group therapy, medication support groups are less often the focus of research but are, nonetheless, common. Psychiatrists can provide secondary prevention with medication support groups. Such groups offer members regular contact with highly trained mental health professionals. Because they are more efficient in terms of numbers of patients seen, visits can be more frequent than individual medication checks. However, they need not meet weekly, because the task is different from that in a therapy group. In a medication support group, the clinician can observe the patient's level of function in an environment that is probably more like the outside world than the environment of dyadic interactions and is not limited by the patient's descriptions of outside events. Additionally, group therapy offers the patient the opportunity to benefit from Yalom's therapeutic factors: universality, altruism, and sharing of information.

Time-limited interpersonal group therapy (TLIGP) is similar to medication support groups in that it is widely used and not commonly the subject of research. Therapists can treat interpersonal difficulties that stem either from an episode of mental illness or from relationships—problems that lead to exacerbations of one's illness. One member may focus on adjusting to the interpersonal stresses of the workplace after a serious depressive episode. Such adjustment might be especially difficult if the depression had been prolonged and modified his or her interpersonal style in an unhealthy way—for example, if the patient tended to withdraw when depressed rather than seeking help. Another patient might have a history of interpersonal difficulties that make him or her susceptible to dismissing the concerns of his or her partner regarding signs of incipient mania. In a sense, TLIGP is generic and requires less effort by the referring providers. They do not need to be as careful matching the patient's illness and the group's purpose. Likewise, the group therapist focuses on helping the patient conceptualize his or her illness in an interpersonal framework rather than focusing on exclusionary or inclusionary criteria. Membership is heterogeneous, and the group therapists can cast a wide net. They can start groups more often simply because there are more eligible patients who can learn to conceptualize their mental illness in an interpersonal framework.

Groups in general lend themselves to more forgiving referral relationships. By *forgiving*, I mean that the referring party can err on the side of referral without worrying about unduly burdening the group therapist. Unlike a patient referred for individual treatment, who will take up a time slot all to him- or herself, a referral to a group takes up a seat rather than a time slot. TLIGP is equally effective for each member when membership is between five and eight or nine persons. Thus, referral to such a group does not need to be as rigorously assessed for its resource utilization. One could even argue that providing a time-limited group after using the patient's crisis benefit should be the standard of care because it may decrease the likelihood and severity of subsequent episodes. Time-limited interpersonal group therapy may be one way to provide benefit to the patient as well as secondary prevention, all at little additional cost.

Resistance

Clinicians are responsible for overcoming not only their patients' reservations but also their own. Prospective group therapists worry about being overwhelmed. They need time before groups to prepare, after them to document the visit for all group members, and at other times during the day to return group members' phone calls. Administrators can plan for this in the clinician's schedule and/or provide additional clerical support (Cox et al. 2000). Some would argue that providing further free time for group therapists is an appropriate reward for being innovative and hard working. After all, the clinic is benefiting in that more patients receive better secondary prevention each day (Dick and Wooff 1986). Perhaps the group therapist will feel sufficiently encouraged by such a reward to start another group.

Clinicians must educate their patients about mental illness, treatment, and group therapy. The fact that group therapy is as effective as individual therapy is not widely known, even among mental health professionals. It is essential that clinicians communicate a sense of certainty about the effectiveness of group therapy to patients. In addition, one must address the patient's fear that the group will reject them. Inexperienced group therapists—even if they are experienced clinicians—are like their patients in that they, too, fear public exposure of and shame about their mistakes. Neophyte group therapists face learning (or at least adapting to) a new set of treatment parameters. Both patients and therapists must learn how group psychotherapy can help them so that they can overcome their initial sense of intimidation.

Group members and therapists alike often feel anxious when starting a group for the first time. In addition to the specter of meeting new people, members may fear sharing shameful experiences and revealing painful feelings. Ironically, the extent to which patients expect humiliation often predicts the degree of relief they feel when they discover that other people have similar problems and fears. Similarly, therapists who are awed by the complexity of running a group and intimidated by the power of the group process may be more likely to recognize opportunities that can influence the group process. At the very least, such therapists may make better use of clinical supervision.

Just like an anxious and eager new group member, a new group therapist should be both excited and daunted by the task ahead. Treatment manuals written by experts and used in their research often focus on specific illnesses or issues and employ a wide variety of theoretical frameworks. Manuals need not be limited to research, and developing such a manual not only permits the outlining of what works well in particular situations but also reduces the neophyte group therapist's anxiety.

The Future

The number of health services studies looking at the economic efficiency of different treatment systems is growing. University researchers and managed care companies alike are seeking to clarify which treatments work under which circumstances. Managed care companies are ahead of universities in the development of information systems and administrative infrastructure for large systems of care that thoroughly test economic and clinical efficiency and efficacy of treatment. Leadership, employee–clinicians, and patient–consumers will all benefit from such infrastructure. Clinic directors, group coordinators, and outpatient clinicians working together will better delineate the benefits of different types of group therapy and patterns of implementation for patients with various disorders. To answer the many remaining questions about helping patients by using group therapy, researchers, clinic administrators, and clinicians will need to collaborate.

Academic medical centers seeking to replace old revenue sources (grants and indirect Medicare funds) are developing new types of relationships with the health care industry. Private sector managed care organizations may work with medical centers or with research consulting companies. Additionally, some academic medical centers have developed their own managed care organizations. These three different models and mixes of academia and industry offer multiple possibilities for how the current challenges can be met. Large group therapy programs should be integrated into mental health care delivery systems and will offer opportunities to test hypotheses. Addressing questions of program structure will require the combination of academic skills and knowledge with private industry's administrative infrastructure and capital.

Even before the ascent of managed care, several prominent authors had written books and articles on developing and maintaining group therapy training programs. Administrative sanction, effective leadership of the group program, and effective coordination of multiple practitioners are some of the essential factors of a successful group therapy training program (Lonergan 1991, 1995, 2000). With the advent of managed care, obtaining administrative support for group programs and even hiring group program coordinators to lead and coordinate such efforts have become easier. Training programs (e.g., in academic medical centers) that are developing the capacity to meet managed care contracts are relying on the efficiency of group therapy to compensate for the inherent inefficiency of some necessary training experiences such as those involving long-term individual treatment of mild to moderately ill patients.

Conclusions

Group therapy is a widely practiced mode of treatment that is used effectively in a vast number of clinical settings. It involves a host of therapeutic factors or mechanisms of change, many of which are unique to group therapy. These mechanisms range from the therapeutic factors widely encountered in many different kinds of groups (such as universality, altruism, catharsis, and the imparting of information) to the potent but often misunderstood factor of interpersonal learning, which requires a skilled and experienced therapist working in a specialized interactional setting. Various constellations of these therapeutic factors operate in different types of groups at any given time. Therapists must understand the particular mechanisms of change at work in different kinds of groups and employ appropriate techniques to facilitate such mechanisms and complete the group task.

Group leaders make use of specific techniques and interventions, and all clinicians should be familiar with the technology used in group therapy. Some of these unique interventions include working in the here and now, therapist transparency, and the use of various procedural aids. These fundamental techniques can be modified to suit any specialized group setting, from the acute inpatient group to the symptom-oriented outpatient group. Indeed, the power of group therapy lies in its adaptability. Highly flexible and efficient, it may be the only mode of psychotherapy that can accommodate an almost infinite variety of settings, goals, and patients.

References

Agazarian YM: Systems-Centered Therapy for Groups. New York, Guilford, 1997

Alonso A, Swiller HI: Introduction: the case for group therapy, in Group Therapy in Clinical Practice. Edited by Alonso A, Swiller HI. Washington, DC, American Psychiatric Press, 1993, pp xxi–xxv

Amaranto EA, Benden S: Individual psychotherapy as an adjunct to group psychotherapy. Int J Group Psychother 40:91–101, 1990

Ansbacher HL: Alfred Adler, in Comprehensive Textbook of Psychiatry/III, 3rd Edition, Vol 1. Edited by Kaplan HI, Freedman AM, Sadock BJ. Baltimore, MD, Williams & Wilkins, 1980, pp 729–740

Baker MN, Baker HS: Self psychological contributions to the theory and practice of group psychotherapy, in Group Therapy in Clinical Practice. Edited by Alonso A, Swiller HI. Washington, DC, American Psychiatric Press, 1993, pp 49–68

Bandura A, Blanchard EB, Ritter B: Relative efficacy of desensitization and modeling approaches for inducing behavioral, affective, and attitudinal changes. J Pers Soc Psychol 13:173–199, 1969

Bandura A: Social Foundations of Thought and Action: A Social Cognitive Theory. Englewood Cliffs, NJ, Prentice-Hall, 1986

Barlow SH, Burlingame GM, Nebeker RS, et al: Meta-analysis of medical self-help groups. Int J Group Psychother 50:53–69, 2000

Bauer MS, McBride L: Structured Group Psychotherapy for Bipolar Disorder: The Life Goals Program. New York, Springer, 1996

Benioff L, Vinogradov S: Group psychotherapy with cancer patients and the terminally ill, in Comprehensive Textbook of Group Psychotherapy, 3rd Edition. Edited by Kaplan HI, Sadock BJ. Baltimore, MD, Williams & Wilkins, 1993, pp 477–489

Bennett MJ: View from the bridge: reflections of a recovering staff model HMO psychiatrist. Psychiatr Q 64:45–75, 1993

Bion WR: Experience in Groups. New York, Basic Books, 1959

Blake-Mortimer J, Gore-Felton C, Kimerling R, et al: Improving the quality and quantity of life among patients with cancer: a review of the effectiveness of group psychotherapy. Eur J Cancer 35:1581–1586, 1999

Bloch S: Therapeutic factors in group psychotherapy, in Psychiatry Update: American Psychiatric Association Annual Review, Vol 5. Edited by Frances AJ, Hales RE. Washington, DC, American Psychiatric Press, 1986, pp 678–698

Bloch S, Crouch E: Therapeutic Factors in Group Psychotherapy. Oxford, UK, Oxford University Press, 1985

Brook DW: Medication groups, in Group Therapy in Clinical Practice. Edited by Alonso A, Swiller HI. Washington, DC, American Psychiatric Press, 1993, pp 155–170

Brook DW: The Use of Medication Groups for the Treatment of Patients with Major Mental Illnesses. Funzione Gamma Journal (a bilingual [Italian and English] telematic journal of Group Psychotherapy), Edited by University of Rome "La Sapienza" 2(4), 2001

Budman SH, Cooley S, Demby A, et al: A model of time-effective group psychotherapy for patients with personality disorders: the clinical model. Int J Group Psychother 46:329–355, 1996

Butler T, Fuhriman A: Patient perspective on the curative process: a comparison of day treatment and outpatient psychotherapy groups. Small Group Behavior 11:371–388, 1980

Butler T, Fuhriman A: Curative factors in group therapy: a review of the recent literature. Small Group Behavior 14:131–142, 1983

Cheifetz DI, Salloway JC: Patterns of mental health services provided by HMOs. Am Psychol 39:495–502, 1984

Connelly JL, Piper WE, De Carufel FL, et al: Premature termination in group psychotherapy: pretherapy and early therapy predictors. Int J Group Psychother 36:145–152, 1986

Corsini R, Rosenberg B: Mechanisms of group psychotherapy: processes and dynamics. J Abnorm Soc Psychol 51:406–411, 1955

Cox PD: Medication Support Groups: Are They "Group Therapy?" Funzione Gamma Journal (a bilingual [Italian and English] telematic journal of Group Psychotherapy), Edited by University of Rome "La Sapienza" 2(4), 2001

Cox PD, Ilfeld F Jr, Ilfeld BS, et al: Group therapy program development: clinician-administrator collaboration in new practice settings. Int J Group Psychother 50:3–24, 2000

Crosby G, Sabin J: Developing and marketing time-limited therapy groups. Psychiatr Serv 46:7–8, 1995

Dick BM, Wooff K: An evaluation of a time-limited programme of dynamic group psychotherapy. Br J Psychiatry 148:159–164, 1986

Dies RR: Group psychotherapy: reflections on three decades of research. Journal of Applied Behavioral Sciences 15:361–373, 1979

Dies RR: Practical, theoretical, and empirical foundations for group psychotherapy, in Psychiatry Update: American Psychiatric Association Annual Review, Vol 5. Edited by Frances AJ, Hales RE. Washington, DC, American Psychiatric Press, 1986, pp 659–667

Dies RR: Research on group psychotherapy: overview and clinical applications, in Group Therapy in Clinical Practice. Edited by Alonso A, Swiller HI. Washington, DC, American Psychiatric Press, 1993, pp 473–518

Dugo JM, Beck AP: Significance and complexity of early phases in the development of the co-therapy relationship. Group Dynamics 1:294–305, 1997

Fawzy FI, Fawzy NW, Hyun CS, et al: Malignant melanoma: effects of an early structured psychiatric intervention, coping, and affective state on recurrence and survival 6 years later. Arch Gen Psychiatry 50:681–689, 1993

Fawzy FI, Fawzy NW, Arndt LA, et al: Critical review of psychosocial interventions in cancer care. Arch Gen Psychiatry 52:100–113, 1995

Flowers JV: The differential outcome effects of simple advice, alternatives and instructions in group psychotherapy. Int J Group Psychother 29:305–316, 1979

Flowers JV, Booraem CD: The frequency and effect on outcome of different types of interpretation in psychodynamic and cognitive-behavioral group psychotherapy. Int J Group Psychother 40:203–214, 1990

Freedman S, Hurley J: Perceptions of helpfulness and behavior in groups. Group 4:51–58, 1980

Fuhriman A, Burlingame GM: Consistency of matter: a comparative analysis of individual and group process variables. The Counseling Psychologist 18:60–63, 1990

Gabbard GO, Lazar SG, Hornberger J, et al: The economic impact of psychotherapy: a review. Am J Psychiatry 154:147–155, 1997

Goffman E: Encounters: Two Studies in the Sociology of Interaction. Indianapolis, IN, Bobbs-Merrill, 1961

Goodman G, Jacobs M: The self-help, mutual support group, in Handbook of Group Psychotherapy: An Empirical and Clinical Synthesis. Edited by Fugheriman A, Burlingame G. New York, Wiley, 1994, pp 489–526

Greenstein M, Breitbart W: Cancer and the experience of meaning: a group psychotherapy program for people with cancer. Am J Psychother 54:486–500, 2000

Harwood I: Towards optimum group placement from the perspective of self and group experience. Group Analysis 29:199–218, 1996

Hoag MJ, Burlingame GM: Evaluating the effectiveness of child and adolescent group treatment: a meta-analytic review. J Clin Child Psychol 26:234–246, 1997

Kahn EM: Group treatment interventions for schizophrenics. Int J Group Psychother 34:149–153, 1984

Kanas N: Inpatient and outpatient group therapy for schizophrenic patients. Am J Psychother 39:431–439, 1985

Kanas N: Group therapy with schizophrenics: a review of controlled studies. Int J Group Psychother 36:339–351, 1986

Kanas N: Group Therapy for Schizophrenic Patients. Washington, DC, American Psychiatric Press, 1996

Kaul TJ, Bednar RL: Experiential group research: results, questions, and suggestions, in Handbook of Psychotherapy and Behavior Change, 3rd Edition. Edited by Garfield SL, Bergin AE. New York, Wiley, 1986, pp 671–714

Kibel HD: Inpatient group psychotherapy, in Group Therapy in Clinical Practice. Edited by Alonso A, Swiller HI. Washington, DC, American Psychiatric Press, 1993, pp 93–111

Laing RD: The Politics of Experience. New York, Pantheon, 1967

Leszcz M, Yalom ID, Norden M: The value of inpatient group psychotherapy: patients' perceptions. Int J Group Psychother 35:411–433, 1985

Lieberman MA: A group therapist perspective on self-help groups. Int J Group Psychother 40:251–278, 1990

Lieberman MA, Borman L: Self-help groups for coping with crisis. San Francisco, CA, Jossey-Bass, 1979

Lieberman MA, Yalom ID, Miles MB: Encounter Groups: First Facts. New York, Basic Books, 1973

Linehan MM: Cognitive-Behavioral Treatment of Borderline Personality Disorder. New York, Guilford, 1993

Lonergan E[C]: Keeping a group psychotherapy program alive and well within a psychiatry residency. Group 15:168–180, 1991

Lonergan EC: Discussion. Group 19:100–107, 1995

Lonergan EC: Discussion of "group therapy program development." Int J Group Psychother 50:43–45, 2000

MacKenzie KR: Time-limited group psychotherapy: has Cinderella found her prince? Group 20:95–111, 1997a

MacKenzie KR: Time-Managed Group Psychotherapy: Effective Clinical Applications. Washington, DC, American Psychiatric Press, 1997b

Mackenzie KR: An Expectation of Radical Changes in the Future of Group Psychotherapy. Int J Group Psychother 51:243–263, 2001a

MacKenzie KR: Personality assessment in clinical practice in Handbook of Personality Disorders: Theory, Research, and Treatment. Edited by Livesley WJ. New York, Guilford, 2001b, pp 307–320

Martindale B, Bateman A, Margison F: Psychosis: Psychological Approaches and Their Effectiveness. London, England, Gaskell/Royal College of Psychiatrists, 2000

McCallum M, Piper WE: Psychological mindedness. Psychiatry: Interpersonal and Biological Processes 59:48–64, 1996

McCallum M, Piper WE, Joyce AS: Dropping out from short-term group therapy. Psychotherapy 29:206–252, 1992

McKay M, Paleg K: Focal Group Psychotherapy. Oakland, CA, New Harbinger, 1992

Orlinsky DE, Howard KI: Process and outcome in psychotherapy, in Handbook of Psychotherapy and Behavior Change, 3rd Edition. Edited by Garfield SL, Bergin AE. New York, Wiley, 1986, pp 311–381

Paleg K, Jongsma AE Jr: The Group Therapy Treatment Planner. New York, Wiley, 2000

Paulson I, Burroughs JC, Gelb CB: Cotherapy: what is the crux of the relationship? Int J Group Psychother 26:213–224, 1976

Pines M, Hutchinson S: Group analysis, in Group Therapy in Clinical Practice. Edited by Alonso A, Swiller HI. Washington, DC, American Psychiatric Press, 1993, pp 29–47

Piper W[E], Joyce A: A consideration of factors influencing the utilization of time-limited, short-term group therapy. Int J Group Psychother 46:311–328, 1996

Piper WE, Perrault EL: Pretherapy preparation for group members. Int J Group Psychother 39:17–34, 1989

Piper WE, Debbane EG, Bienvenu J-P, et al: A study of group pretraining for group psychotherapy. Int J Group Psychother 32:309–325, 1982

Piper WE, McCallum M, Azim HFA: Adaptation to Loss Through Short-Term Group Psychotherapy. New York, Guilford, 1992

Pratt JH: The principles of class treatment and their application to various chronic diseases. Hospital Social Service 6:404, 1922

Rothke S: The role of interpersonal feedback in group psychotherapy. Int J Group Psychother 36:225–240, 1986

Schermer VL, Pines M: Group Psychotherapy of the Psychoses: Concepts, Interventions and Contexts. Bristol, PA, Jessica Kingsley, 1999

Shapiro DA, Shapiro D: Meta-analysis of comparative therapy outcome studies: a replication and refinement. Psychol Bull 92:581–604, 1982

Shapiro JL: Methods of Group Psychotherapy and Encounter. Itasca, IL, Peacock, 1978

Smith ML, Glass GV, Miller TI: The Benefits of Psychotherapy. Baltimore, MD, Johns Hopkins University Press, 1980

Spiegel D, Bloom JR, Kraemer HL, et al: Effect of psychosocial treatment on survival of patients with metastatic breast cancer. Lancet 2:888–891, 1989

Spitz HI: Group Psychotherapy and Managed Mental Health Care: A Clinical Guide for Providers. New York, Brunner/Mazel, 1996

Spitz HI: The effect of managed mental health care and group psychotherapy: treatment, training, and therapist-morale issues. Int J Group Psychother 47:23–30, 1997

Stern MJ: Group therapy with medically ill patients, in Group Therapy in Clinical Practice. Edited by Alonso A, Swiller HI. Washington, DC, American Psychiatric Press, 1993, pp 185–199

Stone W: Group Psychotherapy for People With Chronic Mental Illness. New York, Guilford, 1996

Sullivan HS: The Interpersonal Theory of Psychiatry. New York, WW Norton, 1953

Tasca GA, Russell V, Busby K: Characteristics of patients who choose between two types of group psychotherapy. Int J Group Psychother 44:499–508, 1994

Taylor NT, Burlingame GM, Kristensen KB, et al: A survey of mental health care provider's and managed care organization attitudes toward, familiarity with, and use of group interventions. Int J Group Psychother 51:243–263, 2001

Tillitski CJ: A meta-analysis of estimated effect sizes for group versus individual control treatments. Int J Group Psychother 40:215–224, 1990

Tischler G, Astrachan B: A funny thing happened on the way to reform. Arch Gen Psychiatry 52:959–963, 1996

Toseland RW, Siporin M: When to recommend group treatment: a review of the clinical and the research literature. Int J Group Psychother 36:171–201, 1986

Verhulst J: The role of the psychiatrist: defining methods, theories, and practice in the time of managed care. Acad Psychiatry 20:195–204, 1996

Vinogradov S, Yalom ID: Concise Guide to Group Psychotherapy. Washington, DC, American Psychiatric Press, 1989

Vinogradov S, Yalom ID: Self-disclosure in group psychotherapy, in Self-Disclosure in the Therapeutic Relationship. Edited by Stricker G, Fisher N. New York, Plenum, 1990, pp 191–203

Whitaker DS, Lieberman MAL: Psychotherapy Through the Group Process. New York, Atherton, 1964

Yalom ID: A study of group therapy dropouts. Arch Gen Psychiatry 14:393–414, 1966

Yalom ID: The Theory and Practice of Group Psychotherapy. New York, Basic Books, 1970

Yalom ID: Existential Psychotherapy. New York, Basic Books, 1980

Yalom ID: Inpatient Group Psychotherapy. New York, Basic Books, 1983

Yalom ID: The Theory and Practice of Group Psychotherapy, 3rd Edition. New York, Basic Books, 1985

Yalom ID: Interpersonal learning, in Psychiatry Update: American Psychiatric Association Annual Review, Vol 5. Edited by Frances AJ, Hales RE. Washington, DC, American Psychiatric Press, 1986, pp 699–713

Yalom ID: The Theory and Practice of Group Psychotherapy, 4th Edition. New York, Basic Books, 1995

Yalom ID, Vinogradov S: Bereavement groups: techniques and themes. Int J Group Psychother 38:419–457, 1988

Yalom ID, Vinogradov S: Interpersonal group psychotherapy, in Comprehensive Textbook of Group Psychotherapy, 3rd Edition. Edited by Kaplan HI, Sadock BJ. Baltimore, MD, Williams & Wilkins, 1993, pp 185–195

Yalom I[D], Brown S, Bloch S: The written summary as a group psychotherapy technique. Arch Gen Psychiatry 32:605–613, 1975

Couple and Family Therapy

Laurie Fields, Ph.D.

Thomas L. Morrison, Ph.D.

C. Christian Beels, M.D., M.S.

"Marital and family therapists and researchers can justifiably feel heartened by the considerable accumulated evidence…on the efficacy of marital and family therapy for specific disorders in specific populations. Our field is healthy, strong and growing. In almost every area… outcomes have been found as good as or better than other approaches to psychotherapy." (Pinsof and Wynne 1995a, p. 342)

In modern psychiatry, families and couples are seen in a variety of contexts. Family members may be included in consultation with an identified child or adult patient to obtain collateral information, may be engaged as part of the treatment team to help with medication compliance, and may be included to provide support for the patient. In working with an individual patient, the therapist may discover that some symptoms are influenced by dysfunctional couple or family interaction patterns. In this case, brief therapy including the partner or family of a patient to address relational issues as an adjunct to individual treatment may be provided. As a primary treatment modality, couple or family therapy is indicated for a variety of presenting problems and can be selected on the basis of efficacy research and/or assessment of the problem as relational or maintained by the family system. In all cases, the therapist needs to have knowledge of techniques for engaging the family members, assessing their strengths and needs, and intervening in a helpful way. Thus, even if a therapist does not provide "full fledged" couple or family therapy, family consultation at a variety of levels is a strategic element in general psychiatric practice, and developing some skill with its techniques is important (Wynne et al. 1986).

A word about terminology: *Family therapy* is a general term for consultation with any group of people related by blood, marriage, or cohabitation. It also applies to consultation with one person about his or her family. Pinsof and Wynne (1995b) provide a clear, pragmatic definition: Family therapy is "any psychotherapy that directly involves family members in addition to an index patient and/or explicitly attends to the interaction among family members" (p. 586). *Couple therapy* is an updated term for marital therapy, in that it includes, beyond married couples, gay and lesbian couples and other unmarried but committed couples (Pinsof et al. 1996). It should be noted that the vast majority of outcome research on couples to date has been limited to married couples. The abbreviation CFT refers to couple and/or family therapy. It is derived from MFT, which denoted marital and/or family therapy.

On the basis of progress during the past decade, we can state unequivocally that couple and family therapy (CFT) works, because there is now strong empirical support for its efficacy. Research has clearly demonstrated the superiority of CFT over no treatment, as well as its greater efficacy (with emerging evidence for cost-effectiveness) in comparison with individual therapy for a number of presenting problems. Research, however, has not shown the superiority of any one model of CFT over another in any consistent fashion (Dunn and Schwebel 1995; Hahlweg and Markman 1988; Hazelrigg et al. 1987; Markus et al. 1990; Shadish et al. 1993). The findings from this body of empirical data allow us to move past advocating CFT for every clinical condition. Because many family therapy models evolved from a systemic epistemology, a belief had emerged that *all* psychiatric problems could be understood and treated by addressing the family system. Both individual and systemic conceptualizations of a problem and its treatment are certainly possible; however, research now directs us to be more sophisticated in terms of indications and contraindications for prescribing and administering CFT. Additionally, in the absence of clear empirical evidence of the superiority of specific CFT models, there is now a rationale for moving away from rigid adherence to particular schools of therapy. Instead, selection of CFT techniques on the basis of their clinical utility and identification of universal features that are useful can now be considered. For example, across a number of approaches, two sets of CFT skills—relationship building and session structuring—have been noted as important (Brothers 1992).

In this chapter we first provide a brief overview of the history of CFT to provide context helpful in understanding the current status of the field. We then summarize the indications and contraindications for providing or referring patients for CFT, based on recent empirical findings. We review each of the major schools of family and couple therapy, using an ongoing case example to illustrate application of useful techniques from the various schools. In this way, approaches to handling different aspects of therapy (i.e., stance of the therapist, assessment, intervention) are presented. Finally, we discuss several topics of special importance in today's environment, including cultural diversity and ethical issues inherent in CFT.

History of Couple and Family Therapy

Conjoint family psychotherapy was a development of American social science and social service after World War II. Before that, even in the early 1920s, the child guidance movement, marriage counseling, and orthopsychiatry (an interdisciplinary approach to the child, the family, and the school) were gathering strength. All of these were organized professional efforts to support the family as the primary agency of mental health for both children and adults. But these movements did not

develop a treatment technique with a theory until the 1950s. At that time, American anthropologists began to propose a shift in the boundary of the mind, from the inner pathways of the brain to include as well the outer circuits of behavior patterns between people in the family or the larger social group. They proposed that a natural group such as a family has superordinate dynamics and laws of behavior of its own, independent of its individual constituents' minds: that relationships have a natural history that can be studied. This idea had its prewar American origins in the social psychology of G.H. Mead and others at the University of Chicago, in the interpersonal psychiatry of H.S. Sullivan and in the anthropology of the students of Franz Boas. In the 1940s, research by Ruth Benedict and Margaret Mead began to show the influence of patterns of culture and child rearing on adult behavior and, along with the work of Gregory Bateson, laid the foundations for a theory of relationship patterns upon which an art and science of therapy could be built. In his study of New Guinea society, Bateson described modes of relationships that contributed to the stability or disruption of the group: symmetrical relationships are inherently competitive and therefore disruptive, whereas complementary relationships are inherently stabilizing in the small group (Bateson 1958). Ideas like these, as well as others to be described subsequently, were adopted by therapists from social psychology and anthropology and incorporated into the developing practice of conjoint child–family therapy and of couple therapy.

In the 1960s the paradigm shift continued toward systems and communication theories. By the 1970s— termed the heyday of family therapy (Roy and Frankel 1995)—an extraordinary proliferation of family therapy models had occurred, with many innovators who created schools and aligned adherents. In this process, somewhat of a schism developed between family therapy and psychiatry, with the result that neither group benefited from the other. Although many of its founders were psychiatrists, family therapy developed largely outside of official psychiatry, probably because the psychiatric community during those same years was more focused on psychoanalysis as a general theory of mind and therapy. And although analysts and family therapists have integrated the two fields, the historical antipathy between them had some important consequences. One was a split in the image of the ideal practice of psychotherapy. Psychoanalysis emphasized confidential verbal dialogue between patient and analyst. To facilitate the transference, transactions with the real people in the patient's life and advice about the management of those interpersonal relations were kept to a minimum. Family therapy took a different position: the relational context was seen as most important in the patient's life, and interventions focused on enhancing that context. Family therapists were interested in the mental health issues of the larger society and were eager to tackle a whole new range of contextual problems: child-rearing, marital stability, psychosis, addiction and alcoholism, and the disorganization of family life that comes from poverty. They developed interventions for patients previously thought to be beyond the reach of psychotherapy—those from impoverished backgrounds, with less psychological sophistication and more visible symptoms.

By the 1980s the importance of integrating the concepts of the various schools and professions had become apparent (Becvar and Becvar 1993), and outcome research began in earnest. The 1990s brought increased cross-disciplinary collaboration, some impressive meta-analyses of CFT outcome research, a stronger emphasis on family strengths as well as dysfunction, and a heightened appreciation for human diversity in terms of how family dysfunction was conceptualized and treated. As we move through the first decade of the new millennium, CFT continues to evolve, with an increasing interest in adopting an integrative perspective that highlights some of the more effective factors shared by the different approaches.

Indications and Contraindications for Couple and Family Therapy

A substantial amount of CFT outcome research has been published in recent years, including individual studies, narrative reviews, and meta-analytic reviews. Outcome studies can be classified as either efficacy or effectiveness studies, depending on the settings in which they are conducted. *Effectiveness* refers to the effects of therapy conducted in "normal" settings where therapy is typically provided, whereas *efficacy* refers to a therapy's effects in controlled clinical trials (Pinsof and Wynne 1995b). Because the vast majority of outcome studies to date have been efficacy studies, there is a consensus that more effectiveness research is needed to generalize the findings to settings in which therapy is typically conducted. With that caveat, we have reason to be confident: the research on which the following recommendations are based has been carefully selected by applying rigorous criteria (Carr 2000b; Chambless and Hollon 1998; Pinsof and Wynne 1995b) including only larger, multiple, well-controlled studies that were published with peer review. Together, these studies provide an empirical basis for determining when CFT is indicated. Additionally, Glick et al. (2000c) recently compiled a thoughtful analysis of clinical factors

that aid in clinical decision making about use of CFT. These sources help to answer two important questions: 1) For which disorders, presenting problems, and patients should we provide CFT? and 2) When is it preferable to employ other treatment modalities?

Empirically Informed Indications and Contraindications

Family Therapy for Specific Adult Psychiatric Disorders

Family therapy in combination with medication has been demonstrated to be more effective than medication management alone in the treatment of both schizophrenia and bipolar affective disorders (Carr 2000b; Clarkin et al. 1990; Goldstein and Miklowitz 1995; Miklowitz and Goldstein 1997). For alcoholism, there is good scientific evidence that CFT is more effective than individual treatment in engaging patients in treatment. During the treatment phase and up to 1 year posttreatment, CFT shows some superiority over therapies that do not include family members. In the aftercare phase, CFT also appears to be superior to standard aftercare (i.e., not including family members) up to 2 years posttreatment (Baucom et al. 1998; Carr 2000b; Edwards and Steinglass 1995). For drug abuse in adults, the research is less definitive because of the variety of substances abused, although a review of five studies suggested that adding CFT to standard treatments increases engagement, retention, and positive outcome (Liddle and Dakof 1995). Psychoeducational interventions for family caregivers of dementia patients have been shown to be efficacious (and superior to family support groups) in reducing caregiver burden and depression and can delay institutionalization of dementia patients (Campbell and Patterson 1995).

Couple Therapy

Couple therapy has been shown to be superior to individual therapy for couple relationship distress and conflict, as well as for "unipolar depressed outpatient women in distressed marriages" (Pinsof and Wynne 1995b, p. 603; see also Bray and Jouriles 1995). In contrast, on the basis of studies to date, intensive uncovering couple therapy is contraindicated with married unipolar *inpatient* women (Clarkin et al. 1990), although the positive findings for family psychoeducational interventions for inpatient bipolar patients still hold. Couple therapy in which the spouse serves as a partner in the patient-focused treatment also has demonstrated efficacy in the treatment of obsessive-compulsive disorder and panic disorder with agoraphobia (Baucom et al. 1998; Emmelkamp et al. 1992; Mehta 1990).

Couple therapy for psychosexual problems has been shown to be effective in up to 60% of cases of male erectile dysfunction, up to 80% of cases of premature ejaculation (although this rate is usually lower by follow-up), up to 90% of cases of primary female orgasmic dysfunction, 50% of cases of secondary female orgasmic dysfunction, and between 80% and 100% of cases of vaginismus and dyspareunia (Segraves and Althof 1998). Treatment in which the spouse is included has been shown to be superior to individual psychosexual therapy (Ersner-Hershfield and Kopel 1979; Hurlbert et al. 1993).

Family Therapy for Specific Adolescent Problems

For adolescents, family therapy has been shown to be more effective than individual therapies for conduct disorder, oppositional defiant disorder, and drug abuse (Carr 2000a, 2000c; Chamberlain and Rosicky 1995; Kazdin 1998). Family therapy has also been shown to be effective in treating obesity and anorexia in adolescents (Carr 2000a; Pinsof and Wynne 1995b). In fact, an exclusively individual approach for anorexia or drug abuse is contraindicated, as is group-based treatment for conduct disorder (Carr 2000c).

Family Therapy for Child-Focused Problems

For children, the strongest supportive evidence for the superiority of family treatments is from research on home-based parent training for autistic children (Estrada and Pinsof 1995). Childhood oppositional defiant disorder and conduct disorder are treated more effectively with a combination of family and individual therapy than with either intervention alone (Estrada and Pinsof 1995). A large, well-controlled study has found family therapy to be superior to individual therapies in the treatment of childhood anxiety disorders, particularly separation anxiety and school phobia (Carr 2000c; Pinsof et al. 1996). Family therapy has also been shown to be efficacious in treating the *secondary* symptoms of childhood attention-deficit/hyperactivity disorder: aggressive and noncompliant behaviors. However, it should be noted that medication is clearly superior in treating the core symptoms of inattentiveness and hyperactivity (Estrada and Pinsof 1995). Including family interventions in the treatment of child abuse and neglect has been shown to be important, but family therapy without individual therapy is not effective (Carr 2000a; Edgeworth and Carr 2000). In the treatment of enuresis, the bell and pad method (a nighttime urine alarm) is most effective when paired with parent instruction in immediate reinforcement of the child and avoidance of criticism. Encopresis is successfully treated with family therapy when combined with standard medical intervention (Murphy and Carr 2000). For childhood depression, individual and group approaches are equally efficacious; the addition of parent involvement does *not* appear to be advantageous. An exception is when the depression is related to the death of a parent, in which case family therapy is efficacious (Moore and Carr 2000).

Clarification of Couple and Family Therapy Research Findings

In several studies in which CFT was reported to be more effective than either no treatment or standard or individual treatment, the findings were based on multicomponent treatment packages that included at least one CFT component. Such multicomponent treatment packages have been used in studies of schizophrenia and alcoholism in adults, conduct disorders and drug abuse in adolescents, and autism and conduct disorders in children. Further details of meta-analyses and narrative reviews of CFT interventions can be found in Carr (2000a), Glick et al. (2000b), and Pinsof and Wynne (1995b).

An important finding from the research to date is that CFT appears to have a very low level of risk. There is not a single replicated and controlled study in the literature in which persons receiving CFT fared worse than patients who received no treatment.

In the area of family therapy, despite the diversity of theories and approaches, the existing research gives no consistent indication of any differences in effectiveness among the types of treatment. In the area of couple therapy, most of the research has focused on behavioral or cognitive-behavioral therapy. In a study that compared the effectiveness of behavioral and insight-oriented marital therapy (Snyder et al. 1991), follow-up assessment at 4 years found that 3% of insight-oriented therapy couples versus 38% of behavioral marital therapy couples had separated or divorced (a statistically significant difference). Although this finding suggests that insight-oriented couple therapy is more effective than behavioral couple therapy, it needs to be replicated before definitive conclusions can be drawn.

Although couple therapy has been shown to be more effective than no treatment or individual treatment in reducing marital conflict, the *clinical* significance of the reductions is less than might be desired. Only 40%–50% of couples in clinical trials of marital therapy were found to have shifted from distressed to nondistressed status after treatment (Bray and Jouriles 1995).

Clinically Informed Indications and Contraindications

According to Glick (1999), CFT is indicated when

1. Family or couple treatment is requested.
2. The problem involves two or more family members (e.g., improvement in one family member has resulted in deterioration in another, or symptoms in one family member are reinforced by another member).
3. A sexual problem or sexual dissatisfaction is present.
4. A developmental transition or crisis causes disruption in the family.
5. A child or adolescent is the presenting patient.
6. An adult is being treated for a severe psychiatric illness (in order to obtain history and family support, negotiate treatment, and "clarify how the family interaction is influenced by and has influenced the course of illness" [Glick et al. 2000c, p. 599]).
7. The onset of symptoms is connected to relationship disharmony.

A summary of indications and contraindications is presented in Table 32–1.

CFT is contraindicated in the following circumstances (adapted from Glick et al. 2000c):

1. One family member is very paranoid, manic, psychotic, overtly aggressive, or agitated.
2. The family denies having family problems.
3. Strongly held religious or cultural beliefs against outside intervention in the family system are present.
4. The presenting problem does not have an effect on, or etiology in, the family system.
5. Couple problems are ego syntonic.
6. CFT is used to deny individual responsibility for personal problems.
7. Severe parental pathology is present, indicating that a child should be treated individually.
8. Individuation of a family member who is striving for autonomy requires separate treatment.
9. Another modality of treatment is needed first (e.g., detoxification).
10. A patient is only motivated to be seen alone.
11. Family treatment has stalled and family members still require treatment.
12. Crucial members of the family cannot be included.

Family Therapy in Practice

In the early phase of family therapy, key tasks include evaluation of the family and establishment of the therapeutic alliance. The middle or working phase may involve use of a variety of intervention approaches. As desired goals are reached, the final or termination phase is addressed.

The Family Evaluation and the Therapeutic Alliance

In addition to assessing the symptom presentation of the "identified patient" in usual fashion, important content areas related to family functioning require evaluation. For this task, it is helpful to use an outline analogous to that used in psychiatry for assessing individual patients. Glick et al. (2000a) compiled such an outline from areas of consensual importance across family therapy models (Table 32–2). For many families, the presenting problem can be conceptualized as difficulty in coping with the current family or developmental phase, such as adjusting to new parenthood or retirement (Walsh 1992). Thus, information about the stage of family and individual development is important (e.g., latency, adolescence, children "leaving the nest").

In family therapy there is a fixed hierarchy, parents being responsible for children, and there is the expectation of triangles. The combination of role differentiation and triangles leads to a complex set of structural problems. For example, the triangle of mother, father, and child contains an age and status gradient, with the parents allied on their side of the generation boundary, dealing together with the problems of raising the child. However, this triangle can change its shape in many problematic ways, one of the most familiar involving a covert coalition between the child and one of the parents. The Freudian oedipal triangle is a special case of this type of covert alliance. Triangles also change over the course of the life cycle, as, for example, when the generation gradient begins to reverse as the parents age and become dependent—or try not to become dependent—on the children. Birth order of children, death, divorce, migration, and other changes of social support all involve structural correlates that can alter the shapes of these relationships. Finally, the entire family structure is influenced by cultural expectations, values, and personal history, so that the assessment of a family problem can be very complex indeed.

Assessment interviews can be conjoint (i.e., two or more family members), individual, or both conjoint and individual, depending on the preference of the therapist. Individual interviews are advantageous in that they allow for greater disclosure of feelings, thoughts, and behaviors (e.g., family violence). The disadvantages are that 1) consensual validation of the issues by other family

TABLE 32–1. Indications for and contraindications to couple and family therapy (CFT)

Clinically informed indications: Consider CFT when...

Family or couple treatment is requested.

The presenting problem involves two or more family members.

A sexual problem or dissatisfaction is present.

A family developmental transition or crisis causes disruption in the family.

A child or adolescent is the presenting patient.

An adult is being treated for a severe psychiatric illness.

The onset of symptoms is related to relationship disharmony.

Specific evidence-based indications for CFT:

   Research supports use of family therapy...

In combination with medication for schizophrenia and bipolar disorders.

For alcoholism and drug abuse including engagement, treatment, and aftercare phases.

For family caregivers of dementia patients.

For adolescents with conduct disorder, oppositional defiance, drug abuse, obesity, or anorexia.

As part of in-home parent training for autistic children.

In combination with individual treatment for childhood oppositional defiant disorder and conduct disorder.

For childhood separation anxiety and school phobia.

In combination with medication for children with attention-deficit/hyperactivity disorder.

In combination with individual treatment for child abuse and neglect.

For children with encopresis.

For childhood depression specifically associated with bereavement.

   Research supports use of couple therapy...

For relationship distress.

For unipolar depressed women in distressed relationships.

For couples in which one partner has obsessive-compulsive disorder or panic disorder with agoraphobia.

For psychosexual problems.

Contraindications to CFT

One family member is paranoid, manic, psychotic, overtly aggressive, hostile, or agitated.

The family denies having family problems.

There are strongly held religious or cultural beliefs against outside intervention in the family.

The presenting problem does not have an effect on, or etiology in, the family system.

CFT is used to deny individual responsibility for personal problems.

Severe parental pathology is present.

Individuation of a family member who is striving for autonomy requires separate treatment.

Another modality of treatment is needed first, such as detoxification.

A patient is only motivated to be seen alone.

Family treatment has stalled and family members still require treatment.

Crucial members of the family cannot be included.

Couple problems are ego-syntonic.

There is an obvious lack of commitment to the couple relationship.

One partner is secretly involved and is unwilling to stop the affair or discuss the affair openly.

members is not possible and 2) family members may share "secrets" that the therapist believes must be made known for therapy to be effective. Therefore, the therapist must set clear, specific guidelines about confidentiality early in the treatment (W.C. Nichols 1996). Conjoint assessment sessions are invaluable for observing family interaction patterns. A tool often used to gain perspective on the family within its cultural and historical context is the *genogram*, a structural diagram of several generations of the family (Minuchin 1974). Creating a genogram is a simple, structured exercise to which all family members can contribute in early conjoint sessions. This tool increases family members' sense of shared history or "we-ness." McGoldrick and Gerson (1985) have provided detailed instructions for the use of genograms in family assessment.

Beginning with the initial sessions and extending into the middle phase of therapy, an important task is to build a treatment alliance with the family—a collaborative relationship that creates a favorable climate for change.

TABLE 32–2. Family evaluation outline

I. Identifying data and current phase of family/individual life cycle
II. Interview data
    A. Presenting problem
    B. Recent family events and stressors
    C. History of the presenting problem
    D. History of past treatment attempts, history of problem-solving attempts, other problems
    E. Family's goals and expectations of treatment
    F. Strengths, motivations, and resistances
III. Formulation of family problem areas:
    A. Communication
        1. Which family members can state information clearly and accurately?
        2. Which members can listen to and perceive information accurately?
        3. Tone of communication: Which members are respectful, affirming, demanding, insulting?
    B. Problem solving: Can the family as a group…
        1. State the problem clearly and in behavioral terms?
        2. Formulate—brainstorm possible solutions?
        3. Evaluate the solutions?
        4. Decide on one solution to try?
        5. Assess the effectiveness of the solution?
    C. Roles and coalitions
        1. Refers to patterns of behavior through which family tasks of providing for basic needs, developing a working marital coalition, and raising/socializing offspring are carried out.
        2. Is there a functional and successful marital coalition?
        3. Strength of cross-generational coalitions compared with marital dyad
        4. How is leadership and decision making handled?
        5. Are any family members isolated/fragmented/enmeshed/undifferentiated?
        6. How are their connections with extended family, community?
    D. Affective responsiveness and involvement
        1. Expressive, empathic, spontaneous vs. emotionally dead
        2. Is there an emotional divorce between marital partners?
        3. What is the predominant family mood pattern (suspicion, envy, anger, irritation, frustration, withdrawal, depression)?
        4. What is the family's level of enjoyment, energy, humor?
        5. Degree of emotional interest and investment among family members?
    E. Behavior control
        1. Refers to way of handling physically dangerous situations, needs, and drives
        2. What are the family's limit-setting and discipline practices?
    F. Operative family beliefs and stories
        1. What are the beliefs about how parents and children should be, the family's values?
        2. What are the family history beliefs or beliefs about a certain child?
        3. What are their therapy beliefs: should a person deny or endure problems, accept help, or attempt to solve them on their own?

Source. Adapted from Glick et al. 2000a.

Allying as much as possible with each member of the family by communicating understanding and concern for their well-being is an important process during early sessions. By reframing family members' dysfunctional attempts to deal with problems as well-intentioned, by inquiring about members' understanding of one another's motives, and by conveying a belief that everyone wants things to get better, the therapist can instill hope, reduce hostility, and maintain a positive alliance.

The case example introduced below will be used to illustrate the various approaches to CFT presented in this chapter. We discuss the evolution of this case in terms of the sequence of phases of therapy, with techniques drawn from the various schools to demonstrate their application.

Case Example

Sue and Trent are middle-class parents of two children: Ryan, age 11 years, and Beth, age 8. At the time the family presented for treatment, the sibling conflict between Beth and Ryan had escalated to the point that the two children could not be together in a room or car without displaying extreme agitation or aggressive behavior. Sue worked long hours and was under continual pressure at work, as she was in the middle stages of building her career in engineering. Trent had set his career aspirations in science writing aside to devote his energies to supporting his wife and family. The family had undergone a long series of stressful events and had been in severe financial difficulties for quite some time. The children's behavioral disturbances and intense conflict had been going on for a number of years before the family presented for treatment. In fact, Sue had seen Ryan as dangerous to Beth almost from the time that Beth was born. Ryan reminded Sue of her own brother, who had been regularly aggressive toward her as a child, and Sue felt a strong need to protect Beth. Trent felt that Ryan's needs were neglected by his mother and responded by providing him with regular attention and nurturance. Both parents were very caught up in the children's overwhelming emotional difficulties. Their parenting became polarized, with Trent providing more of the emotional support and Sue making the rules and setting limits. Trent often felt that Sue did not understand him and did not appreciate the practical efforts and sacrifices he made to manage family and home. Sue, in turn, often felt criticized and unappreciated for *her* sacrifices and career efforts on behalf of the family. During the rare times in which they had an opportunity to talk with one another, discussions focused on finding the "right" solution to a problem, and both often wound up feeling frustrated.

In initially considering whether family therapy is indicated for this case, the presenting problem of conflict among two family members and the fact that children are involved support the appropriateness of a family evaluation. After a conjoint family assessment session, a parent meeting, and individual assessment sessions with Beth and Ryan, an initial diagnosis of bipolar affective disorder was given to Ryan. In the assessment sessions, it emerged that Ryan was experiencing psychosis and mixed-mood symptoms and was aggressive toward Beth. Although relational issues and bipolar disorder *are* indications for family therapy, severe depressive, psychotic, agitated, and aggressive symptoms are contraindications. Therefore, initial treatment involved individual medication and supportive therapy, with psychoeducation about bipolar disorder for the parents. After several months, when the more severe symptoms were under control, the family was ready to begin family therapy.

Schools of Family Therapy: Approaches to Intervention

Many family therapists would agree that the simple act of bringing members of a family together to discuss their shared problems is a powerful intervention in and of itself. Increased collaboration and reduced conflict often follow comments such as "I didn't know you felt that way" (Steinglass 1995). There are a number of ways in which family therapy can be conceptualized—metaphors for what the therapist is doing, theories or models of pathology—each of which has been eloquently presented by a different group of adherents. Techniques in couple therapy are useful in family therapy, and vice versa. Indeed, one can easily make too much of the distinction between the two. Certainly couple and family therapy resemble each other more than either resembles individual therapy. As soon as the therapist faces more than one person in the room, many of the assumptions of individual therapy—for example, privacy, confidentiality, neutrality—change radically, to assumptions of disclosure, openness, and shifting alliances. Metaphorically, if therapy is art, then the artistic analogue of individual therapy is literature, in the sense that the patient presents a monologue, a verbal text, and the neutral therapist provides commentary or explication. The artistic analogue of CFT is more like theater, with the therapist as director, arranging scenes, prescribing exercises, dealing with conflicts among the actors, and "getting the show on the road."

The following presentation of family therapy approaches is simplified, as if each model proposed only its own innovation, and it follows a logical order, as they might be considered by a therapist in beginning a treatment. An experienced therapist would likely choose to construct an intuitive blend of these strategies to create a sequence uniquely responsive to the picture that the family presents.

Approaches to family therapy can be conceptualized as lying along a continuum of most to least directive. They are presented in order of increasing indirection, or deviance from the straightforward behavioral approach: First the *behavioral* and *cognitive-behavioral* approaches are discussed, and then the *systems theory–based* approaches (i.e., structural, strategic, communication/ interaction, Milan systemic), which add ways of dealing with resistances to the straight-on approaches. Three types of *psychodynamic* approaches to family therapy are then presented (i.e., contextual, extended family systems, object relations), which assume that resolving current interpersonal family problems requires intrapsychic exploration and resolution of unconscious internalizations from early parent–child relationships. Finally, *experiential*, *psychoeducational*, and *solution-focused/narrative* approaches to family therapy are described. Models of CFT are summarized in Table 32–3.

TABLE 32–3. Models of couple and family therapy

Model (representative schools)	View of dysfunction	Goals of therapy	Strategies and techniques
Behavioral/Cognitive-behavioral *Alexander* *Jacobson* *Patterson* *Weiss*	Maladaptive behavior is reinforced by family attention or other rewards. Desired behaviors are not mutually rewarded; exchanges are coercive or unbalanced. Communication and other social skills are deficient. Family members have faulty beliefs, assumptions, and expectations of one another.	Change contingencies so that desired behaviors receive tangible social reinforcements. Improve communication, problem solving, and social skills. Expose inaccurate assumptions and replace with evidence-based beliefs.	Observe overt behaviors and conduct functional analysis. Guide family to reward desired behaviors. Use contingency contracting between family members. Teach communication, negotiation, and problem-solving skills. Use questioning and logic to expose faulty assumptions and expectations. Teach evidence-testing to examine and replace faulty beliefs.
Structural/Strategic/Systemic *Ackerman* *Aponte* *Bateson* *Haley* *Jackson* *Palazzoli* *Madanes* *Minuchin*	Current family structural imbalance (e.g., weak parental alliance). Inability to adjust to life-cycle transitions. Symptoms are also seen as a communication to control relationships or send a message when other strategies cannot be used.	Reorganize family structure: shift members' relative positions to disrupt malfunctioning pattern and strengthen parental hierarchy. Solve presenting problem with specific behaviorally defined objectives. Create clear, flexible subsystems and boundaries. Shift perspectives by increasing understanding and alternative views of problems.	Assume a pragmatic, focused, action-oriented stance to shift interaction patterns. Map family structure and plan restructuring. Highlight problematic interaction patterns; facilitate communication and sharing of perceptions. Substitute new behaviors to interrupt feedback cycles. Use indirect strategies such as reframing, ordeals, and paradoxical directives to alter frame of reference and allow new choices.
Insight-oriented/Psychodynamic/Emotion-focused *Bowen* *Boszormenyi-Nagy* *Framo* *Greenberg* *Scharff and Scharff* *Susan Johnson*	Symptoms derive from shared family projection processes stemming from unresolved past conflicts, loyalty issues, or losses in family of origin. Expectations including sense of indebtedness or entitlements also arise from experiences in family of origin.	Engender insight and resolution of family-of-origin conflict and losses. Decrease family projection processes. Increase empathic relating. Facilitate relationship reconstruction and reunion.	Employ observation, clarification, and interpretation. Link past and present dynamics. Assist in resolution of conflicts and losses. Facilitate healthier modes of relating by recognizing feelings and defenses aroused by closeness.
Experiential/Existential *Satir* *Whitaker*	Symptoms are nonverbal messages in reaction to current communication dysfunction. Defensive attitudes and feelings of shame arise from experiences in family of origin.	Direct clear communication through immediate shared experience. Genuine nondefensive relating. Individual and family growth.	Demonstrate and create experiences in which family members can sense and express emotions: self-disclosure, direct communication. Experiential techniques include psychodrama, sculpting, and role playing.

TABLE 32–3. Models of couple and family therapy (continued)

Model (representative schools)	View of dysfunction	Goals of therapy	Strategies and techniques
Psychoeducational *Anderson* *Falloon* *Goldstein*	Core biological deficits and environmental factors interact negatively to produce disturbed thinking and behavior.	Reduce levels of negative or intrusive family behaviors toward patient. Reduce stressors in patient's environment and thus reduce relapse. Increase desired behaviors and positive interactions.	Provide information about illness, arrange social support, and furnish management guidelines. Facilitate stress and stigma reduction. Encourage calm, problem-solving approach. For children, provide parent training in application of behavioral procedures (e.g., positive reinforcement, timeouts).
Narrative/Solution-focused *de Shazer* *Epston* *White*	Family members' beliefs about the problem narrow their perspectives in such a way that they become inflexible. The family cannot change, because they believe that the problem controls them.	Assist the family in developing an alternative story about the problem that helps to put them back in control. Discover exceptions to the problem that occur naturally so that family members can develop ways of allowing the desired behaviors to occur.	Pull the family together as a collaborative team to cocreate a new story. Share constructions of the problem to help family members reframe and change their perspectives. Instill a sense that the problem is not within an individual but outside the family to empower the family to work together to handle the problem.

Behavioral and Cognitive-Behavioral Approaches

Behavioral family therapy is based on the principles of operant conditioning and social learning theory. Symptoms are conceptualized as maladaptive behaviors that are learned and maintained by their consequences. The therapist's stance is quite active and directive, and treatment is usually brief and circumscribed. Skills are taught to family members that assist them in eliciting desired behaviors in other members of the family, through techniques such as use of positive reinforcement, communication and problem solving, and behavioral contracting (i.e., agreements between family members: "You do this, and I'll do that"). The presenting problem is defined in terms of antecedents and consequences—those events that trigger the behavior and those that serve to reinforce it. In our case example, the therapist might inquire about how the parents have dealt with sibling conflicts, what they have found most and least effective, and what typically occurs before the conflicts. Reinforcement is provided to parents by giving them credit for having done their best, and to children by giving them credit for what-

ever change in the situation they are willing to make (Griffin and Greene 1999a).

From a behavioral point of view, handling sibling conflict is a matter of extinguishing the behavior by removing factors that serve to reinforce it: in the case presented earlier, Sue and Trent were instructed to isolate Beth and Ryan when they fight and not to reward either child with any victories. Conflict was discussed at length with both children present, and a problem-solving approach was taken to provide them with new, more grown-up ways of negotiating their differences—a quality they both valued. The parents were taught to reward Beth and Ryan for conflict-free periods. For example, in the course of making a list of things he wanted, Ryan said that an important item for him was more time with his father, and this was arranged.

The *cognitive-behavioral* approach adds questioning and logic to expose faulty beliefs, assumptions, meanings, and expectations regarding family members' behaviors. Cognitive-behavioral therapy (CBT) family therapists believe that faulty behavioral patterns reflect faulty cognitions. They teach family members how to examine the fallacy of beliefs and employ standard behavioral change techniques to alter the associated behaviors (Griffin and Greene 1999a). In the case of Beth and Ryan, the therapist uses questions to expose Ryan's beliefs about Beth that escalate his anger and precede aggressive behaviors directed at Beth. These beliefs are that Beth is preferred by their parents and that everyone would be happy if Beth were to kill him and take his place in the family. Ryan had felt abandoned by his mother when Beth was born, and he had projected his anger onto Beth. The CBT therapist would certainly validate these emotions but would also challenge the accuracy of the beliefs through evidence testing, helping other members of the family to express their positive feelings about Ryan so as to alter the inaccurate beliefs. CBT family therapists teach adaptive cognitive and behavioral coping strategies to be used in family interactions, and their use can be increased via parental reinforcement or reward (Fields and Prinz 1997).

Systems Theory–Based Approaches

The systems theory–based approaches have in common the assumption that families tend to act in ways that maintain the status quo or "homeostasis" of the family, which explains why changing a symptom necessarily involves the whole family system. The most directive of the systemic approaches is *structural* family therapy, developed by Minuchin largely as a result of his work with dysfunctional, lower-socioeconomic-status families. Minuchin's research indicated that these families respond best to interventions that employ a directive, concrete, here-and-now approach (Minuchin 1974; Minuchin and Fischman 1981). In structural family therapy, symptoms are perceived as arising because of faulty family structure. For example, power hierarchies are present that determine how members combine forces during times of conflict. Sometimes two family members unite against a third, or all are disengaged from one another. Behavioral techniques and other directives are employed to alter behaviors and interactions rather than to foster insight. A key technique is *enactment*, wherein the therapist directs family members to engage in behavioral patterns that run contrary to the current patterns, either within the therapy session or prescribed for home practice.

In our case example, faulty structure was evident in the cross-generational alliances between mother and daughter and father and son that weakened the parental coalition and contributed to the sibling conflict—and that could also be seen as diverting the parents from addressing their marital conflict (see "Couple Therapy" section later in this chapter). To change this structural problem, mother-to-son, father-to-daughter, and couple interaction was facilitated in session, and each of these dyads were assigned "special time" days during the week when they would engage in pleasant activities together. Although each of the parent–child dyads enjoyed their together times, the couple times led to an uncovering of couple conflicts and sexual dissatisfactions that had previously been obscured by the focus on the children's difficulties.

Strategic family therapists, like behavioral and structural therapists, are directive and assume responsibility for implementing change in problem areas, but they also employ strategies for dealing with resistance, such as paradoxical techniques. Family members may agree to a reasonable assignment of self-reform and clear communication and yet repeatedly find themselves unable to carry out the homework tasks. The therapist recognizes that he or she is dealing with the group homeostasis, the stability of the family system—a property of organization that is stronger than the individual wills to change. The problem from the therapist's point of view is to find a configuration of the forces in the group such that the energies that in the group's homeostatic mode work against change will, in a new arrangement of forces, be liberated to promote the desired change. The intervention involves moving from a demand for change to a no-change position. This difference has been likened to that between wrestling and jujitsu, in which the opponent's own resistant strengths are used to subdue him. Alternatively, one might prefer the less martial metaphor proposed by Milton Erikson: As a boy on the farm, he watched his father try without success to pull a mule head-first into a barn until he realized that the animal would be more likely to go in if he pulled on its tail—that is, in its resistance, the mule would then walk forward into the barn. This image is important, because it reminds us that anyone who tries such a maneuver with a mule must first establish excellent rapport to avoid being kicked.

Therapists in the strategic tradition, Jay Haley (1976), Chloe Madanes (1981), and the Brief Therapy Group at the Mental Research Institute in Palo Alto (Watzlawick et al. 1974), agree on these aspects of the task: Symptoms are seen as a communication to control relationships when all other strategies have failed, and goals for therapy are to alter dysfunctional family interactions. A key technique is the *paradoxical directive*, which uses the patient's resistance in a constructive way—that is, by resisting the directive, the patient ends up abandoning his or her dysfunctional behavior. *Ordeals* are unpleasant tasks assigned to be performed whenever a symptom occurs; their purpose is to facilitate change by making it more difficult to have the symptom than to give it up (Haley 1984).

Ryan's agitation and aggressive behaviors toward Beth could be conceptualized as a way of keeping the family aware of the risk that he might be "killed off," forgotten, or ignored by them. Ryan could be commended for communicating this painful and very important message and praised for his great efforts at not allowing the family to ignore this risk of being forgotten since Beth was born. The therapist might state that he or she appreciates all the hard work Ryan has put into getting the family to this point. It must have been very exhausting and time-consuming, and it certainly could not have been fun getting so upset. But now that his parents are working together, Ryan should not relax and let them take over immediately. To ensure that each of them remains aware of the problem, he should have at least one more outburst each day so that they can practice dealing with it. This might be difficult to do, because he might not feel like being upset, but if he could do a good job of pretending, and above all, not let on whether it is real or pretend, each of them would have a chance to practice. At the next meeting, he could give the therapist criticisms of their technique. This formula does more than just take the wind out of Ryan's sails; it positively connotes his contribution and gives him a positive reason for being in charge of his symptom. By ritualizing the symptom instead of opposing it, the directive makes doing it or not a matter of choice and even introduces the possibility of *not* doing it in defiance of the recommendation.

Redefining Ryan's behavior as a good thing not to be abandoned lightly but rather to be used for practice is an example of "paradoxical" technique, because it characterizes the problem as, in a sense, the opposite of a problem. A considerable literature is available on the formation of paradox (Weeks and L'Abate 1982), but for our purposes, *paradox* should be understood as that aspect of strategy that shifts the problem from a bad to a good category in the family's understanding and in this way brings it under their control. An example of an *ordeal* for Ryan is that he could be prescribed the task of continuing to notice and log in a journal all the times that Beth's behavior feels threatening to him in order to document it for the family so it will not be ignored or forgotten. This is an aversive but constructive activity that may alter the symptom as well.

Communication/interaction family therapy also developed out of the research conducted at the Mental Research Institute in Palo Alto in the 1960s by Gregory Bateson, Jay Haley, Virginia Satir, and others (Satir 1967; Sluzki and Veron 1976; Watzlawick et al. 1974). Their research on communication processes led to recognition of double-bind communication in schizophrenia (in which a family member communicates two messages, one of which contradicts the other, and the patient is inhibited from clarifying the message) and then to the development of a school of family therapy. Assumptions are that all behavior is communicative, even when people are doing nothing, and that communications have both an informational aspect and an aspect that makes a statement about the relationship. The primary goal of therapy is to alter the interactional patterns that maintain the presenting symptoms. Direct techniques (highlighting problematic interaction patterns, teaching communication strategies) and indirect techniques (paradoxical strategies, reframing the problem) are used, both of which alter the family's frame of reference to encourage new ways of attacking the problem.

The *Milan systemic* family therapy approach is systems theory–based but is more concerned with insight and understanding than the others in this model. Milan systemic family therapy was developed by Mara Selvini Palazzoli, who was trained as a child psychoanalyst but altered her therapy techniques when she found a family systems approach to be more effective for treating children with anorexia (Selvini Palazzoli et al. 1978). In this approach, symptoms are conceptualized as resulting from fixed circular patterns that prevent family members from acting creatively or making new choices about their lives (Gelcer et al. 1990). The therapist's stance is neutral, as an ally of the entire family. The goal of therapy is to help family members see their choices and to assist them in implementing those choices by fostering increased understanding and awareness of alternative views of problems. *Circular questioning* is a key technique that helps family members to recognize differences and similarities in their perceptions. For example, to identify differences in perceptions about a recent sibling conflict, each family member might be asked, "Why were Beth and Ryan really fighting?" Such questioning might bring out the following facts: Sue had thought that Ryan's behavior was the result of his being vicious and mean, much like *Sue's* older brother had been, which meant that Sue felt that she needed to protect Beth and did not really understand Ryan's motives; Trent attributed the fights to normal sibling conflicts and felt sorry for Ryan when Sue made him out to be the "bad" one; Beth thought that she needed to protect herself from her angry older brother but sometimes "tested" him by instigating a fight because she felt on edge at the possibility, and also sometimes enjoyed his strong reaction; and Ryan, because of his perception that Beth could kill him, believed that he was protecting himself. When Beth and Ryan were able to hear each other's fears, they were able to shift their behaviors so as to feel less of a need to protect themselves from one another. When Sue listened to

Ryan's fears, she no longer thought of him as cruel but was able to empathize with his feelings of fear. This altered her behaviors in terms of protecting Beth, which reduced Ryan's anger toward Beth.

Milan systemic therapists frequently use directives and have made use of an intriguing technical device for delivering their formulations: the team of consultants. Like other family therapists, they used study groups in which several members watched the treatment from a separate room on the other side of a one-way mirror. Systemic researchers found that the observers behind the mirror not only were a source of new insights but also could serve as the source of the formulations and prescriptions that were delivered to the family, in the form of messages with which the therapist in the room could disagree or not. Use of a separate team of consultants allows the family to consider directives for restraint and directives for change as coming from different sources (Papp 1980), which may have the effect of reducing resistance to change.

Psychodynamic Approaches

Psychodynamic family therapy is concerned with the larger picture of family dynamics and assumes that early parent–child relationships affect and explain the nature of present interpersonal difficulties.

Bowenian family therapy, also called *extended family systems therapy*, is a psychodynamic approach developed by Murray Bowen (1978). Bowenian therapists work with the nuclear family but assume that the emotional systems of previous generations are very much a part of the family and the therapeutic process. A key concept is *differentiation of the self*, which refers both to differentiation of emotions from intellectual processes and to differentiation of self from others. Differentiated family members can feel their own feelings and, although not unaware of the feelings of others, can maintain a degree of objectivity and emotional distance. Problems are not seen as arising in response to stressors but as persisting because of family projection processes in undifferentiated or fused family dyads. In Bowenian family therapy, change occurs through insight into these processes, resulting in the use of cognitive rather than affective coping. Techniques of Bowenian family therapy include family-of-origin work to engender insight and coaching in ways to enhance self-differentiation. They utilize a stance of "researcher of the family process" (Griffin and Greene 1999b). In our case example, much of the family-of-origin work would address Sue's relationship with her brother as a child, in which she felt powerless and victimized. Sue tended to project onto her son Ryan the role of the dangerous and out-of-control brother, thus demonstrating a lack of differentiation from her family of origin as well as acting from an emotional stance in her parenting. Once Sue had gained insight into this dynamic, she would find it much easier to empathize with her son's feelings of fear and to feel less fearful herself of her son's aggressive behaviors.

Contextual family therapy, variously termed an *insight-oriented* and a family-of-origin approach, was developed by Ivan Boszormenyi-Nagy. Boszormenyi-Nagy held that people should not be judged as good or bad, but instead should have their behavior placed in the *context* of their extended family experiences. In collaboration with Geraldine Spark (Boszormenyi-Nagy and Spark 1973), he developed over the years a theory of interpersonal, intergenerational dynamics based on the concept of *exchange of merit*. A balance of indebtedness or entitlement builds up between family members over time, and one of the purposes of therapy is to clarify and resolve these obligations, especially those that are unexpressed or unacknowledged. In essence, the implicit quid pro quo is made explicit. The role of the therapist in this case is to provide a sequential side taking for family members' desires and obligations (Boszormenyi-Nagy and Ulrich 1981). Through the process of therapy, family members begin to gain trust from one another's honest responses, and the therapist promotes an understanding of the other's perspective. The goal is movement from self-serving interests to mutual interests.

From the case example, in Trent's family of origin, his mother tended to take care of everything and everyone, providing for Trent's and his father's needs completely. She had few other activities in her life. This led to Trent's expectation that Sue would easily be able to cater to his needs (a sense of entitlement) without much response on his part. However, Sue felt no such obligation and in fact had become resentful after sacrificing for several years. She strongly felt that Trent had not fulfilled his obligations, considering all that she had done. By uncovering and discussing these issues, Sue and Trent gained insight into and understanding of each other's reactions, and both became more willing to change their behaviors to balance out the giving and receiving.

The *object relations* approach to family therapy expands object relations theory to family functioning. In object relations family therapy, the resolution of current relationship problems requires an intrapsychic focus on internalized object relationships based on early interactions between parents and children. A key concept is *projective identification*, in which one attributes a disliked aspect of oneself to a family member and then reacts to the projected element in the other, attempting to control it (J.S. Scharff 1992). Additionally, family members bring to their relationships expectations based on internal models of how they were treated in childhood by their parents or other caregivers. These processes were evident in the way Trent expected Sue to provide unlimited "holding" or caretaking in the family in much the same way as his mother had provided for him. Projective identification was occurring when Trent saw Sue as always angry and mean toward Ryan, because he could not tolerate those same feelings in himself, especially because of the way his own father had exploded into rage on a regular basis. Trent tried to control Sue's behaviors by demonstrating how a caring parent should handle Ryan's anger and aggression, but he moved away from Sue in the process. In object relations family therapy, the therapist's role is to provide a nurturing environment in which the unconscious object relations that are interfering with current relationships may be understood and resolved. The therapist offers interpretations designed to generate new discussions by revealing hidden motivations or avoided emotions. The process often requires clients to relive and mourn unfulfilling aspects of past relationships and to integrate good and bad objects (D.E. Scharff and Scharff 1987; Slipp 1984).

Experiential Approaches

The *experiential* approaches have their origins in the existential or humanistic orientation of individual psychology, which has here-and-now experiencing as a focus. The presenting problem is defined as the result of defensive attitudes and feelings of shame emanating from experiences in one's family of origin. These emotions remain unexpressed and the associated impulses are denied (Satir 1964). Techniques used in experiential family therapy include psychodrama, sculpting, and role playing. Satir (1967) held that clear communication of feelings and the validation of differences between family members are the beginning points of personal growth. Whitaker's goals included balancing and facilitating both individual autonomy and a sense of togetherness (Whitaker and Keith 1981). The therapist's role is to demonstrate and create experiences whereby family members may overcome their fear of feeling and expressing emotions. Individual and family growth occurs through immediate shared experience.

In our case example, Beth was requested to "sculpt" the family by placing her parents and brother into positions in the therapy room that described the way she experienced them in the family. She placed herself sitting in one corner facing out, with her mother standing over her in a protective stance. She placed her father and

brother in the far corner, with her father sitting and holding Ryan in a nurturing manner as Ryan tried to reach around to attack Beth. Family members were then requested to express their emotional reactions to the sculpture. For example, Ryan's feeling about his mother protecting Beth included shame that he was such an "ogre" that Beth needed to be protected from him, but also enjoyment of the special nurturing he got from his father.

Psychoeducational Approaches

In recent years, family therapists have gained an increased appreciation of the value of psychoeducational approaches for treating and managing serious mental illness in family members and for helping parents manage behavioral disturbances in their children. The psychoeducational model is based on the assumption that the identified patient has a core biological deficit and that environmental factors interact negatively to produce disturbed thinking and behavior. The therapist is quite active and directive, serving as a liaison between the medical treatment team and the family. Psychoeducational family therapy seeks to postpone relapse by reducing the levels of highly negative or excessively intrusive family behaviors and by encouraging a calm and problem-solving approach—a neutral style of interaction—on the part of family members (Goldstein and Miklowitz 1995; McFarlane 1983a, 1983b). Parent training is a form of psychoeducation that incorporates social learning principles; it has been demonstrated to be effective for children with autism, conduct disorder, and behavioral disturbances associated with attention-deficit/hyperactivity disorder (Estrada and Pinsof 1995). Parents learn to recognize problem behaviors and to manage them by applying behavioral procedures such as positive reinforcements, time-outs, and contingency contracting.

In our case example, psychoeducation was provided at the time of Ryan's initial diagnosis of bipolar disorder. Information about the cyclical nature of the illness, the importance of medication compliance, and the necessity of minimizing environmental stressors was related. Signs of relapse and steps to reduce the probability of relapse were discussed as well. Sue and Trent worked on providing clear but reasonable expectations for Ryan given his illness and became aware of the importance of working out their marital conflicts and of disciplining the children without using critical or hostile remarks.

Narrative and Solution-Focused Approaches

Narrative and solution-focused approaches represent newer postmodern poststructuralist/constructivist models of family therapy. These popular models emphasize that perceptions of reality are constructed by the observer and are not inherent in the situation. A family's reality thus derives from its shared narratives and personal stories. It follows that the therapist's beliefs about the family are also uniquely constructed rather than inherent (Doherty 1991). Dysfunctional family patterns arise when the family's stories narrow members' perspectives in such a way that family interactions become inflexible. The therapist brings his or her constructions of the family to a discussion in which old family stories can be modified to allow consideration of new meanings and behaviors. The solution-focused and solution-oriented approaches (de Shazer 1985; O'Hanlon and Weiner-Davis 1989) seek exceptions to the problem that occur naturally and help the family develop ways of allowing the desired behaviors to occur. The narrative approach defines problems as oppressively intruding on people's abilities to lead more fulfilling lives and pulls the whole family in as a collaborative team that co-creates new stories to change the family's relationships with the problems (White and Epston 1990). Altering the story instills a sense that the problem is not within an individual but outside of the family, thus changing the family's perspective about its ability to handle the problem.

In our case example, the family's narrative about the sibling conflict problem revealed that it had started about 5 years before, when the children were playing a game of gunfighting. The gun fighting gradually became a means of expressing anger toward one another and took on a greater meaning in its ability to cause death. In deconstructing this story and considering environmental stressors and parental conflict, the children's fighting could also be understood in terms of their being trapped in the roles of "warriors in a war zone" in which they mistakenly fought with soldiers in their own army. This new narrative created a shared experience of environmental stress that allowed the siblings to experience a sense of shared anger and fear and to empathize with one another. It also placed them on the same team and began a new story in which they developed common interests, such as playing basketball together.

Couple Therapy in Practice

Making couple relationships work is not only the cultural ideal for adult life, it is part of a preventive public health agenda. Couple discord and estrangement are risk factors for disorders of children and for many illnesses of the partners themselves, such as depression and heart disease (Brown and Harris 1978; Lynch 1977). Couples often

present for treatment knowing that they are in need of help that focuses on the relationship rather than on the pathology of one or the other partner. If the therapist, after beginning individual work with one member of a couple, realizes that he or she is working with only one piece of the problem, the therapist may refer the couple for conjoint therapy. When the therapist has not met the partner of a patient who complains of relationship difficulties, the therapist is unable to maintain an objective view of the situation. The frequently used practice of calling that partner in for a short consultation does not solve this problem. Therapists who expect to work with couples should learn couple therapy techniques. They should see the couple together from the beginning or should refer the couple for conjoint therapy if it becomes clear that the relationship is an important problem.

The functioning of the dyad, or two-person relationship, is a special problem in natural groups, and the couple pair is a special case of the dyad. The couple unit is inherently unstable because it is made up of a pair of differing equals: equal in many kinds of responsibilities and rights, but different in personalities, in gender, and in the way society accords power to each. Bateson (1958) defined two modes for such a relationship and described the problem of moving flexibly from one mode to the other: from a *symmetrical* (competitive and equal) relationship, in which the problem is the resolution of conflict between equals, to a *complementary* (caregiving or caretaking and unequal) relationship, in which the problem is knowing who is giving what care to whom and how the roles shift so that the caregiver also has a chance to be the care receiver. These shifts, plus the power implications of the politics of gender, are basic themes in couple therapy. A frequent subtheme involves a third person (parent, child, or rival) appropriated by the couple to make the pair into a triangle and thereby balance the instability of these shifting relationships. Sometimes the therapist may even assume this role. Over time, however, a third person is not the best source of stability for a couple, and couple therapy is concerned with helping the partners discover ways to be united with, yet flexibly different from, one another.

Schools of Couple Therapy: Approaches to Intervention

To illustrate the various approaches to couple therapy, we broaden our case example to address couple issues, and we follow the introduction of each approach to couple therapy with a discussion of its applications to the case example. We start first with the cognitive-behavioral approach, then the insight-oriented approaches, followed by sex therapy, and finally divorce counseling. In general, simple, straightforward approaches such as the behavioral and cognitive can be tried first, because if they work, they can save time and effort, and because trying them out and discovering their limitations can be a good way of getting to know the more complex side of the couple's motivational structure, which often needs to be addressed by other approaches. Table 32–3 summarizes major models of CFT.

Case Example

The couple's relationship distress became apparent when Sue and Trent were given a directive during family therapy to set aside special time to spend together. Previously they had focused their energies on parenting and on the children's conflicts, which had allowed them to avoid facing their marital dissatisfactions. Their communications were often frustrated attempts at problem solving, with a belief that they had to find the only correct answer. Their views on parenting were polarized, with Trent focusing on emotional needs of the children and nurturance and Sue focusing on rules and practical matters. Sue felt that Trent did not back her up in setting limits and rules; Trent felt that Sue was too rigid. Sue aligned with their daughter Beth in protecting her from Ryan, while Trent was very close to Ryan. The couple's sexual relationship had become problematic, with Sue experiencing hypoactive sexual desire related to the mixed emotions intimacy entailed for her (given her frustrations with parenting and being unappreciated), and with Trent having erectile dysfunction related to anxiety. Both had resentments about the sacrifices each felt they made that went unappreciated.

Assessment of couples is similar to that of families, and the family evaluation outline provided in Table 32–2 (Glick et al. 2000a) can be useful in this regard. In addition, asking about each partner's sexual functioning and commitment to the relationship is important, and both conjoint and individual assessment interviews may be needed. If partners are seen for individual meetings, agreements about confidentiality regarding infidelity or other issues that may threaten the relationship or individual well-being need to be made in advance. It can be helpful to indicate that supported disclosure will be necessary because these issues can interfere with the therapy. Additionally, assessing both partners' family-of-origin experiences—through questions about their parents' closeness, anger/conflict, intimacy/affection, emotions, roles, and expectations—can be useful.

Cognitive-Behavioral Approaches

Cognitive-behavioral couple therapy (CBCT), also called behavioral or cognitive-behavioral marital therapy, is based on social learning and cognitive theories and covers a number of specific treatments that have been developed (Jacobson and Holzworth-Monroe 1986). In general, this model teaches couples how to identify and eliminate destructive or unskillful ways of communicating and to rehearse more constructive and rewarding exchanges (Snyder and Wills 1989). The therapist inquires about what each partner wants the other partner to do differently, how each lets the other know his or her preferences, and what kind of influence each partner uses to reinforce his or her messages. CBCT assumes that the partners are each other's strongest behavioral reinforcers. The therapist's job is to clarify each partner's behavioral contingencies and to teach the couple effective and benign ways of influencing each other's behavior by reinforcing it in a positive manner (Jacobson and Holzworth-Monroe 1986).

To do this, the therapist analyzes the fine details of the couple's manner of communication. How are each member's intentions and needs expressed, and how are these understood by the other? In the behavioral model, symmetrical conflict is worked out according to a "bargain" formula: Each partner "gives in order to get" in a conscious turn-taking fashion that emphasizes the fairness, or equal symmetry, of the relationship. Other techniques borrowed directly from the behavior therapy armamentarium, such as listing options, negotiating, and problem solving, are taught as technical skills. The cognitive component adds a focus on both *how* and *what* the partners are thinking that contributes to distress in the relationship. For example, partners will often make assumptions about each other's behaviors that are irrational and cause distress, such as inferring that one is not loved when a spouse appears sad and withdrawn. These beliefs are replaced by more realistic and hopeful ones (Baucom et al. 1989; Weeks and Treat 1992).

In our case example, the couple's communication style was marked by their taking turns stating their opinions about an issue with great conviction. This would often escalate into heated debates that ended with frustration on the part of both partners. Both complained of not feeling understood by the other—in fact, this emerged as the chief complaint. In session, Sue and Trent were asked to practice listening to one another and to rephrase what they heard so as to clarify their understanding of the material presented. Each was also asked to reflect on the underlying emotions being communicated by the other. In the process of learning to listen to and express an understanding of each other, both initially had difficulty inhibiting the urge to immediately counter by stating their own opinion. Gradually, however, the satisfaction of feeling understood fueled their attempts, and repeated practice at home and in further sessions solidified their skills.

Insight-Oriented Approaches

Based on principles derived from psychodynamic theory, insight-oriented approaches have the long-term goal of gradual personal development through the achievement of intimacy and self-understanding. These approaches seek to free the couple to interact in a more mature, autonomous, and congruent manner by resolving hidden or unconscious sources of conflict. Interpretation and clarification are techniques used by the therapist, as well as instruction in listening and empathy.

Object relations couple therapy (D.E. Scharff and Scharff 1991), like object relations family therapy, is based on the work of Fairbairn and other British object relations theorists (Main 1966). There is a focus on exploring the couple's unconscious presuppositions, fears, and hopes—based on early experience—about having a close, intimate relationship. The therapist seeks to provide a "holding environment" in which the partners can work toward discovering and resolving unrecognized motivations and emotions that interfere with intimacy. Where necessary, the therapist attempts to identify and resolve the partners' mutually mistaken and projective responses toward each other (Dicks 1967; Skynner 1981). Morrison (1998) presented a model of couple interaction based on object relations theory and has examined the fit of the model with findings from behavioral research on couples.

In our case example, Trent saw Sue as constantly angry and himself as having the trying task of dealing with her anger. With all the couple's anger safely located in Sue, Trent rarely had to experience his own anger, which could be quite fierce and rejecting but was always perceived by him as the fatigue of having to take care of such a difficult woman.

Emotionally focused couple therapy (Greenberg and Johnson 1986) has the goal of achieving intimacy in parts of the couple's life that are usually dominated by conflict. It is based on attachment theory (Bowlby 1988), which posits that seeking and maintaining contact with a few irreplaceable others is a primary motivating principle in human beings and an innate survival mechanism, providing a safe haven and a secure base in a potentially dangerous world. The two members of a bonding couple naturally seek this kind of attachment, and frustration of their efforts to achieve it lead to absorbing states of negative affect and rigid negative interaction sequences between them (Johnson and Whiffen 1999). This formulation of marital distress has received considerable empirical support from the studies of Gottman (1994), who recorded physiological responses of couples in conflict. From this perspective, work with couples involves recognizing feelings and defenses that are aroused by closeness, vulnerability, and the risk of rejection.

In our case example, as the treatment shifted to an emotional focus, Sue and Trent began to discover the feelings of vulnerability that preceded their defensive maneuvers of attack and retreat. By inhibiting her angry reproaches, Sue was able to experience her fear of abandonment, which was triggered by Trent's difficulty in holding to limits and rules—much like her father, who, in addition to placing no limits, was also distant and aloof. Trent discovered that he felt abandoned when Sue was unable to express empathy for him. Each initially made these discoveries in dialogues with the therapist while the partner was listening. Each then learned ways of introducing his or her need to the other so that a caring bond could be established in place of coercive and defensive responses. Sue learned to listen and to express her understanding of Trent, and she learned that his unstructured style had nothing to do with his love for her.

Sex Therapy

Modern sex therapy originated far from the mainstream of psychotherapy. In 1970, Masters and Johnson published *Human Sexual Inadequacy*, in which they explicated short-term behavioral treatments of common sexual dysfunctions with success rates in the 90% range. Their successes were greeted with amazement by conventional psychotherapists, who had found these problems very difficult to change, despite the fact that sexual "genitality" had a central place in the psychoanalytic value system. Although there has been some debate about the size of the original cure rates, accumulated clinical experience in the past 30 years leaves little question that behaviorally specific sex therapy, sometimes in combination with pharmacotherapy, is the treatment of choice for the sexual dysfunctions listed in DSM-IV (American Psychiatric Association 1994; Segraves and Althof 1998). These included disorders of desire, disorders of arousal, orgasmic disorders, sexual pain disorders, and the paraphilias, as well as substance-induced sexual disorders and sexual disorders due to a general medical condition.

Often it is couples who seek treatment for sexual issues, although individual patients do seek help for sexual disorders as well. Comprehensive assessment, including medical aspects, history, and specific symptoms, is necessary to make a definitive diagnosis, because treatments for the different sexual disorders are quite specific. Treatment may begin with both individual and conjoint interviews to elicit the precise nature of the experience. Each individual is asked about the stimuli that produce arousal or its opposite, about previous sexual experiences, and about beliefs regarding the nature of the dysfunction, with the result that the sexual experience is understood as an enjoyable but nevertheless partly technical phenomenon in which things can easily go wrong through no fault of either partner. The therapist's attitude, plus suggested reading and explanations, helps to lower the high romantic expectations and increase the variety of communication about the subject. This approach is interesting not only because it is effective but also because it provides a model for straight change-oriented therapy in general. Much work goes into defining goals in exact behavioral terms; the problem is then positively characterized as technical and as something about which more can be learned. The steps to solution are subdivided until they are small enough to ensure success; homework assignments are very clear, with alternative strategies if one does not work; and failure is redefined as merely gaining new information. Psychoeducation to normalize the experiences and cognitive restructuring to challenge dysfunctional thoughts (e.g., "sex should always involve orgasm") are useful ways to start the treatment. It is important to address couple-related issues that may underlie the sexual dysfunction, such as affects that are not communicated, conflicts, and past unresolved hurts. Communication training in which partners are helped to state their emotional and sexual needs, desires, and dislikes can be an important component of the treatment (Charlton 1997; LoPiccolo and Hogan 1979). Helen Kaplan, in *The New Sex Therapy* (Kaplan 1979b) and *Disorders of Sexual Desire* (Kaplan 1979a), described cases in which sexual problems were compounded with other kinds of relational and individual difficulties, and presented treatment techniques blended with others from the family, couple, and individual disciplines.

Disorders of desire often present in a couple as one partner having a greater desire for sex than the other. This discrepancy can escalate to an exaggerated projection of the differences over time. Problems with arousal, orgasm, and pain may be present when the root disorder is one of desire. Medical factors to rule out include medications, depression, hormonal levels, chronic pain, and illness. Emotions related to loss of desire include anger at self or partner, shame, fear, and anxiety about performance or rejection. Helping the partners to express underlying emotions and to identify what keeps them from wanting what they want to want is a useful start. Directives to not initiate sex, not have an erection, and not expect orgasm can greatly reduce anxiety (see discussion of sensate focus in paragraph below). Working through painful emotions about past sexual experiences and/or couple relationship issues that interfere with desire may be necessary. Correcting misinformation about sex and promoting new sexual concepts, including adjusting to functional limitations, can be helpful as well (Charlton 1997; Schover and LoPiccolo 1982).

Arousal and orgasmic disorders are the most common sexual disorders and include female arousal disorder, male erectile disorder (impotence), male or female orgasmic disorder, and premature ejaculation. For all of these disorders, the general treatment strategy is the same: 1) assess and alleviate physiological etiological factors (e.g., drug side effects, illness); 2) address inaccurate beliefs, intrusive or distracting thoughts, and the like; 3) address relationship conflicts or emotions from past experiences that interfere with current sexual functioning; and 4) create successful sexual experiences. Masters and Johnson's *sensate focus exercises* are a key component in treating the sexual disorders by creating successful sexual experiences. The idea behind sensate focus is to increase arousal and enjoyment while eliminating as much anxiety and performance demand as possible. The exercises involve setting aside a period of time in which partners are limited to nondemand caressing and touching of the partner's body, excluding the breasts and genitals. Gradually they are permitted to include breasts, then hand-caressing of genitals, then genital-to-genital contact with little movement, and then intercourse without orgasm. The couple is given the reassuring injunction that they should not attempt intercourse until they have been able to learn more about each other's responses; instead, they are to concentrate on successive increases in comfort and pleasure, taking turns doing and communicating to each other (Masters and Johnson 1970).

Effective specific behavioral strategies for the different disorders have been developed. For premature ejaculation, the "stop–start" and "squeeze" techniques; for male erectile dysfunction, medical treatments such as sildenafil (Viagra) or sensate focus exercises, depending on etiology; for male orgasmic disorder, masturbation to orgasm in the presence of partner, then with partner manually followed by insertion; for female orgasmic disorder, the "bridge" technique, including clitoral stimulation; for female arousal, orgasmic, and pain disorders, women's sexuality groups serve to heighten sexual awareness, instruct toward successful experience of arousal and orgasm, and generally provide a form of systematic desensitization along with discussions about positive sexual experiences (Charlton 1997; LoPiccolo and Hogan 1979; Segraves and Althof 1998).

Persons with paraphilias typically seek treatment only after encountering legal troubles or as a result of their partner's demand. Otherwise, the disorder is usually not experienced as ego dystonic. Treatment involves first assessing the patient's degree of control, motivation for change, and history. In establishing an alliance, acceptance of the person can help to counter shame. Covert sensitization, in which the arousing object is paired with an aversive stimulus, and thought blocking, in which paraphilic fantasies are replaced with nonparaphilic thought, are two of the techniques used. Fostering insight into underlying conflicts and developmental roots—usually related to discomfort with or anger at others—can sometimes be worked through.

In our case example, Sue's hypoactive sexual desire often left Trent feeling rejected and resentful. Upon exploration, it became apparent that Sue often felt exhausted after work and parenting responsibilities and that she also wanted to avoid the confusing negative emotions that emerged during sexual activity. Sue's resentments about Trent's lack of limit setting, as transferential affect related to her father and implying lack of love, were worked through in couple therapy. Sue began to feel closer to Trent, and by arranging for special time away from work and children, she began to experience desire to a greater degree. Trent had started to experience erectile dysfunction, for which a physiological cause was ruled out. He was increasingly anxious as he sensed Sue was disapproving of him. Sensate focus exercises were prescribed, which allowed the couple to experience pleasant sensations from one another without pressure, and which eventually led to resolution of their difficulties.

Divorce Counseling

As the divorce rate settles around the 50% mark, separation becomes a rite of passage of almost equal importance with marriage, creating single-parent families, remarried and recombined families, stepparents, half-siblings, joint custody, visitation, and support battles. This is, literally, a whole new subculture—a new way of organizing families, defining adult sexual and financial contracts, and raising children. Many of the traditional expectations concerning the family life cycle and family structure are altered. In the separated or recombined family, dating, courtship, the rearing of small children, and the assumption of adolescent independence are all influenced by the changing family structures.

A subspecialty literature on divorce exists in the family therapy field, and some specialized practice as well, but the most important innovation is the new profession of divorce mediation and counseling. Often these professionals are attorneys with substantial training in family therapy. From their work has come a new way of getting a divorce—a way of avoiding the adversarial two-lawyer battle with its injurious addition of righteousness and revenge to the pain of separation. Studies of the effectiveness of mediation show that it produces a higher level of satisfaction with the agreement, reduction in the amount of later litigation, an increase in joint-custody agreements, and generally a decrease in expense (Gurman et al. 1986). Divorce counselors have been shown to be more effective in reaching agreements when they focus on problem solving, discuss options and solutions rather than facts, maintain flexible control, and are active in structuring the process (Slaikeu et al. 1985). Additionally, they intervene more frequently when conflict is high, helping to shape communication in agreement-oriented directions (Kelly 1996). Therapists should consider divorce counseling or referral for mediation for patients who are planning to divorce. Interparental conflict is reduced with mediation, which in turn reduces the potential for negative effects on children. Because mediation has a higher probability of success when couples have good communication skills, preparing divorcing partners for mediation by providing specific assistance toward improving communication skills is recommended (Hahn and Kleist 2000).

Providing Therapy for Diverse Couples and Families

As we enter the twenty-first century, therapists are confronted with the need for attention to the diversity of patient populations. What many have viewed as the "typical" American family now characterizes a very small proportion of families. For example, 1) by the year 2050, about 40% of the total U.S. population will be African American, Latino American, Asian American, Pacific Islander, or Native American; 2) lesbians, bisexuals, and gay men are estimated to make up about one-tenth of the total population, and a significant proportion of these individuals are parents; 3) half of all marriages currently end in divorce; 4) more than half of the entire population will be part of a stepfamily at some point in their lives; 5) about one-third of all families are headed by single mothers; 6) by 2030, 20% of the population will be over age 65 years; and 7) rates of cohabitation are rising (Crooks and Baur 1990; Larson 1992; U.S. Census Bureau 1997). Diversity can be conceptualized along the lines of ethnicity, race, age, social class, gender, income, sexual preference, marital status, and family form, as well as religion and disability.

Couple and family therapists should be familiar with issues related to the treatment of members of culturally and structurally diverse families. Many of the mental health problems faced by families of diverse ethnic backgrounds may be related to prejudice, discrimination, differing levels of acculturation to the mainstream culture, and other associated stressors. Unique problems are associated with each nontraditional family form, whether it be cohabitation, separation, divorce, remarriage, stepparenting, single parenting, or co-parenting. Ethnic groups differ in terms of what they label as a symptom, what they believe about etiology, how they communicate about pain and symptoms, what their attitude is toward therapists, and what treatment they expect or desire. Compared with the mainstream culture, a number of ethnic minority groups are believed to be more comfortable with family therapy approaches than with individual therapy because of the value their cultures place on interdependence. For example, *familismo* refers to the primacy of the family over the individual in many Latino cultures. Although it is impossible for any therapist to be familiar with the characteristics and difficulties of all groups, certain basic conceptual and operational principles may be implemented across diverse groups and circumstances (Gopaul-McNicol 1997). Culturally sensitive CFT is characterized by responses that acknowledge the family's culture and show appreciation for it (Pontorotto et al. 1995). Sue (1998) provided three guidelines for therapists who wish to be more culturally competent: 1) be careful not to evaluate culturally relevant behaviors as pathology, 2) understand one's own worldview and have some knowledge about the culture of the patient as well as about culture-specific interventions, and 3) do not overgeneralize cultural patterns to all members of a particular group. While being aware of general cultural influences on family organization and functioning, the couple and family therapist needs to remember that the "family culture" of each particular family may be quite different from that of other families in the same ethnic group.

Very often the therapist will be of a different ethnic or other group than the family. Especially at the time of meeting and joining with the family, the fit of the therapist with the culture of the family is crucial. The therapist should not threaten the most important values of the family. Given the above definitions of cultural competence and sensitivity, it is important that the therapist acknowledge the ethnic or other group differences between him- or herself and the family members and ask in a supportive way about their feelings on this issue. Such differences between the therapist and the family members may also become a treatment issue in that they parallel interpersonal relations outside the therapy room and can be worked through in the therapy.

When relevant, level of acculturation (i.e., the degree to which a person adopts the mainstream social and cultural norms) is important to assess early on, because it informs the therapist just how much the family members' backgrounds will influence clinical decisions. For example, less acculturated patients are more likely to continue therapy with an ethnically similar therapist (Sue et al. 1991). Differing levels of acculturation in immigrant families often become great sources of conflict—for example, when younger family members begin to adopt mainstream cultural values. A number of models of identity development have been formulated for various ethnic and sexual (gay or lesbian) minority groups to assist individuals in defining their belief systems and emotional reactions to their world at various stages; these models can be helpful in understanding issues such as cultural paranoia (Helms 1990). Biculturalism, or the ability to function effectively in one's own group or culture as well as the mainstream culture, is held to be the healthiest identity resolution. Goals of CFT thus also include helping to assist culturally diverse families in adapting to their psychosocial environment and to the changing family relationships that result from that environment. One particularly salient form of family therapy has been developed by Szapocznik in his work with Latino families. Intercultural conflict between family members is posited to be the added stressor that, when combined with family structural dysfunction, leads to high rates of behavior problems in adolescents (Kurtines and Szapocznik 1996; Szapocznik et al. 1997). *Bicultural effectiveness training* enhances bicultural skills that parents and youth need to develop, increases competence in managing cultural differences within the family, and "aids successful functioning in their culturally pluralistic milieu" (Szapocznik and Kurtines 1993). Little research has examined which CFT approaches work best with which ethnic groups or family structures, although Bowenian (extended family systems) therapy is compatible with many culturally diverse people's manner of securing help: the multigenerational perspective and stance of the therapist as educator fits well. Minuchin's structural approach, with its concepts of enmeshment and disengagement, is also useful in addressing discrimination and acculturation issues within families—for example, when there are rigid boundaries and disengagement because of differing degrees of acculturation among family members, or when there is enmeshment because the family is isolated from the dominant culture due to discrimination or poverty. Ng (1999) compiled a very insightful overview of helpful models (derived from therapists with

Asian ancestry) of CFT for Asian American families.

These are complex issues, and the clinician is encouraged to make a habit of seeking information and consultation when treating families from diverse backgrounds. The reader is referred to a very useful book, *Ethnicity and Family Therapy* (McGoldrick et al. 1996), which reviews the major ethnic groups and describes value orientations that are crucial to understanding in the therapy process. In addition, Glick et al. (2000b) provide a number of chapters that are quite informative in regard to dealing with nontraditional family forms such as divorced families; stepfamilies; and families of gay men, lesbians, and bisexuals. Family diversity issues are summarized in Table 32–4.

TABLE 32–4. Issues in treating culturally and structurally diverse families

---

1. Consider diversity in terms of ethnicity, race, acculturation, sexual preference, gender identity, age, marital status, parental status, family form, social class, income, religion, and disability.

2. Consider that mental health problems may be related to poverty, discrimination, prejudice, racism, phase of life cycle, and differing levels of acculturation to the mainstream culture.

3. Consider unique problems associated with various family forms including cohabitation, separation, divorce, remarriage, stepparenting, single parenting, and co-parenting.

4. When addressing families, acknowledge—show interest in, demonstrate knowledge of, and express appreciation for—the family's culture. Place their problems in a cultural context.

5. Be careful not to evaluate culturally relevant behaviors as pathology.

6. Obtain information about the culture of the family as well as culture-specific interventions.

7. Be careful not to overgeneralize cultural patterns to all members of a particular group; the "culture of the family" may be quite different.

8. Acknowledge ethnic or other differences between therapist and family members and ask in a supportive way about their feelings on this issue.

9. Assess level of acculturation in immigrant families to understand how much family members' backgrounds will inform clinical decisions. Differing levels of acculturation in immigrant families are often great sources of conflict when some members start to behave according to mainstream values.

10. For immigrant families, biculturalism (the ability to function both in their own culture and in the mainstream culture) is held to be the healthiest goal.

11. Make it a habit to seek information or consultation when treating diverse families.

Ethical, Legal, and Professional Issues Related to Risk Management

The same ethical and legal issues that pertain to treatment of individual patients also pertain to couples and families, although certain issues gain greater complexity when applied to families. Attending to these issues is important, because it will reduce the likelihood of harm and legal problems arising from the therapy. A basic concept that cannot be overemphasized is that the most effective treatment arises from maintaining positive and collaborative relationships with family members. Such relationships are maintained through the use of listening and reflecting skills. Complaints and malpractice suits are increased when there is "impersonal, rushed, and unsatisfactory interpersonal interacting" between the therapist and family members (Weyrauch 1995).

When bringing in family members of an identified patient for education, support, or consultation, the therapist must be aware of the ethical issues implied in involving the family in the treatment process. Confidentiality concerns need to be addressed early on. The patient may need to sign authorization forms permitting the therapist to disclose information to family members, even if the only information to disclose is that the patient is in treatment. All family members should be involved in the informed consent process and should be advised of limits to confidentiality regarding child or elder abuse or danger to self or others. This preliminary discussion may reduce damage to the therapeutic alliance in the event that any of these issues are identified during the course of therapy.

Almost always, therapists will have sessions in which not all members of a family are present, either during initial individual assessment sessions or later, and the issue of disclosure of family secrets arises. Therapists may find themselves in the bind of being the "keeper" of a secret that poses a risk to a family member's well-being or that in some other way is therapeutically burdensome. This situation constitutes an ethical dilemma for therapists, and the best way to circumvent it is to establish a clearly defined policy regarding family secrets at the outset of therapy. Some therapists state that they will not keep any secrets at all; others, particularly in working with adolescents, request that parents allow the adolescent some privacy in the therapy to encourage a stronger therapeutic alliance and disclosure. Clinicians should be aware that legally, both custodial and noncustodial parents have a right to obtain records of their child's therapy, regardless of any agreement. If problems with secrets do arise, it is most appropriate for the therapist to take a stance of helping partners or family members sort out their values, obligations, and options, rather than making a decision for them. In general, a secret should be disclosed if it poses a danger to family members or seriously affects the connections between them (Imber-Black 1993; Knapp 1997). Usually by exploring resistances to disclosure, patients become more comfortable with sharing secrets.

Record keeping is another ethical issue that is more complex in CFT, especially given the potential for child custody and divorce litigation when treating troubled couples and families. Records should be comprehensive and as objective as possible, including all the data pertinent to record keeping for individual patients. The decision of whether to keep a chart on only one identified patient, separate charts for each family member, or one chart for the couple or family has several implications. Keeping separate charts is quite time-consuming, does not easily permit documentation of the family therapy process, and may not be compatible with the practices of many clinics, which base charts on the insured party. Keeping a family chart creates difficulties involving comingled information that raise confidentiality issues if a release is requested. In couple therapy, records should not be released without the consent of both spouses (Magee 1997). The American Psychiatric Association "Guidelines on Confidentiality" state that it may be more practical to keep records in one of the participants' charts, given that most clinics maintain charts this way. However, they also suggest that all involved family members sign a statement at the outset of therapy specifying which signatures will be needed to obtain information from the chart (Committee on Confidentiality 1987). CFT risk management issues are summarized in Table 32–5. A very useful reference for further information about CFT ethical and legal issues is Marsh and Magee's (1997) book, *Ethical and Legal Issues in Professional Practice With Families*.

Conclusions

After reading this chapter, it should be clear that one of the functions of CFT in modern psychiatry is to serve as a reminder that there are many ways of looking at a problem and its solutions in addition to the individual and brain-biological ones that the field is currently developing so successfully. Jay Haley (1980) used a very powerful metaphor to characterize the problem faced by a family with a very disturbed, destructively misbehaving, drug-

TABLE 32–5. Risk management issues relevant to couple and family therapy

1. The most effective treatment arises from maintaining positive and collaborative relationships with family members, maintained through use of listening and reflecting skills and avoiding rushed and impersonal interactions.
2. Confidentiality issues need to be addressed very early in the treatment process. All family members who participate in treatment sessions should be involved in the informed consent process.
3. When bringing in family members after working with a patient individually, the patient should sign an authorization to release information, even to a spouse.
4. Records for CFT should be comprehensive and as objective as possible.
5. The American Psychiatric Association suggests keeping records in one of the participants' charts, but having all involved family members sign a statement at the outset of therapy specifying which signatures will be needed to obtain information from the chart. Couple therapy records should not be released without the consent of both spouses.
6. Be aware that parents have a legal right to obtain information from their children's charts, including both custodial and noncustodial parents.
7. To circumvent the ethical dilemma of keeping family secrets that may be disclosed when meeting with family members individually, it is important at the outset of therapy to clearly define a policy regarding family secrets.
8. If problems with secrets do arise, consider urging disclosure when secrets pose a danger to family members or seriously affect the connections between them. Help to explore options and resistances to disclosure.

abusing, or otherwise ungovernable young person: he said that such a young person is having serious trouble with "leaving home." This description avoids any reference to diagnosis, illness, medication, handicap, and so forth, and it does not imply that the family contributed to the problem by raising the child wrong. In this way, everyone, including the troubled young person, has scope in which to develop without the limitation of a medical prognosis, after the current life crisis is past. It is clear what the parents must do: they must get the youth through his or her difficult transition period as expertly as possible. This will be done by being very clear about expectations and the consequences of misbehavior, with the parents lovingly but very firmly in charge. The approach is highly structural, somewhat behavioral, and even contains some education. The problem is framed in the language of passages in the life cycle, an especially rich storehouse of positive metaphor, as several authors (Carter and McGoldrick 1980; M. Nichols 1984) have noted. Framing the problem as a life cycle issue emphasizes normality rather than illness, development rather than handicap.

Clearly, then, in the treatment of couples and families, the therapist has a wide choice of treatment metaphors, each with its own implications and consequences. The choice of a treatment strategy is a complex one that depends on diagnosis, institutional context, and assessment of the family's capabilities. It is based partly on clinical judgment, partly on intuition and experience, and now increasingly on studies of treatment efficacy.

References

American Psychiatric Association: Diagnostic and Statistical Manual of Mental Disorders, 4th Edition. Washington, DC, American Psychiatric Association, 1994

Bateson G: Naven, 2nd Edition. Stanford, CA, Stanford University Press, 1958

Baucom DH, Epstein N, Sayers S, et al: The role of cognitions in marital relationships: definitional, methodological, and conceptual issues. J Consult Clin Psychol 57:31–38, 1989

Baucom DH, Shoham V, Mueser KT, et al: Empirically supported couple and family interventions for marital distress and adult mental health problems. J Consult Clin Psychol 66:53–88, 1998

Becvar DS, Becvar RJ: The historical perspective, in Family Therapy: A Systemic Integration, 2nd Edition. Boston, MA, Allyn & Bacon, 1993, pp 15–66

Boszormenyi-Nagy I, Spark M: Invisible Loyalties: Reciprocity in Intergenerational Family Therapy. New York, Harper & Row, 1973

Boszormenyi-Nagy I, Ulrich D: Contextual family therapy, in Handbook of Family Therapy. Edited by Gurman AS, Kniskern DP. New York, Brunner/Mazel, 1981, pp 159–186

Bowen M: Family Therapy in Clinical Practice. New York, Jason Aronson, 1978

Bowlby J: A Secure Base. New York, Basic Books, 1988

Bray JH, Jouriles EN: Treatment of marital conflict and prevention of divorce. J Marital Fam Ther 21:461–474, 1995

Brothers BJ (ed): Couples Therapy, Multiple Perspectives: In Search of Universal Threads. New York, Haworth, 1992

Brown GW, Harris T: The Social Origins of Depression. New York, Free Press, 1978

Campbell TL, Patterson JM: The effectiveness of family interventions in the treatment of physical illness. J Marital Fam Ther 21:545–584, 1995

Carr A: Evidence-based practice in family therapy and systemic consultation, I: child-focused problems. Journal of Family Therapy 22:29–60, 2000a

Carr A: Evidence-based practice in family therapy and systemic consultation, II: adult-focused problems. Journal of Family Therapy 22:273–295, 2000b

Carr A: What Works for Children and Adolescents? A Critical Review of Psychological Interventions with Children, Adolescents, and Their Families. London, England, Routledge, 2000c

Carter EA, McGoldrick M: The family life cycle and family therapy: an overview, in The Changing Family Life Cycle: A Framework for Family Therapy. Edited by Carter EA, McGoldrick M. New York, Gardner, 1980, pp 3–28

Chamberlain P, Rosicky JG: The effectiveness of family therapy in the treatment of adolescents with conduct disorders and delinquency. J Marital Fam Ther 21:441–460, 1995

Chambless DL, Hollon SD: Defining empirically supported therapies. J Consult Clin Psychol 66:7–18, 1998

Charlton R (ed): Treating Sexual Disorders. San Francisco, CA, Jossey-Bass, 1997

Clarkin JF, Glick ID, Haas GL, et al: A randomized clinical trial of inpatient family intervention, V: results for affective disorders. J Affect Disord 18:17–28, 1990

Committee on Confidentiality: Guidelines on confidentiality. Am J Psychiatry 144:1522–1526, 1987

Crooks R, Baur K: Our Sexuality. California, Benjamin/Cummings, 1990

de Shazer S: Keys to Solutions in Brief Therapy. New York, WW Norton, 1985

Dicks HV: Marital Tensions. New York, Basic Books, 1967

Doherty WJ: Family therapy goes postmodern. The Family Therapy Networker 15:36–42, 1991

Dunn RL, Schwebel AI: Meta-analytic review of marital therapy outcome research. J Fam Psychol 9:58–68, 1995

Edgeworth J, Carr A: Child abuse, in What Works for Children and Adolescents? A Critical Review of Psychological Interventions with Children, Adolescents, and Their Families. Edited by Carr A. London, England, Routledge, 2000, pp 17–48

Edwards ME, Steinglass P: Family therapy treatment outcomes for alcoholism. J Marital Fam Ther 21:475–510, 1995

Emmelkamp PMG, Van Dyck R, Bitter M, et al: Spouse-aided therapy with agoraphobics. Br J Psychiatry 160:51–56, 1992

Ersner-Hershfield R, Kopel S: Group treatment of pre-orgasmic women. J Consult Clin Psychol 47:750–759, 1979

Estrada AU, Pinsof WM: The effectiveness of family therapies for selected behavioral disorders of childhood. J Marital Fam Ther 21:403–440, 1995

Fields L, Prinz R: Coping and adjustment during childhood and adolescence. Clinical Psychology Review 17:937–976, 1997

Gelcer E, McCabe A, Smith-Resnick C: Milan Family Therapy: Variant and Invariant Methods. New York, Wiley, 1990

Glick ID: Family therapies: efficacy, indications, and treatment outcomes, in Psychotherapy Indications and Outcomes. Washington DC, American Psychiatric Press, 1999, pp 303–321

Glick ID, Berman EM, Clarkin JF, et al: The content of evaluation, in Marital and Family Therapy, 4th Edition. Washington, DC, American Psychiatric Press, 2000a, pp 151–163

Glick ID, Berman EM, Clarkin JF, et al. (eds): Marital and Family Therapy, 4th Edition. Washington, DC, American Psychiatric Press, 2000b

Glick ID, Berman EM, Clarkin JF, et al: Results of and guidelines for recommending family therapy, in Marital and Family Therapy, 4th Edition. Washington, DC, American Psychiatric Press, 2000c, pp 593–651

Goldstein MJ, Miklowitz DJ: The effectiveness of psychoeducational family therapy in the treatment of schizophrenic disorders. J Marital Fam Ther 21:361–376, 1995

Gopaul-McNicol SA: Current major approaches in counseling culturally different families, in A Multicultural/Multimodal/Multisystems Approach to Working With Culturally Different Families. Westport, CT, Praeger, 1997, pp 79–84

Gottman J: An agenda for marital therapy, in The Heart of the Matter: Perspectives on Emotion in Marital Therapy. Edited by Johnson S, Greenberg L. New York, Brunner/Mazel, 1994, pp 256–296

Greenberg LS, Johnson SM: Emotionally focused couples therapy, in Clinical Handbook of Marital Therapy. Edited by Jacobson NS, Gurman AS. New York, Guilford, 1986, pp 253–276

Griffin WA, Greene SM: Behavioral family therapy, in Models of Family Therapy: The Essential Guide. Philadelphia, PA, Taylor & Francis, 1999a, pp 31–40

Griffin WA, Greene SM: Bowen systems therapy, in Models of Family Therapy: The Essential Guide. Philadelphia, PA, Taylor & Francis, 1999b, pp 81–92

Gurman AS, Kniskern DP, Pinsof WM: Research on the process and outcome of marital and family therapy, in Handbook of Psychotherapy and Behavior Change: An Empirical Analysis. Edited by Garfield S, Bergin A. New York, Wiley, 1986, pp 525–623

Hahlweg K, Markman HJ: Effectiveness of behavioral marital therapy: empirical status of behavioral techniques in preventing and alleviating marital distress. J Consult Clin Psychol 56:440–447, 1988

Hahn RA, Kleist DM: Divorce mediation: Research and implications for family and couples counseling. The Family Journal: Counseling and Therapy for Couples and Families 8:165–171, 2000

Haley J: Problem-Solving Therapy. San Francisco, CA, Jossey-Bass, 1976

Haley J: Leaving Home. New York, McGraw Hill, 1980

Haley J: Ordeal Therapy: Unusual Ways to Change Behavior. San Francisco, CA, Jossey-Bass, 1984

Hazelrigg MD, Cooper HM, Borduin CM: Evaluating the effectiveness of family therapies: an integrative review and analysis. Psychol Bull 101:428–442, 1987

Helms JE: Black and White Racial Identity: Theory, Research, and Practice. Westport, CT, Greenwood, 1990

Hurlbert DF, White LC, Powell RD, et al: Orgasm consistency training in the treatment of women reporting hypoactive sexual desire: an outcome comparison of women-only groups and couples-only groups. J Behav Ther Exp Psychiatry 24:3–13, 1993

Imber-Black E (ed): Secrets in Families and Family Therapy. New York, WW Norton, 1993

Jacobson NS, Holzworth-Monroe A: Marital therapy: a social learning-cognitive perspective, in Clinical Handbook of Marital Therapy. Edited by Jacobson NS, Gurman AS. New York, Guilford, 1986, pp 29–70

Johnson SM, Whiffen VE: Made to measure: Adapting emotionally focused couple therapy to partners' attachment styles. Clinical Psychology: Science and Practice 6:366–381, 1999

Kaplan HS: Disorders of Sexual Desire and Other Concepts and Techniques in Sex Therapy. New York, Brunner/Mazel, 1979a

Kaplan HS: The New Sex Therapy: Active Treatment Sexual Dysfunctions. New York, Brunner/Mazel, 1979b

Kazdin A: Psychosocial treatments for conduct disorder in children, in A Guide to Treatments That Work. Edited by Nathan P, Gorman J. New York, Oxford University Press, 1998, pp 65–89

Kelly J: A decade of divorce mediation research. Family and Conciliation Courts Review 34:373–385, 1996

Knapp S: Professional liability and risk management in an era of managed care, in Ethical and Legal Issues in Professional Practice With Families. Edited by Marsh DT, Magee RD. New York, Wiley, 1997, pp 271–288

Kurtines WM, Szapocznik J: Family interaction patterns: structural family therapy in contexts of cultural diversity, in Psychosocial Treatments for Child and Adolescent Disorders: Empirically Based Strategies for Clinical Practice. Edited by Hibbs ED, Jensen PS. Washington DC, American Psychological Association, 1996, pp 671–700

Larson J: Understanding stepfamilies. American Demographics 14:360, 1992

Liddle HA, Dakof GA: Efficacy of family therapy for drug abuse: promising but not definitive. J Marital Fam Ther 21:511–544 1995

LoPiccolo J, Hogan D: Multidimensional behavioral treatment of sexual dysfunction, in Behavioral Medicine. Edited by Pomerlieu O, Brady J. Baltimore, MD, Williams & Wilkins, 1979

Lynch JJ: The Broken Heart. New York, Basic Books, 1977

Madanes C: Strategic Family Therapy. San Francisco, CA, Jossey-Bass, 1981

Magee RD: Ethical issues in couple therapy, in Ethical and Legal Issues in Professional Practice With Families. Edited by Marsh DT, Magee RD. New York, Wiley, 1997, pp 110–119

Main TF: Mutual projection in a marriage. Compr Psychiatry 7:432–439, 1966

Markus E, Lange A, Pettigrew TF: Effectiveness of family therapy: a meta-analysis. Journal of Family Therapy 12:205–221, 1990

Marsh DT, Magee RD: Ethical and Legal Issues in Professional Practice With Families. New York, Wiley, 1997

Masters WH, Johnson VE: Human Sexual Inadequacy. Boston, MA, Little, Brown, 1970

McFarlane WR: Family Therapy in Schizophrenia. New York, Guilford, 1983a

McFarlane WR: Multiple family therapy in schizophrenia, in Family Therapy in Schizophrenia. Edited by McFarlane WR. New York, Guilford, 1983b, pp 141–172

McGoldrick M, Gerson R: Genograms in Family Assessment. New York, WW Norton, 1985

McGoldrick M, Giordano J, Pearce JK: Ethnicity and Family Therapy, 2nd Edition. New York, Guilford, 1996

Mehta M: A comparative study of family-based and patient-based behavioral management in obsessive-compulsive disorder. Br J Psychiatry 157:133–135, 1990

Miklowitz D, Goldstein M: Bipolar Disorder: A Family-Focused Treatment Approach. New York, Guilford, 1997

Minuchin S: Families and Family Therapy. Cambridge, MA, Harvard University Press, 1974

Minuchin S, Fischman HC: Family Therapy Techniques. Cambridge, MA, Harvard University Press, 1981

Moore M, Carr A: Depression and grief, in What Works for Children and Adolescents? A Critical Review of Psychological Interventions With Children, Adolescents, and Their Families. Edited by Carr A. London, England, Routledge, 2000, pp 203–232

Morrison TL: Object relations theory and marital interaction: integrating theory with the known facts, in Couples: A Medley of Models. Edited by Brothers BJ. New York, Haworth, 1998, pp 33–56

Murphy E, Carr A: Enuresis and encopresis, in What Works for Children and Adolescents? A Critical Review of Psychological Interventions With Children, Adolescents, and Their Families. Edited by Carr A. London, England, Routledge, 2000, pp 49–64

Ng KS (ed): Counseling Asian Families From a Systems Perspective. New York, American Counseling Association, 1999

Nichols M: Family Therapy: Concepts and Methods. New York, Gardner, 1984

Nichols WC: Family evaluation and treatment, in Treating People in Families. Edited by Nichols WC. New York, Guilford, 1996, p 107

O'Hanlon WH, Weiner-Davis M: In Search of Solutions: A New Direction in Psychotherapy. New York, WW Norton, 1989

Papp P: The Greek chorus and other techniques of paradoxical therapy. Fam Process 19:45–57, 1980

Pinsof WM, Wynne LC: The effectiveness and efficacy of marital and family therapy: introduction to the special issue. J Marital Fam Ther 21:341–343, 1995a

Pinsof WM, Wynne LC: The efficacy of marital and family therapy: an empirical overview, conclusions, and recommendations. J Marital Fam Ther 21:585–613, 1995b

Pinsof WM, Wynne LC, Hambright AB: The outcomes of couple and family therapy: findings, conclusions, and recommendations. Psychotherapy 33:321–331, 1996

Ponterotto JG, Casas JM, Suzuki LA, et al: Handbook of Multicultural Counseling. Thousand Oaks, CA, Sage, 1995

Roy R, Frankel H: Family therapy: an overview, in How Good is Family Therapy? Toronto, Canada, University of Toronto Press, 1995, pp 3–21

Satir V: Conjoint Family Therapy. Palo Alto, CA, Science and Behavior Books, 1964

Satir V: Conjoint Family Therapy, Revised Edition. Palo Alto, CA, Science and Behavior Books, 1967

Scharff DE, Scharff JS: Object Relations in Family Therapy. Northvale, NJ, Jason Aronson, 1987

Scharff DE, Scharff JS: Object Relations Couple Therapy. Northvale, NJ, Jason Aronson, 1991

Scharff JS: Projective and Introjective Identification and the Use of the Therapist's Self. Northvale, NJ, Jason Aronson, 1992

Schover L, LoPiccolo J: Treatment effectiveness for dysfunctions of sexual desire. J Sex Marital Ther 8:179–197, 1982

Segraves R, Althof S: Psychotherapy and pharmacotherapy for sexual dysfunctions, in A Guide to Treatments that Work. Edited by Nathan P, Gorman J. New York, Oxford University Press, 1998, pp 447–471

Selvini Palazzoli M, Boscolo L, Cecchin G, et al: Paradox and Counterparadox. New York, Jason Aronson, 1978

Shadish WR, Montgomery, LM, Wilson P, et al: Effects of family and marital psychotherapies: a meta-analysis. J Consult Clin Psychol 61:992–1002, 1993

Skynner ACR: An open-systems, group analytic approach to family therapy, in Handbook of Family Therapy. Edited by Gurman AS, Kniskern D. New York, Brunner/Mazel, 1981, pp 39–84

Slaikeu K, Culler R, Pearson J, et al: Process and outcome in divorce mediation. Mediation Quarterly 10:121–134, 1985

Slipp S: Object Relations: A Dynamic Bridge Between Individual and Family Therapy. Northvale, NJ, Jason Aronson, 1984

Sluzki CE, Veron E: The double bind as a universal pathogenic situation, in Double Bind, the Foundation of the Communicational Approach to the Family. Edited by Sluzki CE, Ransome DE. New York, Grune & Stratton, 1976, pp 251–262

Snyder DK, Wills RM: Behavioral versus insight-oriented marital therapy: effects on individual and interspousal functioning. J Consult Clin Psychol 57:39–46, 1989

Snyder DK, Wills RM, Grady-Fletcher A: Long-term effectiveness of behavioral versus insight-oriented marital therapy: a 4-year follow-up study. J Consult Clin Psychol 59:138–141, 1991

Steinglass P: Family Therapy, in Comprehensive Textbook of Psychiatry VI. Edited by Kaplan HI, Saddock BJ. Baltimore, MD, Williams & Wilkins, 1995, pp 1838–1847

Sue S: In search of cultural competence in psychotherapy and counseling. Am Psychol 53:440–448, 1998

Sue S, Fujino DC, Hu LT, et al: Community mental health services for ethnic minority groups: a test of the cultural responsiveness hypothesis. J Consult Clin Psychol 59:533–540, 1991

Szapocznik J, Kurtines WM: Family psychology and cultural diversity: opportunities for theory, research, and application. Am Psychol 48:400–407, 1993

Szapocznik J, Kurtines W, Santiesteban DA, et al: The evolution of a structural ecosystemic theory for working with Latino families, in Psychological Interventions and Research With Latino Populations. Edited by Garcia JG, Zea MC. Boston, MA, Allyn & Bacon, 1997, pp 166–190

U.S. Census Bureau: Statistical Abstract of the United States. Washington DC, U.S. Government Printing Office, 1997

Walsh F (ed): Normal Family Processes, 2nd Edition. New York, Guilford, 1992

Watzlawick P, Weakland J, Fisch R: Change Principle of Problem Formation and Problem Resolution. New York, WW Norton, 1974

Weeks G, L'Abate L: Paradoxical Psychotherapy: Theory and Practice with Individuals, Couples, and Families. New York, Brunner/Mazel, 1982

Weeks GR, Treat S: Cognitive techniques, in Couples in Treatment: Techniques and Approaches for Effective Practice. New York, Brunner/Mazel, 1992, pp 154–170

Weyrauch KF: Malpractice, patient satisfaction, and physician–patient communication (letter). JAMA 274:22–23; discussion 23–24, 1995

Whitaker CA, Keith DV: Symbolic-experiential family therapy, in Handbook of Family Therapy. Edited by Gurman AS, Kniskern DP. New York, Brunner/Mazel, 1981, pp 187–225

White M, Epston D: Narrative Means to Therapeutic Ends. New York, WW Norton, 1990

Wynne LC, McDaniel SH, Weber TT: Systems Consultation: A New Perspective for Family Therapy. Guilford, New York, 1986

CHAPTER 33

Treatment of Children and Adolescents

Stephen J. Cozza, M.D.

Glen C. Crawford, M.D.

Mina K. Dulcan, M.D.

This chapter provides an overview of and an orientation to the psychiatric treatment of children and adolescents. Treatment modalities as they apply to adults are covered in the other chapters in Part III of this textbook. This chapter focuses on what is different or unique in the treatment of children and adolescents. Popper and colleagues, in Chapter 20 ("Disorders Usually First Diagnosed in Infancy, Childhood, or Adolescence"), address childhood psychopathology and outline the treatment methods used for each disorder. Throughout this chapter, the terms child and children refer to children of all ages, including adolescents, unless otherwise stated.

Techniques used in the treatment of child psychiatric conditions have developed from two different sources: the traditions of understanding and treating children based on developmental uniqueness and treatments that were originally designed for adults and were then applied to children and adolescents. Increasingly, more rigorous evaluation and diagnostic procedures have allowed greater specificity in the application of treatments to our younger patients. In addition, expanding research on the efficacy of specific therapeutic approaches continues to enlarge our armamentarium of empirically tested interventions.

The goals of all treatments are to reduce symptoms, to improve emotional and behavioral functioning, to remedy skill deficits, and to remove obstacles to normal development. In contrast to the treatment of adults, a child is usually brought by someone else, and in each case there are at least two clients: the parent and the child, whose needs and desires may conflict. In comparison with adults, children are more dependent on others for meeting their basic needs, they have fewer choices of residence or activities, and they are required to attend school.

Evaluation

Psychiatric treatment should be preceded by a comprehensive clinical evaluation. In an emergency situation, treatment may have to be initiated following a brief expedient assessment of the child's medical and psychological status. A more thorough evaluation should be accomplished as soon as possible. True emergencies are, fortunately, uncommon, and in most cases the evaluation will be completed before treatment is begun. Of course, the process of assessment does not end with the initiation of treatment but continues throughout.

The American Academy of Child and Adolescent Psychiatry (AACAP) has produced a number of practice parameters as guides to evaluation and treatment of specific disorders. Completed practice parameters are listed in Table 33–1.

The purpose of the comprehensive psychiatric assessment of children is similar to the assessment of adults: to determine the presence of one or more psychiatric disorders and to recommend a well-formulated treatment plan that addresses the disorder. Special considerations for children make evaluation different from that for adult

TABLE 33–1. Practice parameters published by the American Academy of Child and Adolescent Psychiatry

Aggressive Behavior in Child and Adolescent Psychiatric Institutions	2002
Attention-Deficit Hyperactivity Disorder	1997
Anxiety Disorders	1997
Assessment of Children and Adolescents	1997
Assessment of Infants and Toddlers	1997
Autism	1999
Bipolar Disorder	1997
Child Custody Evaluations	1997
Conduct Disorder	1997
Depressive Disorders	1998
Enuresis and Encopresis	2002
Forensic Evaluations of Physical or Sexual Abuse	1997
Language and Learning Disorders	1998
Mental Retardation and Comorbid Mental Disorders	1999
Obsessive-Compulsive Disorder	1998
Posttraumatic Stress Disorder	1998
Schizophrenia	2001
Seclusion and Restraint	2002
Sexually Abusive Youth	1999
Stimulant Medications	2002
Substance Use Disorders	1997
Suicide	2001

patients. Practitioners must have a clear understanding of normal development and the differences that may exist among children at the same or different ages in order to distinguish normal from pathological behaviors. Also, practitioners must be able to apply developmental understanding in the diagnostic interview of the child, using approaches like imaginative play or drawings with younger children or with those who are less skilled in verbal communication.

Information from the school is always useful and is essential when there is concern about learning, behavior, or peer functioning. With parental consent, the clinician talks with the teacher; obtains records of testing, grades, and attendance; and requests completion of a standardized checklist, such as the Teacher Report Form of the Child Behavior Checklist (Achenbach 1991). Even better, though less convenient, is a visit to the school to observe the youngster with peers in the classroom and on the playground and to talk with teachers and counselors.

A referral to another provider such as a pediatrician, pediatric neurologist, child psychologist, or speech and language specialist may be necessary to complete the assessment. Psychological evaluation, including an intelligence test and achievement tests, should be obtained when there is any question about learning or IQ, with additional testing as indicated.

Treatment Planning

The planning of a treatment regimen takes into consideration psychiatric diagnosis, target emotional and behavioral symptoms, and the strengths and weaknesses of the patient and family. Resources and risks in the school, neighborhood, and social support network, and any religious group affiliation, also influence the selection of treatment strategies.

In making a plan, the clinician should consider any modality or a combination of the modalities presented in this chapter. The practice of offering a single treatment to all patients, chosen because of the clinician's own training and theoretical beliefs or because that is what the facility offers, is to be avoided, whether that modality is individual therapy, family therapy, pharmacotherapy, hospitalization, or any other form of treatment. Treatments not in the repertoire of the clinician or those requiring additional staff and/or structure should be arranged by referral. Unfortunately, the practical realities of the quality and availability of community resources and the family's ability to pay for treatment often force the clinician to make compromises to an ideal plan.

The clinician must decide which treatment is likely to be the most efficient or to have the highest risk–benefit ratio and whether treatments should be administered simultaneously or in sequence. Unfortunately, very few systematic prospective studies have been conducted comparing well-defined treatments for carefully described groups of child patients.

Parents are best included in the choice of treatment strategies, with the strength of the clinician's recommendation depending on the clarity of the indications. The skilled clinician presents the probable course of the disorder if untreated, as well as the best estimate of benefits and risks of all available treatments for a particular child. The child patient is included in decision making as appropriate. The motivation and ability of the responsible adults to carry out the treatment should be considered because the best treatment has little chance of success without the cooperation of the family.

Treatment planning is an ongoing process, with reevaluations done as interventions are attempted and their results observed and as additional information about the child and family comes to light.

Informed Consent

The implementation of any treatment plan requires carefully obtained informed consent from parents before the plan is initiated. The concept of informed consent is more complicated with children because of legal lack of competency. Although parents provide informed consent for children, clinicians should strive to obtain assent from child patients before initiating any treatment. In obtaining such assent, the clinician should be mindful of the cognitive capacities and developmental level of the patient. The challenge may be even greater when pharmacotherapy is considered (Krener and Mancina 1994). Such a consent should include a general discussion of the selected therapeutic modality, its intended purpose, the availability of any alternative treatments (to include a choice of no treatment), and the nature of any adverse reactions that could result. An open discussion of any questions or concerns not only meets the legal obligations of practice, but also can safeguard the therapeutic alliance should undesirable side effects occur. Although not always necessary, parents' written consent may be useful in some situations. Printed materials to supplement discussion with the physician in educating parents and children regarding a variety of treatments are now available (Bastiaens and Bastiaens 1993; Dulcan and Lizarralde 2002). In addition, the Internet is becoming an increasingly important source of information about medications and treatments for health care consumers. Because the quality of information available on the World Wide Web varies, patients and their families may require guidance as to the best sources of information about mental health issues. Clinicians should also be prepared to respond to questions or concerns about treatments that may arise from a patient's or parent's "surfing" of the Internet. Some potentially useful child psychiatry web sites are listed in Table 33–2.

Confidentiality

It is essential that the guidelines for confidentiality and for sharing information between parent and child be clear. Adolescents are usually more sensitive to this issue than younger children. In general, either party should be told when information from one party's session will be relayed to the other. In some situations, parents and children may participate in the decision. When children are engaged in potentially dangerous activities or have serious thoughts of harming themselves or others, parents must be informed. Carefully planned family sessions in which the therapist coaches and supports a parent or child in sharing information may be more useful than secondhand reports.

An area of rising concern for clinicians is the impingement of managed care practices on the ability to maintain confidentiality. Clinicians should ensure that they inform children and parents of the possible need to share information with third-party entities and make prudent choices sbout what information is appropriate to share.

Psychopharmacology

This necessarily brief and relatively superficial section focuses on how medication treatment of children is different from that of adults (see Chapter 24 for psychopharmacological treatment of adults and shared mechanisms of action and side effects). The reader is referred to other brief (Martin and Scahill 2000) and comprehensive (Green 2001; Werry and Aman 1999) reviews of pediatric psychopharmacology.

Important general principles of pediatric psychopharmacology include minimizing polypharmacy and rarely using medication as the only treatment. Most disorders of children and adolescents that require medication are either chronic (e.g., attention-deficit/hyperactivity disorder [ADHD], autistic disorder, or Tourette's disorder) or likely to have recurrent episodes (e.g., mood disorders), and a long-term relationship with the physician is crucial. It is important to educate the family regarding the disorder, its treatment, and the child's needs at each developmental stage. The physician must consider the meaning of the prescription and administration of a medication to the child, the family, the school, and the child's peer group.

Medication types are classified rather roughly by functional effect (e.g., antidepressant), mechanism of action (e.g., selective serotonin reuptake inhibitor, or SSRI), or chemical structure (e.g., benzodiazepine, tricyclic). Such distinctions ignore the fact that any given agent may affect more than one clinical condition or neurochemical system. In pediatric psychopharmacology, the category name may even be inaccurate for the actual use and clinical effect, as in the treatment of ADHD with "stimulant" medications.

Special Issues for Children and Adolescents

Pharmacokinetics, Pharmacodynamics, and Pharmacogenetics

Pharmacokinetics is the study of the movement of drugs into, around, and out of the body by the processes of absorption, distribution, metabolism, and elimination. Although children share some similarities in the physio-

TABLE 33–2. Useful child psychiatry web sites

About Our Kids	www.aboutourkids.org
Advocates 4 Special Kids	www.a4sk.org
American Academy of Pediatrics	www.aap.org
American Medical Association	www.ama-assn.org
American Psychiatric Association	www.psych.org
American Psychological Association	www.apa.org
American Society of Adolescent Psychiatry	www.adolpsych.org
Autism Society of America	www.autism-society.org
Canadian Mental Health Association	www.cmha.ca
Canadian Paediatric Society	www.cps.ca
Canadian Psychiatric Association	www.cpa-apc.org
Caring for Kids	www.caringforkids.cps.ca
Center for Mental Health Services	www.mentalhealth.org
Child Advocate	www.childadvocate.net
Child and Adolescent Bipolar Foundation	www.bpkids.org
Children and Adults with Attention Deficit/ Hyperactivity Disorder	www.chadd.org
Council of Educators for Students with Disabilities	www.504idea.org
Federation of Families for Children's Mental Health	www.ffcmh.org
Health Canada Mental Health Website	www.hc-sc.gc.ca/hppb/mentalhealth
National Alliance for the Mentally Ill	www.nami.org
National Clearinghouse for Alcohol and Drug Information	www.health.org
National Institute of Mental Health	www.nimh.nih.gov
National Institute on Drug Abuse	www.nida.nih.gov
Online Asperger's Syndrome Information and Support	www.aspergersyndrome.org
Tourette Syndrome Association	www.tsa-usa.org

logical processing of medications with adults, developmental differences are clinically relevant, particularly in regard to drug distribution and metabolism.

Factors that most greatly impact on the developmental differences of distribution of drugs in children are differences in proportion of extracellular water volume and body fat. Extracellular water volume decreases substantially from birth through early adolescence. This decrease results in a larger distribution volume for water-soluble drugs in younger children requiring a relatively higher dose to achieve a comparable plasma concentration (Clein and Riddle 1995).

In general, children have lower proportional body fat than adults, thus reducing the distribution volume for lipid-soluble medications. Although this would result in an expected increase in plasma concentrations of such medications in children compared with adults using weight-adjusted dosages, lower plasma levels in children have been reported. This finding indicates that other pharmacokinetic differences, presumably increased metabolism in children, offset this effect (Clein and Riddle 1995).

From late infancy to early childhood, hepatic metabolic activity is at its peak. This substantially greater metabolic rate is related to the proportionally larger liver size of children compared with adults. Relative to body weight, the liver of a toddler is 40%–50% greater and that of a 6-year-old is 30% greater than the liver of an adult. This greater metabolic rate has been postulated as the principal factor contributing to lower drug plasma concentration levels and shorter drug half-lives in children compared with adults (Clein and Riddle 1995).

An understanding of the cytochrome P450 (CYP) enzyme system is becoming increasingly important for those clinicians who prescribe psychiatric medications to children and adolescents. Many medications are either substrates of, or inhibit or induce one or more of, the CYP isoenzymes. Potentially toxic interactions can result from inappropriate combinations of medications that inhibit CYP enzymes. An excellent source of information on this topic is Flockhart and Oesterheld (2000).

Medication dosage also is determined by pharmacodynamics, or how the biological system responds to the drug. For example, interaction with receptors is determined by receptor number, distribution, structure, function, sensitivity, and mechanism of action. Little is known about the influence of growth and development on these variables.

Pharmacogenetics is the study of how genetics influences the physiological effects of and response to drugs. Genetic variations in the CYP 2D6 isoenzyme, for example, may enhance the metabolism of some of the medications frequently used in child and adolescent psychiatry. Polymorphisms that have been identified in certain isoenzymes of UDP-glucuronosyltransferase may affect the metabolism of almost all psychotherapeutic agents except lithium. Ongoing research is examining genetic variations in drug and neurotransmitter receptor sites important to the field of psychiatry, such as serotonin, norepinephrine, and acetylcholine (G.M. Anderson and Cook 2000).

Ideally, medication doses in children should be derived from studies of children rather than adults, but studies of children often are not possible. Protocols using healthy children are not permitted, and few dosage studies have been done in symptomatic children. Dosage may be determined empirically or by weight or surface area. Generally, children are anticipated to require a higher weight-adjusted dose to achieve the same blood levels and therapeutic effects as adults. However, clinicians should remain alert to the possibility that such practice occasionally results in toxicity.

Side Effects

Side effects are common in children being treated with psychiatric medications. Clinicians must actively look for adverse reactions, as children often will not report them and parents may not notice. Occasionally, children will develop an uncharacteristic or paradoxical response to a particular medication. Such a response may be extremely individual in its manifestation, affecting one child but not another. *Behavioral toxicity* is a term that is used to describe a response to medication in which a child demonstrates behavioral or symptomatic aggravation caused by a particular medication (Van Putten and Marder 1987).

Measurement of Outcome

Effective medication management in children requires the identification of clear target symptoms that are monitored during the course of a medication trial. The physician must obtain emotional, behavioral, and physical baseline and posttreatment data. Therapeutic effects can be assessed by interviews and rating scales, direct observation, collection of data from outside sources (e.g., teachers), or specific tests evaluating attention or learning (Conners 1985). A list of some clinically useful symptom rating scales is presented in Table 33–3.

In reading the psychopharmacology literature, it is important to distinguish between *statistically* significant effects and *clinically* significant ones and to know whether the target symptoms are reduced to near normal levels, or merely changed, and the clinical meaning of the change. The percentage of patients who improve may be more important than changes in group means. Some patients may improve and others worsen, resulting in nonsignificant group data. On the other hand, statistically significant group changes may translate into only modest changes in individual patient functioning that may not be worth the risk of medication. Caution is also advised when drawing conclusions from the results of open trials.

Developmentally Disabled Patients

Medication effects are even more difficult to assess in children and adolescents with mental retardation or pervasive developmental disorders (PDDs). Their impaired ability to verbalize symptoms is relevant to diagnosis, measurement of efficacy, and detection of side effects. These individuals are prone to physical side effects and are at risk for idiosyncratic behavioral effects or simply less prominent therapeutic effects.

Heterogeneity of samples of autistic children in language development, motor activity, severity of stereotypies, affective range and lability, chronological age, and IQ may lead to variable drug effects. Autistic youngsters are even more likely to react differently to specific drugs than do children with other psychiatric disorders, even when the target symptoms seem similar.

Compliance

Taking medication as directed can be particularly problematic for children because the cooperation of two people, parent and child, and often school personnel as well, is required. In general pediatric practice, high compliance to medication regimens is associated with the degree of parental concern about the seriousness of their child's illness, the severity of the child's symptoms, and prior high compliance to treatment (Lewis 1995). Compliance appears to be inversely related to the complexity of the medication regimen (including the number of medicines used and the frequency of dosing). Although experiences in general pediatrics and adult psychiatry indicate that educational efforts may improve compliance, administration of psychotropic medications in children is more complex. Bastiaens (1992) found no correlation between knowledge of medications and compliance in a group of inpatient children and adolescents. In a later study, he found that compliance in a group of inpatient adolescents correlated better with attitudes than with knowledge of pharmacotherapy, indicating a need to examine and

TABLE 33–3. Clinically useful symptom rating scales

Scales for measuring overall symptomatology	Clinical Global Impressions (CGI) Scale
	Child Behavioral Checklist (CBCL)
Scales for measuring specific disorders	
Depression	Children's Depression Inventory
	Children's Depression Rating Scale
	Beck Depression Inventory
	Depressive Self-Rating Scale
	Hamilton Rating Scale for Depression (HRSD)
Mania	Manic-State Rating Scale
	Modified Mania Rating Scale
	Young–Mania Rating Scale (Y-MRS)
Psychosis	Brief Psychiatric Rating Scale (BPRS)
Anxiety disorders	Child Anxiety Frequency Checklist
	Beck Anxiety Inventory
	Hamilton Anxiety Rating Scale
	Multidimensional Anxiety Scale for Children (MASC)
	Leyton Obsessional Inventory—Child Version
	Children's Yale-Brown Obsessive Compulsive Scale (CY-BOCS)
	Post-Traumatic Stress Disorder Reaction Index
	Stress Reaction Index
	Social Phobia Anxiety Inventory for Children
	Screen for Child Anxiety-Related Emotional Disorders (SCARED)
Attention-deficit/hyperactivity disorder	Childhood Attention Problems Scale (CAP)
	Conners Abbreviated Symptom Questionnaire (teacher and parent scales)
Autism and mental retardation	Aberrant Behavior Checklist
	Childhood Autism Rating Scale
	Real Life Rating Scale for Autism
	Timed Stereotypies Rating Scale
Tourette's syndrome	Hopkins Motor/Vocal Tic Scale
	Motor Tic, Obsession and Compulsion and Vocal Tic Evaluation Scale (MOV ES)
	Tourette's Syndrome Symptom List
	Yale Global Tic Severity Scale
Aggression	Overt Aggression Scale

Source. Data from Kutcher 1997.

explore a child's feelings about taking medication (Bastiaens 1995).

Ethical Issues

Those physicians who treat children with pharmacotherapy face significant ethical challenges (Coffey 1995). The practice of pharmacotherapy of children is often modeled on adult treatments because rigorous, controlled double-blind studies in children are few. Pharmaceutical companies often do not go to the expense and trouble of testing drugs in children and adolescents, although a federal (U.S.) law was passed in 1997 to encourage such testing by extending patent protection for 6 months on

drugs studied in children. Additionally, in December 2000 the U.S. Food and Drug Administration (FDA) released guidelines to encourage the clinical investigation of drugs for use in the pediatric population. Although it is important to be aware that FDA guidelines as published in the *Physicians' Desk Reference* (PDR) are not meant to regulate the clinical practice of physicians (Popper 1987), the clinician must be responsible for the careful use of medications in the child population, basing decisions on a thorough understanding of the scientific literature. The lack of knowledge of the potential impact of medications on the neural development of children further complicates the issue. A clinician must balance multiple factors: the risks of the untreated disorder, the relative efficacy of medications, and the potential adverse outcomes or unknowns of medication use.

The interaction between pharmacotherapy and the environment is an issue for adult patients but even more so for children and adolescents because their immature developmental status places them in the care of adults, whether parents, teachers, or staff in an inpatient unit or residential treatment setting. There is a danger of misinterpreting the youngster's response to the family, school, or institutional milieu as an exacerbation requiring medication or as improvement due to a medication. Some adults seek to use medications to eliminate troublesome behavior rather than instituting more time-consuming and difficult therapeutic or behavioral management strategies. The physician must therefore evaluate and monitor the environment as well as the patient.

Stimulants

This category of medications is the most studied and most used in pediatric psychopharmacology and is most often prescribed by non–child psychiatrists such as pediatricians and general practitioners. Traditionally, these medications have included dextroamphetamine, methylphenidate, and magnesium pemoline. More recently, newer mixed-agent medications (Adderall) and medications incorporating innovative delivery systems (Concerta, Metadate-CD) have become increasingly popular as first- and second-line stimulant choices. Magnesium pemoline is no longer a recommended agent even for second- or third-line treatment due to potential life-threatening hepatic toxicity.

Contrary to prevailing mythology, hyperactive boys, healthy boys, and healthy adults have similar cognitive and behavioral responses to comparable doses of stimulants. Although it is clear that stimulants do *not* have a "paradoxical" effect in ADHD, the actual mechanism of action remains unclear. It is likely that stimulant therapeutic effect is related to augmentation of dopaminergic and adrenergic activity in the central nervous system (CNS). Stimulants reduce the performance decrement seen as patients with ADHD perform tasks, perhaps by improving motivation and focusing effort.

Indications and Efficacy

The most established indication for stimulant use is in the treatment of ADHD. The vast majority of the literature on this topic has focused on the efficacy of stimulants in school-age white males. A small literature on the treatment of girls with ADHD suggests equivalent benefit from treatment with stimulant medication (Sharp et al. 1999). Data have been extrapolated to the treatment

of other populations. A relatively limited body of literature is available on preschoolers and adolescents (T. Spencer et al. 1996a). In preschool-age children, stimulant efficacy is more variable, and the rate of side effects, especially sadness, irritability, clinginess, insomnia, and anorexia, is higher (S. B. Campbell 1985). Previous practices calling for discontinuation of stimulant treatment in adolescents have been abandoned. Most recently, T. Spencer et al. (1996a) reviewed studies of stimulant treatment in adolescents and concluded that, although limited, results indicate that stimulants are equally effective in adolescents as in school-age children.

Stimulants have been found to be effective in treating ADHD symptoms in the mentally retarded population (Aman et al. 1991). Of concern, however, is the fact that this population may be prone to more serious side effects, particularly those children who are more severely impaired (Handen et al. 1991). Handen et al. (1999) reported on a double-blind, placebo-controlled, crossover study of the use of methylphenidate in 11 preschool children with developmental disabilities and ADHD. Although the study found a 73% response rate in the subject children, the authors also reported that 45% of the subjects experienced adverse side effects from the medication. Children with fragile X syndrome also have been shown to benefit significantly from stimulant treatment of ADHD symptoms (Hagerman et al. 1988). Despite previous concern about treating children with PDDs with stimulants, Birmaher et al. (1988) described the effective use of this medication in a group of nine autistic children who did not develop significant side effects or show worsening of stereotypies.

The use of stimulants in patients with tics or Tourette's disorder remains controversial. The greatest concern is precipitating new tics. Often, however, patients with Tourette's disorder are far more disabled by their inattention, impulsivity, low frustration tolerance, and oppositional behavior than by the tics. Data suggest that in children who already have Tourette's disorder, methylphenidate improves behavior without significantly worsening tics (Gadow et al. 1995). Law and Schachar (1999) reported the results of a controlled study in a mixed population of boys and girls in which it was concluded that methylphenidate (0.5 mg/kg twice daily) treatment for ADHD was no more likely than placebo to cause or exacerbate tics. Nevertheless, monitoring for tics during stimulant use is still advised.

The short-term efficacy of stimulants in ADHD is well documented. Global judgments by parents, teachers, and clinicians rate 65%–75% of hyperactive children as improved on stimulants, with placebo response reported between 2% and 39% (Wilens and Biederman

1992). Those 25%–35% who are nonresponders demonstrate no change or worsening of symptoms, or they have intolerable side effects to the medications. A study using a wide range of doses of methylphenidate and dextroamphetamine found that 96% of the sample improved behaviorally in response to one or both drugs, although some children did not continue on medication because of adverse effects (Elia et al. 1991). Stimulant effects on various domains (cognitive, behavioral, social) are highly variable within and among individuals. A dose that produces improvement in one domain may have no effect or may even lead to worsening in another. Higher doses of stimulants, in some studies, have been shown to improve behavior but impair cognitive functioning (Sprague and Sleator 1977). Even more puzzling, the response may differ between measures (e.g., math and reading), even in the same domain. Specific effects documented in groups of ADHD stimulant responders are listed in Table 33–4.

TABLE 33–4. Therapeutic effects of stimulant medications in attention-deficit/hyperactivity disorder responders

Cognitive effects[a]
Improve sustained attention
Improve reaction time
Reduce impulsivity
Enhance sensitivity and style of cognitive response
Improve short-term memory
Motor effects
Reduce excessive motor behavior
Improve handwriting
Classroom effects
Decrease off-task behavior
Decrease inappropriate verbalizations
Improve on-task seat work
Improve academic performance
Improve compliance
Effects on aggression
Reduce physical aggression
Reduce verbal aggression
May reduce covert aggression (i.e., vandalism, stealing)
Effects on mother/family–child interaction
Increase maternal warmth
Decrease maternal criticism
Increase verbal interactions
Enhance positive family interactions
Effects on peer relationships
Improve peer cooperation
Partially "normalize" peer interaction

Note. [a]Higher doses of stimulant medications may rarely cause cognitive deterioration.
Source. Data from Greenhill 1995.

Stimulants have been demonstrated to have no effect on learning disabilities in the absence of an attention deficit (Gittelman et al. 1983). The use of stimulants in populations with comorbid ADHD and learning disorders appears to have a role in treating the underlying ADHD-related attentional and behavioral symptoms (Gadow 1983).

The long-term therapeutic effect of stimulant medication remains unclear. Most studies to date have been of short duration and many suffer from poor design. The National Institute of Mental Health Collaborative Multisite Multimodal Treatment Study of ADHD (MTA) was designed to address these areas of weakness (Richters et al. 1995). Analysis of the MTA 14-month-treatment database suggests that combined medication and behavioral treatments provide no greater clinical benefit in treating core ADHD symptoms than systematic medication management alone, although behavioral treatment may offer some added benefit in other areas of social skills and academic performance (Jensen 2000). Behavioral treatments appear to hold added benefit for children suffering from ADHD with comorbid anxiety (Jensen et al. 2001).

Initiation and Maintenance

The decision to medicate a child or adolescent with a stimulant is based on the presence of persistent target symptoms that are sufficiently severe to cause functional impairment at school and usually also at home and with peers. Parents must be willing to monitor medication and to attend appointments. Psychoeducation and school consultation are generally implemented first, unless severe impulsivity and noncompliance create an emergency situation.

Multiple outcome measures, determined by using more than one source, setting, and method of gathering data and including premedication baseline school data on behavior and academic performance, are essential. Education for the child, family, and teacher is helpful before the start of medication (Dulcan and Lizarralde 2002). The physician should explicitly debunk common myths about stimulant treatment—for example, that stimulants have a paradoxical sedative action, that they lead to drug abuse, and that they are not needed or are ineffective after puberty. The physician should work closely with parents on dose adjustments and obtain annual academic testing and more frequent reports from teachers.

No patient characteristics are helpful in suggesting which stimulant drug is best for a particular child. Twenty-five percent of a sample of boys with ADHD taking both methylphenidate and dextroamphetamine were behaviorally positive responders to one of the drugs but not the other. Of the nonresponders to each drug, the majority responded to the other drug (Elia et al. 1991). Methylphenidate is the most commonly used and best studied.

Several longer-acting stimulant preparations (Ritalin-SR, Dexedrine Spansules, Adderall-XR, Metadate-CD, and Concerta) are now available. These particular medications are useful for children who experience a brief duration of action with the standard formulations (2–3 hours), for those who experience severe rebound, or for circumstances when administering medication every 4 hours is inconvenient, stigmatizing, or impossible. Parents and children should be warned by clinicians that breaking or chewing most long-acting preparations will destroy the sustained release packaging and could result in excessively high doses of medication. However, Metadate-CD capsules may be opened and "sprinkled" onto foods such as applesauce. An innovative strategy for difficult-to-manage cases is to combine short-acting and longer-acting medication forms (Fitzpatrick et al. 1992).

Adderall, a racemic mixture of four amphetamine salts (D-amphetamine saccarate, D-amphetamine sulfate, D,L-amphetamine sulfate, and D,L-amphetamine aspartate), has been shown in several randomized double-blind, placebo-controlled studies to be as effective as methylphenidate in treating the behavioral symptoms of ADHD (Pliszka 2000; Swanson et al. 1998a, 1998b). In regard to Adderall's side effects, no significant differences from methylphenidate were noted.

Concerta, a newer long-acting single-daily-dose methylphenidate preparation, uses medication packaging with a slow-release osmotic distribution system. In a recent within-subject double-blind trial (Pelham et al. 2001), it was found to be comparable to three-times-daily dosing of methylphenidate. No additional side effects were noted with Concerta, and many parents preferred its ease of use over methylphenidate's traditional multiple-dosing schedule.

Magnesium pemoline is a longer-acting CNS stimulant that is structurally dissimilar to methylphenidate and dextroamphetamine. In 1996, Abbott Laboratories (manufacturer of the Cylert brand of pemoline) identified 13 cases of acute hepatic failure due to hepatotoxicity that had been reported to the FDA since 1975. As a result of clinician awareness of pemoline hepatotoxicity resulting in death, the United Kingdom and Canada have withdrawn pemoline from their markets. Given the availability of newer and safer long-acting agents, current use of pemoline in children and adolescents appears unsupportable (Safer et al. 2001).

Stimulant medication should be initiated with a low dose and gradually titrated upward within the recommended range every week or two according to response and side effects, with body weight as a rough guide to dosage (Table 33–5). When children reach age 3 years, their absorption, distribution, protein binding, and metabolism of stimulants are similar to those of adults (Coffey et al. 1983), although adults experience more side effects than do children at the same milligrams-per-kilogram dose. Giving medication after meals minimizes anorexia. Preschool-age children or patients with ADHD, predominantly inattentive type; mental retardation; or PDDs may benefit from (and have fewer side effects with) lower doses than those required by patients with ADHD with prominent symptoms of hyperactivity or impulsivity. Starting with only a morning dose may be useful in assessing drug effect by comparing morning and afternoon school performance. The need for an after-school dose or medication on weekends should be individually determined. Results from the MTA study suggest that most children continue to benefit from maintenance medication dosages that are similar to the initial titration dose (Vitiello et al. 2001). However, dosage adjustments were often required in children, indicating the need for ongoing monitoring of treatment response and active medication management (Vitiello et al. 2001).

TABLE 33–5. Clinical use of stimulant medications

	Methylphenidate (Ritalin)	Dextroamphetamine (Dexedrine)	Adderall	Concerta
How supplied (mg)	5, 10, 20 Sustained release 20	5, 10 Elixir (5 mg/5 mL) Spansules 5, 10, 15	5, 10, 20, 30	18, 36
Usual single dose range (mg/kg/dose)	0.3–0.7	0.15–0.50	—	—
Usual daily dosage range (mg/day)	10–60	5–40	5–40	18–54
Usual starting dose (mg)	5–10 qd or bid	2.5 or 5.0 qd or bid	2.5–5.0 qd	18
Maintenance number of doses per day	2–3	2–3	1–2	1

TABLE 33–6. Child Attention Profile (CAP)

Child's name: _____   Child's age: _____

Today's date: _____   Child's sex: M [ ]   F [ ]

Filled out by: _____

Below is a list of items that describes pupils. For each item that describes the pupil **now or within the past week,** check whether the item is **Not True, Somewhat or Sometimes True,** or **Very or Often True.** Please check all items as well as you can, even if some do not seem to apply to this pupil.

	Not true	Somewhat or sometimes true	Very or often true
1. Fails to finish things he/she starts	[ ]	[ ]	[ ]
2. Can't concentrate, can't pay attention for long	[ ]	[ ]	[ ]
3. Can't sit still, restless, or hyperactive	[ ]	[ ]	[ ]
4. Fidgets	[ ]	[ ]	[ ]
5. Daydreams or gets lost in his/her thoughts	[ ]	[ ]	[ ]
6. Impulsive or acts without thinking	[ ]	[ ]	[ ]
7. Difficulty following directions	[ ]	[ ]	[ ]
8. Talks out of turn	[ ]	[ ]	[ ]
9. Messy work	[ ]	[ ]	[ ]
10. Inattentive, easily distracted	[ ]	[ ]	[ ]
11. Talks too much	[ ]	[ ]	[ ]
12. Fails to carry out assigned tasks	[ ]	[ ]	[ ]

Please feel free to write any comments about the pupil's work or behavior in the last week.

Source.   Reprinted with the permission of Craig Edelbrock, Ph.D., University of Massachusetts Medical Center, Worcester, Massachusetts.

TABLE 33–7. Child Attention Profile (CAP) scoring

Each of the 12 items is scored 0, 1, or 2.

Total score = sum of the scores on all items

Subscores:

  Inattention: Sum of scores on items 1, 2, 5, 7, 9, 10, and 12

  Overactivity: Sum of scores on items 3, 4, 6, 8, and 11

Scores recommended as the upper limit of the normal range (93rd percentile):

	Boys	Girls
Inattention	9	7
Overactivity	6	5
Total score	15	11

Source.   Reprinted with the permission of Craig Edelbrock, Ph.D., University of Massachusetts Medical Center, Worcester, Massachusetts.

Behavioral checklists such as the Child Attention Profile (CAP; Edelbrock 1991) (Tables 33–6 and 33–7), the Conners Teacher Rating Scale (CTRS), and the Conners Parent Rating Scale (CPRS; Conners and Barkley 1985) are useful in monitoring the effectiveness of medications in a variety of settings.

If symptoms are not severe outside the school setting, children should have an annual drug-free trial in the summer, at least 2 weeks' duration but longer if possible. If school behavior and academic performance are stable, a carefully monitored trial off medication during the school year (but *not* at the beginning) will provide data on whether medication is still needed.

Tolerance is reported anecdotally, but compliance is often irregular and should be the first possibility considered when medication appears ineffective. Children should not be responsible for their medication because youngsters are impulsive and forgetful at best, and most dislike the idea of taking medication, even when they can verbalize its positive effects and cannot identify any side effects. They will often avoid, "forget," or simply refuse medication. Lower potency or absorption of a generic preparation may be another possibility. Apparent decreased drug effect also may be due to a reaction to a change at home or school. Greenhill (1995) uses the term *pseudotolerance* to define circumstances in which increased symptomatology is inaccurately ascribed to decreased medication efficacy (e.g., when symptoms are exacerbated due to changes in a child's life rather than changes in response to medication). True tolerance may be more likely with the long-acting formulations (Birmaher et al. 1989); if it occurs, another of the stimulants may be substituted.

Risks and Side Effects

Most side effects are similar for all stimulants (Table 33–8). Insomnia may be due to drug effect, to rebound, or to a preexisting sleep problem. Stimulants may worsen or improve irritable mood (Gadow 1992). Black male adolescents who take stimulants may be at higher risk for elevated blood pressure (Brown and Sexson 1989).

Although stimulant-induced growth retardation has been a significant concern, decrease in expected weight gain is small and may be clinically insignificant, despite statistical significance. The magnitude is dose related and appears to be greater with dextroamphetamine than with methylphenidate or pemoline. Effect on height can be minimized by using "drug holidays." The mechanism does not appear to be mediated via effects on growth hormone (Greenhill et al. 1981, 1984). Some authors have suggested that growth delays in ADHD children may be related to dysmaturity inherent to the disorder itself rather than medication effects (T. Spencer et al. 1996b).

Rebound effects, consisting of increased excitability, activity, talkativeness, irritability, and insomnia, beginning 4–15 hours after a dose, may be seen as the last dose of the day wears off or for up to several days after sudden withdrawal of high daily doses of stimulants. This effect may resemble a worsening of the original symptoms (Zahn et al. 1980).

Although psychosis is a well-known side effect of all stimulant medications, psychotic symptoms have not been rigorously studied within the child and adolescent

TABLE 33–8. Side effects of stimulant medications

Common initial side effects (try dose reduction)
Anorexia
Weight loss
Irritability
Abdominal pain
Headaches
Emotional oversensitivity, easy crying
Less common side effects
Insomnia
Dysphoria (especially at higher doses)
Decreased social interest
Impaired cognitive test performance (especially at very high doses)
Less than expected weight gain
Rebound overactivity and irritability (as dose wears off)
Anxiety
Nervous habits (e.g., picking at skin, pulling hair)
Hypersensitivity rash, conjunctivitis, or hives
Withdrawal effects
Insomnia
Rebound ADHD symptoms
Depression (rare)
Rare but potentially serious side effects
Motor or vocal tics
Tourette's disorder
Depression
Growth retardation
Tachycardia
Hypertension
Psychosis with hallucinations
Stereotyped activities or compulsions
Side effects reported with pemoline only
Choreiform movements
Dyskinesias
Night terrors
Lip licking or biting
Chemical hepatitis (potentially fatal)

Note. ADHD = attention-deficit/hyperactivity disorder.

population being treated for ADHD. On chart review, one retrospective study identified 6% of 98 children being treated with methylphenidate who had demonstrated psychotic symptoms (Cherland and Fitzpatrick 1999). While preliminary, these data suggest that, in ADHD children treated with stimulants, psychotic symptoms may be more common than was previously thought.

Attention is required to avoid possible emanative effects of medication—that is, indirect and inadvertent cognitive and social consequences, such as lower self-esteem and self-efficacy; attribution by child, parents, and teachers of both success and failure to the medication rather than to the child's effort; stigmatization by peers; and dependence by parents and teachers on medication rather than making needed changes in the environment (Whalen and Henker 1991). Both patients and relevant adults can be instructed that medication enables the patients to accomplish what they wish to do; it does not *make* them do anything. Children and adolescents should be given full credit for improvement and helped to take an appropriate amount of responsibility for problems.

Although there is a commonly held notion that stimulants lower the seizure threshold, there is no evidence that stimulants produce an increase in seizure activity. Addiction has *not* been found to result from the prescription of stimulants for ADHD. Naturalistic longitudinal data suggest that children with ADHD who are effectively treated with stimulants are less likely to abuse substances than are other children with ADHD (Biederman et al. 1999).

α₂-Noradrenergic Agonists

Clonidine and guanfacine are α₂-noradrenergic agonists approved for the treatment of hypertension.

Indications and Efficacy

Attention-deficit/hyperactivity disorder. Clonidine is useful in modulating mood and activity level and in improving cooperation and frustration tolerance in a subgroup of children with ADHD, especially those who are highly aroused, hyperactive, impulsive, defiant, and labile (Hunt et al. 1990). Steingard et al. (1993) reported that children with ADHD and comorbid tics may have a more positive response to clonidine than do children with ADHD without tics. In a meta-analysis of the literature from 1980 to 1999, Connor et al. (1999) demonstrated an effect size of clonidine on symptoms of ADHD that was intermediate between that of stimulant medication response (stronger) and tricyclic antidepressant (TCA) medication response (weaker). A recent controlled study by Connor et al. (2000) involved 24 ADHD patients with comorbid aggressive oppositional defiant disorder or conduct disorder who were randomized into one of three treatment groups (clonidine, methylphenidate, or the combination). Similar treatment response was observed with clonidine or methylphenidate in this population. No added benefit of combination treatment was noted.

Guanfacine has been shown to be effective in open trials of children with ADHD (Horrigan and Barnhill 1995; Hunt et al. 1995) and children with comorbid ADHD and Tourette's disorder (Chappell et al. 1995). A placebo-controlled study also demonstrated guanfacine's effectiveness in treating children with comorbid ADHD and tic disorders (Scahill et al. 2001).

Tic disorders. In one double-blind study, clonidine was found to modestly decrease complex motor and vocal tics (Leckman et al. 1991), although another study (Singer and Brown 1995) did not support this finding. Clonidine appears to be most useful in reducing subjective distress and the behavioral symptoms of hyperactivity and impulsivity that often accompany Tourette's disorder. As mentioned above, some evidence suggests that guanfacine is a useful agent in treating tics as well (Scahill et al. 2001).

Other uses. Clonidine has been described as beneficial in a small open study of preschool children with severe posttraumatic stress disorder (PTSD) (Harmon and Riggs 1996). Fankhauser et al. (1992) reported a double-blind, placebo-controlled study in which transdermal clonidine was found to reduce hyperarousal and improve social relating in a group of seven children and two adults with autism. These findings are preliminary and require further investigation before clonidine is used routinely for these purposes in children.

Initiation and Maintenance

Because clonidine and guanfacine have similar pharmacological profiles, blood pressure and pulse should be measured before treatment and at regular intervals throughout. An electrocardiogram (ECG) and baseline laboratory blood studies (especially fasting glucose) may be considered. Clonidine is initiated at a low dose of 0.05 mg (one-half of the smallest manufactured tablet) at bedtime. This low dose converts the side effect of initial sedation into a benefit. An alternate strategy is to begin with 0.025 mg four times a day. Either way, the dose is then titrated gradually upward over several weeks to 0.15–0.30 mg/day (0.003–0.01 mg/kg/day) in three or four divided doses. Young children (ages 5–7 years) may require lower initial and maintenance doses. The transdermal form (skin patch) may be useful to improve compliance and reduce variability in blood levels. It lasts only 5 days in children (compared with 7 days in adults) (Hunt et al. 1990). Once the daily dose is determined using pills, an equivalent-size patch may be substituted (0.1, 0.2, 0.3 mg/day). Patches should not be cut to adjust the dose, as this may damage the delivery membrane, potentially causing an increase in the delivered dose of clonidine (Broderick-Cantwell 1999). Unfortunately, patches do not adhere well in hot, humid climates.

For guanfacine, dosages range from 0.5 to 4.0 mg/day,

and a recommended starting regimen is 0.5 mg once or twice a day in children and 1 mg once or twice a day in adolescents, to be increased every 3 or 4 days until therapeutic effect is noted (Silver 1999). Guanfacine is not currently available in a transdermal preparation.

When clonidine or guanfacine is discontinued, it should be tapered over several days to a week, rather than stopped suddenly, to avoid a withdrawal syndrome consisting of increased motor restlessness, headache, agitation, elevated blood pressure and pulse rate, and (in patients with Tourette's disorder) exacerbation of tics (Leckman et al. 1986).

Risks and Side Effects

Sedation and irritability are troublesome side effects of clonidine therapy, although they tend to decrease after several weeks. Dry mouth, nausea, and photophobia have been reported, with hypotension and dizziness possible at high doses. The clonidine skin patch often causes local pruritic dermatitis; daily rotation of the patch site or use of a steroid cream may minimize this. Depression may occur, often in patients with a history of depressive symptoms in themselves or their families (Hunt et al. 1991). Glucose tolerance may decrease, especially in those patients at risk for diabetes. Although guanfacine is less sedating and less hypotensive than clonidine, it shares many of the side effects of this class of medication.

Recent reports of serious adverse drug reactions (including sudden death) in children treated with clonidine, alone or in combination with methylphenidate, have raised concerns about the safety of this medication in the pediatric population (Cantwell et al. 1997; Popper 1995; Swanson et al. 1995, 1999). In all of these cases, the presence of polypharmacy or of other medical conditions made it difficult to implicate clonidine in the adverse events (Wilens and Spencer 1999). Although Popper (1995) identified no clear evidence that the combination of clonidine and methylphenidate is unsafe, he also warned that there was insufficient scientific evidence available on either the potential benefits or the risks of methylphenidate–clonidine treatment and that clinicians should proceed with caution. Cardiovascular screening and monitoring of children treated with clonidine or guanfacine is recommended, as well as gradual titration and tapering of dose to reduce cardiovascular side effects. These medications should not be used unless a parent can supervise them safely and ensure adherence to the prescribed regimen.

Horrigan and Barnhill (1999) described the onset of manic symptoms in 5 of a group of 95 children treated

with guanfacine that resolved with medication discontinuation. Prior treatment with clonidine in 4 of these 5 children had not resulted in manic symptoms. Further study is needed to understand the implications of this finding.

Selective Serotonin Reuptake Inhibitors

Five SSRIs have been approved for use in the United States: citalopram, fluoxetine, fluvoxamine, paroxetine, and sertraline. Of these, only two have FDA-approved indications for use in children: fluvoxamine and sertraline for obsessive-compulsive disorder (OCD). However, all of the SSRIs have been used to treat a wide variety of disorders in children and adolescents.

Indications and Efficacy

Depressive disorders. One rigorous double-blind, placebo-controlled trial in 96 children and adolescents with major depressive episode found that fluoxetine produced significantly greater improvement in depressive symptoms than did placebo, as measured by the Children's Depression Rating Scale and the Clinical Global Impressions scale (Emslie et al. 1997).

Keller et al. (2001) undertook a double-blind, placebo-controlled study of paroxetine in 275 adolescents with major depression, randomizing the patients to paroxetine (20–40 mg/day), imipramine (200–300 mg/day), or placebo. Relative to those taking placebo, patients receiving paroxetine demonstrated significantly greater improvement on several measures of depressive symptomatology. Interestingly, imipramine did not produce statistically significant improvement on any measurement instrument compared with placebo. Open-label studies of sertraline have also shown clinical improvement in symptoms of major depressive disorder in adolescent patients (Ambrosini et al. 1999; McConville et al. 1996).

Obsessive-compulsive disorder. Considerable evidence supports the use of SSRIs in children with OCD. In a study by Riddle et al. (1992), 14 children (ages 8–15 years) diagnosed with OCD demonstrated significant improvement on the Clinical Global Impressions—Obsessive-Compulsive Scale (CGI-OCD), but not the Children's Yale-Brown Obsessive Compulsive Scale (CY-BOCS), with fluoxetine compared with placebo. In a more recent study, D.A. Geller et al. (2001) found that fluoxetine was significantly more effective than placebo, as measured by CY-BOCS scores, in a randomized, controlled study of 103 children and adolescents. March et al.

(1998b) conducted a randomized, double-blind, controlled study of sertraline versus placebo in the treatment of 187 children and adolescents with OCD. Over the 12 weeks of the study, patients treated with sertraline showed a significantly greater improvement on the CY-BOCS than did the placebo group (42% of sertraline group versus 26% of placebo group). Findings from a 52-week open follow-up study (Cook et al. 2001) of this same group suggest that sertraline may be effective in the long-term treatment of OCD symptoms. In another randomized multicenter trial, Riddle et al. (2001) compared fluvoxamine with placebo in 120 children and adolescents diagnosed with OCD. Fluvoxamine-treated subjects demonstrated significantly improved scores on the CY-BOCS throughout the course of the study. Open trials of paroxetine and citalopram have also shown improvements in CY-BOCS scores in children and adolescents with OCD treated with these medications (Rosenberg et al. 1999; Thomsen 1997; Thomsen et al. 2001). In all cited studies, medications were described as generally well tolerated by both child and adolescent subjects.

Other disorders. In a multicenter double-blind, placebo-controlled study, Walkup et al. (2001) demonstrated fluvoxamine's superiority to placebo in treating social phobia, separation anxiety disorder, and generalized anxiety disorder in children and adolescents ages 6–17 years. Over the 8 weeks of the study, the patients who received fluvoxamine had significantly greater decreases in their Pediatric Anxiety Rating Scale scores than did those receiving placebo. In addition, the fluvoxamine group showed a greater response to treatment overall, as measured by the Clinical Global Impressions—Improvement scale. Compton et al. (2001), in an open trial of sertraline in children and adolescents with social anxiety disorder, found treatment response, as measured by the Clinical Global Impressions—Improvement scale, in 65% of patients by the end of the 8-week study. Birmaher et al. (1994) reported marked to moderate improvement in children and adolescents with mixed anxiety disorders who were treated with fluoxetine in an open study. In another open study by Fairbanks et al. (1997), children taking fluoxetine for various anxiety disorders were "much improved," with the most robust response seen in separation anxiety disorder and social phobia, and a lesser response seen in generalized anxiety disorder. A double-blind, placebo-controlled study examining the effectiveness of fluoxetine in the treatment of elective mutism in a small group of children showed mixed results (Black and Uhde 1994). However, in an open trial with fluoxetine in 21 children with selective mutism conducted by Dummit et al. (1996), 76% of children were considered

improved, with decreased anxiety and increased speech in public settings, during the 9-week trial. Dosages of fluoxetine ranged from 10 to 60 mg/day. Further controlled studies are needed to determine the efficacy and safety of the SSRIs in conditions other than depression and OCD in the pediatric population.

Dosage and Administration

Fluoxetine, citalopram, and paroxetine may be started at dosages of 5–10 mg/day, which may be increased as needed to 20 mg/day. Although most children will show an adequate response to 20 mg/day or less of these medications, some children may require dosages in excess of 20 mg/day. All three of these medications are available in a liquid formulation that may facilitate medication administration or dosage titration in small children.

For sertraline and fluvoxamine, doses may be started at 25 mg/day and increased as necessary to a dosage of 100–150 mg/day. Doses may be increased every few days as tolerated. Sertraline is also available in a liquid preparation.

Although children and adolescents usually tolerate this class of medication well, they may experience the same constellation of side effects as seen in adults, such as gastrointestinal complaints or headache. In addition, patients may experience a "withdrawal" phenomenon if the medication is stopped abruptly. Withdrawal symptoms include malaise, myalgias, headache, and anxiety and may occur even if only one dose is missed. This withdrawal phenomenon is not usually noted with fluoxetine because of its active metabolites and long half-life. It is therefore preferable to taper the dosage of medication over several days before cessation rather than discontinuing it abruptly. In a patient who has a recurrence of symptoms after an initial good response, a gentle inquiry about medication compliance should be made before instituting a change in dosage.

Adverse Effects

Several cases of "behavioral activation" and manic symptoms presumed to be caused by treatment with SSRIs have been reported in pediatric patients (Diler and Avci 1999; Grubbs 1997; Guile 1996; Minnery et al. 1995; Oldroyd 1997; Tierney et al. 1995). In many of these cases, the manic symptoms appeared within days to weeks of initiating treatment with an SSRI. Symptoms usually resolved within a few days of reduction in dosage or cessation of medication. In one case (Oldroyd 1997), treatment with a mood stabilizer was necessary. In many of the cases, there was no premorbid or family history of a cyclical mood disorder.

Movement disorders (acute dystonic reactions, akathisia, and ticlike movements) have also been noted in children taking SSRIs (Bates et al. 1998; Boyle 1999; Jones-Fearing 1996; Lenti 1999). Because SSRI-induced movement disorders are thought to be due to serotonin-mediated inhibition of dopaminergic transmission (Lipinski et al. 1989), movement disorders may potentially occur with any of the SSRIs.

Serotonin syndrome is a potentially fatal reaction to serotonergic agents. It is more likely to occur when serotonergic agents are used in combination. Several signs characterize this syndrome: mental status changes, fever, tremor, diaphoresis, and agitation. Although uncommon, serotonin syndrome has been reported in the pediatric population (Gill et al. 1999; Lee and Lee 1999; Mullins and Horowitz 1999; Pao and Tipnis 1997; Spirko and Wiley 1999). It may arise after only one dose of a serotonergic agent. Clinicians should be alert to the possibility of this syndrome occurring in their pediatric patients and should counsel patients and parents as appropriate.

Tricyclic Antidepressants

Until the introduction of the SSRIs into the U.S. market in the late 1980s, TCAs were a mainstay in the pharmacological treatment of a wide variety of disorders in children and adolescents. However, the paucity of clinical studies demonstrating the efficacy of TCAs in children, an increased awareness of the potential cardiac effects of this class of medication, and the availability of alternative medications has resulted in a shift away from using tricyclic agents as first-line agents (Safer 1997). Although TCAs may no longer be considered first line in the treatment of psychiatric conditions in children and adolescents (B. Geller et al. 1999), their continued use and availability warrants their discussion here.

Indications and Efficacy

Depression. Several double-blind, placebo-controlled studies have examined the efficacy of TCAs in treating depressed children and adolescents. Despite promising anecdotal data and results in open trials, only one study has documented superiority of a TCA over placebo (Preskorn et al. 1987). Hypotheses put forward to explain this poor response include suboptimal dosing, an increase in hormone levels in adolescents, a difference in the maturation of the noradrenergic and serotonergic neurotransmitter systems, and speculation that some of the youths studied may have been in the early phase of bipolar disorder (Ambrosini 2000). Given recent findings of the efficacy of SSRIs in the treatment of adolescent depression (Emslie et al. 1997; Keller et al. 2001) and the

consistent lack of data demonstrating the efficacy of TCAs, SSRIs should be considered the treatment of choice for this population.

Attention-deficit/hyperactivity disorder. TCAs may be indicated for patients with ADHD who do not respond to stimulants or who develop significant depression while taking stimulants, or for the treatment of ADHD symptoms in patients with tics or Tourette's disorder. The efficacy of TCAs in improving cognitive symptoms does not appear to be as great as that of stimulants. Because other useful and safe medications are available, TCAs should be a second- or third-line medication for treatment of ADHD in children.

Obsessive-compulsive disorder. Clomipramine, a TCA that inhibits serotonin reuptake, is useful in the treatment of OCD in children (DeVeaugh-Geiss et al. 1992; Leonard et al. 1989). Symptoms are rarely eliminated entirely, but when the medication is effective, the force of obsessions and compulsions is reduced sufficiently to improve quality of life. As in depression, the more favorable side effect and safety profiles of the SSRIs makes clomipramine a second- or third-line treatment of OCD in children.

Autistic disorder. Gordon et al. (1993) reported a double-blind study in which clomipramine was significantly more effective than either placebo or desipramine in improving several autistic symptoms (obsessive-compulsive symptoms, reciprocal social interactions, stereotypies, and self-injury). There was no difference between desipramine and placebo noted. In a recent open study examining the use of clomipramine in treating young children (ages 3.5–8.7 years), Sanchez et al. (1996) reported no therapeutic effect, and significant adverse reactions were noted (urinary retention).

Enuresis. All of the TCAs have been found to be equally effective in the treatment of nocturnal enuresis. In 80% of patients, TCAs reduce the frequency of bed wetting within the first week. Total remission, however, occurs in relatively few cases. Wetting returns when the drug is discontinued. Behavioral treatments that avoid drug side effects and have higher remission and lower relapse rates are the best first choice. Imipramine may be useful on a short-term basis or for special occasions (e.g., overnight camp), although desmopressin is now commonly used for such purposes.

Anxiety disorders. The majority of the literature has examined the use of TCAs for separation anxiety disorder and school absenteeism. Of four double-blind, placebo-

TABLE 33–9. Suggested guidelines for monitoring electrocardiograms and vital signs of children and adolescents receiving tricyclic antidepressants

Parameter	Children	Adolescents
Vital signs		
Heart rate	≤110–130 beats/min[a]	≤110–120 beats/min[a]
Blood pressure	<120/80 mm Hg	<140/90 mm Hg
Electrocardiogram		
P-R interval	<200 msec	<200 msec
QRS interval	≤120 msec ± >30% over baseline	±120 msec
QTc interval	≤460–480 msec	≤460–480 msec

Note. [a]For 2 consecutive weeks.

Source. Reprinted with permission from Wilens TE, Biederman J, Baldessarini RJ, et al.: "Cardiovascular Effects of Therapeutic Doses of Tricyclic Antidepressants in Children and Adolescents." *Journal of the American Academy of Child and Adolescent Psychiatry* 35:1491–1501, 1996. Copyright 1996, American Academy of Child and Adolescent Psychiatry.

controlled studies, only one has demonstrated efficacy of a TCA over placebo in treating separation anxiety disorder and school refusal (Gittelman-Klein and Klein 1971, 1973). Several case studies of the effectiveness of TCAs in treating childhood panic disorder have also been reported (Black and Robbins 1989; Garland and Smith 1990). The efficacy of imipramine in patients with anxiety disorders is controversial (Bernstein et al. 1990; Klein et al. 1992), and other medications are now available. Medication may be useful as an adjunct if psychosocial treatment is ineffective. In a randomized, double-blind trial comparing imipramine plus cognitive-behavioral therapy (CBT) in the treatment of school refusal, imipramine plus CBT was shown to be more effective than CBT plus placebo in decreasing depressive symptoms and improving school attendance (Bernstein et al. 2000).

Initiation and Maintenance

Pharmacokinetics for TCAs is different in children than in adolescents or adults. The smaller fat-to-muscle ratio in children leads to a decreased volume of distribution, and children are not protected from excessive dosage by a large volume of fat in which the drug can be stored. Children have larger livers relative to body size, leading to faster metabolism (Sallee et al. 1986), more rapid absorption, and lower protein binding than in adults (Winsberg et al. 1974). As a result, children are likely to need a higher weight-corrected dose of TCAs than adults. Prepubertal children are prone to rapid dramatic swings in blood levels from toxic to ineffective and should have divided doses to produce more stable levels (Ryan 1992). Parents must be reminded to supervise closely the administration of medication and to keep pills in a safe place, due to the danger of overdose. Guidelines for monitoring the cardiovascular effects of TCAs are given in Table 33–9.

The usefulness of plasma levels is limited by the relative rarity of laboratories able to perform them satisfactorily. Medication cannot be safely titrated by plasma level, as there is no known level below which toxicity can be guaranteed not to occur. Plasma levels (drawn 9–11 hours after the last dose) can identify rapid and slow metabolizers. Determination of levels is recommended for patients who fail to respond to usual doses (possibly low levels) or those who have severe side effects at usual doses (possibly very high levels). If the patient's history suggests head trauma or seizures, an electroencephalogram (EEG) is indicated before starting treatment.

Depression. For imipramine, the starting dose is 25 mg/day, which may be increased every 4 days by 1 mg/kg/day to a maximum dose of 5 mg/kg/day. Optimum plasma level of imipramine appears to be 150–250 ng/mL (Preskorn et al. 1987; Ryan 1990).

Nortriptyline may have fewer side effects and a more precise therapeutic window of 75–150 ng/mL, usually attained at 0.5 to 2.0 mg/kg/day (Ryan 1990). It has a longer half-life than imipramine and may be given twice a day in children. Variability in metabolism is greater for nortriptyline than for imipramine (B. Geller et al. 1986).

Attention-deficit/hyperactivity disorder. Imipramine is begun with 10 or 25 mg/day and increased weekly. The maximum dose is 5 mg/kg/day (given in three divided doses). Plasma levels do not predict efficacy. Some patients respond to a daily dose as low as 2 mg/kg. Nortriptyline is given at 25–75 mg/day in two divided doses (Saul 1985).

Obsessive-compulsive disorder. Doses of clomipramine used to treat OCD are generally lower than TCA doses used for depression. Response is delayed for 10–14 days, as in the treatment of depression, and is unlike the immediate response seen in the treatment of ADHD or enuresis (Rapoport 1986). Clomipramine is started at 25 mg/day (or every other day) and gradually increased over 2 weeks to a maximum of 100 mg/day or 3 mg/kg/day, whichever is less. Divided doses are preferable during titration. Chronic treatment (years) is required.

Enuresis. Daily charting of wet and dry nights is used before starting medication to obtain a baseline and subsequently to monitor progress. Much lower doses are needed than for the treatment of depression. Imipramine is started at 10–25 mg at bedtime and increased by 10- to 25-mg increments weekly to 50 mg (75 mg in preadolescents), if necessary. Maximum dose is 2.5 mg/kg/day (Ryan 1990). Tolerance may develop, requiring a dose increase. For some children, TCAs lose their effect entirely. If medication is used chronically, the child or adolescent should have a drug-free trial at least every 6 months because enuresis has a high spontaneous remission rate.

Anxiety disorders. In separation anxiety disorder and school nonattendance, psychological interventions such as family therapy, consultation with school personnel, and cognitive-behavioral techniques should be used before and along with medication. For children with school phobia, the recommended starting dose is 25 mg/day of imipramine. The dose is titrated upward every 3–5 days, as tolerated, to an expected therapeutic range of 3–5 mg/kg/day. A twice-daily dosing regimen is recommended to minimize side effects from a large single dose.

Risks and Side Effects

The quinidine-like effect of the TCAs slows cardiac conduction time and repolarization. At doses of more than 3 mg/kg/day of imipramine, children and adolescents may develop an increased pulse and small but statistically significant ECG changes (intraventricular conduction defects, such as lengthened P-R interval, that may progress to a first-degree atrioventricular heart block and occasional widening of the QRS complex) (Wilens et al. 1996). Prolongation of the QTc interval may be a sensitive indicator of cardiac effect (Wiles et al. 1991). The tendency of prepubertal children to have wider swings in blood levels may place them at higher risk for serious cardiac conduction changes. A minority of the population has a genetic defect in TCA metabolism, increasing risk for toxicity.

Anticholinergic side effects may occur in children, although less commonly than in adults. Most of these side effects are transient and/or respond to a decrease in dose. Of particular importance for children are dry mouth, which may lead to an increase in dental caries in long-term use (Herskowitz 1987), drying of bronchial secretions (especially problematic for asthmatic children), sedation, anorexia, constipation, nausea, tachycardia, palpitations, and increased diastolic blood pressure.

Other reported side effects include abdominal pain, chest pain, headache, orthostatic hypotension (rare in young patients), syncope, mild tremors of hands and fingers, weight loss, and tics. The seizure threshold may be lowered, with worsening of preexisting EEG abnormalities and rarely a seizure. Seizures appear to be more common with clomipramine. Side effects with a probable allergic mechanism include rash, worsening of eczema, and rarely thrombocytopenia (M. Campbell et al. 1985).

Behavioral toxicity may be manifested by irritability, worsening of psychosis, mania, agitation, anger, aggression, forgetfulness, or confusion. CNS toxicity may be mistaken for exacerbation of the primary condition. A drug blood level is often required to differentiate the two. As depressed children, especially those who are anergic and withdrawn, improve with TCA treatment, crying and verbalizations of sadness and anger may transiently increase.

Sudden cessation of moderate or higher doses results in a flulike anticholinergic withdrawal syndrome, with nausea, cramps, vomiting, headaches, and muscle pains. Other manifestations may include social withdrawal, hyperactivity, depression, agitation, and insomnia (Ryan 1990). TCAs should therefore be tapered over a 2- to 3-week period. The short half-life of TCAs in prepubertal children often produces daily withdrawal symptoms if medication is given only once a day. These symptoms also may indicate that poor compliance is resulting in missed doses. Because of the predictability of TCA-induced ECG changes, a rhythm strip is useful in monitoring compliance.

The physician should be alert to the risk of intentional overdose or accidental poisoning, not only by the patient but by other family members, especially young children.

Cautionary note on the use of desipramine: Six cases of sudden death have been reported in children being treated with desipramine, three of whom died immediately after physical exertion (Riddle et al. 1991, 1993; Varley and McClellan 1997). A causal relationship between the medication and the deaths has not been established. Cardiac etiology has been suspected; however, a recent review of cardiovascular changes in children treated with TCAs (Wilens et al. 1996) concluded that although changes in blood pressure, heart rate, and ECG parameters are identifiable, they are probably of minor significance. In a study of the effects of desipramine on cardiac function during exercise, 9 children and 13 adults were evaluated before and during a course of treatment with desipramine. One 31-year-old subject experienced a brief episode of ventricular tachycardia during exercise while receiving desipramine. The study concluded that desipramine had only minor effects on the cardiovascular response to exercise, and that these effects did not appear to be age related (Waslick et al. 1999). A further study by Walsh et al. (1999) showed that desipramine reduced parasympathetic input to the heart, as measured by R-R interval variability. Although such a reduction in parasympathetic tone could, theoretically, increase vulnerability to cardiac arrhythmias, the R-R interval variability did not differ with age in the 42 subjects studied (who ranged in age from 7 to 66 years). Nevertheless, given that other safe and effective medications are available, the use of desipramine in prepubertal children is discouraged.

Other Antidepressants

Venlafaxine

Venlafaxine is a serotonin-norepinephrine reuptake inhibitor (SNRI) approved for the treatment of depression. Unlike the SSRIs, the SNRIs have both serotonergic and noradrenergic properties. Although some TCAs also possess dual-neurotransmitter activity, the SNRIs do not have α_1-, cholinergic-, or histaminic-blocking properties (Stahl 2000). Few studies have examined the use of venlafaxine in children. In one double-blind, placebo-controlled study, Mandoki et al. (1997) compared venlafaxine and cognitive-behavioral therapy with placebo and therapy in the treatment of 33 pediatric patients (ages 8 to 17 years) diagnosed with major depression. Although no significant differences were found between the two groups, the short treatment time and low dose of venlafaxine used may account for this apparent lack of effect. Olvera et al. (1996) conducted an open trial of venlafaxine in 14 children and adolescents (ages 8–17 years) with ADHD and found that venlafaxine reduced impulsivity and hyperactivity as measured by the Conners Rating Scales. Although initial reports of venlafaxine's use in a variety of disorders are promising, further controlled studies are needed to determine the efficacy and safety of venlafaxine in these disorders.

Bupropion

Bupropion is a compound of the aminoketone class and is structurally unrelated to other antidepressants. Conners et al. (1996) reported the superiority of bupropion to placebo in the treatment of ADHD in children in a mul-

tisite, double-blind, placebo-controlled study. Another study found the efficacy of bupropion in treating ADHD to be not statistically significantly different from methylphenidate (Barrickman et al. 1995). Substance-abusing adolescent patients with ADHD may benefit from treatment with bupropion because of its lack of abuse potential. An open study by Riggs et al. (1998) suggested that bupropion could be useful in treating adolescents with comorbid ADHD, conduct disorder, and a substance use disorder. Bupropion has been reported to exacerbate tics in children with comorbid ADHD and Tourette's disorder and may not be suitable for use in this population (T. Spencer et al. 1993).

Although bupropion is marketed in the United States as an antidepressant and as an aid in smoking cessation, the literature on its use in treating childhood depression is limited. A small open-label study by Arredondo (1993) showed an improvement in 8 of 10 adolescent inpatients treated with bupropion. More recently, Daviss et al. (2001) used bupropion to treat 24 adolescents with ADHD and a mood disorder (major depressive disorder or dysthymic disorder). Patients were treated with the sustained-release preparation of bupropion over 8 weeks. Fourteen of the 24 adolescents showed improvement in both depression and ADHD symptoms, 7 showed improvement in depression only, and one showed improvement in ADHD only. Double-blind, placebo-controlled studies of bupropion's efficacy in childhood mood disorders are needed.

Bupropion is administered in two or three daily doses, beginning with a low dose (37.5 or 50 mg twice daily), with gradual upward titration over 2 weeks to a usual maximum of 250 mg/day (300–400 mg/day in adolescents). A long-acting preparation of this medication is also available that allows once- or twice-daily dosing. The most serious side effect is a decrease in the seizure threshold, seen most frequently in patients with an eating disorder. Bupropion is contraindicated in this population. Other side effects reported in children include skin rash, perioral edema, nausea, increased appetite, agitation, exacerbation of tics, and mania.

Mirtazapine

Mirtazapine is a noradrenergic and specific serotonergic antidepressant that increases norepinephrine and serotonin through α_2 antagonism and blockade of three serotonin receptor subtypes (Stahl 2000). Mirtazapine also blocks H_1 histamine receptors (Stahl 2000). It is indicated for the treatment of depression in adults. Its pharmacological profile includes anxiolytic and antidepressant effects with less gastrointestinal upset and sexual dysfunction than SSRIs. However, somnolence and weight gain are common side effects. There are no published controlled or open-label studies of mirtazapine's use in children.

Monoamine Oxidase Inhibitors

Monoamine oxidase inhibitors (MAOIs) have been useful in the treatment of depressed adolescents who do not respond to TCAs (Ryan et al. 1988b), but the availability of safer effective treatments makes MAOIs a distant therapeutic choice. More recently, case reports have described benefit from MAOIs in children with elective mutism (Golwyn and Sevlie 1999) and in adolescents with severe melancholic depression (Strober et al. 1998). MAOIs should be used with extreme caution, if at all, in suicidal or impulsive outpatients because of the risk of severe reactions with dietary indiscretions or drug interactions. Patients taking MAOIs always require instruction on diet restrictions and potential drug interactions with prescription and over-the-counter medications.

Mood-Stabilizing Agents

Lithium, an element with antimanic properties, has been approved since 1970 in the United States for the treatment of mania in patients 12 years of age and older. The antiepileptic drugs carbamazepine, divalproex sodium, and clonazepam are used for a variety of (non–FDA approved) psychiatric indications, although divalproex sodium has an FDA-approved indication for the treatment of mania in adults. The efficacy of these agents as mood stabilizers may be unrelated to their anticonvulsant effects. Wide variations in the bioavailability and rate of absorption of the available generic mood stabilizers have led to recommendations that the brand name (or at least a single generic) product be prescribed. Data on children and adolescents are far more limited than those from studies of adults, but side effect patterns appear to be similar, and extrapolation may be made from the treatment of children for epilepsy. The anticonvulsants have complex interactions with many other drugs.

Lithium

Indications and efficacy. Lithium may be considered in the treatment of children and adolescents with bipolar affective disorder, mixed or manic (Strober et al. 1990; Varanka et al. 1988). It is not indicated for prophylaxis of bipolar disorder in children and adolescents unless there is well-documented history of recurrent episodes. Lithium augmentation has been effective in some open trials with adolescents who have tricyclic-refractory depression (Ryan et al. 1988a; Strober et al. 1992). How-

ever, fewer adolescents than adults respond to this strategy. Interestingly, in a double-blind, placebo-controlled study of prepubertal children with major depressive disorder without a history of symptoms of mania but with a family history of either bipolar disorder or multigenerational major depressive episodes, B. Geller et al. (1998b) found that lithium was not statistically more effective than placebo in the treatment of depression. It is not yet clear whether lithium is efficacious for the treatment of behavior disorders without an apparent mood disorder in children of bipolar parents or for children and adolescents who have behavior disorders accompanied by mood swings. The combination of lithium and methylphenidate may be more effective in the treatment of combined disruptive behavior disorders (ADHD/conduct disorder) and mood disorders than either medication used alone (Carlson et al. 1992).

In a double-blind, placebo-controlled short-term study of 25 adolescents with bipolar disorder and a substance dependence disorder, B. Geller et al. (1998a) found that lithium significantly improved global functioning and decreased substance use in comparison with placebo. Kowatch et al. (2000) conducted an open study in which 42 children and adolescents with bipolar disorder were randomized to 6 weeks of treatment with lithium, valproic acid, or carbamazepine. All three agents were found to have a large effect size, as measured by a 50% or greater improvement on the Young Mania Rating Scale (Y-MRS) or a score of 1 or 2 on the Bipolar Clinical Global Impression (CGI-BP) scale.

In children with severe impulsive aggression, especially when it was accompanied by explosive affect, lithium was equal or superior to haloperidol in reducing aggression, hostility, and tantrums, with fewer side effects (M. Campbell et al. 1984). These positive findings were replicated in subsequent placebo-controlled studies by M. Campbell et al. (1995) and more recently by Malone et al. (2000). However, a double-blind, placebo-controlled study by Rifkin et al. (1997) of 33 inpatients with conduct disorder failed to demonstrate statistically significant efficacy for lithium in this indication, although the findings may have been influenced by the brief (2-week) duration of the study. Lithium also may be useful in mentally retarded or autistic youths with severe aggression directed toward themselves or others or with symptoms suggestive of bipolar disorder (M. Campbell et al. 1985; Kerbeshian et al. 1987; Steingard and Biederman 1987).

Initiation and maintenance. Lithium should not be prescribed unless the family is willing and able to comply with regular multiple daily doses and with blood monitoring of lithium levels. In addition to the usual detailed medical history and physical examination, complete blood count (CBC) with differential, liver function tests, electrolytes, serum thyroxine and thyroid-stimulating hormone (TSH), blood urea nitrogen (BUN), creatinine, and ECG should be determined before starting lithium. Some clinicians recommend determining renal concentrating ability (urine specific gravity or osmolality after overnight fluid deprivation) (C. Popper, personal communication, 1992). A patient with a history suggesting increased risk of seizures warrants an EEG. Height, weight, TSH, creatinine, and morning urine specific gravity (or osmolality) should be obtained every 3–6 months.

Lithium levels, drawn 10–12 hours after the last dose, should be obtained twice weekly during initial dose adjustment and monthly thereafter. Three to 4 days are required to reach steady-state levels after a dose change. Therapeutic levels are the same as for adults, 0.6–1.2 mEq/L, which can usually be attained with 900–1,200 mg/day, in divided doses, although daily doses of up to 2,000 mg may be required (M. Campbell et al. 1985). The starting dose is 150–300 mg/day, gradually titrated upward in divided doses according to serum levels and clinical effects. Because lithium excretion occurs primarily through the kidney, and most children have more efficient renal function than adults, children may require higher doses for body weight than do adults (Weller et al. 1986). In prepubertal children, dose may be titrated more rapidly with a regimen based on body weight (Weller et al. 1986) or on a serum level drawn 24 hours after a single 600-mg dose (Fetner and Geller 1992). More steady blood levels may be obtained by using a slow-release formulation. Lithium should be taken with food to minimize gastrointestinal distress. Some difference may be present in pharmacokinetics between lithium carbonate and lithium citrate, and clinicians should not assume equal dosing when shifting between the two forms (Reischer and Pfeffer 1996). Given lithium's teratogenicity, the clinician should address this potential with sexually mature female adolescent patients and consider contraceptive options as appropriate.

A naturalistic study of lithium discontinuation in adolescents (Strober et al. 1990), as well as reports of relapse of adolescents in an ongoing double-blind, placebo-controlled study by Keller et al. (as reported in Davanzo and McCracken 2000), suggest that after lithium treatment of an acute manic episode, medication should be continued for at least a year.

Risks and side effects. The younger the child, the more likely the occurrence of side effects (M. Campbell et al. 1991). Autistic children have more frequent and severe side effects from lithium than do children with conduct disorder, even at lower doses (M. Campbell et al. 1991). Children may experience side effects at serum levels that are lower than those in adults: most commonly, weight gain, vomiting, headache, nausea, tremor, enuresis, stomachache, weight loss, sedation, and anorexia (M. Campbell et al. 1991). Common, early onset side effects, which seem to be related to rapid increase in serum level, include nausea, diarrhea, muscle weakness, thirst, urinary frequency, a dazed feeling, and hand tremor. Polydipsia and polyuria secondary to vasopressin-resistant diabetes insipidus may result in enuresis (M. Campbell et al. 1985). In growing children, the consequences of hypothyroidism (which could resemble retarded depression) are potentially more severe than in adults. The calcium mobilization from bones that has been noted in adults might cause a significant problem in growing children (Herskowitz 1987). Lithium's tendency to aggravate acne may be especially significant for adolescents. Lithium's effects on glucose are controversial, but both hyperglycemia and exercise-induced hypoglycemia are possible. Rarely, lithium may cause extrapyramidal side effects (EPS) in children (Samuel 1993).

Toxicity is closely related to serum levels, and the therapeutic margin is narrow. Symptoms of lithium toxicity include vomiting, drowsiness, hyperreflexia, sluggishness, slurred speech, ataxia, anorexia, convulsions, stupor, coma, and death. Adequate salt and fluid intake is necessary to prevent levels rising into the toxic range. The family should be instructed in the importance of preventing dehydration from heat or exercise and in the need to stop the lithium and contact the physician if the child or adolescent develops an illness with fever, vomiting, diarrhea, and/or decreased fluid intake. The erratic consumption of large amounts of salty snack foods may cause fluctuations in lithium levels (Herskowitz 1987). Clinicians should also be aware of potential drug–drug interactions, especially with nonsteroidal anti-inflammatory drugs, antipsychotic agents, SSRIs, and antibiotics (Kowatch and Bucci 1998).

Carbamazepine

Indications and efficacy. Some evidence suggests potential benefit for carbamazepine in the treatment of juvenile bipolar disorder, although no controlled studies have been reported. Woolston (1999) described a case series of three adolescents with bipolar I disorder who were treated effectively and safely with carbamazepine, both for acute mania as well as for maintenance therapy. Kowatch et al. (2000) completed a random-assignment open study that compared the effect sizes of lithium, divalproex sodium and carbamazepine in the treatment of bipolar I and II in children and adolescents. The authors concluded that, similar to lithium and divalproex sodium, carbamazepine had a large effect size and was generally well tolerated. Although preliminary data suggested this drug's efficacy in children with severe explosive aggression (Kafantaris et al. 1992), a later double-blind, placebo-controlled study failed to demonstrate any superiority of carbamazepine over placebo in reducing aggression in this population (Cueva et al. 1996).

Initiation and maintenance. Hemoglobin, hematocrit, white blood cell (WBC) count, platelets, liver function, BUN, and creatinine should all be measured before a patient begins taking carbamazepine. The degree of laboratory monitoring necessary is controversial. A conservative recommendation includes CBC and liver function studies weekly for the first 4 weeks, monthly for 4 months, and every 3 months thereafter (Silverstein et al. 1983). A more modest regimen involves CBC (with differential and platelet count), serum iron, BUN, and creatinine after the first month and then every 3–6 months (Trimble 1990). Tests always should be done if a rash, sore throat, fever, malaise, lethargy, weakness, vomiting, increased urinary frequency, anorexia, jaundice, easy bruising, bleeding, or mouth ulcers develop. If the neutrophil count drops below 1,000, or if hepatitis occurs, the drug should be stopped (Silverstein et al. 1983).

The initial dosage of carbamazepine is 100 mg/day taken with food. Children eliminate carbamazepine more rapidly than do adults (Jatlow 1987), and plasma levels (drawn approximately 12 hours after the last dose) are crucial because dosage calculated by weight correlates poorly with plasma concentration. Titration should be gradual (weekly increase of 100 mg/day), guided by plasma levels, to a usual plateau of 8–12 µg/mL. The usual daily dosage range is 10–50 mg/kg, divided into three doses for children and into two for older adolescents. Autoinduction of hepatic enzymes may lead to declining plasma concentration, especially during the first 6 weeks, requiring an increase in dose. Carbamazepine deteriorates if it is stored under humid conditions.

Risks and side effects. The most common adverse effects of carbamazepine are drowsiness, nausea, rash, diplopia, nystagmus, and reversible dose-related leukopenia. Other side effects include vomiting, vertigo, ataxia, tics, muscle cramps, exacerbation of seizures, rare blood dyscrasias, hepatotoxicity, severe skin reactions (e.g., Stevens-Johnson or systemic lupus–like syndromes), and inappropriate secretion of antidiuretic hormone (in rare cases leading to acute renal failure) (Evans et al. 1987;

Trimble 1990). Teratogenic effects have also been demonstrated. Adverse behavioral reactions, such as extreme irritability, agitation, insomnia, obsessive thinking, hallucinations, delirium, psychosis, paranoia, hyperactivity, aggression, and mania, may be seen during the first 1–4 weeks of treatment (Evans et al. 1987; Herskowitz 1987; Pleak et al. 1988).

Divalproex Sodium

Indications and efficacy. Two open-label, uncontrolled trials of divalproex sodium in the treatment of adolescents with mania have been conducted (Papatheodorou et al. 1995; West et al. 1994); both found that divalproex sodium was generally well tolerated and beneficial. As described earlier, Kowatch et al. (2000) conducted an open study in which children and adolescents with bipolar disorder I and II were randomly assigned to treatment with lithium, divalproex sodium, or carbamazepine. Like carbamazepine and lithium, divalproex sodium had a large effect size and was generally well tolerated. Although divalproex sodium may be beneficial in the treatment of mania in bipolar disorder, larger controlled studies are required.

Initiation and maintenance. The initial laboratory workup for divalproex sodium is the same as that for carbamazepine. Liver function tests and CBC may be repeated weekly for the first month, then every 4–6 months. For children younger than age 10 years, monthly liver function tests are advisable (Trimble 1990). Divalproex sodium may be initiated at 250 mg once or twice daily, depending on the weight of the child. Trough plasma levels should be drawn after reaching a dosage of 15 mg/kg/day dispensed in three divided doses. Dosages should be titrated to achieve a serum level within the therapeutic range (50–120 µg/mL). Clinicians are cautioned that the use of mg/kg loading doses for divalproex sodium may lead to supratherapeutic levels in overweight children (Good et al. 2001).

Risks and side effects. The most frequent adverse effects of divalproex sodium are nausea, vomiting, and gastrointestinal distress (which may be diminished by using enteric-coated divalproex sodium), sedation, weight gain, and tremor (Trimble 1990). Acute hepatic failure is almost always restricted to children younger than age 3 years, especially those with mental retardation or who are on anticonvulsant polytherapy. Other side effects are similar to those seen in adults. Of uncertain significance is a report of menstrual disturbances, polycystic ovaries, and hyperandrogenism in a series of women treated with divalproex sodium for epilepsy (Isojarvi et al. 1993). These findings have been challenged in a recent review of the literature (Genton et al. 2001).

Antipsychotic Medications

Indications and Efficacy

Antipsychotic medications are more fully discussed in Chapter 24. Their use in children and adolescents has been reviewed by Findling et al. (1998) and Bryden et al. (2001). The recent introduction of "atypical" antipsychotic medications (clozapine, risperidone, olanzapine, quetiapine, and ziprasidone) has added significantly to the child and adolescent psychiatrist's pharmaceutical armamentarium. The use of these agents in children and adolescents is specifically reviewed by Toren et al. (1998) and Remschmidt et al. (2000). Studies examining the efficacy and safety of these atypical medications with children and adolescents, although promising, remain limited, particularly with the newer agents.

Schizophrenia. Few studies examining the efficacy of typical antipsychotic medications in schizophrenic children exist (Findling et al. 1996). Of the two investigations with more stringent diagnostic admission criteria, both controlled studies (Pool et al. 1976; Realmuto et al. 1984) demonstrated moderate effectiveness of antipsychotic medication in adolescent schizophrenic patients. Medication-induced side effects in both studies were substantial, particularly sedation (in low-potency agents) and EPS (in high-potency agents), supporting the belief that children may be at higher risk than adults for developing side effects with the typical antipsychotic agents. E.K. Spencer et al. (1992) reported preliminary results of the first double-blind, placebo-controlled trial of haloperidol in schizophrenic prepubertal children. Findings similarly support moderate improvement of symptoms in those taking haloperidol rather than placebo.

The more limited effect of typical antipsychotic medications, coupled with higher side-effect profiles (to include tardive dyskinesia), in children has led clinicians to consider the use of atypical antipsychotics in the treatment of the pediatric population. Open trial and double-blind, controlled studies examining the efficacy of clozapine in treatment-resistant, childhood-onset adolescent schizophrenic patients (Frazier et al. 1994; Kumra et al. 1996; Remschmidt et al. 1994) have demonstrated the superiority of clozapine to standard treatments, specifically haloperidol. As treatment with clozapine is compounded by possible serious side effects (agranulocytosis, seizures, and significant weight gain), its use is reserved for treatment of those select patients who have failed to respond to trials of standard or other atypical antipsychotics.

Information regarding the use of risperidone in the treatment of schizophrenia in the pediatric population is limited to several case reports and open-label studies (Armenteros et al. 1997; Grcevich et al. 1996; Quintana and Keshavan 1995) in which positive and negative symptoms of the disorder appeared to have improved. As an atypical agent, risperidone may eventually prove to have greater efficacy than current standard treatments; however, controlled investigation is required.

The literature on the use of olanzapine in the treatment of schizophrenia in children and adolescents is sparse (Krishanmoorthy and King 1998; Kumra et al. 1998; Mandoki 1997; Sholevar et al. 2000). Reports are limited to retrospective and open-label studies; no controlled trials have been published. Mandoki (1997) described olanzapine's efficacy in this population as similar to that of clozapine; however, Kumra et al. (1998) suggested that although olanzapine was effective in treating refractory schizophrenia, it may not be as effective as clozapine. Krishanmoorthy and King (1998) reported their open-label use of olanzapine in five preadolescent children with varying diagnoses (including schizophrenia). In all five children, medication was discontinued prematurely due either to lack of clinical response or to the development of adverse side effects. Controlled studies examining olanzapine's efficacy and safety in pediatric populations are still needed.

Pervasive developmental disorders. In some hyper- or normoactive autistic children, haloperidol (in doses of 0.5–4.0 mg/day) has been found to decrease behavioral target symptoms such as hyperactivity, aggressiveness, temper tantrums, withdrawal, and stereotypies (L.T. Anderson et al. 1989). Efficacy in enhancing learning is controversial but clearly will not occur in the absence of a highly structured behavioral/educational program. The majority of hypoactive autistic children do not respond well to haloperidol (M. Campbell et al. 1985) but may do better with pimozide (Ernst et al. 1992).

Atypical antipsychotic agents may eventually prove to be more effective and safer in this population. Six open trials have described the effectiveness of risperidone in the treatment of disruptive behavior in children with severe developmental disorders (Fisman and Steele 1996; Hardan et al. 1996; Horrigan and Barnhill 1997; McDougle et al. 1997; Perry et al. 1997; Zuddas et al. 2000). Masi et al. (2001) reported the benefits of low-dose risperidone (0.5 mg/day) in an open trial studying preschool children with PDDs. Risperidone effectively targeted both the disruptive behaviors and the affective dysregulation and was well tolerated. Although controlled studies are still clearly required, these preliminary data suggest that risperidone may be an effective and safe treatment in children of varying ages with PDDs, particularly in targeting serious aggressive behaviors. In two of these studies (Perry et al. 1997; Zuddas et al. 2000), long-term (greater than 6 months) therapeutic benefit was reported.

Two open-label reports of olanzapine (Malone et al. 2001; Potenza et al. 1999) in the treatment of children and adolescents with autism and PDD not otherwise specified (NOS) suggest that olanzapine may be a safe and effective treatment of core symptoms in this population. However, a similar open-label trial of quetiapine in the treatment of six male children and adolescents with autism (Martin et al. 1999) suggested no therapeutic benefit and reported serious side effects in the treatment group. Clearly, further study of the use of atypical agents in this population is required.

Tourette's disorder. Efficacy of antipsychotic medications is often difficult to evaluate in patients with Tourette's disorder because of the natural waxing and waning of symptoms. Haloperidol in low doses is initially effective for up to 70% of patients (Cohen et al. 1992). Unfortunately, side effects often limit haloperidol's usefulness, and withdrawal of the drug may lead to severe exacerbation of symptoms for up to several months. Pimozide, a high-potency antipsychotic that also blocks calcium channels, has been demonstrated to be effective in the treatment of Tourette's disorder. Although considered an alternative medication to haloperidol and clonidine, one study suggests that pimozide may result in less cognitive impairment than haloperidol when prescribed at effective lower doses (Sallee and Rock 1994).

As has occurred in other disorders, atypical agents may eventually prove to be more effective and safer in this population. Risperidone was reported to be effective in reducing symptoms in two open-label studies of chronic tic/Tourette's disorder (Bruun and Budman 1996; Lombroso et al. 1995). In a double-blind, parallel-group study comparison of risperidone versus pimozide in the treatment of adolescents and adults with Tourette's disorder, Bruggeman et al. (2001) reported a favorable efficacy and tolerability profile for risperidone in this population, suggesting its potential benefit as a first-line agent in the treatment of Tourette's disorder.

A pilot study comparing ziprasidone and placebo in the treatment of children and adolescents with Tourette's disorder reported significant clinical improvement with ziprasidone, which was also well tolerated by the study subjects (Sallee et al. 2000). Additional studies are needed to establish this agent's safety and efficacy.

Conduct disorder and aggression. Studies of hospitalized, severely aggressive children, ages 6–12 years, have demonstrated short-term efficacy of haloperidol (1–6 mg/day or 0.04–0.21 mg/kg/day), thioridazine (mean = 170 mg/day), and molindone (mean = 26.8 mg/day) compared with placebo in reducing, although not eliminating, aggression, hostility, negativism, and explosiveness. Chlorpromazine leads to unacceptable sedation at relatively low doses (M. Campbell et al. 1985; Greenhill et al. 1985). A more recent double-blind study of risperidone (up to 3 mg/day) in the treatment of 10 youths with conduct disorder reported significant improvement in aggressive symptoms with risperidone in comparison with placebo, with few side effects (Findling et al. 2000). In a double-blind, parallel-group-design study, Buitelaar et al. (2001) similarly found significant efficacy for risperidone (1.5–4.0 mg/day), compared with placebo, in the treatment of aggression in hospitalized adolescents with disruptive behavior disorders and subaverage cognitive abilities. Risperidone was well tolerated in this study group as well.

Initiation and Maintenance

Medication should not be used as the sole treatment in the aforementioned complex disorders. Before medication is initiated, a complete physical examination and baseline laboratory workup, including CBC, differential, liver profile, and urinalysis, should be done. For those using clozapine, a baseline EEG is recommended, and a weekly WBC count with differential is mandatory. Antipsychotic medication use has been linked to the development of type 2 diabetes mellitus that may or may not be related to weight gain. Patients treated with the atypical agents clozapine and olanzapine should be monitored for changes in weight, as well as changes in fasting glucose levels. Both typical and atypical antipsychotic agents have been shown to increase QT intervals on ECG, potentially leading to dysrhythmias and sudden death. Clinicians should consider ECG monitoring, when appropriate.

Doses must be titrated individually, with careful attention to positive and negative effects. Age, weight, and severity of symptoms do not provide clear guidelines. The initial dose should be very low, with gradual increments no more than once or twice a week. Although divided doses are often used during titration, in most cases, once a therapeutic dosage has been reached, a single daily dose (usually at bedtime) can be used. Children metabolize these drugs more rapidly than do adults but also require lower plasma levels for efficacy (Teicher and Glod 1990). Antipsychotic medications can interact with a wide variety of other drugs (Teicher and Glod 1990).

Schizophrenia. Older adolescents with schizophrenia may require medication dosages in the adult range. Young adolescents fall in between, and doses must be empirically determined because few data exist. It may require several weeks for full therapeutic effect to be achieved. Although data are sparse, they are suggestive of the benefit and safety of atypical antipsychotics as first-line agents in this population. Because of its potentially lethal side effects, clozapine should be used only in cases refractory to treatment with typical or other atypical agents and should be started at very low dosages—12.5 mg/day or 25 mg/day—and titrated slowly upward (to minimize side effects) to an expected dosage range of 25–500 mg/day. Risperidone should also be initiated at low doses (0.5–1.0 mg) and titrated slowly, to prevent development of EPS, up to an expected dosage range of 2.0–4.0 mg/day. Olanzapine may be started at 5.0 mg/day and titrated upward to an expected range of 10.0–20.0 mg/day.

Pervasive developmental disorders. It is important to give a trial of sufficient length to determine if the drug is effective, barring serious side effects requiring immediate discontinuation. Typical daily doses are 0.5–4.0 mg of haloperidol. If the drug appears to be helpful, it should be continued for at least several months. At 3- to 6-month intervals, the drug should be discontinued to observe for withdrawal dyskinesias and to determine if the drug continues to be necessary. Some children may have physical withdrawal symptoms or a rebound phenomenon consisting of worsening of behavior for up to 8 weeks after the medication is stopped (M. Campbell et al. 1985). Developmentally disturbed children treated with risperidone may benefit from dosages as low as 0.5–1.0 mg/day (Fisman and Steele 1996; Masi et al. 2001) but may require doses up to 6.0 mg/day (Perry et al. 1997). Therapeutic daily dosages for olanzapine may range from 5.0 to 20.0 mg.

Tourette's disorder. Careful monitoring of patients with Tourette's disorder for several months before starting medication is possible, since this is a chronic disorder and not usually an emergency. This monitoring permits the clinician to establish a baseline of symptoms and to assess the need for psychological and educational interventions. An initial dose of haloperidol is 0.5 mg/day. It may be slowly increased up to 1–3 mg/day, divided in twice-daily doses (Cohen et al. 1992). Pimozide, which may be given in a single daily dose, is started at 1 mg/day and may be gradually increased to a maximum of 6–10 mg/day (0.2 mg/kg). The usual dose range is 2–6 mg/day (Cohen et al. 1992). Risperidone doses in the range of 1.0–2.5 mg/day appear to be useful (Lombroso et al.

1995). Sallee et al. (2000) initiated ziprasidone at 5 mg/day, titrating as high as 40 mg/day to achieve clinical effect in children with Tourette's disorder.

Risks and Side Effects

Acute EPS, including dystonic reactions, parkinsonian tremor, rigidity and drooling, and akathisia, occur as in adults. Laryngeal dystonia is potentially fatal. Acute dystonia may be treated with oral or intramuscular diphenhydramine, 25 mg or 50 mg, or benztropine mesylate, 0.5–2.0 mg. Adolescent boys seem to be more vulnerable to acute dystonic reactions than are adult patients, so the physician may be more inclined to use prophylactic antiparkinsonian medication. In children, however, reduction of antipsychotic dose is preferable to the use of antiparkinsonian agents (M. Campbell et al. 1985).

For treatment or prevention of parkinsonian symptoms, adolescents may be given the anticholinergic drug benztropine mesylate, 1–2 mg/day, in divided doses. Chronic parkinsonian symptoms are often drastically underrecognized by clinicians (Richardson et al. 1991). The neuromuscular consequences may impair the performance of age-appropriate activities, and the subjective effects may lead to noncompliance with medication. Akathisia may be especially difficult to identify in young patients or those with limited verbal abilities.

Tardive or withdrawal dyskinesias, some transient but others irreversible, seen in 8%–51% of antipsychotic-treated children and adolescents (M. Campbell et al. 1985), mandate caution regarding casual use of these drugs. Tardive dyskinesia has been documented in children and adolescents after as brief a period of treatment as 5 months (Herskowitz 1987) and may appear even during periods of constant medication dose. Cases of tardive dyskinesia have been reported in youths treated with risperidone (Feeney and Klykylo 1996), indicating that atypical antipsychotics may also cause this serious adverse reaction. In children with autism or Tourette's disorder, it may be especially difficult to distinguish medication-induced movements from those characteristic of the disorder. Before patients begin taking an antipsychotic medication, they should be examined carefully for abnormal movements by using a scale such as the Abnormal Involuntary Movement Scale (AIMS 1988) and should be periodically reexamined. Parents and patients (if they are able) should receive regular explanations of the risk of movement disorders.

Potentially fatal neuroleptic malignant syndrome has been reported with antipsychotic agents in children and adolescents (Silva et al. 1999), with a presentation similar to that seen in adults.

Weight gain may be problematic with the long-term use of the low-potency antipsychotics as well as the newer atypical antipsychotic medications. Abnormal laboratory findings seem to be reported less often for children than for adults, but the clinician should be alert to the possibility, especially of agranulocytosis or hepatic dysfunction. If an acute febrile illness or easy bruising occurs, medication should be withheld and CBC with differential and liver enzymes should be determined (M. Campbell et al. 1985).

Another concern is behavioral toxicity, manifested as worsening of preexisting symptoms or development of new symptoms such as hyperactivity or hypoactivity, irritability, apathy, withdrawal, stereotypies, tics, or hallucinations (M. Campbell et al. 1985). Low-potency antipsychotic drugs such as chlorpromazine and thioridazine can produce cognitive dulling and sedation that interfere with the patient's ability to benefit from school (M. Campbell et al. 1985) and are probably best avoided. Children and adolescents are more sensitive than adults to this sedation (Realmuto et al. 1984). Children may be at greater risk of antipsychotic-induced seizures than are adults because of their immature nervous systems and the high prevalence of abnormal EEGs in seriously disturbed children (Teicher and Glod 1990).

Anticholinergic side effects such as hypotension, dry mouth, constipation, nasal congestion, blurred vision, and urinary retention are unusual. Miscellaneous side effects include abdominal pain, enuresis (Realmuto et al. 1984), photosensitivity, and various neuroendocrine effects that may be especially distressing to adolescents.

Kumra et al. (1996) reported a high incidence of serious adverse effects (neutropenia and seizure activity) in children who were treated with clozapine, indicating a need for extremely close monitoring of children treated with this medication.

Side effects are a significant problem of long-term use of haloperidol for Tourette's disorder. Frequent complaints include lethargy, feeling like a "zombie," dysphoria, personality changes, weight gain, parkinsonian symptoms, akathisia, and intellectual dulling (Cohen et al. 1992). Dysphoria and school avoidance also have been reported (Mikkelsen et al. 1981). Pimozide appears to have a similar but less severe side effect profile.

Antipsychotic medications have been associated with prolongation of the QTc interval, torsades de pointes, and sudden death (Glassman 2001). Certain antipsychotics appear to be at greater risk for causing these problems. Recently, the FDA placed a black box warning on the use of thioridazine due to its significantly greater risk for causing QTc prolongation and sudden death. Pimozide and haloperidol have also been associated with torsades

de pointes. Ziprasidone has been shown to have a clear effect on cardiac repolarization, resulting in QTc prolongation greater than that caused by most antipsychotic agents but less than thioridazine. Although no serious cardiac events occurred during the premarketing testing of ziprasidone, its association with sudden death remains unclear at this time (Glassman and Bigger 2001). Clinically, the prudent use of ECG monitoring at baseline and during dosage titration in medications that are of higher risk seems indicated.

For a more detailed discussion of antipsychotic side effects and their management, see Chapter 24 of this textbook.

Anxiolytics, Sedatives, and Hypnotics

There are few data on the safety and efficacy of anxiolytics and sedative-hypnotics in children and adolescents, although they appear to respond similarly to adults (T. Spencer et al. 1995). In most cases, psychosocial interventions should precede and accompany pharmacotherapy.

Benzodiazepines

Indications and efficacy. Little research has examined the use of benzodiazepines in the treatment of pediatric psychiatric conditions. Benzodiazepines may be useful in the short-term treatment of children with severe anticipatory anxiety (Pfefferbaum et al. 1987). Although an open trial of alprazolam for children with avoidant and overanxious disorders was promising, a double-blind study did not find superiority of this drug over placebo in the context of an intensive treatment program (Simeon et al. 1992). Efficacy may have been limited by low doses and the short duration of treatment.

Preliminary evidence suggests that clonazepam may be useful in the treatment of panic disorder and antipsychotic-induced akathisia in adolescents (Biederman 1987; Kutcher et al. 1987, 1989, 1992). In a small open trial, clonazepam was found effective in diminishing tics in children with ADHD and comorbid tic disorders when used adjunctively with clonidine (Steingard et al. 1994). In a double-blind, placebo-controlled study, Graae et al. (1994) reported the clinical effectiveness of clonazepam in the treatment of anxiety disorders (predominantly separation anxiety disorder) in children. However, statistical superiority over placebo was not found, and most children evidenced side effects, notably sedation and disinhibition.

Initiation and maintenance. Infants and children absorb diazepam faster and metabolize it more quickly than do adults (Simeon and Ferguson 1985). Usual daily dose ranges for children and adolescents are as follows: lorazepam, 0.25–6.0 mg; diazepam, 1–20 mg; and alprazolam, 0.25–4.0 mg. Clonazepam has been used at 0.5–3.0 mg/day. Dosage schedule depends on age (more frequent in children) and the specific drug (Coffey 1990; Kutcher et al. 1992). When the medication is being discontinued, the dose needs to be tapered gradually to avoid withdrawal seizures or rebound anxiety.

Risks and side effects. In addition to the risks of substance abuse and physical or psychological dependence, side effects include sedation, cognitive dulling, ataxia, confusion, emotional lability, and worsening of psychosis. Paradoxical or disinhibition reactions may occur, manifested by acute excitation, irritability, increased anxiety, hallucinations, increased aggression and hostility, rage reactions, insomnia, euphoria, and/or incoordination (Coffey 1990; Graae et al. 1994; Reiter and Kutcher 1991; Simeon and Ferguson 1985).

Buspirone

Buspirone is a nonbenzodiazepine anxiolytic that is reported to be less sedating and have less risk of abuse or dependence than do the benzodiazepines. It may also have weak antidepressant efficacy.

Indications and efficacy. All data on buspirone treatment in children are anecdotal. Suggested uses include generalized anxiety disorder (Kutcher et al. 1992), mixed anxiety disorders (Simeon et al. 1994), as a supplementary drug in the treatment of OCD, and for reducing aggression and anxiety in patients with mental retardation (Ratey et al. 1991), PDDs (Buitelaar et al. 1998; Realmuto et al. 1989), or conduct disorder. Pfeffer et al. (1997) conducted an open trial in which buspirone (up to 50 mg/day) was used to treat 25 prepubertal children hospitalized with aggressive behavior and anxiety. Seventy-five percent of the children completed the study, and although improvements were demonstrated in overall functioning (as measured by the Global Assessment of Functioning), only 3 of the children were considered to have derived enough benefit from the medication to continue with treatment after the conclusion of the study. Randomized, controlled clinical studies are needed to assess the safety and efficacy of buspirone for pediatric psychiatric conditions.

Initiation and maintenance. Tentative guidelines for children and adolescents suggest a starting dose of 2.5–5.0 mg/day, increasing to three times a day over 2–3 days (Kutcher et al. 1992). The dose may be increased gradually to a maximum of 20 mg/day in children and 60 mg/day in adolescents, in three divided doses. The therapeutic effects may be delayed for 1–2 weeks after reaching the proper dose, with maximal effects not seen for an additional 2 weeks (Coffey 1990).

Risks and side effects. Reported adverse effects include insomnia, dizziness, anxiety, nausea, headache, restlessness, agitation, depression, and confusion (Coffey 1990). Possible psychotic symptoms were reported in two children treated with buspirone (Soni and Weintraub 1992), indicating that clinicians should closely monitor children who are prescribed this medication.

Beta-Blocking Agents

Indications and Efficacy

β-Adrenergic blockers may be useful in patients with otherwise uncontrollable rage reactions and impulsive aggression or self-injurious behavior, especially those with evidence of organicity. In a comprehensive review of the literature on this topic in 1993, Connor commented on the lack of methodologically controlled studies of these medications in the pediatric population. Little has been added to the literature since then. Propranolol has been found to be effective in daily doses of 50–960 mg, with a median of 160 mg (Williams et al. 1982). Anecdotal reports suggest that propranolol may be effective in the treatment of agitated, hyperaroused children and adolescents with PTSD (Famularo et al. 1988) and children and adolescents with "hyperventilation attacks" (Joorabchi 1977). In an open trial, a single 40-mg dose of propranolol appeared to be helpful in reducing test anxiety and improving performance in high school students (Faigel 1991). Pindolol and nadolol, with fewer side effects and longer half-lives, have been suggested as alternatives. A study by Connor et al. (1997) examined the use of nadolol in the treatment of overt aggression in 12 developmentally delayed youths aged 13–24 years. Seven of the 12 participants received nadolol exclusively. In this open, prospective pilot study, 10 of the 12 patients showed improvement in observer-rated measures of aggression and severity of illness. However, randomized controlled studies are necessary to elucidate the benefit, if any, of this class of medication in pediatric psychiatric populations.

Initiation and Maintenance

Initial workup should include a recent history and physical examination, with particular attention to medical contraindications: asthma, diabetes, bradycardia, heart block, cardiac failure, or hypothyroidism. Fasting blood sugar and glucose tolerance test may be indicated if there is risk of diabetes. An ECG may be considered.

In children and adolescents, the initial dose of propranolol is 10 mg three times a day, increasing by 10–20 mg every 3–4 days, and pulse and blood pressure should be monitored (minimum pulse 50, blood pressure 80/50). The standard daily dose range is 10–120 mg for children and 20–300 mg for adolescents, divided into three doses (2–8 mg/kg/day) (Coffey 1990). The short elimination half-life in children (2–3 hours) may necessitate four doses daily. Dose is titrated to clinical effect or side effects. Maximum improvement at a given dose may not be seen for up to 8 weeks. If a β-blocker is to be discontinued, it should be tapered gradually to avoid rebound hypertension and tachycardia. Because β-blockers may alter the blood levels of other medications, caution must be observed when β-blockers (especially propranolol, which is highly protein bound) are used in combination with other agents.

Risks and Side Effects

Side effects of β-blockers are generally the same as in adults. Tiredness, mild hypotension, and bradycardia are the most common. Decreased sexual interest and performance, dysphoria, insomnia, nightmares, or hypoglycemia (in patients with diabetes) may occur.

Naltrexone

Abnormalities of endogenous opioids have been suggested to occur in persons who have autism and in mentally retarded persons who engage in self-injurious behavior. Naltrexone, a potent opiate antagonist, has been found to be effective in the treatment of hyperactivity in autistic children in several double-blind and placebo-controlled studies (M. Campbell et al. 1993; Kolmen et al. 1995, 1997; Willemsen-Swinkels et al. 1995, 1996). Although earlier reports suggested that naltrexone treatment increased social interaction and decreased self-injury in autistic patients, these later controlled studies failed to demonstrate statistical difference from response to placebo in these behaviors. A recent double-blind, placebo-controlled crossover study in autistic children (Feldman et al. 1999) also failed to demonstrate improvement in communication skills with naltrexone in comparison with placebo. However, the study was limited by a short period of assessment per drug (2 weeks). In their randomized, placebo-controlled crossover study of 25 patients with Rett syndrome who received naltrexone, Percy et al. (1994) showed a worsening of motor function and a more rapid progression of the disorder in

40% of the patients receiving naltrexone, compared with none of those receiving placebo.

Two case reports suggest that naltrexone may be of benefit in alcohol dependence in adolescents. Wold and Kaminer (1997) described a decrease in craving and 30 days of abstinence in a 17-year-old youth. Lifrak et al. (1997) reported on two adolescents who experienced decreased craving and either a reduction in drinking days or successful maintenance of abstinence with naltrexone. All of the patients in the above reports were treated with naltrexone at 50 mg/day. These reports, while anecdotal, suggest that naltrexone may have a place in the treatment of alcohol dependence in adolescents, as it does in adults, although further study is needed.

In doses of 0.5–2.0 mg/kg/day, naltrexone appears to be safe, with only mild side effects noted. No changes in any laboratory measures, ECG, or vital signs have been demonstrated in children or adolescents. Clearly, further controlled trials are needed, but cautious clinical use of naltrexone in patients with severe behavioral symptoms or adolescents with alcohol dependence may be indicated, particularly given its benign side effect profile in this age group.

Desmopressin

Desmopressin is an analogue of antidiuretic hormone administered as a nasal spray or oral tablet to treat nocturnal enuresis. Desmopressin acts by increasing water absorption in the kidneys, thereby reducing the volume of urine. Onset of action is rapid, and side effects are mild (nasal mucosal dryness or irritation, headache, epistaxis, and nausea) in patients with normal electrolyte regulation. In their review of the literature, Thompson and Rey (1995) concluded that desmopressin is superior to placebo in the treatment of nocturnal enuresis. They further noted that behavioral methods are more effective, and that the relapse rate after cessation of desmopressin is high. Most of the studies cited at the time of their review were of brief duration, usually 2 weeks.

In a recent study examining the long-term use of desmopressin, Hjalmas et al. (1998) followed children for 1 year after successful dose titration with nasally administered desmopressin. Three-hundred and ninety-nine children entered the study, and 245 of these (61%) demonstrated at least a 50% reduction in frequency of enuretic episodes after a 6-week period of dosage titration. These 245 patients then entered a 1-year follow-up phase during which treatment was interrupted for 1 week every 3 months. During this follow-up period, 77 children remained dry during the periods off medication, and by the end of the study, another 73 children had obtained a

90% or greater reduction in the frequency of enuretic episodes. The authors of this open study concluded that long-term administration of desmopressin is both safe and effective.

The usual dose is 20–40 µg intranasally at bedtime or 200–400 µg orally. Randomized, double-blind studies have demonstrated that oral desmopressin is just as effective as the intranasal preparation and may be better tolerated (Janknegt et al. 1997; Skoog et al. 1997). Relapse is likely on discontinuation of treatment. Although water intoxication is rare, children should be encouraged to limit fluid intake in the evenings when taking desmopressin.

Electroconvulsive Therapy

Experience in the use of electroconvulsive therapy (ECT) in adolescents is limited, and reports of use in prepubertal children are extremely rare. Rey and Walter (1997) published a review of the literature identifying 60 reports describing 396 patients under 18 years of age who had received ECT. Improvement rates were noted to be 63% for depression, 80% for mania, 42% for schizophrenia, and 80% for catatonia. Although the authors concluded that ECT in adolescents appears to be effective and relatively safe, they noted that many of the published reports were limited by small numbers and lack of consistent diagnostic standardization. No controlled studies were identified.

Walter et al. (1999) surveyed by telephone 26 adolescents who were treated with ECT during 1990–1998. Fifty percent of respondents reported that ECT had been helpful, and the vast majority stated that, if indicated, they would repeat the treatment.

Complications of ECT in the pediatric population include brief cognitive impairment, behavioral disinhibition, and post-ECT anxiety (Bertagnoli and Borchardt 1990). Although Ghaziuddin et al. (2000) identified significant impairments in cognitive functioning between pre-ECT testing and early post-ECT testing (within the first 10 days of treatment), follow-up cognitive testing several months after treatment demonstrated no significant difference from pre-ECT testing. Similarly, Cohen et al. (2000) identified no long-term differences in cognitive functioning when they compared adolescents who had undergone ECT for severe mood disorder (more than 1 year earlier) with a matched control group of adolescents. Limitations of these studies, including small sample size, make it difficult to draw firm conclusions regarding potential long-term impairment.

Psychotherapy

In 1999, the Psychotherapy Task Force of the American Academy of Child and Adolescent Psychiatry addressed, among other issues, matters of psychotherapy research and the clinical use of psychotherapy in children. The importance of psychotherapeutic techniques in the practice of child and adolescent psychiatry is reflected in the first lines of the Task Force's (Ritvo et al. 1999) policy statement:

> Psychotherapy is and must remain a core skill and central to the practice of child and adolescent psychiatry. The psychotherapies remain essential treatment modalities for children's cognitive, emotional and behavioral problems. Additionally, psychotherapy knowledge and skills inform all psychiatric clinical activities, including diagnostic assessment, pharmacotherapy, and consultation to agencies, schools, and other physicians, and well as collaboration with and supervision of staff and trainees.

Although research has shown that psychotherapy can be effective for certain pediatric conditions (Kazdin 2000), methodological challenges arise when studying the efficacy of psychotherapy for children and adolescents. Donenberg (1999) outlined some of these challenges, which include accounting for the many influences in children's lives that affect treatment and functioning and determining what (or who) should be the focus of change (e.g., parent, child, style of parenting). Moreover, how should outcomes in psychotherapy be measured, and who (e.g., parent, child, teacher) should do the measuring? Finally, how does the ongoing development of the child influence the effectiveness of therapy? Several authors (Borkovec and Miranda 1996; Kazdin 2000) have also commented on some of the difficulties inherent in applying research-based techniques of child and adolescent psychotherapy to "real world" clinical practice in which children may be more symptomatic or have other comorbid conditions, and where treatment is often more eclectic. Examining issues related to psychotherapy research will inform our understanding of how the biological, psychological, and social changes brought about by psychotherapy provide relief for suffering children and their families.

Psychotherapies are classified by theoretical model, target of intervention, duration, and goals of treatment (Table 33–10). More data are emerging regarding the use and efficacy of psychotherapy for particular disorders, especially depressive and anxiety disorders.

TABLE 33–10.   Varieties of psychotherapy

Theoretical foundations
Psychoanalytic
Behavioral or social learning
Developmental
Ecological
Family systems
Cognitive
Target of intervention
Individual
Parent
Family
Group
Duration
Short (4–6 sessions)
Intermediate (up to 6 months)
Long (6 months to years)
Goals of therapy
Crisis intervention
Support
Symptom removal/improved functioning
Removing impediments to development

Individual Psychotherapy

All individual therapies have certain common themes (Strupp 1973):

- Relationship with a therapist who is identified as a helping person and who has some degree of control and influence over the patient
- Instillation of hope and improved morale
- Use of attention, encouragement, and suggestion
- Goals of helping the patient to achieve greater control, competence, mastery, and/or autonomy; to improve coping skills; and to abandon or modify unrealistic expectations of himself or herself, others, and the environment

In the treatment of children, it is essential to consider the patients' environment and family dynamics. In most cases, work with parents and school, and often pediatricians, welfare agencies, courts, or recreation leaders, must accompany individual therapy. The cooperation of parents, and often teachers, is required to maintain the child in treatment and to remove any secondary gain resulting from the symptoms. The therapist must be aware of a patient's level of physical, cognitive, and emotional development in order to understand the symptoms, set appropriate goals, and tailor effective interventions.

Communication With Children and Adolescents

Children are less able to use abstract language than are adults. They use play to express feelings, to narrate past events, to work through trauma, and to express wishes and hopes. It is less threatening and anxiety provoking if the therapist uses the metaphor of the play and bases questions and comments on characters in the play rather than on the child (even if the connection is clear to the therapist). Effective communications are tailored to the child's stage of language, cognitive, and affective development. The therapist must be aware that the vocabulary of some bright and precocious children exceeds their emotional understanding of events and concepts.

Dramatic play with dolls or puppets, drawing, painting, or modeling with clay, as well as questions about dreams, wishes, or favorite stories or television shows, can provide access to children's fantasies, emotions, and concerns. Adolescents may prefer creative writing or more complex expressive art techniques.

The Resistant Child or Adolescent

It is not surprising that many children or adolescents do not cooperate in therapy. Most are brought to treatment by adults. These young patients often do not wish to change themselves or their behaviors and view their parents' and teachers' complaints as unreasonable or unfair. In addition, a child or adolescent may refuse to participate in or may attempt to sabotage therapy for a variety of dynamic reasons (Gardner 1979). Effective interventions are tailored to the cause of the resistance.

A child who is anxious or having difficulty separating from a parent may be helped by initially permitting the parent to remain in the therapy room. When a child or adolescent does not talk, whether from anxiety or opposition, the therapist often addresses this reluctance, either directly or through play. Long silences are not generally helpful and tend to increase anxiety or battles for control. Attractive play materials help to make therapy less threatening and to encourage participation while the therapist builds an alliance. However, the therapist must guard against the danger of sessions becoming mere play or recreation instead of therapy. Gardner (1979) has developed a variety of techniques that incorporate therapeutic activities with storytelling, drama, and game boards. Using behavioral contingencies in therapy also may improve motivation, especially of materially deprived children.

The Schizophrenic Child

Certain types of individual psychotherapy may be useful as part of a comprehensive treatment plan for children who are schizophrenic or very fragile (Cantor and Kestenbaum 1986). The therapist must be prepared to provide structure, to limit regression and fantasy, and to focus on reality testing and development of stronger defense mechanisms and healthier coping skills. The relationship with the therapist may be especially crucial for these youngsters.

Types of Individual Psychotherapy

Psychodynamic psychotherapies. In *psychoanalysis*, an infrequently used treatment modality for children and adolescents, neurotic symptoms are viewed as arising from internalized intrapsychic conflict, nonorganic developmental arrest, or regression. The goals are to remove those symptoms that have become independent of their original context, through structural changes in defensive organization and personality. The analyst functions as a transference object. The principal technique for producing change is interpretation of unconscious content, resulting in greater conscious awareness and adaptive control of emotions and behavior. The expense, frequency of sessions, duration of treatment, and often lack of immediate symptom relief have contributed to the decreased use of psychoanalysis.

Psychodynamically oriented psychotherapy is grounded in psychoanalytic theory but is more flexible and emphasizes the real relationship with the therapist and the provision of a corrective emotional experience rather than the transference. Frequency is typically once or twice a week, most commonly over a period of 1–2 years, although shorter, time-limited dynamic psychotherapies are also available (Dulcan 1984). Interaction between the parents and the therapist is more active. Goals of therapy include symptom resolution, change in behavior, and return to normal developmental process. Change occurs via transference interpretation and maturation of defenses, catharsis, development of insight, ego strengthening, improved reality testing, and sublimation (Adams 1982). The therapist forms an alliance with the child or adolescent, reassures, promotes controlled regression, identifies feelings, clarifies thoughts and events, makes interpretations, judiciously educates and advises, and acts as an advocate for the patient (Adams 1982).

Dynamically oriented individual therapy alone is much more likely to be effective for children and adolescents who are in emotional distress or who are struggling to deal with a stressor than for those children with behavior problems. Children and adolescents with attention-deficit, oppositional, or conduct disorders rarely acknowledge their problem behaviors and are usually better treated in family or group therapy, by parent training in behavior management, or in a structured milieu. Youngsters with ADHD have little insight into their behavior and its effect on others, and they may be genuinely unable to report their problems or to reflect on them. However, insight-oriented therapy may be useful for some of these youngsters to address comorbid anxiety or depression or symptoms resulting from psychological trauma. Psychoanalytic therapy is usually considered to be contraindicated in psychotic or very disturbed children.

Supportive therapy. This type of therapy has less ambitious goals than dynamically oriented psychotherapies and is usually focused on a particular crisis or stressor. The therapist provides support to the patient until a stressor resolves, a developmental crisis has passed, or the patient or environment changes sufficiently so that other adults can take on the supportive role. There is a real relationship with the therapist, who facilitates catharsis and provides understanding and judicious advice.

Time-limited therapy. All of the various models of time-limited therapy have in common a planned, relatively brief duration; a predominant focus on the presenting problem; a high degree of structure and attention to specific, limited goals; and active roles for both therapist and patient. Length of treatment varies among models from several sessions to 6 months. The short duration is used to increase patient motivation, participation, and reliance on resources within the patient's world rather than on the therapist (Kisch 1997). Theoretical foundations include psychodynamic, crisis, family systems, cognitive, behavioral or social learning and guidance, or educational theories (Dulcan 1984; Dulcan and Piercy 1985).

The limited outcome data available indicate that time-limited treatment is at least as effective for some patients as longer-term therapy. These methods have been recommended for both multiproblem families in crisis who are unlikely to persist in longer-term treatment and well-functioning children and families with circumscribed problems of relatively recent onset. Although time-limited treatment is designed to be brief, children or families may return to a therapist should other problems or symptoms develop for an additional "round" of treatment. Such intermittent interaction can remain problem-focused and reduce dependency on the therapist (Kisch 1997).

A model of interpersonal psychotherapy has been modified for depressed adolescents (IPT-A; Mufson et al. 1994). This 12-week treatment focuses on improving interpersonal relationships in the lives of depressed adolescents through role clarification and enhanced communication. This modality has been elaborated in a treatment manual and has demonstrated efficacy in preliminary study. In a 12-week study of adolescents with major depression randomized to either weekly treatment with IPT-A or clinical monitoring, 75% of the patients receiving IPT-A, versus 46% of the patients in the clinical monitoring group, had improved (as evidenced by Hamilton Rating Scale for Depression scores of less than 6) at week 12 compared with the clinical monitoring group (Mufson et al. 1999).

Cognitive-behavioral therapy. The CBT techniques developed for the treatment of depression in adults have been adapted for use in children and adolescents. Studies have demonstrated the benefits of CBT for depression in adolescents (Clarke et al. 1999), for OCD in children and adolescents (March 1995), for posttraumatic stress symptoms in children and adolescents (King et al. 2000; March et al. 1998a), for social phobia in female adolescents (Hayward et al. 2000), and for school refusal in children and adolescents (King et al. 1998). Caution is needed to ensure that the homework assignments that are an integral part of this therapy are not perceived as aversive when added to homework assigned in school. Prepubertal children's more concrete cognitive processes may make this rather intellectual model impractical, although creative adaptations and the incorporation of behavioral techniques can render this approach accessible (Emery et al. 1983). Cognitive self-control training may be effective in reducing aggressive behavior in adolescents, although compliance with self-monitoring procedures is often poor (Dangel et al. 1989).

Parent Counseling

Parent counseling or guidance is primarily a psychoeducational intervention, conducted in a mental health setting. It may be conducted with a single parent or couple, or in groups. In counseling sessions, parents learn about normal child and adolescent development. Efforts are made to help parents better understand their child and his or her problems and to modify practices that seem to be contributing to the current difficulties (whatever their original cause). The therapist's understanding of the parents' point of view and of the hardships of living with a disturbed child is crucial to the therapist's successful work with the child. For some parents who have serious difficulties of their own, parent counseling may merge into or pave the way for marital therapy or individual treatment of one or more parents.

Virtually all parents of children with psychiatric or learning problems need and deserve education in the nature of their children's disorders, support of their own emotional needs, and help in selecting treatments and managing difficult behaviors. Parents spend far more time with their children than the therapist and can powerfully assist or impede treatment. Parents of children with chronic problems must become skilled advocates to ensure that their children receive the treatment and schooling they need. Carefully selected reading material and other resources may be extremely useful to parents (see the appendix to this chapter).

Behavior Therapy

In behavior therapy, symptoms are viewed as resulting from bad habits, faulty learning, or inappropriate environmental responses to behavior rather than as stemming from unconscious or intrapsychic motivation. Attention is focused on observable behaviors, psychophysiological responses, and self-report statements. Behavioral approaches are characterized by detailed assessment of problematic responses and the environmental conditions that elicit and maintain them, the development of strategies to produce change in the environment and therefore in the patient's behavior, and repeated assessment to evaluate the success of the intervention.

In an operant approach, positive and negative environmental factors that increase or decrease the frequency of behaviors are identified and then modified in an attempt to decrease problem behaviors and increase adaptive ones. The token economy uses points, stars, or tokens that can be earned for desirable behaviors (and lost for problem behaviors) and exchanged for backup reinforcers. These reinforcers may be money, food, toys, privileges, or time with an adult in a pleasant activity. Token economies can be successfully used by parents, teachers, and therapists (with groups or individuals) and by staff on inpatient units.

Indications and Efficacy

Behavior therapy is by far the most thoroughly evaluated psychological treatment for children. Maximally effective programs require home and school cooperation, focus on specific target behaviors, and ensure that contingencies follow behavior quickly and consistently.

Behavior therapy is the most effective treatment for simple phobias, for enuresis and encopresis, and for the noncompliant behaviors seen in oppositional defiant disorder and conduct disorder. For youngsters with ADHD, behavior modification can improve both academic achievement and behavior, when specifically targeted. Both punishment (time-out and response cost) and reward components are required. Behavior modification is more effective than medication in improving peer interactions, but skills may need to be taught first. Many youngsters require programs that are consistent, intensive, and prolonged (months to years). A wide variety of other childhood problems, such as motor and vocal tics, trichotillomania, and sleep problems, are treated by behavior modification, either alone or in combination with pharmacotherapy.

The greatest weaknesses of behavior therapy are lack of maintenance of improvement over time and failure of changes to generalize to situations other than the ones in which training occurred. Generalization and maintenance can be maximized by conducting training in the settings in which behavior change is desired, at multiple times and places, facilitating transfer to naturally occurring reinforcers and gradually fading reinforcement on an intermittent schedule (Stokes and Baer 1977).

Parent Management Training

Effective training packages, based on social learning theory, have been developed for parents of noncompliant, oppositional, and aggressive children (Barkley and Benton 1998; Forehand and McMahon 1981; Patterson 1975; Webster-Stratton 1992, 2000) and delinquent adolescents (Patterson and Forgatch 1987). Such behaviors in children have been found to lead to inappropriately harsh or ineffective parental responses. Through training, parents are taught to give clear instructions, to positively reinforce good behavior, and to use punishment effectively. One frequently used negative contingency is the time-out, so called because it puts the child in a quiet, boring area where there is a time-out from accidental or naturally occurring positive reinforcement. The most powerful parent training programs use a combination of written materials, verbal instruction, and videotapes in social learning principles and contingency management, modeling by the therapist, and behavioral rehearsal of skills to be used. Families with low socioeconomic status, parental psychopathology (such as depression), marital conflict, and lack of a social support network require maximally potent interventions, with attention to parental problems as necessary. Other families may be able to succeed with written materials only or with manuals supplemented by group lectures. Parent management training was shown to be effective in improving child behavior in a meta-analysis of 26 controlled studies conducted by Serketich and Dumas (1996).

Behavioral intervention can be done in the context of family therapy in which the family learns how to negotiate and to solve problems together. A key technique is parent–child contingency contracting, which entails a written social contract between parent and child to change behaviors in both parties, with specified contingencies (Blechman 1981).

Classroom Behavior Modification

Techniques for behavior modification in schools include token economies, class rules, and attention to positive behavior, as well as response cost programs in which reinforcers are withdrawn in response to undesirable behavior. Although teachers often resist what they perceive as extra work, an effective program for children with attention and conduct problems required only that teachers observe every 30 minutes whether children were on task and provide verbal feedback (Pelham and Murphy 1986). Reinforcers such as positive recognition or stars on a chart may be dispensed by teachers or more tangible rewards or privileges by parents through the use of daily report cards. Even special education teachers rarely have sophisticated skills in behavior modification, and therapists may need to work closely with teachers and other school staff to develop appropriate programs.

Behavioral Treatment of Specific Symptoms

Behavioral treatments are useful for treating enuresis, encopresis, and certain anxiety disorders in children. Particularly in the case of enuresis or encopresis, an evaluation for other psychiatric disorders and sexual abuse as well as a medical history and physical examination should precede behavioral treatment.

Enuresis. In younger children, especially those who wet only at night, enuresis is largely a consequence of delayed maturation. While waiting for the child to outgrow it, the most useful strategy is to minimize secondary symptoms by discouraging the parents from punishing or ridiculing the child. Older children can be taught to change their own beds, thus reducing expectable negative reactions from parents. A simple monitoring and reward procedure that includes a chart with stars to be exchanged for rewards may be effective for some children who are motivated to stop wetting the bed.

Two additional programs found to be effective in treating nocturnal enuresis are the urine alarm device and dry bed training (DBT). The urine alarm is a conditioning treatment that results in dryness in up to 75% of children (Mikkelsen 2001). The success rate can be increased and relapses minimized by the addition of contingencies for wet and dry nights, diminished gradually once urinary control is achieved (Kaplan et al. 1989). DBT (Azrin et al. 1974) is an equally effective, but somewhat more cumbersome, behavioral program that includes positive practice, contingent response, and the urine alarm in combination. A DBT parent training manual is available (see Azrin and Foxx 1974 under "Enuresis" in the appendix).

Children who are secondarily enuretic (having previously been dry) and those who have accompanying psychiatric problems are more difficult to treat. Other interventions may be necessary before they are motivated to participate in or be responsive to behavioral techniques.

Encopresis. The treatment of encopresis is somewhat more complex because encopresis frequently results from chronic constipation and stool withholding, which creates physiological consequences requiring medical treatment. In addition, children with encopresis more commonly have associated psychiatric disorders than do those with enuresis.

Behavioral treatment of encopresis must be integrated into a plan that also includes educational and psychological approaches (Levine 1982). Because encopresis often results in stool retention and impaction, an initial bowel cleanout is sometimes required. This regimen is followed by a bowel "retraining" program using oral mineral oil, a high-roughage diet, ample fluid intake, and a mild suppository. The behavioral program focuses on the development of a regular toileting routine with scheduled positive toilet practicing. Behaviors that progressively approximate the appropriate passing of feces in the toilet are rewarded. Routine pants checks followed by contingent positive or negative response are often included. Administration of enemas by parents is contraindicated, as that alone does not improve bowel function and is toxic to the parent–child relationship.

Anxiety disorders. Desensitization, in vivo or in fantasy, is the treatment of choice for simple phobias, often supplemented by modeling. The principles and techniques are essentially the same as those used with adults, with modification for developmental level. In vivo desensitization, often combined with contingency management and parent guidance, may be effective in the treatment of school avoidance (school phobia) resulting from separation anxiety disorder.

Behavioral approaches using exposure plus response prevention (ERP) appear to be effective in the treatment of OCD in children and adolescents. March et al. (1994) have developed a protocoled, time-limited ERP treatment that has demonstrated therapeutic effect in an open trial with children and adolescents with OCD.

Behavioral Medicine Techniques

Behavioral methods can be used to treat somatic symptoms. These interventions should be carried out in collaboration with the primary physician and any necessary medical specialists. Children are just as sensitive as adults are to implications that their symptoms are not "real," so care must be taken to explain the interaction of psychological processes and physical symptoms and to develop a working alliance.

A variety of techniques have been used for children, in much the same way as for adults, but with adaptations for the children's level of cognitive or emotional development. Especially important is an understanding of any misconceptions youngsters may have about the disease state and its treatment. These notions vary according to a patient's stage of cognitive development and his or her unique experience.

Hypnotherapy. Children are more hypnotizable than are adults (Williams 1979). Although hypnosis is occasionally used to facilitate insight in dynamic psychotherapy or to remove a behavioral symptom or habit, for children the most common uses of hypnosis are in the treatment of physical symptoms with a psychological component or to help a child manage pain or nausea associated with a physical disorder or its treatment. Successful use of hypnosis to reduce pain and anxiety has not been reported in children younger than age 6 years (Varni et al. 1986).

Relaxation training. Four types of relaxation procedures are applicable to children and adolescents: progressive muscle relaxation, meditative breathing, autogenics (i.e., silently repeating commands or statements), and imagery-based techniques (Masek et al. 1984). The choice is determined by the characteristics of the child or adolescent and of the disorder being treated. For example, asthmatic children and adolescents may have difficulty using breathing techniques. Imagery may fit particularly well with most children's interest in fantasy. Relaxation training has been used in the treatment of pediatric migraine, juvenile rheumatoid arthritis, and hemophilia. These techniques, also called cognitive-behavioral self-regulation of pain perception, can result not only in decreased subjective experience of pain and reduced need for analgesics, but also in improved mood, self-esteem, and physical and social functioning (Varni et al. 1986). Similar techniques also have been used in the treatment of children and adolescents with asthma or cystic fibrosis.

Pain behavior management. The strategy of pain behavior management is to use operant techniques in the treatment of chronic pain. For example, the antecedents and consequences of headaches are determined by observation and by keeping a pain diary (if the child is old enough), and then attempts are made to modify those situations and events that seem to precipitate or positively reinforce pain as the therapist works with the patient, parents, teachers, pediatrician, and significant others. Emphasis is placed on stress management techniques (Masek et al. 1984) and on functioning normally despite pain. With reduced pain and pain-related behaviors, patients experience an increased sense of control and mastery and an increase in age-appropriate positive activities (Varni et al. 1986). These techniques have been adapted to the treatment of respiratory symptoms in children and adolescents with asthma or cystic fibrosis.

Stress inoculation. Stress inoculation is a multicomponent cognitive-behavioral approach that combines education, modeling procedures, systematic desensitization, hypnosis, contingency management, and training and practice in coping skills such as imagery and breathing exercises. It is useful in preventing stress and anxiety in children before medical and dental procedures and in chronically ill children for reducing anxiety, pain, or other discomfort related to repeated procedures such as spinal taps, bone marrow aspirations, and chemotherapy injections. Before a therapist implements such a program, the medical procedure is analyzed in detail, including the rationale, details of the procedure and its sensations and side effects, and portions likely to be perceived as uncomfortable or frightening. Also important are the characteristics and previous direct or vicarious experience of the patient (Melamed et al. 1984; Varni et al. 1986).

Family Treatment

Attempts to treat children and adolescents without considering the persons with whom they live and the patients' relationships with other significant persons are doomed to failure. Any change in one family member, whether resulting from a psychiatric disorder, psychiatric treatment, a normal developmental process, or an outside event, is likely to produce change in other family members and in their relationships. Family constellations vary widely from the traditional nuclear family, to single-parent family, a blended or step-family, an adoptive or foster family, or a group home. The term *parents* in this chapter applies to adults filling the parenting role, whatever their actual relationship to the patient.

Evaluation of Families

Data should be gathered on each person living with the patient, as well as on others who may be important or have been so in the past (e.g., noncustodial parents, grandparents, or siblings who are no longer living at home). It is often useful to have at least one session that includes all significant family members. For families with young children, techniques such as the use of family drawings or puppet play or the assignment of family tasks to be carried out in the session are often useful. A variety of schemas exist by which to assess a family's structure and dynamic functioning.

The family's developmental stage offers a clue to predictable transitional crises as children are born, become adolescents, and are launched from the nuclear family (Carter and McGoldrick 1980).

Several different models of family assessment and evaluation exist. Regardless of which model is used, a family assessment should be able to identify the stage of the family life cycle and the challenges encountered therein, indicate problematic areas of family interaction that require intervention, and reveal areas of the child's development that may be at risk because of influences from the family (e.g., difficulties in developing effective communication skills). Other goals of a family assessment should be to define areas of parental problems or psychopathology, identify other vulnerable family members, and determine how the family may be either contributing to or compensating for a child's disorder (Davidson et al. 2001).

Tasks of the initial session of a family assessment include establishing an alliance with family members; gathering data by direct questions, by observing, and by assessing the impact of trial interventions; and proposing a provisional plan for treatment.

Family Therapy

Family therapy addresses primarily the interaction *among* family members rather than the processes *within* an individual. In the most general sense, family therapy is psychological treatment conducted with an identified patient and at least one biological or functional (i.e., by marriage, adoption, and so forth) family member. Related techniques include therapy with an individual patient that takes a family systems perspective or therapy sessions with family members other than the identified patient, based on noncompliance with treatment, severity of illness, or other factors. These days, it is rare for family therapists to insist that all family members attend sessions.

Although some advocate family therapy as the best and only treatment for all disorders, most clinicians would agree that there are some situations in which family therapy is preferred over other treatments, others in which it should be combined with other treatments, and still others in which it is not possible or is relatively contraindicated. Research on this topic is limited, so accumulated clinical judgment and experience must prevail.

Family therapy may be particularly useful when there are dysfunctional interactions or impaired communication within the family, especially when these appear to be related to the presenting problem. It also may be useful when symptoms seem to have been precipitated by difficulty with a developmental stage for an individual or the family or by a change in the family such as divorce or remarriage. If more than one family member is symptomatic, family therapy may be both more efficient and more effective than multiple individual treatments. Family therapy should be considered when one family member improves with treatment but another, not in treatment, worsens. In any case, the family must have, or be induced to have, sufficient motivation to participate. When the identified patient is relatively unmotivated to participate or to change, family therapy is likely to be more effective than individual therapy. Attention to family systems issues also may be useful when progress is blocked in individual therapy or in behavior therapy.

Family therapy is contraindicated as a sole treatment method in cases of clearly organic physical or mental illness or if the family equilibrium is precarious and one or more family members are at serious risk of decompensation. In these situations, family therapy may be useful in combination with other treatments, such as medication or hospitalization. It is counterproductive to include in family therapy sessions a patient who is acutely psychotic, violent, or delusional regarding the family. Family sessions may not be helpful when a parent has severe, intractable, or minimally relevant psychopathology or when the child strongly prefers individual treatment. Children should not be included in sessions in which parents persist (despite redirection) in criticizing the children or in sharing inappropriate information, when the most critical need is marital therapy, or when parents primarily need specific, concrete help with practical affairs.

A variety of family therapies are considered when treating children and adolescents (Table 33–11).

TABLE 33–11. Models of family therapy

Structural
Behavioral
Multigenerational
Psychoeducational
Strategic
Multiple family group

Structural therapy. Structural therapy has been the model most used and studied when a child or adolescent is the identified patient. Developed by Salvador Minuchin and his colleagues at the Philadelphia Child Guidance Clinic, it has been used extensively with families of children and adolescents with eating disorders and psychophysiological disorders such as asthma. Focus is on the present, in which the identified patient's symptoms are presumed to serve a function for the family. The process of assessment includes mapping patterns of communication and the structure of the family, including the location and permeability of boundaries between family members and around the family and its subsystems. Other important variables are the character and flexibility of alignments of family members, including alliances (joining together of two or more members in a common interest or task) and coalitions (joint actions directed against one or more family members). Data are gathered on the distribution of power within the family and on the family's sources of stress and support in the environment.

The therapist uses assigned tasks and his or her interactions with family members to provoke change in the family structure and thereby its functioning. Relabeling (i.e., redefining a behavior or symptom to have a different, less negative meaning) opens alternative pathways for family interactions.

Multigenerational family therapy. Pioneered by Murray Bowen, multigenerational family therapy emphasizes how current patterns in families are repetitions of the past. Change results from insights gained in the exploration of parents' families of origin and the relationships over several generations of the nuclear family to the extended family. Grandparents are often involved indirectly or even included in sessions.

Strategic family therapy. Strategic family therapy, developed by Haley and by Palazolli and her colleagues, produces change through a complex and indirect plan of action that is not fully shared with the family. In practice, paradoxical instructions are devised to upset the family equilibrium and permit change, especially in families resistant to more straightforward techniques. This potentially powerful model should be used only by experienced therapists.

Behavioral family therapy. Models of behavioral family therapy include Patterson's (1975), based on social learning theory, and Alexander's (1992) functional family therapy, both of which are used in the treatment of children and adolescents with conduct disorder. Henggeler et al. (1998) extended this model to a multisystemic approach that uses energetic outreach into the home, neighborhood, and school and adds peer group and school-based interventions to family treatment of adolescent delinquents.

Psychoeducational family therapy. A psychoeducational approach to family therapy has been most extensively developed in the treatment of families of adult schizophrenic patients (C.M. Anderson et al. 1980), but it has been extended to a number of childhood disorders, such as eating disorders, ADHD, and depression. Detailed didactic presentations about the disorder, in the setting of a multiple family group, are designed to improve the family's coping skills through increased understanding of the illness and its treatment, to teach home behavior management techniques, and to enhance family support networks. Ongoing treatment of individual families includes family systems interventions when educational and behavioral techniques are blocked by dysfunctional family structures or processes. The identified patient is included in family sessions when his or her clinical status permits.

Multiple family therapy. The multifamily approach combines features of group and family therapy. Sessions include three to five families with similar problems who may be isolated from other supports and who can benefit from the interaction with other families.

Group Therapy

Indications

Group therapy is particularly appropriate for children, who are often more willing to reveal their thoughts and feelings to peers than to adults. Establishing rewarding social relationships, a crucial developmental task for children of all ages, is especially difficult for those youths with a psychiatric disorder. Group therapy offers unparalleled opportunities for the clinician to evaluate youths' behavior with peers, to model and facilitate practice of important skills, and to provide youngsters with companionship and mutual support. Interventions by peers may be far more acute and powerful in their effect than those by an adult therapist. An additional benefit is the larger number of patients who can benefit from limited therapist time.

Target symptoms include absent or conflictual peer relationships, aggression, withdrawal, timidity, difficulty with separation, and deficient social interactive or problem-solving skills. These problems often are not apparent or accessible to intervention in individual therapy sessions. Group therapy can be a powerful modality in the treatment of adolescents with eating disorders or substance abuse.

On the negative side, forming an outpatient group is often tedious and time consuming. Diverse schedules and lack of transportation make gathering a sufficient number of compatible patients difficult. More space and preparation are required than for individual or family therapy.

Group psychotherapy is contraindicated for those who are acutely psychotic, paranoid, or actively suicidal. Adolescents with sociopathic traits or behaviors should not be included in groups with teenagers who might be victimized or intimidated. Severely aggressive or hyperactive children probably should not be included in outpatient groups because of the difficulty in controlling their behavior, the contagion of problem behaviors, and the intimidation of less assertive children. Groups should *not* be used as a repository for unmotivated, nonverbal, difficult patients.

Although group therapy may be used as the sole treatment modality, it is often used in combination with another intervention. Groups also may serve an evaluation function, particularly for preschool- and school-age children (Scheidlinger 1984).

Technical Considerations

Theoretical models. All of the theoretical models used in individual therapy may be used with groups. Therapy may be exclusively verbal, or it may include expressive arts techniques, psychodrama, arts and crafts, and sports activities; behavioral techniques such as modeling or overt practice; or cognitive-behavioral strategies for depression (Lewinsohn et al. 1990). The skilled group therapist has an understanding of systems theory and group process, whatever the model of intervention. Contingency management (i.e., rewards and consequences) may be an essential adjunct for groups that include children with behavior disorders.

Group size. Groups typically range from 4 to 10 patients, with the number varying according to the number of leaders, the age and type of pathology of the group members, and the number of suitable candidates available.

Group composition. The composition of the group depends on its purpose. Patients in support groups are chosen because they share a single stressor—for example, sexual abuse, parental divorce, or a chronic physical illness. Other groups are specifically targeted to a single disorder. Groups that focus on social skills work best with a mixture of patients.

Groups that are conducted with patients in special schools, inpatient units, or day hospitals typically include all children or adolescents enrolled in the program, although the patients may be divided by age or level of functioning. Special topic groups, such as treatment of substance abuse, or predischarge groups also may be offered in these settings.

It is useful for the group therapist to interview prospective group members individually, to assess suitability for the group, to orient patients to the goals and methods of the group, to learn more about the children or adolescents, and to begin to develop a therapeutic alliance between the patients and the leader. It also is helpful to interview the parent(s) for similar reasons. The younger the child, the more important is parental cooperation.

Group members should be in the same or adjacent developmental stage. Children change so dramatically as they develop that an age span broader than 2–3 years is unlikely to result in a therapeutic group process. In forming groups for pre- and early adolescents, developmental stage is often more important than chronological age because girls are approximately 2 years ahead of boys in physical and social development, and there is great variability among youngsters of the same sex. The dynamic issues differ at various developmental stages.

Opinions on the mixing of boys and girls differ. Although some issues are easier to handle in single-sex groups, children and adolescents need to learn to get along with the opposite sex in school and in the neighborhood and often with siblings. Therefore, mixing boys and girls, although initially more difficult, may be productive.

Frequency, duration, and goals. For convenience, outpatient groups typically meet once a week. Frequency of group meetings on inpatient units varies from one to seven times per week. Groups may have a defined, limited duration from several months to an academic year or may be open ended. Short-term groups focus on "current and explicit behavior, adaptation, coping, competency, strengths and growth…[with] emphasis on the dynamics of the 'here-and-now' corrective emotional experience, [and] on the patients' active participation in the change effort" (Scheidlinger 1984, p. 581). Long-term groups are more likely to aim for the promotion of insight, the resolution of unconscious conflicts, and the removal of developmental arrests. Although there are exceptions, short-term groups generally have a defined membership, with no new members added once the group begins. Long-term groups more often have changing membership, with patients entering and leaving as their clinical status dictates.

Group leadership. Of all modalities of therapy, the need for co-therapists is most clear in group treatment. Groups are complex, with many events occurring simultaneously, and a second observer is valuable. This arrangement also allows continuity of treatment when one leader needs to be absent. In groups of younger children, an extra pair of hands is needed. Coleaders who differ in age, sex, race, or ethnicity expand the opportunity for different types of patient–therapist relationships.

Group rules. The nature of the group and the patients determines the optimal degree of structure. A psychodynamically oriented group composed of depressed or anxious adolescents will need far fewer rules than a group whose goal is to teach social skills to school-age boys with conduct problems. The leaders are responsible for maintaining control of behavior within the group. At times, this control may even require strategies such as the time-out.

The leader(s) must make explicit the rules of confidentiality for the group, as the group setting expands the risk of breach of confidentiality to include the patients' peers. This breach is of most concern to adolescents and preadolescents.

Family contact. Involving parents is especially important for preschool- and school-age children to discover important events in the children's lives and to assess progress. Adolescents are more willing and able to report and are also more sensitive to confidentiality issues. All parents should be kept apprised of the goals of the group, both in general and specifically for their child. Parent education in development and behavior management can be provided efficiently by grouping parents together. Parents also may appreciate the opportunity to meet with others whose children have similar problems.

Developmental Issues

Preschool-age groups. Young children are less able to verbalize and thus require more structure and planned activities. A group can provide a powerful context for the teaching of social skills and language, especially for children who are autistic or severely delayed.

School-age groups. Because school-age children have great difficulty bringing in outside material for discussion or engaging in introspection, verbal portions of the group are best focused on events that occur in the group itself. Games and craft activities can provide a useful framework, but the leaders must ensure that recreation does not become the only function of the group. Behavior modification and cognitive problem-solving techniques are especially useful for children this age.

Many child patients will not spontaneously attempt to relate to other children. Others have been rejected or scapegoated by peers. If the group is successful, the children will use the skills they have learned to form relationships with peers at school and in their neighborhoods.

Children with ADHD are often referred to group therapy because of their difficulty with peer relations and their lack of insight into their difficulties. Those children who are being treated with stimulant medication should receive a dose before the group meets to help them benefit from the therapy and not disrupt it for others.

Adolescent groups.　Scheidlinger (1985) identified four major categories of group work with adolescents:

1. *Group psychotherapy:* treatment of a balanced selection of patients, using the group as the primary modality, with goals of relief of psychological distress, modification of pathological modes of functioning, and amelioration of personality dysfunction
2. *Therapeutic groups for patients in mental health, medical, or residential settings:* used as ancillary treatment or as an aid in rehabilitation
3. *Human development and training groups:* offered to youths who are not psychiatric patients; focus on prevention and enrichment
4. *Self-help and mutual help groups:* may or may not have professional leaders and consist of peers working together to satisfy a shared need or overcome a common handicap; extensively used in the treatment of substance abuse

Although activities may be useful, many adolescent groups can be conducted in an exclusively verbal format. If both boys and girls are included in the same group, the leader must be alert to sexual undercurrents and acting out while facilitating the discussion of sexual concerns and practicing of heterosexual social skills (Scheidlinger 1985). To avoid scapegoating, it is important that the proportion of boys to girls not be too unequal.

Hospital and Residential Treatment

Indications

Because children should be treated in the setting that is least restrictive and disruptive to their lives, hospital or residential treatment is indicated only in emergencies or for youngsters who have not responded to efforts at outpatient treatment because of severity of the disorder, lack of motivation, resistance, or disorganization of patients and/or family. Programs vary widely in their criteria for admission.

Placement in a residential treatment center may be indicated for children and adolescents with chronic behavior problems such as aggression, running away, truancy, substance abuse, school phobia, or self-destructive acts that the family, foster home, and/or community cannot manage or tolerate. Some parents harbor negative attitudes toward their children or adolescents or have severe psychopathology of their own. Children for whom it is not advisable to return home—because of factors in the youngsters, their families, or both—may be referred to a residential treatment center following a hospital stay. Because of the increase in managed care environments, admission criteria have been restricted and lengths of stay have been substantially reduced.

Short-term hospitalization is more often an acute event, stemming from immediate physical danger to self or others, acute psychosis, a crisis in the environment that reduces the ability of the caregiving adults to cope with the child or adolescent, or the need for more intensive, systematic, and detailed evaluation and observation of the patient and family than is possible on an outpatient basis or in a day program. Managed care pressures have forced hospital lengths of stay to decrease significantly, often allowing only clinical stabilization of the patient before his or her discharge from the hospital. Briefer hospitalizations of severely ill child psychiatric patients require well-coordinated transfer to less intense and restrictive levels of care in the clinical continuum (residential, day, and intensive outpatient treatments) to enhance clinical stability.

Longer-term hospitalization may be indicated for those patients who do not improve sufficiently in a brief period and who continue to require a secure setting and intensive treatment.

Efficacy

Systematic outcome evaluation is extremely difficult because of the complexity of the cases and the need for crisis intervention. Controlled studies that would be considered methodologically adequate comparing 24-hour treatment with no treatment or other types of treatment may not be ethical or even feasible. In general, more severely ill patients with fewer individual and family resources have a poorer outcome.

Differences in Settings

Residential treatment centers, compared with hospital units, tend to be longer term, tend to be more open to and integrated with the community, and tend not to use the medical model. Usually, residential centers have a lower staff-to-patient ratio and less highly trained personnel. These centers are more likely to be organized based on a family group model and organized by sections or cottages.

Facilities may be under the auspices of a state, county, or city; part of a medical school; or in a private, a nonprofit, or an investor-owned hospital. Inpatient units may be located in a general hospital, pediatric specialty hospital, or psychiatric hospital. Most settings separate children and adolescents, but others mix age groups. A relatively recent development is the psychosomatic or pediatric medical–psychiatric unit for children and adolescents with coexisting physical and psychiatric problems.

Some units are locked and can accommodate involuntary patients as well as runaways and highly impulsive, psychotic, or actively suicidal youths who require more security. Other units are open and admit only voluntary patients. Intensity of staffing varies widely. Units that are part of a medical school are the most intensively staffed because of the presence of a variety of trainees. Programs operated by state or county governments may have fewer professional staff because of budget restraints and problems in recruiting.

Inpatient units for children can be classified according to the usual length of stay on such units. The lengths of stay on brief-stay or crisis intervention units average 3–10 days. These units emphasize rapid evaluation, triage, stabilization, and development of a treatment plan that will be implemented on an outpatient basis or in another facility. Stays on intermediate units last several weeks to months, and more definitive treatment can be conducted. Children may stay on long-term units from several months to longer than 1 year. On these units, care for the most severely impaired youth is provided. Increasing financial pressures have resulted in reduced overall lengths of stay in all types of units.

Treatment Planning

Ideally, hospitalization forms part of a comprehensive continuum of care for children. With ever-shorter lengths of stay, rapid and efficient planning and execution of evaluation and treatment strategies are essential. The goal is not to eliminate all psychopathology but to address the "focal problem" that precipitated hospitalization and then to discharge the patient to home, residential treatment, or foster placement, where he or she can receive outpatient or day treatment (Harper 1989).

Components of Treatment

The relative emphasis placed on each treatment modality differs according to the philosophy of treatment, the nature of the patient population, the usual length of stay, and the availability of highly specialized staff. All of the following should be present in some form.

Psychopharmacology. Hospitalization offers an ideal opportunity for systematic trials of medication in children or adolescents who have not responded to conventional treatment, who are diagnostically puzzling, who have medical problems complicating pharmacotherapy, or whose parents are noncompliant, disorganized, or unreliable reporters of efficacy or side effects. Systematic drug trials for individual patients can be designed using single- or double-blind methods evaluated by observations on the ward and in the classroom. As-needed (i.e., prn) medications, used to control aggression or other behavior problems, should be used only for brief periods until more effective, ongoing treatments are begun. With increased use of psychopharmacology in children and adolescents, hospitalization now often begins with a drug "washout"—removing patients from complex and ineffective or partially effective polypharmacy regimens.

Individual psychotherapy. As newer treatment methods evolve and hospital stays become ever shorter, individual psychotherapy is less often a primary treatment modality than in the past. However, regularly scheduled individual sessions with a therapist with whom the child or adolescent can develop a special relationship continue to be essential in developing a more complete understanding of the patient's intrapsychic, familial, and social dynamics and in assisting him or her to develop more adaptive methods of coping with strong emotions. The therapist may be able to help the patient to deal with past traumas and losses, to better understand his or her current difficulties, and to make use of the other treatments offered. The confidentiality that is usual in outpatient therapy is not present in a hospital or residential setting, since all staff participate as a treatment team.

Milieu therapy. Milieu therapy includes the total environment of a structured schedule for meals, sleep, tasks of daily living, and a program of recreational and therapeutic activities. The patient can be observed over an extended period of time in school, free play with peers, meals, sleep, and self-care. In the most effective milieus, all activities and interactions with staff are consistent with the treatment plan. Goals of the milieu include promoting a feeling of security, by clarity of rules and regularity of schedule, and increased self-esteem and competence through learning of skills. Most settings include a token economy or levels program, which also may be used for specific treatment, for management of behavior (e.g., encouraging a patient with anorexia nervosa to eat).

Group therapy. In addition to general or special topic groups (e.g., 12-step models, survivors of abuse), group therapy may include community meetings in which privileges and rules are decided, social skills are practiced, and patients learn to observe their own and others' behavior and to recognize the impact of their behavior on others.

Education. Virtually all children who require psychiatric hospitalization have had problems in school. The small classes and highly trained teachers of a hospital unit can provide a detailed evaluation of a youngster's academic strengths and weaknesses, incorporating data from intelligence and achievement tests and special tests for learning disabilities into direct observation of classroom behavior and learning. Educational strategies can be developed and tested. One of the most important parts of discharge planning is arranging for an appropriate educational placement and working with the new teacher to continue progress made in the hospital. The hospitalization often allows child or adolescent patients their first opportunity to experience academic success.

Many residential treatment centers have their own schools on the centers' grounds. As youngsters improve, they are gradually integrated into special education or mainstream programs in local public or private schools.

Family treatment. Work with families is an essential part of hospital treatment, including intensive evaluation of family functioning and deciding where the child should reside. Interventions may include family therapy, parent counseling in behavior management, and education about the nature of their child's disorder. Parents may require marital therapy, individual medical or psychiatric assessment and treatment, or help with housing or income.

Additional services. Medical evaluation and treatment must be provided. The following more specialized resources should be available through consultation as necessary: neurological evaluation and treatment, speech and language assessment and therapy, physical therapy, and occupational therapy.

Disposition planning and aftercare. Disposition planning and follow-up may be the most important parts of the treatment if gains made are to be maintained and continued. A complete disposition plan includes consideration of where the child should live, school placement, and continuation of individual therapy, family therapy, and/or pharmacotherapy. Communication with referring and receiving agencies and professionals is essential.

Day Treatment

Indications

A day program (also called *partial hospitalization*) may be best for the child who requires more intensive intervention than can be provided in outpatient visits but who is able to live at home. Day treatment is less disruptive to the patient and family than hospitalization or residential placement and can offer an opportunity for more intensive work with parents, who may even attend the program on a regular basis. A day program may be used as a transition for a child who has been hospitalized or to avert a hospitalization. It may be implemented in combination with placement in a foster or group home.

Programs

Some programs involve a full day, 5 days a week, and include a school or therapeutic nursery school program. There are decided advantages in being able to integrate the treatment plan and therapeutic focus into the entire day. Other programs may meet in the late afternoon and evening hours, after patients attend community schools. It is desirable to offer all of the treatment modalities that are available on an inpatient unit.

Innovative, intensive summer treatment programs have been developed for children with ADHD and associated behavior and learning problems (Pelham and Hoza 1987). These programs provide positive social and recreational experiences for children who otherwise would not be able to participate in camp, while teaching parents behavior modification techniques, supplementing classroom work, and rigorously assessing medication efficacy and side effects.

Adjunctive Treatments

At times, an intervention that is not a psychiatric treatment may be recommended as part of a treatment plan. These programs may be crucial for the child's well-being and/or the treatment of the psychiatric disorder, or they may be facilitative, speeding progress or improving level of function.

Parent Support Groups

Parents of children with psychiatric disorders, together with mental health professionals and teachers, have established groups that provide education and support for parents, as well as advocacy for services and fundraising for research. National organizations with local chapters include Parents Anonymous, for abusive or potentially abusive parents; the Association for Retarded Citizens; the Autism Society of America; Children and Adults with Attention Deficit/Hyperactivity Disorder (CHADD); and the Learning Disabilities Association of America. The National Alliance for the Mentally Ill (NAMI) established a Child and Adolescent Network (NAMI-CAN) as its concerns broadened to include children and adolescents. Local groups focused on a particular disorder or on more generic issues can provide a powerful adjunct to direct clinical services. The Child and Adolescent Bipolar Foundation is a new addition, offering resources to parents and professionals at its web site (www.bpkids.org).

Special Education

Modified school programs are indicated for those children who cannot perform satisfactorily in regular classrooms or who need special structure or teaching techniques to reach their academic potential. These programs range in intensity from tutoring or resource classrooms several hours a week to special classrooms in mainstream schools to public or private schools that serve only children with special educational needs. Resources differ from community to community, but most communities have programs for mentally retarded youth, for those with learning disabilities (specific developmental disorders), and for those whose emotional and/or behavioral problems require a special setting for learning or for the control of their behavior. Classes are small, with a high teacher-to-student ratio and teachers who are specially trained.

Before being placed in a special class, youngsters must have an individually administered battery of psychological tests, including an intelligence test, achievement tests, and an evaluation for learning disabilities. Federal law requires that all children who need special services receive them and that services be provided in the least-restrictive environment (i.e., as much in the mainstream with other children and adolescents as possible).

Boarding schools may be useful when there is a problem between parent and child that is unresponsive to treatment. Some of these schools have special programs for children with learning disabilities or psychiatric disorders.

Recreation

Learning a sport or skill at which one can do well is an important adjunct in the treatment of a child who lacks positive relationships with peers or adults because of social isolation or withdrawal or who is ignored or actively rejected. A relationship with an adult such as a Big Brother or a YMCA counselor, and an opportunity to interact with a normal peer group under supervision, such as a Girl Scout troop, may provide support and build self-esteem until the child is sufficiently improved to establish relationships independently. Some families have employed a high school or college student one or more afternoons a week to teach social and play skills, develop a relationship, and provide structured time. This approach also gives parents a respite and an opportunity to spend time with their other children.

Day or overnight summer camps may present opportunities for psychological growth in multiple domains. Some youngsters can attend regular camp, whereas others need a special program for children and adolescents with psychiatric or medical problems.

Foster Care

Placement in a foster home may be needed when parents are unwilling or unable to care for a child. Indications are clearest in cases of physical neglect or physical or sexual abuse. Other families may be unable to provide the appropriate emotional or physical environment. Court intervention is required for placement. Although foster placement can be a suitable and effective intervention, children in foster care may have a variety of unmet physical, developmental, and mental health needs, often making foster care less than optimal and clearly unsatisfactory as a long-term solution (Rosenfeld et al. 1997). Unfortunately, child welfare agencies in many communities are overwhelmed, and children and adolescents may require advocacy either to accomplish removal from home to a foster placement or for termination of foster placement and return to parents, group home placement, or release for adoption.

Children with severe behavioral or physical problems and older adolescents who are difficult to place or maintain in foster or adoptive homes may be admitted to group homes. These homes vary in staffing and intensity of their programs. Some approach residential treatment, whereas others simply provide a supervised residence.

Dietary Treatments

Since the mid-1970s, advocates of dietary treatment of behavioral problems have been remarkably persistent, despite the lack of scientific evidence. A variety of food additives and food allergens have been proposed as contributory or even causal in childhood behavior disorders, especially hyperactivity and autism. Reviews of the methodologically adequate studies show that, at most, 5% of hyperactive children may show behavioral or cognitive improvement on the Kaiser Permanente Diet, but these changes are not as dramatic as those induced by stimulants (Wender 1986). The only characteristic associated with greater likelihood of response is age less than 6 years. There are no data to support dietary treatments for autism.

Parents and primary care practitioners find dietary treatment appealing because it is more "natural" than medication. However, special diets demand extra work and often additional expense from a family already disrupted by a child's behavior problems. Given the minimal evidence of efficacy and the extreme difficulty inducing children to comply with restricted diets, such diets should not be recommended. Families who insist on trying a diet should be permitted to do so, provided the diet is nutritionally sound, because initial attempts to dissuade them may disrupt the therapeutic alliance.

Controlled studies have been unable to demonstrate that ingesting sugar has an effect on activity or aggression in healthy or hyperactive children, even those identified by their parents as sugar responsive (Milich et al. 1986; Wender and Solanto 1991). Clinically insignificant effects on attention have been demonstrated only in young children and only after a high-carbohydrate breakfast (Wender and Solanto 1991).

Megavitamin therapy, the prescription of vitamins in quantities greatly in excess of the recommended daily allowance (RDA) guidelines, has been suggested as a treatment for schizophrenia, autism, hyperactivity, and learning disabilities. Extreme claims have been made from uncontrolled studies. Not only is scientific evidence of effectiveness lacking, but toxic effects also are possible (Harley 1980). Parents, particularly those of autistic children, may pursue this treatment out of desperation.

Integration of Multiple Modalities

Sophisticated simultaneous or sequential use of different techniques offers substantial promise of improved treatment outcome. There is a clear need for more power and wider coverage of symptoms than any single treatment alone provides. The following are some examples.

Collaborative Therapy

In general, treatment by a single therapist is most efficient and effective. Indications for collaborative treatment (two or more therapists working as a team) in the outpatient setting include a child who is unusually concerned about confidentiality; the need for several different types of skills (e.g., individual psychotherapy, family therapy and pharmacotherapy), which a single therapist does not have; or clear indications for different qualities in the patient's and parents' therapists (e.g., a boy who would benefit from a male role model but whose mother has great difficulty relating to men).

In collaborative treatment, in order to maintain free and open communication and to discuss and agree on treatment plans, it is essential for the therapists to avoid aligning into competitive teams. Conflicts over relative power and authority of the therapists can sabotage treatment. It is fundamentally important that the child and adolescent psychiatrist not allow him- or herself to be relegated solely to the role of pharmacotherapist without establishing lines of communication with other treating professionals and participation in comprehensive assessment and treatment planning.

Combined Treatments

A clinician must be able to weave together flexibly a treatment that draws from psychodynamic, behavioral, cognitive, family systems, and pharmacotherapeutic approaches in order to address a child's specific disorder at his or her specific developmental level (Lewis 1997).

Combined Psychotherapies

In the treatment of children and adolescents, integrating techniques from different theoretical schools (e.g., play, cognitive-behavioral, psychodynamic) may be more helpful and appropriate than relying on one particular theory or approach (Silverman 1997). Models have been developed that bring together techniques to address specific clinical issues. For example, a highly structured model has been developed from a theoretical framework of ego psychoanalytic object relations theory for children with oppositional or conduct disorders who have some social bonds and a capacity for guilt. Interventions include individual supportive–expressive play psychotherapy, parent training, and play group psychotherapy, according to the child's presenting problems (Kernberg and Chazan 1991).

An ingenious model of child psychotherapy developed by Strayhorn (1988) makes explicit the identification of "psychological skills" or competencies expected for the child's age that are lacking. In this model, specific interventions are designed to address the missing skills, including verbal and play therapy, education of child and parent, and behavioral techniques such as modeling and contingency management.

Medication Plus Psychotherapeutic Intervention

Traditionally, the use of medications and psychotherapy was seen as an either–or phenomenon in which proponents of either modality saw their own as more valuable and the other as unnecessary or even harmful. Increasingly, we are aware of the potential synergistic effect from combining medication with psychotherapeutic interventions, as these treatments may address different aspects of a single disorder (O'Brien and Perlmutter 1997).

Attention-deficit/hyperactivity disorder. The implementation of a multimodal treatment for ADHD has traditionally been clinically encouraged. Such treatment combines medication management (most often stimulants), behavioral interventions, parent management training, appropriate school placement and school-based interventions, as well as child-focused treatments (psychotherapy, cognitive-behavioral treatment, and social skills training). More recent reports from an ongoing multicenter study examining the long-term benefit of multimodal treatments for ADHD have questioned the benefit of multimodal treatment over systematic medication management alone (Jensen 2000).

Autistic disorder. Children with autism require a comprehensive therapeutic plan that may include psychoeducation of the parents and family, special education placement, speech and language therapies, behavioral management approaches, social skills training, and pharmacotherapy. An individualized treatment should take into account the particular deficits of the child, as well as individual and family strengths (M. Campbell et al. 1996).

Depression. Current recommendations for treatment of depression include CBT, interpersonal psychotherapy, and parent and family therapies, as well as pharmacotherapy, either alone or in combination (Birmaher et al. 1996). Treatments should be individualized, based upon presumed etiology, severity of illness, and individual/family strengths.

Anxiety disorders. Recently suggested approaches to treatment of children and adolescents with anxiety disorders include the combined use of behavioral, cognitive-behavioral, and supportive psychotherapies; family therapy; and pharmacotherapy tailored to the child's clinical needs (Bernstein et al. 1996).

Obsessive-compulsive disorder. The combination of CBT and pharmacotherapy appears optimal in the treatment of OCD. One preliminary study suggests that both CBT and pharmacotherapy in the treatment of children and adolescents with OCD may be superior to medication alone (March et al. 1994); however, controlled studies are required.

Conclusions

The treatment of psychiatric disorders in children and adolescents is both an art and a science. Research on assessment and diagnosis, biological correlates of disorders, and outcome of traditional and newly developed techniques will continue to improve the specificity and outcome of treatment. However, a need always will exist for clinical skills in tailoring and applying psychiatric techniques to individual patients and their families.

References

Abbott Laboratories: Press Release: Focus on Cylert, 1996

Abnormal Involuntary Movement Scale (AIMS). Psychopharmacol Bull 24:781–783, 1988

Achenbach TM: Manual for the Teacher's Report Form and 1991 Profile. Burlington, VT, University of Vermont, Department of Psychiatry, 1991

Adams PL: A Primer of Child Psychotherapy, Second Edition. Boston, MA, Little, Brown, 1982

Alexander JF: An integrative model for treating the adolescent who is delinquent/acting out, in Empowering Families, Helping Adolescents: Family-Centered Treatment of Adolescents With Alcohol, Drug Abuse, and Mental Health Problems. Edited by Snyder W, Oooms T. Rockville, MD, U.S. Department of Health and Human Services, 1992, pp 101–110

Aman MG, Marks RE, Turbott SH, et al: Clinical effects of methylphenidate and thioridazine in intellectually subaverage children. J Am Acad Child Adolesc Psychiatry 30:246–256, 1991

Ambrosini PJ: A review of pharmacotherapy of major depression in children and adolescents. Psychiatr Serv 51:627–633, 2000

Ambrosini PJ, Wagner KD, Biederman J, et al: Multicenter open-label sertraline study in adolescent outpatients with major depression. J Am Acad Child Adolesc Psychiatry 38:566–572, 1999

Anderson CM, Hogarty GE, Reiss DJ: Family treatment of adult schizophrenic patients: a psycho-educational approach. Schizophr Bull 6:490–505, 1980

Anderson GM, Cook EH: Pharmacogenetics: promise and potential in child and adolescent psychiatry. Child Adolesc Psychiatr Clin N Am 9:23–42, 2000

Anderson LT, Campbell M, Adams P, et al: The effects of haloperidol on discrimination learning and behavioral symptoms in autistic children. J Autism Dev Disord 19:227–239, 1989

Armenteros JL, Whitaker AH, Welikson M, et al: Risperidone in adolescents with schizophrenia: an open pilot study. J Am Acad Child Adolesc Psychiatry 36:694–700, 1997

Arredondo DE: Bupropion treatment of adolescent depression. Scientific Proceedings of the 146th Meeting of the American Psychiatric Association, San Francisco, CA, May 1993

Azrin NH, Sneed TJ, Foxx RM: Dry-bed training: rapid elimination of childhood enuresis. Behav Res Ther 12:147–156, 1974

Barkley RA, Benton CM: Your Defiant Child. New York, Guilford, 1998

Barrickman LL, Perry PJ, Allen AJ, et al: Bupropion versus methylphenidate in the treatment of attention-deficit hyperactivity disorder. J Am Acad Child Adolesc Psychiatry 34:649–657, 1995

Bastiaens L: Knowledge, expectations and attitudes of hospitalized children and adolescents in psychopharmacological treatment. J Child Adolesc Psychopharmacol 3:157–171, 1992

Bastiaens L: Compliance with pharmacotherapy in adolescents: effects of patients' and parents' knowledge and attitudes toward treatment. J Child Adolesc Psychopharmacol 5:39–48, 1995

Bastiaens L, Bastiaens DK: A manual of psychiatric medications for teenagers. J Child Adolesc Psychopharmacol 3:M1–M59, 1993

Bates GDL, Khin-Maung-Zaw F: Movement disorder with fluoxetine. J Am Acad Child Adolesc Psychiatry 37:14–15, 1998

Bernstein GA, Garfinkel BD, Borchardt CM: Comparative studies of pharmacotherapy for school refusal. J Am Acad Child Adolesc Psychiatry 29:773–781, 1990

Bernstein GA, Borchardt CM, Perwien AR: Anxiety disorders in children and adolescents: a review of the past 10 years. J Am Acad Child Adolesc Psychiatry 35:1110–1119, 1996

Bernstein GA, Borchardt CM, Perwien AR, et al: Imipramine plus cognitive-behavioral therapy in the treatment of school refusal. J Am Acad Child Adolesc Psychiatry 39:276–283, 2000

Bertagnoli MW, Borchardt CM: A review of ECT for children and adolescents. J Am Acad Child Adolesc Psychiatry 29:302–307, 1990

Biederman J: Clonazepam in the treatment of prepubertal children with panic-like symptoms. J Clin Psychiatry 48(suppl):38–41, 1987

Biederman J, Wilens T, Mick E, et al: Pharmacotherapy of attention-deficit/hyperactivity disorder reduces risk for substance use disorder. Pediatrics 104:E20, 1999

Birmaher B, Quintana H, Greenhill LL: Methylphenidate treatment of hyperactive autistic children. J Am Acad Child Adolesc Psychiatry 27:248–251, 1988

Birmaher B, Greenhill LL, Cooper TB, et al: Sustained release methylphenidate: pharmacokinetic studies in ADHD males. J Am Acad Child Adolesc Psychiatry 28:768–772, 1989

Birmaher B, Waterman GS, Ryan N, et al: Fluoxetine for childhood anxiety disorders. J Am Acad Child Adolesc Psychiatry 33:993–999, 1994

Birmaher B, Ryan ND, Williamson DE, et al: Childhood and adolescent depression: a review of the past 10 years, II. J Am Acad Child Adolesc Psychiatry 35:1575–1583, 1996

Black B, Robbins DR: Case study: panic disorder in children and adolescents. J Am Acad Child Adolesc Psychiatry 29:36–44, 1989

Black B, Uhde TW: Treatment of elective mutism with fluoxetine: a double-blind, placebo-controlled study. J Am Acad Child Adolesc Psychiatry 33:1000–1006, 1994

Blechman EA: Toward comprehensive behavioral family intervention: an algorithm for matching families and interventions. Behav Modif 5:221–236, 1981

Borkovec TD, Miranda J: Between-group psychotherapy outcome research and basic science. Psychotherapy and Rehabilitation Research 5:14–20, 1996

Boyle SF: SSRIs and movement disorders. J Am Acad Child Adolesc Psychiatry 38:354–355, 1999

Broderick-Cantwell JJ: Case study: accidental clonidine patch overdose in attention-deficit/hyperactivity disorder patients. J Am Acad Child Adolesc Psychiatry 38:95–98, 1999

Brown RT, Sexson SB: Effects of methylphenidate on cardiovascular responses in attention deficit hyperactivity disordered adolescents. Journal of Adolescent Health Care 10:179–183, 1989

Bruggeman R, van der Linden C, Buitelaar JK, et al: Risperidone versus pimozide in Tourette's disorder: a comparative double-blind parallel-group study. J Clin Psychiatry 62:50–56, 2001

Bruun RD, Budman CL: Risperidone as a treatment for Tourette's disorder. J Clin Psychiatry 57:29–31, 1996

Bryden KE, Carrey NJ, Kutcher SP: Update and recommendations for the use of antipsychotics in early onset psychoses. J Child Adolesc Psychopharmacol 11:113–130, 2001

Buitelaar JK, van der Gaag RJ, van der Hoeven J: Buspirone in the management of anxiety and irritability in children with pervasive developmental disorders: results of an open-label study. J Clin Psychiatry 59:56–59, 1998

Buitelaar JK, van der Gaag RJ, Cohen-Kettenis P, et al: A randomized controlled trial of risperidone in the treatment of aggression in hospitalized adolescents with subaverage cognitive abilities. J Clin Psychiatry 62:239–248, 2001

Campbell M, Small AM, Green WH, et al: Behavioral efficacy of haloperidol and lithium carbonate. Arch Gen Psychiatry 41:650–656, 1984

Campbell M, Green WH, Deutsch SI: Child and Adolescent Psychopharmacology. Beverly Hills, CA, Sage, 1985

Campbell M, Silva RR, Kafantaris V, et al: Predictors of side effects associated with lithium administration in children. Psychopharmacol Bull 27:373–380, 1991

Campbell M, Anderson LT, Small AM, et al: Naltrexone in autistic children: behavioral symptoms and attentional learning. J Am Acad Child Adolesc Psychiatry 32:1283–1291, 1993

Campbell M, Adams PB, Small AM, et al: Lithium in hospitalized aggressive children with conduct disorder: a double-blind and placebo-controlled study. J Am Acad Child Adolesc Psychiatry 34:445–453, 1995

Campbell M, Schopler E, Cueva JE, et al: Treatment of autistic disorder. J Am Acad Child Adolesc Psychiatry 35:134–143, 1996

Campbell SB: Hyperactivity in preschoolers: correlates and prognostic implications. Clin Psychol Rev 5:405–428, 1985

Cantor S, Kestenbaum C: Psychotherapy with schizophrenic children. J Am Acad Child Psychiatry 25:623–630, 1986

Cantwell DP, Swanson J, Connor DF: Case study: adverse response to clonidine. J Am Acad Child Adolesc Psychiatry 36:539–544, 1997

Carlson GA, Rapport MD, Kelly KL, et al: The effects of methylphenidate and lithium on attention and activity level. J Am Acad Child Adolesc Psychiatry 31:262–270, 1992

Carter E, McGoldrick M (eds): The Family Life Cycle: A Framework for Family Therapy. New York, Gardner, 1980

Chappell PB, Riddle MA, Scahill L, et al: Guanfacine treatment of comorbid attention-deficit hyperactivity disorder and Tourette's syndrome: preliminary clinical experience. J Am Acad Child Adolesc Psychiatry 34:1140–1146, 1995

Cherland E, Fitzpatrick R: Psychotic side effects of psychostimulants: a 5-year review. Can J Psychiatry 44:811–813, 1999

Clarke GN, Rohde P, Lewinsohn PM, et al: Cognitive-behavioral treatment of adolescent depression: efficacy of acute group treatment and booster sessions. J Am Acad Child Adolesc Psychiatry 38:272–279, 1999

Clein PD, Riddle MA: Pharmacokinetics in children and adolescents. Child Adolesc Psychiatr Clin N Am 4:59–75, 1995

Coffey BJ: Anxiolytics for children and adolescents: traditional and new drugs. J Child Adolesc Psychopharmacol 1:57–83, 1990

Coffey BJ: Ethical issues in child and adolescent psychopharmacology. Child Adolesc Psychiatr Clin N Am 4:793–807, 1995

Coffey BJ, Shader RI, Greenblatt DJ: Pharmacokinetics of benzodiazepines and psychostimulants in children. J Clin Psychopharmacol 3:217–225, 1983

Cohen D, Taieb O, Flament M, et al: Absence of cognitive impairment at long-term follow-up in adolescents treated with ECT for severe mood disorder. Am J Psychiatry 157:460–462, 2000

Cohen DJ, Riddle MA, Leckman JF: Pharmacotherapy of Tourette's syndrome and associated disorders. Psychiatr Clin North Am 15:109–129, 1992

Compton SN, Grant PJ, Chrisman AK, et al: Sertraline in children and adolescents with social anxiety disorder: an open trial. J Am Acad Child Adolesc Psychiatry 40:564–571, 2001

Conners CK: Methodological and assessment issues in pediatric psychopharmacology, in Diagnosis and Psychopharmacology of Childhood and Adolescent Disorders. Edited by Wiener JM. New York, Wiley, 1985, pp 69–110

Conners CK, Barkley RA: Rating scales and checklists for child psychopharmacology. Psychopharmacol Bull 21:816–832, 1985

Conners CK, Casat CD, Gualtieri CT, et al: Bupropion hydrochloride in attention deficit disorder with hyperactivity. J Am Acad Child Adolesc Psychiatry 35:1314–1321, 1996

Connor DF: Beta blockers for aggression: a review of the pediatric experience. J Child Adolesc Psychopharmacol 3:99–114, 1993

Connor DF, Ozbayrak KR, Benjamin S, et al: A pilot study of nadolol for overt aggression in developmentally delayed individuals. J Am Acad Child Adolesc Psychiatry 36:826–834, 1997

Connor DF, Fletcher KE, Swanson JM: A meta-analysis of clonidine for symptoms of attention-deficit hyperactivity disorder. J Am Acad Child Adolesc Psychiatry 38:1551–1559, 1999

Connor DF, Barkley RA, Davis HT: A pilot study of methylphenidate, clonidine, or the combination in ADHD comorbid with aggressive oppositional defiant or conduct disorder. Clin Pediatr (Phila) 39:15–25, 2000

Cook EH, Wagner KD, March JS, et al: Long-term sertraline treatment of children and adolescents with obsessive-compulsive disorder. J Am Acad Child Adolesc Psychiatry 40:1175–1181, 2001

Cueva JE, Overall JE, Small AM, et al: Carbamazepine in aggressive children with conduct disorder: a double-blind and placebo-controlled study. J Am Acad Child Adolesc Psychiatry 35:480–490, 1996

Dangel RF, Deschner JP, Rasp RR: Anger control training for adolescents in residential treatment. Behav Modif 13:447–458, 1989

Davanzo PA, McCracken JT: Mood stabilizers in the treatment of juvenile bipolar disorder: advances and controversies. Child Adolesc Psychiatr Clin N Am 9:159–182, 2000

Davidson B, Quinn WH, Josephson AM: Assessment of the family: systemic and developmental perspectives. Child Adolesc Psychiatr Clin N Am 10:415–429, 2001

Daviss WB, Bentivoglio P, Racusin R, et al: Bupropion sustained release in adolescents with comorbid attention-deficit/hyperactivity disorder and depression. J Am Acad Child Adolesc Psychiatry 40:307–314, 2001

DeVeaugh-Geiss J, Moroz G, Biederman J, et al: Clomipramine hydrochloride in childhood and adolescent obsessive-compulsive disorder: a multicenter trial. J Am Acad Child Adolesc Psychiatry 31:45–49, 1992

Diler RS, Avci A: SSRI-induced mania in obsessive-compulsive disorder. J Am Acad Child Adolesc Psychiatry 38:6–7, 1999

Donenberg GR: Reconsidering "Between-Group Psychotherapy Outcome Research and Basic Science": applications to child and adolescent psychotherapy outcome research. J Clin Psychol 5:181–190, 1999

Dulcan MK: Brief psychotherapy with children and their families: the state of the art. J Am Acad Child Psychiatry 23:544–551, 1984

Dulcan MK, Lizarralde C (eds): Helping Parents, Youths and Teachers Understand Medications for Emotional and Behavioral Problems: A Resource Book of Medication Information Handouts, 2d Edition. Washington, DC, American Psychiatric Press, 2002

Dulcan MK, Martini DR: Concise Guide to Child and Adolescent Psychiatry, 2nd Edition. Washington, DC, American Psychiatric Press, 1998

Dulcan MK, Piercy PA: A model for teaching and evaluating brief psychotherapy with children and their families. Professional Psychology: Research and Practice 16:689–700, 1985

Dummit ES, Klein RG, Tancer NK, et al: Fluoxetine treatment of children with selective mutism. J Am Acad Child Adolesc Psychiatry 35:615–621, 1996

Edelbrock CS: Child Attention Profile, in Attention-Deficit Hyperactivity Disorder: A Clinical Workbook. Edited by Barkley RA. New York, Guilford, 1991

Elia J, Borcherding BG, Rapoport JL, et al: Methylphenidate and dextroamphetamine treatments of hyperactivity: are there true nonresponders? Psychiatry Res 36:141–155, 1991

Emery G, Bedrosian R, Garber J: Cognitive therapy with depressed children and adolescents, in Affective Disorders in Childhood and Adolescence: An Update. Edited by Cantwell DP, Carlson GA. New York, Spectrum, 1983, pp 445–471

Emslie GJ, Ruch AJ, Weinberg WA, et al: A double-blind, randomized, placebo-controlled trial of fluoxetine in children and adolescents with depression. Arch Gen Psychiatry 54:1031–1037, 1997

Ernst M, Magee HJ, Gonzalez NM, et al: Pimozide in autistic children. Psychopharmacol Bull 28:187–191, 1992

Evans RW, Clay TH, Gualtieri CT: Carbamazepine in pediatric psychiatry. J Am Acad Child Psychiatry 26:2–8, 1987

Faigel HC: The effect of beta blockade on stress-induced cognitive dysfunction in adolescents. Clin Pediatr (Phila) 30:441–445, 1991

Fairbanks JM, Pine DS, Tancer NK, et al: Open fluoxetine treatment of mixed anxiety disorders in children and adolescents. J Child Adolesc Psychopharmacol 7:17–29, 1997

Famularo R, Kinscherff R, Fenton T: Propranolol treatment for childhood posttraumatic stress disorder, acute type. Am J Dis Child 142:1244–1247, 1988

Fankhauser MP, Karumanchi VC, German ML, et al: A double-blind, placebo-controlled study of the efficacy of transdermal clonidine in autism. J Clin Psychiatry 53:77–82, 1992

Feeney DJ, Klykylo W: Risperidone and tardive dyskinesia. J Am Acad Child Adolesc Psychiatry 35:1421–1422, 1996

Feldman HM, Kolmen BK, Gonzaga AM: Naltrexone and communication skills in young children with autism. J Am Acad Child Adolesc Psychiatry 38:587–593, 1999

Fetner HH, Geller B: Lithium and tricyclic antidepressants. Psychiatr Clin North Am 15:223–241, 1992

Findling RL, Grcevich SJ, Lopez I, et al: Antipsychotic medications in children and adolescents. J Clin Psychiatry 57(suppl 9):19–23, 1996

Findling RL, Schulz SC, Reed MD, et al: The antipsychotics: a pediatric perspective. Pediatr Clin North Am 45:1025–1032, 1998

Findling RL, McNamara NK, Branicky LA, et al: A double-blind pilot study of risperidone in the treatment of conduct disorder. J Am Acad Child Adolesc Psychiatry 39:509–516, 2000

Fisman S, Steele M: Use of risperidone in pervasive developmental disorders: a case series. J Child Adolesc Psychopharmacol 6:177–190, 1996

Fitzpatrick PA, Klorman F, Brumaghim JT, et al: Effects of sustained-release and standard preparations of methylphenidate on attention deficit disorder. J Am Acad Child Adolesc Psychiatry 31:226–234, 1992

Fleck S: A general systems approach to severe family pathology. Am J Psychiatry 133:669–673, 1976

Flockhart DA, Oesterheld JR: Cytochrome P450-mediated drug interactions. Child Adolesc Psychiatr Clin N Am 9:43–76, 2000

Forehand RL, McMahon RJ: Helping the Noncompliant Child: A Clinician's Guide to Parent Training. New York, Guilford, 1981

Frazier JA, Gordon CT, McKenna M, et al: An open trial of clozapine in 11 adolescents with childhood-onset schizophrenia. J Am Acad Child Adolesc Psychiatry 33:658–663, 1994

Gadow KD: Effects of stimulant drugs on academic performance in hyperactive and learning disabled children. Journal of Learning Disabilities 16:290–299, 1983

Gadow KD: Pediatric psychopharmacology: a review of recent research. J Child Psychol Psychiatry 33:153–195, 1992

Gadow KD, Sverd J, Sprafkin J, et al: Efficacy of methylphenidate for attention deficit hyperactivity disorder in children with tic disorder. Arch Gen Psychiatry 52:444–455, 1995

Gardner RA: Helping children cooperate in therapy, in Basic Handbook of Child Psychiatry, Vol 3: Therapeutic Interventions. Edited by Harrison SI. New York, Basic Books, 1979, pp 414–433

Garland EJ, Smith DH: Case study: panic disorder on a child psychiatric consultation service. J Am Acad Child Adolesc Psychiatry 29:785–788, 1990

Geller B, Cooper TB, Chestnut EC, et al: Preliminary data on the relationship between nortriptyline plasma level and response in depressed children. Am J Psychiatry 143:1283–1286, 1986

Geller B, Cooper TB, Sun K, et al: Double-blind and placebo-controlled study of lithium for adolescent bipolar disorders with secondary substance dependency. J Am Acad Child Adolesc Psychiatry 37:171–178, 1998a

Geller B, Cooper TB, Zimerman B, et al: Lithium for prepubertal depressed children with family history predictors of future bipolarity: a double-blind, placebo-controlled study. J Affect Disord 51:165–175, 1998b

Geller B, Reising D, Leonard HL, et al: Critical review of tricyclic antidepressant use in children and adolescents. J Am Acad Child Adolesc Psychiatry 38:513–516, 1999

Geller DA, Hoog SL, Heiligenstein JH, et al: Fluoxetine treatment for obsessive compulsive disorder in children and adolescents: a placebo-controlled clinical trial. J Am Acad Child Adolesc Psychiatry 40:773–779, 2001

Genton P, Bauer J, Duncan S, et al: On the association between valproate and polycystic ovary syndrome. Epilepsia 42:305–310, 2001

Ghaziuddin N, Laughrin D, Giordani B: Cognitive side effects of electroconvulsive therapy in adolescents. J Child Adolesc Psychopharmacol 10:269–276, 2000

Gill M, LoVecchio F, Selden B: Serotonin syndrome in a child after a single dose of fluvoxamine. Ann Emerg Med 33:457–459, 1999

Gittelman R, Klein DF, Feingold I: Children with reading disorders, II: effects of methylphenidate in combination with reading remediation. J Child Psychol Psychiatry 24:193–212, 1983

Gittelman-Klein R, Klein DF: Controlled imipramine treatment of school phobia. Arch Gen Psychiatry 25:204–207, 1971

Gittelman-Klein R, Klein DF: School phobia: diagnostic considerations in the light of imipramine effects. J Nerv Ment Dis 156:199–215, 1973

Glassman AH, Bigger JT: Antipsychotic drugs: prolonged QTc interval, torsade de pointes, and sudden death. Am J Psychiatry 158:1774–1782, 2001

Golwyn DH, Sevlie CP: Phenelzine treatment of selective mutism in four prepubertal children. J Child Adolesc Psychopharmacol 9:109–113, 1999

Good CR, Feaster CS, Krecko VF: Tolerability of oral loading of divalproex sodium in child psychiatry inpatients. J Child Adolesc Psychopharmacol 11:53–57, 2001

Gordon CT, State RC, Nelson JE, et al: A double-blind comparison of clomipramine, desipramine, and placebo in the treatment of autistic disorder. Arch Gen Psychiatry 50:441–447, 1993

Graae F, Milner J, Rizzotto L, et al: Clonazepam in childhood anxiety disorders. J Am Acad Child Adolesc Psychiatry 333:372–376, 1994

Grcevich SJ, Findling RL, Rowane WA, et al: Risperidone in the treatment of children and adolescents with schizophrenia: a retrospective study. J Child Adolesc Psychopharmacol 6:251–257, 1996

Green WH: Child and Adolescent Clinical Psychopharmacology, 3rd Edition. Philadelphia, PA, Lippincott Williams & Wilkins, 2001

Greenhill LL: Attention-deficit hyperactivity disorder. Child Adolesc Psychiatr Clin N Am 4:123–168, 1995

Greenhill LL, Puig-Antich J, Chambers W, et al: Growth hormone, prolactin, and growth responses in hyperkinetic males treated with D-amphetamine. J Am Acad Child Adolesc Psychiatry 20:84–103, 1981

Greenhill LL, Puig-Antich J, Novacenko H, et al: Prolactin, growth hormone and growth responses in boys with attention deficit disorder and hyperactivity treated with methylphenidate. J Am Acad Child Adolesc Psychiatry 23:58–67, 1984

Greenhill LL, Solomon M, Pleak R, et al: Molindone hydrochloride treatment of hospitalized children with conduct disorder. J Clin Psychiatry 46:20–25, 1985

Grubbs JH: SSRI-induced mania. J Am Acad Child Adolesc Psychiatry 36:445, 1997

Guile JM: Sertraline-induced behavioral activation during the treatment of an adolescent with major depression. J Child Adolesc Psychopharmacol 6:281–285, 1996

Hagerman RJ, Murphy MA, Wittenberg MD: A controlled trial of stimulant medication in children with the fragile X syndrome. Am J Med Genet 30:377–392, 1988

Handen BL, Feldman H, Gosling A, et al: Adverse side effects of methylphenidate among mentally retarded children with ADHD. J Am Acad Child Adolesc Psychiatry 30:241–245, 1991

Handen BL, Feldman HM, Jurier A, et al: Efficacy of methylphenidate among preschool children with developmental disabilities and ADHD. J Am Acad Child Adolesc Psychiatry 38:944–951, 1999

Hardan A, Johnson K, Johnson C, et al: Case study: risperidone treatment of children and adolescents with developmental disorders. J Am Acad Child Adolesc Psychiatry 35: 1551–1556, 1996

Harley JP: Dietary treatment of behavioral disorders. Advances in Behavioral Pediatrics 1:129–151, 1980

Harmon RJ, Riggs PD: Clonidine for posttraumatic stress disorder in preschool children. J Am Acad Child Adolesc Psychiatry 35:1247–1249, 1996

Harper G: Focal inpatient treatment planning. J Am Acad Child Adolesc Psychiatry 28:31–37, 1989

Hayward C, Varady S, Albano AM, et al: Cognitive-behavioral group therapy for social phobia in female adolescents: results of a pilot study. J Am Acad Child Adolesc Psychiatry 39:721–726, 2000

Henggeler SW, Borduin CM, Schoenwald SK, et al: Multisystemic Treatment of Antisocial Behavior in Children and Adolescents. New York, Guilford, 1998

Herskowitz J: Developmental neurotoxicology, in Psychiatric Pharmacosciences of Children and Adolescents. Edited by Popper C. Washington, DC, American Psychiatric Press, 1987, pp 81–123

Hjalmas KI, Hanson E, Hellstrom AL, et al: Long-term treatment with desmopressin in children with primary monosymptomatic nocturnal enuresis: an open multicentre study. Swedish Enuresis Trial Group (SWEET). Br J Urol 82:704–709, 1998

Horrigan JP, Barnhill LJ: Guanfacine for treatment of attention-deficit hyperactivity disorder in boys. J Child Adolesc Psychopharmacol 5:215–223, 1995

Horrigan JP, Barnhill LJ: Risperidone and explosive aggressive autism. J Autism Dev Disord 27:313–323, 1997

Horrigan JP, Barnhill LJ: Guanfacine and secondary mania in children. J Affect Disord 54:309–314, 1999

Hunt RD, Capper S, O'Connell P: Clonidine in child and adolescent psychiatry. J Child Adolesc Psychopharmacol 1:87–102, 1990

Hunt RD, Lau S, Ryu J: Alternative therapies for ADHD, in Ritalin: Theory and Patient Management. Edited by Greenhill LL, Osman BB. New York, Mary Ann Liebert, 1991, pp 75–95

Hunt RD, Arnsten AF, Asbell MD: An open trial of guanfacine in the treatment of attention-deficit hyperactivity disorder. J Am Acad Child Adolesc Psychiatry 34:50–54, 1995

Isojarvi JI, Laatikainen TJ, Pakarinen AJ, et al: Polycystic ovaries and hyperandrogenism in women taking valproate for epilepsy. N Engl J Med 329:1383–1388, 1993

Janknegt RA, Zweers HMM, Delaere KPJ, et al: Oral desmopressin as a new treatment modality for primary nocturnal enuresis in adolescents and adults: a double-blind, randomized, multicenter study. J Urol 157:513–517, 1997

Jatlow PI: Psychotropic drug disposition during development, in Psychiatric Pharmacosciences of Children and Adolescents. Edited by Popper C. Washington, DC, American Psychiatric Press, 1987, pp 27–44

Jensen PS: Current concepts and controversies in the diagnosis and treatment of attention deficit hyperactivity disorder. Curr Psychiatry Rep 2:102–109, 2000

Jensen PS, Hinshaw SP, Kraemer HC, et al: ADHD comorbidity findings from the MTA study: comparing comorbid subgroups. J Am Acad Child Adolesc Psychiatry 40:147–158, 2001

Jones-Fearing KB: SSRI and EPS with fluoxetine. J Am Acad Child Adolesc Psychiatry 35:1107–1108, 1996

Joorabchi B: Expressions of the hyperventilation syndrome in childhood. Clin Pediatr (Phila) 16:1110–1115, 1977

Kafantaris V, Campbell M, Padron-Gayol MV, et al: Carbamazepine in hospitalized aggressive conduct disorder children: an open pilot study. Psychopharmacol Bull 28:193–199, 1992

Kaplan SL, Breit M, Gauthier B, et al: A comparison of three nocturnal enuresis treatment methods. J Am Acad Child Adolesc Psychiatry 28:282–286, 1989

Kazdin AD: Developing a research agenda for child and adolescent psychotherapy. Arch Gen Psychiatry 57:829–835, 2000

Keller MB, Ryan ND, Strober M, et al: Efficacy of paroxetine in the treatment of adolescent major depression: a randomized, controlled trial. J Am Acad Child Adolesc Psychiatry 40:762–772, 2001

Kerbeshian J, Burd L, Fisher W: Lithium carbonate in the treatment of two patients with infantile autism and atypical bipolar symptomatology. J Clin Psychopharmacol 7:401–405, 1987

Kernberg PF, Chazan SE: Children With Conduct Disorders: A Psychotherapy Manual. New York, Basic Books, 1991

King NJ, Tonge BJ, Heyne D, et al: Cognitive-behavioral treatment of school-refusing children: a controlled evaluation. J Am Acad Child Adolesc Psychiatry 37:395–403, 1998

King NJ, Tonge BJ, Mullen P, et al: Treating sexually abused children with posttraumatic stress symptoms: a randomized clinical trial. J Am Acad Child Adolesc Psychiatry 39:1347–1355, 2000

Kisch EH: Brief psychotherapy with children, adolescents, and their families. Child Adolesc Psychiatr Clin N Am 6:137–150, 1997

Klein RG, Koplewicz HS, Kanner A: Imipramine treatment of children with separation anxiety disorder. J Am Acad Child Adolesc Psychiatry 31:21–28, 1992

Kolmen BK, Feldman HM, Handen BL, et al: Naltrexone in young autistic children: a double-blind, placebo-controlled crossover study. J Am Acad Child Adolesc Psychiatry 34:223–231, 1995

Kolmen BK, Feldman HM, Handen BL, et al: Naltrexone in young autistic children: replication study and learning measures. J Am Acad Child Adolesc Psychiatry 36:1570–1578, 1997

Kowatch RA, Bucci JP: Mood stabilizers and anticonvulsants. Pediatr Clin North Am 45:1173–1186, 1998

Kowatch RA, Suppes T, Carmody TJ, et al: Effect size of lithium, divalproex sodium, and carbamazepine in children and adolescents with bipolar disorder. J Am Acad Child Adolesc Psychiatry 39:713–720, 2000

Krener PK, Mancina RA: Informed consent or informed coercion? Decision-making in pediatric psychopharmacology. J Child Adolesc Psychopharmacol 4:183–200, 1994

Krishanmoorthy J, King BH: Open-label olanzapine treatment in five preadolescent children. J Child Adolesc Psychopharmacol 8:107–113, 1998

Kumra S, Frazier JA, Jacobsen LK, et al: Child-onset schizophrenia: a double-blind clozapine-haloperidol comparison. Arch Gen Psychiatry 53:1090–1097, 1996

Kumra S, Jacobsen LK, Lenane M, et al: Childhood-onset schizophrenia: an open-label study of olanzapine in adolescents. J Am Acad Child Adolesc Psychiatry 37:377–385, 1998

Kutcher SP: Child and Adolescent Psychopharmacology. Philadelphia, PA, WB Saunders, 1997

Kutcher SP, MacKenzie S, Galarraga W, et al: Clonazepam treatment of adolescents with neuroleptic-induced akathisia. Am J Psychiatry 144:823–824, 1987

Kutcher SP, Williamson P, MacKenzie S, et al: Successful clonazepam treatment of neuroleptic-induced akathisia in older adolescents and young adults: a double-blind, placebo-controlled study. J Clin Psychopharmacol 9:403–406, 1989

Kutcher SP, Reiter S, Gardner DM, et al: The pharmacotherapy of anxiety disorders in children and adolescents. Psychiatr Clin North Am 15:41–67, 1992

Law SF, Schachar RJ: Do typical clinical doses of methylphenidate cause tics in children treated for attention-deficit hyperactivity disorder? J Am Acad Child Adolesc Psychiatry 38:40–47, 1999

Leckman JF, Ort S, Caruso KA, et al: Rebound phenomena in Tourette's syndrome after abrupt withdrawal of clonidine: behavioral, cardiovascular, and neurochemical effects. Arch Gen Psychiatry 43:1168–1176, 1986

Leckman JF, Hardin MT, Riddle MA, et al: Clonidine treatment of Gilles de la Tourette's syndrome. Arch Gen Psychiatry 48:324–328, 1991

Lee DO, Lee CD: Serotonin syndrome in a child associated with erythromycin and sertraline. Pharmacotherapy 19:894–896, 1999

Lenti C: Movement disorders associated with fluvoxamine. J Am Acad Child Adolesc Psychiatry 38:942–943, 1999

Leonard HL, Swedo SE, Rapoport JL, et al: Treatment of obsessive-compulsive disorder with clomipramine and desipramine in children and adolescents: a double-blind crossover comparison. Arch Gen Psychiatry 46:1088–1092, 1989

Levine MD: Encopresis: its potentiation, evaluation and alleviation. Pediatr Clin North Am 29:315–330, 1982

Lewinsohn PM, Clarke GN, Hops H, et al: Cognitive-behavioral treatment for depressed adolescents. Behav Ther 21:385–401, 1990

Lewis O: Psychological factors affecting pharmacologic compliance. Child Adolesc Psychiatr Clin North Am 4:15–22, 1995

Lewis O: Integrated psychodynamic psychotherapy with children. Child Adolesc Psychiatr Clin N Am 6:53–68, 1997

Lifrak PD, Alterman AI, O'Brien CP, et al: Naltrexone for alcoholic adolescents. Am J Psychiatry 154:439–440, 1997

Lipinski F, Mallya G, Zimmerman P, et al: Fluoxetine-induced akathisia: clinical and theoretical implications. J Clin Psychiatry 50:339–342, 1989

Lombroso PJ, Scahill L, King RA, et al: Risperidone treatment of children and adolescents with chronic tic disorders: a preliminary report. J Am Acad Child Adolesc Psychiatry 34:1147–1152, 1995

Malone RP, Delaney MA, Luebbert JF, et al: A double-blind placebo-controlled study of lithium in hospitalized aggressive children and adolescents with conduct disorder. Arch Gen Psychiatry 57:649–654, 2000

Malone RP, Cataer J, Sheikh RM, et al: Olanzapine versus haloperidol in children with autistic disorder: an open pilot study. J Am Acad Child Adolesc Psychiatry 40:887–894, 2001

Mandoki M: Olanzapine in the treatment of early onset schizophrenia in children and adolescents. Biol Psychiatry 41:22S, 1997

Mandoki MW, Tapia MR, Tapia MA, et al: Venlafaxine in the treatment of children and adolescents with major depression. Psychopharmacol Bull 33:149–154, 1997

March JS: Cognitive-behavioral psychotherapy for children and adolescents with OCD: a review and recommendations for treatment. J Am Acad Child Adolesc Psychiatry 34:7–18, 1995

March JS, Mulle K, Herbel B: Behavioral psychotherapy for children and adolescents with obsessive-compulsive disorder: an open trial of a new protocol-driven treatment package. J Am Acad Child Adolesc Psychiatry 33:333–341, 1994

March JS, Amaya-Jackson L, Murray MC, et al: Cognitive-behavioral psychotherapy for children and adolescents with posttraumatic stress disorder after a single-incident stressor. J Am Acad Child Adolesc Psychiatry 37:585–593, 1998a

March JS, Biederman J, Wolkow R, et al: Sertraline in children and adolescents with obsessive-compulsive disorder: a multicenter randomized controlled trial. JAMA 280:1752–1756, 1998b

Martin A, Scahill L (eds): Psychopharmacology. Child Adolesc Psychiatr Clin N Am 9(1), 2000

Martin A, Koenig K, Scahill L, et al: Open-label quetiapine in the treatment of children and adolescents with autistic disorder. J Child Adolesc Psychopharmacol 9:99–107, 1999

Masek BJ, Spirito A, Fentress DW: Behavioral treatment of symptoms of childhood illness. Clin Psychol Rev 4:561–570, 1984

Masi G, Cosenza A, Mucci M: Open trial of risperidone in 24 young children with pervasive developmental disorders. J Am Acad Child Adolesc Psychiatry 40:1206–1214, 2001

McConville BJ, Minnery KL, Sorter, MT, et al: An open study of the effects of sertraline on adolescent major depression. J Child Adolesc Psychopharmacol 6:41–51, 1996

McDougle CJ, Holmes JP, Bronson MR, et al: Risperidone treatment of children and adolescents with pervasive developmental disorders: a prospective open-label study. J Am Acad Child Adolesc Psychiatry 36:685–693, 1997

Melamed BG, Klingman A, Siegel LJ: Individualizing cognitive behavioral strategies in the reduction of medical and dental stress, in Cognitive Behavior Therapy With Children. Edited by Meyers AW, Craighead WE. New York, Plenum, 1984, pp 289–313

Mikkelsen EJ: Enuresis and encopresis: ten years of progress. J Am Acad Child Adolesc Psychiatry 40:1146–1158, 2001

Mikkelsen EJ, Detlor J, Cohen DJ: School avoidance and social phobia triggered by haloperidol in patients with Tourette's disorder. Am J Psychiatry 138:1572–1576, 1981

Milich R, Wolraich M, Lindgren S: Sugar and hyperactivity: a critical review of empirical findings. Clin Psychol Rev 6:493–513, 1986

Minnery KL, West SA, McConville BJ, et al: Sertraline-induced mania in an adolescent. J Child Adolesc Psychopharmacol 5:151–153, 1995

Mufson L, Moreau D, Weissman MM, et al: Modification of interpersonal psychotherapy with depressed adolescents (IPT-A): phase I and II studies. J Am Acad Child Adolesc Psychiatry 33:695–705, 1994

Mufson L, Weissman M, Moreau D, et al: Efficacy of interpersonal psychotherapy for depressed adolescents. Arch Gen Psychiatry 56:573–579, 1999

Mullins ME, Horowitz BZ: Serotonin syndrome after a single dose of fluvoxamine (comment). Ann Emerg Med 34:806–807, 1999

O'Brien JD, Perlmutter I: The effect of medication on the process of psychotherapy. Child Adolesc Psychiatr Clin North Am 6:185–196, 1997

Oldroyd J: Paroxetine-induced mania. J Am Acad Child Adolesc Psychiatry 36:721–722, 1997

Olvera RL, Pliszka SR, Luh J, et al: An open trial of venlafaxine in the treatment of attention-deficit/hyperactivity disorder in children and adolescents. J Child Adolesc Psychopharmacol 6:241-250, 1996

Pao M, Tipnis T: Serotonin syndrome after sertraline overdose in a 5-year-old girl. Arch Pediatr Adolesc Med 151:1064–1067, 1997

Papatheodorou G, Kutcher SP, Katic M: The efficacy and safety of divalproex sodium in the treatment of acute mania in adolescents and young adults: an open clinical trial. J Clin Psychopharmacol 15:110–116, 1995

Patterson GR: Families: Applications of Social Learning to Family Life. Champaign, IL, Research Press, 1975

Patterson GR, Forgatch M: Parents and Adolescents Living Together. Eugene, OR, Castalia, 1987

Pelham WE Jr, Hoza J: Behavioral assessment of psychostimulant effects on ADD children in a summer day treatment program, in Advances in Behavioral Assessment of Children and Families, Vol 3. Edited by Prinz R. Greenwich, CT, JAI Press, 1987, pp 3–33

Pelham WE Jr, Murphy HA: Attention deficit and conduct disorders, in Pharmacological and Behavioral Treatment: An Integrative Approach. Edited by Hersen M. New York, Wiley, 1986, pp 108–148

Pelham WE, Gnagy EM, Burrows-Maclean L, et al: Once-a-day Concerta methylphenidate versus three-times-daily methylphenidate in laboratory and natural settings. Pediatrics 107:E105, 2001

Percy AK, Glaze DG, Schultz RJ, et al: Rett syndrome: controlled study of an oral opiate antagonist, naltrexone. Ann Neurol 35:464–470, 1994

Perry R, Pataki C, Monoz-Silva DM, et. Al: Risperidone in children and adolescents with pervasive developmental disorder: pilot trial and follow-up. J Child Adolesc Psychopharmacol 7:167–179, 1997

Pfeffer CR, Jiang H, Domeshek LJ: Buspirone treatment of psychiatrically hospitalized prepubertal children with symptoms of anxiety and moderately severe aggression. J Child Adolesc Psychopharmacol 7:145–155, 1997

Pfefferbaum B, Overall JE, Boron HA, et al: Alprazolam in the treatment of anticipatory and acute situational anxiety in children with cancer. J Am Acad Child Adolesc Psychiatry 26:532–535, 1987

Pleak RR, Birmaher B, Gavrilescu A, et al: Mania and neuropsychiatric excitation following carbamazepine. J Am Acad Child Adolesc Psychiatry 27:500–503, 1988

Pliszka SR: A double-blind, placebo-controlled study of Adderall and methylphenidate in the treatment of attention-deficit/hyperactivity disorder. J Am Acad Child Adolesc Psychiatry 39:619–626, 2000

Pool D, Bloom W, Mielke DH, et al: A controlled evaluation of Loxitane in seventy-five adolescent schizophrenic patients. Curr Ther Res Clin Exp 19:99–104, 1976

Popper C: Medical unknowns and ethical consent: prescribing psychotropic medications for children in the face of uncertainty, in Psychiatric Pharmacosciences of Children and Adolescents. Edited by Popper C. Washington, DC, American Psychiatric Press, 1987, pp 125–161

Popper CW: Combining methylphenidate and clonidine: pharmacologic questions and news reports about sudden death. J Child Adolesc Psychopharmacol 5:157–166, 1995

Potenza MN, Holmes JP, Kanes SJ, et al: Olanzapine treatment of children, adolescents, and adults with pervasive developmental disorders: an open-label pilot study. J Clin Psychopharmacol 19:37–44, 1999

Preskorn SH, Weller EB, Hughes CW, et al: Depression in prepubertal children: dexamethasone nonsuppression predicts differential response to imipramine versus placebo. Psychopharmacol Bull 23:128–133, 1987

Quintana H, Keshavan M: Case study: risperidone in children and adolescents with schizophrenia. J Am Acad Child Adolesc Psychiatry 34:1292–1296, 1995

Rapoport JL: Antidepressants in childhood attention deficit disorder and obsessive-compulsive disorder. Psychosomatics 27(suppl):30–36, 1986

Ratey J, Sovner R, Parks A, et al: Buspirone treatment of aggression and anxiety in mentally retarded patients: a multiple-baseline, placebo lead-in study. J Clin Psychiatry 52:159–162, 1991

Realmuto GM, Erickson WD, Yellin AM, et al: Clinical comparison of thiothixene and thioridazine in schizophrenic adolescents. Am J Psychiatry 141:440–442, 1984

Realmuto GM, August GJ, Garfinkel BD: Clinical effect of buspirone in autistic children. J Clin Psychopharmacol 9:122–125, 1989

Reischer H, Pfeffer CR: Lithium pharmacokinetics. J Am Acad Child Adolesc Psychiatry 35:130–131, 1996

Reiter S, Kutcher SP: Disinhibition and anger outbursts in adolescents treated with clonazepam (letter). J Clin Psychopharmacol 11:268, 1991

Remschmidt H, Schultz E, Martin M: An open trial of clozapine in thirty-six adolescents with schizophrenia. J Child Adolesc Psychopharmacol 4:31–41, 1994

Remschmidt H, Hennighausen K, Clement HW, et al: Atypical neuroleptics in child and adolescent psychiatry. Eur Child Adolesc Psychiatry: 9(suppl 1):I9–I19, 2000

Rey JM, Walter G: Half a century of ECT use in young people. Am J Psychiatry 154:595–602, 1997

Richardson MA, Haugland G, Craig TJ: Neuroleptic use, parkinsonian symptoms, tardive dyskinesia, and associated factors in child and adolescent psychiatric patients. Am J Psychiatry 148:1322–1328, 1991

Richters JE, Arnold E, Jensen PS, et al: NIMH Collaborative Multisite Multimodal Treatment Study of Children with ADHD, I: background and rationale. J Am Acad Child Adolesc Psychiatry 34:987–1000, 1995

Riddle MA, Nelson JC, Kleinman CS, et al: Sudden death in children receiving Norpramin: a review of three reported cases and commentary. J Am Acad Child Adolesc Psychiatry 30:104–108, 1991

Riddle MA, Scahill L, King RA, et al: Double-blind, crossover trial of fluoxetine and placebo in children and adolescents with obsessive-compulsive disorder. J Am Acad Child Adolesc Psychiatry 31:1062–1069, 1992

Riddle MA, Geller B, Ryan N: Another sudden death in a child treated with desipramine. J Am Acad Child Adolesc Psychiatry 32:792–797, 1993

Riddle MA, Reeve, EA, Yaryura-Tobias JA, et al: Fluvoxamine for children and adolescents with obsessive-compulsive disorder: a randomized, controlled, multicenter trial. J Am Acad Child Adolesc Psychiatry 40:222–229, 2001

Rifkin A, Karajgi B, Dicker R, et al: Lithium treatment of conduct disorder in adolescents. Am J Psychiatry 154:554–555, 1997

Riggs PD, Leon SL, Mikulich SK, et al: An open trial of bupropion for ADHD in adolescents with substance use disorders and conduct disorder. J Am Acad Child Adolesc Psychiatry 37:1271–1278, 1998

Ritvo R, Al-Mateen C, Ascherman L, et al: Report of the Psychotherapy Task Force of the American Academy of Child and Adolescent Psychiatry. J Psychother Pract Res 8:93–102, 1999

Rosenberg DR, Stewart CM, Fitzgerald KD, et al: Paroxetine open-label treatment of pediatric outpatients with obsessive-compulsive disorder. J Am Acad Child Adolesc Psychiatry 38:1180–1185, 1999

Rosenfeld AA, Pilowsky DJ, Fine P, et al: Foster care: an update. J Am Acad Child Adolesc Psychiatry 36:448–457, 1997

Ryan ND: Heterocyclic antidepressants in children and adolescents. J Child Adolesc Psychopharmacol 1:21–31, 1990

Ryan ND: The pharmacologic treatment of child and adolescent depression. Psychiatr Clin North Am 15:29–40, 1992

Ryan ND, Meyer V, Dachille S, et al: Lithium antidepressant augmentation in TCA-refractory depression in adolescents. J Am Acad Child Adolesc Psychiatry 27:371–376, 1988a

Ryan ND, Puig-Antich J, Rabinovich H, et al: MAOIs in adolescent major depression unresponsive to tricyclic antidepressants. J Am Acad Child Adolesc Psychiatry 27:755–758, 1988b

Safer DJ: Changing patterns of psychotropic medications prescribed by child psychiatrists in the 1990s. J Child Adolesc Psychopharmacol 7:267–274, 1997

Safer DJ, Zito JM, Gardner JF: Pemoline hepatotoxicity and postmarketing surveillance. J Am Acad Child Adolesc Psychiatry 40:622–629, 2001

Sallee F, Rock CM: Effects of pimozide on cognition in children with Tourette syndrome: interaction with comorbid attention-deficit hyperactivity disorder. Acta Psychiatr Scand 90:4–9, 1994

Sallee F, Stiller R, Perel J, et al: Targeting imipramine dose in children with depression. Clin Pharmacol Ther 40:8–13, 1986

Sallee FR, Kurlan R, Goetz CG, et al: Ziprasidone treatment of children and adolescents with Tourette syndrome: a pilot study. J Am Acad Child Adolesc Psychiatry 39:292–299, 2000

Samuel RZ: EPS with lithium (letter). J Am Acad Child Adolesc Psychiatry 32:1078, 1993

Sanchez LE, Campbell M, Small AM: A pilot study of clomipramine in young autistic children. J Am Acad Child Adolesc Psychiatry 35:537–544, 1996

Saul RC: Nortriptyline in attention deficit disorder. Clin Neuropharmacol 8:382–384, 1985

Scahill L, Chappell PB, Kim YS, et al: A placebo-controlled study of guanfacine in the treatment of children with tic disorders and attention deficit hyperactivity disorder. Am J Psychiatry 158:1067–1074, 2001

Scheidlinger S: Short-term group psychotherapy for children: an overview. Int J Group Psychother 34:573–585, 1984

Scheidlinger S: Group treatment of adolescents: an overview. Am J Orthopsychiatry 55:102–111, 1985

Serketich WJ, Dumas JE: The effectiveness of behavioral parent training to modify antisocial behavior in children: a meta-analysis. Behav Ther 27:171–186, 1996

Sharp WS, Walter JM, Marsh WL, et al: ADHD in girls: clinical comparability of a research sample. J Am Acad Child Adolesc Psychiatry 38:805–812, 1999

Sholevar EH, Baron DA, Hardie TL: Treatment of childhood-onset schizophrenia with olanzapine. J Child Adolesc Psychopharmacol 10:69–78, 2000

Silva RR, Munoz DM, Alpert M, et al: Neuroleptic malignant syndrome in children and adolescents. J Am Acad Child Adolesc Psychiatry 38:187–194, 1999

Silver LB: Alternative (nonstimulant) medications in the treatment of attention-deficit/hyperactivity disorder in children. Pediatr Clin North Am 46:965–975, 1999

Silverman WK: Using what works to help children manage stress and anxiety: an appeal for pragmatism. Session: Psychotherapy in Practice 3:103–108, 1997

Silverstein FS, Boxer L, Johnson MV: Hematological monitoring during therapy with carbamazepine in children. Ann Neurol 13:685–686, 1983

Simeon JG, Ferguson HB: Recent developments in the use of antidepressant and anxiolytic medications. Psychiatr Clin North Am 8:893–907, 1985

Simeon JG, Ferguson HB, Knott V, et al: Clinical, cognitive, and neurophysiological effects of alprazolam in children and adolescents with overanxious and avoidant disorders. J Am Acad Child Adolesc Psychiatry 31:29–33, 1992

Simeon JG, Knott VJ, Dubois C, et al: Buspirone therapy of mixed anxiety disorders in childhood and adolescence: a pilot study. J Child Adolesc Psychopharmacol 4:159–170, 1994

Singer HS, Brown J: The treatment of attention-deficit hyperactivity disorder in Tourette's syndrome: a double-blind placebo-controlled study with clonidine and desipramine. Pediatrics 95:74–81, 1995

Skoog SJ, Stokes A, Turner K: Oral desmopressin: a randomized double-blind placebo controlled study of effectiveness in children with primary nocturnal enuresis. J Urol 158:1035–1040, 1997

Soni P, Weintraub AL: Case study: buspirone-associated mental status changes. J Am Acad Child Adolesc Psychiatry 31:1098–1099, 1992

Spencer EK, Kafantaris V, Padron-Gayol MV, et al: Haloperidol in schizophrenic children: early findings from a study in progress. Psychopharmacol Bull 28:183–186, 1992

Spencer T, Biederman J, Steingard R, et al: Bupropion exacerbates tics in children with attention-deficit hyperactivity disorder and Tourette's syndrome. J Am Acad Child Adolesc Psychiatry 32:211–214, 1993

Spencer T, Wilens T, Biederman J: Psychotropic medication for children and adolescents. Child Adolesc Psychiatr Clin North Am 4:97–121, 1995

Spencer T, Biederman J, Harding M, et al: Growth deficits in ADHD children revisited: evidence for disorder-associated growth delays? J Am Acad Child Adolesc Psychiatry 35:1460–1469, 1996a

Spencer T, Biederman J, Wilens T, et al: Pharmacotherapy of attention-deficit hyperactivity disorder across the life cycle. J Am Acad Child Adolesc Psychiatry 35:409–432, 1996b

Spirko BA, Wiley JF 2d: Serotonin syndrome: a new pediatric intoxication. Pediatr Emerg Care 15:440–443, 1999

Sprague RL, Sleator EK: Methylphenidate in hyperkinetic children: differences in dose effects on learning and social behavior. Science 198:1274–1276, 1977

Stahl SM: Essential Pharmacology: Newer antidepressants and mood stabilizers, in Neuroscientific Basis and Practical Applications, 2nd Edition. New York, Cambridge University Press, 2000, pp 246–255

Steingard R, Biederman J: Lithium responsive manic-like symptoms in two individuals with autism and mental retardation. J Am Acad Child Psychiatry 26:932–935, 1987

Steingard R, Biederman J, Spencer TJ, et al: Comparison of clonidine response in the treatment of attention-deficit hyperactivity disorder with and without comorbid tic disorders. J Am Acad Child Adolesc Psychiatry 32:350–353, 1993

Steingard R, Goldberg M, Lee D, et al: Adjunctive clonazepam treatment of tic symptoms in children with comorbid tic disorders and ADHD. J Am Acad Child Adolesc Psychiatry 33:394–399, 1994

Stokes TF, Baer DM: An implicit technology of generalization. J Appl Behav Anal 10:349–367, 1977

Strayhorn JM Jr: The Competent Child: An Approach to Psychotherapy and Preventive Mental Health. New York, Guilford, 1988

Strober M, Morrell W, Lampert C, et al: Relapse following discontinuation of lithium maintenance therapy in adolescents with bipolar I illness: a naturalistic study. Am J Psychiatry 147:457–461, 1990

Strober M, Freeman R, Rigali J, et al: The pharmacotherapy of depressive illness in adolescence, II: effects of lithium augmentation in nonresponders to imipramine. J Am Acad Child Adolesc Psychiatry 31:16–20, 1992

Strober M, Pataki C, DeAntonio M: Complete remission of 'treatment resistant' severe melancholia in adolescents with phenelzine: two case reports. J Affect Disord 50:55–58, 1998

Strupp HH: Psychotherapy: Clinical, Research, and Theoretical Issues. New York, Jason Aronson, 1973

Swanson JM, Flockhart D, Udrea D, et al: Clonidine in the treatment of ADHD: questions about safety and efficacy. J Child Adolesc Psychopharmacol 5:301–304, 1995

Swanson JM, Wigal S, Greenhill L, et al: Analog classroom assessment of Adderall in children with ADHD. J Am Acad Child Adolesc Psychiatry 37:519–526. 1998a

Swanson J, Wigal S, Greenhill L, et al: Objective and subjective measures of the pharmacodynamic effects of Adderall in the treatment of children with ADHD in a controlled laboratory classroom setting. Psychopharmacol Bull 34:55–60, 1998b

Swanson JM, Connor DF, Cantwell D: Combining methylphenidate and clonidine. J Am Acad Child Adolesc Psychiatry 38:617–619, 1999

Teicher MH, Glod CA: Neuroleptic drugs: indications and guidelines for their rational use in children and adolescents. J Child Adolesc Psychopharmacol 1:33–56, 1990

Thompson S, Rey JM: Functional enuresis: is desmopressin the answer? J Am Acad Child Adolesc Psychiatry 34:266–271, 1995

Thomsen PH: Child and adolescent obsessive-compulsive disorder treated with citalopram: findings from an open trial of 23 cases. J Child Adolesc Psychopharmacol 7:157–166, 1997

Thomsen PH, Ebbesen C, Persson C: Long-term experience with citalopram in the treatment of adolescent OCD. J Am Acad Child Adolesc Psychiatry 40:895–902, 2001

Tierney E, Joshi PT, Llinas JF, et al: Sertraline for major depression in children and adolescents: preliminary clinical experience. J Child Adolesc Psychopharmacol 5:13–27, 1995

Toren P, Laor N, Weizman A: Use of atypical neuroleptics in child and adolescent psychiatry. J Clin Psychiatry 59:644–656, 1998

Trimble MR: Anticonvulsants in children and adolescents. J Child Adolesc Psychopharmacol 1:33–56, 1990

Van Putten T, Marder SR: Behavioral toxicity of antipsychotic drugs. J Clin Psychiatry 48(suppl):13–19, 1987

Varanka TM, Weller RA, Weller EB, et al: Lithium treatment of manic episodes with psychotic features in prepubertal children. Am J Psychiatry 145:1557–1559, 1988

Varni JW, Jay SM, Masek BJ, et al: Cognitive-behavioral assessment and management of pediatric pain, in Handbook of Psychological Treatment Approaches. Edited by Holvman AD, Turk ED. New York, Pergamon, 1986, pp 168–192

Varley C, McClellan J: Case study: two additional sudden deaths with tricyclic antidepressants. J Am Acad Child Adolesc Psychiatry 36:390–394, 1997

Vitiello B, Severe JB, Greenhill LL, et al: Methylphenidate dosage for children with ADHD over time under controlled conditions: lessons from the MTA. J Am Acad Child Adolesc Psychiatry 40:188–196, 2001

Walkup JT, Labellarte MJ, Riddle MA, et al: Fluvoxamine for the treatment of anxiety disorders in children and adolescents. N Engl J Med 344:1279–1285, 2001

Walsh BT, Greenhill LL, Elsa-Grace V, et al: Effects of desipramine on autonomic input to the heart. J Am Acad Child Adolesc Psychiatry 38:1186–1193, 1999

Walter G, Koster K, Rey JM: Electroconvulsive therapy in adolescents: experience, knowledge, and attitudes of recipients. J Am Acad Child Adolesc Psychiatry 38:594–595, 1999

Waslick BD, Walsh BT, Greenhill LL, et al: Cardiovascular effects of desipramine in children and adults during exercise testing. J Am Acad Child Adolesc Psychiatry 38:179–186, 1999

Webster-Stratton C: Incredible Years: A Troubleshooting Guide for Parents of Children Aged 3 to 8. Toronto, ON, Canada, Umbrella Press, 1992

Webster-Stratton C: How to Promote Children's Social and Emotional Competence. London, England, Paul Chapman, 2000

Weller EB, Weller RA, Fristad MA: Lithium dosage guide for prepubertal children: a preliminary report. J Am Acad Child Psychiatry 25:92–95, 1986

Wender EH: The food additive-free diet in the treatment of behavior disorders: a review. J Dev Behav Pediatr 7:35–42, 1986

Wender EH, Solanto MV: Effects of sugar on aggressive and inattentive behavior in children with attention deficit disorder with hyperactivity and normal children. Pediatrics 88:960–966, 1991

Werry JS, Aman MD (eds): Practitioner's Guide to Psychoactive Drugs for Children and Adolescents, 2nd Edition. New York, Plenum, 1999

West SA, Keck PE, McElroy SL: Open trial of valproate in the treatment of adolescent mania. J Child Adolesc Psychopharmacol 4:263–267, 1994

Whalen EH, Henker B: Social impact of stimulant treatment for hyperactive children. Journal of Learning Disabilities 24:231–241, 1991

Wilens TE, Biederman J: The stimulants. Psychiatr Clin North Am 15:191–222, 1992

Wilens TE, Spencer TJ: Combining methylphenidate and clonidine. J Am Acad Child Adolesc Psychiatry 38:614–161, 1999

Wilens TE, Biederman J, Baldessarini RJ, et al: Cardiovascular effects of therapeutic doses of tricyclic antidepressants in children and adolescents. J Am Acad Child Adolesc Psychiatry 35:1491–1501, 1996

Wiles CP, Hardin MT, King RA, et al: Antidepressant-induced prolongation of QTc interval on EKG in two children, in Abstracts of the Annual Meeting of the American Academy of Child and Adolescent Psychiatry. Washington, DC, 1991, p 70

Willemsen-Swinkels SHN, Buitelaar JK, Nijhof GJ, et al: Failure of naltrexone hydrochloride to reduce self-injurious and autistic behavior in mentally retarded adults: double-blind placebo-controlled studies. Arch Gen Psychiatry 52:766–773, 1995

Willemsen-Swinkels SH, Buitelaar JK, van Engeland H: The effects of chronic naltrexone treatment in young autistic children: a double-blind placebo-controlled crossover study. Biol Psychiatry 39:1023–1031, 1996

Williams DT: Hypnosis as a psychotherapeutic adjunct, in Basic Handbook of Child Psychiatry, Vol 3: Therapeutic Interventions. Edited by Harrison SI. New York, Basic Books, 1979, pp 108–116

Williams DT, Mehl R, Yudofsky S, et al: The effect of propranolol on uncontrolled rage outbursts in children and adolescents with organic brain dysfunction. J Am Acad Child Psychiatry 21:129–135, 1982

Winsberg BG, Perel JM, Hurwic MJ, et al: Imipramine protein binding and pharmacokinetics in children, in The Phenothiazines and Structurally Related Drugs. Edited by Forrest IS, Carr CJ, Usdin E. New York, Raven, 1974, pp 425–431

Wold M, Kaminer Y: Naltrexone for alcohol abuse. J Am Acad Child Adolesc Psychiatry 36:6–7, 1997

Woolston JL: Case study: carbamazepine treatment of juvenile-onset bipolar disorder. J Am Acad Child Adolesc Psychiatry 38:335–338, 1999

Zahn TP, Rapoport JL, Thompson CL: Autonomic and behavioral effects of dextroamphetamine and placebo in normal and hyperactive prepubertal boys. J Abnorm Child Psychol 8:145–160, 1980

Zuddas A, Di Martino A, Muglia P, et. Al: Long-term risperidone for pervasive developmental disorder: efficacy, tolerability, and discontinuation. J Child Adolesc Psychopharmacol 10:79–90, 2000

Appendix: Books for Parents

Attention-Deficit/Hyperactivity Disorder

Alexander-Roberts C: ADHD and Teens: A Parent's Guide to Making It Through the Tough Years. Dallas, TX, Taylor, 1995

Barkley RA: Taking Charge of ADHD: The Complete, Authoritative Guide for Parents. New York, Guilford, 2000

Children and Adults with Attention-Deficit/Hyperactivity Disorder: The CHADD Information and Resource Guide for ADHD. Landover, MD, CHADD, 2000

Hallowell EM, Ratey JJ: Driven to Distraction: Recognizing and Coping With Attention Deficit Disorder From Childhood Through Adulthood. New York, Simon & Schuster, 1995

Silver LM, Silver LB: Dr. Larry Silver's Advice to Parents on Attention-Deficit Hyperactivity Disorder. Washington, DC, American Psychiatric Press, 1992

Wender P: The Hyperactive Child, Adolescent and Adult: Attention Deficit Disorder Through the Lifespan. New York, Oxford University Press, 1987

Autism

Gerdtz J, Bregman J: Autism: A Practical Guide for Those Who Help Others. New York, Continuum, 1990

Siegel B: The World of the Autistic Child. New York, Oxford University Press, 1996

Depression

Cytryn L, McKnew DH Jr, Cytryn LW: Growing Up Sad: Childhood Depression and Its Treatment. New York, WW Norton, 1996

Fassler DG, Dumas LS: "Help Me, I'm Sad": Recognizing, Treating, and Preventing Childhood and Adolescent Depression. New York, Viking, 1997

Herskowitz J: Is Your Child Depressed? New York, Pharos, 1988

Enuresis

Azrin N, Foxx R: Toilet Training in Less Than a Day. New York, Simon & Schuster, 1974

Learning Disabilities

Silver LB: The Misunderstood Child: A Guide for Parents of Learning Disabled Children. New York, McGraw-Hill, 1984

Managing Child Behavior

Greenspan SI, Salmon J: The Challenging Child: Understanding, Raising, and Enjoying the Five "Difficult" Types of Children. Reading, MA, Addison-Wesley, 1996

Pruitt D (ed): Your Adolescent: Emotional, Behavioral, and Cognitive Development from Early Adolescence Through the Teen Years. American Academy of Child and Adolescent Psychiatry. San Francisco, CA, Harper-Collins, 2000

Pruitt D (ed): Your Child: Emotional, Behavioral, and Cognitive Development from Birth Through Preadolescence. American Academy of Child and Adolescent Psychiatry. San Francisco, CA, Harper-Collins, 2000

Sears W, Sears M: The Discipline Book: Everything You Need to Know to Have a Better-Behaved Child. For Birth to Age Ten. Boston, MA, Little, Brown, 1995

Turecki S, Tonner L: The Difficult Child. New York, Doubleday Dell, 1989

Mental Illness

McElroy E (ed): Children and Adolescents With Mental Illness: A Parent's Guide. Washington, DC, Woodbine, 1988

Obsessive-Compulsive Disorder

Rapoport JL: The Boy Who Couldn't Stop Washing: The Experience and Treatment of Obsessive-Compulsive Disorder. New York, Penguin, 1990

Posttraumatic Stress Disorder

Terr L: Too Scared to Cry: Psychic Trauma in Childhood. New York, Harper & Row, 1990

Schizophrenia

Cantor S: The Schizophrenic Child: A Primer for Parents and Professionals. Montreal, Quebec, Eden Press, 1982

Tourette's Disorder

Bruun RD, Bruun B: A Mind of Its Own, Tourette's Syndrome: A Story and a Guide. New York, Oxford University Press, 1994

Special Clinical Topics

Suicide

T. Carroll-Ghosh, M.D.

Bruce S. Victor, M.D.

James A. Bourgeois, O.D., M.D.

Suicide can be understood from many different perspectives—from religious, philosophical, and sociological to psychological and biological. Historically, the meaning of suicide has reflected the religious tradition of a given culture (Stevenson 1988). The Judeo-Christian tradition has held that life is a gift from God and that the taking of life is strictly forbidden. These influences still exist and may contribute to the lower suicide rates in more traditionally Catholic countries such as Italy, Spain, and Ireland.

More recently, secular philosophy has influenced how suicide is perceived in our society. Respect for the individual's will and personal rights has led some to view suicide as a rational act, a choice of death over pain. This view has led to movements that support suicide as a right of terminally ill patients and has been taken one step further with physician-assisted suicides in the terminally ill. As of this writing, few communities currently allow for legally sanctioned assisted suicide—Australia's Northern Territory, Canada, Colombia, The Netherlands, and only the state of Oregon in the United States. In these jurisdictions, such actions are expected to meet certain conditions, including the absence of neuromedical or psychiatric conditions that impair the patient's capacity to reason and process pertinent information, the ability of the patient to understand the consequences of his or her decisions based on a realistic view of the situation, and the strong desire of the patient to end his or her suffering from a terminal condition for which there is no hope of reversal, with care to avoid an impulsive decision based on initial diagnosis (Emanuel et al. 2000). Bernat (1997) reviewed the legal and moral issues of physician-assisted suicide and cautioned that that its legalization would

have a negative effect on the practice of palliative care and would be followed by legalization of voluntary and involuntary euthanasia.

The critical issue facing the psychiatric clinician is whether conditions that impair the patient's capacity to reason are truly absent. We know that the overwhelming majority of suicides—more than 90%—occur in individuals who are psychiatrically ill at the time of suicide (Black and Winokur 1990; E. Robins et al. 1959). Thus, our focus in this chapter is to review suicide from a clinical psychiatric viewpoint rather than from a religious, philosophical, or sociological perspective. We review the epidemiology and demographics of suicide and then discuss the psychiatric syndromes and psychological factors most correlated with suicide. We then discuss the emerging neurobiological factors in suicide and review the assessment and management of the suicidal patient.

Epidemiology and Demographics

Knowledge of the epidemiology and demographics of suicide is essential to the clinician assessing the suicidal patient. Suicide is the eighth leading cause of death in the United States. To this end, in a landmark decision, U.S. Surgeon General David Satcher launched a national campaign to combat suicide (Surgeon General of the United States 2001). Despite the development of suicide prevention programs, greater recognition of depression, and advances in biological treatments for depression, the overall rate of suicide has not changed over the past several decades; it has remained in the range of 11–12 per 100,000 annually (Chaudron and Remington 1999; Sainsbury 1986b; Stevenson 1988). One of the few identified factors that correlate with the overall rate of suicide is the availability of the means to suicide. This correlation was first demonstrated in England earlier in the twentieth century: when the toxicity of gas supplied in the homes was reduced, the suicide rate diminished concomitantly. The availability of firearms also appears to correlate with suicide risk. In a study involving five New York counties, Marzuk et al. (1992a) demonstrated that the differences in overall suicide risk among counties were explained by differentially available lethal means of injury. Lambert and Silva (1998) reported a decrease in suicide rates after the implementation of firearms control laws.

With the caveat that "accurate ascertainment of occupation and employment status at the time of suicide is often impossible," Boxer et al. (1997) reviewed the literature on occupation and suicide and concluded that chemistry, farming, law enforcement, and medicine appeared to confer high risk for suicide and that the risk for female physicians may be particularly high. Unemployment has also been shown to increase the rate of suicide for both men and women (Kposowa 2001).

Although the overall rate of suicide has remained constant over the past several decades, rates among subgroups of age, sex, and race have changed. The highly publicized increase in adolescent and youth suicide appears to have been offset by a declining rate of suicide among older adults (L.N. Robins and Kulbok 1988); however, the rates of suicide among the elderly still remain high. The annual suicide rate in the United States in 1990 for persons ages 65–74 and 75–84 were 17.9/100,000 and 24.9/100,000, respectively (Moscicki 1995).

Figure 34–1 provides a breakdown of annual suicide rates in the United States per 100,000 people by age group. The rates for both Caucasian and African American females are relatively constant and low compared with the rates for males. The rate for African American males peaks between ages 20 and 40, declines, and then increases again after age 75. Most strikingly, the high rate of completed suicides in Caucasian males initially peaks between ages 20 and 40, levels off between ages 40 and 65, and then rapidly increases after age 65, becoming extraordinary at age 85 and older (i.e., 50 suicides per 100,000).

The general demographics for persons at low or high risk for completed suicide are presented in Table 34–1. Patients younger than 45 are at low risk compared with patients older than 45; female patients are at low risk compared with male patients. In 1987, the overall annual United States suicide rates for men and women were 24.3/100,000 and 6.5/100,000, respectively (Moscicki

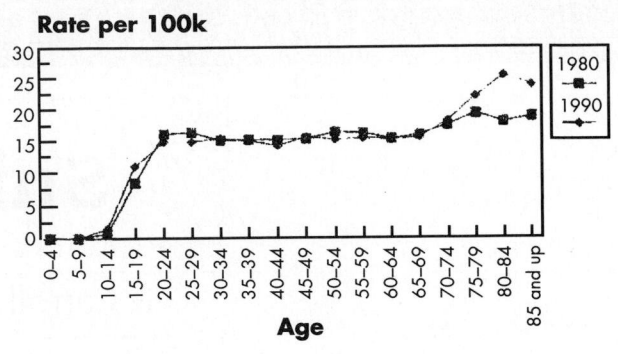

Rate per 100k

FIGURE 34–1. Age-specific suicide rates, United States, 1980 and 1990.
Source. Reprinted with permission from Potter LB, Powell KE, Kachur SP: "Suicide Prevention From a Public Health Perspective." *Suicide and Life-Threatening Behavior* 25:82–91, 1995.

TABLE 34–1. Suicide risk: general demographics

Low risk	High risk
Under age 45	Over age 45
Female	Male
NonCaucasian	Caucasian
Lives with others	Lives alone
Good health	Poor health

1995), and in 1990 they were 20.3/100,000 and 4.7/100,000, respectively (Chaudron and Remington 1999). Olson et al. (1999) found the annual suicide rate among women in New Mexico to be 8.2/100,000; firearms accounted for 46% of these deaths. Sixty-six percent of victims had alcohol or drugs in their systems, and 22% had had a recent fight with or breakup from a male partner. Stack (2000) reported a divergence between 1981 and 1995 in the relative rates for suicide among men and women, primarily due to a decreasing suicide rate among females. The ratio of male:female suicides in the United States increased from 3.1:1 (in 1972) to 4.2:1 (in 1990) (Moscicki 1995).

With regard to ethnicity, most studies demonstrate that Caucasians are at highest risk for suicide, followed by Native Americans, African Americans, Hispanic Americans, and Asian Americans. Patients who live with others or who are married are at lower risk than patients who live alone or who are divorced or widowed. Good health correlates with low risk, and poor health correlates with high risk. The incidence of suicide differs by geographic location in the United States, with mid-Atlantic regions having lower rates compared with the western mountain states. Although this difference may be artifac-

TABLE 34–2. Suicide attempts versus completions: demographics

	Attempts	Completions
Sex	Female	Male
Age	Under 35	Over 60
Means	Low lethality (e.g., wrist laceration)	High lethality (e.g., firearms, hanging)
Setting	High chance of rescue	Low chance of rescue
Diagnosis	Adjustment disorder, personality disorder	Mood disorder, substance abuse

tual and may reflect differential reporting and autopsy examinations, the differences are striking: 18.4 per 100,000 annually in middle-Atlantic states versus 32.2 per 100,000 in western mountain states.

From an international perspective, the United States suicide rate is average and analogous to the rates in Great Britain and Canada. The highest rates are in Germany, Scandinavia, Eastern Europe, and Japan, whereas the lowest rates, as mentioned previously, are in the traditionally Catholic countries (i.e., Italy, Spain, and Ireland) (Sainsbury 1986b). Sartorius (1995) examined suicide rates in 15 European nations and found suicide rates in 1991 or 1992 to vary from a high of 38.7/100,000 annually in Hungary to a low of 14.9/100,000 annually in Poland.

Parasuicide

Self-destructive behavior and nonfatal suicide attempts, although difficult to categorize, have been conceptualized as *parasuicide*. The distinction between parasuicide and completed suicide is important: parasuicidal patients usually recognize that the means are nonlethal, and these patients have different characteristics than patients who display lethal suicidal behavior. Moscicki (1989) reported on the annual rate of suicide attempts found in the National Institute of Mental Health (NIMH) Epidemiologic Catchment Area (ECA) study of more than 18,000 United States residents. Although the rates varied among the sample communities, the overall rate was 0.3%. Extrapolating from the rate of completed suicides (i.e., 12/100,000 annually), one would estimate that about 23 persons attempted suicide for every 1 who completed it.

A 16-center study in 13 European countries found wide variations in rates of parasuicide during the years 1989–1992 (Schmidtke et al. 1996). Age-standardized rates for males varied from 45/100,000 to 314/100,000 attempts annually, whereas the rates for females ranged from 69/100,000 to 462/100,000. The average male:female ratio of attempts was 1:1.5. More than 50% of the attempters made more than one attempt.

The general distinctions between those persons who attempt suicide and those who complete suicide are shown in Table 34–2. Suicide attempts are more likely in females, whereas completions are more likely in males. Suicide attempters are more likely to be young (younger than age 35), whereas completers are more likely to be older (older than age 60). The attempters' methods tend to be of low lethality—for example, so-called pill underdosages or wrist lacerations—compared with highly lethal methods such as firearms or hanging. The setting also distinguishes attempts from completions. The attempter usually makes the suicide attempt at home or in a place where he or she can be discovered, whereas the completer chooses an isolated setting where there is a very low chance for rescue. The method and the setting are important in the determination of the risk-to-rescue fantasy ratio: the higher the ratio, the more serious and potentially lethal the attempt. Finally, certain psychiatric diagnoses in suicidal patients have been found to be associated with either suicide attempt or suicide completion. Suicidal patients with adjustment disorders and personality disorders (especially cluster B personality disorders) are more likely to make nonlethal suicide attempts, whereas suicidal patients with mood disorders, psychoses, and substance abuse problems tend to be completers. One cannot discount the importance of parasuicide, because 10% of attempters ultimately will complete suicide.

Suicide and Psychiatric Illness

In addition to outlining the social factors in suicide, epidemiological surveys have demonstrated that the vast majority of completed suicides are in patients with diagnosable psychiatric conditions. In their classic study, E. Robins et al. (1959) demonstrated that 94% of individuals who completed suicide were psychiatrically ill, mainly from affective disorders or alcoholism. More recently, Black and Winokur (1990) found a similar result based on a review of studies of completed suicides: 90% of those who completed suicide were psychiatrically ill at the time of death. A small percentage of suicides are by people who have suffered a particular interpersonal loss, a financial loss, or a loss in social status. There also is an incidence of suicides in nonpsychiatric patients with terminal medical illness (e.g., cancer), but even suicide in those with terminal illness accounts for only about 5% of the total number of suicides. Most suicides occur in patients with psychiatric disturbances that in most cases are probably treatable. A large meta-analysis by Harris and Barraclough (1997) examined 249 studies of psychiatric disorders and suicide risk with minimum 2-year follow-up. They found that 36 of the 44 psychiatric disorders studied showed an increased risk of suicide. Notably, only mental retardation and dementia did not exhibit an increased suicide risk.

Suicide and Mood Disorders

Mood disorder is the diagnostic category most often represented among persons who suicide. Studies show that the presence of a mood disorder in persons who suicide ranges from 45% to as high as 77% (Barraclough et al. 1974; E. Robins et al. 1959). It has been estimated that about 15% of patients with mood disorders will go on to commit suicide (Sainsbury 1986a). However, many studies that support the 15% figure combined both unipolar depression and bipolar depression. In a review of 30 studies of patients with depressive illness, including "neurotic depression" (now subsumed under the category *dysthymic disorder*), Miles (1977) concluded that 15% ultimately suicided. The suicide rate among persons with dysthymic disorder would be difficult to estimate, given the heterogeneity of the diagnosis and the difficulty in applying this new classification to previous studies of affective illness. Patients with delusional depression have previously been thought to be at greater risk for suicide than are patients with other mood disorders; however, a recent, large study found no correlation between delusionality and suicide risk in major depressive, bipolar, or schizophrenic disorders (Grunebaum et al. 2001). The first 3 months after the onset of a major depressive episode and the first 5 years after the lifetime onset of major depressive disorder represented the highest-risk period for attempted suicide, independent of the severity or duration of depression. Familial and genetic factors, early life loss experiences, and comorbid alcoholism may be causal factors (Malone et al. 1995).

The rate of suicide completion associated with untreated bipolar disorder has been noted to be as high as 20% (Goodwin and Jamison 1990). Another study (Winokur and Tsuang 1975) examined the risk differential between bipolar and unipolar patients. In a 30–40-year follow-up of 76 bipolar patients and 182 unipolar patients,

the suicide rates were 8.5% and 10.6%, respectively. Most authors agree that the predisposing factor is not the manic state itself but rather the presence of depression that accompanies a mixed bipolar state. Clinical experience suggests that the mixed bipolar state is associated with a particularly high risk of suicide because of the dangerous combination of highly dysphoric mood and a high level of energy and perturbation. Also, the bipolar II patient group is frequently associated with suicide (Goldring and Fieve 1984). In the absence of frank mania, the bipolar II patient's condition may be underdiagnosed, and the patient may inadvertently be denied a trial of mood stabilizers; consequently, persistent cycling and affective lability may predispose the patient to suicide.

In summary, about 15%–20% of patients with mood disorders will commit suicide, making these disorders among the most lethal of medical conditions. Many studies that support these conclusions are based on epidemiological data that are drawn from a mixture of treated and untreated populations. Although sparse data are available on the rate of suicide in a treated population, clinical experience suggests that it is significantly less than 15%. For example, in the NIMH Collaborative Program on the Psychobiology of Depression (Fawcett et al. 1990), the rate of completed suicide was only 3% over 10 years.

Suicide and Anxiety

One of the most important findings of recent years is that anxiety, particularly panic attacks, is a major short-term risk factor in suicide. Fawcett et al. (1990) reported results of a 10-year follow-up from the NIMH Collaborative Program on the Psychobiology of Depression. The sample consisted of 954 patients with major affective disorders. The authors outlined nine factors that were correlated with suicide. Six of the factors were correlated with suicide within the first year of the follow-up: panic attacks, severe psychic anxiety, diminished concentration, global insomnia, alcohol abuse, and anhedonia. These factors, including the possibility of alcohol as a self-medication for anxiety, demonstrated the importance of anxiety symptoms as markers of short-term suicide risk. The three factors that were found to correlate with suicide *after* the first year—in the subsequent 9 years of the study—were the risk factors that had been identified in prior studies: history of previous suicide attempts, suicidal ideation, and hopelessness. These findings have a major importance clinically because they are factors that can be modified, which highlights the importance of aggressively treating anxiety, panic, and insomnia in patients with mood disorders.

Weissman et al. (1989), in their analysis of the ECA study, found that 20% of subjects with panic disorder and 12% of subjects with panic attacks had made suicide attempts. These results could not be explained by any coexistence of depression or of substance abuse. Other investigators have challenged the significance of these findings. In a retrospective study of outpatients, Beck et al. (1991) found only one suicide attempt among 151 patients with panic disorder. Friedman et al. (1992) and Henriksson et al. (1996) found that noncomorbid panic disorder in particular appeared to be rare among completed suicides. Suicide in persons with panic disorder is associated with superimposed major depression and substance abuse and with personality disorders. The differences between these studies and Weissman et al.'s study may have to do with clinical versus community sampling. Further research is needed to determine which specific subgroups of panic patients are at higher risk for suicide. At present, when the above findings are considered in conjunction with Fawcett et al.'s (1990) findings, it should be noted that patients with severe anxiety and panic attacks may be at higher risk for suicide, and clinicians should be alert to this possibility.

Suicide and Chemical Dependence

Chemical dependence, on either alcohol or drugs, increases a patient's suicide risk fivefold. It is important to note in this diagnostic group that although alcohol is the single most prevalent substance, most suicides occur in those persons with multiple substance abuse. After mood disorders, chemical dependence represents the most frequently encountered diagnosis among those who suicide (Marzuk and Mann 1988). About 25% of persons who suicide in the United States have been found to have alcoholism (Murphy and Wetzel 1990). Gruenewald et al. (1995) found suicide rates in the United States to correlate with the sale of spirits but not with sales of beer and wine.

Mixed substance abuse is even more closely associated with suicide. In the San Diego Suicide Study (Rich et al. 1986), mixed substance abuse was identified in 67% of completed suicides in youths and young adults and in 46% of suicides in adults ages 30 and older. In recent years, the prevalence of crack cocaine use has increased dramatically, with a subsequent increase in cocaine-related suicide. In a study of completed suicides in New York City, one in five individuals had used cocaine within days of the suicide (Marzuk et al. 1992b). Chemically dependent persons who complete suicide share some general characteristics (Table 34–3). They tend to be young males who use alcohol and other drugs *concur-*

TABLE 34–3. Characteristics of substance abusers who commit suicide

Age: 20s–30s
Sex: Male
Concurrent alcohol abuse and use of multiple substances, especially
 Opiates
 Sedatives
 Amphetamines
 Cocaine
Mean age at onset of disorder: 15 years
Mean duration of disorder: 9 years
Chronic use
History of drug overdoses
Comorbid psychiatric syndromes, especially
 Depression
 Borderline personality disorder
 Psychoses
Recent (< 6 weeks) interpersonal loss
Childhood history of hyperactivity
Incorrigibility
Family financial difficulties
Family suicidal behaviors
Parental abuse
Living in foster homes
Family history of
 Depression
 Suicide
 Alcoholism

Source. Adapted with permission from Marzuk PM, Mann JJ: "Suicide and Substance Abuse." *Psychiatric Annals* 18:639–645, 1988.

rently, who have a history of overdoses, and who have comorbid psychiatric disorders, especially depressive disorders. Although suicide in persons who abuse substances occurs after many years of illness, it tends to occur abruptly, often within 6 weeks of interpersonal loss.

Roy et al. (1990) studied 298 alcoholic subjects who had attempted, but not completed, suicide and compared these findings with data on suicide completers obtained in other studies. Several similarities were found between substance-abusing suicide completers and attempters—namely, the presence of psychiatric diagnoses, especially major depression, antisocial personality disorder, mixed substance abuse, panic disorder, phobic disorder, or generalized anxiety disorder. Like suicide completers, attempters had a family history of alcoholism and had experienced the onset of alcohol-related problems at an earlier age, usually in their early 20s. The main difference between the attempter group in this study and the completer groups reported in other studies was that attempters were more likely to be female. In this study, 30.6% of females attempted suicide compared with 14.6% of males.

Depressive disorder and substance abuse constitute a particularly lethal combination and highlight the importance of recognizing depression in the alcoholic patient. Depressive symptoms may be the result of underlying affective illness but also may result from the direct toxic effects of alcohol, impaired hepatic function, and poor nutrition, as well as organic brain syndromes from head trauma. Another problem is that patients with comorbid psychiatric and substance use disorders exhibit poor compliance with their medication regimen (Drake et al. 1989). Moreover, comorbid psychiatric conditions, especially affective illness, are often undertreated, thus increasing the likelihood of suicidal behavior.

In addition to the underlying risk for suicidal behavior due to alcohol dependence itself, acute intoxication also increases suicide risk. Alcohol and drugs may produce disinhibition and remove the remaining constraints to suicide in a given chemically dependent individual and thus serve as an acute precipitant to suicide. Furthermore, the disinhibition and poor judgment associated with the intoxicated state can result in high-risk behaviors such as auto accidents and drug overdoses. Such events are sometimes considered "accidental" suicidal behavior in this fatalistic population. These accidental suicides occur not only among persons driving while intoxicated, and particularly in accidents involving a single vehicle, but also among pedestrians who are intoxicated; a high percentage of pedestrians killed in traffic accidents were noted to have been intoxicated at the time of the accident (Weiss and Stephens 1992).

Another mechanism for the enhanced suicide risk in the substance-abusing population may be related to serotonergic functioning, as is discussed in more detail later in this chapter. Recent studies have demonstrated the link between hypoactive serotonin function and violent suicide attempts (Brown et al. 1982). There also may be a connection between serotonin dysfunction and alcoholism. Linnoila et al. (1989) noted a high prevalence of alcoholism in impulsive patients and found that those subjects with alcoholic fathers had low cerebrospinal fluid (CSF) levels of 5-hydroxyindoleacetic acid (5-HIAA).

Suicide and Schizophrenia

Approximately 10% of patients with schizophrenia complete suicide (Miles 1977). Most suicides in schizophrenic patients are in young males (Table 34–4): in a review of studies from the 1980s, 73% of those who completed suicide were male, and the mean age at death was 33

(Weiden and Roy 1992). Also of interest is that in schizophrenia, suicide risk is not greatest during the active hallucinatory phase; schizophrenic patients are more likely to complete suicide when the psychosis is under control and they are in a depressive recovery phase of the illness. (In this regard, schizophrenia can be contrasted with depression, in which suicide risk is increased during the psychotic delusional phase.) Schizophrenic patients at greatest risk are young men, usually in the first few years of the illness, who are in remission and nonpsychotic but who remain depressed and perhaps have come to the recognition that their life is fundamentally different than it used to be.

The recognition of loss of functioning, especially in individuals with high premorbid achievement and high self-expectations, appears to correlate with suicide completion. For example, one study found that a higher percentage of schizophrenic patients who suicided had college educations, awareness of the extent of their pathology, and fears of further deterioration compared with schizophrenic patients who had not suicided (Drake and Cotton 1986). These authors also noted that the secondary depression in schizophrenic patients that predisposed them to suicide was better characterized as psychological distress and hopelessness rather than major depressive disorder with vegetative signs. Once again, hopelessness was found to be a key factor in the schizophrenic population and, furthermore, appears to cut across all psychiatric diagnoses as a suicide predictor.

Data on the suicide risk in the actively psychotic schizophrenic patient have been compiled. All clinicians ask the schizophrenic patient about command hallucinations for self-harm and view this state as one of high suicide risk. A meta-analysis of studies (Breier and Astrachan 1984; Drake et al. 1984; Roy 1982) revealed that of 65 completed suicides among schizophrenic patients, only 2 could be attributed to command hallucinations; however, Weiden and Roy (1992) suggested that these meta-analyses may be biased by secondary treatment effects. They noted that clinicians are more likely to hospitalize schizophrenic persons for psychotic symptoms than for depressive symptoms. The net effect of these practices is that the schizophrenic person who is actively experiencing command hallucinations is hospitalized and the suicide is prevented; in contrast, the demoralized psychologically distressed patient tends not to be hospitalized and thus may not be protected from suicidal behavior. The clinical implication of this finding is not to reverse the convention of hospitalizing the command-hallucinating schizophrenic patient but rather to be equally vigilant about the nonpsychotic demoralized schizophrenic patient.

TABLE 34–4. Age and sex ratio in patients with chronic schizophrenia who commit suicide: studies since 1980

Study	Suicides (*n*)	Mean age (*years*)	Male (%)
Cheung 1981	12	31.0	83.3
Roy 1982	30	27.9	80.0
Hogan and Awad 1983	67	35.5	80.6
Breier and Astrachan 1984	20	30.3	90.0
Wilkinson and Bacon 1984	17	42.0	47.0
Allebeck and Wistedt 1986	33	35.9	54.0
Drake and Cotton 1986	15	31.7	60.0
Nyman and Jonsson 1986	10	30.4	90.0
Meta-analysis	204	33.0	73.1

Source. Adapted with permission from Weiden P, Roy A: "General Versus Specific Risk Factors for Suicide in Schizophrenia," in *Suicide and Clinical Practice*. Edited by Jacobs D. Washington, DC, American Psychiatric Press, 1992, pp. 75–100. Copyright 1992 American Psychiatric Press, Inc.

Also of note is that in a recent study of schizophrenic outpatients, although command hallucinations had minimal influence on the outcome of schizophrenia, those in the study that committed suicide had command hallucinations. Therefore, in outpatients with schizophrenia who have a history of suicide attempts, suicidal command hallucinations should be taken seriously (Zisook et al. 1995). In the psychiatric hospital setting, the inpatients most at risk for suicide had previously exhibited suicidal behavior, had schizophrenia, had been admitted involuntarily, and had lived alone. It was noted that the risk of suicide persists among long-stay schizophrenic patients (Roy et al. 1995)

Suicide risk in schizophrenia, as with other disorders, appears to be greatest during the post–inpatient hospitalization period. This finding is consistent with the observation that the greatest risk occurs not during the psychotic period but more often after the psychosis has resolved. At that time, patients actually have more insight into their condition and may more clearly recognize the reality of their situation. Later, in their outpatient course, patients may have developed better coping strategies and adapted to their new life circumstance. The clinical implication is that in the first few weeks up to the first 3 months after discharge, a clinician must be very alert to patients' self-perceptions, recognition of reality, coping strategies, and support systems.

Suicide and Borderline Personality Disorder

Suicidal behavior in a patient with borderline personality disorder represents a particular challenge for the clinician, especially when making the distinction between a potentially lethal attempt on the one hand and chronic self-mutilation or suicide attempts as a way of life on the other. The incidence of completed suicide in borderline patients ranges from 3% to 8% (McGlashan and Heinssen 1988; Stone et al. 1987). Thus, the overall rate of completed suicide in this group is less than that in patients with primary affective disorders, substance abuse, or schizophrenia; however, the borderline personality disorder diagnosis comprises a heterogeneous group of individuals who may have coexisting Axis I disorders, and the literature is inconclusive about whether coexisting Axis I disorders place the borderline patient at higher risk for suicide completion. Moreover, although suicide attempts in patients with personality disorders are often viewed as manipulative, they can be quite serious.

Corbitt et al. (1996) found that subjects with comorbid major depressive disorder and borderline personality disorder were more likely than other patients to have a history of multiple suicide attempts and were equally likely to have made a highly lethal attempt. Number of borderline personality disorder and other cluster B (dramatic/erratic) criteria were better predictors of past suicidal behavior than were depressive symptoms. The authors concluded that patients with borderline personality disorder symptoms are at risk for serious suicide attempts. Hence, severity of comorbid cluster B personality disorder psychopathology should be considered in assessing suicide risk in patients with major depression. Jacobs (1992) proposed a model for the assessment of suicide in the borderline patient that focuses on three areas (Figure 34–2):

1. The specific dynamics of the borderline individual that would place the person at higher risk
2. The coexistence of other psychiatric disorders that would place the individual at high risk
3. The suicide perspective, which includes identification of psychological commonalities of suicide and objectification of suicidal intent and behavior

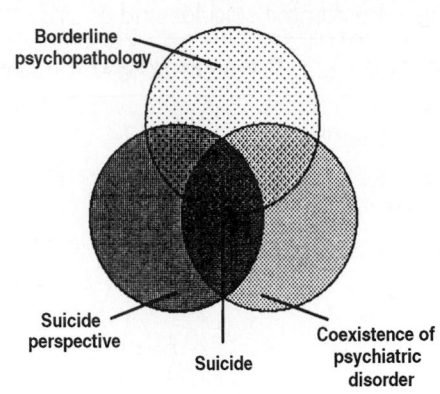

FIGURE 34–2. Tripartite model of suicide assessment in the patient with borderline personality disorder.

Source. Reprinted with permission from Jacobs D: "Evaluating and Treating Suicidal Behavior in the Borderline Patient," in *Suicide and Clinical Practice*. Edited by Jacobs D. Washington, DC, American Psychiatric Press, 1992, pp. 115–130. Copyright 1992 American Psychiatric Press, Inc.

With regard to specific borderline psychopathology, Kernberg (1984) outlined particular characteristics associated with high risk for suicide: impulsivity, hopelessness, despair, antisocial features, and interpersonal aloofness. He also described the characteristics of patients for whom chronic self-mutilation and suicide attempts are a way of life and that thus may predispose patients more to parasuicide than to completed suicide. "Infantile masochistic" patients use suicidal behavior to maintain connection. These behaviors tend to arise at times of intense rage attacks or rage mixed with temporary depressive flare-ups. They are designed to establish control over the environment by evoking guilt in others, such as after the breakup of an interpersonal relationship. At times, the behavior may be an expression of unconscious guilt over success or over the deepening of a psychotherapeutic relationship. Infantile masochistic patients exhibiting this form of negative therapeutic reaction are at particularly high risk for suicide attempts. Another group of patients exhibits suicidal behavior that reflects malignant narcissism. These patients experience increased self-esteem and confirmation of their pathological grandiosity in suicidal behavior. They may convey a sense of calm and "triumph" over the fear of destruction in contrast to the fearful, pleading efforts of staff and relatives to keep the patients from harming themselves (Kernberg 1984).

The second component of the model is evaluation of coexisting psychiatric disorders. Although it is unclear whether comorbid disorders increase suicide risk, it is clinically important to recognize and vigorously treat these conditions in borderline patients. Particular attention should be paid to comorbid affective illness, sub-

stance abuse, eating disorders, and posttraumatic stress disorder (PTSD).

The third component of the tripartite assessment model, the suicide perspective, consists of objectification of suicidal intent and identification of specific psychological commonalities and psychodynamic formulations. After identifying suicidal ideation, it is important that the clinician measure actual suicide intent. The clinician needs to determine the patient's ability to control suicidal thoughts, distinguish between active suicidal thoughts and passive suicidal thoughts, determine the patient's reasons for living and dying, determine the degree to which a suicidal plan has been developed, and evaluate the deterrents to carrying out such a plan (e.g., impact on family, loved ones). Common psychological factors are reviewed later in this chapter.

Along with the tripartite assessment, treatment for the borderline suicidal patient requires a high degree of creativity and individualization for the patient's specific circumstances. First, if there is any doubt about the strength of the therapeutic relationship or of the possibility of a negative therapeutic reaction, the patient should be hospitalized. Hospitalization can be focused on reestablishing the therapeutic alliance. Many clinicians advocate the use of brief hospitalizations to minimize the possibility of institutional dependence in this patient group. Pharmacotherapy is recommended for any overlaying Axis I condition. However, even in the absence of a definable Axis I condition, various psychotropic agents have been useful to help with specific symptoms in borderline patients. Although the psychotropics that have been useful include the entire spectrum of such agents, one study (Cowdry and Gardner 1988) offered guidelines for the differential use of carbamazepine, tranylcypromine, and alprazolam in borderline patients.

Psychological tools in working with the suicidal borderline patient that are particularly important include empathy and development of an antisuicide contract. The so-called no-self-harm contract should not be taken literally as a contract to eliminate suicidal feelings, but rather it serves to communicate the patient's *loss of control over suicidal feelings* and the importance of maintaining communication between patient and psychiatrist.

Psychological Factors in Suicidal Behavior

Given that suicide is not a diagnosis of a specific problem, what are the underlying psychological factors? A central factor is the issue of hopelessness. There is a high association with hopelessness in long-term suicide risk. Not specific to depression, hopelessness can accompany demoralization with a number of other syndromes: schizophrenia, anxiety disorders, and chronic conditions, including medical conditions. This factor can be measured with the Beck Hopelessness Scale, which is a 20-item self-report instrument that assesses the degree to which a person holds negative expectations about the future (Beck and Steer 1988). In a prospective study of 1,958 outpatients, Beck et al. (1990) found that hopelessness was highly correlated with eventual suicide. A scale cutoff score of 9 or above identified 16 (94.2%) of the 17 patients who completed suicide. Assessment of hopelessness is one of the key aspects in the management of the suicidal patient.

In addition to hopelessness, Hendin (1991) identified desperation as another important factor in suicide. Desperation implies not only a sense of hopelessness about change but a sense that life is impossible without such change. Guilt also was found to be another affective component of desperation. In a study of Vietnam veterans with PTSD, guilt was found to be prominent in those veterans exhibiting suicidal behavior. This guilt stemmed from self-hatred and a need for punishment, attributable in part to perceived guilt from actions committed during combat and in part to survivor guilt. These findings can be extended to certain disorders other than PTSD, especially depression, a component of which is the guilt that derives from the self-recriminatory state of the depressed person.

Aggression and violence are important in understanding suicide. Classical psychoanalytic theory postulated the importance of aggression toward the self in suicidal behavior. Freud (1917 [1915]/1957) described suicide as a murderous attack on an internalized object that had become a source of ambivalence. Thus, from a psychological sense, the introjected love object is the focus of the attack. Recent studies, however, demonstrate that aggression toward others—that is, violent behavior—often goes hand in hand with suicidal behavior. Suicide usually was associated with conscious rage in the violent individuals studied, and rage should therefore be viewed as an important psychological factor underlying suicidal behavior (Hendin 1991). Apter et al. (1991) studied suicide risk in patients with a history of violent behavior and in those without a history of violence. Their findings demonstrated that the two groups had similar correlates of suicide risk with regard to several psychological factors: anger, fear, anxiety, impulse dyscontrol, suspiciousness, and rebelliousness. However, of particular note was a correlation found between sadness and suicide risk in the nonviolent patients; no such correlation was found in the violent patients.

Hendin (1991) reviewed some of the common meanings of death ascribed to patients who commit suicide: death as reunion, rebirth, retaliatory abandonment, revenge, and self-punishment or atonement. The fantasy of reunion with a lost object through death may account for the phenomenon of anniversary suicides, as well as suicides that occur during bereavement. The fantasy of rebirth is related to the fantasy of identification with the lost object: patients view themselves as incomplete in the absence of the missing object and view the reunion through suicide as a form of rebirth. Suicide and suicide attempts as retaliatory abandonment are seen in patients who feel that the only way they can have mastery over a situation is through control of living or dying. This illusion of mastery and maintenance of control may account for individuals who keep the means for suicide readily available even if they never attempt suicide. Suicide as revenge correlates with the classical Freudian observation of the unconscious wish to kill the ambivalently regarded lost object. As an extension of this unconscious wish, unconscious rage and murderous impulse are seen as the need for self-punishment or atonement. The patient feels guilty about his or her hatred of the object, and suicide not only serves as revenge but also accomplishes atonement.

Shame and humiliation are two other factors that sometimes underlie suicide. Certain individuals may view suicide as a face-saving mechanism after suffering a social humiliation (e.g., a sudden loss of status or income). This form of suicide is rare in individuals not suffering from psychiatric illness. However, psychiatrically ill patients may feel shame related to suicidal ideation and may be reluctant to seek treatment or rely on support systems. The existence of a support system is not sufficient; the patient must be willing to rely on it. Often, shameful feelings inhibit this process. Therefore, it is important to be alert to these feelings in patients.

Finally, stressors predisposing to suicide coincide with developmental phases over the life cycle (Rich et al. 1991). Three common stressors are 1) conflict, separation, and rejection; 2) economic problems; and 3) medical illness. In the San Diego Suicide Study, interpersonal conflicts, separations, and rejections were the predominant stressors for adolescents and individuals in early adulthood. Although these issues remained as significant stressors for those who completed suicide in middle adulthood, for those in the 40–60-year-old group, economic problems were deemed the principal stressor. In patients older than 60 years, medical illness played an increasingly important role and was considered the most significant predisposing factor in patients older than 80 years of age.

Kessler et al. (1999) examined data from part II of the National Comorbidity Survey, a nationally representative survey carried out from 1990 to 1992 in a sample of 5,877 respondents ages 15–54 years to study prevalences and correlates of DSM-III-R disorders. Of the respondents, 13.5% reported lifetime ideation, 3.9% reported a plan, and 4.6% reported an attempt. Cumulative probabilities were 34% for the transition from ideation to a plan, 72% from a plan to an attempt, and 26% from ideation to an unplanned attempt. About 90% of unplanned and 60% of planned first attempts occurred within 1 year of the onset of ideation. All significant risk factors (female, previously married, age less than 25 years, in a recent cohort, poorly educated, and having one or more of the DSM-III-R disorders assessed in the survey) were more strongly related to ideation than to progression from ideation to a plan or an attempt. The authors noted that intervention efforts should focus on planned attempts because of the rapid onset and unpredictability of unplanned attempts.

Suicide in Special Populations

Suicide and the Elderly

As was shown in Figure 34–1, the suicide rate doubles to quadruples in patients older than age 65, especially among Caucasian males. McIntosh (1995) reported an annual United States suicide rate of 16.9 per 100,000 for persons ages 65–74, 23.5 for persons ages 75–84, and 24.0 for those 85 and older. Adamek and Kaplan (1996) reported an increase in the annual suicide rate among men 65 and older using firearms from a rate of 25.3 in 1979 to 31.3 by 1991. Firearms accounted for 80% of suicides in this study. Factors predisposing older individuals to suicide are social isolation, loss of spouse, anxiety due to financial instability, and undertreated mood disorders. The prevalence of mood disorders is probably not higher in this age group, but the disorders probably are underrecognized and undertreated. In a cross-section of older patients, primary depression was present in about 3.7%, with a total of 14% complaining of a dysphoric state (Blazer and Williams 1980); however, in a cohort of suicidal older individuals, the presence of depression was reported to be as high as 80% (Morgan 1989). Depression may go underrecognized in older persons because of the atypical features in this population, including masked depression (primarily multiple somatic complaints or continued unfounded fearfulness of somatic illness) and pseudodementia (i.e., the artificially reduced cognitive capacities resulting from a primary depressive condition).

Skoog et al. (1996) studied the frequency of suicidal feelings among a population sample of 85-year-olds who did not have dementia. They found that figures for suicidal feelings were significantly higher among subjects with mental disorders. Women who felt that life was not worth living had a higher 3-year mortality rate than did women without these feelings (43.2% versus 14.2%, respectively). This finding was independent of concomitant physical and mental disorders. The substantially higher mortality rate in women who felt that life was not worth living suggests that these feelings must be taken seriously.

Finally, indirect self-destructive behavior is often seen in institutional settings for older individuals when these individuals refuse to accept medications or medical care, refuse to take part in activities, and struggle for control with caregivers. These behaviors should alert the clinician and caregivers to the presence of an underlying depression (Morgan 1989). Because the percentage of older persons in the United States population is growing, the issues of recognizing underlying conditions, implementing vigorous treatment, and managing suicidality in older persons will be increasingly important in the future.

Suicide and Youth

The rate of adolescent suicide has increased dramatically since 1964 (Figure 34–3). The rate of suicide in adolescent males (Caucasian and nonCaucasian) from 1964 to 1996 almost tripled. Adolescent female suicides have increased two- to threefold. The annual suicide rate per 100,000 for African Americans ages 10–19 in the United States increased from 2.1 to 4.5 between 1980 and 1995 (Centers for Disease Control and Prevention 1998). The annual suicide rate per 100,000 for United States residents ages 10–14 and 15–19 increased from 0.8 and 1.7 to 8.5 and 10.9, respectively, between 1980 and 1992 (Centers for Disease Control and Prevention 1995). Gessner (1997) studied the suicide rate in Alaskans ages 14–19 between 1979 and 1993 and found an extremely high overall rate of 31.5 annually. Notably, male Alaska natives had an annual suicide rate of 120.3, one of the highest suicide rates documented. In a recent study, Brener et al. (2000) examined the trends in suicide ideation and behavior over time. They analyzed data from nationally representative samples of high school students from 1991 to 1997. The percentage of students seriously considering suicide and the percentage that had made a suicide plan showed significant linear *decreases*. However, the percentage of students that had made an injurious suicide attempt showed a significant linear *increase*.

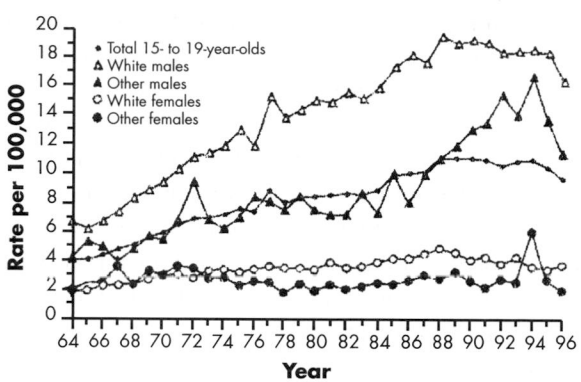

FIGURE 34–3. Adolescent suicide rates (15- to 19-year olds, 1964–1996)

Source. Reprinted with permission from Shaffer D, Craft L: "Methods of Adolescent Suicide Prevention." *Journal of Clinical Psychiatry* 60(suppl):70–74, 1999.

Factors that may have contributed to this increase are the rise in depressive disorders among youths (severe depression is the most prevalent characteristic of the suicidal adolescent), the rise in the divorce rate, the dissolution of the nuclear family, and the availability of firearms (Pfeffer 1988). Males are at greater risk than females and Caucasians are at greater risk than nonCaucasians for completed suicide. In a large, controlled study using psychological autopsy methodology, several other notable risks were identified; these derived from school problems, a family history of suicidal behavior, poor parent–child communication, and stressful life events (Gould et al. 1996).

Exposure to suicide also may be a factor: for certain individuals, experiencing suicide in a family member or friend appears to make suicide more "permissible." This phenomenon may be at play in the cluster suicides observed among youth, although this point is still controversial. Brent et al. (1996), in a 3-year controlled follow-up reported that exposure to suicide does not result in an increased risk of suicidal behavior among friends and acquaintances, but it has a relatively long impact in terms of increased incidence of depression, anxiety, and PTSD.

Although environmental and sociocultural factors exist, the importance of psychopathology in youth suicide cannot be overestimated. In the adolescent, the main diagnoses are depression and conduct disorder, especially with antisocial behaviors. Hostility, aggression, and assaultiveness also are correlated with suicide. Suicide in youth, as in other populations, often goes hand in hand with hostility, not only toward the self but toward others. A correlation between suicidality and aggressive behavior has been found in adolescents in many instances

when there is parental substance abuse. Birckmayer and Hemenway (1999) found a lower suicide rate for 18- to 20-year-olds in U.S. states that had raised the legal drinking age to 21.

Suicide in Patients With HIV/AIDS

Among the most unique medical phenomena identified in the past decade has been the epidemic of infection with HIV and subsequent progression to AIDS. This epidemic also has implications in the field of suicidology because of the unique impact on primarily young people with chronic and life-threatening illness. In clinical practice, there is a high prevalence of suicidal ideation among patients with HIV. Suicidal ideation often comes in the form of a need to maintain control, especially in a syndrome such as AIDS in which a patient can rapidly develop encephalopathy and dementia. These patients often have seen others in their peer group become, over a short period of time, demented and unable to care for themselves. Patients may develop a view of suicide as a legitimate way out before the demise into debilitation or dementia. Clinical experience suggests that suicide appears to have acceptance in the AIDS population. Breitbart et al. (1996) found that HIV-infected patients supported policies favoring physician-assisted suicide at rates comparable with those in the general public. Patients' interest in physician-assisted suicide appeared to be more a function of psychological distress and social factors than physical factors. These findings highlight the importance of psychiatric and psychosocial assessment and intervention in the care of patients who express interest in or request physician-assisted suicide.

However, whether or not the patient actually completes suicide, maintaining suicidal ideation as a source of control over his or her illness appears to be fairly prevalent. The actual risk of suicide in persons with AIDS is greater than that in the general population (Zeck et al. 1988). In an epidemiological study of New York City residents, the suicide rate for men with AIDS was 680 per 100,000 persons per year, whereas for a comparison group of men ages 20–59 without a diagnosis of AIDS the suicide rate was 18 per 100,000 persons per year. The suicide rate in the AIDS patients was 36 times that in age-matched men without AIDS (Marzuk et al. 1988). Interestingly, a later study (McKegney and O'Dowd 1992) found that a group of psychiatric consultation patients with diagnosed AIDS were significantly *less* suicidal than a group of patients who were HIV-positive but had not yet developed AIDS. The authors postulated that the prevalence of delirium and dementia in the AIDS patients may have led to organicity, which might

TABLE 34–6. Postmortem receptor studies of completed suicides: serotonergic receptor findings

Study	Findings
Imipramine binding	
Stanley et al. 1982	↓ [3H]imipramine binding in cortex
Paul et al. 1984	↓ [3H]imipramine binding in hypothalamus
Perry et al. 1983[a]	↓ [3H]imipramine binding in cortex
Crow et al. 1984	↓ [3H]imipramine binding in cortex
Myerson et al. 1982	↑ [3H]imipramine binding in cortex
Owen et al. 1986	No difference in imipramine binding in frontal and occipital cortex and hippocampus
Gross-Isseroff et al. 1989	↑ imipramine binding in pyramidal and molecular layers of cornu ammoni, hippocampal fields, and hilus of dentate gyrus
	↓ imipramine binding in postcentral cortical gyrus, insular cortex, and claustrum
5-HT binding	
Stanley and Mann 1983	↑ 5-HT$_2$ binding in cortex
Mann et al. 1986	↑ 5-HT$_2$ binding in cortex
Meltzer et al. 1987	↑ 5-HT$_2$ binding in cortex
Owen et al. 1983	Nonsignificant ↑ in 5-HT$_2$ binding in cortex
Owen et al. 1986	No differences in 5-HT$_1$ and 5-HT$_2$ binding in frontal and occipital cortex and hippocampus
Cheetam et al. 1987	↓ 5-HT$_2$ binding in cortex
Lawrence et al. 1990	No difference in 5-HT uptake sites
	↓ putamen 5-HT uptake sites in nonviolent suicides
Hrdina et al. 1993	↑ 5-HT$_2$ binding in prefrontal cortex and amygdala
	No ↑ in 5-HT uptake sites in prefrontal cortex and amygdala
Arango et al. 1995	↑ 5-HT$_{1A}$ binding in prefrontal cortex
	↓ 5-HT transporter binding in prefrontal cortex
Mann et al. 1996b	No difference in 5-HT$_3$ binding in temporal cortex
Stockmeier 1997	↑ 5-HT$_{1A}$ binding in venterolateral nucleus of dorsal raphe
Stockmeier et al. 1997	No differences in 5-HT$_{1A}$ or 5-HT$_{2A}$ binding in right prefrontal cortex or hippocampus
Stockmeier et al. 1998	↑ 5-HT$_{1A}$ binding in midbrain dorsal raphe nuclei
Hrdina and Du 2001	↑ 5-HT$_{2A}$ binding in Area 9 of cortex

Note. [a]Depressed patients dying of natural causes.
5-HT = 5-hydroxytryptamine (serotonin).

The initial studies of CSF in depressed patients also attempted to distinguish between biochemically distinct forms of depression. That patients who had made suicide attempts had low levels of 5-HIAA was significant not only from the standpoint of biochemically distinguishing those patients who had attempted suicide, but also from the perspective of predicting future suicidal behavior. One of the initial studies demonstrated that 21% of patients who had been hospitalized after a suicide attempt and had been found to have low levels of CSF 5-HIAA actually committed suicide within 1 year after the original evaluation (Åsberg et al. 1976). Several other studies corroborated the initial finding that depressed patients whose CSF levels of 5-HIAA were subnormal were more likely to have attempted suicide (Agren 1980;

Banki 1981; Träskman et al. 1981).

Interestingly, however, suicidal and nonsuicidal patients with bipolar disorder could not be distinguished on the basis of their CSF 5-HIAA levels (Berrettini et al. 1986). This finding, which contrasts with results from the studies previously discussed regarding patients with unipolar depression, is somewhat perplexing given the high rate of suicide in patients with bipolar disorder. Goodwin (1986) posited that because serotonergic dysregulation is probably central to the genesis of bipolar disorder, this may overshadow any singular relationship between serotonergic hypofunction and suicide in these patients.

Decreases in CSF 5-HIAA also have been shown to distinguish between schizophrenic patients who had attempted suicide and those who had not (Banki et al. 1983; Ninan et al. 1984; Roy et al. 1985). This measure also distinguished suicidal patients with personality disorders as well as alcoholic patients with a history of suicide attempts (Banki et al. 1984; Brown et al. 1979). These findings further support not only the idea that suicidal behavior is not merely an end result of clinical depression but also that serotonergic dysfunction may well underlie suicidal behavior in patients across diagnoses. That low levels of 5-HIAA actually may represent a trait disorder is further suggested by the lack of a temporal relationship between the suicide attempt and the CSF 5-HIAA level.

Both human and animal studies correlate aggressive behavior with serotonergic hypofunction. This hypofunction may not signify a specific diathesis for suicide but rather reflects a decreased threshold for aggressive behavior whether directed against others or oneself. Yet it is clear that successful suicide attempts are often predicated on systematic planning rather than a momentary loss of impulse control; indeed, violent methods of suicide often involve more planning. Thus, it is difficult to determine which aspects of suicidal behavior specifically correlate with decreased levels of CSF 5-HIAA.

Most recently, a study of violent suicide attempters demonstrated not only lower levels of CSF 5-HIAA but also significantly increased CSF levels of 3-methoxy-4-hydroxyphenylglycol (MHPG), the chief metabolic breakdown product of norepinephrine (Träskman-Bendz et al. 1992). This finding appears to corroborate previous research suggesting that serotonin is an inhibitory neurotransmitter of the noradrenergic system and that heightened noradrenergic turnover in the face of diminished serotonergic input may well represent a significant part of the biochemical underpinnings of violent suicide.

In addition, some patients with depression who had attempted suicide also were found to have decreased CSF levels of homovanillic acid (HVA), the metabolite of dopamine. In a 5-year follow-up study, those patients who went on to attempt suicide again after the initial evaluation were found to have significantly lower CSF levels of 5-HIAA and HVA (Roy et al. 1986). It is interesting to note that a recent study also demonstrated that both decreased 5-HIAA and HVA correlated with a history of suicide attempts resulted in greater medical damage (Mann et al. 1996a).

Another biological observation is that major depression and suicide are associated with fewer serotonin transporter (5-HTT) sites. The 5'-flanking promoter region of the 5-HTT gene has a biallelic insertion/deletion (5-HTTLPR). The authors studied the prefrontal cortical 5-HTT binding in major depression and suicide and examined the relationship to the 5-HTTLPR allele. The found that a diffuse reduction of 5-HTT binding in the prefrontal cortex of individuals with major depression may reflect a widespread impairment of serotonergic function consistent with the range of psychopathologic features in major depression. There was a localized reduction in 5-HTT binding in the ventral prefrontal cortex of suicides that may reflect reduced serotonin input to that brain region, underlying the predisposition to act on suicidal thoughts. The 5-HTTLPR genotype was not related to the level of 5-HTT binding and did not explain why 5-HTT binding is lower in major depression or suicide (Mann et al. 2000). Bondy et al. (2000) found a higher incidence of one or two short alleles of 5-HTTLPR in suicide victims compared with control subjects. However, Little et al. (1997) found no differences in 5-HTT binding in the midbrain, hippocampus, and frontal cortex of depressed suicide victims and, similarly, no differences in 5-HTT messenger RNA levels in the dorsal and median raphe nuclei of depressed suicide victims.

Taken together, these findings suggest 1) that it is important to consider more than just serotonergic abnormalities and 2) that increasing the sensitivity and specificity of possible biological predictors of suicidal behavior will involve an analysis of a cluster of biochemical variables.

Further Investigation of the HPA Axis: The Dexamethasone Suppression Test

The DST assesses the responsivity of the HPA axis to an exogenously administered steroid, dexamethasone. The test is considered abnormal if cortisol levels rise above 5 ng/mL at 4:00 P.M. and 11:00 P.M. on the day after the administration of dexamethasone. Ordinarily, the administration of this compound would suppress the rise in cortisol by virtue of providing feedback inhibition at any point in the HPA axis. An abnormal test indicates an "escape" from suppression and thus the presence of HPA dysregulation in the direction of hyperactivity.

Some studies have demonstrated that patients with abnormal DST results are more likely to have made a suicide attempt prior to the evaluation; two studies found that patients who had an abnormal DST at the time of initial evaluation were more likely to make a future suicide attempt. However, there have also been studies that found no statistically significant correlation between the DST and serious suicide attempts.

Although fewer studies have tested HPA axis disturbance as a predictor of completed suicides, the results have been more consistent. Carroll et al. (1980) identified 5 suicide victims among 250 melancholic patients who had undergone the DST and reported that all 5 victims had "escaped from suppression" as measured by serum cortisol at the times noted above. Coryell and Schlesser (2001) noted that all 4 of the suicide completers in their cohort of 205 inpatients with primary unipolar depression had similarly abnormal results; notably, less than half of the remaining melancholic patients were nonsuppressors of cortisol when the DST was administered. However, these authors extended their findings in a study demonstrating that of eight patients who eventually suicided, seven had abnormal DST tests. None of the other demographic predictors of suicide, such as age above 32 years, living alone, feelings of hopelessness, history of delusions, or mania were in any way predictive of suicide risk. Only a serious suicide attempt within the index episode correlated with an increased risk of suicide, generating an odds ratio of 3.8. Dexamethasone nonsuppression increased the likelihood of suicide 14-fold. It should be noted that these results have only applied to depressed patients, but there is also a high rate of DST nonsuppression in alcoholism, chemical dependency, and schizophrenic disorders. Furthermore, in the literature on serotonin hypofunction, some authors (Lopez et al. 1987) hypothesize that HPA dysregulation may actually underlie these abnormalities. Brunner et al. (2001) found suicide attempters to have significantly lower CSF corticotropin-releasing hormone.

Findings in the Periphery: Pharmacological Challenge Tests

Because lumbar puncture is generally not performed in the office, investigators have recently searched for alternative methods of assessing neurochemical functioning. One method of testing the integrity of a patient's serotonergic system is to measure prolactin or cortisol release in response to pharmacological agents such as fenfluramine, precursors such as L-tryptophan or 5-hydroxytryptophan, or serotonin receptor antagonists such as metachlorophenylpiperazine (mCPP) or MK-212. Studies have demonstrated that prolactin response to fenfluramine is blunted in patients who have attempted suicide (Coccaro et al. 1989; De Meo et al. 1988). One study demonstrated a heightened cortisol response to 5-hydroxytryptophan, which may reflect receptor supersensitivity (Mann and Arango 1992).

Platelet

Studies have demonstrated that the number of platelet 5-HT$_2$ receptors is increased in suicidal patients (Pandey et al. 1990, 1995). There also have been studies suggesting platelet manifestations of presynaptic serotonergic hypofunction: specifically, decreased platelet serotonin uptake and ^{3}H imipramine binding in suicide attempters (Marazitti et al. 1995). One study demonstrated that platelet imipramine binding showed significant seasonal variation in adolescents who attempted suicide, with the nadir occurring in late winter/early spring (Pine et al. 1995). These findings are interesting not only because of the consistency with similar changes in the CNS but also because the relative ease of a venipuncture may provide a more accessible avenue for assessment of serotonergic functioning.

Urine

Measuring urine metabolites of neurochemicals might provide another peripheral measure of underlying biological differences among suicidal and nonsuicidal patients. Indeed, one of the first studies of possible biological markers for suicidal behavior found increased amounts of 17-hydroxycorticosteroids in the urine of depressed patients who had attempted suicide (Bunney and Fawcett 1965). Subsequent studies demonstrated increased urinary cortisol, particularly among patients who attempted suicide by violent means (i.e., hanging, firearms). Most recently, one group found that patients with depression who attempted suicide had significantly lowered levels of dopamine, HVA, and dihydrophenylacetic acid compared with nonsuicidal depressed patients (Roy et al. 1992).

Serum

It has been suggested that lowered serum cholesterol is associated with suicide attempts. In one large study, male psychiatric patients with low serum cholesterol levels were twice as likely to have made a serious suicide attempt as men with cholesterol levels above the twenty-fifth percentile (Golier et al. 1995). In an emergency department setting, patients admitted after a suicide attempt were found to have significantly lower serum cholesterol than nonsuicidal psychiatric inpatients (Kunugi et al. 1997). Most recently, a study assessed the "mortality experience" of 11,554 participants in the 1970–1972 Nutrition Canada Survey, wherein 27 patients committed suicide through 1993. The risk of suicide for these subjects increased as cholesterol decreased; specifically, the risk ratios for suicide were 6.39 in the lowest quartile of serum cholesterol, 2.95 in the second quartile, and 1.94 in the third quartile, compared with the highest quartile (Ellison and Morrison 2001). Of additional significance is that, in this study, these risks persisted after patients with clinical depression and those who were unemployed were excluded from the study. Explanations for this finding have included possible modifications of serotonin metabolism and interleukin-2 associated with lower levels of cholesterol, leading to increased impulsive behavior (Alvarez et al. 1999; Kaplan et al. 1997; Penttinen 1995). However, there is conflicting evidence regarding the interrelationship between cholesterol levels and decreased serotonin activity in the brain, perhaps pointing again to the necessity for examining other neurochemical or neuroendocrine processes that might also underlie suicidal behavior. Almeida-Montes et al. (2000) found no significant differences in total cholesterol, low-density lipoprotein, high-density lipoprotein, and triglyceride levels in suicide attempters. They did report lower serotonin and tryptophan levels in suicide attempters.

Brain Weight

Salib and Tadros (2000) reported a finding of increased brain weight (mean weight 1347 g vs. 1238 g) in suicide completers who were over the age of 60, irrespective of method of suicide. The clinical and biochemical significance of this report is unclear at this time.

Cyclic Adenosine Monophosphate

Odagaki et al. (2001) found increases in cyclic adenosine monophosphate (cAMP) response element binding protein in the prefrontal cortex of suicide victims who had not been treated with antidepressants, suggesting that upregulation of cAMP signaling is present in the brains of depressed suicide victims.

Taken together, these findings may one day yield a biological suicide-potential workup for patients who might have other demographic or clinical risk factors. Future research will focus on the identification and prediction of suicidal behavior that may come with consideration of a clustering of these biological variables. It has been proposed that "suicidal behavior is an independent unique behavioral entity with specific neurochemical characteristics" (Gross-Isseroff et al. 1998). As such, research will continue to focus on variations in several neurochemical systems in suicidal behavior regardless of specific psychiatric diagnosis, to describe a "profile" specific to suicidal behavior.

Assessment of the Suicidal Patient

An adage in medicine is that "during a cardiac arrest, the first procedure is to take your own pulse." Facetious as this statement sounds, it exhorts the clinician to monitor his or her own reactions to a potentially life-threatening situation, particularly as they might interfere with his or her ability to assess such a situation accurately. Indeed, the suicidal patient may provoke a panoply of unpleasant emotions, such as hate, fear, and restlessness, in the evaluating clinician that might interfere with the ability to establish adequate rapport. As a result, inquiries regarding suicidal ideation or intent may be rushed, put off until the end of the interview, or not ventured at all. It is of paramount importance, then, that the evaluating clinician acknowledge in a nonjudgmental way his or her own countertransferential reaction to a suicidal patient. In this way, the evaluator can maximize his or her ability to interact with the suicidal patient so as to "blend enough compassion so that the suicidal person experiences the clinician as an ally and enough detachment so that the clinician is not overwhelmed by his or her own responses to the patient's pain" (Doyle 1990).

The evaluation of suicidal ideation or behavior is done in a manner similar to the investigation of any symptom cluster that might have adverse medical consequences. First, the clinician maintains an index of suspicion stemming from the demographic characteristics reviewed earlier in this chapter. Then, the clinician must individualize the assessment to the patient by considering personal and family history, assessing current medical and psychiatric status, determining psychosocial assets and liabilities, and taking into consideration prior response to treatment.

When taking a personal history of a patient to assess suicidal ideation, it is essential to evaluate the patient's level of intention of acting on such ideation and to determine whether the patient has a plan of suicide action, paying particular attention to the steps already taken to implement such a plan and assessing its potential lethality. The availability of means must be assessed, ranging from stockpile medications to firearms, as well as whether the patient has taken any specific actions in preparation for death, such as purchasing a gun, writing a will, or giving away prized objects. It is also important to inquire about the presence of other symptoms that have been associated with a higher suicide risk, including delusional symptoms (particularly command hallucinations), anhedonia, hopelessness, and severe anxiety.

It is essential to obtain a history of prior suicide attempts as well as a history of violence and impulsivity. In addition, the presence of substance abuse should be assessed because, as noted earlier in this chapter, it also has been associated with an increased risk of suicide. A history of suicide as well as violence in the patient's family should also alert the clinician to the presence of a liability to more dangerous suicidal behavior. The clinician

TABLE 34–7. Final set of variables from Risk Estimator Scale for Suicide

Variable	High-risk category	Coefficient (weight)	Standard error	P
Age	Risk increases with age	0.273[a]	0.092	0.001
Occupation	Executive, administrator, owner of business, professional, semiskilled worker	0.515	0.206	0.013
Financial resources	Risk increases with resources	0.373	0.120	0.002
Emotional disorder in family	Depression, alcoholism	0.486	0.195	0.013
Sexual orientation	Bisexual, active; homosexual, inactive	0.692	0.252	0.006
Previous psychiatric hospital admissions	Risk increases with number of admissions	0.228	0.079	0.004
Result of previous efforts to obtain help	Negative or variable	0.593	0.199	0.003
Threatened financial loss	Yes	0.674	0.271	0.013
Special stress	Severe	0.676	0.191	0.000
Sleep (hours per night)	Risk increases with number of hours per night	0.395	0.161	0.014
Weight change, present episode	Gain or 1%–9% loss	0.646	0.241	0.013
Ideas of persecution or reference	Yes	0.636	0.198	0.014
Suicidal impulses	Yes	1.071	0.227	0.000
Seriousness of present suicide attempt—intent	Unambivalent or ambivalent but weighted toward suicide	0.943	0.201	0.000
Interviewer's reaction to subject	Risk increases with negativity of reaction	0.454	0.163	0.006

Note. [a]Applied to square root of age.

Source. Adapted with permission from Motto JA, Heilbron DC, Juster RP: "Development of a Clinical Instrument to Estimate Suicide Risk." *American Journal of Psychiatry* 142:680–686, 1985. Copyright 1985 American Psychiatric Press, Inc.

must inquire about the circumstances of previous violence, as well as whether the patient thinks this behavior is abnormal or unusual, and should attempt to determine whether the violence is tied to a specific mood state.

A complete evaluation for suicide potential also will include the assessment of an individual's strengths. Despite the presence of suicidal behavior, it may well be that an individual has a proven ability not only to control his or her behavior but also to bring familial or financial resources to bear on his or her situation. A motivation to seek help in general, and meaningful psychiatric treatment in particular, should be determined. As part of this assessment, the clinician should become familiar with the patient's prior responses to treatment, including responses to pharmacotherapeutic intervention as well as psychotherapy and psychosocial support.

Several more formal methods of suicide risk assessment have been used in research settings with varying degrees of success. One of the best-developed scales is the Risk Estimator Scale for Suicide (Motto et al. 1985). This scale was the result of a 2-year prospective study of 2,753 patients with depression or suicidality in which completed suicides were noted. Fifteen variables were incorporated into a scale that gives an estimated risk of suicide within 2 years (Table 34–7). These variables included demographics, psychiatric history, and stressors,

as well as interpreted factors such as the interviewer's reaction to the subject. Other scales for the measurement of suicidal ideation include the Scale for Suicidal Ideation and the Suicide Intent Scale, both developed by Beck et al. (1975). Also, because hopelessness has been identified by Beck and his group as being central to suicidal intent, the Beck Hopelessness Scale (Beck and Steer 1988) also might be considered to have clinical utility. These scales also underscore the need to consider a large number of factors that might increase suicide risk; this is particularly true in light of the recent sobering study that suggested that more than three-fourths of patients who ultimately commit suicide do not communicate their intent to do so in appointments with health care professionals occurring within 28 days of the actual suicide.

Treatment of the Suicidal Patient

As mentioned earlier, suicidal behavior is a syndrome that cuts across rigid diagnostic lines. As such, it is important that this behavior be addressed apart from, and in addition to, the ostensible underlying psychiatric condition.

The clinician must first confront his or her own feelings, however unpleasant or embarrassing, regarding the patient. As Doyle (1990) points out, "The clinician's experience of anxiety, anger, sadness, or confusion may reflect the patient's internal milieu and suggest areas for exploration and intervention.... Rather than avoiding or denying feelings, the clinician uses them to form hypotheses about the patient that deserve further investigation" (p. 383).

Initially, it may seem to the patient that his or her alliance with the clinician is his or her only tie to life. Ultimately, the patient and clinician must arrive at a mutually agreeable contract regarding further courses of action to be taken based on their alliance.

Principles of acute intervention, as delineated by Blumenthal (1990), begin with adequate supervision of the suicidal patient. If this supervision cannot be sufficiently accomplished in an outpatient setting, hospitalization, whether on a voluntary or involuntary basis, should be considered. It is also necessary to limit the patient's access to potentially self-destructive methods, principal among which is antidepressant medication. It is a poignant irony that medicinal compounds specifically designed to combat conditions leading to suicide are extremely lethal when taken in overdosage. The clinician should be keenly aware of lethal indexes of medications and prescribe only small amounts at a time. For example, with tricyclic antidepressants, less than 1 g total should be dispensed at any given time. Although the clinician cannot eliminate all other potential means to suicide, he or she must make an effort to reduce the risk. This effort may involve, for example, contracting with the patient for him or her to give up access to firearms that may be in his or her possession and, at times, even convincing the patient to agree to have knives and other sharp instruments under another person's lock and key.

Somatic Treatment

In general, the aim of biological therapy in the treatment of suicidal patients has been to treat the diagnosed psychiatric condition. As a result, few studies describe the response of suicidal behavior per se to specific pharmacotherapeutic interventions.

The role of dopamine in suicidal behavior seemed to be given more weight by two studies that indicated that postsynaptic dopaminergic blocking agents appeared to decrease suicidal behavior in patients with severe character disorders (Cowdry and Gardner 1988; Soloff et al. 1986).

As might be expected, however, much focus has been placed on interventions affecting the serotonergic system. With the advent of medications that selectively affect the serotonergic system, one might expect these medications to be associated with more significant amelioration of suicidal behavior than either tricyclic antidepressants or antidepressants that promote noradrenergic transmission. Some, although not all, of the early comparison studies suggested an earlier improvement in suicidality in the group treated with serotonergic agents (de Wilde et al. 1985; Montgomery et al. 1981; Mullin et al. 1988).

However, Teicher et al. (1990) reported six cases of the emergence of severe suicidal preoccupation in patients undergoing treatment with fluoxetine, a selective serotonin reuptake inhibitor (SSRI). Another study noted the emergence of self-destructive behavior in six children and adolescents receiving fluoxetine (King et al. 1991). The dramatic impact of these studies was to draw attention to the possibility of "paradoxical reactions" of antidepressants: the agents appeared to produce or intensify the symptoms that they were ostensibly introduced to treat. Although the aforementioned studies seemed to popularize the notion of such paradoxical reactions, the emergence of new-onset suicidality, intensification of previously existing suicidality, and increased assaultiveness had already been reported with tricyclic antidepressants (Damluji and Ferguson 1988; Rampling 1978; Soloff et al. 1987), maprotiline (Rouillon et al. 1989), and alprazolam (Gardner and Cowdry 1985).

Larger studies have since assessed the worsening of suicidal ideation on initiation of antidepressant therapy. One study, a retrospective chart review of more than 1,000 patients who were treated with antidepressants, demonstrated no difference in any single antidepressant medication in the seeming production of suicidal ideation (Fava and Rosenbaum 1991), whereas another analysis revealed a worsening of suicidal ideation in fluoxetine-treated patients (Mann and Kapur 1991). Another large study revealed that the emergence of suicidality was less frequent in patients receiving fluoxetine than in patients receiving other antidepressant treatments or placebo (Beasley et al. 1991). In a recent study of more than 600 patients being treated for anxiety disorders, there was no evidence that fluoxetine was associated with increased risk of suicide attempts or gestures; in fact, of those patients who were also diagnosed as having a major depressive disorder at intake, there was a statistically lower probability of suicide attempts or gestures for those taking fluoxetine than for those not taking fluoxetine (Warshaw and Keller 1996). Overall, analyses of clinical trials indicated that paradoxical suicidal ideation emerged less with SSRIs than with tricyclics or placebo (Beasley et al. 1991; Letizia et al. 1996; Montgomery et al. 1995).

It should be evident that the appearance or worsening

of suicidal behavior exists with a wide variety of antidepressants, although this phenomenon probably affects fewer than 6% of the patients treated (Mann and Kapur 1991). What mechanisms might explain the production of this paradoxical effect? One explanation is that this phenomenon occurs as a result of drug-induced akathisia. In fact, neuroleptic-induced akathisia, which is initially indistinguishable from that induced by some antidepressants, has been associated with increased acting-out behaviors and increased suicide attempts (Drake and Ehrlich 1985; Siris 1985). Another possible mechanism might be a paradoxical lowering of serotonin. Electrophysiological studies have demonstrated that medications that block the reuptake of serotonin in the synaptic cleft actually cause an initial decrease in the firing of serotonergic neurons (Blier et al. 1990; de Montigny et al. 1990). It is conceivable that in an unfortunate minority of individuals, this initial phase may be prolonged to a clinically deleterious degree.

Interestingly, other studies suggest that serotonergic agents may selectively decrease suicidality and impulsiveness not only in patients with major depressive disorder (Muijen et al. 1988) but also in patients with borderline personality disorder (Cornelius et al. 1991; Norden 1989). One study compared the relative effectiveness of serotonergic antidepressants with that of noradrenergic antidepressants in the treatment of patients with major depressive disorders who had already made suicide attempts; the serotonergic antidepressants were found to be significantly more effective in the treatment of these patients (Sacchetti et al. 1991). A recent study demonstrated significant reduction in suicidal behavior in a heterogeneous group of patients who had recurrent suicidal behavior but did not have a major depression at the time of the study (Verkes et al. 1998). This is an intriguing finding in light of the posited serotonergic hypofunction in suicidal patients. However, literature to date is too preliminary to support the hypothesis that SSRIs are the antidepressants of choice in the suicidal patient because of their neurotransmitter action. Rather, SSRIs and other new-generation antidepressants may be viewed as more prudent choices over tricyclic antidepressants because of their low lethality index.

Finally, the role of electroconvulsive therapy cannot be overemphasized as a safe and relatively rapid somatic treatment for the acutely suicidal depressed patient.

It is also important to stress that maintenance pharmacotherapy is quintessential to the reduction of suicide risk in patients with mood disorders. Recent studies have shown that suicide risk is enhanced in bipolar patients when lithium is discontinued and is markedly reduced when patients with bipolar disorder maintain their lith-ium regimen (Baldessarini 1999a, 1999b; Tondo et al. 2001). One recent study demonstrated that suicide risk was 24 times as high during periods off, compared with periods on, adequate lithium prophylaxis; conversely, the incidence of patients attempting suicide was similar during the periods before receiving and after discontinuing lithium treatment but was five to six times lower during prophylaxis (Bocchetta et al. 1998). Continuous and adequate lithium prophylaxis should be considered in the presence of high suicide risk, even if the prophylactic effect on the underlying mood disorder may be incomplete.

Psychotherapy With the Suicidal Patient

In his classic treatise on suicide, Durkheim (1897/1951) noted that the risk of suicide varied inversely to the degree of connectedness with family and society as a whole. Indeed, as discussed earlier in this chapter, the risk of suicide seems to correlate inversely with the maintenance of ongoing personal and professional relationships. Thus, one of the daunting tasks in the psychotherapy of the suicidal patient is the realization that the psychotherapist may be perceived as the last ballast of hope that human connectedness may be yet something worth striving for. The establishment of the therapeutic alliance, then, is the single most important task in the treatment of the suicidal patient.

The establishment of the therapeutic alliance is common to all of the psychotherapeutic traditions. Also common to all psychotherapeutic traditions is the role of the empathic method (Jacobs 1989) in the treatment of suicidal patients. There is no "suicide-specific" psychotherapy, and clinicians are increasingly aware of the value of integrating principles from psychodynamic and cognitive-behavioral therapy. An important contribution of cognitive psychology has been the identification of hopelessness as the psychological factor most consistent with suicidal intent—even more so than the subjective experience of depression (Beck et al. 1975; Weisman et al. 1979; Wetzel 1976). The emphasis in cognitive therapy of suicidal behavior is the correction of cognitive distortions that may have resulted in the perception of hopelessness, and the therapist strives to instill hope in this process. Also, to the degree that depression or hopelessness has led to deterioration of problem-solving abilities, therapy is geared to the enhancement of those skills, including increasing the patient's capacity to view options and alternatives to suicide.

Psychodynamic psychotherapies have stemmed from an understanding of the dynamics of the individual's suicidal motivation, as well as of the act of suicide itself

(Dulit and Michels 1992; Hendin 1991). In addition, the psychodynamic literature offers useful insights regarding countertransference pitfalls in the treatment of suicidal patients. It is necessary for therapists to address countertransferential feelings in themselves. Addressing countertransferential feelings is necessary less to expunge oneself of "incorrect" feelings than to realize how one's refusal to acknowledge them might lead to the subversion of the therapeutic alliance (Maltsberger and Buie 1974).

As mentioned previously, psychosocial interventions have had little impact on the rate of suicide. In fact, some of the proposed treatments have been thought to exacerbate suicidal intent (Chowdhury et al. 1973; Liberman and Eckman 1981). As such, psychotherapy per se must be seen as yet another procedure administered to a patient who has a potentially terminal outcome—something that has the capacity to render either better clinical improvement or deterioration. What is necessary, however, is to determine the actual efficacy of specialized psychotherapeutic techniques both alone and in combination with pharmacotherapeutic interventions. Only by determining this efficacy can we expect to have an impact on the suicide rate, a rate that has not changed in 45 years.

Conclusions

Suicide is a complex, multidimensional phenomenon that has been studied from philosophical, sociological, and clinical perspectives. In this chapter we have focused on suicide from a clinical perspective, emphasizing psychiatric illness, psychological factors, and neurobiological correlates of suicidality. We have given an overview of the management of suicidal patients, including risk assessment, pharmacotherapy, and psychotherapy.

As reiterated throughout this chapter, the overall rate of suicide has not changed in 45 years. Indeed, we cannot ultimately prevent suicide in a given patient. However, it is clear that in treated populations the risk of suicide can be reduced. Our role as clinicians is to hone our skills at recognition and treatment to reduce the risk of suicide in a specific patient.

References

Abbar M, Courtet P, Leboyer M, et al: Suicide attempters and the tryptophan hydroxylase gene. Molecular Psychiatry 6:268–273, 2001

Adamek ME, Kaplan MS: Firearm suicide among older men. Psychiatr Serv 47:304–306, 1996

Agren H: Symptom patterns in unipolar and bipolar depression correlating with monoamine metabolites in the cerebrospinal fluid, II: suicide. Psychiatry Res 3:225–236, 1980

Allebeck P, Wistedt B: Mortality in schizophrenia. Arch Gen Psychiatry 43:650–653, 1986

Almeida-Montes LG, Valles-Sanchez V, Moreno-Aguilar J, et al: Relation of serum cholesterol, lipid, serotonin, and tryptophan levels to severity of suicide attempt. J Psychiatry Neurosci 4:371–377, 2000

Alvarez JC, Cremniter D, Lesieur P, et al: Low blood cholesterol and low platelet serotonin levels in violent suicide attempters. Biol Psychiatry 45:1066–1069, 1999

Apter A, Kotler M, Sevy S, et al: Correlates of risk of suicide in violent and nonviolent psychiatric patients. Am J Psychiatry 148:883–887, 1991

Arango V, Underwood M, Gubbi A, et al: Localized alterations in pre- and postsynaptic serotonin binding sites in the ventrolateral prefrontal cortex of suicide victims. Brain Res 688:121–133, 1995

Arranz B, Blennow K, Eriksson A, et al: Serotonergic, noradrenergic, and dopaminergic measures in suicide brains. Biol Psychiatry 41:1000–1009, 1997

Åsberg M, Thorän P, Träskman L, et al: Serotonin depression: a biochemical subgroup within affective disorders? Science 191:478–480, 1976

Bachus SE, Hyde TM, Akil M, et al: Neuropathology of suicide: a review and approach. Ann N Y Acad Sci 863:201–219, 1997

Baldessarini RJ, Tondo L, Hennen J: Antisuicidal effects of lithium in manic-depressive disorders. J Clin Psychiatry 60(suppl):S77–S84, 1999a

Baldessarini RJ, Tondo L, Viguera AC: Effect of discontinuing lithium maintenance treatment. Bipolar Disorder 1:17–24, 1999b

Banki CM: Factors influencing monoamine metabolites and tryptophan in patients with alcohol dependence. J Neural Transm 50:89–101, 1981

Banki CM, Arat M, Papp Z, et al: The effect of dexamethasone on cerebrospinal fluid metabolites in psychiatric patients. Pharmacopsychiatrics 16:77–81, 1983

Banki CM, Arat M, Papp Z, et al: Biochemical markers in suicidal patients: investigations with cerebrospinal fluid amine metabolites and neuroendocrine tests. J Affect Disord 6:341–350, 1984

Barraclough B, Bunch J, Nelson B, et al: A hundred cases of suicide: clinical aspects. Br J Psychiatry 125:355–373, 1974

Baumann B, Danos P, Diekmann S, et al: Tyrosine hydroxylase immunoreactivity in the locus coeruleus is reduced in depressed non-suicidal patients but normal in depressed suicide patients. Eur Arch Psychiatry Clin Neurosci 249:212–219, 1999

Beasley CM Jr, Dornseif BE, Bosomworth JC, et al: Fluoxetine and suicide: a meta-analysis of controlled trials of treatment for depression. Br Med J 303:685–692, 1991

Beck AT, Steer RA: Manual for the Beck Hopelessness Scale. San Antonio, TX, Psychological Corporation, 1988

Beck AT, Beck R, Kovacs M: Classification of suicidal behaviors, I: quantifying intent and medical lethality. Am J Psychiatry 132:285–287, 1975

Beck AT, Brown G, Berchick RJ, et al: Relationship between hopelessness and ultimate suicide: a replication with psychiatric outpatients. Am J Psychiatry 147:190–195, 1990

Beck AT, Steer RA, Sanderson WC, et al: Panic disorder and suicidal ideation and behavior: discrepant findings in psychiatric outpatients. Am J Psychiatry 148:1195–1199, 1991

Berrettini WH, Nurnberger JI Jr, Narrow W, et al: Cerebrospinal fluid studies of bipolar patients with and without a history of suicide attempts. Ann N Y Acad Sci 487:197–201, 1986

Beskow J, Gottfires CG, Roos BE, et al: Determination of monoamine and monoamine metabolites in the human brain: post-mortem studies in a group of suicides and a control group. Acta Psychiatr Scand 53:7–20, 1976

Birckmayer J, Hemenway D: Minimum-age drinking laws and youth suicide, 1970–1990. Am J Public Health 89:1365–1368, 1999

Black DW, Winokur G: Suicide and psychiatric diagnosis, in Suicide Over the Life Cycle: Risk Factors, Assessment, and Treatment of Suicidal Patients. Edited by Blumenthal SJ, Kupfer DJ. Washington, DC, American Psychiatric Press, 1990, pp 135–153

Blazer D, Williams CP: Epidemiology of dysphoria and depression in an elderly population. Am J Psychiatry 137:439–444, 1980

Blier P, de Montigny C, Chaput Y: A role for the serotonin system in the mechanism of action of antidepressant treatments: preclinical evidence. J Clin Psychiatry 51(suppl):14–21, 1990

Bligh-Glover W, Kolli TN, Shapiro-Kulnane L, et al: The serotonin transporter in the midbrain of suicide victims with major depression. Biol Psychiatry 47:1015–1024, 2000

Blumenthal SJ: An overview and synopsis of risk factors, assessment, and treatment of suicidal patients over the life cycle, in Suicide Over the Life Cycle: Risk Factors, Assessment, and Treatment of Suicidal Patients. Edited by Blumenthal SJ, Kupfer DJ. Washington, DC, American Psychiatric Press, 1990, pp 685–733

Bocchetta A, Ardou R, Burrai C, et al: Suicidal behavior on and off lithium prophylaxis in a group of patients with prior suicide attempts. J Clin Psychopharmacol 18:384–389, 1998

Bondy B, Erfurth A, de Jonge S, et al: Possible association of the short allele of the serotonin transporter promoter gene polymorphism (5-HTTLPR) with violent suicide. Mol Psychiatry 5:193–195, 2000

Bourne HR, Bunney WE, Colburn RW, et al: Noradrenaline, 5-hydroxytryptamine, and 5-hydroxyindoleacetic acid in the hindbrains of suicidal patients. Lancet 2:805–808, 1968

Boxer PA, Burnett C, Swanson N: Suicide and occupation: a review of the literature. Journal of Occupational and Environmental Medicine 37:442–452, 1997

Breier A, Astrachan BM: Characterization of schizophrenic patients who commit suicide. Am J Psychiatry 141:206–209, 1984

Brener ND, Krug EG, Simon TR: Trends in suicide ideation and suicidal behavior among high school students in the United States, 1991–1997. Suicide Life Threat Behav 304:304–312, 2000

Breitbart W, Rosenfeld BD, Passik SD: Interest in physician-assisted suicide among ambulatory HIV-infected patients. Am J Psychiatry 153:238–242, 1996

Brent DA, Moritz G, Bridge J, et al: Long-term impact of exposure to suicide: a three-year controlled follow-up. J Am Acad Child Adolesc Psychiatry 35:646–653, 1996

Brown GL, Goodwin FK, Ballenger JC, et al: Aggression in humans correlates with cerebrospinal fluid amine metabolites. Psychiatry Res 1:131–139, 1979

Brown GL, Ebert MH, Goyer PF, et al: Aggression, suicide, and serotonin: relationship to CSF amine metabolites. Am J Psychiatry 139:741–746, 1982

Brunner J, Stalla GK, Stalla J, et al: Decreased corticotropin-releasing hormone (CRH) concentrations in the cerebrospinal fluid of eucortisolemic suicide attempters. J Psychiatr Res 35:1–9, 2001

Bunney WE Jr, Fawcett JA: Possibility of a biochemical test for suicidal potential: an analysis of endocrine findings prior to three suicides. Arch Gen Psychiatry 13:232–239, 1965

Carroll BJ, Greden JF, Feinberg T: Suicide, neuroendocrine dysfunction and CSF 5-HIAA concentrations in depression, in Recent Advances in Neuropsychopharmacology: Proceedings of the 12th CNP Congress. Edited by Angrist B. Oxford, United Kingdom, 1980, pp 307–313

Centers for Disease Control and Prevention: Suicide among children, adolescents, and young adults: United States, 1980–1992. JAMA 274:451–452, 1995

Centers for Disease Control and Prevention: Suicide among black youths: United States, 1980–1995. MMWR Weekly 47:193–196, 1998

Chaudron LH, Remington P: Age and gender differences in suicide trends, Wisconsin and the United States, 1980–1994. Wisconsin Medical Journal 98:35–38, 1999

Cheetam SC, Cross AJ, Crompton MR, et al: Serotonin and GABA function in depressed suicide victims. Paper presented at the International Conference on New Directions in Affective Disorders, Jerusalem, 1987

Cheung HK: Schizophrenics fully remitted on neuroleptics for 3–5 years: to stop or continue drugs? Br J Psychiatry 138:490–494, 1981

Chowdhury N, Hicks RC, Keitman N: Evaluation of an aftercare service for parasuicide (attempted suicide) patients. Social Psychiatry 8:67–81, 1973

Coccaro EF, Siever LJ, Klar HM, et al: Serotonergic studies in patients with affective and personality disorders: correlates with suicidal and impulsive aggressive behavior. Arch Gen Psychiatry 46:587–599, 1989

Cochran E, Robins E, Grote S: Regional serotonin levels in brain: a comparison of depressive suicides and alcoholic suicides with controls. Biol Psychiatry 11:283–294, 1976

Corbitt EM, Malone KM, Haas GL, et al: Suicidal behavior in patients with major depression and comorbid personality disorders. J Affect Disord 39:61–72, 1996

Cornelius JR, Soloff PH, Perel JM, et al: A preliminary trial of fluoxetine in refractory borderline patients. J Clin Psychopharmacol 11:116–120, 1991

Coryell W, Schlesser M: The dexamethasone suppression test and suicide prediction. Am J Psychiatry 158:748–753, 2001

Cowdry RW, Gardner DL: Pharmacotherapy of borderline personality disorder: alprazolam, carbamazepine, trifluoperazine, and tranylcypromine. Arch Gen Psychiatry 45:111–119, 1988

Crow TJ, Cross A, Cooper SJ, et al: Neurotransmitter receptors and monoamine metabolites in the brains of patients with Alzheimer-type dementia and depression, and suicides. Neuropharmacology 23:1561–1569, 1984

Damluji NF, Ferguson JM: Paradoxical worsening of depressive symptomatology caused by antidepressants. J Clin Psychopharmacol 8:347–349, 1988

De Meo MD, McBride PA, Mann JJ, et al: Fenfluramine challenge in major depression, in New Research and Abstracts, 141st annual meeting of the American Psychiatric Association, Montreal, Quebec, Canada, May 1988, NR169, p 91

de Montigny C, Chaput Y, Blier P: Modification of serotonergic neuron properties by long-term treatment with serotonin reuptake blockers. J Clin Psychiatry 51(suppl B):4–8, 1990

de Wilde J, Mertens C, Fredricson Overo K, et al: Citalopram versus mianserin: a controlled, double-blind trial in depressed patients. Acta Psychiatr Scand 72:89–96, 1985

Doyle BB: Crisis management of the suicidal patient, in Suicide Over the Life Cycle: Risk Factors, Assessment, and Treatment of Suicidal Patients. Edited by Blumenthal SJ, Kupfer DJ. Washington, DC, American Psychiatric Press, 1990, pp 381–423

Drake RE, Cotton PG: Depression, hopelessness and suicide in chronic schizophrenia. Br J Psychiatry 148:554–559, 1986

Drake RE, Ehrlich J: Suicide attempts associated with akathisia. Am J Psychiatry 142:499–501, 1985

Drake RE, Gates C, Cotton PG, et al: Suicide among schizophrenics: who is at risk? J Nerv Ment Dis 172:613–617, 1984

Drake RE, Osher FC, Wallach MA: Alcohol use and abuse in schizophrenia: a prospective community study. J Nerv Ment Dis 177:408–414, 1989

Dulit RA, Michels R: Psychodynamics and suicide, in Suicide and Clinical Practice. Edited by Jacobs D. Washington, DC, American Psychiatric Press, 1992, pp 43–53

Durkheim E: Suicide: A Study in Sociology (1897). Translated by Spaulding JA, Simpson G. New York, Free Press, 1951

Ellison L, Morrison H: Low cholesterol is associated with suicide risk. Epidemiology 12:168–172, 2001

Emanuel EJ, Fairclough DL, Emanuel LL: Attitudes and desires related to euthanasia and physician-assisted suicide among terminally ill patients and their caregivers. JAMA 284:2460–2468, 2000

Ettinger R: A follow-up investigation of patients after attempted suicide, in The Suicide Syndrome. Edited by Farmer R, Hirsh S. London, England, Croon Helm, 1980, pp 167–172

Fava M, Rosenbaum JP: Suicidality and fluoxetine: is there a relationship? J Clin Psychiatry 52:108–111, 1991

Fawcett J, Scheftner WA, Fogg L, et al: Time-related predictors of suicide in major affective disorder. Am J Psychiatry 147:1189–1194, 1990

Freud S: Mourning and melancholia (1917[1915]), in Standard Edition of the Complete Psychological Works of Sigmund Freud, Vol 14. Translated and edited by Strachey J. London, England, Hogarth, 1957, pp 237–260

Friedman S, Jones JC, Chernen L, et al: Suicidal ideation and suicide attempts among patients with panic disorder: a survey of two outpatient clinics. Am J Psychiatry 149:680–685, 1992

Gardner DL, Cowdry RW: Alprazolam-induced dyscontrol in borderline personality disorder. Am J Psychiatry 142:98–100, 1985

Gessner BD: Temporal trends and geographic patterns of teen suicide in Alaska, 1979–1993. Suicide and Life-Threatening Behavior 27:264–273, 1997

Goldring N, Fieve RR: Attempted suicide in manic-depressive disorder. Am J Psychother 38:373–383, 1984

Golier J, Marzuk P, Leon A, et al: Low serum cholesterol and attempted suicide. Am J Psychiatry 152:419–423, 1995

Goodwin FK: Suicide, aggression, and depression: a theoretical framework for future research. Ann N Y Acad Sci 487:351–355, 1986

Goodwin FK, Jamison KR: Manic-Depressive Illness. New York, Oxford University Press, 1990

Gould MS, Fisher P, Parides M, et al: Psychosocial risk factors of child and adolescent completed suicide. Arch Gen Psychiatry 53:1155–1162, 1996

Gross-Isseroff R, Israeli M, Biegon A: Autoradiographic analysis of tritiated imipramine binding in the human brain post mortem: effects of suicide. Arch Gen Psychiatry 46:237–241, 1989

Gross-Isseroff R, Biegon A, Voet H, et al: The suicide brain: a review of postmortem receptor/transporter binding studies. Neurosci Biobehav Rev 22:653–661, 1998

Grunebaum MF, Oquendo MA, Harkavy-Friedman JM, et al: Delusions and suicidality. Am J Psychiatry 158:742–747, 2001

Gruenewald PJ, Ponicki WR, Mitchell PR: Suicide rates and alcohol consumption in the United States, 1970–1989. Addiction 90:1063–1075, 1995

Harris EC, Barraclough B: Suicide as an outcome for mental disorders: a meta-analysis. Br J Psychiatry 170:205–228, 1997

Hendin H: Psychodynamics of suicide, with particular reference to the young. Am J Psychiatry 148:1150–1158, 1991

Henriksson MM, Isometsa ET, Kuoppasalmi KI, et al: Panic disorder in completed suicide. J Clin Psychiatry 57:275–281, 1996

Hogan TP, Awad AG: Pharmacotherapy and suicide risk in schizophrenia. Can J Psychiatry 28:277–281, 1983

Hrdina PD, Du L: Levels of serotonin receptor 2A higher in suicide victims? Am J Psychiatry 158:147–148, 2001

Hrdina PD, Demeter E, Vu TB, et al: 5-HT uptake sites and 5-HTs receptors in brain of antidepressant-free suicide victims/depressives: increase in 5-HT2 sites in cortex and amygdala. Brain Res 614:37–44, 1993

Jacobs D: Psychotherapy with suicidal patients, in Suicide: Understanding and Response. Edited by Jacobs D, Brown HN. Madison, CT, International Universities Press, 1989, pp 329–342

Jacobs D: Evaluating and treating suicidal behavior in the borderline patient, in Suicide and Clinical Practice. Edited by Jacobs D. Washington, DC, American Psychiatric Press, 1992, pp 115–130

Kaplan JR, Muldoon MF, Manuck SB, et al: Assessing the observed relationship between low cholesterol and violence-related mortality. Ann N Y Acad Sci 836:57–80, 1997

Kernberg OF: Severe Personality Disorders: Psychotherapeutic Strategies. New Haven, CT, Yale University Press, 1984

Kessler RC, Borges G, Walters EE: Prevalence of and risk factors for lifetime suicide attempts in the National Comorbidity Survey. Arch Gen Psychiatry. 56:7, 1999

King RA, Riddle MA, Chappell PB, et al: Emergence of self-destructive phenomena in children and adolescents during fluoxetine treatment. J Am Acad Child Adolesc Psychiatry 30:179–186, 1991

Korpi ER, Kleinman JE, Goodman SI, et al: Serotonin and 5-hydroxyindoleacetic acid in brains of suicide victims: comparison in chronic schizophrenic patients with suicide as cause of death. Arch Gen Psychiatry 43:594–600, 1986

Kposowa AJ: Unemployment and suicide: a cohort analysis of social factors predicting suicide in the US National Longitudinal Mortality Study. Psychol Med 31:127–138, 2001

Kunugi H, Takei, Aoki H, et al: Low serum cholesterol in suicide attempters. Biol Psychiatry 41:196–200, 1997

Lambert MT, Silva PS: An update on the impact of gun control legislation on suicide. Psychiatr Q 69:127–134, 1998

Lawrence KM, De Paermentier F, Cheetham SC, et al: Brain 5-HT uptake sites, labeled with (3H) paroxetine, in antidepressant-free depressed suicides. Brain Res 526:17–22, 1990

Letizia C, Kapik B, Flanders WD: Suicidal risk during controlled clinical investigations of fluvoxamine. J Clin Psychiatry 57:P415–P421, 1996

Liberman RP, Eckman T: Behavior therapy versus insight-oriented therapy for repeated suicide attempters. Arch Gen Psychiatry 38:1126–1130, 1981

Linnoila M, De Jong J, Virkkunen M: Family history of alcoholism in violent offenders and impulsive fire setters. Arch Gen Psychiatry 46:613–616, 1989

Little KY, McLaughlin DP, Ranc J, et al: Serotonin transporter binding sites and mRNA levels in depressed persons committing suicide. Biol Psychiatry 41:1156–1164, 1997

Lloyd KG, Farley IJ, Deck H, et al: Serotonin and 5-hydroxyindoleacetic acid in discrete areas of the brainstem of suicide victims and control patients. Adv Biochem Psychopharmacol 11:387–397, 1974

Lopez JF, Vasquez DM, Chalmers DT, et al: Regulation of 5-HT receptors and the hypothalamic-pituitary-adrenal axis. Ann NY Acad Sci 836:106–134, 1987

Malone KM, Haas GL, Sweeney JA, et al: Major depression and the risk of attempted suicide. J Affect Disord 34:173–185, 1995

Maltsberger JT, Buie DH: Countertransference hate in the treatment of suicidal patients. Arch Gen Psychiatry 30:625–633, 1974

Mann JJ: The neurobiology of suicide. Nat Med 4:25–30, 1998

Mann JJ, Arango V: Integration of neurobiology and psychopathology in a unified model of suicidal behavior. J Clin Psychopharmacol 12(suppl):2S–7S, 1992

Mann JJ, Kapur S: The emergence of suicidal ideation and behavior during antidepressant pharmacotherapy. Arch Gen Psychiatry 48:1027–1033, 1991

Mann JJ, Stanley M, McBride PA, et al: Increased serotonin$_2$ and β-adrenergic receptor binding in the frontal cortices of suicide victims. Arch Gen Psychiatry 43:954–959, 1986

Mann JJ, Malone K, Psych M, et al: Attempted suicide characteristics and cerebrospinal fluid amine metabolites in depressed inpatients. Neuropsychopharmacology 15:576–586, 1996a

Mann JJ, Arango V, Hentelff RA, et al: Serotonin 5-HT$_3$ receptor binding kinetics in the cortex of suicide victims are normal. J Neural Transm 103:165–171, 1996b

Mann JJ, Huang YY, Underwood MD, et al: A serotonin transporter gene promoter polymorphism (5-HTTLPR) and prefrontal cortical binding in major depression and suicide [see comments]. Arch Gen Psychiatry 57:729–738, 2000

Mann JJ, Brent DA, Arango V: The neurobiology and genetics of suicide and attempted suicide: a focus on the serotonergic system. Neuropsychopharmacology 24:467–477, 2001

Marazitti D, Presta S, Silvestri S, et al: Platelet markers in suicide attempters. Prog Neuropsychopharmacol Biol Psychiatry 19:375–383, 1995

Marzuk PM, Mann JJ: Suicide and substance abuse. Psychiatr Ann 18:639–645, 1988

Marzuk PM, Tierney H, Tardiff K, et al: Increased risk of suicide in persons with AIDS. JAMA 259:1333–1337, 1988

Marzuk PM, Leon AC, Tardiff K, et al: The effect of access to lethal methods of injury on suicide rates. Arch Gen Psychiatry 49:451–458, 1992a

Marzuk PM, Tardiff K, Leon AC, et al: Prevalence of cocaine use among residents of New York City who committed suicide during a one-year period. Am J Psychiatry 149:371–375, 1992b

McGlashan TH, Heinssen RK: Hospital discharge status and long-term outcome for patients with schizophrenia, schizoaffective disorders, borderline personality disorder, and unipolar affective disorder. Arch Gen Psychiatry 45:363–368, 1988

McIntosh JL: Suicide prevention in the elderly (age 65–99). Suicide Life Threat Behav 25:180–192, 1995

McKegney FP, O'Dowd MA: Suicidality and HIV status. Am J Psychiatry 149:396–398, 1992

Meltzer HY, Nash JF, Ohmori T, et al: Neuroendocrine and bio chemical studies in serotonin and dopamine in depression and suicide. Paper presented at the International Conference on New Directions in Affective Disorders, Jerusalem, 1987

Miles CP: Conditions predisposing to suicide: a review. J Nerv Ment Dis 164:231–246, 1977

Montgomery SA, McAuley R, Rani SJ, et al: A double blind comparison of zimelidine and amitriptyline in endogenous depression. Acta Psychiatr Scand Suppl 63(suppl 290):314–329, 1981

Montgomery SA, Dunner DL, Dunbar GC, et al: Reduction of suicidal thoughts with paroxetine in comparison with reference antidepressants and placebo. Eur Neuropsychopharmacol 5:5–13, 1995

Morgan AC: Special issues of assessment and treatment of suicide risk in the elderly, in Suicide: Understanding and Response. Edited by Jacobs D, Brown HN. Madison, CT, International Universities Press, 1989, pp 239–256

Moscicki EK: Epidemiology surveys as tools for studying suicidal behavior: a review. Suicide Life Threat Behav 19:131–146, 1989

Moscicki EK: North American perspectives: epidemiology of suicide. Int Psychogeriatr 7:137–148, 1995

Motto JA, Heilbron DC, Juster RP: Development of a clinical instrument to estimate suicide risk. Am J Psychiatry 142:680–686, 1985

Muijen M, Roy D, Silverstone T, et al: A comparative clinical trial of fluoxetine, mianserin and placebo in depressed outpatients. Acta Psychiatr Scand 78:384–390, 1988

Mullin JM, Pandita-Gunawerdina UR, Whitehead AM: A double-blind comparison of fluvoxamine and dothiepin in the treatment of major affective disorders. Br J Clin Pract 42:51–55, 1988

Murphy GE, Wetzel RD: The lifetime risk of suicide in alcoholism. Arch Gen Psychiatry 47:383–392, 1990

Myerson LR, Wennogle LP, Abel MS, et al: Human brain receptor alterations in suicide victims. Pharmacol Biochem Behav 17:159–163, 1982

Nemeroff CB, Widerlov E, Bissette G, et al: Elevated concentrations of CSF corticotropin releasing factor-like immunoreactivity in depressed patients. Science 226:1342–1344, 1984

Nemeroff CB, Owens MJ, Bissette G, et al: Reduced corticotropin releasing factor binding sites in the frontal cortex of suicide victims. Arch Gen Psychiatry 45:577–579, 1988

Ninan PT, van Kammen DP, Scheinin M, et al: CSF 5-hydroxyindoleacetic acid levels in suicidal schizophrenic patients. Am J Psychiatry 141:566–569, 1984

Nielsen DA, Virkunnen M, Lappalainen J, et al: A tryptophan hydroxyase gene marker for suicidality and alcoholism Arch Gen Psychiatry 5:593–602, 1998

Norden MJ: Fluoxetine in borderline personality disorder. Prog Neuropsychopharmacol Biol Psychiatry 13:885–893, 1989

Nyman A, Jonsson H: Patterns of self-destructive behavior in schizophrenia. Acta Psychiatr Scand 73:252–262, 1986

Odagaki Y, Garcia-Sevilla JA, Huguelet P, et al: Cyclic AMP-mediated signaling components are up-regulated in the prefrontal cortex of depressed suicide victims. Brain Res 898:224–231, 2001

Olson L, Huyler F, Lynch AW, et al: Guns, alcohol, and intimate partner violence: the epidemiology of female suicide in New Mexico. Crisis 20:121–126, 1999

Ordway GA: Pathophysiology of the locus coeruleus in suicide. Ann N Y Acad Sci 836:233–252, 1997

Owen F, Cross A, Crow TJ, et al: Brain 5-HT$_2$ receptors and suicide. Lancet 2:1256–1257, 1983

Owen F, Chambers DR, Cooper SJ: Serotonergic mechanisms in brains of suicide victims. Brain Res 362:185–188, 1986

Pandey GN, Pandey SC, Janicak PG, et al: Platelet serotonin-2 receptor binding sites in depression and suicide. Biol Psychiatry 28:215–222, 1990

Pandey G, Pandey S, Duvivedi Y, et al: Platelet serotonin$_{2A}$ receptors: a potential biological marker for suicidal behavior. Am J Psychiatry 152:850–855, 1995

Pare CMB, Yeung DP, Brice K, et al: 5-Hydroxytryptamine, noradrenaline and dopamine in brainstem, hypothalamus and caudate nucleus of controls and of patients committing suicide by coal gas poisoning. Lancet 2:133–135, 1969

Paul SM, Rehavi M, Skolnick P, et al: High affinity binding of antidepressants to a biogenic amine transport site in human brain and platelet: studies in depression, in Neurobiology of Mood Disorders. Edited by Post RM, Ballenger JC. Baltimore, MD, Williams & Wilkins, 1984, pp 845–853

Perry EK, Marshall EF, Blessed G, et al: Decreased imipramine binding in the brains of patients with depressive illness. Br J Psychiatry 142:188–192, 1983

Penttinen J: Hypothesis: low serum cholesterol, suicide, and interleukin-2. Am J Epidemiol 141:716–718, 1995

Pfeffer CR: Risk factors associated with youth suicide: a clinical perspective. Psychiatr Ann 18:652–656, 1988

Pine D, Trautman P, Shaffer D, et al: Seasonal rhythm of platelet [^{3}H] imipramine binding in adolescents who attempted suicide. Am J Psychiatry 152:923–925, 1995

Potter LB, Powell KE, Kachur SP: Suicide prevention from a public health perspective. Suicide Life Threat Behav 25:82–91, 1995

Rampling D: Aggression: a paradoxical response to tricyclic antidepressants. Am J Psychiatry 135:117–118, 1978

Rich CL, Young D, Fowler RC: San Diego Suicide Study, I: young versus old subjects. Arch Gen Psychiatry 43:577–582, 1986

Rich CL, Warsradt GM, Nemiroff RA, et al: Suicide, stressors, and the life cycle. Am J Psychiatry 148:524–527, 1991

Robins E, Murphy GE, Wilkinson RH, et al: Some clinical considerations in the prevention of suicide based on a study of 134 successful suicides. Am J Public Health 49:888–899, 1959

Robins LN, Kulbok PA: Epidemiological studies in suicide. Psychiatr Ann 18:619, 623–627, 1988

Rouillon F, Phillips R, Seurvier D, et al: Rechutes de depression unipolaire et ellicacite de la maprotiline. Encephale 15:527–534, 1989

Roy A: Suicide in chronic schizophrenia. Br J Psychiatry 141:171–177, 1982

Roy A, Ninan P, Mazonson A, et al: CSF monoamine metabolites in chronic schizophrenic patients who attempt suicide. Psychol Med 15:335–340, 1985

Roy A, Agren H, Pickar D, et al: Reduced CSF concentrations of homovanillic acid and homovanillic acid to 5-hydroxyindoleacetic acid ratios in depressed patients: relationship to suicidal behavior and dexamethasone nonsuppression. Am J Psychiatry 143:1539–1545, 1986

Roy A, Lamparski D, DeJong J, et al: Characteristics of alcoholics who attempt suicide. Am J Psychiatry 147:761–765, 1990

Roy A, Karoum F, Pollack S: Marked reduction in indexes of dopamine metabolism among patients with depression who attempt suicide. Arch Gen Psychiatry 49:447–450, 1992

Roy A, Segal N, Sarchiapone M: Attempted suicide among living co-twins of twin suicide victims. Am J Psychiatry 152:1075–1076, 1995

Sacchetti E, Vita A, Guarneri L, et al: The effectiveness of fluoxetine, clomipramine, nortriptyline, and desipramine in major depressives with suicidal behavior: preliminary findings, in Serotonin Related Psychiatric Syndromes. Edited by Cassano GB, Akiskal HS. London, England, Royal Society of Medicine Services, 1991, pp 47–53

Sainsbury P: Depression, suicide, and suicide prevention, in Suicide. Edited by Roy A. Baltimore, MD, Williams & Wilkins, 1986a, pp 73–88

Sainsbury P: The epidemiology of suicide, in Suicide. Edited by Roy A. Baltimore, MD, Williams & Wilkins, 1986b, pp 17–40

Salib E, Tadros G: Brain weight in suicide: an exploratory study. Br J Psychiatry 177:257–261, 2000

Sartorius N: Recent changes in suicide rates in selected Eastern European and other European countries. Int Psychogeriatr 7:301–308, 1995

Schmidtke A, Bille-Brahe U, DeLo D, et al: Attempted suicide in Europe: rates, trends and sociodemographic characteristics of suicide attempters during the period 1989–1992. Results of the WHO/EURO Multicentre Study on Parasuicide. Acta Psychiatr Scand 93:327–338, 1996

Schulsinger F, Kety SS, Rosenthal D, et al: A family study of suicide, in Origin, Prevention and Treatment of Affective Disorders. Edited by Schon M, Stromgren E. New York, Academic Press, 1979, pp 277–287

Shaffer D, Craft L: Methods of adolescent suicide prevention. J Clin Psychiatry 60(suppl):70–74, 1999

Shaw DM, Camps FE, Eccleston EG: 5-Hydroxytryptamine in the hind-brain of depressive suicides. Br J Psychiatry 113:1407–1411, 1967

Shem S: The House of God. New York, Richard Marek Publishers, 1978

Siris SG: Three cases of akathisia and "acting out." J Clin Psychiatry 46:395–397, 1985

Skoog I, Aevarsson O, Beskow J, et al: Suicide in the elderly. Am J Psychiatry 153:1015–1020, 1996

Soloff PH, George A, Nathan RS, et al: Progress in pharmacotherapy of borderline disorders: a double-blind study of amitriptyline, haloperidol, and placebo. Arch Gen Psychiatry 43:691–697, 1986

Soloff PH, George A, Nathan RS, et al: Behavioral dyscontrol in borderline patients treated with amitriptyline. Psychopharmacol Bull 23:177–181, 1987

Stack S: Suicide: a 15-year review of the sociological literature. Part 1: cultural factors. Suicide Life Threat Behav 30:145–162, 2000

Stanley M, Mann JJ: Increased serotonin-2 binding sites in frontal cortex of suicide victims. Lancet 1:214–216, 1983

Stanley M, Virgilio JJ, Gerson S: Tritiated imipramine binding sites are decreased in the frontal cortex of suicides. Science 216:1337–1339, 1982

Stanley M, McIntyre I, Gershon S: Post-mortem serotonin metabolism in suicide victims. Paper presented at the American College of Neuropsychopharmacology, San Juan, Puerto Rico, December 1983

Stevenson JM: Suicide, in The American Psychiatric Press Textbook of Psychiatry. Edited by Talbot JA, Hales RE, Yudofsky SC. Washington, DC, American Psychiatric Press, 1988, pp 1021–1035

Stockmeier CA: Neurobiology of serotonin in depression and suicide. Ann N Y Acad Sci 836:220–232, 1997

Stockmeier CA, Dilley GE, Shapiro LA, et al: Serotonin receptors in suicide victims with major depression. Neuropsychopharmacology 16:162–173, 1997

Stockmeier CA, Shapiro LA, Dilley GE, et al: Increase in serotonin-1A autoreceptors in the midbrain of suicide victims with major depression: postmortem evidence for decreased serotonin activity. J Neurosci 18:7394–7401, 1998

Stone MH, Stone DK, Hurt SW: Natural history of borderline patients treated by intensive hospitalization. Psychiatr Clin North Am 10:185–206, 1987

Surgeon General of the United States: A National Suicide Prevention Strategy. Washington, DC, U.S. Public Health Service, U.S. Government Printing Office, 2001

Targum SD, Rosen L, Capodanno AE: The dexamethasone suppression test in suicidal patients with unipolar depression. Am J Psychiatry 140:877–879, 1983

Teicher MH, Glod C, Cole JO: Emergence of intense suicidal preoccupation during fluoxetine treatment. Am J Psychiatry 147:207–210, 1990

Tondo L, Hennen J, Baldessarini RJ: Reduced suicide risk with long-term lithium treatment in major affective illness: a meta-analysis. Acta Psychiatr Scand 104:163–172, 2001

Träskman L, Åsberg M, Bertilsson L, et al: Monoamine metabolites in CSF and suicidal behavior. Arch Gen Psychiatry 38:631–636, 1981

Träskman-Bendz L, Alling C, Oreland L, et al: Prediction of suicidal behavior from prologic tests. J Clin Psychopharmacol 12(suppl):21S–26S, 1992

Verkes RJ, Van der Mast RC, Hengeveld MW, et al: Reduction by paroxetine of suicidal behavior in patients with repeated suicide attempts but not major depression. Am J Psychiatry 155:543–547, 1998

Warshaw M, Keller M: The relationship between fluoxetine use and suicidal behavior in 654 subjects with anxiety disorders. J Clin Psychiatry 57:158–166, 1996

Weiden P, Roy A: General versus specific risk factors for suicide in schizophrenia, in Suicide and Clinical Practice. Edited by Jacobs D. Washington, DC, American Psychiatric Press, 1992, pp 75–100

Weisman A, Beck AT, Kovacs M: Drug abuse, hopelessness and suicidal behavior. Int J Addict 14:451–464, 1979

Weiss RD, Stephens PS: Substance abuse and suicide, in Suicide and Clinical Practice. Edited by Jacobs D. Washington, DC, American Psychiatric Press, 1992, pp 101–114

Weissman MM, Klerman GL, Markowitz JS, et al: Suicidal ideation and suicide attempts in panic disorder and attacks. N Engl J Med 321:1209–1214, 1989

Wetzel RD: Hopelessness, depression, and suicide intent. Arch Gen Psychiatry 33:1069–1073, 1976

Wilkinson G, Bacon N: A clinical and epidemiological survey of parasuicide and suicide in Edinburgh schizophrenics. Psychol Med 14:899–912, 1984

Winokur G, Tsuang M: The Iowa 500: suicide in mania, depression, and schizophrenia. Am J Psychiatry 132:650–651, 1975

Zanko MT, Bigeon A: Increased β-adrenergic receptor binding in human frontal cortex of suicide victims. Paper presented at the annual meeting of the Society for Neuroscience, Boston, MA, 1983

Zeck PM, Tierney H, Tardiff K, et al: Increased risk of suicide in persons with AIDS. JAMA 259:1333–1337, 1988

Zisook S, Byrd D, Kuck J, et al: Command hallucinations in outpatients with schizophrenia. J Clin Psychiatry 56:462–465, 1995

Violence

Kenneth J. Tardiff, M.D., M.P.H.

Psychiatrists should be able to evaluate and treat violent patients. A number of studies indicate that approximately 10% of the patients seen in psychiatric hospitals manifested violent behavior toward others just before being admitted to these hospitals (Davis 1991; Tardiff 1983), a finding that is true for private as well as public hospitals. A more recent study found that the percentage of patients who are violent before admission approaches 15% (Tardiff et al. 1997a). Furthermore, the occurrence of violent behavior even among chronic inpatients is still appreciable. Learning how to evaluate and manage violent patients is important not only for the safety of society and of patients in treatment settings but also for the safety of mental health professionals who themselves are at high risk of being assaulted (American Psychiatric Association 1993; Blow et al. 1999; Thackrey 1987).

In this chapter, I discuss the topic of violence from the perspective of the clinician. (For more detailed and extensive coverage of this topic, see Tardiff 1996, 1999a.)

Causes of Violence

Before the clinical aspects of evaluating and managing the violent patient can be discussed, it is important to appreciate that a broad spectrum of factors interact to produce violent behavior in humans. One can conceptualize, although somewhat artificially, a group of internal or innate factors within the individual and external factors present during child development or in the environment that interact to either increase or decrease an individual's propensity for violent behavior. Appreciation of these innate and environmental factors is essential to prepare the clinician to see the evaluation and treatment of the violent patient in the context of society. Conversely, the clinician should realize that much of the violence in society is related to factors such as economics, drug dealing, and other criminal activities not within the usual realm of psychiatric expertise, thus questioning psychiatry's involvement in such matters (Tardiff 1992).

Neurophysiological Factors

Since 1970, researchers have focused on the temporal lobe as the area of the brain responsible for aggressive behavior, based on cases of patients with partial complex seizures who manifested violent behavior (Mark and Ervin 1970; Monroe 1970). Yet the role of the temporal lobe and of epilepsy in violence has remained controversial. Delgado-Escueta et al. (1981) conducted a large international collaborative study and found that violence was rare among epileptic patients. Hermann and Whitman (1984) reviewed the literature and found no overall difference in levels of violence between persons with or without epilepsy. Bogdanovic et al. (2000) found no association between the frequency of epilepsy and violence among a group of institutionalized adults with epilepsy. Interictal and postictal violence among epileptic patients was more related to psychopathology or to attempts to restraint the patients than to epilepsy (Devinsky 1994; Mendez et al. 2000) Despite this, some investigators (Monroe 1985; Weiger and Bear 1988) continue to emphasize the importance of epilepsy and limbic ictus in episodic dyscontrol and violence by maintaining that the surface electroencephalogram (EEG) is a crude and ineffective measurement of subcortical activity and that patients with episodic dyscontrol often respond to anticonvulsant medication. With recent advances in imaging using magnetic resonance, there is evidence that subtle damage to the amygdaloid nucleus is associated with violence (Tonkonogy 1991). Elliot (1992) presented an excellent summary of studies pointing to neurological dysfunction as a factor in violence, and Eichelman (1992) summarized the basic science literature on animal and human aggression.

Genetic Determinants

In the past two decades there has been a great deal of interest and research in sex chromosome abnormalities and violent behavior, particularly the XYY abnormality. Schiavi et al. (1984), having reviewed the literature, conducted a double-blind controlled study and found no association between XYY or XXY chromosome abnormalities and violence. The role of these chromosomal abnormalities is doubtful, and any association with arrest for crimes is probably linked to other factors such as low intelligence. Twin studies showing increased criminal behavior in monozygotic twins were subject to several methodological problems, and a study by Bohman et al. (1982) of adopted men in Sweden failed to show that the violent crimes committed by these men were related to violence in their biological or adoptive parents. Other studies of twins reared apart have found that inheritance is an important factor in the expression of aggression (Tellegen et al. 1988). Thus, genetic determinants deserve further study.

Hormones

Violence may be associated with gross endocrine disease such as Cushing's disease or hyperthyroidism (K.E. Anderson and Silver 1999). The roles of androgens, hypoglycemia, and premenstrual syndrome are more controversial. Studies have not found a relationship between androgens and violent behavior (Rada et al. 1983). This finding leaves us with the probable conclusion that increased rates of violence by men in society are accounted for by other factors such as role expectations in society. Studies of hypoglycemic patients as well as habitually violent offenders have indicated that hypoglycemia may play a role in extreme cases of violence and fire setting (Virkkunen 1982; Virkkunen et al. 1989). Low glucose levels were not found in a later, larger study of violent criminals (De Jong et al. 1992). Perhaps in some individuals with certain personality and environmental precipitants, the hypoglycemic state may tip the balance toward aggressive behavior. Premenstrual syndrome has been used as a defense in crimes of manslaughter, arson, and assault in Europe (Dalton 1980). Reid and Yen (1981) did an extensive search of the literature and found little or no research evidence that premenstrual syndrome is a direct contributing factor to criminal activity or even that it is a nonspecific factor perhaps producing irritability in an individual predisposed to violence.

Neurotransmitters

Brown et al. (1982) found that a history of aggressive behavior and a history of suicidal behavior both were related to decreased cerebrospinal fluid (CSF) 5-hydroxyindoleacetic acid (5-HIAA) levels. Lidberg et al. (1985) found that men who were convicted of criminal homicide and a group of men who committed suicide both had lower levels of 5-HIAA in their CSF than did male control subjects. Lower levels of 5-HIAA in violent individuals is in agreement with other studies of suicide and serotonin metabolism (Apter et al. 1991; Belfrage et al. 1992; Braverman and Pfeiffer 1985; Coccaro et al. 1989; Fishbein et al. 1989; Lidberg et al. 2000). The prefrontal cortex receives a major serotonergic projection that is dysfunctional in persons who are impulsively violent (Davidson et al. 2000). Thus, low CSF 5-HIAA may be a marker of impulsivity rather than of a specific type of violence (i.e., suicide or externally directed aggression). The central serotonergic system has continued to be the focus of attention in research on violent individuals (Coccaro 1992).

Developmental Factors

Kempe and Helfer (1980) found childhood abuse to be related to becoming physically abusive as an adult. In fact, even witnessing intrafamily violence, such as spouse abuse, is related to increased problems with violence among children (Jaffe et al. 1986; Pelcovitz et al. 1994). Studies on the effect of past child abuse and other familial violence have been criticized because of their retrospective designs (Widom 1989a); however, a prospective cohort study confirmed that being abused and neglected as a child does increase one's risk for adult violence (Dodge et al. 1997; Widom 1989b). Others have pointed out that the link could be a genetic one, with abusing parents being criminals and the risk for violence being inherited (Carey 1996; Di Lalla and Gottesman 1991). Violence need not take place in the home to have a possible influence on the child and adolescent; evidence indicates that television violence could be related to later aggressive behavior (National Institute of Mental Health 1982). However, Freedman (1984) criticized this research. Research should be done in naturalistic settings, and the long-term effects of television violence should be studied further. The National Television Violence Study examined thousands of programs and found that more than half contained violence, that in 75% the perpetrator was not punished, and that very few of the victims in those programs appeared to be harmed by the violence

(Federman 1997). Phillips (1999) pointed out that concern about the media and violence by adolescents should extend to rock music as well. In light of the high rate of child abuse, intrafamily violence, and violence depicted in the mass media, there should be great concern that we are raising the next generation of violent adults. Monitoring and regulating violence in the media are essential to prevent this outcome (Centerwall 1992; Phillips 1999).

Social Structure

Messner and Rosenfeld (1999) presented a general review of the social structural approach to violence. They explained that social structure has been linked to violence via the concepts of "social control" and "social strain." *Social control* refers to the process through which a group regulates its members to achieve collective goals, for example, to live in a safe environment free of violence (Horowitz 1990). Social controls can be formal, such as policing, or informal, such as the monitoring of behavior by neighbors. This capacity of neighbors to intervene for purposes of social control has recently been referred to as "collective efficacy" (Morenoff et al. 2001; Sampson et al. 1997). In studies of Chicago neighborhoods, Sampson et al. (1997) interviewed residents about helping and trusting each other to measure collective efficacy. They found that high collective efficacy was related to low violence rates and that low collective efficacy was related to indicators of "concentrated disadvantage" (e.g., poverty, unemployment, racial segregation, disrupted families). In neighborhoods with highly concentrated disadvantage and accompanying low collective efficacy, persons are relatively free to engage in violence and other deviant behaviors.

The second concept linking social structure with violence is that of social strain. *Social strain* refers to negative emotions that are induced when structural conditions make it difficult for people to realize cultural goals and expectations through legitimate means (Agnew 1992, 1999). Whereas social control is a restraint against violence, social strain is a motivation for violence. A given social structural condition might contribute to violence via both kinds of mechanisms. For example, widespread poverty in a neighborhood makes it difficult for neighbors to mobilize to exert informal control, and at the same time such poverty is likely to motivate people to engage in violence and other crimes. A good deal of social structural research on violence has been explained by both control and strain theories. Although the results are sometimes inconsistent, it appears that socioeconomic disadvantage definitely increases the risk of violence in a community

Firearms

Evidence has shown that the number of homicides associated with firearms has increased significantly in the past century, particularly since 1960 (Tardiff et al. 1994). Firearms are important because they can turn what would have been an assault into a homicide. It is difficult to determine whether this rise in homicides is the result of increased availability of firearms, because the import and export of firearms are not accurately measured. There is evidence, however, that gun control legislation is effective in decreasing the rate of homicides involving firearms (Cook 1982). Knowing whether a gun is present in the home is important when evaluating violence potential because guns increase the probability of serious violence and death (Saltzman et al. 1992; U.S. General Accounting Office 1991).

Physical Environment

Physical crowding may relate to violence because it increases contact and decreases defensible space, whereas an increased number of persons without crowding may increase social control and decrease violence (A.C. Anderson 1982; Sampson 1983). These principles in society are similar to what is found on psychiatric inpatient units, namely, that increased numbers of patients are associated with increased violence (Palmstierna et al. 1991). The number of bystanders available for surveillance and intervention may prevent the commission of crimes, including homicide (Messner and Tardiff 1985). Thus, the effect of bystanders on the level of violence in the community may be positive through such programs as Crime Watch and other efforts at community organization.

Bell and Baron (1981), after reviewing several ecological and ethological studies as well as laboratory studies, concluded that a relationship exists between heat and aggression that is curvilinear: moderately uncomfortable ambient temperatures produce an increase in aggression, whereas extremely hot temperatures decrease aggression. The implications of these environmental findings for the community of the inpatient unit are obvious: overcrowding, inadequate numbers of staff, uncomfortable heat, and disruptive rather than supportive patients will likely lead to increased violence.

Psychiatric Disorders

Schizophrenia

Psychosis increases the potential for violent behavior if the patient has thoughts of violence. Schizophrenia is most frequently found in patients with psychosis and violence (Brennan et al. 2000; Link et al. 1992). Patients with schizophrenia can be violent because of delusions, particularly paranoid delusions (Arango et al. 1999; Benjaminsen et al. 1996); however, some authors have not found an increased risk of violence by patients with delusions (Appelbaum et al. 2000). This may be due to differences in methodologies used in these studies. Clinically, we see patients who are violent because they believe others are attempting to harm or have harmed them. These patients regard violence as justifiable self-defense or retaliation. Frequently, the theme of the delusion associated with violence persists throughout the course of the illness. Hallucinations, particularly auditory hallucinations, can be associated with violence by patients with schizophrenia. These may be command auditory hallucinations telling the patient to kill others or harm him or herself; one study found that one-fifth of patients complied with such commands (McNiel et al. 2000). Some have found that an overall increased rate of violence by patients with schizophrenia is due to inadequate treatment with antipsychotic medications (Steinert et al. 2000).

Patients with schizophrenia can be violent for reasons other than psychosis. Violence by these patients may be the result of comorbid alcohol or substance abuse (Lindqvist and Allebeck 1990; Swanson et al. 1990). A superimposed insult to the brain may be present that results in a low threshold for violence, including any of the disorders discussed later in this chapter such as substance abuse, head trauma, AIDS, and other neurologic and systemic medical disorders. Mentally retarded schizophrenic patients may resort to violence out of frustration, in response to either demands from family or staff members or an inability to verbalize their needs and conflicts.

Comorbid antisocial or borderline personality disorder increases the potential for violence (Swanson et al. 1990). Violence can be manipulative—used to control or to express anger by the patient—and not be related to the schizophrenic disorder itself. For example, in one case a paranoid schizophrenic patient with antisocial personality who was no longer psychotic deliberately punched a nurse in the face when he was told that his weekend pass was rescinded.

Delusional Disorder

Delusional disorder can be associated with violent behavior, especially the paranoid and jealous types. Patients with paranoid delusional disorder harbor grudges against those whom they believe have wronged them. Patients with delusional disorders of the jealous type are known to retaliate violently against their spouses or against suspected third persons in the imagined illicit affair.

Mania

Patients experiencing a manic episode can be violent as a result of psychosis and/or gross disorganization of thoughts and/or behavior. Violence by manic patients frequently occurs in the acute phase of the manic episode (Miller et al. 1993). Targets of violence are often random in these cases. Manic patients who are more intact are often violent when they feel restricted or when limits are being set by staff.

Personality Disorders

Some personality disorders, namely the antisocial and borderline types, increase the risk of violence (Johnson and Cohen 2000; Tardiff et al. 1997a, 1997b). Patients with antisocial personality are viciously violent in order to seek revenge or to bolster their images. Frequently the victims are strangers to the patients or superficial acquaintances. Characteristically, these patients show no remorse after the attacks and, instead, regret not inflicting more injury on the victims, whom they believe deserved it. Although these patients may appear glib and/or attractive, the clinician can expect violence if their self-esteems or macho images are threatened.

Patients with borderline personality are violent in several contexts. Violence can be a manifestation of affective instability or manipulation and as such can be unpredictable. Individuals with borderline personality disorders have a pervasive pattern of instability in interpersonal relationships, self-image, emotional states, and marked impulsivity (American Psychiatric Association 1994). They make efforts to avoid real or imagined rejection. They form intense relationships with some people and expect these people to protect and rescue them (Benjamin 1993). When people fail to live up to these unrealistic expectations, these patients react with rage, verbal and/or physical violence, suicidal behavior, or other self-destructive behaviors. Impulsivity is severe in borderline personality and may also result in violence, suicide attempts, and other self-destructive behaviors (Stone 1990).

Patients with paranoid personality frequently threaten violence, because they often feel persecuted and/or discriminated against because of race, gender, or some other personal attribute. This feeling of persecution often leads to arguments with people in their lives. These patients have thoughts or even plans of violence but do not usually act on their violent thoughts; however, if violence occurs it can be catastrophic, as in the case of mass murder.

Intermittent Explosive Disorder

Intermittent explosive disorder is characterized by discrete episodes of loss of control resulting in serious violence toward persons or destruction of property (American Psychiatric Association 1994). The violent episode is not due to the physiological effects of a substance or a general medical condition. The degree of violence is grossly out of proportion to any provocation or environmental stressor. Patients may describe a sense of tension before the violence and a sense of relief afterward. Unlike patients with antisocial personality and borderline personality, after the episode patients with intermittent explosive disorder feel remorseful about their violence. Between episodes of violence, these patients may appear to be stable and model employees or spouses.

Posttraumatic Stress Disorder

Patients with posttraumatic stress disorder (PTSD) can become violent, particularly if the original stressor was related to violence. The violence may be due to the use of alcohol associated with PTSD or may be related to trigger phenomena. It may be diffuse, as part of increased arousal with irritability and anger, or it may be part of intense psychological distress in response to external cues that symbolize or resemble an aspect of the traumatic event.

Substance Abuse

Alcohol has been found to increase the risk of violence in several ways (Coker et al. 2000; Eronen et al. 1996; Tardiff et al. 1997b). Alcohol releases inhibitions such that urges and behaviors that would be unacceptable in sober state—in this case, violence—erupt despite personal and societal restraints against violence. Alcohol produces impairment in tasks associated with the frontal lobes such as assessment, planning, organization of behavior, and ability to abstract. Communication skills may not be sufficient to allow the intoxicated individual to deal with the situation in a verbal rather than physical manner. Cognitive impairment of the brain caused by alcohol may exaggerate provocation through misinterpretation of real events such as perceiving an insult in a bar or in a marital discussion. The intoxicated individual may not appreciate the consequences of violence because of cognitive impairment.

Cocaine produces violent behavior usually during severe intoxication and/or delirium (Giannini et al. 1993; McCormick and Smith 1995). Symptoms of intoxication include auditory, visual, and tactile hallucinations, paranoid and other delusions, irritability, confusion, and psychomotor agitation. Symptoms of intoxication or delirium typically disappear within 2 days after the last dose of cocaine. However, a delusional syndrome may linger for 1 week or longer after the last dose. This syndrome is characterized by persecutory delusions that may elicit violence. Violence may be elicited by cocaine alone; however, in addition to cocaine, alcohol and heroin are frequently used to counter the irritability and other unpleasant effects of cocaine (Denison et al. 1997) and may contribute to the violent behaviors observed. Other stimulants, such as amphetamines, may cause intoxication, delirium, or a delusional disorder; these conditions are clinically indistinguishable from those produced by cocaine. Paranoid delusions may result in assault or homicide.

Phencyclidine (PCP) may be smoked or taken orally, intranasally, or intravenously. Intoxication is manifested by belligerence, assaultiveness, ataxia, dysarthria, muscle rigidity, seizures, and hyperacusis. PCP delirium may last longer than that caused by cocaine, but otherwise it is clinically similar.

Anabolic steroids have been used by athletes and bodybuilders to enhance muscle growth, strength, and performance. Increased irritability and aggressiveness may occur as side effects of these drugs (Pope and Katz 1990). Male athletes demonstrated aggressive behavior and other psychopathology after taking steroids, sometimes at high doses. After several weeks or months of self-medication, the men became irritable and combative and committed violent crimes, including homicide, assault, and robbery. Their irritability and violent outbursts disappeared within several months after steroid discontinuation.

Ecstasy has amphetamine and hallucinogenic properties. It produces confusion, severe anxiety, paranoia, depression, and aggression (National Institute on Drug Abuse 1999). Physical symptoms include muscle tension, involuntary teeth clenching, nausea, blurred vision, rapid eye movement, faintness, chills, sweating, and increased heart rate and blood pressure. It is popular at dance clubs and college scenes.

Polysubstance abuse is very common. Substances may be taken simultaneously, even in the same injection (such as the speedball combination of cocaine and heroin). Alcohol is frequently combined with other drugs of abuse during the same occasion. Polysubstance use may be a deliberate decision on the part of the user or result from a drug supplier's decision to mix several substances together, in which case the user does not necessarily know that he or she is using more than one drug. The combinations of substances result in multiple interactions.

Organicity

Organicity increases the risk of violence (Kutzer 1990; Rao et al. 1985; Tardiff 1998; Zierler et al. 2000). Central nervous system disorders associated with violent behavior include traumatic brain injury, HIV infection, and other intracranial infections (encephalitis, postencephalitic syndrome); tumors; seizures (especially postictally); cerebrovascular disorder; Huntington's disease; Alzheimer's disease; Wilson's disease; multiple sclerosis; and normal pressure hydrocephalus. Systemic disorders that can produce violence include metabolic disorders, electrolyte imbalances, hypoxia, uremia, Cushing's disease, vitamin deficiencies (e.g., pernicious anemia), systemic infections, systemic lupus erythematosus, porphyria, and toxins (K.E. Anderson and Silver 1999).

Summary

Violence is the result of an interaction between characteristics of the individual and factors in the environment. Biological or innate factors such as neurophysiological dysfunction, hormones, inheritance, and neurotransmitter abnormalities are nonspecific in the way they cause violence. Rather than a specific mechanism, they tip the balance by impairing the person's ability to achieve goals through nonviolent means or by increasing impulsivity, irritability, irrationality, or disorganization of behavior. The environment may influence the individual during development, for example, by the child's being subjected to abuse or having to witness violence either within the family or subculture or on television and other mass media. Poverty and other adverse social conditions have a damaging impact on the family and the social network as well as on the individual. Use of alcohol and drugs and the availability of weapons may kindle an explosion of violence. Some biological and environmental factors may be more important than others, but the clinician should weigh all of these factors in the evaluation of the patient and for the purpose of planning and implementing treatment.

Acute Management

Safety

Violence by patients toward clinicians is not uncommon and is a serious problem (Coverdale et al. 2001; Eichelman and Hartwig 1995). All clinicians are faced with the situation—whether in the emergency department, the inpatient unit, or even the outpatient clinic—in which we are summoned to deal with a patient who has struck someone, has thrown something, or is threatening violence. Often, a group of people—staff, police, patients, and other observers—have gathered around the patient. The psychiatrist or other professional in charge of that setting is expected to take control and "do something." When defusing the situation and evaluating future potential for violence, the ideal situation is to be alone with the patient in a closed room. Obviously, this may not always be advisable for safety reasons. Foremost in the psychiatrist's mind should be "Do I feel safe?" (Brasic and Fogelman 1999; Eichelman and Hartwig 1995) The psychiatrist must feel safe with the patient, or this insecurity will interfere with the evaluation and may result in physical injury or death. When talking to the patient, several options should be considered, including interviewing the patient alone with the door closed or open, interviewing the patient with aides outside or inside the room, and interviewing the patient while he or she is in physical restraints. The psychiatrist should not feel omnipotent, even if others expect him or her to have a magical ability to calm violent patients, as is sometimes portrayed in the movies. In addition to relying on his or her own feelings concerning safety, the clinician should consider the possibility of countertransference or other inappropriate reactions, such as denial, that will interfere with the effective management of a particular patient. These reactions are discussed at length later in this chapter.

Instant Differential Diagnosis

When deciding how to proceed, in terms of talking to the patient or using physical means of control, the clinician should make an instant differential diagnosis and categorize the patient's condition into one of three groups:

1. *Organic mental disorders:* For patients with cognitive impairment disorders and substance-related disorders who are having a violent episode, it is frequently impossible to intervene effectively and influence them through verbal means. The underlying medical or other physical disorder should be treated rather than relying on neuroleptics alone to control violence. If the etiology of the disorder is unknown and if there is actual or imminent violence, the patient probably should be restrained while the laboratory tests and evaluation proceed.

2. *Psychotic disorders:* Violent patients with psychotic disorders are usually schizophrenic or manic and are difficult to influence through verbal means. Rapidly

administered neuroleptic medication is the treatment of choice for these patients, although they may have to be restrained or secluded until it takes effect.

3. *Nonpsychotic, nonorganic disorders:* Patients with nonpsychotic, nonorganic disorders are primarily those with personality disorders or intermittent explosive disorder who are often amenable to verbal intervention without seclusion or restraint. It may be desirable to offer medication to the patient and give him or her the option of either accepting or rejecting it, thus giving the patient a sense of control over the situation. When deciding to use a physical means of control, the psychiatrist can assess the patient's degree of impulse control by the patient's compliance with routine requests and procedures in the clinic or emergency department (Table 35–1).

TABLE 35–1. Types of violent patients and emergency responses

Type	Response
Organic mental disorders	Patient generally requires restraint until etiology known. Not usually amenable to talk.
Psychotic disorders	Patient generally requires restraint and neuroleptic. Not usually amenable to talk.
Nonpsychotic, nonorganic disorders	Patient generally responds to talk with de-escalation. Staff for restraint and/or medication should be available nearby.

Verbal Intervention

Verbal means of intervention and even prevention should receive serious consideration (Table 35–2). In terms of prevention, it is essential that an inpatient unit have adequate, well-trained staff to ensure implementation of ongoing treatment programs and also to prevent violence. In an emergency situation, staff should be adequate in number and trained to implement seclusion and restraint techniques effectively, appropriately, and safely. Most important, the staff should be caring and nonauthoritarian yet at the same time should act as part of the ward milieu, demonstrating social norms and limits. This balance is difficult to achieve but is nevertheless essential in the prevention of violent behavior on inpatient units. Staff should talk to patients in a calm, nonprovocative manner and should also listen to patients. As tension increases before violence occurs, even the most psychotic schizophrenic patient may respond to nonprovocative

interpersonal contact and expression of concern and caring. It is important that staff recognize the warning signs of violence that have preceded violent acts in the past for a particular patient. A patient may have a specific pattern of behavior or speech before an explosive episode, such as pacing in front of the nursing station or repeating the same word or phrase.

TABLE 35–2. Verbal management of violent patients

Be concerned for your safety.
Appear calm and in control.
Speak softly in a nonprovocative, nonjudgmental manner.
Both patient and clinician sit, if possible.
Do not tower over patient or stare at the patient.
When the patient begins to talk, listen.

Seclusion and Restraint

In 1982, the Supreme Court ruled in the case of *Youngberg v. Romeo* that Mr. Romeo, a violent, profoundly mentally retarded man who was institutionalized, could be deprived of his liberty in terms of being restrained if it could be justified to protect others or himself and, most important, if the decision was based on a professional's clinical judgment that is not a substantial departure from professional standards. The importance of this case is that the court deferred to professional judgment rather than to a rigid hierarchy of restrictiveness in the management of violence by patients. At the time the decision was rendered, I was chairing a task force of the American Psychiatric Association (APA) to develop guidelines for the psychiatric uses of seclusion and restraint. The guidelines were approved by the APA and published in a Task Force Report (American Psychiatric Association 1984). These guidelines set reasonable, minimal clinical standards for management of violence using seclusion and restraint in the context of verbal intervention, involuntary medication, and other factors in the treatment environment. The guidelines are expanded in a book by members of the task force (Tardiff 1984; see Table 35–3).

Indications for emergency use of seclusion and restraint are as follows:

TABLE 35–3. Indications for seclusion or restraint

To prevent harm to others
To prevent harm to the patient
To prevent serious disruption of treatment environment
As ongoing behavioral treatment

1. To prevent imminent harm to others—namely, staff and other patients—if other means are not effective and appropriate
2. To prevent imminent harm to the patient if other means of control are not effective or appropriate
3. To prevent serious disruption of the treatment program or significant damage to the environment
4. As part of an ongoing behavior treatment program

These indications for emergency use of seclusion and restraint state that violence need not actually occur but that the staff may use these measures for imminent violence, such as when a patient's pattern of escalation to violence is known and in evidence or if it is apparent that a patient is on the verge of exploding.

The decision to use seclusion, restraint, or involuntary medication is clinical and should be based on the individual needs and status of the patient. For example, restraint probably would be preferable if the patient is delirious and the etiology of the delirium is unknown. In this case, it would be better to keep the patient free of drugs, particularly neuroleptics, until the underlying etiology is determined, and seclusion would not be appropriate because the sensory deprivation may worsen the patient's delirium. Restraint also might be preferred if close medical monitoring is necessary, such as for patients with heart disease, infections, metabolic illness, drug overdoses, or other medical problems. On the other hand, seclusion may be the method of choice for a manic person who needs a decrease of stimulation. Involuntary medication may be the preferred method of control, perhaps with seclusion or restraint, for the paranoid schizophrenic patient who has stopped taking medications and has become violent or is imminently so. Emergency medication is discussed later in this chapter. A combination of the control measures may be used, for example, for a violent manic patient with a history of epilepsy. This patient may be secluded and given lower doses of involuntary medication, such as haloperidol, than are usually prescribed because of concern about decreased seizure threshold resulting from neuroleptic medication. The reasons for using seclusion, restraint, or other physical means of control and subsequent monitoring must be documented in the patient's record.

As with any medical procedure, there are contraindications as well as indications (Table 35–4). Seclusion and restraint should never be used to punish a patient as retribution for a particular act. Although this type of retribution may be the philosophy of a penal institution, it has no place in a treatment setting. Seclusion and restraint should never be used solely for the convenience of the staff or of other patients on the inpatient unit, or solely for the sake of the treatment programs on the ward. If seclusion and restraint are used for these reasons, then the treatment plan for the patient should be reviewed and a change of treatment program or setting should be considered. Seclusion and restraint should never be used inappropriately as the result of the dynamics of the ward. Seclusion should not be used if the patient needs close medical monitoring, is self-mutilative, or wants to be secluded so as to avoid participating in the treatment program. Patients should not be secluded if seclusion rooms cannot be cooled, particularly when the patient is taking neuroleptic medication, because hot rooms interfere with regulation of body temperature, resulting in death in some instances on hot days.

TABLE 35–4. Guidelines for seclusion and restraint

Not used to punish a patient or solely for the convenience of staff or other patients.

Psychiatrist/staff must take into consideration the medical and psychiatric status of the patient (e.g., drug overdose, medical disease, self-mutilation).

Psychiatrist/staff must follow written guidelines of institution.

Adequate staff must be present (at least four) for implementation.

When decision is made to use seclusion or restraint, patient should be given seconds to comply by walking to seclusion room.

If patient does not comply, each staff member should grab a limb and bring patient backward to the ground.

Restraint devices are applied, or patient is carried to seclusion by four staff members.

Patient is searched for belts, pins, watches, and other dangerous objects and is placed in gown.

Physician sees patient within 1 hour after beginning of the seclusion or restraint.

Physician sees patient in seclusion or restraint every 4 hours and writes another order.

Nursing staff should observe patient at least every 15 minutes.

Nursing staff should visit patient at least every 2 hours.

Meals (without utensils), fluids, and toileting should be provided at appropriate times and with caution.

With four-point restraints, each limb should be released or restraint loosened every 15 minutes.

Patient should be gradually released from seclusion or restraint.

Each decision, observation, and measurement, as well as care, must be documented in detail in the patient's record or in a log.

Patients and staff should discuss the seclusion or restraint after each episode.

The APA Task Force on Psychiatric Uses of Seclusion and Restraint did not recommend specific techniques for approaching patients or for using restraint devices, but it indicated that seclusion and restraint should be considered analogous to cardiopulmonary resuscitation in an institution in that there should be 1) written, specific guidelines and a manual for the use of these procedure; 2) approval of those guidelines by the administrators of the hospital, their lawyers, and the state; 3) education of the staff in terms of the guidelines and actual rehearsal of the techniques; and 4) feedback from staff regarding problems with the guidelines, with revisions following accordingly.

Generally, states have formulated policies on the use of seclusion and restraint along the lines recommended by the task force in terms of the need for a physician to order seclusion or restraint and to see the patient soon after the seclusion or restraint begins, preferably within an hour. Time parameters were recommended as to how long a patient could be kept in seclusion or restraint before another order was necessary and how frequently nursing assessments and care were administered. Some hospitals objected to these recommendations in terms of the availability of physicians to carry them out.

In 1999, the Health Care Finance Administration (HCFA) issued rules on the use of seclusion and restraint that must be followed for hospitals to receive federal funds. These included mandating an examination of the patient by a physician or other approved, licensed independent health care practitioner (if permitted in a hospital policy) within 1 hour after the seclusion or restraint begins, a limit of 4 hours for seclusion or restraint before another order must be given, and time parameters for nurse physical assessments and care for patients who are in seclusion or restraint. HCFA mandated new requirements that notify families or other individuals, with the patient's consent, about the patient being secluded or restrained; requirements that patients be involved in postseclusion or restraint debriefing; and requirements to monitor the frequency and adverse consequences of seclusion and restraint.

Implementation of Seclusion and Restraint

The APA Task Force described proper procedures for the use of seclusion and restraint. When the decision to seclude or restrain a patient has been made, a clinical staff member should be chosen to be the leader for the procedure. This leader need not be the most senior staff member but should be the most appropriate person for that patient. In addition, sufficient force in the form of four staff members should be assembled behind the leader as the patient is approached. The staff should

appear ready, confident, and emotionally detached but not provocative. If possible, another staff person should be available to clear the area of patients as well as to observe and monitor how the procedure is carried out. Further verbal interchange with the patient is inappropriate, except for a clear statement by the leader that the patient will be secluded or restrained because he or she is out of control. The patient may be asked to walk quietly with or without underarm support to the seclusion room and given a few seconds to respond (Figure 35–1).

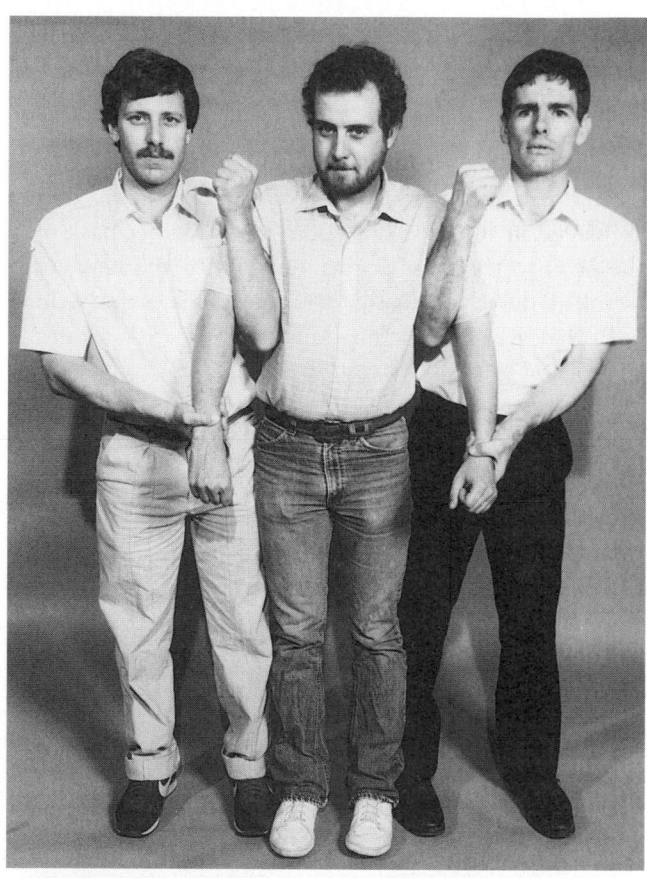

FIGURE 35–1. Walking the patient to the seclusion room with underarm support.
Source. Reprinted with permission from Thackrey M: *Therapeutics for Aggression: Psychological/Physical Crisis Intervention.* New York, Human Sciences Press, 1987. Copyright 1987 Human Sciences Press.

Verbal interchange with the patient at this point often leads to debate, violence by the patient, and a generally chaotic situation and increases the possibility that someone will be injured. If the patient does not immediately respond, each staff member should seize one of the patient's limbs in a plan agreed to beforehand. The patient should be brought backward to the ground and his or her head controlled to avoid biting (see Figure 35–2). Staff should avoid hurting the patient, twisting extremities out of the range of normal motion, sitting on the patient, cursing, or other disrespectful behavior. At this point, restraint devices should be applied or, if the patient is to be taken into seclusion, the staff should grab the patient's legs at the knees and the patient's arms around the elbow with underarm support (see Figure 35–3). Variations on this basic approach have been recommended and illustrated with photographs by Thackrey (1987). These variations may be of interest to clinicians, but again, the specific techniques to be used are the prerogative of each institution and must be clearly stated and rehearsed.

If the patient is to be placed in seclusion, he or she should be searched thoroughly. Belts, pins, rings, matches, and other objects should be removed. It is often advisable to remove the patient's street clothes and place an appropriate gown on the patient. If medication is to be used, it can be injected at this time. The patient should be placed in the seclusion room on his or her back with the head to the door or face down with the head away from the door. Gradually, staff should leave the patient, with the last person controlling the patient's arms and legs.

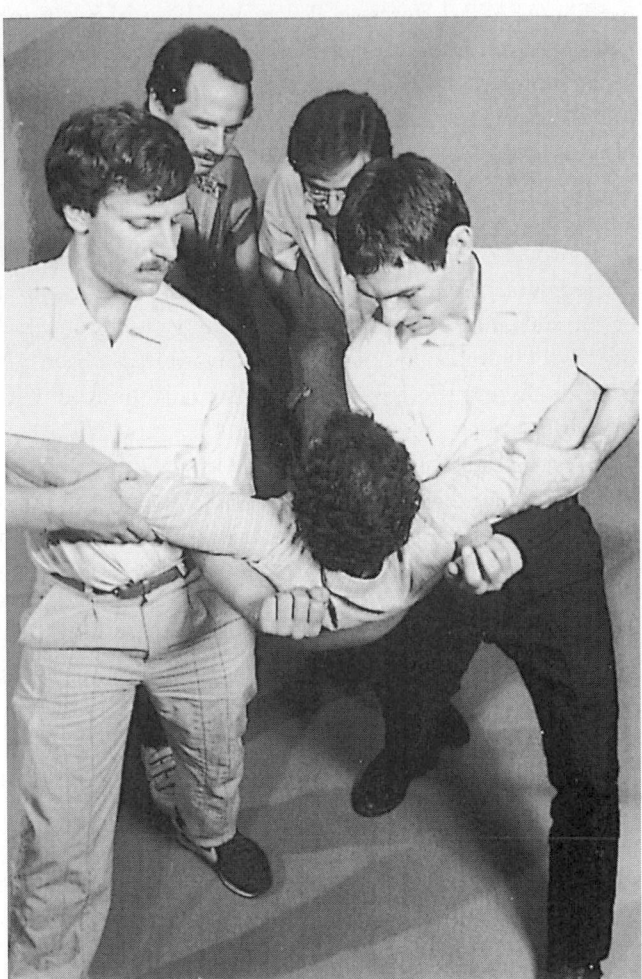

FIGURE 35–3. Transporting the patient to the seclusion room with each limb restrained and support under arms.
Source. Reprinted with permission from Thackrey M: *Therapeutics for Aggression: Psychological/Physical Crisis Intervention.* New York, Human Sciences Press, 1987. Copyright 1987 Human Sciences Press.

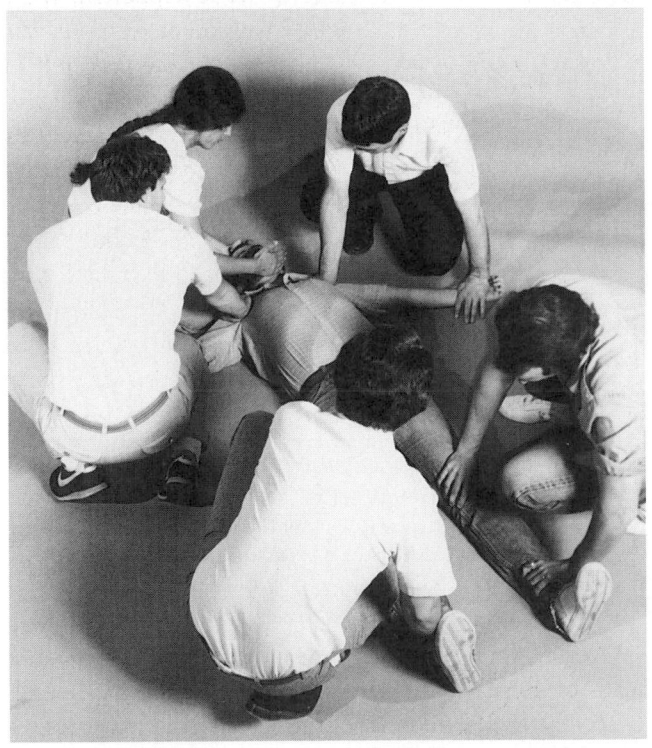

FIGURE 35–2. Patient restrained in supine position with staff holding each limb and controlling head to prevent biting.
Source. Reprinted with permission from Thackrey M: *Therapeutics for Aggression: Psychological/Physical Crisis Intervention.* New York, Human Sciences Press, 1987. Copyright 1987 Human Sciences Press.

In most cases, the seclusion and restraint will take place without the physician being present. HCFA protocol requires that a physician or other licensed independent health practitioner (if approved in a hospital policy) see the patient within 1 hour. This 1-hour time frame is essential because the patient's medical and psychiatric status must be assessed and the appropriateness of seclusion and restraint must be approved, as must be any special monitoring of the patient. A physician should visit a patient and order seclusion or restraint every 4 hours. The patient should be observed by the nursing staff at least every 15 minutes, and the patient's behavior and status should be documented in writing at each observation. In fact, in many units, when a patient is in restraints, constant observation or one-to-one observation by staff is automatically triggered. The placement of a patient in seclusion should not be a reason for abandoning the patient but should increase the amount of attention from staff. A visit and assessment in the room should be made by the nursing staff at least every 2 hours, especially if there is a question of drug overdose or if medication has been given for very agitated persons.

A direct visit with a patient may be dangerous and may require more force and staff equal to the number present when the patient was originally placed in seclusion or restraint. Meals should be served when the ward meals are served. No forks or knives should be provided, even plastic ones, because these can be used as weapons. It is preferable to have a staff member sit with the patient during mealtime, not only for purposes of social interaction but also for evaluation of the degree of control manifested by the patient. The latter point is important in determining when the patient will be removed from seclusion. For four-point restraints of the extremities, each extremity should be released or loosened every 15 minutes, and if the patient is on his or her back, he or she should be constantly observed to prevent aspiration.

The patient is not abruptly removed from seclusion or restraint. Rather, from the very beginning of the episode, staff should be testing the patient's degree of control—for example, whether the patient complies with simple requests, such as to sit in the corner when staff visit or bring meals. As the patient manifests an increased level of control, the seclusion room door may be left open with staff outside the door, and gradually the patient is reintroduced to his or her room and then the general ward setting.

Staff Feelings About Violence

The staff should know their own feelings about violence in general and about specific violent patients based on countertransference reactions or other emotional reactions to patients (Eichelman and Hartwig 1995; Lion and Pasternak 1973). Negative or inappropriate feelings about patients must be recognized so as not to act on them. In addition, the staff should be constantly monitoring ward dynamics, particularly in terms of staff conflict that may translate into inappropriate patient care in the management of violence. The staff know their own past experiences with violence and how this may affect their treatment of patients. Anger toward a patient for a particular act may be justified, or it may be the result of countertransference in which the patient resembles an abusive parent or spouse.

A number of defense mechanisms may interfere with the treatment of violent patients and in fact may pose a danger to the therapist and others. Denial of a patient's dangerousness may occur because of the therapist's past experiences with violence or because the patient may be particularly attractive or interesting. On the other hand, a patient may be viewed as more dangerous than he or she actually is because of staff anxiety that is projected onto the patient. Displacement can occur from one patient who really is dangerous to another who is not dangerous but serves as an acceptable scapegoat.

Negative emotional reactions about patients may exist because of bias and prejudice, which obviously are not acceptable. In addition, ward dynamics may result in the inappropriate treatment of violent patients. For example, nursing staff feeling abandoned by the administration or medical staff inappropriately may seclude or restrain a particular patient so as to activate procedures for which the psychiatrist is required to be on the ward and to examine the patient.

To address some of these concerns, it is important to discuss a violent episode once it has occurred. Contrary to what staff usually wish to do, this discussion should be done among the staff as well as with the patient who was violent and among other patients on the ward. Often, when the episode is finished, staff members are content to forget about or deny it. Instead, the violent episode should be discussed in terms of what happened, what would have prevented it, why seclusion or restraint was used (if it was), and how the patient or the staff felt in terms of using seclusion and restraint. It is important to recognize that most patients will have negative reactions to being secluded and restrained; the most positive reaction from a patient is usually, "I must have really been out of control or crazy to deserve something like that." Among other patients on the ward, it is important to talk about the violent episode and discuss why seclusion and restraint were used for that particular patient so as to allay other patients' fears that they could be secluded or restrained for no apparent reason in the future.

Medication in Emergencies

There are useful reviews of the literature on the use of medication in the emergency situation (Brizer 1988; Dubin et al. 1986; Eichelman 1986; Tardiff 1996, 1999a). The most common types of medication used are the neuroleptics (Table 35–5). In a survey of 20 emergency departments in the United States, the most frequent medications reported to be used for acutely violent patients were haloperidol and lorazepam, often together and intramuscularly (Binder and McNiel 1999). These are most often used for patients with schizophrenia or mania, but they may be used, with some reservations, on an emergency basis for patients with cognitive impairment, organic mental disorders, personality disorders,

TABLE 35–5. Medications in emergencies for violence

Drug	Dosage	Special considerations
Haloperidol	2–5 mg im every 1–4 hours with maximum daily dose of 20 mg	Maximum of 100 mg/day; caution in delirious patients and alcohol/drug toxic or withdrawal states
Chlorpromazine	25 mg im and every 4 hours with increased dose over 1–3 days	Maximum of 400 mg/day; caution in delirium and alcohol/drug states; observe for postural hypotension
Lorazepam	2–4 mg im or orally; repeat every hour if im or every 4–6 hours if oral	Maximum of 10 mg/day

and mental retardation. The following concerns should be borne in mind. In terms of cognitive impairment disorders, the sedative or anticholinergic effects of neuroleptics may aggravate delirious or toxic metabolic confused states. Intoxication with alcohol or sedative drugs is a relative contraindication to the use of neuroleptic medications, particularly in high doses. Overdose with anticholinergic drugs can produce delirium that would be increased by neuroleptics. In such situations and if the etiology of the cognitive impairment disorder is unknown, consider using physical restraint until, in the latter case, the etiology of the disorder can be determined. If the patient is restrained, draw blood for a toxicology screen for alcohol and other drugs.

There is less concern about the short-term use of neuroleptics to control violence among patients with personality disorders or mental retardation; however, prolonged use of this class of medication is ill advised in the absence of psychotic psychopathology because of side effects. Also, in mentally retarded persons there is interference with learning, which is the main problem with this group of patients. Alternate means of management should be seriously considered, including verbal intervention and behavior therapy, as described later in this chapter.

Clinicians today usually prefer to use high-potency antipsychotic medications such as haloperidol rather than low-potency medications such as chlorpromazine to avoid postural hypotension that may result in falls and injuries. Haloperidol can be injected intramuscularly in 2- to 5-mg doses every hour; however, every 4–8 hours is usually satisfactory. The maximum daily intramuscular dose of haloperidol is 20 mg. Chlorpromazine may be injected intramuscularly in a 25-mg dose and, if necessary, a 25- to 50-mg intramuscular dose may be given 1 hour later. Subsequent intramuscular injections may be given every 4 hours and increased in dose over several days; however, the patient is usually quiet in 1 or 2 days and will accept an oral dose. If severe orthostatic hypotension occurs with a low-potency neuroleptic, that medication should be discontinued. If a severe hypoten-

sive crisis occurs, treatment includes intravenous fluids and the use of vasopressors such as metaraminol bitartrate or levarterenol bitartrate. Epinephrine is contraindicated because it may lower blood pressure further in neuroleptic-induced orthostatic hypotension. Another untoward effect of rapid neuroleptics is a paradoxical increase in agitation as the result of akathisia or the feeling that there has been a loss of control as the patient becomes more sedated.

Some authors have not recommended benzodiazepines for management of the acutely violent patient for fear of further decreasing inhibition, particularly in those patients with personality disorders. However, benzodiazepines are the treatment of choice in withdrawal from alcohol, even with associated psychotic psychopathology, because the use of neuroleptic medications in such patients would decrease seizure threshold and increase the risk of seizures. Obviously, restraint or closely monitored seclusion also probably would be indicated in the management of such patients.

For the emergency use of benzodiazepines, lorazepam is the first choice of clinicians because it produces sedation for a longer period of time than diazepam (the former remaining in the circulation rather than being absorbed into tissues) but with a half-life of 12 hours, much shorter than that of diazepam, so accumulation is not as problematic. Intramuscular lorazepam rapidly begins to enter the circulation and produces sedation within 1 hour. Oral lorazepam produces more gradual effects, with sedation occurring between 1 and 4 hours after administration. The dose is 2–4 mg by mouth or intramuscularly. A subsequent 2- to 4-mg dose can be repeated if agitation and aggression continue, with the timing dependent on the route of administration (i.e., in 1 hour or so later if administered intramuscularly or 4–6 hours later if administered orally). Often, this approach is sufficient to manage violence in the emergency situation. After the emergency has subsided, lower maintenance levels of lorazepam with or without neuroleptics, to a maximum of 10 mg/day, can be given.

Potential for Violence in the Near Future

When interviewing the patient who has been violent or who is threatening violence, the evaluator should appear calm and in control and should speak softly in a nonprovocative, nonjudgmental manner. Begin commenting in a neutral, concrete manner about the obvious (e.g., "You look angry" or "Could you tell me what you are concerned about?"). Comments such as "Why did you do that?" or "Act like a man!" should not be used because they are provocative and most certainly will result in further violence. This is not the time for giving the patient insight or dynamic interpretations. The evaluator and the violent patient should both be either sitting or standing. It is important that the evaluator not tower over the patient and that he or she allow enough space between the patient and himself or herself. The evaluator should attempt to project passivity and yet a sense of control in the situation. When the patient begins to talk, the evaluator should listen in an empathic and concerned manner. Again, the evaluator may want to offer medication because it gives the patient a sense of control in terms of choosing whether to accept or reject it.

Evaluation of a given patient's potential to commit violence or homicide is done when determining whether to admit the patient to a hospital, at the time of the patient's discharge, and in outpatient therapy in *Tarasoff*-like situations, with the duty to protect potential victims of the patient (Beck 1985). When deciding a patient's violence potential, the clinician should interview the patient as well as family members, police, and others who have pertinent information about the patient because patients may minimize threats or violent acts that have preceded the interview. The evaluation of violence potential is analogous to that of suicide potential. If the patient does not express thoughts of violence, the evaluation should begin with a subtle question, such as "Have you ever lost your temper?" If the answer is yes, then the evaluation should proceed in terms of how, when, and so on. In the same manner, an evaluation of suicide potential would begin with the question, "Have you ever felt that life was not worth living?" If the answer was yes, the clinician would proceed with the suicide evaluation.

The evaluation of a patient's potential for violence can be relatively accurate if it is made for the near future (Binder 1999). Similar to evaluating suicide potential, evaluating violence potential includes assessing how well planned the threat is (Tardiff 1989, 1996, 1999b). Vague threats of killing someone are not as serious as saying "I'm going to kill my boss because he doesn't appreciate my work and plans to fire me." As is also done in suicide evaluation, determining availability of a means to inflict injury is important in the evaluation of violence potential. For example, if the patient has recently purchased or owns a gun, his or her threats should obviously be taken more seriously. A history of violence or other impulsive behavior is often predictive of future violence. The clinician should ask the patient about injuries to other persons, destruction of property, reckless driving, reckless spending, sexual acting out, and other impulsive behaviors. The degree of the patient's past injuries to self (e.g., broken bones and lacerations) as well as to others and the circumstances of those injuries should be assessed. There is often a pattern of past violent behavior in specific circumstances (e.g., escalation of a dispute between a husband and wife about issues of money, esteem, or sexuality). On an inpatient unit, if a patient has been violent, staff should look for characteristic patterns of behavior before violent episodes or specific situations that have triggered violence.

The presence of alcohol or drug abuse should be determined and should alert the evaluator to an increased risk of violent behavior. Alcohol, sedatives, and minor tranquilizers decrease inhibition and make it more probable that someone will act on his or her thoughts rather than control his or her behavior. (Substance abuse is discussed elsewhere in this chapter.) The importance of immediately getting blood and urine samples for assay in the emergency situation, or unannounced in the more prolonged evaluation of a patient, cannot be overemphasized. The presence of psychosis (in the case of a violent patient, usually paranoid delusional thinking or more disorganized psychosis) should warn the evaluator that threats of violence must be taken seriously and handled accordingly (Table 35–6).

TABLE 35–6. Assessment of violence potential (following increased risk)

How well planned is the threat?

Are means for harming others available?

Is there a history of previous violence or other impulsive behaviors?

If so, what were the precipitants, who were the victims, and how serious were the injuries?

Is there a history of being abused as a child?

Is there alcohol or drug abuse?

Is there psychosis?

TABLE 35–7. Medications for long-term management of violence

Drug	Dosage	Special considerations
Neuroleptics	Doses used for patients with schizophrenia.	Indicated for schizophrenic and other psychotic states. Not for personality disorders or mental retardation. Akathisia may be associated with violence. Depot forms recommended.
Lithium	Doses and blood levels used.	Indicated for violence, especially that accompanying bipolar disorder and mental retardation. Testing for thyroid, renal, and cardiac function.
Anticonvulsants (e.g., carbamazepine, valproate, and clonazepam)	Doses for epilepsy and blood level used.	Indicated for epilepsy and serious episodic violence without electroencephalogram abnormalities. Regular hematological and liver testing.
Propranolol	20 mg three times daily and increase by 60 mg every 4 days. Doses held or cut back if blood pressure below 90/60 mmHg, pulse below 50, or wheezing occurs. Decrease dose gradually.	Contraindications are bronchial asthma, chronic obstructive pulmonary disease, insulin-dependent diabetes, cardiac disease, peripheral vascular disease, renal disease, and hyperthyroidism. Caution with concurrent neuroleptics because propranolol increases blood levels three to four times.

Long-Term Treatment

As with many problems in psychiatry, treatment of violent patients must adhere to the biopsychosocial model. Not all violent patients need medication, but it should be considered in the formulation of the treatment plan. Psychological intervention may be in the form of behavior therapy or psychotherapy. The effect of the patient's violence on various levels of the social order, from the family to society, must be addressed in treatment, as should the role of social factors in causation of the patient's violence.

Long-Term Medication

There is no one drug for treatment of violence because the underlying etiology for violence differs among patients. In the following discussions, I describe drugs that have some proven efficacy in the management of violent behavior, the types of patients in whom these medications have been most effective, the doses and routes of administration, and side effects.

Before medication can be considered, there must be an established baseline for the violence manifested by the patient. A good measure of the frequency, severity, and target of the violent behavior is the Overt Aggression Scale (Yudofsky et al. 1986). Because the build-up, maintenance, and withdrawal phases in the use of medications (particularly propranolol, lithium, and the anticonvulsants) will be long, there must be a quantitative measurement of response (Table 35–7).

Antipsychotics

Antipsychotic medications are used for schizophrenia and mania and in some organic disorders for delusional thinking or control of violence. Antipsychotics are used as long-term medication primarily for patients with schizophrenia. Compliance with medication in such patients is notoriously bad, particularly for patients with paranoid schizophrenia who have manifested violent behavior or made threats of violence (Young et al. 1986). Thus, clinicians should consider using long-acting depot forms of antipsychotic medication. Antipsychotic medication should not be used for violent mentally retarded patients unless there is psychotic symptomatology. Using long-term antipsychotics for these patients raises the risk of side effects (e.g., tardive dyskinesia) and the concern that learning may be impaired in this group of patients for whom learning is already a major problem.

On inpatient units, haloperidol and fluphenazine are popular because they can be administered rapidly in high doses with minimal side effects and without decreasing the seizure threshold in epileptic patients. This latter point is important for patients with schizophrenia and coexisting subictal activity. Equally important as the use of these agents in combating medication noncompliance is the smooth transition from their use in an emergency situation to oral maintenance doses to long-term depot use (Kane 1985).

If the clinician prefers to use an antipsychotic with more sedative side effects or if extrapyramidal side effects are a problem, chlorpromazine or other low-potency antipsychotics are recommended. I do not recommend thioridazine for violent psychotic patients because clinicians also may want to use propranolol for these patients, and as is discussed later, propranolol increases blood levels of thioridazine and the risk of pigmentary retinopathy.

The atypical antipsychotics have been found to be effective for the treatment of violent psychotic patients who do not respond to other antipsychotic medication. Clozapine has been found to be effective in the treatment of psychosis in a third of hospitalized patients with treatment-resistant schizophrenia (Zito et al. 1993). Violent episodes in the hospital decreased significantly over a 6-month period with clozapine treatment (W.H. Wilson and Claussen 1995). In one study, psychotic symptoms were not greatly affected by clozapine but the overall frequency of assaults and self-abuse and of the use of seclusion and restraints were decreased with the use of the drug (Ratey et al. 1993). Clozapine was found to decrease hostility and aggression among patients with schizophrenia (Volavka et al. 1993).

Risperidone has been found effective and safe in the treatment of positive and negative symptoms of schizophrenia (Marder and Meibach 1994). As with clozapine, risperidone decreases hostility separate from its effect on psychosis (Volavka and Meibach 1995). In light of the safer profile of risperidone, it should be considered before clozapine in the treatment of violence. It is hoped that evaluation of other atypical antipsychotics in the treatment of violence will occur in the future.

Benzodiazepines

The use of standard anxiolytic drugs such as diazepam or lorazepam for the control of violence over a long period of time is generally not recommended. This guideline stems from a concern that long-term use of these medications will result in drug abuse, dependency, and tolerance. In addition, these drugs can produce disinhibition and confusion. Buspirone has been shown to be as effective as diazepam and other benzodiazepines in managing anxiety. Buspirone appears to lack the hypnotic effects and abuse potential of other antianxiety agents. It does not appear to interact with other sedating drugs, including alcohol.

There should be clear-cut indications (e.g., anxiety) for the long-term use of anxiolytic agents (Shader and Greenblatt 1993). Indications for long-term use of anxiolytics are distinct from indications for their short-term emergency use, when sedative side effects are sought in the management of violence. I have found clonazepam to be effective in managing episodic violence in patients with intermittent explosive disorder and some personality disorders when there is no serious history of drug abuse. Clonazepam is used to enhance self-control rather than to alleviate anxiety. This drug is used in conjunction with psychotherapy. Low doses in the range of 0.5 mg two or three times daily on a regular basis are often effective. Higher doses may produce disinhibition.

The problems associated with anxiolytic agents and sedatives, particularly in patients with a history of violence and personality disorders, are abuse and dependence. Physical dependence results in a withdrawal reaction if these medications are discontinued rapidly. This withdrawal reaction may involve aggression and violent behavior as well as other symptoms, such as anxiety, irritability, insomnia, tremors, headache, dizziness, anorexia, nausea, vomiting, diarrhea, incoordination, seizures, and depression. The onset of a withdrawal reaction depends on the particular medication and may occur anywhere from 1 day after cessation for a short-acting drug such as lorazepam to up to 1 week after cessation for longer-acting drugs. A gradual reduction of dosage is recommended, namely 5%–10% a day for 10–14 days. A long-acting benzodiazepine may be substituted for shorter-acting benzodiazepines. Patients with a history of seizures, alcohol abuse, or abuse of other drugs should be hospitalized for detoxification.

Carbamazepine and Other Anticonvulsants

A number of case studies and open drug trials have indicated that carbamazepine is probably effective for the management of aggression in several different types of psychiatric patients (Chatham-Showalter 1996; Evans and Gualtieri 1985). In a double-blind, crossover study of 13 chronic psychiatric patients, 10 of whom had schizophrenia, beneficial effects were found in terms of decreased aggressive episodes (Neppe 1983). Although the patients were not epileptic, they did have temporal lobe EEG abnormalities. The patients were treated with antipsychotics, anticholinergics, antidepressants, and benzodiazepines. Luchins (1983) reported on an open carbamazepine trial in seven chronic psychiatric inpatients, six of whom had schizophrenia. None of the patients had EEG abnormalities. He reported that six of the seven patients had fewer aggressive episodes while taking carbamazepine than they did either before or after taking the drug. All of the patients were concurrently treated with antipsychotic drugs. Mattes et al. (1984) found that carbamazepine is effective in decreasing aggression in patients with psychiatric diagnoses other than schizophrenia. These diagnoses include personality disorders, conduct disorders, and some organic disorders. Later uncontrolled studies have confirmed that carbamazepine is effective for violent patients without epilepsy (Mattes 1990; Mattes et al. 1984; Neppe et al. 1991). Evidence has shown that carbamazepine may be effective for managing aggression and irritability in patients with overt seizures, both complex partial and generalized; in schizophrenic patients with and without EEG abnormalities; and in other types of patients with episodic violence but no gross brain damage or mental retardation.

Patients without seizure disorders have benefited from carbamazepine at doses of approximately 600 mg/day. When the therapeutic level (8–12 ng/mL) is reached and a response is obtained, blood levels of carbamazepine should be monitored every month for the first 3 months and then every 3 months thereafter.

Other anticonvulsants have been tried for controlling aggression, with inconsistent results (Brizer 1988). Positive findings have included the use of diphenylhydantoin for the treatment of aggressive mentally retarded children, violent nonepileptic male adults (half of whom had EEG abnormalities), and adults with episodic dyscontrol syndrome (Barratt 1993; Barratt et al. 1991). Valproate has been found to be effective for treating violent patients who cannot be treated with carbamazepine (Brizer 1988).

Propranolol and Other β-blockers

J.M. Silver and Yudofsky (1985) reviewed several control studies, open trials, and case reports on the effectiveness of propranolol in the management of aggressive behavior. Most of the patients studied and responding to propranolol were those with organic brain disease, often with gross impairment secondary to trauma, tumor, alcoholism, encephalitis, Huntington's disease, dementia, Wilson's disease, Korsakoff's psychosis, and mental retardation. In addition, some patients with minimal brain dysfunction or attention deficit also have been reported to respond to propranolol. Nearly all of the patients in these studies were refractory to other medications, including antipsychotics, anxiolytics, anticonvulsants, and lithium. In several cases, concurrent antipsychotic medication was used. β-blockers are effective for violence associated with traumatic brain injury when psychosis is present, because a number of the neurological side effects of antipsychotic drugs may be avoided. On the other hand, propranolol can be used in conjunction with antipsychotic drugs for the management of violence in other types of psychotic disorders.

Before propranolol is given, a thorough medical evaluation of the patient should be performed. Patients with the following diseases should be excluded from treatment with propranolol: bronchial asthma; chronic obstructive pulmonary disease; insulin-dependent diabetes; cardiac diseases, including angina and congestive heart failure; diabetes mellitus; significant peripheral vascular disease; severe renal disease; and hyperthyroidism. Patients with hypertension should be given propranolol with caution because sudden discontinuation of propranolol may result in rebound hypertension.

In other case studies, β-blockers other than propranolol have been used (Ratey et al. 1992; see also Chapter 24). Nadolol is used in the treatment of aggressive patients with chronic paranoid schizophrenia. Pindolol has been reported to be effective in the treatment of aggression in patients with organic brain syndrome. Metoprolol has been reported effective with two patients: one with intermittent explosive disorder related to meningitis and alcohol abuse, and the other with a penetrating brain trauma with temporal lobe epilepsy.

Lithium

Long-term use of lithium helps to prevent manic episodes and associated hyperactive aggressive behavior. In a double-blind trial testing the effectiveness of lithium in the treatment of aggression in adult patients with mental retardation, Craft et al. (1987) found that 73% of patients showed a reduction in aggression during treatment. The use of lithium was the same as that for the management of patients with bipolar disorder. Although reports exist of lithium use in patients with other disorders—including patients with organic brain syndrome or head injury; aggressive schizophrenic patients; nonpsychotic, aggressive prisoners; and delinquents and children with conduct or attention-deficit/hyperactivity disorder (ADHD)—double-blind controlled studies are sparse (Glenn et al. 1989; Luchins and Dojka 1989; Sheard 1975; Sheard et al. 1976; Tupin et al. 1973). Because lithium affects many organ systems in the body, an extensive medical examination is recommended before beginning lithium and during the course of treatment (see Chapter 24).

Psychostimulants

Brizer (1988) reviewed the literature on the use of psychostimulants for the treatment of violent behavior. The use of amphetamines is accepted in controlling aggressive behavior associated with ADHD. Some reports exist of the successful use of amphetamines to control aggression in adults with a history of ADHD as well. In addition, two studies reported the successful use of amphetamines in delinquent youths to control aggression in a group of hospitalized aggressive delinquents (in one study) and to decrease classroom violence for a group of aggressive outpatient boys with antisocial behavior (in the other study). Additional studies are indicated, and clinicians should proceed with caution when prescribing amphetamines because of the great potential for addiction, abuse, and the production of violent behavior through hyperactivity, emotional lability, or delusional thinking as a result of abuse.

Serotonergic Drugs

The development of selective serotonin reuptake inhibitors has opened the door for a clinical test of the theory that serotonin is responsible for impulsive violent behaviors. Earlier, the antidepressant trazodone was found to reduce violence in patients without symptoms of depression (Wilcock 1987). Fluoxetine has been used successfully to treat impulsive, violent patients with personality disorders and patients with chronic schizophrenia (Coccaro et al. 1990; Goldman and Janecek 1990) without depression. With the introduction of sertraline, paroxetine, and other drugs, more research on the use of serotonergic drugs for the treatment of violent patients is anticipated.

Behavior Therapy

Liberman and Wong (1984) described the use of behavioral analysis and therapy in the management of violent behavior. They cautioned that such a program of treatment should be planned and conducted only by clinicians skilled in behavioral analysis and therapy and that there should be standardized policies and review processes to prevent abuse of patients. Programs of behavioral management for patients with violent behavior should definitely not be ad hoc attempts on inadequately staffed and trained general inpatient units.

The target behaviors of the behavioral treatment program must be clearly specified. General terms such as assault or violence are not sufficient; instead, behaviors such as pushing, shoving, hitting, pulling hair, and so forth must be clearly defined. The consequences of such behavior also must be clearly specified; these include a broad spectrum of procedures ranging from a token economy and other means of positive reinforcement and social training skills to more restrictive procedures such as social extinction, sensory extinction, contingent observation, required relaxation, seclusionary time-out, and contingent restraint. Usually, positive reinforcement is tried first, and more restrictive procedures are used as necessary. However, severe, violent behavioral problems usually necessitate use of the more restrictive procedures earlier in the treatment plan.

Positive reinforcement may occur as frequently as every 10–20 seconds in seriously aggressive patients in the manner of giving food and attention to reward and reinforce nonassaultive and nondestructive behavior. This approach is termed *differential reinforcement of other behavior*, and the frequency of reinforcement is gradually spaced out over longer intervals as the patient becomes more cooperative. For less severe violent behavior and more cooperative patients, a token economy program is used to motivate patients toward prosocial behavior. Tokens serving as currency are given for nonviolent and prosocial behavior. These tokens are exchanged for cigarettes, snacks, privileges, and other luxuries.

As noted earlier in this chapter, violent behavior may be the result of an inability to communicate and a lack of other social skills. In social skills training, patients are taught how to satisfy their needs through appropriate behavior rather than violent behavior. Training involves instruction describing a rationale for the behavior desired, demonstration of the desired behavior, rehearsal of the behavior, and reinforcement for performing the behavior. Social extinction is the withdrawal of attention from the patient when the patient manifests some undesirable behavior, such as violence. Obviously, the violent behavior cannot be dangerous, and all members of the treatment team must be consistent in ignoring it. Sensory extinction is used for predominantly self-mutilative or injurious behavior, for example, in patients who bang their heads or scratch their faces. In such patients, helmets and foam-padded gloves are used to protect the patient as well as decrease the sensory consequences of such behavior. Contingent observation is the removal of a patient from an activity for a short period of time following an episode of violence or other inappropriate behavior. This approach is usually taken for minor disruptive behavior such as verbal aggression. It involves placing the patient near the ongoing activity, for example, in a chair for a few minutes while watching the appropriate behavior of other patients.

A more restrictive procedure, required relaxation, involves physically placing a patient in a supine position and restraining the patient's arms, legs, and body, if necessary, while the patient is assisted in relaxation. This process lasts for about 10 minutes. Seclusionary time-out or time-out–form reinforcement involves placing the patient in an area isolated from other patients. In distinction to seclusion used in the emergency situation, seclusionary time-out is often brief, usually 5 minutes and rarely longer than 1 hour. Contingent restraint is also more restrictive in that it involves immobilizing part or all of the patient's body by restraints, such as cuffs and belts, a Posey jacket, or other ties or by a therapist physically holding a patient for a brief period of time after an episode of violent behavior. These seclusionary and restraint-like procedures, in addition to being shorter in duration than the seclusion and restraint used in the emergency situation, need not involve a physician each time they are used because they are part of an ongoing planned treatment program.

Long-Term Outpatient Psychotherapy

The frequency of violence among patients in outpatient treatment settings is less than that for patients admitted to inpatient units. For example, approximately 3% of patients seen in clinics in the New York City area had a history of recent violence toward others. Patients who are violent in outpatient settings are more likely to be those with personality disorders, child or adolescent disorders, or mental retardation. Again, male patients are more likely to be violent than are female patients, and violence is greater among the younger patients. The spouse, mate, or other family members are the targets of violence in more than half of the cases (Tardiff and Koenigsberg 1985).

Although psychotherapy of the violent patient may be on an individual basis, therapists often involve the spouse or family in treatment. This approach is advisable because of the role of the family in the dynamics of violence. Such an approach is intended not to blame the victim(s) but to analyze interactions that lead to violence. In addition, it is important to get information from persons other than the patient to make certain that problems with violence are not minimized by the patient. Finally, even if violence does not appear to be related to the spouse or family, underlying dynamics may be. For example, a young man assaulted an unknown woman. With further analysis of the man's marriage and conflict with his wife, it was apparent that this was a displacement of violence from his wife to the unknown woman.

Some therapists prefer group therapy for violent patients because it is less threatening to the patient than a one-to-one relationship and allows the patient to appreciate that other people have problems with violence. The group is often supportive, yet at the same time the group can confront a patient rather than have the therapist do so. Usually, groups are led by two therapists, which makes it less stressful for each leader.

Lion and Tardiff (1987) reviewed the principles of using psychotherapy for problems with aggression:

1. The motivation of the patient and the patient's reason for psychotherapy must be evaluated. An inappropriate reason to enter psychotherapy is an attempt to impress the court before a trial for some violent crime. A more appropriate reason is because the patient's marriage, job, or another aspect of his or her life is being jeopardized by the violent behavior and/or because the patient feels guilty about his or her behavior.

2. The patient must develop a sense of self-control of emotions and behavior. At first, the patient relies on the strength and self-control of the therapist. The therapist may give the patient his or her telephone number or the telephone number of the emergency department to call if the patient fears impending violence. The therapist and the patient must be aware that, after this honeymoon period in psychotherapy, subsequent violent episodes will occur, and they must be prepared to analyze such episodes without feelings of disappointment. The nature of the transference must be constantly analyzed. Particularly for borderline and psychotic patients, the therapist must look for signs of negative transference that may pose a danger to the therapist. As has been discussed earlier in this chapter, countertransference and negative feelings toward patients are particularly common problems in the treatment of violent patients because violence provokes strong emotions in the therapist that may activate past experience as well as a number of mechanisms of defense. Thus, it is important that the therapist know his or her feelings and not allow them to interfere with treatment.

3. Verbal communication should be facilitated. The patient should be encouraged to talk rather than act when expressing concerns and weaknesses, without fear of the retaliation or humiliation that often occurred when such concerns were shared in the past with spouse, family, or friends.

4. The patient should develop an understanding of the consequences of violent behavior. For example, the patient should be encouraged to fantasize about what it would be like to be in jail or what it would be like to be divorced if spouse abuse continues.

5. The patient should gain insight about the dynamics of violence and early warning signs—for example, flushing of the face, rapid heartbeat, sweating, and a feeling of tension. The patient should be encouraged to

avoid a violent situation at first by taking a walk or by calling the therapist and eventually to develop insight in dealing with a potentially violent situation psychologically.

Special Concerns in the Treatment of Violent Patients

Danger to the Therapist

The first concern when treating violent patients is danger to the therapist. Any threat, even if made in a joking manner, must be taken seriously and evaluated. The therapist should acknowledge to the patient that these threats are frightening, and together they must identify and address the problem if treatment is to continue.

There should be some way for the therapist to communicate to others that he or she is in trouble inside the office or, conversely, for a receptionist to warn the therapist of a potential problem with violence before the patient enters the office (e.g., if a patient is agitated or appears to have been drinking). This warning can be issued through an electrical device such as a buzzer or in other ways such as using code words or prearranged signals to communicate trouble. Even in outpatient settings where few violent patients are seen, a plan of response should be in place for violent situations, including those involving hostage taking. This plan should be written and rehearsed by all involved. In addition, in emergency departments, patients should be searched for weapons. Offices should not contain heavy objects such as ashtrays and should contain pillows or a light chair that may be used as a shield in the event of violence, particularly if the patient has a knife or weapon other than a gun. If a patient appears in the waiting room with a gun and it is possible for the psychiatrist to escape, he or she should do so. If a patient produces a gun in the office and escape is impossible, the therapist should remain outwardly calm and should comply with any requests in the early phase of this emergency. Eventually, the therapist should ask the patient to put the gun on the desk or table rather than reach for the gun or ask the patient to drop the gun, both of which may result in the gun discharging.

Concern for the safety of staff includes injuries caused by patients, particularly on inpatient units or in the emergency room. Thackrey (1987) described and illustrated several physical techniques for self-protection. He included techniques that are effective and safe for the therapist as well as for the patient and that require a minimum amount of training and practice for proficiency. It should be emphasized that reading about these techniques should not replace specific guidelines for, and rehearsal of, physical techniques within each institution.

Thackrey (1987) described one nonthreatening, protective posture that is essentially a sideward stance that minimizes the amount of body area susceptible to violent attack and that is less threatening to a potentially violent patient. The therapist must anticipate a punch, kick, or other form of attack and either escape out of reach of the patient or, conversely, approach the patient so closely that an effective punch or kick is not possible. Thackrey illustrated various ways of deflecting a punch or kick using the arms or legs, and he described various means of escaping from holds. For example, if a patient grabs at the therapist's wrist, the therapist bends the arm at the elbow for added strength and swiftly turns the arm against the patient's thumb, which causes the patient to release. If the patient grabs the therapist's hair, the therapist should establish control on the patient's grabbing hand to minimize further damage and then move the patient's hand into a mechanically inferior position. To escape from a choke-hold the key aspect of survival is to tuck the chin downward, thus protecting critical air and blood circulation structures and making it more difficult for the patient to get a solid grip around the neck. Protection of these structures is essential to avoid losing consciousness and to gain time in terms of release from a choke-hold. Escape from biting, such as of an extremity, is effected by pushing the bitten part deeper into the patient's mouth and closing the patient's nostrils, thus forcing the patient to take a gasp of air and giving the clinician a chance to escape.

Duty to Protect Potential Victims

Another concern is danger to others and the responsibility of the clinician to protect intended victims of violent patients. Mills et al. (1987) reviewed court decisions and legislation in the decade following the *Tarasoff* decision in California. The details and ramifications of this case are discussed in Chapter 39 of this textbook, but a few words about the clinical aspects of the duty to protect are relevant here. A central issue is a balance between the confidentiality and privileged information given to the physician and the duty to protect the community. This balance of responsibility has long been rooted in medical practice. Mills et al. (1987) pointed out that the duty to protect need not involve warning the intended victim or the police but instead should involve change of treatment standards, including civil commitments. A shift of burden of decision making to the courts may be sufficient. The authors argue that a standard of liability for a professional requires that there not be a substantial departure from clinical standards of decision making.

Appelbaum (1985) developed a model for meeting the requirements imposed by the *Tarasoff* doctrine. He recommended viewing the fulfillment of the duty to protect in three stages. First, an assessment of the potential for harm must be made. The therapist must gather and use data relevant to the evaluation of dangerousness. Appelbaum indicated that in many *Tarasoff*-like cases, therapists have been faulted not for inaccurate predictions but for failing to gather data and document how the decision concerning homicide or danger potential was made. The basic model recommended earlier in this chapter in the discussion of short-term evaluation of violence potential could serve in Appelbaum's model. Analogous to assessment of suicide risk, the determination of dangerousness in the immediate future would be made for the next few days or week at most. Reasons for risk of immediate dangerousness should be documented on the patient's record for the specified period of time and reevaluated when the patient is next seen.

The second stage in Appelbaum's model is the formulation of a course of action to protect the intended victim. This course of action may involve changing or increasing the patient's medication, hospitalizing the patient, increasing security on the inpatient unit, or warning the intended victim or the police.

The third stage of this model is directly warning the intended victim. Mills (1984) pointed out the problems in determining which steps in warning an intended victim are reasonable and under what circumstances. Beyond issues of confidentiality and the effect on the therapy of the patient if the victim is warned, there are questions about how to warn a victim (i.e., should the therapist visit, telephone, or send a letter to the intended victim?). Issues about possibly causing needless distress for the intended victim and what actions the victim or police really can take to prevent violence must be considered.

Beck (1985) noted, based on a review of cases (especially those outside of California), that the duty to protect or warn exists only if there is evidence that the patient poses a serious threat to do bodily harm to a specific person. If careful assessment—documented in writing—fails to reveal such evidence, there is no liability for the therapist. In fact, even if *Tarasoff*-like laws do not exist, such documentation should be done as part of professional clinical care.

Conclusions

Violence is a frequent and serious problem in institutions. The causes of violence involve a balance of factors within the patient, usually nonspecific, and factors surrounding the patient. There is never one cause and never one treatment; instead, a balance of biological, social, and psychological factors is responsible for a violent act. Treatment of the violent patient on inpatient units should first address prevention in terms of adequately trained staff who are aware of their feelings and the psychodynamics operating in themselves as well as in the patients. The environment should be therapeutic and uncrowded, with a balance of humanistic caring and a sense of social order. The opportunity for patients to talk to, or at least be with, staff is important. Verbal contact with potentially violent patients should be done in a calm, nonprovocative manner. If a violent episode occurs, there should be an instant differential diagnosis and classification of the patient's condition into one of three categories: organic mental disorders; functional psychotic disorders; or nonpsychotic, nonorganic disorders. The last category is the most amenable to verbal intervention.

If physical controls are used, the decision to use involuntary medication, seclusion, or restraint should be based on the needs of the individual patient and the situation and not on a legal hierarchy of restrictiveness. Seclusion and restraint should be used in keeping with accepted professional guidelines, most notably those of the American Psychiatric Association (Tardiff 1984). If common sense and good professional judgment are used, the therapist is protected under the law for injury to the patient during seclusion or restraint and the number of injuries would be expected to diminish.

When using medication to manage violent patients, rapid neuroleptization is effective for a large proportion of patients in emergency situations, with certain caveats for patients with organic mental disorders with unknown etiology and those with intoxication or withdrawal from alcohol or sedative drugs. For long-term treatment of the violent patient, no single medication is specified, but medication is targeted to the underlying disorder.

Behavioral treatment is effective for the management of violent behaviors in certain types of patients; however, such treatment should be planned by clinicians experienced with behavioral analysis and therapies and implemented by a large number of experienced staff.

There are definite principles and goals of outpatient psychotherapy for the violent patient and his or her family. Issues of transference and countertransference must be monitored and attended to actively.

Two overriding concerns in the treatment of violent patients are fear for the safety of the self and for the safety of others. The treatment of violent patients need not be perilous as long as certain safeguards are kept in mind. The responsibility to protect intended victims of violence should include assessment of a patient's violence potential. This assessment should be documented clearly in the patient's records and reevaluated at the next visit. If the patient is found to pose a substantial threat to others, then in most states the clinician has the duty to protect, although not necessarily warn, intended victims.

Future Directions in Research

Future research should use clear phenomenological definitions of violence—that is, specific behaviors rather than subjective definitions of violence such as "verbal aggression." Research on the biology of violence should include finding more sensitive measures of neurophysiological and biochemical dysfunction of the brain and using technology such as nuclear magnetic resonance imaging, positron emission tomography, single photon emission computed tomography, regional cerebral blood flow, and brain electrical mapping. In addition, studies should be using new techniques for the study of neurotransmitters such as digital subtraction autoradiography for brain dopamine and serotonin receptors (Altar et al. 1985). Drugs that increase serotonin levels should be studied in terms of their effects on violent, and particularly impulsive, behavior. Epidemiological studies should use more sophisticated techniques and data systems concerning crime and violence with the goal of accurate reporting of domestic violence and child abuse and linkage of homicides to detect serial murderers. There should be prospective studies so as to develop a better ability to predict violence in the near and distant future.

Although beyond the scope of psychiatry alone, intervention programs aimed at decreasing child and spouse abuse, relieving poverty and unemployment, and decreasing drug and alcohol use will decrease the incidence of violence in our society. Such efforts must be supported by all citizens of our society.

References

Agnew R: Foundations for a general theory of strain. Criminology 30:47–87, 1992

Agnew R: A general strain theory of community differences in crime rates. Journal of Research in Crime and Delinquency 36:123–155, 1999

Altar CA, O'Neil SO, Walter RJ, et al: Brain dopamine and serotonin receptor sites revealed by digital subtraction autoradiography. Science 228:597–600, 1985

American Psychiatric Association: Report of the American Psychiatric Association Task Force on the Psychiatric Uses of Seclusion and Restraint. Washington, DC, American Psychiatric Association, 1984

American Psychiatric Association: Clinician Safety: Report of the American Psychiatric Association Task Force on Clinician Safety. Washington, DC, American Psychiatric Association, 1993

American Psychiatric Association: Diagnostic and Statistical Manual of Mental Disorders, 4th Edition. Washington, DC, American Psychiatric Association, 1994

Anderson AC: Environmental factors and aggressive behavior. J Clin Psychiatry 43:280–283, 1982

Anderson KE, Silver JM: Neurological and medical diseases and violence, in Medical Management of the Violent Patient. Edited by Tardiff K, New York, Marcel Dekker, 1999, pp 87–124

Appelbaum PS: Tarasoff and the clinician: problems in fulfilling the duty to protect. Am J Psychiatry 142:425–429, 1985

Appelbaum PS, Robbins PC, Monahan J, et al: Violence and delusions: data from the MacArthur Violence Risk Assessment Study. Am J Psychiatry 157:566–572, 2000

Apter A, Kotler M, Sevy S, et al: Correlates of risk of suicide in violent and nonviolent psychiatric patients. Am J Psychiatry 148:883–887, 1991

Arango C, Calcedo B, Alfredo G, et al: Violence in patients with schizophrenia: a prospective study. Schizophr Bull 25:493–503, 1999

Barratt ES: The use of anticonvulsants in aggression and violence. Psychopharmacol Bull 29:75–81, 1993

Barratt ES, Kent TA, Bryant SG, et al: A controlled trial of phenytoin in impulsive aggression. J Clin Psychopharmacol 11:388–389, 1991

Beck JC (ed): The Potentially Violent Patient and the Tarasoff Decision in Psychiatric Practice. Washington, DC, American Psychiatric Press, 1985

Belfrage H, Lidberg L, Oreland L: Platelet monoamine oxidase activity in mentally disordered violent offenders. Acta Psychiatr Scand 85:218–221, 1992

Bell PA, Baron RA: Ambient temperature and human violence, in Multidisciplinary Approaches to Aggression Research. Edited by Brain PF, Benton D. Amsterdam, The Netherlands, Elsevier/North Holland Biomedical, 1981, pp 76–88

Benjamin L: Interpersonal Treatment of Personality Disorders. New York, Guilford, 1993

Benjaminsen S, Botzsche-Laren K, Norrie L, et al: Patient violence in a psychiatric hospital in Denmark: rate of violence and relation to diagnosis. Nord J Psychiatry 50:233–242, 1996

Binder RL: Are the mentally ill dangerous? J Am Acad Psychiatry Law 27:189–201, 1999

Binder RL, McNiel DE: Contemporary practices in managing acutely violent patients in 20 emergency rooms. Psychiatr Serv 50:1553–1554, 1999

Blau JR, Blau PM: The cost of inequality: metropolitan structure and violent crime. Am Sociol Rev 47:114–129, 1982

Blow FC, Barry KL, Copeland LA, et al: Repeated assaults by patients in VA hospital and clinic settings. Psychiatr Serv 50:390–394, 1999

Bogdanovic MD, Mead SH, Duncan JS: Aggressive behaviour at a residential epilepsy centre. Seizure 9:58–64, 2000

Bohman M, Cloninger CR, Sigvardsson S, et al: Predisposition to petty criminality in Swedish adoptees, I: genetic and environmental heterogeneity. Arch Gen Psychiatry 39:1233–1241, 1982

Brasic JR, Fogelman D: Clinician safety. Psychiatr Clin North Am 22:923–940, 1999

Braverman ER, Pfeiffer CC: Suicide and biochemistry. Biol Psychiatry 20:123–124, 1985

Brennan PA, Mednick SA, Hodgins S: Major mental disorders and criminal violence in a Danish birth cohort. Arch Gen Psychiatry 57:494–500, 2000

Brizer DA: Psychopharmacology and the management of violent patients. Psychiatr Clin North Am 11:551–568, 1988

Brown GL, Ebert MH, Goyer PF, et al: Aggression, suicide, and serotonin: relationships to CSF amine metabolites. Am J Psychiatry 139:741–746, 1982

Carey G: Family and genetic epidemiology of aggressive and antisocial behavior, in Aggression and Violence: Genetic, Neurobiological, and Biosocial Perspectives. Edited by Stoff M, Cairns RD. Hillsdale, NJ, Erlbaum, 1996, pp 2–22

Centerwall BS: Race, socioeconomic status and domestic homicide: Atlanta, 1971–1972. Am J Public Health 74:813–815, 1984

Centerwall BS: Television and violence: the scale of the problem and where to go from here. JAMA 267:3059–3063, 1992

Chatham-Showalter PE: Carbamazepine for combativeness in acute traumatic brain injury. J Neuropsychiatry Clin Neurosci 8:96–99, 1996

Coccaro EF: Impulsive aggression and central serotonergic system function in humans: an example of a dimensional brain-behavior relationship. Int Clin Psychopharmacol 7:3–12, 1992

Coccaro EF, Siever LJ, Klar HM, et al: Serotonergic studies in patients with affective and personality disorders: correlates with suicidal and impulsive aggressive behavior. Arch Gen Psychiatry 46:587–599, 1989

Coccaro EF, Astill JL, Herbert JL, et al: Fluoxetine treatment of impulsive aggression in DSM-III-R personality disorder patients. J Clin Psychopharmacol 10:373–375, 1990

Coker AL, Smith PH, McKeown RE, et al: Frequency and correlates of intimate partner violence by type: physical, sexual and psychological battering. Am J Public Health 90:553–559, 2000

Cook PJ: The role of firearms in violent crime: an interpretive review of the literature, in Criminal Violence. Edited by Wolfgang ME, Weiner NA. Beverly Hills, CA, Sage, 1982, pp 236–291

Coverdale J, Gale C, Weeks S, et al: A survey of threats and violent acts by patients against training physicians. Med Educ 35:154–159, 2001

Craft M, Ismail IA, Krishnamurti D, et al: Lithium in the treatment of aggression in mentally handicapped patients: a double-blind trial. Br J Psychiatry 150:685–689, 1987

Dalton K: Cyclical criminal acts in premenstrual syndrome. Lancet 2:1070–1071, 1980

Davidson RJ, Putnam KM, Larson CL: Dysfunction in the neural circuitry of emotion regulation: a possible prelude to violence. Science 289:591–594, 2000

Davis S: Violence by psychiatric inpatients: a review. Hosp Community Psychiatry 42:585–590, 1991

De Jong J, Virkkunen M, Linnoila M: Factors associated with recidivism in a criminal population. J Nerv Ment Dis 180:543–550, 1992

Delgado-Escueta AV, Mattson RH, King L, et al: The nature of aggression during epileptic seizures. N Engl J Med 305:711–716, 1981

Denison MI, Paredes A, Booth JB: Alcohol and cocaine interactions and aggressive behviors. Recent Dev Alcohol 13:283–291, 1997

Devinsky O: Interictal aggression in epilepsy: The Buss-Durkee Hostility Inventory. Epilepsia 35:585, 1994

Di Lalla LF, Gottesman I: Biological and genetic contributors to violence: Widom's untold tale. Psychol Bull 109:125–129, 1991

Dodge A, Lochman JE, Harnish JD, et al: Reactive and proactive aggression in school children and psychiatrically impaired chronically assaultive youth. J Abnorm Psychol 106:37–51, 1997

Dubin WR, Weiss KJ, Dorn JM: Pharmacotherapy of psychiatric emergencies. J Clin Psychopharmacol 6:210–222, 1986

Eichelman BS: Toward a rational pharmacotherapy for aggressive and violent behavior. Hosp Community Psychiatry 39:31–39, 1986

Eichelman BS: Aggressive behavior: from laboratory to clinic: quo vadit? Arch Gen Psychiatry 49:488–492, 1992

Eichelman BS, Hartwig AC (eds): Patient Violence and the Clinician. Washington, DC, American Psychiatric Press, 1995

Elliot FA: Violence: the neurologic contribution. Arch Neurol 49:595–603, 1992

Eronen M, Hakola P, Tihonen J: Mental disorders and homicidal behavior in Finland. Arch Gen Psychiatry 53:497–501, 1996

Evans RW, Gualtieri CT: Carbamazepine: a neuropsychological and psychiatric profile. Clin Neuropharmacol 8:221–241, 1985

Federman J (ed): National Television Violence Study, Vol 2. Santa Barbara, CA, University of California, 1997

Fishbein DH, Lozovsky D, Jaffe JH: Impulsivity, aggression, and neuroendocrine responses to serotonergic stimulation in substance abusers. Biol Psychiatry 25:1049–1066, 1989

Freedman JL: Effects of television violence on aggressiveness. Psychol Bull 96:227–246, 1984

Giannini AJ, Miller NS, Lioselle RH, et al: Cocaine-associated violence and relationship to route of administration. J Subst Abuse Treat 10:67–75, 1993

Glenn MB, Wroblewski B, Parziale J, et al: Lithium carbonate for aggressive behavior or affective instability in ten brain-injured patients. Am J Phys Med Rehabil 68:221–226, 1989

Goldman MB, Janecek HM: Adjunctive fluoxetine improves global function in chronic schizophrenia. J Neuropsychiatry Clin Neurosci 2:429–431, 1990

Health Care Finance Administration: Hospital Interpretive Guidelines. Washington, DC, Health Care Finance Administration, 1999

Hermann BP, Whitman S: Behavioral and personality correlates of epilepsy: a review, methodological critique and conceptual model. Psychol Bull 95:451–497, 1984

Horowitz AV: The Logic of Social Control. New York, Plenum, 1990

Jaffe P, Wolfe D, Wilson SK, et al: Family violence and child adjustment: a comparative analysis of girls' and boys' behavioral symptoms. Am J Psychiatry 143:74–77, 1986

Johnson JG, Cohen P, Smailes E, et al: Adolescent personality disorders associated with violence and criminal behavior during adolescence and early adulthood. Am J Psychiatry 157:1406–1412, 2000

Kane JM: Compliance issues in outpatient treatment. J Clin Psychopharmacol 5(suppl):22S–27S, 1985

Kempe CH, Helfer RE (eds): The Battered Child, 3rd Edition, Revised and Expanded. Chicago, IL, University of Chicago Press, 1980

Kutzer DJ: Psychobiological factors in violent Behavior, in Violent Behavior, Vol I: Assessment and Intervention. Edited by Ostrum GF, Gurvits TV, Huhne AA. New York, PMA, 1990

Liberman RP, Wong SE: Behavior analysis and therapy procedures related to seclusion and restraint, in The Psychiatric Uses of Seclusion and Restraint. Edited by Tardiff K. Washington, DC, American Psychiatric Press, 1984, pp 35–67

Lidberg L, Tuck JR, Åsberg M, et al: Homicide, suicide and CSF 5-HIAA. Acta Psychiatr Scand 71:230–236, 1985

Lidberg L, Belfrage H; Bertilsson L, et al: Suicide attempts and impulse control disorder are related to low cerebrospinal fluid 5-HHIA in mentally disordered violent offenders. Acta Psychiatr Scand 101:L395–L401, 2000

Lindqvist P, Allebeck P: Schizophrenia and crime: a longitudinal follow-up of 644 schizophrenics in Stockholm. Br J Psychiatry 157:345–350, 1990

Link BG, Andrews H, Cullen JT: The violent and illegal behavior of mental patients reconsidered. Am Sociol Rev 57:275–292, 1992

Lion JR, Pasternak SA: Countertransference reactions to violent patients. Am J Psychiatry 130:207–210, 1973

Lion JR, Tardiff K: The long-term treatment of the violent patient, in Psychiatry Update: American Psychiatric Association Annual Review, Vol 6. Edited by Hales RE, Frances AJ. Washington, DC, American Psychiatric Press, 1987, pp 537–548

Luchins DJ: Carbamazepine in violent nonepileptic schizophrenics. Psychopharmacol Bull 20:569–571, 1983

Luchins DJ, Dojka D: Lithium and propranolol in aggression and self-injurious behavior in the mentally retarded. Psychopharmacol Bull 25:372–375, 1989

Marder SR, Meibach RC: Risperidone in the treatment of schizophrenia. Am J Psychiatry 151:825–835, 1994

Mark VH, Ervin FR: Violence and the Brain. New York, Harper & Row, 1970

Mattes JA: Comparative effectiveness of carbamazepine and propranolol for rage outbursts. J Neuropsychiatry Clin Neurosci 2:159–164, 1990

Mattes JA, Rosenberg J, Mays D: Carbamazepine versus propranolol in patients with rage outbursts: a random assignment study. Psychopharmacol Bull 20:98–100, 1984

McCormick RA, Smith M: Aggression and hostility in substance abuser: the relationship to abuse patterns, coping style and relapse triggers. Addict Behav 20: 555–601, 1995

McNiel DE, Eisner JU, Binder RL: The relationship between command hallucinations and violence Psychiatr Serv 51:1288–1292, 2000

Mendez MF, Doss RC, Taylor JL: Interictal violence in epilepsy: relationship to behavior and seizure variables. J Nerv Ment Dis 181:566–573, 2000

Messner S, Rosenfeld R: Social structure and homicide: theory and research, in Homicide: A Sourcebook of Social Research. Edited by Smith MD, Zahn MA. Thousand Oaks, CA, Sage, 1999

Messner S, Tardiff K: The social ecology of urban homicide: an application of the routine activities approach. Criminology 23:241–267, 1985

Messner S, Tardiff K: Economic inequality and levels of homicide: an analysis of urban neighborhoods. Criminology 24:297–317, 1986

Miller RJ, Zadolinnyj K, Hafner RJ, et al: Profiles and predictors of assaultiveness for different psychiatric ward populations. Am J Psychiatry 150:1368–1373, 1993

Mills MJ: The so-called duty to warn: the psychotherapeutic duty to protect third parties from patients' violent acts. Behav Sci Law 2:237–257, 1984

Mills MJ, Sullivan G, Eth S: Protecting third parties: a decade after Tarasoff. Am J Psychiatry 144:68–74, 1987

Monroe RR: Episodic Behavioral Disorders. Cambridge, MA, Harvard University Press, 1970

Monroe RR: Episodic behavioral disorders and limbic ictus. Compr Psychiatry 26:466–479, 1985

Morenoff JD, Sampson RJ, Raudenbush SW: Neighborhood inequality, collective efficacy, and the spatial dynamics of violence. Criminology 39:517–555, 2001

National Institute on Drug Abuse: Facts about Ecstasy, NIDA Notes, Vol 14, No 4. Rockville, MD, National Institute on Drug Abuse, 1999

National Institute of Mental Health: Television and behavior: ten years of scientific progress and implications for the eighties, Vol 1: summary report (DHHS Publ No ADM 82-1195). Rockville, MD, National Institute of Mental Health, 1982

Neppe VM: Carbamazepine as adjunctive treatment in nonepileptic chronic inpatients with EEG temporal lobe abnormalities. J Clin Psychiatry 44:326–331, 1983

Neppe VM, Bourman BR, Lawchuck KS: Carbamazepine for atypical psychosis with episodic hostility. J Nerv Ment Dis 179:439–441, 1991

Palmstierna T, Huitfeldt B, Wistedt B: The relationship of crowding and aggressive behavior on a psychiatric intensive care unit. Hosp Community Psychiatry 42:1237–1240, 1991

Pelcovitz D, Kaplan S: Child witnesses of violence between parents: psychological correlates and implications for treatment. Child Adolesc Psychiatr Clin North Am 3:745–758, 1994

Phillips RTM: Violence in America: Social and Environmental Factors in Medical Management of the Violent Patient. Edited by Tardiff K. New York, Marcel Dekker, 1999

Pope HG, Katz DL: Homicide and near-homicide by anabolic steroid users. J Clin Psychiatry 51:28, 1990

Rada RT, Kellner R, Stivastava C, et al: Plasma androgens in violent and nonviolent sex offenders. Bull Am Acad Psychiatry Law 11:149–158, 1983

Rao N, Jellinek HM, Woolston DC: Agitation in closed head injury: haloperidol effects on rehabilitation outcome. Arch Phys Med Rehabil 66:30–44, 1985

Ratey JJ, Sorgi P, O'Driscoll GA, et al: Nadolol to treat aggression and psychiatric symptomatology in chronic psychiatric inpatients: a double-blind, placebo-controlled study. J Clin Psychiatry 53:41–46, 1992

Ratey JJ, Leveroni C, Kilmer D, et al: The effects of clozapine on severely aggressive psychiatric inpatients in a state hospital. J Clin Psychiatry 54:219–223, 1993

Reid RL, Yen SC: Premenstrual syndrome. Am J Obstet Gynecol 139:85–104, 1981

Saltzman LE, Mercy JA, O'Carroll PW, et al: Weapon involvement and injury outcomes in family and intimates assaults. JAMA 267:3043–3047, 1992

Sampson RJ: Structural density and criminal victimization. Criminology 21:276–293, 1983

Sampson RJ, Raudenbush SW, Earls F: Neighborhoods and violent crime: a multilevel study of collective efficacy. Science 277:918–924, 1997

Schiavi RC, Theilgaard A, Owen DR, et al: Sex chromosome anomalies, hormones, and aggressivity. Arch Gen Psychiatry 41:93–99, 1984

Shader RI, Greenblatt DJ: Drug therapy: use of benzodiazepines in anxiety disorders. N Engl J Med 328:1398–1405, 1993

Sheard MH: Lithium in the treatment of aggression. J Nerv Ment Dis 160:108–118, 1975

Sheard MH, Marini JL, Bridges CI, et al: The effect of lithium in impulsive aggressive behavior in man. Am J Psychiatry 133:1409–1413, 1976

Silver E: Race, neighborhood disadvantage and violence among persons with mental disorders: the importance of contextual measurement. Law Hum Behav 24:449–456, 2000

Silver JM, Yudofsky S: Propranolol for aggression: literature review and clinical guidelines. International Drug Therapy Newsletter 20:9–12, 1985

Steinert T, Sippach T, Gebhardt RP: How common is violence in schizophrenia despite neuroleptic treatment? Pharmacopsychiatry 33:98–102, 2000

Stone MH: The Fate of the Borderline Patient: Successful Outcome in Psychiatric Practice, New York, Guilford, 1990

Swanson JW, Holzer CE, Ganju VK, et al: Violence and psychiatric disorder in the community: evidence from the Epidemiologic Catchment Area surveys. Hosp Community Psychiatry 41:761–770, 1990

Tardiff K: A survey of assault by chronic patients in a state hospital system, in Assaults Within Psychiatric Facilities. Edited by Lion JR, Reid WH. New York, Grune and Stratton, 1983, pp 3–19

Tardiff K (ed): The Psychiatric Uses of Seclusion and Restraint. Washington, DC, American Psychiatric Press, 1984

Tardiff K: A model for the short-term prediction of violence potential, in Current Approaches to the Prediction of Violence. Edited by Brizer DA, Crowner ML. Washington, DC, American Psychiatric Press, 1989, pp 1–12

Tardiff K: The current state of psychiatry in the treatment of violent patients. Arch Gen Psychiatry 49:493–499, 1992

Tardiff K: Concise Guide to Assessment and Management of Violent Patients, 2nd Edition. Washington, DC, American Psychiatric Press, 1996

Tardiff K: Unusual diagnoses among violent patients. Psychiatr Clin North Am 21:567–579, 1998

Tardiff K (ed): Medical Management of the Violent Patient, New York, Marcel Dekker, 1999a

Tardiff K: Prediction of Violence in Medical Management of the Violent Patient, New York, Marcel Dekker, 1999b, pp 201–217

Tardiff K, Koenigsberg HW: Assaultive behavior among psychiatric outpatients. Am J Psychiatry 142:960–963, 1985

Tardiff K, Marzuk PM, Leon AJ, et al: Homicide in New York City: cocaine use and firearms. JAMA 272:43–46, 1994

Tardiff K, Marzuk PM, Leon AJ, et al: Violence by patients admitted to a private psychiatric hospital. Am J Psychiatry 154:88–93, 1997a

Tardiff K, Marzuk PM, Leon AJ, et al: Violence by psychiatric patients after discharge from hospital: a prospective study. Psychiatr Serv 48:678–681, 1997b

Tellegen A, Lykken DT, Bouchard TJ, et al: Personality similarity in twins reared apart and together. J Pers Soc Psychol 54:1031–1039, 1988

Thackrey M: Therapeutics for Aggression: Psychological/Physical Crisis Intervention. New York, Human Sciences Press, 1987

Tonkonogy JM: Violence and temporal lobe lesion: head CT and MRI data. J Neuropsychiatry Clin Neurosci 3:189–196, 1991

Tupin JP, Smith DB, Clanon TL, et al: The long-term use of lithium in aggressive prisoners. Compr Psychiatry 14:311–317, 1973

U.S. General Accounting Office: Many deaths and injuries caused by firearms could be prevented (Publ No GAO/PEMD-91-9). Washington, DC, U.S. Government Printing Office, 1991

Virkkunen M: Reactive hypoglycemia tendency among habitually violent offenders: a further study by means of the glucose tolerance test. Neuropsychobiology 8:35–40, 1982

Virkkunen M, De Jong J, Bartko J, et al: Psychobiological concomitants of history of suicide attempts among violent offenders and impulsive fire setters. Arch Gen Psychiatry 46:604–606, 1989

Volavka J, Meibach RC: Effect of risperidone on hostility in schizophrenia. J Clin Psychopharmacol 15:243–249, 1995

Volavka J, Zito JM, Vitrai J, et al: Clozapine effects on hostility and aggression in schizophrenia. J Clin Psychopharmacol 13:287–288, 1993

Weiger B, Bear D: An approach to the neurology of aggression. J Psychiatr Res 22:85–89, 1988

Widom CS: The cycle of violence. Science 244:160–171, 1989a

Widom CS: Does violence beget violence? A critical examination of the literature. Psychol Bull 106:3–25, 1989b

Wilcock G: Trazodone for aggressive behavior. Lancet 1:929–930, 1987

Williams K: Economic sources of homicide: reestimating the effects of poverty and inequality. Am Sociol Rev 49:283–289, 1984

Wilson WH, Claussen AM: 18-Month outcome of clozapine treatment for 100 patients in a state psychiatric hospital. Psychiatr Serv 46:386–389, 1995

Wilson WJ: The Truly Disadvantaged: The Inner City, The Underclass and Public Policy. Chicago, IL, University of Chicago, 1987

Wolfgang ME: Sociocultural overview of criminal violence, in Violence and the Violent Individual. Edited by Hoys JR, Robert TK, Solway KS. New York, SP Medical and Scientific Books, 1981, pp 153–170

Young JL, Zonana HV, Shepler L: Medication noncompliance in schizophrenia: codification and update. Bull Am Acad Psychiatry Law 14:105–122, 1986

Yudofsky SC, Silver JM, Jackson W: The Overt Aggression Scale: an operationalized rating scale for verbal and physical aggression. Am J Psychiatry 143(suppl):35–39, 1986

Zierler S, Cunningham WE, Andersen R, et al: Violence victimization after HIV infection in a US probability sample of adult patients in primary care. Am J Public Health 90:208–215, 2000

Zito JM, Volavka J, Craig TJ, et al: Pharmacoepidemiology of clozapine in 202 inpatients with schizophrenia. Ann Pharmacother 27:1262–1269, 1993

Women's Mental Health

Vivien K. Burt, M.D., Ph.D.

Victoria C. Hendrick, M.D.

Introduction

There has been a growing awareness of the diagnostic and therapeutic female-specific differences in psychiatric disorders. For example, the prevalence of depressive and anxiety disorders is at least twice as high in women as in men (Kessler et al. 1994; Weissman et al. 1991). Recently published results from the U.S. Burden of Disease and Injury Study revealed that unipolar major depression ranked second in women and tenth in men as the foremost cause of disease burden (Michaud et al. 2001). Psychosocial reasons for women's greater vulnerability to these disorders include their relatively lower income, caregiving responsibilities, greater likelihood of experiencing sexual and domestic violence, and disadvantaged social status. Biologically, gonadal steroids are known to have psychoactive effects and may contribute to gender differences (McGlone 1980; Vogel et al. 1978). For example, estrogen produces antidopaminergic and serotonin-enhancing effects, and progesterone metabolites modulate γ-aminobutyric acid (GABA) receptors (Freeman et al. 1993; Seeman and Lang 1990; Sherwin 1990). It has been suggested that pubertal changes in hormones, adolescent social pressures, and negative life experiences contribute to the emergence of the gender gap in depression that begins at puberty (Cyranowski et al. 2000).

Table 36–1 summarizes female-specific elements of a psychiatric evaluation. These include an assessment of the temporal relationship of symptoms with the patient's menstrual cycle. Thus, for some women treated with psychotropic medications who experience premenstrual exacerbation or recurrence of symptoms, it may be worthwhile to check plasma levels of medication because they may fluctuate

across the menstrual cycle (Kimmel et al. 1992). It is important to consider the possibility that a woman of childbearing age may be pregnant and to assess her use of contraception and her plans for pregnancy because these factors influence treatment recommendations. A history of reproductive-related mood changes (e.g., oral contraceptive dysphoria, premenstrual mood symptoms, postpartum and perimenopausal depression) predicts future reproductive-related mood changes and may guide treatment decisions (Stewart and Boydell 1993). A patient's use of exogenous hormones (e.g., oral contraceptive or hormone replacement therapy) should be assessed because these may influence plasma levels of medications. Estrogen has an inhibitory effect on oxidative hepatic metabolism, thus potentially increasing blood levels of drugs that are oxidatively metabolized (e.g., many tricyclic antidepressants [TCAs], diazepam, clonazepam, chlordiazepoxide). On the other hand, drugs that undergo conjugative metabolism (e.g., lorazepam, oxazepam, temazepam) may be cleared more rapidly, as estrogen appears to induce hepatic conjugative enzymes. For a middle-aged woman reporting sleep impairment, the clinician should inquire about the occurrence of perimenopausal night sweats that may cause sleep disruption. The presence of seasonal affective disorder, which predominates in women, should be explored.

Psychiatric evaluation of female patients should include certain laboratory examinations, particularly a thyroid panel for women reporting changes in energy level, weight, or temperature tolerance. Autoimmune thyroid disorders occur primarily in women and have an estimated prevalence of 16% in women older than age 65 years. A follicle-stimulating hormone (FSH) level may identify perimenopausal/menopausal status in middle-aged women. It is prudent to measure serum beta human chorionic gonadotropin to rule out pregnancy for women

TABLE 36–1. Female-specific elements of a psychiatric evaluation

Component	Consideration
Social and developmental history	Note sexual preference, relationship styles, level of satisfaction with current relationships
	Document tendency to take on certain roles in relationships (e.g., caregiver, nurturer, or dependent and helpless)
	Note current or past sexual, physical, or emotional abuse
Socioeconomic status	Note level of economic support and ability to meet ongoing financial needs
	If parent is a single mother, inquire about child support

of reproductive age who are considering a trial of pharmacotherapy. If menstrual cycling is irregular, serum prolactin and thyroid-stimulating hormone (TSH) levels should be obtained, because both hyperprolactinemia and hypothyroidism may produce amenorrhea or irregular bleeding. Although hyperprolactinemia is a common sequela of antipsychotic medication in female patients, this condition may require an endocrinological evaluation and a brain imaging study to assess for the presence of a prolactin-producing pituitary tumor.

For women with symptoms of an eating disorder, additional laboratory evaluations include serum albumin, total protein, and glucose to assess nutritional status; serum amylase levels to assess the extent of self-induced vomiting; serum electrolytes, blood urea nitrogen, and creatinine to determine fluid/electrolyte abnormalities; and a complete blood count to assess for anemia due to nutritional deficiency and internal bleeding (e.g., due to esophageal tears resulting from self-induced vomiting). An electrocardiogram may reveal cardiac conduction abnormalities from electrolyte imbalance, malnutrition, or ipecac-induced cardiomyopathy.

Premenstrual Dysphoric Disorder

In DSM-IV-TR (American Psychiatric Association 2000), premenstrual dysphoric disorder (PMDD) is listed as a Mood Disorder Not Otherwise Specified and describes the recurrent physical and emotional symptoms restricted to the late luteal phase of the menstrual cycle and remitting within the first day or two following the onset of menstruation. Typical physical symptoms include bloating, breast tenderness, cramping, and headaches, and emotional symptoms include depression, irritability, anxiety,

and insomnia. Although PMDD is best determined by prospective daily symptom ratings over a 2-month interval, in clinical practice PMDD often is provisionally diagnosed and treatment is begun even as prospective daily ratings are in progress. Although most women of childbearing age experience some symptoms of PMDD over the course of some of their menstrual cycles, only about 5%–9% of childbearing-age women meet the criteria needed to establish the diagnosis of PMDD. It is important to identify other psychiatric disorders, including unipolar depression, dysthymia, or an anxiety disorder, that may exacerbate premenstrually, because treatment approaches may necessitate medication or behavioral modification to address premenstrual worsening of symptoms (Hendrick et al. 1996).

Evaluation and Treatment of Premenstrual Dysphoric Disorder

The evaluation for PMDD includes a full psychiatric evaluation, especially documentation of course of presenting symptoms, possible precipitants, and previous treatment approaches and responses. Medical evaluation should rule out physical conditions that may cause symptoms in association with the premenstrual phase of the menstrual cycle (e.g., endometriosis, fibrocystic breast disease, migraine headaches). Family psychiatric history, particularly any history of premenstrual symptoms and effective treatments in female relatives, is useful to guide treatment in the patient with PMDD. Medication use, including over-the-counter medications, should be recorded, and substances that may produce psychiatric side effects should be noted. The use of caffeine, salt, alcohol, and nicotine should be assessed because these may cause symptoms that mimic those of PMDD (e.g., bloating, lethargy, breast tenderness).

Treatment should be based on the severity and nature of symptoms, the patient's desire to be treated continuously throughout the cycle or only on symptomatic days, and the patient's views regarding the use of psychotropic versus other palliative agents. Mild premenstrual symptoms often can be treated with nonpharmacological interventions (e.g., sleep hygiene education, with emphasis on adequate sleep during the symptomatic premenstrual days). Exercise, relaxation therapy, and cognitive-behavioral therapy may also be helpful (Blake et al. 1998). Completion of prospective ratings on a daily basis often alerts the patient to high-risk days during which it is best to avoid difficult decisions and to minimize caffeine, salt, alcohol, and nicotine. Such nonpharmacological interventions are also useful to address symptoms while awaiting the results of prospective symptom rating.

The selective serotonin reuptake inhibitors (SSRIs) fluoxetine, sertraline, paroxetine, and citalopram have been found to effectively treat PMDD (Pearlstein et al. 1999; Steiner et al. 1995; Wikander et al. 1998; Yonkers et al. 1996, 1997). These medications should be given throughout the month, although administration during only the two premenstrual weeks (i.e., the luteal phase) has also met with some success (e.g., Wikander et al. 1998). Other psychotropic medications that have been less studied but appear effective at standard doses include nortriptyline, nefazodone, and clomipramine (Altshuler et al. 1995b). Premenstrual anxiety and irritability may be treated with anxiolytics such as buspirone and alprazolam.

Although progesterone supplementation is a popular treatment, controlled studies have failed to prove its effectiveness in alleviating symptoms of PMDD. Subcutaneous and transdermal estrogen have been somewhat successful but may produce unpleasant side effects, including nausea, weight gain, and breast tenderness. The synthetic androgen danazol and gonadotropin-releasing hormone (GnRH) agonists such as leuprolide produce an anovulatory state by suppressing the hypothalamic-pituitary-ovarian axis and successfully treat the symptoms of PMDD. However, these drugs, in addition to causing significant side effects, produce an hypoestrogenic state and thus increase the risk of osteoporosis and possibly heart disease. Therefore, these treatments are rarely used for PMDD.

Calcium carbonate at a dose of 1,200 mg/day appears to provide some overall improvement in symptoms by the second or third menstrual cycle and is also beneficial for prevention of osteoporosis (Thys-Jacobs 2000). Other pharmacological modalities include vitamin B_6 (pyridoxine) at doses of up to 100 mg/day (Wyatt et al. 1999). Doses greater than 100 mg/day should be avoided because they may cause peripheral neuropathy.

Less clearly useful, but benign and worth a try, are primrose oil, magnesium, and vitamin E. Diuretics (e.g., spironolactone, hydrochlorothiazide) are useful for the treatment of women with premenstrual edema and bloating. The use of the anti-inflammatory prostaglandin inhibitors (e.g., mefenamic acid, naproxen) is effective for the treatment of premenstrual pelvic pain, cramping, and headache. Other medications that have been reported to be helpful include atenolol, clonidine, and naltrexone.

Hormonal Contraception and Effects on Mood

Hormonal contraceptive agents include oral contraceptives, or birth control pills, and long-acting agents (implants and injections). Oral contraceptives are more than 99% effective when properly used, ensure regular menses, and reduce the risks for endometrial and ovarian cancer, ovarian cysts, ectopic pregnancy, and iron deficiency anemia.

Birth control pills are composed of either a combination of an estrogen and progestin or progestin only. Monophasic combination birth control pills contain fixed doses of estrogen and progestin throughout the cycle, whereas biphasic or triphasic agents contain doses of hormones that vary according to different times in the cycle. Although progestin-only pills are somewhat less effective than combination agents and may cause menstrual irregularities, they are nevertheless indicated for breast-feeding women or women for whom estrogen is contraindicated (e.g., hypertension or breast cancer).

Oral contraceptive agents also can be categorized according to their levels of estrogenic, progestational, and androgenic activities. Estrogenic side effects include nausea, breast tenderness, headaches, elevated blood pressure, and uterine fibroid enlargement. Side effects of progestational agents are weight gain, diminished libido, headaches, and irregular bleeding. Androgen-associated side effects include hirsutism, acne, and weight gain.

Recently, the long-acting progestational contraceptive agents Norplant (levonorgestrel implants) and Depo-Provera (medroxyprogesterone acetate injections) have gained acceptance because of their ease of use and long-lasting effectiveness. Norplant, a subdermal implant, provides up to 5 years of contraception, and Depo-Provera, an injectable agent, is administered every 3 months. Like the oral progestational agents, the potential side effects of these long-lasting progestational contraceptives include irregular bleeding and weight gain.

New-onset depression occurring in women without an affective history does not appear to be associated with the use of oral contraceptives (Yonkers and Bradshaw 1999). However, the use of oral contraceptives may precipitate a recurrence in women with a history of depression or premenstrual dysphoria (Bancroft and Sartorius 1990; Kendler et al. 1988). It is also possible that oral contraceptive use may be associated with subclinical depressive syndromes (Bancroft and Sartorius 1990). The triphasic oral contraceptive agents may cause negative moods, especially for women with histories of premenstrual depression (Bancroft and Rennie 1993). Unrelated to depression, diminished libido has been reported in relation to the use of oral contraceptives (Graham and Sherwin 1992). Also, highly progestational contraceptives (e.g., containing 1.5 mg norethindrone acetate) may cause fatigue and lethargy. Norplant and Depo-Provera have been anecdotally associated with depression, but these findings have not been supported by results of controlled studies (Kaunitz 1999; Westhoff et al. 1995).

For women with new-onset mood changes who have recently begun to use hormonal contraception, consideration should be given to switching agents or using another form of birth control. Most women, however, are unlikely to experience these mood changes unless they have histories of depression or premenstrual syndrome.

Psychological Aspects of Infertility, Induced Abortion, and Pregnancy Loss

Infertility

Ten to fifteen percent of all couples in the United States have difficulties in achieving pregnancy. When pregnancy does not occur after 1 year of unprotected intercourse, the couple is said to be infertile (LaPane et al. 1995). Infertility may be caused by ovulatory dysfunction, uterine or tubal disease, cervical problems, infectious disease, and immunological factors. Male factors are believed to underlie infertility in 40%–60% of cases (Jones and Toner 1993; McCartney and Downey 1993; Stephens and Chandra 1998). With the exception of anorexia nervosa, psychiatric syndromes are not believed to contribute significantly to infertility. However, infertility may produce significant psychiatric and psychological symptoms, including a loss of self-esteem and femininity. Women tend to be more emotionally affected than their male partners during treatment for infertility. However, some men experience anxiety and inhibition from the demands to perform sexually at scheduled times. Both members of the couple may have diminished libido and may experience a loss of sexuality. Often there is a sense of isolation from friends whose social activities involve children. The financial burden of the evaluation and treatment for infertility is an additional significant source of stress and may have an impact on major decisions such as the purchase of a home or car or vacations.

Evaluation of infertility involves assessment of both members of the couple and includes screening for sexually transmitted diseases and normal endocrine functioning. The infertility workup includes assessment of ovulation, quantity and quality of sperm, visualization of the woman's anatomy, and determination of patency of ductile systems in the woman and/or man. Tests are often repeated at different intervals over a single menstrual cycle and at subsequent menstrual cycles. The assessment invariably requires substantial reorganization of the day-to-day lives of both partners, with office visits dictated by responses to treatment, dates of ovulation, and physicians' schedules.

Treatment of Infertility

The choice of treatment depends on the etiology of infertility. If mechanical blockage in the female reproductive tract is identified, it can be corrected with surgery or at the time of the laparoscopy. For endometriosis, GnRH agonists such as leuprolide (Lupron) are helpful. If ovulatory dysfunction is identified as etiological, clomiphene citrate can be used to induce ovulation. If clomiphene citrate is unsuccessful, human menopausal gonadotropins (Pergonal [FSH and luteinizing hormone (LH)] or Metrodin [FSH]) are the next step. Unlike clomiphene citrate, which is orally administered, the human menopausal gonadotropins are administered by daily injections. These require daily visits to the physician unless the woman or her partner feel comfortable administering the injections. Side effects may include fatigue, nausea, headache, diarrhea, and weight gain. Clomiphene citrate is associated with a 5% incidence of multiple gestation. This incidence rises to 20% with human menopausal gonadotropins. Pharmacologic induction of ovulation is more likely to succeed if it is combined with intrauterine insemination. The success rate of these two combined procedures approximates 33% (Guzick et al. 1999).

If these treatments do not enable the couple to achieve pregnancy, they may opt for assisted reproductive technology, such as gamete intrafallopian transfer (GIFT) or zygote intrafallopian transfer (ZIFT). In the former method, oocytes and sperm are combined in vitro and immediately deposited in the woman's fallopian tubes; in the latter method, eggs are fertilized in vitro and the resultant zygotes are placed in the fallopian tubes. In the case of in vitro fertilization (IVF), fertilized embryos are placed directly into the uterus. Serial ultrasounds are necessary to monitor ovulation and post-transfer embryological development and to assess for the development of ovarian hyperstimulation. These procedures are expensive and have limited success rates: IVF has a 14% success rate, GIFT a 23% rate, and ZIFT a 15% rate (McCartney and Downey 1993). The risk of multiple gestation is approximately 25%, and there is a 6% chance of severe ovarian hyperstimulation syndrome, a potentially life-threatening complication.

When infertility results from an untreatable male factor, artificial insemination by a donor, also called therapeutic donor insemination, may be attempted. Intracytoplasmic sperm injection followed by artificial insemination is an alternative in cases of male-factor infertility. For a woman who is unable to ovulate, egg donation is an option. Medications are administered to both the donor and the infertile woman in order to synchronize their cycles. The donor eggs are then fertilized with sperm through the procedures of IVF or GIFT and transferred to the infertile woman, who then carries the pregnancy. In the case of a woman who is able to ovulate but cannot carry the pregnancy, a fertilized egg may be inseminated in a surrogate mother who then will carry the pregnancy.

Psychological Implications

Thus, infertility treatment is an arduous and demanding process. The medical interventions into the couple's sexual activities often have a negative impact on intimacy and spontaneity, and the daily monitoring of reproductive-related bodily functions can distract from other aspects of their lives. The relatively modest success rates and the high costs of the procedures add to the stress of treatment. A woman who postponed pregnancy for career concerns may experience significant guilt and self-blame. Complicating this situation, the medications used (clomiphene citrate, human menopausal gonadotropins, GnRH agonists) may produce negative mood changes, anxiety, and insomnia in addition to a number of physical side effects. Infertility is not associated with the development of major depressive disorder (Downey and McKinney 1992), but it does produce negative mood changes and may exacerbate any preexisting psychiatric disorders. Thus, psychiatric evaluation and treatment may be indicated. For mild to moderate psychiatric symptoms, psychotherapy may be sufficient. Group psychological interventions can also be helpful and have been reported to increase pregnancy rates in infertile women (Domar et al. 2000). For major mood or anxiety disorders, treatment should involve psychotherapy and/or psychotropic medication. A psychiatrist also can play a role in exploring alternative parenting options, including adoption. The psychiatrist should encourage both members of the couple to participate in therapy, either jointly or individually. A referral to RESOLVE, the national self-help organization for infertile couples that sponsors groups and workshops, can help the couple feel less isolated and overwhelmed.

Induced Abortion

Since the Supreme Court decision of *Roe v. Wade* in 1973, first-trimester abortions have been a woman's legal right. In the United States, most women who elect to terminate a pregnancy by means of abortion are younger than age 25, single, and have no children. Approximately 1.5 million abortions are performed in the United States each year (Frye et al. 1994).

Most abortions are performed by dilation and evacuation of uterine contents by means of vacuum aspiration or curettage and are associated with a mortality rate of approximately 0.4 per 100,000 procedures. This rate is 25 times lower than the rate associated with carrying a pregnancy to term. Recently, a number of medical methods for inducing abortion have been introduced. In September 2000, a regimen of mifepristone followed 2 days later by the prostaglandin F analogue misoprostol was approved by the FDA for termination of pregnancies of less than 49 days' duration. The off-label use of methotrexate in conjunction with misoprostol has also been used to induce abortion.

Reasons for termination of pregnancy include poor partner support, inability to provide financial support for a child, inability or lack of desire to bear responsibility for a child, and termination for the health of the mother. A woman may be reluctant to carry the pregnancy to term if a fetal congenital anomaly has been diagnosed or if the pregnancy resulted from rape or incest.

For most women, abortion is followed by feelings of relief. Some women, however, may experience depression or other negative psychological outcomes. The strongest predictor of depression after elective abortion is a history of depression before the pregnancy. The risk of adverse psychological sequelae is also higher if there was ambivalence about the decision, if the abortion was performed beyond the first trimester, or if the decision to abort was due to fetal demise or severe deformity (Dagg 1991; Zolese and Blacker 1992). Thus, abortion counseling should be offered before the procedure. Counseling provides an opportunity for a woman and her partner to obtain information regarding the likelihood of pain, discomfort, or other adverse sequelae following the abortion and to learn effective contraceptive methods to prevent future unwanted pregnancies. For women whose pregnancy is the result of a rape, counseling is an important part of the recovery from the trauma of the assault.

For a woman undergoing an abortion because of a fetal diagnosis of congenital deformity or impending fetal demise, feelings may include mourning for the loss of a wished-for baby and self-blame about having produced a deformed fetus. She may experience anxiety and ambivalence about becoming pregnant in the future and will benefit from sensitive education and support. Whenever possible, the woman's partner should be included in therapy, particularly because he also may be grieving.

When a chronically mentally ill woman seeks an abortion, a careful psychiatric evaluation should be undertaken to assess delusions and paranoid feelings that may be influencing her decision. Her ability to understand her condition and the options available to her should be assessed. Before the pregnancy is terminated, the patient's psychiatric condition should be stabilized.

Pregnancy Loss

Approximately 12%–24% of identified pregnancies result in intrauterine death during the first 20 weeks' gestation (miscarriage). However, the rate of miscarriage is probably significantly higher, as many spontaneous abortions occur in women who are unaware that they are pregnant. Miscarriage tends to be a serious traumatic event for expectant parents, and affected couples often feel isolated. In the 6 months following a pregnancy loss, women frequently experience anxiety and depression. Childless women or women with prior histories of depression are at particular risk for major depression after miscarriage (Neugebauer et al. 1997). Normal bereavement should be distinguished from psychopathology, and psychiatric follow-up should be encouraged for couples with depressive histories or who have experienced late-trimester fetal loss. Women who have miscarried and have significant histories of depression should be monitored during the next pregnancy to reduce the risk for subsequent depression.

Psychiatric Disorders in Pregnancy

A growing body of literature shows that pregnancy neither predisposes nor protects against mental illness. When women with psychiatric disorders plan their pregnancies, there is time to discuss treatment options and to switch, if necessary, to medications that appear safer in pregnancy. For patients who become pregnant while taking psychotropic agents, an attempt should be made to discontinue the medication if clinically feasible. Because the uteroplacental circulation does not begin to form until approximately 2 weeks after conception, the developing embryo most likely will not be exposed to a medication taken during the time between conception and the first missed menstrual period.

For the pregnant patient with psychiatric symptoms, nonpharmacological interventions should be attempted whenever possible. Caffeine, nicotine, and alcohol should be discouraged; environmental stressors should be minimized as much as possible; and the need for adequate nutrition and sleep, and strategies to achieve these, should be emphasized and discussed. Psychotherapy, group support, and family and marital counseling should be initiated when appropriate. However, for women with

brittle psychiatric conditions, discontinuation of medication may precipitate a risk of relapse. Although the consequences of relapse vary for different disorders, for many women a relapse may result in alcohol or substance use, impulsive behavior, and inattention to a regimen of good prenatal care.

Before a psychotropic agent is administered to a pregnant patient, risks and benefits to both the mother and the fetus should be evaluated and shared with the patient; her partner, whenever possible; and her obstetrician. The patient and her partner should be informed that both the FDA and the American Medical Association agree that although the FDA does not endorse the safety of any psychiatric medication in pregnancy, physicians may prescribe medications according to data-based knowledge and their own best clinical judgment (Gold 2000). Discussions should be documented, and the clinician should assess and note the patient's understanding and capacity to consent to the treatment plan.

Treatment of Depression During Pregnancy

Approximately 10% of pregnant women experience major or minor depression, a rate similar to that of nonpregnant women. Depression during pregnancy is associated with poor prenatal care, inadequate nutrition, a significantly elevated risk of postpartum depression (O'Hara 1995), suicide, greater incidence of preterm deliveries, and small-for-gestational-age babies (Steer et al. 1992). When depressive symptoms are mild or moderate, it is reasonable to employ nonpharmacological modalities such as individual or conjoint psychotherapy and stress-reduction counseling. If the patient has severe symptoms that do not improve with nonpharmacological means and pose a threat to herself or the pregnancy (i.e., she is suicidal, psychotic, or not gaining weight), it may be necessary to initiate a trial of pharmacotherapy.

Whenever possible, antidepressant medications should be withheld at least during the first trimester, when major organogenesis occurs. However, this may not be possible if a women is experiencing severe depression or if she has a history of chronic depression with severe relapses following medication discontinuation. When a medication is used during pregnancy, the dosage should be kept at the minimum necessary for symptom control.

To date, the most extensive information on the prenatal use of antidepressants involves fluoxetine. Prospective studies have not found an association between the use of fluoxetine during pregnancy and major congenital anomalies in the neonate (Chambers et al. 1996; Ericson et al.

1999; D.J. Goldstein 1995; McElhatton et al. 1996; Nulman et al. 1997). Some (Chambers et al. 1996), but not all (Ericson et al. 1999; D.J. Goldstein 1995; McElhatton et al. 1996; Nulman et al. 1997) studies of fluoxetine use in the third trimester have reported an association with transient perinatal complications such as jitteriness. Studies have also evaluated the use of citalopram, sertraline, paroxetine, and fluvoxamine during pregnancy and have found no link with congenital malformations (Ericson et al. 1999; Kulin et al. 1998). A recent prospective, controlled study of 150 pregnant women taking venlafaxine suggested no increased risk of major congenital anomalies in exposed neonates (Einarson et al. 2001).

Available data show no TCA-associated congenital anomalies, although transient perinatal toxicity or withdrawal symptoms have been reported when these agents are used near the time of birth (Altshuler et al. 1996; Wisner et al. 2001). Symptoms include jitteriness, irritability, lethargy, decreased muscle tone, and anticholinergic effects such as constipation, tachycardia, and urinary retention. If the decision is made to treat with a TCA, nortriptyline or desipramine is preferable because there is less likelihood of anticholinergic and hypotensive side effects. Antidepressant dosages may need to be adjusted over the course of pregnancy as blood levels may fall, particularly after the patient begins the third trimester (Altshuler and Hendrick 1996).

To date, no studies exist on the use of bupropion, trazodone, venlafaxine, mirtazapine or nefazodone in pregnancy. The monoamine oxidase inhibitors (MAOIs) should not be used in pregnant women because of the risk of hypertensive crisis. Additionally, MAOIs interact adversely with tocolytic agents (e.g., terbutaline) that may be necessary to forestall premature labor.

With regard to neurobehavioral sequelae, a prospective study that compared control children with children prenatally exposed to fluoxetine or TCAs found no differences in IQ, temperament, mood, behavior, or attention in children up to age 7 years (Nulman et al. 1997).

Treatment of Bipolar Disorder During Pregnancy

Two recent studies have examined the course of bipolar disorder across pregnancy (Grof et al. 2001; Viguera et al. 2000). One of the studies found that despite not taking medications, lithium-responsive bipolar women experienced fewer relapses during pregnancy than in the 9 months prior to conception, although in a few cases relapses occurred during the last 5 weeks of pregnancy (Grof et al. 2000). The second study of women with bipolar disorder reported that the relapse rate during pregnancy was no different from the rate in nongravid women (Viguera et al. 2000). These inconsistent findings suggest that the history of bipolar illness both with and without mood stabilization may predict the course of the illness in the context of pregnancy and underscore the need for more research on the course of bipolar disorder across pregnancy. In both studies, women who were not treated with mood stabilizers during pregnancy were at increased risk for postpartum decompensation. Furthermore, rapid rather than gradual antepartum discontinuation of lithium appeared to increase the risk for postpartum relapse (Viguera et al. 2000).

With first-trimester use of lithium the incidence of Ebstein's anomaly, a serious defect in the formation of the tricuspid valve of the heart, is raised from the estimated rate of 1 per 20,000 in the general population to a rate of approximately 1 per 1,000 (Altshuler et al. 1996; Cohen et al. 1994). The use of lithium during pregnancy also has been linked with other cardiac malformations, including coarctation of the aorta and mitral atresia. Additional potential adverse consequences to the neonate from lithium use in pregnancy include hypotonia, poor suck reflex, hypoglycemia, cyanosis, neonatal goiter, and diabetes insipidus (Briggs 1998; Miller 1994a).

Use of valproate and carbamazepine in the first trimester is associated with an increased risk of neural tube defects, including spina bifida (up to 5% for valproate and 1% for carbamazepine), and with developmental delay, craniofacial defects, and fingernail hypoplasia. These medications produce antifolate effects that contribute significantly to their embryotoxicity. They can also produce a deficiency in vitamin K–dependent clotting factors, thereby increasing the risk of bleeding disorders in the fetus and neonate. Vitamin K supplementation and folate should therefore be administered to women taking these agents during pregnancy. Hypoglycemia and hepatic dysfunction have also been reported in exposed neonates.

A prospective study of nine epileptic women receiving lamotrigine during pregnancy reported no adverse effects in the infants (Ohman et al. 2000) and a pregnancy registry for this agent also has found no increased risk for congenital anomalies among 53 exposed infants (Morrelli 1996). Little human data exist on gabapentin or topiramate use during pregnancy.

Thus, for patients with relatively stable bipolar disorder, an attempt should be made to discontinue mood-stabilizing medications before conception. Gradual medication taper appears less likely to produce relapse than does abrupt discontinuation (Faedda et al. 1993). However, for women with more brittle illnesses, mood stabilizers may need to be continued during pregnancy. Lithium is preferable to carbamazepine and valproate because it is associated with a lower risk of teratogenicity. It should be administered in multiple daily doses to avoid peak blood levels, and levels should be monitored closely. The lithium dose may require adjustment because blood levels often drop as pregnancy progresses. At week 18, a level-II ultrasound should be obtained to assess for potential cardiovascular anomalies. To reduce the risk of lithium toxicity in the mother due to the rapid drop in plasma volume after childbirth, maternal serum lithium levels should not exceed 1 mEq/L in the 1–2 weeks before the estimated date of delivery.

If carbamazepine or valproate must be continued in pregnancy, an amniotic α-fetoprotein analysis at week 16 and an ultrasound at week 18–22 should be obtained to assess for neural tube defects. For women who experience an exacerbation or escalation of symptoms, electroconvulsive therapy (ECT) is another option.

Treatment of Schizophrenia During Pregnancy

The course of schizophrenia throughout pregnancy is variable and unpredictable. Pregnant women with schizophrenia require close management, because psychotic symptoms have been associated with fetal abuse or neonaticide, failure to obtain prenatal care, paranoid delusions regarding necessary medical procedures that therefore prevent cooperation, impaired self-care, inability to recognize labor, and greater risk of adverse pregnancy outcomes (prematurity, low birth weight, low Apgar scores). Patients should be screened for substance abuse, psychosocial stressors, housing and financial resources, and other factors that negatively affect parenting ability.

As with all psychotropic medications, antipsychotic medications should be used in pregnancy only when necessary (e.g., for patients with psychotic symptoms that pose a risk to the patient or fetus). Use of antipsychotic agents on an as-needed basis may help reduce the overall dose exposure of the fetus. However, daily dosing is often necessary for severely ill patients.

The limited data on antipsychotic medications in pregnancy show no increased risk of congenital malformations with the use of high-potency agents (e.g., haloperidol and trifluoperazine). Low-potency phenothiazines, on the other hand, have been implicated in a higher incidence of nonspecific congenital anomalies and neonatal jaundice. Case reports of clozapine use in pregnancy have shown no adverse sequelae (Trixler and Tenyi 1997), but one child experienced a seizure 8 days after delivery that may have been related to clozapine expo-

sure (Stoner et al. 1997). In a study of 23 pregnant women who took olanzapine during pregnancy, rates of spontaneous abortion, stillbirth, malformation, and prematurity were within the range of the normal population (D.J. Goldstein et al. 2000). No information exists to date on risperidone, quetiapine, or ziprasidone when used during pregnancy. For infants exposed to traditional antipsychotic agents in utero near the time of delivery, a transient syndrome of motor restlessness, tremor, hypertonia, hyperreflexia, irritability, dyskinesia, and poor feeding has been noted (Altshuler et al. 1996; Trixler and Tenyi 1997).

Agents to treat extrapyramidal side effects should be avoided in pregnancy because they are associated with major and minor congenital anomalies. The anticholinergic agents trihexyphenidyl and benztropine have been associated with minor congenital malformations and anticholinergic symptoms in the newborn, including functional bowel obstruction and urinary retention. Diphenhydramine has been linked with a greater risk of orofacial clefts and with perinatal withdrawal symptoms. Animal studies have reported cardiovascular malformations following in utero exposure to amantadine (Altshuler et al. 1996). Alternative strategies for patients who experience extrapyramidal symptoms include reduction of the neuroleptic dose or switching to a lower-potency agent.

Treatment of Anxiety Disorders During Pregnancy

For women with preexisting panic disorder, symptoms may improve during pregnancy, continue unchanged, or worsen. Obsessive-compulsive disorder (OCD) has been reported to worsen during pregnancy (Shear and Mammen 1995). Nonpharmacological interventions for anxiety disorders include cognitive-behavioral therapy, elimination of caffeine and nicotine, reduction of psychosocial stressors, and couples therapy. TCAs and SSRIs are reasonable treatment options for severe intractable symptoms that do not respond to those measures. Until these medications take effect, small, occasional doses of benzodiazepines may be necessary. Intermittent use of low doses of benzodiazepines during pregnancy, particularly after the first trimester, does not appear to increase the risk of adverse neonatal sequelae. Nevertheless, the use of benzodiazepines in pregnancy is controversial, with some researchers noting a significant risk of oral clefts, particularly with diazepam and alprazolam (Altshuler et al. 1996). Other studies, however, have not found this association. Nevertheless, an attempt should be made to avoid benzodiazepines during gestational weeks 5–9, because this is the period when fetal formation of the palate occurs. Transient perinatal syndromes, including hypotonia, failure to feed, temperature dysregulation, apnea, and low Apgar scores, have been noted with last-trimester use of benzodiazepines. Near term, the use of benzodiazepines should generally be kept at a minimum. Whenever possible, benzodiazepine dose changes should be gradual to avoid precipitating in utero withdrawal.

Use of Electroconvulsive Therapy During Pregnancy

ECT is a reasonable treatment option for pregnant patients with severe mood disorders because it appears safe and effective and exposes the developing fetus to a minimum of psychoactive medication (Miller 1994b). Special considerations in the administration of ECT to pregnant women include the need for a pelvic examination and uterine tocodynamometry to exclude uterine contractions and elevation of the right hip to ensure adequate placental perfusion. The muscle relaxant succinylcholine and the anticholinergic agent glycopyrrolate appear relatively safe to use in pregnancy (Miller 1994b). Following the procedure, external fetal monitoring should continue for several hours.

Substance Abuse During Pregnancy

In addition to premature labor, abruptio placentae, stillbirth, and other obstetrical complications, teratogenic effects are associated with alcohol and its metabolite acetaldehyde. Infants exposed in utero to alcohol are at risk for fetal alcohol syndrome, a disorder characterized by mental retardation, microcephaly, hypoplastic philtrum and maxilla, thinned upper vermilion, shortened palpebral fissures, and attention deficit with hyperactivity in childhood. Isolated abnormalities not reaching the full syndrome are described as fetal alcohol effects. No safe quantity of prenatal alcohol consumption has been established.

Cocaine use during pregnancy is associated with reduced placental blood flow, intrauterine growth retardation, and genitourinary tract malformations. Preterm labor, abruptio placentae, and other obstetrical complications may occur as a result of cocaine's vasoconstrictive effect (Ness et al. 1999). Neonates may experience a withdrawal syndrome lasting several months.

Like cocaine, heroin use during pregnancy is frequently associated with obstetrical complications and a perinatal withdrawal syndrome characterized by irritability, poor feeding, respiratory difficulties, and tremulousness. In utero exposure to opiates also has been linked with a greater risk of sudden infant death syndrome (SIDS). Women maintained on methadone and who receive prenatal care have better obstetrical outcomes than women with untreated opiate use (Blume 1994).

While tobacco is not an illegal drug, it can increase the risk of perinatal morbidity when used during pregnancy. Its prenatal use has been linked with intrauterine growth retardation, low birth weight, spontaneous abortion, and preterm delivery (Ness et al. 1999). Similarly, caffeine may increase the risk of early spontaneous abortions (Cnattingius et al. 2000).

Postpartum Psychiatric Disorders

For some women, the weeks after delivery represent a time of increased vulnerability for psychiatric disorders (Kendell et al. 1987). The burden of postpartum illness is significant because it not only affects the mother but also can have a negative affect on family life and infant development. Classically, emotional conditions occurring during the postpartum period include postpartum blues, postpartum depression, and postpartum psychosis. More recently, postpartum anxiety disorders have been recognized. Postpartum panic disorder with or without agoraphobia appears to be the most frequently reported anxiety condition (Shear and Mammen 1995). Postpartum OCD also has been described (Shear and Mammen 1995). Although no specific etiology has been found to explain the onset of psychiatric illness during the postpartum period, the causes probably reside in a combination of biological/endocrinological and psychosocial factors. Because the literature on postpartum anxiety disorders is sparse, the following discussions on postpartum conditions focus on postpartum mood disorders.

Postpartum Blues

Up to 85% of mothers experience postpartum blues (O'Hara 1995), a temporary condition beginning in the first 2–4 days after giving birth, peaking between postpartum days 5–7, and dissipating by the end of the second postpartum week. Symptoms include tearfulness, mood lability, irritability, and anxiety. That this condition is part of the affective spectrum of psychiatric disorders is supported by the findings that risk factors include a history of PMDD and depression (especially during pregnancy) as well as a family history of depression (O'Hara et al. 1991). Because postpartum blues resolve spontaneously, this condition does not require active aggressive treatment. However, because new mothers are generally discharged from the hospital before the onset of postpartum blues, all prospective and new parents should be counseled about its existence. Thus, partners, other family members, and health care providers will be prepared to provide needed support and reassurance.

Postpartum Depression

Although major depression occurring during the 6 months after childbirth has a prevalence of approximately 10%, similar to that of the general population, its rate has been reported to be threefold higher in the first 5 weeks postpartum (Cox et al. 1993). Although many studies of depression after delivery have included women whose symptoms began within 3–12 months following delivery, the "postpartum-onset" specifier in DSM-IV-TR may be applied only for depression with onset in the first 4 weeks after childbirth. Postpartum depression, as well as depression occurring in mothers beyond the postpartum period, affects not only the woman but also her family. Depressed mothers are more likely than nondepressed mothers to engage in negative parenting behaviors, and their children are at risk for behavioral and cognitive deficits from infancy to early childhood (Lyons-Ruth et al. 2000; Murray 1997).

A history of major depression increases the risk for postpartum major depression to 24% (O'Hara 1995) and depression during pregnancy increases the likelihood of postpartum depression to 35% (O'Hara 1995). Women who have had previous postpartum depression are at 50%–60% risk of another episode (Wisner and Wheeler 1994). Other risk factors for postpartum depression include stressful life events and lack of support from a partner or spouse or others.

Treatment of postpartum depression is multimodal and includes individual and group psychotherapy, psychopharmacology, psychoeducation, and support. A combination of individual psychotherapy, particularly in the form of cognitive therapy, and standard pharmacotherapy to treat depression and secondary anxiety is an effective treatment strategy. Lay advocacy groups (e.g., Postpartum Support International, Depression After Delivery) offer assistance in the form of group therapy and mutual support. If there are interpersonal difficulties between the patient and her partner, conjoint therapy provides an important adjunct. Assistance with household duties and childcare is essential, because this provides the patient with opportunities to reduce sleep deprivation. Educating the patient and her family about postpartum disorders—that they are fairly common and treatable—is reassuring and offers everyone the opportunity to talk together about practical strategies to reduce stress in the home and provide assistance with day-to-day household duties. For new mothers with past histories of postpartum depression, studies that have evaluated the effectiveness of prophylaxis with antidepressant medications, begun the day of delivery, have produced mixed results (Wisner and Wheeler 1994; Wisner et al. 2001). Nevertheless, it is prudent for women with histories of depression, particularly postpartum depression, to be treated with the antidepressant that was previously effective. Whether treatment is begun in the last trimester or immediately after delivery, all women with prior affective histories should be carefully monitored throughout pregnancy and the postpartum.

The issue of whether or not to breast-feed should be discussed thoroughly because nursing may alter the treatment modality or may influence the choice of medication should pharmacotherapy be indicated. For patients whose depression is complicated by psychosis or suicidality, ECT is often the treatment of choice to hasten rapid improvement. Such cases generally require hospitalization until stabilization is achieved.

Postpartum Psychosis

The most serious postpartum illness, postpartum psychosis, occurs in 1–2 of every 1,000 births (O'Hara 1995). The condition is characterized by mood lability, agitation, confusion, thought disorganization, hallucinations, and disturbed sleep. Women who have had an episode of postpartum psychosis are at risk for subsequent bipolar disorder, suggesting that postpartum psychosis may be a subcategory of bipolar disorder. A history of bipolar disorder or of a previous postpartum psychosis is associated with approximately a 20%–35% risk of developing postpartum psychosis (Davidson and Robertson 1985; Kendell et al. 1987). Having both bipolar disorder and a prior postpartum psychotic episode increases the risk of subsequent postpartum psychosis to 50% (Kendell et al. 1987). Primiparity and a family history of bipolar disorder also appear to heighten the risk for postpartum psychosis (O'Hara 1995).

Because postpartum psychosis carries with it the risk of suicide, infant neglect, and infanticide (Rohde and Marneros 1993), patients are generally hospitalized. The initial evaluation includes a medical assessment to rule out organic etiologies such as postpartum thyroiditis, Sheehan's syndrome, pregnancy-related autoimmune disorders, HIV–related infection, and intoxication/withdrawal states. Acute pharmacological treatment includes the use of a mood stabilizer, an antipsychotic agent, and a benzodiazepine as needed for agitation. Antidepressants should be administered with great caution because these may provoke rapid cycling (Altshuler et al. 1995a). Maintenance treatment for the patient whose postpartum psychosis was preceded by chronic recurrent affective illness generally involves long-term treatment with a mood stabilizer. For patients without a psychiatric history other than a single episode of postpartum psychosis, medications are often tapered and discontinued by 1 year of treatment, although these women should be monitored because they have approximately a 60% risk of recurrent affective illness (Videbech and Gouliaev 1995). It is prudent for patients with a history of postpartum psychosis who subsequently become pregnant to be placed on a prophylactic mood stabilizer either during the third trimester or at delivery.

Breast-Feeding and Psychotropic Medications

Approximately one-half of new mothers breast-feed, and of these, 10% are estimated to have postpartum depression. Breast-feeding enhances mother–infant bonding and is an excellent source of nutrition for infants. For women who require pharmacological treatment for postpartum psychiatric disorders, the decision of whether to forgo breast-feeding or to proceed with medications can be difficult.

Data regarding the safety of psychotropic medications by breast-feeding mothers have increased substantially in the past decade. Nevertheless, no medication should be taken by a breast-feeding woman without careful assessment of risks and benefits. If it is concluded that the use of psychotropic medication is acceptable during nursing, the treating physician should review the available information with both mother and father.

Guidelines for using psychotropic medication in breast-feeding mothers include apprising the infant's pediatrician of the need to monitor the infant carefully for potential adverse effects. The infant's baseline behavior and sleep and feeding patterns should be assessed before the nursing mother uses the medication. Infant hepatic drug clearance rises from about one-third of the mother's weight-adjusted clearance at birth to 100% at the age of 6 months. Thus, exposure to drugs through breast milk may be riskier in a neonate than in an older infant. In particular, premature infants should not be exposed to psychotropic medications through breast milk until they have reached full maturity. Medication exposure should be minimized by prescribing the lowest dosage of medication that achieves remission of psychiatric

symptoms. Short-acting rather than long-acting medications are preferable, and supplementation of breast milk with formula reduces the infant's exposure to the drug. Because the clinical significance of any exposure to the baby of even small (and nondetectable) doses of psychotropic agents is unknown, the baby's clinical status should be continually monitored.

Most medications, including TCAs, benzodiazepines, and antipsychotic agents, have been classified by the American Academy of Pediatrics as "drugs whose effect on nursing infants is unknown but may be of concern" (American Academy of Pediatrics Committee on Drugs 1994). The data on the use of SSRI antidepressants have been increasingly reassuring (Burt et al. 2001). Because infants nursed by mothers taking SSRIs, particularly paroxetine and sertraline, typically receive low serum levels of medication exposure, routine monitoring of serum concentrations is not necessary (Burt et al. 2001). If the clinician or parent wishes to measure the concentration of an agent in infant serum, steady-state concentrations of both parent drug and metabolite should be determined. If possible, a laboratory should be chosen that is capable of high-sensitivity assays—that is, with limits of detection below 2 ng/mL. MAOIs are best avoided because they may cause hypertension in the infant.

Lithium is contraindicated by the American Academy of Pediatrics Committee on Drugs (1994) because adverse effects, including cyanosis, poor muscle tone, and electrocardiogram changes have been noted in infants exposed to lithium through nursing. Although valproate and carbamazepine are considered by the committee to be compatible with breast-feeding, there are two reported cases of hepatic dysfunction and one possible case of transient seizure-like activity in infants exposed to carbamazepine via breast milk (Brent and Wisner 1998; Frey et al. 1990; Merlob et al. 1992). Although valproate accumulates in breast milk to a lesser extent than carbamazepine (von Unruh et al. 1984), it should be used with caution in breast-feeding mothers because this medication has been associated with infant hepatotoxicity (Dreifuss et al. 1987; Stahl et al. 1997; Trimble 1990).

Perimenopause and Menopause

Menopause refers to the cessation of ovulation and menstrual cycling and usually occurs between ages 44 and 55 (average age, 51.4 years). *Perimenopause* and *climacteric* are interchangeable terms that describe the years before menopause when ovarian function begins to decline.

As ovarian production of estrogen declines, the pituitary hormones LH and FSH rise. An elevated serum FSH level, especially if obtained shortly after the onset of menses (when FSH levels should be at their nadir), suggests a woman is perimenopausal. Elevated FSH levels (i.e., 40 mU/mL or above) obtained later in the cycle can be misleading because this hormone may rise into the menopausal range in premenopausal women, particularly at midcycle. Levels of estradiol, the biologically active form of estrogen, remain under 25 pg/mL following menopause.

Physiological changes resulting from low estrogen levels begin to manifest during the perimenopausal years and include hot flushes and cold sweats. These symptoms occur in 80% of perimenopausal women and may persist for years after the last menstrual period. Hot flushes are sensations of heat that develop in the face and body and last up to several minutes; they often are associated with perspiration, breathlessness, dizziness, and tachycardia. These symptoms may be confused with a panic attack, particularly because they occur unexpectedly and may be associated with some anxiety. Night sweats may produce sleep deprivation, which subsequently may lead to decreased concentration, fatigue, and irritability. Other signs of declining ovarian estrogen production include atrophy of the urogenital tract lining, sometimes leading to infection, urinary frequency and urgency, and occasional stress incontinence. Women may experience painful intercourse and reduced libido. Particularly serious long-term consequences of low estrogen levels are osteoporosis and cardiovascular disease.

Large epidemiological studies have found that most women are not at greater risk for depression during their perimenopausal years compared with other times in their lives (Kaufert et al. 1992; Matthews et al. 1990), thus discrediting the term *involutional melancholia* coined by Kraepelin in 1890 to describe a depressive syndrome occurring in association with menopause.

It appears that there are subgroups of women whose risk for depressive mood rises at perimenopause. These include women with histories of previous reproductive-related mood syndromes (e.g., oral contraceptive–related mood changes, premenstrual dysphoria, and postpartum depression) (Stewart and Boydell 1993) and women who experience severe vasomotor symptoms (hot flushes, night sweats). With the lessening of physical symptoms, mood symptoms tend to resolve. Other risk factors for depressive symptoms at menopause include being divorced, widowed, or separated; having significant caregiving responsibilities; and experiencing a chronic illness (Avis and McKinlay 1991, 1995).

Evaluation of Depression in Perimenopausal Women

Figure 36–1 presents an algorithm for the evaluation and treatment of depression in perimenopausal women. The evaluation of depression in a middle-aged woman should include a descriptive assessment of menstrual status. Thus, the evaluation should document menstrual cycle patterns, vasomotor symptoms, and sexual function. The laboratory workup should include serum FSH and a thyroid panel. A full physical examination will exclude other medical disorders (e.g., autoimmune disorders, endocrine disorders, heart disease, cancer) that may produce depressive symptoms.

Treatment of Depression in Perimenopausal Women

For perimenopausal women with major depression, standard antidepressant treatment, including psychotherapy and/or antidepressants, is essential. If vasomotor symptoms also are present, estrogen replacement will effectively treat this syndrome and reduce sleep disturbance due to middle-of-the-night awakening secondary to the physical symptoms of endogenous estrogen decline. For perimenopausal women with severe hot flushes or night sweats who report subclinical depression and lethargy, administration of hormone replacement therapy (HRT) may relieve the psychological symptoms as the vasomotor symptoms become less distressing. As women experience relief from vasomotor symptoms (usually within 2 weeks of beginning hormone replacement), depressive symptoms also should improve.

Although some studies have suggested that estrogen produces mood-elevating effects in perimenopausal (Schmidt et al. 2000) and surgically menopausal (Sherwin 1988) women, estrogen alone is not currently accepted as effective for clinical depression. Thus, if a patient continues to feel depressed after resolution of the vasomotor symptoms, standard psychiatric treatment should be initiated. Psychosocial factors that may contribute to depressed mood also should be addressed, including caring for aging parents, new-onset health problems in the patient or her spouse, financial difficulties, and changes in sexuality of the patient or her partner.

HRT incurs both benefits and risks. In addition to providing relief of vasomotor symptoms, estrogen replacement helps protect against osteoporotic bony changes and urogenital atrophy. Although estrogen increases the risk of endometrial cancer, the addition of a progestin in women with an intact uterus negates this risk. The effects of hormone replacement on coronary

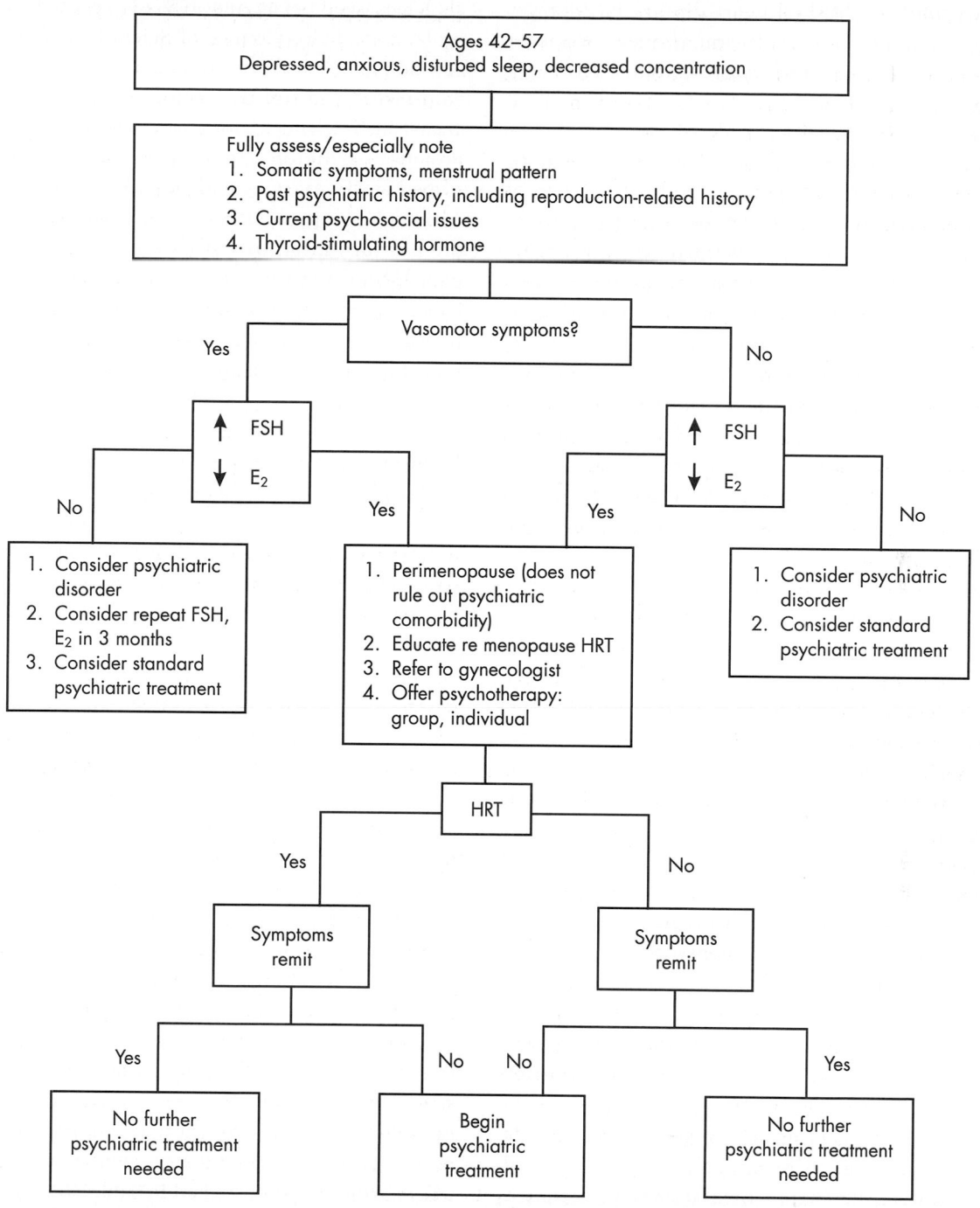

FIGURE 36–1.   Evaluation and treatment of depression in perimenopausal women.

Note.   E$_2$ = estradiol; FSH = follicle stimulating hormone; HRT = hormone replacement therapy.

Source.   Reprinted with permission from Burt VK, Hendrick VC (eds): "Perimenopause and Menopause," in *Concise Guide to Women's Mental Health*, 2nd Edition. Washington, DC, American Psychiatric Publishing, 2001, p. 129. Copyright 2001 American Psychiatric Publishing, Inc.

artery heart disease and breast cancer are currently subjects of intense debate. While epidemiologic studies suggest that hormone replacement may help prevent cardiovascular disease and improve cardiac lipid profiles and other known risk factors for cardiovascular disease in healthy postmenopausal women, results of prospective, randomized, controlled trials have not yet been published (Villablanca 2001). For women with established coronary artery disease, hormone replacement may increase cardiovascular events during the first year of treatment (Schrott et al. 1997). Thus, the role of hormone replacement in reducing the risk of coronary artery disease in women without established heart disease has not yet been proven and hormone replacement does not appear to be effective for the secondary prevention of coronary artery disease.

A recent study of the effect of hormone replacement on breast cancer risks revealed that estrogen increases the risk of breast cancer by 1% per year and the addition of progestin increases that risk to 8% per year (Schairer et al. 2000). The Women's Health Initiative, the largest prospective controlled study to date of hormone use in menopausal women, is currently evaluating the effect of hormone replacement on heart disease, osteoporosis, cancer, and cognitive function. Until the publication of these data, decisions regarding hormone replacement should be made on a case-by-case basis and should address factors such as current health, risk for osteoporosis, cardiac disease, personal and family history of breast cancer, vasomotor discomfort, urogenital dysfunction, and quality of life issues.

For most women, hormone replacement involves the administration of both estrogen and progestin. The purpose of the progestin is to counteract the endometrial proliferation that occurs with estrogen and increases the risk of endometrial cancer. Women who have had a hysterectomy do not require progestin supplementation. The progestin is taken either on a daily basis with the estrogen (continuous regimen) or at a higher dose during only 12–14 days of each month (cyclic regimen). The cyclic regimen produces vaginal bleeding following withdrawal of the progestin. No monthly bleeding occurs with the continuous regimen, but irregular spotting may occur that requires endometrial biopsy to rule out hyperplasia or malignancy.

Estrogen and progesterone supplementation is available in various preparations, including conjugated equine estrogen (Premarin) 0.625–1.25 mg and medroxyprogesterone acetate (Provera) 2.5–10 mg. Numerous alternative preparations of estrogen and progestins are available. In some cases, estrogen formulations include a small amount of testosterone supplementation (e.g., Estratest) and may be helpful for women who have experienced diminished libido.

Women Victims of Violence

Sexual Assault

In 1992 the American Medical Association reported that approximately 20% of all adult women and 12% of adolescent girls have been sexually abused. Despite the serious negative impact of sexual assault on physical and psychological well being, only 10% of assaulted women seek professional help (Council of Scientific Affairs 1992). In addition to physical symptoms such as tremulousness and cold sweats, initial psychological reactions to sexual assault include shock, numbness, withdrawal, and denial. Prolonged symptoms may include startle reactions, disturbed sleep, extreme fatigue, and somatic complaints. Although symptoms tend to dissipate over time, they often return intermittently over the course of ensuing months and even years. Long-term negative sequelae may include sexual dysfunction and aversion, impaired ability to establish healthy interpersonal relationships, and feelings of helplessness, shame, vulnerability, and depression. Posttraumatic stress disorder is particularly common and intense when there is a history of abuse (Stewart and Robinson 1995).

Ideally, initial psychiatric assessment should include an evaluation of current symptoms, preassault level of functioning, and the availability of a healthy support network. Such a detailed evaluation cannot always be obtained in the initial aftermath of an assault but should be completed at a later visit. If needed, provisions should be made for short-term safety. Preexisting psychiatric illnesses, if any, should be treated to reduce the risk for psychiatric decompensation. Although further psychotherapeutic follow-up is often declined, it is important to offer the sexual assault victim the open opportunity for psychiatric follow-up and assistance at a later time. The mental health clinician should provide an empathic "holding environment" in which the patient may safely recount her experience and the ways in which it has altered her sense of self and impairs her ability to function. If needed, medication may be useful to treat depression, posttraumatic stress disorder, or anxiety. Patients should be educated that although disturbing symptoms tend to dissipate over time, they may recur at times of future stress. In such cases a brief return to psychotherapy may be helpful. Female-specific issues associated with the evaluation and treatment of women who have been sexually assaulted are described in Table 36–2.

Domestic Violence

Up to 4 million women are assaulted by their partners each year (Council of Scientific Affairs 1992). The rate of assaults to women by present or former partners is higher than by all other assailants combined. About 7% of pregnant women are victims of domestic violence, and pregnant women who are abused tend to be beaten on the abdomen, in contrast to nonpregnant women who tend to be struck in the face (Stewart and Robinson 1995). In addition to the possibility of serious physical

TABLE 36–2. Special considerations in the evaluation and treatment of women who have been sexually assaulted

Component of examination	Issues to address
Review of symptoms	Assess current symptoms: physical tremulousness, diaphoresis, shortness of breath, palpitations
	Assess psychological symptoms: shock, numbness, withdrawal, isolativeness, denial
	Assess prolonged symptoms: startle reactions, disturbed sleep, fatigue, somatic complaints
	Assess long-term negative sequelae: sexual dysfunction, aversion, impaired interpersonal relationships, depression, posttraumatic stress disorder
Assessment of preassault level of functioning	Interpersonal relationships
	Financial stability
	School and work history
	Ability to cope in times of acute stress
Evaluation of available supports	Assess for short-term safety
	Assess for long-term support system
Evaluation of preassault illness	Preexisting psychiatric illness
	Past treatment
Treatment	If needed, facilitate provisions for short-term safety
	Treat preexisting, ongoing psychiatric illnesses
	Provide a safe place to review the assault and associated events
	Normalize negative effect on sense of self while acknowledging its negative impact
	Establish appropriate cognitive and behavioral mechanisms to restore function and therefore self-esteem
	Consider treatment with psychotropic medications to alleviate depression, posttraumatic stress disorder, anxiety disorder
	Explain that symptom recurrence may occur in the future
	Offer opportunity for psychiatric follow-up in the future

harm or death, female victims of domestic violence are at risk for serious psychological sequelae such as depression, anxiety, eating disorders, and alcoholism (Eisenstat and Bancroft 1999). Furthermore, children of battered mothers are also at risk for physical injury and are more likely to abuse substances, have school problems, exhibit violent and aggressive behaviors toward others or themselves, and experience impaired sleep, enuresis, and chronic somatic disorders (Eisenstat and Bancroft 1999).

Women are often reluctant to spontaneously disclose that they have been battered. It has been proposed that two screening questions should routinely be asked to detect domestic violence: "Do you ever feel unsafe at home?" and "Has anyone at home ever hit you or tried to injure you in any way?" (Eisenstat 1999). All clinicians should be able to provide patients with a list of local hospital and community resources for battered women (available by calling the national clearing house, 1-800-799-SAFE). Legal reporting requirements in the event that a patient is found to have been the victim of domestic abuse vary from state to state.

Typically, during a domestic assault, women fear for their lives. After the assault, experiences include shock, denial, isolation, confusion, psychological numbness, and fear. Long-term sequelae include disturbed sleep and appetite, startle responses, somatic complaints, fatigue, anxiety, and depression (Stewart and Robinson 1995). Treating clinicians should be aware that the existence of legal, financial, and shared parental responsibilities often makes it very difficult for women to leave the setting of their abuse. Treatment should be empathic and supportive. Pharmacotherapy may be needed to treat comorbid psychiatric conditions such as depression and anxiety and to facilitate movement out of the circle of danger. The initial therapeutic modality should be individual, because conjoint therapy tends to precipitate defensive behaviors. After the woman is in a safe setting, if there is the wish for possible resumption of an ongoing relationship between the woman and her partner, conjoint therapy should be instituted.

TABLE 36–3. Gender-specific differences in psychiatric disorders

Disorder	Ratios (female:male)	History, presentation, and course in women	Treatment issues in women
Schizophrenia	Approximately equal	Better premorbid history; more affective symptoms; more positive symptoms; small subgroup with onset in midlife	Better treatment response; increased risk of antipsychotic-induced hyperprolactinemia
Unipolar major depression, dysthymia	1.7:1	Increased risk of exacerbation at times of reproductive transition (i.e., premenstruum, postpartum, perimenopause)	SSRIs advisable in women of childbearing age (more data suggest safety in pregnancy and breast-feeding); early data suggest estrogen may be helpful in perimenopause
Bipolar disorder	Overall, approximately equal	More depressive episodes and more rapid cycling	Increased risk of lithium-induced hypothyroidism and postpartum destabilization
Anxiety disorders	Panic disorder 2.5:1 Social phobia 4:1 Generalized anxiety disorder 1.8:1	Increased risk for exacerbation at times of reproductive transition (i.e., premenstruum, postpartum, perimenopause, pregnancy [OCD])	Increased risk for thyroid disorders, which may produce symptoms similar to those of an anxiety disorder
Substance use disorders	Alcohol dependence 0.4:1 Alcohol abuse without dependence 0.5:1 Drug dependence 0.6:1 Drug abuse without dependence 0.6:1	More likely to develop alcohol-induced medical complications and more likely to become intoxicated	Pregnancy may offer a window for treatment as women have the additional motivation of fetal health
Eating disorders	Anorexia nervosa 10:1 Bulimia 11:1	Anorexia often associated with hypothalamic amenorrhea and secondary infertility	Pregnancy may offer a window for treatment as women have the additional motivation of fetal health
Sleep disorders	Slightly higher	Increased risk for exacerbation at times of reproductive transition (i.e., premenstruum, postpartum, perimenopause)	Differentiate sleep disorder from normative changes in sleep during pregnancy and postpartum or from sleep disruption due to menopausal vasomotor symptoms.

Note. OCD = obsessive-compulsive disorder; SSRI = selective serotonin reuptake inhibitor.

Sex Issues in the Treatment of Major Mental Illness

Although the incidence of schizophrenia does not differ between the sexes, the onset of the disorder tends to occur approximately 5 years later in women (age 20–29 years in women versus age 15–24 years in men). Furthermore, approximately 15% of women develop new-onset symptoms of schizophrenia in their mid-to-late 40s (J.M. Goldstein and Link 1988) (Table 36–3).

Women are less likely to have a poor premorbid history and tend to display more affective and positive symptoms and fewer negative symptoms than do men. Neuroanatomical studies suggest that structural brain abnormalities are more likely to be found in men than in women. More relatives of women with schizophrenia than those of men with schizophrenia are likely to develop the disorder. This suggests that heredity may be more important for women but that environment may play a relatively greater role for men.

Among sex-specific differences in the treatment of schizophrenia, women appear to be more responsive to treatment and to require lower doses of medication than do men. Thus, it has been suggested that estrogen, which in animals has antidopaminergic effects (Bedard et al.

1983), may protect against schizophrenia (Szymanski et al. 1995). This theory is supported by observations that schizophrenia worsens during low-estrogen phases of the menstrual cycle (Seeman and Lang 1990; Szymanski et al. 1995) and in perimenopausal years (Seeman 1986).

Hyperprolactinemia induced by certain antipsychotic agents (e.g., risperidone, haloperidol) frequently causes menstrual irregularities and amenorrhea. Amenorrhea tends to occur with prolactin levels greater than 60 ng/mL (normal prolactin levels = 5–25 ng/mL). If prolactin levels exceed 100 ng/mL, an endocrine consultation should be requested to assess the possibility of a pituitary adenoma.

For antipsychotic-induced hyperprolactinemia, consideration should be given to reducing the dose of medication. If the administered dose is necessary to control psychotic symptoms, the dopamine agonist bromocriptine (2.5–7.5 mg twice daily) or cabergoline (0.5 mg/week) may be given. A third approach is the use of an oral contraceptive, which has the triple effects of restoring menstrual cycle regularity, providing contraception, and protecting against the long-term hypoestrogenic effects of osteoporosis and heart disease.

Women with schizophrenia are at risk for pregnancy because of ineffective use of contraception and high rates of sexual assault. They should therefore be counseled about birth control and provided with behavioral approaches to avoid unwanted sexual advances.

Depression

Depression is more prevalent in women than men by a factor of 1.7 to 2 (Kessler et al. 1993, 1994). Dysthymia is twice as prevalent in women than in men (Kessler et al. 1994). Seasonal affective disorder is also more frequent in women than men (Rosenthal et al. 1992). It appears that women with a history of one or more reproductive-related depressive conditions (e.g., oral contraceptive–induced depression, postpartum depression, PMDD, perimenopausal depression) are at increased risk for other reproductive-related depressive episodes.

Women of childbearing age who are planning to become pregnant and are likely to need continued psychotropic treatment during pregnancy and the postpartum period are best placed on a medication whose safety is such that it will not be necessary to alter medications should pregnancy occur. For those women whose depressive condition occurs throughout the month but with premenstrual exacerbation, charting of symptoms is often a useful way to document those days when an increase in antidepressant dose or addition of another agent may protect recurrence of symptoms. Because

women with histories of depression are at substantial risk for postpartum-onset depression, consideration should be given to prophylactically initiating an antidepressant immediately upon delivery.

Bipolar Disorder

Bipolar disorder is equally prevalent in men and women. However, bipolar women experience more depressions and fewer manic episodes than bipolar men, and mixed states are more common in women than men. Rapid cycling is approximately twice as common in women than men (Tondo and Baldessarini 1998). Because women with bipolar disorder tend to experience recurrent depressions, they are often treated with antidepressants, and this treatment may account for their greater incidence of rapid cycling. Additionally, thyroid dysfunction is more common in women and may precipitate rapid cycling.

For some bipolar women, premenstrual relapse or exacerbation of symptoms occurs. Some reports have indicated that lithium levels fluctuate across the menstrual cycle (Hendrick et al. 1996). If symptoms change over the course of the menstrual cycle, serum lithium levels should be checked during symptomatic days, and adjustments in lithium dosage may be made accordingly.

Because the risk for hypothyroidism is greater for women than for men, particularly in the over-40 age group, women taking lithium should be monitored for thyroid dysfunction at least every 6 months. Carbamazepine induces hormone clearance and metabolism, thereby diminishing oral contraceptive efficacy. In addition, women who take carbamazepine and who receive HRT following menopause may require higher doses of estrogen to treat menopause-related vasomotor symptoms effectively.

Anxiety Disorders

Women are more likely than men to experience anxiety disorders, with comorbid depression being a common complication. Women are twice as likely as men to use anxiolytic medication, in large part because of the predominance of anxiety disorders in women (Baum et al. 1984). For example, women are twice as likely as men to suffer from posttraumatic stress disorder (Kessler et al. 1995) and two to three times as likely to experience panic disorder with agoraphobia (Schneier et al. 1992). Panic disorder with agoraphobia is more common in alcoholic women than alcoholic men (Task Force on Panic Anxiety and Its Treatments 1993). Although OCD prevalence rates are roughly equal between the sexes, the onset of the illness tends to be earlier in women than men (age 25 years in women versus age 20 years in men) (Flament and Rapoport 1984) and women tend to experience more obsessions related to food and weight than do men. The evaluation for anxiety should rule out medical conditions that mimic anxiety symptoms (e.g., cardiovascular disease, thyroid disorders, lupus, and iron deficiency anemia) (Yonkers and Gurguis 1995). Caffeine and nicotine also cause anxiety symptoms in some patients. Medications such as nonsteroidal decongestants, steroids, herbal supplements, and appetite suppressants may precipitate anxiety attacks. In some perimenopausal women, vasomotor symptoms (e.g., heat sensations, sweating, and shortness of breath) may be mistaken for panic attacks. Although lifetime exposure to traumatic events is approximately equal among men and women (Breslau et al. 1997), women are more likely than men to experience rape and sexual assault, whereas men experience more incidents of physical assault.

Substance Abuse

Although the prevalence of alcohol abuse is twice as high in men than in women (Blume 1994), it is not an uncommon disorder in women, with lifetime prevalence rates approximating 6% (Cyr et al. 1990). For an equal amount of alcohol per unit of body weight, women tend to become more intoxicated than men. Complications from alcohol abuse, such as peptic ulcer, liver disease, anemia, and cerebral atrophy, develop more quickly in women, and women are more likely to die from alcoholism than are men (Blume 1994). Risk factors for alcoholism in women include a history of sexual abuse, substance abuse, adult antisocial personality disorder, and depression.

Although hallucinogen and opiate abuse predominates in men, prevalence rates for cocaine and amphetamine abuse are equal. Women often use stimulants for weight control. Substance-abusing women are more likely to experience comorbid psychiatric disorders. Because many women drink to self-medicate premenstrual tension, it is important to assess for premenstrual symptoms in alcohol and drug use (Hendrick et al. 1996). Risk factors for drug abuse in women include a family history of substance abuse, antisocial personality disorder, depression, and being in a relationship with a drug-abusing or dependent partner.

Treatment of substance abuse includes referral to self-help groups such as Alcoholics Anonymous, Cocaine Anonymous, and the all-women support group Women for Sobriety. Family and marital conflicts should be evaluated and addressed carefully, because the likelihood of a woman remaining sober is often dependent on the sobriety of significant others.

Eating Disorders

Anorexia nervosa and bulimia occur in approximately 4% of the population, with over 90% of cases involving women (Becker et al. 1999). These disorders usually begin in adolescence. The symptoms of anorexia nervosa include body weight of less than 85% of expected for age and height; intense fear of gaining weight; distorted body image; and (in postmenarchal females) amenorrhea. Anorexia nervosa is subtyped as either restricting or binge-eating/purge type.

Bulimia nervosa involves repeated episodes of binge eating. Patients feel a lack of control over their eating and are excessively concerned about body image. To compensate for the food intake, patients fast; engage in excessive exercise; use laxatives, diuretics, or enemas; or self-induce vomiting. To meet the DSM-IV-TR criteria for the diagnosis of bulimia nervosa, the binge eating and compensatory behaviors occur at least twice a week for at least 3 months. The disorder is categorized as either purging type (i.e., involving the use of self-induced vomiting, laxatives, diuretics, or enemas) or nonpurging type. Anorexia and bulimia nervosa are frequently complicated by mood, anxiety, personality, and substance use disorders.

The evaluation of women with eating disorders should include assessments of body image; eating habits; actual and desired weight; menstrual patterns; exercise; self-induced vomiting; presence of other psychiatric disturbance; use of laxatives, diuretics, enemas, emetics, and diet pills; and abuse of alcohol and illicit substances. Medical complications that may result from anorexia and bulimia nervosa include electrocardiographic abnormalities, hypotension, atrial and ventricular arrhythmias, esophageal perforation, rectal prolapse, metabolic alkalosis, hypokalemia, amenorrhea, osteoporosis, erosion of dental enamel, parotid and submandibular gland hypertrophy, and anemia (Becker et al. 1999). Therefore, the evaluation should include a physical and dental examination. Laboratory tests should be obtained including albumin, total protein, and glucose levels (to help assess nutritional status), amylase levels (to assess the extent of self-induced vomiting), electrolytes, blood urea nitrogen, and creatinine. An electrocardiogram should be obtained because cardiac conduction abnormalities may result from electrolyte imbalance, malnutrition, and ipecac-induced cardiomyopathy.

The treatment of eating disorders requires an interdisciplinary team of mental health professionals, primary care physicians, nutritionists, and dentists. The initial treatment goal is to stabilize serious medical problems such as malnutrition and electrolyte imbalances. Nasogastric tube feeding may be necessary for life-threatening conditions. When the patient is medically stable, treatment should focus on establishing healthful eating patterns and examining the psychosocial factors contributing to the disorder (Becker et al. 1999). Psychosocial interventions include family counseling, individual/couples psychotherapy, education, and group support. Cognitive-behavioral therapy and interpersonal therapy have been effective for eating disorders, particularly bulimia nervosa (Becker et al. 1999). Serotonergic antidepressant medications at high doses (e.g., 60–80 mg of fluoxetine) have been helpful for bulimia nervosa (Leach 1995). MAOIs (e.g., phenelzine, isocarboxazid) have also been effective but should not be administered to patients with poor impulse control, because all tyramine-containing foods must be avoided.

Antidepressant medications have shown little promise in treating the behavioral symptoms of anorexia nervosa, although they are helpful for associated mood and anxiety disorders. TCAs can be helpful in promoting weight gain. Intensive treatment in an inpatient setting or day program is usually required for patients with anorexia nervosa. These settings allow patients' eating to be supervised and supported. Hospitalization will be necessary for patients who are refusing food or who experience severe medical complications.

Sleep Disorders

Women have a slightly higher rate of insomnia than men, partly because sleep-related difficulties occur more frequently during women's reproductive phases. Sleep disruptions can result from premenstrual cramping, physical discomfort in the third trimester of pregnancy, and perimenopausal night sweats (Millman 1999). Other common causes of insomnia include depression and anxiety disorders, medication side effects (e.g., bronchodilators, blood pressure medications, decongestants), alcohol, caffeine, nicotine, illicit drugs, and medical conditions (e.g., sleep apnea).

In the initial evaluation, the underlying cause of the insomnia should be determined. If the primary cause is a psychiatric or medical problem, this should be treated. The evaluation should also review the patient's daily use of caffeine, nicotine, and alcohol and the occurrence of daytime napping (Millman 1999). If sleep problems are associated with premenstrual discomfort, anti-inflammatory agents or low-dose oral contraceptives may help. For perimenopausal women experiencing sleep disruption as a result of night sweats, hormone replacement is effective (Polo-Kantola et al. 1999). When sleep-promoting interventions have not succeeded, hypnotic medications may be appropriate and include benzodiazepines, zolpidem, and zaleplon. These medications should be administered for short-term use to avoid risks of addiction and rebound insomnia. Sedating antidepressants (e.g., trazodone, doxepin) are another option for treating insomnia.

Female-Specific Cancers

Both breast cancer and gynecological cancers tend to be particularly stressful to women because they affect the organs of reproduction, sexuality, and femininity. Treatment strategies include surgery, radiation therapy, and chemotherapy. Sexual problems may emerge after treatment because of the direct physical effects of these modalities, fears of recurring cancer, or a decreased sense of femininity. Partners' attitudes are particularly important because women with these types of cancer need support and encouragement (Hamilton 1999).

A psychiatric consultation may be requested for women undergoing treatment for breast or gynecological cancer. For women in whom organic etiologies for mood disorders have been excluded, psychotherapy is a useful modality, particularly supportive or cognitive approaches to improve a sense of control. Standard antidepressant medications may be useful to increase appetite and sleep. Additionally, TCAs and SSRIs may be useful to reduce pain. Because tamoxifen may reduce serum TCAs (Jefferson 1995), for antidepressant-treated cancer patients who do not appear to be responding as well as expected, it is prudent to assess serum levels of parent and metabolite compounds and to compare these levels with pretamoxifen-treatment levels. If antidepressant medication is necessary for a tamoxifen-treated cancer patient, consideration should be given to increasing the dose of antidepressant to achieve clinical efficacy.

Many women with breast or gynecological cancer experience anxiety in response to the stress of difficult or uncomfortable treatment regimens and in response to a sense of loss of control with regard to exogenous stressors and toll of the illness. Guided imagery and progressive relaxation techniques, in conjunction with the use of low doses of anxiolytic medication, may be helpful in the acute phase of treatment. For sleep difficulties, reviewing the basic techniques of sleep hygiene are helpful; if insomnia persists, short-acting benzodiazepines or low-dose trazodone also may be useful. Women with cancer who have a history of alcohol or substance abuse or dependence are at risk for a recurrence. Encouraging these women to participate in lay advocacy groups (e.g., Alcoholics Anonymous or Narcotics Anonymous) and providing them with the opportunity to discuss their fear, anger, and sadness in individual therapy are particularly important. Women with breast or gynecological cancer sometimes experience a change in the quality of their sexual or marital relationships. For women whose surgery was extensive, their sense of sexuality and femininity may be called into question. Induced menopause secondary to radical hysterectomy or vasomotor symptoms due to tamoxifen may cause additional discomfort and may cause further sleep disruptions, with depression, irritability, and anxiety. Frequently, the partner also experiences a sense of loss and fear and may have difficulty viewing surgical or radiation scars. Conjoint education and counseling are often helpful.

Group support, in the form of advocacy groups such as Reach to Recovery or groups sponsored by the American Cancer Society, is helpful because it offers group members the opportunity to share common concerns, practical advice, and appreciation of the implications of having a diagnosis of cancer. Participation in support groups has been reported to improve 10-year survival rates for women with metastatic breast cancer (Spiegel et al. 1989).

Summary

When assessing and treating women with psychiatric disorders, it is important that clinicians recognize gender-specific issues related to diagnosis, course, and treatment. These gender-specific differences are undoubtedly due to a combination of biological, genetic, and psychosocial factors. Thus, psychopharmacological and psychotherapeutic treatment modalities should address the special and changing needs of women over the course of their lives.

References

Altshuler LL, Hendrick V: Pregnancy and psychotropic medication: changes in blood levels. J Clin Psychopharmacol 16:78–80, 1996

Altshuler LL, Post RM, Leverich GS, et al: Antidepressant-induced mania and cycle acceleration: a controversy revisited. Am J Psychiatry 152:1124–1129, 1995a

Altshuler LL, Hendrick V, Parry B: Pharmacologic management of premenstrual disorder. Harv Rev Psychiatry 2:223–245, 1995b

Altshuler LL, Cohen L, Szuba MP, et al: Pharmacologic management of psychiatric illness in pregnancy: dilemmas and guidelines. Am J Psychiatry 153:592–606, 1996

American Academy of Pediatrics Committee on Drugs: Transfer of drugs and other chemicals into human milk. Pediatrics 93:137–251, 1994

American Psychiatric Association: Diagnostic and Statistical Manual of Mental Disorders, 4th Edition, Text Revision. Washington, DC, American Psychiatric Association, 2000

Avis NE, McKinlay SM: A longitudinal analysis of women's attitudes towards menopause: results from the Massachusetts Women's Health Study. Maturitas 13:65–79, 1991

Avis NE, McKinlay SM: The Massachusetts Women's Health Study: an epidemiologic investigation of the menopause. J Am Med Womens Assoc 50:45–49, 1995

Bancroft J, Rennie D: The impact of oral contraceptives on the experience of perimenstrual mood, clumsiness, food craving and other symptoms. J Psychosom Res 37:195–202, 1993

Bancroft J, Sartorius N: The effects of oral contraceptives on well-being and sexuality. Oxford Review of Reproductive Biology 12:57–92, 1990

Baum C, Kennedy DL, Forbes MB, et al: Drug use in the United States in 1981. JAMA 251:1293–1297, 1984

Becker AE, Grinspoon SK, Klibanski A, et al: Eating disorders. N Engl J Med 340:1092–1098, 1999

Bedard P, Boucher R, DiPolo T, et al: Biphasic effect of estradiol and domperidone on lingual dyskinesia in monkeys. Exp Neurol 82:172–182, 1983

Blake F, Salkovskis P, Gath D, et al: Cognitive therapy for premenstrual syndrome: a controlled trial. J Psychosom Res 45:307–318, 1998

Blume SB: Gender differences in alcohol-related disorders. Harv Rev Psychiatry 2:7–14, 1994

Brent N, Wisner K: Fluoxetine and carbamazepine concentrations in a nursing mother/infant pair. Clin Pediatr 37:41–44, 1998

Breslau N, Davis GC, Anedereski P, et al: Sex differences in posttraumatic stress disorder in women. Arch Gen Psychiatry 54:1048–1060, 1997

Briggs GG, Freeman RK, Yaffe SJ: Drugs in Pregnancy and Lactation, 5th Edition. Baltimore, MD, Williams & Wilkins, 1998, pp 620–625

Burt VK, Suri R, Altshuler L, et al: The use of psychotropic medications during breast-feeding. Am J Psychiatry 158:1001–1009, 2001

Chambers CD, Johnson KA, Dick LM, et al: Birth outcomes in pregnant women taking fluoxetine. N Engl J Med 155:1010–1015, 1996

Cnattingius S, Signorello LB, Anneren G, et al: Caffeine intake and the risk of first-trimester spontaneous abortion. N Engl J Med 343:1839–1845, 2000

Cohen LS, Friedman JM, Jefferson JW, et al: A re-evaluation of risk of in utero exposure to lithium. JAMA 271:146–150, 1994

Council of Scientific Affairs: Violence against women: relevance for medical practitioners. JAMA 267:3184–3189, 1992

Cox JL, Murray D, Chapman G: A controlled study of the onset, duration and prevalence of postnatal depression. Br J Psychiatry 163:27–31, 1993

Cyr MG, Moulton AW: Substance abuse in women. Obstet Gynecol Clin North Am 17:905–925, 1990

Cyranowski JM, Frank E, Young E, et al: Adolescent onset of the gender differences in lifetime roles of major depression: a theoretical model. Arch Gen Psychiatry 57:21–27, 2000

Dagg PKB: The psychological sequelae of therapeutic abortion: denied and completed. Am J Psychiatry 148:578–585, 1991

Davidson J, Robertson E: A follow-up study of postpartum illness, 1946–1978. Acta Psychiatr Scand 71:451–457, 1985

Domar AD, Clapp D, Slwasby EA, et al: Impact of group psychological interventions on pregnancy rates in infertile women. Fertil Steril 73:805–811, 2000

Downey J, McKinney M: The psychiatric status of women presenting for infertility evaluation. Am J Orthopsychiatry 62:196–205, 1992

Dreifuss FE, Santilli N, Langer DH, et al: Valproic acid hepatic fatalities: a retrospective review. Neurology 37:370–385, 1987

Einarson A, Fatoye B, Sarker M, et al: Pregnancy outcome following gestational exposure to venlafaxine: a multicenter prospective controlled study. Am J Psychiatry 158:1728–1730, 2001

Eisenstat SA, Bancroft L: Domestic violence. N Engl J Med 341:886–892, 1999

Ericson A, Kullen B, Wilholm BE: Delivery outcome after the use of antidepressants in early pregnancy. Eur J Clin Pharmacol 55:503–508, 1999

Eriksson E: Serotonin reuptake inhibitors for the treatment of premenstrual dysphoria. Int Clin Psychopharmacol 14(suppl 2):S27–S33, 1999

Faedda GL, Tondo L, Baldessarini RJ, et al: Outcome after rapid versus gradual discontinuation of lithium treatment in bipolar disorders. Arch Gen Psychiatry 50:448–455, 1993

Flament MF, Rapoport JL: Childhood obsessive-compulsive disorder, in New Findings in Obsessive-Compulsive Disorder. Edited by Insel TR. Washington, DC, American Psychiatric Press, 1984, pp 23–43

Freeman W, Purdy RH, Coutifaris C, et al: Anxiolytic metabolites of progesterone: correlation with mood and performance measures following oral progesterone administration to healthy female volunteers. Clin Neuroendocrinol 58:478–484, 1993

Frey B, Schubiger G, Musy JP: Transient cholestatic hepatitis in a neonate associated with carbamazepine exposure during pregnancy and breastfeeding. Eur J Pediatr 150:136–138, 1990

Frye AA, Atrash HK, Lawson HW, et al: Induced abortion in the United States: a 1994 update. J Am Med Womens Assoc 49:131–136, 1994

Gold LH: Use of psychiatric medication during pregnancy: risk management guidelines. Psychiatr Ann 30:421–432, 2000

Goldstein DJ: Effects of third trimester fluoxetine exposure on the newborn. J Clin Psychopharmacol 15:417–420, 1995

Goldstein DJ, Corbin LA, Fung MC: Olanzapine-exposed pregnancies and lactation: early experience. J Clin Psychopharmacol 20:399–403, 2000

Goldstein JM, Link BG: Gender and the expression of schizophrenia. J Psychiatr Res 22:141–155, 1988

Graham CA, Sherwin BB: A prospective treatment study of premenstrual symptoms using a triphasic oral contraceptive. J Psychosom Res 36:257–266, 1992

Grof P, Robbins W, Aloda M, et al: Protective effect of pregnancy in women with lithium-responsive bipolar disorder. J Affect Disord 61:31–39, 2001

Guzick DS, Carson SA, Coutifaris C, et al: Efficacy of superovulation and intrauterine insemination in the treatment of infertility. National Cooperative Reproductive Medicine Network. N Engl J Med 340:177–183, 1999

Hamilton AB: Psychological aspects of ovarian cancer. Cancer Invest 17:335–341, 1999

Hendrick V, Altshuler LL, Burt VK: Course of psychiatric disorders across the menstrual cycle. Harv Rev Psychiatry 4:200–207, 1996

Jefferson JW: Tamoxifen-associated reduction in tricyclic antidepressant levels in blood. J Clin Psychopharmacol 15:223–224, 1995

Jones HW, Toner JP: The infertile couple. N Engl J Med 23:1710–1715, 1993

Kaufert PA, Gilbert P, Tate R: The Manitoba Project: a reexamination of the link between menopause and depression. Maturitas 14:143–155, 1992

Kaunitz AM: Long-acting hormonal contraception: assessing impact on bone density, weight, and mood. Intl J Fertil Womens Med 44:110–117, 1999

Kendell RE, Chalmers JC, Platz C: Epidemiology of puerperal psychoses. Br J Psychiatry 150:662–673, 1987

Kendler KS, Martin NS, Heath AC, et al: A twin study of the psychiatric side effects of oral contraceptives. J Nerv Ment Dis 176:153–160, 1988

Kessler RC, McGonagle KA, Swartz M, et al: Sex and depression in the National Comorbidity Survey, I: lifetime prevalence, chronicity, and recurrence. J Affect Disord 19:85–96, 1993

Kessler RC, McGonagle KA, Zhao S, et al: Lifetime and 12-month prevalence of DSM-III-R psychiatric disorders in the United States: results from the National Comorbidity Survey. Arch Gen Psychiatry 51:8–19, 1994

Kessler RC, Sonnega A, Bromet E, et al: Posttraumatic stress disorder in the National Comorbidity Survey. Arch Gen Psychiatry 52:1048–1060, 1995

Kimmel S, Gonsalves L, Youngs D, et al: Fluctuating levels of antidepressants. J Psychosom Obstet Gynaecol 2:109–115, 1992

Kulin NA, Pastuszak A, Sage SR, et al: Pregnancy outcome following maternal use of the new selective serotonin reuptake inhibitors: a prospective controlled multicenter study. JAMA 279:609–610, 1998

LaPane KL, Zierler S, Lasater TM, et al: Is a history of depressive symptoms associated with an increased risk of infertility in women? Psychosom Med 57:509–513, 1995

Leach AM: The psychopharmacotherapy of eating disorders. Psychiatr Ann 25:454–462, 1995

Lyons-Ruth K, Wolfe R, Lyubchik A: Depression and the parenting of young children: making the case for early preventive mental health services. Harv Rev Psychiatry 8:148–153, 2000

Matthews KA, Wing RA, Kuller LH: Influences of natural menopause on psychological characteristics and symptoms of middle-aged healthy women. J Consult Clin Psychol 58:345–351, 1990

McCartney CF, Downey J: New reproductive technologies, in Medical Psychiatric Practice. Edited by Stoudemire A, Fogel PS. Washington, DC, American Psychiatric Press, 1993, p 302

McElhatton PR, Garebis HM, Eléfant et al: The outcome of pregnancy in 689 women exposed to therapeutic doses of antidepressants: a collaborative study of the European Network of Teratology Information Service (ENTS). Reprod Toxicol 10:285–289, 1996

McGlone J: Sex differences in human brain asymmetry: a critical survey. Behav Brain Sci 3:215–263, 1980

Merlob P, Mor N, Litwin A: Transient hepatic dysfunction in an infant of an epileptic mother treated with carbamazepine during pregnancy and breastfeeding. Ann Pharmacother 26:1563–1565, 1992

Michaud CM, Murray CJL, Bloom BR: Burden of disease: implications for future research. JAMA 285:535–539, 2001

Miller LJ: Psychiatric medication during pregnancy: understanding and minimizing risks. Psychiatr Ann 24:69–75, 1994a

Miller LJ: Use of electroconvulsive therapy during pregnancy. Hosp Community Psychiatry 45:444–450, 1994b

Millman RP: Coping with insomnia: effective drug and non-drug therapies. Women's Health in Primary Care 1:737–745, 1999

Morrelli MJ: The new antiepileptic drugs and women: efficacy, reproductive health, pregnancy and fetal outcome. Epilepsia 37(suppl):34–44, 1996

Murray L: Postpartum depression and child development. Psychol Med 27:253–260, 1997

Ness RB, Grisso JA, Hirschinger N, et al: Cocaine and tobacco use and the risk of spontaneous abortion. N Engl J Med 340:333–339, 1999

Nulman I, Rovet J, Stewart DE, et al: Neurodevelopment of children exposed in utero to antidepressant drugs. N Engl J Med 336:258–262, 1997

Neugebauer R, Kline J, Shrout P, et al: Major depressive disorder in the 6 months after miscarriage. JAMA 27:383–388, 1997

O'Hara MW: Postpartum Depression: Causes and Consequences. Edited by O'Hara MW. New York, Springer-Verlag, 1995, pp 168–194

O'Hara MW, Schlechte JA, Lewis DA, et al: Prospective study of postpartum blues. Arch Gen Psychiatry 48:801–806, 1991

Ohman I, Vitols S, Tomson T: Lamotrigine in pregnancy: pharmacokinetics during delivery in the neonate and during lactation. Epilepsia 41:709–713, 2000

Pearlstein TB, Stone AB, Lund SA, et al: Comparison of fluoxetine, bupropion and placebo in the treatment of premenstrual dysphoric disorder. J Clin Psychopharmacol 17:261–266, 1999

Polo-Kantola P, Erkkola R, Irjala K, et al: Effect of short-term transdermal estrogen replacement therapy on sleep: a randomized, double-blind crossover trial in postmenopausal women. Fertil Steril 71:873–880, 1999

Rohde A, Marneros A: Postpartum psychoses: onset and long-term course. Psychopathology 26:203–209, 1993

Rosenthal NE, Sack DA, Gillin JC, et al: Seasonal affective disorder: a description of the syndrome and preliminary findings with light therapy. Arch Gen Psychiatry 53:289–292, 1992

Schairer C, Lubin J, Troisi R, et al: Menopausal estrogen and estrogen-progestin replacement therapy and breast cancer risk. JAMA 283:485–491, 2000

Schmidt PJ, Nieman L, Danaceau MA, et al: Estrogen replacement in perimenopause-related depression: a preliminary report. Am J Obstet Gynecol 183:414–420, 2000

Schneier FR, Johnson J, Hornig CD, et al: Social phobia: comorbidity and morbidity in an epidemiologic sample. Arch Gen Psychiatry 49:282–288, 1992

Schrott HG, Bittner V, Vittinnghoff E, et al: Adherence to National Cholesterol Education Program Treatment goals in postmenopausal women with heart disease. The Heart and Estrogen/Progestin Replacement Study (HERS). The HERS Research Group. JAMA 277:1281–1286, 1997

Seeman MV: Current outcome in schizophrenia: women versus men. Acta Psychiatr Scand 73:609–617, 1986

Seeman MV, Lang ML: The role of estrogens in schizophrenia gender differences. Schizophr Bull 16:185–194, 1990

Shear MK, Mammen O: Anxiety disorders in pregnant and postpartum women. Psychopharmacol Bull 31:603–703, 1995

Sherwin BB: Affective changes with estrogen and androgen replacement therapy in surgically menopausal women. J Affect Disord 14:177–187, 1988

Sherwin BB: Up-regulatory effect of estrogen on platelet ^{3}H-imipramine binding sites in surgically menopausal women. Biol Psychiatry 28:339–348, 1990

Spiegel D, Bloom JR, Kraemer HC, et al: Effect of psychosocial treatment on survival of patients with metastatic breast cancer. Lancet 2:888–891, 1989

Stahl MMS, Neiderud J, Vinge E: Thrombocytopenic purpura and anemia in a breast-fed infant whose mother was treated with valproic acid. J Pediatr 130:1001–1003, 1997

Steer RA, Scholl TO, Hediger ML, et al: Self-reported depression and negative pregnancy outcomes. J Clin Epidemiol 45:1093–1099, 1992

Steiner M, Steinberg S, Stewart D, et al: Fluoxetine in the treatment of premenstrual dysphoria. N Engl J Med 332:1529–1534, 1995

Stephens EH, Chandra A: Updated projections of infertility in the United States: 1995–2025. Fertil Steril 70:30–34, 1998

Stewart DE, Boydell KM: Psychologic distress during menopause: associations across the reproductive life cycle. Int J Psychiatry Med 23:157–162, 1993

Stewart DE, Robinson GE: Violence against women, in American Psychiatric Press Review of Psychiatry, Vol 14. Washington DC, American Psychiatric Press, 1995, p 271

Stoner SC, Sommi RW, Marken PA, et al: Clozapine use in two full-term pregnancies. J Clin Psychiatry 58:364–365, 1997

Szymanski S, Lieberman JA, Alvir JM, et al: Gender differences in onset of illness, treatment response, course, and biologic indexes in first-episode schizophrenic patients. Am J Psychiatry 152:698–703, 1995

Task Force on Panic Anxiety and Its Treatments: Panic anxiety and panic disorder, in Panic Anxiety and Its Treatments. Edited by Klerman GL, Hirschfield RMA, Weissman MM, et al. Washington, DC, American Psychiatric Press, 1993, pp 3–38

Thys-Jacobs S: Micronutrients and the premenstrual syndrome: the case for calcium. J Am Coll Nutr 2:220–227, 2000

Tondo L, Baldessarini RJ: Rapid cycling in women and men with bipolar manic-depressive disorders. Am J Psychiatry 155:1434–1436, 1998

Trimble MR: Anticonvulsants in children and adolescents. J Child Adolesc Psychopharmacol 1:107–124, 1990

Trixler M, Tenyi T: Antipsychotic use during pregnancy: what are the best treatment outcomes? Drug Safety 16:403–410, 1997

Videbech P, Gouliaev G: First admission with puerperal psychosis: 7–14 years of follow up. Acta Psychiatr Scand 91:167–173, 1995

Viguera AC, Nomacs R, Cohen LS, et al: Risk of recurrence of bipolar disorder in pregnant and nonpregnant women after discontinuing lithium maintenance. Am J Psychiatr 157:179–184, 2000

Villablanca AC: HRT and cardiovascular risk in women: where do we stand? Women's Health Primary Care 4:121–129, 2001

Vogel W, Klaiber EL, Broverman DM: The role of gonadal steroid hormones in psychiatric depression in men and women. Prog Neuropsychopharmacol 2:487–503, 1978

von Unruh GE, Froescher W, Hoffman F, et al: Valproic acid in breast milk: how much is really there? Ther Drug Monit 6:272–276, 1984

Weissman MM, Bruce MI, Leaf PJ, et al: Affective disorders, in Psychiatric Disorders in America. Edited by Robins LN, Regier DA. New York, Free Press, 1991, pp 53–80

Westhoff C, Wieland D, Tiezzi L: Depression in users of depo-medroxyprogesterone acetate. Contraception 51:351–354, 1995

Wikander I, Sundblad C, Anderssch B, et al: Citalopram in premenstrual dysphoria: is intermittent treatment during luteal phases more effective than continuous medication throughout the menstrual cycle? J Clin Psychopharmacol 18:390–398, 1998

Wisner KL, Wheeler SB: Prevention of recurrent postpartum major depression. Hosp Community Psychiatry 45:1191–1196, 1994

Wisner KL, Perel JM, Peindl KS, et al: Prevention of recurrent postpartum depression: a randomized clinical trial. J Clin Psychiatry 62:82–86, 2001

Wyatt KM, Dimmock PW, Jones PW, et al: Efficacy of vitamin B-6 in the treatment of premenstrual syndrome: systematic review. Br Med J 318:1375–1381, 1999

Yonkers KA, Bradshaw KD: Hormonal replacement and oral contraceptive therapy: do they induce or treat mood symptoms? in Gender Differences in Mood and Anxiety Disorders. Edited by Liebenluft E. Washington, DC, American Psychiatric Press, 1999, pp 91–135

Yonkers KA, Gurguis H: Gender differences in the prevalence and expression of anxiety disorders, in Gender and Psychopathology. Edited by Seeman MV. Washington DC, American Psychiatric Press, 1995, p 120

Yonkers KA, Gullion CA, Williams A, et al: Paroxetine as a treatment for premenstrual dysphoric disorder. J Clin Psychopharmacol 16:3–8, 1996

Yonkers KA, Halbreich U, Freeman E, et al: Symptomatic improvement of premenstrual dysphoric disorder with sertraline treatment. JAMA 278:983–988, 1997

Zolese G, Blacker CVR: The psychological complications of therapeutic abortion. Br J Psychiatry 160:742–749, 1992

Geriatric Psychiatry

Dan G. Blazer, M.D., Ph.D.

Psychiatrists who work with older adults encounter diagnostic and therapeutic problems that are more complex than those encountered in young-adult and middle-aged patients. Most older patients with psychiatric disorders do not fit easily into the diagnostic categories of DSM-IV (American Psychiatric Association 1994) because they experience multiple symptoms that affect both physical and psychiatric functioning. This is especially true when treating the oldest members of this population (Blazer 2000). Once the problem is formulated by the clinician, usual treatment approaches must be modified both to manage the functional disability that results from the psychiatric problem and to reverse the underlying disorder.

Multiple system involvement and functional impairment are not unique to geriatric psychiatry. Geriatricians must manage equally complex disease presentations that involve a range of dysfunctions, from the molecular to the psychosocial. For example, the onset of type 2 diabetes mellitus in an older adult disrupts not only glucose metabolism but also lifelong patterns of food intake and exercise. Educational and psychotherapeutic interventions, as well as diet and medication prescription, are necessary to treat the patient successfully. Type 2 diabetes cannot be cured, so the goal for the clinician is to maintain overall function of the older adult in the presence of the chronic illness.

In an era in which specific disorders are emphasized, psychiatrists working with older adults can benefit from the syndromal approach to impairment, a paradigm shift developed by geriatricians to structure diagnostic and therapeutic strategies for older patients. Geriatricians deemphasize specific *diagnoses* and concentrate instead on *geriatric syndromes*, including incontinence, dizziness, falling, failure to thrive, and constipation. In this chapter, I follow this syndromal approach by identifying seven psychiatric syndromes that are most prevalent among older individuals—acute confusion, memory loss, insomnia, anxiety, suspiciousness, depression, and hypochondriasis—and describing them within the context of managing the resultant impairment (Table 37–1). Because the psychiatric disorders that contribute to these syndromes are described elsewhere in this text, emphasis will be placed on the aspects of the syndromes that are unique to late life and on the management of the older adult with these syndromes.

TABLE 37–1.   Geriatric psychiatric syndromes

Acute confusion	Memory loss
Insomnia	Anxiety
Suspiciousness	Depression
Hypochondriasis	

Acute Confusion

Acute confusion, or delirium, is a transient organic brain syndrome characterized by acute onset and global impairment of cognitive function. The older person with acute confusion exhibits a decreased ability to maintain attention to environmental stimuli and has difficulty shifting attention from one set of stimuli to another. Thinking is disorganized, speech becomes rambling, and a decreased level of consciousness is exhibited. Emotional disturbances often, but not always, accompany acute confusion and may be the presenting problem in late life. These emotional disturbances include anxiety, fear, irritability, and anger. Some older persons, in contrast, are apathetic and withdrawn during an episode of delirium and thus are much more difficult to diagnose (this is sometimes called *hypoactive delirium*). Acute confusion, by definition, is brief, usually lasting a few hours but possibly lasting weeks, such as in the case of confusion secondary to medications.

The frequency of delirium among the older population is difficult to estimate because many episodes are undetected due to their brevity. Most estimates of incidence range from 15% to 25% on medical and surgical wards (Martin et al. 2000). The incidence is higher on intensive care units and among persons recovering from cardiovascular surgery. When delirium is diagnosed in a hospitalized older patient, the hospitalization is usually prolonged, and both in-hospital and posthospital mortality rates are increased. Mortality at 2-year follow-up nears 50%.

Acute confusion in late life is the common outcome of a cascade of biological, cognitive, and environmental contributors. Biological brain function declines with age, although functional capacity varies greatly within age groups. Degenerative changes, such as those characteristic of Alzheimer's disease, render the older person more susceptible to physiological changes secondary to aging and disease. These physiological changes include drug intoxication, electrolyte disturbance, infection, dehydration, hypoalbuminemia, and hypoxia. Visual and hearing impairment may also contribute to delirium. For example, an older adult with early primary degenerative dementia and loss of eyesight may experience congestive heart failure. The vulnerable nervous system cannot adapt to the decreased delivery of oxygen and glucose during failure because of a decreased reserve capacity, and acute confusion emerges. Common external biological stressors that precipitate acute confusion in older adults at risk are listed in Table 37–2.

Cognitive contributors to delirium include a predisposition to hallucinations and delusions, such as that in an aging patient with a history of schizophrenia. Environmental contributors include the unfamiliar surroundings of a hospital or long-term care facility and social isolation. Therefore, the hospital, where the convergence of these contributors is likely, is a high-risk environment for delirium. Additional factors that may contribute to delirium in the hospital include physical restraint and bladder catheter use (Inouye 2000).

General therapy for the confused older individual, to be administered in parallel with specific therapy for the underlying cause of the acute confusion, begins with medical support. Vital signs and level of consciousness should be closely monitored. All medications that are not critical should be discontinued. Vasopressor agents may be needed to increase blood pressure, and excessive fever should be treated with ice baths and alcohol sponges. When the syndrome of acute confusion is recognized and the precipitant of the confusion is established through history, physical examination, and laboratory studies, the clinician can begin therapy. Acute confusion may present

TABLE 37–2. Common external biological stressors that precipitate acute confusion in the at-risk older adult

Intoxication
Drugs (anticholinergic agents, sedative-hypnotics, anxiolytics, hypertensive agents)
Alcohol
Withdrawal symptoms
Medications (sedative, hypnotic, anxiolytic)
Alcohol
Metabolic disorders
Hypoxia
Hypoglycemia
Failure of vital organs, such as the liver and kidney
Nutritional disorders
Vitamin deficiency (thiamine, vitamin B_{12}, folate)
Fluid and electrolyte imbalance
Dehydration
Alkalosis or acidosis
Hypernatremia or hyponatremia
Endocrine disorders
Hyperthyroidism or hypothyroidism
Addison's disease or Cushing's syndrome
Pituitary hypofunction
Cardiovascular disorders
Congestive heart failure
Cardiac arrhythmia
Myocardial infarction
Infections
Pneumonia
Influenza
AIDS
Physical injury
Hyperthermia or hypothermia

as a psychiatric emergency that threatens permanent brain damage. Severe hypoglycemia, hypoxia, and hyperthermia are examples of critical conditions that may present as acute confusion. Therefore, the initial treatment should include the establishment of an adequate airway to ensure that the patient is breathing and the administration of 100 mL 50% dextrose plus 100 mg thiamine intravenously if hypoglycemia and Wernicke's encephalopathy cannot be ruled out.

The clinician also must pay special attention to reducing the demands that excess and conflicting environmental stimuli make on the patient's cerebral function. Order and simplicity in the environment are critical to the management of the confused older patient, who should be maintained in a quiet, simply furnished, and well-lighted room. Lights should be left on at night. Care can best be facilitated by constant attention from familiar persons such as family members, who should frequently orient the patient to time, place, and person. Physicians, nurses, and other hospital personnel should explain all procedures. Restraints should be kept to a minimum. Behavioral agitation generally can be managed by judicious use of antipsychotic medications, such as risperidone, in low doses (administered either intramuscularly or orally).

Memory Loss

The syndrome of memory loss (the dementia syndrome) is one of the more frequent and disabling syndromes experienced by older adults. Late-life memory loss is usually accompanied by a more or less sustained decline in cognitive function from a previously obtained intellectual level, usually with an insidious onset. Other cognitive capacities that decline with memory include language (such as aphasia), spatial or temporal orientation, judgment, executive function, and abstract thought. State of consciousness is usually not altered until very late in the memory loss syndrome, which is in contrast with acute confusion.

Disabling memory loss may begin in midlife, but it is much more frequent in persons older than age 75 years than in those between ages 65 and 74. Prevalence estimates from community samples of memory impairment are generally 5%–15%, with most investigators estimating memory impairment in at least 10% of persons older than age 65 years in the community and in 30%–50% of institutional residents (Small et al. 1997). Alzheimer's disease (AD), the most common disorder contributing to the dementia syndrome, has been estimated to be prevalent in 6%–8% of community-based persons older than age 65 years, with more than 30% of persons age 85 years or older having AD. Prevalence estimates of AD include both mild and severe cases, so significant memory impairment may be found in only a proportion of persons identified as having the condition in community samples. Other causes of memory loss include vascular dementia, Lewy body dementia, dementia associated with Parkinson's disease, and alcohol-related dementias. Although the clinical presentation of memory loss does not always provide clear evidence for the etiology, there are some distinguishing characteristics, such as the increase in visual hallucinations in Lewy body dementia.

Memory loss is usually progressive with the prevalence doubling every 5 years after the age of 60 years. Until age 75, the life expectancy of persons with AD or vascular dementia is reduced by about one-half. After age 75, life expectancy is less affected by memory loss. Some dementing disorders, however, do not lead to inevitable decline in function. For example, alcohol-induced amnestic disorder can be arrested if the older person stops drinking and returns to a nutritional diet. Even those persons who have AD and vascular dementias may experience significant decline over an interval, only to enter a plateau in functioning for a subsequent interval that may last for many months.

More than 50% of persons with chronic memory loss will, at autopsy, exhibit the changes of AD only. The next most common contributors to the syndrome are the vascular dementias, especially vascular dementia. Clinically and pathophysiologically, it is difficult to disaggregate the vascular dementias. (For example, it is difficult to distinguish vascular dementia from Binswanger's disease.) Vascular dementia also frequently is comorbid with AD (Tomlinson et al. 1970). In contrast to AD, however, vascular dementia is more common in males than in females. Many patients with Parkinson's disease develop brain changes late in the course of their disease similar to those changes found in AD. Clinically, except for their parkinsonian symptoms, these patients cannot be distinguished from those with AD. In addition, many patients with AD exhibit changes in the substantia nigra at autopsy. Approximately 5% of older persons experience memory loss as a result of alcohol-induced amnestic disorder.

The primary risk factors for AD are age and family history, with the prevalence of AD, as mentioned previously, being an exponential function of age. Other risk factors for AD include Down's syndrome, head trauma, and possibly lack of education. Use of statins and/or nonsteroidal anti-inflammatory agents (NSAIDS) may be protective. Genetic risk factors have received much attention in recent years, especially the relationship between the disease and apolipoprotein E (*APOE*) genotype (Roses 1994) The *APOE* genotype expresses itself in three alleles (2, 3, and 4). Persons with an *APOE* genotype of 4/4 are at much greater risk for developing AD than are those with a 2/2 genotype, with a range of risk between the most vulnerable (4/4) and the most protective (2/2). Much less common forms of AD have been linked to chromosome 12 among other chromosome sites. Most cases of AD, however, cannot be attributed to one etiological agent. Male sex, hypertension, and possibly black race are risk factors for vascular dementia. Alcohol use regularly over many years is the primary cause of alcohol-induced amnestic disorder.

The diagnostic workup of the older adult with memory loss begins with a history, the most important component of the evaluation. A history should be obtained from both family members and the patient. The nature and severity of memory loss should be assessed in conjunction with a chronological account of the onset of the older adult's problems and specific behavioral changes. Patient and family should be asked about common problems resulting from memory loss, such as becoming lost in a familiar place, having difficulties with driving, becoming repetitive, and losing objects. Medical history should include inquiries about relevant systemic diseases, trauma, surgery, psychiatric problems, diet, and alcohol and drug use. (A thorough documentation of prescription and over-the-counter drugs is essential.) Family history should include questions about relatives who have memory loss, Down syndrome, alcohol problems, and psychiatric disorders. The physical examination should include not only a thorough neurological examination but also a general physical workup to determine the health of the patient.

The nature and degree of the cognitive dysfunction should be assessed by both a thorough mental status examination and objective cognitive testing. Standardized mental status examinations such as the Mini-Mental State Examination (MMSE; Folstein et al. 1975) and the Blessed Information-Memory-Concentration Test (Blessed et al. 1968) are available and are useful quantitative means of documenting memory loss at the initial evaluation.

The in-office or hospital-based initial assessment of memory and cognitive functioning is followed by a more in-depth evaluation of cognition with instruments such as the Reitan Battery, the Trail-Making Test, and tests of functions such as delayed recall and spatial ability (Reitan 1955). Performance on short screening and on more in-depth neuropsychological testing provides a baseline from which decline in function and/or response to therapeutic intervention can be determined. Laboratory tests to assess memory loss, such as that seen in AD, are listed in Table 37–3. Genotyping a patient with AD or a patient's family members cannot be justified at this time, despite the emerging evidence of a hereditary predisposition for certain genotypes such as *APOE 4/4*.

The purpose of the comprehensive diagnostic workup of the older adult with memory loss is to establish the baseline functional impairment as well as to rule out reversible causes of the dementia syndrome. Although screening for reversible causes is essential, the yield from many of these tests is sparse. Reports suggesting that a large percentage of patients who initially see clinicians because of memory loss experience a return to previous function with treatment are misleading.

Most pharmacological therapies are based on the cholinergic hypothesis of memory and include primarily cholinesterase inhibitors. Tacrine, donepezil, and rivastigmine are available to physicians in office-based practice. These drugs have proven moderately effective in reducing decline in memory up to 1 year after administration. Other strategies used frequently with less objective evidence of efficacy include the use of NSAIDS in low doses,

TABLE 37–3. Laboratory tests to assess memory loss

Standard diagnostic tests

Complete blood count, electrolyte panel, screening metabolic panel, thyroid function test (T3, T4, free thyroxine index, thyroid-stimulating hormone)

Vitamin B_{12} and folate levels

Tests for syphilis

Urinalysis

Elective tests

Magnetic resonance imaging or computed tomography (computed tomography scans are usually adequate)

Electroencephalogram

Formal neuropsychological assessment

Cerebral blood flow studies

Lumbar puncture

Event-related potentials

estrogen replacement therapy, and antioxidants such as vitamin E. Patients in late life who have memory loss may be referred to specialized centers (memory disorder clinics) where they can be evaluated and, if they meet criteria, enrolled in a clinical trial where they may receive a number of experimental agents, including estrogens.

Psychotropic medications are used extensively in patients with memory loss, primarily because of secondary symptoms such as verbal or physical aggression, anxiety, depression, psychoses, and severe agitation or regressive behavior. Other secondary behaviors, however, such as wandering, inappropriate verbalization, repetitive activities (touching), obstinacy in following suggestions or commands, hoarding materials, stealing, and inappropriate voiding, are not as amenable to medication. Therefore, the first step for the clinician treating the patient with memory loss is to assess what symptoms might be responsive to a medication.

After determining that the emerging behavioral problem cannot be handled through nonpharmacological means and is ongoing, medication should be prescribed. The specifics of medication use can be found in other portions of this textbook. Agitation and anxiety can be treated with antianxiety agents (such as short-acting benzodiazepines), neuroleptics (such as risperidone and olanzapine), anticonvulsants (such as carbamazepine), β-blockers, lithium, buspirone, and occasionally low doses of antidepressant agents (such as trazodone) at night. Clonazepam has been reported to be of benefit in agitated patients with vascular dementia; however, the episodic mood swings and acute confusion that often accompany such dementia are not as responsive to medications.

The neuroleptics are the most effective psychotropic agents for controlling severe agitation, aggressive behavior, and psychoses. Most neuroleptics are effective but produce side effects, and therefore, the selection of a drug is usually determined by the side effect profile least adverse for a given patient. For this reason the new-generation antipsychotic agents such as olanzapine and risperidone are the preferred drugs at present. The most troublesome side effects that ensue from using neuroleptic agents are postural hypotension (and the risk of falling) and tardive dyskinesia. These side effects may be avoided by using agents such as buspirone and carbamazepine, although the potency of these agents is lower than that of the neuroleptics.

Because depression (even the syndrome of major depression) is frequent among patients with chronic memory loss, the use of an antidepressant agent is often indicated. In general, the antidepressant agent will not lead to an improvement in memory. Postural hypotension and anticholinergic side effects are the major concern when using the antidepressant medications. For this reason, selective serotonin reuptake inhibitors (SSRIs) are usually preferred.

Whatever medication is prescribed to the older adult with memory loss, it should be tapered slowly on a periodic basis to determine whether the medication continues to be required. If the drug is not required, then an unnecessary and potentially dangerous drug can be eliminated from the medication regimen. Careful documentation of the target symptoms for the medication and monitoring of the effectiveness of the medication in reversing these symptoms assists physicians and nursing staff in identifying drugs that can be discontinued.

Behavioral management of the patient with memory loss not only is useful to the patient but also provides the patient's family with a sense of accomplishment in the presence of an illness that tends to leave families feeling helpless and bewildered. The family and the physician should develop behaviors that promote both patient and family security. Familiar routines and consistent repetition of instructions usually enhance security. The family, as much as possible, should provide moments of fun with the patient, even when these brief moments of relief are quickly forgotten by the patient. Families can substitute for the patient's lost abilities by performing tasks for the patient such as putting out clothes in the morning. Families should not hesitate to "do for" these patients, because patients with memory loss are truly more dependent than other elderly persons. Families must also compensate for the loss of impulse control that accompanies memory loss. One means is distraction; the patient who is about to remove his or her clothes or masturbate in public can be distracted with conversation or by being asked to walk with a family member. Patients with mem-

ory loss can usually assist in household tasks, even when the disorder is moderately severe. Although the older adult with memory loss cannot prepare a meal alone, he or she can work with the spouse or other family members in routine tasks.

Management of memory loss must include a review of the patient's environment for problems in safety. Typical safety problems include becoming lost, wandering into busy traffic, erratic or accidental use of medicines, falls (secondary to poor lighting or slippery surfaces), accidents while driving, and leaving things unattended (such as leaving appliances turned on). Home visits by geriatric nurse specialists are most hopeful in reviewing the household for potential problems.

Perhaps the most important long-term component for managing the older adult with memory loss is support of the family. Families are the primary caregivers of elderly persons with memory loss until the memory loss becomes severe enough to lead to institutionalization. With proper support, the older person can remain at home for a longer period of time and the family can function more effectively in the midst of the devastation of the severe memory loss. Education of the family about the expected progression of memory loss and the many behaviors that accompany such loss but that may not be intuitively recognized as resulting from the illness, is key to family support. Excellent educational materials are available and support groups are located throughout the world to assist the family of the patient with memory loss. In addition, families must be monitored for caregiver stress. If the clinician is not sensitive to the potential for stress in caregivers, then family members may exceed their limits and experience burnout, which could lead to neglect and/or abuse of the older adult. Respite for the caregiver, education, and therapy are essential in keeping the care system operative.

Insomnia

Insomnia is more frequent in the elderly population than in any other age group; 28% report difficulty falling asleep and 46% report symptoms of difficulty both falling asleep and staying asleep and use of more sedative-hypnotic medications (Foley et al. 1995). Both the lack of sleep and the subsequent medication use frequently lead to deterioration in daytime alertness and functioning. The most common sleep disturbances leading to insomnia in the elderly are

1. Primary insomnia, which is a persistent difficulty in initiating and maintaining sleep that is not related to

another mental disorder or known organic factor
2. Sleep-disordered breathing (i.e., sleep apnea)
3. Nocturnal myoclonus, or periodic leg movements that disturb sleep
4. Sleep–wake schedule disorder, which is a mismatch between the normal sleep–wake schedule for the elderly person's environment and his or her sleep–wake pattern

Secondary causes of insomnia are frequent in late life and include disorders secondary to medication use, anxiety disorders, depressive disorders, dementing disorders, and physical illnesses such as chronic or obstructive pulmonary disease and, most frequently, nocturia.

Sleep changes characteristic in late life include decreased total sleep time, frequent arousals, increased percentages of Stage 1 and Stage 2 sleep, decreased percentages of Stage 3 and Stage 4 sleep, decreased rapid eye movement (REM) latency, decreased absolute amounts of REM sleep, and a tendency to exhibit a redistribution of sleep across the 24-hour day (e.g., napping during the day). Many of these sleep changes are similar to those that occur in depression and dementing disorders, although not as severe. Older persons are also more likely to phase-advance in the sleep cycle, with a phase tendency toward "morningness."

Approximately 5% of all elderly persons who initially report no sleep problems report new symptoms each year (Anconi-Israel 2000). The proportion of older persons living in long-term care facilities who have sleep problems and take sedative-hypnotic agents is much higher than in the community. Sleep apnea is more prevalent in elderly men than women, with the apnea index (i.e., the number of apneas per hour of sleep) being 5 or greater in 25%–35% of elderly persons in the community. The prevalence of myoclonus probably ranges from 25% to 50% among healthy elderly persons in the community. There is no adequate study of the prevalence of sleep–wake schedule disorder, but the experience of this disorder is frequently reported by elderly persons, especially in long-term care facilities.

The diagnostic workup of an older person with insomnia begins with a recognition of the severity of the sleep disturbance. Screening questions during the interview should include an assessment of the patient's satisfaction with his or her sleep, daytime napping, fatigue during usual daily activities, and complaint by a bed partner or other observer of unusual behavior during sleep (such as snoring, pauses in breathing, or periodic myoclonic movements). A careful medical and psychiatric history is necessary to identify or rule out serious diseases that contribute to the sleep problem.

Medication history is essential in determining the eti-

ology of insomnia. Prescribed medications, especially sedative-hypnotics and anxiolytics, as well as alcohol, have significant effects on sleep and also may impair cardiopulmonary function. Symptoms of the major psychiatric disorders affecting older persons, such as dementia, depression, or severe anxiety, may also lead to insomnia. If a sleep–wake cycle dysfunction is suspected, patients may be asked to keep a log of napping, going to sleep, and awakening. Physical and neurological examinations are necessary, especially when sleep apnea is suspected. Heavy snoring requires a thorough examination of the nose and throat, usually by an otolaryngologist.

Although primary care physicians can usually recognize most sleep disorders and manage them effectively, specialized evaluation of sleep disorders is sometimes required. Referral to a psychiatrist or neurologist with special interest in sleep disorders is indicated. Upon referral, most patients, after a thorough history and physical examination and withdrawal from medication, are evaluated by polysomnography. Polysomnographic techniques have been improved in recent years; patients can now be fitted with a portable recording instrument and returned home to sleep for two evenings. Polysomnography, followed by a multiple sleep latency test, can be used to establish the diagnosis of narcolepsy and to quantify daytime sleepiness as well as to document sleep apnea.

The cornerstones of effective treatment of insomnia in late life are management of the underlying causes of the sleep disturbance and improved sleep hygiene. For example, a significant portion of older adults experiencing chronic insomnia also experience psychiatric disorders, especially depression and alcohol problems. Both of these conditions are responsive to therapy. Physical problems such as hypothyroidism or arthritis may not be reversed, but the symptoms can be relieved with medications or other therapeutic interventions. Nocturnal myoclonus or restless legs syndrome may respond to medication such as tryptophan or clonazepam. Sleep apnea syndrome that does not respond to conservative management may require surgery to improve flow in the nasopharyngeal region.

Institution of good sleep hygiene is the next step in managing insomnia among elderly patients. First, the patient should be encouraged to initiate sleep at the same time every night, preferably at a later rather than an earlier time (to prevent early-morning wakefulness). The bedroom should be used primarily for sleeping and not for napping. Therefore, if the elderly patient has difficulty sleeping at night, the bed should be made up in the morning and the patient should be encouraged not to nap in the bed and to spend as little time as possible in the bedroom during the day. Exercising can facilitate sleep, but exercise should not be initiated after late afternoon. Alcohol and caffeine should be avoided in the evenings, and the evening meal should be moderate and at least 2–3 hours before bedtime. Food intake should also be limited during the 2–3 hours before bedtime (to prevent nocturia).

Bedrooms should generally be maintained at a temperature between 65° and 72°F. To maintain a cool bedroom, many elderly persons who cannot afford air conditioning are forced to leave their windows open at night, possibly exposing them to noises that are likely to disturb sleep. One means for decreasing the potential of noise to disrupt the night's sleep is to institute white noise (such as waterfall or rain sounds) using specially built devices or to run a fan during the night. If the elderly person still cannot sleep at night, he or she is encouraged to get up, go to another room, and engage in some nonstimulating activity (such as reading or listening to music). When the elderly person again becomes drowsy, he or she should return to the bedroom and attempt to initiate sleep once again. If the individual experiences a difficult night of sleep, he or she should make extra efforts the next day to avoid napping.

Methods of relaxation training can be used successfully in enabling the insomniac elderly patient to initiate sleep. Progressive relaxation involves the alternate tensing and relaxing of muscle groups coupled with visualizing a relaxing scene. Elderly patients can be trained in such relaxation techniques by means of training tapes (instructing in progressive relaxation) or directly by a health care professional. However, an elderly patient should not habitually use training tapes to initiate sleep but rather be encouraged to shift to autoregulation of sleep.

A number of medications can be used to facilitate sleep in the elderly population, yet these medications should be used with care. If the elderly patient is taking medications that adversely affect sleep (such as long-term use of a sedative-hypnotic agent), then the pharmacological approach to treatment is to discontinue that medication (usually over about 10 days for a sedative-hypnotic). If the sleep problem is secondary to a medical problem, then optimal management of the medical problem with medications can assist the patient with sleep. For example, adequate treatment of arthritis with analgesics can improve sleep.

The antidepressant agents not only are useful in managing the older adult with insomnia secondary to depression but can be used as sedative agents as well, especially if prescribed in low dose. For example, 25–50 mg of trazodone may be preferable to using a long-term benzodi-azepine if chronic use of a sedative is indicated. Trazodone, however, has not been proven efficacious in clinical trials, and withdrawal may lead to rebound insomnia (in addition, the drug reduces time spent in REM sleep). In general, short- to medium-acting benzodiazepines are preferred over those that are more extended in length of action. For example, flurazepam has been associated with residual daytime sedation, impaired motor coordination, and increased risk for falls and hip fracture. Therefore, shorter-acting agents such as zolpidem (5 mg) and temazepam (15 mg) are preferred to flurazepam (15 mg) as a sedative-hypnotic. A new benzodiazepine receptor agonist, zaleplon (10 mg), has the shortest half-life among these agents and does not appear to cause rebound insomnia or adversely affect psychomotor function (Ancoli-Israel 2000). The benzodiazepines also can be used in individuals with nocturnal myoclonus. This therapy does not suppress the myoclonus but rather overrides the arousal effect of the muscle jerks.

Anxiety

Anxiety is a frequent symptom among older persons secondary to physical illness such as hyperthyroidism, comorbid with other psychiatric disorders such as depression, or as the primary symptom of a disorder such as generalized anxiety disorder (Blazer 1997). Many of the anxiety disorders, however, are relatively less frequent in late life. Although phobia disorders can affect persons at all stages of the life cycle, the more severe phobias, such as agoraphobia and social phobia, begin early in life and are more common in children and young adults than in older persons. Generalized anxiety disorder is a frequent diagnosis regardless of age, yet generalized anxiety is often comorbid with other psychiatric disorders such as major depression. Panic disorder is relatively frequent and severe among younger persons but much less so among older persons (although data documenting a lower prevalence among older persons are sparse). Posttraumatic stress disorder can occur at any age but is found more frequently in younger persons than older persons. Obsessive-compulsive traits are common throughout the life cycle, although the severe manifestations of this disorder are less likely to be observed in older persons. Therefore, the management of anxiety symptoms in older persons usually consists of managing the symptoms of generalized anxiety that are the primary problem or comorbid with other disorders.

Community surveys of individuals with anxiety symptoms estimate that approximately 5% of older persons meet DSM-III (American Psychiatric Association 1980) criteria for the diagnosis of generalized anxiety disorder. (There have been no large community studies of generalized anxiety using DSM-IV criteria, but a comparison of criteria suggests that the prevalence of generalized anxiety would be somewhat lower using the newer criteria.) Approximately 20% of older persons report some cognitive or somatic symptoms of anxiety in community surveys, with somatic symptoms being more prevalent than cognitive symptoms. In a survey in North Carolina, DSM-III simple phobia was found in 10% of persons age 65 years or older compared with 13% of persons in middle age. Agoraphobia was found in 5% of the 65-or-older group compared with 7% of the middle-age group (Blazer et al. 1991). Anxiety and depression are frequently comorbid in community surveys, reaching nearly 50% in some studies (Beekman et al. 2000).

Anxiety results from a number of medical and psychiatric conditions. Hyperthyroidism with an atypical presentation may be mistaken for a psychogenic anxiety disorder. Cardiac arrhythmias may produce palpitations and shortness of breath in older persons in a syndrome resembling generalized anxiety disorder, with episodic exacerbations and remissions depending on the status of the heart. Pulmonary emboli, if not severe, may present as shortness of breath and subjective anxiety.

Many medications lead to symptoms of anxiety. Caffeine is a frequent cause of anxiety, and older persons are frequently not aware of the multiple sources of caffeine in their diet. Over-the-counter sympathomimetic medications (such as ephedrine) may lead to palpitations and subsequent subjective symptoms of anxiety. Anticholinergic agents, when they impair memory, lead to anxiety that is secondary to the memory loss and confusion. Older persons also may experience significant anxiety on withdrawal from certain substances and medications, especially alcohol and anxiolytic agents. Postural hypotension may lead to dizziness and shortness of breath, which may be interpreted by the older person as episodic anxiety. Hypoglycemia 4–5 hours after a large meal is another contributor to anxiety.

Many psychiatric disorders are manifested, in part, by symptoms of anxiety. Moderate to severe acute confusion is usually associated with anxiety and agitation, especially when the older person is in an unfamiliar place. Anxiety is a common accompaniment of major depression; older patients who experience major depression also meet the criteria for generalized anxiety disorder in more than 50% of the cases. Hypochondriasis is associated with anxiety, especially when dependency needs are not met by family and health care professionals. Dementing disorders, especially in the early and middle stages, are associated with anxiety and agitation. Later in the dementing disorder, the agitation is episodic and the cognitive, subjective anxiety is less well documented. Late-life schizophrenia with acute paranoid ideation is usually accompanied by agitation and anxiety, especially in the evenings when the older person is home alone. In addition, some older persons experience acute panic attacks and meet the criteria for panic disorder, and some exhibit symptoms of generalized anxiety without apparent biological or psychosocial causation.

The perceptive clinician must not overlook the possibility that the anxiety symptoms may be secondary to appropriate fear. Many older persons must expose themselves daily to situations that threaten their security. Older adults living in inner cities often fear being attacked as they walk the streets. Those with memory loss who live alone may fear that they will get lost driving to the doctor's office. Individuals who have lost the acuteness of their reflexes fear driving on busy, crowded highways.

The use of nonpharmacological therapies such as relaxation training, cognitive restructuring, and activity structuring for the treatment of anxiety in older adults has not been studied extensively. Nevertheless, the danger of medication, as well as the successful application of cognitive-behavior therapies to other psychiatric disorders in late life (especially depression), suggests that nonpharmacological therapies also may be applicable to anxiety disorders. Older persons who do not have cognitive dysfunction are good candidates for relaxation training and biofeedback. No evidence has been forthcoming to suggest that older persons are less capable of taking advantage of these therapies than are middle-aged persons. Cognitive restructuring, based on the cognitive therapy described originally for depression, has not been adapted for anxiety in older adults to date. However, there is little evidence that nonstructured psychotherapy is of benefit in treating generalized anxiety or panic episodes in late life.

The cornerstone of pharmacological therapy for the anxiety disorders is the benzodiazepines. These drugs repeatedly have been demonstrated to be effective for the control of anxiety when compared with a placebo and are relatively free of side effects. They are generally well tolerated by persons of all ages but present unique problems when prescribed to older persons. For example, the half-life of the benzodiazepines may be increased dramatically in late life, with diazepam (2.5–5 mg) having a half-life nearing 4 days in persons in their 80s. Older persons are also more susceptible to potential side effects of benzodiazepines such as fatigue, drowsiness, motor dysfunction, and memory impairment. Clinicians must be especially careful when prescribing benzodiazepines to older individuals who drive. Therefore, the shorter-acting benzodiazepines, such as alprazolam (0.125 mg), oxazepam (15 mg), and lorazepam (2 mg), given two to three times a day, have been preferred agents in late life. Nevertheless, short-acting drugs in some older patients may lead to brief withdrawal episodes during the day and a rebound of anxiety.

Other agents are generally less effective in controlling late-life anxiety. Buspirone (10 mg three times a day) is relatively safe, with few side effects, and does not appear to lead to abuse or dependency. Nevertheless, it takes 3–4 weeks for the therapeutic effect to become manifest. Older adults who perceive that they have benefited from benzodiazepines generally do not accept buspirone as an alternative. The antidepressant agents are useful in treating anxiety mixed with depression. Nevertheless, in many older persons with a mixed anxiety-depression syndrome, the depressive symptoms improve while the antidepressant is being used, yet the anxiety symptoms persist. Therefore, a combination of a benzodiazepine and an antidepressant is sometimes used. Gabapentin, 100 mg two or three times a day, has been used by some to control symptoms of anxiety in the elderly, but its efficacy has yet to be demonstrated. Some have suggested that β-blockers such as propranolol (10 mg twice daily) are valuable in treating anxiety disorders. These drugs must be monitored carefully, given their propensity to slow the heart rate. Buspirone and the β-blockers may be more effective in controlling agitation and behavioral problems in patients with dementia than in controlling generalized anxiety.

Suspiciousness

A frequent symptom in older adults, especially older adults experiencing cognitive impairment, is suspiciousness, which may range from increased cautiousness and distrust of family and friends to overt paranoid delusions. Among suspicious or paranoid older persons a unique group has been described, especially in the European literature, for many years. *Late-life paraphrenia* has been distinguished from both chronic schizophrenia and dementia and is characterized by marked paranoid delusions in older adults who nevertheless maintain function in the community for months or even years (Almeida et al. 1995). Persons experiencing paraphrenia are predominantly women and often live alone. However, marked suspiciousness and overt psychoses in conjunction with cognitive impairment are a more common manifestation of the syndrome.

The predominant delusions encountered in older persons are persecutory delusions and somatic delusions. Persecutory delusions often revolve around a single theme or a series of connected themes, such as family and neighbors conspiring against the delusional older person or delusions of sexual abuse. Somatic delusions often involve the gastrointestinal tract and frequently reflect the older person's fear that he or she is experiencing cancer. Regardless of the etiology of suspiciousness and paranoid delusions, when older persons believe they are threatened from the social environment, often because they do not understand what is happening in that environment, agitation becomes paramount. Agitation in the suspicious older person is an acute symptom that may require emergency management, as described later in this discussion.

Suspiciousness and paranoid behavior were found in 17% of persons in one community survey (Lowenthal 1964), and a sense of persecution was reported in 4% in another survey (Christenson and Blazer 1984). Thus, the perception by older persons that they live in a hostile social environment is common and represents a much larger proportion of older individuals than those who would be diagnosed as having schizophrenia or even suspiciousness secondary to cognitive impairment. Some of these suspicions may be justified if the older person lives in an unsafe community or has been the victim of fraud. Among persons in the community, fewer than 1% have schizophrenia or a paranoid disorder.

Many different disorders may lead to suspiciousness, delusions, and agitation. Chronic schizophrenic disorder, which has its onset earlier in life and persists into late life, is perhaps the most easily identified cause of late-life suspiciousness. As schizophrenia tends to be characterized by a decline in social function over the life cycle and a shorter life expectancy (although the prognosis of schizophrenia varies greatly from person to person), chronic schizophrenia that persists into late life and yet leaves the older person relatively free of other symptoms is uncommon. Nevertheless, persons may experience severe symptoms of schizophrenia in early or mid-life and then enter a period of remission from which they do not relapse with further schizophrenic behavior until late life. Schizophrenic-like illness also may have its first onset in late life, and the pattern is similar to that described previously for late-life paraphrenia. Usually, depression and organic mental disorders do not contribute to these late-onset schizophrenic-like states. In contrast, organic mental disorders and late-onset depression are frequently associated with some psychotic symptoms.

Late-onset delusional disorder, with mild to moderate symptoms, is a more frequent cause of suspiciousness in late life. Delusions, often of being persecuted by family and friends, usually center on a single theme or a connection of themes. For example, an older woman may become convinced that her daughter was instrumental in the death of her husband (or that the daughter neglected her father during a chronic illness). That woman, in turn, may not listen to reason regarding the daughter's behavior and may never forgive the daughter for the perceived abuse or neglect. These delusions may lead to a withdrawal of affection, financial support, and social contact with the daughter.

Another common cause of suspiciousness in late life is organic delusional syndrome (or dementia with psychosis). These delusions, in contrast to late-onset delusional disorder, wax and wane over time in severity and in content. Persecutory delusions are most common and often emerge when the older person's environment is changed. Organic delusional syndrome often emerges from medications or from localized brain damage (such as in Huntington's chorea and alcohol abuse). Suspiciousness, however, usually results from the dementing disorders. For some persons experiencing AD, paranoid thoughts may dominate other symptoms of the dementing illness, especially in the early stages. Perhaps the most common encounter psychiatrists have with suspicious older persons is with demented patients who have become a management problem because of suspiciousness and agitation.

Despite the range of disorders that may lead to suspiciousness in older persons, some investigators have suggested common psychobiological contributors to the syndrome in late life. A family history of suspiciousness and delusional thought is uncommon among suspicious older persons, and therefore, hereditary contributions are probably less important than at earlier stages of the life cycle. Degeneration of subcortical tissues with aging may disrupt neurotransmission and higher brain functions, which in turn contributes to a deficiency in maintaining attention and filtering information, symptoms that have been associated with psychotic thinking. That women are more likely to experience more severe syndromes of suspiciousness than men in late life (in contrast to the equal sex distribution of psychoses earlier in life) has led some investigators to suggest that menopause and the resultant decrease in estrogen binding to dopamine receptors may place women at risk who were previously protected from developing suspicious thinking. Sensory deprivation also has been identified as a potential risk factor for suspiciousness, regardless of the underlying disorder. Social isolation also may contribute to suspiciousness.

The key to the diagnostic workup of the suspicious older person is the psychiatric evaluation. Delusional thinking and agitation usually render the patient's history inaccurate, and therefore family members should be interviewed to review the patient's behavior, especially any change in behavior. Previous psychotic or delusional episodes should be documented, as well as previous treatment. Clinicians evaluating the suspicious older person should remember that older adults are occasionally abused by family members, and the seemingly delusional description of family behavior by the older individual may contain some truth.

The management of suspiciousness and agitation in older adults requires 1) ensuring a safe environment; 2) initiating a therapeutic alliance; 3) considering and, if appropriate, instituting pharmacological therapy; and 4) managing acute behavioral crises. When the older patient is determined to be suspicious and agitated, the clinician must first decide whether hospitalization is necessary. In general, paranoid older persons do not adapt well to the hospital. Change from familiar surroundings and interaction with strange persons tend to exacerbate the suspiciousness. Nevertheless, older patients often are so disabled in their behavior secondary to schizophrenic or delusional disorder that hospitalization is necessary.

Once the older patient is hospitalized, the clinician must initiate a therapeutic alliance. With the older patient, this alliance is best accomplished by taking a medical approach to the patient and expressing concern about all of the patient's physical and emotional concerns. Most suspicious older patients are quite accepting of medical care and are trusting of physicians. It is rarely necessary for clinicians to confront patients regarding suspicions or delusional thinking; therefore, older patients' responses to questions can be supportive, and clinicians do not need to agree with statements made by the patients that are known to be untrue.

The cornerstone of managing the moderately to severely suspicious older patient is medication, especially antipsychotic agents. Medications most frequently used to treat older persons are risperidone (1–3 mg/day), olanzapine (5–15 mg/day), and haloperidol (0.5–2 mg orally three times a day). Dosage of these agents is relatively small initially, and one-half of the dose should be given during the evening. In a large controlled study, lower doses of risperidone (1 mg/day) significantly improved symptoms of psychosis and aggressive behavior with fewer side effects compared with 2 mg/day (Katz et al. 1999). Doses can be increased if necessary. Physicians who prescribe antipsychotic medications for the treatment of suspiciousness in an older adult should carefully monitor the success of these agents. If the drug is deemed not successful—for example, if the target symptoms do not change with the medication—then it should be discontinued, given the significant side effects that may result. Tardive dyskinesia is five to six times more prevalent in elderly than in younger patients (Jeste 2000).

Finally, the physician must be prepared to deal with severe agitation and violent behavior. Medications alone will not control these behaviors. Physicians must work with the nursing staff to prevent such behavior in patients at risk while they are in the hospital and must instruct families on methods of prevention when these patients are at home. Suggestions for preventing violent behavior are listed in Table 37–4.

TABLE 37–4. Suggestions for preventing aggressive and violent behavior in the suspicious older adult

---

Psychologically disarm the patient by helping him or her to express his or her fears.

Distract the attention of the older patient. One person should calmly speak to the patient to distract attention from perceived threats in the patient's surroundings.

Provide directions to the patient in simple terms for even the most simple behaviors. Suspicious older patients have difficulty interpreting complex procedures.

Communicate clearly and concisely. These patient have decreased ability to receive and organize complex information.

Communicate expectations. A firm command to the patient in simple terms is essential for controlling aggressive behavior.

Avoid arguing and defending. Arguments between staff and an agitated older patient only increase fear and agitation in the patient.

Avoid threatening body language. Staff should move slowly, predictably, and respectfully in the personal space of the patient. Threatening gestures (such as clenched fists) must be avoided.

Remain at a safe distance from the patient until help is available. A staff member should not attempt to single-handedly control even a small agitated older person.

Periods of severe agitation are usually brief and, if managed properly, are soon forgotten by the older patient. Then the physician once more can work toward establishing a sustained therapeutic relationship with the patient.

Depression

Depression is one of the more frequent and the second most disabling geriatric psychiatry syndrome (after memory loss) experienced by older adults. Late-life depression that is not comorbid with physical illness and/or a dementing disorder is characterized by symptoms similar to those experienced at earlier stages of the life cycle, with some significant differences. Depressed mood is usually apparent in the older adult but may not be a spontaneous complaint. Older persons are more likely to experience weight loss (as opposed to weight gain or no change in weight) during a major depressive episode and are less likely to report feelings of worthlessness or guilt. Although older persons experience more difficulty with cognitive performance tests during a depressive episode, they are no more likely than persons in mid-life to report cognitive problems subjectively. Complaints of cognitive dysfunction are common in more severe depressive episodes regardless of the person's age. Persistent anhedonia associated with a lack of response to pleasurable stimuli is a common and central symptom of late-life depression. Older persons are also more likely than younger persons to exhibit psychotic symptoms during a depressive episode. Recent studies have suggested that executive function is impaired in older adults with depression and that this impairment may be associated with a higher likelihood of relapse and recurrence of symptoms (Alexopoulos et al. 2000).

In community surveys, older adults are less likely to be diagnosed as having major depression than are persons in young adulthood or middle age. Depressive symptoms, however, are about equally prevalent across the life cycle. Standardized interviews reveal that 1%–3% of persons in the community are diagnosed as having major depression, and an additional 2% are diagnosed as having dysthymia (Blazer et al. 1987). Major depression is much more prevalent among older persons in the hospital and in long-term care facilities, ranging from 10% to 20% (Koenig et al. 1988).

Late-life depression fits well in the biopsychosocial model of psychiatric disorders. Although a hereditary predisposition to depression is less likely among persons in late life who are experiencing a first onset of depression, a number of biological factors are associated with late-life depression. Poor regulation of the hypothalamic-pituitary-adrenal axis, as well as disruption of the sleep cycle and other circadian rhythms, is more likely to be present among older persons than among younger persons. These problems also have been associated with major depression. In recent years, considerable attention has been directed to the association of depression with lesions in subcortical structures and their frontal projections in the brain (Krishnan 1993). Most older persons are satisfied with their lives and are not psychologically predisposed to depression. Nevertheless, some experience a demoralization and a despair resulting not only from incapacities due to aging but also from a sense of not having fulfilled their life expectations. Older persons must adapt to many adverse life experiences, especially losses of relatives and friends, yet they are often more likely to respond to these losses without difficulty than are persons who are younger. Older persons, for example, expect that they will lose family and friends through death, and those family and friends that they do lose often have suffered chronic illnesses for some time, thus allowing older persons to grieve the loss, in part, before the actual loss.

Major depression is relatively infrequent among older persons yet is the most challenging of the late-life mental disorders to manage. Older persons also may experience bipolar disorder, with a first-onset manic episode after age 65. Psychotic depressions are more common in late life than at other stages of the life cycle. Other common causes of late-life depression include organic mood disorder, such as a depressed mood secondary to antihypertensive medications, and the depression associated with the common dementing disorders, such as primary degenerative dementia and vascular dementia. Medical illness, such as hypothyroidism, frequently leads to an organic mood disorder. An adjustment disorder with depressed mood secondary to physical disability and/or chronic illness is among the most frequent causes of depressed mood among older individuals.

As with the diagnosis of other geriatric psychiatry syndromes, the patient's history and a collateral history from a family member are the keys to making the diagnosis of depression in late life. Although older persons may exhibit some tendency to "mask" their depressive symptoms, a careful interview almost invariably reveals significant depression if it is present. The history should be complemented by a thorough mental status examination with attention to disturbances of motor behavior and perception, presence or absence of hallucinations, disturbances of thinking, and thorough cognitive testing. Psychological testing may be implemented to distinguish depression from dementia but should not be performed in the midst of a severe depressive episode. The laboratory workup of the depressed older adult is presented in Table 37–5.

Some tests, such as the blood count and measurement of B_{12} and folate levels, are useful in screening for medical illnesses that may present with depressive symptoms. The thyroid panel is essential in the diagnosis of the depressed older patient, given that subclinical hypothyroid disorders are frequently uncovered in the workup. The dexamethasone suppression test is not especially valuable in making the diagnosis of late-life depression but may provide information about response to therapy, such as pharmacotherapy or electroconvulsive therapy (ECT), if repeated after the therapy has been in use for a

TABLE 37–5. Laboratory workup of the depressed older adult

Routine
Complete blood cell count
Urinalysis
T3, T4, free thyroxine index, thyroid-stimulating hormone
Venereal Disease Research Laboratory test
Vitamin B_{12} and folate assays
Chemistry screen (sodium, chlorine, potassium, blood urea nitrogen, calcium, glucose, creatinine)
Electrocardiogram
Elective
Dexamethasone suppression test
Polysomnography
Magnetic resonance imaging (or computed tomography)
Thyroid-releasing hormone stimulation test
Screening for HIV

few days. Although the abnormalities in sleep associated with depression frequently parallel those associated with normal aging, experienced polysomnographers can distinguish them. Magnetic resonance imaging is optional despite the association of subcortical white matter hyperintensities with late-life depression. The physician ordering laboratory tests for a depressed older patient also must consider the potential adverse health consequences for an older adult experiencing a severe or chronic mood disorder. For example, major depression is associated with decreased bone mineral density, placing older women with depression at greater risk for osteoporosis (Michelson et al. 1996).

Clinical management involves pharmacotherapy, ECT, psychotherapy, and work with the family. The pharmacological treatment of choice at present is one of the new-generation antidepressant medications. Despite the advent of a new generation of antidepressants, some geriatric psychiatrists still prefer to first administer one of the secondary amines, such as nortriptyline or desipramine, to healthy older adults. Each has relatively low anticholinergic effects and is known to be an effective antidepressant. Postural hypotension and the potential for serious health consequences are the most troublesome side effects that older adults usually encounter when treated with the tricyclic antidepressants. Given that Medicare does not reimburse older adults for medications, the lower cost of the tricyclic antidepressants compared with the cost of newer agents is one factor in prescribing them. The SSRIs fluoxetine, sertraline, paroxetine, and citalopram can be used at a somewhat lower dose than is prescribed at earlier stages of the life cycle (e.g., 10 mg/day for paroxetine). The most common adverse effects that limit the use of SSRIs are agitation and persistent weight loss. Paroxetine has been shown to significantly (but not dramatically) improve the symptoms of minor depression and dysthymia in doses between 10 and 40 mg/day (Williams et al. 2000). The use of antidepressant medications, primarily the SSRIs, has increased dramatically in recent years, with over 10% of elders 75 years and older taking antidepressants at any given time (Blazer et al. 2000).

The older person who does not respond to the antidepressant medications or who experiences significant side effects from the medications may be a candidate for ECT. Depressed older persons who are candidates for ECT should be experiencing a severe depressive episode and are especially likely to respond if they are experiencing psychotic symptoms. With proper medical support, ECT is a safe and effective treatment for older adults. Despite a higher level of physical illness and cognitive impairment, even the oldest patient with severe major depression may tolerate ECT similar to younger patients and demonstrate similar or better acute response (Tew et al. 1999).

Several studies have demonstrated the effectiveness of cognitive and behavioral therapies (including interpersonal psychotherapy) in outpatient treatment of older persons who have major depression without melancholia (Koder et al. 1996). Cognitive therapy also may be an adjunct for severe melancholic depressions that are treated concomitantly with medications. In a large controlled trial of patients over 59 years with major depression, maintenance therapy with interpersonal therapy and nortriptyline was significant in preventing or delaying recurrence (Reynolds et al. 1999). Cognitive-behavioral therapy is well tolerated by older people because of its limited duration and educational orientation, as well as the active interchange between the therapist and the patient.

Any effective therapy for depression in older persons must include work with the family. Families are often the most important allies of the clinician working with depressed older patients. Families should be informed as to the danger signs, such as potential for suicide, in a severely depressed older family member. In addition, the family can provide structure for reengaging a withdrawn and depressed older person into social activities.

Hypochondriasis

Hypochondriasis among older persons is one of the more common and frustrating of the somatoform disorders encountered by health care professionals. An essential feature of hypochondriasis in older persons is their belief that they have one or several serious illnesses. This belief derives from an exaggerated interpretation of physical signs and sensations. The medical workup often will reveal some physical abnormality but does not support a medical diagnosis that can account for the severity and breadth of symptoms experienced. However, hypochondriacal symptoms do not reach the level of somatic delusions. The distinction between a psychotic disorder manifested by somatic delusions and hypochondriasis is usually easy to make because the delusion either is unrelated to any physical sensation or in no way relates to the symptoms reported. To meet criteria for a diagnosis of hypochondriasis, older persons must experience the disorder for at least 6 months; when most physicians encounter hypochondriacal older patients, their symptoms have lasted far longer than 6 months. Hypochondriacal symptoms in older persons usually are described as being in the gastrointestinal or genitourinary area. Exaggerated concerns regarding constipation, difficulty with eating because of gastric problems, abdominal pain, and genitourinary pain are among the most frequent. As with individuals who have hypochondriasis at other stages of life, older persons with this disorder do not experience relief when assured by a physician that the medical problem is not severe.

In community surveys, exaggerated concern about health is found among 10% of older persons (Blazer and Houpt 1979). In contrast, another 10% usually perceive their health as being significantly better than it actually is. Most older persons assessed their health accurately, with no trend for older individuals inaccurately perceiving their health as being worse than it actually is. There are no community surveys that accurately estimate the prevalence of hypochondriasis. That hypochondriacal older persons are frequently encountered by primary care physicians should not lead to the assumption that hypochondriasis is a common problem among this population. Hypochondriacal older persons overuse health care services, and therefore, one or two hypochondriacal older patients in a primary care physician's practice may occupy an appreciable amount of time, leading the physician to believe that hypochondriasis is one of the most common conditions that he or she encounters.

The etiology of hypochondriasis is, by definition, not biological. This does not mean, however, that hypochondriacal older persons do not experience physical illness or that the symptoms reported by some older individuals are not, to some degree, the expression of actual physical problems. Exaggeration of symptoms (as opposed to the invention of symptoms) is the manifestation of hypochondriasis.

Several mechanisms may contribute to hypochondriasis in older persons. First, the symptoms may be used to shift anxiety from specific psychological conflicts to more concrete problems with body functioning. An older person may fear the loss of his or her mind, the loss of a spouse, the loss of personal capabilities, or the loss of a social role. Fear of these losses is then replaced by a preoccupation with physical health in hypochondriasis. Some older persons may use hypochondriacal symptoms as a means of punishing themselves for unacceptable, hostile feelings or behaviors in the past for which they now feel guilty. If an older person has engaged in some type of indiscretion, such as a sexual indiscretion, genitourinary pains or concerns may predominate as hypochondriacal symptoms later in life. Unfortunately, interpreting the connection between past guilt and present concern usually does not alleviate the problem of hypochondriasis.

Social factors are probably the major reason that aging persons are at risk for developing hypochondriasis. Older persons often have difficulty meeting personal and/or social expectations. Family members may wish the older family member to participate in activities that are beyond his or her capability, such as taking a long walk, lifting luggage, or preparing a meal. Failure to meet these family expectations, or perhaps anger at the family for insisting that these expectations be met, can lead the older person to focus on his or her physical problems to the exclusion of facing the issue directly. Older persons also use hypochondriasis as a means of adapting to the real problem of isolation. Preoccupation with physical problems and obtaining help for those physical problems in some cases become the center of the older person's life. Frequent visits to the physician require assistance with transportation from family or friends and provide social contact with persons in the health care professional's office. The older patient also learns that physical complaints facilitate communicating with others because they provide the individual with a topic of conversation. Isolated older persons may feel they have little else to contribute to conversations and, therefore, focus on their physical problems.

The clinician working with a hypochondriacal older patient must be vigilant for the presence of more severe psychopathology. Depression is frequently accompanied by exaggerated physical concerns, regardless of age. If an older person exhibits both significant depressive symptoms and symptoms of hypochondriasis, then the clinician must be alert to the possibility of suicide. Suicide has been demonstrated to be more common in persons exhibiting both depression and exaggerated physical concerns compared with those with depressive symptoms alone. Hypochondriasis also may mask emerging difficulties with memory. Older persons may avoid direct challenges to their cognitive status by focusing on their physical concerns.

The diagnostic workup of the hypochondriacal older patient consists of a thorough history and a routine physical examination. Routine laboratory studies should be performed, but once the clinician is assured that the patient does not have a severe or undetected physical problem that contributes to the symptoms, then he or she should limit further laboratory studies. The differential diagnosis includes major depression and dysthymia, anxiety disorders (both generalized anxiety and panic), schizophrenic disorder (if the exaggerated physical concern expressed by the patient borders on delusional thinking), and dementing disorders. The diagnosis of hypochondriasis does not exclude the diagnosis of other psychiatric disorders. Many older persons with hypochondriasis meet criteria for a somatoform disorder and, for example, a dementing disorder.

Working with the hypochondriacal older patient requires both tact and patience. The development of a management strategy should be based on management goals (see Table 37–6). Older patients with hypochondriasis are best managed by a primary care physician as opposed to a psychiatrist. After the initial evaluation, the hypochondriacal older patient should be seen for relatively brief but regularly scheduled visits, in general lasting no more than 10–20 minutes each. Emphasis during the follow-up visits initially should be on a brief review of interval historical information coupled with a brief physical examination (including checking pulse and blood pressure). The remainder of the visit should be relatively unstructured and should focus on events in the patient's life. The clinician should refrain from interpretations connecting the physical problems with specific life events, instead encouraging the patient to discuss concerns about family, friends, perceived isolation, and so forth. The clinician may prescribe medications but must recognize that older patients with hypochondriasis are at increased risk for becoming dependent on psychotropic medications. Placebos are generally not appropriate because discovery that a placebo has been prescribed undoubtedly will destroy the relationship between patient and doctor.

Medications that can be used for treating the hypochondriacal older patient include those with relatively few side effects and those that have been demonstrated to be at least minimally effective for alleviating the symptoms expressed by the patient. For example, L-tryptophan can be prescribed for problems with sleeping (2 g of this drug at night would be an appropriate dose). Another mildly sedating drug is trazodone, given at 25–50 mg at night. Neither of these drugs will lead to habituation.

The concept of "treatment" for hypochondriasis is actually misleading. Whatever treatment plan is insti-

TABLE 37–6. Goals for managing hypochondriasis in the older adult

Control excessive use of health care services.

Decrease concern and anxiety in the patient.

Assure professional commitment to managing the patient's condition.

Decrease family stress and facilitate the family as social support.

Decrease the anxiety, anger, and frustration of the health care professional treating the patient.

tuted, it is, in fact, a management plan with the goals of 1) controlling and decreasing the use of health services, 2) decreasing the concern and anxiety expressed by the hypochondriacal older person about the availability and commitment of health care professionals, 3) decreasing strain on the family, 4) increasing the capabilities of the family to provide a supportive environment to the hypochondriacal older person, 5) decreasing conflicts within the family, and 6) decreasing anxiety expressed by the health care professional. Given these goals, it is essential that the hypochondriacal older person be treated within the context of the family when family members are available. Hypochondriacal symptoms often disappear during the process of aging. As older persons resolve conflicts with family, and as they accept their one and only life for what it is, anxiety decreases and appropriate social interactions increase.

Conclusions

The seven geriatric syndromes discussed in this chapter account for most of the psychopathology that both psychiatrists and geriatricians encounter while working with older adults. The syndromal approach permits the clinician to focus on the functional impairment that results from psychopathology and on the day-to-day management of the older person in both the hospital and the outpatient clinic. A syndromal approach also provides a more realistic conceptualization of late-life psychopathology, which often is comorbid across psychiatric diagnoses and comorbid with physical illnesses.

References

Alexopoulos GS, Meyers BS, Young RC, et al: Executive dysfunction and long-term outcomes of geriatric depression. Arch Gen Psychiatry 57:285–290, 2000

Almeida OP, Howard RJ, Levy R, et al: Psychotic states arising in late life (late paraphrenia): psychopathology and nosology. Br J Psychiatry 166:205–214, 1995

American Psychiatric Association: Diagnostic and Statistical Manual of Mental Disorders, 3rd Edition. Washington, DC, American Psychiatric Association, 1980

American Psychiatric Association: Diagnostic and Statistical Manual of Mental Disorders, 4th Edition. Washington, DC, American Psychiatric Association, 1994

Anconi-Israel S: Insomnia in the elderly: a review for the primary care practitioner. Sleep 23(suppl 1):S23–S30, 2000

Beekman ATF, de Beurs E, van Balkom AJLM, et al: Anxiety and depression in later life: co-occurrence and communality of risk factors. Am J Psychiatry 157:89–95, 2000

Blazer DG: Generalized anxiety disorder and panic disorder in the elderly: a review. Harv Rev Psychiatry 5:18–27, 1997

Blazer DG: Psychiatry and the oldest old. Am J Psychiatry 157:1915–1924, 2000

Blazer DG, Houpt JL: Perception of poor health in the healthy older adult. J Am Geriatr Soc 27:330–336, 1979

Blazer DG, Hughes DC, George LK: The epidemiology of depression in an elderly community population. Gerontologist 27:281–287, 1987

Blazer DG, George LK, Hughes DC: The epidemiology of anxiety disorders: an age comparison, in Anxiety Disorders in the Elderly. Edited by Salzman C, Lebowitz B. New York, Springer, 1991, pp 17–30

Blazer DG, Hybels CF, Simonsick EM, et al: Marked differences in antidepressant use by race in an elderly community sample: 1986–1996. Am J Psychiatry 157:1089–1094, 2000

Blessed G, Tomlinson BE, Roth M: The association between quantitative measures of dementia and of senile change in the cerebral grey matter of elderly subjects. Br J Psychiatry 114:797–811, 1968

Christenson R, Blazer D: Epidemiology of persecutory ideation in an elderly population in the community. Am J Psychiatry 141:1088–1091, 1984

Foley DY, Monjan AA, Brown SL, et al: Sleep complaints among elderly persons: an epidemiologic study of three communities. Sleep 18:425–432, 1995

Folstein MF, Folstein SE, McHugh PR: Mini-Mental State: a practical method for grading the cognitive state of patients for the clinician. J Psychiatr Res 12:189–198, 1975

Inouye SK: Prevention of delirium in hospitalized older patients: risk factors and targeted intervention. Ann Internal Med 32:257–263, 2000

Jeste DV: Tardive dyskinesia in older patients. J Clin Psychiatry 61(suppl 4):27–32, 2000

Katz IR, Jeste DV, Mintzer JE, et al: Comparison of risperidone and placebo for psychoses and behavioral disturbances with dementia: a randomized, double-blind trial. Risperidone Study Group. J Clin Psychiatry 60:107–115, 1999

Koder D, Brodaty H, Anstey K: Cognitive therapy for depression in the elderly. Int J Geriatr Psychiatry 11:97–107, 1996

Koenig HG, Meador KG, Cohen HJ, et al: Depression in elderly men hospitalized with medical illness. Arch Intern Med 148:1929–1936, 1988

Krishnan KRR: Neuroanatomic substrates of depression in the elderly. J Geriatr Psychiatry Neurol 1:39–58, 1993

Lowenthal MF: Lives in Distress. New York, Basic Books, 1964

Martin NJ, Stones MJ, Young JE, et al: Development of delirium: a prospective cohort study in a community hospital. Int Psychogeriatr 12:117–127, 2000

Michelson D, Stratakis C, Hill L, et al: Bone mineral density in women with depression. N Engl J Med 335:1176–1181, 1996

Reynolds CF III, Frank E, Perel JM, et al: Nortriptyline and interpersonal psychotherapy as maintenance therapies for recurrent major depression: a randomized controlled trial in patients older than 59 years. JAMA 281:39–45, 1999

Reitan R: Validity of the Trail Making Test as an indicator of organic brain disease. Percept Mot Skills 8:271–276, 1958

Roses AD: Apolipoprotein E affects the rate of Alzheimer disease expression: β-amyloid burden is a secondary consequence dependent on APOE genotype and duration of disease. J Neuropathol Exp Neurol 53:429–437, 1994

Small GW, Rabins PV, Barry PP, et al: Diagnosis and treatment of Alzheimer's disease and related disorders: consensus statement of the American Association for Geriatric Psychiatry, the Alzheimer's Association, and American Geriatrics Society. JAMA 278:1363–1371, 1997

Tew JD, Mulsant BH, Haskett RF, et al: Acute efficacy of ECT in the treatment of major depression in the old-old. Am J Psychiatry 156:1865–1870, 1999

Tomlinson E, Blessed G, Roth M: Observations on the brains of demented old people. J Neurol Sci 11:205–242, 1970

Williams JW, Barrett J, Oxman T, et al: Treatment of dysthymia and minor depression in primary care: a randomized controlled trial in older adults. JAMA 284:1519–1526, 2000

Suggested Readings

Anconi-Israel S: Insomnia in the elderly: a review for the primary care practitioner: Sleep 23(suppl 1):S23–S30, 2000

Blazer DG: Hypochondriasis, in A Family Approach to Health Care in the Elderly. Edited by Blazer DG, Siegler IC. Menlo Park, CA, Addison-Wesley, 1984, pp 140–156

Blazer DG: Depression in the elderly. N Engl J Med 320:164–166, 1989

Blazer DG: Depression in Late Life, 3rd Edition. St Louis, MO, CV Mosby, 2002

Blazer DG: Emotional Problems in Later Life: Intervention Strategies for Professional Caregivers, 2nd Edition. New York, Springer, 1996

Blazer DG: Generalized anxiety disorder and panic disorder in the elderly: a review. Harv Rev Psychiatry 5:18–27, 1997

Busse EW: Somatoform and psychosexual disorders, in Geriatric Psychiatry, 2nd Edition. Edited by Busse EW, Blazer DG. Washington, DC, American Psychiatric Press, 1996, pp 291–312

Busse EW, Blazer DG (eds): Geriatric Psychiatry, 2nd Edition. Washington, DC, American Psychiatric Press, 1996

Gublin MJ: Managing sleep disturbance of the elderly without drug therapy. Geriatric Medicine Today 4:72–85, 1985

Gwyther LP: Care of Alzheimer's Patients. New York, Alzheimer's Disease and Related Disease Association/American Health Care Association, 1985

Jeste DV: Tardive dyskinesia in older patients. J Clin Psychiatry 61(suppl 4):27–32, 2000

Koder D, Brodaty H, Anstey K: Cognitive therapy for depression in the elderly. Int J Geriatr Psychiatry 11:97–107, 1996

Krishnan KRR: Neuroanatomic substrates of depression in the elderly. J Geriatr Psychiatry Neurol 1:39–58, 1993

Lipowski ZJ: Delirium in the elderly patient. N Engl J Med 320:578–582, 1989

Reynolds CF III, Frank E, Perel JM, et al: Nortriptyline and interpersonal psychotherapy as maintenance therapies for recurrent major depression: a randomized controlled trial in patients older than 59 years. JAMA 281:39–45, 1999

Roses AD: Apolipoprotein E affects the rate of Alzheimer disease expression: β-amyloid burden is a secondary consequence dependent on APOE genotype and duration of disease. J Neuropathol Exp Neurol 53:429–437, 1994

Small GW, Rabins PV, Barry PP, et al: Diagnosis and treatment of Alzheimer's disease and related disorders: consensus statement of the American Association for Geriatric Psychiatry, the Alzheimer's Association, and American Geriatrics Society. JAMA 278:1363–1371, 1997

CHAPTER 38

Introduction to Cultural Psychiatry

Ezra E. H. Griffith, M.D.

Carlos A. González, M.D.

Howard C. Blue, M.D.

> Culture as it informs contemporary psychiatric diagnosis and practice is not a "visible" or "exotic" difference in symbolic orientation, but rather a subtle all pervasive frame of reference that the psychiatrist may or may not share with his/her patient, and that involves the construction of persons, the assessment of behavior, the choice of a therapeutic rationale and a suitable 'end stage' of adaptive function that is targeted as and/or signals a cure.
>
> *Fabrega 1992, p. 100*

Cultural psychiatry has gained considerable visibility and prestige as a discipline in the past few decades because of an increased recognition that culture plays a significant role in individuals' lives and has a considerable impact on the development of their self-concept. Such understanding has directly resulted from the collaborative efforts of psychiatrists, anthropologists, sociologists, and individuals from other professional groups. The pressure for such interdisciplinary thinking and problem solving has come, too, from society's wish to understand the nature of certain problems that are evidently linked to culture, as well as the important difficulties that are fueled by intercultural differences. How and to what extent, for example, do the differences in lifestyle and values of ethnic groups in the United States account for the varied health and mental health status of these groups? Are there specific cultural elements that determine why certain national groups form suicide squads to perform terrorist actions? Are there cultural determinants of the recently perceived rise in intragroup violence in the United States and intergroup violence abroad? Why is it that certain emotional disorders found in Asia baffle psychiatrists trained in North America? How is it that differences in religious beliefs can seem to fuel protracted strife among groups of people? Such questions reflect the key assumption that their solution lies not simply in some biological framework but at least partly in understanding the role of culture as an integral component of human existence and behavior.

Definitions of Cultural Psychiatry

Certain key concepts, summarized in Table 38–1, have been consistently critical to the understanding of cultural psychiatry. First is *society*, which Leighton and Murphy (1965) defined as a group of human beings who live together in a system of social relationships. Obviously, the structural organization of every group is an important characteristic and influences the values and activities of the group. For example, the organization of the family is often linked to the childrearing practices of the group.

TABLE 38–1. Key definitions

Society	System of social relationships
Culture	Shared patterns of belief, feeling, and knowledge that guide behavior and individuals' definition of reality
Ethnicity	Sense of a shared heritage
Race	Taxonomic schema based on superficial difference, erroneously implying shared genetic heritage
Environment	Physical surroundings, resources and stressors, climate
Cultural difference	Belief that problems between cultures must be approached by looking at both cultures involved, thus avoiding ethnocentric bias
Emic	View of a phenomenon in terms of the culture where it occurs
Etic	Attempts a universal approach to psychological or social phenomena

A second crucial concept is *culture*, which Leighton and Murphy (1965) considered to be an abstract concept that describes a particular society's entire way of living. This notion encompasses shared patterns of belief, feeling, and knowledge that ultimately guide everyone's conduct and definition of reality. Culture refers to a multiplicity of elements that define human life, such as social relationships, religion, technology, and economics. Furthermore, it is an ever-changing concept, one that is learned, taught by one generation to the next, and obviously an integral part of all societies. *Ethnicity* is a somewhat narrower term that encompasses the idea that people identify with each other because of a shared heritage. In a technical sense, distinctions exist between social structure and cultural processes. However, it is often the case in the psychiatric arena that social and cultural components are combined to facilitate conceptualizations.

Race has been a controversial concept since its inception. From the beginning, race has been a taxonomic scheme applied to humans that assumes that certain visible physical characteristics represent a shared genetic heritage (Guthrie 1976; Johnson 1990). Most scientists now reject the use of race as a valid biological variable and the recently completed human genome project further reinforces this rejection by demonstrating that nearly 99% of the code mapped on 23 chromosomes are the same in all humans. No significant racial differences have been revealed in the genetic mapping. Race is therefore best understood as a "sociopolitical designation in which individuals are assigned to a particular racial group based on presumed biological or visible characteristics such as skin color, physical features, and, in some cases, language" (Carter 1995). Smedley (1993) was quite blunt in his assessment when he noted that "race has a reality created in the human mind, not a reflection of objective truths" (p. 22). He further noted that in North America, race was used consciously to "create a social stratification based on visible differences" that became a "major tool by which the dominant whites constructed and maintained social barriers and economic inequalities" (p. 22). Carter (1995) argued that "every person develops a racial component to his or her personality" (p. 227) and that such race-based contexts give "meaning and significance to one's physical features, such as skin color, eye color, facial features, body shape, and hair texture. These physical attributes, in turn, affect one's self-concept and, at the time, influence how others respond to the individual" (p. 228). Although the term *race* is used throughout this chapter, it refers to a sociopolitical construct whose "meaning is derived from prevailing societal attitudes that are invested in defining and characterizing differences between people" (Blue and Griffith 2001, p. 137) in the service of Smedley's aforementioned social stratification.

Another important definition centers on *environment*, which refers to physical circumstances of climate, altitude, natural resources, and the presence or absence of noxious agents. In this context, it is to be understood that, for example, a tropical climate has considerable influence on the games played by adolescents and favors the use of the outdoors. Similarly, a severely cold climate influences the dating practices of young lovers, because activities outdoors would be circumscribed. In the Caribbean, West Indian males have a year-round habit of standing for hours in groups talking about politics, sports, women, and other pressing topics of the day. They call it "liming." West Indians who have lived in cold climates speak disparagingly of the inability to lime where it is cold and snowing. Regarding the effect of noxious agents on those living in a particular area, it is well recognized that persons living in areas plagued by snakes, for example, are preoccupied with protecting themselves from intrusions by reptiles. In addition, special myths and fantasies that carry a central snake theme may then develop in that particular population. Closer to home, various workers have commented about the effect on children of their growing up while being chronically exposed to an environment that is characterized by such noxious agents as violence, crime, poverty, and drug abuse.

These definitions lead to a clearer appreciation of the notion that cultural psychiatry concerns itself with the relationship between psychiatric disorders and the matrix created by the interplay of society, culture, and environment. The more restrictive term *cross-cultural* (or *transcultural*) implies that a psychiatric problem in two different cultures is being compared in some way or that a psychiatric question in a particular culture is being studied or approached by someone who is from another culture.

A concept that may require special attention, despite its seemingly self-explanatory name, is that of *cultural difference*. Although culture is essentially transparent to individuals who share it, cultural difference creates problems in perception, relationships, communication, and ultimately medical diagnosis and treatment. At times, in the interest of abbreviating the term *cultural difference* as *culture*, it is possible to lose sight of the fact that a problem requiring intervention does not belong to the individual from the "other" culture, but may in fact reflect a difference between one cultural worldview and another. Another important consideration in cultural psychiatry is the difference between the *emic* and the *etic* perspective. Simply stated, the term *emic* refers to the ways people in a given culture view a phenomenon occurring within that culture. The term *etic* refers to a culture-general or universal approach to the viewing of psychiatric problems. Westermeyer (1985) warned against thinking that a diagnosable phenomenon is either emic or etic in nature; rather, it is important to determine the extent to which a given diagnostic entity is emic versus the extent to which it is etic. Consequently, observers from culture A may impose their cultural perspectives on their observations about culture B. The result is a "pseudoetic" or "imposed etic" view that may very well include a number of distortions about culture B. Berry (1975) has argued that an observer from culture A should temper this imposed etic view with emic considerations acquired through observation of culture B in order to eventually achieve a "derived etic" view of the specific psychiatric issue that is being considered within culture B.

Scope of the Discipline

Interest in cultural psychiatry has spread around the globe and has led to significant widening of its scope (Table 38–2). Although initially focusing with what has been called a "colonialist" approach (Kirmayer and Minas 2000) on collecting syndromes that appeared exotic to observers, more recent endeavors of cultural psychia-

trists have included studies of the following: the relationship of cultural factors to specific psychiatric disorders; the relationship of psychiatric disorders and processes to human universals such as gender and age; culture and personality development; attempts to understand the so-called culture-bound syndromes; comparative studies of diagnostic entities; culture and healing systems; culture and social roles; the impact of cultural difference on diagnosis and psychotherapy; and the impact of race and ethnicity on response to psychotropic medications.

TABLE 38–2. The scope of cultural psychiatry

Study of people in their natural habitats
Relationship of cultural factors to specific psychiatric disorders
Relationship of psychiatric disorders and processes to human universals such as gender and age
Impact of culture on personality development
Investigation of culture-bound syndromes
Comparative studies of diagnostic entities
Influence of culture on healing systems
Impact of culture on social roles
Interplay of culture and psychotherapy
Impact of race and ethnicity on response to psychotropic medications

---

Brief Historical Review

Early Observations

Although cultural psychiatry's recognition as a discipline may be fairly recent, many examples demonstrate that observers have long been concerned with the relationship of culture and medicine and with the influence of culture on behavior. D.H. Williams (1986) pointed out that data were published in the mid-nineteenth century purportedly showing that free blacks living in Northern states had high rates of admission to state insane asylums. The figures were ultimately intended to show that blacks lacked the ability to exist in a free society and consequently needed slavery to protect them from psychosocial stresses. Such an argument, although deeply flawed, was already clearly linking individuals' experiences with psychosocial institutions and the emergence of mental disorders.

Freud and Other Contributors

In a more formal sense, cultural psychiatry could be properly envisaged as not predating the contributions of Freud. In this regard, Foulks (1977) provided an incisive

In the inner cities, the cultural milieu often includes poverty, chronic exposure to crime, street and domestic violence, and substance abuse as well as a predominance of young, undersupported single mothers who are heads of households. The impact of this upbringing cannot be overlooked when reviewing a child from these origins. It has been stated that traits that are routinely characterized as antisocial may be culturally appropriate and defensive in nature within this culture (Reid 1985). However, other workers (P. Cohen and Brook 1987) have found such phenomena as family instability and parental inconsistency to be risk factors in children for the later development of psychopathology such as immature behavior and conduct disorder, the latter a known precursor to antisocial personality disorder. Canino and Spurlock (2000) commented on the protean effects of drug abuse on children raised in the culture of poverty, stating that neglect, abuse, overly harsh discipline, exposure to violence (domestic and otherwise), and frequent losses contribute greatly to a sense of instability, lack of control, and anger. Similarly, Li et al. (1999) recently examined the specific effect of exposure to drug trafficking itself, aside from any violence associated with the trafficking, as a unique risk factor predisposing toward violence and other risk behaviors in inner city youth. It is unclear what the long-term effects will be of protracted exposure to the chronic stress of such an environment. Nevertheless, Westermeyer (1995) suggested one possibility when he described enculturation as the process by which a well-functioning family passes on its culture to its offspring. He hypothesized that circumstances impairing the family's ability to enculturate their children adequately may result in individuals who are less able to resist substance abuse.

The positive effect of the extended family on the development of otherwise disadvantaged youth has been cited as an important compensatory factor, although its precise long-term effect has yet to be ascertained (Wilson 1989). Comer, in his well-known work about the school's role in the development of children, showed significant enhancement of the self-concept of students participating in his School Development Program (Haynes and Comer 1990).

Despite all we know about the relationship between culture and individual development, longstanding assumptions still deserve constant scrutiny and even occasional revision. This has been particularly evident in recent work on the theories of homosexual development and on the relationship between culture and gender identity. Litzenberger and Buttenheim (1998) have recently pointed out that current dominant cultural assumptions about gender, sexual orientation, and mental health must be reconsidered. This is especially necessary because of the degree to which societal assumptions about heterosexuality have so permeated psychological theories about gender and sexual orientation.

Effect on Intrapsychic Development

The influence of culture on intrapsychic development has been an important theme, and nowhere has this been more evident than in the work generated about the development of self-concept. As would be expected, this has been of special interest to minority groups in this country. It is an old hypothesis that, for example, American blacks possess significant self-hatred. This negative self-concept has been thought to be reinforced by the white-dominant American culture that defines blackness as bad and inferior. Spurlock (1986) reviewed the research that focused on the development of self-concept in black children, pointing out how the early conclusions have been subsequently challenged. Baldwin (1979) also described the theoretical models and research that relate to this important question of black self-hatred and questioned the methodology and subsequent conclusions of the research. Spencer's (1982, 1988) work has been instrumental in our reconceptualization of the influence of the cultural context on the development of self-concept in black children. Much of her research has focused on the nature of the interrelationship among race awareness, race dissonance (white-biased preferences [e.g., black children's preferential selection of white dolls over black dolls]), and self-concept. Prior to Spencer's research, findings of race dissonance in black children had been interpreted as evidence of a negative self-concept among blacks, thus supporting the black self-hatred hypothesis. Her data demonstrated that race dissonance and negative self-concept are not necessarily correlated. Instead, race dissonance among these children may be a product of social learning that attributes negative characteristics to black people and things, rather than an expression of low self-esteem. Close scrutiny has therefore led to a view of the black self-hatred hypothesis as based on incomplete evidence and faulty interpretations of the data.

More recently, Morgan et al. (2000) studied the effect of racism on black women in the workplace and discovered that the experience of racism in the workplace did not necessarily affect women's attitude or approach to work itself, but rather worked to diminish these women's satisfaction with life in general, outside of work. They posited that black women could understand the occurrence of racism at work and thus did not allow racism to color their view of the work environment. However, racism's ability to erode a person's self image may be harder to deter.

Other investigators have written eloquently about the process of developing and refining a positive racial identity (Cross 1991, 1995; Parham 1989; Phinney 1989). Cross (1991) used the term *nigrescence* to refer to a process of resocialization or identity change that ideally leads a person to overcome a negative internalized racial self-concept. He concedes that such a process is not necessary if a black person already possesses a positive racial self-concept or relies on some aspect of personal identity other than race/ethnicity to derive positive self-esteem. However, a black person with a racial attitude ranging from race neutral to antiblack may begin the process of nigrescence after an encounter that challenges his or her racial belief system and values. Whether the encounter is positive in quality (e.g., a trip to an African country) or negative (e.g., the direct experience of racial discrimination), such an event could catalyze initiation of the process and eventually lead to a reconfiguration of the person's racial identity. Cross believed that nigrescence is not necessarily a one-time occurrence; subsequent encounters may initiate new cycles of nigrescence, leading to further progression toward a positive self-image. The theory of racial identity development has been validated through empirical testing and has indeed served as a model for understanding self-concept development among other ethnic groups (Downing and Roush 1985; Finnegan and McNally 1987).

Other equally important issues have been studied with regard to the effect of culture on intrapsychic development. Considerable work has been done on the cultural stimuli in American society that lead women to conceptualize their status as secondary to the male's position (Carmen et al. 1981). The assumption has been that cultural values and stereotypes have been at the core of the notions that women are, for example, unable to be first-rate airplane pilots or surgeons. In general, many workers have taken the position that restructuring such distorted values could lead to significant change in the way future generations of women will think about themselves. Authors such as Gilligan (1982) have shown how previously accepted hypotheses relating to intrapsychic development, identity formation, and even morality have been developed largely from the male perspective, resulting in a view of the female as lacking idealized male qualities rather than as possessing desirable abilities and attributes.

In cultures where the inequities between the sexes are more explicit, more salient, and more rigid, women may resort to alternative ways of developing and wielding power. Constantinides (1985) described the *zar* spirit possession cult in Ethiopia and Sudan as offering such an alternative. A woman possessed by a zar is able to act in a manner that is not routinely acceptable in a nonafflicted woman, and she may make demands of her husband that would not be allowed under any other circumstances.

There are, of course, many values and taboos that a specific culture holds dear. The aggressiveness with which the culture makes clear that the values are important ultimately affects the basic mode of thinking and behavior of the individual. Many Caribbean cultures emphasize that sickness is a manifestation of one's standing with God or other spirits. Such belief enhances the individual's use of projection as an explanatory coping mechanism, but it also finally conditions the help-seeking behavior of the person and influences his or her degree of hope for recovery.

Effect on Interpersonal Relationships

It should follow that the work on culture and its effect on developmental and intrapsychic tasks might be extrapolated to conclusions or hypotheses about interpersonal relationships. Consequently, observations that led to assertions about the development of masculinity in particular societies were also ultimately used to clarify theories about homosexual and transsexual behavior. In the Sambia observations, the powerful and intense initiation rituals, coupled with the values and behavioral interventions of the males, led to the exclusion of transsexual behavior in that culture.

Similarly, females in American culture, who have thought of themselves as unable to perform certain jobs that have traditionally been held by males, have then in turn related hesitantly to the males, who have naturally been viewed as having all the power. Delgado et al. (1985) pointed out that in the business world it has long been assumed that females are submissive, dependent, unadventurous, suggestible, noncompetitive, excitable when facing crises, likely to have their feelings hurt, emotional, and conceited about their appearance. The expectation has also been that such traits render a woman unable to make managerial decisions with confidence and dispatch. Alternatively, it has been argued that the female business manager who, in effect, behaves like a man in this type of job would be considered a "castrating woman."

It is in fact fairly easy to demonstrate that society, through its enunciation of values and beliefs, can affect and order the nature of interpersonal relationships. For example, a group's view of the aging members of their population can influence whether old people are revered or put away to die. The ancient problem of war has also been frequently thought to be a function of how some cultures revere belligerence and the domination of other groups, not to mention how the perception of intergroup differences can lead to hatred and ethnic strife. Similarly, the process whereby specific subgroups such as the deaf population are stigmatized is a culture-mediated process. It is the values and stereotypes held by the hearing majority group that leads to the interpersonal difficulties between stigmatizer and stigmatized.

Nevertheless, it cannot be assumed that one can draw a straight line of linkage from a baby's early experiences with his or her mother, who is the very embodiment of that culture's values, to the specific type of personality that characterizes the adult the baby has become. Schweder (1979) pointed out that it is indeed difficult to be sure how specific childrearing practices can lead to adult behavior that is predictable in a multiplicity of contexts. Such caution is a useful reminder that culture, as a single element, should never be taken as the only determinant of thinking or behavior.

Frequency of Psychiatric Disorders

Attempts to establish the frequency of psychiatric disorders across cultures have been fraught with difficulties. Some of the problems discussed in the section on symptom expression account for the complexities encountered here. Another significant issue arises from the fact that researchers and clinicians have been unable to agree about diagnostic categories. On the one hand, there are country-specific diagnoses, such as the classic *bouffées délirantes* of the French. This is an acute psychotic state that Americans would view as schizophrenia or bipolar illness. On the other hand, it has been well established that schizophrenia tends to be a broader category in the United States than it is in many other countries. Diagnoses such as involutional paraphrenia are used in other countries but do not find currency in the United States. Establishing the frequency of disorders has now become a complex undertaking, because in one culture, for example, the abuse of alcohol may not be viewed in quite the same way as in another culture. Thus, groups may tend to report it with differing frequency. As Westermeyer (1985) pointed out, diagnosis in many countries may be a function of attitudes, political beliefs, historical influences, and even economic factors. Littlewood and Lipsedge (1997) warned that attempts at cross-cultural diagnosis can sometimes lead to "explanation" of symptoms without achieving an understanding of the individual's experience, thus limiting the validity of such an enterprise. Recently, Weissman et al. (1996) published the results of a cross-national epidemiologic study. Their population-based study involved 10 national sites and 38,000 community subjects. The study demonstrated

great variability of the lifetime rates of depression across countries, ranging from 1.5% in Taiwan to 19% in Lebanon; rates of bipolar disorder were more uniform. The high variability of depression rates served to highlight the strong influence of cultural differences on the expression and the detection of symptoms cross-culturally.

In the United States, significant problems have been associated with health care surveys of all the minority populations, specifically those of Native American, Hispanic, African, and Asian heritage. Much has been said about the task of identifying and sampling such groups, the complexity of achieving their cooperation, the tendency among many of the subgroups simply to answer yes to any interviewer's questions, the difficulty in designing valid interview protocols, and the complexity of controlling the bias of interviewers. In addition, there have often been technical difficulties associated with the preparation of interviewers who may not use the language of their respondents. The survey instruments may have been developed and validated using populations other than the minority groups. Even in this country, much of the work done has reflected contradictory results, some of which seem related to either the sampling or the methodologies used. The effects of racism and ethnic bias are also viewed by many (Adebimpe 1999; Fernando et al. 1998; Littlewood and Lipsedge 1997) as having substantial influence and have been addressed elsewhere in this chapter.

D.H. Williams (1986), reviewing the epidemiology of mental illness in black Americans, noted emerging difficulties in the NIMH-sponsored Epidemiologic Catchment Area (ECA) program. For example, the ECA surveys attempted to obtain good samples of blacks by including inner-city communities. However, Williams suggested this was biased in favor of low-income males. Consequently, he questioned whether middle-class and other groups had been surveyed.

There were early claims that depression was rare among American blacks (Schwab 1978), and indeed, conclusions have been drawn from these original data that few blacks commit suicide (Prudhomme 1938). More recent work consistently contradicted such earlier findings (King 1982) and suggested that those earlier conclusions were a function of the bias of the observers who were conducting such work. Serious consideration of all this cross-cultural scholarship leads inevitably to the conclusion that relatively little is understood about the incidence and prevalence of psychiatric disorders across different nations and cultures. It is also equally difficult to sort out in a specific group what influence culture may have on the finding that a particular psychiatric disorder occurs commonly whereas another disorder is

TABLE 38–3.   General trends in cross-cultural diagnosis (International Pilot Study on Schizophrenia)

Diagnostic information	How obtained	Reliability
Symptoms (e.g., hallucinations, delusions)	Patient report	Acceptable
Signs (e.g., flatness of affect, incongruity of affect)	Observation	Unacceptable
Historical data (e.g., work history, social relationships)	Synthesis of cross-cultural exchange	Least acceptable

rarely encountered. Part of the complexity may stem from the fact that it is not clear whether the high rates of one disorder exert a protective effect that results in the low rates of the other disorder, or whether the disorder with high rates masks the expression of the other disorder. This is seen, for example, in some cultures in which extensive alcohol abuse appears to mask the expression of depression or schizophrenia.

Hatch and Friedman (1996) recently argued that, at the level of clinical practice, it may be quite difficult to appreciate the true frequency of a psychiatric disorder because of cultural difference between groups. They gave obsessive-compulsive disorder (OCD) as an example and pointed out that OCD was thought to be evenly distributed across racial groups. Yet black Americans with OCD were difficult to find in clinical settings. The authors suggested that cultural differences influenced both the relatively low help-seeking behavior by blacks and the tendency for underdiagnosis of OCD in the same population. Similarly, a recent survey of individuals diagnosed with Tourette's disorder in Costa Rica (Mathews et al. 2001) revealed that the illness retained its general phenomenology in this cultural setting, but that the perceived impairment of the individuals was much less than would be expected and their social adjustment was remarkably good given the severity of symptoms. This was attributed to cultural difference and actually highlights the question of whether the diagnosis can be made when "marked distress or significant impairment in social, occupational, or other important areas of functioning" (American Psychiatric Association 1994) is absent.

It is hoped that the recent efforts to make DSM-IV a more culturally informed work has led to diagnostic categories that will retain more of their meaning in cross-cultural diagnostic endeavors.

Culture, Symptoms, and Diagnosis

Symptom Expression

The International Pilot Study of Schizophrenia (IPSS) was a transcultural psychiatric investigation of 1,202

patients in nine countries: Colombia, the former Czechoslovakia, Denmark, India, Nigeria, Taiwan, the former Soviet Union, Great Britain, and the United States. Although it was not an epidemiological survey, a major task of the project was to engender methods that might be used in different cultures to evaluate patients (Strauss et al. 1976). Specific interview schedules were used to collect data on patients who had already been admitted to treatment facilities.

Some conclusions from the IPSS merit consideration (Table 38–3). Certain symptoms (e.g., phenomena reported by patients, such as hallucinations and delusions) were the objects of greatest interrater reliability, although the reliability was better for raters from the same center than for raters from different centers. In contrast to this finding, the data showed that the rating of signs gathered by observation rather than by self-report, such as flatness of affect or incongruity of affect, was below acceptable reliability ranges. Historical information, such as that having to do with patients' prior level of functioning, personality traits, work history, and social relationships, showed even more cross-cultural variability. This work suggested that some cross-cultural psychiatric information might be reliable, although it depended on what type of information one was collecting. Symptoms reported by patients would be a more useful reference point for comparison than signs rated by observers, and premorbid history may be misleading when viewed by a clinician from a culture different from the patient's. Consequently, the cross-cultural diagnosis of paranoid schizophrenia (for which there is substantial reliance on symptomatology) might be more reliable than the cross-cultural diagnosis of catatonic schizophrenia (for which the physician relies on observation of signs).

The IPSS project also found that across the nine centers, depressed patients with psychotic symptoms were among the most similar of any diagnostic category. The symptoms that characterized these patients among different centers were depressed mood, gloomy thoughts, hopelessness, early morning waking, delusions of self-depreciation, and sleep problems. These findings demonstrated that through the use of specific interview techniques, it was possible to rely on symptom expression to delineate certain disorders such as paranoid schizophre-

TABLE 38–4. Hypothesized impact of internal (biological) and external (psychosocial) factors on cross-cultural variability of clinical presentation

Clinical entity	Biological factors	Psychosocial factors	Cross-cultural variability
Cerebrovascular accident	***	*	Low
Psychotic disorders	**	**	Moderate
Dissociative disorders	*	***	High

nia and psychotic depression. However, the researchers did point out that better instruments were needed to collect data that could be used in establishing relationships between symptomatology and social functioning.

Adebimpe et al. (1982) participated in a 5-year international study of patients with schizophrenia. Analyzing a subset of the United States data, these authors looked at differences in severity of symptoms between black and white patients and between urban and rural patients. Their patients with schizophrenia included several subtypes, and the raters used the Brief Psychiatric Rating Scale, the Itil-Keskiner Psychopathological Rating Scale, and structured in-person interviews. Black patients were found to exhibit the following severe symptoms when compared with white patients: auditory hallucinations, memory disturbances, disorientation, angry outbursts, and impulsiveness. Urban schizophrenic patients were less angry, aggressive, silly, negativistic, and uncooperative than rural patients, while exhibiting more anxiety, rigidity, ambivalence, posturing, and asocial behavior. Although the authors appropriately expressed caution regarding some of the differential manners in which clinicians perceived black as opposed to white patients or rural as opposed to urban patients, they felt their findings could be seen as reflecting a differentiation of emotional states that was linked to contrasts in the culture of the patients. Studies such as this one have suggested quite strongly that the symptomatic expressions of specific psychiatric disorders may vary as a function of the culture of the patients. This possibility should not be seen as being at odds with the IPSS findings that clinicians from different cultures may be able to agree in their delineation of a subgroup of individuals who carry a similar diagnosis.

Marsella (1988) elaborated a view of the interplay of biology, psychology, and culture that describes an inverse relationship between the extent that a disorder is biologically based (i.e., internal) and the effect of environmental (external) factors on a disorder's clinical presentation (Table 38–4). Marsella posited that a disorder primarily shaped by biological forces will have less variability between cultures than a disorder whose primary causation is social or environmental. Such a model predicts

that the presentation of a cerebrovascular accident, for example, would have much less cross-cultural variability than would a dissociative disorder, the latter having a much larger presumed component from the social and environmental sphere. Psychotic and mood disorders, thought to have a sizable biological determinant but also to be strongly influenced by the sociocultural milieu, should fall between these two extremes with regard to their degree of cross-cultural variability.

With respect to the more basic notion of how culture may affect the expression of distress, studies and other observations of Puerto Ricans have been particularly interesting. Rates of reported symptoms among Puerto Ricans seem to have remained high in all socioeconomic classes and were noted to be higher when compared in the same studies with respondents from other cultural groups. Haberman (1976) specifically attempted to explain the finding that Puerto Ricans living and surveyed in Puerto Rico had higher symptom scores than did Puerto Ricans surveyed in New York City. Also, the severity of the psychiatric symptom scores of the Puerto Ricans in New York lessened as the length of time that the individuals had lived in the city increased. After considering other possible arguments, Haberman concluded that culture seemed to account for the Puerto Ricans' willingness to express their subjective distress; as they acculturated to New York City, their traditional response style was tempered.

The ECA study, conducted in the past decade, appeared to confirm that Puerto Ricans reported somatic symptoms out of proportion to the rest of the population, resulting in a higher mean number of somatization symptoms detected by the Diagnostic Interview Schedule (Escobar 1987). Guarnaccia et al. (1989a) subsequently reviewed these data after having created a measure to quantify the existence of *ataques de nervios*, a culturally accepted syndrome used to express personal distress. Their results implied that the excessive somatic symptoms picked up by the structured interview were related to the presence of *ataques de nervios* in this population, a syndrome that the interview schedule was not looking for and consequently did not find. In a similar way, Malgady et al. (1996) conducted focus groups of

Puerto Rican adults aimed at developing meaningful idioms of expression. They then compared a group of clinic subjects with a group of nonpatients with regard to the presence of idioms of anger. An idiom of vindictive hostility, such as "It pays to remember who your enemies are," was found to correlate weakly with symptoms of anxiety and depression but was not predictive of a person's clinical status. An idiom of aggression, however, such as "At times, it is difficult to control my temper," was more strongly correlated with both anxiety and depression, and also predicted clinical status. It follows that when these idioms are not "seen" by diagnostic tools that do not anticipate their existence, it can influence the rate of diagnosis of anxiety and depressive disorders in this population. Caution therefore suggests that the use of etic diagnostic systems that are not tempered by knowledge of indigenous (i.e., emic) categories may lead to unexplainable or meaningless results. Not only does culture affect the expression of distress, but it can also act to hamper one's ability to identify and characterize distress in an individual from another culture. In other words, culture itself (i.e., the "other" individual's culture) is not the cause of misunderstanding, but rather it is the cultural difference between two interacting individuals that is potentially problematic.

Cultural Difference and Diagnostic Classification

It has been a general assumption that cultural difference has a significant effect on the determination of diagnostic categories. This axiom stems at least partly from the observation that different cultures are often in disagreement as to what behavior they label normal or abnormal. Wig (1983), when suggesting that culture has powerfully influenced diagnostic classification systems, noted that current American and European classification systems have elevated emotions such as anxiety and depression to the level of specific disorders. However, he wondered why other emotions such as jealousy or hatred have not been treated in the same way. Wig was making the point that jealousy and hatred might be treated with much more emphasis in other cultures and therefore in a non-Euro-American system could be considered worthy of consideration as specific disorders.

The categorization or definition of normal behavior is, of course, a culture-bound phenomenon. Thus, someone who suffers from hysterical drop attacks might be considered in one culture to have received a special blessing rather than to be in need of medical or psychiatric attention. Another such example has centered on the phenomenon of homosexuality. Even within the United States, the question of whether homosexuality is abnormal behavior has been the topic of significant discussion and disagreement among the lay public. Psychiatrists have not been exempt from this disagreement, eventually changing the "diagnosis" from homosexuality to ego-dystonic homosexuality (American Psychiatric Association 1980, p. 281), until arriving at the classification of "persistent and marked distress about one's sexual orientation" as a sexual disorder not otherwise specified (NOS) in DSM-III-R (American Psychiatric Association 1987, p. 296), which did not change in DSM-IV. An important criterion that has been reaffirmed by such changes is that any syndrome must be associated with subjective distress and/or help-seeking behavior in order to be classified as a disorder.

Fabrega (1992) warned quite eloquently of the inherent cultural character and possible bias of biomedical psychiatry and introduced, as an alternative to the biomedical "disease" concept, the culturally neutral concept of the "Human Behavioral Breakdown (HBB)" as "sustained anomalies of behavior [that are] not willful and [are] evaluated negatively [from within the culture]" (Fabrega 1992, p. 93). Using this model, he strongly advocated a view of illness that is guided by what he termed "symbolic, culturally relevant parameters of social behavior" (p. 100).

The way in which a particular culture defines hallucinations has also led to extended debate over the years. A Caribbean case example is particularly relevant here. A West Indian child voiced complaints about visual hallucinations that she was experiencing. This young girl was a member of a very fundamentalist religious group. She had been taken by her mother to the pastor of the group because the child had recounted stories of having seen strange figures that no one else could see. The pastor listened attentively to both child and mother and then spent considerable time in calming the mother's fears. Then he reinterpreted the hallucinations and restructured them in a context that was acceptable to the mother and consonant with the religious beliefs of the group to which they all belonged. In fact, the pastor attributed special religious characteristics to the objects that had been perceived in the visual hallucinations and convinced the mother that the child was especially chosen by Christ to have the experience. All of this clearly led to a redefinition of symptomatology that might have been perceived as abnormal. The child was not subsequently referred to a physician, and the whole affair was concluded in a manner that was at least temporarily satisfactory to everyone. The child's experience had been redefined as being normal.

Such differences over the definitions of normal and abnormal are not simply academic and do not relate only to settling what appears at first to be a straightforward disagreement. There are other important implications that flow from the resolution of this basic question. As mentioned above, general health behavior and help-seeking behavior are products of the process that defines normality. Waxler (1974) reminded us that the views of the society not only influence the diagnosis of the disorder but, in fact, also condition the treatment and even the prognosis of what might be ultimately diagnosed as normal. In the case of the West Indian child above, both the mother's help-seeking behavior and her satisfaction with the diagnosis derived from a cultural world view that she accepted. In this case, even the short-term prognosis was a by-product of the cultural context, because the mother, as a result of the pastor's intervention, rejected a sick role for her daughter.

There are, of course, limitations to the power of redefining emotions and behavior in the context of the person's culture in order to "depathologize" them. The idea that all pathology stems from cultural incongruities is just as implausible as attributing all psychopathology to biological processes while ignoring social and environmental influences. Several workers (Levy et al. 1979; Neutra et al. 1977) followed the lives of Navajo persons with epilepsy who presented with "hand-trembling," a symptom viewed by the Navajo as a positive sign of power and ability to become a "shaman-like diagnostician" (Neutra et al. 1977, p. 256). These authors discovered no evidence that the culture provided any protection from physical suffering or that it allowed the sufferer continued privileged status or problem-free function within Navajo society.

Wahass and Kent (1997) investigated differences between the United Kingdom and Saudi Arabia in public attitude toward the etiology of hallucinations and determined that Saudi individuals were more likely to view hallucinations as linked to satanic or evil influences and thus were more likely to avoid an individual with these symptoms and less likely to seek help from mental health treaters for anyone exhibiting these symptoms. These opinions and attitudes seemed relatively unaffected by an individual's level of education, being more dependent on cultural learning.

Culture has possibly influenced diagnostic practices in ways that still await further clarification. For example, little attention has been given to how sociocultural factors such as poverty might influence the expression of psychiatric disorders. Poverty can produce malnutrition that in turn could potentially influence the expression of psychiatric illness. As mentioned earlier, poverty can lead to exposure to a multitude of stressors besides that of material need. Inner-city neighborhoods have more than their share of violence, chemical dependence, crime, and

loss of loved ones by desertion, death, or incarceration. Any of these traumatic events can substantially affect an individual's view of life, and should be encompassed in the focus of a culturally informed clinician.

The issue of diagnostic reliability across different cultures has already been dealt with earlier in the discussion of the World Health Organization's multicenter pilot study of schizophrenia that took place in several countries. It should be reemphasized here that clinicians across cultures can reach agreements in some areas, but, as has been previously noted, they find it difficult to agree in others.

Particular problems have been posed by the phenomenon of bereavement. American psychiatrists have tried to delineate carefully the point at which uncomplicated bereavement ends and clinical depression begins. However, such attempts at categorization seem to fall short when the culture sanctions a recently bereaved individual's hearing the voice or the footsteps of the deceased relative. An appreciation of the specific culture's view of bereavement and a careful delineation of the patient's relationship to the dead relative in the context of the culture can help the psychiatrist avoid the error of diagnosing a psychotic depression when uncomplicated bereavement really exists. Eisenbruch (1984) provided an extensive review of the ethnic and cultural variations in the development of bereavement practices that should be useful to clinicians interested in this complex phenomenon.

Significant cultural variability exists in the manner in which an individual is able or chooses to express inner turmoil. Many workers (Florsheim 1990; Katon et al. 1982; White 1982) have noted that the phenomenon of expressing distress verbally and emotionally, seen predominantly in North American and Western European societies, is not a cultural given for the rest of the world. The experience and expression of distress not only as a mental but also as a bodily dysfunction, dubbed *somatization* by Western cultures, seems to be the global rule, not the exception. "Psychologization," or the experience and expression of distress in primarily mental or psychological terms, seems to be a culture-bound phenomenon in the West, perhaps a vestige of outdated theories of mind–body duality (Goodman 1991). Problems have arisen when individuals subscribing to one of these views attempt to diagnose those individuals whose culture leads them to experience the world differently. Weiss et al. (1995) reported on a group of patients in India who were studied using both the Structured Clinical Interview for DSM-III-R (SCID; Spitzer et al. 1990) and the Explanatory Model Interview Catalogue (EMIC; Weiss et al. 1986), the latter being a semistructured interview designed to produce a view of illness from the patient's perspective. They commented that, although it was the style of most patients to complain of symptoms that were somatic in nature, the SCID, based on the Western diagnostic schema, had a strong tendency to translate these complaints into a diagnosis of depression. Thus, recent Western diagnostic systems and classifications may yield results that reflect their ethnocentric bias at the expense of clinical accuracy.

Language, as a subset of culture, has a more concrete influence on diagnosis. For example, questions have been raised about the existence of depression as a concept in some languages. Some cultures facilitate the expression of complaints, whereas other cultures may inhibit the communication of inner feelings to health professionals. In a transcultural context, language is also thought to have another special influence. This occurs when a health professional assesses a patient whose language is different from that of the clinician. Marcos (1975) found marked distortions when evaluations of patients were conducted through interpreters, even when such interpreters were proficient. Westermeyer (1985) noted that interpreters do fairly well in obtaining the pertinent factual information in a case but do considerably less well when asked to interpret affect. Both minimization and exaggeration of symptoms have been mentioned as results of such interviews. To lessen distortions, translators should be well versed in psychiatry, should not be family members, should be familiar with the patient's culture, and should attempt to translate all utterances of both participants verbatim. In addition, the interviewing clinician should meet with the translator both before and after the interview, as a way of processing some of the intangible, nonverbal components of the interview.

DSM-IV and the Cultural Context

As mentioned earlier, the Task Force on DSM-IV and specifically the large group of cultural advisors to the Task Force labored extensively over the 3 years prior to the work's publication to help produce a diagnostic classification that was more clinically accurate and contained a better integration of biomedical, social, psychological, and cultural concepts of illness and diagnosis.

An important result of these efforts has been the *cultural formulation*, devised as a way of integrating an individual's cultural and experiential context into the scope of diagnosis (Mezzich and Good 1997). An explanatory outline for deriving the cultural formulation can be found in Appendix I of DSM-IV. It focuses the diagnostician's attention on five components of cultural data (Table 38–5), the synthesis of which then produces a more com-

plete view of the individual within the cultural context. These five components include the following:

1. The cultural identity of the individual, including the contrast between culture of origin and host culture in immigrant or ethnic minority individuals
2. Cultural explanations of the individual's illness, such as idioms of distress, culturally based meaning of symptoms, and perceived causes or models for illness
3. Cultural factors related to psychosocial environment, including culturally informed interpretations of problems with social support and environmental stressors
4. Cultural aspects of the relationship between individual and clinician, including potential barriers to understanding and assessing the meaning of symptoms
5. An overall assessment of how the cultural context influences the diagnosis and the approaches to treatment

TABLE 38–5. Components of the cultural formulation

Cultural identity of individual
Cultural explanations of individual's illness
Cultural factors related to psychosocial environment
Cultural aspects of relationship between individual and clinician
Overall cultural influence on diagnosis and approach to treatment

Mezzich (1996) commented that the sparse presentation of the appendix and its somewhat recondite placement in DSM-IV as the ninth appendix (the "I" is a letter, not a roman numeral) has limited the accessibility of clinicians to concepts that are perhaps worthy of their own axis in the multiaxial schema (Guarnaccia 1996; Mezzich 1996; Weiss 1996).

Within the text of DSM-IV, reference to cultural variability was quite explicitly made in sections that describe possible culturally based presentations for each major category of illness. An attempt was therefore made to avoid an ethnocentric approach to diagnosis. For example, the section on mood disorders mentions the variable meaning of somatic complaints, several culturally derived attributions of illness, and warnings about the inappropriateness of interpreting idioms of distress as hallucinations or delusions.

Also important are the comments added to the section on personality disorders, the diagnosis of which is known to have some relative difficulty with interrater reliability. In particular, DSM-IV warns that Cluster A disorders may be overdiagnosed in individuals whose culture, ethnicity, or status as immigrants or minorities may promote a paranoid or schizoid, but nevertheless adaptive, personality style. Antisocial personality disorder, in Cluster B, may also be prone to overuse in oppressed subsets of the population in which such a stance is adaptive. The diagnosis of dependent personality disorder and avoidant personality disorder should also not be made without taking into account cultural norms for behavior and communication and the cultural stressors of migration, respectively.

Race and Diagnosis

Race differs from culture in that, by definition, it is generally outwardly evident and therefore may be the first thing that a clinician usually knows about a patient (and that a patient knows about a clinician). If these two individuals happen to reside in a setting where the race of one is privileged in comparison with the race of the other, then differences take on further clinical significance.

Adebimpe (1981) described how black patients in the United States were overdiagnosed in some categories and underdiagnosed in others. It is an important claim that was suggested earlier by Bell and Mehta (1980) and amplified and reviewed by B.E. Jones and Gray (1986). Adebimpe had reviewed several studies and concluded from the data that the apparent misdiagnosis of blacks in comparison with whites resulted in blacks being found more often to be schizophrenic and less often to have mood disorders. However, Adebimpe realized that the data did not provide an answer to whether black clinicians made the errors less often than white clinicians. There are also obvious implications here that erroneous diagnosing ultimately suggests the execution of inappropriate treatment plans and the communication of negative prognoses to the black patients. In addition, the overdiagnosis of schizophrenic disorders in black patients with bipolar disorder may result in their undue exposure to long-term treatment with antipsychotics, thereby increasing these patients' risk of developing tardive dyskinesia.

Several reasons have been given for these alleged errors in diagnosis (Adebimpe 1981; B.E. Jones and Gray 1986), all of which are related to the amount of social and cultural distance between patient and clinician, which in part is dependent on race. These differences are manifested in the areas of vocabulary, styles of interaction, values, and modes of communicating distress. Stereotypes of black psychopathology have also been evoked as partially responsible. For example, B.E. Jones and Gray (1986) reminded us of the long-held belief that blacks are always cheerful and that having so little, they

are unable to experience object loss. Also, differences in blacks' expression of depression may lead to missing the diagnosis. It has been suggested that black patients somatize a great deal more than white patients. Racial differences can also lead to misperceptions of the clinician by the patient. It is likely that a patient from a nondominant race will react to a clinician from the majority race with feelings of suspicion and anger, which in turn may be interpreted by the clinician as paranoia, lability, or avoidance. It is also possible that a black patient's level of comfort with and feelings of trust about a white physician will lead to some emotional distance, resulting in limited disclosure of symptoms by the patient and limited exploration of possible psychiatric diagnoses by the clinician (Kosch et al. 1998).

An interesting example is the recent case of a black American psychiatrist attempting to diagnose depression in a black African simply by looking at the African's face. The psychiatrist had not talked to the African but pointed out that because the African had to be an oppressed individual, the saddened face was ample proof of a depressive disorder. Such obviously problematic reasoning points out that no particular cultural group is above making arrogant assumptions about another group that eventually lead to erroneous diagnoses and problematic treatment.

Considerable emphasis has been placed on the bias inherent in the instruments used to aid clinicians in making diagnostic conclusions. Black Americans have been noted to score higher than whites on several scales of the Minnesota Multiphasic Personality Inventory (MMPI), including the schizophrenia scale (Gynther 1972). This finding has been used to raise questions about the conclusions clinicians may reach from the use of scales that have not been originally validated on black populations (Greene 1987). Dana and Whatley (1991) cited a number of reasons that the MMPI has limited utility in interracial diagnosis. These include the inventory's lack of social, economic, and political considerations; the intrinsic limitations of comparative norms; the use of stereotypes; and neglect of the impact of the assessor's role on interpretation.

Indeed, extensive arguments have been made on the topic of intelligence testing in the black community, and a most incisive summary was provided by Samuda (1973). C.L. Williams (1987) also summarized the general issues relating to the psychological testing of minority patients. On the one hand, it has been pointed out that the definition of the intelligence quotient is precise and that there is nothing wrong with the use of intelligence tests, even if the tests do nothing but measure the adaptation of a black individual to a white middle-class view of American life. Others have taken opposing views and emphasized that intelligence testing of blacks should be discontinued because the tests were standardized and normalized on white middle-class individuals. Furthermore, such opponents of the use of intelligence testing often have pointed out that the test results are misapplied and that the reference bases for the tests are obscure. Finally, they have frequently underlined the point that the test scores are inappropriately applied to predictions about black Americans that often spell a dim future for this already disadvantaged subgroup of the population.

Neighbors et al. (1989) reviewed research on race and diagnosis and highlighted two opposing viewpoints, neither of which has been unequivocally supported by recent studies. According to these authors, workers have either 1) taken the position that diagnosticians assume racially based differences where none exist, or 2) assumed that racially based differences do exist but are unwittingly ignored by those making a diagnosis. Both hypotheses obviously would result in misdiagnosis, and the authors emphasized the need for further empirical research to resolve this dilemma.

Finally, it is important to remember that the concept of race, based on overt physical differences between groups, cannot be taken to imply clinical uniformity. For example, it would be meaningless to group together people from Japan and China as Asians and expect that they feel, think, and behave in some racially determined pattern. In the same vein, C.I. Cohen et al. (1997) found remarkable differences in clinical presentation between African American and Afro-Caribbean psychiatric outpatients, highlighting the importance of cultural rather than racial factors in symptom expression and presentation.

Gender and Diagnosis

Although a thorough discussion of the impact of gender differences on diagnosis is beyond the scope of this chapter, some mention must be made of recent developments and thinking regarding this topic.

An interesting trend within cultural psychiatry has been to examine gender differences in the presentation of some culture-bound syndromes. Some authors (Constantinides 1985; Littlewood and Lipsedge 1987) have commented that although sexism is a global issue, there are cultural differences in the way that women respond to gender discrimination or oppression. Various others (Bemporad et al. 1988; Gremillion 1992) have viewed anorexia nervosa as a culture-specific manifestation of conflict in women who are reacting to unrealistic expectations imposed by the present Western culture. As previously mentioned, Constantinides (1985) viewed some forms of spirit possession predominant in women in Somalia and Ethiopia as a culturally accepted manner of achieving a modicum of power within an otherwise sexually oppressive society. Littlewood and Lipsedge (1987) hypothesized that, just as the world of the Somali and Ethiopian women is dominated by male-run Islam, the world of Western women is similarly dominated by male-run "biomedicine," in which response to gender differences may tend toward pathologizing women's behavior.

It has been argued that the whole gamut of personality disorders reflects an inherent bias of male psychiatrists against females. Consequently, males in this society would tend to approve the competitive style of male professionals while condemning and labeling the same behavior in females as narcissistic and destructive. Many workers have also felt that the definition of sexual dysfunctions has really been based on male conceptions of female sexuality. Once again, the increasing participation and outspokenness of females in the general society have led to a redefinition and reconsideration of the standards for defining normal sexual functioning in females.

It is commonplace to point out how male therapists, rooted in their culture-bound views of maleness, make errors in dealing with female patients. However, it is also important to emphasize that female therapists can make similar mistakes. For example, American female therapists have difficulty understanding the dependency that women from other cultures show toward their men. Such female therapists may give clear prescriptive guidelines to foreign women to stop being subservient and to treat their men as equals. The clinician in these cases may be unconcerned about the effect that such advice would have on a woman coming from a family that was culturally different from that of the therapist.

Torres (1998) examined the phenomenon of *machismo* in Latino men and pointed out that the literature appears replete with pejorative and widely discrepant "definitions" of *machismo* with little regard for the positive values that such a term originally stood for, including qualities such as self-assertion, self-confidence, respect for others, investment in family, and dignity. He warned that the present, biased view of *machismo* can lead to misunderstanding and errors in diagnosis and treatment of Latino men.

Culture-Specific Syndromes

As part of the initial efforts to study cross-cultural psychiatry, considerable work has been done on the description of syndromes that psychiatrists consider either to be unique to certain cultures or to occur with special frequency among a defined group of people. Although there is historical benefit to mentioning these syndromes, it is important to remember that culture-specific syndromes most likely occur in all cultures. They should not be viewed as foreign curiosities that do not "follow the rules" of Western psychiatric diagnosis, but rather as indications that our diagnostic system is far from complete.

DSM-IV defines *mental disorder* as a "clinically significant behavioral or psychological syndrome or pattern that...is associated with present distress (e.g., a painful symptom) or disability (impairment in...functioning) or with a significantly increased risk of suffering death, pain, disability, or an important loss of freedom" (p. xxi). Recent questions have arisen about why clinically significant and distressing symptom patterns seen as "bound" to non-Western cultures retain the status of syndrome, whereas other symptom patterns, seen as clearly bound to Western culture, are classified as disorders (Hughes 1996). With this in mind, we have included in this section descriptions of syndromes that appear bound to the Western European/North American culture.

It is interesting that many of the syndromes classified as culture bound have components of either somatization, dissociation, or both. Of all diagnostic categories in DSM, those of somatoform and dissociative disorders are the ones most likely to be influenced by environmental and social forces. To make the diagnosis of a somatoform disorder, all biological components must first be excluded. A history of social or environmental trauma or conflict predisposes an individual to dissociative disorders. It therefore makes sense that phenomena that demonstrate either dissociative or somatoform pathology would show the most cross-cultural variability, as theorized by Marsella (1988) and previously shown in Table 38–4.

Difficulty in the clarification and understanding of syndromes thought to be specific or bound to a given culture can be appreciated when attempting to examine anxiety states or the mourning phenomenon across cultures. Most clinicians would agree that anxiety is a ubiquitous human experience. However, its clinical forms are well known to vary considerably from one country to another. It is unclear whether the anxious West Indian who somatizes is experiencing the same condition as the American who panics. Are these two conditions correspondingly equivalent states, and is culture the major differentiating element? Furthermore, there may be a specific cultural belief that strongly permeates the clinical entity. Consequently, a West Indian may see his or her somatic complaints as the result of having been hexed. It is often the existence of a framework of special meaning

in which the symptoms have been couched that makes observers so commonly confident that the clinical syndrome is unique and lacking an equivalent state in another culture.

The following are some examples of culture-bound syndromes (see also Table 38–6).

Ataques de Nervios

Described in Puerto Rican and other Hispanic groups (Guarnaccia et al. 1989a, 1989b), *ataques de nervios* refers to a socially sanctioned display of grief or great conflict characterized by "difficulty moving limbs, loss of consciousness or mind going blank, memory loss, [and symptoms of hyperventilation in which]...the person begins to shout, swear and strike out at others, [then] falls to the ground and either experiences convulsive body movements or lies 'as if dead'" (Guarnaccia et al. 1989a, p. 280). Generally, the episode is self-limited and may last only minutes. At other times, it is severe and extends to a few days, or the victim may suffer frequent attacks with few precipitating stressors, leading to distress and help-seeking behavior. González and Griffith (1996) advocated the classification of this syndrome under the general category of dissociative disorders, whereas others have focused on the somatic and pseudoepileptiform aspects to favor its being classified as a somatoform disorder. The mere fact that a syndrome exists that straddles these two categories questions the wisdom of making hard distinctions between somatoform and dissociative disorders.

"Falling Out"

Seen among black Americans but also called "blacking out" by Bahamians and "indisposition" by Haitians in Miami (Kirmayer et al. 1995; Philippe and Romain 1979), "falling out" characteristically occurs in response to a high degree of emotional excitement, such as may occur in the setting of a religious ceremony, during an argument, in fear-producing situations, or in "profound sexual conflict" (Weidman 1979, p. 99). Those who manifest this syndrome often simply collapse but without biting the tongue or losing the contents of bowel or bladder. There is an accompanying lack of ability to speak or move, although the individual can hear and understand. Although some have favored the addition of trance and possession trance disorder to the section on dissociative disorders in DSM-IV (González et al. 1997), the present decision to include the syndrome's description under dissociative disorder NOS is still a substantial improvement in the manual's cross-cultural scope.

TABLE 38–6. Culture-specific syndromes

Syndrome	Geographic or ethnic distribution	Clinical presentation
Ataques de nervios	The Americas, people of Hispanic heritage	Socially sanctioned display of grief or conflict characterized by agitation, unfocused aggression, lability of mood, fluctuating levels of consciousness, difficulty moving limbs, hyperventilation
"Falling out"	African Americans	Occurs in response to great emotional excitement, characterized by collapse, inability to move, loss of volitional movement without loss of sensory consciousness or of bowel or bladder control
"Blacking out"	Bahamians	
Indisposition	Haitians	
Amok	Various locations and ethnicities, including Asia, Africa, New Guinea	Follows a personal humiliation, characterized by prodromal brooding, followed by sudden, uncontrollable homicidal rage, then full or partial amnesia for the episode
Pibloktoq	Arctic natives	Prodromal lethargic, depressed, anxious state, followed by agitated, seemingly purposeless running, ending in exhaustion, sleep, and amnesia for the episode
Chakore	Ngawbere tribe, Panama Miskito tribe, Nicaragua	
Grisi siknis		
"Frenzy" witchcraft	Navajo, United States	
Koro	Various countries in Asia	Feelings of panic brought about by the conviction that one's genitalia are retracting into the abdomen and that this phenomenon will result in death
Anorexia, bulimia	North America	Bizarre eating patterns, apparently resulting from distorted body image, characterized either by severe caloric restriction, food bingeing and/or purging
Spirit possession	Numerous cases reported in Asia, Africa	Brief, reversible episodes of dissociation, characterized by the victim's behaving as if possessed by a spirit or deity and followed by amnesia for the episode
Multiple personality disorder	Primarily North America, Western Europe	Chronic dissociative syndrome, usually associated with severe abuse in childhood, characterized by the sufferer's experience of two or more "personalities" coexisting and vying for control of the individual
Hwa-byung	Korean nationals and Korean Americans	Ascribed to "excess anger," chronic frustration, adversity; characterized by sensation of an epigastric mass, anorexia, anxiety, dyspnea, epigastric pain
Generalized somatic syndromes ("brain-fag," *ode ori*, *shinkeishitsu*, neurasthenia, *shenjing shuairuo*, chronic fatigue syndrome, others)	Asia, Africa, the Americas	Characterized by low mental and physical energy, poor sleep, vague somatic complaints

Amok

This phenomenon was traditionally associated with Malaya (Carr 1978) but has been described as occurring also in Africa and more rarely in Papua New Guinea (Burton-Bradley 1968). Often, there is a prodromal period of brooding after an incident during which the victim (almost always male) has felt slighted or humiliated. What follows is a sudden, uncontrollable rage that leads to the individual's aimlessly running around with a weapon that is ultimately used to kill a number of people or animals. Sometimes the perpetrator then kills himself. Those captured alive have claimed no memory of the killing (Schmidt et al. 1977). Although some studies have shown the syndrome to be associated with psychotic disorders (Tan and Carr 1977), this does not appear to be a uniform finding. Although some workers (Gaw and Bernstein 1992; D. Spiegel and Cardeña 1991) have favored the inclusion of *amok* as an impulse control disorder, it is mentioned under dissociative disorder NOS in DSM-IV;

a cardinal feature of the syndrome is a temporary alteration in consciousness.

"Running" Syndromes

Simons (1985) used the term *running taxon* to describe several similar syndromes characterized by prodromal lethargy, depression, or anxiety followed by a high level of activity, a trancelike state, potentially dangerous behavior in the form of running or fleeing, and ensuing exhaustion, sleep, and amnesia for the episode. Among such syndromes are *pibloktoq* among native peoples of the Arctic (Gussow 1960), *chakore* in the Ngawbere of Panama (Bletzer 1985), *grisi siknis* among the Miskito of Nicaragua (Dennis 1985), and Navajo "frenzy" witchcraft (Neutra et al. 1977). Although present diagnostic schema are only able to place such syndromes in the sphere of dissociative disorder NOS, it is possible that future versions of DSM will allow for the diagnosis of psychogenic fugue in some of these cases.

Koro

Various reports from Asia, including Hong Kong (Yap 1965), Singapore (Ngui 1969), India (Nandi et al. 1983), China (Tseng et al. 1988), and Malaysia (Adityanjee et al. 1991), have referred to the syndrome of *koro*, or *suoyang*. This syndrome occurs either singly or in epidemics and is characterized by acute and prominent panic-like symptoms brought about by the sudden onset of fear that one's genitalia are retracting into the abdomen and that this will result in death. Although similar syndromes have also been described in Western settings, these have always been associated either with major (Axis I) diagnoses such as schizophrenia (Ede 1976; Edwards 1970) or with neurological/organic etiologies such as brain tumor (Lapierre 1972) or toxic states (Dow and Silver 1973). In contrast, reports from Asia suggest that *koro* presents as a generally benign, time-limited illness without association to additional psychopathology and with a good prognosis. R.L. Bernstein and Gaw (1990) outlined a classification scheme for *koro* as a "genital retraction disorder" under the section of somatoform disorders. The proposed criteria would exclude organic factors and Axis I disorders other than somatoform disorders and would ask for the determination of whether the case occurred within or outside of the cultural context.

Anorexia Nervosa and Bulimia Nervosa

Recently, bulimia nervosa has been argued to be most common among middle-class American white females, although it seems to be appearing also among black females from a similar socioeconomic background. This syndrome is characterized by excessive food intake that is then followed by self-induced vomiting. It is often associated with depression and anorexia. Although classified among the eating disorders by American psychiatrists, these disorders are thought to represent American culture-bound syndromes because of their markedly lower prevalence in other parts of the world. British psychiatrists have also been struck by the infrequent appearance of black subjects among their cases of anorexia nervosa or bulimia nervosa (Thomas and Szmukler 1985).

Spirit Possession and Dissociative Identity Disorder

Globally, there are a number of syndromes of spirit possession or possession trance (Akhtar 1988; Bose 1997; Chandrashekar 1989; Gussler 1973; Kleinman 1980; Salisbury 1968; Sharp 1994; P. Stoller 1989; Suryani 1984; Suwanlert 1976; Yap 1960). These syndromes, which are characterized by the belief that the victim's body is taken over by a spirit, are manifested by identity confusion, an inability to control one's actions, a temporary change in the personality of the victim, and partial or total amnesia for the episode. In India, this disorder appears to be more prevalent among women (Chandrashekar 1989; Saxena and Prasad 1989) and among individuals having experienced chronic or acute interpersonal conflict or a recent loss. It is often reversible, with the longest episodes lasting days to weeks. In many cases, an individual who experiences an episode of possession trance is more likely to be possessed again in the future.

The various accounts of possession trance reveal substantial differences from dissociative identity disorder as described in DSM-IV. The association with childhood abuse has hardly been mentioned with regard to pathological possession trance, but it has also not been systematically studied. Although both dissociative identity disorder and possession trance involve the coexistence within a person of different personalities, a key phenomenological difference between the two is the presumed origin of this other personality: in dissociative identity disorder the personality is understood by the victim as part of him or her, whereas in the possessed person the phenomenon is viewed as the effect of an external supernatural entity. In addition, cases of pathological possession trance are often episodic and remitting, in contrast to the chronic nature of dissociative identity disorder. Furthermore, reports of simultaneous possession by several coconscious "spirits" are rare. The relationship between these two syndromes is presently uncertain, with authors (Adityanjee et al. 1989; Varma et al. 1981) suggesting that the syndromes may share common mechanisms, whereas "the pathoplastic influence of the prevailing culture may be important in causing [the]...differences" in presentation (Adityanjee et al. 1989, p. 1610). The inclusion of dissociative trance disorder in DSM-IV as a criteria set for further study incorporates many of the findings cited previously, so as to allow collection of more data on pathological spirit possession and similar syndromes.

Hwa-Byung

Hwa-byung, a syndrome of somatic complaints ascribed by Korean folklore to excess anger—the word *hwa* means "fire" or "anger," and the word *byung* means "illness"—is typically characterized by a sensation of an epigastric mass, anorexia, anxiety, dyspnea, and epigastric pain (K.-M. Lin 1983). It is said to be primarily an illness of women and to be attributed by the affected persons themselves to adverse social circumstances such as "disappointments, sadness, miseries, hostility, grudges, and unfulfilled dreams and expectations" (Pang 1990, p. 496). Partial response of the syndrome to antidepressants has been reported (K.-M. Lin 1983).

Generalized Somatic Syndromes

The term *generalized somatic syndromes* is meant to cover several illness behaviors that have in common the symptoms of low energy, poor ability to concentrate, poor sleep, headaches, and vague somatic complaints. The Nigerian syndromes of "brain fag" in students, described by Prince (1985), and *ode ori*, described by Makanjuola (1987) among the Yoruba, qualify as part of this group. Sufferers of *ode ori* who were examined with the Present State Examination (Wing et al. 1967) commonly exhibited depressed mood, "tension pains," complaints of ill health, delayed sleep, anxiety, and low energy. In the Western world, chronic fatigue syndrome has been identified as a similar entity, for which no certain biological mechanism has been discovered, and much debate has continued between those who regard it as biological disease being delegitimized by physicians (Richman et al. 2000) and those who comment on the syndrome's strong association with psychiatric morbidity (Skapinakis et al. 2000).

Another generalized somatic syndrome with a strong component of mood dysregulation is that of *shenjing shuairuo*, or *neurasthenia*, in China (Kleinman 1982; Lee 1999; T. Lin 1989; Ming-Yuan 1989), also known in Japan by the name of *shinkeisuijaku*, or "ordinary"

shinkeishitsu (Russell 1989; Suzuki 1989). The term *neurasthenia* was used in the late nineteenth century by the American physician George M. Beard to describe a syndrome of headaches, insomnia, gastrointestinal symptoms, and vague somatic complaints that Beard believed derived from an exhaustion of the victim's nervous system. Although the diagnosis eventually fell into disuse in its country of origin, it quickly caught on in the rest of the world throughout the twentieth century, to the point at which in 1968 it was reinstituted as a type of neurosis in DSM-II (American Psychiatric Association 1968) after having not been listed in DSM-I (American Psychiatric Association 1952; T. Lin 1989). Of note, Kleinman (1982) studied 100 patients diagnosed as neurasthenic in China with the use of a culturally adapted version of the Schedule for Affective Disorders and Schizophrenia (SADS) and determined that the vast majority of these persons, although complaining primarily of somatic ailments, were suffering from clinical depression and could benefit from antidepressant medication. Lee (1999), however, warned that the high prevalence of neurasthenia in China during the Cultural Revolution may have also been a sign of the social and emotional repression enforced on the population during this time, such that it would be a serious error to equate the syndrome with major depressive disorder without understanding the cultural context in which such a syndrome developed.

There are many other culture-specific syndromes excluded here simply because of space limitations. Although they may appear exotic when viewed from outside the culture from which they originate, it is important to remember that understanding each of these syndromes necessitates having a good knowledge of its cultural context.

Significant research is still needed to allow for the eventual elimination of the term *culture-bound* from our diagnostic schema. Clinical and theoretical work must focus on the clear delineation of these syndromes, with the goals of improving our understanding of how patients afflicted with these entities should be treated and enhancing our ability to determine their ultimate prognosis. It should be seen as a step forward that the American Psychiatric Association Task Force on DSM-IV took an interest in improving the cross-cultural scope of the manual by adding material about cultural variation in clinical presentation as well as descriptions of many so-called culture-specific syndromes, both as an appendix and as potential presentations of NOS disorders. This will undoubtedly aid those involved in research on cross-cultural diagnosis.

Migration and Psychiatric Disorders

Effect on Families and Individuals

It is no secret that migration has for many years been regarded as a cause of pathology. The movement of individuals from a cultural context in which they have been surrounded by family, friends, and familiar institutions to a different geographic area that distances these people from their usual support systems has generally been seen as seriously stressful. Such dislocation of human beings from their own cultural groups has frequently been a contributory element to the emergence of psychopathology in the migrating individual. Clinicians have been so confident of this that they have often recommended that the patient then be sent back to his or her hometown or country, presumably with the idea that reentry into the home context would have a therapeutic effect on the patient. However, Hickling (1991) suggested that this reentry into the home environment may also be stressful and problematic.

Littlewood and Lipsedge (1981) described the situation of 16 Caribbean immigrants in London who were socially isolated, working-class women with children. These individuals all experienced a severely traumatic encounter with overt racism, problems with housing, or unemployment. Subsequently, they developed psychological difficulties characterized by rapid mental status changes and the elaboration of persecutory symptoms that involved neighbors. A 3-year follow-up study showed that the women had continued to have significant psychiatric symptoms. These difficulties can be seen as the direct result of an unsuccessful adaptive response to the stress of confronting a new culture. This phenomenon, whereby an individual from one culture comes in contact with another culture, has been termed *psychological acculturation.*

The stress of acculturating to a new sociocultural context can be expected to have serious problems for the families concerned. Canino and Canino (1980) have effectively described the complex process of acculturation for Puerto Rican families who migrated to the United States. Although the authors focused on the urban, low-income Puerto Rican family in the United States, their observations have wide applicability, because most migrants do have at least a temporary drop in their socioeconomic standing as a consequence of moving to a foreign land. Canino and Canino described the traditional pattern of the Puerto Rican family as characterized by the presence of an authoritarian father and a submissive, self-sacrificing mother; a great deal of involvement; dependence; and little emphasis on self-

differentiation. The authors pointed out that independent behavior, especially in adolescent girls, was neither expected nor well tolerated. They emphasized that such a structure in the context of Puerto Rico remains normal and functional. However, the Puerto Rican family that has migrated to the United States then has to confront poverty, discrimination, and minimal political influence, as well as a host of cultural values that are significantly different from those they left behind. The American culture may be hostile to the authoritarian attitudes of the Puerto Rican father, encourage the mother to abandon her submissive style, and foster a sense of autonomy and independence in the adolescent daughter. If the family has to depend on the welfare system, this may further destabilize the prior structure by making the woman the recipient of financial assistance. In an effort to cope with his threatened traditional role, the father may attempt to reassert his authority, resulting in a family structure that is more rigid and less responsive to the stress of adaptation. This renders the family dysfunctional and pathological in this new cultural context.

The problem of migration is most easily conceptualized in terms of movement of families or individuals from one country to another. However, clinicians need to remember that it is also an issue at home in the United States. On several occasions, the lead author (E.E.H.G.) has observed clinicians dealing with black American university students studying in predominantly white universities. The black students previously only frequented predominantly black institutions. In moving to the white university, they felt dislocated, rootless, and overwhelmed by a sensation of inferiority and of being an outsider. This in turn led to their becoming increasingly suspicious, defensive, and withdrawn, and their academic performance suffered. Once the therapist understands the role that is being played by cultural dissonance, he or she can then set about structuring ways of facilitating the adjustment of the student to the new culture.

Process of Acculturation

Anthropologists worked in the early years on the concept of *acculturation* as a way of studying how two groups with different cultures come in contact and interact with each other. Often, one of the groups was numerically, politically, and economically stronger than the other. In recent years, it has been noted that groups, families, and individuals participate in this process of adaptation to a different culture.

The acculturation of groups can have effects that are physically obvious, such as one group's having access only to inferior housing or transportation. Biological changes may result from intermarriage of the two groups in con-

TABLE 38–7. Potential outcome of acculturative interaction between dominant and nondominant groups

Nondominant individual's cultural identity valuable	Positive relations sought with dominant group	Outcome of acculturation
Yes	Yes	Integration
No	No	Marginality
Yes	No	Resistance
No	Yes	Assimilation

Source.   Adapted from Berry and Kim 1988.

tact; political, economic, linguistic, religious, and other changes are equally possible. It was commonly suggested in the past that the stress that resulted from the acculturation phenomenon would be borne principally by the nondominant group. However, we now know that the nature of the interaction between a dominant and a nondominant group depends on a series of elements; consequently, group tension and individual anxieties might be felt by members of both groups.

Berry and Kim (1988) theorized that a systematic course to acculturation existed, characterized by contact of the two groups, conflict between them, and adaptation to the interaction. Conflict occurs especially when either of the two groups is resistant to the process. Such stress ultimately influences the type of acculturative outcome.

The result of acculturation for the groups and the individuals concerned depends on several interacting factors, such as the phase of acculturation, the mode of acculturation, the type of acculturating group, the nature of the dominant cultural group, the social and cultural characteristics of the less dominant group, and the psychological characteristics of the individuals involved in the process.

Berry and Kim constructed a theoretical model (Table 38–7) that is useful when attempting to understand how the various outcomes of the acculturation process differ in the level of stress that they generate for the individual and the group. These theorists suggested that when a nondominant group comes in contact with a dominant group, members of the nondominant group must respond to two important questions. The first is whether the nondominant individual's cultural identity has such value that it should be retained. The second question is whether positive relations with the majority dominant group should be sought. Potentially, the varieties of answers to these two questions would influence the extent of stress present in the acculturative process, both for the individual and for the group.

In the application of this model to acculturation, Berry and Kim carefully asserted that this theoretical framework is still subject to influence by elements such as the psychology of the individuals, economics, and politics. Thus, for example, the minority group may seek to pursue a strategy of *integration* by answering yes to both questions. In doing this, they may be purposefully looking for a style of acculturative adjustment that has minimal stress. Nevertheless, the majority group may simultaneously be following a political goal of blocking such integration because of a wish to deny the importance of the minority group's identity. In such a case, the integration approach would indeed produce significant stress for the nondominant group.

Another possible adaptive response is *marginality*. In this case, both of the questions would be answered in the negative. Marginality represents a hopeless and negative view of life, and individuals who subscribe to this position are most likely to be functioning on the very periphery of the society. By answering no to both questions, these individuals reject any compromise with the dominant group and also see no value in their individual or group identity. It would seem evident that a consequence of this position would be intense identity conflict and confusion, both personally and politically.

In contrast to marginality, integration is characterized by affirmation of the value of the minority group's identity as well as the need to seek positive relations with the majority dominant group. Berry and Kim (1988) hypothesized that this modality represents the least stressful adaptive response to acculturation because it is characterized by healthful ego adaptation and also places a positive premium on minority group institutions. At the same time, the seeking of positive relations with the majority group is a political approach that seeks compromise and consequently sets up a terrain for constructive interaction. This is not to suggest that the integrationist stance may not be full of problems when the dominant group is intent on frustrating the decisions and pursuits of the nondominant group. This is particularly evident in the political arena, as in the case of southern white supremacists who seek to block any political negotiations with African American leaders.

There are two other possibilities of adaptive response to the difficulties of acculturation: *resistance* and *assimilation*. In the context of the theory described above, both of these would be predictive of considerable accultura-tive stress. In the case of resistance, the individual answers affirmatively to the question of whether his or her nondominant group's identity is of value and answers in the negative to the question of whether positive rela-tions should be sought with the majority group. In this situation, resistance implies a state of perpetual conflict with the dominant group. Although it is true that resis-tive acculturation could provide group support and enhancement of self-esteem, opposition to the seeking of positive relations with the dominant group would be expected to take its toll in the political and economic arena. One could argue that the Black Panther party was an example, par excellence, of the resistance pattern.

The posture of assimilation is an adaptive response in which the individual responds in the negative to the ques-tion of whether the nondominant group's identity is of value and answers affirmatively to the question of whether positive relations should be sought with the dominant group. Although resistive acculturation could potentially lead to caustic and difficult interactions with the dominant group, the assimilation stance still leads to a repudiation of the nondominant group's self-esteem and potentially results in what Bush (1976) considered to be the "depreciated character." Clearly, Bush would argue that any refutation of a nondominant group's sense of self would inevitably lead to a pervasive feeling of hopelessness. Consequently, one could argue that the assimilationist position is by definition self-destructive, particularly in the psychological sphere.

The importance of such a model lies in its potential applicability to the study of groups, families, and individ-uals. The model serves to highlight the complexity of the process of acculturation, its influence on the emergence of psychopathology at different unitary levels, and the various adaptive mechanisms available to a group to cope with the stress of migration. The GAP's Committee on Cultural Psychiatry used this model to generate hypoth-eses that explain the suicide rates of certain ethnic groups in the United States who are struggling with the task of adapting to the dominant culture (Group for the Advancement of Psychiatry, Committee on Cultural Psy-chiatry 1989).

Ethnoculture, Race, and Psychiatric Treatment

Culture and Psychotherapy

All societies have developed ways of confronting physical and psychological suffering. Psychotherapy in its broad-

est sense should be seen as a curing system for psycholog-ical ills. The technical ways in which psychotherapy is applied or practiced obviously vary from one culture to another. However, Frank (1963) postulated that six ele-ments lie at the core of all nonmedical healing and should exist independently of the cultural context in which the healing is practiced: 1) the emotional stirring of the indi-vidual, 2) the existence of a healer on whom the individ-ual depends for help and who holds out hope of relief, 3) the arousal of the individual's expectations by the healer's personal attributes, 4) the evocation of hope in the individual, 5) the bolstering of the individual's self-esteem, and 6) the strengthening of the individual's ties with a supportive group (Table 38–8).

TABLE 38–8. Core elements of nonmedical healing

Emotional stirring of the individual

Existence of healer on whom the individual depends

Arousal of individual's expectations by healer's personal attributes

Evocation of hope

Bolstering of self-esteem

Strengthening of the individual's ties with a supportive group

Source. Data from Frank 1963.

Griffith and colleagues (Griffith and Mahy 1984; Griffith et al. 1980) pursued the clarification of mecha-nisms that individuals employ in church for therapeutic purposes. Griffith and Mahy (1984) reported on the cer-emony called "mourning" that is practiced in the Spiri-tual Baptist Church in the West Indies. The ritual involves praying, fasting, and the experiencing of dreams and visions while in isolation. In their analysis of the prac-tice and their interviews of a group of individuals who had gone through the mourning ceremony, the authors concluded that mourning is a viable psychotherapeutic practice for the church members. Griffith and Mahy also were able to show how the mourning experience satisfies the requirements of nonmedical healing established by Frank. Indeed, the authors pointed out that the use of the church as an institution in which one can engage in a psy-chotherapeutic experience requires a specific cultural worldview that includes a view of life and of health as being positively influenced by a special commitment and relationship to God.

The importance of structuring a psychotherapeutic ritual around a belief system has been emphasized by Wittkower and Warnes (1974). These authors under-lined the relevance of cultural factors in the application of psychotherapeutic practices. They showed how a belief in supernatural forces as the cause of psychological suffering would lead the patients away from Western medicine and toward increased reliance on other systems such as churches or other spiritual healing rituals. Numerous authors have emphasized the healing qualities of such native systems as the *Umbanda* cult in Brazil (Pressel 1973), *Espiritismo* in Puerto Rico (Comas-Díaz 1981; Koss 1975), *Vodun* in Haiti (Métraux 1972), and the Native American Church (Calabrese 1997) as being parallel in function and intent to the practice of psychodynamic psychotherapy in North America.

Within the United States, J.P. Spiegel (1976) described the problems created by cultural factors even when traditional psychoanalytically trained psychotherapists were at work. He outlined the problems that confronted middle-class American therapists who were seeking to establish a psychotherapeutic relationship with members of Irish-American families. Spiegel emphasized that the middle-class American therapists held values that were different from those of the Irish-American patients. These therapists approached their work with expectations that the patients would, for example, develop relative independence from their families and from other pressures for conformity to Irish-American values. The therapists also expected to maintain benevolent neutrality in the moral arena while hoping to have their patients be less under the domination of their own superego pressures. There seemed to be a clear expectation that the patients would identify with and accept the goals and values of the therapists. However, this did not happen, and the result of the experimental work was that the therapists ultimately had to modify their own goals and procedures, this being the only alternative to abandoning the research and accepting failure. For example, the therapists had to accept the limitations on autonomy and independence within the general framework of the Irish family.

More recently, Littlewood (1996) and others (Blue and González 1992) have commented on the fallacy of seeing psychodynamic psychotherapy as being independent of culture, noting that psychodynamic thinking is rather a culture unto itself and intimating that even psychodynamic psychotherapy that is intraracial and intraethnic is vulnerable to cross-cultural distortions. Several other workers (Dien 1983; Dwairy 1997; Florsheim 1990; Tung 1991; Yamamoto 1998) have added that the view of the individual as an autonomous, independent being, as idealized by Western-based psychological thought, is not consistent with the prevailing worldview elsewhere, in which considering the individual without looking at how this individual fits into his or her social context is meaningless.

Comas-Díaz and Jacobsen (1991) carefully examined the notable impact of ethnic, racial, and cultural differences on the psychotherapeutic relationship, from the view of both transference and countertransference. Possible signs of interethnic transference include overcompliance, denial of ethnocultural differences, and the more understandable feelings of mistrust and hostility in a patient from an oppressed group. Intraethnic transference, in turn, can be characterized by idealization of the therapist, by viewing the therapist as a "traitor" to his or her race or culture, or by fear of merging with the therapist. Countertransferential reactions in an interethnic psychotherapeutic relationship can be characterized by denial of differences, excessive cultural curiosity, and guilt or pity when the patient is from a highly disadvantaged group. Intraethnic relationships are susceptible to countertransference reactions such as overidentification and collusion, as well as anger, especially when work with the patient touches on the therapist's unresolved feelings about oppression and prejudice.

The successful resolution of many of the difficulties resulting from cultural differences requires from therapists openness, flexibility, curiosity, and a willingness to acknowledge and explore the cross-cultural components of transference and countertransference. However, not all therapists may be capable of such stances. The traditional stance of having the therapist leave value choices ultimately and completely to the patient may only be theoretically possible in a vacuum. As the therapy unfolds, the therapist may indeed be sneaking into the exercise his or her own value representations. Ultimately, the emphasis on individualism and autonomy that is so much a part of American psychotherapy may have to be replaced by what J.P. Spiegel (1976) considered to be horizontal, collaborative decision making.

Psychotherapy and the Social Construct of Race

Whereas workers such as E.E. Jones (1982) have provided significant research impetus to the area of race and psychotherapy, Bradshaw (1982) emphasized effectively the clinical problems that have emerged as a function of the role that race plays in psychotherapy. He concentrated entirely on the problems of the black–white dichotomy. However, the issues that he outlined are applicable to other potential dichotomies in the patient–therapist context. Certain errors seem specific to the white therapist–black patient dyad. Bradshaw showed how the therapist could be influenced by common myths such as that of the black American family as a repository of severe pathology—the one-parent family as leading unavoidably to psychopathology, blacks as having a poor self-image and/or being sexually promiscuous, and black patients as unable to be treated by traditional psychotherapy.

The maintenance of such myths seems partly related to the fact that white therapists are frequently ignorant of the reasons that black patients present themselves as passive and inarticulate. In addition, the situation can be rendered more complex if the therapist's position is countenanced and reinforced by a white supervisor. Obviously, a white therapist's countertransference can be stimulated by antiwhite hostility coming from the patient.

Bradshaw also saw the black therapist–white patient dyad as having the potential for certain difficulties. In this context, both individuals may be unable to deal with the meaning of race in the therapeutic relationship. Blue and González (1992) viewed the stress on black therapists as the result, in part, of their sense of distance from both their culture of origin and the dominant culture, as represented by the patient. For the therapist, the authors advocated careful self-examination and reliance on supervision, with the intent of focusing on racial transference as a way of addressing the patient's conflict rather than as something to be avoided or ignored. Helms (1990), with influence from racial identity theory, proposed a racial identity interaction model for understanding the effect of race and ethnicity on the psychotherapeutic process. Helms hypothesized that whites and people of color undergo racial identity change processes that influence how they handle racial material. There is a continuum of possible attitudes, perspectives, and outcomes of these processes. She suggested that the optimal outcome for whites involved abandoning entitlements associated with being white and relinquishing the myth of white superiority; for people of color, it would involve overcoming internalized racism and negative self-concepts. In a treatment arrangement between a white person and a person of color, the position of each along this racial identity continuum would have a profound effect on the relationship. She theorized that the racial identity stage of each participant in a treatment dyad affects his or her reactions to the other and that the nature of the therapeutic alliance is a function of the interplay of their expressed racial identities. Helms further postulated four types of relationships as possible outcomes of this interplay. She named these relationships parallel, progressive, regressive, and crossed. All of these relationships assume that there is a differential in power between the therapist and the client. In parallel relationships, regardless of the person's racial identity and social power, the participants in the dyad react to and process racialized material in similar ways. In the progressive relationships, the dyad participant with greater social power is able to interpret and respond to racialized material from a more sophisticated status than does the dyad participant with lesser social power. In regressive relationship forms, the dyad participant with greater power operates from a more primitive position than does the person of lesser social power. Crossed relationships are characterized by participants who perceive and react to racialized material in direct opposition to each other. For example, a white therapist whose racial identity stage is manifested by denials that racism has significant impact on people's lives may have difficulty treating a black client whose racial identity stage is characterized by firm beliefs that racism circumscribes his opportunities in life. This would continue to hold true for a dyad consisting of racially similar participants who may differ with regard to their own specific racial identity stage.

For example, the black therapist–black patient dyad is not exempt from having specific difficulties. Black therapists may also accept the myth that black patients are "bad" patients. The patient may be seen as having so many social problems that he or she cannot benefit from psychotherapy. A black therapist who is not of the same social class as his or her black patient may also react negatively to the patient's mannerisms and style that reflect a linkage to the lowest social and educational level. Black therapists and black patients may also establish a quick relationship that can lead to taking certain things for granted. For example, they may collude in attributing all the patient's problems to the white society. Another possibility may be that the black therapist becomes angry at the black patient who expresses negative feelings about black people in general. Carter's (1995) empirical research has validated Helms's racial identity categories as important determinants of the functionality of the dyadic psychotherapeutic relationship. He has confirmed that varying racial identity positions of therapist and client could influence the thoughts and behaviors of both the therapist and the client. Carter's research, in conjunction with Helms's research and theorization, argues convincingly that race alone may be relatively important in the psychotherapy.

Although Bradshaw (1982) limited his comments to the therapeutic process that unfolds in the relationships established by specific types of patients and therapists, the situations are far more complex when the element of economics is introduced. Black patients, for example, may be rich or poor. Similarly, black therapists may come from a variety of socioeconomic backgrounds. The same can be said of white therapists and white patients. Thus, the element of race is likely to be complicated significantly by the element of class and indeed of education. Blumenthal et al. (1985) pointed out that the research conducted on the problems created by these dichotomies remains unfortunately inconclusive.

The white clinician–black patient dyad has served as a useful model for reflecting on countertransference problems in cross-cultural psychotherapy. Indeed, this dyad has been a framework for others, such as the example of Jewish therapist and Arab patient. Gorkin (1986) outlined how to manage certain types of countertransference that emerge in this unique situation. In particular, he noted how a Jewish therapist might experience guilt and aggression while treating an Arab patient. The recently published text *Culture and Psychotherapy: A Guide to Clinical Practice* (Tseng and Streltzer 2001) is an important contribution to the ongoing dialogue about ethnocultural difference and psychotherapy. With the aid of clinical vignettes, the authors reinforce the important notion that "culturally relevant psychotherapy involves the management of cultural influences at multiple levels, including how culture enhances the meaning of the patient's life history, clarifies the nature of any stress that may be encountered, alters coping patterns utilized, and influences the psychopathology present" (p. 11).

Hatch and Friedman (1996) reminded us that relatively little work has been done on the use of cognitive-behavioral treatments with different ethnic and racial groups. In their own clinical work with African Americans and Afro-Caribbean residents in New York City, they recognized that there were certain distinctive elements in their treatment relationships with these patients that forced the authors to develop a unique approach to the care of these patients' OCD. The elements were the patients' secretiveness about their disorder, their reluctance to take medication and to involve their families in the treatment enterprise, their pronounced misunderstanding of the disorder, and their discomfort with white clinicians.

Gender and Psychotherapy

The problems created by the black–white dyad are analogous in many ways to those seen in the male–female therapy dyad. Although some analysts have defended vehemently the idea that social and cultural issues are but peripheral to psychoanalytic treatment, it seems likely that the differences in male and female development, identity formation, and worldview may have a differential impact on the context of therapy. Lester (1990) mentioned that male patients are more likely than female patients to resist transferential feelings to merge with and depend on the analyst. Speaking of countertransference,

she stated that female analysts may be more tolerant of a client's "demands for maternal care" (p. 438), whereas a male therapist might become anxious and be more likely to attempt to distance himself from the patient when he faced such wishes from a patient. Cases in which the therapist is a man and the patient is a woman have also been thought to replicate and reinforce the inequitable power distribution that women have experienced throughout their lives in relationships such as with fathers, husbands, and work associates (Carmen et al. 1981).

Carmen et al. (1981) described the culture-bound view that women's anger is inappropriate. Women themselves may have particular conflict about expressing their own anger, just as men have problems about having women express their anger. It is possible that a male therapist's countertransference will lead him to view an assertive or angry woman as "castrating," whereas this might be less likely to occur to him were he dealing with a male patient who behaved in a similar fashion. There is also the increasingly evident problem of the sexual abuse of female patients by male therapists. Such behavior from therapists has been condemned by the American Psychiatric Association without regard to what role the female patient may have played. Not surprisingly, however, cases are beginning to appear in which male patients have accused female therapists of sexual abuse; similarly, complaints have been made in cases in which patient and therapist are of the same gender.

Bradshaw (1982) raised squarely the problems that are possible in the dyad in which both patient and therapist are black. This makes it worthwhile to speculate that similar problems can occur in the dyadic context in which both patient and therapist are female. For example, a female therapist might encourage women to express inordinate anger against men or to participate in activities that may in fact be expressing the therapist's wishes and value system. One could also expect that the female patient and therapist could collude to project all of the problems onto males in the general society. D.H. Bernstein (1991) posited that a female therapist may overvalue a female patient's efforts in the workplace at the expense of unwittingly contributing to the patient's shame in obtaining pleasure from more traditional female roles, such as mothering. The author also added that therapy with a female patient may awaken within a female therapist the countertransferential reaction of competitiveness with her own mother, to the point where the therapist then injects these feelings into the patient's situation.

Comas-Díaz and Greene (1994) drew attention to the double psychological burden that women of color may face when living in a society dominated by white males. The authors refer to the taxing effort of integrating ethnic and gender identities while dealing with the dominant race and the dominant gender.

Gender and Pharmacotherapy

Recent work has emphasized the influence of culture and culturally derived views of sex and gender on the focus of health research in general and mental health research specifically.

Krieger and Fee (1994) argued that the use of sex and gender as variables has served to restrict the focus of medical research about women to reproductive health, largely ignoring nonreproductive issues such as hypertension, heart disease, cancer, and AIDS. They added that the primary focus on race and sex/gender as variables has impeded investigation of the impact of social class on the health of both women and men.

Weissman and Olfson (1995) commented on current, significant knowledge gaps with regard to the development and treatment of major depression in women, despite the worldwide disproportionate incidence of this disorder in women. They mentioned that, despite well-documented physiological differences between men and women, studies remain to be done to explore differences in drug bioavailability and how they relate to sex-based differential responses to medication. In addition, they cited the potential influence of social and economic factors in promoting gender bias in medical treatment and research. For example, women were more likely than men to suffer disruptions in their medical insurance coverage, in part because a woman insured as a dependent is likely to lose this coverage in the event of divorce or the death of her spouse. Moreover, women may be disproportionately underinsured or uninsured due to their higher representation in part-time work or in positions with companies too small to offer adequate insurance. It is quite possible that these gender-based social and financial inequities result not only in undertreatment but also in a certain amount of invisibility for women in clinical and research settings.

It raises some hope that a recent issue of *CNS Spectrums* (February 2001) focused on female-specific mood disorders, highlighted the relationship of hormonal shifts to the onset of depression (Born and Steiner 2001) and the role of serotonin in premenstrual dysphoria (Eriksson et al. 2001), examined the question of treatment of mood disorders during pregnancy and lactation (Stowe et al. 2001), and reviewed the association of hormonal changes to mood disorders in perimenopause (Soares and Cohen 2001).

Race and Pharmacotherapy

K.-M. Lin et al. (1991) reviewed the response of Asians to various psychotropic agents. They mentioned the well-known enzyme polymorphism of alcohol dehydrogenase and aldehyde dehydrogenase, more prevalent in Asian populations, that are responsible, respectively, for some of the increased sensitivity to alcohol and the flushing response observed in many people of Asian descent or origin. A great majority of Asians are estimated to be "fast acetylators," in comparison with approximately 50% of whites and blacks. This may have an impact on Asians' metabolism of such drugs as clonazepam, caffeine, and phenelzine. In addition, differences in the activity of catechol-O-methyltransferase have been linked to the higher incidence of dyskinesia in Asian parkinsonian patients treated with L-dopa. More recently, Poolsup et al. (2000) reviewed studies that implicate the cytochrome P450 enzyme CYP2C19 (mephenytoin hydroxylase), important in the metabolism of drugs such as diazepam, citalopram, and some tricyclic antidepressants, in that the incidence of poor metabolizers of these substrates is much higher (15–30%) in Asians than in Caucasians (3–6%), serving to explain the possible need to adjust doses downward when treating Asian patients. Interestingly, Asians and blacks have been shown to have a much lower prevalence of CYP2D6 poor metabolizers, although many clinical studies have agreed that blacks and Asians actually achieve higher levels of drugs that are presumed substrates of CYP2D6 than do whites (Poolsup et al. 2000).

Mendoza et al. (1991) reviewed studies on psychopharmacological treatment of Hispanic and Native Americans and stated that although some interesting differences have been found in various pathways of drug metabolism (debrisoquine and S-mephenytoin metabolism, acetylation, protein binding), little in the way of clinical correlation has occurred. In addition, clinical studies have suffered because diagnosis and outcome measures are hampered by wide cultural differences in symptom expression.

Strickland et al. (1991) reviewed psychopharmacological studies in black American populations and commented on the replicated finding that black Americans develop higher plasma levels and faster clinical responses to tricyclic antidepressants than do white populations. More specifically, the intracellular concentration of lithium in red blood cells was higher in blacks than in whites, apparently the result of a less efficient lithium-sodium countertransport system (Strickland et al. 1995). This may necessitate the use of lower doses of lithium in the treatment of bipolar disorder in this group and perhaps the use of alternative antimanic agents such as valproate and carbamazepine. Studies looking at differences in the metabolism of antipsychotics, however, have been inconclusive, in part because of what seems to be a bias toward blacks being diagnosed as schizophrenic more often than whites. Lawson (1996) argued that successful treatment outcomes for black Americans may be compromised by a combination of the aforementioned problem of misdiagnosis, the use of higher dosages of psychotropic medications with the attendant increased likelihood of side effects, the greater use of as-needed medications, poorer treatment compliance, and greater reluctance on the part of this population to seek psychiatric care. Hence, race and ethnicity must be considered seriously if pharmacotherapy is to be maximized and treatment outcomes are to improve.

Dawkins and Potter (1991) commented on the dearth of information available on gender differences in the response to psychopharmacological treatment, given that animal studies have shown important differences related in part to sex hormone levels. These authors attributed the lack of research on women to the delicate issue of the possible far-reaching effects of medication on women of childbearing age.

Medication obviously meets with varying levels of approval among different groups. In the Caribbean, many patients view psychiatrists as medical practitioners and therefore practically demand a prescription for some type of medication regardless of the nature of their complaint. Nevertheless, other Caribbean patients who belong to fundamentalist religious groups see God as the final healer. They refuse to take almost any medication and are convinced that prayer makes it unnecessary to swallow pills of any sort. Still others see the physician as the intermediary through whom God acts. These patients therefore pray and take pills. Such differing responses to pharmacotherapy from patients growing up on the same island show the complexity of the healing enterprise.

Furthermore, all of the foregoing research needs to be reframed in the context of the emerging developments concerning the biology of race. It remains to be seen whether the above biological differences may be explained by other, more biologically sound variables, rather than the presumed racial difference.

Conclusions

It should be clear from this chapter that culture and cultural differences play an important role in psychiatry and all of medicine. The influence of culture extends from the etiological conception of sickness to the implementation of a treatment plan and even the prognosis. Culture, ethnicity, race, and gender require serious consideration by students of psychiatry who wish to become effective healers of mental disorders. Patients present complaints stemming from a matrix that is only partly biological. Culture influences this matrix as powerfully as does biology. Openness to considering the role of culture in the healing process is a hallmark of the thoughtful healer and is the key to a more complete understanding of the individuals we treat.

References

Adebimpe VR: Overview: white norms and psychiatric diagnosis of black patients. Am J Psychiatry 138:279–285, 1981

Adebimpe VR: Participant observer: the experiences of a Black transcultural psychiatrist, in Black Psychiatrists and American Psychiatry. Edited by Spurlock J. Washington, DC, American Psychiatric Association, 1999, pp 77–94

Adebimpe VR, Chu C-C, Klein HE, et al: Racial and geographic differences in the psychopathology of schizophrenia. Am J Psychiatry 139:888–891, 1982

Adityanjee, Raju GSP, Khandelwal SK: Current status of multiple personality disorder in India. Am J Psychiatry 146:1607–1610, 1989

Adityanjee, Zain AM, Subramaniam M: Sporadic koro and marital disharmony. Psychopathology 24:49–52, 1991

Akhtar S: Four culture-bound psychiatric syndromes in India. Int J Soc Psychiatry 34:70–74, 1988

Allen EA: Psychological dependency among students in a "cross-roads" culture. West Indian Medical Journal 34:123–127, 1985

American Psychiatric Association: Diagnostic and Statistical Manual of Mental Disorders. Washington, DC, American Psychiatric Association, 1952

American Psychiatric Association: Diagnostic and Statistical Manual of Mental Disorders, 2nd Edition. Washington, DC, American Psychiatric Association, 1968

American Psychiatric Association: Diagnostic and Statistical Manual of Mental Disorders, 3rd Edition. Washington, DC, American Psychiatric Association, 1980

American Psychiatric Association: Diagnostic and Statistical Manual of Mental Disorders, 3rd Edition, Revised. Washington, DC, American Psychiatric Association, 1987

American Psychiatric Association: Diagnostic and Statistical Manual of Mental Disorders, 4th Edition. Washington, DC, American Psychiatric Association, 1994

American Psychiatric Association: Diagnostic and Statistical Manual of Mental Disorders, 4th Edition, Text Revision. Washington, DC, American Psychiatric Association, 2000

Baldwin JA: Theory and research concerning the notion of black self-hatred: a review and reinterpretation. Journal of Black Psychology 5:51–77, 1979

Bateson G: Some components of socialization for trance. Ethos 3:143–155, 1975

Bell CC, Mehta H: The misdiagnosis of black patients with manic-depressive illness. J Natl Med Assoc 72:141–145, 1980

Bemporad JR, Ratey JJ, O'Driscoll G, et al: Hysteria, anorexia and the culture of self-denial. Psychiatry 51:96–103, 1988

Benedict R: Patterns of Culture. New York, Mentor Books, 1959

Bernstein DH: Gender-specific dangers in the female dyad in treatment. Psychoanal Rev 78:37–48, 1991

Bernstein RL, Gaw AC: Koro: proposed classification for DSM-IV. Am J Psychiatry 147:1670–1674, 1990

Berry JW: Ecology, cultural adaptation and psychological differentiation: traditional patterning and acculturative stress, in Cross-Cultural Perspectives on Learning. Edited by Brislin R, Bochner S, Lonner W. New York, Wiley, 1975, pp 207–231

Berry JW, Kim U: Acculturation and mental health, in Health and Cross-Cultural Psychology: Toward Applications. Edited by Dasen P, Berry JW, Sartorius N. Newbury Park, CA, Sage, 1988, pp 207–236

Bletzer KV: Fleeing hysteria (chakore) among Ngawbere of northwestern Panama: a preliminary analysis and comparison with similar illness phenomena in other settings. Med Anthropol 9:297–318, 1985

Blue HC, González CA: The meaning of ethnocultural difference: its impact on and use in the psychotherapeutic process, in Treating Diverse Disorders With Psychotherapy (New Dir Ment Health Serv No 55). Edited by Greenfeld D. San Francisco, CA, Jossey-Bass, 1992, pp 73–84

Blue HC, Griffith EEH: The African American, in Culture and Psychotherapy: A Guide to Clinical Practice. Edited by Tseng W-S, Streltzer J. Washington, DC, American Psychiatric Publishing, 2001, pp 137–155

Blumenthal SJ, Jones EE, Krupnick JL: The influence of gender and race on the therapeutic alliance, in Psychiatry Update: American Psychiatric Association Annual Review, Vol 4. Edited by Hales RE, Frances AJ. Washington, DC, American Psychiatric Press, 1985, pp 586–606

Born L, Steiner M: The relationship between menarche and depression in adolescence. CNS Spectrums 6:126–138, 2001

Bose R: Psychiatry and the popular conception of possession among the Bangladeshis in London. Int J Soc Psychiatry 43:1–15, 1997

Bradshaw WH Jr: Supervision in black and white: race as a factor in supervision, in Applied Supervision in Psychotherapy. Edited by Blumenfield M. New York, Grune and Stratton, 1982, pp 200–220

Burton-Bradley BG: The amok syndrome in Papua and New Guinea. Med J Aust 1:252–256, 1968

Bush JS: Suicide and blacks: a conceptual framework. Suicide Life Threat Behav 6:216–219, 1976

Calabrese JD: Spiritual healing and human development in the Native American church: toward a cultural psychiatry of peyote. Psychoanal Rev 84:237–255, 1997

Canino IA, Canino G: Impact of stress on the Puerto Rican family: treatment considerations. Am J Orthopsychiatry 50:535–541, 1980

Canino IA, Spurlock J: Culturally Diverse Children and Adolescents: Assessment, Diagnosis, and Treatment. New York, Guilford Press, 2000

Carmen EH, Russo NF, Miller JB: Inequality and women's mental health: an overview. Am J Psychiatry 138:1319–1330, 1981

Carr JE: Ethno-behaviorism and the culture-bound syndromes: the case of amok. Cult Med Psychiatry 2:269–293, 1978

Carter RT: The Influence of Race and Racial Identity in Psychotherapy: Toward a Racially Inclusive Model. New York, John Wiley and Sons, 1995

Chandrashekar CR: Possession syndrome in India, in Altered States of Consciousness and Mental Health. Edited by Ward CA. Newbury Park, CA, Sage, 1989, pp 79–95

Chodoff P: A critique of Freud's theory of infantile sexuality. Am J Psychiatry 123:507–518, 1966

Cohen CI, Berment F, Magai C: A comparison of US-born African-American and African-Caribbean psychiatric outpatients. J Natl Med Assoc 89:117–123, 1997

Cohen P, Brook J: Family factors related to the persistence of psychopathology in childhood and adolescence. Psychiatry 50:332–345, 1987

Comas-Díaz L: Puerto Rican espiritismo and psychotherapy. Am J Orthopsychiatry 51:636–645, 1981

Comas-Díaz L, Greene B (eds): Women of Color: Integrating Ethnic and Gender Identities in Psychotherapy. New York, Guilford Press, 1994

Comas-Díaz L, Jacobsen FM: Ethnocultural transference and countertransference in the therapeutic dyad. Am J Orthopsychiatry 61:392–402, 1991

Constantinides P: Women heal women: spirit possession and sexual segregation in a Muslim society. Soc Sci Med 21:685–692, 1985

Cross WE: Shades of Black: diversity in African American identity. Philadelphia, PA, Temple University Press, 1991

Cross WE: In search of Blackness and Afrocentricity: the psychology of black identity change, in Racial and Ethnic Identity: Psychological Development and Creative Expression. Edited by Harris HW, Blue HC, Griffith EEH. New York, Routledge Publications, 1995, pp 53–72

Dana RH, Whatley PR: When does a difference make a difference? MMPI scores and African Americans. J Clin Psychol 47:400–406, 1991

Dawkins K, Potter WZ: Gender differences in pharmacokinetics and pharmacodynamics of psychotropics: focus on women. Psychopharmacol Bull 27:417–426, 1991

Delgado AK, Griffith EEH, Ruiz P: The black woman mental health executive: problems and perspectives. Administration in Mental Health 12:246–251, 1985

Dennis PA: Grisi Siknis in Miskito culture, in The Culture-Bound Syndromes: Folk Illnesses of Psychiatric and Anthropological Interest. Edited by Simons RC, Hughes CC. Dordrecht, The Netherlands, D Reidel, 1985, pp 289–306

Dien DS: Big Me and Little Me: a Chinese perspective on self. Psychiatry 46:281–286, 1983

Dow TW, Silver DA: Drug-induced koro syndrome. J Fla Med Assoc 60:32–33, 1973

Downing NE, Roush KL: From passive acceptance to active commitment: a model of feminist identity development for women. Journal of Counseling Psychology 13:695–709, 1985

Dwairy M: Addressing the repressed needs of the Arabic client. Cult Divers Ment Health 3:1–12, 1997

Ede A: Koro in an Anglo-Saxon Canadian. Can Psychiatr Assoc J 21:389–392, 1976

Edwards JG: The koro pattern of depersonalization in an American schizophrenic patient. Am J Psychiatry 126:1171–1173, 1970

Eisenbruch M: Cross-cultural aspects of bereavement, II: ethnic and cultural variations in the development of bereavement practices. Cult Med Psychiatry 8:315–347, 1984

Erickson MT: Rethinking oedipus: an evolutionary perspective of incest avoidance. Am J Psychiatry 150:411–416, 1993

Eriksson E, Andersch B, Ho HP, et al: Premenstrual dysphoria: an illustrative example of how serotonin modulates sex-steroid-related behavior. CNS Spectrums 6:141–149, 2001

Escobar JI: Cross-cultural aspects of the somatization trait. Hosp Community Psychiatry 38:174–180, 1987

Fabrega H: The role of culture in a theory of psychiatric illness. Soc Sci Med 35:91–103, 1992

Fernando S, Ndegwa D, Wilson M: Forensic Psychiatry, Race and Culture. London, England, Routledge, 1998

Finnegan DG, McNally EB: Dual Identities: Counseling Chemically Dependent Gay Men and Lesbians. Center City, MN, Hazelton, 1987

Florsheim P: Cross-cultural views of self in the treatment of mental illness: disentangling the curative aspects of myth from the mythic aspects of cure. Psychiatry 53:304–315, 1990

Foulks EF: Anthropology and psychiatry: a new blending of an old relationship, in Current Perspectives in Cultural Psychiatry. Edited by Foulks EF, Wintrob RM, Westermeyer J, et al. New York, Spectrum, 1977, pp 5–18

Frank JD: Persuasion and Healing: A Comparative Study of Psychotherapy. Baltimore, MD, Johns Hopkins University, 1963

Friedman RC, Downey JI: Biology and the oedipus complex. Psychoanal Q 64:234–264, 1995

Gaw AC (ed): Culture, Ethnicity, and Mental Illness. Washington, DC, American Psychiatric Press, 1993

Gaw AC: Concise Guide to Cross-Cultural Psychiatry. Washington, DC, American Psychiatric Press, 2001

Gaw AC, Bernstein RL: Classification of amok in DSM-IV. Hosp Community Psychiatry 43:789–793, 1992

Gilligan C: In a Different Voice: Psychological Theory and Women's Development. Cambridge, MA, Harvard University Press, 1982

González CA, Griffith EEH: Culture and the diagnosis of somatoform and dissociative disorders, in Culture and Psychiatric Diagnosis: A DSM-IV Perspective. Washington, DC, American Psychiatric Press, 1996, pp 137–149

González CA, Griffith EEH, Ruiz P: Cross-cultural issues in psychiatric treatment, in Treatments of Psychiatric Disorders. Edited by Gabbard GO. Washington, DC, American Psychiatric Press, 1995, pp 57–87

González CA, Lewis-Fernández R, Griffith EEH, et al: Impact of culture on dissociation: enhancing the cultural suitability of DSM-IV, in DSM-IV Sourcebook, Vol 3. Edited by Widiger TA, Frances AJ, Pincus HA, et al. Washington, DC, American Psychiatric Press, 1997, pp 943–949

Goodman A: Organic unity theory: the mind-body problem revisited. Am J Psychiatry 148:553–563, 1991

Gorkin M: Countertransference in cross-cultural psychotherapy: the example of Jewish therapist and Arab patient. Psychiatry 49:69–79, 1986

Greene RL: Ethnicity and MMPI performance: a review. J Consult Clin Psychol 55:497–512, 1987

Gremillion H: Psychiatry as social ordering: anorexia nervosa, a paradigm. Soc Sci Med 35:57–71, 1992

Griffith EEH, Mahy GE: Psychological benefits of Spiritual Baptist "mourning." Am J Psychiatry 141:769–773, 1984

Griffith EEH, English T, Mayfield V: Possession, prayer, and testimony: therapeutic aspects of the Wednesday night meeting in a black church. Psychiatry 43:120–128, 1980

Griffith EEH, Young JL, Smith DL: An analysis of the therapeutic elements in a black church service. Hosp Community Psychiatry 35:464–469, 1984

Group for the Advancement of Psychiatry, Committee on Cultural Psychiatry: Suicide and Ethnicity in the United States. New York, Brunner/Mazel, 1989

Group for the Advancement of Psychiatry, Committee on Cultural Psychiatry: Alcoholism in the United States: Racial and Ethnic Considerations. Washington DC, American Psychiatric Press, 1996

Group for the Advancement of Psychiatry, Committee on Cultural Psychiatry: Cultural Assessment in Clinical Psychiatry. Washington DC, American Psychiatric Publishing, 2002

Guarnaccia PJ: Cultural comments on multiaxial issues, in Culture and Psychiatric Diagnosis: A DSM-IV Perspective. Edited by Mezzich JE, Kleinman A, Fabrega H, et al. Washington, DC, American Psychiatric Press, 1996, pp 335–338

Guarnaccia PJ, Rubio-Stipec M, Canino G: Ataques de nervios in the Puerto Rican Diagnostic Interview Schedule: the impact of cultural categories on psychiatric epidemiology. Cult Med Psychiatry 13:275–295, 1989a

Guarnaccia PJ, de la Cancela V, Carrillo E: The multiple meanings of ataques de nervios in the Latino community. Med Anthropol 11:47–62, 1989b

Guarnaccia PJ, Good BJ, Kleinman AM: A critical review of epidemiological studies of Puerto Rican mental health. Am J Psychiatry 147:1449–1456, 1990

Gussler J: Social change, ecology and spirit possession among the South African Nguni, in Religion, Altered States of Consciousness, and Social Change. Edited by Bourguignon E. Columbus, OH, Ohio State University Press, 1973, pp 88–126

Gussow Z: Pibloktoq (hysteria) among the polar Eskimo. The Psychoanalytic Study of Society 1:218–236, 1960

Guthrie RV: Even the Rat Was White: A Historical View of Psychology. New York, Bantam, 1976

Gynther MD: White norms and black MMPIs: a prescription for discrimination? Psychol Bull 78:386–402, 1972

Haberman PW: Psychiatric symptoms among Puerto Ricans in Puerto Rico and New York City. Ethnicity 3:133–144, 1976

Hatch ML, Friedman S: Behavioral treatment of obsessive-compulsive disorder in African Americans. Cognitive and Behavioral Practice 3:303–315, 1996

Haynes NM, Comer JP: The effects of a school development program on self-concept. Yale J Biol Med 63:275–283, 1990

Helms JE: Black and White Racial Identity: Theory, Research, and Practice. Westport, CT, Greenwood, 1990

Hickling FW: Double jeopardy: psychopathology of black mentally ill returned migrants to Jamaica. Int J Soc Psychiatry 37:80–89, 1991

Horney K: The Neurotic Personality of Our Time. New York, Norton, 1937

Hughes CC: The culture-bound syndromes and psychiatric diagnosis, in Culture and Psychiatric Diagnosis: a DSM-IV perspective. Edited by Mezzich JE, Kleinman A, Fabrega H, et al. Washington, DC, American Psychiatric Press, pp 289–305, 1996

Jilek WG: Emil Kraepelin and comparative sociocultural psychiatry. Eur Arch Psychiatry Clin Neurosci 245:231–238, 1995

Johnson SD: Toward clarifying culture, race, and ethnicity in the context of multicultural counseling. Journal of Multicultural Counseling and Development 18:41–50, 1990

Jones BE, Gray BA: Problems in diagnosing schizophrenia and affective disorders among blacks. Hosp Community Psychiatry 37:61–65, 1986

Jones EE: Psychotherapists' impressions of treatment outcome as a function of race. J Clin Psychol 38:722–731, 1982

Katon W, Kleinman A, Rosen G: Depression and somatization: a review. Am J Med 72:127–135, 1982

King LM: Suicide from a "black reality" perspective, in The Afro-American Family: Assessment, Treatment, and Research Issues. Edited by Bass BA, Wyatt GE, Powell GJ. New York, Grune and Stratton, 1982, pp 221–236

Kirmayer LJ, Minas H: The future of cultural psychiatry: an international perspective. Can J Psychiatry 45:438–446, 2000

Kirmayer LJ, Young A, Hayton BC: The cultural context of anxiety disorders. Psychiatr Clin North Am 18:503–521, 1995

Kleinman A: Patients and Healers in the Context of Culture: An Exploration of the Borderland Between Anthropology, Medicine, and Psychiatry. Berkeley, CA, University of California Press, 1980

Kleinman A: Neurasthenia and depression: a study of somatization and culture in China. Cult Med Psychiatry 6:117–189, 1982

Kleinman A: Rethinking Psychiatry: From Cultural Category to Personal Experience. New York, Free Press, 1988

Kosch SG, Burg MA, Podikuju S: Patient ethnicity and diagnosis of emotional disorders in women. Fam Med 30:215–219, 1998

Koss JD: Therapeutic aspects of Puerto Rican cult practices. Psychiatry 38:160–171, 1975

Krieger N, Fee E: Man-made medicine and women's health: the biopolitics of sex/gender and race/ethnicity. Int J Health Serv 24:265–283, 1994

Lapierre YD: Koro in a French Canadian. Can Psychiatr Assoc J 17:333–334, 1972

Lawson WB: Clinical issues in the pharmacotherapy of African Americans. Psychopharmacol Bull 32:275–282, 1996

Lee S: Diagnosis postponed: shenjing shuairuo and the transformation of psychiatry in post-Mao China. Cult Med Psychiatry 23:349–380, 1999

Leighton AH, Murphy JM: Cross-cultural psychiatry, in Approaches to Cross-Cultural Psychiatry. Edited by Murphy JM, Leighton AH. New York, Cornell University Press, 1965, pp 3–20

Lester EP: Gender and identity issues in the analytic process. Int J Psychoanal 71:435–444, 1990

Levy JE, Neutra R, Parker D: Life careers of Navajo epileptics and convulsive hysterics. Soc Sci Med 13B:53–66, 1979

Lewis-Fernández R, Kleinman A: Cultural psychiatry: theoretical, clinical, and research issues. Psychiatr Clin North Am 18:433–448, 1995

Li X, Stanton B, Feigelman S: Exposure to drug trafficking among urban, low-income African American children and adolescents. Arch Pediatr Adolesc Med 153:161–168, 1999

Lin K-M: Hwa-Byung: a Korean culture-bound syndrome? Am J Psychiatry 140:105–107, 1983

Lin K-M, Poland RE, Smith MW, et al: Pharmacokinetic and other related factors affecting psychotropic responses in Asians. Psychopharmacol Bull 27:427–439, 1991

Lin K-M, Anderson D, Poland RE: Ethnicity and psychopharmacology. Psychiatr Clin North Am 18:635–647, 1995

Lin T: Neurasthenia revisited: its place in modern psychiatry. Cult Med Psychiatry 13:105–129, 1989

Littlewood R: Psychiatry's culture. Int J Soc Psychiatry 42:245–268, 1996

Littlewood R, Lipsedge M: Acute psychotic reactions in Caribbean-born patients. Psychol Med 11:303–318, 1981

Littlewood R, Lipsedge M: The butterfly and the serpent: culture, psychopathology and biomedicine. Cult Med Psychiatry 11:289–335, 1987

Littlewood R, Lipsedge M: Aliens and Alienists: Ethnic Minorities and Psychiatry. London, England, Routledge, 1997

Litzenberger BW, Buttenheim MC: Sexual orientation and family development: introduction. Am J Orthopsychiatry 68:344–351, 1998

Makanjuola ROA: "Ode ori": a culture-bound disorder with prominent somatic features in Yoruba Nigerian patients. Acta Psychiatr Scand 75:231–236, 1987

Malgady RG, Rogler LH, Cortés DE: Cultural expressions of psychiatric symptoms: idioms of anger among Puerto Ricans. Psychol Assess 8:265–268, 1996

Manson SM, Walker RD, Kivlahan DR: Psychiatric assessment and treatment of American Indians and Alaska Natives. Hosp Community Psychiatry 38:165–173, 1987

Marcos LR: Effects of interpreters on the evaluation of psychopathology in non–English-speaking patients. Am J Psychiatry 136:171–174, 1975

Marsella AJ: Cross-cultural research on severe mental disorders: issues and findings. Acta Psychiatr Scand Suppl 78:7–22, 1988

Mathews CA, Amighetti LDH, Lowe TL, et al: Cultural influences and perception of Tourette syndrome in Costa Rica. J Am Acad Child Adol Psychiatry 40:456–463, 2001

McGoldrick M, Pearce JK, Giordano J (eds): Ethnicity and Family Therapy. New York, Guilford, 1982

Mendoza R, Smith MW, Poland RE, et al: Ethnic psychopharmacology: the Hispanic and Native American perspective. Psychopharmacol Bull 27:449–461, 1991

Métraux A: Voodoo in Haiti. New York, Schocken Books, 1972

Mezzich JE: Culture and multiaxial diagnosis, in Culture and Psychiatric Diagnosis: A DSM-IV Perspective. Edited by Mezzich JE, Kleinman A, Fabrega H, et al. Washington, DC, American Psychiatric Press, 1996, pp 327–334

Mezzich JE, Good BJ: On culturally enhancing the DSM-IV multiaxial formulation, in DSM-IV Sourcebook, Vol 3. Edited by Widiger TA, Frances AJ, Pincus HA, et al. Washington, DC, American Psychiatric Press, 1997, pp 983–989

Mezzich JE, Kleinman A, Fabrega H, et al: Culture and Psychiatric Diagnosis. Washington, DC, American Psychiatric Press, 1996

Ming-Yuan Z: The diagnosis and phenomenology of neurasthenia: a Shanghai study. Cult Med Psychiatry 13:147–161, 1989

Moffic HS, Kendrick EA, Lomax JW, et al: Education in cultural psychiatry in the United States. Transcultural Psychiatric Research Review 24:167–187, 1987

Morgan LM, Beale RL, Mattis JS, et al: The combined impact of racism at work, non-racial work stress, and financial stress on Black women's psychological well-being. African American Research Perspectives 6:41–50, 2000

Nandi DN, Banerjee G, Saha H, et al: Epidemic koro in West Bengal, India. Int J Soc Psychiatry 29:265–268, 1983

Neighbors HW, Jackson JS, Campbell L, et al: The influence of racial factors on psychiatric diagnosis: a review and suggestions for research. Community Ment Health J 25:301–311, 1989

Ness RC, Wintrob RM: The emotional impact of fundamentalist religious participation: an empirical study of intragroup variation. Am J Orthopsychiatry 50:302–315, 1980

Neutra R, Levy JE, Parker D: Cultural expectations versus reality in Navajo seizure patterns and sick roles. Cult Med Psychiatry 1:255–275, 1977

Ngui PW: The koro epidemic in Singapore. Aust N Z J Psychiatry 3:263–266, 1969

Offer D: The Psychological World of the Teen-Ager: A Study of Normal Adolescent Boys. New York, Basic Books, 1969

Pang KYC: Hwa byung: the construction of a Korean popular illness among Korean elderly immigrant women in the United States. Cult Med Psychiatry 14:495–512, 1990

Parham TA: Cycles of psychological nigrescence. The Counseling Psychologist 17:187–226, 1989

Philippe J, Romain JB: Indisposition in Haiti. Soc Sci Med 13B:129–133, 1979

Phinney J: Stages of ethnic identity development in minority group adolescents. Journal of Early Adolescence 9:34–49, 1989

Poolsup N, Li Wan Po A, Knight TL: Pharmacogenetics and psychopharmacotherapy. J Clin Pharmacol Ther 25:197–220, 2000

Pressel E: Umbanda in Sao Paulo: religious innovation in a developing society, in Religion, Altered States of Consciousness, and Social Change. Edited by Bourguignon E. Columbus, OH, Ohio State University Press, 1973, pp 264–318

Prince R: The concept of culture-bound syndromes: anorexia nervosa and brain-fag. Soc Sci Med 21:197–203, 1985

Prudhomme C: The problem of suicide in the American Negro. Psychoanal Rev 25:372–391, 1938

Reid WH: The antisocial personality: a review. Hosp Community Psychiatry 36:831–837, 1985

Richman JA, Jason LA, Taylor RR, et al: Feminist perspectives on the social construction of chronic fatigue syndrome. Health Care Women Int 21:173–185, 2000

Roelcke V: Biologizing social facts: an early 20th century debate on Kraepelin's concepts of culture, neurasthenia, and degeneration. Cult Med Psychiatry 21:383–403, 1997

Rudorfer MV (ed): Ethnicity in the pharmacologic treatment process. Psychopharmacol Bull 32:181–289, 1996

Ruiz P (ed): Cross-cultural psychiatry (Section IV), in American Psychiatric Press Review of Psychiatry, Vol 14. Edited by Oldham JM, Riba MB. Washington, DC, American Psychiatric Press, 1995, pp 461–630

Ruiz P, Langrod J: Psychiatry and folk healing: a dichotomy? Am J Psychiatry 133:95–97, 1976

Russell JG: Anxiety disorders in Japan: a review of the Japanese literature on Shinkeishitsu and taijinkyofusho. Cult Med Psychiatry 13:391–403, 1989

Salisbury RF: Possession in the New Guinea highlands. Int J Soc Psychiatry 14:85–94, 1968

Samuda RJ: Psychological Testing of American Minorities. New York, Harper and Row, 1973

Saxena S, Prasad KVSR: DSM-III subclassification of dissociative disorders applied to psychiatric outpatients in India. Am J Psychiatry 146:261–262, 1989

Schmidt K, Hill L, Guthrie G: Running amok. Int J Soc Psychiatry 23:264–274, 1977

Schrut AH: The Oedipus complex: some observations and questions regarding its validity and universal existence. J Am Acad Psychoanal 22:727–751, 1994

Schwab JJ: Nineteenth-century studies of mental illness in Southern blacks. Interaction 1:21–25, 1978

Schweder RA: Rethinking culture and personality theory, part 1. Ethos 7:255–278, 1979

Sharp LA: Exorcists, psychiatrists, and the problems of possession in northwest Madagascar. Soc Sci Med 38:525–542, 1994

Shore JH: American Indian suicide: fact and fantasy. Psychiatry 38:86–91, 1975

Simons RC: Sorting the culture-bound syndromes, in The Culture-Bound Syndromes: Folk Illnesses of Psychiatric and Anthropological Interest. Edited by Simons RC, Hughes CC. Dordrecht, The Netherlands, D Reidel, 1985, pp 25–38

Skapinakis P, Lewis G, Meltzer H: Clarifying the relationship between unexplained chronic fatigue and psychiatric morbidity: results from a community survey in Great Britain. Am J Psychiatry 157:1492–1498, 2000

Smedley A: Race in North America: Origin and Evolution of a World View. Boulder, CO, Westview Press, 1993

Soares CN, Cohen LS: Perimenopause and mood disturbance: an update. CNS Spectrums 6:167–174, 2001

Spencer MB: Preschool children's social cognition and cultural cognition: a cognitive developmental interpretation of race dissonance findings. J Psychol 112:275–296, 1982

Spencer MB: Self-concept development, in Perspectives in Black Child Development. Edited by Slaughter DT. San Francisco, CA, Jossey-Bass, 1988, pp 59–72

Spiegel D, Cardeña E: Cultural diversity of dissociative and somatoform disorders. Paper presented at the National Institute of Mental Health Conference on Culture and Diagnosis, Pittsburgh, PA, April 1991

Spiegel JP: Cultural aspects of transference and countertransference revisited. J Am Acad Psychoanal 4:447–467, 1976

Spiegel JP: Community therapy in a Fiji village. Journal of Operational Psychiatry 1:28–34, 1983

Spitzer RL, Williams JBW, Gibbon M, et al: Structured Clinical Interview for DSM-III-R. Washington, DC, American Psychiatric Press, 1990

Spurlock J: Development of self-concept in Afro-American children. Hospital and Community Psychiatry 37:66–70, 1986

Stoller P: Fusion of the Worlds. Chicago, IL, University of Chicago Press, 1989

Stoller RJ, Herdt GH: The development of masculinity: a cross-cultural contribution. J Am Psychoanal Assoc 30:29–59, 1982

Stowe ZN, Calhoun K, Ramsey C, et al: Mood disorders during pregnancy and lactation: defining issues of exposure and treatment. CNS Spectrums 6:150–166, 2001

Strauss JS, Carpenter WT Jr, Bartko JJ: A review of some findings from the international pilot study of schizophrenia, in Annual Review of Schizophrenic Syndrome, Vol 4. Edited by Cancro R. New York, Brunner/Mazel, 1976, pp 74–88

Strickland TL, Ranganath V, Lin K-M, et al: Psychopharmacologic considerations in the treatment of black American populations. Psychopharmacol Bull 27:441–448, 1991

Strickland TL, Lin K-M, Fu P, et al: Comparison of lithium ratio between African American and Caucasian bipolar patients. Biol Psychiatry 37:325–330, 1995

Suryani LK: Culture and mental disorder: the case of bebainan in Bali. Cult Med Psychiatry 8:95–113, 1984

Suwanlert S: Neurotic and psychotic states attributed to Thai "Phii Pob" spirit possession. Aust N Z J Psychiatry 10:119–123, 1976

Suzuki T: The concept of neurasthenia and its treatment in Japan. Cult Med Psychiatry 13:187–202, 1989

Tan EK, Carr JE: Psychiatric sequelae of amok. Cult Med Psychiatry 1:59–67, 1977

Thomas JP, Szmukler GI: Anorexia nervosa in patients of Afro-Caribbean extraction. Br J Psychiatry 146:653–656, 1985

Torres JB: Masculinity and gender roles among Puerto Rican men: machismo on the U.S. mainland. Am J Orthopsychiatry, 68:16–26, 1998

Tseng W-S: The development of psychiatric concepts in traditional Chinese medicine. Arch Gen Psychiatry 29:569–575, 1973

Tseng W-S: Handbook of Cultural Psychiatry. San Diego, CA, Academic Press, 2001

Tseng W-S, Kan-Ming M, Hsu J, et al: A sociocultural study of koro epidemics in Guangdong, China. Am J Psychiatry 145:1538–1543, 1988

Tseng W-S, Streltzer J: Culture and psychotherapy: an overview, in Culture and Psychotherapy: A Guide to Clinical Practice. Edited by Tseng W-S, Streltzer J. Washington, DC, American Psychiatric Publishing, 2001, pp 3–12

Tung M: Insight-oriented psychotherapy and the Chinese patient. Am J Orthopsychiatry 61:186–194, 1991

Varma VK, Bouri M, Wig NN: Multiple personality in India: comparison with hysterical possession state. Am J Psychother 35:113–120, 1981

Wahass S, Kent G: A comparison of public attitudes in Britain and Saudi Arabia towards auditory hallucinations. Int J Soc Psychiatry 43:175–183, 1997

Waxler NE: Culture and mental illness: a social labeling perspective. J Nerv Ment Dis 159:379–395, 1974

Weidman HH: Falling-out: a diagnostic and treatment problem viewed from a transcultural perspective. Soc Sci Med 13B:95–112, 1979

Weiss MG: Cultural comments on somatoform and dissociative disorders, in Culture and Psychiatric Diagnosis: A DSM-IV Perspective. Edited by Mezzich J, Kleinman A, Fabrega H. Washington, DC, American Psychiatric Press, 1996

Weiss MG, Sharma SD, Guar RK, et al: Traditional concepts of mental disorders among Indian psychiatric patients. Soc Sci Med 23:379–386, 1986

Weiss MG, Raguram R, Channabasavanna SM: Cultural dimensions of psychiatric diagnosis: a comparison of DSM-III-R and illness explanatory models in south India. Br J Psychiatry 166:353–359, 1995

Weissman MM, Olfson M: Depression in women: implications for health care research. Science 269:799–801, 1995

Weissman MM, Bland RC, Canino GJ, et al: Cross-national epidemiology of major depression and bipolar disorder. JAMA 276:293–299, 1996

Westermeyer J: Folk concepts of mental disorder among the Lao: continuities with similar concepts in other cultures and in psychiatry. Cult Med Psychiatry 3:301–317, 1979

Westermeyer J: Psychiatric diagnosis across cultural boundaries. Am J Psychiatry 142:798–805, 1985

Westermeyer J: Cultural aspects of substance abuse and alcoholism. Psychiatr Clin North Am 18:589–605, 1995

White GM: The role of cultural explanations in "somatization" and "psychologization." Soc Sci Med 16:1519–1530, 1982

Widiger TA, Frances AJ, Pincus HA, et al (eds): The DSM-IV Sourcebook, Vol 3. Washington, DC, American Psychiatric Press, 1997

Wig NN: DSM-III: a perspective from the third world, in International Perspectives on DSM-III. Edited by Spitzer RL, Williams JBW, Skodol AE. Washington, DC, American Psychiatric Press, 1983, pp 79–89

Wing JK, Birley JLT, Cooper JE, et al: Reliability of a procedure for measuring and classifying "present psychiatric state." Br J Psychiatry 113:499–515, 1967

Williams CL: Issues surrounding psychological testing of minority patients. Hosp Community Psychiatry 38:184–189, 1987

Williams DH: The epidemiology of mental illness in Afro-Americans. Hosp Community Psychiatry 37:42–49, 1986

Wilson MN: Child development in the context of the black extended family. Am Psychol 44:380–385, 1989

Wittkower ED, Warnes H: Cultural aspects of psychotherapy. Am J Psychother 28:566–573, 1974

Yamamoto J: An Asian view of the future of cultural psychiatry, in Current Perspectives in Cultural Psychiatry. Edited by Foulks EF, Wintrob RM, Westermeyer J, et al. New York, Spectrum, 1977, pp 209–215

Yamamoto J: Psychotherapy in the Pacific Rim countries. Psychiatry Clin Neurosci 52(suppl):S233–S235, 1998

Yap PM: The possession syndrome: a comparison of Hong Kong and French findings. J Ment Sci 106:114–137, 1960

Yap PM: Koro: a culture-bound depersonalization syndrome. Br J Psychiatry 111:43–50, 1965

CHAPTER 39

The Law and Psychiatry

Robert I. Simon, M.D.

The body of law applied to the practice of psychiatry does not differ from that of medicine in general. Nevertheless, the diagnosis, treatment, and management of patients with psychiatric disorders present not only unique clinical and ethical concerns but also unique legal considerations. For instance, determination of a patient's competency, as well as the patient's ability to manage his or her personal affairs, may be required to determine the patient's mental capacity to make health care decisions. Currently, competency determinations are particularly relevant for patients with Alzheimer's disease or dementia related to AIDS. Ethical and legal issues such as informed consent, the right to treatment, the right to refuse treatment, substitute decision making, and advance directives are commonly confronted when treating psychiatric patients.

Individuals who have been criminally charged must be legally competent to stand trial. Defendants with psychiatric impairments may not meet the competency standard. Such individuals may require pretrial evaluations of their mental capacity to understand the charges against them and their ability to assist counsel in their own defense. Moreover, depending on the nature and duration of a psychiatric disorder, criminal defendants may seek acquittal or have the charges against them reduced based on the argument that they were legally insane at the time the offense occurred.

Vulnerability to psychiatric malpractice suits has increased, more so in specific areas of psychiatric practice. Table 39–1 reveals the malpractice claims experience of the American Psychiatric Association (APA)–sponsored Professional Liability Insurance Program ("Benefacts" 1996). Somatic therapies, assessment and management of violent patients, techniques to recover memories of sexual abuse, sexual misconduct, boundary violations, premature discharge of potentially violent patients, and managed care settings all represent areas of heightened liability for the psychiatric practitioner.

TABLE 39–1. Recent allegations of malpractice (approximate frequency of claims)

Allegation	Frequency (%)
Incorrect treatment	33
Attempted/completed suicide	20
Incorrect diagnosis	11
Improper supervision	7
Medication error/drug reaction	7
Improper commitment	5
Breach of confidentiality	4
Unnecessary hospitalization	4
Undue familiarity	3
Libel/slander	2
Other (e.g., abandonment, electroconvulsive therapy, third-party injury)	4

Source. Data from "Benefacts" 1996.

The chance of a psychiatrist being sued in the 1980s was 1 in 25 per year ("Benefacts" 1996). Through 1995, however, the odds increased to about 1 of every 12 psychiatrists per year. In some states, psychiatrists are sued at the rate of 1 in 6 per year. The APA Professional Liability Insurance Program identifies several factors to account for the increase in malpractice suits:

1. Psychiatrists are treating "sicker" patients in managed care settings.
2. The media scrutinizes so-called recovered memories and ritual satanic abuse cases.
3. Tort reform legislation has failed.

4. Psychiatrists are specializing in new practice areas such as geriatric psychopharmacology, adolescent addiction medicine, multiple personality disorder, pain management, and adult children of alcoholics.
5. Psychiatrists are providing more primary care, such as in the management of patients with diabetes, hypertension, and a wide variety of acute general medical illnesses.

With the advent of managed care, psychiatrists treat a large volume of patients for brief visits, creating greater liability exposure. When the psychiatrist spends less time with a patient, a working alliance is less likely to develop. Among primary care physicians it was reported that those with no malpractice claims used more statements of orientation, laughed and used more humor, and engaged patients more in a give-and-take dialogue than did colleagues who had been sued (Levinson et al. 1997). Primary care physicians with no claims also spent more time in routine visits than did primary care physicians who had been sued (mean, 18.3 vs. 15.0 minutes). The length of the visit was an independent factor in predicting claims status.

Despite the growth of malpractice claims, psychiatrists prevail in seven out of every eight suits brought against them. The plaintiff has the heavy burden of proving his or her malpractice claim.

Psychiatric Malpractice: Somatic Therapies

Psychiatric malpractice is medical malpractice. *Malpractice* is the provision of substandard professional care that causes a compensable injury to a person with whom a professional relationship existed. Although this concept may seem relatively clear and simple, it has its share of conditions and caveats. For example, the essential issue is *not* the existence of substandard care per se, but whether there is compensable liability.

Medical malpractice is a tort (i.e., a wrong that is noncriminal and not related to a contract): it is a type of civil wrong committed as a result of negligence by a physician that causes injury to a patient in his or her care. *Negligence*, the fundamental concept underlying a malpractice lawsuit, is simply described as either doing something that a physician with a duty of care (to the patient) should not have done or failing to do something that a physician with a duty of care should have done. The fact that a psychiatrist commits an act of negligence does not automatically make him or her liable to the patient bringing the lawsuit.

For a psychiatrist to be found *liable* to a patient for malpractice, four fundamental elements (Table 39–2) must be established by a preponderance of the evidence (more likely than not): 1) that there was a duty of care owed by the defendant, 2) that the duty of care was breached, 3) that the plaintiff (i.e., patient) suffered actual damages, and 4) that the deviation was the direct cause of the damages. Each of these four elements must be met or there can be no finding of liability, regardless of any finding of negligence. A psychiatrist may be negligent but still not found to be liable. For example, if the patient suffered no real injuries because of the negligence, or if there was an injury but it was not directly caused by the psychiatrist's negligence, a claim of malpractice will be defeated.

TABLE 39–2. The four Ds of malpractice

Duty	There was a duty of care owed by the doctor.
Deviation	The duty of care was breached.
Damages	The patient suffered actual damages.
Direct causation	The deviation was the direct cause of the damages.

Critical to establishing a claim of professional negligence is the requirement that the defendant's conduct was substandard or was a deviation in the standard of care owed to the plaintiff. Except in the case of "specialists," the law presumes and holds all physicians to a standard of *ordinary care*, which is measured by its *reasonableness* according to the clinical circumstances in which it is provided.

The use of a somatic therapy, including electroconvulsive therapy (ECT), is evaluated no differently from the use of any other medical treatment or procedure with respect to potential liability. The same general standard of *ordinary* and *reasonable* care governs the assessment of whether a psychiatrist's use of or failure to use a somatic intervention is legally actionable.

It is generally acknowledged within the psychiatric profession that there is no *absolute standard* protocol for the administration of psychotropic medication or ECT. Nevertheless, the existence of professional treatment guidelines and procedures that are generally accepted or used by a significant number of psychiatrists should alert clinicians to consider such guidelines as practice reference sources. For example, the APA has published comprehensive findings and guidelines in the form of task force reports concerning ECT (American Psychiatric Association 1990) and tardive dyskinesia (American Psychiatric Association 1992). Nevertheless, official guidelines must not preempt sound professional judgment in attending to the specific clinical needs of patients.

Official guidelines and procedures publications do not, per se, establish the standard of care by which a court might evaluate a psychiatrist's treatment. They do represent a credible source of information with which a reasonable psychiatrist at least should be familiar and should have considered (*Stone v. Proctor* 1963). In addition to expert testimony, courts generally consider official guidelines and the professional literature that establishes contemporary psychiatric practices in determining the standard of care.

There is less professional autonomy and flexibility associated with the use of ECT. Usually, the "reasonable care" standard applied to psychiatric treatment is construed in a fairly broad manner. However, some psychiatric treatments such as ECT are more rigidly regulated than others. For instance, the Joint Commission on Accreditation of Healthcare Organizations (JCAHO) considers ECT a *special treatment* procedure, to be regulated by written policies. Whenever ECT is used, the procedure must be adequately justified and documented in the patient's medical chart (Joint Commission on Accreditation of Healthcare Organizations 2001a). The ECT policies of treatment facilities as well as judicial decisions and statutory regulation of ECT can also serve as establishing the basis for liability, if violated.

The standard for judging the use and administration of medication, on the other hand, appears to be consistent with the more flexible and general reasonable care requirement. Another reference source is the *Physicians' Desk Reference* (PDR), which may be used to establish or dispute a psychiatrist's pharmacotherapy procedures. The PDR is a commercially distributed and privately published reference of medication products used in the United States. The U.S. Food and Drug Administration (FDA) requires that drug manufacturers have their official package inserts reported in the PDR (Simon 1992a). Accordingly, psychiatrists consult publications such as the PDR as needed to keep abreast of current and accurate medication information. Although numerous courts have cited the PDR as a credible source of medication-related information in the medical profession, the PDR does not by itself establish *the* standard of care (*Gowan v. United States* 1985; *Witherell v. Weimer* 1986/1987). Instead, it may be used as one piece of evidence to establish the standard of care in a particular situation (*Callan v. Norland* 1983; *Doerr v. Hurley Medical Center* 1984). Courts generally follow the reasoning in *Ramon v. Farr* (1989), holding that drug inserts alone do not set the standard of care. They are only one element to be considered, along with previous clinical experience, the scientific literature, approvals in other countries, expert testimony,

and other pertinent factors. The presence of a substantial scientific literature that justifies the clinician's treatment is vastly more persuasive than FDA approval. The PDR or any other reference cannot serve as a substitute for the psychiatrist's sound clinical judgment.

Fortunately, courts recognize the importance of professional judgment and give psychiatrists, like other medical specialists, latitude in explaining special diagnostic or treatment considerations that guide their decision making. For instance, the clinical data regarding pharmacological treatment of rapid cycling bipolar disorder indicate that a variety of potentially useful drug therapies exist, some of which are considered experimental or on the cutting edge (Simon 1997). For instance, various drugs and hormones are clinically useful as mood stabilizers, such as carbamazepine, clozapine, thyroid and estrogen replacement, calcium channel blockers, antihypertensives, neuroleptics, atypical antipsychotics, and other anticonvulsants (lamotrigine, valproate, gabapentin). Valproate is currently the only anticonvulsant approved by the FDA for the management of mania associated with bipolar disorder (Nemeroff 2000).

The courts consider that no one treatment of choice exists and that treatment applications are still being developed. Evidence that a treatment procedure is accepted by at least a respectable minority of professionals in the field can establish that a particular treatment is a reasonable professional practice (Simon 1993). The standard of care associated with the use of a somatic therapy to treat a psychiatric patient, *at a minimum*, should include the following:

Pretreatment

- Complete clinical history (medical, psychiatric)
- Complete physical examination as clinically indicated (preferably performed by another physician or, if necessary, by the psychiatrist)
- Administration of necessary laboratory tests and review of past test results (Daniel et al. 1992)
- Disclosure of sufficient information to the patient to obtain informed consent, including information about the risks and benefits both for receiving treatment and for *not* receiving treatment
- Thorough documentation of all treatment decisions, informed consent information, pertinent patient responses, and other relevant treatment data

Posttreatment

- Careful monitoring of the patient's response to treatment, including adequate follow-up evaluations and

appropriate laboratory testing (Daniel et al. 1992)
- Prompt adjustments in treatment, as clinically indicated
- Arrangement for additional informed consent when treatment is altered appreciably or new treatment is initiated

The final word on treatment interventions is determined by the clinician and the clinical needs of the patient, not the law. The preceding recommendations should be viewed only as general guidelines commonly associated with reasonable care when somatic therapies are implemented.

Theories of Liability

The same basic legal principles are applied to *psychiatric malpractice* as in any other lawsuit alleging malpractice by a physician, regardless of medical subspecialty. Use of descriptive terms such as *psychiatric* or *neuropsychiatric* reflects the general recognition that the theories of liability to be discussed represent the most common areas of malpractice associated with that subspecialty.

The potential for negligence by a psychiatrist appears to be greatest in clinical situations involving the use of psychotropic medication. Although no reliable compilation of malpractice claims data has been published, anecdotal information suggests that medication-related lawsuits constitute a significant share of the litigation filed against psychiatrists. As noted earlier, recent claims data from the APA Professional Liability Insurance Program showed that medication error and drug reaction constituted 7% of malpractice allegations. However, allegations of drug mismanagement are likely a significant contributor to "incorrect treatment," the most common malpractice allegations.

A review of the relevant case law indicates that various mistakes, omissions, and poor medication treatment practices commonly result in malpractice actions brought against psychiatrists. The following discussion, although not intended to be exhaustive, provides a framework for identifying problem areas associated with medication treatment.

Failure to Evaluate Properly

Sound clinical practice requires that, before any form of treatment is initiated, the patient should be properly evaluated. The nature and extent of an evaluation is largely dictated by the type of treatment being contemplated and the medical and psychiatric condition of the patient. A physical examination should be conducted or obtained, if clinically indicated. A recently performed physical examination may suffice, or patients may be referred elsewhere if the psychiatrist does not perform physical examinations. The duty to ensure that proper informed consent is obtained can also be fulfilled at this time.

Several lawsuits have resulted from failure to evaluate a patient properly before administering medications (*Blanchard v. Levine* 1985; *Shaughnessy v. Spray* 1983). As a result of this omission, the patient's condition is misdiagnosed and remains untreated. In addition, the patient is exposed to unnecessary side effects and risks of inappropriate medications.

Failure to Monitor

Probably the most common act of negligence associated with pharmacotherapy is the failure to monitor the patient while he or she is taking medication, including carefully following the patient for adverse side effects.

Once psychotropic medication is prescribed, it is the psychiatrist's duty to monitor the patient. Consultation or referral may be necessary according to the clinical needs of the patient. Monitoring may require the use of laboratory testing. Serum drug levels are obtainable for a number of psychotropic medications. The primary indications for these laboratory tests include assessment of therapeutic and toxic levels of medication and patient compliance with treatment. The use of carbamazepine, valproate, and clozapine requires periodic monitoring of the hematopoietic system and the liver. Failure to supervise patients to ensure that they are taking medications properly can delay or prevent the detection of harmful side effects and a change to more effective treatment. If a patient is harmed, a malpractice action might result (*Chaires v. St. John's Episcopal Hospital* 1984; *Clifford v. United States* 1985; *Kilgore v. County of Santa Clara* 1982).

Split Treatment

Split treatment situations require that the psychiatrist stay fully informed of the patient's clinical status as well as of the nature and quality of treatment the patient is receiving from the nonmedical therapist (Sederer et al. 1998). In a collaborative relationship, responsibility for the patient's care is shared according to the qualifications and limitations of each discipline. The responsibilities of each discipline do not diminish those of the other disciplines. Patients should be informed of the separate responsibilities of each discipline. Periodic evaluation by the psychiatrist and the nonmedical therapist of the patient's clinical condition and needs is necessary to determine whether the collaboration should continue.

On termination of the collaborative relationship, the patient should be informed by the clinicians either separately or jointly. In split treatments, if negligence is claimed on the part of the nonmedical therapist, it is likely that the collaborating psychiatrist will be sued, and vice versa (Woodward et al. 1993).

In managed care or similar treatment settings, the mere prescribing of medication without an informed, working doctor–patient relationship does not meet generally accepted standards of good clinical care. Fragmented care, in which the psychiatrist functions only as a prescriber of medication while remaining uninformed about the patient's overall clinical status, constitutes substandard treatment that may lead to a malpractice action. Such a practice may diminish the efficacy of the drug treatment itself or even lead to the patient's failure to take the prescribed medication.

Psychiatrists who prescribe medications in split treatment arrangements should be able to hospitalize patients if necessary. If the psychiatrist does not have admitting privileges, prearrangements should exist with other psychiatrists who can hospitalize patients if emergencies arise.

Split treatment is increasingly used by managed care companies and is a potential malpractice minefield (Meyer and Simon 1999). In managed care settings, psychiatrists may be required to prescribe medications from a restrictive or closed formulary. For example, selective serotonin reuptake inhibitors (SSRIs) are currently considered first-line treatment for depression. However, a few remaining managed care companies only permit the prescribing of tricyclic antidepressants (TCAs), which have a much greater lethality than SSRIs for suicidal patients who overdose. Psychiatrists, in their professional discretion, should determine which medications will be prescribed according to the special clinical needs of the patient.

Negligent Prescription Practices

The selection of a medication, determination of initial dosage and form of administration, and other related procedures are all decisions left to the professional discretion of the treating psychiatrist. In managed care settings, psychiatrists should vigorously resist attempts to limit their choice of drugs by a restrictive or closed formulary or by therapeutic substitution (interchanging different chemical agents from the same therapeutic class, e.g., a TCA substituted for an SSRI). The prescribing of specific medications should be determined by the psychiatrist and the clinical needs of the patient. An appeal should be filed if a drug that is not formulary approved is

denied. The law recognizes that the physician is in the best position to "know the patient" and to determine what course of treatment is best under the circumstances. The standard by which a psychiatrist's prescription practices will be evaluated is reasonableness. In administering psychotropic medication, psychiatrists need only conform their procedures and decision making to those that are *ordinarily* practiced by other psychiatrists under similar circumstances.

A review of cases involving allegations of negligent prescription procedures reveals several common practices representing potential deviations from generally accepted treatment practice:

- Exceeding recommended dosages without clinical indications
- Negligently prescribing multiple drugs
- Negligently prescribing medication for unapproved uses
- Negligently prescribing unapproved medications
- Negligently failing to disclose medication risks

As stated earlier, any physician who prescribes medication has a duty to first obtain the informed consent of the patient (Table 39–3). Obtaining competent informed consent may be complicated by the fact that some psychiatric patients have a compromised mental capacity for health care decision making as a result of their mental illness. Patients lacking such decision-making capacity require consent for treatment by substitute decision makers (Table 39–4).

TABLE 39–3. Informed consent: reasonable information to be disclosed

Although there exists no consistently accepted set of information to be disclosed for any given medical or psychiatric situation, as a rule of thumb, five areas of information are generally provided:

1.	Diagnosis	Description of the condition or problem
2.	Treatment	Nature and purpose of proposed treatment
3.	Consequences	Risks and benefits of the proposed treatment
4.	Alternatives	Viable alternatives to the proposed treatment including risks and benefits
5.	Prognosis	Projected outcome with and without treatment

Source. Reprinted with permission from Simon RI: *Clinical Psychiatry and the Law,* 2nd Edition. Washington, DC, American Psychiatric Press, 1992. Copyright 1992 American Psychiatric Press, Inc.

TABLE 39–4. Common consent options for patients lacking the mental capacity for health care decisions

Proxy consent of next of kin[a]

Adjudication of incompetence, appointment of a guardian

Institutional administrators or committees

Treatment review panels

Substituted consent of the court

Advance directives (living will, durable power of attorney, health care proxy)

Statutory surrogates (spouse or court-appointed guardian)[a,b]

Note. [a]May be excluded for treatment of mental disorders.
[b]Medical statutory surrogate laws (when treatment wishes of patient are unstated).
Source. Adapted with permission from Simon RI: *Clinical Psychiatry and the Law*, 2nd Edition. Washington, DC, American Psychiatric Press, 1992. Copyright 1992 American Psychiatric Press, Inc.

Each time a medication is changed and a new drug is introduced, informed consent should be obtained. Failure to inform a patient properly of the risks and benefits of a prescribed medication can be grounds for a malpractice action if the patient is injured as a result (*Karasik v. Bird* 1984; *Moran v. Botsford General Hospital* 1984; *Wright v. State* 1986).

Other areas of negligence involving medication that have resulted in legal action include 1) failure to treat side effects after they have been recognized or should have been recognized, 2) failure to monitor a patient's compliance with prescription limits, 3) failure to prescribe medication or appropriate levels of medication according to the treatment needs of the patient, 4) failure to refer a patient for consultation or treatment by a specialist, and 5) negligent withdrawal from medication and unclear or illegible prescriptions.

Tardive Dyskinesia

The development of neuroleptic medications in the mid-1950s dramatically improved the treatment and management of patients with schizophrenia. However, shortly after the introduction of neuroleptic medications as therapeutic agents, researchers and clinicians observed unusual muscle movements in some patients, referred to as *tardive dyskinesia* (TD).

The risk of developing TD is approximately 4%–7% per year of neuroleptic use (Lohr et al. 1986). These projections are even higher for elderly patients (Kane et al. 1982; Klawans and Barr 1982). As the newer antipsychotic drugs are used more frequently, the risk of developing TD is expected to be lower.

Given these data, the potential for TD litigation is clear. Despite the possibility of a large number of TD-related lawsuits, relatively few psychiatrists have been sued under this cause of action. One reason may be that patients who develop TD may not have the physical and psychological stamina required to pursue litigation.

Allegations of negligence after a patient develops TD are based on the same legal elements as any other malpractice action. The bases for negligence mirror those previously identified in general medication cases. These areas include, but are not limited to

- Failure to evaluate and monitor a patient properly.
- Failure to obtain informed consent.
- Negligent diagnosis of a patient's condition. For instance, in *Hyde v. University of Michigan Board of Regents* (1986/1986), a woman was awarded $1 million from a medical center because it misdiagnosed her condition as Huntington's chorea instead of TD; the verdict was later reversed on the basis of a subsequent case that expanded the state's sovereign immunity coverage.
- Wrongful prescription of neuroleptic medication. For example, in *Dovido v. Vasquez* (1986), a net award of $700,000 went to a 42-year-old plaintiff who developed tardive dyskinesia as a result of the defendant psychiatrist's negligent prescription of extremely high doses of fluphenazine.
- Failure to monitor medication side effects. For example, in *Clites v. State* (1982), the plaintiff was a mentally retarded man who had been institutionalized since age 11 and treated with major tranquilizers from age 18 to 23. TD was diagnosed at age 23. The family subsequently sued, claiming the defendants negligently prescribed medication, did not inform the patient of the possibility of developing TD, and failed to monitor and subsequently treat the patient's resulting side effects. The jury returned a verdict for the plaintiff and awarded damages in the amount of $760,165. This award was affirmed on appeal. The court ruled that the defendants were negligent because they deviated from the standards of the industry. Specifically, the court cited various omissions in ordinary psychiatric practice that, they concluded, reasonable psychiatrists would have provided. Among the deviations they noted were failure to conduct regular physical examinations and laboratory tests, failure to intervene at the first sign of TD, inappropriate use of multiple medications at the same time, use of drugs for convenience (e.g., "behavior management") rather than therapy, and failure to obtain informed consent.

Patients receiving neuroleptic medication need to be frequently monitored. No stock answer can be given to the question of how frequently the psychiatrist should see a patient. Generally, psychiatrists should schedule return visits with a frequency that accords with the patient's clinical need. The longer the time between visits, however, the greater the risk of missing adverse drug reactions and untoward developments in the patient's condition. The interval between visits ordinarily should not be longer than 6 months.

The defenses and preventive measures applicable to TD-related malpractice claims are consistent with those used in any case alleging negligent drug treatment. Sound clinical practice accompanied by the patient's competent informed consent, appropriately documented in the medical chart, serves as an effective foil to any allegations of negligence should TD develop (*Frasier v. Department of Health and Human Resources* 1986; *Radank v. Heyl* 1986; *Rivera v. NYC Health and Hospitals* 1988).

For the psychiatrist treating chronic aggression with antipsychotic drugs, it is important to consider the warning by Yudofsky et al. (1987) that

> the use of antipsychotic medications in treating chronic aggression involves a substantial risk of the emergence of tardive dyskinesia, because the prevalence of tardive dyskinesia among patients on long-term neuroleptic treatment is about 25%.... While antipsychotic agents are the treatment of choice for aggression due to psychosis and also may be helpful in the acute short-term management of violence through sedative action, we do *not* recommend their use in the long-term management of aggression, especially that which is secondary to organic brain syndrome. (p. 400)

Electroconvulsive Therapy

It has been estimated that no more than 3%–5% of all psychiatric inpatients in the United States receive ECT (Weiner 1979). With the current shortened length of stay in hospitals, use of ECT appears to be increasing. Legal actions alleging negligence associated with ECT are infrequent (Krouner 1975; Perr 1980). However, lawsuits involving ECT are occasionally brought. Cases involving ECT-related injuries represent a variety of circumstances in which negligence has occurred. These cases can be categorized into three groups: pretreatment, treatment, and posttreatment.

Pretreatment

Although pre-ECT evaluations vary somewhat, the following procedures recommended by the APA Task Force on Electroconvulsive Therapy (American Psychiatric Association 2001) generally should be performed:

1. A psychiatric history and examination to evaluate the indications for ECT
2. A medical examination to determine risk factors
3. Anesthesia evaluation
4. Informed consent (written)
5. An evaluation by a physician privileged to administer ECT

Although these recommendations by the APA Task Force on ECT do not define in absolute terms the standard of care for ECT, they may be proffered as evidence of the standard of care in malpractice suits involving ECT. Official treatment guidelines, however, should not be a substitute for the psychiatrist's sound clinical judgment. Nevertheless, failure to conduct appropriate pretreatment procedures could endanger the welfare of the patient and ultimately result in a lawsuit.

Treatment

It is well established that psychiatrists are not held liable for a mere mistake in judgment, nor is a psychiatrist held to a standard of 100% accuracy or perfect performance (Smith 1986; see also *Holton v. Pfingst* 1976). A bad result does not automatically establish a claim for malpractice (*Howe v. Citizens Memorial Hospital* 1968/1968). Instead, a patient must prove, by a preponderance of the evidence, that the psychiatrist deviated from the standard of care and that the deviation proximately caused the patient injury or damage. The procedure for evaluating the care and treatment afforded a patient when ECT is used is no different. Lawsuits involving ECT-related injuries in which the negligence is related to the actual treatment process include the following errors:

- Failure to use a muscle relaxant to reduce the chance of a bone fracture
- Negligent administration of the procedure
- Failure to conduct an evaluation of the patient, including the use of X rays, before continuing treatment

Posttreatment

It is common for patients treated with ECT to experience side effects such as temporary confusion, disorientation, and memory loss immediately after its administration (O'Connell 1982). Because of these temporary debilitating effects, sound clinical practice requires that psychiatrists provide reasonable posttreatment care and safeguards. Courts have held that the failure to attend properly to a patient for a period of time after administering ECT can result in malpractice liability. The following are examples of posttreatment circumstances that may constitute a basis for a lawsuit:

- Failure to evaluate complaints of pain or discomfort following treatment
- Failure to evaluate a patient's condition before resuming ECT treatments
- Failure to monitor a patient properly to prevent falls
- Failure to supervise properly a patient who was injured as a result of ECT

As a source of civil liability, ECT-related lawsuits today are infrequent and are not likely to represent a significant malpractice risk for psychiatrists. However, as Perlin (1989) cautioned, "recent developments in right-to-refuse treatment law and statutory regulation of intrusive therapy are likely to insure that any future ECT litigation will still be considered carefully" (pp. 47–48).

Right to Refuse Treatment

Buttressed by constitutionally derived rights to privacy and freedom from cruel and unusual punishment, the common law tort of battery, and the doctrine of informed consent, mentally disabled persons are increasingly being afforded protections traditionally reserved for the legally competent. This new freedom often runs counter to the dictates of clinical judgment (i.e., to treat and protect). As a result of this conflict, the courts vary considerably regarding the parameters of this right and the procedures to be followed.

Two landmark cases illustrate this point. In *Rennie v. Klein* (1978), the Third Circuit Court of Appeals recognized a right to refuse treatment in the state of New Jersey. The court, after extended litigation, found that this right could be overridden and antipsychotic drugs administered "whenever, in the exercise of professional judgment, such an action is deemed necessary to prevent the patient from endangering himself or others." In the second case, *Rogers v. Commissioner of Department of Mental Health* (1983), the court decided that in the absence of an emergency (e.g., serious threat of extreme violence or personal injury), any person who has not been adjudicated incompetent has a right to refuse antipsychotic medication. Incompetent persons have a similar right, but it must be exercised through a "substituted judgment treatment plan" that has been reviewed and approved by the court.

These two decisions are often viewed as legal bookends to the issue of the right to refuse treatment. The cases suggest parameters for other courts attempting to define such a right. The *Rennie* case became the model for subsequent legal decisions that adopted a treatment-driven rationale for the right to refuse treatment. *Rogers* became the basis for rights-driven approaches taken by some courts in litigating the right to refuse treatment.

Numerous state and federal decisions have tackled some aspect of this issue. Generally speaking, there is near-judicial recognition of an involuntarily hospitalized patient's right to refuse medication absent an emergency. Case law criteria for emergencies range from a risk of imminent harm to self or others to a deterioration in the patient's mental condition if treatment is halted. Until either more states enact legislation or the United States Supreme Court squarely rules on this issue, jurisdictions will continue to vary regarding the substance of the right to refuse treatment and the procedures by which such a right can be implemented.

The Suicidal Patient

The most common legal action involving psychiatric care is the failure to provide reasonable protection to patients from harming themselves. Theories of negligence involving suicide can be grouped into three broad categories: failure to diagnose properly (i.e., assess the potential for suicide); failure to treat (i.e., use reasonable treatment interventions and precautions); and failure to implement (i.e., carry out treatment properly and not negligently).

These theories, each of which applies to inpatient and outpatient settings, are based on the practitioner's failure to act reasonably in exercising the appropriate duty of care owed to the patient. Wrongful death suits as a result of patient suicides are based on the legal concepts of foreseeability, reasonableness, and causation. A typical lawsuit argues that a patient with the potential for suicide was not diagnosed and treated properly, resulting in the patient's death.

As a general rule, a psychiatrist who exercises reasonable care in compliance with accepted medical practice will not be held liable for any resulting injury. Normally, if a patient's suicide was not reasonably foreseeable, or if the suicide occurred as a result of intervening factors, this rule will apply.

Foreseeable Suicide

The evaluation of suicide risk is one of the most complex, difficult, and challenging clinical tasks in psychiatry. Suicide is a rare event with low specificity (high false-positive rates). A comprehensive assessment of a patient's suicide risk is critical to a sound clinical management plan. Using reasonable care in assessing suicide risk can preempt the problem of predicting the actual occurrence of suicide, for which professional standards do not yet exist. Standard approaches to the assessments of suicide risk are described in the psychiatric literature (Blumenthal 1990; Chiles and Strohsall 1995; Maris et al. 1992; Simon 2000). Short-term suicide risk assessments are more reliable than long-term assessments. Time attenuates suicide risk assessments, requiring that assessment be a process, not an event.

As an accepted standard of care, an evaluation of suicide risk should be done with all patients, regardless of whether they present with overt suicidal complaints. A review of case law shows that reasonable care requires that a patient who is either suspected of being or confirmed to be suicidal must be the subject of certain affirmative precautions. A failure either to assess reasonably a patient's suicidality or to implement an appropriate precautionary plan after the suicide potential becomes foreseeable is likely to render a practitioner liable if the patient is harmed because of a suicide attempt. The law tends to assume that suicide is preventable if it is foreseeable. Foreseeability, however, should not be confused with preventability. In hindsight, many suicides seem preventable that were clearly not foreseeable.

When suicide risk assessments are competently performed and recorded, the psychiatrist demonstrates that he or she was careful and thorough in the management of the suicidal patient. Moreover, evidence of a reasonable suicide risk assessment also demonstrates that the psychiatrist adhered to the prevailing standard of care. Although psychiatrists cannot ensure favorable outcomes with suicidal patients, they can ensure that the process of suicide risk assessment was competently performed (Simon 1998a).

Inpatients

Intervention in an inpatient setting usually requires the following:

- Screening evaluations
- Development of an appropriate treatment plan
- Implementation of that plan
- Ongoing case review by clinical staff

Careful documentation of assessments and management interventions with changes responsive to the patient's clinical situation should be considered evidence of clinically and legally sufficient psychiatric care. Assessing suicide risk is only half of the equation. Documenting the benefits of a psychiatric intervention (e.g., ward change, pass, discharge) against the risk of suicide permits an even-handed approach to the clinical management of the patient. Consideration only of a patient's suicide risk is a manifestation of defensive psychiatry that usually interferes with good clinical care, further exposing the psychiatrist to malpractice liability.

Psychiatrists are more likely to be sued when a psychiatric inpatient commits suicide. The law presumes that the opportunities to foresee (i.e., anticipate) and control (i.e., treat and manage) suicidal patients are greater in the hospital.

Outpatients

Outpatient therapists face a somewhat different situation. Psychiatrists are expected to reasonably assess the severity and imminence of a foreseeable suicidal act. The result of the assessment dictates the duty-of-care options. Courts have reasoned that when an outpatient commits suicide, the therapist has not necessarily breached a duty to safeguard the patient from foreseeable self-harm because of the difficulty in controlling the patient (*Speer v. United States* 1981/1982). Instead, the reasonableness of the psychiatrist's efforts is determinative.

Suicide Prevention Pacts

Suicide prevention contracts created between the clinician and the patient attempt to develop an expressed understanding that the patient will call for help rather than act out suicidal thoughts or impulses. These contracts have no legal authority; although they may be helpful in solidifying the therapeutic alliance, they may falsely reassure the psychiatrist. Suicide prevention agreements between psychiatrists and patients must not be used in place of adequate suicide assessment (Simon 1999).

Legal Defenses

One legal defense that has created a split in the courts involves the use of the "open door" policy in which patients are allowed freedom of movement for therapeutic purposes. In these cases, the individual facts and reasonableness of the staff's application of the "open door" policy appear to be paramount. Nevertheless, courts have difficulty with abstract treatment notions such as personal growth when faced with a dead patient.

Another defense, the doctrine of sovereign or governmental immunity, may statutorily bar a finding of liability against a state or federal facility. An intervening cause of suicide over which the clinician has no control is another valid legal defense. For example, a court may find a psychiatrist not liable for the suicidal act of a borderline patient who experienced a significant rejection between therapy sessions and then impulsively attempted suicide, without trying to contact the psychiatrist. The court may rule that the suicide was caused by the superseding intervening variable of an unforeseen rejection and not by the psychiatrist's negligence. Finally, the best-judgment defense has been used successfully when the patient was properly assessed and treated for suicide risk but he or she committed suicide anyway (J.D. Robertson 1991).

The Violent Patient

As a general rule, one person has no duty to control the conduct of a second person to prevent that person from physically harming a third person (*Restatement [Second] of Torts 315(a)* [1965]). Applying this rule to psychiatric care, psychiatrists traditionally have had only a limited duty to control hospitalized patients and to exercise due care on discharge. After *Tarasoff* (*Tarasoff v. Regents of the University of California* 1976), the therapist's legal duty and potential liability significantly expanded. In *Tarasoff*, the California Supreme Court first recognized that a duty to protect third parties was imposed only when a special relationship existed between the victim, the individual whose conduct created the danger, and the defendant. The court stated that "the single relationship of a doctor to his patient is sufficient to support the duty to exercise reasonable care to protect others [from the violent acts of patients]."

Psychiatrists do not have the ability to predict violence with any accuracy. Violent behaviors are the result of the complex interplay among social, clinical, and personality factors that vary significantly across situations and time (Widiger and Trull 1994). Nonetheless, clinical methods for assessing the risk of violence exist that reflect the current standard of care (Baxter and Beck 1998; Monahan and Steadman 1994; Simon 1992a; Tardiff 1989).

Assessment of risk of violence is essentially a clinical judgment. Because the validity of violence risk assessments is only modestly greater than chance, the Mac-Arthur Violence Risk Assessment Study was established. The purpose of the study was to improve clinical risk assessment validity, to enhance effective clinical risk management, and to provide data on mental disorders and violence for informing mental health law and policy ("The MacArthur Violence Risk Assessment Study" 1996). In this study, violence risk assessments were found to have a validity that was modestly better than chance. Until more studies are available, sound clinical practice requires that thorough violence risk assessments be routinely performed on potentially violent patients on the basis of current knowledge of violence risk factors. Although violence risk assessments need to be made at such critical points as the initiation of ward status changes, passes, and discharge, violence risk assessment is more of a continuing process rather than a solitary event. All such assessments should be duly recorded.

The index of suspicion for potential violence should be high in patients with a past history of violence who are making current, serious threats of harm toward specific individuals. The potential for violence is further heightened if the patient is acutely psychotic, substance abusing, angry, fearful of being harmed, and experiencing delusions of being controlled or influenced (Link and Stueve 1994).

Following *Tarasoff*, courts in other jurisdictions have interpreted the case variously. Some states have adopted the *Tarasoff* holding, whereas others have limited or extended its scope and reach. In most states, psychotherapists have a duty, established by case law or statute, to act affirmatively to protect an endangered third party from a patient's violent or dangerous acts. A few courts have declined to find a *Tarasoff* duty in a specific case, whereas some courts have simply rejected the *Tarasoff* duty (*Evans v. United States* 1995; *Green v. Ross* 1997). In *Thapar v. Zezulka* (1999), the Texas Supreme court ruled that the state statute *permits* but does not *require* disclosures by therapists of threats of harm to endangered third parties by their patients. (*Evans v. United States* 1995; *Green v. Ross* 1997; *Thapar v. Zezulka* 1999).

Most courts have found no duty to protect without an imminent threat of serious harm to a foreseeable victim. Only a small minority of courts have held that a duty to protect exists for the population at large. In some jurisdictions, courts have held that the need to safeguard the public well-being overrides all other considerations, including confidentiality. Although a few courts have declined to find a *Tarasoff* duty in a specific case, a growing number of courts have recognized some variation of the original *Tarasoff* duty. Despite the fact that the *Tarasoff* duty is still not law in some jurisdictions and is subject to different interpretations by individual courts, the duty to protect is, in effect, a national standard of practice.

Several states have enacted immunity statutes that protect the psychiatrist from legal liability caused by a patient's violent acts toward others (Appelbaum et al. 1989). Most of these statutes define the therapist's duty in terms of warning the endangered third party and/or notifying the authorities. The duty-to-protect language stated in some statutes allows for a greater variety of clinical interventions.

Evolving Trends

An important, evolving trend is the application of the *Tarasoff* duty to sexual abuse cases by an alleged pedophile. A psychiatrist was successfully sued for not reporting to the medical school that his patient was a pedophile (*Garamella for Estate of Almonte v. New York Medical College* 1998). The patient, a psychiatric resident, molested a child at a hospital crisis center. The court reasoned that the defendant psychiatrist's control over the psychiatric resident was far greater than in the typical psychiatrist–patient relationship. A *Tarasoff* duty was also found where a spouse had knowledge of her husband's sexually abusive behavior against children in the neighborhood (*JS v. RT* 1998; *Touchette v. Ganal* 1996). In another case, the court found that a *Tarasoff* duty could exist but declined to find the parents of a babysitter liable for his dangerous sexual behavior (*People v. Rose* 1998). The court determined that no evidence existed that the parents knew of their son's proclivity to commit a sexual assault.

Release of Potentially Violent Patients

Under managed care, discharging violent or potentially violent inpatients presents unique challenges for treating psychiatrists (Simon 1998b). The treatment of psychiatric inpatients has changed dramatically in the managed care era (Lazarus and Sharfstein 1994). Most psychiatric units, particularly in general hospitals, have become short-stay, acute care psychiatric facilities. Generally, only suicidal, homicidal, or gravely disabled patients with major psychiatric disorders pass strict precertification review for hospitalization (Tischler 1990). Close scrutiny by utilization reviewers permits only short hospitalization for these patients (Wickizer et al. 1996). The purpose of hospitalization is crisis intervention and management to stabilize patients and to ensure their safety. The treatment of these patients is being provided by a variety of mental health professionals. Nonetheless, the psychiatrist often must bear the ultimate burden of liability for treatments gone awry ("Why Are Liability Premiums Rising?" 1996). Limited opportunity usually exists during the hospital stay to develop a therapeutic alliance with patients. The ability to communicate with patients, the psychiatrist's stock-in-trade, is often severely curtailed. All these factors contribute to a greatly increased risk of

malpractice suits against psychiatrists alleging premature or negligent discharge of patients due to cost-containment policies.

There is more control over the patient in the hospital than is available in an outpatient setting. Courts closely evaluate decisions made by psychiatrists treating inpatients that adversely affect the patient or a third party. Liability imposed on psychiatric facilities that had custody of patients who injured others outside the institution after escape or release is clearly distinguishable from the factual situation of *Tarasoff*. Duty-to-warn cases generally involve patients in outpatient treatment. Liability arises from the inaction of the therapist, who fails to take affirmative measures to warn or protect endangered third parties. In negligent-release cases, liability may arise from the allegation that the institution's affirmative act in releasing the patient caused injury to the third party. Nonetheless, allegations may be made that a psychiatrist or hospital personnel failed, prior to the patient's discharge, to warn individuals known to be at risk of harm from that patient. Lawsuits stemming from the release of foreseeably dangerous patients who subsequently injure or kill others are roughly five to six times more common than outpatient duty-to-warn litigation (Simon 1992b).

The psychiatrist's liability is determined by reference to professional standards. Consultation with other psychiatrists may provide additional protection when the discharge of a potentially violent patient appears problematic. Consulting with an attorney may help clarify legal obligations. However, lawyers tend to be highly risk averse and conservative when making recommendations. Sound legal advice may not necessarily accord with the clinical realities surrounding the management of a specific patient. Clinicians must continue to exercise their professional judgment.

The patient's willingness to cooperate with the psychiatrist is critical to maintaining follow-up treatment. The psychiatrist's obligation focuses on structuring the follow-up visits in such a manner to encourage compliance. A study of Veterans Administration (VA) inpatient referrals to a VA mental health outpatient clinic showed that of 24% of inpatients referred, approximately one-half failed to keep their first appointments (Zeldow and Taub 1981). Nevertheless, limitations do exist on the extent of the psychiatrist's ability to ensure follow-up care. Most patients retain the right to refuse treatment. These limitations must be acknowledged by both the psychiatric and legal communities (Simon 1992a). The American Medical Association Council on Scientific Affairs has developed evidence-based discharge criteria for safe discharge from the hospital (American Medical Association 1996).

In either the outpatient or inpatient situation, psychiatrists are in compliance with the responsibility to warn and protect others from potentially violent patients if they reasonably assess a patient's *risk* for violence and make clinically appropriate interventions based on their findings. Professional standards do exist for assessment of the risk factors for violence (Simon 2001). However, no standard of care exists for the prediction of violent behavior. The clinician should assess the risk of violence frequently, updating the risk assessment at significant clinical junctures (e.g., room and ward changes, passes, discharge). A risk–benefit assessment should be conducted and recorded before a pass or discharge is issued. Assessing the risk of violence is a "here and now" determination performed at the time of discharge. After the patient is discharged, the potential for violence against self or others depends on the nature and course of the mental illness, adequacy of future treatment, adherence to treatment recommendations, and exposure to unforeseeable stressful life events.

Involuntary Hospitalization

A person may be involuntarily hospitalized only if certain statutorily mandated criteria are met. Three main substantive criteria serve as the foundation for all statutory commitment requirements: that the individual 1) be mentally ill, 2) be dangerous to self or others, and/or 3) be unable to provide for his or her basic needs. Generally, each state spells out which criteria are required and what each means. Terms such as *mentally ill* are often loosely described, thus placing the responsibility for proper definition onto the clinical judgment of the petitioner.

In addition to individuals with mental illness, certain states have enacted legislation that permits involuntary hospitalization of three other distinct groups: developmentally disabled (mentally retarded) persons, substance (alcohol, drugs) addicted persons, and mentally disabled minors. Special commitment provisions may exist governing requirements for the admission and discharge of mentally disabled minors as well as numerous due-process rights afforded these individuals (*Parham v. J.R.* 1979).

Involuntary hospitalization of psychiatric patients usually arises when violent behavior threatens to erupt toward the self or others and when patients become unable to care for themselves. These patients frequently manifest mental disorders and conditions that readily meet the substantive criteria for involuntary hospitalization.

Clinicians must remember that they do not commit patients. This is done solely under the jurisdiction of the court. The psychiatrist merely initiates a medical certification that brings the patient before the court, usually after a brief period of hospitalization for evaluation. Clinicians should not attempt to second-guess the court's ultimate decision about involuntary hospitalization. The psychiatrist must be guided by the treatment needs of the patient in seeking medical certification.

Commitment statutes do not require involuntary hospitalization but are permissive (Appelbaum et al. 1989). The statutes enable mental health professionals and others to seek involuntary hospitalization for persons who meet certain substantive criteria. On the other hand, the duty to seek involuntary hospitalization is a standard-of-care issue. Patients who are mentally ill and pose an imminent, serious threat to themselves or others may require involuntary hospitalization as a primary psychiatric intervention.

Liability

The most common cause of a malpractice action involving involuntary hospitalization is the failure of a psychiatrist to adhere in good faith to statutory requirements, leading to a wrongful commitment. Often these lawsuits are brought under the theory of false imprisonment. Other areas of liability that may arise from wrongful commitment include assault and battery, malicious prosecution, abuse of authority, and intentional infliction of emotional distress (Simon 1992a).

In many states, psychiatrists are granted immunity from liability as long as they use reasonable professional judgment and act in good faith when petitioning for commitment (Mishkin 1989). Performing a careful examination of the patient, abiding by the requirements of the law, and ensuring that sound reasoning motivates the certification of the patient is good clinical practice and, only secondarily, good risk management. Evidence of willful, blatant, or gross failure to adhere to statutorily defined commitment procedures may expose a psychiatrist to a lawsuit.

Rights of Involuntarily Hospitalized Patients

Most states recognize the right of inpatients to refuse treatment. Even though the patient is involuntarily hospitalized, that hospitalization does not negate a presumption of competence. In most states, patients involuntarily hospitalized who refuse medication require a separate court hearing for an adjudication of incompetence and the provision of substituted consent by the court. Recently, persons hospitalized under criminal commitment have been accorded the right to refuse treatment. The courts have found that incarcerated patients' constitutional right to due process is adequately protected by the exercise of professional judgment within the medical peer review process of the institution.

Hospitalized patients possess other rights. Patients possess rights of visitation, although these rights can be temporarily suspended for proper cause relating to the patient's care and treatment. Free communications of hospitalized patients through mail, telephone, or visitors are considered a right, unless protection of the patient or others requires supervision of communications. The right to privacy includes allowing patients to have secure locker space, private toilet and shower facilities, and a minimum square footage of floor space. Protection of confidentiality is also included. Economic rights include the right to have and spend money and to handle one's own financial affairs responsibly. In most jurisdictions, involuntarily hospitalized patients do not lose their civil rights, such as the right to manage their own money. Hospitalized patients must be paid for their work in certain jurisdictions unless it is truly therapeutic labor (i.e., work not connected with maintenance of the hospital). "Patients' rights" are not absolute and often must be tempered by the clinical judgment of the mental health professional. Inevitably, disputes over perceived or real violations of patients' rights arise. In some jurisdictions, a civil rights officer or ombudsman is mandated by statute to mediate these disputes.

Recovered Memories Cases

The clamorous controversy concerning recovered memories of sexual abuse threatens to undermine the credibility of the mental health professions. The debate generates intense passions that drive an increasing number of recovered memory cases into the courts. Patients who allege recovered memories of abuse have sued parents and other alleged perpetrators. In a turnabout, the alleged victimizers have sued therapists whom they claim negligently induced false memories of sexual abuse. In some cases, patients have recanted and joined forces with others (usually their parents) to sue their therapists.

The memory debate has polarized many therapists into believers and disbelievers. Most therapists hold personal beliefs about the validity of recovered memories of sexual abuse that are somewhere between the extremes. Strongly held personal biases about recovered memories

represent a new occupational hazard for clinicians that can undermine the therapist's duty of neutrality to patients, creating deviant treatment boundaries and increasing the risk of incurring liability.

Litigation in recovered memory cases is expected to continue. Plaintiffs, alleging induction of false memories, have won multimillion dollar verdicts against mental health practitioners. The basic allegation in these cases is that the therapist abandoned a position of neutrality to suggest, persuade, coerce, and implant false memories of childhood sexual abuse. The guiding principle of clinical risk management in recovered memory cases is to maintain therapist neutrality and establish sound treatment boundaries.

Complicating the situation is the empirical evidence about memory mechanisms. As is typical for any emerging science, contradictory findings exist about how and what persons in various settings retain in memory and forget. Empirical studies frequently fail to distinguish whether allegedly repressed memories are not retrieved or simply not reported to researchers.

Sound risk management rests solidly on a clinical footing and is secondarily informed by awareness of the pertinent legal issues (Gutheil and Simon 1997). Risk management principles that should be considered when evaluating or treating a patient who recovers memories of abuse while in psychotherapy include the following:

- Maintain therapist neutrality—do not suggest abuse.
- Stay clinically focused—provide adequate evaluation and treatment for the patient's presenting problems and symptoms.
- Carefully document the memory recovery process.
- Manage personal biases and countertransference.
- Avoid mixing treater and expert witness roles.
- Closely monitor supervisory and collaborative therapy relationships.
- Clarify nontreatment roles with family members.
- Avoid use of special techniques (e.g., hypnosis or sodium amytal) unless clearly indicated; obtain consultation before proceeding.
- Stay within professional competence—do not take cases beyond personal expertise.
- Distinguish between narrative truth and historical truth; in therapy, the therapist is largely attuned to the patient's perception of reality.
- Obtain consultation in problematic cases.
- Foster patient autonomy and self-determination. Do not suggest lawsuits; this should be the patient's decision after careful consideration.
- In managed care settings, inform patients with recovered memories that more than brief therapy may be required.

- When making public statements, distinguish personal opinions from scientifically established facts.
- If uncomfortable with a patient recovering memories of childhood abuse, stop and refer.
- Do not be reluctant to ask about abuse as part of a competent psychiatric evaluation.

Sexual Misconduct

Therapist–patient sex is usually preceded by progressive boundary violations in treatment (Simon 1989). As a consequence, patients are frequently psychologically damaged by the precursor boundary violations as well as the eventual sexual misconduct of the therapist (Simon 1991). An excellent account of the gradual erosion of treatment boundaries leading to near loss of control with a client is given by Rutter (1989).

General boundary guidelines exist for conducting psychiatric treatment (Simon 1992c). Awareness of these guidelines and of their transgression may help alert the therapist to progressive boundary violations (Simon 1994). Sexual misconduct does not occur in isolation but usually involves a variety of negligent acts of omission and commission.

Civil Liability

Psychiatrists who sexually exploit their patients are subject to civil and criminal actions as well as ethical and professional licensure revocation proceedings. *The Principles of Medical Ethics With Annotations Especially Applicable to Psychiatry* (American Psychiatric Association 2001) states that sex with a current or former patient is unethical (section 2, annotation 1). Malpractice is the most common legal liability.

In a sexual exploitation case, the plaintiff has the difficult burden of proving, by a preponderance of the evidence (i.e., "more likely than not"), that the exploitation actually took place. This burden can be met when the plaintiff provides corroborating evidence to support the claim, such as testimony from other abused (former) patients, letters, pictures, hotel or motel receipts, and identification of incriminating body markings of the exploiter. If the defendant practitioner admits to the exploitation, the plaintiff is left with the responsibility of showing that he or she sustained injuries as a result of the sexual activity. Typically, patient injury occurs in the form of emotional injury (i.e., worsened psychiatric condition, suicide attempts, hospitalization). Expert psychiatric testimony is usually required to establish the type and

extent of psychological damages as well as to establish whether a breach of the standard of care occurred.

An increasing number of states have statutorily made sexual activity both civilly and criminally actionable. For instance, Minnesota enacted legislation that states the following:

> A cause of action against a psychotherapist for sexual exploitation exists for a patient or former patient for injury caused by sexual contact with the psychotherapist if the sexual contact occurred: 1) during the period the patient was receiving psychotherapy…or 2) after the period the patient received psychotherapy…if a) the former patient was emotionally dependent on the psychotherapist; or b) the sexual contact occurred by means of therapeutic deception. (*Minn Stat Ann* 1989)

A few states have enacted civil statutes proscribing sexual misconduct (Simon 1992a). Several states make therapist sexual misconduct a crime (Bisbing et al. 1995). Some states prosecute sexual exploitation suits using their sexual assault statutes. Legislatures in a number of states have enacted statutes that provide civil or criminal remedies to patients who were sexually abused by their therapists (Appelbaum 1990; Strasburger et al. 1991).

Three types of remedies have been codified: reporting, civil liability, and criminal prosecution. *Reporting statutes* require a therapist who learns of any past or current therapist–patient sex to disclose this information. A few states have *civil statutes* proscribing sexual misconduct (Bisbing et al. 1995). Civil statutes incorporate a standard of care and make malpractice suits easier to pursue. For example, Minnesota's statute provides a specific cause of action against psychiatrists and other psychotherapists for injury caused by sexual contact with a patient (Minn Stat Ann 1989). Some of these statutes also restrict unfettered discovery of the plaintiff's past sexual history. *Criminal sanctions* may be the only remedy for exploitative therapists without malpractice insurance, therapists who are unlicensed, or therapists who do not belong to professional organizations.

Other Civil Theories and Defenses

Various causes of action may be asserted by a plaintiff who has been sexually exploited by a psychotherapist. In a minority of states, spouses of the injured patient also have legal standing to initiate their own cause of action against an exploitative practitioner on the grounds of loss of consortium (i.e., interference with the marital relationship).

A variety of defenses have been raised to diminish or protect against liability, but to date, few have been legally successful (Table 39–5). For instance, the contention that the patient was aware that sex was not a part of treatment, that the sex occurred outside the treatment setting, that treatment ended before the sexual relationship began, or that the patient consented to the sexual contact have all been rejected by the courts. Patients cannot consent to malpractice. In sexual misconduct cases, the issue is never patient consent but always breach of fiduciary trust by the therapist.

TABLE 39–5. Legal defenses asserted by defendants in sexual misconduct cases

Denial of plaintiff's allegations of sexual misconduct

Suit barred by statute of limitations

No doctor–patient relationship

Terminated patient—no legal fault under immunity statute

No causation of harm (psychological symptoms reflect inherent course of mental disorder)

No damages (no psychological harm caused by sex with patient)

Superseding intervening variable (not sex with patient) causing harm

Contributory and comparative negligence (plaintiff's "contribution" to sexual misconduct)

Liability in supervision of offending therapist: sexual misconduct of a supervisee is beyond the scope of employment ("detour and frolic")

Marriage to patient

Improper pleading by plaintiff

Consent in sexual assault claims

Source. Reprinted with permission from Simon RI: *Clinical Psychiatry and the Law,* 2nd Edition. Washington, DC, American Psychiatric Press, 1992. Copyright 1992 American Psychiatric Press, Inc.

There is no "respected minority" in the profession that claims sexual relations with patients is therapeutic. This position had a few adherents at one time but is no longer publicly advocated by credible mental health professionals.

Criminal Sanctions

Sexual exploitation of a patient, under certain circumstances, may be considered rape or some analogous sexual offense and may therefore be criminally actionable (Hoge et al. 1995). Typically, the criminality of the exploitation is determined by one of three factors: the practitioner's means of inducement, the age of the victim, or the availability of a relevant state criminal code.

Sex with a current patient may be criminally actionable under sexual assault statutes if the state can prove beyond a reasonable doubt (i.e., with 90%–95% certainty) that the patient was coerced into engaging in the sexual act. Typically, this type of evidence is limited to the use of some form of substance (e.g., medication) either to induce compliance or to reduce resistance. Anesthesia, ECT, hypnosis, drugs, force, and threat of harm have been used to coerce patients into sexual submission (Schoener et al. 1989). To date, claims of psychological coercion through the manipulation of transference phenomena have not been successful in establishing the coercion necessary for a criminal case. In cases involving a minor patient, the issue of consent or coercion is irrelevant because minors and adult incompetent persons are considered unable to provide valid consent. Therefore, sex with a child or an incompetent person is automatically considered a criminal act.

Professional Disciplinary Action

For the purposes of adjudicating allegations of professional misconduct, licensing boards are typically granted certain regulatory and disciplinary authority by state statutes. As a result, state licensing organizations, unlike professional associations, may discipline an offending professional more effectively and punitively by suspending or revoking his or her license. Because licensing boards are not as restrained by rigorous rules of evidence in trial procedures as are the courts in civil and criminal actions, it generally is easier for the patient to seek redress through this means. A review of published reports of sexual misconduct cases adjudicated before licensing boards revealed that, in a vast majority of cases, the evidence was reasonably sufficient to substantiate a claim of exploitation, leading to revocation of the professional's license or suspension from practice for varying lengths of time, including permanent suspension.

Patients can bring ethical charges against psychiatrists before the district branches of the APA. Ethical violators may be reprimanded, suspended, or expelled from the APA. All national organizations of mental health professionals have ethically proscribed sexual relations between therapist and patient. Ethical charges can be filed only against members of a professional group; therefore, this option is not available to patients whose therapists do not belong to a professional organization.

Confidentiality and Testimonial Privilege

Confidentiality refers to the right of a patient to have communications spoken or written in confidence undisclosed to outside parties without implied or expressed authorization. *Privilege*, or more accurately *testimonial privilege*, can be viewed as a derivation of the right of confidentiality. Testimonial privilege is a statutorily created rule of evidence that permits the holder of the privilege (e.g., the patient) to exercise the right to prevent the person to whom confidential information was given (e.g., the psychiatrist) from disclosing it in a judicial proceeding.

Confidentiality

Clinical-Legal Foundation

The basis for recognizing and safeguarding patient confidences is derived from four general sources. First, states have acknowledged this right of protection by including confidentiality provisions in either professional licensure laws or confidentiality and privilege statutes. The second source, and probably the most traditional, comprises the ethical codes of the various mental health professions. Third, the common law recognizes an attorney–client privilege, but developing case law also has carved out this source of protection for physicians and psychotherapists. In 1996, the Supreme Court ruled that communications between psychotherapist and patient are confidential and need not be disclosed in federal trials (*Jaffe v. Redmond* 1996). Fourth, the right of confidentiality may be subsumed under the right of privacy.

Breaching Confidentiality

Regardless of the basis of the right of confidentiality, once the doctor–patient relationship has been created, the professional assumes an automatic duty to safeguard a patient's disclosures. This duty is not absolute, and there are circumstances in which breaching confidentiality is both ethical and legal.

Patients also waive confidentiality in a variety of situations, especially in managed care settings. Medical records are regularly sent to potential employers or to insurance companies when benefits are requested. A limited waiver of confidentiality ordinarily exists when a patient participates in group therapy. Whether one group member can be compelled in court to disclose information shared by another group member during group therapy is still unsettled legally (Slovenko 1998). Many state confidentiality statutes provide statutory exceptions to confidentiality between the psychiatrist and the patient in one or more situations (Brakel et al. 1985) (Table 39–6).

Patients' access to their own records is normally controlled by statutes. These statutory provisions are found under the heading of "medical records" or the much broader term "privilege."

TABLE 39–6. Common statutory exceptions to confidentiality between psychiatrist and patient

Child abuse
Competency proceedings
Court-ordered examination
Dangerousness to self or others
Patient–litigant exception
Intent to commit a crime or harmful act
Civil commitment proceedings
Communication with other treatment providers

If a patient gives the psychiatrist good reason to believe that a warning should be issued to an endangered third party, the confidentiality of the communication that gave rise to the warning may be lost. Psychiatrists who have issued warnings have been compelled to testify in criminal cases (Leong et al. 1992).

Testimonial Privilege

The patient—not the psychiatrist—is the holder of the privilege that controls the release of confidential information. Because the privilege applies only to the judicial setting, it is called *testimonial privilege*. Privilege statutes represent the most common recognition by the state of the importance of protecting information provided by a patient to a psychotherapist. This recognition moves away from the essential purpose of the American system of justice (e.g., "truth finding") by insulating certain information from disclosure in court. This protection is justified on the basis that the special need for privacy in the doctor–patient relationship outweighs the unbridled quest for an accurate outcome in court.

Privilege statutes usually are drafted with reference to one of the following four relationships, depending on the type of practitioner:

- Physician–patient (general)
- Psychiatrist–patient
- Psychologist–patient
- Psychotherapist–patient

Cases have been successfully litigated in which the broader physician–patient category has been applied to the psychotherapist when an applicable statute did not exist.

Privilege statutes also specify exceptions to testimonial privilege. Although exceptions vary, the most common include the following:

- Child abuse reporting
- Civil commitment proceedings

- Court-ordered evaluations
- Cases in which a patient's mental state is in question as a part of litigation

The last exception, known as the *patient–litigant exception*, commonly occurs in will contests, workers' compensation cases, child custody disputes, personal injury actions, and malpractice actions in which the therapist is sued by the patient.

Liability

An unauthorized or unwarranted breach of confidentiality can cause a patient considerable emotional harm. As a result, a psychiatrist typically can be held liable for such a breach on the basis of at least four theories:

- Malpractice (breach of confidentiality)
- Breach of statutory duty
- Invasion of privacy
- Breach of (implied) contract

Informed Consent and the Right to Refuse Treatment

Informed consent is a legal theory in medical malpractice. It provides a patient with a cause of action for not being adequately informed about the nature and consequences of a particular medical treatment or procedure undertaken. This theory is founded on two distinct legal principles. The first is the right of every patient to determine what will or will not be done to his or her body, often referred to as the right of self-determination (*Schloendorff v. Society of New York Hospital* 1914/1957). The second principle emanates from the fiduciary nature of the doctor–patient relationship. Inherent in a physician's duty of fiduciary care is the responsibility to disclose honestly and in good faith all requisite facts concerning a patient's condition. Included among factors to be disclosed are any treatment risks, alternatives, and consequences. The primary purpose of the doctrine of informed consent is to promote individual autonomy; secondarily, it is intended to promote rational decision making (Appelbaum et al. 1987).

There are three essential elements to the doctrine of informed consent:

- Competency
- Information
- Voluntariness

Usually, clinicians provide the first level of screening in identifying patient competency and in deciding whether to accept a patient's treatment decision. The patient or a bona fide representative must be given an adequate description of the treatment. If the patient who refuses treatment appears to lack health care decision-making capacity, it does not mean that the patient cannot be treated. An appropriate substitute decision maker can provide (or withhold) consent. To be able to provide informed consent, the patient or substitute decision maker should be told about the risks, benefits, and prognosis both with and without treatment, as well as alternative treatments and their risks and benefits. In addition, the competent patient must voluntarily consent to or refuse the proposed treatment or procedure.

The legal doctrine of informed consent is consistent with the provision of good clinical care. The informed consent doctrine allows patients to become partners in making treatment determinations that accord with their own needs and values. In the past, physicians operated under the "do no harm" principle. Today, psychiatrists are increasingly required to practice within the model of informed consent and patient autonomy. Most psychiatrists find increased patient autonomy desirable in fostering development of the therapeutic alliance that is so essential to treatment. Furthermore, patient autonomy is the goal of most psychiatric treatments (Beahrs and Gutheil 2001).

Competency

It is clinically useful to distinguish the terms *incompetence* and *incapacity*. *Incompetence* refers to a court adjudication, whereas *incapacity* indicates a functional inability as determined by a clinician (Mishkin 1989). Legally, only competent persons may give informed consent. An adult patient is considered legally competent unless adjudicated incompetent or temporarily incapacitated because of a medical emergency. Incapacity does not prevent treatment; it merely requires the clinician to obtain substitute consent. Treating an incompetent patient without substituted consent is the same as treating a competent patient against his or her will.

Legal competence is narrowly defined in terms of cognitive capacity. The definition derives largely from the laws governing transactions. Important clinical concepts such as affective incompetence are not usually recognized by the law unless cognitive capacity is significantly diminished. For example, a severely depressed but cognitively intact patient may refuse antidepressant medication owing to profound feelings of hopelessness, helplessness, and worthlessness. Manic patients emphasize risks of medications while downplaying benefits. Schizophrenic patients tend to be fearful that medication will cause them serious harm. They are often unable to make a balanced assessment that considers both risks and benefits of a proposed drug. One study, in which three instruments were used to assess competency for treatment decisions, found that the schizophrenia and depression groups demonstrated poorer understanding of treatment disclosures, poorer reasoning in decision making regarding treatment, and a greater likelihood of failing to appreciate their illness or the potential treatment benefits (Grisso and Appelbaum 1995a). Denial of illness often interferes with insight and the ability to appreciate the significance of information provided to the patient. In *In the Guardianship of John Roe* (1992), the Massachusetts Supreme Judicial Court recognized that denial of illness can render a patient incompetent to make treatment decisions.

Competency is not a scientifically determinable state and is situation specific. The issue of competency arises in a number of civil, criminal, and family law contexts. Although there are no hard-and-fast definitions, the patient's ability to do the following is legally germane to determining competency:

- Understand the particular treatment choice being proposed
- Make a treatment choice
- Communicate that choice verbally or nonverbally

This standard obtains only a simple consent from the patient rather than an informed consent, because alternative treatment choices are not provided.

A review of case law and scholarly literature reveals four standards for determining incompetency in decision making (Appelbaum et al. 1987). In order of increasing levels of mental capacity required, these standards include

- Communication of choice
- Understanding of relevant information provided
- Appreciation of available options and consequences
- Rational decision making

Severely mentally disordered patients frequently deny their illnesses. Although they may communicate a choice and understand the information provided, these patients may lack the insight or ability to appreciate the information provided (Grisso and Appelbaum 1995b). Rational decision making is impaired as well. For example, patients with schizophrenia tend to fear some idiosyncratic harm from the treatment while ignoring the actual risk of medication side effects.

Psychiatrists generally feel most comfortable with a rational decision-making standard in determining incompetency. Most courts prefer the first two standards mentioned earlier but often combine competency standards. A truly informed consent that considers the patient's autonomy, personal needs, and values occurs when rational decision making is applied by the patient to the risks and benefits of appropriate treatment options provided by the clinician.

Grisso and Appelbaum (1995a) found that the choice of standards determining competence affected the type and proportion of patients classified as impaired. When compound standards were used, the proportion of patients identified as impaired increased. These authors advised that clinicians be aware of the applicable standards in their jurisdictions.

A valid consent can be either *expressed* (oral or in writing) or *implied* from the patient's actions. The competency issue is particularly sensitive when dealing with minors or mentally disabled persons who lack the requisite cognitive capacity for health care decision making. In both cases, it is generally recognized in the law that an authorized representative or guardian may consent for the patient (see Table 39–4).

Information

The standard for exercising a legally sufficient disclosure varies from state to state. Traditionally, the duty to disclose was measured by a professional standard: either what a reasonable physician would disclose under the circumstances or the customary disclosure practices of physicians in a particular community. In the landmark case *Canterbury v. Spence* (1972), a patient-oriented standard was applied. This standard focused on the "material" information that a *reasonable* person in the patient's position would want to know to make a reasonably informed decision. An increasing number of courts have applied this standard, and some have expanded "material risks" to include information regarding the consequences of not consenting to the treatment or procedure (*Truman v. Thomas* 1980). Even in patient-oriented jurisdictions, there is no duty to disclose every possible risk. A material risk is defined as one in which a physician knows or should know what would be considered significant by a reasonable person in the patient's position. The issue of how much information a patient has to comprehend for consent to be valid is normally resolved by requiring a doctor to convey all appropriate information in terms that the average patient would understand.

Voluntariness

For a consent to be considered legally voluntary, it must be given freely by the patient and without the presence of any form of coercion, fraud, or duress that impinges on the patient's decision-making process. In evaluating whether a consent is truly voluntary, the courts typically examine all the relevant circumstances, including the psychiatrist's manner, the environmental conditions, and the patient's mental state.

Malcolm (1992, p. 241) noted the subtle differences in the concepts of coercion and persuasion. *Persuasion* is defined as the physician's aim "to utilize the patient's reasoning ability to arrive at a desired result." On the other hand, *coercion* occurs "when the doctor aims to manipulate the patient by introducing extraneous elements which have the effect of undermining the patient's ability to reason."

Exceptions and Liability

There are four basic exceptions to the requirement of obtaining informed consent (Table 39–7). When immediate treatment is necessary to save a life or prevent imminent serious harm and it is not possible to obtain either the patient's consent or that of someone authorized to provide consent for the patient, the law typically presumes that the consent would have been granted. Two distinctions must be understood when applying this exception. First, the emergency must be serious and imminent; second, the patient's condition, not the surrounding circumstances (e.g., adverse environmental conditions), determines the existence of an emergency.

TABLE 39–7. Basic exceptions to obtaining informed consent

Emergencies
Incompetency
Therapeutic privilege
Waiver

Source. Reprinted with permission from Simon RI: *Concise Guide to Clinical Psychiatry and the Law.* Washington, DC, American Psychiatric Press, 1992. Copyright 1992 American Psychiatric Press, Inc.

A second exception exists when a patient lacks sufficient mental capacity to give competent consent or is found to be legally incompetent. Someone who is incompetent is incapable of giving informed consent. Under these circumstances, consent must be obtained from a substitute decision maker.

The third exception, *therapeutic privilege*, is the most difficult to apply. Informed consent may not be required if a psychiatrist determines that a complete disclosure of possible risks and alternatives might have a deleterious impact on the patient's health and welfare. Jurisdictions vary in their application of this exception. Absent specific case law or statutes outlining the factors relevant to such a decision, a doctor must substantiate a patient's inability psychologically to withstand being informed of the proposed treatment. Some courts have held that therapeutic privilege may be invoked only if informing the patient will worsen his or her condition or so frighten the patient that rational decision making is precluded (*Canterbury v. Spence* 1972; *Natanson v. Kline* 1960). Therapeutic privilege cannot be used as a means of circumventing the legal requirement for obtaining informed consent from the patient before initiating treatment.

Finally, a physician need not disclose risks of treatment when the patient has competently, knowingly, and voluntarily waived his or her right to be informed (e.g., when the patient does not want to be informed of drug risks).

Absent a situation allowing one of the four exceptions, a psychiatrist who physically treats a patient without first obtaining informed consent is subject to legal liability. In some jurisdictions, a lack-of-informed-consent action may be defeated if case law or statute provides that a reasonable person under the given circumstances would have consented to treatment. As a rule of thumb, treatment without any consent or against a patient's wishes may constitute a battery (intentional tort), whereas treatment commenced with an inadequate consent will be treated as an act of medical negligence.

Seclusion and Restraint

The psychiatric legal issues surrounding seclusion and restraint are complex. Seclusion and restraint have both indications and contraindications as clinical management tools (see Tables 39–8 and 39–9). The legal regulation of seclusion and restraint has become increasingly more stringent over the past decade.

Legal challenges to the use of restraints and seclusion have been made on behalf of the institutionalized mentally ill and the mentally retarded. Normally, these lawsuits do not stand alone but are part of a challenge to a wide range of alleged abuses within a hospital.

Generally, courts hold, or consent decrees provide, that restraints and seclusion can be implemented only when a patient presents a risk of harm to self or others and no less restrictive alternative is available. Additional considerations include the following:

TABLE 39–8. Indications for seclusion and restraint

1. Prevent clear, imminent harm to the patient or others.
2. Prevent significant disruption to treatment program or physical surroundings.
3. Assist in treatment as part of ongoing behavior therapy.
4. Decrease sensory overstimulation (seclusion only).
5. Respond to patient's voluntary reasonable request.[a]

Note. [a]First seclusion; then, if necessary, restraints.
Source. Reprinted with permission from Simon RI: *Concise Guide to Psychiatry and Law for Clinicians*, 3rd Edition. Washington, DC, American Psychiatric Publishing, 2001. Copyright 2001 American Psychiatric Publishing, Inc.

TABLE 39–9. Contraindications to seclusion and restraint

1. Extremely unstable medical and psychiatric conditions[a]
2. Delirious or demented patients unable to tolerate decreased stimulation[a]
3. Overtly suicidal patients[a]
4. Patients with severe drug reactions or overdoses or those patients requiring close monitoring of drug dosages[a]
5. For punishment or for convenience of staff

Note. [a]Unless close supervision and direct observation are provided.
Source. Reprinted with permission from Simon RI: *Concise Guide to Psychiatry and Law for Clinicians*, 3rd Edition. Washington, DC, American Psychiatric Publishing, 2001. Copyright 2001 American Psychiatric Publishing, Inc.

1. Restraint and seclusion can be implemented only by a written order from an appropriate medical official.
2. Orders are to be confined to specific, time-limited periods.
3. A patient's condition must be regularly reviewed and documented.
4. Any extension of an original order must be reviewed and reauthorized.

In addition to these guidelines, some courts and state statutes outline certain due process procedures that must be followed before a restraint or seclusion order can be implemented. Notably, patient due process protections are required only in cases in which restraint and seclusion are used for disciplinary purposes. Typical due process considerations include some form of notice, a hearing, and the involvement of an impartial decision maker. Absent language to the contrary, these procedures may be eased in cases of emergency.

The acceptability of restraint or seclusion for the purposes of training was recognized in the landmark case *Youngberg v. Romeo* (1982/1982). *Youngberg* involved a challenge to the "treatment" practices at the Pennhurst State School and Hospital in Pennsylvania. The United States Supreme Court held that patients could not be restrained except to ensure their safety or, in certain undefined circumstances, "to provide needed training." Although it recognized that the defendant had a liberty interest in safety and freedom from bodily restraint, the court added that these interests were not absolute and were in conflict with the need to provide training. The court also held that decisions made by appropriate professionals regarding restraining the patient would presumptively be considered correct. *Youngberg* is viewed as the first step in the right direction by advocates for the developmentally disabled. In addition, psychiatrists and other mental health professionals have lauded the decision because the court recognized that professionals, rather than the courts, are best able to determine the needs of patients, including when restraint is appropriate.

Most states have enacted statutes regulating the use of restraints, normally specifying the circumstances in which restraints can be used. Most often, those circumstances occur only when a risk of harm to self or danger to others is imminent. Statutory regulation of the use of seclusion is far less common. Most states with laws regarding seclusion and restraint require some type of documentation of their use.

A new federal rule by the Health Care Financing Administration (HCFA) (*42 Code of Federal Regulations* 1999) requires that hospital patients be seen face-to-face by a physician or licensed independent practitioner (LIP) within 1 hour from the time a patient is restrained. An LIP is an individual who is recognized by both state law and hospital policy as having the independent authority to order restraints and seclusion for patients. This requirement is part of expanded policies regulating seclusion and restraint applicable to all hospitals receiving Medicare and Medicaid funds. The 1-hour requirement differs from the corresponding JCAHO mandate because the latter allows nurses to undertake evaluation and management tasks (Joint Commission on Accreditation of Healthcare Organizations 2001b). The JCAHO standard also permits the physician or LIP to conduct an in-person evaluation of the patient within 4 hours of the initiation of restraint or seclusion for patients 18 years old or older. For children and adolescents under age 17, the in-person evaluation must be conducted within 2 hours of the initiation of restraint and seclusion. The 1-hour visit requirement by the HCFA is also recommended by the APA Task Force on the Psychiatric Uses of Seclusion and Restraint (American Psychiatric Association 1984). Regardless of their accreditation status, Medicare- or Medicaid-participating hospitals must meet the standards in the Patient's Rights Condition of Participation

(U.S. Department of Health and Human Services 1999). The HCFA is working with the JCAHO to ensure that the new Medicare requirements are incorporated into JCAHO standards.

The JCAHO made major revisions to its standards for the use of restraint and seclusion, effective January 2001, that seek to reduce the use of restraint and seclusion in order to provide greater assurance of safety and protection of patients with psychiatric or substance abuse disorders. The revised standards restrict the uses of restraints and seclusion to emergency situations in which there is imminent risk that the patient may inflict harm to self or others. Restraints are to be used only as a last resort. The JCAHO has agreed to work with the HCFA to enforce the 1-hour rule in hospitals receiving Medicare and Medicaid funds.

National guidelines for the proper use of seclusion and restraints have been established by the APA Task Force on the Psychiatric Uses of Seclusion and Restraint (American Psychiatric Association 1984). The JCAHO, in cooperation with the HCFA, has promulgated detailed guidelines for hospitals regarding seclusion and restraint requirements. Professional opinion concerning the clinical use of physical restraints and seclusion varies considerably. Unless precluded by state and federal freedom from restraint and seclusion statutes or JCAHO and hospital policies, a variety of uses for seclusion can be justified on both clinical and legal grounds (Simon 1992a).

National Practitioner Data Bank

On September 1, 1990, the National Practitioner Data Bank established by the Health Care Quality Improvement Act of 1986 went into effect. The data bank tracks disciplinary actions, malpractice judgments, and settlements against physicians, dentists, and other health care professionals (Johnson 1991).

Hospitals, health maintenance organizations (HMOs), managed care organizations (MCOs), professional societies, state medical boards, and other health care organizations are required to report any disciplinary action taken against providers lasting more than 30 days. MCOs do not report physicians to the data bank if they do not follow treatment protocols. When a physician is deselected for a quality of care issue, the MCO must report it ("The National Practitioner Data Bank and MCOs" 1999). Disciplinary actions include limitation, suspension, or revocation of privileges or professional society membership. Medical malpractice payments account for approximately three-quarters of reports made to the data bank.

Under the Health Care Quality Improvement Act, immunity from liability is granted for health care entities and providers making peer review reports in good faith (Walzer 1990).

Hospitals are required to request information from the data bank concerning all physicians applying for staff privileges. Every 2 years, a query of the data bank is required concerning each physician or other practitioner on the hospital staff. Hospitals that do not comply face loss of immunity for professional peer review activities.

The public does not have access to the data bank. Plaintiffs' attorneys can have access to the data bank only if they can prove that the hospital failed to query the data bank about the physician in question. The information obtained can be used only to sue the hospital for negligent credentialing. Physicians can request information from the data bank about their own file. A recent study found that hospital reporting of actions taken regarding clinical privileges from 1991–1995 declined, raising concerns about underreporting (Baldwin et al. 1999).

Competency: The Basic Concept

Nearly every area of human endeavor is affected by the law and, as a fundamental condition, requires one to be mentally competent. Essentially, *competency* is defined as "having sufficient capacity, ability...[or] possessing the requisite physical, mental, natural, or legal qualifications" (Black 1990, p. 284). This definition is deliberately vague and ambiguous because the term *competency* is a broad concept encompassing many different legal issues and contexts. As a result, its definition, requirements, and application can vary widely depending on the circumstances in which it is being measured (e.g., health care decisions, executing a will, or confessing to a crime).

In general, competency refers to some *minimal* mental, cognitive, or behavioral ability, trait, or capability required to perform a particular legally recognized act or to assume some legal role. Incompetency is a judicial determination. The term *incapacity*, which is often interchanged with *incompetency*, refers to an individual's functional inability to understand or to form an intention with regard to some act as determined by health care providers (Mishkin 1989).

The legal designation of "incompetent" is applied to an individual who fails one of the mental tests of capacity and is therefore considered *by law* to be not mentally capable of performing a particular act or assuming a particular role. The adjudication of incompetence by a court is subject or issue specific. For example, the fact that a psychiatric patient is adjudicated incompetent to execute a will does not automatically render that patient incompetent to do other things, such as consent to treatment, testify as a witness, marry, drive, or make a legally binding contract.

Generally, the law recognizes only the decisions or choices that have been made by a competent individual. The law seeks to protect incompetent individuals from the harmful effects of their acts. Persons over the age of majority, which is now 18 (U.S. Dept. of Health and Human Services 1981), are presumed to be competent (*Meek v. City of Loveland* 1929). This presumption, however, is rebuttable by evidence of an individual's incapacity (*Scaria v. St. Paul Fire and Marine Insurance Company* 1975). For the psychiatric patient, perception, short- and long-term memory, judgment, language comprehension, verbal fluency, and reality orientation are mental functions that a court will scrutinize regarding "capacity" and "competency."

The issue of competency, whether in a civil or criminal context, is commonly raised in two situations: when the person is a minor and when he or she is mentally disabled. In many situations, minors are not considered legally competent and therefore require the consent of a parent or designated guardian. However, there are exceptions to this general rule, such as when minors are considered emancipated (Smith 1986) or mature (*Gulf S I R Company v. Sullivan* 1928), or in some cases of medical need (e.g., abortion [*Planned Parenthood v. Danforth* 1976]; mental health counseling [*Ill Ann Stat* 1990; *Jehovah's Witnesses v. King County Hospital* 1967/1968]).

The mentally disabled, including mentally impaired psychiatric patients, present a slightly different problem in evaluating competency. Lack of capacity or competency cannot be presumed from either treatment for mental illness (*Wilson v. Lehman* 1964) or institutionalization of such persons (*Rennie v. Klein* 1978). Mental disability or illness does not necessarily render a person incompetent in any or in all areas of functioning. Instead, scrutiny is given to determine whether specific functional incapacities exist that render a person incapable of making a particular kind of decision or performing a particular type of task.

Respect for individual autonomy (*Schloendorff v. Society of New York Hospital* 1914/1957) demands that individuals be allowed to make decisions of which they are capable, even if they are seriously mentally ill, developmentally arrested, or organically impaired. As a rule, a patient with a psychiatric disorder that produces mental incapacity generally must be declared judicially incompetent before exercise of that patient's legal rights can be abridged. The person's current or past history of physical and mental illness is but one factor to be weighed in determining whether a particular test of competency is met.

Health Care Decision Making

Because psychiatric patients frequently have impaired mental capacity, the difficulty associated with obtaining a valid informed consent to proposed diagnostic procedures and treatments can be both challenging and frustrating. The need to obtain competent, informed consent is not negated simply because it "appears" that the patient is in need of medical intervention or would likely benefit from it. Instead, clinicians must assure themselves that the patient or an appropriate substitute decision maker has given a competent consent before proceeding with treatment. An increasing number of states require a judicial determination of incompetence and the court's substituted consent prior to the administration of neuroleptic treatment to a patient who is deemed by a health care provider to lack the functional mental capacity to consent (Simon 1992a).

Only a *competent* person is legally recognized as being able to give informed consent. Competent patients must not be treated against their objections. This is particularly important for health care providers working with patients who sometimes are of questionable competence because of mental illness, narcotic abuse, or alcoholism. When psychiatrists treat patients with neuropsychiatric deficits, the responsibility to obtain a valid informed consent can be clinically daunting because of the vacillating and unpredictable mental states associated with many central nervous system disorders.

Psychiatric patients who have been determined to lack the requisite functional mental capacity to make a treatment decision, except in cases of an emergency (*Frasier v. Department of Health and Human Resources* 1986), must have an authorized representative or guardian appointed to make health care decisions on their behalf (*Aponte v. United States* 1984). A number of consent options may be available for such patients, depending on the jurisdiction (see Table 39–4).

Right to Die

Legal decisions addressing the issue of a patient's "right to die" fall into one of two categories: decisions dealing with individuals who were incompetent at the time removal of life support systems was sought (*In re Conroy* 1985; *In re Quinlin* 1976) and decisions dealing with competent patients.

Incompetent Patients

In what was hoped to be the "final word" on this difficult and personal question of patient autonomy, the United States Supreme Court ruled, in *Cruzan v. Director, Missouri Department of Health* (1990), that the state of Missouri may refuse to remove a food and water tube surgically implanted in the stomach of Nancy Cruzan without clear and convincing evidence of her wishes. Ms. Cruzan was in a persistent vegetative state for 7 years. Without clear and convincing evidence of a patient's decision to have life-sustaining measures withheld in a particular circumstance, the state has the right to maintain that individual's life, even to the exclusion of the family's wishes.

Although it seemed to leave unanswered more questions than it answered, the court's decision buttressed the position of "right-to-refuse" treatment advocates in three significant ways:

1. It seemed to give constitutional status to a competent person's right to refuse treatment: "those competent to express their wishes do enjoy a constitutional right to refuse life-sustaining medical treatment...and...if people appoint relatives or friends to make decisions about medical treatment in the event they become incompetent, states "may well be constitutionally required" to defer to the wishes of such "surrogate decision-makers" (Marcus 1990).
2. It did not distinguish between artificially administered food and water and other life-sustaining measures, such as respirators. This distinction was a hotly contested sticking point in some previous lower-court decisions.
3. It indicated that an incompetent person who makes his or her wishes known in advance, such as through a living will, may have a constitutional right to halt life-sustaining intervention, depending on the proof of those wishes.

The importance of the *Cruzan* decision for physicians treating severely or terminally impaired patients is that physicians must seek clear and competent instructions regarding foreseeable treatment decisions. For example, a psychiatrist treating a patient with progressive degenerative diseases should attempt to ascertain the patient's wishes regarding the use of life-sustaining measures *while that patient can still competently articulate those wishes*. This information is best provided in the form of a living will, durable power-of-attorney agreement, or health care proxy. Any written document that clearly and convincingly sets forth the patient's wishes can serve the same purpose.

Although physicians fear civil or criminal liability for stopping life-sustaining treatment, liability may now arise from overtreating critically or terminally ill patients (Weir and Gostin 1990). Legal liability may occur for providing unwanted treatment to an autonomous patient or treatment that is against the best interests of a nonautonomous patient.

Competent Patients

A growing body of cases has emerged involving *competent* patients—usually with excruciating pain and terminal diseases—who seek the termination of further medical treatment. The single most significant influence in the development of this body of law is the doctrine of informed consent. Beginning with the fundamental tenet that "no right is held more sacred...than the right of every individual to the possession and control of his own person" (*Schloendorff v. Society of New York Hospital* 1914/1957; *Union Pacific Realty Company v. Botsford* 1891), courts have fashioned the present-day informed consent doctrine and applied it to right-to-die cases.

The right to decline life-sustaining medical intervention, even for a competent person, is not absolute. As noted in *In re Conroy* (1985), four countervailing state interests generally exist that may limit the exercise of that right: 1) preservation of life, 2) prevention of suicide, 3) safeguarding the integrity of the medical profession, and 4) protection of innocent third parties (*In re Conroy* 1985). In each of these situations, and depending on the surrounding circumstances, the trend has been to support a competent patient's right to have artificial life-support systems discontinued (*Bartling v. Superior Court* 1984; *Bouvia v. Superior Court* 1986; *In re Farrell* 1987; *In re Jobes* 1987a; *In re Peter* 1987; *Tune v. Walter Reed Army Medical Hospital* 1985).

As a result of the *Cruzan* decision, courts now focus primarily on the reliability of the evidence proffered in establishing the patient's competence, specifically the clarity and certainty with which a decision to withhold medical treatment is made. Assuming that a terminally ill patient has chosen to forgo any further medical intervention *and* the patient is competent at the time this decision is made, courts are unlikely to overrule or subvert the patient's right to privacy and autonomy.

Advance Directives

The use of advance directives such as a living will, health care proxy, or durable medical power of attorney is recommended to avoid ethical and legal complications associated with requests to withhold life-sustaining treatment measures (Simon 1992a; Solnick 1985). The Patient Self-Determination Act, which took effect on December 1, 1991, requires hospitals, nursing homes, hospices, managed care organizations, and home health care agencies to advise patients or family members of their right to accept or refuse medical care and to execute an advance directive (LaPuma et al. 1991). These advance directives provide a method for individuals, while competent, to choose proxy health care decision makers in the event of future incompetency. A living will can be contained as a subsection of a durable power of attorney agreement. In the ordinary power of attorney created for the management of business and financial matters, the power of attorney generally becomes null and void if the person creating it becomes incompetent.

Because federal law does not specify the right to formulate advance directives, state law applies. State legislators have recognized that individuals may want to indicate who should make important health care decisions in case they become incapacitated and unable to act in their own behalf. All 50 states and the District of Columbia permit individuals to create a *durable* power of attorney (i.e., one that endures even if the competence of the creator does not) (*Cruzan v. Director, Missouri Department of Health* 1990). Several states and the District of Columbia have durable power-of-attorney statutes that expressly authorize the appointment of proxies for making health care decisions (*Cruzan v. Director, Missouri Department of Health* 1990).

Generally, durable power of attorney has been construed to empower an agent to make health care decisions. Such a document is much broader and more flexible than a living will, which covers only the period of a diagnosed terminal illness, specifying only that no "extraordinary treatments" be used that would prolong the act of dying (Mishkin 1985). To rectify the sometimes uncertain status of the durable power of attorney as applied to health care decisions, a number of states have passed or are considering passing health care proxy laws. The health care proxy is a legal instrument akin to the durable power of attorney but specifically created for health care decision making. Despite the growing use of advance directives, there is increasing evidence that physician values rather than patient values are more decisive in end-of-life decisions (Orentlicher 1992).

In a durable power of attorney or health care proxy, general or specific directions are set forth about how future decisions should be made in the event a person becomes unable to make these decisions. The determination of a patient's competence is not specified in most durable power-of-attorney and health care proxy statutes. Because this is a medical or psychiatric question, the examination by two physicians to determine the patient's ability to understand the nature and consequences of the proposed treatment or procedure, ability to make a choice, and ability to communicate that choice is usually minimally sufficient. This information, like all significant medical observations, should be clearly documented in the patient's file.

Because of the frequent absence of advance directives, several states have enacted statutory surrogate laws. These laws authorize certain persons, such as a spouse or a court-appointed guardian, to make health care decisions when the patient has not stated his or her wishes in writing.

The application of advance directives to psychiatric patients poses some difficulties. The classic example arises when a currently asymptomatic patient with an organic personality disorder and occasional bouts of severe affective instability draws up a durable power-of-attorney agreement or health care proxy directing the following: "If I become mentally unstable again, administer medications even if I strenuously object or resist." T. G. Gutheil (personal communication, September 1985) described this as the "Ulysses Contract." In Greek mythology, Ulysses was bound to the mast of his ship so he could hear the beautiful, though lethal, sirens' song. All the other sailors covered their ears. When Ulysses heard the irresistible song of the sirens, he tried to struggle loose. When that failed, he demanded to be untied. Similarly, when mental instability recurs, the patient with a recurrent psychiatric disorder may strenuously object to treatment.

Because durable power of attorney agreements or health care proxies can be easily revoked, the treating psychiatrist or institution has no choice but to honor the patient's refusal, even if there is reasonable evidence that the patient is incompetent. Legal consultation should be considered at this point. If the patient is grossly disordered and is an immediate danger to self and others, the physician or hospital is on firmer ground medically and legally to override the patient's treatment refusal temporarily. Otherwise, it is generally better to seek a court order for treatment than risk legal entanglement with the patient by attempting to enforce the original terms of the advance directive. Unless there are compelling medical reasons to do otherwise, courts generally honor the patient's original treatment directions that were given when he or she was competent.

Guardianship

Guardianship is a method of substitute decision making for individuals who have been judicially determined to be unable to act for themselves (Brakel et al. 1985). Historically, the state or sovereign possessed the power and authority to safeguard the estate of incompetent persons (Regan 1972). This traditional role still reflects the purpose of guardianship today. In some states, there are separate provisions for the appointment of a "guardian of one's person" (e.g., health care decision making) and for a "guardian of one's estate" (e.g., authority to make contracts to sell one's property; Sale et al. 1982). The latter type of guardian is frequently referred to as a *conservator*, although this designation is not uniformly used throughout the United States. A further distinction, also found in some jurisdictions, is between *general* (*plenary*) and *specific* guardianship (Sale et al. 1982). As the name implies, the specific guardian is restricted to exercising decisions about a particular subject area. For instance, he or she may be authorized to make decisions about major or emergency medical procedures, with the disabled person retaining the freedom to make decisions about all other medical matters. General guardians, in contrast, have total control over the disabled individual's person, estate, or both (Sale et al. 1982).

Guardianship arrangements are increasingly used with patients who have dementia, particularly AIDS-related dementia and Alzheimer's disease (Overman and Stoudemire 1988). Under the Anglo-American system of law, an individual is presumed to be competent unless adjudicated incompetent. Incompetence is a legal determination made by a court of law on the basis of evidence provided by health care providers and others that the individual's functional mental capacity is significantly impaired. The Uniform Guardianship and Protective Proceeding Act (UGPPA) or the Uniform Probate Code (UPC) is used as a basis for laws governing competency in many states (Mishkin 1989). Drafted by legal scholars and practicing attorneys, the uniform acts serve as models for the purpose of achieving consistency among the state laws by enactment of model laws (*UGPPA § 5–101*). General incompetency is defined by the UGPPA as meaning "impaired by reason of mental illness, mental deficiency, physical illness or disability, advanced age, chronic use of drugs, chronic intoxication, or other cause (except minority) to the extent of lacking sufficient understanding or capacity to make or communicate reasonable decisions."

Some patients with psychiatric disorders may meet the preceding definition. Generally, the appointment of a guardian is limited to situations in which the individual's decision-making capacity is so impaired that he or she is unable to care for personal safety or provide such necessities as food, shelter, clothing, and medical care, with the likely result of physical injury or illness (*In re Boyer* 1981). The standard of proof required for a judicial determination of incompetency is *clear and convincing evidence*. Although the law does not assign percentages to proof, clear and convincing evidence is in the range of 75% certainty (Simon 1992a).

States vary on the extent of their reliance on psychiatric assessments. Nonmedical personnel such as social workers, psychologists, family members, friends, colleagues, and even the individual who is the subject of the proceeding may testify.

Substituted Judgment

Psychiatrists often find that the time required to obtain an adjudication of incompetence is unduly burdensome and that the process frequently interferes with the provision of quality treatment. Moreover, families are often reluctant to face the formal court proceedings necessary to declare their family member incompetent, particularly when sensitive family matters are disclosed. A common solution to both of these problems is to seek the legally authorized proxy consent of a spouse or relative serving as guardian when the refusing patient is believed to be incompetent. Proxy consent, however, is becoming less available as a consent option (Simon 1992a). Many states exclude surrogate authorizations for the treatment of mental disorders.

There are clear advantages associated with having the family serve as decision makers (Perr 1984). First, use of responsible family members as surrogate decision makers maintains the integrity of the family unit and relies on the sources who are most likely to know the patient's wishes. Second, it is more efficient and less costly than an attempt to prove incompetency. There are some disadvantages, however. Proxy decision making requires synthesizing the diverse values, beliefs, practices, and prior statements of the patient for a given specific circumstance (Emanuel and Emanuel 1992). As one judge characterized the problem, any proxy decision making in the absence of specific directions is "at best only an optimistic approximation" (*In re Jobes* 1987b). Ambivalent feelings, conflicts within the family and with the patient, and conflicting economic interests may make certain family members suspect as guardians (Gutheil and Appelbaum 1980). Also, relatives may not be available or may not want to get involved. Moreover, next of kin may possess dubious competence or even less competence than the patient.

The President's Commission for the Study of Ethical Problems in Medicine and Biomedical and Behavioral Research (1982) recommended that the relatives of incompetent patients be selected as proxy decision makers for the following reasons:

1. The family is generally most concerned about the good of the patient.
2. The family is usually most knowledgeable about the patient's goals, preferences, and values.
3. The family deserves recognition as an important social unit, to be treated, within limits, as a single decision maker in matters that intimately affect its members.

Several states permit proxy decision making by statute, mainly through informed consent statutes (Solnick 1985). Some state statutes specify that another person may authorize consent on behalf of the incompetent patient, whereas others mention specific relatives.

Unless proxy consent by a relative is provided by statute or by case law authority in the state where the psychiatrist practices, it is not recommended that the good-faith consent by next of kin be relied on in treating a patient believed to lack health care decision-making capacity (Klein et al. 1983). The legally appropriate procedure to follow is to seek judicial recognition of the family member as the substitute decision maker.

Some patients treated in an emergency are expected to recover competency within a few days. As soon as the patient is able to competently consent to further treatment, such consent should be obtained directly from the patient. For the patient who continues to lack mental capacity for health care decisions, an increasing number of states provide administrative procedures authorized by statute that permit involuntary treatment of incompetent and refusing mentally ill patients who do not meet current standards for involuntary civil commitment (Hassenfeld and Grumet 1984; Zito et al. 1984). In most jurisdictions, a durable power-of-attorney agreement permits the next of kin to consent through durable power-of-attorney statutes (Solnick 1985). However, in some instances, this procedure may not meet judicial challenge. To avoid this problem, several states have created health care proxies specifically for advance health care decision making.

A debate continues about the theory of substitute decision making. Should the substitute decision maker act in the patient's best interest (the "objective test"), or should he or she rely on what the patient would have decided if competent (the "subjective" or "substituted judgment" approach)? The increasingly used subjective test is difficult to implement for patients who have never been competent, who have made improvident or less-than-competent past decisions, or who have never openly stated choices to be implemented by others. Also, the values of substitute decision makers can be easily substituted for the patient regardless of which test is used (Roth 1985). Both the best interest and the substituted judgment standards lead to predictable biases by those who implement them. Use of the best interest standard leads to treatment of patients and sustaining life. Application of the substituted judgment standard favors treatment refusal and the upholding of civil liberties (E.D. Robertson 1989).

The substituted judgment standard has found considerable judicial favor. It is based on the incompetent person's right to privacy translated into the medical context as the right to refuse treatment. The right to privacy is the constitutional expression of the autonomy Americans claim as free persons living in a free society. On this point, courts find authority and inspiration from John Stuart Mill:

> The only purpose for which power can be rightfully exercised over any member of a civilized community against his will, is to prevent harm to others. His own good, either physical or moral, is not a sufficient warrant. He cannot rightfully be compelled to do or forebear because it will be better for him to do so, because it will make him happier, because in the opinion of others, to do so would be wise, or even right. (Mill 1951)

Physician-Assisted Suicide

With increasing legal recognition of physician-assisted suicide (PAS), psychiatrists are likely to be called on to become gatekeepers. Such a role would be a radical departure from the physician's code of ethics, in which doctors are prohibited from participating in any intervention that hastens death. Previously, the Supreme Court ruled in *Cruzan* that terminally ill persons could refuse life-sustaining medical treatment. Courts and legislatures will determine whether hastening death is an unwarranted extension of the right to refuse treatment. Every proposal for PAS requires a psychiatric screening or consultation to determine the terminally ill person's competence to commit suicide. The presence of psychiatric disorders associated with suicide, particularly depression, will have to be ruled out as the driving factor behind PAS. Much controversy rages over the ethics of this gatekeeping function (American Medical Association 1994).

Criminal Proceedings

Individuals charged with committing crimes frequently display significant psychiatric and neurological impairment. A history of severe head injury may be present. The possibility of a neuropsychiatric disorder must be thoroughly investigated. For example, Lewis et al. (1986) examined 15 death-row inmates who were chosen for examination because of imminent execution rather than evidence of neuropathology. In each case, evidence of severe head injury and neurological impairment was found.

The causal connection between brain damage and violence remains frustratingly obscure. Violent behavior spans a wide spectrum from a normal response to a threatening situation to violence emanating directly from an organic brain disorder such as Klüver-Bucy syndrome, hypothalamic tumors, or temporal lobe epilepsy (Strub and Black 1985). Moreover, violent behavior is often the result of the interaction between an individual and a specific situation. Brain damage and mental illness may or may not play a significant role in this equation. Psychiatrists must acknowledge limitations in their expertise concerning the possible connection between brain damage and violence.

Criminal Intent (Mens Rea)

Under the common law, the basic elements of a crime are 1) the mental state or level of intent to commit the act (known as the *mens rea*, or guilty mind), 2) the act itself or conduct associated with committing the crime (known as *actus reus*, or guilty act), and 3) a concurrence in time between the guilty act and the guilty mental state (*Bethea v. United States* 1977). To convict a person of a particular crime, the state must prove beyond a reasonable doubt that the defendant committed the criminal act with the requisite intent. All three elements are necessary to satisfy the threshold requirements for the imposition of criminal sanctions.

The question of intent is a particularly vexing problem for the courts. For example, everyone would agree that killing another person is deplorable conduct. However, should the accidental death of child in a car accident, the heat-of-passion shooting by a husband of his wife's lover, and the cold-blooded murder of a bank teller by a robber all be punished in the same way? The determination of the defendant's intent, or *mens rea*, at the time of the offense is the law's equalizer and trigger mechanism for deciding criminal culpability and the appropriate assessment of retribution. For instance, a person who deliberately plans to commit a crime is more culpable than one who accidentally commits one.

There are two classes of intent used to categorize *mens rea*: specific and general. Specific intent refers to the *mens rea* in crimes in which a *further intention* exists beyond the presence of a general criminal intent. For instance, the courts frequently state that the intent necessary for first-degree murder includes a "specific intent to kill"; on the other hand, a person might commit an assault "with the intent to rape" (Melton et al. 1987). Unlike general criminal intent, specific criminal intent cannot be presumed from the unlawful criminal act but must be proved independently. Because of the imprecision of these categories, modern statutory codes have created more precise criteria for defining mental states (Melton et al. 1997).

General criminal intent is more elusive. Such intent may be presumed from commission of the criminal act. The concept usually is used by the law to explain criminal liability in which a defendant was merely conscious or should have been conscious of his or her physical actions at the time of the offense (Melton et al. 1987). For example, general criminal intent would apply to a person who intended to violate the law by holding up a bank. General criminal intent is presumed by commission of the criminal act. To deal with the vagueness of these two standards, many states have enacted their own definitions of intent.

Persons with certain mental handicaps or impairments represent an interesting challenge for prosecutors, defense counsel, and judges in determining what, if any, retribution is justifiable. Mental impairment often raises serious questions about the intent to commit a crime and the appreciation of its consequences.

In addition to *mens rea*, a person's mental status can play a deciding role in whether he or she is ordered to stand trial to face the criminal charges (*Dusky v. United States* 1960), acquitted of the alleged crime (*M'Naughten's Case* 1843; *United States v. Brawner* 1972/1994), sent to prison, hospitalized (*Commonwealth v. Robinson* 1981; *Mental Aberration and Post Conviction Sanctions* 1981; *State v. Hehman* 1974), or, in some extreme cases, sentenced to death ("Eighth Amendment and the Execution of the Presently Incompetent" 1980; *Ford v. Wainwright* 1986). Before any defendant can be criminally prosecuted, the court must be satisfied that the accused is competent to stand trial—that is, he or she understands the charges brought against him or her and is capable of rationally assisting counsel with the defense.

Competency to Stand Trial

In every situation in which competency is in question, the law seeks to reiterate a common theme: that only the acts of a rational individual are to be given recognition by society (*Neely v. United States* 1945). In doing so, the law attempts to reaffirm the integrity of the individual and of society in general.

The legal standard for assessing pretrial competency was established by the United States Supreme Court in *Dusky v. United States* (1960). Throughout involvement with the trial process, the defendant must have "sufficient present ability to consult with his lawyer with a reasonable degree of rational understanding and whether he has a rational as well as factual understanding of the proceedings against him" (*Dusky v. United States* 1960).

Typically, the impairment that raises the question of the defendant's competence is associated with a mental disease or defect. It is settled, however, that a person may be held to be incompetent to stand trial even if he or she does not suffer from a mental disease or defect as defined by the American Psychiatric Association (1994) in DSM-IV. For example, children under a certain age ordinarily are deemed incompetent to stand trial.

Although most impairments implicated in competency examinations are functional rather than organic (Reich and Wells 1985), various forms of neuropsychiatric impairments typically raise questions about a defendant's competency to stand trial. In *Wilson v. United States* (1968), the defendant had no memory of the time of an alleged robbery because he had permanent retrograde amnesia. This impairment was caused by injuries he suffered in an automobile accident that occurred as he was being pursued by the police following the offense. Of the various criteria that the court established in determining the defendant's competency to stand trial, the following are directly relevant to the issue of neuropsychiatric impairment (*Wilson v. United States* 1968):

1. The extent to which the amnesia affected the defendant's ability to consult with and assist his lawyer
2. The extent to which the amnesia affected the defendant's ability to testify in his own behalf

Any disorder, whether functional or organic, that significantly impairs a defendant's cognitive and communicative abilities is likely to have an impact on competency. Nevertheless, it is the actual *functional* mental capability to meet the minimal standard of trial competency, and not the severity of the deficits, that determines whether an individual is cognitively capable to be tried.

For example, Slovenko (1995) questioned whether psychiatric diagnosis is relevant to competency to stand trial. The presence or absence of a mental illness is irrelevant if the defendant is capable of meeting competency requirements. It is legal criteria, not medical or psychiatric diagnosis, that governs competency. Diagnosis is relevant only to the question of restoring the defendant's competency to stand trial with treatment.

Checklists and structured interviews have been developed to assess specific psychological factors applicable to the competency standards established in *Dusky*. The Interdisciplinary Fitness Interview, designed for use by lawyers and mental health professionals (Schreiber et al. 1987), provides for a detailed examination of psychopathology and legal knowledge using explicit scales for rating each response to the competency evaluation. *Evaluating Competencies: Forensic Assessments and Instruments*, by Thomas Grisso (1986), is a standard reference in the field.

A defendant's impairment in one particular function, however, does not automatically render him or her incompetent. For example, the fact that the defendant is manifesting certain deficits because of damage to the parietal lobe does not necessarily mean that he or she lacks the requisite cognitive ability to aid in his or her own defense at trial (Tranel 1992). The ultimate determination of incompetency is solely for the court to decide (*United States v. David* 1975). Moreover, the impairment must be considered in the context of the particular case or proceeding. Mental impairment may render an individual incompetent to stand trial in a complicated tax fraud case but not incompetent for a misdemeanor trial.

Psychiatrists and psychologists who testify as expert witnesses regarding the effect of psychiatric problems on a defendant's competency to stand trial are most effective if their findings are framed according to the degree to which the defendant is cognitively capable of meeting the standards enunciated in *Dusky*.

Insanity Defense

One of the most controversial issues in American jurisprudence is the insanity defense. Defendants with functional or organic mental disabilities who are found competent to stand trial may seek acquittal on the basis that they were not criminally responsible for their actions because of insanity at the time the offense was committed.

Criminals commit crimes for many reasons, but the law presumes that all of them do so rationally and with their own free will. As a result, the law concludes that they are deserving of some form of punishment. Some offenders, however, are so mentally disturbed in their thinking and behavior that they are thought to be incapable of acting rationally. Under these circumstances, civilized societies have deemed it unjust to punish a "crazy" or insane person (Blackstone 1769; Coke 1680). This is in part due to fundamental principles of fairness and morality. In addition, the punishment of a person who cannot rationally appreciate the consequences of his or her actions thwarts the two major tenets of punishment: retribution and deterrence. The insanity defense is rarely used, and a successful insanity defense is even rarer. Approximately 1% of criminal defendants plead not guilty by reason of insanity; of these, only 10%–25% are successful. The chance of exculpation is greatest when the criminal defendant was found to be psychotic at the time of the crime by the pretrial assessment (Brakel et al. 1985).

A generally accepted, precise definition of legal insanity does not exist. Over the years, tests of insanity have been subject to much controversy, modification, and refinement (Brakel et al. 1985). The development of the insanity defense standard in the United States has had four basic elements (Table 39–10). The existence of a mental disorder has remained a consistent core of the insanity defense, whereas the three other elements have varied over time (Brakel et al. 1985). Thus, there is variability in the insanity defense standard in the United States, depending on which state or jurisdiction has control over the defendant raising the defense.

TABLE 39–10. Basic elements of insanity defense

Presence of a mental disorder
Presence of a defect of reason
A lack of knowledge of the nature or wrongfulness of the act
An incapacity to refrain from the act

Source. Reprinted with permission from Simon RI: "Legal and Ethical Issues in Traumatic Brain Injury," in *Traumatic Brain Injury*. Edited by Silver JM. Washington, DC, American Psychiatric Press, 1994. Copyright 1994 American Psychiatric Press, Inc.

Following the acquittal by reason of insanity of John Hinckley Jr. on charges of attempting to assassinate President Reagan and murder others, an outraged public demanded changes in the insanity defense. Federal and state legislation to accomplish that result ensued. Between 1978 and 1985, approximately 75% of all states made some sort of substantive change in their insanity defense (Perlin 1989). Nevertheless, a number of states continued to adhere to the American Law Institute (ALI) insanity defense standard or a version of it. The ALI test provides that a person is not responsible for criminal conduct if at the time of such conduct as a result of mental disease or defect he lacks substantial capacity either to appreciate the criminality (wrongfulness) of his conduct or to conform his conduct to the requirements of law. As used in this article, the terms *mental disease or defect* do

not include an abnormality manifested only by repeated criminal or otherwise antisocial conduct (*Model Penal Code § 4.01* [1962] ULA 1974).

This standard contains both a cognitive and a volitional prong. The *cognitive prong* derives from the 1843 M'Naughten rule exculpating the defendant who does not know the nature and quality of the alleged act or does not know the act was wrong. The *volitional prong* is a vestige of the irresistible impulse rule, which states that the defendant who is overcome by an irresistible impulse that leads to an alleged act is not responsible for that act. It is on the volitional prong that experts disagree the most in individual cases.

By contrast, defendants tried in a federal court are governed by the standard enunciated in the Comprehensive Crime Control Act (CCCA) of 1984 (*P.L. 1984*). The CCCA provides that it is an affirmative defense to all federal crimes that, at the time of the offense, "the defendant, as a result of a severe mental disease or defect, was unable to appreciate the nature and quality or the wrongfulness of his acts. Mental disease or defect does not otherwise constitute a defense" (*Model Penal Code § 402, 98 Stat*). This codification eliminates the volitional or irresistible impulse portion of the insanity defense—that is, it does not allow an insanity defense based on a defendant's inability to conform his or her conduct to the requirements of the law. The defense is now limited to defendants who are unable to appreciate the wrongfulness of their acts (i.e., the *cognitive portion* of the defense). The federal courts require the defendant to prove insanity by clear and convincing evidence (approximately 75% certainty). The burden of proof varies among the states. In a minority of states, the prosecution has the burden of proving beyond a reasonable doubt that the defendant was sane. In most states, the defendant must bear the burden of proving by a preponderance of the evidence that she or he was insane (Melton et al. 1997). A few states have abolished the special plea of insanity. At the same time, evidence of insanity is admissible to negate *mens rea*.

The threshold issue in making an insanity determination is not the existence of a mental disease or defect per se but the lack of substantial mental capacity because of it. Therefore, the lack of capacity due to mental defects other than mental illness may be sufficient. For instance, mental retardation may represent an adequate basis for the insanity defense under certain circumstances. The impulse disorders—intermittent explosive disorder, kleptomania, pathological gambling, and pyromania—have not fared well under an insanity defense. Persons with these conditions do not meet the criteria for the cognitive prong of an insanity defense. Presumably, the volitional prong would be applicable, but it is usually insufficient by itself. Moreover, courts and juries tend to view criminal acts arising from impulse disorders as impulses not resisted rather than irresistible impulses. Pathological gambling no longer serves as a basis for an insanity defense (Rosenthal and Lorenz 1992). McGarry (1983) pointed out that the lack of volitional control over the isolated act of gambling does not assume a lack of control concerning criminal acts committed in the service of the impulse to gamble. Compulsive gambling, however, is being raised as a mitigating factor at sentencing (Rosenthal and Lorenz 1992). Less severe punishment is feasible through a court's willingness to consider treatment, community service, restitution, and the possibility of probation.

Depending on the severity of the functional or organic mental disorder and its effect on an offender's cognitive and affective processes, a defense of insanity might be warranted. At the least, the presence of a psychiatric disorder should be investigated as a *mitigating* factor that may have caused the offender to have diminished capacity.

Diminished Capacity

It is possible for a person to have the required *mens rea* yet be declared legally insane. For instance, a defendant's actions may be considered so "crazy" as to convince a jury that he or she was criminally insane and therefore not legally responsible, yet his or her knowledge of the criminal act (e.g., committing a murder) was relatively intact. From this distinction, the law recognizes that there are shades of mental impairment that obviously can affect *mens rea*, but not necessarily to the extent of completely nullifying it. In recognition of this fact, the concept of *diminished capacity* was developed (Melton et al. 1997).

Broadly viewed, diminished capacity permits the accused to introduce medical and psychological evidence relating directly to the *mens rea* for the crime charged without having to assert a defense of insanity (Melton et al. 1997). For example, in the crime of assault with the intent to kill, psychiatric testimony would be permitted to address whether the offender acted with the purpose of committing homicide at the time of the assault. When a defendant's *mens rea* for the crime charged is nullified by psychiatric evidence, the defendant is acquitted only of that charge. In the preceding example, the prosecutor may still try to convict the defendant of another offense requiring a lesser *mens rea*, such as manslaughter (Melton et al. 1997). Patients with psychiatric disorders who commit criminal acts may be eligible for a diminished capacity defense.

Guilty but Mentally Ill

In a number of states, an alternative verdict of *guilty but mentally ill* has been established. Under these statutes, if the defendant pleads not guilty by reason of insanity, this alternative verdict is available to the jury (Slovenko 1982). Under an insanity plea, the verdict may be

- Not guilty
- Not guilty by reason of insanity
- Guilty but mentally ill
- Guilty

The problem with guilty but mentally ill is that it is an alternative verdict that is not different from finding the defendant simply guilty. The court must still impose a sentence on the convicted person. Although the convicted person will receive special treatment if necessary, this treatment provision is also available to any other prisoner. Moreover, the frequent unavailability of appropriate psychiatric treatment for prisoners adds an additional element of spuriousness to this verdict.

Exculpatory and Mitigating Disorders

Psychotic disorders of differing etiology form the most common basis for an insanity defense. In addition to the major psychiatric and organic brain disorders, a number of other conditions may provide a foundation for an insanity or diminished capacity defense.

Automatisms

For conviction of a crime, there must be not only a criminal state of mind (*mens rea*) but also the commission of a prohibited act (*actus reus*). The physical movement necessary to satisfy the *actus reus* requirement must be conscious and volitional. In addition to statutory and common law in many jurisdictions, Section 2.01(2) of the *Model Penal Code* (1962) specifically excludes from the *actus reus* the following:

> (a) a reflex or convulsion; (b) a bodily movement during unconsciousness or sleep; (c) conduct during hypnosis or resulting from hypnotic suggestion; [and] (d) a bodily movement that otherwise is not the product of the effort or determination of the actor.

A defense claiming that the commission of a crime was an involuntary act usually is referred to as an "automatism defense." The classic, though rare, example is the person who commits an offense while "sleepwalking." Courts have held that such an individual does not have conscious control of his or her physical actions and therefore acts involuntarily (*Fain v. Commonwealth* 1879; *H.M. Advocate v. Fraser* 1878). A conscious, reflexive action carried out under stressful circumstances may qualify for an automatism defense. For example, a driver who is being attacked in his car by a bee loses control in attempting to swat the insect. The car strikes a pedestrian, who is killed. An automatism defense exists to charges of vehicular homicide. Other situations relevant to psychiatry in which the defense might be used arise when a crime is committed during a state of altered consciousness caused by a concussion after a head injury, involuntary ingestion of drugs or alcohol, hypoxia, metabolic disorders such as hypoglycemia, or epileptic seizures (Low et al. 1982).

There are, however, limitations to the automatism defense. Most notably, some courts have held that if the person asserting the automatism defense was aware of the condition prior to the offense and failed to take reasonable steps to prevent the criminal occurrence, the defense is not available. For example, if a defendant with a known history of uncontrolled epileptic seizures loses control of a car during a seizure and kills someone, that defendant will not be permitted to assert the defense of automatism.

Intoxication

Ordinarily, intoxication is not a defense to a criminal charge. Because intoxication, unlike mental illness, mental retardation, and most neuropsychiatric conditions, is usually the product of a person's own actions, the law is cautious about viewing it as a complete defense or mitigating factor. Most states view voluntary alcoholism as relevant to the issue of whether the defendant possessed the *mens rea* necessary to commit a specific intent crime or whether there was premeditation in a crime of murder. The mere fact that the defendant was voluntarily intoxicated will not justify a finding of automatism or insanity. A distinct difference arises when, because of chronic, heavy use of alcohol, the defendant suffers from an alcohol-induced psychotic disorder, withdrawal delirium, amnestic disorder, or dementia. If competent psychiatric evidence is presented that an alcohol-related neuropsychiatric disorder caused significant cognitive or volitional impairment, a defense of insanity or diminished capacity could be upheld.

Temporal Lobe Seizures

Another "mental state" defense occasionally raised by defendants regarding assault-related crimes is that the assaultive behavior was involuntarily precipitated by abnormal electrical patterns in the defendant's brain.

This condition is frequently diagnosed as temporal lobe epilepsy (Devinsky and Bear 1984). Episodic dyscontrol syndrome (Elliott 1978, 1982) has also been advanced as a neuropsychiatric condition causing involuntary aggression. Studies have hypothesized that there are "centers of aggression" in the temporal lobe or limbic system—primarily the amygdala. This hypothesis has promoted the idea that sustained aggressive behavior by these persons may be primarily the product of an uncontrollable, randomly occurring, abnormal brain dysrhythmia. Hence, the legal argument is raised that these individuals should not be held accountable for their actions. Despite its simplicity and occasional success in the courts, few empirically significant data exist to support this theory at the present time (Blumer 1984).

Metabolic Disorders

Defenses based on metabolic disorders have also been tried. In 1979, the so-called Twinkie defense was used as part of a successful diminished capacity defense of Dan White in the murders of San Francisco Mayor George Moscone and Supervisor Harvey Milk. This defense was based on the theory that the ingestion of large amounts of sugar contributed to a state of temporary insanity (*People v. White* 1981). The forensic psychiatric report stated that the defendant had been "filling himself up with Twinkies and Coca-Cola" (Blinder 1981–1982). A jury found White guilty only of voluntary manslaughter. In 1981, California repealed the defense of diminished capacity (Slovenko 1995).

Hypoglycemic states also may be associated with significant psychiatric impairment (Droba and Whybrow 1989). When substantial glucose depletion occurs, a wide variety of responses may occur including episodic and repetitive dyscontrol, temporary amnesia, depression, and hostility with spontaneous recovery (i.e., quick recovery after the consumption of appropriate nutrients). The degree of mental abnormality associated with hypoglycemic states varies from mild to severe according to the blood glucose level. It is the degree of disturbance, not the mere presence of an etiological metabolic component, that is determinative in a mental state defense. This principle also applies to mental dysfunctions produced by disorders originating in the hepatic, renal, adrenal, and neuroendocrine systems (e.g., premenstrual syndrome; Parry and Berga 1991).

Posttraumatic Stress Disorder

In criminal cases, defendants have pleaded not guilty by reason of insanity secondary to posttraumatic stress disorder (PTSD; Sparr 1990). The diagnosis of PTSD has been alleged in criminal proceedings by prosecutors to bolster the credibility of the victim or by experts who attempt to argue backward from PTSD symptoms to establish the occurrence of a traumatic stressor (e.g., rape). Victims of criminal acts who develop PTSD or other psychiatric disorders may sue under criminal injuries compensation acts. PTSD has bolstered the supporters of "victims rights," whose advocacy poses a threat to the constitutional rights of defendants (Stone 1993). An insanity defense based on PTSD is more likely to succeed if it can be shown that the individual committed a crime while experiencing a dissociative behavioral reenactment of a prior traumatic event. Guidelines for the assessment of PTSD in litigation have been proposed (Simon 1995).

Personal Injury Litigation

Assessment of Sexual Harassment

Psychiatrists perform evaluations of litigants and provide testimony in court in a number of areas of civil litigation. As an example, civil suits alleging sexual harassment are burgeoning. Psychiatrists are being called on to testify in these cases, which present emerging, complex psychological and social issues.

The statutory basis for sexual harassment claims is found in Title VII of the Civil Rights Act of 1964. Section 703(a)(1) of Title VII, 42 U.S.C. § 2000e-2(a), reads as follows: "It shall be an unlawful employment practice for an employer...to fail or refuse to hire or to discharge any individual, or otherwise to discriminate against any individual with respect to his compensation, terms, conditions, or privileges of employment, because of such individual's race, color, religion, sex, or national origin." In 1980, the Equal Employment Opportunity Commission (EEOC) issued guidelines that declared sexual harassment to be a violation of Section 703 of Title VII. The guidelines propounded criteria for determining unwelcome conduct of a sexual nature that constituted sexual harassment, defined the circumstances under which an employer may be held liable, and suggested affirmative steps that an employer should take to prevent sexual harassment (Guidelines on Discrimination Because of Sex).

In defining sexual harassment, Title VII does not proscribe all conduct of a sexual nature in the workplace. Only unwelcome sexual conduct that is a term or condition of employment constitutes a violation. The EEOC's guidelines define two kinds of sexual harassment: "quid pro quo" and "hostile environment." Sexual conduct constitutes sexual harassment when "submission to such conduct is made either explicitly or implicitly a term or condition of an individual's employment" (29 C.F.R. § 1604.11[a][1]). Quid pro quo harassment takes place when "submission or rejection of such conduct by an individual is used as the basis for employment decisions affecting the individual" (29 C.F.R. § 1604.11[a][2]). The EEOC guidelines also recognize that unwelcome sexual conduct that "unreasonably interfere[s] with an individual's job performance" or creates an "intimidating, hostile, or offensive working environment" can constitute sex discrimination, even if it causes no tangible or economic job consequences (29 C.F.R. § 1604.11[a][3]).

The United States Supreme Court, in *Harris v. Forklift Systems, Inc.* (1993), ruled unanimously that a woman who claims she was sexually harassed on the job need not prove she was psychologically injured to win monetary damages. The Court defined unlawful harassment as creating a work environment that a reasonable person would find "hostile or abusive." The broadly written ruling will likely make it easier for employees to bring suits for sexual harassment.

Psychiatrists who become involved in sexual harassment litigation usually are asked to determine the veracity of harassment complaints, the psychological consequences of harassment, and the treatment needs and prognosis for women or men who have been sexually harassed. Binder (1992) presented examples of cases in which psychiatric testimony was provided to help decision making in assessing damages secondary to the psychological effects of sexual harassment. Guidelines have been proposed for conducting a credible forensic psychiatric evaluation in sexual harassment litigation (Simon 1996).

Expert Testimony

Civil litigation in psychic injury and head trauma cases may require the evaluation and testimony of psychiatrists, often working in conjunction with neurologists, other physicians, psychologists, neuropsychologists, and allied mental health professionals. Psychiatrists become involved in litigation as witnesses in one of two ways: as treaters or as forensic experts.

The Treating Clinician

Psychiatrists who venture into the legal arena must be aware of the fundamentally different roles of the treating psychiatrist and the forensic psychiatric expert. Treatment and expert roles do not mix (Greenberg and Shuman 1997; Strasburger et al. 1997). For example, unlike the orthopedist, who possesses objective data such as the X ray of a broken limb to demonstrate physical damages in court, the treating psychiatrist must rely heavily on the subjective reporting of the patient. In the treatment context, psychiatrists are interested primarily in the patient's perception of his or her difficulties, not necessarily the objective reality. As a consequence, treating psychiatrists usually do not speak to third parties or check pertinent records to gain additional information about a patient or to corroborate the patient's statements. The law, however, is interested only in testimony that is based on provable facts. Uncorroborated patient reportage is usually attacked in court as speculative, self-serving, and unreliable. The treating psychiatrist is vulnerable to these charges.

Credibility issues also abound. The treating psychiatrist is, and must be, an ally of the patient. This bias *in favor of* the patient is a proper treatment stance that fosters the therapeutic alliance. Furthermore, to be treated effectively, the patient should be reasonably "liked" by the psychiatrist. No practitioner can treat for very long a patient who is disliked. Moreover, the psychiatrist looks for mental disorders to treat. A treatment, rather than a litigation, agenda is the appropriate stance for the treating psychiatrist.

In court, credibility is a critical commodity to possess when testifying. Opposing counsel will take every opportunity to portray the treating psychiatrist as a subjective mouthpiece for the patient-litigant, which may or may not be true. Also, court testimony by the treating psychiatrist may compel the disclosure of information that is not *legally* privileged but nonetheless is viewed as intimate and confidential by the patient. This disclosure by a trusted therapist is bound to cause psychological damage to the therapeutic relationship (Strasburger 1987). In addition, psychiatrists must be careful to inform patients about the consequences of releasing treatment information, particularly in legal matters. Section 4, Annotation 2, of the *Principles of Medical Ethics with Annotations Especially Applicable to Psychiatry* (American Psychiatric Association 2001) states "The continuing duty of the psychiatrist to protect the patient includes fully apprising him/her of the connotations of waiving the privilege of privacy. This may become an issue when the patient is being investigated by a government agency, is applying for a position, or is involved in legal action."

Finally, when the treating psychiatrist testifies concerning the need for further treatment, a conflict of interest is readily apparent. In making such treatment prognostications, the psychiatrist stands to benefit economically from the recommendation of further treatment. Although this may not be the intention of the psychiatrist, opposing counsel is sure to point out that the psychiatrist has a financial interest in the case.

The American Academy of Psychiatry and the Law (1989/1991), in its ethics statement, advises that "a treating psychiatrist should generally avoid agreeing to be an expert witness or to perform an evaluation of his patient for legal purposes because a forensic evaluation usually requires that other people be interviewed and testimony may adversely affect the therapeutic relationship" (p. xii). The treating psychiatrist should attempt to remain solely in a treatment role. If it becomes necessary to testify on behalf of the patient, the treating psychiatrist should testify only as a fact witness rather than as an expert witness. As a fact witness, the psychiatrist will be asked to describe the number and length of visits, diagnosis, and treatment. Generally, no opinion evidence will be requested about the causation of the injury or the extent of damages. In some jurisdictions, however, the court may convert a fact witness into an expert at the time of the trial. Psychiatrists must remain ever mindful of the many double agent roles that can develop when mixing psychiatry and litigation (Simon 1987, 1992a).

The Forensic Expert

The forensic expert, on the other hand, is usually free from the preceding encumbrances. No doctor–patient relationship, with its treatment biases toward the patient, is created during forensic evaluation. The forensic expert reviews various records and usually speaks to several people who know the litigant. Furthermore, the forensic expert is not as easily distracted from considering exaggeration or malingering because of a clear appreciation of the litigation context and the absence of treatment bias. Finally, the forensic psychiatrist is not placed in a conflict-of-interest position of recommending treatment from which he or she would personally (i.e., financially) benefit. The forensic expert, however, is frequently viewed by opposing counsel as a "hired gun."

Forensic Psychiatry

Definition and Scope

Forensic psychiatry is defined as "a subspecialty of psychiatry in which scientific and clinical expertise is applied to legal issues in legal contexts embracing civil, criminal, correctional or legislative matters" (American Academy of Psychiatry and the Law 1989/1991). The subspecialty of forensic psychiatry is burgeoning. The past decade has witnessed enormous growth in interest in this specialty as demonstrated by the proliferation of journals devoted exclusively to forensic psychiatry, the development of forensic psychiatry fellowships, and established board certification. The American Board of Medical Specialties has recognized forensic psychiatry as a subspecialty of psychiatry. The American Board of Psychiatry and Neurology has conducted examinations for certification in the subspecialty of forensic psychiatry since 1994.

Just a few of the major areas in which forensic psychiatrists evaluate cases and provide testimony include malpractice litigation, will contests, personal injury litigation, competency determinations (both civil and criminal), criminal responsibility, and pre-sentencing hearings. Many other areas of law and psychiatry, too numerous to list here, also require the professional services of the forensic psychiatrist. In the course of practice, the forensic psychiatrist often works on unusual, challenging cases not ordinarily found in the general outpatient or inpatient practice of psychiatry. A list of suggested readings in forensic psychiatry is provided after the references at the end of this chapter.

Forensic Psychiatric Evaluation of the Claimant

The forensic psychiatric evaluation of the injured claimant differs in several significant ways from the traditional psychiatric evaluation. As noted previously, the distinction between the roles of treating psychiatrist and forensic evaluator must be firmly maintained in the litigation context. Problems in both treatment and testimony invariably arise for the clinician when these roles are confused.

The psychiatrist who enters the legal arena must understand that equities usually exist on both sides of a legal case; otherwise the case would probably not have been brought to litigation. The fact that opposing experts disagree does not necessarily mean that one side or the other is wrong. The opinions of opposing experts should be carefully considered.

Team Approach

The comprehensive forensic psychiatric evaluation usually requires cooperation with a number of other practitioners and specialists. The forensic psychiatrist who is evaluating the claimant may require the input of a neurologist, psychologist, neuropsychologist, and internist or general practitioner. Depending on the complexities of the case, representatives of a number of other disciplines may need to be consulted. The forensic evaluator must also consider the findings of other examinations performed at the request of opposing counsel. The burgeon-ing number of ever-more-complicated brain studies currently available makes consultation with a qualified neurologist virtually a necessity in cases involving claims of brain injury.

Absence of Doctor–Patient Relationship

The psychiatrist should inform the claimant at the time of examination that no doctor–patient relationship will be formed. That is, the psychiatrist will not *treat* the claimant in any fashion. The psychiatrist should explain that he or she has been retained by [name the specific party] to perform an independent psychiatric examination. The sole purpose of the examination is to provide information to the party retaining the psychiatrist.

Absence of Confidentiality

The claimant must be informed that, unlike the usual doctor–patient relationship, confidentiality surrounding the forensic evaluation may not exist. Once the retaining attorney decides to disclose the findings of the evaluation in litigation, the information will be available to both sides and can become a public record.

Standard Diagnostic Schema

The diagnostic evaluation of claimants should be made according to the multiaxial classification system contained in DSM-IV. All five axes should be employed. Axis I permits the clinician to consider the major clinical psychiatric syndromes, either singly or multiply. It is not unusual for the claimant to have concurrent Axis I diagnoses. Concurrent Axis I disorders may have preexisted or may be exacerbated.

Axis II forces the clinician to consider personality disorders that are often overlooked or ignored in the forensic evaluation of a claimant. The occurrence of significant head injuries is high in the violent criminal population, where there is a higher incidence of antisocial personality disorder (Lewis et al. 1986; Pétursson and Gudjónsson 1981).

On Axis III, the relationship of medical disorders and their treatments to the patient's clinical presentation on Axis I must be carefully evaluated. The claimant may have a number of injuries requiring extensive pharmacotherapy that may further complicate the clinical picture. Moreover, a host of medical disorders may present with or have associated symptoms of cerebral dysfunction. Prior head injuries or preexisting central nervous system disorders should be considered. For example, young adults who have a history of learning disabilities or attention-deficit disorder are likely to develop serious incapacity when they sustain traumatic brain injury.

Axis IV permits the evaluation of a psychosocial stressor or multiple psychosocial stressors, usually occurring within the year preceding the current evaluation, that may have contributed to the development of a new mental disorder, recurrence of a prior mental disorder, or exacerbation of a preexisting psychiatric disorder. The search for multiple psychosocial stressors must be carefully conducted. It is the rare claimant who has only one psychosocial stressor affecting his or her life. Injury often occurs in the context of other preexisting psychosocial stressors such as sustained interpersonal difficulties, financial problems, occupational distress, or other personal losses.

Finally, functional impairment should be assessed on Axis V according to the Global Assessment of Functioning Scale in combination with other standard methods of evaluation of psychiatric impairment discussed later.

DSM-IV contains a cautionary statement about its use in litigation. Lawyers and courts refer to DSM-IV extensively. Psychiatrists perform an important service to the judicial system by appropriately applying DSM-IV in litigation. Lawyers and courts have a tendency to cloak clinical guidelines and diagnostic manuals with a certainty more properly given to the reading of statutes and codes.

Collateral Sources of Information

In the treatment situation, the psychiatrist relies almost exclusively on the subjective reporting of the patient. The patient, who has a disorder, is presumed to be candid. No conscious, hidden agendas are usually present. In litigation, however, the claimant must naturally be expected to favor his or her own legal case. The possibility of malingering must always be kept in mind (Table 39–11). Malingering is not limited to the fabrication of symptoms. More often, malingering is manifested by the *exaggeration* or even *minimization* of symptoms. Thus, the psychiatrist must consider a broad array of information.

During the course of legal discovery by both parties to the suit, a great deal of information usually is developed. The forensic examiner should request that the retaining lawyer provide all relevant information. Proceeding to court with incomplete information will likely be exposed by opposing counsel, undercutting the psychiatrist's testimony and possibly damaging the claimant's case. The forensic psychiatrist should review all data carefully before coming to a conclusion. The collateral sources of information listed in Table 39–12, although not exhaustive, indicate major areas of inquiry.

TABLE 39–11. Increased index of suspicion for malingering

Litigation context (financial compensation, evading criminal prosecution)
Marked discrepancy between clinical findings and subjective complaints
Lack of cooperation with evaluation and treatment
Antisocial personality traits or disorder
Overdramatization of complaints
History of recurrent accidents or injuries
Evidence of self-induced injuries
Vaguely defined symptoms
Poor work history
Inability to work but retention of capacity for pleasurable activities

Source. Reprinted with permission from Simon RI: "Legal and Ethical Issues in Traumatic Brain Injury," in *Traumatic Brain Injury*. Edited by Silver JM. Washington, DC, American Psychiatric Press, 1994. Copyright 1994 American Psychiatric Press, Inc.

TABLE 39–12. Collateral sources of information

Other physicians and health care providers (reports, direct discussions)
Hospital records
Family
Other third parties
Military records
School records
Police records
Witness information
Work records
Work products (letters, work projects)
Legal discovery (depositions, legal documents)
Prior medical and psychiatric records
Prior psychological and neuropsychological evaluations

Source. Reprinted with permission from Simon RI: "Legal and Ethical Issues in Traumatic Brain Injury," in *Traumatic Brain Injury*. Edited by Silver JM. Washington, DC, American Psychiatric Press, 1994. Copyright 1994 American Psychiatric Press, Inc.

Traumatic Brain Injury

When evaluating the mental status of the traumatic brain injury (TBI) claimant, the psychiatrist must be able to conduct a thorough and reliable mental status examination. Moreover, the mental status assessment is an integral part of the psychiatric examination that cannot be delegated to others. Usually, it is better to conduct the examination in divided sessions over the course of 2 days because of possible fluctuations in the mental status of the TBI claimant. The practice of performing a perfunctory mental status examination or relying solely on the assessment of the neuropsychologist is unwarranted. Neuropsychological assessment can be a valuable adjunct to the neuropsychiatric assessment of the TBI claimant (Becker and Kay 1986). Nevertheless, the psychiatrist will have little basis for critically reviewing the neuropsychological findings unless he or she can perform a competent mental status examination. The mental status examination as described by Strub and Black (1985) provides a scored, comprehensive, reliable format for the evaluation of mental status.

The role of neuropsychological testing must be critically evaluated in each case. Neuropsychological tests are not totally objective. The qualifications and experience of the neuropsychologist constitute a critical variable. Tests of behavior in neuropsychological testing are subject to the control of the person performing the task. Thus, the consideration of motivation is critical. Also, low test scores may be caused by factors other than brain damage (Table 39–13). Doctors, not tests, make diagnoses. A neuropsychological test score by itself cannot be used to point to a specific cause of the litigant's injury. Moreover, in litigation, causation is ultimately a matter for the finder of fact to determine.

TABLE 39–13. Major factors influencing neuropsychological test findings

Original endowment
Environment (e.g., education, occupation, life experiences)
Motivation (effort)
Physical health
Psychological distress
Psychiatric disorders (e.g., depression, dissociative disorders)
Medications (e.g., anticonvulsants, psychotropics)
Qualifications and experience of neuropsychologist
Errors in scoring
Errors in interpretation

Source. Reprinted with permission from Simon RI: "Legal and Ethical Issues in Traumatic Brain Injury," in *Traumatic Brain Injury.* Edited by Silver JM. Washington, DC, American Psychiatric Press, 1994. Copyright 1994 American Psychiatric Press, Inc.

Base rate neuropsychological deficits are typically demonstrated in the normal population. If impairments are noted without evaluation of the claimant's prior history and level of neuropsychological functioning, overinterpretation of the test data is likely. The critical review of school and work records to determine the prior level of intellectual functioning is important in establishing baseline performance. Neuropsychological impairments observed among a normal population increase with the age of the population. Lower IQ score and slower

responses are also associated with normal aging.

Comorbidity and drug effects also must be considered when evaluating the results of neuropsychological test assessments. Questionable results will be obtained in the neuropsychological testing if the impact of concurrent psychiatric disorders and medications on the neuropsychological data is not considered.

Brain Injury Mimics

A number of psychiatric disorders may mimic traumatic brain injury. Some of the more common traumatic brain injury mimics include conversion, factitious, somatization, and depressive disorders presenting with symptoms of neurological and cerebral dysfunction. Conversion disorder symptoms classically mimic neurological disease. Dissociative symptoms may present with amnesia or atypical memory loss. Depressive pseudodementia is a commonly recognized clinical disorder in elderly patients. Posttraumatic stress disorder manifesting symptoms of difficulty in concentration and psychogenic amnesia can also mimic brain injury. Similarly, anxiety disorders may be associated with memory complaints secondary to the inability to concentrate. On the other hand, TBI can cause anxiety and depression.

To complicate matters, litigants may be receiving psychoactive substances. Neuroleptics, antidepressants, lithium, and particularly benzodiazepines can produce side effects that mimic neurological and brain disorders. Psychoactive substances may produce serious memory difficulties, either directly by acting on brain chemistry or indirectly through sedation. Various combinations of medications may interact to produce a host of side effects that involve the central nervous system. Psychoactive drug abuse is also distressingly common in these cases, especially when the litigant complains of persistent pain. Narcotics and barbiturates, when marketed in combination with nonnarcotic pain medications, are commonly abused.

Disability Determinations

In addition to the psychiatric diagnosis, an assessment of functional impairment and disability must be made. In litigation, it is the degree of functional impairment, not the psychiatric diagnosis per se, that determines the monetary damage award. The psychiatrist must also understand the difference between *impairment* and *disability.* An impaired individual may not necessarily be disabled. Psychiatric impairment is considered disabling only when a psychiatric disorder limits a person's capacity to meet the demands of living. A traumatic blow to one eye of a company president that causes mild, uncorrectable visual impairment will not likely significantly impair occupational functioning. The same injury to a major league baseball player will likely be totally disabling and end his career.

Similarly, a patient may have moderate impairment but only mild disability in social or occupational functioning owing to the development of compensatory coping mechanisms. On the other hand, practically every psychiatric clinician has seen patients who have mild impairment but who are seriously disabled. This situation is common in litigation. For claimants presenting such a picture, the psychiatrist should pay particular attention to the possible presence of concurrent Axis IV psychosocial stressors, comorbidity, substance abuse, medication effects, and litigation issues on the clinical presentation of the claimant.

Standard impairment assessment methods should be used in combination with the DSM-IV Axis V global assessment of functioning. The credible psychiatric assessment of functional impairment avoids strictly subjective, conclusory pronouncements about the examinee's impairment and the need for future treatment. Instead, whenever possible, the examinee's functional impairment and future treatment needs should be evaluated according to the American Medical Association's (2000) *Guide to the Evaluation of Permanent Impairment*. The guide closely follows the Social Security Administration's guidelines for the assessment of disability. Assessment of permanent impairment should not be made until maximal medical improvement has been achieved.

Child Custody

Psychiatrists become involved in child custody cases throughout the separation and divorce processes (Billick and Kerry 1994). Psychiatrists may be asked to give opinions in the following situations:

- Custody decisions (request by parents before litigation)
- Child custody litigation
- To assist a *guardian ad litem* (attorney appointed by the court to represent a child)
- Child-care agency (usually court ordered after allegations of abuse have been made)
- Divorce mediation procedures
- Visitation
- Psychiatric treatment of either parent or child

The guiding principle in child custody decisions is the recognition of children's rights through application of the "best interests of the child" standard. Psychiatrists who become involved in child custody decisions should have specialized training in child psychiatry. Adequately trained general psychiatrists may also be able to perform child custody evaluations. However, the general psychiatrist must recognize any limitations in training and experience in performing child psychiatric evaluations (Simon and Wettstein 1997). Consultation with a child psychiatrist may be necessary. The APA provides guidelines for child custody evaluations (American Psychiatric Association 1982).

When performing child custody evaluations, the psychiatrist should see both parties to the litigation. The ethical guidelines of the American Academy of Psychiatry and the Law (Section IV) state the following:

> In custody cases, honesty and striving for objectivity require that all parties be interviewed, if possible, before an opinion is rendered. When this is not possible, or if for any reason not done, this fact should be clearly indicated in the forensic psychiatrist's report and testimony. Where one parent has not been seen, even after deliberate effort, it may be inappropriate to comment on that parent's fitness as a parent. Any comments on that parent's fitness should be qualified and the data for the opinion be clearly indicated.

Child custody disputes often result in "hardball" litigation. If one parent accuses the other of child sexual abuse, a "war" of sorts between the parties breaks out. Many psychiatrists refuse to perform child custody evaluations because they fear being excoriated by aggressive attorneys. Forensically informed psychiatrists are usually able to function effectively in stressful litigation.

Child custody evaluation presents special challenges and rewards. Psychiatrists must be willing to commit the time necessary to do extensive interviewing as well as manage the emotional strain of child custody cases. Evaluators must be careful to identify and correct personal biases and not allow themselves to be influenced by importuning attorneys. Recommendations made by the psychiatrist will likely have a profound influence on the rest of the child's life. The psychiatrist must assiduously maintain a position of advocate for the child's needs. The professional and personal gratifications are great when the psychiatrist's evaluation provides the potential for healthy child development and a sound foundation for adult life.

After a divorce is final, one parent usually is granted custody of any minor children. The custodial parent holds the health care decision-making power. Psychiatrists may be asked to perform an examination or evaluation of a minor child at the request of the noncustodial parent. Psychiatrists who perform such examinations expose themselves to legal action (Simon 1992a). Although no court has found a psychiatrist liable for failure to obtain the custodial parent's consent prior to examination or evaluation, such decisions appear likely (Kuder 1986). Court decisions as well as statutory interpretations of the term *parent* have limited the use of that word to the parent awarded custody under a divorce decree's term (*Gary v. Gary* 1982; *Texas Fam Code Ann* 1990). Before performing an evaluation or examination on a minor child, the psychiatrist should obtain the consent of the parent with legal custody.

Conclusions

The ethical and legal issues surrounding the treatment and management of psychiatric patients are challenging and complex. The legally informed psychiatrist is in a stronger position to provide good clinical care to the patient within the burgeoning regulation of psychiatry by the courts and through governmental legislation. Moreover, psychiatrists will be increasingly required to testify in court concerning psychiatric patients. Familiarity and comfort with the role of a fact or expert witness will facilitate competent psychiatric testimony.

References

American Academy of Psychiatry and the Law: Ethical Guidelines for the Practice of Forensic Psychiatry. Adopted May 1987. Revised October 1989, 1991

American Medical Association: Physician-Assisted Suicide. Code of Medical Ethics Reports, Vol. 5, No. 2. Chicago, IL, American Medical Association, July 1994, pp 269–275

American Medical Association: Report of the Council on Scientific Affairs. Evidence-Based Principles of Discharge and Discharge Criteria (CSA Report 4-A-96), Chicago, IL, American Medical Association, 1996

American Medical Association: Guide to the Evaluation of Permanent Impairment, 5th Edition. Chicago, IL, American Medical Association, 2000

American Psychiatric Association: Child Custody Consultation. Washington, DC, American Psychiatric Association, 1982

American Psychiatric Association: The Psychiatric Uses of Seclusion and Restraint (APA Task Force Report No 22). Washington, DC, American Psychiatric Association, 1984

American Psychiatric Association: The Practice of Electroconvulsive Therapy: Recommendations for Treatment, Training, and Privileging: A Task Force Report of the American Psychiatric Association, 2nd Edition. Edited by Weiner RD. Washington, DC, American Psychiatric Association, 2001

American Psychiatric Association: Tardive Dyskinesia: A Task Force Report of the American Psychiatric Association. Washington, DC, American Psychiatric Association, 1992

American Psychiatric Association: Diagnostic and Statistical Manual of Mental Disorders, 4th Edition. Washington, DC, American Psychiatric Association, 1994

American Psychiatric Association: The Principles of Medical Ethics With Annotations Especially Applicable to Psychiatry, 2001 Edition. Washington, DC, American Psychiatric Association, 2001

Appelbaum PS: Statutes regulating patient–therapist sex. Hosp Community Psychiatry 41:15–16, 1990

Appelbaum PS, Lidz CW, Meisel A: Informed Consent: Legal Theory and Clinical Practice. New York, Oxford University Press, 1987, pp 84–87

Appelbaum PS, Zonana H, Bonnie R, et al: Statutory approaches to limiting psychiatrists' liability for their patients' violent acts. Am J Psychiatry 146:821–828, 1989

Baldwin LM, Hart LG, Oshel RG, et al: Hospital peer review and the National Practitioner Data Bank. JAMA 282:349–355, 1999

Baxter P, Beck JC: The violent patient: minimize your risk, in Practicing Psychiatry Without Fear: Guidelines of Liability Prevention. Edited by Lifson LE, Simon RI. Cambridge, MA, Harvard University Press, 1998

Beahrs JO, Gutheil TG: Informed consent in psychotherapy. Am J Psychiatry 158:4–10, 2001

Becker B, Kay GG: Neuropsychological consultation in psychiatric practice. Psychiatr Clin North Am 9:255–265, 1986

Benefacts. A Message from the APA-sponsored Professional Liability Insurance Program. Psychiatric News, April 19, 1996, pp 1, 26

Billick SB, Kerry CD: Role of the psychiatric evaluator in child custody disputes, in Principles and Practice of Forensic Psychiatry. Edited by Rosner R. New York, Chapman and Hall, 1994, pp 271–281

Binder RL: Sexual harassment: issues for forensic psychiatrists. Bull Am Acad Psychiatry Law 20:109–118, 1992

Bisbing SB, Jorgenson LM, Sutherland PK: Sexual Abuse by Professionals: A Legal Guide. Charlottesville, VA, Michie, 1995

Black HC: Black's Law Dictionary, 6th Edition. St Paul, MN, West Publishing, 1990

Blackstone W: Commentaries, Vol 4, 1769, pp 24–25

Blinder M: My examination of Dan White. Am J Forensic Psychiatry 2:12–22, 1981–1982

Blumenthal SJ: An overview and synopsis of risk factors, assessment, and treatment of suicidal patients over the life cycle, in Suicide Over the Life Cycle. Edited by Blumenthal SJ, Kupfer DJ. Washington, DC, American Psychiatric Press, 1990, pp 685–733

Blumer D: Psychiatric Aspects of Epilepsy. Washington, DC, American Psychiatric Press, 1984

Brakel SJ, Parry J, Weiner BA: The Mentally Disabled and the Law, 3rd Edition. Chicago, IL, American Bar Foundation, 1985

Chiles JH, Strohsall K: The Suicidal Patient: Principles of Assessment, Treatment, and Case Management. Washington, DC, American Psychiatric Press, 1995

Coke E: Third Institute 6, 6th Edition, 1680

Daniel DG, Zigun JR, Weinberger DR: Brain imaging in neuropsychiatry, in The American Psychiatric Press Textbook of Neuropsychiatry, 2nd Edition. Edited by Yudofsky SC, Hales RE. Washington, DC, American Psychiatric Press, 1992, pp 165–186

Devinsky O, Bear D: Varieties of aggressive behavior in temporal lobe epilepsy. Am J Psychiatry 141:651–656, 1984

Droba M, Whybrow PC: Endocrine and metabolic disorders, in Comprehensive Textbook of Psychiatry/V, Vol 2, 5th Edition. Edited by Kaplan HI, Sadock BJ. Baltimore, MD, Williams & Wilkins, 1989, pp 1209–1221

Elliott FA: Neurological aspects of antisocial behavior, in The Psychopath: A Comprehensive Study of Antisocial Disorders and Behaviors. Edited by Reid WH. New York, Brunner/Mazel, 1978, pp 146–189

Elliott FA: Neurological findings in adult minimal brain dysfunction and the dyscontrol syndrome. J Nerv Ment Dis 170:680–687, 1982

Emanuel EJ, Emanuel LL: Proxy decision making for incompetent patients: an ethical and empirical analysis. JAMA 267:2067–2071, 1992

Greenberg SA, Shuman DW: Irreconcilable conflict between therapeutic and forensic roles. Journal of Professional Psychology: Research and Practice 28:50–56, 1997

Grisso T: Evaluating Competencies: Forensic Assessments and Instruments. New York, Plenum, 1986

Grisso T, Appelbaum PS: Comparison of standards for assessing patients' capacities to make treatment decisions. Am J Psychiatry 152:1033–1037, 1995a

Grisso T, Appelbaum PS: The MacArthur treatment competence study, III: abilities of patients to consent to psychiatric and medical treatments. Law and Human Behavior 19:149–174, 1995b

Gutheil TG, Appelbaum PS: Substituted judgement and the physician's ethical dilemma: with special reference to the problem of the psychiatric patient. J Clin Psychiatry 41:303–305, 1980

Gutheil TG, Simon RI: Risk management principles in recovered memory cases: the importance of the clinical foundation. Psychiatr Serv 48:1403–1407, 1997

Hassenfeld IN, Grumet B: A study of the right to refuse treatment. Bull Am Acad Psychiatry Law 12:65–74, 1984

Hoge SK, Jorgenson L, Goldstein N, et al: APA resource document: legal sanctions for mental health professional–patient sexual misconduct. Bull Am Acad Psychiatry Law 23:433–448, 1995

Johnson ID: Reports to the National Practitioner Data Bank. JAMA 265:407–411, 1991

Joint Commission on Accreditation of Healthcare Organizations: Comprehensive Accreditation Manual for Behavioral Health. Oak Brook Terrace, IL, Joint Commission on Accreditation of Healthcare Organizations, 2001a

Joint Commission on Accreditation of Healthcare Organizations: Comprehensive Accreditation Manual for Behavioral Health Care. Restraint and Seclusion Standards for Behavioral Health. Chicago, IL, Joint Commission Accreditation of Healthcare Organizations, 2001b, TX. 7.1.5, TX. 7.1.6.

Kane JM, Weinhold P, Kinon B, et al: Prevalence of abnormal involuntary movements ("spontaneous dyskinesia") in the normal elderly. Psychopharmacology 77:105–108, 1982

Klawans HL, Barr A: Prevalence of spontaneous lingual-facial-buccal dyskinesia in the elderly. Neurology 32:558–559, 1982

Klein J, Onek J, Macbeth J: Seminar on Law in the Practice of Psychiatry. Washington, DC, Onek, Klein and Farr, 1983

Krouner LW: Shock therapy and psychiatric malpractice: the legal accommodation to a controversial treatment. J Forensic Sci 20:404–415, 1975

Kuder A: Legal alert: treatment and consent. Washington Psychiatric Society Newsletter, Summer 1986, pp 8–9

LaPuma J, Orentlicher D, Moss RJ: Advance directives on admission: clinical implications and analysis of the Patient Self-Determination Act of 1990. JAMA 266:402–405, 1991

Lazarus JA, Sharfstein SS: Changes in the economics and ethics of health and mental health care, in American Psychiatric Press Review of Psychiatry, Vol 13. Edited by Oldham JM, Riba MB. Washington, DC, American Psychiatric Press, 1994, pp 389–413

Leong GB, Eth S, Silva JA: The psychotherapist as witness for the prosecution: the criminalization of Tarasoff. Am J Psychiatry 149:1011–1015, 1992

Levinson W, Roter DL, Mullooly JP, et al: Physician–patient communication: the relationship with malpractice claims among primary care physicians and surgeons. JAMA 227:553–559, 1997

Lewis DO, Pincus JH, Feldman M, et al: Psychiatric, neurological, and psychoeducational characteristics of 15 death row inmates in the United States. Am J Psychiatry 143:838–845, 1986

Link BG, Stueve A: Psychotic symptoms and the violent/illegal behavior of mental patients compared to community controls, in Violence and Mental Disorder: Developments in Risk Assessment. Edited by Monahan J, Steadman H. Chicago, IL, University of Chicago Press, 1994, pp 137–159

Lohr JB, Wisinewski A, Jeste DV: Neurological aspects of tardive dyskinesia, in Handbook of Schizophrenia, Vol 1: Neurology of Schizophrenia. Edited by Nasrallah H, Weinberger DR. Amsterdam, The Netherlands, Elsevier, 1986, pp 97–119

Low P, Jeffries J, Bonnie R: Criminal Law: Cases and Materials. Mineola, NY, The Foundation Press, 1982, pp 152–154

The MacArthur Violence Risk Assessment Study. American Psychology Law Society News 16:3, 1996, pp 1–4

Malcolm JG: Informed consent in the practice of psychiatry, in American Psychiatric Press Review of Clinical Psychiatry and the Law, Vol 3. Edited by Simon RI. Washington, DC, American Psychiatric Press, 1992, pp 223–281

Marcus R: Court rules "right to die" depends on patient's intent. Washington Post, June 26, 1990, p A1, 8

Maris RW, Berman AL, Maltsberger JT, et al: Assessment and Prediction of Suicide. New York, Guilford, 1992

McGarry AL: Pathological gambling: a new insanity defense. Bull Am Acad Psychiatry Law 11:301–308, 1983

Melton GB, Petrila J, Poythress NG, et al: Psychological Evaluations for the Courts: A Handbook for Mental Health Professionals and Lawyers. New York, Guilford, 1987

Melton GB, Petrila J, Poythress NG, et al: Psychological Evaluations for the Courts: A Handbook for Mental Health Professionals and Lawyers, 2nd Edition. New York, Guilford, 1997

Meyer DJ, Simon RI: Split treatment: clarity between psychiatrists and psychotherapists. Psychiatr Ann 29:241–245, and 29:327–332, 1999

Mill JS: On liberty, in The World in Literature. Atlanta, GA, Scott, Foresman and Company, 1951, pp 316–333

Mishkin B: Decisions in Hospice. Arlington, VA, The National Hospice Organization, 1985

Mishkin B: Determining the capacity for making health care decisions, in Issues in Geriatric Psychiatry (Advances in Psychosomatic Medicine, Vol 19). Edited by Billig N, Rabins PV. Basel, Switzerland, S Karger, 1989, pp 151–166

Monahan J, Steadman H (eds): Violence and Mental Disorder: Developments in Risk Assessment. Chicago, IL, University of Chicago Press, 1994

The National Practitioner Data Bank and MCOs, in Psychiatric Practice and Managed Care, Vol 5, No 5. Washington, DC, American Psychiatric Association, Sept 1999, pp 1, 9–10

Nemeroff CB: An ever-increasing pharmacopoeia for the management of patients with bipolar disorder. J Clin Psychiatry 61(suppl 13):19–25, 2000

O'Connell RA: A review of the use of electroconvulsive therapy. Hosp Community Psychiatry 33:469–473, 1982

Orentlicher D: The illusion of patient choice in end-of-life decisions. JAMA 267:2101–2104, 1992

Overman W Jr, Stoudemire A: Guidelines for legal and financial counseling of Alzheimer's disease patients and their families. Am J Psychiatry 145:1495–1500, 1988

Parry BL, Berga SL: Neuroendocrine correlates of behavior during the menstrual cycle, in Psychiatry, Vol 3. Edited by Cavenar JO. Philadelphia, PA, JB Lippincott, 1991, pp 1–22

Perlin ML: Mental Disability Law: Civil and Criminal, Vol 3. Charlottesville, VA, Michie, 1989

Perr IN: Liability and electroshock therapy. J Forensic Sci 25:508–513, 1980

Perr IN: The clinical considerations of medication refusal. Legal Aspects of Psychiatric Practice 1:5–8, 1984

Pétursson H, Gudjónsson GH: Psychiatric aspects of homicide. Acta Psychiatr Scand 64:363–372, 1981

President's Commission for the Study of Ethical Problems in Medicine and Biomedical and Behavioral Research: Making Health Care Decisions, Vol 1: A Report on the Ethical and Legal Implications of Informed Consent in the Patient–Practitioner Relationship. Washington, DC, U.S. Government Printing Office, October 1982

Regan M: Protective services for the elderly: commitment, guardianship, and alternatives. William and Mary Law Review 13:569–573, 1972

Reich J, Wells J: Psychiatric diagnosis and competency to stand trial. Compr Psychiatry 26:421–432, 1985

Robertson ED: Is "substituted judgment" a valid legal concept? Issues Law Medicine 5:197–214, 1989

Robertson JD: The trial of a suicide case, in American Psychiatric Press Review of Clinical Psychiatry and the Law, Vol 2. Edited by Simon RI. Washington, DC, American Psychiatric Press, 1991, pp 423–441

Rosenthal RJ, Lorenz VC: The pathological gambler as criminal offender: comments on the evaluation and treatment. Psychiatr Clin North Am 15:647–660, 1992

Roth LH: Informed consent and its applicability for psychiatry, in Psychiatry, Vol 3. Edited by Cavenar JO. Philadelphia, PA, JB Lippincott, 1985, pp 1–17

Rutter P: Sex in the Forbidden Zone: When Therapists, Doctors, Clergy, Teachers and Other Men in Power Betray Women's Trust. Los Angeles, CA, JP Tarcher, 1989

Sale B, Powell DM, Van Duizend R: Disabled Persons and the Law: State Legislative Issues. 1982, p 461

Schoener GR, Milgrom JH, Gonsiorek JC, et al: Psychotherapists' Sexual Involvement With Clients. Minneapolis, MN, Walk-In Counseling Center, 1989

Schreiber J, Roesch R, Golding S: An evaluation of procedures for assessing competency to stand trial. Bull Am Acad Psychiatry Law 155:187–203, 1987

Sederer LI, Ellison J, Keyes C: Guidelines for prescribing psychiatrists in consultative, collaborative, and supervisory relationships. Psychiatr Serv 49:1197–1202, 1998

Simon RI: The psychiatrist as a fiduciary: avoiding the double agent role. Psychiatr Ann 17:622–626, 1987

Simon RI: Sexual exploitation of patients: how it begins before it happens. Psychiatr Ann 19:104–112, 1989

Simon RI: Psychological injury caused by boundary violation precursors to therapist–patient sex. Psychiatr Ann 21:614–619, 1991

Simon RI: Clinical Psychiatry and the Law, 2nd Edition. Washington, DC, American Psychiatric Press, 1992a

Simon RI: Clinical risk management of suicidal patients: assessing the unpredictable, in American Psychiatric Press Review of Clinical Psychiatry and the Law, Vol 3. Edited by Simon RI. Washington, DC, American Psychiatric Press, 1992b, pp 3–63

Simon RI: Treatment boundary violations: clinical, ethical, and legal considerations. Bull Am Acad Psychiatry Law 20:269–288, 1992c

Simon RI: Innovative Psychiatric Therapies and Legal Uncertainty: A Survival Guide for Clinicians. Psychiatr Ann 23:473–479, 1993

Simon RI: Treatment boundaries in psychiatric practice, in Forensic Psychiatry: A Comprehensive Textbook. Edited by Rosner R. New York, Van Nostrand Reinhold, 1994

Simon RI (ed): Posttraumatic Stress Disorder in Litigation: Guidelines for Forensic Assessment. Washington, DC, American Psychiatric Press, 1995

Simon RI: The credible forensic psychiatric evaluation in sexual harassment litigation. Psychiatr Ann 26:139–148, 1996

Simon RI: Clinical Risk Management of the Rapid Cycling Bipolar Patient. Harv Rev Psychiatry 4:245–254, 1997

Simon RI: Psychiatrists awake! Suicide risk assessments are all about a good night's sleep. Psychiatr Ann 28:479–485, 1998a

Simon RI: Psychiatrists' duties in discharging sicker and potentially violent patients in the managed care era. Psychiatr Serv 49:62–67, 1998b

Simon RI: The suicide prevention contract: clinical, legal and risk management issues. J Am Acad Psychiatry Law 27:445–450, 1999

Simon RI: Taking the 'sue' out of suicide: a forensic psychiatrist's perspective. Psychiatr Ann 30:399–407, 2000

Simon RI: Concise Guide to Psychiatry and the Law for Clinicians, 3rd Edition. Washington, DC, American Psychiatric Press, 2001

Simon RI, Wettstein RM: Toward the development of guidelines for the conduct of forensic psychiatric examinations. Journal of American Psychiatry Law 25:17–30, 1997

Slovenko R: Commentaries on psychiatry and law: "guilty but mentally ill." Journal of Psychiatry and Law 10:541–555, 1982

Slovenko R: Assessing competency to stand trial. Psychiatr Ann 26:392–393, 397, 1995

Slovenko R: Psychotherapy And Confidentiality: Testimonial Privileged Communication, Breach of Confidentiality, and Reporting Duties. Springfield, IL, Charles C Thomas, 1998

Smith JT: Medical Malpractice: Psychiatric Care, Colorado Springs, CO, Shepard's/McGraw-Hill, 1986

Solnick PB: Proxy consent for incompetent nonterminally ill adult patients. J Leg Med 6:1–49, 1985

Sparr LF: Legal aspects of posttraumatic stress disorder: uses and abuses, in Posttraumatic Stress Disorder: Etiology, Phenomenology, and Treatment. Edited by Wolf ME, Mosnaim AD. Washington, DC, American Psychiatric Press, 1990, pp 22–34

Stone AA: Posttraumatic stress disorder and the law: critical review of the new frontier. Bull Am Acad Psychiatry Law 21:23–36, 1993

Strasburger LH: "Crudely, without any finesse": the defendant hears his psychiatric evaluation. Bull Am Acad Psychiatry Law 15:229–233, 1987

Strasburger LH, Jorgenson L, Randles R: Criminalization of psychotherapist–patient sex. Am J Psychiatry 148:859–863, 1991

Strasburger LH, Gutheil TG, Brodsky A: On wearing two hats: role conflict in serving as both psychotherapist and expert witness. Am J Psychiatry 154:448–456, 1997

Strub RL, Black FW: The Mental Status Examination in Neurology, 2nd Edition. Philadelphia, PA, FA Davis, 1985

Tardiff K: Concise Guide to Assessment and Management of Violent Patients, 2nd Edition. Washington, DC, American Psychiatric Press, 1989

Tischler GL: Utilization management of mental health services by private third parties. Am J Psychiatry 147:967–973, 1990

Tranel D: Functional neuroanatomy: neuropsychological correlates of cortical and subcortical damage, in The American Psychiatric Press Textbook of Neuropsychiatry, 2nd Edition. Edited by Yudofsky SC, Hales RE. Washington, DC, American Psychiatric Press, 1992, pp 70–75

U.S. Department of Health and Human Services: The Legal Status of Adolescents 1980. Washington, DC, U.S. Department of Health and Human Services, 1981

U.S. Department of Health and Human Services: Medicare and Medicaid Programs; Hospital Conditions of Participation: Patient's Rights; Interim Final Rule. Federal Register. July 2, 1999, pp 36069–36089

Walzer RS: Impaired physicians: an overview and update of legal issues. J Leg Med 11:131–198, 1990

Weiner RD: The psychiatric use of electrically induced seizures. Am J Psychiatry 136:1507–1517, 1979

Weir RF, Gostin L: Decisions to abate life-sustaining treatment for nonautonomous patients: ethical standards and legal liability for physicians after Cruzan. JAMA 264:1846–1853, 1990

Why Are Liability Premiums Rising? Psychiatric News, June 21, 1996, pp 1, 24–25

Wickizer TM, Lessler D, Travis KM: Controlling inpatient psychiatric utilization through managed care. Am J Psychiatry 153:339–345, 1996

Widiger TA, Trull TJ: Personality disorders and violence, in Violence and Mental Disorder: Developments in Risk Assessment. Edited by Monahan J, Steadman H. Chicago, IL, University of Chicago Press, 1994, pp 203–226

Woodward B, Duckworth K, Gutheil TG: The Pharmacotherapist–Psychotherapist Collaboration, in Annual Review of Psychiatry, Vol 12. Edited by Oldham J. Washington, DC, American Psychiatric Press, 1993

Yudofsky SC, Silver JM, Schneider SE: Pharmacologic treatment of aggression. Psychiatr Ann 17:397–407, 1987

Zeldow PB, Taub HA: Evaluating psychiatric discharge and aftercare in a VA medical center. Hosp Community Psychiatry 32:57–58, 1981

Zito JM, Lentz SL, Routt WW, et al: The treatment review panel: a solution to treatment refusal? Bull Am Acad Psychiatry Law 12:349–358, 1984

Legal Citations

Aponte v. United States, 582 FSupp 555, 566–69 (D PR 1984)

Bartling v. Superior Court, 163 Cal App 3d 186, 209 Cal Rptr 220 (1984)

Bethea v. United States, 365 A2d 64 (DC 1976), cert denied, 433 US 911 (1977)

Blanchard v. Levine, No D 014550 Fulton Cty Super Ct (Ga 1985)

Bouvia v. Superior Court, 179 Cal App 3d 1127, 225 Cal Rptr 297 (1986)

Callan v. Norland, 114 Ill App 3d 196, 448 NE2d 651 (1983)

Canterbury v. Spence, 464 F2d 772 (DC Cir), cert denied, Spence v. Canterbury, 409 US 1064 (1972)

Chaires v. St John's Episcopal Hospital, No 808/75 NY Cty Sup Ct (NY Feb 21, 1984)

Clifford v. United States, No 82–5002 USDC (SD 1985)

Clites v. State, 322 NW2d 917 (Iowa Ct App 1982)

42 Code of Federal Regulations 482.13 (f)3 (II) (C) 1999

Commonwealth v. Robinson, 494 Pa 372, 431 A2d 901 (1981)

Cruzan v. Director, Missouri Dept of Health, 497 U.S. 261 (1990)

Doerr v. Hurley Medical Center, No 82–674–39 NM Mich Aug (1984)

Dovido v. Vasquez, No 84–674 CA(L)(H) 15th Jud Dist Cir Ct, Palm Beach Cty (Fl Apr 4, 1986)

Dusky v. United States, 362 U.S. 402 (1960)

Eighth Amendment and the execution of the presently incompetent. Stanford Law Review 32:765, 1980

Evans v. United States, 883 FSupp 124 (5D Miss 1995)

Fain v. Commonwealth, 78 Ky 183 (1879)

Ford v. Wainwright, 477 US 399 (1986)

Frasier v. Department of Health and Human Resources, 500 So 2d 858, 864 (La Ct App 1986)

Garamella for Estate of Almonte v. New York Medical College, 23 F Supp 2d 167 (D Conn 1998)

Gary v. Gary, 631 SW2d 781 (Tex Ct App 1982)

Gowan v. United States, 601 FSupp 1297 (D Or 1985)

Green v. Ross, 691 So2d 542 (Fla App 1997)

Guidelines on Discrimination Because of Sex, 29 C.F.R. § 1604.11

Gulf S I R Co. v. Sullivan, 155 Miss 1, 119 So 501 (1928)

Harris v. Forklift Systems, 510 U.S. 17 (1993)

Health Care Quality Improvement Act of 1986, 42 U.S.C. 11101 (Supp v. 1987)

H M Advocate v. Fraser, 4 Couper 70 (1878)

Holton v. Pfingst, 534 SW2d 786, 789 (Ky 1976)

Howe v. Citizens Memorial Hospital, 426 SW2d 882 (Tex Civ App 1968), rev'd, 436 SW2d 115 (Tex 1968)

Hyde v. University of Michigan Board of Regents, 426 Mich 223, 393 NW2d 847 (1986), revised in accord with Ross v Consumer Power Company, 420 Mich 567, 363 NW2d 641 (1986)

Ill Ann Stat 1990

In re Boyer, 636 P2d 1085, 1089 (Utah 1981)

In re Conroy, 98 NJ 321, 486 A2d 1209, 1222–23 (1985)

In re Farrell, 108 NJ 335, 529 A2d 404 (1987)

In the Guardianship of John Roe, 411 MA 666 (1992)

In re Jobes, 108 NJ 365, 529 A2d 434 (1987a)

In re Jobes, 108 NJ 394 (1987b)

In re Peter, 108 NJ 365, 529 A2d 419 (1987)

In re Quinlin, 70 NJ 10, 355 A2d 647, cert denied, 429 US 922 (1976)

Jaffe v. Redmond, U.S. Lexis 3879 (1996)

Jehovah's Witnesses v. King County Hospital, 278 FSupp 488 (WD Wash 1967), affd, 390 US 598 (1968)

JS v. RT, 714 A2d 924 (NJ 1998)

Karasik v. Bird, 98 AD2d 359, 470 NYS2d 605 (1984)

Kilgore v. County of Santa Clara, No 397–525 (Santa Clara Cty Super Ct Cal 1982)

Meek v. City of Loveland, 85 Colo 346, 276 P 30 (1929)

Mental Aberration and Post Conviction Sanctions, 15 Suffolk UL Rev: 1219 (1981)

Minn Stat Ann 148 A.02 (West 1989)

M'Naughten's Case, 10 Cl F 200, 8 Eng Rep 718 (HL 1843)

Moran v. Botsford General Hospital, No l 81–225–533, Wayne Cty Cir Ct (MI Oct 1, 1984)

Natanson v. Kline, 186 Kan 393, 350 P2d 1093 (1960)

Neely v. United States, 150 F2d 977 (DC Cir), cert denied, 326 US 768 (1945)

P.L. 98–473, 1984

Parham v. JR, 442 US 584 (1979)

People v. Rose, 573 NW 2d 765 (Neb 1998)

People v. White, 117 Cal App 3d 270, 172 Cal Rptr 612 (1981)

Planned Parenthood v. Danforth, 428 US 52, 74 (1976)

Radank v. Heyl, No F4–2316 Wisc Comp Bd (1986)

Ramon v. Farr, 770 P2d 131 (Utah 1989)

Rennie v. Klein, 462 FSupp 1131 (D NJ 1978), remanded, 476 FSupp 1294 (D NJ 1979), affd in part, modified in part and remanded, 653 F2d 836 (3d Cir 1980), vacated and remanded, 458 U.S. 1119 (1982), 720 F2d 266 (3rd Cir 1983)

Restatement [second] of Torts 315(a) [1965]

Rivera v. NYC Health and Hospitals, Reversed, 72 NY2d 1021; 531 N.E.2d 644 (1988)

Rogers v. Commissioner of Dept of Mental Health, 390 Mass 489, 458 NE2d 308 (Mass 1983)

Scaria v. St Paul Fire and Marine Ins Co, 68 Wis 2d 1, 227 NW2d 647 (1975)

Schloendorff v. Society of New York Hospital, 211 NY 125, 105 NE 92 (1914), overruled, Bing v. Thunig, 2 NY2d 656, 143 NE2d 3, 163 NYS2d 3 (1957)

Shaughnessy v. Spray, Reversed and remanded, 55 ORE. App 42; 637 P2d 182 (1983)

Speer v. United States, 512 FSupp 670 (ND Tex 1981), affd, Speer v. United States, 675 F2d 100 (5th Cir 1982)

State v. Hehman, 110 Ariz 459, 520 P2d 507 (1974)

Stone v. Proctor, 259 NC 633, 131 SE2d 297 (1963)

Tarasoff v. Regents of the University of California, 17 Cal 3d 425, 551 P2d 334, 131 Cal Rptr 14 (1976)

Texas Fam Code Ann § 14.08 (C)(I)[Vernon 1990]

Thapar v. Zezulka 944 SW2d 635 (Tx 1999)

Touchette v. Ganal, 922 P2d 347 (Haw 1996)

Truman v. Thomas, 27 Cal 3d 285, 611 P2d 902, 165 Cal Rptr 308 (1980)

Tune v. Walter Reed Army Medical Hospital, 602 FSupp 1452 (DDC 1985)

ULA 1974

Union Pacific Ry Co v. Botsford, 141 US 250, 251 (1891)

United States v. Brawner, 471 F2d 969 (DC Cir 1972), superseded by statute, see Shannon v. United States, 512 U.S. 573 (1994)

United States v. David, 511 F2d 355 (DC Cir 1975)

Wilson v. Lehman, 379 SW2d 478,479 (Ky 1964)

Wilson v. United States, 391 F2d 460, 463 (DC Cir 1968)

Witherell v. Weimer, 148 Ill App 3d 32, 499 NE2d 46 (1986), rev'd on other grounds, 118 Ill 2d 515 NE2d 68 (1987)

Wright v. State, No 83–5035 Orleans Parish Civ Dist Ct (LA April 1986)

Youngberg v. Romeo (457 U.S. 307) (1982), on remand, Romeo v. Youngberg, 687 F2d 33 (3rd Cir 1982)

Suggested Readings in Forensic Psychiatry

Alexander GJ, Scheflin AW: Law and Mental Disorder. Durham, NC, Carolina Academic Press, 1998

American Psychiatric Association: The Principles of Medical Ethics, With Annotations Especially Applicable to Psychiatry. Washington, DC, American Psychiatric Association, 1998

Appelbaum PS: Almost a Revolution: Mental Health Law and the Limits of Change. New York, Oxford University Press, 1994

Appelbaum PS, Gutheil TG: Clinical Handbook of Psychiatry and the Law, 3rd Edition. Baltimore, MD, Lippincott, Williams & Wilkins, 2000

Appelbaum PS, Lidz CW, Meisel A: Informed Consent: Legal Theory and Clinical Practice. New York, Oxford University Press, 1987

Appelbaum PS, Uyehara L, Elin M (eds): Trauma and Memory: Clinical and Legal Controversies. New York, Oxford University Press, 1997

Beck JC (ed): Confidentiality Versus the Duty to Protect: Foreseeable Harm in the Practice of Psychiatry. Washington, DC, American Psychiatric Press, 1990

Blumenthal SJ, Kupfer DJ (eds): Suicide Over the Life Cycle: Risk Factors, Assessment, and Treatment of Suicidal Patients. Washington, DC, American Psychiatric Press, 1990

Chiles JH, Strohsall K: The Suicidal Patient: Principles of Assessment, Treatment and Case Management. Washington, DC, American Psychiatric Press, 1995

Dyer AR: Ethics and Psychiatry: Toward Professional Definition. Washington, DC, American Psychiatric Press, 1988

Gabbard GO (ed): Sexual Exploitation in Professional Relationships. Washington, DC, American Psychiatric Press, 1989

Gutheil TG: The Psychiatrist as Expert Witness. Washington, DC, American Psychiatric Press, 1998

Gutheil TG: The Psychiatrist in Court: A Survival Guide. Washington, DC, American Psychiatric Press, 1998

Gutheil TG, Simon RI: The Psychiatric Expert Witness: Advanced Strategies for Forensic Practice. Washington, DC, American Psychiatric Publishing, 2002

Herbert PB, Young KA: Tarasoff at twenty-five. J Am Acad Psychiatry Law 30:275–281, 2002

Lifson LE, Simon RI: The Mental Health Practitioner and the Law. Cambridge, MA, Harvard University Press, 1998

Maris RW, Berman AL, Maltsberger JT, et al: Assessment and Prediction of Suicide. New York, Guilford, 1992

Melton GB, Petrila NG, et al: Psychological Evaluations for the Courts: A Handbook for Mental Health Practitioners and Lawyers, 2nd Edition. New York, Guilford, 1997

Monahan J, Steadman H (eds): Violence and Mental Disorder: Developments in Risk Assessment. Chicago, IL, University of Chicago Press, 1994

Monahan J. Steadman HJ, Silver E, et al: Rethinking Risk Assessment: The MacArthur Study of Mental Disorder and Violence. New York, Oxford, 2001

Pope KS: Sexual Involvement With Therapist: Patient Assessment, Subsequent Therapy, Forensics. Washington, DC, American Psychological Association, 1994

Pope KS, Brown LS: Recovered Memories of Abuse: Assessment, Therapy, Forensics. Washington, DC, American Psychological Association, 1996

Practice Guideline: Forensic Psychiatric evaluation of defendants raising the insanity defense. J Am Acad Psychiatry Law 30(suppl):3–40, 2002

Rosner R (ed): Principles and Practice of Forensic Psychiatry. New York, Chapman and Hall, 1994

Schoener GR, Milgrom JH, Gonsiorek JC, et al: Psychotherapists' Sexual Involvement With Clients. Minneapolis, MN, Walk-In Counseling Center, 1989

Shafii M, Shafii SL (eds): School Violence: Assessment, Management, Prevention. Washington, DC, American Psychiatric Publishing, 2001

Shrier DK (ed): Sexual Harassment in the Workplace and Academia. Washington, DC, American Psychiatric Press, 1996

Simon RI: Concise Guide to Psychiatry and Law for Clinicians, 3rd Edition. Washington, DC, American Psychiatric Publishing, 2001

Simon RI, Shuman DW: Retrospective Assessment of Mental States in Litigation: Predicting the Past. Washington, DC, American Psychiatric Publishing, 2002

Simon RI: Posttraumatic Stress Disorder in Litigation, 2nd Edition. Washington, DC, American Psychiatric Publishing, 2003

Slovenko R: Psychiatry and Criminal Culpability. New York, Wiley, 1995

Slovenko R: Psychotherapy and Confidentiality. Springfield, IL, Charles C Thomas, 1998

Tardiff K: Concise Guide to Assessment and Management of Violent Patients. Washington, DC, American Psychiatric Press, 1996

CHAPTER 40

Ethics and Psychiatry

Allen R. Dyer, M.D., Ph.D.

Merry N. Miller, M.D.

Ethics is born in conflict. People turn to ethics in the hope of resolving conflict when values clash. Ethics is often used to justify one's own position. Often a decision maker appeals to ethics to resolve a dilemma when torn between alternatives. Some have suggested that one of the roles of ethicists in medical centers is to justify the high technology used to control people's lives—or to call medical practices into question. Others—perhaps those made most uncomfortable by the feelings associated with conflict—hope that rational analysis will solve problems that might otherwise lead to heated emotions. At its best, ethics—like psychotherapy—offers insight into conflict, a clarification of competing motives, drives, and values. At its best, ethics offers insight into the mind and the culture.

Ethics is at the center of human experience. Because it is concerned with what is right and what is wrong, the term *ethics* is often used synonymously with the term *morality*. Sometimes, however, a distinction is made between *ethics*, the systematic approach to understanding right and wrong, and *morality*, the forces that govern right conduct. Ethics is a fundamental aspect of human identity and of one person's relationships with others. It touches on the political, social, psychological, spiritual, and even biological aspects of human existence. In a time of cultural change, the appeal to ethics becomes an important aspect of both civic life and self-understanding. For the professions, psychiatry among them, ethical codes and ethical traditions are important in defining the norms of professional conduct and even in defining what it means for a profession to be a profession. Insofar as

ethics deals with intellectual attempts to understand right and wrong (reason), as well as the affective impact of struggling with moral issues (emotion), psychiatric thinking offers an important perspective on ethics. This chapter deals with both ethics in psychiatry and psychiatry's contributions to ethics.

A Brief History of Medical Ethics

The ethical traditions of the medical profession in Western thought go back some 2,500 years to the fourth century B.C. and the writings of a Pythagorean cult, which have come to be known as the *Hippocratic corpus*.[1] The Oath of Hippocrates, sworn by a band of healer-craftsmen, has come to symbolize the ethical ideals of the medical profession. The Hippocratic oath was not in widespread use until the 19th century, when first the British Medical Association and subsequently the American Medical Association (AMA) and professional organizations in other countries began to adopt formal codes of ethics. These codes of ethics were modeled on the principles first articulated in the Hippocratic body of writings, most notably the principle of patient benefit. Throughout most of the history of medicine, this paternalistic emphasis on patient benefit has been the central tenet of medical ethics, as indicated in Table 40–1.

By the mid-1960s a number of factors in medicine and society had converged in a way that began to change the values underlying the doctor–patient relationship. Most notable was the emergence of new technologies

---

[1]Confucian writings from about the same period in China espouse similar ethical principles, humaneness, compassion, and filial piety.

TABLE 40–1. Brief history of medical ethics

4th century B.C.–1965	Age of medical paternalism
1965–1982	Age of patient autonomy
1982–?	Age of bureaucratic regulation
Twenty-first century–?	Age of partnership and community

that began to change the way people thought about medicine and even what it meant to be human: genetic engineering, organ transplantation, advanced life support, safe abortion and birth control, and medical and surgical treatments based on clinical research. No longer was medical care primarily palliative. No longer could it be assumed that the patient necessarily wanted what the doctor might offer (Dyer 1997b).

Also in this era, several social movements began to change the way society thought about assumed relationships. The civil rights movement, which was about much more than race (landmark: Civil Rights Act of 1964), the women's movement, and the consumer movement all began to place emphasis on the right of the autonomous person to self-determination. Informed consent came to be the key to medical ethics and medical decision making. Autonomy came to be the ethical principle that guided thinking about medical decision making. *Medical ethics* became *bioethics* in this era as it came to be realized that the decisions in medicine were not just decisions faced by doctors but decisions in which society had a stake.

By the 1970s, economics increasingly became a part of thinking about ethics. Benefits were often seen in economic terms, and ethical issues were often translated into economic terms. Allocation of resources became a concern, and the question was often asked, "Can health costs be contained without rationing care?" No longer were the decisions of doctors and patients the only thing to be considered. Society's interests (especially economic interests) became a greater concern. The principle of justice eventually superseded beneficence and autonomy in ethical discourse, and justice was discussed as fair distribution of medical resources (Table 40–2).

In 1975 the Supreme Court rendered a decision, *Goldfarb v. Virginia State Bar Association*, that changed the way professions were to be considered and regulated. *Goldfarb* ended the "learned professions exemption" under the Sherman Antitrust Act. Before 1975 it was held that the Sherman Act applied only to businesses or trades and that learned professions were exempt. Mr. Goldfarb, an attorney himself, sued the Virginia bar because he found that all attorneys in Fairfax County, where he wanted to buy a house, were charging the same fees to conduct a title search. He contended that this was restraint of trade, and the Supreme Court agreed with him.

Not long after the *Goldfarb* decision was announced, the Federal Trade Commission (FTC) sued the AMA, holding that the AMA was in restraint of trade because its code of ethics prohibited advertising. This case was decided by the Supreme Court in 1982 in favor of the FTC, thereby ending any ban on professional advertising and furthermore requiring the AMA to get approval from the FTC for any subsequent additions to its code of ethics (Greenhouse 1982). Medicine in effect ceased to be a profession—at least in the traditional sense of an autonomous association self-regulated by a code of ethics—and became a trade (Table 40–3).

The Ethics of Advertising

Professional organizations such as the AMA can no longer formally constrain physicians from advertising; however, most physicians are not inclined to seek patients though advertising. Health care organizations, however, which employ physicians, may make their appeal through advertising, especially in a market-driven health care economy. The 1957 version of the AMA principles in effect at the time of the Federal Trade Commission suit prohibited "solicitation" of patients, by which was meant "obtaining patients by deception," or making false claims (American Medical Association 1957). The interest of the FTC was primarily in promoting competition and thereby lowering health costs. The FTC was also interested in regulating advertising by requiring that claims be measurable. For example, to claim that a mouthwash "killed germs by millions on contact," it would be necessary to demonstrate a method for measuring millions of killed germs. To claim a success rate, one would need to have both a measurable numerator and a measurable denominator.

Advertising has two basic goals: dissemination of information and product differentiation. For physicians, providing information about services offered and fees charged is consistent with patient benefit, but attempts to differentiate the product are suspect. Licensing, accrediting, and credentialing organizations assume the role of maintaining standards. Beyond the activities of individual practitioners, the larger ethical question for advertising concerns truthfulness. The barrage of advertising in the media says little about the products being sold; instead, products are identified with desirable images, appealing to and manipulating unconscious fantasies of sex, power, status, and pleasure. Much advertising is antithetical to professional goals of patient benefit.

TABLE 40–2. Evolution of ethical priorities

1950s–1960s	1970s–1980s	1990s
Beneficence	Autonomy	Justice
Autonomy	Beneficence	Autonomy
(Justice)	(Justice)	Beneficence

TABLE 40–3. Time line for professional ethics

4th century B.C.	Oath of Hippocrates
1804	Percival's *Medical Ethics* (a basis for British Medical Association and American Medical Association codes)
1847	American Medical Association founded
1895	Sherman Antitrust Act
1975	*Goldfarb* decision ends learned professions exemption
1975	*Federal Trade Commission v. American Medical Association*
1982	Supreme Court decides in favor of Federal Trade Commission

TABLE 40–4. A professional checklist

1. The professional is engaged in social service that is essential and unique.
2. The professional has developed a high degree of knowledge.
3. The professional has developed the ability to apply the special body of knowledge.
4. The professional is part of a group that is autonomous and claims the right to be self-regulating.
5. The professional recognizes and affirms a code of ethics.
6. The professional exhibits strong self-discipline and accepts personal responsibility for actions and decisions.
7. The professional's primary concern and commitment is to communal interest rather than merely to the self.
8. The professional is more concerned with services rendered than with financial rewards.

Source. Modified with permission from Campbell 1982.

Notable is the advertising of unhealthy products, especially alcohol and tobacco, often providing no information but associating the products with strong men, liberated women, and cool teenagers. One of the problems open markets always have to contend with is dangerous drugs. To the extent that dangerous drugs are not regulated and tightly controlled, one is likely to find either commercial promotions or gangsterism—as was the case in the distribution of alcohol during Prohibition and of most other dangerous drugs currently (see Dyer 1985a, 1995, 1997a).

The Place of Ethics in the Definition of a Profession

What makes a profession a profession instead of a trade? What makes medicine a profession? Are medicine (and psychiatry) better considered professions or technologies? Clearly medicine has aspects of business, but medicine should be more than a business. If so, what are the essential characteristics of a profession? The emphasis on the commerce of technology in medicine in recent years may obscure the centrality of an ethical attitude toward the patient that has traditionally been considered the defining feature of a professional life (Table 40–4).

A profession may be defined by its knowledge, technology, and expertise or by its ethics and values. The habits of modern thought might lead one to believe that this is an either/or choice. Clearly for psychiatry, as for most of medicine, technology has become important and perhaps even central in some people's minds. Medicine is usually understood to mean *allopathic* treatment. Drugs and procedures are technologies of choice. The recent primary care thrust has reopened consideration of medicine as a more holistic approach to healing. Talking (communication) again has become a recognized part of healing. Ethics is more fundamental to professional definition than is technology. Technology is useful as long as it serves ethical ends but not as an end in itself. It might be better to recognize that knowledge, technology, and expertise are not merely commodities to be bartered in the marketplace but skills that may be used to ethical ends. Medical technology falls under the purview of professional values.

Ethics is central to professional life. All aspects of professional development involve ethics. Entry into the profession—usually through admission to professional school—involves ethics, at least implicitly, in that candidates are chosen who have demonstrated a work ethic in achieving good grades. Perhaps ethics is involved explicitly as well in attempts to select candidates of character, who reflect the values of the profession. Ethics may be a formal part of the curriculum, but its role is more implicit in the socialization to the norms of the profession. Finally, ethics is involved in professional discipline, which may result in exit (expulsion) from the profession for members who violate the codes of ethics.

The Hippocratic Oath and the Hippocratic Tradition

If one accepts the view that medicine is a profession defined by its ethics, one must make some attempt to articulate those ethics. Although much of a profession's ethics is implicit—the rules of a culture learned by living in it—professional organizations all have formal codes of ethics. Most professional codes of ethics are derived in some way from the Hippocratic oath, which serves as a paradigm code for the organization of a profession. For the medical profession, the Hippocratic oath also serves as a symbol of the profession's ongoing identification with an ethical outlook toward the patient (Figure 40–1).

The Hippocratic oath is a remarkable document, not so much because it answers the ethical questions posed by modern medicine, but because it frames those questions. It is often said that the oath is anachronistic and offers little useful guidance to the modern physician. People who hold this view might expect the oath to function as an administrative list of rules. The oath does indeed offer little to those with such expectations. The oath is much more useful in defining the ends or goals of medicine. It articulates principles, most notably the principle of patient benefit, which is helpful to physicians sorting out where their allegiances lie. Taken together with its corollary, the principle of nonmaleficence (*primum non nocere*—first, do no harm), the principle of beneficence puts the patient at the center of ethical decision making. At a time when many other considerations (especially economic ones) lay claim to the physician's allegiance, the greatest liability of the Hippocratic oath ironically may be its greatest asset, namely its antiquity. The Hippocratic oath provides an ethical perspective that calls into question many of the assumptions of modern culture. It provides a vantage point for an ethical perspective that transcends the pressures of political expediency.

The first paragraph of the oath introduces the idea of sacredness in its invocation of all the gods and goddesses. The oath is not just a list of rules, but a set of ideals that define the character of the healer. It is not just a promise, although it is that, but also a covenant with whatever is held sacred.

In the second paragraph are the origins of what has come to be understood as the professional organization of physician-healers. The profession is organized around its

OATH OF HIPPOCRATES

1. I SWEAR BY Apollo Physician and Asclepius and Hygieia and Panaceia and all the gods and goddesses, making them my witnesses, that I will fulfill according to my ability and judgment this oath and this covenant:
2. To hold him who has taught me this art as equal to my parents and to live my life in partnership with him, and if he is in need of money to give him a share of mine, and to regard his offspring as equal to my brothers in male lineage and to teach them this art—if they desire to learn it—without fee and covenant; to give a share of precepts and oral instruction and all the other learning to my sons and to the sons of him who has instructed me and to pupils who have signed the covenant and have taken an oath according to the medical law, but to no one else.
3. I will apply dietetic measure for the benefit of the sick according to my ability and judgment; I will keep them from harm and injustice.
4. I will neither give a deadly drug to anybody if asked for it, nor will I make a suggestion to this effect. Similarly I will not give to a woman an abortive remedy. In purity and holiness I will guard my life and my art.
5. I will not use the knife, not even on sufferers from the stone, but will withdraw in favor of such men as are engaged in this work.
6. Whatever houses I may visit, I will come for the benefit of the sick, remaining free of all intentional injustice, of all mischief and in particular of sexual relations with both female and male persons, be they free or slaves.
7. What I may see or hear in the course of the treatment or even outside of the treatment in regard to the life of men, which on no account one must spread abroad, I will keep to myself holding such things shameful to be spoken about.
8. If I fulfill this oath and do not violate it, may it be granted to me to enjoy life and art, being honored with fame among all men for all time to come; if I transgress it and swear falsely, may the opposite of all this be my lot.

FIGURE 40–1. Oath of Hippocrates.

Source. Edelstein L: "The Hippocratic Oath: Text, Translation, and Interpretation." *Bulletin of the History of Medicine* (Supplement 1), 1943.

teachers, and the relationship between teacher and student is like family, including the bonds of dependency. The oath is sometimes criticized as exclusionary (by those who view medicine as a commodity) for not making instruction available to everyone. Again, this may be more of a virtue than a shortcoming, for it makes "signing the covenant and taking an oath according to medical law" a requirement of receiving instruction. Entry into the profession requires a commitment to shared values.

The third paragraph provides the context for medical care. Medical care is viewed as primarily dietetic; the main thing the ancient physician had to offer was recommendations about proper diet. Pharmacy (giving drugs) is also mentioned as an acceptable activity of physicians. Cutting is considered an activity that should be left to those trained to do it (i.e., barbers), not an acceptable activity for the physician in Hippocratic times. Talking therapy is not mentioned explicitly in the oath, but therapy of the word (*logos*) was an implicit part of ancient medicine and healing (Laín Entralgo 1970). Doctor and patient related primarily through the medium of language. The patient-benefit principle is stressed here. The physician must strive "according to his ability and judgment" to keep his patients from harm and injustice. The tone is paternalistic; the physician is expected to behave as a benevolent father toward his patients as well as his students.

The fourth paragraph is controversial to modern ears; it requires the physician to forswear euthanasia and abortion. What is striking in this paragraph, seen in historical context, is the emergence of a unique kind of healer. Medicine, emerging from a shamanistic tradition, in which the medicine man might make someone better or worse for moral or social reasons, focuses solely on making people better. More precisely, the physician now focuses on helping the body heal itself through natural means. Anthropologist Margaret Mead noted that this was the first time in the history of the world that the power to heal was vested in a practitioner who was not also a shaman with the power to harm. According to Mead, the Hippocratic oath marked one of the turning points in human history: "For the first time in our tradition there was a complete separation between killing and curing. Throughout the primitive world the doctor and the sorcerer tended to be the same person. He with power to kill had power to cure, including and especially the undoing of his own killing activities. He who had power to cure would necessarily also be able to kill" (Levine 1972, pp. 324–325).

"With the Greeks," according to Mead, "the distinction was made clear. One profession, the followers of Aesculapius, were to be dedicated completely to life under all circumstances, regardless of rank, age, or intellect—the life of a slave, the life of the Emperor, the life of a foreign man, the life of a defective child." Mead observed that "[this] is a priceless possession which we cannot afford to tarnish. However, society is always attempting to make the physician into a killer—to kill the defective child at birth, to leave sleeping pills beside the bed of the cancer patient"—and Mead was convinced that "it is the duty of society to protect the physician from such requests" (Levine 1972, p. 324).

The fifth paragraph, on not using the knife, might also sound antiquated if read as a rule rather than as a principle. Should we understand that the Hippocratic oath does not apply to surgeons or that surgeons should not be considered part of the medical family? The historic meaning of not cutting on the stone is somewhat obscure. It probably refers to gallstones or kidney stones, which caused such great pain that could only be relieved by surgeries with risky outcomes, endangering not only the life of the patient but also the reputation of the practitioner. Some have suggested that cutting the stone refers to castrations, which were performed for nonmedical reasons and thus outside the purview of the Hippocratic physicians, who were known to perform surgery for healing purposes. The contemporary understanding of the principle underlying the admonition not to cut on the stone is that one should practice within the limits of one's competence, doing what one is trained to do. It is not necessary to foreswear surgery to appreciate this principle.

The sixth paragraph speaks to the conduct of physicians in the houses of the sick, introducing character, or virtue, in a way that was unique for the times. The physician was expected to follow forbearance, or restraint, in a way that was not expected of most citizens. The physician entered houses not just for a brief house call but for extended periods of time. He was an itinerant who lived in the household while he tended to the sick. He also advised on preventive measures. In ancient Greece it was common for the master of the house to offer slaves or free men or women or even his own children for sexual companionship as a gesture of hospitality. The oath defines a different relationship between the healer and those served, and the Hippocratic physician forswears such "mischief" and does so equally for males and females.

The seventh paragraph is the confidentiality paragraph. In the context of the oath, secrecy was part of a special relationship between the healer and those with whom he dealt. Spreading secrets is not only prohibited, it is "shameful." The constraint on the physician is not just externally imposed; it is part of self-awareness and self-identity.

The eighth paragraph links with the first to provide the frame for the promises made in the other paragraphs. The reward for following a life of forbearance and restraint is honor and fame, a reputation that defines who one is or how one is perceived. The result of following the code is a reputation for character or predictability, which reflects on the individual and the larger family (the profession as a whole).

The Contemporary Relevance of the Hippocratic Oath

A reading of the Hippocratic oath reveals many phrases that responsible physicians might not want to follow literally. Even in ancient Greece, the oath called the physician to standards of behavior that were not required of ordinary citizens and that might put the physician at odds with the larger society. Medicine was delineated as a higher calling, a covenant with the gods. The oath provided a relationship with a like-minded family of individuals who shared certain values and self-understanding. It defined the physician's life in a beneficial relationship to those served. Its paternalism was questioned when society emphasized individualistic autonomy, but the oath's emphasis on justice foreshadowed a larger concern for community interests.

A physician is a citizen, subject to cultural norms and political forces. The Hippocratic tradition has at various times and places served as an ethical reference, external to immediate expediency, by which physicians may gauge their behavior and to which they can appeal (or by which they may be judged by their colleagues). An extreme example of the lapse of ethical behavior is provided by the activities of Nazi physicians, but there are several other notable examples as well. The World Psychiatric Association has censured the practices of psychiatrists in the former Soviet Union and other Eastern European countries for the detention of political dissidents. Such mislabeling with psychiatric diagnoses, when the profession is used for ends other than patient benefit, is referred to as the "political abuse of psychiatry" (Bloch 1991; Bloch and Reddaway 1977). This is not just an abuse of patients, but also an abuse and misuse of the profession. Military governments in Latin America and elsewhere have used physicians to assist in torture. Medical societies organized as government agencies (rather than independent professional associations) have had difficulty enforcing sanctions against state-supported physician involvement in interrogations. The existence of such extreme abuses makes a case, which is not always appreciated, for autonomous professional organizations self-regulated by a code of ethics rather than serving the interests of political power. Society's interests, as represented by governments, are of necessity conflicted and caught up in striving for power or influence.

Less dramatic examples make a more subtle point. Physicians could be involved in capital punishment—they have the skills to perform lethal injections, and states would be willing to pay them—but such activities are outside the healing role. The forensic psychiatrist, in giving court testimony, does not have the same allegiance to a patient as a treating psychiatrist does. Analogous is the expectation that physicians will be agents of cost containment or rationing of health care. Physicians control much of health expenditures, and their interest should be primarily for patient benefit. The Hippocratic oath is an ever-present reminder that acting in the interest of someone other than the patient creates a conflict, which is often experienced internally by the physician.

Honor in Medicine

The Hippocratic oath speaks of honor, holiness, and purity. All these higher virtues allude to the character, ethics, and integrity of the physician. The good name and respect of both the practitioner and the profession are to be earned through consistent application of the ethical principles, and the code provides guidance. Good conduct becomes "characteristic" of the professional, and a code of conduct is a way of organizing one's thinking about good conduct both symbolically and in practical matters. In this sense medicine is like the military, the profession of arms. The warrior, like the physician, lives by a code that is internalized as a way of life. This code was so deeply internalized that the ancient Japanese samurai warrior understood that violation of the code required death at one's own hand. Physicians often live by a warrior's ideal, and medicine is often spoken of in military analogies. Disease is the enemy. Hard work defends a noble cause. Practice is experienced and described as being "in the trenches."

The role of the military officer, like that of the physician, is not only to win battles but also to provide moral leadership. Thus, honor codes identify the higher principles by which more routine decisions can be made. "An officer will not lie, cheat, or steal," say the codes sworn by military officers, to which is sometimes added the phrase "or tolerate anyone who does" (thereby indicating a responsibility in honor for the reputation of the corps or group, not just oneself). What words can capture such ineffable ideals? How can moral aspirations be articulated? "Thou shalt not kill" (Pentateuch). "Primum non nocere" (Hippocrates). "Do unto others as you would have them do unto you" (Jesus). "Act only according to that maxim that you would at the same time will to be a universal principle" (Kant).

Part of the motivation for acting ethically is the honor of associating with a body that brings high regard and defining purpose for right action. However, the military metaphor is rapidly being replaced by the market metaphor. The market has its own ideals, which create tensions for those with a sense of honor: *caveat emptor*—let the [autonomous] consumer beware.

The Fiduciary Principle

The doctor–patient relationship is understood sacredly as a fiduciary relationship, a relationship based on trust. This sense of honor derives from the sense that the physician must be worthy of the trust, faith, and belief invested in the healer by the patient. That trust must be earned, first by the hard work required to acquire the skills necessary to apply the art. It must also be continuously earned by the consistent application of attentive response ("responsibility") to the patient's needs. There is an important distinction between the fiduciary relationship in medicine and that in law or business, where the trustee may act *for* the client. In medicine the physician must act *with* the patient and with the patient's consent. That action may be paternalistic in the best sense, that of the concern for the child or dependent; if that concern verges on control, however, the modern patient may well lose trust and confidence. In medicine the fiduciary principle is best understood as implying a partnership between doctor and patient.

A Hippocratic Oath for Psychiatrists

Levine (1972) articulated a Hippocratic oath for psychiatrists with some uniquely important insights about the values of this profession. In focusing on high ideals he suggested a standard transcending the minimalist requirements of administrative documents that should be very much part of the self-set moral ideals of any psychiatrist. Levine's oath demands competence but recognizes that human beings are not perfect. His code stresses an important principle about the value of self-knowledge, self-awareness, and constant self-scrutiny. This would be understood in Levine's era and now as recognizing the need for personal therapy or psychoanalysis for those doing such work. Levine stressed the need for psychiatrists to recognize in themselves the feelings that such work can stir up, particularly working with seductive patients, and the importance of getting consultation or supervision, not just in training but whenever it might be necessary. This is a useful reminder at a time when many treatments are briefer and more biologically oriented. Many of the complaints of unethical conduct received by the American Psychiatric Association (APA) come from patients whose doctors did not sufficiently deal with their own feelings and acted out in treatment situations. It might be easier to justify self-disclosure in therapy, giving advice, accepting a gift, or socializing outside of therapy if the therapy were understood as merely a physiological intervention. At the same time, it becomes hard for a psychiatrist to defend against accusations of boundary violations if the feelings involved for both doctor and patient are not carefully considered in the therapy. Self-reflection is an important ethical tradition, not only in psychiatric and psychoanalytic circles but throughout Western culture, dating back to the Socratic admonition to "know thyself." Physician Otto Guttentag (1963) articulated it nicely: "We exist as epistemological peers with our patients; we know no more about our patients than we know about ourselves" (p. 200).

Contemporary Codes of Ethics (AMA and APA)

The second paragraph of the oath of Hippocrates presents the form of a profession organized around its code of ethics. When the AMA was founded in 1847, it adopted a code based largely on the Hippocratic principles of beneficence and honor. This code, *The Principles of Medical Ethics* (Figure 40–2), has been revised every few decades (most recently in 1957 and 1980). When the American Psychiatric Association adopted its first code in 1973, it decided to use the AMA principles (because psychiatrists are physicians) with annotations especially applicable to psychiatry. The preamble of the AMA principles explicitly states that the principles "are not laws but standards of conduct, which define the essentials of honorable behavior for the physician" (Figure 40–2). The principles should be read teleologically as principles, not deontologically as rules. The requirement of honorable behavior of the physician applies to the physician's character and virtue and cannot be reduced to a list of rules. The physician must understand the principles in terms of a higher calling and act in accord with the dictates of conscience. Nonetheless, physicians look to the codes, principles, or annotations for guidance in specific situations. Because there may be sanctions for misconduct, physicians read the perspectives of the AMA (American Medical Association 2000) and the APA (American Psychiatric Association 2001a) to see what may be permitted or prohibited.

Principles of honor transcend the written word, which at best is a distillation of accumulated wisdom, stories, and feelings. To appreciate honor fully, the professional must internalize the norms of a culture by living them and understanding what a teacher or a parent would approve or disapprove of and why. In this sense a code is minimalist but essential. One of the motivating factors for the APA in articulating its annotations in 1973 was to respond to complaints of misconduct against its members. Physicians should know the difference between right and wrong, but if sanctions

Principles of Medical Ethics of the American Medical Association

PREAMBLE The medical profession has long subscribed to a body of ethical statements developed primarily for the benefit of the patient. As a member of this profession, a physician must recognize responsibility not only to patients, but also to society, to other health professionals, and to self. The following Principles adopted by the American Medical Association are not laws but standards of conduct, which define the essentials of honorable behavior for the physician.

SECTION 1 A physician shall be dedicated to providing competent medical service with compassion and respect for human dignity.

SECTION 2 A physician shall deal honestly with patients and colleagues, and strive to expose those physicians deficient in character or competence, or who engage in fraud or deception.

SECTION 3 A physician shall respect the law and also recognize a responsibility to seek changes in those requirements which are contrary to the best interests of the patient.

SECTION 4 A physician shall respect the rights of patients, of colleagues, and of other health professionals, and shall safeguard patient confidences within the constraints of the law.

SECTION 5 A physician shall continue to study, apply, and advance scientific knowledge, make relevant information available to patients, colleagues, and the public, obtain consultation, and use the talents of other health professionals when indicated.

SECTION 6 A physician shall, in the provision of appropriate patient care, except in emergencies, be free to choose whom to serve, with whom to associate, and the environment in which to provide medical services.

SECTION 7 A physician shall recognize a responsibility to participate in activities contributing to an improved community.

FIGURE 40–2. Principles of Medical Ethics, American Medical Association.

Source. Reprinted by permission of American Medical Association: Code of Medical Ethics, in *Current Opinions With Annotations of the Council on Ethical and Judicial Affairs.* Chicago, IL, American Medical Association, 2000. Copyright 2000 American Medical Association.

were to be applied, it would be necessary to spell out the grounds for applying them. Treating the profession as a corps, the code serves as a tool for professional discipline. The entrepreneurial physician may see the medical license licentiously, as sanctioning whatever he or she might choose to do, but ethics provides a fundamental basis for accountability.

The APA (American Psychiatric Association 2001b) may impose four possible sanctions for misconduct:

1. Admonishment—an informal warning
2. Reprimand—a formal censure

3. Suspension (for a period not to exceed 5 years)
4. Expulsion

The Ethics Committee of the APA has given much thought to the procedures needed to ensure due process, particularly the procedures for holding a hearing and the articulation of the various annotations. In the minimalist or legalistic perspective, a psychiatrist should know what is specified in the code because he or she might be subject to sanctions. Membership in the professional organization entails a promise to abide by the code just as it did for the Hippocratic physician. The modern physician should also understand the principles that underlie the code to be able to act in situations that have not been explicitly spelled out. The following discussions illustrate the constant tension between rule and principle and the importance of the physician's acting in the upward perspective to strive for virtuous action.

Sexual Misconduct and Boundary Violations

Sexual contact with a patient is unethical. This is one of the least ambiguous sections of the ethical code. It is a tradition that goes back to the Hippocrates, who speaks of such conduct as "mischief." It is important for psychiatrists because the intimacy of the treatment activates strong feelings and fantasies in the doctor–patient relationship, the discussion of which may be essential to healing. In psychiatry especially, feelings the patient has for the doctor (understood as *transferences*, i.e., derived from significant relationships in the past and activated in the treatment) and feelings the doctor has for the patient (understood as *countertransferences*) receive close scrutiny. Scrutiny of these feelings is no less important for other physicians, other therapists, or other professionals.

It is sometimes argued that sexual contact is proscribed because of the power differential, an argument that applies equally to employers and employees, supervisors and supervisees, teachers and students. Fundamentally, the importance of trust in the therapeutic relationship requires the treater to maintain forbearance, particularly when the mode of therapy is talking to understand rather than acting to alter feelings. Some professionals prefer to think of their relationships with patients (or clients) as contractual (rather than covenantal). This outlook implies more autonomy on the part of the client and gives the client more control and choice in what goes on. In the case of sexual behavior with a professional, however, even the choices of a consenting adult do not justify crossing sexual boundaries. Those more legalistically inclined might wonder whether erotic feel-

TABLE 40–5. Numbers of ethical complaints received by the American Psychiatric Association in three time periods

	1950–1973	1972–1983	1991–1995
Charges made	82	382	211
Number (%) found unethical	12 (15%)	86 (23%)	82 (38%)
Number of expulsions	6	27	8

Source.   Adapted from data of Moore 1985 and J. Lazarus, personal communication, May 1997.

ings may be acted on if the professional relationship were terminated. Because transferences endure over time, the interests of the patient/client can never be served by crossing this boundary. The APA *Principles of Medical Ethics With Annotations Especially Applicable to Psychiatry* (American Psychiatric Association 2001b) spells this out: "Sexual activity with a current or former patient is unethical." How could a psychiatrist who became sexually involved with a patient or former patient ever defend him- or herself against a subsequent claim that the feelings acted on were feelings activated in therapy, which should have been addressed as therapeutic issues? The possible exception to this, which rarely gets consideration (and rarely happens), is when the two parties enter a covenantal relationship of marriage.

Other examples of boundary violations, which rest on similar considerations, are conducting business with a patient, using the professional relationship to make other contacts, and profiting from information gained from the therapeutic relationship. The dramatic sexual and financial boundary violations and the more subtle boundary crossings, which may slide into more serious violations, receive the closest scrutiny in disciplinary actions. However, more subtle examples may go unnoticed by all but the most self-reflective of practitioners. Clues physicians may give to their own religious or political inclinations may in fact be held as articles of true faith, but may nonetheless come across as intimidating or unduly influential to patients dependent on their caregivers. Icons of one's own self in office or waiting room may in fact be boundary violations that would never receive complaint, but nonetheless prevent patient from feeling open or comfortable in such a setting.

Table 40–5 compares the numbers of ethical complaints received by the APA in three periods. The decline in the number of complaints in recent years may suggest that the educational efforts of the APA Ethics Committee are having a beneficial effect.

The Boundary Between Ethics and Law

Ethics and the law share a similar concern for right and wrong, internally or externally enforced. The ethical requirements of professionals are not identical to the requirements of all citizens. The oath of Hippocrates held physicians to a standard that was not required of all citizens. The AMA *Principles* and APA *Annotations* recognize this tension and expect physicians to "respect the law" (Figure 40–2) and "seek changes in those requirements which are contrary to the best interests of the patient" (American Psychiatric Association 2001b, p. xiv). Criminal behavior is usually unethical as well, but there may be situations in which it is not. Civil disobedience against unjust laws is a respected ethical tradition. A physician is a citizen whose professional role requires adherence to principles such as patient benefit. The *Principles* and *Annotations* both recognize an affirmative obligation to take part in activities contributing to the improvement of the community.

Confidentiality and Privacy

Confidentiality, understood as secrecy, in the doctor–patient relationship is one of the most fundamental principles of professional ethics. In the Hippocratic oath it is spoken of as "shameful to noise abroad what I may hear or see in the course of treatment." Confidentiality has its roots in the confidence or trust that is placed in the physician and on which the treatment depends. Confidentiality is one of the most fragile tenets in the contemporary era. As more and more people and agencies are involved in medical treatment and health care, it becomes increasingly difficult to safeguard confidentiality. Insurance companies, managed care organizations, other providers, courts, and sometimes families claim a right to know what is going on in patients' treatments. Mandatory reporting of suspected child abuse is an example in which the interest of the state in protecting children legally supersedes the physician's duty to maintain secrecy. Similarly, the *Tarasoff* decision (now precedent) obligates a psychotherapist who has knowledge that a patient or client may intend harm to a third party to notify that third party of the potential risk. These are examples of principles in conflict, and they speak to the insufficiency of relying absolutely on a principle as a rule. However, in a larger context the erosion of confidentiality threatens to undermine the possibility of a kind of therapy that requires developing openness to another person in which the patient may be confident that what is disclosed is only for his or her benefit.

Confidentiality, trust, and secrecy in the doctor–patient relationship are no longer sufficient to protect patients' privacy needs, interests, and rights. Recently, the U.S. Supreme Court, in its *Redmond v. Jaffee* decision, recognized the necessity of privacy in psychotherapeutic treatment. However the knowledge of what goes on in medical treatments is not just possessed by physicians and therapists but is broadly shared by clinics, hospitals, health care organizations, managed care organizations, insurance companies, and state and federal governments. The ethical behavior of physicians/providers is not enough to ensure patients privacy of essential personal information (such as genetic information). In 2001 the Department of Health and Human Services issued privacy guidelines for federal agencies and agencies receiving federal funds. Such regulations are inevitably political and may not go far enough in providing needed assurances against disclosure and discrimination.

The Double Agent Problem

Double agents work both sides. The whole weight of tradition in professional ethics focuses the physician's responsibility to the patient. The physician works for the patient and is guided by the patient's needs and interests. This is especially the case in fee-for-service financial arrangements, even those buffered by insurance reimbursement. In situations in which the physician works for someone other than the patient, there may be a conflict between the patient and the physician's employer, resulting in a divided allegiance or divided loyalties. The classic case is the physician who works for the military. In such situations confidentiality may be compromised. Psychiatrists dealing with combat neuroses and trying to get soldiers back into combat have faced the ethical dilemma of helping someone get into a situation in which he or she may get killed. This is ethically analogous to treating the psychotic prisoner who is incompetent to face execution. The student health psychiatrist doing an evaluation for the dean and the psychiatrist doing a prearraignment examination have loyalties that go beyond the patient's best interest and require at the least the disclosure of the purpose of the examination and how the information will be used. Increasingly, physicians working for corporations, health maintenance organizations, and managed care organizations have interests that radically transform the nature of the relationship between doctor and patient.

The Ethics of Psychiatric Research

There are several areas of ethical concern for psychiatrists as psychiatric researchers and as practitioners who base decisions on the outcome of that research. First are questions about whether certain research methods such as placebo-controlled designs, medication washout periods, and symptom provocation studies may present with unacceptable risk–benefit ratios for the subjects. The Declaration of Helsinki (World Medical Association 1989), a resolution of the World Medical Association, indicated that the use of a placebo group is contraindicated if an effective treatment is known. This is a subject of scientific debate because use of placebo controls plays an important role in identifying which treatments are truly effective and whether the risk to patients of endorsing ineffective treatments is significant (Quitkin 1999).

Secondly, it has been suggested that many psychiatric patients who become research subjects lack the capacity to give a truly informed consent about their participation in research (Appelbaum 1998). Protections for research subjects have been strengthened across disciplines by the federal government in the aftermath of unfortunate incidents such as the death of an 18-year-old research subject in a gene-transfer trial in which subjects may not have been adequately protected and the subsequent discovery by the National Institutes of Health (NIH) of many unreported adverse events among other research volunteers (Shalala 2000). Although these efforts are well intentioned, one potential consequence for psychiatric patients is a perpetuation of the stigmatization and discrimination that have long been associated with mental illness (Candilis 2001). Evidence demonstrates that even patients with schizophrenia can retain decision-making abilities (Wirshing et al. 1998). As Appelbaum (1998) suggested, one protection for people's rights and interests is to help them make decisions for themselves whenever possible. In research, as in therapy, promoting the goal of patient autonomy is a desirable end.

Also, ethical practice depends on the integrity of the research that informs it. Sciences rests on open communication of knowledge freely shared. This may create a conflict with commercial interests that depend on proprietary information being kept secret for financial gain. A particular example of this is called funnel plots, a publication bias in which positive results are published, but negative results are suppressed, giving a false (unscientific, but commercially advantageous) impression of the efficacy of a particular pharmaceutical agent. This is an issue that affects the psychiatric profession at several levels. Practitioners rely on sound scientific data for clinical decision making. Researchers walk a tightrope of balancing sound scientific research with the inducements of those funding the research. The reputation of any profession depends on the integrity of the judgments it makes. At a time when the effectiveness of pharmacological treatments may be overstated and the cost of time-consuming psychological therapies is closely scrutinized, it is important that the psychiatric profession carefully consider the ways in which it can be most helpful to the patients it serves.

Fees, Billing, and Reimbursement

The financial arrangements for medical service strike at the heart of the ethical issues about how medicine is valued. Not all values are economic, but ethics is often turned into economics. Inevitably there must be some sort of exchange for services rendered, and inescapably there are feelings about the monetary transaction. In the dyadic doctor–patient relationship, there is a direct transaction, although insurance companies, billing clerks, credit cards, or electronic transactions may diffuse the personal nature of that transaction. In Hippocratic times, the physician was likely to be an itinerant who was housed and fed by the families of those he cared for. In horse-and-buggy days, farm produce or manual labor may have substituted for the fee. European academic robes had pockets in the hoods for tuition coins to be placed out of sight, so shameful was the monetary transaction. Not everyone could afford to pay equally, so often the paying patients subsidized the care of the poor. Patient benefit and fee-for-service have traditionally gone hand in hand, and the fee (alongside honor and duty, of course) has helped focus the physician's attention on the recipient of his treatment. One of the general criticisms often leveled against traditional Hippocratic medical ethics is that it does not deal with the physician's larger obligations to society and particularly to the distribution of medical services.

One financial arrangement that sometimes is questioned is the practice of charging for missed sessions. The APA *Annotations* has specifically addressed this issue: "It is ethical for the psychiatrist to make a charge for a missed appointment when this falls within the terms of the specific contractual agreement with the patient" (Section 2, paragraph 6). The idea of patients having responsibility for the treatment and ultimately for their health and wellness is not something usually considered in medical ethics, but it goes beyond the idea of medicine as technology that the doctor delivers, and it stresses the patient's investment and commitment to the healing process.

Another financial arrangement that is addressed throughout the AMA *Opinions* and APA *Annotations* is fee-splitting. Physicians should receive remuneration for the work they do, and they should obtain patients by referral based on the quality of their work and the reputation they earn in the eyes of satisfied patients and other physicians. Any incentive such as splitting the fee with a referring physician is considered unethical. It offers a temptation to place monetary gain above the best interest of the patient. Fee-splitting arrangements have largely been considered in the context of fee-for-service arrangements, but new financial arrangements in physician reimbursement often provide incentives for physicians to be paid for limiting care or otherwise acting in the interest of someone other than their patient.

The Tasks and Methods of Ethics

Throughout the discussion of the codes of professional ethics and their application to particular situations, tension arises between understanding the codes as precise rules and understanding their statements as more general principles. In a homogeneous culture, tribe, or community, morality is tacitly understood with little need for formal reflection or articulation. One learns the rules of culture by living in that culture and not by being taught abstract and explicitly formulated rules. In a heterogeneous group, what is called a "pluralistic society," there may be little adhesion to shared principles. In a stable culture, moral norms are internalized, and ethics are thought of as matters of conscience. In a changing culture, the internalized morality of a particular subgroup or individual may be in conflict with other mores, and people may not trust that the dictates of individual conscience are an adequate safeguard of right conduct.

Increasingly in this society we are moving away from informal standards of both personal and professional ethics, from broad and tacitly indwelling general principles developed over centuries, toward a civilly enforced body of laws and administrative regulations. This change has been interpreted as resulting from a deep mistrust of all "assumed relationships," the breakdown of *gemeinschaft* (a community of feeling that results from likeness and shared life experience) into *gesellschaft* (a more rational, more mechanistic way of life, with greater structure and more written and explicit rules and regulations; Toennies 1940). Broad ethical principles no longer serve as shared values, and there is an attempt to make moral principles explicit as behavioral guidelines.

Deontological Ethical Theories

Ethical theory identifies the tension between rules and principles by the terms *deontological* (rule-based) and *teleological* (from the Greek *telos*, meaning end or goal; Frankena 1963). Deontological ethical theories maintain that there are rules of action that have moral validity independent of the consequences and that one must act in accordance with these rules. Deontological theories assert that there are considerations other than goodness or badness on which to base decisions—such as keeping a promise, maintaining justice, or adhering to a commandment of God or the state—that are important regardless of the consequences of the action. One finds deontological theories in well-defined communities, such as religious communities, where one of the ethical considerations is preservation of the social order. Duty, obligation, obedience, and loyalty are the values that define deontological functioning. Professional standards of ethics have such deontological features, where the rule may be applied to exclude or coerce the deviant member to maintain the reputation of the group. Because of possible ambiguity in interpretation of the laws, there is often a complex corpus of interpretation and devoted study such as in Talmudic scholarship or in American constitutional law or in the opinions concerning professional codes (see the discussion that follows). The problem of interpreting ambiguity can be avoided if an overarching rule that is basic to all situations can be identified. The most successful example of such a pure deontological rule is Kant's famous categorical imperative: "Act only according to that maxim that you would at the same time will to be a universal principle." This formula assumes a highly motivated moral agent who will decide on a course of action by rational reflection.

Teleological Ethical Theories

Teleological theories are based on more general principles. The AMA *Principles* (American Medical Association 2000), on which the APA's standards are based, states explicitly that these principles "are not laws but standards of conduct, which define the essentials of honorable behavior for the physician" (Figure 40–2). Teleological ethical theories hold that the ultimate standard by which an act is judged morally right, wrong, obligatory, or correct is the general happiness of all people concerned or the greatest net balance of good over evil. This is often identified as the principle of utility or beneficence, which implies that good and bad are capable of being measured and balanced in some quantitative or mathematical way ("the greatest good for the greatest number"). Thus teleological theories often go by the name of *utilitarianism*. They are represented by such philosophers as Jeremy Bentham, John Stuart Mill, and G.E. Moore, and more recently by Joseph Fletcher (1966), whose *situation ethics* employs as its central principle "agape, the love for humanity, or general goodwill." Situation ethics is an example of another form of ethical reasoning, called the *consequentialist* approach, in which an action is judged to be morally right or wrong through an assessment of the consequences of the action. Much of clinical medicine is consequentialist in that the goodness of actions is judged by their outcomes. It should be noted, of course, that not all teleologists are utilitarians. Plato, Augustine, and even Aristotle all strove to articulate principles of conduct, but they would be horrified by the mathematical connotations of utilitarianism. Decision trees in Figures 40–3 and 40–4 outline the deontological and consequentialist forms of teleological ethical thinking (modified from Brody 1981).

Deontological and teleological theories are not just options to choose from on an ethical smorgasbord; their use depends greatly on what one is trying to accomplish. In Table 40–6, the first author (A.R.D.) draws a distinction between the upward perspective and the downward perspective in the tasks of ethics (Dyer 1988). The upward perspective is that of the individual moral agent in relation to the larger culture. The downward perspective is the view of the individual from the perspective of the norms of the culture or group. The upward perspective refers to the highest standards of ethical conduct to which anyone might aspire—ethical ideals, ideals of moral perfection. The task of ethics in the downward perspective is the regulation of abuse. In terms of a profession, the downward perspective concerns the profession's policing of itself. The upward perspective is that of the individual (practitioner) seeking to ensure that his or her own conduct is the highest possible. The upward perspective presupposes the mutual trust of the physician and patient in their collaboration. There is no maximum limit on mutual responsibility of the patient and physician in their partnership, but there are minimum limits. The downward perspective is that of the regulatory agency or professional society seeking to ensure that the behavior of a particular individual does not fall below certain minimum standards, which are articulated as well as possible.

Ethics of Virtue and Character

Both teleological and deontological approaches to ethics have one serious shortcoming. They depend on the activities of the rational mind of a motivated moral agent to

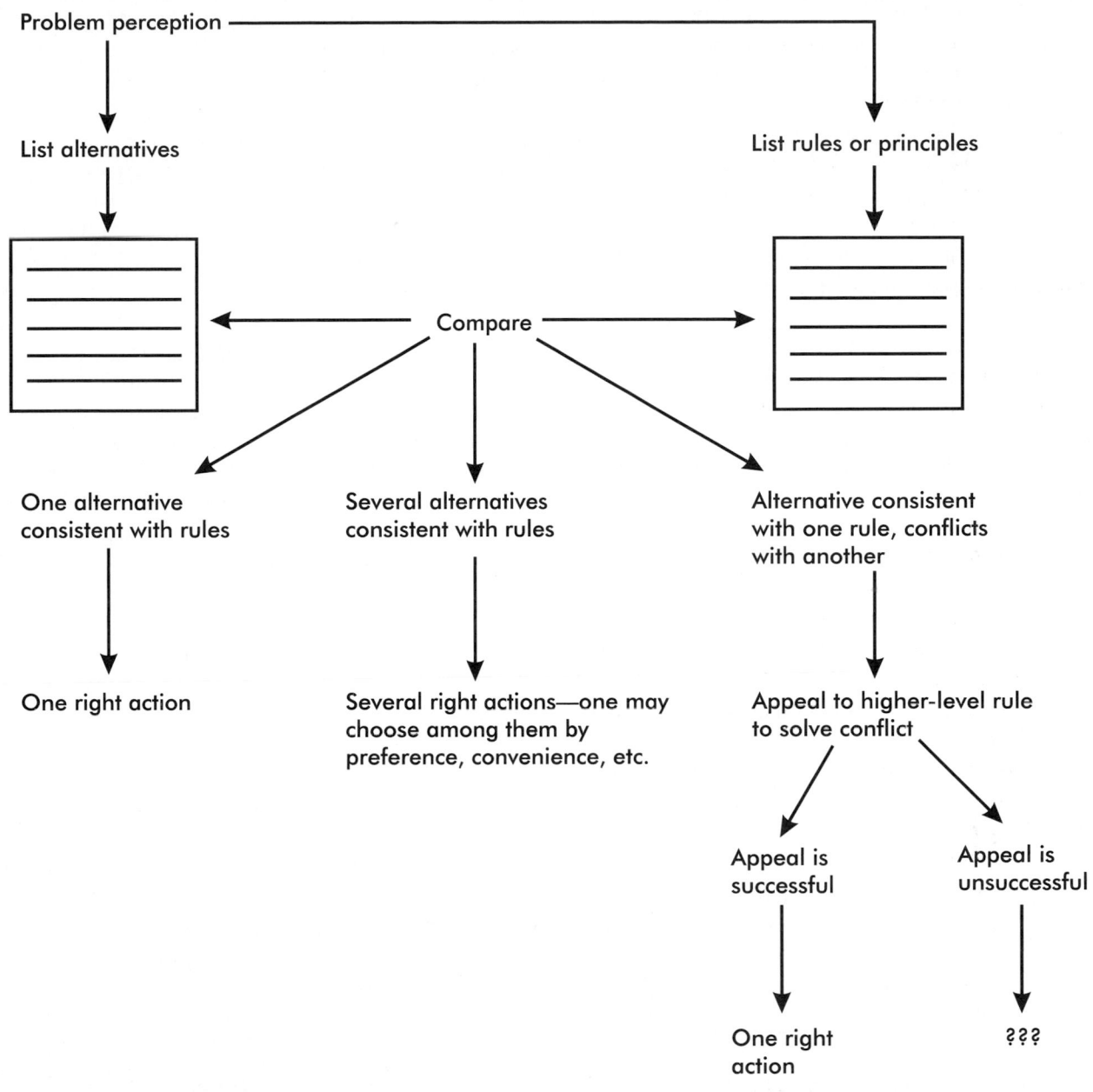

FIGURE 40–3. Deontological ethical method.
Source. Modified with permission from Brody 1981.

apprehend right and wrong. Moral philosophers and psychiatrists alike appreciate that not everyone is motivated to be moral, that even good people sometimes do bad things, and that people are capable of rationalizing self-interest (see Dyer 1985b; Hauerwas 1977, 1981; Pincoffs 1971, 1980). Whatever place Freudian thought assumes in contemporary psychiatry and in modern culture, Freud's explication of moral psychology is inescapable in understanding moral process. Human beings have

impulses that they do not necessarily act on even though they may be tempted to. The urges of the *id* are constrained by the restrictions of society internalized as the *superego* and mediated by the more or less rational *ego*.

A delineation of obligations, however essential, is not the whole picture of ethics. Virtue, character, and integrity are every bit as important in understanding right conduct. For the professions especially, integrity in concrete situations is the hallmark of virtuous life.

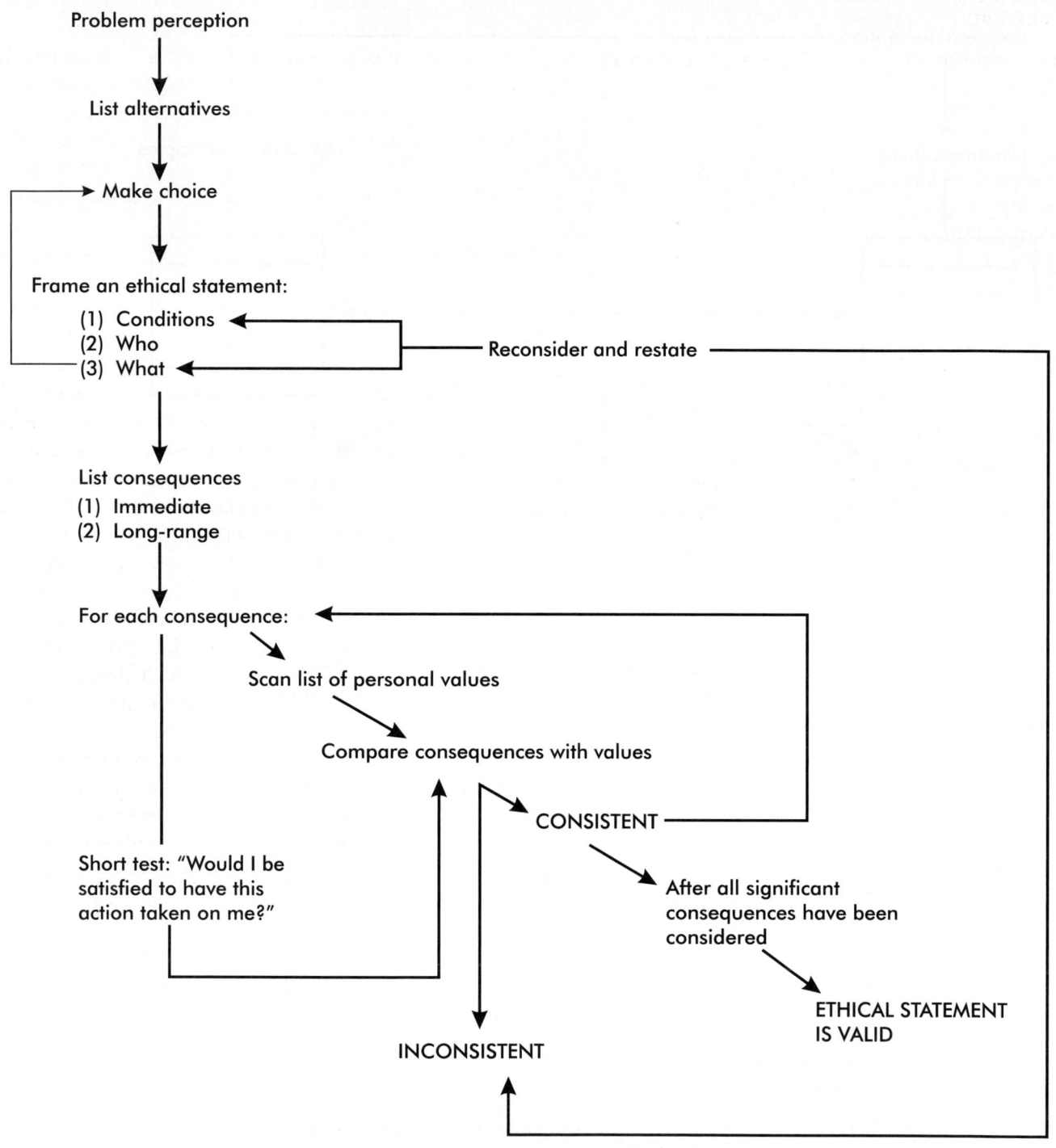

FIGURE 40–4. Teleological ethical method.
Source. Modified with permission from Brody 1981.

The Ethics of Managed Care

The current revolution in health care financing is calling into question many of the traditional assumptions of medical ethics, assumptions about the doctor–patient relationship, the nature of health, and even the role of persons in a society. It is not just about economic values; it is about human values. The most fundamental change to be noted is the departure from a dyadic person-to-person doctor–patient relationship:

doctor ⟷ patient

TABLE 40–6.   The tasks of ethics

Upward perspective	Downward perspective
Moral inspiration	Regulation of abuse
Affective	Cognitive
Self-reflective	Critical
Teleological (end-based, goal-based)	Deontological (rule-based)
Fiduciary relationship (based on trust)	Adversary relationship (based on control)
Tacit	Explicit

Doctors in the new environment are being transformed into "providers"; patients are transformed into "consumers"; health becomes a commodity, and any number of third parties may claim an interest in what goes on in that relationship:

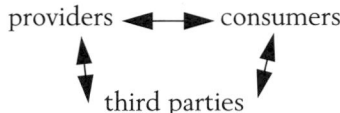

The introduction of third parties in a triad opens the possibility of conflicts of interest and divided allegiances. The metaphor of health care as an industry radically transforms the healing process. In the economic model of marketplace transactions, much more is at stake than how the payment is to be allotted. Health care is reduced to physiological interventions that take place in a delimited period of time. Physicians become not merely providers but technicians, and patients become not merely consumers but recipients of technology. Providers and consumers are likely to be strangers to one another. Medicine is transformed from a human service into a commodity.

In the interest of efficiency or economy (i.e., cost savings), these transformations might seem warranted, but the practices currently witnessed in the name of managed care must themselves be subjected to ethical scrutiny. Certainly much of what is going on is not ethically justifiable, nor are the intended ends served.

The transformation of medicine from a profession to a trade by the FTC was justified as a cost-saving measure on the grounds that increasing consumer choice (through advertising) would lower costs. The value placed on autonomy set the stage for a transformation that reduces the amount of choice consumers have in the health care they receive. Health care has become an investment opportunity in which vast amounts of money have been siphoned away from service delivery into the pockets of executives and shareholders of megacorporations. The market solution has been a nonsolution up until now in

that it has succeeded only in lowering costs without adequately addressing quality of service or the distribution and allocation of services. The current anarchy in health care of the free market or unregulated (or underregulated) market resembles the lawlessness of the post–Civil War American frontier or of the early stages of industrialization, when efficiencies and wealth were achieved by the robber barons at the cost of environmental pollution and human suffering.

The ethical physician is inevitably in tension with a system designed to limit the care given to his or her patients or deny care altogether. Recognizing that resources are finite, the ethical physician must struggle to do the best possible for individual patients without compromising integrity. Many of the practices of managed care are fraudulently unethical, such as gag rules prohibiting physicians from discussing treatment options with their patients. Such policies do not enhance consumer choice (even the choice of paying for treatment out of pocket) but diminish patient autonomy. They are directly counter to the goal of informed consent, which has been such a key feature of the ethics of autonomy. Such gag rules place the physician in the position of a double agent without the possibility of disclosure. It is difficult for the physician to say, "Trust me," and difficult also for him or her to say, "Consumer, beware." Many of the practices of managed care are more subtly unethical, such as use of misleading advertising or incomplete disclosure, and some, such as limiting who may serve on panels, may be in restraint of trade. They are certainly not pro-competitive. Managed care is an ethically unstable response to the health care financing dilemma and must be subjected to thoroughgoing ethical evaluation. A just society must demand accountability for its citizens.

Psychiatry faces unique challenges in the managed care environment. While managed care limits the care of all specialties, it substantially alters the care received by patients with mental illness. It limits the time a psychiatrist is able to spend in empathic discussion and encourages the use of more standardized treatments, particularly pharmacological and behavioral treatments. It encourages treatment of symptoms rather than illnesses, or patients with illnesses. Psychiatrists often are spending less time with more patients, which results in a need for other ancillary support such as community programs; however, managed care does not support such community infrastructure to meet the needs of patients with mental illnesses (Lazarus and Sharfstein 2000; Regestein 2000; Schlesinger et al. 2000).

Psychiatrists and mental health professionals as well as other physicians usually work with a professional self-understanding derived from traditions of professional ethics, such as the Hippocratic tradition. They focus on the fiduciary needs of their patients, one by one. Even within a system of limited resources, it is possible to maintain a patient-benefit ethical focus by advocating for the needs of patients within the economic system. This does not mean ignoring public health goals or the needs of the larger population, but it does mean being mindful of the economic incentives that might compromise patient care.

While individual psychiatrists have responsibilities for individual patients, the profession as a whole has responsibilities for the larger population. Sabin (1994) distinguished these responsibilities as *fiduciary* and *stewardship* responsibilities. As members of a scientifically based profession, psychiatrists should strive for use of the best treatments available and as citizens should strive for the best interests of all and for coordinated systems of care that work to those ends.[2]

Preparing for a Postmodern Future in Medicine and Psychiatry

It is not an exaggeration to suggest that a revolution in health care is taking place. It is probably also true that the revolution in health care is part of a larger revolution in social thinking. Many are suggesting that what is taking place is a paradigm shift of the sort Thomas Kuhn described in *The Structure of Scientific Revolutions* (1970). It is also being suggested that the current cultural change is a transition from modern culture to postmodern culture (see Eberle 1994; Gergen 1991; Jameson 1991; Kolb 1992). There is little consensus, however, as to what postmodern culture might entail. It is too soon to tell. For the medical profession to make an appropriate response to these new challenges, it should begin to reconceptualize the issues it faces. Physicians should do as the great hockey player Wayne Gretzky did: skate to where the puck is going to be. We shall be required to understand historical change as it occurs. We shall be required to understand our own cultural assumptions.

Although there can be no consensus on what the post-

modern future will hold, certain features of modernity can be recognized, as well as the fact that the assumptions of the old modern age are no longer valid. Table 40–7 summarizes features that have come to be associated with modernity: secular society, free market, constitutional democracy, civil rights, nationalism, bureaucratic administration, industrialization/efficiency, capitalism, science and technology, rational thought, and progress. Many of the tensions experienced in professional ethics and bioethics stem from tensions concerning how to think about and experience the process of valuing in the modern paradigm. Whereas many of the features of the old modern age are familiar and comfortable and perhaps worth defending, they cannot be taken for granted.

TABLE 40–7. The old modern age

Secular society
Free market
Constitutional democracy
Civil rights
Nationalism
Bureaucratic administration
Industrialization and efficiency
Capitalism
Science and technology
Rational thought
Progress

There are at least two distinct strains of postmodernism. The intellectual movement most often identified with postmodernism is called *deconstructionism*. Deconstructionism seeks to undermine the unities and certainties found in modern thought on the grounds that they are artificial constructions of a false and impersonal scientism in which human experience is made the object of detached analysis. Often using linguistic innovations, such as talking about "psychiatries" rather than "psychiatry" to emphasize the plurality of opinion within a discipline, deconstructionism seeks to attack traditional values and break traditional restrictions. Deconstructionism's postmodernism is post-individual, postcolonial,

---

[2] We speak of psychiatrists, as members of the medical profession, and of the APA's and AMA's codes of ethics, with full recognition that other professional organizations, notably the American Psychological Association, the National Association of Social Workers, as well as over a hundred allied health professions, have similar codes of ethics based on a similar understanding of what it means to be an autonomous self-regulating profession. The AMA's Principles of Medical Ethics explicitly states in its preamble that "As a member of this profession, a physician must recognize responsibility not only to patients, but also to society, to other health professionals, and to self." The British Medical Association goes a step further in telling physicians that they have an affirmative duty to use the most economic option that achieves clinical objectives on the grounds that efficiency promotes patient benefit by making more of finite resources available to the population.

post-patriarchal, and post-humanist. Deconstructionism is either unnerving or exciting, depending on one's vantage point.

An alternative form of postmodernism may be called "postcritical" after the philosophy of Michael Polanyi (1958). Polanyi recognized that modern science, as it was usually understood, purported to be objective, with a detached, value-neutral observer. In fact, real science never proceeded in this manner but depended on the judgments of a committed knower. Science was neither objective nor subjective, but rather personal. Hence Polanyi called his major work *Personal Knowledge: Toward a Post-Critical Philosophy*. In Polanyi's philosophy, tradition (i.e., scientific tradition) plays an important role in the understanding of the scientific community, and it lays the ground for respecting a variety of cultural traditions.

These epistemological theories have an important bearing on how ethics is to be understood. Ethics explicitly articulated (the deontological ambition) is always in tension with more tacitly understood principles (the teleological tradition). Ethics understood as conflict may be appreciated in the context of the larger cultural tensions of which such conflicts are in fact manifestations.

The goal of autonomy is very much a feature of the modern outlook. The yearning for explicitness is very much a feature of the modern outlook. Yet these approaches—as useful as they are, as far as they go—do not go far enough. Ethics must also deal with the nuances of human experience. Table 40–8 highlights this postmodern outlook. To the list in this figure should be added a key feature of postmodernism, namely, the toleration of ambiguity.

TABLE 40–8. The functions of ethics

Modern account	Postmodern (postcritical) account
Universal	Contextual
Impersonal	Personal
Atemporal	Historical
Acultural	Cultural
Based on obligation	Based on integrity
Enforced by control, suasion, or sanction	Enforced by willing assent, trust in a convivial order, or community

One may anticipate the postmodern by identifying the distinguishing features of modernity. However, the paradigm shift now being experienced may be better appreciated by observing what preceded modernity. Table 40–9 suggests a perspective on this development. Notable in premodern thinking is the focus on human

experience and the human dimension. In the more deconstructive approaches to postmodernism, this dimension drops out; however, in approaches that stress the role of tradition (such as Polanyi's postcritical philosophy), the recovery of the human dimension lost in modernity becomes an important part of the postmodern enterprise. It is notable that in postmodern approaches to art and architecture, one sees the reintroduction of the human form and human scale.

TABLE 40–9. A perspective on modernity

Premodern thinking	Prescientific, ecclesiastical authority, magical thinking, focus on human experience
Modern thinking	Emphasizes the individual and the search for a systematic, scientific *certitude*
Postmodern thinking	*Deconstructive*: undermines the unities and closures found in modern thought *Postcritical*: makes use of modern achievement; offers new freedoms

TABLE 40–10. Modern and postmodern medical practice

Old paradigm (modern)	New paradigm (postmodern)
Acute illness (hospital based)	Chronic illness (community based)
Curative	Preventive
Physician centered	Doctor–patient partnership
Individual patient	Health of population
Prototype: young, white male	Cultural diversity

Premodern art was representational. Pictures told stories. Modern art abandoned these representations in favor of more abstract and expressionistic ideas in painting. Postmodern art reintroduces the human form. Classical (premodern) architecture was built around the human form. Modern architecture, grand and impersonal, forced humans to adapt to monolithic skyscrapers, huge black boxes in which humans were but cogs in the machine. Postmodern architecture reintroduces the human element in building. It does this by whimsical elements such as oversized arches, pediments, columns, and windows, which even in large buildings serve as reminders that the buildings are human meeting places. Postmodern buildings often exist in relationship to their surroundings and community, respecting the traditions of their neighbors by borrowing (mirroring) elements such as classical (Greek) columns, Gothic arches, or Victorian

TABLE 40–11. Ethics on the Web

American Society of Bioethics and Humanities (ASBH)	http://www.asbh.org
American Society of Law, Medicine, and Ethics (ASLME)	http://www.aslme.org
Bioethics.net (The American Journal of Bioethics)	http://www.bioethics.net
Careers in Bioethics	http://www.ethicsjobs.ca
Center for Applied Ethics, University of British Columbia	http://www.ethics.ubc.ca
Duke Center for the Study of Medical Ethics and the Humanities	http://csmeh.mc.duke.edu
East Tennessee State University: Allen R. Dyer	http://faculty.etsu.edu/dyer/
Human Genome Project: Ethical, Legal, and Social Issues (ELSI)	http://www.ornl.gov/hgmis/elsi/elsi.html
International Bioethics Committee	http://www.unesco.org/ibc
Kennedy Institute of Ethics, Georgetown University	http://www.georgetown.edu/research/kie
Midwest Bioethics Center	http://www.midbio.org
National Bioethics Advisory Commission (NBAC)	http://bioethics.gov/cgi-bin/bioeth_counter.pl
National Reference Center for Bioethics Literature	http://www.georgetown.edu/research/nrcbl
The Hastings Center	http://www.thehastingscenter.org
University of Buffalo Center for Clinical Ethics and Humanities in Health Care	http://wings.buffalo.edu/faculty/research/bioethics/nav.html
University of New Mexico Empirical Ethics Group	http://eeg.unm.edu/index.html
University of Pennsylvania School of Medicine Center for Bioethics	http://www.med.upenn.edu/bioethics/index.shtml

ornamentation.

It is such humanistic, communitarian, historical elements in continuity with tradition that offer hopeful and exciting possibilities for the future of medicine (Table 40–10 [see previous page]). Medicine in the modern paradigm has been a technological marvel (Table 40–11), but focusing on the body as a machine has left an impersonal coldness that has created the host of ethical dilemmas now associated with the domain of bioethics; it also has created an economic nightmare. The possibility of recovering the human dimension in medicine suggests a useful direction for postmodernism in medicine. It must be acknowledged, however, that this is not necessarily the way things are headed if present trends are extrapolated into the future. The value of individual life is already threatened by capitated economic systems that focus on the well-being of the population.

Looking back at the contributions of the premodern classical age allows an appreciation for the place of the Hippocratic oath and the Hippocratic tradition in contemporary medicine. Although these ideas are sometimes criticized for being anachronistic, their value becomes apparent. The Hippocratic tradition in medicine provides a perspective of enduring values by which the shortcomings of modern expediency may be judged.

References

American Medical Association: Opinions and Reports of the Judicial Council. Chicago, IL, American Medical Association, 1957

American Medical Association: Code of Medical Ethics: Current Opinions with Annotations of the Council on Ethical and Judicial Affairs. Chicago, IL, American Medical Association, 2000

American Psychiatric Association: Opinions of the Ethics Committee on the Principles of Medical Ethics With Annotations Especially Applicable to Psychiatry, 2001 Edition. Washington, DC, American Psychiatric Publishing, 2001a

American Psychiatric Association: The Principles of Medical Ethics With Annotations Especially Applicable to Psychiatry, 2001 Edition. Washington, DC, American Psychiatric Publishing, 2001b

Appelbaum PS: Missing the boat: competence and consent in psychiatric research. Am J Psychiatry 155:1486–1488, 1998

Bloch S: The political misuse of psychiatry in the Soviet Union, in Psychiatric Ethics, 2nd Edition. Edited by Bloch S, Chodoff P. New York, Oxford University Press, 1991

Bloch S, Reddaway P: Psychiatric Terror: How Soviet Psychiatry is Used to Suppress Dissent. New York, Basic Books, 1977

Brody H: Ethical Decisions in Medicine, 2nd Edition. Boston, MA, Little, Brown, 1981

Campbell D: Doctors, Lawyers, Ministers. Nashville, TN, Abingdon, 1982

Candilis PJ: Advancing the ethics of research. Psychiatr Ann 31:119–124, 2001

Dyer AR: Ethics, advertising, and the definition of a profession. J Med Ethics 11:72–78, 1985a

Dyer AR: Virtue and medicine: a physician's analysis, in Virtue and Medicine. Edited by Shelp E. Dordrecht, The Netherlands, D. Reidel, 1985b, pp 223–235

Dyer AR: Ethics and Psychiatry: Toward Professional Definition. Washington, DC, American Psychiatric Press, 1988

Dyer AR: Advertising, in Encyclopedia of Bioethics, 2nd Edition. Edited by Reich W. New York, Macmillan, 1995

Dyer AR: Ethics, advertising, and assisted reproduction: the goals and methods of advertising. Women's Health Issues 7:143–148, 1997a

Dyer AR: Ethics of human genetic intervention: a postmodern perspective. Exp Neurol 144:168–172, 1997b

Eberle G: The Geography of Nowhere: Finding One's Self in the Postmodern World. Kansas City, MO, Sheed and Ward, 1994

Fletcher J: Situation Ethics. Philadelphia, PA, Westminster Press, 1966

Frankena W: Ethics. Englewood Cliffs, NJ, Prentice-Hall, 1963

Gergen KJ: The Saturated Self: Dilemmas of Identity in Contemporary Life. New York, Basic Books, 1991

Greenhouse J: Justices uphold right of doctors to solicit trade. The New York Times, March 24, 1982, p 10

Guttentag OE: On defining medicine. The Christian Scholar 46:200–211, 1963

Hauerwas S: Truthfulness and Tragedy: Further Investigations Into Christian Ethics. Notre Dame, IN, University of Notre Dame Press, 1977

Hauerwas S: Community and Character. Notre Dame, IN, University of Notre Dame Press, 1981

Jameson F: Postmodernism, or, the Cultural Logic of Late Capitalism. Durham, NC, Duke University Press, 1991

Kolb D: Postmodern Sophistications: Philosophy, Architecture, and Tradition. Chicago, IL, University of Chicago Press, 1992

Kuhn TS: The Structure of Scientific Revolutions, 2nd Edition, enlarged with postscript. Chicago, IL, Chicago University Press, 1970. [2nd Edition includes postscript.]

Laín Entralgo P: The Therapy of the Word in Classical Antiquity. New Haven, CT, Yale University Press, 1970

Lazarus JA, Sharfstein SS: Ethics in Managed Care. Psychiatr Clin North Am 23:269–284, 2000

Levine M: Psychiatry and Ethics. New York, Holt, Rinehart and Winston, 1972

Moore RA: Ethics in the practice of psychiatry: update on the results of enforcement of the code. Am J Psychiatry 142:1043–1046, 1985

Pincoffs E: Quandary Ethics. Mind 75:552–571, 1971

Pincoffs E: Virtue, the quality of life and punishment. The Monist 63:23–27, 1980

Polanyi M: Personal Knowledge: Towards a Post-Critical Philosophy. London, England, Routledge and Kegan Paul, 1958

Quitkin FM: Placebos, drug effects, and study design: a clinician's guide. Am J Psychiatry 156:829–836, 1999

Regestein QR: Psychiatrists' view of managed care and the future of psychiatry. Gen Hosp Psychiatry 22:97–106, 2000

Sabin JE: Caring about patients and caring about money: the American Psychiatric Association Code of Ethics meets managed care. Behavioral Sciences and the Law 12:317–330, 1994

Schlesinger M, Wynia M, Cummins D: Some distinctive features of the impact of managed care on psychiatry. Harv Rev Psychiatry 8:216–230, 2000

Shalala D: Protecting research subjects: what must be done. N Engl J Med 343:808–810, 2000

Toennies F: Fundamental Concepts of Sociology. Translated by Loomis C. New York, American Book Company, 1940

Wirshing DA, Wirshing WC, Marder SR, et al: Informed consent: assessment of comprehension. Am J Psychiatry 155:1508–1511, 1998

World Medical Association: Declaration of Helsinki IV, World Medical Association, 41st World Medical Assembly, Hong Kong, September 1989

Index

Page numbers printed in **boldface** type refer to tables or figures.